W9-CZL-845

VOLUME **III**

Approved Drug Products and Legal Requirements

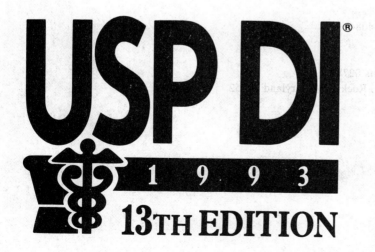

USP DI®

1 9 9 3

13TH EDITION

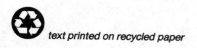

text printed on recycled paper

By authority of the United States Pharmacopeial Convention, Inc.

Turn to the last page for the "Fast-finder" subject guide.

NOTICE AND WARNING

Attention is called to the fact that all volumes of *USP Dispensing Information* are fully copyrighted: Volume I—*Drug Information for the Health Care Professional*; Volume II—*Advice for the Patient*; Volume III—*Approved Drug Products and Legal Requirements*.

For permission to copy or utilize portions of this text, address inquiries to the Secretary of the USPC Board of Trustees, 12601 Twinbrook Parkway, Rockville, Maryland 20852.

This volume contains portions of U.S. Statutes, Federal regulations, and other government publications that are in the public domain. However, their arrangement and compilation, along with other material in this publication, are subject to the copyright notice.

© 1993 The United States Pharmacopeial Convention, Inc.
© 1992, 1991, 1990, 1989, 1988, 1987, 1985, 1984, 1983, 1982, 1981, 1980 The United States Pharmacopeial Convention, Inc., 12601 Twinbrook Parkway, Rockville, MD 20852

All rights reserved.

Library of Congress Catalog Card Number 81-640842
ISBN 0-913595-71-3
ISSN 1045-8298

Printed by Rand McNally, Taunton, Massachusetts 02780.
Distributed by USPC, 12601 Twinbrook Parkway, Rockville, Maryland 20852.

Contents

Turn to the last page for the "Fast-finder" subject guide.

USP DI—Volume III
Approved Drug Products and Legal Requirements

Preface v
The United States Pharmacopeial Convention viii
   Officers of the Convention.. viii
   Board of Trustees viii
   General Committee of Revision... viii
   Executive Committee of Revision x
   Drug Information Division Executive Committee x
   Drug Standards Division Executive Committee x
   Drug Nomenclature Committee.. x
   Drug Information Division Advisory Panels.. xi
   Drug Information Division Additional Contributors xv
   Headquarters Staff... xix
   Members of the Convention as of April 1, 1991 xx

Sections
   I: Approved Drug Products with Therapeutic Equivalence Evaluations....................... I/1
       Contents... I/3
       Preface I/5
       Introduction I/6
       How to Use the Drug Product Lists I/17
       Drug Product Lists... I/20
          Prescription Drug Products.. I/20
          OTC Drug Products I/273
          Drug Products with Approval under Section 505 of the Act
             Administered by the Division of Blood and Blood Products........................... I/283
          Discontinued Drug Products... I/287
          Orphan Drug Product Designations.. I/364
          Drug Products Which Must Demonstrate *in vivo* Bioavailability
             Only If Product Fails to Achieve Adequate Dissolution I/385
          Biopharmaceutic Guidance Availability.. I/386
          ANDA Suitability Petitions I/388
       Appendix A: Product Name Index.. I/405
       Appendix B: Product Name Index Listed by Applicant.................................... I/438
       Appendix C: Uniform Terms I/505
       Patent and Exclusivity Information Addendum.. I/506
   II: Selected USP General Notices and Chapters II/1
       Selected General Notices and Requirements II/1
       Drug and Dosage Form Requirements II/5
       Drug and Dosage Form Information II/9
       Packaging Requirements II/22
       Weights and Measures II/25
       Laws and Regulations... II/30
          Controlled Substances Act Regulations II/30
          Federal Food, Drug, and Cosmetic Act Requirements II/60
          Good Manufacturing Practice for Finished Pharmaceuticals........................... II/79
          Packaging—Child-Safety.. II/91
       Guide to General Chapters.. II/94
   III: Chemistry and Compendial Requirements.. III/1
   IV: The Medicine Chart IV/1
   V: USP-Practitioners' Reporting Network V/1
   VI: Index.. VI/1

Contents

USP DI—Volume III
Approved Drug Products and Legal Requirements

Preface ....

The United States Pharmacopeial Convention
  Officers of the Convention vii
  Board of Trustees vii
  Council (or Committee) of Revision viii
  Executive Committee of Revision ....
  Drug Information Division Executive Committee x
  Drug Standards Division Executive Committee x
  Drug Nomenclature Committee ....
  Drug Information Division Advisory Panel xi
  Drug Information Division Additional Contributors xv
  Headquarters Staff ix
  Members of the Convention as of April 16, 1991 ....

Sections
I. Approved Drug Products with Therapeutic Equivalence Evaluations I/1
      Contents I/1
      Preface I/3
      Introduction I/6
      How to Use the Drug Product Lists ....
      Drug Product Lists I/20
      Prescription Drug Products I/26
      OTC Drug Products ....
      Drug Products with Approval under Section 505 of the Act .....
        Administered by the Division of Blood and Blood Products .... I/25?
      Discontinued Drug Products .... I/26?
      Orphan Drug Product Designations .... I/20?
      Drug Products with Multi-Source (or A) Bioavailability
        Only if Product Fails to Achieve Adequate Dissolution ....
      Bioanalytical Guidance Availability .... I/25?
      ANDA Suitability Petitions .... I/25?
      Appendix A, Product Name Index .... I/25?
      Appendix B, Product Name Index (Index by Applicant) .... I/25?
      Appendix C, Uniform Terms ....
      Patent and Exclusivity Information Addendum ....

II. Selected USP General Notices and Chapters II/1
      Selected General Notices and Requirements ....
      Drug and Dietary Product Equivalence ....
      Drug and Dosage Form Information ....
      Packaging Requirements ....
      Weights and Measures ....
      Tests and Assays ....
      Controlled Substances Act Requirements II/20
      Federal Food, Drug, and Cosmetic Act Requirements ....
      Good Manufacturing Practice for Finished Pharmaceuticals ...
      Packaging—Child Safety, 1991 ....
      Guide to General Chapters ....

III. Chemistry and Compendial Requirements III/1
IV. The Labeling Chart IV/1
V. USP-Dictionary Reporting Network V/1
VI. Index VI/1

Preface

In contrast to "the national consensus" found in Volumes I and II is Volume III of *USP DI*.

Volume III is not a product of the USP Committee of Revision, although some of the Committee's determinations in *USP-NF* are reproduced in it. Rather, Volume III is intended as a service to those who need a convenient source of the legal requirements that affect prescribing/dispensing activities—more convenient, and considerably less expensive than tracking them all down and purchasing them separately.

Volume III contains federal and state requirements relevant to the dispensing situation, including:

• the FDA's "Orange Book," *Approved Drug Products with Therapeutic Equivalence Evaluations.*
• abstracted *USP-NF* monograph requirements relating to strength, quality, purity, packaging, labeling, and storage.
• selected *USP-NF* General Chapters and General Notices particularly applicable to the practice situation.
• selected portions of the federal Controlled Substance Act Regulations.
• the federal Food, Drug and Cosmetic Act requirements as they relate to human drugs, including the recent drug diversion and sampling amendments.
• the FDA's Current Good Manufacturing Practice Regulations for Finished Pharmaceuticals.

Selected portions of each state's pharmacy practice act and regulations for dispensing, including product selection regulations, are included individually in a special Supplement to the subscribers in that state.

The entire Orange Book and those supplements issued up to our printing deadline are directly reproduced in this 1993 Volume III. Subsequent 1992 supplements will be published in the *USP DI Updates* for 1993.

The Poison Prevention and Packaging Act and the Drug Enforcement Administration regulations are also included in Volume III, where it is believed they will be useful in the prescribing/dispensing interface.

Inclusion of these selected federal statutes and regulations should assist in voluntary compliance. Inclusion of drug standards information from the *United States Pharmacopeia* and the *National Formulary* should assist practitioners in obtaining a better understanding of drug product quality requirements overall.

Each 1993 *USP DI Update* will supplement all three volumes of *USP DI*.

Acknowledgments—USP wishes to acknowledge the cooperation of the individual State Boards of Pharmacy and the National Association of Boards of Pharmacy, especially its Executive Director, Carmen A. Catizone, in preparation of the state-related materials.

The Food and Drug Administration, in particular the following individuals, was especially helpful in encouraging and facilitating the publication of this volume: Janet Anderson, Susan Daugherty, Joel S. Davis, Donald B. Hare, James E. Knoben, George Scott, Richard Lipov, Miriam McKee, Theodore E. Rushin, and George R. Scott.

FDA's ORANGE BOOK

The Orange Book—The FDA list, *Approved Drug Products with Therapeutic Equivalence Evaluations,* serves two basic purposes:

(1) it identifies the prescription and nonprescription drug products formally approved by the FDA on the basis of safety and effectiveness; and
(2) it provides the FDA's therapeutic equivalence evaluations for those approved multi-source prescription drug products.

In 1984, the Food, Drug and Cosmetic Act was amended by the Drug Price Competition and Patent Term Restoration Act. This law requires the FDA to publish a list of all currently approved drug products and to update it on a monthly basis. The Orange Book and its supplements satisfy this statutory requirement. An addendum providing patent information and identifying those drugs which qualify under this Act for periods of exclusivity is also included.

The Orange Book is referenced in numerous state laws and regulations governing drug substitution in prescribing/dispensing. These are included in the above-mentioned special state *USP DI Updates*.

The following questions and answers were abstracted and compiled from a survey of questions asked by State Boards of Pharmacy and responded to by FDA representatives at the annual meeting of the National Association of Boards of Pharmacy in 1988.

Question: Does the FDA ever plan to cover all legend drugs authorized for manufacturing in the U.S.A.? If not, why not?

Answer: There are two classes of unapproved prescription* drug products that are presently permitted by the FDA to remain on the market:

(1) copies of drugs first marketed before 1938; and (2) certain DESI ineffective products awaiting completion of the FDA's administrative procedures. FDA is planning to initiate a program to declare all versions of pre-1938 drugs to be new drugs and require an approved application for a drug product to either stay or come on the market. Products deemed ineffective after the administrative and legal procedures of the DESI process are completed will come off the market. There are currently only a few drugs remaining in this category.

Question: How does the FDA revise its evaluation of a product based on adverse reports?

Answer: Adverse events, including therapeutic failures, may be reported for any drug. (Note: The USP reporting form in the Practitioners' Reporting Network section may be used.) Therapeutic failures occur even when the drug product is not changed, as is evident from the reports we receive. Blood pressures can rise on previously effective therapy; heart failure can worsen on a stable digoxin/diuretic regimen; seizures can break through, etc. We would not consider changing our therapeutic equivalence evaluations unless evidence exists that the adverse reports (e.g., therapeutic failures) were due to the specific drug product rather than to a patient or drug substance problem. If such data were presented to us, we would change the code to therapeutically inequivalent or remove the product from the market.

Question: How long does it take for a drug to appear in the Orange Book?

Answer: The Orange Book is updated monthly. Each cumulative supplement indicates the time period covered by it.

Question: Is the Orange Book an official national compendium and authoritative source which can be used to provide protection in civil suits? Does it have force of law?

Answer: The Orange Book is not an official national compendium. The Orange Book displays the FDA's therapeutic equivalence recommendations on approved multiple source drug products. The FDA's evaluation of therapeutic equivalence is a scientific judgment based upon data submitted to the FDA. Generic substitution is a social and economic policy administered at the state level intended to minimize the cost of drugs to consumers. The programs are administered by the states, because the practices of pharmacy and medicine are state functions.

The question of liability is not one in the FDA's area of expertise. We suggest that counsel in your state be consulted. The Orange Book does not have force of law. The preface of the Orange Book addresses this issue.

Question: Provide tips on how to explain to physicians that drugs that are bioequivalent are indeed therapeutically equivalent. Many believe that drugs are not necessarily therapeutically equivalent, just because they are bioequivalent.

Answer: 1. The FDA is not aware of one clinical study that compared two drug products evaluated by the FDA as bioequivalent/therapeutic equivalent that demonstrates therapeutic inequivalence.

2. In the majority of cases the marketed innovator's product is not the formulation that was tested in clinical trials. The marketed innovator's drug product was shown to be therapeutically equivalent to the formulation that was used in the clinical trials by a bioavailability/bioequivalence study. Therefore, a generic drug product and the innovator's drug product stand in the same relationship to the formulation that was originally tested for safety and effectiveness.

Question: How does the Orange Book relate to and/or impact on state formularies?

Answer: It became apparent to the FDA soon after the repeal of the anti-substitution laws by the states that it could not serve the needs of each state on an individual basis in the preparation of their formularies. In 1978 the Commissioner of Food and Drugs notified appropriate officials of all states of the FDA's intention to provide a list of all prescription drug products that had been approved by the FDA for safety and effectiveness, with therapeutic equivalence recommendations being made on all multiple source drug products in the list. This list could be used by each state in implementing its own law and would relieve the FDA of expending an enormous amount of resources to provide individualized service to all states. Three copies of the Orange Book continue to be sent to state officials for their use in implementing their respective state laws. The states are under no mandate to accept the therapeutic equivalence recommendations in the Orange Book.

Question: What is the applicability of the Orange Book in a community pharmacy setting?

Answer: It was never the FDA's intention to have the Orange Book used in community pharmacies. However, a state could implement its law with this as a requirement.

Question: What is the legal status of pharmaceutical substitution of a different dosage form of a given drug entity? Can the FDA provide any assistance in identifying potential therapeutic problems (or therapeutic comparisons) between available dosage forms?

Answer: The Orange Book does not mandate which drug products may or may not be substituted. The therapeutic equivalence evaluations in the Orange Book are recommendations only. However, the FDA does not recommend substitution between different dosage forms. The Agency has very few bioequivalence studies in its files comparing different dosage forms of a given drug entity.

Question: Does the FDA have any way of identifying which distributors are marketing a given manufacturer's product and providing that information in the Orange Book?

Answer: No. Since an approved supplement is not required for an applicant with an approved drug product to license a distributor, FDA has no good mechanism to monitor distributors and to know when they change manufacturers.

A Bioequivalence Hearing was held by the Commissioner of Food and Drugs September 29–October 1, 1986. Following the hearing, the Commissioner appointed a Task Force of high ranking FDA officials and outside consultants to review the testimony, reach conclusions, and recommend actions. Its Report was issued in January 1988.

One of the Task Force recommendations was "that the Orange Book be more widely advertised to pharmacists. This could be accomplished by working more closely with the states. Efforts to decrease the cost should be explored. This could be accomplished by publishing an abbreviated version of the list alone, by selling the Orange Book without the monthly supplements, or by enlisting the assistance of a private organization to make the book available at a lower cost."

By publishing the Orange Book and its supplements as a part of the *USP DI* system, USP is making the Orange Book more widely available at much less expense to health professionals.

USP-NF requirements—The United States Pharmacopeial Convention is the publisher of the *United States Pharmacopeia* and the *National Formulary*. These texts are recognized as official compendia by the pharmacy and medical professions. They contain standards, specifications, and other requirements relating to drugs and other articles used in medical and pharmacy practice that may be enforceable under various statutes. These requirements are applicable not only when drugs are in the possession of the manufacturer, but at the practice level as well.

Although the standards continue to be applicable when drugs are dispensed or sold, it must also be recognized that most prescriptions today are filled with manufactured products and for the most part physicians and pharmacists rarely compound or analyze drug products. On the other hand, dispensers need to be aware of the quality attributes of products, their packaging and storage requirements, and the other applicable standards to which legal consequences may attach.

In recognition of this need, Volume III presents abstracts of the applicable *USP-NF* standards. Similarly, selected portions of the *USP-NF* General Notices and Chapters that are deemed to be especially relevant are reprinted in Volume III.

The incorporation of these official *USP-NF* materials into *USP DI* is for informational purposes only. Because of varying publication schedules, there may occasionally be a time difference between publication of revisions in the *USP-NF* and the appearance of these changes in *USP DI*. Readers are advised that only the standards as written in the *USP-NF* are regarded as official.

The *USP-NF* material included in *USP DI* is not intended to represent nor shall it be interpreted to be the equivalent of or a substitute for the official *United States Pharmacopeia* and/or *National Formulary*. In the event of any difference or discrepancy between the current official *USP* or *NF* standards and the information contained herein, the context and effect of the official compendia shall prevail.

---

*Editor's note: Relatively few nonprescription medications enter the market through the New Drug Application procedures.

The United States Pharmacopeial Convention
1990–1995

Officers

MARK NOVITCH, M.D.
President
Kalamazoo, MI

DONALD R. BENNETT, M.D., PH.D.
Vice-President
Chicago, IL

JOHN T. FAY, JR., PH.D.
Treasurer
Orange, CA

ARTHUR HULL HAYES, JR., M.D.
Past President
New York, NY

JEROME A. HALPERIN
Secretary
Rockville, MD

Board of Trustees

JAMES T. DOLUISIO, PH.D.[2]
Chairman
Austin, TX

DONALD R. BENNETT, M.D., PH.D.
ex officio
Chicago, IL

JOHN V. BERGEN, PH.D.[1]
Vice Chairman
Villanova, PA

EDWIN D. BRANSOME, JR., M.D.[4]
Augusta, GA

JORDAN L. COHEN, PH.D.[2]
Lexington, KY

J. RICHARD CROUT, M.D.[4]
Rockville, MD

JOHN T. FAY, JR., PH.D.
ex officio
Orange, CA

ARTHUR HULL HAYES, JR., M.D.
ex officio
New York, NY

JOSEPH A. MOLLICA, PH.D.[1]
Wilmington, DE

GRACE POWERS MONACO, J.D.[3]
Washington, DC

MARK NOVITCH, M.D.
ex officio
Kalamazoo, MI

---

[1]At large.
[2]Representing pharmacy.
[3]Public member.
[4]Representing medicine.
[5]12601 Twinbrook Parkway, Rockville, MD 20852.

General Committee of Revision

JEROME A. HALPERIN[5], *Executive Director, USPC,*
Chairman

LEE T. GRADY, PH.D.[5], *Director, Drug Standards*
Division

KEITH W. JOHNSON[5], *Director, Drug Information*
Division

LOYD V. ALLEN, JR., PH.D.
Oklahoma City, OK

JERRY R. ALLISON, PH.D.
Syracuse, NY

THOMAS J. AMBROSIO, PH.D.
Somerville, NJ

GREGORY E. AMIDON, PH.D.
Kalamazoo, MI

NORMAN W. ATWATER, PH.D.
Hopewell, NJ

HENRY L. AVALLONE, B.SC.
North Brunswick, NJ

LEONARD C. BAILEY, PH.D.
Piscataway, NJ

JOHN A. BELIS, M.D.
Hershey, PA

LESLIE Z. BENET, PH.D.
San Francisco, CA

JUDY P. BOEHLERT, PH.D.
Nutley, NJ

JAMES C. BOYLAN, PH.D.
Abbott Park, IL

LYNN R. BRADY, PH.D.
Seattle, WA

R. EDWARD BRANSON, PH.D.
Andover, MA

WILLIAM H. BRINER, CAPT., B.S.
Durham, NC

STEPHEN R. BYRN, PH.D.
West Lafayette, IN

PETER R. BYRON, PH.D.
Richmond, VA

HERBERT S. CARLIN, D.SC.
Chappaqua, NY

DENNIS L. CASEY, PH.D.
Raritan, NJ

LESTER CHAFETZ, PH.D.
Kansas City, MO

VIRGINIA C. CHAMBERLAIN, PH.D.
Rockville, MD

WEI-WEI, CHANG, PH.D.
(1992–)
Rockville, MD

MARY BETH CHENAULT, B.S.
Rockville, MD

ZAK T. CHOWHAN, PH.D.
Palo Alto, CA

SEBASTIAN G. CIANCIO, D.D.S.
Buffalo, NY

MURRAY S. COOPER, PH.D.
Islamorada, FL

LLOYD E. DAVIS, PH.D., D.V.M.
Urbana, IL

LEON ELLENBOGEN, PH.D.
Clifton, NJ

R. MICHAEL ENZINGER, PH.D.
(1990–1992)
Kalamazoo, MI

CLYDE R. ERSKINE, B.S., M.B.A.
Newtown Square, PA

EDWARD A. FITZGERALD, PH.D.
Bethesda, MD
EVERETT FLANIGAN, PH.D.
Kankakee, IL
KLAUS G. FLOREY, PH.D.
Princeton, NJ
THOMAS S. FOSTER, PHARM.D.
Lexington, KY
JOSEPH F. GALLELLI, PH.D.
Bethesda, MD
ROBERT L. GARNICK, PH.D.
So. San Francisco, CA
DOUGLAS D. GLOVER, M.D., R.PH.
Morgantown, WV
ALAN M. GOLDBERG, PH.D.
Baltimore, MD
BURTON J. GOLDSTEIN, M.D.
Miami, FL
DENNIS K. J. GORECKI, PH.D.
Saskatoon, Saskatchewan, Canada
MICHAEL J. GROVES, PH.D.
Lake Forest, IL
ROBERT M. GUTHRIE, M.D.
Columbus, OH
SAMIR A. HANNA, PH.D.
Lawrenceville, NJ
STANLEY L. HEM, PH.D.
West Lafayette, IN
JOY HOCHSTADT, PH.D.
New York, NY
DAVID W. HUGHES, PH.D.
Ottawa, Ontario, Canada
NORMAN C. JAMIESON, PH.D.
St. Louis, MO
RICHARD D. JOHNSON, PHARM.D., PH.D.
Kansas City, MO
JUDITH K. JONES, M.D., PH.D.
Arlington, VA
STANLEY A. KAPLAN, PH.D.
Menlo Park, CA
HERBERT E. KAUFMAN, M.D.
New Orleans, LA
DONALD KAYE, M.D.
Philadelphia, PA
PAUL E. KENNEDY, PH.D.
West Conshohocken, PA
JAY S. KEYSTONE, M.D.
Toronto, Ontario, Canada
ROSALYN C. KING, PHARM.D., M.P.H.
Silver Spring, MD
GORDON L. KLEIN, M.D.
Galveston, TX
JOSEPH E. KNAPP, PH.D.
Pittsburgh, PA
JOHN B. LANDIS, PH.D.
(1990–1992)
Kalamazoo, MI
THOMAS P. LAYLOFF, PH.D.
St. Louis, MO
LEWIS J. LEESON, PH.D.
Summit, NJ
JOHN W. LEVCHUK, PH.D.
Rockville, MD
ROBERT D. LINDEMAN, M.D.
Albuquerque, NM
CHARLES H. LOCHMULLER, PH.D.
Durham, NC
EDWARD G. LOVERING, PH.D.
Ottawa, Ontario, Canada
CATHERINE M. MACLEOD, M.D.
Chicago, IL
CAROL S. MARCUS, PH.D., M.D.
Torrance, CA

THOMAS MEDWICK, PH.D.
Piscataway, NJ
ROBERT F. MORRISSEY, PH.D.
New Brunswick, NJ
TERRY E. MUNSON, B.S.
Fairfax, VA
HAROLD S. NELSON, M.D.
Denver, CO
WENDEL L. NELSON, PH.D.
Seattle, WA
MARIA I. NEW, M.D.
New York, NY
SHARON C. NORTHUP, PH.D.
Round Lake, IL
GARNET E. PECK, PH.D.
West Lafayette, IN
ROBERT V. PETERSEN, PH.D.
Salt Lake City, UT
ROSEMARY C. POLOMANO, R.N., M.S.N.
Philadelphia, PA
THOMAS P. REINDERS, PHARM.D.
Richmond, VA
CHRISTOPHER T. RHODES, PH.D.
Kingston, RI
JOSEPH R. ROBINSON, PH.D.
Madison, WI
LARY A. ROBINSON, M.D.
Omaha, NE
DAVID B. ROLL, PH.D.
Salt Lake City, UT
THEODORE J. ROSEMAN, PH.D.
Round Lake, IL
SANFORD H. ROTH, M.D.
Phoenix, AZ
LEONARD P. RYBAK, M.D.
Springfield, IL
RONALD J. SAWCHUK, PH.D.
Minneapolis, MN
GORDON D. SCHIFF, M.D.
Chicago, IL
ANDREW J. SCHMITZ, JR., M.S.
Huntington, NY
RALPH F. SHANGRAW, PH.D.
Baltimore, MD
ALBERT L. SHEFFER, M.D.
Boston, MA
ELI SHEFTER, PH.D.
Boulder, CO
ERIC B. SHEININ, PH.D.
Rockville, MD
ROBERT L. SIEGLE, M.D.
San Antonio, TX
EDWARD B. SILBERSTEIN, M.D.
Cincinnati, OH
JOSEPH E. SINSHEIMER, PH.D.
Ann Arbor, MI
MARILYN DIX SMITH, PH.D.
Dayton, NJ
BURTON E. SOBEL, M.D.
St. Louis, MO
E. JOHN STABA, PH.D.
Minneapolis, MN
ROBERT S. STERN, M.D.
Boston, MA
JAMES T. STEWART, PH.D.
Athens, GA
HENRY S. I. TAN, PH.D.
Cincinnati, OH
THEODORE G. TONG, PHARM.D.
Tucson, AZ
SALVATORE J. TURCO, PHARM.D.
Philadelphia, PA
CLARENCE T. UEDA, PHARM.D., PH.D.
Omaha, NE

ELIZABETH B. VADAS, PH.D.
 Pointe Claire-Dorval, Quebec, Canada
HUIB J. M. VAN DE DONK, PH.D.
 Bilthoven, The Netherlands
STANLEY VAN DEN NOORT, M.D.
 Irvine, CA
VINCENT S. VENTURELLA, PH.D.
 Murray Hill, NJ
ROBERT E. VESTAL, M.D.
 Boise, ID
JAMES A. VISCONTI, PH.D.
 Columbus, OH
EDWARD W. VOSS, JR., PH.D.
 Urbana, IL
PHILIP D. WALSON, M.D.
 Columbus, OH
PAUL F. WHITE, PH.D., M.D.
 Dallas, TX
ROBERT G. WOLFANGEL, PH.D.
 St. Louis, MO
MANFRED E. WOLFF, PH.D.
 San Diego, CA
WESLEY E. WORKMAN, PH.D.
 (1992–)
 St. Louis, MO
JOHN W. YARBRO, M.D., PH.D.
 Springfield, IL
GEORGE ZOGRAFI, PH.D.
 Madison, WI

Executive Committee of Revision (1992–1993)
JEROME A. HALPERIN, *Chairman*
NORMAN W. ATWATER, PH.D.
BURTON J. GOLDSTEIN, M.D.
ROBERT V. PETERSEN, PH.D.
ANDREW J. SCHMITZ, JR.
ROBERT S. STERN, M.D.
PAUL F. WHITE, M.D.

Drug Information Division Executive Committee
JOHN W. YARBRO, M.D., PH.D., *Chairman*
JAMES C. BOYLAN, PH.D.
HERBERT S. CARLIN, D.SC.

SEBASTIAN G. CIANCIO, D.D.S.
LLOYD E. DAVIS, D.V.M., PH.D.
JAY S. KEYSTONE, M.D.
ROBERT D. LINDEMAN, M.D.
MARIA I. NEW, M.D.
ROSEMARY C. POLOMANO, M.S.N.
THOMAS P. REINDERS, PHARM.D.
GORDON D. SCHIFF, M.D.
ALBERT L. SHEFFER, M.D.
THEODORE G. TONG, PHARM.D.
ROBERT E. VESTAL, M.D.

Drug Standards Division Executive Committee
KLAUS G. FLOREY, PH.D., *Chairman*
JERRY R. ALLISON, PH.D.
JUDY P. BOEHLERT, PH.D.
CAPT. WILLIAM H. BRINER
LESTER CHAFETZ, PH.D.
ZAK T. CHOWHAN, PH.D.
MURRAY S. COOPER, PH.D.
JOSEPH F. GALLELLI, PH.D.
ROBERT L. GARNICK, PH.D. (1992–)
DAVID W. HUGHES, PH.D.
JOHN B. LANDIS, PH.D. (1990–1992)
LEWIS J. LEESON, PH.D.
THOMAS MEDWICK, PH.D.
ROBERT F. MORRISSEY, PH.D.
SHARON C. NORTHUP, PH.D.
RALPH F. SHANGRAW, PH.D.
JAMES T. STEWART, PH.D.

Drug Nomenclature Committee
HERBERT S. CARLIN, D.SC., *Chairman*
WILLIAM M. HELLER, PH.D., *Consultant/Advisor*
LESTER CHAFETZ, PH.D.
LLOYD E. DAVIS, D.V.M., PH.D.
EVERETT FLANIGAN, PH.D. (1992–)
DOUGLAS B. GLOVER, M.D.
DAVID W. HUGHES, PH.D.
RICHARD D. JOHNSON, PHARM.D., PH.D.
JOHN B. LANDIS, PH.D. (1990–1992)
ROSEMARY C. POLOMANO, R.N., M.S.N.
THOMAS P. REINDERS, PHARM.D.
ERIC B. SHEININ, PH.D.
PHILIP D. WALSON, M.D.

x

Drug Information Division Advisory Panels
1990–1995

Members who serve as Chairs are listed first.

The information presented in this text represents an ongoing review of the drugs contained herein and represents a consensus of various viewpoints expressed. The individuals listed below have served on the USP Advisory Panels for the 1990–1995 revision period and have contributed to the development of the 1993 USP DI data base. Such listing does not imply that these individuals have reviewed all of the material in this text or that they individually agree with all statements contained herein.

Anesthesiology
Paul F. White, Ph.D., M.D., *Chair*, Dallas, TX; David R. Bevan, M.B., FFARCS, MRCP, Vancouver, British Columbia; Eugene Y. Cheng, M.D., Milwaukee, WI; Charles J. Coté, M.D., Boston, MA; Roy Cronnelly, M.D., Ph.D., Placerville, CA; Peter Glass, M.D., Durham, NC; Michael B. Howie, M.D., Columbus, OH; Beverly A. Krause, C.R.N.A., M.S., St. Louis, MO; Carl Lynch III, M.D., Ph.D., Charlottesville, VA; Carl Rosow, M.D., Ph.D., Boston, MA; Peter S. Sebel, M.B., Ph.D., Atlanta, GA; Walter L. Way, M.D., San Francisco, CA; Matthew B. Weinger, M.D., San Diego, CA; Richard Weiskopf, M.D., San Francisco, CA; David H. Wong, Pharm.D., M.D., Long Beach, CA

Cardiovascular and Renal Drugs
Burton E. Sobel, M.D., *Chair*, St. Louis, MO; William P. Baker, M.D., Ph.D., Bethesda, MD; Nils U. Bang, M.D., Indianapolis, IN; Emmanuel L. Bravo, M.D., Cleveland, OH; Mary Jo Burgess, M.D., Salt Lake City, UT; James H. Chesebro, M.D., Rochester, MN; Peter Corr, Ph.D., St. Louis, MO; Dwain L. Eckberg, M.D., Richmond, VA; Ruth Eshleman, Ph.D., W. Kingston, RI; William H. Frishman, M.D., Bronx, NY; Edward D. Frohlich, M.D., New Orleans, LA; Martha Hill, Ph.D., R.N., Baltimore, MD; Norman M. Kaplan, M.D., Dallas, TX; Michael Lesch, M.D., Ann Arbor, MI; Manuel Martinez-Maldonado, M.D., Decatur, GA; Patrick A. McKee, M.D., Oklahoma City, OK; Dan M. Roden, M.D., Nashville, TN; Michael R. Rosen, M.D., New York, NY; Jane Schultz, R.N., B.S.N., Rochester, MN; Robert L. Talbert, Pharm.D., San Antonio, TX; Raymond L. Woosley, M.D., Ph.D., Washington, DC

Clinical Immunology/Allergy/Rheumatology
Albert L. Sheffer, M.D., *Chair*, Boston, MA; John A. Anderson, M.D., Detroit, MI; Emil Bardana, Jr., M.D., Portland, OR; John Baum, M.D., Rochester, NY; Debra Danoff, M.D., Montreal, Quebec; Daniel G. de Jesus, M.D., Ph.D., Vanier, Ontario; Elliott F. Ellis, M.D., Jacksonville, FL; Patricia A. Fraser, M.D., Boston, MA; Frederick E. Hargreave, M.D., Hamilton, Ontario; Evelyn V. Hess, M.D., Cincinnati, OH; Jean M. Jackson, M.D., Boston, MA; Stephen R. Kaplan, M.D., Buffalo, NY; Sandra M. Koehler, Milwaukee, WI; Richard A. Moscicki, M.D., Boston, MA; Shirley Murphy, M.D., Albuquerque, NM; Gary S. Rachelefsky, M.D., Los Angeles, CA; Robert E. Reisman, M.D., Buffalo, NY; Robert L. Rubin, Ph.D., La Jolla, CA; Daniel J. Stechschulte, M.D., Kansas City, KS; Virginia S. Taggert, Bethesda, MD; Joseph A. Tami, Pharm.D., San Antonio, TX; John H. Toogood, M.D., London, Ontario; Martin D. Valentine, M.D., Baltimore, MD; Michael Weinblatt, M.D., Boston, MA; Dennis Michael Williams, Pharm.D., Chapel Hill, NC; Stewart Wong, Ph.D., Brookfield, CT

Clinical Toxicology/Substance Abuse
Theodore G. Tong, Pharm.D., *Chair*, Tucson, AZ; John Ambre, M.D., Ph.D., Chicago, IL; Usoa E. Busto, Pharm.D., Toronto, Ontario; Darryl Inaba, Pharm.D., San Francisco, CA; Edward P. Krenzelok, Pharm.D., Pittsburgh, PA; Michael Montagne, Ph.D., Boston, MA; Sven A. Normann, Pharm.D., Tampa, FL; Gary M. Oderda, Pharm.D., Salt Lake City, UT; Paul Pentel, M.D., Minneapolis, MN; Rose Ann Soloway, R.N., Washington, DC; Daniel A. Spyker, M.D., Ph.D., Rockville, MD; Anthony R. Temple, M.D., Ft. Washington, PA; Anthony Tommasello, Pharm.D., Baltimore, MD; Joseph C. Veltri, Pharm.D., Salt Lake City, UT; William A. Watson, Pharm.D., Kansas City, MO

Consumer Interest/Health Education
Gordon D. Schiff, M.D., *Chair*, Chicago, IL; Michael J. Ackerman, Ph.D., Bethesda, MD; Barbara Aranda-Naranjo, R.N., San Antonio, TX; Frank J. Ascione, Pharm.D., Ph.D., Ann Arbor, MI; Judith I. Brown, Silver Spring, MD; Jose Camacho, Austin, TX; Margaret A. Charters, Ph.D., Syracuse, NY; Jennifer Cross, San Francisco, CA; William G. Harless, Ph.D., Bethesda, MD; Louis H. Kompare, Lake Buena Vista, FL; Margo Kroshus, R.N., B.S.N., Rochester, MN; Marilyn Lister, Wakefield, Quebec; Margaret Lueders, Seattle, WA; Frederick S. Mayer, R.Ph., M.P.H., Sausalito, CA; Nancy Milio, Ph.D., Chapel Hill, NC; Irving Rubin, Port Washington, NY; T. Donald Rucker, Ph.D., River Forest, IL; Stephen B. Soumerai, Sc.D., Boston, MA; Carol A. Vetter, Rockville, MD

Critical Care Medicine
Catherine M. MacLeod, M.D., *Chair*, Chicago, IL; William Banner, Jr., M.D., Salt Lake City, UT; Philip S. Barie, M.D., New York, NY; Thomas P. Bleck, M.D., Charlottesville, VA; Roger C. Bone, M.D., Chicago, IL; Susan S. Fish, Pharm.D., Boston, MA; Edgar R. Gonzalez, Pharm.D., Richmond, VA; Robert Gottesman, Rockville, MD; Michael Halperin, M.D., Denver, CO; John W. Hoyt, M.D., Pittsburgh, PA; Sheldon A. Magder, M.D., Montreal, Quebec; Henry Masur, M.D., Bethesda, MD; Joseph E. Parrillo, M.D., Chicago, IL; Sharon Peters, M.D., St. John's, Newfoundland; Domenic A. Sica, M.D., Richmond, VA; Martin G. Tweeddale, M.B., Ph.D., Vancouver, British Columbia

Dentistry

Sebastian G. Ciancio, D.D.S., *Chair*, Buffalo, NY; Donald F. Adams, D.D.S., Portland, OR; Karen A. Baker, M.S. Pharm., Iowa City, IA; Stephen A. Cooper, D.M.D., Ph.D., Philadelphia, PA; Frederick A. Curro, D.M.D., Ph.D., Jersey City, NJ; Paul J. Desjardins, D.M.D., Ph.D., Newark, NJ; Tommy W. Gage, D.D.S., Ph.D., Dallas, TX; Stephen F. Goodman, D.D.S., New York, NY; Daniel A. Haas, D.D.S., Ph.D., Toronto, Ontario; Richard E. Hall, D.D.S., Ph.D., Buffalo, NY; Lireka P. Joseph, Dr.P.H., Rockville, MD; Janice Lieberman, Fort Lee, NJ; Laurie Lisowski, Buffalo, NY; Clarence L. Trummel, D.D.S., Ph.D., Farmington, CT; Joel M. Weaver, II, D.D.S., Ph.D., Columbus, OH; Clifford W. Whall, Jr., Ph.D., Chicago, IL; Raymond P. White, Jr., D.D.S., Ph.D., Chapel Hill, NC; Ray C. Williams, D.M.D., Boston, MA

Dermatology

Robert S. Stern, M.D., *Chair*, Boston, MA; Beatrice B. Abrams, Ph.D., Somerville, NJ; Richard D. Baughman, M.D., Hanover, NH; Michael Bigby, M.D., Boston, MA; Janice T. Chussil, R.N., M.S.N., Portland, OR; Stuart Maddin, M.D., Vancouver, British Columbia; Milton Orkin, M.D., Minneapolis, MN; Neil H. Shear, M.D., Toronto, Ontario; Edgar Benton Smith, M.D., Galveston, TX; Dennis P. West, M.S. Pharm., Lincolnshire, IL; Gail M. Zimmerman, Portland, OR

Diagnostic Agents—Nonradioactive

Robert L. Siegle, M.D., *Chair*, San Antonio, TX; Robert C. Brasch, M.D., San Francisco, CA; Jacob J. Fabrikant, M.D., Berkeley, CA; Nicholas Harry Malakis, M.D., Bethesda, MD; Robert F. Mattrey, M.D., San Diego, CA; James A. Nelson, M.D., Seattle, WA; Jovitas Skucas, M.D., Rochester, NY; Gerald L. Wolf, Ph.D., M.D., Charlestown, MA

Drug Information Science

James A. Visconti, Ph.D., *Chair*, Columbus, OH; Marie A. Abate, Pharm.D., Morgantown, WV; Ann B. Amerson, Pharm.D., Lexington, KY; Philip O. Anderson, Pharm.D., San Diego, CA; Danial E. Baker, Pharm.D., Spokane, WA; C. David Butler, Pharm.D., M.B.A., Oak Brook, IL; Linda L. Hart, Pharm.D., San Francisco, CA; Edward J. Huth, M.D., Philadelphia, PA; John M. Kessler, Pharm.D., Chapel Hill, NC; R. David Lauper, Pharm.D., Emeryville, CA; Domingo R. Martinez, Pharm.D., Birmingham, AL; William F. McGhan, Pharm.D., Ph.D., Philadelphia, PA; John K. Murdoch, B.Sc.Phm., Toronto, Ontario; Kurt A. Proctor, Ph.D., Alexandria, VA; Arnauld F. Scafidi, M.D., M.P.H., Rockville, MD; John A. Scarlett, M.D., Princeton, NJ; Gary H. Smith, Pharm.D., Tucson, AZ; Dennis F. Thompson, Pharm.D., Weatherford, OK; William G. Troutman, Pharm.D., Albuquerque, NM; Lee A. Wanke, M.S., Portland, OR

Drug Utilization Review

Judith K. Jones, M.D., Ph.D., *Chair*, Arlington, VA; John F. Beary, III., M.D., Washington, DC; James L. Blackburn, Pharm.D., Saskatoon, Saskatchewan; Richard S. Blum, M.D., East Hills, NY; Amy Cooper-Outlaw, Pharm.D., Atlanta, GA; Joseph W. Cranston, Jr., Ph.D., Chicago, IL; W. Gary Erwin, Pharm.D., Philadelphia, PA; Jere E. Goyan, Ph.D., San Francisco, CA; Duane M. Kirking, Ph.D., Ann Arbor, MI; Karen E. Koch, Pharm.D., Tupelo, MS; Aida A. LeRoy, Pharm.D., Arlington, VA; Jerome Levine, M.D., Baltimore, MD; Richard W. Lindsay, M.D., Charlottesville, VA; Deborah M. Nadzam, R.N., Ph.D., Oak Brook Terrace, IL; William Z. Potter, M.D., Ph.D., Bethesda, MD; Louise R. Rodriquez, M.S., Washington, DC; Stephen P. Spielberg, M.D.,

Ph.D., Gwynedd Valley, PA; Suzan M. Streichenwein, M.D., Houston, TX; Brian L. Strom, M.D., Philadelphia, PA; Michael Weintraub, M.D., Rockville, MD; Antonio Carlos Zanini, M.D., Ph.D., Sao Paulo, Brazil

Endocrinology

Maria I. New, M.D., *Chair*, New York, NY; Ronald D. Brown, M.D., Oklahoma City, OK; R. Keith Campbell, Pharm.D., Pullman, WA; David S. Cooper, M.D., Baltimore, MD; Betty J. Dong, Pharm.D., San Francisco, CA; Andrea Dunaif, M.D., New York, NY; Anke A. Ehrhardt, Ph.D., New York, NY; Nadir R. Farid, M.D., Riyadh, Saudi Arabia; John G. Haddad, Jr., M.D., Philadelphia, PA; Michael M. Kaplan, M.D., Southfield, MI; Harold E. Lebovitz, M.D., Brooklyn, NY; Marvin E. Levin, M.D., St. Louis, MO; Marvin M. Lipman, M.D., Yonkers, NY; Barbara Lippe, M.D., Los Angeles, CA; Barbara J. Maschak-Carey, R.N., M.S.N., Philadelphia, PA; James C. Melby, M.D., Boston, MA; Walter J. Meyer, III., M.D., Galveston, TX; Rita Nemchik, R.N., M.S., C.D.E., Franklin Lakes, NJ; Daniel A. Notterman, M.D., New York, NY; Ron Gershon Rosenfeld, M.D., Stanford, CA; Paul Saenger, M.D., Bronx, NY; Judson J. Van Wyk, M.D., Chapel Hill, NC; Leonard Wartofsky, M.D., Washington, DC

Family Practice

Robert M. Guthrie, M.D., *Chair*, Columbus, OH; Jack A. Brose, D.O., Athens, OH; Jannet M. Carmichael, Pharm.D., Reno, NV; Jacqueline A. Chadwick, M.D., Phoenix, AZ; Mark E. Clasen, M.D., Ph.D., Houston, TX; Lloyd P. Haskell, M.D., West Borough, MA; Luis A. Izquierdo-Mora, M.D., Rio Piedras, PR; Edward L. Langston, M.D., Indianapolis, IN; Charles D. Ponte, Pharm.D., Morgantown, WV; Jack M. Rosenberg, Pharm.D., Ph.D., Brooklyn, NY; John F. Sangster, M.D., London, Ontario; Theodore L. Yarboro, Sr., M.D., M.P.H., Sharon, PA

Gastroenterology

Gordon L. Klein, M.D., *Chair*, Galveston, TX; Karl E. Anderson, M.D., Galveston, TX; William Balistreri, M.D., Cincinnati, OH; Paul Bass, Ph.D., Madison, WI; Rosemary R. Berardi, Pharm.D., Ann Arbor, MI; Raymond F. Burk, M.D., Nashville, TN; Thomas Q. Garvey, III, M.D., Potomac, MD; Donald J. Glotzer, M.D., Boston, MA; Flavio Habal, M.D., Toronto, Ontario; Paul E. Hyman, M.D., Torrance, CA; Bernard Mehl, D.P.S., New York, NY; William J. Snape, Jr., M.D., Torrance, CA; Ronald D. Soltis, M.D., Minneapolis, MN; C. Noel Williams, M.D., Halifax, Nova Scotia; Hyman J. Zimmerman, M.D., Washington, DC

Geriatrics

Robert E. Vestal, M.D., *Chair*, Boise, ID; Darrell R. Abernethy, M.D., Providence, RI; William B. Abrams, M.D., West Point, PA; Jerry Avorn, M.D., Boston, MA; Robert A. Blouin, Pharm.D., Lexington, KY; S. George Carruthers, M.D., Halifax, Nova Scotia; Lynn E. Chaitovitz, Rockville, MD; Terry Fulmer, R.N., Ph.D., New York, NY; Philip P. Gerbino, Pharm.D., Philadelphia, PA; Pearl S. German, Sc.D., Baltimore, MD; David J. Greenblatt, M.D., Boston, MA; Martin D. Higbee, Pharm.D., Tucson, AZ; Brian B. Hoffman, M.D., Palo Alto, CA; J. Edward Jackson, M.D., San Diego, CA; Peter P. Lamy, Ph.D., Baltimore, MD; Joseph V. Levy, Ph.D., San Francisco, CA; Paul A. Mitenko, M.D., FRCPC, Nanaimo, British Columbia; John E. Morley, M.B., B.Ch., St. Louis, MO; Jay Roberts, Ph.D., Philadelphia, PA; Louis J. Rubenstein, R.Ph., Alexandria, VA; Janice B. Schwartz, M.D., San Francisco, CA; Alexander M.M. Shepherd, M.D., San Antonio, TX; William Simonson, Pharm.D., Portland, OR; Daniel S. Sitar, Ph.D., Winnipeg, Manitoba; Mary K.

Walker, R.N., Ph.D., Lexington, KY; Alastair J. J. Wood, M.D., Nashville, TN

Hematologic and Neoplastic Disease
John W. Yarbro, M.D., Ph.D., *Chair*, Springfield, IL; Joseph S. Bailes, M.D., McAllen, TX; Laurence H. Baker, D.O., Detroit, MI; Barbara D. Blumberg, Dallas, TX; Helene G. Brown, B.S., Los Angeles, CA; Nora L. Burnham, Pharm.D., Rochester, MN; William J. Dana, Pharm.D., Houston, TX; Connie Henke-Yarbro, R.N., B.S.N., Springfield, IL; William H. Hryniuk, M.D., San Diego, CA; B. J. Kennedy, M.D., Minneapolis, MN; Barnett Kramer, M.D., Bethesda, MD; Brigid G. Leventhal, M.D., Baltimore, MD; Michael J. Mastrangelo, M.D., Philadelphia, PA; David S. Rosenthal, M.D., Boston, MA; Richard L. Schilsky, M.D., Chicago, IL; Rowena N. Schwartz, Pharm.D., Pittsburgh, PA; Roy L. Silverstein, M.D., New York, NY; Samuel G. Taylor, IV, M.D., Chicago, IL; Raymond B. Weiss, M.D., Washington, DC

Infectious Disease Therapy
Donald Kaye, M.D., *Chair*, Philadelphia, PA; Robert Austrian, M.D., Philadelphia, PA; C. Glenn Cobbs, M.D., Birmingham, AL; Joseph W. Cranston, Jr., Ph.D., Chicago, IL; John J. Dennehy, M.D., Danville, PA; Courtney V. Fletcher, Pharm. D., Minneapolis, MN; Earl H. Freimer, M.D., Toledo, OH; Marla J. Gold, M.D., Philadelphia, PA; Marc LeBel, Pharm.D., Quebec, Quebec; John D. Nelson, M.D., Dallas, TX; Harold C. Neu, M.D., New York, NY; Lindsay E. Nicolle, M.D., Winnipeg, Manitoba; Alvin Novick, M.D., New Haven, CT; Charles G. Prober, M.D., Stanford, CA; Douglas D. Richman, M.D., San Diego, CA; Spotswood L. Spruance, M.D., Salt Lake City, UT; Roy T. Steigbigel, M.D., Stony Brook, NY; Paul F. Wehrle, M.D., San Clemente, CA

International Health
Rosalyn C. King, Pharm.D., M.P.H., *Chair*, Silver Spring, MD; Fernando Antezana, Ph.D., Geneva, Switzerland; Walter M. Batts, Rockville, MD; Eugenie Brown, Pharm.D., Kingston, Jamaica; Alan Cheung, Pharm.D., M.P.H., Washington, DC; Mary Couper, M.D., Geneva, Switzerland; David T. Durack, M.D., Ph.D., Durham, NC; S. Albert Edwards, Pharm.D., Lincolnshire, IL; Enrique Fefer, Ph.D., Washington, DC; Peter H. M. Fontilus, Curacao, Netherlands Antilles; Marcellus Grace, Ph.D., New Orleans, LA; George B. Griffenhagen, Washington, DC; Gan Ee Kiang, Penang, Malaysia; Thomas Langston, Washington, DC; Thomas Lapnet-Moustapha, Yaounde, Cameroon; David Lee, B.A., M.D., Panama City, Panama; Stuart M. MacLeod, M.D., Hamilton, Ontario; Russell E. Morgan, Jr., Dr.P.H., Chevy Chase, MD; David Ofori-Adjei, M.D., Accra, Ghana; S. Ofosu-Amaah, M.D., New York, NY; James Rankin, Boston, MA; Olikoye Ransome-Kuti, M.D., Lagos, Nigeria; Budiono Santoso, M.D., Ph.D., Yogyakarta, Indonesia; Fela Viso-Gurovich, Mexico City, Mexico; William B. Walsh, M.D., Chevy Chase, MD; Lawrence C. Weaver, Ph.D., Minneapolis, MN; Albert I. Wertheimer, Ph.D., Philadelphia, PA

Neurology
Stanley van den Noort, M.D., *Chair*, Irvine, CA; William T. Beaver, M.D., Washington, DC; Elizabeth U. Blalock, M.D., Anaheim, CA; James C. Cloyd, Pharm.D., Minneapolis, MN; David M. Dawson, M.D., West Roxbury, MA; Kevin Farrell, M.D., Vancouver, British Columbia; Kathleen M. Foley, M.D., New York, NY; Anthony E. Lang, M.D., Toronto, Ontario; Ira T. Lott, M.D., Orange, CA; James R. Nelson, M.D., La Jolla, CA; J. Kiffin Penry, M.D., Winston-Salem, NC; Neil H. Raskin, M.D., San Francisco, CA; Alfred J.

Spiro, M.D., Bronx, NY; M. DiAnn Turek, R.N., Lansing, MI

Nursing Practice
Rosemary C. Polomano, R.N., M.S.N., *Chair*, Philadelpia, PA; Mecca S. Cranley, R.N., Ph.D., Buffalo, NY; Jan M. Ellerhorst-Ryan, R.N., M.S.N., Cincinnati, OH; Linda Felver, Ph.D., R.N., Portland, OR; Hector Hugo Gonzalez, R.N., Ph.D., San Antonio, TX; Mary Harper, R.N., Ph.D., Rockville, MD; Ada K. Jacox, R.N., Ph.D., Baltimore, MD; Patricia Kummeth, R.N., M.S., Rochester, MN; Ida M. Martinson, R.N., Ph.D., San Francisco, CA; Carol P. Patton, R.N., Ph.D., J.D., Detroit, MI; Ginette A. Pepper, R.N., Ph.D., Denver, CO; Geraldine A. Peterson, R.N., M.A., Potomac, MD; Linda C. Pugh, R.N., Ph.D., York, PA; Sharon S. Rising, R.N., C.N.M., Cheshire, CT; Marjorie Ann Spiro, R.N., B.S., C.S.N., Scarsdale, NY

Nutrition and Electrolytes
Robert D. Lindeman, M.D., *Chair*, Albuquerque, NM; Hans Fisher, Ph.D., New Brunswick, NJ; Walter H. Glinsmann, M.D., Washington, DC; Helen Andrews Guthrie, M.S., Ph.D., State College, PA; Steven B. Heymsfield, M.D., New York, NY; K. N. Jeejeebhoy, M.D., Toronto, Ontario; Leslie M. Klevay, M.D., Grand Forks, ND; Bonnie Liebman, M.S., Washington, DC; Sudesh K. Mahajan, M.D., Allen Park, MI; Craig J. McClain, M.D., Lexington, KY; Jay M. Mirtallo, M.S., Columbus, OH; Sohrab Mobarhan, M.D., Maywood, IL; Robert M. Russell, M.D., Boston, MA; Harold H. Sandstead, M.D., Galveston, TX; William J. Stone, M.D., Nashville, TN; Carlos A. Vaamonde, M.D., Miami, FL; Stanley Wallach, M.D., Jamaica, NY

Obstetrics and Gynecology
Douglas D. Glover, M.D., *Chair*, Morgantown, WV; Rudi Ansbacher, M.D., Ann Arbor, MI; Florence Comite, M.D., New Haven, CT; James W. Daly, M.D., Columbia, MO; Marilynn C. Frederiksen, M.D., Chicago, IL; Charles B. Hammond, M.D., Durham, NC; Barbara A. Hayes, M.A., New Rochelle, NY; Art Jacknowitz, Pharm.D., Morgantown, WV; William J. Ledger, M.D., New York, NY; Andre-Marie Leroux, M.D., Vanier, Ontario; William A. Nahhas, M.D., Dayton, OH; Warren N. Otterson, M.D., Shreveport, LA; Samuel A. Pasquale, M.D., New Brunswick, NJ; Johanna Perlmutter, M.D., Boston, MA; Robert W. Rebar, M.D., Cincinnati, OH; Richard H. Reindollar, M.D., Boston, MA; G. Millard Simmons, M.D., Morgantown, WV; J. Benjamin Younger, M.D., Birmingham, AL

Ophthalmology
Herbert E. Kaufman, M.D., *Chair*, New Orleans, LA; Steven R. Abel, Pharm.D., Indianapolis, IN; Jules Baum, M.D., Boston, MA; Steven M. Drance, M.D., Vancouver, British Columbia; Lee R. Duffner, M.D., Miami, FL; David L. Epstein, M.D., Durham, NC; Allan J. Flach, Pharm.D., M.D., San Francisco, CA; Vincent H. L. Lee, Ph.D., Los Angeles, CA; Steven M. Podos, M.D., New York, NY; Kirk R. Wilhelmus, M.D., Houston, TX; Thom J. Zimmerman, M.D., Ph.D., Louisville, KY

Otorhinolaryngology
Leonard P. Rybak, M.D., *Chair*, Springfield, IL; Robert E. Brummett, Ph.D., Portland, OR; Robert A. Dobie, M.D., San Antonio, TX; Linda J. Gardiner, M.D., New Haven, CT; David Hilding, M.D., Price, UT; David B. Hom, M.D., Minneapolis, MN; Helen F. Krause, M.D., Pittsburgh, PA; Richard L. Mabry, M.D., Dallas, TX; Lawrence J. Marentette, M.D., Minneapolis, MN; Robert A. Mickel, M.D.,

Ph.D., Los Angeles, CA; Randal A. Otto, M.D., San Antonio, TX; Richard W. Waguespack, M.D., Birmingham, AL; William R. Wilson, M.D., Washington, DC

Parasitic Disease

Jay S. Keystone, M.D., *Chair*, Toronto, Ontario; Michele Barry, M.D., New Haven, CT; Frank J. Bia, M.D., M.P.H., New Haven, CT; David Botero, M.D., Medellin, Colombia; Robert Goldsmith, M.D., Berkeley, CA; Elaine C. Jong, M.D., Seattle, WA; Dennis D. Juranek, M.D., Atlanta, GA; Donald J. Krogstad, M.D., New Orleans, LA; Douglas W. MacPherson, M.D., Hamilton, Ontario; Edward K. Markell, M.D., San Francisco, CA; Theodore Nash, M.D., Bethesda, MD; Murray Wittner, M.D., Bronx, NY

Pediatrics

Philip D. Walson, M.D., *Chair*, Columbus, OH; Jacob V. Aranda, M.D., Ph.D., Montreal, Quebec; Cheston M. Berlin, Jr., M.D., Hershey, PA; Nancy Jo Braden, M.D., Phoenix, AZ; Halyna P. Breslawec, Ph.D., Rockville, MD; Patricia J. Bush, Ph.D., Washington, DC; Marion J. Finkel, M.D., East Hanover, NJ; George S. Goldstein, M.D., Elmsford, NY; Ralph E. Kauffman, M.D., Detroit, MI; Gideon Koren, M.D., Toronto, Ontario; Joan M. Korth-Bradley, Pharm.D., Ph.D., Philadelphia, PA; Richard Leff, Pharm.D., Kansas City, KS; Carolyn Lund, R.N., M.S., Oakland, CA; Wayne Snodgrass, M.D., Galveston, TX; Celia A. Viets, M.D., Ottawa, Canada; John T. Wilson, M.D., Shreveport, LA; Sumner J. Yaffe, M.D., Bethesda, MD; Karin E. Zenk, Pharm.D., Irvine, CA

Pharmacy Practice

Thomas P. Reinders, Pharm.D., *Chair*, Richmond, VA; Olya Duzey, M.S., Reed City, MI; Yves Gariepy, B.Sc.Pharm., Quebec, Quebec; Ned Heltzer, M.S., Philadelphia, PA; Lester S. Hosto, B.S., Little Rock, AR; Martin J. Jinks, Pharm.D., Pullman, WA; Frederick Klein, B.S., Montvale, NJ; Calvin H. Knowlton, Ph.D., Lumberton, NJ; Patricia A. Kramer, B.S., Bismarck, ND; Dennis McCallum, Pharm.D., Rochester, MN; Shirley P. McKee, B.S., Houston, TX; William A. McLean, Pharm.D., Ottawa, Ontario; Gladys Montañez, B.S., San Juan, PR; Donald L. Moore, B.S., Kokomo, IN; John E. Ogden, M.S., Washington, DC; Henry A. Palmer, Ph.D., Storrs, CT; Lorie G. Rice, B.A., M.P.H., San Francisco, CA; Mike R. Sather, M.S., Albuquerque, NM; Albert Sebok, B.S., Twinsburg, OH; William E. Smith, Pharm.D., M.P.H., Auburn, AL; Susan East Torrico, B.S., Orlando, FL; J. Richard Wuest, Pharm.D., Cincinnati, OH; Glenn Y. Yokoyama, Pharm.D., Los Angeles, CA

Psychiatric Disease

Burton J. Goldstein, M.D., *Chair*, Miami, FL; Magda Campbell, M.D., New York, NY; Alex A. Cardoni, M.S. Pharm., Storrs, CT; James L. Claghorn, M.D., Houston, TX; N. Michael Davis, M.S., Miami, FL; Larry Ereshefsky, Pharm.D., San Antonio, TX; W. Edwin Fann, M.D., Houston, TX; Alan J. Gelenberg, M.D., Tucson, AZ; Tracy R. Gordy, M.D., Austin, TX; Paul Grof, M.D., Ottawa, Ontario; Russell T. Joffe, M.D., Toronto, Ontario; Ronald Kartzinel, Ph.D., M.D., Summit, NJ; Harriet P. Lefley, Ph.D., Miami, FL; Nathan Rawls, Pharm.D., Memphis, TN; Jarrett W. Richardson, III, M.D., Rochester, MN; Ruth Robinson, Saskatoon, Saskatchewan; Matthew V. Rudorfer, M.D., Rockville, MD; Karen A. Theesen, Pharm.D., Omaha, NE

Pulmonary Disease

Harold S. Nelson, M.D., *Chair*, Denver, CO; Richard C. Ahrens, M.D., Iowa City, IA; Eugene R. Bleecker, M.D., Baltimore, MD; William W. Busse, M.D., Madison, WI; Christopher Fanta, M.D., Boston, MA; Mary K. Garcia, R.N., Missouri City, TX; Nicholas Gross, M.D., Hines, IL; Leslie Hendeles, Pharm.D., Gainesville, FL; Elliot Israel, M.D., Boston, MA; Susan Janson-Bjerklie, R.N., Ph.D., San Francisco, CA; John W. Jenne, M.D., Hines, IL; H. William Kelly, Pharm.D., Albuquerque, NM; James P. Kemp, M.D., San Diego, CA; Henry Levison, M.D., Toronto, Ontario; Gail Shapiro, M.D., Seattle, WA; Stanley J. Szefler, M.D., Denver, CO

Radiopharmaceuticals

Carol S. Marcus, Ph.D., M.D., *Chair*, Torrance, CA; Capt. William H. Briner, B.S., Durham, NC; Ronald J. Callahan, Ph.D., Boston, MA; Janet F. Eary, M.D., Seattle, WA; Joanna S. Fowler, Ph.D., Upton, NJ; David L. Gilday, M.D., Toronto, Ontario; David A. Goodwin, M.D., Palo Alto, CA; David L. Laven, N.Ph., C.R.Ph., FASCP, Bay Pines, FL; Andrea H. McGuire, M.D., Des Moines, IA; Peter Paras, Ph.D., Rockville, MD; Barry A. Siegel, M.D., St. Louis, MO; Edward B. Silberstein, M.D., Cincinnati, OH; Dennis P. Swanson, M.S., Pittsburgh, PA; Mathew L. Thakur, Ph.D., Philadelphia, PA; Henry N. Wellman, M.D., Indianapolis, IN

Surgical Drugs and Devices

Lary A. Robinson, M.D., *Chair*, Omaha, NE; Greg Alexander, M.D., Rockville, MD; Norman D. Anderson, M.D., Baltimore, MD; Alan R. Dimick, M.D., Birmingham, AL; Jack Hirsh, M.D., Hamilton, Ontario; Manucher J. Javid, M.D., Madison, WI; Henry J. Mann, Pharm.D., Minneapolis, MN; Kurt M. W. Niemann, M.D., Birmingham, AL; Robert P. Rapp, Pharm.D., Lexington, KY; Ronald Rubin, M.D., Boston, MA

Urology

John A. Belis, M.D., *Chair*, Hershey, PA; Culley C. Carson, M.D., Durham, NC; Richard A. Cohen, M.D., Red Bank, NJ; B. J. Reid Czarapata, R.N., Washington, DC; Jean B. de Kernion, M.D., Los Angeles, CA; Warren Heston, Ph.D., New York, NY; Mark V. Jarowenko, M.D., Hershey, PA; Mary Lee, Pharm.D., Chicago, IL; Marguerite C. Lippert, M.D., Charlottesville, VA; Penelope A. Longhurst, Ph.D., Philadelphia, PA; Tom F. Lue, M.D., San Francisco, CA; Michael G. Mawhinney, Ph.D., Morgantown, WV; Martin G. McLoughlin, M.D., Vancouver, British Columbia; Randall G. Rowland, M.D., Ph.D., Indianapolis, IN; J. Patrick Spirnak, M.D., Cleveland, OH; William F. Tarry, M.D., Morgantown, WV; Keith N. Van Arsdalen, M.D., Philadelphia, PA

Veterinary Medicine

Lloyd E. Davis, D.V.M., Ph.D., *Chair*, Urbana, IL; Arthur L. Aronson, D.V.M., Ph.D., Raleigh, NC; Gordon W. Brumbaugh, D.V.M., Ph.D., College Station, TX; Gordon L. Coppoc, D.V.M., Ph.D., West Lafayette, IN; Sidney A. Ewing, D.V.M., Ph.D., Stillwater, OK; Stuart D. Forney, M.S., Fort Collins, CO; Diane K. Gerken, D.V.M., Ph.D., Columbus, OH; William G. Huber, D.V.M., Ph.D., Stillwater, OK; William L. Jenkins, D.V.M., Baton Rouge, LA; V. Corey Langston, D.V.M., Ph.D., Mississippi State, MS; Mark G. Papich, D.V.M., Saskatoon, Saskatchewan; John W. Paul, D.V.M., Somerville, NJ; Thomas E. Powers, D.V.M., Ph.D., Columbus, OH; Charles R. Short, D.V.M., Ph.D., Baton Rouge, LA; Steven L. Sved, Ph.D., Ottawa, Ontario; Richard H. Teske, D.V.M., Ph.D., Rockville, MD; Jeffrey R. Wilcke, D.V.M., M.S., Blacksburg, VA

Drug Information Division
Additional Contributors

The information presented in this text represents an ongoing review of the drugs contained herein and represents a consensus of various viewpoints expressed. In addition to the individuals listed below, many schools, associations, pharmaceutical companies, and governmental agencies have provided comment or otherwise contributed to the development of the 1993 USP DI data base. Such listing does not imply that these individuals have reviewed all of the material in this text or that they individually agree with all statements contained herein.

Donald I. Abrams, M.D., San Francisco, CA
Richard Anderson, M.D., Beltsville, MD
Stephen W. Anderson, M.D., Atlanta, GA
Oscar E. Araujo, Ph.D., Gainesville, FL
Kenneth Arndt, M.D., Boston, MA
Gilbert August, M.D., Washington, DC
Louis V. Avioli, M.D., St. Louis, MO
James R. Ayers, Twinsburg, OH
Martin E. Bacon, M.D., Bethesda, MD
Rick A. Barbarash, Pharm.D., St. Louis, MO
Patsy Barnett, Pharm.D., Bay Pines, FL
Joseph M. Baron, M.D., Chicago, IL
LuAnne Barron, Birmingham, AL
Norman W. Barton, M.D., Phoenix, MD
Ann Bartlett, BSN, Rochester, MN
Rachel Eve Behrman, M.D., Silver Spring, MD
Robert W. Beightol, Pharm.D., Roanoke, VA
William Bell, M.D., Baltimore, MD
Jerry A. Bennett, Pharm.D., Cincinnati, OH
Patricia Bennett, B.S.Pharm., Cincinnati, OH
Edward Bernard, M.D., New York, NY
Ernest Beutler, M.D., La Jolla, CA
David Bickers, M.D., Cleveland, OH
Martin Black, M.D., Philadelphia, PA
Richard Blackwell, M.D., Birmingham, AL
Jack Blaine, M.D., Potomac, MD
Henry G. Bone, M.D., Detroit, MI
John Bonnar, M.D., Dublin, Ireland
Peggy Borum, Ph.D., Gainesville, FL
Wayne E. Bradley, Richmond, VA
Michael Brady, M.D., Columbus, OH
Roscoe O Brady, M.D., Bethesda, MD
Robert E. Braun, D.D.S., Buffalo, NY
Michael S. Burnhill, M.D., New Brunswick, NJ
Louis Buttino, Jr., M.D., Dayton, OH
Wesley G. Byerly, Pharm.D., Winston-Salem, NC
James E. Caldwell, M.D., San Francisco, CA
Karim A. Calis, Pharm.D., Rockville, MD
Jane M. Cardosa, Ph.D., Penang, MALAYSIA
Albert A. Carr, M.D., Augusta, GA
Charles C. J. Carpenter, M.D., Providence, RI
Regina Carson, R.Ph., Randallstown, MD
Jennifer Chan, Pharm.D., San Antonio, TX

Jeffrey Chang, M.D., Davis, CA
Bruce D. Cheson, M.D., Bethesda, MD
James J. Chisolm, Jr., M.D., Baltimore, MD
Cyril R. Clarke, Ph.D., Stillwater, OK
Thomas W. Clarkson, Ph.D., Rochester, NY
Dennis Clifton, Pharm.D., Lexington, KY
Arthur Cocco, M.D., Baltimore, MD
Barry S. Coller, M.D., Stony Brook, NY
James D. Cook, M.D., Kansas City, KS
Timothy P. Cooley, M.D., Boston, MA
Betsy J. Cooper, M.D., Washington, DC
James W. Cooper, Ph.D., Athens, GA
Clinton N. Corder, Ph.D., M.D., Oklahoma City, OK
Corman, M.S.P., Ottawa, Ontario
Donald W. Cox, M.D., Morgantown, WV
Sarah Crabbe-Erush, Pharm.D., Philadelphia, PA
Peter S. Creticos, M.D., Baltimore, MD
Suzanne E. Cronquist, R.Ph., Princeton, NJ
Craig Darby, Twinsburg, OH
Jonathan Davidson, M.D., Durham, NC
Janet Davis, M.D., Miami, FL
Robin L. Davis, Pharm.D., Albuquerque, NM
Thomas D. DeCillis, North Port, FL
Carel P. de Haseth, Netherland Antilles (Caribbean)
John Derry, Toronto, Ont., Canada
Seymour Diamond, M.D., Chicago, IL
Virgil C. Dias, Pharm.D., Kansas City, MO
Barry D. Dickinson, Ph.D., Chicago, IL
James E. Doherty, M.D., Little Rock, AR
Lawrence Dolan, M.D., Cincinnati, OH
Dr. Nacky Dozier, Houston, TX
Marc K. Drezner, M.D., Durham, NC
David J. Durand, M.D., Oakland, CA
Dale R. Dunnihoo, M.D., Ph.D., Shreveport, LA
Johnnie L. Early, II, Ph.D., Tallahassee, FL
Robert Edwards, Pharm.D., Columbus, OH
Charles Ellis, M.D., Ann Arbor, MI
William Fant, Cincinnati, OH
Paul Fenster, M.D., Tucson, AZ
Anne Gilbert Feuer, B.S., Cincinnati, OH
Virginia C. Fielder, M.D., Chicago, IL
Alan J. Fischman, M.D., Ph.D., Boston, MA
Gary Fishbein, M.D., Philadelphia, PA

Greg C. Flaker, M.D., Columbia, MO
Ben Flanigan, R.Ph., Acworth, GA
Linda Franck, RN, MS, Oakland, CA
Rodney Franey, Pharm.D., Gainesville, FL
Rudolph Franklin, M.D., New Orleans, LA
James Freston, M.D., Farmington, CT
Dorothy Friedberg, M.D., New York, NY
Alan H. Friedman, M.D., New York, NY
Carl J. Friedman, M.D., Philadelphia, PA
Barbara L. Fuhrman, Pharm.D., New York, NY
Vincent A. Fulginiti, M.D., Tucson, AZ
Wayne L. Furman, M.D., Memphis, TN
Mike Gasland, Pharm.D., Lexington, KY
Edward Genton, M.D., New Orleans, LA
Anne A. Gershon, M.D., New York, NY
Martin S. Gillieson, M.D., Boston, MA
Michael J. Glade, Ph.D., Chicago, IL
MAJ. John D. Grabenstein, MS, Fort Sam Houston, TX
Nina Graves, Pharm.D., Minneapolis, MN
Martin D. Green, M.D., Rockville, MD
Donald L. Greer, Ph.D., New Orleans, LA
David R. P. Guay, Pharm.D., St. Paul, MN
Harvey Guyda, M.D., Montreal, Quebec
Nortin M. Hadler, M.D., Chapel Hill, NC
Robert M. Hadsell, Ph.D., Richardson, TX
Steven T. Harris, M.D., San Francisco, CA
Edward A. Hartshorn, Ph.D., San Antonio, TX
Patricia Hausman, M.S., Gaithersburg, MD
Robert P. Heaney, M.D., Omaha, NE
Mary Jo Helechek, RN, Baltimore, MD
Victor Henderson, M.D., Los Angeles, CA
Laura A. Hillman, M.D., Columbia, MO
M. E. Hoar, Springfield, MA
Robert Hodgeman, Cincinnati, OH
Paul Hoffer, M.D., New Haven, CT
Gary N. Holland, M.D., Los Angeles, CA
David C. Hooper, M.D., Boston, MA
Rick Horan, M.D., Boston, MA
Herschel S. Horowitz, D.D.S., Bethesda, MD
Colin W. Howden, M.D., Columbia, SC
Stephen Huber, Houston, TX
Bess Dawson Hughes, M.D., Boston, MA
Jeff Hyams, M.D., Hartford, CT
John Iazzetta, Pharm.D., Toronto, Ontario, Canada
Rodney D. Ice, Ph.D., Miami, OK
Kristy Ingebo, M.D., Phoenix, AZ
Cindy Ippoliti, M.D., Houston, TX
Mark Jacobson, M.D., San Francisco, CA
Michael Jamieson, M.D., San Antonio, TX
Ann L. Janer, M.S., Auburn, AL
Janet P. Jaramilla, Pharm.D., Chicago, IL
Alan Jenkins, M.D., Charlottesville, VA
Gerald Johnston, M.D., Baltimore, MD
Hugh F. Kabat, Ph.D., Albuquerque, NM
Henry J. Kaminski, M.D., Cleveland, OH
Thomas G. Kantor, M.D., New York, NY
Selna Kaplan, M.D., Ph.D., San Francisco, CA
Mary Carman Kasparek, Vanier, Ont., Canada

Carol K. Kasper, M.D., Los Angeles, CA
Constance Kasprzak, Pharm.D., Palo Hills, IL
Harry I. Katz, M.D., Minneapolis, MN
John J. Kavanagh, M.D., Houston, TX
Ekkehard Kemmann, M.D., New Brunswick, NJ
Joseph Khoury, M.D., Washington, DC
Patricia Kingsley, MGA, BSN, Brookeville, MD
John M. Kirkwood, M.D., Pittsburgh, PA
Curtis Klaassen, M.D., Kansas City, KS
Michael Kleerekoper, M.D., Detroit, MI
Anne Klibanski, M.D., Boston, MA
Robert A. Knuppel, M.D., Tampa, FL
John Koepke, Pharm.D., Columbus, OH
Joseph Kostick, Rochester MN
Vicki L. Kraus, RN, Iowa City, IA
Lee Kudrow, M.D., Encino, CA
Paul B. Kuehn, Ph.D., Woodinville, WA
Robert Kuhn, Pharm.D., Lexington, KY
Roger Kurlan, M.D., Rochester, NY
Thomas L. Kurt, M.D., Dallas, TX
John S. Lambert, M.D., Rochester, NY
Oscar Laskin, M.D., Rahway, NJ
Belle Lee, Pharm.D., San Francisco, CA
Joseph Levy, M.D., New York, NY
Richard A. Lewis, M.D., Houston, TX
Peter A. Lewitt, M.D., Detroit, MI
Howard A. Liebman, M.D., Los Angeles, CA
Christopher D. Lind, M.D., Nashville, TN
Robert Lindsay, Ph.D., West Havestraw, NY
Nicholas J. Lowe, M.D., Los Angeles, CA
Howard I. Maibach, M.D., San Francisco, CA
Claude Mailhot, Montreal, Quebec
Frank Marcus, M.D., Tucson, AZ
Victor J. Marder, M.D., Rochester, NY
Joseph E. Margarone, D.D.S., Buffalo, NY
Jeffrey Marshall, M.D., Decatur, GA
Jay Mason, Salt Lake City, UT
Leeman P. Maxwell, M.D., Mongantown, WV
J. B. McCormick, M.D., Atlanta, GA
Norman L. McElroy, San Jose, CA
Patrick McGrath, M.D., New York, NY
Ross E. McKinney, M.D., Durham, NC
Carol McManus-Balmer, Pharm.D., Denver, CO
Anne McNulty, M.D., Waterbury, CT
Roland Mertelsmann, M.D., Frgiburg, Germany
Burt Meyers, M.D, New York, NY
Alan M. Miller, Ph.D., M.D., Gainesville, FL
Donald Miller, Pharm.D., Fargo, ND
Larry E. Millikan, M.D., New Orleans, LA
Joel S. Mindel, M.D., Ph.D., New York, NY
Bernard L. Mirkin, M.D., Chicago, IL
Harold Mitty, M.D., New York, NY
John Modlin, M.D., Hanover, NH
Mark Molitch, M.D., Chicago, IL
A. Bruce Montgomery, M.D., South San Francisco, CA
Wayne V. Moore, M.D., Kansas City, KS
Alvaro Morales, M.D., Kingston, Ontario
Mary E. Mortensen, M.D., Columbus, OH

Robyn Mueller, B.S.Pharm., Cincinnati, OH
Geoffrey M. Mukwaya, M.B., Ch.B., M.Sc., Ottawa, Ontario
Michael B. Murphy, M.D., Chicago, IL
John Nemunaitis, M.D., Seattle, WA
Ernest Newbrun, D.M.D., Ph.D., San Francisco, CA
Clarence Nichols, Twinsburg, OH
Kathryn M. Niesen, R.N., M.S.N., Rochester, MN
James O'Donnell, M.D., San Francisco, CA
Linda K. Ohri, Pharm.D., Omaha, NE
Karen S. Oles, Pharm.D., Winston-Salem, NC
Michael J. O'Neil, Twinsburg, OH
James R. Oster, M.D., Miami, FL
Judith M. Ozbun, R.Ph., M.S., Fargo, ND
Charles Y. C. Pak, M.D., Dallas, TX
Michael A. Palmer, M.D., Rochester, MN
David C. Pang, Ph.D., Chicago, IL
Michael F. Para, M.D., Columbus, OH
Robert C. Park, M.D., Washington, DC
Albert Patterson, Hines, IL
Neil A. Petry, M.S., Ann Arbor, MI
Shirley Pfister, R.N., M.S., Denver, CO
Carl Pinsky, M.D., Warren, NJ
Philip A. Pizzo, M.D., Bethesda, MD
Michael A. Polis, M.D., Bethesda, MD
James Ponto, R.Ph., Iowa City, IA
Anthony A. Portale, M.D., San Francisco, CA
Roy E. Pounder, M.D., London England
Richard Price, M.D., Minneapolis, MN
Carol M. Proudfit, Ph.D., Chicago, IL
Mark C. Pugh, Pharm.D., Richmond, VA
Theodore Quilligan, M.D., Orange, CA
Carlos A. Rabito, M.D., Ph.D., Boston, MA
Sharon A. Raimer, M.D., Galveston, TX
Debra L. Rainey, M.D., Birmingham, AL
Norbert P. Rapoza, Ph.D., Chicago, IL
Thomas A. Ratko, Ph.D., Chicago, IL
J. Routt Reigart, M.D., Charleston, SC
Cara Reisenman, Pharm.D., San Antonio, TX
Alfred J. Remillard, Pharm.D., Saskatoon, Saskatchewan
Dr. Louis Ripa, Stony Brook, NY
Daniel Robinson, Pharm.D., Los Angeles, CA
Donald S. Robinson, M.D., Wallingford, CT
Allen Root, M.D., Tampa, FL
Robert L. Rosenfield, M.D., Chicago, IL
Douglas S. Ross, M.D., Boston, MA
Maura K. Roush, M.D., San Antonio, TX
Christian Ruef, M.D., Geneva, Switzerland
Jean A. Rumsfield, Pharm.D., Highland Park, IL
Michael S. Saag, M.D., Birmingham, AL
Joseph R. Sabino, Twinsburg, OH
Eugene L. Saenger, M.D., Cincinnati, OH
Sharon Safrin, M.D., San Francisco, CA
Jan Sahai, M.D., Ottawa, Ont., Canada
Evelyn Salerno, Pharm.D., Hialeah, FL
Jay P. Sanford, M.D., Dallas, TX
Sheila Kelly Scarim, Pharm.D., Indianapolis, IN
Alan F. Schatzberg, M.D., Belmont, MA

I. Herbert Scheinberg, M.D., Bronx, NY
Steven M. Schnittman, M.D., Rockville, MD
Neil R. Schram, M.D., Harbor City, CA
Jerome Seidenfeld, Ph.D., Chicago, IL
Charles F. Seifert, Pharm.D., Oklahoma City, OK
Sandra L. Sessoms, M.D., Houston, TX
Allen F. Shaughnessy, Pharm.D., Harrisburg, PA
Lewis B. Sheiner, M.D., San Francisco, CA
Neil J. Shernoff, M.D., Phoenix, AZ
Yvonne M. Shevchuk, Pharm.D., Saskatoon, Saskatchewan, Canada
Harold M. Silverman, Pharm.D., Silver Spring, MD
Krishna B. Singh, M.D., Shreveport, LA
Michael H. Skinner, M.D., Pharm.D., San Antonio, TX
Dance Smith, Pharm.D., Ft. Steilacoom, WA
Geralynn B. Smith, M.S., Detroit, MI
Samuel Smith, M.D., Baltimore, MD
Steven J. Smith, Ph.D., Chicago, IL
Elliott M. Sogol, Ph.D., Research Triangle Park, NC
Lawrence M. Solomon, M.D., Chicago, IL
Harry Spiera, M.D., New York, NY
William Steers, M.D., Charlottesville, VA
Richard Stiehm, M.D., Los Angeles, CA
Alison Stopeck, M.D., New York, NY
Earnie Stremski, M.D., Minneapolis, MN
David Stuhr, Denver, CO
Mark Summerfield, M.D., Houston, TX
Linda Gore Sutherland, Pharm.D., Laramie, WY
Ronald S. Swerdloff, M.D., Torrance, CA
David A. Taylor, Morgantown, WV
M. E. Teresi, Iowa City, IA
Roger C. Toffle, M.D., Morgantown, WV
Carol Braun Trapnell, M.D., Washington DC
Jayme Trott, Pharm.D., San Antonio, TX
Reginald C. Tsang, M.D., Cincinnati, OH
Eduardo Tschen, M.D., Albuquerque, NM
Barbara S. Turner, RN, Tacoma, WA
Julia Vertrees, Pharm.D., San Antonio, TX
Ronald Vinik, M.D., Birmingham, AL
M. Vohra, Halifax, Nova Scotia, Canada
Paul A. Volberding, M.D., San Francisco, CA
Barbara I. Vuignier, Salt Lake City, UT
Andrea Wall, B.S., R.Ph., West Chester, OH
Bonnie Wallner, Dover, DE
Robert M. Ward, M.D., Salt Lake City, UT
William Warner, Ph.D., New York, NY
R.S. Weinstein, M.D., Augusta, GA
Timothy E. Welty, Pharm.D., Bismarck, ND
Bruce White, M.D., Nashville, TN
George Whitelaw, Cranford, NJ
Gary M. Whitford, M.D., Augusta, GA
Richard J. Whitley, M.D., Birmingham, AL
Catherine Wilfert, M.D., Durham, NC
Craig C. Williams, R.Ph., Cincinnati, OH
Nancy Winiarski, Pharm.D., Chicago, IL
Robert G. Wolfangel, Ph.D., St. Louis, MO
M. Michael Wolfe, M.D., Boston, MA
Richard Wood, Ph.D., Boston, MA

Paul D. Woolf, M.D., Rochester, NY
G. Frederick Wooten, Jr., M.D., Charlottesville, VA
Melvin D. Yahr, M.D., New York, NY
Robert Yarchoan, M.D., Bethesda, MD

Katherine E. Yutzy, Goshen, IN
John M. Zajecka, M.D., Chicago, IL
David Zakin, M.D., New York, NY
William Zipf, M.D., Columbus, OH
Frederic J. Zucchero, M.A., R.Ph., St. Louis, MO

Headquarters Staff

DRUG INFORMATION DIVISION

Director: Keith W. Johnson

Assistant Director: Georgie M. Cathey

Special Assistant for Patient Counseling and Education Programs: Alice E. Kimball

Administrative Staff: Jaime A. Ramirez *(Administrative Assistant),* Albert Crucillo, Mayra L. Martinez

Senior Drug Information Specialists: Nancy Lee Dashiell, Esther H. Klein, Angela Méndez Mayo *(Spanish Publications Coordinator)*

Drug Information Specialists: Ann Corken, Debra A. Edwards, Jymeann King, Doris Lee, Carol A. Pamer

Computer Applications Specialist: Elizabeth Chew

Publications Development Staff: Diana M. Blais *(Supervisor),* David D. Housley *(Associate),* Anne M. Lawrence *(Assistant),* Dorothy Raymond *(Assistant)*

Library Services: Florence A. Hogan *(Coordinator),* Terri Rikhy *(Assistant)*

Research Assistants: Nancy King, Annamarie J. Sibik

Consultants: Sandra Lee Boyer, Henry Fomundan, Marcelo Vernengo, Gordon K. Wurster

Student Interns/Externs: Arthur Bonner, Howard University; Peter D'Orazio, Howard University; Ellen Frank, University of Pittsburgh; Hyun Kim, University of Texas—Austin; Lucy Kim, Philadelphia College of Pharmacy and Science; Amy O'Donnell, Washington State University

Visiting Scholars: Romaldas Maciulaitis, Kaunas, Lithuania; David Ofori-Adjei, Accra, Ghana; Bose Ogunbunmi, Lagos, Nigeria

USPC ADMINISTRATIVE STAFF

Executive Director: Jerome A. Halperin

Associate Executive Director: Joseph G. Valentino

Assistant Executive Director for Professional and Public Affairs: Jacqueline L. Eng

Director, Operations: J. Robert Strang

Director, Personnel: Arlene Bloom

Controller: Russell L. Williams

Fulfillment/Facilities Manager: Drew J. Lutz

DRUG STANDARDS DIVISION

Director: Lee T. Grady

Assistant Directors: Charles H. Barnstein *(Revision),* Barbara B. Hubert, *(Scientific Administration),* Robert H. King *(Technical Services)*

Senior Scientists: Roger Dabbah, Aubrey S. Outschoorn (Ret.), William W. Wright

Scientists: Frank P. Barletta, J. Joseph Belson, Vivian A. Gray, W. Larry Paul, V. Srinivasan

Consultant: Zorach R. Glaser

Hazard Communications: James J. Lenahan, Linda Shear

Technical Editors: Ann K. Ferguson, Melissa Smith

Office Staff: Glenna Etherton, Theresa H. Lee, Cecilia Luna, Anju K. Malhotra, Maureen Rawson, Ernestine Williams

MARKETING

Director: Cathy M. Ferrere

Product Managers: Wendy M. Austin *(Drug Information),* Mitchell A. Lapides *(Electronic Applications)*

Marketing Communications Manager: Amy L. Evans

Marketing Associates: Stacy M. Hartranft, Cara M. Sterling

Marketing Assistant: Susan D. Harmon

PUBLICATION SERVICES

Director: Patricia H. Morgenstern

Managing Editors: A. V. Precup *(USP DI),* Sandra Boynton *(USP-NF)*

Editorial Associates: *USP DI*—Carol M. Griffin, Carol N. Hankin, Ellen R. Loeb, Harriet S. Nathanson, Ellen D. Smith, Barbara A. Visco; *USP-NF*—Jesusa D. Cordova *(Senior Editorial Associate),* Ellen Elovitz, Margaret Kay Walshaw

USAN Staff: Carolyn A. Fleeger *(Editor),* Gerilynne Seigneur

Typesetting Systems Coordinator: Jean E. Dale

Typesetting Staff: Susan L. Entwistle *(Supervisor),* Donna Alie, Deborah R. Connelly, Lauren Taylor Davis, Micheline Tranquille

Graphics: Gail M. Oring *(Manager),* Susan Clagett, Tia C. Morfessis, Mary P. Regan

Word Processing: Barbara A. Bowman *(Supervisor),* Frances Rampp, Susan Schartman, Jane Shulman

Also Contributing: Barbara Arnold, Kay Kessell, and Marie Kotomori, Proofreaders; Dan Edwards and M. T. Samahon, Typesetters; and Terri A. DeIuliis, Graphics.

PRACTITIONER REPORTING PROGRAMS

Assistant Executive Director for Practitioner Reporting Programs: Diane M. McGinnis

Staff: Robin A. Baldwin, Deirdre Beagan, Shawn C. Becker, Alice C. Curtis, Kay E. McClaine, Ilze Mohseni, Joanne Pease, Susmita Samanta, Anne Paula Thompson, Mary Susan Zmuda

Members of the United States Pharmacopeial Convention and the Institutions and Organizations Represented as of April 1, 1991

Current Officers and Board of Trustees

President: Mark Novitch, M.D., Vice Chairman, The Upjohn Company, 7000 Portage Road, Kalamazoo, MI 49001

Vice President: Donald R. Bennett, M.D., Ph.D., Director, Division of Drugs and Toxicology, American Medical Association, 515 North State Street, Chicago, IL 60610

Treasurer: John T. Fay, Jr., Ph.D., Vice President, Corporate Affairs, Bergen Brunswig Corporation, 4000 Metropolitan Drive, Orange, CA 92668

Trustees Representing Medical Sciences: Edwin D. Bransome, Jr., M.D., Division of Metabolic and Endocrine Disease, Medical College of Georgia, Augusta, GA 30912

J. Richard Crout, M.D., Vice President, Medical and Scientific Affairs, Boehringer Mannheim Pharmaceuticals Corporation, 15204 Omega Drive, Rockville, MD 20850-3241

Trustees Representing Pharmaceutical Sciences: Jordan L. Cohen, Ph.D., College of Pharmacy, University of Kentucky, 907 Rose Street, Lexington, KY 40536-0082

James T. Doluisio, Ph.D., Dean, College of Pharmacy, University of Texas at Austin, Austin, TX 78712-1074

Trustee Representing the Public: Grace Powers Monaco, J.D., President, EMPRISE, Inc., 123 C Street, S.E., Washington, DC 20003

Trustees at Large: John V. Bergen, Ph.D., Executive Director, National Committee for Clinical Laboratory Standards, 771 East Lancaster Avenue, Villanova, PA 19085

Joseph A. Mollica, Ph.D., Chief Executive Officer Du Pont Merck Pharmaceuticals, Barley Mill Plaza, Building #25 Willmington, DE 19898

Past President: Arthur Hull Hayes, Jr., M.D., President & Chief Executive Officer, EM Pharmaceuticals, 5 Skyline Drive, Hawthorne, NY 10532

United States Government Services

Department of the Army: Col. Frank A. Cammarata, Falls Church, VA 22041-3258

Food and Drug Administration: Carl C. Peck, M.D., Director, Ctr. for Drug Eval. & Res., FDA, CDER, Room 13B45, 5600 Fishers Lane, Rockville, MD 20857

National Institute of Standards & Technology: Stanley D. Rasberry, B354 Physics Bldg., NIST, Gaithersburg, MD 20899

Office of the Surgeon General, U.S. Air Force: Col. John M. Hammond, USAF/SGHP, Bolling AFB, DC 20332-6188

United States Public Health Service: ASG Richard M. Church, 5600 Fishers Lane, Room 6A-44, Rockville, MD 20857

U.S. Office of Consumer Affairs: Howard Seltzer, Director, Division of Policy Analysis, U.S. Office of Consumer Affairs, 1009 Premier Building, Washington, DC 20201

Department of Veterans Affairs: Mr. John Ogden, Pharmacy Service (119) Dept. of Veterans Affairs, 810 Vermont Avenue, N.W., Washington, DC 20420

Health Care Financing Administration: Robert E. Wren, 6325 Security Blvd, Room 401 EHR, Baltimore, MD 21207

National Organizations

American Association of Pharmaceutical Scientists: Ralph F. Shangraw, Ph.D., School of Pharmacy, University of Maryland, 20 N. Pine Street, Baltimore, MD 21201-1180

American Chemical Society: Norman C. Jamieson, Ph.D., Mallinckrodt, Inc., P.O. Box 5439, St. Louis, MO 63134

American Dental Association: Clifford W. Whall, Ph.D., American Dental Association-CDT, 211 E. Chicago, IL 60611

American Hospital Association: William R. Reid, Community Hospital of Roanoke Valley, Box 12946, Roanoke, VA 24029

American Medical Association: Joseph W. Cranston, Jr., Ph.D., American Medical Association, 535 N. Dearborn Street, Chicago, IL 60610

American Nurses Association: Linda Cronenwett, Ph.D., R.N., F.A.A.N., Director, Nursing Research, Dept of Nursing Administration, Dartmouth-Hitchcock Medical Center, 2 Maynard Street, Hanover, NH 03756

American Pharmaceutical Association: Arthur H. Kibbe, Ph.D., 2215 Constitution Avenue, N.W., Washington, DC 20037

American Society for Clinical Pharmacology & Therapeutics: William J. Mroczek, M.D., Cardiovascular Ctr. of Northern Virginia, 6045 Arlington Boulevard, Falls Church, VA 22044

American Society of Consultant Pharmacists: Mr. Milton S. Moskowitz, 9513 Gerwig Lane, Suites 129-132, Columbia, MD 21046

American Society of Hospital Pharmacists: Stephanie Y. Crawford, Ph.D., American Society of Hospital Pharmacists, 4630 Montgomery Avenue, Bethesda, MD 20814

American Society for Quality Control: Mr. Anthony M. Carfagno, Becton Dickinson and Company, 147 Clinton Road, W. Caldwell, NJ 07006

American Veterinary Medical Association: Dr. Lloyd Davis, 218 Large Animal Clinic, 1102 W. Hazelwood Drive, Urbana, IL 61801

Association of Food and Drug Officials: David R. Work, J.D., Executive Director, North Carolina State Board of Pharmacy, P. O. Box 459, Carrboro, NC 27510

Association of Official Analytical Chemists: Mr. Thomas Layloff, Jr., FDA/Div. of Drug Analysis, 1114 Market Street, Rm. 1002, St. Louis, MO 63101

Chemical Manufacturers Association: Andrew J. Schmitz, Jr., Huntington, NY 11743

Cosmetic, Toiletry & Fragrance Association, Inc.: G.N. McEwen, Jr., Ph.D., J.D., Cosmetic, Toiletry & Fragrance Association, Inc., 1110 Vermont Avenue, N.W., Suite 800, Washington, DC 20005

Drug Information Association: Elizabeth B. D'Angelo, Ph.D., Manager, Quality Assurance and Testing, ICI Pharmaceuticals Group, Wilmington, DE 19897

Generic Pharmaceutical Industry Association: William F. Haddad, Vice Chairman, Danbury Pharmacal, Inc., 12 Stoneleigh Ave., P.O. Box 990, Carmel, NY 10512

Health Industry Manufacturers Association: Ms. Dee Simons, Health Industry Manufacturers Assn., 1030 15th Street, N.W., Washington, DC 20005

National Association of Boards of Pharmacy: Carmen Catizone, Executive Director, National Association of Boards of Pharmacy, 1300 Higgins Road, Suite 103, Park Ridge, IL 60068

National Association of Chain Drug Stores, Inc.: Saul Schneider, Vice President, Pharmacy Director, K & B, Inc., K & B Plaza, Lee Circle, New Orleans, LA 70130-3999

National Association of Retail Druggists: William N. Tindall, Ph.D., 205 Daingerfield Road, Alexandria, VA 22314

National Wholesale Druggists' Association: Bruce R. Siecker, R. Ph., Ph.D., National Wholesale Druggists' Assn., 105 Oronoco St., Alexandria, VA 22314

Nonprescription Drug Manufacturers Association: R. William Soller, Ph.D., Sr. V.P. & Dir., Scientific Affairs, Nonprescription Drug Manufacturers Association, 1150 Connecticut Avenue, N.W., Washington, DC 20036

Parenteral Drug Association, Inc.: Peter E. Manni, Ph.D., Smith Kline Beecham Corp., 1500 Spring Garden Street, Philadelphia, PA 19101

Pharmaceutical Manufacturers Association: Maurice Q. Bectel, Pharmaceutical Manufacturers Association, 1100 Fifteenth Street, N.W., Washington, DC 20005

Other Organizations and Institutions

Alabama

Auburn University, School of Pharmacy: Kenneth N. Barker, Ph.D., Department of Pharmacy Care Systems, School of Pharmacy, Auburn University, Auburn, AL 36849

Samford University School of Pharmacy: H. Anthony McBride, Ph.D., Ingalls Hall, School of Pharmacy, Samford University, 800 Lakeshore Drive, Birmingham, AL 35229

University of South Alabama, College of Medicine: Samuel J. Strada, Ph.D., Department of Pharmacology, University of South Alabama, College of Medicine, 307 University Blvd., 3190 MSB, Mobile, AL 36688

Medical Association of the State of Alabama: Paul A. Palmisano, M.D., The Children's Hospital of Alabama, 1600 7th Avenue, So., Birmingham, AL 35233

Alabama Pharmaceutical Association: Mitchel C. Rothholz, 1211 Carmichael Way, Montgomery, AL 36106-3672

Arizona

University of Arizona, College of Medicine: John D. Palmer, Ph.D., M.D., Department of Pharmacology, College of Medicine, University of Arizona, Tucson, AZ 85724

Arizona Pharmacy Association: Edward Armstrong, Tucson, AZ 85711

University of Arizona, College of Pharmacy: Dr. Michael Mayersohn, College of Pharmacy, University of Arizona, Tucson, AZ 85721

Arkansas

University of Arkansas for Medical Sciences, College of Pharmacy: Kenneth G. Nelson, Ph.D., College of Pharmacy, University of Arkansas for Medical Sciences, 4301 W. Markham St., Little Rock, AR 72205

California

University of California, Davis, School of Medicine: Larry Stark, Ph.D., Dept. of Pharmacology, School of Medicine, University of California, Davis, CA 95616

University of California, San Diego, School of Medicine: Harold J. Simon, M.D., Ph.D., UCSD School of Medicine 0622, La Jolla, CA 92093-0622

University of California, San Francisco, School of Medicine: Walter L. Way, M.D., 521 Parnassus Ave., Rm. C 455, University of California, San Francisco, CA 94143-0418

University of Southern California, School of Medicine: Wayne R. Bidlack, Ph.D., Assoc. Prof of Pharmacology and Nutrition, University of Southern California, School of Medicine, 1975 Zonal Avenue, Los Angeles, CA 90033

University of California, San Francisco, School of Pharmacy: Richard H. Guy, Ph.D., School of Pharmacy, Box 0446, S-926, University of California, San Francisco, CA 94143

University of Southern California, School of Pharmacy: Robert T. Koda, Pharm.D., Ph.D., School of Pharmacy, University of Southern California, 1985 Zonal Avenue, Los Angeles, CA 90033-1086

University of the Pacific, School of Pharmacy: Alice Jean Matuszak, Ph.D., School of Pharmacy, University of the Pacific, 751 Brookside Road, Stockton, CA 95207

California Pharmacists Association: Robert P. Marshall, Pharm.D., California Pharmacists Association, 1112 "I" Street, Sacramento, CA, 95814

Colorado

University of Colorado School of Pharmacy: Eli Shefter, Ph.D., Campus Box 297, University of Colorado, School of Pharmacy, Boulder, CO 80309-0297

Colorado Pharmacal Association: Thomas G. Arthur, R.Ph., Conifer, CO 80433

Connecticut

University of Connecticut, School of Medicine: Paul F. Davern, South Windsor, CT 06074

University of Connecticut, School of Pharmacy: Karl A. Nieforth, Ph.D., School of Pharmacy, University of Connecticut, 372 Fairfield Road, Box U-92, Storrs, CT 06269-2092

Connecticut Pharmaceutical Association: Henry A. Palmer, Ph.D., School of Pharmacy, University of Connecticut, Box U-92, 372 Fairfield Road, Storrs, CT 06269-2092

Delaware

Delaware Pharmaceutical Society: Charles J. O'Connor, Wilmington, DE 19806

Medical Society of Delaware: John M. Levinson, M.D., Wilmington, DE 19806

District of Columbia

George Washington University: Janet Elgert-Madison, Pharm.D., GWU Medical Center, 901 23rd Street, N.W., Washington, DC 20037

Georgetown University, School of Medicine: Arthur Raines, Ph.D., Department of Pharmacology, Georgetown University Medical Center, 3900 Reservoir Road, N.W., Washington, DC 20007

Howard University, College of Medicine: Sonya K. Sobrian, Ph.D., Dept. of Pharmacology, College of Medicine, Howard University, 520 4th Street, N.W., Washington, DC 20059

Howard University, College of Pharmacy & Pharmacal Sciences: Wendell T. Hill, Jr., Pharm.D., Dean, College of Pharmacy, Howard University, 2300 Fourth Street, N.W., Washington, DC 20059

Florida

Southeastern College of Pharmacy: Paul Magalian, Ph.D., Acting Dean, Southeastern College of Pharmacy, 1750 N.E. 168 Street, North Miami Beach, FL 33162

University of Florida, College of Medicine: Thomas F. Muther, Ph.D., College of Medicine, University of Florida, Box J-267, J. Hillis Miller Health Center, Gainesville, FL 32610-0267

University of Florida, College of Pharmacy: Michael A. Schwartz, Ph.D., Dean, College of Pharmacy, Box J-484, J. Hillis Miller Health Center, University of Florida, Gainesville, FL 32610

University of South Florida, College of Medicine: Joseph J. Krzanowski, Jr., Ph.D., Dept. of Pharmacology & Therapeutics, College of Medicine, University of South Florida, Box 9, Tampa, FL 33612

Florida Pharmacy Association: "Red" Camp, Titusville, FL 32796

Georgia

Medical College of Georgia, School of Medicine: David W. Hawkins, Pharm.D., Medical College of Georgia, FI-1087, Augusta, GA 30912

Mercer University School of Medicine: W. Douglas Skelton, M.D., Mercer University School of Medicine, 1550 College Street, Macon, GA 31207

Mercer University, Southern School of Pharmacy: Hewitt W. Matthews, Ph.D., Dean and Professor, Southern School of Pharmacy, Mercer University, 345 Boulevard, N.E., Atlanta, GA 30312

Morehouse School of Medicine: Ralph W. Trottier, Jr., Ph.D., JD, Morehouse School of Medicine, Dept. of Pharmacology, 720 Westview Drive, S.W., Atlanta, GA 30310-1495

University of Georgia, College of Pharmacy: Howard C. Ansel, Ph.D., Dean, College of Pharmacy, University of Georgia, Athens, GA 30602

Medical Association of Georgia: E.D. Bransome, Jr., M.D., Professor of Medicine, Medical College of Georgia, Augusta, GA 30912

Idaho

Idaho State University, College of Pharmacy: Eugene I. Isaacson, Ph.D., College of Pharmacy, Idaho State University, Pocatello, ID 83209

Idaho State Pharmaceutical Association: Doris Denney, Boise, ID 83702

Illinois

Chicago Medical School/University of Health Sciences: Velayudhan Nair, Ph.D., D.Sc., Dean, Graduate Studies & Research, Univ. of Health Sciences/The Chicago Medical School, 3333 Green Bay Road, N. Chicago, IL 60064

Loyola University of Chicago Stritch School of Medicine: Dr. Erwin Coyne, Dept. of Pathology, Loyola University Medical Center, 2160 S. First Avenue, Maywood, IL 60153

Northwestern University Medical School: Marilynn C. Frederiksen, M.D., Northwestern University Medical School, Prentice Pavilion, Room 1176, Chicago, IL 60611

Rush Medical College of Rush University: Paul G. Pierpaoli, M.S., Chicago, IL 60612

Southern Illinois University, School of Medicine: Lionard Rybak, M.D., Ph.D., Dept. of Surgery, Southern Illinois University School of Medicine, P.O. Box 19230, Springfield, IL 62794-9230

University of Illinois, College of Medicine: Marten M. Kernis, Ph.D., UICOM-Dean (M/C 784), Box 6998, Chicago, IL 60680

University of Illinois, College of Pharmacy: Henri R. Manasse, Jr., Ph.D., Dean, College of Pharmacy, Box 6998 m/c 874, University of Illinois-Chicago, Chicago, IL 60680

Illinois Pharmacists Association: Ronald W. Gottrich, Springfield, IL 62761

Illinois State Medical Society: Vincent A. Costanzo, Jr., M.D., Jackson Park Hospital, Chicago, IL 60649

Indiana

Butler University, College of Pharmacy: Wagar H. Bhatti, Ph.D., College of Pharmacy, Butler University, 46th & Sunset Avenue, Indianapolis, IN 46208

Purdue University, School of Pharmacy and Pharmacal Sciences: Garnet E. Peck, Ph.D., School of Pharmacy & Pharmacal Sciences, Purdue University, West Lafayette, IN 47907

Indiana State Medical Association: Edward Langston, M.D., Family Practice Center, 5502 E. 16th St., Indianapolis, IN 46218

Iowa

University of Iowa, College of Medicine: John E. Kasik, M.D., Ph.D., Veterans Administration Medical Center, Iowa City, IA 52242

Drake University, College of Pharmacy: Sidney L. Finn, Ph.D., College of Pharmacy, Drake University, 2507 University Avenue, Des Moines, IA 50311

Iowa Pharmacists Association: Steve C. Firman, Cedar Falls, IA 50613

University of Iowa, College of Pharmacy: Robert A. Wiley, Ph.D., Dean, College of Pharmacy, University of Iowa, Iowa City, IA 52242

Kansas

Kansas Pharmacists Association: Robert R. Williams, 1308 West 10th Street, Topeka, KS 66604

Kentucky

University of Kentucky, College of Medicine: John M. Carney, Ph.D., College of Medicine, University of Kentucky, Lexington, KY 40536

University of Kentucky, College of Pharmacy: Patrick P. DeLuca, Ph.D., College of Pharmacy, University of Kentucky, Lexington, KY 40536-0082

University of Louisville, School of Medicine: Peter P. Rowell, Ph.D., Department of Pharmacology & Toxicology, School of Medicine, University of Louisville, Louisville, KY 40292

Kentucky Medical Association: Ellsworth C. Seeley, M.D., 820 South Limestone, Medical Plaza Annex, Lexington, KY 40536
Kentucky Pharmacists Association: Chester L. Parker, Pharm.D., Lexington, KY 40504

Louisiana

Louisiana State University School of Medicine in New Orleans: Paul L. Kirkendol, Ph.D., New Orleans, LA 70119
Northeast Louisiana University, School of Pharmacy: William M. Bourn, Ph.D., Dean, School of Pharmacy, Northeast Louisiana University, Monroe, LA 71209
Tulane University, School of Medicine: Floyd R. Domer, Ph.D., Department of Pharmacology, School of Medicine, Tulane University, 1430 Tulane Avenue, New Orleans, LA 70112
Xavier University of Louisiana: Barry A. Bleidt, Ph.D., R.Ph. P.O. Box 850665, New Orleans, LA 70185-0665
Louisiana State Medical Society: Henry W. Jolly, Jr., M.D., Baton Rouge, LA 70808

Maryland

Johns Hopkins University, School of Medicine: E. Robert Feroli, Jr., Pharm.D., Lutherville, MD 21093
University of Maryland, School of Medicine: Edson X. Albuquerque, M.D., Ph.D., Professor & Chairman, Dept of Pharmacology, University of Maryland, School of Medicine, 655 West Baltimore St., Rm. 4-0006, Baltimore, MD 21201
Uniformed Services University of the Health Sciences, F. Edward Hebert School of Medicine: Louis R. Cantilena, Jr., M.D., Ph.D., Div. of Clinical Pharmacology, USUHS, 4301 Jones Bridge Road, Bethesda, MD 20814-4799
University of Maryland, School of Pharmacy: Larry L. Augsburger, Ph.D., School of Pharmacy, University of Maryland, 20 North Pine Street, Baltimore, MD 21201
Medical and Chirurgical Faculty of the State of Maryland: Frederick Wilhelm, M.D., Hyattsville, MD 20784
Maryland Pharmacists Association: Nicholas C. Lykos, P.D., 2101 York Road, Timonium, MD 21093

Massachusetts

Harvard Medical School: Peter Goldman, M.D., Dept. of Nutri., School of Public Health, Harvard University, 665 Huntington Ave., Boston, MA 02115
Tufts University, School of Medicine: Dr. John Mazzullo, Boston, MA 02116-1772
Northeastern University, College of Pharmacy and Allied Health Professions: John L. Neumeyer, Ph.D., College of Pharmacy and Allied Health Professions, Northeastern University, 110MU, Boston, MA 02115
University of Massachusetts Medical School: Brian Johnson, M.D., University of Massachusetts Medical Center, 55 Lake Avenue North, Worcester, MA 01655

Michigan

Ferris State College, School of Pharmacy: Gerald W.A. Slywka, Ph.D., School of Pharmacy, Ferris State University, Big Rapids, MI 49307
Michigan State University, College of Human Medicine: John Penner, M.D., Dept. of Medicine, B220 Life Sciences Bldg., Michigan State University, East Lansing, MI 48825
University of Michigan, College of Pharmacy: Ara G. Paul, Ph.D., Dean, College of Pharmacy, University of Michigan, 428 Church Street, Ann Arbor, MI 48109-1065
Wayne State University, School of Medicine: Ralph E. Kauffman, M.D., Children's Hospital of Michigan, 3901 Beaubien Blvd., Detroit, MI 48201
Wayne State University, College of Pharmacy and Allied Health Professions: Janardan B. Nagwekar, Ph.D., College of Pharmacy and Allied Health Professions, Shapero Hall, Room 511, Wayne State University, Detroit, MI 48202
Michigan Pharmacists Association: Patrick L. McKercher, Ph.D., Drug Policy Analysis Director, The Upjohn Company, 7000 Portage Road, Kalamazoo, MI 49001

Minnesota

Mayo Medical School: James J. Lipsky, M.D., Mayo Medical School 200 First Street SW, Rochester, MN 55905
University of Minnesota, College of Pharmacy: E. John Staba, Ph.D., College of Pharmacy 9-106 Health Sciences Unit F, University of Minnesota, 308 Harvard Street, N.E., Minneapolis, MN 55455
University of Minnesota Medical School, Minneapolis: Jack W. Miller, Ph.D., Dept. of Pharmacology, 3-249 Millard Hall, University of Minnesota Medical School, 435 Delaware Street, S.E., Minneapolis, MN 55455
Minnesota Medical Association: Harold Seim, M.D., University Family Practice Clinic, 316 Botany, Box 381, 400 Church Street S.E., Minneapolis, MN 55455
Minnesota State Pharmaceutical Association: Arnold D. Delger, St. Paul, MN 55512

Mississippi

University of Mississippi, School of Medicine: James L. Achord, M.D., University of Mississippi Medical Center, 2500 N. State Street, Jackson, MS 39216
University of Mississippi, School of Pharmacy: Robert W. Cleary, Ph.D., University of Mississippi, University, MS 38677
Mississippi State Medical Association: Charles L. Mathews, Box 5229, Jackson, MS 39296
Mississippi Pharmacists Association: Mike Kelly, 341 Edgewood Terrace Dr., Jackson, MS 39206

Missouri

St. Louis College of Pharmacy: John W. Zuzack, Ph.D., St. Louis College of Pharmacy, 4588 Parkview Place, St. Louis, MO 63110
St. Louis University, School of Medicine: Alvin H. Gold, Ph.D., Dept. of Pharmacology, School of Medicine, St. Louis University, 1402 S. Grand Boulevard, St. Louis, MO 63104
University of Missouri, Columbia, School of Medicine: John W. Yarbro, M.D., Ph.D., School of Medicine, MA434 Medical Science Bldg., University of Missouri-Columbia, Columbia, MO 65212
University of Missouri-Kansas City, School of Medicine: Paul Cuddy, Pharm.D., UMKC School of Medicine, 2411 Holmes, Kansas City, MO 64108
University of Missouri, Kansas City, School of Pharmacy: Lester Chafetz, Ph.D., School of Pharmacy, University of Missouri-Kansas City, 5005 Rockhill Road, Kansas City, MO 64110
Washington University, School of Medicine: H. Mitchell Perry, Jr., M.D., School of Medicine, Washington University, 915 N. Grand Blvd., Bldg. 3, St. Louis, MO 63106
Missouri Pharmaceutical Association: George L. Oestreich, Executive Director, Missouri Pharmaceutical Association, 410 Madison Street, Jefferson City, MO 65101

Nebraska

Creighton University, School of Medicine: Michael C. Makoid, Ph.D., School of Pharmaceutical Sciences and Allied Health, Criss III, Room 460, Creighton University, California Street and 24th Street, Omaha. NE 68178
Creighton University School of Pharmacy and Allied Health Professions: Kenneth R. Keefner, Ph.D., School of Pharmacy & Allied Health Professions, California at 24th Street, Omaha, NE 68178
University of Nebraska, College of Medicine: Manuchair Ebadi, Ph.D., College of Medicine, University of Nebraska, 42nd Street and Dewey Avenue, Omaha, NE 68105
University of Nebraska, College of Pharmacy: Clarence T. Ueda, Pharm.D., Ph.D., Dean, College of Pharmacy, University of Nebraska, 42nd and Dewey Avenues, Omaha, NE 68105-1065
Nebraska Pharmacists Association: Rex C. Higley, R.P., Lincoln, NE 68506

Nevada

Nevada Pharmacists Association: Steven P. Bradford, P.O. Box 504, Minden, NV 89423

New Hampshire

Dartmouth Medical School: James J. Kresel, Ph.D., Mary Hitchcock Memorial Hospital, Hanover, NH 03756
New Hampshire Pharmaceutical Association: William J. Lancaster, P.D., Hanover, NH 03755

New Jersey

University of Medicine and Dentistry of New Jersey, New Jersey Medical School: Sheldon B. Gertner, Ph.D., New Jersey Medical School, UMDNJ, 185 S. Orange Avenue, Newark, NJ 07103-2714
Rutgers, The State University of New Jersey, College of Pharmacy: John L. Colaizzi, Ph.D., Dean, College of Pharmacy, Rutgers-The State University of New Jersey, P.O. Box 789, Piscataway, NJ 08855-0789
Medical Society of New Jersey: Joseph N. Micale, M.D., 914 85th Street, North Bergen, NJ 07047
New Jersey Pharmaceutical Association: Stephen J. Csubak, Ph.D., Washington Crossing, PA 18977

New Mexico

University of New Mexico, College of Pharmacy: William M. Hadley, Ph.D., Dean, College of Pharmacy, University of New Mexico, Albuquerque, NM 87131
New Mexico Pharmaceutical Association: Hugh Kabat, Ph.D., Corrales, NM 87048

New York

Albert Einstein College of Medicine of Yeshiva University: Dr. Walter G. Levine, Albert Einstein College of Medicine, Forchheimer Bldg., Room 230, 1300 Morris Park Avenue, New York, NY 10461
City University of New York, Mt. Sinai School of Medicine: Joel S. Mindel, Mt. Sinai School of Medicine, City University of New York, 1 Gustave L. Levy Place, New York, NY 10029

Columbia Univ. College of Physicians and Surgeons: Michael R. Rosen, M.D., Dept. of Pharmacology, 630 West 168th Street, New York, NY 10032

Cornell University Medical College: Dr. Lorraine J. Gudas, Cornell University Medical College, 1300 York Avenue, New York, NY 10021

Long Island University, Arnold and Marie Schwartz College of Pharmacy and Health Sciences: Jack M. Rosenberg, Ph.D., Arnold & Marie Schwartz College of Pharmacy and Health Sciences, Long Island University, 75 Dekalb Avenue, Brooklyn, NY 11201

New York Medical College: Mario A. Inchiosa, Jr., Ph.D., Department of Pharmacology, New York Medical College, Valhalla, NY 10595

New York University School of Medicine: Norman Altzuler, Ph.D., Dept. of Pharmacology, NYU School of Medicine, 550 First Avenue, New York, NY 10016

State University of New York, Buffalo, School of Medicine: Robert J. McIsaac, Ph.D., Department of Pharmacology and Therapeutics, School of Medicine & Biomedical Sciences, 102 Farber Hall, SUNY at Buffalo, Buffalo, NY 14214

State University of New York, Buffalo, School of Pharmacy: Robert M. Cooper, Assoc. Dean, Getzville, NY 14068

State University of New York, Health Science Center, Syracuse: Oliver M. Brown, Ph.D., Department of Pharmacology, SUNY Health Science Center at Syracuse, 750 East Adams Street, Syracuse, NY 13210

St. John's University, College of Pharmacy and Allied Health Professions: Albert A. Belmonte, Ph.D., College of Pharmacy & Allied Health Professions, St. John's University, Grand Central & Utopia Parkways, Jamaica, NY 11439

Union University, Albany College of Pharmacy: David W. Newton, Ph.D., Albany College of Pharmacy, Union University, 106 New Scotland Avenue, Albany, NY 12208

University of Rochester, School of Medicine and Dentistry: Michael Weintraub, M.D., University of Rochester Medical Center, Box 644, Rochester, NY 14642

Medical Society of the State of New York: Richard S. Blum, M.D., Lake Success, NY 11042

Pharmaceutical Society of the State of New York: Mr. Bruce Moden, West Seneca, NY 14224

North Carolina

Bowman Gray School of Medicine, Wake Forest University: Jack W. Strandhoy, Ph.D., Department of Physiology/Pharmacology, Bowman Gray School of Medicine, Wake Forest University, 300 S. Hawthorne Road, Winston-Salem, NC 27103

Campbell University, School of Pharmacy: Antoine Al-Achi, Ph.D., School of Pharmacy, Campbell University, P.O. Box 1090, Buies Creek, NC 27506

East Carolina University, School of Medicine: A-R. A. Abdel-Rahman, Ph.D., Department of Pharmacology, School of Medicine, East Carolina University, Greenville, NC 27858

University of North Carolina, Chapel Hill, School of Pharmacy: Richard J. Kowalsky, Pharm.D., School of Pharmacy, 24 Beard Hall, CB 7360, University of North Carolina, Chapel Hill, NC 27599

University of North Carolina at Chapel Hill, School of Medicine: Dr. George Hatfield, Director of Pharmacy, UNC Hospitals, CB #7600, NCMH, Chapel Hill, NC 27599-7600

North Carolina Pharmaceutical Association: George H. Cocolas, Ph.D., School of Pharmacy, CB 7360, University of North Carolina, Chapel Hill, NC 27599-7360

North Carolina Medical Society: T. Reginald Harris, M.D., Shelby, NC 28150

North Dakota

North Dakota State University, College of Pharmacy: William M. Henderson, Ph.D., College of Pharmacy, North Dakota State University, Fargo, ND 58105

University of North Dakota, School of Medicine: David W. Hein, Ph.D., Dept. of Pharmacology, Univ of North Dakota, School of Medicine, 501 North Columbia Rd., Grand Forks, ND 58203

North Dakota Medical Association: Vernon E. Wagner, P.O. Box 1198, Bismarck, ND 58502-1198

North Dakota Pharmaceutical Association: William H. Shelver, Ph.D., College of Pharmacy, North Dakota State University, Fargo, ND 58105

Ohio

Case Western Reserve University, School of Medicine: Kenneth A. Scott, Ph.D., Dept. of Pharmacology, School of Medicine, Case Western Reserve University, 2119 Abington Road, Cleveland, OH 44106

Medical College of Ohio at Toledo: R. Douglas Wilkerson, Ph.D., Medical College of Ohio, P.O. Box 10008, Toledo, OH 43699

Northeastern Ohio University, College of Medicine: Ralph E. Berggren, M.D., College of Medicine, Northeastern Ohio University, 4209 State Route 44, Rootstown, OH 44272

Ohio Northern University, College of Pharmacy: Joseph Theodore, Ph.D., Ohio Northern University, Ada, OH 45810

Ohio State University, College of Medicine: Robert Guthrie, M.D., 1142 University Hospitals Clinic, Columbus, OH 43210

Ohio State University, College of Pharmacy: Michael C. Gerald, Ph.D., College of Pharmacy, Ohio State University, 500 West 12th Avenue, Columbus, OH 43210

University of Cincinnati, College of Medicine: Leonard T. Sigell, Ph.D., 231 Bethesda Avenue, Cincinnati, OH 45267-0144

University of Cincinnati, College of Pharmacy: Henry S.I. Tan, Ph.D., College of Pharmacy, University of Cincinnati, 3223 Eden Avenue, Mail Location No. 4, Cincinnati, OH 45267

University of Toledo, College of Pharmacy: Norman F. Billups, Ph.D., Dean, College of Pharmacy, University of Toledo, 2801 W. Bancroft Street, Toledo, OH 43606

Wright State University, School of Medicine: John O. Lindower, M.D., Ph.D., School of Medicine, Wright State University, P.O. Box 927, Dayton, OH 45401-0927

Ohio State Medical Association: Janet K. Bixel, M.D., 289 E. State Street, Suite 200, Columbus, OH 43215

Ohio State Pharmaceutical Association: J. Richard Wuest, Pharm.D., Cincinnati, OH 45219

Oklahoma

Southwestern Oklahoma State University, School of Pharmacy: W. Steven Pray, Ph.D., Southwestern Oklahoma State University, School of Pharmacy, Weatherford, OK 73096

University of Oklahoma, College of Pharmacy: Loyd V. Allen, Jr., Ph.D., College of Pharmacy, University of Oklahoma, P.O. Box 26901, 1110 N. Stonewall, Oklahoma City, OK 73190

Oklahoma Pharmaceutical Association: Carl D. Lyons, Skyline Terrace Nursing Center, 6202 E. 61st, Tulsa, OK 74136

Oklahoma State Medical Association: Clinton Nicholas Corder, M.D., Ph.D., OMRF, 825 N.E. 13th Street, Oklahoma City, OK 73104

Oregon

Oregon Health Sciences University, School of Medicine: Hall Downes, M.D., Ph.D., Oregon Health Sciences University, L221, 3181 S.W. Sam Jackson Park Road, Portland, OR 97201-3098

Oregon State University, College of Pharmacy: Randall L. Vanderveen, Ph.D., College of Pharmacy, Oregon State University, Corvallis, OR 97331-3507

Pennsylvania

Duquesne University, School of Pharmacy: Lawrence H. Block, Ph.D., School of Pharmacy, Duquesne University, Pittsburgh, PA 15282

Hahnemann University, School of Medicine: Vincent J. Zarro, M.D., Broad and Vine Streets, MS 431, Philadelphia, PA 19102

Medical College of Pennsylvania: Athole G. McNeil Jacobi, M.D., Medical College of Pennsylvania, 3300 Henry Avenue, Philadelphia, PA 19129

Pennsylvania State University, College of Medicine: John D. Connor, Ph.D., Milton S. Hershey Medical Center, Pennsylvania State University, P.O. Box 850, Hershey, PA 17033

Philadelphia College of Pharmacy and Science: Alfonso R. Gennaro, Ph.D., Philadelphia College of Pharmacy and Science, Woodland Avenue at 43rd Street, Philadelphia, PA 19104

Temple University, School of Medicine: Ronald J. Tallarida, Ph.D., School of Medicine, Temple University, 3420 N. Broad Street, Philadelphia, PA 19140

Temple University, School of Pharmacy: Murray Tuckerman, Ph.D., P.O. Box 79, Monomonac Drive West, Winchendon Spring, MA 01477

University of Pennsylvania, School of Medicine: Dr. Marilyn E. Hess, School of Medicine, University of Pennsylvania, 36th and Hamilton Walk, Philadelphia, PA 19104

University of Pittsburgh, School of Pharmacy: Terrence L. Schwinghammer, Pharm.D., School of Pharmacy, University of Pittsburgh, 239-B Victoria Hall, Pittsburgh, PA 15261

Pennsylvania Medical Society: Benjamin Calesnick, M.D., Springfield, PA 19064

Pennsylvania Pharmaceutical Association: Joseph A. Mosso R.Ph., Mosso's Pharmacy, 1006 Ligonier Street, Latrobe, PA 15650

Puerto Rico

University of Puerto Rico, College of Pharmacy: Benjamin P. de Gracia, Ph.D., School of Pharmacy, University of Puerto Rico, G.P.O. Box 5067, San Juan, PR 00936-5067

Rhode Island

Brown University Program in Medicine: Darrell R. Abernethy, M.D., Ph.D., Dept. of Medicine, Roger Williams General Hospital, 825 Chalkstone Avenue, Providence, RI 02908

University of Rhode Island, College of Pharmacy: Thomas E. Needham, Ph.D., College of Pharmacy, University of Rhode Island, Kingston, RI 02881

xxiii

South Carolina

Medical University of South Carolina, College of Medicine: Herman B. Daniell, Ph.D., Dept. of Pharmacology, Medical University of South Carolina, 171 Ashley Avenue, Charleston, SC 29425

Medical University of South Carolina, College of Pharmacy: Paul J. Niebergall, Ph.D., College of Pharmacy, Medical University of South Carolina, 171 Ashley Avenue, Charleston, SC 29425

University of South Carolina, College of Pharmacy: Robert L. Beamer, Ph.D., College of Pharmacy, University of South Carolina, Columbia, SC 29208

South Dakota

South Dakota State University, College of Pharmacy: Gary S. Chappell, Ph.D., College of Pharmacy, South Dakota State University, Box 2202c, Brookings, SD 57007

South Dakota Pharmaceutical Association: James Powers, Brookings, SD 57006

Tennessee

East Tennessee State University, Quillen College of Medicine: Ernest A. Daigneault, Ph.D., Dept. of Pharmacology, James H. Quillin College of Medicine, East Tennessee State University, P.O. Box 19810A, Johnson City, TN 37614

Meharry Medical College, School of Medicine: Dolores C. Shockley, Ph.D., Meharry Medical College, Dept. of Pharmacology, 1005 D. B. Todd Jr. Boulevard, Nashville, TN 37208

University of Tennessee College of Pharmacy: Dick R. Gourley, Pharm.D., 847 Monroe, Suite 238, Memphis, TN 38163

Vanderbilt University, School of Medicine: David H. Robertson, M.D., AA-3228, Medical Center North, Vanderbilt School of Medicine, Nashville, TN 37232

Tennessee Pharmacists Association: Roger L. Davis, Pharm.D., 226 Capitol Blvd., Suite 810, Nashville, TN 37219

Texas

Texas A & M University, College of Medicine: Marsha A. Raebel, Pharm.D., Dept. of Internal Medicine, Scott & White Hospital, Temple, TX 76508

Texas Southern University, College of Pharmacy and Health Sciences: Victor Padron, Ph.D., College of Pharmacy & Health Sciences, Texas Southern University, 3100 Cleburne Street, Houston, TX 77004

University of Houston, College of Pharmacy: Mustafa Lokhandwala, Ph.D., Dept. of Pharmacology, College of Pharmacy, University of Houston, Houston, TX 77204-5515

University of Texas, Austin, College of Pharmacy: James T. Doluisio, Ph.D., Dean, College of Pharmacy, University of Texas at Austin, Austin, TX 78712

University of Texas, Medical Branch at Galveston: George T. Bryan, M.D., Dean, University of Texas, Medical Branch at Galveston, 301 University Boulevard, Galveston, TX 77550

University of Texas Medical School, Houston: Jacques E. Chelly, M.D., Ph.D., Dept. of Pharmacology, Medical School at Houston, University of Texas, P.O. Box 20708, Houston, TX 77225

University of Texas Medical School, San Antonio: Alexander M.M. Shepherd, M.D., Ph.D., University of Texas Health Science Center, 7703 Floyd Curl Drive, San Antonio, TX 78284-7764

Texas Medical Association: Robert H. Barr, M.D., P.O. Box 25249, Houston, TX 77265

Texas Pharmaceutical Association: Shirley McKee, R.Ph., Houston, TX 77099

Utah

University of Utah, College of Pharmacy: David B. Roll, Ph.D., College of Pharmacy, University of Utah, Salt Lake City, UT 84109

Utah Pharmaceutical Association: Robert V. Peterson, Ph.D., Murray, UT 84107

Utah Medical Association: David A. Hilding, M.D., Hospital Drive #1, Price, UT 84501

Vermont

University of Vermont, College of Medicine: John J. McCormack, Ph.D., College of Medicine, Room B-322, Given Medical Building, University of Vermont, Burlington, VT 05405

Vermont Pharmacists Association: James S. Craddock, Executive Director, 121 College Street, Montpelier, VT 05602

Virginia

Medical College of Hampton Roads: William J. Cooke, Ph.D., Department of Pharmacology, Eastern Virginia Medical School, P.O. Box 1980, Norfolk, VA 23501

Medical College of Virginia/Virginia Commonwealth University, School of Pharmacy: William H. Barr, Pharm.D., Ph.D., MCV School of Pharmacy, Virginia Commonwealth University, MCV Station Box 581, Richmond, VA 23298-0581

University of Virginia, School of Medicine: Peyton E. Weary, M.D., Chairman, Department of Dermatology, School of Medicine, University of Virginia, Box 134-Medical Center, Charlottesville, VA 22908

Virginia Pharmaceutical Association: Mr. Daniel A. Herbert, Richmond, VA 23228

Washington

University of Washington, School of Pharmacy: Lynn R. Brady, Ph.D., School of Pharmacy, SC-68, University of Washington, Seattle, WA 98195

Washington State University, College of Pharmacy: Martin J. Jinks, Pharm.D., College of Pharmacy, 105 Wegner Hall, Washington State University, Pullman, WA 99164-6510

Washington State Pharmacists Association: Danial E. Baker, Spokane, WA 99203

West Virginia

Marshall University, School of Medicine: John L. Szarek, Ph.D., Marshall University School of Medicine, 1542 Spring Valley Drive, Huntington, WV 25755-9310

West Virginia University, School of Medicine: Douglas D. Glover, M.D., Dept. of Obstetrics & Gynecology, Health Sciences Center North, Rm 4601, West Virginia University, Morgantown, WV 26506

West Virginia University Medical Center, School of Pharmacy: Arthur I. Jacknowitz, Pharm.D., School of Pharmacy, West Virginia University, 1124 Health Sciences North, Morgantown, WV 26506

Wisconsin

University of Wisconsin, Madison, School of Pharmacy: Chester A. Bond, Pharm.D., School of Pharmacy, University of Wisconsin-Madison, 425 N. Charter Street, Madison, WI 53706

University of Wisconsin Medical School, Madison: Joseph M. Benforado, M.D., Madison, WI 53711

State Medical Society of Wisconsin: Thomas L. Adams, CAE, P.O. Box 1109, Madison, WI 53701

Wisconsin Pharmacists Association: Dennis Dziczkowski, R.Ph., Hales Corners, WI 53130

Wyoming

University of Wyoming, School of Pharmacy: Kenneth F. Nelson, Ph.D., School of Pharmacy, Box 3375, University Station, Laramie, WY 82071

Wyoming Medical Society: R. W. Johnson, Jr., P.O. Drawer 4009, Cheyenne, WY 82003

Wyoming Pharmaceutical Association: Linda G. Sutherland, School of Pharmacy, University of Wyoming, P.O. Box 3375, Laramie, WY 82071-3375

Members-at-Large

Norman W. Atwater, Ph.D., Hopewell, NJ 08525

Cheston M. Berlin, Jr., M.D., Chief, Div. of General Pediatrics, Dept. of Pediatrics, The Milton S. Hershey Medical Ctr., P.O. Box 850, Hershey, PA 17033-2396

Mr. Fred S. Brinkley, Jr., Texas State Board of Pharmacy, 8505 Cross Park Drive, Suite 110, Austin, TX 78754-9533

Herbert S. Carlin, D.Sc., Chappaqua, NY 10514

Jordan Cohen, Ph.D., College of Pharmacy, University of Kentucky, Rose Street, Lexington, KY 40536-0082

John L. Cova, Ph.D., Health Insurance Assoc. of America, 1025 Connecticut Ave., N.W., Suite 1200, Washington, DC 20036

Enrique Fefer, Ph.D., Pan American Health Organization, 525 23rd Street, N.W., Washington, DC 20037

Leroy Fevang, Executive Director,* Canadian Pharmaceutical Association, 101-1815 Alta Vista, Ottawa, Ontario K1G 3Y6, Canada

Klaus G. Florey, Ph.D., Squibb Institute for Medical Research, P.O. Box 191, New Brunswick, NJ 08903

Lester Hosto, Ph.D., Executive Director, Arkansas State Board of Pharmacy, 320 W. Capitol, Suite 802, Little Rock, AR 72201

Jay S. Keystone, M.D., Director, Tropical Disease Unit, Toronto General Hospital, 200 Elizabeth Street, Toronto, Ontario, M5G 1L7, Canada

Calvin M. Kunin, M.D.,* Pomerene Professor of Medicine, Ohio State University, Starling-Loving Hall, Rm. M110, 320 W. 10th Avenue, Columbus, OH 43210-1240

Marvin Lipman, M.D., Scarsdale, NY 10583

Joseph A. Mollica, Ph.D., Vice President, Medical Products Dept., E. I. du Pont de Nemours & Co., Inc., Barley Mill Plaza, Bldg. #25, Wilmington, DE 19898

Stuart L. Nightingale, M.D., Assoc. Commissioner for Health Affairs, DHHS, Public Health Service, Food and Drug Administration, 5600 Fishers Lane, Rockville, MD 20857

Daniel A. Nona, Ph.D., Executive Director, The American Council on Pharmaceutical Education, 311 W. Superior Street, Chicago, IL 60610

Mark Novitch, M.D., The Upjohn Company, Kalamazoo, MI 49001

Mr. Charles A. Pergola, President, SmithKline Beecham Consumer Brands, P.O. Box 1467, Pittsburgh, PA 15230

Donald O. Schiffman, Ph.D., Genealogy Unlimited, 538 South Commerce Road, Orem, UT 84058
Carl E. Trinca, Ph.D., Executive Director, Amer. Assoc. of Colleges of Pharmacy, 1426 Prince Street, Alexandria, VA 22314

Members-at-Large (Representing Other Countries That Provide Legal Status To USP or NF)
Prof. T. D. Arias, Apartado 10767, Estafeta Universitaria, Panama, Republica De Panama
Keith Bailey, Ph.D., Director, Bureau of Drug Research, Sir F. Banting Research Centre, Tunney's Pasture, Ottawa K1A OL2, Canada
Quintin L. Kintanar, M.D., Ph.D., Deputy Director General, National Science & Technology Authority, Bicutan, Taguig, Philippines
Marcelo Jorge Vernego, Ph.D., Consultant, Pan American Health Organization, Avenida Brasil no. 4365 - INCQS - sals 103, 21.040 - Rio De Janeiro, Brasil

Members-at-Large (Public)
Clement Bezold, Ph.D., Executive Director, Alternative Futures Association, 108 N. Alfred Street, Alexandria, VA 22314
Alexander Grant, Associate Commissioner for Consumer Affairs, Department of Health & Human Services, Public Health Service, Food and Drug Administration, Parklawn Bldg., Room 16-85, 5600 Fishers Lane, Rockville, MD 20857
Grace Powers Monaco, J.D., President, Emprise, Inc., 123 C Street, S.E., Washington, DC 20003
Paul G. Rogers,* Chairman of the Board, National Council on Patient Information & Education, 666 11th Street, N.W., Washington, DC 20006
Frances M. West, Secretary, State of Delaware, Department of Community Affairs, 156 South State Street, P.O. Box 1401, Dover, DE 19901

Ex-Officio Members
Joseph M. Benforado, M.D., Madison, WI 53711
Joseph P. Buckley, Ph.D., Texas Medical Center, Room 431, University of Houston, 1441 Moursund, Houston, TX 77030

Estelle G. Cohen, M.A., Baltimore, MD 21209
Leo E. Hollister, M.D., Harris County Psychiatric Center, P.O. Box 20249, Houston, TX 77225
Paul F. Parker, D.Sc., Lexington, KY 40504

Committee Chairmen
Credentials Committee: Peyton E. Weary, M.D., Chairman, Dept. of Dermatology, School of Medicine, University of Virginia, Box 134 Medical Center, Charlottesville, VA 22908
Nominating Committee for the General Committee of Revision: Walter L. Way, M.D., 521 Parnassus Ave., Rm. C 455, University of Calif., San Francisco, San Francisco, CA 94143-0418
Nominating Committee for Officers and Trustees: Joseph M. Benforado, M.D., Madison, WI 53711
Resolutions Committee: J. Richard Crout, M.D., Vice President Medical and Scientific Affairs, Boehringer Mannheim Pharmaceuticals Corp., 15204 Omega Drive, Rockville, MD 20850-3241.
General Committee of Revision: Jerome A. Halperin, 12601 Twinbrook Parkway, Rockville, MD 20852
Constitution and Bylaws Committee: John V. Bergen, Ph.D., National Committee for Clinical Laboratory Standards, 771 E. Lancaster Avenue, Villanova, PA 19085

Honorary Members
George F. Archambault, Pharm.D., J.D.,* Bethesda, MD 20814
William J. Kinnard, Jr., Ph.D.,* Acting President, University of Maryland at Baltimore, 20 N. Pine Street, Baltimore, MD 21201
Lloyd C. Miller, Ph.D., Escondido, CA 92025
John H. Moyer, M.D., D.Sc., Palmyra, PA 17078
John A. Owen, Jr., M.D.,* Box 242, University of Virginia Hospital, Charlottesville, VA 22901
Harry C. Shirkey, M.D.,* Cincinnati, OH 45208
Linwood F. Tice, D.Sc., Philadelphia College of Pharmacy & Science, 43rd Street & Kingsessing Avenue, Philadelphia, PA 19104

*Not present at the 1990 Quinquennial Meeting.

Section I

USP DI Volume III Reproduction of

FDA'S APPROVED DRUG PRODUCTS
WITH THERAPEUTIC EQUIVALENCE EVALUATIONS

12th EDITION,
incorporating supplements issued
through August 31, 1992

**The products in this list have been approved under sections
505 and 507 of the Federal Food, Drug, and Cosmetic Act.
This information is current through August 31, 1992.
Later Supplements to the FDA's "Orange Book"
are provided in the monthly *USP DI Update*.**

FOOD AND DRUG ADMINISTRATION
CENTER FOR DRUG EVALUATION AND RESEARCH
APPROVED DRUG PRODUCTS
with
Therapeutic Equivalence Evaluations

CONTENTS

		PAGE
PREFACE TO TWELFTH EDITION		**I/5**
1.	INTRODUCTION	**I/6**
1.1	Content and Exclusion	**I/6**
1.2	Therapeutic Equivalence-Related Terms	**I/7**
1.3	Statistical Criteria for Bioequivalence	**I/7**
1.4	Reference Listed Drug	**I/8**
1.5	General Policies and Legal Status	**I/8**
1.6	Practitioner's Responsibilities	**I/8**
1.7	Therapeutic Equivalence Evaluations Codes	**I/9**
1.8	Description of Special Situations	**I/14**
1.9	Therapeutic Equivalence Code Change for a Drug Entity	**I/14**
1.10	Change of the Therapeutic Equivalence Evaluation for a Single Product	**I/15**
1.11	Availability of Internal Policy and Procedure Guides	**I/15**
1.12	Availability of the Publication and Other FDA Reports and Updating Procedures	**I/15**
2.	HOW TO USE THE DRUG PRODUCT LISTS	**I/17**
2.1	Key Sections for Using the Drug Product Lists	**I/17**
2.2	Drug Product Illustration	**I/18**
2.3	Therapeutic Equivalence Evaluations Illustration	**I/19**
3.	DRUG PRODUCT LISTS	**I/20**
3.1	Prescription Drug Products	**I/20**
3.2	OTC Drug Products	**I/273**
3.3	Drug Products with Approval under Section 505 of the Act Administered by the Division of Blood and Blood Products	**I/283**
3.4	Discontinued Drug Products	**I/287**
3.5	Orphan Drug Product Designations	**I/364**
3.6	Drug Products Which Must Demonstrate *in vivo* Bioavailability Only if Product Fails to Achieve Adequate Dissolution	**I/385**
3.7	Biopharmaceutic Guidance Availability	**I/386**
3.8	ANDA Suitability Petitions	**I/388**
APPENDICES		
A. Product Name Index		**I/405**
B. Product Name Index Listed by Applicant		**I/438**
C. Uniform Terms		**I/505**
PATENT AND EXCLUSIVITY INFORMATION ADDENDUM		**I/506**
A. Exclusivity Terms		**I/507**
B. Patent and Exclusivity Lists		**I/510**

FOOD AND DRUG ADMINISTRATION
CENTER FOR DRUG EVALUATION AND RESEARCH
APPROVED DRUG PRODUCTS
with
Therapeutic Equivalence Evaluations

CONTENTS

	PAGE
PREFACE TO TWELFTH EDITION	1/5
1. INTRODUCTION	1/6
1.1 Content and Exclusion	1/6
1.2 Therapeutic Equivalence-Related Terms	1/7
1.3 Statistical Criteria for Bioequivalence	1/7
1.4 Reference Listed Drug	1/8
1.5 General Policies and Legal Status	1/8
1.6 Practitioner's Responsibilities	1/8
1.7 Therapeutic Equivalence Evaluations Codes	1/9
1.8 Description of Special Situations	1/14
1.9 Therapeutic Equivalence Code Change for a Drug Entity	1/15
1.10 Change of the Therapeutic Equivalence Evaluation for a Single Product	1/15
1.11 Availability of Internal Policy and Procedure Guides	1/15
1.12 Availability of the Publication and Other FDA Reports and Updating Procedures	1/15
2. HOW TO USE THE DRUG PRODUCT LISTS	1/17
2.1 Key Sections for Using the Drug Product Lists	1/17
2.2 Drug Product Illustration	1/18
2.3 Therapeutic Equivalence Evaluations Illustration	1/19
3. DRUG PRODUCT LISTS	1/20
3.1 Prescription Drug Products	1/20
3.2 OTC Drug Products	1/275
3.3 Drug Products with Approval under Section 505 of the Act Administered by the Division of Blood and Blood Products	1/283
3.4 Discontinued Drug Products	1/287
3.5 Orphan Drug Product Designations	1/354
3.6 Drug Products Which Must Demonstrate in vivo Bioavailability Only if Product Fails to Achieve Adequate Dissolution	1/385
3.7 Biopharmaceutic Guidance Availability	1/386
3.8 ANDA Suitability Petitions	1/388
APPENDICES	
A. Product Name Index	1/405
B. Product Name Index Listed by Applicant	1/458
C. Uniform Terms	1/505
PATENT AND EXCLUSIVITY INFORMATION ADDENDUM	1/506
A. Exclusivity Terms	1/507
B. Patent and Exclusivity Lists	1/510

FOOD AND DRUG ADMINISTRATION
CENTER FOR DRUG EVALUATION AND RESEARCH
APPROVED DRUG PRODUCTS
with
Therapeutic Equivalence Evaluations

PREFACE TO TWELFTH EDITION

The *Approved Drug Products with Therapeutic Equivalence Evaluations* publication (the List) identifies drug products approved on the basis of safety and effectiveness by the Food and Drug Administration (FDA) under the Federal Food, Drug, and Cosmetic Act (the Act). Unapproved drugs on the market (covered by the ongoing Drug Efficacy Study Implementation (DESI) review or products not subject to enforcement action as unapproved drugs) are not included in this publication. The main criterion for the inclusion of any product is that the product is the subject of an application with an effective approval that has not been withdrawn for safety or efficacy reasons. Inclusion of products on the List is independent of any current regulatory action through administrative or judicial means against a drug product. In addition, the List contains therapeutic equivalence evaluations for approved multisource prescription drug products. These evaluations have been prepared to serve as public information and advice to state health agencies, prescribers, and pharmacists to promote public education in the area of drug product selection and to foster containment of health costs. Therapeutic equivalence evaluations in this publication are not official FDA actions affecting the legal status of products under the Act.

Background of the Publication. To contain drug costs, virtually every state has adopted laws and/or regulations that encourage the substitution of drug products. These state laws generally require either that substitution be limited to drugs on a specific list (the positive formulary approach) or that it be permitted for all drugs except those prohibited by a particular list (the negative formulary approach). Because of the number of requests in the late 1970s for FDA assistance in preparing both positive and negative formularies, it became apparent that FDA could not serve the needs of each state on an individual basis. The Agency also recognized that providing a single list based on common criteria would be preferable to evaluating drug products on the basis of differing definitions and criteria in various state laws. As a result, on May 31, 1978, the Commissioner of Food and Drugs sent a letter to officials of each state stating FDA's intent to provide a list of all prescription drug products that are approved by FDA for safety and effectiveness, along with therapeutic equivalence determinations for multisource prescription products.

The List was distributed as a proposal in January 1979. It included only currently marketed prescription drug products approved by FDA through new drug applications (NDAs) or abbreviated new drug applications (ANDAs) under the provisions of Section 505 or 507 of the Act.

The therapeutic equivalence evaluations in the List reflect FDA's application of specific criteria to the approved multisource prescription drug products on the List. These evaluations are presented in the form of code letters that indicate the basis for the evaluation made. An explanation of the code appears in the *Introduction*.

A complete discussion of the background and basis of FDA's therapeutic equivalence evaluation policy was published in the *Federal Register* on January 12, 1979 (44 FR 2932). The final rule, which includes FDA's responses to the public comments on the proposal, was published in the *Federal Register* on October 31, 1980 (45 FR 72582). The first publication, October 1980, of the final version of the List incorporated appropriate corrections and additions. Each subsequent edition has included the new approvals and made appropriate changes in data.

On September 24, 1984, the President signed into law the Drug Price Competition and Patent Term Restoration Act (1984 Amendments). The 1984 Amendments require that FDA, among other things, make publicly available a list of approved drug products with monthly supplements. The *Approved Drug Products with Therapeutic Equivalence Evaluations* publication and its monthly Cumulative Supplements satisfy this requirement. The Addendum to this publication identifies drugs that qualify under the 1984 Amendments for periods of exclusivity (during which ANDAs or applications described in Section 505(b)(2) of the Act for those drugs may not be submitted for a specified period of time and if allowed to be submitted would be tentatively approved with a delayed effective date) and provides patent information concerning the listed drugs. The Addendum also provides additional information that may be helpful to those submitting a new drug application to the Agency.

The Agency intends to use this publication to further its objective of obtaining input and comment on the publication itself and related Agency procedures. Therefore, if you have comments on how the publication can be improved, please send them to the Director, Division of Drug Information Resources, Office of Management, Center for Drug Evaluation and Research, HFD-80, 5600 Fishers Lane, Rockville, MD 20857. Comments received are publicly available to the extent allowable under the Freedom of Information regulations.

1. INTRODUCTION

1.1 Content and Exclusion

The List is composed of four parts: (1) approved prescription drug products with therapeutic equivalence evaluations; (2) approved over-the-counter (OTC) drug products for those drugs that may not be marketed without NDA's because they are not covered under the existing OTC monographs; (3) drug products with approval under Section 505 of the Act administered by the Division of Blood and Blood Products, Center for Biologics Evaluation and Research; and (4) products that have never been marketed, have been discontinued from marketing or that have had their approvals withdrawn for other than safety or efficacy reasons. This publication also includes indices of prescription and OTC drug products by trade or established name (if no trade name exists) and by applicant name (holder of the approved application). All established names for active ingredients conform to official compendial names, or *United States Adopted Names* (USAN) as prescribed in 21 CFR 299.4 (e). The latter list includes applicants' names as abbreviated in this publication; in addition, a list of uniform terms is provided. An Addendum contains drug patent and exclusivity information for the Prescription and OTC Drug Product Lists, and for the Drug Products with Approval under Section 505 of the Act Administered by the Division of Blood and Blood Products List.

Prior to the 6th Edition, the publication had excluded OTC drug products and drug products with approval under Section 505 of the Act administered by the Division of Blood and Blood Products, because the main purpose of the publication was to provide information to states regarding FDA's recommendation as to which generic prescription drug products were acceptable candidates for drug product selection. The 1984 Amendments require the Agency to publish an up-to-date list of all marketed drug products, OTC as well as prescription, that have been approved for safety and efficacy and for which new drug applications are required. In general, OTC drug products may be marketed as old drugs not requiring approved NDAs if they meet existing OTC drug monographs. The products included in the OTC Drug Product List are limited to those for which approved applications are currently required as a condition of marketing. Under the 1984 Amendments, some drug products are given tenative approvals with delayed effective dates. Prior to the effective date, the Agency will not represent the drug products with tenative approval in the List. When the tenative approval becomes a full approval through a subsequent letter to the applicant holder, the Agency will list the drug product and the final, effective approval date in the appropriate approved drug product list.

Distributors of the products on the List are not identified. Because distributors are not required to notify FDA when they shift their sources of supply from one approved manufacturer to another, it is not possible to maintain complete information linking the product approval with the distributor or repackager handling the products.

1.2 Therapeutic Equivalence-Related Terms

Pharmaceutical Equivalents. Drug products are considered pharmaceutical equivalents if they contain the same active ingredient(s), are of the same dosage form and are identical in strength or concentration, and route of administration (e.g., chlordiazepoxide hydrochloride, 5mg oral capsules). Pharmaceutically equivalent drug products are formulated to contain the same amount of active ingredient in the same dosage form and to meet the same or compendial or other applicable standards (i.e., strength, quality, purity, and identity), but they may differ in characteristics such as shape, scoring configuration, packaging, excipients (including colors, flavors, preservatives), expiration time, and, within certain limits, labeling.

Pharmaceutical Alternatives. Drug products are considered pharmaceutical alternatives if they contain the same therapeutic moiety, but are different salts, esters, or complexes of that moiety, or are different dosage forms or strengths (e.g., tetracycline hydrochloride, 250mg capsules vs. tetracycline phosphate complex, 250mg capsules; quinidine sulfate, 200mg tablets vs. quinidine sulfate, 200mg capsules). Data are generally not available for FDA to make the determination of the tablet to capsule bioequivalence. Different dosage forms and strengths within a product line by a single manufacturer are thus pharmaceutical alternatives, as are extended-release products when compared with immediate- or standard-release formulations of the same active ingredient.

Therapeutic Equivalents. Drug products are considered to be therapeutic equivalents only if they are pharmaceutical equivalents and if they can be expected to have the same clinical effect when administered to patients under the conditions specified in the labeling.

FDA classifies as therapeutically equivalent those products that meet the following general criteria: (1) they are approved as safe and effective; (2) they are pharmaceutical equivalents in that they (a) contain identical amounts of the same active drug ingredient in the same dosage form and route of administration, and (b) meet compendial or other applicable standards of strength, quality, purity, and identity; (3) they are bioequivalent in that (a) they do not present a known or potential bioequivalence problem, and they meet an acceptable *in vitro* standard, or (b) if they do present such a known or potential problem, they are shown to meet an appropriate bioequivalence standard; (4) they are adequately labeled; and (5) they are manufactured in compliance with Current Good Manufacturing Practice regulations. *The concept of therapeutic equivalence, as used to develop the*

List, *applies only to drug products containing the same active ingredient(s) and does not encompass a comparison of different therapeutic agents used for the same condition (e.g., propoxyphene hydrochloride vs. pentazocine hydrochloride for the treatment of pain).* A single source drug product in the List repackaged and/or distributed by other than the applicant holder is considered to be therapeutically equivalent to the single source drug product.

FDA considers drug products to be therapeutically equivalent if they meet the criteria outlined above, even though they may differ in certain other characteristics such as shape, scoring configuration, packaging, excipients (including colors, flavors, preservatives), expiration time and minor aspects of labeling (e.g., the presence of specific pharmacokinetic information). When such differences are important in the care of a particular patient, it may be appropriate for the prescribing physician to require that a particular brand be dispensed as a medical necessity. With this limitation, however, FDA believes that products classified as therapeutically equivalent can be substituted with the full expectation that the substituted product will produce the same clinical effect as the prescribed product.

Bioavailability. This term describes the rate and extent to which the active drug ingredient or therapeutic ingredient is absorbed from a drug product and becomes available at the site of drug action.

Bioequivalent Drug Products. This term describes pharmaceutically equivalent products that display comparable bioavailability when studied under similar experimental conditions. Section 505 (j)(7)(B) of the Act describes conditions under which a test and reference (listed) drug must be considered bioequivalent:

the rate and extent of absorption of the test drug do not show a significant difference from the rate and extent of absorption of the reference drug when administered at the same molar dose of the therapeutic ingredient under similar experimental conditions in either a single dose or multiple doses; or

the extent of absorption of the test drug does not show a significant difference from the extent of absorption of the reference drug when administered at the same molar dose of the therapeutic ingredient under similar experimental conditions in either a single dose or multiple doses and the difference from the reference drug in the rate of absorption of the drug is intentional, is reflected in its proposed labeling, is not essential to the attainment of effective body drug concentrations on chronic use, and is considered medically insignificant for the drug. Where these above methods are not applicable (e.g., for topically applied products intended for local rather than systemic effect), other *in vivo* tests of bioequivalence may be appropriate.

Bioequivalence may sometimes be demonstrated using an *in vitro* bioequivalence standard, especially when such an *in vitro* test has been correlated with human *in vivo* bioavailability data or in other situations through comparative clinical trials or pharmacodynamic studies.

1.3 Statistical Criteria for Bioequivalence

Under the Drug Price Competition and Patent Term Restoration Act of 1984, manufacturers seeking approval to market a generic drug must submit data demonstrating that the drug product is bioequivalent to the pioneer (innovator) drug product. A major premise underlying the 1984 law is that bioequivalent products are therapeutically equivalent and, therefore, interchangeable.

The standard bioequivalence study is conducted in a crossover fashion in a small number of volunteers, usually with 12 to 24 healthy normal male adults. Single doses of the test and reference drugs are administered and blood or plasma levels of the drug are measured over time. Characteristics of these concentration-time curves, such as the area under the curve (AUC) and the peak blood or plasma concentration (C_{max}), are examined by statistical procedures.

Bioequivalence of different formulations of the same drug substance involves equivalence with respect to the rate and extent of drug absorption. Two formulations whose rate and extent of absorption differ by 20% or less are generally considered bioequivalent. The use of the 20% rule is based on a medical decision that, for most drugs, a 20% difference in the concentration of the active ingredient in blood will not be clinically significant.

In order to verify, for a particular pharmacokinetic parameter, that the ±20% rule is satisfied, two one-sided statistical tests are carried out using the data from the bioequivalence study. One test is used to verify that the average response for the generic product is no more than 20% *below* that for the innovator product; the other test is used to verify that the average response for the generic product is no more than 20% *above* that for the innovator product. The current practice is to carry out the two one-sided tests at the 0.05 level of significance.

Computationally the two one-sided tests are carried out by computing a 90% confidence interval. For approval of abbreviated new drug applications (ANDAs), in most cases, the generic manufacturer must show that a 90% confidence interval of the difference between the mean response (usually AUC and C_{max}) of its product and that of the innovator is within the limits ±20% of the innovator mean. If the true difference between the products is near 20% of the innovator mean, the confidence limit will likely be outside the acceptable range and the product will fail the bioequivalence test. Thus, an approved generic product is likely to differ from that of the innovator by far less than this quantity.

The current practice of carrying out two one-sided tests at the 0.05 level of significance ensures that if the two products truly differ by as much or more than is allowed by the equivalence criteria (usually ±20% of the innovator product average for the bioequivalence parameter, such as AUC or C_{max}) there is no more than a 5% chance that they will be approved as equivalent. This reflects the fact that the primary concern from the regulatory point of view is the protection of the patient against the acceptance of bioequivalence if it does not hold true. The results of a bioequivalence study must usually be acceptable for more than one pharmacokinetic parameter. As such, a generic product that truly differs by 20% or more from the innovator product with respect to one or more pharmacokinetic parameters, would actually have less than a 5% chance of being approved.

1.4 Reference Listed Drug

A reference listed drug means the listed drug identified by FDA as the drug product upon which an applicant relies in seeking approval of its ANDA.

FDA has identified in the Prescription Drug Product List those reference listed drugs to which the *in vivo* bioequivalence of the applicant's product is compared. By designating a single reference listed drug against which all generic versions must be shown to be bioequivalent, FDA hopes to avoid possible significant variations among generic drugs and their brand name counterpart. Such variations could result if generic drugs were compared to different reference listed drugs. The reference listed drug is identified by the symbol "+" in the Prescription Drug Product List. These identified reference listed drugs represent the best judgment of the Division of Bioequivalence at this time. However, it is recommended that a firm planning on conducting an *in vivo* bioequivalence study contact the Division of Bioequivalence to confirm the appropriate referenced drug to use in the study.

1.5 General Policies and Legal Status

The List contains public information and advice. It does not mandate the drug products which may be purchased, prescribed, dispensed, or substituted for one another nor, does it conversely, mandate the products that should be avoided. To the extent that the List sets forth FDA's evaluations of the therapeutic equivalence of drug products that have been approved, it contains FDA's advice to the public, to practitioners and to the states regarding drug product selection. These evaluations do not constitute determinations that any product is in violation of the Act or that any product is preferable to any other. Therapeutic equivalence evaluations are a scientific judgment based upon evidence, while generic substitution may involve social and economic policy administered by the states, intended to reduce the cost of drugs to consumers. To the extent that the List identifies drug products approved under Section 505 or 507 of the Act, it sets forth information that the Agency is required to publish and that the public is entitled to under the Freedom of Information Act. Exclusion of a drug product from the List

does not necessarily mean that the drug product is either in violation of Section 505 or 507 of the Act, or that such a product is not safe or effective, or that such a product is not therapeutically equivalent to other drug products. Rather, the exclusion is based on the fact that FDA has not evaluated the safety, effectiveness, and quality of the drug product.

1.6 Practitioner's Responsibilities

Professional care and judgment should be exercised in using the List. Evaluations of therapeutic equivalence for prescription drugs are based on scientific and medical evaluations by FDA. Products evaluated as therapeutically equivalent can be expected, in the judgment of the FDA, to have equivalent clinical effect and no difference in their potential for adverse effects when used under the conditions of their labeling. However, these products may differ in other characteristics such as shape, scoring configuration, packaging, excipients (including colors, flavors, preservatives), expiration time, and, in some instances, labeling. If products with such differences are substituted for each other, there is a potential for patient confusion due to differences in color or shape of tablets, inability to provide a given dose using a partial tablet if the proper scoring configuration is not available, or decreased patient acceptance of certain products because of flavor. There may also be better stability of one product over another under adverse storage conditions, or allergic reactions in rare cases due to a coloring or a preservative ingredient, as well as differences in cost to the patient.

FDA evaluation of therapeutic equivalence in no way relieves practitioners of their professional responsibilities in prescribing and dispensing such products with due care and with appropriate information to individual patients. In those circumstances where the characteristics of a specific product, other than its active ingredient, are important in the therapy of a particular patient, the physician's specification of that product is appropriate. Pharmacists must also be familiar with the expiration dates and labeling directions for storage of the different products, particularly for reconstituted products, to assure that patients are properly advised when one product is substituted for another.

Multisource and single-source drug products. FDA has evaluated for therapeutic equivalence only multisource prescription drug products, which in virtually all instances means those pharmaceutical equivalents available from more than one manufacturer. For such products, a therapeutic equivalence code is included and, in addition, product information is highlighted in bold face and underlined. Those products with approved applications that are single-source (i.e., there is only one approved product available for that active ingredient, dosage form and route of administration) are also included on the List, but no therapeutic equivalence code is included with such products. However, a single source drug product repackaged and/or distributed by other than the applicant holder is considered therapeutically equivalent to the single source drug product. The details of these codes and the policies underlying them are discussed in Section 1.7, *Therapeutic Equivalence Evaluations Codes.*

Products on the List are identified by the names of the holders of approved applications (applicants) who may not necessarily be the manufacturer of the product. The applicant may have had its product manufactured by a contract manufacturer and may simply be distributing the product for which it has obtained approval. In most instances, however, the manufacturer of the product is also the applicant. The name of the manufacturer is permitted by regulation to appear on the label, even when the manufacturer is not the marketer.

Although the products on the List are identified by the names of the applicants, circumstances, such as changing corporate ownership, have sometimes made identification of the applicant difficult. The Agency believes, based on continuing document review and communication with firms, that the applicant designations on the List are, in most cases, correct.

To relate firm name information on a product label to that on the List, the following should be noted: the applicant's name always appears on the List. This applies whether the applicant (firm name on the Form FDA 356h in the application) is the marketer (firm name in largest letters on the label) or not. However, the applicant's name may not always appear on the label of the product.

If the applicant is the marketer, its name appears on the List and on the label; if the applicant is not the marketer, and the Agency is aware of a corporate relationship (e.g., parent and subsidiary) between the applicant and the marketer, the name of the applicant appears on the List and both firm names may appear on the label. Firms with known corporate relationships are displayed in Appendix B. If there is no known corporate relationship between the applicant and the marketer, the applicant's name appears on the List; however, unless the applicant is the manufacturer, packager or distributor, the applicant's name may not appear on the label. In this case, the practitioner, from labeling alone, will not be able to relate the marketed product to an applicant cited in the List, and hence to a specific approved drug product. In such cases, other references should be used to assure that the product in question is the subject of an approved application.

To relate trade name (proprietary name) information on a product label to that on the List, the following should be noted: if the applicant is the marketer, its name appears on the List and on the label; if the Agency is aware of a corporate relationship between the applicant and the marketer, the trade name (proprietary name) of the drug product (established drug name if no trade name exists) appears on the List. If a corporate relationship exists between an application holder and a marketer and both firms are distributing the drug product, the FDA reserves the right to select the trade name of either the marketer

or the application holder to appear on the List. If there is no known corporate relationship between the applicant and the marketer, the established drug name appears on the List.

Every product on the List is subject at all times to regulatory action. From time to time, approved products may be found in violation of one or more provisions of the Act. In such circumstances, the Agency will commence appropriate enforcement action to correct the violation, if necessary, by securing removal of the product from the market by voluntary recall, seizure, or other enforcement actions. Such regulatory actions are, however, independent of the inclusion of a product on the List. The main criterion for inclusion of a product is that it has an application with an effective approval that has not been withdrawn for safety or efficacy reasons. FDA believes that retention of a violative product on the List will not have any significant adverse health consequences, because other legal mechanisms are available to the Agency to prevent the product's actual marketing. FDA may, however, change a product's therapeutic equivalence rating if the circumstances giving rise to the violation change or otherwise call into question the data upon which the Agency's assessment of whether a product meets the criteria for therapeutic equivalence was made.

1.7 Therapeutic Equivalence Evaluations Codes

The two-letter coding system for therapeutic equivalence evaluations is constructed to allow users to determine quickly whether the Agency has evaluated a particular approved product as therapeutically equivalent to other pharmaceutically equivalent products (first letter) and to provide additional information on the basis of FDA's evaluations (second letter). With few exceptions, the therapeutic equivalence evaluation date is the same as the approval date.

The two basic categories into which multisource drugs have been placed are indicated by the first letter as follows:

A—Drug products that FDA considers to be <u>therapeutically equivalent</u> to other pharmaceutically equivalent products, i.e., drug products for which:

(1)   there are no known or suspected bioequivalence problems. These are designated **AA, AN, AO, AP,** or **AT,** depending on the dosage form; or

(2)   actual or potential bioequivalence problems have been resolved with adequate *in vivo* and/or *in vitro* evidence supporting bioequivalence. These are designated **AB.**

B—Drug products that FDA at this time considers <u>not to be therapeutically equivalent</u> to other pharmaceutically equivalent products, i.e.,

drug products for which actual or potential bioequivalence problems have not been resolved by adequate evidence of bioequivalence. Often the problem is with specific dosage forms rather than with the active ingredients. These are designated **BC, BD, BE, BN, BP, BR, BS, BT, BX, or B***.

Individual drug products have been evaluated as therapeutically equivalent to the reference product in accordance with the definitions and policies outlined below:

"A" CODES

Drug products that are considered to be therapeutically equivalent to other pharmaceutically equivalent products.

Drug products designated with an "A" code fall under one of two main policies:

(1) for those active ingredients for which no bioequivalence issue is known or suspected, the information necessary to show bioequivalence between pharmaceutically equivalent products is presumed for some dosage forms (e.g., solutions) or satisfied for solid oral dosage forms by a showing that an acceptable *in vitro* standard is met. A therapeutically equivalent rating is assigned such products so long as they are manufactured in accordance with Current Good Manufacturing Practice regulations and meet the other requirements of their approved applications (these are designated **AA, AN, AO, AP, or AT**, depending on the dosage form, as described below); or

(2) for those DESI drug products containing active ingredients that have been identified by FDA as having actual or potential bioequivalence problems [21 CFR 320.22, or January 7, 1977 (42 FR 1648), revised July 14, 1981], and for post-1962 drug products, an evaluation of therapeutic equivalence is assigned to pharmaceutical equivalents only if the approved application contains adequate scientific evidence establishing through *in vivo* studies the bioequivalence of the product to a selected reference product.

There are some general principles that may affect the substitution of pharmaceutically equivalent products in specific cases. Prescribers and dispensers of drugs should be alert to these principles so as to deal appropriately with situations that require professional judgment and discretion.

There may be labeling differences among pharmaceutically equivalent products that require attention on the part of the health professional. For example, pharmaceutically equivalent powders to be reconstituted for administration as oral or injectable liquids may vary with respect to their expiration time or storage conditions after reconstitution. An FDA evaluation that such products are therapeutically equivalent is applicable only when each product is reconstituted, stored, and used under the conditions specified in the labeling of that product.

The Agency will use notes in this publication to point out special situations where potential differences between two drug products that have been evaluated as bioequivalent and otherwise therapeutically equivalent should be brought to the attention of health professionals. These notes are contained in Section 1.8, *Description of Special Situations.*

For example, rarely, there may be variations among therapeutically equivalent products in their use or in conditions of administration. Such differences may be due to patent or exclusivity rights associated with such use. When such variations may, in the Agency's opinion, affect prescribing or substitution decisions by health professionals, a note will be added to Section 1.8.

Also, there may occasionally arise a situation in which changes in a listed drug product after its approval (for example, a change in dosing interval) may have an impact on the substitutability of already approved generic versions of that product that were rated by the Agency as therapeutically equivalent to the listed product. When such changes in the listed drug product are considered by the Agency to have a significant impact on therapeutic equivalence, the Agency will change the therapeutic equivalence ratings for other versions of the drug product unless the manufacturers of those other versions of the product provide additional information to assure equivalence under the changed conditions. Pending receipt of the additional data, the Agency may add a note to Section 1.8, or, in rare cases, may even change the therapeutic equivalence rating.

In some cases (e.g., Isolyte® S w/ Dextrose 5% in Plastic Container and Plasma-Lyte® 148 and Dextrose 5% in Plastic Container), closely related products are listed as containing the same active ingredients, but in somewhat different amounts. In determining which of these products are pharmaceutically equivalent, the Agency has considered products to be pharmaceutically equivalent with labeled strengths of an ingredient that do not vary by more than 1%.

Different salts and esters of the same therapeutic moiety are regarded as pharmaceutical alternatives. For the purpose of this publication, such products are not considered to be therapeutically equivalent. There are no instances in this List where pharmaceutical alternatives are evaluated or coded with regard to therapeutic equivalence. Anhydrous and hydrated entities are considered pharmaceutical equivalents and must meet the same standards and, where necessary, as in the case of ampicillin/

ampicillin trihydrate, their equivalence is supported by appropriate bioavailability/bioequivalence studies.

The codes in this book are not intended to preclude health care professionals from converting pharmaceutically different concentrations into pharmaceutical equivalents using accepted professional practice.

Where package size variations have therapeutic implications, products so packaged have not been considered pharmaceutically equivalent. For example, some oral contraceptives are supplied in 21-tablet and 28-tablet packets; the 28-tablet packets contain 7 placebo or iron tablets. These two packaging configurations are not regarded as pharmaceutically equivalent; thus, they are not designated as therapeutically equivalent.

Preservatives may differ among some therapeutically equivalent drug products. Differences in preservatives and other inactive ingredients do not affect FDA's evaluation of therapeutic equivalence except in cases where these components may influence bioequivalence.

The specific sub-codes for those drugs evaluated as therapeutically equivalent and the policies underlying these sub-codes follow:

AA

Products in conventional dosage forms not presenting bioequivalence problems

Products coded as **AA** contain active ingredients and dosage forms that are not regarded as presenting either actual or potential bioequivalence problems or drug quality or standards issues. However, all solid oral dosage forms must, nonetheless, meet an appropriate *in vitro* test for approval.

AB

Products meeting necessary bioequivalence requirements

Products generally will be coded **AB** if a study is submitted demonstrating bioequivalence, even if the study currently is not required for approval. This category also includes those few drugs for which there is more than one approved application but only one manufacturer. Even though drug products of distributors and/or repackagers are not included in the List, they are considered therapeutically equivalent to the application holder's drug product if the application holder's drug product is rated **AB** or is single source in the List. The only instance in which a multisource product will be rated **AB** on the basis of bioavailability rather than bioequivalence is where the innovator product is the only one listed under that drug ingredient heading and has completed an acceptable bioavailability study. It does not signify that this product is therapeutically equivalent to the other drugs under the same heading. Thus, one product under a drug ingredient heading, coded **AB**, is not therapeutically equivalent to a drug product under the same heading that

is coded with a letter "B" in the first field (i.e., **BD** or **BP**). Drugs coded **AB** under an ingredient heading are considered therapeutically equivalent only to other drugs coded **AB** under that heading.

AN

Solutions and powders for aerosolization

Uncertainty regarding the therapeutic equivalence of aerosolized products arises primarily because of differences in the drug delivery system. Solutions and powders intended for aerosolization that are marketed for use in any of several delivery systems are considered to be pharmaceutically and therapeutically equivalent and are coded **AN**. Those products that are compatible only with a specific delivery system or those products that are packaged in and with a specific delivery system are coded **BN**, because drug products in their respective delivery systems are not necessarily pharmaceutically equivalent to each other and, therefore, are not therapeutically equivalent.

AO

Injectable oil solutions

The absorption of drugs in injectable (parenteral) oil solutions may vary substantially with the type of oil employed as a vehicle and the concentration of the active ingredient. Injectable oil solutions are therefore considered to be pharmaceutically and therapeutically equivalent only when the active ingredient, its concentration, and the type of oil used as a vehicle are all identical.

AP

Injectable aqueous solutions

It should be noted that even though injectable (parenteral) products under a specific listing may be evaluated as therapeutically equivalent, there may be important differences among the products in the general category, *Injectable; Injection*. For example, some injectable products that are rated therapeutically equivalent are labeled for different routes of administration. In addition, some products evaluated as therapeutically equivalent may have different preservatives or no preservatives at all. Injectable products available as dry powders for reconstitution, concentrated sterile solutions for dilution, or sterile solutions ready for injection are all considered to be pharmaceutically and therapeutically equivalent provided they are designed to produce the same concentration prior to injection and are similarly labeled. Consistent with accepted professional practice, it is the responsibility of the prescriber, dispenser, or individual administering the product to be familiar with a product's labeling to assure that it is given only by the route(s) of administration stated in the labeling.

Certain commonly used large volume intravenous products in glass containers are not included on the List (e.g., dextrose injection 5%, dextrose injection 10%, sodium chloride injection 0.9%) since these products are on the market without FDA approval and the FDA has not published conditions for marketing such parental products under approved NDAs. When packaged in plastic containers, however, FDA regulations require approved applications prior to marketing. Approval then depends on, among other things, the extent of the available safety data involving the specific plastic component of the product. All large volume parenteral products are manufactured under similar standards, regardless of whether they are packaged in glass or plastic. Thus, FDA has no reason to believe that the packaging container of large volume parenteral drug products that are pharmaceutically equivalent would have any effect on their therapeutic equivalence.

AT

Topical products

There are a variety of topical dosage forms available for dermatologic, ophthalmic, otic, rectal, and vaginal administration, including solutions, creams, ointments, gels, lotions, pastes, sprays, and suppositories. Even though different topical dosage forms may contain the same active ingredient and potency, these dosage forms are not considered pharmaceutically equivalent. Therefore, they are not-considered therapeutically equivalent. All solutions and DESI drug products containing the same active ingredient in the same topical dosage form for which a waiver of *in vivo* bioequivalence has been granted and for which chemistry and manufacturing processes are adequate are considered therapeutically equivalent and coded **AT**. Pharmaceutically equivalent topical products that raise questions of bioequivalence including all post-1962 topical drug products are coded **AB** when supported by adequate bioequivalence data, and **BT** in the absence of such data.

"B" CODES

Drug products that FDA at this time, considers **not to be therapeutically equivalent** to other pharmaceutically equivalent products.

Drug products designated with a **"B"** code fall under one of three main policies:

(1) the drug products contain active ingredients or are manufactured in dosage forms that have been identified by the Agency as having documented bioequivalence problems or a significant potential for such problems and for which no adequate studies demonstrating bioequivalence have been submitted to FDA; or

(2) the quality standards are inadequate or FDA has an insufficient basis to determine therapeutic equivalence; or

(3) the drug products are under regulatory review.

The specific coding definitions and policies for the "B" sub-codes are as follows:

B*

Drug products requiring further FDA investigation and review to determine therapeutic equivalence

The code B* is assigned to products that were previously assigned an A or B code if FDA receives new information that raises a significant question regarding therapeutic equivalence that can be resolved only through further Agency investigation and/or review of data and information submitted by the applicant. The **B*** code signifies that the Agency will take no position regarding the therapeutic equivalence of the product until the Agency completes its investigation and review.

BC

Extended-release tablets, extended-release capsules, and extended-release injectables

An extended-release dosage form is defined by the official compendia as one that allows at least a two-fold reduction in dosing frequency as compared to that drug presented as a conventional dosage form (e.g., as a solution or a prompt drug-releasing, conventional solid dosage form).

Although bioavailability studies have been conducted on these dosage forms, they are subject to bioavailability differences, primarily because firms developing extended-release products for the same active ingredient rarely employ the same formulation approach. FDA, therefore, does not consider different extended-release dosage forms containing the same active ingredient in equal strength to be therapeutically equivalent unless equivalence between individual products in both rate and extent has been specifically demonstrated through appropriate bioequivalence studies. Extended-release products for which such bioequivalence data have not been submitted are coded **BC**, while those for which such data are available have been coded **AB**.

BD

Active ingredients and dosage forms with documented bioequivalence problems

The **BD** code denotes products containing active ingredients with known bioequivalence problems and for which adequate studies have not been submitted to FDA demonstrating bioequivalence. Where such studies showing bioequivalence have been submitted, the product has been coded **AB**.

BE

Delayed-release oral dosage forms

A delayed-release dosage form is defined by the official compendia as one that releases a drug (or drugs) at a time other than promptly after administration. Enteric-coated articles are delayed-release dosage forms.

Drug products in delayed-release dosage forms containing the same active ingredients are subject to significant differences in absorption. Unless otherwise specifically noted, the Agency considers different delayed-release products containing the same active ingredients as presenting a potential bioequivalence problem and codes these products **BE** in the absence of *in vivo* studies showing bioequivalence. If adequate *in vivo* studies have demonstrated the bioequivalence of specific delayed-release products, such products are coded **AB**.

BN

Products in aerosol-nebulizer drug delivery systems

This code applies to drug solutions or powders that are marketed only as a component of, or as compatible with, a specific drug delivery system. There may, for example, be significant differences in the dose of drug and particle size delivered by different products of this type. Therefore, the Agency does not consider different metered aerosol dosage forms containing the same active ingredient(s) in equal strengths to be therapeutically equivalent unless the drug products meet an appropriate bioequivalence standard.

BP

Active ingredients and dosage forms with potential bioequivalence problems

FDA's bioequivalence regulations (21 CFR 320.52) contain criteria and procedures for determining whether a specific active ingredient in a specific dosage form has a potential for causing a bioequivalence problem. It is FDA's policy to consider an ingredient meeting these criteria as having a potential bioequivalence problem even in the absence

of positive data demonstrating inequivalence. Pharmaceutically equivalent products containing these ingredients in oral dosage forms are coded **BP** until adequate *in vivo* bioequivalence data are submitted.

Injectable suspensions containing an active ingredient suspended in an aqueous or oleaginous vehicle have also been coded **BP**. Injectable suspensions are subject to bioequivalence problems because differences in particle size, polymorphic structure of the suspended active ingredient, or the suspension formulation can significantly affect the rate of release and absorption. FDA does not consider pharmaceutical equivalents of these products bioequivalent without adequate evidence of bioequivalence.

BR

Suppositories or enemas that deliver drugs for systemic absorption

The absorption of active ingredients from suppositories or enemas that are intended to have a systemic effect (as distinct from suppositories administered for local effect) can vary significantly from product to product. Therefore, FDA considers pharmaceutically equivalent systemic suppositories or enemas bioequivalent only if *in vivo* evidence of bioequivalence is available. In those cases where *in vivo* evidence is available, the product is coded **AB**. If such evidence is not available, the products are coded **BR**.

BS

Products having drug standard deficiencies

If the drug standards for an active ingredient in a particular dosage form are found by FDA to be deficient so as to prevent an FDA evaluation of either pharmaceutical or therapeutic equivalence, all drug products containing that active ingredient in that dosage form are coded **BS**. For example, if the standards permit a wide variation in pharmacologically active components of the active ingredient such that pharmaceutical equivalence is in question, all products containing that active ingredient in that dosage form are coded **BS**.

BT

Topical products with bioequivalence issues

This code applies mainly to post-1962 dermatologic, ophthalmic, otic, rectal, and vaginal products for topical administration, including creams, ointments, gels, lotions, pastes, and sprays, as well as suppositories not intended for systemic drug absorption. Topical products evaluated as having acceptable clinical performance, but that are not bioequivalent to other pharmaceutically equivalent products or that lack sufficient evidence of bioequivalence will be coded **BT**.

BX
Insufficient data

The code **BX** is assigned to specific drug products for which the data that have been reviewed by the Agency are insufficient to determine therapeutic equivalence under the policies stated in this document. In these situations, the drug products are presumed to be therapeutically inequivalent until the Agency has determined that there is adequate information to make a full evaluation of therapeutic equivalence.

1.8 Description of Special Situations

Certain drugs present special situations that deserve a more complete explanation than can be provided by the two-letter codes used in the List. These drugs have particular problems with standards of identity, analytical methodology, or bioequivalence that are in the process of resolution. The following drugs are in this category:

Amino Acid and Protein Hydrolysate Injections. These products differ in the amount and kinds of amino acids they contain and, therefore, are not considered pharmaceutical equivalents. For this reason, these products are not considered therapeutically equivalent. At the same time, the Agency believes that it is appropriate to point out that where nitrogen balance is the sole therapeutic objective and individual amino acid content is not a consideration, pharmaceutical alternatives with the same total amount of nitrogen content may be considered therapeutically equivalent.

Erythromycin Stearate Tablets. All manufacturers of erythromycin stearate tablet products demonstrated product bioequivalency as a condition of application approval. These bioequivalence studies were performed under fasting conditions and, as a result, all firms were required to label their products to be taken on an empty stomach. Since that time, some firms have demonstrated that their products may be taken immediately before meals, but not with meals, and still achieve acceptable blood levels. On the basis of such studies, FDA has approved those products to be labeled accordingly. At the same time, the Agency stresses that optimal absorption for any erythromycin stearate tablet is achieved when the drug is administered under fasting conditions and recommends that prescriptions include instructions regarding administration in relation to meals. When erythromycin stearate tablets are to be administered under fasting conditions, the Agency believes that any listed product coded **AB** may be considered therapeutically equivalent. If erythromycin stearate is to be taken immediately before meals, only those products with labeling that provides for such administration should be dispensed. Erythromycin stearate tablet products have been designated therapeutically equivalent (**AB**) in the List, because all of the products produce equivalent blood levels provided the drug is prescribed and administered in accordance with the conditions of use in the labeling. This matter is being reviewed by the Agency. Prescribers and dispensers are advised to be familiar with the labeling of these products.

Gaviscon®. Gaviscon® is an OTC product which has been marketed since September 1970. The active ingredients in this product, aluminum hydroxide and magnesium trisilicate, were reviewed by the Agency's OTC Antacid Panel and were considered to be safe and effective ingredients (Category I) by that Panel. However, the tablet failed to pass the antacid test which is required of all antacid products. The Agency, therefore, placed the tablet in Category III for lack of effectiveness. A full NDA with clinical studies was submitted by Marion Laboratories, Inc., and approved by FDA on December 9, 1983. Gaviscon®'s activity in treating reflux acidity is made possible by the physical-chemical properties of the inactive ingredients, sodium bicarbonate and alginic acid. Therefore, *all ANDAs which cite Gaviscon® tablets as the listed drug must contain the inactive ingredients, sodium bicarbonate and alginic acid.* A full NDA will be required to support the effectiveness of the drug product if different inactive ingredients are to be substituted for sodium bicarbonate or alginic acid or if different proportions of these ingredients are to be used.

Theophylline. Studies have suggested that food may significantly alter the absorption of theophylline from some extended-release theophylline drug products. Current research is defining more precisely the relationship between the timing of meals (including type and amount of food) and the rate and extent of absorption of theophylline from the extended-release dosage form. Specific product labeling should be consulted to determine the information available on this subject.

Trazodone Hydrochloride. Generic Trazodone HCl 150mg tablet entries, marked with a "†", are rated as therapeutically equivalent (**AB**) to Mead Johnson's Desyrel® (Trazodone HCl) Dividose 150 mg tablets. The therapeutic equivalence determination was made on the basis, among other things, of an acceptable bioequivalence study and acceptable *in vitro* dissolution testing. A patent that exists on the Desyrel® 150mg tablet scoring design, which enables the patient to break Desyrel® into three 50mg segments, currently prevents a generic firm from copying this feature. Therefore, a patient will not be able to obtain three 50mg segments from the generic tablet. Prescribers and dispensers should be aware of this difference and take it into account when writing a prescription or practicing drug product selection.

1.9 Therapeutic Equivalence Code Change for a Drug Entity

The Agency will use the following procedures when, in response to a petition or on its own initiative, it is considering a change in the therapeutic equivalence code for approved multisource drug products. Such changes will generally occur when the Agency becomes aware of new scientific information affecting the therapeutic equivalence of an entire category of drug products in the List (e.g., information concerning the active ingredient or the dosage form), rather than information concerning a single drug product within the category. These procedures will be used when a change in therapeutic equivalence code is under consideration for all drug products found in the Prescription Drug Product List under a specific drug entity and dosage form. The change may be from the code signifying that the drug does not present a bioequivalence problem (e.g., **AA**) to a code signifying a bioequivalence problem (e.g., **BP**), or vice versa. This procedure does not apply to a change of a particular product code (e.g., a change from **BP** to **AB** or from **AB** to **BX**).

Before making a change in a code for an entire category of drugs, the Agency will announce in the *Introduction* to the Cumulative Supplement that it is considering the change, and will invite comment. Comments, along with scientific data, may be sent to the Director, Division of Bioequivalence, Office of Generic Drugs, Center for Drug Evaluation and Research, (MPN-2) HFD-650, 7500 Standish Place, Rockville, MD 20857. The comment period will generally be 60 days in length, and the closing date for comments will be listed in the description of the proposed change for each drug entity.

The most useful type of scientific data submission is an *in vivo* bioavailability/bioequivalence study conducted on batches of the subject drug products. These submissions should present a full description of the analytical procedures and equipment used, a validation of the analytical methodology, including the standard curve, a description of the method of calculating results, and a description of the pharmacokinetic and statistical models used in analyzing the data. Anecdotal or testimonial information is the least useful to the Agency, and such submissions are discouraged. Copies of supporting reports published in the scientific literature or unpublished material, however, are welcome.

1.10 Change of the Therapeutic Equivalence Evaluation for a Single Product

The aforementioned procedure does not apply to a change in a single drug single product code. For example, a change in a single drug product's code from **BP** to **AB** as a result of the submission of a bioequivalence study will not ordinarily be the subject of notice and comment. Likewise, a change in a single drug product's code from **AB** to **BX** (e.g., as a result of new information raising a significant question as to bioequivalence) does not require notice and comment. The Agency's responsibility to provide the public with the Agency's most current information related to therapeutic equivalence may require a change in a drug product's code prior to any formal notice and opportunity for the applicant to be heard. The publication in the *Federal Register* of a Proposal to withdraw approval of a drug product will ordinarily result in a change in a product's code from **AB** to **BX** if this action has not already been taken.

1.11 Availability of Internal Policy and Procedure Guides

The Office of Generic Drugs maintains internal policy and procedure guides. Although these guides are designed for Office personnel and are subject to change without public notice, they are available to members of the public who may wish to know more about the Office's policies and procedures. Copies of these guides may be obtained from the Executive Secretariat Staff, (MNP-1) HFD-8, FDA, Center for Drug Evaluation and Research, 5600 Fishers Lane, Rockville, MD 20857. The Agency welcomes public comment on the policies, procedures, and practices employed in the approval of generic drugs. Such comments may be sent to the Director, Office of Generic Drugs, (MPN-2) HFD-600, 5600 Fishers Lane, Rockville, MD 20857.

1.12 Availability of the Publication and Other FDA Reports and Updating Procedures

REPORTS AVAILABLE FROM
SUPERINTENDENT OF DOCUMENTS
U.S. GOVERNMENT PRINTING OFFICE
WASHINGTON, DC 20402
(202) 783-3238

- *Approved Drug Products with Therapeutic Equivalence Evaluations, 12th Edition (1992).* This publication and its monthly Cumulative Supplements are provided in the subscription price. The Cumulative Supplements provide new drug approval information and, if necessary, revised therapeutic equivalence evaluations and updated patent and exclusivity information. The publication must be used, therefore, in conjunction with the most current Cumulative Supplement.

An updated magnetic tape containing ONLY the Prescription Drug Product List is available quarterly by subscription. Order from the National Technical Information Service. (See p. xix)

- *Recalls - FDA Enforcement Report.* The FDA Enforcement Report is published weekly and contains information on actions taken in connection with Agency regulatory activities, including recalls and medical device safety alerts voluntarily conducted by firms.

REPORTS AVAILABLE FROM
FREEDOM OF INFORMATION STAFF
5600 FISHERS LANE, HFI-35
ROCKVILLE, MD 20857
(301) 443-6310

- *DESI Drug Products and Known-Related Drug Products that Lack Substantial Evidence of Effectiveness and are Subject to a Notice of Opportunity for Hearing and Those that Already have had Approval Withdrawn.*

- *Inactive Ingredient Guide, 1991.* This guide contains all inactive ingredients present in approved drug products or conditionally approved drug products currently marketed for human use.

- *Phase IV Postapproval Research List.* This report provides monitoring data on the status of postapproval research requested of applicant holders of approved new drug applications.

REPORTS AVAILABLE FROM
FREEDOM OF INFORMATION STAFF
5600 FISHERS LANE, HFI-35
ROCKVILLE, MD 20857
(301) 443-6310

- *Drug Products that may be Subject to the FDA's Prescription Drug Wrap-Up.*

- *Quality Assurance by Manufacturer.* Under Section 510(h) of the Federal Food, Drug, and Cosmetic Act, every drug establishment registered with the FDA must be inspected at least once every two years to determine if the drugs they market are produced in conformance with current GMPs. Copies of the inspection reports generated by the FDA District conducting the inspection or any other inspections conducted are available from the local Districts pursuant to the Freedom of Information regulations.

REPORTS AVAILABLE FROM
NATIONAL TECHNICAL
INFORMATION SERVICE
5285 PORT ROYAL ROAD
SPRINGFIELD, VA 22161
(703) 487-4630 (Subscription Department)
(703) 487-4650 (Order Department)

- *Drug/Biologic Quality Reporting System, Annual DQRS Report.*

REPORTS AVAILABLE FROM
NATIONAL TECHNICAL
INFORMATION SERVICE
5285 PORT ROYAL ROAD
SPRINGFIELD, VA 22161
(703) 487-4630 (Subscription Department)
(703) 487-4650 (Order Department)

- *FDA Drug and Device Product Approvals List.* Official Agency listing of monthly approval data from the Center for Drug Evaluation and Research, Center for Biologics and Research Evaluation, Center for Veterinary Medicine and Center for Devices and Radiological Health.

REPORTS AVAILABLE FROM
EXECUTIVE SECRETARIAT STAFF
CENTER FOR DRUG EVALUATION AND
RESEARCH, FDA
5600 FISHERS LANE (HFD-8)
ROCKVILLE, MD 20857
(301) 295-8012

- *Biopharmaceutic Guidelines.* Individual biopharmaceutic guidelines are available at no charge.

- *Clinical Evaluation Guidelines.* Individual clinical guidelines are available at no charge.

Information about other CDER/FDA publications can be obtained from the CDER Executive Secretariat Staff.

2. HOW TO USE THE DRUG PRODUCT LISTS

2.1 Key Sections for Using the Drug Product Lists

This publication contains the illustrations, along with the Drug Product Lists, indices, and lists of abbreviations and terms which facilitate their use.

Illustrations. The annotated Drug Product Illustration and the Therapeutic Equivalence Evaluations Illustration are offered to provide further clarification. These depict the format found in the Prescription Drug Product List (the only List in which therapeutic equivalence evaluation codes are displayed).

Drug Product Lists. The Drug Product Lists, arranged alphabetically by active ingredient, contain product identification information (active ingredients, dosage forms, routes of administration, product names, application, holders, strengths) for single and multiple ingredient drug products. Also shown is the application number and drug product number (FDA's file numbers) and approval dates for those drug products approved on or after January 1, 1982.

If a prescription drug product is available from more than one source (multisource), a therapeutic equivalence code will appear in front of the applicant's name. If a product is therapeutically equivalent to one or more products or to an appropriate reference, it will be designated with a code beginning with "A" and the entry will be underlined and printed in bold font for emphasis.

Active ingredients in multiple ingredient (combination) drug products are arranged alphabetically. For example, product information for the product labeled as containing methyldopa and chlorothiazide appears under the heading *Chlorothiazide; Methyldopa.* A cross-reference to the product information (for prescription and OTC products) appears for each additional active ingredient in the product. For combination drug products, the ingredient strengths are separated by semicolons and appear in the same relative sequence as the ingredients in the heading. Available strengths of the dosage form from an applicant appear on separate lines.

To use the Drug Product Lists, determine by alphabetical order the ingredient under which the product information is listed, using the Product Name Index, if appropriate. Then, find the ingredient in the applicable

Drug Product List. Proceed to the dosage form and route of administration and compare products within that ingredient heading only. Therapeutic equivalence or inequivalence for prescription products is determined on the basis of the therapeutic equivalence codes provided within that specific dosage form heading. The OTC Drug Product List, Discontinued Drug Product List, and Drug Products with Approval under Section 505 of the Act Administered by the Division of Blood and Blood Products List have their data arranged similarly. The Discontinued Drug Product List contains products that have never been marketed, products discontinued from marketing or products that have had their approval withdrawn for other than safety or effectiveness reasons. All products having a "∂" in the 12th Cumulative Supplement of the 12th Edition List will then be added to the Discontinued Drug Product List appearing in the 13th Edition.

Product Name Index (Prescription and OTC Drug Product Lists). This is an index of drug products by established or trade name. The second term of each entry indicates the active ingredient name under which product information can be found in the appropriate Drug Product List. For those drug products with multiple active ingredients, only the first active ingredient (in alphabetical order) will appear. OTC products are so designated.

Product Name Index Listed by Applicant (Prescription and OTC Drug Product Lists). This is an index that cross-references applicants to drug products. The bolded and underlined entry represents the applicant name abbreviation used in this publication. Each complete applicant name that is represented by the abbreviated name is marked with an asterisk (*). Listed under each complete applicant name is the first alphabetically arranged ingredient under which product information can be found in the appropriate Drug Product List. OTC products are so designated.

Uniform Terms. To improve readability, uniform terms are used to designate dosage forms, routes of administration, and abbreviations used to express strengths. These terms are listed in Appendix C. In some cases, the terms used may differ from those used in product labels and other labeling.

2.2 DRUG PRODUCT ILLUSTRATION

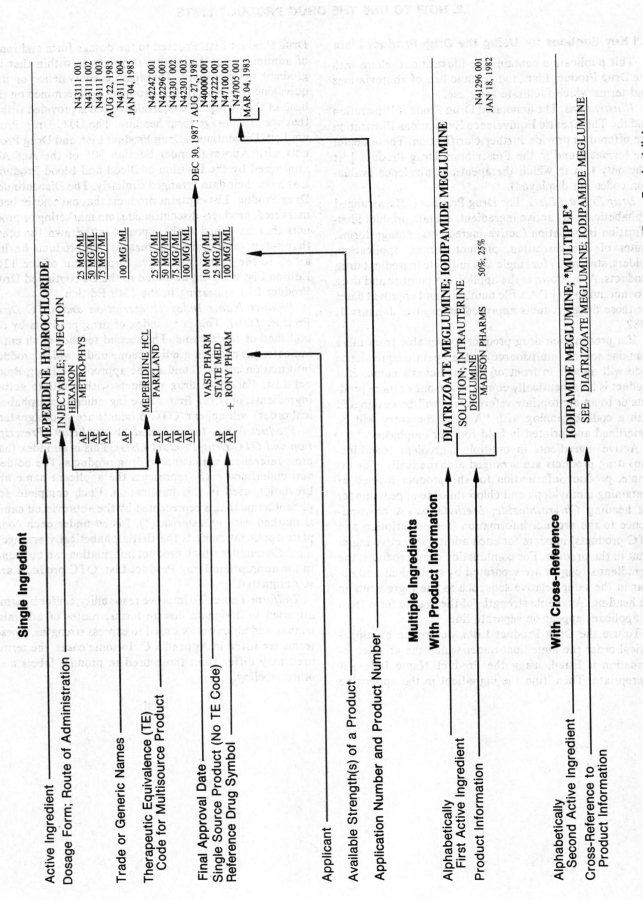

Single Ingredient

MEPERIDINE HYDROCHLORIDE
  INJECTABLE; INJECTION
    HEXANON
      METRO-PHYS

AP	25 MG/ML	N43111 001
AP	50 MG/ML	N43111 002
AP	75 MG/ML	N43111 003
		AUG 22, 1983
AP	100 MG/ML	N43111 004
		JAN 04, 1985

    MEPERIDINE HCL
      PARKLAND

AP	25 MG/ML	N42242 001
AP	50 MG/ML	N42296 001
AP	75 MG/ML	N42301 002
AP	100 MG/ML	N42301 003
		DEC 30, 1987: AUG 27, 1987

      VASD PHARM
      STATE MED
    + RONY PHARM

AP	10 MG/ML	N40000 001
AP	25 MG/ML	N47222 001
	100 MG/ML	N47100 001
		N47005 001
		MAR 04, 1983

Active Ingredient
Dosage Form; Route of Administration

Trade or Generic Names

Therapeutic Equivalence (TE)
Code for Multisource Product

Final Approval Date
Single Source Product (No TE Code)
Reference Drug Symbol

Applicant

Available Strength(s) of a Product

Application Number and Product Number

Multiple Ingredients
With Product Information

DIATRIZOATE MEGLUMINE; IODIPAMIDE MEGLUMINE
  SOLUTION; INTRAUTERINE
    DIGLUMINE
      MADISON PHARMS   50%; 25%   N41296 001
                                    JAN 18, 1982

Alphabetically
First Active Ingredient
Product Information

With Cross-Reference

IODIPAMIDE MEGLUMINE; *MULTIPLE*
  SEE DIATRIZOATE MEGLUMINE; IODIPAMIDE MEGLUMINE

Alphabetically
Second Active Ingredient
Cross-Reference to
Product Information

This example is for purposes of illustration only. It does not represent actual products from the Prescription Drug Product list.

2.3 THERAPEUTIC EQUIVALENCE EVALUATIONS ILLUSTRATION

Drug products coded **AB** (or any code beginning with an "**A**") under an ingredient and dosage form heading are considered therapeutically equivalent only to other products coded **AB** (or any code beginning with an "**A**") and **NOT** to those coded **BP** (or any code beginning with a "**B**") and any products not listed. Drug products coded **BP** (or any code beginning with a "**B**") are **NOT** considered therapeutically equivalent to any other product. For a complete explanation of the TE codes refer to Section 1.5 of the *Introduction.*

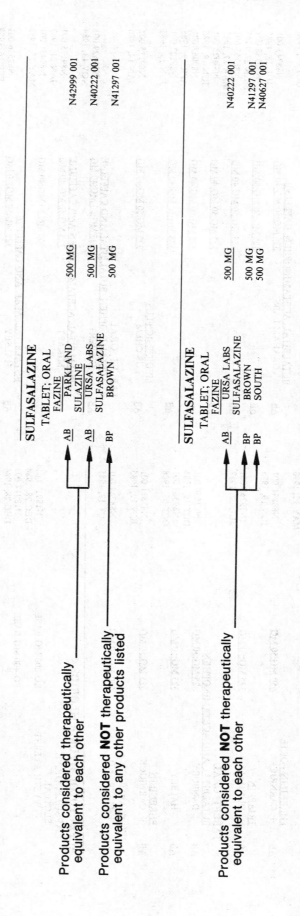

SULFASALAZINE
TABLET; ORAL
  FAZINE
    PARKLAND   500 MG   N42999 001
  SULAZINE
    URSA LABS   500 MG   N40222 001
  SULFASALAZINE
    BROWN   500 MG   N41297 001

AB, AB — Products considered therapeutically equivalent to each other

BP — Products considered **NOT** therapeutically equivalent to any other products listed

SULFASALAZINE
TABLET; ORAL
  FAZINE
    URSA LABS   500 MG   N40222 001
  SULFASALAZINE
    BROWN   500 MG   N41297 001
    SOUTH   500 MG   N40627 001

AB, BP, BP — Products considered **NOT** therapeutically equivalent to each other

NOTE: Underlining denotes multisource products which are considered therapeutically equivalent.

This example is for purposes of illustration only. It does not represent actual products from the Prescription Drug Product list.

PRESCRIPTION DRUG PRODUCTS

ACETAMINOPHEN; BUTALBITAL

CAPSULE; ORAL

BANCAP
AB	+ FOREST PHARMS	325 MG;50 MG	N88889 001	JAN 16, 1986

BUTALBITAL AND ACETAMINOPHEN
AB	GRAHAM LABS	650 MG;50 MG	N88991 001	JUN 28, 1985

CONTEN
AB	GRAHAM LABS	650 MG;50 MG	N89405 001	MAY 15, 1990

PHRENILIN FORTE
AB	+ CARNRICK	650 MG;50 MG	N88831 001	JUN 19, 1985

TRIAPRIN
AB	DUNHALL	325 MG;50 MG	N89268 001	JUL 02, 1987

TABLET; ORAL

BUTALBITAL AND ACETAMINOPHEN
AB	DANBURY	325 MG;50 MG	N87550 001	OCT 19, 1984
AB	HALSEY	325 MG;50 MG	N89568 001	OCT 05, 1988

PHRENILIN
AB	+ CARNRICK	325 MG;50 MG	N87811 001	JUN 19, 1985

SEDAPAP
	+ MAYRAND	650 MG;50 MG	N88944 001	OCT 17, 1985

ACEBUTOLOL HYDROCHLORIDE

CAPSULE; ORAL

SECTRAL
WYETH AYERST	EQ 200 MG BASE	N18917 001	DEC 28, 1984
	EQ 400 MG BASE	N18917 003	DEC 28, 1984
+			

ACETAMINOPHEN; ASPIRIN; CODEINE PHOSPHATE

CAPSULE; ORAL

ACETAMINOPHEN, ASPIRIN, AND CODEINE PHOSPHATE
MIKART	150 MG;180 MG;15 MG	N81095 001	OCT 26, 1990
	150 MG;180 MG;30 MG	N81096 001	OCT 26, 1990
	150 MG;180 MG;60 MG	N81097 001	OCT 26, 1990

ACETAMINOPHEN; BUTALBITAL; CAFFEINE

CAPSULE; ORAL

ACETAMINOPHEN, BUTALBITAL AND CAFFEINE
AB	+ GILBERT	325 MG;50 MG;40 MG	N88825 001	DEC 05, 1984

ACETAMINOPHEN, BUTALBITAL AND CAFFEINE
AB	MIKART	325 MG;50 MG;40 MG	N89007 001	MAR 17, 1986

ANOQUAN
AB	MALLARD	325 MG;50 MG;40 MG	N87628 001	OCT 01, 1986

BUTALBITAL, ACETAMINOPHEN, CAFFEINE
AB	GRAHAM LABS	325 MG;50 MG;40 MG	N88743 001	JUL 18, 1985
AB		325 MG;50 MG;40 MG	N88758 001	MAR 27, 1985
AB		325 MG;50 MG;40 MG	N88765 001	MAR 27, 1985
AB		325 MG;50 MG;40 MG	N89023 001	JUN 19, 1985
AB		325 MG;50 MG;40 MG	N89067 001	APR 19, 1985
AB		325 MG;50 MG;40 MG	N89102 001	JUN 19, 1985

MEDIGESIC PLUS
AB	US CHEM	325 MG;50 MG;40 MG	N89115 001	JAN 14, 1986

TABLET; ORAL

ACETAMINOPHEN, BUTALBITAL AND CAFFEINE
AB	GILBERT	325 MG;50 MG;40 MG	N87629 001	NOV 13, 1984

BUTALBITAL, ACETAMINOPHEN AND CAFFEINE
AB	MIKART	325 MG;50 MG;40 MG	N89175 001	JAN 21, 1987
AB		500 MG;50 MG;40 MG	N89451 001	MAY 23, 1988

BUTALBITAL, APAP, AND CAFFEINE
AB	HALSEY	325 MG;50 MG;40 MG	N89536 001	FEB 16, 1988

ESGIC
AB	FOREST PHARMS	325 MG;50 MG;40 MG	N89660 001	DEC 23, 1988

FIORICET
AB	+ SANDOZ	325 MG;50 MG;40 MG	N88616 001	NOV 09, 1984

REPAN
AB	GRAHAM LABS	325 MG;50 MG;40 MG	N87804 001	JAN 24, 1985

Prescription Drug Products *(continued)*

ACETAMINOPHEN; BUTALBITAL; CAFFEINE; CODEINE PHOSPHATE

CAPSULE; ORAL

TE	Product / Firm	Strength	Appl. No. / Date
	FIORICET W/ CODEINE + SANDOZ	325 MG;50 MG;40 MG;30 MG	N20232 001 JUL 30, 1992

ACETAMINOPHEN; CAFFEINE; DIHYDROCODEINE BITARTRATE

CAPSULE; ORAL

TE	Product / Firm	Strength	Appl. No. / Date
	COMPAL		
AA	SOLVAY	356.4 MG;30 MG;16 MG	N88584 001 MAR 04, 1986
	SYNALGOS-DC-A		
AA	WYETH AYERST	356.4 MG;30 MG;16 MG	N89166 001 MAY 14, 1986

ACETAMINOPHEN; CODEINE PHOSPHATE

CAPSULE; ORAL

TE	Product / Firm	Strength	Appl. No. / Date
	ACETAMINOPHEN W/ CODEINE #3		
	LEMMON	300 MG;30 MG	N88324 001 DEC 29, 1983
	PHENAPHEN W/ CODEINE NO. 2		
	ROBINS	325 MG;15 MG	N84444 001
	PHENAPHEN W/ CODEINE NO. 3		
	ROBINS	325 MG;30 MG	N84445 001
	PHENAPHEN W/ CODEINE NO. 4		
	ROBINS	325 MG;60 MG	N84446 001

ELIXIR; ORAL

TE	Product / Firm	Strength	Appl. No. / Date
	ACETAMINOPHEN AND CODEINE PHOSPHATE		
AA	PHARM ASSOC	120 MG/5 ML;12 MG/5 ML	N87508 001
AA	PHARM BASICS	120 MG/5 ML;12 MG/5 ML	N87006 001
	ACETAMINOPHEN W/ CODEINE		
AA	ROXANE	120 MG/5 ML;12 MG/5 ML	N86366 001
	APAP W/ CODEINE		
AA	BARRE	120 MG/5 ML;12 MG/5 ML	N85861 001
	TYLENOL W/ CODEINE		
AA	JOHNSON RW	120 MG/5 ML;12 MG/5 ML	N85057 001

SUSPENSION; ORAL

TE	Product / Firm	Strength	Appl. No. / Date
	ACETAMINOPHEN W/ CODEINE PHOSPHATE		
AA	BARRE	120 MG/5 ML;12 MG/5 ML	N85883 001
	CAPITAL AND CODEINE		
AA	CARNRICK	120 MG/5 ML;12 MG/5 ML	N86024 001

TABLET; ORAL

TE	Product / Firm	Strength	Appl. No. / Date
	ACETAMINOPHEN AND CODEINE PHOSPHATE		
AA	BARR	300 MG;15 MG	N85795 001
AA		300 MG;30 MG	N85794 001
AA	CHARLOTTE	300 MG;15 MG	N89990 001 SEP 30, 1988
		300 MG;30 MG	N89805 001 SEP 30, 1988
		300 MG;60 MG	N89828 001 SEP 30, 1988

ACETAMINOPHEN; CODEINE PHOSPHATE *(continued)*

TABLET; ORAL

TE	Product / Firm	Strength	Appl. No. / Date
	ACETAMINOPHEN AND CODEINE PHOSPHATE		
	GENEVA	300 MG;30 MG	N81250 001 JUL 16, 1992
AA		300 MG;30 MG	N85291 002
AA		300 MG;60 MG	N81249 001 JUL 16, 1992
AA	HALSEY	300 MG;60 MG	N85964 001
AA		300 MG;60 MG	N86549 001
AA	KV	300 MG;30 MG	N85288 001
AA		300 MG;60 MG	N85365 001
AA	MIKART	325 MG;15 MG	N85364 001
AA		325 MG;45 MG	N85363 001
AA		650 MG;30 MG	N89231 001 MAR 03, 1986
AA	MUTUAL PHARM	650 MG;60 MG	N89363 001 SEP 25, 1991
AA		300 MG;15 MG	N89671 001 FEB 10, 1988
		300 MG;30 MG	N89672 001 FEB 10, 1988
		300 MG;60 MG	N89673 001 FEB 10, 1988
AA	PHARMAFAIR	300 MG;30 MG	N87762 001 DEC 10, 1982
AA	PUREPAC	300 MG;30 MG	N86681 001
		300 MG;60 MG	N86683 001
AA	ROXANE	500 MG;15 MG	N89511 001
		500 MG;30 MG	N89512 001 APR 25, 1989
		500 MG;60 MG	N89513 001 APR 25, 1989
AA	ZENITH	300 MG;60 MG	N87083 001 APR 25, 1989
	ACETAMINOPHEN AND CODEINE PHOSPHATE #2		
AA	SUPERPHARM	300 MG;15 MG	N89183 001 OCT 18, 1985
	ACETAMINOPHEN AND CODEINE PHOSPHATE #3		
AA	MIKART	300 MG;30 MG	N89238 001 FEB 25, 1986
AA	PUREPAC	300 MG;30 MG	N89080 001 JUL 17, 1986
AA	SUPERPHARM	300 MG;30 MG	N89184 001 OCT 18, 1985
	ACETAMINOPHEN AND CODEINE PHOSPHATE #4		
AA	MIKART	300 MG;60 MG	N89244 001 FEB 25, 1986
AA	SUPERPHARM	300 MG;60 MG	N89185 001 OCT 18, 1985
	ACETAMINOPHEN AND CODEINE PHOSPHATE NO. 4		
AA	ROXANE	300 MG;60 MG	N84667 001
	ACETAMINOPHEN W/ CODEINE		
AA	BARR	300 MG;60 MG	N87653 001 APR 13, 1982
	ACETAMINOPHEN W/ CODEINE #2		
AA	LEMMON	300 MG;15 MG	N88627 001 MAR 06, 1985

Prescription Drug Products (continued)

ACETAMINOPHEN; CODEINE PHOSPHATE (continued)

TABLET; ORAL

TE	Brand / Applicant	Strength	Appl. No.	Approval Date
ACETAMINOPHEN W/ CODEINE #3				
AA	LEMMON	300 MG;30 MG	N88628 001	MAR 06, 1985
ACETAMINOPHEN W/ CODEINE #4				
AA	LEMMON	300 MG;60 MG	N88629 001	MAR 06, 1985
ACETAMINOPHEN W/ CODEINE NO. 2				
AA	ROXANE	300 MG;15 MG	N84659 001	
ACETAMINOPHEN W/ CODEINE NO. 3				
AA	ROXANE	300 MG;30 MG	N84656 001	
ACETAMINOPHEN W/ CODEINE PHOSPHATE				
AA	HALSEY	300 MG;15 MG	N83871 001	
AA	HALSEY	300 MG;30 MG	N83872 001	
ACETAMINOPHEN W/ CODEINE PHOSPHATE #3				
AA	ZENITH	300 MG;30 MG	N85868 001	
CAPITAL WITH CODEINE				
AA	CARNRICK	325 MG;30 MG	N83643 001	
PHENAPHEN-650 W/ CODEINE				
AA	ROBINS	650 MG;30 MG	N85856 001	
TYLENOL W/ CODEINE NO. 1				
AA	+ JOHNSON RW	300 MG;7.5 MG	N85055 001	
TYLENOL W/ CODEINE NO. 2				
AA	JOHNSON RW	300 MG;15 MG	N85055 002	
TYLENOL W/ CODEINE NO. 3				
AA	JOHNSON RW	300 MG;30 MG	N85055 003	
TYLENOL W/ CODEINE NO. 4				
AA	JOHNSON RW	300 MG;60 MG	N85055 004	

ACETAMINOPHEN; HYDROCODONE BITARTRATE

CAPSULE; ORAL

TE	Brand / Applicant	Strength	Appl. No.	Approval Date
ACETAMINOPHEN AND HYDROCODONE BITARTRATE				
AA	CENTRAL PHARMS	500 MG;5 MG	N88898 001	MAR 27, 1985
AA	GRAHAM LABS	500 MG;5 MG	N87336 001	JUL 08, 1982
AA	GRAHAM LABS	500 MG;5 MG	N88956 001	JUL 19, 1985
ALLAY				
AA	LUCHEM	500 MG;5 MG	N89907 001	JAN 13, 1989
BANCAP HC				
AA	FOREST PHARMS	500 MG;5 MG	N87961 001	MAR 17, 1983
CO-GESIC				
AA	CENTRAL PHARMS	500 MG;5 MG	N89360 001	MAR 02, 1988
HYDROCET				
AA	GRAHAM LABS	500 MG;5 MG	N89006 001	AUG 09, 1985

ACETAMINOPHEN; HYDROCODONE BITARTRATE (continued)

CAPSULE; ORAL

TE	Brand / Applicant	Strength	Appl. No.	Approval Date
HYDROCODONE BITARTRATE AND ACETAMINOPHEN				
AA	MIKART	500 MG;5 MG	N81067 001	NOV 30, 1989
AA	MIKART	500 MG;5 MG	N81068 001	NOV 30, 1989
AA		500 MG;5 MG	N81069 001	NOV 30, 1989
AA		500 MG;5 MG	N81070 001	NOV 30, 1989
AA		500 MG;5 MG	N89008 001	NOV 30, 1989
AA		500 MG;5 MG		FEB 21, 1986

ELIXIR; ORAL

TE	Brand / Applicant	Strength	Appl. No.	Approval Date
HYDROCODONE BITARTRATE AND ACETAMINOPHEN				
AA	MIKART	500 MG/15 ML,5 MG/15 ML	N89557 001	APR 29, 1992
AA		500 MG/15 ML,7.5 MG/15 ML	N81051 001	AUG 28, 1992

TABLET; ORAL

TE	Brand / Applicant	Strength	Appl. No.	Approval Date
ACETAMINOPHEN AND HYDROCODONE BITARTRATE				
AA	GRAHAM LABS	500 MG;5 MG	N87722 001	JUL 09, 1982
ANEXSIA				
AA	BEECHAM	500 MG;5 MG	N89160 001	APR 23, 1987
ANEXSIA 7.5/650				
AA	BEECHAM	650 MG;7.5 MG	N89725 001	SEP 30, 1987
CO-GESIC				
AA	CENTRAL PHARMS	500 MG;5 MG	N87757 001	MAY 03, 1982
DURADYNE DHC				
AA	FOREST PHARMS	500 MG;5 MG	N87809 001	MAR 17, 1983
HY-PHEN				
AA	ASCHER	500 MG;5 MG	N87677 001	MAY 03, 1982
HYCOPAP				
AA	CHARLOTTE	500 MG;5 MG	N89971 001	DEC 02, 1988
HYDROCODONE BITARTRATE AND ACETAMINOPHEN				
AA	CHARLOTTE	500 MG;5 MG	N89831 001	SEP 07, 1988
AA	HALSEY	500 MG;5 MG	N89554 001	JUN 12, 1987
AA	LUCHEM	500 MG;5 MG	N89696 001	APR 21, 1988

Prescription Drug Products *(continued)*

ACETAMINOPHEN; HYDROCODONE BITARTRATE *(continued)*

TABLET; ORAL

HYDROCODONE BITARTRATE AND ACETAMINOPHEN

	Firm	Strength	Appl. No.	Date
AA	MIKART	500 MG;2.5 MG	N89698 001	AUG 25, 1989
AA		500 MG;5 MG	N89271 001	JUL 16, 1986
AA		500 MG;5 MG	N89697 001	JAN 28, 1992
AA		500 MG;7.5 MG	N89699 001	AUG 25, 1989
AA		650 MG;7.5 MG	N89689 001	JUN 29, 1988
AA		650 MG;10 MG	N81223 001	MAY 29, 1992
AA	WATSON	500 MG;2.5 MG	N81079 001	AUG 30, 1991
AA		500 MG;5 MG	N89883 001	DEC 01, 1988
AA		500 MG;7.5 MG	N81080 001	AUG 30, 1991
AA		750 MG;7.5 MG	N81083 001	AUG 30, 1991

HYDROCODONE BITARTRATE W/ ACETAMINOPHEN

	Firm	Strength	Appl. No.	Date
AA	BARR	500 MG;5 MG	N88577 001	DEC 21, 1984
AA	NORCET / ABANA	500 MG;5 MG	N88871 001	MAY 15, 1986
AA	TYCOLET / JOHNSON RW	500 MG;5 MG	N89385 001	AUG 27, 1986
AA	VICODIN / KNOLL	500 MG;5 MG	N88058 001	JAN 07, 1983
AA	VICODIN ES / KNOLL	750 MG;7.5 MG	N89736 001	DEC 09, 1988

ACETAMINOPHEN; OXYCODONE HYDROCHLORIDE

CAPSULE; ORAL

OXYCODONE AND ACETAMINOPHEN

	Firm	Strength	Appl. No.	Date
AA	HALSEY	500 MG;5 MG	N89994 001	MAY 04, 1989
AA	TYLOX / JOHNSON RW	500 MG;5 MG	N88790 001	DEC 12, 1984

SOLUTION; ORAL

Firm	Strength	Appl. No.	Date
ROXICET / ROXANE	325 MG/5 ML;5 MG/5 ML	N89351 001	DEC 03, 1986

ACETAMINOPHEN; OXYCODONE HYDROCHLORIDE *(continued)*

TABLET; ORAL

OXYCET

	Firm	Strength	Appl. No.	Date
AA	HALSEY	325 MG;5 MG	N87463 001	DEC 07, 1983

OXYCODONE HCL AND ACETAMINOPHEN

	Firm	Strength	Appl. No.	Date
AA	BARR	325 MG;5 MG	N87406 001	

PERCOCET

	Firm	Strength	Appl. No.	Date
AA	DUPONT	325 MG;5 MG	N85106 002	

ROXICET

	Firm	Strength	Appl. No.	Date
AA	ROXANE	325 MG;5 MG	N87003 001	
	ROXICET 5/500 / ROXANE	500 MG;5 MG	N89775 001	JAN 12, 1989

ACETAMINOPHEN; PENTAZOCINE HYDROCHLORIDE

TABLET; ORAL

TALACEN

	Firm	Strength	Appl. No.	Date
AA	+ STERLING	650 MG;EQ 25 MG BASE	N18458 001	SEP 23, 1982

ACETAMINOPHEN; PROPOXYPHENE HYDROCHLORIDE

TABLET; ORAL

PROPOXYPHENE HCL AND ACETAMINOPHEN

	Firm	Strength	Appl. No.	Date
AA	GENEVA	650 MG;65 MG	N89959 001	JUL 18, 1989
AA	MYLAN	650 MG;65 MG	N83978 001	
AA	WYGESIC / WYETH AYERST	650 MG;65 MG	N84999 001	

ACETAMINOPHEN; PROPOXYPHENE NAPSYLATE

TABLET; ORAL

DARVOCET-N 100

	Firm	Strength	Appl. No.	Date
AB	+ LILLY	650 MG;100 MG	N17122 002	

DARVOCET-N 50

	Firm	Strength	Appl. No.	Date
AB	LILLY	325 MG;50 MG	N17122 001	

PROPACET 100

	Firm	Strength	Appl. No.	Date
AB	LEMMON	650 MG;100 MG	N70107 001	JUN 12, 1985

PROPOXYPHENE NAPSYLATE AND ACETAMINOPHEN

	Firm	Strength	Appl. No.	Date
AB	BARR	325 MG;50 MG	N70115 001	JUN 12, 1985
AB		650 MG;100 MG	N70116 001	JUN 12, 1985
AB		650 MG;100 MG	N70615 001	MAR 21, 1986
AB		650 MG;100 MG	N70771 001	MAR 21, 1986
AB		650 MG;100 MG	N70775 001	MAR 21, 1986
AB	GENEVA	650 MG;100 MG	N70443 001	JAN 23, 1986

Prescription Drug Products (continued)

ACETAMINOPHEN; PROPOXYPHENE NAPSYLATE (continued)

TABLET; ORAL

PROPOXYPHENE NAPSYLATE AND ACETAMINOPHEN

TE	Firm	Strength	Appl. No.	Approval Date
AB	HALSEY	325 MG;50 MG	N72105 001	
AB		650 MG;100 MG	N72106 001	MAY 13, 1988
AB		650 MG;100 MG	N70732 001	MAY 13, 1988
AB	LEMMON	650 MG;100 MG	N70145 001	JAN 03, 1986
AB	MYLAN	650 MG;100 MG	N72195 001	JUN 12, 1985
AB		650 MG;100 MG		FEB 16, 1988
AB	PUREPAC	650 MG;100 MG	N70910 001	JAN 02, 1987
AB	SUPERPHARM	650 MG;100 MG	N71319 001	JAN 06, 1987
AB	ZENITH	650 MG;100 MG	N70146 001	AUG 02, 1985

ACETAZOLAMIDE

CAPSULE, EXTENDED RELEASE; ORAL

DIAMOX

TE	Firm	Strength	Appl. No.	Approval Date
+	LEDERLE	500 MG	N12945 001	

TABLET; ORAL

ACETAZOLAMIDE

TE	Firm	Strength	Appl. No.	Approval Date
AB	DANBURY	250 MG	N88882 001	OCT 22, 1985
AB	LANNETT	250 MG	N84840 001	
AB	MUTUAL PHARM	125 MG	N89752 001	JUN 22, 1988
AB		250 MG	N89753 001	JUN 22, 1988

DIAMOX

TE	Firm	Strength	Appl. No.	Approval Date
AB	LEDERLE	125 MG	N08943 001	
AB +		250 MG	N08943 002	

ACETAZOLAMIDE SODIUM

INJECTABLE; INJECTION

ACETAZOLAMIDE SODIUM

TE	Firm	Strength	Appl. No.	Approval Date
AP	QUAD	EQ 500 MG/VIAL	N89619 001	JAN 13, 1988

DIAMOX

TE	Firm	Strength	Appl. No.	Approval Date
AP	LEDERLE	EQ 500 MG/VIAL	N09388 001	DEC 05, 1990

ACETIC ACID, GLACIAL

SOLUTION; IRRIGATION, URETHRAL

ACETIC ACID 0.25% IN PLASTIC CONTAINER

TE	Firm	Strength	Appl. No.	Approval Date
AT	ABBOTT	250 MG/100 ML	N17656 001	
AT	BAXTER	250 MG/100 ML	N18523 001	FEB 19, 1982
AT	MCGAW	250 MG/100 ML	N18161 001	

ACETIC ACID, GLACIAL (continued)

SOLUTION/DROPS; OTIC

ACETASOL

TE	Firm	Strength	Appl. No.	Approval Date
AT	BARRE	2%	N87146 001	

ACETIC ACID

TE	Firm	Strength	Appl. No.	Approval Date
AT	THAMES	2%	N88638 001	SEP 06, 1984

BOROFAIR

TE	Firm	Strength	Appl. No.	Approval Date
AT	PHARMAFAIR	2%	N88606 001	AUG 21, 1985

VOSOL

TE	Firm	Strength	Appl. No.	Approval Date
AT	WALLACE	2%	N12179 001	

ACETIC ACID, GLACIAL; ALUMINUM ACETATE

SOLUTION/DROPS; OTIC

DOMEBORO

Firm	Strength	Appl. No.
MILES	2%;0.79%	N84476 001

ACETIC ACID, GLACIAL; DESONIDE

SOLUTION/DROPS; OTIC

TRIDESILON

Firm	Strength	Appl. No.
MILES	2%;0.05%	N17914 001

ACETIC ACID, GLACIAL; HYDROCORTISONE

SOLUTION/DROPS; OTIC

ACETASOL HC

TE	Firm	Strength	Appl. No.	Approval Date
AT	BARRE	2%;1%	N87143 001	JAN 13, 1982

HYDROCORTISONE AND ACETIC ACID

TE	Firm	Strength	Appl. No.	Approval Date
AT	THAMES	2%;1%	N88759 001	MAR 04, 1985

VOSOL HC

TE	Firm	Strength	Appl. No.
AT	WALLACE	2%;1%	N12770 001

ACETIC ACID, GLACIAL; HYDROCORTISONE; NEOMYCIN SULFATE

SUSPENSION; OTIC

NEO-CORT-DOME

Firm	Strength	Appl. No.
MILES	2%;1%;EQ 0.35% BASE	N50238 001

ACETOHEXAMIDE

TABLET; ORAL

ACETOHEXAMIDE

TE	Firm	Strength	Appl. No.	Approval Date
AB	BARR	250 MG	N70869 001	FEB 09, 1987
AB		500 MG	N70870 001	FEB 09, 1987
AB	DANBURY	250 MG	N71893 001	NOV 25, 1987
AB		500 MG	N71894 001	NOV 25, 1987

DYMELOR

TE	Firm	Strength	Appl. No.
AB	LILLY	250 MG	N13378 002
AB +		500 MG	N13378 001

Prescription Drug Products (continued)

ACETOHYDROXAMIC ACID
TABLET; ORAL
LITHOSTAT

+ MISSION PHARMA	250 MG	N18749 001	MAY 31, 1983

ACETYLCHOLINE CHLORIDE
POWDER FOR RECONSTITUTION; OPHTHALMIC
MIOCHOL

IOLAB	20 MG/VIAL	N16211 001	

ACETYLCYSTEINE
SOLUTION; INHALATION, ORAL
ACETYLCYSTEINE

AN	CETUS BEN VENUE	10%	N72323 001	APR 30, 1992
AN		20%	N72324 001	APR 30, 1992
AN	DUPONT	10%	N71364 001	MAY 01, 1989
AN		20%	N71365 001	MAY 01, 1989

MUCOMYST

AN	MEAD JOHNSON	10%	N13601 002	
AN		20%	N13601 001	

MUCOSOL-10

AN	DEY	10%	N70575 001	OCT 14, 1986

MUCOSOL-20

AN	DEY	20%	N70576 001	OCT 14, 1986

ACYCLOVIR
CAPSULE; ORAL
ZOVIRAX

+ BURROUGHS WELLCOME	200 MG	N18828 001	JAN 25, 1985

OINTMENT; TOPICAL
ZOVIRAX

+ BURROUGHS WELLCOME	5%	N18604 001	MAR 29, 1982

SUSPENSION; ORAL
ZOVIRAX

+ BURROUGHS WELLCOME	200 MG/5 ML	N19909 001	DEC 22, 1989

TABLET; ORAL
ZOVIRAX
BURROUGHS WELLCOME

	400 MG	N20089 001	APR 30, 1991
+	800 MG	N20089 002	APR 30, 1991

ACYCLOVIR SODIUM
INJECTABLE; INJECTION
ZOVIRAX

+ BURROUGHS WELLCOME	EQ 500 MG BASE/VIAL	N18603 001	OCT 22, 1982

ADENOSINE
INJECTABLE; INJECTION
ADENOCARD

MEDCO	3 MG/ML	N19937 002	OCT 30, 1989

ALBUMIN CHROMATED CR-51 SERUM
INJECTABLE; INJECTION
CHROMALBIN

ISO TEX	100 UCI/VIAL	N17835 001	

ALBUMIN IODINATED I-125 SERUM
INJECTABLE; INJECTION
RADIOIODINATED SERUM ALBUMIN (HUMAN) IHSA I 125

MALLINCKRODT	6.67 UCI/ML	N17844 003	
	10 UCI/ML	N17844 001	
	100 UCI/ML	N17844 002	

ALBUMIN IODINATED I-131 SERUM
INJECTABLE; INJECTION
MEGATOPE

ISO TEX	0.5 MCI/VIAL	N17837 001	
	1 MCI/VIAL	N17837 002	

ALBUTEROL
AEROSOL, METERED; INHALATION
PROVENTIL

BN	SCHERING	0.09 MG/INH	N17559 001	

VENTOLIN

BN	+ GLAXO	0.09 MG/INH	N18473 001	

ALBUTEROL SULFATE
CAPSULE; INHALATION
VENTOLIN ROTACAPS

GLAXO	EQ 0.2 MG BASE	N19489 001	MAY 04, 1988

SOLUTION; INHALATION
ALBUTEROL SULFATE

AN	COPLEY	EQ 0.5% BASE	N73307 001	NOV 27, 1991
AN	DEY	EQ 0.083% BASE	N72652 001	FEB 21, 1992

Prescription Drug Products (continued)

ALBUTEROL SULFATE (continued)

SOLUTION; INHALATION

	PROVENTIL			
AN	SCHERING	EQ 0.083% BASE	N19243 002	JAN 14, 1987
AN		EQ 0.5% BASE	N19243 001	JAN 14, 1987
	VENTOLIN			
AN	GLAXO	EQ 0.083% BASE	N19773 001	APR 23, 1992
AN		EQ 0.5% BASE	N19269 002	JAN 16, 1987

SYRUP; ORAL

	ALBUTEROL SULFATE			
AA	LEMMON	EQ 2 MG BASE/5 ML	N73419 001	MAR 30, 1992
	PROVENTIL			
AA	SCHERING	EQ 2 MG BASE/5 ML	N18062 001	JAN 19, 1983
	VENTOLIN			
AA	GLAXO	EQ 2 MG BASE/5 ML	N19621 001	JUN 10, 1987

TABLET; ORAL

	ALBUTEROL SULFATE			
AB	BIOCRAFT	EQ 2 MG BASE	N72619 001	APR 07, 1989
AB		EQ 4 MG BASE	N72620 001	APR 07, 1989
AB	COPLEY	EQ 2 MG BASE	N72966 001	NOV 22, 1991
AB		EQ 4 MG BASE	N72967 001	NOV 22, 1991
AB	DANBURY	EQ 2 MG BASE	N72629 001	JAN 31, 1991
AB		EQ 4 MG BASE	N72630 001	JAN 31, 1991
AB	GENEVA	EQ 2 MG BASE	N72151 001	MAR 23, 1989
AB		EQ 4 MG BASE	N72152 001	MAR 23, 1989
AB	LEDERLE	EQ 2 MG BASE	N72859 001	DEC 20, 1989
AB		EQ 4 MG BASE	N72860 001	DEC 20, 1989
AB	LEMMON	EQ 2 MG BASE	N72938 001	MAR 30, 1990
AB		EQ 4 MG BASE	N72939 001	MAR 30, 1990
AB	MUTUAL PHARM	EQ 2 MG BASE	N72636 001	FEB 01, 1989
AB		EQ 4 MG BASE	N72637 001	FEB 01, 1989

ALBUTEROL SULFATE (continued)

TABLET; ORAL

	ALBUTEROL SULFATE			
AB	MYLAN	EQ 2 MG BASE	N72893 001	JAN 17, 1991
AB		EQ 4 MG BASE	N72894 001	JAN 17, 1991
AB	SIDMAK	EQ 2 MG BASE	N72316 001	JAN 30, 1989
AB		EQ 4 MG BASE	N72317 001	JAN 30, 1989
AB	WARNER CHILCOTT	EQ 2 MG BASE	N72817 001	JAN 09, 1990
AB		EQ 4 MG BASE	N72818 001	JAN 09, 1990
AB	WATSON	EQ 2 MG BASE	N72764 001	AUG 28, 1991
AB		EQ 4 MG BASE	N72765 001	AUG 28, 1991
	PROVENTIL			
AB	SCHERING	EQ 2 MG BASE	N17853 001	MAY 07, 1982
AB		EQ 4 MG BASE	N17853 002	MAY 07, 1982
	VENTOLIN			
AB	GLAXO	EQ 2 MG BASE	N19112 001	JUL 10, 1986
AB		EQ 4 MG BASE	N19112 002	JUL 10, 1986

TABLET, EXTENDED RELEASE; ORAL

	PROVENTIL			
	+ SCHERING	EQ 4 MG BASE	N19383 001	JUL 13, 1987

ALCLOMETASONE DIPROPIONATE

CREAM; TOPICAL

	ACLOVATE			
	+ GLAXO	0.05%	N18707 001	DEC 14, 1982

OINTMENT; TOPICAL

	ACLOVATE			
	+ GLAXO	0.05%	N18702 001	DEC 14, 1982

ALCOHOL

INJECTABLE; INJECTION

	ALCOHOL 10% AND DEXTROSE 5%			
	MCGAW	10 ML/100 ML	N04589 006	
	ALCOHOL 5% AND DEXTROSE 5%			
AP	MCGAW	5 ML/100 ML	N04589 004	
	ALCOHOL 5% IN DEXTROSE 5% IN WATER			
AP	BAXTER	5 ML/100 ML	N83256 001	
	ALCOHOL 5% IN D5-W			
AP	ABBOTT	5 ML/100 ML	N83263 001	

Prescription Drug Products (continued)

ALFENTANIL HYDROCHLORIDE
INJECTABLE; INJECTION
ALFENTA
	JANSSEN	EQ 0.5 MG BASE/ML	N19353 001 DEC 29, 1986

ALGLUCERASE
INJECTABLE; INJECTION
CEREDASE
	GENZYME	10 UNITS/ML	N20057 004 MAY 08, 1992
		80 UNITS/ML	N20057 003 APR 05, 1991

ALLOPURINOL
TABLET; ORAL
ALLOPURINOL
AB	BARR	100 MG	N70466 001 DEC 24, 1985
AB		300 MG	N70467 001 DEC 24, 1985
AB	DANBURY	100 MG	N18832 002 SEP 28, 1984
AB		300 MG	N18877 001 SEP 28, 1984
AB	GENEVA	100 MG	N70268 001 DEC 31, 1985
AB		300 MG	N70269 001 DEC 31, 1985
AB	MUTUAL PHARM	100 MG	N71449 001 JAN 09, 1987
AB		300 MG	N71450 001 JAN 09, 1987
AB	MYLAN	100 MG	N18659 001 OCT 24, 1986
AB		300 MG	N18659 002 OCT 24, 1986
AB	PAR	100 MG	N70150 001 DEC 10, 1985
AB		300 MG	N70147 001 DEC 10, 1985
AB	SUPERPHARM	300 MG	N70951 001 SEP 04, 1986

LOPURIN
AB	BOOTS	100 MG	N71586 001 APR 02, 1987
AB		300 MG	N71587 001 APR 02, 1987

ZYLOPRIM
AB	BURROUGHS WELLCOME	100 MG	N16084 001
AB	+	300 MG	N16084 002

ALPRAZOLAM
TABLET; ORAL
XANAX
	UPJOHN	0.25 MG	N18276 001
		0.5 MG	N18276 002
+		1 MG	N18276 003
		2 MG	N18276 004 NOV 27, 1985

ALPROSTADIL
INJECTABLE; INJECTION
PROSTIN VR PEDIATRIC
	UPJOHN	0.5 MG/ML	N18484 001

ALSEROXYLON
TABLET; ORAL
RAUWILOID
+	3M	2 MG	N08867 001

ALTRETAMINE
CAPSULE; ORAL
HEXALEN
+	US BIOSCIENCE	50 MG	N19926 001 DEC 26, 1990

ALUMINUM ACETATE; *MULTIPLE*
SEE ACETIC ACID, GLACIAL; ALUMINUM ACETATE

AMANTADINE HYDROCHLORIDE
CAPSULE; ORAL
AMANTADINE HCL
AB	BOLAR	100 MG	N71382 001 JAN 21, 1987
AB	INVAMED	100 MG	N71293 001 FEB 18, 1987
AB	PHARM BASICS	100 MG	N70589 001 AUG 05, 1986

SYMADINE
AB	SOLVAY	100 MG	N71000 001 SEP 04, 1986

SYMMETREL
AB	+ DUPONT	100 MG	N16020 001
AB		100 MG	N17117 001

SYRUP; ORAL
AMANTADINE HCL
AA	BARRE	50 MG/5ML	N72655 001 OCT 30, 1990
AA	COPLEY	50 MG/5ML	N73115 001 AUG 23, 1991

SYMMETREL
AA	DUPONT	50 MG/5ML	N16023 002
AA		50 MG/5ML	N17118 001

Prescription Drug Products (continued)

AMANTADINE HYDROCHLORIDE (continued)

TABLET; ORAL

	Strength	Brand / Mfr	NDA	Date
	100 MG	SYMMETREL + DUPONT	N18101 001	

AMBENONIUM CHLORIDE

TABLET; ORAL

	Strength	Brand / Mfr	NDA	Date
	10 MG	MYTELASE STERLING	N10155 002	

AMCINONIDE

CREAM; TOPICAL

	Strength	Brand / Mfr	NDA	Date
	0.025%	CYCLOCORT + LEDERLE	N18116 001	
	0.1%		N18116 002	

LOTION; TOPICAL

	Strength	Brand / Mfr	NDA	Date
	0.1%	CYCLOCORT + LEDERLE	N19729 001	JUN 13, 1988

OINTMENT; TOPICAL

	Strength	Brand / Mfr	NDA	Date
	0.1%	CYCLOCORT + LEDERLE	N18498 001	

AMDINOCILLIN

INJECTABLE; INJECTION

	Strength	Brand / Mfr	NDA	Date
	250 MG/VIAL	COACTIN ROCHE	N50565 001	DEC 21, 1984
	500 MG/VIAL		N50565 002	DEC 21, 1984
	1 GM/VIAL		N50565 003	DEC 21, 1984

AMIKACIN SULFATE

INJECTABLE; INJECTION

AMIKACIN

TE	Strength	Brand / Mfr	NDA	Date
AP	EQ 50 MG BASE/ML	ELKINS SINN	N63274 001	MAY 18, 1992
AP	EQ 250 MG BASE/ML		N63275 001	MAY 18, 1992

AMIKIN

TE	Strength	Brand / Mfr	NDA	Date
AP	EQ 50 MG BASE/ML	BRISTOL	N50495 001	
AP	EQ 50 MG BASE/ML		N62562 001	SEP 20, 1984
AP	EQ 250 MG BASE/ML		N50495 002	
AP	EQ 250 MG BASE/ML		N62562 002	SEP 20, 1984

AMIKIN IN SODIUM CHLORIDE 0.9% IN PLASTIC CONTAINER

	Strength	Brand / Mfr	NDA	Date
	EQ 5 MG BASE/ML	BRISTOL	N50618 002	NOV 30, 1987
	EQ 10 MG BASE/ML		N50618 001	NOV 30, 1987

AMILORIDE HYDROCHLORIDE

TABLET; ORAL

AMILORIDE HCL

TE	Strength	Brand / Mfr	NDA	Date
AB	5 MG	PAR	N70346 001	JAN 22, 1986
AB	5 MG	MIDAMOR + MSD	N18200 001	

AMILORIDE HYDROCHLORIDE; HYDROCHLOROTHIAZIDE

TABLET; ORAL

AMILORIDE HCL AND HYDROCHLOROTHIAZIDE

TE	Strength	Brand / Mfr	NDA	Date
AB	EQ 5 MG ANHYDROUS;50 MG	BARR	N71111 001	MAY 10, 1988
AB	EQ 5 MG ANHYDROUS;50 MG	BIOCRAFT	N70795 001	JUL 15, 1987
AB	EQ 5 MG ANHYDROUS;50 MG	GENEVA	N73357 001	NOV 27, 1991
AB	EQ 5 MG ANHYDROUS;50 MG	MYLAN	N73209 001	OCT 31, 1991
AB	EQ 5 MG ANHYDROUS;50 MG	ROYCE	N73334 001	JUL 19, 1991

HYDRO-RIDE

TE	Strength	Brand / Mfr	NDA	Date
AB	EQ 5 MG ANHYDROUS;50 MG	PAR	N70347 001	AUG 06, 1986

MODURETIC 5-50

TE	Strength	Brand / Mfr	NDA	Date
AB	EQ 5 MG ANHYDROUS;50 MG	+ MSD	N18201 001	

AMINO ACIDS

INJECTABLE; INJECTION

AMINESS 5.2% ESSENTIAL AMINO ACIDS W/ HISTADINE

	Strength	Brand / Mfr	NDA	Date
	5.2%	KABIVITRUM	N18901 001	APR 06, 1984

AMINOSYN II 10%

	Strength	Brand / Mfr	NDA	Date
	10%	ABBOTT	N19438 005	APR 03, 1986

AMINOSYN II 10% IN PLASTIC CONTAINER

	Strength	Brand / Mfr	NDA	Date
	10%	ABBOTT	N20015 001	DEC 19, 1991

AMINOSYN II 15% IN PLASTIC CONTAINER

	Strength	Brand / Mfr	NDA	Date
	15%	ABBOTT	N20041 001	DEC 19, 1991

AMINOSYN II 3.5%

	Strength	Brand / Mfr	NDA	Date
	3.5%	ABBOTT	N19438 001	APR 03, 1986

AMINOSYN II 5%

	Strength	Brand / Mfr	NDA	Date
	5%	ABBOTT	N19438 002	APR 03, 1986

Prescription Drug Products (continued)

AMINO ACIDS (continued)

INJECTABLE; INJECTION

Product		Strength	NDA	Date
AMINOSYN II 7%	ABBOTT	7%	N19438 003	APR 03, 1986
AMINOSYN II 8.5%	ABBOTT	8.5%	N19438 004	APR 03, 1986
AMINOSYN 10%	ABBOTT	10%	N17673 003	
AMINOSYN 10% (PH6)	ABBOTT	10%	N17673 008	NOV 18, 1985
AMINOSYN 3.5%	ABBOTT	3.5%	N17789 004	
AMINOSYN 5%	ABBOTT	5%	N17673 001	
AMINOSYN 7%	ABBOTT	7%	N17673 002	
AMINOSYN 7% (PH6)	ABBOTT	7%	N17673 006	NOV 18, 1985
AMINOSYN 8.5%	ABBOTT	8.5%	N17673 004	
AMINOSYN 8.5% (PH6)	ABBOTT	8.5%	N17673 007	NOV 18, 1985
AMINOSYN-HBC 7%	ABBOTT	7%	N19374 001	JUL 12, 1985
AMINOSYN-PF 10%	ABBOTT	10%	N19492 002	OCT 17, 1986
AMINOSYN-PF 7%	ABBOTT	7%	N19398 001	SEP 06, 1985
AMINOSYN-RF 5.2%	ABBOTT	5.2%	N18429 001	
BRANCHAMIN 4%	BAXTER	4%	N18678 001	SEP 28, 1984
BRANCHAMIN 4% IN PLASTIC CONTAINER	BAXTER	4%	N18684 001	SEP 28, 1984
FREAMINE HBC 6.9%	MCGAW	6.9%	N16822 006	MAY 17, 1983
FREAMINE III 10%	MCGAW	10%	N16822 005	
FREAMINE III 8.5%	MCGAW	8.5%	N16822 004	
HEPATAMINE 8%	MCGAW	8%	N18676 001	AUG 03, 1982

AMINO ACIDS (continued)

INJECTABLE; INJECTION

Product		Strength	NDA	Date
NEPHRAMINE 5.4%	MCGAW	5.4%	N17766 001	
NOVAMINE 11.4%	KABIVITRUM	11.4%	N17957 003	AUG 09, 1982
NOVAMINE 15%	KABIVITRUM	15%	N17957 004	NOV 28, 1986
NOVAMINE 8.5%	KABIVITRUM	8.5%	N17957 002	AUG 09, 1982
RENAMIN W/O ELECTROLYTES	BAXTER	6.5%	N17493 007	OCT 15, 1982
TRAVASOL 10% IN PLASTIC CONTAINER	BAXTER	10%	N18931 004	APR 27, 1988
TRAVASOL 10% W/O ELECTROLYTES	BAXTER	10%	N17493 006	
TRAVASOL 10% W/O ELECTROLYTES IN PLASTIC CONTAINER	BAXTER	10%	N18931 003	AUG 23, 1984
TRAVASOL 5.5% W/O ELECTROLYTES	BAXTER	5.5%	N17493 004	
TRAVASOL 5.5% W/O ELECTROLYTES IN PLASTIC CONTAINER	BAXTER	5.5%	N18931 001	AUG 23, 1984
TRAVASOL 8.5% W/O ELECTROLYTES	BAXTER	8.5%	N17493 005	
TRAVASOL 8.5% W/O ELECTROLYTES IN PLASTIC CONTAINER	BAXTER	8.5%	N18931 002	AUG 23, 1984
TROPHAMINE	MCGAW	6%	N19018 001	JUL 20, 1984
TROPHAMINE 10%	MCGAW	10%	N19018 003	SEP 07, 1988

AMINO ACIDS; CALCIUM ACETATE; GLYCERIN; MAGNESIUM ACETATE; PHOSPHORIC ACID; POTASSIUM CHLORIDE; SODIUM ACETATE; SODIUM CHLORIDE

INJECTABLE; INJECTION

Product		Strength	NDA	Date
PROCALAMINE	MCGAW	3%;26 MG/100 ML;.3 GM/100 ML;.54 MG/100 ML;41 MG/100 ML;150 MG/100 ML;200 MG/100 ML;120 MG/100 ML	N18582 001	MAY 08, 1982

Prescription Drug Products (continued)

AMINO ACIDS; CALCIUM CHLORIDE; DEXTROSE; MAGNESIUM CHLORIDE; POTASSIUM CHLORIDE; POTASSIUM PHOSPHATE, DIBASIC; SODIUM CHLORIDE

INJECTABLE; INJECTION
AMINOSYN II 3.5% W/ ELECTROLYTES IN DEXTROSE 25% W/ CALCIUM IN PLASTIC CONTAINER

ABBOTT	3.5%;36.8 MG/100 ML;25 GM/ 100 ML;51 MG/ 100 ML;22.4 MG/ 100 ML;261 MG/ 100 ML;205 MG/100 ML	N19683 001	NOV 07, 1988
	3.5%;36.8 MG/100 ML;25 GM/ 100 ML;51 MG/ 100 ML;22.4 MG/ 100 ML;261 MG/ 100 ML;205 MG/100 ML	N19714 001	SEP 12, 1988

AMINOSYN II 4.25% W/ ELECTROLYTES IN DEXTROSE 20% W/ CALCIUM IN PLASTIC CONTAINER

ABBOTT	4.25%;36.8 MG/ 100 ML;20 GM/ 100 ML;51 MG/ 100 ML;22.4 MG/ 100 ML;261 MG/ 100 ML;205 MG/100 ML	N19683 002	NOV 07, 1988
	4.25%;36.8 MG/ 100 ML;20 GM/ 100 ML;51 MG/ 100 ML;22.4 MG/ 100 ML;261 MG/ 100 ML;205 MG/100 ML	N19714 002	SEP 12, 1988

AMINOSYN II 4.25% W/ ELECTROLYTES IN DEXTROSE 25% W/ CALCIUM IN PLASTIC CONTAINER

ABBOTT	4.25%;36.8 MG/ 100 ML;25 GM/ 100 ML;51 MG/ 100 ML;22.4 MG/ 100 ML;261 MG/ 100 ML;205 MG/100 ML	N19683 003	NOV 07, 1988
	4.25%;36.8 MG/ 100 ML;25 GM/ 100 ML;51 MG/ 100 ML;22.4 MG/ 100 ML;261 MG/ 100 ML;205 MG/100 ML	N19714 004	SEP 12, 1988

AMINO ACIDS; CALCIUM CHLORIDE; DEXTROSE; MAGNESIUM CHLORIDE; POTASSIUM CHLORIDE; POTASSIUM PHOSPHATE, DIBASIC; SODIUM CHLORIDE (continued)

INJECTABLE; INJECTION
AMINOSYN II 5% W/ ELECTROLYTES IN DEXTROSE 25% W/ CALCIUM IN PLASTIC CONTAINER

ABBOTT	5%;36.8 MG/100 ML;25 GM/ 100 ML;51 MG/ 100 ML;22.4 MG/ 100 ML;261 MG/ 100 ML;205 MG/100 ML	N19683 004	NOV 07, 1988
	5%;36.8 MG/100 ML;25 GM/ 100 ML;51 MG/ 100 ML;22.4 MG/ 100 ML;261 MG/ 100 ML;205 MG/100 ML	N19714 003	SEP 12, 1988

AMINO ACIDS; DEXTROSE

INJECTABLE; INJECTION
AMINOSYN II 3.5% IN DEXTROSE 25% IN PLASTIC CONTAINER

ABBOTT	3.5%;25 GM/100 ML	N19505 002	NOV 07, 1986
	3.5%;25 GM/100 ML	N19681 001	NOV 01, 1988
	3.5%;25 GM/100 ML	N19713 006	SEP 09, 1988

AMINOSYN II 3.5% IN DEXTROSE 5% IN PLASTIC CONTAINER

ABBOTT	3.5%;5 GM/100 ML	N19506 001	NOV 07, 1986
	3.5%;5 GM/100 ML	N19681 002	NOV 01, 1988
	3.5%;5 GM/100 ML	N19713 002	SEP 09, 1988

AMINOSYN II 4.25% IN DEXTROSE 10% IN PLASTIC CONTAINER

ABBOTT	4.25%;10 GM/100 ML	N19681 004	NOV 01, 1988
	4.25%;10 GM/100 ML	N19713 001	SEP 09, 1988

AMINOSYN II 4.25% IN DEXTROSE 20% IN PLASTIC CONTAINER

ABBOTT	4.25%;20 GM/100 ML	N19681 005	NOV 01, 1988
	4.25%;20 GM/100 ML	N19713 004	SEP 09, 1988

AMINOSYN II 4.25% IN DEXTROSE 25% IN PLASTIC CONTAINER

ABBOTT	4.25%;25 GM/100 ML	N19504 002	NOV 07, 1986
	4.25%;25 GM/100 ML	N19681 003	NOV 01, 1988
	4.25%;25 GM/100 ML	N19713 005	SEP 09, 1988

AMINOSYN II 5% IN DEXTROSE 25% IN PLASTIC CONTAINER

ABBOTT	5%;25 GM/100 ML	N19565 001	DEC 17, 1986
	5%;25 GM/100 ML	N19681 006	NOV 01, 1988
	5%;25 GM/100 ML	N19713 003	SEP 09, 1988

Prescription Drug Products (continued)

AMINO ACIDS; DEXTROSE (continued)

INJECTABLE; INJECTION

AMINOSYN 4.25% W/ DEXTROSE 25% IN PLASTIC CONTAINER

ABBOTT	4.25%;25 GM/100 ML	N19119 001	OCT 11, 1984

TRAVASOL 2.75% IN DEXTROSE 10% IN PLASTIC CONTAINER

BAXTER	2.75%;10 GM/100 ML	N19520 002	SEP 23, 1988

TRAVASOL 2.75% IN DEXTROSE 15% IN PLASTIC CONTAINER

BAXTER	2.75%;15 GM/100 ML	N19520 003	SEP 23, 1988

TRAVASOL 2.75% IN DEXTROSE 20% IN PLASTIC CONTAINER

BAXTER	2.75%;20 GM/100 ML	N19520 004	SEP 23, 1988

TRAVASOL 2.75% IN DEXTROSE 25% IN PLASTIC CONTAINER

BAXTER	2.75%;25 GM/100 ML	N19520 005	SEP 23, 1988

TRAVASOL 2.75% IN DEXTROSE 5% IN PLASTIC CONTAINER

BAXTER	2.75%;5 GM/100 ML	N19520 001	SEP 23, 1988

TRAVASOL 4.25% IN DEXTROSE 10% IN PLASTIC CONTAINER

BAXTER	4.25%;10 GM/100 ML	N19520 007	SEP 23, 1988

TRAVASOL 4.25% IN DEXTROSE 15% IN PLASTIC CONTAINER

BAXTER	4.25%;15 GM/100 ML	N19520 008	SEP 23, 1988

TRAVASOL 4.25% IN DEXTROSE 20% IN PLASTIC CONTAINER

BAXTER	4.25%;20 GM/100 ML	N19520 009	SEP 23, 1988

TRAVASOL 4.25% IN DEXTROSE 25% IN PLASTIC CONTAINER

BAXTER	4.25%;25 GM/100 ML	N19520 010	SEP 23, 1988

TRAVASOL 4.25% IN DEXTROSE 5% IN PLASTIC CONTAINER

BAXTER	4.25%;5 GM/100 ML	N19520 006	SEP 23, 1988

AMINO ACIDS; DEXTROSE; MAGNESIUM CHLORIDE; POTASSIUM ACETATE; POTASSIUM CHLORIDE; POTASSIUM PHOSPHATE, DIBASIC; SODIUM CHLORIDE

INJECTABLE; INJECTION

AMINOSYN II 4.25% W/ ELECT AND ADJUSTED PHOSPHATE IN DEXTROSE 10% IN PLASTIC CONTAINER

ABBOTT	4.25%;10 GM/100 ML;51 MG/ 100 ML;176.5 MG/ 100 ML;22.4 MG/ 100 ML;104.5 MG/ 100 ML;205 MG/100 ML	N19682 003	NOV 01, 1988
	4.25%;10 GM/100 ML;51 MG/ 100 ML;176.5 MG/ 100 ML;22.4 MG/ 100 ML;104.5 MG/ 100 ML;205 MG/100 ML	N19712 002	SEP 08, 1988

AMINO ACIDS; DEXTROSE; MAGNESIUM CHLORIDE; POTASSIUM CHLORIDE; SODIUM CHLORIDE; SODIUM PHOSPHATE, DIBASIC

INJECTABLE; INJECTION

AMINOSYN II 3.5% M IN DEXTROSE 5% IN PLASTIC CONTAINER

ABBOTT	3.5%;5 GM/100 ML;30 MG/ 100 ML;97 MG/ 100 ML;120 MG/ 100 ML;49.3 MG/100 MG	N19682 001	NOV 01, 1988
	3.5%;5 GM/100 ML;30 MG/ 100 ML;97 MG/ 100 ML;120 MG/ 100 ML;49.3 MG/100 ML	N19712 001	SEP 08, 1988

AMINOSYN II 4.25% M IN DEXTROSE 10% IN PLASTIC CONTAINER

ABBOTT	4.25%;10 GM/100 ML;30 MG/ 100 ML;97 MG/ 100 ML;120 MG/ 100 ML;49.3 MG/100 ML	N19682 002	NOV 01, 1988

AMINO ACIDS; MAGNESIUM ACETATE; PHOSPHORIC ACID; POTASSIUM ACETATE; POTASSIUM CHLORIDE; SODIUM ACETATE

INJECTABLE; INJECTION

FREAMINE III 8.5% W/ ELECTROLYTES

MCGAW	8.5%;110 MG/ 100 ML;230 MG/ 100 ML;10 MG/ 100 ML;440 MG/ 100 ML;690 MG/100 ML	N16822 007	JUL 01, 1988

AMINO ACIDS; MAGNESIUM ACETATE; PHOSPHORIC ACID; POTASSIUM ACETATE; SODIUM CHLORIDE

INJECTABLE; INJECTION

AMINOSYN 3.5% M

ABBOTT	3.5%;21 MG/100 ML;40 MG/ 100 ML;128 MG/ 100 ML;234 MG/100 ML	N17789 003

AMINO ACIDS; MAGNESIUM ACETATE; PHOSPHORIC ACID; POTASSIUM CHLORIDE; SODIUM ACETATE; SODIUM CHLORIDE

INJECTABLE; INJECTION

FREAMINE III 3% W/ ELECTROLYTES

MCGAW	3%;54 MG/100 ML;40 MG/ 100 ML;150 MG/ 100 ML;200 MG/ 100 ML;120 MG/100 ML	N16822 003

Prescription Drug Products (*continued*)

AMINO ACIDS; MAGNESIUM CHLORIDE; POTASSIUM ACETATE; POTASSIUM CHLORIDE; SODIUM ACETATE
INJECTABLE; INJECTION
VEINAMINE 8%
  KABIVITRUM 8%;61 MG/100 ML;211 MG/
  100 ML;56 MG/
  100 ML;388 MG/100 ML N17957 001

AMINO ACIDS; MAGNESIUM CHLORIDE; POTASSIUM CHLORIDE; POTASSIUM PHOSPHATE, DIBASIC; SODIUM CHLORIDE
INJECTABLE; INJECTION
AMINOSYN II 10% W/ ELECTROLYTES
  ABBOTT 10%;102 MG/100 ML;45 MG/
  100 ML;522 MG/
  100 ML;410 MG/100 ML N19437 004 APR 03, 1986

AMINOSYN II 7% W/ ELECTROLYTES
  ABBOTT 7%;102 MG/100 ML;45 MG/
  100 ML;522 MG/
  100 ML;410 MG/100 ML N19437 006 APR 03, 1986

AMINOSYN II 8.5% W/ ELECTROLYTES
  ABBOTT 8.5%;102 MG/100 ML;45 MG/
  100 ML;522 MG/
  100 ML;410 MG/100 ML N19437 005 APR 03, 1986

AMINO ACIDS; MAGNESIUM CHLORIDE; POTASSIUM CHLORIDE; SODIUM CHLORIDE; SODIUM PHOSPHATE, DIBASIC
INJECTABLE; INJECTION
AMINOSYN II 3.5% M
  ABBOTT 3.5%;30 MG/100 ML;97 MG/
  100 ML;120 MG/
  100 ML;49 MG/100 ML N19437 007 APR 03, 1986

AMINO ACIDS; MAGNESIUM CHLORIDE; POTASSIUM PHOSPHATE, DIBASIC; SODIUM ACETATE; SODIUM CHLORIDE
INJECTABLE; INJECTION
TRAVASOL 3.5% W/ ELECTROLYTES
  BAXTER 3.5%;51 MG/100 ML;131 MG/
  100 ML;218 MG/
  100 ML;35 MG/100 ML N17493 003

TRAVASOL 5.5% W/ ELECTROLYTES
  BAXTER 5.5%;102 MG/
  100 ML;522 MG/
  100 ML;431 MG/
  100 ML;224 MG/100 ML N17493 001

TRAVASOL 8.5% W/ ELECTROLYTES
  BAXTER 8.5%;102 MG/
  100 ML;522 MG/
  100 ML;594 MG/
  100 ML;154 MG/100 ML N17493 002

AMINO ACIDS; MAGNESIUM CHLORIDE; POTASSIUM PHOSPHATE, DIBASIC; SODIUM CHLORIDE
INJECTABLE; INJECTION
AMINOSYN 7% W/ ELECTROLYTES
  ABBOTT 7%;102 MG/100 ML;522 MG/
  100 ML;410 MG/100 ML N17789 002

AMINOSYN 8.5% W/ ELECTROLYTES
  ABBOTT 8.5%;102 MG/
  100 ML;522 MG/
  100 ML;410 MG/100 ML N17673 005

AMINOCAPROIC ACID
INJECTABLE; INJECTION
AMICAR
AP LEDERLE 250 MG/ML N15229 002
AMINOCAPROIC ACID
AP ABBOTT 250 MG/ML N70888 001 JUN 16, 1988
AP ELKINS SINN 250 MG/ML N18590 001 OCT 29, 1982
AP LUITPOLD 250 MG/ML N71192 001 DEC 01, 1987
AP LYPHOMED 250 MG/ML N70522 001 JUN 17, 1986
AMINOCAPROIC ACID IN PLASTIC CONTAINER
AP ABBOTT 250 MG/ML N70010 001 MAR 09, 1987

SYRUP; ORAL
AMICAR
  LEDERLE 1.25 GM/5 ML N15230 002
TABLET; ORAL
AMICAR
+ LEDERLE 500 MG N15197 001

AMINOGLUTETHIMIDE
TABLET; ORAL
CYTADREN
+ CIBA 250 MG N18202 001

AMINOHIPPURATE SODIUM
INJECTABLE; INJECTION
AMINOHIPPURATE SODIUM
  MSD 20% N05619 001

AMINOPHYLLINE
ENEMA; RECTAL
SOMOPHYLLIN
  FISONS 300 MG/5 ML N18232 001 APR 02, 1982

Prescription Drug Products (continued)

AMINOPHYLLINE (continued)

INJECTABLE; INJECTION

AMINOPHYLLIN

TE	Manufacturer	Strength	Appl. No.	Date
AP	SEARLE	25 MG/ML	N87243 001	MAY 24, 1982

AMINOPHYLLINE

TE	Manufacturer	Strength	Appl. No.	Date
AP	ABBOTT	25 MG/ML	N87242 001	OCT 26, 1983
			N87601 001	JUL 23, 1982
AP	BEECHAM	25 MG/ML	N86606 001	
AP	BRISTOL	25 MG/ML	N87431 001	
AP	ELKINS SINN	25 MG/ML	N87239 001	
AP	GENSIA	25 MG/ML	N81142 001	SEP 25, 1991
AP	INTL MEDICATION	25 MG/ML	N87209 001	FEB 01, 1982
AP	LUITPOLD	25 MG/ML	N87240 001	
AP	LYPHOMED	25 MG/ML	N87600 001	
AP		25 MG/ML	N87200 001	
AP		25 MG/ML	N87250 001	JAN 06, 1982
AP		25 MG/ML	N87886 001	AUG 30, 1983
AP		25 MG/ML	N88407 001	JAN 25, 1984
AP	PHARMA SERVE	25 MG/ML	N87387 001	JUN 03, 1983
AP		25 MG/ML	N87392 001	DEC 15, 1983
AP	SMITH NEPHEW SOLOPAK	25 MG/ML	N88749 001	MAY 30, 1985

AMINOPHYLLINE IN SODIUM CHLORIDE 0.45%

TE	Manufacturer	Strength	Appl. No.	Date
AP	ABBOTT	100 MG/100 ML	N88147 002	MAY 03, 1983
			N88147 001	
		200 MG/100 ML	N88147 003	MAY 03, 1982

SOLUTION; ORAL

AMINOPHYLLINE

TE	Manufacturer	Strength	Appl. No.	Date
AA	PHARM BASICS	105 MG/5 ML	N88156 001	DEC 05, 1983
AA	ROXANE	105 MG/5 ML	N88126 001	AUG 19, 1983

AMINOPHYLLINE DYE FREE

TE	Manufacturer	Strength	Appl. No.	Date
AA	BARRE	105 MG/5 ML	N87727 001	APR 16, 1982

SOMOPHYLLIN

TE	Manufacturer	Strength	Appl. No.	Date
AA	FISONS	105 MG/5 ML	N86466 001	

SOMOPHYLLIN-DF

TE	Manufacturer	Strength	Appl. No.	Date
AA	FISONS	105 MG/5 ML	N87045 001	

SUPPOSITORY; RECTAL

TRUPHYLLINE

Manufacturer	Strength	Appl. No.	Date
G AND W	250 MG	N85498 001	MAR 23, 1983
	500 MG	N85498 002	JAN 03, 1983

AMINOPHYLLINE (continued)

TABLET; ORAL

AMINOPHYLLIN

TE	Manufacturer	Strength	Appl. No.
AB +	SEARLE	100 MG	N02386 002
AB +		200 MG	N02386 003

AMINOPHYLLINE

TE	Manufacturer	Strength	Appl. No.	Date
AB	GENEVA	100 MG	N85262 002	
AB		200 MG	N85261 002	
BD	HALSEY	100 MG	N84674 001	
BD	LANNETT	100 MG	N84588 001	
BD		200 MG	N84588 002	
BD	PHOENIX LABS	100 MG	N85409 001	
BD		200 MG	N85410 001	
BD	RICHLYN	100 MG	N84574 001	
BD		200 MG	N84576 001	
AB	ROXANE	100 MG	N87500 001	FEB 09, 1982
		200 MG	N87501 001	FEB 09, 1982
AB	WEST WARD	100 MG	N84540 001	
AB		200 MG	N85003 001	

TABLET, EXTENDED RELEASE; ORAL

PHYLLOCONTIN

Manufacturer	Strength	Appl. No.
+ PURDUE FREDERICK	225 MG	N86760 001

AMINOSALICYLATE SODIUM

POWDER; ORAL

P.A.S. SODIUM

TE	Manufacturer	Strength	Appl. No.
AA	CENTURY	4 GM/PACKET	N80947 001

SODIUM AMINOSALICYLATE

TE	Manufacturer	Strength	Appl. No.
AA	HEXCEL	100%	N80097 001

TABLET; ORAL

SODIUM P.A.S.

Manufacturer	Strength	Appl. No.
+ LANNETT	500 MG	N80138 002

AMINOSALICYLATE SODIUM; AMINOSALICYLIC ACID

TABLET; ORAL

NEOPASALATE

Manufacturer	Strength	Appl. No.
+ WALLACE	846 MG;112 MG	N80059 002

AMINOSALICYLIC ACID; *MULTIPLE*

SEE AMINOSALICYLATE SODIUM; AMINOSALICYLIC ACID

AMIODARONE HYDROCHLORIDE

TABLET; ORAL

CORDARONE

Manufacturer	Strength	Appl. No.	Date
+ WYETH AYERST	200 MG	N18972 001	DEC 24, 1985

Prescription Drug Products (continued)

AMITRIPTYLINE HYDROCHLORIDE

CONCENTRATE; ORAL
  ENDEP

	ROCHE	40 MG/ML	N85749 001

INJECTABLE; INJECTION
  AMITRIPTYLINE HCL

ΔP	STERIS	10 MG/ML	N85594 001

  ELAVIL

ΔP	MSD	10 MG/ML	N12704 001

TABLET; ORAL
  AMITRIPTYLINE HCL

Code	Manufacturer	Strength	Application No.	Date
ΔB	BIOCRAFT	10 MG	N84910 003	
ΔB		25 MG	N85031 001	
ΔB		50 MG	N85032 001	
ΔB		75 MG	N85030 001	
ΔB		100 MG	N85836 001	
ΔB	CHELSEA	10 MG	N85816 001	
ΔB		25 MG	N85817 001	
ΔB		50 MG	N85815 001	
ΔB		75 MG	N85819 001	
BP		100 MG	N85820 001	
ΔB	COPLEY	10 MG	N88421 001	APR 30, 1984
BP		25 MG	N88422 001	APR 30, 1984
BP		50 MG	N88423 001	APR 30, 1984
BP		75 MG	N88424 001	APR 30, 1984
BP		100 MG	N88425 001	APR 30, 1984
BP		150 MG	N88426 001	APR 30, 1984
ΔB	DANBURY	10 MG	N88620 001	
ΔB		25 MG	N88621 001	MAR 02, 1984
ΔB		50 MG	N88622 001	MAR 02, 1984
ΔB		75 MG	N88633 001	MAR 02, 1984
ΔB		100 MG	N88634 001	MAR 02, 1984
ΔB		150 MG	N88635 001	MAR 02, 1984
ΔB	GENEVA	10 MG	N85969 001	
ΔB		25 MG	N85966 001	
ΔB		50 MG	N85968 001	
ΔB		75 MG	N85967 001	
ΔB		100 MG	N85970 001	
ΔB		150 MG	N85971 001	
BP	HALSEY	10 MG	N85923 001	
BP		25 MG	N85922 001	
BP		50 MG	N85925 001	
BP		75 MG	N85926 001	MAY 20, 1983
BP		100 MG	N85927 001	MAY 20, 1983

AMITRIPTYLINE HYDROCHLORIDE (continued)

INJECTABLE; INJECTION
  AMITRIPTYLINE HCL

Code	Manufacturer	Strength	Application No.	Date
ΔB	LEMMON	10 MG	N86610 001	
ΔB		25 MG	N86859 001	
ΔB		50 MG	N86857 001	
ΔB		75 MG	N86860 001	
ΔB		100 MG	N86854 001	
ΔB		150 MG	N86853 001	
ΔB	MD PHARM	10 MG	N85864 001	
ΔB		25 MG	N85935 001	
ΔB		50 MG	N85936 001	
ΔB		75 MG	N86337 001	
ΔB		100 MG	N86336 001	
ΔB		150 MG	N86335 001	
ΔB	MUTUAL PHARM	10 MG	N89398 001	JUL 14, 1987
ΔB		25 MG	N89399 001	JUL 14, 1987
ΔB		50 MG	N89400 001	JUL 14, 1987
ΔB		75 MG	N89401 001	JUL 14, 1987
ΔB		100 MG	N89402 001	JUL 14, 1987
ΔB		150 MG	N89403 001	JUL 14, 1987
ΔB	MYLAN	10 MG	N86157 001	
ΔB		25 MG	N86010 001	
ΔB		50 MG	N86009 001	
ΔB		75 MG	N86011 001	
ΔB		100 MG	N86158 001	
ΔB		150 MG	N86153 001	
ΔB	PUREPAC	10 MG	N88075 001	SEP 16, 1983
ΔB		25 MG	N88076 001	MAY 20, 1983
ΔB		50 MG	N88077 001	SEP 16, 1983
ΔB		75 MG	N88078 001	SEP 16, 1983
ΔB		100 MG	N88079 001	SEP 16, 1983
ΔB	ROXANE	10 MG	N86002 001	
ΔB		25 MG	N85944 001	
ΔB		50 MG	N85945 001	
ΔB		75 MG	N86004 001	
ΔB		100 MG	N86003 001	
ΔB		150 MG	N86090 001	

Prescription Drug Products (continued)

AMITRIPTYLINE HYDROCHLORIDE (continued)
INJECTABLE; INJECTION
AMITRIPTYLINE HCL

	Firm	Strength	Appl. No.	Approval
AB	SIDMAK	10 MG	N88883 001	SEP 26, 1984
AB		25 MG	N88884 001	SEP 26, 1984
AB		50 MG	N88885 001	SEP 26, 1984
AB		75 MG	N88886 001	SEP 26, 1984
AB		100 MG	N88887 001	SEP 26, 1984
AB		150 MG	N88888 001	SEP 26, 1984
AB	SUPERPHARM	10 MG	N88853 001	NOV 13, 1984
AB		25 MG	N88854 001	NOV 13, 1984
AB		50 MG	N88855 001	NOV 13, 1984
AB		75 MG	N88856 001	NOV 13, 1984
AB		100 MG	N88857 001	NOV 13, 1984

ELAVIL

	Firm	Strength	Appl. No.
AB +	MSD	10 MG	N12703 001
AB		25 MG	N12703 003
AB		50 MG	N12703 004
AB		75 MG	N12703 005
AB		100 MG	N12703 006
AB		150 MG	N12703 007

ENDEP

	Firm	Strength	Appl. No.
AB	ROCHE	10 MG	N83639 001
AB		25 MG	N83639 002
AB		50 MG	N83639 003
AB		75 MG	N83639 004
AB		100 MG	N83639 005
AB		150 MG	N85303 001

AMITRIPTYLINE HYDROCHLORIDE; CHLORDIAZEPOXIDE
TABLET; ORAL
CHLORDIAZEPOXIDE AND AMITRIPTYLINE HCL

	Firm	Strength	Appl. No.	Approval
AB	BARR	EQ 12.5 MG BASE;5 MG	N70765 001	DEC 10, 1986
AB		EQ 25 MG BASE;10 MG	N70766 001	DEC 10, 1986
AB	DANBURY	EQ 12.5 MG BASE;5 MG	N70052 001	DEC 16, 1988
AB		EQ 25 MG BASE;10 MG	N70053 001	DEC 16, 1988
AB	MYLAN	EQ 12.5 MG BASE;5 MG	N71296 001	DEC 10, 1986
AB		EQ 25 MG BASE;10 MG	N71297 001	DEC 10, 1986
AB	PAR	EQ 12.5 MG BASE;5 MG	N72277 001	MAY 09, 1988
AB		EQ 25 MG BASE;10 MG	N72278 001	MAY 09, 1988

AMITRIPTYLINE HYDROCHLORIDE; CHLORDIAZEPOXIDE (continued)
TABLET; ORAL
LIMBITROL

	Firm	Strength	Appl. No.
AB +	ROCHE	EQ 12.5 MG BASE;5 MG	N16949 001
AB		EQ 25 MG BASE;10 MG	N16949 002

AMITRIPTYLINE HYDROCHLORIDE; PERPHENAZINE
TABLET; ORAL
ETRAFON 2-10

	Firm	Strength	Appl. No.
BP	SCHERING	10 MG;2 MG	N14713 007

ETRAFON 2-25

	Firm	Strength	Appl. No.
BP	SCHERING	25 MG;2 MG	N14713 004

ETRAFON-A

	Firm	Strength	Appl. No.
BP	SCHERING	10 MG;4 MG	N14713 002

ETRAFON-FORTE

	Firm	Strength	Appl. No.
BP	SCHERING	25 MG;4 MG	N14713 006

PERPHENAZINE AND AMITRIPTYLINE HCL

	Firm	Strength	Appl. No.	Approval
AB	BARR	10 MG;2 MG	N71077 001	NOV 12, 1986
AB		10 MG;4 MG	N71078 001	NOV 12, 1986
AB		25 MG;2 MG	N70297 001	NOV 12, 1986
AB		25 MG;4 MG	N71079 001	NOV 12, 1986
AB	DANBURY	10 MG;2 MG	N72539 001	FEB 15, 1989
AB		10 MG;4 MG	N72540 001	FEB 15, 1989
AB		25 MG;2 MG	N72541 001	FEB 15, 1989
AB		25 MG;4 MG	N72134 001	FEB 15, 1989
AB		50 MG;4 MG	N72135 001	FEB 15, 1989
AB	GENEVA	10 MG;2 MG	N71062 001	NOV 27, 1987
AB		10 MG;4 MG	N71862 001	DEC 21, 1987
AB		25 MG;2 MG	N71063 001	NOV 27, 1987
AB		25 MG;4 MG	N71064 001	NOV 27, 1987
AB		50 MG;4 MG	N71863 001	DEC 21, 1987
AB	MYLAN	10 MG;2 MG	N70336 001	NOV 10, 1988
AB		10 MG;4 MG	N71442 001	NOV 10, 1988
AB		25 MG;2 MG	N70337 001	NOV 10, 1988
AB		25 MG;4 MG	N70338 001	NOV 10, 1988
AB		50 MG;4 MG	N71443 001	NOV 10, 1988

Prescription Drug Products (continued)

AMITRIPTYLINE HYDROCHLORIDE; PERPHENAZINE (continued)

TABLET; ORAL
PERPHENAZINE AND AMITRIPTYLINE HCL

ΔB	PAR	10MG;2MG	N70565 001 SEP 11, 1986
ΔB		10MG;4MG	N70620 001 SEP 11, 1986
ΔB		25MG;2MG	N70621 001 SEP 11, 1986
ΔB		25MG;4MG	N70595 001 SEP 11, 1986
ΔB		50MG;4MG	N70574 001 SEP 11, 1986
ΔB	ROYCE	10MG;2MG	N73007 001 OCT 17, 1991
ΔB		10MG;4MG	N73009 001 OCT 17, 1991
ΔB		25MG;2MG	N73008 001 OCT 17, 1991
ΔB		25MG;4MG	N73010 001 OCT 17, 1991
ΔB	ZENITH	10MG;2MG	N70935 001 SEP 11, 1986
ΔB		10MG;4MG	N70937 001 SEP 11, 1986
ΔB		25MG;2MG	N70936 001 SEP 11, 1986
ΔB		25MG;4MG	N70938 001 SEP 11, 1986
ΔB		50MG;4MG	N70939 001 SEP 12, 1986
ΔB	TRIAVIL 2-10 MSD	10MG;2MG	N14715 004
ΔB	TRIAVIL 2-25 MSD	25MG;2MG	N14715 002
ΔB	TRIAVIL 4-10 MSD	10MG;4MG	N14715 003
ΔB	TRIAVIL 4-25 + MSD	25MG;4MG	N14715 005
ΔB	TRIAVIL 4-50 + MSD	50MG;4MG	N14715 006

AMLODIPINE BESYLATE

TABLET; ORAL
NORVASC

	PFIZER	EQ 2.5 MG BASE	N19787 001 JUL 31, 1992
		EQ 5 MG BASE	N19787 002 JUL 31, 1992
		EQ 10 MG BASE	N19787 003 JUL 31, 1992

AMMONIUM CHLORIDE

INJECTABLE; INJECTION
AMMONIUM CHLORIDE

ΔP	ABBOTT	5 MEQ/ML	N83130 001

AMMONIUM CHLORIDE IN PLASTIC CONTAINER

ΔP	ABBOTT	5 MEQ/ML	N88366 001 JUN 13, 1984

AMMONIUM LACTATE

LOTION; TOPICAL
LAC-HYDRIN

	WESTWOOD SQUIBB	EQ 12% ACID	N19155 001 APR 24, 1985

AMOXAPINE

TABLET; ORAL
AMOXAPINE

ΔB	DANBURY	25 MG	N72688 001 AUG 28, 1992
ΔB		50 MG	N72689 001 AUG 28, 1992
ΔB		100 MG	N72690 001 AUG 28, 1992
ΔB		150 MG	N72691 001 AUG 28, 1992
ΔB	GENEVA	25 MG	N72943 001 JUN 28, 1991
ΔB		50 MG	N72944 001 JUN 28, 1991
ΔB		100 MG	N72878 001 JUN 28, 1991
ΔB		150 MG	N72879 001 JUN 28, 1991
ΔB	WATSON	25 MG	N72418 001 JUN 28, 1991
ΔB		50 MG	N72419 001 MAY 11, 1989
ΔB		100 MG	N72420 001 MAY 11, 1989
ΔB		150 MG	N72421 001 MAY 11, 1989

ASENDIN

ΔB	LEDERLE	25 MG	N18021 001 MAY 11, 1989
ΔB		50 MG	N18021 002
ΔB	+	100 MG	N18021 003
ΔB		150 MG	N18021 004

Prescription Drug Products (continued)

AMOXICILLIN

CAPSULE; ORAL

AMOXICILLIN

TE	Firm / Brand	Strength	Appl. No.	Approval Date
AB	ATRAL	250 MG	N62528 001	AUG 07, 1985
AB		500 MG	N62528 002	AUG 07, 1985
AB	BIOCRAFT	250 MG	N61926 001	
AB		500 MG	N61926 003	
AB	CLONMEL	250 MG	N62884 001	FEB 25, 1988
AB		500 MG	N62881 001	FEB 25, 1988
AB	LEMMON	250 MG	N63030 001	FEB 28, 1989
AB		500 MG	N63031 001	FEB 28, 1989
AB	MYLAN	250 MG	N62067 001	
AB		500 MG	N62067 002	
AB	NOVOPHARM	250 MG	N62853 001	DEC 22, 1987
AB		500 MG	N62854 001	DEC 22, 1987
+	AMOXIL — BEECHAM	250 MG	N50459 001	
+		250 MG	N62216 001	
+		500 MG	N50459 002	
AB	COMOX — COPANOS	250 MG	N62058 001	
AB		500 MG	N62058 002	
AB	LAROTID — BEECHAM	250 MG	N62216 003	
AB		500 MG	N62216 004	
AB	POLYMOX — BRISTOL	250 MG	N61885 001	
AB		500 MG	N61885 002	
AB	BRISTOL MYERS	250 MG	N63099 001	MAR 20, 1992
AB		500 MG	N63099 002	MAR 20, 1992
AB	TRIMOX — SQUIBB	250 MG	N62098 001	
AB		250 MG	N62152 001	
AB		500 MG	N62098 002	
AB		500 MG	N62152 002	
AB	WYMOX — WYETH AYERST	250 MG	N62120 001	
AB		500 MG	N62120 002	

AMOXICILLIN (continued)

POWDER FOR RECONSTITUTION; ORAL

AMOXICILLIN

TE	Firm / Brand	Strength	Appl. No.	Approval Date
AB	BIOCRAFT	125 MG/5 ML	N61931 001	
AB		250 MG/5 ML	N61931 002	
BX	CLONMEL	125 MG/5 ML	N62927 001	NOV 25, 1988
BX		250 MG/5 ML	N62927 002	NOV 25, 1988
AB	MYLAN	125 MG/5 ML	N62090 001	
AB		125 MG/5 ML	N62090 002	
AB	NOVOPHARM	250 MG/5 ML	N62946 001	NOV 01, 1988
AB		250 MG/5 ML	N63001 001	JAN 06, 1989

AMOXICILLIN PEDIATRIC

TE	Firm / Brand	Strength	Appl. No.	Approval Date
AB	BIOCRAFT	50 MG/ML	N61931 003	

AMOXICILLIN TRIHYDRATE

TE	Firm / Brand	Strength	Appl. No.	Approval Date
AB	COPANOS	125 MG/5 ML	N62059 001	DEC 01, 1982
AB		250 MG/5 ML	N62059 002	
AB	AMOXIL — BEECHAM	125 MG/5 ML	N50460 001	
AB		125 MG/5 ML	N62226 001	
+		250 MG/5 ML	N50460 002	
+		50 MG/ML	N50460 005	
AB		250 MG/5 ML	N62226 002	
AB		50 MG/ML	N62226 005	
AB	LAROTID — BEECHAM	125 MG/5 ML	N62226 003	
AB		50 MG/ML	N50460 006	
AB		250 MG/5 ML	N62226 004	
AB	POLYMOX — BRISTOL	125 MG/5 ML	N61851 001	
AB		125 MG/5 ML	N61886 002	
AB		250 MG/5 ML	N62323 001	
AB		250 MG/5 ML	N61851 002	
AB		50 MG/ML	N61886 003	
AB		250 MG/5 ML	N62323 002	
AB	BRISTOL MYERS	125 MG/5 ML	N62885 001	
AB		250 MG/5 ML	N62885 002	MAR 08, 1988
AB	TRIMOX — SQUIBB	125 MG/5 ML	N62099 001	
AB		125 MG/5 ML	N62154 001	
AB		250 MG/5 ML	N62099 002	
AB		250 MG/5 ML	N62154 002	
AB	WYMOX — WYETH AYERST	125 MG/5 ML	N62131 001	
AB		250 MG/5 ML	N62131 002	

TABLET, CHEWABLE; ORAL

AMOXIL — BEECHAM

TE	Strength	Appl. No.
+	125 MG	N50542 002
+	250 MG	N50542 001

Prescription Drug Products (*continued*)

AMOXICILLIN; CLAVULANATE POTASSIUM
POWDER FOR RECONSTITUTION; ORAL

	Strength	Firm	Appl. No.	Date
AUGMENTIN '125'	125 MG/5 ML;EQ 31.25 MG ACID/5 ML	+ BEECHAM	N50575 001	AUG 06, 1984
AUGMENTIN '250'	250 MG/5 ML;EQ 62.5 MG ACID/5 ML	+ BEECHAM	N50575 002	AUG 06, 1984

TABLET; ORAL

	Strength	Firm	Appl. No.	Date
AUGMENTIN '250'	250 MG;EQ 125 MG ACID	+ BEECHAM	N50564 001	AUG 06, 1984
AUGMENTIN '500'	500 MG;EQ 125 MG ACID	+ BEECHAM	N50564 002	AUG 06, 1984

TABLET, CHEWABLE; ORAL

	Strength	Firm	Appl. No.	Date
AUGMENTIN '125'	125 MG;EQ 31.25 MG ACID	+ BEECHAM	N50597 001	JUL 22, 1985
AUGMENTIN '250'	250 MG;EQ 62.5 MG ACID	+ BEECHAM	N50597 002	JUL 22, 1985

AMPHETAMINE ADIPATE; AMPHETAMINE SULFATE; DEXTROAMPHETAMINE ADIPATE; DEXTROAMPHETAMINE SULFATE
CAPSULE; ORAL

	Strength	Firm	Appl. No.
DELCOBESE	1.25 MG;1.25 MG;1.25 MG;1.25 MG	LEMMON	N83564 001
	2.5 MG;2.5 MG;2.5 MG;2.5 MG		N83564 002
	3.75 MG;3.75 MG;3.75 MG;3.75 MG		N83564 003
	5 MG;5 MG;5 MG;5 MG		N83564 004

TABLET; ORAL

	Strength	Firm	Appl. No.
DELCOBESE	1.25 MG;1.25 MG;1.25 MG;1.25 MG	LEMMON	N83563 004
	2.5 MG;2.5 MG;2.5 MG;2.5 MG		N83563 003
	3.75 MG;3.75 MG;3.75 MG;3.75 MG		N83563 002
	5 MG;5 MG;5 MG;5 MG		N83563 001

AMPHETAMINE RESIN COMPLEX; DEXTROAMPHETAMINE RESIN COMPLEX
CAPSULE, EXTENDED RELEASE; ORAL

	Strength	Firm	Appl. No.
BIPHETAMINE 12.5	EQ 6.25 MG BASE;EQ 6.25 MG BASE	FISONS	N10093 007
BIPHETAMINE 20	EQ 10 MG BASE;EQ 10 MG BASE	+ FISONS	N10093 003
BIPHETAMINE 7.5	EQ 3.75 MG BASE;EQ 3.75 MG BASE	FISONS	N10093 009

AMPHETAMINE SULFATE
TABLET; ORAL

	Strength	Firm	Appl. No.	Date
AMPHETAMINE SULFATE	5 MG	LANNETT	N83901 001	AUG 31, 1984
	10 MG		N83901 002	AUG 31, 1984

AMPHETAMINE SULFATE; *MULTIPLE*
SEE AMPHETAMINE ADIPATE; AMPHETAMINE SULFATE; DEXTROAMPHETAMINE ADIPATE; DEXTROAMPHETAMINE SULFATE

AMPHOTERICIN B
CREAM; TOPICAL

	Strength	Firm	Appl. No.
FUNGIZONE	3%	SQUIBB	N50314 001

INJECTABLE; INJECTION

		Strength	Firm	Appl. No.	Date
AMPHOTERICIN B	AP	50 MG/VIAL	LYPHOMED	N62728 001	APR 13, 1987
	AP	50 MG/VIAL	PHARMA TEK	N63206 001	APR 29, 1992
FUNGIZONE	AP	50 MG/VIAL	SQUIBB	N60517 001	

LOTION; TOPICAL

		Strength	Firm	Appl. No.
FUNGIZONE	AP	3%	SQUIBB	N60570 001

OINTMENT; TOPICAL

		Strength	Firm	Appl. No.
FUNGIZONE	AP	3%	SQUIBB	N50313 001

AMPICILLIN SODIUM
INJECTABLE; INJECTION

		Strength	Firm	Appl. No.	Date
AMPICILLIN SODIUM	AP	EQ 125 MG BASE/VIAL	ELKINS SINN	N62692 001	JUN 24, 1986
	AP	EQ 250 MG BASE/VIAL		N62692 002	JUN 24, 1986
	AP	EQ 500 MG BASE/VIAL		N62692 003	JUN 24, 1986
	AP	EQ 1 GM BASE/VIAL		N62692 004	JUN 24, 1986
	AP	EQ 2 GM BASE/VIAL		N62692 005	JUN 24, 1986
	AP	EQ 10 GM BASE/VIAL		N62692 006	JUN 24, 1986
	AP	EQ 250 MG BASE/VIAL	IBI	N62719 001	MAY 12, 1987
	AP	EQ 500 MG BASE/VIAL		N62719 003	MAY 12, 1987
	AP	EQ 1 GM BASE/VIAL		N62719 002	MAY 12, 1987

Prescription Drug Products (continued)

AMPICILLIN SODIUM (continued)

INJECTABLE; INJECTION

AMPICILLIN SODIUM

LILLY

AP	EQ 500 MG BASE/VIAL	N62565 001	APR 04, 1985
AP	EQ 1 GM BASE/VIAL	N62565 002	APR 04, 1985
AP	EQ 2 GM BASE/VIAL	N62565 003	JUN 24, 1986

MARSAM

AP	EQ 125 MG BASE/VIAL	N62816 001	OCT 24, 1988
AP	EQ 250 MG BASE/VIAL	N62816 002	OCT 24, 1988
AP	EQ 500 MG BASE/VIAL	N62816 003	OCT 24, 1988
AP	EQ 1 GM BASE/VIAL	N62816 004	OCT 24, 1988
AP	EQ 2 GM BASE/VIAL	N62816 005	OCT 24, 1988
AP	EQ 10 GM BASE/VIAL	N62994 001	SEP 15, 1988

OMNIPEN-N
WYETH AYERST

AP	EQ 125 MG BASE/VIAL	N60626 001	DEC 16, 1986
AP	EQ 125 MG BASE/VIAL	N62718 001	DEC 16, 1986
AP	EQ 250 MG BASE/VIAL	N60626 002	DEC 16, 1986
AP	EQ 250 MG BASE/VIAL	N62718 002	DEC 16, 1986
AP	EQ 500 MG BASE/VIAL	N60626 003	DEC 16, 1986
AP	EQ 500 MG BASE/VIAL	N62718 003	DEC 16, 1986
AP	EQ 1 GM BASE/VIAL	N60626 004	DEC 16, 1986
AP	EQ 1 GM BASE/VIAL	N62718 004	DEC 16, 1986
AP	EQ 2 GM BASE/VIAL	N60626 005	DEC 16, 1986
AP	EQ 2 GM BASE/VIAL	N62718 005	DEC 16, 1986

PENBRITIN-S
WYETH AYERST

AP	EQ 125 MG BASE/VIAL	N50072 001
AP	EQ 250 MG BASE/VIAL	N50072 002
AP	EQ 500 MG BASE/VIAL	N50072 003
AP	EQ 1 GM BASE/VIAL	N50072 004
AP	EQ 2 GM BASE/VIAL	N50072 005
AP	EQ 4 GM BASE/VIAL	N50072 006

AMPICILLIN SODIUM (continued)

INJECTABLE; INJECTION

POLYCILLIN-N

BRISTOL

AP	EQ 125 MG BASE/VIAL	N61395 001	
AP	EQ 125 MG BASE/VIAL	N62860 001	FEB 05, 1988
AP	EQ 250 MG BASE/VIAL	N61395 002	
AP	EQ 250 MG BASE/VIAL	N62860 002	FEB 05, 1988
AP	EQ 500 MG BASE/VIAL	N61395 003	
AP	EQ 500 MG BASE/VIAL	N62860 003	FEB 05, 1988
AP	EQ 1 GM BASE/VIAL	N61395 004	
AP	EQ 1 GM BASE/VIAL	N62738 001	FEB 19, 1987
AP	EQ 1 GM BASE/VIAL	N62860 004	FEB 05, 1988
AP	EQ 2 GM BASE/VIAL	N61395 005	
AP	EQ 2 GM BASE/VIAL	N62738 002	FEB 19, 1987
AP	EQ 2 GM BASE/VIAL	N62860 005	FEB 05, 1988
AP	EQ 10 GM BASE/VIAL	N61395 006	

TOTACILLIN-N
BEECHAM

AP	EQ 125 MG BASE/VIAL	N60677 001	
AP	EQ 250 MG BASE/VIAL	N60677 002	
AP	EQ 500 MG BASE/VIAL	N60677 003	
AP	EQ 1 GM BASE/VIAL	N60677 004	
AP	EQ 1 GM BASE/VIAL	N62727 001	DEC 19, 1986
AP	EQ 2 GM BASE/VIAL	N60677 005	
AP	EQ 2 GM BASE/VIAL	N62727 002	DEC 19, 1986
AP	EQ 10 GM BASE/VIAL	N60677 006	

AMPICILLIN SODIUM; SULBACTAM SODIUM

INJECTABLE; INJECTION

UNASYN
PFIZER

EQ 500 MG BASE/VIAL;EQ 250 MG BASE/VIAL	N50608 003	DEC 31, 1986
EQ 1 GM BASE/VIAL;EQ 500 MG BASE/VIAL	N50608 002	DEC 31, 1986
EQ 1 GM BASE/VIAL;EQ 500 MG BASE/VIAL	N62901 001	NOV 23, 1988
EQ 2 GM BASE/VIAL;EQ 1 GM BASE/VIAL	N50608 001	DEC 31, 1986

Prescription Drug Products (continued)

AMPICILLIN/AMPICILLIN TRIHYDRATE

CAPSULE; ORAL

TE	Name	Strength	Appl. No.
	AMPICILLIN		
AB	BIOCRAFT	EQ 250 MG BASE	N61502 001
AB		EQ 500 MG BASE	N61502 002
AB	CLONMEL	EQ 250 MG BASE	N62883 001
			FEB 25, 1988
AB		EQ 500 MG BASE	N62882 001
			FEB 25, 1988
AB	ZENITH	EQ 250 MG BASE	N60765 001
AB		EQ 500 MG BASE	N60765 002
	AMPICILLIN TRIHYDRATE		
AB	COPANOS	EQ 250 MG BASE	N61602 001
AB		EQ 500 MG BASE	N61602 002
AB	MYLAN	EQ 250 MG BASE	N61755 001
AB		EQ 250 MG BASE	N61755 002
AB		EQ 500 MG BASE	N61853 002
AB	PUREPAC	EQ 500 MG BASE	
	OMNIPEN (AMPICILLIN)		
AB	WYETH AYERST	250 MG	N60624 001
AB		500 MG	N60624 002
	PFIZERPEN-A		
AB	PFIZER	EQ 250 MG BASE	N62050 001
AB		EQ 500 MG BASE	N62050 002
	POLYCILLIN		
AB	+ BRISTOL	EQ 250 MG BASE	N61392 001
AB		EQ 500 MG BASE	N61392 002
AB	BRISTOL MYERS	EQ 250 MG BASE	N62888 002
			MAR 04, 1988
AB	+	EQ 500 MG BASE	N62888 002
			MAR 04, 1988
	PRINCIPEN '250'		
AB	SQUIBB	EQ 250 MG BASE	N50056 001
AB		EQ 250 MG BASE	N62157 002
	PRINCIPEN '500'		
AB	SQUIBB	EQ 500 MG BASE	N50056 001
AB		EQ 500 MG BASE	N62157 001
	TOTACILLIN		
AB	BEECHAM	EQ 250 MG BASE	N60060 001
AB		EQ 250 MG BASE	N62212 001
AB		EQ 500 MG BASE	N60060 002
AB		EQ 500 MG BASE	N62212 002

POWDER FOR RECONSTITUTION; ORAL

TE	Name	Strength	Appl. No.
	AMPICILLIN		
AB	BIOCRAFT	EQ 125 MG BASE/5 ML	N61370 001
AB		EQ 250 MG BASE/5 ML	N61370 002
AB	CLONMEL	EQ 125 MG BASE/5 ML	N62982 001
			FEB 10, 1989
AB		EQ 250 MG BASE/5 ML	N62982 002
			FEB 10, 1989
	AMPICILLIN TRIHYDRATE		
AB	COPANOS	EQ 125 MG BASE/5 ML	N61601 001
AB		EQ 125 MG BASE/5 ML	N61601 002
AB	MYLAN	EQ 125 MG BASE/5 ML	N61829 002
AB		EQ 250 MG BASE/5 ML	N61829 001
AB	PUREPAC	EQ 250 MG BASE/5 ML	N61980 002

AMPICILLIN/AMPICILLIN TRIHYDRATE (continued)

POWDER FOR RECONSTITUTION; ORAL

TE	Name	Strength	Appl. No.
	OMNIPEN (AMPICILLIN)		
AB	WYETH AYERST	125 MG/5 ML	N60625 002
AB		250 MG/5 ML	N60625 003
AB		100 MG/ML	N60625 001
	PFIZERPEN-A		
AB	PFIZER	EQ 125 MG BASE/5 ML	N62049 001
AB		EQ 250 MG BASE/5 ML	N62049 002
	POLYCILLIN		
AB	BRISTOL	EQ 100 MG BASE/ML	N61394 001
AB	+	EQ 125 MG BASE/5 ML	N50308 001
AB		EQ 125 MG BASE/5 ML	N61394 002
AB		EQ 125 MG BASE/5 ML	N62297 001
AB	+	EQ 250 MG BASE/5 ML	N50308 002
AB		EQ 250 MG BASE/5 ML	N61394 003
AB		EQ 250 MG BASE/5 ML	N62297 002
AB	+	EQ 500 MG BASE/5 ML	N50308 003
	PRINCIPEN '125'		
AB	SQUIBB	EQ 125 MG BASE/5 ML	N60127 002
AB		EQ 125 MG BASE/5 ML	N62151 001
	PRINCIPEN '250'		
AB	SQUIBB	EQ 250 MG BASE/5 ML	N60127 001
AB		EQ 250 MG BASE/5 ML	N62151 002
	TOTACILLIN		
AB	BEECHAM	EQ 125 MG BASE/5 ML	N60666 001
AB		EQ 125 MG BASE/5 ML	N62223 001
AB		EQ 250 MG BASE/5 ML	N60666 002
AB		EQ 250 MG BASE/5 ML	N62223 002

AMPICILLIN/AMPICILLIN TRIHYDRATE; PROBENECID

CAPSULE; ORAL

TE	Name	Strength	Appl. No.
	PRINCIPEN W/ PROBENECID		
	+ SQUIBB	EQ 389 MG BASE;111 MG	N50488 001
		EQ 389 MG BASE;111 MG	N62150 001

POWDER FOR RECONSTITUTION; ORAL

TE	Name	Strength	Appl. No.
	POLYCILLIN-PRB		
AB	+ BRISTOL	EQ 3.5 GM BASE/BOT;1 GM/ BOT	N61898 001
	PROBAMPACIN		
AB	BIOCRAFT	EQ 3.5 GM BASE/BOT;1 GM/ BOT	N61741 001

AMRINONE LACTATE

INJECTABLE; INJECTION

TE	Name	Strength	Appl. No.
	INOCOR		
	STERLING	EQ 5 MG BASE/ML	N18700 001 JUL 31, 1984

ANISINDIONE

TABLET; ORAL

TE	Name	Strength	Appl. No.
	MIRADON		
	SCHERING	50 MG	N10909 003

Prescription Drug Products (continued)

ANISOTROPINE METHYLBROMIDE
TABLET; ORAL
VALPIN 50
DUPONT   50 MG   N13428 001

ANTAZOLINE PHOSPHATE; NAPHAZOLINE HYDROCHLORIDE
SOLUTION/DROPS; OPHTHALMIC
VASOCON-A
IOLAB   0.5%;0.05%   N18746 001 APR 30, 1990

APRACLONIDINE HYDROCHLORIDE
SOLUTION/DROPS; OPHTHALMIC
IOPIDINE
ALCON   EQ 1% BASE   N19779 001 DEC 31, 1987

ARGININE HYDROCHLORIDE
INJECTABLE; INJECTION
R-GENE 10
KABIVITRUM   10 GM/100 ML   N16931 001

ASCORBIC ACID; BIOTIN; CYANOCOBALAMIN; DEXPANTHENOL; ERGOCALCIFEROL; FOLIC ACID; NIACINAMIDE; PYRIDOXINE; RIBOFLAVIN PHOSPHATE SODIUM; THIAMINE; VITAMIN A; VITAMIN E
INJECTABLE; INJECTION
M.V.I.-12 LYOPHILIZED
ASTRA   100 MG/VIAL;0.06 MG/ VIAL;0.005 MG/ VIAL;15 MG/VIAL;5 MCG/ VIAL;0.4 MG/VIAL;40 MG/ VIAL;4 MG/VIAL;3.6 MG/ VIAL;3 MG/VIAL;1 MG/ VIAL;10 MG/VIAL   N18933 002 AUG 08, 1985

ASCORBIC ACID; BIOTIN; CYANOCOBALAMIN; DEXPANTHENOL; ERGOCALCIFEROL; FOLIC ACID; NIACINAMIDE; PYRIDOXINE HYDROCHLORIDE; RIBOFLAVIN PHOSPHATE SODIUM; THIAMINE HYDROCHLORIDE; VITAMIN A; VITAMIN E
INJECTABLE; INJECTION
M.V.C. 9+3
∆P LYPHOMED   10 MG/ML;0.006 MG/ ML;0.5 MCG/ML;1.5 MG/ ML;20 IU/ML;0.04 MG/ ML;4 MG/ML;0.4 MG/ ML;0.36 MG/ML;0.3 MG/ ML;330 UNITS /ML;1 IU/ ML   N18440 002 AUG 08, 1985

ASCORBIC ACID; BIOTIN; CYANOCOBALAMIN; DEXPANTHENOL; ERGOCALCIFEROL; FOLIC ACID; NIACINAMIDE; PYRIDOXINE HYDROCHLORIDE; RIBOFLAVIN PHOSPHATE SODIUM; THIAMINE HYDROCHLORIDE; VITAMIN A; VITAMIN E (continued)
INJECTABLE; INJECTION
M.V.I.-12
∆P ASTRA   10 MG/ML;0.006 MG/ ML;0.5 MCG/ML;1.5 MG/ ML;20 IU/ML;0.04 MG/ ML;4 MG/ML;0.4 MG/ ML;0.36 MG/ML;0.3 MG/ ML;330 UNITS /ML;1 IU/ ML   N08809 004 AUG 08, 1985

MVC PLUS
∆P STERIS   10 MG/ML;0.006 MG/ ML;0.5 MCG/ML;1.5 MG/ ML;20 IU/ML;0.04 MG/ ML;4 MG/ML;0.4 MG/ ML;0.36 MG/ML;0.3 MG/ ML;330 UNITS /ML;1 IU/ ML   N18439 002 AUG 08, 1985

ASPIRIN; *MULTIPLE*
SEE ACETAMINOPHEN; ASPIRIN; CODEINE PHOSPHATE

ASPIRIN; BUTALBITAL
TABLET; ORAL
AXOTAL
+ ADRIA   650 MG;50 MG   N88305 001 OCT 13, 1983

ASPIRIN; BUTALBITAL; CAFFEINE
CAPSULE; ORAL
BUTALBITAL, ASPIRIN AND CAFFEINE
∆B CHELSEA   325 MG;50 MG;40 MG   N86231 002 FEB 12, 1985

FIORINAL
∆B + SANDOZ   325 MG;50 MG;40 MG   N17534 005 APR 16, 1986

LANORINAL
∆B LANNETT   325 MG;50 MG;40 MG   N86996 002 OCT 11, 1985

TABLET; ORAL
ASPIRIN AND CAFFEINE W/ BUTALBITAL
∆B PUREPAC   325 MG;50 MG;40 MG   N86710 002 AUG 23, 1983

BUTAL COMPOUND
∆B GENEVA   325 MG;50 MG;40 MG   N86398 002 APR 06, 1984

Prescription Drug Products *(continued)*

ASPIRIN; BUTALBITAL; CAFFEINE *(continued)*

CAPSULE; ORAL

BUTALBITAL COMPOUND
ΔB	ZENITH	325 MG;50 MG;40 MG	N85441 002 OCT 31, 1984

BUTALBITAL W/ ASPIRIN & CAFFEINE
ΔB	PHARMAFAIR	325 MG;50 MG;40 MG	N87048 002 DEC 09, 1983

BUTALBITAL ASPIRIN & CAFFEINE
ΔB	HALSEY	325 MG;50 MG;40 MG	N89448 001 DEC 01, 1986

BUTALBITAL ASPIRIN AND CAFFEINE
ΔB	CHELSEA	325 MG;50 MG;40 MG	N86237 002 MAR 23, 1984
ΔB	WEST WARD	325 MG;50 MG;40 MG	N86162 002 FEB 16, 1984

FIORINAL
ΔB	+ SANDOZ	325 MG;50 MG;40 MG	N17534 003 APR 16, 1986

LANORINAL
ΔB	LANNETT	325 MG;50 MG;40 MG	N86986 002 OCT 18, 1985

ASPIRIN; BUTALBITAL; CAFFEINE; CODEINE PHOSPHATE

CAPSULE; ORAL

FIORINAL W/ CODEINE NO 3
	+ SANDOZ	325 MG;50 MG;40 MG;30 MG	N19429 003 OCT 26, 1990

ASPIRIN; CAFFEINE; DIHYDROCODEINE BITARTRATE

CAPSULE; ORAL

SYNALGOS-DC
	WYETH AYERST	356.4 MG;30 MG;16 MG	N11483 004 SEP 06, 1983

ASPIRIN; CAFFEINE; ORPHENADRINE CITRATE

TABLET; ORAL

NORGESIC
	3M	385 MG;30 MG;25 MG	N13416 003 OCT 27, 1982

NORGESIC FORTE
	+ 3M	770 MG;60 MG;50 MG	N13416 004 OCT 27, 1982

ASPIRIN; CAFFEINE; PROPOXYPHENE HYDROCHLORIDE

CAPSULE; ORAL

DARVON COMPOUND
ΔB	LILLY	389 MG;32.4 MG;32 MG	N10996 006 MAR 08, 1983

DARVON COMPOUND-65
ΔA	LILLY	389 MG;32.4 MG;65 MG	N10996 007 MAR 08, 1983

PROPOXYPHENE COMPOUND 65
ΔA	LEMMON	389 MG;32.4 MG;65 MG	N89025 001 MAR 29, 1985
ΔA	VITARINE	389 MG;32.4 MG;65 MG	N80044 002 SEP 16, 1983
ΔA	ZENITH	389 MG;32.4 MG;65 MG	N83077 002 DEC 07, 1984

PROPOXYPHENE COMPOUND-65
ΔA	GENEVA	389 MG;32.4 MG;65 MG	N83101 002 JUN 24, 1985

ASPIRIN; CARISOPRODOL

TABLET; ORAL

CARISOPRODOL AND ASPIRIN
ΔB	PAR	325 MG;200 MG	N89594 001 MAR 31, 1989

SOMA COMPOUND
ΔB	+ WALLACE	325 MG;200 MG	N12365 005 JUL 11, 1983

ASPIRIN; CARISOPRODOL; CODEINE PHOSPHATE

TABLET; ORAL

SOMA COMPOUND W/ CODEINE
ΔB	WALLACE	325 MG;200 MG;16 MG	N12366 002 JUL 11, 1983

ASPIRIN; HYDROCODONE BITARTRATE

TABLET; ORAL

AZDONE
	CENTRAL PHARMS	500 MG;5 MG	N89420 001 JAN 25, 1988

ASPIRIN; MEPROBAMATE

TABLET; ORAL

EQUAGESIC
ΔB	+ WYETH AYERST	325 MG;200 MG	N11702 003 DEC 29, 1983

MICRAININ
ΔB	WALLACE	325 MG;200 MG	N84978 001

Prescription Drug Products (continued)

ASPIRIN; METHOCARBAMOL

TABLET; ORAL

METHOCARBAMOL AND ASPIRIN

TE	Firm	Strength	Appl. No.	Date
AB	MCNEIL	325 MG;400 MG	N89193 001	FEB 12, 1986
AB	PAR	325 MG;400 MG	N89657 001	NOV 04, 1988
AB	ZENITH	325 MG;400 MG	N87211 001	DEC 22, 1982
AB	ROBAXISAL + ROBINS	325 MG;400 MG	N12281 001	

ASPIRIN; OXYCODONE HYDROCHLORIDE; OXYCODONE TEREPHTHALATE

TABLET; ORAL

CODOXY

TE	Firm	Strength	Appl. No.	Date
AA	HALSEY	325 MG;4.5 MG;0.38 MG	N87464 001	JUL 01, 1982

OXYCODONE AND ASPIRIN

TE	Firm	Strength	Appl. No.	Date
AA	BARR	325 MG;4.5 MG;0.38 MG	N87794 001	MAY 26, 1982

OXYCODONE AND ASPIRIN (HALF-STRENGTH)

TE	Firm	Strength	Appl. No.	Date
AA	ROXANE	325 MG;2.25 MG;0.19 MG	N87742 001	JUN 04, 1982

PERCODAN

TE	Firm	Strength	Appl. No.	Date
AA	DUPONT	325 MG;4.5 MG;0.38 MG	N07337 006	

PERCODAN-DEMI

TE	Firm	Strength	Appl. No.	Date
AA	DUPONT	325 MG;2.25 MG;0.19 MG	N07337 005	

ROXIPRIN

TE	Firm	Strength	Appl. No.	Date
AA	ROXANE	325 MG;4.5 MG;0.38 MG	N87743 001	JUN 04, 1982

ASPIRIN; PENTAZOCINE HYDROCHLORIDE

TABLET; ORAL

TALWIN COMPOUND

TE	Firm	Strength	Appl. No.	Date
	+ STERLING	325 MG;EQ 12.5 MG BASE	N16891 001	

ASPIRIN; PROPOXYPHENE HYDROCHLORIDE

CAPSULE; ORAL

DARVON W / ASA

TE	Firm	Strength	Appl. No.	Date
	LILLY	325 MG;65 MG	N10996 005	

ASPIRIN; PROPOXYPHENE NAPSYLATE

TABLET; ORAL

DARVON-N W / ASA

TE	Firm	Strength	Appl. No.	Date
	+ LILLY	325 MG;100 MG	N16863 001	

ASTEMIZOLE

TABLET; ORAL

HISMANAL

TE	Firm	Strength	Appl. No.	Date
	+ JANSSEN	10 MG	N19402 001	DEC 29, 1988

ATENOLOL

INJECTABLE; INJECTION

TENORMIN

TE	Firm	Strength	Appl. No.	Date
	ICI	0.5 MG/ML	N19058 001	SEP 13, 1989

TABLET; ORAL

ATENOLOL

TE	Firm	Strength	Appl. No.	Date
AB	APOTHECON	50 MG	N73317 001	MAR 20, 1992
		100 MG	N73318 001	MAR 20, 1992
AB	DANBURY	50 MG	N73352 001	DEC 27, 1991
		100 MG	N73353 001	DEC 27, 1991
AB	GENEVA	25 MG	N74052 001	MAY 01, 1992
		50 MG	N73025 001	SEP 17, 1991
		100 MG	N73026 001	SEP 17, 1991
AB	IPR	25 MG	N73646 001	JUL 31, 1992
		50 MG	N72303 001	JUL 15, 1988
		100 MG	N72304 001	JUL 15, 1988
AB	LEDERLE	25 MG	N74099 001	APR 28, 1992
		50 MG	N73542 001	DEC 19, 1991
		100 MG	N73543 001	DEC 19, 1991
AB	MYLAN	50 MG	N73456 001	JAN 24, 1992
		100 MG	N73457 001	JAN 24, 1992

TENORMIN

TE	Firm	Strength	Appl. No.	Date
AB	ICI	25 MG	N18240 004	APR 09, 1990
AB	+	50 MG	N18240 001	
AB		100 MG	N18240 002	

ATENOLOL; CHLORTHALIDONE

TABLET; ORAL

ATENOLOL AND CHLORTHALIDONE

TE	Firm	Strength	Appl. No.	Date
AB	DANBURY	50 MG;25 MG	N73665 001	JUL 02, 1992
AB		100 MG;25 MG	N73665 002	JUL 02, 1992
AB	IPR	50 MG;25 MG	N72301 001	MAY 31, 1990
AB		100 MG;25 MG	N72302 001	MAY 31, 1990

TENORETIC 100

TE	Firm	Strength	Appl. No.	Date
AB	+ ICI	100 MG;25 MG	N18760 001	JUN 08, 1984

TENORETIC 50

TE	Firm	Strength	Appl. No.	Date
AB	ICI	50 MG;25 MG	N18760 002	JUN 08, 1984

Prescription Drug Products *(continued)*

ATRACURIUM BESYLATE
INJECTABLE; INJECTION
TRACRIUM
BURROUGHS
WELLCOME   10 MG/ML   N18831 001   NOV 23, 1983

ATROPINE
INJECTABLE; INJECTION
ATROPEN
AP   SURVIVAL TECH   EQ 2 MG SULFATE/0.7ML   N17106 001
ATROPINE
AP   KALI DUPHAR   EQ 2 MG SULFATE/0.7ML   N71295 001   JAN 30, 1987

ATROPINE SULFATE
AEROSOL, METERED; INHALATION
ATROPINE SULFATE
US ARMY   EQ 0.36 MG BASE/INH   N20056 001   SEP 19, 1990

ATROPINE SULFATE; DIFENOXIN HYDROCHLORIDE
TABLET; ORAL
MOTOFEN
+ CARNRICK   0.025 MG;1 MG   N17744 002

ATROPINE SULFATE; DIPHENOXYLATE HYDROCHLORIDE
CAPSULE; ORAL
DIPHENOXYLATE HCL W/ ATROPINE SULFATE
SCHERER   0.025 MG;2.5 MG   N86440 001
SOLUTION; ORAL
COLONAID
AA   WALLACE   0.025 MG/5 ML;2.5 MG/5 ML   N85735 001
DIPHENOXYLATE HCL AND ATROPINE SULFATE
AA   ROXANE   0.025 MG/5 ML;2.5 MG/5 ML   N87708 001   MAY 03, 1982
LOMANATE
AA   BARRE   0.025 MG/5 ML;2.5 MG/5 ML   N85746 001
LOMOTIL
AA   SEARLE   0.025 MG/5 ML;2.5 MG/5 ML   N12699 001
TABLET; ORAL
COLONAID
AA   WALLACE   0.025 MG;2.5 MG   N85737 001
DI-ATRO
AA   MD PHARM   0.025 MG;2.5 MG   N85266 001
DIPHENOXYLATE HCL AND ATROPINE SULFATE
AA   BARR   0.025 MG;2.5 MG   N85506 001
AA   INWOOD   0.025 MG;2.5 MG   N85509 001
AA   MYLAN   0.025 MG;2.5 MG   N85762 001
AA   PHARMAFAIR   0.025 MG;2.5 MG   N85035 001
AA   ROXANE   0.025 MG;2.5 MG   N86057 001
AA   WEST WARD   0.025 MG;2.5 MG   N87765 001   MAR 15, 1982

ATROPINE SULFATE; DIPHENOXYLATE HYDROCHLORIDE *(continued)*
TABLET; ORAL
DIPHENOXYLATE HCL W/ ATROPINE SULFATE
ICN   0.025 MG;2.5 MG   N87195 001   FEB 16, 1982
AA   KV   0.025 MG;2.5 MG   N85659 001
AA   PRIVATE FORM   0.025 MG;2.5 MG   N85766 001
AA   ZENITH   0.025 MG;2.5 MG   N86727 001
LOFENE
AA   LANNETT   0.025 MG;2.5 MG   N85372 001
LOGEN
AA   SUPERPHARM   0.025 MG;2.5 MG   N88962 001   MAY 10, 1985
LOMOTIL
AA   SEARLE   0.025 MG;2.5 MG   N12462 001
LONOX
AA   GENEVA   0.025 MG;2.5 MG   N85311 002
LOW-QUEL
AA   HALSEY   0.025 MG;2.5 MG   N85211 001

ATROPINE SULFATE; EDROPHONIUM CHLORIDE
INJECTABLE; INJECTION
ENLON-PLUS
ANAQUEST   0.14 MG/ML;10 MG/ML   N19677 001   NOV 06, 1991
0.14 MG/ML;10 MG/ML   N19678 001   NOV 06, 1991

ATROPINE SULFATE; MEPERIDINE HYDROCHLORIDE
INJECTABLE; INJECTION
ATROPINE AND DEMEROL
STERLING   0.4 MG/ML;50 MG/ML   N87853 001   NOV 26, 1982
0.4 MG/ML;75 MG/ML   N87847 001   NOV 26, 1982
0.4 MG/ML;100 MG/ML   N87848 001   NOV 26, 1982

AURANOFIN
CAPSULE; ORAL
RIDAURA
+ SKF   3 MG   N18689 001   MAY 24, 1985

AZATADINE MALEATE
TABLET; ORAL
OPTIMINE
+ SCHERING   1 MG   N17601 001

Prescription Drug Products *(continued)*

AZATADINE MALEATE; PSEUDOEPHEDRINE SULFATE
TABLET, EXTENDED RELEASE; ORAL
TRINALIN
+ SCHERING   1 MG;120 MG   N18806 001
                                     MAR 23, 1982

AZATHIOPRINE
TABLET; ORAL
IMURAN
+ BURROUGHS
  WELLCOME   50 MG   N16324 001

AZATHIOPRINE SODIUM
INJECTABLE; INJECTION
AZATHIOPRINE
ΔP QUAD   EQ 100 MG BASE/VIAL   N71056 001
                                          JUN 08, 1988
IMURAN
ΔP BURROUGHS
    WELLCOME   EQ 100 MG BASE/VIAL   N17391 001

AZITHROMYCIN DIHYDRATE
CAPSULE; ORAL
ZITHROMAX
+ PFIZER   EQ 250 MG BASE   N50670 001
                                      NOV 01, 1991

AZLOCILLIN SODIUM
INJECTABLE; INJECTION
AZLIN
MILES
EQ 2 GM BASE/VIAL   N50562 001
                         SEP 03, 1982
EQ 2 GM BASE/VIAL   N62388 001
                         SEP 08, 1982
EQ 2 GM BASE/VIAL   N62417 001
                         OCT 12, 1982
EQ 3 GM BASE/VIAL   N50562 002
                         SEP 03, 1982
EQ 3 GM BASE/VIAL   N62388 002
                         SEP 08, 1982
EQ 3 GM BASE/VIAL   N62417 002
                         OCT 12, 1982
EQ 4 GM BASE/VIAL   N50562 003
                         SEP 03, 1982
EQ 4 GM BASE/VIAL   N62388 003
                         SEP 08, 1982
EQ 4 GM BASE/VIAL   N62417 003
                         OCT 12, 1982

AZTREONAM
INJECTABLE; INJECTION
AZACTAM
SQUIBB   500 MG/VIAL   N50580 001
                                 DEC 31, 1986
              1 GM/VIAL   N50580 002
                                 DEC 31, 1986
              2 GM/VIAL   N50580 003
                                 DEC 31, 1986

AZACTAM IN PLASTIC CONTAINER
SQUIBB   10 MG/ML   N50632 003
                              MAY 24, 1989
              20 MG/ML   N50632 002
                              MAY 24, 1989
              40 MG/ML   N50632 001
                              MAY 24, 1989

BACAMPICILLIN HYDROCHLORIDE
POWDER FOR RECONSTITUTION; ORAL
SPECTROBID
+ PFIZER   125 MG/5 ML   N50556 001
                                   MAR 23, 1982

TABLET; ORAL
SPECTROBID
+ PFIZER   400 MG   N50520 001

BACITRACIN
INJECTABLE; INJECTION
BACITRACIN
ΔP PFIZER   50,000 UNITS/VIAL   N60282 001
ΔP UPJOHN   50,000 UNITS/VIAL   N60733 002
                  10,000 UNITS/VIAL   N60733 001

OINTMENT; OPHTHALMIC
BACITRACIN
ΔT ALTANA   500 UNITS/GM   N61212 001
ΔT LILLY   500 UNITS/GM   N60687 001
ΔT PHARMADERM   500 UNITS/GM   N62158 001
ΔT PHARMAFAIR   500 UNITS/GM   N62453 001
                                       MAR 28, 1984

POWDER; FOR RX COMPOUNDING
BACI-RX
ΔA PHARMA TEK   5,000,000 UNITS/BOT   N61580 001
BACITRACIN
ΔA BRAE   5,000,000 UNITS/BOT   N61699 001
ΔA PADDOCK   5,000,000 UNITS/BOT   N62456 001
                                                JUL 27, 1983

BACITRACIN ZINC; NEOMYCIN SULFATE; POLYMYXIN B SULFATE
OINTMENT; OPHTHALMIC
BACITRACIN ZINC-NEOMYCIN SULFATE-POLYMYXIN B SULFATE

ΔT	PHARMAFAIR	400 UNITS/GM;EQ 3.5 MG BASE/GM;10,000 UNITS/GM	N62386 001	SEP 09, 1982

BACITRACIN-NEOMYCIN-POLYMYXIN

ΔT	ALTANA	400 UNITS/GM;EQ 3.5 MG BASE/GM;10,000 UNITS/GM	N60764 002	
	PHARMADERM	400 UNITS/GM;EQ 3.5 MG BASE/GM;5,000 UNITS/GM	N62167 001	
	NEO-POLYCIN DOW	500 UNITS/GM;EQ 3.5 MG BASE/GM;10,000 UNITS/GM	N60647 001	

NEOSPORIN

ΔT	BURROUGHS WELLCOME	400 UNITS/GM;EQ 3.5 MG BASE/GM;10,000 UNITS/GM	N50417 001	

BACITRACIN ZINC; POLYMYXIN B SULFATE
OINTMENT; OPHTHALMIC
OCUMYCIN

ΔT	PHARMAFAIR	500 UNITS/GM;10,000 UNITS/GM	N62430 001	APR 08, 1983

POLYSPORIN

ΔT	BURROUGHS WELLCOME	500 UNITS/GM;10,000 UNITS/GM	N61229 001	

BACLOFEN
INJECTABLE; INJECTION
LIORESAL

	MEDTRONIC	0.5 MG/ML	N20075 001	JUN 17, 1992
		2 MG/ML	N20075 002	JUN 17, 1992

TABLET; ORAL
BACLOFEN

ΔB	BIOCRAFT	10 MG	N73043 001	FEB 27, 1992
ΔB		20 MG	N73044 001	FEB 27, 1992
ΔB	DANBURY	10 MG	N72824 001	SEP 18, 1991
ΔB		20 MG	N72825 001	SEP 18, 1991
ΔB	ZENITH	10 MG	N72234 001	JUL 21, 1988
ΔB		20 MG	N72235 001	JUL 21, 1988

LIORESAL

ΔB	GEIGY	10 MG	N17851 001	
ΔB	+	20 MG	N17851 003	JAN 20, 1982

Prescription Drug Products (continued)

BACITRACIN; HYDROCORTISONE ACETATE; NEOMYCIN SULFATE; POLYMYXIN B SULFATE
OINTMENT; OPHTHALMIC
BACITRACIN-NEOMYCIN-POLYMYXIN W/ HYDROCORTISONE ACETATE

ΔT	ALTANA	400 UNITS/GM;1%;EQ 3.5 MG BASE/GM;10,000 UNITS/GM	N60731 002
ΔT	PHARMADERM	400 UNITS/GM;1%;EQ 3.5 MG BASE/GM;10,000 UNITS/GM	N62166 002

BACITRACIN; NEOMYCIN SULFATE; POLYMYXIN B SULFATE
OINTMENT; OPHTHALMIC
MYCITRACIN

	UPJOHN	500 UNITS/GM;EQ 3.5 MG BASE/GM;10,000 UNITS/GM	N61048 001

BACITRACIN ZINC
POWDER; FOR RX COMPOUNDING
ZIBA-RX

	PHARMA TEK	500,000 UNITS/BOT	N61737 001

BACITRACIN ZINC; HYDROCORTISONE; NEOMYCIN SULFATE; POLYMYXIN B SULFATE
OINTMENT; OPHTHALMIC
CORTISPORIN

ΔT	BURROUGHS WELLCOME	400 UNITS/GM;1%;EQ 3.5 MG BASE/GM;10,000 UNITS/GM	N50416 002	

ZINC BACITRACIN-NEOMYCIN SULFATE-POLYMYXIN B SULFATE & HYDROCORTISONE

ΔT	PHARMAFAIR	400 UNITS/GM;1%;EQ 3.5 MG BASE/GM;10,000 UNITS/GM	N62389 001	JUL 02, 1982

OINTMENT; TOPICAL
CORTISPORIN

ΔT	BURROUGHS WELLCOME	400 UNITS/GM;1%;EQ 3.5 MG BASE/GM;5,000 UNITS/GM	N50168 002	MAY 04, 1984

NEOMYCIN & POLYMYXIN B SULFATES & BACITRACIN ZINC & HYDROCORTISONE

ΔT	PHARMAFAIR	400 UNITS/GM;1%;EQ 3.5 MG BASE/GM;5,000 UNITS/GM	N62381 001	SEP 06, 1985

Prescription Drug Products (continued)

BECLOMETHASONE DIPROPIONATE
AEROSOL, METERED; INHALATION

BECLOVENT				
BN	GLAXO	0.042 MG/INH	N18153 001	
VANCERIL				
BN	+ SCHERING	0.042 MG/INH	N17573 001	

AEROSOL, METERED; NASAL

BECONASE				
BN	+ GLAXO	0.042 MG/INH	N18584 001	
VANCENASE				
BN	SCHERING	0.042 MG/INH	N18521 001	

BECLOMETHASONE DIPROPIONATE MONOHYDRATE
SPRAY, METERED; NASAL

BECONASE AQ				
BN	+ GLAXO	EQ 0.042 MG DIPROP/INH	N19389 001	JUL 27, 1987
VANCENASE AQ				
BN	SCHERING	EQ 0.042 MG DIPROP/INH	N19589 001	DEC 23, 1987

BENAZEPRIL HYDROCHLORIDE
TABLET; ORAL

LOTENSIN				
CIBA		EQ 5 MG BASE	N19851 001	JUN 25, 1991
		EQ 10 MG BASE	N19851 002	JUN 25, 1991
		EQ 20 MG BASE	N19851 003	JUN 25, 1991
+		EQ 40 MG BASE	N19851 004	JUN 25, 1991

BENAZEPRIL HYDROCHLORIDE; HYDROCHLOROTHIAZIDE
TABLET; ORAL

LOTENSIN HCT				
CIBA		5 MG;6.25 MG	N20033 001	MAY 19, 1992
		10 MG;12.5 MG	N20033 002	MAY 19, 1992
		20 MG;12.5 MG	N20033 004	MAY 19, 1992
+		20 MG;25 MG	N20033 003	MAY 19, 1992

BENDROFLUMETHIAZIDE
TABLET; ORAL

NATURETIN-10			
+ SQUIBB	10 MG	N12164 003	
NATURETIN-5			
SQUIBB	5 MG	N12164 002	

BENDROFLUMETHIAZIDE; NADOLOL
TABLET; ORAL

CORZIDE			
SQUIBB	5 MG;40 MG	N18647 001	MAY 25, 1983
+	5 MG;80 MG	N18647 002	MAY 25, 1983

BENTIROMIDE
SOLUTION; ORAL

CHYMEX			
ADRIA	500 MG/7.5 ML	N18366 001	DEC 29, 1983

BENTONITE; SULFUR
POWDER; TOPICAL

BENSULFOID		
POYTHRESS	66.64%;33.32%	N02918 001

BENZONATATE
CAPSULE; ORAL

TESSALON		
+ FOREST LABS	100 MG	N11210 001

BENZOYL PEROXIDE; ERYTHROMYCIN
GEL; TOPICAL

BENZAMYCIN			
+ DERMIK	5%;3%	N50557 001	OCT 26, 1984

BENZPHETAMINE HYDROCHLORIDE
TABLET; ORAL

DIDREX			
UPJOHN	25 MG	N12427 003	
+	50 MG	N12427 002	

BENZQUINAMIDE HYDROCHLORIDE
INJECTABLE; INJECTION

EMETE-CON		
ROERIG	EQ 50 MG BASE/VIAL	N16820 001

SUPPOSITORY; RECTAL

EMETE-CON		
+ ROERIG	EQ 100 MG BASE	N16818 006

BENZTHIAZIDE
TABLET; ORAL

AQUATAG			
BP	SOLVAY	50 MG	N16001 002
EXNA			
BP	+ ROBINS	50 MG	N12489 001

Prescription Drug Products (continued)

BENZTROPINE MESYLATE

INJECTABLE; INJECTION
COGENTIN

	MSD	1 MG/ML	N12015 001

TABLET; ORAL
BENZTROPINE MESYLATE
INVAMED

AA		0.5 MG	N72264 001	FEB 27, 1989
AA		1 MG	N72265 001	FEB 27, 1989
AA		2 MG	N72266 001	FEB 27, 1989

MUTUAL PHARM

AA		1 MG	N81264 001	JAN 23, 1992
AA		2 MG	N81265 001	JAN 23, 1992

PAR

AA		0.5 MG	N88877 001	APR 11, 1985
AA		1 MG	N88894 001	APR 11, 1985
AA		2 MG	N88895 001	APR 11, 1985

SIDMAK

AA		0.5 MG	N89058 001	AUG 10, 1988
AA		1 MG	N89059 001	AUG 10, 1988
AA		2 MG	N89060 001	AUG 10, 1988

COGENTIN

AA	MSD	0.5 MG	N09193 004
AA		1 MG	N09193 003
AA		2 MG	N09193 002

BENZYL BENZOATE

EMULSION; TOPICAL
BENZYL BENZOATE

	LANNETT	50%	N84535 001

BENZYL PENICILLOYL-POLYLYSINE

INJECTABLE; INJECTION
PRE-PEN

	SCHWARZ	60 UMOLAR	N50114 001

BEPRIDIL HYDROCHLORIDE

TABLET; ORAL
BERADIN

AB	WALLACE	200 MG	N19001 001	DEC 28, 1990
AB		300 MG	N19001 002	DEC 28, 1990
AB		400 MG	N19001 003	DEC 28, 1990

BEPRIDIL HYDROCHLORIDE (continued)

TABLET; ORAL
VASCOR

AB	JOHNSON RW	200 MG	N19002 001	DEC 28, 1990
AB		300 MG	N19002 002	DEC 28, 1990
AB		400 MG	N19002 003	DEC 28, 1990

BERACTANT

SUSPENSION; INTRATRACHEAL
SURVANTA

	+ ROSS	25 MG/ML	N20032 001	JUL 01, 1991

BETA-CAROTENE

CAPSULE; ORAL
SOLATENE

	+ ROCHE	30 MG	N17589 001

BETAMETHASONE

SYRUP; ORAL
CELESTONE

	SCHERING	0.6 MG/5 ML	N14215 002

TABLET; ORAL
CELESTONE

	+ SCHERING	0.6 MG	N12657 003

BETAMETHASONE ACETATE; BETAMETHASONE SODIUM PHOSPHATE

INJECTABLE; INJECTION
CELESTONE SOLUSPAN

	+ SCHERING	3 MG/ML;EQ 3 MG BASE/ML	N14602 001

BETAMETHASONE BENZOATE

CREAM; TOPICAL
UTICORT

	+ PARKE DAVIS	0.025%	N16998 002

GEL; TOPICAL
UTICORT

	+ PARKE DAVIS	0.025%	N17244 001

LOTION; TOPICAL
UTICORT

	+ PARKE DAVIS	0.025%	N17528 001

OINTMENT; TOPICAL
UTICORT

	+ PARKE DAVIS	0.025%	N18089 001

Prescription Drug Products *(continued)*

BETAMETHASONE DIPROPIONATE

AEROSOL; TOPICAL
DIPROSONE
+ SCHERING   EQ 0.1% BASE   N17829 001

CREAM; TOPICAL
ALPHATREX
AB   SAVAGE   EQ 0.05% BASE   N19138 001   JUN 26, 1984

BETAMETHASONE DIPROPIONATE
B*   CLAY PARK   EQ 0.05% BASE   N72536 001   JAN 31, 1990
           N19137 001   JUN 26, 1984
AB   FOUGERA   EQ 0.05% BASE   N71476 001   AUG 10, 1987
AB   LEMMON   EQ 0.05% BASE   N70885 001   FEB 03, 1987
AB   NMC   EQ 0.05% BASE   N19136 001   JUN 26, 1984
AB   PHARMADERM   EQ 0.05% BASE   N73552 001   APR 30, 1992
AB   TARO   EQ 0.05% BASE   N71143 001   JUN 17, 1987
AB   THAMES   EQ 0.05% BASE   N17536 001

DIPROSONE
AB   + SCHERING   EQ 0.05% BASE

CREAM, AUGMENTED; TOPICAL
DIPROLENE
AB   + SCHERING   EQ 0.05% BASE   N19408 001   JAN 31, 1986

DIPROLENE AF
AB   + SCHERING   EQ 0.05% BASE   N19555 001   APR 27, 1987

LOTION; TOPICAL
ALPHATREX
AB   SAVAGE   EQ 0.05% BASE   N70273 001   AUG 12, 1985

BETAMETHASONE DIPROPIONATE
AB   BARRE   EQ 0.05% BASE   N70281 001   JUL 31, 1985
AB   CLAY PARK   EQ 0.05% BASE   N72538 001   JAN 31, 1990
AB   COPLEY   EQ 0.05% BASE   N71882 001   JUN 06, 1988
AB   FOUGERA   EQ 0.05% BASE   N70275 001   AUG 12, 1985
AB   LEMMON   EQ 0.05% BASE   N71467 001   AUG 10, 1987
AB   NMC   EQ 0.05% BASE   N71085 001   FEB 03, 1987
AB   PHARMADERM   EQ 0.05% BASE   N70274 001   AUG 12, 1985
AB   THAMES   EQ 0.05% BASE   N72276 001   AUG 24, 1988

DIPROSONE
AB   + SCHERING   EQ 0.05% BASE   N17781 001

BETAMETHASONE DIPROPIONATE *(continued)*

LOTION, AUGMENTED; TOPICAL
DIPROLENE
+ SCHERING   EQ 0.05% BASE   N19716 001   AUG 01, 1988

OINTMENT; TOPICAL
ALPHATREX
AB   SAVAGE   EQ 0.05% BASE   N19143 001   SEP 04, 1984

BETAMETHASONE DIPROPIONATE
B*   CLAY PARK   EQ 0.05% BASE   N72526 001   JAN 31, 1990
           N19141 001   SEP 04, 1984
AB   FOUGERA   EQ 0.05% BASE   N71477 001   AUG 10, 1987
AB   LEMMON   EQ 0.05% BASE   N71012 001   FEB 03, 1987
AB   NMC   EQ 0.05% BASE   N19140 001   SEP 04, 1984
AB   PHARMADERM   EQ 0.05% BASE   N17691 001

DIPROSONE
AB   + SCHERING   EQ 0.05% BASE

OINTMENT, AUGMENTED; TOPICAL
DIPROLENE
AB   + SCHERING   EQ 0.05% BASE   N18741 001   JUL 27, 1983

BETAMETHASONE DIPROPIONATE; CLOTRIMAZOLE

CREAM; TOPICAL
LOTRISONE
+ SCHERING   EQ 0.05% BASE;1%   N18827 001   JUL 10, 1984

BETAMETHASONE SODIUM PHOSPHATE

INJECTABLE; INJECTION
BETAMETHASONE SODIUM PHOSPHATE
AP   STERIS   EQ 3 MG BASE/ML   N85738 001
CELESTONE
AP   SCHERING   EQ 3 MG BASE/ML   N17561 001

BETAMETHASONE SODIUM PHOSPHATE; *MULTIPLE*

SEE   BETAMETHASONE ACETATE; BETAMETHASONE SODIUM
       PHOSPHATE

Prescription Drug Products (continued)

BETAMETHASONE VALERATE

CREAM; TOPICAL

		Strength	Appl. No.	Date
	BETA-VAL			
ΔB	LEMMON	EQ 0.1% BASE	N18642 001	MAR 24, 1983
	BETADERM			
ΔB	ROACO	EQ 0.1% BASE	N18839 001	JUN 30, 1983
	BETAMETHASONE VALERATE			
ΔB	CLAY PARK	EQ 0.1% BASE	N70053 001	JUN 10, 1986
ΔB	FOUGERA	EQ 0.1% BASE	N18861 001	AUG 31, 1983
ΔB	PHARMADERM	EQ 0.1% BASE	N18860 002	AUG 31, 1983
ΔB	THAMES	EQ 0.1% BASE	N70062 001	MAY 14, 1985
	BETATREX			
ΔB	SAVAGE	EQ 0.1% BASE	N18862 001	AUG 31, 1983
	DERMABET			
ΔB	TARO	EQ 0.1% BASE	N72041 001	JAN 06, 1988
	VALISONE			
ΔB	+ SCHERING	EQ 0.1% BASE	N16322 001	
		EQ 0.01% BASE	N16322 002	
	VALNAC			
ΔB	NMC	EQ 0.1% BASE	N70050 001	OCT 10, 1984

LOTION; TOPICAL

		Strength	Appl. No.	Date
	BETA-VAL			
ΔB	LEMMON	EQ 0.1% BASE	N70072 001	JUN 27, 1985
	BETAMETHASONE VALERATE			
ΔB	BARRE	EQ 0.1% BASE	N70052 001	JUL 31, 1985
ΔB	COPLEY	EQ 0.1% BASE	N71883 001	APR 22, 1988
ΔB	FOUGERA	EQ 0.1% BASE	N18866 001	AUG 31, 1983
ΔB	PHARMADERM	EQ 0.1% BASE	N18870 001	AUG 31, 1983
ΔB	PHARMAFAIR	EQ 0.1% BASE	N70484 001	MAY 29, 1987
	BETATREX			
ΔB	SAVAGE	EQ 0.1% BASE	N18867 001	AUG 31, 1983
	VALISONE			
ΔB	+ SCHERING	EQ 0.1% BASE	N16932 001	

OINTMENT; TOPICAL

		Strength	Appl. No.	Date
	BETA-VAL			
ΔB	LEMMON	EQ 0.1% BASE	N70069 001	DEC 19, 1985

BETAMETHASONE VALERATE (continued)

OINTMENT; TOPICAL

		Strength	Appl. No.	Date
	BETAMETHASONE VALERATE			
B*	CLAY PARK	EQ 0.1% BASE	N71478 001	DEC 23, 1987
ΔB	FOUGERA	EQ 0.1% BASE	N18865 001	AUG 31, 1983
ΔB	PHARMADERM	EQ 0.1% BASE	N18864 001	AUG 31, 1983
	BETATREX			
ΔB	SAVAGE	EQ 0.1% BASE	N18863 001	AUG 31, 1983
	VALISONE			
ΔB	+ SCHERING	EQ 0.1% BASE	N16740 001	
	VALNAC			
ΔB	NMC	EQ 0.1% BASE	N70051 001	OCT 10, 1984

BETAXOLOL HYDROCHLORIDE

SOLUTION/DROPS; OPHTHALMIC

		Strength	Appl. No.	Date
	BETOPTIC			
	ALCON	EQ 0.5% BASE	N19270 001	AUG 30, 1985

SUSPENSION/DROPS; OPHTHALMIC

		Strength	Appl. No.	Date
	BETOPTIC S			
	+ ALCON	EQ 0.25% BASE	N19845 001	DEC 29, 1989

TABLET; ORAL

		Strength	Appl. No.	Date
	KERLONE			
	LOREX	10 MG	N19507 001	OCT 27, 1989
	+	20 MG	N19507 002	OCT 27, 1989

BETHANECHOL CHLORIDE

INJECTABLE; INJECTION

		Strength	Appl. No.	Date
	URECHOLINE			
	MSD	5 MG/ML	N06536 001	

TABLET; ORAL

		Strength	Appl. No.	Date
	BETHANECHOL CHLORIDE			
ΔA	DANBURY	5 MG	N84402 001	
ΔA		10 MG	N84408 001	
ΔA		25 MG	N84441 001	
ΔA		50 MG	N87444 001	
ΔA	LANNETT	5 MG	N84702 001	
ΔA		10 MG	N84712 001	
ΔA	SIDMAK	5 MG	N84074 001	
		5 MG	N89095 001	DEC 19, 1985
ΔA		10 MG	N88440 001	MAY 29, 1984
ΔA		25 MG	N88441 001	MAY 29, 1984
ΔA	ZENITH	50 MG	N89096 001	DEC 19, 1985
ΔA		25 MG	N84689 001	

Prescription Drug Products (continued)

BETHANECHOL CHLORIDE (continued)

TABLET; ORAL

DUVOID
ROBERTS

△△	10 MG	N86262 001
△△	25 MG	N86263 001
△△	50 MG	N85882 003

MYOTONACHOL
GLENWOOD

△△	5 MG	N84188 001
△△	10 MG	N84188 003
△△	25 MG	N84188 004

URECHOLINE
MSD

△△	5 MG	N06536 003
△△	10 MG	N06536 002
△△	25 MG	N06536 004
△△	50 MG	N06536 005

BIOTIN; *MULTIPLE*

SEE ASCORBIC ACID: BIOTIN: CYANOCOBALAMIN: DEXPANTHENOL: ERGOCALCIFEROL: FOLIC ACID: NIACINAMIDE: PYRIDOXINE HYDROCHLORIDE: RIBOFLAVIN PHOSPHATE SODIUM: THIAMINE HYDROCHLORIDE: VITAMIN A: VITAMIN E

SEE ASCORBIC ACID: BIOTIN: CYANOCOBALAMIN: DEXPANTHENOL: ERGOCALCIFEROL: FOLIC ACID: NIACINAMIDE: PYRIDOXINE: RIBOFLAVIN PHOSPHATE SODIUM: THIAMINE: VITAMIN A: VITAMIN E

BIPERIDEN HYDROCHLORIDE

TABLET; ORAL

AKINETON
+ KNOLL

	2 MG	N12003 001

BIPERIDEN LACTATE

INJECTABLE; INJECTION

AKINETON
KNOLL

	5 MG/ML	N12418 002

BISOPROLOL FUMARATE

TABLET; ORAL

ZEBETA
LEDERLE

	5 MG	N19982 002	JUL 31, 1992
+	10 MG	N19982 001	JUL 31, 1992

BITOLTEROL MESYLATE

AEROSOL, METERED; INHALATION

TORNALATE
+ STERLING

	0.37 MG/INH	N18770 001	DEC 28, 1984

SOLUTION; INHALATION

TORNALATE
STERLING

	0.2%	N19548 001	FEB 19, 1992

BLEOMYCIN SULFATE

INJECTABLE; INJECTION

BLENOXANE
BRISTOL

	EQ 15 UNITS BASE/VIAL	N50443 001

BRETYLIUM TOSYLATE

INJECTABLE; INJECTION

BRETYLIUM TOSYLATE

△P	ABBOTT	50 MG/ML	N19033 001	APR 16, 1986
△P	ASTRA	50 MG/ML	N71151 001	AUG 10, 1987
		50 MG/ML	N71152 001	AUG 10, 1987
		50 MG/ML	N71153 001	AUG 10, 1987
△P	ELKINS SINN	50 MG/ML	N70545 001	AUG 10, 1987
		50 MG/ML	N70546 001	MAY 14, 1986
△P	INTL MEDICATION	50 MG/ML	N70119 001	MAY 14, 1986
△P	LUITPOLD	50 MG/ML	N70891 001	MAR 06, 1986

BRETYLIUM TOSYLATE IN DEXTROSE 5% IN PLASTIC CONTAINER

△P	ABBOTT	200 MG/100 ML	N19008 002	JUL 26, 1988
		400 MG/100 ML	N19008 003	APR 16, 1986
△P	BAXTER	200 MG/100 ML	N19837 002	APR 16, 1986
		400 MG/100 ML	N19837 001	APR 12, 1989
△P	MCGAW	200 MG/100 ML	N19121 002	APR 12, 1989
		400 MG/100 ML	N19121 003	APR 29, 1986
		100 MG/100 ML	N19121 001	APR 29, 1986

BRETYLIUM TOSYLATE IN PLASTIC CONTAINER

△P	ABBOTT	50 MG/ML	N19030 001	APR 16, 1986

BRETYLOL

△P	DUPONT	50 MG/ML	N17954 001	

BROMOCRIPTINE MESYLATE

CAPSULE; ORAL

PARLODEL
+ SANDOZ

	EQ 5 MG BASE	N17962 002	MAR 01, 1982

TABLET; ORAL

PARLODEL
+ SANDOZ

	EQ 2.5 MG BASE	N17962 001

Prescription Drug Products (continued)

BROMODIPHENHYDRAMINE HYDROCHLORIDE; CODEINE PHOSPHATE

SYRUP; ORAL

AMBENYL
- AA FOREST LABS   12.5 MG/5 ML;10 MG/5 ML   N09319 006   JAN 10, 1984

BROMANYL
- AA BARRE   12.5 MG/5 ML;10 MG/5 ML   N88343 001   AUG 15, 1984

MYBANIL
- AA PHARM BASICS   12.5 MG/5 ML;10 MG/5 ML   N88626 001   OCT 12, 1984

BROMPHENIRAMINE MALEATE

ELIXIR; ORAL

BROMPHENIRAMINE MALEATE
- KV   2 MG/5 ML   N85466 001

INJECTABLE; INJECTION

BROMPHENIRAMINE MALEATE
- AP STERIS   10 MG/ML   N83821 001

DIMETANE-TEN
- AP ROBINS   10 MG/ML   N11418 002

TABLET; ORAL

BROMPHENIRAMINE MALEATE
- AA ANABOLICS   4 MG   N86187 001
- AA DANBURY   4 MG   N83123 001
- AA NEWTRON   4 MG   N86987 001
- AA PHOENIX LABS   4 MG   N85521 001
- AA PRIVATE FORM   4 MG   N85888 001
- AA TABLICAPS   4 MG   N85592 001
- AA ZENITH   4 MG   N84351 001

DIMETANE
- AA ROBINS   4 MG   N10799 003

VELTANE
- AA LANNETT   4 MG   N84088 001

BROMPHENIRAMINE MALEATE; CODEINE PHOSPHATE; PHENYLPROPANOLAMINE HYDROCHLORIDE

SYRUP; ORAL

BROMANATE DC
- AA BARRE   2 MG/5 ML;10 MG/5 ML;12.5 MG/5 ML   N88723 001   FEB 25, 1985

DIMETANE-DC
- AA ROBINS   2 MG/5 ML;10 MG/5 ML;12.5 MG/5 ML   N11694 006   MAR 29, 1984

MYPHETANE DC
- AA PHARM BASICS   2 MG/5 ML;10 MG/5 ML;12.5 MG/5 ML   N88904 001   FEB 21, 1985

BROMPHENIRAMINE MALEATE; DEXTROMETHORPHAN HYDROBROMIDE; PSEUDOEPHEDRINE HYDROCHLORIDE

SYRUP; ORAL

BROMANATE DM
- AA BARRE   2 MG/5 ML;10 MG/5 ML;30 MG/5 ML   N88722 001   MAR 07, 1985

BROMFED-DM
- AA MURO   2 MG/5 ML;10 MG/5 ML;30 MG/5 ML   N89681 001   DEC 22, 1988

DIMETANE-DX
- AA ROBINS   2 MG/5 ML;10 MG/5 ML;30 MG/5 ML   N11694 007   MAR 29, 1984
- AA 2 MG/5 ML;10 MG/5 ML;30 MG/5 ML   N19279 001   AUG 24, 1984

MYPHETANE DX
- AA PHARM BASICS   2 MG/5 ML;10 MG/5 ML;30 MG/5 ML   N88811 001   JUN 07, 1985

BUCLIZINE HYDROCHLORIDE

TABLET; ORAL

BUCLADIN-S
- STUART   50 MG   N10911 006

BUMETANIDE

INJECTABLE; INJECTION

BUMEX
- ROCHE   0.25 MG/ML   N18226 001   FEB 28, 1983

TABLET; ORAL

BUMEX
- ROCHE   0.5 MG   N18225 002   FEB 28, 1983
-         1 MG   N18225 001   FEB 28, 1983
- +   2 MG   N18225 003   JUN 14, 1985

Prescription Drug Products (continued)

BUPIVACAINE HYDROCHLORIDE
INJECTABLE; INJECTION
BUPIVACAINE HCL
ABBOTT

AP	0.25%	N18053 002	
AP	0.25%	N70583 001	FEB 17, 1987
	0.25%	N70586 001	MAR 03, 1987
AP	0.25%	N70590 001	FEB 17, 1987
	0.5%	N18053 001	
AP	0.5%	N70584 001	FEB 17, 1986
	0.5%	N70597 001	MAR 03, 1987
AP	0.5%	N70609 001	MAR 03, 1987
	0.75%	N18053 003	
AP	0.75%	N70585 001	MAR 03, 1987
AP	0.75%	N70587 001	MAR 03, 1987

MARCAINE HCL
STERLING

AP	0.25%	N16964 001
AP	0.5%	N16964 006
AP	0.75%	N16964 009

SENSORCAINE
ASTRA

AP	0.25%	N18304 001	
AP	0.25%	N70552 001	MAY 21, 1986
AP	0.5%	N18304 002	
AP	0.5%	N70553 001	
AP	0.75%	N18304 003	MAY 21, 1986
AP	0.75%	N70554 001	MAY 21, 1986

INJECTABLE; SPINAL
BUPIVACAINE
ABBOTT

AP	0.75%	N71810 001	DEC 11, 1987

MARCAINE
STERLING

AP	0.75%	N16692 001	MAY 04, 1984

SENSORCAINE
ASTRA

AP	0.75%	N71202 001	APR 15, 1987

BUPIVACAINE HYDROCHLORIDE; EPINEPHRINE
INJECTABLE; INJECTION
BUPIVACAINE HCL AND EPINEPHRINE
ABBOTT

0.25%;0.005 MG/ML	N71165 001	JUN 16, 1988
0.25%;0.005 MG/ML	N71166 001	JUN 16, 1988
0.25%;0.005 MG/ML	N71167 001	JUN 16, 1988
0.5%;0.005 MG/ML	N71168 001	JUN 16, 1988
0.5%;0.005 MG/ML	N71169 001	JUN 16, 1988
0.5%;0.005 MG/ML	N71170 001	JUN 16, 1988
0.75%;0.005 MG/ML	N71171 001	JUN 16, 1988

BUPIVACAINE HYDROCHLORIDE; EPINEPHRINE BITARTRATE
INJECTABLE; INJECTION
MARCAINE HCL W/ EPINEPHRINE
STERLING

AP	0.25%;0.0091 MG/ML	N16964 004
AP	0.5%;0.0091 MG/ML	N16964 008
AP	0.75%;0.0091 MG/ML	N16964 010

SENSORCAINE
ASTRA

AP	0.25%;0.0091 MG/ML	N70966 001	OCT 13, 1987
AP	0.25%;0.0091 MG/ML	N70967 001	OCT 13, 1987
AP	0.5%;0.0091 MG/ML	N18304 004	SEP 02, 1983
AP	0.5%;0.0091 MG/ML	N70968 001	OCT 13, 1987
AP	0.75%;0.0091 MG/ML	N18304 005	SEP 02, 1983

BUPRENORPHINE HYDROCHLORIDE
INJECTABLE; INJECTION
BUPRENEX
RECKITT AND COLMAN   EQ 0.3 MG BASE/ML   N18401 001

BUPROPION HYDROCHLORIDE
TABLET; ORAL
WELLBUTRIN
BURROUGHS WELLCOME

	75 MG	N18644 002	DEC 30, 1985
+	100 MG	N18644 003	DEC 30, 1985

Prescription Drug Products (continued)

BUSPIRONE HYDROCHLORIDE
TABLET; ORAL

BUSPAR

	Strength	Appl. No.	Date
BRISTOL	5 MG	N18731 001	SEP 29, 1986
+	10 MG	N18731 002	SEP 29, 1986

BUSULFAN
TABLET; ORAL

MYLERAN

	Strength	Appl. No.
+ BURROUGHS WELLCOME	2 MG	N09386 001

BUTABARBITAL SODIUM
CAPSULE; ORAL

BUTICAPS

	Strength	Appl. No.
WALLACE	15 MG	N85381 001
	30 MG	N85381 002
	50 MG	N85381 003
	100 MG	N85381 004

ELIXIR; ORAL

TE	Product / Company	Strength	Appl. No.
	BUTABARB		
AA	BARRE	30 MG/5 ML	N85873 001
	BUTABARBITAL SODIUM		
AA	PHARM BASICS	30 MG/5 ML	N85383 001
	BUTALAN		
	LANNETT	33.3 MG/5 ML	N85880 001
	BUTISOL SODIUM		
AA	WALLACE	30 MG/5 ML	N85380 001
	SARISOL		
AA	HALSEY	30 MG/5 ML	N84723 001

TABLET; ORAL

TE	Product / Company	Strength	Appl. No.
	BUTABARBITAL		
AA	BUNDY	30 MG	N85550 001
	BUTISOL SODIUM		
AA	WALLACE	15 MG	N00793 002
AA		30 MG	N00793 004
AA		100 MG	N00793 005
		50 MG	N00793 003
	SARISOL NO 1		
AA	HALSEY	15 MG	N84719 001
	SARISOL NO 2		
AA	HALSEY	30 MG	N84719 002
	SODIUM BUTABARBITAL		
AA	LANNETT	15 MG	N85849 001
AA		30 MG	N85866 001
AA		100 MG	N85881 001
	MARSHALL	16.2 MG	N83524 001
		32.4 MG	N83858 001
AA	ZENITH	30 MG	N84040 001

BUTALBITAL; *MULTIPLE*
SEE   ACETAMINOPHEN: BUTALBITAL
SEE   ACETAMINOPHEN: BUTALBITAL: CAFFEINE
SEE   ACETAMINOPHEN: BUTALBITAL: CAFFEINE: CODEINE PHOSPHATE
SEE   ASPIRIN: BUTALBITAL
SEE   ASPIRIN: BUTALBITAL: CAFFEINE
SEE   ASPIRIN: BUTALBITAL: CAFFEINE: CODEINE PHOSPHATE

BUTOCONAZOLE NITRATE
CREAM; VAGINAL

FEMSTAT

	Strength	Appl. No.	Date
SYNTEX	2%	N19215 001	NOV 25, 1985

BUTORPHANOL TARTRATE
INJECTABLE; INJECTION

STADOL

	Strength	Appl. No.
BRISTOL	1 MG/ML	N17857 001
	2 MG/ML	N17857 002

SPRAY, METERED; NASAL

STADOL

	Strength	Appl. No.	Date
+ BRISTOL MYERS SQUIBB	1 MG/INH	N19890 001	DEC 12, 1991

CAFFEINE; *MULTIPLE*
SEE   ACETAMINOPHEN: BUTALBITAL: CAFFEINE
SEE   ACETAMINOPHEN: BUTALBITAL: CAFFEINE: CODEINE PHOSPHATE
SEE   ACETAMINOPHEN: CAFFEINE: DIHYDROCODEINE BITARTRATE
SEE   ASPIRIN: BUTALBITAL: CAFFEINE
SEE   ASPIRIN: BUTALBITAL: CAFFEINE: CODEINE PHOSPHATE
SEE   ASPIRIN: CAFFEINE: DIHYDROCODEINE BITARTRATE
SEE   ASPIRIN: CAFFEINE: ORPHENADRINE CITRATE
SEE   ASPIRIN: CAFFEINE: PROPOXYPHENE HYDROCHLORIDE

CAFFEINE; ERGOTAMINE TARTRATE
SUPPOSITORY; RECTAL

TE	Product / Company	Strength	Appl. No.	Date
	CAFERGOT			
BR	+ SANDOZ	100 MG;2 MG	N09000 002	
	WIGRAINE			
BR	ORGANON	100 MG;2 MG	N86557 001	OCT 04, 1983

Prescription Drug Products (continued)

CAFFEINE; ERGOTAMINE TARTRATE (continued)
TABLET; ORAL
ΔΔ	CAFERGOT SANDOZ	100 MG;1 MG	N06620 001
ΔΔ	ERCATAB GENEVA	100 MG;1 MG	N84294 001
ΔΔ	WIGRAINE ORGANON	100 MG;1 MG	N86562 001

CALCIFEDIOL, ANHYDROUS
CAPSULE; ORAL
CALDEROL UPJOHN	0.02 MG	N18312 001
+	0.05 MG	N18312 002

CALCITONIN, HUMAN
INJECTABLE; INJECTION
CIBACALCIN CIBA	0.5 MG/VIAL	N18470 001	OCT 31, 1986

CALCITONIN, SALMON
INJECTABLE; INJECTION
ΔP	CALCIMAR RHONE POULENC RORER	200 IU/ML	N17769 001	
ΔP	MIACALCIN SANDOZ	200 IU/ML	N17808 002	MAR 29, 1991
		100 IU/ML	N17808 001	JUL 03, 1986

CALCITRIOL
CAPSULE; ORAL
ROCALTROL ROCHE	0.25 UGM	N18044 001
+	0.5 UGM	N18044 002

INJECTABLE; INJECTION
CALCIJEX ABBOTT	0.001 MG/ML	N18874 001	SEP 25, 1986
	0.002 MG/ML	N18874 002	SEP 25, 1986

CALCIUM ACETATE
TABLET; ORAL
PHOSLO			
+ BRAINTREE	EQ 169 MG CALCIUM	N19976 001	DEC 10, 1990

CALCIUM ACETATE; *MULTIPLE*
SEE AMINO ACIDS: CALCIUM ACETATE: GLYCERIN: MAGNESIUM ACETATE: PHOSPHORIC ACID: POTASSIUM CHLORIDE: SODIUM ACETATE: SODIUM CHLORIDE

CALCIUM CHLORIDE; *MULTIPLE*
SEE AMINO ACIDS: CALCIUM CHLORIDE: DEXTROSE: MAGNESIUM CHLORIDE: POTASSIUM CHLORIDE: POTASSIUM PHOSPHATE, DIBASIC: SODIUM CHLORIDE

CALCIUM CHLORIDE; DEXTROSE; GLUTATHIONE DISULFIDE; MAGNESIUM CHLORIDE; POTASSIUM CHLORIDE; SODIUM BICARBONATE; SODIUM CHLORIDE; SODIUM PHOSPHATE
SOLUTION; IRRIGATION

ΔT	BSS PLUS ALCON	0.154 MG/ML;0.92 MG/ML;0.184 MG/ML;0.2 MG/ML;0.38 MG/ML;2.1 MG/ML;7.14 MG/ML;0.42 MG/ML	N18469 001	
ΔT	ENDOSOL PLUS ENTRAVISION	0.154 MG/ML;0.92 MG/ML;0.184 MG/ML;0.2 MG/ML;0.38 MG/ML;2.1 MG/ML;7.14 MG/ML;0.42 MG/ML	N20079 001	NOV 27, 1991

CALCIUM CHLORIDE; DEXTROSE; MAGNESIUM CHLORIDE; POTASSIUM CHLORIDE; SODIUM ACETATE; SODIUM CHLORIDE
INJECTABLE; INJECTION
ISOLYTE R W/ DEXTROSE 5% IN PLASTIC CONTAINER

MCGAW	37 MG/100 ML;5 GM/100 ML;31 MG/100 ML;120 MG/100 ML;330 MG/100 ML;88 MG/100 ML	N18271 001

CALCIUM CHLORIDE; DEXTROSE; MAGNESIUM CHLORIDE; POTASSIUM CHLORIDE; SODIUM ACETATE; SODIUM CHLORIDE; SODIUM CITRATE
INJECTABLE; INJECTION
ISOLYTE E W/ DEXTROSE 5% IN PLASTIC CONTAINER

MCGAW	35 MG/100 ML;5 GM/100 ML;30 MG/100 ML;74 MG/100 ML;640 MG/100 ML;500 MG/100 ML;74 MG/100 ML	N18269 002	JAN 17, 1983

Prescription Drug Products (continued)

CALCIUM CHLORIDE; DEXTROSE; MAGNESIUM CHLORIDE; POTASSIUM CHLORIDE; SODIUM ACETATE; SODIUM CHLORIDE; SODIUM LACTATE

INJECTABLE; INJECTION
PLASMA-LYTE M AND DEXTROSE 5% IN PLASTIC CONTAINER
   BAXTER   37 MG/100 ML;5 GM/
   100 ML;30 MG/
   100 ML;119 MG/
   100 ML;161 MG/
   100 ML;94 MG/
   100 ML;138 MG/100 ML   N17390 001

CALCIUM CHLORIDE; DEXTROSE; MAGNESIUM CHLORIDE; SODIUM ACETATE; SODIUM CHLORIDE

SOLUTION; INTRAPERITONEAL
DIALYTE CONCENTRATE W/ DEXTROSE 30% IN PLASTIC CONTAINER
   MCGAW   510 MG/100 ML;30 GM/
   100 ML;200 MG/
   100 ML;9.2 GM/
   100 ML;9.6 GM/100 ML   N18807 001 AUG 26, 1983

   510 MG/100 ML;30 GM/
   100 ML;200 MG/
   100 ML;9.4 GM/
   100 ML;11 GM/100 ML   N18807 003 AUG 26, 1983

DIALYTE CONCENTRATE W/ DEXTROSE 50% IN PLASTIC CONTAINER
   MCGAW   510 MG/100 ML;50 GM/
   100 ML;200 MG/
   100 ML;9.2 GM/
   100 ML;9.6 GM/100 ML   N18807 002 AUG 26, 1983

   510 MG/100 ML;50 GM/
   100 ML;200 MG/
   100 ML;9.4 GM/
   100 ML;11 GM/100 ML   N18807 004 AUG 26, 1983

CALCIUM CHLORIDE; DEXTROSE; MAGNESIUM CHLORIDE; SODIUM CHLORIDE; SODIUM LACTATE

SOLUTION; INTRAPERITONEAL
DELFLEX W/ DEXTROSE 1.5% IN PLASTIC CONTAINER
AT   DELMED   25.7 MG/100 ML;1.5 GM/
   100 ML;15.2 MG/
   100 ML;567 MG/
   100 ML;392 MG/100 ML   N18883 001 NOV 30, 1984

DELFLEX W/ DEXTROSE 1.5% LOW MAGNESIUM IN PLASTIC CONTAINER
AT   DELMED   25.7 MG/100 ML;1.5 GM/
   100 ML;5.08 MG/
   100 ML;538 MG/
   100 ML;448 MG/100 ML   N18883 004 NOV 30, 1984

CALCIUM CHLORIDE; DEXTROSE; MAGNESIUM CHLORIDE; SODIUM CHLORIDE; SODIUM LACTATE (continued)

SOLUTION; INTRAPERITONEAL
DELFLEX W/ DEXTROSE 1.5% LOW MAGNESIUM LOW CALCIUM IN PLASTIC CONTAINER
   FRESENIUS   18.4 MG/100 ML;1.5 GM/
   100 ML;5.08 MG/
   100 ML;538 MG/
   100 ML;448 MG/100 ML   N20171 001 AUG 19, 1992

DELFLEX W/ DEXTROSE 2.5% IN PLASTIC CONTAINER
AT   DELMED   25.7 MG/100 ML;2.5 GM/
   100 ML;15.2 MG/
   100 ML;567 MG/
   100 ML;392 MG/100 ML   N18883 002 NOV 30, 1984

DELFLEX W/ DEXTROSE 2.5% LOW MAGNESIUM IN PLASTIC CONTAINER
AT   DELMED   25.7 MG/100 ML;2.5 GM/
   100 ML;5.08 MG/
   100 ML;538 MG/
   100 ML;448 MG/100 ML   N18883 005 NOV 30, 1984

DELFLEX W/ DEXTROSE 2.5% LOW MAGNESIUM LOW CALCIUM IN PLASTIC CONTAINER
   FRESENIUS   18.4 MG/100 ML;2.5 GM/
   100 ML;5.08 MG/
   100 ML;538 MG/
   100 ML;448 MG/100 ML   N20171 002 AUG 19, 1992

DELFLEX W/ DEXTROSE 4.25% IN PLASTIC CONTAINER
AT   DELMED   25.7 MG/100 ML;4.25 GM/
   100 ML;15.2 MG/
   100 ML;567 MG/
   100 ML;392 MG/100 ML   N18883 003 NOV 30, 1984

DELFLEX W/ DEXTROSE 4.25% LOW MAGNESIUM IN PLASTIC CONTAINER
AT   DELMED   25.7 MG/100 ML;4.25 GM/
   100 ML;5.08 MG/
   100 ML;538 MG/
   100 ML;448 MG/100 ML   N18883 006 NOV 30, 1984

DELFLEX W/ DEXTROSE 4.25% LOW MAGNESIUM LOW CALCIUM IN PLASTIC CONTAINER
   FRESENIUS   18.4 MG/100 ML;4.25 GM/
   100 ML;5.08 MG/
   100 ML;538 MG/
   100 ML;448 MG/100 ML   N20171 003 AUG 19, 1992

DIALYTE LM/ DEXTROSE 1.5% IN PLASTIC CONTAINER
   MCGAW   26 MG/100 ML;1.5 GM/
   100 ML;5 MG/
   100 ML;530 MG/
   100 ML;450 MG/100 ML   N18460 007 JAN 29, 1986

Prescription Drug Products (continued)

CALCIUM CHLORIDE; DEXTROSE; MAGNESIUM CHLORIDE; SODIUM CHLORIDE; SODIUM LACTATE (continued)

SOLUTION; INTRAPERITONEAL

DIALYTE LM W/ DEXTROSE 2.5% IN PLASTIC CONTAINER
MCGAW   26 MG/100 ML;2.5 GM/
100 ML;5 MG/
100 ML;530 MG/
100 ML;450 MG/100 ML   N18460 005 NOV 02, 1983

DIALYTE LM W/ DEXTROSE 4.25% IN PLASTIC CONTAINER
MCGAW   26 MG/100 ML;4.25 GM/
100 ML;5 MG/
100 ML;530 MG/
100 ML;450 MG/100 ML   N18460 009 JAN 29, 1986

AT DIANEAL PD-1 W/ DEXTROSE 1.5% IN PLASTIC CONTAINER
BAXTER   25.7 MG/100 ML;1.5 GM/
100 ML;15.2 MG/
100 ML;567 MG/
100 ML;392 MG/100 ML   N17512 007 JUL 09, 1984

AT DIANEAL PD-1 W/ DEXTROSE 2.5% IN PLASTIC CONTAINER
BAXTER   25.7 MG/100 ML;2.5 GM/
100 ML;15.2 MG/
100 ML;567 MG/
100 ML;392 MG/100 ML   N17512 008 JUL 09, 1984

AT DIANEAL PD-1 W/ DEXTROSE 3.5% IN PLASTIC CONTAINER
BAXTER   25.7 MG/100 ML;3.5 GM/
100 ML;15.2 MG/
100 ML;567 MG/
100 ML;392 MG/100 ML   N17512 010 NOV 18, 1985

AT DIANEAL PD-2 W/ DEXTROSE 4.25% IN PLASTIC CONTAINER
BAXTER   25.7 MG/100 ML;4.25 GM/
100 ML;15.2 MG/
100 ML;567 MG/
100 ML;392 MG/100 ML   N17512 009 JUL 09, 1984

DIANEAL PD-2 W/ DEXTROSE 1.5% IN PLASTIC CONTAINER
BAXTER   18.3 MG/100 ML;1.5 GM/
100 ML;5.08 MG/
100 ML;538 MG/
100 ML;448 MG/100 ML   N17512 004

AT DIANEAL PD-2 W/ DEXTROSE 2.5% IN PLASTIC CONTAINER
BAXTER   25.7 MG/100 ML;2.5 GM/
100 ML;5.08 MG/
100 ML;538 MG/
100 ML;448 MG/100 ML   N17512 005

AT DIANEAL PD-2 W/ DEXTROSE 3.5% IN PLASTIC CONTAINER
BAXTER   25.7 MG/100 ML;3.5 GM/
100 ML;5.08 MG/
100 ML;538 MG/
100 ML;448 MG/100 ML   N17512 011 NOV 18, 1985

CALCIUM CHLORIDE; DEXTROSE; MAGNESIUM CHLORIDE; SODIUM CHLORIDE; SODIUM LACTATE (continued)

SOLUTION; INTRAPERITONEAL

DIANEAL PD-2 W/ DEXTROSE 4.25% IN PLASTIC CONTAINER
BAXTER   25.7 MG/100 ML;4.25 GM/
100 ML;5.08 MG/
100 ML;538 MG/
100 ML;448 MG/100 ML   N17512 006

AT DIANEAL 137 W/ DEXTROSE 1.5% IN PLASTIC CONTAINER
BAXTER   25.7 MG/100 ML;1.5 MG/
100 ML;15.2 MG/
100 ML;567 MG/
100 ML;392 MG/100 ML   N17512 001

AT DIANEAL 137 W/ DEXTROSE 2.5% IN PLASTIC CONTAINER
BAXTER   25.7 MG/100 ML;2.5 MG/
100 ML;15.2 MG/
100 ML;567 MG/
100 ML;392 MG/100 ML   N17512 003

AT DIANEAL 137 W/ DEXTROSE 4.25% IN PLASTIC CONTAINER
BAXTER   25.7 MG/100 ML;4.25 GM/
100 ML;15.2 MG/
100 ML;567 MG/
100 ML;392 MG/100 ML   N17512 002

AT INPERSOL W/ DEXTROSE 1.5% IN PLASTIC CONTAINER
ABBOTT   25.7 MG/100 ML;1.5 GM/
100 ML;15.2 MG/
100 ML;567 MG/
100 ML;392 MG/100 ML   N18379 002

AT INPERSOL W/ DEXTROSE 2.5% IN PLASTIC CONTAINER
ABBOTT   25.7 MG/100 ML;2.5 GM/
100 ML;15.2 MG/
100 ML;567 MG/
100 ML;392 MG/100 ML   N18379 003

AT INPERSOL W/ DEXTROSE 3.5% IN PLASTIC CONTAINER
ABBOTT   25.7 MG/100 ML;3.5 GM/
100 ML;15.2 MG/
100 ML;567 MG/
100 ML;392 MG/100 ML   N18379 007 JUN 24, 1988

AT INPERSOL-LM W/ DEXTROSE 4.25% IN PLASTIC CONTAINER
ABBOTT   25.7 MG/100 ML;4.25 GM/
100 ML;15.2 MG/
100 ML;567 MG/
100 ML;392 MG/100 ML   N18379 001

AT INPERSOL-LM W/ DEXTROSE 1.5% IN PLASTIC CONTAINER
ABBOTT   25.7 MG/100 ML;1.5 GM/
100 ML;5.08 MG/
100 ML;538 MG/
100 ML;448 MG/100 ML   N18379 004 JUL 07, 1982

AT INPERSOL-LM W/ DEXTROSE 2.5% IN PLASTIC CONTAINER
ABBOTT   25.7 MG/100 ML;2.5 GM/
100 ML;5.08 MG/
100 ML;538 MG/
100 ML;448 MG/100 ML   N18379 005 JUL 07, 1982

Prescription Drug Products (*continued*)

CALCIUM CHLORIDE; DEXTROSE; MAGNESIUM CHLORIDE; SODIUM CHLORIDE; SODIUM LACTATE (*continued*)
SOLUTION; INTRAPERITONEAL
  INPERSOL-LM W/ DEXTROSE 3.5% IN PLASTIC CONTAINER
  ΔT ABBOTT 25.7 MG/100 ML;3.5 GM/100 ML;5.08 MG/100 ML;538 MG/100 ML;448 MG/100 ML   N18379 008 JUN 24, 1988

  INPERSOL-LM W/ DEXTROSE 4.25% IN PLASTIC CONTAINER
  ΔT ABBOTT 25.7 MG/100 ML;4.25 GM/100 ML;5.08 MG/100 ML;538 MG/100 ML;448 MG/100 ML   N18379 006 JUL 07, 1982

CALCIUM CHLORIDE; DEXTROSE; POTASSIUM CHLORIDE; SODIUM ACETATE; SODIUM CHLORIDE
INJECTABLE; INJECTION
  DEXTROSE 5% IN ACETATED RINGER'S IN PLASTIC CONTAINER
  MCGAW 20 MG/100 ML;30 MG/100 ML;380 MG/100 ML;600 MG/100 ML   N18258 001

CALCIUM CHLORIDE; DEXTROSE; POTASSIUM CHLORIDE; SODIUM CHLORIDE
INJECTABLE; INJECTION
  DEXTROSE 5% AND RINGER'S IN PLASTIC CONTAINER
  ΔP ABBOTT 33 MG/100 ML;5 GM/100 ML;30 MG/100 ML;860 MG/100 ML   N18254 001

  DEXTROSE 5% IN RINGER'S IN PLASTIC CONTAINER
  ΔP BAXTER 33 MG/100 ML;5 GM/100 ML;30 MG/100 ML;860 MG/100 ML   N16695 001

  ΔP MCGAW 33 MG/100 ML;5 GM/100 ML;30 MG/100 ML;860 MG/100 ML   N18256 001

  ΔP 33 MG/100 ML;5 GM/100 ML;30 MG/100 ML;860 MG/100 ML   N20000 001 APR 17, 1992

CALCIUM CHLORIDE; DEXTROSE; POTASSIUM CHLORIDE; SODIUM CHLORIDE; SODIUM LACTATE
INJECTABLE; INJECTION
  DEXTROSE 2.5% IN HALF-STRENGTH LACTATED RINGER'S IN PLASTIC CONTAINER
  MCGAW 10 MG/100 ML;2.5 GM/100 ML;15 MG/100 ML;300 MG/100 ML;160 MG/100 ML   N19634 001 FEB 24, 1988

  DEXTROSE 4% IN MODIFIED LACTATED RINGER'S IN PLASTIC CONTAINER
  ΔT MCGAW 4 MG/100 ML;4 GM/100 ML;6 MG/100 ML;120 MG/100 ML;62 MG/100 ML   N19634 002 FEB 24, 1988

  DEXTROSE 5% AND LACTATED RINGER'S IN PLASTIC CONTAINER
  ΔP ABBOTT 20 MG/100 ML;5 GM/100 ML;30 MG/100 ML;600 MG/100 ML;310 MG/100 ML   N17608 001

  DEXTROSE 5% IN LACTATED RINGER'S IN PLASTIC CONTAINER
  ΔP MCGAW 20 MG/100 ML;5 GM/100 ML;30 MG/100 ML;600 MG/100 ML;310 MG/100 ML   N17510 001

  ΔP 20 MG/100 ML;5 GM/100 ML;30 MG/100 ML;600 MG/100 ML;310 MG/100 ML   N19634 003 FEB 24, 1988

  LACTATED RINGER'S AND DEXTROSE 5% IN PLASTIC CONTAINER
  ΔP BAXTER 20 MG/100 ML;5 GM/100 ML;30 MG/100 ML;600 MG/100 ML;310 MG/100 ML   N16679 001

  POTASSIUM CHLORIDE 10 MEQ IN DEXTROSE 5% AND LACTATED RINGER'S IN PLASTIC CONTAINER
  BAXTER 20 MG/100 ML;5 GM/100 ML;105 MG/100 ML;600 MG/100 ML;310 MG/100 ML   N19367 002 APR 05, 1985

  20 MG/100 ML;5 GM/100 ML;179 MG/100 ML;600 MG/100 ML;310 MG/100 ML   N19367 003 APR 05, 1985

  POTASSIUM CHLORIDE 15 MEQ IN DEXTROSE 5% AND LACTATED RINGER'S IN PLASTIC CONTAINER
  ΔP BAXTER 20 MG/100 ML;5 GM/100 ML;254 MG/100 ML;600 MG/100 ML;310 MG/100 ML   N19367 006 APR 05, 1985

Prescription Drug Products (continued)

CALCIUM CHLORIDE; DEXTROSE; POTASSIUM CHLORIDE; SODIUM CHLORIDE; SODIUM LACTATE (continued)

INJECTABLE; INJECTION
POTASSIUM CHLORIDE 20 MEQ IN DEXTROSE 5% AND LACTATED RINGER'S IN PLASTIC CONTAINER

AP ABBOTT   20 MG/100 ML;5 GM/100 ML;179 MG/100 ML;600 MG/100 ML;310 MG/100 ML
N19685 002
OCT 17, 1988

AP   20 MG/100 ML;5 GM/100 ML;328 MG/100 ML;600 MG/100 ML;310 MG/100 ML
N19685 008
OCT 17, 1988

AP BAXTER   20 MG/100 ML;5 GM/100 ML;179 MG/100 ML;600 MG/100 ML;310 MG/100 ML
N19367 004
APR 05, 1985

AP   20 MG/100 ML;5 GM/100 ML;328 MG/100 ML;600 MG/100 ML;310 MG/100 ML
N19367 005
APR 05, 1985

POTASSIUM CHLORIDE 30 MEQ IN DEXTROSE 5% AND LACTATED RINGER'S IN PLASTIC CONTAINER

AP BAXTER   20 MG/100 ML;5 GM/100 ML;254 MG/100 ML;600 MG/100 ML;310 MG/100 ML
N19367 007
APR 05, 1985

POTASSIUM CHLORIDE 40 MEQ IN DEXTROSE 5% AND LACTATED RINGER'S IN PLASTIC CONTAINER

AP ABBOTT   20 MG/100 ML;5 GM/100 ML;328 MG/100 ML;600 MG/100 ML;310 MG/100 ML
N19685 004
OCT 17, 1988

AP BAXTER   20 MG/100 ML;5 GM/100 ML;328 MG/100 ML;600 MG/100 ML;310 MG/100 ML
N19367 008
APR 05, 1985

POTASSIUM CHLORIDE 5 MEQ IN DEXTROSE 5% AND LACTATED RINGER'S IN PLASTIC CONTAINER

BAXTER   20 MG/100 ML;5 GM/100 ML;105 MG/100 ML;600 MG/100 ML;310 MG/100 ML
N19367 001
APR 05, 1985

CALCIUM CHLORIDE; MAGNESIUM CHLORIDE; POTASSIUM CHLORIDE; SODIUM ACETATE; SODIUM CHLORIDE

INJECTABLE; INJECTION
TPN ELECTROLYTES IN PLASTIC CONTAINER

ABBOTT   16.5 MG/ML;25.4 MG/ML;74.6 MG/ML;121 MG/ML;16.1 MG/ML
N18895 001
JUL 20, 1984

CALCIUM CHLORIDE; MAGNESIUM CHLORIDE; POTASSIUM CHLORIDE; SODIUM ACETATE; SODIUM CHLORIDE; SODIUM CITRATE

INJECTABLE; INJECTION
ISOLYTE E IN PLASTIC CONTAINER

MCGAW   35 MG/100 ML;30 MG/100 ML;74 MG/100 ML;640 MG/100 ML;500 MG/100 ML;74 MG/100 ML
N18899 001
OCT 31, 1983

          35 MG/100 ML;30 MG/100 ML;74 MG/100 ML;640 MG/100 ML;500 MG/100 ML;74 MG/100 ML
N19718 001
SEP 29, 1989

CALCIUM CHLORIDE; MAGNESIUM CHLORIDE; POTASSIUM CHLORIDE; SODIUM ACETATE; SODIUM CHLORIDE; SODIUM LACTATE

INJECTABLE; INJECTION
PLASMA-LYTE R IN PLASTIC CONTAINER

BAXTER   36.8 MG/100 ML;30.5 MG/100 ML;74.6 MG/100 ML;640 MG/100 ML;496 MG/100 ML;89.6 MG/100 ML
N17438 001

Prescription Drug Products (continued)

CALCIUM CHLORIDE; MAGNESIUM CHLORIDE; POTASSIUM CHLORIDE; SODIUM CHLORIDE

SOLUTION; PERFUSION, CARDIAC

PLEGISOL IN PLASTIC CONTAINER

	ABBOTT	17.6 MG/100 ML;325.3 MG/ 100 ML;119.3 MG/ 100 ML;643 MG/100 ML	N18608 001	FEB 26, 1982

CALCIUM CHLORIDE; POTASSIUM CHLORIDE; SODIUM CHLORIDE

INJECTABLE; INJECTION

RINGER'S IN PLASTIC CONTAINER

AP	ABBOTT	33 MG/100 ML;30 MG/ 100 ML;860 MG/100 ML	N18251 001	
AP	BAXTER	33 MG/100 ML;30 MG/ 100 ML;860 MG/100 ML	N16693 001	
AP	MCGAW	33 MG/100 ML;30 MG/ 100 ML;860 MG/100 ML	N18721 001	NOV 09, 1982
AP		33 MG/100 ML;30 MG/ 100 ML;860 MG/100 ML	N20002 001	APR 17, 1992

SOLUTION; IRRIGATION

RINGER'S IN PLASTIC CONTAINER

AT	ABBOTT	33 MG/100 ML;30 MG/ 100 ML;860 MG/100 ML	N17635 001	
AT	BAXTER	33 MG/100 ML;30 MG/ 100 ML;860 MG/100 ML	N18495 001	FEB 19, 1982
AT	MCGAW	33 MG/100 ML;30 MG/ 100 ML;860 MG/100 ML	N18156 001	

CALCIUM CHLORIDE; POTASSIUM CHLORIDE; SODIUM CHLORIDE; SODIUM LACTATE

INJECTABLE; INJECTION

LACTATED RINGER'S IN PLASTIC CONTAINER

AP	ABBOTT	20 MG/100 ML;30 MG/ 100 ML;600 MG/ 100 ML;310 MG/100 ML	N17641 001	
AP	BAXTER	20 MG/100 ML;30 MG/ 100 ML;600 MG/ 100 ML;310 MG/100 ML	N16682 001	
AP	MCGAW	20 MG/100 ML;30 MG/ 100 ML;600 MG/ 100 ML;310 MG/100 ML	N18023 001	
AP		20 MG/100 ML;30 MG/ 100 ML;600 MG/ 100 ML;310 MG/100 ML	N19632 001	FEB 29, 1988

CALCIUM CHLORIDE; POTASSIUM CHLORIDE; SODIUM CHLORIDE; SODIUM LACTATE (continued)

SOLUTION; IRRIGATION

LACTATED RINGER'S IN PLASTIC CONTAINER

AT	ABBOTT	20 MG/100 ML;30 MG/ 100 ML;600 MG/ 100 ML;310 MG/100 ML	N19416 001	JAN 17, 1986
AT	BAXTER	20 MG/100 ML;30 MG/ 100 ML;600 MG/ 100 ML;310 MG/100 ML	N18494 001	FEB 19, 1982
AT		20 MG/100 ML;30 MG/ 100 ML;600 MG/ 100 ML;310 MG/100 ML	N18921 001	APR 03, 1984
AT		20 MG/100 ML;30 MG/ 100 ML;600 MG/ 100 ML;310 MG/100 ML	N19933 001	AUG 29, 1989
AT	MCGAW	20 MG/100 ML;30 MG/ 100 ML;600 MG/ 100 ML;310 MG/100 ML	N18681 001	DEC 27, 1982

CALCIUM GLUCEPTATE

INJECTABLE; INJECTION

CALCIUM GLUCEPTATE

AP	ABBOTT	EQ 90 MG CALCIUM/5 ML	N80001 001
AP	LILLY	EQ 90 MG CALCIUM/5 ML	N06470 001
AP	LYPHOMED	EQ 90 MG CALCIUM/5 ML	N89373 001	APR 30, 1987

CANDICIDIN

OINTMENT; VAGINAL

VANOBID

+	MERRELL DOW	0.6 MG/GM	N61596 001

TABLET; VAGINAL

VANOBID

+	MERRELL DOW	3 MG	N61613 001

CAPREOMYCIN SULFATE

INJECTABLE; INJECTION

CAPASTAT SULFATE

	LILLY	EQ 1 GM BASE/VIAL	N50095 001

CAPTOPRIL

TABLET; ORAL

CAPOTEN

BRISTOL MYERS SQUIBB	12.5 MG	N18343 005	JAN 17, 1985
	25 MG	N18343 002	
	50 MG	N18343 001	
	100 MG	N18343 003	

+

Prescription Drug Products (continued)

CAPTOPRIL; HYDROCHLOROTHIAZIDE
TABLET; ORAL

TE	Product	Applicant	Strength	Appl. No.	Date
	CAPOZIDE 25/15	SQUIBB	25 MG;15 MG	N18709 001	OCT 12, 1984
	CAPOZIDE 25/25	SQUIBB	25 MG;25 MG	N18709 002	OCT 12, 1984
	CAPOZIDE 50/15	SQUIBB	50 MG;15 MG	N18709 004	OCT 12, 1984
	CAPOZIDE 50/25	+ SQUIBB	50 MG;25 MG	N18709 003	OCT 12, 1984

CARBACHOL
INJECTABLE; INJECTION

TE	Product	Applicant	Strength	Appl. No.	Date
AP	CARBACHOL	PHARMAFAIR	0.01%	N70292 001	MAY 21, 1986
AP	MIOSTAT	ALCON	0.01%	N16968 001	

CARBAMAZEPINE
SUSPENSION; ORAL

TE	Product	Applicant	Strength	Appl. No.	Date
	TEGRETOL	+ GEIGY	100 MG/5 ML	N18927 001	DEC 18, 1987

TABLET; ORAL

TE	Product	Applicant	Strength	Appl. No.	Date
	CARBAMAZEPINE				
AB		INWOOD	200 MG	N70231 001	AUG 14, 1986
AB		PUREPAC	200 MG	N71696 001	NOV 09, 1987
AB		SIDMAK	200 MG	N71479 001	JUL 24, 1987
	EPITOL				
AB		LEMMON	200 MG	N70541 001	SEP 17, 1986
	TEGRETOL				
AB		+ GEIGY	200 MG	N16608 001	

TABLET, CHEWABLE; ORAL

TE	Product	Applicant	Strength	Appl. No.	Date
	CARBAMAZEPINE				
AB		WARNER CHILCOTT	100 MG	N71940 001	FEB 01, 1988
	EPITOL				
AB		LEMMON	100 MG	N73524 001	JUL 29, 1992
	TEGRETOL				
AB		+ GEIGY	100 MG	N18281 001	

CARBENICILLIN DISODIUM
INJECTABLE; INJECTION

TE	Product	Applicant	Strength	Appl. No.
	GEOPEN	ROERIG		
AP			EQ 1 GM BASE/VIAL	N50306 001
AP			EQ 2 GM BASE/VIAL	N50306 004
AP			EQ 5 GM BASE/VIAL	N50306 002
AP			EQ 10 GM BASE/VIAL	N50306 006
			EQ 30 GM BASE/VIAL	N50306 007
	PYOPEN	BEECHAM		
AP			EQ 1 GM BASE/VIAL	N50298 001
AP			EQ 2 GM BASE/VIAL	N50298 002
AP			EQ 5 GM BASE/VIAL	N50298 003
AP			EQ 10 GM BASE/VIAL	N50298 006
			EQ 20 GM BASE/VIAL	N50298 007

CARBENICILLIN INDANYL SODIUM
TABLET; ORAL

TE	Product	Applicant	Strength	Appl. No.
	GEOCILLIN	+ PFIZER	EQ 382 MG BASE	N50435 001

CARBIDOPA
TABLET; ORAL

TE	Product	Applicant	Strength	Appl. No.
	LODOSYN	+ MSD	25 MG	N17830 001

CARBIDOPA; LEVODOPA
TABLET; ORAL

TE	Product	Applicant	Strength	Appl. No.	Date
	CARBIDOPA AND LEVODOPA	LEMMON			
AB			10 MG:100 MG	N73618 001	AUG 28, 1992
AB			25 MG:100 MG	N73589 001	AUG 28, 1992
			25 MG:250 MG	N73607 001	AUG 28, 1992
	SINEMET	MSD			
AB			10 MG:100 MG	N17555 001	
AB			25 MG:100 MG	N17555 003	
		+	25 MG:250 MG	N17555 002	

TABLET, EXTENDED RELEASE; ORAL

TE	Product	Applicant	Strength	Appl. No.	Date
	SINEMET CR	+ MSD	50 MG:200 MG	N19856 001	MAY 30, 1991

CARBINOXAMINE MALEATE
TABLET; ORAL

TE	Product	Applicant	Strength	Appl. No.
	CLISTIN	JOHNSON RW	4 MG	N08915 001

Prescription Drug Products (continued)

CARBOPLATIN
INJECTABLE; INJECTION
PARAPLATIN

BRISTOL MYERS SQUIBB	50 MG/VIAL	N19880 001	MAR 03, 1989
	150 MG/VIAL	N19880 002	MAR 03, 1989
	450 MG/VIAL	N19880 003	MAR 03, 1989

CARBOPROST TROMETHAMINE
INJECTABLE; INJECTION
HEBAMATE

UPJOHN	EQ 0.25 MG BASE/ML	N17989 001

CARISOPRODOL
CAPSULE; ORAL
SOMA

WALLACE	250 MG	N11792 003

TABLET; ORAL
CARISOPRODOL

△△	CHELSEA	350 MG	N86179 001	
△△	DANBURY	350 MG	N87499 001	APR 20, 1982
B*	EON LABS	350 MG	N89566 001	AUG 30, 1988
△△	GENEVA	350 MG	N81025 001	APR 13, 1989
△△	MUTUAL PHARM	350 MG	N89346 001	OCT 17, 1991
△△	PIONEER PHARMS	350 MG	N89390 001	OCT 13, 1988

RELA

△△	SCHERING	350 MG	N12155 001

SOMA

△△	WALLACE	350 MG	N11792 001

CARISOPRODOL; *MULTIPLE*
SEE ASPIRIN; CARISOPRODOL
SEE ASPIRIN; CARISOPRODOL; CODEINE PHOSPHATE

CARMUSTINE
INJECTABLE; INJECTION
BICNU

BRISTOL	100 MG/VIAL	N17422 001

CARTEOLOL HYDROCHLORIDE
SOLUTION/DROPS; OPHTHALMIC
OPTIPRESS

BURROUGHS WELLCOME	1%	N19972 001	MAY 23, 1990

CARTEOLOL HYDROCHLORIDE (continued)
TABLET; ORAL
CARTROL

ABBOTT	2.5 MG	N19204 001	DEC 28, 1988
+	5 MG	N19204 002	DEC 28, 1988

CEFACLOR
CAPSULE; ORAL
CECLOR

+ LILLY	EQ 250 MG BASE	N50521 001	
	EQ 250 MG BASE	N62206 001	
	EQ 500 MG BASE	N50521 002	
+	EQ 500 MG BASE	N62205 002	APR 20, 1988

POWDER FOR RECONSTITUTION; ORAL
CECLOR

+ LILLY	EQ 125 MG BASE/5 ML	N50522 001	
	EQ 125 MG BASE/5 ML	N62206 001	
	EQ 187 MG BASE/5 ML	N62206 003	APR 20, 1988
+	EQ 250 MG BASE/5 ML	N50522 002	
	EQ 250 MG BASE/5 ML	N62206 002	
+	EQ 375 MG BASE/5 ML	N62206 004	APR 20, 1988

CEFADROXIL/CEFADROXIL HEMIHYDRATE
CAPSULE; ORAL
CEFADROXIL

△B	ZENITH	EQ 500 MG BASE	N62766 001	MAR 03, 1987

DURICEF

△B	+ MEAD JOHNSON	EQ 500 MG BASE	N50512 001

ULTRACEF

△B	BRISTOL	EQ 500 MG BASE	N62291 001

POWDER FOR RECONSTITUTION; ORAL
DURICEF

△B	+ MEAD JOHNSON	EQ 125 MG BASE/5 ML	N50527 002
△B	+	EQ 250 MG BASE/5 ML	N50527 003
△B	+	EQ 500 MG BASE/5 ML	N50527 001

ULTRACEF

△B	BRISTOL	EQ 125 MG BASE/5 ML	N62334 001
△B		EQ 250 MG BASE/5 ML	N62334 002
△B		EQ 500 MG BASE/5 ML	N62334 003

TABLET; ORAL
CEFADROXIL

△B	ZENITH	EQ 1 GM BASE	N62774 001	APR 08, 1987

DURICEF

△B	+ MEAD JOHNSON	EQ 1 GM BASE	N50528 001

ULTRACEF

△B	BRISTOL	EQ 1 GM BASE	N62390 001	JUN 10, 1982

Prescription Drug Products *(continued)*

CEFAMANDOLE NAFATE
INJECTABLE; INJECTION
MANDOL
LILLY

EQ 500 MG BASE/VIAL	N50504 001	
EQ 1 GM BASE/VIAL	N50504 002	
EQ 1 GM BASE/VIAL	N62560 001	SEP 10, 1985
EQ 2 GM BASE/VIAL	N50504 003	
EQ 2 GM BASE/VIAL	N62560 002	SEP 10, 1985

CEFAZOLIN SODIUM
INJECTABLE; INJECTION
ANCEF
SKF

AP	EQ 250 MG BASE/VIAL	N50461 001	
AP	EQ 500 MG BASE/VIAL	N50461 002	
AP	EQ 1 GM BASE/VIAL	N50461 003	
AP	EQ 5 GM BASE/VIAL	N50461 004	
AP	EQ 10 GM BASE/VIAL	N50461 005	

ANCEF IN DEXTROSE 5% IN PLASTIC CONTAINER
BAXTER

EQ 10 MG BASE/ML	N50566 003	JUN 08, 1983
EQ 20 MG BASE/ML	N50566 004	JUN 08, 1983

ANCEF IN PLASTIC CONTAINER
BAXTER

EQ 10 MG BASE/ML	N63002 001	MAR 28, 1991
EQ 20 MG BASE/ML	N63002 002	MAR 28, 1991

CEFAZOLIN SODIUM
BEN VENUE

AP	EQ 250 MG BASE/VIAL	N62894 001	JUL 21, 1988
AP	EQ 500 MG BASE/VIAL	N62894 002	JUL 21, 1988
AP	EQ 1 GM BASE/VIAL	N62894 003	JUL 21, 1988
AP	EQ 5 GM BASE/VIAL	N62894 004	JUL 21, 1988
AP	EQ 10 GM BASE/VIAL	N62894 005	JUL 21, 1988

ELKINS SINN

AP	EQ 250 MG BASE/VIAL	N62807 001	JAN 12, 1988
AP	EQ 500 MG BASE/VIAL	N62807 002	JAN 12, 1988
AP	EQ 1 GM BASE/VIAL	N62807 003	JAN 12, 1988
AP	EQ 5 GM BASE/VIAL	N62807 004	JAN 12, 1988
AP	EQ 10 GM BASE/VIAL	N62807 005	JAN 12, 1988
AP	EQ 20 GM BASE/VIAL	N62807 006	JAN 12, 1988

CEFAZOLIN SODIUM *(continued)*
INJECTABLE; INJECTION
CEFAZOLIN SODIUM
HANFORD

AP	EQ 500 MG BASE/VIAL	N63214 001	DEC 27, 1991
AP	EQ 500 MG BASE/VIAL	N63216 001	DEC 27, 1991
AP	EQ 1 GM BASE/VIAL	N63207 001	DEC 27, 1991
AP	EQ 1 GM BASE/VIAL	N63208 001	DEC 27, 1991
AP	EQ 10 GM BASE/VIAL	N63209 001	DEC 27, 1991

LEMMON

AP	EQ 250 MG BASE/VIAL	N63016 001	MAR 14, 1989
AP	EQ 500 MG BASE/VIAL	N63016 002	MAR 14, 1989
AP	EQ 1 GM BASE/VIAL	N63016 003	MAR 14, 1989
AP	EQ 5 GM BASE/VIAL	N63018 001	MAR 05, 1990
AP	EQ 10 GM BASE/VIAL	N63018 002	MAR 05, 1990

LYPHOMED

AP	EQ 500 MG BASE/VIAL	N62688 002	NOV 17, 1986
AP	EQ 1 GM BASE/VIAL	N62688 003	NOV 17, 1986
AP	EQ 10 GM BASE/VIAL	N62688 004	NOV 17, 1986
AP	EQ 20 GM BASE/VIAL	N62688 005	AUG 03, 1987

MARSAM

AP	EQ 250 MG BASE/VIAL	N62988 001	DEC 29, 1989
AP	EQ 500 MG BASE/VIAL	N62988 002	DEC 29, 1989
AP	EQ 1 GM BASE/VIAL	N62988 003	DEC 29, 1989
AP	EQ 5 GM BASE/VIAL	N62989 001	DEC 29, 1989
AP	EQ 10 GM BASE/VIAL	N62989 002	DEC 29, 1989
AP	EQ 20 GM BASE/VIAL	N62989 003	DEC 29, 1989

KEFZOL
LILLY

AP	EQ 250 MG BASE/VIAL	N61773 001	
AP	EQ 500 MG BASE/VIAL	N61773 002	
AP	EQ 500 MG BASE/VIAL	N62557 001	SEP 10, 1985
AP	EQ 1 GM BASE/VIAL	N61773 003	
AP	EQ 1 GM BASE/VIAL	N62557 002	SEP 10, 1985
AP	EQ 10 GM BASE/VIAL	N61773 004	
AP	EQ 20 GM BASE/VIAL	N61773 005	SEP 08, 1987

ZOLICEF
BRISTOL MYERS

AP	EQ 500 MG BASE/VIAL	N62831 001	DEC 09, 1988
AP	EQ 1 GM BASE/VIAL	N62831 002	DEC 09, 1988

Prescription Drug Products *(continued)*

CEFIXIME
POWDER FOR RECONSTITUTION; ORAL

SUPRAX				
+ LEDERLE	100 MG/5 ML	N50622 001	APR 28, 1989

TABLET; ORAL

SUPRAX				
+ LEDERLE	200 MG	N50621 001	APR 28, 1989
+	400 MG	N50621 002	APR 28, 1989

CEFMENOXIME HYDROCHLORIDE
INJECTABLE; INJECTION

CEFMAX			
TAP	EQ 500 MG BASE/VIAL	N50571 001	DEC 30, 1987
	EQ 1 GM BASE/VIAL	N50571 002	DEC 30, 1987
	EQ 2 GM BASE/VIAL	N50571 003	DEC 30, 1987

CEFMETAZOLE SODIUM
INJECTABLE; INJECTION

ZEFAZONE			
UPJOHN	EQ 1 GM BASE/VIAL	N50637 001	DEC 11, 1989
	EQ 2 GM BASE/VIAL	N50637 002	DEC 11, 1989

CEFONICID SODIUM
INJECTABLE; INJECTION

MONOCID			
SKF	EQ 500 MG BASE/VIAL	N50579 001	MAY 23, 1984
	EQ 1 GM BASE/VIAL	N50579 002	MAY 23, 1984
	EQ 2 GM BASE/VIAL	N50579 003	MAY 23, 1984
	EQ 10 GM BASE/VIAL	N50579 004	MAY 23, 1984

CEFOPERAZONE SODIUM
INJECTABLE; INJECTION

CEFOBID			
PFIZER	EQ 1 GM BASE/VIAL	N50551 001	NOV 18, 1982
	EQ 2 GM BASE/VIAL	N50551 002	NOV 18, 1982
	EQ 10 GM BASE/VIAL	N50551 003	MAR 05, 1990
CEFOBID IN PLASTIC CONTAINER			
PFIZER	EQ 20 MG BASE/ML	N50613 002	JUL 31, 1987
	EQ 40 MG BASE/ML	N50613 001	JUL 22, 1987

CEFORANIDE
INJECTABLE; INJECTION

PRECEF			
BRISTOL	500 MG/VIAL	N50554 001	MAY 24, 1984
	500 MG/VIAL	N62579 001	NOV 26, 1984
	1 GM/VIAL	N50554 002	MAY 24, 1984
	1 GM/VIAL	N62579 002	NOV 26, 1984
	2 GM/VIAL	N50554 003	MAY 24, 1984
	2 GM/VIAL	N62579 003	NOV 26, 1984
	10 GM/VIAL	N50554 004	MAY 24, 1984
	10 GM/VIAL	N62579 004	NOV 26, 1984
	20 GM/VIAL	N50554 005	MAY 24, 1984
	20 GM/VIAL	N62579 005	NOV 26, 1984

CEFOTAXIME SODIUM
INJECTABLE; INJECTION

CLAFORAN			
HOECHST ROUSSEL	EQ 1 GM BASE/VIAL	N50547 002	JAN 13, 1987
	EQ 1 GM BASE/VIAL	N62659 001	JAN 13, 1987
	EQ 2 GM BASE/VIAL	N50547 003	JAN 13, 1987
	EQ 2 GM BASE/VIAL	N62659 002	JAN 13, 1987
	EQ 10 GM BASE/VIAL	N50547 004	DEC 29, 1983
CLAFORAN IN DEXTROSE 5% IN PLASTIC CONTAINER			
HOECHST ROUSSEL	EQ 20 MG BASE/ML	N50596 002	MAY 20, 1985
	EQ 40 MG BASE/ML	N50596 004	MAY 20, 1985
CLAFORAN IN SODIUM CHLORIDE 0.9% IN PLASTIC CONTAINER			
HOECHST ROUSSEL	EQ 20 MG BASE/ML	N50596 001	MAY 20, 1985
	EQ 40 MG BASE/ML	N50596 003	MAY 20, 1985

CEFOTETAN DISODIUM
INJECTABLE; INJECTION

CEFOTAN			
STUART	EQ 1 GM BASE/VIAL	N50588 001	DEC 27, 1985
	EQ 2 GM BASE/VIAL	N50588 002	DEC 27, 1985
	EQ 10 GM BASE/VIAL	N50588 003	APR 25, 1988

Prescription Drug Products *(continued)*

CEFOTIAM HYDROCHLORIDE

INJECTABLE; INJECTION
CERADON

TAKEDA	EQ 1 GM BASE/VIAL	N50601 001	DEC 30, 1988

CEFOXITIN SODIUM

INJECTABLE; INJECTION
MEFOXIN

MSD	EQ 1 GM BASE/VIAL	N50517 001	
	EQ 1 GM BASE/VIAL	N62757 001	JAN 08, 1987
	EQ 2 GM BASE/VIAL	N50517 002	
	EQ 2 GM BASE/VIAL	N62757 002	JAN 08, 1987
	EQ 10 GM BASE/VIAL	N50517 003	JAN 08, 1987

MEFOXIN IN DEXTROSE 5% IN PLASTIC CONTAINER

MSD	EQ 20 MG BASE/ML	N50581 003	SEP 20, 1984
	EQ 40 MG BASE/ML	N50581 004	SEP 20, 1984

MEFOXIN IN SODIUM CHLORIDE 0.9% IN PLASTIC CONTAINER

MSD	EQ 20 MG BASE/ML	N50581 002	SEP 20, 1984
	EQ 40 MG BASE/ML	N50581 001	SEP 20, 1984

CEFPIRAMIDE SODIUM

INJECTABLE; INJECTION
CEFPIRAMIDE SODIUM

WYETH AYERST	EQ 1 GM BASE/VIAL	N50633 002	JAN 31, 1989
	EQ 2 GM BASE/VIAL	N50633 003	JAN 31, 1989
	EQ 10 GM BASE/VIAL	N50633 005	JAN 31, 1989

CEFPODOXIME PROXETIL

GRANULE, FOR RECONSTITUTION; ORAL
BANAN

AB	SANKYO	EQ 50 MG BASE/5 ML	N50688 002	AUG 07, 1992
AB		EQ 100 MG BASE/5 ML	N50688 001	AUG 07, 1992

VANTIN

AB	UPJOHN	EQ 50 MG BASE/5 ML	N50675 001	AUG 07, 1992
AB	+	EQ 100 MG BASE/5 ML	N50675 002	AUG 07, 1992

CEFPODOXIME PROXETIL *(continued)*

TABLET; ORAL
BANAN

AB	SANKYO	EQ 100 MG BASE	N50687 001	AUG 07, 1992
AB		EQ 200 MG BASE	N50687 002	AUG 07, 1992

VANTIN

AB	UPJOHN	EQ 100 MG BASE	N50674 001	AUG 07, 1992
AB	+	EQ 200 MG BASE	N50674 002	AUG 07, 1992

CEFPROZIL

POWDER FOR RECONSTITUTION; ORAL
CEFZIL

BRISTOL MYERS SQUIBB	125 MG/5 ML	N50665 001	DEC 23, 1991
+	250 MG/5 ML	N50665 002	DEC 23, 1991

TABLET; ORAL
CEFZIL

BRISTOL MYERS SQUIBB	250 MG	N50664 001	DEC 23, 1991
+	500 MG	N50664 002	DEC 23, 1991

CEFTAZIDIME

INJECTABLE; INJECTION
FORTAZ

AP	GLAXO	500 MG/VIAL	N50578 001	JUL 19, 1985
AP		1 GM/VIAL	N50578 002	JUL 19, 1985
AP		2 GM/VIAL	N50578 003	JUL 19, 1985
AP		6 GM/VIAL	N50578 004	JUL 19, 1985

TAZICEF

AP	SKF	500 MG/VIAL	N62662 001	MAR 06, 1986
AP		1 GM/VIAL	N62662 002	MAR 06, 1986
AP		2 GM/VIAL	N62662 003	MAR 06, 1986
AP		6 GM/VIAL	N62662 004	MAR 06, 1986

Prescription Drug Products (continued)

CEFTAZIDIME (continued)
INJECTABLE; INJECTION
TAZIDIME
LILLY

	Strength	Number	Date
AP	500 MG/VIAL	N62640 001	NOV 20, 1985
AP	1 GM/VIAL	N62640 002	NOV 20, 1985
AP	1 GM/VIAL	N62655 001	NOV 20, 1985
AP	2 GM/VIAL	N62640 003	NOV 20, 1985
AP	2 GM/VIAL	N62655 002	NOV 20, 1985

TAZIDIME IN PLASTIC CONTAINER
LILLY

	Strength	Number	Date
AP	1 GM/VIAL	N62739 001	JUL 10, 1986
AP	2 GM/VIAL	N62739 002	JUL 10, 1986

CEFTAZIDIME (ARGININE FORMULATION)
INJECTABLE; INJECTION
CEPTAZ
GLAXO

	Strength	Number	Date
AP	1 GM/VIAL	N50646 002	SEP 27, 1990
AP	2 GM/VIAL	N50646 003	SEP 27, 1990
AP	10 GM/VIAL	N50646 004	SEP 27, 1990
	500 MG/VIAL	N50646 001	SEP 27, 1990

PENTACEF
SMITHKLINE BEECHAM

	Strength	Number	Date
AP	1 GM/VIAL	N64006 001	MAR 31, 1992
AP	2 GM/VIAL	N64006 002	MAR 31, 1992
AP	10 GM/VIAL	N64008 002	MAR 31, 1992
AP	6 GM/VIAL	N64008 001	MAR 31, 1992

CEFTAZIDIME SODIUM
INJECTABLE; INJECTION
FORTAZ IN PLASTIC CONTAINER
GLAXO

Strength	Number	Date
EQ 10 MG BASE/ML	N50634 001	APR 28, 1989
EQ 20 MG BASE/ML	N50634 002	APR 28, 1989
EQ 40 MG BASE/ML	N50634 003	APR 28, 1989

CEFTIZOXIME SODIUM
INJECTABLE; INJECTION
CEFIZOX
SKF

Strength	Number	Date
EQ 1 GM BASE/VIAL	N50560 002	SEP 15, 1983
EQ 2 GM BASE/VIAL	N50560 003	SEP 15, 1983

CEFIZOX IN DEXTROSE 5% IN PLASTIC CONTAINER
SKF

Strength	Number	Date
EQ 20 MG BASE/ML	N50589 001	OCT 03, 1984
EQ 40 MG BASE/ML	N50589 002	OCT 03, 1984

CEFTRIAXONE SODIUM
INJECTABLE; INJECTION
ROCEPHIN
ROCHE

Strength	Number	Date
EQ 250 MG BASE/VIAL	N50585 001	DEC 21, 1984
EQ 500 MG BASE/VIAL	N50585 002	DEC 21, 1984
EQ 500 MG BASE/VIAL	N62654 001	APR 30, 1987
EQ 1 GM BASE/VIAL	N50585 003	DEC 21, 1984
EQ 1 GM BASE/VIAL	N62654 002	APR 30, 1987
EQ 2 GM BASE/VIAL	N50585 004	DEC 21, 1984
EQ 2 GM BASE/VIAL	N62654 003	APR 30, 1987
EQ 10 GM BASE/VIAL	N50585 005	DEC 21, 1984

ROCEPHIN W/ DEXTROSE IN PLASTIC CONTAINER
ROCHE

Strength	Number	Date
EQ 10 MG BASE/ML	N50624 001	FEB 11, 1987
EQ 20 MG BASE/ML	N50624 002	FEB 11, 1987
EQ 40 MG BASE/ML	N50624 003	FEB 11, 1987

CEFUROXIME AXETIL
TABLET; ORAL
CEFTIN
GLAXO

	Strength	Number	Date
	EQ 125 MG BASE	N50605 001	DEC 28, 1987
+	EQ 250 MG BASE	N50605 002	DEC 28, 1987
	EQ 500 MG BASE	N50605 003	DEC 28, 1987

Prescription Drug Products (continued)

CEFUROXIME SODIUM
INJECTABLE; INJECTION

KEFUROX
LILLY

ΔP	EQ 750 MG BASE/VIAL	N62591 001	JAN 10, 1986
ΔP	EQ 750 MG BASE/VIAL	N62592 001	JAN 10, 1986
	EQ 1.5 GM BASE/VIAL	N62591 002	JAN 10, 1986
ΔP	EQ 1.5 GM BASE/VIAL	N62592 002	JAN 10, 1986
ΔP	EQ 7.5 GM BASE/VIAL	N62591 003	DEC 17, 1987

KEFUROX IN PLASTIC CONTAINER
LILLY

ΔP	EQ 750 MG BASE/VIAL	N62590 001	JAN 10, 1986
ΔP	EQ 1.5 GM BASE/VIAL	N62590 002	JAN 10, 1986

ZINACEF
GLAXO

ΔP	EQ 750 MG BASE/VIAL	N50558 002	OCT 19, 1983
ΔP	EQ 1.5 GM BASE/VIAL	N50558 003	OCT 19, 1983

ZINACEF IN PLASTIC CONTAINER
GLAXO

	EQ 15 MG BASE/ML	N50643 001	APR 28, 1989
	EQ 30 MG BASE/ML	N50643 002	APR 28, 1989

CELLULOSE SODIUM PHOSPHATE
POWDER; ORAL

CALCIBIND

+	MISSION PHARMA	2.5 GM/PACKET	N18757 002	DEC 28, 1982
+		300 GM/BOT	N18757 003	OCT 16, 1984

CEPHALEXIN
CAPSULE; ORAL

CEFANEX
BRISTOL MYERS

ΔB	EQ 250 MG BASE	N63063 001	SEP 29, 1989
ΔB	EQ 500 MG BASE	N63063 002	SEP 29, 1989

CEPHALEXIN
ATRAL

ΔB	EQ 250 MG BASE	N62713 001	JUL 15, 1988
ΔB	EQ 500 MG BASE	N62713 002	JUL 15, 1988

CEPHALEXIN (continued)
CAPSULE; ORAL

CEPHALEXIN
BARR

ΔB	EQ 250 MG BASE	N62773 001	JUN 26, 1987
ΔB	EQ 500 MG BASE	N62775 001	APR 22, 1987

BIOCRAFT

ΔB	EQ 250 MG BASE	N62702 001	FEB 13, 1987
ΔB	EQ 500 MG BASE	N62702 002	FEB 13, 1987

LEMMON

ΔB	EQ 250 MG BASE	N62821 001	FEB 05, 1988
ΔB	EQ 500 MG BASE	N62823 001	FEB 05, 1988

MJ

ΔB	EQ 250 MG BASE	N62791 001	JUN 11, 1987
ΔB	EQ 500 MG BASE	N62791 002	JUN 11, 1987

NOVOPHARM

ΔB	EQ 250 MG BASE	N62760 001	APR 24, 1987
ΔB	EQ 500 MG BASE	N62761 001	APR 24, 1987

PUREPAC

ΔB	EQ 250 MG BASE	N62809 001	APR 22, 1987
ΔB	EQ 500 MG BASE	N62809 002	APR 22, 1987

SQUIBB MARK

ΔB	EQ 250 MG BASE	N62973 001	NOV 08, 1988
ΔB	EQ 500 MG BASE	N62974 001	NOV 23, 1988

STEVENS

ΔB	EQ 250 MG BASE	N62870 001	MAR 17, 1988
ΔB	EQ 500 MG BASE	N62869 001	MAR 17, 1988

YOSHITOMI

ΔB	EQ 250 MG BASE	N62872 001	JUN 20, 1988
ΔB	EQ 500 MG BASE	N62871 001	JUL 05, 1988

ZENITH

ΔB	EQ 250 MG BASE	N61969 001	
ΔB	EQ 500 MG BASE	N61969 002	

CEPHALEXIN MONOHYDRATE
VITARINE

B*	EQ 250 MG BASE	N62159 001	
B*	EQ 500 MG BASE	N62159 002	

KEFLEX
+ LILLY

ΔB	EQ 250 MG BASE	N50405 002	
ΔB	EQ 250 MG BASE	N62118 001	
ΔB	EQ 500 MG BASE	N50405 003	
ΔB	EQ 500 MG BASE	N62118 002	

Prescription Drug Products (continued)

CEPHALEXIN (continued)

POWDER FOR RECONSTITUTION; ORAL

CEPHALEXIN

TE	Firm	Strength	Appl No	Date
AB	BARR	EQ 125 MG BASE/5 ML	N62778 001	AUG 06, 1987
AB		EQ 250 MG BASE/5 ML	N62777 001	AUG 06, 1987
AB	BIOCRAFT	EQ 125 MG BASE/5 ML	N62703 001	FEB 13, 1987
AB		EQ 250 MG BASE/5 ML	N62703 002	FEB 13, 1987
AB	LEMMON	EQ 125 MG BASE/5 ML	N62873 001	MAY 23, 1988
AB		EQ 250 MG BASE/5 ML	N62867 001	APR 15, 1988
AB	NOVOPHARM	EQ 125 MG BASE/5 ML	N62767 001	JUN 16, 1987
AB		EQ 125 MG BASE/5 ML	N62768 001	JUN 16, 1987
AB	SQUIBB MARK	EQ 125 MG BASE/5 ML	N62986 001	APR 18, 1991
AB		EQ 250 MG BASE/5 ML	N62987 001	JUL 25, 1989

KEFLEX

TE	Firm	Strength	Appl No
AB	+ LILLY	EQ 125 MG BASE/5 ML	N50406 001
AB		EQ 125 MG BASE/5 ML	N62117 002
AB	+	EQ 250 MG BASE/5 ML	N50406 002
AB	+	EQ 250 MG BASE/5 ML	N62117 003
		EQ 100 MG BASE/ML	N50406 003
		EQ 100 MG BASE/ML	N62117 001

TABLET; ORAL

CEPHALEXIN

TE	Firm	Strength	Appl No	Date
AB	BARR	EQ 250 MG BASE	N62826 001	AUG 17, 1987
AB		EQ 500 MG BASE	N62827 001	AUG 17, 1987
AB	BIOCRAFT	EQ 250 MG BASE	N63023 001	JAN 12, 1989
AB		EQ 500 MG BASE	N63024 001	JAN 12, 1989

KEFLET

TE	Firm	Strength	Appl No	Date
AB	+ LILLY	EQ 250 MG BASE	N50440 003	FEB 26, 1987
AB		EQ 250 MG BASE	N62745 001	DEC 01, 1986
AB	+	EQ 500 MG BASE	N50440 001	
AB	+	EQ 500 MG BASE	N62745 002	DEC 01, 1986
	+	EQ 1 GM BASE	N50440 002	

CEPHALEXIN HYDROCHLORIDE

TABLET; ORAL

KEFTAB

TE	Firm	Strength	Appl No	Date
	+ LILLY	EQ 250 MG BASE	N50614 001	OCT 29, 1987
	+	EQ 333 MG BASE	N50614 003	MAY 16, 1988
	+	EQ 500 MG BASE	N50614 002	OCT 29, 1987

CEPHALOGLYCIN

CAPSULE; ORAL

KAFOCIN

TE	Firm	Strength	Appl No
	+ LILLY	250 MG	N50219 001

CEPHALOTHIN SODIUM

INJECTABLE; INJECTION

CEPHALOTHIN SODIUM

TE	Firm	Strength	Appl No	Date
AP	ABBOTT	EQ 1 GM BASE/VIAL	N62547 001	SEP 11, 1985
AP		EQ 1 GM BASE/VIAL	N62548 001	SEP 11, 1985
AP		EQ 2 GM BASE/VIAL	N62547 002	SEP 11, 1985
AP		EQ 2 GM BASE/VIAL	N62548 002	SEP 11, 1985
AP	BRISTOL	EQ 1 GM BASE/VIAL	N62464 001	MAY 07, 1984
AP		EQ 2 GM BASE/VIAL	N62464 002	MAY 07, 1984
AP		EQ 4 GM BASE/VIAL	N62464 003	MAY 07, 1984
AP	LYPHOMED	EQ 1 GM BASE/VIAL	N62666 002	JUN 10, 1987
AP		EQ 2 GM BASE/VIAL	N62666 001	JUN 10, 1987

CEPHALOTHIN SODIUM W/ DEXTROSE IN PLASTIC CONTAINER

TE	Firm	Strength	Appl No	Date
	BAXTER	EQ 20 MG BASE/ML	N62422 003	JAN 31, 1984
		EQ 20 MG BASE/ML	N62422 005	JUL 16, 1991
		EQ 20 MG BASE/ML	N62730 001	MAR 05, 1987
		EQ 40 MG BASE/ML	N62422 004	JAN 31, 1984
		EQ 40 MG BASE/ML	N62422 006	JUL 16, 1991
		EQ 40 MG BASE/ML	N62730 002	MAR 05, 1987

Prescription Drug Products (continued)

CEPHALOTHIN SODIUM (continued)

INJECTABLE; INJECTION
CEPHALOTHIN SODIUM W/ SODIUM CHLORIDE IN PLASTIC CONTAINER

BAXTER
	EQ 20 MG BASE/ML	N62422 001	JAN 31, 1984
	EQ 40 MG BASE/ML	N62422 002	JAN 31, 1984

KEFLIN
LILLY
AP	EQ 1 GM BASE/VIAL	N50482 001	
AP	EQ 2 GM BASE/VIAL	N50482 002	
AP	EQ 4 GM BASE/VIAL	N50482 003	
	EQ 20 GM BASE/VIAL	N50482 007	

KEFLIN IN PLASTIC CONTAINER
LILLY
AP	EQ 1 GM BASE/VIAL	N62549 001	SEP 10, 1985
AP	EQ 2 GM BASE/VIAL	N62549 002	SEP 10, 1985

SEFFIN
GLAXO
AP	EQ 1 GM BASE/VIAL	N62435 001	NOV 15, 1983
AP	EQ 2 GM BASE/VIAL	N62435 002	NOV 15, 1983
AP	EQ 10 GM BASE/VIAL	N62435 003	NOV 15, 1983

CEPHAPIRIN SODIUM

INJECTABLE; INJECTION
CEFADYL

BRISTOL
AP	EQ 500 MG BASE/VIAL	N50446 005	
AP	EQ 1 GM BASE/VIAL	N50446 001	
AP	EQ 1 GM BASE/VIAL	N61769 001	
AP	EQ 1 GM BASE/VIAL	N62724 001	
AP	EQ 2 GM BASE/VIAL	N50446 002	DEC 23, 1986
AP	EQ 2 GM BASE/VIAL	N61769 002	
AP	EQ 2 GM BASE/VIAL	N62724 002	DEC 23, 1986
AP	EQ 4 GM BASE/VIAL	N50446 003	
AP	EQ 4 GM BASE/VIAL	N61769 003	
AP	EQ 20 GM BASE/VIAL	N50446 004	

BRISTOL MYERS
AP	EQ 500 MG BASE/VIAL	N62961 001	SEP 20, 1988
AP	EQ 1 GM BASE/VIAL	N62961 002	SEP 20, 1988
AP	EQ 2 GM BASE/VIAL	N62961 003	SEP 20, 1988
AP	EQ 4 GM BASE/VIAL	N62961 004	SEP 20, 1988

CEPHAPIRIN SODIUM (continued)

INJECTABLE; INJECTION
CEPHAPIRIN SODIUM

ELKINS SINN
AP	EQ 500 MG BASE/VIAL	N62720 001	JUL 02, 1987
AP	EQ 1 GM BASE/VIAL	N62720 002	JUL 02, 1987
AP	EQ 2 GM BASE/VIAL	N62720 003	JUL 02, 1987
AP	EQ 20 GM BASE/VIAL	N62720 004	JUL 02, 1987

LYPHOMED
AP	EQ 500 MG BASE/VIAL	N62723 001	NOV 17, 1986
AP	EQ 1 GM BASE/VIAL	N62723 002	NOV 17, 1986
AP	EQ 2 GM BASE/VIAL	N62723 003	NOV 17, 1986
AP	EQ 4 GM BASE/VIAL	N62723 004	NOV 17, 1986

CEPHRADINE

CAPSULE; ORAL
ANSPOR

SKF
AB	250 MG	N61859 001
AB	500 MG	N61859 002

CEPHRADINE

BARR
AB	250 MG	N62850 001	APR 22, 1988
AB	500 MG	N62851 001	APR 22, 1988

BIOCRAFT
AB	250 MG	N62683 001	JAN 09, 1987
AB	500 MG	N62683 002	JAN 09, 1987

ZENITH
AB	250 MG	N62762 001	MAR 06, 1987
AB	500 MG	N62762 002	MAR 06, 1987

VELOSEF

+ ERSANA +
AB	250 MG	N61764 001
AB	500 MG	N61764 002

INJECTABLE; INJECTION
VELOSEF

SQUIBB
	250 MG/VIAL	N61976 001
	500 MG/VIAL	N61976 002
	1 GM/VIAL	N61976 004
	2 GM/VIAL	N61976 003
	4 GM/VIAL	N61976 005

Prescription Drug Products (continued)

CEPHRADINE (continued)

POWDER FOR RECONSTITUTION; ORAL

	ANSPOR			
AB	SKF	125 MG/5 ML	N61866 001	
AB		250 MG/5 ML	N61866 002	
	CEPHRADINE			
AB	BARR	125 MG/5 ML	N62858 001	MAY 19, 1988
AB		250 MG/5 ML	N62859 001	MAY 19, 1988
AB	BIOCRAFT	125 MG/5 ML	N62693 001	JAN 09, 1987
AB		250 MG/5 ML	N62693 002	JAN 09, 1987
	VELOSEF '125'			
AB	+ ERSANA	125 MG/5 ML	N61763 001	
	VELOSEF '250'			
AB	+ ERSANA	250 MG/5 ML	N61763 002	

TABLET; ORAL

	VELOSEF		
	+ SQUIBB	1 GM	N50530 001

CETYL ALCOHOL; COLFOSCERIL PALMITATE; TYLOXAPOL

POWDER FOR RECONSTITUTION; INTRATRACHEAL

EXOSURF NEONATAL			
BURROUGHS WELLCOME	12 MG/VIAL;108 MG/VIAL;8 MG/VIAL	N20044 001	AUG 02, 1990

CHENODIOL

TABLET; ORAL

CHENIX			
+ SOLVAY	250 MG	N18513 002	JUL 28, 1983

CHLORAMBUCIL

TABLET; ORAL

LEUKERAN			
+ BURROUGHS WELLCOME	2 MG	N10669 002	

CHLORAMPHENICOL

CAPSULE; ORAL

	AMPHICOL		
AB	MK	100 MG	N60058 001
AB		250 MG	N60058 002
	CHLORAMPHENICOL		
AB	ZENITH	250 MG	N62247 001
	CHLOROMYCETIN		
AB	+ PARKE DAVIS	100 MG	N60591 003
AB		250 MG	N60591 002
		50 MG	N60591 001
	MYCHEL		
AB	RACHELLE	250 MG	N60851 001

CHLORAMPHENICOL (continued)

CREAM; TOPICAL

CHLOROMYCETIN			
PARKE DAVIS	1%	N50183 001	

OINTMENT; OPHTHALMIC

	CHLORAMPHENICOL			
AT	ALTANA	1%	N60133 001	
	CHLOROFAIR			
AT	PHARMAFAIR	1%	N62439 001	APR 21, 1983
	CHLOROMYCETIN			
AT	PARKE DAVIS	1%	N50156 001	
	CHLOROPTIC S.O.P.			
AT	ALLERGAN	1%	N61187 001	

POWDER FOR RECONSTITUTION; OPHTHALMIC

CHLOROMYCETIN			
PARKE DAVIS	25 MG/VIAL	N50143 001	

SOLUTION/DROPS; OPHTHALMIC

	CHLORAMPHENICOL			
AT	AKORN	0.5%	N62042 001	
AT	STERIS	0.5%	N62628 001	SEP 25, 1985
	CHLOROFAIR			
AT	PHARMAFAIR	0.5%	N62437 001	APR 14, 1983
	CHLOROPTIC			
AT	ALLERGAN	0.5%	N50091 001	
	OPHTHOCHLOR			
AT	PARKE DAVIS	0.5%	N61220 001	
	OPTOMYCIN			
AT	OPTOPICS	0.5%	N62171 001	MAR 31, 1982

SOLUTION/DROPS; OTIC

CHLOROMYCETIN			
PARKE DAVIS	0.5%	N50205 001	

CHLORAMPHENICOL; DESOXYRIBONUCLEASE; FIBRINOLYSIN

OINTMENT; TOPICAL

ELASE-CHLOROMYCETIN		
PARKE DAVIS	10 MG/GM;666 UNITS/GM;1 UNIT/GM	N50294 001

CHLORAMPHENICOL; HYDROCORTISONE ACETATE

POWDER FOR RECONSTITUTION; OPHTHALMIC

CHLOROMYCETIN HYDROCORTISONE		
PARKE DAVIS	12.5 MG/VIAL;25 MG/VIAL	N50202 001

CHLORAMPHENICOL; HYDROCORTISONE ACETATE; POLYMYXIN B SULFATE

OINTMENT; OPHTHALMIC

OPHTHOCORT		
PARKE DAVIS	10 MG/GM;5 MG/GM;10,000 UNITS/GM	N50201 002

Prescription Drug Products (continued)

CHLORAMPHENICOL PALMITATE

SUSPENSION; ORAL

CHLOROMYCETIN PALMITATE

+ PARKE DAVIS	EQ 150 MG BASE/5 ML	N50152 001	
	EQ 150 MG BASE/5 ML	N62301 001	

CHLORAMPHENICOL SODIUM SUCCINATE

INJECTABLE; INJECTION

CHLORAMPHENICOL

ΔP	ELKINS SINN	EQ 1 GM BASE/VIAL	N62406 001	NOV 09, 1982

CHLORAMPHENICOL SODIUM SUCCINATE

ΔP	GRUPPO LEPETIT	EQ 1 GM BASE/VIAL	N62278 001	
ΔP	LYPHOMED	EQ 1 GM BASE/VIAL	N62365 001	AUG 25, 1982

CHLOROMYCETIN

ΔP	PARKE DAVIS	EQ 1 GM BASE/VIAL	N50155 001

MYCHEL-S

ΔP	RACHELLE	EQ 1 GM BASE/VIAL	N60132 001

CHLORDIAZEPOXIDE

CAPSULE, EXTENDED RELEASE; ORAL

LIBRELEASE

+ ROCHE	30 MG	N17813 001	SEP 12, 1983

TABLET; ORAL

LIBRITABS

ROCHE	5 MG	N85482 001
	10 MG	N85481 001
	25 MG	N85488 001

CHLORDIAZEPOXIDE; *MULTIPLE*

SEE AMITRIPTYLINE HYDROCHLORIDE; CHLORDIAZEPOXIDE

CHLORDIAZEPOXIDE; ESTROGENS, ESTERIFIED

TABLET; ORAL

MENRIUM 10-4

ROCHE	10 MG;0.4 MG	N14740 006

MENRIUM 5-2

ROCHE	5 MG;0.2 MG	N14740 002

MENRIUM 5-4

+ ROCHE	5 MG;0.4 MG	N14740 004

CHLORDIAZEPOXIDE HYDROCHLORIDE

CAPSULE; ORAL

CHLORDIAZACHEL

	RACHELLE	5 MG	N85086 001
		10 MG	N84639 001
		25 MG	N85087 001

CHLORDIAZEPOXIDE HCL

ΔB	BARR	5 MG	N84768 001
ΔB		10 MG	N83116 001
ΔB		25 MG	N84769 001
ΔB	CHELSEA	5 MG	N86383 001
ΔB		10 MG	N86294 001
ΔB		25 MG	N86382 001
ΔB	FERRANTE	5 MG	N85118 001
ΔB		10 MG	N85119 001
ΔB		25 MG	N85120 001
ΔB	GENEVA	5 MG	N84678 001
ΔB		10 MG	N84041 001
ΔB		25 MG	N84679 002
ΔB	HALSEY	5 MG	N85340 001
ΔB		10 MG	N85339 001
ΔB		25 MG	N84685 001
ΔB	MAST	10 MG	N86217 001
ΔB	PHARM BASICS	5 MG	N84644 001
ΔB		10 MG	N84623 001
ΔB		25 MG	N84645 001
ΔB	PIONEER PHARMS	10 MG	N89533 001 JUL 15, 1988
ΔB		25 MG	N89558 001 JUL 15, 1988
ΔB	RICHLYN	5 MG	N86213 001
ΔB		10 MG	N85113 001
ΔB		25 MG	N86212 001
ΔB	ZENITH	5 MG	N83741 001
ΔB		10 MG	N83742 001
ΔB		25 MG	N83570 001

LIBRIUM

ΔB	ROCHE	5 MG	N12249 002
ΔB		5 MG	N85461 001
ΔB		10 MG	N12249 001
ΔB		25 MG	N85472 001
ΔB	+	25 MG	N12249 003
ΔB		25 MG	N85475 001

INJECTABLE; INJECTION

LIBRIUM

ROCHE	100 MG/AMP	N12301 001

CHLORHEXIDINE GLUCONATE

SOLUTION; DENTAL

PERIDEX

+ P AND G	0.12%	N19028 001	AUG 13, 1986

Prescription Drug Products (continued)

CHLORMEZANONE

TABLET; ORAL

TRANCOPAL

	STERLING	100 MG	N11467 003
		200 MG	N11467 005

CHLOROPROCAINE HYDROCHLORIDE

INJECTABLE; INJECTION

CHLOROPROCAINE HCL

ΔP	ABBOTT	2%	N87447 001	APR 16, 1982
ΔP		3%	N87446 001	APR 16, 1982

NESACAINE

	ASTRA	1%	N09435 001
		2%	N09435 002

NESACAINE-MPF

ΔP	ASTRA	2%	N09435 003
ΔP		3%	N09435 004

CHLOROQUINE HYDROCHLORIDE

INJECTABLE; INJECTION

ARALEN HCL

	STERLING	EQ 40 MG BASE/ML	N06002 002

CHLOROQUINE PHOSPHATE

TABLET; ORAL

ARALEN

ΔA	STERLING	EQ 300 MG BASE	N06002 001

CHLOROQUINE PHOSPHATE

ΔA	BIOCRAFT	EQ 150 MG BASE	N87504 001	JAN 13, 1982
ΔA	DANBURY	EQ 150 MG BASE	N87979 001	DEC 21, 1982
ΔA		EQ 300 MG BASE	N88030 001	DEC 21, 1982
ΔA	MD PHARM	EQ 150 MG BASE	N87228 001	
ΔA	RICHLYN	EQ 150 MG BASE	N80880 001	

CHLOROTHIAZIDE

SUSPENSION; ORAL

DIURIL

+ MSD		250 MG/5 ML	N11870 001

CHLOROTHIAZIDE (continued)

TABLET; ORAL

CHLOROTHIAZIDE

ΔB	CAMALL	250 MG	N85569 001	
ΔB	CHELSEA	250 MG	N86795 001	AUG 15, 1983
ΔB	DANBURY	250 MG	N85173 001	
ΔB	MYLAN	500 MG	N84388 001	
ΔB		250 MG	N84217 001	
ΔB	WEST WARD	500 MG	N86028 001	JUL 14, 1982
			N87736 001	JUL 14, 1982

DIURIL

ΔB	MSD	250 MG	N11145 004
ΔB	+	500 MG	N11145 002

CHLOROTHIAZIDE; METHYLDOPA

TABLET; ORAL

ALDOCLOR-150

ΔB	MSD	150 MG;250 MG	N16016 001

ALDOCLOR-250

ΔB	+ MSD	250 MG;250 MG	N16016 002

METHYLDOPA AND CHLOROTHIAZIDE

ΔB	PAR	150 MG;250 MG	N70783 001	NOV 06, 1987
ΔB		250 MG;250 MG	N70654 001	NOV 06, 1987

CHLOROTHIAZIDE; RESERPINE

TABLET; ORAL

CHLOROTHIAZIDE AND RESERPINE

BP	WEST WARD	250 MG;0.125 MG	N88557 001	DEC 22, 1983
BP		500 MG;0.125 MG	N88365 001	DEC 22, 1983

CHLOROTHIAZIDE-RESERPINE

BP	MYLAN	250 MG;0.125 MG	N87744 001	MAY 06, 1982
BP		500 MG;0.125 MG	N87745 001	MAY 06, 1982

DIUPRES-250

BP	MSD	250 MG;0.125 MG	N11635 003	AUG 26, 1987

DIUPRES-500

BP	+ MSD	500 MG;0.125 MG	N11635 006	AUG 26, 1987

CHLOROTHIAZIDE SODIUM

INJECTABLE; INJECTION

DIURIL

	MSD	EQ 500 MG BASE/VIAL	N11145 005

Prescription Drug Products *(continued)*

CHLOROTRIANISENE

	CAPSULE; ORAL		
	CHLOROTRIANISENE		
AA	BANNER GELATIN	12 MG	N84652 001
	TACE		
AA	MERRELL DOW	12 MG	N08102 004
		25 MG	N11444 001
		72 MG	N16235 001

CHLOROXINE

	SHAMPOO; TOPICAL		
	CAPITROL		
	WESTWOOD SQUIBB	2%	N17594 001

CHLORPHENESIN CARBAMATE

	TABLET; ORAL		
	MAOLATE		
	+ UPJOHN	400 MG	N14217 002

CHLORPHENIRAMINE MALEATE

	INJECTABLE; INJECTION		
	CHLOR-TRIMETON		
AP	SCHERING	10 MG/ML	N08826 001
	CHLORPHENIRAMINE MALEATE		
AP	BEL MAR	10 MG/ML	N80821 001
AP	STERIS	10 MG/ML	N83593 001
AP		10 MG/ML	N86096 001
AP		100 MG/ML	N86095 001
	PYRIDAMAL 100		
AP	BEL MAR	100 MG/ML	N83733 001
	TABLET; ORAL		
	CHLORPHENIRAMINE MALEATE		
AA	DANBURY	4 MG	N80696 001
AA	GENEVA	4 MG	N80961 001
AA	ICN	4 MG	N80598 001
AA	KV	4 MG	N87164 001
AA	MARSHALL	4 MG	N83286 001
AA	NEWTRON	4 MG	N86519 001
AA	PHARMAVITE	4 MG	N85104 001
AA	PHOENIX LABS	4 MG	N85522 001
AA	RICHLYN	4 MG	N80809 001
AA	SUPERPHARM	4 MG	N87747 001 APR 20, 1982
AA	TABLICAPS	4 MG	N83394 001
AA	WEST WARD	4 MG	N83787 001
AA	ZENITH	4 MG	N80779 001
	KLOROMIN		
AA	HALSEY	4 MG	N83629 001

CHLORPHENIRAMINE MALEATE; PHENYLPROPANOLAMINE HYDROCHLORIDE

	CAPSULE, EXTENDED RELEASE; ORAL		
	CHLORPHENIRAMINE MALEATE AND PHENYLPROPANOLAMINE HCL		
AB	GENEVA	12 MG;75 MG	N88940 001 JAN 26, 1989
	DRIZE		
BC	ASCHER	12 MG;75 MG	N88359 001 FEB 13, 1986
	ORNADE		
AB	+ SKF	12 MG;75 MG	N12152 004

CHLORPHENIRAMINE POLISTIREX; HYDROCODONE POLISTIREX

	SUSPENION, EXTENDED RELEASE; ORAL		
	TUSSIONEX		
	+ FISONS	EQ 8 MG MALEATE/ 5 ML;EQ 10 MG BITARTRATE/5 ML	N19111 001 DEC 31, 1987

CHLORPROMAZINE

	SUPPOSITORY; RECTAL		
	THORAZINE		
	+ SKF	25 MG	N09149 024
	+	100 MG	N09149 033

CHLORPROMAZINE HYDROCHLORIDE

	CAPSULE, EXTENDED RELEASE; ORAL		
	THORAZINE		
	+ SKF	30 MG	N11120 016
	+	75 MG	N11120 017
	+	150 MG	N11120 018
	+	200 MG	N11120 019
	+	300 MG	N11120 020
	CONCENTRATE; ORAL		
	CHLORPROMAZINE HCL		
AA	BARRE	100 MG/ML	N86863 001
AA	PHARM BASICS	30 MG/ML	N87032 001 JUL 08, 1982
AA		100 MG/ML	N87053 001
	CHLORPROMAZINE HCL INTENSOL		
AA	ROXANE	30 MG/ML	N88157 001 APR 27, 1983
AA		100 MG/ML	N88158 001 APR 27, 1983
	SONAZINE		
AA	GENEVA	30 MG/ML	N80983 004
AA		100 MG/ML	N80983 005
	THORAZINE		
AA	SKF	30 MG/ML	N09149 032
AA		100 MG/ML	N09149 043

Prescription Drug Products *(continued)*

CHLORPROMAZINE HYDROCHLORIDE *(continued)*

INJECTABLE; INJECTION

CHLORPROMAZINE HCL

TE	Firm	Strength	NDC	Approval
AP	ELKINS SINN	25 MG/ML	N83329 001	
AP	LYPHOMED	25 MG/ML	N84911 001	
AP	MARSAM	25 MG/ML	N89563 001	APR 15, 1988
AP	STERIS	25 MG/ML	N80365 001	
AP		25 MG/ML	N85591 001	

THORAZINE

TE	Firm	Strength	NDC	Approval
AP	SKF	25 MG/ML	N09149 011	

SYRUP; ORAL

SONAZINE

TE	Firm	Strength	NDC	Approval
AA	GENEVA	10 MG/5 ML	N83040 001	

THORAZINE

TE	Firm	Strength	NDC	Approval
AA	SKF	10 MG/5 ML	N09149 022	

TABLET; ORAL

CHLORPROMAZINE HCL

TE	Firm	Strength	NDC	Approval
BP	GENEVA	10 MG	N80439 001	
BP		25 MG	N80439 002	
BP		50 MG	N80439 003	
BP		100 MG	N80439 004	
BP		200 MG	N80439 005	
BP	KV	10 MG	N85750 002	JAN 04, 1982
BP		25 MG	N85751 001	
BP		50 MG	N85484 001	
BP		100 MG	N85752 001	
BP		200 MG	N85748 002	JAN 04, 1982
BP	LEDERLE	10 MG	N84803 001	
BP	PHARM BASICS	10 MG	N83386 001	
BP		25 MG	N84112 001	
BP		50 MG	N84113 001	
BP		100 MG	N84114 001	
BP		200 MG	N84115 001	
BP	ZENITH	10 MG	N83549 001	
BP		25 MG	N83549 002	
BP		50 MG	N83549 003	
BP		100 MG	N83574 001	
BP		200 MG	N83575 001	

THORAZINE

TE	Firm	Strength	NDC	Approval
BP	+ SKF	10 MG	N09149 002	
BP		25 MG	N09149 007	
BP		50 MG	N09149 013	
BP	+	100 MG	N09149 018	
BP		200 MG	N09149 020	

CHLORPROPAMIDE

TABLET; ORAL

CHLORPROPAMIDE

TE	Firm	Strength	NDC	Approval
AB	BARR	100 MG	N88812 001	OCT 19, 1984
AB		100 MG	N89446 001	NOV 17, 1986
AB		250 MG	N88813 001	OCT 19, 1984
AB		250 MG	N89447 001	NOV 17, 1986
AB	CHELSEA	250 MG	N86865 001	SEP 24, 1984
AB	DANBURY	100 MG	N88852 001	SEP 26, 1984
AB		250 MG	N88826 001	SEP 26, 1984
AB	GENEVA	100 MG	N88725 001	AUG 31, 1984
AB		250 MG	N88726 001	AUG 31, 1984
AB	HALSEY	100 MG	N89321 001	JAN 16, 1986
AB		250 MG	N88662 001	JAN 09, 1986
AB	LEDERLE	100 MG	N89561 001	SEP 04, 1987
AB		250 MG	N89562 001	SEP 04, 1987
AB	LEMMON	100 MG	N88768 001	OCT 11, 1984
AB	MYLAN	100 MG	N88548 001	JUN 01, 1984
AB		250 MG	N88549 001	JUN 01, 1984
AB	PAR	100 MG	N88175 001	FEB 27, 1984
AB		250 MG	N88176 001	FEB 27, 1984
AB	SIDMAK	100 MG	N88921 001	APR 12, 1985
AB		250 MG	N88922 001	APR 12, 1985
AB	SUPERPHARM	100 MG	N88694 001	SEP 17, 1984
AB		250 MG	N88695 001	SEP 17, 1984
AB	ZENITH	100 MG	N88840 001	SEP 17, 1984
AB		250 MG	N87353 001	OCT 25, 1984

DIABINESE

TE	Firm	Strength	NDC	Approval
AB	PFIZER	100 MG	N11641 003	
AB	+	250 MG	N11641 006	

GLUCAMIDE

TE	Firm	Strength	NDC	Approval
AB	LEMMON	250 MG	N88641 001	OCT 11, 1984

Prescription Drug Products (continued)

CHLORPROTHIXENE

CONCENTRATE; ORAL
TARACTAN

	Firm	Strength	Appl No
	ROCHE	100 MG/5 ML	N16149 002

INJECTABLE; INJECTION
TARACTAN

	Firm	Strength	Appl No
	ROCHE	12.5 MG/ML	N12487 001

TABLET; ORAL
TARACTAN

	Firm	Strength	Appl No
	ROCHE	10 MG	N12486 005
		25 MG	N12486 004
		50 MG	N12486 003
+		100 MG	N12486 001

CHLORTETRACYCLINE HYDROCHLORIDE

OINTMENT; OPHTHALMIC
AUREOMYCIN

	Firm	Strength	Appl No
	LEDERLE	1%	N50404 001

CHLORTHALIDONE

TABLET; ORAL
CHLORTHALIDONE

TE	Firm	Strength	Appl No	Approval Date
AB	ABBOTT	25 MG	N87364 001	
AB		50 MG	N87384 001	
AB	BARR	25 MG	N87292 001	
AB		50 MG	N87293 001	
AB	CHELSEA	25 MG	N87100 001	
AB		50 MG	N87082 001	
AB	DANBURY	25 MG	N87296 001	
AB		25 MG	N87706 001	
AB		50 MG	N87521 001	
AB		50 MG	N87689 001	
AB	EON LABS	50 MG	N87118 001	
AB	GENEVA	25 MG	N87380 001	
AB		50 MG	N87381 001	
AB	KV	25 MG	N87311 001	
AB		25 MG	N87312 001	
AB	LEDERLE	25 MG	N87451 001	
AB		50 MG	N87450 001	
AB	MUTUAL PHARM	25 MG	N89285 001	JUL 21, 1986
			N89738 001	SEP 19, 1988
AB		25 MG	N89286 001	JUL 21, 1986
			N89739 001	SEP 19, 1988
AB		50 MG		
AB	MYLAN	25 MG	N87180 001	
AB		50 MG	N86831 001	
AB	PHARM BASICS	25 MG	N89051 001	JUN 01, 1987
			N89052 001	JUN 01, 1987
AB		50 MG		

CHLORTHALIDONE (continued)
TABLET; ORAL
CHLORTHALIDONE

TE	Firm	Strength	Appl No	Approval Date
AB	PIONEER PHARMS	50 MG	N89591 001	JUL 21, 1988
AB	PUREPAC	25 MG	N88139 001	JUL 16, 1986
AB		50 MG	N88140 001	AUG 11, 1983
AB	SIDMAK	25 MG	N88902 001	SEP 19, 1985
AB		50 MG	N88903 001	SEP 19, 1985
AB	SUPERPHARM	50 MG	N87247 001	FEB 09, 1983
AB	ZENITH	25 MG	N88164 001	JAN 09, 1984
AB		50 MG	N87176 001	
AB		50 MG	N87947 001	FEB 27, 1984

HYGROTON

TE	Firm	Strength	Appl No	Approval Date
AB	RHONE POULENC RORER	25 MG	N12283 004	
AB		50 MG	N12283 003	

THALITONE

TE	Firm	Strength	Appl No	Approval Date
+		25 MG	N88051 001	NOV 12, 1982
BX	HORUS	15 MG	N19574 001	DEC 20, 1988

CHLORTHALIDONE; *MULTIPLE*
SEE ATENOLOL; CHLORTHALIDONE

CHLORTHALIDONE; CLONIDINE HYDROCHLORIDE

TABLET; ORAL
CLONIDINE HCL AND CHLORTHALIDONE

TE	Firm	Strength	Appl No	Approval Date
AB	MYLAN	15 MG;0.1 MG	N71323 001	FEB 09, 1987
AB		15 MG;0.2 MG	N71324 001	FEB 09, 1987
AB		15 MG;0.3 MG	N71325 001	FEB 09, 1987
AB	PAR	15 MG;0.1 MG	N71179 001	DEC 16, 1987
AB		15 MG;0.2 MG	N71178 001	DEC 16, 1987
AB		15 MG;0.3 MG	N71142 001	DEC 16, 1987

COMBIPRES

TE	Firm	Strength	Appl No	Approval Date
AB	BOEHRINGER INGELHEIM	15 MG;0.1 MG	N17503 001	
AB		15 MG;0.2 MG	N17503 002	
+ AB		15 MG;0.3 MG	N17503 003	APR 10, 1984

Prescription Drug Products (continued)

Prescription Drug Products (continued)

CHLORTHALIDONE; METOPROLOL TARTRATE

CAPSULE; ORAL

LOPRESSIDONE

CIBA	25 MG;100 MG	N19451 001	DEC 31, 1987
+	25 MG;200 MG	N19451 002	DEC 31, 1987

CHLORTHALIDONE; RESERPINE

TABLET; ORAL

DEMI-REGROTON

RHONE POULENC RORER	25 MG;0.125 MG	N15103 002

REGROTON

+ RHONE POULENC RORER	50 MG;0.25 MG	N15103 001

CHLORZOXAZONE

TABLET; ORAL

CHLORZOXAZONE

AA	AMIDE PHARM	250 MG	N88928 001	MAY 08, 1987
AA	BARR	500 MG	N89895 001	MAY 04, 1988
AA	DANBURY	250 MG	N86901 001	MAY 04, 1988
AA		500 MG	N81019 001	JUL 29, 1991
AA	GENEVA	250 MG	N89852 001	MAY 04, 1988
AA		500 MG	N89853 001	MAY 04, 1988
AA	LEMMON	500 MG	N89859 001	MAY 04, 1988
AA	MUTUAL PHARM	500 MG	N89970 001	SEP 27, 1990
AA	PAR	250 MG	N87981 001	SEP 20, 1983
AA	PIONEER PHARMS	250 MG	N89592 001	JAN 06, 1989
AA		500 MG	N89948 001	JAN 06, 1989
AA	ROYCE	500 MG	N81040 001	AUG 22, 1989

PARAFLEX

AA	JOHNSON RW	250 MG	N11300 003

PARAFON FORTE DSC

AA	JOHNSON RW	500 MG	N11529 002	JUN 15, 1987

STRIFON FORTE DSC

AA	FERNDALE	500 MG	N81008 001	DEC 23, 1988

CHOLESTYRAMINE

BAR, CHEWABLE; ORAL

CHOLYBAR

+ PARKE DAVIS	EQ 4 GM RESIN/BAR	N71621 001	MAY 26, 1988
	EQ 4 GM RESIN/BAR	N71739 001	MAY 26, 1988

POWDER; ORAL

QUESTRAN

+ BRISTOL MYERS	EQ 4 GM RESIN/PACKET	N16640 001
	EQ 4 GM RESIN/SCOOPFUL	N16640 003

QUESTRAN LIGHT

BRISTOL MYERS	EQ 4 GM RESIN/PACKET	N19669 001	DEC 05, 1988
	EQ 4 GM RESIN/SCOOPFUL	N19669 003	DEC 05, 1988

CHROMIC CHLORIDE

INJECTABLE; INJECTION

CHROMIC CHLORIDE

AP	LYPHOMED	EQ 0.004 MG CHROMIUM/ML	N19271 001	MAY 05, 1987

CHROMIC CHLORIDE IN PLASTIC CONTAINER

AP	ABBOTT	EQ 0.004 MG CHROMIUM/ML	N18961 001	JUN 26, 1986

CHROMIC PHOSPHATE, P-32

INJECTABLE; INJECTION

PHOSPHOCOL P32

MALLINCKRODT	5 MCI/ML	N17084 001

CHYMOPAPAIN

INJECTABLE, INJECTION

CHYMODIACTIN

BOOTS	4,000 UNITS/VIAL	N18663 002	AUG 21, 1984
	10,000 UNITS/VIAL	N18663 001	NOV 10, 1982

CHYMOTRYPSIN

POWDER FOR RECONSTITUTION; OPHTHALMIC

CATARASE

IOLAB	150 UNITS/VIAL	N18121 001
	300 UNITS/VIAL	N16938 001

ZOLYSE

ALCON	750 UNITS/VIAL	N11903 001

Prescription Drug Products (continued)

CICLOPIROX OLAMINE

CREAM; TOPICAL
LOPROX
+ HOECHST ROUSSEL   1%   N18748 001 DEC 30, 1982

LOTION; TOPICAL
LOPROX
+ HOECHST ROUSSEL   1%   N19824 001 DEC 30, 1988

CILASTATIN SODIUM; IMIPENEM

INJECTABLE; INJECTION
PRIMAXIN
MSD

EQ 250 MG BASE/VIAL;250 MG/VIAL	N50587 001	NOV 26, 1985
EQ 250 MG BASE/VIAL;250 MG/VIAL	N62756 001	JAN 08, 1987
EQ 500 MG BASE/VIAL;500 MG/VIAL	N50587 002	NOV 26, 1985
EQ 500 MG BASE/VIAL;500 MG/VIAL	N50630 001	DEC 14, 1990
EQ 500 MG BASE/VIAL;500 MG/VIAL	N62756 002	JAN 08, 1987
EQ 750 MG BASE/VIAL;750 MG/VIAL	N50630 002	DEC 14, 1990

CIMETIDINE

TABLET; ORAL
TAGAMET
SKF

200 MG	N17920 002	
300 MG	N17920 003	
400 MG	N17920 004	DEC 14, 1983
	N17920 005	APR 30, 1986
+ 800 MG		

CIMETIDINE HYDROCHLORIDE

INJECTABLE; INJECTION
TAGAMET
SKF   EQ 300 MG BASE/2 ML   N17939 002
TAGAMET HCL IN SODIUM CHLORIDE 0.9% IN PLASTIC CONTAINER
SKF   EQ 6 MG BASE/ML   N19434 001 OCT 31, 1985

SOLUTION; ORAL
TAGAMET
SKF   EQ 300 MG BASE/5 ML   N17924 001

CINOXACIN

CAPSULE; ORAL
CINOBAC

AB	LILLY	250 MG	N18067 001	
AB	+	500 MG	N18067 002	

CINOXACIN

AB	BIOCRAFT	250 MG	N73005 001	FEB 28, 1992
AB		500 MG	N73006 001	FEB 28, 1992

CIPROFLOXACIN

INJECTABLE; INJECTION
CIPRO
MILES   10 MG/ML   N19847 001 DEC 26, 1990
CIPRO IN DEXTROSE 5% IN PLASTIC CONTAINER
MILES   200 MG/100 ML   N19857 001 DEC 26, 1990
CIPRO IN SODIUM CHLORIDE 0.9% IN PLASTIC CONTAINER
MILES   200 MG/100 ML   N19858 001 DEC 26, 1990

CIPROFLOXACIN HYDROCHLORIDE

SOLUTION/DROPS; OPHTHALMIC
CILOXAN
ALCON   EQ 0.3% BASE   N19992 001 DEC 31, 1990

TABLET; ORAL
CIPRO
MILES

EQ 250 MG BASE	N19537 002	OCT 22, 1987
EQ 500 MG BASE	N19537 003	OCT 22, 1987
+ EQ 750 MG BASE	N19537 004	OCT 22, 1987

CISPLATIN

INJECTABLE; INJECTION
PLATINOL
BRISTOL MYERS   10 MG/VIAL   N18057 001
  50 MG/VIAL   N18057 002
PLATINOL-AQ
BRISTOL MYERS   1 MG/ML   N18057 004 NOV 08, 1988

CITRIC ACID; GLUCONOLACTONE; MAGNESIUM CARBONATE

SOLUTION; IRRIGATION
RENACIDIN
GUARDIAN LABS   6.602 GM/100 ML;198 MG/100 ML;3.177 GM/100 ML   N19481 001 OCT 02, 1990

Prescription Drug Products (continued)

CITRIC ACID; MAGNESIUM OXIDE; SODIUM CARBONATE
SOLUTION; IRRIGATION
IRRIGATING SOLUTION G IN PLASTIC CONTAINER

TE	Applicant	Strength	NDA	Date
AT	BAXTER	3.24 GM/100 ML;380 MG/100 ML;430 MG/100 ML	N18519 001	JUN 22, 1982

UROLOGIC G IN PLASTIC CONTAINER

TE	Applicant	Strength	NDA	Date
AT	ABBOTT	3.24 GM/100 ML;380 MG/100 ML;430 MG/100 ML	N18904 001	MAY 27, 1983

CLARITHROMYCIN
TABLET; ORAL
BIAXIN

Applicant	Strength	NDA	Date
ABBOTT	250 MG	N50662 001	OCT 31, 1991
	500 MG	N50662 002	OCT 31, 1991

CLAVULANATE POTASSIUM; *MULTIPLE*
SEE   AMOXICILLIN; CLAVULANATE POTASSIUM

CLAVULANATE POTASSIUM; TICARCILLIN DISODIUM
INJECTABLE; INJECTION
TIMENTIN

Applicant	Strength	NDA	Date
BEECHAM	EQ 1 GM ACID/VIAL;EQ 30 GM BASE/VIAL	N50590 003	AUG 18, 1987
	EQ 100 MG ACID/VIAL;EQ 3 GM BASE/VIAL	N50590 001	APR 01, 1985
	EQ 100 MG ACID/VIAL;EQ 3 GM BASE/VIAL	N62691 001	DEC 19, 1986
	EQ 200 MG ACID/VIAL;EQ 3 GM BASE/VIAL	N50590 002	APR 01, 1985

TIMENTIN IN PLASTIC CONTAINER

Applicant	Strength	NDA	Date
BEECHAM	EQ 100 MG ACID/100 ML;EQ 3 GM BASE/100 ML	N50658 001	DEC 15, 1989

CLEMASTINE FUMARATE
SYRUP; ORAL
CLEMASTINE FUMARATE

TE	Applicant	Strength	NDA	Date
AA	COPLEY	EQ 0.5 MG BASE/5 ML	N73095 001	APR 21, 1992

TAVIST

TE	Applicant	Strength	NDA	Date
AA	DORSEY	EQ 0.5 MG BASE/5 ML	N18675 001	JUN 28, 1985

CLEMASTINE FUMARATE (continued)
TABLET; ORAL
CLEMASTINE FUMARATE

TE	Applicant	Strength	NDA	Date
AB	LEMMON	2.68 MG	N73283 001	JAN 31, 1992
		1.34 MG	N73282 001	JAN 31, 1992

TAVIST

TE	Applicant	Strength	NDA	Date
AB	+ SANDOZ	2.68 MG	N17661 001	

CLIDINIUM BROMIDE
CAPSULE; ORAL
QUARZAN

Applicant	Strength	NDA	Date
ROCHE	2.5 MG	N10355 001	
	5 MG	N10355 002	

CLINDAMYCIN HYDROCHLORIDE
CAPSULE; ORAL
CLEOCIN

TE	Applicant	Strength	NDA	Date
AB	+ UPJOHN	EQ 75 MG BASE	N61809 001	
AB	+	EQ 150 MG BASE	N61809 002	

CLEOCIN HCL

TE	Applicant	Strength	NDA	Date
	UPJOHN	EQ 300 MG BASE	N50162 003	APR 14, 1988

CLINDAMYCIN HCL

TE	Applicant	Strength	NDA	Date
AB	BIOCRAFT	EQ 75 MG BASE	N63027 001	SEP 20, 1989
AB		EQ 150 MG BASE	N63029 001	SEP 20, 1989
AB	DANBURY	EQ 75 MG BASE	N63082 001	JUL 31, 1991
AB		EQ 150 MG BASE	N63083 001	JUL 31, 1991

CLINDAMYCIN PALMITATE HYDROCHLORIDE
POWDER FOR RECONSTITUTION; ORAL
CLEOCIN

TE	Applicant	Strength	NDA	Date
AA	UPJOHN	EQ 75 MG BASE/5 ML	N61827 001	
AA		EQ 75 MG BASE/5 ML	N62644 001	APR 07, 1986

CLINDAMYCIN PHOSPHATE
CREAM; VAGINAL
CLEOCIN

Applicant	Strength	NDA	Date
+ UPJOHN	EQ 2% BASE	N50680 001	AUG 11, 1992

GEL; TOPICAL
CLEOCIN T

Applicant	Strength	NDA	Date
+ UPJOHN	EQ 1% BASE	N50615 001	JAN 07, 1987

Prescription Drug Products (continued)

CLINDAMYCIN PHOSPHATE (continued)
INJECTABLE; INJECTION

CLEOCIN PHOSPHATE

AP	UPJOHN	EQ 150 MG BASE/ML	N61839 001	
AP		EQ 150 MG BASE/ML	N62803 001	OCT 16, 1987

CLEOCIN PHOSPHATE IN DEXTROSE 5% IN PLASTIC CONTAINER

AP	UPJOHN	EQ 6 MG BASE/ML	N50639 001	AUG 30, 1989
AP		EQ 12 MG BASE/ML	N50639 002	AUG 30, 1989

CLINDAMYCIN PHOSPHATE

AP	ABBOTT	EQ 150 MG BASE/ML	N62800 001	JUL 24, 1987
AP		EQ 150 MG BASE/ML	N62801 001	JUL 24, 1987
AP	ASTRA	EQ 150 MG BASE/ML	N62943 001	SEP 29, 1988
AP	DUPONT	EQ 150 MG BASE/ML	N62928 001	FEB 13, 1989
AP		EQ 150 MG BASE/ML	N62908 001	FEB 01, 1989
AP	ELKINS SINN	EQ 150 MG BASE/ML	N62806 001	OCT 15, 1987
AP		EQ 150 MG BASE/ML	N62953 001	APR 21, 1988
AP	GENSIA	EQ 150 MG BASE/ML	N63041 001	DEC 29, 1989
AP		EQ 150 MG BASE/ML	N63282 001	MAY 29, 1992
AP	LEDERLE	EQ 150 MG BASE/ML	N62889 001	APR 25, 1988
AP		EQ 150 MG BASE/ML	N63068 001	AUG 28, 1989
AP	LOCH	EQ 150 MG BASE/ML	N62905 001	MAY 09, 1988
AP	LYPHOMED	EQ 150 MG BASE/ML	N62747 001	JUN 03, 1988
AP	MARSAM	EQ 150 MG BASE/ML	N62913 001	OCT 20, 1988
AP	QUAD	EQ 150 MG BASE/ML	N62795 001	DEC 21, 1987
AP	SMITH NEPHEW SOLOPAK	EQ 150 MG BASE/ML	N62819 001	MAR 15, 1988
AP		EQ 150 MG BASE/ML	N62852 001	MAR 17, 1988
AP	STERIS	EQ 150 MG BASE/ML	N62900 001	JUN 08, 1988
AP		EQ 150 MG BASE/ML	N63079 001	MAR 05, 1990

CLINDAMYCIN PHOSPHATE (continued)
INJECTABLE; INJECTION

CLINDAMYCIN PHOSPHATE IN DEXTROSE 5%

AP	LYPHOMED	EQ 900 MG BASE/100 ML	N50635 001	DEC 22, 1989
AP		EQ 12 MG BASE/ML	N50636 001	DEC 22, 1989

CLINDAMYCIN PHOSPHATE IN DEXTROSE 5% IN PLASTIC CONTAINER

AP	BAXTER	EQ 6 MG BASE/ML	N50648 001	DEC 29, 1989
AP		EQ 900 MG BASE/100 ML	N50648 003	DEC 29, 1989
AP		EQ 12 MG BASE/ML	N50648 002	DEC 29, 1989

LOTION; TOPICAL

CLEOCIN T

AP	+ UPJOHN	EQ 1% BASE	N50600 001	MAY 31, 1989

SOLUTION; TOPICAL

CLEOCIN T

AT	UPJOHN	EQ 1% BASE	N50537 001	
AT		EQ 1% BASE	N62363 001	FEB 08, 1982

CLINDAMYCIN PHOSPHATE

AT	BARRE	EQ 1% BASE	N62811 001	SEP 01, 1988
AT	COPLEY	EQ 1% BASE	N62944 001	JAN 11, 1989
AT	LEMMON	EQ 1% BASE	N62930 001	JUN 28, 1989

CLIOQUINOL; HYDROCORTISONE
CREAM; TOPICAL

VIOFORM-HYDROCORTISONE

	CIBA	3%;0.5%	N10412 002
		3%;1%	N10412 001

OINTMENT; TOPICAL

VIOFORM-HYDROCORTISONE

	CIBA	3%;1%	N10412 003

CLOBETASOL PROPIONATE
CREAM; TOPICAL

TEMOVATE

	+ GLAXO	0.05%	N19322 001	DEC 27, 1985

OINTMENT; TOPICAL

TEMOVATE

	+ GLAXO	0.05%	N19323 001	DEC 27, 1985

SOLUTION; TOPICAL

TEMOVATE

	GLAXO	0.05%	N19966 001	FEB 22, 1990

Prescription Drug Products *(continued)*

CLOCORTOLONE PIVALATE
CREAM; TOPICAL

CLODERM			
+ HERMAL	0.1%	N17765 001	

CLOFAZIMINE
CAPSULE; ORAL

LAMPRENE			
GEIGY	50 MG	N19500 002	DEC 15, 1986
+	100 MG	N19500 001	DEC 15, 1986

CLOFIBRATE
CAPSULE; ORAL

	ATROMID-S			
	+ WYETH AYERST	500 MG	N16099 002	
	CLOFIBRATE			
AB	CHELSEA	500 MG	N71603 001	SEP 18, 1987
AB		500 MG	N72191 001	MAY 02, 1988
AB	GENEVA	500 MG	N72600 001	JUL 25, 1991
AB	NOVOPHARM	500 MG	N70531 001	JUN 16, 1986
AB	PHARM BASICS	500 MG	N73396 001	JUN 16, 1986
AB	PHARMACAPS	500 MG	N73396 001	MAR 20, 1992

CLOMIPHENE CITRATE
TABLET; ORAL

	CLOMID			
	+ MERRELL DOW	50 MG	N16131 002	
	MILOPHENE			
AB	MILEX	50 MG	N72196 001	DEC 20, 1988
	SEROPHENE			
AB	SERONO	50 MG	N18361 001	MAR 22, 1982

CLOMIPRAMINE HYDROCHLORIDE
CAPSULE; ORAL

	ANAFRANIL			
	CIBA	25 MG	N19906 001	DEC 29, 1989
		50 MG	N19906 002	DEC 29, 1989
	+	75 MG	N19906 003	DEC 29, 1989

CLONAZEPAM
TABLET; ORAL

KLONOPIN			
ROCHE	0.5 MG	N17533 001	
	1 MG	N17533 002	
+	2 MG	N17533 003	

CLONIDINE
FILM, EXTENDED RELEASE; TRANSDERMAL

CATAPRES-TTS-1			
+ BOEHRINGER INGELHEIM	0.1 MG/24 HR	N18891 001	OCT 10, 1984
CATAPRES-TTS-2			
+ BOEHRINGER INGELHEIM	0.2 MG/24 HR	N18891 002	OCT 10, 1984
CATAPRES-TTS-3			
+ BOEHRINGER INGELHEIM	0.3 MG/24 HR	N18891 003	OCT 10, 1984

CLONIDINE HYDROCHLORIDE
TABLET; ORAL

	CATAPRES			
	BOEHRINGER INGELHEIM	0.1 MG	N17407 001	
		0.2 MG	N17407 002	
	+	0.3 MG	N17407 003	
	CLONIDINE HCL			
AB	BARR	0.1 MG	N70925 001	SEP 04, 1987
AB		0.2 MG	N70924 001	SEP 04, 1987
AB		0.3 MG	N70923 001	SEP 04, 1987
AB	BIOCRAFT	0.1 MG	N70747 001	SEP 04, 1987
AB		0.2 MG	N70702 001	MAR 20, 1986
AB		0.3 MG	N70659 001	MAR 20, 1986
AB	DANBURY	0.1 MG	N70965 001	MAR 20, 1986
AB		0.2 MG	N70964 001	JUL 01, 1986
AB		0.3 MG	N70963 001	JUL 01, 1986
AB	GENEVA	0.1 MG	N70887 001	JUL 01, 1986
AB		0.2 MG	N70886 001	AUG 31, 1988
AB		0.3 MG	N71294 001	AUG 31, 1988

Prescription Drug Products (continued)

CLONIDINE HYDROCHLORIDE (continued)

TABLET; ORAL

CLONIDINE HCL

		Strength	Number	Date
AB	LEDERLE	0.1 MG	N71783 001	APR 05, 1988
AB		0.2 MG	N71784 001	APR 05, 1988
AB		0.3 MG	N71785 001	APR 05, 1988
AB	MYLAN	0.1 MG	N70315 001	JUN 09, 1987
AB		0.2 MG	N70316 001	JUN 09, 1987
AB		0.3 MG	N70317 001	JUN 09, 1987
AB	PAR	0.1 MG	N70461 001	NOV 22, 1985
AB		0.2 MG	N70460 001	NOV 22, 1985
AB		0.3 MG	N70459 001	NOV 22, 1985
AB	PUREPAC	0.1 MG	N70974 001	DEC 16, 1986
AB		0.2 MG	N70975 001	DEC 16, 1986
AB		0.3 MG	N70976 001	DEC 16, 1986
AB	WARNER CHILCOTT	0.1 MG	N72138 001	JUN 13, 1988
AB		0.2 MG	N72139 001	JUN 13, 1988
AB		0.3 MG	N72140 001	JUN 13, 1988

CLONIDINE HYDROCHLORIDE; *MULTIPLE*

SEE CHLORTHALIDONE; CLONIDINE HYDROCHLORIDE

CLORAZEPATE DIPOTASSIUM

CAPSULE; ORAL

CLORAZEPATE DIPOTASSIUM

		Strength	Number	Date
AB	ABLE	3.75 MG	N71777 001	JUL 14, 1987
AB		7.5 MG	N71778 001	JUL 14, 1987
AB		15 MG	N71779 001	JUL 14, 1987
AB	GENEVA	3.75 MG	N72219 001	AUG 26, 1988
AB		7.5 MG	N72220 001	AUG 26, 1988
AB		15 MG	N72112 001	AUG 26, 1988
AB	LEDERLE	3.75 MG	N71742 001	DEC 14, 1987
AB		7.5 MG	N71743 001	DEC 14, 1987
AB		15 MG	N71744 001	DEC 14, 1987

CLORAZEPATE DIPOTASSIUM (continued)

CAPSULE; ORAL

CLORAZEPATE DIPOTASSIUM

		Strength	Number	Date
AB	MYLAN	3.75 MG	N71509 001	OCT 19, 1987
AB		7.5 MG	N71510 001	OCT 19, 1987
AB		15 MG	N71511 001	OCT 19, 1987
AB	+	7.5 MG	N71925 001	APR 25, 1988
AB	PUREPAC	7.5 MG	N71926 001	APR 25, 1988
AB		15 MG		APR 25, 1988

TABLET; ORAL

CLORAZEPATE DIPOTASSIUM

		Strength	Number	Date
AB	ABLE	3.75 MG	N71780 001	JUN 26, 1987
AB		7.5 MG	N71781 001	JUN 26, 1987
AB		15 MG	N71782 001	JUN 26, 1987
AB	GENEVA	3.75 MG	N72512 001	MAY 11, 1990
AB		7.5 MG	N72513 001	MAY 11, 1990
AB		15 MG	N72514 001	MAY 11, 1990
AB	MYLAN	3.75 MG	N71856 001	JUL 17, 1987
AB		7.5 MG	N71857 001	JUL 17, 1987
AB		15 MG	N71858 001	JUL 17, 1987
AB	PUREPAC	3.75 MG	N72330 001	AUG 08, 1988
AB		7.5 MG	N72331 001	AUG 08, 1988
AB		15 MG	N72332 001	AUG 08, 1988
AB	WATSON	3.75 MG	N71852 001	FEB 09, 1988
AB		7.5 MG	N71853 001	FEB 09, 1988
AB		15 MG	N71854 001	FEB 09, 1988

GEN-XENE

		Strength	Number	Date
AB	ALRA	3.75 MG	N71787 001	APR 26, 1988
AB		7.5 MG	N71788 001	APR 26, 1988
AB		15 MG	N71789 001	APR 26, 1988

TRANXENE

		Strength	Number	Date
AB	ABBOTT	3.75 MG	N17105 006	
AB		7.5 MG	N17105 007	
AB	+	15 MG	N17105 008	

TRANXENE SD

		Strength	Number	Date
	ABBOTT	11.25 MG	N17105 005	
	+	22.5 MG	N17105 004	

Prescription Drug Products (continued)

CLOTRIMAZOLE
CREAM; TOPICAL
LOTRIMIN
| BT | + SCHERING | 1% | N17619 001 |
MYCELEX
| BT | MILES | 1% | N18183 001 |

CREAM; VAGINAL
GYNE-LOTRIMIN
| BT | SCHERING | 1% | N18052 001 |
MYCELEX-G
| BT | MILES | 1% | N18230 001 |

LOTION; TOPICAL
LOTRIMIN
| BT | + SCHERING | 1% | N18813 001 FEB 17, 1984 |

SOLUTION; TOPICAL
LOTRIMIN
| AT | SCHERING | 1% | N17613 001 |
MYCELEX
| AT | MILES | 1% | N18181 001 |

TABLET; VAGINAL
GYNE-LOTRIMIN
| BT | SCHERING | 100 MG | N17717 001 |
MYCELEX-G
| BT | MILES | 100 MG | N18182 001 |
| BT | | 500 MG | N19069 001 APR 19, 1985 |

TROCHE/LOZENGE; ORAL
MYCELEX
| BT | + MILES | 10 MG | N18713 001 JUN 17, 1983 |

CLOTRIMAZOLE; *MULTIPLE*
SEE BETAMETHASONE DIPROPIONATE: CLOTRIMAZOLE

CLOXACILLIN SODIUM
CAPSULE; ORAL
CLOXACILLIN SODIUM
| AB | BIOCRAFT | EQ 250 MG BASE | N62240 001 |
| AB | | EQ 500 MG BASE | N62240 002 |
CLOXAPEN
AB	BEECHAM	EQ 250 MG BASE	N61806 001
AB		EQ 250 MG BASE	N62233 001
AB		EQ 500 MG BASE	N61806 002
AB		EQ 500 MG BASE	N62233 002
TEGOPEN
AB	+ BRISTOL	EQ 250 MG BASE	N61452 001
AB	+	EQ 500 MG BASE	N61452 002

POWDER FOR RECONSTITUTION; ORAL
CLOXACILLIN SODIUM
| AA | BIOCRAFT | EQ 125 MG BASE/5 ML | N62268 001 |
| AA | NOVOPHARM | EQ 125 MG BASE/5 ML | N62978 001 APR 06, 1989 |
TEGOPEN
| AA | BRISTOL | EQ 125 MG BASE/5 ML | N50192 001 |
| AA | | EQ 125 MG BASE/5 ML | N61453 001 |

CLOZAPINE
TABLET; ORAL
CLOZARIL
SANDOZ	25 MG	N19758 001 SEP 26, 1989
	100 MG	N19758 002 SEP 26, 1989
+		

COBALT CHLORIDE, CO-57; CYANOCOBALAMIN; CYANOCOBALAMIN, CO-57; INTRINSIC FACTOR
N/A; N/A
RUBRATOPE-57 KIT
| SQUIBB | N/A;N/A;N/A;N/A | N16089 001 |

CODEINE PHOSPHATE; *MULTIPLE*
SEE ACETAMINOPHEN: ASPIRIN: CODEINE PHOSPHATE
SEE ACETAMINOPHEN: BUTALBITAL: CAFFEINE: CODEINE PHOSPHATE
SEE ACETAMINOPHEN: CODEINE PHOSPHATE
SEE ASPIRIN: BUTALBITAL: CAFFEINE: CODEINE PHOSPHATE
SEE ASPIRIN: CARISOPRODOL: CODEINE PHOSPHATE
SEE BROMODIPHENHYDRAMINE HYDROCHLORIDE: CODEINE PHOSPHATE
SEE BROMPHENIRAMINE MALEATE: CODEINE PHOSPHATE: PHENYLPROPANOLAMINE HYDROCHLORIDE

CODEINE PHOSPHATE; PHENYLEPHRINE HYDROCHLORIDE; PROMETHAZINE HYDROCHLORIDE
SYRUP; ORAL
PHENERGAN VC W/ CODEINE
| AA | WYETH AYERST | 10 MG/5 ML:5 MG/5 ML:6.25 MG/5 ML | N08306 005 APR 02, 1984 |
PHERAZINE VC W/ CODEINE
| AA | HALSEY | 10 MG/5 ML:5 MG/5 ML:6.25 MG/5 ML | N88870 001 MAR 02, 1987 |
PROMETH VC W/ CODEINE
| AA | BARRE | 10 MG/5 ML:5 MG/5 ML:6.25 MG/5 ML | N88764 001 OCT 31, 1984 |
PROMETHAZINE VC W/ CODEINE
| AA | CENCI | 10 MG/5 ML:5 MG/5 ML:6.25 MG/5 ML | N88816 001 NOV 22, 1985 |
| AA | PHARM BASICS | 10 MG/5 ML:5 MG/5 ML:6.25 MG/5 ML | N88896 001 JAN 04, 1985 |

Prescription Drug Products (continued)

CODEINE PHOSPHATE; PROMETHAZINE HYDROCHLORIDE
SYRUP; ORAL

	PHENERGAN W/ CODEINE			
AA	WYETH AYERST	10 MG/5 ML;6.25 MG/5 ML	N08306 004	APR 02, 1984
	PHERAZINE W/ CODEINE			
AA	HALSEY	10 MG/5 ML;6.25 MG/5 ML	N88739 001	DEC 23, 1988
	PROMETH W/ CODEINE			
AA	BARRE	10 MG/5 ML;6.25 MG/5 ML	N88763 001	OCT 31, 1984
	PROMETHAZINE HCL AND CODEINE PHOSPHATE			
AA	PHARM ASSOC	10 MG/5 ML;6.25 MG/5 ML	N89647 001	DEC 22, 1988
	PROMETHAZINE W/ CODEINE			
AA	CENCI	10 MG/5 ML;6.25 MG/5 ML	N88814 001	NOV 22, 1985
AA	PHARM BASICS	10 MG/5 ML;6.25 MG/5 ML	N88875 001	DEC 17, 1984

CODEINE PHOSPHATE; PSEUDOEPHEDRINE HYDROCHLORIDE; TRIPROLIDINE HYDROCHLORIDE
SYRUP; ORAL

	ACTIFED W/ CODEINE			
AA	BURROUGHS WELLCOME	10 MG/5 ML;30 MG/5 ML;1.25 MG/5 ML	N12575 003	APR 04, 1984
	HISTAFED C			
AA	CENCI	10 MG/5 ML;30 MG/5 ML;1.25 MG/5 ML	N89018 001	JUL 23, 1986
	TRIACIN-C			
AA	BARRE	10 MG/5 ML;30 MG/5 ML;1.25 MG/5 ML	N88704 001	MAR 22, 1985
	TRIPROLIDINE HCL PSEUDOEPHEDRINE HCL AND CODEINE PHOSPHATE			
AA	PHARM BASICS	10 MG/5 ML;30 MG/5 ML;1.25 MG/5 ML	N88833 001	NOV 16, 1984

COLCHICINE; PROBENECID
TABLET; ORAL

	COL-PROBENECID		
BP	DANBURY	0.5 MG;500 MG	N84279 001
	COLBENEMID		
BP	+ MSD	0.5 MG;500 MG	N12383 001
	PROBENECID AND COLCHICINE		
BP	EON LABS	0.5 MG;500 MG	N86130 001
BP	RICHLYN	0.5 MG;500 MG	N83720 002
BP	ZENITH	0.5 MG;500 MG	N83734 001

COLESTIPOL HYDROCHLORIDE
GRANULE; ORAL

	COLESTID		
+	UPJOHN	5 GM/PACKET	N17563 001
		500 GM/BOT	N17563 002

COLFOSCERIL PALMITATE; *MULTIPLE*
SEE <u>CETYL ALCOHOL; COLFOSCERIL PALMITATE; TYLOXAPOL</u>

COLISTIMETHATE SODIUM
INJECTABLE; INJECTION

COLY-MYCIN M		
PARKE DAVIS	EQ 150 MG BASE/VIAL	N50108 002

COLISTIN SULFATE
SUSPENSION; ORAL

COLY-MYCIN S		
PARKE DAVIS	EQ 25 MG BASE/5 ML	N50355 001

COLISTIN SULFATE; HYDROCORTISONE ACETATE; NEOMYCIN SULFATE; THONZONIUM BROMIDE
SUSPENSION; OTIC

COLY-MYCIN S		
PARKE DAVIS	EQ 3 MG BASE/ML;10 MG/ML;EQ 3.3 MG BASE/ML;0.5 MG/ML	N50356 001

COPPER
INTRAUTERINE DEVICE; INTRAUTERINE

COPPER T MODEL TCU 380A			
POPULATION COUNCIL	APPROX 309 MG COPPER	N18680 001	NOV 15, 1984

CORTICOTROPIN
INJECTABLE; INJECTION

	ACTH			
AP	PARKE DAVIS	25 UNITS/VIAL	N08317 002	
AP		40 UNITS/VIAL	N08317 004	
	ACTHAR			
AP	ARMOUR	25 UNITS/VIAL	N07504 002	
AP		40 UNITS/VIAL	N07504 003	
	CORTICOTROPIN			
BC	ORGANICS	40 UNITS/ML	N10831 001	
BC		80 UNITS/ML	N10831 002	
AP	+ STERIS	40 UNITS/VIAL	N88772 001	NOV 21, 1984
	H.P. ACTHAR GEL			
BC	+ ARMOUR	40 UNITS/ML	N08372 006	
BC		80 UNITS/ML	N08372 008	
	PURIFIED CORTROPHIN GEL			
BC	ORGANON	40 UNITS/ML	N08975 001	
BC		80 UNITS/ML	N08975 002	

Prescription Drug Products (continued)

CORTICOTROPIN-ZINC HYDROXIDE
INJECTABLE; INJECTION
CORTROPHIN-ZINC

+ ORGANON	40 UNITS/ML	N09854 001	

CORTISONE ACETATE
INJECTABLE; INJECTION
CORTISONE ACETATE

BP	STERIS	25 MG/ML	N83147 003
BP		25 MG/ML	N85677 001
BP		50 MG/ML	N83147 004
BP		50 MG/ML	N85677 002
BP		25 MG/ML	N08126 002

CORTONE

BP	UPJOHN	25 MG/ML	N07110 002
BP	+ MSD	50 MG/ML	N07110 003

TABLET; ORAL
CORTISONE ACETATE

BP	CHELSEA	25 MG	N85884 001
BP	HEATHER	25 MG	N85736 001
BP	INWOOD	25 MG	N80731 001
BP	PUREPAC	25 MG	N80493 001
BP	RICHLYN	25 MG	N09458 001
BP	UPJOHN	25 MG	N08126 001

CORTONE

BP		5 MG	N08126 003
BP		10 MG	N08126 004
BP	WEST WARD	25 MG	N80776 002

CORTONE

BP	+ MSD	25 MG	N07750 003

COSYNTROPIN
INJECTABLE; INJECTION
CORTROSYN

ORGANON	0.25 MG/VIAL	N16750 001	

CROMOLYN SODIUM
AEROSOL, METERED; INHALATION
INTAL

+ FISONS	0.8 MG/INH	N18887 001	DEC 05, 1985

CAPSULE; INHALATION
INTAL

+ FISONS	20 MG	N16990 001	

CAPSULE; ORAL
GASTROCROM

+ FISONS	100 MG	N19188 001	DEC 22, 1989

CROMOLYN SODIUM (continued)
SOLUTION; INHALATION
INTAL

FISONS	10 MG/ML	N18596 001	MAY 28, 1982

SOLUTION; NASAL
NASALCROM

FISONS	4%	N18306 001	MAR 18, 1983

SOLUTION/DROPS; OPHTHALMIC
OPTICROM

FISONS	4%	N18155 001	OCT 03, 1984

CROTAMITON
CREAM; TOPICAL
EURAX

WESTWOOD SQUIBB	10%	N06927 001	

LOTION; TOPICAL
CROTAN

ΔI	OWEN GALDERMA	10%	N87204 001

EURAX

ΔI	WESTWOOD SQUIBB	10%	N09112 003

CUPRIC CHLORIDE
INJECTABLE; INJECTION
CUPRIC CHLORIDE IN PLASTIC CONTAINER

ABBOTT	EQ 0.4 MG COPPER/ML	N18960 001	JUN 26, 1986

CUPRIC SULFATE
INJECTABLE; INJECTION
CUPRIC SULFATE

LYPHOMED	EQ 0.4 MG COPPER/ML	N19350 001	MAY 05, 1987

CYANOCOBALAMIN
INJECTABLE; INJECTION
BERUBIGEN

AP	UPJOHN	1 MG/ML	N06798 001

BETALIN 12

AP	LILLY	0.1 MG/ML	N80855 001
AP		1 MG/ML	N80855 002

COBAVITE

AP	STERIS	0.1 MG/ML	N83013 001
AP		1 MG/ML	N83064 001

Prescription Drug Products (continued)

CYANOCOBALAMIN (continued)

INJECTABLE; INJECTION

CYANOCOBALAMIN

	Firm	Strength	NDC	
ΔP	AKORN	1MG/ML	N87969 001	NOV 10, 1983
ΔP	DELL	0.03 MG/ML	N80689 001	
ΔP		0.1 MG/ML	N80689 002	
ΔP		1MG/ML	N80689 003	
ΔP	ELKINS SINN	1MG/ML	N80515 002	
ΔP	LUITPOLD	1MG/ML	N80737 001	
ΔP	LYPHOMED	0.1 MG/ML	N80557 002	
ΔP	MERRELL DOW	1MG/ML	N83075 001	
ΔP	SMITH NEPHEW SOLOPAK	1MG/ML	N80564 001	
ΔP	STERIS	1MG/ML	N87551 001	FEB 29, 1984
ΔP		0.1 MG/ML	N80573 002	
ΔP		0.1 MG/ML	N83120 001	
ΔP		1MG/ML	N80573 001	
ΔP		1MG/ML	N83120 002	
ΔP	WYETH AYERST	0.1 MG/ML	N80554 001	
ΔP		1MG/ML	N80554 002	
ΔP	RUBIVITE BEL MAR	0.03 MG/ML	N10791 004	
ΔP		0.1 MG/ML	N10791 002	
ΔP		1MG/ML	N10791 003	
ΔP		0.05 MG/ML	N10791 001	
ΔP		0.12 MG/ML	N10791 005	
ΔP	RUBRAMIN PC SQUIBB	0.1 MG/ML	N06799 002	
ΔP		1MG/ML	N06799 004	
ΔP	RUVITE SAVAGE	1MG/ML	N80570 002	
ΔP	SYTOBEX PARKE DAVIS	1MG/ML	N07085 002	
ΔP	VIBISONE LYPHOMED	1MG/ML	N80557 003	

TABLET; ORAL

	Firm	Strength	NDC
ΔP	CYANOCOBALAMIN + WEST WARD	1 MG	N84264 001

CYANOCOBALAMIN; *MULTIPLE*

SEE   ASCORBIC ACID: BIOTIN: CYANOCOBALAMIN: DEXPANTHENOL: ERGOCALCIFEROL: FOLIC ACID: NIACINAMIDE: PYRIDOXINE HYDROCHLORIDE: RIBOFLAVIN PHOSPHATE SODIUM: THIAMINE HYDROCHLORIDE: VITAMIN A: VITAMIN E

SEE   ASCORBIC ACID: BIOTIN: CYANOCOBALAMIN: DEXPANTHENOL: ERGOCALCIFEROL: FOLIC ACID: NIACINAMIDE: PYRIDOXINE: RIBOFLAVIN PHOSPHATE SODIUM: THIAMINE: VITAMIN A: VITAMIN E

SEE   COBALT CHLORIDE. CO-57: CYANOCOBALAMIN: CYANOCOBALAMIN, CO-57: INTRINSIC FACTOR

CYANOCOBALAMIN; CYANOCOBALAMIN, CO-57; CYANOCOBALAMIN, CO-58

N/A; N/A

DICOPAC KIT

Firm	Strength	NDC
AMERSHAM	N/A;N/A;N/A	N17406 001

CYANOCOBALAMIN; CYANOCOBALAMIN, CO-57; INTRINSIC FACTOR

N/A; N/A

CYANOCOBALAMIN CO 57 SCHILLING TEST KIT

Firm	Strength	NDC
MALLINCKRODT	0.1 MG/ML;0.5 UCI;60 MG	N16635 001

CYANOCOBALAMIN, CO-57

CAPSULE; ORAL

RUBRATOPE-57

Firm	Strength	NDC
SQUIBB	0.5-1 UCI	N16089 002

CYANOCOBALAMIN, CO-57; *MULTIPLE*

SEE   COBALT CHLORIDE, CO-57: CYANOCOBALAMIN: CYANOCOBALAMIN, CO-57: INTRINSIC FACTOR

SEE   CYANOCOBALAMIN: CYANOCOBALAMIN, CO-57: CYANOCOBALAMIN, CO-58

SEE   CYANOCOBALAMIN: CYANOCOBALAMIN, CO-57: INTRINSIC FACTOR

CYANOCOBALAMIN, CO-58; *MULTIPLE*

SEE   CYANOCOBALAMIN: CYANOCOBALAMIN, CO-57: CYANOCOBALAMIN, CO-58

CYCLACILLIN

POWDER FOR RECONSTITUTION; ORAL

CYCLAPEN-W

	Firm	Strength	NDC	
	WYETH AYERST	125 MG/5 ML	N50508 001	
		250 MG/5 ML	N50508 002	
		500 MG/5 ML	N50508 003	
+				

TABLET; ORAL

CYCLACILLIN

	Firm	Strength	NDC	
ΔB	BIOCRAFT	250 MG	N62895 001	AUG 04, 1988
ΔB		500 MG	N62895 002	AUG 04, 1988

CYCLAPEN-W

	Firm	Strength	NDC
ΔB +	WYETH AYERST	250 MG	N50509 001
ΔB +		500 MG	N50509 002

CYCLIZINE LACTATE

INJECTABLE; INJECTION

MAREZINE

Firm	Strength	NDC
BURROUGHS WELLCOME	50 MG/ML	N09495 001

Prescription Drug Products *(continued)*

CYCLOBENZAPRINE HYDROCHLORIDE
TABLET; ORAL

CYCLOBENZAPRINE HCL

ΔB	DANBURY	10 MG	N71611 001	FEB 29, 1988
ΔB	GENEVA	10 MG	N72854 001	NOV 19, 1991
ΔB	MYLAN	10 MG	N73144 001	MAY 31, 1991
ΔB	WATSON	10 MG	N73143 001	NOV 27, 1991

FLEXERIL

ΔB	+ MSD	10 MG	N17821 002

CYCLOPENTOLATE HYDROCHLORIDE
SOLUTION/DROPS; OPHTHALMIC

AK-PENTOLATE

ΔT	AKORN	1%	N85555 001	

CYCLOGYL

ΔT	ALCON	0.5%	N84109 001
ΔT		1%	N84110 001
ΔT		2%	N84108 001

CYCLOPENTOLATE HCL

ΔT	STERIS	1%	N89162 001	JAN 24, 1991

PENTOLAIR

ΔT	PHARMAFAIR	0.5%	N88643 001	FEB 09, 1987
ΔT		1%	N88150 001	FEB 25, 1983

CYCLOPENTOLATE HYDROCHLORIDE; PHENYLEPHRINE HYDROCHLORIDE
SOLUTION/DROPS; OPHTHALMIC

CYCLOMYDRIL

ΔT	ALCON	0.2%;1%	N84300 001

CYCLOPHOSPHAMIDE
INJECTABLE; INJECTION

CYCLOPHOSPHAMIDE

ΔP	ELKINS SINN	100 MG/VIAL	N88371 001	JUL 03, 1986
ΔP		200 MG/VIAL	N88372 001	JUL 03, 1986
ΔP		500 MG/VIAL	N88373 001	JUL 03, 1986
ΔP		1 GM/VIAL	N88374 001	JUL 03, 1986

CYTOXAN

ΔP	BRISTOL	100 MG/VIAL	N12142 001	
ΔP		200 MG/VIAL	N12142 002	
ΔP		500 MG/VIAL	N12142 003	
ΔP		1 GM/VIAL	N12142 004	AUG 30, 1982
ΔP		2 GM/VIAL	N12142 005	AUG 30, 1982

CYCLOPHOSPHAMIDE *(continued)*
INJECTABLE; INJECTION

LYOPHILIZED CYTOXAN

ΔP	BRISTOL	100 MG/VIAL	N12142 006	DEC 05, 1985
ΔP		200 MG/VIAL	N12142 007	DEC 10, 1985
ΔP		500 MG/VIAL	N12142 008	JAN 04, 1984
ΔP		1 GM/VIAL	N12142 010	SEP 24, 1985
ΔP		2 GM/VIAL	N12142 009	DEC 10, 1984

NEOSAR

ΔP	ADRIA	100 MG/VIAL	N87442 001	FEB 16, 1982
ΔP		200 MG/VIAL	N87442 002	FEB 16, 1982
ΔP		500 MG/VIAL	N87442 003	FEB 16, 1982
ΔP		1 GM/VIAL	N87442 004	JUL 08, 1983
ΔP		2 GM/VIAL	N87442 005	MAR 30, 1989

TABLET; ORAL

CYTOXAN

ΔP	BRISTOL	25 MG	N12141 002	
		50 MG	N12141 001	

CYCLOSERINE
CAPSULE; ORAL

SEROMYCIN

+	LILLY	250 MG	N60593 001

CYCLOSPORINE
CAPSULE; ORAL

SANDIMMUNE

	SANDOZ	25 MG	N50625 001	MAR 02, 1990
+		100 MG	N50625 002	MAR 02, 1990

INJECTABLE; INJECTION

SANDIMMUNE

	SANDOZ	50 MG/ML	N50573 001	NOV 14, 1983

SOLUTION; ORAL

SANDIMMUNE

	SANDOZ	100 MG/ML	N50574 001	NOV 14, 1983

Prescription Drug Products (continued)

CYCLOTHIAZIDE

TABLET; ORAL

		Strength	No.	Date
	ANHYDRON			
+	LILLY	2 MG	N13157 002	

CYPROHEPTADINE HYDROCHLORIDE

SYRUP; ORAL

		Strength	No.	Date
	CYPROHEPTADINE HCL			
AA	BARRE	2 MG/5 ML	N86833 001	
AA	HALSEY	2 MG/5 ML	N89199 001	JUL 03, 1986
AA	PHARM BASICS	2 MG/5 ML	N87001 001	NOV 04, 1982
	PERIACTIN			
AA	MSD	2 MG/5 ML	N13220 002	

TABLET; ORAL

		Strength	No.	Date
	CYPROHEPTADINE HCL			
AA	ASCOT	4 MG	N87685 001	OCT 25, 1982
AA	CAMALL	4 MG	N88212 001	MAY 26, 1983
AA	CHELSEA	4 MG	N86165 001	
AA	DANBURY	4 MG	N86580 001	
AA	GENEVA	4 MG	N86808 001	
AA	HALSEY	4 MG	N89057 001	JUL 03, 1986
AA	MD PHARM	4 MG	N87566 001	NOV 10, 1982
AA	MYLAN	4 MG	N86678 001	
AA	PAR	4 MG	N87129 001	
AA	PIONEER PHARMS	4 MG	N87839 001	FEB 08, 1984
AA	SIDMAK	4 MG	N88205 001	JUL 26, 1983
AA	ZENITH	4 MG	N87056 001	
	PERIACTIN			
AA	MSD	4 MG	N12649 001	

CYTARABINE

INJECTABLE; INJECTION

		Strength	No.	Date
	CYTARABINE			
	BULL	20 MG/ML	N71868 001	JUN 04, 1990
		20 MG/ML	N72168 001	AUG 31, 1990
AP	CETUS BEN VENUE	100 MG/VIAL	N71471 001	AUG 02, 1989
AP		500 MG/VIAL	N71472 001	AUG 02, 1989
	CYTOSAR-U			
AP	UPJOHN	100 MG/VIAL	N16793 001	
AP		500 MG/VIAL	N16793 002	
		1 GM/VIAL	N16793 003	DEC 21, 1987
		2 GM/VIAL	N16793 004	DEC 21, 1987

DACARBAZINE

INJECTABLE; INJECTION

		Strength	No.	Date
	DACARBAZINE			
AP	LYPHOMED	100 MG/VIAL	N70962 001	AUG 28, 1986
AP		200 MG/VIAL	N70990 001	AUG 28, 1986
	DTIC-DOME			
AP	MILES	100 MG/VIAL	N17575 001	
AP		200 MG/VIAL	N17575 002	

DACTINOMYCIN

INJECTABLE; INJECTION

		Strength	No.
	COSMEGEN		
	MSD	0.5 MG/VIAL	N60467 001

DANAZOL

CAPSULE; ORAL

		Strength	No.
	DANOCRINE		
	STERLING	50 MG	N17557 003
		100 MG	N17557 004
		200 MG	N17557 002

DANTROLENE SODIUM

CAPSULE; ORAL

		Strength	No.
	DANTRIUM		
	P AND G	25 MG	N17443 001
+		50 MG	N17443 003
		100 MG	N17443 002

INJECTABLE; INJECTION

		Strength	No.
	DANTRIUM		
	P AND G	20 MG/VIAL	N18264 001
+			

DAPIPRAZOLE HYDROCHLORIDE

SOLUTION/DROPS; OPHTHALMIC

		Strength	No.	Date
	REV-EYES			
	ANGELINI	0.5%	N19849 001	DEC 31, 1990

DAPSONE

TABLET; ORAL

		Strength	No.
	DAPSONE		
	JACOBUS	25 MG	N86841 001
+		100 MG	N86842 001

DAUNORUBICIN HYDROCHLORIDE

INJECTABLE; INJECTION

		Strength	No.
	CERUBIDINE		
AP	RHONE POULENC RORER	EQ 20 MG BASE/VIAL	N61876 001
AP	WYETH AYERST	EQ 20 MG BASE/VIAL	N50484 001

Prescription Drug Products *(continued)*

DEFEROXAMINE MESYLATE
INJECTABLE; INJECTION
DESFERAL

CIBA	500 MG/VIAL	N16267 001	

DEMECARIUM BROMIDE
SOLUTION/DROPS; OPHTHALMIC
HUMORSOL

MSD	0.125%	N11860 002
	0.25%	N11860 001

DEMECLOCYCLINE HYDROCHLORIDE
CAPSULE; ORAL
DECLOMYCIN

+ LEDERLE	150 MG	N50262 001

TABLET; ORAL
DECLOMYCIN

LEDERLE	75 MG	N50261 001
	150 MG	N50261 002
+	300 MG	N50261 003

DESERPIDINE
TABLET; ORAL
HARMONYL

+ ABBOTT	0.25 MG	N10796 002

DESERPIDINE; HYDROCHLOROTHIAZIDE
TABLET; ORAL
ORETICYL FORTE

ABBOTT	0.25 MG;25 MG	N12148 002

ORETICYL 25

ABBOTT	0.125 MG;25 MG	N12148 001

ORETICYL 50

+ ABBOTT	0.125 MG;50 MG	N12148 003

DESERPIDINE; METHYCLOTHIAZIDE
TABLET; ORAL
ENDURONYL

ABBOTT	0.25 MG;5 MG	N12775 001

ENDURONYL FORTE

+ ABBOTT	0.5 MG;5 MG	N12775 002

DESIPRAMINE HYDROCHLORIDE
CAPSULE; ORAL
PERTOFRANE
RHONE POULENC

RORER	25 MG	N13621 001
+	50 MG	N13621 002

DESIPRAMINE HYDROCHLORIDE *(continued)*
TABLET; ORAL
DESIPRAMINE HCL

AB	EON LABS	25 MG	N71601 001	JUN 05, 1987
AB		50 MG	N71588 001	JUN 05, 1987
AB		75 MG	N71602 001	JUN 05, 1987
AB		100 MG	N71766 001	OCT 05, 1987
AB	GENEVA	10 MG	N72099 001	OCT 05, 1987
AB		25 MG	N72100 001	MAY 24, 1988
AB		50 MG	N72101 001	MAY 24, 1988
AB		75 MG	N72102 001	MAY 24, 1988
AB		100 MG	N72103 001	JUN 20, 1988
AB		150 MG	N72104 001	JUN 20, 1988
AB	SIDMAK	25 MG	N71800 001	DEC 08, 1987
AB		50 MG	N71801 001	DEC 08, 1987
AB		75 MG	N71802 001	DEC 08, 1987
AB	NORPRAMIN MERRELL DOW	10 MG	N14399 007	FEB 11, 1982
AB		25 MG	N14399 001	
AB		50 MG	N14399 003	
AB +		75 MG	N14399 004	
AB +		100 MG	N14399 005	
AB		150 MG	N14399 006	

DESLANOSIDE
INJECTABLE; INJECTION
CEDILANID-D

SANDOZ	0.2 MG/ML	N09282 002

DESMOPRESSIN ACETATE
INJECTABLE; INJECTION
DDAVP
RHONE POULENC

RORER	0.004 MG/ML	N18938 001	MAR 30, 1984

SOLUTION; NASAL
CONCENTRAID

BX	FERRING	0.01%	N19776 001	DEC 26, 1990

DDAVP

BX	+ RHONE POULENC RORER	0.01%	N17922 001

Prescription Drug Products (continued)

DESONIDE

CREAM; TOPICAL

	DESONIDE		
ΔB	TARO	0.05%	N7548 001 JUN 30, 1992
	DESOWEN		
ΔB	OWEN GALDERMA	0.05%	N19048 001 DEC 14, 1984
	TRIDESILON		
ΔB	+ MILES	0.05%	N17010 001

LOTION; TOPICAL

	DESOWEN		
	OWEN GALDERMA	0.05%	N72354 001 JAN 24, 1992

OINTMENT; TOPICAL

	DESOWEN		
ΔB	OWEN GALDERMA	0.05%	N71425 001 JUN 15, 1988
	TRIDESILON		
ΔB	+ MILES	0.05%	N17426 001

DESONIDE; *MULTIPLE*
SEE ACETIC ACID, GLACIAL; DESONIDE

DESOXIMETASONE

CREAM; TOPICAL

	DESOXIMETASONE		
ΔB	TARO	0.05%	N73210 001 NOV 30, 1990
ΔB	TARO	0.25%	N73193 001 NOV 30, 1990
	TOPICORT		
ΔB	HOECHST ROUSSEL	0.25%	N17856 001
	TOPICORT LP		
ΔB	+ HOECHST ROUSSEL	0.05%	N18309 001

GEL; TOPICAL

	TOPICORT		
ΔB	HOECHST ROUSSEL	0.05%	N18586 001 MAR 29, 1982

OINTMENT; TOPICAL

	TOPICORT		
	HOECHST ROUSSEL	0.25%	N18763 001 SEP 30, 1983

DESOXYCORTICOSTERONE PIVALATE

INJECTABLE; INJECTION

	PERCORTEN		
	CIBA	25 MG/ML	N08822 001

DESOXYRIBONUCLEASE; *MULTIPLE*
SEE CHLORAMPHENICOL; DESOXYRIBONUCLEASE; FIBRINOLYSIN

DEXAMETHASONE

AEROSOL; TOPICAL

	AEROSEB-DEX		
	HERBERT	0.01%	N83296 002
	DECASPRAY		
	MSD	0.4%	N12731 002

ELIXIR; ORAL

	DECADRON		
ΔA	MSD	0.5 MG/5 ML	N12376 002
	DEXAMETHASONE		
ΔA	BARRE	0.5 MG/5 ML	N84754 001
ΔA	NASKA	0.5 MG/5 ML	N88997 001 OCT 10, 1986
	HEXADROL		
ΔA	ORGANON	0.5 MG/5 ML	N12674 001
	MYMETHASONE		
ΔA	PHARM BASICS	0.5 MG/5 ML	N88254 001 JUL 27, 1983

GEL; TOPICAL

	DECADERM		
	MSD	0.1%	N13538 001

SOLUTION; ORAL

	DEXAMETHASONE		
	ROXANE	0.5 MG/5 ML	N88248 001 SEP 01, 1983
	DEXAMETHASONE INTENSOL		
	ROXANE	0.5 MG/0.5 ML	N88252 001 SEP 01, 1983

SUSPENSION/DROPS; OPHTHALMIC

	DEXAMETHASONE		
ΔT	STERIS	0.1%	N89170 001 MAY 09, 1989
	MAXIDEX		
ΔT	ALCON	0.1%	N13422 001

TABLET; ORAL

	DECADRON		
BP	MSD	0.25 MG	N11664 004
BP	MSD	0.5 MG	N11664 001
BP	MSD	0.75 MG	N11664 002
BP	+	1.5 MG	N11664 003
BP	+	4 MG	N11664 005
BP	+	6 MG	N11664 006 JUL 30, 1982

Prescription Drug Products (continued)

DEXAMETHASONE (continued)

TABLET; ORAL

DEXAMETHASONE

			Strength	Number	Date
BP	DANBURY	0.25 MG		N85455 001	
BP		0.5 MG		N85458 001	
BP		0.75 MG		N80968 001	
BP		1.5 MG		N85456 001	
BP	PAR	0.25 MG		N88149 001	APR 28, 1983
BP		0.5 MG		N88148 001	APR 28, 1983
BP		0.75 MG		N88160 001	APR 28, 1983
BP		1.5 MG		N88237 001	APR 28, 1983
BP		4 MG		N88238 001	APR 28, 1983
BP		6 MG		N88481 001	NOV 28, 1983
BP	RICHLYN	0.75 MG		N85376 001	
BP	ROXANE	0.5 MG		N84611 001	
BP		0.75 MG		N84613 001	
BP		1.5 MG		N84610 001	
BP		4 MG		N84612 001	
BP		6 MG		N88316 001	SEP 15, 1983
BP		1 MG		N88306 001	SEP 15, 1983
BP		2 MG		N87916 001	AUG 26, 1982
BP	DEXONE 0.5 SOLVAY	0.5 MG		N84991 001	
BP	DEXONE 0.75 SOLVAY	0.75 MG		N84993 001	
BP	DEXONE 1.5 SOLVAY	1.5 MG		N84990 001	
BP	DEXONE 4 SOLVAY	4 MG		N84992 001	
BP	HEXADROL ORGANON	0.5 MG		N12675 004	
BP		0.75 MG		N12675 007	
BP		1.5 MG		N12675 009	
BP		4 MG		N12675 010	

DEXAMETHASONE; NEOMYCIN SULFATE; POLYMYXIN B SULFATE

OINTMENT; OPHTHALMIC

		Strength	Number	Date
	DEXACIDIN IOLAB	0.1%;EQ 3.5 MG BASE/GM;10,000 UNITS/GM	N62566 001	FEB 22, 1985
AT	DEXASPORIN PHARMAFAIR	0.1%;EQ 3.5 MG BASE/GM;10,000 UNITS/GM	N62411 001	MAY 16, 1983
AT	MAXITROL ALCON	0.1%;EQ 3.5 MG BASE/GM;10,000 UNITS/GM	N50065 002	
AT	NEOMYCIN AND POLYMYXIN B SULFATES AND DEXAMETHASONE FOUGERA	0.1%;EQ 3.5 MG BASE/GM;10,000 UNITS/GM	N62938 001	JUL 31, 1989

SUSPENSION/DROPS; OPHTHALMIC

		Strength	Number	Date
AT	DEXACIDIN IOLAB	0.1%;EQ 3.5 MG BASE/ML;10,000 UNITS/ML	N62544 001	OCT 29, 1984
AT	DEXASPORIN PHARMAFAIR	0.1%;EQ 3.5 MG BASE/ML;10,000 UNITS/ML	N62428 001	MAY 18, 1983
AT	MAXITROL ALCON	0.1%;EQ 3.5 MG BASE/ML;10,000 UNITS/ML	N50023 002	
AT		0.1%;EQ 3.5 MG BASE/ML;10,000 UNITS/ML	N62341 001	MAY 22, 1984
AT	NEOMYCIN AND POLYMYXIN B SULFATES AND DEXAMETHASONE STERIS	0.1%;EQ 3.5 MG BASE/ML;10,000 UNITS/ML	N62721 001	NOV 17, 1986

DEXAMETHASONE; TOBRAMYCIN

OINTMENT; OPHTHALMIC

	Strength	Number	Date
TOBRADEX + ALCON	0.1%;0.3%	N50616 001	SEP 28, 1988

SUSPENSION/DROPS; OPHTHALMIC

	Strength	Number	Date
TOBRADEX + ALCON	0.1%;0.3%	N50592 001	AUG 18, 1988

Prescription Drug Products (continued)

DEXAMETHASONE ACETATE

INJECTABLE; INJECTION

DECADRON-LA

BP	MERCK	EQ 8 MG BASE/ML	N16675 001	

DEXAMETHASONE ACETATE

BP	STERIS	EQ 8 MG BASE/ML	N84315 001	
BP		EQ 16 MG BASE/ML	N87711 001	MAY 24, 1982

DEXAMETHASONE SODIUM PHOSPHATE

AEROSOL; NASAL

DECADRON

	MSD	EQ 0.1 MG PHOSPHATE/INH	N14242 001

AEROSOL, METERED; INHALATION

DECADRON

	MSD	EQ 0.1 MG PHOSPHATE/INH	N13413 001

CREAM; TOPICAL

DECADRON

	MSD	EQ 0.1% PHOSPHATE	N11983 002

INJECTABLE; INJECTION

DECADRON

AP	MSD	EQ 4 MG PHOSPHATE/ML	N12071 002	
AP		EQ 24 MG PHOSPHATE/ML	N12071 004	

DEXAMETHASONE

AP	ELKINS SINN	EQ 4 MG PHOSPHATE/ML	N84282 001	
AP		EQ 10 MG PHOSPHATE/ML	N87702 001	SEP 07, 1982
AP	LYPHOMED	EQ 4 MG PHOSPHATE/ML	N88448 001	JAN 25, 1984
AP		EQ 10 MG PHOSPHATE/ML	N88469 001	JAN 25, 1984

DEXAMETHASONE SODIUM PHOSPHATE

AP	AKORN	EQ 4 MG PHOSPHATE/ML	N84493 001	
AP	BEL MAR	EQ 4 MG PHOSPHATE/ML	N84752 001	
AP	BRISTOL	EQ 4 MG PHOSPHATE/ML	N87065 001	
AP	DELL	EQ 4 MG PHOSPHATE/ML	N83161 001	
AP	GENSIA	EQ 4 MG PHOSPHATE/ML	N81125 001	AUG 31, 1990
AP		EQ 10 MG PHOSPHATE/ML	N81126 001	AUG 31, 1990
AP	LUITPOLD	EQ 4 MG PHOSPHATE/ML	N87440 001	JUL 21, 1982
AP	LYPHOMED	EQ 4 MG PHOSPHATE/ML	N84916 001	
AP	STERIS	EQ 4 MG PHOSPHATE/ML	N83702 001	
AP		EQ 4 MG PHOSPHATE/ML	N84355 001	
AP		EQ 4 MG PHOSPHATE/ML	N89169 001	APR 09, 1986
AP		EQ 10 MG PHOSPHATE/ML	N87668 001	JUL 01, 1982
AP	WYETH AYERST	EQ 24 MG PHOSPHATE/ML	N85606 001	
AP		EQ 4 MG PHOSPHATE/ML	N85641 001	

HEXADROL

AP	ORGANON	EQ 4 MG PHOSPHATE/ML	N14694 002	
AP		EQ 10 MG PHOSPHATE/ML	N14694 003	
AP		EQ 20 MG PHOSPHATE/ML	N14694 004	

DEXAMETHASONE SODIUM PHOSPHATE (continued)

OINTMENT; OPHTHALMIC

DECADRON

AI	MSD	EQ 0.05% PHOSPHATE	N11977 001	

DEXAIR

AI	PHARMAFAIR	EQ 0.05% PHOSPHATE	N88071 001	DEC 28, 1982

MAXIDEX

AI	ALCON	EQ 0.05% PHOSPHATE	N83342 001	

SOLUTION/DROPS; OPHTHALMIC

DEXAIR

	PHARMAFAIR	EQ 0.1% PHOSPHATE	N88433 001	DEC 15, 1983

SOLUTION/DROPS; OPHTHALMIC, OTIC

DECADRON

AI	MSD	EQ 0.1% PHOSPHATE	N11984 001	

DEXAMETHASONE SODIUM PHOSPHATE

AI	AKORN	EQ 0.1% PHOSPHATE	N84855 001	
AI	STERIS	EQ 0.1% PHOSPHATE	N88771 001	JAN 16, 1985

DEXAMETHASONE SODIUM PHOSPHATE; LIDOCAINE HYDROCHLORIDE

INJECTABLE; INJECTION

DECADRON W/ XYLOCAINE

	MSD	EQ 4 MG PHOSPHATE/ML;10 MG/ML	N13334 002

DEXAMETHASONE SODIUM PHOSPHATE; NEOMYCIN SULFATE

OINTMENT; OPHTHALMIC

NEODECADRON

	MSD	EQ 0.05% PHOSPHATE;EQ 3.5 MG BASE/GM	N50324 001

SOLUTION/DROPS; OPHTHALMIC

NEODECADRON

AI	MSD	EQ 0.1% PHOSPHATE;EQ 3.5 MG BASE/ML	N50322 001	

NEOMYCIN SULFATE-DEXAMETHASONE SODIUM PHOSPHATE

AI	PHARMAFAIR	EQ 0.1% PHOSPHATE;EQ 3.5 MG BASE/ML	N62539 001	JAN 10, 1985
AI	STERIS	EQ 0.1% PHOSPHATE;EQ 3.5 MG BASE/ML	N62714 001	JUL 21, 1986

DEXCHLORPHENIRAMINE MALEATE

SYRUP; ORAL

MYLARAMINE

AA	PHARM BASICS	2 MG/5 ML	N88251 001	MAR 23, 1984

POLARAMINE

AA	SCHERING	2 MG/5 ML	N86837 001	JUL 19, 1982

Prescription Drug Products (continued)

DEXCHLORPHENIRAMINE MALEATE (continued)
TABLET; ORAL
DEXCHLORPHENIRAMINE MALEATE
△△ SIDMAK   2 MG   N88682 001   JAN 17, 1986
△△ POLARAMINE
   SCHERING   2 MG   N86835 001

DEXPANTHENOL; *MULTIPLE*
SEE ASCORBIC ACID: BIOTIN: CYANOCOBALAMIN: DEXPANTHENOL: ERGOCALCIFEROL: FOLIC ACID: NIACINAMIDE: PYRIDOXINE HYDROCHLORIDE: RIBOFLAVIN PHOSPHATE SODIUM: THIAMINE HYDROCHLORIDE: VITAMIN A: VITAMIN E
SEE ASCORBIC ACID: BIOTIN: CYANOCOBALAMIN: DEXPANTHENOL: ERGOCALCIFEROL: FOLIC ACID: NIACINAMIDE: PYRIDOXINE: RIBOFLAVIN PHOSPHATE SODIUM: THIAMINE: VITAMIN A: VITAMIN E

DEXTROAMPHETAMINE ADIPATE; *MULTIPLE*
SEE AMPHETAMINE ADIPATE: AMPHETAMINE SULFATE: DEXTROAMPHETAMINE ADIPATE: DEXTROAMPHETAMINE SULFATE

DEXTROAMPHETAMINE RESIN COMPLEX; *MULTIPLE*
SEE AMPHETAMINE RESIN COMPLEX: DEXTROAMPHETAMINE RESIN COMPLEX

DEXTROAMPHETAMINE SULFATE
CAPSULE, EXTENDED RELEASE; ORAL
DEXEDRINE
+ SKF   5 MG   N17078 001
+   10 MG   N17078 002
+   15 MG   N17078 003
ELIXIR; ORAL
DEXEDRINE
  SKF   5 MG/5 ML   N83902 001
TABLET; ORAL
DEXAMPEX
△△ LEMMON   5 MG   N83735 001
△△   10 MG   N83735 002
DEXEDRINE
△△ SKF   5 MG   N84935 001
DEXTROAMPHETAMINE SULFATE
△△ HALSEY   10 MG   N83930 001
△△ LANNETT   5 MG   N83903 001
△△   10 MG   N83903 003
△△   15 MG   N85652 001
△△ MAST   5 MG   N86521 001
△△ REXAR   5 MG   N84051 001
△△   10 MG   N84051 002
FERNDEX
△△ FERNDALE   5 MG   N84001 001

DEXTROAMPHETAMINE SULFATE; *MULTIPLE*
SEE AMPHETAMINE ADIPATE: AMPHETAMINE SULFATE: DEXTROAMPHETAMINE ADIPATE: DEXTROAMPHETAMINE SULFATE

DEXTROMETHORPHAN HYDROBROMIDE; *MULTIPLE*
SEE BROMPHENIRAMINE MALEATE: DEXTROMETHORPHAN HYDROBROMIDE: PSEUDOEPHEDRINE HYDROCHLORIDE

DEXTROMETHORPHAN HYDROBROMIDE; PROMETHAZINE HYDROCHLORIDE
SYRUP; ORAL
PHENERGAN W/ DEXTROMETHORPHAN
△△ WYETH AYERST   15 MG/5 ML:6.25 MG/5 ML   N11265 002   APR 02, 1984
PHERAZINE DM
△△ HALSEY   15 MG/5 ML:6.25 MG/5 ML   N88913 001   MAR 02, 1987
PROMETH W/ DEXTROMETHORPHAN
△△ BARRE   15 MG/5 ML:6.25 MG/5 ML   N88762 001   OCT 31, 1984
PROMETHAZINE W/ DEXTROMETHORPHAN
△△ PHARM BASICS   15 MG/5 ML:6.25 MG/5 ML   N88864 001   JAN 04, 1985

DEXTROSE
INJECTABLE; INJECTION
DEXTROSE 10% IN PLASTIC CONTAINER
AP ABBOTT   10 GM/100 ML   N18080 001
AP BAXTER   10 GM/100 ML   N16694 001
AP MCGAW   10 GM/100 ML   N18046 001
            10 GM/100 ML   N19626 004   FEB 02, 1988
DEXTROSE 2.5% IN PLASTIC CONTAINER
   MCGAW   2.5 GM/100 ML   N18358 001
            2.5 GM/100 ML   N19626 001   FEB 02, 1988
DEXTROSE 20% IN PLASTIC CONTAINER
AP ABBOTT   20 GM/100 ML   N18564 001   MAR 23, 1982
AP BAXTER   20 GM/100 ML   N17521 004
DEXTROSE 30% IN PLASTIC CONTAINER
AP ABBOTT   30 GM/100 ML   N19345 001   JAN 26, 1985
AP BAXTER   30 GM/100 ML   N17521 003

Prescription Drug Products (continued)

DEXTROSE (continued)

INJECTABLE; INJECTION

DEXTROSE 40% IN PLASTIC CONTAINER

TE	Manufacturer	Strength	Appl. No.	Date
AP	ABBOTT	40 GM/100 ML	N18562 001	MAR 23, 1982
AP	BAXTER	40 GM/100 ML	N17521 002	

DEXTROSE 5% IN PLASTIC CONTAINER

TE	Manufacturer	Strength	Appl. No.	Date
AP	ABBOTT	50 MG/ML	N16367 002	
AP		50 MG/ML	N19222 001	JUL 13, 1984
AP		5 GM/100 ML	N19466 001	JUL 15, 1985
AP		5 GM/100 ML	N19479 001	SEP 17, 1985
AP	BAXTER	5 GM/100 ML	N16673 001	
		50 MG/ML	N16673 003	OCT 30, 1985
AP	MCGAW	5 GM/100 ML	N16730 001	
AP		5 GM/100 ML	N19626 002	FEB 02, 1988

DEXTROSE 50% IN PLASTIC CONTAINER

TE	Manufacturer	Strength	Appl. No.	Date
AP	ABBOTT	50 GM/100 ML	N18563 001	MAR 23, 1982
AP		500 MG/ML	N19445 001	JUN 03, 1986
AP		50 GM/100 ML	N19894 001	DEC 26, 1989
AP	BAXTER	50 GM/100 ML	N17521 001	
AP		50 GM/100 ML	N20047 001	JUL 02, 1991

DEXTROSE 60% IN PLASTIC CONTAINER

TE	Manufacturer	Strength	Appl. No.	Date
AP	ABBOTT	60 GM/100 ML	N19346 001	JAN 25, 1985
AP	BAXTER	60 GM/100 ML	N17521 005	MAR 26, 1982
AP		60 GM/100 ML	N20047 002	JUL 02, 1991

DEXTROSE 7.7% IN PLASTIC CONTAINER

TE	Manufacturer	Strength	Appl. No.	Date
	MCGAW	7.7 GM/100 ML	N19626 003	FEB 02, 1988

DEXTROSE 70% IN PLASTIC CONTAINER

TE	Manufacturer	Strength	Appl. No.	Date
AP	ABBOTT	70 GM/100 ML	N18561 001	MAR 23, 1982
AP		70 GM/100 ML	N19893 001	DEC 26, 1989
AP	BAXTER	70 GM/100 ML	N17521 006	MAR 26, 1982
AP		70 GM/100 ML	N20047 003	JUL 02, 1991

DEXTROSE; *MULTIPLE*

SEE AMINO ACIDS; CALCIUM CHLORIDE; DEXTROSE; MAGNESIUM CHLORIDE; POTASSIUM CHLORIDE; POTASSIUM PHOSPHATE, DIBASIC; SODIUM CHLORIDE

SEE AMINO ACIDS; DEXTROSE

SEE AMINO ACIDS; DEXTROSE; MAGNESIUM CHLORIDE; POTASSIUM ACETATE; POTASSIUM CHLORIDE; POTASSIUM PHOSPHATE, DIBASIC; SODIUM CHLORIDE

SEE AMINO ACIDS; DEXTROSE; MAGNESIUM CHLORIDE; POTASSIUM CHLORIDE; SODIUM CHLORIDE; SODIUM PHOSPHATE, DIBASIC

SEE CALCIUM CHLORIDE; DEXTROSE; GLUTATHIONE DISULFIDE; MAGNESIUM CHLORIDE; POTASSIUM CHLORIDE; SODIUM BICARBONATE; SODIUM CHLORIDE; SODIUM PHOSPHATE

SEE CALCIUM CHLORIDE; DEXTROSE; MAGNESIUM CHLORIDE; SODIUM CHLORIDE; SODIUM LACTATE

SEE CALCIUM CHLORIDE; DEXTROSE; MAGNESIUM CHLORIDE; SODIUM ACETATE; SODIUM CHLORIDE

SEE CALCIUM CHLORIDE; DEXTROSE; MAGNESIUM CHLORIDE; POTASSIUM CHLORIDE; SODIUM ACETATE; SODIUM CHLORIDE

SEE CALCIUM CHLORIDE; DEXTROSE; MAGNESIUM CHLORIDE; POTASSIUM CHLORIDE; SODIUM ACETATE; SODIUM CHLORIDE; SODIUM LACTATE

SEE CALCIUM CHLORIDE; DEXTROSE; MAGNESIUM CHLORIDE; POTASSIUM CHLORIDE; SODIUM ACETATE; SODIUM CHLORIDE; SODIUM CITRATE

SEE CALCIUM CHLORIDE; DEXTROSE; MAGNESIUM CHLORIDE; SODIUM CHLORIDE; SODIUM LACTATE

SEE CALCIUM CHLORIDE; DEXTROSE; POTASSIUM CHLORIDE; SODIUM CHLORIDE

SEE CALCIUM CHLORIDE; DEXTROSE; POTASSIUM CHLORIDE; SODIUM CHLORIDE; SODIUM LACTATE

SEE CALCIUM CHLORIDE; DEXTROSE; POTASSIUM CHLORIDE; SODIUM ACETATE; SODIUM CHLORIDE

SEE CALCIUM CHLORIDE; DEXTROSE; POTASSIUM CHLORIDE; SODIUM CHLORIDE; SODIUM LACTATE

DEXTROSE; MAGNESIUM ACETATE; POTASSIUM ACETATE; POTASSIUM CHLORIDE; SODIUM CHLORIDE

INJECTABLE; INJECTION

NORMOSOL-M AND DEXTROSE 5% IN PLASTIC CONTAINER

Manufacturer	Strength	Appl. No.
ABBOTT	5 GM/100 ML;21 MG/ 100 ML;128 MG/ 100 ML;234 MG/100 ML	N17610 001

Prescription Drug Products (*continued*)

DEXTROSE; MAGNESIUM ACETATE TETRAHYDRATE; POTASSIUM ACETATE; SODIUM CHLORIDE

INJECTABLE; INJECTION
PLASMA-LYTE 56 AND DEXTROSE 5% IN PLASTIC CONTAINER
BAXTER
5 GM/100 ML;32 MG/
100 ML;128 MG/
100 ML;234 MG/100 ML   N17385 001

DEXTROSE; MAGNESIUM CHLORIDE; POTASSIUM CHLORIDE; POTASSIUM PHOSPHATE, DIBASIC; SODIUM ACETATE

INJECTABLE; INJECTION
ISOLYTE P W/ DEXTROSE 5% IN PLASTIC CONTAINER
MCGAW
5 GM/100 ML;31 MG/
100 ML;130 MG/
100 ML;26 MG/
100 ML;320 MG/100 ML   N19025 001 DEC 27, 1984

DEXTROSE; MAGNESIUM CHLORIDE; POTASSIUM CHLORIDE; POTASSIUM PHOSPHATE, DIBASIC; SODIUM CHLORIDE; SODIUM LACTATE; SODIUM PHOSPHATE, MONOBASIC

INJECTABLE; INJECTION
IONOSOL B AND DEXTROSE 5% IN PLASTIC CONTAINER
ABBOTT
5 GM/100 ML;53 MG/
100 ML;100 MG/
100 ML;100 MG/
100 ML;180 MG/
100 ML;280 MG/
100 ML;16 MG/100 ML   N19515 001 MAY 08, 1986

DEXTROSE; MAGNESIUM CHLORIDE; POTASSIUM CHLORIDE; POTASSIUM PHOSPHATE, MONOBASIC; SODIUM CHLORIDE; SODIUM LACTATE

INJECTABLE; INJECTION
DEXTROSE 5% AND ELECTROLYTE NO.48 IN PLASTIC CONTAINER
BAXTER
5 GM/100 ML;31 MG/
100 ML;141 MG/
100 ML;20 MG/
100 ML;12 MG/
100 ML;260 MG/100 ML   N17484 001

DEXTROSE; MAGNESIUM CHLORIDE; POTASSIUM CHLORIDE; POTASSIUM PHOSPHATE, MONOBASIC; SODIUM LACTATE; SODIUM PHOSPHATE, MONOBASIC

INJECTABLE; INJECTION
IONOSOL MB AND DEXTROSE 5% IN PLASTIC CONTAINER
ABBOTT
5 GM/100 ML;30 MG/
100 ML;141 MG/
100 ML;15 MG/
100 ML;260 MG/
100 ML;25 MG/100 ML   N19513 001 MAY 08, 1986

DEXTROSE; MAGNESIUM CHLORIDE; POTASSIUM CHLORIDE; SODIUM ACETATE; SODIUM CHLORIDE

INJECTABLE; INJECTION
ISOLYTE H W/ DEXTROSE 5% IN PLASTIC CONTAINER
MCGAW
5 GM/100 ML;30 MG/
100 ML;97 MG/
100 ML;220 MG/
100 ML;140 MG/100 ML   N18273 001

DEXTROSE; MAGNESIUM CHLORIDE; POTASSIUM CHLORIDE; SODIUM ACETATE; SODIUM CHLORIDE; SODIUM GLUCONATE

INJECTABLE; INJECTION
ISOLYTE S W/ DEXTROSE 5% IN PLASTIC CONTAINER
AP MCGAW
5 GM/100 ML;30 MG/
100 ML;37 MG/
100 ML;370 MG/
100 ML;530 MG/
100 ML;500 MG/100 ML   N18274 001

NORMOSOL-R AND DEXTROSE 5% IN PLASTIC CONTAINER
ABBOTT
5 GM/100 ML;30 MG/
100 ML;37 MG/
100 ML;222 MG/
100 ML;526 MG/
100 ML;502 MG/100 ML   N17609 001

PLASMA-LYTE 148 AND DEXTROSE 5% IN PLASTIC CONTAINER
AP BAXTER
5 GM/100 ML;30 MG/
100 ML;37 MG/
100 ML;368 MG/
100 ML;526 MG/
100 ML;502 MG/100 ML   N17451 001

DEXTROSE; POTASSIUM CHLORIDE

INJECTABLE; INJECTION
DEXTROSE 5% AND POTASSIUM CHLORIDE 0.075% IN PLASTIC CONTAINER
AP BAXTER
5 GM/100 ML;75 MG/100 ML   N17634 004

DEXTROSE 5% AND POTASSIUM CHLORIDE 0.15% IN PLASTIC CONTAINER
AP BAXTER
5 GM/100 ML;150 MG/
100 ML   N17634 001

DEXTROSE 5% AND POTASSIUM CHLORIDE 0.224% IN PLASTIC CONTAINER
AP BAXTER
5 GM/100 ML;224 MG/
100 ML   N17634 003

DEXTROSE 5% AND POTASSIUM CHLORIDE 0.3% IN PLASTIC CONTAINER
AP BAXTER
5 GM/100 ML;300 MG/
100 ML   N17634 002

POTASSIUM CHLORIDE 0.037% IN DEXTROSE 5% IN PLASTIC CONTAINER
MCGAW
5 GM/100 ML;37 MG/100 ML   N19699 001 SEP 29, 1989

POTASSIUM CHLORIDE 0.075% IN DEXTROSE 5% IN PLASTIC CONTAINER
AP MCGAW
5 GM/100 ML;75 MG/100 ML   N18744 001 NOV 09, 1982
5 GM/100 ML;75 MG/100 ML   N19699 002 SEP 29, 1989

POTASSIUM CHLORIDE 0.11% IN DEXTROSE 5% IN PLASTIC CONTAINER
AP MCGAW
5 GM/100 ML;110 MG/
100 ML   N19699 003 SEP 29, 1989

Prescription Drug Products *(continued)*

DEXTROSE; POTASSIUM CHLORIDE; POTASSIUM PHOSPHATE, MONOBASIC; SODIUM CHLORIDE; SODIUM LACTATE
INJECTABLE; INJECTION
DEXTROSE 5% AND ELECTROLYTE NO 75 IN PLASTIC CONTAINER

	BAXTER	5 GM/100 ML;205 MG/ 100 ML;100 MG/ 100 ML;120 MG/ 100 ML;220 MG/100 ML	N18840 001 JUN 29, 1983

DEXTROSE; POTASSIUM CHLORIDE; SODIUM CHLORIDE
INJECTABLE; INJECTION
DEXTROSE 5%, SODIUM CHLORIDE 0.2% AND POTASSIUM CHLORIDE 0.15%
IN PLASTIC CONTAINER

AP	MCGAW	5 GM/100 ML;150 MG/ 100 ML;200 MG/100 ML	N18268 004

DEXTROSE 5%, SODIUM CHLORIDE 0.2% AND POTASSIUM CHLORIDE 0.224%
IN PLASTIC CONTAINER

AP	MCGAW	5 GM/100 ML;220 MG/ 100 ML;200 MG/100 ML	N18268 005

DEXTROSE 5%, SODIUM CHLORIDE 0.2% AND POTASSIUM CHLORIDE 0.3%
IN PLASTIC CONTAINER

AP	MCGAW	5 GM/100 ML;300 MG/ 100 ML;200 MG/100 ML	N18268 006

DEXTROSE 5%, SODIUM CHLORIDE 0.2% AND POTASSIUM CHLORIDE
10 MEQ IN PLASTIC CONTAINER

AP	BAXTER	5 GM/100 ML;75 MG/ 100 ML;200 MG/100 ML	N18037 006 APR 13, 1982
AP		5 GM/100 ML;150 MG/ 100 ML;200 MG/100 ML	N18037 007 APR 13, 1982

DEXTROSE 5%, SODIUM CHLORIDE 0.2% AND POTASSIUM CHLORIDE
15 MEQ (K) IN PLASTIC CONTAINER

AP	BAXTER	5 GM/100 ML;224 MG/ 100 ML;200 MG/100 ML	N18037 004

DEXTROSE 5%, SODIUM CHLORIDE 0.2% AND POTASSIUM CHLORIDE
20 MEQ (K) IN PLASTIC CONTAINER

AP	BAXTER	5 GM/100 ML;300 MG/ 100 ML;200 MG/100 ML	N18037 001

DEXTROSE 5%, SODIUM CHLORIDE 0.2% AND POTASSIUM CHLORIDE
20 MEQ IN PLASTIC CONTAINER

AP	BAXTER	5 GM/100 ML;150 MG/ 100 ML;200 MG/100 ML	N18037 008 APR 13, 1982

DEXTROSE 5%, SODIUM CHLORIDE 0.2% AND POTASSIUM CHLORIDE
30 MEQ IN PLASTIC CONTAINER

AP	BAXTER	5 GM/100 ML;224 MG/ 100 ML;200 MG/100 ML	N18037 005 APR 13, 1982

DEXTROSE 5%, SODIUM CHLORIDE 0.2% AND POTASSIUM CHLORIDE
40 MEQ IN PLASTIC CONTAINER

AP	BAXTER	5 GM/100 ML;300 MG/ 100 ML;200 MG/100 ML	N18037 009 APR 13, 1982

Prescription Drug Products *(continued)*

DEXTROSE; POTASSIUM CHLORIDE *(continued)*
INJECTABLE; INJECTION
POTASSIUM CHLORIDE 0.15% IN DEXTROSE 5% IN PLASTIC CONTAINER

AP	MCGAW	5 GM/100 ML;150 MG/ 100 ML	N18744 002 NOV 09, 1982
AP		5 GM/100 ML;150 MG/ 100 ML	N19699 004 SEP 29, 1989

POTASSIUM CHLORIDE 0.22% IN DEXTROSE 5% IN PLASTIC CONTAINER

	MCGAW	5 GM/100 ML;220 MG/ 100 ML	N18744 003 NOV 09, 1982
		5 GM/100 ML;220 MG/ 100 ML	N19699 005 SEP 29, 1989

POTASSIUM CHLORIDE 0.3% IN DEXTROSE 5% IN PLASTIC CONTAINER

AP	MCGAW	5 GM/100 ML;300 MG/ 100 ML	N18744 004 NOV 09, 1982
AP		5 GM/100 ML;300 MG/ 100 ML	N19699 006 SEP 29, 1989

POTASSIUM CHLORIDE 20 MEQ IN DEXTROSE 5% IN PLASTIC CONTAINER

AP	ABBOTT	5 GM/100 ML;149 MG/ 100 ML	N18371 001

POTASSIUM CHLORIDE 30 MEQ IN DEXTROSE 5% IN PLASTIC CONTAINER

AP	ABBOTT	5 GM/100 ML;224 MG/ 100 ML	N18371 003

POTASSIUM CHLORIDE 40 MEQ IN DEXTROSE 5% IN PLASTIC CONTAINER

AP	ABBOTT	5 GM/100 ML;298 MG/ 100 ML	N18371 002

DEXTROSE; POTASSIUM CHLORIDE; POTASSIUM LACTATE; SODIUM CHLORIDE; SODIUM PHOSPHATE, MONOBASIC
INJECTABLE; INJECTION
IONOSOL T AND DEXTROSE 5% IN PLASTIC CONTAINER

	ABBOTT	5 GM/100 ML;111 MG/ 100 ML;256 MG/ 100 ML;146 MG/ 100 ML;207 MG/100 ML	N19514 001 MAY 08, 1986

DEXTROSE; POTASSIUM CHLORIDE; POTASSIUM PHOSPHATE, DIBASIC; SODIUM ACETATE; SODIUM CHLORIDE
INJECTABLE; INJECTION
ISOLYTE M W/ DEXTROSE 5% IN PLASTIC CONTAINER

	MCGAW	5 GM/100 ML;150 MG/ 100 ML;130 MG/ 100 ML;280 MG/ 100 ML;91 MG/100 ML	N18270 001

Prescription Drug Products *(continued)*

DEXTROSE; POTASSIUM CHLORIDE; SODIUM CHLORIDE *(continued)*

INJECTABLE; INJECTION

DEXTROSE 5%, SODIUM CHLORIDE 0.2% AND POTASSIUM CHLORIDE 5 MEQ (K) IN PLASTIC CONTAINER
ΔP BAXTER 5 GM/100 ML;150 MG/100 ML;200 MG/100 ML N18037 003

DEXTROSE 5%, SODIUM CHLORIDE 0.2% AND POTASSIUM CHLORIDE 5 MEQ IN PLASTIC CONTAINER
ΔP BAXTER 5 GM/100 ML;75 MG/100 ML;200 MG/100 ML N18037 002

DEXTROSE 5%, SODIUM CHLORIDE 0.2% AND POTASSIUM CHLORIDE 0.075% IN PLASTIC CONTAINER
ΔP MCGAW 5 GM/100 ML;75 MG/100 ML;200 MG/100 ML N18268 009

DEXTROSE 5%, SODIUM CHLORIDE 0.33% AND POTASSIUM CHLORIDE 10 MEQ IN PLASTIC CONTAINER
ΔP BAXTER 5 GM/100 ML;75 MG/100 ML;330 MG/100 ML N18629 005 MAR 23, 1982

DEXTROSE 5%, SODIUM CHLORIDE 0.33% AND POTASSIUM CHLORIDE 15 MEQ IN PLASTIC CONTAINER
ΔP BAXTER 5 GM/100 ML;150 MG/100 ML;330 MG/100 ML N18629 002 MAR 23, 1982

DEXTROSE 5%, SODIUM CHLORIDE 0.33% AND POTASSIUM CHLORIDE 20 MEQ IN PLASTIC CONTAINER
ΔP BAXTER 5 GM/100 ML;224 MG/100 ML;330 MG/100 ML N18629 003 MAR 23, 1982

DEXTROSE 5%, SODIUM CHLORIDE 0.33% AND POTASSIUM CHLORIDE IN PLASTIC CONTAINER
ΔP BAXTER 5 GM/100 ML;150 MG/100 ML;330 MG/100 ML N18629 004 MAR 23, 1982
ΔP BAXTER 5 GM/100 ML;300 MG/100 ML;330 MG/100 ML N18629 006 MAR 23, 1982

DEXTROSE 5%, SODIUM CHLORIDE 0.33% AND POTASSIUM CHLORIDE 30 MEQ IN PLASTIC CONTAINER
ΔP BAXTER 5 GM/100 ML;224 MG/100 ML;330 MG/100 ML N18629 007 MAR 23, 1982

DEXTROSE 5%, SODIUM CHLORIDE 0.33% AND POTASSIUM CHLORIDE 40 MEQ IN PLASTIC CONTAINER
ΔP BAXTER 5 GM/100 ML;300 MG/100 ML;330 MG/100 ML N18629 008 MAR 23, 1982

DEXTROSE 5%, SODIUM CHLORIDE 0.33% AND POTASSIUM CHLORIDE 5 MEQ IN PLASTIC CONTAINER
ΔP BAXTER 5 GM/100 ML;75 MG/100 ML;330 MG/100 ML N18629 001 MAR 23, 1982

DEXTROSE 5%, SODIUM CHLORIDE 0.33% AND POTASSIUM CHLORIDE 0.075% IN PLASTIC CONTAINER
ΔP MCGAW 5 GM/100 ML;75 MG/100 ML;330 MG/100 ML N18268 011 JAN 18, 1986

DEXTROSE; POTASSIUM CHLORIDE; SODIUM CHLORIDE *(continued)*

INJECTABLE; INJECTION

DEXTROSE 5%, SODIUM CHLORIDE 0.33% AND POTASSIUM CHLORIDE 0.15% IN PLASTIC CONTAINER
ΔP MCGAW 5 GM/100 ML;150 MG/100 ML;330 MG/100 ML N18268 012 JAN 18, 1986

DEXTROSE 5%, SODIUM CHLORIDE 0.33% AND POTASSIUM CHLORIDE 0.22% IN PLASTIC CONTAINER
ΔP MCGAW 5 GM/100 ML;220 MG/100 ML;330 MG/100 ML N18268 013 JAN 18, 1986

DEXTROSE 5%, SODIUM CHLORIDE 0.33% AND POTASSIUM CHLORIDE 0.30% IN PLASTIC CONTAINER
ΔP MCGAW 5 GM/100 ML;300 MG/100 ML;330 MG/100 ML N18268 014 JAN 18, 1986

DEXTROSE 5%, SODIUM CHLORIDE 0.45% AND POTASSIUM CHLORIDE 0.15% IN PLASTIC CONTAINER
ΔP MCGAW 5 GM/100 ML;150 MG/100 ML;450 MG/100 ML N18268 001

DEXTROSE 5%, SODIUM CHLORIDE 0.45% AND POTASSIUM CHLORIDE 0.3% IN PLASTIC CONTAINER
ΔP MCGAW 5 GM/100 ML;300 MG/100 ML;450 MG/100 ML N18268 003

DEXTROSE 5%, SODIUM CHLORIDE 0.45% AND POTASSIUM CHLORIDE 20 MEQ (K) IN PLASTIC CONTAINER
ΔP BAXTER 5 GM/100 ML;300 MG/100 ML;450 MG/100 ML N18008 010

DEXTROSE 5%, SODIUM CHLORIDE 0.45% AND POTASSIUM CHLORIDE 0.075% IN PLASTIC CONTAINER
ΔP MCGAW 5 GM/100 ML;75 MG/100 ML;450 MG/100 ML N18268 010

DEXTROSE 5%, SODIUM CHLORIDE 0.45% AND POTASSIUM CHLORIDE 0.22% IN PLASTIC CONTAINER
ΔP MCGAW 5 GM/100 ML;220 MG/100 ML;450 MG/100 ML N18268 002

POTASSIUM CHLORIDE 0.037% IN DEXTROSE 10% AND SODIUM CHLORIDE 0.2% IN PLASTIC CONTAINER
MCGAW 10 GM/100 ML;37 MG/100 ML;200 MG/100 ML N19630 031 FEB 17, 1988

POTASSIUM CHLORIDE 0.037% IN DEXTROSE 10% AND SODIUM CHLORIDE 0.45% IN PLASTIC CONTAINER
MCGAW 10 GM/100 ML;37 MG/100 ML;450 MG/100 ML N19630 037 FEB 17, 1988

POTASSIUM CHLORIDE 0.037% IN DEXTROSE 10% AND SODIUM CHLORIDE 0.9% IN PLASTIC CONTAINER
MCGAW 10 GM/100 ML;37 MG/100 ML;900 MG/100 ML N19630 043 FEB 17, 1988

POTASSIUM CHLORIDE 0.037% IN DEXTROSE 5% AND SODIUM CHLORIDE 0.11% IN PLASTIC CONTAINER
MCGAW 5 GM/100 ML;37 MG/100 ML;110 MG/100 ML N19630 001 FEB 17, 1988

Prescription Drug Products (continued)

DEXTROSE; POTASSIUM CHLORIDE; SODIUM CHLORIDE (continued)

INJECTABLE; INJECTION

POTASSIUM CHLORIDE 0.037% IN DEXTROSE 5% AND SODIUM CHLORIDE 0.2% IN PLASTIC CONTAINER
  MCGAW   5 GM/100 ML;37 MG/100 ML;200 MG/100 ML   N19630 007   FEB 17, 1988

POTASSIUM CHLORIDE 0.037% IN DEXTROSE 5% AND SODIUM CHLORIDE 0.33% IN PLASTIC CONTAINER
  MCGAW   5 GM/100 ML;37 MG/100 ML;330 MG/100 ML   N19630 013   FEB 17, 1988

POTASSIUM CHLORIDE 0.037% IN DEXTROSE 5% AND SODIUM CHLORIDE 0.45% IN PLASTIC CONTAINER
  MCGAW   5 GM/100 ML;37 MG/100 ML;450 MG/100 ML   N19630 019   FEB 17, 1988

POTASSIUM CHLORIDE 0.037% IN DEXTROSE 5% AND SODIUM CHLORIDE 0.9% IN PLASTIC CONTAINER
  MCGAW   5 GM/100 ML;37 MG/100 ML;900 MG/100 ML   N19630 025   FEB 17, 1988

POTASSIUM CHLORIDE 0.075% IN DEXTROSE 10% AND SODIUM CHLORIDE 0.2% IN PLASTIC CONTAINER
  MCGAW   10 GM/100 ML;75 MG/100 ML;200 MG/100 ML   N19630 032   FEB 17, 1988

POTASSIUM CHLORIDE 0.075% IN DEXTROSE 10% AND SODIUM CHLORIDE 0.45% IN PLASTIC CONTAINER
  MCGAW   10 GM/100 ML;75 MG/100 ML;450 MG/100 ML   N19630 038   FEB 17, 1988

POTASSIUM CHLORIDE 0.075% IN DEXTROSE 10% AND SODIUM CHLORIDE 0.9% IN PLASTIC CONTAINER
  MCGAW   10 GM/100 ML;75 MG/100 ML;900 MG/100 ML   N19630 044   FEB 17, 1988

POTASSIUM CHLORIDE 0.075% IN DEXTROSE 3.3% AND SODIUM CHLORIDE 0.3% IN PLASTIC CONTAINER
  MCGAW   3.3 GM/100 ML;75 MG/100 ML;300 MG/100 ML   N19630 049   MAY 07, 1992

AP POTASSIUM CHLORIDE 0.075% IN DEXTROSE 5% AND SODIUM CHLORIDE 0.2% IN PLASTIC CONTAINER
  MCGAW   5 GM/100 ML;75 MG/100 ML;200 MG/100 ML   N19630 008   FEB 17, 1988

AP POTASSIUM CHLORIDE 0.075% IN DEXTROSE 5% AND SODIUM CHLORIDE 0.33% IN PLASTIC CONTAINER
  MCGAW   5 GM/100 ML;75 MG/100 ML;330 MG/100 ML   N19630 014   FEB 17, 1988

AP POTASSIUM CHLORIDE 0.075% IN DEXTROSE 5% AND SODIUM CHLORIDE 0.45% IN PLASTIC CONTAINER
  MCGAW   5 GM/100 ML;75 MG/100 ML;450 MG/100 ML   N19630 020   FEB 17, 1988

DEXTROSE; POTASSIUM CHLORIDE; SODIUM CHLORIDE (continued)

INJECTABLE; INJECTION

AP POTASSIUM CHLORIDE 0.075% IN DEXTROSE 5% AND SODIUM CHLORIDE 0.9% IN PLASTIC CONTAINER
  MCGAW   5 GM/100 ML;75 MG/100 ML;900 MG/100 ML   N19630 026   FEB 17, 1988

POTASSIUM CHLORIDE 0.075% IN DEXTROSE 5% AND SODIUM CHLORIDE 0.11% IN PLASTIC CONTAINER
  MCGAW   5 GM/100 ML;75 MG/100 ML;110 MG/100 ML   N19630 002   FEB 17, 1988

POTASSIUM CHLORIDE 0.11% IN DEXTROSE 10% AND SODIUM CHLORIDE 0.2% IN PLASTIC CONTAINER
  MCGAW   10 GM/100 ML;110 MG/100 ML;200 MG/100 ML   N19630 033   FEB 17, 1988

POTASSIUM CHLORIDE 0.11% IN DEXTROSE 10% AND SODIUM CHLORIDE 0.45% IN PLASTIC CONTAINER
  MCGAW   10 GM/100 ML;110 MG/100 ML;450 MG/100 ML   N19630 039   FEB 17, 1988

POTASSIUM CHLORIDE 0.11% IN DEXTROSE 10% AND SODIUM CHLORIDE 0.9% IN PLASTIC CONTAINER
  MCGAW   10 GM/100 ML;110 MG/100 ML;900 MG/100 ML   N19630 045   FEB 17, 1988

POTASSIUM CHLORIDE 0.11% IN DEXTROSE 3.3% AND SODIUM CHLORIDE 0.3% IN PLASTIC CONTAINER
  MCGAW   3.3 GM/100 ML;110 MG/100 ML;300 MG/100 ML   N19630 050   MAY 07, 1992

POTASSIUM CHLORIDE 0.11% IN DEXTROSE 5% AND SODIUM CHLORIDE 0.11% IN PLASTIC CONTAINER
  MCGAW   5 GM/100 ML;110 MG/100 ML;110 MG/100 ML   N19630 003   FEB 17, 1988

POTASSIUM CHLORIDE 0.11% IN DEXTROSE 5% AND SODIUM CHLORIDE 0.2% IN PLASTIC CONTAINER
  MCGAW   5 GM/100 ML;110 MG/100 ML;200 MG/100 ML   N19630 009   FEB 17, 1988

POTASSIUM CHLORIDE 0.11% IN DEXTROSE 5% AND SODIUM CHLORIDE 0.33% IN PLASTIC CONTAINER
  MCGAW   5 GM/100 ML;110 MG/100 ML;330 MG/100 ML   N19630 015   FEB 17, 1988

POTASSIUM CHLORIDE 0.11% IN DEXTROSE 5% AND SODIUM CHLORIDE 0.45% IN PLASTIC CONTAINER
  MCGAW   5 GM/100 ML;110 MG/100 ML;450 MG/100 ML   N19630 021   FEB 17, 1988

POTASSIUM CHLORIDE 0.11% IN DEXTROSE 5% AND SODIUM CHLORIDE 0.9% IN PLASTIC CONTAINER
  MCGAW   5 GM/100 ML;110 MG/100 ML;900 MG/100 ML   N19630 027   FEB 17, 1988

Prescription Drug Products (continued)

DEXTROSE; POTASSIUM CHLORIDE; SODIUM CHLORIDE (continued)

INJECTABLE; INJECTION

POTASSIUM CHLORIDE 0.15% IN DEXTROSE 10% AND SODIUM CHLORIDE 0.2% IN PLASTIC CONTAINER
MCGAW   10 GM/100 ML;150 MG/ 100 ML;200 MG/100 ML   N19630 034   FEB 17, 1988

POTASSIUM CHLORIDE 0.15% IN DEXTROSE 10% AND SODIUM CHLORIDE 0.45% IN PLASTIC CONTAINER
MCGAW   10 GM/100 ML;150 MG/ 100 ML;450 MG/100 ML   N19630 040   FEB 17, 1988

POTASSIUM CHLORIDE 0.15% IN DEXTROSE 10% AND SODIUM CHLORIDE 0.9% IN PLASTIC CONTAINER
MCGAW   10 GM/100 ML;150 MG/ 100 ML;900 MG/100 ML   N19630 046   FEB 17, 1988

POTASSIUM CHLORIDE 0.15% IN DEXTROSE 3.3% AND SODIUM CHLORIDE 0.3% IN PLASTIC CONTAINER
MCGAW   3.3 GM/100 ML;150 MG/ 100 ML;300 MG/100 ML   N19630 051   MAY 07, 1992

AP   POTASSIUM CHLORIDE 0.15% IN DEXTROSE 5% AND SODIUM CHLORIDE 0.2% IN PLASTIC CONTAINER
MCGAW   5 GM/100 ML;150 MG/ 100 ML;200 MG/100 ML   N19630 010   FEB 17, 1988

AP   POTASSIUM CHLORIDE 0.15% IN DEXTROSE 5% AND SODIUM CHLORIDE 0.33% IN PLASTIC CONTAINER
MCGAW   5 GM/100 ML;150 MG/ 100 ML;330 MG/100 ML   N19630 016   FEB 17, 1988

AP   POTASSIUM CHLORIDE 0.15% IN DEXTROSE 5% AND SODIUM CHLORIDE 0.45% IN PLASTIC CONTAINER
MCGAW   5 GM/100 ML;150 MG/ 100 ML;450 MG/100 ML   N19630 022   FEB 17, 1988

AP   POTASSIUM CHLORIDE 0.15% IN DEXTROSE 5% AND SODIUM CHLORIDE 0.9% IN PLASTIC CONTAINER
MCGAW   5 GM/100 ML;150 MG/ 100 ML;900 MG/100 ML   N19630 028   FEB 17, 1988

AP   POTASSIUM CHLORIDE 0.15% IN DEXTROSE 5% AND SODIUM CHLORIDE 0.11% IN PLASTIC CONTAINER
MCGAW   5 GM/100 ML;150 MG/ 100 ML;110 MG/100 ML   N19630 004   FEB 17, 1988

POTASSIUM CHLORIDE 0.22% IN DEXTROSE 10% AND SODIUM CHLORIDE 0.2% IN PLASTIC CONTAINER
MCGAW   10 GM/100 ML;220 MG/ 100 ML;200 MG/100 ML   N19630 035   FEB 17, 1988

POTASSIUM CHLORIDE 0.22% IN DEXTROSE 10% AND SODIUM CHLORIDE 0.45% IN PLASTIC CONTAINER
MCGAW   10 GM/100 ML;220 MG/ 100 ML;450 MG/100 ML   N19630 041   FEB 17, 1988

DEXTROSE; POTASSIUM CHLORIDE; SODIUM CHLORIDE (continued)

INJECTABLE; INJECTION

POTASSIUM CHLORIDE 0.22% IN DEXTROSE 10% AND SODIUM CHLORIDE 0.9% IN PLASTIC CONTAINER
MCGAW   10 GM/100 ML;220 MG/ 100 ML;900 MG/100 ML   N19630 047   FEB 17, 1988

POTASSIUM CHLORIDE 0.22% IN DEXTROSE 3.3% AND SODIUM CHLORIDE 0.3% IN PLASTIC CONTAINER
MCGAW   3.3 GM/100 ML;220 MG/ 100 ML;300 MG/100 ML   N19630 052   MAY 07, 1992

POTASSIUM CHLORIDE 0.22% IN DEXTROSE 5% AND SODIUM CHLORIDE 0.2% IN PLASTIC CONTAINER
MCGAW   5 GM/100 ML;220 MG/ 100 ML;200 MG/100 ML   N19630 011   FEB 17, 1988

POTASSIUM CHLORIDE 0.22% IN DEXTROSE 5% AND SODIUM CHLORIDE 0.33% IN PLASTIC CONTAINER
MCGAW   5 GM/100 ML;220 MG/ 100 ML;330 MG/100 ML   N19630 017   FEB 17, 1988

POTASSIUM CHLORIDE 0.22% IN DEXTROSE 5% AND SODIUM CHLORIDE 0.45% IN PLASTIC CONTAINER
MCGAW   5 GM/100 ML;220 MG/ 100 ML;450 MG/100 ML   N19630 023   FEB 17, 1988

POTASSIUM CHLORIDE 0.22% IN DEXTROSE 5% AND SODIUM CHLORIDE 0.11% IN PLASTIC CONTAINER
MCGAW   5 GM/100 ML;220 MG/ 100 ML;110 MG/100 ML   N19630 005   FEB 17, 1988

POTASSIUM CHLORIDE 0.22% IN DEXTROSE 5% AND SODIUM CHLORIDE 0.9% IN PLASTIC CONTAINER
MCGAW   5 GM/100 ML;220 MG/ 100 ML;900 MG/100 ML   N19630 029   FEB 17, 1988

POTASSIUM CHLORIDE 0.3% IN DEXTROSE 10% AND SODIUM CHLORIDE 0.2% IN PLASTIC CONTAINER
MCGAW   10 GM/100 ML;300 MG/ 100 ML;200 MG/100 ML   N19630 036   FEB 17, 1988

POTASSIUM CHLORIDE 0.3% IN DEXTROSE 10% AND SODIUM CHLORIDE 0.45% IN PLASTIC CONTAINER
MCGAW   10 GM/100 ML;300 MG/ 100 ML;450 MG/100 ML   N19630 042   FEB 17, 1988

POTASSIUM CHLORIDE 0.3% IN DEXTROSE 10% AND SODIUM CHLORIDE 0.9% IN PLASTIC CONTAINER
MCGAW   10 GM/100 ML;300 MG/ 100 ML;900 MG/100 ML   N19630 048   FEB 17, 1988

Prescription Drug Products (continued)

DEXTROSE; POTASSIUM CHLORIDE; SODIUM CHLORIDE (continued)

INJECTABLE; INJECTION

POTASSIUM CHLORIDE 0.3% IN DEXTROSE 3.3% AND SODIUM CHLORIDE 0.3% IN PLASTIC CONTAINER
MCGAW   3.3 GM/100 ML;300 MG/100 ML;300 MG/100 ML   N19630 053   MAY 07, 1992

POTASSIUM CHLORIDE 0.3% IN DEXTROSE 5% AND SODIUM CHLORIDE 0.2% IN PLASTIC CONTAINER
AP   MCGAW   5 GM/100 ML;300 MG/100 ML;200 MG/100 ML   N19630 012   FEB 17, 1988

POTASSIUM CHLORIDE 0.3% IN DEXTROSE 5% AND SODIUM CHLORIDE 0.33% IN PLASTIC CONTAINER
AP   MCGAW   5 GM/100 ML;300 MG/100 ML;330 MG/100 ML   N19630 018   FEB 17, 1988

POTASSIUM CHLORIDE 0.3% IN DEXTROSE 5% AND SODIUM CHLORIDE 0.45% IN PLASTIC CONTAINER
AP   MCGAW   5 GM/100 ML;300 MG/100 ML;450 MG/100 ML   N19630 024   FEB 17, 1988

POTASSIUM CHLORIDE 0.3% IN DEXTROSE 5% AND SODIUM CHLORIDE 0.9% IN PLASTIC CONTAINER
AP   MCGAW   5 GM/100 ML;300 MG/100 ML;900 MG/100 ML   N19630 030   FEB 17, 1988

POTASSIUM CHLORIDE 0.3% IN DEXTROSE 5% AND SODIUM CHLORIDE 0.11% IN PLASTIC CONTAINER
MCGAW   5 GM/100 ML;300 MG/100 ML;110 MG/100 ML   N19630 006   FEB 17, 1988

POTASSIUM CHLORIDE 10 MEQ IN DEXTROSE 5% AND SODIUM CHLORIDE 0.225% IN PLASTIC CONTAINER
ABBOTT   5 GM/100 ML;74.5 MG/100 ML;225 MG/100 ML   N18365 002   JUL 05, 1983
   5 GM/100 ML;149 MG/100 ML;225 MG/100 ML   N18365 006   MAR 28, 1988

POTASSIUM CHLORIDE 10 MEQ IN DEXTROSE 5% AND SODIUM CHLORIDE 0.3% IN PLASTIC CONTAINER
ABBOTT   5 GM/100 ML;74.5 MG/100 ML;300 MG/100 ML   N18876 001   JAN 17, 1986
   5 GM/100 ML;149 MG/100 ML;300 MG/100 ML   N18876 006   MAR 28, 1988

POTASSIUM CHLORIDE 10 MEQ IN DEXTROSE 5% AND SODIUM CHLORIDE 0.45% IN PLASTIC CONTAINER
AP   ABBOTT   5 GM/100 ML;74.5 MG/100 ML;450 MG/100 ML   N18362 005   MAR 28, 1988
AP   5 GM/100 ML;74.5 MG/100 ML;450 MG/100 ML   N18362 009   JUL 05, 1983

DEXTROSE; POTASSIUM CHLORIDE; SODIUM CHLORIDE (continued)

INJECTABLE; INJECTION

POTASSIUM CHLORIDE 10 MEQ IN DEXTROSE 5% AND SODIUM CHLORIDE 0.9% IN PLASTIC CONTAINER
AP   ABBOTT   5 GM/100 ML;74.5 MG/100 ML;900 MG/100 ML   N19691 002   MAR 24, 1988
AP   5 GM/100 ML;149 MG/100 ML;900 MG/100 ML   N19691 004   MAR 24, 1988

POTASSIUM CHLORIDE 10 MEQ IN DEXTROSE 5% AND SODIUM CHLORIDE 0.45% IN PLASTIC CONTAINER
BAXTER   5 GM/100 ML;75 MG/100 ML;450 MG/100 ML   N18008 005   APR 28, 1982
AP   5 GM/100 ML;150 MG/100 ML;450 MG/100 ML   N18008 006   APR 28, 1982

POTASSIUM CHLORIDE 10 MEQ IN DEXTROSE 5% AND SODIUM CHLORIDE 0.9% IN PLASTIC CONTAINER
BAXTER   5 GM/100 ML;75 MG/100 ML;900 MG/100 ML   N19308 004   APR 05, 1985
AP   5 GM/100 ML;150 MG/100 ML;900 MG/100 ML   N19308 002   APR 05, 1985

POTASSIUM CHLORIDE 15 MEQ IN DEXTROSE 5% AND SODIUM CHLORIDE 0.225% IN PLASTIC CONTAINER
ABBOTT   5 GM/100 ML;224 MG/100 ML;225 MG/100 ML   N18365 008   MAR 28, 1988

POTASSIUM CHLORIDE 15 MEQ IN DEXTROSE 5% AND SODIUM CHLORIDE 0.3% IN PLASTIC CONTAINER
ABBOTT   5 GM/100 ML;224 MG/100 ML;300 MG/100 ML   N18876 007   MAR 28, 1988

POTASSIUM CHLORIDE 15 MEQ IN DEXTROSE 5% AND SODIUM CHLORIDE 0.45% IN PLASTIC CONTAINER
AP   ABBOTT   5 GM/100 ML;224 MG/100 ML;450 MG/100 ML   N18362 006   MAR 28, 1988

POTASSIUM CHLORIDE 15 MEQ IN DEXTROSE 5% AND SODIUM CHLORIDE 0.9% IN PLASTIC CONTAINER
AP   ABBOTT   5 GM/100 ML;224 MG/100 ML;900 MG/100 ML   N19691 006   MAR 24, 1988

POTASSIUM CHLORIDE 20 MEQ IN DEXTROSE 5% AND SODIUM CHLORIDE 0.225% IN PLASTIC CONTAINER
ABBOTT   5 GM/100 ML;149 MG/100 ML;225 MG/100 ML   N18365 001
   5 GM/100 ML;298 MG/100 ML;225 MG/100 ML   N18365 009   MAR 28, 1988

POTASSIUM CHLORIDE 20 MEQ IN DEXTROSE 5% AND SODIUM CHLORIDE 0.3% IN PLASTIC CONTAINER
ABBOTT   5 GM/100 ML;298 MG/100 ML;300 MG/100 ML   N18876 008   MAR 28, 1988

Prescription Drug Products (continued)

DEXTROSE; POTASSIUM CHLORIDE; SODIUM CHLORIDE (continued)

INJECTABLE; INJECTION

POTASSIUM CHLORIDE 20 MEQ IN DEXTROSE 5% AND SODIUM CHLORIDE 0.45% IN PLASTIC CONTAINER
ΔP ABBOTT   5 GM/100 ML;149 MG/100 ML;450 MG/100 ML   N18362 010   JUL 05, 1983
ΔP   5 GM/100 ML;298 MG/100 ML;450 MG/100 ML   N18362 007   MAR 28, 1988

POTASSIUM CHLORIDE 20 MEQ IN DEXTROSE 5% AND SODIUM CHLORIDE 0.9% IN PLASTIC CONTAINER
ΔP ABBOTT   5 GM/100 ML;149 MG/100 ML;900 MG/100 ML   N19691 005   MAR 24, 1988
ΔP   5 GM/100 ML;298 MG/100 ML;900 MG/100 ML   N19691 008   MAR 24, 1988

POTASSIUM CHLORIDE 20 MEQ IN DEXTROSE 5% AND SODIUM CHLORIDE 0.45% IN PLASTIC CONTAINER
ΔP BAXTER   5 GM/100 ML;150 MG/100 ML;450 MG/100 ML   N18008 007   APR 28, 1982

POTASSIUM CHLORIDE 20 MEQ IN DEXTROSE 5% AND SODIUM CHLORIDE 0.9% IN PLASTIC CONTAINER
ΔP BAXTER   5 GM/100 ML;150 MG/100 ML;900 MG/100 ML   N19308 005   APR 05, 1985
ΔP   5 GM/100 ML;300 MG/100 ML;900 MG/100 ML   N19308 003   APR 05, 1985

POTASSIUM CHLORIDE 20 MEQ IN DEXTROSE 5% IN SODIUM CHLORIDE 0.3% IN PLASTIC CONTAINER
    ABBOTT   5 GM/100 ML;149 MG/100 ML;300 MG/100 ML   N18876 002   JAN 17, 1986

POTASSIUM CHLORIDE 30 MEQ IN DEXTROSE 5% AND SODIUM CHLORIDE 0.225% IN PLASTIC CONTAINER
    ABBOTT   5 GM/100 ML;224 MG/100 ML;225 MG/100 ML   N18365 003   JUL 05, 1983

POTASSIUM CHLORIDE 30 MEQ IN DEXTROSE 5% AND SODIUM CHLORIDE 0.3% IN PLASTIC CONTAINER
    ABBOTT   5 GM/100 ML;224 MG/100 ML;300 MG/100 ML   N18876 003   JAN 17, 1986

POTASSIUM CHLORIDE 30 MEQ IN DEXTROSE 5% AND SODIUM CHLORIDE 0.45% IN PLASTIC CONTAINER
ΔP ABBOTT   5 GM/100 ML;224 MG/100 ML;450 MG/100 ML   N18362 002   JUL 05, 1983

POTASSIUM CHLORIDE 30 MEQ IN DEXTROSE 5% AND SODIUM CHLORIDE 0.9% IN PLASTIC CONTAINER
ΔP ABBOTT   5 GM/100 ML;224 MG/100 ML;900 MG/100 ML   N19691 007   MAR 24, 1988

DEXTROSE; POTASSIUM CHLORIDE; SODIUM CHLORIDE (continued)

INJECTABLE; INJECTION

POTASSIUM CHLORIDE 30 MEQ IN DEXTROSE 5% AND SODIUM CHLORIDE 0.45% IN PLASTIC CONTAINER
    BAXTER   5 GM/100 ML;224 MG/100 ML;450 MG/100 ML   N18008 008   APR 28, 1982

POTASSIUM CHLORIDE 30 MEQ IN DEXTROSE 5% AND SODIUM CHLORIDE 0.9% IN PLASTIC CONTAINER
ΔP BAXTER   5 GM/100 ML;224 MG/100 ML;900 MG/100 ML   N19308 006   APR 05, 1985

POTASSIUM CHLORIDE 40 MEQ IN DEXTROSE 5% AND SODIUM CHLORIDE 0.225% IN PLASTIC CONTAINER
    ABBOTT   5 GM/100 ML;298 MG/100 ML;225 MG/100 ML   N18365 004   JUL 05, 1983

POTASSIUM CHLORIDE 40 MEQ IN DEXTROSE 5% AND SODIUM CHLORIDE 0.3% IN PLASTIC CONTAINER
    ABBOTT   5 GM/100 ML;298 MG/100 ML;300 MG/100 ML   N18876 004   MAR 28, 1988

POTASSIUM CHLORIDE 40 MEQ IN DEXTROSE 5% AND SODIUM CHLORIDE 0.45% IN PLASTIC CONTAINER
ΔP ABBOTT   5 GM/100 ML;298 MG/100 ML;450 MG/100 ML   N18362 003

POTASSIUM CHLORIDE 40 MEQ IN DEXTROSE 5% AND SODIUM CHLORIDE 0.9% IN PLASTIC CONTAINER
ΔP ABBOTT   5 GM/100 ML;298 MG/100 ML;900 MG/100 ML   N19691 009   MAR 24, 1988

POTASSIUM CHLORIDE 40 MEQ IN DEXTROSE 5% AND SODIUM CHLORIDE 0.45% IN PLASTIC CONTAINER
ΔP BAXTER   5 GM/100 ML;300 MG/100 ML;450 MG/100 ML   N18008 009   APR 28, 1982

POTASSIUM CHLORIDE 40 MEQ IN DEXTROSE 5% AND SODIUM CHLORIDE 0.9% IN PLASTIC CONTAINER
ΔP BAXTER   5 GM/100 ML;300 MG/100 ML;900 MG/100 ML   N19308 007   APR 05, 1985

POTASSIUM CHLORIDE 5 MEQ IN DEXTROSE 5% AND SODIUM CHLORIDE 0.225% IN PLASTIC CONTAINER
    ABBOTT   5 GM/100 ML;74.5 MG/100 ML;225 MG/100 ML   N18365 005   MAR 28, 1988
              5 GM/100 ML;149 MG/100 ML;225 MG/100 ML   N18365 007   MAR 28, 1988

POTASSIUM CHLORIDE 5 MEQ IN DEXTROSE 5% AND SODIUM CHLORIDE 0.3% IN PLASTIC CONTAINER
    ABBOTT   5 GM/100 ML;74.5 MG/100 ML;300 MG/100 ML   N18876 005   MAR 28, 1988
              5 GM/100 ML;149 MG/100 ML;300 MG/100 ML   N18876 009   MAR 28, 1988

Prescription Drug Products *(continued)*

DEXTROSE; POTASSIUM CHLORIDE; SODIUM CHLORIDE *(continued)*

INJECTABLE; INJECTION

POTASSIUM CHLORIDE 5 MEQ IN DEXTROSE 5% AND SODIUM CHLORIDE 0.45% IN PLASTIC CONTAINER

	Firm	Strength	Appl. No.	Date
AP	ABBOTT	5 GM/100 ML;74.5 MG/100 ML;450 MG/100 ML	N18362 008	MAR 28, 1988
AP		5 GM/100 ML;149 MG/100 ML;450 MG/100 ML	N18362 004	MAR 28, 1988

POTASSIUM CHLORIDE 5 MEQ IN DEXTROSE 5% AND SODIUM CHLORIDE 0.9% IN PLASTIC CONTAINER

	Firm	Strength	Appl. No.	Date
AP	ABBOTT	5 GM/100 ML;74.5 MG/100 ML;900 MG/100 ML	N19691 001	MAR 24, 1988
AP		5 GM/100 ML;149 MG/100 ML;900 MG/100 ML	N19691 003	MAR 24, 1988

POTASSIUM CHLORIDE 5 MEQ IN DEXTROSE 5% AND SODIUM CHLORIDE 0.45% IN PLASTIC CONTAINER

	Firm	Strength	Appl. No.	Date
AP	BAXTER	5 GM/100 ML;150 MG/100 ML;450 MG/100 ML	N18008 004	

POTASSIUM CHLORIDE 5 MEQ IN DEXTROSE 5% AND SODIUM CHLORIDE 0.9% IN PLASTIC CONTAINER

	Firm	Strength	Appl. No.	Date
AP	BAXTER	5 GM/100 ML;150 MG/100 ML;900 MG/100 ML	N19308 001	APR 05, 1985

DEXTROSE; SODIUM CHLORIDE

INJECTABLE; INJECTION

DEXTROSE 10% AND SODIUM CHLORIDE 0.11% IN PLASTIC CONTAINER

Firm	Strength	Appl. No.	Date
MCGAW	10 GM/100 ML;110 MG/100 ML	N19631 011	FEB 24, 1988

DEXTROSE 10% AND SODIUM CHLORIDE 0.2% IN PLASTIC CONTAINER

Firm	Strength	Appl. No.	Date
MCGAW	10 GM/100 ML;200 MG/100 ML	N18386 001	
	10 GM/100 ML;200 MG/100 ML	N19631 012	FEB 24, 1988

DEXTROSE 10% AND SODIUM CHLORIDE 0.33% IN PLASTIC CONTAINER

Firm	Strength	Appl. No.	Date
MCGAW	10 GM/100 ML;330 MG/100 ML	N19631 013	FEB 24, 1988

DEXTROSE 10% AND SODIUM CHLORIDE 0.45% IN PLASTIC CONTAINER

Firm	Strength	Appl. No.	Date
MCGAW	10 GM/100 ML;450 MG/100 ML	N18229 001	
	10 GM/100 ML;450 MG/100 ML	N19631 014	FEB 24, 1988

DEXTROSE; SODIUM CHLORIDE *(continued)*

INJECTABLE; INJECTION

DEXTROSE 10% AND SODIUM CHLORIDE 0.9% IN PLASTIC CONTAINER

	Firm	Strength	Appl. No.	Date
AP	BAXTER	10 GM/100 ML;900 MG/100 ML	N16696 001	
AP	MCGAW	10 GM/100 ML;900 MG/100 ML	N18047 001	
AP		10 GM/100 ML;900 MG/100 ML	N19631 015	FEB 24, 1988

DEXTROSE 2.5% AND SODIUM CHLORIDE 0.11% IN PLASTIC CONTAINER

	Firm	Strength	Appl. No.	Date
AP	MCGAW	2.5 GM/100 ML;110 MG/100 ML	N19631 001	FEB 24, 1988

DEXTROSE 2.5% AND SODIUM CHLORIDE 0.2% IN PLASTIC CONTAINER

	Firm	Strength	Appl. No.	Date
AP	MCGAW	2.5 GM/100 ML;200 MG/100 ML	N19631 002	FEB 24, 1988

DEXTROSE 2.5% AND SODIUM CHLORIDE 0.33% IN PLASTIC CONTAINER

	Firm	Strength	Appl. No.	Date
AP	MCGAW	2.5 GM/100 ML;330 MG/100 ML	N19631 003	FEB 24, 1988

DEXTROSE 2.5% AND SODIUM CHLORIDE 0.45% IN PLASTIC CONTAINER

	Firm	Strength	Appl. No.	Date
AP	ABBOTT	2.5 GM/100 ML;450 MG/100 ML	N18096 001	
AP	BAXTER	2.5 GM/100 ML;450 MG/100 ML	N16697 001	
AP	MCGAW	2.5 GM/100 ML;450 MG/100 ML	N18030 001	
AP		2.5 GM/100 ML;450 MG/100 ML	N19631 004	FEB 24, 1988

DEXTROSE 2.5% AND SODIUM CHLORIDE 0.9% IN PLASTIC CONTAINER

	Firm	Strength	Appl. No.	Date
AP	MCGAW	2.5 GM/100 ML;900 MG/100 ML	N18376 001	
		2.5 GM/100 ML;900 MG/100 ML	N19631 005	FEB 24, 1988

DEXTROSE 3.3% AND SODIUM CHLORIDE 0.3% IN PLASTIC CONTAINER

Firm	Strength	Appl. No.	Date
MCGAW	3.3 GM/100 ML;300 MG/100 ML	N19631 016	JAN 19, 1990

DEXTROSE 5% AND SODIUM CHLORIDE 0.11% IN PLASTIC CONTAINER

Firm	Strength	Appl. No.	Date
MCGAW	5 GM/100 ML;110 MG/100 ML	N18030 005	
	5 GM/100 ML;110 MG/100 ML	N19631 006	FEB 24, 1988

DEXTROSE 5% AND SODIUM CHLORIDE 0.2% IN PLASTIC CONTAINER

	Firm	Strength	Appl. No.	Date
AP	MCGAW	5 GM/100 ML;200 MG/100 ML	N18030 004	
AP		5 GM/100 ML;200 MG/100 ML	N19631 007	FEB 24, 1988

Prescription Drug Products (continued)

DEXTROSE; SODIUM CHLORIDE (continued)

INJECTABLE; INJECTION

DEXTROSE 5% AND SODIUM CHLORIDE 0.225% IN PLASTIC CONTAINER

	ABBOTT	5 GM/100 ML;225 MG/100 ML	N17606 001	

DEXTROSE 5% AND SODIUM CHLORIDE 0.3% IN PLASTIC CONTAINER

	ABBOTT	5 GM/100 ML;300 MG/100 ML	N17799 001	

DEXTROSE 5% AND SODIUM CHLORIDE 0.33% IN PLASTIC CONTAINER

AP	MCGAW	5 GM/100 ML;330 MG/100 ML	N18030 003	
AP	MCGAW	5 GM/100 ML;330 MG/100 ML	N19631 008	FEB 24, 1988

DEXTROSE 5% AND SODIUM CHLORIDE 0.45% IN PLASTIC CONTAINER

AP	ABBOTT	5 GM/100 ML;450 MG/100 ML	N17607 001	
AP	MCGAW	5 GM/100 ML;450 MG/100 ML	N18030 002	
AP		5 GM/100 ML;450 MG/100 ML	N19631 009	FEB 24, 1988

DEXTROSE 5% AND SODIUM CHLORIDE 0.9% IN PLASTIC CONTAINER

AP	ABBOTT	5 GM/100 ML;900 MG/100 ML	N17585 001	
AP	MCGAW	5 GM/100 ML;900 MG/100 ML	N18026 001	
AP		5 GM/100 ML;900 MG/100 ML	N19631 010	FEB 24, 1988

DEXTROSE 5% IN SODIUM CHLORIDE 0.2% IN PLASTIC CONTAINER

AP	BAXTER	5 GM/100 ML;200 MG/100 ML	N16689 001	

DEXTROSE 5% IN SODIUM CHLORIDE 0.33% IN PLASTIC CONTAINER

AP	BAXTER	5 GM/100 ML;330 MG/100 ML	N16687 001	

DEXTROSE 5% IN SODIUM CHLORIDE 0.45% IN PLASTIC CONTAINER

AP	BAXTER	5 GM/100 ML;450 MG/100 ML	N16683 001	

DEXTROSE 5% IN SODIUM CHLORIDE 0.9% IN PLASTIC CONTAINER

AP	BAXTER	5 GM/100 ML;900 MG/100 ML	N16678 001	

DEXTROTHYROXINE SODIUM

TABLET; ORAL

CHOLOXIN

	BOOTS	1 MG	N12302 005
		2 MG	N12302 002
		4 MG	N12302 004
		6 MG	N12302 006

+

DEZOCINE

INJECTABLE; INJECTION

DALGAN

	ASTRA	5 MG/ML	N19082 001	DEC 29, 1989
		10 MG/ML	N19082 002	DEC 29, 1989
		15 MG/ML	N19082 003	DEC 29, 1989

DIATRIZOATE MEGLUMINE

INJECTABLE; INJECTION

ANGIOVIST 282

AP	BERLEX	60%	N87726 001	SEP 23, 1982

DIATRIZOATE MEGLUMINE

	SQUIBB	76%	N10040 017

HYPAQUE

AP	STERLING	30%	N16403 002
AP		60%	N16403 001

RENO-M-DIP

AP	SQUIBB	30%	N10040 012

RENO-M-60

AP	SQUIBB	60%	N10040 016

UROVIST MEGLUMINE DIU/CT

AP	BERLEX	30%	N87739 001	SEP 23, 1982

SOLUTION; URETERAL

RENO-M-30

AT	SQUIBB	30%	N10040 021

UROVIST CYSTO

AT	BERLEX	30%	N87729 001	SEP 23, 1982

UROVIST CYSTO PEDIATRIC

AT	BERLEX	30%	N87731 001	SEP 23, 1982

SOLUTION; URETHRAL

CYSTOGRAFIN

AT	SQUIBB	30%	N10040 018

CYSTOGRAFIN DILUTE

	SQUIBB	18%	N10040 022	NOV 09, 1982

HYPAQUE-CYSTO

AT	STERLING	30%	N16403 003

Prescription Drug Products (continued)

DIATRIZOATE MEGLUMINE; DIATRIZOATE SODIUM

INJECTABLE; INJECTION

TE	Applicant	Strength	Appl No	Approval
	ANGIOVIST 292			
AP	BERLEX	52%;8%	N87724 001	SEP 23, 1982
	ANGIOVIST 370			
AP	BERLEX	66%;10%	N87723 001	SEP 23, 1982
	HYPAQUE-M,75%			
	STERLING	50%;25%	N10220 003	
	HYPAQUE-M,90%			
	STERLING	60%;30%	N10220 002	
	HYPAQUE-76			
AP	STERLING	66%;10%	N86505 001	
	MD-60			
AP	MALLINCKRODT	52%;8%	N87074 001	
	MD-76			
AP	MALLINCKRODT	66%;10%	N19292 001	SEP 29, 1989
AP		66%;10%	N87073 001	
	RENOCAL-76			
AP	SQUIBB	66%;10%	N89347 001	JUN 01, 1988
	RENOGRAFIN-60			
AP	SQUIBB	52%;8%	N10040 006	
	RENOGRAFIN-76			
AP	SQUIBB	66%;10%	N10040 001	
	RENOVIST			
	SQUIBB	34.3%;35%	N10040 020	
	RENOVIST II			
	SQUIBB	28.5%;29.1%	N10040 019	

SOLUTION; ORAL, RECTAL

TE	Applicant	Strength	Appl No	Approval
	GASTROGRAFIN			
AA	SQUIBB	66%;10%	N11245 003	
	GASTROVIST			
AA	BERLEX	66%;10%	N87728 001	SEP 23, 1982
	MD-GASTROVIEW			
AA	MALLINCKRODT	66%;10%	N87388 001	

DIATRIZOATE MEGLUMINE; IODIPAMIDE MEGLUMINE

SOLUTION; INTRAUTERINE

TE	Applicant	Strength	Appl No	Approval
	SINOGRAFIN			
	SQUIBB	52.7%;26.8%	N11324 002	

DIATRIZOATE SODIUM

INJECTABLE; INJECTION

TE	Applicant	Strength	Appl No	Approval
	HYPAQUE			
AP	STERLING	50%	N09561 001	
		25%	N09561 003	
	UROVIST SODIUM 300			
AP	BERLEX	50%	N87725 001	SEP 23, 1982

DIATRIZOATE SODIUM (continued)

POWDER FOR RECONSTITUTION; ORAL, RECTAL

TE	Applicant	Strength	Appl No	Approval
	HYPAQUE			
	STERLING	100%	N11386 001	

SOLUTION; ORAL, RECTAL

TE	Applicant	Strength	Appl No	Approval
	HYPAQUE			
	STERLING	40%	N11386 003	

SOLUTION; URETERAL

TE	Applicant	Strength	Appl No	Approval
	HYPAQUE SODIUM 20%			
	STERLING	20%	N09561 002	

DIATRIZOATE SODIUM; *MULTIPLE*

SEE DIATRIZOATE MEGLUMINE; DIATRIZOATE SODIUM

DIAZEPAM

CAPSULE, EXTENDED RELEASE; ORAL

TE	Applicant	Strength	Appl No	Approval
	VALRELEASE			
+	ROCHE	15 MG	N18179 001	

CONCENTRATE; ORAL

TE	Applicant	Strength	Appl No	Approval
	DIAZEPAM INTENSOL			
	ROXANE	5 MG/ML	N71415 001	APR 03, 1987

INJECTABLE; INJECTION

TE	Applicant	Strength	Appl No	Approval
	DIAZEPAM			
AP	ABBOTT	5 MG/ML	N71583 001	OCT 13, 1987
AP		5 MG/ML	N71584 001	OCT 13, 1987
AP		5 MG/ML	N70311 001	
AP	ELKINS SINN	5 MG/ML	N70312 001	DEC 16, 1985
AP		5 MG/ML	N70313 001	DEC 16, 1985
AP	LEDERLE	5 MG/ML	N71308 001	DEC 16, 1985
AP		5 MG/ML	N71309 001	JUL 17, 1987
AP		5 MG/ML	N71310 001	JUL 17, 1987
AP	LYPHOMED	5 MG/ML	N70662 001	JUL 17, 1987
AP	STERIS	5 MG/ML	N70296 001	JUN 25, 1986
AP		5 MG/ML	N70911 001	FEB 12, 1986
AP		5 MG/ML	N70912 001	AUG 28, 1986
AP	STERLING	5 MG/ML	N70930 001	AUG 28, 1986
AP		5 MG/ML	N72079 001	DEC 01, 1986
				DEC 20, 1988
	VALIUM			
AP	ROCHE	5 MG/ML	N16087 001	

Prescription Drug Products (continued)

DIAZEPAM (continued)

SOLUTION; ORAL

		Strength	Appl. No.	Date
DIAZEPAM				
ROXANE		5 MG/5 ML	N70928 001	APR 03, 1987

TABLET; ORAL

		Strength	Appl. No.	Date
DIAZEPAM				
BARR				
AB		2 MG	N70152 001	NOV 01, 1985
AB		5 MG	N70153 001	NOV 01, 1985
AB		10 MG	N70154 001	NOV 01, 1985
DANBURY				
AB		2 MG	N71134 001	FEB 03, 1987
AB		5 MG	N71135 001	FEB 03, 1987
AB		10 MG	N71136 001	FEB 03, 1987
GENEVA				
AB		2 MG	N70302 001	DEC 20, 1985
AB		5 MG	N70303 001	DEC 20, 1985
AB		10 MG	N70304 001	DEC 20, 1985
HALSEY				
AB		2 MG	N70987 001	AUG 15, 1986
AB		5 MG	N70996 001	AUG 15, 1986
AB		10 MG	N70956 001	AUG 15, 1986
LEDERLE				
AB		2 MG	N70226 001	SEP 26, 1985
AB		5 MG	N70227 001	SEP 26, 1985
AB		10 MG	N70228 001	SEP 26, 1985
MYLAN				
AB		2 MG	N70323 001	SEP 04, 1985
AB		5 MG	N70324 001	SEP 04, 1985
AB		10 MG	N70325 001	SEP 04, 1985
PAR				
AB		2 MG	N70462 001	FEB 25, 1986
AB		5 MG	N70463 001	FEB 25, 1986
AB		10 MG	N70464 001	FEB 25, 1986
PHARM BASICS				
AB		2 MG	N70903 001	APR 01, 1987
AB		5 MG	N70904 001	APR 01, 1987
AB		10 MG	N70905 001	APR 01, 1987

DIAZEPAM (continued)

TABLET; ORAL

		Strength	Appl. No.	Date
DIAZEPAM				
PUREPAC				
AB		2 MG	N70781 001	MAR 19, 1986
AB		5 MG	N70706 001	MAR 19, 1986
AB		10 MG	N70707 001	MAR 19, 1986
ROXANE				
AB		2 MG	N70356 001	JUN 17, 1986
AB		5 MG	N70357 001	JUN 17, 1986
AB		10 MG	N70358 001	JUN 17, 1986
ZENITH				
AB		2 MG	N70360 001	SEP 04, 1985
AB		2 MG	N71307 001	DEC 10, 1986
AB		5 MG	N70361 001	SEP 04, 1985
AB		5 MG	N71321 001	DEC 10, 1986
AB		10 MG	N70362 001	SEP 04, 1985
AB		10 MG	N71322 001	DEC 10, 1986
VALIUM				
ROCHE				
AB		2 MG	N13263 002	
AB		5 MG	N13263 004	
AB		10 MG	N13263 006 +	

DIAZOXIDE

CAPSULE; ORAL

		Strength	Appl. No.	Date
PROGLYCEM				
+ MEDCL MKTG				
AP		50 MG	N17425 001	

INJECTABLE; INJECTION

		Strength	Appl. No.	Date
DIAZOXIDE				
LYPHOMED				
AP		15 MG/ML	N71519 001	AUG 26, 1987
QUAD				
AP		15 MG/ML	N71908 001	JAN 26, 1988
HYPERSTAT				
SCHERING				
AP		15 MG/ML	N16996 001	

SUSPENSION; ORAL

		Strength	Appl. No.	Date
PROGLYCEM				
+ MEDCL MKTG				
AP		50 MG/ML	N17453 001	

Prescription Drug Products (continued)

DICHLORPHENAMIDE

TABLET; ORAL

	DARANIDE		
	+ MSD	50 MG	N11366 001

DICLOFENAC SODIUM

SOLUTION/DROPS; OPHTHALMIC

	VOLTAREN		
	CIBA	0.1%	N20037 001 MAR 28, 1991

TABLET, DELAYED RELEASE; ORAL

	VOLTAREN		
	GEIGY	25 MG	N19201 001 JUL 28, 1988
		50 MG	N19201 002 JUL 28, 1988
	+	75 MG	N19201 003 JUL 28, 1988

DICLOXACILLIN SODIUM

CAPSULE; ORAL

	DICLOXACILLIN SODIUM		
AB	BIOCRAFT	EQ 250 MG BASE	N62286 001 JUN 03, 1982
AB		EQ 500 MG BASE	N62286 002 JUN 03, 1982
	DYCILL		
AB	BEECHAM	EQ 250 MG BASE	N60254 002
AB		EQ 250 MG BASE	N62238 001
AB		EQ 500 MG BASE	N60254 003
AB		EQ 500 MG BASE	N62238 002
	DYNAPEN		
AB	BRISTOL	EQ 250 MG BASE	N61454 001
AB		EQ 125 MG BASE	N61454 002
	PATHOCIL		
AB	+ WYETH AYERST	EQ 250 MG BASE	N50011 002
AB		EQ 500 MG BASE	N50011 003 MAR 28, 1983

POWDER FOR RECONSTITUTION; ORAL

	DYNAPEN		
AB	BRISTOL	EQ 62.5 MG BASE/5 ML	N61455 001
	PATHOCIL		
AB	+ WYETH AYERST	EQ 62.5 MG BASE/5 ML	N50092 001

DICUMAROL

TABLET; ORAL

	DICUMAROL		
	ABBOTT	25 MG	N05545 003
		50 MG	N05545 004
	+		

DICYCLOMINE HYDROCHLORIDE

CAPSULE; ORAL

	BENTYL		
ΔB	+ MERRELL DOW	10 MG	N07409 003 OCT 15, 1984
	DICYCLOMINE HCL		
ΔB	BARR	10 MG	N84505 001 OCT 21, 1986
ΔB	CHELSEA	10 MG	N85082 001 JUN 19, 1986
ΔB	PIONEER PHARMS	10 MG	N89361 001 JAN 10, 1989

INJECTABLE; INJECTION

	BENTYL		
ΔP	MERRELL DOW	10 MG/ML	N08370 001 OCT 15, 1984
	DICYCLOMINE HCL		
ΔP	STERIS	10 MG/ML	N80614 001 FEB 11, 1986

SYRUP; ORAL

	BENTYL		
ΔA	MERRELL DOW	10 MG/5 ML	N07961 002 OCT 15, 1984
	DICYCLOMINE HCL		
ΔA	BARRE	10 MG/5 ML	N84479 001

TABLET; ORAL

	BENTYL		
ΔB	+ MERRELL DOW	20 MG	N07409 001 OCT 15, 1984
	DICYCLOMINE HCL		
ΔB	BARR	20 MG	N84600 001 JUL 29, 1985
ΔB	CHELSEA	20 MG	N85223 001 JUL 30, 1986
ΔB	PIONEER PHARMS	20 MG	N88585 001 AUG 20, 1986

DIDANOSINE

POWDER FOR RECONSTITUTION; ORAL

	VIDEX		
	BRISTOL MYERS SQUIBB	10 MG/ML	N20156 001 OCT 09, 1991
		100 MG/PACKET	N20155 003 OCT 09, 1991
		167 MG/PACKET	N20155 004 OCT 09, 1991
		250 MG/PACKET	N20155 005 OCT 09, 1991
	+	375 MG/PACKET	N20155 006 OCT 09, 1991

Prescription Drug Products (continued)

DIDANOSINE (continued)

TABLET, CHEWABLE; ORAL
VIDEX
BRISTOL MYERS SQUIBB

	25 MG	N20154 002	OCT 09, 1991
	50 MG	N20154 003	OCT 09, 1991
	100 MG	N20154 004	OCT 09, 1991
+	150 MG	N20154 005	OCT 09, 1991

DIENESTROL

CREAM; VAGINAL
DIENESTROL

AI	JOHNSON RW	0.01%	N06110 005
AI	MERRELL DOW ESTRAGUARD	0.01%	N83518 001
AI	SOLVAY	0.01%	N84436 001

SUPPOSITORY; VAGINAL

DV	MERRELL DOW	0.7 MG	N83517 001

DIETHYLCARBAMAZINE CITRATE

TABLET; ORAL
HETRAZAN

LEDERLE	50 MG	N06459 001

DIETHYLPROPION HYDROCHLORIDE

TABLET; ORAL
DIETHYLPROPION HCL

AA	CAMALL	25 MG	N88267 001	AUG 25, 1983
AA		25 MG	N88268 001	AUG 25, 1983
AA	MD PHARM	25 MG	N85544 001	

TENUATE

AA	MERRELL DOW	25 MG	N11722 002

TEPANIL

AA	3M	25 MG	N11673 001

TABLET, EXTENDED RELEASE; ORAL
TENUATE DOSPAN

BC	+ MERRELL DOW	75 MG	N12546 001

TEPANIL TEN-TAB

BC	3M	75 MG	N17956 001

DIETHYLSTILBESTROL

INJECTABLE; INJECTION
STILBESTROL
SQUIBB

	0.2 MG/ML	N04056 003
	0.5 MG/ML	N04056 004
	1 MG/ML	N04056 005
	5 MG/ML	N04056 006

SUPPOSITORY; VAGINAL
STILBESTROL

	+ SQUIBB	0.1 MG	N04056 001
	+	0.5 MG	N04056 002

TABLET; ORAL
DIETHYLSTILBESTROL

BP	+ LILLY	1 MG	N04041 004
BP	+	5 MG	N04041 005

STILBESTROL

BP	TABLICAPS	1 MG	N83002 001
BP		5 MG	N83006 001
		0.5 MG	N83004 001

TABLET, DELAYED RELEASE; ORAL
DIETHYLSTILBESTROL

BE	+ LILLY	1 MG	N04039 004
BE	+	5 MG	N04039 006

STILBESTROL

BE	TABLICAPS	0.5 MG	N83003 001
BE		1 MG	N83005 001
BE		5 MG	N83007 001

STILBETIN

BE	SQUIBB	0.5 MG	N04056 012
BE		1 MG	N04056 013
BE		5 MG	N04056 014
BE		0.1 MG	N04056 011

DIETHYLSTILBESTROL; METHYLTESTOSTERONE

TABLET; ORAL
TYLOSTERONE

	+ LILLY	0.25 MG;5 MG	N07661 001

DIETHYLSTILBESTROL DIPHOSPHATE

INJECTABLE; INJECTION
STILPHOSTROL

MILES	250 MG/5 ML	N10010 001

TABLET; ORAL
STILPHOSTROL

	+ MILES	50 MG	N10010 002

DIFENOXIN HYDROCHLORIDE; *MULTIPLE*

SEE ATROPINE SULFATE; DIFENOXIN HYDROCHLORIDE

Prescription Drug Products *(continued)*

DIFLORASONE DIACETATE

CREAM; TOPICAL

FLORONE			
+ UPJOHN	0.05%	N17741 001	

OINTMENT; TOPICAL

FLORONE			
+ UPJOHN	0.05%	N17994 001	
PSORCON			
+ UPJOHN	0.05%	N19260 001	AUG 28, 1985

DIFLUNISAL

TABLET; ORAL

	DIFLUNISAL			
	LEMMON			
AB		250 MG	N73679 001	JUL 31, 1992
AB		500 MG	N73673 001	JUL 31, 1992
	DOLOBID			
	MSD			
AB		250 MG	N18445 001	APR 19, 1982
AB	+	500 MG	N18445 002	APR 19, 1982

DIGOXIN

CAPSULE; ORAL

LANOXICAPS			
BURROUGHS WELLCOME			
	0.05 MG	N18118 002	JUL 26, 1982
	0.1 MG	N18118 003	JUL 26, 1982
	0.2 MG	N18118 001	JUL 26, 1982

INJECTABLE; INJECTION

	DIGOXIN		
	ELKINS SINN		
AP	0.25 MG/ML	N83391 001	
	WYETH AYERST		
AP	0.25 MG/ML	N84386 001	
	LANOXIN		
	BURROUGHS WELLCOME		
AP	0.25 MG/ML	N09330 002	
	0.1 MG/ML	N09330 004	

DIHYDROCODEINE BITARTRATE; *MULTIPLE*

SEE   ACETAMINOPHEN; CAFFEINE; DIHYDROCODEINE BITARTRATE

SEE   ASPIRIN; CAFFEINE; DIHYDROCODEINE BITARTRATE

DIHYDROERGOTAMINE MESYLATE

INJECTABLE; INJECTION

D.H.E. 45		
SANDOZ	1 MG/ML	N05929 001

DILTIAZEM HYDROCHLORIDE

CAPSULE, EXTENDED RELEASE; ORAL

	CARDIZEM CD			
	+ MARION MERRELL DOW			
		120 MG	N20062 001	AUG 10, 1992
BC	+	180 MG	N20062 002	DEC 27, 1991
BC	+	240 MG	N20062 003	DEC 27, 1991
	+	300 MG	N20062 004	DEC 27, 1991
	CARDIZEM SR			
	+ MARION MERRELL DOW			
	+	120 MG	N19471 003	JAN 23, 1989
	+	60 MG	N19471 001	JAN 23, 1989
	+	90 MG	N19471 002	JAN 23, 1989
	DILACOR XR			
	RHONE POULENC RORER			
BC		180 MG	N20092 002	MAY 29, 1992
BC		240 MG	N20092 003	MAY 29, 1992

INJECTABLE; INJECTION

CARDIZEM			
MARION MERRELL DOW			
	5 MG/ML	N20027 001	OCT 24, 1991

TABLET; ORAL

	CARDIZEM			
	MARION MERRELL DOW			
		30 MG	N18602 001	NOV 05, 1982
		60 MG	N18602 002	NOV 05, 1982
		90 MG	N18602 003	DEC 08, 1986
	+	120 MG	N18602 004	DEC 08, 1986

DIMENHYDRINATE

INJECTABLE; INJECTION

	DIMENHYDRINATE		
	ELKINS SINN		
AP		50 MG/ML	N84767 001
	STERIS		
AP		50 MG/ML	N80615 001
AP		50 MG/ML	N83531 001
	WYETH AYERST		
AP		50 MG/ML	N84316 001

Prescription Drug Products (continued)

DIMERCAPROL

INJECTABLE; INJECTION

TE	Brand / Labeler	Strength	NDC
	BAL		
	BECTON DICKINSON	10%	N05939 001

DIMETHYL SULFOXIDE

SOLUTION; INTRAVESICAL

TE	Brand / Labeler	Strength	NDC
	RIMSO-50		
	RES INDS	50%	N17788 001

DINOPROSTONE

SUPPOSITORY; VAGINAL

TE	Brand / Labeler	Strength	NDC
	PROSTIN E2		
+	UPJOHN	20 MG	N17810 001

DIPHENHYDRAMINE HYDROCHLORIDE

CAPSULE; ORAL

TE	Brand / Labeler	Strength	NDC
	BENADRYL		
AA	PARKE DAVIS	25 MG	N05845 007
AA		50 MG	N05845 001
	DIPHENHYDRAMINE HCL		
AA	BARR	25 MG	N84506 001
AA		50 MG	N80738 001
AA	CHELSEA	50 MG	N85083 001
AA	DANBURY	25 MG	N80728 001
AA		50 MG	N80727 001
AA	EON LABS	25 MG	N80845 002
AA		50 MG	N80845 001
AA	GENEVA	25 MG	N80832 001
AA		50 MG	N80832 002
AA	HALSEY	50 MG	N87914 001 JUN 04, 1984
AA	ICN	25 MG	N80596 001
AA		50 MG	N80592 001
AA	LANNETT	25 MG	N80868 001
AA		50 MG	N80868 002
AA	LEMMON	25 MG	N85874 001
AA		50 MG	N85874 002
AA	LNK	25 MG	N87977 001 JAN 27, 1983
AA		50 MG	N87978 001 JAN 27, 1983
AA	MK	25 MG	N83087 001
AA		50 MG	N83087 002
AA	MUTUAL PHARM	25 MG	N89488 001 JAN 02, 1987
AA		50 MG	N89489 001 JAN 02, 1987
AA	NEWTRON	25 MG	N86543 001
AA		50 MG	N86544 001
AA	PRIVATE FORM	25 MG	N83027 001
AA		50 MG	N83027 002

DIPHENHYDRAMINE HYDROCHLORIDE (continued)

CAPSULE; ORAL

TE	Brand / Labeler	Strength	NDC
	DIPHENHYDRAMINE HCL		
AA	PUREPAC	25 MG	N85156 001
AA		25 MG	N85150 001
AA	RICHLYN	25 MG	N80807 001
AA		50 MG	N80807 002
AA	ROXANE	50 MG	N80635 001
AA	SUPERPHARM	25 MG	N89040 001 MAY 15, 1985
AA	WEST WARD	50 MG	N83567 001
AA	ZENITH	25 MG	N80762 001
AA		50 MG	N80762 002

ELIXIR; ORAL

TE	Brand / Labeler	Strength	NDC
	BELIX		
AA	HALSEY	12.5 MG/5 ML	N86586 001 OCT 03, 1983
	BENADRYL		
AA	PARKE DAVIS	12.5 MG/5 ML	N05845 004
	DIBENIL		
AA	CENCI	12.5 MG/5 ML	N88304 001 DEC 16, 1983
	DIPHENHYDRAMINE HCL		
AA	BUNDY	12.5 MG/5 ML	N83674 001
AA	CENCI	12.5 MG/5 ML	N87941 001 DEC 17, 1982
AA	LANNETT	12.5 MG/5 ML	N80939 002
AA	MK	12.5 MG/5 ML	N83088 002
AA	PHARM ASSOC	12.5 MG/5 ML	N87513 001 FEB 10, 1982
AA	PUREPAC	12.5 MG/5 ML	N83237 001
AA	ROXANE HYDRAMINE	12.5 MG/5 ML	N80643 001 JAN 25, 1982
AA	BARRE	12.5 MG/5 ML	N80763 002

INJECTABLE; INJECTION

TE	Brand / Labeler	Strength	NDC
	BENADRYL		
AP	PARKE DAVIS	10 MG/ML	N06146 001
AP		50 MG/ML	N06146 002
AP		50 MG/ML	N09486 001
	DIPHENHYDRAMINE HCL		
AP	BEL MAR	10 MG/ML	N80822 001
AP	BRISTOL	10 MG/ML	N87066 001
AP	ELKINS SINN	10 MG/ML	N80817 002
AP	INTL MEDICATION	50 MG/ML	N84094 001
AP	LYPHOMED	50 MG/ML	N80586 002
AP	STERIS	10 MG/ML	N80873 001
AP		50 MG/ML	N83533 001
AP		50 MG/ML	N80873 002
AP	WYETH AYERST	50 MG/ML	N80577 001

DIPHENIDOL HYDROCHLORIDE

TABLET; ORAL

TE	Brand / Labeler	Strength	NDC
	VONTROL		
+	SKF	EQ 25 MG BASE	N16033 001

Prescription Drug Products (continued)

DIPHENOXYLATE HYDROCHLORIDE; *MULTIPLE*
SEE   ATROPINE SULFATE; DIPHENOXYLATE HYDROCHLORIDE

DIPHENYLPYRALINE HYDROCHLORIDE
CAPSULE, EXTENDED RELEASE; ORAL
HISPRIL

+	SMITHKLINE BEECHAM	5 MG	N11945 001	

DIPIVEFRIN HYDROCHLORIDE
SOLUTION/DROPS; OPHTHALMIC
PROPINE

ALLERGAN	0.1%	N18239 001	

DIPYRIDAMOLE
INJECTABLE; INJECTION
IV PERSANTINE

BOEHRINGER INGELHEIM	5 MG/ML	N19817 001	DEC 13, 1990

TABLET; ORAL
DIPYRIDAMOLE

AB	BARR	25 MG	N87184 001	OCT 03, 1990
AB		50 MG	N87716 001	OCT 03, 1990
AB		75 MG	N87717 001	OCT 03, 1990
AB	GENEVA	25 MG	N86944 002	APR 16, 1991
AB		50 MG	N87562 001	FEB 25, 1992
AB		75 MG	N87561 001	FEB 25, 1992
AB	LEDERLE	25 MG	N88999 001	FEB 05, 1991
AB		50 MG	N89000 001	FEB 05, 1991
AB		75 MG	N89001 001	FEB 05, 1991
AB	PUREPAC	25 MG	N89425 001	JUL 12, 1990
AB		50 MG	N89426 001	JUL 12, 1990
AB		75 MG	N89427 001	JUL 12, 1990

PERSANTINE

AB	BOEHRINGER INGELHEIM	25 MG	N12836 003	DEC 22, 1986
AB	+	50 MG	N12836 004	FEB 06, 1987
AB		75 MG	N12836 005	FEB 06, 1987

DISOPYRAMIDE PHOSPHATE
CAPSULE; ORAL
DISOPYRAMIDE PHOSPHATE

AB	BARR	EQ 100 MG BASE	N70351 001	DEC 17, 1985
AB		EQ 150 MG BASE	N70352 001	DEC 17, 1985
AB	BIOCRAFT	EQ 100 MG BASE	N70101 001	FEB 22, 1985
AB		EQ 150 MG BASE	N70102 001	FEB 22, 1985
AB	DANBURY	EQ 100 MG BASE	N70173 001	MAY 31, 1985
AB		EQ 150 MG BASE	N70174 001	MAY 31, 1985
AB	GENEVA	EQ 100 MG BASE	N70470 001	DEC 10, 1985
AB		EQ 150 MG BASE	N70471 001	DEC 10, 1985
AB	SUPERPHARM	EQ 100 MG BASE	N70940 001	FEB 09, 1987
AB	ZENITH	EQ 100 MG BASE	N70186 001	NOV 18, 1985
AB		EQ 150 MG BASE	N70187 001	NOV 18, 1985

NORPACE

AB	SEARLE	EQ 100 MG BASE	N17447 001
AB	+	EQ 150 MG BASE	N17447 002

CAPSULE, EXTENDED RELEASE; ORAL
DISOPYRAMIDE PHOSPHATE

AB	KV	EQ 100 MG BASE	N71929 001	AUG 19, 1988
		EQ 150 MG BASE	N71200 001	DEC 15, 1987

NORPACE CR

AB	SEARLE	EQ 100 MG BASE	N18655 001	JUL 20, 1982
AB	+	EQ 150 MG BASE	N18655 002	JUL 20, 1982

DISULFIRAM
TABLET; ORAL
ANTABUSE

BX	WYETH AYERST	250 MG	N07883 003	
BX	+	500 MG	N07883 002	

DISULFIRAM

BX	DANBURY	250 MG	N86889 001	
BX		500 MG	N86890 001	
BX	PAR	250 MG	N88792 001	AUG 14, 1984
BX		500 MG	N88793 001	AUG 14, 1984
BX	SIDMAK	250 MG	N88482 001	DEC 08, 1983
BX		500 MG	N88483 001	DEC 08, 1983

Prescription Drug Products *(continued)*

DIVALPROEX SODIUM

CAPSULE, DELAYED REL PELLETS; ORAL
DEPAKOTE

	Firm	Strength	NDA	Date
+	ABBOTT	EQ 125 MG BASE	N19680 001	SEP 12, 1989

TABLET, DELAYED RELEASE; ORAL
DEPAKOTE

	Firm	Strength	NDA	Date
	ABBOTT	EQ 250 MG BASE	N18723 001	MAR 10, 1983
+		EQ 500 MG BASE	N18723 002	MAR 10, 1983
		EQ 125 MG BASE	N18723 003	OCT 26, 1984

DEPAKOTE CP

Firm	Strength	NDA	Date
ABBOTT	EQ 250 MG BASE	N19794 001	JUL 11, 1990
	EQ 500 MG BASE	N19794 002	JUL 11, 1990

DOBUTAMINE HYDROCHLORIDE

INJECTABLE; INJECTION
DOBUTREX

Firm	Strength	NDA
LILLY	EQ 12.5 MG BASE/ML	N17820 002

DOPAMINE HYDROCHLORIDE

INJECTABLE; INJECTION
DOPAMINE

TE	Firm	Strength	NDA	Date
AP	ELKINS SINN	40 MG/ML	N18398 001	
AP		80 MG/ML	N18398 002	MAR 22, 1982

DOPAMINE HCL

TE	Firm	Strength	NDA	Date
AP	ABBOTT	80 MG/100 ML	N18132 002	FEB 04, 1982
AP		160 MG/100 ML	N18132 003	FEB 04, 1982
AP		40 MG/ML	N18132 001	
AP		40 MG/ML	N70656 001	JAN 24, 1989
AP		80 MG/ML	N18132 004	JUL 09, 1982
AP		80 MG/ML	N70657 001	JAN 24, 1989
AP	ASTRA	40 MG/ML	N18656 001	JUN 28, 1983
AP		40 MG/ML	N70087 001	OCT 23, 1985
AP		80 MG/ML	N70089 001	OCT 23, 1985
AP		80 MG/ML	N70090 001	OCT 23, 1985
AP		80 MG/ML	N70091 001	OCT 23, 1985
AP		160 MG/ML	N70092 001	OCT 23, 1985
AP		160 MG/ML	N70093 001	OCT 23, 1985
AP		160 MG/ML	N70094 001	OCT 23, 1985

DOPAMINE HYDROCHLORIDE *(continued)*

INJECTABLE; INJECTION
DOPAMINE HCL

TE	Firm	Strength	NDA	Date
AP	BRISTOL	40 MG/ML	N18549 001	MAR 11, 1983
AP	GENSIA	40 MG/ML	N72999 001	OCT 23, 1991
AP		80 MG/ML	N73000 001	OCT 23, 1991
AP	INTL MEDICATION	40 MG/ML	N18014 001	
AP	LUITPOLD	40 MG/ML	N70799 001	FEB 11, 1987
AP		80 MG/ML	N70820 001	FEB 11, 1987
AP	LYPHOMED	160 MG/ML	N70826 001	FEB 11, 1987
AP		40 MG/ML	N70012 001	JUN 12, 1985
AP		80 MG/ML	N70013 001	JUN 12, 1985
AP	SMITH NEPHEW SOLOPAK	40 MG/ML	N70046 001	AUG 29, 1985
AP		80 MG/ML	N70047 001	AUG 29, 1985
AP	WARNER CHILCOTT	40 MG/ML	N18138 001	
AP		40 MG/ML	N70558 001	SEP 20, 1985

DOPAMINE HCL AND DEXTROSE 5%

TE	Firm	Strength	NDA	Date
AP	MCGAW	80 MG/100 ML	N19099 002	OCT 15, 1986
AP		320 MG/100 ML	N19099 004	OCT 15, 1986

DOPAMINE HCL AND DEXTROSE 5% IN PLASTIC CONTAINER

TE	Firm	Strength	NDA	Date
AP	MCGAW	160 MG/100 ML	N19099 003	OCT 15, 1986
		40 MG/100 ML	N19099 001	OCT 15, 1986

DOPAMINE HCL IN DEXTROSE 5% IN PLASTIC CONTAINER

TE	Firm	Strength	NDA	Date
AP	ABBOTT	80 MG/100 ML	N18826 001	SEP 30, 1983
AP		160 MG/100 ML	N18826 002	SEP 30, 1983
AP		320 MG/100 ML	N18826 003	SEP 30, 1983
AP	BAXTER	80 MG/100 ML	N19615 001	MAR 27, 1987
AP		160 MG/100 ML	N19615 002	MAR 27, 1987
AP		320 MG/100 ML	N19615 003	MAR 27, 1987
AP		640 MG/100 ML	N19615 004	MAR 27, 1987

INTROPIN

TE	Firm	Strength	NDA	Date
AP	DUPONT	40 MG/ML	N17395 001	
AP		80 MG/ML	N17395 002	
AP		160 MG/ML	N17395 003	

Prescription Drug Products (continued)

DOXACURIUM CHLORIDE
INJECTABLE; INJECTION
NUROMAX
BURROUGHS WELLCOME
	EQ 1 MG BASE/ML	N19946 001	MAR 07, 1991

DOXAPRAM HYDROCHLORIDE
INJECTABLE; INJECTION
DOPRAM
AP	ROBINS	20 MG/ML	N14879 001

DOXAPRAM HCL
AP	STERIS	20 MG/ML	N73529 001	JAN 30, 1992

DOXAZOSIN MESYLATE
TABLET; ORAL
CARDURA
PFIZER
AB	EQ 1 MG BASE	N19668 001	NOV 02, 1990
AB	EQ 2 MG BASE	N19668 002	NOV 02, 1990
AB	EQ 4 MG BASE	N19668 003	NOV 02, 1990
AB	EQ 8 MG BASE	N19668 004	NOV 02, 1990

DOXEPIN HYDROCHLORIDE
CAPSULE; ORAL
ADAPIN
FISONS
AB	EQ 10 MG BASE	N16987 001	
AB	EQ 25 MG BASE	N16987 002	
AB	EQ 50 MG BASE	N16987 003	
AB	EQ 75 MG BASE	N16987 006	
AB	EQ 100 MG BASE	N16987 004	
AB	EQ 150 MG BASE	N16987 007	APR 13, 1987

DOXEPIN HCL
DANBURY
AB	EQ 10 MG BASE	N71485 001	APR 30, 1987
AB	EQ 25 MG BASE	N71486 001	APR 30, 1987
AB	EQ 50 MG BASE	N71238 001	APR 30, 1987
AB	EQ 75 MG BASE	N71326 001	APR 30, 1987
AB	EQ 100 MG BASE	N71239 001	APR 30, 1987

GENEVA
AB	EQ 10 MG BASE	N71487 001	MAR 02, 1987
AB	EQ 25 MG BASE	N70827 001	MAY 15, 1986
AB	EQ 50 MG BASE	N70828 001	MAY 15, 1986
AB	EQ 75 MG BASE	N70825 001	MAY 15, 1986
AB	EQ 100 MG BASE	N71562 001	MAR 02, 1987

DOXEPIN HYDROCHLORIDE (continued)
CAPSULE; ORAL
DOXEPIN HCL
LEDERLE
AB	EQ 10 MG BASE	N71685 001	JAN 05, 1988
AB	EQ 25 MG BASE	N71686 001	JAN 05, 1988
AB	EQ 50 MG BASE	N71673 001	JAN 05, 1988
AB	EQ 75 MG BASE	N71674 001	JAN 05, 1988
AB	EQ 100 MG BASE	N71675 001	JAN 05, 1988
AB	EQ 150 MG BASE	N71676 001	JAN 05, 1988

MYLAN
AB	EQ 10 MG BASE	N70789 001	MAY 13, 1986
AB	EQ 25 MG BASE	N70790 001	MAY 13, 1986
AB	EQ 50 MG BASE	N70791 001	MAY 13, 1986
AB	EQ 75 MG BASE	N70792 001	MAY 13, 1986
AB	EQ 100 MG BASE	N70793 001	MAY 13, 1986

PAR
AB	EQ 10 MG BASE	N71697 001	NOV 09, 1987
AB	EQ 25 MG BASE	N71437 001	NOV 09, 1987
AB	EQ 50 MG BASE	N71595 001	NOV 09, 1987
AB	EQ 75 MG BASE	N71608 001	NOV 09, 1987
AB	EQ 100 MG BASE	N71422 001	NOV 09, 1987
AB	EQ 150 MG BASE	N71669 001	NOV 09, 1987

PUREPAC
AB	EQ 10 MG BASE	N73054 001	DEC 28, 1990
AB	EQ 25 MG BASE	N72109 001	DEC 28, 1990
AB	EQ 50 MG BASE	N73055 001	DEC 28, 1990
AB	EQ 100 MG BASE	N72110 001	SEP 08, 1988

ROYCE
AB	EQ 10 MG BASE	N72985 001	MAR 29, 1991
AB	EQ 25 MG BASE	N72986 001	MAR 29, 1991
AB	EQ 50 MG BASE	N72987 001	MAR 29, 1991

SINEQUAN
PFIZER
AB	+	EQ 10 MG BASE	N16798 003	
AB	+	EQ 25 MG BASE	N16798 001	
AB		EQ 50 MG BASE	N16798 002	
AB		EQ 75 MG BASE	N16798 006	
AB		EQ 100 MG BASE	N16798 005	
AB		EQ 150 MG BASE	N16798 007	

Prescription Drug Products (continued)

DOXEPIN HYDROCHLORIDE (continued)

CONCENTRATE; ORAL

TE Code	Firm	Strength	Appl No	Approval
DOXEPIN HCL				
AA	COPLEY	EQ 10 MG BASE/ML	N71609 001	NOV 09, 1987
AA	PHARM BASICS	EQ 10 MG BASE/ML	N71918 001	JUL 20, 1988
SINEQUAN				
AA	PFIZER	EQ 10 MG BASE/ML	N17516 001	

DOXORUBICIN HYDROCHLORIDE

INJECTABLE; INJECTION

TE Code	Firm	Strength	Appl No	Approval
ADRIAMYCIN PFS				
AP	ADRIA	2 MG/ML	N50629 001	DEC 23, 1987
AP	ADRIA	200 MG/100 ML	N50629 002	MAY 03, 1988
AP		2 MG/ML	N63165 001	JAN 30, 1991
AP		200 MG/100 ML	N63165 002	JAN 30, 1991
ADRIAMYCIN RDF				
AP	ADRIA	10 MG/VIAL	N50467 001	
AP		20 MG/VIAL	N50467 003	MAY 20, 1985
AP		50 MG/VIAL	N50467 002	
AP		150 MG/VIAL	N50467 004	JUL 22, 1987
DOXORUBICIN HCL				
AP	CETUS BEN VENUE	2 MG/ML	N62975 001	MAR 17, 1989
AP		10 MG/VIAL	N62921 001	MAR 17, 1989
AP		20 MG/VIAL	N62921 002	MAR 17, 1989
AP		50 MG/VIAL	N62921 003	MAR 17, 1989
AP	PHARMACHEMIE	10 MG/VIAL	N63097 001	MAY 21, 1990
AP		20 MG/VIAL	N63097 002	MAY 21, 1990
AP		50 MG/VIAL	N63097 003	MAY 21, 1990
RUBEX				
AP	BRISTOL MYERS	10 MG/VIAL	N62926 001	APR 13, 1989
AP		50 MG/VIAL	N62926 002	APR 13, 1989
		100 MG/VIAL	N62926 003	APR 13, 1989

DOXYCYCLINE

CAPSULE; ORAL

TE Code	Firm	Strength	Appl No	Approval
DOXYCYCLINE MONOHYDRATE				
	+ MEDICOPHARMA	EQ 100 MG BASE	N50641 001	DEC 29, 1989

POWDER FOR RECONSTITUTION; ORAL

TE Code	Firm	Strength	Appl No	Approval
DOXYCHEL				
AB	RACHELLE	EQ 25 MG BASE/5 ML	N61720 001	
VIBRAMYCIN				
AB	+ PFIZER	EQ 25 MG BASE/5 ML	N50006 001	

DOXYCYCLINE CALCIUM

SUSPENSION; ORAL

TE Code	Firm	Strength	Appl No	Approval
VIBRAMYCIN				
	+ PFIZER	EQ 50 MG BASE/5 ML	N50480 001	

DOXYCYCLINE HYCLATE

CAPSULE; ORAL

TE Code	Firm	Strength	Appl No	Approval
DOXY-LEMMON				
AB	LEMMON	EQ 50 MG BASE	N62497 001	AUG 23, 1984
AB		EQ 100 MG BASE	N62497 002	JUN 15, 1984
DOXYCHEL HYCLATE				
AB	RACHELLE	EQ 50 MG BASE	N61717 001	
AB		EQ 100 MG BASE	N61717 002	
DOXYCYCLINE HYCLATE				
AB	BARR	EQ 50 MG BASE	N62418 001	JAN 28, 1983
AB		EQ 100 MG BASE	N62418 002	JAN 28, 1983
AB	CHELSEA	EQ 50 MG BASE	N62142 001	MAR 17, 1989
AB		EQ 100 MG BASE	N62142 002	MAR 17, 1989
AB	DANBURY	EQ 50 MG BASE	N62031 002	OCT 13, 1982
AB		EQ 100 MG BASE	N62031 001	
AB	HALSEY	EQ 50 MG BASE	N62119 002	MAY 24, 1985
AB		EQ 100 MG BASE	N62119 001	MAY 24, 1985
AB	HEATHER	EQ 50 MG BASE	N62463 001	DEC 07, 1983
AB		EQ 100 MG BASE	N62463 002	DEC 07, 1983
AB	MUTUAL PHARM	EQ 50 MG BASE	N62675 001	JUL 10, 1986
AB		EQ 100 MG BASE	N62676 001	JUL 10, 1986
AB	MYLAN	EQ 50 MG BASE	N62337 001	MAR 29, 1982
AB		EQ 100 MG BASE	N62337 002	MAR 29, 1982

Prescription Drug Products (continued)

DOXYCYCLINE HYCLATE (continued)

CAPSULE; ORAL

DOXYCYCLINE HYCLATE

TE	Firm	Strength	Appl. No.	Date
AB	PAR	EQ 50 MG BASE	N62434 001	OCT 19, 1984
AB		EQ 100 MG BASE	N62442 001	DEC 22, 1983
AB	PRIVATE FORM	EQ 50 MG BASE	N62631 001	
AB		EQ 100 MG BASE	N62631 002	JUL 24, 1986
AB	PUREPAC	EQ 50 MG BASE	N62479 001	DEC 23, 1983
AB		EQ 100 MG BASE	N62479 002	DEC 23, 1983
AB	WEST WARD	EQ 50 MG BASE	N62396 002	NOV 07, 1984
AB		EQ 100 MG BASE	N62396 001	MAY 07, 1984
AB	ZENITH	EQ 50 MG BASE	N62500 001	SEP 11, 1984
AB		EQ 100 MG BASE	N62500 002	SEP 11, 1984
AB	VIBRAMYCIN + PFIZER	EQ 50 MG BASE	N50007 001	
AB		EQ 100 MG BASE	N50007 002	

CAPSULE, COATED PELLETS; ORAL

TE	Firm	Strength	Appl. No.	Date
AB	DORYX + FAULDING	EQ 100 MG BASE	N50582 001	JUL 22, 1985
AB	PARKE DAVIS	EQ 100 MG BASE	N62653 001	OCT 30, 1985

DOXYCYCLINE HYCLATE

TE	Firm	Strength	Appl. No.	Date
AB	SIDMAK	EQ 100 MG BASE	N63187 001	JUN 30, 1992

INJECTABLE; INJECTION

TE	Firm	Strength	Appl. No.	Date
AP	DOXY 100 LYPHOMED	EQ 100 MG BASE/VIAL	N62475 001	DEC 09, 1983
AP	DOXY 200 LYPHOMED	EQ 200 MG BASE/VIAL	N62475 002	DEC 09, 1983
AP	DOXYCHEL HYCLATE RACHELLE	EQ 100 MG BASE/VIAL	N61953 001	
AP	DOXYCYCLINE BEN VENUE	EQ 100 MG BASE/VIAL	N62569 001	MAR 09, 1988
AP		EQ 200 MG BASE/VIAL	N62569 002	MAR 09, 1988
AP	ELKINS SINN	EQ 100 MG BASE/VIAL	N62450 001	OCT 27, 1983
AP		EQ 200 MG BASE/VIAL	N62450 002	OCT 27, 1983

DOXYCYCLINE HYCLATE (continued)

INJECTABLE; INJECTION

DOXYCYCLINE HYCLATE

TE	Firm	Strength	Appl. No.	Date
AP	LEDERLE	EQ 100 MG BASE/VIAL	N62992 001	FEB 16, 1989
AP		EQ 200 MG BASE/VIAL	N62992 002	FEB 16, 1989
AP	VIBRAMYCIN PFIZER	EQ 100 MG BASE/VIAL	N50442 002	
AP		EQ 200 MG BASE/VIAL	N50442 001	

TABLET; ORAL

TE	Firm	Strength	Appl. No.	Date
AB	DOXY-LEMMON LEMMON	EQ 100 MG BASE	N62581 001	MAR 15, 1985
AB	DOXY-TABS RACHELLE	EQ 100 MG BASE	N62269 001	
AB		EQ 100 MG BASE	N62269 002	NOV 08, 1982
AB	DOXYCYCLINE HYCLATE BARR	EQ 100 MG BASE	N62391 001	SEP 30, 1982
AB	DANBURY	EQ 100 MG BASE	N62421 001	FEB 02, 1983
AB	HEATHER	EQ 100 MG BASE	N62462 001	MAY 11, 1983
AB	MEDICOPHARMA	EQ 100 MG BASE	N62538 001	APR 07, 1986
AB	MUTUAL PHARM	EQ 100 MG BASE	N62677 001	JUL 10, 1986
AB	MYLAN	EQ 100 MG BASE	N62432 001	FEB 15, 1983
AB	SUPERPHARM	EQ 100 MG BASE	N62494 001	FEB 20, 1985
AB	ZENITH	EQ 100 MG BASE	N62505 001	SEP 11, 1984
AB	VIBRA-TABS + PFIZER	EQ 100 MG BASE	N50533 001	

DRONABINOL

CAPSULE; ORAL

TE	Firm	Strength	Appl. No.	Date
+	MARINOL UNIMED	2.5 MG	N18651 001	MAY 31, 1985
+		5 MG	N18651 002	MAY 31, 1985
+		10 MG	N18651 003	MAY 31, 1985

Prescription Drug Products (continued)

DROPERIDOL

INJECTABLE; INJECTION

DROPERIDOL

TE	Firm	Strength	Appl. No.	Date
AP	ABBOTT	2.5 MG/ML	N71981 001	FEB 29, 1988
AP	ASTRA	2.5 MG/ML	N72018 001	OCT 20, 1988
AP		2.5 MG/ML	N72019 001	OCT 19, 1988
AP	DUPONT	2.5 MG/ML	N72021 001	OCT 19, 1988
AP		2.5 MG/ML	N71645 001	APR 07, 1988
AP	LUITPOLD	2.5 MG/ML	N72123 001	OCT 24, 1988
AP		2.5 MG/ML	N72335 001	OCT 24, 1988
AP	LYPHOMED	2.5 MG/ML	N70992 001	NOV 17, 1986
AP		2.5 MG/ML	N70993 001	NOV 17, 1986
AP	QUAD	2.5 MG/ML	N71941 001	AUG 17, 1988
AP	SMITH NEPHEW SOLOPAK	2.5 MG/ML	N71754 001	SEP 06, 1988
AP		2.5 MG/ML	N71755 001	SEP 06, 1988
AP	STERIS	2.5 MG/ML	N73520 001	NOV 27, 1991
AP		2.5 MG/ML	N73521 001	NOV 27, 1991
AP		2.5 MG/ML	N73523 001	NOV 27, 1991
AP	INAPSINE JANSSEN	2.5 MG/ML	N16796 001	NOV 27, 1991

DROPERIDOL; FENTANYL CITRATE

INJECTABLE; INJECTION

FENTANYL CITRATE AND DROPERIDOL

TE	Firm	Strength	Appl. No.	Date
AP	ABBOTT	2.5 MG/ML;EQ 0.05 MG BASE/ML	N71982 001	MAY 04, 1988
AP	ASTRA	2.5 MG/ML;EQ 0.05 MG BASE/ML	N72026 001	APR 13, 1989
AP		2.5 MG/ML;EQ 0.05 MG BASE/ML	N72027 001	APR 13, 1989
AP		2.5 MG/ML;EQ 0.05 MG BASE/ML	N72028 001	APR 13, 1989
AP	INNOVAR JANSSEN	2.5 MG/ML;EQ 0.05 MG BASE/ML	N16049 001	

DYCLONINE HYDROCHLORIDE

SOLUTION; TOPICAL

DYCLONE

TE	Firm	Strength	Appl. No.
	ASTRA	0.5%	N09925 002
		1%	N09925 001

DYPHYLLINE

INJECTABLE; INJECTION

NEOTHYLLINE

TE	Firm	Strength	Appl. No.
	LEMMON	250 MG/ML	N09088 001

TABLET; ORAL

DILOR

TE	Firm	Strength	Appl. No.
BP	SAVAGE	200 MG	N84514 001

DILOR-400

| BP | SAVAGE | 400 MG | N84751 001 |

LUFYLLIN

| BP | WALLACE | 200 MG | N84566 001 |
| BP | | 400 MG | N84566 002 |

NEOTHYLLINE

| BP | LEMMON | 200 MG | N07794 001 |
| BP | + | 400 MG | N07794 002 |

ECHOTHIOPHATE IODIDE

POWDER FOR RECONSTITUTION; OPHTHALMIC

PHOSPHOLINE IODIDE

TE	Firm	Strength	Appl. No.
	WYETH AYERST	0.03%	N11963 002
		0.06%	N11963 004
		0.125%	N11963 001
		0.25%	N11963 003

ECONAZOLE NITRATE

CREAM; TOPICAL

SPECTAZOLE

TE	Firm	Strength	Appl. No.	Date
	+ JOHNSON RW	1%	N18751 001	DEC 23, 1982

EDETATE CALCIUM DISODIUM

INJECTABLE; INJECTION

CALCIUM DISODIUM VERSENATE

TE	Firm	Strength	Appl. No.
	3M	200 MG/ML	N08922 001

EDETATE DISODIUM

INJECTABLE; INJECTION

DISODIUM EDETATE

TE	Firm	Strength	Appl. No.
AP	STERIS	150 MG/ML	N84356 001

EDETATE DISODIUM

| AP | STERIS | 150 MG/ML | N80391 001 |

ENDRATE

| AP | ABBOTT | 150 MG/ML | N11355 001 |

SODIUM VERSENATE

| AP | 3M | 200 MG/ML | N10573 001 |

Prescription Drug Products *(continued)*

EDROPHONIUM CHLORIDE

INJECTABLE; INJECTION

ENLON

ΔP	ANAQUEST	10MG/ML	N88873 001	AUG 06, 1985

REVERSOL

ΔP	ORGANON	10MG/ML	N89624 001	MAY 13, 1988

TENSILON

ΔP	ROCHE	10MG/ML	N07959 001	

EDROPHONIUM CHLORIDE; *MULTIPLE*

SEE ATROPINE SULFATE; EDROPHONIUM CHLORIDE

EFLORNITHINE HYDROCHLORIDE

INJECTABLE; INJECTION

ORNIDYL

MERRELL DOW	200 MG/ML	N19879 002	NOV 28, 1990

ENALAPRIL MALEATE

TABLET; ORAL

VASOTEC

MERCK	2.5 MG	N18998 005	JUL 26, 1988
	5 MG	N18998 001	DEC 24, 1985
	10 MG	N18998 002	DEC 24, 1985
+	20 MG	N18998 003	DEC 24, 1985

ENALAPRIL MALEATE; HYDROCHLOROTHIAZIDE

TABLET; ORAL

VASERETIC

+	MERCK	10 MG;25 MG	N19221 001	OCT 31, 1986

ENALAPRILAT

INJECTABLE; INJECTION

VASOTEC

MERCK	1.25 MG/ML	N19309 001	FEB 09, 1988

ENCAINIDE HYDROCHLORIDE

CAPSULE; ORAL

ENKAID

BRISTOL	25 MG	N18981 002	DEC 24, 1986
	35 MG	N18981 003	DEC 24, 1986
+	50 MG	N18981 004	DEC 24, 1986

ENFLURANE

LIQUID; INHALATION

ENFLURANE

ΔN	ABBOTT	99.9%	N70803 001	JUL 27, 1987

ETHRANE

ΔN	ANAQUEST	99.9%	N17087 001	

ENOXACIN

TABLET; ORAL

PENETREX

PARKE DAVIS	200 MG	N19616 004	DEC 31, 1991
+	400 MG	N19616 005	DEC 31, 1991

EPINEPHRINE

INJECTABLE; INJECTION

EPIPEN

SURVIVAL TECH	1 MG/ML	N19430 001	DEC 22, 1987

EPIPEN JR.

SURVIVAL TECH	0.5 MG/ML	N19430 002	DEC 22, 1987

SUS-PHRINE

FOREST LABS	5 MG/ML	N07942 001	

EPINEPHRINE; *MULTIPLE*

SEE BUPIVACAINE HYDROCHLORIDE; EPINEPHRINE

EPINEPHRINE; LIDOCAINE HYDROCHLORIDE

INJECTABLE; INJECTION

ALPHACAINE HCL W/ EPINEPHRINE

ΔP	CARLISLE	0.01 MG/ML;2%	N84720 001	
ΔP		0.02 MG/ML;2%	N84732 001	

LIDOCAINE HCL AND EPINEPHRINE

ΔP	ABBOTT	0.005 MG/ML;0.5%	N89635 001	JUN 21, 1988
			N89649 001	JUN 21, 1988
ΔP		0.005 MG/ML;1%	N88571 001	SEP 13, 1985
			N89645 001	JUN 21, 1988
ΔP		0.005 MG/ML;1.5%	N89650 001	JUN 21, 1988
			N89651 001	JUN 21, 1988
ΔP		0.005 MG/ML;1.5%	N89644 001	JUN 21, 1988
ΔP		0.005 MG/ML;2%	N89646 001	JUN 21, 1988
ΔP		0.01 MG/ML;1%		
ΔP		0.01 MG/ML;2%		
ΔP	ELKINS SINN	0.01 MG/ML;1%	N80406 001	
ΔP		0.01 MG/ML;2%	N80406 002	

Prescription Drug Products (continued)

EPINEPHRINE; LIDOCAINE HYDROCHLORIDE (continued)

INJECTABLE; INJECTION

LIDOCAINE HCL W/ EPINEPHRINE

AP	ABBOTT	0.01 MG/ML;1%	N83154 001	
AP	BEL MAR	0.01 MG/ML;1%	N80820 001	
		0.01 MG/ML;2%	N80757 001	
AP	DELL	0.01 MG/ML;1%	N83389 001	
		0.01 MG/ML;2%	N83390 001	
AP	GRAHAM CHEM	0.01 MG/ML;2%	N80504 004	OCT 19, 1983
		0.02 MG/ML;2%	N80504 005	OCT 19, 1983
AP	INTL MEDICATION	0.01 MG/ML;1%	N86402 001	
AP	STERIS	0.01 MG/ML;1%	N80377 003	
AP		0.01 MG/ML;2%	N80377 004	

LIDOCATON

AP	PHARMATON	0.01 MG/ML;2%	N84729 001	AUG 17, 1983
AP		0.02 MG/ML;2%	N84728 001	AUG 17, 1983

OCTOCAINE

AP	NOVOCOL	0.01 MG/ML;2%	N84048 001	
AP		0.02 MG/ML;2%	N84048 002	

XYLOCAINE W/ EPINEPHRINE

AP	ASTRA	0.005 MG/ML;0.5%	N06488 012	
AP		0.005 MG/ML;1%	N06488 018	
			N06488 017	NOV 13, 1986
AP		0.005 MG/ML;1.5%	N06488 019	NOV 13, 1986
AP		0.005 MG/ML;2%	N06488 004	
AP		0.01 MG/ML;1%	N06488 ...	
AP		0.01 MG/ML;2%	N06488 003	

EPINEPHRINE; PROCAINE HYDROCHLORIDE

INJECTABLE; INJECTION

PROCAINE HCL W/ EPINEPHRINE

BEL MAR	0.02 MG/ML;1%	N80758 001	
	0.02 MG/ML;2%	N80759 001	

EPINEPHRINE BITARTRATE; *MULTIPLE*

SEE BUPIVACAINE HYDROCHLORIDE; EPINEPHRINE BITARTRATE

EPINEPHRINE BITARTRATE; ETIDOCAINE HYDROCHLORIDE

INJECTABLE; INJECTION

DURANEST

ASTRA	0.005 MG/ML;1%	N17751 006	
	0.005 MG/ML;1.5%	N17751 007	

EPINEPHRINE BITARTRATE; LIDOCAINE HYDROCHLORIDE

INJECTABLE; INJECTION

LIGNOSPAN FORTE

DEPROCO	EQ 0.02 MG BASE/ML;2%	N88389 001	JAN 22, 1985

LIGNOSPAN STANDARD

DEPROCO	EQ 0.01 MG BASE/ML;2%	N88390 001	JAN 22, 1985

EPINEPHRINE BITARTRATE; PRILOCAINE HYDROCHLORIDE

INJECTABLE; INJECTION

CITANEST FORTE

ASTRA	0.005 MG/ML;4%	N14763 008	

ERGOCALCIFEROL

CAPSULE; ORAL

DELTALIN

AA	LILLY	50,000 IU	N80884 001

DRISDOL

AA	STERLING	50,000 IU	N03444 001

VITAMIN D

AA	LANNETT	50,000 IU	N80825 001
AA	PHARMACAPS	50,000 IU	N80704 001
AA	RICHLYN	50,000 IU	N80951 001
AA	WEST WARD	50,000 IU	N83102 001

ERGOCALCIFEROL; *MULTIPLE*

SEE ASCORBIC ACID; BIOTIN; CYANOCOBALAMIN; DEXPANTHENOL; ERGOCALCIFEROL; FOLIC ACID; NIACINAMIDE; PYRIDOXINE HYDROCHLORIDE; RIBOFLAVIN PHOSPHATE SODIUM; THIAMINE HYDROCHLORIDE; VITAMIN A; VITAMIN E

SEE ASCORBIC ACID; BIOTIN; CYANOCOBALAMIN; DEXPANTHENOL; ERGOCALCIFEROL; FOLIC ACID; NIACINAMIDE; PYRIDOXINE; RIBOFLAVIN PHOSPHATE SODIUM; THIAMINE; VITAMIN A; VITAMIN E

ERGOLOID MESYLATES

CAPSULE; ORAL

HYDERGINE LC

+	SANDOZ	1 MG	N18706 001	JAN 18, 1983

SOLUTION; ORAL

HYDERGINE

SANDOZ	1 MG/ML	N18418 001	

Prescription Drug Products (continued)

ERGOLOID MESYLATES (continued)

TABLET; ORAL

ERGOLOID MESYLATES

TE	Firm	Strength	Appl. No.	Date
AB	BARR	1MG	N88891 001	NOV 01, 1985
AB	DANBURY	1MG	N87244 001	AUG 16, 1982
AB	MUTUAL PHARM	1MG	N81113 001	OCT 31, 1991
AB	HYDERGINE + SANDOZ	1MG	N17993 001	
AB		0.5 MG	N17993 003	

TABLET; SUBLINGUAL

ERGOLOID MESYLATES

TE	Firm	Strength	Appl. No.	Date
AA	BARR	0.5 MG	N87407 001	
AA		1 MG	N87552 001	
AA	DANBURY	0.5 MG	N87233 001	
AA		1 MG	N87183 001	
AA	KV	0.5 MG	N85899 001	
AA		1 MG	N85900 001	
AA	GERIMAL CHELSEA	0.5 MG	N86189 001	
AA		1 MG	N86188 001	
AA	HYDERGINE SANDOZ	0.5 MG	N09087 002	
AA		1 MG	N09087 001	
AA	HYDROGENATED ERGOT ALKALOIDS ZENITH	0.5 MG	N87186 001	
AA		1 MG	N87185 001	

ERGOTAMINE TARTRATE

AEROSOL, METERED; INHALATION

MEDIHALER ERGOTAMINE + 3M

TE	Firm	Strength	Appl. No.	Date
	MEDIHALER ERGOTAMINE + 3M	0.36 MG/INH	N12102 001	

TABLET; SUBLINGUAL

TE	Firm	Strength	Appl. No.	Date
AA	ERGOSTAT PARKE DAVIS	2 MG	N88337 001	JUN 08, 1984
AA	WIGRETTES ORGANON	2 MG	N86750 001	JUL 29, 1982

ERGOTAMINE TARTRATE; *MULTIPLE*

SEE CAFFEINE; ERGOTAMINE TARTRATE

ERYTHROMYCIN

CAPSULE, DELAYED REL PELLETS; ORAL

ERYC

TE	Firm	Strength	Appl. No.	Date
AB	FAULDING	250MG	N50536 001	JUL 25, 1985
AB	+ PARKE DAVIS	250MG	N62338 001	
AB		250MG	N62546 001	
AB		250MG	N62618 001	SEP 25, 1985

ERYTHROMYCIN (continued)

CAPSULE, DELAYED REL PELLETS; ORAL

TE	Firm	Strength	Appl. No.	Date
	ERYC SPRINKLES + FAULDING	125 MG	N50593 001	JUL 22, 1985

ERYTHROMYCIN

TE	Firm	Strength	Appl. No.	Date
AB	ABBOTT	250 MG	N62746 001	DEC 22, 1986
AB	BARR	250 MG	N63098 001	MAY 04, 1989

GEL; TOPICAL

TE	Firm	Strength	Appl. No.	Date
AT	EMGEL GLAXO	2%	N63107 001	AUG 23, 1991
AT	ERYGEL HERBERT	2%	N50617 001	OCT 21, 1987

LOTION; TOPICAL

TE	Firm	Strength	Appl. No.	Date
	E-SOLVE 2 SYOSSET	2%	N62467 001	JUL 03, 1985

OINTMENT; OPHTHALMIC

ERYTHROMYCIN

TE	Firm	Strength	Appl. No.	Date
AT	FOUGERA	5 MG/GM	N62447 001	SEP 26, 1983
AT	PHARMADERM	5 MG/GM	N62446 001	SEP 26, 1983
AT	PHARMAFAIR	5 MG/GM	N62481 001	APR 05, 1984
AT	ILOTYCIN DISTA	5 MG/GM	N50368 001	

OINTMENT; TOPICAL

TE	Firm	Strength	Appl. No.	Date
	AKNE-MYCIN HERMAL	2%	N50584 001	JAN 10, 1985

POWDER; FOR RX COMPOUNDING

ERYTHROMYCIN

TE	Firm	Strength	Appl. No.	Date
	PADDOCK	100%	N50610 001	NOV 07, 1986

SOLUTION; TOPICAL

TE	Firm	Strength	Appl. No.	Date
AT	A/T/S HOECHST ROUSSEL	2%	N62405 001	NOV 18, 1982
AT	C-SOLVE-2 SYOSSET	2%	N62468 001	JUL 03, 1985
AT	ERYDERM ABBOTT	2%	N62290 001	
AT	ERYMAX HERBERT	2%	N62508 002	JUL 11, 1985

Prescription Drug Products (continued)

ERYTHROMYCIN (continued)

SOLUTION; TOPICAL

	ERYTHROMYCIN			
AT	BARRE	1.5%	N62328 001	APR 19, 1982
AT		2%	N62326 001	APR 19, 1982
AT	CLAY PARK	2%	N63038 001	JAN 11, 1991
AT	NASKA	2%	N62957 001	JUL 21, 1988
AT	PHARM BASICS	2%	N62825 001	OCT 23, 1987
AT	PHARMAFAIR	1.5%	N62485 001	JUL 11, 1984
AT		2%	N62616 001	JUL 25, 1985
	ETS-2%			
AT	PADDOCK	2%	N62687 001	FEB 05, 1988
	SANSAC			
AT	OWEN GALDERMA	2%	N62522 001	JAN 24, 1985
	STATICIN			
AT	WESTWOOD SQUIBB	1.5%	N50526 001	
	T-STAT			
AT	WESTWOOD SQUIBB	2%	N62436 001	MAR 09, 1983

SWAB; TOPICAL

	ERYCETTE			
AT	JOHNSON RW	2%	N50594 001	FEB 15, 1985
	T-STAT			
AT	WESTWOOD SQUIBB	2%	N62748 001	JUL 23, 1987

TABLET; ORAL

	ERYTHROMYCIN			
	+ ABBOTT	250 MG	N61621 001	
		500 MG	N61621 002	

TABLET, COATED PARTICLES; ORAL

	PCE			
	+ ABBOTT	333 MG	N50611 001	SEP 09, 1986
			N50611 002	
		500 MG	N50611 002	AUG 22, 1990

ERYTHROMYCIN (continued)

TABLET, DELAYED RELEASE; ORAL

	E-BASE			
AB	BARR	333 MG	N63028 001	MAY 15, 1990
			N63086 001	MAY 15, 1990
AB		500 MG	N62999 001	NOV 25, 1988
	E-MYCIN			
AB	BOOTS	250 MG	N60272 001	
AB	+	333 MG	N60272 002	
	ERY-TAB			
AB	ABBOTT	250 MG	N62298 001	
AB		333 MG	N62298 003	MAR 29, 1982
AB		500 MG	N62298 002	
	ILOTYCIN			
AB	DISTA	250 MG	N61910 001	
	ROBIMYCIN			
AB	ROBINS	250 MG	N61633 001	

ERYTHROMYCIN; *MULTIPLE*

SEE BENZOYL PEROXIDE; ERYTHROMYCIN

ERYTHROMYCIN ESTOLATE

CAPSULE; ORAL

	ERYTHROMYCIN ESTOLATE			
AB	BARR	EQ 125 MG BASE	N62162 001	
AB		EQ 250 MG BASE	N62162 002	
AB	DANBURY	EQ 250 MG BASE	N62087 001	
AB	ZENITH	EQ 250 MG BASE	N62237 001	
	ILOSONE			
AB	DISTA	EQ 125 MG BASE	N61897 001	
AB	+	EQ 250 MG BASE	N61897 002	

DROPS; ORAL

	ILOSONE			
	+ DISTA	EQ 100 MG BASE/ML	N61894 003	

POWDER FOR RECONSTITUTION; ORAL

	ILOSONE			
	+ DISTA	EQ 125 MG BASE/5 ML	N61893 001	

SUSPENSION; ORAL

	ERYTHROMYCIN ESTOLATE			
AB	BARR	EQ 125 MG BASE/5 ML	N62169 001	OCT 17, 1990
		EQ 250 MG BASE/5 ML	N62169 002	OCT 17, 1990
AB	BARRE	EQ 125 MG BASE/5 ML	N62353 001	NOV 18, 1982
AB		EQ 250 MG BASE/5 ML	N62409 001	DEC 16, 1982
	ILOSONE			
AB	DISTA	EQ 125 MG BASE/5 ML	N61894 001	
AB	+	EQ 250 MG BASE/5 ML	N61894 002	

Prescription Drug Products (continued)

ERYTHROMYCIN ESTOLATE (continued)
TABLET; ORAL
ILOSONE
+ DISTA   EQ 500 MG BASE   N61896 001
TABLET, CHEWABLE; ORAL
ILOSONE
DISTA   EQ 125 MG BASE   N61895 001
+   EQ 250 MG BASE   N61895 002

ERYTHROMYCIN ESTOLATE; SULFISOXAZOLE ACETYL
SUSPENSION; ORAL
ILOSONE SULFA
+ LILLY   EQ 125 MG BASE/5 ML;EQ   N50599 001
  600 MG BASE/5 ML   SEP 29, 1989

ERYTHROMYCIN ETHYLSUCCINATE
DROPS; ORAL
PEDIAMYCIN
+ ROSS   EQ 100 MG BASE/2.5 ML   N62305 002
GRANULE; ORAL
E.E.S.
△AB + ABBOTT   EQ 200 MG BASE/5 ML   N50207 001
ERYPED
ABBOTT   EQ 400 MG BASE/5 ML   N50207 002
ERYTHROMYCIN ETHYLSUCCINATE
△AB BARR   EQ 200 MG BASE/5 ML   N62055 001
PEDIAMYCIN
△AB ROSS   EQ 200 MG BASE/5 ML   N62305 001
SUSPENSION; ORAL
E.E.S. 200
△AB ABBOTT   EQ 200 MG BASE/5 ML   N61639 001
E.E.S. 400
△AB + ABBOTT   EQ 400 MG BASE/5 ML   N61639 002
E-MYCIN E
△AB UPJOHN   EQ 200 MG BASE/5 ML   N62198 001
  EQ 400 MG BASE/5 ML   N62198 002
ERYTHROMYCIN ETHYLSUCCINATE
△AB BARRE   EQ 200 MG BASE/5 ML   N62200 001
△AB   EQ 400 MG BASE/5 ML   N62200 002
△AB DISTA   EQ 400 MG BASE/5 ML   N62177 001
△AB   EQ 400 MG BASE/5 ML   N62177 002
△AB KV   EQ 200 MG BASE/5 ML   N62047 001
△AB   EQ 400 MG BASE/5 ML   N62047 002
△AB PARKE DAVIS   EQ 400 MG BASE/5 ML   N62231 001
△AB   EQ 400 MG BASE/5 ML   N62231 002
△AB PHARMAFAIR   EQ 200 MG BASE/5 ML   N62559 001   MAR 15, 1985
△AB   EQ 400 MG BASE/5 ML   N62558 001   MAR 15, 1985
PEDIAMYCIN
△AB ROSS   EQ 200 MG BASE/5 ML   N62304 001
PEDIAMYCIN 400
△AB ROSS   EQ 400 MG BASE/5 ML   N62304 002
WYAMYCIN E
△AB WYETH AYERST   EQ 200 MG BASE/5 ML   N62123 002
△AB   EQ 400 MG BASE/5 ML   N62123 001

ERYTHROMYCIN ETHYLSUCCINATE (continued)
TABLET; ORAL
E.E.S. 400
△AB + ABBOTT   EQ 400 MG BASE   N61905 001
△AB   EQ 400 MG BASE   N61905 002   AUG 12, 1982
ERYTHROMYCIN ETHYLSUCCINATE
△AB BARR   EQ 400 MG BASE   N62256 001
△AB MYLAN   EQ 400 MG BASE   N62847 001   SEP 14, 1988
TABLET, CHEWABLE; ORAL
E.E.S.
△AB + ABBOTT   EQ 200 MG BASE   N50297 002
ERYPED
△AB ABBOTT   EQ 200 MG BASE   N50297 003   JUL 05, 1988
PEDIAMYCIN
△AB ROSS   EQ 200 MG BASE   N62306 001

ERYTHROMYCIN ETHYLSUCCINATE; SULFISOXAZOLE ACETYL
GRANULE; ORAL
ERYTHROMYCIN ETHYLSUCCINATE AND SULFISOXAZOLE ACETYL
△AB BARR   EQ 200 MG BASE/5 ML;EQ 600 MG BASE/5 ML   N62759 001   MAY 20, 1988
ERYZOLE
△AB ALRA   EQ 200 MG BASE/5 ML;EQ 600 MG BASE/5 ML   N62758 001   JUN 15, 1988
PEDIAZOLE
△AB + ROSS   EQ 200 MG BASE/5 ML;EQ 600 MG BASE/5 ML   N50529 001

ERYTHROMYCIN GLUCEPTATE
INJECTABLE; INJECTION
ILOTYCIN GLUCEPTATE
DISTA   EQ 250 MG BASE/VIAL   N50370 001
  EQ 500 MG BASE/VIAL   N50370 002
  EQ 1 GM BASE/VIAL   N50370 003

ERYTHROMYCIN LACTOBIONATE
INJECTABLE; INJECTION
ERYTHROCIN
△AP ABBOTT   EQ 500 MG BASE/VIAL   N50182 002
△AP   EQ 500 MG BASE/VIAL   N50609 001   SEP 24, 1986
△AP   EQ 500 MG BASE/VIAL   N62586 001   JAN 04, 1988
△AP   EQ 500 MG BASE/VIAL   N62638 001   OCT 31, 1986
△AP   EQ 1 GM BASE/VIAL   N50182 003
△AP   EQ 1 GM BASE/VIAL   N50609 002   SEP 24, 1986
△AP   EQ 1 GM BASE/VIAL   N62586 002   JAN 04, 1988
△AP   EQ 1 GM BASE/VIAL   N62638 002   OCT 31, 1986

Prescription Drug Products *(continued)*

ERYTHROMYCIN LACTOBIONATE *(continued)*

INJECTABLE; INJECTION

	Product	Manufacturer	Strength	Appl. No.	Date
	ERYTHROMYCIN				
ΔP		ELKINS SINN	EQ 500 MG BASE/VIAL	N62563 001	MAR 28, 1985
ΔP			EQ 1 GM BASE/VIAL	N62563 002	MAR 28, 1985
	ERYTHROMYCIN LACTOBIONATE				
ΔP		LEDERLE	EQ 500 MG BASE/VIAL	N62993 001	MAY 09, 1989
ΔP			EQ 1 GM BASE/VIAL	N62993 002	MAY 09, 1989
ΔP		LYPHOMED	EQ 500 MG BASE/VIAL	N62604 001	NOV 24, 1986
ΔP			EQ 1 GM BASE/VIAL	N62604 002	NOV 24, 1986

ERYTHROMYCIN STEARATE

TABLET; ORAL

	Product	Manufacturer	Strength	Appl. No.	Date
	ERYPAR				
ΔB		PARKE DAVIS	EQ 250 MG BASE	N62322 001	
	ERYTHROCIN STEARATE				
ΔB	+	ABBOTT	EQ 250 MG BASE	N60359 001	
ΔB			EQ 500 MG BASE	N60359 003	
	ERYTHROMYCIN STEARATE				
ΔB		BARR	EQ 250 MG BASE	N61591 001	
ΔB			EQ 500 MG BASE	N63179 001	MAY 15, 1990
ΔB		CHELSEA	EQ 250 MG BASE	N62121 002	
ΔB			EQ 500 MG BASE	N62121 001	
ΔB		MYLAN	EQ 250 MG BASE	N61505 001	
ΔB			EQ 500 MG BASE	N61505 002	
ΔB		PUREPAC	EQ 250 MG BASE	N61743 001	
ΔB		ZENITH	EQ 250 MG BASE	N61461 001	
ΔB			EQ 500 MG BASE	N61461 002	
	ETHRIL 250				
ΔB		SQUIBB	EQ 250 MG BASE	N61605 001	
	ETHRIL 500				
ΔB		SQUIBB	EQ 500 MG BASE	N61605 002	
	WYAMYCIN S				
ΔB		WYETH AYERST	EQ 250 MG BASE	N61675 001	
ΔB			EQ 500 MG BASE	N61675 002	

ESMOLOL HYDROCHLORIDE

INJECTABLE; INJECTION

	Product	Manufacturer	Strength	Appl. No.	Date
	BREVIBLOC				
		DUPONT	10 MG/ML	N19386 001	AUG 15, 1988
			250 MG/ML	N19386 002	DEC 31, 1986

ESTAZOLAM

TABLET; ORAL

	Product	Manufacturer	Strength	Appl. No.	Date
	PROSOM				
		ABBOTT	1 MG	N19080 001	DEC 26, 1990
			2 MG	N19080 002	DEC 26, 1990

ESTRADIOL

CREAM; VAGINAL

	Product	Manufacturer	Strength	Appl. No.	Date
	ESTRACE				
	+	MEAD JOHNSON	0.01%	N86069 001	JAN 31, 1984

FILM, EXTENDED RELEASE; TRANSDERMAL

	Product	Manufacturer	Strength	Appl. No.	Date
	ESTRADERM				
	+	CIBA	0.05 MG/24 HR	N19081 002	SEP 10, 1986
	+		0.1 MG/24 HR	N19081 003	SEP 10, 1986

TABLET; ORAL

	Product	Manufacturer	Strength	Appl. No.	Date
	ESTRACE				
		MEAD JOHNSON	1 MG	N84499 001	
	+		2 MG	N84500 001	

ESTRADIOL CYPIONATE

INJECTABLE; INJECTION

	Product	Manufacturer	Strength	Appl. No.	Date
	DEPO-ESTRADIOL				
		UPJOHN	5 MG/ML	N85470 003	
ΔO			1 MG/ML	N85470 001	
			3 MG/ML	N85470 002	
	ESTRADIOL CYPIONATE				
		STERIS	5 MG/ML	N85620 001	
ΔO					

ESTRADIOL CYPIONATE; TESTOSTERONE CYPIONATE

INJECTABLE; INJECTION

	Product	Manufacturer	Strength	Appl. No.	Date
	DEPO-TESTADIOL				
		UPJOHN	2 MG/ML;50 MG/ML	N17968 001	
ΔO					
	TESTOSTERONE CYPIONATE-ESTRADIOL CYPIONATE				
		STERIS	2 MG/ML;50 MG/ML	N85603 001	MAR 13, 1986
ΔO					

ESTRADIOL VALERATE

INJECTABLE; INJECTION

	Product	Manufacturer	Strength	Appl. No.	Date
	DELESTROGEN				
		SQUIBB	10 MG/ML	N09402 002	
ΔO			20 MG/ML	N09402 004	
ΔO			40 MG/ML	N09402 003	
	ESTRADIOL VALERATE				
		STERIS	10 MG/ML	N83546 001	
ΔO			20 MG/ML	N83547 001	
ΔO			40 MG/ML	N83714 001	

Prescription Drug Products (continued)

ESTRADIOL VALERATE; TESTOSTERONE ENANTHATE

INJECTABLE; INJECTION

DELADUMONE			
ΔQ	SQUIBB	4 MG/ML;90 MG/ML	N09545 001
DITATE-DS			
	SAVAGE	8 MG/ML;180 MG/ML	N86423 001
TESTOSTERONE ENANTHATE AND ESTRADIOL VALERATE			
ΔQ	STERIS	4 MG/ML;90 MG/ML	N85865 001

ESTRAMUSTINE PHOSPHATE SODIUM

CAPSULE; ORAL

EMCYT			
+	KABI	EQ 140 MG PHOSPHATE	N18045 001

ESTROGENS, CONJUGATED

CREAM; TOPICAL, VAGINAL

PREMARIN			
+	WYETH AYERST	0.625 MG/GM	N83273 001

INJECTABLE; INJECTION

PREMARIN			
	WYETH AYERST	25 MG/VIAL	N10402 001

TABLET; ORAL

PREMARIN			
	WYETH AYERST	0.3 MG	N04782 003
		0.625 MG	N04782 004
		0.9 MG	N04782 005 JAN 26, 1984
+		1.25 MG	N04782 001
		2.5 MG	N04782 002

ESTROGENS, CONJUGATED; MEPROBAMATE

TABLET; ORAL

PMB 200			
+	WYETH AYERST	0.45 MG;200 MG	N10971 005
PMB 400			
+	WYETH AYERST	0.45 MG;400 MG	N10971 003

ESTROGENS, ESTERIFIED

TABLET; ORAL

ESTRATAB			
BS	SOLVAY	0.3 MG	N86715 001
BS		0.625 MG	N83209 001
BS		1.25 MG	N83836 001
BS		2.5 MG	N83857 001
MENEST			
BS	BEECHAM	0.3 MG	N84951 001
BS	+	0.625 MG	N84948 001
BS	+	1.25 MG	N84950 001
BS	+	2.5 MG	N84949 001

ESTROGENS, ESTERIFIED; *MULTIPLE*

SEE CHLORDIAZEPOXIDE; ESTROGENS, ESTERIFIED

ESTRONE

INJECTABLE; INJECTION

ESTROGENIC SUBSTANCE			
	WYETH AYERST	2 MG/ML	N83488 001
ESTRONE			
BP	STERIS	2 MG/ML	N83397 001
BP		5 MG/ML	N85239 001
NATURAL ESTROGENIC SUBSTANCE-ESTRONE			
BP	STERIS	2 MG/ML	N85237 001 NOV 23, 1982
THEELIN			
BP	+ PARKE DAVIS	2 MG/ML	N03977 002

ESTROPIPATE

CREAM; VAGINAL

OGEN			
+	ABBOTT	1.5 MG/GM	N84710 001

TABLET; ORAL

OGEN .625			
ΔB	ABBOTT	0.75 MG	N83220 001
OGEN 1.25			
ΔB	+ ABBOTT	1.5 MG	N83220 002
OGEN 2.5			
	ABBOTT	3 MG	N83220 003
OGEN 5			
	ABBOTT	6 MG	N83220 004
ORTHO-EST			
ΔB	JOHNSON RW	0.75 MG	N89567 001 FEB 27, 1991
ΔB		1.5 MG	N89582 001 JUL 17, 1991

ETHACRYNATE SODIUM

INJECTABLE; INJECTION

EDECRIN			
	MSD	EQ 50 MG ACID/VIAL	N16093 001

ETHACRYNIC ACID

TABLET; ORAL

EDECRIN			
	MSD	25 MG	N16092 001
+		50 MG	N16092 002

ETHAMBUTOL HYDROCHLORIDE

TABLET; ORAL

MYAMBUTOL			
	LEDERLE	100 MG	N16320 001
		200 MG	N16320 002
		400 MG	N16320 003
+		500 MG	N16320 004

Prescription Drug Products (continued)

ETHANOLAMINE OLEATE
INJECTABLE; INJECTION
ETHAMOLIN
  REED AND CARNRICK   50 MG/ML   N19357 001 DEC 22, 1988

ETHCHLORVYNOL
CAPSULE; ORAL
ETHCHLORVYNOL

TE	Product	Strength	NDA
AA	BANNER GELATIN	200 MG	N84463 002
AA		500 MG	N84463 003
AA		750 MG	N84463 004
		100 MG	N84463 001

PLACIDYL

TE	Product	Strength	NDA
AA	ABBOTT	200 MG	N10021 007
AA		500 MG	N10021 002
AA		750 MG	N10021 010

ETHINAMATE
CAPSULE; ORAL
VALMID
  DISTA   500 MG   N09750 001

ETHINYL ESTRADIOL
TABLET; ORAL
ESTINYL

SCHERING	0.02 MG	N05292 001
	0.05 MG	N05292 002
	0.5 MG	N05292 003
+		

ETHINYL ESTRADIOL; ETHYNODIOL DIACETATE
TABLET; ORAL-21

TE	Product	Strength	NDA
AB	DEMULEN 1/35-21 + SEARLE	0.035 MG;1 MG	N18168 001
AB	DEMULEN 1/50-21 + SEARLE	0.05 MG;1 MG	N16927 001
AB	ETHYNODIOL DIACETATE AND ETHINYL ESTRADIOL 1/35-21 WATSON	0.035 MG;1 MG	N72720 001 DEC 30, 1991
AB	ETHYNODIOL DIACETATE AND ETHINYL ESTRADIOL 1/50-21 WATSON	0.05 MG;1 MG	N72722 001 DEC 30, 1991

TABLET; ORAL-28

TE	Product	Strength	NDA
AB	DEMULEN 1/35-28 SEARLE	0.035 MG;1 MG	N18160 001
AB	DEMULEN 1/50-28 SEARLE	0.05 MG;1 MG	N16936 001
AB	ETHYNODIOL DIACETATE AND ETHINYL ESTRADIOL 1/35-28 WATSON	0.035 MG;1 MG	N72721 001 DEC 30, 1991
AB	ETHYNODIOL DIACETATE AND ETHINYL ESTRADIOL 1/50-28 WATSON	0.05 MG;1 MG	N72723 001 DEC 30, 1991

ETHINYL ESTRADIOL; FERROUS FUMARATE; NORETHINDRONE
TABLET; ORAL-28
NORQUEST FE
  + SYNTEX   0.035 MG;75 MG;1 MG   N18926 001 JUL 18, 1986

ETHINYL ESTRADIOL; FERROUS FUMARATE; NORETHINDRONE ACETATE
TABLET; ORAL-28

LOESTRIN FE 1.5/30 + PARKE DAVIS	0.03 MG;75 MG;1.5 MG	N17355 001
LOESTRIN FE 1/20 + PARKE DAVIS	0.02 MG;75 MG;1 MG	N17354 001
NORLESTRIN FE 1/50 + PARKE DAVIS	0.05 MG;75 MG;1 MG	N16766 001
NORLESTRIN FE 2.5/50 + PARKE DAVIS	0.05 MG;75 MG;2.5 MG	N16854 001

ETHINYL ESTRADIOL; FLUOXYMESTERONE
TABLET; ORAL
HALODRIN
  + UPJOHN   0.02 MG;1 MG   N11267 001

ETHINYL ESTRADIOL; LEVONORGESTREL
TABLET; ORAL-21

NORDETTE-21 + WYETH AYERST	0.03 MG;0.15 MG	N18668 001 MAY 10, 1982
TRIPHASIL-21 + WYETH AYERST	0.03 MG,0.04 MG,0.03 MG;0.05 MG,0.075 MG,0.125 MG	N19192 001 NOV 01, 1984

TABLET; ORAL-28

NORDETTE-28 WYETH AYERST	0.03 MG;0.15 MG	N18782 001 JUL 21, 1982
TRIPHASIL-28 WYETH AYERST	0.03 MG,0.04 MG,0.03 MG;0.05 MG,0.075 MG,0.125 MG	N19190 001 NOV 01, 1984

ETHINYL ESTRADIOL; NORETHINDRONE
TABLET; ORAL-21

TE	Product	Strength	NDA
	BREVICON 21-DAY SYNTEX	0.035 MG;0.5 MG	N17566 001
AB	GENCEPT 0.5/35-21 GENCON	0.035 MG;0.5 MG	N72692 001 FEB 28, 1992
AB	GENCEPT 1/35-21 GENCON	0.035 MG;1 MG	N72693 001 FEB 28, 1992
AB	GENCEPT 10/11-21 GENCON	0.035 MG;0.5 MG AND 1 MG	N72694 001 FEB 28, 1992

Prescription Drug Products (continued)

ETHINYL ESTRADIOL; NORETHINDRONE (continued)

TABLET; ORAL-21

TE	Product / Firm	Strength	Appl No	Date
	MODICON 21			
AB	JOHNSON RW	0.035 MG;0.5 MG	N17488 001	
	NORCEPT-E 1/35 21			
AB	GYNOPHARMA	0.035 MG;1 MG	N71545 001	FEB 09, 1989
	NORETHIN 1/35E-21			
AB	SCHIAPPARELLI SEARLE	0.035 MG;1 MG	N71480 001	APR 12, 1988
	NORETHINDRONE AND ETHINYL ESTRADIOL			
AB	WATSON	0.035 MG;1 MG	N70685 001	JAN 29, 1987
AB	WATSON	0.035 MG;0.5 MG	N70684 001	JAN 29, 1987
	NORETHINDRONE AND ETHINYL ESTRADIOL (10/11)			
AB	WATSON	0.035 MG;0.5 MG AND 1 MG	N71043 001	APR 01, 1988
	NORETHINDRONE AND ETHINYL ESTRADIOL (7/14)			
	WATSON	0.035 MG;0.5 MG AND 1 MG	N71041 001	SEP 24, 1991
	NORINYL 1+35 21-DAY			
AB	SYNTEX	0.035 MG;1 MG	N17565 001	
	ORTHO-NOVUM 1/35-21			
AB	+ JOHNSON RW	0.035 MG;1 MG	N17489 002	
	ORTHO-NOVUM 10/11-21			
AB	+ JOHNSON RW	0.035 MG;0.5 MG AND 1 MG	N18354 001	JAN 11, 1982
	ORTHO-NOVUM 7/7/7-21			
	+ JOHNSON RW	0.035 MG;0.5 MG, 0.75 MG AND 1 MG	N18985 001	APR 04, 1984
	OVCON-35			
	+ MEAD JOHNSON	0.035 MG;0.4 MG	N18127 001	
	OVCON-50			
	+ MEAD JOHNSON	0.05 MG;1 MG	N18128 001	
	TRI-NORINYL 21-DAY			
	+ SYNTEX	0.035 MG;0.5 MG AND 1 MG	N18977 001	APR 13, 1984

TABLET; ORAL-28

TE	Product / Firm	Strength	Appl No	Date
	BREVICON 28-DAY			
AB	SYNTEX	0.035 MG;0.5 MG	N17743 001	
	GENCEPT 0.5/35-28			
AB	GENCON	0.035 MG;0.5 MG	N72695 001	FEB 28, 1992
	GENCEPT 1/35-28			
AB	GENCON	0.035 MG;1 MG	N72696 001	FEB 28, 1992
	GENCEPT 10/11-28			
AB	GENCON	0.035 MG;0.5 MG AND 1 MG	N72697 001	FEB 28, 1992

ETHINYL ESTRADIOL; NORETHINDRONE (continued)

TABLET; ORAL-28

TE	Product / Firm	Strength	Appl No	Date
	MODICON 28			
AB	JOHNSON RW	0.035 MG;0.5 MG	N17735 001	
	NORCEPT-E 1/35 28			
AB	GYNOPHARMA	0.035 MG;1 MG	N71546 001	FEB 09, 1989
	NORETHIN 1/35E-28			
AB	SCHIAPPARELLI SEARLE	0.035 MG;1 MG	N71481 001	APR 12, 1988
	NORETHINDRONE AND ETHINYL ESTRADIOL			
AB	WATSON	0.035 MG;1 MG	N70687 001	JAN 29, 1987
AB	WATSON	0.035 MG;0.5 MG	N70686 001	JAN 29, 1987
	NORETHINDRONE AND ETHINYL ESTRADIOL (10/11)			
AB	WATSON	0.035 MG;0.5 MG AND 1 MG	N71044 001	APR 01, 1988
	NORETHINDRONE AND ETHINYL ESTRADIOL (7/14)			
	WATSON	0.035 MG;0.5 MG AND 1 MG	N71042 001	SEP 24, 1991
	NORINYL 1+35 28-DAY			
AB	SYNTEX	0.035 MG;1 MG	N17565 002	
	ORTHO-NOVUM 1/35-28			
AB	JOHNSON RW	0.035 MG;1 MG	N17919 002	
	ORTHO-NOVUM 10/11-28			
AB	JOHNSON RW	0.035 MG;0.5 MG AND 1 MG	N18354 002	JAN 11, 1982
	ORTHO-NOVUM 7/7/7-28			
	JOHNSON RW	0.035 MG;0.5 MG, 0.75 MG AND 1 MG	N18985 002	APR 04, 1984
	OVCON-35			
	MEAD JOHNSON	0.035 MG;0.4 MG	N17716 001	
	OVCON-50			
	MEAD JOHNSON	0.05 MG;1 MG	N17576 001	
	TRI-NORINYL 28-DAY			
	SYNTEX	0.035 MG;0.5 MG AND 1 MG	N18977 002	APR 13, 1984

ETHINYL ESTRADIOL; NORETHINDRONE ACETATE

TABLET; ORAL-21

TE	Product / Firm	Strength	Appl No	Date
	LOESTRIN 21 1.5/30			
	+ PARKE DAVIS	0.03 MG;1.5 MG	N17875 001	
	LOESTRIN 21 1/20			
	+ PARKE DAVIS	0.02 MG;1 MG	N17876 001	
	NORLESTRIN 21 1/50			
	+ PARKE DAVIS	0.05 MG;1 MG	N16749 001	
	NORLESTRIN 21 2.5/50			
	+ PARKE DAVIS	0.05 MG;2.5 MG	N16852 001	

Prescription Drug Products (continued)

ETHINYL ESTRADIOL; NORGESTIMATE

TABLET; ORAL-21

ORTHO CYCLEN-21
+ JOHNSON RW   0.035 MG;0.25 MG   N19653 001 DEC 29, 1989

ORTHO TRI-CYCLEN
+ JOHNSON RW   0.035 MG;0.18 MG,0.215 MG,0.25 MG   N19697 002 JUL 03, 1992

TABLET; ORAL-28

ORTHO CYCLEN-28
JOHNSON RW   0.035 MG;0.25 MG   N19653 002 DEC 29, 1989

ORTHO TRI-CYCLEN
JOHNSON RW   0.035 MG;0.18 MG,0.215 MG,0.25 MG   N19697 001 JUL 03, 1992

ETHINYL ESTRADIOL; NORGESTREL

TABLET; ORAL-21

LO/OVRAL
+ WYETH AYERST   0.03 MG;0.3 MG   N17612 001

OVRAL
+ WYETH AYERST   0.05 MG;0.5 MG   N16672 001

TABLET; ORAL-28

LO/OVRAL-28
WYETH AYERST   0.03 MG;0.3 MG   N17802 001

OVRAL-28
WYETH AYERST   0.05 MG;0.5 MG   N16806 001

ETHIODIZED OIL

OIL; INTRALYMPHATIC, INTRAUTERINE

ETHIODOL
SAVAGE   99%   N09190 001

ETHIONAMIDE

TABLET; ORAL

TRECATOR-SC
WYETH AYERST   250 MG   N13026 002

ETHOPROPAZINE HYDROCHLORIDE

TABLET; ORAL

PARSIDOL
PARKE DAVIS   10 MG   N09078 003
              50 MG   N09078 006
              100 MG   N09078 008

ETHOSUXIMIDE

CAPSULE; ORAL

ZARONTIN
+ PARKE DAVIS   250 MG   N12380 001

SYRUP; ORAL

ZARONTIN
PARKE DAVIS   250 MG/5 ML   N80258 001

ETHOTOIN

TABLET; ORAL

PEGANONE
ABBOTT   250 MG   N10841 001
          500 MG   N10841 003
+

ETHYNODIOL DIACETATE; *MULTIPLE*

SEE ETHINYL ESTRADIOL; ETHYNODIOL DIACETATE

ETHYNODIOL DIACETATE; MESTRANOL

TABLET; ORAL-21

OVULEN-21
+ SEARLE   1 MG;0.1 MG   N16029 003

TABLET; ORAL-28

OVULEN-28
SEARLE   1 MG;0.1 MG   N16705 001

ETIDOCAINE HYDROCHLORIDE

INJECTABLE; INJECTION

DURANEST
ASTRA   1%   N17751 005

ETIDOCAINE HYDROCHLORIDE; *MULTIPLE*

SEE EPINEPHRINE BITARTRATE; ETIDOCAINE HYDROCHLORIDE

ETIDRONATE DISODIUM

INJECTABLE; INJECTION

DIDRONEL
P AND G   50 MG/ML   N19545 001 APR 20, 1987

TABLET; ORAL

DIDRONEL
P AND G   200 MG   N17831 001
           400 MG   N17831 002
+

ETODOLAC

CAPSULE; ORAL

LODINE
WYETH AYERST   200 MG   N18922 002 JAN 31, 1991
                300 MG   N18922 003 JAN 31, 1991
+

ETOMIDATE

INJECTABLE; INJECTION

AMIDATE
ABBOTT   2 MG/ML   N18227 001 SEP 07, 1982

Prescription Drug Products (continued)

ETOPOSIDE

CAPSULE; ORAL

VEPESID

	Strength	Appl. No.	Date
+ BRISTOL	50 MG	N19557 001	DEC 30, 1986

INJECTABLE; INJECTION

VEPESID

	Strength	Appl. No.	Date
BRISTOL	20 MG/ML	N18768 001	NOV 10, 1983

ETRETINATE

CAPSULE; ORAL

TEGISON

	Strength	Appl. No.	Date
ROCHE	10 MG	N19369 001	SEP 30, 1986
+	25 MG	N19369 002	SEP 30, 1986

FAMOTIDINE

INJECTABLE; INJECTION

PEPCID

	Strength	Appl. No.	Date
MERCK	10 MG/ML	N19510 001	NOV 04, 1986

POWDER FOR RECONSTITUTION; ORAL

PEPCID

	Strength	Appl. No.	Date
+ MERCK	40 MG/5 ML	N19527 001	FEB 02, 1987

TABLET; ORAL

PEPCID

	Strength	Appl. No.	Date
MERCK	20 MG	N19462 001	OCT 15, 1986
+	40 MG	N19462 002	OCT 15, 1986

FELODIPINE

TABLET, EXTENDED RELEASE; ORAL

PLENDIL

	Strength	Appl. No.	Date
MERCK	5 MG	N19834 001	JUL 25, 1991
	10 MG	N19834 002	JUL 25, 1991

FENFLURAMINE HYDROCHLORIDE

TABLET; ORAL

PONDIMIN

	Strength	Appl. No.	Date
+ ROBINS	20 MG	N16618 001	

FENOPROFEN CALCIUM

CAPSULE; ORAL

FENOPROFEN CALCIUM

		Strength	Appl. No.	Date
AB	DANBURY	EQ 200 MG BASE	N72981 001	AUG 19, 1991
AB		EQ 300 MG BASE	N72982 001	AUG 19, 1991
AB	GENEVA	EQ 200 MG BASE	N72394 001	OCT 17, 1988
AB		EQ 300 MG BASE	N72395 001	OCT 17, 1988
AB	PAR	EQ 200 MG BASE	N72437 001	AUG 22, 1988
AB		EQ 300 MG BASE	N72438 001	AUG 22, 1988
AB	WARNER CHILCOTT	EQ 200 MG BASE	N72946 001	APR 30, 1991
AB		EQ 300 MG BASE	N72472 001	APR 30, 1991
AB	WATSON	EQ 200 MG BASE	N72294 001	JUL 08, 1988
AB		EQ 300 MG BASE	N72293 001	JUL 08, 1988
AB	NALFON + DISTA	EQ 300 MG BASE	N17604 002	

NALFON 200

		Strength	Appl. No.	Date
AB	DISTA	EQ 200 MG BASE	N17604 003	

TABLET; ORAL

FENOPROFEN CALCIUM

		Strength	Appl. No.	Date
AB	CHELSEA	EQ 600 MG BASE	N72407 001	JUN 13, 1988
AB	DANBURY	EQ 600 MG BASE	N72602 001	OCT 11, 1988
AB	GENEVA	EQ 600 MG BASE	N72396 001	OCT 17, 1988
AB	LEDERLE	EQ 600 MG BASE	N72326 001	APR 20, 1988
AB	MUTUAL PHARM	EQ 600 MG BASE	N72902 001	DEC 21, 1990
AB	MYLAN	EQ 600 MG BASE	N72267 001	JUN 08, 1988
AB	PAR	EQ 600 MG BASE	N72429 001	JUL 19, 1988
AB	PUREPAC	EQ 600 MG BASE	N72274 001	MAY 02, 1988
AB	WATSON	EQ 600 MG BASE	N72165 001	JUL 08, 1988
AB	ZENITH	EQ 600 MG BASE	N72557 001	AUG 29, 1988
AB	NALFON + DISTA	EQ 600 MG BASE	N17710 001	

Prescription Drug Products (continued)

FENTANYL
FILM, EXTENDED RELEASE; TRANSDERMAL
  DURAGESIC
  + ALZA   0.6 MG/24 HR   N19813 004   AUG 07, 1990
  +   1.2 MG/24 HR   N19813 003   AUG 07, 1990
  +   1.8 MG/24 HR   N19813 002   AUG 07, 1990
  +   2.4 MG/24 HR   N19813 001   AUG 07, 1990

FENTANYL CITRATE
INJECTABLE; INJECTION
  FENTANYL CITRATE
AP ABBOTT   EQ 0.05 MG BASE/ML   N19115 001   JAN 12, 1985
AP   EQ 0.05 MG BASE/ML   N70636 001   APR 30, 1990
AP   EQ 0.05 MG BASE/ML   N70637 001   APR 30, 1990
AP ELKINS SINN   EQ 0.05 MG BASE/ML   N19101 001   JUL 11, 1984
AP STERIS   EQ 0.05 MG BASE/ML   N73488 001   JUN 30, 1992
AP STERLING   EQ 0.05 MG BASE/ML   N72786 001   SEP 24, 1991
  SUBLIMAZE
AP JANSSEN   EQ 0.05 MG BASE/ML   N16619 001

FENTANYL CITRATE; *MULTIPLE*
  SEE DROPERIDOL; FENTANYL CITRATE

FERROUS FUMARATE; *MULTIPLE*
  SEE ETHINYL ESTRADIOL; FERROUS FUMARATE; NORETHINDRONE ACETATE
  SEE ETHINYL ESTRADIOL; FERROUS FUMARATE; NORETHINDRONE

FIBRINOGEN, I-125
INJECTABLE; INJECTION
  RADIONUCLIDE-LABELED (125 I) FIBRINOGEN (HUMAN) SENSOR
  ABBOTT   140 UCI/ML   N17787 001

FIBRINOLYSIN; *MULTIPLE*
  SEE CHLORAMPHENICOL; DESOXYRIBONUCLEASE; FIBRINOLYSIN

FINASTERIDE
TABLET; ORAL
  PROSCAR
  + MSD   5 MG   N20180 001   JUN 19, 1992

FLAVOXATE HYDROCHLORIDE
TABLET; ORAL
  URISPAS
  + SKF   100 MG   N16769 001

FLECAINIDE ACETATE
TABLET; ORAL
  TAMBOCOR
  3M   50 MG   N18830 004   AUG 23, 1988
                100 MG   N18830 001   OCT 31, 1985
  +   150 MG   N18830 003   JUN 03, 1988

FLOXURIDINE
INJECTABLE; INJECTION
  FUDR
  ROCHE   500 MG/VIAL   N16929 001

FLUCONAZOLE
INJECTABLE; INJECTION
  DIFLUCAN
  PFIZER   2 MG/ML   N19950 001   JAN 29, 1990
TABLET; ORAL
  DIFLUCAN
  + PFIZER   50 MG   N19949 001   JAN 29, 1990
  +   100 MG   N19949 002   JAN 29, 1990
  +   200 MG   N19949 003   JAN 29, 1990

FLUCYTOSINE
CAPSULE; ORAL
  ANCOBON
  ROCHE   250 MG   N17001 001
  +   500 MG   N17001 002

FLUDARABINE PHOSPHATE
INJECTABLE; INJECTION
  FLUDARA
  BERLEX   50 MG/VIAL   N20038 001   APR 18, 1991

FLUDROCORTISONE ACETATE
TABLET; ORAL
  FLORINEF
  + SQUIBB   0.1 MG   N10060 001

Prescription Drug Products *(continued)*

FLUMAZENIL
INJECTABLE; INJECTION
	MAZICON			
	ROCHE	0.1 MG/ML	N20073 001	DEC 20, 1991

FLUNISOLIDE
AEROSOL, METERED; INHALATION
	AEROBID			
	+ SYNTEX	0.25 MG/INH	N18340 001	AUG 17, 1984

SPRAY, METERED; NASAL
	NASALIDE			
	+ SYNTEX	0.025 MG/INH	N18148 001	

FLUOCINOLONE ACETONIDE
CREAM; TOPICAL
	FLUOCET			
AT	NMC	0.025%	N88360 001	JAN 16, 1984
	FLUOCINOLONE ACETONIDE			
AT	CLAY PARK	0.01%	N86810 001	MAR 04, 1982
AT		0.025%	N86811 001	MAR 04, 1982
AT	FOUGERA	0.01%	N88170 001	DEC 16, 1982
AT		0.025%	N88169 001	DEC 16, 1982
AT	G AND W	0.01%	N89526 001	JUL 26, 1988
AT		0.025%	N89525 001	JUL 26, 1988
AT	NMC	0.01%	N88361 001	JAN 16, 1984
AT	PHARMADERM	0.01%	N88047 001	DEC 16, 1982
AT		0.025%	N88045 001	DEC 16, 1982
AT	PHARMAFAIR	0.01%	N88499 001	AUG 02, 1984
AT		0.025%	N88506 001	AUG 02, 1984
AT	THAMES	0.01%	N87102 001	APR 27, 1982
AT		0.025%	N87104 001	APR 27, 1982
	FLUONID			
AT	ALLERGAN HERBERT	0.025%	N87156 002	SEP 06, 1984
	SYNALAR			
AT	SYNTEX	0.01%	N12787 004	
AT		0.025%	N12787 002	
	SYNALAR-HP			
	SYNTEX	0.2%	N16161 002	
	SYNEMOL			
AT	SYNTEX	0.025%	N12787 005	

FLUOCINOLONE ACETONIDE *(continued)*
OIL; TOPICAL
	DERMA-SMOOTHE/FS			
	HILL DERMAC	0.01%	N19452 001	FEB 03, 1988

OINTMENT; TOPICAL
	FLUOCINOLONE ACETONIDE			
AT	FOUGERA	0.025%	N88168 001	DEC 16, 1982
AT	G AND W	0.025%	N89524 001	JUL 26, 1988
AT	PHARMADERM	0.025%	N88046 001	DEC 16, 1982
AT	PHARMAFAIR	0.025%	N88507 001	FEB 27, 1984
	FLUONID			
AT	HERBERT	0.025%	N87157 001	SEP 06, 1984
	SYNALAR			
AT	SYNTEX	0.025%	N13960 001	

SHAMPOO; TOPICAL
	FS SHAMPOO			
	HILL DERMAC	0.01%	N20001 001	AUG 27, 1990

SOLUTION; TOPICAL
	FLUOCINOLONE ACETONIDE			
AT	BARRE	0.01%	N87159 001	JUN 16, 1982
AT	FOUGERA	0.01%	N88167 001	DEC 16, 1982
AT	PHARM BASICS	0.01%	N88312 001	JAN 27, 1984
AT	PHARMADERM	0.01%	N88048 001	DEC 16, 1982
AT	PHARMAFAIR	0.01%	N88449 001	FEB 08, 1984
AT	THAMES	0.01%	N89124 001	SEP 11, 1985
	FLUONID			
AT	HERBERT	0.01%	N87158 001	MAR 17, 1983
	SYNALAR			
AT	SYNTEX	0.01%	N15296 001	

FLUOCINOLONE ACETONIDE; NEOMYCIN SULFATE
CREAM; TOPICAL
	NEO-SYNALAR			
	SYNTEX	0.025%;EQ 3.5 MG BASE/GM	N60700 001	

Prescription Drug Products (continued)

FLUOCINONIDE

CREAM; TOPICAL
FLUOCINONIDE

TE	Applicant	Strength	Appl. No.	Date
B*	CLAY PARK	0.05%	N71790 001	APR 25, 1988
ΔB	LEMMON	0.05%	N72488 001	FEB 06, 1989
		0.05%	N72490 001	FEB 07, 1989
ΔB	NMC	0.05%	N73085 001	FEB 14, 1992
ΔB	TARO	0.05%	N19117 001	JUN 26, 1984
ΔB	THAMES	0.05%	N71500 001	JUN 10, 1987
ΔB	TICAN	0.05%	N72494 001	JAN 19, 1989
ΔB	LIDEX + SYNTEX	0.05%	N16908 002	
ΔB	LIDEX-E SYNTEX	0.05%	N16908 003	

GEL; TOPICAL
FLUOCINONIDE

TE	Applicant	Strength	Appl. No.	Date
ΔB	LEMMON	0.05%	N72537 001	FEB 07, 1989
ΔB	LIDEX + SYNTEX	0.05%	N17373 001	

OINTMENT; TOPICAL
FLUOCINONIDE

TE	Applicant	Strength	Appl. No.	Date
ΔB	LEMMON	0.05%	N73481 001	DEC 27, 1991
ΔB	LIDEX + SYNTEX	0.05%	N16909 002	

SOLUTION; TOPICAL
FLUOCINONIDE

TE	Applicant	Strength	Appl. No.	Date
ΔI	BARRE	0.05%	N71535 001	DEC 02, 1988
ΔI	COPLEY	0.05%	N72522 001	SEP 28, 1990
ΔI	LEMMON	0.05%	N72511 001	FEB 07, 1989
ΔI	THAMES	0.05%	N72857 001	AUG 02, 1989
ΔI	LIDEX SYNTEX	0.05%	N18849 001	APR 06, 1984

FLUORESCEIN SODIUM

INJECTABLE; INJECTION
FUNDUSCEIN-25

TE	Applicant	Strength	Appl. No.
	IOLAB	25%	N17869 001

FLUOROMETHOLONE

OINTMENT; OPHTHALMIC
FML

TE	Applicant	Strength	Appl. No.	Date
	+ ALLERGAN	0.1%	N17760 001	SEP 04, 1985

SUSPENSION/DROPS; OPHTHALMIC
FLUOR-OP

TE	Applicant	Strength	Appl. No.	Date
ΔB	IOLAB	0.1%	N70185 001	FEB 27, 1986
ΔB	FML + ALLERGAN	0.1%	N16851 002	JUL 28, 1982
ΔB	FML FORTE ALLERGAN	0.25%	N19216 001	APR 23, 1986

FLUOROMETHOLONE; SULFACETAMIDE SODIUM

SUSPENSION/DROPS; OPHTHALMIC
FML-S

TE	Applicant	Strength	Appl. No.	Date
	+ ALLERGAN	0.1%;10%	N19525 001	SEP 29, 1989

FLUOROMETHOLONE ACETATE

SUSPENSION/DROPS; OPHTHALMIC
FLAREX

TE	Applicant	Strength	Appl. No.	Date
	+ ALCON	0.1%	N19079 001	FEB 11, 1986

FLUOROMETHOLONE ACETATE; TOBRAMYCIN

SUSPENSION/DROPS; OPHTHALMIC
TOBRASONE

TE	Applicant	Strength	Appl. No.	Date
	+ ALCON	0.1%;0.3%	N50628 001	JUL 21, 1989

FLUOROURACIL

CREAM; TOPICAL
EFUDEX

TE	Applicant	Strength	Appl. No.
	+ ROCHE	5%	N16831 003
	FLUOROPLEX + HERBERT	1%	N16988 001

INJECTABLE; INJECTION
ADRUCIL

TE	Applicant	Strength	Appl. No.	Date
ΔP	ADRIA	50 MG/ML	N17959 001 / N40023 001	OCT 18, 1991
ΔP		50 MG/ML	N81222 001	JUN 28, 1991
ΔP		50 MG/ML	N81225 001	AUG 28, 1991

Prescription Drug Products (continued)

FLUOROURACIL (continued)

INJECTABLE; INJECTION

FLUOROURACIL

TE	Firm	Strength	Appl. No.	Date
ΔP	ABIC	50 MG/ML	N88929 001	MAR 04, 1986
ΔP	BEN VENUE	50 MG/ML	N89508 001	JAN 26, 1988
ΔP	LYPHOMED	50 MG/ML	N89152 001	MAR 21, 1986
ΔP		50 MG/ML	N89428 001	JAN 12, 1987
ΔP		50 MG/ML	N89519 001	MAR 12, 1987
ΔP	MARCHAR	50 MG/ML	N87791 001	JAN 18, 1983
ΔP		50 MG/ML	N12209 001	
ΔP	ROCHE	50 MG/ML	N88767 001	DEC 28, 1984
ΔP	SMITH NEPHEW SOLOPAK	50 MG/ML	N89434 001	MAR 26, 1987
ΔP	STERIS	50 MG/ML	N87792 001	OCT 13, 1982

SOLUTION; TOPICAL

EFUDEX

Firm	Strength	Appl. No.
ROCHE	2%	N16831 001
	5%	N16831 002

FLUOROPLEX

Firm	Strength	Appl. No.
HERBERT	1%	N16765 001

FLUOXETINE HYDROCHLORIDE

CAPSULE; ORAL

PROZAC

TE	Firm	Strength	Appl. No.	Date
+	LILLY	EQ 20 MG BASE	N18936 001	DEC 29, 1987

SOLUTION; ORAL

PROZAC

Firm	Strength	Appl. No.	Date
LILLY	EQ 20 MG BASE/5 ML	N20101 001	APR 24, 1991

FLUOXYMESTERONE

TABLET; ORAL

ANDROID-F

TE	Firm	Strength	Appl. No.
BP	ICN	10 MG	N87196 001

FLUOXYMESTERONE

TE	Firm	Strength	Appl. No.	Date
BP	ICN	10 MG	N88221 001	MAY 05, 1983
BP	PHARM BASICS	10 MG	N88342 001	OCT 21, 1983

HALOTESTIN

TE	Firm	Strength	Appl. No.
BP	+ UPJOHN	10 MG	N10611 010
		2 MG	N10611 002
		5 MG	N10611 006

FLUOXYMESTERONE; *MULTIPLE*

SEE ETHINYL ESTRADIOL; FLUOXYMESTERONE

FLUPHENAZINE DECANOATE

INJECTABLE; INJECTION

FLUPHENAZINE DECANOATE

TE	Firm	Strength	Appl. No.	Date
ΔO	LYPHOMED	25 MG/ML	N71413 001	JUL 14, 1987

PROLIXIN DECANOATE

TE	Firm	Strength	Appl. No.
ΔO	SQUIBB	25 MG/ML	N16727 001

FLUPHENAZINE ENANTHATE

INJECTABLE; INJECTION

PROLIXIN ENANTHATE

Firm	Strength	Appl. No.
SQUIBB	25 MG/ML	N16110 001

FLUPHENAZINE HYDROCHLORIDE

CONCENTRATE; ORAL

FLUPHENAZINE HCL

TE	Firm	Strength	Appl. No.	Date
ΔA	COPLEY	5 MG/ML	N73058 001	AUG 30, 1991

PERMITIL

TE	Firm	Strength	Appl. No.
ΔA	SCHERING	5 MG/ML	N16008 001

PROLIXIN

TE	Firm	Strength	Appl. No.	Date
ΔA	SQUIBB	5 MG/ML	N70533 001	NOV 07, 1985

ELIXIR; ORAL

PROLIXIN

Firm	Strength	Appl. No.
SQUIBB	2.5 MG/5 ML	N12145 003

INJECTABLE; INJECTION

FLUPHENAZINE HCL

TE	Firm	Strength	Appl. No.	Date
ΔP	LYPHOMED	2.5 MG/ML	N89556 001	APR 16, 1987

PROLIXIN

TE	Firm	Strength	Appl. No.
ΔP	SQUIBB	2.5 MG/ML	N11751 005

TABLET; ORAL

FLUPHENAZINE HCL

TE	Firm	Strength	Appl. No.	Date
ΔB	GENEVA	1 MG	N89583 001	OCT 16, 1987
ΔB		2.5 MG	N89584 001	OCT 16, 1987
ΔB		5 MG	N89585 001	OCT 16, 1987
ΔB		10 MG	N89586 001	OCT 16, 1987
ΔB	MYLAN	1 MG	N89801 001	AUG 12, 1988
ΔB		2.5 MG	N89802 001	AUG 12, 1988
ΔB		5 MG	N89803 001	AUG 12, 1988
ΔB		10 MG	N89804 001	AUG 12, 1988

Prescription Drug Products (continued)

FLUPHENAZINE HYDROCHLORIDE (continued)

TABLET; ORAL
FLUPHENAZINE HCL

AB	PAR	1 MG	N89740 001	AUG 25, 1988
AB		2.5 MG	N89741 001	AUG 25, 1988
AB		5 MG	N89742 001	AUG 25, 1988
AB		10 MG	N89743 001	AUG 25, 1988

PERMITIL

BP	SCHERING	2.5 MG	N12034 004
BP		5 MG	N12034 005
BP		10 MG	N12034 006

PROLIXIN

AB	SQUIBB	1 MG	N11751 004
AB		2.5 MG	N11751 001
AB		5 MG	N11751 003
AB +		10 MG	N11751 002

TABLET, EXTENDED RELEASE; ORAL
PERMITIL

+	SCHERING	1 MG	N12419 004

FLURANDRENOLIDE

CREAM; TOPICAL
CORDRAN SP

	DISTA	0.025%	N12806 003
		0.05%	N12806 002

LOTION; TOPICAL
CORDRAN

AT	DISTA	0.05%	N13790 001	

FLURANDRENOLIDE

AT	BARRE	0.05%	N87203 001	APR 29, 1982

OINTMENT; TOPICAL
CORDRAN

	DISTA	0.025%	N12806 004
		0.05%	N12806 001

TAPE; TOPICAL
CORDRAN

+	DISTA	0.004 MG/SQ CM	N16455 001

FLURANDRENOLIDE; NEOMYCIN SULFATE

CREAM; TOPICAL
CORDRAN-N

	LILLY	0.05%;EQ 3.5 MG BASE/GM	N50346 001

OINTMENT; TOPICAL
CORDRAN-N

	LILLY	0.05%;EQ 3.5 MG BASE/GM	N50345 001

FLURAZEPAM HYDROCHLORIDE

CAPSULE; ORAL
DALMANE

AB	ROCHE	15 MG	N16721 001	
AB +		30 MG	N16721 002	

FLURAZEPAM HCL

AB	BARR	15 MG	N70454 001	AUG 04, 1986
AB		30 MG	N70455 001	AUG 04, 1986
AB	CHELSEA	15 MG	N72368 001	MAR 30, 1989
AB		30 MG	N72369 001	MAR 30, 1989
AB	DANBURY	15 MG	N71205 001	NOV 25, 1986
AB		30 MG	N71068 001	NOV 25, 1986
AB	GENEVA	15 MG	N71716 001	JUL 31, 1991
AB		30 MG	N71717 001	JUL 31, 1991
AB	HALSEY	15 MG	N71808 001	JAN 07, 1988
AB		30 MG	N71809 001	JAN 07, 1988
AB	MYLAN	15 MG	N70344 001	NOV 27, 1985
AB		30 MG	N70345 001	NOV 27, 1985
AB	PAR	15 MG	N70444 001	MAR 20, 1986
AB		30 MG	N70445 001	MAR 20, 1986
AB	PUREPAC	15 MG	N71927 001	SEP 09, 1987
AB		30 MG	N71551 001	SEP 09, 1987
AB	SUPERPHARM	15 MG	N71659 001	AUG 04, 1988
AB		30 MG	N71660 001	AUG 04, 1988
AB	WARNER CHILCOTT	15 MG	N71767 001	DEC 04, 1987
AB		30 MG	N71768 001	DEC 04, 1987
AB	WEST WARD	15 MG	N71107 001	DEC 08, 1986
AB		30 MG	N71108 001	DEC 08, 1986

FLURBIPROFEN

TABLET; ORAL
ANSAID

	UPJOHN	50 MG	N18766 002	OCT 31, 1988
+		100 MG	N18766 003	OCT 31, 1988

Prescription Drug Products (continued)

FLURBIPROFEN SODIUM

SOLUTION/DROPS; OPHTHALMIC
OCUFEN

ALLERGAN	0.03%	N19404 001	DEC 31, 1986

FLUTAMIDE

CAPSULE; ORAL
EULEXIN

+ SCHERING	125 MG	N18554 001	JAN 27, 1989

FLUTICASONE PROPIONATE

CREAM; TOPICAL
CUTIVATE

+ GLAXO	0.05%	N19958 001	DEC 18, 1990

OINTMENT; TOPICAL
CUTIVATE

+ GLAXO	0.005%	N19957 001	DEC 14, 1990

FOLIC ACID

INJECTABLE; INJECTION
FOLIC ACID

AP	LYPHOMED	5 MG/ML	N89202 001	FEB 18, 1986

FOLVITE

AP	LEDERLE	5 MG/ML	N05897 008

TABLET; ORAL
FOLIC ACID

AA	DANBURY	1MG	N80680 001	
AA	HALSEY	1MG	N83598 001	
AA	ICN	1MG	N80903 001	
AA	LANNETT	1MG	N80816 001	
AA	MK	1MG	N83526 001	
AA	PHOENIX LABS	1MG	N86296 001	
AA	PIONEER PHARMS	1MG	N88949 001	SEP 13, 1985
AA	PRIVATE FORM	1MG	N85061 001	
AA	PUREPAC	1MG	N80784 001	
AA	RICHLYN	1MG	N80686 001	
AA	TABLICAPS	1MG	N83133 002	
AA	WEST WARD	1MG	N80600 001	
AA	ZENITH	1MG	N83000 001	

FOLICET

AA	MISSION PHARMA	1MG	N87438 001

FOLVITE

AA	LEDERLE	1MG	N05897 004

FOLIC ACID; *MULTIPLE*

SEE ASCORBIC ACID: BIOTIN: CYANOCOBALAMIN: DEXPANTHENOL: ERGOCALCIFEROL: FOLIC ACID: NIACINAMIDE: PYRIDOXINE HYDROCHLORIDE: RIBOFLAVIN PHOSPHATE SODIUM: THIAMINE HYDROCHLORIDE: VITAMIN A: VITAMIN E

SEE ASCORBIC ACID: BIOTIN: CYANOCOBALAMIN: DEXPANTHENOL: ERGOCALCIFEROL: FOLIC ACID: NIACINAMIDE: PYRIDOXINE: RIBOFLAVIN PHOSPHATE SODIUM: THIAMINE: VITAMIN A: VITAMIN E

FOSCARNET SODIUM

INJECTABLE; INJECTION
FOSCAVIR

ASTRA	24 MG/ML	N20068 001	SEP 27, 1991

FOSINOPRIL SODIUM

TABLET; ORAL
MONOPRIL
BRISTOL MYERS

SQUIBB	10 MG	N19915 002	MAY 16, 1991
		N19915 003	MAY 16, 1991
+	20 MG		

FURAZOLIDONE

SUSPENSION; ORAL
FUROXONE

+ ROBERTS	50 MG/15 ML	N11323 002	

TABLET; ORAL
FUROXONE

+ ROBERTS	100 MG	N11270 002	

FUROSEMIDE

INJECTABLE; INJECTION
FUROSEMIDE

AP	ABBOTT	10 MG/ML	N18667 001	MAY 28, 1982
AP	ASTRA	10 MG/ML	N70014 001	
			N70095 001	SEP 09, 1985
AP		10 MG/ML	N70096 001	SEP 09, 1985
AP		10 MG/ML		SEP 09, 1985
AP	ELKINS SINN	10 MG/ML	N18267 001	SEP 09, 1985
AP	INTL MEDICATION	10 MG/ML	N18025 001	
AP	LEDERLE	10 MG/ML	N71439 001	SEP 14, 1990
AP	LUITPOLD	10 MG/ML	N18579 001	NOV 30, 1983

Prescription Drug Products (continued)

FUROSEMIDE (continued)

INJECTABLE; INJECTION

TE	FUROSEMIDE	Strength	Appl. No.	Date
AP	LYPHOMED	10 MG/ML	N18902 001	MAY 22, 1984
AP	ORGANON	10 MG/ML	N70017 001	DEC 15, 1986
AP	SMITH NEPHEW SOLOPAK	10 MG/ML	N70078 001	FEB 05, 1986
AP	STERIS	10 MG/ML	N70019 001	SEP 22, 1986
AP		10 MG/ML	N70604 001	JAN 02, 1987
AP	STERLING	10 MG/ML	N70578 001	JUL 08, 1987
AP		10 MG/ML	N72080 001	AUG 13, 1991
AP	WARNER CHILCOTT	10 MG/ML	N18420 001	FEB 26, 1982
AP	WYETH AYERST	10 MG/ML	N18670 001	JUL 20, 1982

TE	LASIX	Strength	Appl. No.	Date
AP	HOECHST ROUSSEL	10 MG/ML	N16363 001	

SOLUTION; ORAL

TE	FUROSEMIDE	Strength	Appl. No.	Date
AA	PHARM BASICS	10 MG/ML	N70655 001	OCT 02, 1987
AA	ROXANE	10 MG/ML	N70434 001	APR 22, 1987
		40 MG/5 ML	N70433 001	APR 22, 1987

TE	LASIX	Strength	Appl. No.	Date
AA	HOECHST ROUSSEL	10 MG/ML	N17688 001	

TABLET; ORAL

TE	FUROSEMIDE	Strength	Appl. No.	Date
AB	BARR	20 MG	N70043 001	SEP 26, 1985
AB		40 MG	N18790 001	NOV 29, 1983
AB		80 MG	N70100 001	JAN 26, 1988
AB	DANBURY	20 MG	N70412 001	FEB 26, 1986
AB		40 MG	N70413 001	FEB 26, 1986
AB		80 MG	N71594 001	FEB 09, 1988
AB	GENEVA	20 MG	N18569 002	
AB		40 MG	N18569 001	
AB		80 MG	N18569 005	AUG 14, 1984
AB	INTL MEDICATION	20 MG	N18753 001	FEB 28, 1984
AB		40 MG	N18753 002	FEB 28, 1984

FUROSEMIDE (continued)

TABLET; ORAL

TE	FUROSEMIDE	Strength	Appl. No.	Date
AB	KALAPHARM	20 MG	N18868 001	JUN 28, 1983
AB		40 MG	N18868 002	JUN 28, 1983
AB	LEDERLE	20 MG	N18415 001	JUL 27, 1982
AB		40 MG	N18415 002	JUL 27, 1982
AB		80 MG	N18415 003	NOV 26, 1984
AB	MYLAN	20 MG	N18487 001	
AB		40 MG	N18487 002	
AB		80 MG	N70082 001	OCT 29, 1986
AB	PARKE DAVIS	20 MG	N18419 001	JAN 31, 1983
AB		40 MG	N18419 002	JAN 31, 1983
AB		80 MG	N18419 003	NOV 13, 1984
AB	ROXANE	20 MG	N18823 001	NOV 10, 1983
AB		40 MG	N18823 002	NOV 10, 1983
AB		80 MG	N70086 001	JAN 24, 1986
AB	SUPERPHARM	20 MG	N18370 002	JUN 26, 1984
AB		40 MG	N18370 001	FEB 10, 1983
AB	WATSON	20 MG	N70449 001	NOV 22, 1985
AB		40 MG	N71379 001	JAN 02, 1987
AB		40 MG	N70450 001	NOV 22, 1985
AB		80 MG	N70528 001	JAN 07, 1986
AB	ZENITH	20 MG	N18413 001	NOV 30, 1983
AB		40 MG	N18413 002	NOV 30, 1983

TE	LASIX	Strength	Appl. No.	Date
AB	HOECHST ROUSSEL	20 MG	N16273 002	
AB		40 MG	N16273 001	
AB	+	80 MG	N16273 003	

GADOPENTETATE DIMEGLUMINE

INJECTABLE; INJECTION

	MAGNEVIST	Strength	Appl. No.	Date
	BERLEX	469.01 MG/ML	N19596 001	JUN 02, 1988

Prescription Drug Products (continued)

GALLAMINE TRIETHIODIDE

INJECTABLE; INJECTION

FLAXEDIL

TE	Firm	Strength	Appl. No.
	DAVIS AND GECK	20 MG/ML	N07842 001
		100 MG/ML	N07842 002

GALLIUM CITRATE, GA-67

INJECTABLE; INJECTION

GALLIUM CITRATE GA 67

TE	Firm	Strength	Appl. No.
BS	DUPONT MERCK	2 MCI/ML	N17478 001
BS	MALLINCKRODT	2 MCI/ML	N18058 001

NEOSCAN

TE	Firm	Strength	Appl. No.
BS	MEDI PHYSICS	2 MCI/ML	N17655 001

GALLIUM NITRATE

INJECTABLE; INJECTION

GANITE

TE	Firm	Strength	Appl. No.	Date
	FUJISAWA	25 MG/ML	N19961 002	JAN 17, 1991

GANCICLOVIR SODIUM

INJECTABLE; INJECTION

CYTOVENE

TE	Firm	Strength	Appl. No.	Date
	SYNTEX	EQ 500 MG BASE/VIAL	N19661 001	JUN 23, 1989

GEMFIBROZIL

CAPSULE; ORAL

LOPID

TE	Firm	Strength	Appl. No.
	+ PARKE DAVIS	300 MG	N18422 002

TABLET; ORAL

LOPID

TE	Firm	Strength	Appl. No.	Date
	+ PARKE DAVIS	600 MG	N18422 003	NOV 20, 1986

GENTAMICIN SULFATE

CREAM; TOPICAL

GARAMYCIN

TE	Firm	Strength	Appl. No.	Date
AT	SCHERING	EQ 1 MG BASE/GM	N60462 001	

GENTAFAIR

TE	Firm	Strength	Appl. No.	Date
AT	PHARMAFAIR	EQ 1 MG BASE/GM	N62458 001	SEP 01, 1983

GENTAMICIN

TE	Firm	Strength	Appl. No.	Date
AT	CLAY PARK	EQ 1 MG BASE/GM	N62307 001	
AT	THAMES	EQ 1 MG BASE/GM	N62427 001	MAY 26, 1983

GENTAMICIN SULFATE

TE	Firm	Strength	Appl. No.	Date
AT	FOUGERA	EQ 1 MG BASE/GM	N62531 001	JUL 05, 1984
AT	NMC	EQ 1 MG BASE/GM	N62471 001	SEP 27, 1983
AT	PHARMADERM	EQ 1 MG BASE/GM	N62530 001	JUL 05, 1984

GENTAMICIN SULFATE (continued)

INJECTABLE; INJECTION

APOGEN

TE	Firm	Strength	Appl. No.	Date
AP	BEECHAM	EQ 10 MG BASE/ML	N62289 001	
AP		EQ 40 MG BASE/ML	N62289 002	

BRISTAGEN

TE	Firm	Strength	Appl. No.	Date
AP	BRISTOL	EQ 40 MG BASE/ML	N62288 001	

GARAMYCIN

TE	Firm	Strength	Appl. No.	Date
AP	SCHERING	EQ 1 MG BASE/ML	N61716 002	
AP		EQ 10 MG BASE/ML	N61739 001	
AP		EQ 40 MG BASE/ML	N61716 001	
		EQ 2 MG BASE/ML	N50505 001	

GENTAFAIR

TE	Firm	Strength	Appl. No.	Date
AP	PHARMAFAIR	EQ 40 MG BASE/ML	N62493 001	AUG 28, 1985

GENTAMICIN

TE	Firm	Strength	Appl. No.	Date
AP	INTL MEDICATION	EQ 1 MG BASE/ML	N62325 003	JUN 23, 1982
AP		EQ 100 MG BASE/100 ML	N62325 004	JUN 23, 1982
AP		EQ 40 MG BASE/ML	N62325 001	

GENTAMICIN SULFATE

TE	Firm	Strength	Appl. No.	Date
AP	ABBOTT	EQ 60 MG BASE/100 ML	N62413 006	AUG 11, 1983
AP		EQ 70 MG BASE/100 ML	N62413 007	AUG 11, 1983
AP		EQ 80 MG BASE/100 ML	N62413 008	AUG 11, 1983
AP		EQ 90 MG BASE/100 ML	N62413 009	AUG 11, 1983
AP		EQ 100 MG BASE/100 ML	N62413 010	AUG 11, 1983
AP		EQ 1.2 MG BASE/ML	N62413 001	AUG 11, 1983
AP		EQ 1.4 MG BASE/ML	N62413 002	AUG 11, 1983
AP		EQ 1.6 MG BASE/ML	N62413 003	AUG 11, 1983
AP		EQ 1.8 MG BASE/ML	N62413 004	AUG 11, 1983
AP		EQ 2 MG BASE/ML	N62413 005	AUG 11, 1983
AP		EQ 10 MG BASE/ML	N62420 001	AUG 11, 1983
AP		EQ 40 MG BASE/ML	N62420 002	FEB 20, 1986
AP	ELKINS SINN	EQ 10 MG BASE/ML	N62612 004	AUG 15, 1983
AP	GENSIA	EQ 10 MG BASE/ML	N62251 002	AUG 15, 1983
AP		EQ 40 MG BASE/ML	N62251 001	
AP		EQ 10 MG BASE/ML	N63149 001	NOV 21, 1991
AP		EQ 40 MG BASE/ML	N63106 002	NOV 21, 1991

Prescription Drug Products (continued)

GENTAMICIN SULFATE (continued)

INJECTABLE; INJECTION

GENTAMICIN SULFATE

TE Code	Manufacturer / Strength	Appl No	Approval Date
	KALAPHARM		
AP	EQ 40 MG BASE/ML	N62354 001	APR 05, 1982
	LYPHOMED		
AP	EQ 10 MG BASE/ML	N62356 001	
AP	EQ 40 MG BASE/ML	N62356 002	MAR 04, 1982
AP	EQ 40 MG BASE/ML	N62366 001	MAR 04, 1982
	PHARM SPEC		
AP	EQ 40 MG BASE/ML	N62340 001	AUG 04, 1983
	SMITH NEPHEW SOLOPAK		
AP	EQ 40 MG BASE/ML	N62340 001	MAR 28, 1983
AP	EQ 10 MG BASE/ML	N62507 001	JUN 06, 1985
AP	EQ 40 MG BASE/ML	N62507 002	JUN 06, 1985
	STERIS		
AP	EQ 10 MG BASE/ML	N62318 002	
AP	EQ 40 MG BASE/ML	N62318 001	
	WYETH AYERST		
AP	EQ 10 MG BASE/ML	N62264 001	
AP	EQ 40 MG BASE/ML	N62264 002	

GENTAMICIN SULFATE IN SODIUM CHLORIDE 0.9% IN PLASTIC CONTAINER

TE Code	Manufacturer / Strength	Appl No	Approval Date
	ABBOTT		
AP	EQ 60 MG BASE/100 ML	N62414 006	AUG 15, 1983
AP	EQ 60 MG BASE/100 ML	N62588 006	JAN 06, 1986
AP	EQ 70 MG BASE/100 ML	N62414 007	AUG 15, 1983
AP	EQ 70 MG BASE/100 ML	N62588 007	JAN 06, 1986
AP	EQ 80 MG BASE/100 ML	N62414 008	AUG 15, 1983
AP	EQ 80 MG BASE/100 ML	N62588 008	JAN 06, 1986
AP	EQ 90 MG BASE/100 ML	N62414 009	AUG 15, 1983
AP	EQ 90 MG BASE/100 ML	N62588 009	JAN 06, 1986
AP	EQ 100 MG BASE/100 ML	N62414 010	AUG 15, 1983
AP	EQ 100 MG BASE/100 ML	N62588 010	JAN 06, 1986
AP	EQ 1.2 MG BASE/ML	N62414 001	AUG 15, 1983
AP	EQ 1.2 MG BASE/ML	N62588 001	JAN 06, 1986
AP	EQ 1.4 MG BASE/ML	N62414 002	AUG 15, 1983
AP	EQ 1.4 MG BASE/ML	N62588 002	JAN 06, 1986
AP	EQ 1.6 MG BASE/ML	N62414 003	AUG 15, 1983
AP	EQ 1.6 MG BASE/ML	N62588 003	JAN 06, 1986
AP	EQ 1.8 MG BASE/ML	N62414 004	AUG 15, 1983
AP	EQ 1.8 MG BASE/ML	N62588 004	JAN 06, 1986
AP	EQ 2 MG BASE/ML	N62414 005	AUG 15, 1983
AP	EQ 2 MG BASE/ML	N62588 005	JAN 06, 1986
	MCGAW		
AP	EQ 40 MG BASE/100 ML	N62814 008	AUG 28, 1987
AP	EQ 60 MG BASE/100 ML	N62814 009	AUG 28, 1987
AP	EQ 70 MG BASE/100 ML	N62814 010	AUG 28, 1987
AP	EQ 0.8 MG BASE/ML	N62814 001	AUG 28, 1987
AP	EQ 80 MG BASE/100 ML	N62814 011	AUG 28, 1987
AP	EQ 90 MG BASE/100 ML	N62814 012	AUG 28, 1987
AP	EQ 100 MG BASE/100 ML	N62814 013	AUG 28, 1987
AP	EQ 1.2 MG BASE/ML	N62814 002	AUG 28, 1987
AP	EQ 120 MG BASE/100 ML	N62814 014	AUG 28, 1987
AP	EQ 1.4 MG BASE/ML	N62814 003	AUG 28, 1987
AP	EQ 1.6 MG BASE/ML	N62814 004	AUG 28, 1987
AP	EQ 1.8 MG BASE/ML	N62814 005	AUG 28, 1987
AP	EQ 2 MG BASE/ML	N62814 006	AUG 28, 1987
AP	EQ 2.4 MG BASE/ML	N62814 007	AUG 28, 1987

ISOTONIC GENTAMICIN SULFATE IN PLASTIC CONTAINER

TE Code	Manufacturer / Strength	Appl No	Approval Date
	BAXTER		
AP	EQ 40 MG BASE/100 ML	N62373 003	SEP 07, 1982
AP	EQ 60 MG BASE/100 ML	N62373 004	SEP 07, 1982
AP	EQ 0.8 MG BASE/ML	N62373 001	SEP 07, 1982
AP	EQ 80 MG BASE/100 ML	N62373 002	SEP 07, 1982
AP	EQ 100 MG BASE/100 ML	N62373 005	SEP 07, 1982
AP	EQ 120 MG BASE/100 ML	N62373 006	SEP 07, 1982
AP	EQ 1.2 MG BASE/ML	N62373 007	SEP 07, 1982
AP	EQ 1.6 MG BASE/ML	N62373 008	SEP 07, 1982
AP	EQ 2 MG BASE/ML	N62373 009	SEP 07, 1982
AP	EQ 2.4 MG BASE/ML	N62373 010	SEP 07, 1982

Prescription Drug Products (continued)

GENTAMICIN SULFATE (continued)

INJECTABLE INJECTION
U-GENCIN
  UPJOHN

AP	EQ 10 MG BASE/ML	N62248 001	
AP	EQ 40 MG BASE/ML	N62248 002	

OINTMENT; OPHTHALMIC
GARAMYCIN
  SCHERING

AT	EQ 3 MG BASE/GM	N50425 001	

GENTACIDIN
  IOLAB

AT	EQ 3 MG BASE/GM	N62501 001	JUL 26, 1984

GENTAFAIR
  PHARMAFAIR

AT	EQ 3 MG BASE/GM	N62443 001	MAY 26, 1983

OINTMENT; TOPICAL
GARAMYCIN
  SCHERING

AT	EQ 1 MG BASE/GM	N60463 001	

GENTAFAIR
  PHARMAFAIR

AT	EQ 1 MG BASE/GM	N62444 001	MAY 26, 1983

GENTAMICIN
  CLAY PARK

AT	EQ 1 MG BASE/GM	N62351 001	FEB 18, 1982

GENTAMICIN SULFATE
  FOUGERA

AT	EQ 1 MG BASE/GM	N62533 001	OCT 05, 1984

  NMC

AT	EQ 1 MG BASE/GM	N62496 001	MAR 14, 1984

  PHARMADERM

AT	EQ 1 MG BASE/GM	N62534 001	OCT 10, 1984

  THAMES

AT	EQ 1 MG BASE/GM	N62477 001	DEC 23, 1983

SOLUTION/DROPS; OPHTHALMIC
GARAMYCIN
  SCHERING

AT	EQ 3 MG BASE/ML	N50039 002	

GENOPTIC
  ALLERGAN

AT	EQ 3 MG BASE/ML	N62452 001	OCT 10, 1984

GENTACIDIN
  IOLAB

AT	EQ 3 MG BASE/ML	N62480 001	MAR 30, 1984

GENTAFAIR
  PHARMAFAIR

AT	EQ 3 MG BASE/ML	N62440 001	MAY 03, 1983

GENTAMICIN SULFATE
  AKORN

AT	EQ 3 MG BASE/ML	N62635 001	JAN 08, 1987

  STERIS

AT	EQ 3 MG BASE/ML	N62523 001	NOV 25, 1985

GENTAMICIN SULFATE; PREDNISOLONE ACETATE

OINTMENT; OPHTHALMIC
PRED-G

+ ALLERGAN	EQ 0.3% BASE;0.6%	N50612 001	DEC 01, 1989

GENTAMICIN SULFATE; PREDNISOLONE ACETATE (continued)

SUSPENSION/DROPS; OPHTHALMIC
PRED-G

+ ALLERGAN	EQ 0.3% BASE;1%	N50586 001	JUN 10, 1988

GENTIAN VIOLET

SUPPOSITORY; VAGINAL
GVS
  SAVAGE

0.4%	N83513 001	

GLIPIZIDE

TABLET; ORAL
GLUCOTROL
  ROERIG

	5 MG	N17783 001	MAY 08, 1984
	10 MG	N17783 002	MAY 08, 1984
+		N17783 003	MAY 08, 1984

GLUCAGON HYDROCHLORIDE

INJECTABLE; INJECTION
GLUCAGON
  LILLY

AP	EQ 1 MG BASE/VIAL	N12122 001
	EQ 10 MG BASE/VIAL	N12122 002

  QUAD

AP	EQ 1 MG BASE/VIAL	N71022 001	MAR 04, 1987

GLUCONOLACTONE; *MULTIPLE*

SEE CITRIC ACID; GLUCONOLACTONE; MAGNESIUM CARBONATE

GLUTATHIONE DISULFIDE; *MULTIPLE*

SEE CALCIUM CHLORIDE; DEXTROSE; GLUTATHIONE DISULFIDE; MAGNESIUM CHLORIDE; POTASSIUM CHLORIDE; SODIUM BICARBONATE; SODIUM CHLORIDE; SODIUM PHOSPHATE

GLUTETHIMIDE

CAPSULE; ORAL
DORIDEN
  RHONE POULENC
  RORER

500 MG	N09519 008	

TABLET; ORAL
GLUTETHIMIDE

AA	DANBURY	500 MG	N84362 001	
AA	GENEVA	500 MG	N83234 002	
AA	HALSEY	250 MG	N89458 001	OCT 10, 1986
		500 MG	N89459 001	OCT 10, 1986
AA	LANNETT	250 MG	N83475 001	
		500 MG	N85571 001	
AA	MD PHARM	500 MG	N85171 001	

Prescription Drug Products (continued)

GLUTETHIMIDE (continued)

TABLET; ORAL

		Strength	Appl. No.	
	GLUTETHIMIDE			
AA	DANBURY	500 MG	N84362 001	
AA	GENEVA	500 MG	N83234 002	
AA	HALSEY	250 MG	N89458 001	OCT 10, 1986
AA		500 MG	N89459 001	OCT 10, 1986
AA	LANNETT	250 MG	N83475 001	
AA		500 MG	N85571 001	
AA	MD PHARM	500 MG	N85171 001	

GLYBURIDE

TABLET; ORAL

		Strength	Appl. No.	
	DIABETA			
BX	HOECHST ROUSSEL	1.25 MG	N17532 001	MAY 01, 1984
BX		2.5 MG	N17532 002	MAY 01, 1984
BX		5 MG	N17532 003	MAY 01, 1984
	GLUBATE			
BX	HOECHST ROUSSEL	1.5 MG	N20055 001	APR 17, 1992
BX		3 MG	N20055 002	APR 17, 1992
	GLYNASE			
BX	UPJOHN	1.5 MG	N20051 001	MAR 04, 1992
BX	+	3 MG	N20051 002	MAR 04, 1992
	MICRONASE			
BX	UPJOHN	1.25 MG	N17498 001	MAY 01, 1984
BX		2.5 MG	N17498 002	MAY 01, 1984
BX	+	5 MG	N17498 003	MAY 01, 1984

GLYCOPYRROLATE

INJECTABLE; INJECTION

		Strength	Appl. No.	
	GLYCOPYRROLATE			
AP	ABBOTT	0.2 MG/ML	N89393 001	JUN 15, 1988
AP	GENSIA	0.2 MG/ML	N81169 001	SEP 10, 1991
AP	LUITPOLD	0.2 MG/ML	N89335 001	JUL 23, 1986
AP	LYPHOMED	0.2 MG/ML	N88475 001	JUN 12, 1984
AP	STERIS	0.2 MG/ML	N86947 001	JUN 24, 1983
	ROBINUL			
AP	ROBINS	0.2 MG/ML	N17558 001	

TABLET; ORAL

		Strength	Appl. No.	
	GLYCOPYRROLATE			
AA	DANBURY	1 MG	N86902 001	
AA		2 MG	N86900 001	
	ROBINUL			
AA	ROBINS	1 MG	N12827 001	
	ROBINUL FORTE			
AA	ROBINS	2 MG	N12827 002	

GONADORELIN ACETATE

INJECTABLE; INJECTION

		Strength	Appl. No.	
	LUTREPULSE PUMP KIT			
	FERRING	0.8 MG/VIAL	N19687 001	OCT 10, 1989
		3.2 MG/VIAL	N19687 002	OCT 10, 1989

GONADORELIN HYDROCHLORIDE

INJECTABLE; INJECTION

		Strength	Appl. No.	
	FACTREL			
	WYETH AYERST	EQ 0.1 MG BASE/VIAL	N18123 001	SEP 30, 1982
		EQ 0.5 MG BASE/VIAL	N18123 003	SEP 30, 1982

GONADOTROPIN, CHORIONIC

INJECTABLE; INJECTION

		Strength	Appl. No.
	A.P.L.		
AP	WYETH AYERST	5,000 UNITS/VIAL	N17055 001
AP		10,000 UNITS/VIAL	N17055 002
AP		20,000 UNITS/VIAL	N17055 003

GLYCERIN; *MULTIPLE*

SEE AMINO ACIDS; CALCIUM ACETATE; GLYCERIN; MAGNESIUM ACETATE; PHOSPHORIC ACID; POTASSIUM CHLORIDE; SODIUM ACETATE; SODIUM CHLORIDE

GLYCINE

SOLUTION; IRRIGATION

		Strength	Appl. No.	
	AMINOACETIC ACID 1.5% IN PLASTIC CONTAINER			
AT	BAXTER	1.5 GM/100 ML	N17865 001	
	GLYCINE 1.5% IN PLASTIC CONTAINER			
AT	ABBOTT	1.5 GM/100 ML	N17633 001	
AT		1.5 GM/100 ML	N18315 001	
AT	BAXTER	1.5 GM/100 ML	N18522 001	FEB 19, 1982
AT	MCGAW	1.5 GM/100 ML	N16784 001	

Prescription Drug Products (continued)

GONADOTROPIN, CHORIONIC (continued)

INJECTABLE; INJECTION

CHORIONIC GONADOTROPIN

TE	Firm	Strength	Appl. No.	Date
AP	BEL MAR	5,000 UNITS/VIAL	N17054 001	
AP		10,000 UNITS/VIAL	N17054 002	
AP	LYPHOMED	5,000 UNITS/VIAL	N17067 001	
AP		10,000 UNITS/VIAL	N17067 002	
AP		20,000 UNITS/VIAL	N17067 003	
AP	STERIS	5,000 UNITS/VIAL	N17016 006	
AP		10,000 UNITS/VIAL	N17016 007	
AP		20,000 UNITS/VIAL	N17016 004	
AP		2,000 UNITS/VIAL	N17016 011	FEB 16, 1990
AP		15,000 UNITS/VIAL	N17016 010	FEB 15, 1985

FOLLUTEIN

TE	Firm	Strength	Appl. No.
AP	SQUIBB		

PREGNYL

TE	Firm	Strength	Appl. No.
AP	ORGANON	10,000 UNITS/VIAL	N17056 001
AP		10,000 UNITS/VIAL	N17692 001

GOSERELIN ACETATE

IMPLANT; IMPLANTATION

ZOLADEX

Firm	Strength	Appl. No.	Date
IMPERIAL CHEM	EQ 3.6 MG BASE	N19726 001	DEC 29, 1989

GRAMICIDIN; NEOMYCIN SULFATE; POLYMYXIN B SULFATE

SOLUTION/DROPS; OPHTHALMIC

NEO-POLYCIN

TE	Firm	Strength	Appl. No.
AT	DOW	0.025 MG/ML;EQ 1.75 MG BASE/ML;10,000 UNITS/ML	N60427 001

NEOMYCIN AND POLYMYXIN B SULFATES AND GRAMICIDIN

TE	Firm	Strength	Appl. No.	Date
AT	IPHARM	0.025 MG/ML;EQ 1.75 MG BASE/ML;10,000 UNITS/ML	N62818 001	OCT 11, 1988
AT	STERIS	0.025 MG/ML;EQ 1.75 MG BASE/ML;10,000 UNITS/ML	N62788 001	JUN 11, 1987

NEOMYCIN SULFATE AND POLYMYXIN B SULFATE GRAMICIDIN

TE	Firm	Strength	Appl. No.	Date
AT	PHARMAFAIR	0.025 MG/ML;EQ 1.75 MG BASE/ML;10,000 UNITS/ML	N62383 001	AUG 31, 1982

NEOSPORIN

TE	Firm	Strength	Appl. No.
AT	BURROUGHS WELLCOME	0.025 MG/ML;EQ 1.75 MG BASE/ML;10,000 UNITS/ML	N60582 001

GRISEOFULVIN, MICROCRYSTALLINE

CAPSULE; ORAL

GRISACTIN

TE	Firm	Strength	Appl. No.
	WYETH AYERST	125 MG	N50051 002
		250 MG	N50051 001

SUSPENSION; ORAL

GRIFULVIN V

TE	Firm	Strength	Appl. No.	Date
	+ JOHNSON RW	125 MG/5 ML	N50448 001	
		125 MG/5 ML	N62483 001	JAN 26, 1984

TABLET; ORAL

FULVICIN-U/F

TE	Firm	Strength	Appl. No.
AB	+ SCHERING	250 MG	N60569 002
AB		500 MG	N60569 001

GRIFULVIN V

TE	Firm	Strength	Appl. No.
AB	+ JOHNSON RW	250 MG	N60618 002
AB		250 MG	N62279 002
AB		500 MG	N60618 003
AB		500 MG	N62279 003
AB		125 MG	N60618 001
AB		125 MG	N62279 001

GRISACTIN

TE	Firm	Strength	Appl. No.
AB	WYETH AYERST	500 MG	N60212 001

GRISEOFULVIN, ULTRAMICROCRYSTALLINE

TABLET; ORAL

FULVICIN P/G

TE	Firm	Strength	Appl. No.
AB	+ SCHERING	125 MG	N61996 001
AB		250 MG	N61996 002

FULVICIN P/G 165

TE	Firm	Strength	Appl. No.	Date
AB	+ SCHERING	165 MG	N61996 003	APR 06, 1982

FULVICIN P/G 330

TE	Firm	Strength	Appl. No.	Date
AB	+ SCHERING	330 MG	N61996 004	APR 06, 1982

GRIS-PEG

TE	Firm	Strength	Appl. No.
AB	HERBERT	125 MG	N50475 001
AB		250 MG	N50475 002

GRISACTIN ULTRA

TE	Firm	Strength	Appl. No.	Date
AB	WYETH AYERST	125 MG	N62178 001	
AB		165 MG	N62438 001	
AB		250 MG	N62178 002	NOV 17, 1983
AB		330 MG	N62438 002	NOV 17, 1983

ULTRAGRIS-165

TE	Firm	Strength	Appl. No.	Date
AB	SIDMAK	165 MG	N62645 001	JUN 30, 1992

ULTRAGRIS-330

TE	Firm	Strength	Appl. No.	Date
AB	SIDMAK	330 MG	N62646 001	JUN 30, 1992

Prescription Drug Products (continued)

GUANABENZ ACETATE
TABLET; ORAL
WYTENSIN
WYETH AYERST
EQ 4 MG BASE   N18587 001   SEP 07, 1982
+ EQ 8 MG BASE   N18587 002   SEP 07, 1982

GUANADREL SULFATE
TABLET; ORAL
HYLOREL
UPJOHN
10 MG   N18104 001   DEC 29, 1982
+ 25 MG   N18104 002   DEC 29, 1982

GUANETHIDINE MONOSULFATE
TABLET; ORAL
ISMELIN
CIBA
EQ 10 MG SULFATE   N12329 001
+ EQ 25 MG SULFATE   N12329 002

GUANETHIDINE MONOSULFATE; HYDROCHLOROTHIAZIDE
TABLET; ORAL
ESIMIL
CIBA
10 MG;25 MG   N13553 001

GUANFACINE HYDROCHLORIDE
TABLET; ORAL
TENEX
ROBINS
1 MG   N19032 001   OCT 27, 1986
2 MG   N19032 002   NOV 07, 1988

GUANIDINE HYDROCHLORIDE
TABLET; ORAL
GUANIDINE HCL
KEY PHARMS
125 MG   N01546 001

HALAZEPAM
TABLET; ORAL
PAXIPAM
SCHERING
20 MG   N17736 003
+ 40 MG   N17736 004

HALCINONIDE
CREAM; TOPICAL
HALOG
AT   + WESTWOOD SQUIBB   0.1%   N17556 001
             0.025%   N17818 001
HALOG-E
AT   WESTWOOD SQUIBB   0.1%   N18234 001
OINTMENT; TOPICAL
HALOG
+ WESTWOOD SQUIBB   0.1%   N17824 001
SOLUTION; TOPICAL
HALOG
WESTWOOD SQUIBB   0.1%   N17823 001

HALOBETASOL PROPIONATE
CREAM; TOPICAL
ULTRAVATE
+ WESTWOOD SQUIBB   0.05%   N19967 001   DEC 27, 1990
OINTMENT; TOPICAL
ULTRAVATE
+ WESTWOOD SQUIBB   0.05%   N19968 001   DEC 17, 1990

HALOFANTRINE HYDROCHLORIDE
TABLET; ORAL
HALFAN
+ SMITHKLINE BEECHAM   250 MG   N20250 001   JUL 24, 1992

HALOPERIDOL
TABLET; ORAL
HALDOL
JOHNSON RW
AB   0.5 MG   N15921 001
AB   1 MG   N15921 002
AB   2 MG   N15921 003
AB   + 5 MG   N15921 004
AB   + 10 MG   N15921 005
AB   20 MG   N15921 006   FEB 02, 1982

Prescription Drug Products (continued)

HALOPERIDOL (continued)
TABLET; ORAL
HALOPERIDOL

BARR

	Strength	Number	Date
AB	0.5 MG	N71156 001	JAN 02, 1987
AB	1 MG	N71157 001	JAN 02, 1987
AB	2 MG	N71172 001	JAN 02, 1987
AB	5 MG	N71212 001	JAN 02, 1987
AB	10 MG	N71173 001	JAN 07, 1988
AB	20 MG	N71177 001	JAN 07, 1988

DANBURY

	Strength	Number	Date
AB	0.5 MG	N70981 001	MAR 06, 1987
AB	1 MG	N70982 001	MAR 06, 1987
AB	2 MG	N70983 001	MAR 06, 1987
AB	5 MG	N70984 001	MAR 06, 1987
AB	10 MG	N72113 001	AUG 27, 1991
AB	20 MG	N72353 001	AUG 27, 1991

GENEVA

	Strength	Number	Date
AB	0.5 MG	N71206 001	NOV 17, 1986
AB	1 MG	N71207 001	NOV 17, 1986
AB	2 MG	N71208 001	NOV 17, 1986
AB	5 MG	N71209 001	NOV 17, 1986
AB	10 MG	N71210 001	NOV 17, 1986
AB	20 MG	N71211 001	MAR 11, 1988

LEDERLE

	Strength	Number	Date
AB	0.5 MG	N72727 001	MAR 11, 1988
AB	1 MG	N72728 001	SEP 19, 1989
AB	2 MG	N72729 001	SEP 19, 1989
AB	5 MG	N72730 001	SEP 19, 1989
AB	10 MG	N72731 001	SEP 19, 1989
AB	20 MG	N72732 001	SEP 19, 1989

HALOPERIDOL (continued)
TABLET; ORAL
HALOPERIDOL

MYLAN

	Strength	Number	Date
AB	0.5 MG	N70276 001	JUN 10, 1986
AB	1 MG	N70277 001	JUN 10, 1986
AB	2 MG	N70278 001	JUN 10, 1986
AB	5 MG	N70279 001	JUN 10, 1986

PAR

	Strength	Number	Date
AB	0.5 MG	N71233 001	NOV 03, 1986
AB	1 MG	N71234 001	NOV 03, 1986
AB	2 MG	N71235 001	NOV 03, 1986
AB	5 MG	N71236 001	NOV 03, 1986
AB	10 MG	N71237 001	JUL 20, 1987

PUREPAC

	Strength	Number	Date
AB	0.5 MG	N71071 001	NOV 03, 1986
AB	1 MG	N71072 001	NOV 03, 1986
AB	2 MG	N71073 001	NOV 03, 1986
AB	5 MG	N71074 001	NOV 03, 1986
AB	10 MG	N71075 001	AUG 04, 1987
AB	20 MG	N71076 001	AUG 04, 1987

ROXANE

	Strength	Number	Date
AB	0.5 MG	N71128 001	FEB 17, 1987
AB	1 MG	N71129 001	FEB 17, 1987
AB	2 MG	N71130 001	FEB 17, 1987
AB	5 MG	N71131 001	FEB 17, 1987
AB	10 MG	N71132 001	MAY 12, 1987
AB	20 MG	N71133 001	MAY 12, 1987

SCHIAPPARELLI SEARLE

	Strength	Number	Date
AB	0.5 MG	N70720 001	JUN 10, 1986
AB	1 MG	N70721 001	JUN 10, 1986
AB	2 MG	N70722 001	JUN 10, 1986
AB	5 MG	N70723 001	JUN 10, 1986
AB	10 MG	N70724 001	JUN 10, 1986
AB	20 MG	N70725 001	JUN 10, 1986

Prescription Drug Products *(continued)*

HALOPERIDOL DECANOATE

INJECTABLE; INJECTION
HALDOL DECANOATE 50
JOHNSON RW — EQ 50 MG BASE/ML — N18701 001 — JAN 14, 1986

HALOPERIDOL LACTATE

CONCENTRATE; ORAL

	Name	Strength	Appl. No.	Date
ΔΔ	HALDOL JOHNSON RW	EQ 2 MG BASE/ML	N15922 001	
ΔΔ	HALOPERIDOL BARRE	EQ 2 MG BASE/ML	N70318 001	APR 11, 1986
ΔΔ	COPLEY	EQ 2 MG BASE/ML	N71617 001	DEC 01, 1988
ΔΔ	LEMMON	EQ 2 MG BASE/ML	N71015 001	AUG 25, 1987
ΔΔ	PHARM BASICS	EQ 2 MG BASE/ML	N70710 001	MAR 07, 1986
ΔΔ	SCHIAPPARELLI SEARLE	EQ 2 MG BASE/ML	N70726 001	JUN 10, 1986
ΔΔ	HALOPERIDOL INTENSOL ROXANE	EQ 2 MG BASE/ML	N72045 001	APR 12, 1988

INJECTABLE; INJECTION

	Name	Strength	Appl. No.	Date
ΔP	HALDOL JOHNSON RW	EQ 5 MG BASE/ML	N15923 001	
ΔP	HALOPERIDOL SMITH NEPHEW SOLOPAK	EQ 5 MG BASE/ML	N70800 001	DEC 14, 1987
		EQ 5 MG BASE/ML	N70801 001	DEC 14, 1987
ΔP		EQ 5 MG BASE/ML	N70864 001	DEC 14, 1987
ΔP	STERIS	EQ 5 MG BASE/ML	N70713 001	MAY 17, 1988
ΔP		EQ 5 MG BASE/ML	N70714 001	MAY 17, 1988
ΔP		EQ 5 MG BASE/ML	N70744 001	MAY 17, 1988

HALOPROGIN

CREAM; TOPICAL
HALOTEX
+ WESTWOOD SQUIBB — 1% — N16942 001

SOLUTION; TOPICAL
HALOTEX
WESTWOOD SQUIBB — 1% — N16943 001

HALOTHANE

LIQUID; INHALATION

	Name	Strength	Appl. No.	Date
	FLUOTHANE WYETH AYERST	99.99%	N11338 001	
ΔN	HALOTHANE ABBOTT	99.99%	N83254 001	
ΔN	BH	99.99%	N84977 001	
ΔN	HALOCARBON	99.99%	N80810 001	

HEPARIN CALCIUM

INJECTABLE; INJECTION
CALCIPARINE
DUPONT — 25,000 UNITS/ML — N18237 001

HEPARIN SODIUM

INJECTABLE; INJECTION
HEP FLUSH KIT IN PLASTIC CONTAINER

	Name	Strength	Appl. No.	Date
ΔP	LYPHOMED	10 UNITS/ML	N17029 017	DEC 05, 1985
			N17029 018	DEC 05, 1985
ΔP		100 UNITS/ML		
	HEP-FLUSH 10			
ΔP	LYPHOMED	10 UNITS/ML	N17651 009	JUN 26, 1984
	HEP-LOCK			
ΔP	ELKINS SINN	10 UNITS/ML	N17037 007	
		100 UNITS/ML	N17037 006	
	HEP-LOCK U/P			
ΔP	ELKINS SINN	100 UNITS/ML	N17037 010	JUN 10, 1983
			N17037 011	JUN 10, 1983
	HEPARIN LOCK FLUSH			
ΔP	ABBOTT	10 UNITS/ML	N05264 001	
ΔP	LYPHOMED	10 UNITS/ML	N17029 007	MAY 06, 1982
ΔP	SMITH NEPHEW SOLOPAK	100 UNITS/ML	N17029 006	
ΔP		10 UNITS/ML	N87903 001	APR 20, 1983
ΔP		10 UNITS/ML	N87904 001	APR 20, 1983
ΔP		10 UNITS/ML	N88457 001	OCT 25, 1984
ΔP		10 UNITS/ML	N88458 001	JUL 26, 1984
ΔP		10 UNITS/ML	N88580 001	OCT 25, 1984
ΔP		100 UNITS/ML	N87905 001	APR 20, 1983
ΔP		100 UNITS/ML	N87906 001	APR 20, 1983
ΔP		100 UNITS/ML	N88459 001	JUL 26, 1984
			N88460 001	JUL 26, 1984
ΔP		100 UNITS/ML	N88581 001	OCT 25, 1984
ΔP		100 UNITS/ML		

Prescription Drug Products (continued)

HEPARIN SODIUM (continued)

INJECTABLE; INJECTION

HEPARIN LOCK FLUSH

	Firm	Strength	Appl. No.	Date
AP	STERLING	10 UNITS/ML	N88097 001	APR 28, 1983
AP		10 UNITS/ML	N88346 001	MAY 18, 1983
AP		100 UNITS/ML	N88098 001	APR 28, 1983
AP		100 UNITS/ML	N88347 001	MAY 18, 1983
AP	WYETH AYERST	10 UNITS/ML	N17007 008	
AP		100 UNITS/ML	N17007 009	

HEPARIN LOCK FLUSH IN PLASTIC CONTAINER

	Firm	Strength	Appl. No.	Date
AP	ABBOTT	10 UNITS/ML	N05264 015	MAY 21, 1985
AP		100 UNITS/ML	N05264 016	MAY 21, 1985

HEPARIN SODIUM

	Firm	Strength	Appl. No.	Date
AP	ABBOTT	2,500 UNITS/ML	N05264 014	APR 07, 1986
		2,000 UNITS/ML	N05264 013	APR 07, 1986
AP	AKORN	1,000 UNITS/ML	N17486 001	
AP		5,000 UNITS/ML	N17486 002	
AP		10,000 UNITS/ML	N17486 003	
AP		20,000 UNITS/ML	N17486 004	
AP		40,000 UNITS/ML	N17486 005	
AP	DELL	5,000 UNITS/ML	N17540 001	
AP		10,000 UNITS/ML	N17540 002	
AP		20,000 UNITS/ML	N17540 003	
AP		40,000 UNITS/ML	N17540 004	
AP		1,000 UNITS/ML	N17540 005	
AP	ELKINS SINN	5,000 UNITS/ML	N17037 001	
AP		10,000 UNITS/ML	N17037 002	
AP		10,000 UNITS/ML	N17037 003	
AP		10,000 UNITS/ML	N17037 013	APR 07, 1986
AP	LILLY	1,000 UNITS/ML	N05521 001	
AP		10,000 UNITS/ML	N05521 002	
AP		20,000 UNITS/ML	N05521 004	
AP	LYPHOMED	1,000 UNITS/ML	N17029 001	
AP		1,000 UNITS/ML	N17979 001	
AP		5,000 UNITS/ML	N17651 006	
AP		10,000 UNITS/ML	N17029 003	
AP		10,000 UNITS/ML	N17979 002	
AP	ORGANON	1,000 UNITS/ML	N00552 008	
AP		5,000 UNITS/ML	N00552 009	
AP		10,000 UNITS/ML	N00552 010	
AP	PHARM SPEC	1,000 UNITS/ML	N17780 001	
AP		5,000 UNITS/ML	N17780 003	
AP		10,000 UNITS/ML	N17780 004	
AP	PHARMA SERVE	1,000 UNITS/ML	N86129 001	

HEPARIN SODIUM (continued)

INJECTABLE; INJECTION

HEPARIN SODIUM

	Firm	Strength	Appl. No.	Date
AP	SMITH NEPHEW SOLOPAK	1,000 UNITS/ML	N87043 001	
AP		1,000 UNITS/ML	N88239 001	JUL 26, 1984
AP		5,000 UNITS/ML	N87077 001	
AP		10,000 UNITS/ML	N87107 001	
AP		5,000 UNITS/0.5 ML	N87395 001	
AP		10,000 UNITS/0.5 ML	N87363 001	
AP	STERIS	1,000 UNITS/ML	N17064 002	
AP		5,000 UNITS/ML	N17064 003	
AP		10,000 UNITS/ML	N17064 004	
AP		20,000 UNITS/ML	N17064 005	
AP		40,000 UNITS/ML	N17064 006	
		2,500 UNITS/ML	N88099 001	APR 28, 1983
AP	STERLING	5,000 UNITS/ML	N88100 001	APR 28, 1983
AP	UPJOHN	1,000 UNITS/ML	N04570 001	
AP		5,000 UNITS/ML	N04570 002	
AP		10,000 UNITS/ML	N04570 003	
AP	WYETH AYERST	1,000 UNITS/ML	N17007 001	
AP		2,500 UNITS/ML	N17007 007	
AP		5,000 UNITS/ML	N17007 002	
AP		10,000 UNITS/ML	N17007 004	
AP		20,000 UNITS/ML	N17007 006	
		7,500 UNITS/ML	N17007 003	

HEPARIN SODIUM IN PLASTIC CONTAINER

	Firm	Strength	Appl. No.	Date
AP	LYPHOMED	1,000 UNITS/ML	N17029 013	DEC 05, 1985
		5,000 UNITS/ML	N17029 014	DEC 05, 1985
AP		10,000 UNITS/ML	N17029 015	DEC 05, 1985
AP		20,000 UNITS/ML	N17029 016	DEC 05, 1985

HEPARIN SODIUM PRESERVATIVE FREE

	Firm	Strength	Appl. No.	Date
AP	LYPHOMED	1,000 UNITS/ML	N17029 010	APR 28, 1986
AP	MARSAM	1,000 UNITS/ML	N89464 001	JUN 03, 1986
AP	STERLING	10,000 UNITS/ML	N89522 001	MAY 04, 1987

HEPARIN SODIUM 10,000 UNITS IN DEXTROSE 5%

	Firm	Strength	Appl. No.	Date
AP	ABBOTT	10,000 UNITS/100 ML	N18911 006	JAN 30, 1985

HEPARIN SODIUM 1000 UNITS AND DEXTROSE 5% IN PLASTIC CONTAINER

	Firm	Strength	Appl. No.	Date
AP	MCGAW	200 UNITS/100 ML	N19130 001	DEC 31, 1984

HEPARIN SODIUM 1000 UNITS AND SODIUM CHLORIDE 0.9% IN PLASTIC CONTAINER

	Firm	Strength	Appl. No.	Date
AP	BAXTER	200 UNITS/100 ML	N18609 001	APR 28, 1982

Prescription Drug Products (continued)

HEPARIN SODIUM (continued)
INJECTABLE; INJECTION

HEPARIN SODIUM 1000 UNITS IN SODIUM CHLORIDE 0.9% IN PLASTIC CONTAINER

AP	ABBOTT	200 UNITS/100 ML	N18916 010	JUN 23, 1989
AP	MCGAW	200 UNITS/100 ML	N19042 001	MAR 29, 1985
AP		200 UNITS/100 ML	N19953 001	JUL 20, 1992

HEPARIN SODIUM 12,500 UNITS IN DEXTROSE 5%

AP	ABBOTT	5,000 UNITS/100 ML	N18911 007	JAN 30, 1985

HEPARIN SODIUM 12,500 UNITS IN SODIUM CHLORIDE 0.45% IN PLASTIC CONTAINER

AP	ABBOTT	5,000 UNITS/100 ML	N18916 006	JAN 31, 1984

HEPARIN SODIUM 12500 UNITS IN SODIUM CHLORIDE 0.45% IN PLASTIC CONTAINER

AP	MCGAW	5,000 UNITS/100 ML	N19802 001	JUL 20, 1992

HEPARIN SODIUM 20,000 UNITS AND DEXTROSE 5% IN PLASTIC CONTAINER

AP	BAXTER	4,000 UNITS/100 ML	N18814 001	OCT 31, 1983

HEPARIN SODIUM 20,000 UNITS IN DEXTROSE 5% IN PLASTIC CONTAINER

AP	ABBOTT	4,000 UNITS/100 ML	N19805 001	JAN 25, 1989

HEPARIN SODIUM 2000 UNITS AND SODIUM CHLORIDE 0.9% IN PLASTIC CONTAINER

AP	BAXTER	200 UNITS/100 ML	N18609 002	APR 28, 1982

HEPARIN SODIUM 2000 UNITS IN DEXTROSE 5% IN PLASTIC CONTAINER

AP	MCGAW	200 UNITS/100 ML	N19130 003	DEC 31, 1984

HEPARIN SODIUM 2000 UNITS IN SODIUM CHLORIDE 0.9% IN PLASTIC CONTAINER

AP	ABBOTT	200 UNITS/100 ML	N18916 011	JUN 23, 1989
AP	MCGAW	200 UNITS/100 ML	N19042 002	MAR 29, 1985

HEPARIN SODIUM 20000 UNITS IN DEXTROSE 5% IN PLASTIC CONTAINER

AP	MCGAW	4,000 UNITS/100 ML	N19952 001	JUL 20, 1992

HEPARIN SODIUM 25,000 UNITS AND DEXTROSE 5% IN PLASTIC CONTAINER

AP	BAXTER	5,000 UNITS/100 ML	N18814 003	JUL 09, 1985
AP		10,000 UNITS/100 ML	N18814 004	JUL 02, 1987

HEPARIN SODIUM 25,000 UNITS IN DEXTROSE 5%

AP	ABBOTT	5,000 UNITS/100 ML	N18911 009	JAN 30, 1985
AP		10,000 UNITS/100 ML	N18911 008	JAN 30, 1985

HEPARIN SODIUM (continued)
INJECTABLE; INJECTION

HEPARIN SODIUM 25,000 UNITS IN DEXTROSE 5% IN PLASTIC CONTAINER

AP	ABBOTT	5,000 UNITS/100 ML	N19805 002	JAN 25, 1989

HEPARIN SODIUM 25,000 UNITS IN SODIUM CHLORIDE 0.45% IN PLASTIC CONTAINER

AP	ABBOTT	5,000 UNITS/100 ML	N18916 007	JAN 31, 1984
AP		10,000 UNITS/100 ML	N18916 008	JAN 31, 1984

HEPARIN SODIUM 25000 UNITS IN DEXTROSE 5% IN PLASTIC CONTAINER

AP	MCGAW	5,000 UNITS/100 ML	N19134 001	MAR 29, 1985
AP		5,000 UNITS/100 ML	N19952 004	JUL 20, 1992
AP		10,000 UNITS/100 ML	N19952 005	JUL 20, 1992

HEPARIN SODIUM 25000 UNITS IN SODIUM CHLORIDE 0.45% IN PLASTIC CONTAINER

AP	MCGAW	5,000 UNITS/100 ML	N19802 005	JUL 20, 1992
AP		10,000 UNITS/100 ML	N19802 002	JUL 20, 1992

HEPARIN SODIUM 25000 UNITS IN SODIUM CHLORIDE 0.9% IN PLASTIC CONTAINER

AP	MCGAW	5,000 UNITS/100 ML	N19802 003	JUL 20, 1992

HEPARIN SODIUM 5000 UNITS IN DEXTROSE 5% IN PLASTIC CONTAINER

AP	MCGAW	1,000 UNITS/100 ML	N19130 002	DEC 31, 1984

LIQUAEMIN LOCK FLUSH

AP	ORGANON	100 UNITS/ML	N00552 007

LIQUAEMIN SODIUM

AP	ORGANON	1,000 UNITS/ML	N00552 004
AP		5,000 UNITS/ML	N00552 003
AP		10,000 UNITS/ML	N00552 005
AP		20,000 UNITS/ML	N00552 001
AP		40,000 UNITS/ML	N00552 002

SODIUM HEPARIN

AP	BAXTER	1,000 UNITS/ML	N17036 001

HEXACHLOROPHENE
AEROSOL; TOPICAL

SEPTISOL

	VESTAL	0.23%	N17424 001

TURGEX

	XTTRIUM	3%	N18375 001

EMULSION; TOPICAL

HEXA-GERM

AT	HUNTINGTON	3%	N17411 001

PHISOHEX

AT	STERLING	3%	N06882 001
AT		3%	N08402 001

TURGEX

AT	XTTRIUM	3%	N19055 001	NOV 30, 1984

Prescription Drug Products (continued)

HEXACHLOROPHENE (continued)

SOAP; TOPICAL
GAMOPHEN

	ARBROOK	2%	N06270 003

SOLUTION; TOPICAL
DIAL

ΔT	ARMOUR DIAL	0.25%	N17421 002

GERMA-MEDICA
HUNTINGTON 1% N17412 001

GERMA-MEDICA "MG"

ΔT	HUNTINGTON	0.25%	N17412 002

SPONGE; TOPICAL
E-Z SCRUB
DESERET 450 MG N17452 001
HEXASCRUB

ΔT	PROF DSPLS	3%	N18363 001

PHISO-SCRUB

ΔT	STERLING	3%	N17446 001

PRE-OP

ΔT	DAVIS AND GECK	480 MG	N17433 001

PRE-OP II

ΔT	DAVIS AND GECK	480 MG	N17433 002

SCRUBTEAM SURGICAL SPONGEBRUSH
3M 330 MG N17413 001

HEXAFLUORENIUM BROMIDE

INJECTABLE; INJECTION
MYLAXEN
WALLACE 20 MG/ML N09789 003

HISTAMINE PHOSPHATE

INJECTABLE; INJECTION
HISTAMINE PHOSPHATE

LILLY	EQ 0.1 MG BASE/ML	N00734 003
	EQ 0.2 MG BASE/ML	N00734 002
	EQ 1 MG BASE/ML	N00734 001

HISTRELIN ACETATE

INJECTABLE; INJECTION
SUPPRELIN

JOHNSON RW	EQ 0.2 MG BASE/ML	N19836 001	DEC 24, 1991
	EQ 0.5 MG BASE/ML	N19836 002	DEC 24, 1991
	EQ 1 MG BASE/ML	N19836 003	DEC 24, 1991

HOMATROPINE METHYLBROMIDE

TABLET; ORAL
HOMAPIN-10
MISSION PHARMA 10 MG N86308 001
HOMAPIN-5
MISSION PHARMA 5 MG N86309 001

HOMATROPINE METHYLBROMIDE; HYDROCODONE BITARTRATE

SYRUP; ORAL
HYCODAN

ΔΔ	DUPONT	1.5 MG/5 ML;5 MG/5 ML	N05213 002	JUL 26, 1988

HYDROCODONE COMPOUND

ΔΔ	BARRE	1.5 MG/5 ML;5 MG/5 ML	N88017 001	JUL 05, 1983

HYDROPANE

ΔΔ	HALSEY	1.5 MG/5 ML;5 MG/5 ML	N88066 001	JUN 28, 1985

MYCODONE

ΔΔ	PHARM BASICS	1.5 MG/5 ML;5 MG/5 ML	N88008 001	MAR 03, 1983

TABLET; ORAL
HYCODAN

ΔΔ	DUPONT	1.5 MG;5 MG	N05213 001	JUL 26, 1988

TUSSIGON

ΔΔ	DANIELS	1.5 MG;5 MG	N88508 001	JUL 30, 1985

HYALURONIDASE

INJECTABLE; INJECTION
WYDASE

WYETH AYERST	150 UNITS/ML	N06343 002
	150 UNITS/VIAL	N06343 006
	1,500 UNITS/VIAL	N06343 005

HYDRALAZINE HYDROCHLORIDE

INJECTABLE; INJECTION
APRESOLINE
CIBA 20 MG/ML N08303 003

TABLET; ORAL
APRESOLINE

ΔΔ	CIBA	10 MG	N08303 004
ΔΔ		25 MG	N08303 001
ΔΔ		50 MG	N08303 002
ΔΔ		100 MG	N08303 005

DRALZINE

ΔΔ	LEMMON	25 MG	N84301 001

Prescription Drug Products (continued)

HYDRALAZINE HYDROCHLORIDE (continued)

TABLET; ORAL

HYDRALAZINE HCL

AMIDE PHARM				
AA		25 MG	N88560 001	OCT 04, 1984
AA		50 MG	N88649 001	OCT 18, 1984
BARR				
AA		10 MG	N88728 001	APR 11, 1985
AA		25 MG	N84106 002	
AA		50 MG	N84107 002	
AA		100 MG	N88729 001	APR 11, 1985
CAMALL				
AA		10 MG	N88846 001	FEB 26, 1985
AA		25 MG	N88847 001	FEB 26, 1985
AA		50 MG	N88848 001	FEB 26, 1985
AA		100 MG	N88849 001	FEB 26, 1985
DANBURY				
AA		25 MG	N84504 001	
AA		50 MG	N84503 001	
GENEVA				
AA		10 MG	N83241 001	
AA		25 MG	N83560 001	
AA		50 MG	N83561 001	
HALSEY				
AA		10 MG	N89218 001	JAN 22, 1986
AA		25 MG	N89130 001	
AA		50 MG	N89222 001	JAN 22, 1986
AA		100 MG	N89178 001	JAN 15, 1986
LEDERLE				
AA		25 MG	N86243 001	JAN 15, 1986
AA		50 MG	N86242 002	
MUTUAL PHARM				
AA		10 MG	N89359 001	JUL 25, 1986
AA		25 MG	N89258 001	MAY 05, 1986
PAR				
AA		50 MG	N89259 001	MAY 05, 1986
AA		10 MG	N87836 001	OCT 05, 1982
AA		25 MG	N86961 002	
AA		50 MG	N86962 001	
AA		100 MG	N88391 001	SEP 27, 1983
PUREPAC				
AA		25 MG	N88177 001	JUL 29, 1983

HYDRALAZINE HYDROCHLORIDE (continued)

TABLET; ORAL

HYDRALAZINE HCL

RICHLYN				
AA		25 MG	N84922 001	
AA		50 MG	N84923 001	
SIDMAK				
AA		10 MG	N89097 001	DEC 18, 1985
AA		25 MG	N88467 001	
AA		50 MG	N88468 001	MAY 01, 1984
AA		100 MG	N89098 001	MAY 01, 1984
ZENITH				
AA		10 MG	N84443 001	DEC 18, 1985
AA		25 MG	N84437 001	
AA		50 MG	N84469 002	
AA		100 MG	N84581 001	

HYDRALAZINE HYDROCHLORIDE; HYDROCHLOROTHIAZIDE

CAPSULE; ORAL

APRESAZIDE

CIBA				
AB		25 MG;25 MG	N84735 001	
AB		50 MG;50 MG	N84810 001	
AB		100 MG;50 MG	N84811 001	

HYDRA-ZIDE

PAR				
AB +		25 MG;25 MG	N88957 001	OCT 21, 1985
AB		50 MG;50 MG	N88946 001	OCT 21, 1985
AB		100 MG;50 MG	N88961 001	OCT 21, 1985

HYDRALAZINE HCL AND HYDROCHLOROTHIAZIDE 25/25

SOLVAY				
AB		25 MG;25 MG	N87608 001	FEB 08, 1982
AB		50 MG;50 MG	N87213 001	FEB 08, 1982
SUPERPHARM				
AB		50 MG;50 MG	N89201 001	FEB 09, 1987

HYDRALAZINE HCL W/ HYDROCHLOROTHIAZIDE 25/25

ZENITH				
AB		25 MG;25 MG	N88356 001	APR 10, 1984

HYDRALAZINE HCL W/ HYDROCHLOROTHIAZIDE 50/50

ZENITH				
AB		50 MG;50 MG	N88357 001	APR 10, 1984

TABLET; ORAL

APRESOLINE-ESIDRIX

+ CIBA		25 MG;15 MG	N12026 002	

Prescription Drug Products (continued)

HYDRALAZINE HYDROCHLORIDE; HYDROCHLOROTHIAZIDE; RESERPINE

TABLET; ORAL

TE	Firm	Strength	NDA	Date
	CAM-AP-ES			
	CAMALL	25 MG;15 MG;0.1 MG	N84897 001	
	HYDRALAZINE HCL, HYDROCHLOROTHIAZIDE AND RESERPINE			
BP	ZENITH	25 MG;15 MG;0.1 MG	N84291 001	
	HYDROSERPINE PLUS (R-H-H)			
BP	ZENITH	25 MG;15 MG;0.1 MG	N83877 001	
	RESERPINE/HYDRALAZINE HCL/HYDROCHLOROTHIAZIDE			
BP	DANBURY	25 MG;15 MG;0.1 MG	N85549 001	
BP		25 MG;15 MG;0.1 MG	N87556 001	
	RESERPINE, HYDRALAZINE HCL AND HYDROCHLOROTHIAZIDE			
BP	BARR	25 MG;15 MG;0.1 MG	N88570 001	APR 10, 1984
BP	SOLVAY	25 MG;15 MG;0.1 MG	N88376 001	OCT 28, 1983
	SER-AP-ES			
BP	+ CIBA		N12193 005	
	UNIPRES			
BP	SOLVAY	25 MG;15 MG;0.1 MG	N86298 001	

HYDRALAZINE HYDROCHLORIDE; RESERPINE

TABLET; ORAL

TE	Firm	Strength	NDA	Date
	SERPASIL-APRESOLINE			
	+ CIBA	50 MG;0.2 MG	N09296 002	

HYDROCHLOROTHIAZIDE

SOLUTION; ORAL

TE	Firm	Strength	NDA	Date
	HYDROCHLOROTHIAZIDE			
AA	PHARM BASICS	50 MG/5 ML	N89661 001	JUN 20, 1988
AA	ROXANE	50 MG/5 ML	N88587 001	JUL 02, 1984
	HYDROCHLOROTHIAZIDE INTENSOL			
	ROXANE	100 MG/ML	N88588 001	JUL 02, 1984

TABLET; ORAL

TE	Firm	Strength	NDA	Date
	ESIDRIX			
AB	CIBA	25 MG	N11793 005	
AB		50 MG	N11793 008	
AB		100 MG	N11793 009	
	HYDRO-D			
AB	HALSEY	25 MG	N86504 001	
AB		50 MG	N83891 002	

HYDROCHLOROTHIAZIDE (continued)

TABLET; ORAL

TE	Firm	Strength	NDA	Date
	HYDROCHLOROTHIAZIDE			
AB	ASCOT	50 MG	N87540 001	FEB 03, 1982
AB	BARR	25 MG	N83972 001	
AB		50 MG	N83972 002	
AB		50 MG	N84771 001	
AB		100 MG	N83972 003	
AB	CAMALL	25 MG	N85683 001	
AB		50 MG	N83965 001	
AB		50 MG	N85672 001	
AB	DANBURY	25 MG	N81189 001	JAN 24, 1992
AB		50 MG	N83232 001	
AB		100 MG	N81190 001	JAN 24, 1992
AB	EON LABS	25 MG	N83899 001	
AB	GENEVA	50 MG	N85219 001	
AB		25 MG	N87565 001	MAR 09, 1982
AB	INWOOD	50 MG	N84912 001	
AB		25 MG	N84776 001	
AB	LEDERLE	25 MG	N85067 001	
AB		50 MG	N84776 002	
AB		25 MG	N87059 001	
AB		50 MG	N87068 001	
AB		100 MG	N87060 001	
AB	LEMMON	25 MG	N88924 001	FEB 07, 1985
AB		50 MG	N88923 001	FEB 07, 1985
AB	MAST	25 MG	N86192 001	
AB		50 MG	N86192 002	
AB	PHARMAFAIR	25 MG	N84325 001	
AB		50 MG	N84324 001	
AB	PRIVATE FORM	25 MG	N85181 001	
AB		50 MG	N85182 001	
AB	PUREPAC	50 MG	N86597 001	
AB		25 MG	N85054 002	
AB		50 MG	N85208 001	
AB	RICHLYN	25 MG	N84029 001	
AB		50 MG	N83607 002	
AB		100 MG	N85098 001	
AB	ROXANE	50 MG	N84536 002	
AB	SUPERPHARM	25 MG	N88827 001	DEC 28, 1984
AB		50 MG	N88828 001	DEC 28, 1984
AB		100 MG	N88829 001	DEC 28, 1984
AB	WEST WARD	25 MG	N84899 001	
AB	ZENITH	50 MG	N84878 001	
AB		50 MG	N83177 001	
AB		50 MG	N83177 002	
AB		50 MG	N84658 001	
AB		100 MG	N85022 001	

Prescription Drug Products (continued)

HYDROCHLOROTHIAZIDE (continued)

TABLET; ORAL

HYDRODIURIL
+ MSD
- AB   25 MG   N11835 003
- AB   50 MG   N11835 006
- AB   100 MG   N11835 007

ORETIC
  ABBOTT
- AB   25 MG   N11971 001
- AB   50 MG   N11971 002

HYDROCHLOROTHIAZIDE; *MULTIPLE*

SEE   AMILORIDE HYDROCHLORIDE: HYDROCHLOROTHIAZIDE
SEE   BENAZEPRIL HYDROCHLORIDE: HYDROCHLOROTHIAZIDE
SEE   CAPTOPRIL: HYDROCHLOROTHIAZIDE
SEE   DESERPIDINE: HYDROCHLOROTHIAZIDE
SEE   ENALAPRIL MALEATE: HYDROCHLOROTHIAZIDE
SEE   GUANETHIDINE MONOSULFATE: HYDROCHLOROTHIAZIDE
SEE   HYDRALAZINE HYDROCHLORIDE: HYDROCHLOROTHIAZIDE
SEE   HYDRALAZINE HYDROCHLORIDE: HYDROCHLOROTHIAZIDE: RESERPINE
SEE   HYDRALAZINE HYDROCHLORIDE: HYDROCHLOROTHIAZIDE

HYDROCHLOROTHIAZIDE; METHYLDOPA

TABLET; ORAL

ALDORIL D30
+ MSD
- AB   30 MG;500 MG   N13402 003

ALDORIL D50
+ MSD
- AB   50 MG;500 MG   N13402 004

ALDORIL 15
  MSD
- AB   15 MG;250 MG   N13402 001

ALDORIL 25
  MSD
- AB   25 MG;250 MG   N13402 002

METHYLDOPA AND HYDROCHLOROTHIAZIDE
  DANBURY
- AB   15 MG;250 MG   N70958 001   FEB 06, 1989
- AB   25 MG;250 MG   N70959 001   JAN 19, 1989
- AB   30 MG;500 MG   N71069 001   JAN 19, 1989
- AB   50 MG;500 MG   N70960 001   FEB 06, 1989

  GENEVA
- AB   15 MG;250 MG   N70182 001   JAN 15, 1986
- AB   25 MG;250 MG   N70183 001   JAN 15, 1986
- AB   30 MG;500 MG   N70543 001   JAN 15, 1986
- AB   50 MG;500 MG   N70544 001   JAN 15, 1986

  INVAMED
- AB   15 MG;250 MG   N70829 001   MAR 09, 1987
- AB   25 MG;250 MG   N70830 001   MAR 09, 1987

  LEDERLE
- AB   15 MG;250 MG   N72507 001   JUN 02, 1989
- AB   25 MG;250 MG   N72508 001   JUN 02, 1989
- AB   30 MG;500 MG   N72509 001   JUN 02, 1989
- AB   50 MG;500 MG   N72510 001   JUN 02, 1989

  MYLAN
- AB   15 MG;250 MG   N70264 001   JAN 23, 1986
- AB   25 MG;250 MG   N70265 001   JAN 23, 1986

  NOVOPHARM
- AB   15 MG;250 MG   N71819 001   APR 08, 1988
- AB   25 MG;250 MG   N71820 001   APR 08, 1988
- AB   30 MG;500 MG   N71821 001   APR 08, 1988
- AB   50 MG;500 MG   N71822 001   APR 08, 1988

  PAR
- AB   15 MG;250 MG   N70616 001   FEB 02, 1987
- AB   25 MG;250 MG   N70612 001   FEB 02, 1987
- AB   30 MG;500 MG   N70613 001   FEB 02, 1987
- AB   50 MG;500 MG   N70614 001   FEB 02, 1987

HYDROCHLOROTHIAZIDE; LABETALOL HYDROCHLORIDE

TABLET; ORAL

NORMOZIDE
+ SCHERING
- AB   25 MG;100 MG   N19046 001   APR 06, 1987
- AB   25 MG;200 MG   N19046 002   APR 06, 1987
- AB   25 MG;300 MG   N19046 003   APR 06, 1987

TRANDATE HCT
  GLAXO
- AB   25 MG;100 MG   N19174 001   APR 10, 1987
- AB   25 MG;200 MG   N19174 002   APR 10, 1987
- AB   25 MG;300 MG   N19174 003   APR 10, 1987

HYDROCHLOROTHIAZIDE; LISINOPRIL

TABLET; ORAL

PRINZIDE 12.5
+ MERCK
- AB   12.5 MG;20 MG   N19778 001   FEB 16, 1989

PRINZIDE 25
+ MERCK
- AB   25 MG;20 MG   N19778 002   FEB 16, 1989

ZESTORETIC 20/12.5
  IMPERIAL CHEM
- AB   12.5 MG;20 MG   N19888 001   SEP 20, 1990

ZESTORETIC 20/25
  IMPERIAL CHEM
- AB   25 MG;20 MG   N19888 002   JUL 20, 1989

Prescription Drug Products (continued)

HYDROCHLOROTHIAZIDE; METHYLDOPA (continued)

TABLET; ORAL
METHYLDOPA AND HYDROCHLOROTHIAZIDE

ΔB	PARKE DAVIS	15 MG;250 MG	N71897 001	NOV 23, 1987
ΔB		25 MG;250 MG	N71898 001	NOV 23, 1987
ΔB		30 MG;500 MG	N71899 001	NOV 23, 1987
ΔB		50 MG;500 MG	N71900 001	NOV 23, 1987
ΔB	PUREPAC	15 MG;250 MG	N70853 001	OCT 08, 1986
ΔB		25 MG;250 MG	N70688 001	APR 24, 1986
ΔB		30 MG;500 MG	N70854 001	OCT 08, 1986
ΔB	WATSON	15 MG;250 MG	N71920 001	AUG 29, 1988
ΔB		25 MG;250 MG	N71921 001	AUG 29, 1988
ΔB		30 MG;500 MG	N71922 001	AUG 29, 1988
ΔB		50 MG;500 MG	N71923 001	AUG 29, 1988
ΔB	ZENITH	15 MG;250 MG	N71458 001	MAR 08, 1988
ΔB		25 MG;250 MG	N71459 001	MAR 08, 1988
ΔB		30 MG;500 MG	N71460 001	MAR 08, 1988
ΔB		50 MG;500 MG	N71461 001	MAR 08, 1988

HYDROCHLOROTHIAZIDE; METOPROLOL TARTRATE

TABLET; ORAL

LOPRESSOR HCT 100/25 CIBA	25 MG;100 MG	N18303 002	DEC 31, 1984
LOPRESSOR HCT 100/50 + CIBA	50 MG;100 MG	N18303 003	DEC 31, 1984
LOPRESSOR HCT 50/25 CIBA	25 MG;50 MG	N18303 001	DEC 31, 1984

HYDROCHLOROTHIAZIDE; PROPRANOLOL HYDROCHLORIDE

CAPSULE, EXTENDED RELEASE; ORAL

INDERIDE LA 120/50 + WYETH AYERST	50 MG;120 MG	N19059 002	JUL 03, 1985
INDERIDE LA 160/50 + WYETH AYERST	50 MG;160 MG	N19059 003	JUL 03, 1985
INDERIDE LA 80/50 + WYETH AYERST	50 MG;80 MG	N19059 001	JUL 03, 1985

TABLET; ORAL

ΔB	INDERIDE 40/25 + WYETH AYERST	25 MG;40 MG	N18031 001	
ΔB	INDERIDE 80/25 + WYETH AYERST	25 MG;80 MG	N18031 002	

PROPRANOLOL HCL AND HYDROCHLOROTHIAZIDE

ΔB	BARR	25 MG;40 MG	N70704 001	OCT 01, 1986
		25 MG;80 MG	N70705 001	OCT 01, 1986
ΔB	CHELSEA	25 MG;40 MG	N70301 001	APR 18, 1986
		25 MG;80 MG	N70305 001	APR 18, 1986
ΔB	DANBURY	25 MG;40 MG	N71498 001	DEC 18, 1991
		25 MG;80 MG	N71501 001	DEC 18, 1991
ΔB	GENEVA	25 MG;40 MG	N71060 001	AUG 26, 1987
		25 MG;80 MG	N71061 001	AUG 26, 1987
ΔB	MYLAN	25 MG;40 MG	N70946 001	MAR 04, 1987
ΔB		25 MG;80 MG	N70947 001	APR 01, 1987
ΔB	PUREPAC	25 MG;40 MG	N70851 001	MAY 15, 1986
		25 MG;80 MG	N70852 001	MAY 15, 1986
ΔB	SIDMAK	25 MG;40 MG	N72042 001	MAR 14, 1988
ΔB		25 MG;80 MG	N72043 001	MAR 14, 1988
ΔB	WARNER CHILCOTT	25 MG;40 MG	N71771 001	JAN 26, 1988
ΔB		25 MG;80 MG	N71772 001	JAN 26, 1988
ΔB	ZENITH	25 MG;40 MG	N71552 001	DEC 01, 1988
ΔB		25 MG;80 MG	N71553 001	DEC 01, 1988

Prescription Drug Products (continued)

HYDROCHLOROTHIAZIDE; RESERPINE

TABLET; ORAL

HYDRO-RESERP

BP	CAMALL	50 MG;0.125 MG	N84714 002	JUN 29, 1982

HYDROCHLOROTHIAZIDE W/ RESERPINE

BP	DANBURY	25 MG;0.125 MG	N84466 001
BP		50 MG;0.125 MG	N84467 001
BP		50 MG;0.125 MG	N84603 001
BP	ROXANE	25 MG;0.125 MG	N83571 001
BP	ZENITH	50 MG;0.125 MG	N83573 001
BP		25 MG;0.1 MG	N83572 001
BP		50 MG;0.1 MG	N83568 001

HYDROPRES 25

BP	MSD	25 MG;0.125 MG	N11958 002

HYDROPRES 50

BP	MSD	50 MG;0.125 MG	N11958 003

RESERPINE AND HYDROCHLOROTHIAZIDE-50

BP	WEST WARD	50 MG;0.125 MG	N88189 001	MAY 10, 1984

HYDROCHLOROTHIAZIDE; SPIRONOLACTONE

TABLET; ORAL

ALDACTAZIDE

AB	SEARLE	25 MG;25 MG	N12616 004	DEC 30, 1982
		50 MG;50 MG	N12616 005	DEC 30, 1982

SPIRONOLACTONE AND HYDROCHLOROTHIAZIDE

AB	BARR	25 MG;25 MG	N87267 001	
AB	MUTUAL PHARM	25 MG;25 MG	N89534 001	JUL 02, 1987
AB	MYLAN	25 MG;25 MG	N86513 001	
AB	PUREPAC	25 MG;25 MG	N87999 001	NOV 06, 1985

SPIRONOLACTONE W/ HYDROCHLOROTHIAZIDE

AB	GENEVA	25 MG;25 MG	N86881 001	
AB	PARKE DAVIS	25 MG;25 MG	N87948 001	FEB 22, 1983
AB	UPSHER SMITH	25 MG;25 MG	N87553 001	
AB	ZENITH	25 MG;25 MG	N87004 002	MAY 24, 1982

SPIRONOLACTONE/HYDROCHLOROTHIAZIDE

AB	DANBURY	25 MG;25 MG	N87398 001

HYDROCHLOROTHIAZIDE; TIMOLOL MALEATE

TABLET; ORAL

TIMOLIDE 10-25

+	MSD	25 MG;10 MG	N18061 001

HYDROCHLOROTHIAZIDE; TRIAMTERENE

CAPSULE; ORAL

DYAZIDE

+	SKF	25 MG;50 MG	N16042 002	

TRIAMTERENE AND HYDROCHLOROTHIAZIDE

AB	GENEVA	25 MG;50 MG	N73191 001	JUL 31, 1991

TABLET; ORAL

MAXZIDE

AB	+ MYLAN	50 MG;75 MG	N19129 001	OCT 22, 1984

MAXZIDE-25

AB	MYLAN	25 MG;37.5 MG	N19129 003	MAY 13, 1988

TRIAMTERENE AND HYDROCHLOROTHIAZIDE

AB	BARR	50 MG;75 MG	N71251 001	DEC 08, 1987
AB	DANBURY	50 MG;75 MG	N71969 001	JAN 15, 1988
B*	EON LABS	50 MG;75 MG	N71360 001	DEC 08, 1987
AB	GENEVA	25 MG;37.5 MG	N73281 001	APR 30, 1992
AB		50 MG;75 MG	N72011 001	JUN 17, 1988
B*	PAR	50 MG;75 MG	N72337 001	MAY 11, 1988
AB	WATSON	50 MG;75 MG	N71851 001	NOV 30, 1988

HYDROCODONE BITARTRATE; *MULTIPLE*

SEE   ACETAMINOPHEN; HYDROCODONE BITARTRATE

SEE   ASPIRIN; HYDROCODONE BITARTRATE

SEE   HOMATROPINE METHYLBROMIDE; HYDROCODONE BITARTRATE

HYDROCODONE BITARTRATE; PHENYLPROPANOLAMINE HYDROCHLORIDE

SYRUP; ORAL

HYCOMINE

	DUPONT	5 MG/5 ML;25 MG/5 ML	N19410 001	AUG 17, 1990

HYCOMINE PEDIATRIC

	DUPONT	2.5 MG/5 ML;12.5 MG/5 ML	N19411 001	AUG 17, 1990

HYDROCODONE POLISTIREX; *MULTIPLE*

SEE   CHLORPHENIRAMINE POLISTIREX; HYDROCODONE POLISTIREX

Prescription Drug Products (continued)

HYDROCORTISONE

AEROSOL; TOPICAL

TE	Firm/Product	Strength	Appl. No.	Date
	AEROSEB-HC			
	HERBERT	0.5%	N85805 001	

CREAM; TOPICAL

TE	Firm/Product	Strength	Appl. No.	Date
	ALA-CORT			
AT	DEL RAY	1%	N80706 006	
	ANUSOL HC			
AT	PARKE DAVIS	2.5%	N88250 001	JUN 06, 1984
	CORT-DOME			
AT	MILES	0.5%	N09585 003	
AT		1%	N09585 001	
	DERMACORT			
AT	SOLVAY	1%	N83011 002	
	FLEXICORT			
AT	WESTWOOD SQUIBB	0.5%	N87136 003	
AT		1%	N87136 002	APR 08, 1982
AT		2.5%	N87136 001	APR 08, 1982
	HC (HYDROCORTISONE)			
AT	C AND M	0.5%	N80482 003	
AT		1%	N80482 004	
	HI-COR			
AT	C AND M	2.5%	N80483 001	
	HYDROCORTISONE			
AT	ALTANA	0.5%	N80848 002	
AT		1%	N80848 003	
AT		2.5%	N86080 001	
AT	AMBIX	0.5%	N86271 001	
AT		1%	N80400 002	
AT	BIOCRAFT	2.5%	N80400 003	
AT		0.5%	N80400 004	
AT	CLAY PARK	1%	N84970 002	
AT		2.5%	N85026 001	
AT		0.5%	N85025 001	
AT	EVERYLIFE	1%	N80452 002	
AT	FOUGERA	2.5%	N80693 003	
AT		1%	N89414 001	DEC 16, 1986
AT		2.5%	N84059 001	
AT	G AND W	1%	N80456 002	
AT	INGRAM	0.5%	N80456 003	
AT		1%	N85191 001	
AT	LEMMON	1%	N89682 001	MAR 10, 1988
AT	NASKA	2.5%	N87795 001	MAY 03, 1983
AT	NMC	1%	N89754 001	FEB 01, 1989
AT		2.5%	N88845 001	FEB 27, 1986
AT	PHARMADERM	1%	N89413 001	DEC 16, 1986
AT		2.5%		

HYDROCORTISONE (continued)

CREAM; TOPICAL

TE	Firm/Product	Strength	Appl. No.	Date
	HYDROCORTISONE			
	PHARMAFAIR	1%	N87838 001	JUL 28, 1982
AT	SYOSSET	0.5%	N85527 001	
AT		1%	N85733 001	
AT	THAMES	1%	N86155 001	
AT		2.5%	N88799 001	NOV 09, 1984
AT	TOPIDERM	1%	N89273 001	FEB 17, 1989
	HYTONE			
AT	DERMIK	1%	N80472 003	
AT		2.5%	N80472 004	
	NOGENIC HC			
AT	SYOSSET	1%	N87427 001	APR 04, 1988
	NUTRACORT			
AT	OWEN GALDERMA	0.5%	N80442 002	
AT		1%	N80442 003	
	PENECORT			
AT	HERBERT	1%	N88216 001	JUN 06, 1984
	PROCTOCORT			
AT	SOLVAY	1%	N83011 001	
	SYNACORT			
AT	SYNTEX	1%	N87458 001	
AT		2.5%	N87457 001	

ENEMA; RECTAL

TE	Firm/Product	Strength	Appl. No.	Date
	CORTENEMA			
	SOLVAY	100 MG/60 ML	N16199 001	

GEL; TOPICAL

TE	Firm/Product	Strength	Appl. No.	Date
	NUTRACORT			
AT	OWEN GALDERMA	1%	N84698 001	
	PENECORT			
AT	HERBERT	1%	N88215 001	JUN 06, 1984

INJECTABLE; INJECTION

TE	Firm/Product	Strength	Appl. No.	Date
	CORTEF			
	UPJOHN	50 MG/ML	N09864 001	

LOTION; TOPICAL

TE	Firm/Product	Strength	Appl. No.	Date
	ACTICORT			
AT	KEY PHARMS	1%	N86535 001	
	ALA-CORT			
AT	DEL RAY	1%	N83201 001	
	ALA-SCALP			
	DEL RAY	2%	N83231 001	
	BALNEOL-HC			
AT	SOLVAY	1%	N88041 001	DEC 03, 1982
	BETA-HC			
AT	BETA DERMAC	1%	N89495 001	JAN 25, 1988

Prescription Drug Products (continued)

HYDROCORTISONE (continued)

LOTION; TOPICAL

TE	Name	Strength	Appl. No.	Date
	CETACORT			
AT	OWEN GALDERMA	0.5%	N80426 002	
AT	OWEN GALDERMA	1%	N80426 001	
	DERMACORT			
AT	SOLVAY	0.5%	N84573 002	
AT	SOLVAY	1%	N86462 001	
	EPICORT			
AT	BLULINE	0.5%	N83219 002	
	GLYCORT			
AT	HERAN	1%	N87489 001	OCT 03, 1983
	HYDROCORTISONE			
AT	CLAY PARK	0.5%	N85662 001	
AT	CLAY PARK	0.5%	N85663 001	
AT	CLAY PARK	1%	N85282 001	
			N85282 002	FEB 26, 1987
AT	MERICON	1%	N89024 001	
AT	THAMES	1%	N87644 001	FEB 12, 1986
	HYTONE			
AT	DERMIK	1%	N80473 003	
AT	DERMIK	2.5%	N80473 004	NOV 30, 1982
	NUTRACORT			
AT	OWEN GALDERMA	0.5%	N80443 002	
AT	OWEN GALDERMA	2.5%	N80443 003	
AT	OWEN GALDERMA	1%	N87644 001	AUG 24, 1982
	STIE-CORT			
AT	STIEFEL	1%	N89066 001	NOV 25, 1985
AT	STIEFEL	2.5%	N89074 001	NOV 26, 1985

OINTMENT; TOPICAL

TE	Name	Strength	Appl. No.	Date
	CORTRIL			
AT	PFIPHARMECS	1%	N09176 001	
AT	PFIPHARMECS	2.5%	N09176 002	
	HC (HYDROCORTISONE)			
AT	C AND M	1%	N80481 002	
	HYDROCORTISONE			
AT	ALTANA	1%	N80489 003	
AT	ALTANA	1%	N80692 001	
AT	AMBIX	1%	N86079 001	
AT	AMBIX	2.5%	N86272 001	
AT	CLAY PARK	1%	N85028 001	
AT	CLAY PARK	2.5%	N85027 001	
AT	PHARMADERM	2.5%	N84969 003	
AT	PHARMADERM	0.5%	N88842 001	FEB 09, 1987
AT	THAMES	1%	N86257 001	

HYDROCORTISONE (continued)

OINTMENT; TOPICAL

TE	Name	Strength	Appl. No.	Date
	HYDROCORTISONE IN ABSORBASE			
AT	CAROLINA MEDCL	1%	N88138 001	SEP 06, 1985
	HYMAC			
AT	NMC	1%	N87796 001	OCT 13, 1982
	HYTONE			
AT	DERMIK	1%	N80474 003	
AT	DERMIK	2.5%	N80474 004	
	PENECORT			
AT	HERBERT	2.5%	N88217 001	JUN 06, 1984

POWDER; FOR RX COMPOUNDING

TE	Name	Strength	Appl. No.	Date
	H-CORT			
AA	TORCH LABS	100%	N87834 001	MAR 29, 1982
	HYDROCORTISONE			
AA	PADDOCK	100%	N88082 001	APR 08, 1983
AA	PHARMA TEK	100%	N85982 001	

SOLUTION; TOPICAL

TE	Name	Strength	Appl. No.	Date
	PENECORT			
AT	HERBERT	1%	N88214 001	JUN 06, 1984
	TEXACORT			
AT	GENDERM	1%	N80425 001	
AT	GENDERM	2.5%	N81271 001	APR 17, 1992

TABLET; ORAL

TE	Name	Strength	Appl. No.	Date
	CORTEF			
BP	UPJOHN	10 MG	N08697 001	
BP	UPJOHN	20 MG	N08697 002	
	UPJOHN	5 MG	N08697 003	
	HYDROCORTISONE			
BP	DANBURY	20 MG	N80355 001	
BP	INWOOD	20 MG	N80732 001	
BP	LANNETT	20 MG	N85070 001	
BP	MK	10 MG	N80568 001	
BP	MK	20 MG	N80568 002	
BP	PUREPAC	10 MG	N84247 003	AUG 31, 1982
BP	PUREPAC	20 MG	N84247 002	
BP	RICHLYN	20 MG	N80781 001	
BP	WEST WARD	20 MG	N83365 001	
	HYDROCORTONE			
BP	MSD	10 MG	N08506 007	
BP +	MSD	20 MG	N08506 011	

TABLET; VAGINAL

TE	Name	Strength	Appl. No.	Date
	CORTRIL			
AT	PFIPHARMECS	10 MG	N09796 001	

Prescription Drug Products (continued)

HYDROCORTISONE; *MULTIPLE*
SEE   ACETIC ACID, GLACIAL; HYDROCORTISONE
SEE   ACETIC ACID, GLACIAL; HYDROCORTISONE; NEOMYCIN SULFATE
SEE   BACITRACIN ZINC; HYDROCORTISONE; NEOMYCIN SULFATE; POLYMYXIN B SULFATE
SEE   CLIOQUINOL; HYDROCORTISONE

HYDROCORTISONE; NEOMYCIN SULFATE
CREAM; TOPICAL
NEO-CORT-DOME
  MILES   0.5%;EQ 3.5 MG BASE/GM   N50237 006   JUN 05, 1984
    1%;EQ 3.5 MG BASE/GM   N50237 005   JUN 05, 1984

HYDROCORTISONE; NEOMYCIN SULFATE; POLYMYXIN B SULFATE
SOLUTION/DROPS; OTIC
CORTISPORIN
AT BURROUGHS WELLCOME   1%;EQ 3.5 MG BASE/ML:10,000 UNITS/ML
NEO-OTOSOL-HC
AT STERIS   1%;EQ 3.5 MG BASE/ML:10,000 UNITS/ML   N50479 001

NEOMYCIN SULFATE-POLYMYXIN B SULFATE-HYDROCORTISONE
AT PHARMAFAIR   1%;EQ 3.5 MG BASE/ML:10,000 UNITS/ML   N62423 001   AUG 25, 1983

OTOCORT
AT STERIS   1%;EQ 3.5 MG BASE/ML:10,000 UNITS/ML   N62394 001   SEP 29, 1982   N60730 002

SUSPENSION; OTIC
CORTISPORIN
AT BURROUGHS WELLCOME   1%;EQ 3.5 MG BASE/ML:10,000 UNITS/ML   N60613 001

NEOMYCIN AND POLYMYXIN B SULFATES AND HYDROCORTISONE
AT STERIS   1%;EQ 3.5 MG BASE/ML:10,000 UNITS/ML   N62488 001   NOV 06, 1985

NEOMYCIN SULFATE, POLYMYXIN B SULFATE & HYDROCORTISONE
AT PHARMAFAIR   1%;EQ 3.5 MG BASE/ML:10,000 UNITS/ML   N62617 001   SEP 18, 1985

OTICAIR
AT PHARMAFAIR   1%;EQ 3.5 MG BASE/ML:10,000 UNITS/ML   N62399 001   NOV 18, 1982

HYDROCORTISONE; NEOMYCIN SULFATE; POLYMYXIN B SULFATE (continued)
SUSPENSION; OTIC
OTOBIONE
AT SCHERING   1%;EQ 3.5 MG BASE/ML:10,000 UNITS/ML   N61816 001
OTOCORT
AT STERIS   1%;EQ 3.5 MG BASE/ML:10,000 UNITS/ML   N62521 001   JUL 11, 1985
PEDIOTIC
AT BURROUGHS WELLCOME   1%;EQ 3.5 MG BASE/ML:10,000 UNITS/ML   N62822 001   SEP 29, 1987

SUSPENSION/DROPS; OPHTHALMIC
CORTISPORIN
AT BURROUGHS WELLCOME   1%;EQ 3.5 MG BASE/ML:10,000 UNITS/ML   N50169 001

NEOMYCIN AND POLYMYXIN B SULFATES AND HYDROCORTISONE
AT STERIS   1%;EQ 3.5 MG BASE/ML:10,000 UNITS/ML   N62874 001   MAY 11, 1988

NEOMYCIN SULFATE-POLYMYXIN B SULFATE-HYDROCORTISONE
AT PHARMAFAIR   1%;EQ 3.5 MG BASE/ML:10,000 UNITS/ML   N62623 001   SEP 24, 1985

HYDROCORTISONE; POLYMYXIN B SULFATE
SOLUTION/DROPS; OTIC
OTOBIOTIC
AT SCHERING   5 MG/ML:EQ 10,000 UNITS BASE/ML   N62302 001
PYOCIDIN
AT FOREST LABS   5 MG/ML:EQ 10,000 UNITS BASE/ML   N61606 001

HYDROCORTISONE; TETRACYCLINE HYDROCHLORIDE
OINTMENT; OPHTHALMIC
ACHROMYCIN
AT LEDERLE   1.5%;1%   N50272 001

HYDROCORTISONE; UREA
CREAM; TOPICAL
ALPHADERM
AT VIVAN   1%;10%   N86008 001
CALMURID HC
AT KABI   1%;10%   N83947 001

Prescription Drug Products (continued)

HYDROCORTISONE ACETATE

AEROSOL; RECTAL
CORTIFOAM
REED AND CARNRICK   10%   N17351 001   FEB 10, 1982

CREAM; TOPICAL
HEMSOL-HC
AT   ABLE   1%   N81274 001   JUN 19, 1992

HYDROCORTISONE ACETATE
AT   CENCI   1%   N80419 001   JAN 25, 1982
AT   PARKE DAVIS   1%   N89914 001   JAN 03, 1989
AT   PUREPAC   1%   N86052 001
           0.5%   N86050 001

INJECTABLE; INJECTION
HYDROCORTISONE ACETATE
BP   AKORN   25 MG/ML   N09637 001
BP   50 MG/ML   N09637 002
BP   BEL MAR   25 MG/ML   N83739 001
BP   50 MG/ML   N83739 002
BP   STERIS   25 MG/ML   N83128 001
BP   25 MG/ML   N83759 001
BP   50 MG/ML   N83759 002
BP   50 MG/ML   N85214 001
HYDROCORTONE
BP   MSD   25 MG/ML   N08228 001
BP +   50 MG/ML   N08228 004

LOTION; TOPICAL
DRICORT
INGRAM   0.5%   N86207 001

OINTMENT; OPHTHALMIC
HYDROCORTISONE ACETATE
ALTANA   0.5%   N80828 001

OINTMENT; TOPICAL
CORTEF ACETATE
UPJOHN   EQ 1% BASE   N08917 002
        2.5%   N08917 001

PASTE; TOPICAL
ORABASE HCA
HOYT   0.5%   N83205 001

POWDER; FOR RX COMPOUNDING
HYDROCORTISONE ACETATE
PHARMA TEK   100%   N85981 001

HYDROCORTISONE ACETATE; *MULTIPLE*

SEE   BACITRACIN; HYDROCORTISONE ACETATE; NEOMYCIN SULFATE; POLYMYXIN B SULFATE
SEE   CHLORAMPHENICOL; HYDROCORTISONE ACETATE
SEE   CHLORAMPHENICOL; HYDROCORTISONE ACETATE; POLYMYXIN B SULFATE
SEE   COLISTIN SULFATE; HYDROCORTISONE ACETATE; NEOMYCIN SULFATE; THONZONIUM BROMIDE

HYDROCORTISONE ACETATE; NEOMYCIN SULFATE

CREAM; TOPICAL
NEO-CORTEF
UPJOHN   1%;EQ 3.5 MG BASE/GM   N61049 001
        2.5%;EQ 3.5 MG BASE/GM   N61049 002

OINTMENT; TOPICAL
NEO-CORTEF
UPJOHN   0.5%;EQ 3.5 MG BASE/GM   N60751 001
        1%;EQ 3.5 MG BASE/GM   N60751 002
        2.5%;EQ 3.5 MG BASE/GM   N60751 003

SUSPENSION/DROPS; OPHTHALMIC
COR-OTICIN
AT   AKORN   1.5%;EQ 3.5 MG BASE/ML   N60188 001
NEO-CORTEF
AT   UPJOHN   1.5%;EQ 3.5 MG BASE/ML   N60612 001
          0.5%;EQ 3.5 MG BASE/ML   N60612 002

HYDROCORTISONE ACETATE; NEOMYCIN SULFATE; POLYMYXIN B SULFATE

CREAM; TOPICAL
CORTISPORIN
BURROUGHS WELLCOME   0.5%;EQ 3.5 MG BASE/GM;10,000 UNITS/GM   N50218 001   AUG 09, 1985

HYDROCORTISONE ACETATE; OXYTETRACYCLINE HYDROCHLORIDE

SUSPENSION/DROPS; OPHTHALMIC
TERRA-CORTRIL
PFIZER   1.5%;EQ 5 MG BASE/ML   N61016 001

Prescription Drug Products *(continued)*

HYDROCORTISONE ACETATE; PRAMOXINE HYDROCHLORIDE

AEROSOL; TOPICAL

	EPIFOAM			
BX	REED AND CARNRICK	1%;1%	N86457 001	
	HYDROCORTISONE ACETATE 1% AND PRAMOXINE HCL 1%			
BX	COPLEY	1%;1%	N89440 001	MAY 17, 1988
	PROCTOFOAM HC			
BX	REED AND CARNRICK	1%;1%	N86195 001	

CREAM; TOPICAL

	PRAMOSONE			
	FERNDALE	0.5%;1%	N33778 001	
		1%;1%	N85368 001	

LOTION; TOPICAL

	PRAMOSONE			
	FERNDALE	0.5%;1%	N83213 002	
		1%;1%	N85980 001	
		2.5%;1%	N85979 001	

HYDROCORTISONE ACETATE; UREA

CREAM; TOPICAL

	CARMOL HC			
ΔT	SYNTEX	1%;10%	N80505 001	
	HYDROCORTISONE ACETATE			
ΔT	THAMES	1%;10%	N89472 001	JUN 13, 1988

HYDROCORTISONE BUTYRATE

CREAM; TOPICAL

	LOCOID			
	+ BROCADES PHARMA	0.1%	N18514 001	MAR 31, 1982

OINTMENT; TOPICAL

	LOCOID			
	+ OWEN GALDERMA	0.1%	N19106 001	JUL 03, 1984

SOLUTION; TOPICAL

	LOCOID			
	BROCADES PHARMA	0.1%	N19116 001	FEB 25, 1987

HYDROCORTISONE CYPIONATE

SUSPENSION; ORAL

	CORTEF			
	+ UPJOHN	EQ 10 MG BASE/5 ML	N09900 001	

HYDROCORTISONE SODIUM PHOSPHATE

INJECTABLE; INJECTION

	HYDROCORTONE			
	MSD	EQ 50 MG BASE/ML	N12052 001	

HYDROCORTISONE SODIUM SUCCINATE

INJECTABLE; INJECTION

	A-HYDROCORT			
	ABBOTT			
AP		EQ 100 MG BASE/VIAL	N85928 001	
AP		EQ 100 MG BASE/VIAL	N85929 001	
AP		EQ 100 MG BASE/VIAL	N89577 001	APR 11, 1989
AP		EQ 250 MG BASE/VIAL	N85930 001	
AP		EQ 250 MG BASE/VIAL	N89578 001	APR 11, 1989
		EQ 500 MG BASE/VIAL	N85931 001	
AP		EQ 500 MG BASE/VIAL	N89579 001	APR 11, 1989
AP		EQ 1 GM BASE/VIAL	N85932 001	
AP		EQ 1 GM BASE/VIAL	N89580 001	APR 11, 1989

HYDROCORTISONE SODIUM SUCCINATE

	ELKINS SINN			
AP		EQ 100 MG BASE/VIAL	N86619 001	
AP		EQ 250 MG BASE/VIAL	N87567 001	
AP		EQ 500 MG BASE/VIAL	N87568 001	
AP		EQ 100 MG BASE/VIAL	N87569 001	
	INTL MEDICATION			
AP		EQ 100 MG BASE/VIAL	N87532 001	MAR 19, 1982
	STERIS			
AP		EQ 100 MG BASE/VIAL	N84737 002	
AP		EQ 100 MG BASE/VIAL	N84738 001	
AP		EQ 250 MG BASE/VIAL	N84737 001	
AP		EQ 500 MG BASE/VIAL	N84747 001	
AP		EQ 1 GM BASE/VIAL	N84748 001	
	SOLU-CORTEF			
	UPJOHN			
AP		EQ 100 MG BASE/VIAL	N09866 001	
AP		EQ 250 MG BASE/VIAL	N09866 002	
AP		EQ 500 MG BASE/VIAL	N09866 003	
AP		EQ 1 GM BASE/VIAL	N09866 004	

HYDROCORTISONE VALERATE

CREAM; TOPICAL

	WESTCORT			
	+ WESTWOOD SQUIBB	0.2%	N17950 001	

OINTMENT; TOPICAL

	WESTCORT			
	+ WESTWOOD SQUIBB	0.2%	N18726 001	AUG 08, 1983

HYDROFLUMETHIAZIDE

TABLET; ORAL

	DIUCARDIN			
AB	WYETH AYERST	50 MG	N83383 001	
	HYDROFLUMETHIAZIDE			
AB	PAR	50 MG	N88850 001	MAY 31, 1985
	SALURON			
AB	+ BRISTOL	50 MG	N11949 001	

Prescription Drug Products (continued)

HYDROFLUMETHIAZIDE; RESERPINE

TABLET; ORAL

RESERPINE AND HYDROFLUMETHIAZIDE

TE	Firm	Strength	Appl No	Date
BP	PAR	50 MG;0.125 MG	N88907 001	SEP 20, 1985
BP	ZENITH	50 MG;0.125 MG	N88932 001	JAN 11, 1985

SALUTENSIN

TE	Firm	Strength	Appl No	Date
BP +	BRISTOL	50 MG;0.125 MG	N12359 003	

SALUTENSIN-DEMI

TE	Firm	Strength	Appl No	Date
	BRISTOL	25 MG;0.125 MG	N12359 004	

HYDROMORPHONE HYDROCHLORIDE

INJECTABLE; INJECTION

DILAUDID-HP

Firm	Strength	Appl No	Date
KNOLL	10 MG/ML	N19034 001	JAN 11, 1984

HYDROXOCOBALAMIN

INJECTABLE; INJECTION

ALPHAREDISOL

TE	Firm	Strength	Appl No
AP	MSD	1MG/ML	N80778 001

HYDROXOCOBALAMIN

TE	Firm	Strength	Appl No
AP	STERIS	1MG/ML	N85528 001
AP		1MG/ML	N85998 001

HYDROXOMIN

TE	Firm	Strength	Appl No
AP	BEL MAR	1MG/ML	N84629 001

HYDROXYAMPHETAMINE HYDROBROMIDE

SOLUTION/DROPS; OPHTHALMIC

PAREDRINE

Firm	Strength	Appl No
PHARMICS	1%	N00004 004

HYDROXYAMPHETAMINE HYDROBROMIDE; TROPICAMIDE

SOLUTION/DROPS; OPHTHALMIC

PAREMYD

Firm	Strength	Appl No	Date
ALLERGAN	1%;0.25%	N19261 001	JAN 30, 1992

HYDROXYCHLOROQUINE SULFATE

TABLET; ORAL

PLAQUENIL

Firm	Strength	Appl No
STERLING	EQ 155 MG BASE	N09768 001

HYDROXYPROGESTERONE CAPROATE

INJECTABLE; INJECTION

DELALUTIN

TE	Firm	Strength	Appl No
AO	SQUIBB	125 MG/ML	N10347 004
AO		125 MG/ML	N16911 001
AO		250 MG/ML	N10347 002
AO		250 MG/ML	N16911 002

HYDROXYPROGESTERONE CAPROATE

TE	Firm	Strength	Appl No
AO	AKORN	125 MG/ML	N18004 001
AO	STERIS	125 MG/ML	N17439 001
AO		250 MG/ML	N17439 002

HYDROXYPROPYL CELLULOSE

INSERT; OPHTHALMIC

LACRISERT

Firm	Strength	Appl No
MERCK	5 MG	N18771 001

HYDROXYUREA

CAPSULE; ORAL

HYDREA

Firm	Strength	Appl No
SQUIBB	500 MG	N16295 001

HYDROXYZINE HYDROCHLORIDE

INJECTABLE; INJECTION

HYDROXYZINE

TE	Firm	Strength	Appl No
AP	ELKINS SINN	50 MG/ML	N85551 002

HYDROXYZINE HCL

TE	Firm	Strength	Appl No	Date
AP	ABBOTT	50 MG/ML	N86821 001	
AP	ELKINS SINN	25 MG/ML	N85551 001	
AP	LUITPOLD	25 MG/ML	N87408 001	
AP		50 MG/ML	N87408 002	
AP	LYPHOMED	25 MG/ML	N87329 001	
AP		25 MG/ML	N88184 001	MAR 31, 1983
AP		50 MG/ML	N87329 002	
AP		50 MG/ML	N88185 001	MAR 31, 1983
AP	PHARMAFAIR	50 MG/ML	N88881 001	FEB 14, 1986
AP	SMITH NEPHEW SOLOPAK	25 MG/ML	N86822 001	
AP		25 MG/ML	N87591 001	
AP		50 MG/ML	N87310 001	
AP		50 MG/ML	N87593 001	
AP		50 MG/ML	N87595 001	
AP	STERIS	25 MG/ML	N87596 001	
AP		25 MG/ML	N85778 001	
AP		50 MG/ML	N87274 001	
AP		25 MG/ML	N85779 001	
AP		50 MG/ML	N87274 002	
AP	STERLING	25 MG/ML	N87416 001	
AP		50 MG/ML	N87546 001	
AP	WYETH AYERST	25 MG/ML	N86258 001	
AP		50 MG/ML	N86258 002	

Prescription Drug Products *(continued)*

HYDROXYZINE HYDROCHLORIDE *(continued)*

INJECTABLE; INJECTION

ORGATRAX

TE	Firm	Strength	NDA
ΔP	ORGANON	25 MG/ML	N87014 001
ΔP		50 MG/ML	N87014 002

VISTARIL

TE	Firm	Strength	NDA
ΔP	PFIZER	25 MG/ML	N11111 001
ΔP		50 MG/ML	N11111 002

SYRUP; ORAL

ATARAX

TE	Firm	Strength	NDA
ΔA	ROERIG	10 MG/5 ML	N10485 001

HYDROXYZINE HCL

TE	Firm	Strength	NDA	Date
ΔA	BARRE	10 MG/5 ML	N86880 001	
ΔA	KV	10 MG/5 ML	N87730 001	JUL 01, 1982
ΔA	NASKA	10 MG/5 ML	N88785 001	FEB 03, 1988
ΔA	PHARM BASICS	10 MG/5 ML	N87294 001	APR 12, 1982

TABLET; ORAL

ATARAX

TE	Firm	Strength	NDA
ΔB +	ROERIG	10 MG	N10392 001
ΔB +		25 MG	N10392 004
ΔB +		50 MG	N10392 006
ΔB +		100 MG	N10392 005

HYDROXYZINE HCL

TE	Firm	Strength	NDA	Date
ΔB	AMIDE PHARM	10 MG	N89071 001	JUL 22, 1986
ΔB		25 MG	N89072 001	JUL 22, 1986
ΔB		50 MG	N89073 001	JUL 22, 1986
ΔB	CHELSEA	10 MG	N86827 001	
ΔB		25 MG	N86829 001	
ΔB		50 MG	N86836 001	
ΔB	DANBURY	10 MG	N88348 001	SEP 15, 1983
ΔB		25 MG	N88349 001	SEP 15, 1983
ΔB		50 MG	N88350 001	SEP 15, 1983
ΔB	EON LABS	10 MG	N87246 002	
ΔB		25 MG	N85247 001	
ΔB		50 MG	N87245 001	
ΔB	GENEVA	10 MG	N87869 001	DEC 20, 1982
ΔB		25 MG	N87870 001	
ΔB		50 MG	N87871 001	DEC 20, 1982

HYDROXYZINE HYDROCHLORIDE *(continued)*

TABLET; ORAL

HYDROXYZINE HCL

TE	Firm	Strength	NDA	Date
ΔB	HALSEY	10 MG	N89366 001	MAY 02, 1988
ΔB		25 MG	N89117 001	MAY 02, 1988
ΔB		50 MG	N89396 001	MAY 02, 1988
ΔB	KV	10 MG	N87819 001	JUN 23, 1982
ΔB		25 MG	N87820 001	JUN 23, 1982
ΔB		50 MG	N87821 001	JUN 23, 1982
ΔB		100 MG	N87822 001	JUN 23, 1982
ΔB	MUTUAL PHARM	10 MG	N89381 001	MAY 19, 1986
ΔB		25 MG	N89382 001	MAY 19, 1986
ΔB		50 MG	N89383 001	MAY 19, 1986
ΔB	PAR	10 MG	N87602 001	MAY 19, 1986
ΔB		25 MG	N87603 001	JAN 22, 1982
ΔB		50 MG	N87604 001	JAN 22, 1982
ΔB	PUREPAC	10 MG	N88120 001	JAN 22, 1982
ΔB		25 MG	N88121 001	SEP 25, 1984
ΔB		50 MG	N88122 001	SEP 25, 1984
ΔB	SIDMAK	10 MG	N88617 001	SEP 25, 1984
ΔB		25 MG	N88618 001	JAN 10, 1986
ΔB		50 MG	N88619 001	JAN 10, 1986
ΔB	SUPERPHARM	10 MG	N88794 001	JAN 10, 1986
ΔB		25 MG	N88795 001	DEC 05, 1984
ΔB		50 MG	N88796 001	DEC 05, 1984
ΔB	ZENITH	10 MG	N87216 001	DEC 05, 1984
ΔB		25 MG	N87410 001	
ΔB		50 MG	N87411 001	

Prescription Drug Products (continued)

HYDROXYZINE PAMOATE

CAPSULE; ORAL

HY-PAM
EON LABS

	Firm	Strength	Appl. No.	Date
AB	HYDROXYZINE PAMOATE	EQ 25 MG HCL	N87479 001	
AB	BARR	EQ 25 MG HCL	N88496 001	JUN 15, 1984
AB		EQ 50 MG HCL	N88487 001	JUN 15, 1984
AB		EQ 100 MG HCL	N88488 001	JUN 15, 1984
AB	CHELSEA	EQ 25 MG HCL	N86840 001	JUL 15, 1984
AB		EQ 50 MG HCL	N86705 001	JUL 01, 1982
AB	DANBURY	EQ 25 MG HCL	N81165 001	JUL 01, 1982
AB		EQ 50 MG HCL	N87767 001	JUL 31, 1991
AB		EQ 100 MG HCL	N87790 001	AUG 16, 1982
AB	EON LABS	EQ 50 MG HCL	N86183 001	AUG 16, 1982
AB	GENEVA	EQ 25 MG HCL	N81127 001	JUN 28, 1991
AB		EQ 50 MG HCL	N81128 001	JUN 28, 1991
AB		EQ 100 MG HCL	N81129 001	JUN 28, 1991
AB	VANGARD	EQ 50 MG HCL	N88393 001	SEP 19, 1983
AB	ZENITH	EQ 25 MG HCL	N87761 001	MAR 05, 1982
AB		EQ 50 MG HCL	N87760 001	MAR 05, 1982
AB +	VISTARIL PFIZER	EQ 25 MG HCL	N11459 002	
AB		EQ 50 MG HCL	N11459 004	
AB		EQ 100 MG HCL	N11459 006	

SUSPENSION; ORAL

VISTARIL
PFIZER

		Strength	Appl. No.
	PFIZER	EQ 25 MG HCL/5 ML	N11795 001

IBUPROFEN

SUSPENSION; ORAL

CHILDREN'S ADVIL
WHITEHALL

	Firm	Strength	Appl. No.	Date
BX	WHITEHALL	100 MG/5 ML	N19833 002	SEP 19, 1989
BX	PEDIA PROFEN + MCNEIL	100 MG/5 ML	N19842 001	SEP 19, 1989
BX	RUFEN BOOTS	100 MG/5 ML	N19784 001	DEC 18, 1989

IBUPROFEN (continued)

TABLET; ORAL

IBU-TAB
ALRA

	Firm	Strength	Appl. No.	Date
AB	ALRA	400 MG	N71058 001	AUG 11, 1988
AB		600 MG	N71059 001	AUG 11, 1988
AB		800 MG	N71965 001	AUG 11, 1988
AB	IBUPROFEN BARR	400 MG	N70079 001	JUL 24, 1985
AB		600 MG	N70080 001	JUL 24, 1985
AB		800 MG	N71448 001	FEB 18, 1987
AB	BOOTS	400 MG	N70083 001	FEB 22, 1985
AB		600 MG	N70556 001	JUN 14, 1985
AB	DANBURY	400 MG	N70436 001	AUG 21, 1985
AB		600 MG	N70437 001	AUG 21, 1985
AB		800 MG	N71547 001	JUL 02, 1987
AB	GENEVA	300 MG	N70734 001	JUN 12, 1986
AB		400 MG	N70735 001	JUN 12, 1986
AB		600 MG	N70736 001	JUN 12, 1986
AB		800 MG	N72169 001	DEC 11, 1987
AB	HALSEY	300 MG	N71028 001	MAR 23, 1987
AB		400 MG	N71029 001	MAR 23, 1987
AB		600 MG	N71030 001	MAR 23, 1987
AB		800 MG	N72137 001	FEB 05, 1988
AB	INTERPHARM	400 MG	N71334 001	NOV 25, 1986
AB		600 MG	N71335 001	NOV 25, 1986
AB		800 MG	N71935 001	OCT 13, 1987
AB	INVAMED	400 MG	N72064 001	JAN 14, 1988
AB		600 MG	N72065 001	JAN 14, 1988
AB		800 MG	N71938 001	JAN 14, 1988
AB	LEDERLE	400 MG	N70629 001	SEP 19, 1986
AB		600 MG	N70630 001	SEP 19, 1986

Prescription Drug Products (continued)

IBUPROFEN (continued)
TABLET; ORAL
IBUPROFEN

TE	Firm	Strength	Appl. No.	Date
AB	LEMMON	400 MG	N73343 001	JUN 30, 1992
AB		600 MG	N73344 001	JUN 30, 1992
AB		800 MG	N73345 001	JUN 30, 1992
AB	MEDICOPHARMA	400 MG	N71644 001	FEB 01, 1988
AB	MUTUAL PHARM	300 MG	N71230 001	OCT 22, 1986
AB		400 MG	N71231 001	OCT 22, 1986
AB		600 MG	N71232 001	OCT 22, 1986
AB		800 MG	N72004 001	NOV 18, 1987
AB	MYLAN	400 MG	N70045 001	SEP 24, 1985
AB		600 MG	N70057 001	SEP 24, 1985
AB		800 MG	N71999 001	DEC 03, 1987
AB	OHM	400 MG	N70818 001	DEC 26, 1985
AB	PAR	300 MG	N70328 001	AUG 06, 1985
AB		400 MG	N70329 001	AUG 06, 1985
AB		600 MG	N70330 001	AUG 06, 1985
AB		800 MG	N70986 001	JUL 25, 1986
AB	PRIVATE FORM	300 MG	N71266 001	OCT 15, 1986
AB		400 MG	N71267 001	OCT 15, 1986
AB		600 MG	N71268 001	OCT 15, 1986
AB		800 MG	N72300 001	JUL 01, 1988
AB	PUREPAC	300 MG	N71123 001	SEP 19, 1986
AB		400 MG	N71124 001	SEP 19, 1986
AB		600 MG	N71125 001	SEP 19, 1986
AB		800 MG	N71964 001	FEB 01, 1988
AB	SIDMAK	400 MG	N71666 001	JUN 18, 1987
AB		600 MG	N71667 001	JUN 18, 1987
AB		800 MG	N71668 001	JUN 18, 1987

IBUPROFEN (continued)
TABLET; ORAL
IBUPROHM

TE	Firm	Strength	Appl. No.	Date
AB	OHM	400 MG	N70469 001	AUG 29, 1985

IFEN

TE	Firm	Strength	Appl. No.	Date
AB	LUCHEM	400 MG	N71145 001	SEP 23, 1986
AB		600 MG	N71146 001	SEP 23, 1986
AB		800 MG	N71769 001	MAY 08, 1987

MOTRIN

TE	Firm	Strength	Appl. No.	Date
AB	UPJOHN	300 MG	N17463 003	
AB		400 MG	N17463 002	
AB		600 MG	N17463 004	
AB +		800 MG	N17463 005	MAY 22, 1985

RUFEN

TE	Firm	Strength	Appl. No.	Date
AB	BOOTS	400 MG	N18197 001	
AB		600 MG	N70088 001	FEB 08, 1985
AB		600 MG	N70099 001	MAR 29, 1985
AB		800 MG	N70745 001	JUL 23, 1986

IDARUBICIN HYDROCHLORIDE
INJECTABLE; INJECTION
IDAMYCIN

TE	Firm	Strength	Appl. No.	Date
	ADRIA	5 MG/VIAL	N50661 002	SEP 27, 1990
		10 MG/VIAL	N50661 001	SEP 27, 1990

IDOXURIDINE
OINTMENT; OPHTHALMIC
STOXIL

TE	Firm	Strength	Appl. No.	Date
	+ SKF	0.5%	N15868 001	

SOLUTION/DROPS; OPHTHALMIC
DENDRID

TE	Firm	Strength	Appl. No.	Date
AT	ALCON	0.1%	N14169 001	

HERPLEX

TE	Firm	Strength	Appl. No.	Date
AT	ALLERGAN	0.1%	N13935 002	

STOXIL

TE	Firm	Strength	Appl. No.	Date
AT	SKF	0.1%	N13934 001	

IFOSFAMIDE
INJECTABLE; INJECTION
IFEX

TE	Firm	Strength	Appl. No.	Date
	BRISTOL MYERS SQUIBB	1 GM/VIAL	N19763 001	DEC 30, 1988
		3 GM/VIAL	N19763 002	DEC 30, 1988

Prescription Drug Products (continued)

IMIPENEM; *MULTIPLE*
SEE CILASTATIN SODIUM; IMIPENEM

IMIPRAMINE HYDROCHLORIDE

CONCENTRATE; ORAL

TE Code	Applicant	Strength	Appl. No.	Approval Date
	IMIPRAMINE HCL			
	CIBA	25 MG/ML	N86765 001	

INJECTABLE; INJECTION

TE Code	Applicant	Strength	Appl. No.	Approval Date
	TOFRANIL			
	GEIGY	12.5 MG/ML	N11838 002	

TABLET; ORAL

TE Code	Applicant	Strength	Appl. No.	Approval Date
	IMIPRAMINE HCL			
AB	BIOCRAFT	10 MG	N83729 001	
AB		25 MG	N83729 004	
AB		50 MG	N83729 003	
AB	EON LABS	10 MG	N85200 001	
AB		25 MG	N84869 002	
AB		50 MG	N85133 001	
AB	GENEVA	10 MG	N84936 002	
AB		25 MG	N83745 001	
AB		50 MG	N84937 001	
AB	MUTUAL PHARM	10 MG	N81048 001	JUN 05, 1990
AB		25 MG	N81049 001	JUN 05, 1990
AB		50 MG	N81050 001	JUN 05, 1990
AB	PAR	10 MG	N88292 001	OCT 21, 1983
AB		10 MG	N89422 001	JUL 14, 1987
AB		25 MG	N88262 001	OCT 21, 1983
AB		25 MG	N89497 001	JUL 14, 1987
AB		50 MG	N88276 001	OCT 21, 1983
AB	ROXANE	10 MG	N83799 001	
AB		25 MG	N83799 002	
AB		50 MG	N83799 003	
	JANIMINE			
AB	ABBOTT	10 MG	N17895 001	
AB		25 MG	N17895 002	
AB		50 MG	N17895 003	
	TOFRANIL			
AB	GEIGY	10 MG	N87844 001	MAY 22, 1984
AB		25 MG	N87845 001	MAY 22, 1984
AB +		50 MG	N87846 001	MAY 22, 1984

IMIPRAMINE PAMOATE

CAPSULE; ORAL

Applicant	Strength	Appl. No.
TOFRANIL-PM		
GEIGY	EQ 75 MG HCL	N17090 001
	EQ 100 MG HCL	N17090 004
	EQ 125 MG HCL	N17090 003
	EQ 150 MG HCL	N17090 002

INDAPAMIDE

TABLET; ORAL

Applicant	Strength	Appl. No.	Approval Date
LOZOL			
+ RHONE POULENC RORER	2.5 MG	N18538 001	JUL 06, 1983

INDECAINIDE HYDROCHLORIDE

TABLET, EXTENDED RELEASE; ORAL

Applicant	Strength	Appl. No.	Approval Date
DECABID			
LILLY	EQ 50 MG BASE	N19693 001	DEC 29, 1989
	EQ 75 MG BASE	N19693 002	DEC 29, 1989
+	EQ 100 MG BASE	N19693 003	DEC 29, 1989

INDIUM IN-111 OXYQUINOLINE

INJECTABLE; INJECTION

Applicant	Strength	Appl. No.	Approval Date
INDIUM IN-111 OXYQUINOLINE			
AMERSHAM	1 MCI/ML	N19044 001	DEC 23, 1985

INDIUM IN-111 PENTETATE DISODIUM

INJECTABLE; INTRATHECAL

Applicant	Strength	Appl. No.	Approval Date
MPI INDIUM DTPA IN 111			
MEDI PHYSICS	1 MCI/ML	N17707 001	FEB 18, 1982

INDOCYANINE GREEN

INJECTABLE; INJECTION

Applicant	Strength	Appl. No.
CARDIO-GREEN		
BECTON DICKINSON	25 MG/VIAL	N11525 001
	50 MG/VIAL	N11525 002

Prescription Drug Products (continued)

INDOMETHACIN

CAPSULE; ORAL

		Strength	Application No.	Date
INDO-LEMMON				
	LEMMON			
AB		25 MG	N70266 001	NOV 07, 1985
AB		50 MG	N70267 001	NOV 07, 1985
INDOCIN				
	MERCK			
+	**INDOMETHACIN**			
AB		25 MG	N16059 001	
AB		50 MG	N16059 002	
INDOMETHACIN				
	BARR			
AB		25 MG	N70067 001	OCT 03, 1986
AB		50 MG	N70068 001	OCT 03, 1986
	CHELSEA			
AB		25 MG	N18690 001	JUL 31, 1984
AB		50 MG	N18690 002	JUL 31, 1984
AB		50 MG	N71635 001	MAY 18, 1987
	DANBURY			
AB		25 MG	N72996 001	JUL 31, 1991
AB		50 MG	N72997 001	JUL 31, 1991
	GENEVA			
AB		25 MG	N70673 001	APR 29, 1987
AB		50 MG	N70674 001	APR 29, 1987
	HALSEY			
AB		25 MG	N70782 001	JUN 03, 1987
AB		50 MG	N70635 001	JUN 03, 1987
	LEDERLE			
AB		25 MG	N18851 001	MAY 18, 1984
AB		50 MG	N18851 002	MAY 18, 1984
	MUTUAL PHARM			
AB		25 MG	N70899 001	FEB 09, 1987
AB		50 MG	N70900 001	FEB 09, 1987
	MYLAN			
AB		25 MG	N18858 001	APR 20, 1984
AB		50 MG	N18858 002	APR 20, 1984
	NOVOPHARM			
AB		50 MG	N70624 001	SEP 04, 1985
AB		25 MG	N71342 001	APR 18, 1988
AB		50 MG	N71343 001	APR 18, 1988
	PAR			
AB		25 MG	N18829 001	AUG 06, 1984
AB		50 MG	N18829 002	AUG 06, 1984
AB		50 MG	N70651 001	MAR 05, 1986

INDOMETHACIN (continued)

CAPSULE; ORAL

		Strength	Application No.	Date
INDOMETHACIN				
	PARKE DAVIS			
AB		25 MG	N18806 001	NOV 23, 1984
AB		50 MG	N18806 002	NOV 23, 1984
	PIONEER PHARMS			
AB		25 MG	N70813 001	AUG 11, 1986
AB		50 MG	N70592 001	AUG 11, 1986
	SIDMAK			
AB		25 MG	N71148 001	MAR 18, 1987
AB		50 MG	N71149 001	MAR 18, 1987
	WATSON			
AB		25 MG	N70529 001	OCT 18, 1985
AB		50 MG	N70530 001	OCT 18, 1985
	ZENITH			
AB		25 MG	N70719 001	FEB 12, 1986
AB		50 MG	N70756 001	FEB 12, 1986

CAPSULE, EXTENDED RELEASE; ORAL

		Strength	Application No.	Date
INDOCIN SR				
+	MERCK			
AB		75 MG	N18185 001	FEB 23, 1982
INDOMETHACIN				
	EON LABS			
B*		75 MG	N71531 001	JUL 21, 1987
	INWOOD			
AB		75 MG	N72410 001	MAR 15, 1989

SUPPOSITORY; RECTAL

		Strength	Application No.	Date
INDOCIN				
+	MERCK			
AB		50 MG	N17814 001	AUG 13, 1984
INDOMETHEGAN				
	G AND W			
AB		50 MG	N73314 001	AUG 31, 1992

SUSPENSION; ORAL

		Strength	Application No.	Date
INDOCIN				
+	MERCK			
AB		25 MG/5 ML	N18332 001	OCT 10, 1985
INDOMETHACIN				
	ROXANE			
AB		25 MG/5 ML	N71412 001	MAR 18, 1987

INDOMETHACIN SODIUM

INJECTABLE; INJECTION

		Strength	Application No.	Date
INDOCIN I.V.				
	MERCK		EQ 1 MG BASE/VIAL	N18878 001	JAN 30, 1985

Prescription Drug Products (continued)

INSULIN PORK
INJECTABLE; INJECTION
 ILETIN I
  LILLY   500 UNITS/ML   N17931 001

INSULIN PURIFIED PORK
INJECTABLE; INJECTION
 ILETIN II
  LILLY   500 UNITS/ML   N18344 002

INTRINSIC FACTOR; *MULTIPLE*
 SEE COBALT CHLORIDE, CO-57; CYANOCOBALAMIN; CYANOCOBALAMIN, CO-57; INTRINSIC FACTOR
 SEE CYANOCOBALAMIN; CYANOCOBALAMIN, CO-57; INTRINSIC FACTOR

INULIN
INJECTABLE; INJECTION
 INULIN AND SODIUM CHLORIDE
  ISO TEX   100 MG/ML   N02282 001

INVERT SUGAR
INJECTABLE; INJECTION
 TRAVERT 10% IN PLASTIC CONTAINER
  BAXTER   10 GM/100 ML   N16717 001

IOCETAMIC ACID
TABLET; ORAL
 CHOLEBRINE
  MALLINCKRODT   750 MG   N17129 001

IODAMIDE MEGLUMINE
INJECTABLE; INJECTION
 RENOVUE-DIP
  SQUIBB   24%   N17903 001
 RENOVUE-65
  SQUIBB   65%   N17902 001

IODIPAMIDE MEGLUMINE
INJECTABLE; INJECTION
 CHOLOGRAFIN MEGLUMINE
  SQUIBB   10.3%   N09321 007
                       52%   N09321 003

IODIPAMIDE MEGLUMINE; *MULTIPLE*
 SEE DIATRIZOATE MEGLUMINE; IODIPAMIDE MEGLUMINE

IODOHIPPURATE SODIUM, I-123
INJECTABLE; INJECTION
 NEPHROFLOW
  MEDI PHYSICS   1 MCI/ML   N18289 001   DEC 28, 1984

IODOHIPPURATE SODIUM, I-131
INJECTABLE; INJECTION
 HIPPURAN I 131
  MALLINCKRODT   0.25 MCI/ML   N16666 001
 HIPPUTOPE
  SQUIBB   1-2 MCI/VIAL   N15419 002
 IODOHIPPURATE SODIUM I 131
  CIS   0.2 MCI/ML   N17313 001

IOFETAMINE HYDROCHLORIDE I-123
INJECTABLE; INJECTION
 SPECTAMINE
  IMP   1 MCI/ML   N19432 001 DEC 24, 1987

IOHEXOL
INJECTABLE; INJECTION
 OMNIPAQUE 140
  STERLING   30.2%   N18956 005 NOV 30, 1988
 OMNIPAQUE 180
  STERLING   38.8%   N18956 001 DEC 26, 1985
 OMNIPAQUE 210
  STERLING   45.3%   N18956 006 JUN 30, 1989
SOLUTION; INJECTION, ORAL
 OMNIPAQUE 240
  STERLING   51.8%   N18956 002 DEC 26, 1985
 OMNIPAQUE 300
  STERLING   64.7%   N18956 003 DEC 26, 1985
 OMNIPAQUE 350
  STERLING   75.5%   N18956 004 DEC 26, 1985

Prescription Drug Products (continued)

IOPAMIDOL
INJECTABLE; INJECTION
  ISOVUE-M 200
    SQUIBB — 41% — N18735 001 DEC 31, 1985
  ISOVUE-M 300
    SQUIBB — 61% — N18735 004 DEC 31, 1985
  ISOVUE-128
    SQUIBB — 26% — N18735 005 OCT 21, 1986
  ISOVUE-200
    SQUIBB — 41% — N18735 006 JUL 07, 1987
  ISOVUE-250
    SQUIBB — 51% — N18735 007 JUL 06, 1992
  ISOVUE-300
    SQUIBB — 61% — N18735 002 DEC 31, 1985
  ISOVUE-370
    SQUIBB — 76% — N18735 003 DEC 31, 1985

IOPANOIC ACID
TABLET; ORAL
  TELEPAQUE
    STERLING — 500 MG — N08032 001

IOTHALAMATE MEGLUMINE
INJECTABLE; INJECTION
  CONRAY
    MALLINCKRODT — 60% — N13295 001
  CONRAY 30
    MALLINCKRODT — 30% — N16983 001
  CONRAY 43
    MALLINCKRODT — 43% — N13295 002
SOLUTION; INTRAVESICAL
  CYSTO-CONRAY II
    MALLINCKRODT — 17.2% — N17057 002
SOLUTION; INTRAVESICAL, URETERAL
  CYSTO-CONRAY
    MALLINCKRODT — 43% — N17057 001

IOTHALAMATE MEGLUMINE; IOTHALAMATE SODIUM
INJECTABLE; INJECTION
  VASCORAY
    MALLINCKRODT — 52%;26% — N16783 001

IOTHALAMATE SODIUM
INJECTABLE; INJECTION
  ANGIO-CONRAY
    MALLINCKRODT — 80% — N13319 001
  CONRAY 325
    MALLINCKRODT — 54.3% — N17685 001
  CONRAY 400
    MALLINCKRODT — 66.8% — N14295 001

IOTHALAMATE SODIUM; *MULTIPLE*
  SEE IOTHALAMATE MEGLUMINE; IOTHALAMATE SODIUM

IOTHALAMATE SODIUM, I-125
INJECTABLE; INJECTION
  GLOFIL-125
    ISO TEX — 250-300 UCI/ML — N17279 001

IOTROLAN
INJECTABLE; INTRATHECAL
  OSMOVIST
    BERLEX — EQ 190 MG IODINE/ML — N19580 001 DEC 07, 1989
    — EQ 240 MG IODINE/ML — N19580 002 DEC 07, 1989

IOVERSOL
INJECTABLE; INJECTION
  OPTIRAY 160
    MALLINCKRODT — 34% — N19710 003 DEC 30, 1988
  OPTIRAY 240
    MALLINCKRODT — 51% — N19710 002 DEC 30, 1988
  OPTIRAY 300
    MALLINCKRODT — 64% — N19710 004 JAN 22, 1992
  OPTIRAY 320
    MALLINCKRODT — 68% — N19710 001 DEC 30, 1988
  OPTIRAY 350
    MALLINCKRODT — 74% — N19710 005 JAN 22, 1992

IOXAGLATE MEGLUMINE; IOXAGLATE SODIUM
INJECTABLE; INJECTION
  HEXABRIX
    MALLINCKRODT — 39.3%;19.6% — N18905 002 JUL 26, 1985

Prescription Drug Products (continued)

IOXAGLATE SODIUM; *MULTIPLE*
SEE   IOXAGLATE MEGLUMINE; IOXAGLATE SODIUM

IPODATE CALCIUM
GRANULE; ORAL

	Firm	Strength	Appl No	Date
	ORAGRAFIN CALCIUM			
	SQUIBB	3 GM/PACKET	N12968 001	

IPODATE SODIUM
CAPSULE; ORAL

	Firm	Strength	Appl No	Date
	BILIVIST			
AA	BERLEX	500 MG	N87768 001	AUG 11, 1982
	ORAGRAFIN SODIUM			
AA	SQUIBB	500 MG	N12967 001	

IPRATROPIUM BROMIDE
AEROSOL, METERED; INHALATION

	Firm	Strength	Appl No	Date
	ATROVENT			
	BOEHRINGER INGELHEIM	0.018 MG/INH	N19085 001	DEC 29, 1986

IRON DEXTRAN
INJECTABLE; INJECTION

	Firm	Strength	Appl No	Date
	IMFERON			
AP	FISONS	EQ 50 MG IRON/ML	N10787 002	
	IRON DEXTRAN			
AP	STERIS	EQ 50 MG IRON/ML	N17441 001	

ISOETHARINE HYDROCHLORIDE
SOLUTION; INHALATION

	Firm	Strength	Appl No	Date
	BETA-2			
AN	NEPHRON	1%	N86711 001	
	BRONKOSOL			
AN	STERLING	1%	N12339 008	
	ISOETHARINE HCL			
AN	ASTRA	0.125%	N87938 001	NOV 15, 1982
AN		0.125%	N89615 001	JUN 13, 1991
AN		0.167%	N89616 001	JUN 13, 1991
AN		0.2%	N89617 001	JUN 13, 1991
AN		0.25%	N89618 001	JUN 13, 1991
AN		0.062%	N87937 001	NOV 15, 1982
AN		0.062%	N89614 001	JUN 13, 1991

ISOETHARINE HYDROCHLORIDE (continued)
SOLUTION; INHALATION

	Firm	Strength	Appl No	Date
	ISOETHARINE HCL			
	BARRE			
AN	INTL MEDICATION	1%	N87101 001	
AN		0.08%	N86651 002	
AN		0.1%	N86651 003	
AN		0.167%	N86651 005	
AN		0.2%	N86651 006	
AN		0.25%	N86651 007	
AN		1%	N86651 008	
AN		0.077%	N86651 001	
AN	PARKE DAVIS	0.143%	N86651 004	
AN		1%	N85889 001	
AN	ROXANE	0.5%	N85997 001	
AN		0.1%	N87396 001	
AN		0.125%	N87025 001	
AN		0.167%	N88226 001	SEP 16, 1983
AN		0.2%	N87324 001	
AN		0.25%	N88275 001	
	ISOETHARINE HCL S/F			
AN	DEY	1%	N86899 001	JUN 03, 1983
AN		0.08%	N89817 001	NOV 22, 1988
AN		0.1%	N89818 001	NOV 22, 1988
AN		0.25%	N89820 001	NOV 22, 1988
AN		1%	N89252 001	SEP 15, 1986
AN		0.17%	N89819 001	NOV 22, 1988

ISOETHARINE MESYLATE
AEROSOL, METERED; INHALATION

	Firm	Strength	Appl No	Date
	BRONKOMETER			
BN	+ STERLING	0.34 MG/INH	N12339 007	
	ISOETHARINE MESYLATE			
BN	BARRE	0.34 MG/INH	N87858 001	AUG 21, 1984

ISOFLURANE
LIQUID; INHALATION

	Firm	Strength	Appl No	Date
	FORANE			
	ANAQUEST	99.9%	N17624 001	

ISOFLUROPHATE
OINTMENT; OPHTHALMIC

	Firm	Strength	Appl No	Date
	FLOROPRYL			
	MSD	0.025%	N10656 001	

Prescription Drug Products *(continued)*

ISONIAZID

TE	Firm	Strength	Appl. No.	
INJECTABLE; INJECTION				
	NYDRAZID			
	SQUIBB	100 MG/ML	N08662 001	
SYRUP; ORAL				
	ISONIAZID			
AA	CAROLINA MEDCL	50 MG/5 ML	N88235 001	NOV 10, 1983
	LANIAZID			
AA	LANNETT	50 MG/5 ML	N89243 001	FEB 03, 1986
TABLET; ORAL				
	HYZYD			
AA	MALLINCKRODT	100 MG	N80134 003	
AA		300 MG	N80134 004	
	INH			
AA	CIBA	300 MG	N80935 001	
	ISONIAZID			
AA	BARR	100 MG	N80936 001	
AA		300 MG	N80937 002	
AA	DANBURY	50 MG	N80522 001	
AA		100 MG	N80523 001	
AA		300 MG	N80521 001	
AA	DURAMED	100 MG	N88231 001	MAR 17, 1983
AA		300 MG	N88119 001	MAR 17, 1983
AA	EON LABS	100 MG	N08678 002	
AA		300 MG	N08678 003	
AA	HALSEY	50 MG	N83632 001	
AA		100 MG	N80136 001	
AA	MK	100 MG	N83633 001	
AA		300 MG	N80941 001	
AA	PHARMAVITE	100 MG	N85091 001	
AA	PHOENIX LABS	50 MG	N80368 001	
AA		100 MG	N80368 002	
AA	RICHLYN	100 MG	N80153 001	
AA	WEST WARD	100 MG	N80212 001	
AA		300 MG	N87425 001	
AA	ZENITH	100 MG	N80270 001	
AA		300 MG	N83610 001	
	LANIAZID			
AA	LANNETT	50 MG	N80140 001	
AA		100 MG	N80140 002	
AA		300 MG	N89776 001	JUN 13, 1988
	STANOZIDE			
AA	EVERYLIFE	300 MG	N80126 002	

ISONIAZID; RIFAMPIN

Firm	Strength	Appl. No.
CAPSULE; ORAL		
RIFAMATE		
+ DOW	150 MG;300 MG	N61884 001

ISOPROPAMIDE IODIDE

Firm	Strength	Appl. No.
TABLET; ORAL		
DARBID		
SKF	EQ 5 MG BASE	N10744 001

ISOPROTERENOL HYDROCHLORIDE

TE	Firm	Strength	Appl. No.
AEROSOL, METERED; INHALATION			
	ISOPROTERENOL HCL		
BN	BARRE	0.12 MG/INH	N85904 001
BN	+ 3M	0.12 MG/INH	N10375 004
	ISUPREL		
	STERLING	0.113 MG/INH	N11178 001
INJECTABLE; INJECTION			
	ISOPROTERENOL HCL		
AP	ABBOTT	0.2 MG/ML	N83346 001
AP	ELKINS SINN	0.02 MG/ML	N83283 001
AP	INTL MEDICATION	0.2 MG/ML	N83486 001
	ISUPREL		
AP	STERLING	0.2 MG/ML	N83724 001
SOLUTION; INHALATION			
	AEROLONE		
AN	LILLY	0.2 MG/ML	N10515 001
	ISOPROTERENOL HCL		
AN	PARKE DAVIS	0.25%	N07245 001
	ISUPREL		
AN	STERLING	0.25%	N85994 001
AN		0.5%	N85540 001
	VAPO-ISO		
AN	FISONS	0.5%	N06327 002
		1%	N06327 003
AN		0.5%	N16813 001
TABLET; RECTAL, SUBLINGUAL			
	ISUPREL		
	STERLING	10 MG	N06328 001
		15 MG	N06328 002

ISOPROTERENOL HYDROCHLORIDE; PHENYLEPHRINE BITARTRATE

Firm	Strength	Appl. No.
AEROSOL, METERED; INHALATION		
DUO-MEDIHALER		
3M	0.16 MG/INH;0.24 MG/INH	N13296 001

ISOPROTERENOL SULFATE

Firm	Strength	Appl. No.
AEROSOL, METERED; INHALATION		
MEDIHALER-ISO		
3M	0.08 MG/INH	N10375 003

ISOSORBIDE

Firm	Strength	Appl. No.
SOLUTION; ORAL		
ISMOTIC		
ALCON	100 GM/220 ML	N17063 001

Prescription Drug Products (continued)

ISOSORBIDE DINITRATE

CAPSULE, EXTENDED RELEASE; ORAL

	DILATRATE-SR			
BC	REED AND CARNRICK	40 MG	N19790 001	SEP 02, 1988
	ISORDIL			
BC	+ WYETH AYERST	40 MG	N12882 002	JUL 29, 1988

TABLET; ORAL

	ISORDIL			
AB	WYETH AYERST	5 MG	N12093 007	JUL 29, 1988
AB		10 MG	N12093 002	JUL 29, 1988
AB		20 MG	N12093 006	JUL 29, 1988
AB		30 MG	N12093 005	JUL 29, 1988
AB	+	40 MG	N12093 001	JUL 29, 1988
	ISOSORBIDE DINITRATE			
AB	BARR	5 MG	N86166 002	SEP 19, 1986
AB		10 MG	N86169 001	SEP 19, 1986
AB		20 MG	N86167 001	SEP 19, 1986
AB		30 MG	N87564 001	SEP 18, 1986
AB	DANBURY	5 MG	N86034 001	JAN 06, 1988
AB		10 MG	N86032 001	JAN 07, 1988
AB	GENEVA	5 MG	N86221 001	JAN 07, 1988
AB		10 MG	N86223 001	JAN 07, 1988
AB		20 MG	N89367 001	APR 07, 1988
AB	PAR	5 MG	N86923 001	MAR 12, 1987
AB		10 MG	N86925 001	MAR 12, 1987
AB		20 MG	N87537 001	OCT 02, 1987
AB		30 MG	N87946 001	JAN 12, 1988
AB	WEST WARD	5 MG	N86067 001	OCT 29, 1987
AB		10 MG	N86066 001	OCT 29, 1987
AB		20 MG	N88088 001	NOV 02, 1987

ISOSORBIDE DINITRATE (continued)

TABLET; SUBLINGUAL

	ISORDIL			
AB	WYETH AYERST	2.5 MG	N12940 004	JUL 29, 1988
AB		5 MG	N12940 003	JUL 29, 1988
AB	+	10 MG	N12940 005	JUL 29, 1988
	ISOSORBIDE DINITRATE			
AB	BARR	2.5 MG	N84204 001	SEP 18, 1986
AB		5 MG	N86168 001	SEP 18, 1986
AB		10 MG	N87545 001	SEP 18, 1986
AB	DANBURY	2.5 MG	N86033 001	FEB 26, 1988
AB		5 MG	N86031 001	SEP 29, 1987
AB	GENEVA	2.5 MG	N86225 001	FEB 19, 1988
AB		5 MG	N86222 001	FEB 19, 1988
AB	WEST WARD	2.5 MG	N86054 001	OCT 29, 1987
AB		5 MG	N86055 001	NOV 02, 1987

TABLET, EXTENDED RELEASE; ORAL

	ISORDIL			
	+ WYETH AYERST	40 MG	N12882 001	JUL 29, 1988

ISOSORBIDE MONONITRATE

TABLET; ORAL

	ISMO			
	+ WYETH	20 MG	N19091 001	DEC 30, 1991

ISOSULFAN BLUE

INJECTABLE; INJECTION

	LYMPHAZURIN			
	HIRSCH	1%	N18310 001	

ISOTRETINOIN

CAPSULE; ORAL

	ACCUTANE			
	ROCHE	10 MG	N18662 002	MAY 07, 1982
		20 MG	N18662 004	MAR 28, 1983
	+	40 MG	N18662 003	MAY 07, 1982

Prescription Drug Products (continued)

ISRADIPINE

CAPSULE; ORAL

DYNACIRC

SANDOZ

	Strength	NDA	Date
	2.5 MG	N19546 001	DEC 20, 1990
	5 MG	N19546 002	DEC 20, 1990

KANAMYCIN SULFATE

CAPSULE; ORAL

KANTREX

+ BRISTOL

	Strength	NDA	Date
	EQ 500 MG BASE	N60516 001	
	EQ 500 MG BASE	N61911 001	
	EQ 500 MG BASE	N62726 001	MAR 06, 1987

INJECTABLE; INJECTION

KANAMYCIN

ELKINS SINN

	Strength	NDA
AP	EQ 75 MG BASE/2 ML	N62324 001
AP	EQ 500 MG BASE/2 ML	N62324 002
AP	EQ 1 GM BASE/3 ML	N62324 003

KANAMYCIN SULFATE

LOCH

	Strength	NDA	Date
AP	EQ 75 MG BASE/2 ML	N63021 001	JUL 31, 1992
AP	EQ 500 MG BASE/2 ML	N63022 001	JUL 31, 1992
AP	EQ 1 GM BASE/3 ML	N63025 001	JUL 31, 1992

LYPHOMED

	Strength	NDA	Date
AP	EQ 75 MG BASE/2 ML	N62504 001	APR 05, 1984
AP	EQ 500 MG BASE/2 ML	N62504 002	APR 05, 1984
AP	EQ 1 GM BASE/3 ML	N62504 003	APR 05, 1984

PHARMAFAIR

	Strength	NDA	Date
AP	EQ 75 MG BASE/2 ML	N62668 001	MAY 07, 1987
AP	EQ 500 MG BASE/2 ML	N62672 001	MAY 07, 1987
AP	EQ 1 GM BASE/3 ML	N62669 001	MAY 07, 1987

SMITH NEPHEW

SOLOPAK

	Strength	NDA	Date
AP	EQ 75 MG BASE/2 ML	N62605 003	FEB 26, 1986
AP	EQ 500 MG BASE/2 ML	N62605 001	FEB 26, 1986
AP	EQ 1 GM BASE/3 ML	N62605 002	FEB 26, 1986

STERIS

	Strength	NDA	Date
AP	EQ 1 GM BASE/3 ML	N62520 003	MAY 09, 1985

KANAMYCIN SULFATE (continued)

INJECTABLE; INJECTION

KANTREX

BRISTOL

	Strength	NDA	Date
AP	EQ 75 MG BASE/2 ML	N61655 003	
AP	EQ 75 MG BASE/2 ML	N61901 003	
AP	EQ 75 MG BASE/2 ML	N62564 001	SEP 21, 1984
AP	EQ 500 MG BASE/2 ML	N61655 001	
AP	EQ 500 MG BASE/2 ML	N61901 001	
AP	EQ 500 MG BASE/2 ML	N62564 002	SEP 21, 1984
AP	EQ 1 GM BASE/3 ML	N61655 002	
AP	EQ 1 GM BASE/3 ML	N61901 002	
AP	EQ 1 GM BASE/3 ML	N62564 003	SEP 21, 1984

KLEBCIL

BEECHAM

	Strength	NDA
AP	EQ 75 MG BASE/2 ML	N62170 001
AP	EQ 500 MG BASE/2 ML	N62170 002
AP	EQ 1 GM BASE/3 ML	N62170 003

KETAMINE HYDROCHLORIDE

INJECTABLE; INJECTION

KETALAR

PARKE DAVIS

Strength	NDA
EQ 10 MG BASE/ML	N16812 001
EQ 50 MG BASE/ML	N16812 002
EQ 100 MG BASE/ML	N16812 003

KETOCONAZOLE

CREAM; TOPICAL

NIZORAL

+ JANSSEN

Strength	NDA	Date
2%	N19084 001	DEC 31, 1985
2%	N19576 001	OCT 22, 1987
2%	N19648 001	SEP 25, 1987

SHAMPOO; TOPICAL

NIZORAL

+ JANSSEN

Strength	NDA	Date
2%	N19927 001	AUG 31, 1990

TABLET; ORAL

NIZORAL

+ JANSSEN

Strength	NDA
200 MG	N18533 001

Prescription Drug Products (continued)

KETOPROFEN
CAPSULE; ORAL
ORUDIS
WYETH AYERST

	25 MG	N18754 001	JUL 31, 1987
	50 MG	N18754 002	JAN 09, 1986
+	75 MG	N18754 003	JAN 09, 1986

KETOROLAC TROMETHAMINE
INJECTABLE; INJECTION
TORADOL
SYNTEX

	15 MG/ML	N19698 001	NOV 30, 1989
	30 MG/ML	N19698 002	NOV 30, 1989

TABLET; ORAL
TORADOL
+ SYNTEX

	10 MG	N19645 001	DEC 20, 1991

KRYPTON, KR-81M
GAS; INHALATION
MPI KRYPTON 81M GAS GENERATOR
MEDI PHYSICS

N/A	N18088 001	

LABETALOL HYDROCHLORIDE
INJECTABLE; INJECTION
NORMODYNE

AP	SCHERING	5 MG/ML	N18686 001	AUG 01, 1984

TRANDATE

AP	GLAXO	5 MG/ML	N19425 001	DEC 31, 1985

TABLET; ORAL
NORMODYNE
SCHERING

AB	100 MG	N18687 001	AUG 31, 1987
AB	200 MG	N18687 002	AUG 01, 1984
AB +	300 MG	N18687 003	AUG 01, 1984

TRANDATE
GLAXO

AB	100 MG	N18716 001	MAY 24, 1985
AB	200 MG	N18716 002	AUG 01, 1984
AB	300 MG	N18716 003	AUG 01, 1984

LABETALOL HYDROCHLORIDE; *MULTIPLE*
SEE   HYDROCHLOROTHIAZIDE; LABETALOL HYDROCHLORIDE

LACTULOSE
SYRUP; ORAL
CHRONULAC

	MERRELL DOW	10 GM/15 ML	N17884 001	JUL 26, 1988

CONSTILAC

AA	ALRA	10 GM/15 ML	N71054 001	AUG 15, 1988

CONSTULOSE

AA	BARRE	10 GM/15 ML	N70288 001	

DUPHALAC

AA	SOLVAY	10 GM/15 ML	N72372 001	MAR 22, 1989

LACTULOSE

AA	PACO	10 GM/15 ML	N73160 001	AUG 25, 1992
AA	PHARM BASICS	10 GM/15 ML	N71841 001	SEP 22, 1988
AA	ROXANE	10 GM/15 ML	N73591 001	MAY 29, 1992

SYRUP; ORAL, RECTAL
CEPHULAC

AA	MERRELL DOW	10 GM/15 ML	N17657 001	

CHOLAC

AA	ALRA	10 GM/15 ML	N71331 001	JUL 26, 1988

ENULOSE

AA	BARRE	10 GM/15 ML	N71548 001	AUG 15, 1988

GENERLAC

AA	PHARM BASICS	10 GM/15 ML	N71842 001	SEP 27, 1988

LACTULOSE

AA	PACO	10 GM/15 ML	N72029 001	AUG 25, 1992
AA	ROXANE	10 GM/15 ML	N73590 001	MAY 29, 1992

PORTALAC

AA	SOLVAY	10 GM/15 ML	N72374 001	MAR 22, 1989

Prescription Drug Products (continued)

LEUCOVORIN CALCIUM

INJECTABLE; INJECTION
LEUCOVORIN CALCIUM

TE	Manufacturer	Strength	Appl. No.	Date
AP	ABIC	EQ 3 MG BASE/ML	N89352 001	JUN 01, 1988
AP		EQ 50 MG BASE/VIAL	N89353 001	JUN 01, 1988
AP	BEN VENUE	EQ 50 MG BASE/VIAL	N89384 001	SEP 14, 1987
AP		EQ 100 MG BASE/VIAL	N89717 001	MAR 28, 1988
AP	ELKINS SINN	EQ 50 MG BASE/VIAL	N70480 001	JAN 02, 1987
AP	LEDERLE	EQ 3 MG BASE/ML	N08107 001	
AP		EQ 50 MG BASE/VIAL	N08107 002	
AP		EQ 100 MG BASE/VIAL	N08107 004	MAY 23, 1988
AP		EQ 350 MG BASE/VIAL	N08107 005	APR 05, 1989

WELLCOVORIN

TE	Manufacturer	Strength	Appl. No.	Date
AP	BURROUGHS WELLCOME	EQ 50 MG BASE/VIAL	N89465 001	JAN 23, 1989
AP		EQ 100 MG BASE/VIAL	N89834 001	JAN 23, 1989
		EQ 5 MG BASE/ML	N87439 001	OCT 19, 1982
		EQ 25 MG BASE/VIAL	N89833 001	JAN 23, 1989

POWDER FOR RECONSTITUTION; ORAL
LEUCOVORIN CALCIUM

TE	Manufacturer	Strength	Appl. No.	Date
	LEDERLE	EQ 60 MG BASE/VIAL	N08107 003	JAN 30, 1987

TABLET; ORAL
LEUCOVORIN CALCIUM

TE	Manufacturer	Strength	Appl. No.	Date
AB	BARR	EQ 5 MG BASE	N71198 001	SEP 24, 1987
AB		EQ 25 MG BASE	N71199 001	SEP 24, 1987
BX	LEDERLE	EQ 5 MG BASE	N18459 001	JAN 30, 1986
		EQ 10 MG BASE	N71962 001	NOV 19, 1987
+		EQ 15 MG BASE	N71104 001	MAR 04, 1987

WELLCOVORIN

TE	Manufacturer	Strength	Appl. No.	Date
AB	BURROUGHS WELLCOME	EQ 5 MG BASE	N18342 001	JUL 08, 1983
+		EQ 25 MG BASE	N18342 002	JUL 08, 1983

LEUPROLIDE ACETATE

INJECTABLE; INJECTION
LUPRON

Manufacturer	Strength	Appl. No.	Date
TAP	1 MG/0.2 ML	N19010 001	APR 09, 1985

LUPRON DEPOT

Manufacturer	Strength	Appl. No.	Date
TAP	3.75 MG/VIAL	N20011 001	OCT 22, 1990
TAP	7.5 MG/VIAL	N19732 001	JAN 26, 1989

LEVAMISOLE HYDROCHLORIDE

TABLET; ORAL
ERGAMISOL

Manufacturer	Strength	Appl. No.	Date
JANSSEN	EQ 50 MG BASE	N20035 001	JUN 18, 1990

LEVOBUNOLOL HYDROCHLORIDE

SOLUTION/DROPS; OPHTHALMIC
BETAGAN

Manufacturer	Strength	Appl. No.	Date
ALLERGAN	0.25%	N19814 001	JUN 28, 1989
	0.5%	N19219 002	DEC 19, 1985

LEVOCARNITINE

SOLUTION; ORAL
CARNITOR

Manufacturer	Strength	Appl. No.	Date
SIGMA TAU	1 GM/10 ML	N18948 002	APR 27, 1988
	1 GM/10 ML	N19257 001	APR 10, 1986

TABLET; ORAL
CARNITOR

Manufacturer	Strength	Appl. No.	Date
SIGMA TAU	330 MG	N18948 001	DEC 27, 1985

LEVODOPA

CAPSULE; ORAL
DOPAR

TE	Manufacturer	Strength	Appl. No.
	ROBERTS	100 MG	N16913 003
		250 MG	N16913 001
		500 MG	N16913 002
+			

TABLET; ORAL
DOPAR

TE	Manufacturer	Strength	Appl. No.
BD	ROBERTS	250 MG	N16913 004
BD		500 MG	N16913 005

LARODOPA

TE	Manufacturer	Strength	Appl. No.
BD	ROCHE	250 MG	N16912 003
BD		500 MG	N16912 004
BD		100 MG	N16912 005
+			

Prescription Drug Products *(continued)*

LEVODOPA; *MULTIPLE*
SEE CARBIDOPA;LEVODOPA

LEVONORDEFRIN; MEPIVACAINE HYDROCHLORIDE
INJECTABLE; INJECTION

		Strength	App. No.	Date
	ARESTOCAINE HCL w/ LEVONORDEFRIN			
AP	CARLISLE	0.05 MG/ML;2%	N85010 001	
	CARBOCAINE w/ NEO-COBEFRIN			
AP	COOK WAITE	0.05 MG/ML;2%	N12125 002	
	ISOCAINE HCL w/ LEVONORDEFRIN			
AP	NOVOCOL	0.05 MG/ML;2%	N84697 001	
	MEPIVACAINE HCL w/ LEVONORDEFRIN			
AP	GRAHAM CHEM	0.05 MG/ML;2%	N84850 002	OCT 21, 1983
	POLOCAINE w/ LEVONORDEFRIN			
AP	ASTRA	0.05 MG/ML;2%	N89517 001	APR 14, 1988
	SCANDONEST L			
AP	DEPROCO	0.05 MG/ML;2%	N88388 001	OCT 10, 1984

LEVONORDEFRIN; PROCAINE HYDROCHLORIDE; PROPOXYCAINE HYDROCHLORIDE
INJECTABLE; INJECTION

		Strength	App. No.
	RAVOCAINE AND NOVOCAIN w/ NEO-COBEFRIN		
	COOK WAITE	0.05 MG/ML;2%;0.4%	N08592 007

LEVONORGESTREL
IMPLANT; IMPLANTATION

	Strength	App. No.	Date
NORPLANT SYSTEM			
WYETH AYERST	36 MG/IMPLANT	N20088 001	DEC 10, 1990

LEVONORGESTREL; *MULTIPLE*
SEE ETHINYL ESTRADIOL;LEVONORGESTREL

LEVORPHANOL TARTRATE
INJECTABLE; INJECTION

		Strength	App. No.	Date
	LEVO-DROMORAN			
	ROCHE	2 MG/ML	N08719 001	DEC 19, 1991
	TABLET; ORAL			
	LEVO-DROMORAN			
+	ROCHE	2 MG	N08720 001	DEC 19, 1991

LIDOCAINE

		Strength	App. No.
	AEROSOL; ORAL		
	XYLOCAINE		
	ASTRA	10%	N14394 001
	OINTMENT; TOPICAL		
	ALPHACAINE		
AT	CARLISLE	5%	N84944 001
AT		5%	N84946 001
AT		5%	N84947 001
	LIDOCAINE		
AT	FOUGERA	5%	N80198 001
AT	GRAHAM CHEM	5%	N80210 001
AT	THAMES	5%	N86724 001
	XYLOCAINE		
AT	ASTRA	5%	N08048 001
	SOLUTION; TOPICAL		
	XYLOCAINE		
	ASTRA	5%	N14127 001
	SUPPOSITORY; RECTAL		
	XYLOCAINE		
	ASTRA	100 MG	N13077 001

LIDOCAINE HYDROCHLORIDE
INJECTABLE; INJECTION

		Strength	App. No.	Date
	ALPHACAINE HCL			
AP	CARLISLE	2%	N84721 001	
	LIDOCAINE HCL			
AP	ABBOTT	0.5%	N88328 001	MAY 17, 1984
AP		1%	N80408 001	
AP		1%	N83158 001	
AP		1%	N88329 001	MAY 17, 1984
AP		1.5%	N80408 002	
AP		2%	N83158 002	
AP		2%	N88294 001	MAY 17, 1984
AP		2%	N88331 001	MAY 17, 1984
AP		2%	N88295 001	MAY 17, 1984
AP		4%	N87980 001	MAY 17, 1984
AP		10%		FEB 02, 1983
AP		20%	N89362 001	
AP		20%		MAY 25, 1988
AP	AKORN	1%	N85037 001	
AP		2%	N85037 002	
AP	BEL MAR	1%	N80710 001	
AP		2%	N80760 001	
AP	BRISTOL	1%	N80390 001	
AP		2%	N80390 002	
AP	DELL	1%	N83387 001	
AP		2%	N83388 001	

Prescription Drug Products (continued)

LIDOCAINE HYDROCHLORIDE (continued)

INJECTABLE; INJECTION

LIDOCAINE HCL

TE	Manufacturer	Strength	Number
AP	ELKINS SINN	1%	N80407 001
AP		1%	N84625 001
AP		2%	N80407 002
AP		2%	N84625 002
AP	GRAHAM CHEM	2%	N80504 001
AP	INTL MEDICATION	1%	N17701 002
AP		1%	N83173 001
AP		2%	N17701 001
AP		2%	N83173 002
AP	LUITPOLD	20%	N17702 001
AP		1%	N80850 001
AP	LYPHOMED	1%	N83198 001
AP		1%	N80404 002
AP		2%	N86761 001
AP		2%	N17508 001
AP		2%	N17584 001
AP		2%	N80420 004
AP		2%	N80404 003
AP		4%	N86761 002
AP		4%	N17508 002
AP		20%	N17584 002
AP	STERIS	1%	N17508 004
AP		1%	N80377 001
AP	WYETH AYERST	2%	N80377 002
AP		2%	N83083 001
AP		2%	N83083 002

LIDOCAINE HCL IN PLASTIC CONTAINER

TE	Manufacturer	Strength	Number	Date
AP	ABBOTT	0.5%	N88325 001	JUL 31, 1984
AP		1%	N88299 001	JUL 31, 1984
AP		1.5%	N88326 001	JUL 31, 1984
AP		2%	N88327 001	JUL 31, 1984
AP		10%	N88367 001	JUL 31, 1984
AP		20%	N88368 001	JUL 31, 1984
AP	LYPHOMED	1%	N88586 001	JUL 24, 1985

LIDOCAINE HCL 0.2% AND DEXTROSE 5% IN PLASTIC CONTAINER

TE	Manufacturer	Strength	Number	Date
AP	BAXTER	200 MG/100 ML	N18461 002	
AP	MCGAW	200 MG/100 ML	N18967 001	MAR 30, 1984
AP		200 MG/100 ML	N19830 002	APR 08, 1992

LIDOCAINE HCL 0.2% IN DEXTROSE 5%

TE	Manufacturer	Strength	Number
AP	ABBOTT	200 MG/100 ML	N83158 005

LIDOCAINE HCL 0.2% IN DEXTROSE 5% IN PLASTIC CONTAINER

TE	Manufacturer	Strength	Number
AP	ABBOTT	200 MG/100 ML	N18388 001

LIDOCAINE HYDROCHLORIDE (continued)

INJECTABLE; INJECTION

LIDOCAINE HCL 0.4% AND DEXTROSE 5% IN PLASTIC CONTAINER

TE	Manufacturer	Strength	Number	Date
AP	BAXTER	400 MG/100 ML	N18461 003	
AP	MCGAW	400 MG/100 ML	N18967 002	MAR 30, 1984
AP		400 MG/100 ML	N19830 003	APR 08, 1992

LIDOCAINE HCL 0.4% IN DEXTROSE 5%

TE	Manufacturer	Strength	Number
AP	ABBOTT	400 MG/100 ML	N83158 006

LIDOCAINE HCL 0.4% IN DEXTROSE 5% IN PLASTIC CONTAINER

TE	Manufacturer	Strength	Number
AP	ABBOTT	400 MG/100 ML	N18388 002

LIDOCAINE HCL 0.8% AND DEXTROSE 5% IN PLASTIC CONTAINER

TE	Manufacturer	Strength	Number	Date
AP	BAXTER	800 MG/100 ML	N18461 004	FEB 22, 1982
AP	MCGAW	800 MG/100 ML	N18967 003	MAR 30, 1984
AP		800 MG/100 ML	N19830 004	APR 08, 1992

LIDOCAINE HCL 0.8% IN DEXTROSE 5% IN PLASTIC CONTAINER

TE	Manufacturer	Strength	Number	Date
AP	ABBOTT	800 MG/100 ML	N18388 003	NOV 05, 1982

LIDOCATON

TE	Manufacturer	Strength	Number	Date
AP	PHARMATON	2%	N84727 001	AUG 17, 1983

LIDOPEN

TE	Manufacturer	Strength	Number
AP	SURVIVAL TECH	10%	N17549 001

XYLOCAINE

TE	Manufacturer	Strength	Number	Date
AP	ASTRA	0.5%	N06488 008	
AP		1%	N06488 007	
AP		1%	N16801 005	JAN 19, 1988
AP		1.5%	N06488 010	
AP		2%	N06488 002	
AP		2%	N16801 001	
AP		4%	N16801 002	
AP		10%	N16801 003	
AP		20%	N16801 004	

XYLOCAINE 4%

TE	Manufacturer	Strength	Number
AP	ASTRA	4%	N10417 001

INJECTABLE; SPINAL

LIDOCAINE HCL AND DEXTROSE 7.5%

TE	Manufacturer	Strength	Number
AP	ABBOTT	5%	N83914 001

XYLOCAINE W/ DEXTROSE 7.5%

TE	Manufacturer	Strength	Number
AP	ASTRA	1.5%	N16297 001

XYLOCAINE 5% W/ GLUCOSE 7.5%

TE	Manufacturer	Strength	Number	Date
AP	ASTRA	5%	N10496 002	JUL 07, 1982

JELLY; TOPICAL

LIDOCAINE HCL

TE	Manufacturer	Strength	Number
AT	INTL MEDICATION	2%	N86283 001

XYLOCAINE

TE	Manufacturer	Strength	Number
AT	ASTRA	2%	N08816 001

Prescription Drug Products (continued)

LIDOCAINE HYDROCHLORIDE (continued)

SOLUTION; ORAL

LIDOCAINE HCL VISCOUS			
AT	BARRE	2%	N86578 001
AT	INTL MEDICATION	2%	N86389 001 FEB 02, 1982
LIDOCAINE VISCOUS			
AT	ROXANE	2%	N88802 001 APR 26, 1985
MYLOCAINE			
AT	PHARM BASICS	2%	N87872 001 NOV 18, 1982
XYLOCAINE VISCOUS			
AT	ASTRA	2%	N09470 001

SOLUTION; TOPICAL

ANESTACON			
AT	ALCON	2%	N80429 001
LARYNG-O-JET KIT			
AT	INTL MEDICATION	4%	N86364 001
LIDOCAINE HCL			
AT	ROXANE	4%	N88803 001 APR 03, 1985
LTA II KIT			
AT	ABBOTT	4%	N80409 001
AT		4%	N88542 001 JUL 31, 1984
MYLOCAINE			
AT	PHARM BASICS	4%	N87881 001 NOV 18, 1982
PEDIATRIC LTA KIT			
AT	ABBOTT	2%	N85995 001
AT		2%	N88572 001 JUL 31, 1984
XYLOCAINE 4%			
AT	ASTRA	4%	N10417 002

LIDOCAINE HYDROCHLORIDE; *MULTIPLE*

SEE DEXAMETHASONE SODIUM PHOSPHATE; LIDOCAINE HYDROCHLORIDE

SEE EPINEPHRINE; LIDOCAINE HYDROCHLORIDE

SEE EPINEPHRINE BITARTRATE; LIDOCAINE HYDROCHLORIDE

LINCOMYCIN HYDROCHLORIDE

CAPSULE; ORAL

LINCOCIN			
	UPJOHN	EQ 250 MG BASE	N50316 001
+		EQ 500 MG BASE	N50316 002

INJECTABLE; INJECTION

LINCOCIN			
	UPJOHN	EQ 300 MG BASE/ML	N50317 001
AP	LINCOMYCIN HCL		
AP	STERIS	EQ 300 MG BASE/ML	N63180 001 APR 16, 1991

LINDANE

CREAM; TOPICAL

KWELL			
	REED AND CARNRICK	1%	N06309 001
		1%	N84218 001

LOTION; TOPICAL

KWELL			
AT	REED AND CARNRICK	1%	N06309 003
AT		1%	N84218 002
LINDANE			
AT	BARRE	1%	N87313 001
AT	PHARM BASICS	1%	N88190 001 AUG 16, 1984
SCABENE			
AT	STIEFEL	1%	N86769 001

SHAMPOO; TOPICAL

KWELL			
AT	REED AND CARNRICK	1%	N10718 001
AT		1%	N84219 001
LINDANE			
AT	BARRE	1%	N87266 001
AT	PHARM BASICS	1%	N88191 001 SEP 18, 1984
SCABENE			
AT	STIEFEL	1%	N87940 001 APR 08, 1983

LIOTHYRONINE SODIUM

INJECTABLE; INJECTION

TRIOSTAT			
SMITHKLINE BEECHAM		EQ 0.01 MG BASE/ML	N20105 001 DEC 31, 1991

TABLET; ORAL

CYTOMEL			
	SKF	EQ 0.005 MG BASE	N10379 001
+		EQ 0.025 MG BASE	N10379 002
		EQ 0.05 MG BASE	N10379 003

LIOTRIX (T4;T3)

TABLET; ORAL

EUTHROID-0.5			
	PARKE DAVIS	0.03 MG;0.0075 MG	N16680 001
EUTHROID-1			
	PARKE DAVIS	0.06 MG;0.015 MG	N16680 002
EUTHROID-2			
	PARKE DAVIS	0.12 MG;0.03 MG	N16680 003
EUTHROID-3			
+	PARKE DAVIS	0.18 MG;0.045 MG	N16680 004
THYROLAR-0.25			
	RHONE POULENC RORER	0.0125 MG;0.0031 MG	N16807 001

Prescription Drug Products (continued)

LIOTRIX (T4;T3) (continued)

TABLET; ORAL

TE	Product / Firm	Strength	Appl. No.	Date
	THYROLAR-0.5			
	RHONE POULENC RORER	0.025 MG;0.00625 MG	N16807 005	
	THYROLAR-1			
	RHONE POULENC RORER	0.05 MG;0.0125 MG	N16807 004	
	THYROLAR-2			
	RHONE POULENC RORER	0.1 MG;0.025 MG	N16807 002	
	THYROLAR-3			
+	RHONE POULENC RORER	0.15 MG;0.0375 MG	N16807 003	

LISINOPRIL

TABLET; ORAL

TE	Product / Firm	Strength	Appl. No.	Date
	PRINIVIL			
AB	MERCK	5 MG	N19558 001	DEC 29, 1987
AB		10 MG	N19558 002	DEC 29, 1987
AB		20 MG	N19558 003	DEC 29, 1987
AB		40 MG	N19558 004	DEC 29, 1987
				OCT 25, 1988
	ZESTRIL			
AB	IMPERIAL CHEM	5 MG	N19777 001	MAY 19, 1988
AB		10 MG	N19777 002	MAY 19, 1988
AB		20 MG	N19777 003	MAY 19, 1988
AB +		40 MG	N19777 004	MAY 19, 1988

LISINOPRIL; *MULTIPLE*

SEE HYDROCHLOROTHIAZIDE; LISINOPRIL

LITHIUM CARBONATE

CAPSULE; ORAL

TE	Product / Firm	Strength	Appl. No.	Date
	ESKALITH			
AB +	SKF	300 MG	N16860 001	
	LITHIUM CARBONATE			
AB	ROXANE	300 MG	N17812 001	
		150 MG	N17812 002	
		600 MG	N17812 003	JAN 28, 1987
		300 MG	N17812	JAN 28, 1987
	LITHONATE			
AB	SOLVAY	300 MG	N16782 001	

LITHIUM CARBONATE (continued)

TABLET; ORAL

TE	Product / Firm	Strength	Appl. No.	Date
	ESKALITH			
AB	+ SKF	300 MG	N17971 001	
	LITHANE			
AB	MILES	300 MG	N18833 001	JUL 18, 1985
	LITHIUM CARBONATE			
AB	ROXANE	300 MG	N18558 001	JAN 29, 1982
	LITHOTABS			
AB	SOLVAY	300 MG	N16980 001	

TABLET, EXTENDED RELEASE; ORAL

TE	Product / Firm	Strength	Appl. No.	Date
	ESKALITH CR			
	+ SKF	450 MG	N18152 001	MAR 29, 1982
	LITHOBID			
	+ CIBA	300 MG	N18027 001	

LITHIUM CITRATE

SYRUP; ORAL

TE	Product / Firm	Strength	Appl. No.	Date
	CIBALITH-S			
AA	CIBA	EQ 300 MG CARBONATE/5 ML	N17672 001	
	LITHIUM CITRATE			
AA	PHARM BASICS	EQ 300 MG CARBONATE/5 ML	N70755 001	MAY 21, 1986
AA	ROXANE	EQ 300 MG CARBONATE/5 ML	N18421 001	

LOMEFLOXACIN HYDROCHLORIDE

TABLET; ORAL

TE	Product / Firm	Strength	Appl. No.	Date
	MAXAQUIN			
	+ SEARLE	EQ 400 MG BASE	N20013 001	FEB 21, 1992

LOMUSTINE

CAPSULE; ORAL

TE	Product / Firm	Strength	Appl. No.	Date
	CEENU			
	BRISTOL	10 MG	N17588 001	
+		40 MG	N17588 002	
		100 MG	N17588 003	

Prescription Drug Products (continued)

LOPERAMIDE HYDROCHLORIDE

CAPSULE; ORAL

	IMODIUM			
ΔB	+ JANSSEN	2 MG	N17694 001	
	LOPERAMIDE HCL			
ΔB	GENEVA	2 MG	N72993 001	AUG 28, 1992
ΔB	LEMMON	2 MG	N73192 001	APR 30, 1992
ΔB	MYLAN	2 MG	N72741 001	SEP 18, 1991
ΔB	NOVOPHARM	2 MG	N73122 001	AUG 30, 1991
ΔB	ROXANE	2 MG	N73080 001	NOV 27, 1991

LORACARBEF

CAPSULE; ORAL

	LORABID			
	+ LILLY	200 MG	N50668 001	DEC 31, 1991

POWDER FOR RECONSTITUTION; ORAL

	LORABID			
	LILLY	100 MG/5 ML	N50667 001	DEC 31, 1991
	+	200 MG/5 ML	N50667 002	DEC 31, 1991

LORAZEPAM

CONCENTRATE; ORAL

	LORAZEPAM INTENSOL			
	ROXANE	2 MG/ML	N72755 001	JUN 28, 1991

INJECTABLE; INJECTION

	ATIVAN			
	WYETH AYERST	2 MG/ML	N18140 001	
		4 MG/ML	N18140 002	

TABLET; ORAL

	ATIVAN			
	WYETH AYERST			
ΔB		0.5 MG	N17794 001	DEC 10, 1985
ΔB		1 MG	N17794 002	DEC 10, 1985
ΔB		2 MG	N17794 003	DEC 10, 1985
	LORAZEPAM			
ΔB	BARR	0.5 MG	N70472 001	DEC 10, 1985
ΔB		1 MG	N70473 001	DEC 10, 1985
ΔB		2 MG	N70474 001	DEC 10, 1985

LORAZEPAM (continued)

TABLET; ORAL

	LORAZEPAM			
ΔB	DANBURY	0.5 MG	N71117 001	JUL 24, 1986
ΔB		1 MG	N71118 001	JUL 24, 1986
ΔB		2 MG	N71110 001	JUL 24, 1986
ΔB	GENEVA	0.5 MG	N71193 001	APR 15, 1988
ΔB		1 MG	N71194 001	APR 15, 1988
ΔB		2 MG	N71195 001	APR 15, 1988
ΔB	HALSEY	0.5 MG	N71434 001	SEP 01, 1987
ΔB		1 MG	N71435 001	SEP 01, 1987
ΔB		2 MG	N71436 001	SEP 01, 1987
ΔB	MUTUAL PHARM	0.5 MG	N72553 001	MAR 29, 1991
ΔB		1 MG	N72554 001	MAR 29, 1991
ΔB		2 MG	N72555 001	MAR 29, 1991
ΔB	MYLAN	0.5 MG	N71589 001	OCT 13, 1987
ΔB		1 MG	N71590 001	OCT 13, 1987
ΔB		2 MG	N71591 001	OCT 13, 1987
ΔB	PAR	0.5 MG	N70675 001	DEC 01, 1986
ΔB		1 MG	N70676 001	DEC 01, 1986
ΔB		2 MG	N70677 001	DEC 01, 1986
ΔB	PUREPAC	0.5 MG	N71403 001	APR 21, 1987
ΔB		1 MG	N71404 001	APR 21, 1987
ΔB		2 MG	N71141 001	APR 21, 1987
ΔB	ROYCE	0.5 MG	N72926 001	OCT 31, 1991
ΔB		1 MG	N72927 001	OCT 31, 1991
ΔB		2 MG	N72928 001	OCT 31, 1991
ΔB	SUPERPHARM	0.5 MG	N71245 001	FEB 09, 1987
ΔB		1 MG	N71246 001	FEB 09, 1987
ΔB		2 MG	N71247 001	FEB 09, 1987

Prescription Drug Products (continued)

LORAZEPAM (continued)
TABLET; ORAL
LORAZEPAM

ΔB	WARNER CHILCOTT	1MG	N71038 001	JAN 12, 1988
ΔB		2MG	N71039 001	JAN 12, 1988
ΔB	WATSON	0.5MG	N71086 001	MAR 23, 1987
ΔB		1MG	N71087 001	MAR 23, 1987
ΔB		2MG	N71088 001	MAR 23, 1987

LOVASTATIN
TABLET; ORAL
MEVACOR

	MERCK	10 MG	N19643 002	MAR 28, 1991
		20 MG	N19643 003	AUG 31, 1987
+		40 MG	N19643 004	DEC 14, 1988

LOXAPINE HYDROCHLORIDE
CONCENTRATE; ORAL
LOXITANE C

	LEDERLE	EQ 25 MG BASE/ML	N17658 001

INJECTABLE; INJECTION
LOXITANE IM

	LEDERLE	EQ 50 MG BASE/ML	N18039 001

LOXAPINE SUCCINATE
CAPSULE; ORAL
LOXAPINE SUCCINATE

ΔB	WATSON	EQ 5 MG BASE	N72204 001	JUN 15, 1988
ΔB		EQ 10 MG BASE	N72205 001	JUN 15, 1988
ΔB		EQ 25 MG BASE	N72206 001	JUN 15, 1988
ΔB		EQ 50 MG BASE	N72062 001	JUN 15, 1988

LOXITANE

ΔB	LEDERLE	EQ 5 MG BASE	N17525 001
ΔB		EQ 10 MG BASE	N17525 002
ΔB +		EQ 25 MG BASE	N17525 003
ΔB		EQ 50 MG BASE	N17525 004

LYPRESSIN
SOLUTION; NASAL
DIAPID

	SANDOZ	0.185 MG/ML	N16755 001

MAFENIDE ACETATE
CREAM; TOPICAL
SULFAMYLON

	STERLING	EQ 85 MG BASE/GM	N16763 001

MAGNESIUM ACETATE; *MULTIPLE*
SEE AMINO ACIDS: CALCIUM ACETATE: GLYCERIN: MAGNESIUM ACETATE: PHOSPHORIC ACID: POTASSIUM CHLORIDE: SODIUM ACETATE: SODIUM CHLORIDE

SEE AMINO ACIDS: MAGNESIUM ACETATE: PHOSPHORIC ACID: POTASSIUM ACETATE: POTASSIUM CHLORIDE: SODIUM ACETATE

SEE AMINO ACIDS: MAGNESIUM ACETATE: PHOSPHORIC ACID: POTASSIUM ACETATE: SODIUM CHLORIDE

SEE AMINO ACIDS: MAGNESIUM ACETATE: PHOSPHORIC ACID: POTASSIUM CHLORIDE: SODIUM ACETATE: SODIUM CHLORIDE

SEE AMINO ACIDS: MAGNESIUM ACETATE: POTASSIUM ACETATE: SODIUM CHLORIDE

SEE DEXTROSE: MAGNESIUM ACETATE: POTASSIUM ACETATE: SODIUM CHLORIDE

MAGNESIUM ACETATE TETRAHYDRATE; *MULTIPLE*
SEE DEXTROSE: MAGNESIUM ACETATE TETRAHYDRATE: POTASSIUM ACETATE: SODIUM CHLORIDE

MAGNESIUM ACETATE TETRAHYDRATE; POTASSIUM ACETATE; SODIUM CHLORIDE
INJECTABLE; INJECTION
PLASMA-LYTE 56 IN PLASTIC CONTAINER

	BAXTER	32 MG/100 ML;128 MG/100 ML;234 MG/100 ML	N19047 001 JUN 15, 1984

MAGNESIUM CARBONATE; *MULTIPLE*
SEE CITRIC ACID: GLUCONOLACTONE: MAGNESIUM CARBONATE

Prescription Drug Products (continued)

MAGNESIUM CHLORIDE; *MULTIPLE*

SEE   AMINO ACIDS: CALCIUM CHLORIDE: DEXTROSE: MAGNESIUM CHLORIDE: POTASSIUM CHLORIDE: POTASSIUM PHOSPHATE, DIBASIC: SODIUM CHLORIDE

SEE   AMINO ACIDS: DEXTROSE: MAGNESIUM CHLORIDE: POTASSIUM ACETATE: POTASSIUM CHLORIDE: POTASSIUM PHOSPHATE, DIBASIC: SODIUM CHLORIDE

SEE   AMINO ACIDS: DEXTROSE: MAGNESIUM CHLORIDE: POTASSIUM CHLORIDE: SODIUM CHLORIDE: SODIUM PHOSPHATE, DIBASIC

SEE   AMINO ACIDS: MAGNESIUM CHLORIDE: POTASSIUM ACETATE: POTASSIUM CHLORIDE: SODIUM ACETATE

SEE   AMINO ACIDS: MAGNESIUM CHLORIDE: POTASSIUM CHLORIDE: SODIUM CHLORIDE: SODIUM PHOSPHATE, DIBASIC

SEE   AMINO ACIDS: MAGNESIUM CHLORIDE: POTASSIUM CHLORIDE: POTASSIUM PHOSPHATE, DIBASIC: SODIUM CHLORIDE

SEE   AMINO ACIDS: MAGNESIUM CHLORIDE: POTASSIUM PHOSPHATE, DIBASIC: SODIUM ACETATE: SODIUM CHLORIDE

SEE   AMINO ACIDS: MAGNESIUM CHLORIDE: POTASSIUM PHOSPHATE, DIBASIC: SODIUM CHLORIDE

SEE   CALCIUM CHLORIDE: DEXTROSE: GLUTATHIONE DISULFIDE: MAGNESIUM CHLORIDE: POTASSIUM CHLORIDE: SODIUM BICARBONATE: SODIUM CHLORIDE: SODIUM PHOSPHATE

SEE   CALCIUM CHLORIDE: DEXTROSE: MAGNESIUM CHLORIDE: SODIUM CHLORIDE: SODIUM LACTATE

SEE   CALCIUM CHLORIDE: DEXTROSE: MAGNESIUM CHLORIDE: SODIUM ACETATE: SODIUM CHLORIDE

SEE   CALCIUM CHLORIDE: DEXTROSE: MAGNESIUM CHLORIDE: POTASSIUM CHLORIDE: SODIUM ACETATE: SODIUM CHLORIDE

SEE   CALCIUM CHLORIDE: DEXTROSE: MAGNESIUM CHLORIDE: POTASSIUM CHLORIDE: SODIUM CITRATE

SEE   CALCIUM CHLORIDE: DEXTROSE: MAGNESIUM CHLORIDE: SODIUM CHLORIDE: SODIUM LACTATE

SEE   CALCIUM CHLORIDE: MAGNESIUM CHLORIDE: POTASSIUM CHLORIDE: SODIUM ACETATE: SODIUM CHLORIDE: SODIUM CITRATE

SEE   CALCIUM CHLORIDE: MAGNESIUM CHLORIDE: POTASSIUM CHLORIDE: SODIUM ACETATE: SODIUM CHLORIDE

MAGNESIUM CHLORIDE; *MULTIPLE* (continued)

SEE   CALCIUM CHLORIDE: MAGNESIUM CHLORIDE: POTASSIUM CHLORIDE: SODIUM ACETATE: SODIUM CHLORIDE: SODIUM LACTATE

SEE   CALCIUM CHLORIDE: MAGNESIUM CHLORIDE: POTASSIUM CHLORIDE: SODIUM CHLORIDE

SEE   DEXTROSE: MAGNESIUM CHLORIDE: POTASSIUM CHLORIDE: SODIUM ACETATE: SODIUM CHLORIDE: SODIUM GLUCONATE

SEE   DEXTROSE: MAGNESIUM CHLORIDE: POTASSIUM CHLORIDE: POTASSIUM PHOSPHATE, DIBASIC: SODIUM ACETATE: SODIUM CHLORIDE

SEE   DEXTROSE: MAGNESIUM CHLORIDE: POTASSIUM CHLORIDE: SODIUM ACETATE: SODIUM GLUCONATE: SODIUM CHLORIDE

SEE   DEXTROSE: MAGNESIUM CHLORIDE: POTASSIUM CHLORIDE: POTASSIUM PHOSPHATE, DIBASIC: SODIUM ACETATE

SEE   DEXTROSE: MAGNESIUM CHLORIDE: POTASSIUM CHLORIDE: POTASSIUM PHOSPHATE, DIBASIC: SODIUM CHLORIDE: SODIUM LACTATE: SODIUM PHOSPHATE, MONOBASIC

SEE   DEXTROSE: MAGNESIUM CHLORIDE: POTASSIUM CHLORIDE: POTASSIUM PHOSPHATE, MONOBASIC: SODIUM LACTATE: SODIUM PHOSPHATE, MONOBASIC

SEE   DEXTROSE: MAGNESIUM CHLORIDE: POTASSIUM PHOSPHATE, MONOBASIC: SODIUM CHLORIDE: SODIUM LACTATE

MAGNESIUM CHLORIDE; POTASSIUM CHLORIDE; POTASSIUM PHOSPHATE, MONOBASIC; SODIUM ACETATE; SODIUM CHLORIDE; SODIUM GLUCONATE; SODIUM PHOSPHATE, DIBASIC

INJECTABLE; INJECTION
  ISOLYTE S PH 7.4 IN PLASTIC CONTAINER

MCGAW	30 MG/100 ML;37 MG/100 ML;0.82 MG/100 ML;370 MG/100 ML;530 MG/100 ML;500 MG/100 ML;12 MG/100 ML	N19006 001	APR 04, 1984
	30 MG/100 ML;37 MG/100 ML;0.82 MG/100 ML;370 MG/100 ML;530 MG/100 ML;500 MG/100 ML;12 MG/100 ML	N19696 001	SEP 29, 1989

MAGNESIUM OXIDE; *MULTIPLE*

SEE   CITRIC ACID; MAGNESIUM OXIDE; SODIUM CARBONATE

MAGNESIUM SULFATE

INJECTABLE; INJECTION
MAGNESIUM SULFATE
    LYPHOMED   500 MG/ML   N19916 001   SEP 08, 1986

MAGNESIUM SULFATE; POTASSIUM CHLORIDE; POTASSIUM PHOSPHATE, MONOBASIC; SODIUM CHLORIDE; SODIUM PHOSPHATE

SOLUTION; IRRIGATION
TIS-U-SOL
AT   BAXTER   20 MG/100 ML;40 MG/100 ML;6.25 MG/100 ML;800 MG/100 ML;8.75 MG/100 ML   N18508 001   FEB 19, 1982

TIS-U-SOL IN PLASTIC CONTAINER
AT   BAXTER   20 MG/100 ML;40 MG/100 ML;6.25 MG/100 ML;800 MG/100 ML;8.75 MG/100 ML   N18336 001

MALATHION

LOTION; TOPICAL
OVIDE
    GENDERM   0.5%   N18613 001   AUG 02, 1982

MANGANESE CHLORIDE

INJECTABLE; INJECTION
MANGANESE CHLORIDE IN PLASTIC CONTAINER
    ABBOTT   EQ 0.1 MG MANGANESE/ML   N18962 001   JUN 26, 1986

MANGANESE SULFATE

INJECTABLE; INJECTION
MANGANESE SULFATE
    LYPHOMED   EQ 0.1 MG MANGANESE/ML   N19228 001   MAY 05, 1987

Prescription Drug Products (continued)

MAGNESIUM CHLORIDE; POTASSIUM CHLORIDE; SODIUM ACETATE; SODIUM CHLORIDE; SODIUM GLUCONATE

INJECTABLE; INJECTION
ISOLYTE S IN PLASTIC CONTAINER
AP   MCGAW   30 MG/100 ML;37 MG/100 ML;370 MG/100 ML;530 MG/100 ML;500 MG/100 ML   N18252 001

AP   30 MG/100 ML;37 MG/100 ML;370 MG/100 ML;530 MG/100 ML;500 MG/100 ML   N19711 001   SEP 29, 1989

NORMOSOL-R IN PLASTIC CONTAINER
    ABBOTT   30 MG/100 ML;37 MG/100 ML;222 MG/100 ML;526 MG/100 ML;502 MG/100 ML   N17586 001

PLASMA-LYTE A IN PLASTIC CONTAINER
AP   BAXTER   30 MG/100 ML;37 MG/100 ML;368 MG/100 ML;526 MG/100 ML;502 MG/100 ML   N17378 002   NOV 22, 1982

PLASMA-LYTE 148 IN WATER IN PLASTIC CONTAINER
AP   BAXTER   30 MG/100 ML;37 MG/100 ML;368 MG/100 ML;526 MG/100 ML;502 MG/100 ML   N17378 001

SOLUTION; IRRIGATION
PHYSIOLYTE IN PLASTIC CONTAINER
AT   MCGAW   30 MG/100 ML;37 MG/100 ML;370 MG/100 ML;530 MG/100 ML;500 MG/100 ML   N19024 001   JUN 08, 1984

PHYSIOSOL IN PLASTIC CONTAINER
AT   ABBOTT   30 MG/100 ML;37 MG/100 ML;222 MG/100 ML;526 MG/100 ML;502 MG/100 ML   N17637 002   JUL 08, 1982

PHYSIOSOL PH 7.4 IN PLASTIC CONTAINER
    ABBOTT   30 MG/100 ML;37 MG/100 ML;222 MG/100 ML;526 MG/100 ML;502 MG/100 ML   N18406 002   JUL 08, 1982

SYNOVALYTE IN PLASTIC CONTAINER
AT   BAXTER   30 MG/100 ML;37 MG/100 ML;368 MG/100 ML;526 MG/100 ML;502 MG/100 ML   N19326 001   JAN 25, 1985

Prescription Drug Products *(continued)*

MANNITOL

INJECTABLE; INJECTION

MANNITOL 10%
AP	ABBOTT	10 GM/100 ML	N16269 002
AP	MCGAW	10 GM/100 ML	N16080 002

MANNITOL 10% IN PLASTIC CONTAINER
AP	ABBOTT	10 GM/100 ML	N19603 002 JAN 08, 1987

MANNITOL 10% W/ DEXTROSE 5% IN DISTILLED WATER
AP	MCGAW	10 GM/100 ML	N16080 006

MANNITOL 15%
AP	ABBOTT	15 GM/100 ML	N16269 003
AP	MCGAW	15 GM/100 ML	N16080 003

MANNITOL 15% IN PLASTIC CONTAINER
AP	ABBOTT	15 GM/100 ML	N19603 003 JAN 08, 1990

MANNITOL 15% W/ DEXTROSE 5% IN SODIUM CHLORIDE 0.45%
AP	MCGAW	15 GM/100 ML	N16080 005

MANNITOL 20%
AP	ABBOTT	20 GM/100 ML	N16269 004
AP	MCGAW	20 GM/100 ML	N14738 001
AP	MCGAW	20 GM/100 ML	N16080 004

MANNITOL 20% IN PLASTIC CONTAINER
AP	ABBOTT	20 GM/100 ML	N19603 004 JAN 08, 1990

MANNITOL 25%
AP	ABBOTT	12.5 GM/50 ML	N16269 005
AP	ASTRA	12.5 GM/50 ML	N89239 001 MAY 06, 1987
AP	ASTRA	12.5 GM/50 ML	N89240 001 MAY 06, 1987

INTL MEDICATION
AP	LUITPOLD	12.5 GM/50 ML	N83051 001
AP	LUITPOLD	12.5 GM/50 ML	N87409 001 JAN 21, 1982

LYPHOMED
AP	LYPHOMED	12.5 GM/50 ML	N80677 001
AP	LYPHOMED	12.5 GM/50 ML	N86754 001

STERIS
AP	STERIS	12.5 GM/50 ML	N87460 001 JUN 27, 1983

MANNITOL 5%
AP	ABBOTT	5 GM/100 ML	N16269 001
AP	MCGAW	5 GM/100 ML	N16080 001

MANNITOL 5% IN PLASTIC CONTAINER
AP	ABBOTT	5 GM/100 ML	N19603 001 JAN 08, 1987

MANNITOL 5% W/ DEXTROSE 5% IN SODIUM CHLORIDE 0.12%
AP	MCGAW	5 GM/100 ML	N16080 007

OSMITROL 10% IN WATER
AP	BAXTER	10 GM/100 ML	N13684 002

OSMITROL 10% IN WATER IN PLASTIC CONTAINER
AP	BAXTER	10 GM/100 ML	N13684 006

OSMITROL 15% IN WATER
AP	BAXTER	15 GM/100 ML	N13684 004

OSMITROL 15% IN WATER IN PLASTIC CONTAINER
AP	BAXTER	15 GM/100 ML	N13684 008

MANNITOL *(continued)*

INJECTABLE; INJECTION

OSMITROL 20% IN WATER
AP	BAXTER	20 GM/100 ML	N13684 003

OSMITROL 20% IN WATER IN PLASTIC CONTAINER
AP	BAXTER	20 GM/100 ML	N13684 007

OSMITROL 5% IN WATER
AP	BAXTER	5 GM/100 ML	N13684 001

OSMITROL 5% IN WATER IN PLASTIC CONTAINER
AP	BAXTER	5 GM/100 ML	N13684 005 JAN 08, 1987

SOLUTION; IRRIGATION

RESECTISOL IN PLASTIC CONTAINER
AP	MCGAW	5 GM/100 ML	N16772 002

MANNITOL; SORBITOL

SOLUTION; IRRIGATION

SORBITOL-MANNITOL IN PLASTIC CONTAINER
AT	ABBOTT	540 MG/100 ML;2.7 GM/100 ML	N17636 001
AT	ABBOTT	540 MG/100 ML;2.7 GM/100 ML	N18316 001

MAPROTILINE HYDROCHLORIDE

TABLET; ORAL

LUDIOMIL
AB	CIBA	25 MG	N17543 001
AB	+	50 MG	N17543 002
AB		75 MG	N17543 003 SEP 30, 1982

MAPROTILINE HCL
AB	MYLAN	25 MG	N72284 001 OCT 03, 1988
AB	MYLAN	50 MG	N72285 001 OCT 03, 1988
AB	MYLAN	75 MG	N72286 001 OCT 03, 1988
AB	WATSON	25 MG	N72162 001 JUN 01, 1988
AB	WATSON	50 MG	N72163 001 JUN 01, 1988
AB	WATSON	75 MG	N72164 001 JUN 01, 1988

MAZINDOL

TABLET; ORAL

MAZANOR
BP	WYETH AYERST	1 MG	N17980 002

SANOREX
BP	SANDOZ	1 MG	N17247 001
BP	+	2 MG	N17247 002

Prescription Drug Products (continued)

MEBENDAZOLE
TABLET, CHEWABLE; ORAL

TE	Manufacturer	Strength	Appl. No.	Date
	VERMOX			
	+ JANSSEN	100 MG	N17481 001	

MECAMYLAMINE HYDROCHLORIDE
TABLET; ORAL

TE	Manufacturer	Strength	Appl. No.	Date
	INVERSINE			
	+ MSD	2.5 MG	N10251 001	

MECHLORETHAMINE HYDROCHLORIDE
INJECTABLE; INJECTION

TE	Manufacturer	Strength	Appl. No.	Date
	MUSTARGEN			
	MSD	10 MG/VIAL	N06695 001	

MECLIZINE HYDROCHLORIDE
TABLET; ORAL

TE	Manufacturer	Strength	Appl. No.	Date
	ANTIVERT			
AA	ROERIG	12.5 MG	N10721 006	
AA		25 MG	N10721 004	
AA		50 MG	N10721 001	JAN 20, 1982
	MECLIZINE HCL			
AA	BUNDY	12.5 MG	N84382 001	
AA		25 MG	N84872 001	
AA	CAMALL	12.5 MG	N85253 001	
AA		25 MG	N85252 001	
AA	CHELSEA	12.5 MG	N85269 001	
AA	GENEVA	25 MG	N85740 001	
AA		12.5 MG	N84843 002	MAY 22, 1989
AA		25 MG	N84092 003	MAY 22, 1989
AA	KV	12.5 MG	N85524 001	
AA		25 MG	N85523 001	
AA	PAR	12.5 MG	N87127 001	
AA		25 MG	N87128 001	
AA		50 MG	N89674 001	
AA	SIDMAK	12.5 MG	N88732 001	MAR 31, 1988
AA		25 MG	N88734 001	DEC 11, 1985
AA	ZENITH	12.5 MG	N83784 001	DEC 11, 1985
AA		12.5 MG	N84975 001	
AA		25 MG	N84657 001	

TABLET, CHEWABLE; ORAL

TE	Manufacturer	Strength	Appl. No.	Date
	ANTIVERT			
AA	ROERIG	25 MG	N10721 005	
	MECLIZINE HCL			
AA	SIDMAK	25 MG	N88733 001	DEC 11, 1985
AA	ZENITH	25 MG	N84976 001	

MECLOCYCLINE SULFOSALICYLATE
CREAM; TOPICAL

TE	Manufacturer	Strength	Appl. No.	Date
	MECLAN			
	JOHNSON RW	1%	N50518 001	

MECLOFENAMATE SODIUM
CAPSULE; ORAL

TE	Manufacturer	Strength	Appl. No.	Date
	MECLOFENAMATE SODIUM			
AB	BARR	EQ 50 MG BASE	N72848 001	MAR 20, 1989
AB		EQ 100 MG BASE	N72809 001	MAR 20, 1989
AB	DANBURY	EQ 50 MG BASE	N71468 001	APR 15, 1987
AB		EQ 100 MG BASE	N71469 001	APR 15, 1987
AB	GENEVA	EQ 50 MG BASE	N72262 001	NOV 29, 1988
AB		EQ 100 MG BASE	N72263 001	NOV 29, 1988
AB	MYLAN	EQ 50 MG BASE	N71080 001	SEP 03, 1986
AB		EQ 100 MG BASE	N71081 001	SEP 03, 1986
	MECLOMEN			
AB	PARKE DAVIS	EQ 50 MG BASE	N18006 001	
AB	+	EQ 100 MG BASE	N18006 002	

MEDROXYPROGESTERONE ACETATE
INJECTABLE; INJECTION

TE	Manufacturer	Strength	Appl. No.	Date
	DEPO-PROVERA			
	UPJOHN	100 MG/ML	N12541 002	
		400 MG/ML	N12541 003	

TABLET; ORAL

TE	Manufacturer	Strength	Appl. No.	Date
	AMEN			
BP	CARNRICK	10 MG	N83242 001	
	CURRETAB			
BP	SOLVAY	10 MG	N85686 001	
	CYCRIN			
AB	WYETH AYERST	10 MG	N89386 001	SEP 09, 1987
	MEDROXYPROGESTERONE ACETATE			
	DURAMED	2.5 MG	N89587 001	APR 22, 1992
		5 MG	N89588 001	APR 22, 1992
		10 MG	N89589 001	APR 22, 1992
BP	PHARM BASICS	10 MG	N88484 001	JUL 26, 1984
	PROVERA			
AB	UPJOHN	2.5 MG	N11839 001	
		5 MG	N11839 003	
AB	+	10 MG	N11839 004	

Prescription Drug Products (continued)

MEDRYSONE
SUSPENSION/DROPS; OPHTHALMIC
HMS

TE	Firm	Strength	NDC
+ ALLERGAN		1%	N16624 003

MEFENAMIC ACID
CAPSULE; ORAL
PONSTEL

TE	Firm	Strength	NDC
+ PARKE DAVIS		250 MG	N15034 003

MEFLOQUINE HYDROCHLORIDE
TABLET; ORAL
LARIAM

TE	Firm	Strength	NDC	Date
+ ROCHE		250 MG	N19591 001	MAY 02, 1989

MEGESTROL ACETATE
TABLET; ORAL
MEGACE

TE	Firm	Strength	NDC	Date
AB	+ MEAD JOHNSON	20 MG	N16979 001	
AB	+	40 MG	N16979 002	
	MEGESTROL ACETATE			
AB	PAR	20 MG	N72422 001	AUG 08, 1988
AB		40 MG	N72423 001	AUG 08, 1988

MELPHALAN
TABLET; ORAL
ALKERAN

TE	Firm	Strength	NDC
+ BURROUGHS WELLCOME		2 MG	N14691 002

MENADIOL SODIUM DIPHOSPHATE
INJECTABLE; INJECTION
SYNKAYVITE

TE	Firm	Strength	NDC
	ROCHE	5 MG/ML	N03718 004
		10 MG/ML	N03718 006
		37.5 MG/ML	N03718 008

TABLET; ORAL
SYNKAYVITE

TE	Firm	Strength	NDC
	ROCHE	5 MG	N03718 010

MENOTROPINS
INJECTABLE; INJECTION
PERGONAL

TE	Firm	Strength	NDC	Date
	SERONO	75 IU/AMP	N17646 001	
		150 IU/AMP	N17646 002	MAY 20, 1985

MEPENZOLATE BROMIDE
TABLET; ORAL
CANTIL

TE	Firm	Strength	NDC
	MERRELL DOW	25 MG	N10679 003

MEPERIDINE HYDROCHLORIDE
INJECTABLE; INJECTION
DEMEROL

TE	Firm	Strength	NDC	Date
AP	STERLING	25 MG/ML	N05010 007	
AP		50 MG/ML	N05010 002	
		75 MG/ML	N05010 009	
		100 MG/ML	N05010 003	

MEPERIDINE HCL

TE	Firm	Strength	NDC	Date
AP	ABBOTT	10 MG/ML	N88432 001	AUG 16, 1984
			N89781 001	
AP	ASTRA	25 MG/ML	N89782 001	MAR 31, 1989
		50 MG/ML	N89783 001	MAR 31, 1989
AP		50 MG/ML	N89784 001	MAR 31, 1989
AP		50 MG/ML	N89785 001	MAR 31, 1989
AP		75 MG/ML	N89786 001	MAR 31, 1989
		100 MG/ML	N89787 001	MAR 31, 1989
AP		100 MG/ML	N89788 001	MAR 31, 1989
AP	ELKINS SINN	25 MG/ML	N80445 001	MAR 31, 1989
AP		50 MG/ML	N80445 002	
AP		75 MG/ML	N80445 003	
AP		100 MG/ML	N80445 004	
AP	STERIS	10 MG/ML	N73443 001	MAR 17, 1992
AP		50 MG/ML	N73444 001	MAR 17, 1992
AP		100 MG/ML	N73445 001	MAR 17, 1992
AP	WYETH AYERST	25 MG/ML	N80455 007	
AP		50 MG/ML	N80455 008	
AP		75 MG/ML	N80455 009	
AP		100 MG/ML	N80455 010	

Prescription Drug Products (continued)

MEPERIDINE HYDROCHLORIDE (continued)

SYRUP; ORAL

	DEMEROL			
AA	STERLING	50 MG/5 ML	N05010 005	
	MEPERIDINE HCL			
AA	ROXANE	50 MG/5 ML	N88744 001	JAN 30, 1985

TABLET; ORAL

	DEMEROL			
AA	STERLING	50 MG	N05010 001	
AA		100 MG	N05010 004	
	MEPERIDINE HCL			
AA	BARR	50 MG	N88639 001	JUL 02, 1984
AA		100 MG	N88640 001	SEP 19, 1984
AA	WYETH AYERST	50 MG	N80454 001	
	PETHADOL			
AA	HALSEY	50 MG	N80448 001	
AA		100 MG	N80448 002	

MEPERIDINE HYDROCHLORIDE; *MULTIPLE*
SEE ATROPINE SULFATE; MEPERIDINE HYDROCHLORIDE

MEPERIDINE HYDROCHLORIDE; PROMETHAZINE HYDROCHLORIDE

INJECTABLE; INJECTION

	MEPERGAN		
	WYETH AYERST	25 MG/ML;25 MG/ML	N11730 001

MEPHENTERMINE SULFATE

INJECTABLE; INJECTION

	WYAMINE SULFATE		
	WYETH AYERST	EQ 15 MG BASE/ML	N08248 002
		EQ 30 MG BASE/ML	N08248 001

MEPHENYTOIN

TABLET; ORAL

	MESANTOIN		
	SANDOZ	100 MG	N06008 001

MEPIVACAINE HYDROCHLORIDE

INJECTABLE; INJECTION

	ARESTOCAINE HCL			
AP	CARLISLE	3%	N84777 002	APR 18, 1982
	CARBOCAINE			
AP	COOK WAITE	3%	N12125 003	
AP	STERLING	1%	N12250 001	
AP		1.5%	N12250 005	
AP		2%	N12250 002	
	ISOCAINE HCL			
AP	NOVOCOL	3%	N80925 001	
	MEPIVACAINE HCL			
AP	GRAHAM CHEM	3%	N83559 001	
AP	INTL MEDICATION	1%	N87509 001	OCT 05, 1982
AP	STERIS	1%	N88769 001	NOV 20, 1984
AP		2%	N88770 001	NOV 20, 1984
	POLOCAINE			
AP	ASTRA	1%	N89406 001	DEC 01, 1986
AP		1%	N89407 001	DEC 01, 1986
AP		1.5%	N89408 001	DEC 01, 1986
AP		2%	N89409 001	DEC 01, 1986
AP		2%	N89410 001	DEC 01, 1986
AP		3%	N88653 001	AUG 21, 1984
	SCANDONEST PLAIN			
AP	DEPROCO	3%	N88387 001	OCT 10, 1984

MEPIVACAINE HYDROCHLORIDE; *MULTIPLE*
SEE LEVONORDEFRIN; MEPIVACAINE HYDROCHLORIDE

MEPROBAMATE

CAPSULE, EXTENDED RELEASE; ORAL

	MEPROSPAN		
	WALLACE	200 MG	N11284 001
+		400 MG	N11284 002

Prescription Drug Products (continued)

MEPROBAMATE (continued)

TABLET; ORAL

TE	Manufacturer	Strength	Appl. No.
	AMOSENE		
AA	FERNDALE	400 MG	N84030 001
	EQUANIL		
AA	WYETH AYERST	200 MG	N10028 005
AA		400 MG	N10028 004
	MEPRIAM		
AA	LEMMON	400 MG	N16069 001
	MEPROBAMATE		
AA	BARR	200 MG	N80699 001
AA		400 MG	N80699 002
AA	CHELSEA	400 MG	N84230 001
AA		600 MG	N85720 001
AA		200 MG	N85721 001
AA	DANBURY	400 MG	N83304 001
AA		200 MG	N83308 001
AA		400 MG	N84274 001
AA	EON LABS	600 MG	N14547 002
AA		200 MG	N14547 001
AA		400 MG	N83343 001
AA	FIRST TX	400 MG	N80655 001
AA	GENEVA	400 MG	N16928 003
AA	HEATHER	400 MG	N14882 002
AA		200 MG	N14882 001
AA	LANNETT	400 MG	N89538 001
AA	LEE LABS	400 MG	NOV 25, 1987
AA	MYLAN	200 MG	N14368 004
AA		400 MG	N14368 002
AA	PHARMAVITE	400 MG	N83618 001
AA	PUREPAC	400 MG	N84438 001
AA		200 MG	N84804 001
AA		400 MG	N84804 002
AA	RICHLYN	200 MG	N14322 002
AA		400 MG	N14322 001
AA	ROXANE	400 MG	N84332 001
AA		600 MG	N83494 001
AA	TABLICAPS	400 MG	N15417 003
AA		200 MG	N15417 002
AA	WEST WARD	400 MG	N15438 001
AA		200 MG	N15438 002
AA	ZENITH	400 MG	N84181 001
AA		600 MG	N09698 004
	MILTOWN		
AA	WALLACE	200 MG	N09698 002
AA		400 MG	N83919 001
AA		600 MG	N14359 002
	NEURAMATE		
AA	HALSEY	200 MG	N14359 001
AA		400 MG	N16249 001
	TRANMEP		
AA	SOLVAY	400 MG	

MEPROBAMATE; *MULTIPLE*
SEE ASPIRIN; MEPROBAMATE
SEE ESTROGENS, CONJUGATED; MEPROBAMATE

MERCAPTOPURINE

TABLET; ORAL

Manufacturer	Strength	Appl. No.
PURINETHOL		
+ BURROUGHS WELLCOME	50 MG	N09053 002

MERSALYL SODIUM; THEOPHYLLINE

INJECTABLE; INJECTION

Manufacturer	Strength	Appl. No.
MERSALYL-THEOPHYLLINE		
STERIS	100 MG/ML;50 MG/ML	N84875 001

MESALAMINE

ENEMA; RECTAL

Manufacturer	Strength	Appl. No.	
ROWASA			
+ SOLVAY	4 GM/60 ML	N19618 001	DEC 24, 1987

SUPPOSITORY; RECTAL

Manufacturer	Strength	Appl. No.	
ROWASA			
+ SOLVAY	500 MG	N19919 001	DEC 18, 1990

TABLET, DELAYED RELEASE; ORAL

Manufacturer	Strength	Appl. No.	
ASACOL			
+ P AND G	400 MG	N19651 001	JAN 31, 1992

MESNA

INJECTABLE; INJECTION

Manufacturer	Strength	Appl. No.	
MESNEX			
ASTA	100 MG/ML	N19884 001	DEC 30, 1988

MESORIDAZINE BESYLATE

CONCENTRATE; ORAL

Manufacturer	Strength	Appl. No.
SERENTIL		
SANDOZ	EQ 25 MG BASE/ML	N16997 001

INJECTABLE; INJECTION

Manufacturer	Strength	Appl. No.
SERENTIL		
SANDOZ	EQ 25 MG BASE/ML	N16775 001

TABLET; ORAL

Manufacturer	Strength	Appl. No.
SERENTIL		
+ SANDOZ	EQ 10 MG BASE	N16774 001
	EQ 25 MG BASE	N16774 002
	EQ 50 MG BASE	N16774 003
	EQ 100 MG BASE	N16774 004

Prescription Drug Products (continued)

MESTRANOL; *MULTIPLE*
SEE ETHYNODIOL DIACETATE; MESTRANOL

MESTRANOL; NORETHINDRONE
TABLET; ORAL-20
NORINYL
SYNTEX   0.1 MG;2 MG   N13625 004

TABLET; ORAL-21
NORETHIN 1/50M-21
ΔB SCHIAPPARELLI
SEARLE   0.05 MG;1 MG   N71539 001   APR 12, 1988
NORETHINDRONE AND MESTRANOL
WATSON   0.05 MG;1 MG   N70758 001   JUL 01, 1988
ΔB NORINYL 1+50 21-DAY
SYNTEX   0.05 MG;1 MG   N13625 002
ΔB ORTHO-NOVUM 1/50 21
+ JOHNSON RW   0.05 MG;1 MG   N12728 004

TABLET; ORAL-28
NORETHIN 1/50M-28
ΔB SCHIAPPARELLI
SEARLE   0.05 MG;1 MG   N71540 001   APR 12, 1988
NORETHINDRONE AND MESTRANOL
ΔB WATSON   0.05 MG;1 MG   N70759 001   JUL 01, 1988
ΔB NORINYL 1+50 28-DAY
SYNTEX   0.05 MG;1 MG   N16659 001
ΔB ORTHO-NOVUM 1/50 28
JOHNSON RW   0.05 MG;1 MG   N16709 001

MESTRANOL; NORETHYNODREL
TABLET; ORAL
ENOVID
SEARLE   0.075 MG;5 MG   N10976 008
+   0.15 MG;9.85 MG   N10976 005

METAPROTERENOL SULFATE
AEROSOL, METERED; INHALATION
ALUPENT
+ BOEHRINGER
INGELHEIM   0.65 MG/INH   N16402 001

METAPROTERENOL SULFATE (continued)
SOLUTION; INHALATION
ALUPENT
ΔN BOEHRINGER
INGELHEIM   0.4%   N18761 002   OCT 10, 1986
ΔN   0.6%   N18761 001
ΔN   5%   N18761 001   JUN 30, 1983
N17659 001
METAPROTERENOL SULFATE
ΔN ASTRA   0.4%   N71275 001   JUL 27, 1988
ΔN   0.6%   N71018 001   JUL 27, 1988
ΔN DEY   0.4%   N71786 001   AUG 05, 1988
ΔN   0.6%   N70804 001   AUG 17, 1987
ΔN   5%   N70805 001   AUG 17, 1987
0.5%   N71805 001   AUG 05, 1988
ΔN PACO   0.4%   N71855 001   JUL 14, 1988
ΔN   0.6%   N71726 001   JUL 14, 1988
ΔN PHARM BASICS   5%   N72190 001   JUN 07, 1988
ΔN PROMETA
MURO   5%   N73340 001   MAR 30, 1992

SYRUP; ORAL
ALUPENT
ΔA BOEHRINGER
INGELHEIM   10 MG/5 ML   N17571 001
METAPROTERENOL SULFATE
ΔA BIOCRAFT   10 MG/5 ML   N72761 001   FEB 27, 1992
ΔA COPLEY   10 MG/5 ML   N73034 001   AUG 30, 1991
ΔA PHARM BASICS   10 MG/5 ML   N71656 001   OCT 13, 1987
ΔA SILARX   10 MG/5 ML   N73632 001   JUL 22, 1992
ΔA PROMETA
MURO   10 MG/5 ML   N72023 001   SEP 15, 1988

Prescription Drug Products (continued)

METAPROTERENOL SULFATE (continued)

TABLET; ORAL

	ALUPENT		
	BOEHRINGER INGELHEIM		
AB	10 MG	N15874 002	
AB	20 MG	N15874 001	
+	**METAPROTERENOL SULFATE**		
	BIOCRAFT		
AB	10 MG	N72519 001	MAR 30, 1990
AB	20 MG	N72520 001	MAR 30, 1990
	DANBURY		
AB	10 MG	N73013 001	JAN 31, 1991
AB	20 MG	N72795 001	JAN 31, 1991
	PAR		
AB	10 MG	N72024 001	JUN 28, 1988
AB	20 MG	N72025 001	JUN 28, 1988

METARAMINOL BITARTRATE

INJECTABLE; INJECTION

	ARAMINE		
	MSD		
AP	EQ 10 MG BASE/ML	N09509 002	DEC 22, 1987
	METARAMINOL BITARTRATE		
	LYPHOMED		
AP	EQ 10 MG BASE/ML	N80431 001	
AP	EQ 10 MG BASE/ML	N80722 001	

METAXALONE

TABLET; ORAL

	SKELAXIN		
	CARNRICK	400 MG	N13217 001

METHACHOLINE CHLORIDE

POWDER FOR RECONSTITUTION; INHALATION

	PROVOCHOLINE		
	ROCHE	100 MG/VIAL	N19193 001 OCT 31, 1986

METHACYCLINE HYDROCHLORIDE

CAPSULE; ORAL

	RONDOMYCIN		
	WALLACE	EQ 140 MG BASE	N60641 001
+		EQ 280 MG BASE	N60641 002

SYRUP; ORAL

	RONDOMYCIN		
+	WALLACE	EQ 70 MG BASE/5 ML	N60641 003

METHADONE HYDROCHLORIDE

CONCENTRATE; ORAL

	METHADONE HCL INTENSOL		
	ROXANE		
AA	10 MG/ML	N89897 001	SEP 06, 1988
	METHADOSE		
	MALLINCKRODT		
AA	10 MG/ML	N17116 002	

INJECTABLE; INJECTION

	DOLOPHINE HCL		
	LILLY	10 MG/ML	N06134 006

SOLUTION; ORAL

	METHADONE HCL		
	ROXANE	5 MG/5 ML	N87393 001
		10 MG/5 ML	N87997 001 AUG 30, 1982

SYRUP; ORAL

	DOLOPHINE HCL		
	LILLY	10 MG/30 ML	N06134 004

TABLET; ORAL

	DOLOPHINE HCL		
	LILLY		
AA	5 MG	N06134 002	
AA	10 MG	N06134 010	
	METHADONE HCL		
	ROXANE		
AA	5 MG	N88108 001	MAR 08, 1983
AA	10 MG	N88109 001	MAR 08, 1983

TABLET, DISPERSIBLE; ORAL

	METHADONE HCL		
	LILLY	40 MG	N17058 001

METHAMPHETAMINE HYDROCHLORIDE

TABLET; ORAL

	DESOXYN		
	ABBOTT		
AA	5 MG	N05378 002	
	METHAMPEX		
	LEMMON		
AA	10 MG	N83889 001	
	METHAMPHETAMINE HCL		
	LEMMON		
AA	5 MG	N86359 001	
	REXAR		
AA	5 MG	N84931 001	
AA	10 MG	N84931 002	

TABLET, EXTENDED RELEASE; ORAL

	DESOXYN		
	ABBOTT	5 MG	N05378 004
		10 MG	N05378 003
		15 MG	N05378 005

Prescription Drug Products (continued)

METHANTHELINE BROMIDE
TABLET; ORAL
TE	Trade/Applicant	Strength	NDA
	BANTHINE		
	SCHIAPPARELLI SEARLE	50 MG	N07390 001

METHAZOLAMIDE
TABLET; ORAL
TE	Trade/Applicant	Strength	NDA
	NEPTAZANE		
	LEDERLE	25 MG	N11721 002 NOV 25, 1991
		50 MG	N11721 001

METHDILAZINE
TABLET, CHEWABLE; ORAL
TE	Trade/Applicant	Strength	NDA
	TACARYL		
	WESTWOOD SQUIBB	3.6 MG	N11950 009

METHDILAZINE HYDROCHLORIDE
SYRUP; ORAL
TE	Trade/Applicant	Strength	NDA
	TACARYL		
	WESTWOOD SQUIBB	4 MG/5 ML	N11950 007

TABLET; ORAL
TE	Trade/Applicant	Strength	NDA
	TACARYL		
	WESTWOOD SQUIBB	8 MG	N11950 006

METHENAMINE HIPPURATE
TABLET; ORAL
TE	Trade/Applicant	Strength	NDA
AB +	HIPREX		
	MERRELL DOW	1 GM	N17681 001
AB	UREX		
	3M	1 GM	N16151 001

METHICILLIN SODIUM
INJECTABLE; INJECTION
TE	Trade/Applicant	Strength	NDA
	STAPHCILLIN		
	BRISTOL	EQ 900 MG BASE/VIAL	N61449 001
		EQ 3.6 GM BASE/VIAL	N61449 002
		EQ 5.4 GM BASE/VIAL	N61449 003

METHIMAZOLE
TABLET; ORAL
TE	Trade/Applicant	Strength	NDA
	TAPAZOLE		
	LILLY	5 MG	N07517 002
		10 MG	N07517 004

METHOCARBAMOL
INJECTABLE; INJECTION
TE	Trade/Applicant	Strength	NDA
	METHOCARBAMOL		
AP	MARSAM	100 MG/ML	N89849 001 DEC 27, 1991
	ROBAXIN		
AP	STERIS	100 MG/ML	N86459 001
AP	ROBINS	100 MG/ML	N11790 001

TABLET; ORAL
TE	Trade/Applicant	Strength	NDA
	DELAXIN		
AA	FERNDALE	500 MG	N85454 001
	FORBAXIN		
AA	FOREST LABS	750 MG	N85136 001
	METHOCARBAMOL		
AA	BARR	750 MG	N84486 001
AA	CHELSEA	500 MG	N85180 001
AA		750 MG	N85192 001
AA	DANBURY	750 MG	N84277 001
AA		750 MG	N84276 002
AA	EON LABS	500 MG	N87283 001
AA		750 MG	N87282 001
AA	GENEVA	500 MG	N84616 001
AA		750 MG	N84615 001
AA	INWOOD	500 MG	N85137 001
AA	KV	500 MG	N85660 001
AA	LANNETT	500 MG	N85658 001
AA	LEDERLE	750 MG	N84756 001
AA		500 MG	N85961 001
AA	PAR	500 MG	N85963 001
AA		500 MG	N86989 001
AA		750 MG	N86988 001
AA	PIONEER PHARMS	500 MG	N88731 001 DEC 13, 1985
AA		750 MG	N89082 001 DEC 13, 1985
AA	PUREPAC	500 MG	N85718 001
AA		750 MG	N85718 002
AA	RICHLYN	500 MG	N84927 001
AA		750 MG	N84928 001
AA	SOLVAY	500 MG	N84448 001
AA		750 MG	N84449 001
AA	SUPERPHARM	500 MG	N87589 001 JAN 22, 1982
AA		750 MG	N87590 001 JAN 22, 1982
AA	TABLICAPS	500 MG	N84846 001
AA		750 MG	N85033 001
AA	UPSHER SMITH	500 MG	N87453 001
AA		750 MG	N87454 001
AA	WEST WARD	500 MG	N85159 001
AA		750 MG	N85123 001
AA	ZENITH	500 MG	N84648 001
AA		750 MG	N84649 001
	ROBAXIN		
AA	ROBINS	500 MG	N11011 004
	ROBAXIN-750		
AA	ROBINS	750 MG	N11011 006

Prescription Drug Products (continued)

METHOCARBAMOL; *MULTIPLE*
  SEE   ASPIRIN; METHOCARBAMOL

METHOHEXITAL SODIUM
  INJECTABLE; INJECTION
    BREVITAL SODIUM
      LILLY   500 MG/VIAL   N11559 001
                     2.5 GM/VIAL   N11559 002
                     5 GM/VIAL   N11559 003

METHOTREXATE SODIUM
  INJECTABLE; INJECTION
    ABITREXATE
AP   ABIC   EQ 25 MG BASE/ML   N89161 001   MAR 10, 1987
                                           N89354 001
AP   EQ 50 MG BASE/VIAL   N89355 001   JUL 17, 1987
AP   EQ 100 MG BASE/VIAL   N89356 001   JUL 17, 1987
AP   EQ 250 MG BASE/VIAL   JUL 17, 1987
    FOLEX
AP   ADRIA   EQ 50 MG BASE/VIAL   N87695 002   APR 08, 1983
AP   EQ 100 MG BASE/VIAL   N87695 003   APR 08, 1983
AP   EQ 250 MG BASE/VIAL   N88954 001   OCT 24, 1985
AP   EQ 25 MG BASE/VIAL   N87695 001   APR 08, 1983
    FOLEX PFS
AP   ADRIA   EQ 25 MG BASE/ML   N81242 001   AUG 23, 1991
AP   EQ 25 MG BASE/ML   N89180 001   JAN 03, 1986
    METHOTREXATE
AP   LEDERLE   EQ 25 MG BASE/ML   N11719 005
AP   EQ 20 MG BASE/VIAL   N11719 001
AP   EQ 50 MG BASE/VIAL   N11719 003
AP   EQ 100 MG BASE/VIAL   N11719 006
                     EQ 2.5 MG BASE/ML   N11719 004
                     EQ 1 GM BASE/VIAL   N11719 009   APR 07, 1988
    METHOTREXATE LPF
AP   LEDERLE   EQ 25 MG BASE/ML   N11719 007   MAR 31, 1982

METHOTREXATE SODIUM (*continued*)
  INJECTABLE; INJECTION
    METHOTREXATE SODIUM
AP   AKORN   EQ 25 MG BASE/ML   N88648 001   MAY 09, 1986
AP   BEN VENUE   EQ 25 MG BASE/ML   N89340 001   SEP 16, 1986
                                           N89341 001   SEP 16, 1986
AP   EQ 25 MG BASE/ML   N89342 001   SEP 16, 1986
AP   EQ 25 MG BASE/ML   N89343 001   SEP 16, 1986
AP   EQ 25 MG BASE/ML   N89263 001   JUN 13, 1986
AP   LYPHOMED   EQ 25 MG BASE/ML   N89158 001   JUL 08, 1988
AP   PHARMACHEMIE   EQ 25 MG BASE/ML
    MEXATE
AP   BRISTOL   EQ 20 MG BASE/VIAL   N86358 001
AP   EQ 50 MG BASE/VIAL   N86358 002
AP   EQ 100 MG BASE/VIAL   N86358 003
                     EQ 250 MG BASE/VIAL   N86358 004
    MEXATE-AQ
AP   BRISTOL MYERS EQ 25 MG BASE/ML   N88760 001   FEB 14, 1985
    MEXATE-AQ PRESERVED
AP   BRISTOL MYERS EQ 25 MG BASE/ML   N89887 001   APR 14, 1989
  TABLET; ORAL
    METHOTREXATE
AB   BARR   EQ 2.5 MG BASE   N81099 001   OCT 15, 1990
AB + LEDERLE   EQ 2.5 MG BASE   N08085 002
AB   MYLAN   EQ 2.5 MG BASE   N81235 001   MAY 15, 1992

METHOTRIMEPRAZINE
  INJECTABLE; INJECTION
    LEVOPROME
      LEDERLE   20 MG/ML   N15865 001

METHOXAMINE HYDROCHLORIDE
  INJECTABLE; INJECTION
    VASOXYL
      BURROUGHS
      WELLCOME   20 MG/ML   N06772 001

Prescription Drug Products (continued)

METHOXSALEN

	Brand / Firm	Strength	Appl. No.	Date
	CAPSULE; ORAL			
	8-MOP			
	+ ICN	10 MG	N09048 001	
	CAPSULE, LIQUID FILLED; ORAL			
	OXSORALEN-ULTRA			
	+ ICN	10 MG	N19600 001	OCT 30, 1986
	LOTION; TOPICAL			
	OXSORALEN			
	+ ICN	1%	N09048 002	

METHOXYFLURANE

	Brand / Firm	Strength	Appl. No.
	SOLUTION; INHALATION		
	PENTHRANE		
	ABBOTT	99.9%	N13056 001

METHSCOPOLAMINE BROMIDE

	Brand / Firm	Strength	Appl. No.
	TABLET; ORAL		
	METHSCOPOLAMINE BROMIDE		
∆A	PRIVATE FORM	2.5 MG	N80970 001
	PAMINE		
∆A	UPJOHN	2.5 MG	N08848 001

METHSUXIMIDE

	Brand / Firm	Strength	Appl. No.
	CAPSULE; ORAL		
	CELONTIN		
∆A	PARKE DAVIS	150 MG	N10596 007
∆A	+	300 MG	N10596 008

METHYCLOTHIAZIDE

	Brand / Firm	Strength	Appl. No.	Date
	TABLET; ORAL			
	AQUATENSEN			
∆B	WALLACE	5 MG	N17364 001	
	ENDURON			
∆B	ABBOTT	2.5 MG	N12524 001	
∆B	+	5 MG	N12524 004	
	METHYCLOTHIAZIDE			
∆B	CHELSEA	5 MG	N88724 001	SEP 06, 1984
∆B	GENEVA	2.5 MG	N89835 001	AUG 18, 1988
∆B		5 MG	N89837 001	AUG 18, 1988
∆B	MYLAN	5 MG	N87672 001	AUG 17, 1982
∆B	PAR	2.5 MG	N89135 001	FEB 12, 1986
∆B		5 MG	N89136 001	FEB 12, 1986
∆B	ZENITH	2.5 MG	N87913 001	JUN 03, 1982
∆B		5 MG	N87786 001	MAY 18, 1982

METHYCLOTHIAZIDE; *MULTIPLE*

SEE DESERPIDINE; METHYCLOTHIAZIDE

METHYCLOTHIAZIDE; RESERPINE

	Brand / Firm	Strength	Appl. No.
	TABLET; ORAL		
	DIUTENSEN-R		
	+ WALLACE	2.5 MG;0.1 MG	N12708 005

METHYLDOPA

	Brand / Firm	Strength	Appl. No.	Date
	SUSPENSION; ORAL			
	ALDOMET			
	+ MSD	250 MG/5 ML	N18389 001	
	TABLET; ORAL			
	ALDOMET			
	MSD	125 MG	N13400 003	
		250 MG	N13400 001	
		500 MG	N13400 002	
	+			
	METHYLDOPA			
AB	BARR	125 MG	N70073 001	OCT 09, 1986
AB		250 MG	N70060 001	OCT 09, 1986
AB		500 MG	N70074 001	OCT 09, 1986
AB	DANBURY	250 MG	N70703 001	JUN 06, 1986
AB		500 MG	N70625 001	JUN 06, 1986
AB	GENEVA	125 MG	N71700 001	MAR 02, 1988
AB		250 MG	N18934 001	JUN 29, 1984
AB		500 MG	N18934 002	JUN 29, 1984
AB	HALSEY	125 MG	N71751 001	MAR 28, 1988
AB		250 MG	N71752 001	MAR 28, 1988
AB		500 MG	N71753 001	MAR 28, 1988
AB	LEDERLE	125 MG	N70070 003	OCT 15, 1985
AB		250 MG	N70084 001	OCT 15, 1985
AB		500 MG	N70085 001	OCT 15, 1985
AB	MYLAN	250 MG	N70075 001	APR 18, 1985
AB		500 MG	N70076 001	APR 18, 1985

Prescription Drug Products (continued)

METHYLDOPA (continued)

TABLET; ORAL

METHYLDOPA

	Manufacturer	Strength	Appl. No.	Approval Date
ΔB	NOVOPHARM	125 MG	N71105 001	DEC 05, 1986
ΔB		250 MG	N71106 001	DEC 05, 1986
ΔB		500 MG	N71067 001	DEC 05, 1986
ΔB	PAR	125 MG	N70535 001	JAN 02, 1987
ΔB		250 MG	N70536 001	JAN 02, 1987
ΔB		500 MG	N70537 001	JAN 02, 1987
ΔB	PUREPAC	125 MG	N70749 001	FEB 07, 1986
ΔB		250 MG	N70750 001	FEB 07, 1986
ΔB		500 MG	N70452 001	FEB 07, 1986
ΔB	SIDMAK	125 MG	N72126 001	JUL 07, 1988
ΔB		250 MG	N72127 001	JUL 07, 1988
ΔB		500 MG	N72128 001	JUL 07, 1988
ΔB	SUPERPHARM	250 MG	N70669 001	JUN 23, 1989
ΔB		500 MG	N70670 001	JUN 23, 1989
ΔB	ZENITH	250 MG	N70098 001	FEB 20, 1986
ΔB		500 MG	N70343 001	FEB 20, 1986

METHYLDOPA; *MULTIPLE*

SEE   CHLOROTHIAZIDE; METHYLDOPA
SEE   HYDROCHLOROTHIAZIDE; METHYLDOPA

METHYLDOPATE HYDROCHLORIDE

INJECTABLE; INJECTION

ALDOMET

	Manufacturer	Strength	Appl. No.	Approval Date
ΔP	MSD	50 MG/ML	N13401 001	

METHYLDOPATE HCL

	Manufacturer	Strength	Appl. No.	Approval Date
ΔP	ABBOTT	50 MG/ML	N70698 001	JUN 15, 1987
ΔP		50 MG/ML	N70699 001	JUN 15, 1987

METHYLDOPATE HYDROCHLORIDE (continued)

INJECTABLE; INJECTION

METHYLDOPATE HCL

	Manufacturer	Strength	Appl. No.	Approval Date
ΔP	DUPONT	50 MG/ML	N70691 001	JUN 19, 1987
			N70849 001	JUN 19, 1987
			N70291 001	JUN 19, 1987
ΔP	ELKINS SINN	50 MG/ML	N72974 001	JUL 01, 1986
ΔP	GENSIA	50 MG/ML		NOV 22, 1991
ΔP	LUITPOLD	50 MG/ML	N71279 001	OCT 02, 1987
ΔP	LYPHOMED	50 MG/ML	N70652 001	JUN 03, 1986
ΔP	MARSAM	50 MG/ML	N71812 001	DEC 22, 1987
ΔP	SMITH NEPHEW SOLOPAK	50 MG/ML	N70841 001	JAN 02, 1987

METHYLERGONOVINE MALEATE

INJECTABLE; INJECTION

METHERGINE

	Manufacturer	Strength	Appl. No.
ΔP	SANDOZ	0.2 MG/ML	N06035 004

TABLET; ORAL

METHERGINE

	Manufacturer	Strength	Appl. No.
	SANDOZ	0.2 MG	N06035 003

METHYLPHENIDATE HYDROCHLORIDE

TABLET; ORAL

METHYLPHENIDATE HCL

	Manufacturer	Strength	Appl. No.
ΔB	MD PHARM	5 MG	N86429 001
ΔB		10 MG	N85799 001
ΔB		20 MG	N86428 001

RITALIN

	Manufacturer	Strength	Appl. No.
ΔB	CIBA	5 MG	N10187 003
ΔB		10 MG	N10187 006
ΔB +		20 MG	N10187 010

TABLET, EXTENDED RELEASE; ORAL

METHYLPHENIDATE HCL

	Manufacturer	Strength	Appl. No.	Approval Date
ΔB	MD PHARM	20 MG	N89601 001	JUN 01, 1988

RITALIN-SR

	Manufacturer	Strength	Appl. No.	Approval Date
ΔB +	CIBA	20 MG	N18029 001	MAR 30, 1982

Prescription Drug Products (continued)

METHYLPREDNISOLONE

TABLET; ORAL

MEDROL
UPJOHN

TE	Strength	NDA	Date
AB	4 MG	N11153 001	
AB	16 MG	N11153 003	
AB	24 MG	N11153 005	
AB	32 MG	N11153 006	
+	2 MG	N11153 002	
	8 MG	N11153 004	

METHYLPREDNISOLONE
CHELSEA

TE	Strength	NDA	Date
AB	4 MG	N86161 001	FEB 09, 1982

DURAMED

TE	Strength	NDA	Date
AB	4 MG	N88497 001	FEB 21, 1984

HEATHER
PAR

TE	Strength	NDA	Date
AB	4 MG	N85650 001	
AB	16 MG	N89207 001	APR 25, 1988
AB	24 MG	N89208 001	APR 25, 1988
AB	32 MG	N89209 001	APR 25, 1988

METHYLPREDNISOLONE ACETATE

INJECTABLE; INJECTION

DEPO-MEDROL
UPJOHN

TE	Strength	NDA	Date
BP	20 MG/ML	N11757 002	
BP	40 MG/ML	N11757 001	
BP	80 MG/ML	N11757 004	

M-PREDROL
BEL MAR

TE	Strength	NDA	Date
BP +	40 MG/ML	N86666 001	
BP	80 MG/ML	N87135 001	

METHYLPREDNISOLONE ACETATE
AKORN

TE	Strength	NDA	Date
BP	40 MG/ML	N86903 001	OCT 20, 1982
BP	80 MG/ML	N86903 002	OCT 20, 1982

STERIS

TE	Strength	NDA	Date
BP	20 MG/ML	N85597 001	
BP	40 MG/ML	N85600 001	
BP	80 MG/ML	N85595 001	

OINTMENT; TOPICAL

MEDROL ACETATE
UPJOHN

Strength	NDA
0.25%	N12421 001
1%	N12421 002

METHYLPREDNISOLONE ACETATE; NEOMYCIN SULFATE

CREAM; TOPICAL

NEO-MEDROL ACETATE
UPJOHN

Strength	NDA
0.25%;EQ 3.5 MG BASE/GM	N60611 002
1%;EQ 3.5 MG BASE/GM	N60611 001

METHYLPREDNISOLONE SODIUM SUCCINATE

INJECTABLE; INJECTION

A-METHAPRED
ABBOTT

TE	Strength	NDA	Date
AP	EQ 40 MG BASE/VIAL	N85853 001	
AP	EQ 40 MG BASE/VIAL	N89573 001	FEB 22, 1991
	EQ 125 MG BASE/VIAL	N85855 001	
	EQ 125 MG BASE/VIAL	N89574 001	FEB 22, 1991
AP	EQ 500 MG BASE/VIAL	N85854 001	
AP	EQ 500 MG BASE/VIAL	N89173 001	AUG 18, 1987
	EQ 500 MG BASE/VIAL	N89575 001	FEB 22, 1991
AP	EQ 1 GM BASE/VIAL	N85852 001	
AP	EQ 1 GM BASE/VIAL	N89174 001	AUG 18, 1987
	EQ 1 GM BASE/VIAL	N89576 001	FEB 22, 1991

METHYLPREDNISOLONE
ELKINS SINN

TE	Strength	NDA	Date
AP	EQ 125 MG BASE/VIAL	N86906 002	
AP	EQ 500 MG BASE/VIAL	N86906 003	
AP	EQ 1 GM BASE/VIAL	N86906 004	

ORGANON

TE	Strength	NDA	Date
AP	EQ 500 MG BASE/VIAL	N87535 001	JUN 25, 1982
AP	EQ 1 GM BASE/VIAL	N87535 002	JUN 25, 1982

METHYLPREDNISOLONE SODIUM SUCCINATE
ELKINS SINN

TE	Strength	NDA	Date
AP	EQ 40 MG BASE/VIAL	N86906 001	

LYPHOMED

TE	Strength	NDA	Date
AP	EQ 40 MG BASE/VIAL	N89143 001	MAR 28, 1986
AP	EQ 125 MG BASE/VIAL	N89144 001	MAR 28, 1986
AP	EQ 500 MG BASE/VIAL	N89187 001	MAR 28, 1986
AP	EQ 1 GM BASE/VIAL	N89189 001	MAR 28, 1986

STERIS

TE	Strength	NDA	Date
AP	EQ 40 MG BASE/VIAL	N86953 001	
AP	EQ 125 MG BASE/VIAL	N87030 001	JUL 22, 1982
AP	EQ 500 MG BASE/VIAL	N88523 001	JUL 22, 1982
AP	EQ 1 GM BASE/VIAL	N88524 001	JUL 24, 1984

SOLU-MEDROL
UPJOHN

TE	Strength	NDA	Date
AP	EQ 40 MG BASE/VIAL	N11856 003	
AP	EQ 125 MG BASE/VIAL	N11856 004	
AP	EQ 500 MG BASE/VIAL	N11856 005	
AP	EQ 1 GM BASE/VIAL	N11856 006	
	EQ 2 GM BASE/VIAL	N11856 007	FEB 27, 1985

Prescription Drug Products *(continued)*

METHYLTESTOSTERONE

CAPSULE; ORAL
METHYLTESTOSTERONE
BP + HEATHER 10 MG N84967 001
TESTRED
BP ICN 10 MG N83976 001
VIRILON
BP STAR PHARMS 10 MG N87750 001 NOV 24, 1982

TABLET; BUCCAL
ANDROID 5
ICN 5 MG N87222 001
ORETON
+ SCHERING 10 MG N80281 001

TABLET; BUCCAL/SUBLINGUAL
METHYLTESTOSTERONE
BP + LILLY 10 MG N80256 001
PRIVATE FORM 5 MG N83836 001
BP RICHLYN 10 MG N84287 001
BP TABLICAPS 10 MG N85125 001

TABLET; ORAL
ANDROID 10
AB ICN 10 MG N86450 001
ANDROID 25
AB ICN 25 MG N87147 001
METHYLTESTOSTERONE
BP DANBURY 10 MG N80933 001
BP 25 MG N80931 001
BP INWOOD 10 MG N80839 001
BP 25 MG N80973 001
BP LANNETT 10 MG N87092 001 NOV 05, 1982
BP 25 MG N87111 001 JAN 27, 1983
BP LILLY 25 MG N80256 002
BP PUREPAC 10 MG N80475 002
BP 25 MG N80475 003
BP RICHLYN 10 MG N80767 002
BP 25 MG N84310 001
BP TABLICAPS 10 MG N80313 001
BP 25 MG N85270 001
BP WEST WARD 10 MG N84331 001
BP 25 MG N84331 002
ORETON METHYL
BP SCHERING 10 MG N03158 001
BP + 25 MG N03158 002

METHYLTESTOSTERONE; *MULTIPLE*

SEE DIETHYLSTILBESTROL; METHYLTESTOSTERONE

METHYPRYLON

CAPSULE; ORAL
NOLUDAR
ROCHE 300 MG N09660 008

METHYPRYLON *(continued)*

TABLET; ORAL
NOLUDAR
ROCHE 200 MG N09660 004

METHYSERGIDE MALEATE

TABLET; ORAL
SANSERT
SANDOZ 2 MG N12516 001

METIPRANOLOL HYDROCHLORIDE

SOLUTION/DROPS; OPHTHALMIC
OPTIPRANOLOL
BAUSCH AND LOMB 0.3% N19907 001 DEC 29, 1989

METOCLOPRAMIDE HYDROCHLORIDE

CONCENTRATE; ORAL
METOCLOPRAMIDE INTENSOL
ROXANE EQ 10 MG BASE/ML N72995 001 JAN 30, 1992

INJECTABLE; INJECTION
METOCLOPRAMIDE HCL
AP ABBOTT EQ 10 MG BASE/2 ML N70505 001 JUN 23, 1989
AP EQ 10 MG BASE/2 ML N70506 001 JUN 22, 1989
AP EQ 10 MG BASE/2 ML N73117 001 JAN 17, 1991
AP EQ 10 MG BASE/2 ML N73118 001 JAN 17, 1991
AP AKORN EQ 10 MG BASE/2 ML N70892 001 AUG 26, 1988
AP BULL EQ 10 MG BASE/2 ML N71990 001 JAN 18, 1989
AP CETUS BEN VENUE EQ 10 MG BASE/2 ML N72155 001 MAR 30, 1992
AP EQ 10 MG BASE/2 ML N72244 001 MAR 30, 1992
AP EQ 10 MG BASE/2 ML N72247 001 MAY 18, 1992
AP DUPONT EQ 10 MG BASE/2 ML N70847 001 NOV 07, 1988
AP EQ 10 MG BASE/2 ML N71291 001 MAR 03, 1989
AP GENSIA EQ 10 MG BASE/2 ML N73135 001 NOV 27, 1991
AP LYPHOMED EQ 10 MG BASE/2 ML N70293 001 JAN 24, 1986
AP SMITH NEPHEW SOLOPAK EQ 10 MG BASE/2 ML N70623 001 MAR 02, 1987
REGLAN
AP ROBINS EQ 10 MG BASE/2 ML N17862 001

Prescription Drug Products *(continued)*

METOCLOPRAMIDE HYDROCHLORIDE *(continued)*

SYRUP; ORAL

METOCLOPRAMIDE HCL

AA	BARRE	EQ 5 MG BASE/5 ML	N71340 001	AUG 18, 1988
AA	BIOCRAFT	EQ 5 MG BASE/5 ML	N70819 001	JUL 10, 1987
AA	PHARM ASSOC	EQ 5 MG BASE/5 ML	N72744 001	MAY 28, 1991
AA	PHARM BASICS	EQ 5 MG BASE/5 ML	N70949 001	MAR 06, 1987
AA	ROXANE	EQ 5 MG BASE/5 ML	N72038 001	DEC 05, 1988

REGLAN

AA	ROBINS	EQ 5 MG BASE/5 ML	N18821 001	MAR 25, 1983

TABLET; ORAL

MAXOLON

AB	BEECHAM	EQ 10 MG BASE	N70106 001	MAR 04, 1986

METOCLOPRAMIDE HCL

AB	BIOCRAFT	EQ 10 MG BASE	N70184 001	JUL 29, 1985
AB	DANBURY	EQ 10 MG BASE	N70511 001	JAN 22, 1986
AB	GENEVA	EQ 10 MG BASE	N72215 001	JAN 30, 1990
AB	HALSEY	EQ 10 MG BASE	N70906 001	OCT 28, 1986
AB	INVAMED	EQ 5 MG BASE	N72436 001	JUN 22, 1989
AB	INVAMED	EQ 10 MG BASE	N70850 001	FEB 03, 1987
AB	LEDERLE	EQ 10 MG BASE	N72639 001	MAY 09, 1991
AB	PAR	EQ 10 MG BASE	N70342 001	MAR 25, 1986
AB	PUREPAC	EQ 10 MG BASE	N70581 001	OCT 17, 1985
AB	SCHERING	EQ 10 MG BASE	N70598 001	FEB 02, 1987
AB	SIDMAK	EQ 10 MG BASE	N71250 001	FEB 03, 1988
AB	SUPERPHARM	EQ 10 MG BASE	N70926 001	JUN 26, 1987
AB	WATSON	EQ 10 MG BASE	N70645 001	MAY 11, 1987

REGLAN

AB	ROBINS	EQ 5 MG BASE	N17854 002	MAY 05, 1987
AB	+	EQ 10 MG BASE	N17854 001	

METOCURINE IODIDE

INJECTABLE; INJECTION

METUBINE IODIDE

	LILLY	2 MG/ML	N06632 003

METOLAZONE

TABLET; ORAL

MYKROX

	FISONS	0.5 MG	N19532 001	OCT 30, 1987

ZAROXOLYN

	FISONS	2.5 MG	N17386 001	
	FISONS	5 MG	N17386 002	
	+	10 MG	N17386 003	

METOPROLOL FUMARATE

TABLET, EXTENDED RELEASE; ORAL

LOPRESSOR

	GEIGY	EQ 100 MG TARTRATE	N19786 001	DEC 27, 1989
		EQ 200 MG TARTRATE	N19786 002	DEC 27, 1989
		EQ 300 MG TARTRATE	N19786 003	DEC 27, 1989
	+	EQ 400 MG TARTRATE	N19786 004	DEC 27, 1989

METOPROLOL SUCCINATE

TABLET, EXTENDED RELEASE; ORAL

TOPROL XL

	+ HASSLE	EQ 50 MG TARTRATE	N19962 001	JAN 10, 1992
	+	EQ 100 MG TARTRATE	N19962 002	JAN 10, 1992
	+	EQ 200 MG TARTRATE	N19962 003	JAN 10, 1992

METOPROLOL TARTRATE

INJECTABLE; INJECTION

LOPRESSOR

	GEIGY	1 MG/ML	N18704 001	MAR 30, 1984

TABLET; ORAL

LOPRESSOR

	GEIGY	50 MG	N17963 001
	+	100 MG	N17963 002

METOPROLOL TARTRATE; *MULTIPLE*

SEE CHLORTHALIDONE; METOPROLOL TARTRATE

SEE HYDROCHLOROTHIAZIDE; METOPROLOL TARTRATE

METRIZAMIDE

INJECTABLE; INJECTION

AMIPAQUE

	STERLING	3.75 GM/VIAL	N17982 001
		6.75 GM/VIAL	N17982 002

Prescription Drug Products (continued)

METRONIDAZOLE

TE	Product / Firm	Strength	NDA	Date
GEL; TOPICAL				
	METROGEL + CURATEK	0.75%	N19737 001	NOV 22, 1988
GEL; VAGINAL				
	METROGEL + CURATEK	0.75%	N20208 001	AUG 17, 1992
INJECTABLE; INJECTION				
	FLAGYL I.V. RTU IN PLASTIC CONTAINER			
AP	SCHIAPPARELLI SEARLE	500 MG/100 ML	N18353 002	
AP		500 MG/100 ML	N18657 001	
	METRO I.V.			
AP	MCGAW	500 MG/100 ML	N18674 001	AUG 31, 1982
	METRO I.V. IN PLASTIC CONTAINER			
AP	MCGAW	500 MG/100 ML	N18900 001	SEP 29, 1983
	METRONIDAZOLE			
AP	ABBOTT	500 MG/100 ML	N18889 001	NOV 18, 1983
AP		500 MG/100 ML	N18907 001	MAR 30, 1984
AP	ELKINS SINN	500 MG/100 ML	N70042 001	DEC 20, 1984
AP	STERIS	500 MG/100 ML	N70170 001	APR 01, 1986
	METRONIDAZOLE IN PLASTIC CONTAINER			
AP	ABBOTT	500 MG/100 ML	N18890 002	NOV 18, 1983
TABLET; ORAL				
	FLAGYL			
AB	SEARLE	250 MG	N12623 001	
AB		500 MG	N12623 003	
	METRONIDAZOLE			
AB	BARR	250 MG	N18818 001	FEB 16, 1983
AB		500 MG	N18818 002	FEB 16, 1983
AB	DANBURY	250 MG	N18764 001	SEP 17, 1982
AB		500 MG	N18764 002	DEC 20, 1982
AB	EON LABS	250 MG	N18620 001	MAR 04, 1982
AB		500 MG	N18620 002	JUN 02, 1983

METRONIDAZOLE (continued)

TE	Product / Firm	Strength	NDA	Date
TABLET; ORAL				
	METRONIDAZOLE			
AB	GENEVA	250 MG	N18740 001	OCT 22, 1982
AB		500 MG	N18740 002	OCT 22, 1982
AB	HALSEY	250 MG	N70021 001	APR 02, 1985
AB		500 MG	N70593 001	FEB 27, 1986
AB	LNK	250 MG	N19029 001	APR 10, 1984
AB	MUTUAL PHARM	250 MG	N70772 001	JUL 16, 1986
AB		500 MG	N70773 001	JUL 16, 1986
AB	PAR	250 MG	N18845 001	AUG 18, 1983
AB		250 MG	N70040 001	JAN 29, 1985
AB		500 MG	N18930 001	AUG 18, 1983
AB		500 MG	N70039 001	JAN 29, 1985
AB	SIDMAK	250 MG	N70027 001	NOV 06, 1984
AB		500 MG	N70033 001	DEC 06, 1984
AB	ZENITH	250 MG	N18517 001	
AB		500 MG	N18517 002	MAY 05, 1982
	METRYL			
AB	LEMMON	250 MG	N70035 001	DEC 20, 1984
	METRYL 500			
AB	LEMMON	500 MG	N70044 001	FEB 08, 1985
	PROTOSTAT			
AB	JOHNSON RW	250 MG	N18871 001	MAR 02, 1983
AB		500 MG	N18871 002	MAR 02, 1983
	SATRIC			
AB	SAVAGE	250 MG	N70029 001	MAR 19, 1985
AB		500 MG	N70731 001	JUN 08, 1987

METRONIDAZOLE HYDROCHLORIDE

TE	Product / Firm	Strength	NDA	Date
INJECTABLE; INJECTION				
	FLAGYL I.V.			
	SCHIAPPARELLI SEARLE	EQ 500 MG BASE/VIAL	N18353 001	

Prescription Drug Products *(continued)*

METYRAPONE
TABLET; ORAL
  METOPIRONE
    CIBA   250 MG   N12911 001

METYROSINE
CAPSULE; ORAL
  DEMSER
    + MSD   250 MG   N17871 001

MEXILETINE HYDROCHLORIDE
CAPSULE; ORAL
  MEXITIL
    BOEHRINGER
    INGELHEIM   150 MG   N18873 002 DEC 30, 1985
                   N18873 003 DEC 30, 1985
                  200 MG
  +   250 MG   N18873 004 DEC 30, 1985

MEZLOCILLIN SODIUM MONOHYDRATE
INJECTABLE; INJECTION
  MEZLIN
    MILES   EQ 1 GM BASE/VIAL   N50549 001
               EQ 1 GM BASE/VIAL   N62333 001
               EQ 2 GM BASE/VIAL   N50549 002
               EQ 2 GM BASE/VIAL   N62333 002
               EQ 2 GM BASE/VIAL   N62372 001 MAY 13, 1982
               EQ 3 GM BASE/VIAL   N50549 003
               EQ 3 GM BASE/VIAL   N62333 003
               EQ 3 GM BASE/VIAL   N62372 002 MAY 13, 1982
               EQ 3 GM BASE/VIAL   N62697 001 JAN 22, 1987
               EQ 4 GM BASE/VIAL   N50549 004
               EQ 4 GM BASE/VIAL   N62333 004
               EQ 4 GM BASE/VIAL   N62372 003 MAY 13, 1982
               EQ 4 GM BASE/VIAL   N62697 002 JAN 22, 1987
               EQ 20 GM BASE/VIAL   N50549 005 MAR 02, 1988
               EQ 20 GM BASE/VIAL   N62372 004 MAR 02, 1988

MICONAZOLE
INJECTABLE; INJECTION
  MONISTAT
    JANSSEN   10 MG/ML   N18040 001

MICONAZOLE NITRATE
CREAM; TOPICAL
  MONISTAT-DERM
    + JOHNSON RW   2%   N17494 001
CREAM; VAGINAL
  MONISTAT 7
    JOHNSON RW   2%   N17450 001
LOTION; TOPICAL
  MONISTAT-DERM
    + JOHNSON RW   2%   N17739 001
SUPPOSITORY; VAGINAL
  MONISTAT 3
    + JOHNSON RW   200 MG   N18888 001 AUG 15, 1984
  MONISTAT 7
    JOHNSON RW   100 MG   N18520 001 MAR 15, 1982
TAMPON; VAGINAL
  MONISTAT 5
    + JOHNSON RW   100 MG   N18592 001 OCT 27, 1989

MIDAZOLAM HYDROCHLORIDE
INJECTABLE; INJECTION
  VERSED
    ROCHE   EQ 1 MG BASE/ML   N18654 002 MAY 26, 1987
             EQ 5 MG BASE/ML   N18654 001 DEC 20, 1985

MINOCYCLINE HYDROCHLORIDE
CAPSULE; ORAL
  MINOCIN
  AB   LEDERLE   EQ 50 MG BASE   N50649 001 MAY 31, 1990
  AB   +   EQ 100 MG BASE   N50649 002 MAY 31, 1990
  MINOCYCLINE HCL
  AB   BIOCRAFT   EQ 50 MG BASE   N63011 001 MAR 02, 1992
  AB   EQ 100 MG BASE   N63009 001 MAR 02, 1992
  AB   DANBURY   EQ 50 MG BASE   N63181 001 DEC 30, 1991
  AB   EQ 100 MG BASE   N63065 001 DEC 30, 1991
  AB   WARNER CHILCOTT   EQ 50 MG BASE   N63066 001 AUG 14, 1990
  AB   EQ 100 MG BASE   N63067 001 JUL 31, 1990

Prescription Drug Products (continued)

MINOCYCLINE HYDROCHLORIDE (continued)
INJECTABLE; INJECTION
MINOCIN			
	LEDERLE	EQ 100 MG BASE/VIAL	N50444 001
		EQ 100 MG BASE/VIAL	N62139 001

SUSPENSION; ORAL
MINOCIN			
+	LEDERLE	EQ 50 MG BASE/5 ML	N50445 001

MINOXIDIL
SOLUTION; TOPICAL
ROGAINE			
	UPJOHN	2%	N19501 001
			AUG 17, 1988

TABLET; ORAL
	LONITEN			
△B	UPJOHN	2.5 MG	N18154 001
△B	+	10 MG	N18154 003
	MINOXIDIL			
△B	DANBURY	2.5 MG	N71344 001
			MAR 03, 1987
△B		10 MG	N71345 001
			MAR 03, 1987
△B	PAR	2.5 MG	N71826 001
			NOV 14, 1988
△B		10 MG	N71839 001
			NOV 14, 1988

MISOPROSTOL
TABLET; ORAL
CYTOTEC			
	SEARLE	0.1 MG	N19268 003
			SEP 21, 1990
+		0.2 MG	N19268 001
			DEC 27, 1988

MITOMYCIN
INJECTABLE; INJECTION
	MUTAMYCIN			
△P	BRISTOL	5 MG/VIAL	N50450 001
△P		20 MG/VIAL	N50450 002
△P	BRISTOL MYERS	5 MG/VIAL	N62336 001
△P		20 MG/VIAL	N62336 002
		40 MG/VIAL	N62336 003
			MAR 10, 1988

MITOTANE
TABLET; ORAL
LYSODREN			
+	BRISTOL	500 MG	N16885 001

MITOXANTRONE HYDROCHLORIDE
INJECTABLE; INJECTION
NOVANTRONE			
	LEDERLE	EQ 2 MG BASE/ML	N19297 001
			DEC 23, 1987

MIVACURIUM CHLORIDE
INJECTABLE; INJECTION
MIVACRON			
	BURROUGHS WELLCOME	EQ 2 MG BASE/ML	N20098 001
			JAN 22, 1992
MIVACRON IN DEXTROSE 5% IN PLASTIC CONTAINER			
	BURROUGHS WELLCOME	EQ 0.5 MG BASE/ML	N20098 002
			JAN 22, 1992
		EQ 50 MG BASE/100 ML	N20098 003
			JAN 22, 1992

MOLINDONE HYDROCHLORIDE
CONCENTRATE; ORAL
MOBAN			
	DUPONT	20 MG/ML	N17938 001

TABLET; ORAL
MOBAN			
	DUPONT	5 MG	N17111 004
		10 MG	N17111 005
		25 MG	N17111 006
+		50 MG	N17111 007
+		100 MG	N17111 008

MOMETASONE FUROATE
CREAM; TOPICAL
ELOCON			
+	SCHERING	0.1%	N19625 001
			MAY 06, 1987

LOTION; TOPICAL
ELOCON			
+	SCHERING	0.1%	N19796 001
			MAR 30, 1989

OINTMENT; TOPICAL
ELOCON			
+	SCHERING	0.1%	N19543 001
			APR 30, 1987

MONOBENZONE
CREAM; TOPICAL
BENOQUIN			
	ICN	20%	N08173 003

Prescription Drug Products (continued)

MONOCTANOIN
LIQUID; PERFUSION, BILIARY
  MOCTANIN

	ETHITEK	100%	N19368 001 OCT 29, 1985

MORICIZINE HYDROCHLORIDE
TABLET; ORAL
  ETHMOZINE

	DUPONT	200 MG	N19753 001 JUN 19, 1990
		250 MG	N19753 002 JUN 19, 1990
		300 MG	N19753 003 JUN 19, 1990

MORPHINE SULFATE
INJECTABLE; INJECTION
  ASTRAMORPH PF

AP	ASTRA	0.5 MG/ML	N71050 001 OCT 07, 1986
AP		0.5 MG/ML	N71051 001 OCT 07, 1986
AP		1 MG/ML	N71052 001 OCT 07, 1986
AP		1 MG/ML	N71053 001 OCT 07, 1986

  DURAMORPH PF

AP	ELKINS SINN	0.5 MG/ML	N18565 001 SEP 18, 1984
AP		1 MG/ML	N18565 002 SEP 18, 1984

  INFUMORPH

AP	ELKINS SINN	10 MG/ML	N18565 003 JUL 19, 1991
AP		25 MG/ML	N18565 004 JUL 19, 1991

  MORPHINE SULFATE

AP	ABBOTT	0.5 MG/ML	N71849 001 MAY 11, 1988
AP		1 MG/ML	N71850 001 MAY 11, 1988
AP	STERIS	0.5 MG/ML	N73373 001 SEP 30, 1991
AP		0.5 MG/ML	N73375 001 SEP 30, 1991
AP		1 MG/ML	N73374 001 SEP 30, 1991
AP		1 MG/ML	N73376 001 SEP 30, 1991
	SURVIVAL TECH	15 MG/ML	N19999 001 JUL 12, 1990

MORPHINE SULFATE (continued)
TABLET, EXTENDED RELEASE; ORAL
  MS CONTIN

BC	+ PURDUE FREDERICK	30 MG	N19516 001 MAY 29, 1987
BC	+	60 MG	N19516 002 APR 08, 1988
BC	+	100 MG	N19516 004 JAN 16, 1990
BC	+	15 MG	N19516 003 SEP 12, 1989

  ORAMORPH SR

BC	ROXANE	30 MG	N19977 001 AUG 15, 1991
BC		60 MG	N19977 002 AUG 15, 1991
BC		100 MG	N19977 003 AUG 15, 1991

MOXALACTAM DISODIUM
INJECTABLE; INJECTION
  MOXAM

	LILLY	EQ 250 MG BASE/VIAL	N50550 001
		EQ 500 MG BASE/VIAL	N50550 002
		EQ 1 GM BASE/VIAL	N50550 003
		EQ 2 GM BASE/VIAL	N50550 004
		EQ 10 GM BASE/VIAL	N50550 008

MUPIROCIN
OINTMENT; TOPICAL
  BACTROBAN

	+ BEECHAM	2%	N50591 001 DEC 31, 1987

NABILONE
CAPSULE; ORAL
  CESAMET

	+ LILLY	1 MG	N18677 001 DEC 26, 1985

NABUMETONE
TABLET; ORAL
  RELAFEN

	SMITHKLINE BEECHAM	500 MG	N19583 001 DEC 24, 1991
	+	750 MG	N19583 002 DEC 24, 1991

Prescription Drug Products (continued)

NADOLOL
TABLET; ORAL
CORGARD
SQUIBB

	Strength	Appl. No.	Date
	20 MG	N18063 005	OCT 28, 1986
	40 MG	N18063 001	
	40 MG	N18064 001	
	80 MG	N18063 002	
	80 MG	N18064 002	
	120 MG	N18063 003	
	120 MG	N18064 003	
+	160 MG	N18063 004	
	160 MG	N18064 004	

NADOLOL; *MULTIPLE*
SEE BENDROFLUMETHIAZIDE; NADOLOL

NAFARELIN ACETATE
SPRAY, METERED; NASAL
SYNAREL
+ SYNTEX

	Strength	Appl. No.	Date
	EQ 0.2 MG BASE/INH	N19886 001	FEB 13, 1990
	EQ 0.2 MG BASE/INH	N20109 001	FEB 26, 1992

NAFCILLIN SODIUM
CAPSULE; ORAL
UNIPEN
+ WYETH AYERST

	Strength	Appl. No.	Date
	EQ 250 MG BASE	N50111 001	

INJECTABLE; INJECTION
NAFCIL
BRISTOL

TE	Strength	Appl. No.	Date
AP	EQ 500 MG BASE/VIAL	N61984 001	
AP	EQ 500 MG BASE/VIAL	N62527 001	AUG 02, 1984
	EQ 1 GM BASE/VIAL	N61984 002	
	EQ 1 GM BASE/VIAL	N62527 002	AUG 02, 1984
AP	EQ 1 GM BASE/VIAL	N62732 001	DEC 23, 1986
AP	EQ 2 GM BASE/VIAL	N61984 003	
	EQ 2 GM BASE/VIAL	N62527 003	AUG 02, 1984
AP	EQ 2 GM BASE/VIAL	N62732 002	DEC 23, 1986
AP	EQ 4 GM BASE/VIAL	N61984 005	
AP	EQ 10 GM BASE/VIAL	N62527 004	AUG 02, 1984

NAFCILLIN SODIUM (continued)
INJECTABLE; INJECTION
NAFCILLIN SODIUM
MARSAM

TE	Strength	Appl. No.	Date
AP	EQ 500 MG BASE/VIAL	N62844 001	OCT 26, 1988
AP	EQ 1 GM BASE/VIAL	N62844 002	OCT 26, 1988
AP	EQ 2 GM BASE/VIAL	N62844 004	OCT 26, 1988
AP	EQ 4 GM BASE/VIAL	N62844 005	OCT 26, 1988
AP	EQ 10 GM BASE/VIAL	N63008 001	SEP 29, 1988
	EQ 1.5 GM BASE/VIAL	N62844 003	OCT 26, 1988

NALLPEN
BEECHAM

TE	Strength	Appl. No.	Date
AP	EQ 500 MG BASE/VIAL	N61999 001	
AP	EQ 1 GM BASE/VIAL	N61999 002	
	EQ 1 GM BASE/VIAL	N62755 001	DEC 19, 1986
	EQ 2 GM BASE/VIAL	N61999 003	
AP	EQ 2 GM BASE/VIAL	N62755 002	DEC 19, 1986
AP	EQ 10 GM BASE/VIAL	N61999 004	

NALLPEN IN PLASTIC CONTAINER
BAXTER

	Strength	Appl. No.	Date
	EQ 20 MG BASE/ML	N50655 001	OCT 31, 1989
	EQ 40 MG BASE/ML	N50655 002	OCT 31, 1989

UNIPEN
WYETH AYERST

TE	Strength	Appl. No.	Date
AP	EQ 500 MG BASE/VIAL	N50320 001	
AP	EQ 500 MG BASE/VIAL	N62717 001	DEC 16, 1986
	EQ 1 GM BASE/VIAL	N62717 002	DEC 16, 1986
AP	EQ 2 GM BASE/VIAL	N50320 003	
AP	EQ 2 GM BASE/VIAL	N62717 004	DEC 16, 1986
AP	EQ 4 GM BASE/VIAL	N50320 004	

UNIPEN IN PLASTIC CONTAINER
WYETH AYERST

TE	Strength	Appl. No.	Date
AP	EQ 1 GM BASE/VIAL	N50320 002	

POWDER FOR RECONSTITUTION; ORAL
UNIPEN
+ WYETH AYERST

	Strength	Appl. No.	Date
	EQ 250 MG BASE/5 ML	N50199 001	

TABLET; ORAL
UNIPEN
+ WYETH AYERST

	Strength	Appl. No.	Date
	EQ 500 MG BASE	N50462 001	

Prescription Drug Products (continued)

NAFTIFINE HYDROCHLORIDE

CREAM; TOPICAL
NAFTIN

	+ HERBERT	1%	N19599 001	FEB 29, 1988

GEL; TOPICAL
NAFTIN

	+ ALLERGAN	1%	N19356 001	JUN 18, 1990

NALBUPHINE HYDROCHLORIDE

INJECTABLE; INJECTION
NALBUPHINE HCL

AP	ABBOTT	10 MG/ML	N70914 001	FEB 03, 1989
AP		10 MG/ML	N70915 001	FEB 03, 1989
AP		20 MG/ML	N70916 001	FEB 03, 1989
AP		20 MG/ML	N70917 001	FEB 03, 1989
AP		20 MG/ML	N70918 001	FEB 03, 1989
AP	ASTRA	10 MG/ML	N72070 001	APR 10, 1989
AP		10 MG/ML	N72071 001	APR 10, 1989
AP		10 MG/ML	N72072 001	APR 10, 1989
AP		20 MG/ML	N72073 001	APR 10, 1989
AP		20 MG/ML	N72074 001	APR 10, 1989
AP		20 MG/ML	N72075 001	APR 10, 1989

NUBAIN

AP	DUPONT	10 MG/ML	N18024 001	
AP		20 MG/ML	N18024 002	MAY 27, 1982

NALIDIXIC ACID

SUSPENSION; ORAL
NEGGRAM

	+ STERLING	250 MG/5 ML	N17430 001	

NALIDIXIC ACID (continued)

TABLET; ORAL
NALIDIXIC ACID

AB	BARR	250 MG	N70270 001	MAR 28, 1986
AB		500 MG	N70271 001	MAR 28, 1986
AB		1 GM	N70272 001	MAR 28, 1986
AB	DANBURY	250 MG	N71936 001	JUN 28, 1988
AB		500 MG	N72061 001	JUN 28, 1988
AB		1 GM	N71919 001	JUN 28, 1988

NEGGRAM

AB	STERLING	250 MG	N14214 002	
AB		500 MG	N14214 004	
AB	+	1 GM	N14214 005	

NALOXONE HYDROCHLORIDE

INJECTABLE; INJECTION
NALOXONE

AP	ELKINS SINN	0.4 MG/ML	N70298 001	OCT 22, 1985
AP		0.4 MG/ML	N70299 001	OCT 22, 1985
AP	WYETH AYERST	0.02 MG/ML	N70188 001	OCT 02, 1985
AP		0.02 MG/ML	N70189 001	OCT 02, 1985
AP		0.4 MG/ML	N70190 001	OCT 02, 1985
AP		0.4 MG/ML	N70191 001	OCT 02, 1985

NALOXONE HCL

AP	ABBOTT	0.02 MG/ML	N70252 001	JAN 16, 1987
AP		0.02 MG/ML	N70253 001	JAN 16, 1987
AP		0.4 MG/ML	N70254 001	JAN 07, 1987
AP		0.4 MG/ML	N70255 001	JAN 07, 1987
AP		0.4 MG/ML	N70256 001	JAN 07, 1987
AP		0.4 MG/ML	N70257 001	JAN 07, 1987

Prescription Drug Products *(continued)*

NALOXONE HYDROCHLORIDE *(continued)*
INJECTABLE; INJECTION
NALOXONE HCL

ASTRA

AP	0.02 MG/ML	N72081 001	APR 11, 1989
AP	0.02 MG/ML	N72082 001	APR 11, 1989
AP	0.02 MG/ML	N72083 001	APR 11, 1989
AP	0.02 MG/ML	N72084 001	APR 11, 1989
AP	0.02 MG/ML	N72085 001	APR 11, 1989
AP	0.4 MG/ML	N72086 001	APR 11, 1989
AP	0.4 MG/ML	N72087 001	APR 11, 1989
AP	0.4 MG/ML	N72088 001	APR 11, 1989
AP	0.4 MG/ML	N72089 001	APR 11, 1989
AP	0.4 MG/ML	N72090 001	APR 11, 1989
AP	1 MG/ML	N72091 001	APR 11, 1989
AP	1 MG/ML	N72092 001	APR 11, 1989
AP	1 MG/ML	N72093 001	APR 11, 1989

ELKINS SINN

AP	0.02 MG/ML	N71272 001	MAY 24, 1988
AP	1 MG/ML	N71273 001	MAY 24, 1988
AP	1 MG/ML	N71274 001	MAY 24, 1988
AP	1 MG/ML	N71287 001	MAY 24, 1988

INTL MEDICATION

AP	0.4 MG/ML	N70639 001	JAN 17, 1986
AP	1 MG/ML	N72076 001	MAR 24, 1988

LYPHOMED

AP	0.02 MG/ML	N70648 001	NOV 17, 1986
AP	0.02 MG/ML	N70661 001	NOV 17, 1986
AP	0.4 MG/ML	N70649 001	NOV 17, 1986

MARSAM

AP	0.4 MG/ML	N71811 001	JUL 19, 1988

NALOXONE HYDROCHLORIDE *(continued)*
INJECTABLE; INJECTION
NALOXONE HCL

SMITH NEPHEW SOLOPAK

AP	0.02 MG/ML	N71671 001	NOV 17, 1987
AP	0.02 MG/ML	N71672 001	NOV 17, 1987
AP	0.4 MG/ML	N71681 001	NOV 17, 1987
AP	0.4 MG/ML	N71682 001	NOV 17, 1987
AP	0.4 MG/ML	N71683 001	NOV 17, 1987

STERIS

AP	0.4 MG/ML	N71339 001	NOV 18, 1987

STERLING

AP	0.02 MG/ML	N70171 001	APR 18, 1986
AP	0.4 MG/ML	N70172 001	APR 18, 1986

NARCAN

DUPONT

AP	0.02 MG/ML	N16636 002	
AP	0.4 MG/ML	N16636 001	
AP	0.4 MG/ML	N71083 001	JUL 28, 1988
AP	1 MG/ML	N16636 003	JUN 14, 1982
AP	1 MG/ML	N71084 001	JUL 28, 1988
AP	1 MG/ML	N71311 001	JUL 28, 1988

NALOXONE HYDROCHLORIDE; PENTAZOCINE HYDROCHLORIDE
TABLET; ORAL
TALWIN NX
+ STERLING

	EQ 0.5 MG BASE;EQ 50 MG BASE	N18733 001	DEC 16, 1982

NALTREXONE HYDROCHLORIDE
TABLET; ORAL
TREXAN
+ DUPONT

	50 MG	N18932 001	NOV 20, 1984

Prescription Drug Products (continued)

NANDROLONE DECANOATE
INJECTABLE; INJECTION

DECA-DURABOLIN

	Firm	Strength	Appl. No.	Date
AO	ORGANON	50 MG/ML	N13132 001	JUN 12, 1986
AO		100 MG/ML	N13132 002	JUN 12, 1986
AO		200 MG/ML	N13132 003	JUN 12, 1986

NANDROLONE DECANOATE

	Firm	Strength	Appl. No.	Date
AO	AKORN	100 MG/ML	N87519 001	SEP 28, 1983
AO	LYPHOMED	100 MG/ML	N88290 001	OCT 03, 1983
AO		200 MG/ML	N88317 001	OCT 14, 1983
AO		50 MG/ML	N86385 001	JAN 13, 1984
AO	STERIS	50 MG/ML	N87598 001	OCT 06, 1983
AO		50 MG/ML	N88554 001	FEB 10, 1986
AO		100 MG/ML	N86598 001	JAN 13, 1984
AO		100 MG/ML	N87599 001	OCT 06, 1983
AO		200 MG/ML	N88128 001	DEC 05, 1983

NANDROLONE PHENPROPIONATE
INJECTABLE; INJECTION

DURABOLIN

	Firm	Strength	Appl. No.
AO	ORGANON	25 MG/ML	N11891 001

DURABOLIN-50

	Firm	Strength	Appl. No.
AO	ORGANON	50 MG/ML	N11891 002

NANDROLONE PHENPROPIONATE

	Firm	Strength	Appl. No.	Date
AO	STERIS	25 MG/ML	N86386 001	JUN 17, 1983
AO		50 MG/ML	N87488 001	JUN 17, 1983

NAPHAZOLINE HYDROCHLORIDE
SOLUTION/DROPS; OPHTHALMIC

ALBALON

	Firm	Strength	Appl. No.	Date
AT	ALLERGAN	0.1%	N80248 001	

NAFAZAIR

	Firm	Strength	Appl. No.	Date
AT	PHARMAFAIR	0.1%	N88101 001	APR 15, 1983

NAPHAZOLINE HCL

	Firm	Strength	Appl. No.
AT	AKORN	0.1%	N83590 001

NAPHCON FORTE

	Firm	Strength	Appl. No.
AT	ALCON	0.1%	N80229 001

OPCON

	Firm	Strength	Appl. No.
AT	BAUSCH AND LOMB	0.1%	N87506 001

VASOCON

	Firm	Strength	Appl. No.	Date
AT	IOLAB	0.1%	N80235 002	MAR 24, 1983

NAPHAZOLINE HYDROCHLORIDE; *MULTIPLE*
SEE ANTAZOLINE PHOSPHATE; NAPHAZOLINE HYDROCHLORIDE

NAPROXEN
SUSPENSION; ORAL

NAPROSYN

Firm	Strength	Appl. No.	Date
+ SYNTEX	25 MG/ML	N18965 001	MAR 23, 1987

TABLET; ORAL

NAPROSYN

Firm	Strength	Appl. No.	Date
SYNTEX	250 MG	N17581 002	
	375 MG	N17581 003	
	500 MG	N17581 004	APR 15, 1982

NAPROXEN SODIUM
TABLET; ORAL

ANAPROX

Firm	Strength	Appl. No.
SYNTEX	275 MG	N18164 001

ANAPROX DS

Firm	Strength	Appl. No.	Date
+ SYNTEX	550 MG	N18164 003	SEP 30, 1987

NATAMYCIN
SUSPENSION/DROPS; OPHTHALMIC

NATACYN

Firm	Strength	Appl. No.
+ ALCON	5%	N50514 001

NEOMYCIN SULFATE
INJECTABLE; INJECTION

MYCIFRADIN

	Firm	Strength	Appl. No.
AP	UPJOHN	EQ 350 MG BASE/VIAL	N60477 001

NEOMYCIN SULFATE

	Firm	Strength	Appl. No.
AP	PFIZER	EQ 350 MG BASE/VIAL	N61084 001
AP	SQUBB	EQ 350 MG BASE/VIAL	N60366 001

POWDER; FOR RX COMPOUNDING

NEO-RX

	Firm	Strength	Appl. No.
AA	PHARMA TEK	100%	N61579 001

NEOMYCIN SULFATE

	Firm	Strength	Appl. No.	Date
AA	PADDOCK	100%	N62385 001	JUN 01, 1982

SOLUTION; ORAL

MYCIFRADIN

Firm	Strength	Appl. No.
UPJOHN	EQ 87.5 MG BASE/5 ML	N50285 001

TABLET; ORAL

MYCIFRADIN

	Firm	Strength	Appl. No.
AA	UPJOHN	EQ 350 MG BASE	N60520 001

NEOMYCIN SULFATE

	Firm	Strength	Appl. No.
AA	BIOCRAFT	EQ 350 MG BASE	N60304 001
AA	EON LABS	EQ 350 MG BASE	N61586 001
AA	LANNETT	EQ 350 MG BASE	N60607 001
AA	LILLY	EQ 350 MG BASE	N60385 001

Prescription Drug Products (continued)

NEOMYCIN SULFATE; *MULTIPLE*

SEE ACETIC ACID, GLACIAL; HYDROCORTISONE; NEOMYCIN SULFATE

SEE BACITRACIN; HYDROCORTISONE ACETATE; NEOMYCIN SULFATE; POLYMYXIN B SULFATE

SEE BACITRACIN; NEOMYCIN SULFATE; POLYMYXIN B SULFATE

SEE BACITRACIN ZINC; HYDROCORTISONE; NEOMYCIN SULFATE; POLYMYXIN B SULFATE

SEE BACITRACIN ZINC; NEOMYCIN SULFATE; POLYMYXIN B SULFATE

SEE COLISTIN SULFATE; HYDROCORTISONE ACETATE; NEOMYCIN SULFATE; THONZONIUM BROMIDE

SEE DEXAMETHASONE; NEOMYCIN SULFATE; POLYMYXIN B SULFATE

SEE DEXAMETHASONE SODIUM PHOSPHATE; NEOMYCIN SULFATE

SEE FLUOCINOLONE ACETONIDE; NEOMYCIN SULFATE

SEE FLURANDRENOLIDE; NEOMYCIN SULFATE

SEE GRAMICIDIN; NEOMYCIN SULFATE; POLYMYXIN B SULFATE

SEE HYDROCORTISONE; NEOMYCIN SULFATE

SEE HYDROCORTISONE; NEOMYCIN SULFATE; POLYMYXIN B SULFATE

SEE HYDROCORTISONE ACETATE; NEOMYCIN SULFATE

SEE HYDROCORTISONE ACETATE; NEOMYCIN SULFATE; POLYMYXIN B SULFATE

SEE METHYLPREDNISOLONE ACETATE; NEOMYCIN SULFATE

NEOMYCIN SULFATE; POLYMYXIN B SULFATE

OINTMENT; OPHTHALMIC
STATROL
ALCON   EQ 3.5 MG BASE/GM;10,000 UNITS/GM   N50344 002

SOLUTION; IRRIGATION
NEOMYCIN AND POLYMYXIN B SULFATES
AI STERIS   EQ 40 MG BASE/ML;200,000 UNITS/ML   N62664 001   APR 08, 1986
NEOSPORIN G.U. IRRIGANT
AI BURROUGHS WELLCOME   EQ 40 MG BASE/ML;200,000 UNITS/ML   N60707 001

SOLUTION/DROPS; OPHTHALMIC
STATROL
ALCON   EQ 3.5 MG BASE/ML;16,250 UNITS/ML   N50456 001
EQ 3.5 MG BASE/ML;16,250 UNITS/ML   N62339 001   NOV 30, 1984

NEOMYCIN SULFATE; POLYMYXIN B SULFATE; PREDNISOLONE ACETATE

SUSPENSION/DROPS; OPHTHALMIC
POLY-PRED
ALLERGAN   EQ 0.35% BASE;10,000 UNITS/ML;0.5%   N50081 002

NEOMYCIN SULFATE; PREDNISOLONE ACETATE

SUSPENSION/DROPS; OPHTHALMIC
NEO-DELTA-CORTEF
UPJOHN   EQ 3.5 MG BASE/ML;0.25%   N61037 001

NEOMYCIN SULFATE; PREDNISOLONE SODIUM PHOSPHATE

OINTMENT; OPHTHALMIC
NEO-HYDELTRASOL
MSD   EQ 3.5 MG BASE/GM;EQ 0.25% PHOSPHATE   N50378 001

NETILMICIN SULFATE

INJECTABLE; INJECTION
NETROMYCIN
SCHERING   EQ 100 MG BASE/ML   N50544 003   FEB 28, 1983

NIACIN

CAPSULE; ORAL
WAMPOCAP
WALLACE   500 MG   N11073 003

TABLET; ORAL
NIACIN
AA DANBURY   500 MG   N83305 001
AA HALSEY   500 MG   N83453 001
AA MK   500 MG   N83525 001
AA PUREPAC   500 MG   N83271 001
AA RICHLYN   500 MG   N83115 001
AA TABLICAPS   500 MG   N84237 001
AA WOCKHARDT   500 MG   N81134 001   APR 28, 1992
AA ZENITH   500 MG   N83180 001
NICOLAR
RHONE POULENC RORER   500 MG   N83823 001

NIACINAMIDE; *MULTIPLE*

SEE ASCORBIC ACID; BIOTIN; CYANOCOBALAMIN; DEXPANTHENOL; ERGOCALCIFEROL; FOLIC ACID; NIACINAMIDE; PYRIDOXINE HYDROCHLORIDE; RIBOFLAVIN PHOSPHATE SODIUM; THIAMINE HYDROCHLORIDE; VITAMIN A; VITAMIN E

SEE ASCORBIC ACID; BIOTIN; CYANOCOBALAMIN; DEXPANTHENOL; ERGOCALCIFEROL; FOLIC ACID; NIACINAMIDE; PYRIDOXINE; RIBOFLAVIN PHOSPHATE SODIUM; THIAMINE; VITAMIN A; VITAMIN E

Prescription Drug Products *(continued)*

NICARDIPINE HYDROCHLORIDE

CAPSULE; ORAL

CARDENE

		Strength	Appl. No.	Date
	SYNTEX	20 MG	N19488 001	DEC 21, 1988
+		30 MG	N19488 002	DEC 21, 1988

CAPSULE, EXTENDED RELEASE; ORAL

CARDENE SR

		Strength	Appl. No.	Date
+	SYNTEX	30 MG	N20005 001	FEB 21, 1992
+		45 MG	N20005 002	FEB 21, 1992
+		60 MG	N20005 003	FEB 21, 1992

INJECTABLE; INJECTION

CARDENE

	Strength	Appl. No.	Date
DUPONT MERCK	2.5 MG/ML	N19734 001	JAN 30, 1992

NICLOSAMIDE

TABLET, CHEWABLE; ORAL

NICLOCIDE

		Strength	Appl. No.	Date
+	MILES	500 MG	N18669 001	MAY 14, 1982

NICOTINE

FILM, EXTENDED RELEASE; TRANSDERMAL

HABITROL

TE		Strength	Appl. No.	Date
BC	CIBA GEIGY	7 MG/24 HR	N20076 001	NOV 27, 1991
BC		14 MG/24 HR	N20076 002	NOV 27, 1991
BC		21 MG/24 HR	N20076 003	NOV 27, 1991

NICODERM

TE		Strength	Appl. No.	Date
BC	+ MARION MERRELL DOW	7 MG/24 HR	N20165 001	NOV 07, 1991
BC	+	14 MG/24 HR	N20165 002	NOV 07, 1991
BC	+	21 MG/24 HR	N20165 003	NOV 07, 1991

NICOTROL

		Strength	Appl. No.	Date
+	KABI	5 MG/16 HR	N20150 001	APR 22, 1992
+		10 MG/16 HR	N20150 002	APR 22, 1992
+		15 MG/16 HR	N20150 003	APR 22, 1992

PROSTEP

		Strength	Appl. No.	Date
+	ELAN	11 MG/24 HR	N19983 001	JAN 28, 1992
+		22 MG/24 HR	N19983 002	JAN 28, 1992

NICOTINE POLACRILEX

GUM, CHEWING; BUCCAL

NICORETTE

		Strength	Appl. No.	Date
	MERRELL DOW	EQ 2 MG BASE	N18612 001	JAN 13, 1984

NICORETTE DS

		Strength	Appl. No.	Date
+	MERRELL DOW	EQ 4 MG BASE	N20066 001	JUN 08, 1992

NIFEDIPINE

CAPSULE; ORAL

ADALAT

TE		Strength	Appl. No.	Date
ΔB	MILES	10 MG	N19478 001	NOV 27, 1985
ΔB		20 MG	N19478 002	SEP 17, 1986

NIFEDIPINE

TE		Strength	Appl. No.	Date
ΔB	CHASE	10 MG	N72409 001	JUL 10, 1989
ΔB		20 MG	N73421 001	JUN 19, 1991
ΔB	NOVOPHARM	10 MG	N72651 001	FEB 19, 1992
ΔB	PUREPAC	10 MG	N72579 001	APR 28, 1989
ΔB		20 MG	N72556 001	APR 28, 1989
ΔB	SCHERER	10 MG	N73250 001	OCT 08, 1991
ΔB		20 MG	N74045 001	APR 30, 1992

PROCARDIA

TE		Strength	Appl. No.	Date
ΔB	+ PFIZER	10 MG	N18482 001	
ΔB	+	20 MG	N18482 002	JUL 24, 1986

TABLET, EXTENDED RELEASE; ORAL

PROCARDIA XL

		Strength	Appl. No.	Date
+	PFIZER	30 MG	N19684 001	SEP 06, 1989
+		60 MG	N19684 002	SEP 06, 1989
+		90 MG	N19684 003	SEP 06, 1989

NIMODIPINE

CAPSULE; ORAL

NIMOTOP

		Strength	Appl. No.	Date
+	MILES	30 MG	N18869 001	DEC 28, 1988

Prescription Drug Products (continued)

NITROFURANTOIN

SUSPENSION; ORAL
FURADANTIN
+ P AND G — 25 MG/5 ML — N09175 001

TABLET; ORAL
FURADANTIN
P AND G
ΔB + — 50 MG — N08693 001
ΔB — 100 MG — N08693 002
FURALAN
LANNETT
ΔB — 50 MG — N80017 001
ΔB — 100 MG — N80017 002
NITROFURANTOIN
BOLAR
ΔB — 50 MG — N80447 001
WHITE TOWNE — 100 MG — N84085 002
PAULSEN
ΔB — 50 MG — N80078 002
ZENITH
ΔB — 100 MG — N80078 001

NITROFURANTOIN; NITROFURANTOIN, MACROCRYSTALLINE

CAPSULE, EXTENDED RELEASE; ORAL
MACROBID
+ P AND G — 75 MG;25 MG — N20064 001 DEC 24, 1991

NITROFURANTOIN, MACROCRYSTALLINE

CAPSULE; ORAL
MACRODANTIN
P AND G
+ — 25 MG — N16620 003
— 50 MG — N16620 001
+ — 100 MG — N16620 002

NITROFURANTOIN, MACROCRYSTALLINE; *MULTIPLE*

SEE NITROFURANTOIN; NITROFURANTOIN, MACROCRYSTALLINE

NITROFURAZONE

CREAM; TOPICAL
FURACIN
ROBERTS — 0.2% — N83789 001
DRESSING; TOPICAL
FURACIN
ROBERTS — 0.2% — N05795 001
NITROFURAZONE
THAMES — 0.2% — N86156 001
OINTMENT; TOPICAL
NITROFURAZONE
ΔI AMBIX — 0.2% — N86077 001
ΔI CLAY PARK — 0.2% — N84968 001
ΔI LANNETT — 0.2% — N84393 001
ΔI WENDT — 0.2% — N86766 001

NITROFURAZONE (continued)

POWDER; TOPICAL
FURACIN
ROBERTS — 0.2% — N83791 001
SOLUTION; TOPICAL
NITROFURAZONE
ΔI CLAY PARK — 0.2% — N85130 001
ΔI WENDT — 0.2% — N87081 001

NITROGLYCERIN

AEROSOL; ORAL
NITROLINGUAL
BOSKAMP — 0.4 MG/SPRAY — N18705 001 OCT 31, 1985

INJECTABLE; INJECTION
NITRO IV
ΔP BOSKAMP — 5 MG/ML — N18672 002 AUG 30, 1983
NITRO-BID
MARION MERRELL DOW — 10 MG/ML — N71159 001 FEB 28, 1990
ΔP — 5 MG/ML — N18621 001 JAN 05, 1982
NITROGLYCERIN
ABBOTT
ΔP INTL MEDICATION — 5 MG/ML — N18531 001
ΔP — 5 MG/ML — N70026 001 SEP 10, 1985
ΔP LUITPOLD — 5 MG/ML — N72034 001 MAY 24, 1988
ΔP LYPHOMED — 5 MG/ML — N70077 001 DEC 13, 1985
SMITH NEPHEW
ΔP SOLOPAK — 5 MG/ML — N70633 001 JUN 19, 1986

NITROGLYCERIN IN DEXTROSE 5%
ΔP ABBOTT — 10 MG/100 ML — N71846 001 AUG 31, 1990
ΔP — 20 MG/100 ML — N71847 001 AUG 31, 1990
ΔP — 40 MG/100 ML — N71848 001 AUG 31, 1990
ΔP BAXTER — 10 MG/100 ML — N19970 001 DEC 29, 1989
ΔP — 20 MG/100 ML — N19970 002 DEC 29, 1989
ΔP — 40 MG/100 ML — N19970 003 DEC 29, 1989
NITRONAL
BOSKAMP — 1 MG/ML — N18672 001 AUG 30, 1983

Prescription Drug Products (continued)

NITROGLYCERIN (continued)

INJECTABLE; INJECTION

NITROSTAT

ΔP	PARKE DAVIS	5 MG/ML	N18588 002 DEC 23, 1983
ΔP		5 MG/ML	N70863 001 JAN 08, 1987
ΔP		10 MG/ML	N70871 001 JAN 08, 1987
ΔP		10 MG/ML	N70872 001 JAN 08, 1987
		0.8 MG/ML	N18588 001

TRIDIL

ΔP	DUPONT	5 MG/ML	N18537 001
		0.5 MG/ML	N18537 002 JUN 16, 1983

OINTMENT; TRANSDERMAL

NITROGLYCERIN

	ALTANA	2%	N87355 001 JUL 08, 1988

NIZATIDINE

CAPSULE; ORAL

AXID

	LILLY	150 MG	N19508 001 APR 12, 1988
+		300 MG	N19508 002 APR 12, 1988

NOREPINEPHRINE BITARTRATE

INJECTABLE; INJECTION

LEVOPHED

	STERLING	EQ 1 MG BASE/ML	N07513 001

NOREPINEPHRINE BITARTRATE; PROCAINE HYDROCHLORIDE; PROPOXYCAINE HYDROCHLORIDE

INJECTABLE; INJECTION

RAVOCAINE AND NOVOCAIN W/ LEVOPHED

	COOK WAITE	EQ 0.033 MG BASE/ML,2%;0.4%	N08592 003

NORETHINDRONE

TABLET; ORAL

NOR-Q.D.

	SYNTEX	0.35 MG	N17060 001

NORLUTIN

+	PARKE DAVIS	5 MG	N10895 002

TABLET; ORAL-28

MICRONOR

+	JOHNSON RW	0.35 MG	N16954 001

NORETHINDRONE; *MULTIPLE*

▽ SEE ETHINYL ESTRADIOL; FERROUS FUMARATE; NORETHINDRONE

SEE ETHINYL ESTRADIOL; NORETHINDRONE

SEE MESTRANOL; NORETHINDRONE

NORETHINDRONE ACETATE

TABLET; ORAL

AYGESTIN

ΔB	WYETH AYERST	5 MG	N18405 001 APR 21, 1982

NORLUTATE

ΔB	+ PARKE DAVIS	5 MG	N12184 002

NORETHINDRONE ACETATE; *MULTIPLE*

SEE ETHINYL ESTRADIOL; FERROUS FUMARATE; NORETHINDRONE ACETATE

SEE ETHINYL ESTRADIOL; NORETHINDRONE ACETATE

NORETHYNODREL; *MULTIPLE*

SEE MESTRANOL; NORETHYNODREL

NORFLOXACIN

SOLUTION/DROPS; OPHTHALMIC

CHIBROXIN

	MERCK	0.3%	N19757 001 JUN 17, 1991

TABLET; ORAL

NOROXIN

+	MERCK	400 MG	N19384 002 OCT 31, 1986

NORGESTIMATE; *MULTIPLE*

SEE ETHINYL ESTRADIOL; NORGESTIMATE

NORGESTREL

TABLET; ORAL

OVRETTE

+	WYETH AYERST	0.075 MG	N17031 001

NORGESTREL; *MULTIPLE*

SEE ETHINYL ESTRADIOL; NORGESTREL

Prescription Drug Products (continued)

NORTRIPTYLINE HYDROCHLORIDE

CAPSULE; ORAL

AVENTYL HCL			
BD	LILLY	EQ 10 MG BASE	N14684 001
BD		EQ 25 MG BASE	N14684 002
NORTRIPTYLINE HCL			
AB	DANBURY	EQ 10 MG BASE	N73553 001 MAR 30, 1992
AB		EQ 25 MG BASE	N73554 001 MAR 30, 1992
AB		EQ 50 MG BASE	N73555 001 MAR 30, 1992
AB		EQ 75 MG BASE	N73556 001 MAR 30, 1992
PAMELOR			
AB	SANDOZ	EQ 10 MG BASE	N18013 001
AB		EQ 25 MG BASE	N18013 002
AB		EQ 50 MG BASE	N18013 004
AB		EQ 75 MG BASE	N18013 003

SOLUTION; ORAL

AVENTYL HCL			
AA	LILLY	EQ 10 MG BASE/5 ML	N14685 001
PAMELOR			
AA	SANDOZ	EQ 10 MG BASE/5 ML	N18012 001
+			

NOVOBIOCIN SODIUM

CAPSULE; ORAL

ALBAMYCIN			
+	UPJOHN	EQ 250 MG BASE	N50339 001

NYSTATIN

CREAM; TOPICAL

MYCOSTATIN			
AT	SQUIBB	100,000 UNITS/GM	N60575 001
MYKINAC			
AT	NMC	100,000 UNITS/GM	N62387 001 JUL 29, 1982
NILSTAT			
AT	LEDERLE	100,000 UNITS/GM	N61445 001
NYSTATIN			
AT	ALTANA	100,000 UNITS/GM	N62129 001
AT	CLAY PARK	100,000 UNITS/GM	N62225 001
AT	LEMMON	100,000 UNITS/GM	N61966 001
AT	NASKA	100,000 UNITS/GM	N62949 001 JUN 13, 1988
AT	THAMES	100,000 UNITS/GM	N62457 001 JUL 28, 1983

NYSTATIN (continued)

LOTION; TOPICAL

CANDEX			
	MILES	100,000 UNITS/ML	N50233 001

OINTMENT; TOPICAL

MYCOSTATIN			
AT	SQUIBB	100,000 UNITS/GM	N60571 001
MYKINAC			
AT	NMC	100,000 UNITS/GM	N62731 001 SEP 22, 1986
NILSTAT			
AT	LEDERLE	100,000 UNITS/GM	N61444 001
NYSTATIN			
AT	ALTANA	100,000 UNITS/GM	N62124 002 SEP 23, 1982
AT	CLAY PARK	100,000 UNITS/GM	N62472 001 FEB 13, 1984
AT	NASKA	100,000 UNITS/GM	N62840 001 NOV 13, 1987

PASTILLE; ORAL

MYCOSTATIN			
+	SQUIBB	200,000 UNITS	N50619 001 APR 09, 1987

POWDER; ORAL

BARSTATIN 100			
AA	BARLAN	100%	N62489 001 APR 27, 1988
NILSTAT			
AA	LEDERLE	100%	N50576 001 DEC 22, 1983
NYSTATIN			
AA	PADDOCK	100%	N62613 001 NOV 26, 1985

POWDER; TOPICAL

MYCOSTATIN			
	SQUIBB	100,000 UNITS/GM	N60578 001

SUSPENSION; ORAL

MYCOSTATIN			
AA	SQUIBB	100,000 UNITS/ML	N61533 001
NILSTAT			
AA	LEDERLE	100,000 UNITS/ML	N50299 001
NYSTATIN			
AA	BARRE	100,000 UNITS/ML	N62349 001 JUL 14, 1982
AA	BIOCRAFT	100,000 UNITS/ML	N62670 001 JUN 18, 1987
AA	FOUGERA	100,000 UNITS/ML	N62517 001 JUN 07, 1984
AA	LEMMON	100,000 UNITS/ML	N62776 001 DEC 17, 1987
AA	NASKA	100,000 UNITS/ML	N62571 001 OCT 29, 1985

Prescription Drug Products *(continued)*

NYSTATIN *(continued)*

SUSPENSION; ORAL

NYSTATIN

	Labeler	Strength	Appl No	Date
AA	PHARM BASICS	100,000 UNITS/ML	N62512 001	OCT 29, 1984
AA		100,000 UNITS/ML	N62835 001	NOV 19, 1987
AA	PHARMADERM	100,000 UNITS/ML	N62518 001	JUL 06, 1984
AA	PHARMAFAIR	100,000 UNITS/ML	N62541 001	JAN 16, 1985
AA	ROXANE	100,000 UNITS/ML	N62832 001	DEC 27, 1991
AA	THAMES	100,000 UNITS/ML	N62876 001	FEB 29, 1988

NYSTEX

	Labeler	Strength	Appl No	Date
AA	SAVAGE	100,000 UNITS/ML	N62519 001	JUL 06, 1984

TABLET; ORAL

MYCOSTATIN

	Labeler	Strength	Appl No	Date
AA	SQUIBB	500,000 UNITS	N60574 001	

NILSTAT

	Labeler	Strength	Appl No	Date
AA	LEDERLE	500,000 UNITS	N61151 001	

NYSTATIN

	Labeler	Strength	Appl No	Date
AA	EON LABS	500,000 UNITS	N62065 001	
AA	LEMMON	500,000 UNITS	N62506 001	
AA	MUTUAL PHARM	500,000 UNITS	N62838 001	DEC 22, 1988
AA	PAR	500,000 UNITS	N62474 001	DEC 22, 1983
AA	PHARM BASICS	500,000 UNITS	N62524 001	NOV 26, 1985

TABLET; VAGINAL

KOROSTATIN

	Labeler	Strength	Appl No	Date
AT	HOLLAND RANTOS	100,000 UNITS	N61718 001	

MYCOSTATIN

	Labeler	Strength	Appl No	Date
AT	SQUIBB	100,000 UNITS	N60577 001	

NILSTAT

	Labeler	Strength	Appl No	Date
AT	LEDERLE	100,000 UNITS	N61325 001	

NYSTATIN

	Labeler	Strength	Appl No	Date
AT	FOUGERA	100,000 UNITS	N62459 001	NOV 09, 1983
AT	LEMMON	100,000 UNITS	N62502 001	DEC 23, 1983
AT	PHARMADERM	100,000 UNITS	N62460 001	NOV 09, 1983
AT	SIDMAK	100,000 UNITS	N62615 001	OCT 17, 1985

NYSTATIN; TRIAMCINOLONE ACETONIDE

CREAM; TOPICAL

DERMACOMB

	Labeler	Strength	Appl No	Date
AT	TARO	100,000 UNITS/GM;0.1%	N62364 001	DEC 22, 1987

MYCO-TRIACET II

	Labeler	Strength	Appl No	Date
AT	LEMMON	100,000 UNITS/GM;0.1%	N61954 002	SEP 20, 1985

MYCOLOG-II

	Labeler	Strength	Appl No	Date
AT	SQUIBB	100,000 UNITS/GM;0.1%	N60576 002	MAY 01, 1985
AT		100,000 UNITS/GM;0.1%	N62606 001	MAY 15, 1985

MYKACET

	Labeler	Strength	Appl No	Date
AT	NMC	100,000 UNITS/GM;0.1%	N62367 001	MAY 28, 1985

MYTREX F

	Labeler	Strength	Appl No	Date
AT	SAVAGE	100,000 UNITS/GM;0.1%	N62597 001	OCT 08, 1985

NYSTATIN AND TRIAMCINOLONE ACETONIDE

	Labeler	Strength	Appl No	Date
B*	CLAY PARK	100,000 UNITS/GM;0.1%	N62186 002	JUN 06, 1985
AT	NASKA	100,000 UNITS/GM;0.1%	N63010 001	DEC 20, 1988
AT	PHARMAFAIR	100,000 UNITS/GM;0.1%	N62657 001	JUL 30, 1986

NYSTATIN-TRIAMCINOLONE ACETONIDE

	Labeler	Strength	Appl No	Date
AT	FOUGERA	100,000 UNITS/GM;0.1%	N62599 001	OCT 08, 1985
AT	PHARMADERM	100,000 UNITS/GM;0.1%	N62596 001	OCT 08, 1985
AT	THAMES	100,000 UNITS/GM;0.1%	N62347 001	MAR 30, 1987

OINTMENT; TOPICAL

MYCO-TRIACET II

	Labeler	Strength	Appl No	Date
AT	LEMMON	100,000 UNITS/GM;0.1%	N62045 002	NOV 26, 1985

MYCOLOG-II

	Labeler	Strength	Appl No	Date
AT	SQUIBB	100,000 UNITS/GM;0.1%	N60572 001	JUN 28, 1985

MYKACET

	Labeler	Strength	Appl No	Date
AT	NMC	100,000 UNITS/GM;0.1%	N62733 001	MAR 09, 1987

MYTREX F

	Labeler	Strength	Appl No	Date
AT	SAVAGE	100,000 UNITS/GM;0.1%	N62601 001	OCT 09, 1985

NYSTATIN AND TRIAMCINOLONE ACETONIDE

	Labeler	Strength	Appl No	Date
AT	CLAY PARK	100,000 UNITS/GM;0.1%	N62280 002	OCT 10, 1985
AT	PHARMAFAIR	100,000 UNITS/GM;0.1%	N62656 001	JUL 30, 1986

NYSTATIN-TRIAMCINOLONE ACETONIDE

	Labeler	Strength	Appl No	Date
AT	FOUGERA	100,000 UNITS/GM;0.1%	N62602 001	OCT 09, 1985
AT	PHARMADERM	100,000 UNITS/GM;0.1%	N62603 001	OCT 09, 1985

Prescription Drug Products (continued)

OCTREOTIDE ACETATE
INJECTABLE; INJECTION
SANDOSTATIN
SANDOZ

	EQ 50 MCG BASE/ML	N19667 001 OCT 21, 1988
	EQ 100 MCG BASE/ML	N19667 002 OCT 21, 1988
	EQ 500 MCG BASE/ML	N19667 003 OCT 21, 1988

OFLOXACIN
INJECTABLE; INJECTION
FLOXIN
JOHNSON RW

	20 MG/ML	N20087 002 MAR 31, 1992
	40 MG/ML	N20087 003 MAR 31, 1992

FLOXIN IN DEXTROSE 5%
JOHNSON RW

	400 MG/100 ML	N20087 001 MAR 31, 1992

FLOXIN IN DEXTROSE 5% IN PLASTIC CONTAINER
JOHNSON RW

	4 MG/ML	N20087 004 MAR 31, 1992
	400 MG/100 ML	N20087 005 MAR 31, 1992

TABLET; ORAL
FLOXIN
JOHNSON RW

	200 MG	N19735 001 DEC 28, 1990
	300 MG	N19735 002 DEC 28, 1990
+	400 MG	N19735 003 DEC 28, 1990

OLSALAZINE SODIUM
CAPSULE; ORAL
DIPENTUM
+ KABI

	250 MG	N19715 001 JUL 31, 1990

OMEPRAZOLE
CAPSULE, DELAYED REL PELLETS; ORAL
PRILOSEC
+ MERCK

	20 MG	N19810 001 SEP 14, 1989

ONDANSETRON HYDROCHLORIDE
INJECTABLE; INJECTION
ZOFRAN
GLAXO

	EQ 2 MG BASE/ML	N20007 001 JAN 04, 1991

ORPHENADRINE CITRATE
INJECTABLE; INJECTION
NORFLEX
3M

ΔP		30 MG/ML	N13055 001

ORPHENADRINE CITRATE
STERIS

ΔP		30 MG/ML	N84779 001 MAR 15, 1982
ΔP		30 MG/ML	N87062 001

TABLET, EXTENDED RELEASE; ORAL
NORFLEX
+ 3M

	100 MG	N12157 001

ORPHENADRINE CITRATE; *MULTIPLE*
SEE ASPIRIN; CAFFEINE; ORPHENADRINE CITRATE

ORPHENADRINE HYDROCHLORIDE
TABLET; ORAL
DISIPAL
3M

	50 MG	N10653 001

OXACILLIN SODIUM
CAPSULE; ORAL
BACTOCILL
BEECHAM

ΔB	EQ 250 MG BASE	N61336 001
ΔB	EQ 250 MG BASE	N62241 001
ΔB	EQ 500 MG BASE	N61336 002
ΔB	EQ 500 MG BASE	N62241 002

OXACILLIN SODIUM
BIOCRAFT

ΔB	EQ 250 MG BASE	N62222 001
ΔB	EQ 500 MG BASE	N62222 002

PROSTAPHLIN
BRISTOL
+

ΔB	EQ 250 MG BASE	N61450 002
ΔB	EQ 500 MG BASE	N50118 002
ΔB	EQ 500 MG BASE	N61450 001

INJECTABLE; INJECTION
BACTOCILL
BEECHAM

ΔP	EQ 500 MG BASE/VIAL	N61334 009 MAR 26, 1982
ΔP	EQ 1 GM BASE/VIAL	N61334 006 MAR 26, 1982
ΔP	EQ 1 GM BASE/VIAL	N62736 001 DEC 19, 1986
ΔP	EQ 2 GM BASE/VIAL	N61334 007 MAR 26, 1982
ΔP	EQ 2 GM BASE/VIAL	N62736 002 DEC 19, 1986
ΔP	EQ 4 GM BASE/VIAL	N61334 008 MAR 26, 1982
ΔP	EQ 10 GM BASE/VIAL	N61334 010

Prescription Drug Products *(continued)*

OXACILLIN SODIUM *(continued)*

INJECTABLE; INJECTION

BACTOCILL IN PLASTIC CONTAINER

	BAXTER	EQ 20 MG BASE/ML	N50640 001 OCT 26, 1989
		EQ 40 MG BASE/ML	N50640 002 OCT 26, 1989

OXACILLIN SODIUM

	APOTHECON		
AP		EQ 250 MG BASE/VIAL	N61490 001
AP		EQ 500 MG BASE/VIAL	N61490 002
AP		EQ 1 GM BASE/VIAL	N61490 003
AP		EQ 1 GM BASE/VIAL	N62737 001 DEC 23, 1986
AP		EQ 2 GM BASE/VIAL	N62737 002 DEC 23, 1986
AP		EQ 10 GM BASE/VIAL	N61490 006 MAY 09, 1991
AP	MARSAM	EQ 250 MG BASE/VIAL	N62856 001 OCT 26, 1988
AP		EQ 500 MG BASE/VIAL	N62856 002 OCT 26, 1988
AP		EQ 1 GM BASE/VIAL	N62856 003 OCT 26, 1988
AP		EQ 2 GM BASE/VIAL	N62856 004 OCT 26, 1988
AP		EQ 4 GM BASE/VIAL	N62856 005 OCT 26, 1988
AP		EQ 10 GM BASE/VIAL	N62984 001 SEP 29, 1988

POWDER FOR RECONSTITUTION; ORAL

BACTOCILL

AA	BEECHAM	EQ 250 MG BASE/5 ML	N62321 001

OXACILLIN SODIUM

AA	BIOCRAFT	EQ 250 MG BASE/5 ML	N62252 001

PROSTAPHLIN

AA	BRISTOL	EQ 250 MG BASE/5 ML	N50194 001
AA		EQ 250 MG BASE/5 ML	N61457 001

OXAMNIQUINE

CAPSULE; ORAL

VANSIL

+	PFIZER	250 MG	N18069 001

OXANDROLONE

TABLET; ORAL

OXANDRIN

+	GYNEX	2.5 MG	N13718 001

OXAZEPAM

CAPSULE; ORAL

OXAZEPAM

AB	BARR	10 MG	N70957 001 AUG 10, 1987
AB		15 MG	N71025 001 AUG 10, 1987
AB		30 MG	N71026 001 AUG 10, 1987
AB	DANBURY	10 MG	N72952 001 SEP 28, 1990
AB		15 MG	N72953 001 SEP 28, 1990
AB		30 MG	N72954 001 SEP 28, 1990
AB	GENEVA	10 MG	N71813 001 APR 19, 1988
AB		15 MG	N71756 001 APR 19, 1988
AB		30 MG	N71814 001 APR 19, 1988
AB	PUREPAC	10 MG	N72251 001 APR 14, 1988
AB		15 MG	N72252 001 APR 14, 1988
AB		30 MG	N72253 001 APR 14, 1988
AB	ZENITH	10 MG	N70943 001 AUG 03, 1987
AB		15 MG	N70944 001 AUG 03, 1987
AB		30 MG	N70945 001 AUG 03, 1987

SERAX

AB	WYETH AYERST	10 MG	N15539 002
AB		15 MG	N15539 004
AB +		30 MG	N15539 006

TABLET; ORAL

OXAZEPAM

AB	BARR	15 MG	N70683 001 JAN 16, 1987
AB	DANBURY	15 MG	N71494 001 APR 21, 1987
AB	PARKE DAVIS	15 MG	N71508 001 FEB 02, 1987

SERAX

AB +	WYETH AYERST	15 MG	N15539 008

OXICONAZOLE NITRATE

CREAM; TOPICAL

OXISTAT

+	GLAXO	EQ 1% BASE	N19828 001 DEC 30, 1988

Prescription Drug Products (continued)

OXPRENOLOL HYDROCHLORIDE
CAPSULE; ORAL
TRASICOR

CIBA	20 MG	N18166 001	DEC 28, 1983
	40 MG	N18166 002	DEC 28, 1983
	80 MG	N18166 003	DEC 28, 1983
+	160 MG	N18166 004	DEC 28, 1983

OXTRIPHYLLINE
ELIXIR; ORAL
CHOLEDYL

AA	PARKE DAVIS	100 MG/5 ML	N09268 012	NOV 27, 1984

OXTRIPHYLLINE

AA	PHARM BASICS	100 MG/5 ML	N88243 001	DEC 05, 1983

SYRUP; ORAL
CHOLEDYL

AA	PARKE DAVIS	50 MG/5 ML	N09268 011

OXTRIPHYLLINE PEDIATRIC

AA	PHARM BASICS	50 MG/5 ML	N88242 001	DEC 05, 1983

TABLET, DELAYED RELEASE; ORAL
CHOLEDYL

+ PARKE DAVIS	100 MG	N09268 003	
	200 MG	N09268 007	

TABLET, EXTENDED RELEASE; ORAL
CHOLEDYL SA

+ PARKE DAVIS	400 MG	N87863 001	MAY 24, 1983
+	600 MG	N86742 001	

OXYCODONE HYDROCHLORIDE; *MULTIPLE*
SEE ACETAMINOPHEN; OXYCODONE HYDROCHLORIDE
SEE ASPIRIN; OXYCODONE HYDROCHLORIDE: OXYCODONE TEREPHTHALATE

OXYCODONE TEREPHTHALATE; *MULTIPLE*
SEE ASPIRIN; OXYCODONE HYDROCHLORIDE: OXYCODONE TEREPHTHALATE

OXYMETHOLONE
TABLET; ORAL
ANADROL-50

+ SYNTEX	50 MG	N16848 001

OXYMORPHONE HYDROCHLORIDE
INJECTABLE; INJECTION
NUMORPHAN

DUPONT	1 MG/ML	N11707 002
	1.5 MG/ML	N11707 001

SUPPOSITORY; RECTAL
NUMORPHAN

+ DUPONT	5 MG	N11738 004

OXYPHENCYCLIMINE HYDROCHLORIDE
TABLET; ORAL
DARICON

PFIZER	10 MG	N11612 001

OXYTETRACYCLINE
TABLET; ORAL
TERRAMYCIN

+ PFIZER	250 MG	N50287 001

OXYTETRACYCLINE CALCIUM
SYRUP; ORAL
TERRAMYCIN

+ PFIZER	EQ 125 MG BASE/5 ML	N60595 001

OXYTETRACYCLINE HYDROCHLORIDE
CAPSULE; ORAL
OXY-KESSO-TETRA

	MK	EQ 250 MG BASE	N60179 001

OXYTETRACYCLINE HCL

AB	PROTER	EQ 250 MG BASE	N60869 001
AB	RICHLYN	EQ 250 MG BASE	N60760 001
AB	WEST WARD	EQ 250 MG BASE	N60770 001

TERRAMYCIN

AB	+ PFIZER	EQ 250 MG BASE	N50286 002

OXYBUTYNIN CHLORIDE
SYRUP; ORAL
DITROPAN

	MARION MERRELL DOW	5 MG/5 ML	N18211 001

TABLET; ORAL
DITROPAN

AB	+ MARION MERRELL DOW	5 MG	N17577 001

OXYBUTYNIN CHLORIDE

AB	SIDMAK	5 MG	N71655 001	NOV 14, 1988

Prescription Drug Products (continued)

OXYTETRACYCLINE HYDROCHLORIDE (continued)
INJECTABLE; INJECTION
TERRAMYCIN
PFIZER
EQ 250 MG BASE/VIAL   N60586 001
EQ 500 MG BASE/VIAL   N60586 002

OXYTETRACYCLINE HYDROCHLORIDE; *MULTIPLE*
SEE HYDROCORTISONE ACETATE; OXYTETRACYCLINE HYDROCHLORIDE

OXYTETRACYCLINE HYDROCHLORIDE; POLYMYXIN B SULFATE
OINTMENT; OPHTHALMIC
TERRAMYCIN W/ POLYMYXIN B SULFATE
PFIZER
EQ 5 MG BASE/GM;10,000 UNITS/GM   N61015 001

OINTMENT; OTIC
TERRAMYCIN W/ POLYMYXIN
PFIZER
EQ 5 MG BASE/GM;10,000 UNITS/GM   N61841 001

TABLET; VAGINAL
TERRAMYCIN-POLYMYXIN
PFIZER
EQ 100 MG BASE;100,000 UNITS   N61009 001

OXYTOCIN
INJECTABLE; INJECTION
OXYTOCIN
AP LYPHOMED   10 USP UNITS/ML   N18248 001
AP WYETH AYERST   10 USP UNITS/ML   N18243 001
PITOCIN
AP PARKE DAVIS   10 USP UNITS/ML   N18261 001
SYNTOCINON
AP SANDOZ   10 USP UNITS/ML   N18245 001
SOLUTION; NASAL
SYNTOCINON
SANDOZ   40 USP UNITS/ML   N12285 001

PAMIDRONATE DISODIUM
INJECTABLE; INJECTION
AREDIA
CIBA GEIGY   30 MG/VIAL   N20036 001   OCT 31, 1991

PANCURONIUM BROMIDE
INJECTABLE; INJECTION
PANCURONIUM
ELKINS SINN
AP 1MG/ML   N72058 001   MAR 23, 1988
             N72059 001   MAR 23, 1988
AP 2MG/ML   N72060 001   MAR 23, 1988

PANCURONIUM BROMIDE
ABBOTT
AP 1MG/ML   N72320 001   JAN 19, 1989
AP 2MG/ML   N72321 001   JAN 19, 1989
ASTRA
AP 1MG/ML   N72210 001   MAR 31, 1988
             N72211 001   MAR 31, 1988
AP 2MG/ML   N72212 001   MAR 31, 1988
             N72213 001   MAR 31, 1988
GENSIA
AP 1MG/ML   N72759 001   JUL 31, 1990
AP 2MG/ML   N72760 001   JUL 31, 1990
PAVULON
ORGANON
AP 1MG/ML   N17015 002
AP 2MG/ML   N17015 001

PARAMETHADIONE
CAPSULE; ORAL
PARADIONE
ABBOTT   150 MG   N06800 003
         300 MG   N06800 001

PARAMETHASONE ACETATE
TABLET; ORAL
HALDRONE
LILLY +   1 MG   N12772 005
          2 MG   N12772 006

PARGYLINE HYDROCHLORIDE
TABLET; ORAL
EUTONYL
ABBOTT +   10 MG   N13448 002
           25 MG   N13448 003

Prescription Drug Products (continued)

PAROMOMYCIN SULFATE
CAPSULE; ORAL
HUMATIN

+ PARKE DAVIS	EQ 250 MG BASE	N60521 001
	EQ 250 MG BASE	N62310 001

PEGADEMASE BOVINE
INJECTABLE; INJECTION
ADAGEN

ENZON	250 UNITS/ML	N19818 001	MAR 21, 1990

PEMOLINE
TABLET; ORAL
CYLERT

ABBOTT	18.75 MG	N16832 001
+	37.5 MG	N16832 002
	75 MG	N16832 003

TABLET, CHEWABLE; ORAL
CYLERT

+ ABBOTT	37.5 MG	N17703 001

PENBUTOLOL SULFATE
TABLET; ORAL
LEVATOL

+ REED AND CARNRICK	20 MG	N18976 004	JAN 05, 1989

PENICILLAMINE
CAPSULE; ORAL
CUPRIMINE

MSD	125 MG	N19853 002
+	250 MG	N19853 001

TABLET; ORAL
DEPEN 250

+ WALLACE	250 MG	N19854 001

PENICILLIN G BENZATHINE
INJECTABLE; INJECTION
BICILLIN L-A

BC WYETH AYERST	600,000 UNITS/ML	N50141 001
+	300,000 UNITS/ML	N50131 001
	300,000 UNITS/ML	N50141 003

PERMAPEN

PFIZER	600,000 UNITS/ML	N60014 001

TABLET; ORAL
BICILLIN

BC + WYETH AYERST	200,000 UNITS	N50128 001

PENICILLIN G BENZATHINE; PENICILLIN G PROCAINE
INJECTABLE; INJECTION
BICILLIN C-R

WYETH AYERST	150,000 UNITS/ML;150,000 UNITS/ML	N50138 002
	300,000 UNITS/ML;300,000 UNITS/ML	N50138 001

BICILLIN C-R 900/300

WYETH AYERST	900,000 UNITS/2 ML;300,000 UNITS/2 ML	N50138 003

PENICILLIN G POTASSIUM
INJECTABLE; INJECTION
PENICILLIN G POTASSIUM

AP	LILLY	1,000,000 UNITS/VIAL	N60384 002	
AP		5,000,000 UNITS/VIAL	N60384 001	
AP		20,000,000 UNITS/VIAL	N60384 005	
		20,000,000 UNITS/VIAL	N60601 001	
		200,000 UNITS/VIAL	N60384 004	
		500,000 UNITS/VIAL	N60384 003	
		1,000,000 UNITS/VIAL	N62991 001	SEP 13, 1988
			N62991 002	SEP 13, 1988
AP	MARSAM	5,000,000 UNITS/VIAL	N62991 003	SEP 13, 1988
AP		10,000,000 UNITS/VIAL	N62991 004	SEP 13, 1988
AP		20,000,000 UNITS/VIAL	N60074 003	
AP	PFIZER	20,000,000 UNITS/VIAL	N60362 001	
AP	SQUIBB	1,000,000 UNITS/VIAL	N60362 003	
AP		5,000,000 UNITS/VIAL	N60362 004	
AP		10,000,000 UNITS/VIAL	N60362 002	
AP		20,000,000 UNITS/VIAL		

PENICILLIN G POTASSIUM IN PLASTIC CONTAINER

	BAXTER	20,000 UNITS/ML	N50638 001	JUN 25, 1990
		40,000 UNITS/ML	N50638 002	JUN 25, 1990
		60,000 UNITS/ML	N50638 003	JUN 25, 1990

PFIZERPEN

AP PFIZER	1,000,000 UNITS/VIAL	N60657 001
AP	5,000,000 UNITS/VIAL	N60657 002
AP	20,000,000 UNITS/VIAL	N60657 003

POWDER FOR RECONSTITUTION; ORAL
PENICILLIN

AA BIOCRAFT	200,000 UNITS/5 ML	N60307 002
AA	400,000 UNITS/5 ML	N60307 004

PENICILLIN-2

BIOCRAFT	250,000 UNITS/5 ML	N60307 003

PENTIDS '200'

AA SQUIBB	200,000 UNITS/5 ML	N62149 001

PENTIDS '400'

AA SQUIBB	400,000 UNITS/5 ML	N62149 002

PFIZERPEN G

AA PFIZER	400,000 UNITS/5 ML	N60587 001

Prescription Drug Products (continued)

PENICILLIN G POTASSIUM (continued)

TABLET; ORAL
PENICILLIN G POTASSIUM

	Firm/Name	Strength	Number
AB	BIOCRAFT	200,000 UNITS	N60306 001
AB		250,000 UNITS	N60306 002
AB		400,000 UNITS	N60306 003
AB		500,000 UNITS	N60306 004
AB	DISTA	250,000 UNITS	N60403 001
AB	MYLAN	200,000 UNITS	N60781 001
AB		250,000 UNITS	N60781 002
AB		500,000 UNITS	N60781 003
AB		800,000 UNITS	N60781 005
AB		400,000 UNITS	N60781 004
AB	+ SQUIBB	250,000 UNITS	N60392 003
AB	WYETH AYERST	250,000 UNITS	N60413 001
AB		250,000 UNITS	N60413 002
AB		400,000 UNITS	N60413 003
AB	ZENITH	400,000 UNITS	N60073 004
AB	PENTIDS '200' SQUIBB	200,000 UNITS	N62155 001
AB	PENTIDS '250' SQUIBB	250,000 UNITS	N62155 002
AB	PENTIDS '400' SQUIBB	400,000 UNITS	N60392 004
AB		400,000 UNITS	N62155 003
AB	PENTIDS '800' SQUIBB	800,000 UNITS	N60392 005
AB		800,000 UNITS	N62155 004
AB	PFIZERPEN G PFIZER	200,000 UNITS	N60075 003
AB		250,000 UNITS	N60075 004
AB		400,000 UNITS	N60075 005
AB		800,000 UNITS	N60075 006
AB	+	50,000 UNITS	N60075 001
AB		100,000 UNITS	N60075 002

PENICILLIN G SODIUM

INJECTABLE; INJECTION
PENICILLIN G SODIUM

Firm/Name	Strength	Number	Date
MARSAM	5,000,000 UNITS/VIAL	N63014 001	SEP 13, 1988
UPJOHN	1,000,000 UNITS/VIAL	N61046 001	

PENICILLIN V

POWDER FOR RECONSTITUTION; ORAL
V-CILLIN

	Firm/Name	Strength	Number
	+ LILLY	125 MG/0.6 ML	N60002 001

PENICILLIN V POTASSIUM

POWDER FOR RECONSTITUTION; ORAL

	Firm/Name	Strength	Number	Date
	BEEPEN-VK			
AA	BEECHAM	EQ 125 MG BASE/5 ML	N62270 001	
AA		EQ 250 MG BASE/5 ML	N62270 002	
	BETAPEN-VK			
AA	BRISTOL	EQ 125 MG BASE/5 ML	N61149 001	
AA		EQ 250 MG BASE/5 ML	N61149 002	
	LEDERCILLIN VK			
AA	LEDERLE	EQ 125 MG BASE/5 ML	N60136 001	
AA		EQ 250 MG BASE/5 ML	N60136 002	
	PEN-VEE K			
AA	WYETH AYERST	EQ 125 MG BASE/5 ML	N60007 001	
AA		EQ 250 MG BASE/5 ML	N60007 002	
	PENICILLIN V POTASSIUM			
AA	CLONMEL	EQ 125 MG BASE/5 ML	N62981 001	FEB 10, 1989
AA		EQ 250 MG BASE/5 ML	N62981 002	FEB 10, 1989
AA	COPANOS	EQ 125 MG BASE/5 ML	N61529 001	
AA		EQ 250 MG BASE/5 ML	N61529 002	
AA	MYLAN	EQ 125 MG BASE/5 ML	N61624 002	
AA		EQ 250 MG BASE/5 ML	N61624 001	
	PENICILLIN-VK			
AA	BIOCRAFT	EQ 125 MG BASE/5 ML	N60456 001	
AA		EQ 250 MG BASE/5 ML	N60456 002	
	PFIZERPEN VK			
AA	PFIZER	EQ 125 MG BASE/5 ML	N61815 001	
AA		EQ 250 MG BASE/5 ML	N61815 002	
	V-CILLIN K			
AA	LILLY	EQ 125 MG BASE/5 ML	N60004 001	
AA		EQ 250 MG BASE/5 ML	N60004 002	
	VEETIDS '125'			
AA	SQUIBB	EQ 125 MG BASE/5 ML	N61206 001	
AA		EQ 125 MG BASE/5 ML	N62153 001	
	VEETIDS '250'			
AA	SQUIBB	EQ 250 MG BASE/5 ML	N61206 002	
AA		EQ 250 MG BASE/5 ML	N62153 002	

PENICILLIN G PROCAINE

INJECTABLE; INJECTION

	Firm/Name	Strength	Number
	DURACILLIN A.S.		
AP	LILLY	300,000 UNITS/ML	N60093 001
	PENICILLIN G PROCAINE		
AP	PFIZER	300,000 UNITS/VIAL	N60099 001
		1,500,000 UNITS/VIAL	N60099 002
	PFIZERPEN-AS		
AP	PFIZER	300,000 UNITS/ML	N60286 001
		600,000 UNITS/ML	N60286 002
	WYCILLIN		
AP	WYETH AYERST	300,000 UNITS/ML	N60101 002
AP		600,000 UNITS/ML	N60101 001

PENICILLIN G PROCAINE; *MULTIPLE*
SEE PENICILLIN G BENZATHINE; PENICILLIN G PROCAINE

Prescription Drug Products (continued)

PENICILLIN V POTASSIUM (continued)

TABLET; ORAL

TE	Product / Manufacturer	Strength	Appl. No.	Date
	BEEPEN-VK			
AB	BEECHAM	EQ 250 MG BASE	N62273 001	
AB	BEECHAM	EQ 500 MG BASE	N62273 002	
	BETAPEN-VK			
AB	BRISTOL	EQ 250 MG BASE	N61150 001	
AB	BRISTOL	EQ 250 MG BASE	N61411 001	
AB	BRISTOL	EQ 500 MG BASE	N61150 002	
AB	BRISTOL	EQ 500 MG BASE	N61411 002	
	LEDERCILLIN VK			
AB	LEDERLE	EQ 250 MG BASE	N60134 001	
AB	LEDERLE	EQ 500 MG BASE	N60134 002	
	PEN-VEE K			
AB	WYETH AYERST	EQ 250 MG BASE	N60006 002	
AB	WYETH AYERST	EQ 500 MG BASE	N60006 003	
	PENICILLIN V POTASSIUM			
AB	CLONMEL	EQ 250 MG BASE	N62936 001	NOV 25, 1988
AB	CLONMEL	EQ 500 MG BASE	N62935 001	NOV 23, 1988
AB	COPANOS	EQ 250 MG BASE	N61528 001	
AB	COPANOS	EQ 500 MG BASE	N61528 002	
AB	MYLAN	EQ 250 MG BASE	N61530 001	
AB	MYLAN	EQ 500 MG BASE	N61530 002	
AB	ZENITH	EQ 125 MG BASE	N60518 001	
AB	ZENITH	EQ 250 MG BASE	N60518 002	
AB	ZENITH	EQ 500 MG BASE	N60518 003	
	PENICILLIN-VK			
AB	BIOCRAFT	EQ 250 MG BASE	N60711 002	
AB	BIOCRAFT	EQ 500 MG BASE	N60711 003	
	PFIZERPEN VK			
AB	PFIZER	EQ 250 MG BASE	N61836 001	
AB	PFIZER	EQ 500 MG BASE	N61836 002	
	UTICILLIN VK			
AB	UPJOHN	EQ 250 MG BASE	N61651 001	
AB	UPJOHN	EQ 500 MG BASE	N61651 002	
	V-CILLIN K			
AB+	+ LILLY	EQ 125 MG BASE	N60003 001	
AB+	+	EQ 250 MG BASE	N60003 002	
AB+	+	EQ 500 MG BASE	N60003 003	
	VEETIDS '250'			
AB	SQUIBB	EQ 250 MG BASE	N61164 001	
AB	SQUIBB	EQ 250 MG BASE	N62156 002	
	VEETIDS '500'			
AB	SQUIBB	EQ 500 MG BASE	N61164 002	
AB	SQUIBB	EQ 500 MG BASE	N62156 001	

PENTAGASTRIN

INJECTABLE; INJECTION

TE	Product / Manufacturer	Strength	Appl. No.
	PEPTAVLON		
	WYETH AYERST	0.25 MG/ML	N17048 001

PENTAMIDINE ISETHIONATE

INJECTABLE; INJECTION

TE	Product / Manufacturer	Strength	Appl. No.	Date
	PENTAM 300			
ΔP	FUJISAWA	300 MG/VIAL	N19264 001	OCT 16, 1984
	PENTAMIDINE ISETHIONATE			
ΔP	ABBOTT	300 MG/VIAL	N73479 001	JUN 30, 1992

POWDER FOR RECONSTITUTION; INHALATION

TE	Product / Manufacturer	Strength	Appl. No.	Date
	NEBUPENT			
	FUJISAWA	300 MG/VIAL	N19887 001	JUN 15, 1989

PENTAZOCINE HYDROCHLORIDE; *MULTIPLE*

SEE ACETAMINOPHEN; PENTAZOCINE HYDROCHLORIDE

SEE ASPIRIN; PENTAZOCINE HYDROCHLORIDE

SEE NALOXONE HYDROCHLORIDE; PENTAZOCINE HYDROCHLORIDE

PENTAZOCINE LACTATE

INJECTABLE; INJECTION

TE	Product / Manufacturer	Strength	Appl. No.
	TALWIN		
	STERLING	EQ 30 MG BASE/ML	N16194 001

PENTETATE CALCIUM TRISODIUM YB-169

INJECTABLE; INJECTION

TE	Product / Manufacturer	Strength	Appl. No.
	YTTERBIUM YB 169 DTPA		
	3M	2 MCI/ML	N17518 001

PENTOBARBITAL

ELIXIR; ORAL

TE	Product / Manufacturer	Strength	Appl. No.
	NEMBUTAL		
	ABBOTT	18.2 MG/5 ML	N83244 001

PENTOBARBITAL SODIUM

CAPSULE; ORAL

TE	Product / Manufacturer	Strength	Appl. No.
	NEMBUTAL SODIUM		
AA	ABBOTT	50 MG	N84093 001
AA	ABBOTT	100 MG	N83245 001
	ABBOTT	30 MG	N84095 001
	PENTOBARBITAL SODIUM		
AA	LANNETT	50 MG	N85937 001
AA	LANNETT	100 MG	N85915 001
	SODIUM PENTOBARBITAL		
AA	HALSEY	100 MG	N84677 001
AA	ICN	100 MG	N83264 001
AA	ZENITH	50 MG	N83461 001
AA	ZENITH	100 MG	N83461 002

Prescription Drug Products (continued)

PENTOBARBITAL SODIUM (continued)

INJECTABLE; INJECTION

NEMBUTAL SODIUM
- ΔP   ABBOTT   50 MG/ML   N83246 001

PENTOBARBITAL SODIUM
- ΔP   ELKINS SINN   50 MG/ML   N83270 001

SODIUM PENTOBARBITAL
- ΔP   WYETH AYERST   50 MG/ML   N83261 001

SUPPOSITORY; RECTAL

NEMBUTAL
- + ABBOTT   30 MG   N83247 001   JAN 25, 1982
- +   60 MG   N83247 002   JAN 25, 1982
- +   120 MG   N83247 003   JAN 25, 1982
- +   200 MG   N83247 004   JAN 25, 1982

PENTOSTATIN

INJECTABLE; INJECTION

NIPENT
- PARKE DAVIS   10 MG/VIAL   N20122 001   OCT 11, 1991

PENTOXIFYLLINE

TABLET, EXTENDED RELEASE; ORAL

TRENTAL
- + HOECHST ROUSSEL   400 MG   N18631 001   AUG 30, 1984

PERGOLIDE MESYLATE

TABLET; ORAL

PERMAX
- LILLY   EQ 0.05 MG BASE   N19385 001   DEC 30, 1988
-   EQ 0.25 MG BASE   N19385 002   DEC 30, 1988
- +   EQ 1 MG BASE   N19385 003   DEC 30, 1988

PERMETHRIN

CREAM; TOPICAL

ELIMITE
- BURROUGHS WELLCOME   5%   N19855 001   AUG 25, 1989

LOTION; TOPICAL

NIX
- + BURROUGHS WELLCOME   1%   N19435 001   MAR 31, 1986

PERPHENAZINE

CONCENTRATE; ORAL

TRILAFON
- SCHERING   16 MG/5 ML   N11557 001

INJECTABLE; INJECTION

TRILAFON
- SCHERING   5 MG/ML   N11213 002

TABLET; ORAL

PERPHENAZINE
- ΔB   GENEVA   2 MG   N89683 001   DEC 08, 1988
- ΔB   4 MG   N89684 001   DEC 08, 1988
- ΔB   8 MG   N89685 001   DEC 08, 1988
- ΔB   16 MG   N89686 001   DEC 08, 1988
- ΔB   ZENITH   2 MG   N89707 001   SEP 10, 1987
- ΔB   4 MG   N89708 001   SEP 10, 1987
- ΔB   8 MG   N89456 001   SEP 10, 1987
- ΔB   16 MG   N89457 001   SEP 10, 1987

TRILAFON
- ΔB   SCHERING   2 MG   N10775 001
- ΔB   4 MG   N10775 002
- ΔB   8 MG   N10775 003
- ΔB   16 MG   N10775 004

TABLET, EXTENDED RELEASE; ORAL

TRILAFON
- + SCHERING   8 MG   N11361 002

PERPHENAZINE; *MULTIPLE*

SEE AMITRIPTYLINE HYDROCHLORIDE; PERPHENAZINE

PHENACEMIDE

TABLET; ORAL

PHENURONE
- + ABBOTT   500 MG   N07707 001

PHENAZOPYRIDINE HYDROCHLORIDE; SULFAMETHOXAZOLE

TABLET; ORAL

AZO GANTANOL
- + ROCHE   100 MG;500 MG   N13294 001   SEP 10, 1987

PHENAZOPYRIDINE HYDROCHLORIDE; SULFISOXAZOLE

TABLET; ORAL

AZO GANTRISIN
- + ROCHE   50 MG;500 MG   N19358 001   AUG 31, 1990

Prescription Drug Products (continued)

PHENDIMETRAZINE TARTRATE

CAPSULE; ORAL

	PHENAZINE		
AA	MAST	35 MG	N86523 001
AA		35 MG	N86524 001
AA		35 MG	N86525 001
	PHENDIMETRAZINE TARTRATE		
AA	EON LABS	35 MG	N85633 001
AA		35 MG	N85694 001
AA		35 MG	N85695 001
AA		35 MG	N85702 001
	STATOBEX		
AA	LEMMON	35 MG	N85507 001
	X-TROZINE		
AA	REXAR	35 MG	N87394 001
			SEP 22, 1982

CAPSULE, EXTENDED RELEASE; ORAL

	PHENDIMETRAZINE TARTRATE		
BC	EON LABS	105 MG	N18074 001
BC	+ GENEVA	105 MG	N87378 001
BC	GRAHAM LABS	105 MG	N87214 001
			MAY 26, 1982
BC		105 MG	N88020 001
BC		105 MG	N88021 001
			AUG 16, 1982
BC		105 MG	SEP 21, 1982
BC		105 MG	N88028 001
BC		105 MG	N88062 001
			AUG 16, 1982
BC		105 MG	N88063 001
			SEP 13, 1982
BC		105 MG	N88111 001
			SEP 10, 1982
			OCT 18, 1982
	X-TROZINE L.A.		
BC	REXAR	105 MG	N87371 001
			AUG 24, 1982

TABLET; ORAL

	ADPHEN		
AA	FERNDALE	35 MG	N83655 001
	BONTRIL PDM		
AA	CARNRICK	35 MG	N85272 001
	CAM-METRAZINE		
AA	CAMALL	35 MG	N83922 001
AA		35 MG	N85318 001
AA		35 MG	N85320 001
AA		35 MG	N85321 001
AA		35 MG	N85511 001
AA		35 MG	N85756 001
	MELFIAT		
AA	SOLVAY	35 MG	N83790 002
	METRA		
AA	FOREST PHARMS	35 MG	N83754 001
	PHENAZINE		
AA	MAST	35 MG	N87305 001
	PHENAZINE-35		
AA	CAMALL	35 MG	N85512 001

PHENDIMETRAZINE TARTRATE (continued)

TABLET; ORAL

	PHENDIMETRAZINE TARTRATE		
AA	ANABOLICS	35 MG	N86020 001
AA	CAMALL	35 MG	N85761 001
AA		35 MG	N85941 001
			JUN 27, 1983
AA	EON LABS	35 MG	N85402 001
AA		35 MG	N85830 001
AA	FERNDALE	35 MG	N86834 001
			SEP 15, 1983
AA	GENEVA	35 MG	N83993 001
AA	INWOOD	35 MG	N84740 001
AA		35 MG	N84741 001
AA		35 MG	N84742 001
AA		35 MG	N84743 001
AA		35 MG	N84138 001
AA		35 MG	N84141 001
AA	KV	35 MG	N85525 001
AA		35 MG	N85914 001
AA		35 MG	N89452 001
			OCT 30, 1991
AA	MFG CHEMISTS	35 MG	N84399 001
AA	MIKART	35 MG	N85697 001
AA		35 MG	N85497 001
AA	PHARM BASICS	35 MG	N85588 001
AA	PRIVATE FORM	35 MG	N85611 001
AA	VITARINE	35 MG	
	ZENITH		
	PLEGINE		
AA	WYETH AYERST	35 MG	N12248 001
	STATOBEX		
AA	LEMMON	35 MG	N86013 001
	X-TROZINE		
AA	REXAR	35 MG	N86550 001
AA		35 MG	N86551 001
AA		35 MG	N86552 001
AA		35 MG	N86553 001
AA		35 MG	N86554 001

PHENELZINE SULFATE

TABLET; ORAL

	NARDIL		
+	PARKE DAVIS	EQ 15 MG BASE	N11909 002

PHENMETRAZINE HYDROCHLORIDE

TABLET, EXTENDED RELEASE; ORAL

	PRELUDIN		
+	BOEHRINGER INGELHEIM	75 MG	N11752 003

PHENOXYBENZAMINE HYDROCHLORIDE

CAPSULE; ORAL

	DIBENZYLINE		
+	SKF	10 MG	N08708 001

Prescription Drug Products (continued)

PHENSUXIMIDE

CAPSULE; ORAL

TE	Brand / Firm	Strength	Appl. No.	Date
	MILONTIN			
	+ PARKE DAVIS	500 MG	N08855 004	

PHENTERMINE HYDROCHLORIDE

CAPSULE; ORAL

TE	Brand / Firm	Strength	Appl. No.	Date
	ADIPEX-P			
AA	LEMMON	30 MG	N86911 001	
AA		37.5 MG	N88023 001	
	DAPEX-37.5			
AA	FERNDALE	37.5 MG		AUG 02, 1983
	FASTIN			
AA	BEECHAM	30 MG	N88414 001	OCT 19, 1983
	OBESTIN-30			
AA	FERNDALE	30 MG	N17352 001	
	OBY-TRIM			
AA	REXAR	30 MG	N87144 001	
	ONA-MAST			
AA	MAST	30 MG	N87764 001	MAR 18, 1982
AA		30 MG	N86511 001	
	PHENTERMINE HCL			
AA	CAMALL	30 MG	N86516 001	
AA		15 MG	N86735 001	
AA		30 MG	N85411 001	
AA		30 MG	N85417 001	
AA		30 MG	N86732 002	
AA		30 MG	N87215 001	
AA		37.5 MG	N87226 001	
AA		37.5 MG	N87915 001	DEC 22, 1983
AA		37.5 MG	N87918 001	DEC 22, 1983
AA		37.5 MG	N87930 001	OCT 14, 1983
AA		37.5 MG	N88610 001	JUN 04, 1984
AA		37.5 MG	N88611 001	JUN 04, 1984
AA		37.5 MG	N88625 001	AUG 23, 1984
		18.75 MG	N88576 001	MAY 23, 1984
	EON LABS			
AA		15 MG	N87301 001	
AA		30 MG	N87190 001	
AA		30 MG	N87208 001	
AA		30 MG	N87223 001	
	+ LANNETT	30 MG	N87022 001	FEB 03, 1983

PHENTERMINE HYDROCHLORIDE (continued)

CAPSULE; ORAL

TE	Brand / Firm	Strength	Appl. No.	Date
	PHENTERMINE HCL			
AA	LEMMON	30 MG	N87777 001	NOV 01, 1985
AA		30 MG	N88612 001	
AA		30 MG	N88613 001	APR 04, 1984
AA		30 MG	N88614 001	APR 09, 1984
AA	PHARM BASICS	30 MG	N84487 001	APR 09, 1984
AA		30 MG	N88430 001	APR 09, 1982
AA	VITARINE	30 MG	N88797 001	MAR 27, 1984
AA		30 MG	N86945 001	DEC 10, 1984
AA	ZENITH	30 MG	N86329 001	JUL 20, 1983

TABLET; ORAL

TE	Brand / Firm	Strength	Appl. No.	Date
	ADIPEX-P			
AA	LEMMON	37.5 MG	N85128 001	
	ONA MAST			
AA	MAST	8 MG	N86260 001	
	PHENTERMINE HCL			
AA	CAMALL	8 MG	N83923 001	
AA		8 MG	N85319 001	
AA		37.5 MG	N87805 001	DEC 06, 1982
AA		37.5 MG	N88596 001	APR 04, 1984
AA	PHARM BASICS	8 MG	N83804 001	
AA		37.5 MG	N88910 001	JUL 17, 1985
AA		37.5 MG	N88917 001	JUL 17, 1985
	TORA			
AA	SOLVAY	8 MG	N84035 001	
	UMI-PEX 30			
	FERNDALE	30 MG	N88605 001	SEP 28, 1987

PHENTERMINE RESIN COMPLEX

CAPSULE, EXTENDED RELEASE; ORAL

Brand / Firm	Strength	Appl. No.
IONAMIN-15		
FISONS	EQ 15 MG BASE	N11613 004
IONAMIN-30		
+ FISONS	EQ 30 MG BASE	N11613 002

PHENTOLAMINE MESYLATE

INJECTABLE; INJECTION

Brand / Firm	Strength	Appl. No.
REGITINE		
CIBA	5 MG/VIAL	N08278 003

Prescription Drug Products *(continued)*

PHENYLBUTAZONE

CAPSULE; ORAL

	Firm	Strength	Application No.	Date
	BUTAZOLIDIN			
+	GEIGY	100 MG	N08319 009	
	PHENYLBUTAZONE			
AB	BARR	100 MG	N88994 001	DEC 04, 1985
AB	CHELSEA	100 MG	N88756 001	DEC 17, 1982
AB	GENEVA	100 MG	N87774 001	JUN 16, 1982

TABLET; ORAL

	Firm	Strength	Application No.	Date
	BUTAZOLIDIN			
+	GEIGY	100 MG	N08319 008	
	PHENYLBUTAZONE			
AB	BARR	100 MG	N88863 001	DEC 04, 1985
AB	CHELSEA	100 MG	N86151 001	
AB	DANBURY	100 MG	N87674 001	APR 21, 1982
AB	GENEVA	100 MG	N84339 001	

PHENYLEPHRINE BITARTRATE; *MULTIPLE*

SEE ISOPROTERENOL HYDROCHLORIDE; PHENYLEPHRINE BITARTRATE

PHENYLEPHRINE HYDROCHLORIDE; *MULTIPLE*

SEE CODEINE PHOSPHATE; PHENYLEPHRINE HYDROCHLORIDE; PROMETHAZINE HYDROCHLORIDE

SEE CYCLOPENTOLATE HYDROCHLORIDE; PHENYLEPHRINE HYDROCHLORIDE

PHENYLEPHRINE HYDROCHLORIDE; PROMETHAZINE HYDROCHLORIDE

SYRUP; ORAL

	Firm	Strength	Application No.	Date
	PHENERGAN VC			
AA	WYETH AYERST	5 MG/5 ML;6.25 MG/5 ML	N08604 003	APR 02, 1984
	PHERAZINE VC			
AA	HALSEY	5 MG/5 ML;6.25 MG/5 ML	N88868 001	MAR 02, 1987
	PROMETH VC PLAIN			
AA	BARRE	5 MG/5 ML;6.25 MG/5 ML	N88761 001	NOV 08, 1984
	PROMETHAZINE VC PLAIN			
AA	CENCI	5 MG/5 ML;6.25 MG/5 ML	N88815 001	NOV 22, 1985
AA	PHARM BASICS	5 MG/5 ML;6.25 MG/5 ML	N88897 001	JAN 04, 1985

PHENYLEPHRINE HYDROCHLORIDE; PYRILAMINE MALEATE

SOLUTION/DROPS; OPHTHALMIC

	Firm	Strength	Application No.	Date
	PREFRIN-A			
	ALLERGAN	0.12%;0.1%	N07953 001	

PHENYLPROPANOLAMINE HYDROCHLORIDE; *MULTIPLE*

SEE BROMPHENIRAMINE MALEATE; CODEINE PHOSPHATE; PHENYLPROPANOLAMINE HYDROCHLORIDE

SEE CHLORPHENIRAMINE MALEATE; PHENYLPROPANOLAMINE HYDROCHLORIDE

SEE HYDROCODONE BITARTRATE; PHENYLPROPANOLAMINE HYDROCHLORIDE

PHENYTOIN

SUSPENSION; ORAL

	Firm	Strength	Application No.	Date
	DILANTIN-125			
+	PARKE DAVIS	125 MG/5 ML	N08762 001	
	DILANTIN-30			
	PARKE DAVIS	30 MG/5 ML	N08762 002	

TABLET, CHEWABLE; ORAL

	Firm	Strength	Application No.	Date
	DILANTIN			
+	PARKE DAVIS	50 MG	N84427 001	

PHENYTOIN SODIUM

INJECTABLE; INJECTION

	Firm	Strength	Application No.	Date
	DILANTIN			
AP	PARKE DAVIS	50 MG/ML	N10151 001	
	PHENYTOIN			
AP	ELKINS SINN	50 MG/ML	N84307 001	
	PHENYTOIN SODIUM			
AP	ABBOTT	50 MG/ML	N89521 001	MAR 17, 1987
AP	LYPHOMED	50 MG/ML	N89003 001	MAY 31, 1985
AP	MARSAM	50 MG/ML	N89501 001	OCT 13, 1987
AP	SMITH NEPHEW	50 MG/ML	N88519 001	DEC 19, 1984
	SOLOPAK		N88520 001	DEC 17, 1984
AP	STERIS	50 MG/ML	N85434 001	
AP	WINTHROP	50 MG/ML	N89744 001	DEC 18, 1987

PHENYTOIN SODIUM, EXTENDED

CAPSULE; ORAL

	Firm	Strength	Application No.	Date
	DILANTIN			
+	PARKE DAVIS	30 MG	N84349 001	
		100 MG	N84349 002	

Prescription Drug Products *(continued)*

PHENYTOIN SODIUM, PROMPT
CAPSULE; ORAL

DIPHENYLAN SODIUM

BX	LANNETT	100 MG	N80857 002
		30 MG	N80857 001

PROMPT PHENYTOIN SODIUM

BX	+ DANBURY	100 MG	N80905 001
BX	ZENITH	100 MG	N80259 001

PHOSPHORIC ACID; *MULTIPLE*

SEE AMINO ACIDS: CALCIUM ACETATE: GLYCERIN: MAGNESIUM ACETATE: PHOSPHORIC ACID: POTASSIUM CHLORIDE: SODIUM ACETATE: SODIUM CHLORIDE

SEE AMINO ACIDS: MAGNESIUM ACETATE: PHOSPHORIC ACID: POTASSIUM ACETATE: POTASSIUM CHLORIDE: SODIUM ACETATE

SEE AMINO ACIDS: MAGNESIUM ACETATE: PHOSPHORIC ACID: POTASSIUM ACETATE: SODIUM CHLORIDE

SEE AMINO ACIDS: MAGNESIUM ACETATE: PHOSPHORIC ACID: POTASSIUM CHLORIDE: SODIUM ACETATE: SODIUM CHLORIDE

PHYTONADIONE
INJECTABLE; INJECTION

AQUAMEPHYTON

BP	MSD	1 MG/0.5 ML	N12223 002
BP		10 MG/ML	N12223 001

KONAKION

BP	ROCHE	1 MG/0.5 ML	N11745 001
BP	+	10 MG/ML	N11745 003

PHYTONADIONE

BP	BEECHAM	1 MG/0.5 ML	N84060 001
BP		10 MG/ML	N84060 002
BP	INTL MEDICATION	1 MG/0.5 ML	N83722 001

VITAMIN K1

BP	ABBOTT	1 MG/0.5 ML	N87954 001 JUL 25, 1983
			N87955 001 JUL 25, 1983
BP		10 MG/ML	N10104 003

TABLET; ORAL

MEPHYTON

	+ MSD	5 MG	N17431 001

PILOCARPINE
INSERT, EXTENDED RELEASE; OPHTHALMIC

OCUSERT PILO-20

	+ ALZA	5 MG	N17431 001

OCUSERT PILO-40

	+ ALZA	11 MG	N17548 001

PILOCARPINE HYDROCHLORIDE
GEL; OPHTHALMIC

PILOPINE HS

	+ ALCON	4%	N18796 001 OCT 01, 1984

PIMOZIDE
TABLET; ORAL

ORAP

	+ LEMMON	2 MG	N17473 001 JUL 31, 1984

PINACIDIL
CAPSULE, EXTENDED RELEASE; ORAL

PINDAC

	+ LEO	12.5 MG	N19456 001 DEC 28, 1989
	+	25 MG	N19456 002 DEC 28, 1989

PINDOLOL
TABLET; ORAL

VISKEN

	SANDOZ	5 MG	N18285 001 SEP 03, 1982
	+	10 MG	N18285 002 SEP 03, 1982

PIPECURONIUM BROMIDE
INJECTABLE; INJECTION

ARDUAN

	ORGANON	10 MG/VIAL	N19638 001 JUN 26, 1990

PIPERACILLIN SODIUM
INJECTABLE; INJECTION

PIPRACIL

	LEDERLE	EQ 2 GM BASE/VIAL	N50545 002
		EQ 2 GM BASE/VIAL	N62750 001 OCT 13, 1987
		EQ 3 GM BASE/VIAL	N50545 003
		EQ 3 GM BASE/VIAL	N62750 002 OCT 13, 1987
		EQ 4 GM BASE/VIAL	N50545 004
		EQ 4 GM BASE/VIAL	N62750 003 OCT 13, 1987

Prescription Drug Products *(continued)*

PIPERAZINE CITRATE

SYRUP; ORAL

MULTIFUGE			
AA BLULINE	EQ 500 MG BASE/5 ML	N09452 001	
PIPERAZINE CITRATE			
AA LANNETT	EQ 500 MG BASE/5 ML	N80963 001	
AA LUITPOLD	EQ 500 MG BASE/5 ML	N80671 001	
VERMIDOL			
AA SOLVAY	EQ 500 MG BASE/5 ML	N80992 001	

TABLET; ORAL

PIPERAZINE CITRATE			
RICHLYN	EQ 250 MG BASE	N80874 001	

PIPOBROMAN

TABLET; ORAL

VERCYTE			
+ ABBOTT	25 MG	N16245 002	

PIRBUTEROL ACETATE

AEROSOL, METERED; INHALATION

MAXAIR			
+ 3M	EQ 0.2 MG BASE/INH	N19009 001	DEC 30, 1986

PIROXICAM

CAPSULE; ORAL

FELDENE			
AB PFIZER	10 MG	N18147 002	APR 06, 1982
		N18147 001	
AB +	20 MG	N18147 003	APR 06, 1982
PIROXICAM			
AB COPLEY	10 MG	N74103 001	AUG 28, 1992
AB	20 MG	N74103 002	AUG 28, 1992
AB MYLAN	10 MG	N74102 001	JUL 31, 1992
AB	20 MG	N74102 002	JUL 31, 1992
AB SCHIAPPARELLI SEARLE	10 MG	N74036 001	MAY 29, 1992
AB	20 MG	N74036 002	MAY 29, 1992

PLICAMYCIN

INJECTABLE; INJECTION

MITHRACIN			
PFIZER	2.5 MG/VIAL	N50109 001	

PODOFILOX

SOLUTION; TOPICAL

CONDYLOX			
OCLASSEN	0.5%	N19795 001	DEC 13, 1990

POLYESTRADIOL PHOSPHATE

INJECTABLE; INJECTION

ESTRADURIN			
WYETH AYERST	40 MG/AMP	N10753 001	

POLYETHYLENE GLYCOL 3350; POTASSIUM CHLORIDE; SODIUM BICARBONATE; SODIUM CHLORIDE

POWDER FOR RECONSTITUTION; ORAL

NULYTELY			
BRAINTREE	420 GM/BOT;1.48 GM/BOT;5.72 GM/BOT;11.2 GM/BOT	N19797 001	APR 22, 1991

POLYETHYLENE GLYCOL 3350; POTASSIUM CHLORIDE; SODIUM BICARBONATE; SODIUM CHLORIDE; SODIUM SULFATE

SOLUTION; ORAL

OCL			
ABBOTT	6 GM/100 ML;.75 MG/100 ML;168 MG/100 ML;146 MG/100 ML;1.29 GM/100 ML	N19284 001	APR 30, 1986

POLYETHYLENE GLYCOL 3350; POTASSIUM CHLORIDE; SODIUM BICARBONATE; SODIUM CHLORIDE; SODIUM SULFATE, ANHYDROUS

POWDER FOR RECONSTITUTION; ORAL

CO-LAV			
AA COPLEY	240 GM/BOT;2.98 GM/BOT;6.72 GM/BOT;5.84 GM/BOT;22.72 GM/BOT	N73428 001	JAN 28, 1992
COLOVAGE			
AA DYNAPHARM	227.1 GM/PACKET;2.82 GM/PACKET;6.36 GM/PACKET;5.53 GM/PACKET;21.5 GM/PACKET	N71320 001	APR 20, 1988

Prescription Drug Products (continued)

POLYETHYLENE GLYCOL 3350; POTASSIUM CHLORIDE; SODIUM BICARBONATE; SODIUM CHLORIDE; SODIUM SULFATE, ANHYDROUS (continued)

POWDER FOR RECONSTITUTION; ORAL

COLYTE

AA	REED AND CARNRICK	227.1 GM/BOT;2.82 GM/ BOT:6.36 GM/ BOT:5.53 GM/ BOT:21.5 GM/BOT	N18983 010	JAN 31, 1989
AA		240 GM/BOT:2.98 GM/ BOT:6.72 GM/ BOT:5.84 GM/ BOT:22.72 GM/BOT	N18983 007	JUN 12, 1987

COLYTE-FLAVORED

AA	REED AND CARNRICK	227.1 GM/BOT;2.82 GM/ BOT:6.36 GM/ BOT:5.53 GM/ BOT:21.5 GM/BOT	N18983 008	NOV 14, 1991
AA		240 GM/BOT:2.98 GM/ BOT:6.72 GM/ BOT:5.84 GM/ BOT:22.72 GM/BOT	N18983 009	NOV 14, 1991

E-Z-EM PREP LYTE

AA	E Z EM	236 GM/BOT:2.97 GM/ BOT:6.74 GM/ BOT:5.86 GM/ BOT:22.74 GM/BOT	N71278 001	NOV 21, 1988

GLYCOPREP

AA	GOLDLINE	236 GM/BOT:2.97 GM/ BOT:6.74 GM/ BOT:5.86 GM/ BOT:22.74 GM/BOT	N72319 001	DEC 23, 1988

GO-EVAC

AA	COPLEY	236 GM/BOT:2.97 GM/ BOT:6.74 GM/ BOT:5.86 GM/ BOT:22.74 GM/BOT	N73433 001	APR 28, 1992

GOLYTELY

AA	BRAINTREE	236 GM/BOT:2.97 GM/ BOT:6.74 GM/ BOT:5.86 GM/ BOT:22.74 GM/BOT	N19011 001	JUL 13, 1984

POLYMYXIN B SULFATE

INJECTABLE; INJECTION

AEROSPORIN

AP	BURROUGHS WELLCOME	500,000 UNITS/VIAL	N62036 001
AP	POLYMIXIN B SULFATE PFIZER	500,000 UNITS/VIAL	N60716 001

POWDER; FOR RX COMPOUNDING

POLY-RX

AA	PHARMA TEK	100,000.000 UNITS/BOT	N61578 001	
AA	POLYMIXIN B SULFATE PADDOCK	100,000.000 UNITS/BOT	N62455 001	JUL 27, 1983

POLYMYXIN B SULFATE; *MULTIPLE*

SEE   BACITRACIN; HYDROCORTISONE ACETATE; NEOMYCIN SULFATE; POLYMYXIN B SULFATE

SEE   BACITRACIN; NEOMYCIN SULFATE; POLYMYXIN B SULFATE

SEE   BACITRACIN ZINC; HYDROCORTISONE; NEOMYCIN SULFATE; POLYMYXIN B SULFATE

SEE   BACITRACIN ZINC; NEOMYCIN SULFATE; POLYMYXIN B SULFATE

SEE   BACITRACIN ZINC; POLYMYXIN B SULFATE

SEE   CHLORAMPHENICOL; HYDROCORTISONE ACETATE; POLYMYXIN B SULFATE

SEE   DEXAMETHASONE; NEOMYCIN SULFATE; POLYMYXIN B SULFATE

SEE   GRAMICIDIN; NEOMYCIN SULFATE; POLYMYXIN B SULFATE

SEE   HYDROCORTISONE; NEOMYCIN SULFATE; POLYMYXIN B SULFATE

SEE   HYDROCORTISONE; POLYMYXIN B SULFATE

SEE   HYDROCORTISONE ACETATE; NEOMYCIN SULFATE; POLYMYXIN B SULFATE

SEE   NEOMYCIN SULFATE; POLYMYXIN B SULFATE

SEE   NEOMYCIN SULFATE; POLYMYXIN B SULFATE; PREDNISOLONE ACETATE

SEE   OXYTETRACYCLINE HYDROCHLORIDE; POLYMYXIN B SULFATE

POLYMYXIN B SULFATE; TRIMETHOPRIM SULFATE

SOLUTION/DROPS; OPHTHALMIC

POLYTRIM

	BURROUGHS WELLCOME	10,000 UNITS/ML;EQ 1 MG BASE/ML	N50567 001 OCT 20, 1988

Prescription Drug Products (continued)

POLYTHIAZIDE
TABLET; ORAL
RENESE
PFIZER

1 MG	N12845 001	
2 MG	N12845 002	
4 MG	N12845 003	

+

POLYTHIAZIDE; PRAZOSIN HYDROCHLORIDE
CAPSULE; ORAL
MINIZIDE
PFIZER

0.5 MG;1 MG	N17986 001	
0.5 MG;2 MG	N17986 002	
0.5 MG;5 MG	N17986 003	

+

POLYTHIAZIDE; RESERPINE
TABLET; ORAL
RENESE-R
+ PFIZER

2 MG;0.25 MG	N13636 001	

POTASSIUM ACETATE
INJECTABLE; INJECTION
POTASSIUM ACETATE IN PLASTIC CONTAINER

ABBOTT	2 MEQ/ML	N18896 001	JUL. 20, 1984

POTASSIUM ACETATE; *MULTIPLE*
SEE AMINO ACIDS; DEXTROSE; MAGNESIUM CHLORIDE; POTASSIUM ACETATE; POTASSIUM CHLORIDE; POTASSIUM PHOSPHATE, DIBASIC; SODIUM CHLORIDE

SEE AMINO ACIDS; MAGNESIUM ACETATE; PHOSPHORIC ACID; POTASSIUM CHLORIDE; SODIUM ACETATE

SEE AMINO ACIDS; MAGNESIUM ACETATE; PHOSPHORIC ACID; POTASSIUM ACETATE; SODIUM CHLORIDE

SEE AMINO ACIDS; MAGNESIUM ACETATE; POTASSIUM ACETATE; SODIUM CHLORIDE

SEE AMINO ACIDS; MAGNESIUM CHLORIDE; POTASSIUM ACETATE; POTASSIUM CHLORIDE; SODIUM ACETATE

SEE DEXTROSE; MAGNESIUM ACETATE; POTASSIUM ACETATE; SODIUM CHLORIDE

SEE DEXTROSE; MAGNESIUM ACETATE TETRAHYDRATE; POTASSIUM ACETATE; SODIUM CHLORIDE

SEE MAGNESIUM ACETATE TETRAHYDRATE; POTASSIUM ACETATE; SODIUM CHLORIDE

POTASSIUM AMINOSALICYLATE
CAPSULE; ORAL
PASKALIUM

GLENWOOD	500 MG	N09395 004

TABLET; ORAL
PASKALIUM

GLENWOOD	1 GM	N09395 003

POTASSIUM CHLORIDE
CAPSULE, EXTENDED RELEASE; ORAL
K-LEASE

AB	ADRIA	8 MEQ	N73398 001	JAN 28, 1992
AB		10 MEQ	N72427 001	MAR 28, 1990

MICRO-K

AB	ROBINS	8 MEQ	N18238 001	

MICRO-K 10

AB	+ ROBINS	10 MEQ	N18238 002	MAY 14, 1984

POTASSIUM CHLORIDE

AB	KV	10 MEQ	N70980 001	FEB 17, 1987

GRANULE, FOR RECONSTITUTION ER; ORAL
POTASSIUM CHLORIDE
MICRO-K LS

AB	+ ROBINS	20 MEQ/PACKET	N19561 003	AUG 26, 1988

INJECTABLE; INJECTION
POTASSIUM CHLORIDE

AP	ABBOTT	2 MEQ/ML	N80205 001	
AP		2 MEQ/ML	N83345 002	
		1.5 MEQ/ML	N83345 001	
		2 MEQ/ML	N88286 001	SEP 05, 1985
AP	AKORN	2 MEQ/ML	N85499 001	
		2 MEQ/ML	N80195 001	
AP	BAXTER	4 MEQ/ML	N80195 004	
	CUTTER	2 MEQ/ML	N83163 001	
AP	INTL MEDICATION	2 MEQ/ML	N80221 001	
AP	LUITPOLD	2 MEQ/ML	N80736 001	
AP		2 MEQ/ML	N87584 001	
AP		2 MEQ/ML	N87585 001	
AP		2 MEQ/ML	N80225 001	
AP		2 MEQ/ML	N84290 001	
AP	LYPHOMED	2 MEQ/ML	N87787 001	APR 20, 1982
AP		2 MEQ/ML	N87817 001	OCT 20, 1982
AP		2 MEQ/ML	N87885 001	FEB 03, 1983
AP		3 MEQ/ML	N80225 003	

Prescription Drug Products (continued)

POTASSIUM CHLORIDE (continued)
INJECTABLE; INJECTION
POTASSIUM CHLORIDE

AP	MCGAW	2 MEQ/ML	N85870 001	
AP	PHARMA SERVE	2 MEQ/ML	N86297 001	
AP		2 MEQ/ML	N87362 001	MAR 08, 1983
AP	STERIS	2 MEQ/ML	N86208 001	
AP		2 MEQ/ML	N89163 001	MAR 10, 1988
AP		2 MEQ/ML	N89421 001	JAN 02, 1987
AP		3 MEQ/ML	N86210 001	

POTASSIUM CHLORIDE IN PLASTIC CONTAINER

AP	LYPHOMED	2 MEQ/ML	N88901 001	JAN 25, 1985
AP		2 MEQ/ML	N88908 001	JAN 25, 1985

POTASSIUM CHLORIDE 10 MEQ IN PLASTIC CONTAINER

	BAXTER	14.9 MG/ML	N19904 001	DEC 26, 1989
		746 MG/100 ML	N19904 005	DEC 17, 1990

POTASSIUM CHLORIDE 20 MEQ IN PLASTIC CONTAINER

	BAXTER	1.49 GM/100 ML	N19904 006	DEC 17, 1990
		29.8 MG/ML	N19904 002	DEC 26, 1989

POTASSIUM CHLORIDE 30 MEQ IN PLASTIC CONTAINER

	BAXTER	2.24 GM/100 ML	N19904 003	DEC 26, 1989

POTASSIUM CHLORIDE 40 MEQ IN PLASTIC CONTAINER

	BAXTER	2.98 GM/100 ML	N19904 004	DEC 26, 1989

TABLET, EXTENDED RELEASE; ORAL
K+10

BC	ALRA	10 MEQ	N70999 001	OCT 22, 1987

K-DUR 10

BC	SCHERING	10 MEQ	N19439 002	JUN 13, 1986

K-DUR 20

BC	SCHERING	20 MEQ	N19439 001	JUN 13, 1986

K-TAB

+	ABBOTT	10 MEQ	N18279 001

KAON CL

	ADRIA	6.7 MEQ	N17046 001

KAON CL-10

BC	ADRIA	10 MEQ	N17046 002

POTASSIUM CHLORIDE (continued)
TABLET, EXTENDED RELEASE; ORAL
KLOR-CON

AB	UPSHER SMITH	8 MEQ	N19123 001	APR 17, 1986
BC		10 MEQ	N19123 002	APR 17, 1986

KLOTRIX

BC	APOTHECON	10 MEQ	N17850 001

POTASSIUM CHLORIDE

BC	ABBOTT	8 MEQ	N18279 002	AUG 01, 1988
AB	COPLEY	8 MEQ	N70618 001	SEP 09, 1987

SLOW-K

AB	+ CIBA	8 MEQ	N17476 002

TEN-K

BC	CIBA	10 MEQ	N19381 001	APR 16, 1986

POTASSIUM CHLORIDE; *MULTIPLE*

SEE AMINO ACIDS; CALCIUM ACETATE; GLYCERIN; MAGNESIUM ACETATE; PHOSPHORIC ACID; POTASSIUM CHLORIDE; SODIUM ACETATE; SODIUM CHLORIDE

SEE AMINO ACIDS; CALCIUM CHLORIDE; DEXTROSE; MAGNESIUM CHLORIDE; POTASSIUM CHLORIDE; POTASSIUM PHOSPHATE, DIBASIC; SODIUM CHLORIDE

SEE AMINO ACIDS; DEXTROSE; MAGNESIUM CHLORIDE; POTASSIUM ACETATE; POTASSIUM CHLORIDE; POTASSIUM PHOSPHATE, DIBASIC; SODIUM CHLORIDE

SEE AMINO ACIDS; DEXTROSE; MAGNESIUM CHLORIDE; POTASSIUM CHLORIDE; SODIUM CHLORIDE; SODIUM PHOSPHATE, DIBASIC

SEE AMINO ACIDS; MAGNESIUM ACETATE; PHOSPHORIC ACID; POTASSIUM ACETATE; POTASSIUM CHLORIDE; SODIUM ACETATE

SEE AMINO ACIDS; MAGNESIUM ACETATE; PHOSPHORIC ACID; POTASSIUM CHLORIDE; SODIUM ACETATE; SODIUM CHLORIDE

SEE AMINO ACIDS; MAGNESIUM CHLORIDE; POTASSIUM ACETATE; POTASSIUM CHLORIDE; SODIUM ACETATE

SEE AMINO ACIDS; MAGNESIUM CHLORIDE; POTASSIUM CHLORIDE; SODIUM CHLORIDE; SODIUM PHOSPHATE, DIBASIC

SEE AMINO ACIDS; MAGNESIUM CHLORIDE; POTASSIUM CHLORIDE; POTASSIUM PHOSPHATE, DIBASIC; SODIUM CHLORIDE

SEE CALCIUM CHLORIDE; DEXTROSE; GLUTATHIONE DISULFIDE; MAGNESIUM CHLORIDE; POTASSIUM CHLORIDE; SODIUM BICARBONATE; SODIUM CHLORIDE; SODIUM PHOSPHATE

Prescription Drug Products (continued)

POTASSIUM CHLORIDE; *MULTIPLE* (continued)

SEE   CALCIUM CHLORIDE: DEXTROSE: MAGNESIUM CHLORIDE: POTASSIUM CHLORIDE: SODIUM ACETATE: SODIUM CHLORIDE

SEE   CALCIUM CHLORIDE: DEXTROSE: MAGNESIUM CHLORIDE: POTASSIUM CHLORIDE: SODIUM ACETATE: SODIUM CHLORIDE: SODIUM LACTATE

SEE   CALCIUM CHLORIDE: DEXTROSE: MAGNESIUM CHLORIDE: POTASSIUM CHLORIDE: SODIUM ACETATE: SODIUM CHLORIDE: SODIUM CITRATE

SEE   CALCIUM CHLORIDE: DEXTROSE: POTASSIUM CHLORIDE: SODIUM CHLORIDE

SEE   CALCIUM CHLORIDE: DEXTROSE: POTASSIUM CHLORIDE: SODIUM CHLORIDE: SODIUM LACTATE

SEE   CALCIUM CHLORIDE: DEXTROSE: POTASSIUM CHLORIDE: SODIUM ACETATE: SODIUM CHLORIDE

SEE   CALCIUM CHLORIDE: DEXTROSE: POTASSIUM CHLORIDE: SODIUM CHLORIDE: SODIUM LACTATE

SEE   CALCIUM CHLORIDE: MAGNESIUM CHLORIDE: POTASSIUM CHLORIDE: SODIUM ACETATE: SODIUM CHLORIDE: SODIUM CITRATE

SEE   CALCIUM CHLORIDE: MAGNESIUM CHLORIDE: POTASSIUM CHLORIDE: SODIUM ACETATE: SODIUM CHLORIDE

SEE   CALCIUM CHLORIDE: MAGNESIUM CHLORIDE: POTASSIUM CHLORIDE: SODIUM ACETATE: SODIUM CHLORIDE: SODIUM LACTATE

SEE   CALCIUM CHLORIDE: MAGNESIUM CHLORIDE: POTASSIUM CHLORIDE: SODIUM CHLORIDE

SEE   CALCIUM CHLORIDE: POTASSIUM CHLORIDE: SODIUM CHLORIDE

SEE   CALCIUM CHLORIDE: POTASSIUM CHLORIDE: SODIUM CHLORIDE: SODIUM LACTATE

SEE   DEXTROSE: MAGNESIUM CHLORIDE: POTASSIUM CHLORIDE: SODIUM ACETATE: SODIUM CHLORIDE: SODIUM GLUCONATE

SEE   DEXTROSE: MAGNESIUM CHLORIDE: POTASSIUM CHLORIDE: SODIUM ACETATE: SODIUM CHLORIDE

SEE   DEXTROSE: MAGNESIUM CHLORIDE: POTASSIUM CHLORIDE: SODIUM ACETATE: SODIUM CHLORIDE: SODIUM GLUCONATE

SEE   DEXTROSE: MAGNESIUM CHLORIDE: POTASSIUM CHLORIDE: SODIUM PHOSPHATE, DIBASIC: SODIUM ACETATE

SEE   DEXTROSE: MAGNESIUM CHLORIDE: POTASSIUM CHLORIDE: SODIUM PHOSPHATE, DIBASIC: SODIUM CHLORIDE: SODIUM LACTATE: SODIUM PHOSPHATE, MONOBASIC

SEE   DEXTROSE: MAGNESIUM CHLORIDE: POTASSIUM CHLORIDE: POTASSIUM PHOSPHATE, MONOBASIC: POTASSIUM LACTATE: SODIUM LACTATE: SODIUM PHOSPHATE, MONOBASIC

POTASSIUM CHLORIDE; *MULTIPLE* (continued)

SEE   DEXTROSE: MAGNESIUM CHLORIDE: POTASSIUM CHLORIDE: POTASSIUM PHOSPHATE, MONOBASIC: SODIUM CHLORIDE: SODIUM LACTATE

SEE   DEXTROSE: POTASSIUM CHLORIDE

SEE   DEXTROSE: POTASSIUM CHLORIDE: POTASSIUM LACTATE: SODIUM CHLORIDE: SODIUM PHOSPHATE MONOBASIC

SEE   DEXTROSE: POTASSIUM CHLORIDE: POTASSIUM PHOSPHATE, DIBASIC: SODIUM ACETATE: SODIUM CHLORIDE

SEE   DEXTROSE: POTASSIUM CHLORIDE: POTASSIUM PHOSPHATE, MONOBASIC: SODIUM CHLORIDE: SODIUM LACTATE

SEE   DEXTROSE: POTASSIUM CHLORIDE: SODIUM CHLORIDE

SEE   MAGNESIUM CHLORIDE: POTASSIUM CHLORIDE: POTASSIUM PHOSPHATE, MONOBASIC: SODIUM ACETATE: SODIUM CHLORIDE: SODIUM GLUCONATE: SODIUM PHOSPHATE, DIBASIC

SEE   MAGNESIUM CHLORIDE: POTASSIUM CHLORIDE: SODIUM CHLORIDE: SODIUM GLUCONATE

SEE   MAGNESIUM SULFATE: POTASSIUM CHLORIDE: POTASSIUM PHOSPHATE, MONOBASIC: SODIUM CHLORIDE: SODIUM PHOSPHATE

SEE   POLYETHYLENE GLYCOL 3350: POTASSIUM CHLORIDE: SODIUM BICARBONATE: SODIUM CHLORIDE: SODIUM SULFATE, ANHYDROUS

SEE   POLYETHYLENE GLYCOL 3350: POTASSIUM CHLORIDE: SODIUM BICARBONATE: SODIUM CHLORIDE

SEE   POLYETHYLENE GLYCOL 3350: POTASSIUM CHLORIDE: SODIUM BICARBONATE: SODIUM CHLORIDE: SODIUM SULFATE

SEE   POLYETHYLENE GLYCOL 3350: POTASSIUM CHLORIDE: SODIUM BICARBONATE: SODIUM CHLORIDE: SODIUM SULFATE, ANHYDROUS

POTASSIUM CHLORIDE; SODIUM CHLORIDE

INJECTABLE; INJECTION
POTASSIUM CHLORIDE 0.037% IN SODIUM CHLORIDE 0.9% IN PLASTIC CONTAINER

MCGAW	37 MG/100 ML;900 MG/ 100 ML	N19708 001	SEP 29, 1989

POTASSIUM CHLORIDE 0.075% IN SODIUM CHLORIDE 0.9% IN PLASTIC CONTAINER

MCGAW	75 MG/100 ML;900 MG/ 100 ML	N19708 002	SEP 29, 1989

Prescription Drug Products *(continued)*

POTASSIUM CHLORIDE; SODIUM CHLORIDE *(continued)*

INJECTABLE; INJECTION
POTASSIUM CHLORIDE 0.11% IN SODIUM CHLORIDE 0.9% IN PLASTIC CONTAINER

MCGAW	110 MG/100 ML;900 MG/ 100 ML	N19708 003 SEP 29, 1989

POTASSIUM CHLORIDE 0.15% IN SODIUM CHLORIDE 0.9% IN PLASTIC CONTAINER

AP	MCGAW	150 MG/100 ML;900 MG/ 100 ML	N19708 004 SEP 29, 1989

POTASSIUM CHLORIDE 0.22% IN SODIUM CHLORIDE 0.9% IN PLASTIC CONTAINER

MCGAW	220 MG/100 ML;900 MG/ 100 ML	N19708 005 SEP 29, 1989

POTASSIUM CHLORIDE 0.3% IN SODIUM CHLORIDE 0.9% IN PLASTIC CONTAINER

AP	MCGAW	300 MG/100 ML;900 MG/ 100 ML	N19708 006 SEP 29, 1989

POTASSIUM CHLORIDE 20 MEQ IN SODIUM CHLORIDE 0.9% IN PLASTIC CONTAINER

AP	ABBOTT	149 MG/100 ML;900 MG/ 100 ML	N19686 001 OCT 17, 1988

POTASSIUM CHLORIDE 40 MEQ IN SODIUM CHLORIDE 0.9% IN PLASTIC CONTAINER

AP	ABBOTT	298 MG/100 ML;900 MG/ 100 ML	N19686 002 OCT 17, 1988

SODIUM CHLORIDE 0.9% AND POTASSIUM CHLORIDE 0.15% IN PLASTIC CONTAINER

AP	BAXTER	150 MG/100 ML;900 MG/ 100 ML	N17648 001

SODIUM CHLORIDE 0.9% AND POTASSIUM CHLORIDE 0.224% IN PLASTIC CONTAINER

BAXTER	224 MG/100 ML;900 MG/ 100 ML	N17648 003

SODIUM CHLORIDE 0.9% AND POTASSIUM CHLORIDE 0.3% IN PLASTIC CONTAINER

AP	BAXTER	300 MG/100 ML;900 MG/ 100 ML	N17648 002

POTASSIUM CHLORIDE; SODIUM CHLORIDE; TROMETHAMINE

INJECTABLE; INJECTION
THAM-E

ABBOTT	370 MG/VIAL;1.75 GM/ VIAL;36 GM/VIAL	N13025 001

POTASSIUM CITRATE

POWDER FOR RECONSTITUTION; ORAL
POTASSIUM CITRATE

UNIV TX	10 MEQ/PACKET	N19647 002 OCT 13, 1988
+	20 MEQ/PACKET	N19647 001 OCT 13, 1988

TABLET, EXTENDED RELEASE; ORAL
POTASSIUM CITRATE

+ UNIV TX	5 MEQ	N19071 001 AUG 30, 1985

POTASSIUM LACTATE; *MULTIPLE*

SEE   DEXTROSE; POTASSIUM CHLORIDE; POTASSIUM LACTATE; SODIUM CHLORIDE; SODIUM PHOSPHATE, MONOBASIC

POTASSIUM PERCHLORATE

CAPSULE; ORAL
PERCHLORACAP

MALLINCKRODT	200 MG	N17551 001

POTASSIUM PHOSPHATE, DIBASIC; *MULTIPLE*

SEE   AMINO ACIDS; CALCIUM CHLORIDE; DEXTROSE; MAGNESIUM CHLORIDE; POTASSIUM CHLORIDE; POTASSIUM PHOSPHATE, DIBASIC; SODIUM CHLORIDE

SEE   AMINO ACIDS; DEXTROSE; MAGNESIUM CHLORIDE; POTASSIUM ACETATE; POTASSIUM CHLORIDE; POTASSIUM PHOSPHATE, DIBASIC; SODIUM CHLORIDE

SEE   AMINO ACIDS; MAGNESIUM CHLORIDE; POTASSIUM CHLORIDE; POTASSIUM PHOSPHATE, DIBASIC; SODIUM CHLORIDE

SEE   AMINO ACIDS; MAGNESIUM CHLORIDE; POTASSIUM PHOSPHATE, DIBASIC; SODIUM ACETATE; SODIUM CHLORIDE

SEE   AMINO ACIDS; MAGNESIUM CHLORIDE; POTASSIUM PHOSPHATE, DIBASIC; SODIUM CHLORIDE

SEE   DEXTROSE; MAGNESIUM CHLORIDE; POTASSIUM CHLORIDE; POTASSIUM PHOSPHATE, DIBASIC; SODIUM ACETATE

SEE   DEXTROSE; MAGNESIUM CHLORIDE; POTASSIUM CHLORIDE; POTASSIUM PHOSPHATE, DIBASIC; SODIUM CHLORIDE; SODIUM LACTATE; SODIUM PHOSPHATE, MONOBASIC

SEE   DEXTROSE; POTASSIUM CHLORIDE; POTASSIUM PHOSPHATE, DIBASIC; SODIUM ACETATE; SODIUM CHLORIDE

Prescription Drug Products (continued)

POTASSIUM PHOSPHATE, MONOBASIC; *MULTIPLE*

SEE   DEXTROSE: MAGNESIUM CHLORIDE: POTASSIUM CHLORIDE: POTASSIUM PHOSPHATE, MONOBASIC: SODIUM LACTATE: SODIUM PHOSPHATE, MONOBASIC

SEE   DEXTROSE: MAGNESIUM CHLORIDE: POTASSIUM CHLORIDE: POTASSIUM PHOSPHATE, MONOBASIC: SODIUM CHLORIDE: SODIUM LACTATE

SEE   DEXTROSE: POTASSIUM CHLORIDE: POTASSIUM PHOSPHATE, MONOBASIC: SODIUM CHLORIDE: SODIUM LACTATE

SEE   MAGNESIUM CHLORIDE: POTASSIUM CHLORIDE: POTASSIUM PHOSPHATE, MONOBASIC: SODIUM ACETATE: SODIUM CHLORIDE: SODIUM GLUCONATE: SODIUM PHOSPHATE, DIBASIC

SEE   MAGNESIUM SULFATE: POTASSIUM CHLORIDE: POTASSIUM PHOSPHATE, MONOBASIC: SODIUM CHLORIDE: SODIUM PHOSPHATE

POVIDONE-IODINE

SOLUTION/DROPS; OPHTHALMIC

BETADINE

PURDUE FREDERICK   5%   N18634 001   DEC 17, 1986

PRALIDOXIME CHLORIDE

INJECTABLE; INJECTION

PRALIDOXIME CHLORIDE

SURVIVAL TECH   300 MG/ML   N18986 001   APR 26, 1983

PROTOPAM CHLORIDE

WYETH AYERST   1 GM/VIAL   N14134 001

PRAMOXINE HYDROCHLORIDE; *MULTIPLE*

SEE   HYDROCORTISONE ACETATE: PRAMOXINE HYDROCHLORIDE

PRAVASTATIN SODIUM

TABLET; ORAL

PRAVACHOL

BRISTOL MYERS SQUIBB   10 MG   N19898 002   OCT 31, 1991

+   20 MG   N19898 003   OCT 31, 1991

PRAZEPAM

CAPSULE; ORAL

CENTRAX

PARKE DAVIS   5 MG   N18144 001

+   10 MG   N18144 002

+   20 MG   N18144 003   MAY 10, 1982

PRAZEPAM (continued)

TABLET; ORAL

CENTRAX

+ PARKE DAVIS   10 MG   N17415 001

PRAZIQUANTEL

TABLET; ORAL

BILTRICIDE

+ MILES   600 MG   N18714 001   DEC 29, 1982

PRAZOSIN HYDROCHLORIDE

CAPSULE; ORAL

MINIPRESS

PFIZER   EQ 1 MG BASE   N17442 002

          EQ 2 MG BASE   N17442 003

+   EQ 5 MG BASE   N17442 001

PRAZOSIN HCL

AB DANBURY   EQ 1 MG BASE   N72352 001   JAN 11, 1989
               EQ 2 MG BASE   N72333 001   JAN 11, 1989
AB   EQ 5 MG BASE   N72609 001   JAN 11, 1989

AB GENEVA   EQ 1 MG BASE   N72576 001   APR 10, 1989
               EQ 2 MG BASE   N72577 001   APR 10, 1989
AB   EQ 5 MG BASE   N72578 001   APR 10, 1989

AB LEDERLE   EQ 1 MG BASE   N72705 001   MAR 15, 1989
               EQ 2 MG BASE   N72706 001   MAR 15, 1989
AB   EQ 5 MG BASE   N72707 001   MAR 15, 1989

AB MYLAN   EQ 1 MG BASE   N72573 001   FEB 28, 1989
               EQ 2 MG BASE   N72574 001   FEB 28, 1989
AB   EQ 5 MG BASE   N72575 001   FEB 28, 1989

AB PUREPAC   EQ 1 MG BASE   N72991 001   APR 26, 1989
               EQ 2 MG BASE   N72921 001   APR 26, 1989
AB   EQ 5 MG BASE   N72992 001   APR 26, 1989

AB ZENITH   EQ 1 MG BASE   N71994 001   SEP 12, 1988
               EQ 2 MG BASE   N71995 001   SEP 12, 1988
AB   EQ 5 MG BASE   N71745 001   SEP 12, 1988

Prescription Drug Products (continued)

PRAZOSIN HYDROCHLORIDE (continued)

TABLET, EXTENDED RELEASE; ORAL

MINIPRESS XL

+	PFIZER	2.5 MG	N19775 001	JAN 29, 1992
+		5 MG	N19775 002	JAN 29, 1992

PRAZOSIN HYDROCHLORIDE; *MULTIPLE*

SEE POLYTHIAZIDE; PRAZOSIN HYDROCHLORIDE

PREDNICARBATE

OINTMENT; TOPICAL

DERMATOP

	HOECHST ROUSSEL	0.1%	N19568 001	SEP 23, 1991

PREDNISOLONE

SYRUP; ORAL

PRELONE

	MURO	5 MG/5 ML	N89654 001	JAN 17, 1989
		15 MG/5 ML	N89081 001	FEB 04, 1986

TABLET; ORAL

CORTALONE

BX	HALSEY	1 MG	N80304 003
BX		2.5 MG	N80304 002
BX		5 MG	N80304 001

DELTA-CORTEF

BX +	UPJOHN	5 MG	N09987 004

PREDNISOLONE

BX	BUNDY	5 MG	N83675 001
BX	CHELSEA	5 MG	N85085 002
BX	DANBURY	5 MG	N80354 001
BX	EVERYLIFE	2.5 MG	N84439 002
BX		5 MG	N84439 003
BX	GENEVA	5 MG	N80339 001
BX	ICN	5 MG	N80236 001
BX	INWOOD	5 MG	N80748 001
BX	LANNETT	5 MG	N80531 002
BX	MARSHALL	2.5 MG	N80562 001
BX		5 MG	N80307 001
BX		5 MG	N80562 002
BX	PHOENIX LABS	5 MG	N80322 001
BX	PRIVATE FORM	5 MG	N80211 001
BX	PUREPAC	5 MG	N80325 001
BX	RICHLYN	5 MG	N80780 001
BX	ROXANE	5 MG	N80327 002
BX	SPERTI	1 MG	N80358 001
BX		2.5 MG	N80358 002
BX	TABLICAPS	5 MG	N80358 003
BX	WEST WARD	5 MG	N85170 001
BX	ZENITH	5 MG	N80324 001
BX		5 MG	N80378 001

PREDNISOLONE ACETATE

INJECTABLE; INJECTION

PREDNISOLONE ACETATE

BP	BEL MAR	25 MG/ML	N83738 001
BP		50 MG/ML	N83738 002
BP	STERIS	25 MG/ML	N83398 001
BP		25 MG/ML	N83654 001
BP		50 MG/ML	N83764 001
BP		50 MG/ML	N85781 001
BP		40 MG/ML	N83767 001

SUSPENSION/DROPS; OPHTHALMIC

ECONOPRED

	ALCON	0.125%	N17468 001

ECONOPRED PLUS

AT	ALCON	1%	N17469 001

PRED FORTE

	ALLERGAN	1%	N17011 001

PRED MILD

AT	ALLERGAN	0.12%	N17100 001

PREDNISOLONE ACETATE; *MULTIPLE*

SEE GENTAMICIN SULFATE; PREDNISOLONE ACETATE

SEE NEOMYCIN SULFATE; POLYMYXIN B SULFATE; PREDNISOLONE ACETATE

SEE NEOMYCIN SULFATE; PREDNISOLONE ACETATE

PREDNISOLONE ACETATE; SULFACETAMIDE SODIUM

OINTMENT; OPHTHALMIC

BLEPHAMIDE S.O.P.

	ALLERGAN	0.2%;10%	N8748 001	DEC 03, 1986

PREDSULFAIR

AT	PHARMAFAIR	0.5%;10%	N88032 001	APR 15, 1983

VASOCIDIN

AT	IOLAB	0.5%;10%	N88791 001	OCT 05, 1984

SUSPENSION/DROPS; OPHTHALMIC

BLEPHAMIDE

	ALLERGAN	0.2%;10%	N12813 002

ISOPTO CETAPRED

	ALCON	0.25%;10%	N87547 001

METIMYD

AT	SCHERING	0.5%;10%	N10210 001

PREDAMIDE

AT	AKORN	0.5%;10%	N88059 001	JUL 29, 1983

PREDSULFAIR

AT	PHARMAFAIR	0.5%;10%	N88007 001	APR 19, 1983

SULPHRIN

AT	BAUSCH AND LOMB	0.5%;10%	N88089 001	DEC 28, 1982

Prescription Drug Products (continued)

PREDNISOLONE SODIUM PHOSPHATE

INJECTABLE; INJECTION

HYDELTRASOL
AP	MSD	EQ 20 MG PHOSPHATE/ML	N11583 002	

PREDNISOLONE SODIUM PHOSPHATE
AP	STERIS	EQ 20 MG PHOSPHATE/ML	N80517 001	

SOLUTION; ORAL

PEDIAPRED
	FISONS	EQ 5 MG BASE/5 ML	N19157 001	MAY 28, 1986

SOLUTION/DROPS; OPHTHALMIC

INFLAMASE FORTE
AT	IOLAB	EQ 0.9% PHOSPHATE	N80751 002	

INFLAMASE MILD
AT	IOLAB	EQ 0.11% PHOSPHATE	N80751 001	

PREDAIR
AT	PHARMAFAIR	EQ 0.11% PHOSPHATE	N88415 001	FEB 29, 1984

PREDAIR FORTE
AT	PHARMAFAIR	EQ 0.9% PHOSPHATE	N88165 001	MAR 28, 1983

PREDNISOLONE SODIUM PHOSPHATE
AT	AKORN	EQ 0.11% PHOSPHATE	N83358 001	
AT		EQ 0.9% PHOSPHATE	N83358 002	
AT	STERIS	EQ 0.11% PHOSPHATE	N81043 001	OCT 24, 1991
AT		EQ 0.9% PHOSPHATE	N81044 001	OCT 24, 1991

PREDNISOLONE SODIUM PHOSPHATE; *MULTIPLE*

SEE NEOMYCIN SULFATE; PREDNISOLONE SODIUM PHOSPHATE

PREDNISOLONE SODIUM PHOSPHATE; SULFACETAMIDE SODIUM

SOLUTION/DROPS; OPHTHALMIC

VASOCIDIN
	IOLAB	EQ 0.23% PHOSPHATE;10%	N18988 001	AUG 26, 1988

PREDNISOLONE TEBUTATE

INJECTABLE; INJECTION

HYDELTRA-TBA
BP	MSD	20 MG/ML	N10562 001	

PREDNISOLONE TEBUTATE
BP	STERIS	20 MG/ML	N83362 001	FEB 17, 1984

PREDNISONE

SOLUTION; ORAL

PREDNISONE
AA	PHARM BASICS	5 MG/5 ML	N89726 001	AUG 02, 1988
AA	ROXANE	5 MG/5 ML	N88703 001	NOV 08, 1984

PREDNISONE INTENSOL
	ROXANE	5 MG/ML	N88810 001	FEB 20, 1985

SYRUP; ORAL

LIQUID PRED
	MURO	5 MG/5 ML	N87611 002	SEP 07, 1982

TABLET; ORAL

CORTAN
BX	HALSEY	20 MG	N87480 001	

DELTASONE
AB	UPJOHN	5 MG	N09986 002	
AB		10 MG	N09986 006	
AB		20 MG	N09986 007	
AB		50 MG	N09986 008	
BX		2.5 MG	N09986 005	

METICORTEN
BX	+ SCHERING	1 MG	N09766 002	
BX		5 MG	N09766 001	

ORASONE
AB	SOLVAY	1 MG	N83009 001	
AB		5 MG	N83009 002	
AB		10 MG	N83009 003	
AB		20 MG	N83009 004	
AB		50 MG	N85999 001	

PREDNICEN-M
AB	CENTRAL PHARMS	5 MG	N84655 001	

PREDNISONE
AB	BARR	5 MG	N80701 001	
AB		10 MG	N86595 001	
AB		20 MG	N84634 001	
BX	BUNDY	5 MG	N83676 001	
AB	CHELSEA	5 MG	N85084 002	
AB		10 MG	N87773 001	JUL 13, 1982
AB		20 MG	N86813 001	
AB		50 MG	N87772 001	JUL 13, 1982
AB	DANBURY	5 MG	N80356 001	
AB		10 MG	N85162 001	
BX		20 MG	N85161 001	
BX		50 MG	N86867 001	
BX	EVERYLIFE	1 MG	N84440 001	
BX		2.5 MG	N84440 002	
BX		5 MG	N84440 003	
BX	FIRST TX	5 MG	N80371 001	

Prescription Drug Products (continued)

PREDNISONE (continued)

TABLET; ORAL

PREDNISONE

TE Code	Firm	Strength	Appl. No.	Approval Date
AB	GENEVA	5 MG	N80336 002	
AB		10 MG	N89983 001	JAN 12, 1989
AB		20 MG	N85813 001	
AB		50 MG	N89984 001	JAN 12, 1989
AB	HALSEY	5 MG	N80300 001	
AB	HEATHER	5 MG	N80320 001	
AB		10 MG	N84341 001	
AB		20 MG	N84417 001	
AB		20 MG	N85543 001	
AB		50 MG	N86946 001	
BX	ICN	5 MG	N80237 001	
AB	INTERPHARM	5 MG	N89597 001	OCT 05, 1987
AB		10 MG	N89598 001	OCT 05, 1987
AB		20 MG	N89599 001	OCT 05, 1987
BX	INWOOD	1 MG	N80328 001	
BX		2.5 MG	N80279 001	
BX		5 MG	N84236 001	
BX	KV	5 MG	N80514 001	
BX	LANNETT	20 MG	N84275 001	
BX		5 MG	N80301 001	
BX	MARSHALL	2.5 MG	N80563 001	
BX	MK	5 MG	N80563 002	
BX	MUTUAL PHARM	5 MG	N89245 001	DEC 04, 1985
AB		10 MG	N89246 001	DEC 04, 1985
AB		20 MG	N89247 001	DEC 04, 1985
BX	PHARMAVITE	5 MG	N84662 002	
BX	PHOENIX LABS	5 MG	N80321 001	
AB	PRIVATE FORM	20 MG	N83807 001	
AB	PUREPAC	5 MG	N80209 001	
AB		5 MG	N80353 001	
AB		10 MG	N86062 001	
BX	REXALL	20 MG	N86061 001	
BX	RICHLYN	5 MG	N80232 001	
AB	ROXANE	5 MG	N80782 001	
AB		1 MG	N87800 001	APR 22, 1982
AB		2.5 MG	N87801 001	APR 22, 1982
AB		5 MG	N80352 001	
AB		10 MG	N84122 001	
AB		20 MG	N87342 001	
AB		50 MG	N84283 001	
BX	SPERTI	1 MG	N80359 001	
BX		2.5 MG	N80359 002	
BX		5 MG	N80359 003	

PREDNISONE (continued)

TABLET; ORAL

PREDNISONE

TE Code	Firm	Strength	Appl. No.	Approval Date
AB	SUPERPHARM	5 MG	N88865 001	OCT 25, 1984
AB		10 MG	N88866 001	OCT 25, 1984
AB		20 MG	N88867 001	OCT 25, 1984
BX	TABLICAPS	5 MG	N85115 001	
BX	UPSHER SMITH	5 MG	N87471 001	
BX		20 MG	N87470 001	
AB	WEST WARD	5 MG	N80292 001	
AB		10 MG	N88832 001	DEC 04, 1985
AB		20 MG	N83677 001	
AB		50 MG	N88465 001	JUN 01, 1984
BX	WHITE TOWNE	20 MG	N84913 002	
BX	PAULSEN	5 MG	N80283 001	
BX	ZENITH	10 MG	N84133 001	

PRILOCAINE HYDROCHLORIDE

INJECTABLE; INJECTION

CITANEST PLAIN

TE Code	Firm	Strength	Appl. No.
	ASTRA	4%	N14763 007

PRILOCAINE HYDROCHLORIDE; *MULTIPLE*

SEE   EPINEPHRINE BITARTRATE; PRILOCAINE HYDROCHLORIDE

PRIMAQUINE PHOSPHATE

TABLET; ORAL

PRIMAQUINE

TE Code	Firm	Strength	Appl. No.
	STERLING	EQ 15 MG BASE	N08316 001

PRIMIDONE

SUSPENSION; ORAL

MYSOLINE

TE Code	Firm	Strength	Appl. No.
	WYETH AYERST	250 MG/5 ML	N10401 001

TABLET; ORAL

MYSOLINE

TE Code	Firm	Strength	Appl. No.
AB	+ WYETH AYERST	250 MG	N09170 002
	+	50 MG	N09170 003

PRIMIDONE

TE Code	Firm	Strength	Appl. No.
AB	DANBURY	250 MG	N83551 001
AB	LANNETT	250 MG	N84903 001

Prescription Drug Products (continued)

PROBENECID
TABLET; ORAL

	BENEMID			
	+ MSD	500 MG	N07898 004	
	PROBALAN			
	LANNETT	500 MG	N80966 001	
	PROBENECID			
ΔB	CHELSEA	500 MG	N86150 002	APR 23, 1982
ΔB	DANBURY	500 MG	N84442 004	MAR 29, 1983
ΔB	MYLAN	500 MG	N84211 002	JUN 02, 1982
ΔB	ZENITH	500 MG	N83740 001	MAY 09, 1984

PROBENECID; *MULTIPLE*
SEE   AMPICILLIN/AMPICILLIN TRIHYDRATE; PROBENECID
SEE   COLCHICINE; PROBENECID

PROBUCOL
TABLET; ORAL

	LORELCO		
	MERRELL DOW	250 MG	N17535 001
	+	500 MG	N17535 002	JUL 06, 1988

PROCAINAMIDE HYDROCHLORIDE
CAPSULE; ORAL
PROCAINAMIDE HCL

ΔB	CHELSEA	250 MG	N85167 001	
ΔB		375 MG	N87020 001	
ΔB		500 MG	N87021 001	
ΔB	DANBURY	250 MG	N83287 001	
ΔB		375 MG	N84403 001	
ΔB		500 MG	N84280 001	
ΔB	GENEVA	250 MG	N89219 001	JUL 01, 1986
ΔB		375 MG	N89220 001	JUL 01, 1986
ΔB		500 MG	N89221 001	JUL 01, 1986
ΔB	LANNETT	250 MG	N83693 001	
ΔB		500 MG	N84696 001	
ΔB	ZENITH	250 MG	N84604 001	
ΔB		375 MG	N84595 001	
ΔB		500 MG	N84606 001	
	PRONESTYL			
ΔB	SQUIBB	250 MG	N07335 001	
ΔB		375 MG	N07335 004	
ΔB	+	500 MG	N07335 003	

PROCAINAMIDE HYDROCHLORIDE (continued)
INJECTABLE; INJECTION
PROCAINAMIDE HCL

ΔP	ABBOTT	100 MG/ML	N89069 001	FEB 12, 1986
ΔP		500 MG/ML	N89070 001	FEB 12, 1986
ΔP	ELKINS SINN	100 MG/ML	N89029 001	APR 17, 1986
ΔP		500 MG/ML	N89030 001	APR 17, 1986
ΔP	INTL MEDICATION	100 MG/ML	N88636 001	JUL 31, 1984
ΔP		500 MG/ML	N88637 001	JUL 31, 1984
ΔP	LYPHOMED	100 MG/ML	N89415 001	NOV 17, 1986
ΔP		500 MG/ML	N89416 001	NOV 17, 1986
ΔP	SMITH NEPHEW SOLOPAK	100 MG/ML	N88530 001	MAR 04, 1985
ΔP		500 MG/ML	N88531 001	MAR 04, 1985
ΔP		500 MG/ML	N88532 001	MAR 04, 1985
ΔP	STERIS	100 MG/ML	N87079 001	
ΔP		500 MG/ML	N87080 001	
ΔP	WINTHROP	500 MG/ML	N89537 001	AUG 25, 1987
	PRONESTYL			
ΔP	SQUIBB	100 MG/ML	N07335 002	
ΔP		500 MG/ML	N07335 005	

TABLET; ORAL

	PRONESTYL			
	SQUIBB	250 MG	N17371 001	
		375 MG	N17371 002	
	+	500 MG	N17371 003	

TABLET, EXTENDED RELEASE; ORAL
PROCAINAMIDE HCL

ΔB	COPLEY	500 MG	N88974 001	JUL 22, 1985
ΔB		750 MG	N89438 001	MAR 23, 1987
ΔB	DANBURY	250 MG	N89026 001	OCT 22, 1985
ΔB		500 MG	N89027 001	OCT 22, 1985
ΔB		750 MG	N89042 001	OCT 22, 1985
ΔB	GENEVA	250 MG	N89369 001	AUG 14, 1987
ΔB		500 MG	N89370 001	JAN 09, 1987
ΔB		250 MG	N89371 001	AUG 14, 1987

Prescription Drug Products (continued)

PROCAINAMIDE HYDROCHLORIDE (continued)

TABLET; EXTENDED RELEASE, ORAL

PROCAINAMIDE HCL

ΔB	INVAMED	500 MG	N89284 001	JUN 23, 1986
ΔB	INWOOD	500 MG	N89840 001	MAR 06, 1989
ΔB	SIDMAK	250 MG	N88958 001	DEC 02, 1985
			N88959 001	DEC 02, 1985
ΔB		500 MG	N88959 001	DEC 02, 1985

PROCAN SR

ΔB	PARKE DAVIS	250 MG	N86468 001	
ΔB		500 MG	N86065 001	
ΔB		750 MG	N87510 001	APR 01, 1982
+		1 GM	N88489 001	JAN 16, 1985

PRONESTYL-SR

BC	BRISTOL MYERS SQUIBB	500 MG	N87361 001

PROCAINE HYDROCHLORIDE

INJECTABLE; INJECTION

NOVOCAIN

ΔP	STERLING	1%	N85362 003
ΔP		2%	N85362 004
		10%	N86797 001

PROCAINE HCL

ΔP	ABBOTT	1%	N80416 001
ΔP		2%	N80416 002
ΔP	BEL MAR	1%	N80711 001
ΔP		2%	N80756 001
ΔP	ELKINS SINN	1%	N83315 001
ΔP		2%	N83315 002
ΔP	LYPHOMED	1%	N80421 001
ΔP		1%	N80384 002
ΔP		2%	N80384 003
ΔP			N80421 002
ΔP	STERIS	1%	N80658 001
ΔP		2%	N83535 001
ΔP		2%	N80658 002
			N83535 002

PROCAINE HYDROCHLORIDE; *MULTIPLE*

SEE EPINEPHRINE: PROCAINE HYDROCHLORIDE

SEE LEVONORDEFRIN: PROCAINE HYDROCHLORIDE: PROPOXYCAINE HYDROCHLORIDE:

SEE NOREPINEPHRINE BITARTRATE: PROCAINE HYDROCHLORIDE: PROPOXYCAINE HYDROCHLORIDE

PROCAINE HYDROCHLORIDE; TETRACYCLINE HYDROCHLORIDE

INJECTABLE; INJECTION

ACHROMYCIN

ΔP	LEDERLE	40 MG/VIAL;250 MG/VIAL	N50267 003
		40 MG/VIAL;100 MG/VIAL	N50267 002
		40 MG/VIAL;100 MG/VIAL	N50276 001

TETRACYN

ΔP	PFIZER	40 MG/VIAL;250 MG/VIAL	N60285 003

PROCARBAZINE HYDROCHLORIDE

CAPSULE; ORAL

MATULANE

ΔP	+ ROCHE	EQ 50 MG BASE	N16785 001

PROCHLORPERAZINE

SUPPOSITORY; RECTAL

COMPAZINE

SKF	2.5 MG	N11127 003
	5 MG	N11127 001
	25 MG	N11127 002

PROCHLORPERAZINE EDISYLATE

INJECTABLE; INJECTION

COMPAZINE

ΔP	SKF	EQ 5 MG BASE/ML	N10742 002	

PROCHLORPERAZINE

ΔP	ELKINS SINN	EQ 5 MG BASE/ML	N87759 001	OCT 01, 1982

PROCHLORPERAZINE EDISYLATE

ΔP	ELKINS SINN	EQ 5 MG BASE/ML	N89523 001	MAY 03, 1988
			N89903 001	AUG 29, 1989
ΔP	MARSAM	EQ 5 MG BASE/ML	N89675 001	DEC 05, 1988
ΔP	SMITH NEPHEW SOLOPAK	EQ 5 MG BASE/ML	N89251 001	DEC 04, 1986
ΔP	STERIS	EQ 5 MG BASE/ML	N89530 001	JUL 08, 1987
			N89605 001	JUL 08, 1987
			N89606 001	JUL 08, 1987
ΔP	STERLING	EQ 5 MG BASE/ML	N89703 001	JUL 08, 1987
ΔP	WYETH AYERST	EQ 5 MG BASE/ML	N86348 001	APR 07, 1988

SYRUP; ORAL

COMPAZINE

SKF	EQ 5 MG BASE/5 ML	N11188 001

Prescription Drug Products (continued)

PROCHLORPERAZINE MALEATE

CAPSULE, EXTENDED RELEASE; ORAL
COMPAZINE

	SKF	EQ 10 MG BASE	N11000 001
		EQ 15 MG BASE	N11000 002
		EQ 30 MG BASE	N11000 003

TABLET; ORAL
COMPAZINE

	SKF	EQ 5 MG BASE	N10571 001
		EQ 10 MG BASE	N10571 002
	+	EQ 25 MG BASE	N10571 003

PROCYCLIDINE HYDROCHLORIDE

TABLET; ORAL
KEMADRIN

	BURROUGHS WELLCOME	2 MG	N09818 005
		5 MG	N09818 003

PROGESTERONE

INJECTABLE; INJECTION
PROGESTERONE

AO	LILLY	50 MG/ML	N09238 001
AO	STERIS	50 MG/ML	N17362 002

INSERT, EXTENDED RELEASE; INTRAUTERINE
PROGESTASERT

	ALZA	38 MG	N17553 001

PROMAZINE HYDROCHLORIDE

INJECTABLE; INJECTION
PROMAZINE HCL

AP	STERIS	25 MG/ML	N84510 001
AP		50 MG/ML	N84517 001

SPARINE

AP	WYETH AYERST	25 MG/ML	N10349 008
AP		50 MG/ML	N10349 006

TABLET; ORAL
SPARINE

	WYETH AYERST	25 MG	N10348 001
		50 MG	N10348 002
		100 MG	N10348 003

PROMETHAZINE HYDROCHLORIDE

INJECTABLE; INJECTION
PHENERGAN

AP	WYETH AYERST	25 MG/ML	N08857 002
AP		50 MG/ML	N08857 003

PROMETHAZINE HYDROCHLORIDE (continued)

INJECTABLE; INJECTION
PROMETHAZINE HCL

AP	AKORN	25 MG/ML	N83955 002	
AP		50 MG/ML	N83955 001	
AP	ELKINS SINN	25 MG/ML	N83312 001	
AP		50 MG/ML	N83312 002	
AP	MARSAM	25 MG/ML	N89463 001	MAY 02, 1988
AP		50 MG/ML	N89477 001	MAY 02, 1988
AP	STERIS	25 MG/ML	N83532 001	
AP		50 MG/ML	N84591 001	
AP		50 MG/ML	N80629 002	
AP		50 MG/ML	N83532 002	
AP		50 MG/ML	N83838 002	

SUPPOSITORY; RECTAL
PHENERGAN

BR	WYETH AYERST	25 MG	N10926 001
BR	+	50 MG	N11689 001
		12.5 MG	N10926 002

PROMETHACON

BR	ALCON	25 MG	N84901 001
BR		50 MG	N84902 001

PROMETHEGAN

BR	G AND W	50 MG	N87165 001 AUG 14, 1987

SYRUP; ORAL
PHENERGAN FORTIS

AA	WYETH AYERST	25 MG/5 ML	N08381 003

PHENERGAN PLAIN

AA	WYETH AYERST	6.25 MG/5 ML	N08381 004 APR 18, 1984

PROMETH

AA	BARRE	6.25 MG/5 ML	N85953 001
AA		25 MG/5 ML	N84772 001

PROMETHAZINE

AA	CENCI	6.25 MG/5 ML	N89013 001 SEP 20, 1985

PROMETHAZINE HCL

AA	WHITE TOWNE PAULSEN	6.25 MG/5 ML	N86395 001

PROMETHAZINE PLAIN

AA	PHARM BASICS	6.25 MG/5 ML	N87953 001 NOV 15, 1982

Prescription Drug Products (continued)

PROMETHAZINE HYDROCHLORIDE (continued)

TABLET; ORAL

	PHENERGAN			
BP	WYETH AYERST	12.5 MG		N07935 002
BP		25 MG		N07935 003
BP		50 MG		N07935 004
	+ PROMETHAZINE HCL			
BP	BOLAR	25 MG		N83204 001
BP	DANBURY	12.5 MG		N83712 001
BP		25 MG		N83426 001
BP		50 MG		N83711 001
BP	GENEVA	25 MG		N84234 001
BP		50 MG		N84176 001
BP	LANNETT	12.5 MG		N80949 001
BP		25 MG		N80949 002
BP		50 MG		N80949 003
	PRIVATE FORM			
BP	RICHLYN	25 MG		N83658 001
BP		25 MG		N84214 002
				JUL 07, 1982
BP	TABLICAPS	12.5 MG		N84080 001
BP		25 MG		N84077 001
BP	ZENITH	12.5 MG		N83604 001
BP		25 MG		N83603 001
BP		50 MG		N83613 001
	REMSED			
BP	DUPONT	25 MG		N83176 002

PROMETHAZINE HYDROCHLORIDE; *MULTIPLE*

SEE CODEINE PHOSPHATE; PHENYLEPHRINE HYDROCHLORIDE; PROMETHAZINE HYDROCHLORIDE

SEE CODEINE PHOSPHATE; PROMETHAZINE HYDROCHLORIDE

SEE DEXTROMETHORPHAN HYDROBROMIDE; PROMETHAZINE HYDROCHLORIDE

SEE MEPERIDINE HYDROCHLORIDE; PROMETHAZINE HYDROCHLORIDE

SEE PHENYLEPHRINE HYDROCHLORIDE; PROMETHAZINE HYDROCHLORIDE

PROPAFENONE HYDROCHLORIDE

TABLET; ORAL

	RYTHMOL			
	KNOLL	150 MG		N19151 001
				NOV 27, 1989
	+	300 MG		N19151 002
				NOV 27, 1989

PROPANTHELINE BROMIDE

TABLET; ORAL

	PRO-BANTHINE			
	SCHIAPPARELLI			
AA	SEARLE	7.5 MG		N08732 003
AA		15 MG		N08732 002
	PROPANTHELINE BROMIDE			
AA	DANBURY	15 MG		N83029 002
AA	PAR	15 MG		N88377 001
				DEC 08, 1983
AA	RICHLYN	15 MG		N84541 002
AA	ROXANE	7.5 MG		N80927 001
AA		15 MG		N80927 002
AA	TABLICAPS	15 MG		N84428 001

PROPARACAINE HYDROCHLORIDE

SOLUTION/DROPS; OPHTHALMIC

	ALCAINE			
AT	ALCON	0.5%		N80027 001
	KAINAIR			
AT	PHARMAFAIR	0.5%		N88087 001
				JUN 07, 1983
	OPHTHAINE			
AT	SQUIBB	5 MG/ML		N08883 001
	OPHTHETIC			
AT	ALLERGAN	0.5%		N12583 001
	PARACAINE			
AT	OPTOPICS	0.5%		N87681 001
				AUG 05, 1982

PROPIOLACTONE

SOLUTION; IRRIGATION

	BETAPRONE			
	FOREST LABS	N/A		N11657 001

PROPIOMAZINE HYDROCHLORIDE

INJECTABLE; INJECTION

	LARGON			
	WYETH AYERST	20 MG/ML		N12382 002

PROPOFOL

INJECTABLE; INJECTION

	DIPRIVAN			
	ICI	10 MG/ML		N19627 001
				OCT 02, 1989

PROPOXYCAINE HYDROCHLORIDE; *MULTIPLE*

SEE LEVONORDEFRIN; PROCAINE HYDROCHLORIDE; PROPOXYCAINE HYDROCHLORIDE

SEE NOREPINEPHRINE BITARTRATE; PROCAINE HYDROCHLORIDE; PROPOXYCAINE HYDROCHLORIDE

Prescription Drug Products (continued)

PROPOXYPHENE HYDROCHLORIDE

CAPSULE; ORAL

TE	Brand / Firm	Strength	Appl. No.	Date
	DARVON			
AA	LILLY	32 MG	N10997 001	
AA		65 MG	N10997 003	
	DOLENE			
AA	LEDERLE	65 MG	N80530 001	
	KESSO-GESIC			
AA	MK	65 MG	N83544 001	
	PROPHENE 65			
AA	HALSEY	65 MG	N83538 002	
	PROPOXYPHENE HCL			
AA	DANBURY	65 MG	N80908 002	
AA	GENEVA	65 MG	N83125 002	
AA	ICN	65 MG	N80783 001	
AA	LEMMON	65 MG	N88615 001	OCT 22, 1984
AA	MYLAN	32 MG	N83528 001	
AA	PUREPAC	65 MG	N83278 001	
AA	RICHLYN	65 MG	N83317 001	
AA	ROXANE	32 MG	N83089 001	
AA		65 MG	N83089 002	
AA	WEST WARD	65 MG	N83501 001	
AA	WHITE TOWNE	65 MG	N84551 001	
AA	PAULSEN	32 MG	N83597 001	
AA	ZENITH	65 MG	N80269 001	

PROPOXYPHENE HYDROCHLORIDE; *MULTIPLE*

SEE ACETAMINOPHEN; PROPOXYPHENE HYDROCHLORIDE
SEE ASPIRIN; CAFFEINE; PROPOXYPHENE HYDROCHLORIDE
SEE ASPIRIN; PROPOXYPHENE HYDROCHLORIDE

PROPOXYPHENE NAPSYLATE

SUSPENSION; ORAL

TE	Brand / Firm	Strength	Appl. No.
	DARVON-N		
	+ LILLY	50 MG/5 ML	N16861 001

TABLET; ORAL

TE	Brand / Firm	Strength	Appl. No.
	DARVON-N		
	+ LILLY	100 MG	N16862 002

PROPOXYPHENE NAPSYLATE; *MULTIPLE*

SEE ACETAMINOPHEN; PROPOXYPHENE NAPSYLATE
SEE ASPIRIN; PROPOXYPHENE NAPSYLATE

PROPRANOLOL HYDROCHLORIDE

CAPSULE, EXTENDED RELEASE; ORAL

TE	Brand / Firm	Strength	Appl. No.	Date
	INDERAL LA			
AA	+ WYETH AYERST	60 MG	N18553 004	MAR 18, 1987
AB	+	80 MG	N18553 002	APR 19, 1983
AB	+	120 MG	N18553 003	APR 19, 1983
AB	+	160 MG	N18553 001	APR 19, 1983
	PROPRANOLOL HCL			
AB	INWOOD	60 MG	N72499 001	APR 11, 1989
AB		80 MG	N72500 001	APR 11, 1989
AB		120 MG	N72501 001	APR 11, 1989
AB		160 MG	N72502 001	APR 11, 1989

CONCENTRATE; ORAL

TE	Brand / Firm	Strength	Appl. No.	Date
	PROPRANOLOL HCL INTENSOL			
	ROXANE	80 MG/ML	N71388 001	MAY 15, 1987

INJECTABLE; INJECTION

TE	Brand / Firm	Strength	Appl. No.	Date
	INDERAL			
AP	WYETH AYERST	1MG/ML	N16419 001	
	PROPRANOLOL HCL			
AP	SMITH NEPHEW SOLOPAK	1MG/ML	N70136 001	APR 15, 1986
AP	SOLOPAK	1MG/ML	N70137 001	APR 15, 1986

SOLUTION; ORAL

TE	Brand / Firm	Strength	Appl. No.	Date
	PROPRANOLOL HCL			
	ROXANE	20 MG/5 ML	N70979 001	MAY 15, 1987
		40 MG/5 ML	N70690 001	MAY 15, 1987

SUSPENSION; ORAL

TE	Brand / Firm	Strength	Appl. No.	Date
	INDERAL			
	WYETH AYERST	10 MG/ML	N19536 001	DEC 12, 1986

TABLET; ORAL

TE	Brand / Firm	Strength	Appl. No.	Date
	INDERAL			
AB	+ WYETH AYERST	10 MG	N16418 001	
AB	+	20 MG	N16418 003	
AB	+	40 MG	N16418 002	
AB	+	60 MG	N16418 009	OCT 18, 1982
AB	+	80 MG	N16418 004	

Prescription Drug Products *(continued)*

PROPRANOLOL HYDROCHLORIDE *(continued)*

TABLET; ORAL

PROPRANOLOL HCL

TE Code	Applicant	Strength	Application No.	Approval Date
AB	BARR	10 MG	N70319 001	OCT 22, 1985
AB		20 MG	N70320 001	OCT 22, 1985
AB		40 MG	N70103 001	OCT 22, 1985
AB		60 MG	N70321 001	SEP 15, 1986
AB		80 MG	N70322 001	AUG 04, 1986
AB	DANBURY	10 MG	N70175 001	MAY 13, 1986
AB		20 MG	N70176 001	MAY 13, 1986
AB		40 MG	N70177 001	MAY 13, 1986
AB		60 MG	N71098 001	OCT 06, 1986
AB		80 MG	N70178 001	MAY 13, 1986
AB	GENEVA	10 MG	N70663 001	JUN 13, 1986
AB		20 MG	N70664 001	JUN 13, 1986
AB		40 MG	N70665 001	JUN 13, 1986
AB		60 MG	N70666 001	OCT 10, 1986
AB		80 MG	N70667 001	JUN 13, 1986
AB	INTERPHARM	10 MG	N71368 001	MAY 05, 1987
AB		20 MG	N71369 001	MAY 05, 1987
AB		40 MG	N71370 001	MAY 05, 1987
AB		80 MG	N71371 001	MAY 05, 1987
AB	INVAMED	10 MG	N71658 001	JUL 05, 1988
AB		20 MG	N71687 001	JUL 05, 1988
AB		40 MG	N71688 001	JUL 05, 1988
AB		60 MG	N72197 001	JUL 05, 1988
AB		80 MG	N71689 001	JUL 05, 1988
AB		90 MG	N72198 001	JUL 05, 1988

PROPRANOLOL HYDROCHLORIDE *(continued)*

TABLET; ORAL

PROPRANOLOL HCL

TE Code	Applicant	Strength	Application No.	Approval Date
AB	LEDERLE	10 MG	N70125 001	JUL 30, 1985
AB		20 MG	N70126 001	JUL 30, 1985
AB		40 MG	N70127 001	JUL 30, 1985
AB		60 MG	N71495 001	DEC 31, 1987
AB		80 MG	N70128 001	JUL 30, 1985
AB		90 MG	N71496 001	DEC 31, 1987
AB	LEMMON	40 MG	N70234 001	JUN 23, 1986
AB	MYLAN	10 MG	N70211 001	NOV 19, 1985
AB		20 MG	N70212 001	NOV 19, 1985
AB		40 MG	N70213 001	NOV 19, 1985
AB		60 MG	N72275 001	JUN 09, 1989
AB		80 MG	N70214 001	NOV 19, 1985
AB	PAR	10 MG	N70217 001	AUG 01, 1986
AB		20 MG	N70218 001	AUG 01, 1986
AB		40 MG	N70219 001	AUG 01, 1986
AB		60 MG	N70220 001	AUG 01, 1986
AB		80 MG	N70221 001	JUN 05, 1986
AB		90 MG	N71288 001	APR 14, 1986
AB	PARKE DAVIS	20 MG	N70439 001	OCT 22, 1986
AB		40 MG	N70440 001	SEP 15, 1986
AB		60 MG	N70441 001	SEP 15, 1986
AB		80 MG	N70442 001	SEP 15, 1986
AB	PUREPAC	10 MG	N70814 001	SEP 15, 1986
AB		20 MG	N70815 001	NOV 03, 1986
AB		40 MG	N70816 001	NOV 03, 1986
AB		60 MG	N70817 001	NOV 03, 1986
AB		80 MG	N70757 001	NOV 03, 1986

Prescription Drug Products (continued)

PROPRANOLOL HYDROCHLORIDE (continued)
TABLET; ORAL
PROPRANOLOL HCL

	Manufacturer	Strength	Appl. No.	Date
AB	ROXANE	10 MG	N70516 001	JUL 07, 1986
AB		20 MG	N70517 001	JUL 07, 1986
AB		40 MG	N70518 001	JUL 07, 1986
AB		60 MG	N70519 001	SEP 11, 1986
AB		80 MG	N70520 001	JUL 07, 1986
AB		90 MG	N70521 001	SEP 11, 1986
AB	SCHERING	10 MG	N70120 001	AUG 06, 1985
AB		20 MG	N70121 001	AUG 06, 1985
AB		40 MG	N70122 001	AUG 06, 1985
AB		60 MG	N70123 001	OCT 29, 1986
AB		80 MG	N70124 001	AUG 06, 1985
AB	SIDMAK	10 MG	N71972 001	APR 06, 1988
AB		20 MG	N71973 001	APR 06, 1988
AB		40 MG	N71974 001	APR 06, 1988
AB		60 MG	N71975 001	APR 06, 1988
AB		80 MG	N71976 001	APR 06, 1988
AB		90 MG	N71977 001	APR 06, 1988
AB	WARNER CHILCOTT	10 MG	N70438 001	SEP 15, 1986
AB	WATSON	10 MG	N70548 001	JUL 10, 1986
AB		20 MG	N70549 001	APR 11, 1986
AB		40 MG	N70550 001	APR 11, 1986
AB		60 MG	N71791 001	JUL 15, 1987
AB		80 MG	N70551 001	JUL 10, 1986
AB		90 MG	N71792 001	JUL 15, 1987
AB	ZENITH	10 MG	N72063 001	JUL 29, 1988
AB		20 MG	N72066 001	JUL 29, 1988
AB		40 MG	N72067 001	JUL 29, 1988
AB		80 MG	N72069 001	JUL 29, 1988

PROPRANOLOL HYDROCHLORIDE; *MULTIPLE*
SEE HYDROCHLOROTHIAZIDE; PROPRANOLOL HYDROCHLORIDE

PROPYLIODONE
SUSPENSION; INTRATRACHEAL
DIONOSIL OILY

	Manufacturer	Strength	Appl. No.
	GLAXO	60%	N09309 002

PROPYLTHIOURACIL
TABLET; ORAL
PROPYLTHIOURACIL

	Manufacturer	Strength	Appl. No.
BD	BARR	50 MG	N83982 001
BD	DANBURY	50 MG	N80932 001
BD	HALSEY	50 MG	N80015 001
BD	LANNETT	50 MG	N80016 001
BD	+ LEDERLE	50 MG	N06188 001
BD	LILLY	50 MG	N06213 001
BD	PUREPAC	50 MG	N80172 001
BD	RICHLYN	50 MG	N80159 001
BD	TABLICAPS	50 MG	N80840 001
BD	WEST WARD	50 MG	N80154 001

PROTAMINE SULFATE
INJECTABLE; INJECTION
PROTAMINE SULFATE

	Manufacturer	Strength	Appl. No.	Date
AP	ELKINS SINN	10 MG/ML	N89474 001	NOV 05, 1986
AP		10 MG/ML	N89475 001	NOV 05, 1986
AP	LILLY	10 MG/ML	N06460 002	
AP	LYPHOMED	10 MG/ML	N89454 001	APR 07, 1987
AP	QUAD	10 MG/ML	N89306 001	MAY 30, 1986

PROTIRELIN
INJECTABLE; INJECTION
RELEFACT TRH

	Manufacturer	Strength	Appl. No.
AP	FERRING	0.5 MG/ML	N18087 001

THYPINONE

	Manufacturer	Strength	Appl. No.
AP	ABBOTT	0.5 MG/ML	N17638 001

PROTOKYLOL HYDROCHLORIDE
TABLET; ORAL
VENTAIRE

	Manufacturer	Strength	Appl. No.
	MARION MERRELL DOW	2 MG	N83459 001

PROTRIPTYLINE HYDROCHLORIDE
TABLET; ORAL
VIVACTIL

	Manufacturer	Strength	Appl. No.
	MSD	5 MG	N16012 001
	+	10 MG	N16012 002

Prescription Drug Products (continued)

PSEUDOEPHEDRINE HYDROCHLORIDE
CAPSULE, EXTENDED RELEASE; ORAL
NOVAFED
DOW   120 MG   N17603 001

PSEUDOEPHEDRINE HYDROCHLORIDE; *MULTIPLE*
SEE   BROMPHENIRAMINE MALEATE: DEXTROMETHORPHAN HYDROBROMIDE: PSEUDOEPHEDRINE HYDROCHLORIDE
SEE   CODEINE PHOSPHATE: PSEUDOEPHEDRINE HYDROCHLORIDE: TRIPROLIDINE HYDROCHLORIDE

PSEUDOEPHEDRINE HYDROCHLORIDE; TERFENADINE
TABLET, EXTENDED RELEASE; ORAL
SELDANE-D
MERRELL DOW   120 MG;60 MG   N19664 001   AUG 19, 1991

PSEUDOEPHEDRINE HYDROCHLORIDE; TRIPROLIDINE HYDROCHLORIDE
SYRUP; ORAL
ACTAHIST
AA   CENCI   30 MG/5 ML;1.25 MG/5 ML   N88344 001   FEB 09, 1984
HISTAFED
AA   LIFE LABS   30 MG/5 ML;1.25 MG/5 ML   N88283 001   APR 20, 1984
TRILITRON
AA   NEWTRON   30 MG/5 ML;1.25 MG/5 ML   N88474 001   FEB 12, 1985
TABLET; ORAL
ALLERFED
AA   PRIVATE FORM   60 MG;2.5 MG   N88860 001   JAN 31, 1985
CORPHED
AA   GENEVA   60 MG;2.5 MG   N88602 001   APR 11, 1985
PSEUDOEPHEDRINE HCL AND TRIPROLIDINE HCL
AA   EON LABS   60 MG;2.5 MG   N88193 001   MAY 17, 1983
TRILITRON
AA   NEWTRON   60 MG;2.5 MG   N88515 001   JAN 09, 1985
TRIPHED
AA   LEMMON   60 MG;2.5 MG   N88630 001   MAY 17, 1984
TRIPROLIDINE HCL AND PSEUDOEPHEDRINE HCL
AA   SUPERPHARM   60 MG;2.5 MG   N88578 001   FEB 21, 1985
AA   ZENITH   60 MG;2.5 MG   N85273 001   DEC 12, 1984

PSEUDOEPHEDRINE SULFATE; *MULTIPLE*
SEE   AZATADINE MALEATE: PSEUDOEPHEDRINE SULFATE

PYRANTEL PAMOATE
SUSPENSION; ORAL
ANTIMINTH
+ ROERIG   EQ 250 MG BASE/5 ML   N16883 001

PYRAZINAMIDE
TABLET; ORAL
PYRAZINAMIDE
AB   + LEDERLE   500 MG   N80157 001
AB   + MIKART   500 MG   N81319 001   JUN 30, 1992

PYRIDOSTIGMINE BROMIDE
INJECTABLE; INJECTION
MESTINON
AP   ICN REGONOL   5 MG/ML   N09830 001
AP   ORGANON   5 MG/ML   N17398 001
SYRUP; ORAL
MESTINON
ICN   60 MG/5 ML   N15193 001
TABLET; ORAL
MESTINON
+ ICN   60 MG   N09829 002
PYRIDOSTIGMINE BROMIDE
KALI DUPHAR   30 MG   N89572 001   NOV 27, 1990
TABLET, EXTENDED RELEASE; ORAL
MESTINON
+ ICN   180 MG   N11665 001

PYRIDOXINE; *MULTIPLE*
SEE   ASCORBIC ACID: BIOTIN: CYANOCOBALAMIN: DEXPANTHENOL: ERGOCALCIFEROL: FOLIC ACID: NIACINAMIDE: PYRIDOXINE: RIBOFLAVIN PHOSPHATE SODIUM: THIAMINE: VITAMIN A: VITAMIN E

PYRIDOXINE HYDROCHLORIDE
INJECTABLE; INJECTION
HEXA-BETALIN
AP   LILLY   100 MG/ML   N80854 001
PYRIDOXINE HCL
AP   AKORN   100 MG/ML   N87967 001   OCT 01, 1982
AP   BEL MAR   100 MG/ML   N80761 001
AP   DELL   100 MG/ML   N83772 001
      50 MG/ML   N83771 001
AP   LYPHOMED   100 MG/ML   N80618 001
AP   STERIS   100 MG/ML   N80572 001
      100 MG/ML   N83760 001

Prescription Drug Products (continued)

PYRIDOXINE HYDROCHLORIDE; *MULTIPLE*
SEE   ASCORBIC ACID; BIOTIN; CYANOCOBALAMIN; DEXPANTHENOL; ERGOCALCIFEROL; FOLIC ACID; NIACINAMIDE; PYRIDOXINE HYDROCHLORIDE; RIBOFLAVIN PHOSPHATE SODIUM; THIAMINE HYDROCHLORIDE; VITAMIN A; VITAMIN E

PYRILAMINE MALEATE
TABLET; ORAL
PYRILAMINE MALEATE
RICHLYN   25 MG   N80808 001

PYRILAMINE MALEATE; *MULTIPLE*
SEE   PHENYLEPHRINE HYDROCHLORIDE; PYRILAMINE MALEATE

PYRIMETHAMINE
TABLET; ORAL
DARAPRIM
BURROUGHS WELLCOME   25 MG   N08578 001

PYRIMETHAMINE; SULFADOXINE
TABLET; ORAL
FANSIDAR
+ ROCHE   25 MG;500 MG   N18557 001

QUAZEPAM
TABLET; ORAL
DORAL
BAKER CUMMINS   7.5 MG   N18708 003   FEB 26, 1987
                                            N18708 001
+   15 MG   DEC 27, 1985

QUINAPRIL HYDROCHLORIDE
TABLET; ORAL
ACCUPRIL
PARKE DAVIS   EQ 5 MG BASE   N19885 001   NOV 19, 1991
                      EQ 10 MG BASE   N19885 002   NOV 19, 1991
                      EQ 20 MG BASE   N19885 003   NOV 19, 1991
                      EQ 40 MG BASE   N19885 004   NOV 19, 1991

QUINESTROL
TABLET; ORAL
ESTROVIS
PARKE DAVIS   0.1 MG   N16768 002

QUINETHAZONE
TABLET; ORAL
HYDROMOX
LEDERLE   50 MG   N13264 001

QUINIDINE GLUCONATE
INJECTABLE; INJECTION
QUINIDINE GLUCONATE
LILLY   80 MG/ML   N07529 002   FEB 10, 1989

TABLET, EXTENDED RELEASE; ORAL
DURAQUIN
PARKE DAVIS   330 MG   N17917 001
QUINAGLUTE
+ BERLEX   324 MG   N16647 001
QUINALAN
BC   LANNETT   324 MG   N88081 001   FEB 10, 1986
QUINIDINE GLUCONATE
AB   CHELSEA   324 MG   N87785 001   JAN 24, 1983
AB   DANBURY   324 MG   N87810 001   SEP 29, 1982
AB   GENEVA   324 MG   N89894 001   DEC 15, 1988
AB   HALSEY   324 MG   N89476 001   APR 10, 1987
AB   MUTUAL PHARM   324 MG   N89338 001   FEB 11, 1987

QUINIDINE POLYGALACTURONATE
TABLET; ORAL
CARDIOQUIN
PURDUE FREDERICK   275 MG   N11642 002

QUINIDINE SULFATE
CAPSULE; ORAL
CIN-QUIN
AB   SOLVAY   200 MG   N85296 001
                     300 MG   N85297 001
QUINIDINE SULFATE
AB   + LILLY   200 MG   N85103 001

Prescription Drug Products (continued)

QUINIDINE SULFATE (continued)

TABLET; ORAL

CIN-QUIN

TE	Firm	Strength	Appl. No.	Date
AB	SOLVAY	100 MG	N85299 001	
AB	SOLVAY	200 MG	N84932 001	
AB	SOLVAY	300 MG	N85298 001	

QUINIDINE SULFATE

TE	Firm	Strength	Appl. No.	Date
AB	BARR	200 MG	N84177 001	
AB	BEECHAM	200 MG	N85175 001	
AB	CHELSEA	200 MG	N85140 002	
AB	DANBURY	100 MG	N85584 001	
AB	DANBURY	200 MG	N83288 001	
AB	DANBURY	300 MG	N85583 001	
AB	EON LABS	200 MG	N84631 001	
AB	EON LABS	300 MG	N88072 001	SEP 26, 1983
AB	FIRST TX	200 MG	N85068 001	
AB	GENEVA	200 MG	N84914 001	
AB	GENEVA	300 MG	N89839 001	SEP 29, 1988
AB	HALSEY	200 MG	N83583 001	
AB	ICN	200 MG	N83393 001	
AB	KV	200 MG	N85276 001	
AB	LANNETT	200 MG	N83743 001	
AB	LEDERLE	200 MG	N87011 001	
AB	+ LILLY	200 MG	N85038 001	
AB	MUTUAL PHARM	100 MG	N81029 001	
AB	MUTUAL PHARM	200 MG	N81030 001	APR 14, 1989
AB	MUTUAL PHARM	300 MG	N81031 001	APR 14, 1989
AB	PARKE DAVIS	200 MG	N83879 001	APR 14, 1989
AB	PHARMAVITE	200 MG	N84627 001	
AB	PHOENIX LABS	200 MG	N83963 001	
AB	PRIVATE FORM	200 MG	N83808 001	
AB	PUREPAC	200 MG	N84003 001	
AB	RICHLYN	200 MG	N83347 001	
AB	ROXANE	300 MG	N83640 001	
AB	SUPERPHARM	200 MG	N85632 001	
AB	SUPERPHARM	300 MG	N88973 001	APR 10, 1985
AB	WEST WARD	200 MG	N83862 001	
AB	ZENITH	200 MG	N84549 001	

QUINORA

TE	Firm	Strength	Appl. No.	Date
AB	+ KEY PHARMS	300 MG	N85222 001	

TABLET, EXTENDED RELEASE; ORAL

QUINIDEX

TE	Firm	Strength	Appl. No.	Date
AB	+ ROBINS	300 MG	N12796 002	

RAMIPRIL

CAPSULE; ORAL

ALTACE

Firm	Strength	Appl. No.	Date
HOECHST ROUSSEL	1.25 MG	N19901 001	JAN 28, 1991
	2.5 MG	N19901 002	JAN 28, 1991
	5 MG	N19901 003	JAN 28, 1991
+	10 MG	N19901 004	JAN 28, 1991

RANITIDINE HYDROCHLORIDE

INJECTABLE; INJECTION

ZANTAC

Firm	Strength	Appl. No.	Date
GLAXO	EQ 25 MG BASE/ML	N19090 001	OCT 19, 1984

ZANTAC IN PLASTIC CONTAINER

Firm	Strength	Appl. No.	Date
GLAXO	EQ 1 MG BASE/ML	N19593 002	SEP 27, 1991

SYRUP; ORAL

ZANTAC

Firm	Strength	Appl. No.	Date
GLAXO	EQ 15 MG BASE/ML	N19675 001	DEC 30, 1988

TABLET; ORAL

ZANTAC 150

Firm	Strength	Appl. No.	Date
GLAXO	EQ 150 MG BASE	N18703 001	JUN 09, 1983

ZANTAC 300

Firm	Strength	Appl. No.	Date
+ GLAXO	EQ 300 MG BASE	N18703 002	DEC 09, 1985

RAUWOLFIA SERPENTINA

TABLET; ORAL

HIWOLFIA

TE	Firm	Strength	Appl. No.
BP	BOWMAN	50 MG	N09276 005

RAUDIXIN

TE	Firm	Strength	Appl. No.
BP	SQUIBB	50 MG	N08842 001
BP	+	100 MG	N08842 002

RAUVAL

TE	Firm	Strength	Appl. No.
BP	VALE	50 MG	N09108 002
BP		100 MG	N09108 004

RAUWOLFIA SERPENTINA

TE	Firm	Strength	Appl. No.
BP	DANBURY	50 MG	N80907 001
BP	HALSEY	50 MG	N80498 001
BP		100 MG	N80498 002
BP	RICHLYN	50 MG	N09273 001
BP		100 MG	N09273 002

RESCINNAMINE

TABLET; ORAL

MODERIL

Firm	Strength	Appl. No.
PFIZER	0.25 MG	N10686 003
	0.5 MG	N10686 006

Prescription Drug Products (continued)

RESERPINE
ELIXIR; ORAL
- SERPASIL
  - CIBA — 0.2 MG/4 ML — N09115 005

TABLET; ORAL
- RESERPINE
  - BP EON LABS — 0.1 MG — N09838 001
  - BP — 0.25 MG — N09838 002
  - BP LEMMON — 0.1 MG — N89020 001 — MAR 07, 1985
  - BP — 0.25 MG — N89019 001 — MAR 07, 1985
  - BP PUREPAC — 0.1 MG — N80753 002
  - BP — 0.25 MG — N80753 001
  - BP RICHLYN — 0.1 MG — N09627 001
  - BP — 0.25 MG — N09627 002
  - BP SERPALAN LANNETT — 0.1 MG — N10124 001
  - BP — 0.25 MG — N10124 002
  - BP SERPASIL CIBA — 0.1 MG — N09115 001
  - BP — 0.25 MG — N09115 003
  - BP + SERPIVITE VITARINE — 0.25 MG — N09645 002

RESERPINE; *MULTIPLE*
SEE CHLOROTHIAZIDE: RESERPINE
SEE CHLORTHALIDONE: RESERPINE
SEE HYDRALAZINE HYDROCHLORIDE: HYDROCHLOROTHIAZIDE: RESERPINE
SEE HYDRALAZINE HYDROCHLORIDE: RESERPINE
SEE HYDROCHLOROTHIAZIDE: RESERPINE
SEE HYDROFLUMETHIAZIDE: RESERPINE
SEE METHYCLOTHIAZIDE: RESERPINE
SEE POLYTHIAZIDE: RESERPINE

RESERPINE; TRICHLORMETHIAZIDE
TABLET; ORAL
- METATENSIN #2 MERRELL DOW — 0.1 MG;2 MG — N12972 001
- METATENSIN #4 MERRELL DOW — 0.1 MG;4 MG — N12972 002
- BP NAQUIVAL + SCHERING — 0.1 MG;4 MG — N12265 003

RIBAVIRIN
POWDER FOR RECONSTITUTION; INHALATION
- VIRAZOLE + VIRATEK — 6 GM/VIAL — N18859 001 — DEC 31, 1985

RIBOFLAVIN PHOSPHATE SODIUM; *MULTIPLE*
SEE ASCORBIC ACID: BIOTIN: CYANOCOBALAMIN: DEXPANTHENOL: ERGOCALCIFEROL: FOLIC ACID: NIACINAMIDE: PYRIDOXINE HYDROCHLORIDE: RIBOFLAVIN PHOSPHATE SODIUM: THIAMINE HYDROCHLORIDE: VITAMIN A: VITAMIN E
SEE ASCORBIC ACID: BIOTIN: CYANOCOBALAMIN: DEXPANTHENOL: ERGOCALCIFEROL: FOLIC ACID: NIACINAMIDE: PYRIDOXINE: RIBOFLAVIN PHOSPHATE SODIUM: THIAMINE: VITAMIN A: VITAMIN E

RIFAMPIN
CAPSULE; ORAL
- RIFADIN
  - ΔB + MERRELL DOW — 300 MG — N50420 001
  - — 150 MG — N62303 001
- RIMACTANE
  - ΔB CIBA — 300 MG — N50429 001

INJECTABLE; INJECTION
- RIFADIN MERRELL DOW — 600 MG/VIAL — N50627 001 — MAY 25, 1989

RIFAMPIN; *MULTIPLE*
SEE ISONIAZID: RIFAMPIN

RITODRINE HYDROCHLORIDE
INJECTABLE; INJECTION
- RITODRINE HCL
  - ΔP ABBOTT — 10 MG/ML — N71618 001 — FEB 28, 1991
  - ΔP — 15 MG/ML — N71619 001 — FEB 28, 1991
  - ΔP QUAD — 10 MG/ML — N70700 001 — OCT 06, 1986
- RITODRINE HCL IN DEXTROSE 5% IN PLASTIC CONTAINER
  - ABBOTT — 30 MG/100 ML — N71438 001 — JAN 22, 1991
- YUTOPAR
  - ΔP ASTRA — 10 MG/ML — N18580 001
  - ΔP — 15 MG/ML — N18580 002

TABLET; ORAL
- YUTOPAR
  - BP ASTRA — 10 MG — N18555 001

RUBIDIUM CHLORIDE RB-82
INJECTABLE; INJECTION
- CARDIOGEN-82 SQUIBB — N/A — N19414 001 — DEC 29, 1989

Prescription Drug Products *(continued)*

SAFFLOWER OIL; SOYBEAN OIL

INJECTABLE; INJECTION

Code	Firm	Strength	Appl. No.	Approval
	LIPOSYN II 10%			
	ABBOTT	5%;5%	N18997 001	AUG 27, 1984
	LIPOSYN II 20%			
	ABBOTT	10%;10%	N18991 001	AUG 27, 1984

SCOPOLAMINE

FILM, EXTENDED RELEASE; TRANSDERMAL

Code	Firm	Strength	Appl. No.
	TRANSDERM-SCOP		
	CIBA	0.5 MG/24 HR	N17874 001

SECOBARBITAL SODIUM

CAPSULE; ORAL

Code	Firm	Strength	Appl. No.	Approval
	SECOBARBITAL SODIUM			
AA	EVERYLIFE	100 MG	N85895 001	
AA	ICN	100 MG	N85477 001	
AA	LANNETT	50 MG	N85909 001	
AA	ZENITH	100 MG	N85903 001	
	SECONAL SODIUM			
AA	LILLY	100 MG	N85869 001	
AA	LILLY	50 MG	N86101 001	OCT 03, 1983
		100 MG	N86101 002	OCT 03, 1983
	SODIUM SECOBARBITAL			
AA	HALSEY	100 MG	N84676 001	
AA	WEST WARD	100 MG	N84926 001	

INJECTABLE; INJECTION

Code	Firm	Strength	Appl. No.
	SECOBARBITAL SODIUM		
	ELKINS SINN	100 MG/VIAL	N83281 001
	SODIUM SECOBARBITAL		
	WYETH AYERST	50 MG/ML	N83262 001

SECRETIN

INJECTABLE; INJECTION

Code	Firm	Strength	Appl. No.
	SECRETIN-FERRING		
	FERRING	75CU/VIAL	N18290 001

SELEGILINE HYDROCHLORIDE

TABLET; ORAL

Code	Firm	Strength	Appl. No.	Approval
	ELDEPRYL			
+	SOMERSET	5 MG	N19334 001	JUN 05, 1989

SELENIUM SULFIDE

LOTION/SHAMPOO; TOPICAL

Code	Firm	Strength	Appl. No.	Approval
	EXSEL			
AT	HERBERT	2.5%	N83892 001	
	SELENIUM SULFIDE			
AT	BARRE	2.5%	N84394 001	
AT	CLAY PARK	2.5%	N89996 001	JAN 10, 1991
AT	PHARM BASICS	2.5%	N88228 001	SEP 01, 1983
	SYOSSET			
AT	THAMES	2.5%	N85777 001	
AT		2.5%	N86209 001	
	SELSUN			
AT	ABBOTT	2.5%	N07936 001	

SELENOMETHIONINE, SE-75

INJECTABLE; INJECTION

Code	Firm	Strength	Appl. No.
	SELENOMETHIONINE SE 75		
	CIS	500 UCI/ML	N17322 001

SERACTIDE ACETATE

INJECTABLE; INJECTION

Code	Firm	Strength	Appl. No.
	ACTHAR GEL-SYNTHETIC		
	ARMOUR	40 UNITS/ML	N17861 001
		80 UNITS/ML	N17861 002

SERMORELIN ACETATE

INJECTABLE; INJECTION

Code	Firm	Strength	Appl. No.	Approval
	GEREF			
	SERONO	EQ 0.05 MG BASE/AMP	N19863 001	DEC 28, 1990

SERTRALINE HYDROCHLORIDE

TABLET; ORAL

Code	Firm	Strength	Appl. No.	Approval
	ZOLOFT			
	PFIZER	EQ 50 MG BASE	N19839 001	DEC 30, 1991
		EQ 100 MG BASE	N19839 002	DEC 30, 1991

Prescription Drug Products (continued)

SILVER SULFADIAZINE

CREAM; TOPICAL
SILVADENE
+ MARION MERRELL
   DOW ...... 1% N17381 001
ΔB SSD BOOTS ...... 1% N18578 001
   FEB 25, 1982
ΔB THERMAZENE
SHERWOOD ...... 1% N18810 001
   DEC 23, 1985

DRESSING; TOPICAL
SILDIMAC
MARION MERRELL
   DOW ...... 1% N19608 001
   NOV 30, 1989

SIMVASTATIN

TABLET; ORAL
ZOCOR
MERCK ...... 5 MG N19766 001
   DEC 23, 1991
   10 MG N19766 002
   DEC 23, 1991
   20 MG N19766 003
   DEC 23, 1991
   40 MG N19766 004
   DEC 23, 1991

SINCALIDE

INJECTABLE; INJECTION
KINEVAC
SQUIBB ...... 0.005 MG/VIAL N17697 001

SODIUM ACETATE; *MULTIPLE*

SEE AMINO ACIDS; CALCIUM ACETATE: GLYCERIN: MAGNESIUM
ACETATE: PHOSPHORIC ACID: POTASSIUM CHLORIDE:
SODIUM ACETATE: SODIUM CHLORIDE

SEE AMINO ACIDS: MAGNESIUM ACETATE: PHOSPHORIC ACID:
POTASSIUM ACETATE: POTASSIUM CHLORIDE: SODIUM
ACETATE

SEE AMINO ACIDS: MAGNESIUM ACETATE: PHOSPHORIC ACID:
POTASSIUM CHLORIDE: SODIUM ACETATE: SODIUM
CHLORIDE

SEE AMINO ACIDS: MAGNESIUM CHLORIDE: POTASSIUM
ACETATE: POTASSIUM CHLORIDE: SODIUM ACETATE

SEE AMINO ACIDS: MAGNESIUM CHLORIDE: POTASSIUM
PHOSPHATE, DIBASIC: SODIUM ACETATE: SODIUM CHLORIDE

SEE CALCIUM CHLORIDE: DEXTROSE: MAGNESIUM CHLORIDE:
SODIUM ACETATE: SODIUM CHLORIDE

SODIUM ACETATE; *MULTIPLE* (continued)

SEE CALCIUM CHLORIDE: DEXTROSE: MAGNESIUM CHLORIDE:
POTASSIUM CHLORIDE: SODIUM ACETATE: SODIUM
CHLORIDE

SEE CALCIUM CHLORIDE: DEXTROSE: MAGNESIUM CHLORIDE:
POTASSIUM CHLORIDE: SODIUM ACETATE: SODIUM
CHLORIDE: SODIUM LACTATE

SEE CALCIUM CHLORIDE: DEXTROSE: MAGNESIUM CHLORIDE:
POTASSIUM CHLORIDE: SODIUM ACETATE: SODIUM
CHLORIDE: SODIUM CITRATE

SEE CALCIUM CHLORIDE: DEXTROSE: POTASSIUM CHLORIDE:
SODIUM ACETATE: SODIUM CHLORIDE

SEE CALCIUM CHLORIDE: MAGNESIUM CHLORIDE: POTASSIUM
CHLORIDE: SODIUM ACETATE: SODIUM CHLORIDE: SODIUM
CITRATE

SEE CALCIUM CHLORIDE: MAGNESIUM CHLORIDE: POTASSIUM
CHLORIDE: SODIUM ACETATE: SODIUM CHLORIDE

SEE CALCIUM CHLORIDE: MAGNESIUM CHLORIDE: POTASSIUM
CHLORIDE: SODIUM ACETATE: SODIUM CHLORIDE: SODIUM
LACTATE

SEE DEXTROSE: MAGNESIUM CHLORIDE: POTASSIUM CHLORIDE:
SODIUM ACETATE: SODIUM CHLORIDE: SODIUM GLUCONATE

SEE DEXTROSE: MAGNESIUM CHLORIDE: POTASSIUM CHLORIDE:
SODIUM ACETATE: SODIUM CHLORIDE

SEE DEXTROSE: MAGNESIUM CHLORIDE: POTASSIUM CHLORIDE:
SODIUM ACETATE: SODIUM CHLORIDE: SODIUM GLUCONATE

SEE DEXTROSE: MAGNESIUM CHLORIDE: POTASSIUM CHLORIDE:
POTASSIUM PHOSPHATE, DIBASIC: SODIUM ACETATE

SEE DEXTROSE: POTASSIUM CHLORIDE: POTASSIUM PHOSPHATE,
DIBASIC: SODIUM ACETATE: SODIUM CHLORIDE

SEE MAGNESIUM CHLORIDE: POTASSIUM CHLORIDE: POTASSIUM
PHOSPHATE, MONOBASIC: SODIUM ACETATE: SODIUM
CHLORIDE: SODIUM GLUCONATE: SODIUM PHOSPHATE,
DIBASIC

SEE MAGNESIUM CHLORIDE: POTASSIUM CHLORIDE: SODIUM
ACETATE: SODIUM CHLORIDE: SODIUM GLUCONATE

SODIUM ACETATE, ANHYDROUS

INJECTABLE; INJECTION
SODIUM ACETATE IN PLASTIC CONTAINER
ABBOTT ...... 2 MEQ/ML N18893 001
   MAY 04, 1983

SODIUM BENZOATE; SODIUM PHENYLACETATE

SOLUTION; ORAL
UCEPHAN
MCGAW ...... 100 MG/ML;100 MG/ML N19530 001
   DEC 23, 1987

Prescription Drug Products (continued)

SODIUM BICARBONATE
INJECTABLE; INJECTION
SODIUM BICARBONATE IN PLASTIC CONTAINER

ABBOTT	0.9 MEQ/ML	N19443 001	JUN 03, 1986
	1 MEQ/ML	N19443 002	JUN 03, 1986

SODIUM BICARBONATE; *MULTIPLE*
SEE CALCIUM CHLORIDE; DEXTROSE; GLUTATHIONE DISULFIDE; MAGNESIUM CHLORIDE; POTASSIUM CHLORIDE; SODIUM BICARBONATE; SODIUM CHLORIDE; SODIUM PHOSPHATE

SEE POLYETHYLENE GLYCOL 3350; POTASSIUM CHLORIDE; SODIUM BICARBONATE; SODIUM CHLORIDE; SODIUM SULFATE, ANHYDROUS

SEE POLYETHYLENE GLYCOL 3350; POTASSIUM CHLORIDE; SODIUM BICARBONATE; SODIUM CHLORIDE

SEE POLYETHYLENE GLYCOL 3350; POTASSIUM CHLORIDE; SODIUM BICARBONATE; SODIUM CHLORIDE; SODIUM SULFATE

SEE POLYETHYLENE GLYCOL 3350; POTASSIUM CHLORIDE; SODIUM BICARBONATE; SODIUM CHLORIDE; SODIUM SULFATE, ANHYDROUS

SODIUM BICARBONATE; TARTARIC ACID
GRANULE, EFFERVESCENT; ORAL
BAROS

E Z EM	460 MG/GM;420 MG/GM	N18509 001	AUG 07, 1985

SODIUM CARBONATE; *MULTIPLE*
SEE CITRIC ACID; MAGNESIUM OXIDE; SODIUM CARBONATE

SODIUM CHLORIDE
INJECTABLE; INJECTION
BACTERIOSTATIC SODIUM CHLORIDE 0.9% IN PLASTIC CONTAINER

ABBOTT	9 MG/ML	N18800 001	OCT 29, 1982
		N88911 001	FEB 07, 1985
LYPHOMED	9 MG/ML	N88909 001	FEB 07, 1985

SODIUM CHLORIDE

MCGAW	20 GM/100 ML	N17038 001	

SODIUM CHLORIDE IN PLASTIC CONTAINER

ABBOTT	2.5 MEQ/ML	N18897 001	JUL 20, 1984

SODIUM CHLORIDE (continued)
INJECTABLE; INJECTION
SODIUM CHLORIDE 0.45% IN PLASTIC CONTAINER

AP	ABBOTT	450 MG/100 ML	N18090 001	
AP		450 MG/100 ML	N19759 001	JUN 08, 1988
AP	BAXTER	450 MG/100 ML	N18016 001	
AP	MCGAW	450 MG/100 ML	N18184 001	
AP		450 MG/100 ML	N19635 001	MAR 09, 1988

SODIUM CHLORIDE 0.9% IN PLASTIC CONTAINER

AP	ABBOTT	900 MG/100 ML	N16366 001	
AP		9 MG/ML	N18803 001	OCT 29, 1982
AP		9 MG/ML	N19217 001	JUL 13, 1984
AP		900 MG/100 ML	N19465 001	JUL 15, 1985
AP		900 MG/100 ML	N19480 001	SEP 17, 1985
AP	BAXTER	900 MG/100 ML	N16677 001	
AP		9 MG/ML	N16677 004	OCT 30, 1985
AP	LYPHOMED	9 MG/ML	N88912 001	JAN 10, 1985
AP	MCGAW	900 MG/100 ML	N17464 001	
AP		900 MG/100 ML	N19635 002	MAR 09, 1988

SODIUM CHLORIDE 3% IN PLASTIC CONTAINER

BAXTER	3 GM/100 ML	N19022 001	NOV 01, 1983

SODIUM CHLORIDE 5% IN PLASTIC CONTAINER

BAXTER	5 GM/100 ML	N19022 002	NOV 01, 1983

SOLUTION FOR SLUSH; IRRIGATION
SODIUM CHLORIDE 0.9% IN STERILE PLASTIC CONTAINER

BAXTER	900 MG/100 ML	N19319 002	MAY 17, 1985

SOLUTION; IRRIGATION
SODIUM CHLORIDE 0.45% IN PLASTIC CONTAINER

AT	ABBOTT	450 MG/100 ML	N17670 001	
AT	BAXTER	450 MG/100 ML	N17864 001	
AT		450 MG/100 ML	N18497 001	FEB 19, 1982

SODIUM CHLORIDE 0.9% IN PLASTIC CONTAINER

AT	ABBOTT	900 MG/100 ML	N17514 001	
AT		900 MG/100 ML	N18314 001	
AT	BAXTER	900 MG/100 ML	N17427 001	
AT		900 MG/100 ML	N17867 001	
AT	MCGAW	900 MG/100 ML	N16733 001	

Prescription Drug Products *(continued)*

SODIUM CHLORIDE; *MULTIPLE*

SEE   AMINO ACIDS; CALCIUM ACETATE; GLYCERIN; MAGNESIUM ACETATE; PHOSPHORIC ACID; POTASSIUM CHLORIDE; SODIUM ACETATE; SODIUM CHLORIDE

SEE   AMINO ACIDS; CALCIUM CHLORIDE; DEXTROSE; MAGNESIUM CHLORIDE; POTASSIUM CHLORIDE; POTASSIUM PHOSPHATE, DIBASIC; SODIUM CHLORIDE

SEE   AMINO ACIDS; DEXTROSE; MAGNESIUM CHLORIDE; POTASSIUM ACETATE; POTASSIUM CHLORIDE; POTASSIUM PHOSPHATE, DIBASIC; SODIUM CHLORIDE

SEE   AMINO ACIDS; DEXTROSE; MAGNESIUM CHLORIDE; POTASSIUM CHLORIDE; SODIUM CHLORIDE; SODIUM PHOSPHATE, DIBASIC

SEE   AMINO ACIDS; MAGNESIUM ACETATE; PHOSPHORIC ACID; POTASSIUM ACETATE; SODIUM CHLORIDE

SEE   AMINO ACIDS; MAGNESIUM ACETATE; PHOSPHORIC ACID; POTASSIUM CHLORIDE; SODIUM ACETATE; SODIUM CHLORIDE

SEE   AMINO ACIDS; MAGNESIUM ACETATE; POTASSIUM ACETATE; SODIUM CHLORIDE

SEE   AMINO ACIDS; MAGNESIUM CHLORIDE; POTASSIUM CHLORIDE; SODIUM CHLORIDE; SODIUM PHOSPHATE, DIBASIC

SEE   AMINO ACIDS; MAGNESIUM CHLORIDE; POTASSIUM CHLORIDE; POTASSIUM PHOSPHATE, DIBASIC; SODIUM CHLORIDE

SEE   AMINO ACIDS; MAGNESIUM CHLORIDE; POTASSIUM CHLORIDE; SODIUM ACETATE; SODIUM CHLORIDE; PHOSPHATE, DIBASIC; SODIUM CHLORIDE

SEE   CALCIUM CHLORIDE; DEXTROSE; GLUTATHIONE DISULFIDE; MAGNESIUM CHLORIDE; POTASSIUM CHLORIDE; SODIUM BICARBONATE; SODIUM CHLORIDE; SODIUM PHOSPHATE

SEE   CALCIUM CHLORIDE; DEXTROSE; MAGNESIUM CHLORIDE; SODIUM CHLORIDE; SODIUM LACTATE

SEE   CALCIUM CHLORIDE; DEXTROSE; MAGNESIUM CHLORIDE; SODIUM ACETATE; SODIUM CHLORIDE

SEE   CALCIUM CHLORIDE; DEXTROSE; MAGNESIUM CHLORIDE; POTASSIUM CHLORIDE; SODIUM ACETATE; SODIUM CHLORIDE

SEE   CALCIUM CHLORIDE; DEXTROSE; MAGNESIUM CHLORIDE; POTASSIUM CHLORIDE; SODIUM ACETATE; SODIUM CHLORIDE; SODIUM LACTATE

SEE   CALCIUM CHLORIDE; DEXTROSE; MAGNESIUM CHLORIDE; POTASSIUM CHLORIDE; SODIUM CITRATE

SEE   CALCIUM CHLORIDE; DEXTROSE; MAGNESIUM CHLORIDE; SODIUM CHLORIDE; SODIUM LACTATE

SODIUM CHLORIDE; *MULTIPLE* *(continued)*

SEE   CALCIUM CHLORIDE; DEXTROSE; POTASSIUM CHLORIDE; SODIUM CHLORIDE

SEE   CALCIUM CHLORIDE; DEXTROSE; POTASSIUM CHLORIDE; SODIUM CHLORIDE; SODIUM LACTATE

SEE   CALCIUM CHLORIDE; DEXTROSE; POTASSIUM CHLORIDE; SODIUM ACETATE; SODIUM CHLORIDE

SEE   CALCIUM CHLORIDE; DEXTROSE; POTASSIUM CHLORIDE; SODIUM CHLORIDE; SODIUM LACTATE

SEE   CALCIUM CHLORIDE; MAGNESIUM CHLORIDE; POTASSIUM CHLORIDE; SODIUM ACETATE; SODIUM CHLORIDE; SODIUM CITRATE

SEE   CALCIUM CHLORIDE; MAGNESIUM CHLORIDE; POTASSIUM CHLORIDE; SODIUM ACETATE; SODIUM CHLORIDE

SEE   CALCIUM CHLORIDE; MAGNESIUM CHLORIDE; POTASSIUM CHLORIDE; SODIUM ACETATE; SODIUM CHLORIDE; SODIUM LACTATE

SEE   CALCIUM CHLORIDE; MAGNESIUM CHLORIDE; POTASSIUM CHLORIDE; SODIUM CHLORIDE

SEE   CALCIUM CHLORIDE; POTASSIUM CHLORIDE; SODIUM CHLORIDE

SEE   CALCIUM CHLORIDE; POTASSIUM CHLORIDE; SODIUM CHLORIDE; SODIUM LACTATE

SEE   DEXTROSE; MAGNESIUM ACETATE; POTASSIUM ACETATE; SODIUM CHLORIDE

SEE   DEXTROSE; MAGNESIUM ACETATE TETRAHYDRATE; POTASSIUM ACETATE; SODIUM CHLORIDE

SEE   DEXTROSE; MAGNESIUM CHLORIDE; POTASSIUM CHLORIDE; SODIUM ACETATE; SODIUM CHLORIDE; SODIUM GLUCONATE

SEE   DEXTROSE; MAGNESIUM CHLORIDE; POTASSIUM CHLORIDE; SODIUM ACETATE; SODIUM CHLORIDE

SEE   DEXTROSE; MAGNESIUM CHLORIDE; POTASSIUM CHLORIDE; SODIUM ACETATE; SODIUM CHLORIDE; SODIUM GLUCONATE

SEE   DEXTROSE; MAGNESIUM CHLORIDE; POTASSIUM CHLORIDE; POTASSIUM PHOSPHATE, DIBASIC; SODIUM CHLORIDE; SODIUM LACTATE; SODIUM PHOSPHATE, MONOBASIC

SEE   DEXTROSE; MAGNESIUM CHLORIDE; POTASSIUM CHLORIDE; POTASSIUM PHOSPHATE, MONOBASIC; SODIUM CHLORIDE; SODIUM LACTATE

SEE   DEXTROSE; POTASSIUM CHLORIDE; POTASSIUM LACTATE; SODIUM CHLORIDE; SODIUM PHOSPHATE, MONOBASIC

SEE   DEXTROSE; POTASSIUM CHLORIDE; POTASSIUM PHOSPHATE, DIBASIC; SODIUM ACETATE; SODIUM CHLORIDE

SEE   DEXTROSE; POTASSIUM CHLORIDE; POTASSIUM PHOSPHATE, MONOBASIC; SODIUM CHLORIDE; SODIUM LACTATE

SEE   DEXTROSE; POTASSIUM CHLORIDE; SODIUM CHLORIDE

Prescription Drug Products (continued)

SODIUM CHLORIDE; *MULTIPLE* (continued)

SEE   DEXTROSE: SODIUM CHLORIDE

SEE   MAGNESIUM ACETATE TETRAHYDRATE: POTASSIUM ACETATE: SODIUM CHLORIDE

SEE   MAGNESIUM CHLORIDE: POTASSIUM CHLORIDE: POTASSIUM PHOSPHATE, MONOBASIC: SODIUM ACETATE: SODIUM CHLORIDE: SODIUM GLUCONATE: SODIUM PHOSPHATE, DIBASIC

SEE   MAGNESIUM CHLORIDE: POTASSIUM CHLORIDE: SODIUM ACETATE: SODIUM CHLORIDE: SODIUM GLUCONATE

SEE   MAGNESIUM SULFATE: POTASSIUM CHLORIDE: POTASSIUM PHOSPHATE, MONOBASIC: SODIUM CHLORIDE: SODIUM PHOSPHATE

SEE   POLYETHYLENE GLYCOL 3350: POTASSIUM CHLORIDE: SODIUM BICARBONATE: SODIUM CHLORIDE: SODIUM SULFATE, ANHYDROUS

SEE   POLYETHYLENE GLYCOL 3350: POTASSIUM CHLORIDE: SODIUM BICARBONATE: SODIUM CHLORIDE

SEE   POLYETHYLENE GLYCOL 3350: POTASSIUM CHLORIDE: SODIUM BICARBONATE: SODIUM CHLORIDE: SODIUM SULFATE

SEE   POLYETHYLENE GLYCOL 3350: POTASSIUM CHLORIDE: SODIUM BICARBONATE: SODIUM CHLORIDE: SODIUM SULFATE, ANHYDROUS

SEE   POTASSIUM CHLORIDE: SODIUM CHLORIDE

SEE   POTASSIUM CHLORIDE: SODIUM CHLORIDE: TROMETHAMINE

SODIUM CHROMATE, CR-51

INJECTABLE; INJECTION

CHROMITOPE SODIUM

SQUIBB	250 UCI/VIAL	N13993 001	
	1 MCI/VIAL	N13993 003	
	2 MCI/VIAL	N13993 002	

SODIUM CHROMATE CR 51

MALLINCKRODT	100 UCI/ML	N16708 001	

SODIUM CITRATE; *MULTIPLE*

SEE   CALCIUM CHLORIDE: DEXTROSE: MAGNESIUM CHLORIDE: POTASSIUM CHLORIDE: SODIUM ACETATE: SODIUM CHLORIDE: SODIUM CITRATE

SEE   CALCIUM CHLORIDE: MAGNESIUM CHLORIDE: POTASSIUM CHLORIDE: SODIUM ACETATE: SODIUM CHLORIDE: SODIUM CITRATE

SODIUM GLUCONATE; *MULTIPLE*

SEE   DEXTROSE: MAGNESIUM CHLORIDE: POTASSIUM CHLORIDE: SODIUM ACETATE: SODIUM CHLORIDE: SODIUM GLUCONATE

SEE   MAGNESIUM CHLORIDE: POTASSIUM CHLORIDE: POTASSIUM PHOSPHATE, MONOBASIC: SODIUM ACETATE: SODIUM CHLORIDE: SODIUM GLUCONATE: SODIUM PHOSPHATE, DIBASIC

SEE   MAGNESIUM CHLORIDE: POTASSIUM CHLORIDE: SODIUM ACETATE: SODIUM CHLORIDE: SODIUM GLUCONATE

SODIUM IODIDE, I-123

CAPSULE; ORAL

SODIUM IODIDE I 123

AA	BENEDICT	100 UCI	N18671 001	MAY 27, 1982
AA		200 UCI	N18671 002	MAY 27, 1982
AA	MALLINCKRODT	100 UCI	N71909 001	FEB 28, 1989
AA		200 UCI	N71910 001	FEB 28, 1989
AA	MEDI PHYSICS	100 UCI	N17630 001	

SOLUTION; ORAL

SODIUM IODIDE I 123

MEDI PHYSICS	2 MCI/ML	N17630 002	

SODIUM IODIDE, I-131

CAPSULE; ORAL

IODOTOPE

SQUIBB	8-100 UCI	N10929 001
	1-50 MCI	N10929 003

SODIUM IODIDE I 131

CIS	100 UCI	N17316 002
MALLINCKRODT	15-100 UCI	N16517 002
	0.8-100 MCI	N16517 001

SOLUTION; ORAL

IODOTOPE

SQUIBB	7-106 MCI/BOT	N10929 002

SODIUM IODIDE I 131

CIS	50 MCI/ML	N17315 001
MALLINCKRODT	3.5-150 MCI/VIAL	N16515 001

SODIUM LACTATE

INJECTABLE; INJECTION

SODIUM LACTATE IN PLASTIC CONTAINER

ABBOTT	5 MEQ/ML	N18947 001	SEP 05, 1984

SODIUM LACTATE 0.167 MOLAR IN PLASTIC CONTAINER

AP	ABBOTT	1.87 GM/100 ML	N18249 001
AP	BAXTER	1.87 GM/100 ML	N16692 001
AP	MCGAW	1.87 GM/100 ML	N18186 001

SODIUM LACTATE 1/6 MOLAR IN PLASTIC CONTAINER

AP	MCGAW	1.87 GM/100 ML	N20004 001	APR 21, 1992

Prescription Drug Products (continued)

SODIUM LACTATE; *MULTIPLE*

SEE   CALCIUM CHLORIDE: DEXTROSE: MAGNESIUM CHLORIDE: SODIUM CHLORIDE: SODIUM LACTATE

SEE   CALCIUM CHLORIDE: DEXTROSE: MAGNESIUM CHLORIDE: POTASSIUM CHLORIDE: SODIUM ACETATE: SODIUM CHLORIDE: SODIUM LACTATE

SEE   CALCIUM CHLORIDE: DEXTROSE: MAGNESIUM CHLORIDE: SODIUM CHLORIDE: SODIUM LACTATE

SEE   CALCIUM CHLORIDE: DEXTROSE: POTASSIUM CHLORIDE: SODIUM CHLORIDE: SODIUM LACTATE

SEE   CALCIUM CHLORIDE: MAGNESIUM CHLORIDE: POTASSIUM CHLORIDE: SODIUM ACETATE: SODIUM CHLORIDE: SODIUM LACTATE

SEE   CALCIUM CHLORIDE: POTASSIUM CHLORIDE: SODIUM CHLORIDE: SODIUM LACTATE

SEE   DEXTROSE: MAGNESIUM CHLORIDE: POTASSIUM CHLORIDE: POTASSIUM PHOSPHATE, DIBASIC: SODIUM CHLORIDE: SODIUM LACTATE: SODIUM PHOSPHATE, MONOBASIC

SEE   DEXTROSE: MAGNESIUM CHLORIDE: POTASSIUM CHLORIDE: POTASSIUM PHOSPHATE, MONOBASIC: SODIUM LACTATE: SODIUM PHOSPHATE, MONOBASIC

SEE   DEXTROSE: MAGNESIUM CHLORIDE: POTASSIUM CHLORIDE: POTASSIUM PHOSPHATE, MONOBASIC: SODIUM CHLORIDE: SODIUM LACTATE

SEE   DEXTROSE: POTASSIUM CHLORIDE: POTASSIUM PHOSPHATE, MONOBASIC: SODIUM CHLORIDE: SODIUM LACTATE

SODIUM NITROPRUSSIDE

INJECTABLE; INJECTION
   NIPRIDE

ΔΡ	ROCHE	50 MG/VIAL	N17546 001

   NITROPRESS

ΔΡ	ABBOTT	25 MG/ML	N71961 001 AUG 01, 1988
ΔΡ		50 MG/VIAL	N18450 001
ΔΡ		50 MG/VIAL	N70566 001 JUN 09, 1986
ΔΡ		50 MG/VIAL	N71555 001 NOV 16, 1987

   SODIUM NITROPRUSSIDE

ΔΡ	ELKINS SINN	50 MG/VIAL	N18581 001 JUL 28, 1982
ΔΡ	GENSIA	25 MG/ML	N73465 001 MAR 30, 1992

SODIUM PHENYLACETATE; *MULTIPLE*

SEE   SODIUM BENZOATE: SODIUM PHENYLACETATE

SODIUM PHOSPHATE; *MULTIPLE*

SEE   CALCIUM CHLORIDE: DEXTROSE: GLUTATHIONE DISULFIDE: MAGNESIUM CHLORIDE: POTASSIUM CHLORIDE: SODIUM BICARBONATE: SODIUM CHLORIDE: SODIUM PHOSPHATE

SEE   MAGNESIUM SULFATE: POTASSIUM CHLORIDE: POTASSIUM PHOSPHATE, MONOBASIC:.SODIUM CHLORIDE: SODIUM PHOSPHATE

SODIUM PHOSPHATE, DIBASIC; *MULTIPLE*

SEE   AMINO ACIDS: DEXTROSE: MAGNESIUM CHLORIDE: POTASSIUM CHLORIDE: SODIUM CHLORIDE: SODIUM PHOSPHATE, DIBASIC

SEE   AMINO ACIDS: MAGNESIUM CHLORIDE: POTASSIUM CHLORIDE: SODIUM CHLORIDE: SODIUM PHOSPHATE, DIBASIC

SEE   MAGNESIUM CHLORIDE: POTASSIUM CHLORIDE: POTASSIUM PHOSPHATE, MONOBASIC: SODIUM ACETATE: SODIUM CHLORIDE: SODIUM GLUCONATE: SODIUM PHOSPHATE, DIBASIC

SODIUM PHOSPHATE, DIBASIC; SODIUM PHOSPHATE, MONOBASIC

INJECTABLE; INJECTION
   SODIUM PHOSPHATES IN PLASTIC CONTAINER

	ABBOTT	142 MG/ML;276 MG/ML	N18892 001 MAY 10, 1983

SODIUM PHOSPHATE, MONOBASIC; *MULTIPLE*

SEE   DEXTROSE: MAGNESIUM CHLORIDE: POTASSIUM CHLORIDE: POTASSIUM PHOSPHATE, DIBASIC: SODIUM CHLORIDE: SODIUM LACTATE: SODIUM PHOSPHATE, MONOBASIC

SEE   DEXTROSE: MAGNESIUM CHLORIDE: POTASSIUM CHLORIDE: POTASSIUM PHOSPHATE, MONOBASIC: SODIUM LACTATE: SODIUM PHOSPHATE, MONOBASIC

SEE   DEXTROSE: POTASSIUM CHLORIDE: POTASSIUM LACTATE: SODIUM CHLORIDE: SODIUM PHOSPHATE, MONOBASIC

SEE   SODIUM PHOSPHATE, DIBASIC: SODIUM PHOSPHATE, MONOBASIC

SODIUM PHOSPHATE, P-32

SOLUTION; INJECTION, ORAL
   SODIUM PHOSPHATE P 32

	MALLINCKRODT	0.67 MCI/ML	N11777 001

Prescription Drug Products (continued)

SODIUM POLYSTYRENE SULFONATE

POWDER; ORAL, RECTAL

KAYEXALATE
- STERLING   453.6 GM/BOT   N11287 001

SODIUM POLYSTYRENE SULFONATE
- AA   CAROLINA MEDCL   454 GM/BOT   N89910 001   JAN 19, 1989
- AA   PHARM BASICS   453.6 GM/BOT   N88786 001   SEP 11, 1984

SUSPENSION; ORAL, RECTAL

SODIUM POLYSTYRENE SULFONATE
- AA   PHARM BASICS   15 GM/60 ML   N88717 001   SEP 11, 1984
- AA   ROXANE   15 GM/60 ML   N89049 001   NOV 17, 1986

SPS
- AA   CAROLINA MEDCL   15 GM/60 ML   N87859 001   DEC 08, 1982

SODIUM SULFATE; *MULTIPLE*

SEE POLYETHYLENE GLYCOL 3350: POTASSIUM CHLORIDE: SODIUM BICARBONATE: SODIUM CHLORIDE: SODIUM SULFATE

SODIUM SULFATE, ANHYDROUS; *MULTIPLE*

SEE POLYETHYLENE GLYCOL 3350: POTASSIUM CHLORIDE: SODIUM BICARBONATE: SODIUM CHLORIDE: SODIUM SULFATE, ANHYDROUS

SODIUM TETRADECYL SULFATE

INJECTABLE; INJECTION

SOTRADECOL
- ELKINS SINN   1%   N05970 004
-   3%   N05970 005

SODIUM THIOSULFATE

INJECTABLE; INJECTION

SODIUM THIOSULFATE
- US ARMY   250 MG/ML   N20166 001   FEB 14, 1992

SOMATREM

INJECTABLE; INJECTION

PROTROPIN
- GENENTECH   5 MG/VIAL   N19107 001   OCT 17, 1985
-   10 MG/VIAL   N19107 002   OCT 24, 1989

SOMATROPIN, BIOSYNTHETIC

INJECTABLE; INJECTION

HUMATROPE
- LILLY   5 MG/VIAL   N19640 004   MAR 08, 1987

SORBITOL

SOLUTION; IRRIGATION

SORBITOL 3.3% IN PLASTIC CONTAINER
- MCGAW   3.3 GM/100 ML   N16741 001

SORBITOL 3% IN PLASTIC CONTAINER
- BAXTER   3 GM/100 ML   N17863 001

SORBITOL; *MULTIPLE*

SEE MANNITOL: SORBITOL

SOYBEAN OIL

INJECTABLE; INJECTION

INTRALIPID 10%
- AP   KABIVITRUM   10%   N17643 001

INTRALIPID 20%
- AP   KABIVITRUM   20%   N18449 001

LIPOSYN III 10%
- AP   ABBOTT   10%   N18969 001   SEP 24, 1984

LIPOSYN III 20%
- AP   ABBOTT   20%   N18970 001   SEP 25, 1984

SOYACAL 10%
- AP   ALPHA THERAPEUTIC   10%   N18465 001   JUN 29, 1983

SOYACAL 20%
- AP   ALPHA THERAPEUTIC   20%   N18786 001   JUN 29, 1983

TRAVAMULSION 10%
- AP   BAXTER   10%   N18660 001   FEB 26, 1982

SOYBEAN OIL; *MULTIPLE*

SEE SAFFLOWER OIL: SOYBEAN OIL

SPECTINOMYCIN HYDROCHLORIDE

INJECTABLE; INJECTION

TROBICIN
- UPJOHN   EQ 2 GM BASE/VIAL   N50347 001
-   EQ 4 GM BASE/VIAL   N50347 002

Prescription Drug Products (*continued*)

SPIRONOLACTONE
TABLET; ORAL
  ALDACTONE

△B	+ SEARLE	25 MG	N12151 009 DEC 30, 1983
		50 MG	N12151 008 DEC 30, 1982
		100 MG	N12151 010 DEC 30, 1983

  SPIRONOLACTONE

△B	BARR	25 MG	N87265 001
△B	CHELSEA	25 MG	N87078 001
△B	GENEVA	25 MG	N86809 001
△B	MUTUAL PHARM	25 MG	N89424 001 JUL 23, 1986
△B	MYLAN	25 MG	N87086 001
△B	PUREPAC	25 MG	N87998 001 OCT 14, 1983
△B	SUPERPHARM	25 MG	N89364 001 NOV 07, 1986
△B	UPSHER SMITH	25 MG	N87554 001
△B	ZENITH	25 MG	N87108 001

SPIRONOLACTONE; *MULTIPLE*
  SEE HYDROCHLOROTHIAZIDE; SPIRONOLACTONE

STANOZOLOL
TABLET; ORAL
  WINSTROL

+ STERLING	2 MG	N12885 001 MAY 14, 1984

STREPTOMYCIN SULFATE
INJECTABLE; INJECTION
  STREPTOMYCIN SULFATE

△P	LILLY	EQ 1 GM BASE/2 ML	N60404 001
△P		EQ 1 GM BASE/VIAL	N60107 001
		EQ 5 GM BASE/VIAL	N60107 002
△P	PFIZER	EQ 1 GM BASE/2 ML	N60111 001
△P		EQ 1 GM BASE/VIAL	N60076 001
△P		EQ 5 GM BASE/VIAL	N60076 002

STREPTOZOCIN
INJECTABLE; INJECTION
  ZANOSAR

UPJOHN	1 GM/VIAL	N50577 001 MAY 07, 1982

SUCCIMER
CAPSULE; ORAL
  CHEMET

+ MCNEIL	100 MG	N19998 002 JAN 30, 1991

SUCCINYLCHOLINE CHLORIDE
INJECTABLE; INJECTION
  ANECTINE

△P	BURROUGHS WELLCOME	20 MG/ML	N08453 002
		500 MG/VIAL	N08453 001
		1 GM/VIAL	N08453 004

  QUELICIN

△P	ABBOTT	20 MG/ML	N08845 001
△P		100 MG/ML	N08845 004
		50 MG/ML	N08845 002

  SUCCINYLCHOLINE CHLORIDE

△P	ORGANON	20 MG/ML	N80997 001

  SUCOSTRIN

△P	SQUIBB	20 MG/ML	N08847 001
△P		100 MG/ML	N08847 003

SUCRALFATE
TABLET; ORAL
  CARAFATE

+ BLUE RIDGE	1 GM	N18333 001

SUFENTANIL CITRATE
INJECTABLE; INJECTION
  SUFENTA

JANSSEN	EQ 0.05 MG BASE/ML	N19050 001 MAY 04, 1984

SULBACTAM SODIUM; *MULTIPLE*
  SEE AMPICILLIN SODIUM; SULBACTAM SODIUM

SULCONAZOLE NITRATE
CREAM; TOPICAL
  EXELDERM

WESTWOOD SQUIBB	1%	N18737 001 FEB 28, 1989

SULFACETAMIDE SODIUM
OINTMENT; OPHTHALMIC
  BLEPH-10

△I	ALLERGAN	10%	N84015 001

  CETAMIDE

△I	ALCON	10%	N80021 001

  SODIUM SULAMYD

△I	SCHERING	10%	N05963 002

  SULFACETAMIDE SODIUM

△I	ALTANA	10%	N80029 001

  SULFAIR 10

△I	PHARMAFAIR	10%	N88000 001 DEC 22, 1982

Prescription Drug Products (continued)

SULFACETAMIDE SODIUM (continued)

SOLUTION/DROPS; OPHTHALMIC

	BLEPH-10			
AT	ALLERGAN	10%	N80028 001	
	BLEPH-30			
AT	ALLERGAN	30%	N80028 002	
	ISOPTO CETAMIDE			
AT	ALCON	15%	N80020 002	
	OCUSULE-10			
AT	OPTOPICS	10%	N80660 001	
	OCUSULE-30			
AT	OPTOPICS	30%	N80660 002	
	SODIUM SULAMYD			
AT	SCHERING	10%	N05963 001	
AT		30%	N05963 003	
	SODIUM SULFACETAMIDE			
AT	AKORN	10%	N83021 001	
AT		15%	N83021 002	
AT		30%	N83021 003	
	SULF-10			
AT	IOLAB	10%	N80025 001	
	SULFACEL-15			
AT	OPTOPICS	15%	N80024 001	
	SULFACETAMIDE SODIUM			
AT	PHARMAFAIR	10%	N88947 001	MAY 17, 1985
AT	STERIS	10%	N89560 001	OCT 18, 1988
AT		30%	N89068 001	MAY 05, 1987
	SULFAIR FORTE			
AT	PHARMAFAIR	30%	N88385 001	OCT 13, 1983
	SULFAIR-10			
AT	PHARMAFAIR	10%	N87949 001	DEC 13, 1982
	SULFAIR-15			
AT	PHARMAFAIR	15%	N88186 001	MAY 25, 1983
	SULTEN-10			
AT	BAUSCH AND LOMB	10%	N87818 001	FEB 03, 1983

SULFACETAMIDE SODIUM; *MULTIPLE*

SEE FLUOROMETHOLONE: SULFACETAMIDE SODIUM
SEE PREDNISOLONE ACETATE: SULFACETAMIDE SODIUM
SEE PREDNISOLONE SODIUM PHOSPHATE: SULFACETAMIDE SODIUM

SULFACYTINE

TABLET; ORAL

	RENOQUID		
+	GLENWOOD	250 MG	N17569 001

SULFADIAZINE

TABLET; ORAL

	SULFADIAZINE		
	ABBOTT	300 MG	N04125 005
AB	LANNETT	500 MG	N80084 001
AB	+ LILLY	500 MG	N04122 002
AB	RICHLYN	500 MG	N80081 001

SULFADIAZINE; SULFAMERAZINE

SUSPENSION; ORAL

SULFONAMIDES DUPLEX		
LILLY	250 MG/5 ML;250 MG/5 ML	N06317 007

SULFADIAZINE SODIUM

INJECTABLE; INJECTION

SULFADIAZINE SODIUM		
LEDERLE	250 MG/ML	N04054 002

SULFADOXINE; *MULTIPLE*

SEE PYRIMETHAMINE: SULFADOXINE

SULFAMERAZINE; *MULTIPLE*

SEE SULFADIAZINE: SULFAMERAZINE

SULFAMETHIZOLE

TABLET; ORAL

	THIOSULFIL		
	WYETH AYERST	250 MG	N08565 001
+		500 MG	N08565 004

SULFAMETHOXAZOLE

SUSPENSION; ORAL

	GANTANOL		
	ROCHE	500 MG/5 ML	N13664 002

TABLET; ORAL

	GANTANOL		
AB	+ ROCHE	500 MG	N12715 002
	GANTANOL-DS		
	ROCHE	1 GM	N12715 003
	SULFAMETHOXAZOLE		
AB	GENEVA	500 MG	N85844 001
AB	HEATHER	500 MG	N86163 001

SULFAMETHOXAZOLE; *MULTIPLE*

SEE PHENAZOPYRIDINE HYDROCHLORIDE: SULFAMETHOXAZOLE

Prescription Drug Products (continued)

SULFAMETHOXAZOLE; TRIMETHOPRIM

INJECTABLE; INJECTION

		Strength	Appl. No.	Date
	BACTRIM			
ΔP	ROCHE	80 MG/ML;16 MG/ML	N18374 001	
	SEPTRA			
ΔP	BURROUGHS WELLCOME	80 MG/ML;16 MG/ML	N18452 001	
	SULFAMETHOXAZOLE AND TRIMETHOPRIM			
ΔP	CETUS BEN VENUE	80 MG/ML;16 MG/ML	N72383 001	APR 29, 1992
ΔP	ELKINS SINN	80 MG/ML;16 MG/ML	N70627 001	APR 30, 1987
ΔP		80 MG/ML;16 MG/ML	N70628 001	APR 30, 1987
ΔP	GENSIA	80 MG/ML;16 MG/ML	N73303 001	OCT 31, 1991
ΔP	LYPHOMED	80 MG/ML;16 MG/ML	N70223 001	JAN 16, 1987
ΔP	STERIS	80 MG/ML;16 MG/ML	N71556 001	DEC 17, 1987

SUSPENSION; ORAL

		Strength	Appl. No.	Date
	BACTRIM			
ΔB	+ ROCHE	200 MG/5 ML;40 MG/5 ML	N17560 001	
	BACTRIM PEDIATRIC			
ΔB	ROCHE	200 MG/5 ML;40 MG/5 ML	N17560 002	
	COTRIM PEDIATRIC			
ΔB	LEMMON	200 MG/5 ML;40 MG/5 ML	N70028 001	OCT 29, 1985
	SEPTRA			
ΔB	BURROUGHS WELLCOME	200 MG/5 ML;40 MG/5 ML	N17598 001	
	SEPTRA GRAPE			
ΔB	BURROUGHS WELLCOME	200 MG/5 ML;40 MG/5 ML	N17598 002	FEB 12, 1986
	SMZ-TMP			
ΔB	BIOCRAFT	200 MG/5 ML;40 MG/5 ML	N18812 001	JAN 28, 1983
	SMZ-TMP PEDIATRIC			
ΔB	BIOCRAFT	200 MG/5 ML;40 MG/5 ML	N18812 002	JUN 10, 1983
	SULFATRIM			
ΔB	BARRE	200 MG/5 ML;40 MG/5 ML	N18615 002	JAN 07, 1983
	SULFATRIM PEDIATRIC			
ΔB	BARRE	200 MG/5 ML;40 MG/5 ML	N18615 001	JAN 07, 1983
	TRIMETH/SULFA			
ΔB	NASKA	200 MG/5 ML;40 MG/5 ML	N72289 001	MAY 23, 1988
ΔB		200 MG/5 ML;40 MG/5 ML	N72398 001	MAY 23, 1988
ΔB		200 MG/5 ML;40 MG/5 ML	N72399 001	MAY 23, 1988

SULFAMETHOXAZOLE; TRIMETHOPRIM (continued)

TABLET; ORAL

		Strength	Appl. No.	Date
	BACTRIM			
ΔB	ROCHE	400 MG;80 MG	N17377 001	
	BACTRIM DS			
ΔB	+ ROCHE	800 MG;160 MG	N17377 002	
	COTRIM			
ΔB	LEMMON	400 MG;80 MG	N70034 001	MAY 16, 1985
	COTRIM D.S.			
ΔB	LEMMON	800 MG;160 MG	N70048 001	MAR 18, 1985
	SEPTRA			
ΔB	BURROUGHS WELLCOME	400 MG;80 MG	N17376 001	
	SEPTRA DS			
ΔB	BURROUGHS WELLCOME	800 MG;160 MG	N17376 002	
	SMZ-TMP			
ΔB	BIOCRAFT	400 MG;80 MG	N18242 001	
ΔB		800 MG;160 MG	N18242 002	
	SULFAMETHOPRIM			
ΔB	PAR	400 MG;80 MG	N70022 001	FEB 15, 1985
	SULFAMETHOPRIM-DS			
ΔB	PAR	800 MG;160 MG	N70032 001	FEB 15, 1985
	SULFAMETHOXAZOLE & TRIMETHOPRIM			
ΔB	HEATHER	400 MG;80 MG	N18946 001	AUG 10, 1984
ΔB		800 MG;160 MG	N18946 002	AUG 10, 1984
	SULFAMETHOXAZOLE AND TRIMETHOPRIM			
ΔB	BARR	400 MG;80 MG	N70006 001	NOV 14, 1984
ΔB	CHELSEA	400 MG;80 MG	N70002 001	NOV 07, 1984
ΔB		800 MG;160 MG	N70000 001	NOV 07, 1984
ΔB	DANBURY	400 MG;80 MG	N18852 001	MAY 09, 1983
ΔB	EON LABS	400 MG;80 MG	N18598 003	MAY 19, 1982
ΔB	GENEVA	400 MG;80 MG	N70889 001	NOV 13, 1986
ΔB		800 MG;160 MG	N70890 001	NOV 13, 1986
B*	INTERPHARM	400 MG;80 MG	N71299 001	OCT 27, 1987
B*		800 MG;160 MG	N71300 001	OCT 27, 1987
ΔB	MUTUAL PHARM	400 MG;80 MG	N71016 001	AUG 25, 1986
ΔB		800 MG;160 MG	N71017 001	AUG 25, 1986

Prescription Drug Products (continued)

SULFAMETHOXAZOLE; TRIMETHOPRIM (continued)

TABLET; ORAL

SULFAMETHOXAZOLE AND TRIMETHOPRIM

AB	ROXANE	400 MG;80 MG	N72268 001	AUG 30, 1991
AB	SIDMAK	400 MG;80 MG	N70215 001	SEP 10, 1985
AB		800 MG;160 MG	N70216 001	SEP 10, 1985

SULFAMETHOXAZOLE AND TRIMETHOPRIM DOUBLE STRENGTH

AB	BARR	800 MG;160 MG	N70007 001	NOV 14, 1984
AB	DANBURY	800 MG;160 MG	N18854 001	MAY 09, 1983
AB	EON LABS	800 MG;160 MG	N18598 004	MAY 19, 1982
AB	PLANTEX	800 MG;160 MG	N70037 001	SEP 19, 1985
AB	ROXANE	800 MG;160 MG	N72769 001	AUG 30, 1991

SULFAMETHOXAZOLE AND TRIMETHOPRIM SINGLE STRENGTH

AB	PLANTEX	400 MG;80 MG	N70030 001	SEP 19, 1985

SULFATRIM-DS

AB	SUPERPHARM	800 MG;160 MG	N70066 001	JUN 24, 1985

SULFATRIM-SS

AB	SUPERPHARM	400 MG;80 MG	N70065 002	JUN 24, 1985

UROPLUS DS

AB	SHIONOGI	800 MG;160 MG	N71816 001	SEP 28, 1987

UROPLUS SS

AB	SHIONOGI	400 MG;80 MG	N71815 001	SEP 28, 1987

SULFANILAMIDE

CREAM; VAGINAL

AVC

AT	MERRELL DOW	15%	N06530 003	JAN 27, 1987

SULFANILAMIDE

AT	LEMMON	15%	N88718 001	SEP 19, 1985

SUPPOSITORY; VAGINAL

AVC

	MERRELL DOW	1.05 GM	N06530 004	JAN 27, 1987

SULFAPYRIDINE

TABLET; ORAL

SULFAPYRIDINE

	LILLY	500 MG	N0159 001

SULFASALAZINE

SUSPENSION; ORAL

AZULFIDINE

	+ KABI	250 MG/5 ML	N18605 001
		250 MG/5 ML	N86983 001

TABLET; ORAL

AZULFIDINE

	+ KABI	500 MG	N07073 001

SULFASALAZINE

AB	CHELSEA	500 MG	N85828 001	
AB	DANBURY	500 MG	N87197 001	
AB	LEDERLE	500 MG	N80197 001	
AB	MUTUAL PHARM	500 MG	N89590 001	OCT 19, 1987
AB	SUPERPHARM	500 MG	N89339 001	OCT 26, 1987

TABLET, DELAYED RELEASE; ORAL

AZULFIDINE EN-TABS

	+ KABI	500 MG	N07073 002	APR 06, 1983

SULFINPYRAZONE

CAPSULE; ORAL

ANTURANE

	+ CIBA	200 MG	N11556 004

SULFINPYRAZONE

AB	BARR	200 MG	N87666 001	SEP 17, 1982
AB	PAR	200 MG	N88934 001	SEP 06, 1985
AB	ZENITH	200 MG	N87770 001	NOV 19, 1982

TABLET; ORAL

ANTURANE

	+ CIBA	100 MG	N11556 003

SULFINPYRAZONE

AB	BARR	100 MG	N87665 001	SEP 17, 1982
AB	DANBURY	100 MG	N87667 001	MAY 26, 1982
AB	PAR	100 MG	N88933 001	SEP 06, 1985
AB	ZENITH	100 MG	N87769 001	JUN 01, 1982

Prescription Drug Products *(continued)*

SULFISOXAZOLE
TABLET; ORAL

	GANTRISIN		
	+ ROCHE	500 MG	N06525 001
	SOSOL		
AB	MK	500 MG	N80036 001
	SULFISOXAZOLE		
AB	GENEVA	500 MG	N85628 001
AB	HEATHER	500 MG	N80189 001
AB	ICN	500 MG	N80268 002
AB	LANNETT	500 MG	N80085 001
AB	PUREPAC	500 MG	N80087 001
AB	RICHLYN	500 MG	N80109 001
AB	ROXANE	500 MG	N80082 001
AB	ZENITH	500 MG	N80142 001

SULFISOXAZOLE; *MULTIPLE*
SEE PHENAZOPYRIDINE HYDROCHLORIDE; SULFISOXAZOLE

SULFISOXAZOLE ACETYL
EMULSION; ORAL

	LIPO GANTRISIN		
	ROCHE	EQ 1 GM BASE/5 ML	N09182 009

SUSPENSION; ORAL

	GANTRISIN PEDIATRIC		
	+ ROCHE	EQ 500 MG BASE/5 ML	N09182 004

SYRUP; ORAL

	GANTRISIN		
	+ ROCHE	EQ 500 MG BASE/5 ML	N09182 002

SULFISOXAZOLE ACETYL; *MULTIPLE*
SEE ERYTHROMYCIN ESTOLATE; SULFISOXAZOLE ACETYL
SEE ERYTHROMYCIN ETHYLSUCCINATE; SULFISOXAZOLE ACETYL

SULFISOXAZOLE DIOLAMINE
OINTMENT; OPHTHALMIC

	GANTRISIN		
	ROCHE	EQ 4% BASE	N08414 002

SOLUTION/DROPS; OPHTHALMIC

	GANTRISIN		
	ROCHE	EQ 4% BASE	N07757 002

SULFUR; *MULTIPLE*
SEE BENTONITE; SULFUR

SULINDAC
TABLET; ORAL

	CLINORIL			
AB	MERCK	150 MG	N17911 001	
AB	+	200 MG	N17911 002	
	SULINDAC			
AB	DANBURY	150 MG	N71891 001	MAR 03, 1988
AB		200 MG	N71795 001	MAR 03, 1988
AB	GENEVA	150 MG	N72712 001	AUG 30, 1991
AB		200 MG	N72713 001	AUG 30, 1991
AB	LEDERLE	150 MG	N73261 001	SEP 06, 1991
AB		200 MG	N73262 001	SEP 06, 1991
AB	LEMMON	150 MG	N72972 001	FEB 28, 1992
AB		200 MG	N72973 001	FEB 28, 1992
AB	MUTUAL PHARM	150 MG	N72050 001	APR 17, 1991
AB		200 MG	N72051 001	APR 17, 1991
AB	WARNER CHILCOTT	150 MG	N72710 001	MAR 25, 1991
AB		200 MG	N72711 001	MAR 25, 1991

SUPROFEN
SOLUTION/DROPS; OPHTHALMIC

	PROFENAL			
	ALCON	1%	N19387 001	DEC 23, 1988

SUTILAINS
OINTMENT; TOPICAL

	TRAVASE		
	BOOTS	82,000 UNITS/GM	N12828 001

TAMOXIFEN CITRATE
TABLET; ORAL

	NOLVADEX		
	+ STUART	EQ 10 MG BASE	N17970 001

TARTARIC ACID; *MULTIPLE*
SEE SODIUM BICARBONATE; TARTARIC ACID

Prescription Drug Products (continued)

TECHNETIUM TC-99M ALBUMIN AGGREGATED KIT
INJECTABLE; INJECTION
A-N STANNOUS AGGREGATED ALBUMIN

BS	BENEDICT	N/A	N17916 001
	AN-MAA		
BS	CIS	N/A	N17792 001
BS	MACROTEC	N/A	N17833 001
	SQUIBB		
	PULMOLITE		
BS	DUPONT	N/A	N17776 001
	TECHNESCAN MAA		
BS	MALLINCKRODT	N/A	N17842 001
BS	TECHNETIUM TC-99M ALBUMIN AGGREGATED KIT		
	MSD	N/A	N17881 001
			DEC 30, 1987
	TECHNETIUM TC-99M MAA		
BS	MEDI PHYSICS	N/A	N17773 001

TECHNETIUM TC-99M ALBUMIN COLLOID KIT
INJECTABLE; INJECTION
MICROLITE

	DUPONT	N/A	N18263 001
			MAR 25, 1983

TECHNETIUM TC-99M ALBUMIN KIT
INJECTABLE; INJECTION
TECHNETIUM TC-99M HSA

	MEDI PHYSICS	N/A	N17775 001

TECHNETIUM TC-99M ALBUMIN MICROSPHERES KIT
INJECTABLE; INJECTION
INSTANT MICROSPHERES

	3M	N/A	N17832 001

TECHNETIUM TC-99M DISOFENIN KIT
INJECTABLE; INJECTION
HEPATOLITE

	DUPONT	N/A	N18467 001
			MAR 16, 1982

TECHNETIUM TC-99M ETIDRONATE KIT
INJECTABLE; INJECTION
OSTEOSCAN

	MALLINCKRODT	N/A	N17454 001

TECHNETIUM TC-99M EXAMETAZIME KIT
INJECTABLE; INJECTION
CERETEC

	AMERSHAM	N/A	N19829 001
			DEC 30, 1988

TECHNETIUM TC-99M GLUCEPTATE KIT
INJECTABLE; INJECTION
GLUCOSCAN

ΔP	DUPONT	N/A	N17907 001
	TECHNESCAN GLUCEPTATE		
ΔP	MSD	N/A	N18272 001
			JAN 27, 1982

TECHNETIUM TC-99M LIDOFENIN KIT
INJECTABLE; INJECTION
TECHNESCAN HIDA

	MERCK	N/A	N18489 001
			OCT 31, 1986

TECHNETIUM TC-99M MEBROFENIN KIT
INJECTABLE; INJECTION
CHOLETEC

	SQUIBB	N/A	N18963 001
			JAN 21, 1987

TECHNETIUM TC-99M MEDRONATE KIT
INJECTABLE; INJECTION
AMERSCAN MDP KIT

ΔP	AMERSHAM	N/A	N18335 001
			AUG 05, 1982
	AN-MDP		
ΔP	CIS	N/A	N18124 001
	MDP-SQUIBB		
	SQUIBB	N/A	N18107 001
	OSTEOLITE		
ΔP	DUPONT	N/A	N17972 001
	TECHNESCAN MDP KIT		
ΔP	MSD	N/A	N18035 001
	TECHNETIUM TC 99M MPI MDP		
ΔP	MEDI PHYSICS	N/A	N18141 001

TECHNETIUM TC-99M MERTIATIDE KIT
INJECTABLE; INJECTION
TECHNESCAN MAG3

	MALLINCKRODT	N/A	N19882 001
			JUN 15, 1990

TECHNETIUM TC-99M OXIDRONATE KIT
INJECTABLE; INJECTION
OSTEOSCAN-HDP

	MALLINCKRODT	N/A	N18321 001

Prescription Drug Products (continued)

TECHNETIUM TC-99M PENTETATE KIT
INJECTABLE; INJECTION
AN-DTPA

AP	CIS	N/A	N17714 001
	MPI DTPA KIT - CHELATE		
AP	MEDI PHYSICS	N/A	N17255 001
	TECHNESCAN DTPA KIT		
AP	MERCK	N/A	N18511 001 DEC 29, 1989
	TECHNETIUM TC-99M PENTETATE KIT		
AP	MEDI PHYSICS	N/A	N17264 002

TECHNETIUM TC-99M PYRO/TRIMETA PHOSPHATES KIT
INJECTABLE; INJECTION
PYROLITE

DUPONT	N/A	N17684 001

TECHNETIUM TC-99M PYROPHOSPHATE KIT
INJECTABLE; INJECTION
PHOSPHOTEC

AP	SQUIBB	N/A	N17680 001
	TECHNESCAN PYP KIT		
AP	MALLINCKRODT	N/A	N17538 001

TECHNETIUM TC-99M RED BLOOD CELL KIT
INJECTABLE; INJECTION
RBC-SCAN

CADEMA	N/A	N20063 001 JUN 11, 1992
ULTRATAG		
MALLINCKRODT	N/A	N19981 001 JUN 10, 1991

TECHNETIUM TC-99M SESTAMIBI KIT
INJECTABLE; INJECTION
CARDIOLITE

DUPONT	N/A	N19785 001 DEC 21, 1990

TECHNETIUM TC-99M SODIUM PERTECHNETATE
SOLUTION; INJECTION, ORAL
SODIUM PERTECHNETATE TC 99M

MALLINCKRODT	10-60 MCI/ML	N17725 001

TECHNETIUM TC-99M SODIUM PERTECHNETATE GENERATOR
SOLUTION; INJECTION, ORAL
MINITEC

SQUIBB	0.22-2.22 CI/GENERATOR	N17339 001
TECHNETIUM TC 99M GENERATOR		
DUPONT	0.0083-2.7 CI/GENERATOR	N17771 001
MEDI PHYSICS	830-16,600 MCI/ GENERATOR	N17693 001
ULTRA-TECHNEKOW FM		
MALLINCKRODT	0.25-3 CI/GENERATOR	N17243 002

TECHNETIUM TC-99M SUCCIMER KIT
INJECTABLE; INJECTION
MPI DMSA KIDNEY REAGENT

MEDI PHYSICS	N/A	N17944 001 MAY 18, 1982

TECHNETIUM TC-99M SULFUR COLLOID
SOLUTION; ORAL
TECHNETIUM TC 99M SULFUR COLLOID

MALLINCKRODT	3 MCI/ML	N17724 001

TECHNETIUM TC-99M SULFUR COLLOID KIT
SOLUTION; INJECTION, ORAL
AN-SULFUR COLLOID

AP	CIS	N/A	N17858 001
	TECHNECOLL		
AP	MALLINCKRODT	N/A	N17059 001
	TECHNETIUM TC 99M TSC		
AP	MEDI PHYSICS	N/A	N17784 001
	TESULOID		
AP	SQUIBB	N/A	N16923 001

TECHNETIUM TC-99M TEBOROXIME KIT
INJECTABLE; INJECTION
CARDIOTEC

SQUIBB	N/A	N19928 001 DEC 19, 1990

TEMAZEPAM
CAPSULE; ORAL
RESTORIL

AB	SANDOZ	15 MG	N18163 001
AB	+	30 MG	N18163 002
		7.5 MG	N18163 003 OCT 25, 1991

Prescription Drug Products (continued)

TEMAZEPAM (continued)

CAPSULE; ORAL
TEMAZEPAM

ΔB	BARR	15MG	N71174 001	JUL 10, 1986
ΔB		30MG	N71175 001	JUL 10, 1986
ΔB	GENEVA	15MG	N71427 001	JUL 10, 1986
ΔB		30MG	N71428 001	JAN 12, 1988
ΔB				JAN 12, 1988
ΔB	MYLAN	15MG	N70919 001	JUL 07, 1986
ΔB		30MG	N70920 001	JUL 07, 1986
ΔB	PAR	15MG	N71456 001	APR 21, 1987
ΔB		30MG	N71457 001	APR 21, 1987
ΔB	PUREPAC	15MG	N71638 001	AUG 07, 1987
ΔB		30MG	N71620 001	AUG 07, 1987

TENIPOSIDE

INJECTABLE; INJECTION
VUMON

BRISTOL MYERS SQUIBB	10 MG/ML	N20119 001	JUL 14, 1992

TERAZOSIN HYDROCHLORIDE

TABLET; ORAL
HYTRIN

	ABBOTT	1 MG	N19057 001	AUG 07, 1987
		2 MG	N19057 002	AUG 07, 1987
		5 MG	N19057 003	AUG 07, 1987
+		10 MG	N19057 004	AUG 07, 1987

TERBUTALINE SULFATE

AEROSOL, METERED; INHALATION
BRETHAIRE

GEIGY	0.2 MG/INH	N18762 001	AUG 17, 1984

INJECTABLE; INJECTION
BRETHINE

ΔP	GEIGY	1MG/ML	N18571 001

BRICANYL

ΔP	MERRELL DOW	1MG/ML	N17466 001

TERBUTALINE SULFATE (continued)

TABLET; ORAL
BRETHINE

BP	GEIGY	2.5 MG	N17849 001
BP +		5 MG	N17849 002

BRICANYL

BP	MERRELL DOW	2.5 MG	N17618 001
BP		5 MG	N17618 002

TERCONAZOLE

CREAM; VAGINAL
TERAZOL 3

JOHNSON RW	0.8%	N19964 001	FEB 21, 1991

TERAZOL 7

JOHNSON RW	0.4%	N19579 001	DEC 31, 1987

SUPPOSITORY; VAGINAL
TERAZOL 3

JOHNSON RW	80 MG	N19641 001	MAY 24, 1988

TERFENADINE

TABLET; ORAL
SELDANE

+	MERRELL DOW	60 MG	N18949 001	MAY 08, 1985

TERFENADINE HYDROCHLORIDE; PSEUDOEPHEDRINE HYDROCHLORIDE: *MULTIPLE*
SEE PSEUDOEPHEDRINE HYDROCHLORIDE; TERFENADINE

TERIPARATIDE ACETATE

INJECTABLE; INJECTION
PARATHAR

RHONE POULENC RORER	200 UNITS/VIAL	N19498 001	DEC 23, 1987

TESTOLACTONE

TABLET; ORAL
TESLAC

+	SQUIBB	50 MG	N16118 001

TESTOSTERONE

INJECTABLE; INJECTION
TESTOSTERONE

STERIS	25 MG/ML	N86420 001	MAY 10, 1983
	50 MG/ML	N86419 001	AUG 23, 1983
	100 MG/ML	N86417 001	JUL 07, 1983

Prescription Drug Products (continued)

TESTOSTERONE (continued)

PELLET; IMPLANTATION

		Strength	Number
	TESTOSTERONE		
	BARTOR	75 MG	N80911 001

TESTOSTERONE CYPIONATE

INJECTABLE; INJECTION

		Strength	Number
	DEPO-TESTOSTERONE		
AO	UPJOHN	100 MG/ML	N85635 002
AO		200 MG/ML	N85635 003
		50 MG/ML	N85635 001
	TESTOSTERONE CYPIONATE		
AO	STERIS	100 MG/ML	N84401 001
AO		100 MG/ML	N86029 001
AO		200 MG/ML	N84401 002
AO		200 MG/ML	N86030 001

TESTOSTERONE CYPIONATE; *MULTIPLE*

SEE ESTRADIOL CYPIONATE; TESTOSTERONE CYPIONATE

TESTOSTERONE ENANTHATE

INJECTABLE; INJECTION

		Strength	Number
	DELATESTRYL		
AO	GYNEX	200 MG/ML	N09165 003
	TESTOSTERONE ENANTHATE		
AO	STERIS	200 MG/ML	N83667 002
AO		200 MG/ML	N85598 001
		100 MG/ML	N83667 001
		100 MG/ML	N85599 001

TESTOSTERONE ENANTHATE; *MULTIPLE*

SEE ESTRADIOL VALERATE; TESTOSTERONE ENANTHATE

TESTOSTERONE PROPIONATE

INJECTABLE; INJECTION

		Strength	Number
	TESTOSTERONE PROPIONATE		
AO	BEL MAR	25 MG/ML	N80741 001
AO		50 MG/ML	N80742 001
AO		100 MG/ML	N80743 001
AO	LILLY	50 MG/ML	N80254 002
AO		25 MG/ML	N80188 001
AO	STERIS	25 MG/ML	N85490 001
AO		50 MG/ML	N80188 002
AO		50 MG/ML	N85490 002
AO		100 MG/ML	N80188 003
AO		100 MG/ML	N83595 003

TETRACYCLINE

SYRUP; ORAL

		Strength	Number
	ACHROMYCIN V		
	+ LEDERLE		N50263 002
	SUMYCIN		
AB	SQUIBB	EQ 125 MG HCL/5 ML	N60400 001
	TETRACYCLINE		
AB	BARRE	EQ 125 MG HCL/5 ML	N60633 001
AB	MK	EQ 125 MG HCL/5 ML	N60174 001
	TETRACYCLINE HCL		
AB	PUREPAC	EQ 125 MG HCL/5 ML	N60291 001
	TETRACYN		
AB	PFIPHARMECS	EQ 125 MG HCL/5 ML	N60095 001
	TETRAMED		
AB	ZENITH	EQ 125 MG HCL/5 ML	N61468 001

TETRACYCLINE HYDROCHLORIDE

CAPSULE; ORAL

		Strength	Number
	ACHROMYCIN V		
	+ LEDERLE		
AB		250 MG	N50278 003
AB		500 MG	N50278 001
	BRISTACYCLINE		
	+ BRISTOL		
AB	BRISTOL	250 MG	N61658 001
AB		250 MG	N61888 001
AB		500 MG	N61658 002
AB		500 MG	N61888 002
	PANMYCIN		
AB	UPJOHN	250 MG	N60347 001
	ROBITET		
AB	ROBINS	250 MG	N61734 001
AB		500 MG	N61734 002
	SUMYCIN		
AB	SQUIBB	100 MG	N60429 002
AB		125 MG	N60429 004
AB		250 MG	N60429 001
AB		500 MG	N60429 003
	TETRACHEL		
AB	RACHELLE	250 MG	N60343 001
AB		500 MG	N60343 003
	TETRACYCLINE HCL		
AB	ATRAL	250 MG	N62752 001 AUG 12, 1988
AB		500 MG	N62752 002 AUG 12, 1988
AB	BARR	250 MG	N61837 001
AB		500 MG	N61837 002
AB	DANBURY	500 MG	N62343 001
AB		500 MG	N62343 002
AB	EON LABS	250 MG	N61471 001
AB	HALSEY	250 MG	N60736 001
AB		250 MG	N60736 002
AB	HEATHER	250 MG	N61148 001
AB		250 MG	N61148 002
AB	ICN	250 MG	N60471 001
AB		500 MG	N60471 002
AB	MAST	500 MG	N62085 001
AB	MK	125 MG	N60173 001
AB		250 MG	N60173 002

Prescription Drug Products (continued)

TETRACYCLINE HYDROCHLORIDE (continued)

CAPSULE; ORAL
TETRACYCLINE HCL

TE	Manufacturer	Strength	Appl. No.	Date
AB	MYLAN	250 MG	N60783 001	
AB		500 MG	N60783 002	
AB	PRIVATE FORM	250 MG	N62686 001	
			N62686 002	JUL 24, 1986
AB		500 MG		JUL 24, 1986
AB	PUREPAC	250 MG	N60290 001	
AB		500 MG	N60290 002	
AB	RICHLYN	100 MG	N60469 002	
AB		250 MG	N60469 001	
AB		500 MG	N60469 003	
AB	ROXANE	250 MG	N61214 002	
AB	SUPERPHARM	250 MG	N62540 001	
			N62540 002	MAR 21, 1985
AB		500 MG		MAR 21, 1985
AB	WARNER CHILCOTT	250 MG	N62300 001	
AB		500 MG	N62300 002	
AB	WEST WARD	250 MG	N60768 001	
AB		500 MG	N60768 002	
AB	WYETH AYERST	250 MG	N61685 001	
AB		500 MG	N61685 002	
AB	ZENITH	250 MG	N60704 001	
AB		500 MG	N60704 002	

TETRACYN

TE	Manufacturer	Strength	Appl. No.
AB	PFIPHARMECS	250 MG	N60082 003
AB		500 MG	N60082 004

INJECTABLE; INJECTION
ACHROMYCIN

TE	Manufacturer	Strength	Appl. No.
AP	LEDERLE	250 MG/VIAL	N50273 002
AP		500 MG/VIAL	N50273 003

TETRACYN

TE	Manufacturer	Strength	Appl. No.
AP	PFIZER	250 MG/VIAL	N60096 001
AP		500 MG/VIAL	N60096 002

OINTMENT; OPHTHALMIC, OTIC
ACHROMYCIN

Manufacturer	Strength	Appl. No.
LEDERLE	10 MG/GM	N50266 001

POWDER FOR RECONSTITUTION; TOPICAL
TOPICYCLINE

Manufacturer	Strength	Appl. No.
ROBERTS	2.2 MG/ML	N50493 001

SUSPENSION/DROPS; OPHTHALMIC
ACHROMYCIN

Manufacturer	Strength	Appl. No.
LEDERLE	1%	N50268 001

TABLET; ORAL
PANMYCIN

TE	Manufacturer	Strength	Appl. No.
AB	UPJOHN	500 MG	N61705 002

SUMYCIN

TE	Manufacturer	Strength	Appl. No.
AB	+ SQUIBB	500 MG	N61147 004
		50 MG	N61147 003
		100 MG	N61147 002
		250 MG	N61147 001

TETRACYCLINE HYDROCHLORIDE; *MULTIPLE*

SEE HYDROCORTISONE; TETRACYCLINE HYDROCHLORIDE

SEE PROCAINE HYDROCHLORIDE; TETRACYCLINE HYDROCHLORIDE

TETRACYCLINE PHOSPHATE COMPLEX

CAPSULE; ORAL
TETREX

Manufacturer	Strength	Appl. No.
BRISTOL	EQ 100 MG HCL	N61653 001
	EQ 250 MG HCL	N61653 002
+	EQ 250 MG HCL	N61889 002
	EQ 500 MG HCL	N61653 003
	EQ 500 MG HCL	N61889 001

TETRAHYDROZOLINE HYDROCHLORIDE

SOLUTION; NASAL
TYZINE

Manufacturer	Strength	Appl. No.
KEY PHARMS	0.05%	N86576 002
	0.1%	N86576 001

SPRAY; NASAL
TYZINE

Manufacturer	Strength	Appl. No.
KEY PHARMS	0.1%	N86576 003

THALLOUS CHLORIDE, TL-201

INJECTABLE; INJECTION
THALLOUS CHLORIDE TL 201

TE	Manufacturer	Strength	Appl. No.	Date
AP	DUPONT	1 MCI/ML	N17806 001	
AP	MALLINCKRODT	1 MCI/ML	N18150 001	
	MEDI PHYSICS	2 MCI/ML	N18110 001	FEB 01, 1982
AP	SQUIBB	1 MCI/ML	N18548 001	DEC 30, 1982

THEOPHYLLINE

CAPSULE; ORAL
BRONKODYL

TE	Manufacturer	Strength	Appl. No.	Date
BP	STERLING	100 MG	N85264 001	
BP		200 MG	N85264 002	

ELIXOPHYLLIN

TE	Manufacturer	Strength	Appl. No.	Date
BX	FOREST LABS	100 MG	N85545 001	JUL 31, 1984
BX	+	200 MG	N83921 001	JUL 31, 1984

THEOPHYLLINE

TE	Manufacturer	Strength	Appl. No.
BP	KV	100 MG	N85263 001
BP		200 MG	N85263 002

Prescription Drug Products (continued)

THEOPHYLLINE (continued)
CAPSULE, EXTENDED RELEASE; ORAL

	Product	Strength	Appl. No.	Date
	AEROLATE III + FLEMING	65 MG	N85075 003	NOV 24, 1986
BC	AEROLATE JR FLEMING	130 MG	N85075 002	NOV 24, 1986
BC	AEROLATE SR FLEMING	260 MG	N85075 001	NOV 24, 1986
BC	ELIXOPHYLLIN SR FOREST LABS	125 MG	N86826 001	JAN 29, 1985
BC		250 MG	N86826 002	JAN 29, 1985
BC	SLO-BID + RHONE POULENC RORER	50 MG	N88269 001	JAN 31, 1985
		75 MG	N89539 001	MAY 10, 1989
BC		100 MG	N87892 001	JAN 31, 1985
BC		125 MG	N89540 001	MAY 10, 1989
BC		200 MG	N87893 001	JAN 31, 1985
+		300 MG	N87894 001	JAN 31, 1985
BC	SLO-PHYLLIN RHONE POULENC RORER	125 MG	N85203 001	MAY 24, 1982
		250 MG	N85205 001	MAY 24, 1982
BC		60 MG	N85206 001	MAY 24, 1982
BC	SOMOPHYLLIN-CRT GRAHAM LABS	50 MG	N87763 001	FEB 27, 1985
BC		100 MG	N87194 001	FEB 27, 1985
BC		200 MG	N88382 001	FEB 27, 1985
BC		250 MG	N87193 001	FEB 27, 1985
BC		300 MG	N88383 001	FEB 27, 1985
BC	THEO-DUR KEY PHARMS	50 MG	N88022 001	SEP 10, 1985
BC		75 MG	N88015 001	SEP 10, 1985
BC		125 MG	N88016 001	SEP 10, 1985
BC		200 MG	N87995 001	SEP 10, 1985

THEOPHYLLINE (continued)
CAPSULE, EXTENDED RELEASE; ORAL

	Product	Strength	Appl. No.	Date
BC	THEO-24 WHITBY	100 MG	N87942 001	AUG 22, 1983
BC		200 MG	N87943 001	AUG 22, 1983
BC		300 MG	N87944 001	AUG 22, 1983
		400 MG	N81034 001	FEB 28, 1992
BC	THEOBID + GLAXO	260 MG	N85983 001	MAR 20, 1985
BC	THEOBID JR. + GLAXO	130 MG	N87854 001	MAR 20, 1985
BC	THEOCLEAR L.A.-130 CENTRAL PHARMS	130 MG	N86569 001	MAY 27, 1982
BG	THEOCLEAR L.A.-260 CENTRAL PHARMS	260 MG	N86569 002	MAY 27, 1982
BC	THEOVENT SCHERING	125 MG	N87010 001	JAN 31, 1985
BC		250 MG	N87910 001	JAN 31, 1985

ELIXIR; ORAL

	Product	Strength	Appl. No.	Date
AA	ELIXOMIN CENCI	80 MG/15 ML	N88303 001	JAN 25, 1984
AA	ELIXOPHYLLIN FOREST LABS	80 MG/15 ML	N85186 001	
AA	LANOPHYLLIN LANNETT	80 MG/15 ML	N84578 001	
	THEOPHYL-225 JOHNSON RW	112.5 MG/15 ML	N86485 001	
AA	THEOPHYLLINE BARRE	80 MG/15 ML	N85863 001	
AA	HALSEY	80 MG/15 ML	N85169 001	
AA	LIFE LABS	80 MG/15 ML	N87679 001	APR 15, 1982
AA	NASKA	80 MG/15 ML	N89223 001	
AA	PHARM ASSOC	80 MG/15 ML	N86720 001	MAY 27, 1988
AA	PHARM BASICS	80 MG/15 ML	N86748 001	
	THAMES	80 MG/15 ML	N89626 001	OCT 28, 1988

Prescription Drug Products (continued)

THEOPHYLLINE (continued)

INJECTABLE; INJECTION

THEOPHYLLINE AND DEXTROSE 5% IN PLASTIC CONTAINER

BAXTER

	Strength	Number	Date
AP	40 MG/100 ML	N18649 001	JUL 26, 1982
AP	80 MG/100 ML	N18649 002	JUL 26, 1982
AP	160 MG/100 ML	N18649 003	JUL 26, 1982
AP	200 MG/100 ML	N18649 004	JUL 26, 1982
AP	320 MG/100 ML	N18649 006	NOV 13, 1985
AP	400 MG/100 ML	N18649 005	JUL 26, 1982

THEOPHYLLINE IN DEXTROSE 5% IN PLASTIC CONTAINER

ABBOTT

	Strength	Number	Date
AP	40 MG/100 ML	N19211 001	DEC 14, 1984
AP	80 MG/100 ML	N19211 002	DEC 14, 1984
AP	160 MG/100 ML	N19211 003	DEC 14, 1984
AP	200 MG/100 ML	N19211 004	DEC 14, 1984
AP	320 MG/100 ML	N19211 006	JAN 20, 1988
AP	400 MG/100 ML	N19211 005	DEC 14, 1984

THEOPHYLLINE 0.04% AND DEXTROSE 5% IN PLASTIC CONTAINER

MCGAW

	Strength	Number	Date
AP	40 MG/100 ML	N19083 001	NOV 07, 1984
AP	40 MG/100 ML	N19826 001	AUG 14, 1992

THEOPHYLLINE 0.08% AND DEXTROSE 5% IN PLASTIC CONTAINER

MCGAW

	Strength	Number	Date
AP	80 MG/100 ML	N19083 002	NOV 07, 1984
AP	80 MG/100 ML	N19826 002	AUG 14, 1992

THEOPHYLLINE 0.16% AND DEXTROSE 5% IN PLASTIC CONTAINER

MCGAW

	Strength	Number	Date
AP	160 MG/100 ML	N19083 003	NOV 07, 1984
AP	160 MG/100 ML	N19826 003	AUG 14, 1992

THEOPHYLLINE 0.2% AND DEXTROSE 5% IN PLASTIC CONTAINER

MCGAW

	Strength	Number	Date
AP	200 MG/100 ML	N19212 001	NOV 07, 1984
AP	200 MG/100 ML	N19826 004	AUG 14, 1992

THEOPHYLLINE 0.32% AND DEXTROSE 5% IN PLASTIC CONTAINER

MCGAW

	Strength	Number	Date
AP	320 MG/100 ML	N19826 006	AUG 14, 1992

THEOPHYLLINE 0.4% AND DEXTROSE 5% IN PLASTIC CONTAINER

MCGAW

	Strength	Number	Date
AP	400 MG/100 ML	N19212 002	NOV 07, 1984
AP	400 MG/100 ML	N19826 005	AUG 14, 1992

THEOPHYLLINE (continued)

SOLUTION; ORAL

AEROLATE

		Strength	Number	Date
	FLEMING	150 MG/15 ML	N89141 001	DEC 03, 1986

THEOLAIR

		Strength	Number	Date
	3M	80 MG/15 ML	N86107 001	
ΔΔ	THEOPHYLLINE ROXANE	80 MG/15 ML	N87449 001	SEP 15, 1983

SUSPENSION; ORAL

ELIXICON

		Strength	Number	Date
	FOREST LABS	100 MG/5 ML	N85502 001	

SYRUP; ORAL

ACCURBRON

		Strength	Number	Date
	MERRELL DOW	150 MG/15 ML	N88746 001	NOV 22, 1985
ΔΔ	AQUAPHYLLIN FERNDALE	80 MG/15 ML	N87917 001	JAN 18, 1983
ΔΔ	SLO-PHYLLIN RHONE POULENC RORER	80 MG/15 ML	N85187 001	
ΔΔ	THEOCLEAR-80 CENTRAL PHARMS	80 MG/15 ML	N87095 001	MAR 01, 1982
ΔΔ	THEOPHYLLINE BARRE	80 MG/15 ML	N86001 001	

TABLET; ORAL

QUBRON-T

		Strength	Number	Date
	+ BRISTOL MYERS	300 MG	N88656 001	AUG 22, 1985

SLO-PHYLLIN

		Strength	Number	Date
	+ RHONE POULENC RORER	100 MG	N85202 001	
	+	200 MG	N85204 001	

THEOLAIR

		Strength	Number	Date
	+ 3M	125 MG	N86399 001	
	+	250 MG	N86399 002	

THEOPHYL-225

		Strength	Number	Date
	JOHNSON RW	225 MG	N84726 001	

TABLET, CHEWABLE; ORAL

THEOPHYL

		Strength	Number	Date
	JOHNSON RW	100 MG	N86506 001	SEP 12, 1985

TABLET, EXTENDED RELEASE; ORAL

LABID

		Strength	Number	Date
BC	+ P AND G	250 MG	N87225 001	

QUIBRON-T/SR

		Strength	Number	Date
BC	BRISTOL MYERS	300 MG	N87563 001	JUN 21, 1983

SUSTAIRE

		Strength	Number	Date
BC	ROERIG	100 MG	N85665 001	
BC		300 MG	N85665 002	

T-PHYL

		Strength	Number	Date
BC	PURDUE FREDERICK	200 MG	N88253 001	AUG 17, 1983

Prescription Drug Products (continued)

THEOPHYLLINE (continued)

TABLET, EXTENDED RELEASE; ORAL

THEO-DUR
+ KEY PHARMS

AB	100 MG	N85328 001	
AB	200 MG	N86998 001	
AB	300 MG	N85328 002	
+	450 MG	N89131 001	JUN 25, 1986

THEOCHRON
INWOOD

AB	100 MG	N88320 001	FEB 21, 1985
AB	200 MG	N88321 001	FEB 21, 1985
AB	300 MG	N87400 002	JAN 11, 1983

THEOLAIR-SR
3M

BC	200 MG	N88369 001	JUL 16, 1987
BC	250 MG	N86363 002	JUL 16, 1987
BC	300 MG	N88364 001	JUL 16, 1987
BC	500 MG	N89132 001	JUL 16, 1987

THEOPHYLLINE
SIDMAK

AB	100 MG	N89807 001	APR 30, 1990
AB	200 MG	N89808 001	APR 30, 1990
AB	300 MG	N89763 001	APR 30, 1990

UNIPHYL
+ PURDUE FREDERICK

400 MG	N87571 001	SEP 01, 1982

THEOPHYLLINE; *MULTIPLE*

SEE MERSALYL SODIUM; THEOPHYLLINE

THEOPHYLLINE SODIUM GLYCINATE

ELIXIR; ORAL

SYNOPHYLATE
CENTRAL PHARMS   EQ 165 MG BASE/15 ML   N06333 008

TABLET; ORAL

ASBRON
+ DORSEY   EQ 150 MG BASE   N85148 001

THIABENDAZOLE

SUSPENSION; ORAL

MINTEZOL
+ MSD   500 MG/5 ML   N16097 001

TABLET, CHEWABLE; ORAL

MINTEZOL
MSD   500 MG   N16096 001

THIAMINE; *MULTIPLE*

SEE ASCORBIC ACID; BIOTIN; CYANOCOBALAMIN; DEXPANTHENOL; ERGOCALCIFEROL; FOLIC ACID; NIACINAMIDE; PYRIDOXINE; RIBOFLAVIN PHOSPHATE SODIUM; THIAMINE; VITAMIN A; VITAMIN E

THIAMINE HYDROCHLORIDE

INJECTABLE; INJECTION

BETALIN S
LILLY   100 MG/ML   N80853 001

THIAMINE HCL

AP	AKORN	100 MG/ML	N87968 001	OCT 01, 1982
AP	BEL MAR	100 MG/ML	N80718 001	
		200 MG/ML	N80712 001	
AP	DELL	100 MG/ML	N83775 001	
AP	ELKINS SINN	100 MG/ML	N80575 001	
AP	LYPHOMED	100 MG/ML	N80556 001	
AP	STERIS	100 MG/ML	N80571 001	
AP		100 MG/ML	N83534 001	
AP		200 MG/ML	N80571 002	
AP		200 MG/ML	N83534 002	
AP	WYETH AYERST	100 MG/ML	N80553 001	

THIAMINE HYDROCHLORIDE; *MULTIPLE*

SEE ASCORBIC ACID; BIOTIN; CYANOCOBALAMIN; DEXPANTHENOL; ERGOCALCIFEROL; FOLIC ACID; NIACINAMIDE; PYRIDOXINE HYDROCHLORIDE; RIBOFLAVIN PHOSPHATE SODIUM; THIAMINE HYDROCHLORIDE; VITAMIN A; VITAMIN E

THIAMYLAL SODIUM

INJECTABLE; INJECTION

SURITAL
PARKE DAVIS

1 GM/VIAL	N07600 003	
5 GM/VIAL	N07600 005	
10 GM/VIAL	N07600 009	

THIETHYLPERAZINE MALATE

INJECTABLE; INJECTION

TORECAN
SANDOZ   5 MG/ML   N12754 002

THIETHYLPERAZINE MALEATE

SUPPOSITORY; RECTAL

TORECAN
SANDOZ   10 MG   N13247 001

TABLET; ORAL

TORECAN
SANDOZ   10 MG   N12753 001

Prescription Drug Products (continued)

THIOGUANINE

TABLET; ORAL

TE	Product / Manufacturer	Strength	NDA
	THIOGUANINE		
	BURROUGHS WELLCOME	40 MG	N12429 001

THIOPENTAL SODIUM

SUSPENSION; RECTAL

TE	Product / Manufacturer	Strength	NDA
	PENTOTHAL		
	ABBOTT	400 MG/GM	N11679 001

THIORIDAZINE

SUSPENSION; ORAL

TE	Product / Manufacturer	Strength	NDA
	MELLARIL-S		
	SANDOZ	EQ 25 MG HCL/5 ML	N17923 001
+		EQ 100 MG HCL/5 ML	N17923 002

THIORIDAZINE HYDROCHLORIDE

CONCENTRATE; ORAL

TE	Product / Manufacturer	Strength	NDA	Date
	MELLARIL			
AA	SANDOZ	30 MG/ML	N11808 012	
AA		100 MG/ML	N11808 018	
	THIORIDAZINE HCL			
AA	BARRE	100 MG/ML	N88229 001	AUG 23, 1983
AA	COPLEY	30 MG/ML	N89602 001	NOV 09, 1987
AA		100 MG/ML	N89603 001	NOV 09, 1987
AA	PHARM BASICS	30 MG/ML	N88258 001	JUL 25, 1983
AA		100 MG/ML	N88227 001	JUL 05, 1983
	THIORIDAZINE HCL INTENSOL			
AA	ROXANE	30 MG/ML	N88941 001	DEC 16, 1985
AA		100 MG/ML	N88942 001	DEC 16, 1985

TABLET; ORAL

TE	Product / Manufacturer	Strength	NDA
	MELLARIL		
AB	SANDOZ	10 MG	N11808 003
AB		15 MG	N11808 016
AB +		25 MG	N11808 006
AB		50 MG	N11808 011
AB +		100 MG	N11808 009
AB +		150 MG	N11808 017
AB +		200 MG	N11808 015

THIORIDAZINE HYDROCHLORIDE (continued)

TABLET; ORAL

TE	Product / Manufacturer	Strength	NDA	Date
	THIORIDAZINE HCL			
AB	BARR	10 MG	N88375 001	NOV 18, 1983
AB		15 MG	N88461 001	NOV 18, 1983
AB		25 MG	N87264 001	NOV 18, 1983
AB		50 MG	N88370 001	NOV 18, 1983
AB		100 MG	N88379 001	NOV 16, 1983
AB		150 MG	N88737 001	SEP 26, 1984
AB		200 MG	N88738 001	OCT 16, 1984
AB	BIOCRAFT	10 MG	N88493 001	MAY 17, 1985
AB		100 MG	N88456 001	MAY 17, 1985
AB	CHELSEA	10 MG	N88561 001	MAY 11, 1984
AB		25 MG	N88567 001	MAY 11, 1984
AB		50 MG	N88563 001	MAY 11, 1984
AB		100 MG	N88564 001	MAY 11, 1984
AB	DANBURY	10 MG	N88476 001	NOV 08, 1983
AB		15 MG	N88477 001	NOV 08, 1983
AB		25 MG	N88478 001	NOV 08, 1983
AB		25 MG	N88755 001	JUL 24, 1984
AB		50 MG	N88479 001	NOV 08, 1983
AB		100 MG	N88736 001	NOV 08, 1983
AB		150 MG	N88869 001	JUL 24, 1984
AB		200 MG	N88872 001	JUN 28, 1985
AB	GENEVA	10 MG	N88131 001	APR 26, 1985
AB		15 MG	N88132 001	AUG 30, 1983
AB		25 MG	N88133 001	AUG 30, 1983
AB		50 MG	N88134 001	AUG 30, 1983
AB		100 MG	N88135 001	AUG 30, 1983
AB		150 MG	N88136 001	NOV 20, 1984
AB		200 MG	N88137 001	SEP 17, 1986

Prescription Drug Products (continued)

THIORIDAZINE HYDROCHLORIDE (continued)
TABLET; ORAL
THIORIDAZINE HCL

MUTUAL PHARM				
AB	10 MG		N89431 001	AUG 01, 1986
AB	25 MG		N89432 001	AUG 01, 1986
AB	50 MG		N89433 001	AUG 01, 1986
AB	100 MG		N89953 001	OCT 07, 1988
MYLAN				
AB	10 MG		N88001 001	MAR 15, 1983
AB	25 MG		N88002 001	MAR 15, 1983
AB	50 MG		N88003 001	MAR 15, 1983
AB	100 MG		N88004 001	NOV 18, 1983
PAR				
AB	10 MG		N88351 001	DEC 05, 1983
AB	15 MG		N88352 001	DEC 05, 1983
AB	25 MG		N88336 001	DEC 05, 1983
AB	50 MG		N88322 001	DEC 05, 1983
AB	100 MG		N88480 001	DEC 29, 1983
SUPERPHARM				
AB	10 MG		N89103 001	JUL 02, 1985
AB	25 MG		N89104 001	JUL 02, 1985
AB	50 MG		N89105 001	JUL 02, 1985
ZENITH				
AB	10 MG		N88270 001	APR 14, 1983
AB	15 MG		N88271 001	APR 14, 1983
AB	25 MG		N88272 001	APR 14, 1983
AB	50 MG		N88194 001	APR 14, 1983
AB	100 MG		N88273 001	OCT 03, 1983

THIOTEPA
INJECTABLE; INJECTION
THIO-TEPA

LEDERLE	15 MG/VIAL	N11683 001	

THIOTHIXENE
CAPSULE; ORAL
NAVANE

ROERIG			
AB	1 MG		N16584 001
AB	2 MG	+	N16584 002
AB	5 MG	+	N16584 003
AB	10 MG		N16584 004
AB	20 MG		N16584 005

THIOTHIXENE

DANBURY			
AB	1 MG	N70600 001	JUN 05, 1987
AB	2 MG	N70601 001	JUN 05, 1987
AB	5 MG	N70602 001	JUN 05, 1987
AB	10 MG	N70603 001	JUN 05, 1987
GENEVA			
AB	1 MG	N71610 001	JUN 24, 1987
AB	2 MG	N71570 001	JUN 24, 1987
AB	5 MG	N71529 001	JUN 24, 1987
AB	10 MG	N71530 001	JUN 24, 1987
MYLAN			
AB	1 MG	N71090 001	JUN 23, 1987
AB	2 MG	N71091 001	JUN 23, 1987
AB	5 MG	N71092 001	JUN 23, 1987
AB	10 MG	N71093 001	JUN 23, 1987

THIOTHIXENE HYDROCHLORIDE
CONCENTRATE; ORAL
NAVANE

ROERIG			
AA	EQ 5 MG BASE/ML	N16758 001	

THIOTHIXENE HCL

BARRE			
AA	EQ 5 MG BASE/ML	N70969 001	OCT 16, 1987
COPLEY			
AA	EQ 5 MG BASE/ML	N71554 001	OCT 16, 1987
LEMMON			
AA	EQ 5 MG BASE/ML	N71184 001	JUN 22, 1987

THIOTHIXENE HCL INTENSOL

ROXANE			
AA	EQ 5 MG BASE/ML	N73494 001	JUN 30, 1992

INJECTABLE; INJECTION
NAVANE

ROERIG		
	EQ 2 MG BASE/ML	N16904 001
	EQ 10 MG BASE/VIAL	N16904 002

Prescription Drug Products (continued)

THONZONIUM BROMIDE; *MULTIPLE*
SEE COLISTIN SULFATE; HYDROCORTISONE ACETATE; NEOMYCIN SULFATE; THONZONIUM BROMIDE

THYROGLOBULIN
TABLET; ORAL
  PROLOID
BP + PARKE DAVIS

	Strength	Number
	65 MG	N02245 002
	32 MG	N02245 005
	100 MG	N02245 006
	130 MG	N02245 010
	200 MG	N02245 007

  THYROGLOBULIN
BP RICHLYN 64.8 MG N80151 001

THYROTROPIN
INJECTABLE; INJECTION
  THYTROPAR
  ARMOUR 10 IU/VIAL N08682 001

TICARCILLIN DISODIUM
INJECTABLE; INJECTION
  TICAR
  BEECHAM

	Strength	Number	Date
	EQ 1 GM BASE/VIAL	N50497 001	
	EQ 3 GM BASE/VIAL	N50497 002	
	EQ 3 GM BASE/VIAL	N62690 001	DEC 19, 1986
	EQ 6 GM BASE/VIAL	N50497 003	

TICARCILLIN DISODIUM; *MULTIPLE*
SEE CLAVULANATE POTASSIUM; TICARCILLIN DISODIUM

TICLOPIDINE HYDROCHLORIDE
TABLET; ORAL
  TICLID
  SYNTEX 250 MG N19979 002 OCT 31, 1991

TIMOLOL MALEATE
SOLUTION/DROPS; OPHTHALMIC
  TIMOPTIC
  MERCK

	Strength	Number	Date
	EQ 0.25% BASE	N18086 001	
	EQ 0.5% BASE	N18086 002	

  TIMOPTIC IN OCUDOSE
  MERCK

	Strength	Number	Date
	EQ 0.25% BASE	N19463 001	NOV 05, 1986
	EQ 0.5% BASE	N19463 002	NOV 05, 1986

TIMOLOL MALEATE (continued)
TABLET; ORAL
  BLOCADREN

		Strength	Number	Date
AB	MSD	5 MG	N18017 001	
AB		10 MG	N18017 002	
AB		20 MG	N18017 004	

+
  TIMOLOL MALEATE

		Strength	Number	Date
AB	DANBURY	5 MG	N72917 001	JUL 31, 1991
AB		10 MG	N72918 001	JUL 31, 1991
AB		20 MG	N72919 001	JUL 31, 1991
AB	GENEVA	5 MG	N72550 001	APR 13, 1989
AB		10 MG	N72551 001	APR 13, 1989
AB		20 MG	N72552 001	APR 13, 1989
AB	MYLAN	5 MG	N72666 001	JUN 08, 1990
AB		10 MG	N72667 001	JUN 08, 1990
AB		20 MG	N72668 001	JUN 08, 1990

TIMOLOL MALEATE; *MULTIPLE*
SEE HYDROCHLOROTHIAZIDE; TIMOLOL MALEATE

TIOCONAZOLE
OINTMENT; VAGINAL
  VAGISTAT-1
  BRISTOL MYERS 6.5% N19355 001 DEC 30, 1986

TIOPRONIN
TABLET; ORAL
  TIOPRONIN
  + UNIV TX 100 MG N19569 001 AUG 11, 1988

TOBRAMYCIN
OINTMENT; OPHTHALMIC
  TOBREX
  + ALCON 0.3% N50555 001
SOLUTION/DROPS; OPHTHALMIC
  TOBREX
  ALCON

	Strength	Number	Date
	0.3%	N50541 001	
	0.3%	N62535 001	DEC 13, 1984

Prescription Drug Products (continued)

TOBRAMYCIN; *MULTIPLE*
SEE DEXAMETHASONE:TOBRAMYCIN
SEE FLUOROMETHOLONE ACETATE:TOBRAMYCIN

TOBRAMYCIN SULFATE
INJECTABLE; INJECTION
NEBCIN

TE	Firm	Strength	Appl No	Approval
	LILLY			
AP		EQ 10 MG BASE/ML	N50477 005	
AP		EQ 10 MG BASE/ML	N62008 004	
AP		EQ 10 MG BASE/ML	N62707 001	
		EQ 40 MG BASE/ML	N62008 001	APR 29, 1987
AP		EQ 1.2 GM BASE/VIAL	N50519 001	

TOBRAMYCIN SULFATE

TE	Firm	Strength	Appl No	Approval
AP	ABBOTT	EQ 10 MG BASE/ML	N63080 001	APR 30, 1991
AP		EQ 10 MG BASE/ML	N63112 001	APR 30, 1991
AP		EQ 40 MG BASE/ML	N63111 001	APR 30, 1991
AP		EQ 40 MG BASE/ML	N63116 001	MAY 18, 1992
AP		EQ 40 MG BASE/ML	N63161 001	MAY 29, 1991
AP	ELKINS SINN	EQ 10 MG BASE/ML	N63128 001	NOV 27, 1991
AP		EQ 40 MG BASE/ML	N63127 001	NOV 27, 1991
AP	GENSIA	EQ 40 MG BASE/ML	N63100 001	JAN 30, 1992
AP		EQ 10 MG BASE/ML	N63113 001	APR 26, 1991
AP	LEDERLE	EQ 40 MG BASE/ML	N63117 001	APR 26, 1991
AP		EQ 40 MG BASE/ML	N63118 001	JUL 29, 1991
AP	MARSAM	EQ 10 MG BASE/ML	N62945 001	AUG 09, 1989
AP		EQ 40 MG BASE/ML	N62945 002	AUG 09, 1989

TOBRAMYCIN SULFATE IN SODIUM CHLORIDE 0.9% IN PLASTIC CONTAINER

TE	Firm	Strength	Appl No	Approval
	ABBOTT	EQ 80 MG BASE/100 ML	N63081 001	JUL 31, 1990
		EQ 1.2 MG BASE/ML	N63081 003	JUL 31, 1990

TOCAINIDE HYDROCHLORIDE
TABLET; ORAL
TONOCARD

Firm	Strength	Appl No	Approval
MSD	400 MG	N18257 001	NOV 09, 1984
+	600 MG	N18257 002	NOV 09, 1984

TOLAZAMIDE
TABLET; ORAL
TOLAZAMIDE

TE	Firm	Strength	Appl No	Approval
AB	BARR	100 MG	N70162 001	JAN 14, 1986
AB		250 MG	N70163 001	JAN 14, 1986
AB		500 MG	N70164 001	JAN 14, 1986
AB	DANBURY	100 MG	N70513 001	JAN 09, 1986
AB		250 MG	N70514 001	JAN 09, 1986
AB		500 MG	N70515 001	JAN 09, 1986
AB	GENEVA	100 MG	N71633 001	DEC 09, 1987
AB		250 MG	N70289 001	MAR 13, 1986
AB		500 MG	N70290 001	MAR 13, 1986
B*	INTERPHARM	250 MG	N71270 001	SEP 23, 1986
B*		500 MG	N71271 001	SEP 23, 1986
AB	MUTUAL PHARM	100 MG	N71357 001	JUL 16, 1987
AB		250 MG	N71358 001	JUL 16, 1987
AB		500 MG	N71359 001	JUL 16, 1987
AB	MYLAN	250 MG	N70259 001	JUL 16, 1987
AB		500 MG	N70913 001	JAN 02, 1986
AB	PAR	100 MG	N70159 001	MAR 17, 1986
AB		250 MG	N70160 001	JAN 06, 1986
AB		500 MG	N70161 001	JAN 06, 1986
AB	ZENITH	100 MG	N18894 001	JAN 06, 1986
AB		250 MG	N18894 002	NOV 02, 1984
AB		500 MG	N18894 003	NOV 02, 1984

TOLINASE

TE	Firm	Strength	Appl No
AB	UPJOHN	100 MG	N15500 002
AB +		250 MG	N15500 004
		500 MG	N15500 005

Prescription Drug Products (continued)

TOLAZOLINE HYDROCHLORIDE

INJECTABLE; INJECTION

		Strength	Appl No	Date
	PRISCOLINE			
	CIBA	25 MG/ML	N06403 005	FEB 22, 1985

TOLBUTAMIDE

TABLET; ORAL

		Strength	Appl No	Date
	ORINASE			
+	UPJOHN	500 MG	N10670 001	
		250 MG	N10670 002	
	TOLBUTAMIDE			
ΔB	BARR	500 MG	N87121 001	
ΔB	CHELSEA	500 MG	N86109 001	
ΔB	DANBURY	500 MG	N87318 001	
ΔB	EON LABS	500 MG	N12678 001	
ΔB	GENEVA	500 MG	N86574 001	
ΔB	LEDERLE	500 MG	N86926 001	
ΔB	MYLAN	500 MG	N86445 001	
ΔB	PUREPAC	500 MG	N88950 001	JUN 17, 1985
ΔB	SUPERPHARM	500 MG	N88893 001	NOV 19, 1984
ΔB	ZENITH	500 MG	N87093 001	

TOLBUTAMIDE SODIUM

INJECTABLE; INJECTION

		Strength	Appl No	Date
	ORINASE DIAGNOSTIC			
	UPJOHN	EQ 1 GM BASE/VIAL	N12095 001	

TOLMETIN SODIUM

CAPSULE; ORAL

		Strength	Appl No	Date
	TOLECTIN DS			
+	JOHNSON RW	EQ 400 MG BASE	N18084 001	
	TOLMETIN SODIUM			
ΔB	BAKER CUMMINS	EQ 400 MG BASE	N73392 001	JAN 24, 1992
ΔB	GENEVA	EQ 400 MG BASE	N73462 001	APR 30, 1992
ΔB	LEMMON	EQ 400 MG BASE	N73519 001	MAY 29, 1992
ΔB	MUTUAL PHARM	EQ 400 MG BASE	N73311 001	NOV 27, 1991
ΔB	NOVOPHARM	EQ 400 MG BASE	N73290 001	NOV 27, 1991
ΔB	PUREPAC	EQ 400 MG BASE	N73308 001	JAN 24, 1992

TOLMETIN SODIUM (continued)

TABLET; ORAL

		Strength	Appl No	Date
	TOLECTIN			
	JOHNSON RW	EQ 200 MG BASE	N17628 001	
	TOLECTIN 600			
+	JOHNSON RW	EQ 600 MG BASE	N17628 002	MAR 08, 1989
	TOLMETIN SODIUM			
ΔB	GENEVA	EQ 200 MG BASE	N73588 001	JUL 31, 1992
ΔB	MUTUAL PHARM	EQ 200 MG BASE	N73310 001	NOV 27, 1991
ΔB	PUREPAC	EQ 600 MG BASE	N73527 001	JUN 30, 1992

TRANEXAMIC ACID

INJECTABLE; INJECTION

		Strength	Appl No	Date
	CYKLOKAPRON			
	KABIVITRUM	100 MG/ML	N19281 001	DEC 30, 1986

TABLET; ORAL

		Strength	Appl No	Date
	CYKLOKAPRON			
+	KABIVITRUM	500 MG	N19280 001	DEC 30, 1986

TRAZODONE HYDROCHLORIDE

TABLET; ORAL

		Strength	Appl No	Date
	DESYREL			
ΔB	BRISTOL MYERS	50 MG	N18207 001	
ΔB	+	100 MG	N18207 002	
ΔB	+	150 MG	N18207 003	MAR 25, 1985
		300 MG	N18207 004	NOV 07, 1988
	TRAZODONE HCL			
ΔB	BARR	50 MG	N71258 001	MAR 25, 1987
ΔB		100 MG	N71196 001	MAR 25, 1987
ΔB	DANBURY	50 MG	N70857 001	OCT 10, 1986
ΔB		100 MG	N70858 001	OCT 10, 1986
ΔB	GENEVA	50 MG	N72484 001	APR 30, 1990
ΔB		100 MG	N72483 001	APR 30, 1990
ΔB	LEMMON	50 MG	N72192 001	FEB 02, 1989
ΔB		100 MG	N72193 001	FEB 02, 1989
ΔB	MYLAN	50 MG	N71405 001	FEB 27, 1991
ΔB		100 MG	N71406 001	FEB 27, 1991

Prescription Drug Products (continued)

TRAZODONE HYDROCHLORIDE (continued)

TABLET; ORAL

TE	Product / Company	Strength	Appl. No.	Date
	TRAZODONE HCL			
AB	PUREPAC	50 MG	N71636 001	APR 18, 1988
AB		100 MG	N71514 001	APR 18, 1988
AB	SIDMAK	50 MG	N71523 001	DEC 11, 1987
AB		100 MG	N71524 001	DEC 11, 1987
	TRAZON-150			
AB	SIDMAK	150 MG†	N71525 001	MAR 09, 1988

TRETINOIN

CREAM; TOPICAL

TE	Product / Company	Strength	Appl. No.	Date
	RETIN-A			
	+ JOHNSON RW	0.025%	N19049 001	SEP 16, 1988
	+	0.05%	N17522 001	
	+	0.1%	N17340 001	

GEL; TOPICAL

TE	Product / Company	Strength	Appl. No.	Date
	RETIN-A			
	+ JOHNSON RW	0.01%	N17955 001	
	+	0.025%	N17579 002	

SOLUTION; TOPICAL

TE	Product / Company	Strength	Appl. No.	Date
	RETIN-A			
	JOHNSON RW	0.05%	N16921 001	

SWAB; TOPICAL

TE	Product / Company	Strength	Appl. No.	Date
	RETIN-A			
	+ JOHNSON RW	0.05%	N16921 002	

TRIAMCINOLONE

TABLET; ORAL

TE	Product / Company	Strength	Appl. No.	Date
	ARISTOCORT			
BP	LEDERLE	2 MG	N11161 004	
BP		4 MG	N11161 007	
BP	+	8 MG	N11161 011	
BP		1 MG	N11161 009	
	KENACORT			
BP	SQUIBB	4 MG	N11283 006	
BP		8 MG	N11283 010	
	TRIAMCINOLONE			
BP	DANBURY	4 MG	N84270 001	
BP	LEMMON	4 MG	N84775 001	
BP	MYLAN	2 MG	N84406 001	
BP	PUREPAC	2 MG	N84020 002	
BP		4 MG	N84020 003	
BP	RICHLYN	4 MG	N84340 001	
BP	ROXANE	2 MG	N84708 001	
BP		4 MG	N84709 001	
BP		8 MG	N84707 001	
BP	ZENITH	4 MG	N83750 001	

TRIAMCINOLONE ACETONIDE

AEROSOL; TOPICAL

TE	Product / Company	Strength	Appl. No.	Date
	KENALOG			
	WESTWOOD SQUIBB	0.147 MG/GM	N12104 001	

AEROSOL, METERED; INHALATION

TE	Product / Company	Strength	Appl. No.	Date
	AZMACORT			
	+ RHONE POULENC RORER	0.25 MG/INH	N18117 001	APR 23, 1983

AEROSOL, METERED; NASAL

TE	Product / Company	Strength	Appl. No.	Date
	NASACORT			
	+ RHONE POULENC RORER	0.055 MG/INH	N19798 001	JUL 11, 1991

CREAM; TOPICAL

TE	Product / Company	Strength	Appl. No.	Date
	ARISTOCORT			
AT	LEDERLE	0.025%	N83017 003	
AT		0.1%	N83016 004	
AT		0.5%	N83015 002	
	ARISTOCORT A			
AT	LEDERLE	0.025%	N83017 004	
AT		0.025%	N88818 001	OCT 16, 1984
AT		0.1%	N83016 005	
AT		0.1%	N88819 001	OCT 16, 1984
AT		0.5%	N83015 003	
AT		0.5%	N88820 001	OCT 16, 1984
	FLUTEX			
AT	SYOSSET	0.025%	N85539 001	
AT		0.1%	N85539 002	
AT		0.5%	N85539 003	
	KENALOG			
AT	WESTWOOD SQUIBB	0.025%	N11601 003	
AT		0.1%	N11601 006	
AT		0.5%	N83943 001	
	KENALOG-H			
AT	WESTWOOD SQUIBB	0.1%	N86240 001	
	TRIACET			
AT	LEMMON	0.025%	N84908 001	
AT		0.1%	N84908 002	
AT		0.5%	N84908 003	
	TRIAMCINOLONE ACETONIDE			
AT	ALTANA	0.025%	N85692 001	
AT		0.1%	N85692 003	
AT		0.5%	N85692 002	
AT	AMBIX	0.025%	N87932 001	MAY 09, 1983
AT	CLAY PARK	0.025%	N86415 001	
AT		0.1%	N86414 001	
AT		0.5%	N86413 001	
AT	G AND W	0.025%	N89797 001	MAY 31, 1991
AT		0.1%	N89798 001	MAY 31, 1991

†See Section 1.8 of Introduction.

Prescription Drug Products *(continued)*

TRIAMCINOLONE ACETONIDE *(continued)*

CREAM; TOPICAL
TRIAMCINOLONE ACETONIDE

AT	NMC	0.025%	N87797 001	JUN 07, 1982
AT		0.1%	N87798 001	JUN 04, 1982
AT	PHARMADERM	0.025%	N87990 001	JUL 07, 1983
AT		0.1%	N87991 001	JUL 07, 1983
AT		0.5%	N87992 001	JUL 07, 1983
AT	PHARMAFAIR	0.025%	N87921 001	AUG 10, 1982
AT		0.1%	N87912 001	AUG 10, 1982
AT		0.5%	N87922 001	AUG 10, 1982
AT	THAMES	0.025%	N86277 001	
AT		0.1%	N86276 001	
AT		0.5%	N86275 001	
AT	TOPIDERM	0.025%	N89274 001	FEB 21, 1989
AT		0.1%	N89275 001	FEB 21, 1989
AT		0.5%	N89276 001	FEB 21, 1989
AT	TRIATEX SYOSSET	0.025%	N87430 001	NOV 01, 1988
AT		0.1%	N87429 001	NOV 01, 1988
AT		0.5%	N87428 001	NOV 01, 1988
AT	TRIDERM DEL RAY	0.1%	N88042 001	MAR 19, 1984
AT	TRYMEX SAVAGE	0.025%	N88196 001	MAR 25, 1983
AT		0.1%	N88197 001	MAR 25, 1983

INJECTABLE; INJECTION
KENALOG-10

+	WESTWOOD SQUIBB	10 MG/ML	N12041 001

KENALOG-40

BP	WESTWOOD SQUIBB	40 MG/ML	N14901 001

TRIAMCINOLONE ACETONIDE

	PARNELL	3 MG/ML	N19503 001	OCT 16, 1987
BP	STERIS	40 MG/ML	N85825 001	

TRIAMCINOLONE ACETONIDE *(continued)*

LOTION; TOPICAL
KENALOG

AT	WESTWOOD SQUIBB	0.025%	N84343 001	
AT		0.1%	N84343 002	

TRIAMCINOLONE ACETONIDE

AT	BARRE	0.025%	N87191 001	SEP 08, 1982
AT		0.1%	N87192 001	SEP 08, 1982
AT	PHARM BASICS	0.025%	N88450 001	APR 01, 1985
AT		0.1%	N88451 001	APR 03, 1985
AT	THAMES	0.1%	N89129 001	AUG 14, 1986

OINTMENT; TOPICAL
ARISTOCORT

AT	LEDERLE	0.1%	N80750 004	
AT		0.5%	N80745 002	

ARISTOCORT A

AT	LEDERLE	0.1%	N80750 003	
AT		0.1%	N88780 001	OCT 01, 1984
AT		0.5%	N80745 003	

FLUTEX

AT	SYOSSET	0.025%	N87375 001	NOV 01, 1988
AT		0.1%	N87377 001	NOV 01, 1988
AT		0.5%	N87376 001	NOV 01, 1988

KENALOG

AT	WESTWOOD SQUIBB	0.025%	N11600 003	
AT		0.1%	N11600 001	
AT		0.5%	N83944 001	

TRIAMCINOLONE ACETONIDE

AT	ALTANA	0.025%	N85691 001	
AT		0.1%	N85691 003	
AT		0.5%	N85691 002	
AT	CLAY PARK	0.025%	N87356 001	
AT		0.1%	N87357 001	
AT		0.5%	N87385 001	
AT	G AND W	0.025%	N89795 001	DEC 23, 1988
AT		0.1%	N89796 001	DEC 23, 1988
AT	NASKA	0.5%	N89913 001	DEC 23, 1988
AT	NMC	0.1%	N87799 001	JUN 07, 1982
AT	PHARMADERM	0.025%	N88692 001	AUG 02, 1984
AT		0.1%	N88690 001	AUG 02, 1984
AT	THAMES	0.1%	N87902 001	DEC 27, 1982

Prescription Drug Products (continued)

TRIAMCINOLONE ACETONIDE (continued)

OINTMENT; TOPICAL

	TRYMEX			
ΔT	SAVAGE	0.025%	N88693 001	AUG 02, 1984
ΔT		0.1%	N88691 001	AUG 02, 1984

PASTE; DENTAL

	KENALOG IN ORABASE			
ΔT	SQUIBB	0.1%	N12097 001	
	ORACORT			
ΔT	TARO	0.1%	N70730 001	OCT 01, 1986
	ORALONE			
ΔT	THAMES	0.1%	N71383 001	JUL 06, 1987

TRIAMCINOLONE ACETONIDE; *MULTIPLE*

SEE NYSTATIN; TRIAMCINOLONE ACETONIDE

TRIAMCINOLONE DIACETATE

INJECTABLE; INJECTION

	ARISTOCORT		
BP	+ LEDERLE	25 MG/ML	N11685 003
BP	+	40 MG/ML	N12802 001
	TRIAMCINOLONE DIACETATE		
BP	AKORN	25 MG/ML	N85122 001
BP		40 MG/ML	N86394 001
BP	STERIS	40 MG/ML	N84072 001
BP		40 MG/ML	N85529 001

SYRUP; ORAL

	ARISTOCORT		
	LEDERLE	2 MG/5 ML	N11960 004
	KENACORT		
	SQUIBB	EQ 4 MG BASE/5 ML	N12515 001

TRIAMCINOLONE HEXACETONIDE

INJECTABLE; INJECTION

ARISTOSPAN		
LEDERLE	5 MG/ML	N16466 001
	20 MG/ML	N16466 002

TRIAMTERENE

CAPSULE; ORAL

DYRENIUM		
SKF	50 MG	N13174 001
	100 MG	N13174 002

TRIAMTERENE; *MULTIPLE*

SEE HYDROCHLOROTHIAZIDE; TRIAMTERENE

TRIAZOLAM

TABLET; ORAL

HALCION			
UPJOHN	0.125 MG	N17892 003	APR 26, 1985
	0.25 MG	N17892 001	NOV 15, 1982

TRICHLORMETHIAZIDE

TABLET; ORAL

	METAHYDRIN			
BP	MERRELL DOW	2 MG	N12594 001	JUN 16, 1988
BP		4 MG	N12594 002	JUN 16, 1988
	NAQUA			
BP	SCHERING	2 MG	N12265 001	
BP		4 MG	N12265 002	
	TRICHLOREX			
BP	LANNETT	4 MG	N83436 001	
BP		4 MG	N85630 001	
	TRICHLORMAS			
BP	MAST	4 MG	N86259 001	
	TRICHLORMETHIAZIDE			
BP	CAMALL	4 MG	N85568 001	
BP	DANBURY	2 MG	N83847 001	
BP		4 MG	N83855 001	
BP	PAR	2 MG	N87007 001	
BP		4 MG	N87005 001	
BP	RICHLYN	4 MG	N83967 001	

TRICHLORMETHIAZIDE; *MULTIPLE*

SEE RESERPINE; TRICHLORMETHIAZIDE

TRIENTINE HYDROCHLORIDE

CAPSULE; ORAL

SYPRINE			
+ MSD	250 MG	N19194 001	NOV 08, 1985

TRIETHANOLAMINE POLYPEPTIDE OLEATE CONDENSATE

SOLUTION/DROPS; OTIC

CERUMENEX		
PURDUE FREDERICK	10%	N11340 002

Prescription Drug Products (continued)

TRIFLUOPERAZINE HYDROCHLORIDE

CONCENTRATE; ORAL

		Strength	Application
∆A	STELAZINE		
	SKF	EQ 10 MG BASE/ML	N11552 006
∆A	TFP		
	GENEVA	EQ 10 MG BASE/ML	N85787 001 APR 15, 1982
∆A	TRIFLUOPERAZINE HCL		
	PHARM BASICS	EQ 10 MG BASE/ML	N88143 001 JUL 26, 1983

INJECTABLE; INJECTION

		Strength	Application
	STELAZINE		
	SKF	EQ 2 MG BASE/ML	N11552 005

TABLET; ORAL

		Strength	Application
∆B	STELAZINE		
	SKF	EQ 1 MG BASE	N11552 001
∆B		EQ 2 MG BASE	N11552 002
∆B		EQ 5 MG BASE	N11552 003
∆B		EQ 10 MG BASE	N11552 004
∆B	TFP		
	GENEVA	EQ 1 MG BASE	N85785 001
∆B		EQ 2 MG BASE	N85786 001
∆B		EQ 5 MG BASE	N85789 001
∆B		EQ 10 MG BASE	N85788 001
∆B	TRIFLUOPERAZINE HCL		
	ZENITH	EQ 1 MG BASE	N87612 001 NOV 19, 1982
∆B		EQ 2 MG BASE	N87613 001 NOV 19, 1982
∆B		EQ 5 MG BASE	N87328 001 NOV 19, 1982
∆B		EQ 10 MG BASE	N87614 001 NOV 19, 1982

TRIFLUPROMAZINE

SUSPENSION; ORAL

	Strength	Application
VESPRIN		
SQUIBB	EQ 50 MG HCL/5 ML	N11491 004

TRIFLUPROMAZINE HYDROCHLORIDE

INJECTABLE; INJECTION

	Strength	Application
VESPRIN		
SQUIBB	10 MG/ML	N11325 004
	20 MG/ML	N11325 001

TABLET; ORAL

	Strength	Application
VESPRIN		
SQUIBB	10 MG	N11123 001
	25 MG	N11123 002
	50 MG	N11123 003

TRIFLURIDINE

SOLUTION/DROPS; OPHTHALMIC

	Strength	Application
VIROPTIC		
BURROUGHS WELLCOME	1%	N18299 001

TRIHEXYPHENIDYL HYDROCHLORIDE

CAPSULE, EXTENDED RELEASE; ORAL

		Strength	Application
	ARTANE		
+	LEDERLE	5 MG	N06773 010
		5 MG	N12947 001

ELIXIR; ORAL

		Strength	Application
	ARTANE		
∆A	LEDERLE	2 MG/5 ML	N06773 009
	TRIHEXYPHENIDYL HCL		
∆A	LIQUIPHARM	2 MG/5 ML	N89514 001 APR 07, 1989

TABLET; ORAL

		Strength	Application
	ARTANE		
∆A	LEDERLE	2 MG	N06773 005
∆A		5 MG	N06773 003
	TREMIN		
∆A	SCHERING	2 MG	N80381 001
∆A		5 MG	N80381 003
	TRIHEXYPHENIDYL HCL		
∆A	DANBURY	2 MG	N84363 001
∆A		5 MG	N84364 001
∆A	TABLICAPS	5 MG	N85622 001

TRILOSTANE

CAPSULE; ORAL

		Strength	Application
	MODRASTANE		
	STERLING	30 MG	N18719 002 DEC 31, 1984
+		60 MG	N18719 001 DEC 31, 1984

TRIMEPRAZINE TARTRATE

CAPSULE, EXTENDED RELEASE; ORAL

		Strength	Application
	TEMARIL		
+	HERBERT	EQ 5 MG BASE	N11316 004

SYRUP; ORAL

		Strength	Application
	TEMARIL		
	HERBERT	EQ 2.5 MG BASE/5 ML	N11316 003

TABLET; ORAL

		Strength	Application
	TEMARIL		
	HERBERT	EQ 2.5 MG BASE	N11316 001

TRIMETHADIONE

CAPSULE; ORAL

		Strength	Application
	TRIDIONE		
+	ABBOTT	300 MG	N05856 005

SOLUTION; ORAL

		Strength	Application
	TRIDIONE		
	ABBOTT	200 MG/5 ML	N05856 002

TABLET; ORAL

		Strength	Application
	TRIDIONE		
+	ABBOTT	150 MG	N05856 009

Prescription Drug Products (continued)

TRIMETHAPHAN CAMSYLATE
INJECTABLE; INJECTION

	Firm	Strength	Appl. No.	Date
	ARFONAD			
	ROCHE	50 MG/ML	N08983 001	

TRIMETHOBENZAMIDE HYDROCHLORIDE
INJECTABLE; INJECTION

	Firm	Strength	Appl. No.	Date
	TIGAN			
	BEECHAM	100 MG/ML	N17530 001	
	TRIMETHOBENZAMIDE HCL			
ΔP	SMITH NEPHEW SOLOPAK	100 MG/ML	N88960 001	APR 04, 1986
			N89094 001	APR 04, 1986
ΔP	STERIS	100 MG/ML	N86577 001	OCT 19, 1982
ΔP		100 MG/ML	N87939 001	DEC 28, 1982
ΔP	STERLING	100 MG/ML	N88804 001	APR 03, 1987

TRIMETHOPRIM
TABLET; ORAL

	Firm	Strength	Appl. No.	Date
	PROLOPRIM			
ΔB	BURROUGHS WELLCOME	100 MG	N17943 001	
ΔB		200 MG	N17943 003	JUL 14, 1982
	TRIMETHOPRIM			
ΔB	BARR	100 MG	N70494 001	JAN 22, 1986
ΔB	BIOCRAFT	100 MG	N18679 001	JUL 30, 1982
ΔB		200 MG	N71259 001	JUN 18, 1987
ΔB	DANBURY	100 MG	N70049 001	JUN 06, 1985
	TRIMPEX			
ΔB	ROCHE	100 MG	N17952 001	
ΔB	TRIMPEX 200 + ROCHE	200 MG	N17952 002	NOV 09, 1982

TRIMETHOPRIM; *MULTIPLE*
SEE   SULFAMETHOXAZOLE;TRIMETHOPRIM

TRIMETHOPRIM SULFATE; *MULTIPLE*
SEE   POLYMYXIN B SULFATE;TRIMETHOPRIM SULFATE

TRIMIPRAMINE MALEATE
CAPSULE; ORAL

Firm	Strength	Appl. No.	Date
SURMONTIL			
WYETH AYERST	EQ 25 MG BASE	N16792 001	
	EQ 50 MG BASE	N16792 002	
	EQ 100 MG BASE	N16792 003	SEP 15, 1982
+			

TRIOXSALEN
TABLET; ORAL

Firm	Strength	Appl. No.
TRISORALEN		
ELDER	5 MG	N12697 001

TRIPELENNAMINE CITRATE
ELIXIR; ORAL

Firm	Strength	Appl. No.
PBZ		
GEIGY	EQ 25 MG HCL/5 ML	N05914 004

TRIPELENNAMINE HYDROCHLORIDE
TABLET; ORAL

	Firm	Strength	Appl. No.
	PBZ		
ΔΔ	GEIGY	50 MG	N05914 002
		25 MG	N83149 001
	TRIPELENNAMINE HCL		
ΔΔ	DANBURY	50 MG	N80713 001
ΔΔ	HEATHER	50 MG	N83989 001
ΔΔ	LANNETT	50 MG	N83557 001
ΔΔ	RICHLYN	50 MG	N80785 001
ΔΔ	TABLICAPS	50 MG	N85412 001

TABLET, EXTENDED RELEASE; ORAL

Firm	Strength	Appl. No.
PBZ-SR		
GEIGY	100 MG	N10533 001

TRIPLE SULFA
(SULFABENZAMIDE;SULFACETAMIDE;SULFATHIAZOLE)
CREAM; VAGINAL

	Firm	Strength	Appl. No.	Date
	GYNE-SULF			
ΔI	G AND W	3.7%;2.86%;3.42%	N88607 001	JUN 09, 1986
	SULTRIN			
ΔI	JOHNSON RW	3.7%;2.86%;3.42%	N05794 001	
	TRIPLE SULFA			
ΔI	CLAY PARK	3.7%;2.86%;3.42%	N87285 001	NOV 15, 1982
ΔI	FOUGERA	3.7%;2.86%;3.42%	N86424 001	
ΔI	NMC	3.7%;2.86%;3.42%	N87864 001	SEP 01, 1982
	TRYSUL			
ΔI	SAVAGE	3.7%;2.86%;3.42%	N87887 001	JUL 23, 1982

TABLET; VAGINAL

Firm	Strength	Appl. No.
SULTRIN		
JOHNSON RW	184 MG;143.75 MG;172.5 MG	N05794 002

Prescription Drug Products (continued)

TRIPROLIDINE HYDROCHLORIDE

SYRUP; ORAL

TRIPROLIDINE HCL
HALSEY	1.25 MG/5 ML	N88735 001	JAN 17, 1985

TABLET; ORAL

TRIPROLIDINE HCL
DANBURY	2.5 MG	N85094 001

TRIPROLIDINE HYDROCHLORIDE; *MULTIPLE*

SEE CODEINE PHOSPHATE; PSEUDOEPHEDRINE HYDROCHLORIDE; TRIPROLIDINE HYDROCHLORIDE

SEE PSEUDOEPHEDRINE HYDROCHLORIDE; TRIPROLIDINE HYDROCHLORIDE

TRISULFAPYRIMIDINES

SUSPENSION; ORAL

LANTRISUL			
AB	LANNETT	500 MG/5 ML	N80123 002
NEOTRIZINE			
AB	+ LILLY	500 MG/5 ML	N06317 012
TERFONYL			
AP	SQUIBB	500 MG/5 ML	N06904 002

TABLET; ORAL

NEOTRIZINE			
AB	+ LILLY	500 MG	N06317 011
SULFA-TRIPLE #2			
AB	RICHLYN	500 MG	N80079 001
TERFONYL			
AB	SQUIBB	500 MG	N06904 001
TRIPLE SULFOID			
AB	VALE	500 MG	N80094 001

TROLEANDOMYCIN

CAPSULE; ORAL

TAO
+ ROERIG	EQ 250 MG BASE	N50336 002

TROMETHAMINE

INJECTABLE; INJECTION

THAM
ABBOTT	3.6 GM/100 ML	N13025 002

TROMETHAMINE; *MULTIPLE*

SEE POTASSIUM CHLORIDE; SODIUM CHLORIDE; TROMETHAMINE

TROPICAMIDE

SOLUTION/DROPS; OPHTHALMIC

MYDRIACYL				
AT	ALCON	0.5%	N12111 002	
AT		0.5%	N84305 001	
AT		1%	N12111 004	
AT		1%	N84306 001	
MYDRIAFAIR				
AT	PHARMAFAIR	0.5%	N88274 001	SEP 16, 1983
AT		1%	N88230 001	SEP 16, 1983
TROPICAMIDE				
AT	AKORN	1%	N88447 001	AUG 28, 1985
AT	OPTOPICS	0.5%	N87636 001	JUL 30, 1982
AT		1%	N87637 001	AUG 09, 1982
AT	STERIS	0.5%	N89171 001	DEC 28, 1990
AT		1%	N89172 001	DEC 28, 1990

TROPICAMIDE; *MULTIPLE*

SEE HYDROXYAMPHETAMINE HYDROBROMIDE; TROPICAMIDE

TUBOCURARINE CHLORIDE

INJECTABLE; INJECTION

TUBOCURARINE CHLORIDE				
AP	ABBOTT	3 MG/ML	N06095 001	
AP	LILLY	3 MG/ML	N06325 001	
AP	QUAD	3 MG/ML	N89442 001	AUG 12, 1988
AP	SQUIBB	3 MG/ML	N05657 001	

TYLOXAPOL; *MULTIPLE*

SEE CETYL ALCOHOL; COLFOSCERIL PALMITATE; TYLOXAPOL

TYROPANOATE SODIUM

CAPSULE; ORAL

BILOPAQUE
STERLING	750 MG	N13731 001

URACIL MUSTARD

CAPSULE; ORAL

URACIL MUSTARD
UPJOHN	1 MG	N12892 001

Prescription Drug Products (continued)

UREA

INJECTABLE; INJECTION

UREAPHIL

ABBOTT	40 GM/VIAL	N12154 001	

UREA; *MULTIPLE*

SEE   HYDROCORTISONE: UREA
SEE   HYDROCORTISONE ACETATE: UREA

UROFOLLITROPIN

INJECTABLE; INJECTION

METRODIN

SERONO	75IU/AMP	N19415 002	SEP 18, 1986

URSODIOL

CAPSULE; ORAL

ACTIGALL

+ CIBA	300 MG	N19594 002	DEC 31, 1987

VALPROIC ACID

CAPSULE; ORAL

DEPAKENE

AB	+ ABBOTT	250 MG	N18081 001	

VALPROIC ACID

AB	PAR	250 MG	N70431 001	FEB 28, 1986
		250 MG	N70631 001	JUN 11, 1987
AB	PHARM BASICS	250 MG	N70195 001	JUL 02, 1987
AB	SCHERER	250 MG	N73229 001	OCT 29, 1991
AB		250 MG		

SYRUP; ORAL

DEPAKENE

	ABBOTT	250 MG/5 ML	N18082 001	

MYPROIC ACID

AA	ABBOTT	250 MG/5 ML	N70868 001	JUL 01, 1986
AA	PHARM BASICS	250 MG/5 ML		

VALPROIC ACID

AA	COPLEY	250 MG/5 ML	N73178 001	AUG 25, 1992

VANCOMYCIN HYDROCHLORIDE

CAPSULE; ORAL

VANCOCIN HCL

	LILLY	EQ 125 MG/BASE	N50606 001	APR 15, 1986
+		EQ 250 MG/BASE	N50606 002	APR 15, 1986

INJECTABLE; INJECTION

LYPHOCIN

	LYPHOMED	EQ 500 MG BASE/VIAL	N62663 001	MAR 17, 1987
AP		EQ 1 GM BASE/VIAL	N62663 002	JUL 31, 1987
AP		EQ 5 GM BASE/VIAL	N62663 003	JUN 03, 1988

VANCOCIN HCL

	LILLY	EQ 500 MG BASE/VIAL	N60180 001	
AP		EQ 500 MG BASE/VIAL	N62476 001	MAR 15, 1984
AP		EQ 500 MG BASE/VIAL	N62716 001	MAR 13, 1987
AP		EQ 500 MG BASE/VIAL	N62812 001	NOV 17, 1987
AP		EQ 1 GM BASE/VIAL	N60180 002	MAR 21, 1986
AP		EQ 1 GM BASE/VIAL	N62476 002	MAR 21, 1986
AP		EQ 1 GM BASE/VIAL	N62716 002	MAR 13, 1987
AP		EQ 1 GM BASE/VIAL	N62812 002	NOV 17, 1987
AP		EQ 10 GM BASE/VIAL	N62812 003	NOV 17, 1987

VANCOLED

	LEDERLE	EQ 500 MG BASE/VIAL	N62682 001	JUL 22, 1986
AP		EQ 1 GM BASE/VIAL	N62682 002	MAR 30, 1988
AP		EQ 5 GM BASE/VIAL	N62682 004	MAY 11, 1988
AP		EQ 10 GM BASE/VIAL	N62682 005	MAY 11, 1988
AP		EQ 2 GM BASE/VIAL	N62682 003	MAY 11, 1988

VANCOMYCIN HCL

	ABBOTT	EQ 500 MG BASE/VIAL	N62911 001	AUG 04, 1988
AP		EQ 1 GM BASE/VIAL	N62912 001	AUG 04, 1988
AP		EQ 5 GM BASE/VIAL	N63076 001	DEC 21, 1990
	ELKINS SINN	EQ 500 MG BASE/VIAL	N62879 001	AUG 02, 1988
AP		EQ 1 GM BASE/VIAL	N62879 002	AUG 02, 1988

VANCOR

	ADRIA	EQ 500 MG BASE/VIAL	N62956 001	AUG 01, 1988
AP		EQ 1 GM BASE/VIAL	N62956 002	AUG 01, 1988

Prescription Drug Products (continued)

VANCOMYCIN HYDROCHLORIDE (continued)
POWDER FOR RECONSTITUTION; ORAL
VANCOCIN HCL

		Strength	Number	Date
	LILLY	EQ 250 MG BASE/5 ML	N61667 002	JUL 13, 1983
		EQ 500 MG BASE/6 ML	N61667 001	

VASOPRESSIN TANNATE
INJECTABLE; INJECTION
PITRESSIN TANNATE

		Strength	Number	Date
	PARKE DAVIS	5 PRESSOR UNITS/ML	N03402 001	

VECURONIUM BROMIDE
INJECTABLE; INJECTION
NORCURON

		Strength	Number	Date
	ORGANON	10 MG/VIAL	N18776 002	APR 30, 1984
		20 MG/VIAL	N18776 003	JAN 03, 1992

VERAPAMIL HYDROCHLORIDE
CAPSULE, EXTENDED RELEASE; ORAL
VERELAN

		Strength	Number	Date
+	ELAN	120 MG	N19614 001	MAY 29, 1990
+		180 MG	N19614 003	JAN 09, 1992
+		240 MG	N19614 002	MAY 29, 1990

INJECTABLE; INJECTION
ISOPTIN

		Strength	Number	Date
	KNOLL	2.5 MG/ML	N18485 001	

VERAPAMIL HCL

		Strength	Number	Date
AP	ABBOTT	2.5 MG/ML	N70737 001	MAY 06, 1987
AP		2.5 MG/ML	N70738 001	MAY 06, 1987
AP		2.5 MG/ML	N70739 001	MAY 06, 1987
AP		2.5 MG/ML	N70740 001	MAY 06, 1987
AP	INTL MEDICATION	2.5 MG/ML	N70451 001	DEC 16, 1985
AP		2.5 MG/ML	N70225 001	
AP	LUITPOLD	2.5 MG/ML	N70617 001	NOV 12, 1985
AP		2.5 MG/ML	N70617 001	NOV 12, 1985
AP	SMITH NEPHEW SOLOPAK	2.5 MG/ML	N70695 001	JUL 31, 1987
AP		2.5 MG/ML	N70696 001	JUL 31, 1987
AP	STERLING	2.5 MG/ML	N70577 001	FEB 02, 1987

VERAPAMIL HYDROCHLORIDE (continued)
TABLET; ORAL
CALAN

		Strength	Number	Date
AB	SEARLE	40 MG	N18817 003	FEB 23, 1988
AB		80 MG	N18817 001	SEP 10, 1984
AB		120 MG	N18817 002	SEP 10, 1984

ISOPTIN

		Strength	Number	Date
AB	KNOLL	40 MG	N18593 003	NOV 23, 1987
AB		80 MG	N18593 001	MAR 08, 1982
AB	+	120 MG	N18593 002	MAR 08, 1982

VERAPAMIL HCL

		Strength	Number	Date
AB	BARR	80 MG	N70482 001	SEP 23, 1986
AB		120 MG	N70483 001	SEP 23, 1986
AB	DANBURY	80 MG	N70855 001	SEP 23, 1986
AB		120 MG	N70856 001	SEP 23, 1986
AB	GENEVA	40 MG	N73168 001	JUL 31, 1992
AB		80 MG	N71423 001	MAY 24, 1988
AB		120 MG	N71424 001	MAY 25, 1988
AB	LEDERLE	80 MG	N71880 001	APR 05, 1988
AB		120 MG	N71881 001	APR 05, 1988
AB	MUTUAL PHARM	80 MG	N71488 001	JAN 13, 1988
AB		120 MG	N71489 001	JAN 13, 1988
AB	MYLAN	80 MG	N71482 001	FEB 15, 1989
AB		120 MG	N71483 001	FEB 15, 1989
AB	PUREPAC	80 MG	N71019 001	SEP 23, 1986
AB		120 MG	N70468 001	SEP 23, 1986
AB	SIDMAK	80 MG	N72124 001	JAN 26, 1989
AB		120 MG	N72125 001	JAN 26, 1989
AB	WATSON	80 MG	N70995 001	OCT 01, 1986
AB		80 MG	N71366 001	OCT 01, 1986
AB		120 MG	N70994 001	OCT 01, 1986
AB		120 MG	N71367 001	OCT 01, 1986

Prescription Drug Products *(continued)*

VERAPAMIL HYDROCHLORIDE *(continued)*
TABLET, EXTENDED RELEASE; ORAL

ISOPTIN SR
ΔB	+ KNOLL	240 MG	N19152 001	DEC 16, 1986
	+	120 MG	N19152 003	MAR 06, 1991
	+	180 MG	N19152 002	DEC 15, 1989

VERAPAMIL HCL
ΔB	BAKER CUMMINS	240 MG	N73568 001	JUL 31, 1992

VIDARABINE
INJECTABLE; INJECTION

VIRA-A
	+ PARKE DAVIS	EQ 187.4 MG BASE/ML	N50523 001

OINTMENT; OPHTHALMIC

VIRA-A
	+ PARKE DAVIS	3%	N50486 001

VINBLASTINE SULFATE
INJECTABLE; INJECTION

VELBAN
	LILLY	10 MG/VIAL	N12665 001	

VELSAR
ΔP	BULL	10 MG/VIAL	N89565 001	AUG 18, 1987

VINBLASTINE SULFATE
ΔP	BEN VENUE	10 MG/VIAL	N89395 001	APR 09, 1987
	LYPHOMED	1 MG/ML	N89515 001	APR 29, 1987

VINCRISTINE SULFATE
INJECTABLE; INJECTION

ONCOVIN
ΔP	LILLY	1 MG/ML	N14103 003	MAR 07, 1984

VINCASAR PFS
ΔP	ADRIA	1 MG/ML	N71426 001	JUL 17, 1987

VINCREX
ΔP	BRISTOL	5 MG/VIAL	N70867 001	JUL 12, 1988

VINCRISTINE SULFATE *(continued)*
INJECTABLE; INJECTION

VINCRISTINE SULFATE
ΔP	ABIC	1 MG/ML	N70873 001	FEB 19, 1987
ΔP	BULL	5 MG/VIAL	N71561 001	APR 11, 1988
		1 MG/VIAL	N71559 001	APR 11, 1988
		1 MG/VIAL	N71560 001	APR 11, 1988
		2 MG/VIAL	N70411 001	SEP 10, 1986
ΔP	LYPHOMED	1 MG/ML		

VINCRISTINE SULFATE PFS
ΔP	BULL	1 MG/ML	N71484 001	APR 19, 1988

VITAMIN A
CAPSULE; ORAL

AQUASOL A
ΔΔ	ASTRA	50,000 USP UNITS	N83080 001
		25,000 USP UNITS	N83080 002

VITAMIN A
ΔΔ	PHARMACAPS	50,000 USP UNITS	N83973 001
ΔΔ	RICHLYN	50,000 USP UNITS	N80952 001
ΔΔ	WEST WARD	50,000 USP UNITS	N80985 001

VITAMIN A; *MULTIPLE*
SEE ASCORBIC ACID; BIOTIN; CYANOCOBALAMIN; DEXPANTHENOL; ERGOCALCIFEROL; FOLIC ACID; NIACINAMIDE; PYRIDOXINE HYDROCHLORIDE; RIBOFLAVIN PHOSPHATE SODIUM; THIAMINE HYDROCHLORIDE; VITAMIN A; VITAMIN E

SEE ASCORBIC ACID; BIOTIN; CYANOCOBALAMIN; DEXPANTHENOL; ERGOCALCIFEROL; FOLIC ACID; NIACINAMIDE; PYRIDOXINE; RIBOFLAVIN PHOSPHATE SODIUM; THIAMINE; VITAMIN A; VITAMIN E

VITAMIN A PALMITATE
CAPSULE; ORAL

DEL-VI-A
ΔΔ	DEL RAY	EQ 50,000 UNITS BASE	N80830 001

VITAMIN A
ΔΔ	MK	EQ 50,000 UNITS BASE	N83457 001
		EQ 25,000 UNITS BASE	N83457 002
ΔΔ	PHARMACAPS	EQ 50,000 UNITS BASE	N80702 001
ΔΔ	RICHLYN	EQ 50,000 UNITS BASE	N80953 001
ΔΔ		EQ 50,000 UNITS BASE	N80955 001
ΔΔ	WEST WARD	EQ 50,000 UNITS BASE	N80967 001
ΔΔ	WHARTON	EQ 50,000 UNITS BASE	N83665 001
ΔΔ	ZENITH	EQ 50,000 UNITS BASE	N83035 001
ΔΔ		EQ 50,000 UNITS BASE	N83190 001

Prescription Drug Products (continued)

WATER FOR INJECTION, STERILE (continued)

LIQUID; N/A

STERILE WATER FOR INJECTION IN PLASTIC CONTAINER

AA	ABBOTT	100%	N18233 001
AA		100%	N18801 001
			OCT 27, 1982
			N19869 001
			DEC 26, 1989
AP	BAXTER	100%	N18632 001
			JUN 30, 1982
AP		100%	N18632 002
			APR 19, 1988
			N88400 001
AP	LYPHOMED	100%	JAN 16, 1984
			N19077 001
AP	MCGAW	100%	MAR 02, 1984
AP		100%	N19633 001
			FEB 29, 1988

WATER FOR IRRIGATION, STERILE

LIQUID; IRRIGATION

STERILE WATER

STERILE WATER IN PLASTIC CONTAINER

AT	BAXTER	100%	N17428 001
AT	ABBOTT	100%	N17513 001
AT	BAXTER	100%	N18313 001
AT	MCGAW	100%	N17866 001
			N16734 001

XENON, XE-127

GAS; INHALATION

XENON XE 127

	MALLINCKRODT	5 MCI/VIAL	N18536 001
			OCT 01, 1982
		10 MCI/VIAL	N18536 002
			OCT 01, 1982

XENON, XE-133

GAS; INHALATION

XENON XE 133

AA	DUPONT	10 MCI/VIAL	N17284 001
		20 MCI/VIAL	N17284 002
AA		30 MCI/VIAL	N17284 004
		40 MCI/VIAL	N17284 005
		50 MCI/VIAL	N17284 006
		60 MCI/VIAL	N17284 007
		100 MCI/VIAL	N17284 003
	GENERAL ELECTRIC	1-2.5 CI/AMP	N17550 003
		5 CI/CYLINDER	N17550 001
AA	MALLINCKRODT	10 MCI/VIAL	N18327 001
			MAR 09, 1982
			N18327 002
AA	MEDI PHYSICS	20 MCI/VIAL	MAR 09, 1982
		1 CI/AMP	N17256 002

VITAMIN A PALMITATE (continued)

CAPSULE; ORAL

VITAMIN A PALMITATE

AA	ARCUM	EQ 50,000 UNITS BASE	N83311 001
AA	BANNER GELATIN	EQ 50,000 UNITS BASE	N83321 001
AA	PHARMACAPS	EQ 50,000 UNITS BASE	N83981 001
AA		EQ 50,000 UNITS BASE	N83948 001

INJECTABLE; INJECTION

AQUASOL A

AP	ASTRA	EQ 50,000 UNITS BASE/ML	N06823 001

VITAMIN A PALMITATE

AP	BEL MAR	EQ 50,000 UNITS BASE/ML	N80819 001

VITAMIN E; *MULTIPLE*

SEE ASCORBIC ACID; BIOTIN; CYANOCOBALAMIN;
DEXPANTHENOL; ERGOCALCIFEROL; FOLIC ACID;
NIACINAMIDE; PYRIDOXINE HYDROCHLORIDE; RIBOFLAVIN
PHOSPHATE SODIUM; THIAMINE HYDROCHLORIDE; VITAMIN
A; VITAMIN E

SEE ASCORBIC ACID; BIOTIN; CYANOCOBALAMIN;
DEXPANTHENOL; ERGOCALCIFEROL; FOLIC ACID;
NIACINAMIDE; PYRIDOXINE; RIBOFLAVIN PHOSPHATE
SODIUM; THIAMINE; VITAMIN A; VITAMIN E

WARFARIN SODIUM

TABLET; ORAL

COUMADIN

AB	DUPONT	2 MG	N09218 013
AB		2.5 MG	N09218 018
AB		5 MG	N09218 007
BX	+	7.5 MG	N09218 016
BX	+	10 MG	N09218 005
		1 MG	N09218 022
			MAR 01, 1990

PANWARFIN

BX	ABBOTT	2 MG	N17020 001
BX		2.5 MG	N17020 002
BX		5 MG	N17020 003
BX		7.5 MG	N17020 004
BX		10 MG	N17020 005

WATER FOR INJECTION, STERILE

LIQUID; N/A

BACTERIOSTATIC WATER FOR INJECTION IN PLASTIC CONTAINER

AP	ABBOTT	100%	N18802 001
			OCT 27, 1982
			N89099 001
AP	LYPHOMED	100%	DEC 29, 1987
			N89100 001
AP		100%	DEC 29, 1987

Prescription Drug Products (*continued*)

ZIDOVUDINE (*continued*)

INJECTABLE; INJECTION
  RETROVIR
    BURROUGHS
      WELLCOME   10 MG/ML   N19951 001
                                          FEB 02, 1990

SYRUP; ORAL
  RETROVIR
    BURROUGHS
      WELLCOME   50 MG/5 ML   N19910 001
                                          SEP 28, 1989

ZINC CHLORIDE

INJECTABLE; INJECTION
  ZINC CHLORIDE IN PLASTIC CONTAINER
    ABBOTT   EQ 1 MG ZINC/ML   N18959 001
                                          JUN 26, 1986

ZINC SULFATE

INJECTABLE; INJECTION
  ZINC SULFATE
    LYPHOMED   EQ 1 MG ZINC/ML   N19229 002
                                          MAY 05, 1987
                                          MAY 05, 1987

XENON, XE-133 (*continued*)

SOLUTION; INHALATION, INJECTION
  XENEISOL
    MALLINCKRODT   18-25 MCI/AMP   N17262 002

XYLOSE

POWDER; ORAL
  XYLO-PFAN
ΔΔ ADRIA   25 GM/BOT   N17605 001
  XYLOSE
ΔΔ LYNE   25 GM/BOT   N18856 001
                                          MAR 26, 1987

ZALCITABINE

TABLET; ORAL
  HIVID
    ROCHE   0.375 MG   N20199 001
                                          JUN 19, 1992
    +   0.75 MG   N20199 002
                                          JUN 19, 1992

ZIDOVUDINE

CAPSULE; ORAL
  RETROVIR
  + BURROUGHS
      WELLCOME   100 MG   N19655 001
                                          MAR 19, 1987

OTC DRUG PRODUCTS

ACETAMINOPHEN

SUPPOSITORY; RECTAL

ACEPHEN
- G AND W — 120 MG — N18060 001
- G AND W — 120 MG — N72218 001, MAR 27, 1992
- 325 MG — N18060 003, DEC 18, 1986
- 325 MG — N72344 001, MAR 27, 1992
- 650 MG — N18060 002
- 650 MG — N72237 001, MAR 27, 1992

ACETAMINOPHEN
- ROXANE — 120 MG — N71010 001, MAY 12, 1987
- 650 MG — N71011 001, MAY 12, 1987

SUPPOSITORIA
- 120 MG — N70607 001, APR 06, 1987
- 650 MG — N70608 001, DEC 01, 1986

UPSHER SMITH
- 120 MG — N18337 003, SEP 12, 1983
- 325 MG — N18337 002
- 650 MG — N18337 001

NEOPAP
- ALCON — 120 MG — N16401 001

ACETAMINOPHEN; DEXBROMPHENIRAMINE MALEATE; PSEUDOEPHEDRINE SULFATE

TABLET, EXTENDED RELEASE; ORAL

DRIXORAL PLUS
- SCHERING — 500 MG;3 MG;60 MG — N19453 001, MAY 22, 1987

ALUMINUM HYDROXIDE; MAGNESIUM TRISILICATE

TABLET, CHEWABLE; ORAL

ALUMINUM HYDROXIDE AND MAGNESIUM TRISILICATE
- PENNEX — 80 MG;20 MG — N89449 001, NOV 27, 1987

FOAMCOAT
- GUARDIAN DRUG — 80 MG;20 MG — N71793 001, SEP 04, 1987

FOAMICON
- INVAMED — 80 MG;20 MG — N72687 001, JUN 28, 1989

GAVISCON
- MARION MERRELL DOW — 80 MG;20 MG — N18685 001, DEC 09, 1983

GAVISCON-2
- MARION MERRELL DOW — 160 MG;40 MG — N18685 002, DEC 09, 1983

ASPIRIN

TABLET, EXTENDED RELEASE; ORAL

MEASURIN
- STERLING — 650 MG — N16030 002

8-HOUR BAYER
- STERLING — 650 MG — N16030 001

AVOBENZONE; PADIMATE O

LOTION; TOPICAL

PHOTOPLEX
- HERBERT — 3%;7% — N19459 001, SEP 30, 1988

BACITRACIN

OINTMENT; TOPICAL

BACITRACIN
- COMBE — 500 UNITS/GM — N62799 001, MAY 14, 1987
- NASKA — 500 UNITS/GM — N62857 001, NOV 13, 1987

BACITRACIN; POLYMYXIN B SULFATE

AEROSOL; TOPICAL

LANABIOTIC
- COMBE — 500 UNITS/GM;5,000 UNITS/GM — N50598 001, SEP 22, 1986

BACITRACIN ZINC; LIDOCAINE; NEOMYCIN SULFATE; POLYMYXIN B SULFATE

OINTMENT; TOPICAL

LANABIOTIC
- COMBE — 400 UNITS/GM;40 MG/GM;EQ 5 MG BASE/GM;5,000 UNITS/GM — N62499 001, JUN 03, 1985

BACITRACIN ZINC; NEOMYCIN SULFATE; POLYMYXIN B SULFATE

OINTMENT; TOPICAL

BACITRACIN ZINC-NEOMYCIN SULFATE-POLYMYXIN B SULFATE
- NASKA — 400 UNITS/GM;EQ 3.5 MG BASE/GM;5,000 UNITS/GM — N62833 001, NOV 09, 1987

BACITRACIN ZINC; POLYMYXIN B SULFATE

OINTMENT; TOPICAL

BACITRACIN ZINC-POLYMYXIN B SULFATE
- NASKA — 500 UNITS/GM;10,000 UNITS/GM — N62849 001, NOV 13, 1987

OTC Drug Products *(continued)*

BROMPHENIRAMINE MALEATE
TABLET, EXTENDED RELEASE; ORAL
DIMETANE
ROBINS   8 MG   N10799 010   JUN 10, 1983
          12 MG   N10799 011   JUN 10, 1983

BROMPHENIRAMINE MALEATE; PHENYLPROPANOLAMINE HYDROCHLORIDE
ELIXIR; ORAL
DIMETAPP
ROBINS   2 MG/5 ML;12.5 MG/5 ML   N13087 003   MAR 29, 1984

TABLET, EXTENDED RELEASE; ORAL
BROMATAPP
COPLEY   12 MG;75 MG   N71099 001   JUL 02, 1987

DIMETAPP
ROBINS   12 MG;75 MG   N12436 003   MAY 14, 1985

CHLORHEXIDINE GLUCONATE
AEROSOL; TOPICAL
EXIDINE
XTTRIUM   4%   N19127 001   DEC 24, 1984

SOLUTION; TOPICAL
BRIAN CARE
BRIAN   4%   N71419 001   DEC 17, 1987

CHG SCRUB
HUNTINGTON   4%   N19258 002   JUL 22, 1986

CIDA-STAT
HUNTINGTON   2%   N19258 001   JUL 22, 1986

EXIDINE
XTTRIUM   2%   N19422 001   DEC 17, 1985
           4%   N19125 001   DEC 24, 1984

HIBICLENS
STUART   4%   N17768 001
HIBISTAT
STUART   0.5%   N18300 001
MICROCOL
JOHNSON AND JOHNSON   0.5%   N72292 001   JAN 28, 1992

MICRODERM
JOHNSON AND JOHNSON   4%   N72255 001   APR 15, 1991

STERI-STAT
MATRIX MEDCL   4%   N70104 001   JUL 24, 1986

CHLORHEXIDINE GLUCONATE *(continued)*
SPONGE; TOPICAL
BIOSCRUB
GRIFFEN   4%   N19822 001   MAR 31, 1989

CHLORHEXIDINE GLUCONATE
DESERET   4%   N72525 001   OCT 24, 1989

KENDALL   4%   N19490 001   MAR 27, 1987

HIBICLENS
STUART   4%   N18423 001

MICRODERM
JOHNSON AND JOHNSON   4%   N72295 001   FEB 28, 1991

PHARMASEAL SCRUB CARE
BAXTER   4%   N19793 001   DEC 02, 1988

CHLORPHENIRAMINE MALEATE
CAPSULE, EXTENDED RELEASE; ORAL
CHLORPHENIRAMINE MALEATE
GENEVA   12 MG   N70797 001   AUG 12, 1988

TELDRIN
SKCP   12 MG   N17369 002

TABLET, EXTENDED RELEASE; ORAL
CHLOR-TRIMETON
SCHERING   8 MG   N07638 001
            12 MG   N07638 002

CHLORPHENIRAMINE MALEATE; PHENYLPROPANOLAMINE HYDROCHLORIDE
CAPSULE, EXTENDED RELEASE; ORAL
COLD CAPSULE IV
GRAHAM LABS   12 MG;75 MG   N18793 001   APR 25, 1985

COLD CAPSULE V
GRAHAM LABS   8 MG;75 MG   N18794 001   APR 23, 1985

CONTAC
SKCP   8 MG;75 MG   N18099 001
PHENYLPROPANOLAMINE HCL W/ CHLORPHENIRAMINE MALEATE
CENTRAL PHARMS   8 MG;75 MG   N18809 001   MAY 07, 1984

TABLET, EXTENDED RELEASE; ORAL
DEMAZIN
SCHERING   4 MG;25 MG   N18556 001   MAY 14, 1984

PHENYLPROPANOLAMINE HCL/CHLORPHENIRAMINE
DORSEY   12 MG;75 MG   N19613 001
TRIAMINIC-12
SANDOZ   12 MG;75 MG   N18115 001

OTC Drug Products (continued)

CHLORPHENIRAMINE MALEATE; PSEUDOEPHEDRINE HYDROCHLORIDE

CAPSULE, EXTENDED RELEASE; ORAL

CODIMAL-L.A. 12

| CENTRAL PHARMS | 12 MG;120 MG | N18935 001 | APR 15, 1985 |

ISOCLOR

| FISONS | 8 MG;120 MG | N18747 001 | MAR 06, 1986 |

PSEUDOEPHEDRINE HCL AND CHLORPHENIRAMINE MALEATE

| KV | 12 MG;120 MG | N71455 001 | MAR 01, 1989 |

PSEUDOEPHEDRINE HCL/CHLORPHENIRAMINE MALEATE

| GRAHAM LABS | 8 MG;120 MG | N18844 001 | MAR 20, 1985 |
| | 12 MG;120 MG | N18843 001 | MAR 18, 1985 |

PSEUDOEPHEDRINE HYDROCHLORIDE AND CHLORPHENIRAMINE MALEATE

| CENTRAL PHARMS | 8 MG;120 MG | N19428 001 | AUG 02, 1988 |

CHLORPHENIRAMINE MALEATE; PSEUDOEPHEDRINE SULFATE

TABLET, EXTENDED RELEASE; ORAL

CHLOR-TRIMETON

| SCHERING | 8 MG;120 MG | N18397 001 |

CHLORPHENIRAMINE POLISTIREX; CODEINE POLISTIREX

SUSPENSION, EXTENDED RELEASE; ORAL

PENNTUSS

| FISONS | EQ 4 MG MALEATE/5 ML;EQ 10 MG BASE/5 ML | N18928 001 | AUG 14, 1985 |

CHLORPHENIRAMINE POLISTIREX; PHENYLPROPANOLAMINE POLISTIREX

SUSPENSION, EXTENDED RELEASE; ORAL

CORSYM

| FISONS | EQ 4 MG MALEATE/5 ML;EQ 37.5 MG HCL/5 ML | N18050 001 | JAN 04, 1984 |

CLEMASTINE FUMARATE

TABLET; ORAL

TAVIST-1

| SANDOZ | 1.34 MG | N17661 003 | AUG 21, 1992 |

CLEMASTINE FUMARATE; PHENYLPROPANOLAMINE HYDROCHLORIDE

TABLET, EXTENDED RELEASE; ORAL

TAVIST-D

| SANDOZ | 1.34 MG;75 MG | N18298 002 | AUG 21, 1992 |

CLOTRIMAZOLE

CREAM; TOPICAL

LOTRIMIN AF

| SCHERING | 1% | N17619 002 | OCT 27, 1989 |

MYCELEX

| MILES | 1% | N18183 002 | APR 01, 1991 |

CREAM; VAGINAL

GYNE-LOTRIMIN

| SCHERING | 1% | N18052 002 | NOV 30, 1990 |

MYCELEX-7

| MILES | 1% | N18230 002 | DEC 26, 1991 |

LOTION; TOPICAL

LOTRIMIN AF

| SCHERING | 1% | N18813 002 | OCT 27, 1989 |

SOLUTION; TOPICAL

LOTRIMIN AF

| SCHERING | 1% | N17613 002 | OCT 27, 1989 |

MYCELEX

| MILES | 1% | N18181 002 | APR 01, 1991 |

TABLET; VAGINAL

GYNE-LOTRIMIN

| SCHERING | 100 MG | N17717 002 | NOV 30, 1990 |

MYCELEX-7

| MILES | 100 MG | N18182 002 | DEC 26, 1991 |

CODEINE POLISTIREX; *MULTIPLE*

SEE   CHLORPHENIRAMINE POLISTIREX; CODEINE POLISTIREX

DEXBROMPHENIRAMINE MALEATE; *MULTIPLE*

SEE   ACETAMINOPHEN; DEXBROMPHENIRAMINE MALEATE; PSEUDOEPHEDRINE SULFATE

OTC Drug Products (continued)

DEXBROMPHENIRAMINE MALEATE; PSEUDOEPHEDRINE SULFATE

TABLET, EXTENDED RELEASE; ORAL

BROMPHERIL	COPLEY	6 MG;120 MG	N89116 001	JAN 22, 1987
DISOBROM	GENEVA	6 MG;120 MG	N70770 001	SEP 30, 1991
DISOPHROL	SCHERING	6 MG;120 MG	N13483 004	SEP 13, 1982
DRIXORAL	SCHERING	6 MG;120 MG	N13483 003	SEP 13, 1982

DEXTROMETHORPHAN POLISTIREX

SUSPENSION, EXTENDED RELEASE; ORAL

DELSYM	FISONS	EQ 30 MG HBR/5 ML	N18658 001

DIPHENHYDRAMINE HYDROCHLORIDE

SYRUP; ORAL

ANTITUSSIVE	PERRIGO	12.5 MG/5 ML	N71292 001	APR 10, 1987
BELDIN	HALSEY	12.5 MG/5 ML	N89179 001	JUN 05, 1986
BENYLIN	PARKE DAVIS	12.5 MG/5 ML	N06514 004	
DIPHEN	PHARM BASICS	12.5 MG/5 ML	N70118 001	OCT 01, 1985
DIPHENHYDRAMINE HCL	CUMBERLAND SWAN	12.5 MG/5 ML	N73611 001	AUG 20, 1992
	HI TECH	12.5 MG/5 ML	N72416 001	SEP 28, 1990
	NASKA	12.5 MG/5 ML	N70497 001	APR 25, 1989
HYDRAMINE	BARRE	12.5 MG/5 ML	N70205 001	JAN 28, 1986
SILPHEN	SILARX	12.5 MG/5 ML	N72646 001	FEB 27, 1992
VICKS FORMULA 44	VICKS HEALTH CARE	12.5 MG/5 ML	N70524 001	JAN 14, 1987

DIPHENHYDRAMINE HYDROCHLORIDE; PSEUDOEPHEDRINE HYDROCHLORIDE

SOLUTION; ORAL

BENYLIN	PARKE DAVIS	12.5 MG/5 ML;30 MG/5 ML	N19014 001	JUN 11, 1985

DOXYLAMINE SUCCINATE

CAPSULE; ORAL

UNISOM	PFIZER	25 MG	N19440 001	FEB 05, 1986

TABLET; ORAL

DOXYLAMINE SUCCINATE	COPLEY	25 MG	N88900 002	FEB 12, 1988
UNISOM	PFIZER	25 MG	N18066 001	

EPINEPHRINE

AEROSOL, METERED; INHALATION

BRONKAID MIST	STERLING	0.25 MG/INH	N16803 001	
EPINEPHRINE	BARRE	0.2 MG/INH	N87907 001	MAY 23, 1984
PRIMATENE MIST	WHITEHALL	0.2 MG/INH	N16126 001	

EPINEPHRINE BITARTRATE

AEROSOL, METERED; INHALATION

BRONITIN MIST	WHITEHALL	0.3 MG/INH	N16126 002
MEDIHALER-EPI	3M	0.3 MG/INH	N10374 003

IBUPROFEN

CAPSULE; ORAL

MIDOL	WINTHROP	200 MG	N70626 001	SEP 02, 1987
		200 MG	N71002 001	SEP 02, 1987

OTC Drug Products (continued)

IBUPROFEN (continued)

TABLET; ORAL

Product / Firm	Strength	Appl. No.	Approval Date
ACHES-N-PAIN			
LEDERLE	200 MG	N71065 001	MAY 28, 1987
ADVIL			
WHITEHALL	200 MG	N18989 001	MAY 18, 1984
CAP-PROFEN			
PERRIGO	200 MG	N72097 001	DEC 08, 1987
IBU-TAB 200			
ALRA	200 MG	N71057 001	AUG 11, 1988
IBUPRIN			
SIDMAK	200 MG	N71773 001	JUL 16, 1987
IBUPROFEN			
BARR	200 MG	N70493 001	DEC 24, 1985
	200 MG	N70908 001	SEP 26, 1986
	200 MG	N71462 001	OCT 02, 1986
CHELSEA	200 MG	N70605 001	MAY 07, 1986
DANBURY	200 MG	N70435 001	MAR 05, 1986
	200 MG	N71905 001	MAR 08, 1988
GENEVA	200 MG	N70733 001	SEP 19, 1986
HALSEY	200 MG	N71027 001	SEP 29, 1987
INTERPHARM	200 MG	N71333 001	FEB 17, 1987
	200 MG	N72199 001	MAY 23, 1987
INVAMED	200 MG	N71807 001	FEB 25, 1988
LUCHEM	200 MG	N72901 001	DEC 19, 1991
	200 MG	N72903 001	DEC 19, 1991
MEDICOPHARMA	200 MG	N71639 001	FEB 02, 1988
MUTUAL PHARM	200 MG	N71229 001	APR 01, 1987
	200 MG	N72249 001	JAN 10, 1989
MYLAN	200 MG	N71870 001	MAY 05, 1988
OHM	200 MG	N71163 001	JUL 15, 1986
	200 MG	N71214 001	DEC 01, 1986

IBUPROFEN (continued)

TABLET; ORAL

Product / Firm	Strength	Appl. No.	Approval Date
IBUPROFEN			
PAR	200 MG	N70481 001	OCT 18, 1985
	200 MG	N70985 001	OCT 02, 1987
	200 MG	N71575 001	MAY 08, 1987
PERRIGO	200 MG	N72096 001	DEC 08, 1987
	200 MG	N72098 001	DEC 08, 1987
PRIVATE FORM	200 MG	N71732 001	SEP 10, 1987
	200 MG	N71735 001	SEP 10, 1987
	200 MG	N71299 001	JUL 01, 1988
	200 MG	N71122 001	OCT 03, 1986
PUREPAC	200 MG	N71664 001	FEB 03, 1987
	200 MG	N73141 001	MAY 29, 1992
TAG	200 MG	N71154 001	OCT 27, 1987
ZENITH	200 MG	N70475 001	FEB 06, 1986
MEDIPREN			
MCNEIL	200 MG	N71215 001	JUN 26, 1986
MIDOL			
WINTHROP	200 MG	N70591 001	SEP 02, 1987
	200 MG	N71001 001	SEP 02, 1987
NEUVIL			
LUCHEM	200 MG	N71144 001	JAN 20, 1987
NUPRIN			
BRISTOL MYERS	200 MG	N72035 001	FEB 16, 1988
	200 MG	N72036 001	FEB 16, 1988
PROFEN			
PRIVATE FORM	200 MG	N71265 001	OCT 15, 1986
TAB-PROFEN			
PERRIGO	200 MG	N72095 001	DEC 08, 1987

OTC Drug Products *(continued)*

IBUPROFEN; PSEUDOEPHEDRINE HYDROCHLORIDE
TABLET; ORAL
  ADVIL COLD AND SINUS
    WHITEHALL .... 200 MG;30 MG .... N19771 001 SEP 19, 1989

INSULIN BIOSYNTHETIC HUMAN
INJECTABLE; INJECTION
  HUMULIN BR
    LILLY .... 100 UNITS/ML .... N19529 001 APR 28, 1986
  HUMULIN R
    LILLY .... 100 UNITS/ML .... N18780 001 OCT 28, 1982
  NOVOLIN R
    NOVO NORDISK .... 100 UNITS/ML .... N19938 001 JUN 25, 1991

INSULIN BIOSYNTHETIC HUMAN; INSULIN SUSP ISOPHANE BIOSYNTHETIC HUMAN
INJECTABLE; INJECTION
  HUMULIN 50/50
    LILLY .... 50 UNITS/ML;50 UNITS/ML .... N20100 001 APR 29, 1992
  HUMULIN 70/30
    LILLY .... 30 UNITS/ML;70 UNITS/ML .... N19717 001 APR 25, 1989
  NOVOLIN 70/30
    NOVO NORDISK .... 30 UNITS/ML;70 UNITS/ML .... N19991 001 JUN 25, 1991

INSULIN PORK
INJECTABLE; INJECTION
  INSULIN
    NOVO NORDISK .... 100 UNITS/ML N17926 003

INSULIN PURIFIED BEEF
INJECTABLE; INJECTION
  REGULAR ILETIN II
    LILLY .... 100 UNITS/ML N18478 001

INSULIN PURIFIED PORK
INJECTABLE; INJECTION
  REGULAR ILETIN II (PORK)
    LILLY .... 100 UNITS/ML N18344 001
  REGULAR PURIFIED PORK INSULIN
    NOVO NORDISK .... 100 UNITS/ML N18381 001
  VELOSULIN
    NOVO NORDISK .... 100 UNITS/ML N18193 001

INSULIN PURIFIED PORK; INSULIN SUSP ISOPHANE PURIFIED PORK
INJECTABLE; INJECTION
  INSULIN NORDISK MIXTARD (PORK)
    NOVO NORDISK .... 30 UNITS/ML;70 UNITS/ML N18195 001

INSULIN SEMISYNTHETIC PURIFIED HUMAN
INJECTABLE; INJECTION
  NOVOLIN R
    NOVO NORDISK .... 100 UNITS/ML .... N18778 001 AUG 30, 1983
  VELOSULIN HUMAN
    NOVO NORDISK .... 100 UNITS/ML .... N19450 001 MAY 30, 1986

INSULIN SEMISYNTHETIC PURIFIED HUMAN; INSULIN SUSP ISOPHANE SEMISYNTHETIC PURIFIED HUMAN
INJECTABLE; INJECTION
  MIXTARD HUMAN 70/30
    NOVO NORDISK .... 30 UNITS/ML;70 UNITS/ML .... N19585 001 MAR 11, 1988
  NOVOLIN 70/30
    NOVO NORDISK .... 30 UNITS/ML;70 UNITS/ML .... N19441 001 JUL 11, 1986

INSULIN SUSP ISOPHANE BEEF
INJECTABLE; INJECTION
  NPH INSULIN
    NOVO NORDISK .... 40 UNITS/ML N17929 001
                             100 UNITS/ML N17929 003

INSULIN SUSP ISOPHANE BEEF/PORK
INJECTABLE; INJECTION
  NPH ILETIN I (BEEF-PORK)
    LILLY .... 40 UNITS/ML N17936 001
                      100 UNITS/ML N17936 002

INSULIN SUSP ISOPHANE BIOSYNTHETIC HUMAN
INJECTABLE; INJECTION
  HUMULIN N
    LILLY .... 100 UNITS/ML .... N18781 001 OCT 28, 1982
  NOVOLIN N
    NOVO NORDISK .... 100 UNITS/ML .... N19959 001 JUL 01, 1991

INSULIN SUSP ISOPHANE BIOSYNTHETIC HUMAN; *MULTIPLE*
  SEE INSULIN BIOSYNTHETIC HUMAN; INSULIN SUSP ISOPHANE BIOSYNTHETIC HUMAN

OTC Drug Products (continued)

INSULIN SUSP ISOPHANE PURIFIED BEEF
INJECTABLE; INJECTION
NPH ILETIN II
LILLY — 100 UNITS/ML — N18479 001

INSULIN SUSP ISOPHANE PURIFIED PORK
INJECTABLE; INJECTION
INSULIN INSULATARD NPH NORDISK
NOVO NORDISK — 100 UNITS/ML — N18194 001
NPH PURIFIED PORK ISOPHANE INSULIN
NOVO NORDISK — 100 UNITS/ML — N18623 001

INSULIN SUSP ISOPHANE PURIFIED PORK; *MULTIPLE*
SEE INSULIN PURIFIED PORK: INSULIN SUSP ISOPHANE PURIFIED PORK

INSULIN SUSP ISOPHANE SEMISYNTHETIC PURIFIED HUMAN
INJECTABLE; INJECTION
INSULATARD NPH HUMAN
NOVO NORDISK — 100 UNITS/ML — N19449 001 MAY 30, 1986
NOVOLIN N
NOVO NORDISK — 100 UNITS/ML — N19065 001 JAN 23, 1985

INSULIN SUSP ISOPHANE SEMISYNTHETIC PURIFIED HUMAN; *MULTIPLE*
SEE INSULIN SEMISYNTHETIC PURIFIED HUMAN: INSULIN SUSP ISOPHANE SEMISYNTHETIC PURIFIED HUMAN

INSULIN SUSP PROTAMINE ZINC BEEF/PORK
INJECTABLE; INJECTION
PROTAMINE, ZINC & ILETIN I (BEEF-PORK)
LILLY — 40 UNITS/ML — N17932 001
      — 100 UNITS/ML — N17932 002

INSULIN SUSP PROTAMINE ZINC PURIFIED BEEF
INJECTABLE; INJECTION
PROTAMINE ZINC AND ILETIN II
LILLY — 100 UNITS/ML — N18476 001
PROTAMINE ZINC INSULIN
SQUIBB — 100 UNITS/ML — N17928 003
       — 40 UNITS/ML — N17928 001

INSULIN ZINC SUSP BEEF
INJECTABLE; INJECTION
LENTE INSULIN
NOVO NORDISK — 100 UNITS/ML — N17998 003

INSULIN ZINC SUSP BIOSYNTHETIC HUMAN
INJECTABLE; INJECTION
HUMULIN L
LILLY — 100 UNITS/ML — N19377 002 SEP 30, 1985
NOVOLIN L
NOVO NORDISK — 100 UNITS/ML — N19965 001 JUN 25, 1991

INSULIN ZINC SUSP EXTENDED BEEF
INJECTABLE; INJECTION
ULTRALENTE INSULIN
NOVO NORDISK — 100 UNITS/ML — N17997 003

INSULIN ZINC SUSP EXTENDED BIOSYNTHETIC HUMAN
INJECTABLE; INJECTION
HUMULIN U
LILLY — 100 UNITS/ML — N19571 002 JUN 10, 1987

INSULIN ZINC SUSP EXTENDED PURIFIED BEEF
INJECTABLE; INJECTION
ULTRALENTE
NOVO NORDISK — 100 UNITS/ML — N18385 001

INSULIN ZINC SUSP PROMPT BEEF
INJECTABLE; INJECTION
SEMILENTE INSULIN
NOVO NORDISK — 100 UNITS/ML — N17996 003

INSULIN ZINC SUSP PROMPT PURIFIED PORK
INJECTABLE; INJECTION
SEMILENTE
NOVO NORDISK — 100 UNITS/ML — N18382 001

INSULIN ZINC SUSP PURIFIED BEEF
INJECTABLE; INJECTION
LENTE ILETIN II
LILLY — 100 UNITS/ML — N18477 001

INSULIN ZINC SUSP PURIFIED PORK
INJECTABLE; INJECTION
LENTE
NOVO NORDISK — 100 UNITS/ML — N18383 001
LENTE ILETIN II (PORK)
LILLY — 100 UNITS/ML — N18347 001

OXYMETAZOLINE HYDROCHLORIDE
SOLUTION/DROPS; OPHTHALMIC
  OCUCLEAR
    SCHERING   0.025%   N18471 001
                                          MAY 30, 1986
  VISINE L.R.
    PFIZER   0.025%   N19407 001
                                          MAR 31, 1989

PADIMATE O; *MULTIPLE*
  SEE   AVOBENZONE: PADIMATE O

PERMETHRIN
LOTION; TOPICAL
  NIX
    BURROUGHS
    WELLCOME   1%   N19918 001
                                          MAY 02, 1990

PHENYLPROPANOLAMINE HYDROCHLORIDE; *MULTIPLE*
  SEE   BROMPHENIRAMINE MALEATE: PHENYLPROPANOLAMINE
        HYDROCHLORIDE
  SEE   CHLORPHENIRAMINE MALEATE: PHENYLPROPANOLAMINE
        HYDROCHLORIDE
  SEE   CLEMASTINE FUMARATE: PHENYLPROPANOLAMINE
        HYDROCHLORIDE

PHENYLPROPANOLAMINE POLISTIREX; *MULTIPLE*
  SEE   CHLORPHENIRAMINE POLISTIREX: PHENYLPROPANOLAMINE
        POLISTIREX

POLYMYXIN B SULFATE; *MULTIPLE*
  SEE   BACITRACIN: POLYMYXIN B SULFATE
  SEE   BACITRACIN ZINC: LIDOCAINE: NEOMYCIN SULFATE:
        POLYMYXIN BSULFATE
  SEE   BACITRACIN ZINC: NEOMYCIN SULFATE: POLYMYXIN B
        SULFATE
  SEE   BACITRACIN ZINC: POLYMYXIN B SULFATE

POTASSIUM IODIDE
SOLUTION; ORAL
  POTASSIUM IODIDE
    ROXANE   1 GM/ML   N18551 001
                                          FEB 19, 1982

OTC Drug Products *(continued)*

INSULIN ZINC SUSP SEMISYNTHETIC PURIFIED HUMAN
INJECTABLE; INJECTION
  NOVOLIN L
    NOVO NORDISK   100 UNITS/ML N18777 001
                                          AUG 30, 1983

LIDOCAINE; *MULTIPLE*
  SEE   BACITRACIN ZINC: LIDOCAINE: NEOMYCIN SULFATE:
        POLYMYXIN BSULFATE

LOPERAMIDE HYDROCHLORIDE
SOLUTION; ORAL
  IMODIUM A-D
    MCNEIL   1 MG/5 ML   N19487 001
                                          MAR 01, 1988
  LOPERAMIDE HCL
    PERRIGO   1 MG/5 ML   N73243 001
                                          JAN 21, 1992
    ROXANE   1 MG/5 ML   N73079 001
                                          APR 30, 1992
TABLET; ORAL
  IMODIUM A-D
    MCNEIL   2 MG   N19860 001
                                          NOV 22, 1989

MAGNESIUM TRISILICATE; *MULTIPLE*
  SEE   ALUMINUM HYDROXIDE: MAGNESIUM TRISILICATE

MICONAZOLE NITRATE
CREAM; VAGINAL
  MONISTAT 7
    JOHNSON RW   2%   N17450 002
                                          FEB 15, 1991
SUPPOSITORY; VAGINAL
  MONISTAT 7
    JOHNSON RW   100 MG   N18520 002
                                          FEB 15, 1991

NEOMYCIN SULFATE; *MULTIPLE*
  SEE   BACITRACIN ZINC: LIDOCAINE: NEOMYCIN SULFATE:
        POLYMYXIN BSULFATE
  SEE   BACITRACIN ZINC: NEOMYCIN SULFATE: POLYMYXIN B
        SULFATE

NONOXYNOL-9
SPONGE; VAGINAL
  TODAY
    WHITEHALL   1 GM   N18683 001
                                          APR 01, 1983

OTC Drug Products (continued)

POTASSIUM IODIDE (continued)

TABLET; ORAL

IOSAT			
ANBEX	130 MG	N18664 001	OCT 14, 1982
THYRO-BLOCK			
WALLACE	130 MG	N18307 001	

POVIDONE-IODINE

SOLUTION; TOPICAL

E-Z PREP			
BECTON DICKINSON	10%	N19382 001	JUL 25, 1989
POVIDONE IODINE			
BAXTER	1%	N19522 001	MAR 31, 1989

SPONGE; TOPICAL

E-Z PREP			
BECTON DICKINSON	5%	N19382 002	JUL 25, 1989
E-Z PREP 220			
BECTON DICKINSON	5%	N19382 003	JUL 25, 1989
E-Z SCRUB 201			
BECTON DICKINSON	20%	N19240 001	NOV 29, 1985
E-Z SCRUB 241			
BECTON DICKINSON	10%	N19476 001	JAN 07, 1987

PSEUDOEPHEDRINE HYDROCHLORIDE

CAPSULE, EXTENDED RELEASE; ORAL

SUDAFED 12 HOUR			
BURROUGHS WELLCOME	120 MG	N17941 002	

TABLET, EXTENDED RELEASE; ORAL

SUDAFED 12 HOUR			
BURROUGHS WELLCOME	120 MG	N73585 001	OCT 31, 1991

PSEUDOEPHEDRINE HYDROCHLORIDE; *MULTIPLE*

SEE   CHLORPHENIRAMINE MALEATE; PSEUDOEPHEDRINE HYDROCHLORIDE

SEE   DIPHENHYDRAMINE HYDROCHLORIDE; PSEUDOEPHEDRINE HYDROCHLORIDE

SEE   IBUPROFEN; PSEUDOEPHEDRINE HYDROCHLORIDE

PSEUDOEPHEDRINE HYDROCHLORIDE; TRIPROLIDINE HYDROCHLORIDE

CAPSULE; ORAL

ACTIFED			
BURROUGHS WELLCOME	60 MG;2.5 MG	N19208 001	JAN 15, 1985

CAPSULE, EXTENDED RELEASE; ORAL

ACTIFED			
BURROUGHS WELLCOME	120 MG;5 MG	N18996 001	JUN 17, 1985
TRIPROLIDINE AND PSEUDOEPHRINE HCL			
KV	120 MG;5 MG	N71798 001	MAR 16, 1989

SYRUP; ORAL

ACTIFED			
BURROUGHS WELLCOME	30 MG/5 ML;1.25 MG/5 ML	N11935 003	NOV 26, 1982
TRIOFED			
BARRE	30 MG/5 ML;1.25 MG/5 ML	N88115 001	MAR 04, 1983
TRIPOSED			
HALSEY	30 MG/5 ML;1.25 MG/5 ML	N88213 002	MAR 30, 1984

TABLET; ORAL

ACTIFED			
BURROUGHS WELLCOME	60 MG;2.5 MG	N11936 002	NOV 26, 1982
TRI-SUDO			
MD PHARM	60 MG;2.5 MG	N85024 002	JAN 10, 1984
TRIPODRINE			
DANBURY	60 MG;2.5 MG	N88112 001	JAN 20, 1983
TRIPOSED			
HALSEY	60 MG;2.5 MG	N88192 002	MAY 01, 1984
TRIPROLIDINE HCL AND PSEUDOEPHEDRINE HCL			
CHELSEA	60 MG;2.5 MG	N88118 002	JAN 26, 1984

TABLET, EXTENDED RELEASE; ORAL

TRIPROLIDINE AND PSEUDOEPHEDRINE HCL			
KV	120 MG;5 MG	N72758 001	NOV 25, 1991

PSEUDOEPHEDRINE POLISTIREX

SUSPENION, EXTENDED RELEASE; ORAL

PSEUDO-12			
FISONS	EQ 60 MG HCL/5 ML	N19401 001	JUN 19, 1987

OTC Drug Products (continued)

PSEUDOEPHEDRINE SULFATE
TABLET, EXTENDED RELEASE; ORAL
AFRINOL
   SCHERING   120 MG   N18191 001

PSEUDOEPHEDRINE SULFATE; *MULTIPLE*
SEE ACETAMINOPHEN: DEXBROMPHENIRAMINE MALEATE: PSEUDOEPHEDRINE SULFATE
SEE CHLORPHENIRAMINE MALEATE: PSEUDOEPHEDRINE SULFATE
SEE DEXBROMPHENIRAMINE MALEATE: PSEUDOEPHEDRINE SULFATE

PYRITHIONE ZINC
LOTION; TOPICAL
HEAD & SHOULDERS CONDITIONER
   P AND G   0.3%   N19412 004 MAR 10, 1986

SODIUM MONOFLUOROPHOSPHATE
GEL; DENTAL
EXTRA-STRENGTH AIM
   CHESEBROUGH PONDS   1.2%   N19518 002 AUG 06, 1986

SODIUM MONOFLUOROPHOSPHATE (continued)
PASTE; DENTAL
EXTRA-STRENGTH AIM
   CHESEBROUGH PONDS   1.2%   N19518 001 JUN 03, 1987

TRIPROLIDINE HYDROCHLORIDE
SYRUP; ORAL
ACTIDIL
   BURROUGHS WELLCOME   1.25 MG/5 ML   N11496 002 JUL 01, 1983

TABLET; ORAL
ACTIDIL
   BURROUGHS WELLCOME   2.5 MG   N11110 002 JUL 01, 1983

TRIPROLIDINE HYDROCHLORIDE; *MULTIPLE*
SEE PSEUDOEPHEDRINE HYDROCHLORIDE: TRIPROLIDINE HYDROCHLORIDE

DRUG PRODUCTS WITH APPROVAL UNDER SECTION 505 OF THE ACT ADMINISTERED BY THE DIVISION OF BLOOD AND BLOOD PRODUCTS

ANTICOAGULANT CITRATE DEXTROSE SOLUTION USP
INJECTABLE; INJECTION
  NONE
    CUTTER BIO   N 71497

ANTICOAGULANT CITRATE DEXTROSE SOLUTION USP
INJECTABLE; INJECTION
  NONE
    CUTTER BIO   N 10102

ANTICOAGULANT CITRATE DEXTROSE SOLUTION USP
INJECTABLE; INJECTION
  NONE
    DELMED   N 11912

ANTICOAGULANT CITRATE DEXTROSE SOLUTION USP
INJECTABLE; INJECTION
  NONE
    TRAVENOL LABS   N 10855

ANTICOAGULANT CITRATE DEXTROSE SOLUTION USP
INJECTABLE; INJECTION
  NONE
    TRAVENOL LABS   N 16918

ANTICOAGULANT CITRATE PHOSPHATE DEXTROSE ADENINE SOLUTION
INJECTABLE; INJECTION
  NONE
    DELMED   N 78519

ANTICOAGULANT CITRATE PHOSPHATE DEXTROSE ADENINE SOLUTION
INJECTABLE; INJECTION
  NONE
    TERUMO   N 82528
                                                           NOV 03, 1982

ANTICOAGULANT CITRATE PHOSPHATE DEXTROSE ADENINE SOLUTION
INJECTABLE; INJECTION
  NONE
    TRAVENOL LABS   N 77420

ANTICOAGULANT CITRATE PHOSPHATE DEXTROSE ADENINE-1
SOLUTION
INJECTABLE; INJECTION
  NONE
    CUTTER BIO   N 08077

ANTICOAGULANT CITRATE PHOSPHATE DEXTROSE SOLUTION USP
INJECTABLE; INJECTION
  NONE
    CUTTER BIO   N 16527

ANTICOAGULANT CITRATE PHOSPHATE DEXTROSE SOLUTION USP
INJECTABLE; INJECTION
  NONE
    CUTTER BIO   N 80222
                                                           AUG 23, 1982

ANTICOAGULANT CITRATE PHOSPHATE DEXTROSE SOLUTION USP
INJECTABLE; INJECTION
  NONE
    DELMED   N 16907

ANTICOAGULANT CITRATE PHOSPHATE DEXTROSE SOLUTION USP
INJECTABLE; INJECTION
  NONE
    TERUMO   N 781211

ANTICOAGULANT CITRATE PHOSPHATE DEXTROSE SOLUTION USP
INJECTABLE; INJECTION
  NONE
    TRAVENOL LABS   N 17401

ANTICOAGULANT CITRATE PHOSPHATE DEXTROSE SOLUTION USP
INJECTABLE; INJECTION
  NONE
    TRAVENOL LABS   N 811012
                                                           JUN 28, 1983

ANTICOAGULANT CITRATE PHOSPHATE DEXTROSE SOLUTION USP
WITH: AS-1: DEXTROSE USP; SODIUM CHLORIDE USP; MANNITOL USP;
ADENINE
INJECTABLE; INJECTION
  ADSOL RED BLOOD CELL PRESERVATIVE SOLUTION
    TRAVENOL LABS   2.2 GM/100 ML;0.9 GM/
                         100 ML;0.75 GM/
                         100 ML;0.027 GM/100 ML   N 811104
                                                           MAY 16, 1983

Drug Products with Approval Under Section 505 of the Act Administered by the Division of Blood and Blood Products *(continued)*

ANTICOAGULANT CITRATE PHOSPHATE DEXTROSE SOLUTION USP WITH: AS-5: DEXTROSE USP; SODIUM CHLORIDE USP; MANNITOL USP; ADENINE
INJECTABLE; INJECTION
OPTISOL RED BLOOD CELL PRESERVATIVE SOLUTION
   TERUMO   0.9 GM/100 ML;0.877 GM/
         100 ML;0.525 GM/   N 880217
         100 ML;0.03 GM/100 ML   OCT 07, 1988

ANTICOAGULANT CITRATE PHOSPHATE DOUBLE DEXTROSE SOLUTION WITH: AS-2: CITRIC ACID USP; DIBASIC SODIUM PHOSPHATE USP; SODIUM CHLORIDE USP; ADENINE; DEXTROSE USP; SODIUM CITRATE USP
INJECTABLE; INJECTION
AS-2 NUTRICEL ADDITIVE SYSTEM
   CUTTER BIO   0.042 GM/100 ML;0.285 GM/
         100 ML;0.718 GM/
         100 ML;0.017 GM/
         100 ML;0.396 GM/   N 82915
         100 ML;0.588 GM/100 ML   SEP 22, 1983

ANTICOAGULANT CITRATE PHOSPHATE DOUBLE DEXTROSE SOLUTION WITH: AS-3: CITRIC ACID USP; MONOBASIC SODIUM PHOSPHATE USP; SODIUM CHLORIDE USP; ADENINE; DEXTROSE USP; SODIUM CITRATE USP
INJECTABLE; INJECTION
AS-3 NUTRICEL ADDITIVE SYSTEM
   CUTTER BIO   0.042 GM/100 ML;0.276 GM/
         100 ML;0.410 GM/
         100 ML;0.30 GM/
         100 ML;1.10 GM/   N 82915
         100 ML;0.588 GM/100 ML   OCT 19, 1984

ANTICOAGULANT HEPARIN SOLUTION USP
INJECTABLE; INJECTION
   NONE
      DELMED   N 77822

ANTICOAGULANT HEPARIN SOLUTION USP
INJECTABLE; INJECTION
   NONE
      TRAVENOL LABS   N 811217
                        MAY 16, 1983

ANTICOAGULANT SODIUM CITRATE SOLUTION USP
INJECTABLE; INJECTION
   NONE
      ALPHA THERPTC   N 81416
                        OCT 12, 1983

ANTICOAGULANT SODIUM CITRATE SOLUTION USP
INJECTABLE; INJECTION
   NONE
      CUTTER BIO   N 76305

ANTICOAGULANT SODIUM CITRATE SOLUTION USP
INJECTABLE; INJECTION
   NONE
      DELMED   N 16702

ANTICOAGULANT SODIUM CITRATE SOLUTION USP
INJECTABLE; INJECTION
   NONE
      TERUMO   N 781214

ANTICOAGULANT SODIUM CITRATE SOLUTION USP
INJECTABLE; INJECTION
   NONE
      TRAVENOL LABS   N 77923

CDP BLOOD BAG UNIT
INJECTABLE; INJECTION
CDP BLOOD BAG UNIT IN PLASTIC CONTAINER
   BAXTER HLTHCARE   N900224
                       DEC 27, 1991

DEXTRAN 1 IN SODIUM CHLORIDE 0.6%
INJECTABLE; INJECTION
   PROMIT
      PHARMACIA LABS   150 MG/ML;6 MG/ML   N 83715
                       OCT 30, 1984

DEXTRAN 40, 10% IN DEXTROSE 5%
INJECTABLE; INJECTION
   NONE
      ABBOTT LABS   10 GM/100 ML;5 GM/100 ML   N 16375

DEXTRAN 40, 10% IN DEXTROSE 5%
INJECTABLE; INJECTION
   NONE
      AMERICAN MCGAW   10 GM/100 ML;5 GM/100 ML   N 16767

Drug Products with Approval Under Section 505 of the Act Administered by the Division of Blood and Blood Products (continued)

DEXTRAN 40, 10% IN DEXTROSE 5%
INJECTABLE; INJECTION
NONE
   CUTTER BIO   10 GM/100 ML;5 GM/100 ML   N 16653

DEXTRAN 40, 10% IN DEXTROSE 5%
INJECTABLE; INJECTION
NONE
   PHARMACHEM   10 GM/100 ML;5 GM/100 ML   N 16836

DEXTRAN 40, 10% IN DEXTROSE 5%
INJECTABLE; INJECTION
RHEOMACRODEX
   PHARMACIA LABS   10 GM/100 ML;5 GM/100 ML   N 14716

DEXTRAN 40, 10% IN DEXTROSE 5%
INJECTABLE; INJECTION
GENTRAN 40
   TRAVENOL LABS   10 GM/100 ML;5 GM/100 ML   N 16628

DEXTRAN 40, 10% IN DEXTROSE 5%
INJECTABLE; INJECTION
GENTRAN 40
   TRAVENOL LABS   10 GM/100 ML;5 GM/100 ML   N 84619 FEB 22, 1985

DEXTRAN 40, 10% IN DEXTROSE SODIUM CHLORIDE 0.9%
INJECTABLE; INJECTION
NONE
   CUTTER BIO   10 GM/100 ML;0.9 GM/100 ML   N 16653

DEXTRAN 40, 10% IN SODIUM CHLORIDE 0.9%
INJECTABLE; INJECTION
NONE
   ABBOTT LABS   10 GM/100 ML;0.9 GM/100 ML   N 16375

DEXTRAN 40, 10% IN SODIUM CHLORIDE 0.9%
INJECTABLE; INJECTION
NONE
   AMERICAN MCGAW   10 GM/100 ML;0.9 GM/100 ML   N 16767

DEXTRAN 40, 10% IN SODIUM CHLORIDE 0.9%
INJECTABLE; INJECTION
NONE
   PHARMACHEM   10 GM/100 ML;0.9 GM/100 ML   N 16836

DEXTRAN 40, 10% IN SODIUM CHLORIDE 0.9%
INJECTABLE; INJECTION
RHEOMACRODEX
   PHARMACIA LABS   10 GM/100 ML;0.9 GM/100 ML   N 14716

DEXTRAN 40, 10% IN SODIUM CHLORIDE 0.9%
INJECTABLE; INJECTION
GENTRAN 40
   TRAVENOL LABS   10 GM/100 ML;0.9 GM/100 ML   N 16628

DEXTRAN 40, 10% IN SODIUM CHLORIDE 0.9%
INJECTABLE; INJECTION
GENTRAN 40
   TRAVENOL LABS   10 GM/100 ML;0.9 GM/100 ML   N 84620 FEB 22, 1985

DEXTRAN 70, 6% IN DEXTROSE 5%
INJECTABLE; INJECTION
MACRODEX
   PHARMACIA INC   6 GM/100 ML;5 GM/100 ML   N 06826

DEXTRAN 70, 6% IN SODIUM CHLORIDE 0.9%
INJECTABLE; INJECTION
MACRODEX
   PHARMACIA INC   6 GM/100 ML;0.9 GM/100 ML   N 06826

DEXTRAN 70, 6% IN SODIUM CHLORIDE 0.9%
INJECTABLE; INJECTION
NONE
   AMERICAN MCGAW   6 GM/100 ML;0.9 GM/100 ML   N 09024

DEXTRAN 70, 6% IN SODIUM CHLORIDE 0.9%
INJECTABLE; INJECTION
NONE
   CUTTER BIO   6 GM/100 ML;0.9 GM/100 ML   N 08716

DEXTRAN 75, 6% IN DEXTROSE 5%
INJECTABLE; INJECTION
NONE
   ABBOTT LABS   6 GM/100 ML;5 GM/100 ML   N 08819

Drug Products with Approval Under Section 505 of the Act Administered by the Division of Blood and Blood Products (*continued*)

DEXTRAN 75, 6% IN SODIUM CHLORIDE 0.9%
INJECTABLE; INJECTION
NONE
ABBOTT LABS   6 GM/100 ML;0.9 GM/100 ML   N 08819

DEXTRAN 75, 6% IN SODIUM CHLORIDE 0.9%
INJECTABLE; INJECTION
NONE
ABBOTT LABS   6 GM/100 ML;0.9 GM/100 ML   N 18253 FEB 04, 1983

DEXTRAN 75, 6% IN SODIUM CHLORIDE 0.9%
INJECTABLE; INJECTION
NONE
PHARMACHEM   6 GM/100 ML;0.9 GM/100 ML   N 08564

DEXTRAN 75, 6% IN SODIUM CHLORIDE 0.9%
INJECTABLE; INJECTION
NONE
PHARMACHEM   6 GM/100 ML;0.9 GM/100 ML   N 16759

DEXTRAN 75, 6% IN SODIUM CHLORIDE 0.9%
INJECTABLE; INJECTION
GENTRAN 75
TRAVENOL LABS   6 GM/100 ML;0.9 GM/100 ML   N 16607

DEXTRAN 75, 6% INVERTED SUGAR 10% IN SODIUM CHLORIDE 0.9%
INJECTABLE; INJECTION
6% GENTRAN 75 AND 10% TRAVERT
TRAVENOL LABS   6 GM/100 ML;10 GM/100 ML;0.9 GM/100 ML   N 08788

HETASTARCH 6% IN SODIUM CHLORIDE 0.9%
INJECTABLE; INJECTION
HESPAN
AM CRITICAL CARE   6 GM/100 ML;0.9 GM/100 ML   N 16889

HETASTARCH 6% IN SODIUM CHLORIDE 0.9%
INJECTABLE; INJECTION
HESPAN IN PLASTIC CONTAINER
DUPONT MERCK PHARM   6 GM/ 100 ML;0.9 GM/ 100 ML   N 890105 APR 04, 1991

PENTASTARCH 10% IN SODIUM CHLORIDE 0.9%
INJECTABLE; INJECTION
PENTASPAN
DUPONT CRI CARE   10 GM/100 ML;0.9 GM/ 100 ML   N 841207 MAY 19, 1987

PENTASTARCH 10% IN SODIUM CHLORIDE 0.9%
INJECTABLE; INJECTION
PENTASPAN IN PLASTIC CONTAINER
DUPONT MERCK PHARM   10 GM/100 ML;0.9 GM/ 100 ML   N 890104 APR 04, 1991

PERFLUORODECALIN; PERFLUOOROTRI-N-PROPYLAMINE
INJECTABLE; INJECTION
FLUOSOL
ALPHA THERPTC   17.5 GM/100 ML;7.5 GM/ 100 ML   N 860909 DEC 26, 1989

RED CELL PRESERVATION SOLUTION SYSTEM
INJECTABLE; INJECTION
ADSOL IN PLASTIC CONTAINER
BAXTER HLTH CARE   N900223 DEC 27, 1991

UROKINASE
INJECTABLE; INJECTION
ABBOKINASE OPEN-CATHETER
ABBOTT LABS   5000 IU/VIAL   N 761021 DEC 15, 1983

UROKINASE
INJECTABLE; INJECTION
ABBOKINASE
ABBOTT LABS   250,000 IU/VIAL   N 761021

UROKINASE
INJECTABLE; INJECTION
BREOKINASE
STERLING DRUG   250,000 IU/VIAL   N 17873

DISCONTINUED DRUG PRODUCTS

ACETAMINOPHEN

INJECTABLE; INJECTION

INJECTAPAP

JOHNSON RW	100 MG/ML	N17785 001	MAR 07, 1986

SUPPOSITORY; RECTAL

TYLENOL

MCNEIL	120 MG	N17756 002
	650 MG	N17756 001

ACETAMINOPHEN; ASPIRIN; CODEINE PHOSPHATE

CAPSULE; ORAL

CODEINE, ASPIRIN, APAP FORMULA NO. 2

FIRST TX	150 MG;180 MG;15 MG	N85640 001

CODEINE, ASPIRIN, APAP FORMULA NO. 3

FIRST TX	150 MG;180 MG;30 MG	N85639 001

CODEINE, ASPIRIN, APAP FORMULA NO. 4

FIRST TX	150 MG;180 MG;60 MG	N85638 001

ACETAMINOPHEN; CODEINE PHOSPHATE

CAPSULE; ORAL

ACETAMINOPHEN W/ CODEINE #2

LEMMON	300 MG;15 MG	N88537 001	JUN 04, 1984

ACETAMINOPHEN W/ CODEINE #4

LEMMON	300 MG;60 MG	N88599 001	JUN 01, 1984

PROVAL #3

SOLVAY	325 MG;30 MG	N85685 001

TYLENOL W/ CODEINE NO. 3

JOHNSON RW	300 MG;30 MG	N87422 001

TYLENOL W/ CODEINE NO. 4

JOHNSON RW	300 MG;60 MG	N87421 001

TABLET; ORAL

ACETAMINOPHEN AND CODEINE PHOSPHATE

DURAMED	300 MG;15 MG	N88353 001	FEB 06, 1984
	300 MG;30 MG	N88354 001	FEB 06, 1984
	300 MG;60 MG	N88355 001	FEB 06, 1984
EON LABS	300 MG;15 MG	N87433 001	
	300 MG;30 MG	N85917 001	
	300 MG;60 MG	N87423 001	
PARKE DAVIS	300 MG;15 MG	N85992 001	
	300 MG;30 MG	N85218 002	

ACETAMINOPHEN AND CODEINE PHOSPHATE #3

SUPERPHARM	300 MG;30 MG	N89253 001	MAY 19, 1986

ACETAMINOPHEN AND CODEINE PHOSPHATE #4

SUPERPHARM	300 MG;60 MG	N89254 001	MAY 19, 1986

ACETAMINOPHEN; CODEINE PHOSPHATE (*continued*)

TABLET; ORAL

ACETAMINOPHEN AND CODEINE PHOSPHATE NO. 2

AM THERAP	300 MG;15 MG	N89478 001	MAR 03, 1987
		N89481 001	MAR 03, 1987

ACETAMINOPHEN AND CODEINE PHOSPHATE NO. 3

AM THERAP	300 MG;30 MG	N89479 001	MAR 03, 1987
		N89482 001	MAR 03, 1987

ACETAMINOPHEN AND CODEINE PHOSPHATE NO. 4

AM THERAP	300 MG;60 MG	N89480 001	MAR 03, 1987
		N89483 001	MAR 03, 1987

ACETAMINOPHEN W/ CODEINE

LEDERLE	300 MG;30 MG	N87141 001

ACETAMINOPHEN W/ CODEINE PHOSPHATE

CHELSEA	300 MG;15 MG	N87277 001	MAY 26, 1982
	300 MG;30 MG	N87276 001	MAY 26, 1982
	300 MG;60 MG	N87275 001	MAY 26, 1982
PHARM BASICS	300 MG;30 MG	N87919 001	JUN 22, 1982
	300 MG;60 MG	N87920 001	JUN 22, 1982
VITARINE	300 MG;30 MG	N85676 001	
WARNER CHILCOTT	300 MG;60 MG	N87306 001	
WHITE TOWNE	300 MG;30 MG	N84360 001	
PAULSEN	300 MG;60 MG	N85607 001	

APAP W/ CODEINE PHOSPHATE

EVERYLIFE	325 MG;30 MG	N85217 001

CODEINE PHOSPHATE AND ACETAMINOPHEN

ICN	300 MG;30 MG	N85896 001

EMPRACET W/ CODEINE PHOSPHATE #3

BURROUGHS WELLCOME	300 MG;30 MG	N83951 001

EMPRACET W/ CODEINE PHOSPHATE #4

BURROUGHS WELLCOME	300 MG;60 MG	N83951 002

PAPA-DEINE #3

VANGARD	300 MG;30 MG	N88037 001	MAR 20, 1984

PAPA-DEINE #4

VANGARD	300 MG;60 MG	N88715 001	MAR 20, 1984

TYLENOL W/ CODEINE

JOHNSON RW	325 MG;30 MG	N85056 003
	325 MG;7.5 MG	N85056 001
	325 MG;15 MG	N85056 002
	325 MG;60 MG	N85056 004

Discontinued Drug Products (continued)

ACETAMINOPHEN; HYDROCODONE BITARTRATE
TABLET; ORAL
 HYDROCODONE BITARTRATE AND ACETAMINOPHEN
  PHARM BASICS   500 MG;5 MG   N89290 001
                                 MAY 29, 1987
                 500 MG;5 MG   N89291 001
                                 MAY 29, 1987
 VICODIN
  KNOLL   500 MG;5 MG   N85667 001

ACETAMINOPHEN; OXYCODONE HYDROCHLORIDE
CAPSULE; ORAL
 TYLOX-325
  JOHNSON RW   325 MG;5 MG   N88246 001
                                 NOV 08, 1984
TABLET; ORAL
 OXYCODONE 2.5/APAP 500
  DUPONT   500 MG;2.5 MG   N85910 001
 OXYCODONE 5/APAP 500
  DUPONT   500 MG;5 MG   N85911 001

ACETAMINOPHEN; OXYCODONE HYDROCHLORIDE; OXYCODONE TEREPHTHALATE
CAPSULE; ORAL
 TYLOX
  JOHNSON RW   500 MG;4.5 MG;0.38 MG   N85375 001

ACETAMINOPHEN; PROPOXYPHENE HYDROCHLORIDE
TABLET; ORAL
 DARVOCET
  LILLY   325 MG;32.5 MG   N16844 001
 DOLENE AP-65
  LEDERLE   650 MG;65 MG   N85100 001
 PROPOXYPHENE HCL AND ACETAMINOPHEN
  MYLAN   325 MG;32 MG   N83689 001

ACETAMINOPHEN; PROPOXYPHENE NAPSYLATE
TABLET; ORAL
 PROPOXYPHENE NAPSYLATE AND ACETAMINOPHEN
  BOLAR   325 MG;50 MG   N70398 001
                                  DEC 18, 1986
                 650 MG;100 MG   N70399 001
                                  DEC 18, 1986

ACETAZOLAMIDE
TABLET; ORAL
 ACETAZOLAMIDE
  ALRA   250 MG   N83320 001
  ASCOT   250 MG   N87686 001
                           OCT 20, 1982
  BOLAR   250 MG   N84498 002
  VANGARD   250 MG   N87654 001
                           FEB 05, 1982

ACETIC ACID, GLACIAL
SOLUTION/DROPS; OTIC
 ACETIC ACID
  KV   2%   N85493 001
  ORLEX   2%   N86845 001
  P AND G

ACETIC ACID, GLACIAL; HYDROCORTISONE
SOLUTION/DROPS; OTIC
 ACETIC ACID W/ HYDROCORTISONE
  KV   2%;1%   N85492 001
  ORLEX HC   2%;1%   N86844 001
  P AND G

ACETOHEXAMIDE
TABLET; ORAL
 ACETOHEXAMIDE
  PHARM BASICS   250 MG   N70753 001
                           NOV 03, 1986
                 500 MG   N70754 001
                           NOV 03, 1986

ACETOPHENAZINE MALEATE
TABLET; ORAL
 TINDAL
  SCHERING   20 MG   N12254 002

ACETRIZOATE SODIUM
SOLUTION; INTRAUTERINE
 SALPIX
  JOHNSON RW   53%   N09008 001

ACETYLCYSTEINE
SOLUTION; INHALATION, ORAL
 ACETYLCYSTEINE
  QUAD   10%   N71740 001
                        AUG 11, 1987
                 20%   N71741 001
                        AUG 11, 1987

ACETYLCYSTEINE; ISOPROTERENOL HYDROCHLORIDE
SOLUTION; INHALATION
 MUCOMYST W/ ISOPROTERENOL
  MEAD JOHNSON   10%;0.05%   N17366 001

ACETYLDIGITOXIN
TABLET; ORAL
 ACYLANID
  SANDOZ   0.1 MG   N09436 001

Discontinued Drug Products *(continued)*

ACRISORCIN
CREAM; TOPICAL
AKRINOL
| SCHERING | 2 MG/GM | N12470 001 |

ALBUMIN CHROMATED CR-51 SERUM
INJECTABLE; INJECTION
CHROMALBIN
| ISO TEX | 250 UCI/VIAL | N17835 002 |
| | 500 UCI/VIAL | N17835 003 |

ALBUMIN IODINATED I-125 SERUM
INJECTABLE; INJECTION
ALBUMOTOPE 125 I
| ISO TEX | 5-50 UCI/AMP | N17836 001 |

RADIO-IODINATED (I 125) SERUM ALBUMIN (HUMAN)
| MILES | 2.5 UCI/AMP | N17846 001 |

ALBUMIN IODINATED I-131 SERUM
INJECTABLE; INJECTION
MEGATOPE
ISO TEX	5 UCI/AMP	N17837 004
	20 UCI/AMP	N17837 005
	2 MCI/VIAL	N17837 003

ALBUTEROL SULFATE
TABLET; ORAL
ALBUTEROL SULFATE
| AM THERAP | EQ 2 MG BASE | N72449 001 | FEB 01, 1989 |
| | EQ 4 MG BASE | N72450 001 | FEB 01, 1989 |

ALCOHOL
INJECTABLE; INJECTION
ALCOHOL 5% IN DEXTROSE 5%
| CUTTER | 5 ML/100 ML | N83483 001 |

ALKAVERVIR
TABLET; ORAL
VERILOID
| 3M | 2 MG | N07336 002 |
| | 3 MG | N07336 003 |

ALLOPURINOL
TABLET; ORAL
ALLOPURINOL
BOLAR	100 MG	N18241 001	NOV 16, 1984
	300 MG	N18241 002	NOV 16, 1984
CHELSEA	100 MG	N18785 001	SEP 28, 1984
	300 MG	N18785 002	SEP 28, 1984
PUREPAC	100 MG	N70579 001	APR 14, 1986
	300 MG	N70580 001	APR 14, 1986
SUPERPHARM	100 MG	N70950 001	SEP 04, 1986

LOPURIN
| BOOTS | 100 MG | N18297 001 |
| | 300 MG | N18297 002 |

ALSEROXYLON
TABLET; ORAL
RAUTENSIN
| DORSEY | 2 MG | N09215 001 |

AMINO ACIDS
INJECTABLE; INJECTION
AMINOSYN II 3.5% IN PLASTIC CONTAINER
| ABBOTT | 3.5% | N19491 001 | OCT 10, 1986 |

AMINOSYN 3.5% IN PLASTIC CONTAINER
| ABBOTT | 3.5% | N18804 001 | MAY 15, 1984 |
| | 3.5% | N18875 001 | AUG 08, 1984 |

AMINOSYN-HBC 7% IN PLASTIC CONTAINER
| ABBOTT | 7% | N19400 001 | JUL 23, 1986 |

FREAMINE II 8.5%
| MCGAW | 8.5% | N16822 002 |

FREAMINE 8.5%
| MCGAW | 8.5% | N16822 001 |

NEOPHAM 6.4%
| KABIVITRUM | 6.4% | N18792 001 | JAN 17, 1984 |

AMINO ACIDS; DEXTROSE
INJECTABLE; INJECTION
AMINOSYN 3.5% W/ DEXTROSE 25% IN PLASTIC CONTAINER
| ABBOTT | 3.5%;25 GM/100 ML | N19118 001 | OCT 11, 1984 |

AMINOSYN 3.5% W/ DEXTROSE 5% IN PLASTIC CONTAINER
| ABBOTT | 3.5%;5 GM/100 ML | N19120 001 | OCT 11, 1984 |

Discontinued Drug Products (continued)

AMINO ACIDS; DEXTROSE; MAGNESIUM CHLORIDE; POTASSIUM CHLORIDE; POTASSIUM PHOSPHATE, DIBASIC; SODIUM CHLORIDE
INJECTABLE; INJECTION
AMINOSYN II 3.5% W/ ELECTROLYTES IN DEXTROSE 25% IN PLASTIC CONTAINER
  ABBOTT   3.5%;25 GM/100 ML;51 MG/
                  100 ML;22.4 MG/
                  100 ML;261 MG/
                  100 ML;205 MG/100 ML   N19564 002
                                              DEC 16, 1986
AMINOSYN II 4.25% W/ ELECTROLYTES IN DEXTROSE 25% IN PLASTIC CONTAINER
  ABBOTT   4.25%;25 GM/100 ML;51 MG/
                  100 ML;22.4 MG/
                  100 ML;261 MG/
                  100 ML;205 MG/100 ML   N19564 004
                                              DEC 16, 1986

AMINO ACIDS; DEXTROSE; MAGNESIUM CHLORIDE; POTASSIUM CHLORIDE; SODIUM CHLORIDE; SODIUM PHOSPHATE, DIBASIC
INJECTABLE; INJECTION
AMINOSYN II 3.5% M IN DEXTROSE 5% IN PLASTIC CONTAINER
  ABBOTT   3.5%;5 GM/100 ML;30 MG/
                  100 ML;97 MG/
                  100 ML;120 MG/
                  100 ML;49.3 MG/100 ML   N19564 001
                                              DEC 16, 1986
AMINOSYN II 4.25% M IN DEXTROSE 10% IN PLASTIC CONTAINER
  ABBOTT   4.25%;10 GM/100 ML;30 MG/
                  100 ML;97 MG/
                  100 ML;120 MG/
                  100 ML;49.3 MG/100 ML   N19564 003
                                              DEC 16, 1986

AMINO ACIDS; MAGNESIUM ACETATE; PHOSPHORIC ACID; POTASSIUM ACETATE; SODIUM CHLORIDE
INJECTABLE; INJECTION
AMINOSYN 3.5% M IN PLASTIC CONTAINER
  ABBOTT   3.5%;21 MG/100 ML;40 MG/
                  100 ML;128 MG/
                  100 ML;234 MG/100 ML   N18804 002
                                              MAY 15, 1984
                  3.5%;21 MG/100 ML;40 MG/
                  100 ML;128 MG/
                  100 ML;234 MG/100 ML   N18875 002
                                              AUG 08, 1984

AMINO ACIDS; MAGNESIUM ACETATE; POTASSIUM ACETATE; SODIUM CHLORIDE
INJECTABLE; INJECTION
AMINOSYN 3.5% M
  ABBOTT   3.5%;21 MG/100 ML;128 MG/
                  100 ML;234 MG/100 ML   N17789 001

AMINO ACIDS; MAGNESIUM ACETATE; POTASSIUM ACETATE; SODIUM CHLORIDE; SODIUM PHOSPHATE, DIBASIC
INJECTABLE; INJECTION
AMINOSYN II 3.5% M IN PLASTIC CONTAINER
  ABBOTT   3.5%;32 MG/100 ML;128 MG/
                  100 ML;222 MG/
                  100 ML;49 MG/100 ML   N19493 001
                                              OCT 16, 1986

AMINOCAPROIC ACID
INJECTABLE; INJECTION
AMINOCAPROIC ACID
  QUAD   250 MG/ML   N70694 001
                                              MAR 04, 1986

AMINOHIPPURATE SODIUM
INJECTABLE; INJECTION
AMINOHIPPURATE SODIUM
  QUAD   20%   N89821 001
                                              JUL 14, 1988

AMINOPHYLLINE
INJECTABLE; INJECTION
AMINOPHYLLIN
  SEARLE   25 MG/ML   N87621 001
                                              MAY 24, 1982
AMINOPHYLLINE
  INTL MEDICATION 25 MG/ML   N87867 001
                                              NOV 10, 1983
                  25 MG/ML   N87868 001
                                              NOV 10, 1983
  LYPHOMED   25 MG/ML   N84568 001
                                              NOV 10, 1983
  SMITH NEPHEW
  SOLOPAK   25 MG/ML   N88429 001
                                              MAY 30, 1985
AMINOPHYLLINE IN SODIUM CHLORIDE 0.45% IN PLASTIC CONTAINER
  ABBOTT   100 MG/100 ML   N18924 001
                                              DEC 12, 1984
                  200 MG/100 ML   N18924 002
                                              DEC 12, 1984
                  400 MG/100 ML   N18924 003
                                              DEC 12, 1984
                  500 MG/100 ML   N18924 004
                                              DEC 12, 1984

Discontinued Drug Products (continued)

AMINOPHYLLINE (continued)

TABLET; ORAL

AMINOPHYLLINE

Firm	Strength	Appl. No.	Date
ASCOT	100 MG	N87522 001	FEB 12, 1982
	200 MG	N87523 001	FEB 12, 1982
BARR	100 MG	N88297 001	AUG 19, 1983
	200 MG	N88298 001	AUG 19, 1983
CHELSEA	100 MG	N85567 001	
	200 MG	N85564 001	
DURAMED	100 MG	N88182 001	MAR 31, 1983
	200 MG	N88183 001	MAR 31, 1983
GENEVA	100 MG	N85261 003	
ICN	200 MG	N84563 001	
KV	100 MG	N85284 001	
	200 MG	N85289 001	
PAL PAK	100 MG	N84533 001	
PANRAY	100 MG	N84552 001	
	200 MG	N84552 002	
PUREPAC	100 MG	N84699 001	
	200 MG	N85333 001	
VANGARD	100 MG	N88314 001	OCT 03, 1983
	200 MG	N88319 001	OCT 03, 1983

TABLET, DELAYED RELEASE; ORAL

AMINOPHYLLINE

Firm	Strength	Appl. No.
RICHLYN	100 MG	N84577 001
	200 MG	N84575 001
TABLICAPS	100 MG	N84632 002
VALE	100 MG	N84531 001
	200 MG	N84530 001

AMINOSALICYLATE SODIUM

TABLET; ORAL

PARASAL SODIUM

Firm	Strength	Appl. No.
PANRAY	500 MG	N06811 006
	1 GM	N06811 011

TEEBACIN

Firm	Strength	Appl. No.
CONSOLIDATED MIDLAND	500 MG	N07320 002

AMINOSALICYLIC ACID

TABLET; ORAL

PARASAL

Firm	Strength	Appl. No.
PANRAY	500 MG	N06811 001
	1 GM	N06811 002

AMINOSALICYLIC ACID RESIN COMPLEX

POWDER; ORAL

REZIPAS

Firm	Strength	Appl. No.
SQUIBB	EQ 500 MG BASE/GM	N09052 001

AMITRIPTYLINE HYDROCHLORIDE

TABLET; ORAL

AMITID

Firm	Strength	Appl. No.
SQUIBB	10 MG	N86454 001
	25 MG	N86454 002
	50 MG	N86454 003
	75 MG	N86454 004
	100 MG	N86454 005

AMITRIL

Firm	Strength	Appl. No.
WARNER CHILCOTT	10 MG	N83939 001
	25 MG	N83937 001
	50 MG	N83938 002
	75 MG	N84957 001
	100 MG	N85093 001
	150 MG	N86295 001

AMITRIPTYLINE HCL

Firm	Strength	Appl. No.	Date
AM THERAP	25 MG	N88672 001	NOV 20, 1984
	50 MG	N88673 001	NOV 20, 1984
	75 MG	N88674 001	NOV 20, 1984
	100 MG	N88675 001	NOV 20, 1984
BARR	10 MG	N85744 001	
	25 MG	N85627 001	
	50 MG	N85745 001	
	75 MG	N85743 001	
	100 MG	N85742 002	MAY 11, 1982
	150 MG	N89423 001	FEB 17, 1987
CHELSEA	150 MG	N85821 001	
LEDERLE	10 MG	N86744 001	
	10 MG	N87366 001	JAN 04, 1982
	25 MG	N86746 001	
	25 MG	N87367 001	MAY 03, 1982
	50 MG	N86743 001	
	50 MG	N87181 001	JAN 04, 1982
	75 MG	N86745 001	
	75 MG	N87369 001	JAN 04, 1982
	100 MG	N86747 001	
	100 MG	N87368 001	MAY 03, 1982
	150 MG	N87370 001	JAN 04, 1982

Discontinued Drug Products (continued)

AMITRIPTYLINE HYDROCHLORIDE; PERPHENAZINE
TABLET; ORAL

PERPHENAZINE AND AMITRIPTYLINE HCL

Firm	Strength	Appl. No.	Date
BOLAR	50 MG;4 MG	N70377 001	NOV 04, 1986
	10 MG;2 MG	N70373 001	AUG 25, 1986
	10 MG;4 MG	N70375 001	AUG 25, 1986
	25 MG;2 MG	N70374 001	AUG 25, 1986
	25 MG;4 MG	N70376 001	AUG 25, 1986
CHELSEA	50 MG;4 MG	N71558 001	MAR 02, 1987

AMMONIUM CHLORIDE
INJECTABLE; INJECTION

AMMONIUM CHLORIDE

Firm	Strength	Appl. No.
SEARLE	3 MEQ/ML	N86205 001

AMMONIUM CHLORIDE 0.9% IN NORMAL SALINE

Firm	Strength	Appl. No.
MCGAW	900 MG/100 ML	N06580 001

AMMONIUM CHLORIDE 2.14%

Firm	Strength	Appl. No.
MCGAW	40 MEQ/100 ML	N85734 001

AMODIAQUINE HYDROCHLORIDE
TABLET; ORAL

CAMOQUIN HCL

Firm	Strength	Appl. No.
PARKE DAVIS	EQ 200 MG BASE	N06441 001

AMOXICILLIN
CAPSULE; ORAL

UTIMOX

Firm	Strength	Appl. No.
PARKE DAVIS	250 MG	N62107 001
	500 MG	N62107 002

POWDER FOR RECONSTITUTION; ORAL

UTIMOX

Firm	Strength	Appl. No.
PARKE DAVIS	125 MG/5 ML	N62127 001
	250 MG/5 ML	N62127 002

AMPICILLIN SODIUM
INJECTABLE; INJECTION

AMPICILLIN SODIUM

Firm	Strength	Appl. No.	Date
COPANOS	EQ 125 MG BASE/VIAL	N61936 005	
	EQ 250 MG BASE/VIAL	N61936 001	
	EQ 500 MG BASE/VIAL	N61936 002	
	EQ 1 GM BASE/VIAL	N61936 003	
	EQ 2 GM BASE/VIAL	N61936 004	
INTL MEDICATION	EQ 1 GM BASE/VIAL	N62634 002	JAN 09, 1987
	EQ 2 GM BASE/VIAL	N62634 003	JAN 09, 1987

AMITRIPTYLINE HYDROCHLORIDE (continued)
TABLET; ORAL

AMITRIPTYLINE HCL

Firm	Strength	Appl. No.	Date
PAR	10 MG	N88697 001	SEP 25, 1984
	25 MG	N88698 001	SEP 25, 1984
	50 MG	N88699 001	SEP 25, 1984
	75 MG	N88700 001	SEP 25, 1984
	100 MG	N88701 001	SEP 25, 1984
	150 MG	N88702 001	SEP 25, 1984
PHARM BASICS	25 MG	N87775 001	FEB 10, 1982
PUREPAC	10 MG	N88084 001	JUL 18, 1983
	25 MG	N88085 001	JUL 18, 1983
	50 MG	N88105 001	JUL 18, 1983
	75 MG	N88106 001	JUL 18, 1983
	100 MG	N88107 001	JUL 18, 1983
ROXANE	10 MG	N86144 001	
	25 MG	N86145 001	
	50 MG	N86143 001	
	75 MG	N86147 001	
	100 MG	N86146 001	
	150 MG	N86148 001	
VANGARD	10 MG	N87632 001	FEB 01, 1982
	50 MG	N87616 001	FEB 08, 1982
	75 MG	N87617 001	FEB 08, 1982
	100 MG	N87639 001	FEB 05, 1982
WEST WARD	10 MG	N87647 001	FEB 08, 1982
	25 MG	N87278 001	MAR 05, 1982
	50 MG	N87557 001	MAR 05, 1982

AMITRIPTYLINE HYDROCHLORIDE; CHLORDIAZEPOXIDE
TABLET; ORAL

CHLORDIAZEPOXIDE AND AMITRIPTYLINE HCL

Firm	Strength	Appl. No.	Date
PHARM BASICS	EQ 12.5 MG BASE;5 MG	N70477 001	JAN 12, 1988
	EQ 25 MG BASE;10 MG	N70478 001	JAN 12, 1988

Discontinued Drug Products (continued)

AMPICILLIN SODIUM (continued)
INJECTABLE; INJECTION
POLYCILLIN-N

BRISTOL	EQ 125 MG BASE/VIAL	N50309 001
	EQ 250 MG BASE/VIAL	N50309 002
	EQ 500 MG BASE/VIAL	N50309 003
	EQ 1 GM BASE/VIAL	N50309 004
	EQ 2 GM BASE/VIAL	N50309 005

AMPICILLIN/AMPICILLIN TRIHYDRATE
CAPSULE; ORAL
AMCILL

PARKE DAVIS	EQ 250 MG BASE	N62041 001
	EQ 500 MG BASE	N62041 002

AMPICILLIN

LEDERLE	EQ 250 MG BASE	N62208 001
	EQ 500 MG BASE	N62208 002
VITARINE	EQ 250 MG BASE	N61387 001
	EQ 500 MG BASE	N61387 003

AMPICILLIN TRIHYDRATE

PUREPAC	EQ 250 MG BASE	N61853 001

PENBRITIN

WYETH AYERST	EQ 250 MG BASE	N60908 001
	EQ 500 MG BASE	N60908 002

POLYCILLIN

BRISTOL	EQ 250 MG BASE	N50310 001
	EQ 500 MG BASE	N50310 002

POWDER FOR RECONSTITUTION; ORAL
AMCILL

PARKE DAVIS	EQ 125 MG BASE/5 ML	N62030 001
	EQ 250 MG BASE/5 ML	N62030 002

AMPICILLIN TRIHYDRATE

PUREPAC	EQ 125 MG BASE/5 ML	N61980 001

OMNIPEN (AMPICILLIN)

WYETH AYERST	500 MG/5 ML	N60625 004

PENBRITIN

WYETH AYERST	EQ 125 MG BASE/5 ML	N50019 002
	EQ 250 MG BASE/5 ML	N50019 003
	EQ 100 MG BASE/ML	N50019 001

POLYCILLIN

BRISTOL	EQ 100 MG BASE/ML	N50308 004

TABLET, CHEWABLE; ORAL
POLYCILLIN

BRISTOL	EQ 125 MG BASE	N50093 001

AMPICILLIN/AMPICILLIN TRIHYDRATE; PROBENECID
POWDER FOR RECONSTITUTION; ORAL
POLYCILLIN-PRB

BRISTOL	EQ 3.5 GM BASE/BOT;1 GM/BOT	N50457 001

ANILERIDINE HYDROCHLORIDE
TABLET; ORAL
LERITINE

MSD	EQ 25 MG BASE	N10585 002

ANILERIDINE PHOSPHATE
INJECTABLE; INJECTION
LERITINE

MSD	EQ 25 MG BASE/ML	N10520 003

ANISOTROPINE METHYLBROMIDE
TABLET; ORAL
ANISOTROPINE METHYLBROMIDE

BOLAR	50 MG	N86046 001

ASCORBIC ACID; BIOTIN; CYANOCOBALAMIN; DEXPANTHENOL; ERGOCALCIFEROL; FOLIC ACID; NIACINAMIDE; PYRIDOXINE HYDROCHLORIDE; RIBOFLAVIN PHOSPHATE SODIUM; THIAMINE HYDROCHLORIDE; VITAMIN A PALMITATE; VITAMIN E
INJECTABLE; INJECTION
BEROCCA PN

ROCHE	50 MG/ML;0.03 MG/ML;0.0025 MG/ML;7.5 MG/ML;100 IU/ML;0.2 MG/ML;20 MG/ML;2 MG/ML;1.8 MG/ML;1.5 MG/ML;1,650 IU/ML;5 IU/ML	N06071 003	OCT 10, 1985

ASPIRIN; *MULTIPLE*
SEE ACETAMINOPHEN; ASPIRIN; CODEINE PHOSPHATE

ASPIRIN; BUTALBITAL; CAFFEINE
TABLET; ORAL
BUTALBITAL ASPIRIN AND CAFFEINE

QUANTUM PHARMICS	325 MG;50 MG;40 MG	N88972 001	JUN 18, 1985

ASPIRIN; CAFFEINE; ORPHENADRINE CITRATE
TABLET; ORAL
ORPHENADRINE COMPOUND

EON LABS	385 MG;30 MG;25 MG	N71564 001	JUN 23, 1988

ORPHENADRINE COMPOUND DOUBLE STRENGTH

EON LABS	770 MG;60 MG;50 MG	N71565 001	JUN 23, 1988

ORPHENGESIC

PAR	385 MG;30 MG;25 MG	N71642 001	JUN 23, 1987

ORPHENGESIC FORTE

PAR	770 MG;60 MG;50 MG	N71643 001	JUN 23, 1987

Discontinued Drug Products *(continued)*

ASPIRIN; CAFFEINE; PROPOXYPHENE HYDROCHLORIDE
CAPSULE; ORAL
COMPOUND 65

ALRA	389 MG;32.4 MG;65 MG	N84553 002	AUG 17, 1983

PROPOXYPHENE HCL W/ ASPIRIN AND CAFFEINE

CHELSEA	389 MG;32.4 MG;65 MG	N85732 002	SEP 03, 1984

ASPIRIN; CARISOPRODOL
TABLET; ORAL
CARISOPRODOL COMPOUND

BOLAR	325 MG;200 MG	N88809 001	OCT 03, 1985

ASPIRIN; HYDROCODONE BITARTRATE
TABLET; ORAL
VICOPRIN

KNOLL	500 MG;5 MG	N86333 001	SEP 14, 1983

ASPIRIN; MEPROBAMATE
TABLET; ORAL
MEPRO-ASPIRIN

EON LABS	325 MG;200 MG	N89127 001	MAR 02, 1987

MEPROBAMATE AND ASPIRIN

PAR	325 MG;200 MG	N89126 001	AUG 19, 1986

Q-GESIC

QUANTUM PHARMICS	325 MG;200 MG	N88740 001	JUN 01, 1984

ASPIRIN; PROPOXYPHENE NAPSYLATE
CAPSULE; ORAL
DARVON-N W/ ASA

LILLY	325 MG;100 MG	N16829 001

ATROPINE SULFATE; DIFENOXIN HYDROCHLORIDE
TABLET; ORAL
MOTOFEN HALF-STRENGTH

CARNRICK	0.025 MG;0.5 MG	N17744 001

ATROPINE SULFATE; DIPHENOXYLATE HYDROCHLORIDE
TABLET; ORAL
DIPHENOXYLATE HCL AND ATROPINE SULFATE

ASCOT	0.025 MG;2.5 MG	N87934 001	JUL 19, 1983
CHELSEA	0.025 MG;2.5 MG	N85876 001	
HEATHER	0.025 MG;2.5 MG	N86798 001	
LEDERLE	0.025 MG;2.5 MG	N86950 001	
PARKE DAVIS	0.025 MG;2.5 MG	N87131 001	

DIPHENOXYLATE HCL W/ ATROPINE SULFATE

EON LABS	0.025 MG;2.5 MG	N86173 001	
PHARM BASICS	0.025 MG;2.5 MG	N87842 001	MAR 29, 1982

LO-TROL

VANGARD	0.025 MG;2.5 MG	N88009 001	MAR 25, 1983

ATROPINE SULFATE; MEPERIDINE HYDROCHLORIDE
INJECTABLE; INJECTION
MEPERIDINE AND ATROPINE SULFATE

WYETH AYERST	0.4 MG/ML;50 MG/ML	N85121 001	
	0.4 MG/ML;75 MG/ML	N85121 002	
	0.4 MG/ML;100 MG/ML	N85121 003	

AZATHIOPRINE
TABLET; ORAL
IMURAN

BURROUGHS WELLCOME	25 MG	N16324 002

BACAMPICILLIN HYDROCHLORIDE
TABLET; ORAL
SPECTROBID

PFIZER	800 MG	N50520 002	SEP 12, 1983

BACITRACIN
INJECTABLE; INJECTION
BACITRACIN

QUAD	10,000 UNITS/VIAL	N62696 001	APR 17, 1987
	50,000 UNITS/VIAL	N62696 002	APR 17, 1987

OINTMENT; OPHTHALMIC
BACIGUENT

UPJOHN	500 UNITS/GM	N60734 001

BETAMETHASONE

CREAM; TOPICAL
  CELESTONE
    SCHERING   0.2%   N14762 001

BETAMETHASONE VALERATE

CREAM; TOPICAL
  BETAMETHASONE VALERATE
    PHARMAFAIR   EQ 0.1% BASE   N70485 001 MAY 29, 1987
OINTMENT; TOPICAL
  BETAMETHASONE VALERATE
    PHARMAFAIR   EQ 0.1% BASE   N70486 001 MAY 29, 1987

BETAZOLE HYDROCHLORIDE

INJECTABLE; INJECTION
  HISTALOG
    LILLY   50 MG/ML   N09344 001

BETHANECHOL CHLORIDE

INJECTABLE; INJECTION
  BETHANECHOL CHLORIDE
    QUAD   5 MG/ML   N89815 001 APR 12, 1988
TABLET; ORAL
  BETHANECHOL CHLORIDE
    ASCOT   10 MG   N88288 001 JUN 08, 1983
             25 MG   N88289 001 JUN 08, 1983
    BOLAR   5 MG   N85230 002
             10 MG   N85228 001
             25 MG   N85229 001
             50 MG   N87397 001
    CHELSEA 5 MG   N85841 001
             10 MG   N85842 001
             25 MG   N85839 001
    VITARINE 5 MG   N84353 001
             10 MG   N84378 001
             10 MG   N84379 001
             25 MG   N84383 001
             25 MG   N84384 001

BETHANIDINE SULFATE

TABLET; ORAL
  TENATHAN
    ROBINS   10 MG   N17675 001
              25 MG   N17675 002

Discontinued Drug Products (continued)

BACLOFEN

TABLET; ORAL
  BACLOFEN
    EON LABS   10 MG   N71901 001 APR 13, 1988
                   20 MG   N71902 001 APR 13, 1988
    PHARM BASICS   10 MG   N71260 001 MAY 06, 1988
                   20 MG   N71261 001 MAY 06, 1988

BENDROFLUMETHIAZIDE

TABLET; ORAL
  NATURETIN-2.5
    SQUIBB   2.5 MG   N12164 001

BENOXINATE HYDROCHLORIDE

SOLUTION/DROPS; OPHTHALMIC
  BENOXINATE HCL
    SOLA BARNES HIND   0.4%   N84149 001

BENZTHIAZIDE

TABLET; ORAL
  AQUATAG
    SOLVAY   25 MG   N16001 001
  BENZTHIAZIDE
    PRIVATE FORM   50 MG   N83206 001
  FOVANE
    PFIZER   50 MG   N12128 002
  URESE
    PFIZER   25 MG   N12128 003

BENZTROPINE MESYLATE

TABLET; ORAL
  BENZTROPINE MESYLATE
    PHARM BASICS   0.5 MG   N89211 001 JUN 14, 1988
                       1 MG   N89212 001 JUN 14, 1988
                       2 MG   N89213 001 JUN 14, 1988
    QUANTUM PHARMICS   0.5 MG   N88514 001 JAN 31, 1984
                       1 MG   N88510 001 JAN 31, 1984
                       2 MG   N88511 001 JAN 31, 1984

Discontinued Drug Products *(continued)*

BIOTIN; *MULTIPLE*
SEE   ASCORBIC ACID; BIOTIN; CYANOCOBALAMIN;
       DEXPANTHENOL; ERGOCALCIFEROL; FOLIC ACID;
       NIACINAMIDE; PYRIDOXINE HYDROCHLORIDE; RIBOFLAVIN
       PHOSPHATE SODIUM; THIAMINE HYDROCHLORIDE; VITAMIN
       A PALMITATE; VITAMIN E

BRETYLIUM TOSYLATE
INJECTABLE; INJECTION

BRETYLIUM TOSYLATE		
LYPHOMED	50 MG/ML	N70134 001 FEB 12, 1986
	100 MG/ML	N71298 001 FEB 13, 1987
QUAD	50 MG/ML	N71181 001 FEB 16, 1988

BRETYLIUM TOSYLATE IN DEXTROSE 5%		
ABBOTT	800 MG/100 ML	N19005 001 APR 16, 1986
	200 MG/100 ML	N19005 002 APR 16, 1986
	400 MG/100 ML	N19005 003 APR 16, 1986

BRETYLIUM TOSYLATE IN DEXTROSE 5% IN PLASTIC CONTAINER		
ABBOTT	800 MG/100 ML	N19008 001 APR 16, 1986

BROMODIPHENHYDRAMINE HYDROCHLORIDE
CAPSULE; ORAL

AMBODRYL		
PARKE DAVIS	25 MG	N07984 001

BROMPHENIRAMINE MALEATE
ELIXIR; ORAL

BROMPHENIRAMINE MALEATE		
BARRE	2 MG/5 ML	N86936 001
PHARM ASSOC	2 MG/5 ML	N87517 001
PHARM BASICS	2 MG/5 ML	N87964 001 JAN 25, 1983

INJECTABLE; INJECTION

BROMPHENIRAMINE MALEATE		
STERIS	100 MG/ML	N83820 001

TABLET; ORAL

BROMPHENIRAMINE MALEATE		
BARR	4 MG	N84468 001
CHELSEA	4 MG	N85769 001
GENEVA	4 MG	N83215 001
PAR	4 MG	N87009 001
PIONEER PHARMS	4 MG	N88604 001 JUL 13, 1984
VITARINE	4 MG	N85850 001

BROMPHENIRAMINE MALEATE; PHENYLPROPANOLAMINE HYDROCHLORIDE
ELIXIR; ORAL

BIPHETAP		
PHARM BASICS	4 MG/5 ML;25 MG/5 ML	N88687 001 SEP 26, 1984
BROMANATE		
BARRE	4 MG/5 ML;25 MG/5 ML	N88688 001 FEB 06, 1985

BUPROPION HYDROCHLORIDE
TABLET; ORAL

WELLBUTRIN		
BURROUGHS WELLCOME	50 MG	N18644 001 DEC 30, 1985

BUTABARBITAL SODIUM
TABLET; ORAL

BUTABARBITAL SODIUM		
CHELSEA	15 MG	N85764 001
	30 MG	N85772 001
EON LABS	15 MG	N85938 001
	30 MG	N85934 001
GENEVA	15 MG	N84292 003 FEB 09, 1982
	30 MG	N84272 002
	15 MG	N88632 001 MAY 18, 1985
LEMMON	30 MG	N88631 001 MAY 01, 1985
SOLVAY	16.2 MG	N83606 001
	32.4 MG	N83898 001
	48.6 MG	N83897 001
	97.2 MG	N83896 001
WHITE TOWNE	15 MG	N83325 002
PAULSEN	30 MG	N83337 001
SODIUM BUTABARBITAL		
WEST WARD	15 MG	N85418 001
	30 MG	N85432 001
ZENITH	15 MG	N83484 001

BUTALBITAL; *MULTIPLE*
SEE   ASPIRIN; BUTALBITAL; CAFFEINE

BUTOCONAZOLE NITRATE
SUPPOSITORY; VAGINAL

FEMSTAT		
SYNTEX	100 MG	N19359 001 NOV 25, 1985

Discontinued Drug Products (continued)

CAFFEINE; *MULTIPLE*
SEE   ASPIRIN; BUTALBITAL; CAFFEINE
SEE   ASPIRIN; CAFFEINE; ORPHENADRINE CITRATE
SEE   ASPIRIN; CAFFEINE; PROPOXYPHENE HYDROCHLORIDE

CALCITONIN, SALMON
INJECTABLE; INJECTION
CALCIMAR
RHONE POULENC
RORER   400 IU/VIAL   N17497 001

CALCIUM; MEGLUMINE; METRIZOIC ACID
INJECTABLE; INJECTION
ISOPAQUE 280
STERLING   0.35 MG/ML;140.1 MG/
                ML;461.8 MG/ML   N17506 001

CALCIUM CHLORIDE; DEXTROSE; MAGNESIUM CHLORIDE; SODIUM ACETATE; SODIUM CHLORIDE
SOLUTION; INTRAPERITONEAL
DIALYTE W/ DEXTROSE 2.5% IN PLASTIC CONTAINER
MCGAW   29 MG/100 ML;2.5 GM/
            100 ML;15 MG/
            100 ML;610 MG/
            100 ML;560 MG/100 ML   N18460 006   JAN 29, 1986

DIALYTE W/ DEXTROSE 1.5% IN PLASTIC CONTAINER
MCGAW   29 MG/100 ML;1.5 GM/
            100 ML;15 MG/
            100 ML;610 MG/
            100 ML;560 MG/100 ML   N18460 001

DIALYTE W/ DEXTROSE 4.25% IN PLASTIC CONTAINER
MCGAW   29 MG/100 ML;4.25 GM/
            100 ML;15 MG/
            100 ML;610 MG/
            100 ML;560 MG/100 ML   N18460 003

CALCIUM CHLORIDE; DEXTROSE; MAGNESIUM CHLORIDE; SODIUM CHLORIDE; SODIUM LACTATE
SOLUTION; INTRAPERITONEAL
DIALYTE LM/ DEXTROSE 1.5% IN PLASTIC CONTAINER
MCGAW   26 MG/100 ML;1.5 GM/
            100 ML;15 MG/
            100 ML;560 MG/
            100 ML;390 MG/100 ML   N18460 002

DIALYTE LM/ DEXTROSE 2.5% IN PLASTIC CONTAINER
MCGAW   26 MG/100 ML;2.5 GM/
            100 ML;530 MG/
            100 ML;5 MG/
            100 ML;450 MG/100 ML   N18460 008   JAN 29, 1986

CALCIUM CHLORIDE; DEXTROSE; MAGNESIUM CHLORIDE; SODIUM CHLORIDE; SODIUM LACTATE (continued)
SOLUTION; INTRAPERITONEAL
DIALYTE LM/ DEXTROSE 4.25% IN PLASTIC CONTAINER
MCGAW   26 MG/100 ML;4.25 GM/
            100 ML;15 MG/
            100 ML;560 MG/
            100 ML;390 MG/100 ML   N18460 004

CALCIUM CHLORIDE; DEXTROSE; POTASSIUM CHLORIDE; SODIUM CHLORIDE; SODIUM LACTATE
INJECTABLE; INJECTION
DEXTROSE 5% IN LACTATED RINGER'S IN PLASTIC CONTAINER
CUTTER   20 MG/100 ML;5 GM/
            100 ML;30 MG/
            100 ML;600 MG/
            100 ML;310 MG/100 ML   N18499 001

POTASSIUM CHLORIDE 10 MEQ IN DEXTROSE 5% AND LACTATED RINGER'S IN PLASTIC CONTAINER
ABBOTT   20 MG/100 ML;5 GM/
            100 ML;104 MG/
            100 ML;600 MG/
            100 ML;310 MG/100 ML   N19685 005   OCT 17, 1988

            20 MG/100 ML;5 GM/
            100 ML;179 MG/
            100 ML;600 MG/
            100 ML;310 MG/100 ML   N19685 006   OCT 17, 1988

POTASSIUM CHLORIDE 15 MEQ IN DEXTROSE 5% AND LACTATED RINGER'S IN PLASTIC CONTAINER
ABBOTT   20 MG/100 ML;5 GM/
            100 ML;254 MG/
            100 ML;600 MG/
            100 ML;310 MG/100 ML   N19685 007   OCT 17, 1988

POTASSIUM CHLORIDE 30 MEQ IN DEXTROSE 5% AND LACTATED RINGER'S IN PLASTIC CONTAINER
ABBOTT   20 MG/100 ML;5 GM/
            100 ML;254 MG/
            100 ML;600 MG/
            100 ML;310 MG/100 ML   N19685 003   OCT 17, 1988

POTASSIUM CHLORIDE 5 MEQ IN DEXTROSE 5% AND LACTATED RINGER'S IN PLASTIC CONTAINER
ABBOTT   20 MG/100 ML;5 GM/
            100 ML;104 MG/
            100 ML;600 MG/
            100 ML;310 MG/100 ML   N19685 001   OCT 17, 1988

Discontinued Drug Products (continued)

CALCIUM CHLORIDE; DEXTROSE; SODIUM CHLORIDE; SODIUM LACTATE
SOLUTION; INTRAPERITONEAL
INPERSOL-ZM W/ DEXTROSE 1.5% IN PLASTIC CONTAINER
ABBOTT   25.7 MG/100 ML;1.5 GM/100 ML;538 MG/100 ML;448 MG/100 ML   N19395 001   MAR 26, 1986

INPERSOL-ZM W/ DEXTROSE 2.5% IN PLASTIC CONTAINER
ABBOTT   25.7 MG/100 ML;2.5 GM/100 ML;538 MG/100 ML;448 MG/100 ML   N19395 002   MAR 26, 1986

INPERSOL-ZM W/ DEXTROSE 4.25% IN PLASTIC CONTAINER
ABBOTT   25.7 MG/100 ML;4.25 GM/100 ML;538 MG/100 ML;448 MG/100 ML   N19395 003   MAR 26, 1986

CALCIUM CHLORIDE; MAGNESIUM CHLORIDE; POTASSIUM CHLORIDE; SODIUM ACETATE; SODIUM CHLORIDE
INJECTABLE; INJECTION
TPN ELECTROLYTES IN PLASTIC CONTAINER
ABBOTT   16.5 MG/ML;25.4 MG/ML;74.6 MG/ML;121 MG/ML;16.1 MG/ML   N19399 001   JUN 16, 1986

CALCIUM CHLORIDE; POTASSIUM CHLORIDE; SODIUM ACETATE; SODIUM CHLORIDE
INJECTABLE; INJECTION
ACETATED RINGER'S IN PLASTIC CONTAINER
MCGAW   20 MG/100 ML;30 MG/100 ML;380 MG/100 ML;600 MG/100 ML   N18725 001   NOV 29, 1982

CALCIUM CHLORIDE; POTASSIUM CHLORIDE; SODIUM CHLORIDE
SOLUTION; IRRIGATION
RINGER'S IN PLASTIC CONTAINER
ABBOTT   33 MG/100 ML;30 MG/100 ML;860 MG/100 ML   N18462 001

CALCIUM CHLORIDE; POTASSIUM CHLORIDE; SODIUM CHLORIDE; SODIUM LACTATE
INJECTABLE; INJECTION
LACTATED RINGER'S IN PLASTIC CONTAINER
ABBOTT   20 MG/100 ML;30 MG/100 ML;600 MG/100 ML;310 MG/100 ML   N19485 001   OCT 24, 1985
CUTTER   20 MG/100 ML;30 MG/100 ML;600 MG/100 ML;310 MG/100 ML   N18417 001

CALCIUM GLUCEPTATE
INJECTABLE; INJECTION
CALCIUM GLUCEPTATE
ABBOTT   EQ 90 MG CALCIUM/5 ML   N83159 001

CALCIUM METRIZOATE; MAGNESIUM METRIZOATE; MEGLUMINE METRIZOATE; METRIZOATE SODIUM
INJECTABLE; INJECTION
ISOPAQUE 440
STERLING   0.78 MG/ML;0.15 MG/ML;75.9 MG/ML;16.6 MG/ML   N16847 001

CAPTOPRIL
TABLET; ORAL
CAPOTEN
BRISTOL MYERS SQUIBB   37.5 MG   N18343 006   SEP 17, 1986

CARBAMAZEPINE
TABLET; ORAL
CARBAMAZEPINE
PHARM BASICS   200 MG   N70300 001   MAY 15, 1986   N70429 001   JAN 02, 1987
WARNER CHILCOTT   200 MG

CARISOPRODOL
TABLET; ORAL
CARISOPRODOL
BOLAR   350 MG   N85433 001

CARISOPRODOL; *MULTIPLE*
SEE   ASPIRIN; CARISOPRODOL

CARPHENAZINE MALEATE
CONCENTRATE; ORAL
PROKETAZINE
WYETH AYERST   50 MG/ML   N14173 001
TABLET; ORAL
PROKETAZINE
WYETH AYERST   12.5 MG   N12768 001
  25 MG   N12768 002
  50 MG   N12768 004

Discontinued Drug Products *(continued)*

CARPROFEN
TABLET; ORAL
RIMADYL

Applicant	Strength	Appl. No.	Date
ROCHE	100 MG	N18550 002	DEC 31, 1987
	150 MG	N18550 003	DEC 31, 1987

CARTEOLOL HYDROCHLORIDE
TABLET; ORAL
CARTROL

Applicant	Strength	Appl. No.	Date
ABBOTT	10 MG	N19204 003	DEC 28, 1988

CEFADROXIL/CEFADROXIL HEMIHYDRATE
CAPSULE; ORAL
CEFADROXIL

Applicant	Strength	Appl. No.	Date
BIOCRAFT	EQ 500 MG BASE	N62695 001	FEB 10, 1989
PUREPAC	EQ 500 MG BASE	N63017 001	JAN 05, 1989

DURICEF

Applicant	Strength	Appl. No.	Date
MEAD JOHNSON	EQ 250 MG BASE	N50512 002	

ULTRACEF

Applicant	Strength	Appl. No.	Date
BRISTOL	EQ 500 MG BASE	N62378 001	MAR 16, 1982

POWDER FOR RECONSTITUTION; ORAL
CEFADROXIL

Applicant	Strength	Appl. No.	Date
BIOCRAFT	EQ 125 MG BASE/5 ML	N62698 001	MAR 01, 1989
	EQ 250 MG BASE/5 ML	N62698 002	MAR 01, 1989
	EQ 500 MG BASE/5 ML	N62698 003	MAR 01, 1989

ULTRACEF

Applicant	Strength	Appl. No.	Date
BRISTOL	EQ 125 MG BASE/5 ML	N62376 001	MAR 16, 1982
	EQ 250 MG BASE/5 ML	N62376 002	MAR 16, 1982
	EQ 500 MG BASE/5 ML	N62376 003	MAR 16, 1982

TABLET; ORAL
ULTRACEF

Applicant	Strength	Appl. No.	Date
BRISTOL	EQ 1 GM BASE	N62408 001	AUG 31, 1982

CEFAZOLIN SODIUM
INJECTABLE; INJECTION
ANCEF IN SODIUM CHLORIDE 0.9% IN PLASTIC CONTAINER

Applicant	Strength	Appl. No.	Date
BAXTER	EQ 10 MG BASE/ML	N50566 001	JUN 08, 1983
	EQ 20 MG BASE/ML	N50566 002	JUN 08, 1983

CEFTRIAXONE SODIUM
INJECTABLE; INJECTION
ROCEPHIN

Applicant	Strength	Appl. No.	Date
ROCHE	EQ 250 MG BASE/VIAL	N62510 001	MAR 12, 1985
	EQ 500 MG BASE/VIAL	N62510 002	MAR 12, 1985
	EQ 1 GM BASE/VIAL	N62510 003	MAR 12, 1985

CEPHALEXIN
POWDER FOR RECONSTITUTION; ORAL
CEPHALEXIN

Applicant	Strength	Appl. No.	Date
VITARINE	EQ 125 MG BASE/5 ML	N62779 001	DEC 22, 1987
	EQ 250 MG BASE/5 ML	N62781 001	DEC 22, 1987

TABLET; ORAL
CEPHALEXIN

Applicant	Strength	Appl. No.	Date
VITARINE	EQ 250 MG BASE	N62863 001	AUG 11, 1988
	EQ 500 MG BASE	N62863 002	AUG 11, 1988
	EQ 1 GM BASE	N62863 003	AUG 11, 1988

CEPHALOTHIN SODIUM
INJECTABLE; INJECTION
CEPHALOTHIN

Applicant	Strength	Appl. No.	Date
INTL MEDICATION	EQ 500 MG BASE/VIAL	N62426 001	MAY 03, 1985
	EQ 1 GM BASE/VIAL	N62426 002	MAY 03, 1985
	EQ 2 GM BASE/VIAL	N62426 003	MAY 03, 1985
	EQ 4 GM BASE/VIAL	N62426 004	MAY 03, 1985

CEPHAPIRIN SODIUM
INJECTABLE; INJECTION
CEPHAPIRIN SODIUM

Applicant	Strength	Appl. No.	Date
LYPHOMED	EQ 20 GM BASE/VIAL	N62723 005	NOV 17, 1986

CEPHRADINE
CAPSULE; ORAL
CEPHRADINE

Applicant	Strength	Appl. No.	Date
VITARINE	250 MG	N62813 001	FEB 25, 1988
	500 MG	N62813 002	FEB 25, 1988

Discontinued Drug Products (continued)

CEPHRADINE (continued)

CAPSULE; ORAL

Brand	Manufacturer	Strength	Number
VELOSEF '250'	ERSANA	250 MG	N50548 001
VELOSEF '500'	ERSANA	500 MG	N50548 002

CERULETIDE DIETHYLAMINE

INJECTABLE; INJECTION

Brand	Manufacturer	Strength	Number
TYMTRAN	ADRIA	0.02 MG/ML	N18296 001

CHLOPHEDIANOL HYDROCHLORIDE

SYRUP; ORAL

Brand	Manufacturer	Strength	Number
ULO	3M	25 MG/5 ML	N12126 001

CHLORAMPHENICOL

INJECTABLE; INJECTION

Brand	Manufacturer	Strength	Number
CHLOROMYCETIN	PARKE DAVIS	250 MG/ML	N50153 001

OINTMENT; OPHTHALMIC

Brand	Manufacturer	Strength	Number
ECONOCHLOR	ALCON	1%	N61648 001

SOLUTION/DROPS; OPHTHALMIC

Brand	Manufacturer	Strength	Number
ECONOCHLOR	ALCON	0.5%	N61645 001

CHLORAMPHENICOL; POLYMYXIN B SULFATE

OINTMENT; OPHTHALMIC

Brand	Manufacturer	Strength	Number
CHLOROMYXIN	PARKE DAVIS	1%;10,000 UNITS/GM	N50203 002

CHLORAMPHENICOL; PREDNISOLONE

OINTMENT; OPHTHALMIC

Brand	Manufacturer	Strength	Number
CHLOROPTIC-P S.O.P.	ALLERGAN	1%;0.5%	N61188 001

CHLORDIAZEPOXIDE; *MULTIPLE*

SEE   AMITRIPTYLINE HYDROCHLORIDE; CHLORDIAZEPOXIDE

CHLORDIAZEPOXIDE HYDROCHLORIDE

CAPSULE; ORAL

Brand	Manufacturer	Strength	Number	Date
A-POXIDE	ABBOTT	5 MG	N85447 001	
		5 MG	N85517 001	
		10 MG	N85447 002	
		10 MG	N85518 001	
		25 MG	N85447 003	
		25 MG	N85513 001	
CHLORDIAZEPOXIDE HCL	ASCOT	5 MG	N87525 001	JAN 07, 1982
		10 MG	N87524 001	JAN 07, 1982
		25 MG	N87512 001	JAN 07, 1982
	EON LABS	5 MG	N84919 001	JAN 07, 1982
		10 MG	N84920 001	
		25 MG	N84823 001	
	LEDERLE	5 MG	N86892 001	
		5 MG	N87234 001	
		10 MG	N86876 001	
		10 MG	N87037 001	
		25 MG	N86893 001	
		25 MG	N87231 001	
	LEMMON	5 MG	N88705 001	JAN 18, 1985
		10 MG	N88706 001	JAN 18, 1985
		25 MG	N86494 001	JAN 18, 1985
		25 MG	N88707 001	JAN 18, 1985
	MYLAN	5 MG	N84886 001	
		10 MG	N84601 001	
		25 MG	N84887 001	
	PARKE DAVIS	5 MG	N85163 001	
		10 MG	N84598 001	
		25 MG	N85164 001	
	PUREPAC	5 MG	N85155 001	
		10 MG	N84939 002	
		25 MG	N85144 001	
	ROXANE	5 MG	N84706 001	
		10 MG	N84700 001	
		25 MG	N84705 001	
	SUPERPHARM	5 MG	N88987 001	APR 25, 1985
		10 MG	N88986 001	APR 25, 1985
		25 MG	N88988 001	APR 25, 1985
	VANGARD	5 MG	N88129 001	MAR 28, 1983
		10 MG	N88010 001	MAR 28, 1983
		25 MG	N88130 001	MAR 28, 1983
	WEST WARD	5 MG	N85014 001	MAR 28, 1983
		10 MG	N85000 001	
		25 MG	N85294 001	

Discontinued Drug Products (continued)

CHLORDIAZEPOXIDE HYDROCHLORIDE (continued)
CAPSULE; ORAL
- LYGEN
- ALRA
  - 5 MG   N85107 001
  - 10 MG   N85009 001
  - 25 MG   N85108 001

CHLORHEXIDINE GLUCONATE
SOLUTION; TOPICAL
- EXIDINE
- XTTRIUM   2.5%   N19421 001   DEC 17, 1985

TINCTURE; TOPICAL
- HIBITANE
- STUART   0.5%   N18049 001

CHLORMERODRIN, HG-197
INJECTABLE; INJECTION
- CHLORMERODRIN HG 197
- SQUIBB   0.6-1.4 MCI/ML   N17269 001

CHLOROQUINE PHOSPHATE
TABLET; ORAL
- CHLOROQUINE PHOSPHATE
- PUREPAC   EQ 150 MG BASE   N80886 001
- WEST WARD   EQ 150 MG BASE   N83082 001

CHLOROQUINE PHOSPHATE; PRIMAQUINE PHOSPHATE
TABLET; ORAL
- ARALEN PHOSPHATE W/ PRIMAQUINE PHOSPHATE
- STERLING   EQ 300 MG BASE;EQ 45 MG BASE   N14860 002

CHLOROTHIAZIDE
TABLET; ORAL
- CHLOROTHIAZIDE
- BOLAR
  - 250 MG   N85165 001
  - 500 MG   N84026 001   SEP 01, 1982
- CHELSEA   500 MG   N86796 001   AUG 15, 1983
- EON LABS   250 MG   N85485 001
- LEDERLE
  - 250 MG   N86940 001
  - 500 MG   N86938 001

CHLOROTHIAZIDE; RESERPINE
TABLET; ORAL
- CHLOROTHIAZIDE W/ RESERPINE
- BOLAR
  - 250 MG;0.125 MG   N84853 001
  - 500 MG;0.125 MG   N88151 001   JUN 09, 1983

CHLORPHENIRAMINE MALEATE
CAPSULE, EXTENDED RELEASE; ORAL
- TELDRIN
- SKCP   8 MG   N17369 001

INJECTABLE; INJECTION
- CHLOR-TRIMETON
- SCHERING   100 MG/ML   N08794 001
- CHLORPHENIRAMINE MALEATE
- ELKINS SINN   10 MG/ML   N80797 001

SYRUP; ORAL
- CHLOR-TRIMETON
- SCHERING   2 MG/5 ML   N06921 006
- CHLORPHENIRAMINE MALEATE
- PHARM ASSOC   2 MG/5 ML   N87520 001   FEB 10, 1982

TABLET; ORAL
- ANTAGONATE
- MILES   4 MG   N83381 001
- CHLOR-TRIMETON
- SCHERING   4 MG   N06921 002
- CHLORPHENIRAMINE MALEATE
- ANABOLICS   4 MG   N83078 001
- BARR   4 MG   N80700 001
- BELL PHARMA   4 MG   N83062 001
- BOLAR   4 MG   N80791 001
- CHELSEA   4 MG   N85139 001
- ELKINS SINN   4 MG   N80938 001
- LEDERLE   4 MG   N86941 001
- PANRAY   4 MG   N83243 001
- PHARMAFAIR   4 MG   N83753 001
- PIONEER PHARMS   4 MG   N88556 001   JUL 13, 1984
- PRIVATE FORM   4 MG   N80786 001
- PUREPAC   4 MG   N86306 001
- ROXANE   4 MG   N80626 001
- VITARINE   4 MG   N85837 001
- PHENETRON
- LANNETT   4 MG   N80846 001

CHLORPHENIRAMINE MALEATE; PHENYLPROPANOLAMINE HYDROCHLORIDE
CAPSULE, EXTENDED RELEASE; ORAL
- CHLORPHENIRAMINE MALEATE AND PHENYLPROPANOLAMINE HCL
- CHELSEA   12 MG;75 MG   N88681 001   SEP 29, 1987

CHLORPHENTERMINE HYDROCHLORIDE
TABLET; ORAL
- PRE-SATE
- PARKE DAVIS   EQ 65 MG BASE   N14696 001

Discontinued Drug Products *(continued)*

CHLORPROMAZINE HYDROCHLORIDE

INJECTABLE; INJECTION

CHLORPROMAZINE HCL

Firm	Strength	NDA	Date
WYETH AYERST	25 MG/ML	N80370 001	

SYRUP; ORAL

CHLORPROMAZINE HCL

Firm	Strength	NDA	Date
BARRE	10 MG/5 ML	N86712 001	

TABLET; ORAL

CHLORPROMAZINE HCL

Firm	Strength	NDA	Date
BOOTS	10 MG	N84414 001	
	25 MG	N84415 001	
	50 MG	N84411 001	
	100 MG	N84412 001	
	200 MG	N84413 001	
CHELSEA	10 MG	N85959 001	
	25 MG	N85956 001	
	50 MG	N85960 001	
	100 MG	N85957 001	
	200 MG	N85958 001	
LEDERLE	25 MG	N84801 001	
	50 MG	N84800 001	
	100 MG	N84789 001	
	200 MG	N84802 001	
PRIVATE FORM	25 MG	N80340 001	
	50 MG	N80340 002	
	200 MG	N80340 003	
PUREPAC	10 MG	N80340 004	
	25 MG	N80403 001	
	50 MG	N80403 002	
	100 MG	N80403 003	
	200 MG	N80403 005	
ROXANE	10 MG	N85331 001	
	25 MG	N85331 002	
	50 MG	N85331 003	
	100 MG	N85331 004	
	200 MG	N85331 005	
VANGARD	10 MG	N88038 001	AUG 16, 1982
	25 MG	N87645 001	
	50 MG	N87646 001	
WEST WARD	10 MG	N87783 001	SEP 16, 1982
	25 MG	N87865 001	SEP 16, 1982
	50 MG	N87878 001	SEP 16, 1982
	100 MG	N87884 001	SEP 15, 1982
	200 MG	N87880 001	SEP 16, 1982

PROMAPAR

Firm	Strength	NDA	Date
PARKE DAVIS	10 MG	N86886 001	
	25 MG	N84423 001	
	50 MG	N86887 001	
	100 MG	N86888 001	
	200 MG	N86885 001	

CHLORPROPAMIDE

TABLET; ORAL

CHLORPROPAMIDE

Firm	Strength	NDA	Date
BOLAR	100 MG	N88608 001	APR 12, 1984
	250 MG	N88568 001	APR 12, 1984
CHELSEA	250 MG	N86866 001	APR 12, 1984
DURAMED	100 MG	N88918 001	OCT 16, 1984
	250 MG	N88919 001	OCT 16, 1984
EON LABS	250 MG	N84669 001	OCT 16, 1984
PHARM BASICS	100 MG	N88708 001	AUG 30, 1984
	250 MG	N88709 001	AUG 30, 1984

CHLORTHALIDONE

TABLET; ORAL

CHLORTHALIDONE

Firm	Strength	NDA	Date
ASCOT	25 MG	N87698 001	OCT 20, 1982
	50 MG	N87699 001	OCT 20, 1982
BOLAR	25 MG	N87050 001	
	50 MG	N87029 001	
LEMMON	50 MG	N88651 001	MAY 30, 1985
SUPERPHARM	25 MG	N87473 001	FEB 09, 1983
VANGARD	25 MG	N88012 001	JUL 14, 1982
	50 MG	N88073 001	MAR 25, 1983
WARNER CHILCOTT	25 MG	N87515 001	JAN 24, 1983
	50 MG	N87516 001	FEB 09, 1983
ZENITH	25 MG	N87555 001	

CHLORZOXAZONE

TABLET; ORAL

CHLORZOXAZONE

Firm	Strength	NDA	Date
CHELSEA	250 MG	N86948 001	AUG 09, 1982

CHYMOPAPAIN

INJECTABLE; INJECTION

DISCASE

Firm	Strength	NDA	Date
BOOTS	12,500 UNITS/VIAL	N18625 001	JAN 18, 1984

Discontinued Drug Products (continued)

CHYMOTRYPSIN

POWDER FOR RECONSTITUTION; OPHTHALMIC

ALPHA CHYMAR

SOLA BARNES HIND	750 UNITS/VIAL	N11837 001	

CISPLATIN

INJECTABLE; INJECTION

PLATINOL-AQ

BRISTOL MYERS	0.5 MG/ML	N18057 003	JUL 18, 1984

CLEMASTINE FUMARATE

TABLET; ORAL

TAVIST-1

SANDOZ	1.34 MG	N17661 002	

CLEMASTINE FUMARATE; PHENYLPROPANOLAMINE HYDROCHLORIDE

TABLET, EXTENDED RELEASE; ORAL

TAVIST D

SANDOZ	EQ 1 MG BASE;75 MG	N18298 001	DEC 15, 1982

CLINDAMYCIN HYDROCHLORIDE

CAPSULE; ORAL

CLINDAMYCIN HCL

EON LABS	EQ 75 MG BASE	N62910 001	JUL 05, 1988
	EQ 150 MG BASE	N62910 002	JUL 05, 1988

CLINDAMYCIN PHOSPHATE

INJECTABLE; INJECTION

CLINDAMYCIN PHOSPHATE

QUAD	EQ 150 MG BASE/ML	N62877 001	MAR 15, 1988

CLIOQUINOL; HYDROCORTISONE

OINTMENT; TOPICAL

VIOFORM-HYDROCORTISONE

CIBA	3%;0.5%	N10412 004	

CLIOQUINOL; NYSTATIN

OINTMENT; TOPICAL

NYSTAFORM

MILES	10 MG/GM;100,000 UNITS/GM	N50235 001	

CLONIDINE HYDROCHLORIDE

TABLET; ORAL

CLONIDINE HCL

AM THERAP	0.1 MG	N70881 001	MAY 27, 1986
	0.2 MG	N70882 001	MAY 27, 1986
	0.3 MG	N70883 001	MAY 27, 1986
BOLAR	0.1 MG	N70395 001	MAR 23, 1987
	0.2 MG	N70396 001	MAR 23, 1987
	0.3 MG	N70397 001	MAR 23, 1987
DURAMED	0.1 MG	N71103 001	AUG 14, 1986
	0.2 MG	N71102 001	AUG 14, 1986
	0.3 MG	N71101 001	AUG 14, 1986
INTERPHARM	0.1 MG	N71252 001	OCT 01, 1986
	0.2 MG	N71253 001	OCT 01, 1986
	0.3 MG	N71254 001	OCT 01, 1986

CLORAZEPATE DIPOTASSIUM

CAPSULE; ORAL

CLORAZEPATE DIPOTASSIUM

AM THERAP	3.75 MG	N71429 001	JAN 08, 1987
	7.5 MG	N71430 001	JAN 08, 1987
	15 MG	N71431 001	JAN 08, 1987
CHELSEA	3.75 MG	N71878 001	JAN 08, 1987
	7.5 MG	N71879 001	MAR 15, 1988
	15 MG	N71860 001	MAR 15, 1988
PHARM BASICS	3.75 MG	N71242 001	MAR 15, 1988
	7.5 MG	N71243 001	MAY 20, 1987
	15 MG	N71244 001	MAY 20, 1987
PUREPAC	3.75 MG	N71924 001	MAY 20, 1987
QUANTUM PHARMICS	3.75 MG	N71549 001	APR 25, 1988
	7.5 MG	N71550 001	SEP 12, 1988
	15 MG	N71522 001	SEP 12, 1988

Discontinued Drug Products (continued)

CLORAZEPATE DIPOTASSIUM (continued)

CAPSULE; ORAL

CLORAZEPATE DIPOTASSIUM

SEARLE	3.75 MG	N71727 001	DEC 18, 1987
	7.5 MG	N71728 001	DEC 18, 1987
	15 MG	N71729 001	DEC 18, 1987
WARNER CHILCOTT	3.75 MG	N71774 001	DEC 18, 1987
	7.5 MG	N71775 001	MAR 01, 1988
	15 MG	N71776 001	MAR 01, 1988

TRANXENE

ABBOTT	3.75 MG	N17105 001
	7.5 MG	N17105 002
	15 MG	N17105 003

TABLET; ORAL

CLORAZEPATE DIPOTASSIUM

AM THERAP	3.75 MG	N71747 001	JUN 09, 1987
	7.5 MG	N71748 001	JUN 09, 1987
	15 MG	N71749 001	JUN 09, 1987
LEDERLE	3.75 MG	N72013 001	DEC 15, 1987
	7.5 MG	N72014 001	DEC 15, 1987
	15 MG	N72015 001	DEC 15, 1987
QUANTUM PHARMICS	3.75 MG	N71730 001	OCT 26, 1987
	7.5 MG	N71731 001	OCT 26, 1987
	15 MG	N71702 001	OCT 26, 1987
WARNER CHILCOTT	3.75 MG	N71828 001	MAR 03, 1988
	7.5 MG	N71829 001	MAR 03, 1988
	15 MG	N71830 001	MAR 03, 1988

COBALT CHLORIDE, CO-60; CYANOCOBALAMIN; CYANOCOBALAMIN, CO-60; INTRINSIC FACTOR

N/A; N/A

RUBRATOPE-60 KIT

SQUIBB	N/A;N/A;N/A;N/A	N16090 001

CODEINE PHOSPHATE; *MULTIPLE*

SEE   ACETAMINOPHEN; ASPIRIN; CODEINE PHOSPHATE

SEE   ACETAMINOPHEN; CODEINE PHOSPHATE

COLCHICINE; PROBENECID

TABLET; ORAL

PROBEN-C

CHELSEA	0.5 MG;500 MG	N85552 001

PROBENECID AND COLCHICINE

BEECHAM	0.5 MG;500 MG	N84321 001

PROBENECID W/ COLCHICINE

BOLAR	0.5 MG;500 MG	N83221 001
LEDERLE	0.5 MG;500 MG	N86954 001

COPPER

INTRAUTERINE DEVICE; INTRAUTERINE

CU-7

SEARLE	89 MG	N17408 001

TATUM-T

SEARLE	120 MG	N18205 001

CORTISONE ACETATE

TABLET; ORAL

CORTISONE ACETATE

BARR	25 MG	N83471 001
ELKINS SINN	25 MG	N80836 001
EVERYLIFE	25 MG	N84246 001
LANNETT	25 MG	N80694 001
PANRAY	25 MG	N08284 001
	5 MG	N08284 002
VITARINE	25 MG	N80333 001
WHITE TOWNE	25 MG	N80341 001
PAULSEN	25 MG	N80630 001
ZENITH	25 MG	N83536 001

CRYPTENAMINE ACETATES

INJECTABLE; INJECTION

UNITENSEN

WALLACE	260 CSR UNITS/ML	N08814 001

CRYPTENAMINE TANNATES

TABLET; ORAL

UNITENSEN

WALLACE	260 CSR UNITS	N09217 001

Discontinued Drug Products (continued)

CYANOCOBALAMIN
INJECTABLE; INJECTION
CYANOCOBALAMIN

LUITPOLD	0.03 MG/ML	N80668 001
LYPHOMED	0.03 MG/ML	N80510 003
	1 MG/ML	N80510 002
	0.1 MG/ML	N80510 001
REDISOL	1 MG/ML	N06668 010
MSD		
VI-TWEL		
BERLEX	1 MG/ML	N07012 002

CYANOCOBALAMIN; *MULTIPLE*
SEE ASCORBIC ACID; BIOTIN; CYANOCOBALAMIN; DEXPANTHENOL; ERGOCALCIFEROL; FOLIC ACID; NIACINAMIDE; PYRIDOXINE HYDROCHLORIDE; RIBOFLAVIN PHOSPHATE SODIUM; THIAMINE HYDROCHLORIDE; VITAMIN A PALMITATE; VITAMIN E

SEE COBALT CHLORIDE, CO-60; CYANOCOBALAMIN; CYANOCOBALAMIN, CO-60; INTRINSIC FACTOR

CYANOCOBALAMIN; TANNIC ACID; ZINC ACETATE
INJECTABLE; INJECTION
DEPINAR

ARMOUR	0.5 MG/ML;2.3 MG/ML;1 MG/ML	N11208 001

CYANOCOBALAMIN, CO-60
CAPSULE; ORAL
RUBRATOPE-60

SQUIBB	0.5-1 UCI	N16090 002

CYANOCOBALAMIN, CO-60; *MULTIPLE*
SEE COBALT CHLORIDE, CO-60; CYANOCOBALAMIN; CYANOCOBALAMIN, CO-60; INTRINSIC FACTOR

CYCLOBENZAPRINE HYDROCHLORIDE
TABLET; ORAL
FLEXERIL

MSD	5 MG	N17821 001

CYCLOPENTOLATE HYDROCHLORIDE
SOLUTION/DROPS; OPHTHALMIC
CYCLOPENTOLATE HCL

SOLA BARNES HIND	1%	N84150 001
	1%	N84863 001

CYCLOTHIAZIDE
TABLET; ORAL
FLUIDIL

ADRIA	2 MG	N18173 001

CYCRIMINE HYDROCHLORIDE
TABLET; ORAL
PAGITANE

LILLY	1.25 MG	N08951 001
	2.5 MG	N08951 002

CYPROHEPTADINE HYDROCHLORIDE
SYRUP; ORAL
CYPROHEPTADINE HCL

NASKA	2 MG/5 ML	N89021 001	DEC 21, 1987

TABLET; ORAL
CYPROHEPTADINE HCL

AM THERAP	4 MG	N88798 001	FEB 15, 1985
BOLAR	4 MG	N85245 001	
DURAMED	4 MG	N88232 001	OCT 25, 1983
KV	4 MG	N86737 001	
SUPERPHARM	4 MG	N87405 001	
VITARINE	4 MG	N87284 001	

CYSTEINE HYDROCHLORIDE
INJECTABLE; INJECTION
CYSTEINE HCL

KABIVITRUM	7.25%	N19523 001	OCT 22, 1986

CYTARABINE
INJECTABLE; INJECTION
CYTARABINE

QUAD	100 MG/VIAL	N71248 001	DEC 30, 1987
	500 MG/VIAL	N71249 001	DEC 30, 1987

DACARBAZINE
INJECTABLE; INJECTION
DACARBAZINE

QUAD	100 MG/VIAL	N70821 001	OCT 09, 1986
	200 MG/VIAL	N70822 001	OCT 09, 1986
	500 MG/VIAL	N71563 001	MAY 06, 1988

Discontinued Drug Products (continued)

DANAZOL

CAPSULE; ORAL

DANAZOL			
AM THERAP	200 MG	N71569 001	DEC 30, 1987

DECAMETHONIUM BROMIDE

INJECTABLE; INJECTION

SYNCURINE		
BURROUGHS WELLCOME	1 MG/ML	N06931 002

DEMECLOCYCLINE HYDROCHLORIDE

SYRUP; ORAL

DECLOMYCIN		
LEDERLE	75 MG/5 ML	N50257 001

DESERPIDINE

TABLET; ORAL

HARMONYL		
ABBOTT	0.1 MG	N10796 001

DESERPIDINE; METHYCLOTHIAZIDE

TABLET; ORAL

METHYCLOTHIAZIDE AND DESERPIDINE			
BOLAR	0.25 MG;5 MG	N88486 001	AUG 10, 1984
	0.5 MG;5 MG	N88452 001	AUG 10, 1984

DESIPRAMINE HYDROCHLORIDE

TABLET; ORAL

DESIPRAMINE HCL			
EON LABS	10 MG	N72167 001	FEB 03, 1988
	150 MG	N72254 001	FEB 03, 1988
PHARM BASICS	25 MG	N71864 001	SEP 09, 1987
	50 MG	N71865 001	SEP 09, 1987
	75 MG	N71866 001	SEP 09, 1987
	100 MG	N71867 001	SEP 09, 1987

DESOXIMETASONE

OINTMENT; TOPICAL

TOPICORT			
HOECHST ROUSSEL	0.05%	N18594 001	JAN 17, 1985

DESOXYCORTICOSTERONE ACETATE

INJECTABLE; INJECTION

DOCA		
ORGANON	5 MG/ML	N01104 001

PELLET; IMPLANTATION

PERCORTEN		
CIBA	125 MG	N05151 001

DEXAMETHASONE

TABLET; ORAL

DEXAMETHASONE		
BARR	0.25 MG	N84013 001
	0.25 MG	N84764 001
	0.5 MG	N84084 001
	0.5 MG	N84766 001
	0.75 MG	N84081 001
	0.75 MG	N84765 001
	1.5 MG	N84086 001
	1.5 MG	N84763 001
BOLAR	0.75 MG	N84457 001
CHELSEA	0.75 MG	N85818 001
	1.5 MG	N85840 001
GENEVA	0.75 MG	N80399 001
PHOENIX LABS	0.75 MG	N83806 001
PRIVATE FORM	0.75 MG	N83420 001
ROXANE	0.25 MG	N84614 001
UPSHER SMITH	0.75 MG	N87534 001
	1.5 MG	N87533 001
WHITE TOWNE		
PAULSEN	0.75 MG	N84327 001

DEXAMETHASONE SODIUM PHOSPHATE

INJECTABLE; INJECTION

DEXACEN-4			
CENTRAL PHARMS	EQ 4 MG PHOSPHATE/ML	N84342 001	

DEXAMETHASONE SODIUM PHOSPHATE			
INTL MEDICATION	EQ 20 MG PHOSPHATE/ML	N88522 001	FEB 17, 1984
	EQ 4 MG PHOSPHATE/ML	N89280 001	MAR 18, 1987
QUAD	EQ 4 MG PHOSPHATE/ML	N89282 001	MAR 18, 1987
	EQ 20 MG PHOSPHATE/ML	N89281 001	MAR 18, 1987
	EQ 10 MG PHOSPHATE/ML	N89372 001	MAR 18, 1987
	EQ 24 MG PHOSPHATE/ML	N84173 001	MAR 18, 1987

SOLUTION/DROPS; OPHTHALMIC

DEXAMETHASONE SODIUM PHOSPHATE		
SOLA BARNES HIND	EQ 0.1% PHOSPHATE	N84170 001
	EQ 0.1% PHOSPHATE	N84173 001

Discontinued Drug Products (continued)

DEXBROMPHENIRAMINE MALEATE
SYRUP; ORAL
- DISOMER
  - SCHERING   2 MG/5 ML   N11814 002

TABLET; ORAL
- DISOMER
  - SCHERING   2 MG   N11814 001

DEXBROMPHENIRAMINE MALEATE; PSEUDOEPHEDRINE SULFATE
TABLET; ORAL
- DISOPHROL
  - SCHERING   2 MG;60 MG   N12394 002

TABLET, EXTENDED RELEASE; ORAL
- RESPORAL
  - PIONEER PHARMS   6 MG;120 MG   N89139 001   JUN 16, 1988

DEXPANTHENOL; *MULTIPLE*
SEE   ASCORBIC ACID; BIOTIN; CYANOCOBALAMIN; DEXPANTHENOL; ERGOCALCIFEROL; FOLIC ACID; NIACINAMIDE; PYRIDOXINE HYDROCHLORIDE; RIBOFLAVIN PHOSPHATE SODIUM; THIAMINE HYDROCHLORIDE; VITAMIN A PALMITATE; VITAMIN E

DEXTROAMPHETAMINE SULFATE
CAPSULE; ORAL
- DEXAMPEX
  - LEMMON   15 MG   N85355 001

TABLET; ORAL
- DEXTROAMPHETAMINE SULFATE
  - GENEVA   5 MG   N85370 001
  -    10 MG   N85371 001
  - PUREPAC   5 MG   N84125 001
  - VITARINE   5 MG   N84986 001
  -    10 MG   N85892 001

DEXTROSE
INJECTABLE; INJECTION
- DEXTROSE 10% IN PLASTIC CONTAINER
  - CUTTER   10 GM/100 ML   N18504 001
- DEXTROSE 38.5% IN PLASTIC CONTAINER
  - ABBOTT   38.5 GM/100 ML   N18923 001   SEP 19, 1984
- DEXTROSE 60%
  - MCGAW   60 GM/100 ML   N17995 002   SEP 22, 1982
- DEXTROSE 60% IN PLASTIC CONTAINER
  - MCGAW   60 GM/100 ML   N17995 001

DEXTROSE; *MULTIPLE*
SEE   AMINO ACIDS; DEXTROSE

SEE   AMINO ACIDS; DEXTROSE; MAGNESIUM CHLORIDE; POTASSIUM CHLORIDE; SODIUM CHLORIDE; SODIUM PHOSPHATE, DIBASIC

SEE   AMINO ACIDS; DEXTROSE; MAGNESIUM CHLORIDE; POTASSIUM CHLORIDE; POTASSIUM PHOSPHATE, DIBASIC; SODIUM CHLORIDE

SEE   CALCIUM CHLORIDE; DEXTROSE; MAGNESIUM CHLORIDE; SODIUM ACETATE; SODIUM CHLORIDE

SEE   CALCIUM CHLORIDE; DEXTROSE; MAGNESIUM CHLORIDE; SODIUM CHLORIDE; SODIUM LACTATE

SEE   CALCIUM CHLORIDE; DEXTROSE; POTASSIUM CHLORIDE; SODIUM CHLORIDE; SODIUM LACTATE

SEE   CALCIUM CHLORIDE; DEXTROSE; SODIUM CHLORIDE; SODIUM LACTATE

DEXTROSE; POTASSIUM CHLORIDE; SODIUM CHLORIDE
INJECTABLE; INJECTION
- DEXTROSE 5%, SODIUM CHLORIDE 0.45% AND POTASSIUM CHLORIDE 15 MEQ IN PLASTIC CONTAINER
  - BAXTER   5 GM/100 ML;224 MG/100 ML; 450 MG/100 ML   N18008 003
- DEXTROSE 5%, SODIUM CHLORIDE 0.45% AND POTASSIUM CHLORIDE 20 MEQ (K) IN PLASTIC CONTAINER
  - BAXTER   5 GM/100 ML;300 MG/100 ML; 450 MG/100 ML   N18008 001
- DEXTROSE 5%, SODIUM CHLORIDE 0.45% AND POTASSIUM CHLORIDE 5 MEQ IN PLASTIC CONTAINER
  - BAXTER   5 GM/100 ML;75 MG/100 ML; 450 MG/100 ML   N18008 002

DEXTROSE; SODIUM CHLORIDE
INJECTABLE; INJECTION
- DEXTROSE 3.3% AND SODIUM CHLORIDE 0.3% IN PLASTIC CONTAINER
  - ABBOTT   3.3 GM/100 ML;300 MG/100 ML   N18055 001
- DEXTROSE 5% AND SODIUM CHLORIDE 0.2% IN PLASTIC CONTAINER
  - CUTTER   5 GM/100 ML;200 MG/100 ML   N18399 001
- DEXTROSE 5% AND SODIUM CHLORIDE 0.225% IN PLASTIC CONTAINER
  - ABBOTT   5 GM/100 ML;225 MG/100 ML   N19482 001   OCT 04, 1985
- DEXTROSE 5% AND SODIUM CHLORIDE 0.3% IN PLASTIC CONTAINER
  - ABBOTT   5 GM/100 ML;300 MG/100 ML   N19486 001   OCT 04, 1985
  - CUTTER   5 GM/100 ML;300 MG/100 ML   N18501 001

Discontinued Drug Products (continued)

DEXTROSE; SODIUM CHLORIDE (continued)

INJECTABLE; INJECTION
DEXTROSE 5% AND SODIUM CHLORIDE 0.45% IN PLASTIC CONTAINER
- ABBOTT — 5 GM/100 ML;450 MG/100 ML — N19484 001
- CUTTER — 5 GM/100 ML;450 MG/100 ML — N18400 001 — OCT 04, 1985

DEXTROSE 5% AND SODIUM CHLORIDE 0.9% IN PLASTIC CONTAINER
- ABBOTT — 5 GM/100 ML;900 MG/100 ML — N19483 001
- CUTTER — 5 GM/100 ML;900 MG/100 ML — N18500 001 — OCT 04, 1985

DIATRIZOATE MEGLUMINE

INJECTABLE; INJECTION
CARDIOGRAFIN
- SQUIBB — 85% — N11620 002

DIATRIZOATE MEGLUMINE; DIATRIZOATE SODIUM

INJECTABLE; INJECTION
DIATRIZOATE-60
- INTL MEDICATION — 52%;8% — N88166 001 — JUN 17, 1983

DIATRIZOATE SODIUM

INJECTABLE; INJECTION
MD-50
- MALLINCKRODT — 50% — N87075 001

DIATRIZOATE SODIUM; *MULTIPLE*

SEE   DIATRIZOATE MEGLUMINE; DIATRIZOATE SODIUM

DIAZEPAM

INJECTABLE; INJECTION
DIAZEPAM
- PARKE DAVIS — 5 MG/ML — N71613 001 — OCT 22, 1987
- — 5 MG/ML — N71614 001 — OCT 22, 1987
- US ARMY — 5 MG/ML — N20124 001 — DEC 05, 1990

TABLET; ORAL
DIAZEPAM
- CHELSEA — 2 MG — N70456 001 — NOV 01, 1985
- — 5 MG — N70457 001 — NOV 01, 1985
- — 10 MG — N70458 001 — NOV 01, 1985
- DURAMED — 2 MG — N70894 001 — AUG 27, 1986
- — 5 MG — N70895 001 — AUG 27, 1986

DIAZEPAM (continued)

TABLET; ORAL
DIAZEPAM
- MARTEC — 10 MG — N72402 001 — APR 25, 1989
- — 2 MG — N70787 001 — AUG 02, 1988
- PIONEER PHARMS — 2 MG — N70788 001 — AUG 02, 1988
- — 5 MG — N70776 001 — AUG 02, 1988
- — 10 MG — N70209 001 — AUG 02, 1988
- WARNER CHILCOTT — 2 MG — N70210 001 — SEP 04, 1985
- — 5 MG — N70222 001 — SEP 04, 1985
- — 10 MG — SEP 04, 1985

Q-PAM
- QUANTUM PHARMICS — 2 MG — N70423 001 — DEC 12, 1985
- — 2 MG — N70431 001 — APR 29, 1988
- — 5 MG — N70424 001 — DEC 12, 1985
- — 5 MG — N70432 001 — APR 29, 1988
- — 10 MG — N70425 001 — DEC 12, 1985
- — 10 MG — N70433 001 — APR 29, 1988

DIAZOXIDE

CAPSULE; ORAL
PROGLYCEM
- MEDCL MKTG — 100 MG — N17425 002

DIBUCAINE HYDROCHLORIDE

INJECTABLE; INJECTION
HEAVY SOLUTION NUPERCAINE
- CIBA — 2.5 MG/ML — N06203 001

DICLOXACILLIN SODIUM

POWDER FOR RECONSTITUTION; ORAL
DYNAPEN
- BRISTOL — EQ 62.5 MG BASE/5 ML — N50337 002

DICUMAROL

CAPSULE; ORAL
DICUMAROL
- LILLY — 25 MG — N05509 003
- — 50 MG — N05509 001

TABLET; ORAL
DICUMAROL
- ABBOTT — 100 MG — N05545 005

Discontinued Drug Products (continued)

DICYCLOMINE HYDROCHLORIDE

CAPSULE; ORAL
DICYCLOMINE HCL

	Strength	Appl. No.
BOLAR	10 MG	N83179 001 FEB 12, 1986

TABLET; ORAL
DICYCLOMINE HCL

	Strength	Appl. No.
BOLAR	20 MG	N84361 001 FEB 06, 1986

DIETHYLPROPION HYDROCHLORIDE

TABLET; ORAL
DIETHYLPROPION HCL

	Strength	Appl. No.
CHELSEA	25 MG	N85741 001
EON LABS	25 MG	N85916 001
LEMMON	25 MG	N88642 001 SEP 20, 1984

TENUATE

	Strength	Appl. No.
MERRELL DOW	25 MG	N17668 001

TABLET, EXTENDED RELEASE; ORAL
TENUATE

	Strength	Appl. No.
MERRELL DOW	75 MG	N17669 001

DIETHYLSTILBESTROL

SUPPOSITORY; VAGINAL
DIETHYLSTILBESTROL

	Strength	Appl. No.
LILLY	0.1 MG	N04040 001
	0.5 MG	N04040 002

TABLET; ORAL
DIETHYLSTILBESTROL

	Strength	Appl. No.
LILLY	0.1 MG	N04041 002
	0.5 MG	N04041 003

STILBETIN

	Strength	Appl. No.
SQUIBB	0.1 MG	N04056 007
	0.5 MG	N04056 008
	0.25 MG	N04056 017
	1 MG	N04056 009
	5 MG	N04056 010

TABLET, DELAYED RELEASE; ORAL
DIETHYLSTILBESTROL

	Strength	Appl. No.
LILLY	0.1 MG	N04039 002
	0.25 MG	N04039 005
	0.5 MG	N04039 003

DIFENOXIN HYDROCHLORIDE; *MULTIPLE*

SEE   ATROPINE SULFATE; DIFENOXIN HYDROCHLORIDE

DIFLORASONE DIACETATE

CREAM; TOPICAL
DIFLORASONE DIACETATE

	Strength	Appl. No.
UPJOHN	0.05%	N19259 001 AUG 28, 1985

DIGITOXIN

INJECTABLE; INJECTION
CRYSTODIGIN

	Strength	Appl. No.
LILLY	0.2 MG/ML	N84100 005

DIGOXIN

CAPSULE; ORAL
LANOXICAPS

	Strength	Appl. No.
BURROUGHS WELLCOME	0.15 MG	N18118 004 SEP 24, 1984

INJECTABLE; INJECTION
DIGOXIN

	Strength	Appl. No.
LYPHOMED	0.25 MG/ML	N83217 001

DIHYDROERGOTAMINE MESYLATE; HEPARIN SODIUM; LIDOCAINE HYDROCHLORIDE

INJECTABLE; INJECTION
EMBOLEX

	Strength	Appl. No.
SANDOZ	0.5 MG/0.7 ML;5,000 UNITS/0.7 ML;7.46 MG/0.7 ML	N18885 002 NOV 30, 1984
	0.5 MG/0.5 ML;2,500 UNITS/0.5 ML;5.33 MG/0.5 ML	N18885 001 NOV 30, 1984

DILTIAZEM HYDROCHLORIDE

CAPSULE, EXTENDED RELEASE; ORAL
CARDIZEM SR

	Strength	Appl. No.
MARION MERRELL DOW	180 MG	N19471 004 JAN 23, 1989

DILACOR XR

	Strength	Appl. No.
RHONE POULENC RORER	120 MG	N20092 001 MAY 29, 1992

DIMENHYDRINATE

LIQUID; ORAL
DIMENHYDRINATE

	Strength	Appl. No.
ALRA	12.5 MG/4 ML	N80715 001

TABLET; ORAL
DIMENHYDRINATE

	Strength	Appl. No.
ANABOLICS	50 MG	N85985 001
CHELSEA	50 MG	N85166 001
HEATHER	50 MG	N80841 001

DINOPROST TROMETHAMINE

INJECTABLE; INJECTION
PROSTIN F2 ALPHA

	Strength	Appl. No.
UPJOHN	EQ 5 MG BASE/ML	N17434 001

I/310

Approved Drug Products with Therapeutic Equivalence Evaluations

Discontinued Drug Products (continued)

DIPHEMANIL METHYLSULFATE

TABLET; ORAL

PRANTAL			
SCHERING	100 MG	N08114 004	

DIPHENHYDRAMINE HYDROCHLORIDE

CAPSULE; ORAL

DIPHENHYDRAMINE HCL

ALRA	25 MG	N80519 004	
	50 MG	N80519 003	
ANABOLICS	25 MG	N83634 001	
	50 MG	N83275 001	
BOLAR	25 MG	N83797 001	
	50 MG	N83797 002	
CHELSEA	25 MG	N85138 001	
ELKINS SINN	25 MG	N85701 001	
	50 MG	N85701 002	
HEATHER	25 MG	N84524 001	
	50 MG	N83953 001	
LEDERLE	25 MG	N86874 001	
	50 MG	N86875 001	
PERRIGO	25 MG	N83061 001	
	50 MG	N83061 002	
PIONEER PHARMS	25 MG	N89101 001	DEC 20, 1985
	50 MG	N88880 001	DEC 20, 1985
SUPERPHARM	50 MG	N89041 001	MAY 15, 1985
VANGARD	25 MG	N88034 001	OCT 27, 1982
	50 MG	N87630 001	
WHITE TOWNE PAULSEN	25 MG	N83441 001	
	50 MG	N80800 001	MAY 31, 1985

ELIXIR; ORAL

DIPHEN			
PHARM BASICS	12.5 MG/5 ML	N84640 001	

DIPHENHYDRAMINE HCL

KV	12.5 MG/5 ML	N85621 001	
LEDERLE	12.5 MG/5 ML	N86937 001	
NASKA	12.5 MG/5 ML	N88680 001	MAY 31, 1985
PERRIGO	12.5 MG/5 ML	N83063 001	
PRIVATE FORM	12.5 MG/5 ML	N85287 001	

INJECTABLE; INJECTION

DIPHENHYDRAMINE HCL

ELKINS SINN	50 MG/ML	N83183 001	

DIPHENOXYLATE HYDROCHLORIDE; *MULTIPLE*

SEE ATROPINE SULFATE: DIPHENOXYLATE HYDROCHLORIDE

DISOPYRAMIDE PHOSPHATE

CAPSULE; ORAL

DISOPYRAMIDE PHOSPHATE

BOLAR	EQ 100 MG BASE	N70240 001	FEB 02, 1986
	EQ 150 MG BASE	N70241 001	FEB 02, 1986
INTERPHARM	EQ 100 MG BASE	N71190 001	JAN 15, 1987
	EQ 150 MG BASE	N71191 001	JAN 15, 1987
MYLAN	EQ 100 MG BASE	N70138 001	JUN 14, 1985
	EQ 150 MG BASE	N70139 001	JUN 14, 1985
SUPERPHARM	EQ 150 MG BASE	N70941 001	FEB 09, 1987

DISULFIRAM

TABLET; ORAL

DISULFIRAM

CHELSEA	250 MG	N87973 001	AUG 05, 1983
	500 MG	N87974 001	AUG 05, 1983

DOPAMINE HYDROCHLORIDE

INJECTABLE; INJECTION

DOPAMINE HCL

LYPHOMED	40 MG/ML	N70058 001	MAR 20, 1985
	80 MG/ML	N70059 001	MAR 20, 1985
	160 MG/ML	N70364 001	DEC 04, 1985
SMITH NEPHEW SOLOPAK	40 MG/ML	N70011 001	AUG 29, 1985
WARNER CHILCOTT	80 MG/ML	N70559 001	SEP 20, 1985

DOXEPIN HYDROCHLORIDE

CAPSULE; ORAL

DOXEPIN HCL

BARR	EQ 25 MG BASE	N71502 001	FEB 18, 1988
	EQ 50 MG BASE	N71653 001	FEB 18, 1988
	EQ 75 MG BASE	N71654 001	FEB 18, 1988
	EQ 100 MG BASE	N71521 001	FEB 18, 1988

Discontinued Drug Products (continued)

DOXEPIN HYDROCHLORIDE (continued)

CAPSULE; ORAL

DOXEPIN HCL

CHELSEA

Strength	Appl. No.	Date
EQ 10 MG BASE	N70952 001	MAR 04, 1987
EQ 25 MG BASE	N70953 001	MAY 15, 1986
EQ 50 MG BASE	N70954 001	MAY 15, 1986
EQ 75 MG BASE	N71763 001	FEB 09, 1988
EQ 100 MG BASE	N70955 001	MAY 15, 1986
EQ 150 MG BASE	N71764 001	FEB 09, 1988

PUREPAC

Strength	Appl. No.	Date
EQ 75 MG BASE	N72386 001	SEP 08, 1988
EQ 150 MG BASE	N72387 001	SEP 08, 1988

QUANTUM PHARMICS

Strength	Appl. No.	Date
EQ 10 MG BASE	N70972 001	SEP 29, 1987
EQ 25 MG BASE	N70973 001	SEP 29, 1987
EQ 50 MG BASE	N70931 001	SEP 29, 1987
EQ 75 MG BASE	N70932 001	SEP 29, 1987
EQ 100 MG BASE	N72375 001	MAR 15, 1989
EQ 150 MG BASE	N72376 001	MAR 15, 1989

DOXYCYCLINE HYCLATE

CAPSULE; ORAL

DOXYCYCLINE HYCLATE

EON LABS

Strength	Appl. No.	Date
EQ 50 MG BASE	N62780 001	APR 12, 1988
EQ 100 MG BASE	N62227 001	
EQ 50 MG BASE	N62763 001	SEP 02, 1988

INTERPHARM

Strength	Appl. No.	Date
EQ 100 MG BASE	N62763 002	SEP 02, 1988

SUPERPHARM

Strength	Appl. No.	Date
EQ 50 MG BASE	N62469 001	OCT 31, 1984
EQ 100 MG BASE	N62469 002	OCT 31, 1984

WARNER CHILCOTT

Strength	Appl. No.	Date
EQ 50 MG BASE	N62594 001	DEC 05, 1985
EQ 100 MG BASE	N62594 002	DEC 05, 1985

INJECTABLE; INJECTION

DOXYCYCLINE HYCLATE

QUAD

Strength	Appl. No.	Date
EQ 100 MG BASE/VIAL	N62643 001	FEB 13, 1986
EQ 200 MG BASE/VIAL	N62643 002	FEB 13, 1986

DOXYCYCLINE HYCLATE (continued)

TABLET; ORAL

DOXYCYCLINE HYCLATE

CHELSEA

Strength	Appl. No.	Date
EQ 100 MG BASE	N62392 002	MAR 31, 1983
EQ 50 MG BASE	N62392 001	MAR 31, 1983

INTERPHARM

Strength	Appl. No.	Date
EQ 100 MG BASE	N62764 001	SEP 02, 1988

WARNER CHILCOTT

Strength	Appl. No.	Date
EQ 100 MG BASE	N62593 001	AUG 28, 1985

DOXYLAMINE SUCCINATE

TABLET; ORAL

DECAPRYN

MERRELL DOW

Strength	Appl. No.	Date
25 MG	N06412 014	
12.5 MG	N06412 015	

DOXY-SLEEP-AID

PAR

Strength	Appl. No.	Date
25 MG	N70156 001	JUL 02, 1987

DOXYLAMINE SUCCINATE

QUANTUM PHARMICS

Strength	Appl. No.	Date
25 MG	N88603 001	AUG 07, 1984

DROMOSTANOLONE PROPIONATE

INJECTABLE; INJECTION

DROLBAN

LILLY

Strength	Appl. No.	Date
50 MG/ML	N12936 001	

DROPERIDOL

INJECTABLE; INJECTION

DROPERIDOL

ASTRA

Strength	Appl. No.	Date
2.5 MG/ML	N72020 001	OCT 19, 1988

QUAD

Strength	Appl. No.	Date
2.5 MG/ML	N71942 001	AUG 17, 1988

SMITH NEPHEW SOLOPAK

Strength	Appl. No.	Date
2.5 MG/ML	N71750 001	SEP 06, 1988

DYDROGESTERONE

TABLET; ORAL

GYNOREST

SOLVAY

Strength	Appl. No.	Date
5 MG	N17388 001	
10 MG	N17388 002	

DYPHYLLINE

ELIXIR; ORAL

NEOTHYLLINE

LEMMON

Strength	Appl. No.	Date
160 MG/15 ML	N07794 003	

Discontinued Drug Products (continued)

EDETATE CALCIUM DISODIUM
TABLET; ORAL
CALCIUM DISODIUM VERSENATE

3M	500 MG	N08922 002

EPINEPHRINE; ETIDOCAINE HYDROCHLORIDE
INJECTABLE; INJECTION
DURANEST

ASTRA	0.005 MG/ML;0.5%	N17751 004

EPINEPHRINE; LIDOCAINE HYDROCHLORIDE
INJECTABLE; INJECTION
LIDOCAINE HCL W/ EPINEPHRINE

STERIS	0.01 MG/ML;1%	N85463 001

XYLOCAINE W/ EPINEPHRINE

ASTRA	0.005 MG/ML;1%	N10418 006
	0.005 MG/ML;1.5%	N10418 010
	0.005 MG/ML;2%	N10418 008
	0.02 MG/ML;2%	N06488 005

ERGOCALCIFEROL
CAPSULE; ORAL
VITAMIN D

CHASE	50,000 IU	N80747 001
EVERYLIFE	50,000 IU	N80956 001
VITARINE	50,000 IU	N84053 001

ERGOCALCIFEROL; *MULTIPLE*
SEE ASCORBIC ACID; BIOTIN; CYANOCOBALAMIN; DEXPANTHENOL; ERGOCALCIFEROL; FOLIC ACID; NIACINAMIDE; PYRIDOXINE HYDROCHLORIDE; RIBOFLAVIN PHOSPHATE SODIUM; THIAMINE HYDROCHLORIDE; VITAMIN A PALMITATE; VITAMIN E

ERGOLOID MESYLATES
TABLET; ORAL
ERGOLOID MESYLATES

BOLAR	1 MG	N86433 001 MAY 27, 1982
GERIMAL		
CHELSEA	1 MG	N88207 001 MAR 22, 1984

TABLET; SUBLINGUAL
ALKERGOT

EON LABS	0.5 MG	N85153 001
	1 MG	N87417 001

CIRCANOL

3M	0.5 MG	N84868 001
	1 MG	N85809 001

DEAPRIL-ST

BRISTOL MYERS SQUIBB	1 MG	N85020 002

ERGOLOID MESYLATES (continued)
TABLET; SUBLINGUAL
ERGOLOID MESYLATES

BOLAR	0.5 MG	N84930 001
	1 MG	N85177 001
KV	0.5 MG	N86265 001
	1 MG	N86264 001
LEDERLE	0.5 MG	N86984 001
	1 MG	N86985 001
SUPERPHARM	0.5 MG	N89233 001 SEP 23, 1986
	1 MG	N89234 001 SEP 23, 1986
VANGARD	0.5 MG	N88013 001 SEP 20, 1982
	1 MG	N88014 001 SEP 20, 1982

ERGOTAMINE TARTRATE
TABLET; SUBLINGUAL
ERGOMAR

FISONS	2 MG	N87693 001 FEB 24, 1983

ERYTHROMYCIN
CAPSULE, DELAYED REL PELLETS; ORAL
ERYC 125

PARKE DAVIS	125 MG	N62648 001 OCT 24, 1985

SOLUTION; TOPICAL
ERYTHROMYCIN

BARRE	2%	N62327 001 APR 19, 1982
	2%	N62342 001 FEB 25, 1982
LILLY	2%	N50532 001

TABLET, DELAYED RELEASE; ORAL
R-P MYCIN

SOLVAY	250 MG	N61659 001

ERYTHROMYCIN ETHYLSUCCINATE
SUSPENSION; ORAL
ERYTHROMYCIN ETHYLSUCCINATE

NASKA	EQ 400 MG BASE/5 ML	N62674 001 MAR 10, 1987

ERYTHROMYCIN LACTOBIONATE
INJECTABLE; INJECTION
ERYTHROMYCIN LACTOBIONATE

QUAD	EQ 500 MG BASE/VIAL	N62660 001 NOV 24, 1986
	EQ 1 GM BASE/VIAL	N62660 003 NOV 24, 1986

Discontinued Drug Products (continued)

ERYTHROMYCIN STEARATE

TABLET; ORAL

Product / Firm	Strength	Appl. No.
BRISTAMYCIN — BRISTOL	EQ 250 MG BASE	N61304 001
	EQ 250 MG BASE	N61887 001
ERYPAR — PARKE DAVIS	EQ 250 MG BASE	N62032 001
	EQ 500 MG BASE	N62032 002
ERYTHROCIN STEARATE — ABBOTT	EQ 125 MG BASE	N60359 002
ERYTHROMYCIN STEARATE — LEDERLE	EQ 250 MG BASE	N62089 001
	EQ 500 MG BASE	N62089 002
PFIZER-E — PFIZER	EQ 250 MG BASE	N61791 001
	EQ 500 MG BASE	N61791 002

ESMOLOL HYDROCHLORIDE

INJECTABLE; INJECTION

Product / Firm	Strength	Appl. No.	Date
BREVIBLOC — DUPONT	100 MG/ML	N19386 003	DEC 31, 1986

ESTRADIOL CYPIONATE

INJECTABLE; INJECTION

Product / Firm	Strength	Appl. No.	Date
ESTRADIOL CYPIONATE — QUAD	5 MG/ML	N89310 001	FEB 09, 1987

ESTRADIOL VALERATE; TESTOSTERONE ENANTHATE

INJECTABLE; INJECTION

Product / Firm	Strength	Appl. No.
DELADUMONE OB — SQUIBB	8 MG/ML;180 MG/ML	N09545 002
TESTOSTERONE ENANTHATE AND ESTRADIOL VALERATE — STERIS	8 MG/ML;180 MG/ML	N85860 001

ESTROGENS, CONJUGATED

TABLET; ORAL

Product / Firm	Strength	Appl. No.	Date
CONJUGATED ESTROGENS — ZENITH	0.3 MG	N88569 001	NOV 29, 1984
	0.625 MG	N83373 001	
	1.25 MG	N83601 001	
	2.5 MG	N83602 001	

ESTROGENS, CONJUGATED; MEPROBAMATE

TABLET; ORAL

Product / Firm	Strength	Appl. No.
MILPREM-200 — WALLACE	0.45 MG;200 MG	N11045 002
MILPREM-400 — WALLACE	0.45 MG;400 MG	N11045 001

ESTROGENS, ESTERIFIED

TABLET; ORAL

Product / Firm	Strength	Appl. No.
AMNESTROGEN — SQUIBB	0.625 MG	N83266 002
	1.25 MG	N83266 003
	2.5 MG	N83266 004
	0.3 MG	N83266 001
ESTERIFIED ESTROGENS — GENEVA (PRIVATE FORM)	1.25 MG	N85302 001
	0.625 MG	N83414 001
	1.25 MG	N83765 001
	2.5 MG	N85907 001
EVEX — SYNTEX	0.625 MG	N84215 001
	1.25 MG	N83376 002
FEMOGEN — PRIVATE FORM	0.625 MG	N85076 001
	1.25 MG	N85008 001
	2.5 MG	N85007 001

ESTRONE

INJECTABLE; INJECTION

Product / Firm	Strength	Appl. No.
THEELIN — PARKE DAVIS	1 MG/ML	N03977 001
	5 MG/ML	N03977 003

ETHCHLORVYNOL

CAPSULE; ORAL

Product / Firm	Strength	Appl. No.
PLACIDYL — ABBOTT	100 MG	N10021 004

ETHINYL ESTRADIOL

TABLET; ORAL

Product / Firm	Strength	Appl. No.
FEMINONE — UPJOHN	0.05 MG	N16649 001
LYNORAL — ORGANON	0.05 MG	N05490 002
	0.01 MG	N05490 003

ETHINYL ESTRADIOL; NORETHINDRONE

TABLET; ORAL-21

Product / Firm	Strength	Appl. No.	Date
N.E.E. 1/35 21 — LPI	0.035 MG;1 MG	N71541 001	DEC 14, 1987
ORTHO-NOVUM 7/14-21 — JOHNSON RW	0.035 MG;0.5 MG AND 1 MG	N19004 001	APR 04, 1984

TABLET; ORAL-28

Product / Firm	Strength	Appl. No.	Date
N.E.E. 1/35 28 — LPI	0.035 MG;1 MG	N71542 001	DEC 14, 1987
ORTHO-NOVUM 7/14-28 — JOHNSON RW	0.035 MG;0.5 MG AND 1 MG	N19004 002	APR 04, 1984

Discontinued Drug Products (continued)

ETHINYL ESTRADIOL; NORETHINDRONE ACETATE

TABLET; ORAL-28

NORLESTRIN 28 1/50			
PARKE DAVIS	0.05 MG;1 MG	N16723 001	

ETHOXZOLAMIDE

TABLET; ORAL

CARDASE			
UPJOHN	62.5 MG	N11047 002	
CARDRASE			
UPJOHN	125 MG	N11047 001	
ETHAMIDE			
ALLERGAN	125 MG	N16144 001	

ETHYLESTRENOL

ELIXIR; ORAL

MAXIBOLIN			
ORGANON	2 MG/5 ML	N14006 002	

TABLET; ORAL

MAXIBOLIN			
ORGANON	2 MG	N14005 002	

ETHYNODIOL DIACETATE; MESTRANOL

TABLET; ORAL-20

OVULEN			
SEARLE	1 MG;0.1 MG	N16029 002	

ETIDOCAINE HYDROCHLORIDE

INJECTABLE; INJECTION

DURANEST			
ASTRA	0.5%	N17751 003	

ETIDOCAINE HYDROCHLORIDE; *MULTIPLE*

SEE EPINEPHRINE; ETIDOCAINE HYDROCHLORIDE

ETOPOSIDE

CAPSULE; ORAL

VEPESID			
BRISTOL	100 MG	N19557 002	DEC 30, 1986

FENFLURAMINE HYDROCHLORIDE

TABLET, EXTENDED RELEASE; ORAL

PONDIMIN			
ROBINS	60 MG	N16618 003	JUL 27, 1982

FENOPROFEN CALCIUM

CAPSULE; ORAL

FENOPROFEN CALCIUM			
AM THERAP	EQ 200 MG BASE	N72307 001	AUG 22, 1988
	EQ 300 MG BASE	N72308 001	AUG 22, 1988
HALSEY	EQ 200 MG BASE	N72355 001	JUL 05, 1988
	EQ 300 MG BASE	N72356 001	JUL 05, 1988
QUANTUM PHARMICS	EQ 200 MG BASE	N72214 001	APR 14, 1988
	EQ 300 MG BASE	N71738 001	APR 14, 1988

TABLET; ORAL

FENOPROFEN CALCIUM			
AM THERAP	EQ 600 MG BASE	N72309 001	JUN 16, 1988
HALSEY	EQ 600 MG BASE	N72357 001	JUL 05, 1988
PHARM BASICS	EQ 600 MG BASE	N72362 001	JUN 16, 1988
QUANTUM PHARMICS	EQ 600 MG BASE	N72194 001	APR 14, 1988

FERROUS CITRATE, FE-59

INJECTABLE; INJECTION

FERROUS CITRATE FE 59			
MALLINCKRODT	25 UCI/ML	N16729 001	

FERROUS SULFATE; FOLIC ACID

CAPSULE; ORAL

FOLVRON			
LEDERLE	182 MG;0.33 MG	N06012 003	

FIBRINOGEN, I-125

INJECTABLE; INJECTION

IBRIN			
AMERSHAM	154 UCI/VIAL	N17879 001	

FLOXURIDINE

INJECTABLE; INJECTION

FLOXURIDINE			
QUAD	500 MG/VIAL	N71055 001	AUG 24, 1987

FLUMETHASONE PIVALATE

CREAM; TOPICAL

LOCORTEN			
CIBA	0.03%	N16379 001	

Discontinued Drug Products *(continued)*

FLUOCINOLONE ACETONIDE

CREAM; TOPICAL

FLUOCINOLONE ACETONIDE
- PHARM BASICS
  - 0.01% — N88757 001 — FEB 11, 1985
  - 0.025% — N88756 001 — MAR 28, 1985
- FLUOTREX
- SAVAGE
  - 0.01% — N88174 001 — MAY 06, 1983
  - 0.025% — N88173 001 — MAR 09, 1983

GEL; TOPICAL

FLUONID
- HERBERT
  - 0.025% — N87300 001 — MAY 27, 1982

OINTMENT; TOPICAL

FLUOCINOLONE ACETONIDE
- PHARM BASICS
  - 0.025% — N88742 001 — FEB 08, 1985
- FLUOTREX
- SAVAGE
  - 0.025% — N88172 001 — MAR 09, 1983

SOLUTION; TOPICAL

FLUOTREX
- SAVAGE
  - 0.01% — N88171 001 — MAR 09, 1983

FLUOROMETHOLONE

CREAM; TOPICAL

OXYLONE
- UPJOHN
  - 0.025% — N11748 001

FLUOROURACIL

INJECTABLE; INJECTION

FLUOROURACIL
- QUAD
  - 50 MG/ML — N89368 001 — FEB 03, 1987
  - 50 MG/ML — N89455 001 — FEB 03, 1987
- SMITH NEPHEW SOLOPAK
  - 50 MG/ML — N88766 001 — DEC 28, 1984

FLUOXYMESTERONE

TABLET; ORAL

FLUOXYMESTERONE
- BOLAR
  - 2 MG — N88260 001 — DEC 06, 1983
  - 5 MG — N88265 001 — DEC 06, 1983
  - 10 MG — N88309 001 — DEC 06, 1983
- ORA-TESTRYL
- SQUIBB
  - 2 MG — N11359 001
  - 5 MG — N11359 002

FLUPHENAZINE DECANOATE

INJECTABLE; INJECTION

FLUPHENAZINE
- QUAD
  - 25 MG/ML — N70762 001 — FEB 20, 1986

FLUPHENAZINE HYDROCHLORIDE

INJECTABLE; INJECTION

FLUPHENAZINE HCL
- QUAD
  - 2.5 MG/ML — N89800 001 — JUN 08, 1988

TABLET; ORAL

FLUPHENAZINE HCL
- BOLAR
  - 1 MG — N88555 001 — DEC 18, 1987
  - 2.5 MG — N88544 001 — DEC 18, 1987
  - 5 MG — N88527 001 — DEC 18, 1987
  - 10 MG — N88550 001 — DEC 18, 1987
- PERMITIL
- SCHERING
  - 0.25 MG — N12034 001

FLUPREDNISOLONE

TABLET; ORAL

ALPHADROL
- UPJOHN
  - 1.5 MG — N12259 002

FLURAZEPAM HYDROCHLORIDE

CAPSULE; ORAL

FLURAZEPAM HCL
- PHARM BASICS
  - 15 MG — N70562 001 — JUL 09, 1987
  - 30 MG — N70563 001 — JUL 09, 1987

FOLIC ACID

TABLET; ORAL

FOLIC ACID
- ANABOLICS
  - 1 MG — N84915 001
- BARR
  - 1 MG — N89177 001 — JAN 08, 1986
- BOLAR
  - 1 MG — N83141 001
- BOOTS
  - 1 MG — N84158 001
- CHELSEA
  - 1 MG — N85141 002
- EON LABS
  - 1 MG — N84472 001
- EVERYLIFE
  - 1 MG — N80755 001
- LILLY
  - 1 MG — N06135 003
- PHARM BASICS
  - 1 MG — N87828 001 — MAY 13, 1982

GENTAMICIN SULFATE

SOLUTION/DROPS; OPHTHALMIC
GENTAMICIN SULFATE
PACO   EQ 3 MG BASE/ML   N62932 001   NOV 07, 1988

GENTIAN VIOLET

TAMPON; VAGINAL
GENAPAX
KEY PHARMS   5 MG   N85017 001

GLUCAGON HYDROCHLORIDE

INJECTABLE; INJECTION
GLUCAGON
QUAD   EQ 10 MG BASE/VIAL   N71023 001   MAR 04, 1987

GLUTETHIMIDE

TABLET; ORAL
DORIDEN
RHONE POULENC RORER   500 MG   N09519 005
     250 MG   N09519 002
GLUTETHIMIDE
CHELSEA   500 MG   N85763 001
VITARINE   500 MG   N87297 001

GLYCOPYRROLATE

INJECTABLE; INJECTION
GLYCOPYRROLATE
QUAD   0.2 MG/ML   N89397 001   DEC 09, 1986
ROBINUL
ROBINS   0.2 MG/ML   N14764 001
TABLET; ORAL
GLYCOPYRROLATE
BOLAR   2 MG   N85563 001
     1 MG   N85562 001
CHELSEA   2 MG   N86178 001

GONADORELIN HYDROCHLORIDE

INJECTABLE; INJECTION
FACTREL
WYETH AYERST   EQ 0.2 MG BASE/VIAL   N18123 002   SEP 30, 1982

Discontinued Drug Products (continued)

FOLIC ACID (continued)

TABLET; ORAL
FOLIC ACID
UDL   1 MG   N88199 001   MAR 29, 1983
VANGARD   1 MG   N88730 001   MAR 23, 1984
WHITE TOWNE PAULSEN   1 MG   N80691 002

FOLIC ACID; *MULTIPLE*

SEE   ASCORBIC ACID; BIOTIN; CYANOCOBALAMIN; DEXPANTHENOL; ERGOCALCIFEROL; FOLIC ACID; NIACINAMIDE; PYRIDOXINE HYDROCHLORIDE; RIBOFLAVIN PHOSPHATE SODIUM; THIAMINE HYDROCHLORIDE; VITAMIN A PALMITATE; VITAMIN E

SEE   FERROUS SULFATE; FOLIC ACID

FUROSEMIDE

INJECTABLE; INJECTION
FUROSEMIDE
LYPHOMED   10 MG/ML   N18507 001   JUL 30, 1982
     10 MG/ML   N19036 001   AUG 13, 1984
SMITH NEPHEW SOLOPAK   10 MG/ML   N70023 001   FEB 05, 1986
TABLET; ORAL
FUROSEMIDE
CHELSEA   40 MG   N18369 002   MAY 14, 1982
     20 MG   N18369 001   MAY 14, 1982
EON LABS   40 MG   N18750 002   JUL 30, 1984

GALLIUM CITRATE, GA-67

INJECTABLE; INJECTION
GALLIUM CITRATE GA 67
MEDI PHYSICS   1 MCI/ML   N17700 001

GEMFIBROZIL

CAPSULE; ORAL
LOPID
PARKE DAVIS   200 MG   N18422 001

Discontinued Drug Products (continued)

GONADOTROPIN, CHORIONIC

INJECTABLE; INJECTION

CHORIONIC GONADOTROPIN	Strength	Appl. No.	Date
LYPHOMED	15,000 UNITS/VIAL	N17067 004	
QUAD	5,000 UNITS/VIAL	N89312 001	DEC 04, 1986
	5,000 UNITS/VIAL	N89313 001	DEC 04, 1986
	10,000 UNITS/VIAL	N89314 001	DEC 04, 1986
	10,000 UNITS/VIAL	N89315 001	DEC 04, 1986
	20,000 UNITS/VIAL	N89316 001	DEC 04, 1986
		N17016 009	DEC 04, 1986
STERIS	2,000 UNITS/VIAL		DEC 27, 1984

GUANABENZ ACETATE

TABLET; ORAL

WYTENSIN	Strength	Appl. No.	Date
WYETH AYERST	EQ 16 MG BASE	N18587 003	SEP 07, 1982

GUANETHIDINE MONOSULFATE

TABLET; ORAL

GUANETHIDINE MONOSULFATE	Strength	Appl. No.	Date
BOLAR	EQ 10 MG SULFATE	N86113 001	MAR 26, 1985
	EQ 25 MG SULFATE	N86114 001	MAR 26, 1985

GUANFACINE HYDROCHLORIDE

TABLET; ORAL

TENEX	Strength	Appl. No.	Date
ROBINS	3 MG	N19032 003	NOV 07, 1988

HALCINONIDE

OINTMENT; TOPICAL

HALOG	Strength	Appl. No.	Date
SQUIBB	0.025%	N18125 001	

HALOPERIDOL

TABLET; ORAL

Product / Manufacturer	Strength	Appl. No.	Date
HALDOL SOLUTAB			
JOHNSON RW	1 MG	N17079 001	
HALOPERIDOL			
BOLAR	0.5 MG	N71571 001	JUN 03, 1988
	1 MG	N71572 001	JUN 03, 1988
	2 MG	N71573 001	JUN 03, 1988
	5 MG	N71374 001	JUN 03, 1988
	10 MG	N71375 001	JUN 03, 1988
	20 MG	N71376 001	JUN 03, 1988
DURAMED	0.5 MG	N71216 001	DEC 04, 1986
	1 MG	N71217 001	DEC 04, 1986
	2 MG	N71218 001	DEC 04, 1986
	5 MG	N71219 001	DEC 04, 1986
	10 MG	N71220 001	DEC 04, 1986
	20 MG	N71221 001	JUL 07, 1987
PAR	20 MG	N71328 001	JUL 07, 1987
QUANTUM PHARMICS	0.5 MG	N71255 001	JUL 20, 1987
	1 MG	N71269 001	FEB 17, 1987
	2 MG	N71256 001	FEB 17, 1987
	5 MG	N71257 001	FEB 17, 1987
ROYCE	0.5 MG	N71722 001	FEB 17, 1987
	1 MG	N71723 001	DEC 24, 1987
	2 MG	N71724 001	DEC 24, 1987
	5 MG	N71725 001	DEC 24, 1987
	10 MG	N72121 001	DEC 24, 1987
	20 MG	N72122 001	DEC 24, 1987

Discontinued Drug Products (continued)

HALOPERIDOL LACTATE
INJECTABLE; INJECTION
HALOPERIDOL
- LYPHOMED — EQ 5 MG BASE/ML — N71187 001 — JAN 20, 1987
- QUAD — EQ 5 MG BASE/ML — N71082 001 — JAN 02, 1987
- SMITH NEPHEW SOLOPAK — EQ 5 MG BASE/ML — N70802 001 — DEC 14, 1987

HEPARIN SODIUM
INJECTABLE; INJECTION
HEPARIN LOCK FLUSH
- ABBOTT — 100 UNITS/ML — N05264 010
- INTL MEDICATION — 10 UNITS/ML — N86357 001
- — 500 UNITS/ML — N86357 002
- LUITPOLD — 10 UNITS/ML — N89063 001 — OCT 09, 1985
- — 100 UNITS/ML — N89064 001 — OCT 09, 1985
- LYPHOMED — 100 UNITS/ML — N17651 010
- PARKE DAVIS — 10 UNITS/ML — N17346 006
- SMITH NEPHEW SOLOPAK — 10 UNITS/ML — N87958 001 — APR 20, 1983
- — 100 UNITS/ML — N87959 001 — APR 20, 1983
- STERIS — 100 UNITS/ML — N17064 001

HEPARIN LOCK FLUSH PRESERVATIVE FREE
- LYPHOMED — 10 UNITS/ML — N17029 011 — SEP 22, 1987
- — 100 UNITS/ML — N17029 012 — SEP 22, 1987

HEPARIN LOCK FLUSH PRESERVATIVE FREE IN PLASTIC CONTAINER
- LYPHOMED — 10 UNITS/ML — N17029 008 — SEP 22, 1987
- — 100 UNITS/ML — N17029 009 — SEP 22, 1987

HEPARIN SODIUM
- CHAMBERLIN — 1,000 UNITS/ML — N17130 001
- — 5,000 UNITS/ML — N17130 002
- — 10,000 UNITS/ML — N17130 003
- — 20,000 UNITS/ML — N17130 004
- LUITPOLD — 1,000 UNITS/ML — N87452 001 — OCT 31, 1983
- LYPHOMED — 1,000 UNITS/ML — N17033 001
- — 1,000 UNITS/ML — N17651 005
- — 5,000 UNITS/ML — N17029 002
- — 5,000 UNITS/ML — N17979 003
- — 10,000 UNITS/ML — N17651 003
- — 20,000 UNITS/ML — N17651 008
- PARKE DAVIS — 1,000 UNITS/ML — N17346 001
- — 5,000 UNITS/ML — N17346 002
- — 7,500 UNITS/ML — N17346 003
- — 10,000 UNITS/ML — N17346 004
- — 20,000 UNITS/ML — N17346 005

HEPARIN SODIUM (continued)
INJECTABLE; INJECTION
HEPARIN SODIUM
- PHARM SPEC STERIS — 40,000 UNITS/ML — N17780 005
- — 7,500 UNITS/ML — N17064 019
- — 2,500 UNITS/ML — N17064 015
- — 3,000 UNITS/ML — N17064 016
- — 4,000 UNITS/ML — N17064 017
- — 6,000 UNITS/ML — N17064 018
- WYETH AYERST — 15,000 UNITS/ML — N17007 005

HEPARIN SODIUM 10,000 UNITS IN DEXTROSE 5% IN PLASTIC CONTAINER
- ABBOTT — 10,000 UNITS/100 ML — N19339 003 — MAR 27, 1985
- BAXTER — 2,000 UNITS/100 ML — N18814 002 — JUL 09, 1985

HEPARIN SODIUM 10,000 UNITS IN SODIUM CHLORIDE 0.45%
- ABBOTT — 10,000 UNITS/100 ML — N18911 001 — JAN 30, 1985

HEPARIN SODIUM 10,000 UNITS IN SODIUM CHLORIDE 0.45% IN PLASTIC CONTAINER
- ABBOTT — 10,000 UNITS/100 ML — N18916 005 — JAN 31, 1984

HEPARIN SODIUM 10,000 UNITS IN SODIUM CHLORIDE 0.9%
- ABBOTT — 10,000 UNITS/100 ML — N18911 003 — JAN 30, 1985

HEPARIN SODIUM 10,000 UNITS IN SODIUM CHLORIDE 0.9% IN PLASTIC CONTAINER
- ABBOTT — 10,000 UNITS/100 ML — N18916 002 — JAN 31, 1984

HEPARIN SODIUM 12,500 UNITS IN DEXTROSE 5% IN PLASTIC CONTAINER
- ABBOTT — 5,000 UNITS/100 ML — N19339 001 — MAR 27, 1985

HEPARIN SODIUM 12,500 UNITS IN SODIUM CHLORIDE 0.9%
- ABBOTT — 5,000 UNITS/100 ML — N18911 005 — JAN 30, 1985

HEPARIN SODIUM 12,500 UNITS IN SODIUM CHLORIDE 0.9% IN PLASTIC CONTAINER
- ABBOTT — 5,000 UNITS/100 ML — N18916 003 — JAN 31, 1984

HEPARIN SODIUM 25,000 UNITS IN DEXTROSE 5% IN PLASTIC CONTAINER
- ABBOTT — 5,000 UNITS/100 ML — N19339 004 — MAR 27, 1985
- — 10,000 UNITS/100 ML — N19339 002 — MAR 27, 1985

HEPARIN SODIUM 25,000 UNITS IN SODIUM CHLORIDE 0.9%
- ABBOTT — 5,000 UNITS/100 ML — N18911 004 — JAN 30, 1985

HEPARIN SODIUM 25,000 UNITS IN SODIUM CHLORIDE 0.9% IN PLASTIC CONTAINER
- ABBOTT — 5,000 UNITS/100 ML — N18916 009 — JAN 31, 1984

HEPARIN SODIUM 25000 UNITS IN SODIUM CHLORIDE 0.9% IN PLASTIC CONTAINER
- MCGAW — 5,000 UNITS/100 ML — N19135 001 — MAR 29, 1985

Discontinued Drug Products (continued)

HEPARIN SODIUM (continued)

INJECTABLE; INJECTION

HEPARIN SODIUM 5,000 UNITS IN SODIUM CHLORIDE 0.45% IN PLASTIC CONTAINER

ABBOTT	100 UNITS/ML	N18916 004	JAN 31, 1984

HEPARIN SODIUM 5000 UNITS AND SODIUM CHLORIDE 0.9% IN PLASTIC CONTAINER

BAXTER	500 UNITS/100 ML	N18609 003	APR 28, 1982

HEPARIN SODIUM 5000 UNITS IN SODIUM CHLORIDE 0.45%

ABBOTT	100 UNITS/ML	N18911 002	JAN 30, 1985

HEPARIN SODIUM 5000 UNITS IN SODIUM CHLORIDE 0.9% IN PLASTIC CONTAINER

ABBOTT	1,000 UNITS/100 ML	N18916 001	JAN 31, 1984
MCGAW	1,000 UNITS/100 ML	N19042 004	MAR 29, 1985

LIPO-HEPIN

3M	1,000 UNITS/ML	N17027 006
	5,000 UNITS/ML	N17027 008
	5,000 UNITS/0.5 ML	N17027 002
	10,000 UNITS/ML	N17027 009
	7,500 UNITS/0.5 ML	N17027 010
	10,000 UNITS/0.5 ML	N17027 003
	20,000 UNITS/ML	N17027 007
	20,000 UNITS/0.5 ML	N17027 004
	40,000 UNITS/ML	N17027 005
	1,000 UNITS/0.5 ML	N17027 001
	15,000 UNITS/0.5 ML	N17027 011

LIQUAEMIN SODIUM PRESERVATIVE FREE

ORGANON	1,000 UNITS/ML	N00552 011	APR 11, 1986
	5,000 UNITS/ML	N00552 012	APR 11, 1986
	10,000 UNITS/ML	N00552 013	APR 11, 1986

PANHEPRIN

ABBOTT	1,000 UNITS/ML	N05264 004
	5,000 UNITS/ML	N05264 006
	10,000 UNITS/ML	N05264 007
	20,000 UNITS/ML	N05264 008
	40,000 UNITS/ML	N05264 009

SODIUM HEPARIN

LYPHOMED	5,000 UNITS/ML	N17033 002
	10,000 UNITS/ML	N17033 003
	20,000 UNITS/ML	N17033 004

HEPARIN SODIUM; *MULTIPLE*

SEE DIHYDROERGOTAMINE MESYLATE; HEPARIN SODIUM; LIDOCAINE HYDROCHLORIDE

HETACILLIN

POWDER FOR RECONSTITUTION; ORAL

VERSAPEN

BRISTOL	EQ 112.5 MG AMPICIL/ML	N50060 003
	EQ 112.5 MG AMPICIL/ML	N61398 001
	EQ 112.5 MG AMPICIL/5 ML	N50060 001
	EQ 225 MG AMPICIL/5 ML	N61398 002

HETACILLIN POTASSIUM

CAPSULE; ORAL

VERSAPEN-K

BRISTOL	EQ 450 MG AMPICIL	N61396 002
	EQ 225 MG AMPICIL	N61396 001

HEXACHLOROPHENE

EMULSION; TOPICAL

SOY-DOME

MILES	3%	N17405 001

SOLUTION; TOPICAL

SEPTI-SOFT

CALGON	0.25%	N17460 001

SEPTISOL

VESTAL	0.25%	N17423 001

HEXOCYCLIUM METHYLSULFATE

TABLET; ORAL

TRAL

ABBOTT	25 MG	N10599 001

HEXYLCAINE HYDROCHLORIDE

SOLUTION; TOPICAL

CYCLAINE

MSD	5%	N08472 001

HOMATROPINE METHYLBROMIDE

TABLET, CHEWABLE; ORAL

EQUIPIN

MISSION PHARMA	3 MG	N86310 001

HYDRALAZINE HYDROCHLORIDE

INJECTABLE; INJECTION

HYDRALAZINE HCL

LYPHOMED	20 MG/ML	N89532 001	AUG 11, 1987
SMITH NEPHEW	20 MG/ML	N88517 001	AUG 22, 1985
SOLOPAK	20 MG/ML	N88518 001	APR 20, 1984

Discontinued Drug Products (continued)

HYDRALAZINE HYDROCHLORIDE (continued)
TABLET; ORAL

HYDRALAZINE HCL

Firm	Strength	Appl No	Date
ASCOT	25 MG	N88310 001	DEC 19, 1984
	50 MG	N88311 001	DEC 19, 1984
CHELSEA	25 MG	N85532 002	MAY 24, 1982
	50 MG	N85533 002	MAY 25, 1982
EON LABS	50 MG	N85088 001	
PHARM BASICS	25 MG	N87780 001	MAR 29, 1982
	50 MG	N87751 001	MAR 29, 1982
PUREPAC	50 MG	N88178 001	AUG 15, 1983
QUANTUM PHARMICS	10 MG	N86671 001	
	25 MG	N88657 001	MAY 01, 1984
	50 MG	N88652 001	JUN 15, 1984
	100 MG	N88686 001	MAY 08, 1984
SUPERPHARM	10 MG	N88787 001	MAY 01, 1984
	25 MG	N88788 001	AUG 28, 1984
	50 MG	N88789 001	AUG 28, 1984
VANGARD	25 MG	N87712 001	AUG 28, 1984
	50 MG	N87908 001	
VITARINE	25 MG	N86088 001	MAY 07, 1982
WEST WARD	25 MG	N88240 001	MAY 27, 1983
	50 MG	N88241 001	MAY 27, 1983

HYDRALAZINE HYDROCHLORIDE; HYDROCHLOROTHIAZIDE
CAPSULE; ORAL

HYDRALAZINE HCL AND HYDROCHLOROTHIAZIDE

Firm	Strength	Appl No	Date
BOLAR	25 MG;25 MG	N85457 001	MAR 04, 1982
	100 MG;50 MG	N85440 001	MAR 04, 1982
CHELSEA	50 MG;50 MG	N85446 001	MAR 04, 1982
SOLVAY	100 MG;50 MG	N87609 001	FEB 08, 1982
SUPERPHARM	25 MG;25 MG	N89200 001	FEB 09, 1987

HYDRALAZINE HCL W/ HYDROCHLOROTHIAZIDE 100/50

Firm	Strength	Appl No	Date
ZENITH	100 MG;50 MG	N88358 001	APR 10, 1984

HYDRALAZINE HYDROCHLORIDE; HYDROCHLOROTHIAZIDE
(continued)
TABLET; ORAL

HYDRALAZINE AND HYDROCHLORTHIAZIDE

Firm	Strength	Appl No
CHELSEA	25 MG;15 MG	N85827 001

HYDROCHLOROTHIAZIDE W/ HYDRALAZINE

Firm	Strength	Appl No
BOLAR	25 MG;15 MG	N85373 001

HYDRALAZINE HYDROCHLORIDE; HYDROCHLOROTHIAZIDE; RESERPINE
TABLET; ORAL

HYDRALAZINE HCL-HYDROCHLOROTHIAZIDE-RESERPINE

Firm	Strength	Appl No
MYLAN	25 MG;15 MG;0.1 MG	N87085 001

HYDRALAZINE, HYDROCHLOROTHIAZIDE W/ RESERPINE

Firm	Strength	Appl No
CHELSEA	25 MG;15 MG;0.1 MG	N85771 001

HYDRAP-ES

Firm	Strength	Appl No
EON LABS	25 MG;15 MG;0.1 MG	N84876 001

HYDROCHLOROTHIAZIDE W/ RESERPINE AND HYDRALAZINE

Firm	Strength	Appl No
BOLAR	25 MG;15 MG;0.1 MG	N83770 001

RESERPINE, HYDROCHLOROTHIAZIDE, AND HYDRALAZINE HCL

Firm	Strength	Appl No	Date
LEDERLE	25 MG;15 MG;0.1 MG	N87709 001	MAY 13, 1982

SER-A-GEN

Firm	Strength	Appl No
SOLVAY	25 MG;15 MG;0.1 MG	N87210 001

UNIPRES

Firm	Strength	Appl No
SOLVAY	25 MG;15 MG;0.1 MG	N85893 001

HYDRALAZINE HYDROCHLORIDE; RESERPINE
TABLET; ORAL

DRALSERP

Firm	Strength	Appl No
EON LABS	25 MG;0.1 MG	N84617 001

HYDROCHLOROTHIAZIDE
TABLET; ORAL

HYDROCHLOROTHIAZIDE

Firm	Strength	Appl No	Date
ALRA	25 MG	N86369 001	
	50 MG	N83554 001	
ASCOT	25 MG	N87539 001	FEB 03, 1982
BOLAR	25 MG	N83458 001	
	50 MG	N83456 001	
	100 MG	N85099 001	
CHELSEA	25 MG	N85232 002	
	50 MG	N85233 001	
	50 MG	N86087 001	
	50 MG	N86594 001	
	100 MG	N87002 001	
ELKINS SINN	50 MG	N85152 002	
HEATHER	50 MG	N84135 001	
MYLAN	25 MG	N84880 001	
	50 MG	N85112 001	
PHARM BASICS	25 MG	N87827 001	APR 19, 1982
		N87752 001	APR 19, 1982
	50 MG		APR 19, 1982

Discontinued Drug Products (continued)

HYDROCHLOROTHIAZIDE (continued)

TABLET; ORAL

HYDROCHLOROTHIAZIDE

Manufacturer	Strength	Number	Date
ROXANE	25 MG	N85004 001	
	50 MG	N85005 001	
SOLVAY	25 MG	N85323 001	
VANGARD	25 MG	N87638 001	
	50 MG	N87610 001	
WARNER CHILCOTT	25 MG	N87586 001	MAY 03, 1982
	50 MG	N87587 001	MAY 03, 1982
WHITE TOWNE PAULSEN	25 MG	N83809 002	
	50 MG	N83809 001	
	100 MG	N85347 001	
ZIDE SOLVAY	50 MG	N83925 001	

HYDROCHLOROTHIAZIDE; *MULTIPLE*

SEE HYDRALAZINE HYDROCHLORIDE; HYDROCHLOROTHIAZIDE
SEE HYDRALAZINE HYDROCHLORIDE; HYDROCHLOROTHIAZIDE; RESERPINE
SEE HYDRALAZINE HYDROCHLORIDE; HYDROCHLOROTHIAZIDE

HYDROCHLOROTHIAZIDE; LABETALOL HYDROCHLORIDE

TABLET; ORAL

Manufacturer	Strength	Number	Date
NORMOZIDE SCHERING	25 MG;400 MG	N19046 004	APR 06, 1987
TRANDATE HCT GLAXO	25 MG;400 MG	N19174 004	APR 10, 1987

HYDROCHLOROTHIAZIDE; METHYLDOPA

TABLET; ORAL

METHYLDOPA AND HYDROCHLOROTHIAZIDE

Manufacturer	Strength	Number	Date
BOLAR	50 MG;500 MG	N70368 001	APR 16, 1986
	15 MG;250 MG	N70365 001	MAR 19, 1986
	25 MG;250 MG	N70366 001	APR 16, 1986
	30 MG;500 MG	N70367 001	MAR 19, 1986
PUREPAC	50 MG;500 MG	N70689 001	APR 24, 1986

HYDROCHLOROTHIAZIDE; PINDOLOL

TABLET; ORAL

VISKAZIDE

Manufacturer	Strength	Number	Date
SANDOZ	25 MG;5 MG	N18872 001	JUL 22, 1987
	25 MG;10 MG	N18872 002	JUL 22, 1987

HYDROCHLOROTHIAZIDE; PROPRANOLOL HYDROCHLORIDE

TABLET; ORAL

PROPRANOLOL HCL & HYDROCHLOROTHIAZIDE

Manufacturer	Strength	Number	Date
DURAMED	25 MG;40 MG	N71126 001	MAR 02, 1987
	25 MG;80 MG	N71127 001	MAR 02, 1987

HYDROCHLOROTHIAZIDE; RESERPINE

TABLET; ORAL

Manufacturer	Strength	Number	Date
H.R.-50 WHITE TOWNE PAULSEN	50 MG;0.125 MG	N85338 001	
HYDRO-SERP "25" EON LABS	25 MG;0.125 MG	N84827 001	
HYDRO-SERP "50" EON LABS	50 MG;0.125 MG	N85213 001	

HYDROCHLOROTHIAZIDE W/ RESERPINE

Manufacturer	Strength	Number	Date
BOLAR	25 MG;0.125 MG	N85317 001	
	25 MG;0.125 MG	N83666 001	
CHELSEA	50 MG;0.125 MG	N86330 002	
	25 MG;0.125 MG	N86331 001	
PHARMAFAIR	25 MG;0.125 MG	N85421 001	
	50 MG;0.125 MG	N85420 001	

RESERPINE AND HYDROCHLOROTHIAZIDE

Manufacturer	Strength	Number	Date
BARR	25 MG;0.125 MG	N84580 001	
	50 MG;0.125 MG	N84579 001	
GENEVA	50 MG;0.125 MG	N88200 001	JAN 31, 1984
SERPASIL-ESIDRIX #1 CIBA	25 MG;0.1 MG	N11878 003	
SERPASIL-ESIDRIX #2 CIBA	50 MG;0.1 MG	N11878 005	

HYDROCHLOROTHIAZIDE; SPIRONOLACTONE

TABLET; ORAL

SPIRONOLACTONE + HYDROCHLOROTHIAZIDE

Manufacturer	Strength	Number	Date
ASCOT	25 MG;25 MG	N88025 001	NOV 23, 1984

SPIRONOLACTONE AND HYDROCHLOROTHIAZIDE

Manufacturer	Strength	Number	Date
SUPERPHARM	25 MG;25 MG	N89137 001	AUG 26, 1985

SPIRONOLACTONE W/ HYDROCHLOROTHIAZIDE

Manufacturer	Strength	Number	Date
BOLAR	25 MG;25 MG	N85974 001	
CHELSEA	25 MG;25 MG	N86026 001	
LEDERLE	25 MG;25 MG	N87511 001	
PHARM BASICS	25 MG;25 MG	N87651 001	
PUREPAC	25 MG;25 MG	N88054 001	AUG 18, 1983
VANGARD	25 MG;25 MG	N87655 001	

Discontinued Drug Products *(continued)*

HYDROCHLOROTHIAZIDE; TRIAMTERENE

CAPSULE; ORAL
TRIAMTERENE AND HYDROCHLOROTHIAZIDE

VITARINE	25 MG;50 MG	N71737 001	FEB 12, 1988

TABLET; ORAL
TRIAMTERENE AND HYDROCHLOROTHIAZIDE

AM THERAP	50 MG;75 MG	N72022 001	NOV 03, 1987
		N71980 001	
QUANTUM PHARMICS	50 MG;75 MG		FEB 01, 1988

HYDROCODONE BITARTRATE; *MULTIPLE*

SEE   ACETAMINOPHEN; HYDROCODONE BITARTRATE
SEE   ASPIRIN; HYDROCODONE BITARTRATE

HYDROCORTAMATE HYDROCHLORIDE

OINTMENT; TOPICAL
MAGNACORT

PFIZER	0.5%	N10554 001

HYDROCORTISONE

CREAM; TOPICAL
ELDECORT

ELDER	1%	N80459 001	
	2.5%	N84055 001	
H-CORT			
PHARM ASSOC	0.5%	N86823 001	
HC #1			
MILES	0.5%	N80438 001	
HC #4			
MILES	1%	N80438 002	
HYDROCORTISONE			
EVERYLIFE	0.5%	N80452 001	
NASKA	1%	N89706 001	MAR 10, 1988
PHARM BASICS	1%	N88027 001	SEP 27, 1983
	2.5%	N88029 001	SEP 27, 1983
STIEFEL	1%	N86170 001	
THAMES	0.5%	N86154 001	
WHITE TOWNE	1%	N80496 002	
PAULSEN			
SYNACORT			
SYNTEX	0.5%	N87459 001	

HYDROCORTISONE *(continued)*

LOTION; TOPICAL
CORT-DOME

MILES	0.5%	N09895 003	
	1%	N09895 001	
H-CORT			
PHARM ASSOC	0.5%	N86824 001	
HYDROCORTISONE			
BARRE	0.5%	N87317 001	JUN 07, 1982
	1%	N87315 001	JUN 07, 1982
NASKA	1%	N89705 001	APR 25, 1988

OINTMENT; TOPICAL
HC (HYDROCORTISONE)

C AND M	0.5%	N80481 001

HYDROCORTISONE

ALTANA	0.5%	N80489 002	
NASKA	1%	N89704 001	MAR 10, 1988
PHARM BASICS	1%	N88061 001	SEP 27, 1983
	2.5%	N88039 001	SEP 27, 1983
THAMES	0.5%	N86256 001	

TABLET; ORAL
CORTRIL

PFIZER	10 MG	N09127 005	
	20 MG	N09127 003	
HYDROCORTISONE			
ANABOLICS	20 MG	N83140 001	
BARR	20 MG	N83999 001	
ELKINS SINN	20 MG	N80624 001	
EON LABS	20 MG	N80642 002	
PANRAY	10 MG	N09659 001	
	20 MG	N09659 002	
PARKE DAVIS	20 MG	N84243 001	
PUREPAC	20 MG	N80395 001	
ROXANE	10 MG	N88539 001	MAR 21, 1984
WHITE TOWNE	10 MG	N80344 001	
PAULSEN	20 MG	N80344 002	

HYDROCORTISONE; *MULTIPLE*

SEE   ACETIC ACID, GLACIAL; HYDROCORTISONE
SEE   CLIOQUINOL; HYDROCORTISONE

Discontinued Drug Products *(continued)*

HYDROCORTISONE ACETATE
INJECTABLE; INJECTION

CORTEF ACETATE			
UPJOHN	50 MG/ML	N09378 002	
CORTRIL			
PFIZER	25 MG/ML	N09164 001	

OINTMENT; OPHTHALMIC, OTIC

HYDROCORTONE			
MSD	1.5%	N09018 003	

HYDROCORTISONE ACETATE; NEOMYCIN SULFATE
OINTMENT; OPHTHALMIC

NEO-CORTEF			
UPJOHN	0.5%;EQ 3.5 MG BASE/GM	N60610 001	
	1.5%;EQ 3.5 MG BASE/GM	N60610 002	

HYDROCORTISONE BUTYRATE
CREAM; TOPICAL

LOCOID			
OWEN GALDERMA	0.1%	N18795 001	JAN 07, 1983

OINTMENT; TOPICAL

LOCOID			
BROCADES PHARMA	0.1%	N18652 001	OCT 29, 1982

SOLUTION; TOPICAL

LOCOID			
OWEN GALDERMA	0.1%	N19819 001	SEP 15, 1988

HYDROCORTISONE SODIUM PHOSPHATE
INJECTABLE; INJECTION

HYDROCORTISONE SODIUM PHOSPHATE			
QUAD	EQ 50 MG BASE/ML	N89581 001	MAY 28, 1987

HYDROCORTISONE SODIUM SUCCINATE
INJECTABLE; INJECTION

HYDROCORTISONE SODIUM SUCCINATE			
LYPHOMED	EQ 100 MG BASE/VIAL	N88667 001	JUN 08, 1984
	EQ 100 MG BASE/VIAL	N88712 001	JUN 08, 1984
	EQ 250 MG BASE/VIAL	N88668 001	JUN 08, 1984
	EQ 500 MG BASE/VIAL	N88669 001	JUN 08, 1984
	EQ 1 GM BASE/VIAL	N88670 001	JUN 08, 1984

HYDROFLUMETHIAZIDE
TABLET; ORAL

HYDROFLUMETHIAZIDE			
BOLAR	50 MG	N88031 001	APR 06, 1983
CHELSEA	50 MG	N88528 001	AUG 15, 1984

HYDROFLUMETHIAZIDE; RESERPINE
TABLET; ORAL

HYDROFLUMETHIAZIDE AND RESERPINE			
PHARM BASICS	50 MG;0.125 MG	N88195 001	OCT 26, 1983
HYDROFLUMETHIAZIDE W/ RESERPINE			
BOLAR	50 MG;0.125 MG	N88110 001	MAR 22, 1983
	25 MG;0.125 MG	N88127 001	MAR 22, 1983

HYDROXOCOBALAMIN
INJECTABLE; INJECTION

HYDROXOCOBALAMIN			
LYPHOMED	1 MG/ML	N84921 001	

HYDROXYPROGESTERONE CAPROATE
INJECTABLE; INJECTION

HYDROXYPROGESTERONE CAPROATE			
QUAD	125 MG/ML	N89330 001	JAN 02, 1987
	250 MG/ML	N89331 001	JAN 02, 1987

HYDROXYSTILBAMIDINE ISETHIONATE
INJECTABLE; INJECTION

HYDROXYSTILBAMIDINE ISETHIONATE			
MERRELL DOW	225 MG/AMP	N09166 001	

HYDROXYZINE HYDROCHLORIDE
INJECTABLE; INJECTION

HYDROXYZINE HCL			
ALTANA	25 MG/ML	N87273 001	APR 20, 1982
	50 MG/ML	N87273 002	APR 20, 1982
PHARMAFAIR	25 MG/ML	N88862 001	FEB 14, 1986
	25 MG/ML	N89106 001	FEB 14, 1986
	50 MG/ML	N89107 001	FEB 14, 1986
SMITH NEPHEW SOLOPAK	25 MG/ML	N87592 001	

Discontinued Drug Products *(continued)*

HYDROXYZINE HYDROCHLORIDE *(continued)*

TABLET; ORAL
HYDROXYZINE HCL

Firm	Strength	Appl. No.	Approval Date
BARR	10 MG	N88409 001	NOV 15, 1983
	25 MG	N87857 001	APR 18, 1983
	50 MG	N87860 001	APR 18, 1983
	100 MG	N87862 001	APR 18, 1983
PHARM BASICS	10 MG	N89121 001	MAR 20, 1986
	25 MG	N89122 001	MAR 20, 1986
	50 MG	N89123 001	MAR 20, 1986
QUANTUM PHARMICS	10 MG	N88540 001	OCT 22, 1985
	25 MG	N88551 001	OCT 22, 1985
	50 MG	N88529 001	OCT 22, 1985

HYDROXYZINE PAMOATE

CAPSULE; ORAL
HY-PAM "25"

Firm	Strength	Appl. No.	Approval Date
LEMMON	EQ 25 MG HCL	N88713 001	MAR 04, 1985

HYDROXYZINE PAMOATE

Firm	Strength	Appl. No.	Approval Date
BOLAR	EQ 25 MG HCL	N86698 001	
	EQ 50 MG HCL	N86695 001	
	EQ 100 MG HCL	N86697 001	
	EQ 100 MG HCL	N86728 001	OCT 05, 1982
CHELSEA	EQ 25 MG HCL	N88593 001	FEB 29, 1984
DURAMED	EQ 50 MG HCL	N88594 001	FEB 29, 1984
	EQ 100 MG HCL	N88595 001	FEB 29, 1984
PAR	EQ 25 MG HCL	N87656 001	JUN 11, 1982
	EQ 25 MG HCL	N89145 001	MAR 17, 1986
	EQ 50 MG HCL	N87657 001	
	EQ 50 MG HCL	N89146 001	JUN 11, 1982
	EQ 100 MG HCL	N87658 001	MAR 17, 1986
SUPERPHARM	EQ 25 MG HCL	N89031 001	JUN 11, 1982
	EQ 50 MG HCL	N89032 001	JAN 02, 1987
	EQ 100 MG HCL	N89033 001	JAN 02, 1987
VANGARD	EQ 25 MG HCL	N88392 001	SEP 19, 1983

IBUPROFEN

TABLET; ORAL
IBUPROFEN

Firm	Strength	Appl. No.	Approval Date
BOOTS	800 MG	N71264 001	JUL 25, 1986
CHELSEA	200 MG	N71765 001	SEP 04, 1987
	400 MG	N70038 001	SEP 06, 1985
	600 MG	N70041 001	SEP 06, 1985
	800 MG	N71911 001	OCT 13, 1987
MCNEIL	300 MG	N71338 001	DEC 01, 1986
	400 MG	N70081 001	JUN 16, 1986
	600 MG	N70476 001	JUN 16, 1986
SUPERPHARM	600 MG	N70709 001	APR 25, 1986
ZENITH	200 MG	N72040 001	APR 29, 1988

NUPRIN

Firm	Strength	Appl. No.	Approval Date
UPJOHN	200 MG	N19012 001	MAY 18, 1984
	200 MG	N19012 003	JUL 29, 1987

RUFEN

Firm	Strength	Appl. No.	Approval Date
BOOTS	600 MG	N18197 002	MAR 05, 1984

IMIPRAMINE HYDROCHLORIDE

TABLET; ORAL
IMIPRAMINE HCL

Firm	Strength	Appl. No.	Approval Date
BOLAR	10 MG	N85220 001	
	25 MG	N84252 002	
	50 MG	N85221 001	
CHELSEA	10 MG	N85875 001	
	25 MG	N85878 001	
	50 MG	N85877 001	
LEDERLE	10 MG	N86269 001	
	25 MG	N86267 001	
	50 MG	N86268 001	
PHARM BASICS	25 MG	N87776 001	FEB 10, 1982
VANGARD	10 MG	N88036 001	NOV 03, 1982
	25 MG	N87619 001	FEB 09, 1982
	50 MG	N87631 001	JAN 04, 1982
WEST WARD	25 MG	N88222 001	MAY 26, 1983
	50 MG	N88223 001	MAY 26, 1983

Discontinued Drug Products (continued)

IMIPRAMINE HYDROCHLORIDE (continued)
TABLET; ORAL
PRAMINE
ALRA

10 MG	N83827 001
25 MG	N83827 002
50 MG	N83827 003

PRESAMINE
RHONE POULENC RORER

10 MG	N11836 006
25 MG	N11836 003
50 MG	N11836 007

INDOCYANINE GREEN
INJECTABLE; INJECTION
CARDIO-GREEN
BECTON DICKINSON

10 MG/VIAL	N11525 003
40 MG/VIAL	N11525 004

INDOMETHACIN
CAPSULE; ORAL
INDOMETHACIN
BOLAR

25 MG	N70784 001	AUG 20, 1986
50 MG	N70785 001	AUG 20, 1986

DURAMED

25 MG	N70326 001	OCT 18, 1985
50 MG	N70327 001	OCT 18, 1985

EON LABS

25 MG	N71711 001	JUL 05, 1988
50 MG	N71712 001	JUL 05, 1988

ROXANE

25 MG	N70353 001	JUN 18, 1985
50 MG	N70354 001	JUN 18, 1985

SUPERPHARM

25 MG	N70487 001	OCT 10, 1986
50 MG	N70488 001	OCT 10, 1986

ZENITH

25 MG	N18730 001	MAY 04, 1984
50 MG	N18730 002	MAY 04, 1984

INSULIN PORK
INJECTABLE; INJECTION
INSULIN
NOVO NORDISK

40 UNITS/ML	N17926 001

INSULIN SUSP ISOPHANE PURIFIED PORK
INJECTABLE; INJECTION
NPH ILETIN II (PORK)
LILLY

100 UNITS/ML	N18345 001

INSULIN SUSP PROTAMINE ZINC PURIFIED PORK
INJECTABLE; INJECTION
PROTAMINE ZINC AND ILETIN II (PORK)
LILLY

100 UNITS/ML	N18346 001

INSULIN ZINC SUSP BEEF
INJECTABLE; INJECTION
LENTE INSULIN
NOVO NORDISK

40 UNITS/ML	N17998 001

INSULIN ZINC SUSP EXTENDED BIOSYNTHETIC HUMAN
INJECTABLE; INJECTION
HUMULIN U
LILLY

40 UNITS/ML	N19571 001	JUN 10, 1987

INSULIN ZINC SUSP PURIFIED BEEF/PORK
INJECTABLE; INJECTION
LENTARD
NOVO NORDISK

100 UNITS/ML	N18384 001

INTRINSIC FACTOR; *MULTIPLE*
SEE   COBALT CHLORIDE, CO-60; CYANOCOBALAMIN; CYANOCOBALAMIN, CO-60; INTRINSIC FACTOR

IODIPAMIDE SODIUM
INJECTABLE; INJECTION
CHOLOGRAFIN SODIUM
SQUIBB

20%	N09321 001

IODOXAMATE MEGLUMINE
INJECTABLE; INJECTION
CHOLOVUE
SQUIBB

9.9%	N18077 001
40.3%	N18076 001

IOPHENDYLATE
INJECTABLE; INJECTION
PANTOPAQUE
ALCON

100%	N05319 001

ISONIAZID (continued)

TABLET; ORAL

ISONIAZID			
ANABOLICS	100 MG	N84050 001	
BOLAR	100 MG	N80401 001	
	300 MG	N83178 001	
CHELSEA	100 MG	N85790 001	
	300 MG	N85784 001	
LILLY	100 MG	N08499 002	
	300 MG	N08499 003	
PANRAY	50 MG	N08428 001	
	100 MG	N08428 002	
	300 MG	N08428 003	
PERRIGO	100 MG	N83060 001	
PUREPAC	50 MG	N80132 003	JUL 14, 1982
	100 MG	N80132 004	JUL 14, 1982
WHITE TOWNE			
PAULSEN	100 MG	N80120 002	
NYDRAZID			
SQUIBB	100 MG	N08392 003	
STANOZIDE			
EVERYLIFE	100 MG	N80126 001	

ISOPROTERENOL HYDROCHLORIDE

AEROSOL; INHALATION

NORISODRINE AEROTROL		
ABBOTT	0.25%	N16814 001

INJECTABLE; INJECTION

ISOPROTERENOL HCL		
LYPHOMED	0.2 MG/ML	N83431 001

SOLUTION; INHALATION

ISOPROTERENOL HCL			
ARMOUR	0.031%	N87935 001	NOV 18, 1982
	0.062%	N87936 001	NOV 18, 1982
DEY	0.5%	N86764 001	JAN 04, 1982

ISOPROTERENOL HYDROCHLORIDE; *MULTIPLE*

SEE ACETYLCYSTEINE; ISOPROTERENOL HYDROCHLORIDE

ISOPROTERENOL SULFATE

POWDER; INHALATION

NORISODRINE		
ABBOTT	10%	N06905 003
	25%	N06905 002

Discontinued Drug Products (continued)

IRON DEXTRAN

INJECTABLE; INJECTION

PROFERDEX		
FISONS	EQ 50 MG IRON/ML	N17807 001

ISOETHARINE HYDROCHLORIDE

SOLUTION; INHALATION

BRONKOSOL			
STERLING	0.25%	N12339 009	
ISOETHARINE HCL			
ASTRA	0.25%	N88472 001	MAR 14, 1984
	0.25%	N88470 001	
	0.167%	N88471 001	MAR 14, 1984
	0.2%	N88144 001	MAR 14, 1984
BAXTER	0.08%	N88146 001	JUL 29, 1983
	0.25%	N88145 001	AUG 01, 1983
	0.14%	N88187 001	MAR 26, 1984
DEY	0.08%	N88188 001	DEC 03, 1982
	0.25%	N87389 001	DEC 03, 1982
	0.1%	N87390 001	
	0.17%	N86763 001	
	1%		

ISONIAZID

INJECTABLE; INJECTION

ISONIAZID			
QUAD	100 MG/ML	N89816 001	OCT 28, 1988
RIMIFON			
ROCHE	100 MG/ML	N08420 003	
	25 MG/ML	N08420 002	

SYRUP; ORAL

RIMIFON		
ROCHE	50 MG/5 ML	N08420 001

TABLET; ORAL

DOW-ISONIAZID		
DOW	300 MG	N80330 002

Discontinued Drug Products (continued)

ISOSORBIDE DINITRATE
TABLET; ORAL
ISOSORBIDE DINITRATE

SUPERPHARM	5 MG	N89190 001	FEB 17, 1987
	10 MG	N89191 001	FEB 17, 1987
	20 MG	N89192 001	FEB 17, 1987

KANAMYCIN SULFATE
INJECTABLE; INJECTION
KANAMYCIN SULFATE

INTL MEDICATION	EQ 500 MG BASE/2 ML	N62466 001	SEP 30, 1983
	EQ 1 GM BASE/3 ML	N62466 002	SEP 30, 1983
QUAD	EQ 500 MG BASE/2 ML	N62642 002	FEB 03, 1986
	EQ 1 GM BASE/3 ML	N62642 003	FEB 03, 1986
	EQ 75 MG BASE/2 ML	N62642 001	FEB 03, 1986
WARNER CHILCOTT	EQ 1 GM BASE/3 ML	N63092 001	OCT 11, 1989

KETAMINE HYDROCHLORIDE
INJECTABLE; INJECTION
KETAMINE HCL

QUAD	EQ 10 MG BASE/ML	N71949 001	APR 11, 1988
	EQ 50 MG BASE/ML	N71950 001	APR 11, 1988
	EQ 100 MG BASE/ML	N71951 001	APR 11, 1988

KETOCONAZOLE
SUSPENSION; ORAL
NIZORAL

JANSSEN	100 MG/5 ML	N70767 001	NOV 07, 1986

LABETALOL HYDROCHLORIDE
TABLET; ORAL
NORMODYNE

SCHERING	400 MG	N18687 004	AUG 01, 1984

TRANDATE

GLAXO	400 MG	N18716 004	AUG 01, 1984

LABETALOL HYDROCHLORIDE; *MULTIPLE*
SEE HYDROCHLOROTHIAZIDE; LABETALOL HYDROCHLORIDE

LACTULOSE
SYRUP; ORAL, RECTAL
LACTULOSE

SOLVAY	10 GM/15 ML	N17906 001

LEUCOVORIN CALCIUM
INJECTABLE; INJECTION
LEUCOVORIN CALCIUM

LYPHOMED	EQ 50 MG BASE/VIAL	N88939 001	DEC 01, 1986
QUAD	EQ 50 MG BASE/VIAL	N89496 001	MAR 05, 1987
	EQ 5 MG BASE/ML	N89503 001	OCT 05, 1987
	EQ 5 MG BASE/ML	N89504 001	DEC 22, 1987
	EQ 100 MG BASE/VIAL	N89636 001	DEC 24, 1987

TABLET; ORAL
LEUCOVORIN CALCIUM

PAR	EQ 5 MG BASE	N71600 001	OCT 14, 1987
	EQ 25 MG BASE	N71598 001	OCT 14, 1987

LEVALLORPHAN TARTRATE
INJECTABLE; INJECTION
LORFAN

ROCHE	1 MG/ML	N10423 001

LEVODOPA
CAPSULE; ORAL
BENDOPA

ICN	100 MG	N16948 003
	250 MG	N16948 001
	500 MG	N16948 002

LARODOPA

ROCHE	100 MG	N16912 002
	250 MG	N16912 001
	500 MG	N16912 006

LEVONORGESTREL
IMPLANT; IMPLANTATION
NORPLANT

POPULATION COUNCIL	36 MG/IMPLANT	N19897 001	DEC 10, 1990

Discontinued Drug Products (continued)

LEVOPROPOXYPHENE NAPSYLATE, ANHYDROUS

CAPSULE; ORAL
NOVRAD

LILLY	EQ 50 MG BASE	N12928 006
	EQ 100 MG BASE	N12928 004

SUSPENSION; ORAL
NOVRAD

LILLY	EQ 50 MG BASE/5 ML	N12928 002

LIDOCAINE HYDROCHLORIDE

INJECTABLE; INJECTION
LIDOCAINE HCL

ABBOTT	1.5%	N88330 001	MAY 17, 1984
CUTTER	1%	N80414 001	
	2%	N80414 002	
ELKINS SINN	4%	N84626 001	
	0.5%	N85131 001	
INTL MEDICATION	4%	N17702 002	
	1 GM/VIAL	N18543 001	
	2 GM/VIAL	N18543 002	
LYPHOMED	1%	N80420 001	
	1.5%	N80420 005	
	2%	N80420 002	
SEARLE	1%	N83135 001	
	2%	N83135 002	
STERIS	1%	N83627 001	
	2%	N83627 002	

LIDOCAINE HCL 0.1% AND DEXTROSE 5% IN PLASTIC CONTAINER

BAXTER	100 MG/100 ML	N18461 001

LIDOCAINE HCL 0.2% IN DEXTROSE 5% IN PLASTIC CONTAINER

ABBOTT	200 MG/100 ML	N18954 001	JUL 09, 1985

XYLOCAINE

ASTRA	1%	N10418 005
	1.5%	N10418 009
	2%	N10418 007

SOLUTION; TOPICAL
LARYNGOTRACHEAL ANESTHESIA KIT

KENDALL	4%	N87931 001	JUN 10, 1983

LIDOCAINE HCL

PACO	4%	N89688 001	JUN 30, 1989

LIDOCAINE HYDROCHLORIDE; *MULTIPLE*

SEE   DIHYDROERGOTAMINE MESYLATE; HEPARIN SODIUM; LIDOCAINE HYDROCHLORIDE

SEE   EPINEPHRINE; LIDOCAINE HYDROCHLORIDE

LIDOCAINE HYDROCHLORIDE; OXYTETRACYCLINE

INJECTABLE; INJECTION
TERRAMYCIN

PFIZER	2%;50 MG/ML	N60567 001
	2%;125 MG/ML	N60567 002

LINCOMYCIN HYDROCHLORIDE

INJECTABLE; INJECTION
LINCOMYCIN HCL

QUAD	EQ 300 MG BASE/ML	N62784 001	MAR 14, 1988

LINDANE

LOTION; TOPICAL
GAMENE

SOLA BARNES HIND	1%	N84989 001

SHAMPOO; TOPICAL
GAMENE

SOLA BARNES HIND	1%	N84988 001

LIOTHYRONINE SODIUM

TABLET; ORAL
LIOTHYRONINE SODIUM

BOLAR	EQ 0.025 MG BASE	N85755 001	JAN 25, 1982
	EQ 0.05 MG BASE	N85753 001	FEB 03, 1982

LIOTRIX (T4;T3)

TABLET; ORAL
THYROLAR-5
RHONE POULENC

RORER	0.25 MG;0.0625 MG	N16807 006

LITHIUM CARBONATE

CAPSULE; ORAL
LITHIUM CARBONATE

BOLAR	300 MG	N70407 001	MAR 19, 1987
PHARM BASICS	300 MG	N72542 001	FEB 01, 1989

TABLET; ORAL
LITHANE

ROERIG	300 MG	N16834 001

Discontinued Drug Products (continued)

LOPERAMIDE HYDROCHLORIDE
CAPSULE; ORAL
  IMODIUM
    JANSSEN   2 MG   N17690 001
SOLUTION; ORAL
  IMODIUM
    JANSSEN   1 MG/5 ML   N19037 001 JUL 31, 1984

LORAZEPAM
TABLET; ORAL
  LORAZ
    QUANTUM PHARMICS   0.5 MG   N70200 001 AUG 09, 1985
                        1 MG   N70201 001 AUG 09, 1985
                        2 MG   N70202 001 AUG 09, 1985
  LORAZEPAM
    AM THERAP   0.5 MG   N70727 001 MAR 07, 1986
                 1 MG   N70728 001 MAR 07, 1986
                 2 MG   N70729 001 MAR 07, 1986
    PHARM BASICS   1 MG   N70539 001 DEC 22, 1986
                    2 MG   N70540 001 DEC 22, 1986

LOXAPINE SUCCINATE
TABLET; ORAL
  LOXITANE
    LEDERLE   EQ 10 MG BASE   N17525 006
               EQ 25 MG BASE   N17525 007
               EQ 50 MG BASE   N17525 008

MAGNESIUM ACETATE; *MULTIPLE*
SEE AMINO ACIDS: MAGNESIUM ACETATE: PHOSPHORIC ACID: POTASSIUM ACETATE: SODIUM CHLORIDE
SEE AMINO ACIDS: MAGNESIUM ACETATE: POTASSIUM ACETATE: SODIUM CHLORIDE
SEE AMINO ACIDS: MAGNESIUM ACETATE: POTASSIUM ACETATE: SODIUM CHLORIDE: SODIUM PHOSPHATE, DIBASIC

MAGNESIUM CHLORIDE; *MULTIPLE*
SEE AMINO ACIDS: DEXTROSE: MAGNESIUM CHLORIDE: POTASSIUM CHLORIDE: SODIUM CHLORIDE: SODIUM PHOSPHATE, DIBASIC
SEE AMINO ACIDS: DEXTROSE: MAGNESIUM CHLORIDE: POTASSIUM CHLORIDE: POTASSIUM PHOSPHATE, DIBASIC: SODIUM CHLORIDE
SEE CALCIUM CHLORIDE: DEXTROSE: MAGNESIUM CHLORIDE: SODIUM ACETATE: SODIUM CHLORIDE
SEE CALCIUM CHLORIDE: DEXTROSE: MAGNESIUM CHLORIDE: SODIUM CHLORIDE: SODIUM LACTATE
SEE CALCIUM CHLORIDE: MAGNESIUM CHLORIDE: POTASSIUM CHLORIDE: SODIUM ACETATE: SODIUM CHLORIDE

MAGNESIUM CHLORIDE; POTASSIUM CHLORIDE; SODIUM ACETATE; SODIUM CHLORIDE; SODIUM GLUCONATE
SOLUTION; IRRIGATION
  PHYSIOSOL IN PLASTIC CONTAINER
    ABBOTT   14 MG/100 ML;37 MG/100 ML;222 MG/100 ML;526 MG/100 ML;502 MG/100 ML   N18406 001

MAGNESIUM METRIZOATE; *MULTIPLE*
SEE CALCIUM METRIZOATE: MAGNESIUM METRIZOATE: MEGLUMINE METRIZOATE: METRIZOATE SODIUM

MANNITOL
INJECTABLE; INJECTION
  MANNITOL 10%
    CUTTER   10 GM/100 ML   N16472 002
  MANNITOL 15%
    CUTTER   15 GM/100 ML   N16472 005
  MANNITOL 20%
    CUTTER   20 GM/100 ML   N16472 004
  MANNITOL 25%
    MSD   12.5 GM/50 ML   N05620 001
SOLUTION; IRRIGATION
  RESECTISOL
    MCGAW   5 GM/100 ML   N16704 002

MANNITOL; SORBITOL
SOLUTION; IRRIGATION
  SORBITOL-MANNITOL
    ABBOTT   540 MG/100 ML;2.7 GM/100 ML   N80224 001

Discontinued Drug Products *(continued)*

MAPROTILINE HYDROCHLORIDE

TABLET; ORAL

MAPROTILINE HCL

Firm	Strength	Appl. No.	Approval Date
AM THERAP	25 MG	N72129 001	JAN 14, 1988
	50 MG	N72130 001	JAN 14, 1988
	75 MG	N72131 001	JAN 14, 1988
BOLAR	25 MG	N71943 001	DEC 30, 1987
	50 MG	N71944 001	DEC 30, 1987
	75 MG	N71945 001	DEC 30, 1987

MAZINDOL

TABLET; ORAL

MAZANOR

Firm	Strength	Appl. No.	Approval Date
WYETH AYERST	2 MG	N17980 001	

MEBUTAMATE

TABLET; ORAL

DORMATE

Firm	Strength	Appl. No.	Approval Date
WALLACE	600 MG	N17374 001	

MECLIZINE HYDROCHLORIDE

TABLET; ORAL

MECLIZINE HCL

Firm	Strength	Appl. No.	Approval Date
ANABOLICS	25 MG	N85891 001	
	12.5 MG	N85195 001	
BOLAR	12.5 MG	N89113 001	AUG 20, 1985
SUPERPHARM	25 MG	N89114 001	AUG 20, 1985
UDL	12.5 MG	N88256 001	
	25 MG	N88257 001	JUN 13, 1983
VANGARD	12.5 MG	N87877 001	JUN 13, 1983
	25 MG	N87620 001	APR 20, 1982
			JAN 04, 1982

TABLET, CHEWABLE; ORAL

MECLIZINE HCL

Firm	Strength	Appl. No.	Approval Date
ANABOLICS	25 MG	N86392 001	

MECLOFENAMATE SODIUM

CAPSULE; ORAL

MECLODIUM

Firm	Strength	Appl. No.	Approval Date
QUANTUM PHARMICS	EQ 50 MG BASE	N71380 001	JUL 14, 1987
	EQ 100 MG BASE	N71381 001	JUL 14, 1987

MECLOFENAMATE SODIUM

Firm	Strength	Appl. No.	Approval Date
AM THERAP	EQ 50 MG BASE	N71362 001	FEB 10, 1987
	EQ 100 MG BASE	N71363 001	FEB 10, 1987
BOLAR	EQ 50 MG BASE	N70400 001	NOV 25, 1986
	EQ 100 MG BASE	N70401 001	NOV 25, 1986
CHELSEA	EQ 50 MG BASE	N71640 001	AUG 11, 1987
	EQ 100 MG BASE	N71641 001	AUG 11, 1987
PAR	EQ 50 MG BASE	N72077 001	MAR 10, 1988
	EQ 100 MG BASE	N72078 001	MAR 10, 1988
PHARM BASICS	EQ 50 MG BASE	N71007 001	MAR 25, 1988
	EQ 100 MG BASE	N71008 001	MAR 25, 1988
VITARINE	EQ 50 MG BASE	N71710 001	JUN 15, 1988
	EQ 100 MG BASE	N71684 001	JUN 15, 1988

MEFENAMIC ACID

CAPSULE; ORAL

MEFENAMIC ACID

Firm	Strength	Appl. No.	Approval Date
EON LABS	250 MG	N72179 001	APR 21, 1988

MEFLOQUINE HYDROCHLORIDE

TABLET; ORAL

MEFLOQUINE HCL

Firm	Strength	Appl. No.	Approval Date
US ARMY	250 MG	N19578 001	MAY 02, 1989

MEGESTROL ACETATE

TABLET; ORAL

MEGESTROL ACETATE

Firm	Strength	Appl. No.	Approval Date
PHARM BASICS	20 MG	N70646 001	OCT 02, 1987
	40 MG	N70647 001	OCT 02, 1987

Discontinued Drug Products (continued)

MEGLUMINE; *MULTIPLE*
SEE   CALCIUM: MEGLUMINE: METRIZOIC ACID

MEGLUMINE METRIZOATE; *MULTIPLE*
SEE   CALCIUM METRIZOATE: MAGNESIUM METRIZOATE: MEGLUMINE METRIZOATE: METRIZOATE SODIUM

MENADIOL SODIUM DIPHOSPHATE
INJECTABLE; INJECTION
  KAPPADIONE
    LILLY   10 MG/ML   N05725 001

MENADIONE
TABLET; ORAL
  MENADIONE
    LILLY   5 MG   N02139 003

MEPENZOLATE BROMIDE
SOLUTION; ORAL
  CANTIL
    MERRELL DOW   25 MG/5 ML   N10679 004

MEPERIDINE HYDROCHLORIDE
INJECTABLE; INJECTION
  MEPERIDINE HCL
    ELKINS SINN   25 MG/ML   N88279 001   JUN 15, 1984
       50 MG/ML   N88280 001   JUN 15, 1984
       75 MG/ML   N88281 001   JUN 15, 1984
       100 MG/ML   N88282 001   JUN 15, 1984
  INTL MEDICATION
    KNOLL   10 MG/ML   N86332 001
       25 MG/ML   N80388 001
       50 MG/ML   N80385 001
       50 MG/ML   N80387 001
       75 MG/ML   N80389 001
       100 MG/ML   N80386 001
    PARKE DAVIS   50 MG/ML   N80364 002
       75 MG/ML   N80364 003
       100 MG/ML   N80364 001

MEPERIDINE HYDROCHLORIDE; *MULTIPLE*
SEE   ATROPINE SULFATE: MEPERIDINE HYDROCHLORIDE

MEPREDNISONE
TABLET; ORAL
  BETAPAR
    SCHERING   4 MG   N16053 002

MEPROBAMATE
CAPSULE; ORAL
  EQUANIL
    WYETH AYERST   400 MG   N12455 002
TABLET; ORAL
  BAMATE
    ALRA   200 MG   N80380 001
       400 MG   N80380 002
  MEPROBAMATE
    ANABOLICS   200 MG   N84220 001
       400 MG   N84589 001
       600 MG   N85719 001
    CHELSEA   200 MG   N15426 002
    ELKINS SINN   400 MG   N15426 001
    HEATHER   600 MG   N84329 001
    ICN   200 MG   N15139 006
       400 MG   N15139 005
    LEDERLE   400 MG   N86299 001
    MALLARD   400 MG   N15072 002
    PARKE DAVIS   200 MG   N84744 001
       400 MG   N84744 002
    PERRIGO   200 MG   N84546 001
       400 MG   N84547 001
    PHARM BASICS   200 MG   N87825 001   MAR 18, 1982
       400 MG   N87826 001   MAR 18, 1982
    PHARMAFAIR   400 MG   N84153 001
    PRIVATE FORM   400 MG   N14601 001
    SOLVAY   200 MG   N84435 001
    STANLABS   200 MG   N14474 002
    VANGARD   400 MG   N14474 004
       400 MG   N88011 001
    WHITE TOWNE PAULSEN   200 MG   JUL 14, 1982
       400 MG   N83830 001
         N83442 001
  TRANMEP
    SOLVAY   400 MG   N84369 001

MEPROBAMATE; *MULTIPLE*
SEE   ASPIRIN: MEPROBAMATE
SEE   ESTROGENS, CONJUGATED: MEPROBAMATE

Discontinued Drug Products (continued)

MESTRANOL; *MULTIPLE*
SEE   ETHYNODIOL DIACETATE; MESTRANOL

MESTRANOL; NORETHINDRONE
TABLET; ORAL-21
NORINYL 1+80 21-DAY		
SYNTEX	0.08 MG;1 MG	N16724 001
ORTHO-NOVUM 1/80 21		
JOHNSON RW	0.08 MG;1 MG	N16715 001
ORTHO-NOVUM 10-21		
JOHNSON RW	0.06 MG;10 MG	N12728 001
ORTHO-NOVUM 2-21		
JOHNSON RW	0.1 MG;2 MG	N12728 005

TABLET; ORAL-28
NORINYL 1+80 28-DAY		
SYNTEX	0.08 MG;1 MG	N16725 001
ORTHO-NOVUM 1/80 28		
JOHNSON RW	0.08 MG;1 MG	N16715 002

MESTRANOL; NORETHYNODREL
TABLET; ORAL-20
ENOVID		
SEARLE	0.075 MG;5 MG	N10976 004
ENOVID-E		
SEARLE	0.1 MG;2.5 MG	N10976 006

TABLET; ORAL-21
| ENOVID-E 21 | | |
| SEARLE | 0.1 MG;2.5 MG | N10976 007 |

METAPROTERENOL SULFATE
SOLUTION; INHALATION
METAPROTERENOL SULFATE		
DEY	0.33%	N71806 001
		AUG 05, 1988

TABLET; ORAL
METAPROTERENOL SULFATE		
AM THERAP	10 MG	N72054 001
		JUN 23, 1988
	20 MG	N72055 001
		JUN 23, 1988
PHARM BASICS	10 MG	N71013 001
		JAN 25, 1988
	20 MG	N71014 001
		JAN 25, 1988

METARAMINOL BITARTRATE
INJECTABLE; INJECTION
METARAMINOL BITARTRATE		
ELKINS SINN	EQ 10 MG BASE/ML	N83363 001
SEARLE	EQ 10 MG BASE/ML	N86418 001
	EQ 20 MG BASE/ML	N86418 002

METHADONE HYDROCHLORIDE
TABLET, DISPERSIBLE; ORAL
WESTADONE		
EON LABS	2.5 MG	N17108 001
	5 MG	N17108 002
	10 MG	N17108 003
	40 MG	N17108 004

METHARBITAL
TABLET; ORAL
| GEMONIL | | |
| ABBOTT | 100 MG | N08322 001 |

METHDILAZINE HYDROCHLORIDE
SYRUP; ORAL
| METHDILAZINE HCL | | |
| BARRE | 4 MG/5 ML | N87122 001 |

METHICILLIN SODIUM
INJECTABLE; INJECTION
STAPHCILLIN		
BRISTOL	EQ 900 MG BASE/VIAL	N50117 001
	EQ 3.6 GM BASE/VIAL	N50117 002
	EQ 5.4 GM BASE/VIAL	N50117 003

METHIXENE HYDROCHLORIDE
TABLET; ORAL
| TREST | | |
| SANDOZ | 1 MG | N13420 001 |

METHOCARBAMOL
TABLET; ORAL
METHOCARBAMOL		
AM THERAP	500 MG	N89417 001
		FEB 11, 1987
	750 MG	N89418 001
		FEB 11, 1987
ASCOT	500 MG	N87660 001
		OCT 27, 1982
	750 MG	N87661 001
		OCT 27, 1982
BARR	500 MG	N84488 001
BOLAR	500 MG	N83605 001
	750 MG	N83605 002
HEATHER	500 MG	N84675 001
	750 MG	N84924 001
MYLAN	500 MG	N84259 001
	750 MG	N84323 001
PHARMAFAIR	500 MG	N84231 002
	750 MG	N84471 001
ROXANE	500 MG	N88646 001
		FEB 29, 1984
	750 MG	N88647 001
		FEB 29, 1984

Discontinued Drug Products (continued)

METHOTREXATE SODIUM
INJECTABLE; INJECTION
METHOTREXATE SODIUM

Firm	Strength	Number	Date
LYPHOMED	EQ 25 MG BASE/ML	N89322 001	JUN 13, 1986
	EQ 20 MG BASE/VIAL	N88935 001	OCT 11, 1985
	EQ 50 MG BASE/VIAL	N88936 001	OCT 11, 1985
	EQ 100 MG BASE/VIAL	N88937 001	OCT 11, 1985
	EQ 2.5 MG BASE/ML	N89323 001	JUN 13, 1986
QUAD	EQ 25 MG BASE/ML	N89308 001	JUL 10, 1986
	EQ 25 MG BASE/ML	N89309 001	JUL 10, 1986
	EQ 20 MG BASE/VIAL	N89293 001	JUL 10, 1986
	EQ 50 MG BASE/VIAL	N89294 001	JUL 10, 1986
	EQ 100 MG BASE/VIAL	N89295 001	JUL 10, 1986
	EQ 250 MG BASE/VIAL	N89296 001	JUL 10, 1986

METHOXAMINE HYDROCHLORIDE
INJECTABLE; INJECTION
VASOXYL

Firm	Strength	Number	Date
BURROUGHS WELLCOME	10 MG/ML	N06772 002	

METHOXSALEN
CAPSULE; ORAL
METHOXSALEN

Firm	Strength	Number	Date
GENEVA	10 MG	N87781 001	JUN 08, 1982

METHYCLOTHIAZIDE
TABLET; ORAL
METHYCLOTHIAZIDE

Firm	Strength	Number	Date
BOLAR	2.5 MG	N85487 001	MAR 11, 1982
	5 MG	N85476 001	MAR 11, 1982
CHELSEA	2.5 MG	N88750 001	SEP 06, 1984
MYLAN	2.5 MG	N87671 001	AUG 17, 1982
PHARM BASICS	5 MG	N88745 001	MAR 21, 1985

METHYCLOTHIAZIDE; *MULTIPLE*
SEE DESERPIDINE; METHYCLOTHIAZIDE

METHYCLOTHIAZIDE; PARGYLINE HYDROCHLORIDE
TABLET; ORAL
EUTRON

Firm	Strength	Number	Date
ABBOTT	5 MG;25 MG	N16047 001	

METHYLDOPA
TABLET; ORAL
METHYLDOPA

Firm	Strength	Number	Date
BOLAR	125 MG	N70245 001	FEB 25, 1986
	250 MG	N70246 001	FEB 25, 1986
	500 MG	N70247 001	FEB 25, 1986
CHELSEA	125 MG	N70260 001	JUN 24, 1985
	250 MG	N70261 001	JUN 24, 1985
	500 MG	N70262 001	JUN 24, 1985
DURAMED	250 MG	N71006 001	DEC 16, 1986
	500 MG	N71009 001	DEC 16, 1986
PARKE DAVIS	125 MG	N70331 001	APR 15, 1986
	250 MG	N70332 001	APR 15, 1986
	500 MG	N70333 001	APR 15, 1986
ROXANE	125 MG	N70192 001	APR 25, 1986
	250 MG	N70193 001	APR 25, 1986
	500 MG	N70194 001	APR 25, 1986

METHYLDOPA; *MULTIPLE*
SEE HYDROCHLOROTHIAZIDE; METHYLDOPA

METHYLDOPATE HYDROCHLORIDE
INJECTABLE; INJECTION
METHYLDOPATE HCL

Firm	Strength	Number	Date
QUAD	50 MG/ML	N71024 001	SEP 18, 1986

Discontinued Drug Products (continued)

METHYLPREDNISOLONE

TABLET; ORAL

METHYLPREDNISOLONE

Firm	Strength	Appl. No.	Date
CHELSEA	16 MG	N86159 001	FEB 09, 1982
EON LABS	4 MG	N87341 001	

METHYLPREDNISOLONE; NEOMYCIN SULFATE

OINTMENT; OPHTHALMIC

NEO-MEDROL

Firm	Strength	Appl. No.
UPJOHN	0.1%;EQ 3.5 MG BASE/GM	N60645 001

METHYLPREDNISOLONE ACETATE

ENEMA; RECTAL

MEDROL

Firm	Strength	Appl. No.
UPJOHN	40 MG/BOT	N18102 001

INJECTABLE; INJECTION

METHYLPREDNISOLONE ACETATE

Firm	Strength	Appl. No.
STERIS	20 MG/ML	N87248 001
	40 MG/ML	N85374 001
	80 MG/ML	N86507 001

METHYLPREDNISOLONE SODIUM SUCCINATE

INJECTABLE; INJECTION

METHYLPREDNISOLONE SODIUM SUCCINATE

Firm	Strength	Appl. No.	Date
INTL MEDICATION	EQ 40 MG BASE/VIAL	N87812 001	FEB 09, 1983
	EQ 125 MG BASE/VIAL	N87813 001	FEB 09, 1983
	EQ 500 MG BASE/VIAL	N87851 001	FEB 09, 1983
	EQ 1 GM BASE/VIAL	N87852 001	FEB 09, 1983
LYPHOMED	EQ 40 MG BASE/VIAL	N88676 001	JUN 08, 1984
	EQ 125 MG BASE/VIAL	N88677 001	JUN 08, 1984
	EQ 500 MG BASE/VIAL	N88678 001	JUN 08, 1984
	EQ 500 MG BASE/VIAL	N89186 001	JUN 08, 1984
	EQ 1 GM BASE/VIAL	N88679 001	MAR 28, 1986
	EQ 1 GM BASE/VIAL	N89188 001	JUN 08, 1984
QUAD	EQ 40 MG BASE/VIAL	N89264 001	MAR 28, 1986
	EQ 125 MG BASE/VIAL	N89265 001	JAN 22, 1986
	EQ 500 MG BASE/VIAL	N89266 001	JAN 22, 1986
	EQ 1 GM BASE/VIAL	N89267 001	JAN 22, 1986

METHYLTESTOSTERONE

TABLET; BUCCAL/SUBLINGUAL

METANDREN

Firm	Strength	Appl. No.
CIBA	10 MG	N03240 005
	5 MG	N03240 004

METHYLTESTOSTERONE

Firm	Strength	Appl. No.
PHARM BASICS	10 MG	N80271 001
PUREPAC	10 MG	N80308 001
	10 MG	N80475 001

TABLET; ORAL

METANDREN

Firm	Strength	Appl. No.
CIBA	10 MG	N03240 001
	25 MG	N03240 003

METHYLTESTOSTERONE

Firm	Strength	Appl. No.
KV	10 MG	N84312 001
PARKE DAVIS	10 MG	N84244 001
	25 MG	N84241 001
PRIVATE FORM	10 MG	N80214 002
	25 MG	N80214 003
	5 MG	N80214 001
PUREPAC	10 MG	N80309 001
	25 MG	N80310 001
WEST WARD	25 MG	N84642 001

METHYPRYLON

ELIXIR; ORAL

NOLUDAR

Firm	Strength	Appl. No.
ROCHE	50 MG/5 ML	N09660 007

TABLET; ORAL

NOLUDAR

Firm	Strength	Appl. No.
ROCHE	50 MG	N09660 002

METOCLOPRAMIDE HYDROCHLORIDE

INJECTABLE; INJECTION

METOCLOPRAMIDE HCL

Firm	Strength	Appl. No.	Date
QUAD	EQ 10 MG BASE/2 ML	N70671 001	MAY 27, 1986
SMITH NEPHEW SOLOPAK	EQ 10 MG BASE/2 ML	N70622 001	MAR 02, 1987

REGLAN

Firm	Strength	Appl. No.	Date
ROBINS	EQ 10 MG BASE/ML	N17862 004	MAY 28, 1987

SYRUP; ORAL

METOCLOPRAMIDE HCL

Firm	Strength	Appl. No.	Date
PACO	EQ 5 MG BASE/5 ML	N71665 001	DEC 05, 1988

Discontinued Drug Products *(continued)*

METOCLOPRAMIDE HYDROCHLORIDE *(continued)*

TABLET; ORAL

CLOPRA			
QUANTUM PHARMICS	EQ 10 MG BASE	N70294 001	JUL 29, 1985
	EQ 5 MG BASE	N72384 001	JUN 02, 1988
CLOPRA-"YELLOW"			
QUANTUM PHARMICS	EQ 10 MG BASE	N70632 001	OCT 28, 1985
METOCLOPRAMIDE HCL			
BARR	EQ 10 MG BASE	N70660 001	FEB 10, 1987
BOLAR	EQ 10 MG BASE	N70363 001	MAR 02, 1987
CHELSEA	EQ 10 MG BASE	N70453 001	JUN 06, 1986
INTERPHARM	EQ 10 MG BASE	N71213 001	SEP 24, 1986
PHARM BASICS	EQ 10 MG BASE	N70339 001	JUL 29, 1985

METOCURINE IODIDE

INJECTABLE; INJECTION

METOCURINE IODIDE			
QUAD	2 MG/ML	N89443 001	JUN 01, 1988

METOLAZONE

TABLET; ORAL

DIULO			
SCHIAPPARELLI			
SEARLE	2.5 MG	N18535 001	
	5 MG	N18535 002	
	10 MG	N18535 003	

METRIZAMIDE

INJECTABLE; INJECTION

AMIPAQUE			
STERLING	2.5 GM/VIAL	N17982 003	SEP 12, 1983
	13.5 GM/VIAL	N17982 004	SEP 12, 1983

METRIZOATE SODIUM; *MULTIPLE*

SEE CALCIUM METRIZOATE; MAGNESIUM METRIZOATE;
MEGLUMINE METRIZOATE; METRIZOATE SODIUM

METRIZOIC ACID; *MULTIPLE*

SEE CALCIUM METRIZOATE; MEGLUMINE; METRIZOIC ACID

METRONIDAZOLE

INJECTABLE; INJECTION

METRONIDAZOLE			
INTL MEDICATION	500 MG/100 ML	N70004 001	MAY 08, 1985
LYPHOMED	500 MG/100 ML	N70071 001	DEC 03, 1984

TABLET; ORAL

METRONIDAZOLE			
CHELSEA	250 MG	N18599 001	SEP 17, 1982
	500 MG	N18599 002	FEB 13, 1984
SUPERPHARM	250 MG	N70008 001	DEC 11, 1984
	500 MG	N70009 001	DEC 11, 1984

METRONIDAZOLE HYDROCHLORIDE

INJECTABLE; INJECTION

METRONIDAZOLE HCL			
LYPHOMED	EQ 500 MG BASE/VIAL	N70295 001	OCT 15, 1985

MILRINONE LACTATE

INJECTABLE; INJECTION

MILRINONE LACTATE			
STERLING	EQ 1 MG BASE/ML	N19436 001	DEC 31, 1987

MINOCYCLINE HYDROCHLORIDE

CAPSULE; ORAL

MINOCIN			
LEDERLE	EQ 50 MG BASE	N50315 002	
	EQ 100 MG BASE	N50315 001	

TABLET; ORAL

MINOCIN			
LEDERLE	EQ 50 MG BASE	N50451 003	AUG 10, 1982
	EQ 100 MG BASE	N50451 002	AUG 10, 1982

Discontinued Drug Products (continued)

MINOXIDIL
TABLET; ORAL
MINODYL
QUANTUM PHARMICS   2.5 MG   N72153 001   JUL 13, 1988
  10 MG   N71534 001   MAR 19, 1987
MINOXIDIL
PHARM BASICS   2.5 MG   N71537 001   DEC 16, 1988
  N71799 001
ROYCE   2.5 MG   N71796 001   NOV 10, 1987
  10 MG   N71799 001   NOV 10, 1987

MOLINDONE HYDROCHLORIDE
CAPSULE; ORAL
MOBAN
DUPONT   5 MG   N17111 001
  10 MG   N17111 002
  25 MG   N17111 003

NALBUPHINE HYDROCHLORIDE
INJECTABLE; INJECTION
NALBUPHINE
LYPHOMED   10 MG/ML   N70751 001   JUL 02, 1986
  20 MG/ML   N70752 001   JUL 02, 1986
QUAD   10 MG/ML   N70692 001   MAR 25, 1986
  20 MG/ML   N70693 001   MAR 25, 1986

NALOXONE HYDROCHLORIDE
INJECTABLE; INJECTION
NALOXONE
ELKINS SINN   0.4 MG/ML   N70496 001   OCT 22, 1985
NALOXONE HCL
INTL MEDICATION   0.4 MG/ML   N70417 001   NOV 06, 1985
  1 MG/ML   N72115 001   APR 27, 1988
LYPHOMED   1 MG/ML   N71604 001   DEC 16, 1988
  0.4 MG/ML   N70679 001   DEC 18, 1986
QUAD   1 MG/ML   N70680 001   DEC 18, 1986
  0.02 MG/ML   N70678 001   DEC 18, 1986

NANDROLONE DECANOATE
INJECTABLE; INJECTION
NANDROLONE DECANOATE
QUAD   50 MG/ML   N89248 001   JUN 25, 1986
  100 MG/ML   N89249 001   JUN 25, 1986
  200 MG/ML   N89250 001   JUN 25, 1986

NANDROLONE PHENPROPIONATE
INJECTABLE; INJECTION
NANDROLONE PHENPROPIONATE
QUAD   25 MG/ML   N89297 001   OCT 01, 1986
  50 MG/ML   N89298 001   OCT 01, 1986

NEOMYCIN SULFATE
POWDER; FOR RX COMPOUNDING
NEOMYCIN SULFATE
ELKINS SINN   100%   N61698 001
TABLET; ORAL
NEOBIOTIC
PFIZER   EQ 350 MG BASE   N60475 001
NEOMYCIN SULFATE
ROXANE   EQ 350 MG BASE   N62173 001
SQUIBB   EQ 350 MG BASE   N60365 001

NEOMYCIN SULFATE; *MULTIPLE*
SEE   HYDROCORTISONE ACETATE; NEOMYCIN SULFATE
SEE   METHYLPREDNISOLONE; NEOMYCIN SULFATE

NEOMYCIN SULFATE; PREDNISOLONE ACETATE
OINTMENT; OPHTHALMIC
NEO-DELTA-CORTEF
UPJOHN   EQ 3.5 MG BASE/GM;0.25%   N61039 002
  EQ 3.5 MG BASE/GM;0.5%   N61039 001

NEOMYCIN SULFATE; TRIAMCINOLONE ACETONIDE
CREAM; TOPICAL
MYTREX A
SAVAGE   EQ 3.5 MG BASE/GM;0.1%   N62598 001   JUL 21, 1986
NEOMYCIN SULFATE-TRIAMCINOLONE ACETONIDE
FOUGERA   EQ 3.5 MG BASE/GM;0.1%   N62600 001   JUL 21, 1986
PHARMADERM   EQ 3.5 MG BASE/GM;0.1%   N62595 001   JUL 21, 1986

Discontinued Drug Products (continued)

NEOMYCIN SULFATE; TRIAMCINOLONE ACETONIDE (continued)
OINTMENT; TOPICAL
MYTREX A

SAVAGE	EQ 3.5 MG BASE/GM;0.1%	N62609 001	MAY 23, 1986

NEOMYCIN SULFATE-TRIAMCINOLONE ACETONIDE

FOUGERA	EQ 3.5 MG BASE/GM;0.1%	N62608 001	MAY 23, 1986
PHARMADERM	EQ 3.5 MG BASE/GM;0.1%	N62607 001	MAY 23, 1986

NETILMICIN SULFATE
INJECTABLE; INJECTION
NETROMYCIN

SCHERING	EQ 10 MG BASE/ML	N50544 001	FEB 28, 1983
	EQ 25 MG BASE/ML	N50544 002	FEB 28, 1983

NIACIN
TABLET; ORAL
NIACIN

BOLAR	500 MG	N83136 001
CHELSEA	500 MG	N85172 001
EVERYLIFE	500 MG	N83203 001
GENEVA	500 MG	N83306 001
WEST WARD	500 MG	N83718 001

NIACINAMIDE; *MULTIPLE*
SEE ASCORBIC ACID; BIOTIN; CYANOCOBALAMIN; DEXPANTHENOL; ERGOCALCIFEROL; FOLIC ACID; NIACINAMIDE; PYRIDOXINE HYDROCHLORIDE; RIBOFLAVIN PHOSPHATE SODIUM; THIAMINE HYDROCHLORIDE; VITAMIN A PALMITATE; VITAMIN E

NITROFURANTOIN
CAPSULE; ORAL
NITROFURANTOIN

BOLAR	50 MG	N84326 001
	100 MG	N84326 002

TABLET; ORAL
NITROFURANTOIN

BOLAR	100 MG	N80447 002
CHELSEA	50 MG	N85797 001
	100 MG	N85796 001
ELKINS SINN	50 MG	N80003 002
	100 MG	N80003 001
EON LABS	50 MG	N80043 001
	100 MG	N80043 002

NITROFURANTOIN SODIUM
INJECTABLE; INJECTION
IVADANTIN

P AND G	EQ 180 MG BASE/VIAL	N12402 001

NITROFURANTOIN, MACROCRYSTALLINE
CAPSULE; ORAL
NITROFURANTOIN MACROCRYSTALLINE

BOLAR	50 MG	N70248 001	JUN 24, 1988
	100 MG	N70249 001	JUN 24, 1988

NITROFURAZONE
DRESSING; TOPICAL
ACTIN-N

SHERWOOD	0.2%	N17343 001

NITROGLYCERIN
INJECTABLE; INJECTION
NITROGLYCERIN

LUITPOLD	5 MG/ML	N71492 001	MAY 24, 1988
LYPHOMED	5 MG/ML	N71203 001	MAY 08, 1987
QUAD	5 MG/ML	N71094 001	JUL 31, 1987
QUAD	10 MG/ML	N71095 001	JUL 31, 1987
SMITH NEPHEW SOLOPAK	5 MG/ML	N70634 001	JUN 19, 1986
NITROL RORER	0.8 MG/ML	N18774 001	JAN 19, 1983

NORETHINDRONE; *MULTIPLE*
SEE ETHINYL ESTRADIOL; NORETHINDRONE
SEE MESTRANOL; NORETHINDRONE

NORETHINDRONE ACETATE; *MULTIPLE*
SEE ETHINYL ESTRADIOL; NORETHINDRONE ACETATE

NORETHYNODREL; *MULTIPLE*
SEE MESTRANOL; NORETHYNODREL

NYSTATIN
CREAM; TOPICAL
CANDEX

MILES	100,000 UNITS/GM	N61810 001

Discontinued Drug Products (continued)

NYSTATIN (continued)

SUPPOSITORY; VAGINAL
NYSERT

NYSTATIN			
P AND G	100,000 UNITS	N50478 001	

TABLET; ORAL

NYSTATIN			
CHELSEA	500,000 UNITS	N62402 001	DEC 16, 1982
QUANTUM PHARMICS	500,000 UNITS	N62525 001	OCT 29, 1984

TABLET; VAGINAL

NYSTATIN			
CHELSEA	100,000 UNITS	N62176 001	
EON LABS	100,000 UNITS	N61965 001	
QUANTUM PHARMICS	100,000 UNITS	N62509 001	APR 03, 1984

NYSTATIN; *MULTIPLE*
SEE CLIOQUINOL; NYSTATIN

ORPHENADRINE CITRATE

TABLET, EXTENDED RELEASE; ORAL

ORPHENADRINE CITRATE			
ASCOT	100 MG	N88067 001	APR 06, 1983
BOLAR	100 MG	N84303 001	
GENEVA	100 MG	N85046 001	AUG 25, 1983

ORPHENADRINE CITRATE; *MULTIPLE*
SEE ASPIRIN; CAFFEINE; ORPHENADRINE CITRATE

OXACILLIN SODIUM

INJECTABLE; INJECTION

OXACILLIN SODIUM			
APOTHECON	EQ 250 MG BASE/VIAL	N50195 001	
	EQ 500 MG BASE/VIAL	N50195 002	
	EQ 1 GM BASE/VIAL	N50195 003	
	EQ 2 GM BASE/VIAL	N50195 004	
	EQ 4 GM BASE/VIAL	N50195 005	
ELKINS SINN	EQ 250 MG BASE/VIAL	N62711 001	FEB 03, 1989
	EQ 500 MG BASE/VIAL	N62711 002	FEB 03, 1989
	EQ 1 GM BASE/VIAL	N62711 003	FEB 03, 1989
	EQ 2 GM BASE/VIAL	N62711 004	FEB 03, 1989
	EQ 4 GM BASE/VIAL	N62711 005	FEB 03, 1989
	EQ 10 GM BASE/VIAL	N62711 006	FEB 03, 1989

OXAZEPAM

CAPSULE; ORAL

OXAZEPAM			
AM THERAP	10 MG	N71955 001	MAR 03, 1988
	15 MG	N71956 001	MAR 03, 1988
	30 MG	N71957 001	MAR 03, 1988
MYLAN	10 MG	N71713 001	OCT 20, 1987
	15 MG	N71714 001	OCT 20, 1987
	30 MG	N71715 001	OCT 20, 1987

ZAXOPAM

QUANTUM PHARMICS	10 MG	N70650 001	MAR 01, 1988
	15 MG	N70640 001	MAR 01, 1988
	30 MG	N70641 001	MAR 01, 1988

OXTRIPHYLLINE

TABLET, DELAYED RELEASE; ORAL

OXTRIPHYLLINE			
BOLAR	100 MG	N87866 001	AUG 25, 1983
	200 MG	N87835 001	AUG 25, 1983

OXYBUTYNIN CHLORIDE

TABLET; ORAL

OXYBUTYNIN CHLORIDE			
BOLAR	5 MG	N72485 001	APR 19, 1989
PHARM BASICS	5 MG	N70746 001	MAR 10, 1988
QUANTUM PHARMICS	5 MG	N72296 001	DEC 08, 1988

OXYCODONE HYDROCHLORIDE; *MULTIPLE*
SEE ACETAMINOPHEN; OXYCODONE HYDROCHLORIDE
SEE ACETAMINOPHEN; OXYCODONE HYDROCHLORIDE; OXYCODONE TEREPHTHALATE

OXYCODONE TEREPHTHALATE; *MULTIPLE*
SEE ACETAMINOPHEN; OXYCODONE HYDROCHLORIDE; OXYCODONE TEREPHTHALATE

Discontinued Drug Products (continued)

OXYPHENBUTAZONE
TABLET; ORAL
OXYPHENBUTAZONE
BOLAR   100 MG   N8399 001 SEP 17, 1984
TANDEARIL
RHONE POULENC RORER   100 MG   N12542 004 SEP 03, 1982

OXYPHENONIUM BROMIDE
TABLET; ORAL
ANTRENYL
CIBA   5 MG   N08492 002

OXYTETRACYCLINE; *MULTIPLE*
SEE LIDOCAINE HYDROCHLORIDE; OXYTETRACYCLINE

OXYTETRACYCLINE HYDROCHLORIDE
CAPSULE; ORAL
OXYTETRACYCLINE HCL
PUREPAC   EQ 250 MG BASE   N60634 001
TERRAMYCIN
PFIZER   EQ 125 MG BASE   N50286 001

OXYTOCIN
INJECTABLE; INJECTION
OXYTOCIN 10 USP UNITS IN DEXTROSE 5%
ABBOTT   1 USP UNIT/100 ML   N19185 004 MAR 29, 1985
   2 USP UNITS/100 ML   N19185 003 MAR 29, 1985
OXYTOCIN 20 USP UNITS IN DEXTROSE 5%
ABBOTT   2 USP UNITS/100 ML   N19185 002 MAR 29, 1985
OXYTOCIN 5 USP UNITS IN DEXTROSE 5%
ABBOTT   1 USP UNIT/100 ML   N19185 001 MAR 29, 1985

PANCURONIUM BROMIDE
INJECTABLE; INJECTION
PANCURONIUM BROMIDE
QUAD   1 MG/ML   N72209 001 JUN 03, 1988
   2 MG/ML   N72208 001 JUN 03, 1988

PARAMETHADIONE
SOLUTION; ORAL
PARADIONE
ABBOTT   300 MG/ML   N06800 002

PARGYLINE HYDROCHLORIDE
TABLET; ORAL
EUTONYL
ABBOTT   50 MG   N13448 004

PARGYLINE HYDROCHLORIDE; *MULTIPLE*
SEE METHYCLOTHIAZIDE; PARGYLINE HYDROCHLORIDE

PAROMOMYCIN SULFATE
SYRUP; ORAL
HUMATIN
PARKE DAVIS   EQ 125 MG BASE/5 ML   N60522 001

PENBUTOLOL SULFATE
TABLET; ORAL
LEVATOL
REED AND CARNRICK   10 MG   N18976 001 DEC 30, 1987

PENICILLIN G BENZATHINE
SUSPENSION; ORAL
BICILLIN
WYETH AYERST   300,000 UNITS/5 ML   N50126 002

PENICILLIN G POTASSIUM
INJECTABLE; INJECTION
PENICILLIN G POTASSIUM
COPANOS   1,000,000 UNITS/VIAL   N60806 002
   5,000,000 UNITS/VIAL   N60806 003
   500,000 UNITS/VIAL   N60806 001
   10,000,000 UNITS/VIAL   N60806 004
PARKE DAVIS   1,000,000 UNITS/VIAL   N62003 001
   5,000,000 UNITS/VIAL   N62003 002
POWDER FOR RECONSTITUTION; ORAL
PENICILLIN G POTASSIUM
MYLAN   250,000 UNITS/5 ML   N60752 002
   400,000 UNITS/5 ML   N60752 001
   200,000 UNITS/5 ML   N60752 003
PUREPAC   250,000 UNITS/5 ML   N61740 001
   400,000 UNITS/5 ML   N61740 002
TABLET; ORAL
PENICILLIN G POTASSIUM
PUREPAC   200,000 UNITS   N61588 001
   250,000 UNITS   N61588 002
   400,000 UNITS   N61588 003

Discontinued Drug Products (continued)

PENICILLIN G PROCAINE
INJECTABLE; INJECTION
  PENICILLIN G PROCAINE
    COPANOS   300,000 UNITS/ML   N60800 001
       600,000 UNITS/1.2 ML   N60800 002
    PARKE DAVIS   300,000 UNITS/ML   N62029 001

PENICILLIN G SODIUM
INJECTABLE; INJECTION
  PENICILLIN G SODIUM
    COPANOS   5,000,000 UNITS/VIAL   N61051 001
    SQUIBB   5,000,000 UNITS/VIAL   N61935 001

PENICILLIN V POTASSIUM
POWDER FOR RECONSTITUTION; ORAL
  PENAPAR-VK
    PARKE DAVIS   EQ 125 MG BASE/5 ML   N62002 001
       EQ 250 MG BASE/5 ML   N62002 002
  PENICILLIN V POTASSIUM
    PUREPAC   EQ 125 MG BASE/5 ML   N61758 001
       EQ 250 MG BASE/5 ML   N61758 002
TABLET; ORAL
  PEN-VEE K
    WYETH AYERST   EQ 125 MG BASE   N60006 001
  PENAPAR-VK
    PARKE DAVIS   EQ 250 MG BASE   N62001 001
       EQ 500 MG BASE   N62001 002
  PENICILLIN V POTASSIUM
    PUREPAC   EQ 125 MG BASE   N61571 001
       EQ 250 MG BASE   N61571 002
       EQ 500 MG BASE   N61571 003

PENTAZOCINE HYDROCHLORIDE
TABLET; ORAL
  TALWIN 50
    STERLING   EQ 50 MG BASE   N16732 001

PENTOBARBITAL SODIUM
CAPSULE; ORAL
  PENTOBARBITAL SODIUM
    VITARINE   100 MG   N83284 001
    WHITE TOWNE   100 MG
    PAULSEN   100 MG   N83338 001
  SODIUM PENTOBARBITAL
    ANABOLICS   100 MG   N84590 001
    CHELSEA   100 MG   N85791 001
    ELKINS SINN   100 MG   N83368 001
    EVERYLIFE   100 MG   N83259 001
    PARKE DAVIS   100 MG   N84156 001
    PERRIGO   100 MG   N84560 001
    PUREPAC   100 MG   N83301 001
    WYETH AYERST   100 MG   N83239 001

PENTOBARBITAL SODIUM (continued)
TABLET; ORAL
  PENTOBARBITAL SODIUM
    VITARINE   100 MG   N83285 001
  SODIUM PENTOBARBITAL
    ANABOLICS   100 MG   N84238 001

PENTOLINIUM TARTRATE
INJECTABLE; INJECTION
  ANSOLYSEN
    WYETH AYERST   10 MG/ML   N09372 001

PERPHENAZINE
SYRUP; ORAL
  TRILAFON
    SCHERING   2 MG/5 ML   N11294 002

PERPHENAZINE; *MULTIPLE*
SEE   AMITRIPTYLINE HYDROCHLORIDE; PERPHENAZINE

PHENDIMETRAZINE TARTRATE
CAPSULE; ORAL
  PHENDIMETRAZINE TARTRATE
    VITARINE   35 MG   N85634 001
       35 MG   N85645 001
       35 MG   N85670 001
       35 MG   N86403 001
       35 MG   N86408 001
       35 MG   N86410 001
       35 MG   N87424 001
  SPRX-3
    SOLVAY   35 MG   N85897 001
CAPSULE, EXTENDED RELEASE; ORAL
  MELFIAT-105
    SOLVAY   105 MG   N87487 001   OCT 13, 1982
  SPRX-105
    SOLVAY   105 MG   N88024 001   DEC 22, 1982
TABLET; ORAL
  ALPHAZINE
    EON LABS   35 MG   N85034 001
  DI-METREX
    PRIVATE FORM   35 MG   N85698 001

Discontinued Drug Products (continued)

PHENDIMETRAZINE TARTRATE (continued)

TABLET; ORAL

PHENDIMETRAZINE TARTRATE		
BARR	35 MG	N83644 001
	35 MG	N83684 001
	35 MG	N83686 001
	35 MG	N83687 001
	35 MG	N84831 001
	35 MG	N84834 001
	35 MG	N84835 001
CHELSEA	35 MG	N85767 001
	35 MG	N85768 001
	35 MG	N85770 001
	35 MG	N85773 001
GENEVA	35 MG	N86365 001
	35 MG	N86370 001
PHARM BASICS	35 MG	N83805 001
	35 MG	N84398 001
PRIVATE FORM	35 MG	N85199 001
SOLVAY	35 MG	N83790 001
VITARINE	35 MG	N85519 001
	35 MG	N86005 001
	35 MG	N86106 001
ZENITH	35 MG	N83682 001
	35 MG	N85612 001

STATOBEX-G		
LEMMON	35 MG	N85095 001

PHENINDIONE

TABLET; ORAL

HEDULIN		
MERRELL DOW	50 MG	N08767 002

PHENMETRAZINE HYDROCHLORIDE

TABLET; ORAL

PRELUDIN		
BOEHRINGER INGELHEIM	25 MG	N10460 005

TABLET, EXTENDED RELEASE; ORAL

PRELUDIN		
BOEHRINGER INGELHEIM	50 MG	N11752 004

PHENPROCOUMON

TABLET; ORAL

LIQUAMAR		
ORGANON	3 MG	N11228 001

PHENTERMINE HYDROCHLORIDE

CAPSULE; ORAL

PHENTERMINE HCL			
CHELSEA	30 MG	N86740 001	MAR 21, 1985
DURAMED	30 MG	N88948 001	APR 25, 1986
LEMMON	30 MG	N87126 001	
VITARINE	30 MG	N87202 001	
	30 MG	N87235 001	

TABLET; ORAL

PHENTERMINE HCL		
CHELSEA	8 MG	N85739 001
EON LABS	8 MG	N85671 001
	8 MG	N85689 001
VITARINE	8 MG	N86453 001
	8 MG	N86456 001
ZENITH	8 MG	N85553 001

PHENTERMINE RESIN COMPLEX

CAPSULE, EXTENDED RELEASE; ORAL

PHENTERMINE RESIN 30			
QUANTUM PHARMICS	EQ 30 MG BASE	N89120 001	FEB 04, 1988

PHENYL AMINOSALICYLATE

POWDER; ORAL

PHENY-PAS-TEBAMIN		
PURDUE FREDERICK	50%	N11695 002

TABLET; ORAL

PHENY-PAS-TEBAMIN		
PURDUE FREDERICK	500 MG	N11695 003

PHENYLBUTAZONE

CAPSULE; ORAL

AZOLID		
RHONE POULENC RORER	100 MG	N87260 001

PHENYLBUTAZONE			
ZENITH	100 MG	N88218 001	JUN 24, 1983

TABLET; ORAL

AZOLID		
RHONE POULENC RORER	100 MG	N87091 001

Discontinued Drug Products (continued)

PHENYLPROPANOLAMINE HYDROCHLORIDE; *MULTIPLE*
  SEE BROMPHENIRAMINE MALEATE: PHENYLPROPANOLAMINE HYDROCHLORIDE
  SEE CHLORPHENIRAMINE MALEATE: PHENYLPROPANOLAMINE HYDROCHLORIDE
  SEE CLEMASTINE FUMARATE: PHENYLPROPANOLAMINE HYDROCHLORIDE

PHENYTOIN SODIUM
  INJECTABLE; INJECTION
    PHENYTOIN SODIUM
      SMITH NEPHEW
        SOLOPAK   50 MG/ML   N88521 001   DEC 18, 1984
      WARNER CHILCOTT   50 MG/ML   N89900 001   MAR 30, 1990

PHENYTOIN SODIUM, EXTENDED
  CAPSULE; ORAL
    EXTENDED PHENYTOIN SODIUM
      SIDMAK   100 MG   N89441 001   DEC 18, 1986
    PHENYTEX
      BOLAR   100 MG   N88711 001   DEC 21, 1984

PHENYTOIN SODIUM, PROMPT
  CAPSULE; ORAL
    PHENYTOIN SODIUM
      CHELSEA   100 MG   N85894 001
      PHARMAFAIR   100 MG   N85435 001

PHOSPHORIC ACID; *MULTIPLE*
  SEE AMINO ACIDS: MAGNESIUM ACETATE: PHOSPHORIC ACID: POTASSIUM ACETATE: SODIUM CHLORIDE

PHYTONADIONE
  INJECTABLE; INJECTION
    VITAMIN K1
      ABBOTT   10 MG/ML   N87956 001   JUL 25, 1983

PINDOLOL; *MULTIPLE*
  SEE HYDROCHLOROTHIAZIDE: PINDOLOL

PIPERACETAZINE
  TABLET; ORAL
    QUIDE
      DOW   10 MG   N13615 001
           25 MG   N13615 002

PIPERAZINE CITRATE
  SYRUP; ORAL
    ANTEPAR
      BURROUGHS WELLCOME   EQ 500 MG BASE/5 ML   N09102 001
    BRYREL
      STERLING   EQ 500 MG BASE/5 ML   N17796 001
    PIPERAZINE CITRATE
      BARRE   EQ 500 MG BASE/5 ML   N80774 001
  TABLET; ORAL
    ANTEPAR
      BURROUGHS WELLCOME   EQ 500 MG BASE   N09102 003

PIPOBROMAN
  TABLET; ORAL
    VERCYTE
      ABBOTT   10 MG   N16245 001

POLYETHYLENE GLYCOL 3350; POTASSIUM CHLORIDE; SODIUM BICARBONATE; SODIUM CHLORIDE; SODIUM SULFATE, ANHYDROUS
  POWDER FOR RECONSTITUTION; ORAL
    COLYTE
      REED AND CARNRICK   120 GM/PACKET;1.49 GM/PACKET;3.36 GM/PACKET;2.92 GM/PACKET;11.36 GM/PACKET   N18983 005   OCT 26, 1984
                   227.1 GM/PACKET;2.82 GM/PACKET;6.36 GM/PACKET;5.53 GM/PACKET;21.5 GM/PACKET   N18983 004   OCT 26, 1984
                   360 GM/PACKET;4.47 GM/PACKET;10.08 GM/PACKET;8.76 GM/PACKET;34.08 GM/PACKET   N18983 006   OCT 26, 1984

POTASSIUM CHLORIDE; *MULTIPLE* (continued)

SEE   CALCIUM CHLORIDE: MAGNESIUM CHLORIDE: POTASSIUM CHLORIDE: SODIUM ACETATE: SODIUM CHLORIDE

POTASSIUM ACETATE; *MULTIPLE*

SEE   CALCIUM CHLORIDE: POTASSIUM CHLORIDE: SODIUM CHLORIDE: SODIUM LACTATE

SEE   CALCIUM CHLORIDE: POTASSIUM CHLORIDE: SODIUM ACETATE: SODIUM CHLORIDE

SEE   CALCIUM CHLORIDE: POTASSIUM CHLORIDE: SODIUM CHLORIDE

SEE   DEXTROSE: POTASSIUM CHLORIDE: SODIUM CHLORIDE

SEE   MAGNESIUM CHLORIDE: POTASSIUM CHLORIDE: SODIUM ACETATE: SODIUM CHLORIDE: SODIUM GLUCONATE

SEE   POLYETHYLENE GLYCOL 3350: POTASSIUM CHLORIDE: SODIUM BICARBONATE: SODIUM CHLORIDE: SODIUM SULFATE, ANHYDROUS

POTASSIUM CHLORIDE; SODIUM CHLORIDE

INJECTABLE; INJECTION

SODIUM CHLORIDE 0.9% AND POTASSIUM CHLORIDE 0.075% IN PLASTIC CONTAINER

BAXTER	75 MG/100 ML;900 MG/ 100 ML	N17648 004	
MCGAW	75 MG/100 ML;900 MG/ 100 ML	N18722 001	NOV 09, 1982

SODIUM CHLORIDE 0.9% AND POTASSIUM CHLORIDE 0.15% IN PLASTIC CONTAINER

MCGAW	150 MG/100 ML;900 MG/ 100 ML	N18722 002	NOV 09, 1982

SODIUM CHLORIDE 0.9% AND POTASSIUM CHLORIDE 0.22% IN PLASTIC CONTAINER

MCGAW	220 MG/100 ML;900 MG/ 100 ML	N18722 003	NOV 09, 1982

SODIUM CHLORIDE 0.9% AND POTASSIUM CHLORIDE 0.3% IN PLASTIC CONTAINER

MCGAW	300 MG/100 ML;900 MG/ 100 ML	N18722 004	NOV 09, 1982

POTASSIUM PHOSPHATE, DIBASIC; *MULTIPLE*

SEE   AMINO ACIDS: DEXTROSE: MAGNESIUM CHLORIDE: POTASSIUM CHLORIDE: POTASSIUM PHOSPHATE, DIBASIC: SODIUM CHLORIDE

PRALIDOXIME CHLORIDE

INJECTABLE; INJECTION

PRALIDOXIME CHLORIDE

QUAD	1 GM/VIAL	N72224 001	NOV 23, 1988
WYETH AYERST	300 MG/ML	N18799 001	DEC 13, 1982

Discontinued Drug Products (continued)

POLYMYXIN B SULFATE; *MULTIPLE*

SEE   CHLORAMPHENICOL: POLYMYXIN B SULFATE

POTASSIUM ACETATE; *MULTIPLE*

SEE   AMINO ACIDS: MAGNESIUM ACETATE: PHOSPHORIC ACID: POTASSIUM ACETATE: SODIUM CHLORIDE

SEE   AMINO ACIDS: MAGNESIUM ACETATE: POTASSIUM ACETATE: SODIUM CHLORIDE

SEE   AMINO ACIDS: MAGNESIUM ACETATE: POTASSIUM ACETATE: SODIUM CHLORIDE: SODIUM PHOSPHATE, DIBASIC

POTASSIUM AMINOSALICYLATE

POWDER; ORAL

POTASSIUM AMINOSALICYLATE

HEXCEL	100%	N80098 001

POTASSIUM CHLORIDE

INJECTABLE; INJECTION

POTASSIUM CHLORIDE

ABBOTT	1 MEQ/ML	N80205 003
	1 MEQ/ML	N83345 003
	2.4 MEQ/ML	N80205 004
	3.2 MEQ/ML	N80205 005
CUTTER	1 MEQ/ML	N80195 002
	2 MEQ/ML	N80195 001
	3 MEQ/ML	N80195 003
ELKINS SINN	2 MEQ/ML	N80203 001
LILLY	2 MEQ/ML	N07865 002
LYPHOMED	2 MEQ/ML	N80204 001
	2 MEQ/ML	N86713 001
	2 MEQ/ML	N86714 001
SEARLE	1 MEQ/ML	N86219 001
	2 MEQ/ML	N86219 002
	2 MEQ/ML	N86220 002
	3 MEQ/ML	N86219 003
	3 MEQ/ML	N86220 001
	4 MEQ/ML	N86219 004

POTASSIUM CHLORIDE; *MULTIPLE*

SEE   AMINO ACIDS: DEXTROSE: MAGNESIUM CHLORIDE: POTASSIUM CHLORIDE: SODIUM CHLORIDE: SODIUM PHOSPHATE, DIBASIC

SEE   AMINO ACIDS: DEXTROSE: MAGNESIUM CHLORIDE: POTASSIUM CHLORIDE: POTASSIUM PHOSPHATE, DIBASIC: SODIUM CHLORIDE

SEE   CALCIUM CHLORIDE: DEXTROSE: POTASSIUM CHLORIDE: SODIUM CHLORIDE: SODIUM LACTATE

PREDNISOLONE; *MULTIPLE*
SEE CHLORAMPHENICOL; PREDNISOLONE

PREDNISOLONE ACETATE
INJECTABLE; INJECTION

METICORTELONE		
SCHERING	25 MG/ML	N10255 002
PREDNISOLONE ACETATE		
AKORN	25 MG/ML	N83032 001
	50 MG/ML	N84492 001
CENTRAL PHARMS	25 MG/ML	N84717 001
	50 MG/ML	N84717 002
STERANE		
PFIZER	25 MG/ML	N11446 001

PREDNISOLONE ACETATE; *MULTIPLE*
SEE NEOMYCIN SULFATE; PREDNISOLONE ACETATE

PREDNISOLONE ACETATE; SULFACETAMIDE SODIUM
SUSPENSION/DROPS; OPHTHALMIC

PREDSULFAIR II			
PHARMAFAIR	0.2%;10%	N88837 001	DEC 24, 1985

PREDNISOLONE SODIUM PHOSPHATE
OINTMENT; OPHTHALMIC, OTIC

HYDELTRASOL		
MSD	EQ 0.25% PHOSPHATE	N11028 001

SOLUTION/DROPS; OPHTHALMIC

METRETON		
SCHERING	EQ 0.5% PHOSPHATE	N83834 001
PREDNISOLONE SODIUM PHOSPHATE		
SOLA BARNES HIND	EQ 0.11% PHOSPHATE	N84171 001
	EQ 0.9% PHOSPHATE	N84168 001
	EQ 0.9% PHOSPHATE	N84169 001
	EQ 0.9% PHOSPHATE	N84172 001

PREDNISONE
TABLET; ORAL

DELTA-DOME		
MILES	5 MG	N80293 001
FERNISONE		
FERNDALE	5 MG	N83364 001
METICORTEN		
SCHERING	5 MG	N09766 003
PARACORT		
PARKE DAVIS	5 MG	N10962 002

Discontinued Drug Products (continued)

PRALIDOXIME CHLORIDE (continued)
TABLET; ORAL

PROTOPAM CHLORIDE		
WYETH AYERST	500 MG	N14122 002

PRAZEPAM
CAPSULE; ORAL

PRAZEPAM			
PHARM BASICS	5 MG	N70427 001	NOV 06, 1987
	10 MG	N70428 001	NOV 06, 1987

PRAZOSIN HYDROCHLORIDE
CAPSULE; ORAL

PRAZOSIN HCL			
AM THERAP	EQ 1 MG BASE	N72782 001	APR 11, 1989
	EQ 2 MG BASE	N72783 001	APR 11, 1989
	EQ 5 MG BASE	N72784 001	APR 11, 1989

PREDNISOLONE
CREAM; TOPICAL

METI-DERM		
SCHERING	0.5%	N10209 002

TABLET; ORAL

FERNISOLONE-P			
FERNDALE	5 MG	N83941 001	
PREDNISOLONE			
BARR	5 MG	N84426 002	
CHELSEA	5 MG	N85415 001	
	5 MG	N85416 001	
ELKINS SINN	5 MG	N80625 001	
EON LABS	5 MG	N84773 001	
EVERYLIFE	1 MG	N84439 001	
	5 MG	N80326 001	
HEATHER	5 MG	N80398 001	
LEMMON	5 MG	N80351 001	
PANRAY	1 MG	N80351 002	
	5 MG	N84542 001	
PERRIGO	5 MG	N88892 001	FEB 26, 1985
SUPERPHARM	5 MG	N87987 001	JAN 18, 1983
UDL	5 MG	N80534 001	
VITARINE	5 MG		
WHITE TOWNE	5 MG	N80342 001	
PAULSEN	5 MG		
STERANE			
PFIZER	5 MG	N09996 001	

Discontinued Drug Products (continued)

PREDNISONE (continued)

TABLET; ORAL

PREDNISONE

AM THERAP	5 MG	N89387 001	NOV 06, 1986
	10 MG	N89388 001	NOV 06, 1986
	20 MG	N89389 001	NOV 06, 1986
BARR	50 MG	N86596 001	
DURAMED	5 MG	N88394 001	OCT 04, 1983
		N88395 001	
	10 MG		OCT 04, 1983
	20 MG	N88396 001	OCT 04, 1983
		N80491 001	
ELKINS SINN	5 MG	N85811 001	
	20 MG	N84774 001	
EON LABS	5 MG	N86968 001	
LEDERLE	5 MG	N80397 001	
LEMMON	5 MG	N80350 002	
PANRAY	2.5 MG	N80350 003	
	5 MG	N80350 001	
	1 MG	N83059 001	
PERRIGO	5 MG	N85151 001	
PRIVATE FORM	20 MG	N17109 001	
ROXANE	20 MG	N87833 001	
	25 MG		MAY 04, 1982
UDL	5 MG	N87984 001	JAN 18, 1983
		N87985 001	JAN 18, 1983
	10 MG	N87986 001	JAN 18, 1983
	20 MG	N87682 001	JAN 15, 1982
VANGARD	5 MG	N87701 001	JAN 15, 1982
	20 MG	N80334 001	
VITARINE	5 MG	N80506 001	
	5 MG		
WHITE TOWNE	2.5 MG	N84913 001	
PAULSEN	5 MG	N80343 001	
	10 MG	N89028 001	JUL 24, 1986
ZENITH	20 MG	N84134 001	

SERVISONE

LEDERLE	5 MG	N80223 001	

PRILOCAINE HYDROCHLORIDE

INJECTABLE; INJECTION

CITANEST

ASTRA	1%	N14763 004	
	2%	N14763 005	
	3%	N14763 003	

PRIMAQUINE PHOSPHATE; *MULTIPLE*

SEE CHLOROQUINE PHOSPHATE: PRIMAQUINE PHOSPHATE

PRIMIDONE

TABLET; ORAL

PRIMIDONE

BOLAR	250 MG	N85052 001	

PROBENECID

TABLET; ORAL

PROBENECID

LEDERLE	500 MG	N86917 001	

PROBENECID; *MULTIPLE*

SEE AMPICILLIN/AMPICILLIN TRIHYDRATE: PROBENECID
SEE COLCHICINE: PROBENECID

PROCAINAMIDE HYDROCHLORIDE

CAPSULE; ORAL

PROCAINAMIDE HCL

ASCOT	250 MG	N87542 001	JAN 08, 1982
	375 MG	N87697 001	MAR 01, 1983
	500 MG	N87543 001	JAN 08, 1982
BOLAR	250 MG	N83795 001	
	500 MG	N84357 001	
LEDERLE	250 MG	N86942 001	
	375 MG	N86952 001	
	500 MG	N86943 001	
ROXANE	250 MG	N88989 001	APR 26, 1985
	500 MG	N88990 001	APR 26, 1985
VANGARD	250 MG	N87643 001	JUN 01, 1982
	500 MG	N87875 001	JUN 01, 1982

PROCAN

PARKE DAVIS	250 MG	N85804 001	
	375 MG	N87502 001	
	500 MG	N85079 001	

PROCAPAN

PANRAY	250 MG	N83553 002	

Discontinued Drug Products (continued)

PROCAINAMIDE HYDROCHLORIDE (continued)

INJECTABLE; INJECTION

PROCAINAMIDE HCL

Firm	Strength	Appl. No.	Date
PHARMAFAIR	100 MG/ML	N88824 001	NOV 20, 1985
	500 MG/ML	N88830 001	NOV 20, 1985
QUAD	100 MG/ML	N89256 001	MAY 30, 1986
		N89257 001	MAY 30, 1986
	500 MG/ML	N89528 001	MAY 30, 1986
WARNER CHILCOTT	100 MG/ML	N89529 001	MAY 03, 1988
	500 MG/ML	N89520 001	MAY 03, 1988

TABLET, EXTENDED RELEASE; ORAL

PROCAINAMIDE HCL

Firm	Strength	Appl. No.	Date
BOLAR	250 MG	N88533 001	DEC 03, 1984
	500 MG	N88534 001	DEC 03, 1984
	750 MG	N88535 001	NOV 03, 1984
	1 GM	N89520 001	JAN 15, 1987

PROCAINE HYDROCHLORIDE

INJECTABLE; INJECTION

PROCAINE HCL

Firm	Strength	Appl. No.
CUTTER	1%	N80415 001
	2%	N80415 002
SEARLE	1%	N86202 001
	2%	N86202 002

PROCAINE HYDROCHLORIDE; TETRACYCLINE HYDROCHLORIDE

INJECTABLE; INJECTION

TETRACYN

Firm	Strength	Appl. No.
PFIZER	40 MG/VIAL;100 MG/VIAL	N60285 002

PROCAINE MERETHOXYLLINE; THEOPHYLLINE

INJECTABLE; INJECTION

DICURIN PROCAINE

Firm	Strength	Appl. No.
LILLY	100 MG/ML;50 MG/ML	N08869 001

PROCHLORPERAZINE EDISYLATE

CONCENTRATE; ORAL

COMPAZINE

Firm	Strength	Appl. No.	Date
SKF	EQ 10 MG BASE/ML	N11276 001	

PROCHLORPERAZINE

Firm	Strength	Appl. No.	Date
BARRE	EQ 10 MG BASE/ML	N87153 001	JUN 08, 1982

PROCHLORPERAZINE EDISYLATE

Firm	Strength	Appl. No.	Date
PHARM BASICS	EQ 10 MG BASE/ML	N88598 001	OCT 25, 1984

INJECTABLE; INJECTION

PROCHLORPERAZINE EDISYLATE

Firm	Strength	Appl. No.	Date
QUAD	EQ 5 MG BASE/ML	N89637 001	FEB 01, 1988
	EQ 5 MG BASE/ML	N89638 001	FEB 01, 1988

SYRUP; ORAL

PROCHLORPERAZINE EDISYLATE

Firm	Strength	Appl. No.	Date
BARRE	EQ 5 MG BASE/5 ML	N87154 001	SEP 01, 1982
PHARM BASICS	EQ 5 MG BASE/5 ML	N88597 001	OCT 25, 1984

PROCHLORPERAZINE MALEATE

CAPSULE, EXTENDED RELEASE; ORAL

COMPAZINE

Firm	Strength	Appl. No.
SKF	EQ 75 MG BASE	N11000 004

TABLET; ORAL

PROCHLORPERAZINE

Firm	Strength	Appl. No.
BOLAR	EQ 5 MG BASE	N85580 001
	EQ 10 MG BASE	N85178 001
	EQ 25 MG BASE	N85579 001

PROCHLORPERAZINE MALEATE

Firm	Strength	Appl. No.	Date
DURAMED	EQ 5 MG BASE	N89484 001	JAN 20, 1987
	EQ 10 MG BASE	N89485 001	JAN 20, 1987
	EQ 25 MG BASE	N89486 001	JAN 20, 1987

PROGESTERONE

INJECTABLE; INJECTION

PROGESTERONE

Firm	Strength	Appl. No.
LILLY	25 MG/ML	N09238 002

Discontinued Drug Products (continued)

PROMAZINE HYDROCHLORIDE
CONCENTRATE; ORAL
- SPARINE
  - WYETH AYERST   30 MG/ML   N10942 001
  -   100 MG/ML   N10942 004

SYRUP; ORAL
- SPARINE
  - WYETH AYERST   10 MG/5 ML   N10942 003

TABLET; ORAL
- SPARINE
  - WYETH AYERST   10 MG   N10348 006
  -   200 MG   N10348 004

PROMETHAZINE HYDROCHLORIDE
INJECTABLE; INJECTION
- PROMETHAZINE HCL
  - KNOLL   25 MG/ML   N84223 001
  -   50 MG/ML   N84222 001
- ZIPAN-25
  - ALTANA   25 MG/ML   N83997 001
- ZIPAN-50
  - ALTANA   50 MG/ML   N83997 002

SYRUP; ORAL
- MYMETHAZINE FORTIS
  - PHARM BASICS   25 MG/5 ML   N87996 001   JAN 18, 1983
- PROMETHAZINE HCL
  - KV   6.25 MG/5 ML   N85388 001
  -   25 MG/5 ML   N85385 001
  - PHARM ASSOC   6.25 MG/5 ML   N87518 001

TABLET; ORAL
- PROMETHAZINE HCL
  - BARR   12.5 MG   N84555 001
  -   25 MG   N84554 001
  -   50 MG   N84557 001
  - BOLAR   12.5 MG   N83401 001
  -   50 MG   N83403 001
  - BOOTS   12.5 MG   N84160 001
  -   25 MG   N84166 001
  -   50 MG   N84539 001
  - CHELSEA   12.5 MG   N85986 001
  -   25 MG   N85684 001
  -   50 MG   N85664 001
  - EON LABS   25 MG   N85146 001
  -   50 MG   N85146 002
  - GENEVA   12.5 MG   N84233 001
  - LEMMON   25 MG   N89109 001   SEP 10, 1985
  - PRIVATE FORM
    - REMSED   12.5 MG   N83214 001
    - DUPONT   50 MG   N83176 001

PROPANTHELINE BROMIDE
INJECTABLE; INJECTION
- PRO-BANTHINE
  - SEARLE   30 MG/VIAL   N08843 001

TABLET; ORAL
- PROPANTHELINE BROMIDE
  - ASCOT   15 MG   N87663 001   OCT 25, 1982
  - BOLAR   15 MG   N83151 001
  - GENEVA   15 MG   N80928 001
  - HEATHER   15 MG   N85780 001
  - MYLAN   15 MG   N83706 001
  - PRIVATE FORM   15 MG   N80977 001

PROPARACAINE HYDROCHLORIDE
SOLUTION/DROPS; OPHTHALMIC
- PROPARACAINE HCL
  - SOLA BARNES HIND   0.5%   N84144 001
  -   0.5%   N84151 001

PROPOXYPHENE HYDROCHLORIDE
CAPSULE; ORAL
- PROPOXYPHENE HCL
  - ALRA   65 MG   N83184 001
  - ANABOLICS   65 MG   N83185 001
  - BARR   65 MG   N83186 001
  - CHELSEA   65 MG   N85190 001
  - EON LABS   65 MG   N83870 002
  - MYLAN   65 MG   N86495 001
  - PRIVATE FORM   32 MG   N83299 001
  -   65 MG   N83464 001
  - VITARINE   32 MG   N83113 001
  -   65 MG   N84014 001
  - PROPOXYPHENE HCL 65   N83688 001
  - WARNER CHILCOTT   65 MG   N83786 001

PROPOXYPHENE HYDROCHLORIDE; *MULTIPLE*
SEE   ACETAMINOPHEN; PROPOXYPHENE HYDROCHLORIDE
SEE   ASPIRIN; CAFFEINE; PROPOXYPHENE HYDROCHLORIDE

PROPOXYPHENE NAPSYLATE; *MULTIPLE*
SEE   ACETAMINOPHEN; PROPOXYPHENE NAPSYLATE
SEE   ASPIRIN; PROPOXYPHENE NAPSYLATE

Discontinued Drug Products (continued)

PROPRANOLOL HYDROCHLORIDE

INJECTABLE; INJECTION

PROPRANOLOL HCL			
SMITH NEPHEW SOLOPAK	1 MG/ML	N70135 001	APR 15, 1986

SOLUTION; ORAL

PROPRANOLOL HCL			
PHARM BASICS	20 MG/5 ML	N71984 001	MAR 03, 1989
	40 MG/5 ML	N71985 001	MAR 03, 1989

TABLET; ORAL

INDERAL			
WYETH AYERST	90 MG	N16418 010	OCT 18, 1982

PROPRANOLOL HCL			
BOLAR	10 MG	N70378 001	MAR 19, 1987
	20 MG	N70379 001	MAR 19, 1987
	40 MG	N70380 001	MAR 19, 1987
	60 MG	N70381 001	MAR 19, 1987
	80 MG	N70382 001	MAR 19, 1987
CHELSEA	10 MG	N70140 001	MAR 19, 1987
	20 MG	N70141 001	JUL 30, 1985
	40 MG	N70142 001	JUL 30, 1985
	60 MG	N70143 001	JUL 30, 1985
	80 MG	N70144 001	JAN 15, 1987
	90 MG	N71183 001	JUL 30, 1985
DANBURY	10 MG	N70306 001	OCT 06, 1986
DURAMED	20 MG	N70307 001	SEP 09, 1985
	40 MG	N70308 001	SEP 09, 1985
	60 MG	N70309 001	SEP 09, 1985
	80 MG	N70310 001	OCT 01, 1986
	90 MG	N71327 001	SEP 09, 1985
			OCT 01, 1986

PROPRANOLOL HYDROCHLORIDE (continued)

TABLET; ORAL

PROPRANOLOL HCL			
LEDERLE	10 MG	N72117 001	JUN 23, 1988
	20 MG	N72118 001	JUN 23, 1988
		N72119 001	JUN 23, 1988
	40 MG	N72120 001	JUN 23, 1988
	80 MG		
LEMMON	10 MG	N70232 001	OCT 07, 1987
	20 MG	N70233 001	JUN 23, 1986
SUPERPHARM	10 MG	N71515 001	JUN 23, 1986
	20 MG	N71516 001	JUN 08, 1988
	40 MG	N71517 001	JUN 08, 1988
	80 MG	N71518 001	JUN 08, 1988
ZENITH	60 MG	N72068 001	JUN 08, 1988
			JUL 29, 1988

PROPRANOLOL HYDROCHLORIDE; *MULTIPLE*

SEE HYDROCHLOROTHIAZIDE; PROPRANOLOL HYDROCHLORIDE

PROPYLIODONE

SUSPENSION; INTRATRACHEAL

DIONOSIL AQUEOUS		
GLAXO	50%	N09309 001

PROPYLTHIOURACIL

TABLET; ORAL

PROPYLTHIOURACIL		
ANABOLICS	50 MG	N80285 001
BOOTS	50 MG	N84075 001
CHELSEA	50 MG	N85201 001
PERRIGO	50 MG	N84543 001
ZENITH	50 MG	N80215 001

PYRVINIUM PAMOATE
SUSPENSION; ORAL
  POVAN

PARKE DAVIS	EQ 50 MG BASE/5 ML	N11964 001

TABLET; ORAL
  POVAN

PARKE DAVIS	EQ 50 MG BASE	N12485 002

QUINESTROL
TABLET; ORAL
  ESTROVIS

PARKE DAVIS	0.2 MG	N16768 003

QUINETHAZONE; RESERPINE
TABLET; ORAL
  HYDROMOX R

LEDERLE	50 MG;0.125 MG	N13927 001

QUINIDINE GLUCONATE
TABLET; ORAL
  QUINACT

BERLEX	266 MG	N85978 001	
	400 MG	N86099 001	

TABLET, EXTENDED RELEASE; ORAL
  QUINATIME

BOLAR	324 MG	N87448 001	

  QUINIDINE GLUCONATE

ASCOT	324 MG	N88582 001	JUN 17, 1985
ROXANE	324 MG	N88431 001	JAN 06, 1984
SUPERPHARM	324 MG	N89164 001	NOV 21, 1985

QUINIDINE SULFATE
TABLET; ORAL
  QUINIDINE SULFATE

ELKINS SINN	200 MG	N83622 001	
EVERYLIFE	200 MG	N83439 001	
LEDERLE	200 MG	N86176 001	
PERRIGO	200 MG	N85322 001	
PHARM BASICS	200 MG	N87837 001	APR 14, 1982
VANGARD	200 MG	N87909 001	JUL 13, 1982
WHITE TOWNE			
PAULSEN	200 MG	N85444 001	

  QUINORA

KEY PHARMS	200 MG	N83576 001	

Discontinued Drug Products *(continued)*

PROTAMINE SULFATE
INJECTABLE; INJECTION
  PROTAMINE SULFATE

QUAD	50 MG/VIAL	N89307 001	MAY 30, 1986
UPJOHN	50 MG/VIAL	N07413 001	
	250 MG/VIAL	N07413 002	AUG 02, 1984

PROTEIN HYDROLYSATE
INJECTABLE; INJECTION
  AMINOSOL 5%

ABBOTT	5%	N05932 012	JAN 31, 1985

  HYPROTIGEN 5%

MCGAW	5%	N06170 003	JAN 10, 1984

PSEUDOEPHEDRINE HYDROCHLORIDE; TRIPROLIDINE HYDROCHLORIDE
SYRUP; ORAL
  MYFED

PHARM BASICS	30 MG/5 ML;1.25 MG/5 ML	N88116 001	MAR 04, 1983

TABLET; ORAL
  TRIPROLIDINE AND PSEUDOEPHEDRINE

BOLAR	60 MG;2.5 MG	N88318 002	JAN 13, 1984
WEST WARD	60 MG;2.5 MG	N88117 001	APR 19, 1983

PSEUDOEPHEDRINE SULFATE; *MULTIPLE*
SEE DEXBROMPHENIRAMINE MALEATE; PSEUDOEPHEDRINE SULFATE

PYRIDOXINE HYDROCHLORIDE
INJECTABLE; INJECTION
  PYRIDOXINE HCL

ELKINS SINN	100 MG/ML	N80581 001
LUITPOLD	100 MG/ML	N80669 001

PYRIDOXINE HYDROCHLORIDE; *MULTIPLE*
SEE ASCORBIC ACID; BIOTIN; CYANOCOBALAMIN; DEXPANTHENOL; ERGOCALCIFEROL; FOLIC ACID; NIACINAMIDE; PYRIDOXINE HYDROCHLORIDE; RIBOFLAVIN PHOSPHATE SODIUM; THIAMINE HYDROCHLORIDE; VITAMIN A PALMITATE; VITAMIN E

PYRILAMINE MALEATE
TABLET; ORAL
  PYRILAMINE MALEATE

CHELSEA	25 MG	N85231 001

Discontinued Drug Products (continued)

RANITIDINE HYDROCHLORIDE

INJECTABLE; INJECTION

ZANTAC IN PLASTIC CONTAINER

GLAXO	EQ 50 MG BASE/100 ML	N19593 001	DEC 17, 1986

RAUWOLFIA SERPENTINA

TABLET; ORAL

Brand / Manufacturer	Strength	Appl. No.
HIWOLFIA		
BOWMAN	50 MG	N09276 003
	100 MG	N09276 004
HYSERPIN		
PHYSICIANS PRODS	50 MG	N10581 001
KOGLUCOID		
PANRAY	50 MG	N09278 001
	100 MG	N09278 002
RAUSERPIN		
FERNDALE	50 MG	N09926 002
	100 MG	N09926 004
RAUWOLFIA SERPENTINA		
BUNDY	50 MG	N09477 001
	100 MG	N09477 002
DANBURY	100 MG	N80914 001
ICN	50 MG	N09668 001
	100 MG	N09668 002
PRIVATE FORM	50 MG	N80583 001
	100 MG	N80583 002
PUREPAC	50 MG	N80842 001
	100 MG	N80842 002
SOLVAY	50 MG	N80500 001
	100 MG	N80500 002
TABLICAPS	50 MG	N83867 001
	100 MG	N83444 001
ZENITH	50 MG	N11521 001
	100 MG	N11521 002
WOLFINA		
FOREST PHARMS	50 MG	N09255 008
	100 MG	N09255 006

RESCINNAMINE

CAPSULE; ORAL

Brand / Manufacturer	Strength	Appl. No.
CINNASIL		
PANRAY	0.5 MG	N84736 001

RESERPINE

INJECTABLE; INJECTION

Brand / Manufacturer	Strength	Appl. No.
SANDRIL		
LILLY	2.5 MG/ML	N10012 001
SERPASIL		
CIBA	2.5 MG/ML	N09434 002

RESERPINE (continued)

TABLET; ORAL

Brand / Manufacturer	Strength	Appl. No.
HISERPIA		
BOWMAN	0.1 MG	N09631 002
	0.25 MG	N09631 004
RAU-SED		
SQUIBB	0.1 MG	N09357 001
	0.25 MG	N09357 004
	0.5 MG	N09357 006
	1 MG	N09357 008
RESERPINE		
BARR	0.25 MG	N80721 002
BELL PHARMA	0.1 MG	N83058 001
	0.25 MG	N83058 002
BUNDY	0.1 MG	N09663 001
	0.25 MG	N09663 003
CHELSEA	0.1 MG	N85401 001
DANBURY	0.1 MG	N80679 001
	0.25 MG	N80393 001
	1 MG	N80749 001
ELKINS SINN	0.1 MG	N83145 001
	0.25 MG	N83145 002
EVERYLIFE	0.1 MG	N10441 001
	0.25 MG	N10441 002
	0.5 MG	N10441 003
	1 MG	N10441 004
HALSEY	0.1 MG	N80457 002
	0.25 MG	N80457 001
	1 MG	N80457 003
ICN	0.1 MG	N09667 001
	0.25 MG	N09667 002
MARSHALL	0.1 MG	N80492 001
	0.25 MG	N80492 002
MK	0.1 MG	N80525 002
	0.25 MG	N80525 001
	1 MG	N84974 001
MYLAN	0.25 MG	N84663 001
PHARMAVITE	0.1 MG	N86117 001
PRIVATE FORM	0.25 MG	N80582 001
	0.25 MG	N85775 001
	1 MG	N80582 002
REXALL	0.25 MG	N80637 001
ROXANE	0.1 MG	N09859 001
	0.25 MG	N09859 002
SOLVAY	0.25 MG	N80446 001
TABLICAPS	0.25 MG	N85207 001
WEST WARD	0.1 MG	N80975 001
	0.25 MG	N80975 002
	1 MG	N80975 003
WHITE TOWNE PAULSEN	0.1 MG	N80723 001
	0.25 MG	N80723 002
	1 MG	N80723 003
ZENITH	0.1 MG	N11185 001
	0.25 MG	N11185 002

Discontinued Drug Products (continued)

RESERPINE (continued)
TABLET; ORAL
SANDRIL
  LILLY   0.1 MG   N09376 004
                   0.25 MG   N09376 001
SERPANRAY
  PANRAY   0.1 MG   N09391 001
                   0.25 MG   N09391 002
                   1 MG   N09391 004
SERPASIL
  CIBA   1 MG   N09115 004
SERPATE
  VALE   0.1 MG   N09453 001
                   0.25 MG   N09453 002

RESERPINE; *MULTIPLE*
SEE CHLOROTHIAZIDE; RESERPINE
SEE HYDRALAZINE HYDROCHLORIDE; HYDROCHLOROTHIAZIDE; RESERPINE
SEE HYDRALAZINE HYDROCHLORIDE; RESERPINE
SEE HYDROCHLOROTHIAZIDE; RESERPINE
SEE HYDROFLUMETHIAZIDE; RESERPINE
SEE QUINETHAZONE; RESERPINE

RESERPINE; TRICHLORMETHIAZIDE
TABLET; ORAL
TRICHLORMETHIAZIDE W/ RESERPINE
  BOLAR   0.1 MG;4 MG   N85248 001

RIBOFLAVIN PHOSPHATE SODIUM; *MULTIPLE*
SEE ASCORBIC ACID; BIOTIN; CYANOCOBALAMIN; DEXPANTHENOL; ERGOCALCIFEROL; FOLIC ACID; NIACINAMIDE; PYRIDOXINE HYDROCHLORIDE; RIBOFLAVIN PHOSPHATE SODIUM; THIAMINE HYDROCHLORIDE; VITAMIN A PALMITATE; VITAMIN E

RITODRINE HYDROCHLORIDE
INJECTABLE; INJECTION
RITODRINE HCL
  LYPHOMED   15 MG/ML   N71189 001   JUL 23, 1987
                   10 MG/ML   N71188 001   JUL 23, 1987
  QUAD   15 MG/ML   N70701 001   OCT 06, 1986

ROSE BENGAL SODIUM, I-131
INJECTABLE; INJECTION
ROBENGATOPE
  SQUIBB   0.5 MCI/VIAL   N16224 001
                   1 MCI/VIAL   N16224 002
                   2 MCI/VIAL   N16224 003
SODIUM ROSE BENGAL I 131
  SORIN   0.5 MCI/ML   N17318 001

SAFFLOWER OIL
INJECTABLE; INJECTION
LIPOSYN 10%
  ABBOTT   10%   N18203 001
LIPOSYN 20%
  ABBOTT   20%   N18614 001

SARALASIN ACETATE
INJECTABLE; INJECTION
SARENIN
  P AND G   EQ 0.6 MG BASE/ML   N18009 001

SECOBARBITAL SODIUM
CAPSULE; ORAL
SECOBARBITAL SODIUM
  PARKE DAVIS   100 MG   N84762 001
  PUREPAC   100 MG   N85867 001
  VITARINE   100 MG   N85898 001
                   100 MG   N86273 001
  WHITE TOWNE   100 MG   N85798 001
  PAULSEN   100 MG   N86390 001
SODIUM SECOBARBITAL
  WYETH AYERST   100 MG   N84422 001
  ANABOLICS   100 MG   N84225 001
  BARR   100 MG   N85792 001
  CHELSEA   100 MG   N85285 001
  KV   100 MG   N84561 001
  PERRIGO   100 MG
INJECTABLE; INJECTION
SECONAL SODIUM
  LILLY   50 MG/ML   N07392 002
SUPPOSITORY; RECTAL
SECONAL SODIUM
  LILLY   30 MG   N86530 001
                   60 MG   N86530 002
                   120 MG   N86530 003
                   200 MG   N86530 004

Discontinued Drug Products *(continued)*

SELENOMETHIONINE, SE-75
INJECTABLE; INJECTION
SELENOMETHIONINE SE 75
MALLINCKRODT	100 UCI/ML	N17098 001
MEDI PHYSICS	250 UCI/ML	N17257 001
SETHOTOPE		
SQUIBB	85-550 UCI/ML	N17047 001

SERTRALINE HYDROCHLORIDE
TABLET; ORAL
ZOLOFT
PFIZER	EQ 150 MG BASE	N19839 003 DEC 30, 1991
	EQ 200 MG BASE	N19839 004 DEC 30, 1991

SODIUM ACETATE; *MULTIPLE*
SEE   CALCIUM CHLORIDE: DEXTROSE: MAGNESIUM CHLORIDE: SODIUM ACETATE: SODIUM CHLORIDE

SEE   CALCIUM CHLORIDE: MAGNESIUM CHLORIDE: POTASSIUM CHLORIDE: SODIUM ACETATE: SODIUM CHLORIDE

SEE   CALCIUM CHLORIDE: POTASSIUM CHLORIDE: SODIUM ACETATE: SODIUM CHLORIDE

SEE   MAGNESIUM CHLORIDE: POTASSIUM CHLORIDE: SODIUM ACETATE: SODIUM CHLORIDE: SODIUM GLUCONATE

SODIUM BICARBONATE; *MULTIPLE*
SEE   POLYETHYLENE GLYCOL 3350: POTASSIUM CHLORIDE: SODIUM BICARBONATE: SODIUM CHLORIDE: SODIUM SULFATE, ANHYDROUS

SODIUM CHLORIDE
INJECTABLE; INJECTION
SODIUM CHLORIDE
ABBOTT	20 GM/100 ML	N17013 001

SODIUM CHLORIDE 0.45% IN PLASTIC CONTAINER
CUTTER	450 MG/100 ML	N18503 001

SODIUM CHLORIDE 0.9% IN PLASTIC CONTAINER
ABBOTT	9 MG/ML	N19218 001 JUL 13, 1984
CUTTER	900 MG/100 ML	N18502 001

SODIUM CHLORIDE 23.4% IN PLASTIC CONTAINER
LYPHOMED	234 MG/ML	N19329 001 APR 22, 1987

SODIUM CHLORIDE 3% IN PLASTIC CONTAINER
MCGAW	3 GM/100 ML	N19635 003 MAR 09, 1988

SODIUM CHLORIDE 5% IN PLASTIC CONTAINER
MCGAW	5 GM/100 ML	N19635 004 MAR 09, 1988

SODIUM CHLORIDE *(continued)*
SOLUTION; IRRIGATION
SODIUM CHLORIDE IN PLASTIC CONTAINER
CUTTER	900 MG/100 ML	N18247 001

SODIUM CHLORIDE 0.45% IN PLASTIC CONTAINER
ABBOTT	450 MG/100 ML	N18380 001

SODIUM CHLORIDE; *MULTIPLE*
SEE   AMINO ACIDS: DEXTROSE: MAGNESIUM CHLORIDE: POTASSIUM CHLORIDE: SODIUM CHLORIDE: SODIUM PHOSPHATE, DIBASIC

SEE   AMINO ACIDS: DEXTROSE: MAGNESIUM CHLORIDE: POTASSIUM CHLORIDE: POTASSIUM PHOSPHATE, DIBASIC: SODIUM CHLORIDE

SEE   AMINO ACIDS: MAGNESIUM ACETATE: PHOSPHORIC ACID: POTASSIUM ACETATE: SODIUM CHLORIDE

SEE   AMINO ACIDS: MAGNESIUM ACETATE: POTASSIUM ACETATE: SODIUM CHLORIDE

SEE   AMINO ACIDS: MAGNESIUM ACETATE: POTASSIUM ACETATE: SODIUM CHLORIDE: SODIUM PHOSPHATE, DIBASIC

SEE   CALCIUM CHLORIDE: DEXTROSE: MAGNESIUM CHLORIDE: SODIUM ACETATE: SODIUM CHLORIDE

SEE   CALCIUM CHLORIDE: DEXTROSE: MAGNESIUM CHLORIDE: SODIUM CHLORIDE: SODIUM LACTATE

SEE   CALCIUM CHLORIDE: DEXTROSE: POTASSIUM CHLORIDE: SODIUM CHLORIDE: SODIUM LACTATE

SEE   CALCIUM CHLORIDE: DEXTROSE: SODIUM CHLORIDE: SODIUM LACTATE

SEE   CALCIUM CHLORIDE: MAGNESIUM CHLORIDE: POTASSIUM CHLORIDE: SODIUM ACETATE: SODIUM CHLORIDE

SEE   CALCIUM CHLORIDE: POTASSIUM CHLORIDE: SODIUM CHLORIDE: SODIUM LACTATE

SEE   CALCIUM CHLORIDE: POTASSIUM CHLORIDE: SODIUM ACETATE: SODIUM CHLORIDE

SEE   CALCIUM CHLORIDE: POTASSIUM CHLORIDE: SODIUM CHLORIDE

SEE   DEXTROSE: POTASSIUM CHLORIDE: SODIUM CHLORIDE

SEE   DEXTROSE: SODIUM CHLORIDE

SEE   MAGNESIUM CHLORIDE: POTASSIUM CHLORIDE: SODIUM ACETATE: SODIUM CHLORIDE: SODIUM GLUCONATE

SEE   POLYETHYLENE GLYCOL 3350: POTASSIUM CHLORIDE: SODIUM BICARBONATE: SODIUM CHLORIDE: SODIUM SULFATE, ANHYDROUS

SEE   POTASSIUM CHLORIDE: SODIUM CHLORIDE

Discontinued Drug Products (continued)

SODIUM GLUCONATE; *MULTIPLE*
SEE   MAGNESIUM CHLORIDE: POTASSIUM CHLORIDE: SODIUM
       ACETATE: SODIUM CHLORIDE: SODIUM GLUCONATE

SODIUM IODIDE, I-123
CAPSULE; ORAL
  SODIUM IODIDE I 123
    BENEDICT   400 UCI   N18671 003
                                         MAY 27, 1982

SODIUM IODIDE, I-131
CAPSULE; ORAL
  SODIUM IODIDE I 131
    CIS   50 UCI   N17316 001
    MALLINCKRODT   0.8-100 MCI   N16515 002

SODIUM LACTATE; *MULTIPLE*
SEE   CALCIUM CHLORIDE: DEXTROSE: MAGNESIUM CHLORIDE:
       SODIUM CHLORIDE: SODIUM LACTATE
SEE   CALCIUM CHLORIDE: DEXTROSE: POTASSIUM CHLORIDE:
       SODIUM CHLORIDE: SODIUM LACTATE
SEE   CALCIUM CHLORIDE: DEXTROSE: SODIUM CHLORIDE:
       SODIUM LACTATE
SEE   CALCIUM CHLORIDE: POTASSIUM CHLORIDE: SODIUM
       CHLORIDE: SODIUM LACTATE

SODIUM NITROPRUSSIDE
INJECTABLE; INJECTION
  SODIUM NITROPRUSSIDE
    LYPHOMED   50 MG/VIAL   N70031 001
                                         JAN 17, 1985

SODIUM PHOSPHATE, DIBASIC; *MULTIPLE*
SEE   AMINO ACIDS: DEXTROSE: MAGNESIUM CHLORIDE:
       POTASSIUM CHLORIDE: SODIUM CHLORIDE: SODIUM
       PHOSPHATE, DIBASIC
SEE   AMINO ACIDS: MAGNESIUM ACETATE: POTASSIUM ACETATE:
       SODIUM CHLORIDE: SODIUM PHOSPHATE, DIBASIC

SODIUM PHOSPHATE, P-32
SOLUTION; INJECTION, ORAL
  PHOSPHOTOPE
    SQUIBB   1-8 MCI/VIAL   N10927 001
  SODIUM PHOSPHATE P 32
    MALLINCKRODT   1.5 MCI/VIAL   N11777 002

SODIUM POLYSTYRENE SULFONATE
SUSPENSION; ORAL, RECTAL
  SODIUM POLYSTYRENE SULFONATE
    ROXANE   15 GM/60 ML   N8453 001
                                         NOV 17, 1983

SODIUM SUCCINATE
INJECTABLE; INJECTION
  SODIUM SUCCINATE
    ELKINS SINN   30%   N80516 001

SODIUM SULFATE, ANHYDROUS; *MULTIPLE*
SEE   POLYETHYLENE GLYCOL 3350: POTASSIUM CHLORIDE:
       SODIUM BICARBONATE: SODIUM CHLORIDE: SODIUM
       SULFATE, ANHYDROUS

SOMATROPIN
INJECTABLE; INJECTION
  ASELLACRIN 10
    SERONO   10 IU/VIAL   N17726 001
  ASELLACRIN 2
    SERONO   2 IU/VIAL   N17726 002
                                         JUL 21, 1983
  CRESCORMON
    GENENTECH   4 IU/VIAL   N17992 001

SOMATROPIN, BIOSYNTHETIC
INJECTABLE; INJECTION
  HUMATROPE
    LILLY   2 MG/VIAL   N19640 001
                                         JUN 23, 1987

SORBITOL
SOLUTION; IRRIGATION
  SORBITOL 3% IN PLASTIC CONTAINER
    BAXTER   3 GM/100 ML   N18512 001
                                         MAY 27, 1982

SORBITOL; *MULTIPLE*
SEE   MANNITOL: SORBITOL

SOYBEAN OIL
INJECTABLE; INJECTION
  TRAVAMULSION 20%
    BAXTER   20%   N18758 001
                                         FEB 15, 1983

Discontinued Drug Products *(continued)*

SPIRONOLACTONE
TABLET; ORAL
SPIRONOLACTONE

ASCOT	25 MG	N87687 001	OCT 20, 1982
BOLAR	25 MG	N88898 002	MAR 02, 1982
LEDERLE	25 MG	N87634 001	
PUREPAC	25 MG	N88053 001	AUG 25, 1983
VANGARD	25 MG	N87648 001	FEB 01, 1982
WARNER CHILCOTT	25 MG	N87952 001	NOV 18, 1982

SPIRONOLACTONE; *MULTIPLE*
SEE   HYDROCHLOROTHIAZIDE; SPIRONOLACTONE

STREPTOMYCIN SULFATE
INJECTABLE; INJECTION
STREPTOMYCIN SULFATE

COPANOS	EQ 500 MG BASE/ML	N60684 001

SUCCINYLCHOLINE CHLORIDE
INJECTABLE; INJECTION
ANECTINE

BURROUGHS WELLCOME	50 MG/ML	N08453 003	

SUCCINYLCHOLINE CHLORIDE

INTL MEDICATION	100 MG/VIAL	N85400 001	FEB 04, 1982

SULCONAZOLE NITRATE
SOLUTION; TOPICAL
EXELDERM

WESTWOOD SQUIBB	1%	N18738 001	AUG 30, 1985

SULFACETAMIDE SODIUM
SOLUTION/DROPS; OPHTHALMIC
SODIUM SULFACETAMIDE

SOLA BARNES HIND	10%	N84143 001
	10%	N84145 001
	30%	N84146 001
	30%	N84147 001

SULFACETAMIDE SODIUM; *MULTIPLE*
SEE   PREDNISOLONE ACETATE; SULFACETAMIDE SODIUM

SULFADIAZINE
TABLET; ORAL
SULFADIAZINE

EVERYLIFE	500 MG	N80088 001
LEDERLE	500 MG	N04054 001

SULFAMETER
TABLET; ORAL
SULLA

BERLEX	500 MG	N16000 002

SULFAMETHIZOLE
TABLET; ORAL
MICROSUL

FOREST PHARMS	1 GM	N86012 001

PROKLAR

FOREST PHARMS	500 MG	N80273 001

SULFAMETHOXAZOLE
TABLET; ORAL
SULFAMETHOXAZOLE

ASCOT	500 MG	N87662 001	OCT 20, 1982
BARR	500 MG	N87189 001	JUL 25, 1983
BOLAR	500 MG	N85053 001	
	1 GM	N86000 001	

UROBAK

SHIONOGI	500 MG	N87307 001

SULFAMETHOXAZOLE; TRIMETHOPRIM
INJECTABLE; INJECTION
SULFAMETHOPRIM

QUAD	80 MG/ML;16 MG/ML	N71341 001	AUG 07, 1987

SUSPENSION; ORAL
SULMEPRIM

PHARM BASICS	200 MG/5 ML;40 MG/5 ML	N70063 001	AUG 01, 1986

SULMEPRIM PEDIATRIC

PHARM BASICS	200 MG/5 ML;40 MG/5 ML	N70064 001	AUG 01, 1986

TABLET; ORAL
SULFAMETHOXAZOLE AND TRIMETHOPRIM

MARTEC	400 MG;80 MG	N72408 001	DEC 07, 1988
PHARM BASICS	400 MG;80 MG	N70203 001	NOV 08, 1985
	800 MG;160 MG	N70204 001	NOV 08, 1985

SULFAMETHOXAZOLE AND TRIMETHOPRIM DOUBLE STRENGTH

MARTEC	800 MG;160 MG	N72417 001	DEC 07, 1988

Discontinued Drug Products (continued)

SULFAPHENAZOLE
SUSPENSION; ORAL
SULFABID
PURDUE FREDERICK   500 MG/5 ML   N13093 001

TABLET; ORAL
SULFABID
PURDUE FREDERICK   500 MG   N13092 002

SULFASALAZINE
TABLET; ORAL
S.A.S.-500
SOLVAY   500 MG   N83450 001

SULFASALAZINE
BOLAR   500 MG   N84964 001
EON LABS   500 MG   N86184 001

TABLET, DELAYED RELEASE; ORAL
SULFASALAZINE
BOLAR   500 MG   N88052 001
MAY 24, 1983

SULFINPYRAZONE
CAPSULE; ORAL
SULFINPYRAZONE
VANGARD   200 MG   N88666 001
FEB 17, 1984

SULFISOXAZOLE
TABLET; ORAL
SOXAZOLE
ALRA   500 MG   N80366 001

SULFALAR
PARKE DAVIS   500 MG   N84955 001

SULFISOXAZOLE
BARR   500 MG   N84031 001
CHELSEA   500 MG   N85534 001
LEDERLE   500 MG   N87649 001
PHARMAFAIR   500 MG   N84385 001
VITARINE   500 MG   N87332 001
WEST WARD   500 MG   N80379 001

SULSOXIN
SOLVAY   500 MG   N80040 001

SULFISOXAZOLE DIOLAMINE
INJECTABLE; INJECTION
GANTRISIN
ROCHE   EQ 400 MG BASE/ML   N06917 001

SOLUTION/DROPS; OPHTHALMIC
SULFISOXAZOLE DIOLAMINE
SOLA BARNES HIND   EQ 4% BASE   N84148 001

SULFOXONE SODIUM
TABLET, DELAYED RELEASE; ORAL
DIASONE SODIUM
ABBOTT   165 MG   N06044 003

SUPROFEN
CAPSULE; ORAL
SUPROL
JOHNSON RW   200 MG   N18217 001
DEC 24, 1985

TALBUTAL
TABLET; ORAL
LOTUSATE
STERLING   120 MG   N09410 005

TANNIC ACID; *MULTIPLE*
SEE   CYANOCOBALAMIN; TANNIC ACID; ZINC ACETATE

TECHNETIUM TC-99M ALBUMIN AGGREGATED
INJECTABLE; INJECTION
TC 99M-LUNGAGGREGATE
MEDI PHYSICS   5 MCI/ML   N17848 001

TECHNETIUM TC-99M ALBUMIN AGGREGATED KIT
INJECTABLE; INJECTION
LUNGAGGREGATE REAGENT
MEDI PHYSICS   N/A   N17838 001

TECHNETIUM TC-99M ETIDRONATE KIT
INJECTABLE; INJECTION
CINTICHEM TECHNETIUM 99M HEDSPA
MEDI PHYSICS   N/A   N17653 001
MPI STANNOUS DIPHOSPHONATE
MEDI PHYSICS   N/A   N17667 001
TECHNETIUM TC 99M DIPHOSPHONATE-TIN KIT
MEDI PHYSICS   N/A   N17562 001

TECHNETIUM TC-99M FERPENTETATE KIT
INJECTABLE; INJECTION
RENOTEC
SQUIBB   N/A   N17045 001

TECHNETIUM TC-99M POLYPHOSPHATE KIT
INJECTABLE; INJECTION
SODIUM POLYPHOSPHATE-TIN KIT
MEDI PHYSICS   N/A   N17664 001

Discontinued Drug Products *(continued)*

TECHNETIUM TC-99M PYROPHOSPHATE KIT
INJECTABLE; INJECTION
AN-PYROTEC
CIS	N/A	N19039 001	JUN 30, 1987

TECHNETIUM TC-99M SODIUM PERTECHNETATE
SOLUTION; INJECTION, ORAL
SODIUM PERTECHNETATE TC-99M

CIS	12 MCI/ML	N17321 001
	24 MCI/ML	N17321 002
	48 MCI/ML	N17321 003
MEDI PHYSICS	2-100 MCI/ML	N17471 001

TECHNETIUM TC-99M SULFUR COLLOID
SOLUTION; INJECTION, ORAL
TECHNETIUM TC 99M SULFUR COLLOID

MEDI PHYSICS	4 MCI/ML	N17456 001

TEMAFLOXACIN HYDROCHLORIDE
TABLET; ORAL
OMNIFLOX

ABBOTT	EQ 400 MG BASE	N20043 003	JAN 30, 1992
	EQ 600 MG BASE	N20043 004	JAN 30, 1992

TEMAZEPAM
CAPSULE; ORAL
TEMAZ

QUANTUM PHARMICS	15 MG	N70564 001	OCT 15, 1985
	30 MG	N70547 001	OCT 15, 1985

TEMAZEPAM

BOLAR	15 MG	N70383 001	MAR 23, 1987
	30 MG	N70384 001	MAR 23, 1987
DURAMED	15 MG	N71708 001	SEP 29, 1988
	30 MG	N71709 001	SEP 29, 1988
PHARM BASICS	15 MG	N70489 001	JUL 07, 1986
	30 MG	N70490 001	JUL 07, 1986

TERBUTALINE SULFATE
AEROSOL, METERED; INHALATION
BRICANYL

MERRELL DOW	0.2 MG/INH	N18000 001	MAR 19, 1985

TESTOLACTONE
INJECTABLE; INJECTION
TESLAC

SQUIBB	100 MG/ML	N16119 001

TABLET; ORAL
TESLAC

SQUIBB	250 MG	N16118 002

TESTOSTERONE CYPIONATE
INJECTABLE; INJECTION
TESTOSTERONE CYPIONATE

QUAD	100 MG/ML	N89326 001	OCT 28, 1988
	200 MG/ML	N89327 001	OCT 28, 1988

TESTOSTERONE ENANTHATE
INJECTABLE; INJECTION
DELATESTRYL

GYNEX	200 MG/ML	N09165 001

TESTOSTERONE ENANTHATE

QUAD	200 MG/ML	N89325 001	SEP 16, 1986
	100 MG/ML	N89324 001	SEP 16, 1986

TESTOSTERONE ENANTHATE; *MULTIPLE*
SEE ESTRADIOL VALERATE; TESTOSTERONE ENANTHATE

TESTOSTERONE PROPIONATE
INJECTABLE; INJECTION
TESTOSTERONE PROPIONATE

ELKINS SINN	25 MG/ML	N80276 001	
QUAD	100 MG/ML	N89283 001	NOV 03, 1986

TETRACYCLINE HYDROCHLORIDE
CAPSULE; ORAL
CYCLOPAR

WARNER CHILCOTT	250 MG	N61725 001
	250 MG	N62175 001
	250 MG	N62332 001
	500 MG	N61725 002
	500 MG	N62332 002

RETET

SOLVAY	250 MG	N61443 001
	500 MG	N61443 002

TETRACYCLINE HCL

BOOTS	250 MG	N61802 001	
	500 MG	N61802 002	
CHELSEA	250 MG	N62103 001	
	500 MG	N62103 002	
ELKINS SINN	250 MG	N60059 001	
EON LABS	500 MG	N61471 002	SEP 06, 1988

THEOPHYLLINE (continued)

SYRUP; ORAL
  THEOPHYLLINE
    BARRE   150 MG/15 ML   N86545 001

TABLET; ORAL
  THEOCLEAR-100
    CENTRAL PHARMS   100 MG   N85353 002
  THEOCLEAR-200
    CENTRAL PHARMS   200 MG   N85353 001

TABLET, EXTENDED RELEASE; ORAL
  DURAPHYL
    FOREST LABS   100 MG   N88503 001; APR 03, 1985
               200 MG   N88504 001; APR 03, 1985
               300 MG   N88505 001; APR 03, 1985

THEOPHYLLINE; *MULTIPLE*

SEE PROCAINE MERETHOXYLLINE; THEOPHYLLINE

THIAMINE HYDROCHLORIDE

INJECTABLE; INJECTION
  THIAMINE HCL
    LUITPOLD   100 MG/ML   N80667 001
    LYPHOMED   100 MG/ML   N80509 001
    PARKE DAVIS   100 MG/ML   N80770 001

THIAMINE HYDROCHLORIDE; *MULTIPLE*

SEE ASCORBIC ACID; BIOTIN; CYANOCOBALAMIN; DEXPANTHENOL; ERGOCALCIFEROL; FOLIC ACID; NIACINAMIDE; PYRIDOXINE HYDROCHLORIDE; RIBOFLAVIN PHOSPHATE SODIUM; THIAMINE HYDROCHLORIDE; VITAMIN A PALMITATE; VITAMIN E

THIORIDAZINE HYDROCHLORIDE

CONCENTRATE; ORAL
  THIORIDAZINE HCL
    BARRE   30 MG/ML   N87766 001; APR 26, 1983
    GENEVA   30 MG/ML   N88307 001; NOV 23, 1983
              100 MG/ML   N88308 001; NOV 23, 1983

Discontinued Drug Products (continued)

TETRACYCLINE HYDROCHLORIDE; *MULTIPLE*

SEE PROCAINE HYDROCHLORIDE; TETRACYCLINE HYDROCHLORIDE

TETRACYCLINE PHOSPHATE COMPLEX

CAPSULE; ORAL
  TETREX
    BRISTOL   EQ 250 MG HCL   N50212 002
            EQ 500 MG HCL   N50212 003

THEOPHYLLINE

CAPSULE; ORAL
  SOMOPHYLLIN-T
    FISONS   100 MG   N87155 001; FEB 25, 1985
          200 MG   N87155 002; FEB 25, 1985
          250 MG   N87155 003; FEB 25, 1985
  THEOPHYLLINE
    SCHERER   100 MG   N84731 002; NOV 07, 1986
           200 MG   N84731 001; NOV 07, 1986
           250 MG   N84731 003; NOV 07, 1986

CAPSULE, EXTENDED RELEASE; ORAL
  THEOPHYL-SR
    JOHNSON RW   125 MG   N86480 001; FEB 08, 1985
              250 MG   N86471 001; FEB 08, 1985
  THEOPHYLLINE
    CENTRAL PHARMS   125 MG   N88654 001; FEB 12, 1985
                  250 MG   N88689 001; FEB 12, 1985
    EON LABS   260 MG   N87462 001; MAY 11, 1982
  THEOPHYLLINE-SR
    SCHERER   300 MG   N88255 001; JUN 12, 1986

ELIXIR; ORAL
  THEOLIXIR
    PANRAY   80 MG/15 ML   N84559 001
  THEOPHYLLINE
    PERRIGO   80 MG/15 ML   N85952 001
    ROXANE   80 MG/15 ML   N84739 001

Discontinued Drug Products (continued)

THIORIDAZINE HYDROCHLORIDE (continued)

TABLET; ORAL
THIORIDAZINE HCL

Firm	Strength	Number	Date
BOLAR	10 MG	N88412 001	SEP 12, 1983
	15 MG	N88345 001	JUL 28, 1983
	25 MG	N88296 001	JUL 28, 1983
	50 MG	N88323 001	JUL 28, 1983
	100 MG	N88284 001	AUG 25, 1983
	150 MG	N88410 001	MAR 05, 1984
	200 MG	N88381 001	MAR 14, 1984
CHELSEA	15 MG	N88562 001	MAY 11, 1984
MYLAN	10 MG	N88332 001	JUN 27, 1983
	25 MG	N88333 001	JUN 27, 1983
	50 MG	N88334 001	JUN 27, 1983
	100 MG	N88335 001	NOV 18, 1983
PAR	150 MG	N89764 001	FEB 09, 1988
	200 MG	N89765 001	FEB 09, 1988
ROXANE	10 MG	N88663 001	MAR 15, 1984
	25 MG	N88664 001	MAR 15, 1984
	50 MG	N88665 001	MAR 15, 1984
	100 MG	N89048 001	FEB 26, 1985
WEST WARD	10 MG	N88658 001	MAR 26, 1984
	15 MG	N88659 001	MAR 26, 1984
	25 MG	N88660 001	MAR 26, 1984
	50 MG	N88661 001	MAR 26, 1984

THIOTHIXENE

CAPSULE; ORAL
THIOTHIXENE

Firm	Strength	Number	Date
AM THERAP	2 MG	N71885 001	AUG 12, 1987
	5 MG	N71886 001	AUG 12, 1987
	10 MG	N71887 001	AUG 12, 1987
	1 MG	N71884 001	AUG 12, 1987
	20 MG	N72200 001	DEC 17, 1987
CHELSEA	2 MG	N71626 001	JUN 25, 1987
	5 MG	N71627 001	JUN 25, 1987
	10 MG	N71628 001	JUN 25, 1987

THIOTHIXENE HYDROCHLORIDE

CONCENTRATE; ORAL
THIOTHIXENE HCL

Firm	Strength	Number	Date
PACO	EQ 1 MG BASE/ML	N71917 001	SEP 20, 1989
	EQ 5 MG BASE/ML	N71939 001	DEC 16, 1988

THYROGLOBULIN

TABLET; ORAL
PROLOID

Firm	Strength	Number
PARKE DAVIS	16 MG	N00245 009
	325 MG	N00245 004

TIMOLOL MALEATE

TABLET; ORAL
TIMOLOL MALEATE

Firm	Strength	Number	Date
BOLAR	5 MG	N72269 001	MAR 14, 1989
	10 MG	N72270 001	MAR 14, 1989
	20 MG	N72271 001	MAR 14, 1989
PHARM BASICS	5 MG	N72001 001	JAN 10, 1989
	10 MG	N72002 001	JAN 10, 1989
	20 MG	N72003 001	JAN 10, 1989
QUANTUM PHARMICS	5 MG	N72466 001	MAY 19, 1989
	10 MG	N72467 001	MAY 19, 1989
	20 MG	N72468 001	MAY 19, 1989

Discontinued Drug Products (continued)

TIOCONAZOLE

CREAM; TOPICAL

TZ-3			
PFIZER	1%	N18682 001	FEB 18, 1983

TOLAZAMIDE

TABLET; ORAL

TOLAZAMIDE			
BOLAR	100 MG	N70242 001	AUG 01, 1986
	250 MG	N70243 001	AUG 01, 1986
	500 MG	N70244 001	AUG 01, 1986
DURAMED	100 MG	N70165 001	JAN 10, 1986
	250 MG	N70166 001	JAN 10, 1986
	500 MG	N70167 001	JAN 10, 1986
PHARM BASICS	100 MG	N71355 001	JAN 11, 1988
	250 MG	N70168 001	APR 02, 1986
	500 MG	N70169 001	APR 02, 1986
SUPERPHARM	250 MG	N70763 001	JUN 16, 1986
	500 MG	N70764 001	JUN 16, 1986

TOLBUTAMIDE

TABLET; ORAL

TOLBUTAMIDE			
ALRA	500 MG	N86141 001	
ASCOT	500 MG	N87541 001	MAR 01, 1983
BOLAR	500 MG	N89111 001	
	250 MG	N89110 001	MAY 29, 1987
PARKE DAVIS	500 MG	N86047 001	MAY 29, 1987
VANGARD	500 MG	N87876 001	APR 20, 1982

TRAZODONE HYDROCHLORIDE

TABLET; ORAL

TRAZODONE HCL			
AM THERAP	50 MG	N71139 001	OCT 29, 1986
	100 MG	N71140 001	OCT 29, 1986
BOLAR	50 MG	N71112 001	NOV 17, 1986
	100 MG	N71113 001	NOV 17, 1986
PHARM BASICS	50 MG	N70491 001	APR 29, 1987
	100 MG	N70492 001	APR 29, 1987
QUANTUM PHARMICS	100 MG	N70921 001	DEC 01, 1986
TRIALODINE			
QUANTUM PHARMICS	50 MG	N70942 001	DEC 01, 1986

TRIAMCINOLONE

TABLET; ORAL

ARISTOCORT			
LEDERLE	16 MG	N11161 010	
KENACORT			
SQUIBB	2 MG	N11283 008	
	1 MG	N11283 003	
TRIAMCINOLONE			
BARR	2 MG	N84286 001	
	2 MG	N84318 001	
	4 MG	N84267 001	
	4 MG	N84319 001	
	8 MG	N84268 001	
	8 MG	N84320 001	
CHELSEA	4 MG	N85834 001	
GENEVA	4 MG	N85601 001	

TRIAMCINOLONE ACETONIDE

CREAM; TOPICAL

TRIACORT			
SOLVAY	0.1%	N87113 001	
TRIAMCINOLONE ACETONIDE			
PHARM BASICS	0.1%	N88095 001	SEP 01, 1983
	0.5%	N88096 001	SEP 01, 1983
	0.025%	N88094 001	SEP 01, 1983
TRYMEX			
SAVAGE	0.5%	N88198 001	MAR 25, 1983

Discontinued Drug Products (continued)

TRIAMCINOLONE ACETONIDE (continued)

GEL; TOPICAL
ARISTOGEL
   LEDERLE   0.1%   N83380 001

LOTION; TOPICAL
KENALOG
   WESTWOOD SQUIBB   0.025%   N11602 003
       0.1%   N11602 001

OINTMENT; TOPICAL
ARISTOCORT A
   LEDERLE   0.5%   N88781 001   OCT 05, 1984

TRIAMCINOLONE ACETONIDE
   PHARM BASICS   0.5%   N88092 001   SEP 01, 1983
       0.025%   N88090 001   SEP 01, 1983
       0.1%   N88091 001   SEP 01, 1983

TRIAMCINOLONE ACETONIDE; *MULTIPLE*
SEE   NEOMYCIN SULFATE: TRIAMCINOLONE ACETONIDE

TRIAMTERENE; *MULTIPLE*
SEE   HYDROCHLOROTHIAZIDE: TRIAMTERENE

TRIAZOLAM

TABLET; ORAL
HALCION
   UPJOHN   0.5 MG   N17892 002   NOV 15, 1982

TRICHLORMETHIAZIDE

TABLET; ORAL
TRICHLORMETHIAZIDE
   BOLAR   4 MG   N83462 001
   CHELSEA   4 MG   N85962 001
       2 MG   N86458 001
   EON LABS   4 MG   N86171 001

TRICHLORMETHIAZIDE; *MULTIPLE*
SEE   RESERPINE: TRICHLORMETHIAZIDE

TRICLOFOS SODIUM

SOLUTION; ORAL
TRICLOS
   MERRELL DOW   1.5 GM/15 ML   N16830 001

TABLET; ORAL
TRICLOS
   MERRELL DOW   750 MG   N16809 002

TRIDIHEXETHYL CHLORIDE

INJECTABLE; INJECTION
PATHILON
   LEDERLE   10 MG/ML   N09729 001

TABLET; ORAL
PATHILON
   LEDERLE   25 MG   N09489 005

TRIFLUOPERAZINE HYDROCHLORIDE

INJECTABLE; INJECTION
TRIFLUOPERAZINE HCL
   QUAD   EQ 2 MG BASE/ML   N89893 001   OCT 17, 1988

TABLET; ORAL
TRIFLUOPERAZINE HCL
   BOLAR   EQ 1 MG BASE   N85975 001   JUN 23, 1988
       EQ 2 MG BASE   N85976 001   JUN 23, 1988
       EQ 5 MG BASE   N85973 001   JUN 23, 1988
       EQ 10 MG BASE   N88710 001   JUN 23, 1988
   DURAMED   EQ 1 MG BASE   N88967 001   APR 23, 1985
       EQ 2 MG BASE   N88968 001   APR 23, 1985
       EQ 5 MG BASE   N88969 001   APR 23, 1985
       EQ 10 MG BASE   N88970 001   APR 23, 1985

TRIFLUPROMAZINE HYDROCHLORIDE

INJECTABLE; INJECTION
VESPRIN
   SQUIBB   3 MG/ML   N11325 005

TRIHEXYPHENIDYL HYDROCHLORIDE

TABLET; ORAL
TRIHEXYPHENIDYL HCL
   BOLAR   2 MG   N85117 001
       5 MG   N85105 001
   VANGARD   2 MG   N88035 001   JUL 30, 1982

TRIMEPRAZINE TARTRATE

SYRUP; ORAL
TRIMEPRAZINE TARTRATE
   BARRE   EQ 2.5 MG BASE/5 ML   N85015 001   FEB 18, 1982
   PHARM BASICS   EQ 2.5 MG BASE/5 ML   N88285 001   APR 11, 1985

Discontinued Drug Products (continued)

TRIMETHOBENZAMIDE HYDROCHLORIDE
INJECTABLE; INJECTION
  TRIMETHOBENZAMIDE HCL
    SMITH NEPHEW
      SOLOPAK   100 MG/ML   N89043 001   APR 04, 1986

TRIMETHOPRIM
TABLET; ORAL
  TRIMETHOPRIM
    BARR   200 MG   N70495 001   MAR 14, 1986

TRIMETHOPRIM; *MULTIPLE*
SEE   SULFAMETHOXAZOLE: TRIMETHOPRIM

TRIMIPRAMINE MALEATE
CAPSULE; ORAL
  TRIMIPRAMINE MALEATE
    EON LABS   EQ 25 MG BASE   N71832 001   SEP 10, 1987
       EQ 50 MG BASE   N71833 001   SEP 10, 1987
       EQ 100 MG BASE   N71834 001   SEP 10, 1987
    PHARM BASICS   EQ 25 MG BASE   N71283 001   DEC 08, 1987
       EQ 50 MG BASE   N71284 001   DEC 08, 1987
       EQ 100 MG BASE   N71285 001   DEC 08, 1987

TRIPELENNAMINE HYDROCHLORIDE
TABLET; ORAL
  TRIPELENNAMINE HCL
    ANABOLICS   50 MG   N83037 001
    BARR   50 MG   N80744 001
    BOLAR   50 MG   N80790 001
    CHELSEA   50 MG   N85188 001
    PARKE DAVIS   50 MG   N83626 001
       25 MG   N83625 001
TABLET, EXTENDED RELEASE; ORAL
  PBZ-SR
    GEIGY   50 MG   N10533 002

TRIPLE SULFA (SULFABENZAMIDE; SULFACETAMIDE; SULFATHIAZOLE)
CREAM; VAGINAL
  VAGILIA
    LEMMON   3.7%;2.86%;3.42%   N88821 001   NOV 09, 1987
TABLET; VAGINAL
  TRIPLE SULFA
    FOUGERA   184 MG;143.75 MG;172.5 MG   N88463 001   JAN 03, 1985
    PHARMADERM   184 MG;143.75 MG;172.5 MG   N88462 001   JAN 03, 1985

TRIPROLIDINE HYDROCHLORIDE
SYRUP; ORAL
  MYIDYL
    PHARM BASICS   1.25 MG/5 ML   N87963 001   JAN 18, 1983
  TRIPROLIDINE HCL
    BARRE   1.25 MG/5 ML   N85940 001
    PHARM ASSOC   1.25 MG/5 ML   N87514 001   FEB 10, 1982
TABLET; ORAL
  TRIPROLIDINE HCL
    VITARINE   2.5 MG   N85610 001

TRIPROLIDINE HYDROCHLORIDE; *MULTIPLE*
SEE   PSEUDOEPHEDRINE HYDROCHLORIDE: TRIPROLIDINE HYDROCHLORIDE

TRISULFAPYRIMIDINES
SUSPENSION; ORAL
  SULFALOID
    FOREST PHARMS   500 MG/5 ML   N80100 001
  SULFOSE
    WYETH AYERST   500 MG/5 ML   N80013 002
  TRIPLE SULFA
    BARRE   500 MG/5 ML   N80280 001
  TRIPLE SULFAS
    LEDERLE   500 MG/5 ML   N06920 003
TABLET; ORAL
  SULFALOID
    FOREST PHARMS   500 MG   N80099 001
  SULFOSE
    WYETH AYERST   500 MG   N80013 001
  TRIPLE SULFA
    PUREPAC   500 MG   N80086 001
  TRIPLE SULFAS
    LEDERLE   500 MG   N06920 002

Discontinued Drug Products (continued)

VERAPAMIL HYDROCHLORIDE (continued)
TABLET; ORAL
- CALAN
  - SEARLE — 160 MG — N18817 004 — FEB 23, 1988
- VERAPAMIL HCL
  - CHELSEA — 40 MG — N72799 001 — APR 28, 1989
  - PARKE DAVIS — 80 MG — N70340 001 — AUG 20, 1986
  - 120 MG — N70341 001 — AUG 20, 1986

VERATRUM VIRIDE
TABLET; ORAL
- VERTAVIS
  - WALLACE — 130 CSR UNITS — N05691 002

VINBLASTINE SULFATE
INJECTABLE; INJECTION
- VINBLASTINE SULFATE
  - LYPHOMED — 10 MG/VIAL — N89011 001 — NOV 18, 1985
  - N89365 001 — AUG 07, 1986
  - QUAD — 10 MG/VIAL — N89311 001
  - 1 MG/ML — MAR 23, 1987

VINCRISTINE SULFATE
INJECTABLE; INJECTION
- ONCOVIN
  - LILLY — 1 MG/VIAL — N14103 001
  - 5 MG/VIAL — N14103 002
- VINCRISTINE SULFATE
  - QUAD — 1 MG/VIAL — N71222 001 — MAR 07, 1988
  - 5 MG/VIAL — N71937 001 — MAR 07, 1988
  - 1 MG/ML — N70777 001 — APR 29, 1986
  - 1 MG/ML — N70778 001 — MAY 01, 1986
  - 2 MG/VIAL — N71223 001 — MAR 07, 1988

VIOMYCIN SULFATE
INJECTABLE; INJECTION
- VIOCIN SULFATE
  - PFIZER — EQ 1 GM BASE/VIAL — N61086 001
  - EQ 5 GM BASE/VIAL — N61086 002

TROLEANDOMYCIN
SUSPENSION; ORAL
- TAO
  - PFIZER — EQ 125 MG BASE/5 ML — N50332 001

UNDECOYLIUM CHLORIDE; UNDECOYLIUM CHLORIDE IODINE COMPLEX
SOLUTION; TOPICAL
- VIRAC REX
  - CHESEBROUGH PONDS — 0.5%;1.8% — N11914 001

UNDECOYLIUM CHLORIDE IODINE COMPLEX; *MULTIPLE*
SEE UNDECOYLIUM CHLORIDE; UNDECOYLIUM CHLORIDE IODINE COMPLEX

UREA
INJECTABLE; INJECTION
- STERILE UREA
  - ABBOTT — 40 GM/VIAL — N17698 001

URSODIOL
CAPSULE; ORAL
- ACTIGALL
  - CIBA — 150 MG — N19594 001 — DEC 31, 1987

VANCOMYCIN HYDROCHLORIDE
INJECTABLE; INJECTION
- VANCOMYCIN HCL
  - QUAD — EQ 500 MG BASE/VIAL — N62845 001 — JUL 15, 1988
  - EQ 1 GM BASE/VIAL — N62845 002 — JUL 15, 1988

VERAPAMIL HYDROCHLORIDE
INJECTABLE; INJECTION
- CALAN
  - SEARLE — 2.5 MG/ML — N18925 001 — MAR 30, 1984
  - 2.5 MG/ML — N19038 001 — MAR 30, 1984
- VERAPAMIL HCL
  - LYPHOMED — 2.5 MG/ML — N70348 001 — MAY 01, 1986
  - QUAD — 2.5 MG/ML — N70672 001 — MAR 07, 1986
  - SMITH NEPHEW SOLOPAK — 2.5 MG/ML — N70697 001 — JUL 31, 1987

Discontinued Drug Products (continued)

VITAMIN A

CAPSULE; ORAL

VITAMIN A

CHASE	50,000 IU	N83351 001
EVERYLIFE	50,000 IU	N83134 001

VITAMIN A PALMITATE

CAPSULE; ORAL

VITAMIN A

ALPHALIN		
LILLY	EQ 50,000 UNITS BASE	N80883 001
VI-DOM-A		
MILES	EQ 50,000 UNITS BASE	N80972 001
VITAMIN A		
CHASE	EQ 50,000 UNITS BASE	N80746 001
	EQ 50,000 UNITS BASE	N83207 001
	EQ 50,000 UNITS BASE	N85479 001
ELKINS SINN	EQ 50,000 UNITS BASE	N80943 001
EVERYLIFE	EQ 50,000 UNITS BASE	N83114 001
SQUIBB	EQ 50,000 UNITS BASE	N80860 001
VITAMIN A SOLUBILIZED		
LEMMON	EQ 50,000 UNITS BASE	N80921 001

VITAMIN A PALMITATE; *MULTIPLE*

SEE ASCORBIC ACID; BIOTIN; CYANOCOBALAMIN; DEXPANTHENOL; ERGOCALCIFEROL; FOLIC ACID; NIACINAMIDE; PYRIDOXINE HYDROCHLORIDE; RIBOFLAVIN PHOSPHATE SODIUM; THIAMINE HYDROCHLORIDE; VITAMIN A PALMITATE; VITAMIN E

VITAMIN E; *MULTIPLE*

SEE ASCORBIC ACID; BIOTIN; CYANOCOBALAMIN; DEXPANTHENOL; ERGOCALCIFEROL; FOLIC ACID; NIACINAMIDE; PYRIDOXINE HYDROCHLORIDE; RIBOFLAVIN PHOSPHATE SODIUM; THIAMINE HYDROCHLORIDE; VITAMIN A PALMITATE; VITAMIN E

WARFARIN POTASSIUM

TABLET; ORAL

ATHROMBIN-K

PURDUE FREDERICK	2 MG	N11771 007
	5 MG	N11771 004
	10 MG	N11771 005
	25 MG	N11771 006

WARFARIN SODIUM

INJECTABLE; INJECTION

COUMADIN

DUPONT	50 MG/VIAL	N09218 020
	75 MG/VIAL	N09218 012

TABLET; ORAL

ATHROMBIN

PURDUE FREDERICK	5 MG	N11771 003
	10 MG	N11771 002
	25 MG	N11771 001

WARFARIN SODIUM

BOLAR	2 MG	N86123 001	AUG 17, 1982
	2.5 MG	N86120 001	AUG 17, 1982
	5 MG	N86119 001	AUG 17, 1982
	10 MG	N86122 001	AUG 17, 1982
	7.5 MG	N86118 001	AUG 17, 1982
PHARM BASICS	2 MG	N88719 001	JUN 27, 1985
	2.5 MG	N88720 001	AUG 06, 1985
	5 MG	N88721 001	JUL 02, 1985

WATER FOR IRRIGATION, STERILE

LIQUID; IRRIGATION

STERILE WATER IN PLASTIC CONTAINER

CUTTER	100%	N18246 001

XENON, XE-133

GAS; INHALATION

XENON XE 133-V.S.S.

MEDI PHYSICS	10 MCI/VIAL	N17687 001

INJECTABLE; INJECTION

XENON XE 133

DUPONT	6.3 MCI/ML	N17283 001
MEDI PHYSICS	1.3-1.7 CI/AMP	N17256 001

ZINC ACETATE; *MULTIPLE*

SEE CYANOCOBALAMIN; TANNIC ACID; ZINC ACETATE

ORPHAN DRUG PRODUCT DESIGNATIONS

THE FOLLOWING DRUGS AND BIOLOGICALS HAVE BEEN GRANTED ORPHAN DRUG DESIGNATION PURSUANT TO SECTION 526 OF THE FOOD, DRUG, AND COSMETIC ACT AS AMENDED BY THE ORPHAN DRUG ACT [PUB. L. 97-414].

TWO PARAGRAPHS EXCERPTED FROM THE SUPPLEMENTARY INFORMATION SECTION OF THE CUMULATIVE LIST OF ORPHAN DRUG AND BIOLOGICAL DESIGNATIONS, PUBLISHED IN THE *FEDERAL REGISTER* OF FEBRUARY 16, 1989 [VOL. 54, NO. 31, P. 7100], STATE:

"THE ORPHAN-DRUG DESIGNATION OF A DRUG OR BIOLOGICAL PRODUCT APPLIES ONLY TO THE SPONSOR THAT REQUESTED THE DESIGNATION. EACH SPONSOR INTERESTED IN DEVELOPING AN ORPHAN DRUG OR ORPHAN BIOLOGICAL PRODUCT MUST APPLY FOR ORPHAN-DRUG DESIGNATION TO OBTAIN EXCLUSIVE MARKETING RIGHTS."

"THE NAMES USED IN THE LIST TO IDENTIFY DRUG AND BIOLOGICAL PRODUCTS THAT HAVE NOT BEEN APPROVED/LICENSED FOR MARKETING MAY NOT BE THE ESTABLISHED/PROPER NAMES APPROVED BY FDA FOR THESE PRODUCTS IF THEY ARE EVENTUALLY APPROVED-LICENSED FOR MARKETING. BECAUSE THESE PRODUCTS ARE INVESTIGATIONAL, SOME MAY NOT YET HAVE BEEN REVIEWED FOR PURPOSES OF ASSIGNING THE MOST APPROPRIATE ESTABLISHED/PROPER NAME."

BIOLOGICAL DESIGNATIONS
[Approved for Marketing*]
[Exclusive Approval**]

NAME OF BIOLOGICAL	DESIGNATED USE [EXCLUSIVITY EXPIRATION DATE]	SPONSOR NAME
GENERIC: AEROSOLIZED POOLED IMMUNE GLOBULIN TRADE: NOT ESTABLISHED	TREATMENT OF RESPIRATORY SYNCYTIAL VIRUS LOWER RESPIRATORY TRACT DISEASE.	PPI HOLDING COMPANY, INC
GENERIC: ALDESLEUKIN TRADE: PROLEUKIN*/**	TREATMENT OF METASTATIC RENAL CELL CARCINOMA. TREATMENT OF PRIMARY IMMUNODEFICIENCY DISEASE ASSOCIATED WITH T-CELL DEFECTS.*/** [MAY 05, 1999]	CETUS
GENERIC: ALPHA-GALACTOSIDASE A TRADE: CC-GALACTOSIDASE	TREATMENT OF ALPHA-GALACTOSIDASE A DEFICIENCY. (FABRY'S DISEASE).	DAVID H. CALHOUN, PH.D. NEW YORK, NY
GENERIC: ALPHA-1-ANTITRYPSIN (RECOMBINANT DNA ORIGIN) TRADE: NOT ESTABLISHED	SUPPLEMENTATION THERAPY FOR ALPHA-1 ANTITRYPSIN DEFICIENCY IN THE ZZ PHENOTYPE POPULATION.	COOPER DEVELOPMENT COMPANY
GENERIC: ALPHA-1-PROTEINASE INHIBITOR TRADE: PROLASTIN*/**	REPLACEMENT THERAPY IN THE ALPHA-1 PROTEINASE CONGENITAL DEFICIENCY STATE. [DEC 02, 1994]	CUTTER
GENERIC: ANANAIN, COMOSAIN TRADE: VIANAIN	FOR THE ENZYMATIC DEBRIDEMENT OF SEVERE BURNS.	GENZYME CORPORATION
GENERIC: ANCROD TRADE: ARVIN	FOR USE AS AN ANTITHROMBOTIC IN PATIENTS WITH HEPARIN-INDUCED THROMBOCYTOPENIA OR THROMBOSIS, WHO REQUIRE IMMEDIATE AND CONTINUED ANTICOAGULATION.	KNOLL PHARMACEUTICALS
GENERIC: ANTI PAN T LYMPHOCYTE MONOCLONAL TRADE: ANTI-T LYMPHOCYTE IMMUNOTOXIN XMMLY-H65-RTA	FOR EX-VIVO TREATMENT TO ELIMINATE MATURE T CELLS FROM POTENTIAL BONE MARROW GRAFTS. FOR IN-VIVO TREATMENT OF BONE MARROW RECIPIENTS TO PREVENT GRAFT REJECTION AND GRAFT VS. HOST DISEASE (GVHD).	XOMA CORPORATION
GENERIC: ANTIHEMOPHILIC FACTOR (RECOMBINANT) (BHK) TRADE: RFVIII	PROPHYLAXIS AND TREATMENT OF BLEEDING IN INDIVIDUALS WITH HEMOPHILIA A OR FOR PROPHYLAXIS WHEN SURGERY IS REQUIRED IN INDIVIDUALS WITH HEMOPHILIA A.	MILES, INC
GENERIC: ANTIMELANOMA ANTIBODY XMMME-0001-DTPA 111 INDIUM TRADE: ANTIMELANOMA ANTIBODY XMMME-0001-DTPA 111 INDIUM	DIAGNOSTIC USE IN IMAGING SYSTEMIC AND NODAL MELANOMA METASTASES.	XOMA CORPORATION
GENERIC: ANTIMELANOMA ANTIBODY XMMME-001-RTA TRADE: ANTIMELANOMA ANTIBODY XMMME-001-RTA	TREATMENT OF STAGE III MELANOMA NOT AMENABLE TO SURGICAL RESECTION.	XOMA CORPORATION
GENERIC: ANTI-CYTOMEGALOVIRUS MONOCLONAL ANTIBODIES TRADE: NOT ESTABLISHED	PREVENTION OF HUMAN CYTOMEGALOVIRUS INFECTION IN BONE MARROW AND ORGAN TRANSPLANT PATIENTS. TREATMENT OF HUMAN CYTOMEGALOVIRUS INFECTION IN BONE MARROW AND ORGAN TRANSPLANT PATIENTS. PREVENTION OF HUMAN CYTOMEGALOVIRUS INFECTION IN PATIENTS DIAGNOSED WITH AIDS. TREATMENT OF HUMAN CYTOMEGALOVIRUS INFECTION IN PATIENTS DIAGNOSED WITH AIDS.	BIOMEDICAL RESEARCH INSTITUTE

BIOLOGICAL DESIGNATIONS (continued)

NAME OF BIOLOGICAL	DESIGNATED USE [EXCLUSIVITY EXPIRATION DATE]	SPONSOR NAME
GENERIC: ANTI-TAP-72 IMMUNO-TOXIN TRADE: XOMAZYME-791	TREATMENT OF METASTATIC COLORECTAL ADENOCARCINOMA.	XOMA CORPORATION
GENERIC: ANTITHROMBIN III TRADE: THROMBATE III*/***	USE AS REPLACEMENT THERAPY IN CONGENITAL DEFICIENCY OF ANTITHROMBIN-III FOR PREVENTION AND TREATMENT OF THROMBOSIS AND PULMONARY EMBOLI.	CUTTER
GENERIC: ANTITHROMBIN III CONCENTRATE I.V. TRADE: KYBERNIN	PROPHYLAXIS AND TREATMENT OF THROMBOEMBOLIC EPISODES IN PATIENTS WITH GENETIC AT-III DEFICIENCY.	HOECHST ROUSSEL PHARMACEUTICAL
GENERIC: ANTITHROMBIN III (HUMAN) TRADE: ANTITHROMBIN III (HUMAN)	PREVENTING OR ARRESTING EPISODES OF THROMBOSIS IN PATIENTS WITH CONGENITAL ANTITHROMBIN III DEFICIENCY AND/OR TO PREVENT THE OCCURRENCE OF THROMBOSIS IN PATIENTS WITH ANTITHROMBIN III DEFICIENCY WHO HAVE UNDERGONE TRAUMA OR WHO ARE ABOUT TO UNDERGO SURGERY OR PARTURITION.	AMERICAN NATIONAL RED CROSS
GENERIC: ANTITHROMBIN III (HUMAN) TRADE: ATNATIV*/**	HEREDITARY AT-III DEFICIENCY IN CONNECTION WITH SURGICAL OR OBSTETRICAL PROCEDURES OR WHEN THEY SUFFER FROM THROMBOEMBOLISM. [DEC 13, 1996]	KABIVITRUM
GENERIC: ANTIVENOM (CROTALIDAE) PURIFIED (AVIAN) TRADE: NOT ESTABLISHED	TREATMENT OF ENVENOMATION BY POISONOUS SNAKES BELONGING TO THE CROTALIDE FAMILY.	OPHIDIAN PHARMA
GENERIC: BENZYLPENICILLIN, BENZYLPENICILLOIC, BENZYLPENILLOIC ACID TRADE: PRE-PEN/MDM	ASSESSING THE RISK OF ADMINISTRATING PENICILLIN WHEN IT IS THE PREFERRED DRUG OF CHOICE IN ADULT PATIENTS WHO HAVE PREVIOUSLY RECEIVED PENICILLIN AND HAVE A HISTORY OF CLINICAL SENSITIVITY.	KREMERS-URBAN COMPANY
GENERIC: BOTULINUM TOXIN TYPE A TRADE: OCULINUM*/**	TREATMENT OF STRABISMUS ASSOCIATED WITH DYSTONIA IN ADULTS (PATIENTS 12 YEARS OF AGE AND ABOVE).*/** [DEC 29, 1996] TREATMENT OF BLEPHAROSPASM ASSOCIATED WITH DYSTONIA IN ADULTS (PATIENTS 12 YEARS OF AGE AND ABOVE).*/** [DEC 29, 1996] TREATMENT OF CERVICAL DYSTONIA. TREATMENT OF DYNAMIC MUSCLE CONTRACTURE IN PEDIATIC CEREBRAL PALSY PATIENTS.	ALLERGAN
GENERIC: BOTULINUM, TOXIN TYPE A TRADE: DYSPORT	TREATMENT OF ESSENTIAL BLEPHAROSPASM.	PORTON INTERNATIONAL, INC
GENERIC: BOTULINUM TOXIN TYPE B TRADE: NOT ESTABLISHED	TREATMENT OF CERVICAL DYSTONIA.	ATHENA NEUROSCIENCES, INC
GENERIC: BOTULINUM TOXIN TYPE F TRADE: NOT ESTABLISHED	TREATMENT OF SPASMODIC TORTICOLLIS. TREATMENT OF ESSENTIAL BLEPHAROSPASM.	PORTON PRODUCTS LIMITED
GENERIC: BOTULISM IMMUNE GLOBULIN TRADE: NOT ESTABLISHED	TREATMENT OF INFANT BOTULISM.	CALIFORNIA DEPT HEALTH SERVICE
GENERIC: BOVINE COLOSTRUM TRADE: NOT ESTABLISHED	TREATMENT OF AIDS-RELATED DIARRHEA.	DONALD H. HASTINGS, D.V.M. BISMARCK, ND
GENERIC: CHIMERIC M-T412 (HUMAN-MURINE) IGG MONOCLONAL ANTI-CD4 ANTIBODY TRADE: NOT ESTABLISHED	TREATMENT OF MULTIPLE SCLEROSIS.	CENTOCOR, INC
GENERIC: CILIARY NEUROTROPHIC FACTOR TRADE: NOT ESTABLISHED	TREATMENT OF AMYOTROPHIC LATERAL SCLEROSIS.	ROGENERON PHARMACEUTICALS, INC
GENERIC: CILIARY NEUROTROPHIC FACTOR, RECOMBINANT HUMAN TRADE: NOT ESTABLISHED	TREATMENT OF SPINAL MUSCULAR ATROPHIES. TREATMENT OF MOTOR NEURON DISEASE (INCLUDING AMYOTROPHIC LATERAL SCLEROSIS, PROGRESSIVE MUSCULAR ATROPHY, PROGRESSIVE BULBAR PALSY, AND PRIMARY LATERAL SCLEROSIS).	SYNTEX-SYNERGEN NEUROSCIENCE
GENERIC: COAGULATION FACTOR IX (HUMAN) TRADE: ALPHANINE*/**	FOR USE AS REPLACEMENT THERAPY IN PATIENTS WITH HEMOPHILIA B FOR THE PREVENTION AND CONTROL OF BLEEDING EPISODES, AND DURING SURGERY TO CORRECT DEFECTIVE HEMOSTASIS. [DEC 31, 1997]	ALPHA THERAPEUTIC
GENERIC: COAGULATION FACTOR IX TRADE: MONONINE*/**	REPLACEMENT TREATMENT AND PROPHYLAXIS OF THE HEMORRHAGIC COMPLICATIONS OF HEMOPHILIA B. [AUG 20, 1999]	ARMOUR PHARMACEUTICAL

BIOLOGICAL DESIGNATIONS *(continued)*

NAME OF BIOLOGICAL	DESIGNATED USE [EXCLUSIVITY EXPIRATION DATE]	SPONSOR NAME
GENERIC: CRYPTOSPORIDIUM HYPERIMMUNE BOVINE COLOSTRUM IGG TRADE: NOT ESTABLISHED	TREATMENT OF DIARRHEA IN AIDS PATIENTS CAUSED BY INFECTION WITH CRYPTOSPORIDIUM PARVUM.	IMMUCELL CORPORATION
GENERIC: CYSTIC FIBROSIS GENE THERAPY TRADE: NOT ESTABLISHED	TREATMENT OF CYSTIC FIBROSIS.	GENZYME CORPORATION
GENERIC: CYSTIC FIBROSIS TRANSMEMBRANE CONDUCTANCE REGULATOR TRADE: NOT ESTABLISHED	FOR CYSTIC FIBROSIS TRANSMEMBRANE CONDUCTANCE REGULATOR PROTEIN REPLACEMENT THERAPY IN CYSTIC FIBROSIS PATIENTS.	GENZYME CORPORATION
GENERIC: CYTOMEGALOVIRUS IMMUNE GLOBULIN (HUMAN) TRADE: NOT ESTABLISHED*/**	PREVENTION OR ATTENUATION OF PRIMARY CYTOMEGALOVIRUS DISEASE IN IMMUNOSUPPRESSED RECIPIENTS OF ORGAN TRANSPLANTS. [APR 17, 1997]	MA PUB HLTH BIOLOGICAL LABS
GENERIC: CYTOMEGALOVIRUS IMMUNE GLOBULIN INTRAVENOUS (HUMAN) TRADE: NOT ESTABLISHED	USE IN CONJUNCTION WITH GANCICLOVIR SODIUM FOR THE TREATMENT OF CYTOMEGALOVIRUS PNEUMONIA IN BONE MARROW TRANSPLANT PATIENTS.	MILES, INC
GENERIC: C1-INHIBITOR TRADE: C1-INHIBITOR (HUMAN) VAPOR HEATED, IMMUNO	PREVENTION OF ACUTE ATTACKS OF ANGIOEDEMA, INCLUDING SHORT-TERM PROPHYLAXIS FOR PATIENTS REQUIRING DENTAL OR OTHER SURGICAL PROCEDURES. TREATMENT OF ACUTE ATTACKS OF ANGIOEDEMA.	IMMUNO CLINICAL RESEARCH CORP
GENERIC: CD4, HUMAN-RECOMBINANT SOLUBLE TRADE: NOT ESTABLISHED	TREATMENT OF AIDS RESULTING FROM INFECTION WITH HIV.	GENENTECH, INC
GENERIC: CD4, HUMAN-RECOMBINANT SOLUBLE TRADE: RECEPTIN	TREATMENT OF ACQUIRED IMMUNODEFICIENCY SYNDROME (AIDS).	BIOGEN, INC
GENERIC: CD4, HUMAN TRUNCATED-369 AA POLYPEPTIDE TRADE: SOLUBLE T4	TREATMENT OF ACQUIRED IMMUNODEFICIENCY SYNDROME (AIDS).	SMITHKLINE BEECHAM
GENERIC: CD4 IMMUNOGLOBULIN G (RECOMBINANT-HUMAN) TRADE: NOT ESTABLISHED	TREATMENT OF ACQUIRED IMMUNODEFICIENCY SYNDROME (AIDS) RESULTING FROM INFECTION WITH THE HUMAN IMMUNODEFICIENCY VIRUS (HIV-1).	GENENTECH
GENERIC: CD5-T LYMPHOCYTE IMMUNOTOXIN TRADE: XOMAZYME-H65	FOR TREATMENT OF GRAFT VS HOST DISEASE (GVHD) AND/OR REJECTION IN PATIENTS WHO HAVE RECEIVED BONE MARROW TRANSPLANTS.	XOMA CORPORATION
GENERIC: CD-45 MONOCLONAL ANTIBODIES TRADE: NOT ESTABLISHED	PREVENTION OF ACUTE GRAFT REJECTION OF HUMAN ORGAN TRANSPLANTS.	BAXTER HEALTHCARE CORPORATION
GENERIC: DIGOXIN IMMUNE FAB (OVINE) TRADE: DIGIBIND*/**	TREATMENT OF POTENTIALLY LIFE-THREATENING DIGITALIS INTOXICATION IN PATIENTS WHO ARE REFRACTORY TO MANAGEMENT BY CONVENTIONAL THERAPY. [APR 22, 1993]	BURROUGHS WELLCOME
GENERIC: DIGOXIN IMMUNE FAB (OVINE) TRADE: DIGIDOTE	LIFE-THREATENING ACUTE CARDIAC GLYCOSIDE INTOXICATION MANIFESTED CONDUCTION DISORDERS, ECTOPIC VENTRICULAR ACTIVITY AND (IN SOME CASES) HYPERKALEMIA.	BOEHRINGER MANNHEIM CORP
GENERIC: DISACCHARIDE TRIPEPTIDE GLYCEROL DIPALMITOYL (DTP-GDP) TRADE: IMMTHER	TREATMENT OF PULMONARY AND HEPATIC METASTASES IN COLORECTAL ADENOCARCINOMA PATIENTS.	IMMUNO THERAPEUTICS, INC
GENERIC: EPOETIN ALFA (RECOMBINANT-HUMAN) TRADE: EPOGEN*/**	TREATMENT OF ANEMIA ASSOCIATED WITH CHRONIC RENAL FAILURE, INCLUDING PATIENTS ON DIALYSIS (END STAGE RENAL DISEASE) AND PATIENTS NOT ON DIALYSIS.*/** [JUN 01, 1996] TREATMENT OF ANEMIA ASSOCIATED WITH HIV INFECTION OR HIV TREATMENT. [TREATMENT OF AZT-INDUCED ANEMIA IN HIV INFECTED PATIENTS.*/**] [DEC 31, 1997]	AMGEN
GENERIC: EPOETIN BETA TRADE: MAROGEN	TREATMENT OF ANEMIA ASSOCIATED WITH END STAGE RENAL DISEASE (ESRD).	CHUGAI-UPJOHN, INC
GENERIC: ERWINIA L-ASPARAGINASE TRADE: ERWINASE	TREATMENT OF ACUTE LYMPHOCYTIC LEUKEMIA (ALL).	PORTON PRODUCTS, LTD
GENERIC: ERYTHROPOIETIN (RECOMBINANT-HUMAN) TRADE: PROCRIT	TREATMENT OF ANEMIA ASSOCIATED WITH END STAGE RENAL DISEASE (ESRD). TREATMENT OF ANEMIA OF PREMATURITY IN PRETERM INFANTS. TREATMENT OF HIV ASSOCIATED ANEMIA RELATED TO HIV INFECTION OR HIV TREATMENT.	R.W. JOHNSON RESEARCH INSTITUTE

BIOLOGICAL DESIGNATIONS *(continued)*

NAME OF BIOLOGICAL	DESIGNATED USE [EXCLUSIVITY EXPIRATION DATE]	SPONSOR NAME
GENERIC: ERYTHROPOIETIN (RECOMBINANT-HUMAN) TRADE: NOT ESTABLISHED	TREATMENT OF ANEMIA ASSOCIATED WITH END STAGE RENAL DISEASE (ESRD).	MCDONNELL DOUGLAS CORP
GENERIC: FACTOR VIIa (RECOMBINANT, DNA ORIGIN) TRADE: NOT ESTABLISHED	TREATMENT OF PATIENTS WITH HEMOPHILIA A & B WITH AND WITHOUT ANTIBODIES AGAINST FACTOR VIII/IX AND TREATMENT OF PATIENTS WITH VON WILLEBRAND'S DISEASE.	NOVO LABORATORIES
GENERIC: FACTOR XIII (PLACENTA-DERIVED) TRADE: FIBROGAMMIN	CONGENITAL FACTOR XIII DEFICIENCY.	HOECHST-ROUSSEL PHARMACEUTICAL
GENERIC: FIBRONECTIN (HUMAN PLASMA DERIVED) TRADE: NOT ESTABLISHED	TREATMENT OF NON-HEALING CORNEAL ULCERS OR EPITHELIAL DEFECTS WHICH HAVE BEEN UNRESPONSIVE TO CONVENTIONAL THERAPY AND THE UNDERLYING CAUSE HAS BEEN ELIMINATED.	NEW YORK BLOOD CENTER
GENERIC: FIBRONECTIN (PLASMA DERIVED) TRADE: NOT ESTABLISHED	TREATMENT OF NON-HEALING CORNEAL ULCERS OR EPITHELIAL DEFECTS WHICH HAVE BEEN UNRESPONSIVE TO CONVENTIONAL THERAPY AND FOR WHICH ANY INFECTIOUS CAUSE HAS BEEN ELIMINATED.	CHIRON OPHTHALMICS, INC
GENERIC: FILGRASTIM TRADE: NEUPOGEN	TREATMENT OF MYELODYSPLASTIC SYNDROME. TREATMENT OF NEUTROPENIA ASSOCIATED WITH BONE MARROW TRANSPLANTS. TREATMENT OF PATIENTS WITH SEVERE CHRONIC NEUTROPENIA (ABSOLUTE NEUTROPHIL COUNT LESS THAN 500 PER CUBIC MILLIMETER.) TREATMENT OF PATIENTS WITH ACQUIRED IMMUNODEFICIENCY SYNDROME (AIDS) WHO, IN ADDITION, ARE AFFLICTED WITH CYTOMEGALOVIRUS RETINITIS (CMV RETINITIS) AND ARE BEING TREATED WITH GANCICLOVIR.	AMGEN, INC
GENERIC: GRANULOCYTE MACROPHAGE-COLONY STIMULATING FACTOR TRADE: LEUCOMAX	TREATMENT OF AIDS PATIENTS WITH NEUTROPENIA DUE TO EITHER THE DISEASE ITSELF, ZIDOVUDINE (AZIDOTHYMIDINE) [AZT], OR GANCICLOVIR (DHPG). TREATMENT OF PATIENTS WITH MYELODYSPLASTIC SYNDROME. TREATMENT OF APLASTIC ANEMIA.	SCHERING CORPORATION
GENERIC: GROUP B STREPTOCOCCUS IMMUNE GLOBULIN TRADE: NOT ESTABLISHED	TREATMENT OF NEONATES WITH DISSEMINATED GROUP B STREPTOCOCCAL INFECTION.	UNIVAX CORPORATION
GENERIC: HEME ARGINATE TRADE: NORMOSANG	TREATMENT OF SYMPTOMATIC STAGE OF ACUTE PORPHYRIA.	HUHTAMAKI OY LEIRAS
GENERIC: HEMIN TRADE: PANHEMATIN*/**	AMELIORATION OF RECURRENT ATTACKS OF ACUTE INTERMITTENT PORPHYRIA TEMPORARILY RELATED TO THE MENSTRUAL CYCLE IN SUSCEPTIBLE WOMEN AND SIMILAR SYMPTOMS WHICH OCCUR IN OTHER PATIENTS WITH ACUTE INTERMITTENT PORPHYRIA, PORPHYRIA VARIEGATA AND HEREDITARY COPROPORPHYRIA. [JUL 20, 1990]	ABBOTT
GENERIC: HIV NEUTRALIZING ANTIBODIES TRADE: IMMUPATH	TREATMENT OF ACQUIRED IMMUNODEFICIENCY SYNDROME (AIDS).	HEMACARE CORPORATION
GENERIC: HUMAN IGM MONOCLONAL ANTIBODY (C-58) TO CYTOMEGALOVIRUS (CMV) TRADE: CENTOVIR	TREATMENT OF CYTOMEGALOVIRUS (CMV) INFECTIONS IN BONE MARROW TRANSPLANT PATIENTS. PROPHYLAXIS OF CMV INFECTIONS IN BONE MARROW TRANSPLANT PATIENTS.	CENTOCOR, INC
GENERIC: HUMAN IMMUNODEFICIENCY VIRUS IMMUNE GLOBULIN TRADE: NOT ESTABLISHED	TREATMENT OF ACQUIRED IMMUNODEFICIENCY SYNDROME (AIDS). TREATMENT OF HIV-INFECTED PREGNANT WOMEN AND INFANTS OF HIV-INFECTED MOTHERS.	ABBOTT LABORATORIES
GENERIC: HUMAN MONOCLONAL ANTIBODY AGAINST HEPATITIS B VIRUS TRADE: NOT ESTABLISHED	PROPHYLAXIS OF HEPATITIS B REINFECTION IN PATIENTS UNDERGOING LIVER TRANSPLANTATION SECONDARY TO END-STAGE CHRONIC HEPATITIS B INFECTION.	SANDOX PHARMACEUTICALS CORPORATION
GENERIC: HUMAN T-LYMPHOTROPIC VIRUS TYPE III gp160 ANTIGENS, RECOMBINANT VACCINE, ALUM ABSORBED TRADE: VAXSYN HIV-1	TREATMENT OF ACQUIRED IMMUNODEFICIENCY SYNDROME (AIDS).	MICRO GENE SYSTEMS, INC
GENERIC: IMPORTED FIRE ANT VENOM, ALLERGENIC EXTRACT TRADE: NOT ESTABLISHED	FOR SKIN TESTING OF VICTIMS OF FIRE ANT STINGS TO CONFIRM FIRE ANT SENSITIVITY AND IF POSITIVE, FOR USE AS IMMUNOTHERAPY FOR THE PREVENTION OF IgE-MEDIATED ANAPHYLACTIC REACTIONS.	ALK LABORATORIES, INC

BIOLOGICAL DESIGNATIONS *(continued)*

NAME OF BIOLOGICAL	DESIGNATED USE [EXCLUSIVITY EXPIRATION DATE]	SPONSOR NAME
GENERIC: [INDIUM 111 MURINE ANTI-CEA MONOCLONAL ANTIBODY TYPE ZCE 025] TRADE: CEAKER	FOR THE DETECTION OF SUSPECTED AND PREVIOUSLY UN-IDENTIFIED TUMOR FOCI OF RECURRENT COLORECTAL CARCINOMA.	HYBRITECH, INC
GENERIC: INDIUM IN 111 MURINE MONOCLONAL ANTIBODY B72.3 TRADE: ONCOSCINT OV103	DETECTION OF OVARIAN CANCER.	CYTOGEN CORPORATION
GENERIC: INDIUM IN 111 MURINE MONOCLONAL ANTIBODY FAB TO MYOSIN TRADE: MYOSCINT	DETECTING EARLY NECROSIS AS AN INDICATOR OF REJECTION OF ORTHOTOPIC CARDIAC TRANSPLANTS. DIAGNOSIS OF MYOCARDITIS.	CENTOCOR, INC
GENERIC: INSULIN-LIKE GROWTH FACTOR-1 TRADE: MYOTROPHIN	TREATMENT OF AMYOTROPHIC LATERAL SCLEROSIS.	CEPHALON, INC
GENERIC: INTERFERON (RECOMBINANT HUMAN, BETA) TRADE: BETASERON	TREATMENT OF ACQUIRED IMMUNE DEFICIENCY SYNDROME (AIDS). TREATMENT OF MULTIPLE SCLEROSIS (MS).	TRITON BIOSCIENCES, INC
GENERIC: INTERFERON (RECOMBINANT HUMAN, BETA) TRADE: NOT ESTABLISHED	SYSTEMIC TREATMENT OF METASTATIC RENAL CELL CARCINOMA. SYSTEMIC TREATMENT OF CUTANEOUS T-CELL LYMPHOMA. SYSTEMIC TREATMENT OF CUTANEOUS MALIGNANT MELANOMA. INTRALESIONAL AND/OR SYSTEMIC TREATMENT OF AIDS-RELATED KAPOSI'S SARCOMA. TREATMENT OF MULTIPLE SCLEROSIS. TREATMENT OF ACUTE NON-A, NON-B HEPATITIS.	BIOGEN
GENERIC: INTERFERON ALPHA-NL TRADE: WELLFERON	TREATMENT OF ACQUIRED IMMUNE DEFICIENCY SYNDROME (AIDS)-RELATED KAPOSI'S SARCOMA. TREATMENT OF HUMAN PAPILLOMAVIRUS (HPV) IN PATIENTS WITH SEVERE RESISTANT/RECURRENT RESPIRATORY (LARYNGEAL) PAPILLOMATOSIS.	BURROUGHS WELLCOME COMPANY
GENERIC: INTERFERON ALFA-2A (RECOMBINANT) TRADE: ROFERON-A*/**	TREATMENT OF SELECTED PATIENTS WITH ACQUIRED IMMUNE DEFICIENCY SYNDROME (AIDS)-RELATED KAPOSI'S SARCOMA.*/** [NOV 21, 1995] TREATMENT OF RENAL CELL CARCINOMA. TREATMENT OF CHRONIC MYELOGENOUS LEUKEMIA (CML). FOR USE IN COMBINATION WITH FLUOROURACIL FOR THE TREATMENT OF ESOPHAGEAL CARCINOMA. TREATMENT OF METASTATIC RENAL CELL CARCINOMA IN COMBINATION WITH TECELEUKIN. TREATMENT OF METASTATIC MALIGNANT MELANOMA IN COMBINATION WITH TECELEUKIN. CONCOMITANT ADMINISTRATION WITH FLUOROURACIL FOR THE TREATMENT OF PATIENTS WITH ADVANCED COLORECTAL CANCER.	ROCHE
GENERIC: INTERFERON ALPHA-2B (RECOMBINANT) TRADE: INTRON A*/**	TREATMENT OF CHRONIC MYELOGENOUS LEUKEMIA (CML). TREATMENT OF SELECTED PATIENTS WITH AIDS-RELATED KAPOSI'S SARCOMA.*/** [NOV 21, 1995] TREATMENT OF ACUTE HEPATITIS B. TREATMENT OF PATIENTS WITH CHRONIC DELTA HEPATITIS.	SCHERING
GENERIC: INTERFERON GAMMA-1B TRADE: ACTIMMUNE*/**	TREATMENT OF CHRONIC GRANULOMATOUS DISEASE (CGD). [DEC 20, 1997]	GENENTECH
GENERIC: INTERLEUKIN-1, ALPHA, HUMAN RECOMBINANT TRADE: NOT ESTABLISHED	FOR THE PROMOTION OF EARLY ENGRAFTMENT IN BONE MARROW TRANSPLANTATION. FOR HEMATOPOIETIC POTENTIATION IN APLASTIC ANEMIA.	IMMUNEX CORPORATION
GENERIC: INTERLEUKIN-1 RECEPTOR ANTAGONIST, HUMAN RECOMBINANT TRADE: ANTRIL	TREATMENT OF JUVENILE RHEUMATOID ARTHRITIS.	SYNERGEN, INC
GENERIC: INTERLEUKIN-2 POLYETHYLENE CONJUGATE; RECOMBINANT E. COLI TRADE: NOT ESTABLISHED	TREATMENT OF PRIMARY IMMUNODEFICIENCY DISEASE ASSOCIATED WITH T-CELL DEFECTS.	CETUS CORPORATION
GENERIC: INTERLEUKIN-3, RECOMBINANT HUMAN TRADE: NOT ESTABLISHED	PROMOTION OF ERYTHROPOIESIS IN DIAMOND-BLACKFAN ANEMIA (CONGENITAL PURE CELL RED APLASIA).	IMMUNEX CORPORATION
GENERIC: IODINE I 123 MURINE MONOCLONAL ANTIBODY TO HUMAN ALPHA-FETOPROTEIN TRADE: NOT ESTABLISHED	DETECTION OF HEPATOCELLULAR CARCINOMA AND HEPATOBLASTOMA. DETECTION OF ALPHA-FETOPROTEIN PRODUCING GERM CELL TUMORS.	IMMUNOMEDICS, INC

BIOLOGICAL DESIGNATIONS *(continued)*

NAME OF BIOLOGICAL	DESIGNATED USE [EXCLUSIVITY EXPIRATION DATE]	SPONSOR NAME
GENERIC: IODINE I 123 MURINE MONOCLONAL ANTIBODY TO HUMAN CHORIONIC GONADOTROPIN (HCG) TRADE: NOT ESTABLISHED	DETECTION OF HCG PRODUCING TUMORS SUCH AS GERM CELL AND TROPHOBLASTIC CELL TUMORS.	IMMUNOMEDICS, INC
GENERIC: IODINE I 131 LYM-1 MONOCLONAL ANTIBODY TRADE: NOT ESTABLISHED	TREATMENT OF B-CELL LYMPHOMA.	LEDERLE LABORATORIES DIVISION AMERICAN CYANAMIDE COMPANY
GENERIC: IODINE I 131 MURINE MONOCLONAL ANTIBODY IGG2A TO B CELL TRADE: IMMURAIT, LL-2-I-131	TREATMENT OF B-CELL LEUKEMIA AND B-CELL LYMPHOMA.	IMMUNOMEDICS, INC
GENERIC: IODINE I 131 MURINE MONOCLONAL ANTIBODY TO HUMAN ALPHA-FETOPROTEIN TRADE: NOT ESTABLISHED	TREATMENT OF HEPATOCELLULAR CARCINOMA AND HEPATOBLASTOMA. TREATMENT OF ALPHA-FETOPROTEIN PRODUCING GERM CELL TUMORS.	IMMUNOMEDICS, INC
GENERIC: LACTOBIN TRADE: LACTOBIN	TREATMENT OF AIDS ASSOCIATED DIARRHEA UNRESPONSIVE TO INITIAL ANTIDIARRHEAL THERAPY.	ROXANE LABORATORIES
GENERIC: LEUPEPTIN TRADE: NOT ESTABLISHED	ADJUNCT TO MICROSURGICAL PERIPHERAL NERVE REPAIR.	LAWRENCE C. HURST, M.D. STATE UNIVERSITY OF NEW YORK
GENERIC: LIPOSOME ENCAPSULATED RECOMBINANT INTERLEUKIN-2 TRADE: NOT ESTABLISHED	TREATMENT OF BRAIN AND CNS TUMORS.	ONCOTHERAPEUTICS, INC
GENERIC: MELANOMA VACCINE TRADE: MELACCINE	TREATMENT OF STAGE III-IV MELANOMA.	RIBI IMMUNOCHEM RESEARCH, INC
GENERIC: MONOCLONAL ANTIBODIES (MURINE OR HUMAN) B-CELL LYMPHOMA TRADE: NOT ESTABLISHED	TREATMENT OF B-CELL LYMPHOMA.	IDEC PHARMACEUTICAL CORP
GENERIC: MONOCLONAL ANTIBODY PM-81 TRADE: NOT ESTABLISHED	ADJUNCTIVE TREATMENT OF ACUTE MYELOGENOUS LEUKEMIA.	MEDAREX, INC
GENERIC: MONOCLONAL ANTIBODIES PM-81 AND AML 2-23 TRADE: NOT ESTABLISHED	FOR EXOGENOUS DEPLETION OF CD14 AND CD15 POSITIVE ACUTE MYELOID LEUKEMIC BONE MARROW CELLS FROM PATIENTS UNDERGOING BONE MARROW TRANSPLANTATION.	MEDAREX, INC
GENERIC: MONOCLONAL ANTIBODY 17-1A TRADE: PANOREX	TREATMENT OF PANCREATIC CANCER.	CENTOCOR, INC
GENERIC: MONOCLONAL FACTOR IX TRADE: MONONINE	REPLACEMENT TREATMENT AND PROPHYLAXIS OF HEMORRHAGIC COMPLICATIONS OF HEMOPHILIA B.	ARMOUR PHARMACEUTICAL COMPANY
GENERIC: MUCOID EXOPOLYSACCHARIDE PSEUDOMONAS HYPERIMMUNE GLOBULIN TRADE: MEPIG	PREVENTION OF PULMONARY INFECTIONS DUE TO PSEUDOMONAS AERUGINOSA IN PATIENTS WITH CYSTIC FIBROSIS. TREATMENT OF PULMONARY INFECTIONS DUE TO PSEUDOMONAS AERUGINOSA IN PATIENTS WITH CYSTIC FIBROSIS.	UNIVAX BIOLOGICS, INC
GENERIC: MYELIN TRADE: NOT ESTABLISHED	TREATMENT OF MULTIPLE SCLEROSIS	AUTOIMMUNE, INC
GENERIC: ONCORAD OV103 TRADE: NOT ESTABLISHED	TREATMENT OF OVARIAN CARCINOMA.	CYTOGEN CORPORATION
GENERIC: PEG-INTERLEUKIN-2 TRADE: NOT ESTABLISHED	TREATMENT OF PRIMARY IMMUNODEFICIENCIES ASSOCIATED WITH T-CELL DEFECTS.	CETUS CORPORATION
GENERIC: PEG-L-ASPARAGINASE TRADE: NOT ESTABLISHED	TREATMENT OF ACUTE LYMPHOCYTIC LEUKEMIA (ALL).	ENZON, INC
GENERIC: PENTASTARCH TRADE: PENTASPAN*/**	FOR USE AS AN ADJUNCT IN LEUKOPHERESIS, TO IMPROVE THE HARVESTING AND INCREASE THE YIELD OF LEUKOCYTES BY CENTRIFUGAL MEANS. [MAY 19, 1994]	DUPONT
GENERIC: POLY I; POLY C$_{12}$U TRADE: AMPLIGEN	TREATMENT OF RENAL CELL CARCINOMA TREATMENT OF ACQUIRED IMMUNODEFICIENCY SYNDROME (AIDS).	HEM RESEARCH, INC

BIOLOGICAL DESIGNATIONS *(continued)*

NAME OF BIOLOGICAL	DESIGNATED USE [EXCLUSIVITY EXPIRATION DATE]	SPONSOR NAME
GENERIC: PROTEIN C CONCENTRATE TRADE: PROTEIN C CONCENTRATE (HUMAN) VAPOR HEATED, IMMUNO	FOR REPLACEMENT THERAPY IN PATIENTS WITH CONGENITAL OR ACQUIRED PROTEIN C DEFICIENCY FOR THE PREVENTION AND TREATMENT OF WARFARIN-INDUCED SKIN NECROSIS DURING ORAL ANTICOAGULATION. FOR REPLACEMENT THERAPY IN CONGENITAL PROTEIN C DEFICIENCY FOR THE PREVENTION AND TREATMENT OF THROMBOSIS, PULMONARY EMBOLI, AND PURPURA FULMINANS.	IMMUNO CLINICAL RESEARCH CORPORATION
GENERIC: RECOMBINANT HUMAN DEOXYRIBONUCLEASE (RHDNASE) TRADE: NOT ESTABLISHED	TO REDUCE MUCOUS VISCOSITY AND ENABLE CLEARANCE OF AIRWAY SECRETIONS IN PATIENTS WITH CYSTIC FIBROSIS.	GENENTECH, INC
GENERIC: RECOMBINANT SECRETORY LEUCOCYTE PROTEASE INHIBITOR TRADE: NOT ESTABLISHED	TREATMENT OF CONGENTIAL ALPHA-1 ANTITRYPSIN DEFICIENCY. TREATMENT OF CYSTIC FIBROSIS.	SYNERGEN, INC
GENERIC: RESPIRATORY SYNCYTIAL VIRUS IMMUNE GLOBULIN (HUMAN) TRADE: HYPERMUNE RSV	PROPHYLAXIS OF RESPIRATORY SYNCYTIAL VIRUS (RSV) LOWER RESPIRATORY INFECTIONS IN INFANTS AND YOUNG CHILDREN AT HIGH RISK OF SEROUS RSV DISEASE. TREATMENT OF RESPIRATORY SYNCYTIAL VIRUS (RSV) LOWER (RSV) RESPIRATORY INFECTIONS IN HOSPITALIZED INFANTS AND YOUNG CHILDREN.	MEDIMMUNE, INC
GENERIC: RICIN (BLOCKED) CONJUGATED MURINE MCA (ANTI-B4) TRADE: NOT ESTABLISHED	TREATMENT OF B-CELL LEUKEMIA AND B-CELL LYMPHOMA. FOR THE EX-VIVO PURGING OF LEUKEMIC CELLS FROM THE BONE MARROW OF NON-T CELL ACUTE LYMPHOCYTIC LEUKEMIA PATIENTS WHO ARE IN COMPLETE REMISSION.	IMMUNOGEN, INC
GENERIC: RICIN (BLOCKED) CONJUGATED MURINE MCA (ANTI-MY^9) TRADE: NOT ESTABLISHED	TREATMENT OF MYELOID LEUKEMIA, INCLUDING AML, AND BLAST CRISIS OF CML. FOR USE IN THE EX VIVO TREATMENT OF AUTOLOGOUS BONE MARROW AND SUBSEQUENT REINFUSION IN PATIENTS WITH ACUTE MYELOGENOUS LEUKEMIA.	IMMUNOGEN, INC
GENERIC: RICIN (BLOCKED) CONJUGATED MURINE MCA (N901) TRADE: NOT ESTABLISHED	TREATMENT OF SMALL CELL LUNG CANCER.	IMMUNOGEN, INC
GENERIC: SARGRAMOSTIM TRADE: LEUKINE*/**	TREATMENT OF NEUTROPENIA ASSOCIATED WITH BONE MARROW TRANSPLANT, FOR THE PROMOTION OF EARLY ENGRAFTMENT, AND FOR THE TREATMENT OF GRAFT FAILURE AND DELAY OF ENGRAFTMENT.*/** [DEC 31, 1998] TREATMENT OF NEUTROPENIA ASSOCIATED WITH BONE MARROW TRANSPLANTS IN PATIENTS WITH NON-HODGKIN'S LYMPHOMA, HODGKIN'S DISEASE AND ACUTE LYMPHOBLASTIC LEUKEMIA.*/** [MAR 5, 1998]	IMMUNEX
GENERIC: SEPTOMONAB TRADE: CENTOXIN	TREATMENT OF PATIENTS WITH GRAM-NEGATIVE BACTEREMIA WHICH HAS PROGRESSED TO ENDOTOXIN SHOCK.	CENTOCOR
GENERIC: SERRATIA MARCESCENS EXTRACT (POLY-RIBOSOMES) TRADE: IMUVERT	TREATMENT OF PRIMARY BRAIN MALIGNANCIES.	CELL TECHNOLOGY, INC
GENERIC: ST1-RTA IMMUNOTOXIN (SR 44163) TRADE: NOT ESTABLISHED	PREVENTION OF ACUTE GRAFT VS HOST DISEASE (GVHD) IN ALLOGENEIC BONE MARROW TRANSPLANTATION. TREATMENT OF PATIENTS WITH B-CHRONIC LYMPHOCYTIC LEUKEMIA (CLL).	SANOFI, INC
GENERIC: TECELEUKIN TRADE: NOT ESTABLISHED	TREATMENT OF METASTATIC MALIGNANT MELANOMA. TREATMENT OF METASTATIC RENAL CELL CARCINOMA. TREATMENT OF METASTATIC MALIGNANT MELANOMA IN COMBINATION WITH ROFERON-A. TREATMENT OF METASTATIC RENAL CELL CARCINOMA IN COMBINATION WITH ROFERON-A (INTERFERON ALPHA-2A, RECOMBINANT/ROCHE).	HOFFMANN-LA ROCHE, INC
GENERIC: TECHNETIUM TC 99M ANTI-MELANOMA MURINE MONOCLONAL ANTIBODY KIT TRADE: NOT ESTABLISHED	FOR USE IN DETECTING, BY IMAGING, METASTASES OF MALIGNANT MELANOMA.	NEORX CORPORATION
GENERIC: TECHNETIUM TC 99M MURINE MONOCLONAL ANTIBODY TO HUMAN ALPHA-FETOPROTEIN TRADE: IMMURAID, AFP-TC99M	DETECTION OF HEPATOCELLULAR CARCINOMA AND HEPATOBLASTOMA. DETECTION OF ALPHA-FETOPROTEIN (AFP) PRODUCING GERM CELL TUMORS.	IMMUNOMEDICS, INC

BIOLOGICAL DESIGNATIONS (continued)

NAME OF BIOLOGICAL	DESIGNATED USE [EXCLUSIVITY EXPIRATION DATE]	SPONSOR NAME
GENERIC: TECHNETIUM TC 99M MURINE MONOCLONAL ANTIBODY (IGG2A) TO BCE TRADE: IMMURAID-LL-2[99mTc]	DIAGNOSTIC IMAGING IN THE EVALUATION OF THE EXTENT OF DISEASE IN PATIENTS WITH HISTOLOGICALLY CONFIRMED DIAGNOSIS OF NON-HODGKIN'S B-CELL LYMPHOMA, ACUTE B-CELL LYMPHOBLASTIC LEUKEMIA (IN CHILDREN AND ADULTS), AND CHRONIC B-CELL LYMPHOCYTIC LEUKEMIA.	IMMUNOMEDICS, INC
GENERIC: TECHNETIUM TC 99M MURINE MONOCLONAL ANTIBODY TO HUMAN CHORIONIC GONADOTROPIN (HCG) TRADE: IMMURAID, HCG-TC99M	DETECTION OF HCG PRODUCING TUMORS SUCH AS GERM CELL TUMORS AND TROPHOBLASTIC CELL TUMORS.	IMMUNOMEDICS, INC
GENERIC: THYMOSIN ALPHA-1 TRADE: NOT ESTABLISHED	ADJUNCTIVE TREATMENT OF CHRONIC ACTIVE HEPATITIS B.	ALPHA 1 BIOMEDICALS, INC
GENERIC: TRISACCHARIDES A & B TRADE: BIOSYNJECT	TREATMENT OF MODERATE TO SEVERE CLINICAL FORMS OF HEMOLYTIC DISEASE OF THE NEWBORN ARISING FROM PLACENTAL TRANSFER OF ANTIBODIES AGAINST BLOOD GROUP SUBSTANCES A & B. FOR USE IN ABO-INCOMPATIBLE SOLID ORGAN TRANSPLANTATION INCLUDING KIDNEY, HEART, LIVER, AND PANCREAS. PREVENTION OF ABO MEDICAL HEMOLYTIC REACTIONS ARISING FROM ABO-INCOMPATIBLE BONE MARROW TRANSPLANTATION.	CHEMBIOMED, LTD
GENERIC: T4 ENDONUCLEASE V, LIPOSOME ENCAPSULATED TRADE: T4N5	TO PREVENT CUTANEOUS NEOPLASMS AND OTHER SKIN ABNORMALITIES ASSOCIATED WITH PATIENTS DIAGNOSED WITH XERODERMA PIGMENTOSUM (XP).	APPLIED GENETICS, INC

DRUG DESIGNATIONS
[Approved for Marketing*]
[Exclusive Approval**]

NAME OF DRUG	DESIGNATED USE [EXCLUSIVITY EXPIRATION DATE]	SPONSOR NAME
GENERIC: ACETYLCYSTEINE TRADE: MUCOMYST/MUCOMYST 10 I.V.	INTRAVENOUS TREATMENT OF PATIENTS PRESENTING WITH MODERATE TO SEVERE ACETAMINOPHEN OVERDOSE.	APOTHECON
GENERIC: ACONIAZIDE TRADE: NOT ESTABLISHED	TREATMENT OF TUBERCULOSIS.	LINCOLN DIAGNOSTICS
GENERIC: ADENOSINE TRADE: NOT ESTABLISHED	FOR USE IN CONJUNCTION WITH BCNU IN THE TREATMENT OF BRAIN TUMORS.	MEDCO RESEARCH, INC
GENERIC: ALGLUCERASE TRADE: CEREDASE*/**	REPLACEMENT THERAPY IN PATIENTS WITH GAUCHER'S DISEASE TYPE I. [APR 5, 1988]	GENZYME
GENERIC: ALLOPURINOL SODIUM TRADE: ZYLOPRIM	EX-VIVO PRESERVATION OF CADAVERIC KIDNEYS FOR TRANSPLANTATION.	BURROUGHS WELLCOME COMPANY
GENERIC: ALLOPURINOL RIBOSIDE TRADE: NOT ESTABLISHED	TREATMENT OF CUTANEOUS VISCERAL LEISHMANIASIS. TREATMENT OF CHAGAS' DISEASE.	BURROUGHS WELLCOME COMPANY
GENERIC: ALL-TRANS RETINOIC ACID TRADE: VEASNOID	TREATMENT OF ACUTE PROMYELOCYTIC LEUKEMIA.	HOFFMANN-LA ROCHE, INC
GENERIC: ALPHA-GALACTOSIDASE A TRADE: FABRASE	TREATMENT OF FABRY'S DISEASE.	ROBERT J. DESNICK, M.D. MOUNT SINAI SCHOOL OF MEDICINE
GENERIC: ALTRETAMINE TRADE: HEXALEN*/**	TREATMENT OF ADVANCED ADENOCARCINOMA OF THE OVARY. [DEC 26, 1997]	US BIOSCIENCE
GENERIC: AMILORIDE HCL SOLUTION FOR INHALATION TRADE: NOT ESTABLISHED	TREATMENT OF CYSTIC FIBROSIS.	GLAXO, INC
GENERIC: AMPHOTERICIN B LIPID COMPLEX TRADE: NOT ESTABLISHED	TREATMENT OF CRYPTOCOCCAL MENINGITIS.	BRISTOL MYERS SQUIBB
GENERIC: AMSACRINE TRADE: AMSIDYL	TREATMENT OF ACUTE ADULT LEUKEMIA.	WARNER-LAMBERT COMPANY
GENERIC: ANAGRELIDE TRADE: NOT ESTABLISHED	TREATMENT OF THROMBOCYTOSIS IN CHRONIC MYELOGENOUS LEUKEMIA. TREATMENT OF ESSENTIAL THROMBOCYTHEMIA (ET). TREATMENT OF POLYCYTHEMIA VERA.	ROBERTS PHARMACEUTICAL CORP.
GENERIC: ANTIEPILEPSIRINE TRADE: NOT ESTABLISHED	TREATMENT OF DRUG-RESISTANT GENERALIZED TONIC-CLONIC (GTC) EPILEPSY IN CHILDREN AND IN ADULTS.	COLUMBUS CHILDREN'S HOSPITAL

DRUG DESIGNATIONS (continued)

NAME OF DRUG	DESIGNATED USE [EXCLUSIVITY EXPIRATION DATE]	SPONSOR NAME
GENERIC: ANTIPYRINE TRADE: NOT ESTABLISHED	ANTIPYRINE TEST AS AN INDEX OF HEPATIC DRUG-METABOLIZING CAPACITY.	UPSHER-SMITH LABORATORIES, INC
GENERIC: ARGININE BUTYRATE TRADE: NOT ESTABLISHED	TREATMENT OF BETA-HEMOGLOBINOPATHIES AND BETA-THALASSEMIA.	SUSAN P. PERRINE, M.D.
GENERIC: AS-101 TRADE: NOT ESTABLISHED	TREATMENT OF ACQUIRED IMMUNODEFICIENCY SYNDROME (AIDS).	NPDC-AS101, INC
GENERIC: BACITRACIN TRADE: ALTRACIN	ANTIBIOTIC-ASSOCIATED PSEUDOMEMBRANOUS ENTEROCOLITIS CAUSED BY TOXINS A & B ELABORATED BY CLOSTRIDIUM DIFFICILE.	AL LABORATORIES, INC
GENERIC: BACLOFEN (INTRATHECAL) TRADE: LIORESAL	TREATMENT OF INTRACTABLE SPASTICITY CAUSED BY SPINAL CORD INJURY, MULTIPLE SCLEROSIS, AND OTHER SPINAL DISEASES [JUN 17, 1999].	MEDTRONIC, INC
GENERIC: BACLOFEN TRADE: NOT ESTABLISHED	TREATMENT OF INTRACTABLE SPASTICITY DUE TO MULTIPLE SCLEROSIS OR SPINAL CORD INJURY.	INFUSAID, INC
GENERIC: BERACTANT TRADE: SURVANTA*/**	PREVENTION OF NEONATAL RESPIRATORY DISTRESS SYNDROME (RDS).*/** [JUL 01, 1998] TREATMENT OF NEONATAL RESPIRATORY DISTRESS SYNDROME (RDS).*/** [JUL 01, 1998]	ROSS
GENERIC: BETHANIDINE SULFATE TRADE: NOT ESTABLISHED	TREATMENT OF PRIMARY VENTRICULAR FIBRILLATION. PREVENTION OF RECURRENCE OF PRIMARY VENTRICULAR FIBRILLATION.	MEDCO RESEARCH, INC
GENERIC: BIODEGRADABLE POLYMER IMPLANT CONTAINING CARMUSTINE TRADE: BIODEL IMPLANT CONTIANING BCNU	FOR THE LOCALIZED PLACEMENT IN THE BRAIN FOR THE TREATMENT OF RECURRENT MALIGNANT GLIOMA.	NOVA PHARMACEUTICAL COMPANY
GENERIC: BUTYRYLCHOLINESTERASE TRADE: NOT ESTABLISHED	FOR THE REDUCTION AND CLEARANCE OF TOXIC BLOOD LEVELS OF COCAINE ENCOUNTERED DURING A DRUG OVERDOSE.	PHARMAVENE, INC
GENERIC: BRANCHED CHAIN AMINO ACIDS TRADE: NOT ESTABLISHED	TREATMENT OF AMYOTROPHIC LATERAL SCLEROSIS.	MOUNT SINAI MEDICAL CENTER
GENERIC: BROMHEXINE TRADE: NOT ESTABLISHED	TREATMENT OF MILD TO MODERATE KERATOCONJUNCTIVITIS SICCA IN PATIENTS WITH SJOGREN'S SYNDROME.	BOEHRINGER INGELHEIM
GENERIC: BW B759U (DHPG) TRADE: NOT ESTABLISHED	TREATMENT OF SEVERE HUMAN CYTOMEGALOVIRUS INFECTIONS (HCMV) IN SPECIFIC IMMUNOSUPPRESSED PATIENT POPULATIONS (e.g., BONE MARROW TRANSPLANT RECIPIENTS AND ACQUIRED IMMUNODEFICIENCY SYNDROME PATIENTS).	SYNTEX
GENERIC: BW 12C TRADE: NOT ESTABLISHED	TREATMENT OF SICKLE CELL DISEASE.	BURROUGHS WELLCOME COMPANY
GENERIC: CAFFEINE TRADE: NEOCAF	TREATMENT OF APNEA OF PREMATURITY.	PEDIATRIC PHARMACEUTICS, INC
GENERIC: CALCITONIN (HUMAN) TRADE: CIBACALCIN*/**	TREATMENT OF SYMPTOMATIC PAGET'S DISEASE OF BONE (OSTEITIS DEFORMANS). [OCT 31, 1993]	CIBA
GENERIC: CALCITONIN SALMON NASAL SPRAY TRADE: MIACALCIN NASAL SPRAY	TREATMENT OF SYMPTOMATIC PAGET'S DISEASE OF BONE (OSTEITIS DEFORMANS).	SANDOZ RESEARCH INSTITUTE
GENERIC: CALCIUM ACETATE TRADE: NOT ESTABLISHED	TREATMENT OF HYPERPHOSPHATEMIA IN END STAGE RENAL DISEASE (ESRD).	PHARMEDIC COMPANY
GENERIC: CALCIUM ACETATE TRADE: PHOSLO*/**	TREATMENT OF HYPERPHOSPHATEMIA IN END STAGE RENAL DISEASE. [DEC 10, 1997]	BRAINTREE
GENERIC: CALCIUM CARBONATE TRADE: R & D CALCIUM CARBONATE/600	TREATMENT OF HYPERPHOSPHATEMIA IN PATIENTS WITH END STAGE RENAL DISEASE (ESRD).	R & D LABORATORIES, INC
GENERIC: CALCIUM GLUCONATE GEL TRADE: H-F GEL	FOR USE IN THE EMERGENCY TOPICAL TREATMENT OF HYDROGEN FLUORIDE (HYDROFLUORIC ACID) BURNS.	LTR PHARMACEUTICALS, INC
GENERIC: CALCIUM GLUCONATE GEL 2.5% TRADE: NOT ESTABLISHED	EMERGENCY TOPICAL TREATMENT OF HYDROGEN FLUORIDE (HYDROFLUORIC ACID) BURNS.	PADDOCK LABORATORIES, INC
GENERIC: CARBOVIR TRADE: NOT ESTABLISHED	TREATMENT OF PERSONS WITH AIDS AND IN THE TREATMENT OF PERSONS WITH SYMPTOMATIC HIV INFECTION AND A CD4 COUNT OF LESS THAN 200/MM³.	GLAXO, INC

DRUG DESIGNATIONS *(continued)*

NAME OF DRUG	DESIGNATED USE [EXCLUSIVITY EXPIRATION DATE]	SPONSOR NAME
GENERIC: CASCARA SAGRADA FLUID EXTRACT TRADE: NOT ESTABLISHED	TREATMENT OF ORAL DRUG OVERDOSAGE TO SPEED LOWER BOWEL EVACUATION.	INTRAMED CORPORATION
GENERIC: CERAMIDE TRIHEXOSIDASE/ALPHA-GALACTOSIDASE A TRADE: NOT ESTABLISHED	TREATMENT OF FABRY'S DISEASE.	GENZYME CORPORATION
GENERIC: CETYL ALCOHOL; COLFOSCERIL PALMITATE; TYLOXAPOL TRADE: EXOSURF NEONATAL*/**	PREVENTION OF HYALINE MEMBRANE DISEASE (HMD), ALSO KNOWN AS RESPIRATORY DISTRESS SYNDROME (RDS), IN INFANTS BORN AT 32 WEEKS GESTATION OR LESS.*/** [AUG 02, 1997] TREATMENT OF ESTABLISHED HMD AT ALL GESTATIONAL AGES.*/** [AUG 02, 1997]	BURROUGHS WELLCOME
GENERIC: CHENODIOL TRADE: CHENIX*/**	FOR PATIENTS WITH RADIOLUCENT STONES IN WELL OPACIFYING GALLBLADDERS, IN WHOM ELECTIVE SURGERY WOULD BE UNDERTAKEN EXCEPT FOR THE PRESENCE OF INCREASED SURGICAL RISK DUE TO SYSTEMIC DISEASE OR AGE. [JUL 28, 1990]	SOLVAY
GENERIC: CHLORHEXIDINE GLUCONATE MOUTHRINSE TRADE: PERIDEX	FOR USE IN THE AMELIORATION OF ORAL MUCOSITIS ASSOCIATED WITH CYTOREDUCTIVE THERAPY USED IN CONDITIONING PATIENTS FOR BONE MARROW TRANSPLANTATION THERAPY.	PROCTER & GAMBLE COMPANY
GENERIC: CITRIC ACID, GLUCONO-DELTA-LACTONE, AND MAGNESIUM CARBONATE TRADE: RENACIDIN	TREATMENT OF RENAL AND BLADDER CALCULI OF THE APATITE OR STRUVITE VARIETY.	UNITED-GUARDIAN, INC
GENERIC: CLINDAMYCIN TRADE: CLEOCIN	TREATMENT OF PNEUMOCYSTIS CARINII PNEUMONIA (PCP) ASSOCIATED WITH THE ACQUIRED IMMUNODEFICIENCY SYNDROME (AIDS). PREVENTION OF PCP ASSOCIATED WITH AIDS.	UPJOHN COMPANY
GENERIC: CLOFAZIMINE TRADE: LAMPRENE*/**	TREATMENT OF LEPROMATOUS LEPROSY, INCLUDING DAPSONE-RESISTANT LEPROMATOUS LEPROSY AND LEPROMATOUS LEPROSY COMPLICATED BY ERYTHEMA NODOSUM LEPROSUM. [DEC 15, 1993]	GEIGY
GENERIC: CLONIDINE HYDROCHLORIDE TRADE: NOT ESTABLISHED	BY THE EPIDURAL ROUTE FOR THE TREATMENT OF PAIN IN CANCER PATIENTS TOLERANT TO, OR UNRESPONSIVE TO, INTRASPINAL OPIATES.	FUKISAWA PHARMACEUTICAL CO
GENERIC: COLCHICINE TRADE: NOT ESTABLISHED	FOR USE IN ARRESTING THE PROGRESSION OF NEUROLOGIC DISABILITY CAUSED BY CHRONIC PROGRESSIVE MULTIPLE SCLEROSIS (MS).	PHARMACONTROL CORPORATION
GENERIC: COPOLYMER 1 (COP 1) TRADE: NOT ESTABLISHED	TREATMENT OF MULTIPLE SCLEROSIS (MS).	TAG PHARMACEUTICALS INC c/o LEMMON COMPANY
GENERIC: CROMOLYN SODIUM TRADE: GASTROCROM*/**	TREATMENT OF MASTOCYTOSIS. [DEC 22, 1996]	FISONS
GENERIC: CROMOLYN SODIUM TRADE: OPTICROM*/**	TREATMENT OF VERNAL KERATOCONJUNCTIVITIS (VKC). [OCT 03, 1991]	FISONS
GENERIC: CYCLOSPORINE OPHTHALMIC TRADE: OPTIMMUNE	TREATMENT OF SEVERE KERATOCONJUNCTIVITIS SICCA. ASSOCIATED WITH SJOGREN'S SYNDROME.	UNIVERSITY OF GEORGIA
GENERIC: CYCLOSPORINE 2% OPHTHALMIC OINTMENT TRADE: SANDIMMUNE	TREATMENT OF PATIENTS AT HIGH RISK OF GRAFT REJECTION FOLLOWING PENETRATING KERATOPLASTY. USE IN CORNEAL MELTING SYNDROMES OF KNOWN OR PRESUMED IMMUNOLOGIC ETIOPATHOGENESIS INCLUDING MOOREN'S ULCER.	SANDOZ PHARMACEUTICALS CORP
GENERIC: CYPROTERONE ACETATE TRADE: ANDROCUR	TREATMENT OF SEVERE HIRSUTISM.	BERLEX LABORATORIES, INC
GENERIC: CYSTEAMINE (2-AMINOETHANETHIOL) TRADE: NOT ESTABLISHED	TREATMENT OF NEPHROPATHIC CYSTINOSIS.	JESS G. THOENE, M.D. UNIVERSITY OF MICHIGAN
GENERIC: CYSTEAMINE HCL TRADE: NOT ESTABLISHED	TREATMENT OF NEPHROPATHIC CYSTINOSIS.	WARNER-LAMBERT COMPANY
GENERIC: DANTROLENE SODIUM TRADE: DANTRIUM	TREATMENT OF NEUROLEPTIC MALIGNANT SYNDROME.	NORWICH EATON PHARMACEUTICALS
GENERIC: DAPSONE TRADE: DAPSONE	PROPHYLAXIS OF PNEUMOCYSTIS CARINII PNEUMONIA. FOR THE COMBINATION TREATMENT OF PNEUMOCYSTIS CARINII PNEUMONIA IN CONJUNCTION WITH TRIMETHOPRIM)	JACOBUS PHARMACEUTICAL COMPANY

DRUG DESIGNATIONS *(continued)*

NAME OF DRUG	DESIGNATED USE [EXCLUSIVITY EXPIRATION DATE]	SPONSOR NAME
GENERIC: DEFEROXAMINE AND DEXTRAN TRADE: BIO-RESCUE	TREATMENT OF ACUTE IRON POISONING.	BIOMEDICAL FRONTIERS, INC
GENERIC: DEFIBROTIDE TRADE: NOT ESTABLISHED	TREATMENT OF THROMBOTIC THROMBOCYTOPENIC PURPURA.	CRINOS INTERNATIONAL
GENERIC: DEHYDREX TRADE: NOT ESTABLISHED	TREATMENT OF RECURRENT CORNEAL EROSION UNRESPONSIVE TO CONVENTIONAL THERAPY.	HOLLES LABS
GENERIC: DESLORELIN TRADE: SOMAGARD	TREATMENT OF CENTRAL PRECOCIOUS PUBERTY.	ROBERTS LABORATORIES, INC
GENERIC: DESMOPRESSIN ACETATE TRADE: DDAVP HIGH CONCENTRATION	TREATMENT OF MILD HEMOPHILIA A AND VON WILLEBRAND'S DISEASE.	RORER PHARMACEUTICAL CORP
GENERIC: DEXRAZOXONE TRADE: ZINECARD	PREVENTION OF CARDIOMYOPATHY ASSOCIATED WITH DOXORUBICIN ADMINISTRATION.	ADRIA LABORATORIES
GENERIC: DEXTRAN SULFATE (INHALED, AEROSOLIZED) TRADE: UENDEX	ADJUNCT TO THE TREATMENT OF CYSTIC FIBROSIS.	THOMAS P. KENNEDY, M.D. J. HOIDAL, M.D. RICHMOND, VA
GENERIC: DEXTRAN SULFATE SODIUM TRADE: NOT ESTABLISHED	TREATMENT OF ACQUIRED IMMUNODEFICIENCY SYNDROME (AIDS).	UENO FINE CHEMICALS
GENERIC: DIANEAL PD-2 PERITONEAL DIALYSIS SOLN WITH 1.1% AMINO ACIDS TRADE: NUTRINEAL PD-2 PERITONEAL DIALYSIS SOLN WITH 1.1% AMINO ACIDS	FOR USE AS A NUTRITIONAL SUPPLEMENT FOR THE TREATMENT OF MALNOURISHMENT IN PATIENTS UNDERGOING CONTINUOUS AMBULATORY PERITONEAL DIALYSIS.	BAXTER HEALTHCARE CORPORATION
GENERIC: DIAZEPAM VISCOUS SOLUTION FOR RECTAL ADMINISTRATION TRADE: DIASTAT	TREATMENT OF ACUTE REPETITIVE SEIZURES.	UPSHER SMITH LABORATORIES, INC
GENERIC: DIETHYLDITHIOCARBAMATE TRADE: IMUTHIOL	TREATMENT OF ACQUIRED IMMUNODEFICIENCY SYNDROME (AIDS).	CONNAUGHT LABORATORIES, INC
GENERIC: DIHEMATOPORPHYRIN ETHERS TRADE: PHOTOFRIN	USE IN THE PHOTODYNAMIC THERAPY OF PATIENTS WITH TRANSITIONAL CELL CARCINOMA IN SITU OF THE URINARY BLADDER. USE FOR THE PHOTODYNAMIC THERAPY OF PATIENTS WITH PRIMARY OR RECURRENT OBSTRUCTING (PARTIALLY OR COMPLETELY) ESOPHAGEAL CARCINOMA.	QLT PHOTOTHERAPEUTICS, INC
GENERIC: DIMETHYL SULFOXIDE (DMSO) TRADE: SCLEROSOL	TREATMENT OF CUTANEOUS MANIFESTATIONS OF SCLERODERMA.	RESEARCH MEDICAL, INC
GENERIC: DIPALMITOYLPHOSPHATIDYLCHOLINE/PHOSPHATIDYLGLYCEROL TRADE: ALEC	PREVENTION AND TREATMENT OF NEONATAL RESPIRATORY DISTRESS SYNDROME.	BRITANNIA PHARMACEUTICALS
GENERIC: DISODIUM CLODRONATE TETRAHYDRATE TRADE: BONEFOS	TREATMENT OF INCREASED BONE RESORPTION DUE TO MALIGNANCY.	LEIRAS PHARMACEUTICALS, INC
GENERIC: DISODIUM SILIBININ DIHEMISUCCINATE TRADE: LEGALON	TREATMENT OF HEPATIC INTOXICATION BY AMANITA PHALLOIDES (MUSHROOM POISONING).	PHARMAQUEST CORPORATION
GENERIC: DRONABINOL TRADE: MARINOL	STIMULATION OF APPETITE AND PREVENTION OF WEIGHT LOSS IN PATIENTS WITH A CONFIRMED DIAGNOSIS OF ACQUIRED IMMUNODEFICIENCY SYNDROME (AIDS).	UNIMED, INC
GENERIC: DYNAMINE TRADE: NOT ESTABLISHED	TREATMENT OF LAMBERT-EATON MYASTHENIC SYNDROME.	MAYO FOUNDATION
GENERIC: EFLORNITHINE HCL TRADE: ORNIDYL*/**	TREATMENT OF TRYPANOSOMA BRUCEI GAMBIENSE SLEEPING SICKNESS.*/** [NOV 28, 1997] TREATMENT OF PNEUMOCYSTIS CARINII PNEUMONIA (PCP) IN ACQUIRED IMMUNODEFICIENCY SYNDROME (AIDS) PATIENTS.	MERRELL DOW
GENERIC: ENISOPROST TRADE: NOT ESTABLISHED	FOR CO-ADMINISTRATION WITH CYCLOSPORINE IN ORGAN TRANSPLANT RECIPIENTS TO REDUCE ACUTE TRANSPLANT REJECTION. FOR CO-ADMINISTRATION WITH CYCLOSPORINE IN ORGAN TRANSPLANT RECIPIENTS TO DIMINISH THE NEPHROTOXICITY INDUCED BY CYCLOSPORINE.	G.D. SEARLE & COMPANY

DRUG DESIGNATIONS *(continued)*

NAME OF DRUG	DESIGNATED USE [EXCLUSIVITY EXPIRATION DATE]	SPONSOR NAME
GENERIC: EPIDERMAL GROWTH FACTOR (HUMAN) TRADE: NOT ESTABLISHED	ACCELERATION OF CORNEAL EPITHELIAL REGENERATION AND HEALING OF STROMAL INCISIONS FROM CORNEAL TRANSPLANT SURGERY. ACCELERATION OF CORNEAL EPITHELIAL REGENERATION AND THE HEALING OF STROMAL TISSUE IN THE CONDITION OF NON-HEALING CORNEAL DEFECTS.	CHIRON CORPORATION
GENERIC: EPOPROSTENOL TRADE: CYCLO-PROSTIN	REPLACEMENT OF HEPARIN IN PATIENTS REQUIRING HEMO-DIALYSIS AND WHO ARE AT INCREASED RISK OF HEMOR-RHAGE.	UPJOHN COMPANY
GENERIC: EPOPROSTENOL, PROSTA-CYCLIN TRADE: FLOLAN	REPLACEMENT OF HEPARIN IN PATIENTS REQUIRING HEMO-DIALYSIS AND WHO ARE AT INCREASED RISK OF HEMOR-RHAGE. TREATMENT OF PRIMARY PULMONARY HYPERTENSION (PPH).	BURROUGHS WELLCOME COMPANY
GENERIC: ETHANOLAMINE OLEATE TRADE: ETHAMOLIN*/**	TREATMENT OF PATIENTS WITH ESOPHAGEAL VARICES THAT HAVE RECENTLY BLED, TO PREVENT REBLEEDING. [DEC 22, 1995]	REED AND CARNICK
GENERIC: ETHINYL ESTRADIOL TRADE: NOT ESTABLISHED	TREATMENT OF TURNER'S SYNDROME.	GYNEX, INC
GENERIC: ETHIOFOS TRADE: ETHYOL	FOR USE AS A CHEMOPROTECTIVE AGENT FOR CISPLATIN IN THE TREATMENT OF ADVANCED OVARIAN CARCINOMA. FOR USE AS A CHEMOPROTECTIVE AGENT FOR CYCLOPHOS-PHAMIDE IN THE TREATMENT OF ADVANCED OVARIAN CAR-CINOMA. FOR USE AS A CHEMOPROTECTIVE AGENT FOR CISPLATIN IN THE TREATMENT OF METASTATIC MELANOMA.	US BIOSCIENCE
GENERIC: ETIDRONATE DISODIUM TRADE: DIDRONEL	PREVENTION OF DEGENERATIVE METABOLIC BONE DISEASE OCCURRING IN PATIENTS WHO REQUIRE LONG TERM (6 MONTHS OR GREATER) TOTAL PARENTERAL NUTRITION. TREATMENT OF DEGENERATIVE METABOLIC BONE DISEASE OCCURRING IN PATIENTS WHO REQUIRE LONG TERM (6 MONTHS OR GREATER) TOTAL PARENTERAL NUTRITION.	MGI PHARMA, INC
GENERIC: ETIDRONATE DISODIUM TRADE: DIDRONEL*/**	TREATMENT OF HYPERCALCEMIA OF A MALIGNANCY MAN-AGED BY DIETARY MODIFICATION AND/OR ORAL HYDRA-TION. [APR 20, 1994]	NORWICH EATON
GENERIC: FIAU TRADE: NOT ESTABLISHED	ADJUNCTIVE TREATMENT OF CHRONIC ACTIVE HEPATITIS B.	OCLASSEN PHARMACEUTI-CALS, INC
GENERIC: FELBAMATE TRADE: NOT ESTABLISHED	TREATMENT OF LENNOX-GASTAUT SYNDROME.	WALLACE LABORATORIES
GENERIC: FLUDARABINE PHOSPHATE TRADE: FLUDARA*/**	TREATMENT OF REFRACTORY CHRONIC LYMPHOCYTIC LEU-KEMIA.*/** [APR 18, 1998] TREATMENT AND MANAGEMENT OF NON-HODGKIN'S LYM-PHOMA (NHL).	BERLEX
GENERIC: FLUMECINOL TRADE: ZIXORYN	HYPERBILIRUBINEMIA IN NEWBORN INFANTS UNRESPON-SIVE TO PHOTOTHERAPY.	FARMACON, INC
GENERIC: FLUNARIZINE TRADE: SIBELIUM	TREATMENT OF ALTERNATING HEMIPLEGIA.	JANSSEN PHARMACEUTICA
GENERIC: FLUOROURACIL TRADE: NOT ESTABLISHED	FOR USE IN COMBINATION WITH INTERFERON ALFA-2A RE-COMBINANT FOR THE TREATMENT OF ESOPHAGEAL CARCI-NOMA. CONCOMITANT ADMINISTRATION WITH INTERFERON ALFA-2A FOR THE TREATMENT OF PATIENTS WITH ADVANCED CO-LORECTAL CANCER.	HOFFMAN-LA ROCHE, INC
GENERIC: FLUOROURACIL TRADE: ADRUCIL	FOR USE IN COMBINATION WITH LEUCOVORIN FOR THER-APY OF METASTATIC ADENOCARCINOMA OF THE COLON AND RECTUM.	LEDERLE LABORATORIES DI-VISION AMERICAN CYANA-MIDE COMPANY
GENERIC: FOSPHENYTOIN TRADE: NOT ESTABLISHED	ACUTE TREATMENT OF PATIENTS WITH STATUS EPILEPTI-CUS OF THE GRAND MAL TYPE.	WARNER-LAMBERT COM-PANY
GENERIC: GALLIUM NITRATE TRADE: GANITE*/**	TREATMENT OF HYPERCALCEMIA OF MALIGNANCY. [JAN 17, 1998]	FUJISAWA
GENERIC: GANGLIOSIDES AS SODIUM SALTS TRADE: CRONASSIAL	TREATMENT OF RETINITIS PIGMENTOSA.	FIDIA PHARMACEUTICAL CORP
GENERIC: GENTAMICIN IMPREG-NATED PMMA BEADS ON SURGICAL WIRE TRADE: SEPTOPAL	TREATMENT OF CHRONIC OSTEOMYELITIS OF POST-TRAU-MATIC, POSTOPERATIVE OR HEMATOGENOUS ORIGIN.	E. MERCK, DARMSTADT
GENERIC: GENTAMICIN LIPOSOME TRADE: NOT ESTABLISHED	TREATMENT OF DISSEMINATED MYCOBACTERIUM AVIUM-INTRACELLULARE INFECTION.	LIPOSOME COMPANY

DRUG DESIGNATIONS *(continued)*

NAME OF DRUG	DESIGNATED USE [EXCLUSIVITY EXPIRATION DATE]	SPONSOR NAME
GENERIC: GM 6001 TRADE: NOT ESTABLISHED	TREATMENT OF CORNEAL ULCERS.	GLYCOMED, INC.
GENERIC: GONADORELIN ACETATE TRADE: LUTREPULSE PUMP KIT*/**	TREATMENT OF PRIMARY HYPOTHALAMIC AMENORRHEA. [OCT 10, 1996]	RW JOHNSON
GENERIC: GOSSYPOL TRADE: NOT ESTABLISHED	TREATMENT OF CANCER OF THE ADRENAL CORTEX.	MARCUS M. REIDENBERG, M.D. NEW YORK, NY
GENERIC: GUANETHIDINE MONOSUL- FATE TRADE: ISMELIN I.V.	TREATMENT OF MODERATE TO SEVERE REFLEX SYMPA- THETIC DYSTROPHY AND CAUSALGIA.	CIBA-GEIGY CORPORATION
GENERIC: HALOFANTRINE HCL TRADE: HALFAN*/**	TREATMENT OF MILD TO MODERATE ACUTE MALARIA CAUSED BY SUSCEPTIBLE STRAINS OF P. FALCIPARUM AND P. VIVAX. [JUL 24, 1999]	SMITHKLINE BEECHAM
GENERIC: HISTRELIN TRADE: NOT ESTABLISHED	TREATMENT OF ACUTE INTERMITTENT PORPHYRIA, HEREDI- TARY CORPROPORPHYRIA, AND VARIEGATE PORPHYRIA.	KARL E. ANDERSON, M.D. UNIVERSITY OF TEXAS
GENERIC: HISTRELIN ACETATE TRADE: SUPPRELIN*/**	TREATMENT OF CENTRAL PRECOCIOUS PUBERTY. [DEC 24, 1998]	RW JOHNSON
GENERIC: HPA-23 TRADE: NOT ESTABLISHED	TREATMENT OF ACQUIRED IMMUNODEFICIENCY SYNDROME (AIDS).	RHONE-POULENC, INC
GENERIC: HUMAN GROWTH HOR- MONE, RELEASING FAC- TOR (1-44) AMIDE TRADE: NOT ESTABLISHED	FOR THE LONG TERM TREATMENT OF CHILDREN WHO HAVE GROWTH FAILURE DUE TO A LACK OF ADEQUATE ENDOGE- NOUS GROWTH HORMONE SECRETION.	FUJISAWA PHARMACEUTI- CAL CO
GENERIC: HUMAN THYROID STIMU- LATING HORMONE (TSH) TRADE: THYROGEN	AS AN ADJUNCT IN THE DIAGNOSIS OF THYROID CANCER	GENZYME CORPORATION
GENERIC: HYDROXYCOBALAMIN/SO- DIUM THIOSULFATE TRADE: NOT ESTABLISHED	TREATMENT OF SEVERE ACUTE CYANIDE POISONING.	EVREKA, INC
GENERIC: HYDROXYUREA TRADE: HYDREA	TREATMENT OF SICKLE CELL ANEMIA AS SHOWN BY THE PRESENCE OF HEMOGLOBIN S.	BRISTOL-MYERS SQUIBB
GENERIC: IDARUBICIN HCL TRADE: IDAMYCIN*/**	TREATMENT OF ACUTE MYELOGENOUS LEUKEMIA (AML), ALSO REFERRED TO AS ACUTE NONLYMPHOCYTIC LEUKE- MIA (ANLL).*/** [SEP 27, 1990] TREATMENT OF ACUTE LYMPHOBLASTIC LEUKEMIA (ALL) IN PEDIATRIC PATIENTS.	ADRIA
GENERIC: IFOSFAMIDE TRADE: IFEX*/**	TREATMENT OF SOFT TISSUE SARCOMA. TREATMENT OF BONE SARCOMA. TO BE USED IN COMBINATION WITH OTHER APPROVED ANTI- NEOPLASTIC AGENTS, FOR THIRD LINE CHEMOTHERAPY OF GERM CELL TESTICULAR CANCER.*/** [DEC 30, 1995]	BRISTOL MYERS SQUIBB
GENERIC: ILOPROST TRADE: NOT ESTABLISHED	TREATMENT OF RAYNAUD'S PHENOMENON SECONDARY TO SYSTEMIC SCLEROSIS. TREATMENT OF HEPARIN-ASSOCIATED THROMBOCYTO- PENIA.	BERLEX LABORATORIES, INC
GENERIC: INOSINE PRANOBEX TRADE: ISOPRINOSINE	TREATMENT OF SUBACUTE SCLEROSING PANENCEPHALITIS.	NEWPORT PHARMACEUTI- CALS
GENERIC: IODINE I 131 META-IODO- BENZYLGUANIDINE (NP-59) TRADE: NOT ESTABLISHED	DIAGNOSTIC ADJUNCT IN PATIENTS WITH PHEOCHROMOCY- TOMA.	WILLIAM BEIERWALTES, M.D. ANN ARBOR, MI
GENERIC: IODINE I 131 6B-IODO- METHYL-19-NORCHOLES- TEROL TRADE: NOT ESTABLISHED	ADRENAL CORTICAL IMAGING.	WILLIAM BEIERWALTES, M.D. ANN ARBOR, MI
GENERIC: KETOCONAZOLE TRADE: NIZORAL	FOR USE WITH CYCLOSPORIN A TO DIMINISH THE NEPHRO- TOXICITY INDUCED BY CYCLOSPORIN IN ORGAN TRANS- PLANTATION.	PHARAMEDIC COMPANY
GENERIC: L-ALPHA-ACETYL-METHA- DOL (LAAM) TRADE: NOT ESTABLISHED	TREATMENT OF HEROIN ADDICTS SUITABLE FOR MAINTE- NANCE ON OPIATE AGONISTS.	BIOMETRIC RESEARCH IN- STITUTE
GENERIC: L-BACLOFEN TRADE: NEURALGON	TREATMENT OF INTRACTABLE SPASTICITY ASSOCIATED WITH SPINAL CORD INJURY OR MULTIPLE SCLEROSIS. TREATMENT OF INTRACTABLE SPASTICITY IN CHILDREN WITH CEREBRAL PALSY.	WTD, INC
GENERIC: L-BACLOFEN TRADE: NOT ESTABLISHED	TREATMENT OF TRIGEMINAL NEURALGIA.	GERHARD H. FROMM, M.D. UNIV OF PITTSBURGH

DRUG DESIGNATIONS *(continued)*

NAME OF DRUG	DESIGNATED USE [EXCLUSIVITY EXPIRATION DATE]	SPONSOR NAME
GENERIC: L-CYCLOSERINE TRADE: NOT ESTABLISHED	TREATMENT OF GAUCHER'S DISEASE.	CITY UNIV, NY MEDICAL SCHOOL
GENERIC: L-LEUCOVORIN CALCIUM TRADE: ISOVORIN	FOR USE IN COMBINATION CHEMOTHERAPY WITH THE AP-PROVED AGENT 5-FLUOROURACIL IN THE PALLIATIVE. TREATMENT OF ADVANCED METASTATIC ADENOCARCI-NOMA OF THE COLON AND RECTUM. USE IN CONJUNCTION WITH HIGH-DOSE METHOTREXATE IN THE TREATMENT OF OSTEOSARCOMA.	LEDERLE LABORATORIES
GENERIC: LEUCOVORIN CALCIUM TRADE: LEUCOVORIN CALCIUM*/**	FOR USE IN COMBINATION WITH 5-FLOROURACIL FOR THE TREATMENT OF METASTATIC COLORECTAL CANCER. (USE IN COMBINATION WITH 5-FLUOROURACIL TO PROLONG SUR-VIVAL IN THE PALLIATIVE TREATMENT OF PATIENTS WITH ADVANCED COLORECTAL CANCER.*/** [DEC 12, 1998) FOR RESCUE USE AFTER HIGH DOSE METHOTREXATE THERAPY IN THE TREATMENT OF OSTEOSARCOMA.*/** [AUG 31, 1995]	LEDERLE
GENERIC: LEUCOVORIN CALCIUM TRADE: WELLCOVORIN	FOR USE IN COMBINATION WITH 5-FLUOROURACIL FOR THE TREATMENT OF METASTATIC COLORECTAL CANCER.	BURROUGHS WELLCOME COMPANY
GENERIC: LEUPROLIDE ACETATE TRADE: LUPRON	TREATMENT OF CENTRAL PRECOCIOUS PUBERTY.	TAP PHARMACEUTICALS, INC
GENERIC: LEVOCABASTINE HCL TRADE: NOT ESTABLISHED	TREATMENT OF VERNAL KERATOCONJUNCTIVITIS (VKC).	IOLAB PHARMACEUTICALS
GENERIC: LEVOCARNITINE TRADE: CARNITOR*/**	TREATMENT OF PRIMARY AND SECONDARY CARNITINE DE-FICIENCY OF GENETIC ORIGIN.*/** [DEC 27, 1992] TREATMENT OF MANIFESTATIONS OF CARNITINE DEFI-CIENCY IN PATIENTS WITH END STAGE RENAL DISEASE (ESRD) WHO REQUIRE DIALYSIS.	SIGMA TAU
GENERIC: LEVOCARNITINE TRADE: CARNITOR*/**	GENETIC CARNITINE DEFICIENCY.* TREATMENT OF MANIFESTATIONS OF CARNITINE DEFI-CIENCY IN PATIENTS WITH END STAGE RENAL DISEASE (ESRD) WHO REQUIRE DIALYSIS. PREVENTION OF SECONDARY CARNITINE DEFICIENCY IN VALPROIC ACID TOXICITY. TREATMENT OF SECONDARY CARNITINE DEFICIENCY IN VALPROIC ACID TOXICITY.	SIGMA TAU
GENERIC: LIOTHYRONINE SODIUM TRADE: TRIOSTAT	TREATMENT OF MYXEDEMA COMA/PRE-COMA. [DEC 31, 1998]	SMITHKLINE BEECHAM
GENERIC: LODOXAMIDE TROMETH-AMINE TRADE: ALOMIDE	TREATMENT OF VERNAL KERATOCONJUNCTIVITIS.	ALCON LABORATORIES, INC
GENERIC: LOXORIBINE TRADE: NOT ESTABLISHED	TREATMENT OF COMMON VARIABLE IMMUNODEFICIENCY.	R.W. JOHNSON RESEARCH INSTITUTE
GENERIC: L-THREONINE TRADE: NOT ESTABLISHED	TREATMENT OF SPASTICITY ASSOCIATED WITH FAMILIAL SPASTIC PARAPARESIS.	INTERNEURON PHARMACEUTICALS, INC
GENERIC: L-THREONINE TRADE: THREOSTAT	TREATMENT OF AMYOTROPHIC LATERAL SCLEROSIS (ALS).	TYSON AND ASSOCIATES
GENERIC: L-5 HYDROXYTRYPTOPHAN (L-5HTP) TRADE: NOT ESTABLISHED	TREATMENT OF POSTANOXIC INTENTION MYOCLONUS.	BOLAR PHARMACEUTICAL COMPANY
GENERIC: MAFENIDE ACETATE TRADE: SULFAMYLON	FOR USE IN THE PREVENTION OF GRAFT LOSS OF MESHED AUTOGRAFTS ON EXCISED BURN WOUNDS.	DOW B. HICKAM, INC
GENERIC: MAZINDOL TRADE: SANOREX	TREATMENT OF DUCHENNE MUSCULAR DYSTROPHY (DMD).	PLATON J. COLLIP, M.D. JESSUP, GA
GENERIC: MEFLOQUINE HCL TRADE: LARIAM*/**	TREATMENT OF ACUTE MALARIA DUE TO PLASMODIUM FAL-CIPARUM AND PLASMODIUM VIVAX.*/** [MAY 02, 1996] PROPHYLAXIS OF PLASMODIUM FALCIPARUM MALARIA WHICH IS RESISTANT TO OTHER AVAILABLE DRUGS.*/** [MAY 02, 1996]	ROCHE
GENERIC: MEFLOQUINE HCL TRADE: MEPHAQUIN	PREVENTION OF CHLOROQUINE-RESISTANT FALCIPARUM MALARIA. TREATMENT OF CHLOROQUINE-RESISTANT FALCIPARUM MALARIA.	MEPHRA AG
GENERIC: MEGESTROL ACETATE TRADE: MEGACE	TREATMENT OF PATIENTS WITH ANOREXIA, CACHEXIA, OR SIGNIFICANT WEIGHT LOSS (=/>10% OF BASELINE BODY WEIGHT) AND CONFIRMED DIAGNOSIS OF AIDS.	BRISTOL-MYERS SQUIBB
GENERIC: MELPHALAN TRADE: ALKERAN FOR INJECTION	TREATMENT OF PATIENTS WITH MULTIPLE MYELOMA FOR WHOM ORAL THERAPY IS INAPPROPRIATE. FOR USE IN HY-PERTHERMIC REGIONAL LIMB PERFUSION TO TREAT META-STATIC MELANOMA OF THE EXTREMITY.	BURROUGHS WELLCOME COMPANY

DRUG DESIGNATIONS *(continued)*

NAME OF DRUG	DESIGNATED USE [EXCLUSIVITY EXPIRATION DATE]	SPONSOR NAME
GENERIC: MESNA TRADE: MESNEX*/**	FOR USE AS A PROPHYLACTIC AGENT IN REDUCING THE INCIDENCE OF IFOSFAMIDE-INDUCED HEMORRHAGIC CYSTITIS. [DEC 30, 1995]	ASTA
GENERIC: MESNA TRADE: NOT ESTABLISHED	INHIBITION OF THE UROTOXIC EFFECTS INDUCED BY OXAZAPHOSPHORINE COMPOUNDS SUCH AS CYCLOPHOSPHAMIDE.	ADRIA LABORATORIES
GENERIC: METHOTREXATE SODIUM TRADE: METHOTREXATE*/**	FOR USE WITH LEUCOVORIN RESCUE IN COMBINATION WITH OTHER CHEMOTHERAPEUTIC AGENTS TO DELAY RECURRENCE IN PATIENTS WITH NON-METASTATIC OSTEOSARCOMA WHO HAVE UNDERGONE SURGICAL RESECTION OR AMPUTATION FOR THE PRIMARY TUMOR. [APR 07, 1995]	LEDERLE
GENERIC: METHOTREXATE USP WITH LAUROCAPRAM TRADE: NOT ESTABLISHED	TOPICAL TREATMENT OF MYCOSIS FUNGOIDES.	WHITBY RESEARCH, INC
GENERIC: METRONIDAZOLE (TOPICAL) TRADE: FLAGYL	TREATMENT OF GRADE III AND IV, ANAEROBICALLY INFECTED, DECUBITUS ULCERS.	G.D. SEARLE & COMPANY
GENERIC: METRONIDAZOLE TRADE: METROGEL*/**	TREATMENT OF ACNE ROSACEA. */** [NOV 22, 1995] TREATMENT OF PERIORAL DERMATITIS.	CURATEK
GENERIC: MICROBUBBLE CONTRAST AGENT TRADE: FILMIX (NEUROSONOGRAPHIC CONTRAST AGENT)	INTRAOPERATIVE AID IN THE IDENTIFICATION AND LOCALIZATION OF INTRACRANIAL TUMORS.	CAV-CON, INC
GENERIC: MIDODRINE HCL TRADE: AMATINE	TREATMENT OF IDIOPATHIC ORTHOSTATIC HYPOTENSION.	ROBERTS PHARMACEUTICAL CORP
GENERIC: MINOCYCLINE HCL TRADE: MINOCIN	TREATMENT OF CHRONIC MALIGNANT PLEURAL EFFUSION.	LEDERLE LABORATORIES
GENERIC: MITOLACTOL TRADE: DIBROMODULCITOL	TREATMENT OF RECURRENT INVASIVE OR METASTATIC SQUAMOUS CARCINOMA OF THE CERVIX.	AMSWISS PHARMACEUTICALS
GENERIC: MITOXANTRONE HCL TRADE: NOVANTRONE*/**	TREATMENT OF ACUTE MYELOGENOUS LEUKEMIA (AML), ALSO REFERRED TO AS ACUTE NONLYMPHOCYTIC LEUKEMIA (ANLL). [DEC 23, 1994]	LEDERLE
GENERIC: MONOCTANOIN TRADE: MOCTANIN*/**	DISSOLUTION OF CHOLESTEROL GALLSTONES RETAINED IN THE COMMON BILE DUCT. [OCT 29, 1992]	ETHITEK
GENERIC: MORPHINE SULFATE TRADE: INFUMORPH*/**	FOR USE IN MICROINFUSION DEVICES FOR INTRASPINAL ADMINISTRATION IN THE TREATMENT OF INTRACTABLE CHRONIC PAIN. [JULY 19, 1998]	ELKINS SINN
GENERIC: MULTI-VITAMIN INFUSION-NEONATAL FORMULA TRADE: NOT ESTABLISHED	FOR THE ESTABLISHMENT AND MAINTENANCE OF TOTAL PARENTERAL NUTRITION IN VERY LOW BIRTH WEIGHT INFANTS (LESS THAN 1500 GRAMS).	ASTRA PHARMACEUTICAL PRODUCTS
GENERIC: NAFARELIN ACETATE TRADE: SYNAREL	TREATMENT OF CENTRAL PRECOCIOUS PUBERTY.	SYNTEX (USA), INC
GENERIC: NALTREXONE HCL TRADE: TREXAN*/**	BLOCKADE OF THE PHARMACOLOGICAL EFFECTS OF EXOGENOUSLY ADMINISTERED OPIOIDS AS AN ADJUNCT TO THE MAINTENANCE OF THE OPIOID-FREE STATE IN DETOXIFIED FORMERLY OPIOID-DEPENDENT INDIVIDUALS. [NOV 20, 1991]	DUPONT
GENERIC: N-ACETYLPROCAINAMIDE TRADE: NAPA	TO LOWER THE DEFIBRILLATION ENERGY REQUIREMENT SUFFICIENTLY TO ALLOW AUTOMATIC IMPLANTABLE CARDIOVERTER DEFIBRILLATOR (AICD) THERAPY IN THOSE PATIENTS WHO COULD OTHERWISE NOT USE THE DEVICE.	MEDCO RESEARCH, INC
GENERIC: NG-29 TRADE: SOMATREL	FOR THE ASSESSMENT OF THE CAPACITY OF THE PITUITARY GLAND TO RELEASE GH IN CHILDREN OF SHORT STATURE POSSIBLY DUE TO GH DEFICIENCY.	FERRING LABORATORIES, INC
GENERIC: NIFEDIPINE TRADE: NOT ESTABLISHED	TREATMENT OF INTERSTITIAL CYSTITIS.	JONATHAN FLEISCHMANN, M.D. CLEVELAND METROHEALTH
GENERIC: OFLOXACIN TRADE: NOT ESTABLISHED	TREATMENT OF BACTERIAL CORNEAL ULCERS.	ALLERGAN, INC
GENERIC: OM 401 TRADE: DREPANOL	PROPHYLACTIC TREATMENT OF SICKLE CELL DISEASE.	OMEX INTERNATIONAL, INC
GENERIC: OVINE CORTICOTROPIN RELEASING HORMONE TRADE: ACTHREL	USE IN DIFFERENTIATING PITUITARY AND ECTOPIC PRODUCTION OF ACTH IN PATIENTS WITH ACTH-DEPENDENT CUSHING'S SYNDROME.	FERRING LABORATORIES, INC

DRUG DESIGNATIONS (continued)

NAME OF DRUG	DESIGNATED USE [EXCLUSIVITY EXPIRATION DATE]	SPONSOR NAME
GENERIC: OXANDROLONE TRADE: OXANDRIN	TREATMENT OF CONSTITUTIONAL DELAY OF GROWTH AND PUBERTY. TREATMENT OF SHORT STATURE ASSOCIATED WITH TURNER'S SYNDROME. ADJUNCTIVE THERAPY FOR AIDS PATIENTS SUFFERING FROM HIV-WASTING SYNDROME.	GYNEX, INC
GENERIC: OXYMORPHONE HCL TRADE: NUMORPHAN H.P.	RELIEF OF SEVERE INTRACTABLE PAIN IN NARCOTIC-TOLERANT PATIENTS.	DUPONT PHARMACEUTICALS, INC
GENERIC: PAPAVERINE (TOPICAL GEL) TRADE: NOT ESTABLISHED	TREATMENT OF SEXUAL DYSFUNCTION IN SPINAL CORD INJURY PATIENTS.	PHARMEDIC COMPANY
GENERIC: PARA-AMINOSALICYLIC ACID TRADE: NOT ESTABLISHED	TREATMENT OF TUBERCULOSIS INFECTIONS.	JACOBUS PHARMACEUTICAL COMPANY
GENERIC: PEGADEMASE BOVINE TRADE: ADAGEN*/**	USE AS ENZYME REPLACEMENT THERAPY FOR ADENOSINE DEAMINASE (ADA) DEFICIENCY IN PATIENTS WITH SEVERE COMBINED IMMUNODEFICIENCY (SCID) WHO ARE NOT SUITABLE CANDIDATES FOR (OR WHO HAVE FAILED) BONE MARROW TRANSPLANTATION.[MAR 21, 1997]	ENZON
GENERIC: PENTAMIDINE ISETHIONATE TRADE: NEBUPENT*/**	PREVENTION OF PNEUMOCYSTIS CARINII PNEUMONIA (PCP) IN PATIENTS AT HIGH RISK OF DEVELOPING THIS DISEASE. [JUN 15, 1996]	FUJISAWA
GENERIC: PENTAMIDINE ISETHIONATE TRADE: NOT ESTABLISHED	TREATMENT OF PNEUMOCYSTIS CARINII PNEUMONIA (PCP).	RHONE-POULENC, INC
GENERIC: PENTAMIDINE ISETHIONATE TRADE: PENTAM 300*/**	TREATMENT OF PNEUMOCYSTIS CARINII PNEUMONIA (PCP). [OCT 16, 1991]	FUJISAWA
GENERIC: PENTAMIDINE ISETHIONATE TRADE: NOT ESTABLISHED	PREVENTION OF PNEUMOCYSTIS CARINII PNEUMONIA (PCP) IN PATIENTS AT HIGH RISK OF DEVELOPING THIS DISEASE.	FISONS CORPORATION
GENERIC: PENTOSTATIN TRADE: NIPENT*/**	TREATMENT OF HAIRY CELL LEUKEMIA. (SINGLE AGENT TREATMENT FOR ADULT PATIENTS WITH ALPHA-INTERFERON-REFRACTORY HAIRY CELL LEUKEMIA.*/** [OCT 11, 1998]) TREATMENT OF PATIENTS WITH CHRONIC LYMPHOCYTIC LEUKEMIA.	PARKE DAVIS
GENERIC: PHOSPHOCYSTEAMINE TRADE: NOT ESTABLISHED	TREATMENT OF CYSTINOSIS.	MEDEA RESEARCH LABORATORIES
GENERIC: PHYSOSTIGMINE SALICYLATE TRADE: ANTILIRIUM	FRIEDREICH'S AND OTHER INHERITED ATAXIAS.	FOREST PHARMACEUTICALS, INC
GENERIC: PILOCARPINE HCL TRADE: NOT ESTABLISHED	TREATMENT OF XEROSTOMIA INDUCED BY RADIATION THERAPY FOR HEAD AND NECK CANCER. TREATMENT OF XEROSTOMIA AND KERATOCONJUNCTIVITIS SICCA IN SJOGREN'S SYNDROME PATIENTS.	MGI PHARMA, INC
GENERIC: PIRACETAM TRADE: NOOTROPYL	TREATMENT OF MYOCLONUS.	UCB SECTEUR PHARMACEUTIQUE
GENERIC: PIRITREXIM ISETHIONATE (BW 301U) TRADE: NOT ESTABLISHED	TREATMENT OF INFECTIONS CAUSED BY PNEUMOCYSTIS CARINII, TOXOPLASMA GONDII, AND MYCOBACTERIUM AVIUM-INTRACELLULARE.	BURROUGHS WELLCOME COMPANY
GENERIC: POLOXAMER 188 TRADE: RHEOTHRX COPOLYMER	TREATMENT OF SICKLE CELL CRISIS. TREATMENT OF SEVERE BURNS REQUIRING HOSPITALIZATION.	BURROUGHS WELLCOME COMPANY
GENERIC: POLOXAMER 331 TRADE: PROTOX	INITIAL THERAPY OF TOXOPLASMOSIS IN PATIENTS WITH ACQUIRED IMMUNODEFICIENCY SYNDROME (AIDS).	BURROUGHS WELLCOME COMPANY
GENERIC: POLYMERIC OXYGEN TRADE: NOT ESTABLISHED	TREATMENT OF SICKLE CELL ANEMIA.	CAPMED, USA
GENERIC: POTASSIUM CITRATE TRADE: POTASSIUM CITRATE*/**	PREVENTION OF CALCIUM RENAL STONES IN PATIENTS WITH HYPOCITRATURIA.*/** [AUG 30, 1992] AVOIDANCE OF THE COMPLICATION OF CALCIUM STONE FORMATION IN PATIENTS WITH URIC ACID LITHIASIS.*/** [AUG 30, 1992] PREVENTION OF URIC ACID NEPHROLITHIASIS.*/** [AUG 30, 1992]	UNIV TX
GENERIC: POTASSIUM CITRATE AND CITRIC ACID TRADE: POLYCITRA-K	DISSOLUTION AND CONTROL OF URIC ACID AND CYSTINE CALCULI IN THE URINARY TRACT.	WILLEN DRUG COMPANY

DRUG DESIGNATIONS (*continued*)

NAME OF DRUG	DESIGNATED USE [EXCLUSIVITY EXPIRATION DATE]	SPONSOR NAME
GENERIC: PPI-002 TRADE: NOT ESTABLISHED	TREATMENT OF MALIGNANT MESOTHELIOMA	PLEXUS PHARMACEUTICALS, INC
GENERIC: PRAMIRACETAM SULFATE TRADE: NOT ESTABLISHED	FOR THE MANAGEMENT OF COGNITIVE DYSFUNCTION AND ENHANCEMENT OF ANTIDEPRESSANT ACTIVITY ASSOCIATED WITH ELECTROCONVULSIVE THERAPY.	CAMBRIDGE NEUROSCIENCE, INC
GENERIC: PRAZIQUANTEL TRADE: CYSTICIDE	TREATMENT OF NEUROCYSTICERCOSIS.	EM PHARMACEUTICALS, INC
GENERIC: PREDNIMUSTINE TRADE: STERECYT	TREATMENT OF MALIGNANT NON-HODGKIN'S LYMPHOMAS.	KAVI PHARMACIA, INC
GENERIC: PROPAMIDINE ISETHIONATE TRADE: BROLENE	TREATMENT OF ACANTHAMOEBA KERATITIS.	BAUSCH & LOMB PHARMACEUTICALS
GENERIC: PROTIRELIN (TRH) TRADE: THYMONE	AMYOTROPHIC OF AMYOTROPHIC LATERAL SCLEROSIS (ALS)	ABBOTT LABORATORIES
GENERIC: PR-122 (REDOX-PHENYTOIN) TRADE: NOT ESTABLISHED	FOR THE EMERGENCY RESCUE TREATMENT OF STATUS EPILEPTICUS, GRAND MAL TYPE.	PHARMATEC, INC
GENERIC: PR-225 (REDOX ACYCLOVIR) TRADE: NOT ESTABLISHED	TREATMENT OF HERPES SIMPLEX ENCEPHALITIS IN INDIVIDUALS AFFLICTED WITH AIDS.	PHARMATEC, INC
GENERIC: PR-239 (REDOX PENICILLIN G) TRADE: NOT ESTABLISHED	TREATMENT OF AIDS ASSOCIATED NEUROSYPHILIS.	PHARMATEC, INC
GENERIC: PR-320 (MOLECUSOL-CARBAMAZEPINE) TRADE: NOT ESTABLISHED	FOR THE EMERGENCY RESCUE TREATMENT OF STATUS EPILEPTICUS, GRAND MAL TYPE.	PHARMATEC, INC
GENERIC: PULMONARY SURFACTANT REPLACEMENT TRADE: NOT ESTABLISHED	PREVENTION AND TREATMENT OF INFANT RESPIRATORY DISTRESS SYNDROME (RDS).	CALIFORNIA BIOTECHNOLOGY, INC
GENERIC: RECOMBINANT BETA-GLUCOCEREBROSIDASE TRADE: NOT ESTABLISHED	FOR REPLACEMENT THERAPY IN PATIENTS WITH TYPES I, II, AND III GAUCHER'S DISEASE.	GENZYME CORPORATION
GENERIC: RECOMBINANT HUMAN SUPEROXIDE DISMUTASE TRADE: NOT ESTABLISHED	PREVENTION OF BRONCHOPULMONARY DYSPLASIA IN PREMATURE NEONATES WEIGHING LESS THAN 1500 GRMS.	BIO TECHNOLOGY GENERAL CORP
GENERIC: RIBAVIRIN TRADE: VIRAZOLE	TREATMENT OF HEMORRHAGIC FEVER WITH RENAL SYNDROME.	ICN PHARMACEUTICALS, INC
GENERIC: RIFABUTIN TRADE: NOT ESTABLISHED	PREVENTION OF MYCOBACTERIUM AVIUM COMPLEX (MAC) DISEASE IN PATIENTS WITH AIDS AND IN PATIENTS WITH CD4 COUNTS LESS THAN 200/MM³. TREATMENT OF DISSEMINATED MYCOBACTERIUM AVIUM COMPLEX (MAC) DISEASE.	ADRIA LABORATORIES
GENERIC: RIFAMPIN TRADE: RIFADIN I.V.*/**	ANTITUBERCULOSIS TREATMENT WHERE USE OF THE ORAL FORM OF THE DRUG IS NOT FEASIBLE. [MAY 25, 1996]	MERRELL DOW
GENERIC: RIFAMPIN, ISONIAZID, PYRAZINAMIDE TRADE: RIFATER	SHORT COURSE TREATMENT OF TUBERCULOSIS.	MERRELL DOW RESEARCH
GENERIC: SELEGILINE HCL TRADE: ELDEPRYL*/**	ADJUVANT TO LEVODOPA AND CARBIDOPA TREATMENT OF IDIOPATHIC PARKINSON'S DISEASE (PARALYSIS AGITANS), POSTENCEPHALITIC PARKINSONISM, AND SYMPTOMATIC PARKINSONISM. [JUN 5, 1996]	SOMERSET
GENERIC: SERMORELIN ACETATE TRADE: GEREF	TREATMENT OF IDIOPATHIC AND ORGANIC GROWTH HORMONE DEFICIENCY IN CHILDREN WITH GROWTH FAILURE. AS AN ADJUNCT TO GONADOTROPIN THERAPY IN THE INDUCTION OF OVULATION IN WOMEN WITH ANOVULATORY OR OLIGO-OVULATORY INFERTILITY WHO FAIL TO OVULATE IN RESPONSE TO ADEQUATE TREATMENT WITH CLOMIPHENE CITRATE ALONE AND GONADOTROPIN THERAPY ALONE. TREATMENT OF AIDS-ASSOCIATED CATABOLISM/WEIGHT LOSS.	SERONO
GENERIC: SHORT CHAIN FATTY ACID SOLUTION TRADE: NOT ESTABLISHED	TREATMENT OF THE ACTIVE PHASE OF ULCERATIVE COLITIS WITH INVOLVEMENT RESTRICTED TO THE LEFT SIDE OF THE COLON.	RICHARD I. BREUER, M.D. EVANSTON, IL
GENERIC: SK&F 110679 TRADE: NOT ESTABLISHED	LONG TERM TREATMENT OF CHILDREN WHO HAVE GROWTH FAILURE DUE TO A LACK OF ADEQUATE ENDOGENOUS GROWTH HORMONE SECRETION.	SMITHKLINE BEECHAM

DRUG DESIGNATIONS *(continued)*

NAME OF DRUG	DESIGNATED USE [EXCLUSIVITY EXPIRATION DATE]	SPONSOR NAME
GENERIC: SODIUM BENZOATE/SODIUM PHENYLACETATE TRADE: UCEPHAN*/**	FOR ADJUNCTIVE THERAPY IN THE PREVENTION AND TREATMENT OF HYPERAMMONEMIA IN PATIENTS WITH UREA CYCLE ENZYMOPATHY (UCME) DUE TO CARBAMYL-PHOSPHATE SYNTHESTASE, ORNITHINE, TRANSCARBAMYL-ASE, OR ARGINOSUCCINATE SYNTHETASE DEFICIENCY. [DEC 23, 1994]	MCGAW
GENERIC: SODIUM DICHLOROACE-TATE TRADE: NOT ESTABLISHED	TREATMENT OF CONGENITAL LACTIC ACIDOSIS. TREATMENT OF HOMOZYGOUS FAMILIAL HYPERCHOLES-TEROLEMIA.	PETER STACPOOLE, M.D., PH.D. UNIVERSITY OF FLORIDA
GENERIC: SODIUM MONOMERCAP-TOUNDECAHYDRO-CLOSO-DODECABORATE TRADE: BOROCELL	FOR USE IN BORON NEUTRON CAPTURE THERAPY IN THE TREATMENT OF GLIOBLASTOMA MULTIFORME.	NEUTRON TECHNOLOGY CORPORATION
GENERIC: SODIUM OXYBATE (GAM-MAHYDROXYBUTYRATE) TRADE: NOT ESTABLISHED	TREATMENT OF NARCOLEPSY AND THE AUXILIARY SYMPTOMS OF CATAPLEXY, SLEEP PARALYSIS, HYPNAGOGIC HALLUCINATIONS AND AUTOMATIC BEHAVIOR.	BIOCRAFT LABORATORIES, INC
GENERIC: SODIUM PENTOSAN POLY-SULFATE TRADE: ELMIRON	TREATMENT OF INTERSTITIAL CYSTITIS.	BAKER CUMMINS PHARMA-CEUTICALS
GENERIC: SODIUM PHENYLBUTY-RATE TRADE: NOT ESTABLISHED	TREATMENT OF SICKLING DISORDERS, WHICH INCLUDE S-S HEMOGLOBINOPATHY, S-C HEMOGLOBINOPATHY, AND S-THALASSEMIA HEMOGLOBINOPATHY.	JOHNS HOPKINS MEDICAL INSTITUTIONS
GENERIC: SODIUM TETRADECYL SULFATE TRADE: SOTRADECOL	TREATMENT OF BLEEDING ESOPHAGEAL VARICES.	ELKINS-SINN, INC
GENERIC: SOMATOSTATIN TRADE: REDUCIN	ADJUNCT TO THE NONOPERATIVE MANAGEMENT OF SE-CRETING CUTANEOUS FISTULAS OF THE STOMACH, DUO-DENUM, SMALL INTESTINE (JEJUNUM AND ILEUM), OR PAN-CREAS.	FERRING LABORATORIES, INC
GENERIC: SOMATREM TRADE: PROTROPIN*/**	LONG-TERM TREATMENT OF CHILDREN WHO HAVE GROWTH FAILURE DUE TO A LACK OF ADEQUATE ENDOGENOUS GROWTH HORMONE SECRETION.*/** [OCT 17, 1992] SHORT STATURE ASSOCIATED WITH TURNER'S SYNDROME.	GENENTECH
GENERIC: SOMATROPIN, BIOSYN-THETIC TRADE: HUMATROPE*/**	LONG-TERM TREATMENT OF CHILDREN WHO HAVE GROWTH FAILURE DUE TO INADEQUATE SECRETION OF NORMAL EN-DOGENOUS GROWTH HORMONE.*/** [MAR 08, 1994] TREATMENT OF SHORT STATURE ASSOCIATED WITH TURN-ER'S SYNDROME.	LILLY
GENERIC: SOMATROPIN TRADE: NORDITROPIN	TREATMENT OF GROWTH FAILURE IN CHILDREN DUE TO IN-ADEQUATE GROWTH HORMONE SECRETION. FOR ADJUNCTIVE USE IN THE INDUCTION OF OVULATION IN WOMEN WITH INFERTILITY DUE TO 1) HYPOGONADOTROPIC HYPOGONADISM, AND 2) BILATERAL TUBAL OCCLUSION OR UNEXPLAINED INFERTILITY, WHO ARE UNDERGOING IN VIVO FERTILIZATION PROCEDURES OR IN VITRO FERTILIZA-TION WITH EMBRYO TRANSFER PROCEDURES, RESPEC-TIVELY, AND WHO FAIL TO OVULATE IN RESPONSE TO GO-NADOTROPIN THERAPY ALONE. TREATMENT OF SHORT STATURE ASSOCIATED WITH TURN-ER'S SYNDROME.	NORDISK-USA
GENERIC: SOMATROPIN TRADE: NUTROPIN	LONG-TERM TREATMENT OF CHILDREN WHO HAVE GROWTH FAILURE DUE TO A LACK OF ADEQUATE ENDOGENOUS GROWTH HORMONE SECRETION. TREATMENT OF SHORT STATURE ASSOCIATED WITH TURN-ER'S SYNDROME. TREATMENT OF GROWTH RETARDATION ASSOCIATED WITH CHRONIC RENAL FAILURE.	GENENTECH, INC
GENERIC: SOMATROPIN TRADE: SAIZEN	ENHANCEMENT OF NITROGEN RETENTION IN HOSPITAL-IZED PATIENTS SUFFERING FROM SEVERE BURNS. TREATMENT OF IDIOPATHIC OR ORGANIC GROWTH HOR-MONE DEFICIENCY IN CHILDREN WITH GROWTH FAILURE. TREATMENT OF AIDS-ASSOCIATED CATABOLISM/WEIGHT LOSS.	SERONO LABORATORIES, INC
GENERIC: SOTALOL HCL TRADE: BETAPACE	PREVENTION OF LIFE-THREATENING VENTRICULAR TACHY-ARRHYTHMIAS. TREATMENT OF LIFE-THREATENING VENTRICULAR TACHY-ARRHYTHMIAS.	BRISTOL-MYERS SQUIBB
GENERIC: SPIRAMYCIN TRADE: ROVAMYCINE	SYMPTOMATIC RELIEF AND PARASITIC CURE OF CHRONIC CRYPTOSPORIDIOSIS IN PATIENTS WITH IMMUNODEFI-CIENCY.	RHONE-POULENC, INC

DRUG DESIGNATIONS *(continued)*

NAME OF DRUG	DESIGNATED USE [EXCLUSIVITY EXPIRATION DATE]	SPONSOR NAME
GENERIC: SUCCIMER TRADE: CHEMET*/**	TREATMENT OF LEAD POISONING IN CHILDREN*/** [JAN 30, 1998] TREATMENT OF MERCURY INTOXICATION. PREVENTION OF CYSTINE KIDNEY STONE FORMATION IN PATIENTS WITH HOMOZYGOUS CYSTINURIA WHO ARE PRONE TO STONE DEVELOPMENT.	MCNEIL
GENERIC: SUCRALFATE TRADE: NOT ESTABLISHED	TREATMENT OF ORAL COMPLICATIONS OF CHEMOTHERAPY IN BONE MARROW TRANSPLANT RECIPIENTS. TREATMENT OF ORAL ULCERATIONS AND DYSPHAGIA IN PATIENTS WITH EPIDERMOLYSIS BULLOSA.	NASKA PHARMACAL CO
GENERIC: SULFAPYRIDINE TRADE: NOT ESTABLISHED	TREATMENT OF DERMATITIS HERPETIFORMIS.	JACOBUS PHARMACEUTICAL COMPANY
GENERIC: SUPEROXIDE DISMUTASE (RECOMBINANT-HUMAN) TRADE: NOT ESTABLISHED	PREVENTION OF REPERFUSION INJURY TO DONOR ORGAN TISSUE.	BRISTOL-MYERS SQUIBB
GENERIC: SUPEROXIDE DISMUTASE (RECOMBINANT-HUMAN) TRADE: NOT ESTABLISHED	PROTECTION OF DONOR ORGAN TISSUE FROM DAMAGE OR INJURY MEDIATED BY OXYGEN-DERIVED FREE RADICALS THAT ARE GENERATED DURING THE NECESSARY PERIODS OF ISCHEMIA (HYPOXIA, ANOXIA), AND ESPECIALLY REPERFUSION, ASSOCIATED WITH THE OPERATIVE PROCEDURE.	PHARMACIA-CHIRON PARTNERSHIP
GENERIC: SURFACE ACTIVE EXTRACT OF SALINE LAVAGE OF BOVINE LUNGS TRADE: INFASURF	TREATMENT AND PREVENTION OF RESPIRATORY FAILURE DUE TO PULMONARY SURFACTANT DEFICIENCY IN PRETERM INFANTS.	ONY, INC
GENERIC: SURFACTANT (HUMAN) (AMNIOTIC FLUID DERIVED) TRADE: HUMAN SURF	PREVENTION AND TREATMENT OF NEONATAL RESPIRATORY DISTRESS SYNDROME (RDS).	T. ALLEN MERRITT, M.D. UNIVERSITY OF CALIFORNIA
GENERIC: TENIPOSIDE TRADE: VUMON */**	TREATMENT OF REFRACTORY CHILDHOOD ACUTE LYMPHOCYTIC LEUKEMIA (ALL). [JUL 14, 1999]	BRISTOL-MYERS SQUIBB
GENERIC: TERIPARATIDE ACETATE TRADE: PARATHAR*/**	DIAGNOSTIC AGENT TO ASSIST IN ESTABLISHING THE DIAGNOSIS IN PATIENTS PRESENTING WITH CLINCIAL AND LABORATORY EVIDENCE OF HYPOCALCEMIA DUE TO EITHER HYPOPARATHYROIDISM OR PSEUDOHYPOPARATHYROIDISM. [DEC 23, 1994]	RHONE POULENC RORER
GENERIC: TERLIPRESSIN TRADE: GLYPRESSIN	TREATMENT OF BLEEDING ESOPHAGEAL VARICES.	FERRING AB
GENERIC: TESTOSTERONE PROPIONATE TRADE: NOT ESTABLISHED	TREATMENT OF VULVAR DYSTROPHIES.	STAR PHARMACEUTICALS, INC
GENERIC: TESTOSTERONE SUBLINGUAL TRADE: NOT ESTABLISHED	TREATMENT OF CONSTITUTIONAL DELAY OF GROWTH AND PUBERTY IN BOYS.	GYNEX, INC
GENERIC: THALIDOMIDE TRADE: NOT ESTABLISHED	TREATMENT OF GRAFT VERSUS HOST DISEASE (GVHD) IN PATIENTS RECEIVING BONE MARROW TRANSPLANTATION (BMT). PREVENTION OF GVHD IN PATIENTS RECEIVING BMT.	ANDRULIS RESEARCH CORPORATION
GENERIC: THALIDOMIDE TRADE: NOT ESTABLISHED	TREATMENT OF GRAFT VS HOST DISEASE (GVHD) IN PATIENTS RECEIVING BONE MARROW TRANSPLANTATION (BMT). PREVENTION OF GVHD IN PATIENTS RECEIVING BMT. TREATMENT AND MAINTENANCE OF REACTIONAL LEPROMATOUS LEPROSY.	PEDIATRIC PHARMACEUTICS
GENERIC: THYMOXAMINE HCL TRADE: NOT ESTABLISHED	REVERSAL OF PHENYLEPHRINE-INDUCED MYDRIASIS IN PATIENTS WHO HAVE NARROW ANTERIOR ANGLES AND ARE AT RISK OF DEVELOPING AN ACUTE ATTACK OF ANGLE-CLOSURE GLAUCOMA FOLLOWING MYDRIASIS.	IOLAB PHARMACEUTICALS
GENERIC: TIOPRONIN TRADE: THIOLA*/**	PREVENTION OF CYSTINE NEPHROLITHIASIS IN PATIENTS WITH HOMOZYGOUS CYSTINURIA. [AUG 11, 1995]	UNIV TX
GENERIC: TIRATRICOL TRADE: TRIACANA	USE IN COMBINATION WITH LEVO-THYROXINE TO SUPPRESS THYROID STIMULATING HORMONE (TSH) IN PATIENTS WITH WELL-DIFFERENTIATED THYROID CANCER WHO ARE INTOLERANT TO ADEQUATE DOSES OF LEVO-THYROXINE ALONE.	MEDGENIX GROUP
GENERIC: TOREMIFENE TRADE: NOT ESTABLISHED	HORMONAL THERAPY OF METASTATIC CARCINOMA OF THE BREAST.	ADRIA LABORATORIES, INC

DRUG DESIGNATIONS (continued)

NAME OF DRUG	DESIGNATED USE [EXCLUSIVITY EXPIRATION DATE]	SPONSOR NAME
GENERIC: TRANEXAMIC ACID TRADE: CYKLOKAPRON*/**	TREATMENT OF HEREDITARY ANGIONEUROTIC EDEMA. TREATMENT OF PATIENTS UNDERGOING PROSTATECTOMY WHERE THERE IS HEMORRHAGE OR RISK OF HEMORRHAGE AS A RESULT OF INCREASED FIBRINOLYSIS OR FIBRINOGEN-OLYSIS. TREATMENT OF PATIENTS WITH CONGENITAL COAGULOPA-THIES WHO ARE UNDERGOING DENTAL SURGICAL PROCE-DURES (e.g., DENTAL EXTRACTIONS).*/** [DEC 30, 1993]	KABIVITRUM
GENERIC: TRETINOIN TRADE: NOT ESTABLISHED	TREATMENT OF SQUAMOUS METAPLASIA OF THE OCULAR SURFACE EPITHELIA (CONJUNCTIVA AND/OR CORNEA) WITH MUCOUS DEFICIENCY AND KERATINIZATION.	SPECTRA PHARMACEUTI-CALS
GENERIC: TRIENTINE HCL TRADE: SYPRINE*/**	TREATMENT OF PATIENTS WITH WILSON'S DISEASE WHO ARE INTOLERANT, OR INADEQUATELY RESPONSIVE TO PENI-CILLAMINE. [NOV 08, 1992]	MSD
GENERIC: TRIMETREXATE GLUCU-RONATE TRADE: NOT ESTABLISHED	TREATMENT OF METASTATIC COLORECTAL ADENOCARCI-NOMA. TREATMENT OF METASTATIC CARCINOMA OF THE HEAD AND NECK (i.e., BUCCAL CAVITY, PHARYNX AND LARYNX). TREATMENT OF PANCREATIC ADENOCARCINOMA. TREATMENT OF PNEUMOCYSTIS CARINII PNEUMONIA (PCP) IN AIDS PATIENTS. TREATMENT OF PATIENTS WITH ADVANCED NONSMALL CELL CARCINOMA OF THE LUNG.	US BIOSCIENCE
GENERIC: TRIPTORELIN PAMOATE TRADE: DECAPEPTYL INJECTION	FOR USE IN THE PALLIATIVE TREATMENT OF ADVANCED OVARIAN CARCINOMA OF EPITHELIAL ORIGIN.	ORGANON, INC
GENERIC: TROLEANDOMYCIN TRADE: NOT ESTABLISHED	TREATMENT OF SEVERE STEROID-REQUIRING ASTHMA.	STANLEY SZEFLER, M.D. NATIONAL JEWISH CENTER FOR IMMUNOLOGY AND RESPIRATORY MEDICINE
GENERIC: UROFOLLITROPIN TRADE: METRODIN*/**	INDUCTION OF OVULATION IN PATIENTS WITH POLYCYSTIC OVARIAN DISEASE WHO HAVE AN ELEVATED LH/FSH RATIO AND WHO HAVE FAILED TO RESPOND TO ADEQUATE CLOMI-PHENE CITRATE THERAPY. [SEP 18, 1993]	SERONO
GENERIC: URSODEOXYCHOLIC ACID TRADE: ACTIGALL	MANAGEMENT OF THE CLINICAL SIGNS AND SYMPTOMS AS-SOCIATED WITH PRIMARY BILIARY CIRRHOSIS.	CIBA GEIGY
GENERIC: URSODEOXYCHOLIC ACID TRADE: URSOFALK	TREATMENT OF PATIENTS WITH PRIMARY BILIARY CIRRHO-SIS.	INTERFALK U.S., INC
GENERIC: ZALCITABINE TRADE: HIVID	TREATMENT OF ACQUIRED IMMUNODEFICIENCY SYNDROME (AIDS). [JUN 19, 1999]	ROCHE
GENERIC: ZIDOVUDINE (AZT) TRADE: RETROVIR*/**	TREATMENT OF ACQUIRED IMMUNODEFICIENCY SYNDROME AIDS).*/** [MAR 19, 1994] TREATMENT OF CERTAIN PATIENTS WITH AIDS RELATED COMPLEX (ARC).*/** [MAR 19, 1994]	BURROUGHS WELLCOME
GENERIC: ZINC ACETATE TRADE: NOT ESTABLISHED	TREATMENT OF WILSON'S DISEASE.	LEMMON COMPANY
GENERIC: 2-CHLORODEOXYA-DENOSINE TRADE: NOT ESTABLISHED	TREATMENT OF HAIRY CELL LEUKEMIA. TREATMENT OF CHRONIC LYMPHOCYTIC LEUKEMIA.	R.W. JOHNSON PHARM RE-SEARCH
GENERIC: 2-CHLORO-2'-DEOXYADENO-SINE TRADE: NOT ESTABLISHED	TREATMENT OF ACUTE MYELOID LEUKEMIA.	ST JUDE CHILDRENS' HOSPI-TAL
GENERIC: 2'-3'-DIDEOXYCYTIDINE TRADE: NOT ESTABLISHED	TREATMENT OF ACQUIRED IMMUNODEFICIENCY SYNDROME (AIDS).	NATIONAL CANCER INSTI-TUTE
GENERIC: 3'AZIDO-2', 3'DIDEOXYURIDINE TRADE: NOT ESTABLISHED	TREATMENT OF ACQUIRED IMMUNODEFICIENCY SYNDROME (AIDS).	TRITON BIOSCIENCES, INC
GENERIC: 3,4-DIAMINOPYRIDINE TRADE: NOT ESTABLISHED	TREATMENT OF LAMBERT-EATON MYASTHENIC SYNDROME.	JACOBUS PHARMACEUTICAL COMPANY
GENERIC: 3,4-DIAMINOPYRIDINE TRADE: DYNAMINE	TREATMENT OF HEREDITARY MOTOR AND SENSORY NEU-ROPATHY TYPE I (CHARCOT-MARIE-TOOTH DISEASE).	MAYO CLINIC
GENERIC: 4-AMINOPYRIDINE TRADE: NOT ESTABLISHED	RELIEF OF SYMPTOMS OF MULTIPLE SCLEROSIS (MS).	ELAN PHARMACEUTICAL RE-SEARCH
GENERIC: 4-AMINOSALICYLIC ACID TRADE: PAMISYL (P-D), REZIPAS	TREATMENT OF MILD TO MODERATE ULCERATIVE COLITIS WHO ARE INTOLERANT TO SULFASALAZINE.	WARREN L. BEEKEN, M.D. UNIVERSITY OF VERMONT
GENERIC: 4-HYDROPEROXYCYCLO-PHOSPHAMIDE (4-HC) TRADE: NOT ESTABLISHED	FOR USE IN THE EX VIVO TREATMENT OF AUTOLOGOUS BONE MARROW AND SUBSEQUENT REINFUSION IN PA-TIENTS WITH ACUTE MYELOGENOUS LEUKEMIA (AML), ALSO REFERRED TO AS ACUTE NONLYMPHOCYTIC LEUKE-MIA (ANLL).	NOVA PHARMACEUTICAL CORP

DRUG DESIGNATIONS (*continued*)

NAME OF DRUG	DESIGNATED USE [EXCLUSIVITY EXPIRATION DATE]	SPONSOR NAME
GENERIC: 4-METHYLPYRAZOLE TRADE: 4-MP	TREATMENT OF METHANOL, ETHYLENE GLYCOL POISONING.	LOUISIANA STATE UNIVERSITY
GENERIC: 5-AZA-2'-DEOXYCYTIDINE TRADE: NOT ESTABLISHED	TREATMENT OF ACUTE LEUKEMIA.	PHARMACHEMIE U.S.A. INC
GENERIC: 6-METHYLENANDROSTA- 1,4-DIENE-3,17-DIONE TRADE: NOT ESTABLISHED	HORMONAL THERAPY OF METASTATIC CARCINOMA OF THE BREAST.	ADRIA LABORATORIES, INC
GENERIC: 9-CIS RETINOIC ACID NOT ESTABLISHED TRADE:	TREATMENT OF ACUTE PROMYELOCYTIC LEUKEMIA.	LIGAND PHARMACEUTICALS, INC
GENERIC: 24,25 DIHYDROXY-CHOLE- CALCIFEROL TRADE: NOT ESTABLISHED	TREATMENT OF UREMIC OSTEODYSTROPHY.	LEMMON COMPANY
GENERIC: 566C80 TRADE: NOT ESTABLISHED	TREATMENT OF AIDS ASSOCIATED PNEUMOCYSTIS CARINII PNEUMONIA (PCP). PREVENTION OF PNEUMOCYSTIS CARINII PNEUMONIA (PCP) IN HIGH-RISK, HIV-INFECTED PATIENTS DEFINED BY A HISTORY OF ONE OR MORE EPISODES OF PCP AND/OR A PERIPHERAL CD4+ (T4 HELPER/INDUCER) LYMPHOCYTE COUNT LESS THAN OR EQUAL TO 200/MM³.	BURROUGHS WELLCOME COMPANY

DRUG PRODUCTS WHICH MUST DEMONSTRATE *IN VIVO* BIOAVAILABILITY ONLY IF PRODUCT FAILS TO ACHIEVE ADEQUATE DISSOLUTION

Acetaminophen; Aspirin;
Butalbital
Capsule or Tablet; Oral
160-165 mg; 160-165 mg; 50 mg

Acetaminophen; Aspirin;
Butalbital
Capsule or Tablet; Oral
325 mg; 325 mg; 50 mg

Acetaminophen; Aspirin;
Butalbital; Caffeine
Capsule or Tablet; Oral
160-165 mg; 160-165 mg; 50 mg; 40 mg

Acetaminophen; Aspirin;
Butalbital; Caffeine
Capsule or Tablet; Oral
325 mg; 325 mg; 50 mg; 40 mg

Acetaminophen; Butalbital
Capsule or Tablet; Oral
325 mg; 50 mg
650 mg; 50 mg

Acetaminophen; Butalbital;
Caffeine
Capsule or Tablet; Oral
325 mg; 50 mg; 40 mg
650 mg; 50 mg; 40 mg

Aminophylline
Tablet; Oral
100 mg
200 mg

Aspirin; Butalbital;
Capsule or Tablet; Oral
325 mg; 50 mg
650 mg; 50 mg

Aspirin; Butalbital; Caffeine
Capsule or Tablet; Oral
325 mg; 50 mg; 40 mg
650 mg; 50 mg; 40 mg

Aspirin; Caffeine;
Carisoprodol
Tablet; Oral
160 mg; 32 mg; 200 mg

Aspirin; Caffeine;
Carisoprodol; Codeine Phosphate
Tablet; Oral
160 mg; 32 mg; 200 mg; 16 mg

Aspirin; Carisoprodol
Tablet; Oral
325 mg; 200 mg

Aspirin; Carisoprodol;
Codeine Phosphate
Tablet; Oral
325 mg; 200 mg; 16 mg

Aspirin; Meprobamate
Tablet; Oral
325 mg; 200 mg

Aspirin; Methocarbamol
Tablet; Oral
325 mg; 400 mg

Chlorothiazide
Tablet; Oral
250 mg

Hydroxyzine Hydrochloride
Tablet; Oral
10 mg; 25 mg; 50 mg; 100 mg

Prednisone
Tablet; Oral
1 mg; 2.5 mg; 5 mg; 10 mg;
20 mg; 25 mg; 50 mg

BIOPHARMACEUTIC GUIDANCE AVAILABILITY

THE FOLLOWING IS A LIST OF GUIDANCES AVAILABLE FOR *IN VIVO* BIOEQUIVALENCE STUDIES AND *IN VITRO* DISSOLUTION TESTING. COMMENTS AND SUGGESTIONS CONCERNING THESE GUIDANCES ARE ENCOURAGED AND SHOULD BE SENT TO THE DIVISION OF BIOEQUIVALENCE (HFD-650, MPN-2 ROOM 279) 5600 FISHERS LANE, ROCKVILLE, MD 20857.

DRUG NAME (DOSAGE FORM)	DATE	REVISED DATE
ACETOHEXAMIDE (TABLET)	NOV 15, 1985	AUG 01, 1988
ACETAMINOPHEN WITH PROPOXYPHENE NAPSYLATE (TABLET)	MAR 26, 1980	
ALBUTEROL; SULFATE (TABLET)	MAY 29, 1987	
ALBUTEROL AND METAPROTERENOL SULFATE (METERED DOSE INHALER - *IN VITRO*)	JUN 27, 1989	
ALLOPURINOL (TABLET)	JUL 15, 1985	
AMILORIDE HYDROCHLORIDE (TABLET)	MAR 29, 1985	
AMINOPHYLLINE (SUPPOSITORY)	JUL 05, 1983	
AMITRIPTYLINE HYDROCHLORIDE (TABLET)	JUL 05, 1983	
AMITRIPTYLINE AND PERPHENAZINE (TABLET)	AUG 27,1987	
AMOXAPINE (TABLET)	SEP 10, 1987	AUG 05, 1988
AMOXICILLIN (CAPSULE, SUSPENSION AND TABLET)	AUG 18, 1987	JUN 10, 1988
ANTIFUNGAL (DRAFT GUIDANCE) (TOPICAL)	FEB 24, 1990	
ANTIFUNGAL (DRAFT GUIDANCE) (VAGINAL)	FEB 24, 1990	
ATENOLOL (TABLET)	OCT 06, 1988	
BACLOFEN (TABLET)	MAY 05, 1986	
CARBAMAZEPINE (TABLET)	SEP 30, 1987	JAN 20, 1988
CARBIDOPA AND LEVODOPA (TABLET)	JUN 19, 1992	
CEFADROXIL (CAPSULE, SUSPENSION, AND TABLET)	OCT 07, 1986	
CEPHALEXIN (CAPSULE AND TABLET)	AUG 13, 1986	MAR 19, 1987
CEPHRADINE (CAPSULE AND SUSPENSION)	SEP 10, 1986	
CHLORDIAZEPOXIDE (TABLET)	JUL 05, 1983	
CHLORDIAZEPOXIDE HYDROCHLORIDE (CAPSULE)	JUL 05, 1983	
CHLORPROPAMIDE (TABLET)	JUL 05, 1983	
CHLORTHALIDONE (TABLET)	JUL 05, 1983	
CIMETIDINE (TABLET)	JUN 12, 1992	
CLINDAMYCIN HYDROCHLORIDE(CAPSULE)	MAY 31, 1988	
CLOFIBRATE (CAPSULE)	APR 07, 1986	
CLONIDINE HYDROCHLORIDE (TABLET)	DEC 05, 1984	
CLORAZEPATE DIPOTASSIUM (CAPSULE AND TABLET)	MAR 10, 1986	FEB 17, 1987
CORTICOSTEROID *IN VITRO* AND *IN VIVO* INTERIM (TOPICAL)	JUL 01, 1992	
CYCLOBENZAPRINE HYDROCHLORIDE (TABLET)	DEC 18, 1987	JAN 25, 1988
DESIPRAMINE HYDROCHLORIDE (TABLET)	APR 28, 1987	SEP 22, 1987
DIAZEPAM (TABLET)	JUL 08, 1985	
DICYCLOMINE HYDROCHLORIDE (CAPSULE AND TABLET)	AUG 10, 1984	
DIFLUNISAL (TABLET)	MAY 16, 1992	
DILTIAZEM HYDROCHLORIDE (TABLET)	MAY 16, 1992	
DIPYRIDAMOLE (TABLET)	JUL 05, 1983	SEP 25, 1987
DISOPYRAMIDE PHOSPHATE (CAPSULE)	JUL 09, 1985	
DISSOLUTION TESTING (GENERAL)	APR 01, 1978	
DOXEPIN HYDROCHLORIDE (CAPSULE)	APR 02, 1985	OCT 09, 1986
DOXYCYCLINE HYCLATE (CAPSULE AND TABLET)	APR 11, 1988	
ERYTHROMYCIN (CAPSULE, DELAYED RELEASE PELLETS)	SEP 21, 1988	
ESTROGENS, CONJUGATED (TABLET)	AUG 21, 1991	
ETHINYL ESTRADIOL AND NORETHINDRONE (TABLET)	MAR 18, 1988	
FENOPROFEN (CAPSULE AND TABLET)	AUG 27, 1987	FEB 03, 1988
FLURAZEPAM HYDROCHLORIDE (CAPSULE)	OCT 15, 1985	
GEMFIBROZIL (CAPSULE AND TABLET)	JUN 23, 1989	JUN 15, 1992
HALOPERIDOL (TABLET)	APR 30, 1987	
HYDROCHLOROTHIAZIDE (TABLET)	JUL 25, 1983	SEP 28, 1987
HYDROXYZINE HYDROCHLORIDE (TABLET, DISSOLUTION ONLY)	JAN 27, 1981	
HYDROXYZINE PAMOATE (CAPSULE)	JUL 26, 1983	SEP 28, 1987
INDOMETHACIN (CAPSULE)	APR 06, 1985	JAN 27, 1988
ISOPROPAMIDE IODIDE (TABLET)	MAY 12, 1982	
ISOSORBIDE DINITRATE (CAPSULE, EXTENDED RELEASE AND TABLET, EXTENDED RELEASE)	NOV 06, 1985	
ISOSORBIDE DINITRATE (CHEWABLE TABLET, ORAL TABLET, AND SUBLINGUAL TABLET)	JUN 04, 1985	SEP 22, 1987
LEUCOVORIN CALCIUM (TABLET)	APR 28, 1987	AUG 04, 1988
LORAZEPAM (TABLET)	DEC 03, 1984	SEP 16, 1987

LOXAPINE SUCCINATE (CAPSULE)	SEP 10, 1987	
MAPROTILINE HYDROCHLORIDE (TABLET)	AUG 27, 1987	
MECLOFENAMATE SODIUM (CAPSULE)	NOV 12, 1986	
MEDROXYPROGESTERONE ACETATE (TABLET)	DEC 24, 1986	SEP 17, 1987
MEGESTROL ACETATE (TABLET)	AUG 17, 1987	
MESTRANOL AND NORETHINDRONE (TABLET)	MAY 13, 1988	
METAPROTERENOL SULFATE (TABLET)	MAR 18, 1988	
METHYLPREDNISOLONE (TABLET)	JUN 12, 1986	
METOCLOPRAMIDE HYDROCHLORIDE (TABLET)	DEC 27, 1984	
METOPROLOL TARTRATE (TABLET)	JUN 12, 1992	
MINOXIDIL (TABLET)	APR 02, 1986	
NADOLOL (TABLET)	MAY 16, 1992	
NAFCILLIN SODIUM (CAPSULE AND TABLET)	SEP 10, 1987	
NALIDIXIC ACID (TABLET)	AUG 19, 1987	
NAPROXEN (TABLET)	JUN 12, 1992	
NITROFURANTOIN (CAPSULE, MACROCRYSTALLINE)	OCT 29, 1985	
NITROGLYCERIN (OINTMENT)	DEC 17, 1986	
NORTRIPTYLINE HYDROCHLORIDE (CAPSULE)	JUN 15, 1992	
ORPHENADRINE CITRATE (TABLET)	JUL 22, 1983	
PERPHENAZINE (TABLET)	AUG 27, 1987	
PHENYLBUTAZONE (CAPSULE AND TABLET)	JUL 15, 1983	SEP 28, 1987
PIROXICAM (CAPSULE)	JUN 15, 1992	
POTASSIUM CHLORIDE (CAPSULE, SLOW RELEASE AND TABLET, SLOW RELEASE)	JAN 17, 1987	
PRAZEPAM (CAPSULE AND TABLET)	JUL 26, 1988	
PREDNISONE (TABLET–DISSOLUTION ONLY)	JUL 10, 1985	
PROBENECID (TABLET)	JUL 26, 1983	
PROCAINAMIDE HYDROCHLORIDE (TABLET)	JUL 25, 1983	SEP 28, 1987
PROPRANOLOL HYDROCHLORIDE (TABLET)	MAY 19, 1984	
PROPYLTHIOURACIL (TABLET)	AUG 13, 1986	
QUINIDINE GLUCONATE (TABLET, EXTENDED RELEASE)	JUN 15, 1981	SEP 22, 1987
RIFAMPIN (CAPSULE)	SEP 08, 1988	
RITODRINE HYDROCHLORIDE (TABLET)	AUG 27, 1987	
SILVER SULFADIAZINE (CREAM)	MAY 07, 1987	
SPIRONOLACTONE (TABLET)	JUL 25, 1983	
STATISTICAL PROCEDURE FOR BIOEQUIVALENCE STUDIES USING A STANDARD TWO-TREATMENT CROSSOVER DESIGN	JUL 01, 1992	
SULFASALAZINE (TABLET)	OCT 08, 1987	
SULFINPYRAZONE (CAPSULE AND TABLET)	JUL 15, 1983	SEP 25, 1987
SULFONES (TABLET)	NOV 07, 1986	
SULINDAC (TABLET)	SEP 28, 1987	JUL 18, 1988
TEMAZEPAM (CAPSULE)	AUG 08, 1985	
TERFENADINE (TABLET)	JUN 12, 1992	
THEOPHYLLINE (TABLET)	NOV 01, 1984	
TIMOLOL MALEATE (TABLET)	AUG 09, 1988	
TOLAZAMIDE (TABLET)	AUG 22, 1984	
TOLBUTAMIDE (TABLET)	DEC 01, 1983	
TOLMETIN SODIUM (CAPSULE AND TABLET)	APR 20, 1989	
TRAZODONE HYDROCHLORIDE (TABLET)	NOV 15, 1985	APR 30, 1986
TRIMIPRAMINE MALEATE (CAPSULE)	NOV 03, 1986	AUG 18, 1987
VERAPAMIL (TABLET)	JUL 18, 1985	
WAIVER POLICY (DRAFT GUIDANCE)	JUN 23, 1989	

ANDA SUITABILITY PETITIONS

THE FOLLOWING ARE TWO LISTS OF PETITIONS FILED UNDER SECTION 505(j)(2)(C) OF THE ACT WHERE THE AGENCY HAS DETERMINED THAT THE REFERENCED PRODUCT: (1) IS SUITABLE FOR SUBMISSION AS AN ANDA (PETITIONS APPROVED) OR (2) IS NOT SUITABLE FOR SUBMISSION AS AN ANDA (PETITIONS DENIED). THE DETERMINATION THAT AN ANDA WILL BE APPROVED IS NOT MADE UNTIL THE ANDA ITSELF IS SUBMITTED AND REVIEWED BY THE AGENCY. A COPY OF EACH PETITION IS LISTED BY DOCKET NUMBER ON PUBLIC DISPLAY IN FDA'S DOCKETS MANAGEMENT BRANCH, HFA-305, ROOM 4-62, 5600 FISHERS LANE, ROCKVILLE, MD 20857.

PETITIONS APPROVED

DRUG NAME DOSAGE FORM; ROUTE	STRENGTH (CONTAINER SIZE)	DOCKET NUMBER	PETITIONER	REASON FOR PETITION	STATUS
ACETAMINOPHEN SUPPOSITORY; RECTAL	80 MG	85 P-0403/CP	UPSHER SMITH	NEW STRENGTH	APPROVED OCT 16, 1985
ACETAMINOPHEN; ASPIRIN; CODEINE PHOSPHATE TABLET; ORAL	325 MG 325 MG 30 MG	86 P-0361/CP	BOCK PHARMA	NEW DOSAGE FORM NEW STRENGTH	APPROVED DEC 16, 1987
ACETAMINOPHEN; BUTALBITAL; CAFFEINE CAPSULE; ORAL	500 MG 50 MG 40 MG	89 P-0345/CP	MALLARD	NEW DOSAGE FORM	APPROVED OCT 27, 1989
ACETAMINOPHEN; BUTALBITAL; CAFFEINE CODEINE PHOSPHATE CAPSULE; ORAL	325 MG 50 MG 40 MG 30 MG	91 P-069/CP2	KING & SPAULDING	NEW COMBINATION	APPROVED DEC 10, 1991
ACETAMINOPHEN; CODEINE PHOSPHATE CAPSULE; ORAL	500 MG 30 MG	84 P-0228/CP	RW JOHNSON	NEW DOSAGE FORM NEW STRENGTH	APPROVED JUN 02, 1986
ACETAMINOPHEN; CODEINE PHOSPHATE CAPSULE; ORAL	500 MG 60 MG	84 P-0228/CP	RW JOHNSON	NEW DOSAGE FORM NEW STRENGTH	APPROVED JUN 02, 1986
ACETAMINOPHEN; CODEINE PHOSPHATE CAPSULE; ORAL	650 MG 15 MG	86 P-0200/CP	MIKART	NEW DOSAGE FORM NEW STRENGTH	APPROVED OCT 03, 1986
ACETAMINOPHEN; CODEINE PHOSPHATE SOFT GELATIN CAPSULE; ORAL	300 MG 30 MG	85 P-0543/CP	SOFTAN	NEW DOSAGE FORM	APPROVED MAR 18, 1986
ACETAMINOPHEN; CODEINE PHOSPHATE SOFT GELATIN CAPSULE; ORAL	500 MG 7.5 MG	85 P-0543/ CP0002	SOFTAN	NEW DOSAGE FORM NEW STRENGTH	APPROVED MAR 19, 1986
ACETAMINOPHEN; CODEINE PHOSPHATE SOFT GELATIN CAPSULE; ORAL	500 MG 15 MG	85 P-0543/ CP0002	SOFTAN	NEW DOSAGE FORM NEW STRENGTH	APPROVED MAR 19, 1986
ACETAMINOPHEN; CODEINE PHOSPHATE SOLUTION; ORAL	160 MG/5 ML 6 MG/5 ML	86 P-0133/CP	KLEINFELD, KAPLAN AND BECKER	NEW STRENGTH	APPROVED MAY 21, 1986
ACETAMINOPHEN; CODEINE PHOSPHATE SYRUP; ORAL	160 MG/5 ML 6 MG/5 ML	87 P-0323/CP	KLEINFELD, KAPLAN AND BECKER	NEW DOSAGE FORM NEW STRENGTH	APPROVED NOV 04, 1987
ACETAMINOPHEN; CODEINE PHOSPHATE TABLET; ORAL	500 MG 7.5 MG	91 P-0514/CP1	SOFTAN	NEW STRENGTH	APPROVED JUN 03, 1992
ACETAMINOPHEN; CODEINE PHOSPHATE TABLET; ORAL	650 MG 15 MG	86 P-0200/CP	MIKART	NEW STRENGTH	APPROVED OCT 03, 1986

ANDA SUITABILITY PETITIONS

PETITIONS APPROVED *(continued)*

DRUG NAME DOSAGE FORM; ROUTE	STRENGTH (CONTAINER SIZE)	DOCKET NUMBER	PETITIONER	REASON FOR PETITION	STATUS
ACETAMINOPHEN; HYDROCODONE BITARTRATE CAPSULE; ORAL	650 MG 7.5 MG	85 P-0390/CP	UAD LABS	NEW DOSAGE FORM NEW STRENGTH	APPROVED MAR 17, 1987
ACETAMINOPHEN; HYDROCODONE BITARTRATE ELIXIR; ORAL	500 MG/15 ML 7.5 MG/15 ML	85 P-0439/ CP0003	RUSS PHARMS	NEW DOSAGE FORM NEW STRENGTH	APPROVED APR 01, 1987
ACETAMINOPHEN; HYDROCODONE BITARTRATE SOLUTION; ORAL	325 MG/15 ML 2.5 MG/15 ML	87 P-0129/ CP0002	MIKART	NEW STRENGTH	APPROVED JUN 08, 1987
ACETAMINOPHEN; HYDROCODONE BITARTRATE SOLUTION; ORAL	325 MG/15 ML 5 MG/15 ML	87 P-0129/ CP0002	MIKART	NEW STRENGTH	APPROVED JUN 08, 1987
ACETAMINOPHEN; HYDROCODONE BITARTRATE SOLUTION; ORAL	325 MG/15 ML 7.5 MG/15 ML	87 P-0129/ CP0002	MIKART	NEW STRENGTH	APPROVED JUN 08, 1987
ACETAMINOPHEN; HYDROCODONE BITARTRATE SOLUTION; ORAL	325 MG/15 ML 10 MG/15 ML	87 P-0129/ CP0002	MIKART	NEW STRENGTH	APPROVED JUN 08, 1987
ACETAMINOPHEN; HYDROCODONE BITARTRATE SOLUTION; ORAL	500 MG/15 ML 5 MG/15 ML	84 P-0391/CP	UAD LABS	NEW DOSAGE FORM	APPROVED JUL 02, 1985
ACETAMINOPHEN; HYDROCODONE BITARTRATE TABLET; ORAL	325 MG 2.5 MG	87 P-0129/CP	MIKART	NEW STRENGTH	APPROVED JUN 08, 1987
ACETAMINOPHEN; HYDROCODONE BITARTRATE TABLET; ORAL	325 MG 5 MG	87 P-0129/CP	MIKART	NEW STRENGTH	APPROVED JUN 08, 1987
ACETAMINOPHEN; HYDROCODONE BITARTRATE TABLET; ORAL	325 MG 7.5 MG	87 P-0129/CP	MIKART	NEW STRENGTH	APPROVED JUN 08, 1987
ACETAMINOPHEN; HYDROCODONE BITARTRATE TABLET; ORAL	325 MG 10 MG	87 P-0129/CP	MIKART	NEW STRENGTH	APPROVED JUN 08, 1987
ACETAMINOPHEN; HYDROCODONE BITARTRATE TABLET; ORAL	500 MG 10 MG	87 P-0170/CP	LUCHEM	NEW STRENGTH	APPROVED JUL 07, 1987
ACETAMINOPHEN; HYDROCODONE BITARTRATE TABLET; ORAL	650 MG 10 MG	88 P-0416/CP	MORAVEC	NEW STRENGTH	APPROVED MAR 01, 1989
ACETAMINOPHEN; OXYCODONE HYDROCHLO- RIDE SOFT GELATIN CAPSULE; ORAL	500 MG 5 MG	85 P-0543/ CP0003	SOFTAN	NEW DOSAGE FORM	APPROVED MAR 18, 1986
ACETAMINOPHEN; PROPOXYPHENE HYDROCHLO- RIDE SOFT GELATIN CAPSULE; ORAL	500 MG 32 MG	85 P-0581/CP	SOFTAN	NEW DOSAGE FORM NEW STRENGTH	APPROVED MAR 18, 1986
ACETYLCYSTEINE SOLUTION; INHALATION	20%	88 P-0237/CP	DEY	NEW STRENGTH	APPROVED NOV 29, 1988
ALBUTEROL SULFATE CAPSULE, EXTENDED RELEASE; ORAL	EQ 4 MG BASE	91 P-0348/CP1	HAMER	NEW DOSAGE FORM	APPROVED MAR 17, 1992
ALBUTEROL SULFATE SOLUTION; ORAL	2 MG/5 ML	89 P-0447/CP	BIOCRAFT	NEW DOSAGE FORM	APPROVED MAR 15, 1990
AMINOCAPROIC ACID INJECTABLE; INJECTION	500 MG/ML (10 ML/VIAL)	85 P-0308/CP	ABBOTT	NEW STRENGTH	APPROVED FEB 12, 1986

ANDA SUITABILITY PETITIONS

PETITIONS APPROVED (*continued*)

DRUG NAME DOSAGE FORM; ROUTE	STRENGTH (CONTAINER SIZE)	DOCKET NUMBER	PETITIONER	REASON FOR PETITION	STATUS
AMINOPHYLLINE INJECTABLE; INJECTION	10 MG/ML (10 ML/VIAL)	85 P-0459/CP	ABBOTT	NEW STRENGTH	APPROVED FEB 12, 1986
AMINOPHYLLINE INJECTABLE; INJECTION	10 MG/ML (10 ML/VIAL)	87 P-0103/CP	LYPHOMED	NEW STRENGTH	APPROVED JUL 07, 1987
AMINOPHYLLINE INJECTABLE; INJECTION	50 MG/ML (20 ML/VIAL)	85 P-0459/CP	ABBOTT	NEW STRENGTH	APPROVED FEB 12, 1986
ASPIRIN; CAFFEINE; DIHYDROCODEINE BITAR- TRATE TABLET; ORAL	356.4 MG 30 MG 16 MG	86 P-0359/CP	CENTRAL PHARMS	NEW DOSAGE FORM	APPROVED SEP 29, 1986
ASPIRIN; HYDROCODONE BITARTRATE TABLET; ORAL	325 MG 5 MG	87 P-0376/ CP0002	ANABOLIC	NEW STRENGTH	APPROVED FEB 12, 1988
ASPIRIN; HYDROCODONE BITARTRATE TABLET; ORAL	500 MG 7.5 MG	87 P-0100/CP	KING AND SPAULDING	NEW STRENGTH	APPROVED APR 24, 1987
ASPIRIN; HYDROCODONE BITARTRATE TABLET; ORAL	650 MG 5 MG	87 P-0376/CP	ANABOLIC	NEW STRENGTH	APPROVED FEB 12, 1988
ASPIRIN; HYDROCODONE BITARTRATE TABLET; ORAL	650 MG 7.5 MG	90 P-0050/CP	MASON PHARMS	NEW STRENGTH	APPROVED JUN 01, 1990
AZATADINE MALEATE; PHENYLPROPANOLAMINE HY- DROCHLORIDE CAPSULE, EXTENDED RE- LEASE; ORAL	1 MG 75 MG	85 P-0492/CP	SKF	NEW COMBINATION NEW DOSAGE FORM	APPROVED JAN 28, 1986
BENZTROPINE MESYLATE SYRUP; ORAL	0.5 MG/5 ML	85 P-0423/CP	RIM CONSULTING	NEW DOSAGE FORM	APPROVED OCT 16, 1985
BRETYLIUM TOSYLATE INJECTABLE; INJECTION	200 MG/ML (5 ML/CONTAINER)	87 P-0228/CP	ASTRA	NEW STRENGTH	APPROVED OCT 06, 1987
BRETYLIUM TOSYLATE INJECTABLE; INJECTION	200 MG/ML (10 ML/CONTAINER)	85 P-0546/CP	INTL MEDI- CATION	NEW STRENGTH	APPROVED JAN 20, 1987
BRETYLIUM TOSYLATE IN DEXTROSE 5% INJECTABLE; INJECTION	10 MG/ML (50 ML/CONTAINER)	87 P-0065/CP	LYPHOMED	NEW STRENGTH	APPROVED APR 27, 1987
BRETYLIUM TOSYLATE IN DEXTROSE 5% INJECTABLE; INJECTION	10 MG/ML (100 ML/CONTAINER)	87 P-0128/CP	LYPHOMED	NEW STRENGTH	APPROVED JUL 22, 1987
BROMPHENIRAMINE MALEATE; PSEUDOEPHEDRINE HYDRO- CHLORIDE CAPSULE, EXTENDED RE- LEASE; ORAL	12 MG 120 MG	85 P-0095/CP	UAD LABS	NEW COMBINATION NEW DOSAGE FORM	APPROVED DEC 13, 1985
CARBAMAZINE SUSPENSION; ORAL	200 MG/5 ML	89 P-0399/CP	GUIDELINES	NEW DOSAGE FORM	APPROVED MAY 16, 1991
CARMUSTINE, STERILE INJECTABLE; INJECTION	200 MG/VIAL	88 P-0410/CP	QUAD	NEW STRENGTH	APPROVED FEB 13, 1989
CHLORHEXIDINE GLUCONATE SOLUTION; TOPICAL	1.5%	84 P-0417/CP	PARKE DAVIS	NEW STRENGTH	APPROVED SEP 18, 1985
CHLORHEXIDINE GLUCONATE SPRAY; TOPICAL	0.5%	88 P-0036/CP	ARENT, FOX, KINTNER, PLOTKIN & KAHN	NEW DOSAGE FORM	APPROVED AUG 19, 1988
CHLORHEXIDINE GLUCONATE TOWELETTE; TOPICAL	4%	88 P-0295/CP	BRIAN	NEW STRENGTH	APPROVED NOV 03, 1988

ANDA SUITABILITY PETITIONS

PETITIONS APPROVED (continued)

DRUG NAME DOSAGE FORM; ROUTE	STRENGTH (CONTAINER SIZE)	DOCKET NUMBER	PETITIONER	REASON FOR PETITION	STATUS
CHLORPHENIRAMINE MALEATE; PHENYLPROPANOLAMINE HYDROCHLORIDE CAPSULE, EXTENDED RELEASE; ORAL	10 MG 75 MG	85 P-0149/CP	DURA PHARMS	NEW STRENGTH	APPROVED DEC 13, 1985
CHLORPHENIRAMINE MALEATE; PSEUDOEPHEDRINE HYDROCHLORIDE TABLET, EXTENDED RELEASE; ORAL	12 MG 120 MG	87 P-0165/CP	SANDOZ	NEW DOSAGE FORM	APPROVED MAY 19, 1987
CHLORZOXAZONE CAPSULE; ORAL	250 MG	90 P-0084/ CP0001	MIKART	NEW DOSAGE FORM	APPROVED MAY 24, 1990
CHLORZOXAZONE CAPSULE; ORAL	500 MG	82 N-0032/ CP0006	MIKART	NEW DOSAGE FORM	APPROVED JAN 13, 1988
CHLORZOXAZONE TABLET; ORAL	750 MG	91 P-0153/CP1	MIKART	NEW STRENGTH	APPROVED JUN 03, 1992
CHOLESTYRAMINE CAPSULE; ORAL	EQ 500 MG RESIN	86 P-0474/CP	BRISTOL MYERS	NEW DOSAGE FORM NEW STRENGTH	APPROVED JAN 30, 1987
CHOLESTYRAMINE GEL; ORAL	EQ 4 GM RESIN/ CONTAINER	87 P-0301/CP	CIBA	NEW DOSAGE FORM	APPROVED NOV 04, 1987
CHOLESTYRAMINE TABLET; ORAL	EQ 800 MG RESIN	86 P-0475/CP	BRISTOL MYERS	NEW DOSAGE FORM NEW STRENGTH	APPROVED JAN 30, 1987
CHOLESTYRAMINE TABLET; ORAL	EQ 1 GM RESIN	87 P-0324/CP	BRISTOL MYERS	NEW DOSAGE FORM NEW STRENGTH	APPROVED DEC 08, 1987
CISPLATIN INJECTABLE; INJECTION	1 MG/ML (10 ML/VIAL) (50 ML/VIAL) (100 ML/VIAL)	87 P-0421/CP	BULL	NEW DOSAGE FORM NEW STRENGTH	APPROVED FEB 29, 1988
CISPLATIN INJECTABLE; INJECTION	1 MG/ML (20 ML/VIAL)	88 P-0010/CP	LYPHOMED	NEW DOSAGE FORM NEW STRENGTH	APPROVED APR 01, 1988
CISPLATIN INJECTABLE; INJECTION	1 MG/ML (100 ML/VIAL) (500 ML/VIAL)	87 P-0130/CP	BAXTER	NEW DOSAGE FORM NEW STRENGTH	APPROVED OCT 06, 1987
CISPLATIN INJECTABLE; INJECTION	20 MG/VIAL	87 P-0291/CP	LYPHOMED	NEW STRENGTH	APPROVED NOV 03, 1987
CISPLATIN INJECTABLE; INJECTION	100 MG/VIAL	86 P-0395/CP	BEN VENUE	NEW STRENGTH	APPROVED DEC 08, 1986
CLEMASTINE FUMARATE; PHENYLPROPANOLAMINE HYDROCHLORIDE CAPSULE, EXTENDED RELEASE; ORAL	1.34 MG 75 MG	88 P-0350/CP	SCI CONSULTING	NEW DOSAGE FORM	APPROVED DEC 13, 1988
CLEMASTINE FUMARATE; PSEUDOEPHEDRINE HYDROCHLORIDE TABLET, EXTENDED RELEASE; ORAL	EQ 1 MG BASE 120 MG	87 P-0314/CP	DORSEY	NEW COMBINATION	APPROVED NOV 03, 1987
CLOBETASOL PROPIONATE LOTION; TOPICAL	0.05%	90 P-0198/ CP1	KROSS	NEW DOSAGE FORM	APPROVED MAR 14, 1991

ANDA SUITABILITY PETITIONS

PETITIONS APPROVED *(continued)*

DRUG NAME DOSAGE FORM; ROUTE	STRENGTH (CONTAINER SIZE)	DOCKET NUMBER	PETITIONER	REASON FOR PETITION	STATUS
CODEINE PHOSPHATE; DEXBROMPHENIRAMINE MALEATE; PHENYLPROPANOLAMINE HYDROCHLORIDE SYRUP; ORAL	10 MG/5 ML 1 MG/5 ML 12.5 MG/5 ML	85 P-0269/CP	BOCK PHARMA	NEW COMBINATION	APPROVED DEC 06, 1985
CYCLOPHOSPHAMIDE INJECTABLE; INJECTION	20 MG/ML (250 ML/CONTAINER)	88 P-0379/CP	BAXTER	NEW DOSAGE FORM NEW STRENGTH	APPROVED MAR 01, 1989
CYCLOPHOSPHAMIDE INJECTABLE; INJECTION	20 MG/ML (500 ML/CONTAINER)	88 P-0011/CP	BAXTER	NEW DOSAGE FORM	APPROVED JUN 10, 1988
CYCLOPHOSPHAMIDE INJECTABLE; INJECTION	100 MG/VIAL	90 P-0250/CP1	PHARMA-CHEMIE	NEW DOSAGE FORM	APPROVED MAY 07, 1991
CYCLOPHOSPHAMIDE INJECTABLE; INJECTION	200 MG/VIAL	90 P-0250/CP2	PHARMA-CHEMIE	NEW DOSAGE FORM	APPROVED MAY 07, 1991
CYCLOPHOSPHAMIDE INJECTABLE; INJECTION	500 MG/VIAL	90 P-0250/CP3	PHARMA-CHEMIE	NEW DOSAGE FORM	APPROVED MAY 07, 1991
CYCLOPHOSPHAMIDE INJECTABLE; INJECTION	1 GM/VIAL	90 P-0250/CP4	PHARMA-CHEMIE	NEW DOSAGE FORM	APPROVED MAY 07, 1991
CYTARABINE INJECTABLE; INJECTION	20 MG/ML (5 ML/VIAL)	86 P-0130/CP	QUAD	NEW DOSAGE FORM	APPROVED AUG 21, 1986
CYTARABINE INJECTABLE; INJECTION	20 MG/ML (25 ML/VIAL)	86 P-0130/CP	QUAD	NEW DOSAGE FORM	APPROVED AUG 21, 1986
CYTARABINE INJECTABLE; INJECTION	20 MG/ML (50 ML/CONTAINER)	86 P-0428/CP0002	ADRIA	NEW DOSAGE FORM NEW STRENGTH	APPROVED MAY 07, 1987
CYTARABINE INJECTABLE; INJECTION	20 MG/ML (100 ML/CONTAINER)	86 P-0428/CP0005	ADRIA	NEW DOSAGE FORM	APPROVED OCT 28, 1991
CYTARABINE INJECTABLE; INJECTION	1 GM/VIAL	86 P-0313/CP	QUAD	NEW STRENGTH	APPROVED MAY 07, 1987
DESONIDE LOTION; TOPICAL	0.05%	87 P-0105/CP	OWEN	NEW DOSAGE FORM	APPROVED SEP 10, 1987
DEXBROMPHENIRAMINE MALEATE; PHENYLPROPANOLAMINE HYDROCHLORIDE CAPSULE, EXTENDED RELEASE; ORAL	6 MG 75 MG	85 P-0238/CP0002	BOCK PHARMA	NEW COMBINATION	APPROVED DEC 13, 1985
DEXBROMPHENIRAMINE MALEATE; PHENYLPROPANOLAMINE HYDROCHLORIDE CAPSULE, EXTENDED RELEASE; ORAL	6 MG 75 MG	87 P-0265/CP	BOCK PHARMA	NEW COMBINATION NEW DOSAGE FORM	APPROVED NOV 04, 1987
DEXBROMPHENIRAMINE MALEATE; PSEUDOEPHEDRINE HYDROCHLORIDE CAPSULE, EXTENDED RELEASE; ORAL	6 MG 120 MG	85 P-0140/CP	CENTRAL PHARMS	NEW COMBINATION NEW DOSAGE FORM	APPROVED DEC 13, 1985
DEXBROMPHENIRAMINE MALEATE; PSEUDOEPHEDRINE SULFATE CAPSULE, EXTENDED RELEASE; ORAL	6 MG 120 MG	85 P-0140/CP0002	CENTRAL PHARMS	NEW DOSAGE FORM	APPROVED JAN 22, 1986
DEXTROMETHORPHAN POLISTIREX SUSPENSION, EXTENDED RELEASE; ORAL	EQ 15 MG HBR/5 ML	87 P-0088/CP	KING AND SPAULDING	NEW STRENGTH	APPROVED APR 27, 1987

ANDA SUITABILITY PETITIONS

PETITIONS APPROVED *(continued)*

DRUG NAME DOSAGE FORM; ROUTE	STRENGTH (CONTAINER SIZE)	DOCKET NUMBER	PETITIONER	REASON FOR PETITION	STATUS
DIAZEPAM INTENSOL SOLUTION (CONCENTRATE); ORAL	5 MG/ML	85 P-0566/CP	ROXANE	NEW DOSAGE FORM	APPROVED MAR 18, 1986
DIAZEPAM SYRUP; ORAL	2 MG/5 ML	85 P-0499/CP	CAROLINA MEDCL	NEW DOSAGE FORM	APPROVED FEB 28, 1986
DIPHENHYDRAMINE HYDRO-CHLORIDE CONCENTRATE; ORAL	50 MG/ML	84 P-0174/CP	ROXANE	NEW STRENGTH	APPROVED SEP 11, 1985
DISOPYRAMIDE PHOSPHATE TABLET, EXTENDED RELEASE; ORAL	200 MG 300 MG	84 N-0116/CP	BIOCRAFT	NEW DOSAGE FORM NEW STRENGTH	APPROVED JUN 03, 1986
DISULFIRAM SUSPENSION; ORAL	500 MG/30 ML	85 P-0215/CP	PADDOCK	NEW DOSAGE FORM	APPROVED OCT 08, 1985
DOPAMINE HYDROCHLORIDE INJECTABLE; INJECTION	5 MG/ML	90 P-0137/CP1	ABBOTT	NEW STRENGTH	APPROVED APR 10, 1991
ESTRADIOL FILM, EXTENDED RELEASE; TRANSDERMAL	0.067 MG/24 HR	90 P-0125/CP1	NOVEN PHARMS	NEW STRENGTH	APPROVED MAR 14, 1991
ESTRADIOL FILM, EXTENDED RELEASE; TRANSDERMAL	0.084 MG/24 HR	90 P-0125/CP2	NOVEN PHARMS	NEW STRENGTH	APPROVED MAR 14, 1991
ESTRADIOL TABLET; ORAL	0.5 MG	84 P-0308/CP	KEY PHARMS	NEW STRENGTH	APPROVED MAR 24, 1986
ETOPOSIDE INJECTABLE; INJECTION	20 MG/ML (25 ML/VIAL)	91 P-0041/CP1	ADRIA	NEW STRENGTH	APPROVED MAY 22, 1991
FENOPROFEN CALCIUM TABLET; ORAL	EQ 200 MG BASE EQ 300 MG BASE	87 P-0133/CP	BARR	NEW STRENGTH	APPROVED AUG 04, 1987
FLOXURIDINE INJECTABLE; INJECTION	100 MG/ML	86 P-0242/CP	QUAD	NEW DOSAGE FORM	APPROVED AUG 15, 1986
FLUOCINONIDE LOTION; TOPICAL	0.05%	87 P-0004/CP	HAMER	NEW DOSAGE FORM	APPROVED SEP 10, 1987
FLUOROURACIL INJECTABLE; INJECTION	25 MG/ML	85 P-0208/CP	INTL PHARM	NEW STRENGTH	APPROVED OCT 08, 1985
FLUOROURACIL INJECTABLE; INJECTION	50 MG/ML (5 ML/VIAL)	88 P-0052/CP	BEN VENUE	NEW STRENGTH	APPROVED MAR 21, 1988
FLUOROURACIL INJECTABLE; INJECTION	50 MG/ML (20 ML/VIAL)	86 P-0080/CP	BEN VENUE	NEW STRENGTH	APPROVED APR 02, 1986
FLUOROURACIL INJECTABLE; INJECTION	50 MG/ML (50 ML/VIAL)	86 P-0490/CP	ADRIA	NEW STRENGTH	APPROVED JAN 09, 1987
FLUOROURACIL INJECTABLE; INJECTION	50 MG/ML (100 ML/VIAL)	85 P-0221/CP	LYPHOMED	NEW STRENGTH	APPROVED FEB 18, 1986
FLUOROURACIL INJECTABLE; INJECTION	50 MG/ML (250 ML/VIAL)	88 P-0146/CP	BAXTER	NEW STRENGTH	APPROVED JUN 10, 1988
FLURAZEPAM HYDROCHLO-RIDE CONCENTRATE; ORAL	30 MG/ML	85 P-0081/CP	ROXANE	NEW DOSAGE FORM	APPROVED JUL 10, 1985
FLURAZEPAM HYDROCHLO-RIDE SOLUTION; ORAL	15 MG/5 ML	85 P-0091/CP	ROXANE	NEW DOSAGE FORM	APPROVED OCT 25, 1985
FUROSEMIDE SOLUTION; ORAL	40 MG/5 ML	85 P-0106/CP0002	ROXANE	NEW STRENGTH	APPROVED SEP 19, 1985
FUROSEMIDE CONCENTRATE; ORAL	80 MG/ML	85 P-0106/CP	ROXANE	NEW STRENGTH	APPROVED SEP 19, 1985
GLUCAGON HYDROCHLORIDE INJECTABLE; INJECTION	EQ 2 MG BASE/VIAL	86 P-0411/CP	KING AND SPAULDING	NEW STRENGTH	APPROVED OCT 30, 1986
HALOPERIDOL CONCENTRATE; ORAL	EQ 0.5 MG/5 ML	89 P-0088/CP	UDL	NEW STRENGTH	APPROVED MAY 11, 1989

ANDA SUITABILITY PETITIONS

PETITIONS APPROVED *(continued)*

DRUG NAME DOSAGE FORM; ROUTE	STRENGTH (CONTAINER SIZE)	DOCKET NUMBER	PETITIONER	REASON FOR PETITION	STATUS
HALOPERIDOL DECANOATE INJECTABLE; INJECTION	EQ 50 MG BASE/ML (2 ML/CONTAINER)	88 P-0411/CP	QUAD	NEW STRENGTH	APPROVED FEB 13, 1989
HALOPERIDOL LACTATE SOLUTION; ORAL	EQ 2 MG BASE/5 ML	85 P-0076/ CP0002	ROXANE	NEW STRENGTH	APPROVED MAR 28, 1986
HALOPERIDOL LACTATE SOLUTION; ORAL	EQ 5 MG BASE/5 ML	85 P-0080/CP	ROXANE	NEW DOSAGE FORM	APPROVED SEP 19, 1985
HALOPERIDOL LACTATE IN-TENSOL CONCENTRATE; ORAL	EQ 5 MG BASE/ML	85 P-0076/CP	ROXANE	NEW STRENGTH	APPROVED DEC 08, 1986
HOMATROPINE METHYLBROMIDE; HYDROCODONE BITARTRATE SOFT GELATIN CAPSULE; ORAL	1.5 MG 5 MG	88 P-0061/CP	KLEINFELD, KAPLAN AND BECKER	NEW DOSAGE FORM	APPROVED MAY 12, 1988
HYDRALAZINE HYDROCHLO-RIDE SOLUTION; ORAL	25 MG/5 ML	85 P-0074/CP	ROXANE	NEW DOSAGE FORM	APPROVED JUL 03, 1985
HYDROCHLOROTHIAZIDE; PROPRANOLOL HYDROCHLO-RIDE SOLUTION; ORAL	25 MG/5 ML 40 MG/5 ML	87 P-0399/CP	BURDITT, BOWLES, RADZIUS AND RUBERRY	NEW DOSAGE FORM	APPROVED FEB 16, 1988
HYDROCHLOROTHIAZIDE; PROPRANOLOL HYDROCHLO-RIDE SOLUTION; ORAL	25 MG/5 ML 80 MG/5 ML	87 P-0399/CP	BURDITT, BOWLES, RADZIUS AND RUBERRY	NEW DOSAGE FORM	APPROVED FEB 16, 1988
HYDROCHLOROTHIAZIDE; TRIAMTERENE CAPSULE; ORAL	50 MG 75 MG	86 P-0427/CP	PAR	NEW DOSAGE FORM	APPROVED DEC 11, 1986
HYDROCHLOROTHIAZIDE; TRIAMTERENE TABLET; ORAL	25 MG 50 MG	87 P-0335/CP	PAR	NEW DOSAGE FORM	APPROVED FEB 26, 1988
HYDROCORTISONE SOLUTION; TOPICAL	2.5%	89 P-0175/CP	GENDERM	NEW STRENGTH	APPROVED JAN 11, 1990
HYDROCORTISONE ACETATE AEROSOL; TOPICAL	2.5%	92 P-0101/CP1	HOGAN & HARTSON	NEW DOSAGE FORM	APPROVED JUL 08, 1992
HYDROCORTISONE ACETATE CREAM; TOPICAL	2.5%	90 P-0049/CP	FERNDALE	NEW STRENGTH	APPROVED JUN 22, 1990
HYDROCORTISONE ACETATE LOTION; TOPICAL	1%	90 P-0049/CP	FERNDALE	NEW DOSAGE FORM	APPROVED JUN 22, 1990
HYDROCORTISONE ACETATE LOTION; TOPICAL	2.5%	90 P-0049/CP	FERNDALE	NEW DOSAGE FORM	APPROVED JUN 22, 1990
HYDROCORTISONE ACETATE OINTMENT; TOPICAL	1%	90 P-0154/ CP1	FERNDALE	NEW DOSAGE FORM	APPROVED DEC 07, 1990
HYDROCORTISONE VALERATE LOTION; TOPICAL	0.2%	89 P-0028/CP	MCKENNA, CONNER & CUNEO	NEW DOSAGE FORM	APPROVED MAY 10, 1989
HYDROCORTISONE VALERATE SOLUTION; TOPICAL	0.2%	89 P-0029/CP	MCKENNA, CONNER & CUNEO	NEW DOSAGE FORM	APPROVED MAY 10, 1989
IBUPROFEN CAPSULE; ORAL	200 MG	84 P-0383/CP	STERLING	NEW DOSAGE FORM	APPROVED JUN 25, 1985
IBUPROFEN SOFT GELATIN CAPSULE; ORAL	200 MG	87 P-0232/CP	SIDMAK	NEW DOSAGE FORM	APPROVED OCT 06, 1987
IBUPROFEN SOFT GELATIN CAPSULE; ORAL	300 MG 400 MG 600 MG	85 P-0563/CP	SOFTAN	NEW DOSAGE FORM	APPROVED MAR 19, 1986

ANDA SUITABILITY PETITIONS

PETITIONS APPROVED (continued)

DRUG NAME DOSAGE FORM; ROUTE	STRENGTH (CONTAINER SIZE)	DOCKET NUMBER	PETITIONER	REASON FOR PETITION	STATUS
IBUPROFEN SOFT GELATIN CAPSULE; ORAL	800 MG	87 P-0242/CP	SIDMAK	NEW DOSAGE FORM	APPROVED OCT 06, 1987
ISONIAZID CONCENTRATE; ORAL	50 MG/ML	85 P-0468/CP	CAROLINA MEDCL	NEW STRENGTH	APPROVED DEC 13, 1985
ISOSORBIDE DINITRATE TABLET, EXTENDED RELEASE; ORAL	60 MG	89 P-0485/CP	ADRIA	NEW STRENGTH	APPROVED JUN 01, 1990
LEUCOVORIN CALCIUM INJECTABLE; INJECTION	EQ 1 MG BASE/ML	86 P-0149/CP	ROXANE	NEW DOSAGE FORM	APPROVED JUL 25, 1988
LEUCOVORIN CALCIUM INJECTABLE; INJECTION	EQ 5 MG BASE/ML (10 ML/VIAL)	86 P-0241/CP	QUAD	NEW STRENGTH	APPROVED JUL 28, 1987
LEUCOVORIN CALCIUM INJECTABLE; INJECTION	EQ 5 MG BASE/ML (20 ML/VIAL)	86 P-0241/CP	QUAD	NEW STRENGTH	APPROVED JUL 28, 1987
LEUCOVORIN CALCIUM INJECTABLE; INJECTION	EQ 200 MG BASE/VIAL	91 P-0235/CP1	CETUS	NEW STRENGTH	APPROVED DEC 10, 1991
LOPERAMIDE HYDROCHLORIDE TABLET; ORAL	2 MG	87 P-0268/CP	KROSS	NEW DOSAGE FORM	APPROVED OCT 06, 1987
LORAZEPAM SOFT GELATIN CAPSULE; ORAL	0.5 MG 1 MG 2 MG	87 P-0037/CP	APPLIED LABS	NEW DOSAGE FORM	APPROVED MAR 10, 1987
LORAZEPAM SOLUTION; ORAL	1 MG/5 ML	86 P-0292/CP	ROXANE	NEW DOSAGE FORM	APPROVED OCT 15, 1986
LORAZEPAM SOLUTION (CONCENTRATE); ORAL	2 MG/ML	86 P-0291/CP	ROXANE	NEW DOSAGE FORM	APPROVED OCT 15, 1986
LORAZEPAM TABLET; ORAL	0.5 MG 1 MG 2 MG	85 P-0515/CP	WYETH AYERST	NEW DOSAGE FORM	APPROVED FEB 25, 1986
MEPERIDINE HYDROCHLORIDE CONCENTRATE; ORAL	100 MG/ML	84 P-0175/CP	ROXANE	NEW STRENGTH	APPROVED JUN 07, 1985
MEPERIDINE HYDROCHLORIDE INJECTABLE; INJECTION	10 MG/ML (50 ML/CONTAINER)	88 P-0008/CP	LYPHOMED	NEW STRENGTH	APPROVED APR 01, 1988
METHYLDOPATE HYDROCHLORIDE IN DEXTROSE 5% INJECTABLE; INJECTION	2.5 MG/ML (100 ML/CONTAINER)	86 P-0410/CP0002	KING AND SPAULDING	NEW STRENGTH	APPROVED MAR 10, 1987
METHYLDOPATE HYDROCHLORIDE IN DEXTROSE 5% INJECTABLE; INJECTION	5 MG/ML (100 ML/CONTAINER)	86 P-0410/CP0003	KING AND SPAULDING	NEW STRENGTH	APPROVED MAR 10, 1987
METHYLTESTOSTERONE CAPSULE; ORAL	25 MG	85 P-0067/CP	STAR PHARMS	NEW DOSAGE FORM	APPROVED AUG 23, 1985
METOCLOPRAMIDE HYDROCHLORIDE INJECTABLE; INJECTION	5 MG/ML (20 ML/VIAL)	86 P-0036/CP	DUPONT	NEW STRENGTH	APPROVED MAR 18, 1986
METOCLOPRAMIDE HYDROCHLORIDE INJECTABLE; INJECTION	5 MG/ML (50 ML/VIAL)	85 P-0545/CP	LYPHOMED	NEW STRENGTH	APPROVED FEB 28, 1986
METOCLOPRAMIDE HYDROCHLORIDE INJECTABLE; INJECTION	5 MG/ML (50 ML/VIAL) (100 ML/VIAL)	85 P-0540/CP	QUAD	NEW STRENGTH	APPROVED FEB 28, 1986
METOCLOPRAMIDE HYDROCHLORIDE INTENSOL CONCENTRATE; ORAL	10 MG/ML	88 P-0164/CP	ROXANE	NEW STRENGTH	APPROVED JUN 28, 1988

ANDA SUITABILITY PETITIONS

PETITIONS APPROVED *(continued)*

DRUG NAME DOSAGE FORM; ROUTE	STRENGTH (CONTAINER SIZE)	DOCKET NUMBER	PETITIONER	REASON FOR PETITION	STATUS
MICONAZOLE NITRATE CREAM; VAGINAL	4%	84 P-0398/CP	RW JOHNSON	NEW STRENGTH	APPROVED MAR 31, 1986
MORPHINE SULFATE CAPSULE, EXTENDED RELEASE; ORAL	30 MG	89 P-0071/CP	OXFORD RES INTL	NEW DOSAGE FORM	APPROVED MAY 10, 1989
NIFEDIPINE CAPSULE; ORAL	10 MG	88 P-0072/ CP0002	MARTEC	NEW DOSAGE FORM	APPROVED MAY 11, 1988
NIFEDIPINE CAPSULE; ORAL	20 MG	88 P-0072/CP	MARTEC	NEW DOSAGE FORM	APPROVED MAY 11, 1988
NIFEDIPINE CAPSULE, EXTENDED RELEASE; ORAL	30 MG 60 MG 90 MG	90 P-0436/CP1	KV	NEW DOSAGE FORM	APPROVED OCT 23, 1991
NIFEDIPINE TABLET; ORAL	10 MG 20 MG	87 P-0340/CP	PAR	NEW DOSAGE FORM	APPROVED DEC 11, 1987
NITROGLYCERIN IN DEXTROSE 5% INJECTABLE; INJECTION	0.5 MG/ML (100 ML/CONTAINER)	86 P-0099/ CP0004	ABBOTT	NEW STRENGTH	APPROVED FEB 02, 1987
NITROGLYCERIN IN DEXTROSE 5% INJECTABLE; INJECTION	5 MG/ML (50 ML/CONTAINER)	91 P-0387/CP1	ABBOTT	NEW STRENGTH	APPROVED FEB 18, 1992
NITROGLYCERIN IN DEXTROSE 5% INJECTABLE; INJECTION	10 MG/ML (100 ML/CONTAINER)	91 P-0387/CP1	ABBOTT	NEW STRENGTH	APPROVED FEB 18, 1992
NITROGLYCERIN IN DEXTROSE 5% INJECTABLE; INJECTION	10 MG/100 ML (500 ML/CONTAINER)	86 P-0099/CP	ABBOTT	NEW STRENGTH	APPROVED APR 01, 1986
NITROGLYCERIN IN DEXTROSE 5% INJECTABLE; INJECTION	40 MG/100 ML (500 ML/CONTAINER)	86 P-0099/ CP0003	ABBOTT	NEW STRENGTH	APPROVED APR 01, 1986
NITROGLYCERIN IN DEXTROSE 5% INJECTABLE; INJECTION	0.05 MG/ML (500 ML/CONTAINER)	89 P-0422/CP	LYPHOMED	NEW STRENGTH	APPROVED APR 20, 1990
NITROGLYCERIN IN DEXTROSE 5% INJECTABLE; INJECTION	0.2 MG/ML (500 ML/CONTAINER)	89 P-0422/CP	LYPHOMED	NEW STRENGTH	APPROVED APR 20, 1990
NITROGLYCERIN OINTMENT; TOPICAL	4%	87 P-0184/CP	FOREST	NEW STRENGTH	APPROVED SEP 15, 1987
OXAZEPAM TABLET; ORAL	15 MG 30 MG	85 P-0516/CP	WYETH AYERST	NEW DOSAGE FORM	APPROVED FEB 25, 1986
PENTAMIDINE ISETHIONATE INJECTABLE; INJECTION	100 MG/ML (3 ML/VIAL)	89 P-0435/CP	ASTRA	NEW DOSAGE FORM	APPROVED JAN 18, 1990
PENTETATE PENTASODIUM; STANNOUS CHLORIDE (TECHNETIUM TC-99M PENTETATE KIT) INJECTABLE; INJECTION	10 MG 0.55 MG	89 P-0113/CP	CADEMA MED PRODS	NEW STRENGTH	APPROVED JUL 14, 1989
PHENYTOIN SODIUM INJECTABLE; INJECTION	100 MG/VIAL 250 MG/VIAL	87 P-0367/CP	LYPHOMED	NEW DOSAGE FORM	APPROVED FEB 16, 1988
POLYETHYLENE GLYCOL 3350; POTASSIUM CHLORIDE; SODIUM BICARBONATE; SODIUM CHLORIDE; SODIUM SULFATE IN PLASTIC CONTAINER POWDER FOR RECONSTITUTION; ORAL	59 GM/PACKET 0.7425 GM/PACKET 1.685 GM/PACKET 1.465 GM/PACKET 5.685 GM/PACKET	88 P-0419/CP	GUIDELINES	NEW STRENGTH	APPROVED MAR 01, 1989

ANDA SUITABILITY PETITIONS

PETITIONS APPROVED (continued)

DRUG NAME DOSAGE FORM; ROUTE	STRENGTH (CONTAINER SIZE)	DOCKET NUMBER	PETITIONER	REASON FOR PETITION	STATUS
PREDNISOLONE SODIUM PHOS-PHATE SOLUTION; ORAL	EQ 5 MG BASE/ML	88 P-0235/CP	PAN AM PHARMS	NEW STRENGTH	APPROVED AUG 24, 1988
PREDNISOLONE SODIUM PHOS-PHATE SOLUTION; ORAL	EQ 15 MG BASE/5 ML	87 P-0235/CP	FISONS	NEW STRENGTH	APPROVED NOV 04, 1987
PREDNISONE CAPSULE; ORAL	1 MG 2.5 MG 5 MG 10 MG 20 MG 25 MG 50 MG	88 P-0391/CP	ASCHER	NEW DOSAGE FORM	APPROVED MAR 01, 1989
PROBUCOL TABLET; ORAL	500 MG	85 P-0337/CP	MERRELL DOW	NEW STRENGTH	APPROVED OCT 25, 1985
PROCAINAMIDE HYDROCHLO-RIDE TABLET, EXTENDED RELEASE; ORAL	375 MG	85 P-0125/CP	KEY PHARMS	NEW STRENGTH	APPROVED SEP 19, 1985
PROMETHAZINE HYDROCHLO-RIDE INJECTABLE; INJECTION	25 MG/ML (2 ML/VIAL)	87 P-0087/CP	LYPHOMED	NEW STRENGTH	APPROVED MAY 01, 1987
PROMETHAZINE HYDROCHLO-RIDE INJECTABLE; INJECTION	50 MG/ML (2 ML/VIAL)	87 P-0087/ CP0002	LYPHOMED	NEW STRENGTH	APPROVED MAY 01, 1987
PROPRANOLOL HYDROCHLO-RIDE CAPSULE; ORAL	10 MG 20 MG 40 MG 60 MG 80 MG 90 MG	86 P-0045/CP	NUTRIPHARM LABS	NEW DOSAGE FORM	APPROVED MAR 19, 1986
PROPRANOLOL HYDROCHLO-RIDE TABLET, EXTENDED RELEASE; ORAL	80 MG 120 MG 160 MG	85 P-0197/CP	FOREST	NEW DOSAGE FORM	APPROVED SEP 27, 1985
PROPRANOLOL HYDROCHLO-RIDE TABLET, EXTENDED RELEASE; ORAL	160 MG	85 P-0129/CP	VEREX LABS	NEW DOSAGE FORM	APPROVED SEP 25, 1985
PROTIRELIN INJECTABLE; INJECTION	0.2 MG/ML	90 P-0214/ CP1	FERRING	NEW STRENGTH	APPROVED DEC 21, 1990
PSEUDOEPHEDRINE HYDRO-CHLORIDE TABLET, EXTENDED RELEASE; ORAL	120 MG	87 P-0297/CP	HLTH PLCY NTWK	NEW DOSAGE FORM	APPROVED NOV 03, 1987
PSEUDOEPHEDRINE HYDRO-CHLORIDE; TRIPROLIDINE HYDROCHLO-RIDE TABLET, EXTENDED RELEASE; ORAL	120 MG 5 MG	87 P-0296/CP	HLTH PLCY NTWK	NEW DOSAGE FORM	APPROVED NOV 03, 1987
QUINIDINE GLUCONATE TABLET, EXTENDED RELEASE; ORAL	648 MG	87 P-0276/CP	FOREST	NEW STRENGTH	APPROVED NOV 22, 1988
QUINIDINE SULFATE CAPSULE, EXTENDED RE-LEASE; ORAL	300 MG	88 P-0277/CP	ROBINS	NEW DOSAGE FORM	APPROVED DEC 13, 1988
RITODRINE HYDROCHLORIDE IN DEXTROSE 5% INJECTABLE; INJECTION	30 MG/100 ML (500 ML/CONTAINER)	86 P-0100/CP	ABBOTT	NEW STRENGTH	APPROVED MAY 07, 1986

ANDA SUITABILITY PETITIONS

PETITIONS APPROVED *(continued)*

DRUG NAME DOSAGE FORM; ROUTE	STRENGTH (CONTAINER SIZE)	DOCKET NUMBER	PETITIONER	REASON FOR PETITION	STATUS
SCOPOLAMINE TRANSDERMAL SYSTEM/24 HOUR FILM, EXTENDED RELEASE; PERCUTANEOUS	1 MG	85 P-0168/CP	CIBA	NEW STRENGTH (DOSING INTERVAL)	APPROVED SEP 27, 1985
SODIUM CHLORIDE 0.9% IN PLASTIC CONTAINER INJECTABLE; INJECTION	900 MG/100 ML (100 ML/VIAL)	87 P-0391/CP	LYPHOMED	NEW STRENGTH	APPROVED AUG 11, 1988
SODIUM NITROPRUSSIDE INJECTABLE; INJECTION	0.5 MG/ML	90 P-0179/ CP1	ABBOTT	NEW STRENGTH	APPROVED DEC 21, 1990
SPIRONOLACTONE SUSPENSION; ORAL	25 MG/5 ML	86 P-0055/CP	CAROLINA MEDCL	NEW DOSAGE FORM	APPROVED MAR 28, 1986
SPIRONOLACTONE SYRUP; ORAL	25 MG/5 ML	85 P-0510/CP	CAROLINA MEDCL	NEW DOSAGE FORM	APPROVED JAN 22, 1986
STERILE WATER IN PLASTIC CONTAINER INJECTABLE; INJECTION	100% (100 ML/CONTAINER)	87 P-0392/CP	LYPHOMED	NEW STRENGTH	APPROVED AUG 11, 1988
TECHNETIUM TC99 MEDRONATE KIT INJECTABLE: INJECTION	N/A	91 P-0040/CP1	ABARIS	NEW STRENGTH	APPROVED OCT 28, 1991
TERFENADINE CAPSULE: ORAL	60 MG	91 P-0087/CP1	ARTHUR A. CHECCHI	NEW DOSAGE FORM	APPROVED OCT 28, 1991
THEOPHYLLINE CAPSULE; ORAL	150 MG 300 MG	85 P-0175/CP	MEAD JOHNSON	NEW STRENGTH	APPROVED OCT 08, 1985
THEOPHYLLINE CAPSULE, EXTENDED RE-LEASE; ORAL	400 MG	86 P-0471/ CP0002	SEARLE	NEW STRENGTH	APPROVED MAR 10, 1987
THEOPHYLLINE CAPSULE, EXTENDED RE-LEASE; ORAL	450 MG	88 P-0119/CP	RIKER LABS	NEW STRENGTH	APPROVED MAY 11, 1988
THEOPHYLLINE CAPSULE, EXTENDED RE-LEASE; ORAL	500 MG	88 P-0226/CP	SAVAGE	NEW STRENGTH	APPROVED AUG 25, 1988
THEOPHYLLINE SOLUTION; ORAL	160 MG/15 ML	88 P-0301/CP	FLEMING	NEW STRENGTH	APPROVED NOV 04, 1988
THEOPHYLLINE TABLET; ORAL	150 MG	89 P-0499/CP	SCI CONSULTING	NEW STRENGTH	APPROVED MAY 03, 1990
THEOPHYLLINE TABLET, EXTENDED RELEASE; ORAL	600 MG	85 P-0580/CP	PURDUE FREDERICK	NEW STRENGTH	APPROVED OCT 24, 1986
THEOPHYLLINE TABLET, EXTENDED RELEASE; ORAL	800 MG	91 P-0209/CP1	PURDUE FREDERICK	NEW STRENGTH	APPROVED DEC 10, 1991
THIOTEPA, STERILE INJECTABLE; INJECTION	30 MG/VIAL 60 MG/VIAL	88 P-0412/CP	QUAD	NEW STRENGTH	APPROVED MAR 01, 1989
THIOTEPA, STERILE (WITH DILUENT) INJECTABLE; INJECTION	15 MG/VIAL	87 P-0382/CP	LYPHOMED	NEW DOSAGE FORM	APPROVED MAY 12, 1988
THIOTHIXENE HYDROCHLO-RIDE SOLUTION; ORAL	5 MG/5 ML	86 P-0178/CP	ELLIS PHARM	NEW STRENGTH	APPROVED JUN 04, 1986
TOLMETIN SODIUM TABLET; ORAL	EQ 400 MG BASE	90 P-0011/CP	QUANTUM PHARMICS	NEW STRENGTH	APPROVED MAY 03, 1990
TRIAMCINOLONE ACETONIDE CREAM; TOPICAL	0.05%	86 P-0360/CP	CAROLINA MEDCL	NEW STRENGTH	APPROVED OCT 15, 1986
TRIAMCINOLONE ACETONIDE LOTION; TOPICAL	0.5%	87 P-0019/CP	HAMER	NEW STRENGTH	APPROVED SEP 11, 1987
TRIAMCINOLONE ACETONIDE OINTMENT; TOPICAL	0.05%	86 P-0360/CP	CAROLINA MEDCL	NEW STRENGTH	APPROVED OCT 15, 1986

ANDA SUITABILITY PETITIONS

PETITIONS APPROVED (continued)

DRUG NAME DOSAGE FORM; ROUTE	STRENGTH (CONTAINER SIZE)	DOCKET NUMBER	PETITIONER	REASON FOR PETITION	STATUS
VERAPAMIL HYDROCHLORIDE CAPSULE, EXTENDED RE-LEASE; ORAL	120 MG 240 MG	87 P-0233/CP	SEARLE	NEW DOSAGE FORM NEW STRENGTH	APPROVED FEB 26, 1988
VERAPAMIL HYDROCHLORIDE SOLUTION; ORAL	40 MG/5 ML 80 MG/5 ML	87 P-0101/CP	PHARM BASICS	NEW DOSAGE FORM	APPROVED SEP 10, 1987
VERAPAMIL HYDROCHLORIDE TABLET, EXTENDED RELEASE; ORAL	120 MG	89 P-0220/CP	LEDERLE	NEW STRENGTH	APPROVED JAN 11, 1990
VINBLASTINE SULFATE INJECTABLE; INJECTION	1 MG/ML (10 ML/VIAL)	86 P-0056/CP	QUAD	NEW DOSAGE FORM	APPROVED MAR 28, 1986
VINBLASTINE SULFATE INJECTABLE; INJECTION	1 MG/ML (25 ML/VIAL)	87 P-0112/CP	QUAD	NEW DOSAGE FORM NEW STRENGTH	APPROVED JUN 08, 1987
VINBLASTINE SULFATE INJECTABLE; INJECTION	1 MG/ML (30 ML/VIAL)	87 P-0211/CP	LYPHOMED	NEW STRENGTH	APPROVED JUL 28, 1987
VINCRISTINE SULFATE INJECTABLE; INJECTION	1 MG/ML (1.5 ML/CONTAINER)	87 P-0210/CP	LYPHOMED	NEW STRENGTH	APPROVED JUL 28, 1987
XENON XE 133 GAS; INHALATION	150 MCI/VIAL 250 MCI/VIAL	86 P-0041/CP	MEDI NUCLR	NEW STRENGTH	APPROVED OCT 15, 1986
XENON XE 133 INJECTABLE; INJECTION	60 MCI/VIAL 150 MCI/VIAL	86 P-0342/CP	MEDI NUCLR	NEW STRENGTH	APPROVED SEP 11, 1987

ANDA SUITABILITY PETITIONS

PETITIONS DENIED

DRUG NAME DOSAGE FORM; ROUTE	STRENGTH (CONTAINER SIZE)	DOCKET NUMBER	PETITIONER	REASON FOR PETITION	STATUS
ACETAMINOPHEN; DIHYDROCODEINE BITARTRATE CAPSULE; ORAL	356.4 MG 20 MG	86 P-0040/CP	DUNHALL	NEW COMBINATION NEW STRENGTH	DENIED FEB 12, 1987
ACETAMINOPHEN; HYDROCODONE BITARTRATE TABLET; ORAL	650 MG 10 MG	85 P-0015/CP	APPLIED LABS	NEW STRENGTH	DENIED NOV 07, 1985
ACETAMINOPHEN; METHOCARBAMOL TABLET; ORAL	325 MG 400 MG	85 P-0102/CP	RW JOHNSON	NEW COMBINATION	DENIED JUN 24, 1986
ALBUTEROL SULFATE CAPSULE, EXTENDED RELEASE; ORAL	EQ 4 MG BASE	89 P-0207/CP	PARTICLE DYNAMICS	NEW DOSAGE FORM	DENIED DEC 13, 1991
ALLOPURINOL SODIUM INJECTABLE; INJECTION	500 MG (30 ML/VIAL)	89 P-0103/CP	BURROUGHS WELLCOME	NEW DOSAGE FORM NEW INGREDIENT (NEW SALT) NEW ROUTE OF ADMINISTRATION	DENIED JUL 14, 1989
AMINOCAPROIC ACID INJECTABLE; INJECTION	500 MG/ML	85 P-0064/CP	ABBOTT	NEW STRENGTH	DENIED MAY 29, 1985
AMINOPHYLLINE INJECTABLE; INJECTION	10 MG/ML 50 MG/ML	85 P-0066/CP	ABBOTT	NEW STRENGTH	DENIED MAY 03, 1985
5-AMINOSALICYLIC ACID SUPPOSITORY; RECTAL	500 MG	84 P-0425/CP	REID ROWELL	NEW INGREDIENT	DENIED JUN 05, 1986
ASPIRIN; BUTALBITAL; CAFFEINE; CODEINE PHOSPHATE CAPSULE; ORAL	325 MG 50 MG 40 MG 7.5 MG	85 P-0101/CP	SANDOZ	NEW COMBINATION	DENIED SEP 11, 1985
ASPIRIN; BUTALBITAL; CAFFEINE; CODEINE PHOSPHATE CAPSULE; ORAL	325 MG 50 MG 40 MG 15 MG	85 P-0101/CP	SANDOZ	NEW COMBINATION	DENIED SEP 11, 1985
ASPIRIN; BUTALBITAL; CAFFEINE; CODEINE PHOSPHATE CAPSULE; ORAL	325 MG 50 MG 40 MG 30 MG	85 P-0101/CP	SANDOZ	NEW COMBINATION	DENIED SEP 11, 1985
ASPIRIN; BUTALBITAL; CAFFEINE; CODEINE PHOSPHATE CAPSULE; ORAL	325 MG 50 MG 40 MG 60 MG	85 P-0101/ CP0002	SANDOZ	NEW COMBINATION	DENIED SEP 11, 1985
ASPIRIN; CAFFEINE; HYDROCODONE BITARTRATE TABLET; ORAL	224 MG 32 MG 5 MG	86 P-0243/CP	MASON PHARMS	NEW COMBINATION NEW DOSAGE FORM NEW STRENGTH	DENIED JUN 12, 1987
ASPIRIN; CAFFEINE; HYDROCODONE BITARTRATE TABLET; ORAL	325 MG 30 MG 5 MG	85 P-0455/CP	CENTRAL PHARMS	NEW COMBINATION NEW DOSAGE FORM NEW STRENGTH	DENIED JUN 08, 1987
ASPIRIN; CAFFEINE; HYDROCODONE BITARTRATE TABLET; ORAL	356.4 MG 30 MG 5 MG	86 P-0243/ CP0002	MASON PHARMS	NEW COMBINATION NEW DOSAGE FORM	DENIED JUN 16, 1987

ANDA SUITABILITY PETITIONS

PETITIONS DENIED *(continued)*

DRUG NAME DOSAGE FORM; ROUTE	STRENGTH (CONTAINER SIZE)	DOCKET NUMBER	PETITIONER	REASON FOR PETITION	STATUS
ASPIRIN; CHLORZOXAZONE TABLET; ORAL	325 MG 250 MG	85 P-0071/CP	RW JOHNSON	NEW COMBINATION	DENIED SEP 03, 1985
BENZOYL METRONIDAZOLE SUSPENSION; ORAL	200 MG/5 ML	85 P-0258/CP	APKON LABS	NEW INGREDIENT (NEW ESTER)	DENIED MAR 19, 1986
BETAMETHASONE DIPROPIO-NATE; MICONAZOLE NITRATE CREAM; TOPICAL	0.05% 2%	85 P-0271/CP	RW JOHNSON	NEW COMBINATION	DENIED APR 18, 1986
BRETYLIUM TOSYLATE INJECTABLE; INJECTION	2 MG/ML	85 P-0063/CP	ABBOTT	NEW STRENGTH	DENIED MAY 29, 1985
BRETYLIUM TOSYLATE INJECTABLE; INJECTION	4 MG/ML	85 P-0063/ CP0002	ABBOTT	NEW STRENGTH	DENIED MAY 29, 1985
BRETYLIUM TOSYLATE INJECTABLE; INJECTION	8 MG/ML	85 P-0063/ CP0003	ABBOTT	NEW STRENGTH	DENIED MAY 29, 1985
BRETYLIUM TOSYLATE INJECTABLE; INJECTION	10 MG/ML	85 P-0063/ CP0004	ABBOTT	NEW STRENGTH	DENIED MAY 29, 1985
BROMDIPHENHYDRAMINE HY-DROCHLORIDE; HYDROCODONE BITARTRATE SOLUTION; ORAL	12.5 MG/5 ML 2.5 MG/5 ML	85 P-0255/CP	MIKART	NEW COMBINATION	DENIED MAY 11, 1988
BROMDIPHENHYDRAMINE HY-DROCHLORIDE; HYDROCODONE BITARTRATE SYRUP; ORAL	12.5 MG/5 ML 2.5 MG/5 ML	85 P-0255/CP	MIKART	NEW COMBINATION	DENIED MAY 11, 1988
BROMPHENIRAMINE MALEATE; HYDROCODONE BITARTRATE; PHENYLPROPANOLAMINE HY-DROCHLORIDE SYRUP; ORAL	2 MG/5 ML 2.5 MG/5 ML 12.5 MG/5 ML	85 P-0237/CP	MIKART	NEW COMBINATION	DENIED MAY 11, 1988
CAFFEINE; ERGOTAMINE TARTRATE; PENTOBARBITAL SODIUM SUPPOSITORY; RECTAL	200 MG 2 MG 60 MG	85 P-0433/ CP0002	SANDOZ	NEW COMBINATION	DENIED NOV 08, 1985
CAFFEINE; ERGOTAMINE TARTRATE; PENTOBARBITAL SODIUM TABLET; ORAL	100 MG 1 MG 30 MG	85 P-0433/CP	SANDOZ	NEW COMBINATION	DENIED NOV 08, 1985
CHOLECALCIFEROL CAPSULE; ORAL	1.25 MG	84 P-0161/CP	PHARMACAPS	NEW INGREDIENT	DENIED FEB 13, 1986
CHOLINE MAGNESIUM TRISALICYLATE; CODEINE PHOSPHATE TABLET; ORAL	500 MG 30 MG	85 P-0142/CP	PURDUE FREDERICK	NEW COMBINATION	DENIED JUL 21, 1986
CHOLINE MAGNESIUM TRISALICYLATE; CODEINE PHOSPHATE TABLET; ORAL	500 MG 60 MG	85 P-0142/CP	PURDUE FREDERICK	NEW COMBINATION	DENIED JUL 21, 1986
CLONIDINE HYDROCHLORIDE CAPSULE, EXTENDED RE-LEASE; ORAL	0.2 MG	88 P-0365/CP	BOEHRINGER INGELHEIM	NEW DOSAGE FORM	DENIED JAN 11, 1990
CODEINE PHOSPHATE; IBUPROFEN CAPSULE; ORAL	30 MG 200 MG	84 P-0388/CP	RW JOHNSON	NEW COMBINATION	DENIED SEP 16, 1985
CODEINE PHOSPHATE; IBUPROFEN CAPSULE; ORAL	60 MG 200 MG	84 P-0388/CP	RW JOHNSON	NEW COMBINATION	DENIED SEP 16, 1985

ANDA SUITABILITY PETITIONS

PETITIONS DENIED *(continued)*

DRUG NAME DOSAGE FORM; ROUTE	STRENGTH (CONTAINER SIZE)	DOCKET NUMBER	PETITIONER	REASON FOR PETITION	STATUS
CODEINE PHOSPHATE; IBUPROFEN TABLET; ORAL	30 MG 200 MG	84 P-0388/CP	RW JOHNSON	NEW COMBINATION	DENIED SEP 16, 1985
CODEINE PHOSPHATE; IBUPROFEN TABLET; ORAL	60 MG 200 MG	84 P-0388/CP	RW JOHNSON	NEW COMBINATION	DENIED SEP 16, 1985
CYCLOBENZAPRINE HYDRO-CHLORIDE TABLET; ORAL	15 MG	86 P-0386/CP	CENTRAL PHARMS	NEW STRENGTH	DENIED AUG 15, 1988
CYCLOPHOSPHAMIDE INJECTABLE; INJECTION	100 MG/ML (1 ML/VIAL) (2 ML/VIAL)	87 P-0283/CP	LYPHOMED	NEW DOSAGE FORM NEW STRENGTH	DENIED JAN 21, 1988
CYCLOPHOSPHAMIDE INJECTABLE; INJECTION	500 MG/ML (1 ML/VIAL) (2 ML/VIAL) (4 ML/VIAL)	87 P-0283/CP	LYPHOMED	NEW DOSAGE FORM NEW STRENGTH	DENIED JAN 21, 1988
DEXTROMETHORPHAN HY-DROBROMIDE TABLET, EXTENDED RELEASE; ORAL	60 MG	85 P-0135/CP	CIBA	NEW DOSAGE FORM NEW INGREDIENT	DENIED JUL 17, 1986
DIATRIZOATE MEGLUMINE; LIDOCAINE HYDROCHLORIDE INJECTABLE; INJECTION	60% 1.5 MG/ML	84 P-0325/CP	COOK	NEW COMBINATION	DENIED SEP 03, 1985
DIAZEPAM INTENSOL CONCENTRATE; ORAL	10 MG/ML	85 P-0075/CP	ROXANE	NEW DOSAGE FORM	DENIED SEP 24, 1985
DIPHENHYDRAMINE HYDRO-CHLORIDE CAPSULE, EXTENDED RE-LEASE; ORAL	75 MG	87 P-0355/CP	PARKE DAVIS	NEW DOSAGE FORM NEW STRENGTH	DENIED MAY 11, 1988
TRI-PHASIC CONTRACEPTIVE TABLET; ORAL (21 AND 28 DAYS) ETHINYL ESTRADIOL; NORETHINDRONE ETHINYL ESTRADIOL; NORETHINDRONE ETHINYL ESTRADIOL; NORETHINDRONE	0.05 MG 0.5 MG 0.05 MG 0.75 MG 0.05 MG 1 MG	84 P-0443/CP	RW JOHNSON	NEW STRENGTH (DOSE SCHEDULE)	DENIED SEP 03, 1985
ETOPOSIDE INJECTABLE; INJECTION	20 MG/ML (50 ML/VIAL)	91 P-0076/CP1	ADRIA	NEW STRENGTH	DENIED FEB 19, 1992
FLUPHENAZINE HYDROCHLO-RIDE INJECTABLE; INJECTION	5 MG/ML	85 P-0019/CP	SQUIBB	NEW STRENGTH	DENIED OCT 25, 1985
FUROSEMIDE INJECTABLE; INJECTION	1 MG/ML	90 P-0313/CP1	LYPHOMED	NEW STRENGTH	DENIED OCT 28, 1991
HEPARIN SODIUM INJECTABLE; INJECTION	2,000 UNITS/ML 4,000 UNITS/ML	85 P-0065/CP	ABBOTT	NEW STRENGTH	DENIED MAY 29, 1985
HYDROCHLOROTHIAZIDE; PROPRANOLOL HYDROCHLO-RIDE; TRIAMTERENE CAPSULE, EXTENDED RE-LEASE; ORAL	50 MG 80 MG 75 MG	85 P-0571/CP	WYETH AYERST	NEW COMBINATION	DENIED MAY 16, 1986
HYDROCHLOROTHIAZIDE; PROPRANOLOL HYDROCHLO-RIDE; TRIAMTERENE CAPSULE, EXTENDED RE-LEASE; ORAL	50 MG 120 MG 75 MG	85 P-0571/CP	WYETH AYERST	NEW COMBINATION	DENIED MAY 16, 1986

ANDA SUITABILITY PETITIONS

PETITIONS DENIED *(continued)*

DRUG NAME DOSAGE FORM; ROUTE	STRENGTH (CONTAINER SIZE)	DOCKET NUMBER	PETITIONER	REASON FOR PETITION	STATUS
HYDROCHLOROTHIAZIDE; PROPRANOLOL HYDROCHLORIDE; TRIAMTERENE CAPSULE, EXTENDED RELEASE; ORAL	50 MG 160 MG 75 MG	85 P-0571/CP	WYETH AYERST	NEW COMBINATION	DENIED MAY 16, 1986
HYDROCODONE BITARTRATE; PHENYLEPHRINE HYDROCHLORIDE; PROMETHAZINE HYDROCHLORIDE SYRUP; ORAL	1.66 MG/5 ML 5 MG/5 ML 6.25 MG/5 ML	85 P-0389/CP	UAD LABS	NEW COMBINATION	DENIED MAY 11, 1988
HYDROCODONE BITARTRATE; PROMETHAZINE HYDROCHLORIDE SOLUTION; ORAL	2.5 MG/5 ML 6.25 MG/5 ML	85 P-0256/CP	MIKART	NEW COMBINATION	DENIED MAY 11, 1988
HYDROCORTISONE; SALICYLIC ACID; SULFUR CREAM; TOPICAL	0.25% 2.35% 4%	86 P-0439/CP	C&M PHARMA	NEW COMBINATION	DENIED MAY 06, 1987
HYDROCORTISONE ACETATE SUPPOSITORY; RECTAL	1%	85 P-0088/CP	PARKE DAVIS	NEW DOSAGE FORM NEW ROUTE OF ADMINISTRATION	DENIED SEP 16, 1986
IBUPROFEN LIQUID; ORAL	200 MG/5 ML	88 P-0291/ CP0001	BIOCRAFT	NEW DOSAGE FORM	DENIED DEC 15, 1988
IBUPROFEN LIQUID; ORAL	400 MG/10 ML	88 P-0291/ CP0002	BIOCRAFT	NEW DOSAGE FORM	DENIED DEC 15, 1988
IBUPROFEN; OXYCODONE HYDROCHLORIDE CAPSULE; ORAL	200 MG 5 MG	85 P-0141/CP	DUPONT	NEW COMBINATION	DENIED SEP 27, 1985
IBUPROFEN; OXYCODONE HYDROCHLORIDE TABLET; ORAL	200 MG 5 MG	85 P-0141/CP	DUPONT	NEW COMBINATION	DENIED SEP 27, 1985
INDOMETHACIN TABLET; ORAL	25 MG 50 MG	85 P-0025/CP	VEREX LABS	NEW DOSAGE FORM	DENIED MAR 31, 1986
INDOMETHACIN TABLET, EXTENDED RELEASE; ORAL	75 MG	85 P-0026/CP	VEREX LABS	NEW DOSAGE FORM	DENIED SEP 16, 1985
INDOMETHACIN TABLET, EXTENDED RELEASE; ORAL	75 MG	85 P-0180/CP	FOREST	NEW DOSAGE FORM	DENIED APR 07, 1986
INDOMETHACIN INTENSOL SOLUTION (CONCENTRATE); ORAL	50 MG/ML	85 P-0077/CP	ROXANE	NEW DOSAGE FORM	DENIED APR 07, 1986
MAGNESIUM ASCORBATE INJECTABLE; INJECTION	10% 20%	88 P-0200/CP	RIM CONSULTING	NEW INGREDIENT	DENIED JUN 10, 1988
METOCLOPRAMIDE HYDROCHLORIDE INJECTABLE; INJECTION	1 MG/ML (50 ML/VIAL) (75 ML/VIAL) (100 ML/VIAL)	86 P-0015/CP	INTL MEDICATION	NEW STRENGTH	DENIED APR 25, 1986
METOCLOPRAMIDE HYDROCHLORIDE INJECTABLE; INJECTION	1 MG/ML (50 ML/VIAL) (75 ML/VIAL) (100 ML/VIAL)	87 P-0090/CP	INTL MEDICATION	NEW STRENGTH	DENIED FEB 08, 1988
METOCLOPRAMIDE HYDROCHLORIDE INJECTABLE; INJECTION	10 MG/ML	85 P-0062/CP	ABBOTT	NEW STRENGTH	DENIED MAY 29, 1985

ANDA SUITABILITY PETITIONS

PETITIONS DENIED *(continued)*

DRUG NAME DOSAGE FORM; ROUTE	STRENGTH (CONTAINER SIZE)	DOCKET NUMBER	PETITIONER	REASON FOR PETITION	STATUS
METOCLOPRAMIDE HYDROCHLORIDE INJECTABLE; INJECTION	10 MG/ML	85 P-0457/CP	ABBOTT	NEW STRENGTH	DENIED APR 18, 1986
METOCLOPRAMIDE HYDROCHLORIDE INJECTABLE; INJECTION	20 MG/ML	85 P-0062/ CP0002	ABBOTT	NEW STRENGTH	DENIED MAY 29, 1985
METOCLOPRAMIDE HYDROCHLORIDE INJECTABLE; INJECTION	20 MG/ML	85 P-0457/ CP0002	ABBOTT	NEW STRENGTH	DENIED APR 18, 1986
METRONIDAZOLE SPONGE; VAGINAL	50-125 MG/SPONGE	85 P-0117/CP	VLI	NEW DOSAGE FORM	DENIED OCT 08, 1985
NITROGLYCERIN FILM, EXTENDED RELEASE; PERCUTANEOUS	NONE GIVEN	84 P-0302/CP	KEY PHARMS	NEW DOSAGE FORM (NEW MATRIX)	DENIED JUL 29, 1985
PHENYLEPHRINE HYDROCHLORIDE; SULFATHIAZOLE NASAL SUSPENSION; TOPICAL	0.5% 5%	85 P-0205/CP	TANYA W ROSS	NEW COMBINATION NEW DOSAGE FORM	DENIED NOV 14, 1985
PHENYLPROPANOLAMINE HYDROCHLORIDE FILM, EXTENDED RELEASE; PERCUTANEOUS	150 MG	88 P-0265/CP	BIO AMERICAN	NEW DOSAGE FORM NEW STRENGTH	DENIED OCT 07, 1988
PROCAINAMIDE HYDROCHLORIDE TABLET, EXTENDED RELEASE; ORAL	500 MG 750 MG 1,000 MG	85 P-0181/CP	FOREST	NEW DOSAGE FORM	DENIED APR 21, 1987
PROCAINAMIDE HYDROCHLORIDE TABLET, EXTENDED RELEASE; ORAL	500 MG 750 MG 1,000 MG	86 P-0328/CP	KV	NEW DOSAGE FORM	DENIED APR 21, 1987
PSEUDOEPHEDRINE POLISTEREX CAPSULE, EXTENDED RELEASE; ORAL	60 MG	85 P-0334/CP	PENNWALT	NEW INGREDIENT NEW SALT	DENIED MAR 19, 1986
TEMAZEPAM SOFT GELATIN CAPSULE; ORAL	10 MG 20 MG	85 P-0016/CP	WYETH AYERST	NEW DOSAGE FORM NEW STRENGTH	DENIED SEP 29, 1986
TRIAMCINOLONE ACETONIDE SUSPENSION; INJECTION	2.5 MG/ML	85 P-0001/CP	GENDERM	NEW STRENGTH	DENIED MAR 04, 1985
TRIAMCINOLONE ACETONIDE SUSPENSION; INJECTION	3 MG/ML	84 P-0240/CP	PHARM BASICS	NEW STRENGTH	DENIED MAR 04, 1985

APPENDIX A
PRODUCT NAME INDEX

A

A.P.L., GONADOTROPIN, CHORIONIC
A-HYDROCORT, HYDROCORTISONE SODIUM SUCCINATE
A-METHAPRED, METHYLPREDNISOLONE SODIUM
    SUCCINATE
A-N STANNOUS AGGREGATED ALBUMIN, TECHNETIUM
    TC-99M ALBUMIN AGGREGATED KIT
A-POXIDE, CHLORDIAZEPOXIDE HYDROCHLORIDE
A/T/S, ERYTHROMYCIN
ABITREXATE, METHOTREXATE SODIUM
ACCUPRIL, QUINAPRIL HYDROCHLORIDE
ACCURBRON, THEOPHYLLINE
ACCUTANE, ISOTRETINOIN
ACEPHEN, ACETAMINOPHEN (OTC)
ACETAMINOPHEN, ACETAMINOPHEN (OTC)
ACETAMINOPHEN AND CODEINE PHOSPHATE,
    ACETAMINOPHEN
ACETAMINOPHEN AND CODEINE PHOSPHATE #2,
    ACETAMINOPHEN
ACETAMINOPHEN AND CODEINE PHOSPHATE #3,
    ACETAMINOPHEN
ACETAMINOPHEN AND CODEINE PHOSPHATE #4,
    ACETAMINOPHEN
ACETAMINOPHEN AND CODEINE PHOSPHATE NO. 2,
    ACETAMINOPHEN
ACETAMINOPHEN AND CODEINE PHOSPHATE NO. 3,
    ACETAMINOPHEN
ACETAMINOPHEN AND CODEINE PHOSPHATE NO. 4,
    ACETAMINOPHEN
ACETAMINOPHEN AND HYDROCODONE BITARTRATE,
    ACETAMINOPHEN
ACETAMINOPHEN W/ CODEINE, ACETAMINOPHEN
ACETAMINOPHEN W/ CODEINE #2, ACETAMINOPHEN
ACETAMINOPHEN W/ CODEINE #3, ACETAMINOPHEN
ACETAMINOPHEN W/ CODEINE #4, ACETAMINOPHEN
ACETAMINOPHEN W/ CODEINE NO. 2, ACETAMINOPHEN
ACETAMINOPHEN W/ CODEINE NO. 3, ACETAMINOPHEN
ACETAMINOPHEN W/ CODEINE PHOSPHATE,
    ACETAMINOPHEN
ACETAMINOPHEN W/ CODEINE PHOSPHATE #3,
    ACETAMINOPHEN
ACETAMINOPHEN, ASPIRIN, AND CODEINE PHOSPHATE,
    ACETAMINOPHEN
ACETAMINOPHEN, BUTALBITAL AND CAFFEINE,
    ACETAMINOPHEN
ACETAMINOPHEN, BUTALBITAL, AND CAFFEINE,
    ACETAMINOPHEN
ACETASOL, ACETIC ACID, GLACIAL
ACETASOL HC, ACETIC ACID, GLACIAL
ACETATED RINGER'S IN PLASTIC CONTAINER, CALCIUM
    CHLORIDE
ACETAZOLAMIDE, ACETAZOLAMIDE
ACETAZOLAMIDE SODIUM, ACETAZOLAMIDE SODIUM
ACETIC ACID, ACETIC ACID, GLACIAL
ACETIC ACID W/ HYDROCORTISONE, ACETIC ACID,
    GLACIAL
ACETIC ACID 0.25% IN PLASTIC CONTAINER, ACETIC
    ACID, GLACIAL
ACETOHEXAMIDE, ACETOHEXAMIDE
ACETYLCYSTEINE, ACETYLCYSTEINE
ACHES-N-PAIN, IBUPROFEN (OTC)
ACHROMYCIN, HYDROCORTISONE
ACHROMYCIN, PROCAINE HYDROCHLORIDE
ACHROMYCIN, TETRACYCLINE HYDROCHLORIDE
ACHROMYCIN V, TETRACYCLINE

ACHROMYCIN V, TETRACYCLINE HYDROCHLORIDE
ACLOVATE, ALCLOMETASONE DIPROPIONATE
ACTAHIST, PSEUDOEPHEDRINE HYDROCHLORIDE
ACTH, CORTICOTROPIN
ACTHAR, CORTICOTROPIN
ACTHAR GEL-SYNTHETIC, SERACTIDE ACETATE
ACTICORT, HYDROCORTISONE
ACTIDIL, TRIPROLIDINE HYDROCHLORIDE (OTC)
ACTIFED, PSEUDOEPHEDRINE HYDROCHLORIDE (OTC)
ACTIFED W/ CODEINE, CODEINE PHOSPHATE
ACTIGALL, URSODIOL
ACTIN-N, NITROFURAZONE
ACYLANID, ACETYLDIGITOXIN
ADAGEN, PEGADEMASE BOVINE
ADALAT, NIFEDIPINE
ADAPIN, DOXEPIN HYDROCHLORIDE
ADENOCARD, ADENOSINE
ADIPEX-P, PHENTERMINE HYDROCHLORIDE
ADPHEN, PHENDIMETRAZINE TARTRATE
ADRIAMYCIN PFS, DOXORUBICIN HYDROCHLORIDE
ADRIAMYCIN RDF, DOXORUBICIN HYDROCHLORIDE
ADRUCIL, FLUOROURACIL
ADVIL, IBUPROFEN (OTC)
ADVIL COLD AND SINUS, IBUPROFEN (OTC)
AEROBID, FLUNISOLIDE
AEROLATE, THEOPHYLLINE
AEROLATE III, THEOPHYLLINE
AEROLATE JR, THEOPHYLLINE
AEROLATE SR, THEOPHYLLINE
AEROLONE, ISOPROTERENOL HYDROCHLORIDE
AEROSEB-DEX, DEXAMETHASONE
AEROSEB-HC, HYDROCORTISONE
AEROSPORIN, POLYMYXIN B SULFATE
AFRINOL, PSEUDOEPHEDRINE SULFATE (OTC)
AK-PENTOLATE, CYCLOPENTOLATE HYDROCHLORIDE
AKINETON, BIPERIDEN HYDROCHLORIDE
AKINETON, BIPERIDEN LACTATE
AKNE-MYCIN, ERYTHROMYCIN
AKRINOL, ACRISORCIN
ALA-CORT, HYDROCORTISONE
ALA-SCALP, HYDROCORTISONE
ALBALON, NAPHAZOLINE HYDROCHLORIDE
ALBAMYCIN, NOVOBIOCIN SODIUM
ALBUMOTOPE 125 I, ALBUMIN IODINATED I-125 SERUM
ALBUTEROL SULFATE, ALBUTEROL SULFATE
ALCAINE, PROPARACAINE HYDROCHLORIDE
ALCOHOL 10% AND DEXTROSE 5%, ALCOHOL
ALCOHOL 5% AND DEXTROSE 5%, ALCOHOL
ALCOHOL 5% IN DEXTROSE 5%, ALCOHOL
ALCOHOL 5% IN DEXTROSE 5% IN WATER, ALCOHOL
ALCOHOL 5% IN D5-W, ALCOHOL
ALDACTAZIDE, HYDROCHLOROTHIAZIDE
ALDACTONE, SPIRONOLACTONE
ALDOCLOR-150, CHLOROTHIAZIDE
ALDOCLOR-250, CHLOROTHIAZIDE
ALDOMET, METHYLDOPA
ALDOMET, METHYLDOPATE HYDROCHLORIDE
ALDORIL D30, HYDROCHLOROTHIAZIDE
ALDORIL D50, HYDROCHLOROTHIAZIDE
ALDORIL 15, HYDROCHLOROTHIAZIDE
ALDORIL 25, HYDROCHLOROTHIAZIDE
ALFENTA, ALFENTANIL HYDROCHLORIDE
ALKERAN, MELPHALAN
ALKERGOT, ERGOLOID MESYLATES
ALLAY, ACETAMINOPHEN
ALLERFED, PSEUDOEPHEDRINE HYDROCHLORIDE
ALLOPURINOL, ALLOPURINOL

APPENDIX A
PRODUCT NAME INDEX *(continued)*

ALPHA CHYMAR, CHYMOTRYPSIN
ALPHACAINE, LIDOCAINE
ALPHACAINE HCL, LIDOCAINE HYDROCHLORIDE
ALPHACAINE HCL W/ EPINEPHRINE, EPINEPHRINE
ALPHADERM, HYDROCORTISONE
ALPHADROL, FLUPREDNISOLONE
ALPHALIN, VITAMIN A PALMITATE
ALPHAREDISOL, HYDROXOCOBALAMIN
ALPHATREX, BETAMETHASONE DIPROPIONATE
ALPHAZINE, PHENDIMETRAZINE TARTRATE
ALTACE, RAMIPRIL
ALUMINUM HYDROXIDE AND MAGNESIUM
    TRISILICATE, ALUMINUM HYDROXIDE (OTC)
ALUPENT, METAPROTERENOL SULFATE
AMANTADINE HCL, AMANTADINE HYDROCHLORIDE
AMBENYL, BROMODIPHENHYDRAMINE
    HYDROCHLORIDE
AMBODRYL, BROMODIPHENHYDRAMINE
    HYDROCHLORIDE
AMCILL, AMPICILLIN/AMPICILLIN TRIHYDRATE
AMEN, MEDROXYPROGESTERONE ACETATE
AMERSCAN MDP KIT, TECHNETIUM TC-99M
    MEDRONATE KIT
AMICAR, AMINOCAPROIC ACID
AMIDATE, ETOMIDATE
AMIKACIN, AMIKACIN SULFATE
AMIKIN, AMIKACIN SULFATE
AMIKIN IN SODIUM CHLORIDE 0.9%, AMIKACIN
    SULFATE
AMILORIDE HCL, AMILORIDE HYDROCHLORIDE
AMILORIDE HCL AND HYDROCHLOROTHIAZIDE,
    AMILORIDE HYDROCHLORIDE
AMINESS 5.2% ESSENTIAL AMINO ACIDS W/ HISTADINE,
    AMINO ACIDS
AMINOACETIC ACID 1.5% IN PLASTIC CONTAINER,
    GLYCINE
AMINOCAPROIC ACID, AMINOCAPROIC ACID
AMINOHIPPURATE SODIUM, AMINOHIPPURATE SODIUM
AMINOPHYLLIN, AMINOPHYLLINE
AMINOPHYLLINE, AMINOPHYLLINE
AMINOPHYLLINE DYE FREE, AMINOPHYLLINE
AMINOPHYLLINE IN SODIUM CHLORIDE 0.45%,
    AMINOPHYLLINE
AMINOPHYLLINE IN SODIUM CHLORIDE 0.45% IN
    PLASTIC CONTAINER, AMINOPHYLLINE
AMINOSOL 5%, PROTEIN HYDROLYSATE
AMINOSYN II 10%, AMINO ACIDS
AMINOSYN II 10% W/ ELECTROLYTES, AMINO ACIDS
AMINOSYN II 15%, AMINO ACIDS
AMINOSYN II 3.5%, AMINO ACIDS
AMINOSYN II 3.5% IN DEXTROSE 25%, AMINO ACIDS
AMINOSYN II 3.5% IN DEXTROSE 5%, AMINO ACIDS
AMINOSYN II 3.5% M, AMINO ACIDS
AMINOSYN II 3.5% M IN DEXTROSE 5%, AMINO ACIDS
AMINOSYN II 3.5% W/ ELECTROLYTES IN DEXTROSE
    25%, AMINO ACIDS
AMINOSYN II 3.5% W/ ELECTROLYTES IN DEXTROSE 25%
    W/ CALCIUM, AMINO ACIDS
AMINOSYN II 4.25% IN DEXTROSE 10%, AMINO ACIDS
AMINOSYN II 4.25% IN DEXTROSE 20%, AMINO ACIDS
AMINOSYN II 4.25% IN DEXTROSE 25%, AMINO ACIDS
AMINOSYN II 4.25% M IN DEXTROSE 10%, AMINO ACIDS
AMINOSYN II 4.25% W/ ELECT AND ADJUSTED
    PHOSPHATE IN DEXTROSE 10%, AMINO ACIDS
AMINOSYN II 4.25% W/ ELECTROLYTES IN DEXTROSE
    20% W/ CALCIUM, AMINO ACIDS
AMINOSYN II 4.25% W/ ELECTROLYTES IN DEXTROSE
    25%, AMINO ACIDS
AMINOSYN II 4.25% W/ ELECTROLYTES IN DEXTROSE
    25% W/ CALCIUM, AMINO ACIDS
AMINOSYN II 5%, AMINO ACIDS
AMINOSYN II 5% IN DEXTROSE 25%, AMINO ACIDS

AMINOSYN II 5% W/ ELECTROLYTES IN DEXTROSE 25%
    W/ CALCIUM, AMINO ACIDS
AMINOSYN II 7%, AMINO ACIDS
AMINOSYN II 7% W/ ELECTROLYTES, AMINO ACIDS
AMINOSYN II 8.5%, AMINO ACIDS
AMINOSYN II 8.5% W/ ELECTROLYTES, AMINO ACIDS
AMINOSYN 10%, AMINO ACIDS
AMINOSYN 10% (PH6), AMINO ACIDS
AMINOSYN 3.5%, AMINO ACIDS
AMINOSYN 3.5% IN PLASTIC CONTAINER, AMINO ACIDS
AMINOSYN 3.5% M, AMINO ACIDS
AMINOSYN 3.5% M IN PLASTIC CONTAINER, AMINO
    ACIDS
AMINOSYN 3.5% W/ DEXTROSE 25% IN PLASTIC
    CONTAINER, AMINO ACIDS
AMINOSYN 3.5% W/ DEXTROSE 5% IN PLASTIC
    CONTAINER, AMINO ACIDS
AMINOSYN 4.25% W/ DEXTROSE 25% IN PLASTIC
    CONTAINER, AMINO ACIDS
AMINOSYN 5%, AMINO ACIDS
AMINOSYN 7%, AMINO ACIDS
AMINOSYN 7% (PH6), AMINO ACIDS
AMINOSYN 7% W/ ELECTROLYTES, AMINO ACIDS
AMINOSYN 8.5%, AMINO ACIDS
AMINOSYN 8.5% (PH6), AMINO ACIDS
AMINOSYN 8.5% W/ ELECTROLYTES, AMINO ACIDS
AMINOSYN-HBC 7%, AMINO ACIDS
AMINOSYN-HBC 7% IN PLASTIC CONTAINER, AMINO
    ACIDS
AMINOSYN-PF 10%, AMINO ACIDS
AMINOSYN-PF 7%, AMINO ACIDS
AMINOSYN-RF 5.2%, AMINO ACIDS
AMIPAQUE, METRIZAMIDE
AMITID, AMITRIPTYLINE HYDROCHLORIDE
AMITRIL, AMITRIPTYLINE HYDROCHLORIDE
AMITRIPTYLINE HCL, AMITRIPTYLINE
    HYDROCHLORIDE
AMMONIUM CHLORIDE, AMMONIUM CHLORIDE
AMMONIUM CHLORIDE IN PLASTIC CONTAINER,
    AMMONIUM CHLORIDE
AMMONIUM CHLORIDE 0.9% IN NORMAL SALINE,
    AMMONIUM CHLORIDE
AMMONIUM CHLORIDE 2.14%, AMMONIUM CHLORIDE
AMNESTROGEN, ESTROGENS, ESTERIFIED
AMOSENE, MEPROBAMATE
AMOXAPINE, AMOXAPINE
AMOXICILLIN, AMOXICILLIN
AMOXICILLIN PEDIATRIC, AMOXICILLIN
AMOXICILLIN TRIHYDRATE, AMOXICILLIN
AMOXIL, AMOXICILLIN
AMPHETAMINE SULFATE, AMPHETAMINE SULFATE
AMPHICOL, CHLORAMPHENICOL
AMPHOTERICIN B, AMPHOTERICIN B
AMPICILLIN, AMPICILLIN/AMPICILLIN TRIHYDRATE
AMPICILLIN SODIUM, AMPICILLIN SODIUM
AMPICILLIN TRIHYDRATE, AMPICILLIN/AMPICILLIN
    TRIHYDRATE
AN-DTPA, TECHNETIUM TC-99M PENTETATE KIT
AN-MAA, TECHNETIUM TC-99M ALBUMIN AGGREGATED
    KIT
AN-MDP, TECHNETIUM TC-99M MEDRONATE KIT
AN-PYROTEC, TECHNETIUM TC-99M PYROPHOSPHATE
    KIT
AN-SULFUR COLLOID, TECHNETIUM TC-99M SULFUR
    COLLOID KIT
ANADROL-50, OXYMETHOLONE
ANAFRANIL, CLOMIPRAMINE HYDROCHLORIDE
ANAPROX, NAPROXEN SODIUM
ANAPROX DS, NAPROXEN SODIUM
ANCEF, CEFAZOLIN SODIUM
ANCEF IN DEXTROSE 5% IN PLASTIC CONTAINER,
    CEFAZOLIN SODIUM

APPENDIX A
PRODUCT NAME INDEX *(continued)*

ANCEF IN SODIUM CHLORIDE 0.9% IN PLASTIC
  CONTAINER, CEFAZOLIN SODIUM
ANCOBON, FLUCYTOSINE
ANDROID 10, METHYLTESTOSTERONE
ANDROID 25, METHYLTESTOSTERONE
ANDROID 5, METHYLTESTOSTERONE
ANDROID-F, FLUOXYMESTERONE
ANECTINE, SUCCINYLCHOLINE CHLORIDE
ANESTACON, LIDOCAINE HYDROCHLORIDE
ANEXSIA, ACETAMINOPHEN
ANEXSIA 7.5/650, ACETAMINOPHEN
ANGIO-CONRAY, IOTHALAMATE SODIUM
ANGIOVIST 282, DIATRIZOATE MEGLUMINE
ANGIOVIST 292, DIATRIZOATE MEGLUMINE
ANGIOVIST 370, DIATRIZOATE MEGLUMINE
ANHYDRON, CYCLOTHIAZIDE
ANISOTROPINE METHYLBROMIDE, ANISOTROPINE
  METHYLBROMIDE
ANOQUAN, ACETAMINOPHEN
ANSAID, FLURBIPROFEN
ANSOLYSEN, PENTOLINIUM TARTRATE
ANSPOR, CEPHRADINE
ANTABUSE, DISULFIRAM
ANTAGONATE, CHLORPHENIRAMINE MALEATE
ANTEPAR, PIPERAZINE CITRATE
ANTIMINTH, PYRANTEL PAMOATE
ANTITUSSIVE, DIPHENHYDRAMINE HYDROCHLORIDE
  (OTC)
ANTIVERT, MECLIZINE HYDROCHLORIDE
ANTRENYL, OXYPHENONIUM BROMIDE
ANTURANE, SULFINPYRAZONE
ANUSOL HC, HYDROCORTISONE
APAP W/ CODEINE, ACETAMINOPHEN
APAP W/ CODEINE PHOSPHATE, ACETAMINOPHEN
APOGEN, GENTAMICIN SULFATE
APRESAZIDE, HYDRALAZINE HYDROCHLORIDE
APRESOLINE, HYDRALAZINE HYDROCHLORIDE
APRESOLINE-ESIDRIX, HYDRALAZINE HYDROCHLORIDE
AQUAMEPHYTON, PHYTONADIONE
AQUAPHYLLIN, THEOPHYLLINE
AQUASOL A, VITAMIN A
AQUASOL A, VITAMIN A PALMITATE
AQUATAG, BENZTHIAZIDE
AQUATENSEN, METHYCLOTHIAZIDE
ARALEN, CHLOROQUINE PHOSPHATE
ARALEN HCL, CHLOROQUINE HYDROCHLORIDE
ARALEN PHOSPHATE W/ PRIMAQUINE PHOSPHATE,
  CHLOROQUINE PHOSPHATE
ARAMINE, METARAMINOL BITARTRATE
ARDUAN, PIPECURONIUM BROMIDE
AREDIA, PAMIDRONATE DISODIUM
ARESTOCAINE HCL, MEPIVACAINE HYDROCHLORIDE
ARESTOCAINE HCL W/ LEVONORDEFRIN,
  LEVONORDEFRIN
ARFONAD, TRIMETHAPHAN CAMSYLATE
ARISTOCORT, TRIAMCINOLONE
ARISTOCORT, TRIAMCINOLONE ACETONIDE
ARISTOCORT, TRIAMCINOLONE DIACETATE
ARISTOCORT A, TRIAMCINOLONE ACETONIDE
ARISTOGEL, TRIAMCINOLONE ACETONIDE
ARISTOSPAN, TRIAMCINOLONE HEXACETONIDE
ARTANE, TRIHEXYPHENIDYL HYDROCHLORIDE
ASACOL, MESALAMINE
ASBRON, THEOPHYLLINE SODIUM GLYCINATE
ASELLACRIN 10, SOMATROPIN
ASELLACRIN 2, SOMATROPIN
ASENDIN, AMOXAPINE
ASPIRIN AND CAFFEINE W/ BUTALBITAL, ASPIRIN
ASTRAMORPH PF, MORPHINE SULFATE
ATARAX, HYDROXYZINE HYDROCHLORIDE
ATENOLOL, ATENOLOL
ATENOLOL AND CHLORTHALIDONE, ATENOLOL

ATHROMBIN, WARFARIN SODIUM
ATHROMBIN-K, WARFARIN POTASSIUM
ATIVAN, LORAZEPAM
ATROMID-S, CLOFIBRATE
ATROPEN, ATROPINE
ATROPINE, ATROPINE
ATROPINE AND DEMEROL, ATROPINE SULFATE
ATROPINE SULFATE, ATROPINE SULFATE
ATROVENT, IPRATROPIUM BROMIDE
AUGMENTIN '125', AMOXICILLIN
AUGMENTIN '250', AMOXICILLIN
AUGMENTIN '500', AMOXICILLIN
AUREOMYCIN, CHLORTETRACYCLINE HYDROCHLORIDE
AVC, SULFANILAMIDE
AVENTYL HCL, NORTRIPTYLINE HYDROCHLORIDE
AXID, NIZATIDINE
AXOTAL, ASPIRIN
AYGESTIN, NORETHINDRONE ACETATE
AZACTAM, AZTREONAM
AZATHIOPRINE, AZATHIOPRINE SODIUM
AZDONE, ASPIRIN
AZLIN, AZLOCILLIN SODIUM
AZMACORT, TRIAMCINOLONE ACETONIDE
AZO GANTANOL, PHENAZOPYRIDINE HYDROCHLORIDE
AZO GANTRISIN, PHENAZOPYRIDINE HYDROCHLORIDE
AZOLID, PHENYLBUTAZONE
AZULFIDINE, SULFASALAZINE
AZULFIDINE EN-TABS, SULFASALAZINE

B

BACI-RX, BACITRACIN
BACIGUENT, BACITRACIN
BACITRACIN, BACITRACIN
BACITRACIN, BACITRACIN (OTC)
BACITRACIN ZINC-NEOMYCIN SULFATE-POLYMYXIN B
  SULFATE, BACITRACIN ZINC
BACITRACIN ZINC-NEOMYCIN SULFATE-POLYMYXIN B
  SULFATE, BACITRACIN ZINC (OTC)
BACITRACIN ZINC-POLYMYXIN B SULFATE, BACITRACIN
  ZINC (OTC)
BACITRACIN-NEOMYCIN-POLYMYXIN, BACITRACIN
  ZINC
BACITRACIN-NEOMYCIN-POLYMYXIN W/
  HYDROCORTISONE ACETATE, BACITRACIN
BACLOFEN, BACLOFEN
BACTERIOSTATIC SODIUM CHLORIDE 0.9% IN PLASTIC
  CONTAINER, SODIUM CHLORIDE
BACTERIOSTATIC WATER FOR INJECTION, WATER FOR
  INJECTION, STERILE
BACTOCILL, OXACILLIN SODIUM
BACTRIM, SULFAMETHOXAZOLE
BACTRIM DS, SULFAMETHOXAZOLE
BACTRIM PEDIATRIC, SULFAMETHOXAZOLE
BACTROBAN, MUPIROCIN
BAL, DIMERCAPROL
BALNEOL-HC, HYDROCORTISONE
BAMATE, MEPROBAMATE
BANAN, CEFPODOXIME PROXETIL
BANCAP, ACETAMINOPHEN
BANCAP HC, ACETAMINOPHEN
BANTHINE, METHANTHELINE BROMIDE
BAROS, SODIUM BICARBONATE
BARSTATIN 100, NYSTATIN
BECLOVENT, BECLOMETHASONE DIPROPIONATE
BECONASE, BECLOMETHASONE DIPROPIONATE
BECONASE AQ, BECLOMETHASONE DIPROPIONATE
  MONOHYDRATE
BEEPEN-VK, PENICILLIN V POTASSIUM
BELDIN, DIPHENHYDRAMINE HYDROCHLORIDE (OTC)

APPENDIX A
PRODUCT NAME INDEX *(continued)*

BELIX, DIPHENHYDRAMINE HYDROCHLORIDE
BENADRYL, DIPHENHYDRAMINE HYDROCHLORIDE
BENDOPA, LEVODOPA
BENEMID, PROBENECID
BENOQUIN, MONOBENZONE
BENOXINATE HCL, BENOXINATE HYDROCHLORIDE
BENSULFOID, BENTONITE
BENTYL, DICYCLOMINE HYDROCHLORIDE
BENYLIN, DIPHENHYDRAMINE HYDROCHLORIDE (OTC)
BENZAMYCIN, BENZOYL PEROXIDE
BENZTHIAZIDE, BENZTHIAZIDE
BENZTROPINE MESYLATE, BENZTROPINE MESYLATE
BENZYL BENZOATE, BENZYL BENZOATE
BEPADIN, BEPRIDIL HYDROCHLORIDE
BEROCCA PN, ASCORBIC ACID
BERUBIGEN, CYANOCOBALAMIN
BETA-HC, HYDROCORTISONE
BETA-VAL, BETAMETHASONE VALERATE
BETA-2, ISOETHARINE HYDROCHLORIDE
BETADERM, BETAMETHASONE VALERATE
BETADINE, POVIDONE-IODINE
BETAGAN, LEVOBUNOLOL HYDROCHLORIDE
BETALIN S, THIAMINE HYDROCHLORIDE
BETALIN 12, CYANOCOBALAMIN
BETAMETHASONE DIPROPIONATE, BETAMETHASONE
    DIPROPIONATE
BETAMETHASONE SODIUM PHOSPHATE,
    BETAMETHASONE SODIUM PHOSPHATE
BETAMETHASONE VALERATE, BETAMETHASONE
    VALERATE
BETAPAR, MEPREDNISONE
BETAPEN-VK, PENICILLIN V POTASSIUM
BETAPRONE, PROPIOLACTONE
BETATREX, BETAMETHASONE VALERATE
BETHANECHOL CHLORIDE, BETHANECHOL CHLORIDE
BETOPTIC, BETAXOLOL HYDROCHLORIDE
BETOPTIC S, BETAXOLOL HYDROCHLORIDE
BIAXIN, CLARITHROMYCIN
BICILLIN, PENICILLIN G BENZATHINE
BICILLIN C-R, PENICILLIN G BENZATHINE
BICILLIN C-R 900/300, PENICILLIN G BENZATHINE
BICILLIN L-A, PENICILLIN G BENZATHINE
BICNU, CARMUSTINE
BILIVIST, IPODATE SODIUM
BILOPAQUE, TYROPANOATE SODIUM
BILTRICIDE, PRAZIQUANTEL
BIOSCRUB, CHLORHEXIDINE GLUCONATE (OTC)
BIPHETAMINE 12.5, AMPHETAMINE RESIN COMPLEX
BIPHETAMINE 20, AMPHETAMINE RESIN COMPLEX
BIPHETAMINE 7.5, AMPHETAMINE RESIN COMPLEX
BIPHETAP, BROMPHENIRAMINE MALEATE
BLENOXANE, BLEOMYCIN SULFATE
BLEPH-10, SULFACETAMIDE SODIUM
BLEPH-30, SULFACETAMIDE SODIUM
BLEPHAMIDE, PREDNISOLONE ACETATE
BLEPHAMIDE S.O.P., PREDNISOLONE ACETATE
BLOCADREN, TIMOLOL MALEATE
BONTRIL PDM, PHENDIMETRAZINE TARTRATE
BOROFAIR, ACETIC ACID, GLACIAL
BRANCHAMIN 4%, AMINO ACIDS
BRETHAIRE, TERBUTALINE SULFATE
BRETHINE, TERBUTALINE SULFATE
BRETYLIUM TOSYLATE, BRETYLIUM TOSYLATE
BRETYLIUM TOSYLATE IN DEXTROSE 5%, BRETYLIUM
    TOSYLATE
BRETYLIUM TOSYLATE IN DEXTROSE 5% IN PLASTIC
    CONTAINER, BRETYLIUM TOSYLATE
BRETYLOL, BRETYLIUM TOSYLATE
BREVIBLOC, ESMOLOL HYDROCHLORIDE
BREVICON 21-DAY, ETHINYL ESTRADIOL
BREVICON 28-DAY, ETHINYL ESTRADIOL
BREVITAL SODIUM, METHOHEXITAL SODIUM

BRIAN CARE, CHLORHEXIDINE GLUCONATE (OTC)
BRICANYL, TERBUTALINE SULFATE
BRISTACYCLINE, TETRACYCLINE HYDROCHLORIDE
BRISTAGEN, GENTAMICIN SULFATE
BRISTAMYCIN, ERYTHROMYCIN STEARATE
BROMANATE, BROMPHENIRAMINE MALEATE
BROMANATE DC, BROMPHENIRAMINE MALEATE
BROMANATE DM, BROMPHENIRAMINE MALEATE
BROMANYL, BROMODIPHENHYDRAMINE
    HYDROCHLORIDE
BROMATAPP, BROMPHENIRAMINE MALEATE (OTC)
BROMFED-DM, BROMPHENIRAMINE MALEATE
BROMPHENIRAMINE MALEATE, BROMPHENIRAMINE
    MALEATE
BROMPHERIL, DEXBROMPHENIRAMINE MALEATE (OTC)
BRONITIN MIST, EPINEPHRINE BITARTRATE (OTC)
BRONKAID MIST, EPINEPHRINE (OTC)
BRONKODYL, THEOPHYLLINE
BRONKOMETER, ISOETHARINE MESYLATE
BRONKOSOL, ISOETHARINE HYDROCHLORIDE
BRYREL, PIPERAZINE CITRATE
BSS PLUS, CALCIUM CHLORIDE
BUCLADIN-S, BUCLIZINE HYDROCHLORIDE
BUMEX, BUMETANIDE
BUPIVACAINE, BUPIVACAINE HYDROCHLORIDE
BUPIVACAINE HCL, BUPIVACAINE HYDROCHLORIDE
BUPIVACAINE HCL AND EPINEPHRINE, BUPIVACAINE
    HYDROCHLORIDE
BUPRENEX, BUPRENORPHINE HYDROCHLORIDE
BUSPAR, BUSPIRONE HYDROCHLORIDE
BUTABARB, BUTABARBITAL SODIUM
BUTABARBITAL, BUTABARBITAL SODIUM
BUTABARBITAL SODIUM, BUTABARBITAL SODIUM
BUTAL COMPOUND, ASPIRIN
BUTALAN, BUTABARBITAL SODIUM
BUTALBITAL AND ACETAMINOPHEN, ACETAMINOPHEN
BUTALBITAL ASPIRIN AND CAFFEINE, ASPIRIN
BUTALBITAL COMPOUND, ASPIRIN
BUTALBITAL W/ ASPIRIN & CAFFEINE, ASPIRIN
BUTALBITAL, ACETAMINOPHEN AND CAFFEINE,
    ACETAMINOPHEN
BUTALBITAL, ACETAMINOPHEN, CAFFEINE,
    ACETAMINOPHEN
BUTALBITAL, APAP, AND CAFFEINE, ACETAMINOPHEN
BUTALBITAL, ASPIRIN & CAFFEINE, ASPIRIN
BUTALBITAL, ASPIRIN AND CAFFEINE, ASPIRIN
BUTAZOLIDIN, PHENYLBUTAZONE
BUTICAPS, BUTABARBITAL SODIUM
BUTISOL SODIUM, BUTABARBITAL SODIUM

C

C-SOLVE-2, ERYTHROMYCIN
CAFERGOT, CAFFEINE
CALAN, VERAPAMIL HYDROCHLORIDE
CALCIBIND, CELLULOSE SODIUM PHOSPHATE
CALCIJEX, CALCITRIOL
CALCIMAR, CALCITONIN, SALMON
CALCIPARINE, HEPARIN CALCIUM
CALCIUM DISODIUM VERSENATE, EDETATE CALCIUM
    DISODIUM
CALCIUM GLUCEPTATE, CALCIUM GLUCEPTATE
CALDEROL, CALCIFEDIOL, ANHYDROUS
CALMURID HC, HYDROCORTISONE
CAM-AP-ES, HYDRALAZINE HYDROCHLORIDE
CAM-METRAZINE, PHENDIMETRAZINE TARTRATE
CAMOQUIN HCL, AMODIAQUINE HYDROCHLORIDE
CANDEX, NYSTATIN
CANTIL, MEPENZOLATE BROMIDE
CAP-PROFEN, IBUPROFEN (OTC)

APPENDIX A
PRODUCT NAME INDEX *(continued)*

CAPASTAT SULFATE, CAPREOMYCIN SULFATE
CAPITAL AND CODEINE, ACETAMINOPHEN
CAPITAL WITH CODEINE, ACETAMINOPHEN
CAPITROL, CHLOROXINE
CAPOTEN, CAPTOPRIL
CAPOZIDE 25/15, CAPTOPRIL
CAPOZIDE 25/25, CAPTOPRIL
CAPOZIDE 50/15, CAPTOPRIL
CAPOZIDE 50/25, CAPTOPRIL
CARAFATE, SUCRALFATE
CARBACHOL, CARBACHOL
CARBAMAZEPINE, CARBAMAZEPINE
CARBIDOPA AND LEVODOPA, CARBIDOPA
CARBOCAINE, MEPIVACAINE HYDROCHLORIDE
CARBOCAINE W/ NEO-COBEFRIN, LEVONORDEFRIN
CARDASE, ETHOXZOLAMIDE
CARDENE, NICARDIPINE HYDROCHLORIDE
CARDENE SR, NICARDIPINE HYDROCHLORIDE
CARDIO-GREEN, INDOCYANINE GREEN
CARDIOGEN-82, RUBIDIUM CHLORIDE RB-82
CARDIOGRAFIN, DIATRIZOATE MEGLUMINE
CARDIOLITE, TECHNETIUM TC-99M SESTAMIBI KIT
CARDIOQUIN, QUINIDINE POLYGALACTURONATE
CARDIOTEC, TECHNETIUM TC-99M TEBOROXIME KIT
CARDIZEM, DILTIAZEM HYDROCHLORIDE
CARDIZEM CD, DILTIAZEM HYDROCHLORIDE
CARDIZEM SR, DILTIAZEM HYDROCHLORIDE
CARDRASE, ETHOXZOLAMIDE
CARDURA, DOXAZOSIN MESYLATE
CARISOPRODOL, CARISOPRODOL
CARISOPRODOL AND ASPIRIN, ASPIRIN
CARISOPRODOL COMPOUND, ASPIRIN
CARMOL HC, HYDROCORTISONE ACETATE
CARNITOR, LEVOCARNITINE
CARTROL, CARTEOLOL HYDROCHLORIDE
CATAPRES, CLONIDINE HYDROCHLORIDE
CATAPRES-TTS-1, CLONIDINE
CATAPRES-TTS-2, CLONIDINE
CATAPRES-TTS-3, CLONIDINE
CATARASE, CHYMOTRYPSIN
CECLOR, CEFACLOR
CEDILANID-D, DESLANOSIDE
CEENU, LOMUSTINE
CEFADROXIL, CEFADROXIL/CEFADROXIL
  HEMIHYDRATE
CEFADYL, CEPHAPIRIN SODIUM
CEFANEX, CEPHALEXIN
CEFAZOLIN SODIUM, CEFAZOLIN SODIUM
CEFIZOX, CEFTIZOXIME SODIUM
CEFIZOX IN DEXTROSE 5% IN PLASTIC CONTAINER,
  CEFTIZOXIME SODIUM
CEFMAX, CEFMENOXIME HYDROCHLORIDE
CEFOBID, CEFOPERAZONE SODIUM
CEFOTAN, CEFOTETAN DISODIUM
CEFPIRAMIDE SODIUM, CEFPIRAMIDE SODIUM
CEFTIN, CEFUROXIME AXETIL
CEFZIL, CEFPROZIL
CELESTONE, BETAMETHASONE
CELESTONE, BETAMETHASONE SODIUM PHOSPHATE
CELESTONE SOLUSPAN, BETAMETHASONE ACETATE
CELONTIN, METHSUXIMIDE
CENTRAX, PRAZEPAM
CEPHALEXIN, CEPHALEXIN
CEPHALEXIN MONOHYDRATE, CEPHALEXIN
CEPHALOTHIN, CEPHALOTHIN SODIUM
CEPHALOTHIN SODIUM, CEPHALOTHIN SODIUM
CEPHALOTHIN SODIUM W/ DEXTROSE, CEPHALOTHIN
  SODIUM
CEPHALOTHIN SODIUM W/ SODIUM CHLORIDE,
  CEPHALOTHIN SODIUM
CEPHAPIRIN SODIUM, CEPHAPIRIN SODIUM
CEPHRADINE, CEPHRADINE

CEPHULAC, LACTULOSE
CEPTAZ, CEFTAZIDIME (ARGININE FORMULATION)
CERADON, CEFOTIAM HYDROCHLORIDE
CEREDASE, ALGLUCERASE
CERETEC, TECHNETIUM TC-99M EXAMETAZIME KIT
CERUBIDINE, DAUNORUBICIN HYDROCHLORIDE
CERUMENEX, TRIETHANOLAMINE POLYPEPTIDE
  OLEATE CONDENSATE
CESAMET, NABILONE
CETACORT, HYDROCORTISONE
CETAMIDE, SULFACETAMIDE SODIUM
CHEMET, SUCCIMER
CHENIX, CHENODIOL
CHG SCRUB, CHLORHEXIDINE GLUCONATE (OTC)
CHIBROXIN, NORFLOXACIN
CHILDREN'S ADVIL, IBUPROFEN
CHLOR-TRIMETON, CHLORPHENIRAMINE MALEATE
CHLOR-TRIMETON, CHLORPHENIRAMINE MALEATE
  (OTC)
CHLORAMPHENICOL, CHLORAMPHENICOL
CHLORAMPHENICOL, CHLORAMPHENICOL SODIUM
  SUCCINATE
CHLORAMPHENICOL SODIUM SUCCINATE,
  CHLORAMPHENICOL SODIUM SUCCINATE
CHLORDIAZACHEL, CHLORDIAZEPOXIDE
  HYDROCHLORIDE
CHLORDIAZEPOXIDE AND AMITRIPTYLINE HCL,
  AMITRIPTYLINE HYDROCHLORIDE
CHLORDIAZEPOXIDE HCL, CHLORDIAZEPOXIDE
  HYDROCHLORIDE
CHLORHEXIDINE GLUCONATE, CHLORHEXIDINE
  GLUCONATE (OTC)
CHLORMERODRIN HG 197, CHLORMERODRIN, HG-197
CHLOROFAIR, CHLORAMPHENICOL
CHLOROMYCETIN, CHLORAMPHENICOL
CHLOROMYCETIN, CHLORAMPHENICOL SODIUM
  SUCCINATE
CHLOROMYCETIN HYDROCORTISONE,
  CHLORAMPHENICOL
CHLOROMYCETIN PALMITATE, CHLORAMPHENICOL
  PALMITATE
CHLOROMYXIN, CHLORAMPHENICOL
CHLOROPROCAINE HCL, CHLOROPROCAINE
  HYDROCHLORIDE
CHLOROPTIC, CHLORAMPHENICOL
CHLOROPTIC S.O.P., CHLORAMPHENICOL
CHLOROPTIC-P S.O.P., CHLORAMPHENICOL
CHLOROQUINE PHOSPHATE, CHLOROQUINE PHOSPHATE
CHLOROTHIAZIDE, CHLOROTHIAZIDE
CHLOROTHIAZIDE AND RESERPINE, CHLOROTHIAZIDE
CHLOROTHIAZIDE W/ RESERPINE, CHLOROTHIAZIDE
CHLOROTHIAZIDE-RESERPINE, CHLOROTHIAZIDE
CHLOROTRIANISENE, CHLOROTRIANISENE
CHLORPHENIRAMINE MALEATE, CHLORPHENIRAMINE
  MALEATE
CHLORPHENIRAMINE MALEATE, CHLORPHENIRAMINE
  MALEATE (OTC)
CHLORPHENIRAMINE MALEATE AND
  PHENYLPROPANOLAMINE HCL, CHLORPHENIRAMINE
  MALEATE
CHLORPROMAZINE HCL, CHLORPROMAZINE
  HYDROCHLORIDE
CHLORPROMAZINE HCL INTENSOL, CHLORPROMAZINE
  HYDROCHLORIDE
CHLORPROPAMIDE, CHLORPROPAMIDE
CHLORTHALIDONE, CHLORTHALIDONE
CHLORZOXAZONE, CHLORZOXAZONE
CHOLAC, LACTULOSE
CHOLEBRINE, IOCETAMIC ACID
CHOLEDYL, OXTRIPHYLLINE
CHOLEDYL SA, OXTRIPHYLLINE
CHOLETEC, TECHNETIUM TC-99M MEBROFENIN KIT

APPENDIX A
PRODUCT NAME INDEX *(continued)*

CHOLOGRAFIN MEGLUMINE, IODIPAMIDE MEGLUMINE
CHOLOGRAFIN SODIUM, IODIPAMIDE SODIUM
CHOLOVUE, IODOXAMATE MEGLUMINE
CHOLOXIN, DEXTROTHYROXINE SODIUM
CHOLYBAR, CHOLESTYRAMINE
CHORIONIC GONADOTROPIN, GONADOTROPIN, CHORIONIC
CHROMALBIN, ALBUMIN CHROMATED CR-51 SERUM
CHROMIC CHLORIDE, CHROMIC CHLORIDE
CHROMITOPE SODIUM, SODIUM CHROMATE, CR-51
CHRONULAC, LACTULOSE
CHYMEX, BENTIROMIDE
CHYMODIACTIN, CHYMOPAPAIN
CIBACALCIN, CALCITONIN, HUMAN
CIBALITH-S, LITHIUM CITRATE
CIDA-STAT, CHLORHEXIDINE GLUCONATE (OTC)
CILOXAN, CIPROFLOXACIN HYDROCHLORIDE
CIN-QUIN, QUINIDINE SULFATE
CINNASIL, RESCINNAMINE
CINOBAC, CINOXACIN
CINOXACIN, CINOXACIN
CINTICHEM TECHNETIUM 99M HEDSPA, TECHNETIUM TC-99M ETIDRONATE KIT
CIPRO, CIPROFLOXACIN
CIPRO, CIPROFLOXACIN HYDROCHLORIDE
CIPRO IN DEXTROSE 5%, CIPROFLOXACIN
CIPRO IN SODIUM CHLORIDE 0.9%, CIPROFLOXACIN
CIRCANOL, ERGOLOID MESYLATES
CITANEST, PRILOCAINE HYDROCHLORIDE
CITANEST FORTE, EPINEPHRINE BITARTRATE
CITANEST PLAIN, PRILOCAINE HYDROCHLORIDE
CLAFORAN, CEFOTAXIME SODIUM
CLAFORAN IN DEXTROSE 5%, CEFOTAXIME SODIUM
CLAFORAN IN SODIUM CHLORIDE 0.9%, CEFOTAXIME SODIUM
CLEMASTINE FUMARATE, CLEMASTINE FUMARATE
CLEOCIN, CLINDAMYCIN HYDROCHLORIDE
CLEOCIN, CLINDAMYCIN PALMITATE HYDROCHLORIDE
CLEOCIN, CLINDAMYCIN PHOSPHATE
CLEOCIN HCL, CLINDAMYCIN HYDROCHLORIDE
CLEOCIN PHOSPHATE, CLINDAMYCIN PHOSPHATE
CLEOCIN PHOSPHATE IN DEXTROSE 5%, CLINDAMYCIN PHOSPHATE
CLEOCIN T, CLINDAMYCIN PHOSPHATE
CLINDAMYCIN HCL, CLINDAMYCIN HYDROCHLORIDE
CLINDAMYCIN PHOSPHATE, CLINDAMYCIN PHOSPHATE
CLINDAMYCIN PHOSPHATE IN DEXTROSE 5%, CLINDAMYCIN PHOSPHATE
CLINORIL, SULINDAC
CLISTIN, CARBINOXAMINE MALEATE
CLODERM, CLOCORTOLONE PIVALATE
CLOFIBRATE, CLOFIBRATE
CLOMID, CLOMIPHENE CITRATE
CLONIDINE HCL, CLONIDINE HYDROCHLORIDE
CLONIDINE HCL AND CHLORTHALIDONE, CHLORTHALIDONE
CLOPRA, METOCLOPRAMIDE HYDROCHLORIDE
CLOPRA-"YELLOW", METOCLOPRAMIDE HYDROCHLORIDE
CLORAZEPATE DIPOTASSIUM, CLORAZEPATE DIPOTASSIUM
CLOXACILLIN SODIUM, CLOXACILLIN SODIUM
CLOXAPEN, CLOXACILLIN SODIUM
CLOZARIL, CLOZAPINE
CO-GESIC, ACETAMINOPHEN
CO-LAV, POLYETHYLENE GLYCOL 3350
COACTIN, AMDINOCILLIN
COBAVITE, CYANOCOBALAMIN
CODEINE PHOSPHATE AND ACETAMINOPHEN, ACETAMINOPHEN
CODEINE, ASPIRIN, APAP FORMULA NO. 2, ACETAMINOPHEN

CODEINE, ASPIRIN, APAP FORMULA NO. 3, ACETAMINOPHEN
CODEINE, ASPIRIN, APAP FORMULA NO. 4, ACETAMINOPHEN
CODIMAL-L.A. 12, CHLORPHENIRAMINE MALEATE (OTC)
CODOXY, ASPIRIN
COGENTIN, BENZTROPINE MESYLATE
COL-PROBENECID, COLCHICINE
COLBENEMID, COLCHICINE
COLD CAPSULE IV, CHLORPHENIRAMINE MALEATE (OTC)
COLD CAPSULE V, CHLORPHENIRAMINE MALEATE (OTC)
COLESTID, COLESTIPOL HYDROCHLORIDE
COLONAID, ATROPINE SULFATE
COLOVAGE, POLYETHYLENE GLYCOL 3350
COLY-MYCIN M, COLISTIMETHATE SODIUM
COLY-MYCIN S, COLISTIN SULFATE
COLYTE, POLYETHYLENE GLYCOL 3350
COLYTE-FLAVORED, POLYETHYLENE GLYCOL 3350
COMBIPRES, CHLORTHALIDONE
COMOX, AMOXICILLIN
COMPAL, ACETAMINOPHEN
COMPAZINE, PROCHLORPERAZINE
COMPAZINE, PROCHLORPERAZINE EDISYLATE
COMPAZINE, PROCHLORPERAZINE MALEATE
COMPOUND 65, ASPIRIN
CONCENTRAID, DESMOPRESSIN ACETATE
CONDYLOX, PODOFILOX
CONJUGATED ESTROGENS, ESTROGENS, CONJUGATED
CONRAY, IOTHALAMATE MEGLUMINE
CONRAY 30, IOTHALAMATE MEGLUMINE
CONRAY 325, IOTHALAMATE SODIUM
CONRAY 400, IOTHALAMATE SODIUM
CONRAY 43, IOTHALAMATE MEGLUMINE
CONSTILAC, LACTULOSE
CONSTULOSE, LACTULOSE
CONTAC, CHLORPHENIRAMINE MALEATE (OTC)
CONTEN, ACETAMINOPHEN
COPPER T MODEL TCU 380A, COPPER
COR-OTICIN, HYDROCORTISONE ACETATE
CORDARONE, AMIODARONE HYDROCHLORIDE
CORDRAN, FLURANDRENOLIDE
CORDRAN SP, FLURANDRENOLIDE
CORDRAN-N, FLURANDRENOLIDE
CORGARD, NADOLOL
CORPHED, PSEUDOEPHEDRINE HYDROCHLORIDE
CORSYM, CHLORPHENIRAMINE POLISTIREX (OTC)
CORT-DOME, HYDROCORTISONE
CORTALONE, PREDNISOLONE
CORTAN, PREDNISONE
CORTEF, HYDROCORTISONE
CORTEF, HYDROCORTISONE CYPIONATE
CORTEF ACETATE, HYDROCORTISONE ACETATE
CORTENEMA, HYDROCORTISONE
CORTICOTROPIN, CORTICOTROPIN
CORTIFOAM, HYDROCORTISONE ACETATE
CORTISONE ACETATE, CORTISONE ACETATE
CORTISPORIN, BACITRACIN ZINC
CORTISPORIN, HYDROCORTISONE
CORTISPORIN, HYDROCORTISONE ACETATE
CORTONE, CORTISONE ACETATE
CORTRIL, HYDROCORTISONE
CORTRIL, HYDROCORTISONE ACETATE
CORTROPHIN-ZINC, CORTICOTROPIN-ZINC HYDROXIDE
CORTROSYN, COSYNTROPIN
CORZIDE, BENDROFLUMETHIAZIDE
COSMEGEN, DACTINOMYCIN
COTRIM, SULFAMETHOXAZOLE
COTRIM D.S., SULFAMETHOXAZOLE
COTRIM PEDIATRIC, SULFAMETHOXAZOLE
COUMADIN, WARFARIN SODIUM

APPENDIX A
PRODUCT NAME INDEX *(continued)*

CRESCORMON, SOMATROPIN
CROTAN, CROTAMITON
CRYSTODIGIN, DIGITOXIN
CU-7, COPPER
CUPRIC CHLORIDE, CUPRIC CHLORIDE
CUPRIC SULFATE, CUPRIC SULFATE
CUPRIMINE, PENICILLAMINE
CURRETAB, MEDROXYPROGESTERONE ACETATE
CUTIVATE, FLUTICASONE PROPIONATE
CYANOCOBALAMIN, CYANOCOBALAMIN
CYANOCOBALAMIN CO 57 SCHILLING TEST KIT,
    CYANOCOBALAMIN
CYCLACILLIN, CYCLACILLIN
CYCLAINE, HEXYLCAINE HYDROCHLORIDE
CYCLAPEN-W, CYCLACILLIN
CYCLOBENZAPRINE HCL, CYCLOBENZAPRINE
    HYDROCHLORIDE
CYCLOCORT, AMCINONIDE
CYCLOGYL, CYCLOPENTOLATE HYDROCHLORIDE
CYCLOMYDRIL, CYCLOPENTOLATE HYDROCHLORIDE
CYCLOPAR, TETRACYCLINE HYDROCHLORIDE
CYCLOPENTOLATE HCL, CYCLOPENTOLATE
    HYDROCHLORIDE
CYCLOPHOSPHAMIDE, CYCLOPHOSPHAMIDE
CYCRIN, MEDROXYPROGESTERONE ACETATE
CYKLOKAPRON, TRANEXAMIC ACID
CYLERT, PEMOLINE
CYPROHEPTADINE HCL, CYPROHEPTADINE
    HYDROCHLORIDE
CYSTEINE HCL, CYSTEINE HYDROCHLORIDE
CYSTO-CONRAY, IOTHALAMATE MEGLUMINE
CYSTO-CONRAY II, IOTHALAMATE MEGLUMINE
CYSTOGRAFIN, DIATRIZOATE MEGLUMINE
CYSTOGRAFIN DILUTE, DIATRIZOATE MEGLUMINE
CYTADREN, AMINOGLUTETHIMIDE
CYTARABINE, CYTARABINE
CYTOMEL, LIOTHYRONINE SODIUM
CYTOSAR-U, CYTARABINE
CYTOTEC, MISOPROSTOL
CYTOVENE, GANCICLOVIR SODIUM
CYTOXAN, CYCLOPHOSPHAMIDE

D

D.H.E. 45, DIHYDROERGOTAMINE MESYLATE
DACARBAZINE, DACARBAZINE
DALGAN, DEZOCINE
DALMANE, FLURAZEPAM HYDROCHLORIDE
DANAZOL, DANAZOL
DANOCRINE, DANAZOL
DANTRIUM, DANTROLENE SODIUM
DAPEX-37.5, PHENTERMINE HYDROCHLORIDE
DAPSONE, DAPSONE
DARANIDE, DICHLORPHENAMIDE
DARAPRIM, PYRIMETHAMINE
DARBID, ISOPROPAMIDE IODIDE
DARICON, OXYPHENCYCLIMINE HYDROCHLORIDE
DARVOCET, ACETAMINOPHEN
DARVOCET-N 100, ACETAMINOPHEN
DARVOCET-N 50, ACETAMINOPHEN
DARVON, PROPOXYPHENE HYDROCHLORIDE
DARVON COMPOUND, ASPIRIN
DARVON COMPOUND-65, ASPIRIN
DARVON W/ ASA, ASPIRIN
DARVON-N, PROPOXYPHENE NAPSYLATE
DARVON-N W/ ASA, ASPIRIN
DDAVP, DESMOPRESSIN ACETATE
DEAPRIL-ST, ERGOLOID MESYLATES
DECA-DURABOLIN, NANDROLONE DECANOATE
DECABID, INDECAINIDE HYDROCHLORIDE

DECADERM, DEXAMETHASONE
DECADRON, DEXAMETHASONE
DECADRON, DEXAMETHASONE SODIUM PHOSPHATE
DECADRON W/ XYLOCAINE, DEXAMETHASONE SODIUM
    PHOSPHATE
DECADRON-LA, DEXAMETHASONE ACETATE
DECAPRYN, DOXYLAMINE SUCCINATE
DECASPRAY, DEXAMETHASONE
DECLOMYCIN, DEMECLOCYCLINE HYDROCHLORIDE
DEL-VI-A, VITAMIN A PALMITATE
DELADUMONE, ESTRADIOL VALERATE
DELADUMONE OB, ESTRADIOL VALERATE
DELALUTIN, HYDROXYPROGESTERONE CAPROATE
DELATESTRYL, TESTOSTERONE ENANTHATE
DELAXIN, METHOCARBAMOL
DELCOBESE, AMPHETAMINE ADIPATE
DELESTROGEN, ESTRADIOL VALERATE
DELFLEX W/ DEXTROSE 1.5% IN PLASTIC CONTAINER,
    CALCIUM CHLORIDE
DELFLEX W/ DEXTROSE 1.5% LOW MAGNESIUM IN
    PLASTIC CONTAINER, CALCIUM CHLORIDE
DELFLEX W/ DEXTROSE 1.5% LOW MAGNESIUM LOW
    CALCIUM, CALCIUM CHLORIDE
DELFLEX W/ DEXTROSE 2.5% IN PLASTIC CONTAINER,
    CALCIUM CHLORIDE
DELFLEX W/ DEXTROSE 2.5% LOW MAGNESIUM IN
    PLASTIC CONTAINER, CALCIUM CHLORIDE
DELFLEX W/ DEXTROSE 2.5% LOW MAGNESIUM LOW
    CALCIUM, CALCIUM CHLORIDE
DELFLEX W/ DEXTROSE 4.25% IN PLASTIC CONTAINER,
    CALCIUM CHLORIDE
DELFLEX W/ DEXTROSE 4.25% LOW MAGNESIUM IN
    PLASTIC CONTAINER, CALCIUM CHLORIDE
DELFLEX W/ DEXTROSE 4.25% LOW MAGNESIUM LOW
    CALCIUM, CALCIUM CHLORIDE
DELSYM, DEXTROMETHORPHAN POLISTIREX (OTC)
DELTA-CORTEF, PREDNISOLONE
DELTA-DOME, PREDNISONE
DELTALIN, ERGOCALCIFEROL
DELTASONE, PREDNISONE
DEMAZIN, CHLORPHENIRAMINE MALEATE (OTC)
DEMEROL, MEPERIDINE HYDROCHLORIDE
DEMI-REGROTON, CHLORTHALIDONE
DEMSER, METYROSINE
DEMULEN 1/35-21, ETHINYL ESTRADIOL
DEMULEN 1/35-28, ETHINYL ESTRADIOL
DEMULEN 1/50-21, ETHINYL ESTRADIOL
DEMULEN 1/50-28, ETHINYL ESTRADIOL
DENDRID, IDOXURIDINE
DEPAKENE, VALPROIC ACID
DEPAKOTE, DIVALPROEX SODIUM
DEPAKOTE CP, DIVALPROEX SODIUM
DEPEN 250, PENICILLAMINE
DEPINAR, CYANOCOBALAMIN
DEPO-ESTRADIOL, ESTRADIOL CYPIONATE
DEPO-MEDROL, METHYLPREDNISOLONE ACETATE
DEPO-PROVERA, MEDROXYPROGESTERONE ACETATE
DEPO-TESTADIOL, ESTRADIOL CYPIONATE
DEPO-TESTOSTERONE, TESTOSTERONE CYPIONATE
DERMA-SMOOTHE/FS, FLUOCINOLONE ACETONIDE
DERMABET, BETAMETHASONE VALERATE
DERMACOMB, NYSTATIN
DERMACORT, HYDROCORTISONE
DERMATOP, PREDNICARBATE
DESFERAL, DEFEROXAMINE MESYLATE
DESIPRAMINE HCL, DESIPRAMINE HYDROCHLORIDE
DESONIDE, DESONIDE
DESOWEN, DESONIDE
DESOXIMETASONE, DESOXIMETASONE
DESOXYN, METHAMPHETAMINE HYDROCHLORIDE
DESYREL, TRAZODONE HYDROCHLORIDE
DEXACEN-4, DEXAMETHASONE SODIUM PHOSPHATE

APPENDIX A
PRODUCT NAME INDEX *(continued)*

DEXACIDIN, DEXAMETHASONE
DEXAIR, DEXAMETHASONE SODIUM PHOSPHATE
DEXAMETHASONE, DEXAMETHASONE
DEXAMETHASONE, DEXAMETHASONE SODIUM
   PHOSPHATE
DEXAMETHASONE ACETATE, DEXAMETHASONE
   ACETATE
DEXAMETHASONE INTENSOL, DEXAMETHASONE
DEXAMETHASONE SODIUM PHOSPHATE,
   DEXAMETHASONE SODIUM PHOSPHATE
DEXAMPEX, DEXTROAMPHETAMINE SULFATE
DEXASPORIN, DEXAMETHASONE
DEXCHLORPHENIRAMINE MALEATE,
   DEXCHLORPHENIRAMINE MALEATE
DEXEDRINE, DEXTROAMPHETAMINE SULFATE
DEXONE 0.5, DEXAMETHASONE
DEXONE 0.75, DEXAMETHASONE
DEXONE 1.5, DEXAMETHASONE
DEXONE 4, DEXAMETHASONE
DEXTROAMPHETAMINE SULFATE,
   DEXTROAMPHETAMINE SULFATE
DEXTROSE 10%, DEXTROSE
DEXTROSE 10% AND SODIUM CHLORIDE 0.11%,
   DEXTROSE
DEXTROSE 10% AND SODIUM CHLORIDE 0.2%, DEXTROSE
DEXTROSE 10% AND SODIUM CHLORIDE 0.33%,
   DEXTROSE
DEXTROSE 10% AND SODIUM CHLORIDE 0.45%,
   DEXTROSE
DEXTROSE 10% AND SODIUM CHLORIDE 0.9%, DEXTROSE
DEXTROSE 10% AND SODIUM CHLORIDE 0.9% IN PLASTIC
   CONTAINER, DEXTROSE
DEXTROSE 10% IN PLASTIC CONTAINER, DEXTROSE
DEXTROSE 2.5%, DEXTROSE
DEXTROSE 2.5% AND SODIUM CHLORIDE 0.11%,
   DEXTROSE
DEXTROSE 2.5% AND SODIUM CHLORIDE 0.2%,
   DEXTROSE
DEXTROSE 2.5% AND SODIUM CHLORIDE 0.33%,
   DEXTROSE
DEXTROSE 2.5% AND SODIUM CHLORIDE 0.45%,
   DEXTROSE
DEXTROSE 2.5% AND SODIUM CHLORIDE 0.45% IN
   PLASTIC CONTAINER, DEXTROSE
DEXTROSE 2.5% AND SODIUM CHLORIDE 0.9%,
   DEXTROSE
DEXTROSE 2.5% IN HALF-STRENGTH LACTATED
   RINGER'S, CALCIUM CHLORIDE
DEXTROSE 20% IN PLASTIC CONTAINER, DEXTROSE
DEXTROSE 3.3% AND SODIUM CHLORIDE 0.3%,
   DEXTROSE
DEXTROSE 3.3% AND SODIUM CHLORIDE 0.3% IN
   PLASTIC CONTAINER, DEXTROSE
DEXTROSE 30% IN PLASTIC CONTAINER, DEXTROSE
DEXTROSE 38.5% IN PLASTIC CONTAINER, DEXTROSE
DEXTROSE 4% IN MODIFIED LACTATED RINGER'S,
   CALCIUM CHLORIDE
DEXTROSE 40% IN PLASTIC CONTAINER, DEXTROSE
DEXTROSE 5%, DEXTROSE
DEXTROSE 5% AND ELECTROLYTE NO 75, DEXTROSE
DEXTROSE 5% AND ELECTROLYTE NO.48 IN PLASTIC
   CONTAINER, DEXTROSE
DEXTROSE 5% AND LACTATED RINGER'S IN PLASTIC
   CONTAINER, CALCIUM CHLORIDE
DEXTROSE 5% AND POTASSIUM CHLORIDE 0.075% IN
   PLASTIC CONTAINER, DEXTROSE
DEXTROSE 5% AND POTASSIUM CHLORIDE 0.15% IN
   PLASTIC CONTAINER, DEXTROSE
DEXTROSE 5% AND POTASSIUM CHLORIDE 0.224% IN
   PLASTIC CONTAINER, DEXTROSE
DEXTROSE 5% AND POTASSIUM CHLORIDE 0.3% IN
   PLASTIC CONTAINER, DEXTROSE

DEXTROSE 5% AND RINGER'S IN PLASTIC CONTAINER,
   CALCIUM CHLORIDE
DEXTROSE 5% AND SODIUM CHLORIDE 0.11%, DEXTROSE
DEXTROSE 5% AND SODIUM CHLORIDE 0.11% IN PLASTIC
   CONTAINER, DEXTROSE
DEXTROSE 5% AND SODIUM CHLORIDE 0.2%, DEXTROSE
DEXTROSE 5% AND SODIUM CHLORIDE 0.2% IN PLASTIC
   CONTAINER, DEXTROSE
DEXTROSE 5% AND SODIUM CHLORIDE 0.225%,
   DEXTROSE
DEXTROSE 5% AND SODIUM CHLORIDE 0.225% IN
   PLASTIC CONTAINER, DEXTROSE
DEXTROSE 5% AND SODIUM CHLORIDE 0.3%, DEXTROSE
DEXTROSE 5% AND SODIUM CHLORIDE 0.3% IN PLASTIC
   CONTAINER, DEXTROSE
DEXTROSE 5% AND SODIUM CHLORIDE 0.33%, DEXTROSE
DEXTROSE 5% AND SODIUM CHLORIDE 0.33% IN PLASTIC
   CONTAINER, DEXTROSE
DEXTROSE 5% AND SODIUM CHLORIDE 0.45%, DEXTROSE
DEXTROSE 5% AND SODIUM CHLORIDE 0.45% IN PLASTIC
   CONTAINER, DEXTROSE
DEXTROSE 5% AND SODIUM CHLORIDE 0.9%, DEXTROSE
DEXTROSE 5% AND SODIUM CHLORIDE 0.9% IN PLASTIC
   CONTAINER, DEXTROSE
DEXTROSE 5% IN ACETATED RINGER'S IN PLASTIC
   CONTAINER, CALCIUM CHLORIDE
DEXTROSE 5% IN LACTATED RINGER'S, CALCIUM
   CHLORIDE
DEXTROSE 5% IN LACTATED RINGER'S IN PLASTIC
   CONTAINER, CALCIUM CHLORIDE
DEXTROSE 5% IN PLASTIC CONTAINER, DEXTROSE
DEXTROSE 5% IN RINGER'S, CALCIUM CHLORIDE
DEXTROSE 5% IN RINGER'S IN PLASTIC CONTAINER,
   CALCIUM CHLORIDE
DEXTROSE 5% IN SODIUM CHLORIDE 0.2% IN PLASTIC
   CONTAINER, DEXTROSE
DEXTROSE 5% IN SODIUM CHLORIDE 0.33% IN PLASTIC
   CONTAINER, DEXTROSE
DEXTROSE 5% IN SODIUM CHLORIDE 0.45% IN PLASTIC
   CONTAINER, DEXTROSE
DEXTROSE 5% IN SODIUM CHLORIDE 0.9% IN PLASTIC
   CONTAINER, DEXTROSE
DEXTROSE 5%, SODIUM CHLORIDE 0.2% AND POTASSIUM
   CHLORIDE 0.15%, DEXTROSE
DEXTROSE 5%, SODIUM CHLORIDE 0.2% AND POTASSIUM
   CHLORIDE 0.224%, DEXTROSE
DEXTROSE 5%, SODIUM CHLORIDE 0.2% AND
   POTASSIUMCHLORIDE 0.3%, DEXTROSE
DEXTROSE 5%, SODIUM CHLORIDE 0.2% AND POTASSIUM
   CHLORIDE 0.075%, DEXTROSE
DEXTROSE 5%, SODIUM CHLORIDE 0.2% AND POTASSIUM
   CHLORIDE 10 MEQ, DEXTROSE
DEXTROSE 5%, SODIUM CHLORIDE 0.2% AND POTASSIUM
   CHLORIDE 15 MEQ (K), DEXTROSE
DEXTROSE 5%, SODIUM CHLORIDE 0.2% AND POTASSIUM
   CHLORIDE 20 MEQ (K), DEXTROSE
DEXTROSE 5%, SODIUM CHLORIDE 0.2% AND POTASSIUM
   CHLORIDE 20 MEQ, DEXTROSE
DEXTROSE 5%, SODIUM CHLORIDE 0.2% AND POTASSIUM
   CHLORIDE 30 MEQ, DEXTROSE
DEXTROSE 5%, SODIUM CHLORIDE 0.2% AND POTASSIUM
   CHLORIDE 40 MEQ, DEXTROSE
DEXTROSE 5%, SODIUM CHLORIDE 0.2% AND POTASSIUM
   CHLORIDE 5 MEQ (K), DEXTROSE
DEXTROSE 5%, SODIUM CHLORIDE 0.2% AND POTASSIUM
   CHLORIDE 5 MEQ, DEXTROSE
DEXTROSE 5%, SODIUM CHLORIDE 0.33% AND
   POTASSIUM CHLORIDE 0.075%, DEXTROSE
DEXTROSE 5%, SODIUM CHLORIDE 0.33% AND
   POTASSIUM CHLORIDE 0.15%, DEXTROSE
DEXTROSE 5%, SODIUM CHLORIDE 0.33% AND
   POTASSIUM CHLORIDE 0.22%, DEXTROSE

APPENDIX A
PRODUCT NAME INDEX (continued)

DEXTROSE 5%, SODIUM CHLORIDE 0.33% AND
POTASSIUM CHLORIDE 0.30%, DEXTROSE
DEXTROSE 5%, SODIUM CHLORIDE 0.33% AND
POTASSIUM CHLORIDE 10 MEQ, DEXTROSE
DEXTROSE 5%, SODIUM CHLORIDE 0.33% AND
POTASSIUM CHLORIDE 15 MEQ, DEXTROSE
DEXTROSE 5%, SODIUM CHLORIDE 0.33% AND
POTASSIUM CHLORIDE 20 MEQ, DEXTROSE
DEXTROSE 5%, SODIUM CHLORIDE 0.33% AND
POTASSIUM CHLORIDE 30 MEQ, DEXTROSE
DEXTROSE 5%, SODIUM CHLORIDE 0.33% AND
POTASSIUM CHLORIDE 40 MEQ, DEXTROSE
DEXTROSE 5%, SODIUM CHLORIDE 0.33% AND
POTASSIUM CHLORIDE 5 MEQ, DEXTROSE
DEXTROSE 5%, SODIUM CHLORIDE 0.45% AND
POTASSIUM CHLORIDE 0.15%, DEXTROSE
DEXTROSE 5%, SODIUM CHLORIDE 0.45% AND
POTASSIUM CHLORIDE 0.3%, DEXTROSE
DEXTROSE 5%, SODIUM CHLORIDE 0.45% AND
POTASSIUM CHLORIDE 0.075%, DEXTROSE
DEXTROSE 5%, SODIUM CHLORIDE 0.45% AND
POTASSIUM CHLORIDE 0.22%, DEXTROSE
DEXTROSE 5%, SODIUM CHLORIDE 0.45% AND
POTASSIUM CHLORIDE 15 MEQ, DEXTROSE
DEXTROSE 5%, SODIUM CHLORIDE 0.45% AND
POTASSIUM CHLORIDE 20 MEQ (K), DEXTROSE
DEXTROSE 5%, SODIUM CHLORIDE 0.45% AND
POTASSIUM CHLORIDE 5 MEQ, DEXTROSE
DEXTROSE 50%, DEXTROSE
DEXTROSE 50% IN PLASTIC CONTAINER, DEXTROSE
DEXTROSE 60%, DEXTROSE
DEXTROSE 60% IN PLASTIC CONTAINER, DEXTROSE
DEXTROSE 7.7%, DEXTROSE
DEXTROSE 70%, DEXTROSE
DEXTROSE 70% IN PLASTIC CONTAINER, DEXTROSE
DI-ATRO, ATROPINE SULFATE
DI-METREX, PHENDIMETRAZINE TARTRATE
DIABETA, GLYBURIDE
DIABINESE, CHLORPROPAMIDE
DIAL, HEXACHLOROPHENE
DIALYTE CONCENTRATE W/ DEXTROSE 30% IN PLASTIC
CONTAINER, CALCIUM CHLORIDE
DIALYTE CONCENTRATE W/ DEXTROSE 50% IN PLASTIC
CONTAINER, CALCIUM CHLORIDE
DIALYTE LM/ DEXTROSE 1.5%, CALCIUM CHLORIDE
DIALYTE LM/ DEXTROSE 2.5%, CALCIUM CHLORIDE
DIALYTE LM/ DEXTROSE 4.25%, CALCIUM CHLORIDE
DIALYTE W/ DEXTROSE 1.5% IN PLASTIC CONTAINER,
CALCIUM CHLORIDE
DIALYTE W/ DEXTROSE 4.25% IN PLASTIC CONTAINER,
CALCIUM CHLORIDE
DIAMOX, ACETAZOLAMIDE
DIAMOX, ACETAZOLAMIDE SODIUM
DIANEAL PD-1 W/ DEXTROSE 1.5% IN PLASTIC
CONTAINER, CALCIUM CHLORIDE
DIANEAL PD-1 W/ DEXTROSE 2.5% IN PLASTIC
CONTAINER, CALCIUM CHLORIDE
DIANEAL PD-1 W/ DEXTROSE 3.5%, CALCIUM CHLORIDE
DIANEAL PD-1 W/ DEXTROSE 4.25% IN PLASTIC
CONTAINER, CALCIUM CHLORIDE
DIANEAL PD-2 W/ DEXTROSE 1.5% IN PLASTIC
CONTAINER, CALCIUM CHLORIDE
DIANEAL PD-2 W/ DEXTROSE 2.5% IN PLASTIC
CONTAINER, CALCIUM CHLORIDE
DIANEAL PD-2 W/ DEXTROSE 3.5%, CALCIUM CHLORIDE
DIANEAL PD-2 W/ DEXTROSE 4.25% IN PLASTIC
CONTAINER, CALCIUM CHLORIDE
DIANEAL 137 W/ DEXTROSE 1.5% IN PLASTIC
CONTAINER, CALCIUM CHLORIDE
DIANEAL 137 W/ DEXTROSE 2.5% IN PLASTIC
CONTAINER, CALCIUM CHLORIDE
DIANEAL 137 W/ DEXTROSE 4.25% IN PLASTIC
CONTAINER, CALCIUM CHLORIDE

DIAPID, LYPRESSIN
DIASONE SODIUM, SULFOXONE SODIUM
DIATRIZOATE MEGLUMINE, DIATRIZOATE MEGLUMINE
DIATRIZOATE-60, DIATRIZOATE MEGLUMINE
DIAZEPAM, DIAZEPAM
DIAZEPAM INTENSOL, DIAZEPAM
DIAZOXIDE, DIAZOXIDE
DIBENIL, DIPHENHYDRAMINE HYDROCHLORIDE
DIBENZYLINE, PHENOXYBENZAMINE HYDROCHLORIDE
DICLOXACILLIN SODIUM, DICLOXACILLIN SODIUM
DICOPAC KIT, CYANOCOBALAMIN
DICUMAROL, DICUMAROL
DICURIN PROCAINE, PROCAINE MERETHOXYLLINE
DICYCLOMINE HCL, DICYCLOMINE HYDROCHLORIDE
DIDREX, BENZPHETAMINE HYDROCHLORIDE
DIDRONEL, ETIDRONATE DISODIUM
DIENESTROL, DIENESTROL
DIETHYLPROPION HCL, DIETHYLPROPION
HYDROCHLORIDE
DIETHYLSTILBESTROL, DIETHYLSTILBESTROL
DIFLORASONE DIACETATE, DIFLORASONE DIACETATE
DIFLUCAN, FLUCONAZOLE
DIFLUNISAL, DIFLUNISAL
DIGOXIN, DIGOXIN
DILACOR XR, DILTIAZEM HYDROCHLORIDE
DILANTIN, PHENYTOIN
DILANTIN, PHENYTOIN SODIUM
DILANTIN, PHENYTOIN SODIUM, EXTENDED
DILANTIN-125, PHENYTOIN
DILANTIN-30, PHENYTOIN
DILATRATE-SR, ISOSORBIDE DINITRATE
DILAUDID-HP, HYDROMORPHONE HYDROCHLORIDE
DILOR, DYPHYLLINE
DILOR-400, DYPHYLLINE
DIMENHYDRINATE, DIMENHYDRINATE
DIMETANE, BROMPHENIRAMINE MALEATE
DIMETANE, BROMPHENIRAMINE MALEATE (OTC)
DIMETANE-DC, BROMPHENIRAMINE MALEATE
DIMETANE-DX, BROMPHENIRAMINE MALEATE
DIMETANE-TEN, BROMPHENIRAMINE MALEATE
DIMETAPP, BROMPHENIRAMINE MALEATE (OTC)
DIONOSIL AQUEOUS, PROPYLIODONE
DIONOSIL OILY, PROPYLIODONE
DIPENTUM, OLSALAZINE SODIUM
DIPHEN, DIPHENHYDRAMINE HYDROCHLORIDE
DIPHEN, DIPHENHYDRAMINE HYDROCHLORIDE (OTC)
DIPHENHYDRAMINE HCL, DIPHENHYDRAMINE
HYDROCHLORIDE
DIPHENHYDRAMINE HCL, DIPHENHYDRAMINE
HYDROCHLORIDE (OTC)
DIPHENOXYLATE HCL AND ATROPINE SULFATE,
ATROPINE SULFATE
DIPHENOXYLATE HCL W/ ATROPINE SULFATE,
ATROPINE SULFATE
DIPHENYLAN SODIUM, PHENYTOIN SODIUM, PROMPT
DIPRIVAN, PROPOFOL
DIPROLENE, BETAMETHASONE DIPROPIONATE
DIPROLENE AF, BETAMETHASONE DIPROPIONATE
DIPROSONE, BETAMETHASONE DIPROPIONATE
DIPYRIDAMOLE, DIPYRIDAMOLE
DISCASE, CHYMOPAPAIN
DISIPAL, ORPHENADRINE HYDROCHLORIDE
DISOBROM, DEXBROMPHENIRAMINE MALEATE (OTC)
DISODIUM EDETATE, EDETATE DISODIUM
DISOMER, DEXBROMPHENIRAMINE MALEATE
DISOPHROL, DEXBROMPHENIRAMINE MALEATE (OTC)
DISOPYRAMIDE PHOSPHATE, DISOPYRAMIDE
PHOSPHATE
DISULFIRAM, DISULFIRAM
DITATE-DS, ESTRADIOL VALERATE
DITROPAN, OXYBUTYNIN CHLORIDE
DIUCARDIN, HYDROFLUMETHIAZIDE

APPENDIX A
PRODUCT NAME INDEX *(continued)*

DIULO, METOLAZONE
DIUPRES-250, CHLOROTHIAZIDE
DIUPRES-500, CHLOROTHIAZIDE
DIURIL, CHLOROTHIAZIDE
DIURIL, CHLOROTHIAZIDE SODIUM
DIUTENSEN-R, METHYCLOTHIAZIDE
DOBUTREX, DOBUTAMINE HYDROCHLORIDE
DOCA, DESOXYCORTICOSTERONE ACETATE
DOLENE, PROPOXYPHENE HYDROCHLORIDE
DOLENE AP-65, ACETAMINOPHEN
DOLOBID, DIFLUNISAL
DOLOPHINE HCL, METHADONE HYDROCHLORIDE
DOMEBORO, ACETIC ACID, GLACIAL
DOPAMINE, DOPAMINE HYDROCHLORIDE
DOPAMINE HCL, DOPAMINE HYDROCHLORIDE
DOPAMINE HCL AND DEXTROSE 5%, DOPAMINE
  HYDROCHLORIDE
DOPAMINE HCL IN DEXTROSE 5%, DOPAMINE
  HYDROCHLORIDE
DOPAR, LEVODOPA
DOPRAM, DOXAPRAM HYDROCHLORIDE
DORAL, QUAZEPAM
DORIDEN, GLUTETHIMIDE
DORMATE, MEBUTAMATE
DORYX, DOXYCYCLINE HYCLATE
DOW-ISONIAZID, ISONIAZID
DOXAPRAM HCL, DOXAPRAM HYDROCHLORIDE
DOXEPIN HCL, DOXEPIN HYDROCHLORIDE
DOXORUBICIN HCL, DOXORUBICIN HYDROCHLORIDE
DOXY 100, DOXYCYCLINE HYCLATE
DOXY 200, DOXYCYCLINE HYCLATE
DOXY-LEMMON, DOXYCYCLINE HYCLATE
DOXY-SLEEP-AID, DOXYLAMINE SUCCINATE (OTC)
DOXY-TABS, DOXYCYCLINE HYCLATE
DOXYCHEL, DOXYCYCLINE
DOXYCHEL HYCLATE, DOXYCYCLINE HYCLATE
DOXYCYCLINE, DOXYCYCLINE HYCLATE
DOXYCYCLINE HYCLATE, DOXYCYCLINE HYCLATE
DOXYCYCLINE MONOHYDRATE, DOXYCYCLINE
DOXYLAMINE SUCCINATE, DOXYLAMINE SUCCINATE
DOXYLAMINE SUCCINATE, DOXYLAMINE SUCCINATE
  (OTC)
DRALSERP, HYDRALAZINE HYDROCHLORIDE
DRALZINE, HYDRALAZINE HYDROCHLORIDE
DRICORT, HYDROCORTISONE ACETATE
DRISDOL, ERGOCALCIFEROL
DRIXORAL, DEXBROMPHENIRAMINE MALEATE (OTC)
DRIXORAL PLUS, ACETAMINOPHEN (OTC)
DRIZE, CHLORPHENIRAMINE MALEATE
DROLBAN, DROMOSTANOLONE PROPIONATE
DROPERIDOL, DROPERIDOL
DTIC-DOME, DACARBAZINE
DUO-MEDIHALER, ISOPROTERENOL HYDROCHLORIDE
DUPHALAC, LACTULOSE
DURABOLIN, NANDROLONE PHENPROPIONATE
DURABOLIN-50, NANDROLONE PHENPROPIONATE
DURACILLIN A.S., PENICILLIN G PROCAINE
DURADYNE DHC, ACETAMINOPHEN
DURAGESIC, FENTANYL
DURAMORPH PF, MORPHINE SULFATE
DURANEST, EPINEPHRINE
DURANEST, EPINEPHRINE BITARTRATE
DURANEST, ETIDOCAINE HYDROCHLORIDE
DURAPHYL, THEOPHYLLINE
DURAQUIN, QUINIDINE GLUCONATE
DURICEF, CEFADROXIL/CEFADROXIL HEMIHYDRATE
DUVOID, BETHANECHOL CHLORIDE
DV, DIENESTROL
DYAZIDE, HYDROCHLOROTHIAZIDE
DYCILL, DICLOXACILLIN SODIUM
DYCLONE, DYCLONINE HYDROCHLORIDE
DYMELOR, ACETOHEXAMIDE

DYNACIRC, ISRADIPINE
DYNAPEN, DICLOXACILLIN SODIUM
DYRENIUM, TRIAMTERENE

E

E.E.S., ERYTHROMYCIN ETHYLSUCCINATE
E.E.S. 200, ERYTHROMYCIN ETHYLSUCCINATE
E.E.S. 400, ERYTHROMYCIN ETHYLSUCCINATE
E-BASE, ERYTHROMYCIN
E-MYCIN, ERYTHROMYCIN
E-MYCIN E, ERYTHROMYCIN ETHYLSUCCINATE
E-SOLVE 2, ERYTHROMYCIN
E-Z PREP, POVIDONE-IODINE (OTC)
E-Z PREP 220, POVIDONE-IODINE (OTC)
E-Z SCRUB, HEXACHLOROPHENE
E-Z SCRUB 201, POVIDONE-IODINE (OTC)
E-Z SCRUB 241, POVIDONE-IODINE (OTC)
E-Z-EM PREP LYTE, POLYETHYLENE GLYCOL 3350
ECONOCHLOR, CHLORAMPHENICOL
ECONOPRED, PREDNISOLONE ACETATE
ECONOPRED PLUS, PREDNISOLONE ACETATE
EDECRIN, ETHACRYNATE SODIUM
EDECRIN, ETHACRYNIC ACID
EDETATE DISODIUM, EDETATE DISODIUM
EFUDEX, FLUOROURACIL
ELASE-CHLOROMYCETIN, CHLORAMPHENICOL
ELAVIL, AMITRIPTYLINE HYDROCHLORIDE
ELDECORT, HYDROCORTISONE
ELDEPRYL, SELEGILINE HYDROCHLORIDE
ELIMITE, PERMETHRIN
ELIXICON, THEOPHYLLINE
ELIXOMIN, THEOPHYLLINE
ELIXOPHYLLIN, THEOPHYLLINE
ELIXOPHYLLIN SR, THEOPHYLLINE
ELOCON, MOMETASONE FUROATE
EMBOLEX, DIHYDROERGOTAMINE MESYLATE
EMCYT, ESTRAMUSTINE PHOSPHATE SODIUM
EMETE-CON, BENZQUINAMIDE HYDROCHLORIDE
EMGEL, ERYTHROMYCIN
EMPRACET W/ CODEINE PHOSPHATE #3,
  ACETAMINOPHEN
EMPRACET W/ CODEINE PHOSPHATE #4,
  ACETAMINOPHEN
ENDEP, AMITRIPTYLINE HYDROCHLORIDE
ENDOSOL PLUS, CALCIUM CHLORIDE
ENDRATE, EDETATE DISODIUM
ENDURON, METHYCLOTHIAZIDE
ENDURONYL, DESERPIDINE
ENDURONYL FORTE, DESERPIDINE
ENFLURANE, ENFLURANE
ENKAID, ENCAINIDE HYDROCHLORIDE
ENLON, EDROPHONIUM CHLORIDE
ENLON-PLUS, ATROPINE SULFATE
ENOVID, MESTRANOL
ENOVID-E, MESTRANOL
ENOVID-E 21, MESTRANOL
ENULOSE, LACTULOSE
EPICORT, HYDROCORTISONE
EPIFOAM, HYDROCORTISONE ACETATE
EPINEPHRINE, EPINEPHRINE (OTC)
EPIPEN, EPINEPHRINE
EPIPEN JR., EPINEPHRINE
EPITOL, CARBAMAZEPINE
EQUAGESIC, ASPIRIN
EQUANIL, MEPROBAMATE
EQUIPIN, HOMATROPINE METHYLBROMIDE
ERCATAB, CAFFEINE
ERGAMISOL, LEVAMISOLE HYDROCHLORIDE
ERGOLOID MESYLATES, ERGOLOID MESYLATES

APPENDIX A
PRODUCT NAME INDEX *(continued)*

ERGOMAR, ERGOTAMINE TARTRATE
ERGOSTAT, ERGOTAMINE TARTRATE
ERY-TAB, ERYTHROMYCIN
ERYC, ERYTHROMYCIN
ERYC SPRINKLES, ERYTHROMYCIN
ERYC 125, ERYTHROMYCIN
ERYCETTE, ERYTHROMYCIN
ERYDERM, ERYTHROMYCIN
ERYGEL, ERYTHROMYCIN
ERYMAX, ERYTHROMYCIN
ERYPAR, ERYTHROMYCIN STEARATE
ERYPED, ERYTHROMYCIN ETHYLSUCCINATE
ERYTHROCIN, ERYTHROMYCIN LACTOBIONATE
ERYTHROCIN STEARATE, ERYTHROMYCIN STEARATE
ERYTHROMYCIN, ERYTHROMYCIN
ERYTHROMYCIN, ERYTHROMYCIN LACTOBIONATE
ERYTHROMYCIN ESTOLATE, ERYTHROMYCIN ESTOLATE
ERYTHROMYCIN ETHYLSUCCINATE, ERYTHROMYCIN
    ETHYLSUCCINATE
ERYTHROMYCIN ETHYLSUCCINATE AND
    SULFISOXAZOLE ACETYL, ERYTHROMYCIN
    ETHYLSUCCINATE
ERYTHROMYCIN LACTOBIONATE, ERYTHROMYCIN
    LACTOBIONATE
ERYTHROMYCIN STEARATE, ERYTHROMYCIN
    STEARATE
ERYZOLE, ERYTHROMYCIN ETHYLSUCCINATE
ESGIC, ACETAMINOPHEN
ESIDRIX, HYDROCHLOROTHIAZIDE
ESIMIL, GUANETHIDINE MONOSULFATE
ESKALITH, LITHIUM CARBONATE
ESKALITH CR, LITHIUM CARBONATE
ESTERIFIED ESTROGENS, ESTROGENS, ESTERIFIED
ESTINYL, ETHINYL ESTRADIOL
ESTRACE, ESTRADIOL
ESTRADERM, ESTRADIOL
ESTRADIOL CYPIONATE, ESTRADIOL CYPIONATE
ESTRADIOL VALERATE, ESTRADIOL VALERATE
ESTRADURIN, POLYESTRADIOL PHOSPHATE
ESTRAGUARD, DIENESTROL
ESTRATAB, ESTROGENS, ESTERIFIED
ESTROGENIC SUBSTANCE, ESTRONE
ESTRONE, ESTRONE
ESTROVIS, QUINESTROL
ETHAMIDE, ETHOXZOLAMIDE
ETHAMOLIN, ETHANOLAMINE OLEATE
ETHCHLORVYNOL, ETHCHLORVYNOL
ETHIODOL, ETHIODIZED OIL
ETHMOZINE, MORICIZINE HYDROCHLORIDE
ETHRANE, ENFLURANE
ETHRIL 250, ERYTHROMYCIN STEARATE
ETHRIL 500, ERYTHROMYCIN STEARATE
ETHYNODIOL DIACETATE AND ETHINYL ESTRADIOL 1/
    35-21, ETHINYL ESTRADIOL
ETHYNODIOL DIACETATE AND ETHINYL ESTRADIOL 1/
    35-28, ETHINYL ESTRADIOL
ETHYNODIOL DIACETATE AND ETHINYL ESTRADIOL 1/
    50-21, ETHINYL ESTRADIOL
ETHYNODIOL DIACETATE AND ETHINYL ESTRADIOL 1/
    50-28, ETHINYL ESTRADIOL
ETRAFON 2-10, AMITRIPTYLINE HYDROCHLORIDE
ETRAFON 2-25, AMITRIPTYLINE HYDROCHLORIDE
ETRAFON-A, AMITRIPTYLINE HYDROCHLORIDE
ETRAFON-FORTE, AMITRIPTYLINE HYDROCHLORIDE
ETS-2%, ERYTHROMYCIN
EULEXIN, FLUTAMIDE
EURAX, CROTAMITON
EUTHROID-0.5, LIOTRIX (T4; T3)
EUTHROID-1, LIOTRIX (T4; T3)
EUTHROID-2, LIOTRIX (T4; T3)
EUTHROID-3, LIOTRIX (T4; T3)
EUTONYL, PARGYLINE HYDROCHLORIDE

EUTRON, METHYCLOTHIAZIDE
EVEX, ESTROGENS, ESTERIFIED
EXELDERM, SULCONAZOLE NITRATE
EXIDINE, CHLORHEXIDINE GLUCONATE (OTC)
EXNA, BENZTHIAZIDE
EXOSURF NEONATAL, CETYL ALCOHOL
EXSEL, SELENIUM SULFIDE
EXTENDED PHENYTOIN SODIUM, PHENYTOIN SODIUM,
    EXTENDED
EXTRA-STRENGTH AIM, SODIUM
    MONOFLUOROPHOSPHATE (OTC)

F

FACTREL, GONADORELIN HYDROCHLORIDE
FANSIDAR, PYRIMETHAMINE
FASTIN, PHENTERMINE HYDROCHLORIDE
FELDENE, PIROXICAM
FEMINONE, ETHINYL ESTRADIOL
FEMOGEN, ESTROGENS, ESTERIFIED
FEMSTAT, BUTOCONAZOLE NITRATE
FENOPROFEN CALCIUM, FENOPROFEN CALCIUM
FENTANYL CITRATE, FENTANYL CITRATE
FENTANYL CITRATE AND DROPERIDOL, DROPERIDOL
FERNDEX, DEXTROAMPHETAMINE SULFATE
FERNISOLONE-P, PREDNISOLONE
FERNISONE, PREDNISONE
FERROUS CITRATE FE 59, FERROUS CITRATE, FE-59
FIORICET, ACETAMINOPHEN
FIORICET W/ CODEINE, ACETAMINOPHEN
FIORINAL, ASPIRIN
FIORINAL W/CODEINE NO 3, ASPIRIN
FLAGYL, METRONIDAZOLE
FLAGYL I.V., METRONIDAZOLE HYDROCHLORIDE
FLAGYL I.V. RTU, METRONIDAZOLE
FLAGYL I.V. RTU IN PLASTIC CONTAINER,
    METRONIDAZOLE
FLAREX, FLUOROMETHOLONE ACETATE
FLAXEDIL, GALLAMINE TRIETHIODIDE
FLEXERIL, CYCLOBENZAPRINE HYDROCHLORIDE
FLEXICORT, HYDROCORTISONE
FLORINEF, FLUDROCORTISONE ACETATE
FLORONE, DIFLORASONE DIACETATE
FLOROPRYL, ISOFLUROPHATE
FLOXIN, OFLOXACIN
FLOXIN IN DEXTROSE 5%, OFLOXACIN
FLOXURIDINE, FLOXURIDINE
FLUDARA, FLUDARABINE PHOSPHATE
FLUIDIL, CYCLOTHIAZIDE
FLUOCET, FLUOCINOLONE ACETONIDE
FLUOCINOLONE ACETONIDE, FLUOCINOLONE
    ACETONIDE
FLUOCINONIDE, FLUOCINONIDE
FLUONID, FLUOCINOLONE ACETONIDE
FLUOR-OP, FLUOROMETHOLONE
FLUOROPLEX, FLUOROURACIL
FLUOROURACIL, FLUOROURACIL
FLUOTHANE, HALOTHANE
FLUOTREX, FLUOCINOLONE ACETONIDE
FLUOXYMESTERONE, FLUOXYMESTERONE
FLUPHENAZINE, FLUPHENAZINE DECANOATE
FLUPHENAZINE DECANOATE, FLUPHENAZINE
    DECANOATE
FLUPHENAZINE HCL, FLUPHENAZINE HYDROCHLORIDE
FLURANDRENOLIDE, FLURANDRENOLIDE
FLURAZEPAM HCL, FLURAZEPAM HYDROCHLORIDE
FLUTEX, TRIAMCINOLONE ACETONIDE
FML, FLUOROMETHOLONE
FML FORTE, FLUOROMETHOLONE
FML-S, FLUOROMETHOLONE

APPENDIX A
PRODUCT NAME INDEX (*continued*)

FOAMCOAT, ALUMINUM HYDROXIDE (OTC)
FOAMICON, ALUMINUM HYDROXIDE (OTC)
FOLEX, METHOTREXATE SODIUM
FOLEX PFS, METHOTREXATE SODIUM
FOLIC ACID, FOLIC ACID
FOLICET, FOLIC ACID
FOLLUTEIN, GONADOTROPIN, CHORIONIC
FOLVITE, FOLIC ACID
FOLVRON, FERROUS SULFATE
FORANE, ISOFLURANE
FORBAXIN, METHOCARBAMOL
FORTAZ, CEFTAZIDIME
FORTAZ, CEFTAZIDIME SODIUM
FOSCAVIR, FOSCARNET SODIUM
FOVANE, BENZTHIAZIDE
FREAMINE HBC 6.9%, AMINO ACIDS
FREAMINE II 8.5%, AMINO ACIDS
FREAMINE III 10%, AMINO ACIDS
FREAMINE III 3% W/ ELECTROLYTES, AMINO ACIDS
FREAMINE III 8.5%, AMINO ACIDS
FREAMINE III 8.5% W/ ELECTROLYTES, AMINO ACIDS
FREAMINE 8.5%, AMINO ACIDS
FS SHAMPOO, FLUOCINOLONE ACETONIDE
FUDR, FLOXURIDINE
FULVICIN P/G, GRISEOFULVIN,
    ULTRAMICROCRYSTALLINE
FULVICIN P/G 165, GRISEOFULVIN,
    ULTRAMICROCRYSTALLINE
FULVICIN P/G 330, GRISEOFULVIN,
    ULTRAMICROCRYSTALLINE
FULVICIN-U/F, GRISEOFULVIN, MICROCRYSTALLINE
FUNDUSCEIN-25, FLUORESCEIN SODIUM
FUNGIZONE, AMPHOTERICIN B
FURACIN, NITROFURAZONE
FURADANTIN, NITROFURANTOIN
FURALAN, NITROFURANTOIN
FUROSEMIDE, FUROSEMIDE
FUROXONE, FURAZOLIDONE

G

GALLIUM CITRATE GA 67, GALLIUM CITRATE, GA-67
GAMENE, LINDANE
GAMOPHEN, HEXACHLOROPHENE
GANITE, GALLIUM NITRATE
GANTANOL, SULFAMETHOXAZOLE
GANTANOL-DS, SULFAMETHOXAZOLE
GANTRISIN, SULFISOXAZOLE
GANTRISIN, SULFISOXAZOLE ACETYL
GANTRISIN, SULFISOXAZOLE DIOLAMINE
GANTRISIN PEDIATRIC, SULFISOXAZOLE ACETYL
GARAMYCIN, GENTAMICIN SULFATE
GASTROCROM, CROMOLYN SODIUM
GASTROGRAFIN, DIATRIZOATE MEGLUMINE
GASTROVIST, DIATRIZOATE MEGLUMINE
GAVISCON, ALUMINUM HYDROXIDE (OTC)
GAVISCON-2, ALUMINUM HYDROXIDE (OTC)
GEMONIL, METHARBITAL
GEN-XENE, CLORAZEPATE DIPOTASSIUM
GENAPAX, GENTIAN VIOLET
GENCEPT 0.5/35-21, ETHINYL ESTRADIOL
GENCEPT 0.5/35-28, ETHINYL ESTRADIOL
GENCEPT 1/35-21, ETHINYL ESTRADIOL
GENCEPT 1/35-28, ETHINYL ESTRADIOL
GENCEPT 10/11-21, ETHINYL ESTRADIOL
GENCEPT 10/11-28, ETHINYL ESTRADIOL
GENERLAC, LACTULOSE
GENOPTIC, GENTAMICIN SULFATE
GENTACIDIN, GENTAMICIN SULFATE
GENTAFAIR, GENTAMICIN SULFATE

GENTAMICIN, GENTAMICIN SULFATE
GENTAMICIN SULFATE, GENTAMICIN SULFATE
GENTAMICIN SULFATE IN SODIUM CHLORIDE 0.9%,
    GENTAMICIN SULFATE
GEOCILLIN, CARBENICILLIN INDANYL SODIUM
GEOPEN, CARBENICILLIN DISODIUM
GEREF, SERMORELIN ACETATE
GERIMAL, ERGOLOID MESYLATES
GERMA-MEDICA, HEXACHLOROPHENE
GERMA-MEDICA "MG", HEXACHLOROPHENE
GLOFIL-125, IOTHALAMATE SODIUM, I-125
GLUBATE, GLYBURIDE
GLUCAGON, GLUCAGON HYDROCHLORIDE
GLUCAMIDE, CHLORPROPAMIDE
GLUCOSCAN, TECHNETIUM TC-99M GLUCEPTATE KIT
GLUCOTROL, GLIPIZIDE
GLUTETHIMIDE, GLUTETHIMIDE
GLYCINE 1.5%, GLYCINE
GLYCINE 1.5% IN PLASTIC CONTAINER, GLYCINE
GLYCOPREP, POLYETHYLENE GLYCOL 3350
GLYCOPYRROLATE, GLYCOPYRROLATE
GLYCORT, HYDROCORTISONE
GLYNASE, GLYBURIDE
GO-EVAC, POLYETHYLENE GLYCOL 3350
GOLYTELY, POLYETHYLENE GLYCOL 3350
GRIFULVIN V, GRISEOFULVIN, MICROCRYSTALLINE
GRIS-PEG, GRISEOFULVIN, ULTRAMICROCRYSTALLINE
GRISACTIN, GRISEOFULVIN, MICROCRYSTALLINE
GRISACTIN ULTRA, GRISEOFULVIN,
    ULTRAMICROCRYSTALLINE
GUANETHIDINE MONOSULFATE, GUANETHIDINE
    MONOSULFATE
GUANIDINE HCL, GUANIDINE HYDROCHLORIDE
GVS, GENTIAN VIOLET
GYNE-LOTRIMIN, CLOTRIMAZOLE
GYNE-LOTRIMIN, CLOTRIMAZOLE (OTC)
GYNE-SULF, TRIPLE SULFA (SULFABENZAMIDE;
    SULFACETAMIDE; SULFATHIAZOLE)
GYNOREST, DYDROGESTERONE

H

H.P. ACTHAR GEL, CORTICOTROPIN
H.R.-50, HYDROCHLOROTHIAZIDE
H-CORT, HYDROCORTISONE
HABITROL, NICOTINE
HALCION, TRIAZOLAM
HALDOL, HALOPERIDOL
HALDOL, HALOPERIDOL LACTATE
HALDOL DECANOATE 50, HALOPERIDOL DECANOATE
HALDOL SOLUTAB, HALOPERIDOL
HALDRONE, PARAMETHASONE ACETATE
HALFAN, HALOFANTRINE HYDROCHLORIDE
HALODRIN, ETHINYL ESTRADIOL
HALOG, HALCINONIDE
HALOG-E, HALCINONIDE
HALOPERIDOL, HALOPERIDOL
HALOPERIDOL, HALOPERIDOL LACTATE
HALOPERIDOL INTENSOL, HALOPERIDOL LACTATE
HALOTESTIN, FLUOXYMESTERONE
HALOTEX, HALOPROGIN
HALOTHANE, HALOTHANE
HARMONYL, DESERPIDINE
HC (HYDROCORTISONE), HYDROCORTISONE
HC (HYDROCORTISONE), HYDROCORTISONE (OTC)
HC #1, HYDROCORTISONE
HC #4, HYDROCORTISONE
HEAD & SHOULDERS CONDITIONER, PYRITHIONE ZINC
    (OTC)
HEAVY SOLUTION NUPERCAINE, DIBUCAINE
    HYDROCHLORIDE

APPENDIX A
PRODUCT NAME INDEX (continued)

HEBAMATE, CARBOPROST TROMETHAMINE
HEDULIN, PHENINDIONE
HEMSOL-HC, HYDROCORTISONE ACETATE
HEP FLUSH KIT, HEPARIN SODIUM
HEP-FLUSH 10, HEPARIN SODIUM
HEP-LOCK, HEPARIN SODIUM
HEP-LOCK U/P, HEPARIN SODIUM
HEPARIN LOCK FLUSH, HEPARIN SODIUM
HEPARIN LOCK FLUSH PRESERVATIVE FREE, HEPARIN
    SODIUM
HEPARIN SODIUM, HEPARIN SODIUM
HEPARIN SODIUM PRESERVATIVE FREE, HEPARIN
    SODIUM
HEPARIN SODIUM 10,000 UNITS IN DEXTROSE 5%,
    HEPARIN SODIUM
HEPARIN SODIUM 10,000 UNITS IN DEXTROSE 5% IN
    PLASTIC CONTAINER, HEPARIN SODIUM
HEPARIN SODIUM 10,000 UNITS IN SODIUM CHLORIDE
    0.45%, HEPARIN SODIUM
HEPARIN SODIUM 10,000 UNITS IN SODIUM CHLORIDE
    0.9%, HEPARIN SODIUM
HEPARIN SODIUM 1000 UNITS AND DEXTROSE 5% IN
    PLASTIC CONTAINER, HEPARIN SODIUM
HEPARIN SODIUM 1000 UNITS AND SODIUM CHLORIDE
    0.9%, HEPARIN SODIUM
HEPARIN SODIUM 1000 UNITS IN SODIUM CHLORIDE
    0.9%, HEPARIN SODIUM
HEPARIN SODIUM 12,500 UNITS IN DEXTROSE 5%,
    HEPARIN SODIUM
HEPARIN SODIUM 12,500 UNITS IN DEXTROSE 5% IN
    PLASTIC CONTAINER, HEPARIN SODIUM
HEPARIN SODIUM 12,500 UNITS IN SODIUM CHLORIDE
    0.45%, HEPARIN SODIUM
HEPARIN SODIUM 12,500 UNITS IN SODIUM CHLORIDE
    0.9%, HEPARIN SODIUM
HEPARIN SODIUM 12500 UNITS IN SODIUM CHLORIDE
    0.45%, HEPARIN SODIUM
HEPARIN SODIUM 20,000 UNITS AND DEXTROSE 5% IN
    PLASTIC CONTAINER, HEPARIN SODIUM
HEPARIN SODIUM 20,000 UNITS IN DEXTROSE 5%,
    HEPARIN SODIUM
HEPARIN SODIUM 2000 UNITS AND SODIUM CHLORIDE
    0.9%, HEPARIN SODIUM
HEPARIN SODIUM 2000 UNITS IN DEXTROSE 5% IN
    PLASTIC CONTAINER, HEPARIN SODIUM
HEPARIN SODIUM 2000 UNITS IN SODIUM CHLORIDE
    0.9%, HEPARIN SODIUM
HEPARIN SODIUM 20000 UNITS IN DEXTROSE 5%,
    HEPARIN SODIUM
HEPARIN SODIUM 25,000 UNITS AND DEXTROSE 5%,
    HEPARIN SODIUM
HEPARIN SODIUM 25,000 UNITS IN DEXTROSE 5%,
    HEPARIN SODIUM
HEPARIN SODIUM 25,000 UNITS IN DEXTROSE 5% IN
    PLASTIC CONTAINER, HEPARIN SODIUM
HEPARIN SODIUM 25,000 UNITS IN SODIUM CHLORIDE
    0.45%, HEPARIN SODIUM
HEPARIN SODIUM 25,000 UNITS IN SODIUM CHLORIDE
    0.9%, HEPARIN SODIUM
HEPARIN SODIUM 25000 UNITS IN DEXTROSE 5%,
    HEPARIN SODIUM
HEPARIN SODIUM 25000 UNITS IN DEXTROSE 5% IN
    PLASTIC CONTAINER, HEPARIN SODIUM
HEPARIN SODIUM 25000 UNITS IN SODIUM CHLORIDE
    0.45%, HEPARIN SODIUM
HEPARIN SODIUM 25000 UNITS IN SODIUM CHLORIDE
    0.9%, HEPARIN SODIUM
HEPARIN SODIUM 5,000 UNITS IN SODIUM CHLORIDE
    0.45%, HEPARIN SODIUM
HEPARIN SODIUM 5000 UNITS AND SODIUM CHLORIDE
    0.9%, HEPARIN SODIUM
HEPARIN SODIUM 5000 UNITS IN DEXTROSE 5% IN
    PLASTIC CONTAINER, HEPARIN SODIUM

HEPARIN SODIUM 5000 UNITS IN SODIUM CHLORIDE
    0.45%, HEPARIN SODIUM
HEPARIN SODIUM 5000 UNITS IN SODIUM CHLORIDE
    0.9%, HEPARIN SODIUM
HEPATAMINE 8%, AMINO ACIDS
HEPATOLITE, TECHNETIUM TC-99M DISOFENIN KIT
HERPLEX, IDOXURIDINE
HETRAZAN, DIETHYLCARBAMAZINE CITRATE
HEXA-BETALIN, PYRIDOXINE HYDROCHLORIDE
HEXA-GERM, HEXACHLOROPHENE
HEXABRIX, IOXAGLATE MEGLUMINE
HEXADROL, DEXAMETHASONE
HEXADROL, DEXAMETHASONE SODIUM PHOSPHATE
HEXALEN, ALTRETAMINE
HEXASCRUB, HEXACHLOROPHENE
HI-COR, HYDROCORTISONE
HIBICLENS, CHLORHEXIDINE GLUCONATE (OTC)
HIBISTAT, CHLORHEXIDINE GLUCONATE (OTC)
HIBITANE, CHLORHEXIDINE GLUCONATE (OTC)
HIPPURAN I 131, IODOHIPPURATE SODIUM, I-131
HIPPUTOPE, IODOHIPPURATE SODIUM, I-131
HIPREX, METHENAMINE HIPPURATE
HISERPIA, RESERPINE
HISMANAL, ASTEMIZOLE
HISPRIL, DIPHENYLPYRALINE HYDROCHLORIDE
HISTAFED, PSEUDOEPHEDRINE HYDROCHLORIDE
HISTAFED C, CODEINE PHOSPHATE
HISTALOG, BETAZOLE HYDROCHLORIDE
HISTAMINE PHOSPHATE, HISTAMINE PHOSPHATE
HIVID, ZALCITABINE
HIWOLFIA, RAUWOLFIA SERPENTINA
HMS, MEDRYSONE
HOMAPIN-10, HOMATROPINE METHYLBROMIDE
HOMAPIN-5, HOMATROPINE METHYLBROMIDE
HUMATIN, PAROMOMYCIN SULFATE
HUMATROPE, SOMATROPIN, BIOSYNTHETIC
HUMORSOL, DEMECARIUM BROMIDE
HUMULIN BR, INSULIN BIOSYNTHETIC HUMAN (OTC)
HUMULIN L, INSULIN ZINC SUSP BIOSYNTHETIC
    HUMAN (OTC)
HUMULIN N, INSULIN SUSP ISOPHANE BIOSYNTHETIC
    HUMAN (OTC)
HUMULIN R, INSULIN BIOSYNTHETIC HUMAN (OTC)
HUMULIN U, INSULIN ZINC SUSP EXTENDED
    BIOSYNTHETIC HUMAN (OTC)
HUMULIN 50/50, INSULIN BIOSYNTHETIC HUMAN (OTC)
HUMULIN 70/30, INSULIN BIOSYNTHETIC HUMAN (OTC)
HY-PAM, HYDROXYZINE PAMOATE
HY-PAM "25", HYDROXYZINE PAMOATE
HY-PHEN, ACETAMINOPHEN
HYCODAN, HOMATROPINE METHYLBROMIDE
HYCOMINE, HYDROCODONE BITARTRATE
HYCOMINE PEDIATRIC, HYDROCODONE BITARTRATE
HYCOPAP, ACETAMINOPHEN
HYDELTRA-TBA, PREDNISOLONE TEBUTATE
HYDELTRASOL, PREDNISOLONE SODIUM PHOSPHATE
HYDERGINE, ERGOLOID MESYLATES
HYDERGINE LC, ERGOLOID MESYLATES
HYDRA-ZIDE, HYDRALAZINE HYDROCHLORIDE
HYDRALAZINE AND HYDROCHLORTHIAZIDE,
    HYDRALAZINE HYDROCHLORIDE
HYDRALAZINE HCL, HYDRALAZINE HYDROCHLORIDE
HYDRALAZINE HCL AND HYDROCHLOROTHIAZIDE,
    HYDRALAZINE HYDROCHLORIDE
HYDRALAZINE HCL W/ HYDROCHLOROTHIAZIDE 100/50,
    HYDRALAZINE HYDROCHLORIDE
HYDRALAZINE HCL W/ HYDROCHLOROTHIAZIDE 25/25,
    HYDRALAZINE HYDROCHLORIDE
HYDRALAZINE HCL W/ HYDROCHLOROTHIAZIDE 50/50,
    HYDRALAZINE HYDROCHLORIDE
HYDRALAZINE HCL-HYDROCHLOROTHIAZIDE-
    RESERPINE, HYDRALAZINE HYDROCHLORIDE

APPENDIX A
PRODUCT NAME INDEX (continued)

HYDRALAZINE HCL, HYDROCHLOROTHIAZIDE AND
   RESERPINE, HYDRALAZINE HYDROCHLORIDE
HYDRALAZINE, HYDROCHLOROTHIAZIDE W/
   RESERPINE, HYDRALAZINE HYDROCHLORIDE
HYDRAMINE, DIPHENHYDRAMINE HYDROCHLORIDE
HYDRAMINE, DIPHENHYDRAMINE HYDROCHLORIDE
   (OTC)
HYDRAP-ES, HYDRALAZINE HYDROCHLORIDE
HYDREA, HYDROXYUREA
HYDRO-D, HYDROCHLOROTHIAZIDE
HYDRO-RESERP, HYDROCHLOROTHIAZIDE
HYDRO-RIDE, AMILORIDE HYDROCHLORIDE
HYDRO-SERP "25", HYDROCHLOROTHIAZIDE
HYDRO-SERP "50", HYDROCHLOROTHIAZIDE
HYDROCET, ACETAMINOPHEN
HYDROCHLOROTHIAZIDE, HYDROCHLOROTHIAZIDE
HYDROCHLOROTHIAZIDE INTENSOL,
   HYDROCHLOROTHIAZIDE
HYDROCHLOROTHIAZIDE W/ HYDRALAZINE,
   HYDRALAZINE HYDROCHLORIDE
HYDROCHLOROTHIAZIDE W/ RESERPINE,
   HYDROCHLOROTHIAZIDE
HYDROCHLOROTHIAZIDE W/ RESERPINE AND
   HYDRALAZINE, HYDRALAZINE HYDROCHLORIDE
HYDROCODONE BITARTRATE AND ACETAMINOPHEN,
   ACETAMINOPHEN
HYDROCODONE BITARTRATE W/ ACETAMINOPHEN,
   ACETAMINOPHEN
HYDROCODONE COMPOUND, HOMATROPINE
   METHYLBROMIDE
HYDROCORTISONE, HYDROCORTISONE
HYDROCORTISONE ACETATE, HYDROCORTISONE
   ACETATE
HYDROCORTISONE ACETATE 1% AND PRAMOXINE HCL
   1%, HYDROCORTISONE ACETATE
HYDROCORTISONE AND ACETIC ACID, ACETIC ACID,
   GLACIAL
HYDROCORTISONE IN ABSORBASE, HYDROCORTISONE
HYDROCORTISONE SODIUM PHOSPHATE,
   HYDROCORTISONE SODIUM PHOSPHATE
HYDROCORTISONE SODIUM SUCCINATE,
   HYDROCORTISONE SODIUM SUCCINATE
HYDROCORTONE, HYDROCORTISONE
HYDROCORTONE, HYDROCORTISONE ACETATE
HYDROCORTONE, HYDROCORTISONE SODIUM
   PHOSPHATE
HYDRODIURIL, HYDROCHLOROTHIAZIDE
HYDROFLUMETHIAZIDE, HYDROFLUMETHIAZIDE
HYDROFLUMETHIAZIDE AND RESERPINE,
   HYDROFLUMETHIAZIDE
HYDROFLUMETHIAZIDE W/ RESERPINE,
   HYDROFLUMETHIAZIDE
HYDROGENATED ERGOT ALKALOIDS, ERGOLOID
   MESYLATES
HYDROMOX, QUINETHAZONE
HYDROMOX R, QUINETHAZONE
HYDROPANE, HOMATROPINE METHYLBROMIDE
HYDROPRES 25, HYDROCHLOROTHIAZIDE
HYDROPRES 50, HYDROCHLOROTHIAZIDE
HYDROSERPINE PLUS (R-H-H), HYDRALAZINE
   HYDROCHLORIDE
HYDROXOCOBALAMIN, HYDROXOCOBALAMIN
HYDROXOMIN, HYDROXOCOBALAMIN
HYDROXYPROGESTERONE CAPROATE,
   HYDROXYPROGESTERONE CAPROATE
HYDROXYSTILBAMIDINE ISETHIONATE,
   HYDROXYSTILBAMIDINE ISETHIONATE
HYDROXYZINE, HYDROXYZINE HYDROCHLORIDE
HYDROXYZINE HCL, HYDROXYZINE HYDROCHLORIDE
HYDROXYZINE PAMOATE, HYDROXYZINE PAMOATE
HYGROTON, CHLORTHALIDONE
HYLOREL, GUANADREL SULFATE

HYMAC, HYDROCORTISONE
HYPAQUE, DIATRIZOATE MEGLUMINE
HYPAQUE, DIATRIZOATE SODIUM
HYPAQUE SODIUM 20%, DIATRIZOATE SODIUM
HYPAQUE-CYSTO, DIATRIZOATE MEGLUMINE
HYPAQUE-M,75%, DIATRIZOATE MEGLUMINE
HYPAQUE-M,90%, DIATRIZOATE MEGLUMINE
HYPAQUE-76, DIATRIZOATE MEGLUMINE
HYPERSTAT, DIAZOXIDE
HYPROTIGEN 5%, PROTEIN HYDROLYSATE
HYSERPIN, RAUWOLFIA SERPENTINA
HYTONE, HYDROCORTISONE
HYTRIN, TERAZOSIN HYDROCHLORIDE
HYZYD, ISONIAZID

I

IBRIN, FIBRINOGEN, I-125
IBU-TAB, IBUPROFEN
IBU-TAB 200, IBUPROFEN (OTC)
IBUPRIN, IBUPROFEN (OTC)
IBUPROFEN, IBUPROFEN
IBUPROFEN, IBUPROFEN (OTC)
IBUPROHM, IBUPROFEN
IDAMYCIN, IDARUBICIN HYDROCHLORIDE
IFEN, IBUPROFEN
IFEX, IFOSFAMIDE
ILETIN I, INSULIN PORK
ILETIN II, INSULIN PURIFIED PORK
ILOSONE, ERYTHROMYCIN ESTOLATE
ILOSONE SULFA, ERYTHROMYCIN ESTOLATE
ILOTYCIN, ERYTHROMYCIN
ILOTYCIN GLUCEPTATE, ERYTHROMYCIN GLUCEPTATE
IMFERON, IRON DEXTRAN
IMIPRAMINE HCL, IMIPRAMINE HYDROCHLORIDE
IMODIUM, LOPERAMIDE HYDROCHLORIDE
IMODIUM A-D, LOPERAMIDE HYDROCHLORIDE (OTC)
IMURAN, AZATHIOPRINE
IMURAN, AZATHIOPRINE SODIUM
INAPSINE, DROPERIDOL
INDERAL, PROPRANOLOL HYDROCHLORIDE
INDERAL LA, PROPRANOLOL HYDROCHLORIDE
INDERIDE LA 120/50, HYDROCHLOROTHIAZIDE
INDERIDE LA 160/50, HYDROCHLOROTHIAZIDE
INDERIDE LA 80/50, HYDROCHLOROTHIAZIDE
INDERIDE-40/25, HYDROCHLOROTHIAZIDE
INDERIDE-80/25, HYDROCHLOROTHIAZIDE
INDIUM IN-111 OXYQUINOLINE, INDIUM IN-111
   OXYQUINOLINE
INDO-LEMMON, INDOMETHACIN
INDOCIN, INDOMETHACIN
INDOCIN I.V., INDOMETHACIN SODIUM
INDOCIN SR, INDOMETHACIN
INDOMETHACIN, INDOMETHACIN
INDOMETHEGAN, INDOMETHACIN
INFLAMASE FORTE, PREDNISOLONE SODIUM
   PHOSPHATE
INFLAMASE MILD, PREDNISOLONE SODIUM PHOSPHATE
INFUMORPH, MORPHINE SULFATE
INH, ISONIAZID
INJECTAPAP, ACETAMINOPHEN
INNOVAR, DROPERIDOL
INOCOR, AMRINONE LACTATE
INPERSOL W/ DEXTROSE 1.5%, CALCIUM CHLORIDE
INPERSOL W/ DEXTROSE 2.5% IN PLASTIC CONTAINER,
   CALCIUM CHLORIDE
INPERSOL W/ DEXTROSE 3.5%, CALCIUM CHLORIDE
INPERSOL W/ DEXTROSE 4.25%, CALCIUM CHLORIDE
INPERSOL-LM W/ DEXTROSE 1.5%, CALCIUM CHLORIDE
INPERSOL-LM W/ DEXTROSE 2.5%, CALCIUM CHLORIDE

APPENDIX A
PRODUCT NAME INDEX (continued)

INPERSOL-LM W/ DEXTROSE 3.5%, CALCIUM CHLORIDE
INPERSOL-LM W/ DEXTROSE 4.25%, CALCIUM CHLORIDE
INPERSOL-ZM W/ DEXTROSE 1.5% IN PLASTIC
  CONTAINER, CALCIUM CHLORIDE
INPERSOL-ZM W/ DEXTROSE 2.5% IN PLASTIC
  CONTAINER, CALCIUM CHLORIDE
INPERSOL-ZM W/ DEXTROSE 4.25% IN PLASTIC
  CONTAINER, CALCIUM CHLORIDE
INSTANT MICROSPHERES, TECHNETIUM TC-99M
  ALBUMIN MICROSPHERES KIT
INSULATARD NPH HUMAN, INSULIN SUSP ISOPHANE
  SEMISYNTHETIC PURIFIED HUMAN (OTC)
INSULIN, INSULIN PORK (OTC)
INSULIN INSULATARD NPH NORDISK, INSULIN SUSP
  ISOPHANE PURIFIED PORK (OTC)
INSULIN NORDISK MIXTARD (PORK), INSULIN PURIFIED
  PORK (OTC)
INTAL, CROMOLYN SODIUM
INTRALIPID 10%, SOYBEAN OIL
INTRALIPID 20%, SOYBEAN OIL
INTROPIN, DOPAMINE HYDROCHLORIDE
INULIN AND SODIUM CHLORIDE, INULIN
INVERSINE, MECAMYLAMINE HYDROCHLORIDE
IODOHIPPURATE SODIUM I 131, IODOHIPPURATE
  SODIUM, I-131
IODOTOPE, SODIUM IODIDE, I-131
IONAMIN-15, PHENTERMINE RESIN COMPLEX
IONAMIN-30, PHENTERMINE RESIN COMPLEX
IONOSOL B AND DEXTROSE 5%, DEXTROSE
IONOSOL MB AND DEXTROSE 5%, DEXTROSE
IONOSOL T AND DEXTROSE 5%, DEXTROSE
IOPIDINE, APRACLONIDINE HYDROCHLORIDE
IOSAT, POTASSIUM IODIDE (OTC)
IRON DEXTRAN, IRON DEXTRAN
IRRIGATING SOLUTION G IN PLASTIC CONTAINER,
  CITRIC ACID
ISMELIN, GUANETHIDINE MONOSULFATE
ISMO, ISOSORBIDE MONONITRATE
ISMOTIC, ISOSORBIDE
ISOCAINE HCL, MEPIVACAINE HYDROCHLORIDE
ISOCAINE HCL W/ LEVONORDEFRIN, LEVONORDEFRIN
ISOCLOR, CHLORPHENIRAMINE MALEATE (OTC)
ISOETHARINE HCL, ISOETHARINE HYDROCHLORIDE
ISOETHARINE HCL S/F, ISOETHARINE HYDROCHLORIDE
ISOETHARINE MESYLATE, ISOETHARINE MESYLATE
ISOLYTE E, CALCIUM CHLORIDE
ISOLYTE E IN PLASTIC CONTAINER, CALCIUM
  CHLORIDE
ISOLYTE E W/ DEXTROSE 5% IN PLASTIC CONTAINER,
  CALCIUM CHLORIDE
ISOLYTE H W/ DEXTROSE 5% IN PLASTIC CONTAINER,
  DEXTROSE
ISOLYTE M W/ DEXTROSE 5% IN PLASTIC CONTAINER,
  DEXTROSE
ISOLYTE P W/ DEXTROSE 5% IN PLASTIC CONTAINER,
  DEXTROSE
ISOLYTE R W/ DEXTROSE 5% IN PLASTIC CONTAINER,
  CALCIUM CHLORIDE
ISOLYTE S, MAGNESIUM CHLORIDE
ISOLYTE S IN PLASTIC CONTAINER, MAGNESIUM
  CHLORIDE
ISOLYTE S PH 7.4, MAGNESIUM CHLORIDE
ISOLYTE S PH 7.4 IN PLASTIC CONTAINER, MAGNESIUM
  CHLORIDE
ISOLYTE S W/ DEXTROSE 5% IN PLASTIC CONTAINER,
  DEXTROSE
ISONIAZID, ISONIAZID
ISOPAQUE 280, CALCIUM
ISOPAQUE 440, CALCIUM METRIZOATE
ISOPROTERENOL HCL, ISOPROTERENOL
  HYDROCHLORIDE
ISOPTIN, VERAPAMIL HYDROCHLORIDE

ISOPTIN SR, VERAPAMIL HYDROCHLORIDE
ISOPTO CETAMIDE, SULFACETAMIDE SODIUM
ISOPTO CETAPRED, PREDNISOLONE ACETATE
ISORDIL, ISOSORBIDE DINITRATE
ISOSORBIDE DINITRATE, ISOSORBIDE DINITRATE
ISOTONIC GENTAMICIN SULFATE IN PLASTIC
  CONTAINER, GENTAMICIN SULFATE
ISOVUE-M 200, IOPAMIDOL
ISOVUE-M 300, IOPAMIDOL
ISOVUE-128, IOPAMIDOL
ISOVUE-200, IOPAMIDOL
ISOVUE-250, IOPAMIDOL
ISOVUE-300, IOPAMIDOL
ISOVUE-370, IOPAMIDOL
ISUPREL, ISOPROTERENOL HYDROCHLORIDE
IV PERSANTINE, DIPYRIDAMOLE
IVADANTIN, NITROFURANTOIN SODIUM

J

JANIMINE, IMIPRAMINE HYDROCHLORIDE

K

K+10, POTASSIUM CHLORIDE
K-DUR 10, POTASSIUM CHLORIDE
K-DUR 20, POTASSIUM CHLORIDE
K-LEASE, POTASSIUM CHLORIDE
K-TAB, POTASSIUM CHLORIDE
KAFOCIN, CEPHALOGLYCIN
KAINAIR, PROPARACAINE HYDROCHLORIDE
KANAMYCIN, KANAMYCIN SULFATE
KANAMYCIN SULFATE, KANAMYCIN SULFATE
KANTREX, KANAMYCIN SULFATE
KAON CL, POTASSIUM CHLORIDE
KAON CL-10, POTASSIUM CHLORIDE
KAPPADIONE, MENADIOL SODIUM DIPHOSPHATE
KAYEXALATE, SODIUM POLYSTYRENE SULFONATE
KEFLET, CEPHALEXIN
KEFLEX, CEPHALEXIN
KEFLIN, CEPHALOTHIN SODIUM
KEFTAB, CEPHALEXIN HYDROCHLORIDE
KEFUROX, CEFUROXIME SODIUM
KEFUROX IN PLASTIC CONTAINER, CEFUROXIME
  SODIUM
KEFZOL, CEFAZOLIN SODIUM
KEMADRIN, PROCYCLIDINE HYDROCHLORIDE
KENACORT, TRIAMCINOLONE
KENACORT, TRIAMCINOLONE DIACETATE
KENALOG, TRIAMCINOLONE ACETONIDE
KENALOG IN ORABASE, TRIAMCINOLONE ACETONIDE
KENALOG-H, TRIAMCINOLONE ACETONIDE
KENALOG-10, TRIAMCINOLONE ACETONIDE
KENALOG-40, TRIAMCINOLONE ACETONIDE
KERLONE, BETAXOLOL HYDROCHLORIDE
KESSO-GESIC, PROPOXYPHENE HYDROCHLORIDE
KETALAR, KETAMINE HYDROCHLORIDE
KETAMINE HCL, KETAMINE HYDROCHLORIDE
KINEVAC, SINCALIDE
KLEBCIL, KANAMYCIN SULFATE
KLONOPIN, CLONAZEPAM
KLOR-CON, POTASSIUM CHLORIDE
KLOROMIN, CHLORPHENIRAMINE MALEATE
KLOTRIX, POTASSIUM CHLORIDE
KOGLUCOID, RAUWOLFIA SERPENTINA
KONAKION, PHYTONADIONE
KOROSTATIN, NYSTATIN
KWELL, LINDANE

APPENDIX A
PRODUCT NAME INDEX (continued)

L

LABID, THEOPHYLLINE
LAC-HYDRIN, AMMONIUM LACTATE
LACRISERT, HYDROXYPROPYL CELLULOSE
LACTATED RINGER'S, CALCIUM CHLORIDE
LACTATED RINGER'S AND DEXTROSE 5% IN PLASTIC
    CONTAINER, CALCIUM CHLORIDE
LACTATED RINGER'S IN PLASTIC CONTAINER, CALCIUM
    CHLORIDE
LACTULOSE, LACTULOSE
LAMPRENE, CLOFAZIMINE
LANABIOTIC, BACITRACIN (OTC)
LANABIOTIC, BACITRACIN ZINC (OTC)
LANIAZID, ISONIAZID
LANOPHYLLIN, THEOPHYLLINE
LANORINAL, ASPIRIN
LANOXICAPS, DIGOXIN
LANOXIN, DIGOXIN
LANTRISUL, TRISULFAPYRIMIDINES
LARGON, PROPIOMAZINE HYDROCHLORIDE
LARIAM, MEFLOQUINE HYDROCHLORIDE
LARODOPA, LEVODOPA
LAROTID, AMOXICILLIN
LARYNG-O-JET KIT, LIDOCAINE HYDROCHLORIDE
LARYNGOTRACHEAL ANESTHESIA KIT, LIDOCAINE
    HYDROCHLORIDE
LASIX, FUROSEMIDE
LEDERCILLIN VK, PENICILLIN V POTASSIUM
LENTARD, INSULIN ZINC SUSP PURIFIED BEEF/PORK
    (OTC)
LENTE, INSULIN ZINC SUSP PURIFIED PORK (OTC)
LENTE ILETIN II, INSULIN ZINC SUSP PURIFIED BEEF
    (OTC)
LENTE ILETIN II (PORK), INSULIN ZINC SUSP PURIFIED
    PORK (OTC)
LENTE INSULIN, INSULIN ZINC SUSP BEEF (OTC)
LERITINE, ANILERIDINE HYDROCHLORIDE
LERITINE, ANILERIDINE PHOSPHATE
LEUCOVORIN CALCIUM, LEUCOVORIN CALCIUM
LEUKERAN, CHLORAMBUCIL
LEVATOL, PENBUTOLOL SULFATE
LEVO-DROMORAN, LEVORPHANOL TARTRATE
LEVOPHED, NOREPINEPHRINE BITARTRATE
LEVOPROME, METHOTRIMEPRAZINE
LIBRELEASE, CHLORDIAZEPOXIDE
LIBRITABS, CHLORDIAZEPOXIDE
LIBRIUM, CHLORDIAZEPOXIDE HYDROCHLORIDE
LIDEX, FLUOCINONIDE
LIDEX-E, FLUOCINONIDE
LIDOCAINE, LIDOCAINE
LIDOCAINE HCL, LIDOCAINE HYDROCHLORIDE
LIDOCAINE HCL AND DEXTROSE 7.5%, LIDOCAINE
    HYDROCHLORIDE
LIDOCAINE HCL AND EPINEPHRINE, EPINEPHRINE
LIDOCAINE HCL IN PLASTIC CONTAINER, LIDOCAINE
    HYDROCHLORIDE
LIDOCAINE HCL VISCOUS, LIDOCAINE
    HYDROCHLORIDE
LIDOCAINE HCL W/ EPINEPHRINE, EPINEPHRINE
LIDOCAINE HCL 0.1% AND DEXTROSE 5% IN PLASTIC
    CONTAINER, LIDOCAINE HYDROCHLORIDE
LIDOCAINE HCL 0.2% AND DEXTROSE 5%, LIDOCAINE
    HYDROCHLORIDE
LIDOCAINE HCL 0.2% AND DEXTROSE 5% IN PLASTIC
    CONTAINER, LIDOCAINE HYDROCHLORIDE
LIDOCAINE HCL 0.2% IN DEXTROSE 5%, LIDOCAINE
    HYDROCHLORIDE
LIDOCAINE HCL 0.2% IN DEXTROSE 5% IN PLASTIC
    CONTAINER, LIDOCAINE HYDROCHLORIDE
LIDOCAINE HCL 0.4% AND DEXTROSE 5%, LIDOCAINE
    HYDROCHLORIDE

LIDOCAINE HCL 0.4% AND DEXTROSE 5% IN PLASTIC
    CONTAINER, LIDOCAINE HYDROCHLORIDE
LIDOCAINE HCL 0.4% IN DEXTROSE 5%, LIDOCAINE
    HYDROCHLORIDE
LIDOCAINE HCL 0.4% IN DEXTROSE 5% IN PLASTIC
    CONTAINER, LIDOCAINE HYDROCHLORIDE
LIDOCAINE HCL 0.8% AND DEXTROSE 5%, LIDOCAINE
    HYDROCHLORIDE
LIDOCAINE HCL 0.8% AND DEXTROSE 5% IN PLASTIC
    CONTAINER, LIDOCAINE HYDROCHLORIDE
LIDOCAINE HCL 0.8% IN DEXTROSE 5% IN PLASTIC
    CONTAINER, LIDOCAINE HYDROCHLORIDE
LIDOCAINE VISCOUS, LIDOCAINE HYDROCHLORIDE
LIDOCATON, EPINEPHRINE
LIDOCATON, LIDOCAINE HYDROCHLORIDE
LIDOPEN, LIDOCAINE HYDROCHLORIDE
LIGNOSPAN FORTE, EPINEPHRINE BITARTRATE
LIGNOSPAN STANDARD, EPINEPHRINE BITARTRATE
LIMBITROL, AMITRIPTYLINE HYDROCHLORIDE
LINCOCIN, LINCOMYCIN HYDROCHLORIDE
LINCOMYCIN HCL, LINCOMYCIN HYDROCHLORIDE
LINDANE, LINDANE
LIORESAL, BACLOFEN
LIOTHYRONINE SODIUM, LIOTHYRONINE SODIUM
LIPO GANTRISIN, SULFISOXAZOLE ACETYL
LIPO-HEPIN, HEPARIN SODIUM
LIPOSYN II 10%, SAFFLOWER OIL
LIPOSYN II 20%, SAFFLOWER OIL
LIPOSYN III 10%, SOYBEAN OIL
LIPOSYN III 20%, SOYBEAN OIL
LIPOSYN 10%, SAFFLOWER OIL
LIPOSYN 20%, SAFFLOWER OIL
LIQUAEMIN LOCK FLUSH, HEPARIN SODIUM
LIQUAEMIN SODIUM, HEPARIN SODIUM
LIQUAEMIN SODIUM PRESERVATIVE FREE, HEPARIN
    SODIUM
LIQUAMAR, PHENPROCOUMON
LIQUID PRED, PREDNISONE
LITHANE, LITHIUM CARBONATE
LITHIUM CARBONATE, LITHIUM CARBONATE
LITHIUM CITRATE, LITHIUM CITRATE
LITHOBID, LITHIUM CARBONATE
LITHONATE, LITHIUM CARBONATE
LITHOSTAT, ACETOHYDROXAMIC ACID
LITHOTABS, LITHIUM CARBONATE
LO-TROL, ATROPINE SULFATE
LO/OVRAL, ETHINYL ESTRADIOL
LO/OVRAL-28, ETHINYL ESTRADIOL
LOCOID, HYDROCORTISONE BUTYRATE
LOCORTEN, FLUMETHASONE PIVALATE
LODINE, ETODOLAC
LODOSYN, CARBIDOPA
LOESTRIN FE 1.5/30, ETHINYL ESTRADIOL
LOESTRIN FE 1/20, ETHINYL ESTRADIOL
LOESTRIN 21 1.5/30, ETHINYL ESTRADIOL
LOESTRIN 21 1/20, ETHINYL ESTRADIOL
LOFENE, ATROPINE SULFATE
LOGEN, ATROPINE SULFATE
LOMANATE, ATROPINE SULFATE
LOMOTIL, ATROPINE SULFATE
LONITEN, MINOXIDIL
LONOX, ATROPINE SULFATE
LOPERAMIDE HCL, LOPERAMIDE HYDROCHLORIDE
LOPERAMIDE HCL, LOPERAMIDE HYDROCHLORIDE
    (OTC)
LOPID, GEMFIBROZIL
LOPRESSIDONE, CHLORTHALIDONE
LOPRESSOR, METOPROLOL FUMARATE
LOPRESSOR, METOPROLOL TARTRATE
LOPRESSOR HCT 100/25, HYDROCHLOROTHIAZIDE
LOPRESSOR HCT 100/50, HYDROCHLOROTHIAZIDE
LOPRESSOR HCT 50/25, HYDROCHLOROTHIAZIDE

APPENDIX A
PRODUCT NAME INDEX *(continued)*

LOPROX, CICLOPIROX OLAMINE
LOPURIN, ALLOPURINOL
LORABID, LORACARBEF
LORAZ, LORAZEPAM
LORAZEPAM, LORAZEPAM
LORAZEPAM INTENSOL, LORAZEPAM
LORELCO, PROBUCOL
LORFAN, LEVALLORPHAN TARTRATE
LOTENSIN, BENAZEPRIL HYDROCHLORIDE
LOTENSIN HCT, BENAZEPRIL HYDROCHLORIDE
LOTRIMIN, CLOTRIMAZOLE
LOTRIMIN AF, CLOTRIMAZOLE (OTC)
LOTRISONE, BETAMETHASONE DIPROPIONATE
LOTUSATE, TALBUTAL
LOW-QUEL, ATROPINE SULFATE
LOXAPINE SUCCINATE, LOXAPINE SUCCINATE
LOXITANE, LOXAPINE SUCCINATE
LOXITANE C, LOXAPINE HYDROCHLORIDE
LOXITANE IM, LOXAPINE HYDROCHLORIDE
LOZOL, INDAPAMIDE
LTA II KIT, LIDOCAINE HYDROCHLORIDE
LUDIOMIL, MAPROTILINE HYDROCHLORIDE
LUFYLLIN, DYPHYLLINE
LUNGAGGREGATE REAGENT, TECHNETIUM TC-99M
    ALBUMIN AGGREGATED KIT
LUPRON, LEUPROLIDE ACETATE
LUPRON DEPOT, LEUPROLIDE ACETATE
LUTREPULSE PUMP KIT, GONADORELIN ACETATE
LYGEN, CHLORDIAZEPOXIDE HYDROCHLORIDE
LYMPHAZURIN, ISOSULFAN BLUE
LYNORAL, ETHINYL ESTRADIOL
LYOPHILIZED CYTOXAN, CYCLOPHOSPHAMIDE
LYPHOCIN, VANCOMYCIN HYDROCHLORIDE
LYSODREN, MITOTANE

M

M.V.C. 9+3, ASCORBIC ACID
M.V.I.-12, ASCORBIC ACID
M.V.I.-12 LYOPHILIZED, ASCORBIC ACID
M-PREDROL, METHYLPREDNISOLONE ACETATE
MACROBID, NITROFURANTOIN
MACRODANTIN, NITROFURANTOIN,
    MACROCRYSTALLINE
MACROTEC, TECHNETIUM TC-99M ALBUMIN
    AGGREGATED KIT
MAGNACORT, HYDROCORTAMATE HYDROCHLORIDE
MAGNESIUM SULFATE, MAGNESIUM SULFATE
MAGNEVIST, GADOPENTETATE DIMEGLUMINE
MANDOL, CEFAMANDOLE NAFATE
MANGANESE CHLORIDE, MANGANESE CHLORIDE
MANGANESE SULFATE, MANGANESE SULFATE
MANNITOL 10%, MANNITOL
MANNITOL 10% W/ DEXTROSE 5% IN DISTILLED WATER,
    MANNITOL
MANNITOL 15%, MANNITOL
MANNITOL 15% W/ DEXTROSE 5% IN SODIUM CHLORIDE
    0.45%, MANNITOL
MANNITOL 20%, MANNITOL
MANNITOL 25%, MANNITOL
MANNITOL 5%, MANNITOL
MANNITOL 5% W/ DEXTROSE 5% IN SODIUM CHLORIDE
    0.12%, MANNITOL
MAOLATE, CHLORPHENESIN CARBAMATE
MAPROTILINE HCL, MAPROTILINE HYDROCHLORIDE
MARCAINE, BUPIVACAINE HYDROCHLORIDE
MARCAINE HCL, BUPIVACAINE HYDROCHLORIDE
MARCAINE HCL W/ EPINEPHRINE, BUPIVACAINE
    HYDROCHLORIDE
MAREZINE, CYCLIZINE LACTATE

MARINOL, DRONABINOL
MATULANE, PROCARBAZINE HYDROCHLORIDE
MAXAIR, PIRBUTEROL ACETATE
MAXAQUIN, LOMEFLOXACIN HYDROCHLORIDE
MAXIBOLIN, ETHYLESTRENOL
MAXIDEX, DEXAMETHASONE
MAXIDEX, DEXAMETHASONE SODIUM PHOSPHATE
MAXITROL, DEXAMETHASONE
MAXOLON, METOCLOPRAMIDE HYDROCHLORIDE
MAXZIDE, HYDROCHLOROTHIAZIDE
MAXZIDE-25, HYDROCHLOROTHIAZIDE
MAZANOR, MAZINDOL
MAZICON, FLUMAZENIL
MD-GASTROVIEW, DIATRIZOATE MEGLUMINE
MD-50, DIATRIZOATE SODIUM
MD-60, DIATRIZOATE MEGLUMINE
MD-76, DIATRIZOATE MEGLUMINE
MDP-SQUIBB, TECHNETIUM TC-99M MEDRONATE KIT
MEASURIN, ASPIRIN (OTC)
MECLAN, MECLOCYCLINE SULFOSALICYLATE
MECLIZINE HCL, MECLIZINE HYDROCHLORIDE
MECLODIUM, MECLOFENAMATE SODIUM
MECLOFENAMATE SODIUM, MECLOFENAMATE SODIUM
MECLOMEN, MECLOFENAMATE SODIUM
MEDIGESIC PLUS, ACETAMINOPHEN
MEDIHALER ERGOTAMINE, ERGOTAMINE TARTRATE
MEDIHALER-EPI, EPINEPHRINE BITARTRATE (OTC)
MEDIHALER-ISO, ISOPROTERENOL SULFATE
MEDIPREN, IBUPROFEN (OTC)
MEDROL, METHYLPREDNISOLONE
MEDROL, METHYLPREDNISOLONE ACETATE
MEDROL ACETATE, METHYLPREDNISOLONE ACETATE
MEDROXYPROGESTERONE ACETATE,
    MEDROXYPROGESTERONE ACETATE
MEFENAMIC ACID, MEFENAMIC ACID
MEFLOQUINE HCL, MEFLOQUINE HYDROCHLORIDE
MEFOXIN, CEFOXITIN SODIUM
MEFOXIN IN DEXTROSE 5% IN PLASTIC CONTAINER,
    CEFOXITIN SODIUM
MEFOXIN IN SODIUM CHLORIDE 0.9% IN PLASTIC
    CONTAINER, CEFOXITIN SODIUM
MEGACE, MEGESTROL ACETATE
MEGATOPE, ALBUMIN IODINATED I-131 SERUM
MEGESTROL ACETATE, MEGESTROL ACETATE
MELFIAT, PHENDIMETRAZINE TARTRATE
MELFIAT-105, PHENDIMETRAZINE TARTRATE
MELLARIL, THIORIDAZINE HYDROCHLORIDE
MELLARIL-S, THIORIDAZINE
MENADIONE, MENADIONE
MENEST, ESTROGENS, ESTERIFIED
MENRIUM 10-4, CHLORDIAZEPOXIDE
MENRIUM 5-2, CHLORDIAZEPOXIDE
MENRIUM 5-4, CHLORDIAZEPOXIDE
MEPERGAN, MEPERIDINE HYDROCHLORIDE
MEPERIDINE AND ATROPINE SULFATE, ATROPINE
    SULFATE
MEPERIDINE HCL, MEPERIDINE HYDROCHLORIDE
MEPHYTON, PHYTONADIONE
MEPIVACAINE HCL, MEPIVACAINE HYDROCHLORIDE
MEPIVACAINE HCL W/ LEVONORDEFRIN,
    LEVONORDEFRIN
MEPRIAM, MEPROBAMATE
MEPRO-ASPIRIN, ASPIRIN
MEPROBAMATE, MEPROBAMATE
MEPROBAMATE AND ASPIRIN, ASPIRIN
MEPROSPAN, MEPROBAMATE
MERSALYL-THEOPHYLLINE, MERSALYL SODIUM
MESANTOIN, MEPHENYTOIN
MESNEX, MESNA
MESTINON, PYRIDOSTIGMINE BROMIDE
METAHYDRIN, TRICHLORMETHIAZIDE
METANDREN, METHYLTESTOSTERONE

APPENDIX A
PRODUCT NAME INDEX (continued)

METAPROTERENOL SULFATE, METAPROTERENOL
  SULFATE
METARAMINOL BITARTRATE, METARAMINOL
  BITARTRATE
METATENSIN #2, RESERPINE
METATENSIN #4, RESERPINE
METHADONE HCL, METHADONE HYDROCHLORIDE
METHADONE HCL INTENSOL, METHADONE
  HYDROCHLORIDE
METHADOSE, METHADONE HYDROCHLORIDE
METHAMPEX, METHAMPHETAMINE HYDROCHLORIDE
METHAMPHETAMINE HCL, METHAMPHETAMINE
  HYDROCHLORIDE
METHDILAZINE HCL, METHDILAZINE HYDROCHLORIDE
METHERGINE, METHYLERGONOVINE MALEATE
METHOCARBAMOL, METHOCARBAMOL
METHOCARBAMOL AND ASPIRIN, ASPIRIN
METHOTREXATE, METHOTREXATE SODIUM
METHOTREXATE LPF, METHOTREXATE SODIUM
METHOTREXATE SODIUM, METHOTREXATE SODIUM
METHOXSALEN, METHOXSALEN
METHSCOPOLAMINE BROMIDE, METHSCOPOLAMINE
  BROMIDE
METHYCLOTHIAZIDE, METHYCLOTHIAZIDE
METHYCLOTHIAZIDE AND DESERPIDINE, DESERPIDINE
METHYLDOPA, METHYLDOPA
METHYLDOPA AND CHLOROTHIAZIDE,
  CHLOROTHIAZIDE
METHYLDOPA AND HYDROCHLOROTHIAZIDE,
  HYDROCHLOROTHIAZIDE
METHYLDOPATE HCL, METHYLDOPATE
  HYDROCHLORIDE
METHYLPHENIDATE HCL, METHYLPHENIDATE
  HYDROCHLORIDE
METHYLPREDNISOLONE, METHYLPREDNISOLONE
METHYLPREDNISOLONE, METHYLPREDNISOLONE
  SODIUM SUCCINATE
METHYLPREDNISOLONE ACETATE,
  METHYLPREDNISOLONE ACETATE
METHYLPREDNISOLONE SODIUM SUCCINATE,
  METHYLPREDNISOLONE SODIUM SUCCINATE
METHYLTESTOSTERONE, METHYLTESTOSTERONE
METI-DERM, PREDNISOLONE
METICORTELONE, PREDNISOLONE ACETATE
METICORTEN, PREDNISONE
METIMYD, PREDNISOLONE ACETATE
METOCLOPRAMIDE HCL, METOCLOPRAMIDE
  HYDROCHLORIDE
METOCLOPRAMIDE INTENSOL, METOCLOPRAMIDE
  HYDROCHLORIDE
METOCURINE IODIDE, METOCURINE IODIDE
METOPIRONE, METYRAPONE
METRA, PHENDIMETRAZINE TARTRATE
METRETON, PREDNISOLONE SODIUM PHOSPHATE
METRO I.V., METRONIDAZOLE
METRO I.V. IN PLASTIC CONTAINER, METRONIDAZOLE
METRODIN, UROFOLLITROPIN
METROGEL, METRONIDAZOLE
METRONIDAZOLE, METRONIDAZOLE
METRONIDAZOLE HCL, METRONIDAZOLE
  HYDROCHLORIDE
METRYL, METRONIDAZOLE
METRYL 500, METRONIDAZOLE
METUBINE IODIDE, METOCURINE IODIDE
MEVACOR, LOVASTATIN
MEXATE, METHOTREXATE SODIUM
MEXATE-AQ, METHOTREXATE SODIUM
MEXATE-AQ PRESERVED, METHOTREXATE SODIUM
MEXITIL, MEXILETINE HYDROCHLORIDE
MEZLIN, MEZLOCILLIN SODIUM MONOHYDRATE
MIACALCIN, CALCITONIN, SALMON
MICRAININ, ASPIRIN

MICRO-K, POTASSIUM CHLORIDE
MICRO-K LS, POTASSIUM CHLORIDE
MICRO-K 10, POTASSIUM CHLORIDE
MICROCOL, CHLORHEXIDINE GLUCONATE (OTC)
MICRODERM, CHLORHEXIDINE GLUCONATE (OTC)
MICROLITE, TECHNETIUM TC-99M ALBUMIN COLLOID
  KIT
MICRONASE, GLYBURIDE
MICRONOR, NORETHINDRONE
MICROSUL, SULFAMETHIZOLE
MIDAMOR, AMILORIDE HYDROCHLORIDE
MIDOL, IBUPROFEN (OTC)
MILONTIN, PHENSUXIMIDE
MILOPHENE, CLOMIPHENE CITRATE
MILPREM-200, ESTROGENS, CONJUGATED
MILPREM-400, ESTROGENS, CONJUGATED
MILRINONE LACTATE, MILRINONE LACTATE
MILTOWN, MEPROBAMATE
MINIPRESS, PRAZOSIN HYDROCHLORIDE
MINIPRESS XL, PRAZOSIN HYDROCHLORIDE
MINITEC, TECHNETIUM TC-99M SODIUM
  PERTECHNETATE GENERATOR
MINIZIDE, POLYTHIAZIDE
MINOCIN, MINOCYCLINE HYDROCHLORIDE
MINOCYCLINE HCL, MINOCYCLINE HYDROCHLORIDE
MINODYL, MINOXIDIL
MINOXIDIL, MINOXIDIL
MINTEZOL, THIABENDAZOLE
MIOCHOL, ACETYLCHOLINE CHLORIDE
MIOSTAT, CARBACHOL
MIRADON, ANISINDIONE
MITHRACIN, PLICAMYCIN
MIVACRON, MIVACURIUM CHLORIDE
MIVACRON IN DEXTROSE 5%, MIVACURIUM CHLORIDE
MIXTARD HUMAN 70/30, INSULIN SEMISYNTHETIC
  PURIFIED HUMAN (OTC)
MOBAN, MOLINDONE HYDROCHLORIDE
MOCTANIN, MONOCTANOIN
MODERIL, RESCINNAMINE
MODICON 21, ETHINYL ESTRADIOL
MODICON 28, ETHINYL ESTRADIOL
MODRASTANE, TRILOSTANE
MODURETIC 5-50, AMILORIDE HYDROCHLORIDE
MONISTAT, MICONAZOLE
MONISTAT 3, MICONAZOLE NITRATE
MONISTAT 5, MICONAZOLE NITRATE
MONISTAT 7, MICONAZOLE NITRATE
MONISTAT 7, MICONAZOLE NITRATE (OTC)
MONISTAT-DERM, MICONAZOLE NITRATE
MONOCID, CEFONICID SODIUM
MONOPRIL, FOSINOPRIL SODIUM
MORPHINE SULFATE, MORPHINE SULFATE
MOTOFEN, ATROPINE SULFATE
MOTOFEN HALF-STRENGTH, ATROPINE SULFATE
MOTRIN, IBUPROFEN
MOXAM, MOXALACTAM DISODIUM
MPI DMSA KIDNEY REAGENT, TECHNETIUM TC-99M
  SUCCIMER KIT
MPI DTPA KIT - CHELATE, TECHNETIUM TC-99M
  PENTETATE KIT
MPI INDIUM DTPA IN 111, INDIUM IN-111 PENTETATE
  DISODIUM
MPI KRYPTON 81M GAS GENERATOR, KRYPTON, KR-81M
MPI STANNOUS DIPHOSPHONATE, TECHNETIUM TC-99M
  ETIDRONATE KIT
MS CONTIN, MORPHINE SULFATE
MUCOMYST, ACETYLCYSTEINE
MUCOMYST W/ ISOPROTERENOL, ACETYLCYSTEINE
MUCOSOL-10, ACETYLCYSTEINE
MUCOSOL-20, ACETYLCYSTEINE
MULTIFUGE, PIPERAZINE CITRATE
MUSTARGEN, MECHLORETHAMINE HYDROCHLORIDE

APPENDIX A
PRODUCT NAME INDEX (continued)

MUTAMYCIN, MITOMYCIN
MVC PLUS, ASCORBIC ACID
MYAMBUTOL, ETHAMBUTOL HYDROCHLORIDE
MYBANIL, BROMODIPHENHYDRAMINE
   HYDROCHLORIDE
MYCELEX, CLOTRIMAZOLE
MYCELEX, CLOTRIMAZOLE (OTC)
MYCELEX-G, CLOTRIMAZOLE
MYCELEX-7, CLOTRIMAZOLE (OTC)
MYCHEL, CHLORAMPHENICOL
MYCHEL-S, CHLORAMPHENICOL SODIUM SUCCINATE
MYCIFRADIN, NEOMYCIN SULFATE
MYCITRACIN, BACITRACIN
MYCO-TRIACET II, NYSTATIN
MYCODONE, HOMATROPINE METHYLBROMIDE
MYCOLOG-II, NYSTATIN
MYCOSTATIN, NYSTATIN
MYDRIACYL, TROPICAMIDE
MYDRIAFAIR, TROPICAMIDE
MYFED, PSEUDOEPHEDRINE HYDROCHLORIDE (OTC)
MYIDYL, TRIPROLIDINE HYDROCHLORIDE
MYKACET, NYSTATIN
MYKINAC, NYSTATIN
MYKROX, METOLAZONE
MYLARAMINE, DEXCHLORPHENIRAMINE MALEATE
MYLAXEN, HEXAFLUORENIUM BROMIDE
MYLERAN, BUSULFAN
MYLOCAINE, LIDOCAINE HYDROCHLORIDE
MYMETHASONE, DEXAMETHASONE
MYMETHAZINE FORTIS, PROMETHAZINE
   HYDROCHLORIDE
MYOTONACHOL, BETHANECHOL CHLORIDE
MYPHETANE DC, BROMPHENIRAMINE MALEATE
MYPHETANE DX, BROMPHENIRAMINE MALEATE
MYPROIC ACID, VALPROIC ACID
MYSOLINE, PRIMIDONE
MYTELASE, AMBENONIUM CHLORIDE
MYTREX A, NEOMYCIN SULFATE
MYTREX F, NYSTATIN

N

N.E.E. 1/35 21, ETHINYL ESTRADIOL
N.E.E. 1/35 28, ETHINYL ESTRADIOL
NAFAZAIR, NAPHAZOLINE HYDROCHLORIDE
NAFCIL, NAFCILLIN SODIUM
NAFCILLIN SODIUM, NAFCILLIN SODIUM
NAFTIN, NAFTIFINE HYDROCHLORIDE
NALBUPHINE, NALBUPHINE HYDROCHLORIDE
NALBUPHINE HCL, NALBUPHINE HYDROCHLORIDE
NALFON, FENOPROFEN CALCIUM
NALFON 200, FENOPROFEN CALCIUM
NALIDIXIC ACID, NALIDIXIC ACID
NALLPEN, NAFCILLIN SODIUM
NALOXONE, NALOXONE HYDROCHLORIDE
NALOXONE HCL, NALOXONE HYDROCHLORIDE
NANDROLONE DECANOATE, NANDROLONE DECANOATE
NANDROLONE PHENPROPIONATE, NANDROLONE
   PHENPROPIONATE
NAPHAZOLINE HCL, NAPHAZOLINE HYDROCHLORIDE
NAPHCON FORTE, NAPHAZOLINE HYDROCHLORIDE
NAPROSYN, NAPROXEN
NAQUA, TRICHLORMETHIAZIDE
NAQUIVAL, RESERPINE
NARCAN, NALOXONE HYDROCHLORIDE
NARDIL, PHENELZINE SULFATE
NASACORT, TRIAMCINOLONE ACETONIDE
NASALCROM, CROMOLYN SODIUM
NASALIDE, FLUNISOLIDE
NATACYN, NATAMYCIN

NATURAL ESTROGENIC SUBSTANCE-ESTRONE, ESTRONE
NATURETIN-10, BENDROFLUMETHIAZIDE
NATURETIN-2.5, BENDROFLUMETHIAZIDE
NATURETIN-5, BENDROFLUMETHIAZIDE
NAVANE, THIOTHIXENE
NAVANE, THIOTHIXENE HYDROCHLORIDE
NEBCIN, TOBRAMYCIN SULFATE
NEBUPENT, PENTAMIDINE ISETHIONATE
NEGGRAM, NALIDIXIC ACID
NEMBUTAL, PENTOBARBITAL
NEMBUTAL, PENTOBARBITAL SODIUM
NEMBUTAL SODIUM, PENTOBARBITAL SODIUM
NEO-CORT-DOME, ACETIC ACID, GLACIAL
NEO-CORT-DOME, HYDROCORTISONE
NEO-CORTEF, HYDROCORTISONE ACETATE
NEO-DELTA-CORTEF, NEOMYCIN SULFATE
NEO-HYDELTRASOL, NEOMYCIN SULFATE
NEO-MEDROL, METHYLPREDNISOLONE
NEO-MEDROL ACETATE, METHYLPREDNISOLONE
   ACETATE
NEO-OTOSOL-HC, HYDROCORTISONE
NEO-POLYCIN, BACITRACIN ZINC
NEO-POLYCIN, GRAMICIDIN
NEO-RX, NEOMYCIN SULFATE
NEO-SYNALAR, FLUOCINOLONE ACETONIDE
NEOBIOTIC, NEOMYCIN SULFATE
NEODECADRON, DEXAMETHASONE SODIUM
   PHOSPHATE
NEOMYCIN & POLYMYXIN B SULFATES & BACITRACIN
   ZINC & HYDROCORTISONE, BACITRACIN ZINC
NEOMYCIN AND POLYMYXIN B SULFATES, NEOMYCIN
   SULFATE
NEOMYCIN AND POLYMYXIN B SULFATES AND
   DEXAMETHASONE, DEXAMETHASONE
NEOMYCIN AND POLYMYXIN B SULFATES AND
   GRAMICIDIN, GRAMICIDIN
NEOMYCIN AND POLYMYXIN B SULFATES AND
   HYDROCORTISONE, HYDROCORTISONE
NEOMYCIN SULFATE, NEOMYCIN SULFATE
NEOMYCIN SULFATE AND POLYMYXIN B SULFATE
   GRAMICIDIN, GRAMICIDIN
NEOMYCIN SULFATE-DEXAMETHASONE SODIUM
   PHOSPHATE, DEXAMETHASONE SODIUM PHOSPHATE
NEOMYCIN SULFATE-POLYMYXIN B SULFATE-
   HYDROCORTISONE, HYDROCORTISONE
NEOMYCIN SULFATE-TRIAMCINOLONE ACETONIDE,
   NEOMYCIN SULFATE
NEOMYCIN SULFATE, POLYMYXIN B SULFATE &
   HYDROCORTISONE, HYDROCORTISONE
NEOPAP, ACETAMINOPHEN (OTC)
NEOPASALATE, AMINOSALICYLATE SODIUM
NEOPHAM 6.4%, AMINO ACIDS
NEOSAR, CYCLOPHOSPHAMIDE
NEOSCAN, GALLIUM CITRATE, GA-67
NEOSPORIN, BACITRACIN ZINC
NEOSPORIN, GRAMICIDIN
NEOSPORIN G.U. IRRIGANT, NEOMYCIN SULFATE
NEOTHYLLINE, DYPHYLLINE
NEOTRIZINE, TRISULFAPYRIMIDINES
NEPHRAMINE 5.4%, AMINO ACIDS
NEPHROFLOW, IODOHIPPURATE SODIUM, I-123
NEPTAZANE, METHAZOLAMIDE
NESACAINE, CHLOROPROCAINE HYDROCHLORIDE
NESACAINE-MPF, CHLOROPROCAINE HYDROCHLORIDE
NETROMYCIN, NETILMICIN SULFATE
NEURAMATE, MEPROBAMATE
NEUVIL, IBUPROFEN (OTC)
NIACIN, NIACIN
NICLOCIDE, NICLOSAMIDE
NICODERM, NICOTINE
NICOLAR, NIACIN
NICORETTE, NICOTINE POLACRILEX

APPENDIX A
PRODUCT NAME INDEX (continued)

NICORETTE DS, NICOTINE POLACRILEX
NICOTROL, NICOTINE
NIFEDIPINE, NIFEDIPINE
NILSTAT, NYSTATIN
NIMOTOP, NIMODIPINE
NIPENT, PENTOSTATIN
NIPRIDE, SODIUM NITROPRUSSIDE
NITRO IV, NITROGLYCERIN
NITRO-BID, NITROGLYCERIN
NITROFURANTOIN, NITROFURANTOIN
NITROFURANTOIN MACROCRYSTALLINE,
　　NITROFURANTOIN, MACROCRYSTALLINE
NITROFURAZONE, NITROFURAZONE
NITROGLYCERIN, NITROGLYCERIN
NITROGLYCERIN IN DEXTROSE 5%, NITROGLYCERIN
NITROL, NITROGLYCERIN
NITROLINGUAL, NITROGLYCERIN
NITRONAL, NITROGLYCERIN
NITROPRESS, SODIUM NITROPRUSSIDE
NITROSTAT, NITROGLYCERIN
NIX, PERMETHRIN
NIX, PERMETHRIN (OTC)
NIZORAL, KETOCONAZOLE
NOGENIC HC, HYDROCORTISONE
NOLUDAR, METHYPRYLON
NOLVADEX, TAMOXIFEN CITRATE
NOR-Q.D., NORETHINDRONE
NORCEPT-E 1/35 21, ETHINYL ESTRADIOL
NORCEPT-E 1/35 28, ETHINYL ESTRADIOL
NORCET, ACETAMINOPHEN
NORCURON, VECURONIUM BROMIDE
NORDETTE-21, ETHINYL ESTRADIOL
NORDETTE-28, ETHINYL ESTRADIOL
NORETHIN 1/35E-21, ETHINYL ESTRADIOL
NORETHIN 1/35E-28, ETHINYL ESTRADIOL
NORETHIN 1/50M-21, MESTRANOL
NORETHIN 1/50M-28, MESTRANOL
NORETHINDRONE AND ETHINYL ESTRADIOL, ETHINYL
　　ESTRADIOL
NORETHINDRONE AND ETHINYL ESTRADIOL (10/11),
　　ETHINYL ESTRADIOL
NORETHINDRONE AND ETHINYL ESTRADIOL (7/14),
　　ETHINYL ESTRADIOL
NORETHINDRONE AND MESTRANOL, MESTRANOL
NORFLEX, ORPHENADRINE CITRATE
NORGESIC, ASPIRIN
NORGESIC FORTE, ASPIRIN
NORINYL, MESTRANOL
NORINYL 1+35 21-DAY, ETHINYL ESTRADIOL
NORINYL 1+35 28-DAY, ETHINYL ESTRADIOL
NORINYL 1+50 21-DAY, MESTRANOL
NORINYL 1+50 28-DAY, MESTRANOL
NORINYL 1+80 21-DAY, MESTRANOL
NORINYL 1+80 28-DAY, MESTRANOL
NORISODRINE, ISOPROTERENOL SULFATE
NORISODRINE AEROTROL, ISOPROTERENOL
　　HYDROCHLORIDE
NORLESTRIN FE 1/50, ETHINYL ESTRADIOL
NORLESTRIN FE 2.5/50, ETHINYL ESTRADIOL
NORLESTRIN 21 1/50, ETHINYL ESTRADIOL
NORLESTRIN 21 2.5/50, ETHINYL ESTRADIOL
NORLESTRIN 28 1/50, ETHINYL ESTRADIOL
NORLUTATE, NORETHINDRONE ACETATE
NORLUTIN, NORETHINDRONE
NORMODYNE, LABETALOL HYDROCHLORIDE
NORMOSOL-M AND DEXTROSE 5%, DEXTROSE
NORMOSOL-R AND DEXTROSE 5% IN PLASTIC
　　CONTAINER, DEXTROSE
NORMOSOL-R IN PLASTIC CONTAINER, MAGNESIUM
　　CHLORIDE
NORMOZIDE, HYDROCHLOROTHIAZIDE
NOROXIN, NORFLOXACIN

NORPACE, DISOPYRAMIDE PHOSPHATE
NORPACE CR, DISOPYRAMIDE PHOSPHATE
NORPLANT, LEVONORGESTREL
NORPLANT SYSTEM, LEVONORGESTREL
NORPRAMIN, DESIPRAMINE HYDROCHLORIDE
NORQUEST FE, ETHINYL ESTRADIOL
NORTRIPTYLINE HCL, NORTRIPTYLINE
　　HYDROCHLORIDE
NORVASC, AMLODIPINE BESYLATE
NOVAFED, PSEUDOEPHEDRINE HYDROCHLORIDE
NOVAMINE 11.4%, AMINO ACIDS
NOVAMINE 15%, AMINO ACIDS
NOVAMINE 8.5%, AMINO ACIDS
NOVANTRONE, MITOXANTRONE HYDROCHLORIDE
NOVOCAIN, PROCAINE HYDROCHLORIDE
NOVOLIN L, INSULIN ZINC SUSP BIOSYNTHETIC
　　HUMAN (OTC)
NOVOLIN L, INSULIN ZINC SUSP SEMISYNTHETIC
　　PURIFIED HUMAN (OTC)
NOVOLIN N, INSULIN SUSP ISOPHANE BIOSYNTHETIC
　　HUMAN (OTC)
NOVOLIN N, INSULIN SUSP ISOPHANE SEMISYNTHETIC
　　PURIFIED HUMAN (OTC)
NOVOLIN R, INSULIN BIOSYNTHETIC HUMAN (OTC)
NOVOLIN R, INSULIN SEMISYNTHETIC PURIFIED
　　HUMAN (OTC)
NOVOLIN 70/30, INSULIN BIOSYNTHETIC HUMAN (OTC)
NOVOLIN 70/30, INSULIN SEMISYNTHETIC PURIFIED
　　HUMAN (OTC)
NOVRAD, LEVOPROPOXYPHENE NAPSYLATE,
　　ANHYDROUS
NPH ILETIN I (BEEF-PORK), INSULIN SUSP ISOPHANE
　　BEEF/PORK (OTC)
NPH ILETIN II, INSULIN SUSP ISOPHANE PURIFIED BEEF
　　(OTC)
NPH ILETIN II (PORK), INSULIN SUSP ISOPHANE
　　PURIFIED PORK (OTC)
NPH INSULIN, INSULIN SUSP ISOPHANE BEEF (OTC)
NPH PURIFIED PORK ISOPHANE INSULIN, INSULIN SUSP
　　ISOPHANE PURIFIED PORK (OTC)
NUBAIN, NALBUPHINE HYDROCHLORIDE
NULYTELY, POLYETHYLENE GLYCOL 3350
NUMORPHAN, OXYMORPHONE HYDROCHLORIDE
NUPRIN, IBUPROFEN (OTC)
NUROMAX, DOXACURIUM CHLORIDE
NUTRACORT, HYDROCORTISONE
NYDRAZID, ISONIAZID
NYSERT, NYSTATIN
NYSTAFORM, CLIOQUINOL
NYSTATIN, NYSTATIN
NYSTATIN AND TRIAMCINOLONE ACETONIDE,
　　NYSTATIN
NYSTATIN-TRIAMCINOLONE ACETONIDE, NYSTATIN
NYSTEX, NYSTATIN

O

OBESTIN-30, PHENTERMINE HYDROCHLORIDE
OBY-TRIM, PHENTERMINE HYDROCHLORIDE
OCL, POLYETHYLENE GLYCOL 3350
OCTOCAINE, EPINEPHRINE
OCUCLEAR, OXYMETAZOLINE HYDROCHLORIDE (OTC)
OCUFEN, FLURBIPROFEN SODIUM
OCUMYCIN, BACITRACIN ZINC
OCUSERT PILO-20, PILOCARPINE
OCUSERT PILO-40, PILOCARPINE
OCUSULF-10, SULFACETAMIDE SODIUM
OCUSULF-30, SULFACETAMIDE SODIUM
OGEN, ESTROPIPATE
OGEN .625, ESTROPIPATE

APPENDIX A
PRODUCT NAME INDEX (continued)

OGEN 1.25, ESTROPIPATE
OGEN 2.5, ESTROPIPATE
OGEN 5, ESTROPIPATE
OMNIFLOX, TEMAFLOXACIN HYDROCHLORIDE
OMNIPAQUE 140, IOHEXOL
OMNIPAQUE 180, IOHEXOL
OMNIPAQUE 210, IOHEXOL
OMNIPAQUE 240, IOHEXOL
OMNIPAQUE 300, IOHEXOL
OMNIPAQUE 350, IOHEXOL
OMNIPEN (AMPICILLIN), AMPICILLIN/AMPICILLIN
    TRIHYDRATE
OMNIPEN-N, AMPICILLIN SODIUM
ONA MAST, PHENTERMINE HYDROCHLORIDE
ONA-MAST, PHENTERMINE HYDROCHLORIDE
ONCOVIN, VINCRISTINE SULFATE
OPCON, NAPHAZOLINE HYDROCHLORIDE
OPHTHAINE, PROPARACAINE HYDROCHLORIDE
OPHTHETIC, PROPARACAINE HYDROCHLORIDE
OPHTHOCHLOR, CHLORAMPHENICOL
OPHTHOCORT, CHLORAMPHENICOL
OPTICROM, CROMOLYN SODIUM
OPTIMINE, AZATADINE MALEATE
OPTIPRANOLOL, METIPRANOLOL HYDROCHLORIDE
OPTIPRESS, CARTEOLOL HYDROCHLORIDE
OPTIRAY 160, IOVERSOL
OPTIRAY 240, IOVERSOL
OPTIRAY 300, IOVERSOL
OPTIRAY 320, IOVERSOL
OPTIRAY 350, IOVERSOL
OPTOMYCIN, CHLORAMPHENICOL
ORA-TESTRYL, FLUOXYMESTERONE
ORABASE HCA, HYDROCORTISONE ACETATE
ORACORT, TRIAMCINOLONE ACETONIDE
ORAGRAFIN CALCIUM, IPODATE CALCIUM
ORAGRAFIN SODIUM, IPODATE SODIUM
ORALONE, TRIAMCINOLONE ACETONIDE
ORAMORPH SR, MORPHINE SULFATE
ORAP, PIMOZIDE
ORASONE, PREDNISONE
ORETIC, HYDROCHLOROTHIAZIDE
ORETICYL FORTE, DESERPIDINE
ORETICYL 25, DESERPIDINE
ORETICYL 50, DESERPIDINE
ORETON, METHYLTESTOSTERONE
ORETON METHYL, METHYLTESTOSTERONE
ORGATRAX, HYDROXYZINE HYDROCHLORIDE
ORINASE, TOLBUTAMIDE
ORINASE DIAGNOSTIC, TOLBUTAMIDE SODIUM
ORLEX, ACETIC ACID, GLACIAL
ORLEX HC, ACETIC ACID, GLACIAL
ORNADE, CHLORPHENIRAMINE MALEATE
ORNIDYL, EFLORNITHINE HYDROCHLORIDE
ORPHENADRINE CITRATE, ORPHENADRINE CITRATE
ORPHENADRINE COMPOUND, ASPIRIN
ORPHENADRINE COMPOUND DOUBLE STRENGTH,
    ASPIRIN
ORPHENGESIC, ASPIRIN
ORPHENGESIC FORTE, ASPIRIN
ORTHO CYCLEN-21, ETHINYL ESTRADIOL
ORTHO CYCLEN-28, ETHINYL ESTRADIOL
ORTHO TRI-CYCLEN, ETHINYL ESTRADIOL
ORTHO-EST, ESTROPIPATE
ORTHO-NOVUM 1/35-21, ETHINYL ESTRADIOL
ORTHO-NOVUM 1/35-28, ETHINYL ESTRADIOL
ORTHO-NOVUM 1/50 21, MESTRANOL
ORTHO-NOVUM 1/50 28, MESTRANOL
ORTHO-NOVUM 1/80 21, MESTRANOL
ORTHO-NOVUM 10-21, MESTRANOL
ORTHO-NOVUM 10/11-21, ETHINYL ESTRADIOL
ORTHO-NOVUM 10/11-28, ETHINYL ESTRADIOL
ORTHO-NOVUM 2-21, MESTRANOL

ORTHO-NOVUM 7/14-21, ETHINYL ESTRADIOL
ORTHO-NOVUM 7/14-28, ETHINYL ESTRADIOL
ORTHO-NOVUM 7/7/7-21, ETHINYL ESTRADIOL
ORTHO-NOVUM 7/7/7-28, ETHINYL ESTRADIOL
ORTHO-N0VUM 1/80 28, MESTRANOL
ORUDIS, KETOPROFEN
OSMITROL 10% IN WATER, MANNITOL
OSMITROL 10% IN WATER IN PLASTIC CONTAINER,
    MANNITOL
OSMITROL 15% IN WATER, MANNITOL
OSMITROL 15% IN WATER IN PLASTIC CONTAINER,
    MANNITOL
OSMITROL 20% IN WATER, MANNITOL
OSMITROL 20% IN WATER IN PLASTIC CONTAINER,
    MANNITOL
OSMITROL 5% IN WATER, MANNITOL
OSMITROL 5% IN WATER IN PLASTIC CONTAINER,
    MANNITOL
OSMOVIST, IOTROLAN
OSTEOLITE, TECHNETIUM TC-99M MEDRONATE KIT
OSTEOSCAN, TECHNETIUM TC-99M ETIDRONATE KIT
OSTEOSCAN-HDP, TECHNETIUM TC-99M OXIDRONATE
    KIT
OTICAIR, HYDROCORTISONE
OTOBIONE, HYDROCORTISONE
OTOBIOTIC, HYDROCORTISONE
OTOCORT, HYDROCORTISONE
OVCON-35, ETHINYL ESTRADIOL
OVCON-50, ETHINYL ESTRADIOL
OVIDE, MALATHION
OVRAL, ETHINYL ESTRADIOL
OVRAL-28, ETHINYL ESTRADIOL
OVRETTE, NORGESTREL
OVULEN, ETHYNODIOL DIACETATE
OVULEN-21, ETHYNODIOL DIACETATE
OVULEN-28, ETHYNODIOL DIACETATE
OXACILLIN SODIUM, OXACILLIN SODIUM
OXANDRIN, OXANDROLONE
OXAZEPAM, OXAZEPAM
OXISTAT, OXICONAZOLE NITRATE
OXSORALEN, METHOXSALEN
OXSORALEN-ULTRA, METHOXSALEN
OXTRIPHYLLINE, OXTRIPHYLLINE
OXTRIPHYLLINE PEDIATRIC, OXTRIPHYLLINE
OXY-KESSO-TETRA, OXYTETRACYCLINE
    HYDROCHLORIDE
OXYBUTYNIN CHLORIDE, OXYBUTYNIN CHLORIDE
OXYCET, ACETAMINOPHEN
OXYCODONE AND ACETAMINOPHEN, ACETAMINOPHEN
OXYCODONE AND ASPIRIN, ASPIRIN
OXYCODONE AND ASPIRIN (HALF-STRENGTH), ASPIRIN
OXYCODONE HCL AND ACETAMINOPHEN,
    ACETAMINOPHEN
OXYCODONE 2.5/APAP 500, ACETAMINOPHEN
OXYCODONE 5/APAP 500, ACETAMINOPHEN
OXYLONE, FLUOROMETHOLONE
OXYPHENBUTAZONE, OXYPHENBUTAZONE
OXYTETRACYCLINE HCL, OXYTETRACYCLINE
    HYDROCHLORIDE
OXYTOCIN, OXYTOCIN
OXYTOCIN 10 USP UNITS IN DEXTROSE 5%, OXYTOCIN
OXYTOCIN 20 USP UNITS IN DEXTROSE 5%, OXYTOCIN
OXYTOCIN 5 USP UNITS IN DEXTROSE 5%, OXYTOCIN

P

P.A.S. SODIUM, AMINOSALICYLATE SODIUM
PAGITANE, CYCRIMINE HYDROCHLORIDE
PAMELOR, NORTRIPTYLINE HYDROCHLORIDE
PAMINE, METHSCOPOLAMINE BROMIDE

APPENDIX A
PRODUCT NAME INDEX (continued)

PANCURONIUM, PANCURONIUM BROMIDE
PANCURONIUM BROMIDE, PANCURONIUM BROMIDE
PANHEPRIN, HEPARIN SODIUM
PANMYCIN, TETRACYCLINE HYDROCHLORIDE
PANTOPAQUE, IOPHENDYLATE
PANWARFIN, WARFARIN SODIUM
PAPA-DEINE #3, ACETAMINOPHEN
PAPA-DEINE #4, ACETAMINOPHEN
PARACAINE, PROPARACAINE HYDROCHLORIDE
PARACORT, PREDNISONE
PARADIONE, PARAMETHADIONE
PARAFLEX, CHLORZOXAZONE
PARAFON FORTE DSC, CHLORZOXAZONE
PARAPLATIN, CARBOPLATIN
PARASAL, AMINOSALICYLIC ACID
PARASAL SODIUM, AMINOSALICYLATE SODIUM
PARATHAR, TERIPARATIDE ACETATE
PAREDRINE, HYDROXYAMPHETAMINE HYDROBROMIDE
PAREMYD, HYDROXYAMPHETAMINE HYDROBROMIDE
PARLODEL, BROMOCRIPTINE MESYLATE
PARSIDOL, ETHOPROPAZINE HYDROCHLORIDE
PASKALIUM, POTASSIUM AMINOSALICYLATE
PATHILON, TRIDIHEXETHYL CHLORIDE
PATHOCIL, DICLOXACILLIN SODIUM
PAVULON, PANCURONIUM BROMIDE
PAXIPAM, HALAZEPAM
PBZ, TRIPELENNAMINE CITRATE
PBZ, TRIPELENNAMINE HYDROCHLORIDE
PBZ-SR, TRIPELENNAMINE HYDROCHLORIDE
PCE, ERYTHROMYCIN
PEDIA PROFEN, IBUPROFEN
PEDIAMYCIN, ERYTHROMYCIN ETHYLSUCCINATE
PEDIAMYCIN 400, ERYTHROMYCIN ETHYLSUCCINATE
PEDIAPRED, PREDNISOLONE SODIUM PHOSPHATE
PEDIATRIC LTA KIT, LIDOCAINE HYDROCHLORIDE
PEDIAZOLE, ERYTHROMYCIN ETHYLSUCCINATE
PEDIOTIC, HYDROCORTISONE
PEGANONE, ETHOTOIN
PEN-VEE K, PENICILLIN V POTASSIUM
PENAPAR-VK, PENICILLIN V POTASSIUM
PENBRITIN, AMPICILLIN/AMPICILLIN TRIHYDRATE
PENBRITIN-S, AMPICILLIN SODIUM
PENECORT, HYDROCORTISONE
PENETREX, ENOXACIN
PENICILLIN, PENICILLIN G POTASSIUM
PENICILLIN G POTASSIUM, PENICILLIN G POTASSIUM
PENICILLIN G PROCAINE, PENICILLIN G PROCAINE
PENICILLIN G SODIUM, PENICILLIN G SODIUM
PENICILLIN V POTASSIUM, PENICILLIN V POTASSIUM
PENICILLIN-VK, PENICILLIN V POTASSIUM
PENICILLIN-2, PENICILLIN G POTASSIUM
PENNTUSS, CHLORPHENIRAMINE POLISTIREX (OTC)
PENTACEF, CEFTAZIDIME (ARGININE FORMULATION)
PENTAM 300, PENTAMIDINE ISETHIONATE
PENTAMIDINE ISETHIONATE, PENTAMIDINE
    ISETHIONATE
PENTHRANE, METHOXYFLURANE
PENTIDS '200', PENICILLIN G POTASSIUM
PENTIDS '250', PENICILLIN G POTASSIUM
PENTIDS '400', PENICILLIN G POTASSIUM
PENTIDS '800', PENICILLIN G POTASSIUM
PENTOBARBITAL SODIUM, PENTOBARBITAL SODIUM
PENTOLAIR, CYCLOPENTOLATE HYDROCHLORIDE
PENTOTHAL, THIOPENTAL SODIUM
PEPCID, FAMOTIDINE
PEPTAVLON, PENTAGASTRIN
PERCHLORACAP, POTASSIUM PERCHLORATE
PERCOCET, ACETAMINOPHEN
PERCODAN, ASPIRIN
PERCODAN-DEMI, ASPIRIN
PERCORTEN, DESOXYCORTICOSTERONE ACETATE
PERCORTEN, DESOXYCORTICOSTERONE PIVALATE

PERGONAL, MENOTROPINS
PERIACTIN, CYPROHEPTADINE HYDROCHLORIDE
PERIDEX, CHLORHEXIDINE GLUCONATE
PERMAPEN, PENICILLIN G BENZATHINE
PERMAX, PERGOLIDE MESYLATE
PERMITIL, FLUPHENAZINE HYDROCHLORIDE
PERPHENAZINE, PERPHENAZINE
PERPHENAZINE AND AMITRIPTYLINE HCL,
    AMITRIPTYLINE HYDROCHLORIDE
PERSANTINE, DIPYRIDAMOLE
PERTOFRANE, DESIPRAMINE HYDROCHLORIDE
PETHADOL, MEPERIDINE HYDROCHLORIDE
PFIZER-E, ERYTHROMYCIN STEARATE
PFIZERPEN, PENICILLIN G POTASSIUM
PFIZERPEN G, PENICILLIN G POTASSIUM
PFIZERPEN VK, PENICILLIN V POTASSIUM
PFIZERPEN-A, AMPICILLIN/AMPICILLIN TRIHYDRATE
PFIZERPEN-AS, PENICILLIN G PROCAINE
PHARMASEAL SCRUB CARE, CHLORHEXIDINE
    GLUCONATE (OTC)
PHENAPHEN W/ CODEINE NO. 2, ACETAMINOPHEN
PHENAPHEN W/ CODEINE NO. 3, ACETAMINOPHEN
PHENAPHEN W/ CODEINE NO. 4, ACETAMINOPHEN
PHENAPHEN-650 W/ CODEINE, ACETAMINOPHEN
PHENAZINE, PHENDIMETRAZINE TARTRATE
PHENAZINE-35, PHENDIMETRAZINE TARTRATE
PHENDIMETRAZINE TARTRATE, PHENDIMETRAZINE
    TARTRATE
PHENERGAN, PROMETHAZINE HYDROCHLORIDE
PHENERGAN FORTIS, PROMETHAZINE HYDROCHLORIDE
PHENERGAN PLAIN, PROMETHAZINE HYDROCHLORIDE
PHENERGAN VC, PHENYLEPHRINE HYDROCHLORIDE
PHENERGAN VC W/ CODEINE, CODEINE PHOSPHATE
PHENERGAN W/ CODEINE, CODEINE PHOSPHATE
PHENERGAN W/ DEXTROMETHORPHAN,
    DEXTROMETHORPHAN HYDROBROMIDE
PHENETRON, CHLORPHENIRAMINE MALEATE
PHENTERMINE HCL, PHENTERMINE HYDROCHLORIDE
PHENTERMINE RESIN 30, PHENTERMINE RESIN
    COMPLEX
PHENURONE, PHENACEMIDE
PHENY-PAS-TEBAMIN, PHENYL AMINOSALICYLATE
PHENYLBUTAZONE, PHENYLBUTAZONE
PHENYLPROPANOLAMINE HCL W/
    CHLORPHENIRAMINE MALEATE,
    CHLORPHENIRAMINE MALEATE (OTC)
PHENYLPROPANOLAMINE HCL/CHLORPHENIRAMINE,
    CHLORPHENIRAMINE MALEATE (OTC)
PHENYTEX, PHENYTOIN SODIUM, EXTENDED
PHENYTOIN, PHENYTOIN SODIUM
PHENYTOIN SODIUM, PHENYTOIN SODIUM
PHENYTOIN SODIUM, PHENYTOIN SODIUM, PROMPT
PHERAZINE DM, DEXTROMETHORPHAN
    HYDROBROMIDE
PHERAZINE VC, PHENYLEPHRINE HYDROCHLORIDE
PHERAZINE VC W/ CODEINE, CODEINE PHOSPHATE
PHERAZINE W/ CODEINE, CODEINE PHOSPHATE
PHISO-SCRUB, HEXACHLOROPHENE
PHISOHEX, HEXACHLOROPHENE
PHOSLO, CALCIUM ACETATE
PHOSPHOCOL P32, CHROMIC PHOSPHATE, P-32
PHOSPHOLINE IODIDE, ECHOTHIOPHATE IODIDE
PHOSPHOTEC, TECHNETIUM TC-99M PYROPHOSPHATE
    KIT
PHOSPHOTOPE, SODIUM PHOSPHATE, P-32
PHOTOPLEX, AVOBENZONE (OTC)
PHRENILIN, ACETAMINOPHEN
PHRENILIN FORTE, ACETAMINOPHEN
PHYLLOCONTIN, AMINOPHYLLINE
PHYSIOLYTE IN PLASTIC CONTAINER, MAGNESIUM
    CHLORIDE
PHYSIOSOL IN PLASTIC CONTAINER, MAGNESIUM
    CHLORIDE

APPENDIX A
PRODUCT NAME INDEX *(continued)*

PHYSIOSOL PH 7.4, MAGNESIUM CHLORIDE
PHYTONADIONE, PHYTONADIONE
PILOPINE HS, PILOCARPINE HYDROCHLORIDE
PINDAC, PINACIDIL
PIPERAZINE CITRATE, PIPERAZINE CITRATE
PIPRACIL, PIPERACILLIN SODIUM
PIROXICAM, PIROXICAM
PITOCIN, OXYTOCIN
PITRESSIN TANNATE, VASOPRESSIN TANNATE
PLACIDYL, ETHCHLORVYNOL
PLAQUENIL, HYDROXYCHLOROQUINE SULFATE
PLASMA-LYTE A IN PLASTIC CONTAINER, MAGNESIUM
   CHLORIDE
PLASMA-LYTE M AND DEXTROSE 5% IN PLASTIC
   CONTAINER, CALCIUM CHLORIDE
PLASMA-LYTE R IN PLASTIC CONTAINER, CALCIUM
   CHLORIDE
PLASMA-LYTE 148 AND DEXTROSE 5% IN PLASTIC
   CONTAINER, DEXTROSE
PLASMA-LYTE 148 IN WATER IN PLASTIC CONTAINER,
   MAGNESIUM CHLORIDE
PLASMA-LYTE 56 AND DEXTROSE 5% IN PLASTIC
   CONTAINER, DEXTROSE
PLASMA-LYTE 56 IN PLASTIC CONTAINER, MAGNESIUM
   ACETATE TETRAHYDRATE
PLATINOL, CISPLATIN
PLATINOL-AQ, CISPLATIN
PLEGINE, PHENDIMETRAZINE TARTRATE
PLEGISOL, CALCIUM CHLORIDE
PLENDIL, FELODIPINE
PMB 200, ESTROGENS, CONJUGATED
PMB 400, ESTROGENS, CONJUGATED
POLARAMINE, DEXCHLORPHENIRAMINE MALEATE
POLOCAINE, MEPIVACAINE HYDROCHLORIDE
POLOCAINE W/ LEVONORDEFRIN, LEVONORDEFRIN
POLY-PRED, NEOMYCIN SULFATE
POLY-RX, POLYMYXIN B SULFATE
POLYCILLIN, AMPICILLIN/AMPICILLIN TRIHYDRATE
POLYCILLIN-N, AMPICILLIN SODIUM
POLYCILLIN-PRB, AMPICILLIN TRIHYDRATE
POLYMIXIN B SULFATE, POLYMYXIN B SULFATE
POLYMOX, AMOXICILLIN
POLYSPORIN, BACITRACIN ZINC
POLYTRIM, POLYMYXIN B SULFATE
PONDIMIN, FENFLURAMINE HYDROCHLORIDE
PONSTEL, MEFENAMIC ACID
PORTALAC, LACTULOSE
POTASSIUM ACETATE IN PLASTIC CONTAINER,
   POTASSIUM ACETATE
POTASSIUM AMINOSALICYLATE, POTASSIUM
   AMINOSALICYLATE
POTASSIUM CHLORIDE, POTASSIUM CHLORIDE
POTASSIUM CHLORIDE IN PLASTIC CONTAINER,
   POTASSIUM CHLORIDE
POTASSIUM CHLORIDE 0.037% IN DEXTROSE 10% AND
   SODIUM CHLORIDE 0.2%, DEXTROSE
POTASSIUM CHLORIDE 0.037% IN DEXTROSE 10% AND
   SODIUM CHLORIDE 0.45%, DEXTROSE
POTASSIUM CHLORIDE 0.037% IN DEXTROSE 10% AND
   SODIUM CHLORIDE 0.9%, DEXTROSE
POTASSIUM CHLORIDE 0.037% IN DEXTROSE 5%,
   DEXTROSE
POTASSIUM CHLORIDE 0.037% IN DEXTROSE 5% AND
   SODIUM CHLORIDE 0.11%, DEXTROSE
POTASSIUM CHLORIDE 0.037% IN DEXTROSE 5% AND
   SODIUM CHLORIDE 0.2%, DEXTROSE
POTASSIUM CHLORIDE 0.037% IN DEXTROSE 5% AND
   SODIUM CHLORIDE 0.33%, DEXTROSE
POTASSIUM CHLORIDE 0.037% IN DEXTROSE 5% AND
   SODIUM CHLORIDE 0.45%, DEXTROSE
POTASSIUM CHLORIDE 0.037% IN DEXTROSE 5% AND
   SODIUM CHLORIDE 0.9%, DEXTROSE

POTASSIUM CHLORIDE 0.037% IN SODIUM CHLORIDE
   0.9%, POTASSIUM CHLORIDE
POTASSIUM CHLORIDE 0.075% IN DEXTROSE 10% AND
   SODIUM CHLORIDE 0.2%, DEXTROSE
POTASSIUM CHLORIDE 0.075% IN DEXTROSE 10% AND
   SODIUM CHLORIDE 0.45%, DEXTROSE
POTASSIUM CHLORIDE 0.075% IN DEXTROSE 10% AND
   SODIUM CHLORIDE 0.9%, DEXTROSE
POTASSIUM CHLORIDE 0.075% IN DEXTROSE 3.3% AND
   SODIUM CHLORIDE 0.3%, DEXTROSE
POTASSIUM CHLORIDE 0.075% IN DEXTROSE 5%,
   DEXTROSE
POTASSIUM CHLORIDE 0.075% IN DEXTROSE 5% AND
   SODIUM CHLORIDE 0.11%, DEXTROSE
POTASSIUM CHLORIDE 0.075% IN DEXTROSE 5% AND
   SODIUM CHLORIDE 0.2%, DEXTROSE
POTASSIUM CHLORIDE 0.075% IN DEXTROSE 5% AND
   SODIUM CHLORIDE 0.33%, DEXTROSE
POTASSIUM CHLORIDE 0.075% IN DEXTROSE 5% AND
   SODIUM CHLORIDE 0.45%, DEXTROSE
POTASSIUM CHLORIDE 0.075% IN DEXTROSE 5% AND
   SODIUM CHLORIDE 0.9%, DEXTROSE
POTASSIUM CHLORIDE 0.075% IN SODIUM CHLORIDE
   0.9%, POTASSIUM CHLORIDE
POTASSIUM CHLORIDE 0.11% IN DEXTROSE 10% AND
   SODIUM CHLORIDE 0.2%, DEXTROSE
POTASSIUM CHLORIDE 0.11% IN DEXTROSE 10% AND
   SODIUM CHLORIDE 0.45%, DEXTROSE
POTASSIUM CHLORIDE 0.11% IN DEXTROSE 10% AND
   SODIUM CHLORIDE 0.9%, DEXTROSE
POTASSIUM CHLORIDE 0.11% IN DEXTROSE 3.3% AND
   SODIUM CHLORIDE 0.3%, DEXTROSE
POTASSIUM CHLORIDE 0.11% IN DEXTROSE 5%,
   DEXTROSE
POTASSIUM CHLORIDE 0.11% IN DEXTROSE 5% AND
   SODIUM CHLORIDE 0.11%, DEXTROSE
POTASSIUM CHLORIDE 0.11% IN DEXTROSE 5% AND
   SODIUM CHLORIDE 0.2%, DEXTROSE
POTASSIUM CHLORIDE 0.11% IN DEXTROSE 5% AND
   SODIUM CHLORIDE 0.33%, DEXTROSE
POTASSIUM CHLORIDE 0.11% IN DEXTROSE 5% AND
   SODIUM CHLORIDE 0.45%, DEXTROSE
POTASSIUM CHLORIDE 0.11% IN DEXTROSE 5% AND
   SODIUM CHLORIDE 0.9%, DEXTROSE
POTASSIUM CHLORIDE 0.11% IN SODIUM CHLORIDE 0.9%,
   POTASSIUM CHLORIDE
POTASSIUM CHLORIDE 0.15% IN DEXTROSE 10% AND
   SODIUM CHLORIDE 0.2%, DEXTROSE
POTASSIUM CHLORIDE 0.15% IN DEXTROSE 10% AND
   SODIUM CHLORIDE 0.45%, DEXTROSE
POTASSIUM CHLORIDE 0.15% IN DEXTROSE 10% AND
   SODIUM CHLORIDE 0.9%, DEXTROSE
POTASSIUM CHLORIDE 0.15% IN DEXTROSE 3.3% AND
   SODIUM CHLORIDE 0.3%, DEXTROSE
POTASSIUM CHLORIDE 0.15% IN DEXTROSE 5%,
   DEXTROSE
POTASSIUM CHLORIDE 0.15% IN DEXTROSE 5% AND
   SODIUM CHLORIDE 0.11%, DEXTROSE
POTASSIUM CHLORIDE 0.15% IN DEXTROSE 5% AND
   SODIUM CHLORIDE 0.2%, DEXTROSE
POTASSIUM CHLORIDE 0.15% IN DEXTROSE 5% AND
   SODIUM CHLORIDE 0.33%, DEXTROSE
POTASSIUM CHLORIDE 0.15% IN DEXTROSE 5% AND
   SODIUM CHLORIDE 0.45%, DEXTROSE
POTASSIUM CHLORIDE 0.15% IN DEXTROSE 5% AND
   SODIUM CHLORIDE 0.9%, DEXTROSE
POTASSIUM CHLORIDE 0.15% IN SODIUM CHLORIDE 0.9%,
   POTASSIUM CHLORIDE
POTASSIUM CHLORIDE 0.22% IN DEXTROSE 10% AND
   SODIUM CHLORIDE 0.2%, DEXTROSE
POTASSIUM CHLORIDE 0.22% IN DEXTROSE 10% AND
   SODIUM CHLORIDE 0.45%, DEXTROSE

APPENDIX A
PRODUCT NAME INDEX (*continued*)

POTASSIUM CHLORIDE 0.22% IN DEXTROSE 10% AND SODIUM CHLORIDE 0.9%, DEXTROSE

POTASSIUM CHLORIDE 0.22% IN DEXTROSE 3.3% AND SODIUM CHLORIDE 0.3%, DEXTROSE

POTASSIUM CHLORIDE 0.22% IN DEXTROSE 5%, DEXTROSE

POTASSIUM CHLORIDE 0.22% IN DEXTROSE 5% AND SODIUM CHLORIDE 0.11%, DEXTROSE

POTASSIUM CHLORIDE 0.22% IN DEXTROSE 5% AND SODIUM CHLORIDE 0.2%, DEXTROSE

POTASSIUM CHLORIDE 0.22% IN DEXTROSE 5% AND SODIUM CHLORIDE 0.33%, DEXTROSE

POTASSIUM CHLORIDE 0.22% IN DEXTROSE 5% AND SODIUM CHLORIDE 0.45%, DEXTROSE

POTASSIUM CHLORIDE 0.22% IN DEXTROSE 5% AND SODIUM CHLORIDE 0.9%, DEXTROSE

POTASSIUM CHLORIDE 0.22% IN SODIUM CHLORIDE 0.9%, POTASSIUM CHLORIDE

POTASSIUM CHLORIDE 0.3% IN DEXTROSE 10% AND SODIUM CHLORIDE 0.2%, DEXTROSE

POTASSIUM CHLORIDE 0.3% IN DEXTROSE 10% AND SODIUM CHLORIDE 0.45%, DEXTROSE

POTASSIUM CHLORIDE 0.3% IN DEXTROSE 10% AND SODIUM CHLORIDE 0.9%, DEXTROSE

POTASSIUM CHLORIDE 0.3% IN DEXTROSE 3.3% AND SODIUM CHLORIDE 0.3%, DEXTROSE

POTASSIUM CHLORIDE 0.3% IN DEXTROSE 5%, DEXTROSE

POTASSIUM CHLORIDE 0.3% IN DEXTROSE 5% AND SODIUM CHLORIDE 0.11%, DEXTROSE

POTASSIUM CHLORIDE 0.3% IN DEXTROSE 5% AND SODIUM CHLORIDE 0.2%, DEXTROSE

POTASSIUM CHLORIDE 0.3% IN DEXTROSE 5% AND SODIUM CHLORIDE 0.33%, DEXTROSE

POTASSIUM CHLORIDE 0.3% IN DEXTROSE 5% AND SODIUM CHLORIDE 0.45%, DEXTROSE

POTASSIUM CHLORIDE 0.3% IN DEXTROSE 5% AND SODIUM CHLORIDE 0.9%, DEXTROSE

POTASSIUM CHLORIDE 0.3% IN SODIUM CHLORIDE 0.9%, POTASSIUM CHLORIDE

POTASSIUM CHLORIDE 10 MEQ, POTASSIUM CHLORIDE

POTASSIUM CHLORIDE 10 MEQ IN DEXTROSE 5% AND LACTATED RINGER'S, CALCIUM CHLORIDE

POTASSIUM CHLORIDE 10 MEQ IN DEXTROSE 5% AND SODIUM CHLORIDE 0.225%, DEXTROSE

POTASSIUM CHLORIDE 10 MEQ IN DEXTROSE 5% AND SODIUM CHLORIDE 0.3%, DEXTROSE

POTASSIUM CHLORIDE 10 MEQ IN DEXTROSE 5% AND SODIUM CHLORIDE 0.45%, DEXTROSE

POTASSIUM CHLORIDE 10 MEQ IN DEXTROSE 5% AND SODIUM CHLORIDE 0.9%, DEXTROSE

POTASSIUM CHLORIDE 15 MEQ IN DEXTROSE 5% AND LACTATED RINGER'S, CALCIUM CHLORIDE

POTASSIUM CHLORIDE 15 MEQ IN DEXTROSE 5% AND SODIUM CHLORIDE 0.225%, DEXTROSE

POTASSIUM CHLORIDE 15 MEQ IN DEXTROSE 5% AND SODIUM CHLORIDE 0.3%, DEXTROSE

POTASSIUM CHLORIDE 15 MEQ IN DEXTROSE 5% AND SODIUM CHLORIDE 0.45%, DEXTROSE

POTASSIUM CHLORIDE 15 MEQ IN DEXTROSE 5% AND SODIUM CHLORIDE 0.9%, DEXTROSE

POTASSIUM CHLORIDE 20 MEQ, POTASSIUM CHLORIDE

POTASSIUM CHLORIDE 20 MEQ IN DEXTROSE 5%, DEXTROSE

POTASSIUM CHLORIDE 20 MEQ IN DEXTROSE 5% AND LACTATED RINGER'S, CALCIUM CHLORIDE

POTASSIUM CHLORIDE 20 MEQ IN DEXTROSE 5% AND SODIUM CHLORIDE 0.225%, DEXTROSE

POTASSIUM CHLORIDE 20 MEQ IN DEXTROSE 5% AND SODIUM CHLORIDE 0.3%, DEXTROSE

POTASSIUM CHLORIDE 20 MEQ IN DEXTROSE 5% AND SODIUM CHLORIDE 0.45%, DEXTROSE

POTASSIUM CHLORIDE 20 MEQ IN DEXTROSE 5% AND SODIUM CHLORIDE 0.9%, DEXTROSE

POTASSIUM CHLORIDE 20 MEQ IN DEXTROSE 5% IN SODIUM CHLORIDE 0.3%, DEXTROSE

POTASSIUM CHLORIDE 20 MEQ IN SODIUM CHLORIDE 0.9%, POTASSIUM CHLORIDE

POTASSIUM CHLORIDE 30 MEQ, POTASSIUM CHLORIDE

POTASSIUM CHLORIDE 30 MEQ IN DEXTROSE 5%, DEXTROSE

POTASSIUM CHLORIDE 30 MEQ IN DEXTROSE 5% AND LACTATED RINGER'S, CALCIUM CHLORIDE

POTASSIUM CHLORIDE 30 MEQ IN DEXTROSE 5% AND SODIUM CHLORIDE 0.225%, DEXTROSE

POTASSIUM CHLORIDE 30 MEQ IN DEXTROSE 5% AND SODIUM CHLORIDE 0.3%, DEXTROSE

POTASSIUM CHLORIDE 30 MEQ IN DEXTROSE 5% AND SODIUM CHLORIDE 0.45%, DEXTROSE

POTASSIUM CHLORIDE 30 MEQ IN DEXTROSE 5% AND SODIUM CHLORIDE 0.9%, DEXTROSE

POTASSIUM CHLORIDE 40 MEQ, POTASSIUM CHLORIDE

POTASSIUM CHLORIDE 40 MEQ IN DEXTROSE 5%, DEXTROSE

POTASSIUM CHLORIDE 40 MEQ IN DEXTROSE 5% AND LACTATED RINGER'S, CALCIUM CHLORIDE

POTASSIUM CHLORIDE 40 MEQ IN DEXTROSE 5% AND SODIUM CHLORIDE 0.225%, DEXTROSE

POTASSIUM CHLORIDE 40 MEQ IN DEXTROSE 5% AND SODIUM CHLORIDE 0.3%, DEXTROSE

POTASSIUM CHLORIDE 40 MEQ IN DEXTROSE 5% AND SODIUM CHLORIDE 0.45%, DEXTROSE

POTASSIUM CHLORIDE 40 MEQ IN DEXTROSE 5% AND SODIUM CHLORIDE 0.9%, DEXTROSE

POTASSIUM CHLORIDE 40 MEQ IN SODIUM CHLORIDE 0.9%, POTASSIUM CHLORIDE

POTASSIUM CHLORIDE 5 MEQ IN DEXTROSE 5% AND LACTATED RINGER'S, CALCIUM CHLORIDE

POTASSIUM CHLORIDE 5 MEQ IN DEXTROSE 5% AND SODIUM CHLORIDE 0.225%, DEXTROSE

POTASSIUM CHLORIDE 5 MEQ IN DEXTROSE 5% AND SODIUM CHLORIDE 0.3%, DEXTROSE

POTASSIUM CHLORIDE 5 MEQ IN DEXTROSE 5% AND SODIUM CHLORIDE 0.45%, DEXTROSE

POTASSIUM CHLORIDE 5 MEQ IN DEXTROSE 5% AND SODIUM CHLORIDE 0.9%, DEXTROSE

POTASSIUM CITRATE, POTASSIUM CITRATE

POTASSIUM IODIDE, POTASSIUM IODIDE (OTC)

POVAN, PYRVINIUM PAMOATE

POVIDONE IODINE, POVIDONE-IODINE (OTC)

PRALIDOXIME CHLORIDE, PRALIDOXIME CHLORIDE

PRAMINE, IMIPRAMINE HYDROCHLORIDE

PRAMOSONE, HYDROCORTISONE ACETATE

PRANTAL, DIPHEMANIL METHYLSULFATE

PRAVACHOL, PRAVASTATIN SODIUM

PRAZEPAM, PRAZEPAM

PRAZOSIN HCL, PRAZOSIN HYDROCHLORIDE

PRE-OP, HEXACHLOROPHENE

PRE-OP II, HEXACHLOROPHENE

PRE-PEN, BENZYL PENICILLOYL-POLYLYSINE

PRE-SATE, CHLORPHENTERMINE HYDROCHLORIDE

PRECEF, CEFORANIDE

PRED FORTE, PREDNISOLONE ACETATE

PRED MILD, PREDNISOLONE ACETATE

PRED-G, GENTAMICIN SULFATE

PREDAIR, PREDNISOLONE SODIUM PHOSPHATE

PREDAIR FORTE, PREDNISOLONE SODIUM PHOSPHATE

PREDAMIDE, PREDNISOLONE ACETATE

PREDNICEN-M, PREDNISONE

PREDNISOLONE, PREDNISOLONE

PREDNISOLONE ACETATE, PREDNISOLONE ACETATE

PREDNISOLONE SODIUM PHOSPHATE, PREDNISOLONE SODIUM PHOSPHATE

PREDNISOLONE TEBUTATE, PREDNISOLONE TEBUTATE

APPENDIX A
PRODUCT NAME INDEX (continued)

PREDNISONE, PREDNISONE
PREDNISONE INTENSOL, PREDNISONE
PREDSULFAIR, PREDNISOLONE ACETATE
PREDSULFAIR II, PREDNISOLONE ACETATE
PREFRIN-A, PHENYLEPHRINE HYDROCHLORIDE
PREGNYL, GONADOTROPIN, CHORIONIC
PRELONE, PREDNISOLONE
PRELUDIN, PHENMETRAZINE HYDROCHLORIDE
PREMARIN, ESTROGENS, CONJUGATED
PRESAMINE, IMIPRAMINE HYDROCHLORIDE
PRILOSEC, OMEPRAZOLE
PRIMAQUINE, PRIMAQUINE PHOSPHATE
PRIMATENE MIST, EPINEPHRINE (OTC)
PRIMAXIN, CILASTATIN SODIUM
PRIMIDONE, PRIMIDONE
PRINCIPEN '125', AMPICILLIN/AMPICILLIN TRIHYDRATE
PRINCIPEN '250', AMPICILLIN/AMPICILLIN TRIHYDRATE
PRINCIPEN '500', AMPICILLIN/AMPICILLIN TRIHYDRATE
PRINCIPEN W/ PROBENECID, AMPICILLIN TRIHYDRATE
PRINIVIL, LISINOPRIL
PRINZIDE 12.5, HYDROCHLOROTHIAZIDE
PRINZIDE 25, HYDROCHLOROTHIAZIDE
PRISCOLINE, TOLAZOLINE HYDROCHLORIDE
PRO-BANTHINE, PROPANTHELINE BROMIDE
PROBALAN, PROBENECID
PROBAMPACIN, AMPICILLIN TRIHYDRATE
PROBEN-C, COLCHICINE
PROBENECID, PROBENECID
PROBENECID AND COLCHICINE, COLCHICINE
PROBENECID W/ COLCHICINE, COLCHICINE
PROCAINAMIDE HCL, PROCAINAMIDE HYDROCHLORIDE
PROCAINE HCL, PROCAINE HYDROCHLORIDE
PROCAINE HCL W/ EPINEPHRINE, EPINEPHRINE
PROCALAMINE, AMINO ACIDS
PROCAN, PROCAINAMIDE HYDROCHLORIDE
PROCAN SR, PROCAINAMIDE HYDROCHLORIDE
PROCAPAN, PROCAINAMIDE HYDROCHLORIDE
PROCARDIA, NIFEDIPINE
PROCARDIA XL, NIFEDIPINE
PROCHLORPERAZINE, PROCHLORPERAZINE EDISYLATE
PROCHLORPERAZINE, PROCHLORPERAZINE MALEATE
PROCHLORPERAZINE EDISYLATE, PROCHLORPERAZINE
  EDISYLATE
PROCHLORPERAZINE MALEATE, PROCHLORPERAZINE
  MALEATE
PROCTOCORT, HYDROCORTISONE
PROCTOFOAM HC, HYDROCORTISONE ACETATE
PROFEN, IBUPROFEN (OTC)
PROFENAL, SUPROFEN
PROFERDEX, IRON DEXTRAN
PROGESTASERT, PROGESTERONE
PROGESTERONE, PROGESTERONE
PROGLYCEM, DIAZOXIDE
PROKETAZINE, CARPHENAZINE MALEATE
PROKLAR, SULFAMETHIZOLE
PROLIXIN, FLUPHENAZINE HYDROCHLORIDE
PROLIXIN DECANOATE, FLUPHENAZINE DECANOATE
PROLIXIN ENANTHATE, FLUPHENAZINE ENANTHATE
PROLOID, THYROGLOBULIN
PROLOPRIM, TRIMETHOPRIM
PROMAPAR, CHLORPROMAZINE HYDROCHLORIDE
PROMAZINE HCL, PROMAZINE HYDROCHLORIDE
PROMETA, METAPROTERENOL SULFATE
PROMETH, PROMETHAZINE HYDROCHLORIDE
PROMETH VC PLAIN, PHENYLEPHRINE
  HYDROCHLORIDE
PROMETH VC W/ CODEINE, CODEINE PHOSPHATE
PROMETH W/ CODEINE, CODEINE PHOSPHATE
PROMETH W/ DEXTROMETHORPHAN,
  DEXTROMETHORPHAN HYDROBROMIDE
PROMETHACON, PROMETHAZINE HYDROCHLORIDE
PROMETHAZINE, PROMETHAZINE HYDROCHLORIDE

PROMETHAZINE HCL, PROMETHAZINE
  HYDROCHLORIDE
PROMETHAZINE HCL AND CODEINE PHOSPHATE,
  CODEINE PHOSPHATE
PROMETHAZINE PLAIN, PROMETHAZINE
  HYDROCHLORIDE
PROMETHAZINE VC PLAIN, PHENYLEPHRINE
  HYDROCHLORIDE
PROMETHAZINE VC W/ CODEINE, CODEINE PHOSPHATE
PROMETHAZINE W/ CODEINE, CODEINE PHOSPHATE
PROMETHAZINE W/ DEXTROMETHORPHAN,
  DEXTROMETHORPHAN HYDROBROMIDE
PROMETHEGAN, PROMETHAZINE HYDROCHLORIDE
PROMPT PHENYTOIN SODIUM, PHENYTOIN SODIUM,
  PROMPT
PRONESTYL, PROCAINAMIDE HYDROCHLORIDE
PRONESTYL-SR, PROCAINAMIDE HYDROCHLORIDE
PROPACET 100, ACETAMINOPHEN
PROPANTHELINE BROMIDE, PROPANTHELINE BROMIDE
PROPARACAINE HCL, PROPARACAINE HYDROCHLORIDE
PROPHENE 65, PROPOXYPHENE HYDROCHLORIDE
PROPINE, DIPIVEFRIN HYDROCHLORIDE
PROPOXYPHENE COMPOUND 65, ASPIRIN
PROPOXYPHENE COMPOUND-65, ASPIRIN
PROPOXYPHENE HCL, PROPOXYPHENE
  HYDROCHLORIDE
PROPOXYPHENE HCL AND ACETAMINOPHEN,
  ACETAMINOPHEN
PROPOXYPHENE HCL W/ ASPIRIN AND CAFFEINE,
  ASPIRIN
PROPOXYPHENE HCL 65, PROPOXYPHENE
  HYDROCHLORIDE
PROPOXYPHENE NAPSYLATE AND ACETAMINOPHEN,
  ACETAMINOPHEN
PROPRANOLOL HCL, PROPRANOLOL HYDROCHLORIDE
PROPRANOLOL HCL & HYDROCHLOROTHIAZIDE,
  HYDROCHLOROTHIAZIDE
PROPRANOLOL HCL AND HYDROCHLOROTHIAZIDE,
  HYDROCHLOROTHIAZIDE
PROPRANOLOL HCL INTENSOL, PROPRANOLOL
  HYDROCHLORIDE
PROPYLTHIOURACIL, PROPYLTHIOURACIL
PROSCAR, FINASTERIDE
PROSOM, ESTAZOLAM
PROSTAPHLIN, OXACILLIN SODIUM
PROSTEP, NICOTINE
PROSTIN E2, DINOPROSTONE
PROSTIN F2 ALPHA, DINOPROST TROMETHAMINE
PROSTIN VR PEDIATRIC, ALPROSTADIL
PROTAMINE SULFATE, PROTAMINE SULFATE
PROTAMINE ZINC AND ILETIN II, INSULIN SUSP
  PROTAMINE ZINC PURIFIED BEEF (OTC)
PROTAMINE ZINC AND ILETIN II (PORK), INSULIN SUSP
  PROTAMINE ZINC PURIFIED PORK (OTC)
PROTAMINE ZINC INSULIN, INSULIN SUSP PROTAMINE
  ZINC PURIFIED BEEF (OTC)
PROTAMINE, ZINC & ILETIN I (BEEF-PORK), INSULIN
  SUSP PROTAMINE ZINC BEEF/PORK (OTC)
PROTOPAM CHLORIDE, PRALIDOXIME CHLORIDE
PROTOSTAT, METRONIDAZOLE
PROTROPIN, SOMATREM
PROVAL #3, ACETAMINOPHEN
PROVENTIL, ALBUTEROL
PROVENTIL, ALBUTEROL SULFATE
PROVERA, MEDROXYPROGESTERONE ACETATE
PROVOCHOLINE, METHACHOLINE CHLORIDE
PROZAC, FLUOXETINE HYDROCHLORIDE
PSEUDO-12, PSEUDOEPHEDRINE POLISTIREX (OTC)
PSEUDOEPHEDRINE HCL AND CHLORPHENIRAMINE
  MALEATE, CHLORPHENIRAMINE MALEATE (OTC)
PSEUDOEPHEDRINE HCL AND TRIPROLIDINE HCL,
  PSEUDOEPHEDRINE HYDROCHLORIDE

APPENDIX A
PRODUCT NAME INDEX *(continued)*

PSEUDOEPHEDRINE HCL/CHLORPHENIRAMINE
    MALEATE, CHLORPHENIRAMINE MALEATE (OTC)
PSEUDOEPHEDRINE HYDROCHLORIDE AND
    CHLORPHENIRAMINE MALEATE,
    CHLORPHENIRAMINE MALEATE (OTC)
PSORCON, DIFLORASONE DIACETATE
PULMOLITE, TECHNETIUM TC-99M ALBUMIN
    AGGREGATED KIT
PURIFIED CORTROPHIN GEL, CORTICOTROPIN
PURINETHOL, MERCAPTOPURINE
PYOCIDIN, HYDROCORTISONE
PYOPEN, CARBENICILLIN DISODIUM
PYRAZINAMIDE, PYRAZINAMIDE
PYRIDAMAL 100, CHLORPHENIRAMINE MALEATE
PYRIDOSTIGMINE BROMIDE, PYRIDOSTIGMINE
    BROMIDE
PYRIDOXINE HCL, PYRIDOXINE HYDROCHLORIDE
PYRILAMINE MALEATE, PYRILAMINE MALEATE
PYROLITE, TECHNETIUM TC-99M PYRO/TRIMETA
    PHOSPHATES KIT

Q

Q-GESIC, ASPIRIN
Q-PAM, DIAZEPAM
QUARZAN, CLIDINIUM BROMIDE
QUELICIN, SUCCINYLCHOLINE CHLORIDE
QUESTRAN, CHOLESTYRAMINE
QUESTRAN LIGHT, CHOLESTYRAMINE
QUIBRON-T, THEOPHYLLINE
QUIBRON-T/SR, THEOPHYLLINE
QUIDE, PIPERACETAZINE
QUINACT, QUINIDINE GLUCONATE
QUINAGLUTE, QUINIDINE GLUCONATE
QUINALAN, QUINIDINE GLUCONATE
QUINATIME, QUINIDINE GLUCONATE
QUINIDEX, QUINIDINE SULFATE
QUINIDINE GLUCONATE, QUINIDINE GLUCONATE
QUINIDINE SULFATE, QUINIDINE SULFATE
QUINORA, QUINIDINE SULFATE

R

R-GENE 10, ARGININE HYDROCHLORIDE
R-P MYCIN, ERYTHROMYCIN
RADIO-IODINATED (I 125) SERUM ALBUMIN (HUMAN),
    ALBUMIN IODINATED I-125 SERUM
RADIOIODINATED SERUM ALBUMIN (HUMAN) IHSA I
    125, ALBUMIN IODINATED I-125 SERUM
RADIONUCLIDE-LABELED (125 I) FIBRINOGEN (HUMAN)
    SENSOR, FIBRINOGEN, I-125
RAU-SED, RESERPINE
RAUDIXIN, RAUWOLFIA SERPENTINA
RAUSERPIN, RAUWOLFIA SERPENTINA
RAUTENSIN, ALSEROXYLON
RAUVAL, RAUWOLFIA SERPENTINA
RAUWILOID, ALSEROXYLON
RAUWOLFIA SERPENTINA, RAUWOLFIA SERPENTINA
RAVOCAINE AND NOVOCAIN W/ LEVOPHED,
    NOREPINEPHRINE BITARTRATE
RAVOCAINE AND NOVOCAIN W/ NEO-COBEFRIN,
    LEVONORDEFRIN
RBC-SCAN, TECHNETIUM TC-99M RED BLOOD CELL KIT
REDISOL, CYANOCOBALAMIN
REGITINE, PHENTOLAMINE MESYLATE
REGLAN, METOCLOPRAMIDE HYDROCHLORIDE
REGONOL, PYRIDOSTIGMINE BROMIDE
REGROTON, CHLORTHALIDONE
REGULAR ILETIN II, INSULIN PURIFIED BEEF (OTC)

REGULAR ILETIN II (PORK), INSULIN PURIFIED PORK
    (OTC)
REGULAR PURIFIED PORK INSULIN, INSULIN PURIFIED
    PORK (OTC)
RELA, CARISOPRODOL
RELAFEN, NABUMETONE
RELEFACT TRH, PROTIRELIN
REMSED, PROMETHAZINE HYDROCHLORIDE
RENACIDIN, CITRIC ACID
RENAMIN W/O ELECTROLYTES, AMINO ACIDS
RENESE, POLYTHIAZIDE
RENESE-R, POLYTHIAZIDE
RENO-M-DIP, DIATRIZOATE MEGLUMINE
RENO-M-30, DIATRIZOATE MEGLUMINE
RENO-M-60, DIATRIZOATE MEGLUMINE
RENOCAL-76, DIATRIZOATE MEGLUMINE
RENOGRAFIN-60, DIATRIZOATE MEGLUMINE
RENOGRAFIN-76, DIATRIZOATE MEGLUMINE
RENOQUID, SULFACYTINE
RENOTEC, TECHNETIUM TC-99M FERPENTETATE KIT
RENOVIST, DIATRIZOATE MEGLUMINE
RENOVIST II, DIATRIZOATE MEGLUMINE
RENOVUE-DIP, IODAMIDE MEGLUMINE
RENOVUE-65, IODAMIDE MEGLUMINE
REPAN, ACETAMINOPHEN
RESECTISOL, MANNITOL
RESERPINE, RESERPINE
RESERPINE AND HYDROCHLOROTHIAZIDE,
    HYDROCHLOROTHIAZIDE
RESERPINE AND HYDROCHLOROTHIAZIDE-50,
    HYDROCHLOROTHIAZIDE
RESERPINE AND HYDROFLUMETHIAZIDE,
    HYDROFLUMETHIAZIDE
RESERPINE/HYDRALAZINE HCL/
    HYDROCHLOROTHIAZIDE, HYDRALAZINE
    HYDROCHLORIDE
RESERPINE, HYDRALAZINE HCL AND
    HYDROCHLOROTHIAZIDE, HYDRALAZINE
    HYDROCHLORIDE
RESERPINE, HYDROCHLOROTHIAZIDE, AND
    HYDRALAZINE HCL, HYDRALAZINE
    HYDROCHLORIDE
RESPORAL, DEXBROMPHENIRAMINE MALEATE (OTC)
RESTORIL, TEMAZEPAM
RETET, TETRACYCLINE HYDROCHLORIDE
RETIN-A, TRETINOIN
RETROVIR, ZIDOVUDINE
REV-EYES, DAPIPRAZOLE HYDROCHLORIDE
REVERSOL, EDROPHONIUM CHLORIDE
REZIPAS, AMINOSALICYLIC ACID RESIN COMPLEX
RIDAURA, AURANOFIN
RIFADIN, RIFAMPIN
RIFAMATE, ISONIAZID
RIMACTANE, RIFAMPIN
RIMADYL, CARPROFEN
RIMIFON, ISONIAZID
RIMSO-50, DIMETHYL SULFOXIDE
RINGER'S, CALCIUM CHLORIDE
RINGER'S IN PLASTIC CONTAINER, CALCIUM CHLORIDE
RITALIN, METHYLPHENIDATE HYDROCHLORIDE
RITALIN-SR, METHYLPHENIDATE HYDROCHLORIDE
RITODRINE HCL, RITODRINE HYDROCHLORIDE
RITODRINE HCL IN DEXTROSE 5% IN PLASTIC CON-
    TAINER, RITODRINE HYDROCHLORIDE
ROBAXIN, METHOCARBAMOL
ROBAXIN-750, METHOCARBAMOL
ROBAXISAL, ASPIRIN
ROBENGATOPE, ROSE BENGAL SODIUM, I-131
ROBIMYCIN, ERYTHROMYCIN
ROBINUL, GLYCOPYRROLATE
ROBINUL FORTE, GLYCOPYRROLATE

APPENDIX A
PRODUCT NAME INDEX (continued)

ROBITET, TETRACYCLINE HYDROCHLORIDE
ROCALTROL, CALCITRIOL
ROCEPHIN, CEFTRIAXONE SODIUM
ROCEPHIN W/ DEXTROSE, CEFTRIAXONE SODIUM
ROGAINE, MINOXIDIL
RONDOMYCIN, METHACYCLINE HYDROCHLORIDE
ROWASA, MESALAMINE
ROXICET, ACETAMINOPHEN
ROXICET 5/500, ACETAMINOPHEN
ROXIPRIN, ASPIRIN
RUBEX, DOXORUBICIN HYDROCHLORIDE
RUBIVITE, CYANOCOBALAMIN
RUBRAMIN PC, CYANOCOBALAMIN
RUBRATOPE-57, CYANOCOBALAMIN, CO-57
RUBRATOPE-57 KIT, COBALT CHLORIDE, CO-57
RUBRATOPE-60, CYANOCOBALAMIN, CO-60
RUBRATOPE-60 KIT, COBALT CHLORIDE, CO-60
RUFEN, IBUPROFEN
RUVITE, CYANOCOBALAMIN
RYTHMOL, PROPAFENONE HYDROCHLORIDE

S

S.A.S.-500, SULFASALAZINE
SALPIX, ACETRIZOATE SODIUM
SALURON, HYDROFLUMETHIAZIDE
SALUTENSIN, HYDROFLUMETHIAZIDE
SALUTENSIN-DEMI, HYDROFLUMETHIAZIDE
SANDIMMUNE, CYCLOSPORINE
SANDOSTATIN, OCTREOTIDE ACETATE
SANDRIL, RESERPINE
SANOREX, MAZINDOL
SANSAC, ERYTHROMYCIN
SANSERT, METHYSERGIDE MALEATE
SARENIN, SARALASIN ACETATE
SARISOL, BUTABARBITAL SODIUM
SARISOL NO. 1, BUTABARBITAL SODIUM
SARISOL NO. 2, BUTABARBITAL SODIUM
SATRIC, METRONIDAZOLE
SCABENE, LINDANE
SCANDONEST L, LEVONORDEFRIN
SCANDONEST PLAIN, MEPIVACAINE HYDROCHLORIDE
SCRUBTEAM SURGICAL SPONGEBRUSH,
    HEXACHLOROPHENE
SECOBARBITAL SODIUM, SECOBARBITAL SODIUM
SECONAL SODIUM, SECOBARBITAL SODIUM
SECRETIN-FERRING, SECRETIN
SECTRAL, ACEBUTOLOL HYDROCHLORIDE
SEDAPAP, ACETAMINOPHEN
SEFFIN, CEPHALOTHIN SODIUM
SELDANE, TERFENADINE
SELDANE-D, PSEUDOEPHEDRINE HYDROCHLORIDE
SELENIUM SULFIDE, SELENIUM SULFIDE
SELENOMETHIONINE SE 75, SELENOMETHIONINE, SE-75
SELSUN, SELENIUM SULFIDE
SEMILENTE, INSULIN ZINC SUSP PROMPT PURIFIED
    PORK (OTC)
SEMILENTE INSULIN, INSULIN ZINC SUSP PROMPT BEEF
    (OTC)
SENSORCAINE, BUPIVACAINE HYDROCHLORIDE
SEPTI-SOFT, HEXACHLOROPHENE
SEPTISOL, HEXACHLOROPHENE
SEPTRA, SULFAMETHOXAZOLE
SEPTRA DS, SULFAMETHOXAZOLE
SEPTRA GRAPE, SULFAMETHOXAZOLE
SER-A-GEN, HYDRALAZINE HYDROCHLORIDE
SER-AP-ES, HYDRALAZINE HYDROCHLORIDE
SERAX, OXAZEPAM
SERENTIL, MESORIDAZINE BESYLATE
SEROMYCIN, CYCLOSERINE

SEROPHENE, CLOMIPHENE CITRATE
SERPALAN, RESERPINE
SERPANRAY, RESERPINE
SERPASIL, RESERPINE
SERPASIL-APRESOLINE, HYDRALAZINE
    HYDROCHLORIDE
SERPASIL-ESIDRIX #1, HYDROCHLOROTHIAZIDE
SERPASIL-ESIDRIX #2, HYDROCHLOROTHIAZIDE
SERPATE, RESERPINE
SERPIVITE, RESERPINE
SERVISONE, PREDNISONE
SETHOTOPE, SELENOMETHIONINE, SE-75
SILDIMAC, SILVER SULFADIAZINE
SILPHEN, DIPHENHYDRAMINE HYDROCHLORIDE (OTC)
SILVADENE, SILVER SULFADIAZINE
SINEMET, CARBIDOPA
SINEMET CR, CARBIDOPA
SINEQUAN, DOXEPIN HYDROCHLORIDE
SINOGRAFIN, DIATRIZOATE MEGLUMINE
SKELAXIN, METAXALONE
SLO-BID, THEOPHYLLINE
SLO-PHYLLIN, THEOPHYLLINE
SLOW-K, POTASSIUM CHLORIDE
SMZ-TMP, SULFAMETHOXAZOLE
SMZ-TMP PEDIATRIC, SULFAMETHOXAZOLE
SODIUM ACETATE IN PLASTIC CONTAINER, SODIUM
    ACETATE, ANHYDROUS
SODIUM AMINOSALICYLATE, AMINOSALICYLATE
    SODIUM
SODIUM BICARBONATE IN PLASTIC CONTAINER,
    SODIUM BICARBONATE
SODIUM BUTABARBITAL, BUTABARBITAL SODIUM
SODIUM CHLORIDE, SODIUM CHLORIDE
SODIUM CHLORIDE IN PLASTIC CONTAINER, SODIUM
    CHLORIDE
SODIUM CHLORIDE 0.45%, SODIUM CHLORIDE
SODIUM CHLORIDE 0.45% IN PLASTIC CONTAINER,
    SODIUM CHLORIDE
SODIUM CHLORIDE 0.9%, SODIUM CHLORIDE
SODIUM CHLORIDE 0.9% AND POTASSIUM CHLORIDE
    0.075%, POTASSIUM CHLORIDE
SODIUM CHLORIDE 0.9% AND POTASSIUM CHLORIDE
    0.15%, POTASSIUM CHLORIDE
SODIUM CHLORIDE 0.9% AND POTASSIUM CHLORIDE
    0.22%, POTASSIUM CHLORIDE
SODIUM CHLORIDE 0.9% AND POTASSIUM CHLORIDE
    0.224%, POTASSIUM CHLORIDE
SODIUM CHLORIDE 0.9% AND POTASSIUM CHLORIDE
    0.3%, POTASSIUM CHLORIDE
SODIUM CHLORIDE 0.9% IN PLASTIC CONTAINER,
    SODIUM CHLORIDE
SODIUM CHLORIDE 0.9% IN STERILE PLASTIC
    CONTAINER, SODIUM CHLORIDE
SODIUM CHLORIDE 23.4%, SODIUM CHLORIDE
SODIUM CHLORIDE 3%, SODIUM CHLORIDE
SODIUM CHLORIDE 3% IN PLASTIC CONTAINER, SODIUM
    CHLORIDE
SODIUM CHLORIDE 5%, SODIUM CHLORIDE
SODIUM CHLORIDE 5% IN PLASTIC CONTAINER, SODIUM
    CHLORIDE
SODIUM CHROMATE CR 51, SODIUM CHROMATE, CR-51
SODIUM HEPARIN, HEPARIN SODIUM
SODIUM IODIDE I 123, SODIUM IODIDE, I-123
SODIUM IODIDE I 131, SODIUM IODIDE, I-131
SODIUM LACTATE IN PLASTIC CONTAINER, SODIUM
    LACTATE
SODIUM LACTATE 0.167 MOLAR IN PLASTIC CONTAINER,
    SODIUM LACTATE
SODIUM LACTATE 1/6 MOLAR, SODIUM LACTATE
SODIUM NITROPRUSSIDE, SODIUM NITROPRUSSIDE
SODIUM P.A.S., AMINOSALICYLATE SODIUM
SODIUM PENTOBARBITAL, PENTOBARBITAL SODIUM

APPENDIX A
PRODUCT NAME INDEX *(continued)*

SODIUM PERTECHNETATE TC 99M, TECHNETIUM TC-99M SODIUM PERTECHNETATE
SODIUM PHOSPHATE P 32, SODIUM PHOSPHATE, P-32
SODIUM PHOSPHATES IN PLASTIC CONTAINER, SODIUM PHOSPHATE, DIBASIC
SODIUM POLYPHOSPHATE-TIN KIT, TECHNETIUM TC-99M POLYPHOSPHATE KIT
SODIUM POLYSTYRENE SULFONATE, SODIUM POLYSTYRENE SULFONATE
SODIUM ROSE BENGAL I 131, ROSE BENGAL SODIUM, I-131
SODIUM SECOBARBITAL, SECOBARBITAL SODIUM
SODIUM SUCCINATE, SODIUM SUCCINATE
SODIUM SULAMYD, SULFACETAMIDE SODIUM
SODIUM SULFACETAMIDE, SULFACETAMIDE SODIUM
SODIUM THIOSULFATE, SODIUM THIOSULFATE
SODIUM VERSENATE, EDETATE DISODIUM
SOLATENE, BETA-CAROTENE
SOLU-CORTEF, HYDROCORTISONE SODIUM SUCCINATE
SOLU-MEDROL, METHYLPREDNISOLONE SODIUM SUCCINATE
SOMA, CARISOPRODOL
SOMA COMPOUND, ASPIRIN
SOMA COMPOUND W/ CODEINE, ASPIRIN
SOMOPHYLLIN, AMINOPHYLLINE
SOMOPHYLLIN-CRT, THEOPHYLLINE
SOMOPHYLLIN-DF, AMINOPHYLLINE
SOMOPHYLLIN-T, THEOPHYLLINE
SONAZINE, CHLORPROMAZINE HYDROCHLORIDE
SORBITOL 3.3% IN PLASTIC CONTAINER, SORBITOL
SORBITOL 3% IN PLASTIC CONTAINER, SORBITOL
SORBITOL-MANNITOL, MANNITOL
SORBITOL-MANNITOL IN PLASTIC CONTAINER, MANNITOL
SOSOL, SULFISOXAZOLE
SOTRADECOL, SODIUM TETRADECYL SULFATE
SOXAZOLE, SULFISOXAZOLE
SOY-DOME, HEXACHLOROPHENE
SOYACAL 10%, SOYBEAN OIL
SOYACAL 20%, SOYBEAN OIL
SPARINE, PROMAZINE HYDROCHLORIDE
SPECTAMINE, IOFETAMINE HYDROCHLORIDE I-123
SPECTAZOLE, ECONAZOLE NITRATE
SPECTROBID, BACAMPICILLIN HYDROCHLORIDE
SPIRONOLACTONE, SPIRONOLACTONE
SPIRONOLACTONE + HYDROCHLOROTHIAZIDE, HYDROCHLOROTHIAZIDE
SPIRONOLACTONE AND HYDROCHLOROTHIAZIDE, HYDROCHLOROTHIAZIDE
SPIRONOLACTONE W/ HYDROCHLOROTHIAZIDE, HYDROCHLOROTHIAZIDE
SPIRONOLACTONE/HYDROCHLOROTHIAZIDE, HYDROCHLOROTHIAZIDE
SPRX-105, PHENDIMETRAZINE TARTRATE
SPRX-3, PHENDIMETRAZINE TARTRATE
SPS, SODIUM POLYSTYRENE SULFONATE
SSD, SILVER SULFADIAZINE
STADOL, BUTORPHANOL TARTRATE
STANOZIDE, ISONIAZID
STAPHCILLIN, METHICILLIN SODIUM
STATICIN, ERYTHROMYCIN
STATOBEX, PHENDIMETRAZINE TARTRATE
STATOBEX-G, PHENDIMETRAZINE TARTRATE
STATROL, NEOMYCIN SULFATE
STELAZINE, TRIFLUOPERAZINE HYDROCHLORIDE
STERANE, PREDNISOLONE
STERANE, PREDNISOLONE ACETATE
STERI-STAT, CHLORHEXIDINE GLUCONATE (OTC)
STERILE UREA, UREA
STERILE WATER, WATER FOR IRRIGATION, STERILE
STERILE WATER FOR INJECTION, WATER FOR INJECTION, STERILE

STERILE WATER FOR INJECTION IN PLASTIC CONTAINER, WATER FOR INJECTION, STERILE
STERILE WATER IN PLASTIC CONTAINER, WATER FOR IRRIGATION, STERILE
STIE-CORT, HYDROCORTISONE
STILBESTROL, DIETHYLSTILBESTROL
STILBETIN, DIETHYLSTILBESTROL
STILPHOSTROL, DIETHYLSTILBESTROL DIPHOSPHATE
STOXIL, IDOXURIDINE
STREPTOMYCIN SULFATE, STREPTOMYCIN SULFATE
STRIFON FORTE DSC, CHLORZOXAZONE
SUBLIMAZE, FENTANYL CITRATE
SUCCINYLCHOLINE CHLORIDE, SUCCINYLCHOLINE CHLORIDE
SUCOSTRIN, SUCCINYLCHOLINE CHLORIDE
SUDAFED 12 HOUR, PSEUDOEPHEDRINE HYDROCHLORIDE (OTC)
SUFENTA, SUFENTANIL CITRATE
SULF-10, SULFACETAMIDE SODIUM
SULFA-TRIPLE #2, TRISULFAPYRIMIDINES
SULFABID, SULFAPHENAZOLE
SULFACEL-15, SULFACETAMIDE SODIUM
SULFACETAMIDE SODIUM, SULFACETAMIDE SODIUM
SULFADIAZINE, SULFADIAZINE
SULFADIAZINE SODIUM, SULFADIAZINE SODIUM
SULFAIR FORTE, SULFACETAMIDE SODIUM
SULFAIR 10, SULFACETAMIDE SODIUM
SULFAIR-15, SULFACETAMIDE SODIUM
SULFALAR, SULFISOXAZOLE
SULFALOID, TRISULFAPYRIMIDINES
SULFAMETHOPRIM, SULFAMETHOXAZOLE
SULFAMETHOPRIM-DS, SULFAMETHOXAZOLE
SULFAMETHOXAZOLE, SULFAMETHOXAZOLE
SULFAMETHOXAZOLE & TRIMETHOPRIM, SULFAMETHOXAZOLE
SULFAMETHOXAZOLE AND TRIMETHOPRIM, SULFAMETHOXAZOLE
SULFAMETHOXAZOLE AND TRIMETHOPRIM DOUBLE STRENGTH, SULFAMETHOXAZOLE
SULFAMETHOXAZOLE AND TRIMETHOPRIM SINGLE STRENGTH, SULFAMETHOXAZOLE
SULFAMYLON, MAFENIDE ACETATE
SULFANILAMIDE, SULFANILAMIDE
SULFAPYRIDINE, SULFAPYRIDINE
SULFASALAZINE, SULFASALAZINE
SULFATRIM, SULFAMETHOXAZOLE
SULFATRIM PEDIATRIC, SULFAMETHOXAZOLE
SULFATRIM-DS, SULFAMETHOXAZOLE
SULFATRIM-SS, SULFAMETHOXAZOLE
SULFINPYRAZONE, SULFINPYRAZONE
SULFISOXAZOLE, SULFISOXAZOLE
SULFISOXAZOLE DIOLAMINE, SULFISOXAZOLE DIOLAMINE
SULFONAMIDES DUPLEX, SULFADIAZINE
SULFOSE, TRISULFAPYRIMIDINES
SULINDAC, SULINDAC
SULLA, SULFAMETER
SULMEPRIM, SULFAMETHOXAZOLE
SULMEPRIM PEDIATRIC, SULFAMETHOXAZOLE
SULPHRIN, PREDNISOLONE ACETATE
SULSOXIN, SULFISOXAZOLE
SULTEN-10, SULFACETAMIDE SODIUM
SULTRIN, TRIPLE SULFA (SULFABENZAMIDE; SULFACETAMIDE; SULFATHIAZOLE)
SUMYCIN, TETRACYCLINE
SUMYCIN, TETRACYCLINE HYDROCHLORIDE
SUPPRELIN, HISTRELIN ACETATE
SUPRAX, CEFIXIME
SUPROL, SUPROFEN
SURITAL, THIAMYLAL SODIUM
SURMONTIL, TRIMIPRAMINE MALEATE
SURVANTA, BERACTANT

APPENDIX A
PRODUCT NAME INDEX *(continued)*

SUS-PHRINE, EPINEPHRINE
SUSTAIRE, THEOPHYLLINE
SYMADINE, AMANTADINE HYDROCHLORIDE
SYMMETREL, AMANTADINE HYDROCHLORIDE
SYNACORT, HYDROCORTISONE
SYNALAR, FLUOCINOLONE ACETONIDE
SYNALAR-HP, FLUOCINOLONE ACETONIDE
SYNALGOS-DC, ASPIRIN
SYNALGOS-DC-A, ACETAMINOPHEN
SYNAREL, NAFARELIN ACETATE
SYNCURINE, DECAMETHONIUM BROMIDE
SYNEMOL, FLUOCINOLONE ACETONIDE
SYNKAYVITE, MENADIOL SODIUM DIPHOSPHATE
SYNOPHYLATE, THEOPHYLLINE SODIUM GLYCINATE
SYNOVALYTE IN PLASTIC CONTAINER, MAGNESIUM
    CHLORIDE
SYNTOCINON, OXYTOCIN
SYPRINE, TRIENTINE HYDROCHLORIDE
SYTOBEX, CYANOCOBALAMIN

T

T-PHYL, THEOPHYLLINE
T-STAT, ERYTHROMYCIN
TAB-PROFEN, IBUPROFEN (OTC)
TACARYL, METHDILAZINE
TACARYL, METHDILAZINE HYDROCHLORIDE
TACE, CHLOROTRIANISENE
TAGAMET, CIMETIDINE
TAGAMET, CIMETIDINE HYDROCHLORIDE
TAGAMET HCL IN SODIUM CHLORIDE 0.9%, CIMETIDINE
    HYDROCHLORIDE
TALACEN, ACETAMINOPHEN
TALWIN, PENTAZOCINE LACTATE
TALWIN COMPOUND, ASPIRIN
TALWIN NX, NALOXONE HYDROCHLORIDE
TALWIN 50, PENTAZOCINE HYDROCHLORIDE
TAMBOCOR, FLECAINIDE ACETATE
TANDEARIL, OXYPHENBUTAZONE
TAO, TROLEANDOMYCIN
TAPAZOLE, METHIMAZOLE
TARACTAN, CHLORPROTHIXENE
TATUM-T, COPPER
TAVIST, CLEMASTINE FUMARATE
TAVIST D, CLEMASTINE FUMARATE
TAVIST-D, CLEMASTINE FUMARATE (OTC)
TAVIST-1, CLEMASTINE FUMARATE
TAVIST-1, CLEMASTINE FUMARATE (OTC)
TAZICEF, CEFTAZIDIME
TAZIDIME, CEFTAZIDIME
TC 99M-LUNGAGGREGATE, TECHNETIUM TC-99M
    ALBUMIN AGGREGATED
TECHNECOLL, TECHNETIUM TC-99M SULFUR COLLOID
    KIT
TECHNESCAN DTPA KIT, TECHNETIUM TC-99M
    PENTETATE KIT
TECHNESCAN GLUCEPTATE, TECHNETIUM TC-99M
    GLUCEPTATE KIT
TECHNESCAN HIDA, TECHNETIUM TC-99M LIDOFENIN
    KIT
TECHNESCAN MAA, TECHNETIUM TC-99M ALBUMIN
    AGGREGATED KIT
TECHNESCAN MAG3, TECHNETIUM TC-99M MERTIATIDE
    KIT
TECHNESCAN MDP KIT, TECHNETIUM TC-99M
    MEDRONATE KIT
TECHNESCAN PYP KIT, TECHNETIUM TC-99M
    PYROPHOSPHATE KIT
TECHNETIUM TC 99M ALBUMIN AGGREGATED KIT,
    TECHNETIUM TC-99M ALBUMIN AGGREGATED KIT

TECHNETIUM TC 99M DIPHOSPHONATE-TIN KIT,
    TECHNETIUM TC-99M ETIDRONATE KIT
TECHNETIUM TC 99M GENERATOR, TECHNETIUM
    TC-99M SODIUM PERTECHNETATE GENERATOR
TECHNETIUM TC 99M HSA, TECHNETIUM TC-99M
    ALBUMIN KIT
TECHNETIUM TC 99M MAA, TECHNETIUM TC-99M
    ALBUMIN AGGREGATED KIT
TECHNETIUM TC 99M MPI MDP, TECHNETIUM TC-99M
    MEDRONATE KIT
TECHNETIUM TC 99M SULFUR COLLOID, TECHNETIUM
    TC-99M SULFUR COLLOID
TECHNETIUM TC 99M TSC, TECHNETIUM TC-99M
    SULFUR COLLOID KIT
TECHNETIUM TC-99M PENTETATE KIT, TECHNETIUM
    TC-99M PENTETATE KIT
TEEBACIN, AMINOSALICYLATE SODIUM
TEGISON, ETRETINATE
TEGOPEN, CLOXACILLIN SODIUM
TEGRETOL, CARBAMAZEPINE
TELDRIN, CHLORPHENIRAMINE MALEATE (OTC)
TELEPAQUE, IOPANOIC ACID
TEMARIL, TRIMEPRAZINE TARTRATE
TEMAZ, TEMAZEPAM
TEMAZEPAM, TEMAZEPAM
TEMOVATE, CLOBETASOL PROPIONATE
TEN-K, POTASSIUM CHLORIDE
TENATHAN, BETHANIDINE SULFATE
TENEX, GUANFACINE HYDROCHLORIDE
TENORETIC 100, ATENOLOL
TENORETIC 50, ATENOLOL
TENORMIN, ATENOLOL
TENSILON, EDROPHONIUM CHLORIDE
TENUATE, DIETHYLPROPION HYDROCHLORIDE
TENUATE DOSPAN, DIETHYLPROPION HYDROCHLORIDE
TEPANIL, DIETHYLPROPION HYDROCHLORIDE
TEPANIL TEN-TAB, DIETHYLPROPION HYDROCHLORIDE
TERAZOL 3, TERCONAZOLE
TERAZOL 7, TERCONAZOLE
TERFONYL, TRISULFAPYRIMIDINES
TERRA-CORTRIL, HYDROCORTISONE ACETATE
TERRAMYCIN, LIDOCAINE HYDROCHLORIDE
TERRAMYCIN, OXYTETRACYCLINE
TERRAMYCIN, OXYTETRACYCLINE CALCIUM
TERRAMYCIN, OXYTETRACYCLINE HYDROCHLORIDE
TERRAMYCIN W/ POLYMYXIN, OXYTETRACYCLINE
    HYDROCHLORIDE
TERRAMYCIN W/ POLYMYXIN B SULFATE,
    OXYTETRACYCLINE HYDROCHLORIDE
TERRAMYCIN-POLYMYXIN, OXYTETRACYCLINE
    HYDROCHLORIDE
TESLAC, TESTOLACTONE
TESSALON, BENZONATATE
TESTOSTERONE, TESTOSTERONE
TESTOSTERONE CYPIONATE, TESTOSTERONE
    CYPIONATE
TESTOSTERONE CYPIONATE-ESTRADIOL CYPIONATE,
    ESTRADIOL CYPIONATE
TESTOSTERONE ENANTHATE, TESTOSTERONE
    ENANTHATE
TESTOSTERONE ENANTHATE AND ESTRADIOL
    VALERATE, ESTRADIOL VALERATE
TESTOSTERONE PROPIONATE, TESTOSTERONE
    PROPIONATE
TESTRED, METHYLTESTOSTERONE
TESULOID, TECHNETIUM TC-99M SULFUR COLLOID KIT
TETRACHEL, TETRACYCLINE HYDROCHLORIDE
TETRACYCLINE, TETRACYCLINE
TETRACYCLINE HCL, TETRACYCLINE
TETRACYCLINE HCL, TETRACYCLINE HYDROCHLORIDE
TETRACYN, PROCAINE HYDROCHLORIDE
TETRACYN, TETRACYCLINE

APPENDIX A
PRODUCT NAME INDEX *(continued)*

TETRACYN, TETRACYCLINE HYDROCHLORIDE
TETRAMED, TETRACYCLINE
TETREX, TETRACYCLINE PHOSPHATE COMPLEX
TEXACORT, HYDROCORTISONE
TFP, TRIFLUOPERAZINE HYDROCHLORIDE
THALITONE, CHLORTHALIDONE
THALLOUS CHLORIDE TL 201, THALLOUS CHLORIDE, TL-201
THAM, TROMETHAMINE
THAM-E, POTASSIUM CHLORIDE
THEELIN, ESTRONE
THEO-DUR, THEOPHYLLINE
THEO-24, THEOPHYLLINE
THEOBID, THEOPHYLLINE
THEOBID JR., THEOPHYLLINE
THEOCHRON, THEOPHYLLINE
THEOCLEAR L.A.-130, THEOPHYLLINE
THEOCLEAR L.A.-260, THEOPHYLLINE
THEOCLEAR-100, THEOPHYLLINE
THEOCLEAR-200, THEOPHYLLINE
THEOCLEAR-80, THEOPHYLLINE
THEOLAIR, THEOPHYLLINE
THEOLAIR-SR, THEOPHYLLINE
THEOLIXIR, THEOPHYLLINE
THEOPHYL, THEOPHYLLINE
THEOPHYL-SR, THEOPHYLLINE
THEOPHYL-225, THEOPHYLLINE
THEOPHYLLINE, THEOPHYLLINE
THEOPHYLLINE AND DEXTROSE 5%, THEOPHYLLINE
THEOPHYLLINE IN DEXTROSE 5%, THEOPHYLLINE
THEOPHYLLINE IN DEXTROSE 5% IN PLASTIC CONTAINER, THEOPHYLLINE
THEOPHYLLINE 0.04% AND DEXTROSE 5%, THEOPHYLLINE
THEOPHYLLINE 0.04% AND DEXTROSE 5% IN PLASTIC CONTAINER, THEOPHYLLINE
THEOPHYLLINE 0.08% AND DEXTROSE 5%, THEOPHYLLINE
THEOPHYLLINE 0.08% AND DEXTROSE 5% IN PLASTIC CONTAINER, THEOPHYLLINE
THEOPHYLLINE 0.16% AND DEXTROSE 5%, THEOPHYLLINE
THEOPHYLLINE 0.16% AND DEXTROSE 5% IN PLASTIC CONTAINER, THEOPHYLLINE
THEOPHYLLINE 0.2% AND DEXTROSE 5%, THEOPHYLLINE
THEOPHYLLINE 0.2% AND DEXTROSE 5% IN PLASTIC CONTAINER, THEOPHYLLINE
THEOPHYLLINE 0.32% AND DEXTROSE 5%, THEOPHYLLINE
THEOPHYLLINE 0.4% AND DEXTROSE 5%, THEOPHYLLINE
THEOPHYLLINE 0.4% AND DEXTROSE 5% IN PLASTIC CONTAINER, THEOPHYLLINE
THEOPHYLLINE-SR, THEOPHYLLINE
THEOVENT, THEOPHYLLINE
THERMAZENE, SILVER SULFADIAZINE
THIAMINE HCL, THIAMINE HYDROCHLORIDE
THIO-TEPA, THIOTEPA
THIOGUANINE, THIOGUANINE
THIORIDAZINE HCL, THIORIDAZINE HYDROCHLORIDE
THIORIDAZINE HCL INTENSOL, THIORIDAZINE HYDROCHLORIDE
THIOSULFIL, SULFAMETHIZOLE
THIOTHIXENE, THIOTHIXENE
THIOTHIXENE HCL, THIOTHIXENE HYDROCHLORIDE
THIOTHIXENE HCL INTENSOL, THIOTHIXENE HYDROCHLORIDE
THORAZINE, CHLORPROMAZINE
THORAZINE, CHLORPROMAZINE HYDROCHLORIDE
THYPINONE, PROTIRELIN
THYRO-BLOCK, POTASSIUM IODIDE (OTC)

THYROGLOBULIN, THYROGLOBULIN
THYROLAR-0.25, LIOTRIX (T4; T3)
THYROLAR-0.5, LIOTRIX (T4; T3)
THYROLAR-1, LIOTRIX (T4; T3)
THYROLAR-2, LIOTRIX (T4; T3)
THYROLAR-3, LIOTRIX (T4; T3)
THYROLAR-5, LIOTRIX (T4; T3)
THYTROPAR, THYROTROPIN
TICAR, TICARCILLIN DISODIUM
TICLID, TICLOPIDINE HYDROCHLORIDE
TIGAN, TRIMETHOBENZAMIDE HYDROCHLORIDE
TIMENTIN, CLAVULANATE POTASSIUM
TIMOLIDE 10-25, HYDROCHLOROTHIAZIDE
TIMOLOL MALEATE, TIMOLOL MALEATE
TIMOPTIC, TIMOLOL MALEATE
TIMOPTIC IN OCUDOSE, TIMOLOL MALEATE
TINDAL, ACETOPHENAZINE MALEATE
TIOPRONIN, TIOPRONIN
TIS-U-SOL, MAGNESIUM SULFATE
TIS-U-SOL IN PLASTIC CONTAINER, MAGNESIUM SULFATE
TOBRADEX, DEXAMETHASONE
TOBRAMYCIN SULFATE, TOBRAMYCIN SULFATE
TOBRAMYCIN SULFATE IN SODIUM CHLORIDE 0.9%, TOBRAMYCIN SULFATE
TOBRASONE, FLUOROMETHOLONE ACETATE
TOBREX, TOBRAMYCIN
TODAY, NONOXYNOL-9 (OTC)
TOFRANIL, IMIPRAMINE HYDROCHLORIDE
TOFRANIL-PM, IMIPRAMINE PAMOATE
TOLAZAMIDE, TOLAZAMIDE
TOLBUTAMIDE, TOLBUTAMIDE
TOLECTIN, TOLMETIN SODIUM
TOLECTIN DS, TOLMETIN SODIUM
TOLECTIN 600, TOLMETIN SODIUM
TOLINASE, TOLAZAMIDE
TOLMETIN SODIUM, TOLMETIN SODIUM
TONOCARD, TOCAINIDE HYDROCHLORIDE
TOPICORT, DESOXIMETASONE
TOPICORT LP, DESOXIMETASONE
TOPICYCLINE, TETRACYCLINE HYDROCHLORIDE
TOPROL XL, METOPROLOL SUCCINATE
TORA, PHENTERMINE HYDROCHLORIDE
TORADOL, KETOROLAC TROMETHAMINE
TORECAN, THIETHYLPERAZINE MALATE
TORECAN, THIETHYLPERAZINE MALEATE
TORNALATE, BITOLTEROL MESYLATE
TOTACILLIN, AMPICILLIN/AMPICILLIN TRIHYDRATE
TOTACILLIN-N, AMPICILLIN SODIUM
TPN ELECTROLYTES IN PLASTIC CONTAINER, CALCIUM CHLORIDE
TRACRIUM, ATRACURIUM BESYLATE
TRAL, HEXOCYCLIUM METHYLSULFATE
TRANCOPAL, CHLORMEZANONE
TRANDATE, LABETALOL HYDROCHLORIDE
TRANDATE HCT, HYDROCHLOROTHIAZIDE
TRANMEP, MEPROBAMATE
TRANSDERM-SCOP, SCOPOLAMINE
TRANXENE, CLORAZEPATE DIPOTASSIUM
TRANXENE SD, CLORAZEPATE DIPOTASSIUM
TRASICOR, OXPRENOLOL HYDROCHLORIDE
TRAVAMULSION 10%, SOYBEAN OIL
TRAVAMULSION 20%, SOYBEAN OIL
TRAVASE, SUTILAINS
TRAVASOL 10%, AMINO ACIDS
TRAVASOL 10% W/O ELECTROLYTES, AMINO ACIDS
TRAVASOL 10% W/O ELECTROLYTES IN PLASTIC CONTAINER, AMINO ACIDS
TRAVASOL 2.75% IN DEXTROSE 10%, AMINO ACIDS
TRAVASOL 2.75% IN DEXTROSE 15%, AMINO ACIDS
TRAVASOL 2.75% IN DEXTROSE 20%, AMINO ACIDS
TRAVASOL 2.75% IN DEXTROSE 25%, AMINO ACIDS

APPENDIX A
PRODUCT NAME INDEX *(continued)*

TRAVASOL 2.75% IN DEXTROSE 5%, AMINO ACIDS
TRAVASOL 3.5% W/ ELECTROLYTES, AMINO ACIDS
TRAVASOL 4.25% IN DEXTROSE 10%, AMINO ACIDS
TRAVASOL 4.25% IN DEXTROSE 15%, AMINO ACIDS
TRAVASOL 4.25% IN DEXTROSE 20%, AMINO ACIDS
TRAVASOL 4.25% IN DEXTROSE 25%, AMINO ACIDS
TRAVASOL 4.25% IN DEXTROSE 5%, AMINO ACIDS
TRAVASOL 5.5% W/ ELECTROLYTES, AMINO ACIDS
TRAVASOL 5.5% W/O ELECTROLYTES, AMINO ACIDS
TRAVASOL 5.5% W/O ELECTROLYTES IN PLASTIC
    CONTAINER, AMINO ACIDS
TRAVASOL 8.5% W/ ELECTROLYTES, AMINO ACIDS
TRAVASOL 8.5% W/O ELECTROLYTES, AMINO ACIDS
TRAVASOL 8.5% W/O ELECTROLYTES IN PLASTIC
    CONTAINER, AMINO ACIDS
TRAVERT 10%, INVERT SUGAR
TRAZODONE HCL, TRAZODONE HYDROCHLORIDE
TRAZON-150, TRAZODONE HYDROCHLORIDE
TRECATOR-SC, ETHIONAMIDE
TREMIN, TRIHEXYPHENIDYL HYDROCHLORIDE
TRENTAL, PENTOXIFYLLINE
TREST, METHIXENE HYDROCHLORIDE
TREXAN, NALTREXONE HYDROCHLORIDE
TRI-NORINYL 21-DAY, ETHINYL ESTRADIOL
TRI-NORINYL 28-DAY, ETHINYL ESTRADIOL
TRI-SUDO, PSEUDOEPHEDRINE HYDROCHLORIDE (OTC)
TRIACET, TRIAMCINOLONE ACETONIDE
TRIACIN-C, CODEINE PHOSPHATE
TRIACORT, TRIAMCINOLONE ACETONIDE
TRIALODINE, TRAZODONE HYDROCHLORIDE
TRIAMCINOLONE, TRIAMCINOLONE
TRIAMCINOLONE ACETONIDE, TRIAMCINOLONE
    ACETONIDE
TRIAMCINOLONE DIACETATE, TRIAMCINOLONE
    DIACETATE
TRIAMINIC-12, CHLORPHENIRAMINE MALEATE (OTC)
TRIAMTERENE AND HYDROCHLOROTHIAZIDE,
    HYDROCHLOROTHIAZIDE
TRIAPRIN, ACETAMINOPHEN
TRIATEX, TRIAMCINOLONE ACETONIDE
TRIAVIL 2-10, AMITRIPTYLINE HYDROCHLORIDE
TRIAVIL 2-25, AMITRIPTYLINE HYDROCHLORIDE
TRIAVIL 4-10, AMITRIPTYLINE HYDROCHLORIDE
TRIAVIL 4-25, AMITRIPTYLINE HYDROCHLORIDE
TRIAVIL 4-50, AMITRIPTYLINE HYDROCHLORIDE
TRICHLOREX, TRICHLORMETHIAZIDE
TRICHLORMAS, TRICHLORMETHIAZIDE
TRICHLORMETHIAZIDE, TRICHLORMETHIAZIDE
TRICHLORMETHIAZIDE W/ RESERPINE, RESERPINE
TRICLOS, TRICLOFOS SODIUM
TRIDERM, TRIAMCINOLONE ACETONIDE
TRIDESILON, ACETIC ACID, GLACIAL
TRIDESILON, DESONIDE
TRIDIL, NITROGLYCERIN
TRIDIONE, TRIMETHADIONE
TRIFLUOPERAZINE HCL, TRIFLUOPERAZINE
    HYDROCHLORIDE
TRIHEXYPHENIDYL HCL, TRIHEXYPHENIDYL
    HYDROCHLORIDE
TRILAFON, PERPHENAZINE
TRILITRON, PSEUDOEPHEDRINE HYDROCHLORIDE
TRIMEPRAZINE TARTRATE, TRIMEPRAZINE TARTRATE
TRIMETH/SULFA, SULFAMETHOXAZOLE
TRIMETHOBENZAMIDE HCL, TRIMETHOBENZAMIDE
    HYDROCHLORIDE
TRIMETHOPRIM, TRIMETHOPRIM
TRIMIPRAMINE MALEATE, TRIMIPRAMINE MALEATE
TRIMOX, AMOXICILLIN
TRIMPEX, TRIMETHOPRIM
TRIMPEX 200, TRIMETHOPRIM
TRINALIN, AZATADINE MALEATE
TRIOFED, PSEUDOEPHEDRINE HYDROCHLORIDE (OTC)

TRIOSTAT, LIOTHYRONINE SODIUM
TRIPELENNAMINE HCL, TRIPELENNAMINE
    HYDROCHLORIDE
TRIPHASIL-21, ETHINYL ESTRADIOL
TRIPHASIL-28, ETHINYL ESTRADIOL
TRIPHED, PSEUDOEPHEDRINE HYDROCHLORIDE
TRIPLE SULFA, TRIPLE SULFA
    (SULFABENZAMIDE; SULFACETAMIDE; SULFATHIAZOLE)
TRIPLE SULFA, TRISULFAPYRIMIDINES
TRIPLE SULFAS, TRISULFAPYRIMIDINES
TRIPLE SULFOID, TRISULFAPYRIMIDINES
TRIPODRINE, PSEUDOEPHEDRINE HYDROCHLORIDE
    (OTC)
TRIPOSED, PSEUDOEPHEDRINE HYDROCHLORIDE (OTC)
TRIPROLIDINE AND PSEUDOEPHEDRINE,
    PSEUDOEPHEDRINE HYDROCHLORIDE
TRIPROLIDINE AND PSEUDOEPHEDRINE,
    PSEUDOEPHEDRINE HYDROCHLORIDE (OTC)
TRIPROLIDINE AND PSEUDOEPHEDRINE HCL,
    PSEUDOEPHEDRINE HYDROCHLORIDE (OTC)
TRIPROLIDINE AND PSEUDOEPHRINE HCL,
    PSEUDOEPHEDRINE HYDROCHLORIDE (OTC)
TRIPROLIDINE HCL, TRIPROLIDINE HYDROCHLORIDE
TRIPROLIDINE HCL AND PSEUDOEPHEDRINE HCL,
    PSEUDOEPHEDRINE HYDROCHLORIDE
TRIPROLIDINE HCL AND PSEUDOEPHEDRINE HCL,
    PSEUDOEPHEDRINE HYDROCHLORIDE (OTC)
TRIPROLIDINE HCL, PSEUDOEPHEDRINE HCL AND
    CODEINE PHOSPHATE, CODEINE PHOSPHATE
TRISORALEN, TRIOXSALEN
TROBICIN, SPECTINOMYCIN HYDROCHLORIDE
TROPHAMINE, AMINO ACIDS
TROPHAMINE 10%, AMINO ACIDS
TROPICAMIDE, TROPICAMIDE
TRUPHYLLINE, AMINOPHYLLINE
TRYMEX, TRIAMCINOLONE ACETONIDE
TRYSUL, TRIPLE SULFA
    (SULFABENZAMIDE; SULFACETAMIDE; SULFATHIAZOLE)
TUBOCURARINE CHLORIDE, TUBOCURARINE
    CHLORIDE
TURGEX, HEXACHLOROPHENE
TUSSIGON, HOMATROPINE METHYLBROMIDE
TUSSIONEX, CHLORPHENIRAMINE POLISTIREX
TYCOLET, ACETAMINOPHEN
TYLENOL, ACETAMINOPHEN (OTC)
TYLENOL W/ CODEINE, ACETAMINOPHEN
TYLENOL W/ CODEINE NO. 1, ACETAMINOPHEN
TYLENOL W/ CODEINE NO. 2, ACETAMINOPHEN
TYLENOL W/ CODEINE NO. 3, ACETAMINOPHEN
TYLENOL W/ CODEINE NO. 4, ACETAMINOPHEN
TYLOSTERONE, DIETHYLSTILBESTROL
TYLOX, ACETAMINOPHEN
TYLOX-325, ACETAMINOPHEN
TYMTRAN, CERULETIDE DIETHYLAMINE
TYZINE, TETRAHYDROZOLINE HYDROCHLORIDE
TZ-3, TIOCONAZOLE (OTC)

U

U-GENCIN, GENTAMICIN SULFATE
UCEPHAN, SODIUM BENZOATE
ULO, CHLOPHEDIANOL HYDROCHLORIDE
ULTRA-TECHNEKOW FM, TECHNETIUM TC-99M SODIUM
    PERTECHNETATE GENERATOR
ULTRACEF, CEFADROXIL/CEFADROXIL HEMIHYDRATE
ULTRAGRIS-165, GRISEOFULVIN,
    ULTRAMICROCRYSTALLINE
ULTRAGRIS-330, GRISEOFULVIN,
    ULTRAMICROCRYSTALLINE
ULTRALENTE, INSULIN ZINC SUSP EXTENDED PURIFIED
    BEEF (OTC)

APPENDIX A
PRODUCT NAME INDEX (continued)

ULTRALENTE INSULIN, INSULIN ZINC SUSP EXTENDED
  BEEF (OTC)
ULTRATAG, TECHNETIUM TC-99M RED BLOOD CELL KIT
ULTRAVATE, HALOBETASOL PROPIONATE
UMI-PEX 30, PHENTERMINE HYDROCHLORIDE
UNASYN, AMPICILLIN SODIUM
UNIPEN, NAFCILLIN SODIUM
UNIPHYL, THEOPHYLLINE
UNIPRES, HYDRALAZINE HYDROCHLORIDE
UNISOM, DOXYLAMINE SUCCINATE (OTC)
UNITENSEN, CRYPTENAMINE ACETATES
UNITENSEN, CRYPTENAMINE TANNATES
URACIL MUSTARD, URACIL MUSTARD
UREAPHIL, UREA
URECHOLINE, BETHANECHOL CHLORIDE
URESE, BENZTHIAZIDE
UREX, METHENAMINE HIPPURATE
URISPAS, FLAVOXATE HYDROCHLORIDE
UROBAK, SULFAMETHOXAZOLE
UROLOGIC G IN PLASTIC CONTAINER, CITRIC ACID
UROPLUS DS, SULFAMETHOXAZOLE
UROPLUS SS, SULFAMETHOXAZOLE
UROVIST CYSTO, DIATRIZOATE MEGLUMINE
UROVIST CYSTO PEDIATRIC, DIATRIZOATE MEGLUMINE
UROVIST MEGLUMINE DIU/CT, DIATRIZOATE
  MEGLUMINE
UROVIST SODIUM 300, DIATRIZOATE SODIUM
UTICILLIN VK, PENICILLIN V POTASSIUM
UTICORT, BETAMETHASONE BENZOATE
UTIMOX, AMOXICILLIN

V

V-CILLIN, PENICILLIN V
V-CILLIN K, PENICILLIN V POTASSIUM
VAGILIA, TRIPLE SULFA
  (SULFABENZAMIDE; SULFACETAMIDE; SULFATHIAZOLE)
  VAGISTAT-1, TIOCONAZOLE
VALISONE, BETAMETHASONE VALERATE
VALIUM, DIAZEPAM
VALMID, ETHINAMATE
VALNAC, BETAMETHASONE VALERATE
VALPIN 50, ANISOTROPINE METHYLBROMIDE
VALPROIC ACID, VALPROIC ACID
VALRELEASE, DIAZEPAM
VANCENASE, BECLOMETHASONE DIPROPIONATE
VANCENASE AQ, BECLOMETHASONE DIPROPIONATE
  MONOHYDRATE
VANCERIL, BECLOMETHASONE DIPROPIONATE
VANCOCIN HCL, VANCOMYCIN HYDROCHLORIDE
VANCOLED, VANCOMYCIN HYDROCHLORIDE
VANCOMYCIN HCL, VANCOMYCIN HYDROCHLORIDE
VANCOR, VANCOMYCIN HYDROCHLORIDE
VANOBID, CANDICIDIN
VANSIL, OXAMNIQUINE
VANTIN, CEFPODOXIME PROXETIL
VAPO-ISO, ISOPROTERENOL HYDROCHLORIDE
VASCOR, BEPRIDIL HYDROCHLORIDE
VASCORAY, IOTHALAMATE MEGLUMINE
VASERETIC, ENALAPRIL MALEATE
VASOCIDIN, PREDNISOLONE ACETATE
VASOCIDIN, PREDNISOLONE SODIUM PHOSPHATE
VASOCON, NAPHAZOLINE HYDROCHLORIDE
VASOCON-A, ANTAZOLINE PHOSPHATE
VASOTEC, ENALAPRIL MALEATE
VASOTEC, ENALAPRILAT
VASOXYL, METHOXAMINE HYDROCHLORIDE
VEETIDS '125', PENICILLIN V POTASSIUM
VEETIDS '250', PENICILLIN V POTASSIUM
VEETIDS '500', PENICILLIN V POTASSIUM

VEINAMINE 8%, AMINO ACIDS
VELBAN, VINBLASTINE SULFATE
VELOSEF, CEPHRADINE
VELOSEF '125', CEPHRADINE
VELOSEF '250', CEPHRADINE
VELOSEF '500', CEPHRADINE
VELOSULIN, INSULIN PURIFIED PORK (OTC)
VELOSULIN HUMAN, INSULIN SEMISYNTHETIC
  PURIFIED HUMAN (OTC)
VELSAR, VINBLASTINE SULFATE
VELTANE, BROMPHENIRAMINE MALEATE
VENTAIRE, PROTOKYLOL HYDROCHLORIDE
VENTOLIN, ALBUTEROL
VENTOLIN, ALBUTEROL SULFATE
VENTOLIN ROTACAPS, ALBUTEROL SULFATE
VEPESID, ETOPOSIDE
VERAPAMIL HCL, VERAPAMIL HYDROCHLORIDE
VERCYTE, PIPOBROMAN
VERELAN, VERAPAMIL HYDROCHLORIDE
VERILOID, ALKAVERVIR
VERMIDOL, PIPERAZINE CITRATE
VERMOX, MEBENDAZOLE
VERSAPEN, HETACILLIN
VERSAPEN-K, HETACILLIN POTASSIUM
VERSED, MIDAZOLAM HYDROCHLORIDE
VERTAVIS, VERATRUM VIRIDE
VESPRIN, TRIFLUPROMAZINE
VESPRIN, TRIFLUPROMAZINE HYDROCHLORIDE
VI-DOM-A, VITAMIN A PALMITATE
VI-TWEL, CYANOCOBALAMIN
VIBISONE, CYANOCOBALAMIN
VIBRA-TABS, DOXYCYCLINE HYCLATE
VIBRAMYCIN, DOXYCYCLINE
VIBRAMYCIN, DOXYCYCLINE CALCIUM
VIBRAMYCIN, DOXYCYCLINE HYCLATE
VICKS FORMULA 44, DIPHENHYDRAMINE
  HYDROCHLORIDE (OTC)
VICODIN, ACETAMINOPHEN
VICODIN ES, ACETAMINOPHEN
VICOPRIN, ASPIRIN
VIDEX, DIDANOSINE
VINBLASTINE SULFATE, VINBLASTINE SULFATE
VINCASAR PFS, VINCRISTINE SULFATE
VINCREX, VINCRISTINE SULFATE
VINCRISTINE SULFATE, VINCRISTINE SULFATE
VINCRISTINE SULFATE PFS, VINCRISTINE SULFATE
VIOCIN SULFATE, VIOMYCIN SULFATE
VIOFORM-HYDROCORTISONE, CLIOQUINOL
VIRA-A, VIDARABINE
VIRAC REX, UNDECOYLIUM CHLORIDE
VIRAZOLE, RIBAVIRIN
VIRILON, METHYLTESTOSTERONE
VIROPTIC, TRIFLURIDINE
VISINE L.R., OXYMETAZOLINE HYDROCHLORIDE (OTC)
VISKAZIDE, HYDROCHLOROTHIAZIDE
VISKEN, PINDOLOL
VISTARIL, HYDROXYZINE HYDROCHLORIDE
VISTARIL, HYDROXYZINE PAMOATE
VITAMIN A, VITAMIN A
VITAMIN A, VITAMIN A PALMITATE
VITAMIN A PALMITATE, VITAMIN A PALMITATE
VITAMIN A SOLUBILIZED, VITAMIN A PALMITATE
VITAMIN D, ERGOCALCIFEROL
VITAMIN K1, PHYTONADIONE
VIVACTIL, PROTRIPTYLINE HYDROCHLORIDE
VOLTAREN, DICLOFENAC SODIUM
VONTROL, DIPHENIDOL HYDROCHLORIDE
VOSOL, ACETIC ACID, GLACIAL
VOSOL HC, ACETIC ACID, GLACIAL
VUMON, TENIPOSIDE

APPENDIX A
PRODUCT NAME INDEX *(continued)*

W

WAMPOCAP, NIACIN
WARFARIN SODIUM, WARFARIN SODIUM
WELLBUTRIN, BUPROPION HYDROCHLORIDE
WELLCOVORIN, LEUCOVORIN CALCIUM
WESTADONE, METHADONE HYDROCHLORIDE
WESTCORT, HYDROCORTISONE VALERATE
WIGRAINE, CAFFEINE
WIGRETTES, ERGOTAMINE TARTRATE
WINSTROL, STANOZOLOL
WOLFINA, RAUWOLFIA SERPENTINA
WYAMINE SULFATE, MEPHENTERMINE SULFATE
WYAMYCIN E, ERYTHROMYCIN ETHYLSUCCINATE
WYAMYCIN S, ERYTHROMYCIN STEARATE
WYCILLIN, PENICILLIN G PROCAINE
WYDASE, HYALURONIDASE
WYGESIC, ACETAMINOPHEN
WYMOX, AMOXICILLIN
WYTENSIN, GUANABENZ ACETATE

X

X-TROZINE, PHENDIMETRAZINE TARTRATE
X-TROZINE L.A., PHENDIMETRAZINE TARTRATE
XANAX, ALPRAZOLAM
XENEISOL, XENON, XE-133
XENON XE 127, XENON, XE-127
XENON XE 133, XENON, XE-133
XENON XE 133-V.S.S., XENON, XE-133
XYLO-PFAN, XYLOSE
XYLOCAINE, LIDOCAINE
XYLOCAINE, LIDOCAINE HYDROCHLORIDE
XYLOCAINE VISCOUS, LIDOCAINE HYDROCHLORIDE
XYLOCAINE W/ DEXTROSE 7.5%, LIDOCAINE
    HYDROCHLORIDE
XYLOCAINE W/ EPINEPHRINE, EPINEPHRINE
XYLOCAINE 4%, LIDOCAINE HYDROCHLORIDE
XYLOCAINE 5% W/ GLUCOSE 7.5%, LIDOCAINE
    HYDROCHLORIDE
XYLOSE, XYLOSE

Y

YTTERBIUM YB 169 DTPA, PENTETATE CALCIUM
    TRISODIUM YB-169
YUTOPAR, RITODRINE HYDROCHLORIDE

Z

ZANOSAR, STREPTOZOCIN
ZANTAC, RANITIDINE HYDROCHLORIDE
ZANTAC 150, RANITIDINE HYDROCHLORIDE
ZANTAC 300, RANITIDINE HYDROCHLORIDE
ZARONTIN, ETHOSUXIMIDE
ZAROXOLYN, METOLAZONE
ZAXOPAM, OXAZEPAM
ZEBETA, BISOPROLOL FUMARATE
ZEFAZONE, CEFMETAZOLE SODIUM
ZESTORETIC 20/12.5, HYDROCHLOROTHIAZIDE
ZESTORETIC 20/25, HYDROCHLOROTHIAZIDE
ZESTRIL, LISINOPRIL
ZIBA-RX, BACITRACIN ZINC
ZIDE, HYDROCHLOROTHIAZIDE
ZINACEF, CEFUROXIME SODIUM
ZINC BACITRACIN,NEOMYCIN SULFATE,POLYMYXIN B
    SULFATE & HYDROCORTISONE, BACITRACIN ZINC
ZINC CHLORIDE, ZINC CHLORIDE
ZINC SULFATE, ZINC SULFATE
ZIPAN-25, PROMETHAZINE HYDROCHLORIDE
ZIPAN-50, PROMETHAZINE HYDROCHLORIDE
ZITHROMAX, AZITHROMYCIN DIHYDRATE
ZOCOR, SIMVASTATIN
ZOFRAN, ONDANSETRON HYDROCHLORIDE
ZOLADEX, GOSERELIN ACETATE
ZOLICEF, CEFAZOLIN SODIUM
ZOLOFT, SERTRALINE HYDROCHLORIDE
ZOLYSE, CHYMOTRYPSIN
ZOVIRAX, ACYCLOVIR
ZOVIRAX, ACYCLOVIR SODIUM
ZYLOPRIM, ALLOPURINOL

8

8-HOUR BAYER, ASPIRIN (OTC)
8-MOP, METHOXSALEN

APPENDIX B
PRODUCT NAME INDEX
LISTED BY APPLICANT

A

ABANA
* ABANA PHARMACEUTICALS INC
  NORCET, ACETAMINOPHEN

ABBOTT
* ABBOTT LABORATORIES
  PENTAMIDINE ISETHIONATE, PENTAMIDINE
  ISETHIONATE
* ABBOTT LABORATORIES HOSP PRODUCTS DIV
  A-HYDROCORT, HYDROCORTISONE SODIUM
  SUCCINATE
  A-METHAPRED, METHYLPREDNISOLONE SODIUM
  SUCCINATE
  AMINOCAPROIC ACID, AMINOCAPROIC ACID
  AMINOSYN II 10%, AMINO ACIDS
  AMINOSYN II 15%, AMINO ACIDS
  AMINOSYN II 3.5% IN DEXTROSE 25%, AMINO ACIDS
  AMINOSYN II 3.5% IN DEXTROSE 5%, AMINO ACIDS
  AMINOSYN II 3.5% M IN DEXTROSE 5%, AMINO ACIDS
  AMINOSYN II 3.5% W/ ELECTROLYTES IN DEXTROSE
  25% W/ CALCIUM, AMINO ACIDS
  AMINOSYN II 4.25% IN DEXTROSE 10%, AMINO ACIDS
  AMINOSYN II 4.25% IN DEXTROSE 20%, AMINO ACIDS
  AMINOSYN II 4.25% IN DEXTROSE 25%, AMINO ACIDS
  AMINOSYN II 4.25% M IN DEXTROSE 10%, AMINO
  ACIDS
  AMINOSYN II 4.25% W/ ELECT AND ADJUSTED
  PHOSPHATE IN DEXTROSE 10%, AMINO ACIDS
  AMINOSYN II 4.25% W/ ELECTROLYTES IN DEXTROSE
  20% W/ CALCIUM, AMINO ACIDS
  AMINOSYN II 4.25% W/ ELECTROLYTES IN DEXTROSE
  25% W/ CALCIUM, AMINO ACIDS
  AMINOSYN II 5% IN DEXTROSE 25%, AMINO ACIDS
  AMINOSYN II 5% W/ ELECTROLYTES IN DEXTROSE
  25% W/ CALCIUM, AMINO ACIDS
  BUPIVACAINE HCL AND EPINEPHRINE,
  BUPIVACAINE HYDROCHLORIDE
  CLINDAMYCIN PHOSPHATE, CLINDAMYCIN
  PHOSPHATE
  DEXTROSE 50%, DEXTROSE
  DEXTROSE 70%, DEXTROSE
  DIAZEPAM, DIAZEPAM
  DOPAMINE HCL, DOPAMINE HYDROCHLORIDE
  FENTANYL CITRATE, FENTANYL CITRATE
  FENTANYL CITRATE AND DROPERIDOL,
  DROPERIDOL
  HEPARIN SODIUM 20,000 UNITS IN DEXTROSE 5%,
  HEPARIN SODIUM
  HEPARIN SODIUM 25,000 UNITS IN DEXTROSE 5%,
  HEPARIN SODIUM
  INPERSOL W/ DEXTROSE 1.5%, CALCIUM CHLORIDE
  INPERSOL W/ DEXTROSE 2.5% IN PLASTIC
  CONTAINER, CALCIUM CHLORIDE
  INPERSOL W/ DEXTROSE 3.5%, CALCIUM CHLORIDE
  INPERSOL W/ DEXTROSE 4.25%, CALCIUM CHLORIDE
  INPERSOL-LM W/ DEXTROSE 1.5%, CALCIUM
  CHLORIDE
  INPERSOL-LM W/ DEXTROSE 2.5%, CALCIUM
  CHLORIDE
  INPERSOL-LM W/ DEXTROSE 3.5%, CALCIUM
  CHLORIDE
  INPERSOL-LM W/ DEXTROSE 4.25%, CALCIUM
  CHLORIDE

LIDOCAINE HCL, LIDOCAINE HYDROCHLORIDE
LIDOCAINE HCL AND EPINEPHRINE, EPINEPHRINE
METOCLOPRAMIDE HCL, METOCLOPRAMIDE
  HYDROCHLORIDE
MORPHINE SULFATE, MORPHINE SULFATE
NALBUPHINE HCL, NALBUPHINE HYDROCHLORIDE
NITROGLYCERIN IN DEXTROSE 5%, NITROGLYCERIN
NITROPRESS, SODIUM NITROPRUSSIDE
PANCURONIUM BROMIDE, PANCURONIUM BROMIDE
POTASSIUM CHLORIDE 10 MEQ IN DEXTROSE 5% AND
  LACTATED RINGER'S, CALCIUM CHLORIDE
POTASSIUM CHLORIDE 15 MEQ IN DEXTROSE 5% AND
  LACTATED RINGER'S, CALCIUM CHLORIDE
POTASSIUM CHLORIDE 20 MEQ IN DEXTROSE 5% AND
  LACTATED RINGER'S, CALCIUM CHLORIDE
POTASSIUM CHLORIDE 20 MEQ IN SODIUM
  CHLORIDE 0.9%, POTASSIUM CHLORIDE
POTASSIUM CHLORIDE 30 MEQ IN DEXTROSE 5% AND
  LACTATED RINGER'S, CALCIUM CHLORIDE
POTASSIUM CHLORIDE 40 MEQ IN DEXTROSE 5% AND
  LACTATED RINGER'S, CALCIUM CHLORIDE
POTASSIUM CHLORIDE 40 MEQ IN SODIUM
  CHLORIDE 0.9%, POTASSIUM CHLORIDE
POTASSIUM CHLORIDE 5 MEQ IN DEXTROSE 5% AND
  LACTATED RINGER'S, CALCIUM CHLORIDE
RITODRINE HCL, RITODRINE HYDROCHLORIDE
RITODRINE HCL IN DEXTROSE 5% IN PLASTIC
  CONTAINER, RITODRINE HYDROCHLORIDE
SODIUM CHLORIDE 0.45%, SODIUM CHLORIDE
STERILE WATER FOR INJECTION, WATER FOR
  INJECTION, STERILE
TOBRAMYCIN SULFATE, TOBRAMYCIN SULFATE
TOBRAMYCIN SULFATE IN SODIUM CHLORIDE 0.9%,
  TOBRAMYCIN SULFATE
VANCOMYCIN HCL, VANCOMYCIN HYDROCHLORIDE
* ABBOTT LABORATORIES PHARMACEUTICAL
PRODUCTS DIV
  A-HYDROCORT, HYDROCORTISONE SODIUM
  SUCCINATE
  A-METHAPRED, METHYLPREDNISOLONE SODIUM
  SUCCINATE
  A-POXIDE, CHLORDIAZEPOXIDE HYDROCHLORIDE
  ACETIC ACID 0.25% IN PLASTIC CONTAINER, ACETIC
  ACID, GLACIAL
  ALCOHOL 5% IN D5-W, ALCOHOL
  AMIDATE, ETOMIDATE
  AMINOCAPROIC ACID, AMINOCAPROIC ACID
  AMINOPHYLLINE, AMINOPHYLLINE
  AMINOPHYLLINE IN SODIUM CHLORIDE 0.45%,
  AMINOPHYLLINE
  AMINOPHYLLINE IN SODIUM CHLORIDE 0.45% IN
  PLASTIC CONTAINER, AMINOPHYLLINE
  AMINOSOL 5%, PROTEIN HYDROLYSATE
  AMINOSYN II 10%, AMINO ACIDS
  AMINOSYN II 10% W/ ELECTROLYTES, AMINO ACIDS
  AMINOSYN II 3.5%, AMINO ACIDS
  AMINOSYN II 3.5% IN DEXTROSE 25%, AMINO ACIDS
  AMINOSYN II 3.5% IN DEXTROSE 5%, AMINO ACIDS
  AMINOSYN II 3.5% M, AMINO ACIDS
  AMINOSYN II 3.5% M IN DEXTROSE 5%, AMINO ACIDS
  AMINOSYN II 3.5% W/ ELECTROLYTES IN DEXTROSE
  25%, AMINO ACID
  AMINOSYN II 4.25% IN DEXTROSE 25%, AMINO ACIDS
  AMINOSYN II 4.25% M IN DEXTROSE 10%, AMINO
  ACIDS
  AMINOSYN II 4.25% W/ ELECTROLYTES IN DEXTROSE
  25%, AMINO ACIDS

APPENDIX B
PRODUCT NAME INDEX
LISTED BY APPLICANT (continued)

AMINOSYN II 5%, AMINO ACIDS
AMINOSYN II 5% IN DEXTROSE 25%, AMINO ACIDS
AMINOSYN II 7%, AMINO ACIDS
AMINOSYN II 7% W/ ELECTROLYTES, AMINO ACIDS
AMINOSYN II 8.5%, AMINO ACIDS
AMINOSYN II 8.5% W/ ELECTROLYTES, AMINO ACIDS
AMINOSYN 10%, AMINO ACIDS
AMINOSYN 10% (PH6), AMINO ACIDS
AMINOSYN 3.5%, AMINO ACIDS
AMINOSYN 3.5% IN PLASTIC CONTAINER, AMINO
   ACIDS
AMINOSYN 3.5% M, AMINO ACIDS
AMINOSYN 3.5% M IN PLASTIC CONTAINER, AMINO
   ACIDS
AMINOSYN 3.5% W/ DEXTROSE 25% IN PLASTIC
   CONTAINER, AMINO ACIDS
AMINOSYN 3.5% W/ DEXTROSE 5% IN PLASTIC
   CONTAINER, AMINO ACIDS
AMINOSYN 4.25% W/ DEXTROSE 25% IN PLASTIC
   CONTAINER, AMINO ACIDS
AMINOSYN 5%, AMINO ACIDS
AMINOSYN 7%, AMINO ACIDS
AMINOSYN 7% (PH6), AMINO ACIDS
AMINOSYN 7% W/ ELECTROLYTES, AMINO ACIDS
AMINOSYN 8.5%, AMINO ACIDS
AMINOSYN 8.5% (PH6), AMINO ACIDS
AMINOSYN 8.5% W/ ELECTROLYTES, AMINO ACIDS
AMINOSYN-HBC 7%, AMINO ACIDS
AMINOSYN-HBC 7% IN PLASTIC CONTAINER, AMINO
   ACIDS
AMINOSYN-PF 10%, AMINO ACIDS
AMINOSYN-PF 7%, AMINO ACIDS
AMINOSYN-RF 5.2%, AMINO ACIDS
AMMONIUM CHLORIDE, AMMONIUM CHLORIDE
AMMONIUM CHLORIDE IN PLASTIC CONTAINER,
   AMMONIUM CHLORIDE
BACTERIOSTATIC SODIUM CHLORIDE 0.9% IN
   PLASTIC CONTAINER, SODIUM CHLORIDE
BACTERIOSTATIC WATER FOR INJECTION, WATER
   FOR INJECTION, STERILE
BIAXIN, CLARITHROMYCIN
BRETYLIUM TOSYLATE, BRETYLIUM TOSYLATE
BRETYLIUM TOSYLATE IN DEXTROSE 5%,
   BRETYLIUM TOSYLATE
BRETYLIUM TOSYLATE IN DEXTROSE 5% IN PLASTIC
   CONTAINER, BRETYLIUM TOSYLATE
BUPIVACAINE, BUPIVACAINE HYDROCHLORIDE
BUPIVACAINE HCL, BUPIVACAINE HYDROCHLORIDE
CALCIJEX, CALCITRIOL
CALCIUM GLUCEPTATE, CALCIUM GLUCEPTATE
CARTROL, CARTEOLOL HYDROCHLORIDE
CEPHALOTHIN SODIUM, CEPHALOTHIN SODIUM
CHLOROPROCAINE HCL, CHLOROPROCAINE
   HYDROCHLORIDE
CHLORTHALIDONE, CHLORTHALIDONE
CHROMIC CHLORIDE, CHROMIC CHLORIDE
CLINDAMYCIN PHOSPHATE, CLINDAMYCIN
   PHOSPHATE
CUPRIC CHLORIDE, CUPRIC CHLORIDE
CYLERT, PEMOLINE
DEPAKENE, VALPROIC ACID
DEPAKOTE, DIVALPROEX SODIUM
DEPAKOTE CP, DIVALPROEX SODIUM
DESOXYN, METHAMPHETAMINE HYDROCHLORIDE
DEXTROSE 10% IN PLASTIC CONTAINER, DEXTROSE
DEXTROSE 2.5% AND SODIUM CHLORIDE 0.45% IN
   PLASTIC CONTAINER, DEXTROSE
DEXTROSE 20% IN PLASTIC CONTAINER, DEXTROSE
DEXTROSE 3.3% AND SODIUM CHLORIDE 0.3% IN
   PLASTIC CONTAINER, DEXTROSE

DEXTROSE 30% IN PLASTIC CONTAINER, DEXTROSE
DEXTROSE 38.5% IN PLASTIC CONTAINER, DEXTROSE
DEXTROSE 40% IN PLASTIC CONTAINER, DEXTROSE
DEXTROSE 5%, DEXTROSE
DEXTROSE 5% AND LACTATED RINGER'S IN PLASTIC
   CONTAINER, CALCIUM CHLORIDE
DEXTROSE 5% AND RINGER'S IN PLASTIC
   CONTAINER, CALCIUM CHLORIDE
DEXTROSE 5% AND SODIUM CHLORIDE 0.225%,
   DEXTROSE
DEXTROSE 5% AND SODIUM CHLORIDE 0.225% IN
   PLASTIC CONTAINER, DEXTROSE
DEXTROSE 5% AND SODIUM CHLORIDE 0.3%,
   DEXTROSE
DEXTROSE 5% AND SODIUM CHLORIDE 0.3% IN
   PLASTIC CONTAINER, DEXTROSE
DEXTROSE 5% AND SODIUM CHLORIDE 0.45%,
   DEXTROSE
DEXTROSE 5% AND SODIUM CHLORIDE 0.45% IN
   PLASTIC CONTAINER, DEXTROSE
DEXTROSE 5% AND SODIUM CHLORIDE 0.9%,
   DEXTROSE
DEXTROSE 5% AND SODIUM CHLORIDE 0.9% IN
   PLASTIC CONTAINER, DEXTROSE
DEXTROSE 5% IN PLASTIC CONTAINER, DEXTROSE
DEXTROSE 50% IN PLASTIC CONTAINER, DEXTROSE
DEXTROSE 60% IN PLASTIC CONTAINER, DEXTROSE
DEXTROSE 70% IN PLASTIC CONTAINER, DEXTROSE
DIASONE SODIUM, SULFOXONE SODIUM
DICUMAROL, DICUMAROL
DOPAMINE HCL, DOPAMINE HYDROCHLORIDE
DOPAMINE HCL IN DEXTROSE 5%, DOPAMINE
   HYDROCHLORIDE
DROPERIDOL, DROPERIDOL
E.E.S., ERYTHROMYCIN ETHYLSUCCINATE
E.E.S. 200, ERYTHROMYCIN ETHYLSUCCINATE
E.E.S. 400, ERYTHROMYCIN ETHYLSUCCINATE
ENDRATE, EDETATE DISODIUM
ENDURON, METHYCLOTHIAZIDE
ENDURONYL, DESERPIDINE
ENDURONYL FORTE, DESERPIDINE
ENFLURANE, ENFLURANE
ERY-TAB, ERYTHROMYCIN
ERYDERM, ERYTHROMYCIN
ERYPED, ERYTHROMYCIN ETHYLSUCCINATE
ERYTHROCIN, ERYTHROMYCIN LACTOBIONATE
ERYTHROCIN STEARATE, ERYTHROMYCIN
   STEARATE
ERYTHROMYCIN, ERYTHROMYCIN
EUTONYL, PARGYLINE HYDROCHLORIDE
EUTRON, METHYCLOTHIAZIDE
FENTANYL CITRATE, FENTANYL CITRATE
FUROSEMIDE, FUROSEMIDE
GEMONIL, METHARBITAL
GENTAMICIN SULFATE, GENTAMICIN SULFATE
GENTAMICIN SULFATE IN SODIUM CHLORIDE 0.9%,
   GENTAMICIN SULFATE
GLYCINE 1.5%, GLYCINE
GLYCINE 1.5% IN PLASTIC CONTAINER, GLYCINE
GLYCOPYRROLATE, GLYCOPYRROLATE
HALOTHANE, HALOTHANE
HARMONYL, DESERPIDINE
HEPARIN LOCK FLUSH, HEPARIN SODIUM
HEPARIN SODIUM, HEPARIN SODIUM
HEPARIN SODIUM 10,000 UNITS IN DEXTROSE 5%,
   HEPARIN SODIUM
HEPARIN SODIUM 10,000 UNITS IN DEXTROSE 5% IN
   PLASTIC CONTAINER, HEPARIN SODIUM
HEPARIN SODIUM 10,000 UNITS IN SODIUM
   CHLORIDE 0.45%, HEPARIN SODIUM

APPENDIX B
PRODUCT NAME INDEX
LISTED BY APPLICANT (continued)

HEPARIN SODIUM 10,000 UNITS IN SODIUM
CHLORIDE 0.9%, HEPARIN SODIUM
HEPARIN SODIUM 1000 UNITS IN SODIUM CHLORIDE
0.9%, HEPARIN SODIUM
HEPARIN SODIUM 12,500 UNITS IN DEXTROSE 5%,
HEPARIN SODIUM
HEPARIN SODIUM 12,500 UNITS IN DEXTROSE 5% IN
PLASTIC CONTAINER, HEPARIN SODIUM
HEPARIN SODIUM 12,500 UNITS IN SODIUM
CHLORIDE 0.45%, HEPARIN SODIUM
HEPARIN SODIUM 12,500 UNITS IN SODIUM
CHLORIDE 0.9%, HEPARIN SODIUM
HEPARIN SODIUM 2000 UNITS IN SODIUM CHLORIDE
0.9%, HEPARIN SODIUM
HEPARIN SODIUM 25,000 UNITS IN DEXTROSE 5%,
HEPARIN SODIUM
HEPARIN SODIUM 25,000 UNITS IN DEXTROSE 5% IN
PLASTIC CONTAINER, HEPARIN SODIUM
HEPARIN SODIUM 25,000 UNITS IN SODIUM
CHLORIDE 0.45%, HEPARIN SODIUM
HEPARIN SODIUM 25,000 UNITS IN SODIUM
CHLORIDE 0.9%, HEPARIN SODIUM
HEPARIN SODIUM 5,000 UNITS IN SODIUM CHLORIDE
0.45%, HEPARIN SODIUM
HEPARIN SODIUM 5000 UNITS IN SODIUM CHLORIDE
0.45%, HEPARIN SODIUM
HEPARIN SODIUM 5000 UNITS IN SODIUM CHLORIDE
0.9%, HEPARIN SODIUM
HYDROXYZINE HCL, HYDROXYZINE
HYDROCHLORIDE
HYTRIN, TERAZOSIN HYDROCHLORIDE
INPERSOL-ZM W/ DEXTROSE 1.5% IN PLASTIC
CONTAINER, CALCIUM CHLORIDE
INPERSOL-ZM W/ DEXTROSE 2.5% IN PLASTIC
CONTAINER, CALCIUM CHLORIDE
INPERSOL-ZM W/ DEXTROSE 4.25% IN PLASTIC
CONTAINER, CALCIUM CHLORIDE
IONOSOL B AND DEXTROSE 5%, DEXTROSE
IONOSOL MB AND DEXTROSE 5%, DEXTROSE
IONOSOL T AND DEXTROSE 5%, DEXTROSE
ISOPROTERENOL HCL, ISOPROTERENOL
HYDROCHLORIDE
JANIMINE, IMIPRAMINE HYDROCHLORIDE
K-TAB, POTASSIUM CHLORIDE
LACTATED RINGER'S, CALCIUM CHLORIDE
LACTATED RINGER'S IN PLASTIC CONTAINER,
CALCIUM CHLORIDE
LIDOCAINE HCL, LIDOCAINE HYDROCHLORIDE
LIDOCAINE HCL AND DEXTROSE 7.5%, LIDOCAINE
HYDROCHLORIDE
LIDOCAINE HCL AND EPINEPHRINE, EPINEPHRINE
LIDOCAINE HCL IN PLASTIC CONTAINER,
LIDOCAINE HYDROCHLORIDE
LIDOCAINE HCL W/ EPINEPHRINE, EPINEPHRINE
LIDOCAINE HCL 0.2% IN DEXTROSE 5%, LIDOCAINE
HYDROCHLORIDE
LIDOCAINE HCL 0.2% IN DEXTROSE 5% IN PLASTIC
CONTAINER, LIDOCAINE HYDROCHLORIDE
LIDOCAINE HCL 0.4% IN DEXTROSE 5%, LIDOCAINE
HYDROCHLORIDE
LIDOCAINE HCL 0.4% IN DEXTROSE 5% IN PLASTIC
CONTAINER, LIDOCAINE HYDROCHLORIDE
LIDOCAINE HCL 0.8% IN DEXTROSE 5% IN PLASTIC
CONTAINER, LIDOCAINE HYDROCHLORIDE
LIPOSYN II 10%, SAFFLOWER OIL
LIPOSYN II 20%, SAFFLOWER OIL
LIPOSYN III 10%, SOYBEAN OIL
LIPOSYN III 20%, SOYBEAN OIL
LIPOSYN 10%, SAFFLOWER OIL
LIPOSYN 20%, SAFFLOWER OIL

LTA II KIT, LIDOCAINE HYDROCHLORIDE
MANGANESE CHLORIDE, MANGANESE CHLORIDE
MANNITOL 10%, MANNITOL
MANNITOL 15%, MANNITOL
MANNITOL 20%, MANNITOL
MANNITOL 25%, MANNITOL
MANNITOL 5%, MANNITOL
MEPERIDINE HCL, MEPERIDINE HYDROCHLORIDE
METHYLDOPATE HCL, METHYLDOPATE
HYDROCHLORIDE
METRONIDAZOLE, METRONIDAZOLE
NALOXONE HCL, NALOXONE HYDROCHLORIDE
NEMBUTAL, PENTOBARBITAL
NEMBUTAL, PENTOBARBITAL SODIUM
NEMBUTAL SODIUM, PENTOBARBITAL SODIUM
NITROGLYCERIN, NITROGLYCERIN
NITROPRESS, SODIUM NITROPRUSSIDE
NORISODRINE, ISOPROTERENOL SULFATE
NORISODRINE AEROTROL, ISOPROTERENOL
HYDROCHLORIDE
NORMOSOL-M AND DEXTROSE 5%, DEXTROSE
NORMOSOL-R AND DEXTROSE 5% IN PLASTIC
CONTAINER, DEXTROSE
NORMOSOL-R IN PLASTIC CONTAINER, MAGNESIUM
CHLORIDE
OCL, POLYETHYLENE GLYCOL 3350
OGEN, ESTROPIPATE
OGEN .625, ESTROPIPATE
OGEN 1.25, ESTROPIPATE
OGEN 2.5, ESTROPIPATE
OGEN 5, ESTROPIPATE
OMNIFLOX, TEMAFLOXACIN HYDROCHLORIDE
ORETIC, HYDROCHLOROTHIAZIDE
ORETICYL FORTE, DESERPIDINE
ORETICYL 25, DESERPIDINE
ORETICYL 50, DESERPIDINE
OXYTOCIN 10 USP UNITS IN DEXTROSE 5%,
OXYTOCIN
OXYTOCIN 20 USP UNITS IN DEXTROSE 5%,
OXYTOCIN
OXYTOCIN 5 USP UNITS IN DEXTROSE 5%, OXYTOCIN
PANHEPRIN, HEPARIN SODIUM
PANWARFIN, WARFARIN SODIUM
PARADIONE, PARAMETHADIONE
PCE, ERYTHROMYCIN
PEDIATRIC LTA KIT, LIDOCAINE HYDROCHLORIDE
PEGANONE, ETHOTOIN
PENTHRANE, METHOXYFLURANE
PENTOTHAL, THIOPENTAL SODIUM
PHENURONE, PHENACEMIDE
PHENYTOIN SODIUM, PHENYTOIN SODIUM
PHYSIOSOL IN PLASTIC CONTAINER, MAGNESIUM
CHLORIDE
PHYSIOSOL PH 7.4, MAGNESIUM CHLORIDE
PLACIDYL, ETHCHLORVYNOL
PLEGISOL, CALCIUM CHLORIDE
POTASSIUM ACETATE IN PLASTIC CONTAINER,
POTASSIUM ACETATE
POTASSIUM CHLORIDE, POTASSIUM CHLORIDE
POTASSIUM CHLORIDE 10 MEQ IN DEXTROSE 5% AND
SODIUM CHLORIDE 0.225%, DEXTROSE
POTASSIUM CHLORIDE 10 MEQ IN DEXTROSE 5% AND
SODIUM CHLORIDE 0.3%, DEXTROSE
POTASSIUM CHLORIDE 10 MEQ IN DEXTROSE 5% AND
SODIUM CHLORIDE 0.45%, DEXTROSE
POTASSIUM CHLORIDE 10 MEQ IN DEXTROSE 5% AND
SODIUM CHLORIDE 0.9%, DEXTROSE
POTASSIUM CHLORIDE 15 MEQ IN DEXTROSE 5% AND
SODIUM CHLORIDE 0.225%, DEXTROSE
POTASSIUM CHLORIDE 15 MEQ IN DEXTROSE 5% AND
SODIUM CHLORIDE 0.3%, DEXTROSE

APPENDIX B
PRODUCT NAME INDEX
LISTED BY APPLICANT (continued)

POTASSIUM CHLORIDE 15 MEQ IN DEXTROSE 5% AND SODIUM CHLORIDE 0.45%, DEXTROSE

POTASSIUM CHLORIDE 15 MEQ IN DEXTROSE 5% AND SODIUM CHLORIDE 0.9%, DEXTROSE

POTASSIUM CHLORIDE 20 MEQ IN DEXTROSE 5%, DEXTROSE

POTASSIUM CHLORIDE 20 MEQ IN DEXTROSE 5% AND SODIUM CHLORIDE 0.225%, DEXTROSE

POTASSIUM CHLORIDE 20 MEQ IN DEXTROSE 5% AND SODIUM CHLORIDE 0.3%, DEXTROSE

POTASSIUM CHLORIDE 20 MEQ IN DEXTROSE 5% AND SODIUM CHLORIDE 0.45%, DEXTROSE

POTASSIUM CHLORIDE 20 MEQ IN DEXTROSE 5% AND SODIUM CHLORIDE 0.9%, DEXTROSE

POTASSIUM CHLORIDE 20 MEQ IN DEXTROSE 5% IN SODIUM CHLORIDE 0.3%, DEXTROSE

POTASSIUM CHLORIDE 30 MEQ IN DEXTROSE 5%, DEXTROSE

POTASSIUM CHLORIDE 30 MEQ IN DEXTROSE 5% AND SODIUM CHLORIDE 0.225%, DEXTROSE

POTASSIUM CHLORIDE 30 MEQ IN DEXTROSE 5% AND SODIUM CHLORIDE 0.3%, DEXTROSE

POTASSIUM CHLORIDE 30 MEQ IN DEXTROSE 5% AND SODIUM CHLORIDE 0.45%, DEXTROSE

POTASSIUM CHLORIDE 30 MEQ IN DEXTROSE 5% AND SODIUM CHLORIDE 0.9%, DEXTROSE

POTASSIUM CHLORIDE 40 MEQ IN DEXTROSE 5%, DEXTROSE

POTASSIUM CHLORIDE 40 MEQ IN DEXTROSE 5% AND SODIUM CHLORIDE 0.225%, DEXTROSE

POTASSIUM CHLORIDE 40 MEQ IN DEXTROSE 5% AND SODIUM CHLORIDE 0.3%, DEXTROSE

POTASSIUM CHLORIDE 40 MEQ IN DEXTROSE 5% AND SODIUM CHLORIDE 0.45%, DEXTROSE

POTASSIUM CHLORIDE 40 MEQ IN DEXTROSE 5% AND SODIUM CHLORIDE 0.9%, DEXTROSE

POTASSIUM CHLORIDE 5 MEQ IN DEXTROSE 5% AND SODIUM CHLORIDE 0.225%, DEXTROSE

POTASSIUM CHLORIDE 5 MEQ IN DEXTROSE 5% AND SODIUM CHLORIDE 0.3%, DEXTROSE

POTASSIUM CHLORIDE 5 MEQ IN DEXTROSE 5% AND SODIUM CHLORIDE 0.45%, DEXTROSE

POTASSIUM CHLORIDE 5 MEQ IN DEXTROSE 5% AND SODIUM CHLORIDE 0.9%, DEXTROSE

PROCAINAMIDE HCL, PROCAINAMIDE HYDROCHLORIDE

PROCAINE HCL, PROCAINE HYDROCHLORIDE

PROSOM, ESTAZOLAM

QUELICIN, SUCCINYLCHOLINE CHLORIDE

RADIONUCLIDE-LABELED (125 I) FIBRINOGEN (HUMAN) SENSOR, FIBRINOGEN, I-125

RINGER'S IN PLASTIC CONTAINER, CALCIUM CHLORIDE

SELSUN, SELENIUM SULFIDE

SODIUM ACETATE IN PLASTIC CONTAINER, SODIUM ACETATE, ANHYDROUS

SODIUM BICARBONATE IN PLASTIC CONTAINER, SODIUM BICARBONATE

SODIUM CHLORIDE, SODIUM CHLORIDE

SODIUM CHLORIDE IN PLASTIC CONTAINER, SODIUM CHLORIDE

SODIUM CHLORIDE 0.45% IN PLASTIC CONTAINER, SODIUM CHLORIDE

SODIUM CHLORIDE 0.9%, SODIUM CHLORIDE

SODIUM CHLORIDE 0.9% IN PLASTIC CONTAINER, SODIUM CHLORIDE

SODIUM LACTATE IN PLASTIC CONTAINER, SODIUM LACTATE

SODIUM LACTATE 0.167 MOLAR IN PLASTIC CONTAINER, SODIUM LACTATE

SODIUM PHOSPHATES IN PLASTIC CONTAINER, SODIUM PHOSPHATE, DIBASIC

SORBITOL-MANNITOL, MANNITOL

SORBITOL-MANNITOL IN PLASTIC CONTAINER, MANNITOL

STERILE UREA, UREA

STERILE WATER, WATER FOR IRRIGATION, STERILE

STERILE WATER FOR INJECTION, WATER FOR INJECTION, STERILE

STERILE WATER IN PLASTIC CONTAINER, WATER FOR IRRIGATION, STERILE

SULFADIAZINE, SULFADIAZINE

THAM, TROMETHAMINE

THAM-E, POTASSIUM CHLORIDE

THEOPHYLLINE IN DEXTROSE 5%, THEOPHYLLINE

THEOPHYLLINE IN DEXTROSE 5% IN PLASTIC CONTAINER, THEOPHYLLINE

THYPINONE, PROTIRELIN

TPN ELECTROLYTES IN PLASTIC CONTAINER, CALCIUM CHLORIDE

TRAL, HEXOCYCLIUM METHYLSULFATE

TRANXENE, CLORAZEPATE DIPOTASSIUM

TRANXENE SD, CLORAZEPATE DIPOTASSIUM

TRIDIONE, TRIMETHADIONE

TUBOCURARINE CHLORIDE, TUBOCURARINE CHLORIDE

UREAPHIL, UREA

UROLOGIC G IN PLASTIC CONTAINER, CITRIC ACID

VERAPAMIL HCL, VERAPAMIL HYDROCHLORIDE

VERCYTE, PIPOBROMAN

VITAMIN K1, PHYTONADIONE

ZINC CHLORIDE, ZINC CHLORIDE

ABIC
* ABIC LTD

ABITREXATE, METHOTREXATE SODIUM

FLUOROURACIL, FLUOROURACIL

LEUCOVORIN CALCIUM, LEUCOVORIN CALCIUM

VINCRISTINE SULFATE, VINCRISTINE SULFATE

ABLE
* ABLE LABORATORIES INC

CLORAZEPATE DIPOTASSIUM, CLORAZEPATE DIPOTASSIUM

HEMSOL-HC, HYDROCORTISONE ACETATE

ADRIA
* ADRIA LABORATORIES DIV ERBAMONT INC

ADRIAMYCIN PFS, DOXORUBICIN HYDROCHLORIDE

ADRIAMYCIN RDF, DOXORUBICIN HYDROCHLORIDE

ADRUCIL, FLUOROURACIL

AXOTAL, ASPIRIN

CHYMEX, BENTIROMIDE

FLUIDIL, CYCLOTHIAZIDE

FOLEX, METHOTREXATE SODIUM

FOLEX PFS, METHOTREXATE SODIUM

IDAMYCIN, IDARUBICIN HYDROCHLORIDE

K-LEASE, POTASSIUM CHLORIDE

KAON CL, POTASSIUM CHLORIDE

KAON CL-10, POTASSIUM CHLORIDE

NEOSAR, CYCLOPHOSPHAMIDE

TYMTRAN, CERULETIDE DIETHYLAMINE

VANCOR, VANCOMYCIN HYDROCHLORIDE

VINCASAR PFS, VINCRISTINE SULFATE

XYLO-PFAN, XYLOSE

AKORN
* AKORN INC

AK-PENTOLATE, CYCLOPENTOLATE HYDROCHLORIDE

CHLORAMPHENICOL, CHLORAMPHENICOL

COR-OTICIN, HYDROCORTISONE ACETATE

APPENDIX B
PRODUCT NAME INDEX
LISTED BY APPLICANT (continued)

CYANOCOBALAMIN, CYANOCOBALAMIN
DEXAMETHASONE SODIUM PHOSPHATE,
  DEXAMETHASONE SODIUM PHOSPHATE
GENTAMICIN SULFATE, GENTAMICIN SULFATE
HEPARIN SODIUM, HEPARIN SODIUM
HYDROCORTISONE ACETATE, HYDROCORTISONE
  ACETATE
HYDROXYPROGESTERONE CAPROATE,
  HYDROXYPROGESTERONE CAPROATE
LIDOCAINE HCL, LIDOCAINE HYDROCHLORIDE
METHOTREXATE SODIUM, METHOTREXATE SODIUM
METHYLPREDNISOLONE ACETATE,
  METHYLPREDNISOLONE ACETATE
METOCLOPRAMIDE HCL, METOCLOPRAMIDE
  HYDROCHLORIDE
NANDROLONE DECANOATE, NANDROLONE
  DECANOATE
NAPHAZOLINE HCL, NAPHAZOLINE
  HYDROCHLORIDE
POTASSIUM CHLORIDE, POTASSIUM CHLORIDE
PREDAMIDE, PREDNISOLONE ACETATE
PREDNISOLONE ACETATE, PREDNISOLONE ACETATE
PREDNISOLONE SODIUM PHOSPHATE,
  PREDNISOLONE SODIUM PHOSPHATE
PROMETHAZINE HCL, PROMETHAZINE
  HYDROCHLORIDE
PYRIDOXINE HCL, PYRIDOXINE HYDROCHLORIDE
SODIUM SULFACETAMIDE, SULFACETAMIDE SODIUM
THIAMINE HCL, THIAMINE HYDROCHLORIDE
TRIAMCINOLONE DIACETATE, TRIAMCINOLONE
  DIACETATE
TROPICAMIDE, TROPICAMIDE

ALCON
* ALCON LABORATORIES INC
  ALCAINE, PROPARACAINE HYDROCHLORIDE
  ANESTACON, LIDOCAINE HYDROCHLORIDE
  BETOPTIC, BETAXOLOL HYDROCHLORIDE
  BETOPTIC S, BETAXOLOL HYDROCHLORIDE
  BSS PLUS, CALCIUM CHLORIDE
  CETAMIDE, SULFACETAMIDE SODIUM
  CILOXAN, CIPROFLOXACIN HYDROCHLORIDE
  CYCLOGYL, CYCLOPENTOLATE HYDROCHLORIDE
  CYCLOMYDRIL, CYCLOPENTOLATE
    HYDROCHLORIDE
  DENDRID, IDOXURIDINE
  ECONOCHLOR, CHLORAMPHENICOL
  ECONOPRED, PREDNISOLONE ACETATE
  ECONOPRED PLUS, PREDNISOLONE ACETATE
  FLAREX, FLUOROMETHOLONE ACETATE
  IOPIDINE, APRACLONIDINE HYDROCHLORIDE
  ISMOTIC, ISOSORBIDE
  ISOPTO CETAMIDE, SULFACETAMIDE SODIUM
  ISOPTO CETAPRED, PREDNISOLONE ACETATE
  MAXIDEX, DEXAMETHASONE
  MAXIDEX, DEXAMETHASONE SODIUM PHOSPHATE
  MAXITROL, DEXAMETHASONE
  MIOSTAT, CARBACHOL
  MYDRIACYL, TROPICAMIDE
  NAPHCON FORTE, NAPHAZOLINE HYDROCHLORIDE
  NATACYN, NATAMYCIN
  NEOPAP, ACETAMINOPHEN (OTC)
  PANTOPAQUE, IOPHENDYLATE
  PILOPINE HS, PILOCARPINE HYDROCHLORIDE
  PROFENAL, SUPROFEN
  PROMETHACON, PROMETHAZINE HYDROCHLORIDE
  STATROL, NEOMYCIN SULFATE
  TOBRADEX, DEXAMETHASONE
  TOBRASONE, FLUOROMETHOLONE ACETATE
  TOBREX, TOBRAMYCIN
  ZOLYSE, CHYMOTRYPSIN

ALLERGAN
* ALLERGAN PHARMACEUTICALS DIV ALLERGAN INC
  ALBALON, NAPHAZOLINE HYDROCHLORIDE
  BETAGAN, LEVOBUNOLOL HYDROCHLORIDE
  BLEPH-10, SULFACETAMIDE SODIUM
  BLEPH-30, SULFACETAMIDE SODIUM
  BLEPHAMIDE, PREDNISOLONE ACETATE
  BLEPHAMIDE S.O.P., PREDNISOLONE ACETATE
  CHLOROPTIC, CHLORAMPHENICOL
  CHLOROPTIC S.O.P., CHLORAMPHENICOL
  CHLOROPTIC-P S.O.P., CHLORAMPHENICOL
  ETHAMIDE, ETHOXZOLAMIDE
  FML, FLUOROMETHOLONE
  FML FORTE, FLUOROMETHOLONE
  FML-S, FLUOROMETHOLONE
  GENOPTIC, GENTAMICIN SULFATE
  HERPLEX, IDOXURIDINE
  HMS, MEDRYSONE
  NAFTIN, NAFTIFINE HYDROCHLORIDE
  OCUFEN, FLURBIPROFEN SODIUM
  OPHTHETIC, PROPARACAINE HYDROCHLORIDE
  PAREMYD, HYDROXYAMPHETAMINE
    HYDROBROMIDE
  POLY-PRED, NEOMYCIN SULFATE
  PRED FORTE, PREDNISOLONE ACETATE
  PRED MILD, PREDNISOLONE ACETATE
  PRED-G, GENTAMICIN SULFATE
  PREFRIN-A, PHENYLEPHRINE HYDROCHLORIDE
  PROPINE, DIPIVEFRIN HYDROCHLORIDE

ALLERGAN HERBERT
* ALLERGAN HERBERT SKIN CARE DIV ALLERGAN INC
  FLUONID, FLUOCINOLONE ACETONIDE

ALPHA THERAPEUTIC
* ALPHA THERAPEUTIC CORP
  SOYACAL 10%, SOYBEAN OIL
  SOYACAL 20%, SOYBEAN OIL

ALRA
* ALRA LABORATORIES INC
  ACETAZOLAMIDE, ACETAZOLAMIDE
  BAMATE, MEPROBAMATE
  CHOLAC, LACTULOSE
  COMPOUND 65, ASPIRIN
  CONSTILAC, LACTULOSE
  DIMENHYDRINATE, DIMENHYDRINATE
  DIPHENHYDRAMINE HCL, DIPHENHYDRAMINE
    HYDROCHLORIDE
  ERYZOLE, ERYTHROMYCIN ETHYLSUCCINATE
  GEN-XENE, CLORAZEPATE DIPOTASSIUM
  HYDROCHLOROTHIAZIDE, HYDROCHLOROTHIAZIDE
  IBU-TAB, IBUPROFEN
  IBU-TAB 200, IBUPROFEN (OTC)
  K+10, POTASSIUM CHLORIDE
  LYGEN, CHLORDIAZEPOXIDE HYDROCHLORIDE
  PRAMINE, IMIPRAMINE HYDROCHLORIDE
  PROPOXYPHENE HCL, PROPOXYPHENE
    HYDROCHLORIDE
  SOXAZOLE, SULFISOXAZOLE
  TOLBUTAMIDE, TOLBUTAMIDE

ALTANA
* ALTANA INC
  BACITRACIN, BACITRACIN
  BACITRACIN-NEOMYCIN-POLYMYXIN, BACITRACIN
    ZINC
  BACITRACIN-NEOMYCIN-POLYMYXIN W/
    HYDROCORTISONE ACETATE, BACITRACIN
  CHLORAMPHENICOL, CHLORAMPHENICOL
  HYDROCORTISONE, HYDROCORTISONE
  HYDROCORTISONE ACETATE, HYDROCORTISONE
    ACETATE

APPENDIX B
PRODUCT NAME INDEX
LISTED BY APPLICANT (continued)

HYDROXYZINE HCL, HYDROXYZINE
  HYDROCHLORIDE
NITROGLYCERIN, NITROGLYCERIN
NYSTATIN, NYSTATIN
SULFACETAMIDE SODIUM, SULFACETAMIDE SODIUM
TRIAMCINOLONE ACETONIDE, TRIAMCINOLONE
  ACETONIDE
ZIPAN-25, PROMETHAZINE HYDROCHLORIDE
ZIPAN-50, PROMETHAZINE HYDROCHLORIDE

ALZA
* ALZA CORP
  DURAGESIC, FENTANYL
  OCUSERT PILO-20, PILOCARPINE
  OCUSERT PILO-40, PILOCARPINE
  PROGESTASERT, PROGESTERONE

AM THERAP
* AMERICAN THERAPEUTICS INC
  ACETAMINOPHEN AND CODEINE PHOSPHATE NO. 2,
    ACETAMINOPHEN
  ACETAMINOPHEN AND CODEINE PHOSPHATE NO. 3,
    ACETAMINOPHEN
  ACETAMINOPHEN AND CODEINE PHOSPHATE NO. 4,
    ACETAMINOPHEN
  ALBUTEROL SULFATE, ALBUTEROL SULFATE
  AMITRIPTYLINE HCL, AMITRIPTYLINE
    HYDROCHLORIDE
  CLONIDINE HCL, CLONIDINE HYDROCHLORIDE
  CLORAZEPATE DIPOTASSIUM, CLORAZEPATE
    DIPOTASSIUM
  CYPROHEPTADINE HCL, CYPROHEPTADINE
    HYDROCHLORIDE
  DANAZOL, DANAZOL
  FENOPROFEN CALCIUM, FENOPROFEN CALCIUM
  LORAZEPAM, LORAZEPAM
  MAPROTILINE HCL, MAPROTILINE HYDROCHLORIDE
  MECLOFENAMATE SODIUM, MECLOFENAMATE
    SODIUM
  METAPROTERENOL SULFATE, METAPROTERENOL
    SULFATE
  METHOCARBAMOL, METHOCARBAMOL
  OXAZEPAM, OXAZEPAM
  PRAZOSIN HCL, PRAZOSIN HYDROCHLORIDE
  PREDNISONE, PREDNISONE
  THIOTHIXENE, THIOTHIXENE
  TRAZODONE HCL, TRAZODONE HYDROCHLORIDE
  TRIAMTERENE AND HYDROCHLOROTHIAZIDE,
    HYDROCHLOROTHIAZIDE

AMBIX
* AMBIX LABORATORIES DIV ORGANICS CORP AMERICA
  HYDROCORTISONE, HYDROCORTISONE
  NITROFURAZONE, NITROFURAZONE
  TRIAMCINOLONE ACETONIDE, TRIAMCINOLONE
    ACETONIDE

AMERSHAM
* AMERSHAM CORP SUB RADIOCHEMICAL CENTER
  AMERSCAN MDP KIT, TECHNETIUM TC-99M
    MEDRONATE KIT
  CERETEC, TECHNETIUM TC-99M EXAMETAZIME KIT
  DICOPAC KIT, CYANOCOBALAMIN
  IBRIN, FIBRINOGEN, I-125
  INDIUM IN-111 OXYQUINOLINE, INDIUM IN-111
    OXYQUINOLINE

AMIDE PHARM
* AMIDE PHARMACEUTICAL INC
  CHLORZOXAZONE, CHLORZOXAZONE
  HYDRALAZINE HCL, HYDRALAZINE
    HYDROCHLORIDE

HYDROXYZINE HCL, HYDROXYZINE
  HYDROCHLORIDE

ANABOLICS
* ANABOLICS INC
  BROMPHENIRAMINE MALEATE, BROMPHENIRAMINE
    MALEATE
  CHLORPHENIRAMINE MALEATE,
    CHLORPHENIRAMINE MALEATE
  DIMENHYDRINATE, DIMENHYDRINATE
  DIPHENHYDRAMINE HCL, DIPHENHYDRAMINE
    HYDROCHLORIDE
  FOLIC ACID, FOLIC ACID
  HYDROCORTISONE, HYDROCORTISONE
  ISONIAZID, ISONIAZID
  MECLIZINE HCL, MECLIZINE HYDROCHLORIDE
  MEPROBAMATE, MEPROBAMATE
  PHENDIMETRAZINE TARTRATE, PHENDIMETRAZINE
    TARTRATE
  PROPOXYPHENE HCL, PROPOXYPHENE
    HYDROCHLORIDE
  PROPYLTHIOURACIL, PROPYLTHIOURACIL
  SODIUM PENTOBARBITAL, PENTOBARBITAL SODIUM
  SODIUM SECOBARBITAL, SECOBARBITAL SODIUM
  TRIPELENNAMINE HCL, TRIPELENNAMINE
    HYDROCHLORIDE

ANAQUEST
* ANAQUEST DIV BOC INC
  ENLON-PLUS, ATROPINE SULFATE
* ANAQUEST INC
  ENLON, EDROPHONIUM CHLORIDE
  ETHRANE, ENFLURANE
  FORANE, ISOFLURANE

ANBEX
* ANBEX INC
  IOSAT, POTASSIUM IODIDE (OTC)

ANGELINI
* ANGELINI PHARMACEUTICALS INC
  REV-EYES, DAPIPRAZOLE HYDROCHLORIDE

APOTHECON
* APOTHECON SUB BRISTOL MYERS SQUIBB CO
  ATENOLOL, ATENOLOL
  KLOTRIX, POTASSIUM CHLORIDE
  OXACILLIN SODIUM, OXACILLIN SODIUM

ARBROOK
* ARBROOK INC
  GAMOPHEN, HEXACHLOROPHENE

ARCUM
* ARCUM PHARMACEUTICAL CORP
  VITAMIN A PALMITATE, VITAMIN A PALMITATE

ARMOUR
* ARMOUR PHARMACEUTICAL CO
  ACTHAR, CORTICOTROPIN
  ACTHAR GEL-SYNTHETIC, SERACTIDE ACETATE
  DEPINAR, CYANOCOBALAMIN
  H.P. ACTHAR GEL, CORTICOTROPIN
  ISOPROTERENOL HCL, ISOPROTERENOL
    HYDROCHLORIDE
  THYTROPAR, THYROTROPIN

ARMOUR DIAL
* ARMOUR DIAL INC DIV ARMOUR AND CO
  DIAL, HEXACHLOROPHENE

ASCHER
* BF ASCHER AND CO INC
  DRIZE, CHLORPHENIRAMINE MALEATE
  HY-PHEN, ACETAMINOPHEN

APPENDIX B
PRODUCT NAME INDEX
LISTED BY APPLICANT *(continued)*

ASCOT
* ASCOT HOSP PHARMACEUTICALS INC DIV TRAVENOL LABORATORIES I
  ACETAZOLAMIDE, ACETAZOLAMIDE
  AMINOPHYLLINE, AMINOPHYLLINE
  BETHANECHOL CHLORIDE, BETHANECHOL CHLORIDE
  CHLORDIAZEPOXIDE HCL, CHLORDIAZEPOXIDE HYDROCHLORIDE
  CHLORTHALIDONE, CHLORTHALIDONE
  CYPROHEPTADINE HCL, CYPROHEPTADINE HYDROCHLORIDE
  DIPHENOXYLATE HCL AND ATROPINE SULFATE, ATROPINE SULFATE
  HYDRALAZINE HCL, HYDRALAZINE HYDROCHLORIDE
  HYDROCHLOROTHIAZIDE, HYDROCHLOROTHIAZIDE
  METHOCARBAMOL, METHOCARBAMOL
  ORPHENADRINE CITRATE, ORPHENADRINE CITRATE
  PROCAINAMIDE HCL, PROCAINAMIDE HYDROCHLORIDE
  PROPANTHELINE BROMIDE, PROPANTHELINE BROMIDE
  QUINIDINE GLUCONATE, QUINIDINE GLUCONATE
  SPIRONOLACTONE, SPIRONOLACTONE
  SPIRONOLACTONE + HYDROCHLOROTHIAZIDE, HYDROCHLOROTHIAZIDE
  SULFAMETHOXAZOLE, SULFAMETHOXAZOLE
  TOLBUTAMIDE, TOLBUTAMIDE

ASTA
* ASTA PHARMA AG
  MESNEX, MESNA

ASTRA
* ASTRA PHARMACEUTICAL PRODUCTS INC
  AQUASOL A, VITAMIN A
  AQUASOL A, VITAMIN A PALMITATE
  ASTRAMORPH PF, MORPHINE SULFATE
  BRETYLIUM TOSYLATE, BRETYLIUM TOSYLATE
  CITANEST, PRILOCAINE HYDROCHLORIDE
  CITANEST FORTE, EPINEPHRINE BITARTRATE
  CITANEST PLAIN, PRILOCAINE HYDROCHLORIDE
  CLINDAMYCIN PHOSPHATE, CLINDAMYCIN PHOSPHATE
  DALGAN, DEZOCINE
  DOPAMINE HCL, DOPAMINE HYDROCHLORIDE
  DROPERIDOL, DROPERIDOL
  DURANEST, EPINEPHRINE
  DURANEST, EPINEPHRINE BITARTRATE
  DURANEST, ETIDOCAINE HYDROCHLORIDE
  DYCLONE, DYCLONINE HYDROCHLORIDE
  FENTANYL CITRATE AND DROPERIDOL, DROPERIDOL
  FOSCAVIR, FOSCARNET SODIUM
  FUROSEMIDE, FUROSEMIDE
  ISOETHARINE HCL, ISOETHARINE HYDROCHLORIDE
  M.V.I.-12, ASCORBIC ACID
  M.V.I.-12 LYOPHILIZED, ASCORBIC ACID
  MANNITOL 25%, MANNITOL
  MEPERIDINE HCL, MEPERIDINE HYDROCHLORIDE
  METAPROTERENOL SULFATE, METAPROTERENOL SULFATE
  NALBUPHINE HCL, NALBUPHINE HYDROCHLORIDE
  NALOXONE HCL, NALOXONE HYDROCHLORIDE
  NESACAINE, CHLOROPROCAINE HYDROCHLORIDE
  NESACAINE-MPF, CHLOROPROCAINE HYDROCHLORIDE
  PANCURONIUM BROMIDE, PANCURONIUM BROMIDE
  POLOCAINE, MEPIVACAINE HYDROCHLORIDE
  POLOCAINE W/ LEVONORDEFRIN, LEVONORDEFRIN

SENSORCAINE, BUPIVACAINE HYDROCHLORIDE
XYLOCAINE, LIDOCAINE
XYLOCAINE, LIDOCAINE HYDROCHLORIDE
XYLOCAINE VISCOUS, LIDOCAINE HYDROCHLORIDE
XYLOCAINE W/ DEXTROSE 7.5%, LIDOCAINE HYDROCHLORIDE
XYLOCAINE W/ EPINEPHRINE, EPINEPHRINE
XYLOCAINE 4%, LIDOCAINE HYDROCHLORIDE
XYLOCAINE 5% W/ GLUCOSE 7.5%, LIDOCAINE HYDROCHLORIDE
YUTOPAR, RITODRINE HYDROCHLORIDE

ATRAL
* LABORATORIOS ATRAL SARL
  AMOXICILLIN, AMOXICILLIN
  CEPHALEXIN, CEPHALEXIN
  TETRACYCLINE HCL, TETRACYCLINE HYDROCHLORIDE

B

BAKER CUMMINS
* BAKER CUMMINS PHARMACEUTICALS INC
  DORAL, QUAZEPAM
  TOLMETIN SODIUM, TOLMETIN SODIUM
  VERAPAMIL HCL, VERAPAMIL HYDROCHLORIDE

BANNER GELATIN
* BANNER GELATIN PRODUCTS CORP
  CHLOROTRIANISENE, CHLOROTRIANISENE
  ETHCHLORVYNOL, ETHCHLORVYNOL
  VITAMIN A PALMITATE, VITAMIN A PALMITATE

BARLAN
* BARLAN PHARMACAL CO INC
  BARSTATIN 100, NYSTATIN

BARR
* BARR LABORATORIES INC
  ACETAMINOPHEN AND CODEINE PHOSPHATE, ACETAMINOPHEN
  ACETAMINOPHEN W/ CODEINE, ACETAMINOPHEN
  ACETOHEXAMIDE, ACETOHEXAMIDE
  ALLOPURINOL, ALLOPURINOL
  AMILORIDE HCL AND HYDROCHLOROTHIAZIDE, AMILORIDE HYDROCHLORIDE
  AMINOPHYLLINE, AMINOPHYLLINE
  AMITRIPTYLINE HCL, AMITRIPTYLINE HYDROCHLORIDE
  BROMPHENIRAMINE MALEATE, BROMPHENIRAMINE MALEATE
  CEPHALEXIN, CEPHALEXIN
  CEPHRADINE, CEPHRADINE
  CHLORDIAZEPOXIDE AND AMITRIPTYLINE HCL, AMITRIPTYLINE HYDROCHLORIDE
  CHLORDIAZEPOXIDE HCL, CHLORDIAZEPOXIDE HYDROCHLORIDE
  CHLORPHENIRAMINE MALEATE, CHLORPHENIRAMINE MALEATE
  CHLORPROPAMIDE, CHLORPROPAMIDE
  CHLORTHALIDONE, CHLORTHALIDONE
  CHLORZOXAZONE, CHLORZOXAZONE
  CLONIDINE HCL, CLONIDINE HYDROCHLORIDE
  CORTISONE ACETATE, CORTISONE ACETATE
  DEXAMETHASONE, DEXAMETHASONE
  DIAZEPAM, DIAZEPAM
  DICYCLOMINE HCL, DICYCLOMINE HYDROCHLORIDE
  DIPHENHYDRAMINE HCL, DIPHENHYDRAMINE HYDROCHLORIDE

APPENDIX B
PRODUCT NAME INDEX
LISTED BY APPLICANT (continued)

DIPHENOXYLATE HCL AND ATROPINE SULFATE, ATROPINE SULFATE
DIPYRIDAMOLE, DIPYRIDAMOLE
DISOPYRAMIDE PHOSPHATE, DISOPYRAMIDE PHOSPHATE
DOXEPIN HCL, DOXEPIN HYDROCHLORIDE
DOXYCYCLINE HYCLATE, DOXYCYCLINE HYCLATE
E-BASE, ERYTHROMYCIN
ERGOLOID MESYLATES, ERGOLOID MESYLATES
ERYTHROMYCIN, ERYTHROMYCIN
ERYTHROMYCIN ESTOLATE, ERYTHROMYCIN ESTOLATE
ERYTHROMYCIN ETHYLSUCCINATE, ERYTHROMYCIN ETHYLSUCCINATE
ERYTHROMYCIN ETHYLSUCCINATE AND SULFISOXAZOLE ACETYL, ERYTHROMYCIN ETHYLSUCCINATE
ERYTHROMYCIN STEARATE, ERYTHROMYCIN STEARATE
FLURAZEPAM HCL, FLURAZEPAM HYDROCHLORIDE
FOLIC ACID, FOLIC ACID
FUROSEMIDE, FUROSEMIDE
HALOPERIDOL, HALOPERIDOL
HYDRALAZINE HCL, HYDRALAZINE HYDROCHLORIDE
HYDROCHLOROTHIAZIDE, HYDROCHLOROTHIAZIDE
HYDROCODONE BITARTRATE W/ ACETAMINOPHEN, ACETAMINOPHEN
HYDROCORTISONE, HYDROCORTISONE
HYDROXYZINE HCL, HYDROXYZINE HYDROCHLORIDE
HYDROXYZINE PAMOATE, HYDROXYZINE PAMOATE
IBUPROFEN, IBUPROFEN
IBUPROFEN, IBUPROFEN (OTC)
INDOMETHACIN, INDOMETHACIN
ISONIAZID, ISONIAZID
ISOSORBIDE DINITRATE, ISOSORBIDE DINITRATE
LEUCOVORIN CALCIUM, LEUCOVORIN CALCIUM
LORAZEPAM, LORAZEPAM
MECLOFENAMATE SODIUM, MECLOFENAMATE SODIUM
MEPERIDINE HCL, MEPERIDINE HYDROCHLORIDE
MEPROBAMATE, MEPROBAMATE
METHOCARBAMOL, METHOCARBAMOL
METHOTREXATE, METHOTREXATE SODIUM
METHYLDOPA, METHYLDOPA
METOCLOPRAMIDE HCL, METOCLOPRAMIDE HYDROCHLORIDE
METRONIDAZOLE, METRONIDAZOLE
NALIDIXIC ACID, NALIDIXIC ACID
OXAZEPAM, OXAZEPAM
OXYCODONE AND ASPIRIN, ASPIRIN
OXYCODONE HCL AND ACETAMINOPHEN, ACETAMINOPHEN
PERPHENAZINE AND AMITRIPTYLINE HCL, AMITRIPTYLINE HYDROCHLORIDE
PHENDIMETRAZINE TARTRATE, PHENDIMETRAZINE TARTRATE
PHENYLBUTAZONE, PHENYLBUTAZONE
PREDNISOLONE, PREDNISOLONE
PREDNISONE, PREDNISONE
PROMETHAZINE HCL, PROMETHAZINE HYDROCHLORIDE
PROPOXYPHENE HCL, PROPOXYPHENE HYDROCHLORIDE
PROPOXYPHENE NAPSYLATE AND ACETAMINOPHEN, ACETAMINOPHEN
PROPRANOLOL HCL, PROPRANOLOL HYDROCHLORIDE
PROPRANOLOL HCL AND HYDROCHLOROTHIAZIDE, HYDROCHLOROTHIAZIDE

PROPYLTHIOURACIL, PROPYLTHIOURACIL
QUINIDINE SULFATE, QUINIDINE SULFATE
RESERPINE, RESERPINE
RESERPINE AND HYDROCHLOROTHIAZIDE, HYDROCHLOROTHIAZIDE
RESERPINE, HYDRALAZINE HCL AND HYDROCHLOROTHIAZIDE, HYDRALAZINE HYDROCHLORIDE
SODIUM SECOBARBITAL, SECOBARBITAL SODIUM
SPIRONOLACTONE, SPIRONOLACTONE
SPIRONOLACTONE AND HYDROCHLOROTHIAZIDE, HYDROCHLOROTHIAZIDE
SULFAMETHOXAZOLE, SULFAMETHOXAZOLE
SULFAMETHOXAZOLE AND TRIMETHOPRIM, SULFAMETHOXAZOLE
SULFAMETHOXAZOLE AND TRIMETHOPRIM DOUBLE STRENGTH, SULFAMETHOXAZOLE
SULFINPYRAZONE, SULFINPYRAZONE
SULFISOXAZOLE, SULFISOXAZOLE
TEMAZEPAM, TEMAZEPAM
TETRACYCLINE HCL, TETRACYCLINE HYDROCHLORIDE
THIORIDAZINE HCL, THIORIDAZINE HYDROCHLORIDE
TOLAZAMIDE, TOLAZAMIDE
TOLBUTAMIDE, TOLBUTAMIDE
TRAZODONE HCL, TRAZODONE HYDROCHLORIDE
TRIAMCINOLONE, TRIAMCINOLONE
TRIAMTERENE AND HYDROCHLOROTHIAZIDE, HYDROCHLOROTHIAZIDE
TRIMETHOPRIM, TRIMETHOPRIM
TRIPELENNAMINE HCL, TRIPELENNAMINE HYDROCHLORIDE
VERAPAMIL HCL, VERAPAMIL HYDROCHLORIDE

BARRE
* BARRE NATIONAL INC
ACETAMINOPHEN W/ CODEINE PHOSPHATE, ACETAMINOPHEN
ACETASOL, ACETIC ACID, GLACIAL
ACETASOL HC, ACETIC ACID, GLACIAL
AMANTADINE HCL, AMANTADINE HYDROCHLORIDE
AMINOPHYLLINE DYE FREE, AMINOPHYLLINE
APAP W/ CODEINE, ACETAMINOPHEN
BETAMETHASONE DIPROPIONATE, BETAMETHASONE DIPROPIONATE
BETAMETHASONE VALERATE, BETAMETHASONE VALERATE
BROMANATE, BROMPHENIRAMINE MALEATE
BROMANATE DC, BROMPHENIRAMINE MALEATE
BROMANATE DM, BROMPHENIRAMINE MALEATE
BROMANYL, BROMODIPHENHYDRAMINE HYDROCHLORIDE
BROMPHENIRAMINE MALEATE, BROMPHENIRAMINE MALEATE
BUTABARB, BUTABARBITAL SODIUM
CHLORPROMAZINE HCL, CHLORPROMAZINE HYDROCHLORIDE
CLINDAMYCIN PHOSPHATE, CLINDAMYCIN PHOSPHATE
CONSTULOSE, LACTULOSE
CYPROHEPTADINE HCL, CYPROHEPTADINE HYDROCHLORIDE
DEXAMETHASONE, DEXAMETHASONE
DICYCLOMINE HCL, DICYCLOMINE HYDROCHLORIDE
ENULOSE, LACTULOSE
EPINEPHRINE, EPINEPHRINE (OTC)
ERYTHROMYCIN, ERYTHROMYCIN
ERYTHROMYCIN ESTOLATE, ERYTHROMYCIN ESTOLATE

APPENDIX B
PRODUCT NAME INDEX
LISTED BY APPLICANT (continued)

ERYTHROMYCIN ETHYLSUCCINATE,
 ERYTHROMYCIN ETHYLSUCCINATE
FLUOCINOLONE ACETONIDE, FLUOCINOLONE
 ACETONIDE
FLUOCINONIDE, FLUOCINONIDE
FLURANDRENOLIDE, FLURANDRENOLIDE
HALOPERIDOL, HALOPERIDOL LACTATE
HYDRAMINE, DIPHENHYDRAMINE HYDROCHLORIDE
 (OTC)
HYDRAMINE, DIPHENHYDRAMINE HYDROCHLORIDE
HYDROCODONE COMPOUND, HOMATROPINE
 METHYLBROMIDE
HYDROCORTISONE, HYDROCORTISONE
HYDROXYZINE HCL, HYDROXYZINE
 HYDROCHLORIDE
ISOETHARINE HCL, ISOETHARINE HYDROCHLORIDE
ISOETHARINE MESYLATE, ISOETHARINE MESYLATE
ISOPROTERENOL HCL, ISOPROTERENOL
 HYDROCHLORIDE
LIDOCAINE HCL VISCOUS, LIDOCAINE
 HYDROCHLORIDE
LINDANE, LINDANE
LOMANATE, ATROPINE SULFATE
METHDILAZINE HCL, METHDILAZINE
 HYDROCHLORIDE
METOCLOPRAMIDE HCL, METOCLOPRAMIDE
 HYDROCHLORIDE
NYSTATIN, NYSTATIN
PIPERAZINE CITRATE, PIPERAZINE CITRATE
PROCHLORPERAZINE, PROCHLORPERAZINE
 EDISYLATE
PROCHLORPERAZINE EDISYLATE,
 PROCHLORPERAZINE EDISYLATE
PROMETH, PROMETHAZINE HYDROCHLORIDE
PROMETH VC PLAIN, PHENYLEPHRINE
 HYDROCHLORIDE
PROMETH VC W/ CODEINE, CODEINE PHOSPHATE
PROMETH W/ CODEINE, CODEINE PHOSPHATE
PROMETH W/ DEXTROMETHORPHAN,
 DEXTROMETHORPHAN HYDROBROMIDE
SELENIUM SULFIDE, SELENIUM SULFIDE
SULFATRIM, SULFAMETHOXAZOLE
SULFATRIM PEDIATRIC, SULFAMETHOXAZOLE
TETRACYCLINE, TETRACYCLINE
THEOPHYLLINE, THEOPHYLLINE
THIORIDAZINE HCL, THIORIDAZINE
 HYDROCHLORIDE
THIOTHIXENE HCL, THIOTHIXENE HYDROCHLORIDE
TRIACIN-C, CODEINE PHOSPHATE
TRIAMCINOLONE ACETONIDE, TRIAMCINOLONE
 ACETONIDE
TRIMEPRAZINE TARTRATE, TRIMEPRAZINE
 TARTRATE
TRIOFED, PSEUDOEPHEDRINE HYDROCHLORIDE
 (OTC)
TRIPLE SULFA, TRISULFAPYRIMIDINES
TRIPROLIDINE HCL, TRIPROLIDINE
 HYDROCHLORIDE

BARTOR
* BARTOR PHARMACAL CO
 TESTOSTERONE, TESTOSTERONE

BAUSCH AND LOMB
* BAUSCH AND LOMB INC
 OPCON, NAPHAZOLINE HYDROCHLORIDE
 SULPHRIN, PREDNISOLONE ACETATE
 SULTEN-10, SULFACETAMIDE SODIUM
* BAUSCH AND LOMB PHARMACEUTICALS INC
 OPTIPRANOLOL, METIPRANOLOL HYDROCHLORIDE

BAXTER
* BAXTER HEALTHCARE CORP
 ACETIC ACID 0.25% IN PLASTIC CONTAINER, ACETIC
  ACID, GLACIAL
 ALCOHOL 5% IN DEXTROSE 5% IN WATER, ALCOHOL
 AMINOACETIC ACID 1.5% IN PLASTIC CONTAINER,
  GLYCINE
 ANCEF, CEFAZOLIN SODIUM
 ANCEF IN DEXTROSE 5% IN PLASTIC CONTAINER,
  CEFAZOLIN SODIUM
 ANCEF IN SODIUM CHLORIDE 0.9% IN PLASTIC
  CONTAINER, CEFAZOLIN SODIUM
 BACTOCILL, OXACILLIN SODIUM
 BRANCHAMIN 4%, AMINO ACIDS
 BRETYLIUM TOSYLATE IN DEXTROSE 5%,
  BRETYLIUM TOSYLATE
 CEPHALOTHIN SODIUM W/ DEXTROSE,
  CEPHALOTHIN SODIUM
 CEPHALOTHIN SODIUM W/ SODIUM CHLORIDE,
  CEPHALOTHIN SODIUM
 CLINDAMYCIN PHOSPHATE IN DEXTROSE 5%,
  CLINDAMYCIN PHOSPHATE
 DEXTROSE 10% AND SODIUM CHLORIDE 0.9% IN
  PLASTIC CONTAINER, DEXTROSE
 DEXTROSE 10% IN PLASTIC CONTAINER, DEXTROSE
 DEXTROSE 2.5% AND SODIUM CHLORIDE 0.45% IN
  PLASTIC CONTAINER, DEXTROSE
 DEXTROSE 20% IN PLASTIC CONTAINER, DEXTROSE
 DEXTROSE 30% IN PLASTIC CONTAINER, DEXTROSE
 DEXTROSE 40% IN PLASTIC CONTAINER, DEXTROSE
 DEXTROSE 5%, DEXTROSE
 DEXTROSE 5% AND ELECTROLYTE NO 75, DEXTROSE
 DEXTROSE 5% AND ELECTROLYTE NO.48 IN PLASTIC
  CONTAINER, DEXTROSE
 DEXTROSE 5% AND POTASSIUM CHLORIDE 0.075% IN
  PLASTIC CONTAINER, DEXTROSE
 DEXTROSE 5% AND POTASSIUM CHLORIDE 0.15% IN
  PLASTIC CONTAINER, DEXTROSE
 DEXTROSE 5% AND POTASSIUM CHLORIDE 0.224% IN
  PLASTIC CONTAINER, DEXTROSE
 DEXTROSE 5% AND POTASSIUM CHLORIDE 0.3% IN
  PLASTIC CONTAINER, DEXTROSE
 DEXTROSE 5% IN RINGER'S IN PLASTIC CONTAINER,
  CALCIUM CHLORIDE
 DEXTROSE 5% IN SODIUM CHLORIDE 0.2% IN
  PLASTIC CONTAINER, DEXTROSE
 DEXTROSE 5% IN SODIUM CHLORIDE 0.33% IN
  PLASTIC CONTAINER, DEXTROSE
 DEXTROSE 5% IN SODIUM CHLORIDE 0.45% IN
  PLASTIC CONTAINER, DEXTROSE
 DEXTROSE 5% IN SODIUM CHLORIDE 0.9% IN
  PLASTIC CONTAINER, DEXTROSE
 DEXTROSE 5%, SODIUM CHLORIDE 0.2% AND
  POTASSIUM CHLORIDE 10 MEQ, DEXTROSE
 DEXTROSE 5%, SODIUM CHLORIDE 0.2% AND
  POTASSIUM CHLORIDE 15 MEQ (K), DEXTROSE
 DEXTROSE 5%, SODIUM CHLORIDE 0.2% AND
  POTASSIUM CHLORIDE 20 MEQ, DEXTROSE
 DEXTROSE 5%, SODIUM CHLORIDE 0.2% AND
  POTASSIUM CHLORIDE 20 MEQ (K), DEXTROSE
 DEXTROSE 5%, SODIUM CHLORIDE 0.2% AND
  POTASSIUM CHLORIDE 30 MEQ, DEXTROSE
 DEXTROSE 5%, SODIUM CHLORIDE 0.2% AND
  POTASSIUM CHLORIDE 40 MEQ, DEXTROSE
 DEXTROSE 5%, SODIUM CHLORIDE 0.2% AND
  POTASSIUM CHLORIDE 5 MEQ, DEXTROSE
 DEXTROSE 5%, SODIUM CHLORIDE 0.2% AND
  POTASSIUM CHLORIDE 5 MEQ (K), DEXTROSE
 DEXTROSE 5%, SODIUM CHLORIDE 0.33% AND
  POTASSIUM CHLORIDE 10 MEQ, DEXTROSE

APPENDIX B
PRODUCT NAME INDEX
LISTED BY APPLICANT *(continued)*

DEXTROSE 5%, SODIUM CHLORIDE 0.33% AND POTASSIUM CHLORIDE 15 MEQ, DEXTROSE
DEXTROSE 5%, SODIUM CHLORIDE 0.33% AND POTASSIUM CHLORIDE 20 MEQ, DEXTROSE
DEXTROSE 5%, SODIUM CHLORIDE 0.33% AND POTASSIUM CHLORIDE 30 MEQ, DEXTROSE
DEXTROSE 5%, SODIUM CHLORIDE 0.33% AND POTASSIUM CHLORIDE 40 MEQ, DEXTROSE
DEXTROSE 5%, SODIUM CHLORIDE 0.33% AND POTASSIUM CHLORIDE 5 MEQ, DEXTROSE
DEXTROSE 5%, SODIUM CHLORIDE 0.45% AND POTASSIUM CHLORIDE 15 MEQ, DEXTROSE
DEXTROSE 5%, SODIUM CHLORIDE 0.45% AND POTASSIUM CHLORIDE 20 MEQ (K), DEXTROSE
DEXTROSE 5%, SODIUM CHLORIDE 0.45% AND POTASSIUM CHLORIDE 5 MEQ, DEXTROSE
DEXTROSE 50%, DEXTROSE
DEXTROSE 60%, DEXTROSE
DEXTROSE 60% IN PLASTIC CONTAINER, DEXTROSE
DEXTROSE 70%, DEXTROSE
DEXTROSE 70% IN PLASTIC CONTAINER, DEXTROSE
DIANEAL PD-1 W/ DEXTROSE 1.5% IN PLASTIC CONTAINER, CALCIUM CHLORIDE
DIANEAL PD-1 W/ DEXTROSE 2.5% IN PLASTIC CONTAINER, CALCIUM CHLORIDE
DIANEAL PD-1 W/ DEXTROSE 3.5%, CALCIUM CHLORIDE
DIANEAL PD-1 W/ DEXTROSE 4.25% IN PLASTIC CONTAINER, CALCIUM CHLORIDE
DIANEAL PD-2 W/ DEXTROSE 1.5% IN PLASTIC CONTAINER, CALCIUM CHLORIDE
DIANEAL PD-2 W/ DEXTROSE 2.5% IN PLASTIC CONTAINER, CALCIUM CHLORIDE
DIANEAL PD-2 W/ DEXTROSE 3.5%, CALCIUM CHLORIDE
DIANEAL PD-2 W/ DEXTROSE 4.25% IN PLASTIC CONTAINER, CALCIUM CHLORIDE
DIANEAL 137 W/ DEXTROSE 1.5% IN PLASTIC CONTAINER, CALCIUM CHLORIDE
DIANEAL 137 W/ DEXTROSE 2.5% IN PLASTIC CONTAINER, CALCIUM CHLORIDE
DIANEAL 137 W/ DEXTROSE 4.25% IN PLASTIC CONTAINER, CALCIUM CHLORIDE
DOPAMINE HCL IN DEXTROSE 5%, DOPAMINE HYDROCHLORIDE
GLYCINE 1.5%, GLYCINE
HEPARIN SODIUM 10,000 UNITS IN DEXTROSE 5%, HEPARIN SODIUM
HEPARIN SODIUM 1000 UNITS AND SODIUM CHLORIDE 0.9%, HEPARIN SODIUM
HEPARIN SODIUM 20,000 UNITS AND DEXTROSE 5% IN PLASTIC CONTAINER, HEPARIN SODIUM
HEPARIN SODIUM 2000 UNITS AND SODIUM CHLORIDE 0.9%, HEPARIN SODIUM
HEPARIN SODIUM 25,000 UNITS AND DEXTROSE 5%, HEPARIN SODIUM
HEPARIN SODIUM 5000 UNITS AND SODIUM CHLORIDE 0.9%, HEPARIN SODIUM
IRRIGATING SOLUTION G IN PLASTIC CONTAINER, CITRIC ACID
ISOETHARINE HCL, ISOETHARINE HYDROCHLORIDE
ISOTONIC GENTAMICIN SULFATE IN PLASTIC CONTAINER, GENTAMICIN SULFATE
LACTATED RINGER'S, CALCIUM CHLORIDE
LACTATED RINGER'S AND DEXTROSE 5% IN PLASTIC CONTAINER, CALCIUM CHLORIDE
LACTATED RINGER'S IN PLASTIC CONTAINER, CALCIUM CHLORIDE
LIDOCAINE HCL 0.1% AND DEXTROSE 5% IN PLASTIC CONTAINER, LIDOCAINE HYDROCHLORIDE
LIDOCAINE HCL 0.2% AND DEXTROSE 5% IN PLASTIC CONTAINER, LIDOCAINE HYDROCHLORIDE
LIDOCAINE HCL 0.4% AND DEXTROSE 5% IN PLASTIC CONTAINER, LIDOCAINE HYDROCHLORIDE
LIDOCAINE HCL 0.8% AND DEXTROSE 5% IN PLASTIC CONTAINER, LIDOCAINE HYDROCHLORIDE
NALLPEN, NAFCILLIN SODIUM
NITROGLYCERIN IN DEXTROSE 5%, NITROGLYCERIN
OSMITROL 10% IN WATER, MANNITOL
OSMITROL 10% IN WATER IN PLASTIC CONTAINER, MANNITOL
OSMITROL 15% IN WATER, MANNITOL
OSMITROL 15% IN WATER IN PLASTIC CONTAINER, MANNITOL
OSMITROL 20% IN WATER, MANNITOL
OSMITROL 20% IN WATER IN PLASTIC CONTAINER, MANNITOL
OSMITROL 5% IN WATER, MANNITOL
OSMITROL 5% IN WATER IN PLASTIC CONTAINER, MANNITOL
PENICILLIN G POTASSIUM, PENICILLIN G POTASSIUM
PLASMA-LYTE A IN PLASTIC CONTAINER, MAGNESIUM CHLORIDE
PLASMA-LYTE M AND DEXTROSE 5% IN PLASTIC CONTAINER, CALCIUM CHLORIDE
PLASMA-LYTE R IN PLASTIC CONTAINER, CALCIUM CHLORIDE
PLASMA-LYTE 148 AND DEXTROSE 5% IN PLASTIC CONTAINER, DEXTROSE
PLASMA-LYTE 148 IN WATER IN PLASTIC CONTAINER, MAGNESIUM CHLORIDE
PLASMA-LYTE 56 AND DEXTROSE 5% IN PLASTIC CONTAINER, DEXTROS
PLASMA-LYTE 56 IN PLASTIC CONTAINER, MAGNESIUM ACETATE TETRAHYDRATE
POTASSIUM CHLORIDE, POTASSIUM CHLORIDE
POTASSIUM CHLORIDE 10 MEQ, POTASSIUM CHLORIDE
POTASSIUM CHLORIDE 10 MEQ IN DEXTROSE 5% AND LACTATED RINGER'S, CALCIUM CHLORIDE
POTASSIUM CHLORIDE 10 MEQ IN DEXTROSE 5% AND SODIUM CHLORIDE 0.45%, DEXTROSE
POTASSIUM CHLORIDE 10 MEQ IN DEXTROSE 5% AND SODIUM CHLORIDE 0.9%, DEXTROSE
POTASSIUM CHLORIDE 15 MEQ IN DEXTROSE 5% AND LACTATED RINGER'S, CALCIUM CHLORIDE
POTASSIUM CHLORIDE 20 MEQ, POTASSIUM CHLORIDE
POTASSIUM CHLORIDE 20 MEQ IN DEXTROSE 5% AND LACTATED RINGER'S, CALCIUM CHLORIDE
POTASSIUM CHLORIDE 20 MEQ IN DEXTROSE 5% AND SODIUM CHLORIDE 0.45%, DEXTROSE
POTASSIUM CHLORIDE 20 MEQ IN DEXTROSE 5% AND SODIUM CHLORIDE 0.9%, DEXTROSE
POTASSIUM CHLORIDE 30 MEQ, POTASSIUM CHLORIDE
POTASSIUM CHLORIDE 30 MEQ IN DEXTROSE 5% AND LACTATED RINGER'S, CALCIUM CHLORIDE
POTASSIUM CHLORIDE 30 MEQ IN DEXTROSE 5% AND SODIUM CHLORIDE 0.45%, DEXTROSE
POTASSIUM CHLORIDE 30 MEQ IN DEXTROSE 5% AND SODIUM CHLORIDE 0.9%, DEXTROSE
POTASSIUM CHLORIDE 40 MEQ, POTASSIUM CHLORIDE
POTASSIUM CHLORIDE 40 MEQ IN DEXTROSE 5% AND LACTATED RINGER'S, CALCIUM CHLORIDE
POTASSIUM CHLORIDE 40 MEQ IN DEXTROSE 5% AND SODIUM CHLORIDE 0.45%, DEXTROSE
POTASSIUM CHLORIDE 40 MEQ IN DEXTROSE 5% AND SODIUM CHLORIDE 0.9%, DEXTROSE

APPENDIX B
PRODUCT NAME INDEX
LISTED BY APPLICANT (continued)

POTASSIUM CHLORIDE 5 MEQ IN DEXTROSE 5% AND
    LACTATED RINGER'S, CALCIUM CHLORIDE
POTASSIUM CHLORIDE 5 MEQ IN DEXTROSE 5% AND
    SODIUM CHLORIDE 0.45%, DEXTROSE
POTASSIUM CHLORIDE 5 MEQ IN DEXTROSE 5% AND
    SODIUM CHLORIDE 0.9%, DEXTROSE
RENAMIN W/O ELECTROLYTES, AMINO ACIDS
RINGER'S IN PLASTIC CONTAINER, CALCIUM
    CHLORIDE
SODIUM CHLORIDE 0.45%, SODIUM CHLORIDE
SODIUM CHLORIDE 0.45% IN PLASTIC CONTAINER,
    SODIUM CHLORIDE
SODIUM CHLORIDE 0.9%, SODIUM CHLORIDE
SODIUM CHLORIDE 0.9% AND POTASSIUM CHLORIDE
    0.075%, POTASSIUM CHLORIDE
SODIUM CHLORIDE 0.9% AND POTASSIUM CHLORIDE
    0.15%, POTASSIUM CHLORIDE
SODIUM CHLORIDE 0.9% AND POTASSIUM CHLORIDE
    0.224%, POTASSIUM CHLORIDE
SODIUM CHLORIDE 0.9% AND POTASSIUM CHLORIDE
    0.3%, POTASSIUM CHLORIDE
SODIUM CHLORIDE 0.9% IN PLASTIC CONTAINER,
    SODIUM CHLORIDE
SODIUM CHLORIDE 0.9% IN STERILE PLASTIC
    CONTAINER, SODIUM CHLORIDE
SODIUM CHLORIDE 3% IN PLASTIC CONTAINER,
    SODIUM CHLORIDE
SODIUM CHLORIDE 5% IN PLASTIC CONTAINER,
    SODIUM CHLORIDE
SODIUM HEPARIN, HEPARIN SODIUM
SODIUM LACTATE 0.167 MOLAR IN PLASTIC
    CONTAINER, SODIUM LACTATE
SORBITOL 3% IN PLASTIC CONTAINER, SORBITOL
STERILE WATER, WATER FOR IRRIGATION, STERILE
STERILE WATER FOR INJECTION, WATER FOR
    INJECTION, STERILE
STERILE WATER FOR INJECTION IN PLASTIC
    CONTAINER, WATER FOR INJECTION, STERILE
STERILE WATER IN PLASTIC CONTAINER, WATER
    FOR IRRIGATION, STERILE
SYNOVALYTE IN PLASTIC CONTAINER, MAGNESIUM
    CHLORIDE
THEOPHYLLINE AND DEXTROSE 5%, THEOPHYLLINE
TIS-U-SOL, MAGNESIUM SULFATE
TIS-U-SOL IN PLASTIC CONTAINER, MAGNESIUM
    SULFATE
TRAVAMULSION 10%, SOYBEAN OIL
TRAVAMULSION 20%, SOYBEAN OIL
TRAVASOL 10%, AMINO ACIDS
TRAVASOL 10% W/O ELECTROLYTES, AMINO ACIDS
TRAVASOL 10% W/O ELECTROLYTES IN PLASTIC
    CONTAINER, AMINO ACIDS
TRAVASOL 2.75% IN DEXTROSE 10, AMINO ACIDS
TRAVASOL 2.75% IN DEXTROSE 15, AMINO ACIDS
TRAVASOL 2.75% IN DEXTROSE 20, AMINO ACIDS
TRAVASOL 2.75% IN DEXTROSE 25, AMINO ACIDS
TRAVASOL 2.75% IN DEXTROSE 5, AMINO ACIDS
TRAVASOL 3.5% W/ ELECTROLYTES, AMINO ACIDS
TRAVASOL 4.25% IN DEXTROSE 10, AMINO ACIDS
TRAVASOL 4.25% IN DEXTROSE 15, AMINO ACIDS
TRAVASOL 4.25% IN DEXTROSE 20, AMINO ACIDS
TRAVASOL 4.25% IN DEXTROSE 25, AMINO ACIDS
TRAVASOL 4.25% IN DEXTROSE 5, AMINO ACIDS
TRAVASOL 5.5% W/ ELECTROLYTES, AMINO ACIDS
TRAVASOL 5.5% W/O ELECTROLYTES, AMINO ACIDS
TRAVASOL 5.5% W/O ELECTROLYTES IN PLASTIC
    CONTAINER, AMINO ACIDS
TRAVASOL 8.5% W/ ELECTROLYTES, AMINO ACIDS
TRAVASOL 8.5% W/O ELECTROLYTES, AMINO ACIDS
TRAVASOL 8.5% W/O ELECTROLYTES IN PLASTIC
    CONTAINER, AMINO ACIDS

TRAVERT 10%, INVERT SUGAR
* BAXTER HEALTHCARE CORP PHARMASEAL DIV
    PHARMASEAL SCRUB CARE, CHLORHEXIDINE
      GLUCONATE (OTC)
    POVIDONE IODINE, POVIDONE-IODINE (OTC)

BECTON DICKINSON
* BECTON DICKINSON AND CO
    E-Z PREP, POVIDONE-IODINE (OTC)
    E-Z PREP 220, POVIDONE-IODINE (OTC)
    E-Z SCRUB 201, POVIDONE-IODINE (OTC)
    E-Z SCRUB 241, POVIDONE-IODINE (OTC)
* BECTON DICKINSON MICROBIOLOGY SYSTEMS
    BAL, DIMERCAPROL
    CARDIO-GREEN, INDOCYANINE GREEN

BEECHAM
* BEECHAM LABORATORIES DIV BEECHAM INC
    AMINOPHYLLINE, AMINOPHYLLINE
    AMOXIL, AMOXICILLIN
    ANEXSIA, ACETAMINOPHEN
    ANEXSIA 7.5/650, ACETAMINOPHEN
    APOGEN, GENTAMICIN SULFATE
    AUGMENTIN '125', AMOXICILLIN
    AUGMENTIN '250', AMOXICILLIN
    AUGMENTIN '500', AMOXICILLIN
    BACTOCILL, OXACILLIN SODIUM
    BACTROBAN, MUPIROCIN
    BEEPEN-VK, PENICILLIN V POTASSIUM
    CLOXAPEN, CLOXACILLIN SODIUM
    DYCILL, DICLOXACILLIN SODIUM
    FASTIN, PHENTERMINE HYDROCHLORIDE
    KLEBCIL, KANAMYCIN SULFATE
    LAROTID, AMOXICILLIN
    MAXOLON, METOCLOPRAMIDE HYDROCHLORIDE
    MENEST, ESTROGENS, ESTERIFIED
    NALLPEN, NAFCILLIN SODIUM
    PHYTONADIONE, PHYTONADIONE
    PROBENECID AND COLCHICINE, COLCHICINE
    PYOPEN, CARBENICILLIN DISODIUM
    QUINIDINE SULFATE, QUINIDINE SULFATE
    TICAR, TICARCILLIN DISODIUM
    TIGAN, TRIMETHOBENZAMIDE HYDROCHLORIDE
    TIMENTIN, CLAVULANATE POTASSIUM
    TOTACILLIN, AMPICILLIN/AMPICILLIN TRIHYDRATE
    TOTACILLIN-N, AMPICILLIN SODIUM

BEL MAR
* BEL MAR LABORATORIES INC
    CHLORPHENIRAMINE MALEATE,
      CHLORPHENIRAMINE MALEATE
    CHORIONIC GONADOTROPIN, GONADOTROPIN,
      CHORIONIC
    DEXAMETHASONE SODIUM PHOSPHATE,
      DEXAMETHASONE SODIUM PHOSPHATE
    DIPHENHYDRAMINE HCL, DIPHENHYDRAMINE
      HYDROCHLORIDE
    HYDROCORTISONE ACETATE, HYDROCORTISONE
      ACETATE
    HYDROXOMIN, HYDROXOCOBALAMIN
    LIDOCAINE HCL, LIDOCAINE HYDROCHLORIDE
    LIDOCAINE HCL W/ EPINEPHRINE, EPINEPHRINE
    M-PREDROL, METHYLPREDNISOLONE ACETATE
    PREDNISOLONE ACETATE, PREDNISOLONE ACETATE
    PROCAINE HCL, PROCAINE HYDROCHLORIDE
    PROCAINE HCL W/ EPINEPHRINE, EPINEPHRINE
    PYRIDAMAL 100, CHLORPHENIRAMINE MALEATE
    PYRIDOXINE HCL, PYRIDOXINE HYDROCHLORIDE
    RUBIVITE, CYANOCOBALAMIN
    TESTOSTERONE PROPIONATE, TESTOSTERONE
      PROPIONATE

APPENDIX B
PRODUCT NAME INDEX
LISTED BY APPLICANT (continued)

THIAMINE HCL, THIAMINE HYDROCHLORIDE
VITAMIN A PALMITATE, VITAMIN A PALMITATE

BELL PHARMA
* BELL PHARMACAL CORP
CHLORPHENIRAMINE MALEATE,
CHLORPHENIRAMINE MALEATE
RESERPINE, RESERPINE

BEN VENUE
* BEN VENUE LABORATORIES INC
CEFAZOLIN SODIUM, CEFAZOLIN SODIUM
DOXYCYCLINE, DOXYCYCLINE HYCLATE
FLUOROURACIL, FLUOROURACIL
LEUCOVORIN CALCIUM, LEUCOVORIN CALCIUM
METHOTREXATE SODIUM, METHOTREXATE SODIUM
VINBLASTINE SULFATE, VINBLASTINE SULFATE

BENEDICT
* BENEDICT NUCLEAR PHARMACEUTICALS INC
A-N STANNOUS AGGREGATED ALBUMIN,
TECHNETIUM TC-99M ALBUMIN AGGREGATED KIT
SODIUM IODIDE I 123, SODIUM IODIDE, I-123

BERLEX
* BERLEX LABORATORIES INC
ANGIOVIST 282, DIATRIZOATE MEGLUMINE
ANGIOVIST 292, DIATRIZOATE MEGLUMINE
ANGIOVIST 370, DIATRIZOATE MEGLUMINE
BILIVIST, IPODATE SODIUM
FLUDARA, FLUDARABINE PHOSPHATE
GASTROVIST, DIATRIZOATE MEGLUMINE
QUINACT, QUINIDINE GLUCONATE
QUINAGLUTE, QUINIDINE GLUCONATE
SULLA, SULFAMETER
UROVIST CYSTO, DIATRIZOATE MEGLUMINE
UROVIST CYSTO PEDIATRIC, DIATRIZOATE
MEGLUMINE
UROVIST MEGLUMINE DIU/CT, DIATRIZOATE
MEGLUMINE
UROVIST SODIUM 300, DIATRIZOATE SODIUM
VI-TWEL, CYANOCOBALAMIN
* BERLEX LABORATORIES INC SUB SCHERING AG
MAGNEVIST, GADOPENTETATE DIMEGLUMINE
OSMOVIST, IOTROLAN

BETA DERMAC
* BETA DERMACEUTICALS INC
BETA-HC, HYDROCORTISONE

BH
* BH CHEMICALS INC
HALOTHANE, HALOTHANE

BIOCRAFT
* BIOCRAFT LABORATORIES INC
ALBUTEROL SULFATE, ALBUTEROL SULFATE
AMILORIDE HCL AND HYDROCHLOROTHIAZIDE,
AMILORIDE HYDROCHLORIDE
AMITRIPTYLINE HCL, AMITRIPTYLINE
HYDROCHLORIDE
AMOXICILLIN, AMOXICILLIN
AMOXICILLIN PEDIATRIC, AMOXICILLIN
AMPICILLIN, AMPICILLIN/AMPICILLIN TRIHYDRATE
BACLOFEN, BACLOFEN
CEFADROXIL, CEFADROXIL/CEFADROXIL
HEMIHYDRATE
CEPHALEXIN, CEPHALEXIN
CEPHRADINE, CEPHRADINE
CHLOROQUINE PHOSPHATE, CHLOROQUINE
PHOSPHATE
CINOXACIN, CINOXACIN

CLINDAMYCIN HCL, CLINDAMYCIN
HYDROCHLORIDE
CLONIDINE HCL, CLONIDINE HYDROCHLORIDE
CLOXACILLIN SODIUM, CLOXACILLIN SODIUM
CYCLACILLIN, CYCLACILLIN
DICLOXACILLIN SODIUM, DICLOXACILLIN SODIUM
DISOPYRAMIDE PHOSPHATE, DISOPYRAMIDE
PHOSPHATE
HYDROCORTISONE, HYDROCORTISONE
IMIPRAMINE HCL, IMIPRAMINE HYDROCHLORIDE
METAPROTERENOL SULFATE, METAPROTERENOL
SULFATE
METOCLOPRAMIDE HCL, METOCLOPRAMIDE
HYDROCHLORIDE
MINOCYCLINE HCL, MINOCYCLINE
HYDROCHLORIDE
NEOMYCIN SULFATE, NEOMYCIN SULFATE
NYSTATIN, NYSTATIN
OXACILLIN SODIUM, OXACILLIN SODIUM
PENICILLIN, PENICILLIN G POTASSIUM
PENICILLIN G POTASSIUM, PENICILLIN G
POTASSIUM
PENICILLIN-VK, PENICILLIN V POTASSIUM
PENICILLIN-2, PENICILLIN G POTASSIUM
PROBAMPACIN, AMPICILLIN TRIHYDRATE
SMZ-TMP, SULFAMETHOXAZOLE
SMZ-TMP PEDIATRIC, SULFAMETHOXAZOLE
THIORIDAZINE HCL, THIORIDAZINE
HYDROCHLORIDE
TRIMETHOPRIM, TRIMETHOPRIM

BLUE RIDGE
* BLUE RIDGE LABORATORIES INC
CARAFATE, SUCRALFATE

BLULINE
* BLULINE LABORATORIES INC
EPICORT, HYDROCORTISONE
MULTIFUGE, PIPERAZINE CITRATE

BOEHRINGER INGELHEIM
* BOEHRINGER INGELHEIM PHARMACEUTICALS INC
ALUPENT, METAPROTERENOL SULFATE
ATROVENT, IPRATROPIUM BROMIDE
CATAPRES, CLONIDINE HYDROCHLORIDE
CATAPRES-TTS-1, CLONIDINE
CATAPRES-TTS-2, CLONIDINE
CATAPRES-TTS-3, CLONIDINE
COMBIPRES, CHLORTHALIDONE
IV PERSANTINE, DIPYRIDAMOLE
MEXITIL, MEXILETINE HYDROCHLORIDE
PERSANTINE, DIPYRIDAMOLE
PRELUDIN, PHENMETRAZINE HYDROCHLORIDE

BOLAR
* BOLAR PHARMACEUTICAL CO INC
ACETAZOLAMIDE, ACETAZOLAMIDE
ALLOPURINOL, ALLOPURINOL
AMANTADINE HCL, AMANTADINE HYDROCHLORIDE
ANISOTROPINE METHYLBROMIDE, ANISOTROPINE
METHYLBROMIDE
BETHANECHOL CHLORIDE, BETHANECHOL
CHLORIDE
CARISOPRODOL, CARISOPRODOL
CARISOPRODOL COMPOUND, ASPIRIN
CHLOROTHIAZIDE, CHLOROTHIAZIDE
CHLOROTHIAZIDE W/ RESERPINE, CHLOROTHIAZIDE
CHLORPHENIRAMINE MALEATE,
CHLORPHENIRAMINE MALEATE
CHLORPROPAMIDE, CHLORPROPAMIDE
CHLORTHALIDONE, CHLORTHALIDONE
CLONIDINE HCL, CLONIDINE HYDROCHLORIDE

APPENDIX B
PRODUCT NAME INDEX
LISTED BY APPLICANT (continued)

CYPROHEPTADINE HCL, CYPROHEPTADINE
  HYDROCHLORIDE
DEXAMETHASONE, DEXAMETHASONE
DICYCLOMINE HCL, DICYCLOMINE
  HYDROCHLORIDE
DIPHENHYDRAMINE HCL, DIPHENHYDRAMINE
  HYDROCHLORIDE
DISOPYRAMIDE PHOSPHATE, DISOPYRAMIDE
  PHOSPHATE
ERGOLOID MESYLATES, ERGOLOID MESYLATES
FLUOXYMESTERONE, FLUOXYMESTERONE
FLUPHENAZINE HCL, FLUPHENAZINE
  HYDROCHLORIDE
FOLIC ACID, FOLIC ACID
GLYCOPYRROLATE, GLYCOPYRROLATE
GUANETHIDINE MONOSULFATE, GUANETHIDINE
  MONOSULFATE
HALOPERIDOL, HALOPERIDOL
HYDRALAZINE HCL AND HYDROCHLOROTHIAZIDE,
  HYDRALAZINE HYDROCHLORIDE
HYDROCHLOROTHIAZIDE, HYDROCHLOROTHIAZIDE
HYDROCHLOROTHIAZIDE W/ HYDRALAZINE,
  HYDRALAZINE HYDROCHLORID
HYDROCHLOROTHIAZIDE W/ RESERPINE,
  HYDROCHLOROTHIAZIDE
HYDROCHLOROTHIAZIDE W/ RESERPINE AND
  HYDRALAZINE, HYDRALAZINE HYDROCHLORIDE
HYDROFLUMETHIAZIDE, HYDROFLUMETHIAZIDE
HYDROFLUMETHIAZIDE W/ RESERPINE,
  HYDROFLUMETHIAZIDE
HYDROXYZINE PAMOATE, HYDROXYZINE PAMOATE
IMIPRAMINE HCL, IMIPRAMINE HYDROCHLORIDE
INDOMETHACIN, INDOMETHACIN
ISONIAZID, ISONIAZID
LIOTHYRONINE SODIUM, LIOTHYRONINE SODIUM
LITHIUM CARBONATE, LITHIUM CARBONATE
MAPROTILINE HCL, MAPROTILINE HYDROCHLORIDE
MECLIZINE HCL, MECLIZINE HYDROCHLORIDE
MECLOFENAMATE SODIUM, MECLOFENAMATE
  SODIUM
METHOCARBAMOL, METHOCARBAMOL
METHYCLOTHIAZIDE, METHYCLOTHIAZIDE
METHYCLOTHIAZIDE AND DESERPIDINE,
  DESERPIDINE
METHYLDOPA, METHYLDOPA
METHYLDOPA AND HYDROCHLOROTHIAZIDE,
  HYDROCHLOROTHIAZIDE
METOCLOPRAMIDE HCL, METOCLOPRAMIDE
  HYDROCHLORIDE
NIACIN, NIACIN
NITROFURANTOIN, NITROFURANTOIN
NITROFURANTOIN MACROCRYSTALLINE,
  NITROFURANTOIN, MACROCRYSTALLINE
ORPHENADRINE CITRATE, ORPHENADRINE CITRATE
OXTRIPHYLLINE, OXTRIPHYLLINE
OXYBUTYNIN CHLORIDE, OXYBUTYNIN CHLORIDE
OXYPHENBUTAZONE, OXYPHENBUTAZONE
PERPHENAZINE AND AMITRIPTYLINE HCL,
  AMITRIPTYLINE HYDROCHLORIDE
PHENYTEX, PHENYTOIN SODIUM, EXTENDED
PRIMIDONE, PRIMIDONE
PROBENECID W/ COLCHICINE, COLCHICINE
PROCAINAMIDE HCL, PROCAINAMIDE
  HYDROCHLORIDE
PROCHLORPERAZINE, PROCHLORPERAZINE
  MALEATE
PROMETHAZINE HCL, PROMETHAZINE
  HYDROCHLORIDE
PROPANTHELINE BROMIDE, PROPANTHELINE
  BROMIDE

PROPOXYPHENE NAPSYLATE AND ACETAMINOPHEN,
  ACETAMINOPHEN
PROPRANOLOL HCL, PROPRANOLOL
  HYDROCHLORIDE
QUINATIME, QUINIDINE GLUCONATE
SPIRONOLACTONE, SPIRONOLACTONE
SPIRONOLACTONE W/ HYDROCHLOROTHIAZIDE,
  HYDROCHLOROTHIAZIDE
SULFAMETHOXAZOLE, SULFAMETHOXAZOLE
SULFASALAZINE, SULFASALAZINE
TEMAZEPAM, TEMAZEPAM
THIORIDAZINE HCL, THIORIDAZINE
  HYDROCHLORIDE
TIMOLOL MALEATE, TIMOLOL MALEATE
TOLAZAMIDE, TOLAZAMIDE
TOLBUTAMIDE, TOLBUTAMIDE
TRAZODONE HCL, TRAZODONE HYDROCHLORIDE
TRICHLORMETHIAZIDE, TRICHLORMETHIAZIDE
TRICHLORMETHIAZIDE W/ RESERPINE, RESERPINE
TRIFLUOPERAZINE HCL, TRIFLUOPERAZINE
  HYDROCHLORIDE
TRIHEXYPHENIDYL HCL, TRIHEXYPHENIDYL
  HYDROCHLORIDE
TRIPELENNAMINE HCL, TRIPELENNAMINE
  HYDROCHLORIDE
TRIPROLIDINE AND PSEUDOEPHEDRINE,
  PSEUDOEPHEDRINE HYDROCHLORIDE (OTC)
WARFARIN SODIUM, WARFARIN SODIUM

BOOTS
* BOOTS PHARMACEUTICALS INC
  CHLORPROMAZINE HCL, CHLORPROMAZINE
    HYDROCHLORIDE
  CHOLOXIN, DEXTROTHYROXINE SODIUM
  CHYMODIACTIN, CHYMOPAPAIN
  DISCASE, CHYMOPAPAIN
  E-MYCIN, ERYTHROMYCIN
  FOLIC ACID, FOLIC ACID
  IBUPROFEN, IBUPROFEN
  LOPURIN, ALLOPURINOL
  PROMETHAZINE HCL, PROMETHAZINE
    HYDROCHLORIDE
  PROPYLTHIOURACIL, PROPYLTHIOURACIL
  RUFEN, IBUPROFEN
  SSD, SILVER SULFADIAZINE
  TETRACYCLINE HCL, TETRACYCLINE
    HYDROCHLORIDE
  TRAVASE, SUTILAINS

BOSKAMP
* G POHL BOSKAMP GMBH AND CO
  NITRO IV, NITROGLYCERIN
  NITROLINGUAL, NITROGLYCERIN
  NITRONAL, NITROGLYCERIN

BOWMAN
* BOWMAN PHARMACEUTICALS INC
  HISERPIA, RESERPINE
  HIWOLFIA, RAUWOLFIA SERPENTINA

BRAE
* BRAE LABORATORIES INC DIV INTERNATIONAL
MINERALS AND CHEMI
  BACITRACIN, BACITRACIN

BRAINTREE
* BRAINTREE LABORATORIES INC
  GOLYTELY, POLYETHYLENE GLYCOL 3350
  NULYTELY, POLYETHYLENE GLYCOL 3350
  PHOSLO, CALCIUM ACETATE

BRIAN
* BRIAN PHARMAEUTICALS
  BRIAN CARE, CHLORHEXIDINE GLUCONATE (OTC)

APPENDIX B
PRODUCT NAME INDEX
LISTED BY APPLICANT (continued)

BRISTOL
* BRISTOL LABORATORIES DIV BRISTOL MYERS CO
  AMIKIN, AMIKACIN SULFATE
  AMIKIN IN SODIUM CHLORIDE 0.9%, AMIKACIN
    SULFATE
  AMINOPHYLLINE, AMINOPHYLLINE
  BETAPEN-VK, PENICILLIN V POTASSIUM
  BICNU, CARMUSTINE
  BLENOXANE, BLEOMYCIN SULFATE
  BRISTACYCLINE, TETRACYCLINE HYDROCHLORIDE
  BRISTAGEN, GENTAMICIN SULFATE
  BRISTAMYCIN, ERYTHROMYCIN STEARATE
  BUSPAR, BUSPIRONE HYDROCHLORIDE
  CEENU, LOMUSTINE
  CEFADYL, CEPHAPIRIN SODIUM
  CEPHALOTHIN SODIUM, CEPHALOTHIN SODIUM
  CYTOXAN, CYCLOPHOSPHAMIDE
  DEXAMETHASONE SODIUM PHOSPHATE,
    DEXAMETHASONE SODIUM PHOSPHATE
  DIPHENHYDRAMINE HCL, DIPHENHYDRAMINE
    HYDROCHLORIDE
  DOPAMINE HCL, DOPAMINE HYDROCHLORIDE
  DYNAPEN, DICLOXACILLIN SODIUM
  ENKAID, ENCAINIDE HYDROCHLORIDE
  KANTREX, KANAMYCIN SULFATE
  LIDOCAINE HCL, LIDOCAINE HYDROCHLORIDE
  LYOPHILIZED CYTOXAN, CYCLOPHOSPHAMIDE
  LYSODREN, MITOTANE
  MEXATE, METHOTREXATE SODIUM
  MUTAMYCIN, MITOMYCIN
  NAFCIL, NAFCILLIN SODIUM
  POLYCILLIN, AMPICILLIN/AMPICILLIN TRIHYDRATE
  POLYCILLIN-N, AMPICILLIN SODIUM
  POLYCILLIN-PRB, AMPICILLIN TRIHYDRATE
  POLYMOX, AMOXICILLIN
  PRECEF, CEFORANIDE
  PROSTAPHLIN, OXACILLIN SODIUM
  SALURON, HYDROFLUMETHIAZIDE
  SALUTENSIN, HYDROFLUMETHIAZIDE
  SALUTENSIN-DEMI, HYDROFLUMETHIAZIDE
  STADOL, BUTORPHANOL TARTRATE
  STAPHCILLIN, METHICILLIN SODIUM
  TEGOPEN, CLOXACILLIN SODIUM
  TETREX, TETRACYCLINE PHOSPHATE COMPLEX
  ULTRACEF, CEFADROXIL/CEFADROXIL
    HEMIHYDRATE
  VEPESID, ETOPOSIDE
  VERSAPEN, HETACILLIN
  VERSAPEN-K, HETACILLIN POTASSIUM
  VINCREX, VINCRISTINE SULFATE
* BRISTOL LABORATORIES INC
  POLYCILLIN, AMPICILLIN/AMPICILLIN TRIHYDRATE

BRISTOL MYERS
* BRISTOL MYERS CO
  CEFANEX, CEPHALEXIN
  DESYREL, TRAZODONE HYDROCHLORIDE
  MEXATE-AQ, METHOTREXATE SODIUM
  MEXATE-AQ PRESERVED, METHOTREXATE SODIUM
  MUTAMYCIN, MITOMYCIN
  PLATINOL, CISPLATIN
  PLATINOL-AQ, CISPLATIN
  QUESTRAN, CHOLESTYRAMINE
  QUESTRAN LIGHT, CHOLESTYRAMINE
  QUIBRON-T, THEOPHYLLINE
  QUIBRON-T/SR, THEOPHYLLINE
  VAGISTAT-1, TIOCONAZOLE
  ZOLICEF, CEFAZOLIN SODIUM
* BRISTOL MYERS INDUSTRIAL DIV
  CEFADYL, CEPHAPIRIN SODIUM
  POLYCILLIN, AMPICILLIN/AMPICILLIN TRIHYDRATE
  POLYMOX, AMOXICILLIN

* BRISTOL MYERS PRODUCTS DIV BRISTOL MYERS CO
  NUPRIN, IBUPROFEN (OTC)
* BRISTOL MYERS US PHARMACEUTICAL AND
  NUTRITION GROUP
  RUBEX, DOXORUBICIN HYDROCHLORIDE

BRISTOL MYERS SQUIBB
* BRISTOL MYERS SQUIBB CO
  CAPOTEN, CAPTOPRIL
  MONOPRIL, FOSINOPRIL SODIUM
  PRAVACHOL, PRAVASTATIN SODIUM
  PRONESTYL-SR, PROCAINAMIDE HYDROCHLORIDE
* BRISTOL MYERS SQUIBB CO PHARMACEUTICAL
  RESEARCH AND DEVELO
  CEFZIL, CEFPROZIL
  STADOL, BUTORPHANOL TARTRATE
  VIDEX, DIDANOSINE
* BRISTOL MYERS SQUIBB CO PHARMACEUTICAL
  RESEARCH INSTITUTE
  DEAPRIL-ST, ERGOLOID MESYLATES
  IFEX, IFOSFAMIDE
  PARAPLATIN, CARBOPLATIN
* BRISTOL MYERS SQUIBB PHARMACEUTICAL
  RESEARCH INSTITUTE
  VUMON, TENIPOSIDE

BROCADES PHARMA
* BROCADES PHARMA BV DIV YAMANOUCHI GROUP
  LOCOID, HYDROCORTISONE BUTYRATE

BULL
* DAVID BULL LABORATORIES PARTY LTD
  CYTARABINE, CYTARABINE
  METOCLOPRAMIDE HCL, METOCLOPRAMIDE
    HYDROCHLORIDE
  VELSAR, VINBLASTINE SULFATE
  VINCRISTINE SULFATE, VINCRISTINE SULFATE
  VINCRISTINE SULFATE PFS, VINCRISTINE SULFATE

BUNDY
* CM BUNDY CO
  BUTABARBITAL, BUTABARBITAL SODIUM
  DIPHENHYDRAMINE HCL, DIPHENHYDRAMINE
    HYDROCHLORIDE
  MECLIZINE HCL, MECLIZINE HYDROCHLORIDE
  PREDNISOLONE, PREDNISOLONE
  PREDNISONE, PREDNISONE
  RAUWOLFIA SERPENTINA, RAUWOLFIA SERPENTINA
  RESERPINE, RESERPINE

BURROUGHS WELLCOME
* BURROUGHS WELLCOME CO
  ACTIDIL, TRIPROLIDINE HYDROCHLORIDE (OTC)
  ACTIFED, PSEUDOEPHEDRINE HYDROCHLORIDE
    (OTC)
  ACTIFED W/ CODEINE, CODEINE PHOSPHATE
  AEROSPORIN, POLYMYXIN B SULFATE
  ALKERAN, MELPHALAN
  ANECTINE, SUCCINYLCHOLINE CHLORIDE
  ANTEPAR, PIPERAZINE CITRATE
  CORTISPORIN, BACITRACIN ZINC
  CORTISPORIN, HYDROCORTISONE
  CORTISPORIN, HYDROCORTISONE ACETATE
  DARAPRIM, PYRIMETHAMINE
  ELIMITE, PERMETHRIN
  EMPRACET W/ CODEINE PHOSPHATE #3,
    ACETAMINOPHEN
  EMPRACET W/ CODEINE PHOSPHATE #4,
    ACETAMINOPHEN
  EXOSURF NEONATAL, CETYL ALCOHOL
  IMURAN, AZATHIOPRINE
  IMURAN, AZATHIOPRINE SODIUM

APPENDIX B
PRODUCT NAME INDEX
LISTED BY APPLICANT (continued)

KEMADRIN, PROCYCLIDINE HYDROCHLORIDE
LANOXICAPS, DIGOXIN
LANOXIN, DIGOXIN
LEUKERAN, CHLORAMBUCIL
MAREZINE, CYCLIZINE LACTATE
MIVACRON, MIVACURIUM CHLORIDE
MIVACRON IN DEXTROSE 5%, MIVACURIUM
    CHLORIDE
MYLERAN, BUSULFAN
NEOSPORIN, BACITRACIN ZINC
NEOSPORIN, GRAMICIDIN
NEOSPORIN G.U. IRRIGANT, NEOMYCIN SULFATE
NIX, PERMETHRIN
NIX, PERMETHRIN (OTC)
NUROMAX, DOXACURIUM CHLORIDE
OPTIPRESS, CARTEOLOL HYDROCHLORIDE
PEDIOTIC, HYDROCORTISONE
POLYSPORIN, BACITRACIN ZINC
POLYTRIM, POLYMYXIN B SULFATE
PROLOPRIM, TRIMETHOPRIM
PURINETHOL, MERCAPTOPURINE
RETROVIR, ZIDOVUDINE
SEPTRA, SULFAMETHOXAZOLE
SEPTRA DS, SULFAMETHOXAZOLE
SEPTRA GRAPE, SULFAMETHOXAZOLE
SUDAFED 12 HOUR, PSEUDOEPHEDRINE
    HYDROCHLORIDE (OTC)
SYNCURINE, DECAMETHONIUM BROMIDE
THIOGUANINE, THIOGUANINE
TRACRIUM, ATRACURIUM BESYLATE
VASOXYL, METHOXAMINE HYDROCHLORIDE
VIROPTIC, TRIFLURIDINE
WELLBUTRIN, BUPROPION HYDROCHLORIDE
WELLCOVORIN, LEUCOVORIN CALCIUM
ZOVIRAX, ACYCLOVIR
ZOVIRAX, ACYCLOVIR SODIUM
ZYLOPRIM, ALLOPURINOL

C

C AND M
* C AND M PHARMACAL INC
    HC (HYDROCORTISONE), HYDROCORTISONE
    HC (HYDROCORTISONE), HYDROCORTISONE (OTC)
    HI-COR, HYDROCORTISONE

CADEMA
* CADEMA MEDICAL PRODUCTS INC
    RBC-SCAN, TECHNETIUM TC-99M RED BLOOD CELL
        KIT

CALGON
* CALGON CORP DIV MERCK AND CO INC
    SEPTI-SOFT, HEXACHLOROPHENE

CAMALL
* CAMALL CO
    CAM-AP-ES, HYDRALAZINE HYDROCHLORIDE
    CAM-METRAZINE, PHENDIMETRAZINE TARTRATE
    CHLOROTHIAZIDE, CHLOROTHIAZIDE
    CYPROHEPTADINE HCL, CYPROHEPTADINE
        HYDROCHLORIDE
    DIETHYLPROPION HCL, DIETHYLPROPION
        HYDROCHLORIDE
    HYDRALAZINE HCL, HYDRALAZINE
        HYDROCHLORIDE
    HYDRO-RESERP, HYDROCHLOROTHIAZIDE
    HYDROCHLOROTHIAZIDE, HYDROCHLOROTHIAZIDE
    MECLIZINE HCL, MECLIZINE HYDROCHLORIDE

PHENAZINE-35, PHENDIMETRAZINE TARTRATE
PHENDIMETRAZINE TARTRATE, PHENDIMETRAZINE
    TARTRATE
PHENTERMINE HCL, PHENTERMINE
    HYDROCHLORIDE
TRICHLORMETHIAZIDE, TRICHLORMETHIAZIDE

CARLISLE
* CARLISLE LABORATORIES INC
    ALPHACAINE, LIDOCAINE
    ALPHACAINE HCL, LIDOCAINE HYDROCHLORIDE
    ALPHACAINE HCL W/ EPINEPHRINE, EPINEPHRINE
    ARESTOCAINE HCL, MEPIVACAINE HYDROCHLORIDE
    ARESTOCAINE HCL W/ LEVONORDEFRIN,
        LEVONORDEFRIN

CARNRICK
* CARNRICK LABORATORIES DIV GW CARNRICK CO
    AMEN, MEDROXYPROGESTERONE ACETATE
    BONTRIL PDM, PHENDIMETRAZINE TARTRATE
    CAPITAL AND CODEINE, ACETAMINOPHEN
    CAPITAL WITH CODEINE, ACETAMINOPHEN
    MOTOFEN, ATROPINE SULFATE
    MOTOFEN HALF-STRENGTH, ATROPINE SULFATE
    PHRENILIN, ACETAMINOPHEN
    PHRENILIN FORTE, ACETAMINOPHEN
    SKELAXIN, METAXALONE

CAROLINA MEDCL
* CAROLINA MEDICAL PRODUCTS CO
    HYDROCORTISONE IN ABSORBASE,
        HYDROCORTISONE
    ISONIAZID, ISONIAZID
    SODIUM POLYSTYRENE SULFONATE, SODIUM
        POLYSTYRENE SULFONATE
    SPS, SODIUM POLYSTYRENE SULFONATE

CENCI
* HR CENCI LABORATORIES INC
    ACTAHIST, PSEUDOEPHEDRINE HYDROCHLORIDE
    DIBENIL, DIPHENHYDRAMINE HYDROCHLORIDE
    DIPHENHYDRAMINE HCL, DIPHENHYDRAMINE
        HYDROCHLORIDE
    ELIXOMIN, THEOPHYLLINE
    HISTAFED C, CODEINE PHOSPHATE
    HYDROCORTISONE ACETATE, HYDROCORTISONE
        ACETATE
    PROMETHAZINE, PROMETHAZINE HYDROCHLORIDE
    PROMETHAZINE VC PLAIN, PHENYLEPHRINE
        HYDROCHLORIDE
    PROMETHAZINE VC W/ CODEINE, CODEINE
        PHOSPHATE
    PROMETHAZINE W/ CODEINE, CODEINE PHOSPHATE

CENTRAL PHARMS
* CENTRAL PHARMACEUTICALS INC
    ACETAMINOPHEN AND HYDROCODONE
        BITARTRATE, ACETAMINOPHEN
    AZDONE, ASPIRIN
    CO-GESIC, ACETAMINOPHEN
    CODIMAL-L.A. 12, CHLORPHENIRAMINE MALEATE
        (OTC)
    DEXACEN-4, DEXAMETHASONE SODIUM PHOSPHATE
    PHENYLPROPANOLAMINE HCL W/
        CHLORPHENIRAMINE MALEATE,
        CHLORPHENIRAMINE MALEATE (OTC)
    PREDNICEN-M, PREDNISONE
    PREDNISOLONE ACETATE, PREDNISOLONE ACETATE
    PSEUDOEPHEDRINE HYDROCHLORIDE AND
        CHLORPHENIRAMINE MALEATE,
        CHLORPHENIRAMINE MALEATE (OTC)
    SYNOPHYLATE, THEOPHYLLINE SODIUM GLYCINATE

APPENDIX B
PRODUCT NAME INDEX
LISTED BY APPLICANT (continued)

THEOCLEAR L.A.-130, THEOPHYLLINE
THEOCLEAR L.A.-260, THEOPHYLLINE
THEOCLEAR-100, THEOPHYLLINE
THEOCLEAR-200, THEOPHYLLINE
THEOCLEAR-80, THEOPHYLLINE
THEOPHYLLINE, THEOPHYLLINE

CENTURY
* CENTURY PHARMACEUTICALS INC
P.A.S. SODIUM, AMINOSALICYLATE SODIUM

CETUS BEN VENUE
* CETUS BEN VENUE THERAPEUTICS
ACETYLCYSTEINE, ACETYLCYSTEINE
CYTARABINE, CYTARABINE
DOXORUBICIN HCL, DOXORUBICIN
   HYDROCHLORIDE
METOCLOPRAMIDE HCL, METOCLOPRAMIDE
   HYDROCHLORIDE
SULFAMETHOXAZOLE AND TRIMETHOPRIM,
   SULFAMETHOXAZOLE

CHAMBERLIN
* CHAMBERLIN PARENTERAL CORP
HEPARIN SODIUM, HEPARIN SODIUM

CHARLOTTE
* CHARLOTTE PHARMACEUTICALS INC
ACETAMINOPHEN AND CODEINE PHOSPHATE,
   ACETAMINOPHEN
HYCOPAP, ACETAMINOPHEN
HYDROCODONE BITARTRATE AND
   ACETAMINOPHEN, ACETAMINOPHEN

CHASE
* CHASE CHEMICAL CO
VITAMIN A, VITAMIN A
VITAMIN A, VITAMIN A PALMITATE
VITAMIN D, ERGOCALCIFEROL
* CHASE LABORATORIES
NIFEDIPINE, NIFEDIPINE

CHELSEA
* CHELSEA LABORATORIES INC
ACETAMINOPHEN W/ CODEINE PHOSPHATE,
   ACETAMINOPHEN
ALLOPURINOL, ALLOPURINOL
AMINOPHYLLINE, AMINOPHYLLINE
AMITRIPTYLINE HCL, AMITRIPTYLINE
   HYDROCHLORIDE
BETHANECHOL CHLORIDE, BETHANECHOL
   CHLORIDE
BROMPHENIRAMINE MALEATE, BROMPHENIRAMINE
   MALEATE
BUTABARBITAL SODIUM, BUTABARBITAL SODIUM
BUTALBITAL, ASPIRIN AND CAFFEINE, ASPIRIN
CARISOPRODOL, CARISOPRODOL
CHLORDIAZEPOXIDE HCL, CHLORDIAZEPOXIDE
   HYDROCHLORIDE
CHLOROTHIAZIDE, CHLOROTHIAZIDE
CHLORPHENIRAMINE MALEATE,
   CHLORPHENIRAMINE MALEATE
CHLORPHENIRAMINE MALEATE AND
   PHENYLPROPANOLAMINE HCL,
   CHLORPHENIRAMINE MALEATE
CHLORPROMAZINE HCL, CHLORPROMAZINE
   HYDROCHLORIDE
CHLORPROPAMIDE, CHLORPROPAMIDE
CHLORTHALIDONE, CHLORTHALIDONE
CHLORZOXAZONE, CHLORZOXAZONE
CLOFIBRATE, CLOFIBRATE
CLORAZEPATE DIPOTASSIUM, CLORAZEPATE
   DIPOTASSIUM

CORTISONE ACETATE, CORTISONE ACETATE
CYPROHEPTADINE HCL, CYPROHEPTADINE
   HYDROCHLORIDE
DEXAMETHASONE, DEXAMETHASONE
DIAZEPAM, DIAZEPAM
DICYCLOMINE HCL, DICYCLOMINE
   HYDROCHLORIDE
DIETHYLPROPION HCL, DIETHYLPROPION
   HYDROCHLORIDE
DIMENHYDRINATE, DIMENHYDRINATE
DIPHENHYDRAMINE HCL, DIPHENHYDRAMINE
   HYDROCHLORIDE
DIPHENOXYLATE HCL AND ATROPINE SULFATE,
   ATROPINE SULFATE
DISULFIRAM, DISULFIRAM
DOXEPIN HCL, DOXEPIN HYDROCHLORIDE
DOXYCYCLINE HYCLATE, DOXYCYCLINE HYCLATE
ERYTHROMYCIN STEARATE, ERYTHROMYCIN
   STEARATE
FENOPROFEN CALCIUM, FENOPROFEN CALCIUM
FLURAZEPAM HCL, FLURAZEPAM HYDROCHLORIDE
FOLIC ACID, FOLIC ACID
FUROSEMIDE, FUROSEMIDE
GERIMAL, ERGOLOID MESYLATES
GLUTETHIMIDE, GLUTETHIMIDE
GLYCOPYRROLATE, GLYCOPYRROLATE
HYDRALAZINE AND HYDROCHLORTHIAZIDE,
   HYDRALAZINE HYDROCHLORID
HYDRALAZINE HCL, HYDRALAZINE
   HYDROCHLORIDE
HYDRALAZINE, HYDROCHLOROTHIAZIDE W/
   RESERPINE, HYDRALAZINE HYDROCHLORIDE
HYDROCHLOROTHIAZIDE, HYDROCHLOROTHIAZIDE
HYDROCHLOROTHIAZIDE W/ RESERPINE,
   HYDROCHLOROTHIAZIDE
HYDROFLUMETHIAZIDE, HYDROFLUMETHIAZIDE
HYDROXYZINE HCL, HYDROXYZINE
   HYDROCHLORIDE
HYDROXYZINE PAMOATE, HYDROXYZINE PAMOATE
IBUPROFEN, IBUPROFEN
IBUPROFEN, IBUPROFEN (OTC)
IMIPRAMINE HCL, IMIPRAMINE HYDROCHLORIDE
INDOMETHACIN, INDOMETHACIN
ISONIAZID, ISONIAZID
MECLIZINE HCL, MECLIZINE HYDROCHLORIDE
MECLOFENAMATE SODIUM, MECLOFENAMATE
   SODIUM
MEPROBAMATE, MEPROBAMATE
METHOCARBAMOL, METHOCARBAMOL
METHYCLOTHIAZIDE, METHYCLOTHIAZIDE
METHYLDOPA, METHYLDOPA
METHYLPREDNISOLONE, METHYLPREDNISOLONE
METOCLOPRAMIDE HCL, METOCLOPRAMIDE
   HYDROCHLORIDE
METRONIDAZOLE, METRONIDAZOLE
NIACIN, NIACIN
NITROFURANTOIN, NITROFURANTOIN
NYSTATIN, NYSTATIN
PERPHENAZINE AND AMITRIPTYLINE HCL,
   AMITRIPTYLINE HYDROCHLORIDE
PHENDIMETRAZINE TARTRATE, PHENDIMETRAZINE
   TARTRATE
PHENTERMINE HCL, PHENTERMINE
   HYDROCHLORIDE
PHENYLBUTAZONE, PHENYLBUTAZONE
PHENYTOIN SODIUM, PHENYTOIN SODIUM, PROMPT
PREDNISOLONE, PREDNISOLONE
PREDNISONE, PREDNISONE
PROBEN-C, COLCHICINE
PROBENECID, PROBENECID

APPENDIX B
PRODUCT NAME INDEX
LISTED BY APPLICANT (*continued*)

PROCAINAMIDE HCL, PROCAINAMIDE
  HYDROCHLORIDE
PROMETHAZINE HCL, PROMETHAZINE
  HYDROCHLORIDE
PROPOXYPHENE HCL, PROPOXYPHENE
  HYDROCHLORIDE
PROPOXYPHENE HCL W/ ASPIRIN AND CAFFEINE,
  ASPIRIN
PROPRANOLOL HCL, PROPRANOLOL
  HYDROCHLORIDE
PROPRANOLOL HCL AND HYDROCHLOROTHIAZIDE,
  HYDROCHLOROTHIAZIDE
PROPYLTHIOURACIL, PROPYLTHIOURACIL
PYRILAMINE MALEATE, PYRILAMINE MALEATE
QUINIDINE GLUCONATE, QUINIDINE GLUCONATE
QUINIDINE SULFATE, QUINIDINE SULFATE
RESERPINE, RESERPINE
SODIUM PENTOBARBITAL, PENTOBARBITAL SODIUM
SODIUM SECOBARBITAL, SECOBARBITAL SODIUM
SPIRONOLACTONE, SPIRONOLACTONE
SPIRONOLACTONE W/ HYDROCHLOROTHIAZIDE,
  HYDROCHLOROTHIAZIDE
SULFAMETHOXAZOLE AND TRIMETHOPRIM,
  SULFAMETHOXAZOLE
SULFASALAZINE, SULFASALAZINE
SULFISOXAZOLE, SULFISOXAZOLE
TETRACYCLINE HCL, TETRACYCLINE
  HYDROCHLORIDE
THIORIDAZINE HCL, THIORIDAZINE
  HYDROCHLORIDE
THIOTHIXENE, THIOTHIXENE
TOLBUTAMIDE, TOLBUTAMIDE
TRIAMCINOLONE, TRIAMCINOLONE
TRICHLORMETHIAZIDE, TRICHLORMETHIAZIDE
TRIPELENNAMINE HCL, TRIPELENNAMINE
  HYDROCHLORIDE
TRIPROLIDINE HCL AND PSEUDOEPHEDRINE HCL,
  PSEUDOEPHEDRINE HYDROCHLORIDE (OTC)
VERAPAMIL HCL, VERAPAMIL HYDROCHLORIDE

CHESEBROUGH PONDS
* CHESEBROUGH PONDS INC
  EXTRA-STRENGTH AIM, SODIUM
    MONOFLUOROPHOSPHATE (OTC)
  VIRAC REX, UNDECOYLIUM CHLORIDE

CIBA
* CIBA PHARMACEUTICAL CO DIV CIBA GEIGY CORP
  ACTIGALL, URSODIOL
  ANAFRANIL, CLOMIPRAMINE HYDROCHLORIDE
  ANTRENYL, OXYPHENONIUM BROMIDE
  ANTURANE, SULFINPYRAZONE
  APRESAZIDE, HYDRALAZINE HYDROCHLORIDE
  APRESOLINE, HYDRALAZINE HYDROCHLORIDE
  APRESOLINE-ESIDRIX, HYDRALAZINE
    HYDROCHLORIDE
  CIBACALCIN, CALCITONIN, HUMAN
  CIBALITH-S, LITHIUM CITRATE
  CYTADREN, AMINOGLUTETHIMIDE
  DESFERAL, DEFEROXAMINE MESYLATE
  ESIDRIX, HYDROCHLOROTHIAZIDE
  ESIMIL, GUANETHIDINE MONOSULFATE
  ESTRADERM, ESTRADIOL
  HEAVY SOLUTION NUPERCAINE, DIBUCAINE
    HYDROCHLORIDE
  IMIPRAMINE HCL, IMIPRAMINE HYDROCHLORIDE
  INH, ISONIAZID
  ISMELIN, GUANETHIDINE MONOSULFATE
  LITHOBID, LITHIUM CARBONATE
  LOCORTEN, FLUMETHASONE PIVALATE
  LOPRESSIDONE, CHLORTHALIDONE

LOPRESSOR HCT 100/25, HYDROCHLOROTHIAZIDE
LOPRESSOR HCT 100/50, HYDROCHLOROTHIAZIDE
LOPRESSOR HCT 50/25, HYDROCHLOROTHIAZIDE
LOTENSIN, BENAZEPRIL HYDROCHLORIDE
LOTENSIN HCT, BENAZEPRIL HYDROCHLORIDE
LUDIOMIL, MAPROTILINE HYDROCHLORIDE
METANDREN, METHYLTESTOSTERONE
METOPIRONE, METYRAPONE
PERCORTEN, DESOXYCORTICOSTERONE ACETATE
PERCORTEN, DESOXYCORTICOSTERONE PIVALATE
PRISCOLINE, TOLAZOLINE HYDROCHLORIDE
REGITINE, PHENTOLAMINE MESYLATE
RIMACTANE, RIFAMPIN
RITALIN, METHYLPHENIDATE HYDROCHLORIDE
RITALIN-SR, METHYLPHENIDATE HYDROCHLORIDE
SER-AP-ES, HYDRALAZINE HYDROCHLORIDE
SERPASIL, RESERPINE
SERPASIL-APRESOLINE, HYDRALAZINE
  HYDROCHLORIDE
SERPASIL-ESIDRIX #1, HYDROCHLOROTHIAZIDE
SERPASIL-ESIDRIX #2, HYDROCHLOROTHIAZIDE
SLOW-K, POTASSIUM CHLORIDE
TEN-K, POTASSIUM CHLORIDE
TRANSDERM-SCOP, SCOPOLAMINE
TRASICOR, OXPRENOLOL HYDROCHLORIDE
VIOFORM-HYDROCORTISONE, CLIOQUINOL
VOLTAREN, DICLOFENAC SODIUM

CIBA GEIGY
* CIBA GEIGY CORP PHARMACEUTICAL DIV
  AREDIA, PAMIDRONATE DISODIUM
  HABITROL, NICOTINE

CIS
* CIS US INC
  AN-DTPA, TECHNETIUM TC-99M PENTETATE KIT
  AN-MAA, TECHNETIUM TC-99M ALBUMIN
    AGGREGATED KIT
  AN-MDP, TECHNETIUM TC-99M MEDRONATE KIT
  AN-PYROTEC, TECHNETIUM TC-99M PYROPHOSPHATE
    KIT
  AN-SULFUR COLLOID, TECHNETIUM TC-99M SULFUR
    COLLOID KIT
  IODOHIPPURATE SODIUM I 131, IODOHIPPURATE
    SODIUM, I-131
  SELENOMETHIONINE SE 75, SELENOMETHIONINE,
    SE-75
  SODIUM IODIDE I 131, SODIUM IODIDE, I-131
  SODIUM PERTECHNETATE TC 99M, TECHNETIUM TC-
    99M SODIUM PERTECHNETATE

CLAY PARK
* CLAY PARK LABORATORIES INC
  BETAMETHASONE DIPROPIONATE, BETAMETHASONE
    DIPROPIONATE
  BETAMETHASONE VALERATE, BETAMETHASONE
    VALERATE
  ERYTHROMYCIN, ERYTHROMYCIN
  FLUOCINOLONE ACETONIDE, FLUOCINOLONE
    ACETONIDE
  FLUOCINONIDE, FLUOCINONIDE
  GENTAMICIN, GENTAMICIN SULFATE
  HYDROCORTISONE, HYDROCORTISONE
  NITROFURAZONE, NITROFURAZONE
  NYSTATIN, NYSTATIN
  NYSTATIN AND TRIAMCINOLONE ACETONIDE,
    NYSTATIN
  SELENIUM SULFIDE, SELENIUM SULFIDE
  TRIAMCINOLONE ACETONIDE, TRIAMCINOLONE
    ACETONIDE
  TRIPLE SULFA, TRIPLE SULFA
    (SULFABENZAMIDE; SULFACETAMIDE; SULFATHIAZOLE)

APPENDIX B
PRODUCT NAME INDEX
LISTED BY APPLICANT (continued)

CLONMEL
* CLONMEL CHEMICALS CO LTD
  AMOXICILLIN, AMOXICILLIN
  AMPICILLIN, AMPICILLIN/AMPICILLIN TRIHYDRATE
  PENICILLIN V POTASSIUM, PENICILLIN V
    POTASSIUM

COMBE
* COMBE INC
  BACITRACIN, BACITRACIN (OTC)
  LANABIOTIC, BACITRACIN (OTC)
  LANABIOTIC, BACITRACIN ZINC (OTC)

CONSOLIDATED MIDLAND
* CONSOLIDATED MIDLAND CORP
  TEEBACIN, AMINOSALICYLATE SODIUM

COOK WAITE
* COOK WAITE LABORATORIES INC SUB STERLING
DRUG INC
  CARBOCAINE, MEPIVACAINE HYDROCHLORIDE
  CARBOCAINE W/ NEO-COBEFRIN, LEVONORDEFRIN
  RAVOCAINE AND NOVOCAIN W/ LEVOPHED,
    NOREPINEPHRINE BITARTRAT
  RAVOCAINE AND NOVOCAIN W/ NEO-COBEFRIN,
    LEVONORDEFRIN

COPANOS
* JOHN D COPANOS INC
  AMOXICILLIN TRIHYDRATE, AMOXICILLIN
  AMPICILLIN SODIUM, AMPICILLIN SODIUM
  AMPICILLIN TRIHYDRATE, AMPICILLIN/AMPICILLIN
    TRIHYDRATE
  COMOX, AMOXICILLIN
  PENICILLIN G POTASSIUM, PENICILLIN G
    POTASSIUM
  PENICILLIN G PROCAINE, PENICILLIN G PROCAINE
  PENICILLIN G SODIUM, PENICILLIN G SODIUM
  PENICILLIN V POTASSIUM, PENICILLIN V
    POTASSIUM
  STREPTOMYCIN SULFATE, STREPTOMYCIN SULFATE

COPLEY
* COPLEY PHARMACEUTICAL INC
  ALBUTEROL SULFATE, ALBUTEROL SULFATE
  AMANTADINE HCL, AMANTADINE HYDROCHLORIDE
  AMITRIPTYLINE HCL, AMITRIPTYLINE
    HYDROCHLORIDE
  BETAMETHASONE DIPROPIONATE, BETAMETHASONE
    DIPROPIONATE
  BETAMETHASONE VALERATE, BETAMETHASONE
    VALERATE
  BROMATAPP, BROMPHENIRAMINE MALEATE (OTC)
  BROMPHERIL, DEXBROMPHENIRAMINE MALEATE
    (OTC)
  CLEMASTINE FUMARATE, CLEMASTINE FUMARATE
  CLINDAMYCIN PHOSPHATE, CLINDAMYCIN
    PHOSPHATE
  CO-LAV, POLYETHYLENE GLYCOL 3350
  DOXEPIN HCL, DOXEPIN HYDROCHLORIDE
  DOXYLAMINE SUCCINATE, DOXYLAMINE
    SUCCINATE (OTC)
  FLUOCINONIDE, FLUOCINONIDE
  FLUPHENAZINE HCL, FLUPHENAZINE
    HYDROCHLORIDE
  GO-EVAC, POLYETHYLENE GLYCOL 3350
  HALOPERIDOL, HALOPERIDOL LACTATE
  HYDROCORTISONE ACETATE 1% AND PRAMOXINE
    HCL 1%, HYDROCORTISONE ACETATE
  METAPROTERENOL SULFATE, METAPROTERENOL
    SULFATE
  PIROXICAM, PIROXICAM

  POTASSIUM CHLORIDE, POTASSIUM CHLORIDE
  PROCAINAMIDE HCL, PROCAINAMIDE
    HYDROCHLORIDE
  THIORIDAZINE HCL, THIORIDAZINE
    HYDROCHLORIDE
  THIOTHIXENE HCL, THIOTHIXENE HYDROCHLORIDE
  VALPROIC ACID, VALPROIC ACID

CUMBERLAND SWAN
* CUMBERLAND SWAN INC
  DIPHENHYDRAMINE HCL, DIPHENHYDRAMINE
    HYDROCHLORIDE (OTC)

CURATEK
* CURATEK PHARMACEUTICALS INC
  METROGEL, METRONIDAZOLE
* CURATEK PHARMACEUTICALS LTD PARTNERSHIP
  METROGEL, METRONIDAZOLE

CUTTER
* CUTTER BIOLOGICAL DIV MILES LABORATORIES INC
  ALCOHOL 5% IN DEXTROSE 5%, ALCOHOL
  DEXTROSE 10% IN PLASTIC CONTAINER, DEXTROSE
  DEXTROSE 5% AND SODIUM CHLORIDE 0.2% IN
    PLASTIC CONTAINER, DEXTROSE
  DEXTROSE 5% AND SODIUM CHLORIDE 0.3% IN
    PLASTIC CONTAINER, DEXTROSE
  DEXTROSE 5% AND SODIUM CHLORIDE 0.45% IN
    PLASTIC CONTAINER, DEXTROSE
  DEXTROSE 5% AND SODIUM CHLORIDE 0.9% IN
    PLASTIC CONTAINER, DEXTROSE
  DEXTROSE 5% IN LACTATED RINGER'S IN PLASTIC
    CONTAINER, CALCIUM CHLORIDE
  LACTATED RINGER'S IN PLASTIC CONTAINER,
    CALCIUM CHLORIDE
  LIDOCAINE HCL, LIDOCAINE HYDROCHLORIDE
  MANNITOL 10%, MANNITOL
  MANNITOL 15%, MANNITOL
  MANNITOL 20%, MANNITOL
  POTASSIUM CHLORIDE, POTASSIUM CHLORIDE
  PROCAINE HCL, PROCAINE HYDROCHLORIDE
  SODIUM CHLORIDE IN PLASTIC CONTAINER,
    SODIUM CHLORIDE
  SODIUM CHLORIDE 0.45% IN PLASTIC CONTAINER,
    SODIUM CHLORIDE
  SODIUM CHLORIDE 0.9% IN PLASTIC CONTAINER,
    SODIUM CHLORIDE
  STERILE WATER IN PLASTIC CONTAINER, WATER
    FOR IRRIGATION, STERILE

D

DANBURY
* DANBURY PHARMACAL INC
  ACETAZOLAMIDE, ACETAZOLAMIDE
  ACETOHEXAMIDE, ACETOHEXAMIDE
  ALBUTEROL SULFATE, ALBUTEROL SULFATE
  ALLOPURINOL, ALLOPURINOL
  AMITRIPTYLINE HCL, AMITRIPTYLINE
    HYDROCHLORIDE
  AMOXAPINE, AMOXAPINE
  ATENOLOL, ATENOLOL
  ATENOLOL AND CHLORTHALIDONE, ATENOLOL
  BACLOFEN, BACLOFEN
  BETHANECHOL CHLORIDE, BETHANECHOL
    CHLORIDE
  BROMPHENIRAMINE MALEATE, BROMPHENIRAMINE
    MALEATE
  BUTALBITAL AND ACETAMINOPHEN,
    ACETAMINOPHEN

APPENDIX B
PRODUCT NAME INDEX
LISTED BY APPLICANT *(continued)*

CARISOPRODOL, CARISOPRODOL
CHLORDIAZEPOXIDE AND AMITRIPTYLINE HCL, AMITRIPTYLINE HYDROCHLORIDE
CHLOROQUINE PHOSPHATE, CHLOROQUINE PHOSPHATE
CHLOROTHIAZIDE, CHLOROTHIAZIDE
CHLORPHENIRAMINE MALEATE, CHLORPHENIRAMINE MALEATE
CHLORPROPAMIDE, CHLORPROPAMIDE
CHLORTHALIDONE, CHLORTHALIDONE
CHLORZOXAZONE, CHLORZOXAZONE
CLINDAMYCIN HCL, CLINDAMYCIN HYDROCHLORIDE
CLONIDINE HCL, CLONIDINE HYDROCHLORIDE
COL-PROBENECID, COLCHICINE
CYCLOBENZAPRINE HCL, CYCLOBENZAPRINE HYDROCHLORIDE
CYPROHEPTADINE HCL, CYPROHEPTADINE HYDROCHLORIDE
DEXAMETHASONE, DEXAMETHASONE
DIAZEPAM, DIAZEPAM
DIPHENHYDRAMINE HCL, DIPHENHYDRAMINE HYDROCHLORIDE
DISOPYRAMIDE PHOSPHATE, DISOPYRAMIDE PHOSPHATE
DISULFIRAM, DISULFIRAM
DOXEPIN HCL, DOXEPIN HYDROCHLORIDE
DOXYCYCLINE HYCLATE, DOXYCYCLINE HYCLATE
ERGOLOID MESYLATES, ERGOLOID MESYLATES
ERYTHROMYCIN ESTOLATE, ERYTHROMYCIN ESTOLATE
FENOPROFEN CALCIUM, FENOPROFEN CALCIUM
FLURAZEPAM HCL, FLURAZEPAM HYDROCHLORIDE
FOLIC ACID, FOLIC ACID
FUROSEMIDE, FUROSEMIDE
GLUTETHIMIDE, GLUTETHIMIDE
GLYCOPYRROLATE, GLYCOPYRROLATE
HALOPERIDOL, HALOPERIDOL
HYDRALAZINE HCL, HYDRALAZINE HYDROCHLORIDE
HYDROCHLOROTHIAZIDE, HYDROCHLOROTHIAZIDE
HYDROCHLOROTHIAZIDE W/ RESERPINE, HYDROCHLOROTHIAZIDE
HYDROCORTISONE, HYDROCORTISONE
HYDROXYZINE HCL, HYDROXYZINE HYDROCHLORIDE
HYDROXYZINE PAMOATE, HYDROXYZINE PAMOATE
IBUPROFEN, IBUPROFEN
IBUPROFEN, IBUPROFEN (OTC)
INDOMETHACIN, INDOMETHACIN
ISONIAZID, ISONIAZID
ISOSORBIDE DINITRATE, ISOSORBIDE DINITRATE
LORAZEPAM, LORAZEPAM
MECLOFENAMATE SODIUM, MECLOFENAMATE SODIUM
MEPROBAMATE, MEPROBAMATE
METAPROTERENOL SULFATE, METAPROTERENOL SULFATE
METHOCARBAMOL, METHOCARBAMOL
METHYLDOPA, METHYLDOPA
METHYLDOPA AND HYDROCHLOROTHIAZIDE, HYDROCHLOROTHIAZIDE
METHYLTESTOSTERONE, METHYLTESTOSTERONE
METOCLOPRAMIDE HCL, METOCLOPRAMIDE HYDROCHLORIDE
METRONIDAZOLE, METRONIDAZOLE
MINOCYCLINE HCL, MINOCYCLINE HYDROCHLORIDE
MINOXIDIL, MINOXIDIL
NALIDIXIC ACID, NALIDIXIC ACID

NIACIN, NIACIN
NORTRIPTYLINE HCL, NORTRIPTYLINE HYDROCHLORIDE
OXAZEPAM, OXAZEPAM
PERPHENAZINE AND AMITRIPTYLINE HCL, AMITRIPTYLINE HYDROCHLORIDE
PHENYLBUTAZONE, PHENYLBUTAZONE
PRAZOSIN HCL, PRAZOSIN HYDROCHLORIDE
PREDNISOLONE, PREDNISOLONE
PREDNISONE, PREDNISONE
PRIMIDONE, PRIMIDONE
PROBENECID, PROBENECID
PROCAINAMIDE HCL, PROCAINAMIDE HYDROCHLORIDE
PROMETHAZINE HCL, PROMETHAZINE HYDROCHLORIDE
PROMPT PHENYTOIN SODIUM, PHENYTOIN SODIUM, PROMPT
PROPANTHELINE BROMIDE, PROPANTHELINE BROMIDE
PROPOXYPHENE HCL, PROPOXYPHENE HYDROCHLORIDE
PROPRANOLOL HCL, PROPRANOLOL HYDROCHLORIDE
PROPRANOLOL HCL AND HYDROCHLOROTHIAZIDE, HYDROCHLOROTHIAZIDE
PROPYLTHIOURACIL, PROPYLTHIOURACIL
QUINIDINE GLUCONATE, QUINIDINE GLUCONATE
QUINIDINE SULFATE, QUINIDINE SULFATE
RAUWOLFIA SERPENTINA, RAUWOLFIA SERPENTINA
RESERPINE, RESERPINE
RESERPINE/HYDRALAZINE HCL/ HYDROCHLOROTHIAZIDE, HYDRALAZINE HYDROCHLORIDE
SPIRONOLACTONE/HYDROCHLOROTHIAZIDE, HYDROCHLOROTHIAZIDE
SULFAMETHOXAZOLE AND TRIMETHOPRIM, SULFAMETHOXAZOLE
SULFAMETHOXAZOLE AND TRIMETHOPRIM DOUBLE STRENGTH, SULFAMETHOXAZOLE
SULFASALAZINE, SULFASALAZINE
SULFINPYRAZONE, SULFINPYRAZONE
SULINDAC, SULINDAC
TETRACYCLINE HCL, TETRACYCLINE HYDROCHLORIDE
THIORIDAZINE HCL, THIORIDAZINE HYDROCHLORIDE
THIOTHIXENE, THIOTHIXENE
TIMOLOL MALEATE, TIMOLOL MALEATE
TOLAZAMIDE, TOLAZAMIDE
TOLBUTAMIDE, TOLBUTAMIDE
TRAZODONE HCL, TRAZODONE HYDROCHLORIDE
TRIAMCINOLONE, TRIAMCINOLONE
TRIAMTERENE AND HYDROCHLOROTHIAZIDE, HYDROCHLOROTHIAZIDE
TRICHLORMETHIAZIDE, TRICHLORMETHIAZIDE
TRIHEXYPHENIDYL HCL, TRIHEXYPHENIDYL HYDROCHLORIDE
TRIMETHOPRIM, TRIMETHOPRIM
TRIPELENNAMINE HCL, TRIPELENNAMINE HYDROCHLORIDE
TRIPODRINE, PSEUDOEPHEDRINE HYDROCHLORIDE (OTC)
TRIPROLIDINE HCL, TRIPROLIDINE HYDROCHLORIDE
VERAPAMIL HCL, VERAPAMIL HYDROCHLORIDE

DANIELS
* DANIELS PHARMACEUTICALS INC
TUSSIGON, HOMATROPINE METHYLBROMIDE

APPENDIX B
PRODUCT NAME INDEX
LISTED BY APPLICANT (continued)

DAVIS AND GECK
* DAVIS AND GECK DIV AMERICAN CYANAMID CO
  FLAXEDIL, GALLAMINE TRIETHIODIDE
  PRE-OP, HEXACHLOROPHENE
  PRE-OP II, HEXACHLOROPHENE

DEL RAY
* DEL RAY LABORATORIES INC
  ALA-CORT, HYDROCORTISONE
  ALA-SCALP, HYDROCORTISONE
  DEL-VI-A, VITAMIN A PALMITATE
  TRIDERM, TRIAMCINOLONE ACETONIDE

DELL
* DELL LABORATORIES INC
  CYANOCOBALAMIN, CYANOCOBALAMIN
  DEXAMETHASONE SODIUM PHOSPHATE,
    DEXAMETHASONE SODIUM PHOSPHATE
  HEPARIN SODIUM, HEPARIN SODIUM
  LIDOCAINE HCL, LIDOCAINE HYDROCHLORIDE
  LIDOCAINE HCL W/ EPINEPHRINE, EPINEPHRINE
  PYRIDOXINE HCL, PYRIDOXINE HYDROCHLORIDE
  THIAMINE HCL, THIAMINE HYDROCHLORIDE

DELMED
* DELMED INC
  DELFLEX W/ DEXTROSE 1.5% IN PLASTIC
    CONTAINER, CALCIUM CHLORIDE
  DELFLEX W/ DEXTROSE 1.5% LOW MAGNESIUM IN
    PLASTIC CONTAINER, CALCIUM CHLORIDE
  DELFLEX W/ DEXTROSE 2.5% IN PLASTIC
    CONTAINER, CALCIUM CHLORIDE
  DELFLEX W/ DEXTROSE 2.5% LOW MAGNESIUM IN
    PLASTIC CONTAINER, CALCIUM CHLORIDE
  DELFLEX W/ DEXTROSE 4.25% IN PLASTIC
    CONTAINER, CALCIUM CHLORIDE
  DELFLEX W/ DEXTROSE 4.25% LOW MAGNESIUM IN
    PLASTIC CONTAINER, CALCIUM CHLORIDE

DEPROCO
* DEPROCO INC
  LIGNOSPAN FORTE, EPINEPHRINE BITARTRATE
  LIGNOSPAN STANDARD, EPINEPHRINE BITARTRATE
  SCANDONEST L, LEVONORDEFRIN
  SCANDONEST PLAIN, MEPIVACAINE
    HYDROCHLORIDE

DERMIK
* DERMIK LABORATORIES INC SUB RORER
  BENZAMYCIN, BENZOYL PEROXIDE
  HYTONE, HYDROCORTISONE

DESERET
* DESERET MEDICAL INC DIV BECTON DICKINSON AND
CO
  CHLORHEXIDINE GLUCONATE, CHLORHEXIDINE
    GLUCONATE (OTC)
  E-Z SCRUB, HEXACHLOROPHENE

DEY
* DEY LABORATORIES INC
  ALBUTEROL SULFATE, ALBUTEROL SULFATE
  ISOETHARINE HCL, ISOETHARINE HYDROCHLORIDE
  ISOETHARINE HCL S/F, ISOETHARINE
    HYDROCHLORIDE
  ISOPROTERENOL HCL, ISOPROTERENOL
    HYDROCHLORIDE
  METAPROTERENOL SULFATE, METAPROTERENOL
    SULFATE
  MUCOSOL-10, ACETYLCYSTEINE
  MUCOSOL-20, ACETYLCYSTEINE

DISTA
* DISTA PRODUCTS CO DIV ELI LILLY AND CO
  CORDRAN, FLURANDRENOLIDE
  CORDRAN SP, FLURANDRENOLIDE
  ERYTHROMYCIN ETHYLSUCCINATE,
    ERYTHROMYCIN ETHYLSUCCINATE
  ILOSONE, ERYTHROMYCIN ESTOLATE
  ILOTYCIN, ERYTHROMYCIN
  ILOTYCIN GLUCEPTATE, ERYTHROMYCIN
    GLUCEPTATE
  NALFON, FENOPROFEN CALCIUM
  NALFON 200, FENOPROFEN CALCIUM
  PENICILLIN G POTASSIUM, PENICILLIN G
    POTASSIUM
  VALMID, ETHINAMATE

DORSEY
* DORSEY LABORATORIES DIV SANDOZ INC
  ASBRON, THEOPHYLLINE SODIUM GLYCINATE
  PHENYLPROPANOLAMINE HCL/
    CHLORPHENIRAMINE, CHLORPHENIRAMINE
    MALEATE (OTC)
  RAUTENSIN, ALSEROXYLON
  TAVIST, CLEMASTINE FUMARATE

DOW
* DOW PHARMACEUTICALS SUB DOW CHEMICAL CO
  DOW-ISONIAZID, ISONIAZID
  NEO-POLYCIN, BACITRACIN ZINC
  NEO-POLYCIN, GRAMICIDIN
  NOVAFED, PSEUDOEPHEDRINE HYDROCHLORIDE
  QUIDE, PIPERACETAZINE
  RIFAMATE, ISONIAZID

DUNHALL
* DUNHALL PHARMACEUTICALS INC
  TRIAPRIN, ACETAMINOPHEN

DUPONT
* DUPONT PHARMACEUTICALS
  ACETYLCYSTEINE, ACETYLCYSTEINE
  BRETYLOL, BRETYLIUM TOSYLATE
  BREVIBLOC, ESMOLOL HYDROCHLORIDE
  CALCIPARINE, HEPARIN CALCIUM
  CLINDAMYCIN PHOSPHATE, CLINDAMYCIN
    PHOSPHATE
  COUMADIN, WARFARIN SODIUM
  DROPERIDOL, DROPERIDOL
  ETHMOZINE, MORICIZINE HYDROCHLORIDE
  HYCODAN, HOMATROPINE METHYLBROMIDE
  HYCOMINE, HYDROCODONE BITARTRATE
  HYCOMINE PEDIATRIC, HYDROCODONE BITARTRATE
  INTROPIN, DOPAMINE HYDROCHLORIDE
  METHYLDOPATE HCL, METHYLDOPATE
    HYDROCHLORIDE
  METOCLOPRAMIDE HCL, METOCLOPRAMIDE
    HYDROCHLORIDE
  MOBAN, MOLINDONE HYDROCHLORIDE
  NARCAN, NALOXONE HYDROCHLORIDE
  NUBAIN, NALBUPHINE HYDROCHLORIDE
  NUMORPHAN, OXYMORPHONE HYDROCHLORIDE
  OXYCODONE 2.5/APAP 500, ACETAMINOPHEN
  OXYCODONE 5/APAP 500, ACETAMINOPHEN
  PERCOCET, ACETAMINOPHEN
  PERCODAN, ASPIRIN
  PERCODAN-DEMI, ASPIRIN
  REMSED, PROMETHAZINE HYDROCHLORIDE
  SYMMETREL, AMANTADINE HYDROCHLORIDE
  TREXAN, NALTREXONE HYDROCHLORIDE
  TRIDIL, NITROGLYCERIN
  VALPIN 50, ANISOTROPINE METHYLBROMIDE

APPENDIX B
PRODUCT NAME INDEX
LISTED BY APPLICANT (continued)

* DUPONT RADIOPHARMACEUTICALS
  CARDIOLITE, TECHNETIUM TC-99M SESTAMIBI KIT
  GLUCOSCAN, TECHNETIUM TC-99M GLUCEPTATE KIT
  HEPATOLITE, TECHNETIUM TC-99M DISOFENIN KIT
  MICROLITE, TECHNETIUM TC-99M ALBUMIN
    COLLOID KIT
  OSTEOLITE, TECHNETIUM TC-99M MEDRONATE KIT
  PULMOLITE, TECHNETIUM TC-99M ALBUMIN
    AGGREGATED KIT
  PYROLITE, TECHNETIUM TC-99M PYRO/TRIMETA
    PHOSPHATES KIT
  TECHNETIUM TC 99M GENERATOR, TECHNETIUM TC-
    99M SODIUM PERTECHNETATE GENERATOR
  THALLOUS CHLORIDE TL 201, THALLOUS CHLORIDE,
    TL-201
  XENON XE 133, XENON, XE-133

DUPONT MERCK
* DUPONT MERCK PHARMACEUTICAL CO
  CARDENE, NICARDIPINE HYDROCHLORIDE
  GALLIUM CITRATE GA 67, GALLIUM CITRATE, GA-67

DURAMED
* DURAMED PHARMACEUTICALS INC
  ACETAMINOPHEN AND CODEINE PHOSPHATE,
    ACETAMINOPHEN
  AMINOPHYLLINE, AMINOPHYLLINE
  CHLORPROPAMIDE, CHLORPROPAMIDE
  CLONIDINE HCL, CLONIDINE HYDROCHLORIDE
  CYPROHEPTADINE HCL, CYPROHEPTADINE
    HYDROCHLORIDE
  DIAZEPAM, DIAZEPAM
  HALOPERIDOL, HALOPERIDOL
  HYDROXYZINE PAMOATE, HYDROXYZINE PAMOATE
  INDOMETHACIN, INDOMETHACIN
  ISONIAZID, ISONIAZID
  MEDROXYPROGESTERONE ACETATE,
    MEDROXYPROGESTERONE ACETATE
  METHYLDOPA, METHYLDOPA
  METHYLPREDNISOLONE, METHYLPREDNISOLONE
  PHENTERMINE HCL, PHENTERMINE
    HYDROCHLORIDE
  PREDNISONE, PREDNISONE
  PROCHLORPERAZINE MALEATE,
    PROCHLORPERAZINE MALEATE
  PROPRANOLOL HCL, PROPRANOLOL
    HYDROCHLORIDE
  PROPRANOLOL HCL & HYDROCHLOROTHIAZIDE,
    HYDROCHLOROTHIAZIDE
  TEMAZEPAM, TEMAZEPAM
  TOLAZAMIDE, TOLAZAMIDE
  TRIFLUOPERAZINE HCL, TRIFLUOPERAZINE
    HYDROCHLORIDE

DYNAPHARM
* DYNAPHARM INC
  COLOVAGE, POLYETHYLENE GLYCOL 3350

E

E Z EM
* E Z EM CO INC
  BAROS, SODIUM BICARBONATE
  E-Z-EM PREP LYTE, POLYETHYLENE GLYCOL 3350

ELAN
* ELAN PHARMACEUTICAL RESEARCH CORP
  PROSTEP, NICOTINE
  VERELAN, VERAPAMIL HYDROCHLORIDE

ELDER
* ELDER PHARMACEUTICALS LTD
  ELDECORT, HYDROCORTISONE
  TRISORALEN, TRIOXSALEN

ELKINS SINN
* ELKINS SINN INC SUB AH ROBINS CO
  AMIKACIN, AMIKACIN SULFATE
  AMINOCAPROIC ACID, AMINOCAPROIC ACID
  AMINOPHYLLINE, AMINOPHYLLINE
  AMPICILLIN SODIUM, AMPICILLIN SODIUM
  BRETYLIUM TOSYLATE, BRETYLIUM TOSYLATE
  CEFAZOLIN SODIUM, CEFAZOLIN SODIUM
  CEPHAPIRIN SODIUM, CEPHAPIRIN SODIUM
  CHLORAMPHENICOL, CHLORAMPHENICOL SODIUM
    SUCCINATE
  CHLORPHENIRAMINE MALEATE,
    CHLORPHENIRAMINE MALEATE
  CHLORPROMAZINE HCL, CHLORPROMAZINE
    HYDROCHLORIDE
  CLINDAMYCIN PHOSPHATE, CLINDAMYCIN
    PHOSPHATE
  CORTISONE ACETATE, CORTISONE ACETATE
  CYANOCOBALAMIN, CYANOCOBALAMIN
  CYCLOPHOSPHAMIDE, CYCLOPHOSPHAMIDE
  DEXAMETHASONE, DEXAMETHASONE SODIUM
    PHOSPHATE
  DIAZEPAM, DIAZEPAM
  DIGOXIN, DIGOXIN
  DIMENHYDRINATE, DIMENHYDRINATE
  DIPHENHYDRAMINE HCL, DIPHENHYDRAMINE
    HYDROCHLORIDE
  DOPAMINE, DOPAMINE HYDROCHLORIDE
  DOXYCYCLINE, DOXYCYCLINE HYCLATE
  DURAMORPH PF, MORPHINE SULFATE
  ERYTHROMYCIN, ERYTHROMYCIN LACTOBIONATE
  FENTANYL CITRATE, FENTANYL CITRATE
  FUROSEMIDE, FUROSEMIDE
  GENTAMICIN SULFATE, GENTAMICIN SULFATE
  HEP-LOCK, HEPARIN SODIUM
  HEP-LOCK U/P, HEPARIN SODIUM
  HEPARIN SODIUM, HEPARIN SODIUM
  HYDROCHLOROTHIAZIDE, HYDROCHLOROTHIAZIDE
  HYDROCORTISONE, HYDROCORTISONE
  HYDROCORTISONE SODIUM SUCCINATE,
    HYDROCORTISONE SODIUM SUCCINATE
  HYDROXYZINE, HYDROXYZINE HYDROCHLORIDE
  HYDROXYZINE HCL, HYDROXYZINE
    HYDROCHLORIDE
  INFUMORPH, MORPHINE SULFATE
  ISOPROTERENOL HCL, ISOPROTERENOL
    HYDROCHLORIDE
  KANAMYCIN, KANAMYCIN SULFATE
  LEUCOVORIN CALCIUM, LEUCOVORIN CALCIUM
  LIDOCAINE HCL, LIDOCAINE HYDROCHLORIDE
  LIDOCAINE HCL AND EPINEPHRINE, EPINEPHRINE
  MEPERIDINE HCL, MEPERIDINE HYDROCHLORIDE
  MEPROBAMATE, MEPROBAMATE
  METARAMINOL BITARTRATE, METARAMINOL
    BITARTRATE
  METHYLDOPATE HCL, METHYLDOPATE
    HYDROCHLORIDE
  METHYLPREDNISOLONE, METHYLPREDNISOLONE
    SODIUM SUCCINATE
  METHYLPREDNISOLONE SODIUM SUCCINATE,
    METHYLPREDNISOLONE SODIUM SUCCINATE
  METRONIDAZOLE, METRONIDAZOLE
  NALOXONE, NALOXONE HYDROCHLORIDE
  NALOXONE HCL, NALOXONE HYDROCHLORIDE
  NEOMYCIN SULFATE, NEOMYCIN SULFATE
  NITROFURANTOIN, NITROFURANTOIN

APPENDIX B
PRODUCT NAME INDEX
LISTED BY APPLICANT (continued)

OXACILLIN SODIUM, OXACILLIN SODIUM
PANCURONIUM, PANCURONIUM BROMIDE
PENTOBARBITAL SODIUM, PENTOBARBITAL SODIUM
PHENYTOIN, PHENYTOIN SODIUM
POTASSIUM CHLORIDE, POTASSIUM CHLORIDE
PREDNISOLONE, PREDNISOLONE
PREDNISONE, PREDNISONE
PROCAINAMIDE HCL, PROCAINAMIDE
    HYDROCHLORIDE
PROCAINE HCL, PROCAINE HYDROCHLORIDE
PROCHLORPERAZINE, PROCHLORPERAZINE
    EDISYLATE
PROCHLORPERAZINE EDISYLATE,
    PROCHLORPERAZINE EDISYLATE
PROMETHAZINE HCL, PROMETHAZINE
    HYDROCHLORIDE
PROTAMINE SULFATE, PROTAMINE SULFATE
PYRIDOXINE HCL, PYRIDOXINE HYDROCHLORIDE
QUINIDINE SULFATE, QUINIDINE SULFATE
RESERPINE, RESERPINE
SECOBARBITAL SODIUM, SECOBARBITAL SODIUM
SODIUM NITROPRUSSIDE, SODIUM NITROPRUSSIDE
SODIUM PENTOBARBITAL, PENTOBARBITAL SODIUM
SODIUM SUCCINATE, SODIUM SUCCINATE
SOTRADECOL, SODIUM TETRADECYL SULFATE
SULFAMETHOXAZOLE AND TRIMETHOPRIM,
    SULFAMETHOXAZOLE
TESTOSTERONE PROPIONATE, TESTOSTERONE
    PROPIONATE
TETRACYCLINE HCL, TETRACYCLINE
    HYDROCHLORIDE
THIAMINE HCL, THIAMINE HYDROCHLORIDE
TOBRAMYCIN SULFATE, TOBRAMYCIN SULFATE
VANCOMYCIN HCL, VANCOMYCIN HYDROCHLORIDE
VITAMIN A, VITAMIN A PALMITATE

ENTRAVISION
* ENTRAVISION INC
    ENDOSOL PLUS, CALCIUM CHLORIDE

ENZON
* ENZON INC
    ADAGEN, PEGADEMASE BOVINE

EON LABS
* EON LABORATORIES MANUFACTURING INC
    ACETAMINOPHEN AND CODEINE PHOSPHATE,
      ACETAMINOPHEN
    ALKERGOT, ERGOLOID MESYLATES
    ALPHAZINE, PHENDIMETRAZINE TARTRATE
    BACLOFEN, BACLOFEN
    BUTABARBITAL SODIUM, BUTABARBITAL SODIUM
    CARISOPRODOL, CARISOPRODOL
    CHLORDIAZEPOXIDE HCL, CHLORDIAZEPOXIDE
      HYDROCHLORIDE
    CHLOROTHIAZIDE, CHLOROTHIAZIDE
    CHLORPROPAMIDE, CHLORPROPAMIDE
    CHLORTHALIDONE, CHLORTHALIDONE
    CLINDAMYCIN HCL, CLINDAMYCIN
      HYDROCHLORIDE
    DESIPRAMINE HCL, DESIPRAMINE HYDROCHLORIDE
    DIETHYLPROPION HCL, DIETHYLPROPION
      HYDROCHLORIDE
    DIPHENHYDRAMINE HCL, DIPHENHYDRAMINE
      HYDROCHLORIDE
    DIPHENOXYLATE HCL W/ ATROPINE SULFATE,
      ATROPINE SULFATE
    DOXYCYCLINE HYCLATE, DOXYCYCLINE HYCLATE
    DRALSERP, HYDRALAZINE HYDROCHLORIDE
    FOLIC ACID, FOLIC ACID
    FUROSEMIDE, FUROSEMIDE

HY-PAM, HYDROXYZINE PAMOATE
HYDRALAZINE HCL, HYDRALAZINE
    HYDROCHLORIDE
HYDRAP-ES, HYDRALAZINE HYDROCHLORIDE
HYDRO-SERP "25", HYDROCHLOROTHIAZIDE
HYDRO-SERP "50", HYDROCHLOROTHIAZIDE
HYDROCHLOROTHIAZIDE, HYDROCHLOROTHIAZIDE
HYDROCORTISONE, HYDROCORTISONE
HYDROXYZINE HCL, HYDROXYZINE
    HYDROCHLORIDE
HYDROXYZINE PAMOATE, HYDROXYZINE PAMOATE
IMIPRAMINE HCL, IMIPRAMINE HYDROCHLORIDE
INDOMETHACIN, INDOMETHACIN
ISONIAZID, ISONIAZID
MEFENAMIC ACID, MEFENAMIC ACID
MEPRO-ASPIRIN, ASPIRIN
MEPROBAMATE, MEPROBAMATE
METHOCARBAMOL, METHOCARBAMOL
METHYLPREDNISOLONE, METHYLPREDNISOLONE
METRONIDAZOLE, METRONIDAZOLE
NEOMYCIN SULFATE, NEOMYCIN SULFATE
NITROFURANTOIN, NITROFURANTOIN
NYSTATIN, NYSTATIN
ORPHENADRINE COMPOUND, ASPIRIN
ORPHENADRINE COMPOUND DOUBLE STRENGTH,
    ASPIRIN
PHENDIMETRAZINE TARTRATE, PHENDIMETRAZINE
    TARTRATE
PHENTERMINE HCL, PHENTERMINE
    HYDROCHLORIDE
PREDNISOLONE, PREDNISOLONE
PREDNISONE, PREDNISONE
PROBENECID AND COLCHICINE, COLCHICINE
PROMETHAZINE HCL, PROMETHAZINE
    HYDROCHLORIDE
PROPOXYPHENE HCL, PROPOXYPHENE
    HYDROCHLORIDE
PSEUDOEPHEDRINE HCL AND TRIPROLIDINE HCL,
    PSEUDOEPHEDRINE HYDROCHLORIDE
QUINIDINE SULFATE, QUINIDINE SULFATE
RESERPINE, RESERPINE
SULFAMETHOXAZOLE AND TRIMETHOPRIM,
    SULFAMETHOXAZOLE
SULFAMETHOXAZOLE AND TRIMETHOPRIM DOUBLE
    STRENGTH, SULFAMETHOXAZOLE
SULFASALAZINE, SULFASALAZINE
TETRACYCLINE HCL, TETRACYCLINE
    HYDROCHLORIDE
THEOPHYLLINE, THEOPHYLLINE
TOLBUTAMIDE, TOLBUTAMIDE
TRIAMTERENE AND HYDROCHLOROTHIAZIDE,
    HYDROCHLOROTHIAZIDE
TRICHLORMETHIAZIDE, TRICHLORMETHIAZIDE
TRIMIPRAMINE MALEATE, TRIMIPRAMINE MALEATE
WESTADONE, METHADONE HYDROCHLORIDE

ERSANA
* ERSANA INC SUB ER SQUIBB AND SONS
    VELOSEF, CEPHRADINE
    VELOSEF '125', CEPHRADINE
    VELOSEF '250', CEPHRADINE
    VELOSEF '500', CEPHRADINE

ETHITEK
* ETHITEK PHARMACEUTICALS CO
    MOCTANIN, MONOCTANOIN

EVERYLIFE
* EVERYLIFE
    APAP W/ CODEINE PHOSPHATE, ACETAMINOPHEN
    CORTISONE ACETATE, CORTISONE ACETATE
    FOLIC ACID, FOLIC ACID

APPENDIX B
PRODUCT NAME INDEX
LISTED BY APPLICANT *(continued)*

HYDROCORTISONE, HYDROCORTISONE
NIACIN, NIACIN
PREDNISOLONE, PREDNISOLONE
PREDNISONE, PREDNISONE
QUINIDINE SULFATE, QUINIDINE SULFATE
RESERPINE, RESERPINE
SECOBARBITAL SODIUM, SECOBARBITAL SODIUM
SODIUM PENTOBARBITAL, PENTOBARBITAL SODIUM
STANOZIDE, ISONIAZID
SULFADIAZINE, SULFADIAZINE
VITAMIN A, VITAMIN A
VITAMIN A, VITAMIN A PALMITATE
VITAMIN D, ERGOCALCIFEROL

F

FAULDING
* FH FAULDING AND CO LTD
 DORYX, DOXYCYCLINE HYCLATE
 ERYC, ERYTHROMYCIN
 ERYC SPRINKLES, ERYTHROMYCIN

FERNDALE
* FERNDALE LABORATORIES INC
 ADPHEN, PHENDIMETRAZINE TARTRATE
 AMOSENE, MEPROBAMATE
 AQUAPHYLLIN, THEOPHYLLINE
 DAPEX-37.5, PHENTERMINE HYDROCHLORIDE
 DELAXIN, METHOCARBAMOL
 FERNDEX, DEXTROAMPHETAMINE SULFATE
 FERNISOLONE-P, PREDNISOLONE
 FERNISONE, PREDNISONE
 OBESTIN-30, PHENTERMINE HYDROCHLORIDE
 PHENDIMETRAZINE TARTRATE, PHENDIMETRAZINE
  TARTRATE
 PRAMOSONE, HYDROCORTISONE ACETATE
 RAUSERPIN, RAUWOLFIA SERPENTINA
 STRIFON FORTE DSC, CHLORZOXAZONE
 UMI-PEX 30, PHENTERMINE HYDROCHLORIDE

FERRANTE
* FERRANTE JOHN J
 CHLORDIAZEPOXIDE HCL, CHLORDIAZEPOXIDE
  HYDROCHLORIDE

FERRING
* FERRING LABORATORIES INC
 CONCENTRAID, DESMOPRESSIN ACETATE
 LUTREPULSE PUMP KIT, GONADORELIN ACETATE
 RELEFACT TRH, PROTIRELIN
 SECRETIN-FERRING, SECRETIN

FIRST TX
* FIRST TEXAS PHARMACEUTICALS INC SUB SCHERER
LABORATORIES I
 CODEINE, ASPIRIN, APAP FORMULA NO. 2,
  ACETAMINOPHEN
 CODEINE, ASPIRIN, APAP FORMULA NO. 3,
  ACETAMINOPHEN
 CODEINE, ASPIRIN, APAP FORMULA NO. 4,
  ACETAMINOPHEN
 MEPROBAMATE, MEPROBAMATE
 PREDNISONE, PREDNISONE
 QUINIDINE SULFATE, QUINIDINE SULFATE

FISONS
* FISONS CORP
 ADAPIN, DOXEPIN HYDROCHLORIDE
 BIPHETAMINE 12.5, AMPHETAMINE RESIN COMPLEX
 BIPHETAMINE 20, AMPHETAMINE RESIN COMPLEX

BIPHETAMINE 7.5, AMPHETAMINE RESIN COMPLEX
CORSYM, CHLORPHENIRAMINE POLISTIREX (OTC)
DELSYM, DEXTROMETHORPHAN POLISTIREX (OTC)
ERGOMAR, ERGOTAMINE TARTRATE
GASTROCROM, CROMOLYN SODIUM
IMFERON, IRON DEXTRAN
INTAL, CROMOLYN SODIUM
IONAMIN-15, PHENTERMINE RESIN COMPLEX
IONAMIN-30, PHENTERMINE RESIN COMPLEX
ISOCLOR, CHLORPHENIRAMINE MALEATE (OTC)
MYKROX, METOLAZONE
NASALCROM, CROMOLYN SODIUM
OPTICROM, CROMOLYN SODIUM
PEDIAPRED, PREDNISOLONE SODIUM PHOSPHATE
PENNTUSS, CHLORPHENIRAMINE POLISTIREX (OTC)
PROFERDEX, IRON DEXTRAN
PSEUDO-12, PSEUDOEPHEDRINE POLISTIREX (OTC)
SOMOPHYLLIN, AMINOPHYLLINE
SOMOPHYLLIN-DF, AMINOPHYLLINE
SOMOPHYLLIN-T, THEOPHYLLINE
TUSSIONEX, CHLORPHENIRAMINE POLISTIREX
VAPO-ISO, ISOPROTERENOL HYDROCHLORIDE
ZAROXOLYN, METOLAZONE

FLEMING
* FLEMING AND CO
 AEROLATE, THEOPHYLLINE
 AEROLATE III, THEOPHYLLINE
 AEROLATE JR, THEOPHYLLINE
 AEROLATE SR, THEOPHYLLINE

FOREST LABS
* FOREST LABORATORIES INC
 AMBENYL, BROMODIPHENHYDRAMINE
  HYDROCHLORIDE
 BETAPRONE, PROPIOLACTONE
 DURAPHYL, THEOPHYLLINE
 ELIXICON, THEOPHYLLINE
 ELIXOPHYLLIN, THEOPHYLLINE
 ELIXOPHYLLIN SR, THEOPHYLLINE
 FORBAXIN, METHOCARBAMOL
 PYOCIDIN, HYDROCORTISONE
 SUS-PHRINE, EPINEPHRINE
 TESSALON, BENZONATATE

FOREST PHARMS
* FOREST PHARMACEUTICALS INC
 BANCAP, ACETAMINOPHEN
 BANCAP HC, ACETAMINOPHEN
 DURADYNE DHC, ACETAMINOPHEN
 ESGIC, ACETAMINOPHEN
 METRA, PHENDIMETRAZINE TARTRATE
 MICROSUL, SULFAMETHIZOLE
 PROKLAR, SULFAMETHIZOLE
 SULFALOID, TRISULFAPYRIMIDINES
 WOLFINA, RAUWOLFIA SERPENTINA

FOUGERA
* E FOUGERA DIV ALTANA INC
 BETAMETHASONE DIPROPIONATE, BETAMETHASONE
  DIPROPIONATE
 BETAMETHASONE VALERATE, BETAMETHASONE
  VALERATE
 ERYTHROMYCIN, ERYTHROMYCIN
 FLUOCINOLONE ACETONIDE, FLUOCINOLONE
  ACETONIDE
 GENTAMICIN SULFATE, GENTAMICIN SULFATE
 HYDROCORTISONE, HYDROCORTISONE
 LIDOCAINE, LIDOCAINE
 NEOMYCIN AND POLYMYXIN B SULFATES AND
  DEXAMETHASONE, DEXAMETHASONE
 NEOMYCIN SULFATE-TRIAMCINOLONE ACETONIDE,
  NEOMYCIN SULFATE

APPENDIX B
PRODUCT NAME INDEX
LISTED BY APPLICANT *(continued)*

NYSTATIN, NYSTATIN
NYSTATIN-TRIAMCINOLONE ACETONIDE, NYSTATIN
TRIPLE SULFA, TRIPLE SULFA
  (SULFABENZAMIDE; SULFACETAMIDE; SULFATHIAZOLE)

FRESENIUS
* FRESENIUS USA INC
  DELFLEX W/ DEXTROSE 1.5% LOW MAGNESIUM LOW
    CALCIUM, CALCIUM CHLORIDE
  DELFLEX W/ DEXTROSE 2.5% LOW MAGNESIUM LOW
    CALCIUM, CALCIUM CHLORIDE
  DELFLEX W/ DEXTROSE 4.25% LOW MAGNESIUM
    LOW CALCIUM, CALCIUM CHLORIDE

FUJISAWA
* FUJISAWA PHARMACEUTICAL CO
  GANITE, GALLIUM NITRATE
  NEBUPENT, PENTAMIDINE ISETHIONATE
  PENTAM 300, PENTAMIDINE ISETHIONATE

G

G AND W
* G AND W LABORATORIES INC
  ACEPHEN, ACETAMINOPHEN (OTC)
  FLUOCINOLONE ACETONIDE, FLUOCINOLONE
    ACETONIDE
  GYNE-SULF, TRIPLE SULFA
    (SULFABENZAMIDE; SULFACETAMIDE; SULFATHIAZOLE)
  HYDROCORTISONE, HYDROCORTISONE
  INDOMETHEGAN, INDOMETHACIN
  PROMETHEGAN, PROMETHAZINE HYDROCHLORIDE
  TRIAMCINOLONE ACETONIDE, TRIAMCINOLONE
    ACETONIDE
  TRUPHYLLINE, AMINOPHYLLINE

GEIGY
* GEIGY PHARMACEUTICALS DIV CIBA GEIGY CORP
  BRETHAIRE, TERBUTALINE SULFATE
  BRETHINE, TERBUTALINE SULFATE
  BUTAZOLIDIN, PHENYLBUTAZONE
  LAMPRENE, CLOFAZIMINE
  LIORESAL, BACLOFEN
  LOPRESSOR, METOPROLOL FUMARATE
  LOPRESSOR, METOPROLOL TARTRATE
  PBZ, TRIPELENNAMINE CITRATE
  PBZ, TRIPELENNAMINE HYDROCHLORIDE
  PBZ-SR, TRIPELENNAMINE HYDROCHLORIDE
  TEGRETOL, CARBAMAZEPINE
  TOFRANIL, IMIPRAMINE HYDROCHLORIDE
  TOFRANIL-PM, IMIPRAMINE PAMOATE
  VOLTAREN, DICLOFENAC SODIUM

GENCON
* GENCON PHARMACEUTICALS INC
  GENCEPT 0.5/35-21, ETHINYL ESTRADIOL
  GENCEPT 0.5/35-28, ETHINYL ESTRADIOL
  GENCEPT 1/35-21, ETHINYL ESTRADIOL
  GENCEPT 1/35-28, ETHINYL ESTRADIOL
  GENCEPT 10/11-21, ETHINYL ESTRADIOL
  GENCEPT 10/11-28, ETHINYL ESTRADIOL

GENDERM
* GENDERM CORP
  OVIDE, MALATHION
  TEXACORT, HYDROCORTISONE

GENENTECH
* GENENTECH INC
  CRESCORMON, SOMATROPIN
  PROTROPIN, SOMATREM

GENERAL ELECTRIC
* GENERAL ELECTRIC CO
  XENON XE 133, XENON, XE-133

GENEVA
* GENEVA PHARMACEUTICALS INC
  ACETAMINOPHEN AND CODEINE PHOSPHATE,
    ACETAMINOPHEN
  ALBUTEROL SULFATE, ALBUTEROL SULFATE
  ALLOPURINOL, ALLOPURINOL
  AMILORIDE HCL AND HYDROCHLOROTHIAZIDE,
    AMILORIDE HYDROCHLORIDE
  AMINOPHYLLINE, AMINOPHYLLINE
  AMITRIPTYLINE HCL, AMITRIPTYLINE
    HYDROCHLORIDE
  AMOXAPINE, AMOXAPINE
  ATENOLOL, ATENOLOL
  BROMPHENIRAMINE MALEATE, BROMPHENIRAMINE
    MALEATE
  BUTABARBITAL SODIUM, BUTABARBITAL SODIUM
  BUTAL COMPOUND, ASPIRIN
  CARISOPRODOL, CARISOPRODOL
  CHLORDIAZEPOXIDE HCL, CHLORDIAZEPOXIDE
    HYDROCHLORIDE
  CHLORPHENIRAMINE MALEATE,
    CHLORPHENIRAMINE MALEATE (OTC)
  CHLORPHENIRAMINE MALEATE,
    CHLORPHENIRAMINE MALEATE
  CHLORPHENIRAMINE MALEATE AND
    PHENYLPROPANOLAMINE HCL,
    CHLORPHENIRAMINE MALEATE
  CHLORPROMAZINE HCL, CHLORPROMAZINE
    HYDROCHLORIDE
  CHLORPROPAMIDE, CHLORPROPAMIDE
  CHLORTHALIDONE, CHLORTHALIDONE
  CHLORZOXAZONE, CHLORZOXAZONE
  CLOFIBRATE, CLOFIBRATE
  CLONIDINE HCL, CLONIDINE HYDROCHLORIDE
  CLORAZEPATE DIPOTASSIUM, CLORAZEPATE
    DIPOTASSIUM
  CORPHED, PSEUDOEPHEDRINE HYDROCHLORIDE
  CYCLOBENZAPRINE HCL, CYCLOBENZAPRINE
    HYDROCHLORIDE
  CYPROHEPTADINE HCL, CYPROHEPTADINE
    HYDROCHLORIDE
  DESIPRAMINE HCL, DESIPRAMINE HYDROCHLORIDE
  DEXAMETHASONE, DEXAMETHASONE
  DEXTROAMPHETAMINE SULFATE,
    DEXTROAMPHETAMINE SULFATE
  DIAZEPAM, DIAZEPAM
  DIPHENHYDRAMINE HCL, DIPHENHYDRAMINE
    HYDROCHLORIDE
  DIPYRIDAMOLE, DIPYRIDAMOLE
  DISOBROM, DEXBROMPHENIRAMINE MALEATE (OTC)
  DISOPYRAMIDE PHOSPHATE, DISOPYRAMIDE
    PHOSPHATE
  DOXEPIN HCL, DOXEPIN HYDROCHLORIDE
  ERCATAB, CAFFEINE
  ESTERIFIED ESTROGENS, ESTROGENS, ESTERIFIED
  FENOPROFEN CALCIUM, FENOPROFEN CALCIUM
  FLUPHENAZINE HCL, FLUPHENAZINE
    HYDROCHLORIDE
  FLURAZEPAM HCL, FLURAZEPAM HYDROCHLORIDE
  FUROSEMIDE, FUROSEMIDE
  GLUTETHIMIDE, GLUTETHIMIDE
  HALOPERIDOL, HALOPERIDOL
  HYDRALAZINE HCL, HYDRALAZINE
    HYDROCHLORIDE
  HYDROCHLOROTHIAZIDE, HYDROCHLOROTHIAZIDE
  HYDROXYZINE HCL, HYDROXYZINE
    HYDROCHLORIDE

APPENDIX B
PRODUCT NAME INDEX
LISTED BY APPLICANT (continued)

HYDROXYZINE PAMOATE, HYDROXYZINE PAMOATE
IBUPROFEN, IBUPROFEN
IBUPROFEN, IBUPROFEN (OTC)
IMIPRAMINE HCL, IMIPRAMINE HYDROCHLORIDE
INDOMETHACIN, INDOMETHACIN
ISOSORBIDE DINITRATE, ISOSORBIDE DINITRATE
LONOX, ATROPINE SULFATE
LOPERAMIDE HCL, LOPERAMIDE HYDROCHLORIDE
LORAZEPAM, LORAZEPAM
MECLIZINE HCL, MECLIZINE HYDROCHLORIDE
MECLOFENAMATE SODIUM, MECLOFENAMATE
  SODIUM
MEPROBAMATE, MEPROBAMATE
METHOCARBAMOL, METHOCARBAMOL
METHOXSALEN, METHOXSALEN
METHYCLOTHIAZIDE, METHYCLOTHIAZIDE
METHYLDOPA, METHYLDOPA
METHYLDOPA AND HYDROCHLOROTHIAZIDE,
  HYDROCHLOROTHIAZIDE
METOCLOPRAMIDE HCL, METOCLOPRAMIDE
  HYDROCHLORIDE
METRONIDAZOLE, METRONIDAZOLE
NIACIN, NIACIN
ORPHENADRINE CITRATE, ORPHENADRINE CITRATE
OXAZEPAM, OXAZEPAM
PERPHENAZINE, PERPHENAZINE
PERPHENAZINE AND AMITRIPTYLINE HCL,
  AMITRIPTYLINE HYDROCHLORIDE
PHENDIMETRAZINE TARTRATE, PHENDIMETRAZINE
  TARTRATE
PHENYLBUTAZONE, PHENYLBUTAZONE
PRAZOSIN HCL, PRAZOSIN HYDROCHLORIDE
PREDNISOLONE, PREDNISOLONE
PREDNISONE, PREDNISONE
PROCAINAMIDE HCL, PROCAINAMIDE
  HYDROCHLORIDE
PROMETHAZINE HCL, PROMETHAZINE
  HYDROCHLORIDE
PROPANTHELINE BROMIDE, PROPANTHELINE
  BROMIDE
PROPOXYPHENE COMPOUND-65, ASPIRIN
PROPOXYPHENE HCL, PROPOXYPHENE
  HYDROCHLORIDE
PROPOXYPHENE HCL AND ACETAMINOPHEN,
  ACETAMINOPHEN
PROPOXYPHENE NAPSYLATE AND ACETAMINOPHEN,
  ACETAMINOPHEN
PROPRANOLOL HCL, PROPRANOLOL
  HYDROCHLORIDE
PROPRANOLOL HCL AND HYDROCHLOROTHIAZIDE,
  HYDROCHLOROTHIAZIDE
QUINIDINE GLUCONATE, QUINIDINE GLUCONATE
QUINIDINE SULFATE, QUINIDINE SULFATE
RESERPINE AND HYDROCHLOROTHIAZIDE,
  HYDROCHLOROTHIAZIDE
SONAZINE, CHLORPROMAZINE HYDROCHLORIDE
SPIRONOLACTONE, SPIRONOLACTONE
SPIRONOLACTONE W/ HYDROCHLOROTHIAZIDE,
  HYDROCHLOROTHIAZIDE
SULFAMETHOXAZOLE, SULFAMETHOXAZOLE
SULFAMETHOXAZOLE AND TRIMETHOPRIM,
  SULFAMETHOXAZOLE
SULFISOXAZOLE, SULFISOXAZOLE
SULINDAC, SULINDAC
TEMAZEPAM, TEMAZEPAM
TFP, TRIFLUOPERAZINE HYDROCHLORIDE
THIORIDAZINE HCL, THIORIDAZINE
  HYDROCHLORIDE
THIOTHIXENE, THIOTHIXENE
TIMOLOL MALEATE, TIMOLOL MALEATE

TOLAZAMIDE, TOLAZAMIDE
TOLBUTAMIDE, TOLBUTAMIDE
TOLMETIN SODIUM, TOLMETIN SODIUM
TRAZODONE HCL, TRAZODONE HYDROCHLORIDE
TRIAMCINOLONE, TRIAMCINOLONE
TRIAMTERENE AND HYDROCHLOROTHIAZIDE,
  HYDROCHLOROTHIAZIDE
VERAPAMIL HCL, VERAPAMIL HYDROCHLORIDE

GENSIA
* GENSIA PHARMACEUTICAL INC
  AMINOPHYLLINE, AMINOPHYLLINE
  CLINDAMYCIN PHOSPHATE, CLINDAMYCIN
    PHOSPHATE
  DEXAMETHASONE SODIUM PHOSPHATE,
    DEXAMETHASONE SODIUM PHOSPHATE
  DOPAMINE HCL, DOPAMINE HYDROCHLORIDE
  GENTAMICIN SULFATE, GENTAMICIN SULFATE
  GLYCOPYRROLATE, GLYCOPYRROLATE
  METHYLDOPATE HCL, METHYLDOPATE
    HYDROCHLORIDE
  METOCLOPRAMIDE HCL, METOCLOPRAMIDE
    HYDROCHLORIDE
  PANCURONIUM BROMIDE, PANCURONIUM BROMIDE
  SODIUM NITROPRUSSIDE, SODIUM NITROPRUSSIDE
  SULFAMETHOXAZOLE AND TRIMETHOPRIM,
    SULFAMETHOXAZOLE
  TOBRAMYCIN SULFATE, TOBRAMYCIN SULFATE

GENZYME
* GENZYME CORP
  CEREDASE, ALGLUCERASE

GILBERT
* GILBERT LABORATORIES
  ACETAMINOPHEN, BUTALBITAL AND CAFFEINE,
    ACETAMINOPHEN

GLAXO
* GLAXO INC
  ACLOVATE, ALCLOMETASONE DIPROPIONATE
  BECLOVENT, BECLOMETHASONE DIPROPIONATE
  BECONASE, BECLOMETHASONE DIPROPIONATE
  BECONASE AQ, BECLOMETHASONE DIPROPIONATE
    MONOHYDRATE
  CEFTIN, CEFUROXIME AXETIL
  CEPTAZ, CEFTAZIDIME (ARGININE FORMULATION)
  CUTIVATE, FLUTICASONE PROPIONATE
  DIONOSIL AQUEOUS, PROPYLIODONE
  DIONOSIL OILY, PROPYLIODONE
  EMGEL, ERYTHROMYCIN
  FORTAZ, CEFTAZIDIME
  FORTAZ, CEFTAZIDIME SODIUM
  OXISTAT, OXICONAZOLE NITRATE
  SEFFIN, CEPHALOTHIN SODIUM
  TEMOVATE, CLOBETASOL PROPIONATE
  THEOBID, THEOPHYLLINE
  THEOBID JR., THEOPHYLLINE
  TRANDATE, LABETALOL HYDROCHLORIDE
  TRANDATE HCT, HYDROCHLOROTHIAZIDE
  VENTOLIN, ALBUTEROL
  VENTOLIN, ALBUTEROL SULFATE
  VENTOLIN ROTACAPS, ALBUTEROL SULFATE
  ZANTAC, RANITIDINE HYDROCHLORIDE
  ZANTAC 150, RANITIDINE HYDROCHLORIDE
  ZANTAC 300, RANITIDINE HYDROCHLORIDE
  ZINACEF, CEFUROXIME SODIUM
  ZOFRAN, ONDANSETRON HYDROCHLORIDE

GLENWOOD
* GLENWOOD INC
  MYOTONACHOL, BETHANECHOL CHLORIDE
  PASKALIUM, POTASSIUM AMINOSALICYLATE
  RENOQUID, SULFACYTINE

APPENDIX B
PRODUCT NAME INDEX
LISTED BY APPLICANT *(continued)*

GOLDLINE
* GOLDLINE LABORATORIES
  GLYCOPREP, POLYETHYLENE GLYCOL 3350

GRAHAM CHEM
* GRAHAM CHEMICAL CORP
  LIDOCAINE, LIDOCAINE
  LIDOCAINE HCL, LIDOCAINE HYDROCHLORIDE
  LIDOCAINE HCL W/ EPINEPHRINE, EPINEPHRINE
  MEPIVACAINE HCL, MEPIVACAINE HYDROCHLORIDE
  MEPIVACAINE HCL W/ LEVONORDEFRIN,
    LEVONORDEFRIN

GRAHAM LABS
* DM GRAHAM LABORATORIES INC
  ACETAMINOPHEN AND HYDROCODONE
    BITARTRATE, ACETAMINOPHEN
  BUTALBITAL AND ACETAMINOPHEN,
    ACETAMINOPHEN
  BUTALBITAL, ACETAMINOPHEN, CAFFEINE,
    ACETAMINOPHEN
  COLD CAPSULE IV, CHLORPHENIRAMINE MALEATE
    (OTC)
  COLD CAPSULE V, CHLORPHENIRAMINE MALEATE
    (OTC)
  CONTEN, ACETAMINOPHEN
  HYDROCET, ACETAMINOPHEN
  PHENDIMETRAZINE TARTRATE, PHENDIMETRAZINE
    TARTRATE
  PSEUDOEPHEDRINE HCL/CHLORPHENIRAMINE
    MALEATE, CHLORPHENIRAMINE MALEATE (OTC)
  REPAN, ACETAMINOPHEN
  SOMOPHYLLIN-CRT, THEOPHYLLINE

GRIFFEN
* KW GRIFFEN CO
  BIOSCRUB, CHLORHEXIDINE GLUCONATE (OTC)

GRUPPO LEPETIT
* GRUPPO LEPETIT SPA
  CHLORAMPHENICOL SODIUM SUCCINATE,
    CHLORAMPHENICOL SODIUM SUCCINATE

GUARDIAN DRUG
* GUARDIAN DRUG CO INC
  FOAMCOAT, ALUMINUM HYDROXIDE (OTC)

GUARDIAN LABS
* GUARDIAN LABORATORIES DIV UNITED GUARDIAN
INC
  RENACIDIN, CITRIC ACID

GYNEX
* GYNEX INC
  DELATESTRYL, TESTOSTERONE ENANTHATE
  OXANDRIN, OXANDROLONE

GYNOPHARMA
* GYNOPHARMA INC
  NORCEPT-E 1/35 21, ETHINYL ESTRADIOL
  NORCEPT-E 1/35 28, ETHINYL ESTRADIOL

H

HALOCARBON
* HALOCARBON LABORATORIES INC
  HALOTHANE, HALOTHANE

HALSEY
* HALSEY DRUG CO INC
  ACETAMINOPHEN AND CODEINE PHOSPHATE,
    ACETAMINOPHEN
  ACETAMINOPHEN W/ CODEINE PHOSPHATE,
    ACETAMINOPHEN

AMINOPHYLLINE, AMINOPHYLLINE
AMITRIPTYLINE HCL, AMITRIPTYLINE
  HYDROCHLORIDE
BELDIN, DIPHENHYDRAMINE HYDROCHLORIDE
  (OTC)
BELIX, DIPHENHYDRAMINE HYDROCHLORIDE
BUTALBITAL AND ACETAMINOPHEN,
  ACETAMINOPHEN
BUTALBITAL, APAP, AND CAFFEINE,
  ACETAMINOPHEN
BUTALBITAL, ASPIRIN & CAFFEINE, ASPIRIN
CHLORDIAZEPOXIDE HCL, CHLORDIAZEPOXIDE
  HYDROCHLORIDE
CHLORPROPAMIDE, CHLORPROPAMIDE
CODOXY, ASPIRIN
CORTALONE, PREDNISOLONE
CORTAN, PREDNISONE
CYPROHEPTADINE HCL, CYPROHEPTADINE
  HYDROCHLORIDE
DEXTROAMPHETAMINE SULFATE,
  DEXTROAMPHETAMINE SULFATE
DIAZEPAM, DIAZEPAM
DIPHENHYDRAMINE HCL, DIPHENHYDRAMINE
  HYDROCHLORIDE
DOXYCYCLINE HYCLATE, DOXYCYCLINE HYCLATE
FENOPROFEN CALCIUM, FENOPROFEN CALCIUM
FLURAZEPAM HCL, FLURAZEPAM HYDROCHLORIDE
FOLIC ACID, FOLIC ACID
GLUTETHIMIDE, GLUTETHIMIDE
HYDRALAZINE HCL, HYDRALAZINE
  HYDROCHLORIDE
HYDRO-D, HYDROCHLOROTHIAZIDE
HYDROCODONE BITARTRATE AND
  ACETAMINOPHEN, ACETAMINOPHEN
HYDROPANE, HOMATROPINE METHYLBROMIDE
HYDROXYZINE HCL, HYDROXYZINE
  HYDROCHLORIDE
IBUPROFEN, IBUPROFEN
IBUPROFEN, IBUPROFEN (OTC)
INDOMETHACIN, INDOMETHACIN
ISONIAZID, ISONIAZID
KLOROMIN, CHLORPHENIRAMINE MALEATE
LORAZEPAM, LORAZEPAM
LOW-QUEL, ATROPINE SULFATE
METHYLDOPA, METHYLDOPA
METOCLOPRAMIDE HCL, METOCLOPRAMIDE
  HYDROCHLORIDE
METRONIDAZOLE, METRONIDAZOLE
NEURAMATE, MEPROBAMATE
NIACIN, NIACIN
OXYCET, ACETAMINOPHEN
OXYCODONE AND ACETAMINOPHEN,
  ACETAMINOPHEN
PETHADOL, MEPERIDINE HYDROCHLORIDE
PHERAZINE DM, DEXTROMETHORPHAN
  HYDROBROMIDE
PHERAZINE VC, PHENYLEPHRINE HYDROCHLORIDE
PHERAZINE VC W/ CODEINE, CODEINE PHOSPHATE
PHERAZINE W/ CODEINE, CODEINE PHOSPHATE
PREDNISONE, PREDNISONE
PROPHENE 65, PROPOXYPHENE HYDROCHLORIDE
PROPOXYPHENE NAPSYLATE AND ACETAMINOPHEN,
  ACETAMINOPHEN
PROPYLTHIOURACIL, PROPYLTHIOURACIL
QUINIDINE GLUCONATE, QUINIDINE GLUCONATE
QUINIDINE SULFATE, QUINIDINE SULFATE
RAUWOLFIA SERPENTINA, RAUWOLFIA SERPENTINA
RESERPINE, RESERPINE
SARISOL, BUTABARBITAL SODIUM
SARISOL NO. 1, BUTABARBITAL SODIUM

APPENDIX B
PRODUCT NAME INDEX
LISTED BY APPLICANT (continued)

SARISOL NO. 2, BUTABARBITAL SODIUM
SODIUM PENTOBARBITAL, PENTOBARBITAL SODIUM
SODIUM SECOBARBITAL, SECOBARBITAL SODIUM
TETRACYCLINE HCL, TETRACYCLINE
 HYDROCHLORIDE
THEOPHYLLINE, THEOPHYLLINE
TRIPOSED, PSEUDOEPHEDRINE HYDROCHLORIDE
 (OTC)
TRIPROLIDINE HCL, TRIPROLIDINE
 HYDROCHLORIDE

HANFORD
* GC HANFORD MFG CO
 CEFAZOLIN SODIUM, CEFAZOLIN SODIUM

HASSLE
* AB HASSLE
 TOPROL XL, METOPROLOL SUCCINATE

HEATHER
* HEATHER DRUG CO INC
 CORTISONE ACETATE, CORTISONE ACETATE
 DIMENHYDRINATE, DIMENHYDRINATE
 DIPHENHYDRAMINE HCL, DIPHENHYDRAMINE
  HYDROCHLORIDE
 DIPHENOXYLATE HCL AND ATROPINE SULFATE,
  ATROPINE SULFATE
 DOXYCYCLINE HYCLATE, DOXYCYCLINE HYCLATE
 HYDROCHLOROTHIAZIDE, HYDROCHLOROTHIAZIDE
 MEPROBAMATE, MEPROBAMATE
 METHOCARBAMOL, METHOCARBAMOL
 METHYLPREDNISOLONE, METHYLPREDNISOLONE
 METHYLTESTOSTERONE, METHYLTESTOSTERONE
 PREDNISOLONE, PREDNISOLONE
 PREDNISONE, PREDNISONE
 PROPANTHELINE BROMIDE, PROPANTHELINE
  BROMIDE
 SULFAMETHOXAZOLE, SULFAMETHOXAZOLE
 SULFAMETHOXAZOLE & TRIMETHOPRIM,
  SULFAMETHOXAZOLE
 SULFISOXAZOLE, SULFISOXAZOLE
 TETRACYCLINE HCL, TETRACYCLINE
  HYDROCHLORIDE
 TRIPELENNAMINE HCL, TRIPELENNAMINE
  HYDROCHLORIDE

HERAN
* HERAN PHARMACEUTICAL INC
 GLYCORT, HYDROCORTISONE

HERBERT
* HERBERT LABORATORIES DIV SMITH KLINE AND
FRENCH CO
 AEROSEB-DEX, DEXAMETHASONE
 AEROSEB-HC, HYDROCORTISONE
 ERYGEL, ERYTHROMYCIN
 ERYMAX, ERYTHROMYCIN
 EXSEL, SELENIUM SULFIDE
 FLUONID, FLUOCINOLONE ACETONIDE
 FLUOROPLEX, FLUOROURACIL
 GRIS-PEG, GRISEOFULVIN,
  ULTRAMICROCRYSTALLINE
 NAFTIN, NAFTIFINE HYDROCHLORIDE
 PENECORT, HYDROCORTISONE
 PHOTOPLEX, AVOBENZONE (OTC)
 TEMARIL, TRIMEPRAZINE TARTRATE

HERMAL
* HERMAL PHARMACEUTICAL LABORATORIES INC
 AKNE-MYCIN, ERYTHROMYCIN
 CLODERM, CLOCORTOLONE PIVALATE

HEXCEL
* HEXCEL CHEMICAL PRODUCTS
 POTASSIUM AMINOSALICYLATE, POTASSIUM
  AMINOSALICYLATE
 SODIUM AMINOSALICYLATE, AMINOSALICYLATE
  SODIUM

HI TECH
* HI TECH PHARMACAL CO INC
 DIPHENHYDRAMINE HCL, DIPHENHYDRAMINE
  HYDROCHLORIDE (OTC)

HILL DERMAC
* HILL DERMACEUTICALS INC
 DERMA-SMOOTHE/FS, FLUOCINOLONE ACETONIDE
 FS SHAMPOO, FLUOCINOLONE ACETONIDE

HIRSCH
* HIRSCH INDUSTRIES INC
 LYMPHAZURIN, ISOSULFAN BLUE

HOECHST ROUSSEL
* HOECHST ROUSSEL PHARMACEUTICALS INC
 A/T/S, ERYTHROMYCIN
 ALTACE, RAMIPRIL
 CLAFORAN, CEFOTAXIME SODIUM
 CLAFORAN IN DEXTROSE 5%, CEFOTAXIME SODIUM
 CLAFORAN IN SODIUM CHLORIDE 0.9%, CEFOTAXIME
  SODIUM
 DERMATOP, PREDNICARBATE
 DIABETA, GLYBURIDE
 GLUBATE, GLYBURIDE
 LASIX, FUROSEMIDE
 LOPROX, CICLOPIROX OLAMINE
 TOPICORT, DESOXIMETASONE
 TOPICORT LP, DESOXIMETASONE
 TRENTAL, PENTOXIFYLLINE

HOLLAND RANTOS
* HOLLAND RANTOS CO INC
 KOROSTATIN, NYSTATIN

HORUS
* HORUS THERAPEUTICS INC
 THALITONE, CHLORTHALIDONE

HOYT
* HOYT LABORATORIES DIV COLGATE PALMOLIVE CO
 ORABASE HCA, HYDROCORTISONE ACETATE

HUNTINGTON
* HUNTINGTON LABORATORIES INC
 CHG SCRUB, CHLORHEXIDINE GLUCONATE (OTC)
 CIDA-STAT, CHLORHEXIDINE GLUCONATE (OTC)
 GERMA-MEDICA, HEXACHLOROPHENE
 GERMA-MEDICA "MG", HEXACHLOROPHENE
 HEXA-GERM, HEXACHLOROPHENE

I

IBI
* ISTITUTO BIOCHIMICO ITALIANO GIOVANNI
LORENZINI
 AMPICILLIN SODIUM, AMPICILLIN SODIUM

ICI
* ICI AMERICAS INC
 DIPRIVAN, PROPOFOL
* ICI PHARMA
 TENORETIC 100, ATENOLOL
 TENORETIC 50, ATENOLOL

APPENDIX B
PRODUCT NAME INDEX
LISTED BY APPLICANT (continued)

* ICI PHARMACEUTICALS GROUP DIV ICI AMERICAS
   TENORMIN, ATENOLOL

ICN
* ICN PHARMACEUTICALS INC
   AMINOPHYLLINE, AMINOPHYLLINE
   ANDROID 10, METHYLTESTOSTERONE
   ANDROID 25, METHYLTESTOSTERONE
   ANDROID 5, METHYLTESTOSTERONE
   ANDROID-F, FLUOXYMESTERONE
   BENDOPA, LEVODOPA
   BENOQUIN, MONOBENZONE
   CHLORPHENIRAMINE MALEATE,
     CHLORPHENIRAMINE MALEATE
   CODEINE PHOSPHATE AND ACETAMINOPHEN,
     ACETAMINOPHEN
   DIPHENHYDRAMINE HCL, DIPHENHYDRAMINE
     HYDROCHLORIDE
   DIPHENOXYLATE HCL W/ ATROPINE SULFATE,
     ATROPINE SULFATE
   FLUOXYMESTERONE, FLUOXYMESTERONE
   FOLIC ACID, FOLIC ACID
   MEPROBAMATE, MEPROBAMATE
   MESTINON, PYRIDOSTIGMINE BROMIDE
   OXSORALEN, METHOXSALEN
   OXSORALEN-ULTRA, METHOXSALEN
   PREDNISOLONE, PREDNISOLONE
   PREDNISONE, PREDNISONE
   PROPOXYPHENE HCL, PROPOXYPHENE
     HYDROCHLORIDE
   QUINIDINE SULFATE, QUINIDINE SULFATE
   RAUWOLFIA SERPENTINA, RAUWOLFIA SERPENTINA
   RESERPINE, RESERPINE
   SECOBARBITAL SODIUM, SECOBARBITAL SODIUM
   SODIUM PENTOBARBITAL, PENTOBARBITAL SODIUM
   SULFISOXAZOLE, SULFISOXAZOLE
   TESTRED, METHYLTESTOSTERONE
   TETRACYCLINE HCL, TETRACYCLINE
     HYDROCHLORIDE
   8-MOP, METHOXSALEN

IMP
* IMP INC
   SPECTAMINE, IOFETAMINE HYDROCHLORIDE I-123

IMPERIAL CHEM
* IMPERIAL CHEMICAL INDUSTRIES PLC
   ZESTORETIC 20/12.5, HYDROCHLOROTHIAZIDE
   ZESTORETIC 20/25, HYDROCHLOROTHIAZIDE
   ZESTRIL, LISINOPRIL
   ZOLADEX, GOSERELIN ACETATE

INGRAM
* INGRAM PHARMACEUTICAL CO
   DRICORT, HYDROCORTISONE ACETATE
   HYDROCORTISONE, HYDROCORTISONE

INTERPHARM
* INTERPHARM INC
   CLONIDINE HCL, CLONIDINE HYDROCHLORIDE
   DISOPYRAMIDE PHOSPHATE, DISOPYRAMIDE
     PHOSPHATE
   DOXYCYCLINE HYCLATE, DOXYCYCLINE HYCLATE
   IBUPROFEN, IBUPROFEN
   IBUPROFEN, IBUPROFEN (OTC)
   METOCLOPRAMIDE HCL, METOCLOPRAMIDE
     HYDROCHLORIDE
   PREDNISONE, PREDNISONE
   PROPRANOLOL HCL, PROPRANOLOL
     HYDROCHLORIDE
   SULFAMETHOXAZOLE AND TRIMETHOPRIM,
     SULFAMETHOXAZOLE

   TOLAZAMIDE, TOLAZAMIDE

INTL MEDICATION
* INTERNATIONAL MEDICATION SYSTEMS LTD
   AMINOPHYLLINE, AMINOPHYLLINE
   AMPICILLIN SODIUM, AMPICILLIN SODIUM
   BRETYLIUM TOSYLATE, BRETYLIUM TOSYLATE
   CEPHALOTHIN, CEPHALOTHIN SODIUM
   DEXAMETHASONE SODIUM PHOSPHATE,
     DEXAMETHASONE SODIUM PHOSPHATE
   DIATRIZOATE-60, DIATRIZOATE MEGLUMINE
   DIPHENHYDRAMINE HCL, DIPHENHYDRAMINE
     HYDROCHLORIDE
   DOPAMINE HCL, DOPAMINE HYDROCHLORIDE
   FUROSEMIDE, FUROSEMIDE
   GENTAMICIN, GENTAMICIN SULFATE
   HEPARIN LOCK FLUSH, HEPARIN SODIUM
   HYDROCORTISONE SODIUM SUCCINATE,
     HYDROCORTISONE SODIUM SUCCINATE
   ISOETHARINE HCL, ISOETHARINE HYDROCHLORIDE
   ISOPROTERENOL HCL, ISOPROTERENOL
     HYDROCHLORIDE
   KANAMYCIN SULFATE, KANAMYCIN SULFATE
   LARYNG-O-JET KIT, LIDOCAINE HYDROCHLORIDE
   LIDOCAINE HCL, LIDOCAINE HYDROCHLORIDE
   LIDOCAINE HCL VISCOUS, LIDOCAINE
     HYDROCHLORIDE
   LIDOCAINE HCL W/ EPINEPHRINE, EPINEPHRINE
   MANNITOL 25%, MANNITOL
   MEPERIDINE HCL, MEPERIDINE HYDROCHLORIDE
   MEPIVACAINE HCL, MEPIVACAINE HYDROCHLORIDE
   METHYLPREDNISOLONE SODIUM SUCCINATE,
     METHYLPREDNISOLONE SODIUM SUCCINATE
   METRONIDAZOLE, METRONIDAZOLE
   NALOXONE HCL, NALOXONE HYDROCHLORIDE
   NITROGLYCERIN, NITROGLYCERIN
   PHYTONADIONE, PHYTONADIONE
   POTASSIUM CHLORIDE, POTASSIUM CHLORIDE
   PROCAINAMIDE HCL, PROCAINAMIDE
     HYDROCHLORIDE
   SUCCINYLCHOLINE CHLORIDE, SUCCINYLCHOLINE
     CHLORIDE
   VERAPAMIL HCL, VERAPAMIL HYDROCHLORIDE

INVAMED
* INVAMED INC
   AMANTADINE HCL, AMANTADINE HYDROCHLORIDE
   BENZTROPINE MESYLATE, BENZTROPINE MESYLATE
   FOAMICON, ALUMINUM HYDROXIDE (OTC)
   IBUPROFEN, IBUPROFEN
   IBUPROFEN, IBUPROFEN (OTC)
   METHYLDOPA AND HYDROCHLOROTHIAZIDE,
     HYDROCHLOROTHIAZIDE
   METOCLOPRAMIDE HCL, METOCLOPRAMIDE
     HYDROCHLORIDE
   PROCAINAMIDE HCL, PROCAINAMIDE
     HYDROCHLORIDE
   PROPRANOLOL HCL, PROPRANOLOL
     HYDROCHLORIDE

INWOOD
* INWOOD LABORATORIES INC SUB FOREST
LABORATORIES INC
   CARBAMAZEPINE, CARBAMAZEPINE
   CORTISONE ACETATE, CORTISONE ACETATE
   DIPHENOXYLATE HCL AND ATROPINE SULFATE,
     ATROPINE SULFATE
   HYDROCHLOROTHIAZIDE, HYDROCHLOROTHIAZIDE
   HYDROCORTISONE, HYDROCORTISONE
   INDOMETHACIN, INDOMETHACIN
   METHOCARBAMOL, METHOCARBAMOL

APPENDIX B
PRODUCT NAME INDEX
LISTED BY APPLICANT (continued)

METHYLTESTOSTERONE, METHYLTESTOSTERONE
PHENDIMETRAZINE TARTRATE, PHENDIMETRAZINE TARTRATE
PREDNISOLONE, PREDNISOLONE
PREDNISONE, PREDNISONE
PROCAINAMIDE HCL, PROCAINAMIDE HYDROCHLORIDE
PROPRANOLOL HCL, PROPRANOLOL HYDROCHLORIDE
THEOCHRON, THEOPHYLLINE

IOLAB
* IOLAB PHARMACEUTICALS SUB JOHNSON AND JOHNSON CO
CATARASE, CHYMOTRYPSIN
DEXACIDIN, DEXAMETHASONE
FLUOR-OP, FLUOROMETHOLONE
FUNDUSCEIN-25, FLUORESCEIN SODIUM
GENTACIDIN, GENTAMICIN SULFATE
INFLAMASE FORTE, PREDNISOLONE SODIUM PHOSPHATE
INFLAMASE MILD, PREDNISOLONE SODIUM PHOSPHATE
MIOCHOL, ACETYLCHOLINE CHLORIDE
SULF-10, SULFACETAMIDE SODIUM
VASOCIDIN, PREDNISOLONE ACETATE
VASOCIDIN, PREDNISOLONE SODIUM PHOSPHATE
VASOCON, NAPHAZOLINE HYDROCHLORIDE
VASOCON-A, ANTAZOLINE PHOSPHATE

IPHARM
* IPHARM DIV LYPHOMED INC
NEOMYCIN AND POLYMYXIN B SULFATES AND GRAMICIDIN, GRAMICIDIN

IPR
* IPR PHARMACEUTICALS INC
ATENOLOL, ATENOLOL
ATENOLOL AND CHLORTHALIDONE, ATENOLOL

ISO TEX
* ISO TEX DIAGNOSTICS INC
ALBUMOTOPE 125 I, ALBUMIN IODINATED I-125 SERUM
CHROMALBIN, ALBUMIN CHROMATED CR-51 SERUM
GLOFIL-125, IOTHALAMATE SODIUM, I-125
INULIN AND SODIUM CHLORIDE, INULIN MEGATOPE, ALBUMIN IODINATED I-131 SERUM

J

JACOBUS
* JACOBUS PHARMACEUTICAL CO
DAPSONE, DAPSONE

JANSSEN
* JANSSEN PHARMACEUTICA INC
ALFENTA, ALFENTANIL HYDROCHLORIDE
HISMANAL, ASTEMIZOLE
IMODIUM, LOPERAMIDE HYDROCHLORIDE
INAPSINE, DROPERIDOL
INNOVAR, DROPERIDOL
MONISTAT, MICONAZOLE
NIZORAL, KETOCONAZOLE
SUBLIMAZE, FENTANYL CITRATE
SUFENTA, SUFENTANIL CITRATE
* JANSSEN RESEARCH FOUNDATION DIV JOHNSON AND JOHNSON
ERGAMISOL, LEVAMISOLE HYDROCHLORIDE
NIZORAL, KETOCONAZOLE
VERMOX, MEBENDAZOLE

JOHNSON AND JOHNSON
* JOHNSON AND JOHNSON MEDICAL INC
MICROCOL, CHLORHEXIDINE GLUCONATE (OTC)
MICRODERM, CHLORHEXIDINE GLUCONATE (OTC)

JOHNSON RW
* RW JOHNSON PHARMACEUTICAL RESEARCH INSTITUTE DIV MCNEILAB
CLISTIN, CARBINOXAMINE MALEATE
HALDOL, HALOPERIDOL
HALDOL, HALOPERIDOL LACTATE
HALDOL DECANOATE 50, HALOPERIDOL DECANOATE
HALDOL SOLUTAB, HALOPERIDOL
INJECTAPAP, ACETAMINOPHEN
PARAFLEX, CHLORZOXAZONE
PARAFON FORTE DSC, CHLORZOXAZONE
SUPROL, SUPROFEN
THEOPHYL, THEOPHYLLINE
THEOPHYL-SR, THEOPHYLLINE
THEOPHYL-225, THEOPHYLLINE
TOLECTIN, TOLMETIN SODIUM
TOLECTIN DS, TOLMETIN SODIUM
TOLECTIN 600, TOLMETIN SODIUM
TYCOLET, ACETAMINOPHEN
TYLENOL W/ CODEINE, ACETAMINOPHEN
TYLENOL W/ CODEINE NO. 1, ACETAMINOPHEN
TYLENOL W/ CODEINE NO. 2, ACETAMINOPHEN
TYLENOL W/ CODEINE NO. 3, ACETAMINOPHEN
TYLENOL W/ CODEINE NO. 4, ACETAMINOPHEN
TYLOX, ACETAMINOPHEN
TYLOX-325, ACETAMINOPHEN
VASCOR, BEPRIDIL HYDROCHLORIDE
* RW JOHNSON PHARMACEUTICAL RESEARCH INSTITUTE DIV ORTHO PHA
DIENESTROL, DIENESTROL
ERYCETTE, ERYTHROMYCIN
FLOXIN, OFLOXACIN
FLOXIN IN DEXTROSE 5%, OFLOXACIN
GRIFULVIN V, GRISEOFULVIN, MICROCRYSTALLINE
MECLAN, MECLOCYCLINE SULFOSALICYLATE
MICRONOR, NORETHINDRONE
MODICON 21, ETHINYL ESTRADIOL
MODICON 28, ETHINYL ESTRADIOL
MONISTAT 3, MICONAZOLE NITRATE
MONISTAT 5, MICONAZOLE NITRATE
MONISTAT 7, MICONAZOLE NITRATE
MONISTAT 7, MICONAZOLE NITRATE (OTC)
MONISTAT-DERM, MICONAZOLE NITRATE
ORTHO CYCLEN-21, ETHINYL ESTRADIOL
ORTHO CYCLEN-28, ETHINYL ESTRADIOL
ORTHO TRI-CYCLEN, ETHINYL ESTRADIOL
ORTHO-EST, ESTROPIPATE
ORTHO-NOVUM 1/35-21, ETHINYL ESTRADIOL
ORTHO-NOVUM 1/35-28, ETHINYL ESTRADIOL
ORTHO-NOVUM 1/50 21, MESTRANOL
ORTHO-NOVUM 1/50 28, MESTRANOL
ORTHO-NOVUM 1/80 21, MESTRANOL
ORTHO-NOVUM 10-21, MESTRANOL
ORTHO-NOVUM 10/11-21, ETHINYL ESTRADIOL
ORTHO-NOVUM 10/11-28, ETHINYL ESTRADIOL
ORTHO-NOVUM 2-21, MESTRANOL
ORTHO-NOVUM 7/14-21, ETHINYL ESTRADIOL
ORTHO-NOVUM 7/14-28, ETHINYL ESTRADIOL
ORTHO-NOVUM 7/7/7-21, ETHINYL ESTRADIOL
ORTHO-NOVUM 7/7/7-28, ETHINYL ESTRADIOL
ORTHO-NOVUM 1/80 28, MESTRANOL
PROTOSTAT, METRONIDAZOLE
RETIN-A, TRETINOIN
SALPIX, ACETRIZOATE SODIUM
SPECTAZOLE, ECONAZOLE NITRATE

APPENDIX B
PRODUCT NAME INDEX
LISTED BY APPLICANT (continued)

SULTRIN, TRIPLE SULFA
  (SULFABENZAMIDE; SULFACETAMIDE; SULFATHIAZOLE)
  SUPPRELIN, HISTRELIN ACETATE
  TERAZOL 3, TERCONAZOLE
  TERAZOL 7, TERCONAZOLE

K

KABI
* KABI PHARMACIA INC
  AZULFIDINE, SULFASALAZINE
  AZULFIDINE EN-TABS, SULFASALAZINE
  CALMURID HC, HYDROCORTISONE
  DIPENTUM, OLSALAZINE SODIUM
  EMCYT, ESTRAMUSTINE PHOSPHATE SODIUM
  NICOTROL, NICOTINE

KABIVITRUM
* KABIVITRUM INC
  AMINESS 5.2% ESSENTIAL AMINO ACIDS W/
    HISTADINE, AMINO ACIDS
  CYKLOKAPRON, TRANEXAMIC ACID
  CYSTEINE HCL, CYSTEINE HYDROCHLORIDE
  INTRALIPID 10%, SOYBEAN OIL
  INTRALIPID 20%, SOYBEAN OIL
  NEOPHAM 6.4%, AMINO ACIDS
  NOVAMINE 11.4%, AMINO ACIDS
  NOVAMINE 15%, AMINO ACIDS
  NOVAMINE 8.5%, AMINO ACIDS
  R-GENE 10, ARGININE HYDROCHLORIDE
  VEINAMINE 8%, AMINO ACIDS

KALAPHARM
* KALAPHARM INC
  FUROSEMIDE, FUROSEMIDE
  GENTAMICIN SULFATE, GENTAMICIN SULFATE

KALI DUPHAR
* KALI DUPHAR INC
  ATROPINE, ATROPINE
  PYRIDOSTIGMINE BROMIDE, PYRIDOSTIGMINE
    BROMIDE

KENDALL
* KENDALL CO
  CHLORHEXIDINE GLUCONATE, CHLORHEXIDINE
    GLUCONATE (OTC)
  LARYNGOTRACHEAL ANESTHESIA KIT, LIDOCAINE
    HYDROCHLORIDE

KEY PHARMS
* KEY PHARMACEUTICALS INC SUB SCHERING PLOUGH
CORP
  ACTICORT, HYDROCORTISONE
  GENAPAX, GENTIAN VIOLET
  GUANIDINE HCL, GUANIDINE HYDROCHLORIDE
  QUINORA, QUINIDINE SULFATE
  THEO-DUR, THEOPHYLLINE
  TYZINE, TETRAHYDROZOLINE HYDROCHLORIDE

KNOLL
* KNOLL PHARMACEUTICAL CO UNIT BASF K AND CORP
  AKINETON, BIPERIDEN HYDROCHLORIDE
  AKINETON, BIPERIDEN LACTATE
  DILAUDID-HP, HYDROMORPHONE HYDROCHLORIDE
  ISOPTIN, VERAPAMIL HYDROCHLORIDE
  ISOPTIN SR, VERAPAMIL HYDROCHLORIDE
  MEPERIDINE HCL, MEPERIDINE HYDROCHLORIDE
  PROMETHAZINE HCL, PROMETHAZINE
    HYDROCHLORIDE

RYTHMOL, PROPAFENONE HYDROCHLORIDE
VICODIN, ACETAMINOPHEN
VICODIN ES, ACETAMINOPHEN
VICOPRIN, ASPIRIN

KV
* KV PHARMACEUTICAL CO
  ACETAMINOPHEN AND CODEINE PHOSPHATE,
    ACETAMINOPHEN
  ACETIC ACID, ACETIC ACID, GLACIAL
  ACETIC ACID W/ HYDROCORTISONE, ACETIC ACID,
    GLACIAL
  AMINOPHYLLINE, AMINOPHYLLINE
  BROMPHENIRAMINE MALEATE, BROMPHENIRAMINE
    MALEATE
  CHLORPHENIRAMINE MALEATE,
    CHLORPHENIRAMINE MALEATE
  CHLORPROMAZINE HCL, CHLORPROMAZINE
    HYDROCHLORIDE
  CHLORTHALIDONE, CHLORTHALIDONE
  CYPROHEPTADINE HCL, CYPROHEPTADINE
    HYDROCHLORIDE
  DIPHENHYDRAMINE HCL, DIPHENHYDRAMINE
    HYDROCHLORIDE
  DIPHENOXYLATE HCL W/ ATROPINE SULFATE,
    ATROPINE SULFATE
  DISOPYRAMIDE PHOSPHATE, DISOPYRAMIDE
    PHOSPHATE
  ERGOLOID MESYLATES, ERGOLOID MESYLATES
  ERYTHROMYCIN ETHYLSUCCINATE, ERYTHROMYCIN
    ETHYLSUCCINATE
  HYDROXYZINE HCL, HYDROXYZINE
    HYDROCHLORIDE
  MECLIZINE HCL, MECLIZINE HYDROCHLORIDE
  METHOCARBAMOL, METHOCARBAMOL
  METHYLTESTOSTERONE, METHYLTESTOSTERONE
  PHENDIMETRAZINE TARTRATE, PHENDIMETRAZINE
    TARTRATE
  POTASSIUM CHLORIDE, POTASSIUM CHLORIDE
  PREDNISONE, PREDNISONE
  PROMETHAZINE HCL, PROMETHAZINE
    HYDROCHLORIDE
  PSEUDOEPHEDRINE HCL AND CHLORPHENIRAMINE
    MALEATE, CHLORPHENIRAMINE MALEATE (OTC)
  QUINIDINE SULFATE, QUINIDINE SULFATE
  SODIUM SECOBARBITAL, SECOBARBITAL SODIUM
  THEOPHYLLINE, THEOPHYLLINE
  TRIPROLIDINE AND PSEUDOEPHEDRINE HCL,
    PSEUDOEPHEDRINE HYDROCHLORIDE (OTC)
  TRIPROLIDINE AND PSEUDOEPHRINE HCL,
    PSEUDOEPHEDRINE HYDROCHLORIDE (OTC)

L

LANNETT
* LANNETT CO INC
  ACETAZOLAMIDE, ACETAZOLAMIDE
  AMINOPHYLLINE, AMINOPHYLLINE
  AMPHETAMINE SULFATE, AMPHETAMINE SULFATE
  BENZYL BENZOATE, BENZYL BENZOATE
  BETHANECHOL CHLORIDE, BETHANECHOL CHLORIDE
  BUTALAN, BUTABARBITAL SODIUM
  CORTISONE ACETATE, CORTISONE ACETATE
  DEXTROAMPHETAMINE SULFATE,
    DEXTROAMPHETAMINE SULFATE
  DIPHENHYDRAMINE HCL, DIPHENHYDRAMINE
    HYDROCHLORIDE
  DIPHENYLAN SODIUM, PHENYTOIN SODIUM, PROMPT
  FOLIC ACID, FOLIC ACID

APPENDIX B
PRODUCT NAME INDEX
LISTED BY APPLICANT *(continued)*

FURALAN, NITROFURANTOIN
GLUTETHIMIDE, GLUTETHIMIDE
HYDROCORTISONE, HYDROCORTISONE
LANIAZID, ISONIAZID
LANOPHYLLIN, THEOPHYLLINE
LANORINAL, ASPIRIN
LANTRISUL, TRISULFAPYRIMIDINES
LOFENE, ATROPINE SULFATE
MEPROBAMATE, MEPROBAMATE
METHOCARBAMOL, METHOCARBAMOL
METHYLTESTOSTERONE, METHYLTESTOSTERONE
NEOMYCIN SULFATE, NEOMYCIN SULFATE
NITROFURAZONE, NITROFURAZONE
PENTOBARBITAL SODIUM, PENTOBARBITAL SODIUM
PHENETRON, CHLORPHENIRAMINE MALEATE
PHENTERMINE HCL, PHENTERMINE
   HYDROCHLORIDE
PIPERAZINE CITRATE, PIPERAZINE CITRATE
PREDNISOLONE, PREDNISOLONE
PREDNISONE, PREDNISONE
PRIMIDONE, PRIMIDONE
PROBALAN, PROBENECID
PROCAINAMIDE HCL, PROCAINAMIDE
   HYDROCHLORIDE
PROMETHAZINE HCL, PROMETHAZINE
   HYDROCHLORIDE
PROPYLTHIOURACIL, PROPYLTHIOURACIL
QUINALAN, QUINIDINE GLUCONATE
QUINIDINE SULFATE, QUINIDINE SULFATE
SECOBARBITAL SODIUM, SECOBARBITAL SODIUM
SERPALAN, RESERPINE
SODIUM BUTABARBITAL, BUTABARBITAL SODIUM
SODIUM P.A.S., AMINOSALICYLATE SODIUM
SULFADIAZINE, SULFADIAZINE
SULFISOXAZOLE, SULFISOXAZOLE
TRICHLOREX, TRICHLORMETHIAZIDE
TRIPELENNAMINE HCL, TRIPELENNAMINE
   HYDROCHLORIDE
VELTANE, BROMPHENIRAMINE MALEATE
VITAMIN D, ERGOCALCIFEROL

LEDERLE
* LEDERLE LABORATORIES DIV AMERICAN CYANAMID
CO
ACETAMINOPHEN W/ CODEINE, ACETAMINOPHEN
ACHES-N-PAIN, IBUPROFEN (OTC)
ACHROMYCIN, HYDROCORTISONE
ACHROMYCIN, PROCAINE HYDROCHLORIDE
ACHROMYCIN, TETRACYCLINE HYDROCHLORIDE
ACHROMYCIN V, TETRACYCLINE
ACHROMYCIN V, TETRACYCLINE HYDROCHLORIDE
ALBUTEROL SULFATE, ALBUTEROL SULFATE
AMICAR, AMINOCAPROIC ACID
AMITRIPTYLINE HCL, AMITRIPTYLINE
   HYDROCHLORIDE
AMPICILLIN, AMPICILLIN/AMPICILLIN TRIHYDRATE
ARISTOCORT, TRIAMCINOLONE
ARISTOCORT, TRIAMCINOLONE ACETONIDE
ARISTOCORT, TRIAMCINOLONE DIACETATE
ARISTOCORT A, TRIAMCINOLONE ACETONIDE
ARISTOGEL, TRIAMCINOLONE ACETONIDE
ARISTOSPAN, TRIAMCINOLONE HEXACETONIDE
ARTANE, TRIHEXYPHENIDYL HYDROCHLORIDE
ASENDIN, AMOXAPINE
ATENOLOL, ATENOLOL
AUREOMYCIN, CHLORTETRACYCLINE
   HYDROCHLORIDE
CHLORDIAZEPOXIDE HCL, CHLORDIAZEPOXIDE
   HYDROCHLORIDE
CHLOROTHIAZIDE, CHLOROTHIAZIDE
CHLORPHENIRAMINE MALEATE,
   CHLORPHENIRAMINE MALEATE

CHLORPROMAZINE HCL, CHLORPROMAZINE
   HYDROCHLORIDE
CHLORPROPAMIDE, CHLORPROPAMIDE
CHLORTHALIDONE, CHLORTHALIDONE
CLONIDINE HCL, CLONIDINE HYDROCHLORIDE
CLORAZEPATE DIPOTASSIUM, CLORAZEPATE
   DIPOTASSIUM
CYCLOCORT, AMCINONIDE
DECLOMYCIN, DEMECLOCYCLINE HYDROCHLORIDE
DIAMOX, ACETAZOLAMIDE
DIAMOX, ACETAZOLAMIDE SODIUM
DIAZEPAM, DIAZEPAM
DIPHENHYDRAMINE HCL, DIPHENHYDRAMINE
   HYDROCHLORIDE
DIPHENOXYLATE HCL AND ATROPINE SULFATE,
   ATROPINE SULFATE
DIPYRIDAMOLE, DIPYRIDAMOLE
DOLENE, PROPOXYPHENE HYDROCHLORIDE
DOLENE AP-65, ACETAMINOPHEN
DOXEPIN HCL, DOXEPIN HYDROCHLORIDE
ERGOLOID MESYLATES, ERGOLOID MESYLATES
ERYTHROMYCIN STEARATE, ERYTHROMYCIN
   STEARATE
FENOPROFEN CALCIUM, FENOPROFEN CALCIUM
FOLVITE, FOLIC ACID
FOLVRON, FERROUS SULFATE
FUROSEMIDE, FUROSEMIDE
HALOPERIDOL, HALOPERIDOL
HETRAZAN, DIETHYLCARBAMAZINE CITRATE
HYDRALAZINE HCL, HYDRALAZINE
   HYDROCHLORIDE
HYDROCHLOROTHIAZIDE, HYDROCHLOROTHIAZIDE
HYDROMOX, QUINETHAZONE
HYDROMOX R, QUINETHAZONE
IBUPROFEN, IBUPROFEN
IMIPRAMINE HCL, IMIPRAMINE HYDROCHLORIDE
INDOMETHACIN, INDOMETHACIN
LEDERCILLIN VK, PENICILLIN V POTASSIUM
LEUCOVORIN CALCIUM, LEUCOVORIN CALCIUM
LEVOPROME, METHOTRIMEPRAZINE
LOXITANE, LOXAPINE SUCCINATE
LOXITANE C, LOXAPINE HYDROCHLORIDE
LOXITANE IM, LOXAPINE HYDROCHLORIDE
MEPROBAMATE, MEPROBAMATE
METHOCARBAMOL, METHOCARBAMOL
METHOTREXATE, METHOTREXATE SODIUM
METHOTREXATE LPF, METHOTREXATE SODIUM
METHYLDOPA, METHYLDOPA
METHYLDOPA AND HYDROCHLOROTHIAZIDE,
   HYDROCHLOROTHIAZIDE
METOCLOPRAMIDE HCL, METOCLOPRAMIDE
   HYDROCHLORIDE
MINOCIN, MINOCYCLINE HYDROCHLORIDE
MYAMBUTOL, ETHAMBUTOL HYDROCHLORIDE
NEPTAZANE, METHAZOLAMIDE
NILSTAT, NYSTATIN
NOVANTRONE, MITOXANTRONE HYDROCHLORIDE
PATHILON, TRIDIHEXETHYL CHLORIDE
PIPRACIL, PIPERACILLIN SODIUM
PRAZOSIN HCL, PRAZOSIN HYDROCHLORIDE
PREDNISONE, PREDNISONE
PROBENECID, PROBENECID
PROBENECID W/ COLCHICINE, COLCHICINE
PROCAINAMIDE HCL, PROCAINAMIDE
   HYDROCHLORIDE
PROPRANOLOL HCL, PROPRANOLOL
   HYDROCHLORIDE
PROPYLTHIOURACIL, PROPYLTHIOURACIL
PYRAZINAMIDE, PYRAZINAMIDE
QUINIDINE SULFATE, QUINIDINE SULFATE

APPENDIX B
PRODUCT NAME INDEX
LISTED BY APPLICANT (continued)

RESERPINE, HYDROCHLOROTHIAZIDE, AND
  HYDRALAZINE HCL, HYDRALAZINE
  HYDROCHLORIDE
SERVISONE, PREDNISONE
SPIRONOLACTONE, SPIRONOLACTONE
SPIRONOLACTONE W/ HYDROCHLOROTHIAZIDE,
  HYDROCHLOROTHIAZIDE
SULFADIAZINE, SULFADIAZINE
SULFADIAZINE SODIUM, SULFADIAZINE SODIUM
SULFASALAZINE, SULFASALAZINE
SULFISOXAZOLE, SULFISOXAZOLE
SULINDAC, SULINDAC
SUPRAX, CEFIXIME
THIO-TEPA, THIOTEPA
TOLBUTAMIDE, TOLBUTAMIDE
TRIPLE SULFAS, TRISULFAPYRIMIDINES
VANCOLED, VANCOMYCIN HYDROCHLORIDE
VERAPAMIL HCL, VERAPAMIL HYDROCHLORIDE
ZEBETA, BISOPROLOL FUMARATE
* LEDERLE PARENTERALS INC
  CLINDAMYCIN PHOSPHATE, CLINDAMYCIN
    PHOSPHATE
  DOXYCYCLINE HYCLATE, DOXYCYCLINE HYCLATE
  ERYTHROMYCIN LACTOBIONATE, ERYTHROMYCIN
    LACTOBIONATE
  FUROSEMIDE, FUROSEMIDE
  TOBRAMYCIN SULFATE, TOBRAMYCIN SULFATE
* LEDERLE PIPERACILLIN INC
  PIPRACIL, PIPERACILLIN SODIUM

LEE LABS
* KM LEE LABORATORIES
  MEPROBAMATE, MEPROBAMATE

LEMMON
* LEMMON CO
  ACETAMINOPHEN W/ CODEINE #2, ACETAMINOPHEN
  ACETAMINOPHEN W/ CODEINE #3, ACETAMINOPHEN
  ACETAMINOPHEN W/ CODEINE #4, ACETAMINOPHEN
  ADIPEX-P, PHENTERMINE HYDROCHLORIDE
  ALBUTEROL SULFATE, ALBUTEROL SULFATE
  AMITRIPTYLINE HCL, AMITRIPTYLINE
    HYDROCHLORIDE
  AMOXICILLIN, AMOXICILLIN
  BETA-VAL, BETAMETHASONE VALERATE
  BETAMETHASONE DIPROPIONATE, BETAMETHASONE
    DIPROPIONATE
  BUTABARBITAL SODIUM, BUTABARBITAL SODIUM
  CARBIDOPA AND LEVODOPA, CARBIDOPA
  CEFAZOLIN SODIUM, CEFAZOLIN SODIUM
  CEPHALEXIN, CEPHALEXIN
  CHLORDIAZEPOXIDE HCL, CHLORDIAZEPOXIDE
    HYDROCHLORIDE
  CHLORPROPAMIDE, CHLORPROPAMIDE
  CHLORTHALIDONE, CHLORTHALIDONE
  CHLORZOXAZONE, CHLORZOXAZONE
  CLEMASTINE FUMARATE, CLEMASTINE FUMARATE
  CLINDAMYCIN PHOSPHATE, CLINDAMYCIN
    PHOSPHATE
  COTRIM, SULFAMETHOXAZOLE
  COTRIM D.S., SULFAMETHOXAZOLE
  COTRIM PEDIATRIC, SULFAMETHOXAZOLE
  DELCOBESE, AMPHETAMINE ADIPATE
  DEXAMPEX, DEXTROAMPHETAMINE SULFATE
  DIETHYLPROPION HCL, DIETHYLPROPION
    HYDROCHLORIDE
  DIFLUNISAL, DIFLUNISAL
  DIPHENHYDRAMINE HCL, DIPHENHYDRAMINE
    HYDROCHLORIDE
  DOXY-LEMMON, DOXYCYCLINE HYCLATE

DRALZINE, HYDRALAZINE HYDROCHLORIDE
EPITOL, CARBAMAZEPINE
FLUOCINONIDE, FLUOCINONIDE
GLUCAMIDE, CHLORPROPAMIDE
HALOPERIDOL, HALOPERIDOL LACTATE
HY-PAM "25", HYDROXYZINE PAMOATE
HYDROCHLOROTHIAZIDE, HYDROCHLOROTHIAZIDE
HYDROCORTISONE, HYDROCORTISONE
IBUPROFEN, IBUPROFEN
INDO-LEMMON, INDOMETHACIN
LOPERAMIDE HCL, LOPERAMIDE HYDROCHLORIDE
MEPRIAM, MEPROBAMATE
METHAMPEX, METHAMPHETAMINE
  HYDROCHLORIDE
METHAMPHETAMINE HCL, METHAMPHETAMINE
  HYDROCHLORIDE
METRYL, METRONIDAZOLE
METRYL 500, METRONIDAZOLE
MYCO-TRIACET II, NYSTATIN
NEOTHYLLINE, DYPHYLLINE
NYSTATIN, NYSTATIN
ORAP, PIMOZIDE
PHENTERMINE HCL, PHENTERMINE
  HYDROCHLORIDE
PREDNISOLONE, PREDNISOLONE
PREDNISONE, PREDNISONE
PROMETHAZINE HCL, PROMETHAZINE
  HYDROCHLORIDE
PROPACET 100, ACETAMINOPHEN
PROPOXYPHENE COMPOUND 65, ASPIRIN
PROPOXYPHENE HCL, PROPOXYPHENE
  HYDROCHLORIDE
PROPOXYPHENE NAPSYLATE AND ACETAMINOPHEN,
  ACETAMINOPHEN
PROPRANOLOL HCL, PROPRANOLOL
  HYDROCHLORIDE
RESERPINE, RESERPINE
STATOBEX, PHENDIMETRAZINE TARTRATE
STATOBEX-G, PHENDIMETRAZINE TARTRATE
SULFANILAMIDE, SULFANILAMIDE
SULINDAC, SULINDAC
THIOTHIXENE HCL, THIOTHIXENE HYDROCHLORIDE
TOLMETIN SODIUM, TOLMETIN SODIUM
TRAZODONE HCL, TRAZODONE HYDROCHLORIDE
TRIACET, TRIAMCINOLONE ACETONIDE
TRIAMCINOLONE, TRIAMCINOLONE
TRIPHED, PSEUDOEPHEDRINE HYDROCHLORIDE
VAGILIA, TRIPLE SULFA
  (SULFABENZAMIDE; SULFACETAMIDE; SULFATHIAZOLE)
  VITAMIN A SOLUBILIZED, VITAMIN A PALMITATE

LEO
* LEO PHARMACEUTICAL PRODUCTS LTD
  PINDAC, PINACIDIL

LIFE LABS
* LIFE LABORATORIES INC
  HISTAFED, PSEUDOEPHEDRINE HYDROCHLORIDE
  THEOPHYLLINE, THEOPHYLLINE

LILLY
* ELI LILLY AND CO
  AEROLONE, ISOPROTERENOL HYDROCHLORIDE
  ALPHALIN, VITAMIN A PALMITATE
  AMPICILLIN SODIUM, AMPICILLIN SODIUM
  ANHYDRON, CYCLOTHIAZIDE
  AVENTYL HCL, NORTRIPTYLINE HYDROCHLORIDE
  AXID, NIZATIDINE
  BACITRACIN, BACITRACIN
  BETALIN S, THIAMINE HYDROCHLORIDE
  BETALIN 12, CYANOCOBALAMIN

APPENDIX B
PRODUCT NAME INDEX
LISTED BY APPLICANT (continued)

BREVITAL SODIUM, METHOHEXITAL SODIUM
CALCIUM GLUCEPTATE, CALCIUM GLUCEPTATE
CAPASTAT SULFATE, CAPREOMYCIN SULFATE
CECLOR, CEFACLOR
CESAMET, NABILONE
CINOBAC, CINOXACIN
CORDRAN-N, FLURANDRENOLIDE
CRYSTODIGIN, DIGITOXIN
DARVOCET, ACETAMINOPHEN
DARVOCET-N 100, ACETAMINOPHEN
DARVOCET-N 50, ACETAMINOPHEN
DARVON-N, PROPOXYPHENE NAPSYLATE
DARVON-N W/ ASA, ASPIRIN
DECABID, INDECAINIDE HYDROCHLORIDE
DELTALIN, ERGOCALCIFEROL
DICUMAROL, DICUMAROL
DICURIN PROCAINE, PROCAINE MERETHOXYLLINE
DIETHYLSTILBESTROL, DIETHYLSTILBESTROL
DOBUTREX, DOBUTAMINE HYDROCHLORIDE
DOLOPHINE HCL, METHADONE HYDROCHLORIDE
DROLBAN, DROMOSTANOLONE PROPIONATE
DURACILLIN A.S., PENICILLIN G PROCAINE
ERYTHROMYCIN, ERYTHROMYCIN
FOLIC ACID, FOLIC ACID
GLUCAGON, GLUCAGON HYDROCHLORIDE
HALDRONE, PARAMETHASONE ACETATE
HEPARIN SODIUM, HEPARIN SODIUM
HEXA-BETALIN, PYRIDOXINE HYDROCHLORIDE
HISTALOG, BETAZOLE HYDROCHLORIDE
HISTAMINE PHOSPHATE, HISTAMINE PHOSPHATE
HUMATROPE, SOMATROPIN, BIOSYNTHETIC
HUMULIN BR, INSULIN BIOSYNTHETIC HUMAN (OTC)
HUMULIN L, INSULIN ZINC SUSP BIOSYNTHETIC HUMAN (OTC)
HUMULIN N, INSULIN SUSP ISOPHANE BIOSYNTHETIC HUMAN (OTC)
HUMULIN R, INSULIN BIOSYNTHETIC HUMAN (OTC)
HUMULIN U, INSULIN ZINC SUSP EXTENDED BIOSYNTHETIC HUMAN (OTC)
HUMULIN 50/50, INSULIN BIOSYNTHETIC HUMAN (OTC)
HUMULIN 70/30, INSULIN BIOSYNTHETIC HUMAN (OTC)
ILETIN I, INSULIN PORK
ILETIN II, INSULIN PURIFIED PORK
ILOSONE SULFA, ERYTHROMYCIN ESTOLATE
ISONIAZID, ISONIAZID
KAFOCIN, CEPHALOGLYCIN
KAPPADIONE, MENADIOL SODIUM DIPHOSPHATE
KEFLET, CEPHALEXIN
KEFLEX, CEPHALEXIN
KEFLIN, CEPHALOTHIN SODIUM
KEFTAB, CEPHALEXIN HYDROCHLORIDE
KEFUROX, CEFUROXIME SODIUM
KEFUROX IN PLASTIC CONTAINER, CEFUROXIME SODIUM
KEFZOL, CEFAZOLIN SODIUM
LENTE ILETIN II, INSULIN ZINC SUSP PURIFIED BEEF (OTC)
LENTE ILETIN II (PORK), INSULIN ZINC SUSP PURIFIED PORK (OTC
LORABID, LORACARBEF
MANDOL, CEFAMANDOLE NAFATE
MENADIONE, MENADIONE
METHADONE HCL, METHADONE HYDROCHLORIDE
METHYLTESTOSTERONE, METHYLTESTOSTERONE
METUBINE IODIDE, METOCURINE IODIDE
MOXAM, MOXALACTAM DISODIUM
NEBCIN, TOBRAMYCIN SULFATE

NEOMYCIN SULFATE, NEOMYCIN SULFATE
NEOTRIZINE, TRISULFAPYRIMIDINES
NPH ILETIN I (BEEF-PORK), INSULIN SUSP ISOPHANE BEEF/PORK (OTC)
NPH ILETIN II, INSULIN SUSP ISOPHANE PURIFIED BEEF (OTC)
NPH ILETIN II (PORK), INSULIN SUSP ISOPHANE PURIFIED PORK (OTC)
ONCOVIN, VINCRISTINE SULFATE
PAGITANE, CYCRIMINE HYDROCHLORIDE
PENICILLIN G POTASSIUM, PENICILLIN G POTASSIUM
PERMAX, PERGOLIDE MESYLATE
POTASSIUM CHLORIDE, POTASSIUM CHLORIDE
PROGESTERONE, PROGESTERONE
PROPYLTHIOURACIL, PROPYLTHIOURACIL
PROTAMINE SULFATE, PROTAMINE SULFATE
PROTAMINE ZINC AND ILETIN II, INSULIN SUSP PROTAMINE ZINC PURIFIED BEEF (OTC)
PROTAMINE ZINC AND ILETIN II (PORK), INSULIN SUSP PROTAMINE ZINC PURIFIED PORK (OTC)
PROTAMINE, ZINC & ILETIN I (BEEF-PORK), INSULIN SUSP PROTAMINE ZINC BEEF/PORK (OTC)
PROZAC, FLUOXETINE HYDROCHLORIDE
QUINIDINE GLUCONATE, QUINIDINE GLUCONATE
QUINIDINE SULFATE, QUINIDINE SULFATE
REGULAR ILETIN II, INSULIN PURIFIED BEEF (OTC)
REGULAR ILETIN II (PORK), INSULIN PURIFIED PORK (OTC)
SANDRIL, RESERPINE
SECONAL SODIUM, SECOBARBITAL SODIUM
SEROMYCIN, CYCLOSERINE
STREPTOMYCIN SULFATE, STREPTOMYCIN SULFATE
SULFADIAZINE, SULFADIAZINE
SULFAPYRIDINE, SULFAPYRIDINE
SULFONAMIDES DUPLEX, SULFADIAZINE
TAPAZOLE, METHIMAZOLE
TAZIDIME, CEFTAZIDIME
TESTOSTERONE PROPIONATE, TESTOSTERONE PROPIONATE
TUBOCURARINE CHLORIDE, TUBOCURARINE CHLORIDE
TYLOSTERONE, DIETHYLSTILBESTROL
V-CILLIN, PENICILLIN V
V-CILLIN K, PENICILLIN V POTASSIUM
VANCOCIN HCL, VANCOMYCIN HYDROCHLORIDE
VELBAN, VINBLASTINE SULFATE
* ELI LILLY INDUSTRIES INC
  DARVON, PROPOXYPHENE HYDROCHLORIDE
  DARVON COMPOUND, ASPIRIN
  DARVON COMPOUND-65, ASPIRIN
  DARVON W/ ASA, ASPIRIN
  DARVON-N, PROPOXYPHENE NAPSYLATE
  DYMELOR, ACETOHEXAMIDE
  NOVRAD, LEVOPROPOXYPHENE NAPSYLATE, ANHYDROUS
* LILLY RESEARCH LABORATORIES DIV ELI LILLY CO
  PROZAC, FLUOXETINE HYDROCHLORIDE

LIQUIPHARM
* LIQUIPHARM INC
  TRIHEXYPHENIDYL HCL, TRIHEXYPHENIDYL HYDROCHLORIDE

LNK
* LNK INTERNATIONAL INC
  DIPHENHYDRAMINE HCL, DIPHENHYDRAMINE HYDROCHLORIDE
  METRONIDAZOLE, METRONIDAZOLE

APPENDIX B
PRODUCT NAME INDEX
LISTED BY APPLICANT (continued)

LOCH
* LOCH PHARMACEUTICALS INC
  CLINDAMYCIN PHOSPHATE, CLINDAMYCIN
    PHOSPHATE
  KANAMYCIN SULFATE, KANAMYCIN SULFATE

LOREX
* LOREX PHARMACEUTICALS INC
  KERLONE, BETAXOLOL HYDROCHLORIDE

LPI
* LPI HOLDINGS INC
  N.E.E. 1/35 21, ETHINYL ESTRADIOL
  N.E.E. 1/35 28, ETHINYL ESTRADIOL

LUCHEM
* LUCHEM PHARMACEUTICALS INC
  ALLAY, ACETAMINOPHEN
  HYDROCODONE BITARTRATE AND
    ACETAMINOPHEN, ACETAMINOPHEN
  IBUPROFEN, IBUPROFEN (OTC)
  IFEN, IBUPROFEN
  NEUVIL, IBUPROFEN (OTC)

LUITPOLD
* LUITPOLD PHARMACEUTICALS INC
  AMINOCAPROIC ACID, AMINOCAPROIC ACID
  AMINOPHYLLINE, AMINOPHYLLINE
  BRETYLIUM TOSYLATE, BRETYLIUM TOSYLATE
  CYANOCOBALAMIN, CYANOCOBALAMIN
  DEXAMETHASONE SODIUM PHOSPHATE,
    DEXAMETHASONE SODIUM PHOSPHATE
  DOPAMINE HCL, DOPAMINE HYDROCHLORIDE
  DROPERIDOL, DROPERIDOL
  FUROSEMIDE, FUROSEMIDE
  GLYCOPYRROLATE, GLYCOPYRROLATE
  HEPARIN LOCK FLUSH, HEPARIN SODIUM
  HEPARIN SODIUM, HEPARIN SODIUM
  HYDROXYZINE HCL, HYDROXYZINE
    HYDROCHLORIDE
  LIDOCAINE HCL, LIDOCAINE HYDROCHLORIDE
  MANNITOL 25%, MANNITOL
  METHYLDOPA HCL, METHYLDOPA
    HYDROCHLORIDE
  NITROGLYCERIN, NITROGLYCERIN
  PIPERAZINE CITRATE, PIPERAZINE CITRATE
  POTASSIUM CHLORIDE, POTASSIUM CHLORIDE
  PYRIDOXINE HCL, PYRIDOXINE HYDROCHLORIDE
  THIAMINE HCL, THIAMINE HYDROCHLORIDE
  VERAPAMIL HCL, VERAPAMIL HYDROCHLORIDE

LYNE
* LYNE LABORATORIES INC
  XYLOSE, XYLOSE

LYPHOMED
* LYPHOMED DIV FUJISAWA USA INC
  AMINOCAPROIC ACID, AMINOCAPROIC ACID
  AMINOPHYLLINE, AMINOPHYLLINE
  AMPHOTERICIN B, AMPHOTERICIN B
  BACTERIOSTATIC SODIUM CHLORIDE 0.9% IN
    PLASTIC CONTAINER, SODIUM CHLORIDE
  BACTERIOSTATIC WATER FOR INJECTION, WATER
    FOR INJECTION, STERILE
  BRETYLIUM TOSYLATE, BRETYLIUM TOSYLATE
  CALCIUM GLUCEPTATE, CALCIUM GLUCEPTATE
  CEFAZOLIN SODIUM, CEFAZOLIN SODIUM
  CEPHALOTHIN SODIUM, CEPHALOTHIN SODIUM
  CEPHAPIRIN SODIUM, CEPHAPIRIN SODIUM
  CHLORAMPHENICOL SODIUM SUCCINATE,
    CHLORAMPHENICOL SODIUM SUCCINATE
  CHLORPROMAZINE HCL, CHLORPROMAZINE
    HYDROCHLORIDE

CHORIONIC GONADOTROPIN, GONADOTROPIN,
  CHORIONIC
CHROMIC CHLORIDE, CHROMIC CHLORIDE
CLINDAMYCIN PHOSPHATE, CLINDAMYCIN
  PHOSPHATE
CLINDAMYCIN PHOSPHATE IN DEXTROSE 5%,
  CLINDAMYCIN PHOSPHATE
CUPRIC SULFATE, CUPRIC SULFATE
CYANOCOBALAMIN, CYANOCOBALAMIN
DACARBAZINE, DACARBAZINE
DEXAMETHASONE, DEXAMETHASONE SODIUM
  PHOSPHATE
DEXAMETHASONE SODIUM PHOSPHATE,
  DEXAMETHASONE SODIUM PHOSPHATE
DIAZEPAM, DIAZEPAM
DIAZOXIDE, DIAZOXIDE
DIGOXIN, DIGOXIN
DIPHENHYDRAMINE HCL, DIPHENHYDRAMINE
  HYDROCHLORIDE
DOPAMINE HCL, DOPAMINE HYDROCHLORIDE
DOXY 100, DOXYCYCLINE HYCLATE
DOXY 200, DOXYCYCLINE HYCLATE
DROPERIDOL, DROPERIDOL
ERYTHROMYCIN LACTOBIONATE, ERYTHROMYCIN
  LACTOBIONATE
FLUOROURACIL, FLUOROURACIL
FLUPHENAZINE DECANOATE, FLUPHENAZINE
  DECANOATE
FLUPHENAZINE HCL, FLUPHENAZINE
  HYDROCHLORIDE
FOLIC ACID, FOLIC ACID
FUROSEMIDE, FUROSEMIDE
GENTAMICIN SULFATE, GENTAMICIN SULFATE
GLYCOPYRROLATE, GLYCOPYRROLATE
HALOPERIDOL, HALOPERIDOL LACTATE
HEP FLUSH KIT, HEPARIN SODIUM
HEP-FLUSH 10, HEPARIN SODIUM
HEPARIN LOCK FLUSH, HEPARIN SODIUM
HEPARIN LOCK FLUSH PRESERVATIVE FREE,
  HEPARIN SODIUM
HEPARIN SODIUM, HEPARIN SODIUM
HEPARIN SODIUM PRESERVATIVE FREE, HEPARIN
  SODIUM
HYDRALAZINE HCL, HYDRALAZINE
  HYDROCHLORIDE
HYDROCORTISONE SODIUM SUCCINATE,
  HYDROCORTISONE SODIUM SUCCINATE
HYDROXOCOBALAMIN, HYDROXOCOBALAMIN
HYDROXYZINE HCL, HYDROXYZINE
  HYDROCHLORIDE
ISOPROTERENOL HCL, ISOPROTERENOL
  HYDROCHLORIDE
KANAMYCIN SULFATE, KANAMYCIN SULFATE
LEUCOVORIN CALCIUM, LEUCOVORIN CALCIUM
LIDOCAINE HCL, LIDOCAINE HYDROCHLORIDE
LIDOCAINE HCL IN PLASTIC CONTAINER,
  LIDOCAINE HYDROCHLORIDE
LYPHOCIN, VANCOMYCIN HYDROCHLORIDE
M.V.C. 9+3, ASCORBIC ACID
MAGNESIUM SULFATE, MAGNESIUM SULFATE
MANGANESE SULFATE, MANGANESE SULFATE
MANNITOL 25%, MANNITOL
METARAMINOL BITARTRATE, METARAMINOL
  BITARTRATE
METHOTREXATE SODIUM, METHOTREXATE SODIUM
METHYLDOPA HCL, METHYLDOPA
  HYDROCHLORIDE
METHYLPREDNISOLONE SODIUM SUCCINATE,
  METHYLPREDNISOLONE SODIUM SUCCINATE
METOCLOPRAMIDE HCL, METOCLOPRAMIDE
  HYDROCHLORIDE

APPENDIX B
PRODUCT NAME INDEX
LISTED BY APPLICANT *(continued)*

METRONIDAZOLE, METRONIDAZOLE
METRONIDAZOLE HCL, METRONIDAZOLE
HYDROCHLORIDE
NALBUPHINE, NALBUPHINE HYDROCHLORIDE
NALOXONE HCL, NALOXONE HYDROCHLORIDE
NANDROLONE DECANOATE, NANDROLONE
DECANOATE
NITROGLYCERIN, NITROGLYCERIN
OXYTOCIN, OXYTOCIN
PHENYTOIN SODIUM, PHENYTOIN SODIUM
POTASSIUM CHLORIDE, POTASSIUM CHLORIDE
POTASSIUM CHLORIDE IN PLASTIC CONTAINER,
POTASSIUM CHLORIDE
PROCAINAMIDE HCL, PROCAINAMIDE
HYDROCHLORIDE
PROCAINE HCL, PROCAINE HYDROCHLORIDE
PROTAMINE SULFATE, PROTAMINE SULFATE
PYRIDOXINE HCL, PYRIDOXINE HYDROCHLORIDE
RITODRINE HCL, RITODRINE HYDROCHLORIDE
SODIUM CHLORIDE 0.9% IN PLASTIC CONTAINER,
SODIUM CHLORIDE
SODIUM CHLORIDE 23.4%, SODIUM CHLORIDE
SODIUM HEPARIN, HEPARIN SODIUM
SODIUM NITROPRUSSIDE, SODIUM NITROPRUSSIDE
STERILE WATER FOR INJECTION IN PLASTIC
CONTAINER, WATER FOR INJECTION, STERILE
SULFAMETHOXAZOLE AND TRIMETHOPRIM,
SULFAMETHOXAZOLE
THIAMINE HCL, THIAMINE HYDROCHLORIDE
VERAPAMIL HCL, VERAPAMIL HYDROCHLORIDE
VIBISONE, CYANOCOBALAMIN
VINBLASTINE SULFATE, VINBLASTINE SULFATE
VINCRISTINE SULFATE, VINCRISTINE SULFATE
ZINC SULFATE, ZINC SULFATE

M

MALLARD
* MALLARD INC
ANOQUAN, ACETAMINOPHEN
MEPROBAMATE, MEPROBAMATE

MALLINCKRODT
* MALLINCKRODT INC
ANGIO-CONRAY, IOTHALAMATE SODIUM
CHOLEBRINE, IOCETAMIC ACID
CONRAY, IOTHALAMATE MEGLUMINE
CONRAY 30, IOTHALAMATE MEGLUMINE
CONRAY 325, IOTHALAMATE SODIUM
CONRAY 400, IOTHALAMATE SODIUM
CONRAY 43, IOTHALAMATE MEGLUMINE
FERROUS CITRATE FE 59, FERROUS CITRATE, FE-59
HEXABRIX, IOXAGLATE MEGLUMINE
HYZYD, ISONIAZID
MD-GASTROVIEW, DIATRIZOATE MEGLUMINE
MD-50, DIATRIZOATE SODIUM
MD-60, DIATRIZOATE MEGLUMINE
MD-76, DIATRIZOATE MEGLUMINE
OPTIRAY 160, IOVERSOL
OPTIRAY 240, IOVERSOL
OPTIRAY 300, IOVERSOL
OPTIRAY 320, IOVERSOL
OPTIRAY 350, IOVERSOL
OSTEOSCAN, TECHNETIUM TC-99M ETIDRONATE KIT
SELENOMETHIONINE SE 75, SELENOMETHIONINE,
SE-75
SODIUM IODIDE I 123, SODIUM IODIDE, I-123
TECHNESCAN MAA, TECHNETIUM TC-99M ALBUMIN
AGGREGATED KIT

VASCORAY, IOTHALAMATE MEGLUMINE
XENEISOL, XENON, XE-133
* MALLINCKRODT MEDICAL INC
CYANOCOBALAMIN CO 57 SCHILLING TEST KIT,
CYANOCOBALAMIN
CYSTO-CONRAY, IOTHALAMATE MEGLUMINE
CYSTO-CONRAY II, IOTHALAMATE MEGLUMINE
GALLIUM CITRATE GA 67, GALLIUM CITRATE, GA-67
HIPPURAN I 131, IODOHIPPURATE SODIUM, I-131
OSTEOSCAN-HDP, TECHNETIUM TC-99M OXIDRONATE
KIT
PERCHLORACAP, POTASSIUM PERCHLORATE
PHOSPHOCOL P32, CHROMIC PHOSPHATE, P-32
RADIOIODINATED SERUM ALBUMIN (HUMAN) IHSA I
125, ALBUMIN IODINATED I-125 SERUM
SODIUM CHROMATE CR 51, SODIUM CHROMATE, CR-
51
SODIUM IODIDE I 131, SODIUM IODIDE, I-131
SODIUM PERTECHNETATE TC 99M, TECHNETIUM TC-
99M SODIUM PERTECHNETATE
SODIUM PHOSPHATE P 32, SODIUM PHOSPHATE, P-32
TECHNECOLL, TECHNETIUM TC-99M SULFUR
COLLOID KIT
TECHNESCAN MAG3, TECHNETIUM TC-99M
MERTIATIDE KIT
TECHNESCAN PYP KIT, TECHNETIUM TC-99M
PYROPHOSPHATE KIT
TECHNETIUM TC 99M SULFUR COLLOID,
TECHNETIUM TC-99M SULFUR COLLOID
THALLOUS CHLORIDE TL 201, THALLOUS CHLORIDE,
TL-201
ULTRA-TECHNEKOW FM, TECHNETIUM TC-99M
SODIUM PERTECHNETATE GENERATOR
ULTRATAG, TECHNETIUM TC-99M RED BLOOD CELL
KIT
XENON XE 127, XENON, XE-127
XENON XE 133, XENON, XE-133
* MALLINCKRODT SPECIALTY CHEMICALS CO
METHADOSE, METHADONE HYDROCHLORIDE

MARCHAR
* MARCHAR LABORATORIES INC LTD
FLUOROURACIL, FLUOROURACIL

MARION MERRELL DOW
* MARION MERRELL DOW INC
CARDIZEM, DILTIAZEM HYDROCHLORIDE
CARDIZEM CD, DILTIAZEM HYDROCHLORIDE
CARDIZEM SR, DILTIAZEM HYDROCHLORIDE
DITROPAN, OXYBUTYNIN CHLORIDE
GAVISCON, ALUMINUM HYDROXIDE (OTC)
GAVISCON-2, ALUMINUM HYDROXIDE (OTC)
NICODERM, NICOTINE
NITRO-BID, NITROGLYCERIN
SILDIMAC, SILVER SULFADIAZINE
SILVADENE, SILVER SULFADIAZINE
VENTAIRE, PROTOKYLOL HYDROCHLORIDE

MARSAM
* MARSAM PHARMACEUTICALS INC
AMPICILLIN SODIUM, AMPICILLIN SODIUM
CEFAZOLIN SODIUM, CEFAZOLIN SODIUM
CHLORPROMAZINE HCL, CHLORPROMAZINE
HYDROCHLORIDE
CLINDAMYCIN PHOSPHATE, CLINDAMYCIN
PHOSPHATE
HEPARIN SODIUM PRESERVATIVE FREE, HEPARIN
SODIUM
METHOCARBAMOL, METHOCARBAMOL
METHYLDOPATE HCL, METHYLDOPATE
HYDROCHLORIDE

APPENDIX B
PRODUCT NAME INDEX
LISTED BY APPLICANT (continued)

NAFCILLIN SODIUM, NAFCILLIN SODIUM
NALOXONE HCL, NALOXONE HYDROCHLORIDE
OXACILLIN SODIUM, OXACILLIN SODIUM
PENICILLIN G POTASSIUM, PENICILLIN G
   POTASSIUM
PENICILLIN G SODIUM, PENICILLIN G SODIUM
PHENYTOIN SODIUM, PHENYTOIN SODIUM
PROCHLORPERAZINE EDISYLATE,
   PROCHLORPERAZINE EDISYLATE
PROMETHAZINE HCL, PROMETHAZINE
   HYDROCHLORIDE
TOBRAMYCIN SULFATE, TOBRAMYCIN SULFATE

MARSHALL
* MARSHALL PHARMACAL CORP
   CHLORPHENIRAMINE MALEATE,
      CHLORPHENIRAMINE MALEATE
   PREDNISOLONE, PREDNISOLONE
   PREDNISONE, PREDNISONE
   RESERPINE, RESERPINE
   SODIUM BUTABARBITAL, BUTABARBITAL SODIUM

MARTEC
* MARTEC PHARMACEUTICALS INC
   DIAZEPAM, DIAZEPAM
   SULFAMETHOXAZOLE AND TRIMETHOPRIM,
      SULFAMETHOXAZOLE
   SULFAMETHOXAZOLE AND TRIMETHOPRIM DOUBLE
      STRENGTH, SULFAMETHOXAZOLE

MAST
* MM MAST AND CO
   CHLORDIAZEPOXIDE HCL, CHLORDIAZEPOXIDE
      HYDROCHLORIDE
   DEXTROAMPHETAMINE SULFATE,
      DEXTROAMPHETAMINE SULFATE
   HYDROCHLOROTHIAZIDE, HYDROCHLOROTHIAZIDE
   ONA MAST, PHENTERMINE HYDROCHLORIDE
   ONA-MAST, PHENTERMINE HYDROCHLORIDE
   PHENAZINE, PHENDIMETRAZINE TARTRATE
   TETRACYCLINE HCL, TETRACYCLINE
      HYDROCHLORIDE
   TRICHLORMAS, TRICHLORMETHIAZIDE

MATRIX MEDCL
* MATRIX MEDICAL CORP
   STERI-STAT, CHLORHEXIDINE GLUCONATE (OTC)

MAYRAND
* MAYRAND INC
   SEDAPAP, ACETAMINOPHEN

MCGAW
* MCGAW INC
   ACETATED RINGER'S IN PLASTIC CONTAINER,
      CALCIUM CHLORIDE
   ACETIC ACID 0.25% IN PLASTIC CONTAINER, ACETIC
      ACID, GLACIAL
   ALCOHOL 10% AND DEXTROSE 5%, ALCOHOL
   ALCOHOL 5% AND DEXTROSE 5%, ALCOHOL
   AMMONIUM CHLORIDE 0.9% IN NORMAL SALINE,
      AMMONIUM CHLORIDE
   AMMONIUM CHLORIDE 2.14%, AMMONIUM
      CHLORIDE
   BRETYLIUM TOSYLATE IN DEXTROSE 5%,
      BRETYLIUM TOSYLATE
   DEXTROSE 10%, DEXTROSE
   DEXTROSE 10% AND SODIUM CHLORIDE 0.11%,
      DEXTROSE
   DEXTROSE 10% AND SODIUM CHLORIDE 0.2%,
      DEXTROSE
   DEXTROSE 10% AND SODIUM CHLORIDE 0.33%,
      DEXTROSE

DEXTROSE 10% AND SODIUM CHLORIDE 0.45%,
   DEXTROSE
DEXTROSE 10% AND SODIUM CHLORIDE 0.9%,
   DEXTROSE
DEXTROSE 10% AND SODIUM CHLORIDE 0.9% IN
   PLASTIC CONTAINER, DEXTROSE
DEXTROSE 10% IN PLASTIC CONTAINER, DEXTROSE
DEXTROSE 2.5%, DEXTROSE
DEXTROSE 2.5% AND SODIUM CHLORIDE 0.11%,
   DEXTROSE
DEXTROSE 2.5% AND SODIUM CHLORIDE 0.2%,
   DEXTROSE
DEXTROSE 2.5% AND SODIUM CHLORIDE 0.33%,
   DEXTROSE
DEXTROSE 2.5% AND SODIUM CHLORIDE 0.45%,
   DEXTROSE
DEXTROSE 2.5% AND SODIUM CHLORIDE 0.45% IN
   PLASTIC CONTAINER, DEXTROSE
DEXTROSE 2.5% AND SODIUM CHLORIDE 0.9%,
   DEXTROSE
DEXTROSE 2.5% IN HALF-STRENGTH LACTATED
   RINGER'S, CALCIUM CHLORIDE
DEXTROSE 3.3% AND SODIUM CHLORIDE 0.3%,
   DEXTROSE
DEXTROSE 4% IN MODIFIED LACTATED RINGER'S,
   CALCIUM CHLORIDE
DEXTROSE 5%, DEXTROSE
DEXTROSE 5% AND SODIUM CHLORIDE 0.11%,
   DEXTROSE
DEXTROSE 5% AND SODIUM CHLORIDE 0.11% IN
   PLASTIC CONTAINER, DEXTROSE
DEXTROSE 5% AND SODIUM CHLORIDE 0.2%,
   DEXTROSE
DEXTROSE 5% AND SODIUM CHLORIDE 0.2% IN
   PLASTIC CONTAINER, DEXTROSE
DEXTROSE 5% AND SODIUM CHLORIDE 0.33%,
   DEXTROSE
DEXTROSE 5% AND SODIUM CHLORIDE 0.33% IN
   PLASTIC CONTAINER, DEXTROSE
DEXTROSE 5% AND SODIUM CHLORIDE 0.45%,
   DEXTROSE
DEXTROSE 5% AND SODIUM CHLORIDE 0.45% IN
   PLASTIC CONTAINER, DEXTROSE
DEXTROSE 5% AND SODIUM CHLORIDE 0.9%,
   DEXTROSE
DEXTROSE 5% IN ACETATED RINGER'S IN PLASTIC
   CONTAINER, CALCIUM CHLORIDE
DEXTROSE 5% IN LACTATED RINGER'S, CALCIUM
   CHLORIDE
DEXTROSE 5% IN LACTATED RINGER'S IN PLASTIC
   CONTAINER, CALCIUM CHLORIDE
DEXTROSE 5% IN PLASTIC CONTAINER, DEXTROSE
DEXTROSE 5% IN RINGER'S, CALCIUM CHLORIDE
DEXTROSE 5% IN RINGER'S IN PLASTIC CONTAINER,
   CALCIUM CHLORIDE
DEXTROSE 5%, SODIUM CHLORIDE 0.2% AND
   POTASSIUM CHLORIDE 0.15%, DEXTROSE
DEXTROSE 5%, SODIUM CHLORIDE 0.2% AND
   POTASSIUM CHLORIDE 0.224%, DEXTROSE
DEXTROSE 5%, SODIUM CHLORIDE 0.2% AND
   POTASSIUM CHLORIDE 0.3%, DEXTROSE
DEXTROSE 5%, SODIUM CHLORIDE 0.2% AND
   POTASSIUM CHLORIDE 0.075%, DEXTROSE
DEXTROSE 5%, SODIUM CHLORIDE 0.33% AND
   POTASSIUM CHLORIDE 0.075%, DEXTROSE
DEXTROSE 5%, SODIUM CHLORIDE 0.33% AND
   POTASSIUM CHLORIDE 0.15%, DEXTROSE
DEXTROSE 5%, SODIUM CHLORIDE 0.33% AND
   POTASSIUM CHLORIDE 0.22%, DEXTROSE
DEXTROSE 5%, SODIUM CHLORIDE 0.33% AND
   POTASSIUM CHLORIDE 0.30%, DEXTROSE

APPENDIX B
PRODUCT NAME INDEX
LISTED BY APPLICANT (continued)

DEXTROSE 5%, SODIUM CHLORIDE 0.45%AND
POTASSIUM CHLORIDE 0.15%, DEXTROSE
DEXTROSE 5%, SODIUM CHLORIDE 0.45% AND
POTASSIUM CHLORIDE 0.3%, DEXTROSE
DEXTROSE 5%, SODIUM CHLORIDE 0.45% AND
POTASSIUM CHLORIDE 0.075%, DEXTROSE
DEXTROSE 5%, SODIUM CHLORIDE 0.45% AND
POTASSIUM CHLORIDE 0.22%, DEXTROSE
DEXTROSE 60%, DEXTROSE
DEXTROSE 60% IN PLASTIC CONTAINER, DEXTROSE
DEXTROSE 7.7%, DEXTROSE
DIALYTE CONCENTRATE W/ DEXTROSE 30% IN
PLASTIC CONTAINER, CALCIUM CHLORIDE
DIALYTE CONCENTRATE W/ DEXTROSE 50% IN
PLASTIC CONTAINER, CALCIUM CHLORIDE
DIALYTE LM/ DEXTROSE 1.5%, CALCIUM CHLORIDE
DIALYTE LM/ DEXTROSE 2.5%, CALCIUM CHLORIDE
DIALYTE LM/ DEXTROSE 4.25%, CALCIUM CHLORIDE
DIALYTE W/ DEXTROSE 1.5% IN PLASTIC
CONTAINER, CALCIUM CHLORIDE
DIALYTE W/ DEXTROSE 4.25% IN PLASTIC
CONTAINER, CALCIUM CHLORIDE
DOPAMINE HCL AND DEXTROSE 5%, DOPAMINE
HYDROCHLORIDE
FREAMINE HBC 6.9%, AMINO ACIDS
FREAMINE II 8.5%, AMINO ACIDS
FREAMINE III 10%, AMINO ACIDS
FREAMINE III 3% W/ ELECTROLYTES, AMINO ACIDS
FREAMINE III 8.5%, AMINO ACIDS
FREAMINE III 8.5% W/ ELECTROLYTES, AMINO ACIDS
FREAMINE 8.5%, AMINO ACIDS
GENTAMICIN SULFATE IN SODIUM CHLORIDE 0.9%,
GENTAMICIN SULFATE
GLYCINE 1.5% IN PLASTIC CONTAINER, GLYCINE
HEPARIN SODIUM 1000 UNITS AND DEXTROSE 5% IN
PLASTIC CONTAINER, HEPARIN SODIUM
HEPARIN SODIUM 1000 UNITS IN SODIUM CHLORIDE
0.9%, HEPARIN SODIUM
HEPARIN SODIUM 12500 UNITS IN SODIUM
CHLORIDE 0.45%, HEPARIN SODIUM
HEPARIN SODIUM 2000 UNITS IN DEXTROSE 5% IN
PLASTIC CONTAINER, HEPARIN SODIUM
HEPARIN SODIUM 2000 UNITS IN SODIUM CHLORIDE
0.9%, HEPARIN SODIUM
HEPARIN SODIUM 20000 UNITS IN DEXTROSE 5%,
HEPARIN SODIUM
HEPARIN SODIUM 25000 UNITS IN DEXTROSE 5%,
HEPARIN SODIUM
HEPARIN SODIUM 25000 UNITS IN DEXTROSE 5% IN
PLASTIC CONTAINER, HEPARIN SODIUM
HEPARIN SODIUM 25000 UNITS IN SODIUM
CHLORIDE 0.45%, HEPARIN SODIUM
HEPARIN SODIUM 25000 UNITS IN SODIUM
CHLORIDE 0.9%, HEPARIN SODIUM
HEPARIN SODIUM 5000 UNITS IN DEXTROSE 5% IN
PLASTIC CONTAINER, HEPARIN SODIUM
HEPARIN SODIUM 5000 UNITS IN SODIUM CHLORIDE
0.9%, HEPARIN SODIUM
HEPATAMINE 8%, AMINO ACIDS
HYPROTIGEN 5%, PROTEIN HYDROLYSATE
ISOLYTE E, CALCIUM CHLORIDE
ISOLYTE E IN PLASTIC CONTAINER, CALCIUM
CHLORIDE
ISOLYTE E W/ DEXTROSE 5% IN PLASTIC
CONTAINER, CALCIUM CHLORIDE
ISOLYTE H W/ DEXTROSE 5% IN PLASTIC
CONTAINER, DEXTROSE
ISOLYTE M W/ DEXTROSE 5% IN PLASTIC
CONTAINER, DEXTROSE
ISOLYTE P W/ DEXTROSE 5% IN PLASTIC
CONTAINER, DEXTROSE

ISOLYTE R W/ DEXTROSE 5% IN PLASTIC
CONTAINER, CALCIUM CHLORIDE
ISOLYTE S, MAGNESIUM CHLORIDE
ISOLYTE S IN PLASTIC CONTAINER, MAGNESIUM
CHLORIDE
ISOLYTE S PH 7.4, MAGNESIUM CHLORIDE
ISOLYTE S PH 7.4 IN PLASTIC CONTAINER,
MAGNESIUM CHLORIDE
ISOLYTE S W/ DEXTROSE 5% IN PLASTIC
CONTAINER, DEXTROSE
LACTATED RINGER'S, CALCIUM CHLORIDE
LACTATED RINGER'S IN PLASTIC CONTAINER,
CALCIUM CHLORIDE
LIDOCAINE HCL 0.2% AND DEXTROSE 5%, LIDOCAINE
HYDROCHLORIDE
LIDOCAINE HCL 0.2% AND DEXTROSE 5% IN PLASTIC
CONTAINER, LIDOCAINE HYDROCHLORIDE
LIDOCAINE HCL 0.4% AND DEXTROSE 5%, LIDOCAINE
HYDROCHLORIDE
LIDOCAINE HCL 0.4% AND DEXTROSE 5% IN PLASTIC
CONTAINER, LIDOCAINE HYDROCHLORIDE
LIDOCAINE HCL 0.8% AND DEXTROSE 5%, LIDOCAINE
HYDROCHLORIDE
LIDOCAINE HCL 0.8% AND DEXTROSE 5% IN PLASTIC
CONTAINER, LIDOCAINE HYDROCHLORIDE
MANNITOL 10%, MANNITOL
MANNITOL 10% W/ DEXTROSE 5% IN DISTILLED
WATER, MANNITOL
MANNITOL 15%, MANNITOL
MANNITOL 15% W/ DEXTROSE 5% IN SODIUM
CHLORIDE 0.45%, MANNITOL
MANNITOL 20%, MANNITOL
MANNITOL 5%, MANNITOL
MANNITOL 5% W/ DEXTROSE 5% IN SODIUM
CHLORIDE 0.12%, MANNITO
METRO I.V., METRONIDAZOLE
METRO I.V. IN PLASTIC CONTAINER,
METRONIDAZOLE
NEPHRAMINE 5.4%, AMINO ACIDS
PHYSIOLYTE IN PLASTIC CONTAINER, MAGNESIUM
CHLORIDE
POTASSIUM CHLORIDE, POTASSIUM CHLORIDE
POTASSIUM CHLORIDE 0.037% IN DEXTROSE 10% AND
SODIUM CHLORIDE 0.2%, DEXTROSE
POTASSIUM CHLORIDE 0.037% IN DEXTROSE 10% AND
SODIUM CHLORIDE 0.45%, DEXTROSE
POTASSIUM CHLORIDE 0.037% IN DEXTROSE 10% AND
SODIUM CHLORIDE 0.9%, DEXTROSE
POTASSIUM CHLORIDE 0.037% IN DEXTROSE 5%,
DEXTROSE
POTASSIUM CHLORIDE 0.037% IN DEXTROSE 5% AND
SODIUM CHLORIDE 0.11%, DEXTROSE
POTASSIUM CHLORIDE 0.037% IN DEXTROSE 5% AND
SODIUM CHLORIDE 0.2%, DEXTROSE
POTASSIUM CHLORIDE 0.037% IN DEXTROSE 5% AND
SODIUM CHLORIDE 0.33%, DEXTROSE
POTASSIUM CHLORIDE 0.037% IN DEXTROSE 5% AND
SODIUM CHLORIDE 0.45%, DEXTROSE
POTASSIUM CHLORIDE 0.037% IN DEXTROSE 5% AND
SODIUM CHLORIDE 0.9%, DEXTROSE
POTASSIUM CHLORIDE 0.037% IN SODIUM CHLORIDE
0.9%, POTASSIUM CHLORIDE
POTASSIUM CHLORIDE 0.075% IN DEXTROSE 10% AND
SODIUM CHLORIDE 0.2%, DEXTROSE
POTASSIUM CHLORIDE 0.075% IN DEXTROSE 10% AND
SODIUM CHLORIDE 0.45%, DEXTROSE
POTASSIUM CHLORIDE 0.075% IN DEXTROSE 10% AND
SODIUM CHLORIDE 0.9%, DEXTROSE
POTASSIUM CHLORIDE 0.075% IN DEXTROSE 3.3%
AND SODIUM CHLORIDE 0.3%, DEXTROSE

APPENDIX B
PRODUCT NAME INDEX
LISTED BY APPLICANT *(continued)*

POTASSIUM CHLORIDE 0.075% IN DEXTROSE 5%, DEXTROSE

POTASSIUM CHLORIDE 0.075% IN DEXTROSE 5% AND SODIUM CHLORIDE 0.11%, DEXTROSE

POTASSIUM CHLORIDE 0.075% IN DEXTROSE 5% AND SODIUM CHLORIDE 0.2%, DEXTROSE

POTASSIUM CHLORIDE 0.075% IN DEXTROSE 5% AND SODIUM CHLORIDE 0.33%, DEXTROSE

POTASSIUM CHLORIDE 0.075% IN DEXTROSE 5% AND SODIUM CHLORIDE 0.45%, DEXTROSE

POTASSIUM CHLORIDE 0.075% IN DEXTROSE 5% AND SODIUM CHLORIDE 0.9%, DEXTROSE

POTASSIUM CHLORIDE 0.075% IN SODIUM CHLORIDE 0.9%, POTASSIUM CHLORIDE

POTASSIUM CHLORIDE 0.11% IN DEXTROSE 10% AND SODIUM CHLORIDE 0.2%, DEXTROSE

POTASSIUM CHLORIDE 0.11% IN DEXTROSE 10% AND SODIUM CHLORIDE 0.45%, DEXTROSE

POTASSIUM CHLORIDE 0.11% IN DEXTROSE 10% AND SODIUM CHLORIDE 0.9%, DEXTROSE

POTASSIUM CHLORIDE 0.11% IN DEXTROSE 3.3% AND SODIUM CHLORIDE 0.3%, DEXTROSE

POTASSIUM CHLORIDE 0.11% IN DEXTROSE 5%, DEXTROSE

POTASSIUM CHLORIDE 0.11% IN DEXTROSE 5% AND SODIUM CHLORIDE 0.11%, DEXTROSE

POTASSIUM CHLORIDE 0.11% IN DEXTROSE 5% AND SODIUM CHLORIDE 0.2%, DEXTROSE

POTASSIUM CHLORIDE 0.11% IN DEXTROSE 5% AND SODIUM CHLORIDE 0.33%, DEXTROSE

POTASSIUM CHLORIDE 0.11% IN DEXTROSE 5% AND SODIUM CHLORIDE 0.45%, DEXTROSE

POTASSIUM CHLORIDE 0.11% IN DEXTROSE 5% AND SODIUM CHLORIDE 0.9%, DEXTROSE

POTASSIUM CHLORIDE 0.11% IN SODIUM CHLORIDE 0.9%, POTASSIUM CHLORIDE

POTASSIUM CHLORIDE 0.15% IN DEXTROSE 10% AND SODIUM CHLORIDE 0.2%, DEXTROSE

POTASSIUM CHLORIDE 0.15% IN DEXTROSE 10% AND SODIUM CHLORIDE 0.45%, DEXTROSE

POTASSIUM CHLORIDE 0.15% IN DEXTROSE 10% AND SODIUM CHLORIDE 0.9%, DEXTROSE

POTASSIUM CHLORIDE 0.15% IN DEXTROSE 3.3% AND SODIUM CHLORIDE 0.3%, DEXTROSE

POTASSIUM CHLORIDE 0.15% IN DEXTROSE 5%, DEXTROSE

POTASSIUM CHLORIDE 0.15% IN DEXTROSE 5% AND SODIUM CHLORIDE 0.11%, DEXTROSE

POTASSIUM CHLORIDE 0.15% IN DEXTROSE 5% AND SODIUM CHLORIDE 0.2%, DEXTROSE

POTASSIUM CHLORIDE 0.15% IN DEXTROSE 5% AND SODIUM CHLORIDE 0.33%, DEXTROSE

POTASSIUM CHLORIDE 0.15% IN DEXTROSE 5% AND SODIUM CHLORIDE 0.45%, DEXTROSE

POTASSIUM CHLORIDE 0.15% IN DEXTROSE 5% AND SODIUM CHLORIDE 0.9%, DEXTROSE

POTASSIUM CHLORIDE 0.15% IN SODIUM CHLORIDE 0.9%, POTASSIUM CHLORIDE

POTASSIUM CHLORIDE 0.22% IN DEXTROSE 10% AND SODIUM CHLORIDE 0.2%, DEXTROSE

POTASSIUM CHLORIDE 0.22% IN DEXTROSE 10% AND SODIUM CHLORIDE 0.45%, DEXTROSE

POTASSIUM CHLORIDE 0.22% IN DEXTROSE 10% AND SODIUM CHLORIDE 0.9%, DEXTROSE

POTASSIUM CHLORIDE 0.22% IN DEXTROSE 3.3% AND SODIUM CHLORIDE 0.3%, DEXTROSE

POTASSIUM CHLORIDE 0.22% IN DEXTROSE 5%, DEXTROSE

POTASSIUM CHLORIDE 0.22% IN DEXTROSE 5% AND SODIUM CHLORIDE 0.11%, DEXTROSE

POTASSIUM CHLORIDE 0.22% IN DEXTROSE 5% AND SODIUM CHLORIDE 0.2%, DEXTROSE

POTASSIUM CHLORIDE 0.22% IN DEXTROSE 5% AND SODIUM CHLORIDE 0.33%, DEXTROSE

POTASSIUM CHLORIDE 0.22% IN DEXTROSE 5% AND SODIUM CHLORIDE 0.45%, DEXTROSE

POTASSIUM CHLORIDE 0.22% IN DEXTROSE 5% AND SODIUM CHLORIDE 0.9%, DEXTROSE

POTASSIUM CHLORIDE 0.22% IN SODIUM CHLORIDE 0.9%, POTASSIUM CHLORIDE

POTASSIUM CHLORIDE 0.3% IN DEXTROSE 10% AND SODIUM CHLORIDE 0.2%, DEXTROSE

POTASSIUM CHLORIDE 0.3% IN DEXTROSE 10% AND SODIUM CHLORIDE 0.45%, DEXTROSE

POTASSIUM CHLORIDE 0.3% IN DEXTROSE 10% AND SODIUM CHLORIDE 0.9%, DEXTROSE

POTASSIUM CHLORIDE 0.3% IN DEXTROSE 3.3% AND SODIUM CHLORIDE 0.3%, DEXTROSE

POTASSIUM CHLORIDE 0.3% IN DEXTROSE 5%, DEXTROSE

POTASSIUM CHLORIDE 0.3% IN DEXTROSE 5% AND SODIUM CHLORIDE 0.11%, DEXTROSE

POTASSIUM CHLORIDE 0.3% IN DEXTROSE 5% AND SODIUM CHLORIDE 0.2%, DEXTROSE

POTASSIUM CHLORIDE 0.3% IN DEXTROSE 5% AND SODIUM CHLORIDE 0.33%, DEXTROSE

POTASSIUM CHLORIDE 0.3% IN DEXTROSE 5% AND SODIUM CHLORIDE 0.45%, DEXTROSE

POTASSIUM CHLORIDE 0.3% IN DEXTROSE 5% AND SODIUM CHLORIDE 0.9%, DEXTROSE

POTASSIUM CHLORIDE 0.3% IN SODIUM CHLORIDE 0.9%, POTASSIUM CHLORIDE

PROCALAMINE, AMINO ACIDS

RESECTISOL, MANNITOL

RINGER'S, CALCIUM CHLORIDE

RINGER'S IN PLASTIC CONTAINER, CALCIUM CHLORIDE

SODIUM CHLORIDE, SODIUM CHLORIDE

SODIUM CHLORIDE 0.45%, SODIUM CHLORIDE

SODIUM CHLORIDE 0.45% IN PLASTIC CONTAINER, SODIUM CHLORIDE

SODIUM CHLORIDE 0.9%, SODIUM CHLORIDE

SODIUM CHLORIDE 0.9% AND POTASSIUM CHLORIDE 0.075%, POTASSIUM CHLORIDE

SODIUM CHLORIDE 0.9% AND POTASSIUM CHLORIDE 0.15%, POTASSIUM CHLORIDE

SODIUM CHLORIDE 0.9% AND POTASSIUM CHLORIDE 0.22%, POTASSIUM CHLORIDE

SODIUM CHLORIDE 0.9% AND POTASSIUM CHLORIDE 0.3%, POTASSIUM CHLORIDE

SODIUM CHLORIDE 0.9% IN PLASTIC CONTAINER, SODIUM CHLORIDE

SODIUM CHLORIDE 3%, SODIUM CHLORIDE

SODIUM CHLORIDE 5%, SODIUM CHLORIDE

SODIUM LACTATE 0.167 MOLAR IN PLASTIC CONTAINER, SODIUM LACTATE

SODIUM LACTATE 1/6 MOLAR, SODIUM LACTATE

SORBITOL 3.3% IN PLASTIC CONTAINER, SORBITOL

STERILE WATER FOR INJECTION, WATER FOR INJECTION, STERILE

STERILE WATER FOR INJECTION IN PLASTIC CONTAINER, WATER FOR INJECTION, STERILE

STERILE WATER IN PLASTIC CONTAINER, WATER FOR IRRIGATION, STERILE

THEOPHYLLINE 0.04% AND DEXTROSE 5%, THEOPHYLLINE

THEOPHYLLINE 0.04% AND DEXTROSE 5% IN PLASTIC CONTAINER, THEOPHYLLINE

THEOPHYLLINE 0.08% AND DEXTROSE 5%, THEOPHYLLINE

THEOPHYLLINE 0.08% AND DEXTROSE 5% IN PLASTIC
  CONTAINER, THEOPHYLLINE
THEOPHYLLINE 0.16% AND DEXTROSE 5%,
  THEOPHYLLINE
THEOPHYLLINE 0.16% AND DEXTROSE 5% IN PLASTIC
  CONTAINER, THEOPHYLLINE
THEOPHYLLINE 0.2% AND DEXTROSE 5%,
  THEOPHYLLINE
THEOPHYLLINE 0.2% AND DEXTROSE 5% IN PLASTIC
  CONTAINER, THEOPHYLLINE
THEOPHYLLINE 0.32% AND DEXTROSE 5%,
  THEOPHYLLINE
THEOPHYLLINE 0.4% AND DEXTROSE 5%,
  THEOPHYLLINE
THEOPHYLLINE 0.4% AND DEXTROSE 5% IN PLASTIC
  CONTAINER, THEOPHYLLINE
TROPHAMINE, AMINO ACIDS
TROPHAMINE 10%, AMINO ACIDS
UCEPHAN, SODIUM BENZOATE

MCNEIL
* MCNEIL CONSUMER PRODUCTS CO DIV MCNEILAB
INC
  CHEMET, SUCCIMER
  IBUPROFEN, IBUPROFEN
  IMODIUM A-D, LOPERAMIDE HYDROCHLORIDE (OTC)
  MEDIPREN, IBUPROFEN (OTC)
  METHOCARBAMOL AND ASPIRIN, ASPIRIN
  PEDIA PROFEN, IBUPROFEN
  TYLENOL, ACETAMINOPHEN (OTC)

MD PHARM
* MD PHARMACEUTICAL INC
  AMITRIPTYLINE HCL, AMITRIPTYLINE
    HYDROCHLORIDE
  CHLOROQUINE PHOSPHATE, CHLOROQUINE
    PHOSPHATE
  CYPROHEPTADINE HCL, CYPROHEPTADINE
    HYDROCHLORIDE
  DI-ATRO, ATROPINE SULFATE
  DIETHYLPROPION HCL, DIETHYLPROPION
    HYDROCHLORIDE
  GLUTETHIMIDE, GLUTETHIMIDE
  METHYLPHENIDATE HCL, METHYLPHENIDATE
    HYDROCHLORIDE
  TRI-SUDO, PSEUDOEPHEDRINE HYDROCHLORIDE
    (OTC)

MEAD JOHNSON
* MEAD JOHNSON AND CO SUB BRISTOL MYERS CO
  DURICEF, CEFADROXIL/CEFADROXIL HEMIHYDRATE
  ESTRACE, ESTRADIOL
  MEGACE, MEGESTROL ACETATE
  MUCOMYST, ACETYLCYSTEINE
  MUCOMYST W/ ISOPROTERENOL, ACETYLCYSTEINE
  OVCON-35, ETHINYL ESTRADIOL
  OVCON-50, ETHINYL ESTRADIOL

MEDCL MKTG
* MEDICAL MARKETING SPECIALTIES INC
  PROGLYCEM, DIAZOXIDE

MEDCO
* MEDCO RESEARCH INC
  ADENOCARD, ADENOSINE

MEDI PHYSICS
* MEDI PHYSICS INC
  CINTICHEM TECHNETIUM 99M HEDSPA,
    TECHNETIUM TC-99M ETIDRONATE KIT
  GALLIUM CITRATE GA 67, GALLIUM CITRATE, GA-67
  LUNGAGGREGATE REAGENT, TECHNETIUM TC-99M
    ALBUMIN AGGREGATED KIT

MPI DMSA KIDNEY REAGENT, TECHNETIUM TC-99M
  SUCCIMER KIT
MPI DTPA KIT - CHELATE, TECHNETIUM TC-99M
  PENTETATE KIT
MPI INDIUM DTPA IN 111, INDIUM IN-111 PENTETATE
  DISODIUM
MPI KRYPTON 81M GAS GENERATOR, KRYPTON, KR-
  81M
MPI STANNOUS DIPHOSPHONATE, TECHNETIUM TC-
  99M ETIDRONATE KIT
NEOSCAN, GALLIUM CITRATE, GA-67
NEPHROFLOW, IODOHIPPURATE SODIUM, I-123
SELENOMETHIONINE SE 75, SELENOMETHIONINE,
  SE-75
SODIUM IODIDE I 123, SODIUM IODIDE, I-123
SODIUM PERTECHNETATE TC 99M, TECHNETIUM TC-
  99M SODIUM PERTECHNETATE
SODIUM POLYPHOSPHATE-TIN KIT, TECHNETIUM TC-
  99M POLYPHOSPHATE KIT
TC 99M-LUNGAGGREGATE, TECHNETIUM TC-99M
  ALBUMIN AGGREGATED
TECHNETIUM TC 99M DIPHOSPHONATE-TIN KIT,
  TECHNETIUM TC-99M ETIDRONATE KIT
TECHNETIUM TC 99M GENERATOR, TECHNETIUM TC-
  99M SODIUM PERTECHNETATE GENERATOR
TECHNETIUM TC 99M HSA, TECHNETIUM TC-99M
  ALBUMIN KIT
TECHNETIUM TC 99M MAA, TECHNETIUM TC-99M
  ALBUMIN AGGREGATED KIT
TECHNETIUM TC 99M MPI MDP, TECHNETIUM TC-99M
  MEDRONATE KIT
TECHNETIUM TC 99M SULFUR COLLOID,
  TECHNETIUM TC-99M SULFUR COLLOID
TECHNETIUM TC 99M TSC, TECHNETIUM TC-99M
  SULFUR COLLOID KIT
TECHNETIUM TC-99M PENTETATE KIT, TECHNETIUM
  TC-99M PENTETATE KIT
THALLOUS CHLORIDE TL 201, THALLOUS CHLORIDE,
  TL-201
XENON XE 133, XENON, XE-133
XENON XE 133-V.S.S., XENON, XE-133

MEDICOPHARMA
* MEDICOPHARMA INC
  DOXYCYCLINE HYCLATE, DOXYCYCLINE HYCLATE
  DOXYCYCLINE MONOHYDRATE, DOXYCYCLINE
  IBUPROFEN, IBUPROFEN
  IBUPROFEN, IBUPROFEN (OTC)

MEDTRONIC
* MEDTRONIC INC
  LIORESAL, BACLOFEN

MERCK
* MERCK RESEARCH LABORATORIES DIV MERCK AND
CO INC
  CHIBROXIN, NORFLOXACIN
  CLINORIL, SULINDAC
  DECADRON-LA, DEXAMETHASONE ACETATE
  INDOCIN, INDOMETHACIN
  INDOCIN I.V., INDOMETHACIN SODIUM
  INDOCIN SR, INDOMETHACIN
  LACRISERT, HYDROXYPROPYL CELLULOSE
  MEVACOR, LOVASTATIN
  NOROXIN, NORFLOXACIN
  PEPCID, FAMOTIDINE
  PLENDIL, FELODIPINE
  PRILOSEC, OMEPRAZOLE
  PRINIVIL, LISINOPRIL
  PRINZIDE 12.5, HYDROCHLOROTHIAZIDE
  PRINZIDE 25, HYDROCHLOROTHIAZIDE

APPENDIX B
PRODUCT NAME INDEX
LISTED BY APPLICANT (continued)

TECHNESCAN DTPA KIT, TECHNETIUM TC-99M
  PENTETATE KIT
TECHNESCAN HIDA, TECHNETIUM TC-99M
  LIDOFENIN KIT
TIMOPTIC, TIMOLOL MALEATE
TIMOPTIC IN OCUDOSE, TIMOLOL MALEATE
VASERETIC, ENALAPRIL MALEATE
VASOTEC, ENALAPRIL MALEATE
VASOTEC, ENALAPRILAT
ZOCOR, SIMVASTATIN

MERICON
* MERICON INDUSTRIES INC
  HYDROCORTISONE, HYDROCORTISONE

MERRELL DOW
* MERRELL DOW PHARMACEUTICALS INC SUB MARION
MERRELL DOW INC
  ACCURBRON, THEOPHYLLINE
  AVC, SULFANILAMIDE
  BENTYL, DICYCLOMINE HYDROCHLORIDE
  BRICANYL, TERBUTALINE SULFATE
  CANTIL, MEPENZOLATE BROMIDE
  CEPHULAC, LACTULOSE
  CHRONULAC, LACTULOSE
  CLOMID, CLOMIPHENE CITRATE
  CYANOCOBALAMIN, CYANOCOBALAMIN
  DECAPRYN, DOXYLAMINE SUCCINATE
  DV, DIENESTROL
  HEDULIN, PHENINDIONE
  HIPREX, METHENAMINE HIPPURATE
  HYDROXYSTILBAMIDINE ISETHIONATE,
    HYDROXYSTILBAMIDINE ISETHIONATE
  LORELCO, PROBUCOL
  METAHYDRIN, TRICHLORMETHIAZIDE
  METATENSIN #2, RESERPINE
  METATENSIN #4, RESERPINE
  NICORETTE, NICOTINE POLACRILEX
  NICORETTE DS, NICOTINE POLACRILEX
  NORPRAMIN, DESIPRAMINE HYDROCHLORIDE
  ORNIDYL, EFLORNITHINE HYDROCHLORIDE
  RIFADIN, RIFAMPIN
  SELDANE, TERFENADINE
  SELDANE-D, PSEUDOEPHEDRINE HYDROCHLORIDE
  TACE, CHLOROTRIANISENE
  TENUATE, DIETHYLPROPION HYDROCHLORIDE
  TENUATE DOSPAN, DIETHYLPROPION
    HYDROCHLORIDE
  TRICLOS, TRICLOFOS SODIUM
  VANOBID, CANDICIDIN

MFG CHEMISTS
* MANUFACTURING CHEMISTS INC
  PHENDIMETRAZINE TARTRATE, PHENDIMETRAZINE
    TARTRATE

MIKART
* MIKART INC
  ACETAMINOPHEN AND CODEINE PHOSPHATE,
    ACETAMINOPHEN
  ACETAMINOPHEN AND CODEINE PHOSPHATE #3,
    ACETAMINOPHEN
  ACETAMINOPHEN AND CODEINE PHOSPHATE #4,
    ACETAMINOPHEN
  ACETAMINOPHEN, ASPIRIN, AND CODEINE
    PHOSPHATE, ACETAMINOPHEN
  ACETAMINOPHEN, BUTALBITAL, AND CAFFEINE,
    ACETAMINOPHEN
  BUTALBITAL, ACETAMINOPHEN AND CAFFEINE,
    ACETAMINOPHEN
  HYDROCODONE BITARTRATE AND
    ACETAMINOPHEN, ACETAMINOPHEN

PHENDIMETRAZINE TARTRATE, PHENDIMETRAZINE
  TARTRATE
PYRAZINAMIDE, PYRAZINAMIDE

MILES
* MILES PHARMACEUTICAL DIV MILES INC
  ADALAT, NIFEDIPINE
  ANTAGONATE, CHLORPHENIRAMINE MALEATE
  AZLIN, AZLOCILLIN SODIUM
  BILTRICIDE, PRAZIQUANTEL
  CANDEX, NYSTATIN
  CIPRO, CIPROFLOXACIN
  CIPRO, CIPROFLOXACIN HYDROCHLORIDE
  CIPRO IN DEXTROSE 5%, CIPROFLOXACIN
  CIPRO IN SODIUM CHLORIDE 0.9%, CIPROFLOXACIN
  CORT-DOME, HYDROCORTISONE
  DELTA-DOME, PREDNISONE
  DOMEBORO, ACETIC ACID, GLACIAL
  DTIC-DOME, DACARBAZINE
  HC #1, HYDROCORTISONE
  HC #4, HYDROCORTISONE
  LITHANE, LITHIUM CARBONATE
  MEZLIN, MEZLOCILLIN SODIUM MONOHYDRATE
  MYCELEX, CLOTRIMAZOLE
  MYCELEX, CLOTRIMAZOLE (OTC)
  MYCELEX-G, CLOTRIMAZOLE
  MYCELEX-7, CLOTRIMAZOLE (OTC)
  NEO-CORT-DOME, ACETIC ACID, GLACIAL
  NEO-CORT-DOME, HYDROCORTISONE
  NICLOCIDE, NICLOSAMIDE
  NIMOTOP, NIMODIPINE
  NYSTAFORM, CLIOQUINOL
  RADIO-IODINATED (I 125) SERUM ALBUMIN
    (HUMAN), ALBUMIN IODINATED I-125 SERUM
  SOY-DOME, HEXACHLOROPHENE
  STILPHOSTROL, DIETHYLSTILBESTROL
    DIPHOSPHATE
  TRIDESILON, ACETIC ACID, GLACIAL
  TRIDESILON, DESONIDE
  VI-DOM-A, VITAMIN A PALMITATE

MILEX
* MILEX PRODUCTS INC
  MILOPHENE, CLOMIPHENE CITRATE

MISSION PHARMA
* MISSION PHARMACAL CO
  CALCIBIND, CELLULOSE SODIUM PHOSPHATE
  EQUIPIN, HOMATROPINE METHYLBROMIDE
  FOLICET, FOLIC ACID
  HOMAPIN-10, HOMATROPINE METHYLBROMIDE
  HOMAPIN-5, HOMATROPINE METHYLBROMIDE
  LITHOSTAT, ACETOHYDROXAMIC ACID

MJ
* MJ PHARMACEUTICALS LTD
  CEPHALEXIN, CEPHALEXIN

MK
* MK LABORATORIES INC
  AMPHICOL, CHLORAMPHENICOL
  DIPHENHYDRAMINE HCL, DIPHENHYDRAMINE
    HYDROCHLORIDE
  FOLIC ACID, FOLIC ACID
  HYDROCORTISONE, HYDROCORTISONE
  ISONIAZID, ISONIAZID
  KESSO-GESIC, PROPOXYPHENE HYDROCHLORIDE
  MEPROBAMATE, MEPROBAMATE
  NIACIN, NIACIN
  OXY-KESSO-TETRA, OXYTETRACYCLINE
    HYDROCHLORIDE
  PREDNISONE, PREDNISONE

APPENDIX B
PRODUCT NAME INDEX
LISTED BY APPLICANT (continued)

RESERPINE, RESERPINE
SOSOL, SULFISOXAZOLE
TETRACYCLINE, TETRACYCLINE
TETRACYCLINE HCL, TETRACYCLINE
  HYDROCHLORIDE
VITAMIN A, VITAMIN A PALMITATE

MSD
* MERCK SHARP AND DOHME DIV MERCK AND CO INC
ALDOCLOR-150, CHLOROTHIAZIDE
ALDOCLOR-250, CHLOROTHIAZIDE
ALDOMET, METHYLDOPA
ALDOMET, METHYLDOPATE HYDROCHLORIDE
ALDORIL D30, HYDROCHLOROTHIAZIDE
ALDORIL D50, HYDROCHLOROTHIAZIDE
ALDORIL 15, HYDROCHLOROTHIAZIDE
ALDORIL 25, HYDROCHLOROTHIAZIDE
ALPHAREDISOL, HYDROXOCOBALAMIN
AMINOHIPPURATE SODIUM, AMINOHIPPURATE
  SODIUM
AQUAMEPHYTON, PHYTONADIONE
ARAMINE, METARAMINOL BITARTRATE
BENEMID, PROBENECID
BLOCADREN, TIMOLOL MALEATE
COGENTIN, BENZTROPINE MESYLATE
COLBENEMID, COLCHICINE
CORTONE, CORTISONE ACETATE
COSMEGEN, DACTINOMYCIN
CUPRIMINE, PENICILLAMINE
CYCLAINE, HEXYLCAINE HYDROCHLORIDE
DARANIDE, DICHLORPHENAMIDE
DECADERM, DEXAMETHASONE
DECADRON, DEXAMETHASONE
DECADRON, DEXAMETHASONE SODIUM PHOSPHATE
DECADRON W/ XYLOCAINE, DEXAMETHASONE
  SODIUM PHOSPHATE
DECASPRAY, DEXAMETHASONE
DEMSER, METYROSINE
DIUPRES-250, CHLOROTHIAZIDE
DIUPRES-500, CHLOROTHIAZIDE
DIURIL, CHLOROTHIAZIDE
DIURIL, CHLOROTHIAZIDE SODIUM
DOLOBID, DIFLUNISAL
EDECRIN, ETHACRYNATE SODIUM
EDECRIN, ETHACRYNIC ACID
ELAVIL, AMITRIPTYLINE HYDROCHLORIDE
FLEXERIL, CYCLOBENZAPRINE HYDROCHLORIDE
FLOROPRYL, ISOFLUROPHATE
HUMORSOL, DEMECARIUM BROMIDE
HYDELTRA-TBA, PREDNISOLONE TEBUTATE
HYDELTRASOL, PREDNISOLONE SODIUM PHOSPHATE
HYDROCORTONE, HYDROCORTISONE
HYDROCORTONE, HYDROCORTISONE ACETATE
HYDROCORTONE, HYDROCORTISONE SODIUM
  PHOSPHATE
HYDRODIURIL, HYDROCHLOROTHIAZIDE
HYDROPRES 25, HYDROCHLOROTHIAZIDE
HYDROPRES 50, HYDROCHLOROTHIAZIDE
INVERSINE, MECAMYLAMINE HYDROCHLORIDE
LERITINE, ANILERIDINE HYDROCHLORIDE
LERITINE, ANILERIDINE PHOSPHATE
LODOSYN, CARBIDOPA
MANNITOL 25%, MANNITOL
MEFOXIN, CEFOXITIN SODIUM
MEFOXIN IN DEXTROSE 5% IN PLASTIC CONTAINER,
  CEFOXITIN SODIU
MEFOXIN IN SODIUM CHLORIDE 0.9% IN PLASTIC
  CONTAINER, CEFOXITIN SODIUM
MEPHYTON, PHYTONADIONE
MIDAMOR, AMILORIDE HYDROCHLORIDE
MINTEZOL, THIABENDAZOLE

MODURETIC 5-50, AMILORIDE HYDROCHLORIDE
MUSTARGEN, MECHLORETHAMINE
  HYDROCHLORIDE
NEO-HYDELTRASOL, NEOMYCIN SULFATE
NEODECADRON, DEXAMETHASONE SODIUM
  PHOSPHATE
PERIACTIN, CYPROHEPTADINE HYDROCHLORIDE
PRIMAXIN, CILASTATIN SODIUM
PROSCAR, FINASTERIDE
REDISOL, CYANOCOBALAMIN
SINEMET, CARBIDOPA
SINEMET CR, CARBIDOPA
SYPRINE, TRIENTINE HYDROCHLORIDE
TECHNESCAN GLUCEPTATE, TECHNETIUM TC-99M
  GLUCEPTATE KIT
TECHNESCAN MDP KIT, TECHNETIUM TC-99M
  MEDRONATE KIT
TECHNETIUM TC 99M ALBUMIN AGGREGATED KIT,
  TECHNETIUM TC-99M ALBUMIN AGGREGATED KIT
TIMOLIDE 10-25, HYDROCHLOROTHIAZIDE
TONOCARD, TOCAINIDE HYDROCHLORIDE
TRIAVIL 2-10, AMITRIPTYLINE HYDROCHLORIDE
TRIAVIL 2-25, AMITRIPTYLINE HYDROCHLORIDE
TRIAVIL 4-10, AMITRIPTYLINE HYDROCHLORIDE
TRIAVIL 4-25, AMITRIPTYLINE HYDROCHLORIDE
TRIAVIL 4-50, AMITRIPTYLINE HYDROCHLORIDE
URECHOLINE, BETHANECHOL CHLORIDE
VIVACTIL, PROTRIPTYLINE HYDROCHLORIDE

MURO
* MURO PHARMACEUTICAL INC
BROMFED-DM, BROMPHENIRAMINE MALEATE
LIQUID PRED, PREDNISONE
PRELONE, PREDNISOLONE
PROMETA, METAPROTERENOL SULFATE

MUTUAL PHARM
* MUTUAL PHARMACEUTICAL CO INC
ACETAMINOPHEN AND CODEINE PHOSPHATE,
  ACETAMINOPHEN
ACETAZOLAMIDE, ACETAZOLAMIDE
ALBUTEROL SULFATE, ALBUTEROL SULFATE
ALLOPURINOL, ALLOPURINOL
AMITRIPTYLINE HCL, AMITRIPTYLINE
  HYDROCHLORIDE
BENZTROPINE MESYLATE, BENZTROPINE MESYLATE
CARISOPRODOL, CARISOPRODOL
CHLORTHALIDONE, CHLORTHALIDONE
CHLORZOXAZONE, CHLORZOXAZONE
DIPHENHYDRAMINE HCL, DIPHENHYDRAMINE
  HYDROCHLORIDE
DOXYCYCLINE HYCLATE, DOXYCYCLINE HYCLATE
ERGOLOID MESYLATES, ERGOLOID MESYLATES
FENOPROFEN CALCIUM, FENOPROFEN CALCIUM
HYDRALAZINE HCL, HYDRALAZINE
  HYDROCHLORIDE
HYDROXYZINE HCL, HYDROXYZINE
  HYDROCHLORIDE
IBUPROFEN, IBUPROFEN
IBUPROFEN, IBUPROFEN (OTC)
IMIPRAMINE HCL, IMIPRAMINE HYDROCHLORIDE
INDOMETHACIN, INDOMETHACIN
LORAZEPAM, LORAZEPAM
METRONIDAZOLE, METRONIDAZOLE
NYSTATIN, NYSTATIN
PREDNISONE, PREDNISONE
QUINIDINE GLUCONATE, QUINIDINE GLUCONATE
QUINIDINE SULFATE, QUINIDINE SULFATE
SPIRONOLACTONE, SPIRONOLACTONE
SPIRONOLACTONE AND HYDROCHLOROTHIAZIDE,
  HYDROCHLOROTHIAZIDE

APPENDIX B
PRODUCT NAME INDEX
LISTED BY APPLICANT *(continued)*

SULFAMETHOXAZOLE AND TRIMETHOPRIM,
   SULFAMETHOXAZOLE
SULFASALAZINE, SULFASALAZINE
SULINDAC, SULINDAC
THIORIDAZINE HCL, THIORIDAZINE
   HYDROCHLORIDE
TOLAZAMIDE, TOLAZAMIDE
TOLMETIN SODIUM, TOLMETIN SODIUM
VERAPAMIL HCL, VERAPAMIL HYDROCHLORIDE

MYLAN
* MYLAN PHARMACEUTICALS INC
   ALBUTEROL SULFATE, ALBUTEROL SULFATE
   ALLOPURINOL, ALLOPURINOL
   AMILORIDE HCL AND HYDROCHLOROTHIAZIDE,
      AMILORIDE HYDROCHLORIDE
   AMITRIPTYLINE HCL, AMITRIPTYLINE
      HYDROCHLORIDE
   AMOXICILLIN, AMOXICILLIN
   AMPICILLIN TRIHYDRATE, AMPICILLIN/AMPICILLIN
      TRIHYDRATE
   ATENOLOL, ATENOLOL
   CHLORDIAZEPOXIDE AND AMITRIPTYLINE HCL,
      AMITRIPTYLINE HYDROCHLORIDE
   CHLORDIAZEPOXIDE HCL, CHLORDIAZEPOXIDE
      HYDROCHLORIDE
   CHLOROTHIAZIDE, CHLOROTHIAZIDE
   CHLOROTHIAZIDE-RESERPINE, CHLOROTHIAZIDE
   CHLORPROPAMIDE, CHLORPROPAMIDE
   CHLORTHALIDONE, CHLORTHALIDONE
   CLONIDINE HCL, CLONIDINE HYDROCHLORIDE
   CLONIDINE HCL AND CHLORTHALIDONE,
      CHLORTHALIDONE
   CLORAZEPATE DIPOTASSIUM, CLORAZEPATE
      DIPOTASSIUM
   CYCLOBENZAPRINE HCL, CYCLOBENZAPRINE
      HYDROCHLORIDE
   CYPROHEPTADINE HCL, CYPROHEPTADINE
      HYDROCHLORIDE
   DIAZEPAM, DIAZEPAM
   DIPHENOXYLATE HCL AND ATROPINE SULFATE,
      ATROPINE SULFATE
   DISOPYRAMIDE PHOSPHATE, DISOPYRAMIDE
      PHOSPHATE
   DOXEPIN HCL, DOXEPIN HYDROCHLORIDE
   DOXYCYCLINE HYCLATE, DOXYCYCLINE HYCLATE
   ERYTHROMYCIN ETHYLSUCCINATE,
      ERYTHROMYCIN ETHYLSUCCINATE
   ERYTHROMYCIN STEARATE, ERYTHROMYCIN
      STEARATE
   FENOPROFEN CALCIUM, FENOPROFEN CALCIUM
   FLUPHENAZINE HCL, FLUPHENAZINE
      HYDROCHLORIDE
   FLURAZEPAM HCL, FLURAZEPAM HYDROCHLORIDE
   FUROSEMIDE, FUROSEMIDE
   HALOPERIDOL, HALOPERIDOL
   HYDRALAZINE HCL-HYDROCHLOROTHIAZIDE-
      RESERPINE, HYDRALAZINE HYDROCHLORIDE
   HYDROCHLOROTHIAZIDE, HYDROCHLOROTHIAZIDE
   IBUPROFEN, IBUPROFEN
   IBUPROFEN, IBUPROFEN (OTC)
   INDOMETHACIN, INDOMETHACIN
   LOPERAMIDE HCL, LOPERAMIDE HYDROCHLORIDE
   LORAZEPAM, LORAZEPAM
   MAPROTILINE HCL, MAPROTILINE HYDROCHLORIDE
   MAXZIDE, HYDROCHLOROTHIAZIDE
   MAXZIDE-25, HYDROCHLOROTHIAZIDE
   MECLOFENAMATE SODIUM, MECLOFENAMATE
      SODIUM
   MEPROBAMATE, MEPROBAMATE
   METHOCARBAMOL, METHOCARBAMOL

   METHOTREXATE, METHOTREXATE SODIUM
   METHYCLOTHIAZIDE, METHYCLOTHIAZIDE
   METHYLDOPA, METHYLDOPA
   METHYLDOPA AND HYDROCHLOROTHIAZIDE,
      HYDROCHLOROTHIAZIDE
   OXAZEPAM, OXAZEPAM
   PENICILLIN G POTASSIUM, PENICILLIN G
      POTASSIUM
   PENICILLIN V POTASSIUM, PENICILLIN V
      POTASSIUM
   PERPHENAZINE AND AMITRIPTYLINE HCL,
      AMITRIPTYLINE HYDROCHLORIDE
   PIROXICAM, PIROXICAM
   PRAZOSIN HCL, PRAZOSIN HYDROCHLORIDE
   PROBENECID, PROBENECID
   PROPANTHELINE BROMIDE, PROPANTHELINE
      BROMIDE
   PROPOXYPHENE HCL, PROPOXYPHENE
      HYDROCHLORIDE
   PROPOXYPHENE HCL AND ACETAMINOPHEN,
      ACETAMINOPHEN
   PROPOXYPHENE NAPSYLATE AND ACETAMINOPHEN,
      ACETAMINOPHEN
   PROPRANOLOL HCL, PROPRANOLOL
      HYDROCHLORIDE
   PROPRANOLOL HCL AND HYDROCHLOROTHIAZIDE,
      HYDROCHLOROTHIAZIDE
   RESERPINE, RESERPINE
   SPIRONOLACTONE, SPIRONOLACTONE
   SPIRONOLACTONE AND HYDROCHLOROTHIAZIDE,
      HYDROCHLOROTHIAZIDE
   TEMAZEPAM, TEMAZEPAM
   TETRACYCLINE HCL, TETRACYCLINE
      HYDROCHLORIDE
   THIORIDAZINE HCL, THIORIDAZINE
      HYDROCHLORIDE
   THIOTHIXENE, THIOTHIXENE
   TIMOLOL MALEATE, TIMOLOL MALEATE
   TOLAZAMIDE, TOLAZAMIDE
   TOLBUTAMIDE, TOLBUTAMIDE
   TRAZODONE HCL, TRAZODONE HYDROCHLORIDE
   TRIAMCINOLONE, TRIAMCINOLONE
   VERAPAMIL HCL, VERAPAMIL HYDROCHLORIDE

N

NASKA
* NASKA PHARMACAL CO INC
   BACITRACIN, BACITRACIN (OTC)
   BACITRACIN ZINC-NEOMYCIN SULFATE-POLYMYXIN
      B SULFATE, BACITRACIN ZINC (OTC)
   BACITRACIN ZINC-POLYMYXIN B SULFATE,
      BACITRACIN ZINC (OTC)
   CYPROHEPTADINE HCL, CYPROHEPTADINE
      HYDROCHLORIDE
   DEXAMETHASONE, DEXAMETHASONE
   DIPHENHYDRAMINE HCL, DIPHENHYDRAMINE
      HYDROCHLORIDE (OTC)
   DIPHENHYDRAMINE HCL, DIPHENHYDRAMINE
      HYDROCHLORIDE
   ERYTHROMYCIN, ERYTHROMYCIN
   ERYTHROMYCIN ETHYLSUCCINATE,
      ERYTHROMYCIN ETHYLSUCCINATE
   HYDROCORTISONE, HYDROCORTISONE
   HYDROXYZINE HCL, HYDROXYZINE
      HYDROCHLORIDE
   NYSTATIN, NYSTATIN
   NYSTATIN AND TRIAMCINOLONE ACETONIDE,
      NYSTATIN

APPENDIX B
PRODUCT NAME INDEX
LISTED BY APPLICANT *(continued)*

THEOPHYLLINE, THEOPHYLLINE
TRIAMCINOLONE ACETONIDE, TRIAMCINOLONE
   ACETONIDE
TRIMETH/SULFA, SULFAMETHOXAZOLE

NEPHRON
* NEPHRON CORP
   BETA-2, ISOETHARINE HYDROCHLORIDE

NEWTRON
* NEWTRON PHARMACEUTICALS INC
   BROMPHENIRAMINE MALEATE, BROMPHENIRAMINE
     MALEATE
   CHLORPHENIRAMINE MALEATE,
     CHLORPHENIRAMINE MALEATE
   DIPHENHYDRAMINE HCL, DIPHENHYDRAMINE
     HYDROCHLORIDE
   TRILITRON, PSEUDOEPHEDRINE HYDROCHLORIDE

NMC
* NMC LABORATORIES INC
   BETAMETHASONE DIPROPIONATE, BETAMETHASONE
     DIPROPIONATE
   FLUOCET, FLUOCINOLONE ACETONIDE
   FLUOCINOLONE ACETONIDE, FLUOCINOLONE
     ACETONIDE
   FLUOCINONIDE, FLUOCINONIDE
   GENTAMICIN SULFATE, GENTAMICIN SULFATE
   HYDROCORTISONE, HYDROCORTISONE
   HYMAC, HYDROCORTISONE
   MYKACET, NYSTATIN
   MYKINAC, NYSTATIN
   TRIAMCINOLONE ACETONIDE, TRIAMCINOLONE
     ACETONIDE
   TRIPLE SULFA, TRIPLE SULFA
     (SULFABENZAMIDE; SULFACETAMIDE; SULFATHIAZOLE)
   VALNAC, BETAMETHASONE VALERATE

NOVO NORDISK
* NOVO NORDISK PHARMACEUTICALS INC
   INSULATARD NPH HUMAN, INSULIN SUSP ISOPHANE
     SEMISYNTHETIC PURIFIED HUMAN (OTC)
   INSULIN, INSULIN PORK (OTC)
   INSULIN INSULATARD NPH NORDISK, INSULIN SUSP
     ISOPHANE PURIFIED PORK (OTC)
   INSULIN NORDISK MIXTARD (PORK), INSULIN
     PURIFIED PORK (OTC)
   LENTARD, INSULIN ZINC SUSP PURIFIED BEEF/PORK
     (OTC)
   LENTE, INSULIN ZINC SUSP PURIFIED PORK (OTC)
   LENTE INSULIN, INSULIN ZINC SUSP BEEF (OTC)
   MIXTARD HUMAN 70/30, INSULIN SEMISYNTHETIC
     PURIFIED HUMAN (OTC)
   NOVOLIN L, INSULIN ZINC SUSP BIOSYNTHETIC
     HUMAN (OTC)
   NOVOLIN L, INSULIN ZINC SUSP SEMISYNTHETIC
     PURIFIED HUMAN (OTC)
   NOVOLIN N, INSULIN SUSP ISOPHANE
     SEMISYNTHETIC PURIFIED HUMAN (OTC)
   NOVOLIN N, INSULIN SUSP ISOPHANE
     BIOSYNTHETIC HUMAN (OTC)
   NOVOLIN R, INSULIN BIOSYNTHETIC HUMAN (OTC)
   NOVOLIN R, INSULIN SEMISYNTHETIC PURIFIED
     HUMAN (OTC)
   NOVOLIN 70/30, INSULIN BIOSYNTHETIC HUMAN
     (OTC)
   NOVOLIN 70/30, INSULIN SEMISYNTHETIC PURIFIED
     HUMAN (OTC)
   NPH INSULIN, INSULIN SUSP ISOPHANE BEEF (OTC)
   NPH PURIFIED PORK ISOPHANE INSULIN, INSULIN
     SUSP ISOPHANE PURIFIED PORK (OTC)
   REGULAR PURIFIED PORK INSULIN, INSULIN
     PURIFIED PORK (OTC)

SEMILENTE, INSULIN ZINC SUSP PROMPT PURIFIED
   PORK (OTC)
SEMILENTE INSULIN, INSULIN ZINC SUSP PROMPT
   BEEF (OTC)
ULTRALENTE, INSULIN ZINC SUSP EXTENDED
   PURIFIED BEEF (OTC)
ULTRALENTE INSULIN, INSULIN ZINC SUSP
   EXTENDED BEEF (OTC)
VELOSULIN, INSULIN PURIFIED PORK (OTC)
VELOSULIN HUMAN, INSULIN SEMISYNTHETIC
   PURIFIED HUMAN (OTC)

NOVOCOL
* NOVOCOL PHARMACEUTICAL INC
   ISOCAINE HCL, MEPIVACAINE HYDROCHLORIDE
   ISOCAINE HCL W/ LEVONORDEFRIN,
     LEVONORDEFRIN
   OCTOCAINE, EPINEPHRINE

NOVOPHARM
* NOVOPHARM LTD
   AMOXICILLIN, AMOXICILLIN
   CEPHALEXIN, CEPHALEXIN
   CLOFIBRATE, CLOFIBRATE
   CLOXACILLIN SODIUM, CLOXACILLIN SODIUM
   INDOMETHACIN, INDOMETHACIN
   LOPERAMIDE HCL, LOPERAMIDE HYDROCHLORIDE
   METHYLDOPA, METHYLDOPA
   METHYLDOPA AND HYDROCHLOROTHIAZIDE,
     HYDROCHLOROTHIAZIDE
   NIFEDIPINE, NIFEDIPINE
   TOLMETIN SODIUM, TOLMETIN SODIUM

O

OCLASSEN
* OCLASSEN PHARMACEUTICALS INC
   CONDYLOX, PODOFILOX

OHM
* OHM LABORATORIES INC
   IBUPROFEN, IBUPROFEN
   IBUPROFEN, IBUPROFEN (OTC)
   IBUPROHM, IBUPROFEN

OPTOPICS
* OPTOPICS LABORATORIES CORP
   OCUSULF-10, SULFACETAMIDE SODIUM
   OCUSULF-30, SULFACETAMIDE SODIUM
   OPTOMYCIN, CHLORAMPHENICOL
   PARACAINE, PROPARACAINE HYDROCHLORIDE
   SULFACEL-15, SULFACETAMIDE SODIUM
   TROPICAMIDE, TROPICAMIDE

ORGANICS
* ORGANICS DIV LA GRANGE INC
   CORTICOTROPIN, CORTICOTROPIN

ORGANON
* ORGANON INC SUB AKZONA INC
   ARDUAN, PIPECURONIUM BROMIDE
   CORTROPHIN-ZINC, CORTICOTROPIN-ZINC
     HYDROXIDE
   CORTROSYN, COSYNTROPIN
   DECA-DURABOLIN, NANDROLONE DECANOATE
   DOCA, DESOXYCORTICOSTERONE ACETATE
   DURABOLIN, NANDROLONE PHENPROPIONATE
   DURABOLIN-50, NANDROLONE PHENPROPIONATE
   FUROSEMIDE, FUROSEMIDE
   HEPARIN SODIUM, HEPARIN SODIUM

APPENDIX B
PRODUCT NAME INDEX
LISTED BY APPLICANT (continued)

HEXADROL, DEXAMETHASONE
HEXADROL, DEXAMETHASONE SODIUM PHOSPHATE
LIQUAEMIN LOCK FLUSH, HEPARIN SODIUM
LIQUAEMIN SODIUM, HEPARIN SODIUM
LIQUAEMIN SODIUM PRESERVATIVE FREE, HEPARIN
    SODIUM
LIQUAMAR, PHENPROCOUMON
LYNORAL, ETHINYL ESTRADIOL
MAXIBOLIN, ETHYLESTRENOL
METHYLPREDNISOLONE, METHYLPREDNISOLONE
    SODIUM SUCCINATE
NORCURON, VECURONIUM BROMIDE
ORGATRAX, HYDROXYZINE HYDROCHLORIDE
PAVULON, PANCURONIUM BROMIDE
PREGNYL, GONADOTROPIN, CHORIONIC
PURIFIED CORTROPHIN GEL, CORTICOTROPIN
REGONOL, PYRIDOSTIGMINE BROMIDE
REVERSOL, EDROPHONIUM CHLORIDE
SUCCINYLCHOLINE CHLORIDE, SUCCINYLCHOLINE
    CHLORIDE
WIGRAINE, CAFFEINE
WIGRETTES, ERGOTAMINE TARTRATE

OWEN GALDERMA
* OWEN GALDERMA LABORATORIES INC
    CETACORT, HYDROCORTISONE
    CROTAN, CROTAMITON
    DESOWEN, DESONIDE
    LOCOID, HYDROCORTISONE BUTYRATE
    NUTRACORT, HYDROCORTISONE
    SANSAC, ERYTHROMYCIN

P

P AND G
* PROCTER AND GAMBLE CO
    HEAD & SHOULDERS CONDITIONER, PYRITHIONE
      ZINC (OTC)
    PERIDEX, CHLORHEXIDINE GLUCONATE
* PROCTER AND GAMBLE PHARMACEUTICALS INC SUB
PROCTER AND GAM
    ASACOL, MESALAMINE
    DANTRIUM, DANTROLENE SODIUM
    DIDRONEL, ETIDRONATE DISODIUM
    FURADANTIN, NITROFURANTOIN
    IVADANTIN, NITROFURANTOIN SODIUM
    LABID, THEOPHYLLINE
    MACROBID, NITROFURANTOIN
    MACRODANTIN, NITROFURANTOIN,
      MACROCRYSTALLINE
    NYSERT, NYSTATIN
    ORLEX, ACETIC ACID, GLACIAL
    ORLEX HC, ACETIC ACID, GLACIAL
    SARENIN, SARALASIN ACETATE

PACO
* PACO PHARMACEUTICAL SERVICES INC
    LACTULOSE, LACTULOSE
* PACO RESEARCH CORP
    GENTAMICIN SULFATE, GENTAMICIN SULFATE
    LIDOCAINE HCL, LIDOCAINE HYDROCHLORIDE
    METAPROTERENOL SULFATE, METAPROTERENOL
      SULFATE
    METOCLOPRAMIDE HCL, METOCLOPRAMIDE
      HYDROCHLORIDE
    THIOTHIXENE HCL, THIOTHIXENE HYDROCHLORIDE

PADDOCK
* PADDOCK LABORATORIES
    BACITRACIN, BACITRACIN
    ERYTHROMYCIN, ERYTHROMYCIN

ETS-2%, ERYTHROMYCIN
HYDROCORTISONE, HYDROCORTISONE
NEOMYCIN SULFATE, NEOMYCIN SULFATE
NYSTATIN, NYSTATIN
POLYMIXIN B SULFATE, POLYMYXIN B SULFATE

PAL PAK
* PAL PAK INC
    AMINOPHYLLINE, AMINOPHYLLINE

PANRAY
* PANRAY CORP SUB ORMONT DRUG AND CHEMICAL CO
INC
    AMINOPHYLLINE, AMINOPHYLLINE
    CHLORPHENIRAMINE MALEATE,
      CHLORPHENIRAMINE MALEATE
    CINNASIL, RESCINNAMINE
    CORTISONE ACETATE, CORTISONE ACETATE
    HYDROCORTISONE, HYDROCORTISONE
    ISONIAZID, ISONIAZID
    KOGLUCOID, RAUWOLFIA SERPENTINA
    PARASAL, AMINOSALICYLIC ACID
    PARASAL SODIUM, AMINOSALICYLATE SODIUM
    PREDNISOLONE, PREDNISOLONE
    PREDNISONE, PREDNISONE
    PROCAPAN, PROCAINAMIDE HYDROCHLORIDE
    SERPANRAY, RESERPINE
    THEOLIXIR, THEOPHYLLINE

PAR
* PAR PHARMACEUTICAL INC
    ALLOPURINOL, ALLOPURINOL
    AMILORIDE HCL, AMILORIDE HYDROCHLORIDE
    AMITRIPTYLINE HCL, AMITRIPTYLINE
      HYDROCHLORIDE
    BENZTROPINE MESYLATE, BENZTROPINE MESYLATE
    BROMPHENIRAMINE MALEATE, BROMPHENIRAMINE
      MALEATE
    CARISOPRODOL AND ASPIRIN, ASPIRIN
    CHLORDIAZEPOXIDE AND AMITRIPTYLINE HCL,
      AMITRIPTYLINE HYDROCHLORIDE
    CHLORPROPAMIDE, CHLORPROPAMIDE
    CHLORZOXAZONE, CHLORZOXAZONE
    CLONIDINE HCL, CLONIDINE HYDROCHLORIDE
    CLONIDINE HCL AND CHLORTHALIDONE,
      CHLORTHALIDONE
    CYPROHEPTADINE HCL, CYPROHEPTADINE
      HYDROCHLORIDE
    DEXAMETHASONE, DEXAMETHASONE
    DIAZEPAM, DIAZEPAM
    DISULFIRAM, DISULFIRAM
    DOXEPIN HCL, DOXEPIN HYDROCHLORIDE
    DOXY-SLEEP-AID, DOXYLAMINE SUCCINATE (OTC)
    DOXYCYCLINE HYCLATE, DOXYCYCLINE HYCLATE
    FENOPROFEN CALCIUM, FENOPROFEN CALCIUM
    FLUPHENAZINE HCL, FLUPHENAZINE
      HYDROCHLORIDE
    FLURAZEPAM HCL, FLURAZEPAM HYDROCHLORIDE
    HALOPERIDOL, HALOPERIDOL
    HYDRA-ZIDE, HYDRALAZINE HYDROCHLORIDE
    HYDRALAZINE HCL, HYDRALAZINE
      HYDROCHLORIDE
    HYDRO-RIDE, AMILORIDE HYDROCHLORIDE
    HYDROFLUMETHIAZIDE, HYDROFLUMETHIAZIDE
    HYDROXYZINE HCL, HYDROXYZINE
      HYDROCHLORIDE
    HYDROXYZINE PAMOATE, HYDROXYZINE PAMOATE
    IBUPROFEN, IBUPROFEN
    IBUPROFEN, IBUPROFEN (OTC)
    IMIPRAMINE HCL, IMIPRAMINE HYDROCHLORIDE
    INDOMETHACIN, INDOMETHACIN
    ISOSORBIDE DINITRATE, ISOSORBIDE DINITRATE

APPENDIX B
PRODUCT NAME INDEX
LISTED BY APPLICANT (continued)

LEUCOVORIN CALCIUM, LEUCOVORIN CALCIUM
LORAZEPAM, LORAZEPAM
MECLIZINE HCL, MECLIZINE HYDROCHLORIDE
MECLOFENAMATE SODIUM, MECLOFENAMATE
  SODIUM
MEGESTROL ACETATE, MEGESTROL ACETATE
MEPROBAMATE AND ASPIRIN, ASPIRIN
METAPROTERENOL SULFATE, METAPROTERENOL
  SULFATE
METHOCARBAMOL, METHOCARBAMOL
METHOCARBAMOL AND ASPIRIN, ASPIRIN
METHYCLOTHIAZIDE, METHYCLOTHIAZIDE
METHYLDOPA, METHYLDOPA
METHYLDOPA AND CHLOROTHIAZIDE,
  CHLOROTHIAZIDE
METHYLDOPA AND HYDROCHLOROTHIAZIDE,
  HYDROCHLOROTHIAZIDE
METHYLPREDNISOLONE, METHYLPREDNISOLONE
METOCLOPRAMIDE HCL, METOCLOPRAMIDE
  HYDROCHLORIDE
METRONIDAZOLE, METRONIDAZOLE
MINOXIDIL, MINOXIDIL
NYSTATIN, NYSTATIN
ORPHENGESIC, ASPIRIN
ORPHENGESIC FORTE, ASPIRIN
PERPHENAZINE AND AMITRIPTYLINE HCL,
  AMITRIPTYLINE HYDROCHLORIDE
PROPANTHELINE BROMIDE, PROPANTHELINE
  BROMIDE
PROPRANOLOL HCL, PROPRANOLOL
  HYDROCHLORIDE
RESERPINE AND HYDROFLUMETHIAZIDE,
  HYDROFLUMETHIAZIDE
SULFAMETHOPRIM, SULFAMETHOXAZOLE
SULFAMETHOPRIM-DS, SULFAMETHOXAZOLE
SULFINPYRAZONE, SULFINPYRAZONE
TEMAZEPAM, TEMAZEPAM
THIORIDAZINE HCL, THIORIDAZINE
  HYDROCHLORIDE
TOLAZAMIDE, TOLAZAMIDE
TRIAMTERENE AND HYDROCHLOROTHIAZIDE,
  HYDROCHLOROTHIAZIDE
TRICHLORMETHIAZIDE, TRICHLORMETHIAZIDE
VALPROIC ACID, VALPROIC ACID

PARKE DAVIS
* PARKE DAVIS DIV WARNER LAMBERT CO
ACETAMINOPHEN AND CODEINE PHOSPHATE,
  ACETAMINOPHEN
ACTH, CORTICOTROPIN
AMBODRYL, BROMODIPHENHYDRAMINE
  HYDROCHLORIDE
AMCILL, AMPICILLIN/AMPICILLIN TRIHYDRATE
ANUSOL HC, HYDROCORTISONE
BENADRYL, DIPHENHYDRAMINE HYDROCHLORIDE
BENYLIN, DIPHENHYDRAMINE HYDROCHLORIDE
  (OTC)
CAMOQUIN HCL, AMODIAQUINE HYDROCHLORIDE
CELONTIN, METHSUXIMIDE
CENTRAX, PRAZEPAM
CHLORDIAZEPOXIDE HCL, CHLORDIAZEPOXIDE
  HYDROCHLORIDE
CHLOROMYCETIN, CHLORAMPHENICOL
CHLOROMYCETIN, CHLORAMPHENICOL SODIUM
  SUCCINATE
CHLOROMYCETIN HYDROCORTISONE,
  CHLORAMPHENICOL
CHLOROMYCETIN PALMITATE, CHLORAMPHENICOL
  PALMITATE
CHLOROMYXIN, CHLORAMPHENICOL
CHOLEDYL, OXTRIPHYLLINE

CHOLEDYL SA, OXTRIPHYLLINE
CHOLYBAR, CHOLESTYRAMINE
COLY-MYCIN M, COLISTIMETHATE SODIUM
COLY-MYCIN S, COLISTIN SULFATE
DIAZEPAM, DIAZEPAM
DILANTIN, PHENYTOIN
DILANTIN, PHENYTOIN SODIUM
DILANTIN, PHENYTOIN SODIUM, EXTENDED
DILANTIN-125, PHENYTOIN
DILANTIN-30, PHENYTOIN
DIPHENOXYLATE HCL AND ATROPINE SULFATE,
  ATROPINE SULFATE
DORYX, DOXYCYCLINE HYCLATE
DURAQUIN, QUINIDINE GLUCONATE
ELASE-CHLOROMYCETIN, CHLORAMPHENICOL
ERGOSTAT, ERGOTAMINE TARTRATE
ERYC, ERYTHROMYCIN
ERYC 125, ERYTHROMYCIN
ERYPAR, ERYTHROMYCIN STEARATE
ERYTHROMYCIN ETHYLSUCCINATE,
  ERYTHROMYCIN ETHYLSUCCINATE
ESTROVIS, QUINESTROL
EUTHROID-0.5, LIOTRIX (T4; T3)
EUTHROID-1, LIOTRIX (T4; T3)
EUTHROID-2, LIOTRIX (T4; T3)
EUTHROID-3, LIOTRIX (T4; T3)
FUROSEMIDE, FUROSEMIDE
HEPARIN LOCK FLUSH, HEPARIN SODIUM
HEPARIN SODIUM, HEPARIN SODIUM
HUMATIN, PAROMOMYCIN SULFATE
HYDROCORTISONE, HYDROCORTISONE
HYDROCORTISONE ACETATE, HYDROCORTISONE
  ACETATE
INDOMETHACIN, INDOMETHACIN
ISOETHARINE HCL, ISOETHARINE HYDROCHLORIDE
ISOPROTERENOL HCL, ISOPROTERENOL
  HYDROCHLORIDE
KETALAR, KETAMINE HYDROCHLORIDE
LOESTRIN FE 1.5/30, ETHINYL ESTRADIOL
LOESTRIN FE 1/20, ETHINYL ESTRADIOL
LOESTRIN 21 1.5/30, ETHINYL ESTRADIOL
LOESTRIN 21 1/20, ETHINYL ESTRADIOL
LOPID, GEMFIBROZIL
MECLOMEN, MECLOFENAMATE SODIUM
MEPERIDINE HCL, MEPERIDINE HYDROCHLORIDE
MEPROBAMATE, MEPROBAMATE
METHYLDOPA, METHYLDOPA
METHYLDOPA AND HYDROCHLOROTHIAZIDE,
  HYDROCHLOROTHIAZIDE
METHYLTESTOSTERONE, METHYLTESTOSTERONE
MILONTIN, PHENSUXIMIDE
NARDIL, PHENELZINE SULFATE
NITROSTAT, NITROGLYCERIN
OPHTHOCHLOR, CHLORAMPHENICOL
OPHTHOCORT, CHLORAMPHENICOL
OXAZEPAM, OXAZEPAM
PARACORT, PREDNISONE
PARSIDOL, ETHOPROPAZINE HYDROCHLORIDE
PENAPAR-VK, PENICILLIN V POTASSIUM
PENICILLIN G POTASSIUM, PENICILLIN G
  POTASSIUM
PENICILLIN G PROCAINE, PENICILLIN G PROCAINE
PITOCIN, OXYTOCIN
PITRESSIN TANNATE, VASOPRESSIN TANNATE
POVAN, PYRVINIUM PAMOATE
PRE-SATE, CHLORPHENTERMINE HYDROCHLORIDE
PROCAN, PROCAINAMIDE HYDROCHLORIDE
PROCAN SR, PROCAINAMIDE HYDROCHLORIDE
PROLOID, THYROGLOBULIN
PROMAPAR, CHLORPROMAZINE HYDROCHLORIDE

APPENDIX B
PRODUCT NAME INDEX
LISTED BY APPLICANT (continued)

PROPRANOLOL HCL, PROPRANOLOL
   HYDROCHLORIDE
QUINIDINE SULFATE, QUINIDINE SULFATE
SECOBARBITAL SODIUM, SECOBARBITAL SODIUM
SODIUM PENTOBARBITAL, PENTOBARBITAL SODIUM
SPIRONOLACTONE W/ HYDROCHLOROTHIAZIDE,
   HYDROCHLOROTHIAZIDE
SULFALAR, SULFISOXAZOLE
SURITAL, THIAMYLAL SODIUM
SYTOBEX, CYANOCOBALAMIN
THEELIN, ESTRONE
THIAMINE HCL, THIAMINE HYDROCHLORIDE
TOLBUTAMIDE, TOLBUTAMIDE
TRIPELENNAMINE HCL, TRIPELENNAMINE
   HYDROCHLORIDE
UTICORT, BETAMETHASONE BENZOATE
UTIMOX, AMOXICILLIN
VERAPAMIL HCL, VERAPAMIL HYDROCHLORIDE
VIRA-A, VIDARABINE
ZARONTIN, ETHOSUXIMIDE
* PARKE DAVIS DIV WARNER LAMBERT INC
   NORLUTATE, NORETHINDRONE ACETATE
   NORLUTIN, NORETHINDRONE
   PONSTEL, MEFENAMIC ACID
* PARKE DAVIS LABORATORIES DIV WARNER LAMBERT
CO
   NORLESTRIN FE 1/50, ETHINYL ESTRADIOL
   NORLESTRIN FE 2.5/50, ETHINYL ESTRADIOL
   NORLESTRIN 21 1/50, ETHINYL ESTRADIOL
   NORLESTRIN 21 2.5/50, ETHINYL ESTRADIOL
   NORLESTRIN 28 1/50, ETHINYL ESTRADIOL
* PARKE DAVIS PHARMACEUTICAL RESEARCH DIV
WARNER LAMBERT CO
   ACCUPRIL, QUINAPRIL HYDROCHLORIDE
   NIPENT, PENTOSTATIN
   PENETREX, ENOXACIN

PARNELL
* PARNELL PHARMACEUTICALS INC
   TRIAMCINOLONE ACETONIDE, TRIAMCINOLONE
     ACETONIDE

PENNEX
* PENNEX PRODUCTS CO INC
   ALUMINUM HYDROXIDE AND MAGNESIUM
     TRISILICATE, ALUMINUM HYDROXIDE (OTC)

PERRIGO
* L PERRIGO CO
   ANTITUSSIVE, DIPHENHYDRAMINE
     HYDROCHLORIDE (OTC)
   CAP-PROFEN, IBUPROFEN (OTC)
   DIPHENHYDRAMINE HCL, DIPHENHYDRAMINE
     HYDROCHLORIDE
   IBUPROFEN, IBUPROFEN (OTC)
   ISONIAZID, ISONIAZID
   LOPERAMIDE HCL, LOPERAMIDE HYDROCHLORIDE
     (OTC)
   MEPROBAMATE, MEPROBAMATE
   PREDNISOLONE, PREDNISOLONE
   PREDNISONE, PREDNISONE
   PROPYLTHIOURACIL, PROPYLTHIOURACIL
   QUINIDINE SULFATE, QUINIDINE SULFATE
   SODIUM PENTOBARBITAL, PENTOBARBITAL SODIUM
   SODIUM SECOBARBITAL, SECOBARBITAL SODIUM
   TAB-PROFEN, IBUPROFEN (OTC)
   THEOPHYLLINE, THEOPHYLLINE

PFIPHARMECS
* PFIPHARMECS DIV PFIZER INC
   CORTRIL, HYDROCORTISONE
   TETRACYN, TETRACYCLINE
   TETRACYN, TETRACYCLINE HYDROCHLORIDE

PFIZER
* PFIZER CENTRAL RESEARCH
   DIFLUCAN, FLUCONAZOLE
   NORVASC, AMLODIPINE BESYLATE
   ZITHROMAX, AZITHROMYCIN DIHYDRATE
   ZOLOFT, SERTRALINE HYDROCHLORIDE
* PFIZER INC
   MINIPRESS XL, PRAZOSIN HYDROCHLORIDE
* PFIZER LABORATORIES DIV PFIZER INC
   BACITRACIN, BACITRACIN
   CARDURA, DOXAZOSIN MESYLATE
   CEFOBID, CEFOPERAZONE SODIUM
   CORTRIL, HYDROCORTISONE
   CORTRIL, HYDROCORTISONE ACETATE
   DARICON, OXYPHENCYCLIMINE HYDROCHLORIDE
   DIABINESE, CHLORPROPAMIDE
   FELDENE, PIROXICAM
   FOVANE, BENZTHIAZIDE
   GEOCILLIN, CARBENICILLIN INDANYL SODIUM
   MAGNACORT, HYDROCORTAMATE HYDROCHLORIDE
   MINIPRESS, PRAZOSIN HYDROCHLORIDE
   MINIZIDE, POLYTHIAZIDE
   MITHRACIN, PLICAMYCIN
   MODERIL, RESCINNAMINE
   NEOBIOTIC, NEOMYCIN SULFATE
   NEOMYCIN SULFATE, NEOMYCIN SULFATE
   PENICILLIN G POTASSIUM, PENICILLIN G
     POTASSIUM
   PENICILLIN G PROCAINE, PENICILLIN G PROCAINE
   PERMAPEN, PENICILLIN G BENZATHINE
   PFIZER-E, ERYTHROMYCIN STEARATE
   PFIZERPEN, PENICILLIN G POTASSIUM
   PFIZERPEN G, PENICILLIN G POTASSIUM
   PFIZERPEN VK, PENICILLIN V POTASSIUM
   PFIZERPEN-A, AMPICILLIN/AMPICILLIN
     TRIHYDRATE
   PFIZERPEN-AS, PENICILLIN G PROCAINE
   POLYMIXIN B SULFATE, POLYMYXIN B SULFATE
   PROCARDIA, NIFEDIPINE
   PROCARDIA XL, NIFEDIPINE
   RENESE, POLYTHIAZIDE
   RENESE-R, POLYTHIAZIDE
   SINEQUAN, DOXEPIN HYDROCHLORIDE
   SPECTROBID, BACAMPICILLIN HYDROCHLORIDE
   STERANE, PREDNISOLONE
   STERANE, PREDNISOLONE ACETATE
   STREPTOMYCIN SULFATE, STREPTOMYCIN SULFATE
   TAO, TROLEANDOMYCIN
   TERRA-CORTRIL, HYDROCORTISONE ACETATE
   TERRAMYCIN, LIDOCAINE HYDROCHLORIDE
   TERRAMYCIN, OXYTETRACYCLINE
   TERRAMYCIN, OXYTETRACYCLINE CALCIUM
   TERRAMYCIN, OXYTETRACYCLINE
     HYDROCHLORIDE
   TERRAMYCIN W/ POLYMYXIN, OXYTETRACYCLINE
     HYDROCHLORIDE
   TERRAMYCIN W/ POLYMYXIN B SULFATE,
     OXYTETRACYCLINE HYDROCHLORIDE
   TERRAMYCIN-POLYMYXIN, OXYTETRACYCLINE
     HYDROCHLORIDE
   TETRACYN, PROCAINE HYDROCHLORIDE
   TETRACYN, TETRACYCLINE HYDROCHLORIDE
   TZ-3, TIOCONAZOLE (OTC)
   UNASYN, AMPICILLIN SODIUM
   UNISOM, DOXYLAMINE SUCCINATE (OTC)
   URESE, BENZTHIAZIDE
   VANSIL, OXAMNIQUINE
   VIBRA-TABS, DOXYCYCLINE HYCLATE
   VIBRAMYCIN, DOXYCYCLINE
   VIBRAMYCIN, DOXYCYCLINE CALCIUM

APPENDIX B
PRODUCT NAME INDEX
LISTED BY APPLICANT (continued)

VIBRAMYCIN, DOXYCYCLINE HYCLATE
VIOCIN SULFATE, VIOMYCIN SULFATE
VISINE L.R., OXYMETAZOLINE HYDROCHLORIDE
  (OTC)
VISTARIL, HYDROXYZINE HYDROCHLORIDE
VISTARIL, HYDROXYZINE PAMOATE

PHARM ASSOC
* PHARMACEUTICAL ASSOCIATES INC DIV BEACH
PRODUCTS
  ACETAMINOPHEN AND CODEINE PHOSPHATE,
    ACETAMINOPHEN
  BROMPHENIRAMINE MALEATE, BROMPHENIRAMINE
    MALEATE
  CHLORPHENIRAMINE MALEATE,
    CHLORPHENIRAMINE MALEATE
  DIPHENHYDRAMINE HCL, DIPHENHYDRAMINE
    HYDROCHLORIDE
  H-CORT, HYDROCORTISONE
  METOCLOPRAMIDE HCL, METOCLOPRAMIDE
    HYDROCHLORIDE
  PROMETHAZINE HCL, PROMETHAZINE
    HYDROCHLORIDE
  PROMETHAZINE HCL AND CODEINE PHOSPHATE,
    CODEINE PHOSPHATE
  THEOPHYLLINE, THEOPHYLLINE
  TRIPROLIDINE HCL, TRIPROLIDINE
    HYDROCHLORIDE

PHARM BASICS
* PHARMACEUTICAL BASICS INC
  ACETAMINOPHEN AND CODEINE PHOSPHATE,
    ACETAMINOPHEN
  ACETAMINOPHEN W/ CODEINE PHOSPHATE,
    ACETAMINOPHEN
  ACETOHEXAMIDE, ACETOHEXAMIDE
  AMANTADINE HCL, AMANTADINE HYDROCHLORIDE
  AMINOPHYLLINE, AMINOPHYLLINE
  AMITRIPTYLINE HCL, AMITRIPTYLINE
    HYDROCHLORIDE
  BACLOFEN, BACLOFEN
  BENZTROPINE MESYLATE, BENZTROPINE MESYLATE
  BIPHETAP, BROMPHENIRAMINE MALEATE
  BROMPHENIRAMINE MALEATE, BROMPHENIRAMINE
    MALEATE
  BUTABARBITAL SODIUM, BUTABARBITAL SODIUM
  CARBAMAZEPINE, CARBAMAZEPINE
  CHLORDIAZEPOXIDE AND AMITRIPTYLINE HCL,
    AMITRIPTYLINE HYDROCHLORIDE
  CHLORDIAZEPOXIDE HCL, CHLORDIAZEPOXIDE
    HYDROCHLORIDE
  CHLORPROMAZINE HCL, CHLORPROMAZINE
    HYDROCHLORIDE
  CHLORPROPAMIDE, CHLORPROPAMIDE
  CHLORTHALIDONE, CHLORTHALIDONE
  CLOFIBRATE, CLOFIBRATE
  CLORAZEPATE DIPOTASSIUM, CLORAZEPATE
    DIPOTASSIUM
  CYPROHEPTADINE HCL, CYPROHEPTADINE
    HYDROCHLORIDE
  DESIPRAMINE HCL, DESIPRAMINE HYDROCHLORIDE
  DIAZEPAM, DIAZEPAM
  DIPHEN, DIPHENHYDRAMINE HYDROCHLORIDE
    (OTC)
  DIPHEN, DIPHENHYDRAMINE HYDROCHLORIDE
  DIPHENOXYLATE HCL W/ ATROPINE SULFATE,
    ATROPINE SULFATE
  DOXEPIN HCL, DOXEPIN HYDROCHLORIDE
  ERYTHROMYCIN, ERYTHROMYCIN
  FENOPROFEN CALCIUM, FENOPROFEN CALCIUM
  FLUOCINOLONE ACETONIDE, FLUOCINOLONE
    ACETONIDE

FLUOXYMESTERONE, FLUOXYMESTERONE
FLURAZEPAM HCL, FLURAZEPAM HYDROCHLORIDE
FOLIC ACID, FOLIC ACID
FUROSEMIDE, FUROSEMIDE
GENERLAC, LACTULOSE
HALOPERIDOL, HALOPERIDOL LACTATE
HYDRALAZINE HCL, HYDRALAZINE
  HYDROCHLORIDE
HYDROCHLOROTHIAZIDE, HYDROCHLOROTHIAZIDE
HYDROCODONE BITARTRATE AND
  ACETAMINOPHEN, ACETAMINOPHEN
HYDROCORTISONE, HYDROCORTISONE
HYDROFLUMETHIAZIDE AND RESERPINE,
  HYDROFLUMETHIAZIDE
HYDROXYZINE HCL, HYDROXYZINE
  HYDROCHLORIDE
IMIPRAMINE HCL, IMIPRAMINE HYDROCHLORIDE
LACTULOSE, LACTULOSE
LINDANE, LINDANE
LITHIUM CARBONATE, LITHIUM CARBONATE
LITHIUM CITRATE, LITHIUM CITRATE
LORAZEPAM, LORAZEPAM
MECLOFENAMATE SODIUM, MECLOFENAMATE
  SODIUM
MEDROXYPROGESTERONE ACETATE,
  MEDROXYPROGESTERONE ACETATE
MEGESTROL ACETATE, MEGESTROL ACETATE
MEPROBAMATE, MEPROBAMATE
METAPROTERENOL SULFATE, METAPROTERENOL
  SULFATE
METHYCLOTHIAZIDE, METHYCLOTHIAZIDE
METHYLTESTOSTERONE, METHYLTESTOSTERONE
METOCLOPRAMIDE HCL, METOCLOPRAMIDE
  HYDROCHLORIDE
MINOXIDIL, MINOXIDIL
MYBANIL, BROMODIPHENHYDRAMINE
  HYDROCHLORIDE
MYCODONE, HOMATROPINE METHYLBROMIDE
MYFED, PSEUDOEPHEDRINE HYDROCHLORIDE (OTC)
MYIDYL, TRIPROLIDINE HYDROCHLORIDE
MYLARAMINE, DEXCHLORPHENIRAMINE MALEATE
MYLOCAINE, LIDOCAINE HYDROCHLORIDE
MYMETHASONE, DEXAMETHASONE
MYMETHAZINE FORTIS, PROMETHAZINE
  HYDROCHLORIDE
MYPHETANE DC, BROMPHENIRAMINE MALEATE
MYPHETANE DX, BROMPHENIRAMINE MALEATE
MYPROIC ACID, VALPROIC ACID
NYSTATIN, NYSTATIN
OXTRIPHYLLINE, OXTRIPHYLLINE
OXTRIPHYLLINE PEDIATRIC, OXTRIPHYLLINE
OXYBUTYNIN CHLORIDE, OXYBUTYNIN CHLORIDE
PHENDIMETRAZINE TARTRATE, PHENDIMETRAZINE
  TARTRATE
PHENTERMINE HCL, PHENTERMINE
  HYDROCHLORIDE
PRAZEPAM, PRAZEPAM
PREDNISONE, PREDNISONE
PROCHLORPERAZINE EDISYLATE,
  PROCHLORPERAZINE EDISYLATE
PROMETHAZINE PLAIN, PROMETHAZINE
  HYDROCHLORIDE
PROMETHAZINE VC PLAIN, PHENYLEPHRINE
  HYDROCHLORIDE
PROMETHAZINE VC W/ CODEINE, CODEINE
  PHOSPHATE
PROMETHAZINE W/ CODEINE, CODEINE PHOSPHATE
PROMETHAZINE W/ DEXTROMETHORPHAN,
  DEXTROMETHORPHAN HYDROBROMIDE
PROPRANOLOL HCL, PROPRANOLOL
  HYDROCHLORIDE

APPENDIX B
PRODUCT NAME INDEX
LISTED BY APPLICANT (continued)

QUINIDINE SULFATE, QUINIDINE SULFATE
SELENIUM SULFIDE, SELENIUM SULFIDE
SODIUM POLYSTYRENE SULFONATE, SODIUM
    POLYSTYRENE SULFONATE
SPIRONOLACTONE W/ HYDROCHLOROTHIAZIDE,
    HYDROCHLOROTHIAZIDE
SULFAMETHOXAZOLE AND TRIMETHOPRIM,
    SULFAMETHOXAZOLE
SULMEPRIM, SULFAMETHOXAZOLE
SULMEPRIM PEDIATRIC, SULFAMETHOXAZOLE
TEMAZEPAM, TEMAZEPAM
THEOPHYLLINE, THEOPHYLLINE
THIORIDAZINE HCL, THIORIDAZINE
    HYDROCHLORIDE
TIMOLOL MALEATE, TIMOLOL MALEATE
TOLAZAMIDE, TOLAZAMIDE
TRAZODONE HCL, TRAZODONE HYDROCHLORIDE
TRIAMCINOLONE ACETONIDE, TRIAMCINOLONE
    ACETONIDE
TRIFLUOPERAZINE HCL, TRIFLUOPERAZINE
    HYDROCHLORIDE
TRIMEPRAZINE TARTRATE, TRIMEPRAZINE
    TARTRATE
TRIMIPRAMINE MALEATE, TRIMIPRAMINE MALEATE
TRIPROLIDINE HCL, PSEUDOEPHEDRINE HCL AND
    CODEINE PHOSPHATE, CODEINE PHOSPHATE
VALPROIC ACID, VALPROIC ACID
WARFARIN SODIUM, WARFARIN SODIUM

PHARM SPEC
* PHARMACEUTICAL SPECIALIST ASSOCIATES
    GENTAMICIN SULFATE, GENTAMICIN SULFATE
    HEPARIN SODIUM, HEPARIN SODIUM

PHARMA SERVE
* PHARMA SERVE INC
    AMINOPHYLLINE, AMINOPHYLLINE
    HEPARIN SODIUM, HEPARIN SODIUM
    POTASSIUM CHLORIDE, POTASSIUM CHLORIDE

PHARMA TEK
* PHARMA TEK INC
    AMPHOTERICIN B, AMPHOTERICIN B
    BACI-RX, BACITRACIN
    HYDROCORTISONE, HYDROCORTISONE
    HYDROCORTISONE ACETATE, HYDROCORTISONE
      ACETATE
    NEO-RX, NEOMYCIN SULFATE
    POLY-RX, POLYMYXIN B SULFATE
    ZIBA-RX, BACITRACIN ZINC

PHARMACAPS
* PHARMACAPS INC
    CLOFIBRATE, CLOFIBRATE
    VITAMIN A, VITAMIN A
    VITAMIN A, VITAMIN A PALMITATE
    VITAMIN A PALMITATE, VITAMIN A PALMITATE
    VITAMIN D, ERGOCALCIFEROL

PHARMACHEMIE
* PHARMACHEMIE BV
    DOXORUBICIN HCL, DOXORUBICIN
      HYDROCHLORIDE
* PHARMACHEMIE USA INC
    METHOTREXATE SODIUM, METHOTREXATE SODIUM

PHARMADERM
* PHARMADERM DIV ALTANA INC
    BACITRACIN, BACITRACIN
    BACITRACIN-NEOMYCIN-POLYMYXIN, BACITRACIN
      ZINC
    BACITRACIN-NEOMYCIN-POLYMYXIN W/
      HYDROCORTISONE ACETATE, BACITRACIN

BETAMETHASONE DIPROPIONATE, BETAMETHASONE
    DIPROPIONATE
BETAMETHASONE VALERATE, BETAMETHASONE
    VALERATE
ERYTHROMYCIN, ERYTHROMYCIN
FLUOCINOLONE ACETONIDE, FLUOCINOLONE
    ACETONIDE
GENTAMICIN SULFATE, GENTAMICIN SULFATE
HYDROCORTISONE, HYDROCORTISONE
NEOMYCIN SULFATE-TRIAMCINOLONE ACETONIDE,
    NEOMYCIN SULFATE
NYSTATIN, NYSTATIN
NYSTATIN-TRIAMCINOLONE ACETONIDE, NYSTATIN
TRIAMCINOLONE ACETONIDE, TRIAMCINOLONE
    ACETONIDE
TRIPLE SULFA, TRIPLE SULFA
    (SULFABENZAMIDE; SULFACETAMIDE; SULFATHIAZOLE)

PHARMAFAIR
* PHARMAFAIR INC
    ACETAMINOPHEN AND CODEINE PHOSPHATE,
      ACETAMINOPHEN
    BACITRACIN, BACITRACIN
    BACITRACIN ZINC-NEOMYCIN SULFATE-POLYMYXIN
      B SULFATE, BACITRACIN ZINC
    BETAMETHASONE VALERATE, BETAMETHASONE
      VALERATE
    BOROFAIR, ACETIC ACID, GLACIAL
    BUTALBITAL W/ ASPIRIN & CAFFEINE, ASPIRIN
    CARBACHOL, CARBACHOL
    CHLOROFAIR, CHLORAMPHENICOL
    CHLORPHENIRAMINE MALEATE,
      CHLORPHENIRAMINE MALEATE
    DEXAIR, DEXAMETHASONE SODIUM PHOSPHATE
    DEXASPORIN, DEXAMETHASONE
    DIPHENOXYLATE HCL AND ATROPINE SULFATE,
      ATROPINE SULFATE
    ERYTHROMYCIN, ERYTHROMYCIN
    ERYTHROMYCIN ETHYLSUCCINATE,
      ERYTHROMYCIN ETHYLSUCCINATE
    FLUOCINOLONE ACETONIDE, FLUOCINOLONE
      ACETONIDE
    GENTAFAIR, GENTAMICIN SULFATE
    HYDROCHLOROTHIAZIDE, HYDROCHLOROTHIAZIDE
    HYDROCHLOROTHIAZIDE W/ RESERPINE,
      HYDROCHLOROTHIAZIDE
    HYDROCORTISONE, HYDROCORTISONE
    HYDROXYZINE HCL, HYDROXYZINE
      HYDROCHLORIDE
    KAINAIR, PROPARACAINE HYDROCHLORIDE
    KANAMYCIN SULFATE, KANAMYCIN SULFATE
    MEPROBAMATE, MEPROBAMATE
    METHOCARBAMOL, METHOCARBAMOL
    MYDRIAFAIR, TROPICAMIDE
    NAFAZAIR, NAPHAZOLINE HYDROCHLORIDE
    NEOMYCIN & POLYMYXIN B SULFATES &
      BACITRACIN ZINC & HYDROCORTISONE,
      BACITRACIN ZINC
    NEOMYCIN SULFATE AND POLYMYXIN B SULFATE
      GRAMICIDIN, GRAMICIDIN
    NEOMYCIN SULFATE-DEXAMETHASONE SODIUM
      PHOSPHATE, DEXAMETHASONE SODIUM
      PHOSPHATE
    NEOMYCIN SULFATE-POLYMYXIN B SULFATE-
      HYDROCORTISONE, HYDROCORTISONE
    NEOMYCIN SULFATE, POLYMYXIN B SULFATE &
      HYDROCORTISONE, HYDROCORTISONE
    NYSTATIN, NYSTATIN
    NYSTATIN AND TRIAMCINOLONE ACETONIDE,
      NYSTATIN
    OCUMYCIN, BACITRACIN ZINC

APPENDIX B
PRODUCT NAME INDEX
LISTED BY APPLICANT (*continued*)

OTICAIR, HYDROCORTISONE
PENTOLAIR, CYCLOPENTOLATE HYDROCHLORIDE
PHENYTOIN SODIUM, PHENYTOIN SODIUM, PROMPT
PREDAIR, PREDNISOLONE SODIUM PHOSPHATE
PREDAIR FORTE, PREDNISOLONE SODIUM
    PHOSPHATE
PREDSULFAIR, PREDNISOLONE ACETATE
PREDSULFAIR II, PREDNISOLONE ACETATE
PROCAINAMIDE HCL, PROCAINAMIDE
    HYDROCHLORIDE
SULFACETAMIDE SODIUM, SULFACETAMIDE SODIUM
SULFAIR FORTE, SULFACETAMIDE SODIUM
SULFAIR 10, SULFACETAMIDE SODIUM
SULFAIR-15, SULFACETAMIDE SODIUM
SULFISOXAZOLE, SULFISOXAZOLE
TRIAMCINOLONE ACETONIDE, TRIAMCINOLONE
    ACETONIDE
ZINC BACITRACIN,NEOMYCIN SULFATE,POLYMYXIN
    B SULFATE & HYDROCORTISONE, BACITRACIN
    ZINC

PHARMATON
* PHARMATON LTD
    LIDOCATON, EPINEPHRINE
    LIDOCATON, LIDOCAINE HYDROCHLORIDE

PHARMAVITE
* PHARMAVITE PHARMACEUTICALS
    CHLORPHENIRAMINE MALEATE,
        CHLORPHENIRAMINE MALEATE
    ISONIAZID, ISONIAZID
    MEPROBAMATE, MEPROBAMATE
    PREDNISONE, PREDNISONE
    QUINIDINE SULFATE, QUINIDINE SULFATE
    RESERPINE, RESERPINE

PHARMICS
* PHARMICS INC
    PAREDRINE, HYDROXYAMPHETAMINE
        HYDROBROMIDE

PHOENIX LABS
* PHOENIX LABORATORIES INC
    AMINOPHYLLINE, AMINOPHYLLINE
    BROMPHENIRAMINE MALEATE, BROMPHENIRAMINE
        MALEATE
    CHLORPHENIRAMINE MALEATE,
        CHLORPHENIRAMINE MALEATE
    DEXAMETHASONE, DEXAMETHASONE
    FOLIC ACID, FOLIC ACID
    ISONIAZID, ISONIAZID
    PREDNISOLONE, PREDNISOLONE
    PREDNISONE, PREDNISONE
    QUINIDINE SULFATE, QUINIDINE SULFATE

PHYSICIANS PRODS
* PHYSICIANS PRODUCTS CO INC DIV INTERNATIONAL
LATEX CORP
    HYSERPIN, RAUWOLFIA SERPENTINA

PIONEER PHARMS
* PIONEER PHARMACEUTICALS INC
    BROMPHENIRAMINE MALEATE, BROMPHENIRAMINE
        MALEATE
    CARISOPRODOL, CARISOPRODOL
    CHLORDIAZEPOXIDE HCL, CHLORDIAZEPOXIDE
        HYDROCHLORIDE
    CHLORPHENIRAMINE MALEATE,
        CHLORPHENIRAMINE MALEATE
    CHLORTHALIDONE, CHLORTHALIDONE
    CHLORZOXAZONE, CHLORZOXAZONE
    CYPROHEPTADINE HCL, CYPROHEPTADINE
        HYDROCHLORIDE

DIAZEPAM, DIAZEPAM
DICYCLOMINE HCL, DICYCLOMINE
    HYDROCHLORIDE
DIPHENHYDRAMINE HCL, DIPHENHYDRAMINE
    HYDROCHLORIDE
FOLIC ACID, FOLIC ACID
INDOMETHACIN, INDOMETHACIN
METHOCARBAMOL, METHOCARBAMOL
RESPORAL, DEXBROMPHENIRAMINE MALEATE (OTC)

PLANTEX
* PLANTEX USA INC DIV IKAPHARM INC
    SULFAMETHOXAZOLE AND TRIMETHOPRIM DOUBLE
        STRENGTH, SULFAMETHOXAZOLE
    SULFAMETHOXAZOLE AND TRIMETHOPRIM SINGLE
        STRENGTH, SULFAMETHOXAZOLE

POPULATION COUNCIL
* POPULATION COUNCIL
    NORPLANT, LEVONORGESTREL
* POPULATION COUNCIL CENTER FOR BIOMEDICAL
RESEARCH
    COPPER T MODEL TCU 380A, COPPER

POYTHRESS
* WILLIAM P POYTHRESS AND CO INC
    BENSULFOID, BENTONITE

PRIVATE FORM
* PRIVATE FORMULATIONS INC
    ALLERFED, PSEUDOEPHEDRINE HYDROCHLORIDE
    BENZTHIAZIDE, BENZTHIAZIDE
    BROMPHENIRAMINE MALEATE, BROMPHENIRAMINE
        MALEATE
    CHLORPHENIRAMINE MALEATE,
        CHLORPHENIRAMINE MALEATE
    CHLORPROMAZINE HCL, CHLORPROMAZINE
        HYDROCHLORIDE
    DEXAMETHASONE, DEXAMETHASONE
    DI-METREX, PHENDIMETRAZINE TARTRATE
    DIPHENHYDRAMINE HCL, DIPHENHYDRAMINE
        HYDROCHLORIDE
    DIPHENOXYLATE HCL W/ ATROPINE SULFATE,
        ATROPINE SULFATE
    DOXYCYCLINE HYCLATE, DOXYCYCLINE HYCLATE
    ESTERIFIED ESTROGENS, ESTROGENS, ESTERIFIED
    FEMOGEN, ESTROGENS, ESTERIFIED
    FOLIC ACID, FOLIC ACID
    HYDROCHLOROTHIAZIDE, HYDROCHLOROTHIAZIDE
    IBUPROFEN, IBUPROFEN
    IBUPROFEN, IBUPROFEN (OTC)
    MEPROBAMATE, MEPROBAMATE
    METHSCOPOLAMINE BROMIDE, METHSCOPOLAMINE
        BROMIDE
    METHYLTESTOSTERONE, METHYLTESTOSTERONE
    PHENDIMETRAZINE TARTRATE, PHENDIMETRAZINE
        TARTRATE
    PREDNISOLONE, PREDNISOLONE
    PREDNISONE, PREDNISONE
    PROFEN, IBUPROFEN (OTC)
    PROMETHAZINE HCL, PROMETHAZINE
        HYDROCHLORIDE
    PROPANTHELINE BROMIDE, PROPANTHELINE
        BROMIDE
    PROPOXYPHENE HCL, PROPOXYPHENE
        HYDROCHLORIDE
    QUINIDINE SULFATE, QUINIDINE SULFATE
    RAUWOLFIA SERPENTINA, RAUWOLFIA SERPENTINA
    RESERPINE, RESERPINE
    TETRACYCLINE HCL, TETRACYCLINE
        HYDROCHLORIDE

APPENDIX B
PRODUCT NAME INDEX
LISTED BY APPLICANT (continued)

PROF DSPLS
* PROFESSIONAL DISPOSABLES INC
  HEXASCRUB, HEXACHLOROPHENE

PROTER
* PROTER LABORATORY SPA
  OXYTETRACYCLINE HCL, OXYTETRACYCLINE
  HYDROCHLORIDE

PURDUE FREDERICK
* PURDUE FREDERICK CO
  ATHROMBIN, WARFARIN SODIUM
  ATHROMBIN-K, WARFARIN POTASSIUM
  BETADINE, POVIDONE-IODINE
  CARDIOQUIN, QUINIDINE POLYGALACTURONATE
  CERUMENEX, TRIETHANOLAMINE POLYPEPTIDE
    OLEATE CONDENSATE
  MS CONTIN, MORPHINE SULFATE
  PHENY-PAS-TEBAMIN, PHENYL AMINOSALICYLATE
  PHYLLOCONTIN, AMINOPHYLLINE
  SULFABID, SULFAPHENAZOLE
  T-PHYL, THEOPHYLLINE
  UNIPHYL, THEOPHYLLINE

PUREPAC
* PUREPAC PHARMACEUTICAL CO
  TOLMETIN SODIUM, TOLMETIN SODIUM
* PUREPAC PHARMACEUTICAL CO DIV KALIPHARMA
INC
  ACETAMINOPHEN AND CODEINE PHOSPHATE,
    ACETAMINOPHEN
  ACETAMINOPHEN AND CODEINE PHOSPHATE #3,
    ACETAMINOPHEN
  ALLOPURINOL, ALLOPURINOL
  AMINOPHYLLINE, AMINOPHYLLINE
  AMITRIPTYLINE HCL, AMITRIPTYLINE
    HYDROCHLORIDE
  AMPICILLIN TRIHYDRATE, AMPICILLIN/AMPICILLIN
    TRIHYDRATE
  ASPIRIN AND CAFFEINE W/ BUTALBITAL, ASPIRIN
  CARBAMAZEPINE, CARBAMAZEPINE
  CEFADROXIL, CEFADROXIL/CEFADROXIL
    HEMIHYDRATE
  CEPHALEXIN, CEPHALEXIN
  CHLORDIAZEPOXIDE HCL, CHLORDIAZEPOXIDE
    HYDROCHLORIDE
  CHLOROQUINE PHOSPHATE, CHLOROQUINE
    PHOSPHATE
  CHLORPHENIRAMINE MALEATE,
    CHLORPHENIRAMINE MALEATE
  CHLORPROMAZINE HCL, CHLORPROMAZINE
    HYDROCHLORIDE
  CHLORTHALIDONE, CHLORTHALIDONE
  CLONIDINE HCL, CLONIDINE HYDROCHLORIDE
  CLORAZEPATE DIPOTASSIUM, CLORAZEPATE
    DIPOTASSIUM
  CORTISONE ACETATE, CORTISONE ACETATE
  DEXTROAMPHETAMINE SULFATE,
    DEXTROAMPHETAMINE SULFATE
  DIAZEPAM, DIAZEPAM
  DIPHENHYDRAMINE HCL, DIPHENHYDRAMINE
    HYDROCHLORIDE
  DIPYRIDAMOLE, DIPYRIDAMOLE
  DOXEPIN HCL, DOXEPIN HYDROCHLORIDE
  DOXYCYCLINE HYCLATE, DOXYCYCLINE HYCLATE
  ERYTHROMYCIN STEARATE, ERYTHROMYCIN
    STEARATE
  FENOPROFEN CALCIUM, FENOPROFEN CALCIUM
  FLURAZEPAM HCL, FLURAZEPAM HYDROCHLORIDE
  FOLIC ACID, FOLIC ACID
  HALOPERIDOL, HALOPERIDOL

HYDRALAZINE HCL, HYDRALAZINE
  HYDROCHLORIDE
HYDROCHLOROTHIAZIDE, HYDROCHLOROTHIAZIDE
HYDROCORTISONE, HYDROCORTISONE
HYDROCORTISONE ACETATE, HYDROCORTISONE
  ACETATE
HYDROXYZINE HCL, HYDROXYZINE
  HYDROCHLORIDE
IBUPROFEN, IBUPROFEN
IBUPROFEN, IBUPROFEN (OTC)
ISONIAZID, ISONIAZID
LORAZEPAM, LORAZEPAM
MEPROBAMATE, MEPROBAMATE
METHOCARBAMOL, METHOCARBAMOL
METHYLDOPA, METHYLDOPA
METHYLDOPA AND HYDROCHLOROTHIAZIDE,
  HYDROCHLOROTHIAZIDE
METHYLTESTOSTERONE, METHYLTESTOSTERONE
METOCLOPRAMIDE HCL, METOCLOPRAMIDE
  HYDROCHLORIDE
NIACIN, NIACIN
NIFEDIPINE, NIFEDIPINE
OXAZEPAM, OXAZEPAM
OXYTETRACYCLINE HCL, OXYTETRACYCLINE
  HYDROCHLORIDE
PENICILLIN G POTASSIUM, PENICILLIN G
  POTASSIUM
PENICILLIN V POTASSIUM, PENICILLIN V
  POTASSIUM
PRAZOSIN HCL, PRAZOSIN HYDROCHLORIDE
PREDNISOLONE, PREDNISOLONE
PREDNISONE, PREDNISONE
PROPOXYPHENE HCL, PROPOXYPHENE
  HYDROCHLORIDE
PROPOXYPHENE NAPSYLATE AND ACETAMINOPHEN,
  ACETAMINOPHEN
PROPRANOLOL HCL, PROPRANOLOL
  HYDROCHLORIDE
PROPRANOLOL HCL AND HYDROCHLOROTHIAZIDE,
  HYDROCHLOROTHIAZIDE
PROPYLTHIOURACIL, PROPYLTHIOURACIL
QUINIDINE SULFATE, QUINIDINE SULFATE
RAUWOLFIA SERPENTINA, RAUWOLFIA SERPENTINA
RESERPINE, RESERPINE
SECOBARBITAL SODIUM, SECOBARBITAL SODIUM
SODIUM PENTOBARBITAL, PENTOBARBITAL SODIUM
SPIRONOLACTONE, SPIRONOLACTONE
SPIRONOLACTONE AND HYDROCHLOROTHIAZIDE,
  HYDROCHLOROTHIAZIDE
SPIRONOLACTONE W/ HYDROCHLOROTHIAZIDE,
  HYDROCHLOROTHIAZIDE
SULFISOXAZOLE, SULFISOXAZOLE
TEMAZEPAM, TEMAZEPAM
TETRACYCLINE HCL, TETRACYCLINE
TETRACYCLINE HCL, TETRACYCLINE
  HYDROCHLORIDE
TOLBUTAMIDE, TOLBUTAMIDE
TOLMETIN SODIUM, TOLMETIN SODIUM
TRAZODONE HCL, TRAZODONE HYDROCHLORIDE
TRIAMCINOLONE, TRIAMCINOLONE
TRIPLE SULFA, TRISULFAPYRIMIDINES
VERAPAMIL HCL, VERAPAMIL HYDROCHLORIDE

Q

QUAD
* QUAD PHARMACEUTICALS
  ACETAZOLAMIDE SODIUM, ACETAZOLAMIDE
    SODIUM
  ACETYLCYSTEINE, ACETYLCYSTEINE

APPENDIX B
PRODUCT NAME INDEX
LISTED BY APPLICANT *(continued)*

AMINOCAPROIC ACID, AMINOCAPROIC ACID
AMINOHIPPURATE SODIUM, AMINOHIPPURATE
  SODIUM
AZATHIOPRINE, AZATHIOPRINE SODIUM
BACITRACIN, BACITRACIN
BETHANECHOL CHLORIDE, BETHANECHOL
  CHLORIDE
BRETYLIUM TOSYLATE, BRETYLIUM TOSYLATE
CHORIONIC GONADOTROPIN, GONADOTROPIN,
  CHORIONIC
CLINDAMYCIN PHOSPHATE, CLINDAMYCIN
  PHOSPHATE
CYTARABINE, CYTARABINE
DACARBAZINE, DACARBAZINE
DEXAMETHASONE SODIUM PHOSPHATE,
  DEXAMETHASONE SODIUM PHOSPHATE
DIAZOXIDE, DIAZOXIDE
DOXYCYCLINE HYCLATE, DOXYCYCLINE HYCLATE
DROPERIDOL, DROPERIDOL
ERYTHROMYCIN LACTOBIONATE, ERYTHROMYCIN
  LACTOBIONATE
ESTRADIOL CYPIONATE, ESTRADIOL CYPIONATE
FLOXURIDINE, FLOXURIDINE
FLUOROURACIL, FLUOROURACIL
FLUPHENAZINE, FLUPHENAZINE DECANOATE
FLUPHENAZINE HCL, FLUPHENAZINE
  HYDROCHLORIDE
GLUCAGON, GLUCAGON HYDROCHLORIDE
GLYCOPYRROLATE, GLYCOPYRROLATE
HALOPERIDOL, HALOPERIDOL LACTATE
HYDROCORTISONE SODIUM PHOSPHATE,
  HYDROCORTISONE SODIUM PHOSPHATE
HYDROXYPROGESTERONE CAPROATE,
  HYDROXYPROGESTERONE CAPROATE
ISONIAZID, ISONIAZID
KANAMYCIN SULFATE, KANAMYCIN SULFATE
KETAMINE HCL, KETAMINE HYDROCHLORIDE
LEUCOVORIN CALCIUM, LEUCOVORIN CALCIUM
LINCOMYCIN HCL, LINCOMYCIN HYDROCHLORIDE
METHOTREXATE SODIUM, METHOTREXATE SODIUM
METHYLDOPATE HCL, METHYLDOPATE
  HYDROCHLORIDE
METHYLPREDNISOLONE SODIUM SUCCINATE,
  METHYLPREDNISOLONE SODIUM SUCCINATE
METOCLOPRAMIDE HCL, METOCLOPRAMIDE
  HYDROCHLORIDE
METOCURINE IODIDE, METOCURINE IODIDE
NALBUPHINE, NALBUPHINE HYDROCHLORIDE
NALOXONE HCL, NALOXONE HYDROCHLORIDE
NANDROLONE DECANOATE, NANDROLONE
  DECANOATE
NANDROLONE PHENPROPIONATE, NANDROLONE
  PHENPROPIONATE
NITROGLYCERIN, NITROGLYCERIN
PANCURONIUM BROMIDE, PANCURONIUM BROMIDE
PRALIDOXIME CHLORIDE, PRALIDOXIME CHLORIDE
PROCAINAMIDE HCL, PROCAINAMIDE
  HYDROCHLORIDE
PROCHLORPERAZINE EDISYLATE,
  PROCHLORPERAZINE EDISYLATE
PROTAMINE SULFATE, PROTAMINE SULFATE
RITODRINE HCL, RITODRINE HYDROCHLORIDE
SULFAMETHOPRIM, SULFAMETHOXAZOLE
TESTOSTERONE CYPIONATE, TESTOSTERONE
  CYPIONATE
TESTOSTERONE ENANTHATE, TESTOSTERONE
  ENANTHATE
TESTOSTERONE PROPIONATE, TESTOSTERONE
  PROPIONATE
TRIFLUOPERAZINE HCL, TRIFLUOPERAZINE
  HYDROCHLORIDE

TUBOCURARINE CHLORIDE, TUBOCURARINE
  CHLORIDE
VANCOMYCIN HCL, VANCOMYCIN HYDROCHLORIDE
VERAPAMIL HCL, VERAPAMIL HYDROCHLORIDE
VINBLASTINE SULFATE, VINBLASTINE SULFATE
VINCRISTINE SULFATE, VINCRISTINE SULFATE

QUANTUM PHARMICS
* QUANTUM PHARMICS LTD
  BENZTROPINE MESYLATE, BENZTROPINE MESYLATE
  BUTALBITAL ASPIRIN AND CAFFEINE, ASPIRIN
  CLOPRA, METOCLOPRAMIDE HYDROCHLORIDE
  CLOPRA-"YELLOW", METOCLOPRAMIDE
    HYDROCHLORIDE
  CLORAZEPATE DIPOTASSIUM, CLORAZEPATE
    DIPOTASSIUM
  DOXEPIN HCL, DOXEPIN HYDROCHLORIDE
  DOXYLAMINE SUCCINATE, DOXYLAMINE
    SUCCINATE
  FENOPROFEN CALCIUM, FENOPROFEN CALCIUM
  HALOPERIDOL, HALOPERIDOL
  HYDRALAZINE HCL, HYDRALAZINE
    HYDROCHLORIDE
  HYDROXYZINE HCL, HYDROXYZINE
    HYDROCHLORIDE
  LORAZ, LORAZEPAM
  MECLODIUM, MECLOFENAMATE SODIUM
  MINODYL, MINOXIDIL
  NYSTATIN, NYSTATIN
  OXYBUTYNIN CHLORIDE, OXYBUTYNIN CHLORIDE
  PHENTERMINE RESIN 30, PHENTERMINE RESIN
    COMPLEX
  Q-GESIC, ASPIRIN
  Q-PAM, DIAZEPAM
  TEMAZ, TEMAZEPAM
  TIMOLOL MALEATE, TIMOLOL MALEATE
  TRAZODONE HCL, TRAZODONE HYDROCHLORIDE
  TRIALODINE, TRAZODONE HYDROCHLORIDE
  TRIAMTERENE AND HYDROCHLOROTHIAZIDE,
    HYDROCHLOROTHIAZIDE
  ZAXOPAM, OXAZEPAM

R

RACHELLE
* RACHELLE LABORATORIES INC
  CHLORDIAZACHEL, CHLORDIAZEPOXIDE
    HYDROCHLORIDE
  DOXY-TABS, DOXYCYCLINE HYCLATE
  DOXYCHEL, DOXYCYCLINE
  DOXYCHEL HYCLATE, DOXYCYCLINE HYCLATE
  MYCHEL, CHLORAMPHENICOL
  MYCHEL-S, CHLORAMPHENICOL SODIUM
    SUCCINATE
  TETRACHEL, TETRACYCLINE HYDROCHLORIDE

RECKITT AND COLMAN
* RECKITT AND COLMAN PHARMACEUTICALS INC
  BUPRENEX, BUPRENORPHINE HYDROCHLORIDE

REED AND CARNRICK
* REED AND CARNRICK
  CORTIFOAM, HYDROCORTISONE ACETATE
* REED AND CARNRICK DIV BLOCK DRUG CO INC
  LEVATOL, PENBUTOLOL SULFATE
* REED AND CARNRICK PHARMACEUTICALS DIV BLOCK
DRUG CO INC
  COLYTE, POLYETHYLENE GLYCOL 3350
  COLYTE-FLAVORED, POLYETHYLENE GLYCOL 3350
  DILATRATE-SR, ISOSORBIDE DINITRATE

APPENDIX B
PRODUCT NAME INDEX
LISTED BY APPLICANT (continued)

EPIFOAM, HYDROCORTISONE ACETATE
ETHAMOLIN, ETHANOLAMINE OLEATE
KWELL, LINDANE
PROCTOFOAM HC, HYDROCORTISONE ACETATE

RES INDS
* RESEARCH INDUSTRIES CORP
    RIMSO-50, DIMETHYL SULFOXIDE

REXALL
* REXALL DRUG CO
    PREDNISONE, PREDNISONE
    RESERPINE, RESERPINE

REXAR
* REXAR PHARMACAL CORP
    DEXTROAMPHETAMINE SULFATE,
        DEXTROAMPHETAMINE SULFATE
    METHAMPHETAMINE HCL, METHAMPHETAMINE
        HYDROCHLORIDE
    OBY-TRIM, PHENTERMINE HYDROCHLORIDE
    X-TROZINE, PHENDIMETRAZINE TARTRATE
    X-TROZINE L.A., PHENDIMETRAZINE TARTRATE

RHONE POULENC RORER
* RHONE POULENC RORER PHARMACEUTICALS INC
    AZMACORT, TRIAMCINOLONE ACETONIDE
    AZOLID, PHENYLBUTAZONE
    CALCIMAR, CALCITONIN, SALMON
    CERUBIDINE, DAUNORUBICIN HYDROCHLORIDE
    DDAVP, DESMOPRESSIN ACETATE
    DEMI-REGROTON, CHLORTHALIDONE
    DILACOR XR, DILTIAZEM HYDROCHLORIDE
    DORIDEN, GLUTETHIMIDE
    HYGROTON, CHLORTHALIDONE
    LOZOL, INDAPAMIDE
    NASACORT, TRIAMCINOLONE ACETONIDE
    NICOLAR, NIACIN
    PARATHAR, TERIPARATIDE ACETATE
    PERTOFRANE, DESIPRAMINE HYDROCHLORIDE
    PRESAMINE, IMIPRAMINE HYDROCHLORIDE
    REGROTON, CHLORTHALIDONE
    SLO-BID, THEOPHYLLINE
    SLO-PHYLLIN, THEOPHYLLINE
    TANDEARIL, OXYPHENBUTAZONE
    THYROLAR-0.25, LIOTRIX (T4; T3)
    THYROLAR-0.5, LIOTRIX (T4; T3)
    THYROLAR-1, LIOTRIX (T4; T3)
    THYROLAR-2, LIOTRIX (T4; T3)
    THYROLAR-3, LIOTRIX (T4; T3)
    THYROLAR-5, LIOTRIX (T4; T3)

RICHLYN
* RICHLYN LABORATORIES INC
    AMINOPHYLLINE, AMINOPHYLLINE
    CHLORDIAZEPOXIDE HCL, CHLORDIAZEPOXIDE
        HYDROCHLORIDE
    CHLOROQUINE PHOSPHATE, CHLOROQUINE
        PHOSPHATE
    CHLORPHENIRAMINE MALEATE,
        CHLORPHENIRAMINE MALEATE
    CORTISONE ACETATE, CORTISONE ACETATE
    DEXAMETHASONE, DEXAMETHASONE
    DIPHENHYDRAMINE HCL, DIPHENHYDRAMINE
        HYDROCHLORIDE
    FOLIC ACID, FOLIC ACID
    HYDRALAZINE HCL, HYDRALAZINE
        HYDROCHLORIDE
    HYDROCHLOROTHIAZIDE, HYDROCHLOROTHIAZIDE
    HYDROCORTISONE, HYDROCORTISONE
    ISONIAZID, ISONIAZID
    MEPROBAMATE, MEPROBAMATE

METHOCARBAMOL, METHOCARBAMOL
METHYLTESTOSTERONE, METHYLTESTOSTERONE
NIACIN, NIACIN
OXYTETRACYCLINE HCL, OXYTETRACYCLINE
    HYDROCHLORIDE
PIPERAZINE CITRATE, PIPERAZINE CITRATE
PREDNISOLONE, PREDNISOLONE
PREDNISONE, PREDNISONE
PROBENECID AND COLCHICINE, COLCHICINE
PROMETHAZINE HCL, PROMETHAZINE
    HYDROCHLORIDE
PROPANTHELINE BROMIDE, PROPANTHELINE
    BROMIDE
PROPOXYPHENE HCL, PROPOXYPHENE
    HYDROCHLORIDE
PROPYLTHIOURACIL, PROPYLTHIOURACIL
PYRILAMINE MALEATE, PYRILAMINE MALEATE
QUINIDINE SULFATE, QUINIDINE SULFATE
RAUWOLFIA SERPENTINA, RAUWOLFIA SERPENTINA
RESERPINE, RESERPINE
SULFA-TRIPLE #2, TRISULFAPYRIMIDINES
SULFADIAZINE, SULFADIAZINE
SULFISOXAZOLE, SULFISOXAZOLE
TETRACYCLINE HCL, TETRACYCLINE
    HYDROCHLORIDE
THYROGLOBULIN, THYROGLOBULIN
TRIAMCINOLONE, TRIAMCINOLONE
TRICHLORMETHIAZIDE, TRICHLORMETHIAZIDE
TRIPELENNAMINE HCL, TRIPELENNAMINE
    HYDROCHLORIDE
VITAMIN A, VITAMIN A
VITAMIN A, VITAMIN A PALMITATE
VITAMIN D, ERGOCALCIFEROL

ROACO
* TJ ROACO LTD
    BETADERM, BETAMETHASONE VALERATE

ROBERTS
* ROBERTS LABORATORIES INC
    DOPAR, LEVODOPA
    DUVOID, BETHANECHOL CHLORIDE
    FURACIN, NITROFURAZONE
    FUROXONE, FURAZOLIDONE
    TOPICYCLINE, TETRACYCLINE HYDROCHLORIDE

ROBINS
* AH ROBINS CO
    DIMETANE, BROMPHENIRAMINE MALEATE
    DIMETANE, BROMPHENIRAMINE MALEATE (OTC)
    DIMETANE-DC, BROMPHENIRAMINE MALEATE
    DIMETANE-DX, BROMPHENIRAMINE MALEATE
    DIMETANE-TEN, BROMPHENIRAMINE MALEATE
    DIMETAPP, BROMPHENIRAMINE MALEATE (OTC)
    DOPRAM, DOXAPRAM HYDROCHLORIDE
    EXNA, BENZTHIAZIDE
    MICRO-K, POTASSIUM CHLORIDE
    MICRO-K LS, POTASSIUM CHLORIDE
    MICRO-K 10, POTASSIUM CHLORIDE
    PHENAPHEN W/ CODEINE NO. 2, ACETAMINOPHEN
    PHENAPHEN W/ CODEINE NO. 3, ACETAMINOPHEN
    PHENAPHEN W/ CODEINE NO. 4, ACETAMINOPHEN
    PHENAPHEN-650 W/ CODEINE, ACETAMINOPHEN
    PONDIMIN, FENFLURAMINE HYDROCHLORIDE
    QUINIDEX, QUINIDINE SULFATE
    REGLAN, METOCLOPRAMIDE HYDROCHLORIDE
    ROBAXIN, METHOCARBAMOL
    ROBAXIN-750, METHOCARBAMOL
    ROBAXISAL, ASPIRIN
    ROBIMYCIN, ERYTHROMYCIN
    ROBINUL, GLYCOPYRROLATE

ROBINUL FORTE, GLYCOPYRROLATE
ROBITET, TETRACYCLINE HYDROCHLORIDE
TENATHAN, BETHANIDINE SULFATE
TENEX, GUANFACINE HYDROCHLORIDE

ROCHE
* HOFFMANN LA ROCHE INC
ACCUTANE, ISOTRETINOIN
ANCOBON, FLUCYTOSINE
ARFONAD, TRIMETHAPHAN CAMSYLATE
AZO GANTANOL, PHENAZOPYRIDINE
    HYDROCHLORIDE
AZO GANTRISIN, PHENAZOPYRIDINE
    HYDROCHLORIDE
BACTRIM, SULFAMETHOXAZOLE
BACTRIM DS, SULFAMETHOXAZOLE
BACTRIM PEDIATRIC, SULFAMETHOXAZOLE
BEROCCA PN, ASCORBIC ACID
BUMEX, BUMETANIDE
COACTIN, AMDINOCILLIN
EFUDEX, FLUOROURACIL
ENDEP, AMITRIPTYLINE HYDROCHLORIDE
FANSIDAR, PYRIMETHAMINE
FLUOROURACIL, FLUOROURACIL
FUDR, FLOXURIDINE
GANTANOL, SULFAMETHOXAZOLE
GANTANOL-DS, SULFAMETHOXAZOLE
GANTRISIN, SULFISOXAZOLE
GANTRISIN, SULFISOXAZOLE ACETYL
GANTRISIN, SULFISOXAZOLE DIOLAMINE
GANTRISIN PEDIATRIC, SULFISOXAZOLE ACETYL
HIVID, ZALCITABINE
KLONOPIN, CLONAZEPAM
KONAKION, PHYTONADIONE
LARIAM, MEFLOQUINE HYDROCHLORIDE
LARODOPA, LEVODOPA
LEVO-DROMORAN, LEVORPHANOL TARTRATE
LIBRELEASE, CHLORDIAZEPOXIDE
LIBRIUM, CHLORDIAZEPOXIDE HYDROCHLORIDE
LIMBITROL, AMITRIPTYLINE HYDROCHLORIDE
LIPO GANTRISIN, SULFISOXAZOLE ACETYL
LORFAN, LEVALLORPHAN TARTRATE
MATULANE, PROCARBAZINE HYDROCHLORIDE
MAZICON, FLUMAZENIL
MENRIUM 10-4, CHLORDIAZEPOXIDE
MENRIUM 5-2, CHLORDIAZEPOXIDE
MENRIUM 5-4, CHLORDIAZEPOXIDE
NIPRIDE, SODIUM NITROPRUSSIDE
NOLUDAR, METHYPRYLON
PROVOCHOLINE, METHACHOLINE CHLORIDE
QUARZAN, CLIDINIUM BROMIDE
RIMADYL, CARPROFEN
RIMIFON, ISONIAZID
ROCALTROL, CALCITRIOL
ROCEPHIN, CEFTRIAXONE SODIUM
ROCEPHIN W/ DEXTROSE, CEFTRIAXONE SODIUM
SOLATENE, BETA-CAROTENE
SYNKAYVITE, MENADIOL SODIUM DIPHOSPHATE
TARACTAN, CHLORPROTHIXENE
TEGISON, ETRETINATE
TENSILON, EDROPHONIUM CHLORIDE
TRIMPEX, TRIMETHOPRIM
TRIMPEX 200, TRIMETHOPRIM
VALIUM, DIAZEPAM
VALRELEASE, DIAZEPAM
VERSED, MIDAZOLAM HYDROCHLORIDE
* ROCHE PRODUCTS INC
DALMANE, FLURAZEPAM HYDROCHLORIDE
LIBRITABS, CHLORDIAZEPOXIDE
LIBRIUM, CHLORDIAZEPOXIDE HYDROCHLORIDE

ROERIG
* ROERIG DIV PFIZER INC
ANTIMINTH, PYRANTEL PAMOATE
ANTIVERT, MECLIZINE HYDROCHLORIDE
ATARAX, HYDROXYZINE HYDROCHLORIDE
EMETE-CON, BENZQUINAMIDE HYDROCHLORIDE
GEOPEN, CARBENICILLIN DISODIUM
GLUCOTROL, GLIPIZIDE
LITHANE, LITHIUM CARBONATE
NAVANE, THIOTHIXENE
NAVANE, THIOTHIXENE HYDROCHLORIDE
SUSTAIRE, THEOPHYLLINE
TAO, TROLEANDOMYCIN

RORER
* RORER PHARMACEUTICAL CORP SUB RORER GROUP
NITROL, NITROGLYCERIN

ROSS
* ROSS LABORATORIES DIV ABBOTT LABORATORIES INC
PEDIAMYCIN, ERYTHROMYCIN ETHYLSUCCINATE
PEDIAMYCIN 400, ERYTHROMYCIN
    ETHYLSUCCINATE
PEDIAZOLE, ERYTHROMYCIN ETHYLSUCCINATE
SURVANTA, BERACTANT

ROXANE
* ROXANE LABORATORIES INC
ACETAMINOPHEN, ACETAMINOPHEN (OTC)
ACETAMINOPHEN AND CODEINE PHOSPHATE,
    ACETAMINOPHEN
ACETAMINOPHEN AND CODEINE PHOSPHATE NO. 4,
    ACETAMINOPHEN
ACETAMINOPHEN W/ CODEINE, ACETAMINOPHEN
ACETAMINOPHEN W/ CODEINE NO. 2,
    ACETAMINOPHEN
ACETAMINOPHEN W/ CODEINE NO. 3,
    ACETAMINOPHEN
AMINOPHYLLINE, AMINOPHYLLINE
AMITRIPTYLINE HCL, AMITRIPTYLINE
    HYDROCHLORIDE
CHLORDIAZEPOXIDE HCL, CHLORDIAZEPOXIDE
    HYDROCHLORIDE
CHLORPHENIRAMINE MALEATE,
    CHLORPHENIRAMINE MALEATE
CHLORPROMAZINE HCL, CHLORPROMAZINE
    HYDROCHLORIDE
CHLORPROMAZINE HCL INTENSOL,
    CHLORPROMAZINE HYDROCHLORIDE
DEXAMETHASONE, DEXAMETHASONE
DEXAMETHASONE INTENSOL, DEXAMETHASONE
DIAZEPAM, DIAZEPAM
DIAZEPAM INTENSOL, DIAZEPAM
DIPHENHYDRAMINE HCL, DIPHENHYDRAMINE
    HYDROCHLORIDE
DIPHENOXYLATE HCL AND ATROPINE SULFATE,
    ATROPINE SULFATE
FUROSEMIDE, FUROSEMIDE
HALOPERIDOL, HALOPERIDOL
HALOPERIDOL INTENSOL, HALOPERIDOL LACTATE
HYDROCHLOROTHIAZIDE, HYDROCHLOROTHIAZIDE
HYDROCHLOROTHIAZIDE INTENSOL,
    HYDROCHLOROTHIAZIDE
HYDROCHLOROTHIAZIDE W/ RESERPINE,
    HYDROCHLOROTHIAZIDE
HYDROCORTISONE, HYDROCORTISONE
IMIPRAMINE HCL, IMIPRAMINE HYDROCHLORIDE
INDOMETHACIN, INDOMETHACIN
ISOETHARINE HCL, ISOETHARINE HYDROCHLORIDE
LACTULOSE, LACTULOSE
LIDOCAINE HCL, LIDOCAINE HYDROCHLORIDE

APPENDIX B
PRODUCT NAME INDEX
LISTED BY APPLICANT *(continued)*

LIDOCAINE VISCOUS, LIDOCAINE HYDROCHLORIDE
LITHIUM CARBONATE, LITHIUM CARBONATE
LITHIUM CITRATE, LITHIUM CITRATE
LOPERAMIDE HCL, LOPERAMIDE HYDROCHLORIDE
 (OTC)
LOPERAMIDE HCL, LOPERAMIDE HYDROCHLORIDE
LORAZEPAM INTENSOL, LORAZEPAM
MEPERIDINE HCL, MEPERIDINE HYDROCHLORIDE
MEPROBAMATE, MEPROBAMATE
METHADONE HCL, METHADONE HYDROCHLORIDE
METHADONE HCL INTENSOL, METHADONE
 HYDROCHLORIDE
METHOCARBAMOL, METHOCARBAMOL
METHYLDOPA, METHYLDOPA
METOCLOPRAMIDE HCL, METOCLOPRAMIDE
 HYDROCHLORIDE
METOCLOPRAMIDE INTENSOL, METOCLOPRAMIDE
 HYDROCHLORIDE
NEOMYCIN SULFATE, NEOMYCIN SULFATE
NYSTATIN, NYSTATIN
ORAMORPH SR, MORPHINE SULFATE
OXYCODONE AND ASPIRIN (HALF-STRENGTH),
 ASPIRIN
POTASSIUM IODIDE, POTASSIUM IODIDE (OTC)
PREDNISOLONE, PREDNISOLONE
PREDNISONE, PREDNISONE
PREDNISONE INTENSOL, PREDNISONE
PROCAINAMIDE HCL, PROCAINAMIDE
 HYDROCHLORIDE
PROPANTHELINE BROMIDE, PROPANTHELINE
 BROMIDE
PROPOXYPHENE HCL, PROPOXYPHENE
 HYDROCHLORIDE
PROPRANOLOL HCL, PROPRANOLOL
 HYDROCHLORIDE
PROPRANOLOL HCL INTENSOL, PROPRANOLOL
 HYDROCHLORIDE
QUINIDINE GLUCONATE, QUINIDINE GLUCONATE
QUINIDINE SULFATE, QUINIDINE SULFATE
RESERPINE, RESERPINE
ROXICET, ACETAMINOPHEN
ROXICET 5/500, ACETAMINOPHEN
ROXIPRIN, ASPIRIN
SODIUM POLYSTYRENE SULFONATE, SODIUM
 POLYSTYRENE SULFONATE
SULFAMETHOXAZOLE AND TRIMETHOPRIM,
 SULFAMETHOXAZOLE
SULFAMETHOXAZOLE AND TRIMETHOPRIM DOUBLE
 STRENGTH, SULFAMETHOXAZOLE
SULFISOXAZOLE, SULFISOXAZOLE
TETRACYCLINE HCL, TETRACYCLINE
 HYDROCHLORIDE
THEOPHYLLINE, THEOPHYLLINE
THIORIDAZINE HCL, THIORIDAZINE
 HYDROCHLORIDE
THIORIDAZINE HCL INTENSOL, THIORIDAZINE
 HYDROCHLORIDE
THIOTHIXENE HCL INTENSOL, THIOTHIXENE
 HYDROCHLORIDE
TRIAMCINOLONE, TRIAMCINOLONE

ROYCE
* ROYCE LABORATORIES
 AMILORIDE HCL AND HYDROCHLOROTHIAZIDE,
  AMILORIDE HYDROCHLORIDE
 CHLORZOXAZONE, CHLORZOXAZONE
 DOXEPIN HCL, DOXEPIN HYDROCHLORIDE
 HALOPERIDOL, HALOPERIDOL
 LORAZEPAM, LORAZEPAM
 MINOXIDIL, MINOXIDIL
 PERPHENAZINE AND AMITRIPTYLINE HCL,
  AMITRIPTYLINE HYDROCHLORIDE

S

SANDOZ
* SANDOZ PHARMACEUTICALS CORP
 ACYLANID, ACETYLDIGITOXIN
 CAFERGOT, CAFFEINE
 CEDILANID-D, DESLANOSIDE
 CLOZARIL, CLOZAPINE
 D.H.E. 45, DIHYDROERGOTAMINE MESYLATE
 DIAPID, LYPRESSIN
 DYNACIRC, ISRADIPINE
 EMBOLEX, DIHYDROERGOTAMINE MESYLATE
 FIORICET, ACETAMINOPHEN
 FIORINAL, ASPIRIN
 FIORINAL W/CODEINE NO 3, ASPIRIN
 HYDERGINE, ERGOLOID MESYLATES
 HYDERGINE LC, ERGOLOID MESYLATES
 MELLARIL, THIORIDAZINE HYDROCHLORIDE
 MELLARIL-S, THIORIDAZINE
 MESANTOIN, MEPHENYTOIN
 METHERGINE, METHYLERGONOVINE MALEATE
 MIACALCIN, CALCITONIN, SALMON
 PAMELOR, NORTRIPTYLINE HYDROCHLORIDE
 PARLODEL, BROMOCRIPTINE MESYLATE
 RESTORIL, TEMAZEPAM
 SANDIMMUNE, CYCLOSPORINE
 SANDOSTATIN, OCTREOTIDE ACETATE
 SANOREX, MAZINDOL
 SANSERT, METHYSERGIDE MALEATE
 SERENTIL, MESORIDAZINE BESYLATE
 SYNTOCINON, OXYTOCIN
 TAVIST, CLEMASTINE FUMARATE
 TAVIST D, CLEMASTINE FUMARATE
 TAVIST-D, CLEMASTINE FUMARATE (OTC)
 TAVIST-1, CLEMASTINE FUMARATE
 TAVIST-1, CLEMASTINE FUMARATE (OTC)
 TORECAN, THIETHYLPERAZINE MALEATE
 TORECAN, THIETHYLPERAZINE MALATE
 TORECAN, THIETHYLPERAZINE MALEATE
 TREST, METHIXENE HYDROCHLORIDE
 VISKAZIDE, HYDROCHLOROTHIAZIDE
 VISKEN, PINDOLOL
* SANDOZ PHARMACEUTICALS CORP DIV SANDOZ INC
 FIORICET W/ CODEINE, ACETAMINOPHEN
 TRIAMINIC-12, CHLORPHENIRAMINE MALEATE (OTC)

SANKYO
* SANKYO USA CORP
 BANAN, CEFPODOXIME PROXETIL

SAVAGE
* SAVAGE LABORATORIES DIV ALTANA INC
 ALPHATREX, BETAMETHASONE DIPROPIONATE
 BETATREX, BETAMETHASONE VALERATE
 DILOR, DYPHYLLINE
 DILOR-400, DYPHYLLINE
 DITATE-DS, ESTRADIOL VALERATE
 ETHIODOL, ETHIODIZED OIL
 FLUOTREX, FLUOCINOLONE ACETONIDE
 GVS, GENTIAN VIOLET
 MYTREX A, NEOMYCIN SULFATE
 MYTREX F, NYSTATIN
 NYSTEX, NYSTATIN
 RUVITE, CYANOCOBALAMIN
 SATRIC, METRONIDAZOLE
 TRYMEX, TRIAMCINOLONE ACETONIDE
 TRYSUL, TRIPLE SULFA
  (SULFABENZAMIDE; SULFACETAMIDE; SULFATHIAZOLE)

SCHERER
* RP SCHERER
 NIFEDIPINE, NIFEDIPINE

APPENDIX B
PRODUCT NAME INDEX
LISTED BY APPLICANT (continued)

* RP SCHERER NORTH AMERICA
  NIFEDIPINE, NIFEDIPINE
  VALPROIC ACID, VALPROIC ACID
* RP SCHERER NORTH AMERICA DIV RP SCHERER CORP
  DIPHENOXYLATE HCL W/ ATROPINE SULFATE,
    ATROPINE SULFATE
  THEOPHYLLINE, THEOPHYLLINE
  THEOPHYLLINE-SR, THEOPHYLLINE
  VALPROIC ACID, VALPROIC ACID

SCHERING
* SCHERING CORP SUB SCHERING PLOUGH CORP
  AFRINOL, PSEUDOEPHEDRINE SULFATE (OTC)
  AKRINOL, ACRISORCIN
  BETAPAR, MEPREDNISONE
  CELESTONE, BETAMETHASONE
  CELESTONE, BETAMETHASONE SODIUM PHOSPHATE
  CELESTONE SOLUSPAN, BETAMETHASONE ACETATE
  CHLOR-TRIMETON, CHLORPHENIRAMINE MALEATE
  CHLOR-TRIMETON, CHLORPHENIRAMINE MALEATE
    (OTC)
  CHLOR-TRIMETON, CHLORPHENIRAMINE MALEATE
  CHLOR-TRIMETON, CHLORPHENIRAMINE MALEATE
    (OTC)
  DEMAZIN, CHLORPHENIRAMINE MALEATE (OTC)
  DIPROLENE, BETAMETHASONE DIPROPIONATE
  DIPROLENE AF, BETAMETHASONE DIPROPIONATE
  DIPROSONE, BETAMETHASONE DIPROPIONATE
  DISOMER, DEXBROMPHENIRAMINE MALEATE
  DISOPHROL, DEXBROMPHENIRAMINE MALEATE
    (OTC)
  DRIXORAL, DEXBROMPHENIRAMINE MALEATE (OTC)
  DRIXORAL PLUS, ACETAMINOPHEN (OTC)
  ELOCON, MOMETASONE FUROATE
  ESTINYL, ETHINYL ESTRADIOL
  ETRAFON 2-10, AMITRIPTYLINE HYDROCHLORIDE
  ETRAFON 2-25, AMITRIPTYLINE HYDROCHLORIDE
  ETRAFON-A, AMITRIPTYLINE HYDROCHLORIDE
  ETRAFON-FORTE, AMITRIPTYLINE HYDROCHLORIDE
  EULEXIN, FLUTAMIDE
  FULVICIN P/G, GRISEOFULVIN,
    ULTRAMICROCRYSTALLINE
  FULVICIN P/G 165, GRISEOFULVIN,
    ULTRAMICROCRYSTALLINE
  FULVICIN P/G 330, GRISEOFULVIN,
    ULTRAMICROCRYSTALLINE
  FULVICIN-U/F, GRISEOFULVIN, MICROCRYSTALLINE
  GARAMYCIN, GENTAMICIN SULFATE
  GYNE-LOTRIMIN, CLOTRIMAZOLE
  GYNE-LOTRIMIN, CLOTRIMAZOLE (OTC)
  HYPERSTAT, DIAZOXIDE
  K-DUR 10, POTASSIUM CHLORIDE
  K-DUR 20, POTASSIUM CHLORIDE
  LOTRIMIN, CLOTRIMAZOLE
  LOTRIMIN AF, CLOTRIMAZOLE (OTC)
  LOTRISONE, BETAMETHASONE DIPROPIONATE
  METI-DERM, PREDNISOLONE
  METICORTELONE, PREDNISOLONE ACETATE
  METICORTEN, PREDNISONE
  METIMYD, PREDNISOLONE ACETATE
  METOCLOPRAMIDE HCL, METOCLOPRAMIDE
    HYDROCHLORIDE
  METRETON, PREDNISOLONE SODIUM PHOSPHATE
  MIRADON, ANISINDIONE
  NAQUA, TRICHLORMETHIAZIDE
  NAQUIVAL, RESERPINE
  NETROMYCIN, NETILMICIN SULFATE
  NORMODYNE, LABETALOL HYDROCHLORIDE
  NORMOZIDE, HYDROCHLOROTHIAZIDE
  OCUCLEAR, OXYMETAZOLINE HYDROCHLORIDE
    (OTC)

OPTIMINE, AZATADINE MALEATE
ORETON, METHYLTESTOSTERONE
ORETON METHYL, METHYLTESTOSTERONE
OTOBIONE, HYDROCORTISONE
OTOBIOTIC, HYDROCORTISONE
PAXIPAM, HALAZEPAM
PERMITIL, FLUPHENAZINE HYDROCHLORIDE
POLARAMINE, DEXCHLORPHENIRAMINE MALEATE
PRANTAL, DIPHEMANIL METHYLSULFATE
PROPRANOLOL HCL, PROPRANOLOL
  HYDROCHLORIDE
PROVENTIL, ALBUTEROL
PROVENTIL, ALBUTEROL SULFATE
RELA, CARISOPRODOL
SODIUM SULAMYD, SULFACETAMIDE SODIUM
THEOVENT, THEOPHYLLINE
TINDAL, ACETOPHENAZINE MALEATE
TREMIN, TRIHEXYPHENIDYL HYDROCHLORIDE
TRILAFON, PERPHENAZINE
TRINALIN, AZATADINE MALEATE
VALISONE, BETAMETHASONE VALERATE
VANCENASE, BECLOMETHASONE DIPROPIONATE
VANCENASE AQ, BECLOMETHASONE DIPROPIONATE
  MONOHYDRATE
VANCERIL, BECLOMETHASONE DIPROPIONATE

SCHIAPPARELLI SEARLE
* SCHIAPPARELLI SEARLE
  BANTHINE, METHANTHELINE BROMIDE
  DIULO, METOLAZONE
  FLAGYL I.V., METRONIDAZOLE HYDROCHLORIDE
  FLAGYL I.V. RTU, METRONIDAZOLE
  FLAGYL I.V. RTU IN PLASTIC CONTAINER,
    METRONIDAZOLE
  HALOPERIDOL, HALOPERIDOL
  HALOPERIDOL, HALOPERIDOL LACTATE
  NORETHIN 1/35E-21, ETHINYL ESTRADIOL
  NORETHIN 1/35E-28, ETHINYL ESTRADIOL
  NORETHIN 1/50M-21, MESTRANOL
  NORETHIN 1/50M-28, MESTRANOL
  PIROXICAM, PIROXICAM
  PRO-BANTHINE, PROPANTHELINE BROMIDE

SCHWARZ
* SCHWARZ PHARMACEUTICALS INC
  PRE-PEN, BENZYL PENICILLOYL-POLYLYSINE

SEARLE
* GD SEARLE AND CO
  ALDACTAZIDE, HYDROCHLOROTHIAZIDE
  ALDACTONE, SPIRONOLACTONE
  AMINOPHYLLIN, AMINOPHYLLINE
  AMMONIUM CHLORIDE, AMMONIUM CHLORIDE
  CALAN, VERAPAMIL HYDROCHLORIDE
  CLORAZEPATE DIPOTASSIUM, CLORAZEPATE
    DIPOTASSIUM
  CU-7, COPPER
  CYTOTEC, MISOPROSTOL
  DEMULEN 1/35-21, ETHINYL ESTRADIOL
  DEMULEN 1/35-28, ETHINYL ESTRADIOL
  DEMULEN 1/50-21, ETHINYL ESTRADIOL
  DEMULEN 1/50-28, ETHINYL ESTRADIOL
  ENOVID, MESTRANOL
  ENOVID-E, MESTRANOL
  ENOVID-E 21, MESTRANOL
  FLAGYL, METRONIDAZOLE
  LIDOCAINE HCL, LIDOCAINE HYDROCHLORIDE
  LOMOTIL, ATROPINE SULFATE
  MAXAQUIN, LOMEFLOXACIN HYDROCHLORIDE
  METARAMINOL BITARTRATE, METARAMINOL
    BITARTRATE

APPENDIX B
PRODUCT NAME INDEX
LISTED BY APPLICANT *(continued)*

NORPACE, DISOPYRAMIDE PHOSPHATE
NORPACE CR, DISOPYRAMIDE PHOSPHATE
OVULEN, ETHYNODIOL DIACETATE
OVULEN-21, ETHYNODIOL DIACETATE
OVULEN-28, ETHYNODIOL DIACETATE
POTASSIUM CHLORIDE, POTASSIUM CHLORIDE
PRO-BANTHINE, PROPANTHELINE BROMIDE
PROCAINE HCL, PROCAINE HYDROCHLORIDE
TATUM-T, COPPER

SERONO
* SERONO LABORATORIES INC
  ASELLACRIN 10, SOMATROPIN
  ASELLACRIN 2, SOMATROPIN
  GEREF, SERMORELIN ACETATE
  METRODIN, UROFOLLITROPIN
  PERGONAL, MENOTROPINS
  SEROPHENE, CLOMIPHENE CITRATE

SHERWOOD
* SHERWOOD MEDICAL CO
  ACTIN-N, NITROFURAZONE
  THERMAZENE, SILVER SULFADIAZINE

SHIONOGI
* SHIONOGI USA INC
  UROBAK, SULFAMETHOXAZOLE
  UROPLUS DS, SULFAMETHOXAZOLE
  UROPLUS SS, SULFAMETHOXAZOLE

SIDMAK
* SIDMAK LABORATORIES INC
  ALBUTEROL SULFATE, ALBUTEROL SULFATE
  AMITRIPTYLINE HCL, AMITRIPTYLINE
    HYDROCHLORIDE
  BENZTROPINE MESYLATE, BENZTROPINE MESYLATE
  BETHANECHOL CHLORIDE, BETHANECHOL
    CHLORIDE
  CARBAMAZEPINE, CARBAMAZEPINE
  CHLORPROPAMIDE, CHLORPROPAMIDE
  CHLORTHALIDONE, CHLORTHALIDONE
  CYPROHEPTADINE HCL, CYPROHEPTADINE
    HYDROCHLORIDE
  DESIPRAMINE HCL, DESIPRAMINE HYDROCHLORIDE
  DEXCHLORPHENIRAMINE MALEATE,
    DEXCHLORPHENIRAMINE MALEATE
  DISULFIRAM, DISULFIRAM
  DOXYCYCLINE HYCLATE, DOXYCYCLINE HYCLATE
  EXTENDED PHENYTOIN SODIUM, PHENYTOIN
    SODIUM, EXTENDED
  HYDRALAZINE HCL, HYDRALAZINE
    HYDROCHLORIDE
  HYDROXYZINE HCL, HYDROXYZINE
    HYDROCHLORIDE
  IBUPRIN, IBUPROFEN (OTC)
  IBUPROFEN, IBUPROFEN
  INDOMETHACIN, INDOMETHACIN
  MECLIZINE HCL, MECLIZINE HYDROCHLORIDE
  METHYLDOPA, METHYLDOPA
  METOCLOPRAMIDE HCL, METOCLOPRAMIDE
    HYDROCHLORIDE
  METRONIDAZOLE, METRONIDAZOLE
  NYSTATIN, NYSTATIN
  OXYBUTYNIN CHLORIDE, OXYBUTYNIN CHLORIDE
  PROCAINAMIDE HCL, PROCAINAMIDE
    HYDROCHLORIDE
  PROPRANOLOL HCL, PROPRANOLOL
    HYDROCHLORIDE
  PROPRANOLOL HCL AND HYDROCHLOROTHIAZIDE,
    HYDROCHLOROTHIAZIDE
  SULFAMETHOXAZOLE AND TRIMETHOPRIM,
    SULFAMETHOXAZOLE

THEOPHYLLINE, THEOPHYLLINE
TRAZODONE HCL, TRAZODONE HYDROCHLORIDE
TRAZON-150, TRAZODONE HYDROCHLORIDE
ULTRAGRIS-165, GRISEOFULVIN,
  ULTRAMICROCRYSTALLINE
ULTRAGRIS-330, GRISEOFULVIN,
  ULTRAMICROCRYSTALLINE
VERAPAMIL HCL, VERAPAMIL HYDROCHLORIDE

SIGMA TAU
* SIGMA TAU PHARMACEUTICALS INC
  CARNITOR, LEVOCARNITINE

SILARX
* SILARX PHARMACEUTICALS INC
  METAPROTERENOL SULFATE, METAPROTERENOL
    SULFATE
  SILPHEN, DIPHENHYDRAMINE HYDROCHLORIDE
    (OTC)

SKCP
* SMITH KLINE CONSUMER PRODUCTS DIV SMITH
KLINE AND FRENCH L
  CONTAC, CHLORPHENIRAMINE MALEATE (OTC)
  TELDRIN, CHLORPHENIRAMINE MALEATE (OTC)

SKF
* SMITH KLINE AND FRENCH LABORATORIES DIV
SMITHKLINE BECKMAN
  ANCEF, CEFAZOLIN SODIUM
  ANSPOR, CEPHRADINE
  CEFIZOX, CEFTIZOXIME SODIUM
  CEFIZOX IN DEXTROSE 5% IN PLASTIC CONTAINER,
    CEFTIZOXIME SODIUM
  COMPAZINE, PROCHLORPERAZINE
  COMPAZINE, PROCHLORPERAZINE EDISYLATE
  COMPAZINE, PROCHLORPERAZINE MALEATE
  CYTOMEL, LIOTHYRONINE SODIUM
  DARBID, ISOPROPAMIDE IODIDE
  DEXEDRINE, DEXTROAMPHETAMINE SULFATE
  DIBENZYLINE, PHENOXYBENZAMINE
    HYDROCHLORIDE
  DYAZIDE, HYDROCHLOROTHIAZIDE
  DYRENIUM, TRIAMTERENE
  ESKALITH, LITHIUM CARBONATE
  ESKALITH CR, LITHIUM CARBONATE
  MONOCID, CEFONICID SODIUM
  ORNADE, CHLORPHENIRAMINE MALEATE
  RIDAURA, AURANOFIN
  STELAZINE, TRIFLUOPERAZINE HYDROCHLORIDE
  STOXIL, IDOXURIDINE
  TAGAMET, CIMETIDINE
  TAGAMET, CIMETIDINE HYDROCHLORIDE
  TAGAMET HCL IN SODIUM CHLORIDE 0.9%,
    CIMETIDINE HYDROCHLORID
  TAZICEF, CEFTAZIDIME
  THORAZINE, CHLORPROMAZINE
  THORAZINE, CHLORPROMAZINE HYDROCHLORIDE
  URISPAS, FLAVOXATE HYDROCHLORIDE
  VONTROL, DIPHENIDOL HYDROCHLORIDE

SMITH NEPHEW SOLOPAK
* SMITH AND NEPHEW SOLOPAK DIV SMITH AND
NEPHEW
  AMINOPHYLLINE, AMINOPHYLLINE
  CLINDAMYCIN PHOSPHATE, CLINDAMYCIN
    PHOSPHATE
  CYANOCOBALAMIN, CYANOCOBALAMIN
  DOPAMINE HCL, DOPAMINE HYDROCHLORIDE
  DROPERIDOL, DROPERIDOL
  FLUOROURACIL, FLUOROURACIL
  FUROSEMIDE, FUROSEMIDE

APPENDIX B
PRODUCT NAME INDEX
LISTED BY APPLICANT (continued)

GENTAMICIN SULFATE, GENTAMICIN SULFATE
HALOPERIDOL, HALOPERIDOL LACTATE
HEPARIN LOCK FLUSH, HEPARIN SODIUM
HEPARIN SODIUM, HEPARIN SODIUM
HYDRALAZINE HCL, HYDRALAZINE
    HYDROCHLORIDE
HYDROXYZINE HCL, HYDROXYZINE
    HYDROCHLORIDE
KANAMYCIN SULFATE, KANAMYCIN SULFATE
METHYLDOPATE HCL, METHYLDOPATE
    HYDROCHLORIDE
METOCLOPRAMIDE HCL, METOCLOPRAMIDE
    HYDROCHLORIDE
NALOXONE HCL, NALOXONE HYDROCHLORIDE
NITROGLYCERIN, NITROGLYCERIN
PHENYTOIN SODIUM, PHENYTOIN SODIUM
PROCAINAMIDE HCL, PROCAINAMIDE
    HYDROCHLORIDE
PROCHLORPERAZINE EDISYLATE,
    PROCHLORPERAZINE EDISYLATE
PROPRANOLOL HCL, PROPRANOLOL
    HYDROCHLORIDE
TRIMETHOBENZAMIDE HCL, TRIMETHOBENZAMIDE
    HYDROCHLORIDE
VERAPAMIL HCL, VERAPAMIL HYDROCHLORIDE

SMITHKLINE BEECHAM
* SMITHKLINE BEECHAM PHARMACEUTICALS
    HALFAN, HALOFANTRINE HYDROCHLORIDE
    HISPRIL, DIPHENYLPYRALINE HYDROCHLORIDE
    PENTACEF, CEFTAZIDIME (ARGININE
        FORMULATION)
    RELAFEN, NABUMETONE
    TRIOSTAT, LIOTHYRONINE SODIUM

SOLA BARNES HIND
* SOLA BARNES HIND
    ALPHA CHYMAR, CHYMOTRYPSIN
    BENOXINATE HCL, BENOXINATE HYDROCHLORIDE
    CYCLOPENTOLATE HCL, CYCLOPENTOLATE
        HYDROCHLORIDE
    DEXAMETHASONE SODIUM PHOSPHATE,
        DEXAMETHASONE SODIUM PHOSPHATE
    GAMENE, LINDANE
    PREDNISOLONE SODIUM PHOSPHATE,
        PREDNISOLONE SODIUM PHOSPHATE
    PROPARACAINE HCL, PROPARACAINE
        HYDROCHLORIDE
    SODIUM SULFACETAMIDE, SULFACETAMIDE SODIUM
    SULFISOXAZOLE DIOLAMINE, SULFISOXAZOLE
        DIOLAMINE

SOLVAY
* SOLVAY PHARMACEUTICALS
    AQUATAG, BENZTHIAZIDE
    BALNEOL-HC, HYDROCORTISONE
    BUTABARBITAL SODIUM, BUTABARBITAL SODIUM
    CHENIX, CHENODIOL
    CIN-QUIN, QUINIDINE SULFATE
    COMPAL, ACETAMINOPHEN
    CORTENEMA, HYDROCORTISONE
    CURRETAB, MEDROXYPROGESTERONE ACETATE
    DERMACORT, HYDROCORTISONE
    DEXONE 0.5, DEXAMETHASONE
    DEXONE 0.75, DEXAMETHASONE
    DEXONE 1.5, DEXAMETHASONE
    DEXONE 4, DEXAMETHASONE
    DUPHALAC, LACTULOSE
    ESTRAGUARD, DIENESTROL
    ESTRATAB, ESTROGENS, ESTERIFIED
    GYNOREST, DYDROGESTERONE

HYDRALAZINE HCL AND HYDROCHLOROTHIAZIDE,
    HYDRALAZINE HYDROCHLORIDE
HYDROCHLOROTHIAZIDE, HYDROCHLOROTHIAZIDE
LACTULOSE, LACTULOSE
LITHONATE, LITHIUM CARBONATE
LITHOTABS, LITHIUM CARBONATE
MELFIAT, PHENDIMETRAZINE TARTRATE
MELFIAT-105, PHENDIMETRAZINE TARTRATE
MEPROBAMATE, MEPROBAMATE
METHOCARBAMOL, METHOCARBAMOL
ORASONE, PREDNISONE
PHENDIMETRAZINE TARTRATE, PHENDIMETRAZINE
    TARTRATE
PORTALAC, LACTULOSE
PROCTOCORT, HYDROCORTISONE
PROVAL #3, ACETAMINOPHEN
R-P MYCIN, ERYTHROMYCIN
RAUWOLFIA SERPENTINA, RAUWOLFIA SERPENTINA
RESERPINE, RESERPINE
RESERPINE, HYDRALAZINE HCL AND
    HYDROCHLOROTHIAZIDE, HYDRALAZINE
    HYDROCHLORIDE
RETET, TETRACYCLINE HYDROCHLORIDE
ROWASA, MESALAMINE
S.A.S.-500, SULFASALAZINE
SER-A-GEN, HYDRALAZINE HYDROCHLORIDE
SPRX-105, PHENDIMETRAZINE TARTRATE
SPRX-3, PHENDIMETRAZINE TARTRATE
SULSOXIN, SULFISOXAZOLE
SYMADINE, AMANTADINE HYDROCHLORIDE
TORA, PHENTERMINE HYDROCHLORIDE
TRANMEP, MEPROBAMATE
TRIACORT, TRIAMCINOLONE ACETONIDE
UNIPRES, HYDRALAZINE HYDROCHLORIDE
VERMIDOL, PIPERAZINE CITRATE
ZIDE, HYDROCHLOROTHIAZIDE

SOMERSET
* SOMERSET PHARMACEUTICALS INC
    ELDEPRYL, SELEGILINE HYDROCHLORIDE

SORIN
* SORIN BIOMEDICA SPA
    SODIUM ROSE BENGAL I 131, ROSE BENGAL SODIUM,
        I-131

SPERTI
* SPERTI DRUG PRODUCTS INC
    PREDNISOLONE, PREDNISOLONE
    PREDNISONE, PREDNISONE

SQUIBB
* ER SQUIBB AND SONS INC
    AMITID, AMITRIPTYLINE HYDROCHLORIDE
    AMNESTROGEN, ESTROGENS, ESTERIFIED
    AZACTAM, AZTREONAM
    CAPOZIDE 25/15, CAPTOPRIL
    CAPOZIDE 25/25, CAPTOPRIL
    CAPOZIDE 50/15, CAPTOPRIL
    CAPOZIDE 50/25, CAPTOPRIL
    CARDIOGRAFIN, DIATRIZOATE MEGLUMINE
    CHLORMERODRIN HG 197, CHLORMERODRIN, HG-197
    CHOLOGRAFIN MEGLUMINE, IODIPAMIDE
        MEGLUMINE
    CHOLOGRAFIN SODIUM, IODIPAMIDE SODIUM
    CHOLOVUE, IODOXAMATE MEGLUMINE
    CHROMITOPE SODIUM, SODIUM CHROMATE, CR-51
    CORGARD, NADOLOL
    CORZIDE, BENDROFLUMETHIAZIDE
    DELADUMONE, ESTRADIOL VALERATE
    DELADUMONE OB, ESTRADIOL VALERATE
    DELALUTIN, HYDROXYPROGESTERONE CAPROATE

APPENDIX B
PRODUCT NAME INDEX
LISTED BY APPLICANT (continued)

DELESTROGEN, ESTRADIOL VALERATE
ETHRIL 250, ERYTHROMYCIN STEARATE
ETHRIL 500, ERYTHROMYCIN STEARATE
FLORINEF, FLUDROCORTISONE ACETATE
FOLLUTEIN, GONADOTROPIN, CHORIONIC
FUNGIZONE, AMPHOTERICIN B
HALOG, HALCINONIDE
HYDREA, HYDROXYUREA
IODOTOPE, SODIUM IODIDE, I-131
KENACORT, TRIAMCINOLONE
KENACORT, TRIAMCINOLONE DIACETATE
KENALOG IN ORABASE, TRIAMCINOLONE ACETONIDE
MACROTEC, TECHNETIUM TC-99M ALBUMIN AGGRE-
  GATED KIT
MDP-SQUIBB, TECHNETIUM TC-99M MEDRONATE KIT
MYCOLOG-II, NYSTATIN
MYCOSTATIN, NYSTATIN
NATURETIN-10, BENDROFLUMETHIAZIDE
NATURETIN-2.5, BENDROFLUMETHIAZIDE
NATURETIN-5, BENDROFLUMETHIAZIDE
NEOMYCIN SULFATE, NEOMYCIN SULFATE
NYDRAZID, ISONIAZID
OPHTHAINE, PROPARACAINE HYDROCHLORIDE
ORA-TESTRYL, FLUOXYMESTERONE
ORAGRAFIN CALCIUM, IPODATE CALCIUM
ORAGRAFIN SODIUM, IPODATE SODIUM
PENICILLIN G POTASSIUM, PENICILLIN G POTASSIUM
PENTIDS '200', PENICILLIN G POTASSIUM
PENTIDS '250', PENICILLIN G POTASSIUM
PENTIDS '400', PENICILLIN G POTASSIUM
PENTIDS '800', PENICILLIN G POTASSIUM
PHOSPHOTOPE, SODIUM PHOSPHATE, P-32
PRINCIPEN '125', AMPICILLIN/AMPICILLIN TRIHYDRATE
PRINCIPEN '250', AMPICILLIN/AMPICILLIN TRIHYDRATE
PRINCIPEN '500', AMPICILLIN/AMPICILLIN TRIHYDRATE
PRINCIPEN W/ PROBENECID, AMPICILLIN TRIHYDRATE
PROLIXIN, FLUPHENAZINE HYDROCHLORIDE
PROLIXIN DECANOATE, FLUPHENAZINE DECANOATE
PROLIXIN ENANTHATE, FLUPHENAZINE ENANTHATE
PRONESTYL, PROCAINAMIDE HYDROCHLORIDE
PROTAMINE ZINC INSULIN, INSULIN SUSP PROTAMINE
  ZINC PURIFIED BEEF (OTC)
RAU-SED, RESERPINE
RAUDIXIN, RAUWOLFIA SERPENTINA
RENOTEC, TECHNETIUM TC-99M FERPENTETATE KIT
RENOVUE-65, IODAMIDE MEGLUMINE
REZIPAS, AMINOSALICYLIC ACID RESIN COMPLEX
ROBENGATOPE, ROSE BENGAL SODIUM, I-131
RUBRAMIN PC, CYANOCOBALAMIN
RUBRATOPE-57, CYANOCOBALAMIN, CO-57
RUBRATOPE-57 KIT, COBALT CHLORIDE, CO-57
RUBRATOPE-60, CYANOCOBALAMIN, CO-60
RUBRATOPE-60 KIT, COBALT CHLORIDE, CO-60
SETHOTOPE, SELENOMETHIONINE, SE-75
SINOGRAFIN, DIATRIZOATE MEGLUMINE
STILBESTROL, DIETHYLSTILBESTROL
STILBETIN, DIETHYLSTILBESTROL
SUCOSTRIN, SUCCINYLCHOLINE CHLORIDE
SUMYCIN, TETRACYCLINE
SUMYCIN, TETRACYCLINE HYDROCHLORIDE
TERFONYL, TRISULFAPYRIMIDINES
TESLAC, TESTOLACTONE
TESULOID, TECHNETIUM TC-99M SULFUR COLLOID KIT
TRIMOX, AMOXICILLIN
TUBOCURARINE CHLORIDE, TUBOCURARINE CHLORIDE
VEETIDS '125', PENICILLIN V POTASSIUM
VEETIDS '250', PENICILLIN V POTASSIUM
VEETIDS '500', PENICILLIN V POTASSIUM
VELOSEF, CEPHRADINE
VESPRIN, TRIFLUPROMAZINE
VESPRIN, TRIFLUPROMAZINE HYDROCHLORIDE

VITAMIN A, VITAMIN A PALMITATE
* SQUIBB DIAGNOSTICS
  CARDIOGEN-82, RUBIDIUM CHLORIDE RB-82
  CARDIOTEC, TECHNETIUM TC-99M TEBOROXIME KIT
  CHOLETEC, TECHNETIUM TC-99M MEBROFENIN KIT
  CYSTOGRAFIN, DIATRIZOATE MEGLUMINE
  CYSTOGRAFIN DILUTE, DIATRIZOATE MEGLUMINE
  DIATRIZOATE MEGLUMINE, DIATRIZOATE MEGLU-
    MINE
  GASTROGRAFIN, DIATRIZOATE MEGLUMINE
  HIPPUTOPE, IODOHIPPURATE SODIUM, I-131
  ISOVUE-M 200, IOPAMIDOL
  ISOVUE-M 300, IOPAMIDOL
  ISOVUE-128, IOPAMIDOL
  ISOVUE-200, IOPAMIDOL
  ISOVUE-250, IOPAMIDOL
  ISOVUE-300, IOPAMIDOL
  ISOVUE-370, IOPAMIDOL
  KINEVAC, SINCALIDE
  MINITEC, TECHNETIUM TC-99M SODIUM PERTECHNE-
    TATE GENERATOR
  PHOSPHOTEC, TECHNETIUM TC-99M PYROPHOSPHATE
    KIT
  RENO-M-DIP, DIATRIZOATE MEGLUMINE
  RENO-M-30, DIATRIZOATE MEGLUMINE
  RENO-M-60, DIATRIZOATE MEGLUMINE
  RENOCAL-76, DIATRIZOATE MEGLUMINE
  RENOGRAFIN-60, DIATRIZOATE MEGLUMINE
  RENOGRAFIN-76, DIATRIZOATE MEGLUMINE
  RENOVIST, DIATRIZOATE MEGLUMINE
  RENOVIST II, DIATRIZOATE MEGLUMINE
  RENOVUE-DIP, IODAMIDE MEGLUMINE
  THALLOUS CHLORIDE TL 201, THALLOUS CHLORIDE,
    TL-201
* SQUIBB SPA
  PENICILLIN G SODIUM, PENICILLIN G SODIUM

SQUIBB MARK
* SQUIBB MARK DIV ER SQUIBB AND SONS INC
  CEPHALEXIN, CEPHALEXIN

STANLABS
* STANLABS PHARMACEUTICAL CO SUB SIMPAK CORP
  MEPROBAMATE, MEPROBAMATE

STAR PHARMS
* STAR PHARMACEUTICALS INC
  VIRILON, METHYLTESTOSTERONE

STERIS
* STERIS LABORATORIES INC
  AMITRIPTYLINE HCL, AMITRIPTYLINE
    HYDROCHLORIDE
  BETAMETHASONE SODIUM PHOSPHATE,
    BETAMETHASONE SODIUM PHOSPHATE
  BROMPHENIRAMINE MALEATE, BROMPHENIRAMINE
    MALEATE
  CHLORAMPHENICOL, CHLORAMPHENICOL
  CHLORPHENIRAMINE MALEATE,
    CHLORPHENIRAMINE MALEATE
  CHLORPROMAZINE HCL, CHLORPROMAZINE
    HYDROCHLORIDE
  CHORIONIC GONADOTROPIN, GONADOTROPIN,
    CHORIONIC
  CLINDAMYCIN PHOSPHATE, CLINDAMYCIN
    PHOSPHATE
  COBAVITE, CYANOCOBALAMIN
  CORTICOTROPIN, CORTICOTROPIN
  CORTISONE ACETATE, CORTISONE ACETATE
  CYANOCOBALAMIN, CYANOCOBALAMIN
  CYCLOPENTOLATE HCL, CYCLOPENTOLATE
    HYDROCHLORIDE

APPENDIX B
PRODUCT NAME INDEX
LISTED BY APPLICANT *(continued)*

DEXAMETHASONE, DEXAMETHASONE
DEXAMETHASONE ACETATE, DEXAMETHASONE
   ACETATE
DEXAMETHASONE SODIUM PHOSPHATE,
   DEXAMETHASONE SODIUM PHOSPHATE
DIAZEPAM, DIAZEPAM
DICYCLOMINE HCL, DICYCLOMINE
   HYDROCHLORIDE
DIMENHYDRINATE, DIMENHYDRINATE
DIPHENHYDRAMINE HCL, DIPHENHYDRAMINE
   HYDROCHLORIDE
DISODIUM EDETATE, EDETATE DISODIUM
DOXAPRAM HCL, DOXAPRAM HYDROCHLORIDE
DROPERIDOL, DROPERIDOL
EDETATE DISODIUM, EDETATE DISODIUM
ESTRADIOL CYPIONATE, ESTRADIOL CYPIONATE
ESTRADIOL VALERATE, ESTRADIOL VALERATE
ESTRONE, ESTRONE
FENTANYL CITRATE, FENTANYL CITRATE
FLUOROURACIL, FLUOROURACIL
FUROSEMIDE, FUROSEMIDE
GENTAMICIN SULFATE, GENTAMICIN SULFATE
GLYCOPYRROLATE, GLYCOPYRROLATE
HALOPERIDOL, HALOPERIDOL LACTATE
HEPARIN LOCK FLUSH, HEPARIN SODIUM
HEPARIN SODIUM, HEPARIN SODIUM
HYDROCORTISONE ACETATE, HYDROCORTISONE
   ACETATE
HYDROCORTISONE SODIUM SUCCINATE,
   HYDROCORTISONE SODIUM SUCCINATE
HYDROXOCOBALAMIN, HYDROXOCOBALAMIN
HYDROXYPROGESTERONE CAPROATE,
   HYDROXYPROGESTERONE CAPROATE
HYDROXYZINE HCL, HYDROXYZINE
   HYDROCHLORIDE
IRON DEXTRAN, IRON DEXTRAN
KANAMYCIN SULFATE, KANAMYCIN SULFATE
LIDOCAINE HCL, LIDOCAINE HYDROCHLORIDE
LIDOCAINE HCL W/ EPINEPHRINE, EPINEPHRINE
LINCOMYCIN HCL, LINCOMYCIN HYDROCHLORIDE
MANNITOL 25%, MANNITOL
MEPERIDINE HCL, MEPERIDINE HYDROCHLORIDE
MEPIVACAINE HCL, MEPIVACAINE HYDROCHLORIDE
MERSALYL-THEOPHYLLINE, MERSALYL SODIUM
METHOCARBAMOL, METHOCARBAMOL
METHYLPREDNISOLONE ACETATE,
   METHYLPREDNISOLONE ACETATE
METHYLPREDNISOLONE SODIUM SUCCINATE,
   METHYLPREDNISOLONE SODIUM SUCCINATE
METRONIDAZOLE, METRONIDAZOLE
MORPHINE SULFATE, MORPHINE SULFATE
MVC PLUS, ASCORBIC ACID
NALOXONE HCL, NALOXONE HYDROCHLORIDE
NANDROLONE DECANOATE, NANDROLONE
   DECANOATE
NANDROLONE PHENPROPIONATE, NANDROLONE
   PHENPROPIONATE
NATURAL ESTROGENIC SUBSTANCE-ESTRONE,
   ESTRONE
NEO-OTOSOL-HC, HYDROCORTISONE
NEOMYCIN AND POLYMYXIN B SULFATES,
   NEOMYCIN SULFATE
NEOMYCIN AND POLYMYXIN B SULFATES AND
   DEXAMETHASONE, DEXAMETHASONE
NEOMYCIN AND POLYMYXIN B SULFATES AND
   GRAMICIDIN, GRAMICIDIN
NEOMYCIN AND POLYMYXIN B SULFATES AND
   HYDROCORTISONE, HYDROCORTISONE
NEOMYCIN SULFATE-DEXAMETHASONE SODIUM
   PHOSPHATE, DEXAMETHASONE SODIUM
   PHOSPHATE

ORPHENADRINE CITRATE, ORPHENADRINE CITRATE
OTOCORT, HYDROCORTISONE
PHENYTOIN SODIUM, PHENYTOIN SODIUM
POTASSIUM CHLORIDE, POTASSIUM CHLORIDE
PREDNISOLONE ACETATE, PREDNISOLONE ACETATE
PREDNISOLONE SODIUM PHOSPHATE,
   PREDNISOLONE SODIUM PHOSPHATE
PREDNISOLONE TEBUTATE, PREDNISOLONE
   TEBUTATE
PROCAINAMIDE HCL, PROCAINAMIDE
   HYDROCHLORIDE
PROCAINE HCL, PROCAINE HYDROCHLORIDE
PROCHLORPERAZINE EDISYLATE,
   PROCHLORPERAZINE EDISYLATE
PROGESTERONE, PROGESTERONE
PROMAZINE HCL, PROMAZINE HYDROCHLORIDE
PROMETHAZINE HCL, PROMETHAZINE
   HYDROCHLORIDE
PYRIDOXINE HCL, PYRIDOXINE HYDROCHLORIDE
SULFACETAMIDE SODIUM, SULFACETAMIDE SODIUM
SULFAMETHOXAZOLE AND TRIMETHOPRIM,
   SULFAMETHOXAZOLE
TESTOSTERONE, TESTOSTERONE
TESTOSTERONE CYPIONATE, TESTOSTERONE
   CYPIONATE
TESTOSTERONE CYPIONATE-ESTRADIOL CYPIONATE,
   ESTRADIOL CYPIONATE
TESTOSTERONE ENANTHATE, TESTOSTERONE
   ENANTHATE
TESTOSTERONE ENANTHATE AND ESTRADIOL
   VALERATE, ESTRADIOL VALERATE
TESTOSTERONE PROPIONATE, TESTOSTERONE
   PROPIONATE
THIAMINE HCL, THIAMINE HYDROCHLORIDE
TRIAMCINOLONE ACETONIDE, TRIAMCINOLONE
   ACETONIDE
TRIAMCINOLONE DIACETATE, TRIAMCINOLONE
   DIACETATE
TRIMETHOBENZAMIDE HCL, TRIMETHOBENZAMIDE
   HYDROCHLORIDE
TROPICAMIDE, TROPICAMIDE

STERLING
* STERLING DRUG INC
   AMIPAQUE, METRIZAMIDE
   ARALEN, CHLOROQUINE PHOSPHATE
   ARALEN HCL, CHLOROQUINE HYDROCHLORIDE
   ARALEN PHOSPHATE W/ PRIMAQUINE PHOSPHATE,
      CHLOROQUINE PHOSPHATE
   ATROPINE AND DEMEROL, ATROPINE SULFATE
   BILOPAQUE, TYROPANOATE SODIUM
   BRONKAID MIST, EPINEPHRINE (OTC)
   BRONKODYL, THEOPHYLLINE
   BRONKOMETER, ISOETHARINE MESYLATE
   BRONKOSOL, ISOETHARINE HYDROCHLORIDE
   BRYREL, PIPERAZINE CITRATE
   CARBOCAINE, MEPIVACAINE HYDROCHLORIDE
   DANOCRINE, DANAZOL
   DEMEROL, MEPERIDINE HYDROCHLORIDE
   DIAZEPAM, DIAZEPAM
   DRISDOL, ERGOCALCIFEROL
   FENTANYL CITRATE, FENTANYL CITRATE
   FUROSEMIDE, FUROSEMIDE
   HEPARIN LOCK FLUSH, HEPARIN SODIUM
   HEPARIN SODIUM, HEPARIN SODIUM
   HEPARIN SODIUM PRESERVATIVE FREE, HEPARIN
      SODIUM
   HYDROXYZINE HCL, HYDROXYZINE
      HYDROCHLORIDE
   HYPAQUE, DIATRIZOATE MEGLUMINE
   HYPAQUE, DIATRIZOATE SODIUM

APPENDIX B
PRODUCT NAME INDEX
LISTED BY APPLICANT (continued)

HYPAQUE SODIUM 20%, DIATRIZOATE SODIUM
HYPAQUE-CYSTO, DIATRIZOATE MEGLUMINE
HYPAQUE-M,75%, DIATRIZOATE MEGLUMINE
HYPAQUE-M,90%, DIATRIZOATE MEGLUMINE
HYPAQUE-76, DIATRIZOATE MEGLUMINE
INOCOR, AMRINONE LACTATE
ISOPAQUE 280, CALCIUM
ISOPAQUE 440, CALCIUM METRIZOATE
ISUPREL, ISOPROTERENOL HYDROCHLORIDE
KAYEXALATE, SODIUM POLYSTYRENE SULFONATE
LEVOPHED, NOREPINEPHRINE BITARTRATE
LOTUSATE, TALBUTAL
MARCAINE, BUPIVACAINE HYDROCHLORIDE
MARCAINE HCL, BUPIVACAINE HYDROCHLORIDE
MARCAINE HCL W/ EPINEPHRINE, BUPIVACAINE
   HYDROCHLORIDE
MEASURIN, ASPIRIN (OTC)
MILRINONE LACTATE, MILRINONE LACTATE
MODRASTANE, TRILOSTANE
MYTELASE, AMBENONIUM CHLORIDE
NALOXONE HCL, NALOXONE HYDROCHLORIDE
NEGGRAM, NALIDIXIC ACID
NOVOCAIN, PROCAINE HYDROCHLORIDE
OMNIPAQUE 140, IOHEXOL
OMNIPAQUE 180, IOHEXOL
OMNIPAQUE 210, IOHEXOL
OMNIPAQUE 240, IOHEXOL
OMNIPAQUE 300, IOHEXOL
OMNIPAQUE 350, IOHEXOL
PHISO-SCRUB, HEXACHLOROPHENE
PHISOHEX, HEXACHLOROPHENE
PLAQUENIL, HYDROXYCHLOROQUINE SULFATE
PRIMAQUINE, PRIMAQUINE PHOSPHATE
PROCHLORPERAZINE EDISYLATE,
   PROCHLORPERAZINE EDISYLATE
PROMETHAZINE HCL, PROMETHAZINE
   HYDROCHLORIDE
SULFAMYLON, MAFENIDE ACETATE
TALACEN, ACETAMINOPHEN
TALWIN, PENTAZOCINE LACTATE
TALWIN COMPOUND, ASPIRIN
TALWIN NX, NALOXONE HYDROCHLORIDE
TALWIN 50, PENTAZOCINE HYDROCHLORIDE
TELEPAQUE, IOPANOIC ACID
TORNALATE, BITOLTEROL MESYLATE
TRANCOPAL, CHLORMEZANONE
TRIMETHOBENZAMIDE HCL, TRIMETHOBENZAMIDE
   HYDROCHLORIDE
VERAPAMIL HCL, VERAPAMIL HYDROCHLORIDE
WINSTROL, STANOZOLOL
8-HOUR BAYER, ASPIRIN (OTC)

STEVENS
* JEROME STEVENS PHARMACEUTICALS INC
   CEPHALEXIN, CEPHALEXIN

STIEFEL
* STIEFEL LABORATORIES INC
   HYDROCORTISONE, HYDROCORTISONE
   SCABENE, LINDANE
   STIE-CORT, HYDROCORTISONE

STUART
* STUART PHARMACEUTICALS DIV ICI AMERICAS
   BUCLADIN-S, BUCLIZINE HYDROCHLORIDE
   CEFOTAN, CEFOTETAN DISODIUM
   HIBICLENS, CHLORHEXIDINE GLUCONATE (OTC)
   HIBISTAT, CHLORHEXIDINE GLUCONATE (OTC)
   HIBITANE, CHLORHEXIDINE GLUCONATE (OTC)
   NOLVADEX, TAMOXIFEN CITRATE

SUPERPHARM
* SUPERPHARM CORP
   ACETAMINOPHEN AND CODEINE PHOSPHATE #2,
     ACETAMINOPHEN
   ACETAMINOPHEN AND CODEINE PHOSPHATE #3,
     ACETAMINOPHEN
   ACETAMINOPHEN AND CODEINE PHOSPHATE #4,
     ACETAMINOPHEN
   ALLOPURINOL, ALLOPURINOL
   AMITRIPTYLINE HCL, AMITRIPTYLINE
     HYDROCHLORIDE
   CHLORDIAZEPOXIDE HCL, CHLORDIAZEPOXIDE
     HYDROCHLORIDE
   CHLORPHENIRAMINE MALEATE,
     CHLORPHENIRAMINE MALEATE
   CHLORPROPAMIDE, CHLORPROPAMIDE
   CHLORTHALIDONE, CHLORTHALIDONE
   CYPROHEPTADINE HCL, CYPROHEPTADINE
     HYDROCHLORIDE
   DIPHENHYDRAMINE HCL, DIPHENHYDRAMINE
     HYDROCHLORIDE
   DISOPYRAMIDE PHOSPHATE, DISOPYRAMIDE
     PHOSPHATE
   DOXYCYCLINE HYCLATE, DOXYCYCLINE HYCLATE
   ERGOLOID MESYLATES, ERGOLOID MESYLATES
   FLURAZEPAM HCL, FLURAZEPAM HYDROCHLORIDE
   FUROSEMIDE, FUROSEMIDE
   HYDRALAZINE HCL, HYDRALAZINE
     HYDROCHLORIDE
   HYDRALAZINE HCL AND HYDROCHLOROTHIAZIDE,
     HYDRALAZINE HYDROCHLORIDE
   HYDROCHLOROTHIAZIDE, HYDROCHLOROTHIAZIDE
   HYDROXYZINE HCL, HYDROXYZINE
     HYDROCHLORIDE
   HYDROXYZINE PAMOATE, HYDROXYZINE PAMOATE
   IBUPROFEN, IBUPROFEN
   INDOMETHACIN, INDOMETHACIN
   ISOSORBIDE DINITRATE, ISOSORBIDE DINITRATE
   LOGEN, ATROPINE SULFATE
   LORAZEPAM, LORAZEPAM
   MECLIZINE HCL, MECLIZINE HYDROCHLORIDE
   METHOCARBAMOL, METHOCARBAMOL
   METHYLDOPA, METHYLDOPA
   METOCLOPRAMIDE HCL, METOCLOPRAMIDE
     HYDROCHLORIDE
   METRONIDAZOLE, METRONIDAZOLE
   PREDNISOLONE, PREDNISOLONE
   PREDNISONE, PREDNISONE
   PROPOXYPHENE NAPSYLATE AND ACETAMINOPHEN,
     ACETAMINOPHEN
   PROPRANOLOL HCL, PROPRANOLOL
     HYDROCHLORIDE
   QUINIDINE GLUCONATE, QUINIDINE GLUCONATE
   QUINIDINE SULFATE, QUINIDINE SULFATE
   SPIRONOLACTONE, SPIRONOLACTONE
   SPIRONOLACTONE AND HYDROCHLOROTHIAZIDE,
     HYDROCHLOROTHIAZIDE
   SULFASALAZINE, SULFASALAZINE
   SULFATRIM-DS, SULFAMETHOXAZOLE
   SULFATRIM-SS, SULFAMETHOXAZOLE
   TETRACYCLINE HCL, TETRACYCLINE
     HYDROCHLORIDE
   THIORIDAZINE HCL, THIORIDAZINE
     HYDROCHLORIDE
   TOLAZAMIDE, TOLAZAMIDE
   TOLBUTAMIDE, TOLBUTAMIDE
   TRIPROLIDINE HCL AND PSEUDOEPHEDRINE HCL,
     PSEUDOEPHEDRINE HYDROCHLORIDE

SUPPOSITORIA
* SUPPOSITORIA LABORATORIES INC
   ACETAMINOPHEN, ACETAMINOPHEN (OTC)

APPENDIX B
PRODUCT NAME INDEX
LISTED BY APPLICANT (continued)

SURVIVAL TECH
* SURVIVAL TECHNOLOGY INC
  ATROPEN, ATROPINE
  EPIPEN, EPINEPHRINE
  EPIPEN JR., EPINEPHRINE
  LIDOPEN, LIDOCAINE HYDROCHLORIDE
  MORPHINE SULFATE, MORPHINE SULFATE
  PRALIDOXIME CHLORIDE, PRALIDOXIME CHLORIDE

SYNTEX
* SYNTEX (FP) INC
  ANAPROX, NAPROXEN SODIUM
  ANAPROX DS, NAPROXEN SODIUM
  BREVICON 21-DAY, ETHINYL ESTRADIOL
  BREVICON 28-DAY, ETHINYL ESTRADIOL
  NAPROSYN, NAPROXEN
  NOR-Q.D., NORETHINDRONE
  NORINYL 1+35 21-DAY, ETHINYL ESTRADIOL
  NORINYL 1+35 28-DAY, ETHINYL ESTRADIOL
  NORINYL 1+50 28-DAY, MESTRANOL
  NORINYL 1+80 21-DAY, MESTRANOL
  NORINYL 1+80 28-DAY, MESTRANOL
  NORQUEST FE, ETHINYL ESTRADIOL
  TRI-NORINYL 21-DAY, ETHINYL ESTRADIOL
  TRI-NORINYL 28-DAY, ETHINYL ESTRADIOL
* SYNTEX LABORATORIES INC SUB SYNTEX CORP
  AEROBID, FLUNISOLIDE
  ANADROL-50, OXYMETHOLONE
  CARDENE, NICARDIPINE HYDROCHLORIDE
  CARDENE SR, NICARDIPINE HYDROCHLORIDE
  CARMOL HC, HYDROCORTISONE ACETATE
  CYTOVENE, GANCICLOVIR SODIUM
  EVEX, ESTROGENS, ESTERIFIED
  FEMSTAT, BUTOCONAZOLE NITRATE
  LIDEX, FLUOCINONIDE
  LIDEX-E, FLUOCINONIDE
  NASALIDE, FLUNISOLIDE
  NEO-SYNALAR, FLUOCINOLONE ACETONIDE
  NORINYL, MESTRANOL
  NORINYL 1+50 21-DAY, MESTRANOL
  SYNACORT, HYDROCORTISONE
  SYNALAR, FLUOCINOLONE ACETONIDE
  SYNALAR-HP, FLUOCINOLONE ACETONIDE
  SYNAREL, NAFARELIN ACETATE
  SYNEMOL, FLUOCINOLONE ACETONIDE
  TICLID, TICLOPIDINE HYDROCHLORIDE
  TORADOL, KETOROLAC TROMETHAMINE

SYOSSET
* SYOSSET LABORATORIES INC
  C-SOLVE-2, ERYTHROMYCIN
  E-SOLVE 2, ERYTHROMYCIN
  FLUTEX, TRIAMCINOLONE ACETONIDE
  HYDROCORTISONE, HYDROCORTISONE
  NOGENIC HC, HYDROCORTISONE
  SELENIUM SULFIDE, SELENIUM SULFIDE
  TRIATEX, TRIAMCINOLONE ACETONIDE

T

TABLICAPS
* TABLICAPS INC
  AMINOPHYLLINE, AMINOPHYLLINE
  BROMPHENIRAMINE MALEATE, BROMPHENIRAMINE
    MALEATE
  CHLORPHENIRAMINE MALEATE,
    CHLORPHENIRAMINE MALEATE
  FOLIC ACID, FOLIC ACID
  MEPROBAMATE, MEPROBAMATE

METHOCARBAMOL, METHOCARBAMOL
METHYLTESTOSTERONE, METHYLTESTOSTERONE
NIACIN, NIACIN
PREDNISOLONE, PREDNISOLONE
PREDNISONE, PREDNISONE
PROMETHAZINE HCL, PROMETHAZINE
  HYDROCHLORIDE
PROPANTHELINE BROMIDE, PROPANTHELINE
  BROMIDE
PROPYLTHIOURACIL, PROPYLTHIOURACIL
RAUWOLFIA SERPENTINA, RAUWOLFIA SERPENTINA
RESERPINE, RESERPINE
STILBESTROL, DIETHYLSTILBESTROL
TRIHEXYPHENIDYL HCL, TRIHEXYPHENIDYL
  HYDROCHLORIDE
TRIPELENNAMINE HCL, TRIPELENNAMINE
  HYDROCHLORIDE

TAG
* TAG PHARMACEUTICALS INC
  IBUPROFEN, IBUPROFEN (OTC)

TAKEDA
* TAKEDA CHEMICAL INDUSTRIES LTD
  CERADON, CEFOTIAM HYDROCHLORIDE

TAP
* TAP PHARMACEUTICALS INC
  CEFMAX, CEFMENOXIME HYDROCHLORIDE
  LUPRON, LEUPROLIDE ACETATE
  LUPRON DEPOT, LEUPROLIDE ACETATE

TARO
* TARO PHARMACEUTICALS INC
  BETAMETHASONE DIPROPIONATE, BETAMETHASONE
    DIPROPIONATE
  DERMABET, BETAMETHASONE VALERATE
  DERMACOMB, NYSTATIN
  DESONIDE, DESONIDE
  DESOXIMETASONE, DESOXIMETASONE
  FLUOCINONIDE, FLUOCINONIDE
  ORACORT, TRIAMCINOLONE ACETONIDE

THAMES
* THAMES PHARMACAL CO INC
  ACETIC ACID, ACETIC ACID, GLACIAL
  BETAMETHASONE DIPROPIONATE, BETAMETHASONE
    DIPROPIONATE
  BETAMETHASONE VALERATE, BETAMETHASONE
    VALERATE
  FLUOCINOLONE ACETONIDE, FLUOCINOLONE
    ACETONIDE
  FLUOCINONIDE, FLUOCINONIDE
  GENTAMICIN, GENTAMICIN SULFATE
  GENTAMICIN SULFATE, GENTAMICIN SULFATE
  HYDROCORTISONE, HYDROCORTISONE
  HYDROCORTISONE ACETATE, HYDROCORTISONE
    ACETATE
  HYDROCORTISONE AND ACETIC ACID, ACETIC ACID,
    GLACIAL
  LIDOCAINE, LIDOCAINE
  NITROFURAZONE, NITROFURAZONE
  NYSTATIN, NYSTATIN
  NYSTATIN-TRIAMCINOLONE ACETONIDE, NYSTATIN
  ORALONE, TRIAMCINOLONE ACETONIDE
  SELENIUM SULFIDE, SELENIUM SULFIDE
  THEOPHYLLINE, THEOPHYLLINE
  TRIAMCINOLONE ACETONIDE, TRIAMCINOLONE
    ACETONIDE

TICAN
* TICAN PHARMACEUTICALS LTD
  FLUOCINONIDE, FLUOCINONIDE

APPENDIX B
PRODUCT NAME INDEX
LISTED BY APPLICANT (continued)

TOPIDERM
* TOPIDERM INC
    HYDROCORTISONE, HYDROCORTISONE
    TRIAMCINOLONE ACETONIDE, TRIAMCINOLONE
      ACETONIDE

TORCH LABS
* TORCH LABORATORIES INC
    H-CORT, HYDROCORTISONE

U

UDL
* UDL LABORATORIES INC
    FOLIC ACID, FOLIC ACID
    MECLIZINE HCL, MECLIZINE HYDROCHLORIDE
    PREDNISOLONE, PREDNISOLONE
    PREDNISONE, PREDNISONE

UNIMED
* UNIMED INC
    MARINOL, DRONABINOL

UNIV TX
* UNIV TEXAS HEALTH SCIENCE CENTER
    POTASSIUM CITRATE, POTASSIUM CITRATE
    TIOPRONIN, TIOPRONIN

UPJOHN
* UPJOHN CO
    ALBAMYCIN, NOVOBIOCIN SODIUM
    ALPHADROL, FLUPREDNISOLONE
    ANSAID, FLURBIPROFEN
    BACIGUENT, BACITRACIN
    BACITRACIN, BACITRACIN
    BERUBIGEN, CYANOCOBALAMIN
    CALDEROL, CALCIFEDIOL, ANHYDROUS
    CARDASE, ETHOXZOLAMIDE
    CARDRASE, ETHOXZOLAMIDE
    CLEOCIN, CLINDAMYCIN PALMITATE
      HYDROCHLORIDE
    CLEOCIN, CLINDAMYCIN PHOSPHATE
    CLEOCIN HCL, CLINDAMYCIN HYDROCHLORIDE
    CLEOCIN PHOSPHATE, CLINDAMYCIN PHOSPHATE
    CLEOCIN PHOSPHATE IN DEXTROSE 5%,
      CLINDAMYCIN PHOSPHATE
    CLEOCIN T, CLINDAMYCIN PHOSPHATE
    COLESTID, COLESTIPOL HYDROCHLORIDE
    CORTEF, HYDROCORTISONE
    CORTEF, HYDROCORTISONE CYPIONATE
    CORTEF ACETATE, HYDROCORTISONE ACETATE
    CORTISONE ACETATE, CORTISONE ACETATE
    CYTOSAR-U, CYTARABINE
    DELTA-CORTEF, PREDNISOLONE
    DELTASONE, PREDNISONE
    DEPO-ESTRADIOL, ESTRADIOL CYPIONATE
    DEPO-MEDROL, METHYLPREDNISOLONE ACETATE
    DEPO-PROVERA, MEDROXYPROGESTERONE ACETATE
    DEPO-TESTADIOL, ESTRADIOL CYPIONATE
    DEPO-TESTOSTERONE, TESTOSTERONE CYPIONATE
    DIDREX, BENZPHETAMINE HYDROCHLORIDE
    DIFLORASONE DIACETATE, DIFLORASONE
      DIACETATE
    E-MYCIN E, ERYTHROMYCIN ETHYLSUCCINATE
    FEMINONE, ETHINYL ESTRADIOL
    FLORONE, DIFLORASONE DIACETATE
    GLYNASE, GLYBURIDE
    HALCION, TRIAZOLAM
    HALODRIN, ETHINYL ESTRADIOL
    HALOTESTIN, FLUOXYMESTERONE

    HEBAMATE, CARBOPROST TROMETHAMINE
    HEPARIN SODIUM, HEPARIN SODIUM
    HYLOREL, GUANADREL SULFATE
    LINCOCIN, LINCOMYCIN HYDROCHLORIDE
    LONITEN, MINOXIDIL
    MAOLATE, CHLORPHENESIN CARBAMATE
    MEDROL, METHYLPREDNISOLONE
    MEDROL, METHYLPREDNISOLONE ACETATE
    MEDROL ACETATE, METHYLPREDNISOLONE
      ACETATE
    MICRONASE, GLYBURIDE
    MOTRIN, IBUPROFEN
    MYCIFRADIN, NEOMYCIN SULFATE
    MYCITRACIN, BACITRACIN
    NEO-CORTEF, HYDROCORTISONE ACETATE
    NEO-DELTA-CORTEF, NEOMYCIN SULFATE
    NEO-MEDROL, METHYLPREDNISOLONE
    NEO-MEDROL ACETATE, METHYLPREDNISOLONE
      ACETATE
    NUPRIN, IBUPROFEN (OTC)
    ORINASE, TOLBUTAMIDE
    ORINASE DIAGNOSTIC, TOLBUTAMIDE SODIUM
    OXYLONE, FLUOROMETHOLONE
    PAMINE, METHSCOPOLAMINE BROMIDE
    PANMYCIN, TETRACYCLINE HYDROCHLORIDE
    PENICILLIN G SODIUM, PENICILLIN G SODIUM
    PROSTIN E2, DINOPROSTONE
    PROSTIN F2 ALPHA, DINOPROST TROMETHAMINE
    PROSTIN VR PEDIATRIC, ALPROSTADIL
    PROTAMINE SULFATE, PROTAMINE SULFATE
    PROVERA, MEDROXYPROGESTERONE ACETATE
    PSORCON, DIFLORASONE DIACETATE
    ROGAINE, MINOXIDIL
    SOLU-CORTEF, HYDROCORTISONE SODIUM
      SUCCINATE
    SOLU-MEDROL, METHYLPREDNISOLONE SODIUM
      SUCCINATE
    TOLINASE, TOLAZAMIDE
    TROBICIN, SPECTINOMYCIN HYDROCHLORIDE
    U-GENCIN, GENTAMICIN SULFATE
    URACIL MUSTARD, URACIL MUSTARD
    UTICILLIN VK, PENICILLIN V POTASSIUM
    XANAX, ALPRAZOLAM
    ZANOSAR, STREPTOZOCIN
    ZEFAZONE, CEFMETAZOLE SODIUM
* UPJOHN MANUFACTURING CO
    CLEOCIN, CLINDAMYCIN HYDROCHLORIDE
    CLEOCIN, CLINDAMYCIN PALMITATE
      HYDROCHLORIDE
    CLEOCIN PHOSPHATE, CLINDAMYCIN PHOSPHATE
* UPJOHN TRADING CORP
    VANTIN, CEFPODOXIME PROXETIL

UPSHER SMITH
* UPSHER SMITH LABORATORIES INC
    ACETAMINOPHEN, ACETAMINOPHEN (OTC)
    DEXAMETHASONE, DEXAMETHASONE
    KLOR-CON, POTASSIUM CHLORIDE
    METHOCARBAMOL, METHOCARBAMOL
    PREDNISONE, PREDNISONE
    SPIRONOLACTONE, SPIRONOLACTONE
    SPIRONOLACTONE W/ HYDROCHLOROTHIAZIDE,
      HYDROCHLOROTHIAZIDE

US ARMY
* OFFICE SURGEON GENERAL DEPT ARMY
    SODIUM THIOSULFATE, SODIUM THIOSULFATE
* UNITED STATES ARMY
    ATROPINE SULFATE, ATROPINE SULFATE
    DIAZEPAM, DIAZEPAM
* WALTER REED ARMY INSTITUTE RESEARCH
    MEFLOQUINE HCL, MEFLOQUINE HYDROCHLORIDE

APPENDIX B
PRODUCT NAME INDEX
LISTED BY APPLICANT (continued)

US BIOSCIENCE
* US BIOSCIENCE
  HEXALEN, ALTRETAMINE

US CHEM
* US CHEMICAL MARKETING GROUP INC
  MEDIGESIC PLUS, ACETAMINOPHEN

V

VALE
* VALE CHEMICAL CO INC
  AMINOPHYLLINE, AMINOPHYLLINE
  RAUVAL, RAUWOLFIA SERPENTINA
  SERPATE, RESERPINE
  TRIPLE SULFOID, TRISULFAPYRIMIDINES

VANGARD
* VANGARD LABORATORIES DIV MIDWAY MED CO
  ACETAZOLAMIDE, ACETAZOLAMIDE
  AMINOPHYLLINE, AMINOPHYLLINE
  AMITRIPTYLINE HCL, AMITRIPTYLINE
    HYDROCHLORIDE
  CHLORDIAZEPOXIDE HCL, CHLORDIAZEPOXIDE
    HYDROCHLORIDE
  CHLORPROMAZINE HCL, CHLORPROMAZINE
    HYDROCHLORIDE
  CHLORTHALIDONE, CHLORTHALIDONE
  DIPHENHYDRAMINE HCL, DIPHENHYDRAMINE
    HYDROCHLORIDE
  ERGOLOID MESYLATES, ERGOLOID MESYLATES
  FOLIC ACID, FOLIC ACID
  HYDRALAZINE HCL, HYDRALAZINE
    HYDROCHLORIDE
  HYDROCHLOROTHIAZIDE, HYDROCHLOROTHIAZIDE
  HYDROXYZINE PAMOATE, HYDROXYZINE PAMOATE
  IMIPRAMINE HCL, IMIPRAMINE HYDROCHLORIDE
  LO-TROL, ATROPINE SULFATE
  MECLIZINE HCL, MECLIZINE HYDROCHLORIDE
  MEPROBAMATE, MEPROBAMATE
  PAPA-DEINE #3, ACETAMINOPHEN
  PAPA-DEINE #4, ACETAMINOPHEN
  PREDNISONE, PREDNISONE
  PROCAINAMIDE HCL, PROCAINAMIDE
    HYDROCHLORIDE
  QUINIDINE SULFATE, QUINIDINE SULFATE
  SPIRONOLACTONE, SPIRONOLACTONE
  SPIRONOLACTONE W/ HYDROCHLOROTHIAZIDE,
    HYDROCHLOROTHIAZIDE
  SULFINPYRAZONE, SULFINPYRAZONE
  TOLBUTAMIDE, TOLBUTAMIDE
  TRIHEXYPHENIDYL HCL, TRIHEXYPHENIDYL
    HYDROCHLORIDE

VESTAL
* VESTAL LABORATORIES DIV CHEMED CORP
  SEPTISOL, HEXACHLOROPHENE

VICKS HEALTH CARE
* VICKS HEALTH CARE DIV RICHARDSON VICKS INC
  VICKS FORMULA 44, DIPHENHYDRAMINE
    HYDROCHLORIDE (OTC)

VIRATEK
* VIRATEK INC
  VIRAZOLE, RIBAVIRIN

VITARINE
* VITARINE PHARMACEUTICALS INC
  ACETAMINOPHEN W/ CODEINE PHOSPHATE,
    ACETAMINOPHEN
  AMPICILLIN, AMPICILLIN/AMPICILLIN TRIHYDRATE

BETHANECHOL CHLORIDE, BETHANECHOL
  CHLORIDE
BROMPHENIRAMINE MALEATE, BROMPHENIRAMINE
  MALEATE
CEPHALEXIN, CEPHALEXIN
CEPHALEXIN MONOHYDRATE, CEPHALEXIN
CEPHRADINE, CEPHRADINE
CHLORPHENIRAMINE MALEATE,
  CHLORPHENIRAMINE MALEATE
CORTISONE ACETATE, CORTISONE ACETATE
CYPROHEPTADINE HCL, CYPROHEPTADINE
  HYDROCHLORIDE
DEXTROAMPHETAMINE SULFATE,
  DEXTROAMPHETAMINE SULFATE
GLUTETHIMIDE, GLUTETHIMIDE
HYDRALAZINE HCL, HYDRALAZINE
  HYDROCHLORIDE
MECLOFENAMATE SODIUM, MECLOFENAMATE
  SODIUM
PENTOBARBITAL SODIUM, PENTOBARBITAL SODIUM
PHENDIMETRAZINE TARTRATE, PHENDIMETRAZINE
  TARTRATE
PHENTERMINE HCL, PHENTERMINE
  HYDROCHLORIDE
PREDNISOLONE, PREDNISOLONE
PREDNISONE, PREDNISONE
PROPOXYPHENE COMPOUND 65, ASPIRIN
PROPOXYPHENE HCL, PROPOXYPHENE
  HYDROCHLORIDE
SECOBARBITAL SODIUM, SECOBARBITAL SODIUM
SERPIVITE, RESERPINE
SULFISOXAZOLE, SULFISOXAZOLE
TRIAMTERENE AND HYDROCHLOROTHIAZIDE,
  HYDROCHLOROTHIAZIDE
TRIPROLIDINE HCL, TRIPROLIDINE
  HYDROCHLORIDE
VITAMIN D, ERGOCALCIFEROL

VIVAN
* VIVAN PHARMACOL INC DIV ELLIS PHARMACEUTICAL
CONSULTING IN
  ALPHADERM, HYDROCORTISONE

W

WALLACE
* WALLACE LABORATORIES DIV CARTER WALLACE INC
  AQUATENSEN, METHYCLOTHIAZIDE
  BEPADIN, BEPRIDIL HYDROCHLORIDE
  BUTICAPS, BUTABARBITAL SODIUM
  BUTISOL SODIUM, BUTABARBITAL SODIUM
  COLONAID, ATROPINE SULFATE
  DEPEN 250, PENICILLAMINE
  DIUTENSEN-R, METHYCLOTHIAZIDE
  LUFYLLIN, DYPHYLLINE
  MYLAXEN, HEXAFLUORENIUM BROMIDE
  NEOPASALATE, AMINOSALICYLATE SODIUM
  RONDOMYCIN, METHACYCLINE HYDROCHLORIDE
  SOMA, CARISOPRODOL
  THYRO-BLOCK, POTASSIUM IODIDE (OTC)
  UNITENSEN, CRYPTENAMINE ACETATES
  UNITENSEN, CRYPTENAMINE TANNATES
  VERTAVIS, VERATRUM VIRIDE
  VOSOL, ACETIC ACID, GLACIAL
  VOSOL HC, ACETIC ACID, GLACIAL
  WAMPOCAP, NIACIN
* WALLACE PHARMACEUTICALS DIV CARTER WALLACE
INC
  DORMATE, MEBUTAMATE
  MEPROSPAN, MEPROBAMATE
  MICRAININ, ASPIRIN

APPENDIX B
PRODUCT NAME INDEX
LISTED BY APPLICANT (continued)

MILPREM-200, ESTROGENS, CONJUGATED
MILPREM-400, ESTROGENS, CONJUGATED
MILTOWN, MEPROBAMATE
SOMA COMPOUND, ASPIRIN
SOMA COMPOUND W/ CODEINE, ASPIRIN

WARNER CHILCOTT
* WARNER CHILCOTT DIV WARNER LAMBERT CO
ACETAMINOPHEN W/ CODEINE PHOSPHATE,
   ACETAMINOPHEN
ALBUTEROL SULFATE, ALBUTEROL SULFATE
AMITRIL, AMITRIPTYLINE HYDROCHLORIDE
CARBAMAZEPINE, CARBAMAZEPINE
CHLORTHALIDONE, CHLORTHALIDONE
CLONIDINE HCL, CLONIDINE HYDROCHLORIDE
CLORAZEPATE DIPOTASSIUM, CLORAZEPATE
   DIPOTASSIUM
CYCLOPAR, TETRACYCLINE HYDROCHLORIDE
DIAZEPAM, DIAZEPAM
DOPAMINE HCL, DOPAMINE HYDROCHLORIDE
DOXYCYCLINE HYCLATE, DOXYCYCLINE HYCLATE
FENOPROFEN CALCIUM, FENOPROFEN CALCIUM
FLURAZEPAM HCL, FLURAZEPAM HYDROCHLORIDE
FUROSEMIDE, FUROSEMIDE
HYDROCHLOROTHIAZIDE, HYDROCHLOROTHIAZIDE
KANAMYCIN SULFATE, KANAMYCIN SULFATE
LORAZEPAM, LORAZEPAM
MINOCYCLINE HCL, MINOCYCLINE
   HYDROCHLORIDE
PHENYTOIN SODIUM, PHENYTOIN SODIUM
PROCAINAMIDE HCL, PROCAINAMIDE
   HYDROCHLORIDE
PROPOXYPHENE HCL 65, PROPOXYPHENE
   HYDROCHLORIDE
PROPRANOLOL HCL, PROPRANOLOL
   HYDROCHLORIDE
PROPRANOLOL HCL AND HYDROCHLOROTHIAZIDE,
   HYDROCHLOROTHIAZIDE
SPIRONOLACTONE, SPIRONOLACTONE
SULINDAC, SULINDAC
TETRACYCLINE HCL, TETRACYCLINE
   HYDROCHLORIDE

WATSON
* WATSON LABORATORIES INC
ALBUTEROL SULFATE, ALBUTEROL SULFATE
AMOXAPINE, AMOXAPINE
CLORAZEPATE DIPOTASSIUM, CLORAZEPATE
   DIPOTASSIUM
CYCLOBENZAPRINE HCL, CYCLOBENZAPRINE
   HYDROCHLORIDE
ETHYNODIOL DIACETATE AND ETHINYL ESTRADIOL
   1/35-21, ETHINYL ESTRADIOL
ETHYNODIOL DIACETATE AND ETHINYL ESTRADIOL
   1/35-28, ETHINYL ESTRADIOL
ETHYNODIOL DIACETATE AND ETHINYL ESTRADIOL
   1/50-21, ETHINYL ESTRADIOL
ETHYNODIOL DIACETATE AND ETHINYL ESTRADIOL
   1/50-28, ETHINYL ESTRADIOL
FENOPROFEN CALCIUM, FENOPROFEN CALCIUM
FUROSEMIDE, FUROSEMIDE
HYDROCODONE BITARTRATE AND
   ACETAMINOPHEN, ACETAMINOPHEN
INDOMETHACIN, INDOMETHACIN
LORAZEPAM, LORAZEPAM
LOXAPINE SUCCINATE, LOXAPINE SUCCINATE
MAPROTILINE HCL, MAPROTILINE HYDROCHLORIDE
METHYLDOPA AND HYDROCHLOROTHIAZIDE,
   HYDROCHLOROTHIAZIDE
METOCLOPRAMIDE HCL, METOCLOPRAMIDE
   HYDROCHLORIDE

NORETHINDRONE AND ETHINYL ESTRADIOL,
   ETHINYL ESTRADIOL
NORETHINDRONE AND ETHINYL ESTRADIOL (10/11),
   ETHINYL ESTRADIOL
NORETHINDRONE AND ETHINYL ESTRADIOL (7/14),
   ETHINYL ESTRADIOL
NORETHINDRONE AND MESTRANOL, MESTRANOL
PROPRANOLOL HCL, PROPRANOLOL
   HYDROCHLORIDE
TRIAMTERENE AND HYDROCHLOROTHIAZIDE,
   HYDROCHLOROTHIAZIDE
VERAPAMIL HCL, VERAPAMIL HYDROCHLORIDE

WENDT
* WENDT LABORATORIES INC
NITROFURAZONE, NITROFURAZONE

WEST WARD
* WEST WARD PHARMACEUTICAL CORP
AMINOPHYLLINE, AMINOPHYLLINE
AMITRIPTYLINE HCL, AMITRIPTYLINE
   HYDROCHLORIDE
BUTALBITAL, ASPIRIN AND CAFFEINE, ASPIRIN
CHLORDIAZEPOXIDE HCL, CHLORDIAZEPOXIDE
   HYDROCHLORIDE
CHLOROQUINE PHOSPHATE, CHLOROQUINE
   PHOSPHATE
CHLOROTHIAZIDE, CHLOROTHIAZIDE
CHLOROTHIAZIDE AND RESERPINE,
   CHLOROTHIAZIDE
CHLORPHENIRAMINE MALEATE,
   CHLORPHENIRAMINE MALEATE
CHLORPROMAZINE HCL, CHLORPROMAZINE
   HYDROCHLORIDE
CORTISONE ACETATE, CORTISONE ACETATE
CYANOCOBALAMIN, CYANOCOBALAMIN
DIPHENHYDRAMINE HCL, DIPHENHYDRAMINE
   HYDROCHLORIDE
DIPHENOXYLATE HCL AND ATROPINE SULFATE,
   ATROPINE SULFATE
DOXYCYCLINE HYCLATE, DOXYCYCLINE HYCLATE
FLURAZEPAM HCL, FLURAZEPAM HYDROCHLORIDE
FOLIC ACID, FOLIC ACID
HYDRALAZINE HCL, HYDRALAZINE
   HYDROCHLORIDE
HYDROCHLOROTHIAZIDE, HYDROCHLOROTHIAZIDE
HYDROCORTISONE, HYDROCORTISONE
IMIPRAMINE HCL, IMIPRAMINE HYDROCHLORIDE
ISONIAZID, ISONIAZID
ISOSORBIDE DINITRATE, ISOSORBIDE DINITRATE
MEPROBAMATE, MEPROBAMATE
METHOCARBAMOL, METHOCARBAMOL
METHYLTESTOSTERONE, METHYLTESTOSTERONE
NIACIN, NIACIN
OXYTETRACYCLINE HCL, OXYTETRACYCLINE
   HYDROCHLORIDE
PREDNISOLONE, PREDNISOLONE
PREDNISONE, PREDNISONE
PROPOXYPHENE HCL, PROPOXYPHENE
   HYDROCHLORIDE
PROPYLTHIOURACIL, PROPYLTHIOURACIL
QUINIDINE SULFATE, QUINIDINE SULFATE
RESERPINE, RESERPINE
RESERPINE AND HYDROCHLOROTHIAZIDE-50,
   HYDROCHLOROTHIAZIDE
SODIUM BUTABARBITAL, BUTABARBITAL SODIUM
SODIUM SECOBARBITAL, SECOBARBITAL SODIUM
SULFISOXAZOLE, SULFISOXAZOLE
TETRACYCLINE HCL, TETRACYCLINE
   HYDROCHLORIDE
THIORIDAZINE HCL, THIORIDAZINE
   HYDROCHLORIDE

APPENDIX B
PRODUCT NAME INDEX
LISTED BY APPLICANT (continued)

TRIPROLIDINE AND PSEUDOEPHEDRINE,
  PSEUDOEPHEDRINE HYDROCHLORIDE
VITAMIN A, VITAMIN A
VITAMIN A, VITAMIN A PALMITATE
VITAMIN D, ERGOCALCIFEROL

WESTWOOD SQUIBB
* WESTWOOD SQUIBB PHARMACEUTICALS INC
  CAPITROL, CHLOROXINE
  EURAX, CROTAMITON
  EXELDERM, SULCONAZOLE NITRATE
  FLEXICORT, HYDROCORTISONE
  HALOG, HALCINONIDE
  HALOG-E, HALCINONIDE
  HALOTEX, HALOPROGIN
  KENALOG, TRIAMCINOLONE ACETONIDE
  KENALOG-H, TRIAMCINOLONE ACETONIDE
  KENALOG-10, TRIAMCINOLONE ACETONIDE
  KENALOG-40, TRIAMCINOLONE ACETONIDE
  LAC-HYDRIN, AMMONIUM LACTATE
  STATICIN, ERYTHROMYCIN
  T-STAT, ERYTHROMYCIN
  TACARYL, METHDILAZINE
  TACARYL, METHDILAZINE HYDROCHLORIDE
  ULTRAVATE, HALOBETASOL PROPIONATE
  WESTCORT, HYDROCORTISONE VALERATE

WHARTON
* WHARTON LABORATORIES INC DIV US ETHICALS
  VITAMIN A, VITAMIN A PALMITATE

WHITBY
* WHITBY PHARMACEUTICALS INC
  THEO-24, THEOPHYLLINE

WHITE TOWNE PAULSEN
* WHITEWORTH TOWNE PAULSEN INC
  ACETAMINOPHEN W/ CODEINE PHOSPHATE,
    ACETAMINOPHEN
  BUTABARBITAL SODIUM, BUTABARBITAL SODIUM
  CORTISONE ACETATE, CORTISONE ACETATE
  DEXAMETHASONE, DEXAMETHASONE
  DIPHENHYDRAMINE HCL, DIPHENHYDRAMINE
    HYDROCHLORIDE
  FOLIC ACID, FOLIC ACID
  H.R.-50, HYDROCHLOROTHIAZIDE
  HYDROCHLOROTHIAZIDE, HYDROCHLOROTHIAZIDE
  HYDROCORTISONE, HYDROCORTISONE
  ISONIAZID, ISONIAZID
  MEPROBAMATE, MEPROBAMATE
  NITROFURANTOIN, NITROFURANTOIN
  PENTOBARBITAL SODIUM, PENTOBARBITAL SODIUM
  PREDNISOLONE, PREDNISOLONE
  PREDNISONE, PREDNISONE
  PROMETHAZINE HCL, PROMETHAZINE
    HYDROCHLORIDE
  PROPOXYPHENE HCL, PROPOXYPHENE
    HYDROCHLORIDE
  QUINIDINE SULFATE, QUINIDINE SULFATE
  RESERPINE, RESERPINE
  SECOBARBITAL SODIUM, SECOBARBITAL SODIUM

WHITEHALL
* WHITEHALL LABORATORIES DIV AMERICAN HOME
PRODUCTS CORP
  ADVIL, IBUPROFEN (OTC)
  ADVIL COLD AND SINUS, IBUPROFEN (OTC)
  BRONITIN MIST, EPINEPHRINE BITARTRATE (OTC)
  CHILDREN'S ADVIL, IBUPROFEN
  PRIMATENE MIST, EPINEPHRINE (OTC)
  TODAY, NONOXYNOL-9 (OTC)

WINTHROP
* WINTHROP PHARMACEUTICALS DIV STERLING DRUG
INC
  MIDOL, IBUPROFEN (OTC)
  PHENYTOIN SODIUM, PHENYTOIN SODIUM
  PROCAINAMIDE HCL, PROCAINAMIDE
    HYDROCHLORIDE

WOCKHARDT
* WOCKHARDT LTD
  NIACIN, NIACIN

WYETH
* WYETH LABORATORIES INC
  ISMO, ISOSORBIDE MONONITRATE

WYETH AYERST
* WYETH AYERST LABORATORIES
  A.P.L., GONADOTROPIN, CHORIONIC
  ANSOLYSEN, PENTOLINIUM TARTRATE
  ANTABUSE, DISULFIRAM
  ATIVAN, LORAZEPAM
  ATROMID-S, CLOFIBRATE
  AYGESTIN, NORETHINDRONE ACETATE
  BICILLIN, PENICILLIN G BENZATHINE
  BICILLIN C-R, PENICILLIN G BENZATHINE
  BICILLIN C-R 900/300, PENICILLIN G BENZATHINE
  BICILLIN L-A, PENICILLIN G BENZATHINE
  CEFPIRAMIDE SODIUM, CEFPIRAMIDE SODIUM
  CHLORPROMAZINE HCL, CHLORPROMAZINE
    HYDROCHLORIDE
  CORDARONE, AMIODARONE HYDROCHLORIDE
  CYANOCOBALAMIN, CYANOCOBALAMIN
  CYCLAPEN-W, CYCLACILLIN
  CYCRIN, MEDROXYPROGESTERONE ACETATE
  DEXAMETHASONE SODIUM PHOSPHATE,
    DEXAMETHASONE SODIUM PHOSPHATE
  DIGOXIN, DIGOXIN
  DIMENHYDRINATE, DIMENHYDRINATE
  DIPHENHYDRAMINE HCL, DIPHENHYDRAMINE
    HYDROCHLORIDE
  DIUCARDIN, HYDROFLUMETHIAZIDE
  EQUAGESIC, ASPIRIN
  EQUANIL, MEPROBAMATE
  ESTRADURIN, POLYESTRADIOL PHOSPHATE
  ESTROGENIC SUBSTANCE, ESTRONE
  FACTREL, GONADORELIN HYDROCHLORIDE
  FLUOTHANE, HALOTHANE
  FUROSEMIDE, FUROSEMIDE
  GENTAMICIN SULFATE, GENTAMICIN SULFATE
  GRISACTIN, GRISEOFULVIN, MICROCRYSTALLINE
  GRISACTIN ULTRA, GRISEOFULVIN,
    ULTRAMICROCRYSTALLINE
  HEPARIN LOCK FLUSH, HEPARIN SODIUM
  HEPARIN SODIUM, HEPARIN SODIUM
  HYDROXYZINE HCL, HYDROXYZINE
    HYDROCHLORIDE
  INDERAL, PROPRANOLOL HYDROCHLORIDE
  INDERAL LA, PROPRANOLOL HYDROCHLORIDE
  INDERIDE LA 120/50, HYDROCHLOROTHIAZIDE
  INDERIDE LA 160/50, HYDROCHLOROTHIAZIDE
  INDERIDE LA 80/50, HYDROCHLOROTHIAZIDE
  INDERIDE-40/25, HYDROCHLOROTHIAZIDE
  INDERIDE-80/25, HYDROCHLOROTHIAZIDE
  ISORDIL, ISOSORBIDE DINITRATE
  LARGON, PROPIOMAZINE HYDROCHLORIDE
  LIDOCAINE HCL, LIDOCAINE HYDROCHLORIDE
  LO/OVRAL, ETHINYL ESTRADIOL
  LO/OVRAL-28, ETHINYL ESTRADIOL
  LODINE, ETODOLAC
  MAZANOR, MAZINDOL

APPENDIX B
PRODUCT NAME INDEX
LISTED BY APPLICANT (continued)

MEPERGAN, MEPERIDINE HYDROCHLORIDE
MEPERIDINE AND ATROPINE SULFATE, ATROPINE
  SULFATE
MEPERIDINE HCL, MEPERIDINE HYDROCHLORIDE
MYSOLINE, PRIMIDONE
NALOXONE, NALOXONE HYDROCHLORIDE
NORDETTE-21, ETHINYL ESTRADIOL
NORDETTE-28, ETHINYL ESTRADIOL
NORPLANT SYSTEM, LEVONORGESTREL
OMNIPEN (AMPICILLIN), AMPICILLIN/AMPICILLIN
  TRIHYDRATE
OMNIPEN-N, AMPICILLIN SODIUM
ORUDIS, KETOPROFEN
OVRAL, ETHINYL ESTRADIOL
OVRAL-28, ETHINYL ESTRADIOL
OVRETTE, NORGESTREL
OXYTOCIN, OXYTOCIN
PATHOCIL, DICLOXACILLIN SODIUM
PEN-VEE K, PENICILLIN V POTASSIUM
PENBRITIN, AMPICILLIN/AMPICILLIN TRIHYDRATE
PENBRITIN-S, AMPICILLIN SODIUM
PENICILLIN G POTASSIUM, PENICILLIN G
  POTASSIUM
PEPTAVLON, PENTAGASTRIN
PHENERGAN, PROMETHAZINE HYDROCHLORIDE
PHENERGAN FORTIS, PROMETHAZINE
  HYDROCHLORIDE
PHENERGAN PLAIN, PROMETHAZINE
  HYDROCHLORIDE
PHENERGAN VC, PHENYLEPHRINE HYDROCHLORIDE
PHENERGAN VC W/ CODEINE, CODEINE PHOSPHATE
PHENERGAN W/ CODEINE, CODEINE PHOSPHATE
PHENERGAN W/ DEXTROMETHORPHAN,
  DEXTROMETHORPHAN HYDROBROMIDE
PHOSPHOLINE IODIDE, ECHOTHIOPHATE IODIDE
PLEGINE, PHENDIMETRAZINE TARTRATE
PMB 200, ESTROGENS, CONJUGATED
PMB 400, ESTROGENS, CONJUGATED
PRALIDOXIME CHLORIDE, PRALIDOXIME CHLORIDE
PREMARIN, ESTROGENS, CONJUGATED
PROCHLORPERAZINE EDISYLATE,
  PROCHLORPERAZINE EDISYLATE
PROKETAZINE, CARPHENAZINE MALEATE
PROTOPAM CHLORIDE, PRALIDOXIME CHLORIDE
SECOBARBITAL SODIUM, SECOBARBITAL SODIUM
SECTRAL, ACEBUTOLOL HYDROCHLORIDE
SERAX, OXAZEPAM
SODIUM PENTOBARBITAL, PENTOBARBITAL SODIUM
SODIUM SECOBARBITAL, SECOBARBITAL SODIUM
SPARINE, PROMAZINE HYDROCHLORIDE
SULFOSE, TRISULFAPYRIMIDINES
SURMONTIL, TRIMIPRAMINE MALEATE
SYNALGOS-DC, ASPIRIN
SYNALGOS-DC-A, ACETAMINOPHEN
TETRACYCLINE HCL, TETRACYCLINE
  HYDROCHLORIDE
THIAMINE HCL, THIAMINE HYDROCHLORIDE
THIOSULFIL, SULFAMETHIZOLE
TRECATOR-SC, ETHIONAMIDE
TRIPHASIL-21, ETHINYL ESTRADIOL
TRIPHASIL-28, ETHINYL ESTRADIOL
UNIPEN, NAFCILLIN SODIUM
WYAMINE SULFATE, MEPHENTERMINE SULFATE
WYAMYCIN E, ERYTHROMYCIN ETHYLSUCCINATE
WYAMYCIN S, ERYTHROMYCIN STEARATE
WYCILLIN, PENICILLIN G PROCAINE
WYDASE, HYALURONIDASE
WYGESIC, ACETAMINOPHEN
WYMOX, AMOXICILLIN
WYTENSIN, GUANABENZ ACETATE

* WYETH AYERST RESEARCH
  CERUBIDINE, DAUNORUBICIN HYDROCHLORIDE

X

XTTRIUM
* XTTRIUM LABORATORIES INC
  EXIDINE, CHLORHEXIDINE GLUCONATE (OTC)
  TURGEX, HEXACHLOROPHENE

Y

YOSHITOMI
* YOSHITOMI PHARMACEUTICAL INDUSTRIES LTD
  CEPHALEXIN, CEPHALEXIN

Z

ZENITH
* ZENITH LABORATORIES INC
  ACETAMINOPHEN AND CODEINE PHOSPHATE,
    ACETAMINOPHEN
  ACETAMINOPHEN W/ CODEINE PHOSPHATE #3,
    ACETAMINOPHEN
  AMPICILLIN, AMPICILLIN/AMPICILLIN TRIHYDRATE
  BACLOFEN, BACLOFEN
  BETHANECHOL CHLORIDE, BETHANECHOL
    CHLORIDE
  BROMPHENIRAMINE MALEATE, BROMPHENIRAMINE
    MALEATE
  BUTALBITAL COMPOUND, ASPIRIN
  CEFADROXIL, CEFADROXIL/CEFADROXIL
    HEMIHYDRATE
  CEPHALEXIN, CEPHALEXIN
  CEPHRADINE, CEPHRADINE
  CHLORAMPHENICOL, CHLORAMPHENICOL
  CHLORDIAZEPOXIDE HCL, CHLORDIAZEPOXIDE
    HYDROCHLORIDE
  CHLORPHENIRAMINE MALEATE,
    CHLORPHENIRAMINE MALEATE
  CHLORPROMAZINE HCL, CHLORPROMAZINE
    HYDROCHLORIDE
  CHLORPROPAMIDE, CHLORPROPAMIDE
  CHLORTHALIDONE, CHLORTHALIDONE
  CONJUGATED ESTROGENS, ESTROGENS,
    CONJUGATED
  CORTISONE ACETATE, CORTISONE ACETATE
  CYPROHEPTADINE HCL, CYPROHEPTADINE
    HYDROCHLORIDE
  DIAZEPAM, DIAZEPAM
  DIPHENHYDRAMINE HCL, DIPHENHYDRAMINE
    HYDROCHLORIDE
  DIPHENOXYLATE HCL W/ ATROPINE SULFATE,
    ATROPINE SULFATE
  DISOPYRAMIDE PHOSPHATE, DISOPYRAMIDE
    PHOSPHATE
  DOXYCYCLINE HYCLATE, DOXYCYCLINE HYCLATE
  ERYTHROMYCIN ESTOLATE, ERYTHROMYCIN
    ESTOLATE
  ERYTHROMYCIN STEARATE, ERYTHROMYCIN
    STEARATE
  FENOPROFEN CALCIUM, FENOPROFEN CALCIUM
  FOLIC ACID, FOLIC ACID
  FUROSEMIDE, FUROSEMIDE

APPENDIX B
PRODUCT NAME INDEX
LISTED BY APPLICANT (continued)

HYDRALAZINE HCL, HYDRALAZINE
  HYDROCHLORIDE
HYDRALAZINE HCL W/ HYDROCHLOROTHIAZIDE
  100/50, HYDRALAZINE HYDROCHLORIDE
HYDRALAZINE HCL W/ HYDROCHLOROTHIAZIDE 25/
  25, HYDRALAZINE HYDROCHLORIDE
HYDRALAZINE HCL W/ HYDROCHLOROTHIAZIDE 50/
  50, HYDRALAZINE HYDROCHLORIDE
HYDRALAZINE HCL, HYDROCHLOROTHIAZIDE AND
  RESERPINE, HYDRALAZINE HYDROCHLORIDE
HYDROCHLOROTHIAZIDE, HYDROCHLOROTHIAZIDE
HYDROCHLOROTHIAZIDE W/ RESERPINE,
  HYDROCHLOROTHIAZIDE
HYDROGENATED ERGOT ALKALOIDS, ERGOLOID
  MESYLATES
HYDROSERPINE PLUS (R-H-H), HYDRALAZINE
  HYDROCHLORIDE
HYDROXYZINE HCL, HYDROXYZINE
  HYDROCHLORIDE
HYDROXYZINE PAMOATE, HYDROXYZINE PAMOATE
IBUPROFEN, IBUPROFEN (OTC)
INDOMETHACIN, INDOMETHACIN
ISONIAZID, ISONIAZID
MECLIZINE HCL, MECLIZINE HYDROCHLORIDE
MEPROBAMATE, MEPROBAMATE
METHOCARBAMOL, METHOCARBAMOL
METHOCARBAMOL AND ASPIRIN, ASPIRIN
METHYCLOTHIAZIDE, METHYCLOTHIAZIDE
METHYLDOPA, METHYLDOPA
METHYLDOPA AND HYDROCHLOROTHIAZIDE,
  HYDROCHLOROTHIAZIDE
METRONIDAZOLE, METRONIDAZOLE
NIACIN, NIACIN
NITROFURANTOIN, NITROFURANTOIN
OXAZEPAM, OXAZEPAM
PENICILLIN G POTASSIUM, PENICILLIN G
  POTASSIUM
PENICILLIN V POTASSIUM, PENICILLIN V
  POTASSIUM
PERPHENAZINE, PERPHENAZINE
PERPHENAZINE AND AMITRIPTYLINE HCL,
  AMITRIPTYLINE HYDROCHLORIDE
PHENDIMETRAZINE TARTRATE, PHENDIMETRAZINE
  TARTRATE
PHENTERMINE HCL, PHENTERMINE
  HYDROCHLORIDE
PHENYLBUTAZONE, PHENYLBUTAZONE
PRAZOSIN HCL, PRAZOSIN HYDROCHLORIDE
PREDNISOLONE, PREDNISOLONE
PREDNISONE, PREDNISONE
PROBENECID, PROBENECID
PROBENECID AND COLCHICINE, COLCHICINE
PROCAINAMIDE HCL, PROCAINAMIDE
  HYDROCHLORIDE
PROMETHAZINE HCL, PROMETHAZINE
  HYDROCHLORIDE
PROMPT PHENYTOIN SODIUM, PHENYTOIN SODIUM,
  PROMPT
PROPOXYPHENE COMPOUND 65, ASPIRIN
PROPOXYPHENE HCL, PROPOXYPHENE
  HYDROCHLORIDE
PROPOXYPHENE NAPSYLATE AND ACETAMINOPHEN,
  ACETAMINOPHEN
PROPRANOLOL HCL, PROPRANOLOL
  HYDROCHLORIDE
PROPRANOLOL HCL AND HYDROCHLOROTHIAZIDE,
  HYDROCHLOROTHIAZIDE
PROPYLTHIOURACIL, PROPYLTHIOURACIL

QUINIDINE SULFATE, QUINIDINE SULFATE
RAUWOLFIA SERPENTINA, RAUWOLFIA SERPENTINA
RESERPINE, RESERPINE
RESERPINE AND HYDROFLUMETHIAZIDE,
  HYDROFLUMETHIAZIDE
SECOBARBITAL SODIUM, SECOBARBITAL SODIUM
SODIUM BUTABARBITAL, BUTABARBITAL SODIUM
SODIUM PENTOBARBITAL, PENTOBARBITAL SODIUM
SPIRONOLACTONE, SPIRONOLACTONE
SPIRONOLACTONE W/ HYDROCHLOROTHIAZIDE,
  HYDROCHLOROTHIAZIDE
SULFINPYRAZONE, SULFINPYRAZONE
SULFISOXAZOLE, SULFISOXAZOLE
TETRACYCLINE HCL, TETRACYCLINE
  HYDROCHLORIDE
TETRAMED, TETRACYCLINE
THIORIDAZINE HCL, THIORIDAZINE
  HYDROCHLORIDE
TOLAZAMIDE, TOLAZAMIDE
TOLBUTAMIDE, TOLBUTAMIDE
TRIAMCINOLONE, TRIAMCINOLONE
TRIFLUOPERAZINE HCL, TRIFLUOPERAZINE
  HYDROCHLORIDE
TRIPROLIDINE HCL AND PSEUDOEPHEDRINE HCL,
  PSEUDOEPHEDRINE HYDROCHLORIDE
VITAMIN A, VITAMIN A PALMITATE

3

3M
* 3M
  SCRUBTEAM SURGICAL SPONGEBRUSH,
    HEXACHLOROPHENE
* 3M MEDICAL PRODUCTS DIV
  INSTANT MICROSPHERES, TECHNETIUM TC-99M
    ALBUMIN MICROSPHERES KIT
  YTTERBIUM YB 169 DTPA, PENTETATE CALCIUM
    TRISODIUM YB-169
* 3M PHARMACEUTICALS
  CALCIUM DISODIUM VERSENATE, EDETATE
    CALCIUM DISODIUM
  CIRCANOL, ERGOLOID MESYLATES
  DISIPAL, ORPHENADRINE HYDROCHLORIDE
  DUO-MEDIHALER, ISOPROTERENOL
    HYDROCHLORIDE
  ISOPROTERENOL HCL, ISOPROTERENOL
    HYDROCHLORIDE
  LIPO-HEPIN, HEPARIN SODIUM
  MAXAIR, PIRBUTEROL ACETATE
  MEDIHALER ERGOTAMINE, ERGOTAMINE TARTRATE
  MEDIHALER-EPI, EPINEPHRINE BITARTRATE (OTC)
  MEDIHALER-ISO, ISOPROTERENOL SULFATE
  NORFLEX, ORPHENADRINE CITRATE
  NORGESIC, ASPIRIN
  NORGESIC FORTE, ASPIRIN
  RAUWILOID, ALSEROXYLON
  SODIUM VERSENATE, EDETATE DISODIUM
  TAMBOCOR, FLECAINIDE ACETATE
  TEPANIL, DIETHYLPROPION HYDROCHLORIDE
  TEPANIL TEN-TAB, DIETHYLPROPION
    HYDROCHLORIDE
  THEOLAIR, THEOPHYLLINE
  THEOLAIR-SR, THEOPHYLLINE
  ULO, CHLOPHEDIANOL HYDROCHLORIDE
  UREX, METHENAMINE HIPPURATE
  VERILOID, ALKAVERVIR

APPENDIX C
UNIFORM TERMS

DOSAGE FORMS

AEROSOL
AEROSOL, METERED
BAR, CHEWABLE
CAPSULE
CAPSULE, COATED PELLETS
CAPSULE, DELAYED REL PELLETS
CAPSULE, EXTENDED RELEASE
CAPSULE, LIQUID FILLED
CONCENTRATE
CREAM
CREAM, AUGMENTED
DRESSING
DROPS
ELIXIR
EMULSION
ENEMA
FILM, EXTENDED RELEASE
GAS
GEL
GRANULE
GRANULE, EFFERVESCENT
GRANULE FOR RECONSTITUTION, ER
GUM, CHEWING
IMPLANT
INJECTABLE
INSERT
INSERT, EXTENDED RELEASE
INTRAUTERINE DEVICE
JELLY
LIQUID
LOTION
LOTION, AUGMENTED
OIL
OINTMENT
OINTMENT, AUGMENTED
PASTE
PASTILLE
PELLET
POWDER
POWDER FOR RECONSTITUTION*
SHAMPOO
SOAP
SOLUTION
SOLUTION FOR SLUSH
SPONGE
SPRAY
SPRAY, METERED
SUPPOSITORY
SUSPENSION
SUSPENSION, EXTENDED RELEASE
SWAB
SYRUP
TABLET
TABLET, CHEWABLE
TABLET, COATED PARTICLES
TABLET, DELAYED RELEASE
TABLET, DISPERSABLE
TABLET, EXTENDED RELEASE
TAMPON
TAPE
TINCTURE
TROCHE/LOZENGE

ROUTES OF ADMINISTRATION

BUCCAL
DENTAL
FOR RX COMPOUNDING
IMPLANTATION
INHALATION
INJECTION
INTRALYMPHATIC
INTRAPERITONEAL
INTRATHECAL
INTRATRACHEAL
INTRAUTERINE
INTRAVESICAL
IRRIGATION
NASAL
OPHTHALMIC
ORAL
ORAL-20
ORAL-21
ORAL-28
OTIC
PERFUSION, BILIARY
PERFUSION, CARDIAC
RECTAL
SPINAL
SUBLINGUAL
TOPICAL
TRANSDERMAL
URETERAL
URETHRAL
VAGINAL

ABBREVIATIONS

AMP	AMPULE
AMPICIL	AMPICILLIN
APPROX	APPROXIMATELY
BOT	BOTTLE
CI	CURIE
CSR	CAROTID SINUS REFLEX
CU	CLINICAL UNITS
DIPROP	DIPROPIONATE
EQ	EQUIVALENT TO
ELECT	ELECTROLYTE
ER	EXTENDED RELEASE
GM	GRAM
HBR	HYDROBROMIDE
HCL	HYDROCHLORIDE
HR	HOUR
INH	INHALATION
IU	INTERNATIONAL UNITS
MCG	MICROGRAM
MCI	MILLICURIE
MEQ	MILLIEQUIVALENT
MG	MILLIGRAM
ML	MILLILITER
N/A	NOT APPLICABLE
REL	RELEASE
SQ CM	SQUARE CENTIMETER
UCI	MICROCURIE
UGM	MICROGRAM
UMOLAR	MICROMOLAR
USP	UNITED STATES PHARMACOPEIA

* FOR ORAL, OPHTHALMIC, INTRATRACHEAL OR INHALATION USE ONLY

PATENT AND EXCLUSIVITY INFORMATION ADDENDUM

This *Addendum* identifies drugs that qualify under the Drug Price Competition and Patent Term Restoration Act (1984 Amendments) for periods of exclusivity, during which abbreviated new drug applications (ANDAs) and applications described in Section 505(b)(2) of the Federal Food, Drug, and Cosmetic Act (the Act) for those drug products may not be submitted or made effective as described below, and provides patent information concerning the listed drug products. Those drugs that have qualified for Orphan Drug Exclusivity pursuant to Section 527 of the Act are also included in this *Addendum*. This section is arranged in alphabetical order by active ingredient name. For those drug products with multiple active ingredients, only the first active ingredient (in alphabetical order) will appear. For an explanation of the codes used in the *Addendum*, see the *Exclusivity Terms* page. Exclusivity prevents the submission or effective approval of ANDAs or applications described in Section 505(b)(2) of the Act. It does not prevent the submission or approval of a second full NDA. Applications qualifying for periods of exclusivity are:

(1) A new drug application approved between January 1, 1982 and September 24, 1984, for a drug product all active ingredients (including any ester or salt of the active ingredient) of which had never been approved in any other application under Section 505(b) of the Act. Approval of an ANDA or an application described in Section 505(b)(2) of the Act for the same drug may not be *made effective* for a period of *ten years* from the date of the approval of the original application.

(2) A new drug application approved after September 24, 1984, for a drug product all active ingredients (including any ester or salt of the active ingredient) of which had never been approved in any other new drug application under Section 505(b) of the Act. No subsequent ANDA or application described in Section 505(b)(2) of the Act for the same drug may be *submitted* for a period of *five years* from the date of approval of the original application, except that such an application may be *submitted* after *four years* if it contains a certification that a patent claiming the drug is invalid or will not be infringed by the product for which approval is sought.

(3) A new drug application approved after September 24, 1984, for a drug product containing an active ingredient (including any ester or salt of that active ingredient) that has been approved in an earlier new drug application and that includes reports of new clinical investigations (other than bioavailability studies). Such investigations must have been conducted or sponsored by the applicant and must have been essential to approval of the application. If these requirements are met, the approval of a subsequent ANDA or an application described in Section 505(b)(2) of the Act may not be *made effective* for the same drug or use, if for a new indication, before the expiration of *three years* from the date of approval of the original application. If an applicant has exclusivity for a new use or indication, this does not preclude the approval of an ANDA application or 505(b)(2) application for the drug product with indications not covered by the exclusivity.

(4) A supplement to a new drug application for a drug containing a previously approved active ingredient (including any ester or salt of the active ingredient) approved after September 24, 1984, that contains reports of new clinical investigations (other than bioavailability studies) essential to the approval of the supplement and conducted or sponsored by the applicant. The approval of a subsequent application for a change approved in the supplement may not be *made effective* for *three years* from the date of approval of the original supplement.

The Act requires approved new drug applications to be supplemented with certain patent information by October 24, 1984, and that patent information must now be filed with all newly submitted drug applications, and no NDA may be approved after September 24, 1984, without the submission of pertinent patent information to the Agency. The patent numbers and the expiration dates of appropriate patents claiming drug products that are the subject of approved applications will be published in this *Addendum* or in the monthly Cumulative Supplement to this publication. Patent information on unapproved applications or on patents (i.e., process or manufacturing patents) beyond the scope of the Act will not be published.

The patents that FDA regards as covered by the statutory provisions for submission of patent information are: patents that claim the active ingredient or ingredients; drug product patents, which include formulation/composition patents; and use patents for a particular approved indication or method of using the product. NDA holders or applicants amending or supplementing applications with formulation/composition patent information are asked to certify that the patent(s) is appropriate for publication and refers to an approved product or one for which approval is being sought. The Agency asks all applicants or application holders with use patents to provide information as to the approved indications or uses covered by such patents. This information will be included in the Cumulative Supplement to the List as it becomes available.

Title I of the 1984 Amendments does not apply to drug products submitted or approved under Section 507 of the Federal Food, Drug, and Cosmetic Act (antibiotic products). Therefore, (1) applicants submitting abbreviated applications for antibiotic products are not required to provide the patent certification statement that must be included in ANDAs, (2) antibiotic products are not eligible for exclusivity protection, and (3) holders of approved applications for antibiotic products need not submit the patent information as required of NDA application holders.

Since all parts of this publication are subject to changes, additions, or deletions, the *Addendum* must be used in conjunction with the most current Cumulative Supplement.

EXCLUSIVITY TERMS

DUE TO SPACE LIMITATIONS IN THE EXCLUSIVITY COLUMN, THE FOLLOWING ABBREVIATIONS HAVE BEEN DEVELOPED. PLEASE REFER BACK TO THIS PAGE FOR AN EXPLANATION OF THE EXCLUSIVITY ABBREVIATIONS FOUND IN THE ADDENDUM.

ABBREVIATIONS

D	NEW DOSING SCHEDULE (SEE REFERENCES, BELOW)
I	NEW INDICATION (SEE REFERENCES, BELOW)
NC	NEW COMBINATION
NCE	NEW CHEMICAL ENTITY
NDF	NEW DOSAGE FORM
NE	NEW ESTER OR SALT OF AN ACTIVE INGREDIENT
NP	NEW PRODUCT
NR	NEW ROUTE
NS	NEW STRENGTH
ODE	ORPHAN DRUG EXCLUSIVITY
PC	PATENT CHALLENGE
U	PATENT USE CODE (SEE REFERENCES, BELOW)

REFERENCES
NEW DOSING SCHEDULE

D-1	ONCE A DAY APPLICATION
D-2	ONCE DAILY DOSING
D-3	SEVEN DAYS/SEVEN DAYS/SEVEN DAYS DOSING SCHEDULE
D-4	SEVEN DAYS/FOURTEEN DAYS DOSING SCHEDULE
D-5	TEN DAYS/ELEVEN DAYS DOSING SCHEDULE
D-6	SEVEN DAYS/NINE DAYS/FIVE DAYS DOSING SCHEDULE
D-7	BID DOSING
D-8	INTRAVENOUS, EPIDURAL AND INTRATHECAL DOSING
D-9	NARCOTIC OVERDOSE IN ADULTS
D-10	NARCOTIC OVERDOSE IN CHILDREN
D-11	POSTOPERATIVE NARCOTIC DEPRESSION IN CHILDREN
D-12	BEDTIME DOSING OF 800 MG FOR TREATMENT OF ACTIVE DUODENAL ULCER
D-13	INCREASED MAXIMUM DAILY DOSAGE RECOMMENDATION
D-14	BEDTIME DOSING OF 800 MG FOR TREATMENT OF ACTIVE BENIGN GASTRIC ULCER
D-15	SINGLE DAILY DOSE OF 25 MG/37.5 MG
D-16	CONTINUOUS INTRAVENOUS INFUSION
D-17	400 MQ EVERY 12 HOURS FOR THREE DAYS FOR UNCOMPLICATED URINARY TRACT INFECTIONS

REFERENCES
NEW INDICATION

I-1	DYSMENORRHEA
I-2	CHOLANGIOPANCREATOGRAPHY
I-3	INTRAVENOUS DIGITAL SUBTRACTION ANGIOGRAPHY
I-4	PERIPHERAL VENOGRAPHY (PHLEBOGRAPHY)
I-5	HYSTEROSALPINGOGRAPHY
I-6	TREATMENT OF JUVENILE ARTHRITIS
I-7	BIOPSY PROVEN MINIMAL CHANGE NEPHROTIC SYNDROME IN CHILDREN
I-8	ADULT INTRAVENOUS CONTRAST-ENHANCED COMPUTED TOMOGRAPHY OF THE HEAD AND BODY
I-9	PREVENTION OF POSTOPERATIVE NAUSEA AND VOMITING
I-10	PREVENTION OF POSTOPERATIVE DEEP VENOUS THROMBOSIS AND PULMONARY EMBOLISM IN TOTAL HIP REPLACEMENT SURGERY
I-11	RELIEF OF MILD TO MODERATE PAIN
I-12	TREATMENT OF CUTANEOUS CANDIDIASIS
I-13	URINARY TRACT INFECTION (UTI) PREVENTION FOR PERIODS UP TO FIVE MONTHS IN WOMEN WITH A HISTORY OF RECURRENT UTI
I-14	SEBORRHEIC DERMATITIS
I-15	PHOTOPHERESIS IN THE PALLIATIVE TREATMENT OF SKIN MANIFESTATIONS OF CUTANEOUS T-CELL LYMPHOMA IN PERSONS NOT RESPONSIVE TO OTHER TREATMENT
I-16	STIMULATE THE DEVELOPMENT OF MULTIPLE FOLLICLES/OOCYTES IN OVULATORY PATIENTS PARTICIPATING IN AN *IN VITRO* FERTILIZATION PROGRAM
I-17	MANAGEMENT OF CONGESTIVE HEART FAILURE
I-18	ENDOSCOPIC RETROGRADE PANCREATOGRAPHY
I-19	HERNIOGRAPHY
I-20	KNEE ARTHROGRAPHY
I-21	HIGH DOSE METHOTREXATE WITH LEUCOVORIN RESCUE IN COMBINATION WITH OTHER CHEMOTHERAPEUTIC AGENTS TO DELAY RECURRENCE IN PATIENTS WITH NONMETASTATIC OSTEOSARCOMA WHO HAVE UNDERGONE SURGICAL RESECTION OR AMPUTATION FOR THE PRIMARY TUMOR
I-22	RESCUE AFTER HIGH-DOSE METHOTREXATE THERAPY IN OSTEOSARCOMA
I-23	SHORT-TERM TREATMENT OF ACTIVE BENIGN GASTRIC ULCER
I-24	TREATMENT OF RHEUMATOID ARTHRITIS
I-25	ADULT INTRA-ARTERIAL DIGITAL SUBTRACTION ANGIOGRAPHY OF THE HEAD, NECK, ABDOMINAL, RENAL AND PERIPHERAL VESSELS

EXCLUSIVITY TERMS

NEW INDICATION (continued)

I-26	TREATMENT OF LIVER FLUKES
I-27	ADJUNCTIVE THERAPY TO DIET TO REDUCE THE RISK OF CORONARY ARTERY DISEASE
I-28	SELECTIVE ADULT VISCERAL ARTERIOGRAPHY
I-29	METASTATIC BREAST CANCER IN PREMENOPAUSAL WOMEN AS AN ALTERNATIVE TO OOPHOREC-TOMY OR OVARIAN IRRADIATION
I-30	TREATMENT OF TINEA PEDIS
I-31	CONTRAST ENHANCEMENT AGENT TO FACILITATE VISUALIZATION OF LESIONS IN THE SPINE AND ASSOCIATED TISSUES
I-32	PEDIATRIC MYELOGRAPHY
I-33	ORAL USE OF DILUTED OMNIPAQUE INJECTION IN ADULTS FOR CONTRAST ENHANCED COMPUTED TOMOGRAPHY OF THE ABDOMEN
I-34	ORAL USE IN ADULTS FOR PASS-THROUGH EXAMINATION OF THE GASTROINTESTINAL TRACT
I-35	PEDIATRIC CONTRAST ENHANCEMENT OF COMPUTED TOMOGRAPHIC HEAD IMAGING
I-36	ARTHROGRAPHY OF THE SHOULDER JOINTS IN ADULTS
I-37	RADIOGRAPHY OF THE TEMPOROMANDIBULAR JOINT IN ADULTS
I-38	CONTRAST ENHANCEMENT AGENT TO FACILITATE VISUALIZATION OF LESIONS OF THE CENTRAL NERVOUS SYSTEM IN CHILDREN (2 YEARS OF AGE AND OLDER)
I-39	TREATMENT OF ACUTE MYOCARDIAL INFARCTION
I-40	PRIMARY NOCTURNAL ENURESIS
I-41	MIGRAINE HEADACHE PROPHYLAXIS
I-42	HERPES ZOSTER
I-43	HERPES SIMPLEX ENCEPHALITIS
I-44	MAINTENANCE THERAPY IN HEALED DUODENAL ULCER PATIENTS AT DOSE OF 1 GRAM TWICE DAILY
I-45	ACUTE TREATMENT OF VARICELLA ZOSTER VIRUS
I-46	USE IN PEDIATRIC COMPUTED TOMOGRAPHIC HEAD AND BODY IMAGING
I-47	TREATMENT OF PEDIATRIC PATIENTS WITH SYMPTOMATIC HUMAN IMMUNODEFICIENCY VIRUS (HIV) DISEASE
I-48	PEDIATRIC ANGIOCARDIOGRAPHY
I-49	TREATMENT OF TRAVELERS' DIARRHEA DUE TO SUSCEPTIBLE STRAINS OF ENTEROTOXIGENIC ESCH-ERICHIA COLI
I-50	FOR USE IN WOMEN WITH AXILLARY NODE-NEGATIVE BREAST CANCER
I-51	TREATMENT OF PRIMARY DYSMENORRHEA AND FOR THE TREATMENT OF IDIOPATHIC HEAVY MEN-STRUAL BLOOD LOSS.
I-52	PEDIATRIC EXCRETORY UROGRAPHY
I-53	TREATMENT OF PANIC DISORDER, WITH OR WITHOUT AGORAPHOBIA
I-54	RENAL CONCENTRATION CAPACITY TEST
I-55	HYPERTENSION
I-56	EROSIVE GASTROESOPHAGEAL REFLUX DISEASE
I-57	SHORT-TERM TREATMENT OF ACTIVE DUODENAL ULCER
I-58	INITIAL TREATMENT OF ADVANCED OVARIAN CARCINOMA IN COMBINATION WITH OTHER AP-PROVED CHEMOTHERAPEUTIC AGENTS
I-59	ENDOSCOPICALLY DIAGNOSED ESOPHAGITIS, INCLUDING EROSIVE AND ULCERATIVE ESOPHAGITIS, AND ASSOCIATED HEARTBURN DUE TO GASTROESOPHAGEAL REFLUX DISEASE
I-60	SINGLE APPLICATION TREATMENT OF HEAD LICE IN CHILDREN TWO MONTHS TO TWO YEARS IN AGE
I-61	FEMALE ADROGENETIC ALOPECIA
I-62	PREVENTION AND TREATMENT OF POSTMENOPAUSAL OSTEOPOROSIS
I-63	ONCE DAILY TREATMENT AS INITIAL THERAPY IN THE TREATMENT OF HYPERTENSION
I-64	PREVENTION OF SUPRAVENTRICULAR TACHYCARDIAS
I-65	PREVENTION OF UPPER GASTROINTESTINAL BLEEDING IN CRITICALLY ILL PATIENTS
I-66	UNCOMPLICATED GONORRHEA
I-67	TREATMENT OF ACUTE ASTHMATIC ATTACKS IN CHILDREN SIX YEARS OF AGE AND OLDER
I-68	CENTRAL PRECOCIOUS PUBERTY
I-69	SHORT TERM TREATMENT OF PATIENTS WITH SYMPTOMS OF GASTROESOPHAGEAL REFLUX DISEASE (GERD), AND FOR THE SHORT TERM TREATMENT OF ESOPHAGITIS DUE TO GERD INCLUDING UL-CERATIVE DISEASE DIAGNOSED BY ENDOSCOPY
I-70	USE IN COMBINATION WITH 5-FLUOROURACIL TO PROLONG SURVIVAL IN THE PALLIATIVE TREAT-MENT OF PATIENTS WITH ADVANCED COLORECTAL CANCER
I-71	VARICELLA INFECTIONS (CHICKENPOX)
I-72	PREVENTION OF CMV DISEASE IN TRANSPLANT PATIENTS AT RISK FOR CMV DISEASE
I-73	INITIATE AND MAINTAIN MONITORED ANESTHESIA CARE (MAC) SEDATION DURING DIAGNOSTIC PROCEDURES
I-74	INTRAVENOUS DIGITAL SUBTRACTION ANGIOGRAPHY
I-75	TREATMENT OF ENDOSCOPICALLY DIAGNOSED EROSIVE ESOPHAGITIS

PATENT USE CODE

U-1	PREVENTION OF PREGNANCY
U-2	TREATMENT OR PROPHYLAXIS OF ANGINA PECTORIS AND ARRHYTHMIA
U-3	TREATMENT OF HYPERTENSION
U-4	PROVIDING PREVENTION AND TREATMENT OF EMESIS AND NAUSEA IN MAMMALS
U-5	METHOD OF PRODUCING BRONCHODILATION
U-6	METHOD OF PRODUCING SYMPATHOMIMETIC EFFECTS
U-7	INCREASING CARDIAC CONTRACTILITY

EXCLUSIVITY TERMS

PATENT USE CODE (continued)

U-8	ACUTE MYOCARDIAL INFARCTION
U-9	CONTROL OF EMESIS ASSOCIATED WITH ANY CANCER CHEMOTHERAPY AGENT
U-10	DIAGNOSTIC METHOD FOR DISTINGUISHING BETWEEN HYPOTHALMIC MALFUNCTIONS OR LESIONS IN HUMANS
U-11	TREATMENT OR PROPHYLAXIS OF CARDIAC DISORDERS
U-12	METHOD OF TREATING [A] HUMAN SUFFERING FROM DEPRESSION
U-13	A METHOD FOR TREATING ANXIETY IN A HUMAN SUBJECT IN NEED OF SUCH TREATMENT
U-14	ADJUNCTIVE THERAPY FOR THE PREVENTION AND TREATMENT OF HYPERAMMONEMIA IN THE CHRONIC MANAGEMENT OF PATIENTS WITH UREA CYCLE ENZYMOPATHIES
U-15	METHOD OF LOWERING INTRAOCULAR PRESSURE
U-16	USE IN LUNG SCANNING PROCEDURES
U-17	TREATMENT OF VENTRICULAR AND SUPRAVENTRICULAR ARRHYTHMIAS
U-18	METHOD FOR INHIBITING GASTRIC SECRETION IN MAMMALS
U-19	TREATMENT OF INFLAMMATION
U-20	A PROCESS FOR TREATING A PATIENT SUFFERING FROM PARKINSON'S SYNDROME AND IN NEED OF TREATMENT
U-21	TREATMENT OF HUMANS SUFFERING UNDESIRED UROTOXIC SIDE EFFECTS CAUSED BY CYTOSTATICALLY ACTIVE ALKYLATING AGENTS
U-22	METHOD OF COMBATING PATHOLOGICALLY REDUCED CEREBRAL FUNCTIONS AND PERFORMANCE WEAKNESSES, CEREBRAL INSUFFICIENCY AND DISORDERS IN CEREBRAL CIRCULATION AND METABOLISM IN WARM-BLOODED ANIMALS
U-23	METHOD FOR TREATING PROSTATIC CARCINOMA COMPRISING ADMINISTERING FLUTAMIDE
U-24	METHOD FOR TREATING PROSTATE ADENOCARCINOMA COMPRISING ADMINISTERING AN ANTIANDROGEN INCLUDING FLUTAMIDE AND AN LHRH AGONIST
U-25	REDUCING CHOLESTEROL IN CHOLELITHIASIS PATIENTS
U-26	REDUCING CHOLESTEROL GALLSTONES AND/OR FRAGMENTS THEREOF
U-27	DISSOLVING CHOLESTEROL GALLSTONES AND/OR FRAGMENTS THEREOF
U-28	CEREBRAL, CORONARY, PERIPHERAL, VISCERAL AND RENAL ARTERIOGRAPHY, AORTOGRAPHY AND LEFT VENTRICULOGRAPHY
U-29	CT IMAGING OF THE HEAD AND BODY, AND INTRAVENOUS EXCRETORY UROGRAPHY
U-30	CEREBRAL ANGIOGRAPHY, AND VENOGRAPHY
U-31	INTRA-ARTERIAL DIGITAL SUBTRACTION ANGIOGRAPHY
U-32	PALLIATIVE TREATMENT OF PATIENTS WITH OVARIAN CARCINOMA RECURRENT AFTER PRIOR CHEMOTHERAPY, INCLUDING PATIENTS WHO HAVE BEEN PREVIOUSLY TREATED WITH CISPLATIN
U-33	TREATING VIRAL INFECTIONS IN A MAMMAL
U-34	TREATING VIRAL INFECTIONS IN A WARM-BLOODED ANIMAL
U-35	TREATING CYTOMEGALOVIRUS IN A HUMAN WITH AN INJECTABLE COMPOSITION
U-36	METHODS OF TREATING BACTERIAL ILLNESSES
U-37	METHOD OF TREATING GASTROINTESTINAL DISEASE
U-38	TREATMENT OF PAROXYSMAL SUPRAVENTRICULAR TACHYCARDIA
U-39	ANGINA PECTORIS
U-40	METHOD OF TREATMENT OF BURNS
U-41	METHOD OF TREATING CARDIAC ARRHYTHMIAS
U-42	ADJUVANT TREATMENT IN COMBINATION WITH FLUOROURACIL AFTER SURGICAL RESECTION IN PATIENTS WITH DUKES' STAGE C COLON CANCER.
U-43	MANAGEMENT OF CHRONIC PAIN IN PATIENTS REQUIRING OPIOID ANALGESIA
U-44	RELIEF OF NAUSEA AND VOMITING
U-45	TREATMENT OF INFLAMMATION AND ANALGESIA
U-46	TREATMENT OF PANIC DISORDER
U-47	STIMULATION OF THE RELEASE OF GROWTH HORMONE
U-48	ANALGESIA
U-49	SYMPTOMATIC CANCER-RELATED HYPERCALCEMIA
U-50	USE IN TREATING INFLAMMATORY DERMATOSES
U-51	BLOOD POOL IMAGING, INCLUDING CARDIAC FIRST PASS AND GATED EQUILIBRIUM IMAGING AND FOR DETECTION OF SITES OF GASTROINTESTINAL BLEEDING
U-52	TREATMENT OF ADULT AND PEDIATRIC PATIENTS (OVER SIX MONTHS OF AGE) WITH ADVANCED HIV INFECTION
U-53	HYPERCALCEMIA OF MALIGNANCY
U-54	REVERSAL AGENT OR ANTAGONIST OF NONDEPOLARIZING NEUROMUSCULAR BLOCKING AGENTS
U-55	TREATMENT OF PAIN
U-56	AID TO SMOKING CESSATION
U-57	OPHTHALMIC USE OF NORFLOXACIN
U-58	METHOD OF TREATING INFLAMMATORY INTESTINAL DISEASES
U-59	METHOD OF TREATING HYPERCHOLESTEROLEMIA
U-60	NASAL ADMINISTRATION OF BUTORPHANOL
U-61	CEREBRAL AND PERIPHERAL ARTERIOGRAPHY AND CT IMAGING OF THE HEAD
U-62	CORONARY ARTERIOGRAPHY, LEFT VENTRICULOGRAPHY, CT IMAGING OF THE BODY, INTRAVENOUS EXCRETORY UROGRAPHY, INTRAVENOUS DIGITAL SUBTRACTION ANGIOGRAPHY AND VENOGRAPHY
U-63	ISOPRENALINE ANTAGONISM ON THE HEART RATE OR BLOOD PRESSURE
U-64	TREATMENT OF VIRAL INFECTIONS

PRESCRIPTION AND OTC DRUG PRODUCT
PATENT AND EXCLUSIVITY DATA

APPL/ PROD NUMBER	INGREDIENT NAME; TRADE NAME	PATENT NUMBER	PATENT EXPIRES	USE CODE	EX- CLUS CODE	EXCLUS EXPIRES
18917 001	ACEBUTOLOL HYDROCHLORIDE; SECTRAL	3857952	DEC 31, 1993	U-2		
18917 003	ACEBUTOLOL HYDROCHLORIDE; SECTRAL	3857952	DEC 31, 1993	U-2		
18458 001	ACETAMINOPHEN; TALACEN	4105659	AUG 08, 1995			
20232 001	ACETAMINOPHEN; FIORICET W/CODEINE				NC	OCT 26, 1993
18749 001	ACETOHYDROXAMIC ACID; LITHOSTAT				NCE	MAY 31, 1993
18604 001	ACYCLOVIR; ZOVIRAX	4199574	APR 22, 1997		NCE	MAR 29, 1992
18828 001	ACYCLOVIR; ZOVIRAX	4199574	APR 22, 1997		NCE	MAR 29, 1992
					I-45	APR 20, 1993
					I-71	FEB 26, 1995
19909 001	ACYCLOVIR; ZOVIRAX	4199574	APR 22, 1997		NCE	MAR 29, 1992
					I-45	APR 26, 1993
					I-71	FEB 26, 1995
20089 001	ACYCLOVIR; ZOVIRAX	4199574	APR 22, 1997		I-45	APR 26, 1993
					NCE	MAR 29, 1992
					I-71	FEB 26, 1995
20089 002	ACYCLOVIR; ZOVIRAX	4199574	APR 22, 1997		I-45	APR 26, 1993
					NCE	MAR 29, 1992
					I-71	FEB 26, 1995
18603 001	ACYCLOVIR SODIUM; ZOVIRAX	4199574	APR 22, 1997		NCE	MAR 29, 1992
					I-43	FEB 09, 1993
					I-42	FEB 09, 1993
19937 002	ADENOSINE; ADENOCARD	4673563	JUN 16, 2004	U-38	NCE	OCT 30, 1994
18062 001	ALBUTEROL SULFATE; PROVENTIL	4499108	FEB 12, 2002			
18702 001	ALCLOMETASONE DIPROPIONATE; ACLOVATE	4124707	NOV 07, 1995		NCE	DEC 14, 1992
18707 001	ALCLOMETASONE DIPROPIONATE; ACLOVATE	4124707	NOV 07, 1995		NCE	DEC 14, 1992
19353 001	ALFENTANIL HYDROCHLORIDE; ALFENTA	4167574	SEP 11, 1998			
20057 003	ALGLUCERASE; CEREDASE				NCE	APR 05, 1996
					ODE	APR 05, 1998
18276 001	ALPRAZOLAM; XANAX	3987052	APR 02, 2002	U-46		
		4508726	OCT 19, 1993			
		3980789	SEP 14, 1993		I-53	NOV 06, 1993
18276 002	ALPRAZOLAM; XANAX	4508726	APR 02, 2002	U-46		
		3987052	OCT 19, 1993			
		3980789	SEP 14, 1993		I-53	NOV 06, 1993
18276 003	ALPRAZOLAM; XANAX	4508726	APR 02, 2002	U-46		
		3987052	OCT 19, 1993			
		3980789	SEP 14, 1993		I-53	NOV 06, 1993
18276 004	ALPRAZOLAM; XANAX	4508726	APR 02, 2002	U-46		
		3987052	OCT 19, 1993		I-53	NOV 06, 1993
		3980789	SEP 14, 1993			
19926 001	ALTRETAMINE; HEXALEN				NCE	DEC 26, 1995
					ODE	DEC 26, 1997
18116 002	AMCINONIDE; CYCLOCORT	4158055	JUN 12, 1996	U-19		
18498 001	AMCINONIDE; CYCLOCORT	4158055	JUN 12, 1996	U-19		
19729 001	AMCINONIDE; CYCLOCORT	4158055	JUN 12, 1996	U-34		
18676 001	AMINO ACIDS; HEPATAMINE 8%	3950529	APR 13, 1993			
18678 001	AMINO ACIDS; BRANCHAMIN 4%	4438144	MAR 20, 2001			
18684 001	AMINO ACIDS; BRANCHAMIN 4%	4438144	MAR 20, 2001			
18202 001	AMINOGLUTETHIMIDE; CYTADREN	3944671	MAR 16, 1993			
16949 001	AMITRIPTYLINE HYDROCHLORIDE; LIMBITROL	4316897	FEB 23, 1999			
16949 002	AMITRIPTYLINE HYDROCHLORIDE; LIMBITROL	4316897	FEB 23, 1999			
19787 001	AMLODIPINE BESYLATE; NORVASC	4572909	FEB 25, 2003		NCE	JUL 31, 1997
19787 002	AMLODIPINE BESYLATE; NORVASC	4572909	FEB 25, 2003		NCE	JUL 31, 1997
19787 003	AMLODIPINE BESYLATE; NORVASC	4572909	FEB 25, 2003		NCE	JUL 31, 1997
19155 001	AMMONIUM LACTATE; LAC-HYDRIN	4105783	OCT 26, 1995			
18700 001	AMRINONE LACTATE; INOCOR	4072746	APR 23, 1998	U-7	NCE	JUL 31, 1994
18746 001	ANTAZOLINE PHOSPHATE; VASOCON-A				NC	APR 30, 1993
19779 001	APRACLONIDINE HYDROCHLORIDE; IOPIDINE	4517199	MAY 14, 2002	U-15	NCE	DEC 31, 1992
12365 005	ASPIRIN; SOMA COMPOUND	4534973	AUG 13, 2002			
12366 002	ASPIRIN; SOMA COMPOUND W/ CODEINE	4534974	AUG 13, 2002			
16891 001	ASPIRIN; TALWIN COMPOUND	4105659	AUG 08, 1995			
19429 003	ASPIRIN; FIORINAL W/CODEINE NO 3				NC	OCT 26, 1993
19402 001	ASTEMIZOLE; HISMANAL	4219559	AUG 26, 1997		NCE	DEC 29, 1993
18240 001	ATENOLOL; TENORMIN	3934032	JAN 20, 1993	U-3	I-39	SEP 13, 1992
18240 002	ATENOLOL; TENORMIN	3934032	JAN 20, 1993	U-3	I-39	SEP 13, 1992
18240 004	ATENOLOL; TENORMIN	3934032	JAN 20, 1993	U-3	I-39	SEP 13, 1992

PRESCRIPTION AND OTC DRUG PRODUCT
PATENT AND EXCLUSIVITY DATA *(continued)*

APPL/ PROD NUMBER	INGREDIENT NAME; TRADE NAME	PATENT NUMBER	PATENT EXPIRES	USE CODE	EX- CLUS CODE	EXCLUS EXPIRES
18760 001	ATENOLOL; TENORETIC 100	3934032	JAN 20, 1993			
18760 002	ATENOLOL; TENORETIC 50	3934032	JAN 20, 1993			
19058 001	ATENOLOL; TENORMIN				NDF	
72303 001	ATENOLOL; ATENOLOL	3934032	JAN 20, 1993	U-3	I-39	SEP 13, 1992
72304 001	ATENOLOL; ATENOLOL	3934032	JAN 20, 1993	U-3	I-39	SEP 13, 1992
18831 001	ATRACURIUM BESYLATE; TRACRIUM	4179507	DEC 18, 1996		NCE	NOV 23, 1993
19677 001	ATROPINE SULFATE; ENLON-PLUS	4952586	AUG 28, 2007	U-54	NC	NOV 06, 1994
19678 001	ATROPINE SULFATE; ENLON-PLUS	4952586	AUG 28, 2007	U-54	NC	NOV 06, 1994
20056 001	ATROPINE SULFATE; ATROPINE SULFATE				NDF	SEP 19, 1993
18689 001	AURANOFIN; RIDAURA	3708579	JAN 02, 1992			
19459 001	AVOBENZONE; PHOTOPLEX	4387089	JUN 07, 2002		NCE	SEP 30, 1993
20075 001	BACLOFEN; LIORESAL				ODE	JUN 17, 1999
					NDF	JUN 17, 1995
20075 002	BACLOFEN; LIORESAL				ODE	JUN 17, 1999
					NDF	JUN 17, 1995
17573 001	BECLOMETHASONE DIPROPIONATE; VANCERIL	4414209	AUG 23, 1994			
		4364923	OCT 29, 1999			
		4225597	SEP 30, 1997			
18153 001	BECLOMETHASONE DIPROPIONATE; BECLOVENT	4414209	AUG 23, 1994			
		4364923	DEC 21, 1999			
18521 001	BECLOMETHASONE DIPROPIONATE; VANCENASE	4414209	AUG 23, 1994			
		4364923	OCT 29, 1999			
		4225597	SEP 30, 1997			
18584 001	BECLOMETHASONE DIPROPIONATE; BECONASE	4414209	AUG 23, 1994			
		4364923	DEC 21, 1999			
19851 001	BENAZEPRIL HYDROCHLORIDE; LOTENSIN	4410520	OCT 18, 2000		NCE	JUN 25, 1996
19851 002	BENAZEPRIL HYDROCHLORIDE; LOTENSIN	4410520	OCT 18, 2000		NCE	JUN 25, 1996
19851 003	BENAZEPRIL HYDROCHLORIDE; LOTENSIN	4410520	OCT 18, 2000		NCE	JUN 25, 1996
19851 004	BENAZEPRIL HYDROCHLORIDE; LOTENSIN	4410520	OCT 18, 2000		NCE	JUN 25, 1996
20033 001	BENAZEPRIL HYDROCHLORIDE; LOTENSIN HCT	4410520	OCT 18, 2002		NCE	JUN 25, 1996
					NC	MAY 19, 1995
20033 002	BENAZEPRIL HYDROCHLORIDE; LOTENSIN HCT	4410520	OCT 18, 2002		NCE	JUN 25, 1996
					NC	MAY 19, 1995
20033 003	BENAZEPRIL HYDROCHLORIDE; LOTENSIN HCT	4410520	OCT 18, 2002		NCE	JUN 25, 1996
					NC	MAY 19, 1995
20033 004	BENAZEPRIL HYDROCHLORIDE; LOTENSIN HCT	4410520	OCT 18, 2002		NCE	JUN 25, 1996
					NC	MAY 19, 1995
18647 001	BENDROFLUMETHIAZIDE; CORZIDE	3982021	SEP 21, 1993			
		3935267	JAN 27, 1993			
18647 002	BENDROFLUMETHIAZIDE; CORZIDE	3982021	SEP 21, 1993			
		3935267	JAN 27, 1993			
18366 001	BENTIROMIDE; CHYMEX				NCE	DEC 29, 1993
19001 001	BEPRIDIL HYDROCHLORIDE; BEPADIN	RE30577	JUN 08, 1993		NCE	DEC 28, 1995
19001 002	BEPRIDIL HYDROCHLORIDE; BEPADIN	RE30577	JUN 08, 1993		NCE	DEC 28, 1995
19001 003	BEPRIDIL HYDROCHLORIDE; BEPADIN	RE30577	JUN 08, 1993		NCE	DEC 28, 1995
19002 001	BEPRIDIL HYDROCHLORIDE; VASCOR	RE30577	JUN 08, 1995		NCE	DEC 28, 1995
19002 002	BEPRIDIL HYDROCHLORIDE; VASCOR	RE30577	JUN 08, 1995		NCE	DEC 28, 1995
19002 003	BEPRIDIL HYDROCHLORIDE; VASCOR	RE30577	JUN 08, 1995		NCE	DEC 28, 1995
20032 001	BERACTANT; SURVANTA	4397839	AUG 10, 2000		NCE	JUL 01, 1996
					ODE	JUL 01, 1998
18741 001	BETAMETHASONE DIPROPIONATE; DIPROLENE	4070462	JAN 24, 1995			
18827 001	BETAMETHASONE DIPROPIONATE; LOTRISONE	4298604	NOV 03, 1998			
19408 001	BETAMETHASONE DIPROPIONATE; DIPROLENE	4489070	DEC 18, 2001			
		4482539	NOV 03, 2001			
19555 001	BETAMETHASONE DIPROPIONATE; DIPROLENE AF	4489071	DEC 18, 2001			
19716 001	BETAMETHASONE DIPROPIONATE; DIPROLENE	4775529	OCT 04, 2005			
19270 001	BETAXOLOL HYDROCHLORIDE; BETOPTIC	4911920	MAR 27, 2007			
		4342783	AUG 03, 1999			
		4311708	JAN 19, 1999			
		4252984	AUG 30, 1999			
19507 001	BETAXOLOL HYDROCHLORIDE; KERLONE	4311708	JAN 19, 1999	U-3		
		4252984	AUG 30, 1999		NDF	OCT 27, 1992
19507 002	BETAXOLOL HYDROCHLORIDE; KERLONE	4311708	JAN 19, 1999	U-3		
		4252984	AUG 30, 1999		NDF	OCT 27, 1992
19845 001	BETAXOLOL HYDROCHLORIDE; BETOPTIC S	4911920	MAR 27, 2007			
		4342783	AUG 03, 1999			
		4311708	JAN 19, 1999		NDF	DEC 29, 1992
		4252984	AUG 30, 1999			
19982 001	BISOPROLOL FUMARATE; ZEBETA	4258062	MAR 24, 1998	U-63	NCE	JUL 31, 1997

PRESCRIPTION AND OTC DRUG PRODUCT
PATENT AND EXCLUSIVITY DATA (continued)

APPL/ PROD NUMBER	INGREDIENT NAME; TRADE NAME	PATENT NUMBER	PATENT EXPIRES	USE CODE	EX- CLUS CODE	EXCLUS EXPIRES
19982 002	BISOPROLOL FUMARATE; ZEBETA	4258062	MAR 24, 1988	U-63	NCE	JUL 31, 1997
18770 001	BITOLTEROL MESYLATE; TORNALATE	4336400	JUN 22, 1999	U-5		
		4336400	JUN 22, 1999	U-6		
		4138581	FEB 06, 1998			
19548 001	BITOLTEROL MESYLATE; TORNALATE	4336400	JUN 22, 1999	U-5		
		4138581	FEB 06, 1998		NDF	FEB 19, 1995
18225 001	BUMETANIDE; BUMEX				NCE	FEB 28, 1993
18225 002	BUMETANIDE; BUMEX				NCE	FEB 28, 1993
18225 003	BUMETANIDE; BUMEX				NCE	FEB 28, 1993
18226 001	BUMETANIDE; BUMEX				NCE	FEB 28, 1993
18644 001	BUPROPION HYDROCHLORIDE; WELLBUTRIN	4507323	MAR 26, 2002			
		4438138	MAR 20, 2001			
		4435449	MAR 06, 2001			
		4425363	JAN 10, 2001			
		4393078	JUL 12, 2000			
		4347257	AUG 31, 1999			
		3885046	MAY 20, 1994	U-12		
18644 002	BUPROPION HYDROCHLORIDE; WELLBUTRIN	4507323	MAR 26, 2002			
		4438138	MAR 20, 2001			
		4435449	MAR 06, 2001			
		4425363	JAN 10, 2001			
		4393078	JUL 12, 2000			
		4347257	AUG 31, 1999			
		3885046	MAY 20, 1994	U-12		
18644 003	BUPROPION HYDROCHLORIDE; WELLBUTRIN	4507323	MAR 26, 2002			
		4438138	MAR 20, 2001			
		4435449	MAR 06, 2001			
		4425363	JAN 10, 2001			
		4393078	JUL 12, 2000			
		4347257	AUG 31, 1999			
		3885046	MAY 20, 1994	U-12		
18731 001	BUSPIRONE HYDROCHLORIDE; BUSPAR	4182763	JAN 08, 1999			
18731 002	BUSPIRONE HYDROCHLORIDE; BUSPAR	4182763	JAN 08, 1999			
19215 001	BUTOCONAZOLE NITRATE; FEMSTAT	4078071	MAR 07, 1997			
19359 001	BUTOCONAZOLE NITRATE; FEMSTAT	4078071	MAR 07, 1997			
19890 001	BUTORPHANOL TARTRATE; STADOL	4464378	AUG 07, 2001	U-60	NDF	DEC 12, 1994
18470 001	CALCITONIN, HUMAN; CIBACALCIN	RE32347	JUN 30, 1998		ODE	OCT 31, 1991
18044 001	CALCITRIOL; ROCALTROL	4391802	JUL 05, 2000			
		4341774	JUL 27, 1999			
		4225596	SEP 30, 1997			
18044 002	CALCITRIOL; ROCALTROL	4391802	JUL 05, 2000			
		4341774	JUL 27, 1999			
		4225596	SEP 30, 1997			
18874 001	CALCITRIOL; CALCIJEX	4308264	DEC 29, 1998			
18874 002	CALCITRIOL; CALCIJEX	4308264	DEC 29, 1998			
19976 001	CALCIUM ACETATE; PHOSLO	4870105	SEP 26, 2006		NDF	DEC 10, 1993
					ODE	DEC 10, 1997
18469 001	CALCIUM CHLORIDE; BSS PLUS	4550022	OCT 29, 2002			
		4443432	APR 17, 2001			
18343 001	CAPTOPRIL; CAPOTEN	4105776	AUG 08, 1995			
18343 002	CAPTOPRIL; CAPOTEN	4105776	AUG 08, 1995			
18343 003	CAPTOPRIL; CAPOTEN	4105776	AUG 08, 1995			
18343 005	CAPTOPRIL; CAPOTEN	4105776	AUG 08, 1995			
18709 001	CAPTOPRIL; CAPOZIDE 25/15	4217347	AUG 12, 1997			
		4105776	AUG 08, 1995		I-63	OCT 24, 1994
18709 002	CAPTOPRIL; CAPOZIDE 25/25	4217347	AUG 12, 1997			
		4105776	AUG 08, 1995		I-63	OCT 24, 1994
18709 003	CAPTOPRIL; CAPOZIDE 50/25	4217347	AUG 12, 1997			
		4105776	AUG 08, 1995		I-63	OCT 24, 1994
18709 004	CAPTOPRIL; CAPOZIDE 50/15	4217347	AUG 12, 1997			
		4105776	AUG 08, 1995		I-63	OCT 24, 1994
16608 001	CARBAMAZEPINE; TEGRETOL	4409212	OCT 11, 2000			
18281 001	CARBAMAZEPINE; TEGRETOL	4409212	OCT 11, 2000			
18927 001	CARBAMAZEPINE; TEGRETOL	4409212	OCT 11, 2000			
19856 001	CARBIDOPA; SINEMET CR	4900755	MAY 23, 2006		NDF	MAY 30, 1994
		4832957	MAY 23, 2006			
19880 001	CARBOPLATIN; PARAPLATIN	4657927	APR 14, 2004	U-32	NCE	MAR 03, 1994
		4140707	AUG 25, 1998		I-58	JUL 05, 1994

PRESCRIPTION AND OTC DRUG PRODUCT
PATENT AND EXCLUSIVITY DATA (continued)

APPL/ PROD NUMBER	INGREDIENT NAME; TRADE NAME	PATENT NUMBER	PATENT EXPIRES	USE CODE	EX- CLUS CODE	EXCLUS EXPIRES
19880 002	CARBOPLATIN; PARAPLATIN	4657927	APR 14, 2004	U-32	NCE	MAR 03, 1994
		4140707	AUG 25, 1998		I-58	JUL 05, 1994
19880 003	CARBOPLATIN; PARAPLATIN	4657927	APR 14, 2004	U-32	NCE	MAR 03, 1994
		4140707	AUG 25, 1998		I-58	JUL 05, 1994
18550 002	CARPROFEN; RIMADYL	3896145	JUL 22, 1994		NCE	DEC 31, 1992
18550 003	CARPROFEN; RIMADYL	3896145	JUL 22, 1994		NCE	DEC 31, 1992
19204 001	CARTEOLOL HYDROCHLORIDE; CARTROL	3910924	OCT 07, 1994		NCE	DEC 28, 1993
19204 002	CARTEOLOL HYDROCHLORIDE; CARTROL	3910924	OCT 07, 1994		NCE	DEC 28, 1993
19204 003	CARTEOLOL HYDROCHLORIDE; CARTROL	3910924	OCT 07, 1994		NCE	DEC 28, 1993
19972 001	CARTEOLOL HYDROCHLORIDE; OPTIPRESS	4309432	JAN 05, 1999		NDF	MAY 23, 1993
		3910924	OCT 07, 1994		NCE	DEC 28, 1993
18757 002	CELLULOSE SODIUM PHOSPHATE; CALCIBIND				NCE	DEC 28, 1992
20044 001	CETYL ALCOHOL; EXOSURF NEONATAL	4826821	MAY 02, 2006		ODE	AUG 02, 1997
		4312860	NOV 23, 2001		NC	AUG 02, 1993
18513 002	CHENODIOL; CHENIX				NCE	JUL 28, 1993
13071 007	CHLORDIAZEPOXIDE; LIBRITABS	4316897	FEB 23, 1999			
13071 008	CHLORDIAZEPOXIDE; LIBRITABS	4316897	FEB 23, 1999			
13071 009	CHLORDIAZEPOXIDE; LIBRITABS	4316897	FEB 23, 1999			
14740 002	CHLORDIAZEPOXIDE; MENRIUM 5-2	4316897	FEB 23, 1999			
14740 004	CHLORDIAZEPOXIDE; MENRIUM 5-4	4316897	FEB 23, 1999			
14740 006	CHLORDIAZEPOXIDE; MENRIUM 10-4	4316897	FEB 23, 1999			
17813 001	CHLORDIAZEPOXIDE; LIBRELEASE	4316897	FEB 23, 1999			
12249 001	CHLORDIAZEPOXIDE HYDROCHLORIDE; LIBRIUM	4316897	FEB 23, 1999			
12249 002	CHLORDIAZEPOXIDE HYDROCHLORIDE; LIBRIUM	4316897	FEB 23, 1999			
12249 003	CHLORDIAZEPOXIDE HYDROCHLORIDE; LIBRIUM	4316897	FEB 23, 1999			
12301 001	CHLORDIAZEPOXIDE HYDROCHLORIDE; LIBRIUM	4316897	FEB 23, 1999			
12750 001	CHLORDIAZEPOXIDE HYDROCHLORIDE; LIBRAX	4316897	FEB 23, 1999			
17594 001	CHLOROXINE; CAPITROL	3886277	MAY 27, 1992			
18050 001	CHLORPHENIRAMINE POLISTIREX; CORSYM	4221778	SEP 09, 1997			
18928 001	CHLORPHENIRAMINE POLISTIREX; PENNTUSS	4221778	SEP 09, 1997			
19111 001	CHLORPHENIRAMINE POLISTIREX; TUSSIONEX	4221778	SEP 09, 1997			
19451 001	CHLORTHALIDONE; LOPRESSIDONE	3998790	DEC 21, 1993			
19451 002	CHLORTHALIDONE; LOPRESSIDONE	3998790	DEC 21, 1993			
71621 001	CHOLESTYRAMINE; CHOLYBAR	4778676	OCT 18, 2005			
71739 001	CHOLESTYRAMINE; CHOLYBAR	4778676	OCT 18, 2005			
18625 001	CHYMOPAPAIN; DISCASE				NCE	NOV 10, 1992
18663 001	CHYMOPAPAIN; CHYMODIACTIN	4439423	MAR 26, 2001		NCE	NOV 10, 1992
18663 002	CHYMOPAPAIN; CHYMODIACTIN	4439423	MAR 26, 2001		NCE	NOV 10, 1992
18748 001	CICLOPIROX OLAMINE; LOPROX	3883545	MAY 13, 1992		NCE	DEC 30, 1992
19824 001	CICLOPIROX OLAMINE; LOPROX	3883545	MAY 13, 1992		NCE	DEC 30, 1992
17920 002	CIMETIDINE; TAGAMET	4024271	MAY 17, 1994			
		3950333	APR 13, 1993		I-56	MAR 07, 1994
17920 003	CIMETIDINE; TAGAMET	4024271	MAY 17, 1994			
		3950333	APR 13, 1993		I-56	MAR 07, 1994
17920 004	CIMETIDINE; TAGAMET	4024271	MAY 17, 1994			
		3950333	APR 13, 1993		I-56	MAR 07, 1994
17920 005	CIMETIDINE; TAGAMET	4024271	MAY 17, 1994			
		3950333	APR 13, 1993		I-56	MAR 07, 1994
17924 001	CIMETIDINE HYDROCHLORIDE; TAGAMET	4024271	MAY 17, 1994			
		3950333	APR 13, 1993		I-56	MAR 07, 1994
17939 002	CIMETIDINE HYDROCHLORIDE; TAGAMET	4024271	MAY 17, 1994		I-65	NOV 13, 1994
		3950333	APR 13, 1993		D-16	NOV 13, 1992
19434 001	CIMETIDINE HYDROCHLORIDE; TAGAMET HCL IN SODIUM CHLORIDE 0.9%	4024271	MAY 17, 1994			
		3950333	APR 13, 1993			
19847 001	CIRPOFLOXACIN; CIPRO	4808583	FEB 28, 2006			
		4705789	NOV 10, 2004			
		4670444	OCT 01, 2002		NCE	OCT 22, 1992
19857 001	CIPROFLOXACIN; CIPRO IN DEXTROSE 5%	4957922	SEP 18, 2007			
		4808583	FEB 28, 2006			
		4705789	NOV 10, 2004			
		4670444	OCT 01, 2002		NCE	OCT 22, 1992
19858 001	CIPROFLOXACIN; CIPRO IN SODIUM CHLORIDE 0.9%	4957922	SEP 18, 2007			
		4808583	FEB 28, 2006			
		4705789	NOV 10, 2004			
		4670444	OCT 01, 2002		NCE	OCT 22, 1992
19537 002	CIPROFLOXACIN HYDROCHLORIDE; CIPRO	4670444	OCT 01, 2002	U-36	NCE	OCT 22, 1992
19537 003	CIPROFLOXACIN HYDROCHLORIDE; CIPRO	4670444	OCT 01, 2002	U-36	NCE	OCT 22, 1992
19537 004	CIPROFLOXACIN HYDROCHLORIDE; CIPRO	4670444	OCT 01, 2002	U-36	NCE	OCT 22, 1992

PRESCRIPTION AND OTC DRUG PRODUCT
PATENT AND EXCLUSIVITY DATA *(continued)*

APPL/ PROD NUMBER	INGREDIENT NAME; TRADE NAME	PATENT NUMBER	PATENT EXPIRES	USE CODE	EX- CLUS CODE	EXCLUS EXPIRES
19992 001	CIPROFLOXACIN HYDROCHLORIDE; CILOXAN	4670444	OCT 01, 2002		NDF	DEC 31, 1993
					NCE	OCT 22, 1992
18057 001	CISPLATIN; PLATINOL	4177263	DEC 04, 1996			
18057 002	CISPLATIN; PLATINOL	4177263	DEC 04, 1996			
18057 003	CISPLATIN; PLATINOL-AQ	4310515	JAN 12, 1999			
		4177263	DEC 04, 1996			
18057 004	CISPLATIN; PLATINOL-AQ	4310515	JAN 12, 1999			
		4177263	DEC 04, 1996			
19481 001	CITRIC ACID; RENACIDIN				ODE	OCT 02, 1997
18298 001	CLEMASTINE FUMARATE; TAVIST D	3933999	JAN 20, 1993			
19322 001	CLOBETASOL PROPIONATE; TEMOVATE	3721687	MAR 20, 1992			
19323 001	CLOBETASOL PROPIONATE; TEMOVATE	3721687	MAR 20, 1992			
19966 001	CLOBETASOL PROPIONATE; TEMOVATE	3721687	MAR 20, 1992		NP	FEB 22, 1993
19500 001	CLOFAZIMINE; LAMPRENE				ODE	DEC 15, 1991
19500 002	CLOFAZIMINE; LAMPRENE				ODE	DEC 15, 1991
19906 001	CLOMIPRAMINE HYDROCHLORIDE; ANAFRANIL				NCE	DEC 29, 1994
19906 002	CLOMIPRAMINE HYDROCHLORIDE; ANAFRANIL				NCE	DEC 29, 1994
19906 003	CLOMIPRAMINE HYDROCHLORIDE; ANAFRANIL				NCE	DEC 29, 1994
17533 001	CLONAZEPAM; KLONOPIN	4316897	FEB 23, 1999			
17533 002	CLONAZEPAM; KLONOPIN	4316897	FEB 23, 1999			
17533 003	CLONAZEPAM; KLONOPIN	4316897	FEB 23, 1999			
18891 001	CLONIDINE; CATAPRES-TTS-1	4559222	DEC 17, 2002			
		4201211	MAY 06, 1997			
		4060084	JUN 28, 1994			
		3996934	JUL 29, 1992			
18891 002	CLONIDINE; CATAPRES-TTS-2	4559222	DEC 17, 2002			
		4201211	MAY 06, 1997			
		4060084	JUN 28, 1994			
		3996934	JUL 29, 1992			
18891 003	CLONIDINE; CATAPRES-TTS-3	4559222	DEC 17, 2002			
		4201211	MAY 06, 1997			
		4060084	JUN 28, 1994			
		3996934	JUL 29, 1992			
19758 001	CLOZAPINE; CLOZARIL				NCE	SEP 26, 1994
19758 002	CLOZAPINE; CLOZARIL				NCE	SEP 26, 1994
17408 001	COPPER; CU-7	4040417	AUG 09, 1994			
		RE28399	APR 29, 1992			
18205 001	COPPER; TATUM-T	4040417	AUG 09, 1994			
		RE28399	APR 29, 1992			
16990 001	CROMOLYN SODIUM; INTAL	3957965	MAY 18, 1993			
		3860618	JAN 14, 1992			
18155 001	CROMOLYN SODIUM; OPTICROM	4053628	OCT 11, 1994			
		3975536	AUG 17, 1993			
18306 001	CROMOLYN SODIUM; NASALCROM	4053628	OCT 11, 1994			
		3975536	AUG 17, 1993			
18596 001	CROMOLYN SODIUM; INTAL	3975536	AUG 17, 1993			
18887 001	CROMOLYN SODIUM; INTAL	4405598	SEP 20, 2000			
		3860618	JAN 14, 1992			
19188 001	CROMOLYN SODIUM; GASTROCROM	4395421	JUL 26, 2000		ODE	DEC 22, 1996
12142 006	CYCLOPHOSPHAMIDE; LYOPHILIZED CYTOXAN	4537883	AUG 27, 2002			
12142 007	CYCLOPHOSPHAMIDE; LYOPHILIZED CYTOXAN	4537883	AUG 27, 2002			
12142 008	CYCLOPHOSPHAMIDE; LYOPHILIZED CYTOXAN	4537883	AUG 27, 2002			
12142 009	CYCLOPHOSPHAMIDE; LYOPHILIZED CYTOXAN	4537883	AUG 27, 2002			
12142 010	CYCLOPHOSPHAMIDE; LYOPHILIZED CYTOXAN	4537883	AUG 27, 2002			
19849 001	DAPIPRAZOLE HYDROCHLORIDE; REV-EYES	4252721	JAN 06, 2002		NCE	DEC 31, 1995
17922 001	DESMOPRESSIN ACETATE; DDAVP			I-40		NOV 28, 1992
19776 001	DESMOPRESSIN ACETATE; CONCENTRATAID			I-54		DEC 26, 1993
18658 001	DEXTROMETHORPHAN POLISTIREX; DELSYM	4221778	SEP 09, 1997			
19082 001	DEZOCINE; DALGAN	4605671	AUG 12, 2003			
		4001331	JAN 04, 1996		NCE	DEC 29, 1994
19082 002	DEZOCINE; DALGAN	4605671	AUG 12, 2003			
		4001331	JAN 04, 1996		NCE	DEC 29, 1994
19082 003	DEZOCINE; DALGAN	4605671	AUG 12, 2003			
		4001331	JAN 04, 1996		NCE	DEC 29, 1994
13263 002	DIAZEPAM; VALIUM	4316897	FEB 23, 1999			
13263 004	DIAZEPAM; VALIUM	4316897	FEB 23, 1999			
13263 006	DIAZEPAM; VALIUM	4316897	FEB 23, 1999			
16087 001	DIAZEPAM; VALIUM	4316897	FEB 23, 1999			
18179 001	DIAZEPAM; VALRELEASE	4316897	FEB 23, 1999			

PRESCRIPTION AND OTC DRUG PRODUCT
PATENT AND EXCLUSIVITY DATA (continued)

APPL/ PROD NUMBER	INGREDIENT NAME; TRADE NAME	PATENT NUMBER	PATENT EXPIRES	USE CODE	EX- CLUS CODE	EXCLUS EXPIRES
19201 001	DICLOFENAC SODIUM; VOLTAREN				NCE	JUL 28, 1993
19201 002	DICLOFENAC SODIUM; VOLTAREN				NCE	JUL 28, 1993
19201 003	DICLOFENAC SODIUM; VOLTAREN				NCE	JUL 28, 1993
20037 001	DICLOFENAC SODIUM; VOLTAREN	4960799	OCT 02, 2007		NDF	MAR 28, 1994
20154 002	DIDANOSINE, VIDEX	4861759	AUG 29, 2006	U-52	NCE	OCT 09, 1996
20154 003	DIDANOSINE, VIDEX	4861759	AUG 29, 2006	U-52	NCE	OCT 09, 1996
20154 004	DIDANOSINE, VIDEX	4861759	AUG 29, 2006	U-52	NCE	OCT 09, 1996
20154 005	DIDANOSINE, VIDEX	4861759	AUG 29, 2006	U-52	NCE	OCT 09, 1996
20155 003	DIDANOSINE, VIDEX	4861759	AUG 29, 2006	U-52	NCE	OCT 09, 1996
20155 004	DIDANOSINE, VIDEX	4861759	AUG 29, 2006	U-52	NCE	OCT 09, 1996
20155 005	DIDANOSINE, VIDEX	4861759	AUG 29, 2006	U-52	NCE	OCT 09, 1996
20155 006	DIDANOSINE, VIDEX	4861759	AUG 29, 2006	U-52	NCE	OCT 09, 1996
20156 001	DIDANOSINE, VIDEX	4861759	AUG 29, 2006	U-52	NCE	OCT 09, 1996
17741 001	DIFLORASONE DIACETATE; FLORONE	3980778	SEP 14, 1993			
17994 001	DIFLORASONE DIACETATE; FLORONE	3980778	SEP 14, 1993			
19259 001	DIFLORASONE DIACETATE; DIFLORASONE DIACETATE	3980778	SEP 14, 1993			
19260 001	DIFLORASONE DIACETATE; PSORCON	3980778	SEP 14, 1993			
18445 001	DIFLUNISAL; DOLOBID				NCE	APR 19, 1992
18445 002	DIFLUNISAL; DOLOBID				NCE	APR 19, 1992
18118 001	DIGOXIN; LANOXICAPS	4088750	MAY 09, 1995			
18118 002	DIGOXIN; LANOXICAPS	4088750	MAY 09, 1995			
18118 003	DIGOXIN; LANOXICAPS	4088750	MAY 09, 1995			
18118 004	DIGOXIN; LANOXICAPS	4088750	MAY 09, 1995			
18885 001	DIHYDROERGOTAMINE MESYLATE; EMBOLEX	4451458	MAY 29, 2001			
		4402949	SEP 06, 2000			
18885 002	DIHYDROERGOTAMINE MESYLATE; EMBOLEX	4451458	MAY 29, 2001			
		4402949	SEP 06, 2000			
18602 001	DILTIAZEM HYDROCHLORIDE; CARDIZEM				NCE	NOV 05, 1992
18602 002	DILTIAZEM HYDROCHLORIDE; CARDIZEM				NCE	NOV 05, 1992
18602 003	DILTIAZEM HYDROCHLORIDE; CARDIZEM				NCE	NOV 05, 1992
18602 004	DILTIAZEM HYDROCHLORIDE; CARDIZEM				NCE	NOV 05, 1992
19471 001	DILTIAZEM HYDROCHLORIDE; CARDIZEM SR	4721619	JAN 26, 2005		NCE	NOV 05, 1992
					NP	JAN 23, 1992
19471 002	DILTIAZEM HYDROCHLORIDE; CARDIZEM SR	4721619	JAN 26, 2005		NCE	NOV 05, 1992
					NP	JAN 23, 1992
19471 003	DILTIAZEM HYDROCHLORIDE; CARDIZEM SR	4721619	JAN 26, 2005		NCE	NOV 05, 1992
					NP	JAN 23, 1992
19471 004	DILTIAZEM HYDROCHLORIDE; CARDIZEM SR	4721619	JAN 26, 2005		NCE	NOV 05, 1992
					NP	JAN 23, 1992
20027 001	DILTIAZEM HYDROCHLORIDE; CARDIZEM				NDF	OCT 24, 1994
					NCE	NOV 05, 1992
20027 002	DILTIAZEM HYDROCHLORIDE; CARDIZEM				NDF	OCT 24, 1994
					NCE	NOV 05, 1992
20062 001	DILTIAZEM HYDROCHLORIDE; CARDIZEM CD	5002776	MAR 26, 2008		NCE	NOV 05, 1992
		4894240	JAN 16, 2007		NP	DEC 27, 1994
20062 002	DILTIAZEM HYDROCHLORIDE; CARDIZEM CD	5002776	MAR 26, 2008		NCE	NOV 05, 1992
		4894240	JAN 16, 2007		NP	DEC 27, 1994
20062 003	DILTIAZEM HYDROCHLORIDE; CARDIZEM CD	5002776	MAR 26, 2008		NCE	NOV 05, 1992
		4894240	JAN 16, 2007		NP	DEC 27, 1994
20062 004	DILTIAZEM HYDROCHLORIDE; CARDIZEM CD	5002776	MAR 26, 2008		NCE	NOV 05, 1992
		4894240	JAN 16, 2007		NP	DEC 27, 1994
20092 001	DILTIAZEM HYDROCHLORIDE; DILACOR XR				NP	DEC 27, 1994
					NCE	NOV 05, 1992
20092 002	DILTIAZEM HYDROCHLORIDE; DILACOR XR				NP	DEC 27, 1994
					NCE	NOV 05, 1992
20092 003	DILTIAZEM HYDROCHLORIDE; DILACOR XR				NP	DEC 27, 1994
					NCE	NOV 05, 1992
17810 001	DINOPROSTONE; PROSTIN E2	3899587	AUG 12, 1992			
19817 001	DIPYRIDAMOLE; IV PERSANTINE				NDF	DEC 13, 1993
18723 001	DIVALPROEX SODIUM; DEPAKOTE	4988731	JAN 29, 2008			
18723 002	DIVALPROEX SODIUM; DEPAKOTE	4988731	JAN 29, 2008			
18723 003	DIVALPROEX SODIUM; DEPAKOTE	4988731	JAN 29, 2008			
19680 001	DIVALPROEX SODIUM; DEPAKOTE	4988731	JAN 29, 2008			
19794 001	DIVALPROEX SODIUM; DEPAKOTE CP	4988731	JAN 29, 2008			
19794 002	DIVALPROEX SODIUM; DEPAKOTE CP	4988731	JAN 29, 2008			
17820 002	DOBUTAMINE HYDROCHLORIDE; DOBUTREX	3987200	OCT 19, 1993	U-7		
19946 001	DOXACURIUM CHLORIDE; NUROMAX	4701460	MAR 06, 2005		NCE	MAR 07, 1996
19668 001	DOXAZOSIN MESYLATE; CARDURA	4188390	FEB 12, 1999		NCE	NOV 02, 1995

PRESCRIPTION AND OTC DRUG PRODUCT
PATENT AND EXCLUSIVITY DATA *(continued)*

APPL/ PROD NUMBER	INGREDIENT NAME; TRADE NAME	PATENT NUMBER	PATENT EXPIRES	USE CODE	EX- CLUS CODE	EXCLUS EXPIRES
19668 002	DOXAZOSIN MESYLATE; CARDURA	4188390	FEB 12, 1999		NCE	NOV 02, 1995
19668 003	DOXAZOSIN MESYLATE; CARDURA	4188390	FEB 12, 1999		NCE	NOV 02, 1995
19668 004	DOXAZOSIN MESYLATE; CARDURA	4188390	FEB 12, 1999		NCE	NOV 02, 1995
18751 001	ECONAZOLE NITRATE; SPECTAZOLE				NCE	DEC 23, 1992
19879 002	EFLORNITHINE HYDROCHLORIDE; ORNIDYL	4413141	NOV 01, 2000		ODE	NOV 28, 1997
		4339151	AUG 16, 2000		NCE	NOV 28, 1995
18998 001	ENALAPRIL MALEATE; VASOTEC	4374829	FEB 22, 2000			
18998 002	ENALAPRIL MALEATE; VASOTEC	4374829	FEB 22, 2000			
18998 003	ENALAPRIL MALEATE; VASOTEC	4374829	FEB 22, 2000			
18998 005	ENALAPRIL MALEATE; VASOTEC	4374829	FEB 22, 2000			
19221 001	ENALAPRIL MALEATE; VASERETIC	4472380	SEP 18, 2001			
		4374829	FEB 22, 2000			
19309 001	ENALAPRILAT; VASOTEC	4374829	FEB 22, 2000			
18981 002	ENCAINIDE HYDROCHLORIDE; ENKAID	3931195	JAN 06, 1993			
		RE30811	DEC 20, 1996	U-17		
18981 003	ENCAINIDE HYDROCHLORIDE; ENKAID	3931195	JAN 06, 1993			
		RE30811	DEC 20, 1996	U-17		
18981 004	ENCAINIDE HYDROCHLORIDE; ENKAID	3931195	JAN 06, 1993			
		RE30811	DEC 20, 1996	U-17		
19616 004	ENOXACIN; PENETREX	4442101	APR 10, 2001			
		4359578	NOV 16, 1999		NCE	DEC 31, 1996
		4352803	OCT 05, 1999	U-36		
19616 005	ENOXACIN; PENETREX	4442101	APR 10, 2001			
		4359578	NOV 16, 1999		NCE	DEC 31, 1996
		4352803	OCT 05, 1999	U-36		
17751 004	EPINEPHRINE; DURANEST	3862321	JAN 21, 1992			
17751 006	EPINEPHRINE BITARTRATE; DURANEST	3862321	JAN 21, 1992			
17751 007	EPINEPHRINE BITARTRATE; DURANEST	3862321	JAN 21, 1992			
18418 001	ERGOLOID MESYLATES; HYDERGINE	4138565	FEB 06, 1996			
18706 001	ERGOLOID MESYLATES; HYDERGINE LC	4366145	DEC 28, 1999			
19386 001	ESMOLOL HYDROCHLORIDE; BREVIBLOC	4593119	JUN 03, 2003			
		4387103	JUN 07, 2000	U-11		
19386 002	ESMOLOL HYDROCHLORIDE; BREVIBLOC	4593119	JUN 03, 2003			
		4387103	JUN 07, 2000	U-11		
19386 003	ESMOLOL HYDROCHLORIDE; BREVIBLOC	4387103	JUN 07, 2000	U-11		
19080 001	ESTAZOLAM; PROSOM	3987052	OCT 19, 1993		NCE	DEC 26, 1995
19080 002	ESTAZOLAM; PROSOM	3987052	OCT 19, 1993		NCE	DEC 26, 1995
19081 002	ESTRADIOL; ESTRADERM	4379454	APR 12, 2000		I-62	OCT 24, 1994
		4144317	SEP 09, 1992			
		3948262	JUL 29, 1992			
19081 003	ESTRADIOL; ESTRADERM	4379454	APR 12, 2000		I-62	OCT 24, 1994
		4144317	SEP 09, 1992			
		3948262	JUL 29, 1992			
86069 001	ESTRADIOL; ESTRACE	4436738	MAR 13, 2001			
19357 001	ETHANOLAMINE OLEATE; ETHAMOLIN				ODE	DEC 22, 1995
18977 001	ETHINYL ESTRADIOL; TRI-NORINYL 21-DAY	4390531	JUN 28, 2000			
18977 002	ETHINYL ESTRADIOL; TRI-NORINYL 28-DAY	4390531	JUN 28, 2000			
18985 001	ETHINYL ESTRADIOL; ORTHO-NOVUM 7/7/7-21	4616006	OCT 07, 2003			
		4544554	JUL 23, 2002			
		4530839	JUL 23, 2002			
18985 002	ETHINYL ESTRADIOL; ORTHO-NOVUM 7/7/7-28	4616006	OCT 07, 2003			
		4544554	JUL 23, 2002			
		4530839	JUL 23, 2002			
19190 001	ETHINYL ESTRADIOL; TRIPHASIL-28	3957982	MAY 18, 1993	U-1		
19192 001	ETHINYL ESTRADIOL; TRIPHASIL-21	3957982	MAY 18, 1993	U-1		
19653 001	ETHINYL ESTRADIOL; ORTHO CYCLEN-21	4027019	MAY 31, 1996		NC	DEC 29, 1992
19653 002	ETHINYL ESTRADIOL; ORTHO CYCLEN-28	4027019	MAY 31, 1996		NC	DEC 29, 1992
19697 001	ETHINYL ESTRADIOL; ORTHO TRI-CYCLEN				NP	JUL 03, 1995
19697 002	ETHINYL ESTRADIOL; ORTHO TRI-CYCLEN				NP	JUL 03, 1995
17751 003	ETIDOCAINE HYDROCHLORIDE; DURANEST	3862321	JAN 21, 1992			
17751 005	ETIDOCAINE HYDROCHLORIDE; DURANEST	3862321	JAN 21, 1992			
17831 001	ETIDRONATE DISODIUM; DIDRONEL	4254114	MAR 03, 1998			
		4216211	AUG 05, 1997			
		4137309	JAN 30, 1996			
17831 002	ETIDRONATE DISODIUM; DIDRONEL	4254114	MAR 03, 1998			
		4216211	AUG 05, 1997			
		4137309	JAN 30, 1996			

PRESCRIPTION AND OTC DRUG PRODUCT
PATENT AND EXCLUSIVITY DATA (continued)

APPL/ PROD NUMBER	INGREDIENT NAME; TRADE NAME	PATENT NUMBER	PATENT EXPIRES	USE CODE	EX- CLUS CODE	EXCLUS EXPIRES
19545 001	ETIDRONATE DISODIUM; DIDRONEL	4254114	MAR 03, 1998			
		4216211	AUG 05, 1997			
		4137309	JAN 30, 1996		ODE	APR 20, 1994
18922 002	ETODOLAC; LODINE					
		3939178	FEB 17, 1993		NCE	JAN 31, 1996
18922 003	ETODOLAC; LODINE					
		3939178	FEB 17, 1993		NCE	JAN 31, 1996
18227 001	ETOMIDATE; AMIDATE				NCE	SEP 07, 1992
18768 001	ETOPOSIDE; VEPESID				NCE	NOV 10, 1993
19557 001	ETOPOSIDE; VEPESID				NCE	NOV 10, 1993
19557 002	ETOPOSIDE; VEPESID				NCE	NOV 10, 1993
19369 001	ETRETINATE; TEGISON	4215215	JUL 29, 1999			
		4200647	APR 29, 1997			
19369 002	ETRETINATE; TEGISON	4215215	JUL 29, 1999			
		4200647	APR 29, 1997			
19462 001	FAMOTIDINE; PEPCID	4283408	AUG 11, 2000	I-69		DEC 10, 1994
19462 002	FAMOTIDINE; PEPCID	4283408	AUG 11, 2000	I-69		DEC 10, 1994
19510 001	FAMOTIDINE; PEPCID	4283408	AUG 11, 2000			
19527 001	FAMOTIDINE; PEPCID	4283408	AUG 11, 2000	I-69		DEC 10, 1991
19834 001	FELODIPINE; PLENDIL	4264611	APR 28, 1998		NCE	JUL 25, 1996
19834 002	FELODIPINE; PLENDIL	4264611	APR 28, 1998		NCE	JUL 25, 1996
19813 001	FENTANYL; DURAGESIC	4588580	MAY 13, 2003	U-43		
		4144317	SEP 09, 1992			
		4060084	JUN 28, 1994	U-43	NDF	AUG 07, 1993
19813 002	FENTANYL; DURAGESIC	4588580	MAY 13, 2003	U-43		
		4144317	SEP 09, 1992			
		4060084	JUN 28, 1994	U-43	NDF	AUG 07, 1993
19813 003	FENTANYL; DURAGESIC	4588580	MAY 13, 2003	U-43		
		4144317	SEP 09, 1992			
		4060084	JUN 28, 1994	U-43	NDF	AUG 07, 1993
19813 004	FENTANYL; DURAGESIC	4588580	MAY 13, 2003	U-43		
		4144317	SEP 09, 1992			
		4060084	JUN 28, 1994	U-43	NDF	AUG 07, 1993
20180 001	FINASTERIDE; PROSCAR	4760071	JUL 26, 2005			
		4377584	MAR 22, 2000		NCE	JUN 19, 1997
18830 001	FLECAINIDE ACETATE; TAMBOCOR	4005209	JAN 25, 1996			
		3900481	AUG 19, 1992	I-64		OCT 23, 1994
18830 003	FLECAINIDE ACETATE; TAMBOCOR	4005209	JAN 25, 1996			
		3900481	AUG 19, 1992	I-64		OCT 23, 1994
18830 004	FLECAINIDE ACETATE; TAMBOCOR	4005209	JAN 25, 1996	I-64		OCT 23, 1994
		3900481	AUG 19, 1992			
19949 001	FLUCONAZOLE; DIFLUCAN	4416682	NOV 22, 2000			
		4404216	OCT 16, 2003		NCE	JAN 29, 1995
19949 002	FLUCONAZOLE; DIFLUCAN	4416682	NOV 22, 2000			
		4404216	OCT 16, 2003		NCE	JAN 29, 1995
19949 003	FLUCONAZOLE; DIFLUCAN	4416682	NOV 22, 2000			
		4404216	OCT 16, 2003		NCE	JAN 29, 1995
19950 001	FLUCONAZOLE; DIFLUCAN	4416682	NOV 22, 2000			
		4404216	OCT 16, 2003		NCE	JAN 29, 1995
20038 001	FLUDARABINE PHOSPHATE; FLUDARA	4357324	NOV 02, 1999		NCE	APR 18, 1996
					ODE	APR 18, 1998
20073 001	FLUMAZENIL; MAZICON	4316839	FEB 23, 1999		NCE	DEC 20, 1996
20001 001	FLUOCINOLONE ACETONIDE; FS SHAMPOO				NDF	AUG 27, 1993
16909 002	FLUOCINONIDE; LIDEX	4017615	APR 12, 1994			
18936 001	FLUOXETINE HYDROCHLORIDE; PROZAC	4314081	FEB 02, 2001			
		4194009	APR 19, 1994			
		4018895	APR 19, 1994	U-12	NCE	DEC 29, 1992
20101 001	FLUOXETINE HYDROCHLORIDE; PROZAC	4626549	DEC 02, 2003			
		4314081	FEB 02, 2001		NCE	DEC 29, 1992
		4194009	APR 19, 1994			
		4018895	APR 19, 1994	U-12		
16721 001	FLURAZEPAM HYDROCHLORIDE; DALMANE	4316897	FEB 23, 1999			
16721 002	FLURAZEPAM HYDROCHLORIDE; DALMANE	4316897	FEB 23, 1999			
18766 002	FLURBIPROFEN; ANSAID	3793457	FEB 19, 1993			
18766 003	FLURBIPROFEN; ANSAID	3793457	FEB 19, 1993			
19404 001	FLURBIPROFEN SODIUM; OCUFEN	3793457	FEB 19, 1993			
18554 001	FLUTAMIDE; EULEXIN	4474813	NOV 30, 1993		NCE	JAN 27, 1994
		4472382	JAN 27, 2003	U-24		
		4329364	MAY 11, 2001	U-23		

PRESCRIPTION AND OTC DRUG PRODUCT
PATENT AND EXCLUSIVITY DATA *(continued)*

APPL/ PROD NUMBER	INGREDIENT NAME; TRADE NAME	PATENT NUMBER	PATENT EXPIRES	USE CODE	EX- CLUS CODE	EXCLUS EXPIRES
19957 001	FLUTICASONE PROPIONATE; CUTIVATE	4335121	MAR 16, 2002		NCE	DEC 14, 1995
19958 001	FLUTICASONE PROPIONATE; CUTIVATE	4335121	MAR 16, 2002		NCE	DEC 14, 1995
20068 001	FOSCARNET SODIUM; FOSCAVIR	4771041	JUL 29, 1997			
		4665062	JUL 29, 1997			
		4339445	JUL 29, 1997	U-64		
		4215113	JUL 29, 1997	U-64	NCE	SEP 27, 1996
19915 002	FOSINOPRIL SODIUM; MONOPRIL	4384123	MAY 17, 2000			
		4337201	JUN 29, 1999		NCE	MAY 16, 1996
19915 003	FOSINOPRIL SODIUM; MONOPRIL	4384123	MAY 17, 2000			
		4337201	JUN 29, 2001		NCE	MAY 16, 1996
19596 001	GADOPENTETATE DIMEGLUMINE; MAGNEVIST	4963344	MAR 03, 2004	I-38		AUG 10, 1992
		4957939	MAR 03, 2004	I-31		APR 28, 1992
		4647447	MAR 03, 2004		NCE	JUN 02, 1993
19961 002	GALLIUM NITRATE; GANITE	4529593	JAN 17, 2005	U-49	NCE	JAN 17, 1996
					ODE	JAN 17, 1998
19661 001	GANCICLOVIR SODIUM; CYTOVENE	4507305	OCT 19, 1999	U-35	I-72	MAY 15, 1995
		4423050	OCT 19, 1999	U-34		
		4355032	MAR 16, 2003	U-33	NCE	JUN 23, 1994
18422 001	GEMFIBROZIL; LOPID	3674836	JAN 04, 1993	I-27		JAN 17, 1992
18422 002	GEMFIBROZIL; LOPID	3674836	JAN 04, 1993	I-27		JAN 17, 1992
18422 003	GEMFIBROZIL; LOPID	3674836	JAN 04, 1993	I-27		JAN 17, 1992
17783 001	GLIPIZIDE; GLUCOTROL	3669966	APR 21, 1992		NCE	MAY 08, 1994
17783 002	GLIPIZIDE; GLUCOTROL	3669966	APR 21, 1992		NCE	MAY 08, 1994
17498 001	GLYBURIDE; MICRONASE	3507961	APR 21, 1992			
		3507954	APR 21, 1992			
		3454635	APR 21, 1992			
		3426067	APR 21, 1992		NCE	MAY 01, 1994
17498 002	GLYBURIDE; MICRONASE	3507961	APR 21, 1992			
		3507954	APR 21, 1992			
		3454635	APR 21, 1992			
		3426067	APR 21, 1992		NCE	MAY 01, 1994
17498 003	GLYBURIDE; MICRONASE	3507961	APR 21, 1992			
		3507954	APR 21, 1992			
		3454635	APR 21, 1992			
		3426067	APR 21, 1992		NCE	MAY 01, 1994
17532 001	GLYBURIDE; DIABETA	4060634	SEP 07, 1993			
		3507961	APR 21, 1992			
		3507954	APR 21, 1992			
		3454635	APR 21, 1992			
		3426067	APR 21, 1992		NCE	MAY 01, 1994
17532 002	GLYBURIDE; DIABETA	4060634	SEP 07, 1993			
		3507961	APR 21, 1992			
		3507954	APR 21, 1992			
		3454635	APR 21, 1992			
		3426067	APR 21, 1992		NCE	MAY 01, 1994
17532 003	GLYBURIDE; DIABETA	4060634	SEP 07, 1993			
		3507961	APR 21, 1992			
		3507954	APR 21, 1992			
		3454635	APR 21, 1992			
		3426067	APR 21, 1992		NCE	MAY 01, 1994
20051 001	GLYBURIDE; GLYNASE	4916163	APR 10, 2007			
		4735805	APR 05, 2005		NCE	MAY 01, 1994
		3507961	APR 21, 1992		NP	MAR 04, 1995
		3507954	APR 21, 1992			
		3454635	APR 21, 1992			
		3426067	APR 21, 1992			
20051 002	GLYBURIDE; GLYNASE	4916163	APR 10, 2007			
		4735805	APR 05, 2005		NCE	MAY 01, 1994
		3507961	APR 21, 1992		NP	MAR 04, 1995
		3507954	APR 21, 1992			
		3454635	APR 21, 1992			
		3426067	APR 21, 1992			
20055 001	GLYBURIDE; GLUBATE				NP	MAR 04, 1995
					NCE	MAY 01, 1994
20055 002	GLYBURIDE; GLUBATE				NP	MAR 04, 1995
					NCE	MAY 01, 1994
19687 001	GONADORELIN ACETATE; LUTREPULSE PUMP KIT				NE	OCT 10, 1992
19687 002	GONADORELIN ACETATE; LUTREPULSE PUMP KIT				NE	OCT 10, 1992
18123 001	GONADORELIN HYDROCHLORIDE; FACTREL	3947569	MAR 30, 1993	U-10	NCE	SEP 30, 1992

PRESCRIPTION AND OTC DRUG PRODUCT
PATENT AND EXCLUSIVITY DATA *(continued)*

APPL/ PROD NUMBER	INGREDIENT NAME; TRADE NAME	PATENT NUMBER	PATENT EXPIRES	USE CODE	EX-CLUS CODE	EXCLUS EXPIRES
18123 002	GONADORELIN HYDROCHLORIDE; FACTREL	3947569	MAR 30, 1993	U-10	NCE	SEP 30, 1992
18123 003	GONADORELIN HYDROCHLORIDE; FACTREL	3947569	MAR 30, 1993	U-10	NCE	SEP 30, 1992
19726 001	GOSERELIN ACETATE; ZOLADEX	4100274	JUL 10, 1997		NCE	DEC 29, 1994
18587 001	GUANABENZ ACETATE; WYTENSIN				NCE	SEP 07, 1992
18587 002	GUANABENZ ACETATE; WYTENSIN				NCE	SEP 07, 1992
18587 003	GUANABENZ ACETATE; WYTENSIN				NCE	SEP 07, 1992
18104 001	GUANADREL SULFATE; HYLOREL				NCE	DEC 29, 1992
18104 002	GUANADREL SULFATE; HYLOREL				NCE	DEC 29, 1992
17556 001	HALCINONIDE; HALOG	3892857	JUL 01, 1992			
17818 001	HALCINONIDE; HALOG	3892857	JUL 01, 1992			
17824 001	HALCINONIDE; HALOG	3892856	JUL 01, 1992			
18234 001	HALCINONIDE; HALOG-E	4048310	SEP 13, 1994			
19967 001	HALOBETASOL PROPIONATE, ULTRAVATE	4619921	DEC 17, 2004		NCE	DEC 17, 1995
					D-1	DEC 31, 1994
19968 001	HALOBETASOL PROPIONATE; ULTRAVATE	4619921	DEC 17, 2004		NCE	DEC 17, 1995
20250 001	HALOFANTRINE HYDROCHLORIDE; HALFAN				D-1	DEC 31, 1994
19836 001	HISTRELIN ACETATE; SUPPRELIN	4244946	JAN 13, 1998		NCE	DEC 24, 1996
					ODE	DEC 24, 1998
19836 002	HISTRELIN ACETATE; SUPPRELIN	4244946	JAN 13, 1998		NCE	DEC 24, 1996
					ODE	DEC 24, 1998
19836 003	HISTRELIN ACETATE; SUPPRELIN	4244946	JAN 13, 1998		NCE	DEC 24, 1996
					ODE	DEC 24, 1998
18061 001	HYDROCHLOROTHIAZIDE; TIMOLIDE 10-25	4238485	DEC 09, 1997			
18303 001	HYDROCHLOROTHIAZIDE; LOPRESSOR HCT 50/25	3998790	DEC 21, 1993			
		3876802	APR 08, 1992			
18303 002	HYDROCHLOROTHIAZIDE; LOPRESSOR HCT 100/25	3998790	DEC 21, 1993			
		3876802	APR 08, 1992			
18303 003	HYDROCHLOROTHIAZIDE; LOPRESSOR HCT 100/50	3998790	DEC 21, 1993			
		3876802	APR 08, 1992			
18872 001	HYDROCHLOROTHIAZIDE; VISKAZIDE				NCE	SEP 03, 1992
18872 002	HYDROCHLOROTHIAZIDE; VISKAZIDE				NCE	SEP 03, 1992
19046 001	HYDROCHLOROTHIAZIDE; NORMOZIDE	4066755	JAN 03, 1995			
		4012444	MAR 15, 1994		NCE	AUG 01, 1994
19046 002	HYDROCHLOROTHIAZIDE; NORMOZIDE	4066755	JAN 03, 1995			
		4012444	MAR 15, 1994		NCE	AUG 01, 1994
19046 003	HYDROCHLOROTHIAZIDE; NORMOZIDE	4066755	JAN 03, 1995			
		4012444	MAR 15, 1994		NCE	AUG 01, 1994
19046 004	HYDROCHLOROTHIAZIDE; NORMOZIDE	4066755	JAN 03, 1995			
		4012444	MAR 15, 1994		NCE	AUG 01, 1994
19059 001	HYDROCHLOROTHIAZIDE; INDERIDE LA 80/50	4138475	FEB 06, 1996			
19059 002	HYDROCHLOROTHIAZIDE; INDERIDE LA 120/50	4138475	FEB 06, 1996			
19059 003	HYDROCHLOROTHIAZIDE; INDERIDE LA 160/50	4138475	FEB 06, 1996			
19129 001	HYDROCHLOROTHIAZIDE; MAXZIDE	4444769	APR 24, 2001			
19129 003	HYDROCHLOROTHIAZIDE; MAXZIDE-25	4444769	APR 24, 2001			
19174 001	HYDROCHLOROTHIAZIDE; TRANDATE HCT	4066755	JAN 03, 1995			
		4012444	MAR 15, 1994		NCE	AUG 01, 1994
19174 002	HYDROCHLOROTHIAZIDE; TRANDATE HCT	4066755	JAN 03, 1995			
		4012444	MAR 15, 1994		NCE	AUG 01, 1994
19174 003	HYDROCHLOROTHIAZIDE; TRANDATE HCT	4066755	JAN 03, 1995			
		4012444	MAR 15, 1994		NCE	AUG 01, 1994
19174 004	HYDROCHLOROTHIAZIDE; TRANDATE HCT	4066755	JAN 03, 1995			
		4012444	MAR 15, 1994		NCE	AUG 01, 1994
19778 001	HYDROCHLOROTHIAZIDE; PRINZIDE 12.5	4472380	SEP 18, 2001		NCE	DEC 29, 1992
		4374829	DEC 30, 2001		NC	FEB 16, 1992
19778 002	HYDROCHLOROTHIAZIDE; PRINZIDE 25	4472380	SEP 18, 2001		NCE	DEC 29, 1992
		4374829	DEC 30, 2001		NC	FEB 16, 1992
19888 002	HYDROCHLOROTHIAZIDE; ZESTORETIC 20/25	4472380	SEP 18, 2001			
		4374829	DEC 30, 2001		NCE	DEC 29, 1992
19034 001	HYDROMORPHONE HYDROCHLORIDE; DILAUDID-HP				NCE	JAN 11, 1994
19261 001	HYDROXYAMPHETAMINE HYDROBROMIDE; PARE-MYD				NC	JAN 30, 1995
16295 001	HYDROXYUREA; HYDREA	3968249	JUL 06, 1993			
19771 001	IBUPROFEN; ADVIL COLD AND SINUS				NC	SEP 19, 1992
19784 001	IBUPROFEN; RUFEN				NDF	SEP 19, 1992
19833 002	IBUPROFEN; CHILDREN'S ADVIL	4788220	NOV 29, 2005		NDF	SEP 19, 1992
19842 001	IBUPROFEN; PEDIA PROFEN				NDF	SEP 19, 1992
50661 001	IDARUBICIN HYDROCHLORIDE; IDAMYCIN				ODE	SEP 27, 1997
50661 002	IDARUBICIN HYDROCHLORIDE; IDAMYCIN				ODE	SEP 27, 1997

PRESCRIPTION AND OTC DRUG PRODUCT
PATENT AND EXCLUSIVITY DATA *(continued)*

APPL/ PROD NUMBER	INGREDIENT NAME; TRADE NAME	PATENT NUMBER	PATENT EXPIRES	USE CODE	EX- CLUS CODE	EXCLUS EXPIRES
19763 001	IFOSFAMIDE; IFEX	3732340	MAY 08, 1992		ODE	DEC 30, 1995
					NCE	DEC 30, 1993
19763 002	IFOSFAMIDE; IFEX	3732340	MAY 08, 1992		ODE	DEC 30, 1995
					NCE	DEC 30, 1993
18538 001	INDAPAMIDE; LOZOL				NCE	JUL 06, 1993
19693 001	INDECAINIDE HYDROCHLORIDE; DECABID	4452745	JUN 05, 2003		NCE	DEC 29, 1994
		4389393	JUN 21, 2000			
		4382093	MAY 03, 2000			
		4197313	APR 08, 1997	U-41		
19693 002	INDECAINIDE HYDROCHLORIDE; DECABID	4452745	JUN 05, 2003		NCE	DEC 29, 1994
		4389393	JUN 21, 2000			
		4382093	MAY 03, 2000			
		4197313	APR 08, 1997	U-41		
19693 003	INDECAINIDE HYDROCHLORIDE; DECABID	4452745	JUN 05, 2003		NCE	DEC 29, 1994
		4389393	JUN 21, 2000			
		4382093	MAY 03, 2000			
		4197313	APR 08, 1997	U-41		
19044 001	INDIUM IN-111 OXYQUINOLINE; INDIUM IN-111 OXYQUINOLINE	4335095	JUN 15, 1999			
17707 001	INDIUM IN-111 PENTETATE DISODIUM; MPI INDIUM DTPA IN 111				NCE	FEB 18, 1992
18185 001	INDOMETHACIN; INDOCIN SR	4173626	NOV 06, 1996			
20100 001	INSULIN BIOSYNTHETIC HUMAN; HUMULIN 50/50				NP	APR 29, 1995
19432 001	IOFETAMINE HYDROCHLORIDE I-123; SPECTAMINE	4360511	NOV 23, 2001		NCE	DEC 24, 1992
18956 001	IOHEXOL; OMNIPAQUE 180	4396597	JUL 14, 1998	I-32		JUN 30, 1992
		4250113	DEC 26, 1999			
		4021481	MAY 03, 1994			
18956 002	IOHEXOL; OMNIPAQUE 240	4396597	JUL 14, 1998	I-35		JUL 28, 1992
		4250113	DEC 26, 1999	I-33		JUN 30, 1992
		4021481	MAY 03, 1994		NR	JUN 30, 1992
					I-36	JUL 28, 1992
18956 003	IOHEXOL; OMNIPAQUE 300	4396597	JUL 14, 1998	I-35		JUL 28, 1992
		4250113	DEC 26, 1999	I-33		JUN 30, 1992
		4021481	MAY 03, 1994	I-28		MAR 31, 1992
					NR	JUN 30, 1992
					I-37	JUL 28, 1992
18956 004	IOHEXOL; OMNIPAQUE 350	4396597	JUL 14, 1998	I-33		JUN 30, 1992
		4250113	DEC 26, 1999		NR	JUN 30, 1992
		4021481	MAY 03, 1994	I-28		MAR 31, 1992
					I-34	JUN 30, 1992
18956 005	IOHEXOL; OMNIPAQUE 140	4396597	JUL 14, 1998	I-25		NOV 30, 1991
		4250113	DEC 26, 1999			
		4021481	MAY 03, 1994			
18956 006	IOHEXOL; OMNIPAQUE 210	4396597	JUL 14, 1998			
		4250113	DEC 26, 1999		I-36	JUL 28, 1992
		4021481	MAY 03, 1994		NS	JUN 30, 1992
18735 001	IOPAMIDOL; ISOVUE-M 200	4001323	JAN 04, 1996			
18735 002	IOPAMIDOL; ISOVUE-300	4001323	JAN 04, 1996		I-46	MAY 30, 1993
					I-52	SEP 21, 1993
18735 003	IOPAMIDOL; ISOVUE-370	4001323	JAN 04, 1996		I-48	OCT 04, 1992
18735 004	IOPAMIDOL; ISOVUE-M 300	4001323	JAN 04, 1996			
19580 001	IOTROLAN; OSMOVIST	4239747	DEC 16, 1999		NCE	DEC 07, 1994
19580 002	IOTROLAN; OSMOVIST	4239747	DEC 16, 1999		NCE	DEC 07, 1994
19710 001	IOVERSOL; OPTIRAY 320	4396598	OCT 26, 2002	U-28	NCE	DEC 30, 1993
		4396598	OCT 26, 2002	U-29		
19710 002	IOVERSOL; OPTIRAY 240	4396598	OCT 26, 2002	U-30	NCE	DEC 30, 1993
19710 003	IOVERSOL; OPTIRAY 160	4396598	OCT 26, 2002	U-31	NCE	DEC 30, 1993
19710 004	IOVERSOL; OPTIRAY 300	4396598	OCT 26, 2002	U-61	NS	JAN 22, 1995
19710 005	IOVERSOL; OPTIRAY 350	4396598	OCT 26, 2002	U-62	NS	JAN 22, 1995
					I-74	JAN 22, 1995
18905 002	IOXAGLATE MEGLUMINE; HEXABRIX	4094966	JUN 13, 1995			
		4065554	DEC 27, 1994			
		4065553	DEC 27, 1994			
		4014986	MAR 29, 1996			
17624 001	ISOFLURANE; FORANE	3535425	JAN 24, 1993			
		3535388	JAN 24, 1993			
19091 001	ISOSORBIDE MONONITRATE; ISMO				NCE	DEC 30, 1996

PRESCRIPTION AND OTC DRUG PRODUCT
PATENT AND EXCLUSIVITY DATA *(continued)*

APPL/ PROD NUMBER	INGREDIENT NAME; TRADE NAME	PATENT NUMBER	PATENT EXPIRES	USE CODE	EX- CLUS CODE	EXCLUS EXPIRES
18662 002	ISOTRETINOIN; ACCUTANE	4464394	AUG 07, 2001			
		4322438	MAR 30, 1999			
		4200647	APR 29, 1997		NCE	MAY 07, 1992
18662 003	ISOTRETINOIN; ACCUTANE	4464394	AUG 07, 2001			
		4322438	MAR 30, 1999			
		4200647	APR 29, 1997		NCE	MAY 07, 1992
18662 004	ISOTRETINOIN; ACCUTANE	4464394	AUG 07, 2001			
		4322438	MAR 30, 1999			
		4200647	APR 29, 1997		NCE	MAY 07, 1992
19546 001	ISRADIPINE; DYNACIRC	4466972	AUG 21, 2003	U-3	NCE	DEC 20, 1995
19546 002	ISRADIPINE; DYNACIRC	4466972	AUG 21, 2003	U-3	NCE	DEC 20, 1995
18533 001	KETOCONAZOLE; NIZORAL	4335125	JUN 15, 1999			
19084 001	KETOCONAZOLE; NIZORAL	4335125	JUN 15, 1999			
19576 001	KETOCONAZOLE; NIZORAL	4335125	JUN 15, 1999			
19648 001	KETOCONAZOLE; NIZORAL	4335125	JUN 15, 1999			
19927 001	KETOCONAZOLE; NIZORAL	4335125	JUN 15, 1999		NDF	AUG 31, 1993
19645 001	KETOROLAC TROMETHAMINE; TORADOL	4089969	MAY 16, 1997	U-55	NDF	DEC 20, 1994
					NCE	NOV 30, 1994
19698 001	KETOROLAC TROMETHAMINE; TORADOL	4089969	MAY 16, 1997	U-55	NCE	NOV 30, 1994
19698 002	KETOROLAC TROMETHAMINE; TORADOL	4089969	MAY 16, 1997	U-55	NCE	NOV 30, 1994
18686 001	LABETALOL HYDROCHLORIDE; NORMODYNE	4328213	MAY 04, 1999			
		4066755	JAN 03, 1995			
18687 001	LABETALOL HYDROCHLORIDE; NORMODYNE	4012444	AUG 2, 1998		NCE	AUG 01, 1994
		4066755	JAN 03, 1995			
18687 002	LABETALOL HYDROCHLORIDE; NORMODYNE	4012444	AUG 2, 1998		NCE	AUG 01, 1994
		4066755	JAN 03, 1995			
18687 003	LABETALOL HYDROCHLORIDE; NORMODYNE	4012444	AUG 2, 1998		NCE	AUG 01, 1994
		4066755	JAN 03, 1995			
18687 004	LABETALOL HYDROCHLORIDE; NORMODYNE	4012444	AUG 2, 1998		NCE	AUG 01, 1994
		4066755	JAN 03, 1995			
18716 001	LABETALOL HYDROCHLORIDE; TRANDATE	4012444	AUG 2, 1998		NCE	AUG 01, 1994
		4066755	JAN 03, 1995			
18716 002	LABETALOL HYDROCHLORIDE; TRANDATE	4012444	AUG 2, 1998		NCE	AUG 01, 1994
		4066755	JAN 03, 1995			
18716 003	LABETALOL HYDROCHLORIDE; TRANDATE	4012444	AUG 2, 1998		NCE	AUG 01, 1994
		4066755	JAN 03, 1995			
18716 004	LABETALOL HYDROCHLORIDE; TRANDATE	4012444	AUG 02, 1998		NCE	AUG 01, 1994
		4066755	JAN 03, 1995			
19425 001	LABETALOL HYDROCHLORIDE; TRANDATE	4012444	AUG 02, 1998		NCE	AUG 01, 1994
		4066755	JAN 03, 1995			
17657 001	LACTULOSE; CEPHULAC	4012444	AUG 02, 1998		NCE	AUG 01, 1994
		3867524	FEB 18, 1992			
		3860708	JAN 14, 1992			
		3860707	JAN 14, 1992			
08107 001	LEUCOVORIN CALCIUM; LEUCOVORIN CALCIUM				ODE	AUG 31, 1995
					I-22	AUG 31, 1995
					ODE	DEC 12, 1998
					I-70	DEC 12, 1994
08107 002	LEUCOVORIN CALCIUM; LEUCOVORIN CALCIUM				ODE	AUG 31, 1995
					I-22	AUG 31, 1995
					ODE	DEC 12, 1998
					I-70	DEC 12, 1994
08107 003	LEUCOVORIN CALCIUM; LEUCOVORIN CALCIUM				ODE	AUG 31, 1995
					I-22	AUG 31, 1995
08107 002	LEUCOVORIN CALCIUM; LEUCOVORIN CALCIUM				ODE	DEC 12, 1998
					I-70	DEC 12, 1994
					ODE	AUG 31, 1995
					I-22	AUG 31, 1995
08107 003	LEUCOVORIN CALCIUM; LEUCOVORIN CALCIUM				ODE	AUG 31, 1995
					I-22	AUG 31, 1995
08107 004	LEUCOVORIN CALCIUM; LEUCOVORIN CALCIUM				ODE	AUG 31, 1995
					I-22	AUG 31, 1995
19010 001	LEUPROLIDE ACETATE; LUPRON	4005063	JAN 25, 1996			
		4917893	MAR 24, 2004			
		4849228	JUL 18, 2006			
		4728721	MAR 01, 2005			
		4677191	JUN 30, 2004			
		4652441	MAR 24, 2004			

PRESCRIPTION AND OTC DRUG PRODUCT
PATENT AND EXCLUSIVITY DATA *(continued)*

APPL/ PROD NUMBER	INGREDIENT NAME; TRADE NAME	PATENT NUMBER	PATENT EXPIRES	USE CODE	EX- CLUS CODE	EXCLUS EXPIRES
19732 001	LEUPROLIDE ACETATE; LUPRON DEPOT	4005063	JAN 25, 1996		NP	JAN 26, 1992
		4917893	MAR 24, 2004			
		4849228	JUL 18, 2006			
		4728721	MAR 01, 2005			
		4677191	JUN 30, 2004			
		4652441	MAR 24, 2004			
20011 001	LEUPROLIDE ACETATE; LUPRON DEPOT	4005063	JAN 25, 1996		NP	OCT 22, 1993
20035 001	LEVAMISOLE HYDROCHLORIDE; ERGAMISOL	4584305	JUN 19, 2004	U-42	NCE	JUN 18, 1995
19814 001	LEVOBUNOLOL HYDROCHLORIDE; BETAGAN				NS	JUN 28, 1992
18948 001	LEVOCARNITINE; CARNITOR				ODE	DEC 27, 1992
19257 001	LEVOCARNITINE; CARNITOR				ODE	DEC 27, 1992
19897 001	LEVONORGESTREL; NORPLANT				NP	DEC 10, 1993
20088 001	LEVONORGESTREL; NORPLANT SYSTEM				NP	DEC 10, 1993
20105 001	LIOTHYRONINE SODIUM; TRIOSTAT				NDF	DEC 31, 1994
					ODE	DEC 31, 1998
19558 001	LISINOPRIL; PRINIVIL	4374829	DEC 30, 2001		NCE	DEC 29, 1992
19558 002	LISINOPRIL; PRINIVIL	4374829	DEC 30, 2001		NCE	DEC 29, 1992
19558 003	LISINOPRIL; PRINIVIL	4374829	DEC 30, 2001		NCE	DEC 29, 1992
19558 004	LISINOPRIL; PRINIVIL	4374829	DEC 30, 2001		NCE	DEC 29, 1992
19777 001	LISINOPRIL; ZESTRIL	4374829	DEC 30, 2001		NCE	DEC 29, 1992
19777 002	LISINOPRIL; ZESTRIL	4374829	DEC 30, 2001		NCE	DEC 29, 1992
19777 003	LISINOPRIL; ZESTRIL	4374829	DEC 30, 2001		NCE	DEC 29, 1992
19777 004	LISINOPRIL; ZESTRIL	4374829	DEC 30, 2001		NCE	DEC 29, 1992
18027 001	LITHIUM CARBONATE; LITHOBID	4264573	APR 28, 1998			
20013 001	LOMEFLOXACIN HYDROCHLORIDE; MAXAQUIN	4528287	JUL 09, 2002	U-36	NCE	FEB 21, 1997
18140 001	LORAZEPAM; ATIVAN	4017616	APR 12, 1994			
18140 001	LORAZEPAM; ATIVAN	4017616	APR 12, 1994			
19643 003	LOVASTATIN; MEVACOR	4231938	NOV 04, 1999		NCE	AUG 31, 1992
19643 004	LOVASTATIN; MEVACOR	4231938	NOV 04, 1999		NCE	AUG 31, 1992
17658 001	LOXAPINE HYDROCHLORIDE; LOXITANE C	4049809	SEP 20, 1994			
18613 001	MALATHION; OVIDE				NCE	AUG 02, 1992
18006 001	MECLOFENAMATE SODIUM; MECLOMEN				I-51	JUL 23, 1993
18006 002	MECLOFENAMATE SODIUM; MECLOMEN				I-51	JUL 23, 1993
12541 002	MEDROXYPROGESTERONE ACETATE; DEPO-PROVERA	4038389	JUL 26, 1994			
12541 003	MEDROXYPROGESTERONE ACETATE; DEPO-PROVERA	4038389	JUL 26, 1994			
19578 001	MEFLOQUINE HYDROCHLORIDE; MEFLOQUINE HCL				NCE	MAY 02, 1994
19591 001	MEFLOQUINE HYDROCHLORIDE; LARIAM				NCE	MAY 02, 1994
					ODE	MAY 02, 1996
17646 001	MENOTROPINS; PERGONAL				I-16	AUG 23, 1992
17646 002	MENOTROPINS; PERGONAL				I-16	AUG 23, 1992
19618 001	MESALAMINE; ROWASA				NCE	DEC 24, 1992
19651 001	MESALAMINE; ASACOL				NCE	DEC 24, 1992
					NDF	JAN 31, 1995
19919 001	MESALAMINE; ROWASA				NCE	DEC 24, 1992
19884 001	MESNA; MESNEX	4220660	DEC 02, 1999	U-21	ODE	DEC 30, 1995
					NCE	DEC 30, 1993
17659 001	METAPROTERENOL SULFATE; ALUPENT				I-67	NOV 14, 1994
11719 001	METHOTREXATE SODIUM; METHOTREXATE				ODE	APR 07, 1995
					I-21	APR 07, 1995
11719 003	METHOTREXATE SODIUM; METHOTREXATE				ODE	APR 07, 1995
					I-21	APR 07, 1995
11719 006	METHOTREXATE SODIUM; METHOTREXATE				ODE	APR 07, 1995
					I-21	APR 07, 1995
11719 007	METHOTREXATE SODIUM; METHOTREXATE LPF				ODE	APR 07, 1995
					I-21	APR 07, 1995
11719 009	METHOTREXATE SODIUM; METHOTREXATE				ODE	APR 07, 1995
					I-21	APR 07, 1995
19600 001	METHOXSALEN; OXSORALEN-ULTRA	4454152	JUN 12, 2001			
18389 001	METHYLDOPA; ALDOMET	4404193	SEP 13, 2000			
18029 001	METHYLPHENIDATE HYDROCHLORIDE; RITALIN-SR	4137300	JAN 30, 1996			
19907 001	METIPRANOLOL HYDROCHLOIDE; OPTIPRANOLOL				NCE	DEC 29, 1994
17862 001	METOCLOPRAMIDE HYDROCHLORIDE; REGLAN	4536386	AUG 20, 2002	U-9		
17862 004	METOCLOPRAMIDE HYDROCHLORIDE; REGLAN	4536386	AUG 20, 2002	U-9		
19532 001	METOLAZONE; MYKROX	4517179	MAY 14, 2002			

PRESCRIPTION AND OTC DRUG PRODUCT
PATENT AND EXCLUSIVITY DATA (continued)

APPL/ PROD NUMBER	INGREDIENT NAME; TRADE NAME	PATENT NUMBER	PATENT EXPIRES	USE CODE	EX- CLUS CODE	EXCLUS EXPIRES
19786 001	METOPROLOL FUMARATE; LOPRESSOR	3998790	DEC 21, 1993			
		3916899	NOV 04, 1992			
		3876802	APR 08, 1992		NP	DEC 27, 1992
19786 002	METOPROLOL FUMARATE; LOPRESSOR	3998790	DEC 21, 1993			
		3916899	NOV 04, 1992			
		3876802	APR 08, 1992		NP	DEC 27, 1992
19786 003	METOPROLOL FUMARATE; LOPRESSOR	4892739	JAN 09, 2007			
		3998790	DEC 21, 1993			
		3916899	NOV 04, 1992			
		3876802	APR 08, 1992		NP	DEC 27, 1992
19786 004	METOPROLOL FUMARATE; LOPRESSOR	4892739	JAN 09, 2007			
		3998790	DEC 21, 1993			
		3916899	NOV 04, 1992			
		3876802	APR 08, 1992		NP	DEC 27, 1992
19962 001	METOPROLOL SUCCINATE; TOPROL XL	3998790	APR 08, 1992		NE	JAN 10, 1995
		3876802	APR 08, 1992			
19962 002	METOPROLOL SUCCINATE; TOPROL XL	3998790	APR 08, 1992		NE	JAN 10, 1995
		3876802	APR 08, 1992			
19962 003	METOPROLOL SUCCINATE; TOPROL XL	3998790	APR 08, 1992		NE	JAN 10, 1995
		3876802	APR 08, 1992			
17963 001	METOPROLOL TARTRATE; LOPRESSOR	3998790	DEC 21, 1993			
		3876802	APR 08, 1992			
17963 002	METOPROLOL TARTRATE; LOPRESSOR	3998790	DEC 21, 1993			
		3876802	APR 08, 1992			
18704 001	METOPROLOL TARTRATE; LOPRESSOR	3998790	DEC 21, 1993			
		3876802	APR 08, 1992			
19737 001	METRONIDAZOLE; METROGEL				ODE	NOV 22, 1991
20208 001	METRONIDAZOLE; METROGEL				NDF	AUG 17, 1995
18873 002	MEXILETINE HYDROCHLORIDE; MEXITIL	4031244	JUN 21, 1994			
		3954872	MAY 04, 1995			
18873 003	MEXILETINE HYDROCHLORIDE; MEXITIL	4031244	JUN 21, 1994			
		3954872	MAY 04, 1995			
18873 004	MEXILETINE HYDROCHLORIDE; MEXITIL	4031244	JUN 21, 1994			
		3954872	MAY 04, 1995			
18592 001	MICONAZOLE NITRATE; MONISTAT 5				NDF	OCT 27, 1992
18654 001	MIDAZOLAM HYDROCHLORIDE; VERSED	4280957	DEC 20, 1999			
18654 002	MIDAZOLAM HYDROCHLORIDE; VERSED	4280957	DEC 20, 1999			
19436 001	MILRINONE LACTATE; MILRINONE LACTATE	4313951	FEB 02, 2001		NCE	DEC 31, 1992
19501 001	MINOXIDIL; ROGAINE	4596812	FEB 13, 1996	I-61		AUG 13, 1994
		4139619	FEB 13, 1996			
19268 001	MISOPROSTOL; CYTOTEC	4301146	NOV 17, 1998			
		4060691	JUN 22, 1993			
		3965143	JUN 22, 1995		NCE	DEC 27, 1993
19297 001	MITOXANTRONE HYDROCHLORIDE; NOVANTRONE	4278689	JUL 14, 2000			
		4197249	APR 08, 1997		NCE	DEC 23, 1992
		4138415	FEB 06, 1996		ODE	DEC 23, 1994
20098 001	MIVACURIUM CHLORIDE; MIVACRON	4761418	AUG 02, 2005		NCE	JAN 22, 1997
20098 002	MIVACURIUM CHLORIDE; MIVACRON IN DEX- TROSE 5%	4761418	AUG 02, 2005		NCE	JAN 22, 1997
19543 001	MOMETASONE FUROATE; ELOCON	4472393	SEP 18, 2001		NCE	APR 30, 1992
19625 001	MOMETASONE FUROATE; ELOCON	4808610	FEB 28, 2006			
		4472393	SEP 18, 2001		NCE	APR 30, 1992
19796 001	MOMETASONE FUROATE; ELOCON	4775529	OCT 04, 2005		NCE	APR 30, 1992
		4472393	SEP 18, 2001		NDF	MAR 30, 1992
19368 001	MONOCTANOIN; MOCTANIN	4205086	MAY 27, 1997		ODE	OCT 29, 1992
19753 001	MORICIZINE HYDROCHLORIDE; ETHMOZINE	3864487	FEB 04, 1994		NCE	JUN 19, 1995
19753 002	MORICIZINE HYDROCHLORIDE; ETHMOZINE	3864487	FEB 04, 1994		NCE	JUN 19, 1995
19753 003	MORICIZINE HYDROCHLORIDE; ETHMOZINE	3864487	FEB 04, 1994		NCE	JUN 19, 1995
18565 003	MORPHINE SULFATE; INFUMORPH				ODE	JUL 19, 1998
18565 004	MORPHINE SULFATE; INFUMORPH				ODE	JUL 19, 1998
18677 001	NABILONE; CESAMET	4087545	MAY 02, 1997	U-4		
		3920809	NOV 18, 1992			
19583 001	NABUMETONE; RELAFEN	4420639	DEC 13, 200		NCE	DEC 24, 1996
		4061779	DEC 06, 1994	U-19		
19583 002	NABUMETONE; RELAFEN	4420639	DEC 13, 2000		NCE	DEC 24, 1996
		4061779	DEC 06, 1994	U-19		
18063 001	NADOLOL; CORGARD	3982021	SEP 21, 1993			
		3935267	JAN 27, 1993			

PRESCRIPTION AND OTC DRUG PRODUCT
PATENT AND EXCLUSIVITY DATA *(continued)*

APPL/ PROD NUMBER	INGREDIENT NAME; TRADE NAME	PATENT NUMBER	PATENT EXPIRES	USE CODE	EX-CLUS CODE	EXCLUS EXPIRES
18063 002	NADOLOL; CORGARD	3982021	SEP 21, 1993			
		3935267	JAN 27, 1993			
18063 003	NADOLOL; CORGARD	3982021	SEP 21, 1993			
		3935267	JAN 27, 1993			
18063 004	NADOLOL; CORGARD	3982021	SEP 21, 1993			
		3935267	JAN 27, 1993			
18063 005	NADOLOL; CORGARD	3982021	SEP 21, 1993			
		3935267	JAN 27, 1993			
18064 001	NADOLOL; CORGARD	3982021	SEP 21, 1993			
		3935267	JAN 27, 1993			
18064 002	NADOLOL; CORGARD	3982021	SEP 21, 1993			
		3935267	JAN 27, 1993			
18064 003	NADOLOL; CORGARD	3982021	SEP 21, 1993			
		3935267	JAN 27, 1993			
18064 004	NADOLOL; CORGARD	3982021	SEP 21, 1993			
		3935267	JAN 27, 1993			
19886 001	NAFARELIN ACETATE; SYNAREL	4234571	NOV 18, 1999		NCE	FEB 13, 1995
					I-68	FEB 26, 1995
20109 001	NAFARELIN ACETATE; SYNAREL	4234571	NOV 18, 1997		NCE	FEB 13, 1995
					I-68	FEB 26, 1995
20109 001	NAFARELIN ACETATE; SYNAREL	4234571	NOV 18, 1997		NCE	FEB 13, 1995
					I-68	FEB 26, 1995
19356 001	NAFTIFINE HYDROCHLORIDE; NAFTIN	4282251	AUG 04, 1998		NCE	MAR 01, 1993
					NDF	JUN 18, 1993
19599 001	NAFTIFINE HYDROCHLORIDE; NAFTIN	4282251	AUG 04, 2000		NCE	MAR 01, 1993
					I-30	APR 05, 1992
					D-1	JUL 05, 1993
18733 001	NALOXONE HYDROCHLORIDE; TALWIN NX	4105659	AUG 08, 1995			
17581 001	NAPROXEN; NAPROSYN	4009197	SEP 09, 1992			
17581 002	NAPROXEN; NAPROSYN	4009197	SEP 09, 1992			
		4001301	SEP 09, 1992			
		3998966	DEC 21, 1993			
		3904682	SEP 09, 1992			
17581 003	NAPROXEN; NAPROSYN	4009197	SEP 09, 1992			
		4001301	SEP 09, 1992			
		3998966	DEC 21, 1993			
		3904682	SEP 09, 1992			
17581 004	NAPROXEN; NAPROSYN	4009197	SEP 09, 1992			
		4001301	SEP 09, 1992			
		3998966	DEC 21, 1993			
		3904682	SEP 09, 1992			
18965 001	NAPROXEN; NAPROSYN	4009197	SEP 09, 1992			
		4001301	SEP 09, 1992			
		3998966	DEC 21, 1993			
		3904682	SEP 09, 1992			
18164 001	NAPROXEN SODIUM; ANAPROX	4009197	SEP 09, 1992			
		4001301	SEP 09, 1992			
		3998966	DEC 21, 1993			
18164 003	NAPROXEN SODIUM; ANAPROX DS	4009197	SEP 09, 1992			
		4001301	SEP 09, 1992			
		3998966	DEC 21, 1993			
19488 001	NICARDIPINE HYDROCHLORIDE; CARDENE	3985758	OCT 12, 1995		NCE	DEC 21, 1993
19488 002	NICARDIPINE HYDROCHLORIDE; CARDENE	3985758	OCT 12, 1995		NCE	DEC 21, 1993
19734 001	NICARDIPINE HYDROCHLORIDE; CARDENE				NDF	JAN 30, 1995
					NCE	DEC 21, 1993
20005 001	NICARDIPINE HYDROCHLORIDE; CARDENE SR	3985758	OCT 12, 1995		NDF	FEB 21, 1995
					NCE	DEC 21, 1993
20005 002	NICARDIPINE HYDROCHLORIDE; CARDENE SR	3985758	OCT 12, 1995		NDF	FEB 21, 1995
					NCE	DEC 21, 1993
20005 003	NICARDIPINE HYDROCHLORIDE; CARDENE SR	3985758	OCT 12, 1995		NDF	FEB 21, 1995
					NCE	DEC 21, 1993
18669 001	NICLOSAMIDE; NICLOCIDE				NCE	MAY 14, 1992
19983 001	NICOTINE; PROSTEP	4946853	AUG 07, 2007	U-56	NS	JAN 28, 1995
19983 002	NICTOINE; PROSTEP	4946853	AUG 07, 2007	U-56	NS	JAN 28, 1995
20076 001	NICOTINE; HABITROL	5016652	MAY 21, 2008			
		4597961	JUL 01, 2003	U-56	NDF	NOV 07, 1994
20076 002	NICOTINE; HABITROL	5016652	MAY 21, 2008			
		4597961	JUL 01, 2003	U-56	NDF	NOV 07, 1994

PRESCRIPTION AND OTC DRUG PRODUCT
PATENT AND EXCLUSIVITY DATA (*continued*)

APPL/ PROD NUMBER	INGREDIENT NAME; TRADE NAME	PATENT NUMBER	PATENT EXPIRES	USE CODE	EX-CLUS CODE	EXCLUS EXPIRES
20076 003	NICOTINE; HABITROL	5016652	MAY 21, 2008			
		4597961	JUL 01, 2003	U-56	NDF	NOV 07, 1994
20150 001	NICOTINE; NICOTROL				NP	APR 22, 1995
20150 002	NICOTINE; NICOTROL				NP	APR 22, 1995
20150 003	NICOTINE; NICOTROL				NP	APR 22, 1995
20165 001	NICOTINE; NICODERM	5004610	APR 02, 2008			
		4144317	SEP 09, 1992		NDF	NOV 07, 1994
20165 002	NICOTINE; NICODERM	5004610	APR 02, 2008			
		4144317	SEP 09, 1992		NDF	NOV 07, 1994
20165 003	NICOTINE; NICODERM	5004610	APR 02, 2008			
		4144317	SEP 09, 1992		NDF	NOV 07, 1994
18612 001	NICOTINE POLACRILEX; NICORETTE	3901248	AUG 26, 1992		NCE	JAN 13, 1994
19684 001	NIFEDIPINE; PROCARDIA XL	4783337	SEP 16, 2003	I-55		SEP 06, 1992
		4765989	SEP 16, 2003		D-2	SEP 06, 1992
		4612008	SEP 16, 2003		NDF	SEP 06, 1992
		4327725	MAY 04, 1997			
19684 002	NIFEDIPINE; PROCARDIA XL	4783337	SEP 16, 2003	I-55		SEP 06, 1992
		4765989	SEP 16, 2003		D-2	SEP 06, 1992
		4612008	SEP 16, 2003		NDF	SEP 06, 1992
		4327725	MAY 04, 1997			
19684 003	NIFEDIPINE; PROCARDIA XL	4783337	SEP 16, 2003	I-55		SEP 06, 1992
		4765989	SEP 16, 2003		D-2	SEP 06, 1992
		4612008	SEP 16, 2003		NDF	SEP 06, 1992
		4327725	MAY 04, 1997			
18869 001	NIMODIPINE; NIMOTOP	4406906	SEP 27, 2002	U-22	NCE	DEC 28, 1993
					NCE	DEC 28, 1993
20064 001	NITROFURANTOIN; MACROBID	4798725	JAN 17, 2006			
		4772473	SEP 20, 2005		NDF	DEC 24, 1994
19508 001	NIZATIDINE; AXID	4760075	MAY 03, 2000	U-18		
		4382090	MAY 03, 2000	U-18	I-59	JUL 26, 1994
		4375547	MAR 01, 2002		NCE	APR 12, 1993
19508 002	NIZATIDINE; AXID	4760075	MAY 03, 2000	U-18		
		4382090	MAY 03, 2000	U-18	I-59	JUL 26, 1994
		4375547	MAR 01, 2002		NCE	APR 12, 1993
18683 001	NONOXYNOL-9; TODAY	4393871	JUL 19, 2000			
19384 002	NORFLOXACIN; NOROXIN	4639458	JAN 27, 2004		I-66	NOV 26, 1994
		4146719	MAR 27, 1998		D-17	NOV 26, 1994
19757 001	NORFLOXACIN; CHIBROXIN	4551456	NOV 05, 2002	U-57		
		4146719	MAR 27, 1998		NDF	JUN 17, 1994
14684 001	NORTRIPTYLINE HYDROCHLORIDE; AVENTYL HCL	3922305	NOV 25, 1992			
14684 002	NORTRIPTYLINE HYDROCHLORIDE; AVENTYL HCL	3922305	NOV 25, 1992			
14685 001	NORTRIPTYLINE HYDROCHLORIDE; AVENTYL HCL	3922305	NOV 25, 1992			
18012 001	NORTRIPTYLINE HYDROCHLORIDE; PAMELOR	3922305	NOV 25, 1992			
18013 001	NORTRIPTYLINE HYDROCHLORIDE; PAMELOR	3922305	NOV 25, 1992			
18013 002	NORTRIPTYLINE HYDROCHLORIDE; PAMELOR	3922305	NOV 25, 1992			
18013 003	NORTRIPTYLINE HYDROCHLORIDE; PAMELOR	3922305	NOV 25, 1992			
18013 004	NORTRIPTYLINE HYDROCHLORIDE; PAMELOR	3922305	NOV 25, 1992			
19667 001	OCTREOTIDE ACETATE; SANDOSTATIN	4395403	JUL 26, 2002		NCE	OCT 21, 1993
19667 002	OCTREOTIDE ACETATE; SANDOSTATIN	4395403	JUL 26, 2002		NCE	OCT 21, 1993
19667 003	OCTREOTIDE ACETATE; SANDOSTATIN	4395403	JUL 26, 2002		NCE	OCT 21, 1993
19735 001	OFLOXACIN; FLOXIN	4382892	MAY 10, 2000		NCE	DEC 28, 1995
19735 002	OFLOXACIN; FLOXIN	4382892	MAY 10, 2000		NCE	DEC 28, 1995
19735 003	OFLOXACIN, FLOXIN	4382892	MAY 10, 2000		NCE	DEC 28, 1995
20087 001	OFLOXACIN; FLOXIN IN DEXTROSE 5%	4382892	MAY 10, 2000		NCE	DEC 28, 1995
20087 002	OFLOXACIN; FLOXIN	4382892	MAY 10, 2000		NCE	DEC 28, 1995
20087 003	OFLOXACIN; FLOXIN	4382892	MAY 10, 2000		NCE	DEC 28, 1995
20087 004	OFLOXACIN; FLOXIN IN DEXTROSE 5%	4382892	MAY 10, 2000		NCE	DEC 28, 1995
20087 005	OFLOXACIN; FLOXIN IN DEXTROSE 5%	4382892	MAY 10, 2000		NCE	DEC 28, 1995
19715 001	OLSALAZINE SODIUM; DIPENTUM	4559330	AUG 04, 2004	U-58	NCE	JUL 31, 1995
19810 001	OMEPRAZOLE; PRILOSEC	4786505	NOV 22, 2005	U-37	NCE	SEP 14, 1994
		4255431	MAR 10, 2000		I-57	JUN 12, 1994
20007 001	ONDANSETRON HYDROCHLORIDE; ZOFRAN	4753789	JUN 28, 2005	U-44	NCE	JAN 04, 1996
		4695578	SEP 22, 2004			
18069 001	OXAMNIQUINE; VANSIL	3925391	DEC 09, 1992			
		3903283	SEP 02, 1992			
15539 002	OXAZEPAM; SERAX	4620974	NOV 04, 2003			
15539 004	OXAZEPAM; SERAX	4620974	NOV 04, 2003			
15539 006	OXAZEPAM; SERAX	4620974	NOV 04, 2003			
19828 001	OXICONAZOLE NITRATE; OXISTAT				NCE	DEC 30, 1993

PRESCRIPTION AND OTC DRUG PRODUCT
PATENT AND EXCLUSIVITY DATA *(continued)*

APPL/ PROD NUMBER	INGREDIENT NAME; TRADE NAME	PATENT NUMBER	PATENT EXPIRES	USE CODE	EX- CLUS CODE	EXCLUS EXPIRES
18166 001	OXPRENOLOL HYDROCHLORIDE; TRASICOR				NCE	DEC 28, 1993
18166 002	OXPRENOLOL HYDROCHLORIDE; TRASICOR				NCE	DEC 28, 1993
18166 003	OXPRENOLOL HYDROCHLORIDE; TRASICOR				NCE	DEC 28, 1993
18166 004	OXPRENOLOL HYDROCHLORIDE; TRASICOR				NCE	DEC 28, 1993
20036 001	PAMIDRONATE DISODIUM; AREDIA	4711880	DEC 08, 2004		NCE	OCT 03, 1996
		3962432	JUN 08, 1993	U-53		
19818 001	PEGADEMASE BOVINE; ADAGEN	4179337	DEC 18, 1996		ODE	MAR 21, 1997
					NCE	MAR 21, 1995
18976 001	PENBUTOLOL SULFATE; LEVATOL				NCE	DEC 30, 1992
17048 001	PENTAGASTRIN; PEPTAVLON	3896103	JUL 22, 1992			
19887 001	PENTAMIDINE ISETHIONATE; NEBUPENT				ODE	JUN 15, 1996
					NDF	JUN 15, 1992
16194 003	PENTAZOCINE LACTATE; TALWIN	4105659	AUG 08, 1995			
20122 001	PENTOSTATIN; NIPENT	3923785	DEC 02, 1992		ODE	OCT 11, 1998
					NCE	OCT 11, 1996
18631 001	PENTOXIFYLLINE; TRENTAL	4189469	FEB 02, 1997			
		3737433	APR 03, 1997		NCE	AUG 30, 1994
19385 001	PERGOLIDE MESYLATE; PERMAX	4797405	JAN 10, 2006			
		4180582	DEC 25, 1996	U-20		
		4166182	AUG 28, 1998		NCE	DEC 30, 1993
19385 002	PERGOLIDE MESYLATE; PERMAX	4797405	JAN 10, 2006			
		4180582	DEC 25, 1996	U-20		
		4166182	AUG 28, 1998		NCE	DEC 30, 1993
19385 003	PERGOLIDE MESYLATE; PERMAX	4797405	JAN 10, 2006			
		4180582	DEC 25, 1996	U-20		
		4166182	AUG 28, 1998		NCE	DEC 30, 1993
19435 001	PERMETHRIN; NIX	4024163	MAY 17, 1996			
19855 001	PERMETHRIN; ELIMITE	4024163	MAY 17, 1996		NDF	AUG 25, 1992
19918 001	PERMETHRIN; NIX	4024163	MAY 17, 1996		I-60	MAY 02, 1993
18796 001	PILOCARPINE HYDROCHLORIDE; PILOPINE HS	4271143	JUN 02, 1998			
17473 001	PIMOZIDE; ORAP				NCE	JUL 31, 1994
19456 001	PINACIDIL; PINDAC	RE31244	NOV 08, 1996	U-3	NCE	DEC 28, 1994
19456 002	PINACIDIL; PINDAC	RE31244	NOV 08, 1996	U-3	NCE	DEC 28, 1994
18285 001	PINDOLOL; VISKEN				NCE	SEP 03, 1992
18285 002	PINDOLOL; VISKEN				NCE	SEP 03, 1992
18285 003	PINDOLOL; VISKEN				NCE	SEP 03, 1992
19638 001	PIPECURONIUM BROMIDE; ARDUAN				NCE	JUN 26, 1995
19009 001	PIRBUTEROL ACETATE; MAXAIR	4175128	NOV 20, 1996			
		3786160	JAN 15, 1993			
18147 002	PIROXICAM; FELDENE	3862319	JAN 21, 1992		NCE	APR 06, 1992
18147 003	PIROXICAM; FELDENE	3862319	JAN 21, 1992		NCE	APR 06, 1992
19797 001	POLYETHYLENE GLYCOL 3350; NULYTELY				NP	APR 22, 1994
17986 001	POLYTHIAZIDE; MINIZIDE	4130647	DEC 19, 1995			
17986 002	POLYTHIAZIDE; MINIZIDE	4130647	DEC 19, 1995			
17986 003	POLYTHIAZIDE; MINIZIDE	4130647	DEC 19, 1995			
17850 001	POTASSIUM CHLORIDE; KLOTRIX	4140756	FEB 20, 1996			
18238 001	POTASSIUM CHLORIDE; MICRO-K	4259315	MAR 31, 1998			
18238 002	POTASSIUM CHLORIDE; MICRO-K 10	4259315	MAR 31, 1998			
19561 003	POTASSIUM CHLORIDE; MICRO-K LS	4259315	MAR 31, 1998			
19071 001	POTASSIUM CITRATE; POTASSIUM CITRATE				ODE	AUG 30, 1992
19647 001	POTASSIUM CITRATE; POTASSIUM CITRATE				ODE	AUG 30, 1992
19647 002	POTASSIUM CITRATE; POTASSIUM CITRATE				ODE	AUG 30, 1992
19898 002	PRAVASTATIN SODIUM; PRAVACHOL	4346227	AUG 24, 1999		NCE	OCT 31, 1996
19898 003	PRAVASTATIN SODIUM; PRAVACHOL	4346227	AUG 24, 1999		NCE	OCT 31, 1996
18714 001	PRAZIQUANTEL; BILTRICIDE	4001411	JAN 04, 1994		NCE	DEC 29, 1992
17442 001	PRAZOSIN HYDROCHLORIDE; MINIPRESS	4130647	DEC 19, 1995			
		4092315	MAY 30, 1995			
17442 002	PRAZOSIN HYDROCHLORIDE; MINIPRESS	4130647	DEC 19, 1995			
		4092315	MAY 30, 1995			
17442 003	PRAZOSIN HYDROCHLORIDE; MINIPRESS	4130647	DEC 19, 1995			
		4092315	MAY 30, 1995			
19775 001	PRAZOSIN HYDROCHLORIDE; MINIPRESS XL	5082668	SEP 16, 2003			
		4783337	SEP 16, 2003			
		4765989	SEP 16, 2003			
		4612008	SEP 16, 2003			
		4327725	MAY 04, 1999			
		4092315	MAY 30, 1995		NDF	JAN 29, 1995

PRESCRIPTION AND OTC DRUG PRODUCT
PATENT AND EXCLUSIVITY DATA (continued)

APPL/ PROD NUMBER	INGREDIENT NAME; TRADE NAME	PATENT NUMBER	PATENT EXPIRES	USE CODE	EX- CLUS CODE	EXCLUS EXPIRES
19775 002	PRAZOSIN HYDROCHLORIDE; MINIPRESS XL	5082668	SEP 16, 2003			
		4783337	SEP 16, 2003			
		4765989	SEP 16, 2003			
		4612008	SEP 16, 2003			
		4327725	MAY 04, 1999			
		4092315	MAY 30, 1995		NDF	JAN 29, 1995
19568 001	PREDNICARBATE; DERMATOP	4242334	DEC 30, 1997	U-50	NE	SEP 23, 1994
19157 001	PREDNISOLONE SODIUM PHOSPHATE; PEDIAPRED	4448774	MAY 15, 2001			
17535 001	PROBUCOL; LORELCO	3862332	JAN 21, 1992			
17535 002	PROBUCOL; LORELCO	3862332	JAN 21, 1992			
87361 001	PROCAINAMIDE HYDROCHLORIDE; PRONESTYL-SR	4252786	FEB 24, 1998			
19151 001	PROPAFENONE HYDROCHLORIDE; RYTHMOL				NCE	NOV 27, 1994
19151 002	PROPAFENONE HYDROCHLORIDE; RYTHMOL				NCE	NOV 27, 1994
19627 001	PROPOFOL; DIPRIVAN	4798846	NOV 01, 1996	I-73		DEC 31, 1994
		4056635	NOV 01, 1996		NCE	OCT 02, 1994
18553 001	PROPRANOLOL HYDROCHLORIDE; INDERAL LA	4138475	FEB 06, 1996			
18553 002	PROPRANOLOL HYDROCHLORIDE; INDERAL LA	4138475	FEB 06, 1996			
18553 003	PROPRANOLOL HYDROCHLORIDE; INDERAL LA	4138475	FEB 06, 1996			
18553 004	PROPRANOLOL HYDROCHLORIDE; INDERAL LA	4138475	FEB 06, 1996			
19536 001	PROPRANOLOL HYDROCHLORIDE; INDERAL	4600708	JUL 15, 2003			
19664 001	PSEUDOEPHEDRINE HYDROCHLORIDE; SELDANE-D	3878217	APR 15, 1994		NC	AUG 19, 1994
18708 001	QUAZEPAM; DORAL	3920818	NOV 18, 1994			
18708 003	QUAZEPAM; DORAL	3920818	NOV 18, 1994			
19885 001	QUINAPRIL HYDROCHLORIDE; ACCUPRIL	4743450	MAY 10, 2005			
		4344949	AUG 17, 1999	U-3	NCE	NOV 19, 1996
19885 002	QUINAPRIL HYDROCHLORIDE; ACCUPRIL	4743450	MAY 10, 2005			
		4344949	AUG 17, 1999	U-3	NCE	NOV 19, 1996
19885 003	QUINAPRIL HYDROCHLORIDE; ACCUPRIL	4743450	MAY 10, 2005			
		4344949	AUG 17, 1999	U-3	NCE	NOV 19, 1996
19885 004	QUINAPRIL HYDROCHLORIDE; ACCUPRIL	4743450	MAY 10, 2005			
		4344949	AUG 17, 1999	U-3	NCE	NOV 19, 1996
19901 001	RAMIPRIL; ALTACE	4587258	JAN 29, 2005		NCE	JAN 28, 1996
19901 002	RAMIPRIL; ALTACE	4587258	JAN 29, 2005		NCE	JAN 28, 1996
19901 003	RAMIPRIL; ALTACE	4587258	JAN 29, 2005		NCE	JAN 28, 1996
19901 004	RAMIPRIL; ALTACE	4587258	JAN 29, 2005		NCE	JAN 28, 1996
18703 001	RANITIDINE HYDROCHLORIDE; ZANTAC 150	4521431	JUN 04, 2002	I-75		MAY 19, 1995
		4128658	DEC 05, 1995		NCE	JUN 09, 1993
18703 002	RANITIDINE HYDROCHLORIDE; ZANTAC 300	4521431	JUN 04, 2002	I-75		MAY 19, 1995
		4128658	DEC 05, 1995		NCE	JUN 09, 1993
19090 001	RANITIDINE HYDROCHLORIDE; ZANTAC	4585790	APR 29, 2003			
		4521431	JUN 04, 2002			
		4128658	DEC 05, 1995		NCE	JUN 09, 1993
19593 001	RANITIDINE HYDROCHLORIDE; ZANTAC	4585790	APR 29, 2003			
		4521431	JUN 04, 2002			
		4128658	DEC 05, 1995		NCE	JUN 09, 1993
19675 001	RANITIDINE HYDROCHLORIDE; ZANTAC	4585790	APR 29, 2003		NCE	JUN 09, 1993
		4521431	JUN 04, 2002			
		4128658	DEC 05, 1995	I-75		MAY 19, 1995
18859 001	RIBAVIRIN; VIRAZOLE	4211771	JUL 08, 1999			
50627 001	RIFAMPIN; RIFADIN				ODE	MAY 25, 1996
19414 001	RUBIDIUM CHLORIDE RB-82; CARDIOGEN-82	4400358	AUG 23, 2002		NCE	DEC 29, 1994
18009 001	SARALASIN ACETATE; SARENIN	3932624	JAN 13, 1993			
		3886134	MAY 27, 1992			
17874 001	SCOPOLAMINE; TRANSDERM-SCOP	4436741	APR 14, 1998			
		4262003	APR 14, 1998			
		4031894	JUN 28, 1994			
19334 001	SELEGILINE HYDROCHLORIDE; ELDEPRYL				NCE	JUN 05, 1994
					ODE	JUN 05, 1996
19863 001	SERMORELIN ACETATE; GEREF	4703035	MAY 14, 2002	U-47	NCE	DEC 28, 1995
		4517181	MAY 14, 2002		NCE	DEC 28, 1995
19839 001	SERTRALINE HYDROCHLORIDE; ZOLOFT	4536518	AUG 20, 2002		NCE	DEC 30, 1996
19839 002	SERTRALINE HYDROCHLORIDE; ZOLOFT	4536518	AUG 20, 2002		NCE	DEC 30, 1996
19839 003	SERTRALINE HYDROCHLORIDE; ZOLOFT	4536518	AUG 20, 2002		NCE	DEC 30, 1996
19839 004	SERTRALINE HYDROCHLORIDE; ZOLOFT	4536518	AUG 20, 2002		NCE	DEC 30, 1996
19608 001	SILVER SULFADIAZINE; SILDIMAC	4563184	JAN 07, 2003		NP	NOV 30, 1992
19766 001	SIMVASTATIN; ZOCOR	4444784	APR 24, 2001	U-59	NCE	DEC 23, 1997
19766 002	SIMVASTATIN; ZOCOR	4444784	APR 24, 2001	U-59	NCE	DEC 23, 1997
19766 003	SIMVASTATIN; ZOCOR	4444784	APR 24, 2001	U-59	NCE	DEC 23, 1997
19766 004	SIMVASTATIN; ZOCOR	4444784	APR 24, 2001	U-59	NCE	DEC 23, 1997

PRESCRIPTION AND OTC DRUG PRODUCT
PATENT AND EXCLUSIVITY DATA *(continued)*

APPL/ PROD NUMBER	INGREDIENT NAME; TRADE NAME	PATENT NUMBER	PATENT EXPIRES	USE CODE	EX- CLUS CODE	EXCLUS EXPIRES
19530 001	SODIUM BENZOATE; UCEPHAN	4284647	AUG 18, 2000	U-14	NCE	DEC 23, 1992
					ODE	DEC 23, 1994
10929 001	SODIUM IODIDE, I-131; IODOTOPE	4349529	SEP 14, 1999			
10929 002	SODIUM IODIDE, I-131; IODOTOPE	4349529	SEP 14, 1999			
10929 003	SODIUM IODIDE, I-131; IODOTOPE	4349529	SEP 14, 1999			
20166 001	SODIUM THIOSULFATE; SODIUM THIOSULFATE				NCE	FEB 14, 1997
19107 001	SOMATREM; PROTROPIN	4658021	APR 14, 2004			
					ODE	OCT 17, 1992
19640 001	SOMATROPIN, BIOSYNTHETIC; HUMATROPE				ODE	MAR 08, 1994
					NR	MAY 10, 1992
19640 004	SOMATROPIN, BIOSYNTHETIC; HUMATROPE				ODE	MAR 08, 1994
					NR	MAY 10, 1992
17961 001	STREPTOZOCIN; ZANOSAR				NCE	MAY 07, 1992
19998 002	SUCCIMER; CHEMET				NCE	JAN 30, 1996
					ODE	JAN 30, 1998
18333 001	SUCRALFATE; CARAFATE				I-44	MAY 11, 1993
19050 001	SUFENTANIL CITRATE; SUFENTA	3998834	DEC 21, 1993		NCE	MAY 04, 1994
18737 001	SULCONAZOLE NITRATE; EXELDERM	4055652	OCT 25, 1996		NDF	FEB 28, 1992
18738 001	SULCONAZOLE NITRATE; EXELDERM	4055652	OCT 25, 1996			
17376 001	SULFAMETHOXAZOLE; SEPTRA	4209513	JUN 24, 1997		I-49	JUN 15, 1993
17376 002	SULFAMETHOXAZOLE; SEPTRA DS	4209513	JUN 24, 1997		I-49	JUN 15, 1993
17377 001	SULFAMETHOXAZOLE; BACTRIM				I-49	JUN 15, 1993
17377 002	SULFAMETHOXAZOLE; BACTRIM DS				I-49	JUN 15, 1993
17560 001	SULFAMETHOXAZOLE; BACTRIM				I-49	JUN 15, 1993
17560 002	SULFAMETHOXAZOLE; BACTRIM PEDIATRIC				I-49	JUN 15, 1993
17598 001	SULFAMETHOXAZOLE; SEPTRA				I-49	JUN 15, 1993
17598 002	SULFAMETHOXAZOLE; SEPTRA GRAPE				I-49	JUN 15, 1993
18217 001	SUPROFEN; SUPROL	4035376	JUL 12, 1996			
19387 001	SUPROFEN; PROFENAL	4559343	DEC 17, 2002			
		4035376	JUL 12, 1996			
17970 001	TAMOXIFEN CITRATE; NOLVADEX	4536516	AUG 20, 2002		I-50	JUN 21, 1993
					I-29	MAR 16, 1992
17881 001	TECHNETIUM TC-99M ALBUMIN AGGREGATED KIT; TECHNETIUM TC 99M A	3872226	MAR 18, 1992			
		3863004	JAN 28, 1992	U-16		
19829 001	TECHNETIUM TC-99M EXAMETAZIME KIT; CERETEC	4789736	DEC 06, 2005		NCE	DEC 30, 1993
18489 001	TECHNETIUM TC-99M LIDOFENIN KIT; TECHNESCAN HIDA	RE31463	APR 12, 1994			
18963 001	TECHNETIUM TC-99M MEBROFENIN KIT; CHOLETEC	4418208	JAN 21, 2001		NCE	JAN 21, 1992
18107 001	TECHNETIUM TC-99M MEDRONATE KIT; MDP-SQUIBB	4115541	SEP 19, 1995			
19882 001	TECHNETIUM TC-99M MERTIATIDE KIT; TECHNESCAN MAG3				NCE	JUN 15, 1995
18321 001	TECHNETIUM TC-99M OXIDRONATE KIT; OSTEOSCAN-HDP	4497744	FEB 05, 2002			
		4432963	FEB 21, 2001			
		4247534	JAN 27, 1998			
		4233284	NOV 11, 1997			
19981 001	TECHNETIUM TC-99M RED BLOOD CELL KIT; UL-TRATAG	4755375	JUL 05, 2005	U-51	NP	JUN 10, 1994
20063 001	TECHNETIUM TC-99M RED BLOOD CELL KIT; RBC-SCAN				NP	JUN 11, 1995
19785 001	TECHNETIUM TC-99M SESTAMIBI KIT; CARDIOLITE	4452774	SEP 09, 2004		NCE	DEC 21, 1995
19785 002	TECHNETIUM TC-99M SESTAMIBI KIT; CARDIOLITE	4452774	SEP 09, 2004		NCE	DEC 21, 1995
17339 001	TECHNETIUM TC-99M SODIUM PERTECHNETATE GENERATOR; MINITEC	4041317	AUG 09, 1994			
		3920995	NOV 18, 1992			
17944 001	TECHNETIUM TC-99M SUCCIMER KIT; MPI DMSA KIDNEY REAGENT	4233285	NOV 11, 1997			
		4208398	JUN 17, 1997			
19928 001	TECHNETIUM TC-99M TEBOROXIME KIT; CARDI-OTEC	4705849	NOV 10, 2004		NCE	DEC 19, 1995
20043 003	TEMAFLOXACIN HYDROCHLORIDE; OMNIFLOX	4730000	MAR 08, 2005	U-36	NCE	JAN 30, 1997
20043 004	TEMAFLOXACIN HYDROCHLORIDE; OMNIFLOX	4730000	MAR 08, 2005	U-36	NCE	JAN 30, 1997
18163 003	TEMAZEPAM; RESTORIL				NS	OCT 25, 1994
20119 001	TENIPOSIDE; VUMON				NCE	JUL 14, 1997
					ODE	JUL 14, 1999

PRESCRIPTION AND OTC DRUG PRODUCT
PATENT AND EXCLUSIVITY DATA *(continued)*

APPL/ PROD NUMBER	INGREDIENT NAME; TRADE NAME	PATENT NUMBER	PATENT EXPIRES	USE CODE	EX- CLUS CODE	EXCLUS EXPIRES
19057 001	TERAZOSIN HYDROCHLORIDE; HYTRIN	4251532	FEB 17, 2000	U-3	NCE	AUG 07, 1992
		4112097	SEP 05, 1995	U-3		
		4026894	MAY 31, 1994			
19057 002	TERAZOSIN HYDROCHLORIDE; HYTRIN	4251532	FEB 17, 2000	U-3	NCE	AUG 07, 1992
		4112097	SEP 05, 1995	U-3		
		4026894	MAY 31, 1994			
19057 003	TERAZOSIN HYDROCHLORIDE; HYTRIN	4251532	FEB 17, 2000	U-3	NCE	AUG 07, 1992
		4112097	SEP 05, 1995	U-3		
		4026894	MAY 31, 1994			
19057 004	TERAZOSIN HYDROCHLORIDE; HYTRIN	4251532	FEB 17, 2000	U-3	NCE	AUG 07, 1992
		4112097	SEP 05, 1995	U-3		
		4026894	MAY 31, 1994			
17466 001	TERBUTALINE SULFATE; BRICANYL	4011258	MAR 08, 1994			
		3937838	FEB 10, 1993			
17618 001	TERBUTALINE SULFATE; BRICANYL	4011258	MAR 08, 1994			
		3937838	FEB 10, 1993			
17618 002	TERBUTALINE SULFATE; BRICANYL	4011258	MAR 08, 1994			
		3937838	FEB 10, 1993			
17849 001	TERBUTALINE SULFATE; BRETHINE	4011258	MAR 08, 1994			
		3937838	FEB 10, 1993			
17849 002	TERBUTALINE SULFATE; BRETHINE	4011258	MAR 08, 1994			
		3937838	FEB 10, 1993			
18000 001	TERBUTALINE SULFATE; BRICANYL	4011258	MAR 08, 1994			
		3937838	FEB 10, 1993			
18571 001	TERBUTALINE SULFATE; BRETHINE	4011258	MAR 08, 1994			
		3937838	FEB 10, 1993			
18762 001	TERBUTALINE SULFATE; BRETHAIRE	4011258	MAR 08, 1994			
		3937838	FEB 10, 1993			
19579 001	TERCONAZOLE; TERAZOL 7	4358449	NOV 09, 2001		NCE	DEC 31, 1992
19641 001	TERCONAZOLE; TERAZOL 3	4358449	NOV 09, 2001		NCE	DEC 31, 1992
					NDF	MAY 24, 1991
18949 001	TERFENADINE; SELDANE	3878217	APR 15, 1994			
19498 001	TERIPARATIDE ACETATE; PARATHAR				NCE	DEC 23, 1992
					ODE	DEC 23, 1994
87563 001	THEOPHYLLINE; QUIBRON-T/SR	4465660	AUG 14, 2001			
19979 001	TICLOPIDINE HYDROCHLORIDE; TICLID	4591592	MAY 27, 2003			
		4051141	SEP 27, 1994		NCE	OCT 31, 1996
19979 002	TICLOPIDINE HYDROCHLORIDE; TICLID	4591592	MAY 27, 2003			
		4051141	SEP 27, 1994		NCE	OCT 31, 1996
18017 001	TIMOLOL MALEATE; BLOCADREN				I-41	MAR 03, 1993
18017 002	TIMOLOL MALEATE; BLOCADREN				I-41	MAR 03, 1993
18017 004	TIMOLOL MALEATE; BLOCADREN				I-41	MAR 03, 1993
18086 001	TIMOLOL MALEATE; TIMOPTIC	4195085	MAR 25, 1997			
18086 002	TIMOLOL MALEATE; TIMOPTIC	4195085	MAR 25, 1997			
19463 001	TIMOLOL MALEATE; TIMOPTIC IN OCUDOSE	4195085	MAR 25, 1997			
19463 002	TIMOLOL MALEATE; TIMOPTIC IN OCUDOSE	4195085	MAR 25, 1997			
18682 001	TIOCONAZOLE; TZ-3	4062966	DEC 13, 1994		NCE	FEB 18, 1993
19355 001	TIOCONAZOLE; VAGISTAT	4062966	DEC 13, 1994		NCE	FEB 18, 1993
19569 001	TIOPRONIN; TIOPRONIN				NCE	AUG 11, 1993
					ODE	AUG 11, 1995
18257 001	TOCAINIDE HYDROCHLORIDE; TONOCARD	4237068	NOV 09, 1998			
		4218477	AUG 19, 1997			
18257 002	TOCAINIDE HYDROCHLORIDE; TONOCARD	4237068	NOV 09, 1998			
		4218477	AUG 19, 1997			
19280 001	TRANEXAMIC ACID; CYKLOKAPRON	3950405	APR 13, 1993		ODE	DEC 30, 1993
19281 001	TRANEXAMIC ACID; CYKLOKAPRON	3950405	APR 13, 1993		ODE	DEC 30, 1993
18207 003	TRAZODONE HYDROCHLORIDE; DESYREL	4258027	MAR 24, 1998			
		4215104	JUL 29, 1997			
17340 001	TRETINOIN; RETIN-A	3906108	SEP 16, 1992			
17522 001	TRETINOIN; RETIN-A	3906108	SEP 16, 1992			
17579 002	TRETINOIN; RETIN-A	4247547	JAN 27, 1998			
17955 001	TRETINOIN; RETIN-A	4247547	JAN 27, 1998			
19049 001	TRETINOIN; RETIN-A	3906108	SEP 16, 1992			
18117 001	TRIAMCINOLONE ACETONIDE; AZMACORT	3927806	DEC 23, 1992			
		3897779	AUG 05, 1992			
19798 001	TRIAMCINOLONE ACETONIDE; NASACORT				NR	JUL 11, 1994
86240 001	TRIAMCINOLONE ACETONIDE; KENALOG-H	4048310	SEP 13, 1994			

PRESCRIPTION AND OTC DRUG PRODUCT
PATENT AND EXCLUSIVITY DATA *(continued)*

APPL/ PROD NUMBER	INGREDIENT NAME; TRADE NAME	PATENT NUMBER	PATENT EXPIRES	USE CODE	EX- CLUS CODE	EXCLUS EXPIRES
17892 001	TRIAZOLAM; HALCION	3987052	OCT 19, 1993			
		3980790	SEP 14, 1993		NCE	NOV 15, 1992
17892 002	TRIAZOLAM; HALCION	3987052	OCT 19, 1993			
		3980790	SEP 14, 1993		NCE	NOV 15, 1992
17892 003	TRIAZOLAM; HALCION	3987052	OCT 19, 1993			
		3980790	SEP 14, 1993		NCE	NOV 15, 1992
19194 001	TRIENTINE HYDROCHLORIDE; SYPRINE				ODE	NOV 11, 1992
19415 002	UROFOLLITROPIN; METRODIN				ODE	SEP 18, 1993
					I-16	MAR 01, 1991
19594 001	URSODIOL; ACTIGALL	RE30910	JAN 07, 1994	U-25		
		RE30910	JAN 07, 1994	U-26		
		RE30910	JAN 07, 1994	U-27	NCE	DEC 31, 1992
19594 002	URSODIOL; ACTIGALL	RE30910	JAN 07, 1994	U-25		
		RE30910	JAN 07, 1994	U-26		
		RE30910	JAN 07, 1994	U-27	NCE	DEC 31, 1992
18776 002	VECURONIUM BROMIDE; NORCURON	4297351	OCT 27, 1998			
		4237126	DEC 02, 1997		NCE	APR 30, 1994
19152 002	VERAPAMIL HYDROCHLORIDE; ISOPTIN SR				NS	DEC 15, 1992
19614 001	VERAPAMIL HYDROCHLORIDE; VERELAN	4863742	SEP 05, 2006	U-3	NDF	MAY 29, 1993
19614 002	VERAPAMIL HYDROCHLORIDE; VERELAN	4863742	SEP 05, 2006	U-3	NDF	MAY 29, 1993
19614 003	VERAPAMIL HYDROCHLORIDE; VERELAN	4863742	SEP 05, 2006	U-3	NDF	MAY 29, 1993
14103 003	VINCRISTINE SULFATE; ONCOVIN	4619935	OCT 28, 2003			
18536 001	XENON, XE-127; XENON XE 127				NCE	OCT 01, 1992
18536 002	XENON, XE-127; XENON XE 127				NCE	OCT 01, 1992
20199 001	ZALCITABINE; HIVID				NCE	JUN 19, 1997
					ODE	JUN 19, 1999
20199 002	ZALCITABINE; HIVID				NCE	JUN 19, 1997
					ODE	JUN 19, 1999
19655 001	ZIDOVUDINE; RETROVIR	4837208	FEB 02, 2005			
		4833130	FEB 02, 2005	I-47		MAY 02, 1993
		4828838	FEB 02, 2005		ODE	MAR 19, 1994
		4724232	FEB 02, 2005		NCE	MAR 19, 1992
19910 001	ZIDOVUDINE; RETROVIR	4837208	FEB 02, 2005			
		4833130	FEB 02, 2005		ODE	MAR 19, 1994
		4818538	FEB 02, 2005	I-47		MAY 02, 1993
		4724232	FEB 02, 2005		NCE	MAR 19, 1992
19951 001	ZIDOVUDINE; RETROVIR	4837208	FEB 02, 2005			
		4833130	FEB 02, 2005		NCE	MAR 19, 1992
		4818538	FEB 02, 2005			
		4724232	FEB 02, 2005		ODE	MAR 19, 1994

DRUG PRODUCTS WITH APPROVAL UNDER SECTION 505 OF THE ACT ADMINISTERED BY THE DIVISION OF BLOOD AND BLOOD PRODUCTS LIST PATENT AND EXCLUSIVITY DATA

II

APPL/ PROD NUMBER	INGREDIENT NAME; TRADE NAME	PATENT NUMBER	PATENT EXPIRES	USE CODE	EX- CLUS CODE	EXCLUS EXPIRES
841207 001	PENTASTARCH 10% IN SODIUM CHLORIDE 0.9%; PENTASPAN				ODE	MAY 19, 1994
860909 001	PERFLUORODECALIN; FLUOSOL	3911138	OCT 07, 1994		NCE	DEC 26, 1994
		4252827	FEB 24, 1998			

Section II

SELECTED USP GENERAL NOTICES AND CHAPTERS

Selected General Notices and Requirements

Applying to Standards, Tests, Assays, and Other Specifications of the United States Pharmacopeia

"OFFICIAL" AND "OFFICIAL ARTICLES"

The word "official," as used in this Pharmacopeia or with reference hereto, is synonymous with "Pharmacopeial," with "USP," and with "compendial."

The designation USP in conjunction with the official title on the label of an article is a reminder that the article purports to comply with USP standards; such specific designation on the label does not constitute a representation, endorsement, or incorporation by the manufacturer's labeling of the informational material contained in the USP monograph, nor does it constitute assurance by USP that the article is known to comply with USP standards. The standards apply equally to articles bearing the official titles or names derived by transposition of the definitive words of official titles or transposition in the order of the names of two or more active ingredients in official titles, whether or not the added designation "USP" is used. Names considered to be synonyms of the official titles may not be used for official titles.

Where an article differs from the standards of strength, quality, and purity, as determined by the application of the assays and tests, set forth for it in the Pharmacopeia, its difference shall be plainly stated on its label. Where an article fails to comply in identity with the identity prescribed in the USP, or contains an added substance that interferes with the prescribed assays and tests, such article shall be designated by a name that is clearly distinguishing and differentiating from any name recognized in the Pharmacopeia.

Articles listed herein are official and the standards set forth in the monographs apply to them only when the articles are intended or labeled for use as drugs or as medical devices and when bought, sold, or dispensed for these purposes or when labeled as conforming to this Pharmacopeia.

An article is deemed to be recognized in this Pharmacopeia when a monograph for the article is published in it, including its supplements, addenda, or other interim revisions, and an official date is generally or specifically assigned to it.

The following terminology is used for distinguishing the articles for which monographs are provided: an *official substance* is an active drug entity or a pharmaceutic ingredient (see also NF XVII) or a component of a finished device for which the monograph title includes no indication of the nature of the finished form; an *official preparation* is a *drug product* or a *finished device*. It is the finished or partially finished (e.g., as in the case of a sterile solid to be constituted into a solution for administration) preparation or product of one or more official substances formulated for use on or for the patient; an *article* is an item for which a monograph is provided, whether an official substance or an official preparation.

TOLERANCES

Tolerances—The limits specified in the monographs for Pharmacopeial articles are established with a view to the use of these articles as drugs, except where the monograph indicates

otherwise. The use of the molecular formula for the active ingredient(s) named in defining the required strength of a Pharmacopeial article is intended to designate the chemical entity or entities, as given in the complete chemical name of the article, having absolute (100 percent) purity.

A dosage form shall be formulated with the intent to provide 100 percent of the quantity of each ingredient declared on the label. Where the content of an ingredient is known to decrease with time, an amount in excess of that declared on the label may be introduced into the dosage form at the time of manufacture to assure compliance with the content requirements of the monograph throughout the expiration period. The tolerances and limits stated in the definitions in the monographs for Pharmacopeial articles allow for such overages, and for analytical error, for unavoidable variations in manufacturing and compounding, and for deterioration to an extent considered insignificant under practical conditions.

The specified tolerances are based upon such attributes of quality as might be expected to characterize an article produced from suitable raw materials under recognized principles of good manufacturing practice.

The existence of compendial limits or tolerances does not constitute a basis for a claim that an official substance that more nearly approaches 100 percent purity "exceeds" the Pharmacopeial quality. Similarly, the fact that an article has been prepared to closer tolerances than those specified in the monograph does not constitute a basis for a claim that the article "exceeds" the Pharmacopeial requirements.

ALCOHOL

All statements of percentages of alcohol, such as under the heading, Alcohol content, refer to percentage, by volume, of C_2H_5OH at 15.56 °C. Where reference is made to "C_2H_5OH," the chemical entity possessing absolute (100 percent) strength is intended.

Alcohol—Where "alcohol" is called for in formulas, tests, and assays, the monograph article *Alcohol* is to be used.

Denatured Alcohol—Specially denatured alcohol formulas are available for use in accordance with federal statutes and regulations of the Internal Revenue Service. A suitable formula of specially denatured alcohol may be substituted for Alcohol in the manufacture of Pharmacopeial preparations intended for internal or topical use, provided that the denaturant is volatile and does not remain in the finished product. A finished product that is intended for topical application to the skin may contain specially denatured alcohol, provided that the denaturant is either a normal ingredient or a permissible added substance; in either case the denaturant must be identified on the label of the topical preparation. Where a process is given in the individual monograph, the preparation so made must be identical with that prepared by the given process.

UNITS OF POTENCY

For those products for which it is necessary to express the potency in terms of units by reference to a suitable working standard (usually a USP Reference Standard), the individual monographs refer to USP Units of activity. Unless otherwise indicated, USP Units are equivalent to the corresponding international units, where such exist or formerly existed, or to the

II

units of activity established by the Food and Drug Administration in the case of antibiotics and biological products.

INGREDIENTS AND PROCESSES

Official preparations are prepared from ingredients that meet the requirements of the compendial monographs for those individual ingredients for which monographs are provided (see also NF XVII). Water used as an ingredient of official preparations meets the requirements for *Purified Water*, for *Water for Injection*, or for one of the sterile forms of water covered by a monograph in this Pharmacopeia.

Potable water meeting the requirements for drinking water as set forth in the regulations of the federal Environmental Protection Agency may be used in the preparation of official substances.

Official substances are prepared according to recognized principles of good manufacturing practice and from ingredients complying with specifications designed to assure that the resultant substances meet the requirements of the compendial monographs (see also *Foreign Substances and Impurities* under *Tests and Assays*).

Preparations for which a complete composition is given in this Pharmacopeia, unless specifically exempted herein or in the individual monograph, are to contain only the ingredients named in the formulas. However, there may be deviation from the specified processes or methods of compounding, though not from the ingredients or proportions thereof, provided the finished preparation conforms to the relevant standards laid down herein and to preparations produced by following the specified process.

Where a monograph on a preparation calls for an ingredient in an amount expressed on the dried basis, the ingredient need not be dried prior to use if due allowance is made for the water or other volatile substances present in the quantity taken.

Unless specifically exempted elsewhere in this Pharmacopeia, the identity, strength, quality, and purity of an official article are determined by the definition, physical properties, tests, assays, and other specifications relating to the article, whether incorporated in the monograph itself, in the General Notices, or in the section, *General Chapters*.

Added Substances—An official substance, as distinguished from an official preparation, contains no added substances except where specifically permitted in the individual monograph. Where such addition is permitted, the label indicates the name(s) and amount(s) of any added substance(s).

Unless otherwise specified in the individual monograph, or elsewhere in the General Notices, suitable substances such as bases, carriers, coatings, colors, flavors, preservatives, stabilizers, and vehicles may be added to an official preparation to enhance its stability, usefulness, or elegance or to facilitate its preparation. Such substances are regarded as unsuitable and are prohibited unless (a) they are harmless in the amounts used, (b) they do not exceed the minimum quantity required to provide their intended effect, (c) their presence does not impair the bioavailability or the therapeutic efficacy or safety of the official preparation, and (d) they do not interfere with the assays and tests prescribed for determining compliance with the Pharmacopeial standards.

Inert Headspace Gases—The air in a container of an article for parenteral use may be evacuated or be replaced by carbon dioxide, helium, or nitrogen, or by a mixture of these gases, which fact need not be declared on the label unless otherwise specified in the individual monograph.

Colors—Added substances employed solely to impart color may be incorporated into official preparations, except those intended for parenteral or ophthalmic use, in accordance with the regulations pertaining to the use of colors issued by the Food and Drug Administration, provided such added substances

are otherwise appropriate in all respects. (See also *Added Substances* under *Injections* ⟨1⟩.)

Ointments and Suppositories—In the preparation of ointments and suppositories, the proportions of the substances constituting the base may be varied to maintain a suitable consistency under different climatic conditions, provided the concentrations of active ingredients are not varied.

TESTS AND ASSAYS

Foreign Substances and Impurities—Tests for the presence of foreign substances and impurities are provided to limit such substances to amounts that are unobjectionable under conditions in which the article is customarily employed (see also *Impurities in Official Articles* ⟨1086⟩).

While one of the primary objectives of the Pharmacopeia is to assure the user of official articles of their identity, strength, quality, and purity, it is manifestly impossible to include in each monograph a test for every impurity, contaminant, or adulterant that might be present, including microbial contamination. These may arise from a change in the source of material or from a change in the processing, or may be introduced from extraneous sources. Tests suitable for detecting such occurrences, the presence of which is inconsistent with good pharmaceutical practice, should be employed in addition to the tests provided in the individual monograph.

Procedures—Assay and test procedures are provided for determining compliance with the Pharmacopeial standards of identity, strength, quality, and purity.

In performing the assay or test procedures in this Pharmacopeia, it is expected that safe laboratory practices will be followed. This includes the utilization of precautionary measures, protective equipment, and work practices consistent with the chemicals and procedures utilized. Prior to undertaking any assay or procedure described in this Pharmacopeia, the individual should be aware of the hazards associated with the chemicals and the procedures and means of protecting against them. This Pharmacopeia is not designed to describe such hazards or protective measures.

Every compendial article in commerce shall be so constituted that when examined in accordance with these assay and test procedures, it meets all of the requirements in the monograph defining it. However, it is not to be inferred that application of every analytical procedure in the monograph to samples from every production batch is necessarily a prerequisite for assuring compliance with Pharmacopeial standards before the batch is released for distribution. Data derived from manufacturing process validation studies and from in-process controls sometimes may provide greater assurance that a batch meets a particular monograph requirement than analytical data derived from an examination of finished units drawn from that batch. On the basis of such assurances, the analytical procedures in the monograph may be omitted by the manufacturer in judging compliance of the batch with the Pharmacopeial standards.

Automated procedures employing the same basic chemistry as those assay and test procedures given in the monograph are recognized as being equivalent in their suitability for determining compliance. Conversely, where an automated procedure is given in the monograph, manual procedures employing the same basic chemistry are recognized as being equivalent in their suitability for determining compliance. Compliance may be determined also by the use of alternative methods, chosen for advantages in accuracy, sensitivity, precision, selectivity, or adaptability to automation or computerized data reduction or in other special circumstances. However, Pharmacopeial standards and procedures are interrelated; therefore, where a difference appears or in the event of dispute, only the result obtained by the procedure given in this Pharmacopeia is conclusive.

Odor—Terms such as "odorless," "practically odorless," "a faint characteristic odor," or variations thereof, apply to examination, after exposure to the air for 15 minutes, of either a freshly opened package of the article (for packages containing not more than 25 g) or (for larger packages) of a portion of about 25 g of the article that has been removed from its package to an open evaporating dish of about 100-mL capacity. An odor designation is descriptive only and is not to be regarded as a standard of purity for a particular lot of an article.

Description—Information on the "description" pertaining to an article, which is relatively general in nature, is provided in the reference table, *Description and Relative Solubility of USP and NF Articles*, in this Pharmacopeia for those who use, prepare, and dispense drugs and/or related articles, solely to indicate properties of an article complying with monograph standards. The properties are not in themselves standards or tests for purity even though they may indirectly assist in the preliminary evaluation of an article.

Solubility—The statements concerning solubilities given in the reference table, *Description and Relative Solubility of USP and NF Articles*, for Pharmacopeial articles are not standards or tests for purity but are provided primarily as information for those who use, prepare, and dispense drugs and/or related articles. Only where a quantitative solubility test is given, and is designated as such, is it a test for purity.

The approximate solubilities of Pharmacopeial substances are indicated by the descriptive terms in the accompanying table.

Descriptive Term	Parts of Solvent Required for 1 Part of Solute
Very soluble	Less than 1
Freely soluble	From 1 to 10
Soluble	From 10 to 30
Sparingly soluble	From 30 to 100
Slightly soluble	From 100 to 1000
Very slightly soluble	From 1000 to 10,000
Practically insoluble, or Insoluble	10,000 and over

Soluble Pharmacopeial articles, when brought into solution, may show traces of physical impurities, such as minute fragments of filter paper, fibers, and other particulate matter, unless limited or excluded by definite tests or other specifications in the individual monographs.

PRESERVATION, PACKAGING, STORAGE, AND LABELING

Containers—The *container* is that which holds the article and is or may be in direct contact with the article. The *immediate container* is that which is in direct contact with the article at all times. The *closure* is a part of the container.

Prior to its being filled, the container should be clean. Special precautions and cleaning procedures may be necessary to ensure that each container is clean and that extraneous matter is not introduced into or onto the article.

The container does not interact physically or chemically with the article placed in it so as to alter the strength, quality, or purity of the article beyond the official requirements.

The Pharmacopeial requirements for the use of specified containers apply also to articles as packaged by the pharmacist or other dispenser, unless otherwise indicated in the individual monograph.

Tamper-resistant Packaging—The container or individual carton of a sterile article intended for ophthalmic or otic use, except where extemporaneously compounded for immediate dispensing on prescription, shall be so sealed that the contents cannot be used without obvious destruction of the seal.

Articles intended for sale without prescription are also required to comply with the tamper-resistant packaging and labeling requirements of the Food and Drug Administration where applicable.

Preferably, the immediate container and/or the outer container or protective packaging utilized by a manufacturer or distributor for all dosage forms that are not specifically exempt is designed so as to show evidence of any tampering with the contents.

Light-resistant Container (see *Light Transmission* under *Containers* ⟨661⟩)—A light-resistant container protects the contents from the effects of light by virtue of the specific properties of the material of which it is composed, including any coating applied to it. Alternatively, a clear and colorless or a translucent container may be made light-resistant by means of an opaque covering, in which case the label of the container bears a statement that the opaque covering is needed until the contents are to be used or administered. Where it is directed to "protect from light" in an individual monograph, preservation in a light-resistant container is intended.

Where an article is required to be packaged in a light-resistant container, and if the container is made light-resistant by means of an opaque covering, a single-use, unit-dose container or mnemonic pack for dispensing may not be removed from the outer opaque covering prior to dispensing.

Well-closed Container—A well-closed container protects the contents from extraneous solids and from loss of the article under the ordinary or customary conditions of handling, shipment, storage, and distribution.

Tight Container—A tight container protects the contents from contamination by extraneous liquids, solids, or vapors, from loss of the article, and from efflorescence, deliquescence, or evaporation under the ordinary or customary conditions of handling, shipment, storage, and distribution, and is capable of tight reclosure. Where a tight container is specified, it may be replaced by a hermetic container for a single dose of an article.

A gas cylinder is a metallic tight container designed to hold a gas under pressure. As a safety measure, for carbon dioxide, cyclopropane, helium, nitrous oxide, and oxygen, the Pin-index Safety System of matched fittings is recommended for cylinders of Size E or smaller.

NOTE—Where packaging and storage in a *tight container* or a *well-closed container* is specified in the individual monograph, the container utilized for an article when dispensed on prescription meets the requirements under *Containers—Permeation* ⟨671⟩.

Hermetic Container—A hermetic container is impervious to air or any other gas under the ordinary or customary conditions of handling, shipment, storage, and distribution.

Single-unit Container—A single-unit container is one that is designed to hold a quantity of drug product intended for administration as a single dose or a single finished device intended for use promptly after the container is opened. Preferably, the immediate container and/or the outer container or protective packaging shall be so designed as to show evidence of any tampering with the contents. Each single-unit container shall be labeled to indicate the identity, quantity and/or strength, name of the manufacturer, lot number, and expiration date of the article.

Single-dose Container (see also *Containers for Injections* under *Injections* ⟨1⟩)—A single-dose container is a single-unit container for articles intended for parenteral administration only. A single-dose container is labeled as such. Examples of single-dose containers include pre-filled syringes, cartridges, fusion-sealed containers, and closure-sealed containers when so labeled.

Unit-dose Container—A unit-dose container is a single-unit container for articles intended for administration by other than the parenteral route as a single dose, direct from the container.

Multiple-unit Container—A multiple-unit container is a container that permits withdrawal of successive portions of the contents without changing the strength, quality, or purity of the remaining portion.

Multiple-dose Container (see also *Containers for Injections* under *Injections* ⟨1⟩)—A multiple-dose container is a multiple-unit container for articles intended for parenteral administration only.

Storage Temperature—Specific directions are stated in some monographs with respect to the temperatures at which Pharmacopeial articles shall be stored, when stability data indicate that storage at a lower or a higher temperature produces undesirable results. Such directions apply except where the label on an article states a different storage temperature on the basis of stability studies of that particular formulation. The conditions are defined by the following terms.

Cold—Any temperature not exceeding 8° (46°F). A *refrigerator* is a cold place in which the temperature is maintained thermostatically between 2° and 8° (36° and 46 °F). A *freezer* is a cold place in which the temperature is maintained thermostatically between −20° and −10° (−4° and 14°F).

Cool—Any temperature between 8° and 15° (46° and 59°F). An article for which storage in a cool place is directed may, alternatively, be stored in a *refrigerator*, unless otherwise specified in the individual monograph.

Room Temperature—The temperature prevailing in a working area. *Controlled room temperature* is a temperature maintained thermostatically between 15° and 30° (59° and 86 °F).

Warm—Any temperature between 30° and 40° (86° and 104°F).

Excessive Heat—Any temperature above 40° (104°F).

Protection from Freezing—Where, in addition to the risk of breakage of the container, freezing subjects an article to loss of strength or potency, or to destructive alteration of its characteristics, the container label bears an appropriate instruction to protect the article from freezing.

Storage under Nonspecific Conditions—For articles, regardless of quantity, where no specific storage directions or limitations are provided in the individual monograph, it is to be understood that conditions of storage and distribution include protection from moisture, freezing, and excessive heat.

Labeling—The term "labeling" designates all labels and other written, printed, or graphic matter upon an immediate container of an article or upon, or in, any package or wrapper in which it is enclosed, except any outer shipping container. The term "label" designates that part of the labeling upon the immediate container.

A shipping container, unless such container is also essentially the immediate container or the outside of the consumer package, is exempt from the labeling requirements of this Pharmacopeia.

Articles in this Pharmacopeia are subject to compliance with such labeling requirements as may be promulgated by governmental bodies in addition to the Pharmacopeial requirements set forth for the articles.

Amount of Ingredient per Dosage Unit—The strength of a drug product is preferably expressed in terms of μg or mg of the therapeutically active moiety. The full name of the chemical compound is also used in the content declaration.

Pharmacopeial articles in capsule, tablet, or other unit dosage form shall be labeled to express the quantity of each active ingredient contained in each such unit. Pharmacopeial drug products not in unit dosage form shall be labeled to express the quantity of each active ingredient in each mL or in each g, or to express the percentage of each such ingredient (see *Percentage Measurements*), except that oral liquids or solids intended to be constituted to yield oral liquids may, alternatively, be labeled in terms of each 5-mL portion of the liquid or resulting liquid.

In order to help minimize the possibility of errors in the dispensing and administration of drugs, the quantity of active ingredient when expressed in whole numbers shall be shown without a decimal point that is followed by a terminal zero (e.g., express as 4 mg [not 4.0 mg]).

Labeling of Salts of Drugs—It is an established principle that Pharmacopeial articles shall have only one official name. For purposes of saving space on labels, and because chemical symbols for the most common inorganic salts of drugs are well known to practitioners as synonymous with the written forms, the following alternatives are permitted in labeling official articles that are salts: HCl for hydrochloride; HBr for hydrobromide; Na for sodium; and K for potassium.

Labeling Vitamin-containing Products—The vitamin content of Pharmacopeial preparations shall be stated on the label in metric units per dosage unit. The amounts of vitamins A, D, and E may be stated also in USP Units. Quantities of vitamin A declared in metric units refer to the equivalent amounts of retinol (vitamin A alcohol).

Labeling Parenteral and Topical Preparations—The label of a preparation intended for parenteral or topical use states the names of all added substances (see *Added Substances* in these General Notices, and see *Labeling* under *Injections* ⟨1⟩), and, in the case of parenteral preparations, also their amounts or proportions, except that for substances added for adjustment of pH or to achieve isotonicity, the label may indicate only their presence and the reason for their addition.

Labeling Electrolytes—The concentration and dosage of electrolytes for replacement therapy (e.g., sodium chloride or potassium chloride) shall be stated on the label in milliequivalents (mEq). The label of the product shall indicate also the quantity of ingredient(s) in terms of weight or percentage concentration.

Special Capsules and Tablets—The label of any form of Capsule or Tablet intended for administration other than by swallowing intact bears a prominent indication of the manner in which it is to be used.

Expiration Date—The label of an official drug product shall bear an expiration date. The monographs for some preparations specify the expiration date that shall appear on the label. In the absence of a specific requirement in the individual monograph for a drug product, the label shall bear an expiration date assigned for the particular formulation and package of the article, with the following exception: the label need not show an expiration date in the case of a drug product packaged in a container that is intended for sale without prescription and the labeling of which states no dosage limitations, and which is stable for not less than 3 years when stored under the prescribed conditions.

Where an official article is required to bear an expiration date, such article shall be dispensed solely in, or from, a container labeled with an expiration date, and the date on which the article is dispensed shall be within the labeled expiry period. The expiration date identifies the time during which the article may be expected to meet the requirements of the Pharmacopeial monograph provided it is kept under the prescribed storage conditions. The expiration date limits the time during which the article may be dispensed or used. Where an expiration date is stated only in terms of the month and the year, it is a representation that the intended expiration date is the last day of the stated month.

For articles requiring constitution prior to use, a suitable beyond-use date for the constituted product shall be identified in the labeling.

In determining an appropriate period of time during which a prescription drug may be retained by a patient after its dispensing, the dispenser shall take into account, in addition to any other relevant factors, the nature of the drug; the container in which it was packaged by the manufacturer and the expiration date thereon; the characteristics of the patient's container, if the article is repackaged for dispensing; the expected storage conditions to which the article may be exposed; and the expected length of time of the course of therapy. Unless otherwise required, the dispenser may, on taking into account the foregoing, place on the label of a multiple-unit container a suitable beyond-use date to limit the patient's use of the article. Unless otherwise specified in the individual monograph, such beyond-use date shall be not later than (a) the expiration date on the manufacturer's container, or (b) one year from the date the drug is dispensed, whichever is earlier.

WEIGHTS AND MEASURES

The metric system of weights and measures is used in this Pharmacopeia. The metric and other units, and the abbreviations commonly employed, are as follows:

Ci=curie	Eq=gram-equivalent weight (equivalent)
mCi=millicurie	
μCi=microcurie	mEq=milliequivalent
nCi=nanocurie	mol=gram-molecular weight (mole)
Mrad=megarad	
m=meter	mmol=millimole
dm=decimeter	Osmol=osmole
cm=centimeter	mOsmol=milliosmole
mm=millimeter	Hz=hertz
μm=micrometer (0.001 mm)	kHz=kilohertz
	MHz=megahertz
nm=nanometer*	MeV=million electron volts
kg=kilogram	
g=gram	keV=kilo-electron volt
mg=milligram	mV=millivolt
μg; mcg=microgram†	psi=pounds per square inch
ng=nanogram	
pg=picogram	Pa=pascal
dL=deciliter	kPa=kilopascal
L=liter	g=gravity (in centrifugation)
mL=milliliter; ‡	
μL=microliter	

*Formerly the abbreviation mμ (for millimicron) was used.

†Formerly the abbreviation mcg was used in the Pharmacopeial monographs; however, the symbol μg now is more widely accepted and thus is used in this Pharmacopeia. The term "gamma," symbolized by γ, is frequently used for microgram in biochemical literature.

‡One milliliter (mL) is used herein as the equivalent of 1 cubic centimeter (cc).

The International System of Units (SI) is also used in all radiopharmaceutical monographs. The abbreviations commonly employed are as follows.

Bq=becquerel	GBq=gigabecquerel
kBq=kilobecquerel	Gy=gray
MBq=megabecquerel	mGy=milligray

NOTE—The abbreviation mcg is still commonly employed to denote microgram(s) in labeling and in prescription writing. Therefore, for purposes of labeling, "mcg" may be used to denote microgram(s).

CONCENTRATIONS

Percentage Measurements—Percentage concentrations are expressed as follows:

Percent weight in weight—(w/w) expresses the number of g of a constituent in 100 g of solution or mixture.

Percent weight in volume—(w/v) expresses the number of g of a constituent in 100 mL of solution, and is used regardless of whether water or another liquid is the solvent.

Percent volume in volume—(v/v) expresses the number of mL of a constituent in 100 mL of solution.

The term *percent* used without qualification means, for mixtures of solids and semisolids, percent weight in weight; for solutions or suspensions of solids in liquids, percent weight in volume; for solutions of liquids in liquids, percent volume in volume; and for solutions of gases in liquids, percent weight in volume. For example, a 1 percent solution is prepared by dissolving 1 g of a solid or semisolid, or 1 mL of a liquid, in sufficient solvent to make 100 mL of the solution.

In the dispensing of prescription medications, slight changes in volume owing to variations in room temperatures may be disregarded.

Drug and Dosage Form Requirements

⟨1⟩ INJECTIONS

Every care should be exercised in the preparation of all products intended for injection, to prevent contamination with microorganisms and foreign material. Good pharmaceutical practice requires also that each final container of Injection be subjected individually to a physical inspection, whenever the nature of the container permits, and that every container whose contents show evidence of contamination with visible foreign material be rejected.

Definitions—In this Pharmacopeia, the sterile preparations for parenteral use are grouped into five distinct classes, defined as follows: (1) medicaments or solutions or emulsions thereof suitable for injection, bearing titles of the form, _____*Injection;* (2) dry solids or liquid concentrates containing no buffers, diluents, or other added substances, and which, upon the addition of suitable solvents, yield solutions conforming in all respects to the requirements for Injections, and which are distinguished by titles of the form, *Sterile* _____; (3) preparations the same as those described under (2) except that they contain one or more buffers, diluents, or other added substances, and which are distinguished by titles of the form, _____*for Injection;* (4) solids which are suspended in a suitable fluid medium and which are not to be injected intravenously or into the spinal canal, distinguished by titles of the form, *Sterile* _____*Suspension;* and (5) dry solids which, upon the addition of suitable vehicles, yield preparations conforming in all respects to the requirements for Sterile Suspensions, and which are distinguished by titles of the form, *Sterile* _____*for Suspension.*

A *Pharmacy bulk package* is a container of a sterile preparation for parenteral use that contains many single doses. The contents are intended for use in a pharmacy admixture program and are restricted to the preparation of admixtures for infusion or, through a sterile transfer device, for the filling of empty sterile syringes.

The closure shall be penetrated only one time after constitution with a suitable sterile transfer device or dispensing set which allows measured dispensing of the contents. The *Pharmacy bulk package* is to be used only in a suitable work area such as a laminar flow hood (or an equivalent clean air compounding area).

Designation as a *Pharmacy bulk package* is limited to preparations from classes 1, 2, or 3 as defined above. *Pharmacy bulk packages*, although containing more than one single dose, are exempt from the multiple-dose container volume limit of 30 mL and the requirement that they contain a substance or suitable mixture of substances to prevent the growth of microorganisms.

Where a container is offered as a *Pharmacy bulk package*, the label shall (a) state prominently "Pharmacy Bulk Package—Not for direct infusion," (b) contain or refer to information on proper techniques to help assure safe use of the product, and (c) bear a statement limiting the time frame in which the container may be used once it has been entered, provided it is held under the labeled storage conditions.

Where used in this Pharmacopeia, the designation *Large-volume intravenous solution* applies to a single-dose injection that is intended for intravenous use and is packaged in containers labeled as containing more than 100 mL. The designation *Small-volume Injection* applies to an Injection that is packaged in containers labeled as containing 100 mL or less.

The Pharmacopeial definitions for sterile preparations for parenteral use generally do not apply in the case of the biologics, because of their special nature and licensing requirements (see *Biologics* ⟨1041⟩).

Aqueous Vehicles—The vehicles for aqueous Injections meet the requirements of the *Pyrogen Test* ⟨151⟩ or the *Bacterial Endotoxins Test* ⟨85⟩, whichever is specified. *Water for Injection* generally is used as the vehicle, unless otherwise specified in the individual monograph. Sodium chloride may be added in amounts sufficient to render the resulting solution isotonic; and *Sodium Chloride Injection*, or *Ringer's Injection*, may be used in whole or in part instead of *Water for Injection* unless otherwise specified in the individual monograph. For conditions applying to other adjuvants, see *Added Substances*, in this chapter.

Other Vehicles—Fixed oils used as vehicles for nonaqueous injections are of vegetable origin, are odorless or nearly so, and have no odor or taste suggesting rancidity. They meet the requirements of the test for *Solid paraffin* under *Mineral Oil*, the cooling bath being maintained at 10 °C, have a *Saponification value* of between 185 and 200 (see *Fats and Fixed Oils* ⟨401⟩), have an *Iodine value* of between 79 and 128 (see *Fats and Fixed Oils* ⟨401⟩), and meet the requirements of the following tests.

Unsaponifiable Matter—Reflux on a steam bath 10 mL of the oil with 15 mL of sodium hydroxide solution (1 in 6) and 30 mL of alcohol, with occasional shaking until the mixture becomes clear. Transfer the solution to a shallow dish, evaporate the alcohol on a steam bath, and mix the residue with 100 mL of water: a clear solution results.

Free Fatty Acids—The free fatty acids in 10 g of oil require for neutralization not more than 2.0 mL of 0.020 N sodium hydroxide (see *Fats and Fixed Oils* ⟨401⟩).

Synthetic mono- or diglycerides of fatty acids may be used as vehicles, provided they are liquid and remain clear when cooled to 10 °C and have an *Iodine value* of not more than 140 (see *Fats and Fixed Oils* ⟨401⟩).

These and other nonaqueous vehicles may be used, provided they are safe in the volume of injection administered, and also provided they do not interfere with the therapeutic efficacy of the preparation or with its response to prescribed assays and tests.

Added Substances—Suitable substances may be added to preparations intended for injection to increase stability or usefulness, unless proscribed in the individual monograph, provided they are harmless in the amounts administered and do not interfere with the therapeutic efficacy or with the responses to the specified assays and tests. No coloring agent may be added, solely for the purpose of coloring the finished preparation, to a solution intended for parenteral administration (see also *Added Substances* under *General Notices and Requirements* and *Antimicrobial Preservatives—Effectiveness* ⟨51⟩).

Observe special care in the choice and use of added substances in preparations for injection that are administered in a volume exceeding 5 mL. The following maximum limits prevail unless otherwise directed: for agents containing mercury and the cationic, surface-active compounds, 0.01%; for those of the types of chlorobutanol, cresol, and phenol, 0.5%; and for sulfur dioxide, or an equivalent amount of the sulfite, bisulfite, or metabisulfite of potassium or sodium, 0.2%.

A suitable substance or mixture of substances to prevent the growth of microorganisms must be added to preparations intended for injection that are packaged in multiple-dose containers, regardless of the method of sterilization employed, unless otherwise directed in the individual monograph, or unless the active ingredients are themselves antimicrobial. Such substances are used in concentrations that will prevent the growth of or kill microorganisms in the preparations for injection. Such substances also meet the requirements of *Antimicrobial Preservatives—Effectiveness* ⟨51⟩ and *Antimicrobial Agents—Content* ⟨341⟩. Sterilization processes are employed even though such substances are used (see also *Parenteral and Topical Preparations* in the section, *Added Substances*, under *General Notices and Requirements* and *Sterilization and Sterility Assurance of Compendial Articles* ⟨1211⟩). The air in the container may be evacuated or be displaced by a chemically inert gas. If the injection is oxygen-sensitive, that information must appear in the labeling.

Containers for Injections—Containers, including the closures, for preparations for injection do not interact physically or chemically with the preparations in any manner to alter the strength, quality, or purity beyond the official requirements under the ordinary or customary conditions of handling, shipment, storage, sale, and use. The container is made of material that permits inspection of the contents. The type of glass preferable for each parenteral preparation is usually stated in the individual monograph.

For definitions of single-dose and multiple-dose containers, see *Containers* under *General Notices and Requirements*. Containers meet the requirements under *Containers* ⟨661⟩.

Containers are closed by fusion, or by application of suitable closures, in such manner as to prevent contamination or loss of contents. Closures for multiple-dose containers permit the withdrawal of the contents without removal or destruction of the closure. The closure permits penetration by a needle, and, upon withdrawal of the needle, at once recloses the container against contamination.

Containers for Sterile Solids—Containers, including the closures, for dry solids intended for parenteral use do not interact physically or chemically with the preparation in any manner to alter the strength, quality, or purity beyond the official requirements under the ordinary or customary conditions of handling, shipment, storage, sale, and use.

A container for a sterile solid permits the addition of a suitable solvent and withdrawal of portions of the resulting solution or suspension in such manner that the sterility of the product is maintained.

Where the *Assay* in a monograph provides a procedure for *Assay preparation* in which the total withdrawable contents are to be withdrawn from a single-dose container with a hypodermic needle and syringe, the contents are to be withdrawn as completely as possible into a dry hypodermic syringe of a rated capacity not exceeding three times the volume to be withdrawn and fitted with a 21-gauge needle not less than 2.5 cm (1 inch) in length, care being taken to expel any air bubbles, and discharged into a container for dilution and assay.

Volume in Container—Each container of an Injection is filled with a volume in slight excess of the labeled "size" or that volume which is to be withdrawn. The excess volumes recommended in the accompanying table are usually sufficient to permit withdrawal and administration of the labeled volumes.

DETERMINATION OF VOLUME OF INJECTION IN CONTAINERS—Select 1 or more containers if the volume is 10 mL or more, 3 or more if the volume is more than 3 mL and less than 10 mL, or 5 or more if the volume is 3 mL or less. Take up individually the contents of each container selected into a dry hypodermic syringe of a rated capacity not exceeding three times the volume to be measured, and fitted with a 21-gauge needle not less than 2.5 cm (1 inch) in length. Expel any air bubbles from the syringe and needle, and then discharge the contents of the syringe, without emptying the needle, into a standardized, dry cylinder (graduated to contain rather than to deliver the designated volumes) of such size that the volume to be measured occupies at least 40% of its rated volume. Alternatively, the contents of the syringe may be discharged into a dry, tared beaker, the volume, in mL, being calculated as the weight, in g, of Injection taken divided by its density. The contents of two or three 1-mL or 2-mL containers may be pooled for the measurement, provided that a separate, dry syringe assembly is used for each container. The content of containers holding 10 mL or more may be determined by means of opening them and emptying the contents directly into the graduated cylinder or tared beaker.

Labeled Size	Recommended Excess Volume For Mobile Liquids	For Viscous Liquids
0.5 mL	0.10 mL	0.12 mL
1.0 mL	0.10 mL	0.15 mL
2.0 mL	0.15 mL	0.25 mL
5.0 mL	0.30 mL	0.50 mL
10.0 mL	0.50 mL	0.70 mL
20.0 mL	0.60 mL	0.90 mL
30.0 mL	0.80 mL	1.20 mL
50.0 mL or more	2%	3%

The volume is not less than the labeled volume in the case of containers examined individually or, in the case of 1-mL and 2-mL containers, is not less than the sum of the labeled volumes of the containers taken collectively.

For Injections in multiple-dose containers labeled to yield a specific number of doses of a stated volume, proceed as directed in the foregoing, using the same number of separate syringes as the number of doses specified. The volume is such that each syringe delivers not less than the stated dose.

For Injections containing oil, warm the containers, if necessary, and thoroughly shake them immediately before removing the contents. Cool to 25 °C before measuring the volume.

Particulate Matter—All large-volume Injections for single-dose infusion, and those small-volume Injections for which the monographs specify such requirements, are subject to the particulate matter limits set forth under *Particulate Matter in Injections* ⟨788⟩. An article packaged as both a large-volume and a small-volume Injection meets the requirements set forth for *Small-volume Injections* where the container is labeled as containing 100 mL or less if the individual monograph includes a test for *Particulate matter;* it meets the requirements set forth for *Large-volume Injections for Single-dose Infusion* where the container is labeled as containing more than 100 mL. Injections packaged and labeled for use as irrigating solutions are exempt from requirements for *Particulate matter.*

Sterility Tests—Preparations for injection meet the requirements under *Sterility Tests* ⟨71⟩.

Labeling—[NOTE—See definitions of "label" and "labeling" under *Labeling* in the section *Preservation, Packaging, Storage, and Labeling* of the *General Notices and Requirements.*]

The label states the name of the preparation; in the case of a liquid preparation, the percentage content of drug or amount of drug in a specified volume; in the case of a dry preparation, the amount of *active* ingredient; the route of administration; a statement of storage conditions and an expiration date; the name of the manufacturer and distributor; and an identifying lot number. The lot number is capable of yielding the complete manufacturing history of the specific package, including all manufacturing, filling, sterilizing, and labeling operations.

Where the individual monograph permits varying concentrations of active ingredients in the large-volume parenteral, the concentration of each ingredient named in the official title is stated as if part of the official title, e.g., Dextrose Injection 5%, or Dextrose (5%) and Sodium Chloride (0.2%) Injection.

The labeling includes the following information, if the complete formula is not specified in the individual monograph: (1) In the case of a liquid preparation, the percentage content of each ingredient or the amount of each ingredient in a specified volume, except that ingredients added to adjust to a given pH or to make the solution isotonic may be declared by name and a statement of their effect; and (2) in the case of a dry preparation or other preparation to which a diluent is intended to be added before use, the amount of each ingredient, the composition of recommended diluent(s) [the name(s) alone, if the formula is specified in the individual monograph], the amount to be used to attain a specific concentration of active ingredient and the final volume of solution so obtained, a brief description of the physical appearance of the constituted solution, directions for proper storage of the constituted solution, and an expiration date limiting the period during which the constituted solution may be expected to have the required or labeled potency if it has been stored as directed.

Containers for Injections that are intended for use as dialysis, hemofiltration, or irrigation solutions and that contain a volume of more than 1 liter are labeled to indicate that the contents are not intended for use by intravenous infusion.

Injections intended for veterinary use are labeled to that effect.

The container is so labeled that a sufficient area of the container remains uncovered for its full length or circumference to permit inspection of the contents.

Packaging and Storage—The volume of Injection in single-dose containers provides the amount specified for parenteral administration at one time and in no case is more than sufficient to permit the withdrawal and administration of 1 liter.

Preparations intended for intraspinal, intracisternal, or peridural administration are packaged only in single-dose containers.

Unless otherwise specified in the individual monograph, no multiple-dose container contains a volume of Injection more than sufficient to permit the withdrawal of 30 mL.

Injections packaged for use as irrigation solutions or for hemofiltration or dialysis or for parenteral nutrition are exempt from the 1-liter restriction of the foregoing requirements relating to packaging. Containers for Injections packaged for use as hemofiltration or irrigation solutions may be designed to empty rapidly and may contain a volume of more than 1 liter.

Injections labeled for veterinary use are exempt from packaging and storage requirements concerning the limitation to single-dose containers and the limitation on the volume of multiple-dose containers.

CONSTITUTED SOLUTIONS

Sterile dosage forms from which constituted solutions are prepared for injection bear titles of the form, *Sterile ____ or ____ for Injection.* Since these dosage forms are constituted at the time of use by the health-care practitioner, tests and standards pertaining to the solution as constituted for administration are not included in the individual monographs on sterile dry solids or liquid concentrates. However, in the interest of assuring the quality of injection preparations as they are actually administered, the following nondestructive tests are provided for demonstrating the suitability of constituted solutions when they are prepared just prior to use.

Completeness and Clarity of Solution—Constitute the solution as directed in the labeling supplied by the manufacturer for the sterile dry dosage form.

A: The solid dissolves completely, leaving no visible residue as undissolved matter.

B: The constituted solution is not significantly less clear than an equal volume of the diluent or of Purified Water contained in a similar vessel and examined similarly.

Particulate Matter—Constitute the solution as directed in the labeling supplied by the manufacturer for the sterile dry dosage form: the solution is essentially free from particles of foreign matter that can be observed on visual inspection.

⟨771⟩ OPHTHALMIC OINTMENTS

Added Substances—Suitable substances may be added to ophthalmic ointments to increase stability or usefulness, unless proscribed in the individual monograph, provided they are harmless in the amounts administered and do not interfere with the therapeutic efficacy or with the responses to the specified assays and tests. No coloring agent may be added, solely for the purpose of coloring the finished preparation, to an article intended for ophthalmic use (see also *Added Substances* under *General Notices,* and *Antimicrobial Preservatives—Effectiveness* ⟨51⟩).

A suitable substance or mixture of substances to prevent the growth of microorganisms must be added to ophthalmic ointments that are packaged in multiple-use containers, regardless of the method of sterilization employed, unless otherwise directed in the individual monograph, or unless the formula itself is bacteriostatic. Such substances are used in concentrations that will prevent the growth of or kill microorganisms in the ophthalmic ointments (see also *Antimicrobial Preservatives—Effectiveness* ⟨51⟩ and *Antimicrobial Agents—Content* ⟨341⟩). Sterilization processes are employed for the finished ointment or for all ingredients, if the ointment is manufactured under rigidly aseptic conditions, even though such substances are used (see also *Parenteral and Topical Preparations* in the section *Added Substances,* under *General Notices,* and *Sterilization and Sterility Assurance of Compendial Articles* ⟨1211⟩). Ophthalmic ointments that are packaged in single-use containers are not required to contain antibacterial agents; however, they meet the requirements for *Sterility Tests* ⟨71⟩.

Containers—Containers, including the closures, for ophthalmic ointments do not interact physically or chemically with the preparation in any manner to alter the strength, quality, or purity beyond the official requirements under the ordinary or customary conditions of handling, shipment, storage, sale, and use (see also *Containers for Articles Intended for Ophthalmic Use,* under *General Notices*).

Metal Particles—Follow the *Procedure* set forth under *Metal Particles in Ophthalmic Ointments* ⟨751⟩.

Leakage—Select 10 tubes of the Ointment, with seals applied when specified. Thoroughly clean and dry the exterior surfaces of each tube with an absorbent cloth. Place the tubes in a horizontal position on a sheet of absorbent blotting paper in an oven maintained at a temperature of 60 ± 3 °C for 8 hours. No significant leakage occurs during or at the completion of the test (disregard traces of ointment presumed to originate externally from within the crimp of the tube or from the thread of the cap). If leakage is observed from one, but not more than one, of the tubes, repeat the test with 20 additional tubes of the Ointment. The requirement is met if no leakage is observed from the first 10 tubes tested, or if leakage is observed from not more than one of 30 tubes tested.

⟨785⟩ OSMOLARITY

Osmotic pressure is fundamentally related to all biological processes that involve diffusion of solutes or transfer of fluids through membranes. Thus, knowledge of the osmolar concentrations of parenteral fluids is essential. The labels of Pharmacopeial solutions that provide intravenous replenishment of fluid, nutrient(s), or electrolyte(s), as well as of the osmotic

diuretic Mannitol Injection, are required to state the osmolar concentration.

The declaration of osmolar concentration on the label of a parenteral solution serves primarily to inform the practitioner whether the solution is hypo-osmotic, iso-osmotic, or hyper-osmotic. A quantitative statement facilitates calculation of the dilution required to render a hyper-osmotic solution iso-osmotic. It also simplifies many calculations involved in peritoneal dialysis and hemodialysis procedures. The osmolar concentration of an extemporaneously compounded intravenous solution prepared in the pharmacy (e.g., a hyperalimentation solution) from osmolar-labeled solutions also can be obtained simply by summing the osmoles contributed by each constituent.

The units of osmolar concentration are usually expressed as milliosmoles (abbreviation: mOsmol) of solute per liter of solution. In general terms, the weight of an osmole is the gram molecular weight of a substance divided by the number of ions or chemical species (n) formed upon dissolution. In ideal solutions, for example, $n = 1$ for glucose, $n = 2$ for sodium chloride or magnesium sulfate, $n = 3$ for calcium chloride, and $n = 4$ for sodium citrate.

The ideal osmolar concentration may be determined according to the formula:

osmolar concentration (mOsmol/liter) = mOsM

$$= \frac{\text{wt. of substance (g/liter)}}{\text{mol. wt. (g)}} \times \text{number of species} \times 1000.$$

As the concentration of the solute increases, interaction among solute particles increases, and actual osmolar values decrease when compared to ideal values. Deviation from ideal conditions is usually slight in solutions within the physiologic range and for more dilute solutions, but for highly concentrated solutions the actual osmolarities may be appreciably lower than ideal values. For example, the ideal osmolarity of 0.9% Sodium Chloride Injection is $9/58.4 \times 2 \times 1000 = 308$ milliosmoles per liter. In fact, however, n is slightly less than 2 for solutions of sodium chloride at this concentration, and the actual measured osmolarity of 0.9% Sodium Chloride Injection is about 286 milliosmoles per liter.

The theoretical osmolarity of a complex mixture, such as Protein Hydrolysate Injection, cannot be readily calculated. In such instances, actual values of osmolar concentration are to be used to meet the labeling requirement set forth in the individual monograph. They are determined by calculating the osmolarity from measured values of osmolal concentration and water content. Each osmole of solute added to 1 kg of water lowers the freezing point approximately 1.86 °C and lowers the vapor pressure approximately 0.3 mm of mercury (at 25 °C). These physical changes are measurable, and they permit accurate estimations of osmolal concentrations.

Where osmometers that measure the freezing-point depression are employed, a measured volume of solution (usually 2 mL) is placed in a glass tube immersed in a temperature-controlled bath. A thermistor and a vibrator are lowered into the mixture, and the temperature of the bath is decreased until the mixture is super-cooled. The vibrator is activated to induce crystallization of the water in the test solution, and the released heat of fusion raises the temperature of the mixture to its freezing point. By means of a Wheatstone bridge, the recorded freezing point is converted to a measurement in terms of milliosmolality, or its near equivalent for dilute solutions, milliosmolarity. The instrument is calibrated by using two standard solutions of sodium chloride that span the expected range of osmolarities.

Osmometers that measure the vapor pressures of solutions are less frequently employed. They require a smaller volume of specimen (generally about 5 μL), but the accuracy and precision of the resulting osmolality determination are comparable to those obtained by the use of osmometers that depend upon the observed freezing points of solutions.

Labeling—Where an osmolarity declaration is required in the individual monograph, the label states the total osmolar concentration in milliosmoles per liter. Where the contents are less than 100 mL, or where the label states that the article is not for direct injection but is to be diluted before use, the label alternatively may state the total osmolar concentration in milliosmoles per milliliter.

Drug and Dosage Form Information

⟨1151⟩ PHARMACEUTICAL DOSAGE FORMS

Dosage forms are provided for most of the Pharmacopeial drug substances, but the processes for the preparation of many of them are, in general, beyond the scope of the Pharmacopeia. In addition to defining the dosage forms, this section presents the general principles involved in the manufacture of some of them, particularly on a small scale. Other information that is given bears on the use of the Pharmacopeial substances in extemporaneous compounding of dosage forms.

BIOAVAILABILITY

Bioavailability, or the extent to which the therapeutic constituent of a pharmaceutical dosage form intended for oral or topical use is available for absorption is influenced by a variety of factors. Among the inherent factors known to affect absorption are the method of manufacture or method of compounding; the particle size and crystal form or polymorph of the drug substance; and the diluents and excipients used in formulating the dosage form, including fillers, binders, disintegrating agents, lubricants, coatings, solvents, suspending agents, and dyes. Lubricants and coatings are foremost among these. The maintenance of a demonstrably high degree of bioavailability requires particular attention to all aspects of production and quality control that may affect the nature of the finished dosage form.

STABILITY

The term "stability," with respect to a drug dosage form, refers to the chemical and physical integrity of the dosage unit, and, when appropriate, the ability of the dosage unit to maintain protection against microbiological contamination. The shelf life of the dosage form is the time lapse from initial preparation and packaging to the specified expiration date. The monograph specifications of identity, strength, quality, and purity apply throughout the shelf life of the product. Stability of manufactured dosage forms must be demonstrated by the manufacturer by the use of methods adequate for the purpose. Monograph assays may be used for stability testing if they are stability-indicating, i.e., if they accurately differentiate between the intact drug molecules and their degradation products. Stability considerations should include not only the specific compendial requirements, but also changes in physical appearance of the product that would warn users that the product's continued integrity is questionable.

Typically, stability studies are conducted on a packaged product stored at conditions to which it might be exposed during shipping and storage, including temperature, humidity, light, etc. Ordinarily, long-term studies are conducted at a specific temperature, such as 25 °C, representing average storage conditions, as given in the product labeling. Conducting studies at exaggerated conditions may be helpful in determining or predicting expiration dates.

The stability parameters of a drug dosage form can be influenced by environmental conditions of storage (temperature, light, air, and humidity), as well as the package components.

Pharmacopeial articles should include required storage conditions on their labeling. These are the conditions under which the expiration date shall apply. The storage requirements specified in the labeling for the article must be observed throughout the distribution of the article, i.e., beyond the time it leaves the manufacturer up to and including its handling by the dispenser or seller of the article to the consumer. Although labeling for the consumer should indicate proper storage conditions, it is recognized that control beyond the dispenser or seller is difficult.

A discussion of aspects of drug product stability that are of primary concern to the pharmacist in the dispensing of medications may be found under *Stability Considerations in Dispensing Practice* ⟨1191⟩.

Inasmuch as this chapter is for purposes of general information only, no statement herein is intended to modify or supplant any of the specific requirements pertinent to pharmaceutical preparations, which are given elsewhere in this Pharmacopeia.

Terminology

Occasionally it is necessary to add solvent to the contents of a container just prior to use, usually because of instability of some drugs in the diluted form. Thus, a solid diluted to yield a suspension is called "_____ for Suspension;" a solid dissolved and diluted to yield a solution is called "_____ for Solution;" and a solution or suspension diluted to yield a more dilute form of the drug is called "_____ Oral Concentrate" or "_____ Injection Concentrate" as appropriate for the route of administration of the drug. After dilution, it is important that the drug be homogeneously dispersed before administration.

Aerosols

Pharmaceutical aerosols are products that are packaged under pressure and contain therapeutically active ingredients that are released upon activation of an appropriate valve system. They are intended for topical application to the skin as well as local application into the nose (nasal aerosols), mouth (lingual aerosols), or lungs (inhalation aerosols).

The term "aerosol" refers to the fine mist of spray that results from most pressurized systems. However, the term has been broadly misapplied to all self-contained pressurized products, some of which deliver foams or semisolid fluids. In the case of *Inhalation Aerosols*, the particle size of the delivered medication must be carefully controlled and the average size of the particles should be under 10 μm. These products are also known as metered-dose inhalers (MDIs). (See *Inhalations*.) Other aerosol sprays may contain particles up to several hundred micrometers in diameter.

The basic components of an aerosol system are the container, the propellant, the concentrate containing the active ingredient(s), the valve, and the actuator. The nature of these components determines such characteristics as particle size distribution, uniformity of valve delivery for metered valves, delivery rate, wetness and temperature of the spray, foam density, or fluid viscosity.

TYPES OF AEROSOLS

Aerosols consist of two-phase (gas and liquid) or three-phase (gas, liquid, and solid or liquid) systems. The two-phase aerosol consists of a solution of active ingredients in liquefied propellant and the vaporized propellant. The solvent is composed of the propellant or a mixture of the propellant and co-solvents such as alcohol, propylene glycol, and polyethylene glycols, which are often used to enhance the solubility of the active ingredients.

Three-phase systems consist of a suspension or emulsion of the active ingredient(s) in addition to the vaporized propellants. A suspension consists of the active ingredient(s) that may be dispersed in the propellant system with the aid of suitable excipients such as wetting agents and/or solid carriers such as talc or colloidal silicas.

A foam aerosol is an emulsion containing one or more active ingredients, surfactants, aqueous or nonaqueous liquids, and the propellants. If the propellant is in the internal (discontinuous) phase (i.e., of the oil-in-water type), a stable foam is discharged; and if the propellant is in the external (continuous) phase (i.e., of the water-in-oil type), a spray or a quick-breaking foam is discharged.

PROPELLANTS

The propellant supplies the necessary pressure within an aerosol system to expel material from the container and, in combination with other components, to convert the material into the desired physical form. Propellants may be broadly classified as liquefied or compressed gases having vapor pressures generally exceeding atmospheric pressure. Propellants within this definition include various hydrocarbons, especially fluorochloroderivatives of methane and ethane, low molecular weight hydrocarbons such as the butanes and pentanes, and compressed gases such as carbon dioxide, nitrogen, and nitrous oxide. Mixtures of propellants are frequently used to obtain desirable pressure, delivery, and spray characteristics. A good propellant system should have the proper vapor pressure characteristics consistent with the other aerosol components.

VALVES

The primary function of the valve is to regulate the flow of the therapeutic agent and propellant from the container. The spray characteristics of the aerosol are influenced by orifice dimension, number, and location. Most aerosol valves provide for continuous spray operation and are used on most topical products. However, pharmaceutical products for oral or nasal inhalation often utilize metered-dose valves that must deliver a uniform quantity of spray upon each valve activation. The accuracy and reproducibility of the doses delivered from metering valves are generally good, comparing favorably to the uniformity of solid dosage forms such as tablets and capsules. However, when aerosol packages are stored improperly, or when they have not been used for long periods of time, valves must be primed before use. Materials used for the manufacture of valves should be inert to the formulations used. Plastic, rubber, aluminum, and stainless steel valve components are commonly used. Metered-dose valves must deliver an accurate dose within specified tolerances.

ACTUATORS

An actuator is the fitting attached to an aerosol valve stem which, when depressed or moved, opens the valve, and directs the spray containing the drug preparation to the desired area. The actuator usually indicates the direction in which the preparation is dispensed and protects the hand or finger from the refrigerant effects of the propellant. Actuators incorporate an orifice which may vary widely in size and shape. The size of this orifice, the expansion chamber design, and the nature of the propellant and formulation influence the physical characteristics of the spray, foam, or stream of solid particles dispensed. For inhalation or oral dose aerosols, an actuator capable of delivering the medication in the proper particle size range is utilized.

CONTAINERS

Aerosol containers usually are made of glass, plastic, or metal, or a combination of these materials. Glass containers must be precisely engineered to provide the maximum in pressure safety and impact resistance. Plastics may be employed to coat glass containers for improved safety characteristics, or to coat metal containers to improve corrosion resistance and enhance stability

of the formulation. Suitable metals include stainless steel, aluminum, and tin-plated steel.

MANUFACTURE

Aerosols are usually prepared by one of two general processes. In the "cold-fill" process, the concentrate (generally cooled to a temperature below 0 °C) and the refrigerated propellant are measured into open containers (usually chilled). The valve-actuator assembly is then crimped onto the container to form a pressure-tight seal. During the interval between propellant addition and crimping, sufficient volatilization of propellant occurs to displace air from the container. In the "pressure-fill" method, the concentrate is placed in the container, and either the propellant is forced under pressure through the valve orifice after the valve is sealed, or the propellant is allowed to flow under the valve cap and then the valve assembly is sealed ("under-the-cap" filling). In both cases of the "pressure-fill" method, provision must be made for evacuation of air by means of vacuum or displacement with a small amount of propellant. Manufacturing process controls usually include monitoring of proper formulation and propellant fill weight, and pressure testing and leak testing of the finished aerosol.

LABELING

Medicinal aerosols should contain at least the following warning information on the label as in accordance with appropriate regulations.

Warning—Avoid inhaling. Keep away from eyes or other mucous membranes.

The statement "Avoid inhaling" is not necessary for preparations specifically designed for use by inhalation.

The phrase "or other mucous membranes" is not necessary for preparations specifically designed for use on mucous membranes.

Warning—Contents under pressure. Do not puncture or incinerate container. Do not expose to heat or store at temperatures above 120 °CF (49 °CC). Keep out of reach of children.

In addition to the aforementioned warnings, the label of a drug packaged in an aerosol container in which the propellant consists in whole or in part of a halocarbon or hydrocarbon shall, where required under regulations of the Food and Drug Administration, bear the following warning:

Warning—Do not inhale directly; deliberate inhalation of contents can cause death.

or

Warning—Use only as directed; intentional misuse by deliberately concentrating and inhaling the contents can be harmful or fatal.

Capsules

Capsules are solid dosage forms in which the drug is enclosed within either a hard or soft soluble container or "shell." The shells are usually formed from gelatin; however, they also may be made from starch or other suitable substances. Hard shell capsule sizes range from No. 5, the smallest, to No. 000, which is the largest, except for veterinary sizes. However, size No. 00 generally is the largest size acceptable to patients. Size 0 hard gelatin capsules having an elongated body (known as size OE) also are available, which provide greater fill capacity without an increase in diameter. Hard gelatin capsules consist of two, telescoping cap and body pieces. Generally, there are unique grooves or indentations molded into the cap and body portions to provide a positive closure when fully engaged, which helps prevent the accidental separation of the filled capsules during shipping and handling. Positive closure also may be affected by spot fusion ("welding") of the cap and body pieces together through direct thermal means or by application of ultrasonic energy. Factory-filled hard gelatin capsules may be completely sealed by banding, a process in which one or more layers of gelatin are applied over the seam of the cap and body, or by a liquid fusion process wherein the filled capsules are wetted with a hydroalcoholic solution that penetrates into the space where the cap overlaps the body, and then dried. Hard shell capsules made from starch consist of two fitted cap and body pieces. Since the two pieces do not telescope or interlock positively, they are sealed together at the time of filling to prevent their separation. Starch capsules are sealed by the application of a hydroalcoholic solution to the recessed section of the cap immediately prior to its being placed onto the body.

The banding of hard shell gelatin capsules or the liquid sealing of hard shell starch capsules enhances consumer safety by making the capsules difficult to open without causing visible, obvious damage, and may improve the stability of contents by limiting O_2 penetration. Industrially filled hard shell capsules also are often of distinctive color and shape or are otherwise marked to identify them with the manufacturer. Additionally, such capsules may be printed axially or radially with strengths, product codes, etc. Pharmaceutical grade printing inks are usually based on shellac and employ FDA-approved pigments and lake dyes.

In extemporaneous prescription practice, hard shell capsules may be hand-filled; this permits the prescriber a latitude of choice in selecting either a single drug or a combination of drugs at the exact dosage level considered best for the individual patient. This flexibility gives hard shell capsules an advantage over compressed tablets and soft shell capsules as a dosage form. Hard shell capsules are usually formed from gelatins having relatively high gel strength. Either type may be used, but blends of pork skin and bone gelatin are often used to optimize shell clarity and toughness. Hard shell capsules also may be formed from starch or other suitable substances. Hard shell capsules may also contain colorants, such as D&C and FD&C dyes or the various iron oxides, opaquing agents such as titanium dioxide, dispersing agents, hardening agents such as sucrose, and preservatives. They normally contain between 10% and 15% water.

Hard gelatin capsules are made by a process that involves dipping shaped pins into gelatin solutions, after which the gelatin films are dried, trimmed, and removed from the pins, and the body and cap pieces are joined. Starch capsules are made by injection molding a mixture of starch and water, after which the capsules are dried. A separate mold is used for caps and bodies, and the two parts are supplied separately. The empty capsules should be stored in tight containers until they are filled. Since gelatin is of animal origin and starch is of vegetable origin, capsules made with these materials should be protected from potential sources of microbial contamination.

Hard shell capsules typically are filled with powder, beads, or granules. Inert sugar beads (nonpareils) may be coated with active ingredients and coating compositions that provide extended-release profiles or enteric properties. Alternatively, larger dose active ingredients themselves may be suitably formed into pellets and then coated. Semisolids or liquids also may be filled into hard shell capsules; however, when the latter are encapsulated, one of the sealing techniques must be employed to prevent leakage.

In hard gelatin capsule filling operations, the body and cap of the shell are separated prior to dosing. In hard starch shell filling operations, the bodies and caps are supplied separately and are fed into separate hoppers of the filling machine. Machines employing various dosing principles may be employed to fill powders into hard shell capsules; however, most fully automatic machines form powder plugs by compression and eject them into empty capsule bodies. Accessories to these machines generally are available for the other types of fills. Powder formulations often require adding fillers, lubricants, and glidants to the active ingredients to facilitate encapsulation. The formulation, as well as the method of filling, particularly the degree of compaction, may influence the rate of drug release. The addition of wetting agents to the powder mass is common where the active ingredient is hydrophobic. Disintegrants also may be included in powder formulations to facilitate deaggregation and dispersal of capsule plugs in the gut. Powder formulations often may be produced by dry blending; however, bulky formulations may require densification by roll compaction or other suitable granulation techniques.

Powder mixtures that tend to liquefy may be dispensed in hard shell capsules if an absorbent such as magnesium carbonate, colloidal silicon dioxide, or other suitable substance is used. Potent drugs are often mixed with an inert diluent before being filled into capsules. Where two mutually incompatible drugs are prescribed together, it is sometimes possible to place one in a small capsule and then enclose it with the second drug in a larger capsule. Incompatible drugs also can be separated by placing coated pellets or tablets, or soft shell capsules of one drug into the capsule shell before adding the second drug.

Thixotropic semisolids may be formed by gelling liquid drugs or vehicles with colloidal silicas or powdered high molecular weight polyethylene glycols. Various waxy or fatty compounds may be used to prepare semisolid matrices by fusion.

Soft shell capsules made from gelatin (sometimes called softgels) or other suitable material require large-scale production methods. The soft gelatin shell is somewhat thicker than that of hard shell capsules and may be plasticized by the addition of a polyol such as sorbitol or glycerin. The ratio of dry plasticizer to dry gelatin determines the "hardness" of the shell and may be varied to accommodate environmental conditions as well as the nature of the contents. Like hard shells, the shell composition may include approved dyes and pigments, opaquing agents such as titanium dioxide, and preservatives. Flavors may be added and up to 5% sucrose may be included for its sweetness and to produce a chewable shell. Soft gelatin shells normally contain 6% to 13% water. Soft shell capsules also may be printed with a product code, strength, etc. In most cases, soft shell capsules are filled with liquid contents. Typically, active ingredients are dissolved or suspended in a liquid vehicle. Classically, an oleaginous vehicle such as a vegetable oil was used; however, nonaqueous, water-miscible liquid vehicles such as the lower molecular weight polyethylene glycols are more common today due to fewer bioavailability problems.

Available in a wide variety of sizes and shapes, soft shell capsules are both formed, filled, and sealed in the same machine; typically, this is a rotary die process, although a plate process or reciprocating die process also may be employed. Soft shell capsules also may be manufactured in a bubble process that forms seamless spherical capsules. With suitable equipment, powders and other dry solids also may be filled into soft shell capsules.

Liquid-filled capsules of either type involve similar formulation technology and offer similar advantages and limitations. For instance, both may offer advantages over dry-filled capsules and tablets in content uniformity and drug dissolution. Greater homogeneity is possible in liquid systems, and liquids can be metered more accurately. Drug dissolution may benefit because the drug may already be in solution or at least suspended in a hydrophilic vehicle. However, the contact between the hard or soft shell and its liquid content is more intimate than exists with dry-filled capsules, and this may enhance the chances for undesired interactions. The liquid nature of capsule contents presents different technological problems than dry-filled capsules in regard to disintegration and dissolution testing. From formulation, technological, and biopharmaceutical points of view, liquid-filled capsules of either type have more in common than liquid-filled and dry-filled capsules having the same shell composition. Thus, for compendial purposes, standards and methods should be established based on capsule contents rather than on whether the contents are filled into hard or soft shell capsules.

Enteric-coated Capsules—Capsules may be coated, or, more commonly, encapsulated granules may be coated to resist releasing the drug in the gastric fluid of the stomach where a delay is important to alleviate potential problems of drug inactivation or gastric mucosal irritation. The term "delayed-release" is used for Pharmacopeial monographs on enteric-coated capsules that are intended to delay the release of medicament until the capsule has passed through the stomach, and the individual monographs include tests and specifications for *Drug release* (see *Drug Release* ⟨724⟩).

Extended-release Capsules—Extended-release capsules are formulated in such manner as to make the contained medicament available over an extended period of time following ingestion. Expressions such as "prolonged-action," "repeat-action," and "sustained-release" have also been used to describe such dosage forms. However, the term "extended-release" is used for Pharmacopeial purposes and requirements for *Drug release* (see *Drug Release* ⟨724⟩) typically are specified in the individual monographs.

Creams

Creams are semisolid dosage forms containing one or more drug substances dissolved or dispersed in a suitable base. This term has traditionally been applied to semisolids that possess a relatively fluid consistency formulated as either water-in-oil (e.g., *Cold Cream*) or oil-in-water (e.g., *Fluocinolone Acetonide Cream*) emulsions. However, more recently the term has been restricted to products consisting of oil-in-water emulsions or aqueous microcrystalline dispersions of long chain fatty acids or alcohols that are water washable and more cosmetically and aesthetically acceptable. Creams can be used for administering drugs via the vaginal route (e.g., *Triple Sulfa Vaginal Cream*).

Elixirs

See *Solutions*.

Emulsions

Emulsions are two-phase systems in which one liquid is dispersed throughout another liquid in the form of small droplets. Where oil is the dispersed phase and an aqueous solution is the continuous phase, the system is designated as an oil-in-water emulsion. Conversely, where water or an aqueous solution is the dispersed phase and oil or oleaginous material is the continuous phase, the system is designated as a water-in-oil emulsion. Emulsions are stabilized by emulsifying agents that prevent coalescence, the merging of small droplets into larger droplets and, ultimately, into a single separated phase. Emulsifying agents (surfactants) do this by concentrating in the interface between the droplet and external phase and by providing a physical barrier around the particle to coalescence. Surfactants also reduce the interfacial tension between the phases, thus increasing the ease of emulsification upon mixing.

Natural, semisynthetic, and synthetic hydrophilic polymers may be used in conjunction with surfactants in oil-in-water emulsions as they accumulate at interfaces and also increase the viscosity of the aqueous phase, thereby decreasing the rate of formation of aggregates of droplets. Aggregation is generally accompanied by a relatively rapid separation of an emulsion into a droplet-rich and droplet-poor phase. Normally the density of an oil is lower than that of water, in which case the oil droplets and droplet aggregates rise, a process referred to as creaming. The greater the rate of aggregation, the greater the droplet size and the greater the rate of creaming. The water droplets in a water-in-oil emulsion generally sediment because of their greater density.

The consistency of emulsions varies widely, ranging from easily pourable liquids to semisolid creams. Generally oil-in-water creams are prepared at high temperature, where they are fluid, and cooled to room temperature, whereupon they solidify as a result of solidification of the internal phase. When this is the case, a high internal-phase volume to external-phase volume ratio is not necessary for semisolid character, and, for example, stearic acid creams or vanishing creams are semisolid with as little as 15% internal phase. Any semisolid character with water-in-oil emulsions generally is attributable to a semisolid external phase.

All emulsions require an antimicrobial agent because the aqueous phase is favorable to the growth of microorganisms. The presence of a preservative is particularly critical in oil-in-water emulsions where contamination of the external phase occurs readily. Since fungi and yeasts are found with greater frequency than bacteria, fungistatic as well as bacteriostatic properties are desirable. Bacteria have been shown to degrade nonionic and anionic emulsifying agents, glycerin, and many natural stabilizers such as tragacanth and guar gum.

Complications arise in preserving emulsion systems, as a result of partitioning of the antimicrobial agent out of the aqueous phase where it is most needed, or of complexation with emulsion ingredients that reduce effectiveness. Therefore, the effectiveness of the preservative system should always be tested in the final product. Preservatives commonly used in emulsions include methyl-, ethyl-, propyl-, and butyl-parabens, benzoic acid, and quaternary ammonium compounds.

See also *Creams* and *Ointments*.

Extracts and Fluidextracts

Extracts are concentrated preparations of vegetable or animal drugs obtained by removal of the active constituents of the respective drugs with suitable menstrua, by evaporation of all or nearly all of the solvent, and by adjustment of the residual masses or powders to the prescribed standards.

In the manufacture of most extracts, the drugs are extracted by percolation. The entire percolates are concentrated, generally by distillation under reduced pressure in order to subject the drug principles to as little heat as possible.

Fluidextracts are liquid preparations of vegetable drugs, containing alcohol as a solvent or as a preservative, or both, and so made that, unless otherwise specified in an individual monograph, each mL contains the therapeutic constituents of 1 g of the standard drug that it represents.

A fluidextract that tends to deposit sediment may be aged and filtered or the clear portion decanted, provided the resulting clear liquid conforms to the Pharmacopeial standards.

Fluidextracts may be prepared from suitable extracts.

Gels

Gels (sometimes called Jellies) are semisolid systems consisting of either suspensions made up of small inorganic particles or large organic molecules interpenetrated by a liquid. Where the gel mass consists of a network of small discrete particles, the gel is classified as a two-phase system (e.g., *Aluminum Hydroxide Gel*). In a two-phase system, if the particle size of the dispersed phase is relatively large, the gel mass is sometimes referred to as a magma (e.g., *Bentonite Magma*). Both gels and magmas may be thixotropic, forming semisolids on standing and becoming liquid on agitation. They should be shaken before use to ensure homogeneity and should be labeled to that effect. (See *Suspensions*.)

Single-phase gels consist of organic macromolecules uniformly distributed throughout a liquid in such a manner that no apparent boundaries exist between the dispersed macromolecules and the liquid. Single-phase gels may be made from synthetic macromolecules (e.g., *Carbomer*) or from natural gums (e.g., *Tragacanth*). The latter preparations are also called mucilages. Although these gels are commonly aqueous, alcohols and oils may be used as the continuous phase. For example, mineral oil can be combined with a polyethylene resin to form an oleaginous ointment base.

Gels can be used to administer drugs topically or into body cavities (e.g., *Phenylephrine Hydrochloride Nasal Jelly*).

Implants (Pellets)

Implants or pellets are small sterile solid masses consisting of a highly purified drug (with or without excipients) made by compression or molding. They are intended for implantation in the body (usually subcutaneously) for the purpose of providing continuous release of the drug over long periods of time. Implants are administered by means of a suitable special injector or surgical incision. This dosage form has been used to administer hormones such as testosterone or estradiol. They are packaged individually in sterile vials or foil strips.

Infusions, Intramammary

Intramammary infusions are suspensions of drugs in suitable oil vehicles. These preparations are intended for veterinary use only, and are administered by instillation via the teat canals into the udders of milk-producing animals.

Inhalations

Inhalations are drugs or solutions or suspensions of one or more drug substances administered by the nasal or oral respiratory route for local or systemic effect.

Solutions of drug substances in sterile water for inhalation or in sodium chloride inhalation solution may be nebulized by use of inert gases. Nebulizers are suitable for the administration of inhalation solutions only if they give droplets sufficiently fine and uniform in size so that the mist reaches the bronchioles. Nebulized solutions may be breathed directly from the nebulizer or the nebulizer may be attached to a plastic face mask, tent, or intermittent positive pressure breathing (IPPB) machine.

Another group of products, also known as metered-dose inhalers (MDIs) are propellant driven drug suspensions or solutions in liquified gas propellant with or without a cosolvent and are intended for delivering metered doses of the drug to the respiratory tract. An MDI contains multiple doses, often exceeding several hundred. The most common single-dose volumes delivered are from 25 to 100 μL (also expressed as mg) per actuation.

Examples of MDIs containing drug solutions and suspensions in this pharmacopeia are *Epinephrine Inhalation Aerosol* and *Isoproterenol Hydrochloride and Phenylephrine Bitartrate Inhalation Aerosol*, respectively.

Powders may also be administered by mechanical devices that require manually produced pressure or a deep inhalation by the patient (e.g., *Cromolyn Sodium for Inhalation.*)

A special class of inhalations termed inhalants consists of drugs or combination of drugs, that by virtue of their high vapor pressure, can be carried by an air current into the nasal passage where they exert their effect. The container from which the inhalant generally is administered is known as an inhaler.

Injections

See *Injections* ⟨1⟩.

Irrigations

Irrigations are sterile solutions intended to bathe or flush open wounds or body cavities. They are used topically, never parenterally. They are labeled to indicate that they are not intended for injection.

Lotions

See *Solutions* or *Suspensions*.

Lozenges

Lozenges are solid preparations, which are intended to dissolve or disintegrate slowly in the mouth. They contain one or more medicaments, usually in a flavored, sweetened base. They can be prepared by molding (gelatin and/or fused sucrose or sorbitol base) or by compression of sugar based tablets. Molded lozenges are sometimes referred to as pastilles while compressed lozenges are often referred to as troches. They are usually intended for treatment of local irritation or infections of the mouth or throat but may contain active ingredients intended for systemic absorption after swallowing.

Ointments

Ointments are semisolid preparations intended for external application to the skin or mucous membranes.

Ointment bases recognized for use as vehicles fall into four general classes: the hydrocarbon bases, the absorption bases, the water-removable bases, and the water-soluble bases. Each therapeutic ointment possesses as its base a representative of one of these four general classes.

Hydrocarbon Bases—These bases, which are known also as "oleaginous ointment bases," are represented by *White Petrolatum* and *White Ointment*. Only small amounts of an aqueous component can be incorporated into them. They serve to keep medicaments in prolonged contact with the skin and act as occlusive dressings. Hydrocarbon bases are used chiefly for their emollient effects, and are difficult to wash off. They do not "dry out" or change noticeably on aging.

Absorption Bases—This class of bases may be divided into two groups: the first group consisting of bases that permit the incorporation of aqueous solutions with the formation of a water-in-oil emulsion (*Hydrophilic Petrolatum* and *Anhydrous Lanolin*), and the second group consisting of water-in-oil emulsions that permit the incorporation of additional quantities of aqueous solutions (*Lanolin*). Absorption bases are useful also as emollients.

Water-removable Bases—Such bases are oil-in-water emulsions, e.g., *Hydrophilic Ointment*, and are more correctly called "creams." (See *Creams*.) They are also described as "water-washable," since they may be readily washed from the skin or clothing with water, an attribute that makes them more acceptable for cosmetic reasons. Some medicaments may be more effective in these bases than in hydrocarbon bases. Other advantages of the water-removable bases are that they may be diluted with water and that they favor the absorption of serous discharges in dermatological conditions.

Water-soluble Bases—This group of so-called "greaseless ointment bases" is comprised of water-soluble constituents. *Polyethylene Glycol Ointment* is the only Pharmacopeial preparation in this group. Bases of this type offer many of the advantages of the water-removable bases and, in addition, contain no water-insoluble substances such as petrolatum, anhydrous lanolin, or waxes. They are more correctly called "Gels." (See *Gels*.)

Choice of Base—The choice of an ointment base depends upon many factors, such as the action desired, the nature of the medicament to be incorporated and its bioavailability and stability, and the requisite shelf-life of the finished product. In some cases, it is necessary to use a base that is less than ideal in order to achieve the stability required. Drugs that hydrolyze rapidly, for example, are more stable in hydrocarbon bases than in bases containing water, even though they may be more effective in the latter.

Ophthalmic Preparations

Drugs are administered to the eyes in a wide variety of dosage forms, some of which require special consideration. They are discussed in the following paragraphs.

Ointments—Ophthalmic ointments are ointments for application to the eye. Special precautions must be taken in the preparation of ophthalmic ointments. They are manufactured from sterilized ingredients under rigidly aseptic conditions and meet the requirements under *Sterility Tests* ⟨71⟩. If the specific ingredients used in the formulation do not lend themselves to routine sterilization techniques, ingredients that meet the sterility requirements described under *Sterility Tests* ⟨71⟩, along with aseptic manufacture, may be employed. Ophthalmic ointments must contain a suitable substance or mixture of substances to prevent growth of, or to destroy, microorganisms accidentally introduced when the container is opened during use, unless otherwise directed in the individual monograph, or unless the formula itself is bacteriostatic (see *Added Substances* under *Ophthalmic Ointments* ⟨771⟩). The medicinal agent is added to the ointment base either as a solution or as a micronized powder. The finished ointment must be free from large particles and must meet the requirements for *Leakage* and for *Metal Particles* under *Ophthalmic Ointments* ⟨771⟩. The immediate containers for ophthalmic ointments shall be sterile at the time of filling and closing. It is mandatory that the immediate containers for ophthalmic ointments be sealed and tamper-proof so that sterility is assured at time of first use.

The ointment base that is selected must be nonirritating to the eye, permit diffusion of the drug throughout the secretions bathing the eye, and retain the activity of the medicament for a reasonable period under proper storage conditions.

Petrolatum is mainly used as a base for ophthalmic drugs. Some absorption bases, water-removable bases, and water-soluble bases may be desirable for water-soluble drugs. Such bases allow for better dispersion of water-soluble medicaments, but they must be nonirritating to the eye.

Solutions—Ophthalmic solutions are sterile solutions, essentially free from foreign particles, suitably compounded and packaged for instillation into the eye. Preparation of an ophthalmic solution requires careful consideration of such factors as the inherent toxicity of the drug itself, isotonicity value, the need for buffering agents, the need for a preservative (and, if needed, its selection), sterilization, and proper packaging. Similar considerations are also made for nasal and otic products.

Isotonicity Value—Lacrimal fluid is isotonic with blood, having an isotonicity value corresponding to that of a 0.9% sodium chloride solution. Ideally, an ophthalmic solution should have this isotonicity value; but the eye can tolerate isotonicity values as low as that of a 0.6% sodium chloride solution and as high as that of a 2.0% sodium chloride solution without marked discomfort.

Some ophthalmic solutions are necessarily hypertonic in order to enhance absorption and provide a concentration of the active ingredient(s) strong enough to exert a prompt and effective action. Where the amount of such solutions used is small, dilution with lacrimal fluid takes place rapidly so that discomfort from the hypertonicity is only temporary. However, any adjustment toward isotonicity by dilution with tears is negligible where large volumes of hypertonic solutions are used as collyria to wash the eyes; it is therefore important that solutions used for this purpose be approximately isotonic.

Buffering—Many drugs, notably alkaloidal salts, are most effective at pH levels that favor the undissociated free bases. At such pH levels, however, the drug may be unstable so that compromise levels must be found and held by means of buffers. One purpose of buffering some ophthalmic solutions is to prevent an increase in pH caused by the slow release of hydroxyl ions by glass. Such a rise in pH can affect both the solubility and the stability of the drug. The decision whether or not buffering agents should be added in preparing an ophthalmic solution must be based on several considerations. Normal tears have a pH of about 7.4 and possess some buffer capacity. The application of a solution to the eye stimulates the flow of tears and the rapid neutralization of any excess hydrogen or hydroxyl ions within the buffer capacity of the tears. Many ophthalmic drugs, such as alkaloidal salts, are weakly acidic and have only weak buffer capacity. Where only 1 or 2 drops of a solution containing them are added to the eye, the buffering action of

the tears is usually adequate to raise the pH and prevent marked discomfort. In some cases pH may vary between 3.5 and 8.5. Some drugs, notably pilocarpine hydrochloride and epinephrine bitartrate, are more acid and overtax the buffer capacity of the lacrimal fluid. Ideally, an ophthalmic solution should have the same pH, as well as the same isotonicity value, as lacrimal fluid. This is not usually possible since, at pH 7.4, many drugs are not appreciably soluble in water. Most alkaloidal salts precipitate as the free alkaloid at this pH. Additionally, many drugs are chemically unstable at pH levels approaching 7.4. This instability is more marked at the high temperatures employed in heat sterilization. For this reason, the buffer system should be selected that is nearest to the physiological pH of 7.4 and does not cause precipitation of the drug or its rapid deterioration.

An ophthalmic preparation with a buffer system approaching the physiological pH can be obtained by mixing a sterile solution of the drug with a sterile buffer solution using aseptic technique. Even so, the possibility of a shorter shelf-life at the higher pH must be taken into consideration, and attention must be directed toward the attainment and maintenance of sterility throughout the manipulations.

Many drugs, when buffered to a therapeutically acceptable pH, would not be stable in solution for long periods of time. These products are lyophilized and are intended for reconstitution immediately before use (e.g., *Acetylcholine Chloride for Ophthalmic Solution*).

Sterilization—The sterility of solutions applied to an injured eye is of the greatest importance. Sterile preparations in special containers for individual use on one patient should be available in every hospital, office, or other installation where accidentally or surgically traumatized eyes are treated. The method of attaining sterility is determined primarily by the character of the particular product (see *Sterilization and Sterility Assurance of Compendial Articles* ⟨1211⟩).

Whenever possible, sterile membrane filtration under aseptic conditions is the preferred method. If it can be shown that product stability is not adversely affected, sterilization by autoclaving in the final container is also a preferred method.

Buffering certain drugs near the physiological pH range makes them quite unstable at high temperature.

Avoiding the use of heat by employing a bacteria-retaining filter is a valuable technique, provided caution is exercised in the selection, assembly, and use of the equipment. Single-filtration, presterilized disposable units are available and should be utilized wherever possible.

Preservation—Ophthalmic solutions may be packaged in multiple-dose containers when intended for the individual use of one patient and where the ocular surfaces are intact. It is mandatory that the immediate containers for ophthalmic solutions be sealed and tamper-proof so that sterility is assured at time of first use. Each solution must contain a suitable substance or mixture of substances to prevent the growth of, or to destroy, microorganisms accidentally introduced when the container is opened during use.

Where intended for use in surgical procedures, ophthalmic solutions, although they must be sterile, should not contain antibacterial agents, since they may be irritating to the ocular tissues.

Thickening agent—A pharmaceutical grade of methylcellulose (e.g., 1% if the viscosity is 25 centipoises, or 0.25% if 4000 centipoises) or other suitable thickening agents such as hydroxypropyl methylcellulose or polyvinyl alcohol occasionally are added to ophthalmic solutions to increase the viscosity and prolong contact of the drug with the tissue. The thickened ophthalmic solution must be free from visible particles.

Suspensions—Ophthalmic suspensions are sterile liquid preparations containing solid particles dispersed in a liquid vehicle intended for application to the eye (see *Suspensions*). It is imperative that such suspensions contain the drug in a micronized form to prevent irritation and/or scratching of the cornea. Ophthalmic suspensions should never be dispensed if there is evidence of caking or aggregation.

Strips—Fluorescein sodium solution should be dispensed in a sterile, single-use container or in the form of a sterile, impregnated paper strip. The strip releases a sufficient amount of the drug for diagnostic purposes when touched to the eye being examined for a foreign body or a corneal abrasion. Contact of the paper with the eye may be avoided by leaching the drug from the strip onto the eye with the aid of sterile water or sterile sodium chloride solution.

Pastes

Pastes are semisolid dosage forms that contain one or more drug substances intended for topical application. One class is made from a single phase aqueous gel (e.g., *Carboxymethylcellulose Sodium Paste*). The other class, the fatty pastes (e.g., *Zinc Oxide Paste*), consists of thick, stiff ointments that do not ordinarily flow at body temperature, and therefore serve as protective coatings over the areas to which they are applied.

The fatty pastes appear less greasy and more absorptive than ointments by reason of a high proportion of drug substance(s) having an affinity for water. These pastes tend to absorb serous secretions, and are less penetrating and less macerating than ointments, so that they are preferred for acute lesions that have a tendency towards crusting, vesiculation, or oozing.

A dental paste is intended for adhesion to the mucous membrane for local effect (e.g., *Triamcinolone Acetonide Dental Paste*).

Pellets

See *Implants*.

Powders

Powders are intimate mixtures of dry, finely divided drugs and/or chemicals that may be intended for internal (Oral Powders) or external (Topical Powders) use. Because of their greater specific surface area, powders disperse and dissolve more readily than compacted dosage forms. Children and those adults who experience difficulty in swallowing tablets or capsules may find powders more acceptable. Drugs that are too bulky to be formed into tablets or capsules of convenient size may be administered as powders. Immediately prior to use, oral powders are mixed in a beverage or apple sauce.

Often, stability problems encountered in liquid dosage forms are avoided in powdered dosage forms. Drugs that are unstable in aqueous suspensions or solutions may be prepared in the form of granules or powders. These are intended to be constituted by the pharmacist by the addition of a specified quantity of water just prior to dispensing. Because these constituted products have limited stability, they are required to have a specified expiration date after constitution and may require storage in a refrigerator.

Oral powders may be dispensed in doses premeasured by the pharmacist, i.e., divided powders, or in bulk. Traditionally, divided powders have been wrapped in materials such as bond paper and parchment. However, the pharmacist may provide greater protection from the environment by sealing individual doses in small cellophane or polyethylene envelopes.

Bulk oral powders are limited to relatively nonpotent drugs such as laxatives, antacids, dietary supplements, and certain analgesics that the patient may safely measure by the teaspoonful or capful. Other bulky powders include douche powders, tooth powders, and dusting powders. Bulk powders are best dispensed in tight, wide-mouth glass containers to afford maximum protection from the atmosphere and to prevent the loss of volatile constituents.

Dusting powders are impalpable powders intended for topical application. They may be dispensed in sifter-top containers to facilitate dusting onto the skin. In general, dusting powders should be passed through at least a 100-mesh sieve to assure freedom from grit that could irritate traumatized areas (see *Powder Fineness* ⟨811⟩).

Solutions

Solutions are liquid preparations that contain one or more chemical substances dissolved, i.e., molecularly dispersed, in a suitable solvent or mixture of mutually miscible solvents. Since molecules in solutions are uniformly dispersed, the use of solutions as dosage forms generally provides for the assurance of uniform dosage upon administration, and good accuracy when diluting or otherwise mixing solutions.

Substances in solutions, however, are more susceptible to chemical instability than the solid state and dose for dose, generally require more bulk and weight in packaging relative to solid dosage forms. For all solutions, but particularly those containing volatile solvents, tight containers, stored away from excessive heat, should be used. Consideration should also be given to the use of light-resistant containers when photolytic chemical degradation is a potential stability problem. Dosage forms categorized as "Solutions" are classified according to route of administration, such as "Oral Solutions" and "Topical Solutions," or by their solute and solvent systems, such as "Spirits," "Tinctures," and "Waters." Solutions intended for parenteral administration are officially entitled, "Injections" (see *Injections* ⟨1⟩).

Oral Solutions—Oral Solutions are liquid preparations, intended for oral administration, that contain one or more substances with or without flavoring, sweetening, or coloring agents dissolved in water or cosolvent-water mixtures. Oral Solutions may be formulated for direct oral administration to the patient or they may be dispensed in a more concentrated form that must be diluted prior to administration. It is important to recognize that dilution with water of Oral Solutions containing cosolvents, such as alcohol, could lead to precipitation of some ingredients. Hence, great care must be taken in diluting concentrated solutions when cosolvents are present. Preparations dispensed as soluble solids or soluble mixtures of solids, with the intent of dissolving them in a solvent and administering them orally, are designated "for Oral Solution" (e.g., *Potassium Chloride for Oral Solution*).

Oral Solutions containing high concentrations of sucrose or other sugars traditionally have been designated as Syrups. A near-saturated solution of sucrose in purified water, for example, is known as Syrup or "Simple Syrup." Through common usage the term, syrup, also has been used to include any other liquid dosage form prepared in a sweet and viscid vehicle, including oral suspensions.

In addition to sucrose and other sugars, certain polyols such as sorbitol or glycerin may be present in Oral Solutions to inhibit crystallization and to modify solubility, taste, mouth-feel, and other vehicle properties. Antimicrobial agents to prevent the growth of bacteria, yeasts, and molds are generally also present. Some sugarless Oral Solutions contain sweetening agents such as sorbitol or aspartame, as well as thickening agents such as the cellulose gums. Such viscid sweetened solutions, containing no sugars, are occasionally prepared as vehicles for administration of drugs to diabetic patients.

Many oral solutions, which contain alcohol as a cosolvent, have been traditionally designated as Elixirs. Many others, however, designated as Oral Solutions, also contain significant amounts of alcohol. Since high concentrations of alcohol can produce a pharmacologic effect when administered orally, other cosolvents, such as glycerin and propylene glycol, should be used to minimize the amount of alcohol required. To be designated as an Elixir, however, the solution must contain alcohol.

Topical Solutions—Topical Solutions are solutions, usually aqueous but often containing other solvents, such as alcohol and polyols, intended for topical application to the skin, or as in the case of Lidocaine Oral Topical Solution, to the oral mucosal surface. The term "lotion" is applied to solutions or suspensions applied topically.

Otic Solutions—Otic Solutions, intended for instillation in the outer ear, are aqueous, or they are solutions prepared with glycerin or other solvents and dispersing agents (e.g., *Antipyrine and Benzocaine Otic Solution* and *Neomycin and Polymyxin B Sulfates and Hydrocortisone Otic Solution*).

Ophthalmic Solutions (See *Ophthalmic Preparations*.)

Spirits—Spirits are alcoholic or hydroalcoholic solutions of volatile substances prepared usually by simple solution or by admixture of the ingredients. Some spirits serve as flavoring agents while others have medicinal value. Reduction of the high alcoholic content of spirits by admixture with aqueous preparations often causes turbidity.

Spirits require storage in tight, light-resistant containers to prevent loss by evaporation and to limit oxidative changes.

Tinctures—Tinctures are alcoholic or hydroalcoholic solutions prepared from vegetable materials or from chemical substances.

The proportion of drug represented in the different chemical tinctures is not uniform but varies according to the established standards for each. Traditionally, tinctures of potent vegetable drugs essentially represent the activity of 10 g of the drug in each 100 mL of tincture, the potency being adjusted following assay. Most other vegetable tinctures represent 20 g of the respective vegetable material in each 100 mL of tincture.

Process P—Carefully mix the ground drug or mixture of drugs with a sufficient quantity of the prescribed solvent or solvent mixture to render it evenly and distinctly damp, allow it to stand for 15 minutes, transfer it to a suitable percolator, and pack the drug firmly. Pour on enough of the prescribed solvent or solvent mixture to saturate the drug, cover the top of the percolator and, when the liquid is about to drip from the percolator, close the lower orifice, and allow the drug to macerate for 24 hours or for the time specified in the monograph. If no assay is directed, allow the percolation to proceed slowly, or at the specified rate, gradually adding sufficient solvent or solvent mixture to produce 1000 mL of tincture, and mix (for definitions of flow rates, see under *Fluidextracts*). If an assay is directed, collect only 950 mL of percolate, mix this, and assay a portion of it as directed. Dilute the remainder with such quantity of the prescribed solvent or solvent mixture as calculation from the assay indicates is necessary to produce a tincture that conforms to the prescribed standard, and mix.

Process M—Macerate the drug with 750 mL of the prescribed solvent or solvent mixture in a container that can be closed, and put in a warm place. Agitate it frequently during 3 days or until the soluble matter is dissolved. Transfer the mixture to a filter, and when most of the liquid has drained away, wash the residue on the filter with a sufficient quantity of the prescribed solvent or solvent mixture, combining the filtrates, to produce 1000 mL of tincture, and mix.

Tinctures require storage in tight, light-resistant containers, away from direct sunlight and excessive heat.

Waters, Aromatic—Aromatic waters are clear, saturated aqueous solutions (unless otherwise specified) of volatile oils or other aromatic or volatile substances. Their odors and tastes are similar, respectively, to those of the drugs or volatile substances from which they are prepared, and they are free from empyreumatic and other foreign odors. Aromatic waters may be prepared by distillation or solution of the aromatic substance, with or without the use of a dispersing agent.

Aromatic waters require protection from intense light and excessive heat.

Suppositories

Suppositories are solid bodies of various weights and shapes, adapted for introduction into the rectal, vaginal, or urethral orifice of the human body. They usually melt, soften, or dissolve at body temperature. A suppository may act as a protectant or palliative to the local tissues at the point of introduction or as a carrier of therapeutic agents for systemic or local action. Suppository bases usually employed are cocoa butter, glycerinated gelatin, hydrogenated vegetable oils, mixtures of polyethylene glycols of various molecular weights, and fatty acid esters of polyethylene glycol.

The suppository base employed has a marked influence on the release of the active ingredient incorporated in it. While cocoa butter melts quickly at body temperature, it is immiscible with body fluids and this inhibits the diffusion of fat-soluble drugs to the affected sites. Polyethylene glycol is a suitable base for some antiseptics. In cases where systemic action is expected, it is preferable to incorporate the ionized rather than the nonionized form of the drug, in order to maximize bioavailability. Although un-ionized drugs partition more readily out of water-miscible bases such as glycerinated gelatin and polyethylene glycol, the bases themselves tend to dissolve very slowly and thus retard release in this manner. Oleaginous vehicles such as cocoa butter are seldom used in vaginal preparations because of the nonabsorbable residue formed, while glycerinated gelatin is seldom used rectally because of its slow dissolution. Cocoa butter and its substitutes (Hard Fat) are superior for allaying irritation, as in preparations intended for treating internal hemorrhoids.

Cocoa Butter Suppositories—Suppositories having cocoa butter as the base may be made by means of incorporating the finely divided medicinal substance into the solid oil at room temperature and suitably shaping the resulting mass, or by working with the oil in the melted state and allowing the resulting suspension to cool in molds. A suitable quantity of hardening agents may be added to counteract the tendency of some medicaments such as chloral hydrate and phenol to soften the base. It is important that the finished suppository melt at body temperature.

The approximate weights of suppositories prepared with cocoa butter are given below. Suppositories prepared from other bases vary in weight and generally are heavier than the weights indicated here.

Rectal Suppositories for adults are tapered at one or both ends and usually weigh about 2 g each.

Vaginal Suppositories are usually globular or oviform and weigh about 5 g each. They are made from water soluble or water miscible vehicles such as polyethylene glycol or glycerinated gelatin.

Suppositories with cocoa butter base require storage in well-closed containers, preferably at a temperature below 30 °C (controlled room temperature).

Cocoa Butter Substitutes—Fat-type suppository bases can be produced from a variety of vegetable oils, such as coconut or palm kernel, which are modified by esterification, hydrogenation, and fractionation to obtain products of varying composition and melting temperatures (e.g., *Hydrogenated Vegetable Oil* and *Hard Fat*). These products can be so designed as to reduce rancidity. At the same time, desired characteristics such as narrow intervals between melting and solidification temperatures, and melting ranges to accommodate various formulation and climatic conditions, can be built in.

Glycerinated Gelatin Suppositories—Medicinal substances may be incorporated into glycerinated gelatin bases by addition of the prescribed quantities to a vehicle consisting of about 70 parts of glycerin, 20 parts of gelatin, and 10 parts of water.

Glycerinated gelatin suppositories require storage in tight containers, preferably at a temperature below 35 °C.

Polyethylene Glycol–Base Suppositories—Several combinations of polyethylene glycols having melting temperatures that are above body temperature have been used as suppository bases. Inasmuch as release from these bases depends on dissolution rather than on melting, there are significantly fewer problems in preparation and storage than exist with melting-type vehicles. However, high concentrations of higher molecular weight polyethylene glycols may lengthen dissolution time, resulting in problems with retention. Labels on polyethylene glycol suppositories should contain directions that they be moistened with water before inserting. Although they can be stored without refrigeration, they should be packaged in tightly closed containers.

Surfactant Suppository Bases—Several nonionic surface-active agents closely related chemically to the polyethylene glycols can be used as suppository vehicles. Examples of such surfactants are polyoxyethylene sorbitan fatty acid esters and the polyoxyethylene stearates. These surfactants are used alone or in combination with other suppository vehicles to yield a wide range of melting temperatures and consistencies. One of the major advantages of such vehicles is their water-dispersibility. However, care must be taken with the use of surfactants, because they may either increase the rate of drug absorption or interact with drug molecules, causing a decrease in therapeutic activity.

Tableted Suppositories or Inserts—Vaginal suppositories occasionally are prepared by the compression of powdered materials into a suitable shape. They are prepared also by encapsulation in soft gelatin.

Suspensions

Suspensions are liquid preparations that consist of solid particles dispersed throughout a liquid phase in which the particles are not soluble. Dosage forms officially categorized as Suspensions are designated as such if they are not included in other more specific categories of suspensions, such as Oral Suspensions, Topical Suspensions, etc. (see these other categories). Some suspensions are prepared and ready for use, while others are prepared as solid mixtures intended for constitution just before use with an appropriate vehicle. Such products are designated "for Oral Suspension," etc. The term, Milk, is sometimes used for suspensions in aqueous vehicles intended for oral administration (e.g., *Milk of Magnesia*). The term, Magma, is often used to describe suspensions of inorganic solids such as clays in water, where there is a tendency for strong hydration and aggregation of the solid, giving rise to gel-like consistency and thixotropic rheological behavior (e.g., *Bentonite Magma*). The term, Lotion, has been used to categorize many topical suspensions and emulsions intended for application to the skin (e.g., *Calamine Lotion*). Some suspensions are prepared in sterile form and are used as Injectables, as well as for ophthalmic and otic administration. These may be of two types, ready to use or intended for constitution with a prescribed amount of Water for Injection or other suitable diluent before use by the designated route. Suspensions should not be injected intravenously or intrathecally.

Suspensions intended for any route of administration should contain suitable antimicrobial agents to protect against bacteria, yeast, and mold contamination (see *Emulsions* for some consideration of antimicrobial preservative properties that apply also to Suspensions). By its very nature, the particular matter in a suspension may settle or sediment to the bottom of the container upon standing. Such sedimentation may also lead to caking and solidification of the sediment with a resulting difficulty in redispersing the suspension upon agitation. To prevent such problems, suitable ingredients that increase viscosity and the gel state of the suspension, such as clays, surfactants, polyols, polymers, or sugars, should be added. It is important that suspensions always be shaken well before use to ensure uniform distribution of the solid in the vehicle, thereby ensuring uniform and proper dosage. Suspensions require storage in tight containers.

Oral Suspensions—Oral Suspensions are liquid preparations containing solid particles dispersed in a liquid vehicle, with suitable flavoring agents, intended for oral administration. Some suspensions labeled as Milks or Magmas fall into this category.

Topical Suspensions—Topical Suspensions are liquid preparations containing solid particles dispersed in a liquid vehicle, intended for application to the skin. Some suspensions labeled as Lotions fall into this category.

Otic Suspensions—Otic Suspensions are liquid preparations containing micronized particles intended for instillation in the outer ear.

Ophthalmic Suspensions—(See *Ophthalmic Preparations*).

Syrups

See *Solutions*.

Systems

In recent years, a number of dosage forms have been developed using modern technology that allows for the uniform release or targeting of drugs to the body. These products are commonly called delivery systems. The most widely used of these are Transdermal Systems.

Transdermal Systems—Transdermal drug delivery systems are self-contained, discrete dosage forms that, when applied to intact skin, are designed to deliver the drug(s) through the skin to the systemic circulation. Systems typically comprise an outer covering (barrier), a drug reservoir, which may have a rate controlling membrane, a contact adhesive applied to some or all parts of the system and the system/skin interface, and a protective liner that is removed before applying the system. The activity of these systems is defined in terms of the release rate of the drug(s) from the system. The total duration of drug release from the system and the system surface area may also be stated.

Transdermal drug delivery systems work by diffusion: the drug diffuses from the drug reservoir, directly or through the rate controlling membrane and/or contact adhesive if present, and then through the skin into the general circulation. Typically, modified-release systems are designed to provide drug delivery at a constant rate, such that a true steady state blood concentration is achieved and maintained until the system is removed. At that time, blood concentration declines at a rate consistent with the pharmacokinetics of the drug.

Transdermal drug delivery systems are applied to body areas consistent with the labeling for the product(s). As long as drug concentration at the system/skin interface remains constant, the amount of drug in the dosage form does not influence plasma concentrations. The functional lifetime of the system is defined by the initial amount of drug in the reservoir and the release rate from the reservoir.

NOTE—Drugs for local rather than systemic effect are commonly applied to the skin embedded in glue on a cloth or plastic backing. These products are defined traditionally as plasters or tapes.

Ocular System—Another type of system is the ocular system, which is intended for placement in the lower conjunctival fornix from which the drug diffuses through a membrane at a constant rate over a seven-day period (e.g., *Pilocarpine Ocular System*).

Intrauterine System—An intrauterine system, based on a similar principle but intended for release of drug over a much longer period of time, i.e., one year, is also available (e.g., *Progesterone Intrauterine Contraceptive System*).

Tablets

Tablets are solid dosage forms containing medicinal substances with or without suitable diluents. They may be classed, according to the method of manufacture, as molded tablets or compressed tablets.

The vast majority of all tablets manufactured are made by compression, and compressed tablets are the most widely used dosage form in this country. Compressed tablets are prepared by the application of high pressures, utilizing steel punches and dies, to powders or granulations. Tablets can be produced in a wide variety of sizes, shapes, and surface markings, depending upon the design of the punches and dies. Capsule-shaped tablets are commonly referred to as caplets. Boluses are large tablets intended for veterinary use, usually for large animals.

Molded tablets are prepared by forcing dampened powders under low pressure into die cavities. Solidification depends upon crystal bridges built up during the subsequent drying process, and not upon the compaction force.

Tablet triturates are small, usually cylindrical, molded or compressed tablets. Tablet triturates were traditionally used as dispensing tablets in order to provide a convenient, measured quantity of a potent drug for compounding purposes. Such tablets are rarely used today. Hypodermic tablets are molded tablets made from completely and readily water-soluble ingredients and formerly were intended for use in making preparations for hypodermic injection. They are employed orally, or where rapid drug availability is required such as in the case of *Nitroglycerin Tablets*, sublingually.

Buccal tablets are intended to be inserted in the buccal pouch, and sublingual tablets are intended to be inserted beneath the tongue, where the active ingredient is absorbed directly through the oral mucosa. Few drugs are readily absorbed in this way, but for those that are (such as nitroglycerin and certain steroid hormones), a number of advantages may result.

Soluble, effervescent tablets are prepared by compression and contain, in addition to active ingredients, mixtures of acids (citric acid, tartaric acid) and sodium bicarbonate, which release carbon dioxide when dissolved in water. They are intended to be dissolved or dispersed in water before administration. Effervescent tablets should be stored in tightly closed containers or moisture-proof packs and labeled to indicate that they are not to be swallowed directly.

CHEWABLE TABLETS

Chewable tablets are intended to be chewed, producing a pleasant tasting residue in the oral cavity that is easily swallowed and does not leave a bitter or unpleasant after-taste. These tablets have been used in tablet formulations for children, especially multivitamin formulations, and for the administration of antacids and selected antibiotics. Chewable tablets are prepared by compression, usually utilizing mannitol, sorbitol, or sucrose as binders and fillers, and containing colors and flavors to enhance their appearance and taste.

PREPARATION OF MOLDED TABLETS

Molded tablets are prepared from mixtures of medicinal substances and a diluent usually consisting of lactose and powdered sucrose in varying proportions. The powders are dampened with solutions containing high percentages of alcohol. The concentration of alcohol depends upon the solubility of the active ingredients and fillers in the solvent system and the desired degree of hardness of the finished tablets. The dampened powders are pressed into molds, removed, and allowed to dry. Molded tablets are quite friable and care must be taken in packaging and dispensing.

FORMULATION OF COMPRESSED TABLETS

Most compressed tablets consist of the active ingredient and a diluent (filler), binder, disintegrating agent, and lubricant. Approved FD&C and D&C dyes or lakes (dyes adsorbed onto insoluble aluminum hydroxide), flavors, and sweetening agents may also be present. Diluents are added where the quantity of active ingredient is small or difficult to compress. Common tablet fillers include lactose, starch, dibasic calcium phosphate, and microcrystalline cellulose. Chewable tablets often contain sucrose, mannitol, or sorbitol as a filler. Where the amount of active ingredient is small, the overall tableting properties are in large measure determined by the filler. Because of problems encountered with bioavailability of hydrophobic drugs of low water-solubility, water-soluble diluents are used as fillers for these tablets.

Binders give adhesiveness to the powder during the preliminary granulation and to the compressed tablet. They add to the cohesive strength already available in the diluent. While binders may be added dry, they are more effective when added out of solution. Common binders include acacia, gelatin, sucrose, povidone, methylcellulose, carboxymethylcellulose, and hydrolyzed starch pastes. The most effective dry binder is microcrystalline cellulose, which is commonly used for this purpose in tablets prepared by direct compression.

A disintegrating agent serves to assist in the fragmentation of the tablet after administration. The most widely used tablet disintegrating agent is starch. Chemically modified starches and cellulose, alginic acid, microcrystalline cellulose, and cross-linked povidone, are also used for this purpose. Effervescent mixtures are used in soluble tablet systems as disintegrating agents. The concentration of the disintegrating agent, method of addition, and degree of compaction play a role in effectiveness.

Lubricants reduce friction during the compression and ejection cycle. In addition, they aid in preventing adherence of tablet material to the dies and punches. Metallic stearates, stearic acid, hydrogenated vegetable oils, and talc are used as lubricants. Because of the nature of this function, most lubricants are hydrophobic, and as such tend to reduce the rates of tablet disintegration and dissolution. Consequently, excessive concentrations of lubricant should be avoided. Polyethylene glycols and some lauryl sulfate salts have been used as soluble lubricants, but such agents generally do not possess optimal lubricating properties, and comparatively high concentrations are usually required.

Glidants are agents that improve powder fluidity, and they are commonly employed in direct compression where no granulation step is involved. The most effective glidants are the colloidal pyrogenic silicas.

Colorants are often added to tablet formulations for esthetic value or for product identification. Both D&C and FD&C dyes and lakes are used. Most dyes are photosensitive and they fade when exposed to light. The federal Food and Drug Administration regulates the colorants employed in drugs.

MANUFACTURE

Tablets are prepared by three general methods: wet granulation, dry granulation (roll compaction or slugging), and direct compression. The purpose of both wet and dry granulation is to improve flow of the mixture and/or to enhance its compressibility.

Dry granulation (slugging) involves the compaction of powders at high pressures into large, often poorly formed tablet compacts. These compacts are then milled and screened to form a granulation of the desired particle size. The advantage of dry granulation is the elimination of both heat and moisture in the processing. Dry granulations can be produced also by extruding powders between hydraulically operated rollers to produce thin cakes which are subsequently screened or milled to give the desired granule size.

Excipients are available that allow production of tablets at high speeds without prior granulation steps. These directly compressible excipients consist of special physical forms of substances such as lactose, sucrose, dextrose, or cellulose, which possess the desirable properties of fluidity and compressibility.

The most widely used direct-compaction fillers are microcrystalline cellulose, anhydrous lactose, spray-dried lactose, compressible sucrose, and some forms of modified starches. Direct compression avoids many of the problems associated with wet and dry granulations. However, the inherent physical properties of the individual filler materials are highly critical, and minor variations can alter flow and compression characteristics so as to make them unsuitable for direct compression.

Physical evidence of poor tablet quality is discussed under *Stability Considerations in Dispensing Practice* ⟨1191⟩.

Weight Variation and Content Uniformity—Tablets are required to meet a weight variation test (see *Uniformity of Dosage Units* ⟨905⟩) where the active ingredient comprises a major portion of the tablet and where control of weight may be presumed to be an adequate control of drug content uniformity. Weight variation is not an adequate indication of content uniformity where the drug substance comprises a relatively minor portion of the tablet, or where the tablet is sugar-coated. Thus, the Pharmacopeia generally requires that coated tablets and tablets containing 50 mg or less of active ingredient, comprising less than 50% by weight of the dosage-form unit, pass a content uniformity test (see *Uniformity of Dosage Units* ⟨905⟩), wherein individual tablets are assayed for actual drug content.

Disintegration and Dissolution—Disintegration is an essential attribute of tablets intended for administration by mouth, except those intended to be chewed before being swallowed and except some types of extended-release tablets. A disintegration test is provided (see *Disintegration* ⟨701⟩), and limits on the times in which disintegration is to take place, appropriate for the types of tablets concerned, are given in the individual monographs.

For drugs of limited water-solubility, dissolution may be a more meaningful quality attribute than disintegration. A dissolution test (see *Dissolution* ⟨711⟩) is required in a number of monographs on tablets. In many cases, it is possible to correlate dissolution rates with biological availability of the active ingredient. However, such tests are useful mainly as a means of screening preliminary formulations and as a routine quality-control procedure.

COATINGS

Tablets may be coated for a variety of reasons, including protection of the ingredients from air, moisture, or light, masking of unpleasant tastes and odors, improvement of appearance, and control of the site of drug release in the gastrointestinal tract.

Plain Coated Tablets—Classically, tablets have been coated with sugar applied from aqueous suspensions containing insoluble powders such as starch, calcium carbonate, talc, or titanium dioxide, suspended by means of acacia or gelatin. For purposes of identification and esthetic value, the outside coatings may be colored. The finished coated tablets are polished by application of dilute solutions of wax in solvents such as chloroform or powdered mix. Water-protective coatings consisting of substances such as shellac or cellulose acetate phthalate are often applied out of nonaqueous solvents prior to application of sugar coats. Excessive quantities should be avoided. Drawbacks of sugar coating include the lengthy time necessary for application, the need for waterproofing, which also adversely affects dissolution, and the increased bulk of the finished tablet. These factors have resulted in increased acceptance of film coatings. Film coatings consist of water-soluble or dispersible materials such as hydroxypropyl methylcellulose, methylcellulose, hydroxypropylcellulose, carboxymethylcellulose sodium, and mixtures of cellulose acetate phthalate and polyethylene glycols applied out of nonaqueous or aqueous solvents. Evaporation of the solvents leaves a thin film that adheres directly to the tablet and allows it to retain the original shape, including grooves or identification codes.

Enteric-coated Tablets—Where the drug may be destroyed or inactivated by the gastric juice or where it may irritate the gastric mucosa, the use of "enteric" coatings is indicated. Such coatings are intended to delay the release of the medication until the tablet has passed through the stomach. The term "delayed-release" is used for Pharmacopeial purposes, and the individual monographs include tests and specifications for *Drug release* (see *Drug Release* ⟨724⟩).

Extended-release Tablets—Extended-release tablets are formulated in such manner as to make the contained medicament available over an extended period of time following ingestion. Expressions such as "prolonged-action," "repeat-action," and "sustained-release" have also been used to describe such dosage forms. However, the term "extended-release" is used for Pharmacopeial purposes, and requirements for *Drug release* typically are specified in the individual monographs.

⟨1191⟩ STABILITY CONSIDERATIONS IN DISPENSING PRACTICE

NOTE—Inasmuch as this chapter is for purposes of general information only, no statement in the chapter is intended to modify or supplant any of the specific requirements pertinent to Pharmacopeial articles, which are given elsewhere in this Pharmacopeia.

Aspects of drug product stability that are of primary concern to the pharmacist in the dispensing of medications are discussed herein.

Stability is defined as the extent to which a product retains, within specified limits, and throughout its period of storage and use, i.e., its shelf-life, the same properties and characteristics that it possessed at the time of its manufacture. Five types of stability generally recognized are shown in the accompanying table.

Factors Affecting Product Stability

Each ingredient, whether therapeutically active or inactive, in a dosage form can affect stability. Environmental factors, such as temperature, radiation, light, air (specifically oxygen, carbon dioxide, and water vapor), and humidity also can affect stability. Similarly, such factors as particle size, pH, the properties of water and other solvents employed, the nature of the container, and the presence of other chemicals resulting from contamination or from the intentional mixing of different products can influence stability.

Criteria for Acceptable Levels of Stability

Type of Stability	Conditions Maintained Throughout the Shelf-Life of the Drug Product
Chemical	Each active ingredient retains its chemical integrity and labeled potency, within the specified limits.
Physical	The original physical properties, including appearance, palatability, uniformity, dissolution, and suspendability are retained.
Microbiological	Sterility or resistance to microbial growth is retained according to the specified requirements. Antimicrobial agents that are present retain effectiveness within the specified limits.
Therapeutic	The therapeutic effect remains unchanged.
Toxicological	No significant increase in toxicity occurs.

Stability Studies in Manufacturing

The scope and design of a stability study vary according to the product and the manufacturer concerned. Ordinarily the formulator of a product first determines the effects of temperature, light, air, pH, moisture, and trace metals, and commonly used excipients or solvents on the active ingredient(s). From this information, one or more formulations of each dosage form are prepared, packaged in suitable containers, and stored under a variety of environmental conditions, both exaggerated and normal. At appropriate time intervals, samples of the product are assayed for potency by use of a stability-indicating method, observed for physical changes, and, where applicable, tested for sterility and/or for resistance to microbial growth and for toxicity and bioavailability. Such a study in combination with clinical and toxicological results enables the manufacturer to select the optimum formulation and container, and to assign recommended storage conditions and an expiration date for each dosage form in its package.

Responsibility of the Pharmacist

The pharmacist helps to ensure that the products under his supervision meet acceptable criteria of stability by (1) dispensing oldest stock first and observance of expiration dates; (2) storing products under the environmental conditions stated in the individual monographs and/or in the labeling; (3) observing products for evidence of instability; (4) properly treating and labeling products that are repackaged, diluted, or mixed with other products; (5) dispensing in the proper container with the proper closure; and (6) informing and educating patients concerning the proper storage and use of the products, including the disposition of outdated or excessively aged prescriptions.

Rotating Stock and Observance of Expiration Dates—Proper rotation of stock is necessary to ensure the dispensing of suitable products. A product that is dispensed on an infrequent basis should be closely monitored so that old stocks are given special attention, particularly with regard to expiration dates. The manufacturer can guarantee the quality of a product up to the time designated as its expiration date only if the product has been stored in the original container under recommended storage conditions.

Storage under Recommended Environmental Conditions—In most instances, the recommended storage conditions are stated on the label, in which case it is imperative to adhere to those conditions. They may include a specified temperature range or a designated storage place or condition (e.g., "refrigerator," or "controlled room temperature") as defined in the General Notices. Supplemental instructions, such as a direction to protect the product from light, also should be followed carefully. Where a product is required to be protected from light and is in a clear or translucent container enclosed in an opaque outer covering, such outer covering is not to be removed and discarded until the contents have been used. In the absence of specific instructions, the product should be stored at controlled room temperature (see *Storage Temperature* in the *General Notices*). The product should be stored away from locations where excessive or variable heat, cold, or light prevails, such as near heating pipes or fluorescent lighting.

Observing Products for Evidence of Instability—Loss of potency usually results from a chemical change, the most common reactions being hydrolysis, oxidation-reduction, and photolysis. Chemical changes may occur also through interaction between ingredients within a product, or rarely between product and container. An apparent loss of potency in the active ingredient(s) may result from diffusion of the drug into or its combination with the surface of the container-closure system. An apparent gain in potency usually is caused by solvent evaporation or by leaching of materials from the container-closure system.

The chemical potency of the active ingredient(s) is required to remain within the limits specified in the monograph definition. Potency is determined by means of an assay procedure that differentiates between the intact molecule and its degradation products; and chemical stability data should be available from the manufacturer. Although chemical degradation ordinarily cannot be detected by the pharmacist, excessive chemical degradation sometimes is accompanied by observable physical

changes. In addition, some physical changes not necessarily related to chemical potency, such as change in color and odor, or formation of a precipitate, or clouding of solution, may serve to alert the pharmacist to the possibility of a stability problem. It should be assumed that a product that has undergone a physical change not explained in the labeling may also have undergone a chemical change and such a product is never to be dispensed. Excessive microbial growth and/or contamination also may appear as a physical change. A gross change in a physical characteristic such as color or odor is a sign of instability in any product. Other common physical signs of deterioration of dosage forms include the following.

SOLID DOSAGE FORMS—Many solid dosage forms are designed for storage under low-moisture conditions. They require protection from environmental water, and therefore should be stored in tight containers (see *Containers* in the *General Notices*) or in the container supplied by the manufacturer. The appearance of fog or liquid droplets, or clumping of the product, inside the container signifies improper conditions. The presence of a desiccant inside the manufacturer's container indicates that special care should be taken in dispensing. Some degradation products, for example, salicylic acid from aspirin, may sublime and be deposited as crystals on the outside of the dosage form or on the walls of the container.

Hard and Soft Gelatin Capsules—Since the capsule formulation is encased in a gelatin shell, a change in gross physical appearance or consistency, including hardening or softening of the shell, is the primary evidence of instability. Evidence of release of gas, such as a distended paper seal, is another sign of instability.

Uncoated Tablets—Evidence of physical instability in uncoated tablets may be shown by excessive powder and/or pieces (i.e., crumbling as distinct from breakage) of tablet at the bottom of the container (from abraded, crushed, or broken tablets); cracks or chips in tablet surfaces; swelling; mottling; discoloration; fusion between tablets; or the appearance of crystals that obviously are not part of the tablet itself on the container walls or on the tablets.

Coated Tablets—Evidence of physical instability in coated tablets is shown by cracks, mottling, or tackiness in the coating and the clumping of tablets.

Dry Powders and Granules—Dry powders and granules that are not intended for constitution into a liquid form in the original container may cake into hard masses or change color, which may render them unacceptable.

Powders and Granules Intended for Constitution as Solutions or Suspensions—Dry powders and granules intended for constitution into solutions or suspensions require special attention. Usually such forms are those antibiotics or vitamins that are particularly sensitive to moisture. Since they are always dispensed in the original container, they generally are not subject to contamination by moisture. However, an unusual caked appearance necessitates careful evaluation, and the presence of a fog or liquid droplets inside the container generally renders the preparation unfit for use. Presence of an objectionable odor also may be evidence of instability.

Effervescent Tablets, Granules, and Powders—Effervescent products are particularly sensitive to moisture. Swelling of the mass or development of gas pressure is a specific sign of instability, indicating that some of the effervescent action has occurred prematurely.

LIQUID DOSAGE FORMS—Of primary concern with respect to liquid dosage forms are homogeneity and freedom from excessive microbial contamination and growth. Instability may be indicated by cloudiness or precipitation in a solution, breaking of an emulsion, non-resuspendable caking of a suspension, or organoleptic changes. Microbial growth may be accompanied by discoloration, turbidity, or gas formation.

Solutions, Elixirs, and Syrups—Precipitation and evidence of microbial or chemical gas formation are the two major signs of instability.

Emulsions—The breaking of an emulsion, i.e., separation of an oil phase that is not easily dispersed, is a characteristic sign of instability; this is not to be confused with creaming, an easily redispersible separation of the oil phase that is a common occurrence with stable emulsions.

Suspensions—A caked solid phase that cannot be resuspended by a reasonable amount of shaking is a primary indication of instability in a suspension. The presence of relatively large particles may mean that excessive crystal growth has occurred.

Tinctures and Fluidextracts—Tinctures, fluidextracts, and similar preparations usually are dark in color because they are concentrated, and thus they should be scrutinized carefully for evidence of precipitation.

Sterile Liquids—Maintenance of sterility is of course critical for sterile liquids. The presence of microbial contamination in sterile liquids usually cannot be detected visually, but any haze, color change, cloudiness, surface film, particulate or flocculent matter, or gas formation is sufficient reason to suspect possible contamination. Clarity of sterile solutions intended for ophthalmic or parenteral use is of utmost importance. Evidence that the integrity of the seal has been violated on such products should make them suspect.

SEMISOLIDS (CREAMS, OINTMENTS, AND SUPPOSITORIES)—For creams, ointments, and suppositories, the primary indication of instability is often either discoloration or a noticeable change in consistency or odor.

Creams—Unlike ointments, creams usually are emulsions containing water and oil. Indications of instability in creams are emulsion breakage, crystal growth, shrinking due to evaporation of water, and gross microbial contamination.

Ointments—Common signs of instability in ointments are a change in consistency and excessive "bleeding," i.e., separation of excessive amounts of liquid; and formation of granules or grittiness.

Suppositories—Excessive softening is the major indication of instability in suppositories, although some suppositories may dry out and harden or shrivel. Evidence of oil stains on packaging material should warn the pharmacist to examine individual suppositories more closely by removing any foil covering if necessary. As a general rule (although there are exceptions), suppositories should be stored in a refrigerator (see *Storage Temperature* in the *General Notices*).

Proper Treatment of Products Subjected to Additional Manipulations—In repackaging, diluting, or mixing a product with another product, the pharmacist may become responsible for its stability.

REPACKAGING—In general, repackaging is inadvisable. However, if repackaging is necessary, the manufacturer should be consulted concerning potential problems. In the filling of prescriptions, it is essential that suitable containers be used. Appropriate storage conditions and, where appropriate, an expiration date, should be indicated on the label of the prescription container. Single-unit packaging calls for care and judgment, and for strict observance of the following guidelines: (1) use appropriate packaging materials; (2) where stability data on the new package are not available, repackage at any one time only sufficient stock for a limited time; (3) include on the unit-dose label a lot number and an appropriate expiration date; (4) where a sterile product is repackaged from a multiple-dose vial into unit-dose (disposable) syringes, discard the latter if not used within 24 hours, unless data are available to support longer storage; (5) where quantities are repackaged in advance of immediate needs, maintain suitable repackaging records showing name of manufacturer, lot number, date, and designation of persons responsible for repackaging and for checking; (6) where

safety closures are required, use container closure systems that ensure compliance with compendial and regulatory standards for storage.

DILUTION OR MIXING—Where a product is diluted, or where two products are mixed, the pharmacist should observe good professional and scientific procedures to guard against incompatibility and instability. For example, tinctures such as those of belladonna and digitalis contain high concentrations of alcohol to dissolve the active ingredient(s), and they may develop a precipitate if they are diluted or mixed with aqueous systems. Pertinent technical literature and labeling should be consulted routinely; it should be current literature, because at times formulas are changed by the manufacturer. If a particular combination is commonly used, consultation with the manufacturer(s) is advisable. Since the chemical stability of extemporaneously prepared mixtures is unknown, the use of such combinations should be discouraged; if such a mixture involved an incompatibility, the pharmacist might be responsible. Oral antibiotic preparations constituted from powder into liquid form should never be mixed with other products.

Combining parenteral products necessitates special care, particularly in the case of intravenous solutions, primarily because of the route of administration. This area of practice demands the utmost in care, aseptic technique, judgment, and diligence. Because of potential unobservable problems with respect to sterility and chemical stability, all extemporaneous parenteral preparations should be used within 24 hours unless data are available to support longer storage.

Informing and Educating the Patient—As a final step in meeting responsibility for the stability of drugs dispensed, the pharmacist is obligated to inform the patient regarding the proper storage conditions (for example, in a cool, dry place—not in the bathroom), for both prescription and nonprescription products, and to suggest a reasonable estimate of the time after which the medication should be discarded. Where expiration dates are applied, the pharmacist should emphasize to the patient that the dates are applicable only when proper storage conditions are used. Patients should be encouraged to clean out their drug storage cabinets periodically.

⟨1231⟩ WATER FOR PHARMACEUTICAL PURPOSES

Water is the most copiously and widely used substance in pharmaceutical manufacturing. Control of the chemical and microbiological quality of water for pharmaceutical purposes is difficult because its basic sources—municipal and non-municipal water systems—are influenced by many factors.

Monitoring of quality parameters in source water is necessary to ensure an acceptable water supply.

Water is required for a variety of purposes ranging from the needs of manufacturing processes to the final preparation of therapeutic agents just prior to their administration to patients.

Drinking water, which is subject to federal Environmental Protection Agency regulations and which is delivered by the municipal or other local public system or drawn from a private well or reservoir, is the starting material for most forms of water covered by Pharmacopeial monographs. Water prepared from other starting material may have to be processed to meet drinking water standards. Drinking water may be used in the preparation of USP drug substances but not in the preparation of dosage forms, or in the preparation of reagents or test solutions.

The Pharmacopeia provides several monographs for water. Of these, *Purified Water* and *Water for Injection* represent ingredient materials, while the other monographs for water provide standards for compendial pharmaceutical articles in themselves.

Purified Water (see USP monograph)—This article represents water rendered suitable for pharmaceutical purposes by processes such as distillation, ion-exchange treatment (deionization or demineralization), or reverse osmosis. It meets rigid specifications for chemical purity, the requirements of the federal Environmental Protection Agency with respect to drinking water, and it contains no added substances. However, the various methods of production each present different potential for contaminating products. Purified Water produced by distillation is sterile, provided the production equipment is suitable and is sterile. On the other hand, ion-exchange columns and reverse osmosis units require special attention in that they afford sites for microorganisms to foul the system and to contaminate the effluent water. Thus, frequent monitoring may be called for, particularly with the use of these units following periods of shutdown of more than a few hours.

Water for Injection (see USP monograph)—By definition, this article is water purified by distillation or by reverse osmosis, and it meets the purity requirements under *Purified Water*. Although not intended to be sterile, it meets a test for a limit of bacterial endotoxin. It must be produced, stored, and distributed under conditions designed to prevent production of endotoxin.

Sterile Water for Injection (see USP monograph)—As a form in which water is distributed in sterile packages, Sterile Water for Injection is intended mainly for use as a solvent for parenteral products such as sterile solids that must be distributed dry because of limited stability of their solutions. It must be packaged only in single-dose containers of not larger than 1-liter size.

Bacteriostatic Water for Injection (see USP monograph)—Inasmuch as it serves the same purposes as Sterile Water for Injection, it meets the same standards, with the exception that it may be packaged in either single-dose or multiple-dose containers of not larger than 30-mL size.

Sterile Water for Irrigation (see USP monograph)—This form of water meets most, but not all, of the requirements for Sterile Water for Injection. The exceptions are with respect to the following: (1) container size (i.e., the container may contain a volume of more than 1 liter of Sterile Water for Irrigation), (2) container design (i.e., the container may be designed so as to empty rapidly the contents as a single dose), (3) *Particulate matter* requirements (i.e., it need not meet the requirement for particulate matter for Large-volume Injections for single-dose infusions), and (4) *Labeling* requirements (e.g., the designations "For irrigation only" and "Not for injection" appear prominently on the label).

ACTION GUIDELINES FOR THE MICROBIAL CONTROL OF INGREDIENT WATER—Criteria for controlling the microbial quality of Purified Water and Water for Injection may vary according to the method of production, distribution and/or storage and use. The suitability of water systems to produce water of acceptable microbiological quality should be validated prior to production. Suitable microbiological, chemical, and operating controls should be in place. The compendial *Microbial Limit Tests* ⟨61⟩ have not been designed for testing of ingredient waters. Suitable standard methods are found elsewhere. (Standard Methods for the Examination of Water and Wastewater—American Public Health Association, Current Edition, Washington, DC 20005.)

A total microbial (aerobic) count that may be used for source drinking water is 500 colony-forming units (cfu) per mL. Since *Purified Water* is used to manufacture a variety of products, the action limit set should be based on the intended use of the water, the nature of the product to be made, and the effect of the manufacturing process on the fate of the microorganisms. A general guideline for *Purified Water* may be 100 cfu/mL. Since ingredient waters are not produced as a lot or batch, these numbers, when exceeded or approached, serve as an alert for corrective action. In practice, the supply of ingredient water and manufacture of pharmaceutical articles are usually carried

out concurrently, and the results of the microbial tests made may be available only after some pharmaceutical articles have already been manufactured. The actions to be taken to bring the microbial quality of the ingredient water into desired conformance may include sanitization of the system, for example, flushing with hot water, steam, or suitable disinfectants. Further sampling and monitoring to ensure that the corrective action has been adequate should be conducted.

Packaging Requirements
⟨661⟩ CONTAINERS

Many Pharmacopeial articles are of such nature as to require the greatest attention to the containers in which they are stored or maintained even for short periods of time. While the needs vary widely and some of them are not fully met by the containers available, objective standards are essential. It is the purpose of this chapter to provide such standards as have been developed for the materials of which pharmaceutical containers principally are made, i.e., glass and plastic.

A container intended to provide protection from light or offered as a "light-resistant" container meets the requirements for *Light Transmission*, where such protection or resistance is by virtue of the specific properties of the material of which the container is composed, including any coating applied thereto. A clear and colorless or a translucent container that is made light-resistant by means of an opaque enclosure (see *General Notices and Requirements*) is exempt from the requirements for *Light Transmission*.

Containers composed of glass meet the requirements for *Chemical Resistance—Glass Containers*, and containers composed of plastic and intended for packaging products prepared for parenteral use meet the requirements under *Biological Tests—Plastics* and *Physicochemical Tests—Plastics*.

Where dry oral dosage forms, not meant for constitution into solution, are intended to be packaged in a container defined in the section *Polyethylene Containers*, the requirements given in that section are to be met.

Guidelines and requirements under *Single-unit Containers and Unit-dose Containers for Nonsterile Solid and Liquid Dosage Forms* apply to official dosage forms that are repackaged into single-unit or unit-dose containers or mnemonic packs for dispensing pursuant to prescription.

LIGHT TRANSMISSION
Table 1. Limits for Glass Types I, II, and III and Plastic Classes I–VI.

Nominal Size (in mL)	Maximum Percentage of Light Transmission at Any Wavelength Between 290 and 450 nm	
	Flame-sealed Containers	Closure-sealed Containers
1	50	25
2	45	20
5	40	15
10	35	13
20	30	12
50	15	10

NOTE—Any container of a size intermediate to those listed above exhibits a transmission not greater than that of the next larger size container listed in the table. For containers larger than 50 mL, the limits for 50 mL apply.

CHEMICAL RESISTANCE—GLASS CONTAINERS

Glass Types—Glass containers suitable for packaging Pharmacopeial preparations may be classified as in Table 2 on the basis of the tests set forth in this section. Containers of Type I borosilicate glass are generally used for preparations that are intended for parenteral administration. Containers of Type I glass, or of Type II glass, i.e., soda-lime glass that is suitably dealkalized, are usually used for packaging acidic and neutral parenteral preparations. Type I glass containers, or Type II glass containers (where stability data demonstrate their suitability), are used for alkaline parenteral preparations. Type III soda-lime glass containers usually are not used for parenteral preparations, except where suitable stability test data indicate that Type III glass is satisfactory for the parenteral preparations that are packaged therein. Containers of Type NP glass are intended for packaging nonparenteral articles; i.e., those intended for oral or topical use.

Table 2.   Glass Types and Test Limits.

Type	General Description[a]	Type of Test	Size,[b] mL	Limits mL of 0.020 N Acid
I	Highly resistant, borosilicate glass	*Powdered Glass*	All	1.0
II	Treated soda-lime glass	*Water Attack*	100 or less	0.7
			Over 100	0.2
III	Soda-lime glass	*Powdered Glass*	All	8.5
NP	General-purpose soda-lime glass	*Powdered Glass*	All	15.0

[a]The description applies to containers of this type of glass usually available.
[b]Size indicates the overflow capacity of the container.

SINGLE-UNIT CONTAINERS AND UNIT-DOSE CONTAINERS FOR NONSTERILE SOLID AND LIQUID DOSAGE FORMS

An official dosage form is required to bear on its label an expiration date assigned for the particular formulation and package of the article. This date limits the time during which the product may be dispensed or used. Because the expiration date stated on the manufacturer's or distributor's package has been determined for the drug in that particular package and may not be applicable to the product where it has been repackaged in a different container, repackaged drugs dispensed pursuant to a prescription are exempt from this label requirement. It is necessary, therefore, that other precautions be taken by the dispenser to preserve the strength, quality, and purity of drugs that are repackaged for ultimate distribution or sale to patients.

The following guidelines and requirements are applicable where official dosage forms are repackaged into single-unit or unit-dose containers or mnemonic packs for dispensing pursuant to prescription.

Labeling—It is the responsibility of the dispenser, taking into account the nature of the drug repackaged, the characteristics of the containers, and the storage conditions to which the article may be subjected, to determine a suitable beyond-use date to be placed on the label. In the absence of stability data to the contrary, such date should not exceed (1) 25% of the remaining time between the date of repackaging and the expiration date on the original manufacturer's bulk container, or (2) a six-month period from the date the drug is repackaged, whichever is earlier. Each single-unit or unit-dose container bears a separate label, unless the device holding the unit-dose form does not allow for the removal or separation of the intact single-unit or unit-dose container therefrom.

Storage—Store the repackaged article in a humidity-controlled environment and at the temperature specified in the individual monograph or in the product labeling. Where no temperature or humidity is specified in the monograph or in the labeling of the product, controlled room temperature and a relative humidity corresponding to 75% at 23 °C are not to be exceeded during repackaging or storage.

A refrigerator or freezer shall not be considered to be a humidity-controlled environment, and drugs that are to be stored at a cold temperature in a refrigerator or freezer shall be placed within an outer container that meets the monograph requirements for the drug contained therein.

CUSTOMIZED PATIENT MEDICATION PACKAGES

In lieu of dispensing two or more prescribed drug products in separate containers, a pharmacist may, with the consent of the patient, the patient's caregiver, or a prescriber, provide a customized patient medication package (patient med pak). [NOTE: It should be noted that there is no special exemption for patient med paks from the requirements of the Poison Prevention Packaging Act. Thus the patient med pak, if it does not meet child-resistant standards, shall be placed in an outer package that does comply, or the necessary consent of the purchaser or physician, to dispense in a container not intended to be child-resistant, shall be obtained.]

A patient med pak is a package prepared by a pharmacist for a specific patient comprising a series of containers and containing two or more prescribed solid oral dosage forms. The patient med pak is so designed or each container is so labeled as to indicate the day and time, or period of time, that the contents within each container are to be taken.

It is the responsibility of the dispenser to instruct the patient or caregiver on the use of the patient med pak.

Label—
(A) The patient med pak shall bear a label stating:
(1) the name of the patient;
(2) a serial number for the patient med pak itself and a separate identifying serial number for each of the prescription orders for each of the drug products contained therein;
(3) the name, strength, physical description or identification, and total quantity of each drug product contained therein;
(4) the directions for use and cautionary statements, if any, contained in the prescription order for each drug product therein;
(5) any storage instructions or cautionary statements required by the official compendia;
(6) the name of the prescriber of each drug product;
(7) the date of preparation of the patient med pak and the beyond-use date or period of time assigned to the patient med pak (such beyond-use date or period of time shall be not longer then the shortest recommended beyond-use date for any dosage form included therein or not longer than 60 days from the date of preparation of the patient med pak and shall not exceed the shortest expiration date on the original manufacturer's bulk containers for the dosage forms included therein); alternatively, the package label shall state the date of the prescription(s) or the date of preparation of the patient med pak, provided the package is accompanied by a record indicating the start date and the beyond-use date;
(8) the name, address, and telephone number of the dispenser (and the dispenser's registration number where necessary); and
(9) any other information, statements, or warnings required for any of the drug products contained therein.
(B) If the patient med pak allows for the removal or separation of the intact containers therefrom, each individual container shall bear a label identifying each of the drug products contained therein.

Labeling—The patient med pak shall be accompanied by a patient package insert, in the event that any medication therein is required to be dispensed with such insert as accompanying labeling. Alternatively, such required information may be incorporated into a single, overall educational insert provided by the pharmacist for the total patient med pak.

Packaging—In the absence of more stringent packaging requirements for any of the drug products contained therein, each container of the patient med pak shall comply with the moisture permeation requirements for a Class B single-unit or unit-dose container (see *Containers—Permeation* ⟨671⟩). Each container shall be either not reclosable or so designed as to show evidence of having been opened.

Guidelines—It is the responsibility of the dispenser, when preparing a patient med pak, to take into account any applicable compendial requirements or guidelines and the physical and chemical compatibility of the dosage forms placed within each container, as well as any therapeutic incompatibilities that may attend the simultaneous administration of the medications. In this regard, pharmacists are encouraged to report to USP headquarters any observed or reported incompatibilities.

Recordkeeping—In addition to any individual prescription filing requirements, a record of each patient med pak shall be made and filed. Each record shall contain, as a minimum:

(1) the name and address of the patient;

(2) the serial number of the prescription order for each drug product contained therein;

(3) the name of the manufacturer or labeler and lot number for each drug product contained therein;

(4) information identifying or describing the design, characteristics, or specifications of the patient med pak sufficient to allow subsequent preparation of an identical patient med pak for the patient;

(5) the date of preparation of the patient med pak and the beyond-use date that was assigned;

(6) any special labeling instructions; and

(7) the name or initials of the pharmacist who prepared the patient med pak.

⟨671⟩ CONTAINERS—PERMEATION

This test is provided to determine the moisture permeability of a container utilized for a drug when dispensed on prescription where packaging and storage in a *tight container* or a *well-closed container* is specified in the individual monograph. It is applicable to multiple-unit containers (see *Preservation, Packaging, Storage, and Labeling* under *General Notices and Requirements*). As used herein, the term "container" refers to the entire system comprising, usually, the container itself, the liner (if used), and the closure. Where the manufacturer's container, previously unopened, is utilized for dispensing the drug, such container is exempt from the requirements of this test.

Desiccant—Place a quantity of 4- to 8-mesh, anhydrous calcium chloride in a shallow container, taking care to exclude any fine powder, then dry at 110 °C for 1 hour, and cool in a desiccator. [NOTE: Suitable 4- to 8-mesh, anhydrous calcium chloride is available commercially as Item JT1313-1 from VWR Scientific. Consult the VWR Scientific catalog for ordering information or call 1-800-932-5000.]

Procedure—Select 12 containers of a uniform size and type, clean the sealing surfaces with a lint-free cloth, and close and open each container 30 times. Apply the closure firmly and uniformly each time the container is closed. Close screw-capped containers with a torque that is within the range of tightness specified in the accompanying table. Add *Desiccant* to 10 of the containers, designated *test containers*, filling each to within 13 mm of the closure if the container volume is 20 mL or more, or filling each to two-thirds of capacity if the container volume is less than 20 mL. If the interior of the container is more than 63 mm in depth, an inert filler or spacer may be placed in the bottom to minimize the total weight of the container and *Desiccant;* the layer of *Desiccant* in such a container shall be not less than 5 cm in depth. Close each immediately after adding

Desiccant, applying the torque designated in the accompanying table when closing screw-capped containers. To each of the remaining 2 containers, designated *controls*, add a sufficient number of glass beads to attain a weight approximately equal to that of each of the *test containers*, and close, applying the torque designated in the accompanying table when closing screw-capped containers. Record the weight of the individual containers so prepared to the nearest 0.1 mg if the container volume is less than 20 mL; to the nearest mg if the container volume is 20 mL or more but less than 200 mL; or to the nearest centigram (10 mg) if the container volume is 200 mL or more; and store at 75 ± 3% relative humidity and a temperature of 23 ± 2 °C. [NOTE—A saturated system of 35 g of sodium chloride with each 100 mL of water placed in the bottom of a desiccator maintains the specified humidity. Other methods may be employed to maintain these conditions.] After 336 ± 1 hours (14 days), record the weight of the individual containers in the same manner. Completely fill 5 empty containers of the same size and type as the containers under test with water or a noncompressible, free-flowing solid such as well-tamped fine glass beads, to the level indicated by the closure surface when in place. Transfer the contents of each to a graduated cylinder, and determine the average container volume, in mL. Calculate the rate of moisture permeability, in mg per day per liter, by the formula:

$$(1000/14V)[(T_f - T_i) - (C_f - C_i)],$$

in which V is the volume, in mL, of the container, $(T_f - T_i)$ is the difference, in mg, between the final and initial weights of each *test container*, and $(C_f - C_i)$ is the average of the differences, in mg, between the final and initial weights of the 2 *controls*. The containers so tested are *tight containers* if not more than one of the 10 *test containers* exceeds 100 mg per day per liter in moisture permeability, and none exceeds 200 mg per day per liter.

Torque Applicable to Screw-Type Container

Closure Diameter[1] (mm)	Suggested Tightness Range with Manually Applied Torque[2] (inch-pounds)
8	5
10	6
13	8
15	5–9
18	7–10
20	8–12
22	9–14
24	10–18
28	12–21
30	13–23
33	15–25
38	17–26
43	17–27
48	19–30
53	21–36
58	23–40
63	25–43
66	26–45
70	28–50
83	32–65
86	40–65
89	40–70
100	45–70
110	45–70
120	55–95
132	60–95

[1]The torque designated for the next larger closure diameter is to be applied in testing containers having a closure diameter intermediate to the diameters listed.

[2]A suitable apparatus is available from Owens-Illinois, Toledo, OH 43666. (Model 25 torque tester is used for testing between 0 and 25; Model 50 for testing between 0 and 50; and Model 100 for testing between 0 and 100 inch-pounds of torque.) The torque values refer to application, not removal, of the closure. For further detail regarding instructions, reference may be made to "Standard Method of Measuring Application and Removal Torque of Threaded Closures," ASTM Designation D 3198-73, published by the American Society for Testing and Materials, 1916 Race St., Philadelphia, PA 19103.

The containers are *well-closed containers* if not more than one of the 10 *test containers* exceeds 2000 mg per day per liter in moisture permeability, and none exceeds 3000 mg per day per liter.

SINGLE-UNIT CONTAINERS AND UNIT-DOSE CONTAINERS FOR CAPSULES AND TABLETS

To permit an informed judgment regarding the suitability of the packaging for a particular type of product, the following procedure and classification scheme are provided for evaluating the moisture-permeation characteristics of single-unit and unit-dose containers. Inasmuch as equipment and operator performance may affect the moisture permeation of a container formed or closed, the moisture-permeation characteristics of the packaging system being utilized shall be determined.

Desiccant—Dry suitable desiccant pellets at 110 °C for 1 hour prior to use. Use pellets weighing approximately 400 mg each and having a diameter of approximately 8 mm. (NOTE: Suitable moisture-indicating desiccant pellets are available commercially from sources such as Medical Packaging, Inc., 11-10 Ilene Court, Belle Mead, NJ 08502[Telephone 800-257-5282; in NJ, 609-767-3604 telex: WUI 6851151 medpack atco; FAX: 609-753-0143cb, as Indicating Desiccant Pellets, item No. TK-1002.)

Procedure—

Method I—Seal not less than 10 unit-dose containers with 1 pellet in each, and seal 10 additional, empty unit-dose containers to provide the controls, using finger cots or padded forceps to handle the sealed containers. Number the containers, and record the individual weights to the nearest mg. Weigh the controls as a unit, and divide the total weight by the number of controls to obtain the average. Store all of the containers at 75 ± 3% relative humidity and at a temperature of 23 ± 2 °C. [NOTE—A saturated system of 35 g of sodium chloride with each 100 mL of water placed in the bottom of a desiccator maintains the specified humidity. Other methods may be employed to maintain these conditions.] After a 24-hour interval, or a multiple thereof (see *Results*), remove the containers from the chamber, and allow them to equilibrate for 15 to 60 minutes in the weighing area. Again record the weight of the individual containers and the combined controls in the same manner. [NOTE—If any indicating pellets turn pink during this procedure, or if the pellet weight increase exceeds 10%, terminate the test, and regard only earlier determinations as valid.] Return the containers to the humidity chamber. Calculate the rate of moisture permeation, in mg per day, of each container by the formula:

$$(1/N)[(W_f - W_i) - (C_f - C_i)],$$

in which N is the number of days expired in the test period, $(W_f - W_i)$ is the difference, in mg, between the final and initial weights of each test container, and $(C_f - C_i)$ is the average of the difference, in mg, between the final and initial weights of the controls, the data being calculated to two significant figures. [NOTE—Where the permeations measured are less than 5 mg per day, and where the controls are observed to reach a steady state in 7 days, the individual permeations may be determined more accurately after an initial 7 days of equilibration by using that weight as W_i, zero time, in the calculation. NOTE: Accurate

comparisons of *Class A* containers may require test periods in excess of 28 days if weighings are performed on a *Class A* prescription balance (see *Prescription Balances and Volumetric Apparatus* ⟨1176⟩). The use of an analytical balance on which weights can be recorded to 4 or 5 decimal places may permit more precise characterization between containers and/or shorter test periods.]

Method II—Use this procedure for packs (e.g., punch-out cards) that incorporate a number of separately sealed unit-dose containers or blisters. Seal a sufficient number of packs, such that not less than 4 packs and a total of not less than 10 unit-dose containers or blisters filled with 1 pellet in each unit are tested. Seal a corresponding number of empty packs, each pack containing the same number of unit-dose containers or blisters as used in the test packs, to provide the controls. Store all of the containers at 75 ± 3% relative humidity and at a temperature of 23 ± 2 °C. [See *Note* under *Method I*.] After 24 hours, and at multiples thereof (see *Results*), remove the packs from the chamber, and allow them to equilibrate for approximately 45 minutes. Record the weights of the individual packs, and return them to the chamber. Weigh the control packs as a unit, and divide the total weight by the number of control packs to obtain the average empty pack weight. [NOTE—If any indicating pellets turn pink during the procedure, or if the average pellet weight increase in any pack exceeds 10%, terminate the test, and regard only earlier determinations as valid.] Calculate the average rate of moisture permeation, in mg per day, for each unit-dose container or blister in each pack by the formula:

$$(1/NX)[(W_f - W_i) - (C_f - C_i)],$$

in which N is the number of days expired in the test period (beginning after the initial 24 hour equilibration period), X is the number of separately sealed units per pack, $(W_f - W_i)$ is the difference, in mg, between the final and initial weights of each test pack, and $(C_f - C_i)$ is the average of the difference, in mg, between the final and initial weights of the control packs, the rates being calculated to two significant figures.

Results—The individual unit-dose containers as tested in *Method I* are designated *Class A* if not more than 1 of 10 containers tested exceeds 0.5 mg per day in moisture permeation rate and none exceeds 1 mg per day; they are designated *Class B* if not more than 1 of 10 containers tested exceeds 5 mg per day and none exceeds 10 mg per day; they are designated *Class C* if not more than 1 of 10 containers tested exceeds 20 mg per day and none exceeds 40 mg per day; and they are designated *Class D* if the containers tested meet none of the moisture permeation rate requirements.

The packs as tested in *Method II* are designated *Class A* if no pack tested exceeds 0.5 mg per day in average blister moisture permeation rate; they are designated *Class B* if no pack tested exceeds 5 mg per day in average blister moisture permeation rate; they are designated *Class C* if no pack tested exceeds 20 mg per day in average blister moisture permeation rate; and they are designated *Class D* if the packs tested meet none of the above average blister moisture permeation rate requirements.

With the use of the *Desiccant* described herein, suitable test intervals for the final weighings, W_f, are: 24 hours for *Class D;* 48 hours for *Class C;* 7 days for *Class B;* and not less than 28 days for *Class A.*

Weights and Measures

⟨1176⟩ PRESCRIPTION BALANCES AND VOLUMETRIC APPARATUS

Prescription Balances

NOTE—Balances other than the type described herein may be used provided these afford equivalent or better accuracy.

This includes micro-, semimicro-, or electronic single-pan balances (see *Weights and Balances* ⟨41⟩). Some balances offer digital or direct-reading features. All balances should be calibrated and tested frequently using appropriate test weights, both singly and in combination.

Description—A prescription balance is a scale or balance adapted to weighing medicinal and other substances required in prescriptions or in other pharmaceutical compounding. It is constructed so as to support its full capacity without developing undue stresses, and its adjustment is not altered by repeated weighings of the capacity load. The removable pans or weighing vessels should be of equal weight. The balance should have leveling feet or screws. The balance may feature dial-in weights and also a precision spring and dial instead of a weighbeam. A balance that has a graduated weighbeam must have a stop that halts the rider or poise at the "zero" reading. The reading edge of the rider is parallel to the graduations on the weighbeam. The distance from the face of the index plate to the indicator pointer or pointers should be not more than 1.0 mm (0.04 inch), the points should be sharp, and when there are two, their ends should be separated by not more than 1.0 mm (0.04 inch) when the scale is in balance. The indicating elements and the lever system should be protected against drafts, and the balance lid should permit free movement of the loaded weighing pans when the lid is closed. The balance must have a mechanical arresting device.

Definitions—

Capacity—Maximum weight, including the weight of tares, to be placed on one pan. The *N.B.S. Handbook 44*, 4th ed., states: "*In the absence of information to the contrary*, the nominal capacity of a Class *A* balance shall be assumed to be 15.5 g (½ apothecaries' ounce)." Most of the commercially available Class *A* balances have a capacity of 120 g (4 ounces) and bear a statement to that effect.

Weighbeam or Beam—A graduated bar equipped with a movable poise or rider. Metric graduations are in 0.01-g increments up to a maximum of 1.0 g; apothecaries' graduations are in ⅛-grain increments up to a maximum of 15 ⅜-grains. The bar may be graduated in both systems.

Tare Bar—An auxiliary ungraduated weighbeam bar with a movable poise. This can be used to correct for variations in weighing-glasses or papers.

Balance Indicator—A combination of elements, one or both of which will oscillate with respect to the other, to indicate the equilibrium state of the balance during weighing.

Rest Point—The point on the index plate at which the indicator or pointer stops when the oscillations of the balance cease; or the index plate position of the indicator or pointer calculated from recorded consecutive oscillations in both directions past the "zero" of the index plate scale. If the balance has a two-pointer indicating mechanism, the position or the oscillations of only one of the pointers need be recorded or used to determine the rest point.

Sensitivity Requirements (SR)—The maximum change in load that will cause a specified change, one subdivision on the index plate, in the position of rest of the indicating element or elements of the balance.

Class A Prescription Balance—A balance that meets the tests for this type of balance has a sensitivity requirement of 6 mg or less with no load and with a load of 10 g on each pan. The Class *A* balance should be used for all of the weighing operations required in prescription compounding.

In order to avoid errors of 5 percent or more that might be due to the limit of sensitivity of the Class *A* prescription balance, do not weigh less than 120 mg (2 grains) of any material. If a smaller weight of dry material is required, mix a larger known weight of the ingredient with a known weight of dry diluent, and weigh an aliquot portion of the mixture for use.

Testing the Prescription Balance—A Class *A* prescription balance meets the following four basic tests. Use a set of test weights, and keep the rider on the weighbeam at zero unless directed to change its position.

1. *Sensitivity Requirement*—Level the balance, determine the rest point, and place a 6-mg weight on one of the empty pans. Repeat the operation with a 10-g weight in the center of each pan. The rest point is shifted not less than one division on the index plate each time the 6-mg weight is added.

2. *Arm Ratio Test*—This test is designed to check the equality of length of both arms of the balance. Determine the rest point of the balance with no weight on the pans. Place in the center of each pan a 30-g test weight, and determine the rest point. If the second rest point is not the same as the first, place a 20-mg weight on the lighter side; the rest point should move back to the original place on the index plate scale or farther.

3. *Shift Tests*—These tests are designed to check the arm and lever components of the balance.

A. Determine the rest point of the indicator without any weights on the pans.

B. Place one of the 10-g weights in the center of the left pan, and place the other 10-g weight successively toward the right, left, front, and back of the right pan, noting the rest point in each case. If in any case the rest point differs from the rest point determined in Step *A*, add a 10-mg weight to the lighter side; this should cause the rest point to shift back to the rest point determined in Step *A* or farther.

C. Place a 10-g weight in the center of the right pan, and place a 10-g weight successively toward the right, left, front, and back of the left pan, noting the rest point in each case. If in any case the rest point is different from that obtained with no weights on the pans, this difference should be overcome by addition of the 10-mg weight to the lighter side.

D. Make a series of observations in which both weights are simultaneously shifted to off-center positions on their pans, both toward the outside, both toward the inside, one toward the outside, and the other toward the inside, both toward the back, and so on until all combinations have been checked. If in any case the rest point differs from that obtained with no weights on the pan, the addition of the 10-mg weight to the lighter side should overcome this difference.

A balance that does not meet the requirements of these tests must be adjusted.

4. *Rider and Graduated Beam Tests*—Determine the rest point for the balance with no weight on the pans. Place on the left pan the 500-mg test weight, move the rider to the 500-mg point on the beam, and determine the rest point. If it is different from the zero rest point, add a 6-mg weight to the lighter side. This should bring the rest point back to its original position or farther. Repeat this test, using the 1-g test weight and moving the rider to the 1-g division on the beam. If the rest point is different, it should be brought back at least to the zero rest point position by addition of 6 mg to the lighter pan. If the balance does not meet this test, the weighbeam graduations or the rider must be corrected.

Metric or apothecaries' weights for use with a prescription balance should be kept in a special rigid and compartmentalized box and handled with plastic or plastic-tipped forceps to prevent scratching or soiling. For prescription use, analytical weights (Class P or better) are recommended. However, Class Q weights have tolerances well within the limits of accuracy of the prescription balance, and they retain their accuracy for a long time with proper care. Apothecaries' weights should have the same general (cylindrical) construction as metric weights. Coin-type (or disk-shaped) weights should not be used.

Test weights consisting of two 20-g or two 30-g, two 10-g, one 1-g, one 500-mg, one 20-mg, one 10-mg, and one 6-mg (or suitable combination totaling 6 mg) weights, adjusted to N.B.S. tolerances for analytical weights (Class P or better) should be used for testing the prescription balances. These weights should be kept in a tightly closed box and should be handled only with plastic or plastic-tipped forceps. The set of test weights should be used only for testing the balance or constantly used weights. If properly cared for, the set lasts indefinitely.

Volumetric Apparatus

Pharmaceutical devices for measuring volumes of liquids, including burets, pipets, and cylinders graduated either in metric or apothecary units meet the standard specifications for glass volumetric apparatus described in NTIS COM-73-10504 of the National Technical Information Service. Conical graduates meet the standard specifications described in Handbook 44, 4th Edition, of the National Institute of Standards and Technology. Graduated medicine droppers meet the specifications (see *Medicine Dropper* ⟨1101⟩). An acceptable ungraduated medicine dropper has a delivery end 3 mm in external diameter and delivers 20 drops of water, weighing 1 g at a temperature of 15 °C. A tolerance of ±10% of the delivery specification is reasonable. [NOTE: NTIS COM-73-10504 is for sale by the National Technical Information Service, Springfield, VA 22151. N.B.S. Handbook 44, 4th ed. (1971) is for sale by the Superintendent of Documents, U. S. Government Printing Office, Washington, DC 20402.]

Selection and Use of Graduates—

Capacity—The capacity of a graduate is the designated volume, at the maximum graduation, that the graduate will contain, or deliver, as indicated, at the specified temperature.

Cylindrical and Conical Graduates—The error in a measured volume caused by a deviation of ±1 mm, in reading the lower meniscus in a graduated cylinder, remains constant along the height of the uniform column. The same deviation of ±1 mm causes a progressively larger error in a conical graduate, the extent of the error being further dependent upon the angle of the flared sides to the perpendicular of the upright graduate. A deviation of ±1 mm in the meniscus reading causes an error of approximately 0.5 mL in the measured volume at any mark on the uniform 100-mL cylinder graduate. The same deviation of ±1 mm can cause an error of 1.8 mL at the 100-mL mark on an acceptable conical graduate marked for 125 mL (4 fluid ounces).

A general rule for selection of a graduate for use is to use the graduate with a capacity equal to or *just exceeding* the volume to be measured. Measurement of small volumes in large graduates tends to increase errors, because the larger diameter increases the volume error in a deviation of ±1 mm from the mark. The relation of the volume error to the internal diameters of graduated cylinders is based upon the equation $V = \pi r^2 h$. An acceptable 10-mL cylinder having an internal diameter of 1.18 cm holds 109 μL in 1 mm of the column. Reading 4.5 mL in this graduate with a deviation of ±1 mm from the mark causes an error of about ±2.5%, while the same deviation in a volume of 2.2 mL in the same graduate causes an error of about ±5%. Minimum volumes that can be measured within certain limits of error in graduated cylinders of different capacities are

incorporated in the design details of graduates in Handbook 44, 4th ed., of the National Bureau of Standards. Conical graduates having a capacity of less than 25 mL should not be used in prescription compounding.

⟨1101⟩ MEDICINE DROPPER

The Pharmacopeial medicine dropper consists of a tube made of glass or other suitable transparent material that generally is fitted with a collapsible bulb and, while varying in capacity, is constricted at the delivery end to a round opening having an external diameter of about 3 mm. The dropper, when held vertically, delivers water in drops each of which weighs between 45 mg and 55 mg.

In using a medicine dropper, one should keep in mind that few medicinal liquids have the same surface and flow characteristics as water, and therefore the size of drops varies materially from one preparation to another.

Where accuracy of dosage is important, a dropper that has been calibrated especially for the preparation with which it is supplied should be employed. The volume error incurred in measuring any liquid by means of a calibrated dropper should not exceed 15%, under normal use conditions.

⟨1221⟩ TEASPOON

For household purposes, an American Standard Teaspoon has been established by the American National Standards Institute (1430 Broadway, New York, NY 10018) as containing 4.93 ± 0.24 mL. In view of the almost universal practice of employing teaspoons ordinarily available in the household for the administration of medicine, the teaspoon may be regarded as representing 5 mL. Preparations intended for administration by teaspoon should be formulated on the basis of dosage in 5-mL units. Any dropper, syringe, medicine cup, special spoon, or other device used to administer liquids should deliver 5 mL wherever a teaspoon calibration is indicated. Under ideal conditions of use, the volume error incurred in measuring liquids for individual dose administration by means of such calibrated devices should be not greater than 10% of the indicated amount.

Household units are used often to inform the patient of the size of the dose. Fifteen milliliters should be considered 1 standard tablespoonful; 10 mL, 2 standard teaspoonfuls; and 5 mL, 1 standard teaspoonful. Doses of less than 5 mL are frequently stated as fractions of a teaspoonful or in drops.

Because of the difficulties involved in measuring liquids under normal conditions of use, patients should be cautioned that household spoons are not appropriate for measuring medicines. They should be directed to use the standard measures in the cooking-and-baking measuring spoon sets or, preferably, oral dosing devices that may be provided by the practitioner. It must be kept in mind that the actual volume of a spoonful of any given liquid is related to the latter's viscosity and surface tension, among other influencing factors. These factors can also cause variability in the true volumes contained in or delivered by medicine cups. Where accurate dosage is required, a calibrated syringe or dropper should be used.

EQUIVALENTS OF WEIGHTS AND MEASURES

Metric, Avoirdupois, and Apothecaries

NOTE—These values are for water at the temperature of 4 °C (39.2 °F) in vacuum. For practical purposes the values may be used without correction.

This table of exact equivalents should not be confused with the table of *approximate* dose equivalents, which appears on the next page. The latter table is provided only as a convenience to physicians for prescribing.

For the conversion of specific quantities in pharmaceutical formulas, use the exact equivalents. For prescription compounding, use the exact equivalents rounded to three significant figures.

Weights					Metric Equivalents	Measures		
Apothecaries		Avoirdupois					Fluid	Decimal
oz	grains	lb	oz	grains	g or mL	ounces	minims	Equivalent
32	72.4	2	3	119.9	1000	33	391.1	33.815
30	204.1	2	1	166.6	946.333	32	....	32
29	80.0	2	..	....	907.185	30	324.6	30.676
16	36.2	1	1	278.7	500	16	435.6	16.907
15	102.1	1	..	302.1	473.167	16	....	16
14	280.0	1	..	....	453.592	15	162.3	15.338
12	....	..	13	72.5	373.242	12	298.1	12.621
8	....	..	8	340.0	248.828	8	198.7	8.414
7	291.0	..	8	151.0	236.583	8	....	8
7	140.0	..	8	....	226.796	7	321.1	7.669
6	206.5	..	7	24.0	200	6	366.2	6.763
4	....	..	4	170.0	124.414	4	99.4	4.207
3	385.5	..	4	75.5	118.292	4	....	4
3	310.0	..	4	....	113.398	3	400.6	3.835
3	103.2	..	3	230.7	100	3	183.1	3.381
2	....	..	2	85.0	62.207	2	49.7	2.104
1	432.8	..	2	37.8	59.146	2	....	2
1	395.0	..	2	....	56.699	1	440.3	1.917
1	291.6	..	1	334.1	50	1	331.5	1.691
1	....	..	1	42.5	31.1035	1	24.9	1.052
..	456.380	..	1	18.88	29.5729	1	....	1
..	437.5	..	1	....	28.350	..	460.15	0.959
..	385.8	..	..	....	25	..	405.78	0.845
..	308.6	..	..	....	20	..	324.62	0.676
..	154.3	..	..	....	10	..	162.31	0.338
..	19.02	..	..	....	1.232	..	20	....
..	15.4324	..	..	....	1	..	16.23	....
..	9.51	..	..	....	0.616	..	10	....
..	5	..	..	....	0.324	..	....	....
..	4.75	..	..	....	0.308	..	5	....
..	1	..	..	....	0.06480	..	1.0517	....

Approximate Metric Equivalents of Grains (5 Grains and Less)

Grains	Milligrams	Grains	Milligrams	Grains	Milligrams
5	324	1/2	32.4	1/30	2.2
4	259	2/5	25.9	1/40	1.6
3	194	1/4	16.2	1/50	1.3
2	130	1/8	8.1	1/60	1.1
1½	97	1/10	6.5	1/64	1.0
1	65	1/16	4.0	1/100	0.6
3/4	48.6	1/20	3.2	1/128	0.5

TABLE OF METRIC—APOTHECARY

Approximate Dose Equivalents

When prepared dosage forms such as tablets, capsules, etc., are prescribed in the metric system, the pharmacist may dispense the corresponding *approximate* equivalent in the apothecary system, and vice versa, as indicated in this table.

However, to calculate quantities required in pharmaceutical formulas, use the *exact* equivalents. For prescription compounding, use the exact equivalents rounded to three significant figures. Where expressed in the metric and apothecary systems, statements of quantity or strength in the labeling of drug products shall utilize the *exact* equivalents. (Also see *Volumetric Apparatus* ⟨31⟩, *Weights and Balances* ⟨41⟩, and *Prescription Balances and Volumetric Apparatus* ⟨1176⟩.)

NOTE—A milliliter (mL) is the *approximate* equivalent of a cubic centimeter (cc).

LIQUID MEASURE

Metric		Apothecary	
1000	mL	1	quart
750	mL	$1^1/_2$	pints
500	mL	1	pint
250	mL	8	fluid ounces
200	mL	7	fluid ounces
100	mL	$3^1/_2$	fluid ounces
50	mL	$1^3/_4$	fluid ounces
30	mL	1	fluid ounce
15	mL	4	fluid drams
10	mL	$2^1/_2$	fluid drams
8	mL	2	fluid drams
5	mL	$1^1/_4$	fluid drams
4	mL	1	fluid dram
3	mL	45	minims
2	mL	30	minims
1	mL	15	minims
0.75	mL	12	minims
0.6	mL	10	minims
0.5	mL	8	minims
0.3	mL	5	minims
0.25	mL	4	minims
0.2	mL	3	minims
0.1	mL	$1^1/_2$	minims
0.06	mL	1	minim
0.05	mL	$^3/_4$	minim
0.03	mL	$^1/_2$	minim

WEIGHT

Metric		Apothecary		
30	g	1	ounce	
15	g	4	drams	
10	g	$2^1/_2$	drams	
7.5	g	2	drams	
6	g	90	grains	
5	g	75	grains	
4	g	60	grains	(1 dram)
3	g	45	grains	
2	g	30	grains	($^1/_2$ dram)
1.5	g	22	grains	
1	g	15	grains	
750	mg	12	grains	
600	mg	10	grains	
500	mg	$7^1/_2$	grains	
400	mg	6	grains	
300	mg	5	grains	
250	mg	4	grains	
200	mg	3	grains	
150	mg	$2^1/_2$	grains	
125	mg	2	grains	
100	mg	$1^1/_2$	grains	
75	mg	$1^1/_4$	grains	
60	mg	1	grain	
50	mg	$^3/_4$	grain	
40	mg	$^2/_3$	grain	
30	mg	$^1/_2$	grain	
25	mg	$^3/_8$	grain	
20	mg	$^1/_3$	grain	
15	mg	$^1/_4$	grain	
12	mg	$^1/_5$	grain	
10	mg	$^1/_6$	grain	
8	mg	$^1/_8$	grain	
6	mg	$^1/_{10}$	grain	
5	mg	$^1/_{12}$	grain	
4	mg	$^1/_{15}$	grain	
3	mg	$^1/_{20}$	grain	
2	mg	$^1/_{30}$	grain	
1.5	mg	$^1/_{40}$	grain	
1.2	mg	$^1/_{50}$	grain	
1	mg	$^1/_{60}$	grain	
800	mcg	$^1/_{80}$	grain	
600	mcg	$^1/_{100}$	grain	
500	mcg	$^1/_{120}$	grain	
400	mcg	$^1/_{150}$	grain	
300	mcg	$^1/_{200}$	grain	
250	mcg	$^1/_{250}$	grain	
200	mcg	$^1/_{300}$	grain	
150	mcg	$^1/_{400}$	grain	
120	mcg	$^1/_{500}$	grain	
100	mcg	$^1/_{600}$	grain	

Laws and Regulations

⟨1071⟩ CONTROLLED SUBSTANCES ACT REGULATIONS

NOTE: A complete set of the regulations appears in Volume 21, part 1300 to end, of the *Code of Federal Regulations*, revised annually, and covers regulations pertaining to manufacturers, distributors, researchers, exporters, and importers.

Information regarding procedures under these regulations and instructions implementing them are obtainable from the Drug Enforcement Administration, Department of Justice, 1405 I Street, N.W., Washington, DC 20537.

Selected portions of the regulations promulgated under the Controlled Substances Act that are believed to be of most concern to practitioners and students of pharmacy and medicine are presented here as a service to the professions and at the suggestion of the Drug Enforcement Administration in accordance with its registrant information and self-regulation program.

The publication of these regulations in The United States Pharmacopeia is for purposes of information and does not impart to them any legal effect.

The Drug Enforcement Administration was established July 1, 1973, through the merging of various Bureaus and offices of the federal government with the Bureau of Narcotics and Dangerous Drugs.

INDEX TO THE PORTIONS OF CONTROLLED SUBSTANCES ACT REGULATIONS PRESENTED HEREIN

General Provisions
290.05   Drugs; statement of required warning
290.06   Spanish-language version of required warning
290.10   Definition of emergency situation

General Information
1301.01   Scope of part 1301
1301.02   Definitions
1301.03   Information; special instructions

Fees for Registration and Reregistration
1301.11   Fee amounts
1301.12   Time and method of payment; refund

Requirements for Registration
1301.21   Persons required to register
1301.22   Separate registration for independent activities
1301.23   Separate registrations for separate locations
1301.24   Exemption of agents and employees; affiliated practitioners
1301.25   Exemption of certain military and other personnel
1301.28   Registration regarding ocean vessels
1301.29   Provisional registration of narcotic treatment programs; compounders

Applications for Registration
1301.31   Time for application for registration; expiration date
1301.32   Application forms; contents; signature
1301.34   Filing of application; joint filings
1301.35   Acceptance for filing; defective applications
1301.36   Additional information
1301.37   Amendments to and withdrawal of applications
1301.38   Special procedures for certain applications

Action on Applications for Registration: Revocation or Suspension of Registration
1301.41   Administrative review generally
1301.44   Certificate of registration; denial of registration
1301.47   Extension of registration pending final order

Modification, Transfer and Termination of Registration
1301.61   Modification in registration
1301.62   Termination of registration
1301.63   Transfer of registration

Security Requirements
1301.71   Security requirements generally
1301.72   Physical security controls for non-practitioners; narcotic treatment programs and compounders for narcotic treatment programs; storage areas
1301.73   Physical security controls for non-practitioners; compounders for narcotic treatment programs; manufacturing and compounding areas
1301.74   Other security controls for non-practitioners; narcotic treatment programs and compounders for narcotic treatment programs
1301.75   Physical security controls for practitioners
1301.76   Other security controls for practitioners

Labeling and Packaging Requirements for Controlled Substances
1302.02   Definitions
1302.03   Symbol required; exceptions
1302.04   Location and size of symbol on label
1302.05   Location and size of symbol on labeling
1302.07   Sealing of controlled substances

Records and Reports of Registrants
1304.02   Definitions
1304.03   Persons required to keep records and file reports
1304.04   Maintenance of records and inventories

Inventory Requirements
1304.11   General requirements for inventories
1304.12   Initial inventory date
1304.13   Biennial inventory date
1304.14   Inventory date for newly controlled substances
1304.15   Inventories of manufacturers
1304.17   Inventories of dispensers and researchers

Continuing Records
1304.21   General requirements for continuing records
1304.23   Records for distribution
1304.24   Records for dispensers and researchers
1304.28   Records for maintenance treatment programs and detoxification treatment programs
1304.29   Records for treatment programs which compound narcotics for treatment programs and other locations

Order Forms
1305.02   Definitions
1305.03   Distributions requiring order forms
1305.04   Persons entitled to obtain and execute order forms
1305.05   Procedure for obtaining order forms
1305.06   Procedure for executing order forms
1305.07   Power of attorney
1305.08   Persons entitled to fill order forms
1305.09   Procedure for filling order forms
1305.10   Procedure for endorsing order forms
1305.11   Unaccepted and defective order forms
1305.12   Lost and stolen order forms
1305.13   Preservation of order forms
1305.14   Return of unused order forms
1305.15   Cancellation and voiding of order forms

Prescriptions
1306.02   Definitions
1306.03   Persons entitled to issue prescriptions
1306.04   Purpose of issue of prescription
1306.05   Manner of issuance of prescriptions
1306.06   Persons entitled to fill prescriptions
1306.07   Administering or dispensing of narcotic drugs

Controlled Substances Listed in Schedule II

1306.11   Requirement of prescription
1306.12   Refilling prescriptions
1306.13   Partial filling of prescriptions
1306.14   Labeling of substances
1306.15   Filing of prescriptions

Controlled Substances Listed in Schedules III and IV

1306.21   Requirement of prescription
1306.22   Refilling of prescriptions
1306.23   Partial filling of prescriptions
1306.24   Labeling of substances
1306.25   Filing of prescriptions
1306.26   Transfer between pharmacies of prescription information for schedules III, IV, and V controlled substances for refill purposes

Controlled Substances Listed in Schedule V

1306.31   Requirement of prescription
1306.32   Dispensing without prescription

Miscellaneous

1307.02   Application of State law and other Federal law
1307.03   Exceptions to regulations

Special Exceptions for Manufacture and Distribution of Controlled Substances

1307.11   Distribution by dispenser to another practitioner
1307.12   Manufacture and distribution of narcotic solutions and compounds by a pharmacist
1307.13   Distribution to supplier
1307.14   Distribution upon discontinuation or transfer of business

Disposal of Controlled Substances

1307.21   Procedure for disposing of controlled substances

Schedules of Controlled Substances

1308.02   Definitions
1308.11   Schedule I
1308.12   Schedule II
1308.13   Schedule III
1308.14   Schedule IV
1308.15   Schedule V

Inspections

1316.02   Definitions
1316.03   Authority to make inspections
1316.04   Exclusion from inspection
1316.05   Entry
1316.06   Notice of inspection
1316.07   Requirement for administrative inspection warrant; exceptions
1316.08   Consent to inspection
1316.11   Execution of warrants
1316.12   Refusal to allow inspection with an administrative warrant
1316.13   Frequency of administrative inspections

General Provisions

§ 290.05   Drugs; statement of required warning.

The label of any drug listed as a "controlled substance" in schedule II, III, or IV of the Federal Controlled Substances Act shall, when dispensed to or for a patient, contain the following warning: "Caution: Federal law prohibits the transfer of this drug to any person other than the patient for whom it was prescribed." This statement is not required to appear on the label of a controlled substance dispensed for use in clinical investigations which are "blind."

§ 290.06   Spanish-language version of required warning.

By direction of section 305(c) of the Federal Controlled Substances Act, § 290.05, promulgated under section 503(b) of the Federal Food, Drug, and Cosmetic Act, requires the following warning on the label of certain drugs when dispensed to or for a patient: "Caution: Federal law prohibits the transfer of this drug to any person other than the patient for whom it was prescribed." The Spanish version of this is: "Precaucion: La ley Federal prohibe el transferir de esta droga a otra persona que no sea el paciente para quien fue recetada." (Secs. 502, 503; 53 Stat. 854, 65 Stat. 648; 21 U.S.C. 352, 353)

§ 290.10   Definition of emergency situation.

For the purposes of authorizing an oral prescription of a controlled substance listed in Schedule II of the Federal Controlled Substances Act, the term "emergency situation" means those situations in which the prescribing practitioner determines:

(a) That immediate administration of the controlled substance is necessary, for proper treatment of the intended ultimate user; and

(b) That no appropriate alternative treatment is available, including administration of a drug which is not a controlled substance under Schedule II of the Act, and

(c) That it is not reasonably possible for the prescribing practitioner to provide a written prescription to be presented to the person dispensing the substance, prior to the dispensing.

General Information

§ 1301.01   Scope of Part 1301.

Procedures governing the registration of manufacturers, distributors, and dispensers of controlled substances pursuant to sections 1301 through 1304 of the Act (21 U.S.C. 821–824) are set forth generally by those sections and specifically by the sections of this part.

§ 1301.02   Definitions.

As used in this part, the following terms shall have the meanings specified:

(a) The term "Act" means the Controlled Substances Act (84 Stat. 1242; 21 U.S.C. 801) and/or the Controlled Substances Import and Export Act (84 Stat. 1285; 21 U.S.C. 951).

(b) The term "basic class" means, as to controlled substances listed in schedules I and II:

(1) Each of the opiates, including its isomers, esters, ethers, salts, and salts of isomers, esters, and ethers whenever the existence of such isomers, esters, ethers, and salts is possible within the specific chemical designation, listed in § 1308.11(b) of this chapter;

(2) Each of the opium derivatives, including its salts, isomers, and salts of isomers whenever the existence of such salts, isomers, and salts of isomers is possible within the specific chemical designation, listed in § 1308.11(c) of this chapter;

(3) Each of the hallucinogenic substances, including its salts, isomers, and salts of isomers whenever the existence of such salts, isomers, and salts of isomers is possible within the specific chemical designation, listed in § 1308.11(d) of this chapter;

(4) Each of the following substances, whether produced directly or indirectly by extraction from substances of vegetable origin, or independently by means of chemical synthesis, or by a combination of extraction and chemical synthesis:

(i) Opium, including raw opium, opium extracts, opium fluid extracts, powdered opium, granulated opium, deodorized opium and tincture of opium;

(ii) Apomorphine;

(iii) Codeine;

(iv) Etorphine hydrochloride;

(v) Ethylmorphine;

(vi) Hydrocodone;

(vii) Hydromorphone;

(viii) Metopon;

(ix) Morphine;

(x) Oxycodone;

(xi) Oxymorphone;

(xii) Thebaine;

(xiii) Mixed alkaloids of opium listed in § 1308.12(b) (2) of this chapter;

(xiv) Cocaine; and

(xv) Ecgonine;

(5) Each of the opiates, including its isomers, esters, ethers, salts, and salts of isomers, esters, and ethers whenever the existence of such isomers, esters, ethers, and salts is possible within the specific chemical designation, listed in § 1308.12(c) of this chapter; and

(6) Methamphetamine, its salts, isomers, and salts of its isomers;

(7) Amphetamine, its salts, optical isomers, and salts of its optical isomers;

(8) Phenmetrazine and its salts;

(9) Methylphenidate;

(10) Each of the substances having a depressant effect on the central nervous system, including its salts, isomers, and salts of isomers whenever the existence of such salts, isomers, and salts of isomers is possible within the specific chemical designation, listed in § 1308.12(e) of this chapter.

(c) The term "Administration" means the Drug Enforcement Administration.

(d) The term "compounder" means any person engaging in maintenance or detoxification treatment who also mixes, prepares, packages or changes the dosage form of a narcotic drug listed in Schedules II, III, IV or V for use in maintenance or detoxification treatment by another narcotic treatment program.

(e) The term *detoxification treatment* means the dispensing, for a period of time as specified below, of a narcotic drug or narcotic drugs in decreasing doses to an individual to alleviate adverse physiological or psychological effects incident to withdrawal from the continuous or sustained use of a narcotic drug and as a method of bringing the individual to a narcotic drug-free state within such period of time. There are two types of detoxification treatments: Short-term detoxification treatment and long-term detoxification treatment.

(1) *Short-term detoxification treatment* is for a period not in excess of 30 days.

(2) *Long-term detoxification treatment* is for a period more than 30 days but not in excess of 180 days.

(f) The term "Administrator" means the Administrator of the Drug Enforcement Administration. The Administrator has been delegated authority under the Act by the Attorney General (28 CFR 0.100).

(g) The term "hearing" means any hearing held pursuant to this part for the granting, denial, revocation, or suspension of a registration pursuant to sections 303 and 304 of the Act (21 U.S.C. 823–824).

(h) The term "maintenance treatment" means the dispensing for a period in excess of twenty-one days, of a narcotic drug or narcotic drugs in the treatment of an individual for dependence upon heroin or other morphine-like drug.

(i) The term "narcotic treatment program" means a program engaged in maintenance and/or detoxification treatment with narcotic drugs.

(j) The term "person" includes any individual, corporation, government or governmental subdivision or agency, business trust, partnership, association, or other legal entity.

(k) The terms "register" and "registration" refer only to registration required and permitted by section 303 of the Act (21 U.S.C. 823).

(l) The term "registrant" means any person who is registered pursuant to either section 303 or section 1008 of the Act (21 U.S.C. 823 or 958).

(m) Any term not defined in this section shall have the definition set forth in section 102 of the Act (21 U.S.C. 802).

§ 1301.03   Information; special instructions.

Information regarding procedures under these rules and instructions supplementing these rules will be furnished upon request by writing to the Registration Unit, Drug Enforcement Administration, Department of Justice, Post Office Box 28083, Central Station, Washington, D. C. 20005.

Fees for Registration and Reregistration

§ 1301.11   Fee amounts.

(c) For each registration or reregistration to dispense, or to conduct instructional activities with, controlled substances listed in Schedules II through V, the registrant shall pay an application fee of $60 for a three-year registration.

(d) For each registration to conduct research or instructional activities with a controlled substance listed in Schedule I, or to conduct research with a controlled substance in Schedules II through V, the registrant shall pay an application fee of $20.

(f) For each registration or reregistration to engage in a narcotic treatment program, including a compounder, the registrant shall pay an application fee of $5.

§ 1301.12   Time and method of payment; refund.

Application fees shall be paid at the time when the application for registration or reregistration is submitted for filing. Payments should be made in the form of a personal, certified, or cashier's check or money order made payable to "Drug Enforcement Administration." Payments made in the form of stamps, foreign currency, or third party endorsed checks will not be accepted. These application fees are not refundable.

Requirements for Registration

§ 1301.21   Persons required to register.

Every person who manufactures, distributes, or dispenses any controlled substance or who proposes to engage in the manufacture, distribution, or dispensing of any controlled substance shall obtain annually a registration unless exempted by law or pursuant to §§ 1301.24–1301.29. Only persons actually engaged in such activities are required to obtain a registration; related or affiliated persons who are not engaged in such activities are not required to be registered. (For example, a stockholder or parent corporation of a corporation manufacturing controlled substances is not required to obtain a registration.)

§ 1301.22   Separate registration for independent activities.

(a) The following groups of activities are deemed to be independent of each other:

(1) Manufacturing controlled substances;

(2) Distributing controlled substances;

(3) Dispensing controlled substances listed in Schedules II through V;

(4) Conducting research with controlled substances listed in Schedules II through V;

(5) Conducting instructional activities with controlled substances listed in Schedules II through V;

(6) Conducting a narcotic treatment program using any narcotic drug listed in Schedules II, III, IV or V, however, pursuant to § 1301.24, employees, agents, or affiliated practitioners, in programs, need not register separately. Each program site located away from the principal location and at which place narcotic drugs are stored or dispensed must be separately registered and obtain narcotic drugs by use of order forms pursuant to § 1305.03;

(7) Conducting research and instructional activities with controlled substances listed in Schedule I;

(8) Conducting chemical analysis with controlled substances listed in any schedule;

(9) Importing controlled substances; and

(10) Exporting controlled substances; and

(11) A compounder as defined by § 1301.02(d).

(b) Every person who engages in more than one group of independent activities shall obtain a separate registration for each group of activities, except as provided in this paragraph. Any person, when registered to engage in the group of activities described in each subparagraph in this paragraph, shall be authorized to engage in the coincident activities described in that subparagraph without obtaining a registration to engage in such coincident activities, provided that, unless specifically exempted, he complies with all requirements and duties prescribed by law for persons registered to engage in such coincident activities;

(6) A person registered to dispense controlled substances listed in Schedules II through V shall be authorized to conduct research and to conduct instructional activities with those substances.

(c) A single registration to engage in any group of independent activities may include one or more controlled substances listed in the schedules authorized in that group of independent activities. A person registered to conduct research with controlled substances listed in Schedule I may conduct research with any substance listed in Schedule I for which he has filed and had approved a research protocol.

§ 1301.23   Separate registrations for separate locations.

(a) A separate registration is required for each principal place of business or professional practice at one general physical location where controlled substances are manufactured, distributed, or dispensed by a person.

(b) The following locations shall be deemed not to be places where controlled substances are manufactured, distributed, or dispensed:

(1) A warehouse where controlled substances are stored by or on behalf of a registered person, unless such substances are distributed directly from such warehouse to registered locations other than the registered location from which the substances were delivered or to persons not required to register by virtue of subsection 302(c) (2) of the Act (21 U.S.C. 822(c) (2));

(2) An office used by agents of a registrant where sales of controlled substances are solicited, made, or supervised but which neither contains such substances (other than substances for display purposes or lawful distribution as samples only) nor serves as a distribution point for filling sales orders; and

(3) An office used by a practitioner (who is registered at another location) where controlled substances are prescribed but neither administered nor otherwise dispensed as a regular part of the professional practice of the practitioner at such office, and where no supplies of controlled substances are maintained.

§ 1301.24   Exemption of agents and employees; affiliated practitioners.

(a) The requirement of registration is waived for any agent or employee of a person who is registered to engage in any group of independent activities, if such agent or employee is acting in the usual course of his business or employment.

(b) An individual practitioner, as defined in § 1304.02 of this chapter (other than an intern, resident, foreign-trained physician, or physician on the staff of a Veterans Administration facility or physician who is an agent or employee of the Health Bureau of the Canal Zone Government), who is an agent or employee of another practitioner registered to dispense controlled substances may, when acting in the usual course of his employment, administer and dispense (other than by issuance of prescription) controlled substances if and to the extent that such individual practitioner is authorized or permitted to do so by the jurisdiction in which he practices, under the registration of the employer or principal practitioner in lieu of being registered himself. (For example, a staff physician employed by a hospital need not be registered individually to administer and dispense, other than by prescribing, controlled substances within the hospital.)

(c) An individual practitioner, as defined in § 1304.02 of this chapter, who is an intern, resident, or foreign-trained physician or physician on the staff of a Veterans Administration facility or physician who is an agent or employee of the Health Bureau of the Canal Zone Government, may dispense, administer and prescribe controlled substances under the registration of the hospital or other institution which is registered and by whom he is employed in lieu of being registered himself, provided that:

(1) Such dispensing, administering or prescribing is done in the usual course of his professional practice;

(2) Such individual practitioner is authorized or permitted to do so by the jurisdiction in which he is practicing;

(3) The hospital or other institution by whom he is employed has verified that the individual practitioner is so permitted to dispense, administer, or prescribe drugs within the jurisdiction;

(4) Such individual practitioner is acting only within the scope of his employment in the hospital or institution;

(5) The hospital or other institution authorizes the intern, resident, or foreign-trained physician to dispense or prescribe under the hospital registration and designates a specific internal code number for each intern, resident, or foreign-trained physician so authorized. The code number shall consist of numbers, letters, or a combination thereof and shall be a suffix to the institution's DEA registration number, preceded by a hyphen (e.g., APO 123456-10 or APO 123456-A12); and

(6) A current list of internal codes and the corresponding individual practitioners is kept by the hospital or other institution and is made available at all times to other registrants and law enforcement agencies upon request for the purpose of verifying the authority of the prescribing individual practitioner.

§ 1301.25   Exemption of certain military and other personnel.

(a) The requirement of registration is waived for any official of the U. S. Army, Navy, Marine Corps, Air Force, Coast Guard, Public Health Service, or Bureau of Prisons who is authorized to prescribe, dispense, or administer, but not to procure or purchase, controlled substances in the course of his official duties. Such officials shall follow procedures set forth in Part 1306 of this chapter regarding prescriptions, but shall state the branch of service or agency (e.g., "U. S. Army" or "Public Health Service") and the service identification number of the issuing official in lieu of the registration number required on prescription forms. The service identification number for a Public Health Service employee is his Social Security identification number.

(b) If any official exempted by this section also engages as a private individual in any activity or group of activities for which registration is required, such official shall obtain a registration for such private activities.

§ 1301.28   Registration regarding ocean vessels.

(a) If acquired by and dispensed under the general supervision of a medical officer described in paragraph (b) of this section, or the master or first officer of the vessel under the circumstances described in paragraph (d) of this section, controlled substances may be held for stocking, be maintained in, and dispensed from medicine chests, first aid packets, or dispensaries:

(1) On board any vessel engaged in international trade or in trade between ports of the United States and any merchant vessel belonging to the U. S. Government;

(2) On board any aircraft operated by an air carrier under a certificate of permit issued pursuant to the Federal Aviation Act of 1958 (49 U.S.C. 1301); and

(3) In any other entity of fixed or transient location approved by the Administrator as appropriate for application of this section (e.g., emergency kits at field sites of an industrial firm).

(b) A medical officer shall be:
(1) Licensed in a state as a physician;

(2) Employed by the owner or operator of the vessel, aircraft or other entity; and

(3) Registered under the Act at either of the following locations:

(i) The principal office of the owner or operator of the vessel, aircraft or other entity or

(ii) At any other location provided that the name, address, registration number and expiration date as they appear on his Certificate of Registration (DEA Form 223) for this location are maintained for inspection at said principal office in a readily retrievable manner.

(c) A registered medical officer may serve as medical officer for more than one vessel, aircraft, or other entity under a single registration, unless he serves as medical officer for more than one owner or operator, in which case he shall either maintain a separate registration at the location of the principal office of each such owner or operator or utilize one or more registrations pursuant to paragraph (b)(3)(ii) of this section.

(d) If no medical officer is employed by the owner or operator of a vessel, or in the event such medical officer is not accessible and the acquisition of controlled substances is required, the master or first officer of the vessel, who shall not be registered under the Act, may purchase controlled substances from a registered manufacturer or distributor, or from an authorized pharmacy as described in paragraph (f) of this section, by following the procedure outlined below:

(1) The master or first officer of the vessel must personally appear at the vendor's place of business, present proper identification (e.g., Seaman's photographic identification card) and a written requisition for the controlled substances.

(2) The written requisition must be on the vessel's official stationery or purchase order form and must include the name and address of the vendor, the name of the controlled substance, description of the controlled substance (dosage form, strength and number or volume per container), number of containers ordered, the name of the vessel, the vessel's official number and country of registry, the owner or operator of the vessel, the port at which the vessel is located, signature of the vessel's officer who is ordering the controlled substances and the date of the requisition.

(3) The vendor may, after verifying the identification of the vessel's officer requisitioning the controlled substances, deliver the control substances to that officer. The transaction shall be documented, in triplicate, on a record of sale in a format similar to that outlined in paragraph (d)(4) of this section. The vessel's requisition shall be attached to copy 1 of the record of sale and filed with the controlled substances records of the vendor, copy 2 of the record of sale shall be furnished to the officer of the vessel and retained aboard the vessel, copy 3 of the record of sale shall be forwarded to the nearest DEA Division Office within 15 days after the end of the month in which the sale is made.

(4) The vendor's record of sale should be similar to, and must include all the information contained in, the below listed format.

Sale of Controlled Substances to Vessels

(Name of registrant)_____
(Address of registrant)_____
(DEA registration number)_____

Line No.	Number of packages ordered	Size of packages	Name of product	Packages distributed	Date distributed
1					
2					
3					

Line numbers may be continued according to needs of the vendor.

Number of lines completed_____
Name of vessel_____
Vessel's official number_____
Vessel's country of registry_____
Owner or operator of the vessel_____
Name and title of vessel's officer who presented the requisition_____
Signature of vessel's officer who presented the requisition_____

(e) Any medical officer described in paragraph (b) of this section shall, in addition to complying with all requirements and duties prescribed for registrants generally, prepare an annual report as of the date on which his registration expires, which shall give in detail an accounting for each vessel, aircraft, or other entity, and a summary accounting for all vessels, aircraft, or other entities under his supervision for all controlled substances purchased, dispensed or disposed of during the year. The medical officer shall maintain this report with other records required to be kept under the Act and, upon request, deliver a copy of the report to the Administration. The medical officer need not be present when controlled substances are dispensed, if the person who actually dispensed the controlled substances is responsible to the medical officer to justify his actions.

(f) Any registered pharmacy which wishes to distribute controlled substances pursuant to this section shall be authorized to do so, provided that:

(1) The registered pharmacy notifies the nearest Division Office of the Administration of its intention to so distribute

controlled substances prior to the initiation of such activity. This notification shall be by registered mail and shall contain the name, address, and registration number of the pharmacy as well as the date upon which such activity will commence; and

(2) Such activity is authorized by state law; and

(3) The total number of dosage units of all controlled substances distributed by the pharmacy during any calendar year in which the pharmacy is registered to dispense does not exceed the limitations imposed upon such distribution by § 1307.11(a)(4) and (b) of this chapter.

(g) Owners or operators of vessels, aircraft, or other entities described in this section shall not be deemed to possess or dispense any controlled substance acquired, stored and dispensed in accordance with this section.

(h) The Master of a vessel shall prepare a report for each calendar year which shall give in detail an accounting for all controlled substances purchased, dispensed, or disposed of during the year. The Master shall file this report with the medical officer employed by the owner or operator of his vessel, if any, or, if not, he shall maintain this report with other records required to be kept under the Act and, upon request, deliver a copy of the report to the Administration.

(i) Controlled substances acquired and possessed in accordance with this section shall not be distributed to persons not under the general supervision of the medical officer employed by the owner or operator of the vessel, aircraft, or other entity, except in accordance with § 1307.21 of this chapter.

§ 1301.29 Provisional registration of narcotic treatment programs; compounders.

(a) All persons currently approved by the Food and Drug Administration under § 310.505 (formerly § 130.44) of this title to conduct a methadone treatment program and who are registered by the Drug Enforcement Administration under this section will be granted a Provisional Narcotic Treatment Program Registration.

(b) The provisions of §§ 1301.45–1301.57 relating to revocation and suspension of registration, shall apply to a provisional registration.

(c) Unless sooner revoked or suspended under paragraph (b) of this section, a provisional registration shall remain in effect until (1) the date on which such person has registered under this section or has had his registration denied, or (2) such date as may be prescribed by written notification to the person from the Drug Enforcement Administration for the person to become registered to conduct a narcotic treatment program, whichever occurs first.

Applications for Registration

§ 1301.31 Time for application for registration; expiration date.

(a) Any person who is required to be registered and who is not so registered may apply for registration at any time. No person required to be registered shall engage in any activity for which registration is required until the application for registration is granted and a Certificate of Registration is issued by the Administrator to such person.

(b) Any person who is registered may apply to be reregistered not more than 60 days before the expiration date of his registration.

(c) At the time a manufacturer, distributor, researcher, analytical lab, importer, exporter or narcotic treatment program is first registered, that business activity shall be assigned to one of twelve groups, which shall correspond to the months of the year. The expiration date of the registrations of all registrants within any group will be the last date of the month designated for that group. In assigning any of the above business activities to a group, the Administration may select a group the expiration date of which is less than one year from the date such business activity was registered. If the business activity is assigned to a group which has an expiration date less than three months from the date on which the business activity is registered, the registration shall not expire until one year from that expiration date; in all other cases, the registration shall expire on the expiration date following the date on which the business activity is registered.

(d) At the time a retail pharmacy, hospital/clinic, practitioner or teaching institution is first registered, that business activity shall be assigned to one of twelve groups, which shall correspond to the months of the year. The expiration date of the registrations of all registrants within any group will be the last day of the month designated for that group. In assigning any of the above business activities to a group, the Administration may select a group the expiration date of which is not less than 28 months nor more than 39 months from the date such business activity was registered. After the initial registration period, the registration shall expire 36 months from the initial expiration date.

§ 1301.32 Application forms; contents; signature.

(a) If any person is required to be registered, and is not so registered and is applying for registration:

(1) To manufacture or distribute controlled substances, he shall apply on DEA Form 225;

(2) To dispense controlled substances listed in schedules II through V, he shall apply on DEA Form 224;

(9) To conduct a narcotic treatment program, including a compounder, he shall apply on DEA Form 363.

(b) If any person is registered and is applying for reregistration:

(1) To manufacture or distribute controlled substances, he shall apply on DEA Form 225a;

(2) To dispense controlled substances listed in schedules II through V, he shall apply on DEA Form 224a;

(9) To conduct a narcotic treatment program, including a compounder, he shall apply on DEA Form 363a (Renewal Form).

(c) DEA Forms 224 and 225 may be obtained at any regional office of the Administration or by writing to the Registration Unit, Drug Enforcement Administration, Department of Justice, Post Office Box 28083, Central Station, Washington, D. C. 20005. DEA (or BND) Forms 224a, 225a and 363a will be mailed, as applicable, to each registered person approximately 60 days before the expiration date of his registration; if any registered person does not receive such forms within 45 days before the expiration date of his registration, he must promptly give notice of such fact and request such forms by writing to the Registration Unit of the Administration at the foregoing address.

(d) Each application for registration to handle any basic class of controlled substance listed in Schedule I (except to conduct chemical analysis with such classes) and each application for registration to manufacture a basic class of controlled substance listed in Schedule II shall include the Administration Controlled Substances Code Number, as set forth in Part 1308 of this chapter, for each basic class to be covered by such registration.

(e) Each application for registration to conduct research with any basic class of controlled substance listed in Schedule II shall include the Administration Controlled Substances Code Number, as set forth in Part 1308 of this chapter, for each such basic class to be manufactured or imported as a coincident activity of that registration. A statement listing the quantity of each such basic class or controlled substance to be imported or manufactured during the registration period for which application is being made shall be included with each such application. For purposes of this paragraph only, manufacturing is defined as the production of a controlled substance by synthesis, extraction or by agricultural/horticultural means.

(f) Each application shall include all information called for in the form, unless the item is not applicable, in which case this fact shall be indicated.

(g) Each application, attachment, or other document filed as part of an application, shall be signed by the applicant, if an individual; by a partner of the applicant, if a partnership; or by an officer of the applicant, if a corporation, corporate division, association, trust or other entity. An applicant may authorize one or more individuals, who would not otherwise be authorized to do so, to sign applications for the applicant by filing with the Registration Unit of the Administration a power of attorney for each such individual. The power of attorney shall be signed by a person who is authorized to sign applications under this paragraph and shall contain the signature of the individual being authorized to sign applications. The power of attorney shall be valid until revoked by the applicant.

§ 1301.34 Filing of application; joint filings.

(a) All applications for registration shall be submitted for filing to the Registration Unit, Drug Enforcement Administration, Department of Justice, Post Office Box 28083, Central Station, Washington, D. C. 20005. The appropriate registration fee and any required attachments must accompany the application.

(b) Any person required to obtain more than one registration may submit all applications in one package. Each application must be complete and should not refer to any accompanying application for required information.

§ 1301.35 Acceptance for filing; defective applications.

(a) Applications submitted for filing are dated upon receipt. If found to be complete, the application will be accepted for filing. Applications failing to comply with the requirements of this part will not generally be accepted for filing. In the case of minor defects as to completeness, the Administrator may accept the application for filing with a request to the applicant for additional information. A defective application will be returned to the applicant within 10 days following its receipt with a statement of the reason for not accepting the application for filing. A defective application may be corrected and resubmitted for filing at any time; the Administrator shall accept for filing any application upon resubmission by the applicant, whether complete or not.

(b) Accepting an application for filing does not preclude any subsequent request for additional information pursuant to § 1301.36 and has no bearing on whether the application will be granted.

§ 1301.36 Additional information.

The Administrator may require an applicant to submit such documents or written statements of fact relevant to the application as he deems necessary to determine whether the application should be granted. The failure of the applicant to provide such documents or statements within a reasonable time after being requested to do so shall be deemed to be a waiver by the applicant of an opportunity to present such documents or facts for consideration by the Administrator in granting or denying the application.

§ 1301.37 Amendments to and withdrawal of applications.

(a) An application may be amended or withdrawn without permission of the Administrator at any time before the date on which the applicant receives an order to show cause pursuant to § 1301.48, or before the date on which a notice of hearing on the application is published pursuant to § 1301.43, whichever is sooner. An application may be amended or withdrawn with permission of the Administrator at any time where good cause is shown by the applicant or where the amendment or withdrawal is in the public interest.

(b) After an application has been accepted for filing, the request by the applicant that it be returned or the failure of the applicant to respond to official correspondence regarding the application, when sent by registered or certified mail, return receipt requested, shall be deemed to be a withdrawal of the application.

§ 1301.38 Special procedures for certain applications.

(a) If, at the time of application for registration of a new pharmacy, the pharmacy has been issued a license from the appropriate State licensing agency, the applicant may include with his application an affidavit as to the existence of the State license in the following form:

AFFIDAVIT FOR NEW PHARMACY

I,_____, the_____
(Title of officer, official, partner,
_____of_____
or other position)   (Corporation, partnership, or sole
_____, doing business as_____at_____
proprietor)   (Store name)   (Number
_____
and Street)   (City)   (State)   (Zip code)
hereby certify that said store was issued a pharmacy permit
No. by the_____
(Board of Pharmacy or Licensing Agency)
of the State of_____on_____
(Date)

This statement is submitted in order to obtain a Drug Enforcement Administration registration number. I understand that if any information is false, the Administration may immediately suspend the registration for this store and commence proceedings to revoke under 21 U.S.C. 824(a) because of the danger to public health and safety. I further understand that any false information contained in this affidavit may subject me personally and the above-named corporation/partnership/business to prosecution under 21 U.S.C. 843, the penalties for conviction of which include imprisonment for up to 4 years, a fine of not more than $30,000 or both.

_____
Signature (Person who signs
Application for Registration)
State of_____
County of_____
Subscribed to and sworn before me this_____day
of _____, 19____.

_____
Notary Public

(b) Whenever the ownership of a pharmacy is being transferred from one person to another, if the transferee owns at least one other pharmacy licensed in the same State as the one the ownership of which is being transferred, the transferee may apply for registration prior to the date of transfer. The Administrator may register the applicant and authorize him to obtain controlled substances at the time of transfer. Such registration shall not authorize the transferee to dispense controlled substances until the pharmacy has been issued a valid State license. The transferee shall include with his application the following affidavit:

AFFIDAVIT FOR TRANSFER OF PHARMACY

I,_____, the_____
(Title of officer, official, partner,
_____of_____
or other position)   (Corporation, partnership, or sole
_____, doing business as_____,
proprietor)   (Store name)
hereby certify:
(1) That said company was issued a pharmacy permit
No._____by the_____
(Board of Pharmacy or Licensing Agency)
of the State of_____and a DEA Registration Number
_____for a pharmacy located at_____
(Number and Street)
_____; and
(City)   (State)   (Zip code)
(2) That said company is acquiring the pharmacy business
of_____doing business as_____
(Name of Seller)
with DEA Registration Number_____on or about
_____and that said company has applied (or
(Date of Transfer)
will apply) on_____for a pharmacy permit from
(Date)
the board of pharmacy (or licensing agency) of the State of
_____to do business as_____
(Store name)
at_____
(Number and Street)   (City)   (State)   (Zip code)

This statement is submitted in order to obtain a Drug Enforcement Administration registration number.

I understand that if a DEA registration number is issued, the pharmacy may acquire controlled substances but may not dispense them until a pharmacy permit or license is issued by the State board of pharmacy or licensing agency.

I understand that if any information is false, the Administration may immediately suspend the registration for this store and commence proceedings to revoke under 21 U.S.C. 824(a) because of the danger to public health and safety. I further understand that any false information contained in this affidavit may subject me personally to prosecution under 21 U.S.C. 843, the penalties for conviction of which include imprisonment for up to 4 years, a fine of not more than $30,000 or both.

_____
Signature (Person who signs
Application for Registration)

State of_____

County of_____

Subscribed to and sworn before me this_____day of _____, 19_____.

_____
Notary Public

(c) The Administrator shall follow the normal procedures for approving an application to verify the statements in the affidavit. If the statements prove to be false, the Administrator may revoke the registration on the basis of section 1304(a) (1) of the Act (21 U.S.C. 824(a) (1)) and suspend the registration immediately by pending revocation on the basis of section 1304(d) of the Act (21 U.S.C. 824(d)). At the same time, the Administrator may seize and place under seal all controlled substances possessed by the applicant under section 1304(f) of the Act (21 U.S.C. 824(f)). Intentional misuse of the affidavit procedure may subject the applicant to prosecution for fraud under section 403(a) (4) of the Act (21 U.S.C. 843(a) (4)), and obtaining controlled substances under a registration fraudulently gotten may subject the applicant to prosecution under section 403(a) (3) of the Act (21 U.S.C. 843(a) (3)). The penalties for conviction of either offense include imprisonment for up to 4 years, a fine not exceeding $30,000 or both.

Action on Applications for Registration: Revocation or Suspension of Registration

§ 1301.41 Administrative review generally.

The Administrator may inspect, or cause to be inspected, the establishment of an applicant or registrant, pursuant to Subpart A of Part 1316 of this chapter. The Administrator shall review the application for registration and other information gathered by the Administrator regarding an applicant in order to determine whether the applicable standards of section 1303 of the Act (21 U.S.C. 823) have been met by the applicant.

§ 1301.44 Certificate of registration; denial of registration.

(a) The Administrator shall issue a Certificate of Registration (DEA Form 223) to an applicant if the issuance of registration or reregistration is required under the applicable provisions of section 303 of the Act (21 U.S.C. 823). In the event that the issuance of registration or reregistration is not required, the Administrator shall deny the application. Before denying any application, the Administrator shall issue an order to show cause pursuant to § 1301.48 and, if requested by the applicant, shall hold a hearing on the application pursuant to § 1301.51.

(b) The Certificate of Registration (DEA Form 223) shall contain the name, address, and registration number of the registrant, the activity authorized by the registration, the schedules and/or Administration Controlled Substances Code Number (as set forth in Part 1308 of this chapter) of the controlled substances which the registrant is authorized to handle, the

amount of fee paid (or exemption), and the expiration date of the registration. The registrant shall maintain the certificate of registration at the registered location in a readily retrievable manner and shall permit inspection of the certificate by any official, agent or employee of the Administration or of any Federal, State, or local agency engaged in enforcement of laws relating to controlled substances.

§ 1301.47 Extension of registration pending final order.

In the event that an applicant for reregistration (who is doing business under a registration previously granted and not revoked or suspended) has applied for reregistration at least 45 days before the date on which the existing registration is due to expire, and the Administrator has issued no order on the application on the date on which the existing registration is due to expire, the existing registration of the applicant shall automatically be extended and continue in effect until the date on which the Administrator so issues his order. The Administrator may extend any other existing registration under the circumstances contemplated in this section even though the registrant failed to apply for reregistration at least 45 days before expiration of the existing registration, with or without request by the registrant, if the Administrator finds that such extension is not inconsistent with the public health and safety.

Modification, Transfer and Termination of Registration

§ 1301.61 Modification in registration.

Any registrant may apply to modify his registration to authorize the handling of additional controlled substances or to change his name or address, by submitting a letter of request to the Registration Unit, Drug Enforcement Administration, Department of Justice, Post Office Box 28083, Central Station, Washington, D. C. 20005. The letter shall contain the registrant's name, address, and registration number as printed on the certificate of registration, and the substances and/or schedules to be added to his registration or the new name or address and shall be signed in accordance with § 1301.32(f). If the registrant is seeking to handle additional controlled substances listed in Schedule I for the purpose of research or instructional activities, he shall attach three copies of a research protocol describing each research project involving the additional substances, or two copies of a statement describing the nature, extent, and duration of such instructional activities, as appropriate. No fee shall be required to be paid for the modification. The request for modification shall be handled in the same manner as an application for registration. If the modification in registration is approved, the Administrator shall issue a new certificate of registration (DEA Form 223) to the registrant, who shall maintain it with the old certificate of registration until expiration.

§ 1301.62 Termination of registration.

The registration of any person shall terminate if and when such person dies, ceases legal existence, or discontinues business or professional practice. Any registrant who ceases legal existence or discontinues business or professional practice shall notify the Administrator promptly of such fact.

§ 1301.63 Transfer of registration.

No registration or any authority conferred thereby shall be assigned or otherwise transferred except upon such conditions as the Administrator may specifically designate and then only pursuant to his written consent.

Security Requirements

§ 1301.71 Security requirements generally.

(a) All applicants and registrants shall provide effective controls and procedures to guard against theft and diversion of controlled substances. In order to determine whether a registrant has provided effective controls against diversion, the Administrator shall use the security requirements set forth in §§ 1301.72–1301.76 as standards for the physical security controls and operating procedures necessary to prevent diversion. Materials and construction which will provide a structural equivalent to the physical security controls set forth in §§ 1301.72, 1301.73 and 1301.75 may be used in lieu of the materials and construction described in those sections.

§ 1301.72 Physical security controls for non-practitioners; narcotic treatment programs and compounders for narcotic treatment programs; storage areas.

(a) *Schedules I and II.* Raw materials, bulk materials awaiting further processing, and finished products which are controlled substances listed in Schedule I or II shall be stored in one of the following secure storage areas:

(1) Where small quantities permit, a safe or steel cabinet:

(i) Which safe or steel cabinet shall have the following specifications or the equivalent: 30 man-minutes against surreptitious entry, 10 man-minutes against forced entry, 20 man-hours against lock manipulation, and 20 man-hours against radiological techniques;

(ii) Which safe or steel cabinet, if it weighs less than 750 pounds, is bolted or cemented to the floor or wall in such a way that it cannot be readily removed; and

(iii) Which safe or steel cabinet, if necessary, depending upon the quantities and type of controlled substances stored, is equipped with an alarm system which, upon attempted unauthorized entry, shall transmit a signal directly to a central protection company or a local or State police agency which has a legal duty to respond, or a 24-hour control station operated by the registrant, or such other protection as the Administrator may approve.

(2) A vault constructed before, or under construction on, September 1, 1971, which is of substantial construction with a steel door, combination or key lock, and an alarm system; or

(3) A vault constructed after September 1, 1971:

(i) The walls, floors, and ceilings of which vault are constructed of at least 8 inches of reinforced concrete or other substantial masonry, reinforced vertically and horizontally with ½-inch steel rods tied 6 inches on center, or the structural equivalent to such reinforced walls, floors, and ceilings;

(ii) The door and frame unit of which vault shall conform to the following specifications or the equivalent: 30 man-minutes against surreptitious entry, 10 man-minutes against forced entry, 20 man-hours against lock manipulation, and 20 man-hours against radiological techniques;

(iii) Which vault, if operations require it to remain open for frequent access, is equipped with a "day-gate" which is self-closing and self-locking, or the equivalent, for use during the hours of operation in which the vault door is open;

(iv) The walls or perimeter of which vault are equipped with an alarm, which upon unauthorized entry shall transmit a signal directly to a central station protection company, or a local or State police agency which has a legal duty to respond, or a 24-hour control station operated by the registrant, or such other protection as the Administrator may approve, and, if necessary, holdup buttons at strategic points of entry to the perimeter area of the vault;

(v) The door of which vault is equipped with contact switches; and

(vi) Which vault has one of the following: complete electrical lacing of the walls, floor and ceilings; sensitive ultrasonic equipment within the vault; a sensitive sound accumulator system; or such other device designed to detect illegal entry as may be approved by the Administration.

(b) *Schedules III, IV, and V.* Raw materials, bulk materials awaiting further processing, and finished products which are

controlled substances listed in Schedules III, IV, and V shall be stored in the following secure storage areas:

(1) A safe or steel cabinet as described in paragraph (a) (1) of this section;

(2) A vault as described in paragraph (a) (2) or (3) of this section equipped with an alarm system as described in paragraph (b) (4) (v) of this section;

(3) A building used for storage of Schedules III through V controlled substances with perimeter security which limits access during working hours and provides security after working hours and meets the following specifications:

(i) Has an electronic alarm system as described in paragraph (b) (4) (v) of this section,

(ii) Is equipped with self-closing, self-locking doors constructed of substantial material commensurate with the type of building construction, provided, however, a door which is kept closed and locked at all times when not in use and when in use is kept under direct observation of a responsible employee or agent of the registrant is permitted in lieu of a self-closing, self-locking door. Doors may be sliding or hinged. Regarding hinged doors, where hinges are mounted on the outside, such hinges shall be sealed, welded or otherwise constructed to inhibit removal. Locking devices for such doors shall be either of the multiple-position combination or key lock type and:

(a) In the case of key locks, shall require key control which limits access to a limited number of employees, or;

(b) In the case of combination locks, the combination shall be limited to a minimum number of employees and can be changed upon termination of employment of an employee having knowledge of the combination;

(4) A cage, located within a building on the premises, meeting the following specifications:

(i) Having walls constructed of not less than No. 10 gauge steel fabric mounted on steel posts, which posts are:

(a) At least one inch in diameter;

(b) Set in concrete or installed with lay bolts that are pinned or brazed; and

(c) Which are placed no more than ten feet apart with horizontal one and one-half inch reinforcements every sixty inches.

(ii) Having a mesh construction with openings of not more than two and one-half inches across the square,

(iii) Having a ceiling constructed of the same material, or in the alternative, a cage shall be erected which reaches and is securely attached to the structural ceiling of the building. A lighter gauge mesh may be used for the ceilings of large enclosed areas if walls are at least 14 feet in height,

(iv) Is equipped with a door constructed of No. 10 gauge steel fabric on a metal door frame in a metal door flange, and in all other respects conforms to all the requirements of 21 CFR 1301.72(b) (3) (ii), and

(v) Is equipped with an alarm system which upon unauthorized entry shall transmit a signal directly to a central station protection agency or a local or State police agency, each having a legal duty to respond, or to a 24-hour control station operated by the registrant, or to such other source of protection as the Administrator may approve;

(5) An enclosure of masonry or other material, approved in writing by the Administrator as providing security comparable to a cage;

(6) A building or enclosure within a building which has been inspected and approved by DEA or its predecessor agency, BNDD, and continues to provide adequate security against the diversion of Schedule III through V controlled substance, of which fact written acknowledgment has been made by the Special Agent in Charge of DEA for the area in which such building or enclosure is situated;

(7) Such other secure storage areas as may be approved by the Administrator after considering the factors listed in § 1301.71(b), (1) through (14);

(8) (i) Schedule III through V controlled substances may be stored with Schedules I and II controlled substances under security measures provided by 21 CFR 1301.72(a);

(ii) Non-controlled drugs, substances and other materials may be stored with Schedule III through V controlled substances in any of the secure storage areas required by 21 CFR 1301.72(b), provided that permission for such storage of non-controlled items is obtained in advance, in writing, from the Special Agent in Charge of DEA for the area in which such storage area is situated. Any such permission tendered must be upon the Special Agent in Charge's written determination that such non-segregated storage does not diminish security effectiveness for Schedule III through V controlled substances.

(c) *Multiple storage areas.* Where several types or classes of controlled substances are handled separately by the registrant or applicant for different purposes (e.g., returned goods, or goods in process), the controlled substances may be stored separately, provided that each storage area complies with the requirements set forth in this section.

(d) *Accessibility to storage areas.* The controlled substances storage areas shall be accessible only to an absolute minimum number of specifically authorized employees. When it is necessary for employee maintenance personnel, nonemployee maintenance personnel, business guests, or visitors to be present in or pass through controlled substances storage areas, the registrant shall provide for adequate observation of the area by an employee specifically authorized in writing.

§ 1301.73 Physical security controls for non-practitioners; compounders for narcotic treatment programs; manufacturing and compounding areas.

All manufacturing activities (including processing, packaging and labeling) involving controlled substances listed in any schedule and all activities of compounders shall be conducted in accordance with the following:

(a) All in-process substances shall be returned to the controlled substances storage area at the termination of the process. If the process is not terminated at the end of a workday (except where a continuous process or other normal manufacturing operation should not be interrupted), the processing area or tanks, vessels, bins or bulk containers containing such substances shall be securely locked, with adequate security for the area or building. If such security requires an alarm, such alarm, upon unauthorized entry, shall transmit a signal directly to a central station protection company, or local or State police agency which has a legal duty to respond, or a 24-hour control station operated by the registrant.

(b) Manufacturing activities with controlled substances shall be conducted in an area or areas of clearly defined limited access which is under surveillance by an employee or employees designated in writing as responsible for the area. "Limited access" may be provided, in the absence of physical dividers such as walls or partitions, by traffic control lines or restricted space designation. The employee designated as responsible for the area may be engaged in the particular manufacturing operation being conducted: *Provided,* That he is able to provide continuous surveillance of the area in order that unauthorized persons may not enter or leave the area without his knowledge.

(c) During the production of controlled substances, the manufacturing areas shall be accessible to only those employees required for efficient operation. When it is necessary for employee maintenance personnel, nonemployee maintenance personnel, business guests, or visitors to be present in or pass through manufacturing areas during production of controlled substances, the registrant shall provide for adequate observation of the area by an employee specifically authorized in writing.

§ 1301.74 Other security controls for non-practitioners; narcotic treatment programs and compounders for narcotic treatment programs.

(c) The registrant shall notify the Field Division Office of the Administration in his area of any theft or significant loss of any controlled substances upon discovery of such theft or loss. The supplier shall be responsible for reporting in-transit losses of controlled substances by the common or contract carrier selected pursuant to § 1301.74(e), upon discovery of such theft or loss. The registrant shall also complete DEA Form 106 regarding such theft or loss. Thefts must be reported whether or not the controlled substances are subsequently recovered and/or the responsible parties are identified and action taken against them.

(h) The acceptance of delivery of narcotic substances by a narcotic treatment program shall be made only by a licensed practitioner employed at the facility or other authorized individuals designated in writing. At the time of delivery, the licensed practitioner or other authorized individual designated in writing (excluding persons currently or previously dependent on narcotic drugs), shall sign for the narcotics and place his specific title (if any) on any invoice. Copies of these signed invoices shall be kept by the distributor.

(i) Narcotics dispensed or administered at a narcotic treatment program will be dispensed or administered directly to the patient by either (1) the licensed practitioner, (2) a registered nurse under the direction of the licensed practitioner, (3) a licensed practical nurse under the direction of the licensed practitioner, or (4) a pharmacist under the direction of the licensed practitioner.

(j) Persons enrolled in a narcotic treatment program will be required to wait in an area physically separated from the narcotic storage and dispensing area. This requirement will be enforced by the program physician and employees.

(k) All narcotic treatment programs must comply with standards established by the Secretary of Health and Human Services (after consultation with the Administration) respecting the quantities of narcotic drugs which may be provided to persons enrolled in a narcotic treatment program for unsupervised use.

(l) DEA may exercise discretion regarding the degree of security required in narcotic treatment programs based on such factors as the location of a program, the number of patients enrolled in a program and the number of physicians, staff members and security guards. Similarly, such factors will be taken into consideration when evaluating existing security or requiring new security at a narcotic treatment program.

§ 1301.75 Physical security controls for practitioners.

(a) Controlled substances listed in Schedule I shall be stored in a securely locked, substantially constructed cabinet.

(b) Controlled substances listed in Schedules II, III, IV, and V shall be stored in a securely locked, substantially constructed cabinet. However, pharmacies and institutional practitioners (as defined in § 1304.02(e) of this chapter) may disperse such substances throughout the stock of noncontrolled substances in such a manner as to obstruct the theft or diversion of the controlled substances.

(d) Carfentanil, etorphine hydrochloride and diprenorphine shall be stored in a safe or steel cabinet equivalent to a U. S. Government Class V security container.

§ 1301.76 Other security controls for practitioners.

(a) The registrant shall not employ, as an agent or employee who has access to controlled substances, any person who has been convicted of a felony offense relating to controlled substances or who, at any time, had an application for registration with the DEA denied, had a DEA registration revoked or has surrendered a DEA registration for cause. For purposes of this subsection, the term "for cause" means a surrender in lieu of, or as a consequence of, any federal or state administrative, civil or criminal action resulting from an investigation of the individual's handling of controlled substances.

(b) The registrant shall notify the Field Division Office of the Administration in his area of the theft or significant loss of any controlled substances upon discovery of such loss or theft. The registrant shall also complete DEA (or BND) Form 106 regarding such loss or theft.

(c) Whenever the registrant distributes a controlled substance (without being registered as a distributor, as permitted in § 1301.22(b) and/or §§ 1307.11–1307.14), he shall comply with the requirements imposed on nonpractitioners in § 1301.74 (a), (b), and (e).

Labeling and Packaging Requirements for Controlled Substances

§ 1302.02   Definitions.

As used in this part, the following terms shall have the meanings specified:

(a) The term "commercial container" means any bottle, jar, tube, ampule, or other receptacle in which a substance is held for distribution or dispensing to an ultimate user, and in addition, any box or package in which the receptacle is held for distribution or dispensing to an ultimate user. The term "commercial container" does not include any package liner, package insert or other material kept with or within a commercial container, nor any carton, crate, drum, or other package in which commercial containers are stored or are used for shipment of controlled substances.

(b) The term "label" means any display of written, printed, or graphic matter placed upon the commercial container of any controlled substance by any manufacturer of such substance.

(c) The term "labeling" means all labels and other written, printed, or graphic matter (1) upon any controlled substance or any of its commercial containers or wrappers, or (2) accompanying such controlled substance.

(d) The term "manufacture" means the producing, preparation, propagation, compounding, or processing of a drug or other substance or the packaging or repackaging of such substance, or the labeling or relabeling of the commercial container of such substance, but does not include the activities of a practitioner who, as an incident to his administration or dispensing such substance in the course of his professional practice, prepares, compounds, packages or labels such substance. The term "manufacturer" means a person who manufactures a drug or other substance, whether under a registration as a manufacturer or under authority of registration as a researcher or chemical analyst.

§ 1302.03   Symbol required; exceptions.

(a) Each commercial container of a controlled substance (except for a controlled substance excepted by the Administrator pursuant to § 1308.31 of this chapter) shall have printed on the label the symbol designating the schedule in which such controlled substance is listed. Each such commercial container, if it otherwise has no label, must bear a label complying with the requirement of this part.

(b) Each manufacturer shall print upon the labeling of each controlled substance distributed by him the symbol designating the schedule in which such controlled substance is listed.

(c) The following symbols shall designate the schedule corresponding thereto:

Schedule	Symbol
Schedule I	CI or C-I.
Schedule II	CII or C-II.
Schedule III	CIII or C-III.
Schedule IV	CIV or C-IV.
Schedule V	CV or C-V.

The word "schedule" need not be used. No distinction need be made between narcotic and nonnarcotic substances.

(d) The symbol is not required on a carton or wrapper in which a commercial container is held if the symbol is easily legible through such carton or wrapper.

(e) The symbol is not required on a commercial container too small or otherwise unable to accommodate a label, if the symbol is printed on the box or package from which the commercial container is removed upon dispensing to an ultimate user.

(f) The symbol is not required on a commercial container containing, or on the labeling of, a controlled substance being utilized in clinical research involving blind and double blind studies.

§ 1302.04   Location and size of symbol on label.

(a) The symbol shall be prominently located on the right upper corner of the principal panel of the label of the commercial container and/or the panel of the commercial container normally displayed to dispensers of any controlled substance listed in Schedules I through V. The symbol must be at least two times as large as the largest type otherwise printed on the label.

(b) In lieu of locating the symbol in the corner of the label, as prescribed in paragraph (a) of this section, the symbol may be overprinted on the label, in which case the symbol must be printed at least one-half the height of the label and in a contrasting color providing clear visibility against the background color of the label.

(c) In all cases the symbol shall be clear and large enough to afford easy identification of the schedule of the controlled substance upon inspection without removal from the dispenser's shelf.

§ 1302.05   Location and size of symbol on labeling.

The symbol shall be prominently located on all labeling other than labels covered by § 1302.04. In all cases the symbol shall be clear and large enough to afford prompt identification of the controlled substance upon inspection of the labeling.

§ 1302.07   Sealing of controlled substances.

(a) On each bottle, multiple dose vial, or other commercial container of any controlled substance listed in Schedule I or II or of any narcotic controlled substance listed in Schedule III or IV, there shall be securely affixed to the stopper, cap, lid, covering, or wrapper of such container a seal to disclose upon inspection any tampering or opening of the container.

Records and Reports of Registrants

§ 1304.02   Definitions.

As used in this part, the following terms shall have the meanings specified:

(a) The term "Act" means the Controlled Substances Act (84 Stat. 1242; 21 U.S.C. 801) and/or the Controlled Substances Import and Export Act (84 Stat. 1285; 21 U.S.C. 951).

(b) The term "commercial container" means any bottle, jar, tube, ampule, or other receptable in which a substance is held for distribution or dispensing to an ultimate user, and in addition, any box or package in which the receptacle is held for distribution or dispensing to an ultimate user. The term "commercial container" does not include any package liner, package insert or other material kept with or within a commercial container, nor any carton, crate, drum, or other package in which commercial containers are stored or are used for shipment of controlled substances.

(c) The term "dispenser" means an individual practitioner, institutional practitioner, pharmacy or pharmacist who dispenses a controlled substance.

(d) The term "individual practitioner" means a physician, dentist, veterinarian, or other individual licensed, registered, or otherwise permitted, by the United States or the jurisdiction in which he practices, to dispense a controlled substance in the course of professional practice, but does not include a pharmacist, a pharmacy, or an institutional practitioner.

(e) The term "institutional practitioner" means a hospital or other person (other than an individual) licensed, registered, or otherwise permitted, by the United States or the jurisdiction in which it practices, to dispense a controlled substance in the course of professional practice, but does not include a pharmacy.

(f) The term "name" means the official name, common or usual name, chemical name, or brand name of a substance.

(g) The term "pharmacist" means any pharmacist licensed by a State to dispense controlled substances, and shall include any other person (e.g., pharmacist intern) authorized by a State to dispense controlled substances under the supervision of a pharmacist licensed by such State.

(h) The term "readily retrievable" means that certain records are kept by automatic data processing systems or other electronic or mechanized record-keeping systems in such a manner that they can be separated out from all other records in a reasonable time and/or records are kept on which certain items are asterisked, redlined, or in some other manner visually identifiable apart from other items appearing on the records.

§ 1304.03 Persons required to keep records and file reports.

(a) Each registrant shall maintain the records and inventories and shall file the reports required by this part, except as exempted by this section. Any registrant who is authorized to conduct other activities without being registered to conduct those activities, either pursuant to § 1301.22(b) of this chapter or pursuant to §§ 1307.11–1307.15 of this chapter, shall maintain the records and inventories and shall file the reports required by this part for persons registered to conduct such activities. This latter requirement should not be construed as requiring stocks of controlled substances being used in various activities under one registration to be stored separately, nor that separate records are required for each activity. The intent of the Administration is to permit the registrant to keep one set of records which are adapted by the registrant to account for controlled substances used in any activity. Also, the Administration does not wish to require separate stocks of the same substance to be purchased and stored for separate activities. Otherwise, there is no advantage gained by permitting several activities under one registration. Thus, when a researcher manufactures a controlled item, he must keep a record of the quantity manufactured; when he distributes a quantity of the item, he must use and keep invoices or order forms to document the transfer; when he imports a substance, he keeps as part of his records the documentation required of an importer; and when substances are used in chemical analysis, he need not keep a record of this because such a record would not be required of him under a registration to do chemical analysis. All of these records may be maintained in one consolidated record system. Similarly, the researcher may store all of his controlled items in one place, and every two years take inventory of all items on hand, regardless of whether the substances were manufactured by him, imported by him, or purchased domestically by him, or whether the substances will be administered to subjects, distributed to other researchers, or destroyed during chemical analysis.

(b) A registered individual practitioner is required to keep records, as described in § 1304.04 of controlled substances in Schedules II, III, IV, and V which are dispensed, other than by prescribing or administering in the lawful course of professional practice.

(c) A registered individual practitioner is not required to keep records of controlled substances in Schedules II, III, IV, and V which are prescribed in the lawful course of professional practice, unless such substances are prescribed in the course of maintenance or detoxification treatment of an individual.

(d) A registered individual practitioner is not required to keep records of controlled substances listed in Schedules II, III, IV and V which are administered in the lawful course of professional practice unless the practitioner regularly engages in the dispensing or administering of controlled substances and charges patients, either separately or together with charges for other professional services, for substances so dispensed or administered. Records are required to be kept for controlled substances administered in the course of maintenance or detoxification treatment of an individual.

§ 1304.04 Maintenance of records and inventories.

(a) Every inventory and other records required to be kept under this Part shall be kept by the registrant and be available, for at least 2 years from the date of such inventory or records, for inspection and copying by authorized employees of the Administration, except that financial and shipping records (such as invoices and packing slips but not executed order forms subject to paragraph 1305.13 of this chapter) may be kept at a central location, rather than at the registered location, if the registrant has notified the Administration of his intention to keep central records. Written notification must be submitted by registered or certified mail, return receipt requested, in triplicate, to the Special Agent in Charge of the Administration in the area in which the registrant is located. Unless the registrant is informed by the Special Agent in Charge that permission to keep central records is denied, the registrant may maintain central records commencing 14 days after receipt of his notification by the Special Agent in Charge.

All notifications must include:

(1) The nature of the records to be kept centrally.

(2) The exact location where the records will be kept.

(3) The name, address, DEA registration number and type of DEA registration of the registrant whose records are being maintained centrally.

(4) Whether central records will be maintained in a manual, or computer readable form.

(b) All registrants that are authorized to maintain a central recordkeeping system shall be subject to the following conditions:

(1) The records to be maintained at the central record location shall not include executed order forms, prescriptions and/or inventories which shall be maintained at each registered location.

(2) If the records are kept on microfilm, computer media or in any form requiring special equipment to render the records easily readable, the registrant shall provide access to such equipment with the records. If any code system is used (other than pricing information), a key to the code shall be provided to make the records understandable.

(3) The registrant agrees to deliver all or any part of such records to the registered location within two business days upon receipt of a written request from the Administration for such records, and if the Administration chooses to do so in lieu of requiring delivery of such records to the registered location, to allow authorized employees of the Administration to inspect such records at the central location upon request by such employees without a warrant of any kind.

(4) In the event that a registrant fails to comply with these conditions, the Special Agent in Charge may cancel such central recordkeeping authorization, and all other central recordkeeping authorizations held by the registrant without a hearing or other procedures. In the event of a cancellation of central recordkeeping authorizations under this sub-paragraph the registrant shall, within the time specified by the Special Agent in Charge, comply with the requirements of this section that all records be kept at the registered location.

(c) Registrants need not notify the Special Agent in Charge or obtain central recordkeeping approval in order to maintain records on an in-house computer system.

II/42 Selected USP General Notices and Chapters

(d) ARCOS participants who desire authorization to report from other than their registered locations must obtain a separate central reporting identifier. Request for central reporting identifiers will be submitted to: ARCOS Unit, P. O. Box 28293, Central Station, Washington, D. C. 20005.

(e) All central recordkeeping permits previously issued by the Administration will expire on September 30, 1980. Registrants who desire to continue maintaining central records will make notification to the local Special Agent in Charge as provided in (a) above.

(f) Each registered manufacturer, distributor, importer, exporter, narcotic treatment program and compounder for narcotic treatment program shall maintain inventories and records of controlled substances as follows:

(1) Inventories and records of controlled substances listed in Schedules I and II shall be maintained separately from all of the records of the registrant; and

(2) Inventories and records of controlled substances listed in Schedules III, IV, and V shall be maintained either separately from all other records of the registrant or in such form that the information required is readily retrievable from the ordinary business records of the registrant.

(g) Each registered individual practitioner required to keep records and institutional practitioner shall maintain inventories and records of controlled substances in the manner prescribed in paragraph (f) of this section.

(h) Each registered pharmacy shall maintain the inventories and records of controlled substances as follows:

(1) Inventories and records of all controlled substances listed in Schedules I and II shall be maintained separately from all other records of the pharmacy, and prescriptions for such substances shall be maintained in a separate prescription file; and

(2) Inventories and records of controlled substances listed in Schedules III, IV, and V shall be maintained either separately from all other records of the pharmacy or in such form that the information required is readily retrievable from ordinary business records of the pharmacy, and prescriptions for such substances shall be maintained either in a separate prescription file for controlled substances listed in Schedules III, IV, and V only or in such form that they are readily retrievable from the other prescription records of the pharmacy. Prescriptions will be deemed readily retrievable if, at the time they are initially filed, the face of the prescription is stamped in red ink in the lower right corner with the letter "C" no less than 1-inch high and filed either in the prescription file for controlled substances listed in Schedules I and II or in the usual consecutively numbered prescription file for non-controlled substances.

Inventory Requirements

§ 1304.11   General requirements for inventories.

(a) Each inventory shall contain a complete and accurate record of all controlled substances on hand on the date the inventory is taken. Controlled substances shall be deemed to be "on hand" if they are in the possession of or under the control of the registrant, including substances returned by a customer, substances ordered by a customer but not yet invoiced, substances stored in a warehouse on behalf of the registrant, and substances in the possession of employees of the registrant and intended for distribution as complimentary samples.

(b) A separate inventory shall be made by a registrant for each registered location. In the event controlled substances are in the possession or under the control of the registrant at a location for which he is not registered, the substances shall be included in the inventory of the registered location to which they are subject to control or to which the person possessing the substance is responsible. Each inventory for a registered location shall be kept at the registered location.

(c) A separate inventory shall be made by a registrant for each independent activity for which he is registered, except as provided in § 1304.18.

(d) A registrant may take an inventory on a date that is within 4 days of his biennial inventory date pursuant to § 1304.13 if he notifies in advance the Special Agent in Charge of the Administration in his area of the date on which he will take the inventory. A registrant may take an inventory either as of the opening of business or as of the close of business on the inventory date. The registrant shall indicate on the inventory records whether the inventory is taken as of the opening or as of the close of business and the date the inventory is taken.

(e) An inventory must be maintained in a written, typewritten or printed form. An inventory taken by use of an oral recording device must be promptly transcribed.

§ 1304.12   Initial inventory date.

(b) Every person required to keep records who is registered after May 1, 1971, and who was not provisionally registered on that date, shall take an inventory of all stocks of controlled substances on hand on the date he first engages in the manufacture, distribution, or dispensing of controlled substances, in accordance with §§ 1304.15–1304.19, as applicable. In the event a person commences business with no controlled substances on hand, he shall record this fact as his initial inventory.

§ 1304.13   Biennial inventory date.

Every 2 years following the date on which the initial inventory is taken by a registrant pursuant to § 1304.12, the registrant shall take a new inventory of all stocks of controlled substances on hand. The biennial inventory may be taken (a) on the day of the year on which the initial inventory was taken or (b) on the registrant's regular general physical inventory date, if any, which is nearest to and does not vary by more than 6 months from the biennial date that would otherwise apply or (c) on any other fixed date which does not vary by more than 6 months from the biennial date that would otherwise apply. If the registrant elects to take the biennial inventory on his regular general physical inventory date or another fixed date, he shall notify the Administration of this election and of the date on which the biennial inventory will be taken.

§ 1304.14   Inventory date for newly controlled substances.

On the effective date of a rule by the Administrator pursuant to §§ 1308.48–1308.49, or 1308.50 of this chapter adding a substance to any schedule of controlled substances, which substance was, immediately prior to that date, not listed on any such schedule, every registrant required to keep records who possesses that substance shall take an inventory of all stocks of the substance on hand. Thereafter such substance shall be included in each inventory made by the registrant pursuant to § 1304.13.

§ 1304.15   Inventories of manufacturers.

Each person registered or authorized (by § 1301.22(b), § 1307.12, or § 1307.15 of this chapter) to manufacture controlled substances shall include the following information in his inventory:

(a) For each controlled substance in bulk form to be used in (or capable of use in) the manufacture of the same or other controlled or non-controlled substances in finished form:

(1) The name of the substance; and

(2) The total quantity of the substance to the nearest metric unit weight consistent with unit size (except that for inventories made in 1971, avoirdupois weights may be utilized where metric weights are not readily available).

(b) For each controlled substance in the process of manufacture on the inventory date:

(1) The name of the substance;

(2) The quantity of the substance in each batch and/or stage of manufacture, identified by the batch number or other appropriate identifying number;

(3) The physical form which the substance is to take upon completion of the manufacturing process (e.g., granulations, tablets, capsules, or solutions), identified by the batch number or other appropriate identifying number, and if possible the finished form of the substance (e.g., 10-milligram tablet or 10-milligram concentration per fluid ounce or milliliter) and the number or volume thereof; and

(c) For each controlled substance in finished form:

(1) The name of the substance;

(2) Each finished form of the substance (e.g., 10-milligram tablet or 10-milligram concentration per fluid ounce or milliliter);

(3) The number of units or volume of each finished form in each commercial container (e.g., 100-tablet bottle or 3-milliliter vial); and

(4) The number of commercial containers of each such finished form (e.g., four 100-tablet bottles or six 3-milliliter vials).

(d) For each controlled substance not included in paragraphs (a), (b) or (c) of this section (e.g., damaged, defective or impure substances awaiting disposal, substances held for quality control purposes, or substances maintained for extemporaneous compoundings):

(1) The name of the substance;

(2) The total quantity of the substance to the nearest metric unit weight or the total number of units of finished form; and

(3) The reason for the substance being maintained by the registrant and whether such substance is capable of use in the manufacture of any controlled substance in finished form.

§ 1304.17   Inventories of dispensers and researchers.

Each person registered or authorized (by § 1301.22(b) of this chapter) to dispense or conduct research with controlled substances and required to keep records pursuant to § 1304.03 shall include in his inventory the same information required of manufacturers pursuant to § 1304.15(c) and (d). In determining the number of units of each finished form of a controlled substance in a commercial container which has been opened, the dispenser shall do as follows:

(a) If the substance is listed in Schedule I or II, he shall make an exact count or measure of the contents; and

(b) If the substance is listed in Schedule III, IV, or V, he shall make an estimated count or measure of the contents, unless the container holds more than 1,000 tablets or capsules in which case he must make an exact count of the contents.

Continuing Records

§ 1304.21   General requirements for continuing records.

(a) On and after May 1, 1971, every registrant required to keep records pursuant to § 1304.03 shall maintain on a current basis a complete and accurate record of each such substance manufactured, imported, received, sold, delivered, exported, or otherwise disposed of by him, except that no registrant shall be required to maintain a perpetual inventory.

(b) Separate records shall be maintained by a registrant for each registered location except as provided in § 1304.04(a). In the event controlled substances are in the possession or under the control of a registrant at a location for which he is not registered, the substances shall be included in the records of the registered location to which they are subject to control or to which the person possessing the substance is responsible.

(c) Separate records shall be maintained by a registrant for each independent activity for which he is registered, except as provided in §§ 1304.25 and 1304.26.

(d) In recording dates of receipt, importation, distribution, exportation, or other transfers, the date on which the controlled substances are actually received, imported, distributed, exported, or otherwise transferred shall be used as the date of receipt or distribution of any documents of transfer (e.g., invoices or packing slips).

§ 1304.23   Records for distributors.

Each person registered or authorized (by § 1301.22(b) or §§ 1307.11–1307.14 of this chapter) to distribute controlled substances shall maintain records with the following information for each controlled substance:

(a) The name of the substance;

(b) Each finished form (e.g., 10-milligram tablet or 10-milligram concentration per fluid ounce or milliliter) and the number of units or volume of finished form in each commercial container (e.g., 100-tablet bottle or 3-milliliter vial);

(c) The number of commercial containers of each such finished form received from other persons, including the date of and number of containers in each receipt and the name, address, and registration number of the person from whom the containers were received;

(d) The number of commercial containers of each such finished form imported directly by the person (under a registration or authorization to import), including the date of, the number of commercial containers in, and the import permit or declaration number for, each importation;

(e) The number of commercial containers of each such finished form distributed to other persons, including the date of and number of containers in each distribution and the name, address, and registration number of the person to whom the containers were distributed;

(f) The number of commercial containers of each such finished form exported directly by the person (under a registration or authorization to export), including the date of, the number of commercial containers in, and the export permit or declaration number for, each exportation; and

(g) The number of units or volume of finished forms and/or commercial containers distributed or disposed of in any other manner by the person (e.g., by distribution as complimentary samples or by destruction) including the date and manner of distribution or disposal, the name, address, and registration number of the person to whom distributed, and the quantity of the substance in finished form distributed or disposed.

§ 1304.24   Records for dispensers and researchers.

Each person registered or authorized (by § 1301.22(b) of this chapter) to dispense or conduct research with controlled substances and required to keep records pursuant to § 1304.03 shall maintain records with the following information for each controlled substance:

(a) The name of the substance;

(b) Each finished form (e.g., 10-milligram tablet or 10-milligram concentration per fluid ounce or milliliter) and the number of units or volume of finished form in each commercial container (e.g., 100-tablet bottle or 3-milliliter vial);

(c) The number of commercial containers of each such finished form received from other persons, including the date of and number of containers in each receipt and the name, address, and registration number of the person from whom the containers were received;

(d) The number of units or volume of such finished form dispensed, including the name and address of the person to whom it was dispensed, the date of dispensing, the number of units or volume dispensed, and the written or typewritten name or initials of the individual who dispensed or administered the substance on behalf of the dispenser; and

(e) The number of units or volume of such finished forms and/or commercial containers disposed of in any other manner by the registrant, including the date and manner of disposal and the quantity of the substance in finished form disposed.

§ 1304.28   Records for maintenance treatment programs and detoxification treatment programs.

(a) Each person registered or authorized (by § 1301.22 of this chapter) to maintain and/or detoxify controlled substance users in a narcotic treatment program shall maintain records with the following information for each narcotic controlled substance:

(1) Name of substance;

(2) Strength of substance;

(3) Dosage form;

(4) Date dispensed;

(5) Adequate identification of patient (consumer);

(6) Amount consumed;

(7) Amount and dosage form taken home by patient; and

(8) Dispenser's initials.

(b) The records required by paragraph (a) of this section will be maintained in a dispensing log at the narcotic treatment program site and will be maintained in compliance with § 1304.24 without reference to § 1304.03.

(c) All sites which compound a bulk narcotic solution from bulk narcotic powder to liquid for on-site use must keep a separate batch record of the compounding.

(d) Records of identity, diagnosis, prognosis, or treatment of any patients which are maintained in connection with the performance of a narcotic treatment program shall be confidential, except that such records may be disclosed for purposes and under the circumstances authorized by Part 310 and Part 1401 of this title.

§ 1304.29 Records for treatment programs which compound narcotics for treatment programs and other locations.

Each person registered or authorized by § 1301.22 of this chapter to compound narcotic drugs for off-site use in a narcotic treatment program shall maintain records which include the following information for each narcotic drug:

(a) For each narcotic controlled substance in bulk form to be used in, or capable of use in, or being used in, the compounding of the same or other non-controlled substances in finished form:

(1) The name of the substance;

(2) The quantity compounded in bulk form by the registrant, including the date, quantity and batch or other identifying number of each batch compounded;

(3) The quantity received from other persons, including the date and quantity of each receipt and the name, address and registration number of the other person from whom the substance was received;

(4) The quantity imported directly by the registrant (under a registration as an importer) for use in compounding by him, including the date, quantity and import permit or declaration number of each importation;

(5) The quantity used to compound the same substance in finished form, including:

(i) The date and batch or other identifying number of each compounding;

(ii) The quantity used in the compound;

(iii) The finished form (e.g., 10-milligram tablets or 10-milligram concentration per fluid ounce or milliliter);

(iv) The number of units of finished form compounded;

(v) The quantity used in quality control;

(vi) The quantity lost during compounding and the causes therefore, if known;

(vii) The total quantity of the substance contained in the finished form;

(viii) The theoretical and actual yields; and

(ix) Such other information as is necessary to account for all controlled substances used in the compounding process;

(6) The quantity used to manufacture other controlled and non-controlled substances; including the name of each substance manufactured and the information required in paragraph (a)(5) of this section;

(7) The quantity distributed in bulk form to other programs, including the date and quantity of each distribution and the name, address and registration number of each program to whom a distribution was made;

(8) The quantity exported directly by the registrant (under a registration as an exporter), including the date, quantity, and export permit or declaration number of each exportation; and

(9) The quantity disposed of by destruction, including the reason, date and manner of destruction. All other destruction of narcotic controlled substances will comply with § 1307.22.

(b) For each narcotic controlled substance in finished form:

(1) The name of the substance;

(2) Each finished form (e.g., 10-milligram tablet or 10-milligram concentration per fluid ounce or milliliter) and the number of units or volume or finished form in each commercial container (e.g., 100-tablet bottle or 3-milliliter vial);

(3) The number of containers of each such commercial finished form compounded from bulk form by the registrant, including the information required pursuant to paragraph (a)(5) of this section;

(4) The number of units of finished forms and/or commercial containers received from other persons, including the date of and number of units and/or commercial containers in each receipt and the name, address and registration number of the person from whom the units were received;

(5) The number of units of finished forms and/or commercial containers imported directly by the person (under a registration or authorization to import), including the date of, the number of units and/or commercial containers in, and the import permit or declaration number for, each importation;

(6) The number of units and/or commercial containers compounded by the registrant from units in finished form received from others or imported, including:

(i) The date and batch or other identifying number of each compounding;

(ii) The operation performed (e.g., repackaging or relabeling);

(iii) The number of units of finished form used in the compound, the number compounded and the number lost during compounding, with the causes for such losses, if known; and

(iv) Such other information as is necessary to account for all controlled substances used in the compounding process;

(7) The number of containers distributed to other programs, including the date, the number of containers in each distribution, and the name, address and registration number of the program to whom the containers were distributed;

(8) The number of commercial containers exported directly by the registrant (under a registration as an exporter), including the date, number of containers and export permit or declaration number for each exportation; and

(9) The number of units of finished forms and/or commercial containers destroyed in any manner by the registrant, including the reason, the date and manner of destruction. All other destruction of narcotic controlled substances will comply with §1307.22.

Order Forms

§ 1305.02 Definitions.

As used in this part, the following terms shall have the meanings specified:

(b) The term "purchaser" means any registered person entitled to obtain and execute order forms pursuant to § 1305.04 and § 1305.06.

(c) The term "supplier" means any registered person entitled to fill order forms pursuant to § 1305.08.

Change to read:

§ 1305.03 Distributions requiring order forms.

An order form (DEA Form 222) is required for each distribution of a controlled substance listed in Schedule I or II, except for the following:

(a) The exportation of such substances from the United States in conformity with the Act;

(b) The delivery of such substances to or by a common or contract carrier for carriage in the lawful and usual course of its business, or to or by a warehouseman for storage in the lawful and usual course of its business (but excluding such carriage or storage by the owner of the substance in connection with the distribution to a third person);

(c) The procurement of a sample of such substances by an exempt law enforcement official pursuant to § 1301.26(b) of this chapter, provided that the receipt required by that section is used and is preserved in the manner prescribed in this part for order forms;

(d) The procurement of such substances by a civil defense or disaster relief organization, pursuant to § 1301.27 of this chapter, provided that the Civil Defense Emergency Order Form required by that section is used and is preserved with other records of the registrant; and

(e) The purchase of such substances by the master or first officer of a vessel pursuant to § 1301.28 of this chapter: Provided, that copies of the record of sale are generated, distributed and preserved by the vendor according to that section.

(f) The delivery of such substances to a registered analytical laboratory, or its agent approved by DEA, from an anonymous source for the analysis of the drug sample, provided the laboratory has obtained a written waiver of the order form requirement from the Regional Director[1] of the Region in which the laboratory is located, which waiver may be granted upon agreement of the laboratory to conduct its activities in accordance with Administration guidelines.

§ 1305.04   Persons entitled to obtain and execute order forms.

(a) Order forms may be obtained only by persons who are registered under section 303 of the Act (21 U.S.C. 823) to handle controlled substances listed in Schedules I and II, and by persons who are registered under section 1008 of the Act (21 U.S.C. 958) to export such substances. Persons not registered to handle controlled substances listed in Schedule I or II and persons registered only to import controlled substances listed in any schedule are not entitled to obtain order forms.

(b) An order form may be executed only on behalf of the registrant named thereon and only if his registration as to the substances being purchased has not expired or been revoked or suspended.

§ 1305.05   Procedure for obtaining order forms.

(a) Order forms are issued in mailing envelopes containing either seven or fourteen forms, each form containing an original duplicate and triplicate copy (respectively, Copy 1, Copy 2, and Copy 3). A limit, which is based on the business activity of the registrant, will be imposed on the number of order forms which will be furnished on any requisition unless additional forms are specifically requested and a reasonable need for such additional forms is shown.

(b) Any person applying for a registration which would entitle him to obtain order forms may requisition such forms by so indicating on the application form; order forms will be supplied upon the registration of the applicant. Any person holding a registration entitling him to obtain order forms may requisition such forms for the first time by contacting any Division Officer or the Registration Unit of the Administration. Any person already holding order forms may requisition additional forms on DEA Form 222a which is mailed to a registrant approximately 30 days after each shipment of order forms to that registrant or by contacting any Division Office or the Registration Unit of the Administration. All forms requisition (DEA Form 222a) shall be submitted to the Registration Unit, Drug Enforcement Administration, Department of Justice, Post Office Box 28083, Central Station, Washington, D. C. 20005.

(c) Each requisition shall show the name, address, and registration number of the registrant and the number of books of order forms desired. Each requisition shall be signed and dated by the same person who signed the most recent application for registration or for reregistration, or by any person authorized to obtain and execute order forms by a power of attorney pursuant to § 1305.07.

(d) Order forms will be serially numbered and issued with the name, address and registration number of the registrant, the authorized activity and schedules of the registrant. This information cannot be altered or changed by the registrant; any errors must be corrected by the Registration Unit of the Administration by returning the forms with notification of the error.

§ 1305.06   Procedure for executing order forms.

(a) Order forms shall be prepared and executed by the purchaser simultaneously in triplicate by means of interleaved carbon sheets which are part of the DEA Form 222. Order forms shall be prepared by use of a typewriter, pen, or indelible pencil.

(b) Only one item shall be entered on each numbered line. There are ten lines on each order form. If one order form is not sufficient to include all items in an order, additional forms shall be used. Order forms for carfentanil, etorphine hydrochloride and diprenorphine shall contain only these substances. The total number of items ordered shall be noted on that form in the space provided.

(c) An item shall consist of one or more commercial or bulk containers of the same finished or bulk form and quantity of the same substance; a separate item shall be made for each commercial or bulk container of different finished or bulk form, quantity or substance. For each item the form shall show the name of the article ordered, the finished or bulk form of the article (e.g., 10-milligram tablet, 10-milligram concentration per fluid ounce or milliliter, or USP), the number of units or volume in each commercial or bulk container (e.g., 100-tablet bottle or 3-milliliter vial) or the quantity or volume of each bulk container (e.g., 10 kilograms), the number of commercial or bulk containers ordered, and the name and quantity per unit of the controlled substance or substances contained in the article if not in pure form. The catalogue number of the article may be included at the discretion of the purchaser.

(d) The name and address of the supplier from whom the controlled substances are being ordered shall be entered on the form. Only one supplier may be listed on any one form.

(e) Each order form shall be signed and dated by a person authorized to sign a requisition for order forms on behalf of the purchaser pursuant to § 1305.05(c). The name of the purchaser, if different from the individual signing the order form, shall also be inserted in the signature space. Unexecuted order forms may be kept and may be executed at a location other than the registered location printed on the form, provided that all unexecuted forms are delivered promptly to the registered location upon an inspection of such location by any officer authorized to make inspections, or to enforce, any Federal, State, or local law regarding controlled substances.

§ 1305.07   Power of attorney.

Any purchaser may authorize one or more individuals, whether or not located at the registered location of the purchaser, to obtain and execute order forms on his behalf by executing a power of attorney for each such individual. The power of attorney shall be signed by the same person who signed (or was authorized to sign, pursuant to § 1301.32(f) of this chapter or § 1311.32(f) of this chapter) the most recent application for registration or reregistration and by the individual being authorized to obtain and execute order forms. The power of attorney shall be filed with the executed order forms of the purchaser, and shall be retained for the same period as any order form bearing the signature of the attorney. The power of attorney shall be available for inspection together with other order form records. Any power of attorney may be revoked at any time by executing a notice of revocation, signed by the person who signed (or was authorized to sign) the power of attorney or by a successor, whoever signed the most recent application for registration or reregistration, and filing it with the power of attorney being revoked. The form for the power of attorney and notice of revocation shall be similar to the following:

POWER OF ATTORNEY FOR DEA ORDER FORMS

_____
(Name of registrant)

_____
(Address of registrant)

_____
(DEA registration
number)

I, _____, the undersigned,
(name of person granting power)

who is authorized to sign the current application for registration of the above-named registrant under the Controlled Substances Act or Controlled Substances Import and Export Act, have made, constituted, and appointed, and by these presents, do make, constitute, and appoint _____ my true
(name of attorney-in-fact)

and lawful attorney for me in my name, place, and stead, to execute applications for books of official order forms and to sign such order forms in requisition for Schedule I and II controlled substances, in accordance with section 308 of the Controlled Substances Act (21 U.S.C. 828) and Part 305 of Title 21 of the Code of Federal Regulations. I hereby ratify and confirm all that said attorney shall lawfully do or cause to be done by virtue hereof.

_____
(Signature of person
granting power)

I, _____, hereby affirm that
(name of attorney-in-fact)

I am the person named herein as attorney-in-fact and that the signature affixed hereto is my signature.

_____
(Signature of
attorney-in-fact)

Witnesses:

1. _____

2. _____

Signed and dated on the _____ day of _____, 19___,

at _____

NOTICE OF REVOCATION

The foregoing power of attorney is hereby revoked by the undersigned, who is authorized to sign the current application for registration of the above-named registrant under the Controlled Substances Act or the Controlled Substances Import and Export Act. Written notice of this revocation has been given to the attorney-in-fact_____ this same day.

_____
(Signature of person
revoking power)

Witnesses:

1. _____

2. _____

Signed and dated on the _____ day of _____, 19___,

at _____

§ 1305.08   Persons entitled to fill order forms.

An order form may be filled only by a person registered as a manufacturer or distributor of controlled substances listed in Schedule I or II under section 303 of the Act (21 U.S.C. 823)

or as an importer of such substances under section 1008 of the Act (21 U.S.C. 958), except for the following:

(a) A person registered to dispense such substances under section 303 of the Act, or to export such substances under section 1008 of the Act, if he is discontinuing business or if his registration is expiring without reregistration, may dispose of any controlled substances listed in Schedule I or II in his possession pursuant to order forms in accordance with § 1307.14 of this chapter;

(b) A person who has obtained any controlled substance in Schedule I or II by order form may return such substance, or portion thereof, to the person from whom he obtained the substance or the manufacturer of the substance pursuant to the order form of the latter person;

(c) A person registered to dispense such substances may distribute such substances to another dispenser pursuant to, and only in the circumstances described in, § 1307.11 of this chapter; and

(d) A person registered or authorized to conduct chemical analysis or research with controlled substances may distribute a controlled substance listed in Schedule I or II to another person registered or authorized to conduct chemical analysis, instructional activities, or research with such substances pursuant to the order form of the latter person, if such distribution is for the purpose of furthering such chemical analysis, instructional activities, or research.

(e) A person registered as a compounder of narcotic substances for use at off-site locations in conjunction with a narcotic treatment program at the compounding location, who is authorized to handle Schedule II narcotics, is authorized to fill order forms for distribution of narcotic drugs to off-site narcotic treatment programs only.

§ 1305.09   Procedure for filling order forms.

(a) The purchaser shall submit Copy 1 and Copy 2 of the order form to the supplier, and retain Copy 3 in his own files.

(b) The supplier shall fill the order, if possible and if he desires to do so, and record on Copies 1 and 2 the number of commercial or bulk containers furnished on each item and the date on which such containers are shipped to the purchaser. If an order cannot be filled in its entirety, it may be filled in part and the balance supplied by additional shipments within 60 days following the date of the order form. No order form shall be valid more than 60 days after its execution by the purchaser, except as specified in paragraph (f) of this section.

(c) The controlled substances shall only be shipped to the purchaser and at the location printed by the Administration on the order form, except as specified in paragraph (f) of this section.

(d) The supplier shall retain Copy 1 of the order form for his own files and forward Copy 2 to the Special Agent in Charge of the Drug Enforcement Administration in the area in which the supplier is located. Copy 2 shall be forwarded at the close of the month during which the order is filled; if an order is filled by partial shipments, Copy 2 shall be forwarded at the close of the month during which the final shipment is made or during which the 60-day validity period expires.

(e) The purchaser shall record on Copy 3 of the order form the number of commercial or bulk containers furnished on each item and the dates on which such containers are received by the purchaser.

(f) Order forms submitted by registered procurement officers of the Defense Personnel Support Center of Defense Supply Agency for delivery to armed services establishments within the United States may be shipped to locations other than the location printed on the order form, and in partial shipments at different times not to exceed six months from the date of the order, as designated by the procurement officer when submitting the order.

§ 1305.10   Procedure for endorsing order forms.

(a) An order form made out to any supplier who cannot fill all or a part of the order within the time limitation set forth in § 1305.09 may be endorsed to another supplier for filling. The endorsement shall be made only by the supplier to whom the order form was first made, shall state (in the spaces provided on the reverse sides of Copies 1 and 2 of the order form) the name and address of the second supplier, and shall be signed by a person authorized to obtain and execute order forms on behalf of the first supplier. The first supplier may not fill any part of an order on an endorsed form. The second supplier shall fill the order, if possible and if he desires to do so, in accordance with § 1305.09 (b), (c), and (d), including shipping all substances directly to the purchaser.

(b) Distributions made on endorsed order forms shall be reported by the second supplier in the same manner as all other distributions except that where the name of the supplier is requested on the reporting form, the second supplier shall record the name, address and registration number of the first supplier.

§ 1305.11   Unaccepted and defective order forms.

(a) No order form shall be filled if it:

(1) Is not complete, legible, or properly prepared, executed, or endorsed; or

(2) Shows any alteration, erasure, or change of any description.

(b) If an order form cannot be filled for any reason under this section, the supplier shall return Copies 1 and 2 to the purchaser with a statement as to the reason (e.g., illegible or altered). A supplier may for any reason refuse to accept any order and if a supplier refuses to accept the order, a statement that the order is not accepted shall be sufficient for purposes of this paragraph.

(c) When received by the purchaser, Copies 1 and 2 of the order form and the statement shall be attached to Copy 3 and retained in the files of the purchaser in accordance with § 1305.13. A defective order form may not be corrected; it must be replaced by a new order form in order for the order to be filled.

§ 1305.12   Lost and stolen order forms.

(a) If a purchaser ascertains that an unfilled order form has been lost, he shall execute another in triplicate and a statement containing the serial number and date of the lost form, and stating that the goods covered by the first order form were not received through loss of that order form. Copy 3 of the second form and a copy of the statement shall be retained with Copy 3 of the order form first executed. A copy of the statement shall be attached to Copies 1 and 2 of the second order form sent to the supplier. If the first order form is subsequently received by the supplier to whom it was directed, the supplier shall mark upon the face thereof "Not accepted" and return Copies 1 and 2 to the purchaser, who shall attach it to Copy 3 and the statement.

(b) Whenever any used or unused order forms are stolen from or lost (otherwise than in the course of transmission) by any purchaser or supplier, he shall immediately upon discovery of such theft or loss, report the same to the Registration Unit, Drug Enforcement Administration, Department of Justice, Post Office Box 28083, Central Station, Washington, D. C. 20005, stating the serial number of each form stolen or lost. If the theft or loss includes any original order forms received from purchasers and the supplier is unable to state the serial numbers of such order forms, he shall report the date or approximate date of receipt thereof and the names and addresses of the purchasers. If an entire book of order forms is lost or stolen, and the purchaser is unable to state the serial numbers of the order forms contained therein, he shall report, in lieu of the numbers of the forms contained in such book, the date or approximate date of issuance thereof. If any unused order form

reported stolen or lost is subsequently recovered or found, the Registration Unit of the Administration shall immediately be notified.

§ 1305.13   Preservation of order forms.

(a) The purchaser shall retain Copy 3 of each order form which has been filled. He shall also retain in his files all copies of each unaccepted or defective order form and each statement attached thereto.

(b) The supplier shall retain Copy 1 of each order form which he has filled.

(c) Order forms must be maintained separately from all other records of the registrant. Order forms are required to be kept available for inspection for a period of 2 years. If a purchaser has several registered locations, he must retain Copy 3 of the executed order forms and any attached statements or other related documents (not including unexecuted order forms which may be kept elsewhere pursuant to § 1305.06(e)) at the registered location printed on the order form.

(d) The supplier of carfentanil, etorphine hydrochloride and diprenorphine shall maintain order forms for these substances separately from all other order forms and records required to be maintained by the registrant.

§ 1305.14   Return of unused order forms.

If the registration of any purchaser terminates (because the purchaser dies, ceases legal existence, discontinues business or professional practice, or changes his name or address as shown on his registration) or is suspended or revoked pursuant to §§ 1301.45 or 1301.46 of this chapter as to all controlled substances listed in Schedules I and II for which he is registered, he shall return all unused order forms for such substance to the nearest office of the Administration.

§ 1305.15   Cancellation and voiding of order forms.

(a) A purchaser may cancel part or all of an order on an order form by notifying the supplier in writing of such cancellation. The supplier shall indicate the cancellation on Copies 1 and 2 of the order form by drawing a line through the canceled items and printing "canceled" in the space provided for number of items shipped.

(b) A supplier may void part or all of an order on an order form by notifying the purchaser in writing of such voiding. The supplier shall indicate the voiding in the manner prescribed for cancellation in paragraph (a) of this section.

(c) No cancellation or voiding permitted by this section shall affect in any way contract rights of either the purchaser or the supplier.

Prescriptions

§ 1306.02   Definitions.

As used in this part, the following terms shall have the meanings specified:

(b) The term "individual practitioner" means a physician, dentist, veterinarian, or other individual licensed, registered, or otherwise permitted, by the United States or the jurisdiction in which he practices, to dispense a controlled substance in the course of professional practice, but does not include a pharmacist, a pharmacy, or an institutional practitioner.

(c) The term "institutional practitioner" means a hospital or other person (other than an individual) licensed, registered, or otherwise permitted, by the United States or the jurisdiction in which it practices, to dispense a controlled substance in the course of professional practice, but does not include a pharmacy.

(d) The term "pharmacist" means any pharmacist licensed by a State to dispense controlled substances, and shall include any other person (e.g., a pharmacist intern) authorized by a State to dispense controlled substances under the supervision of a pharmacist licensed by such State.

(e) A "Long Term Care Facility" (LTCF) means a nursing home, retirement care, mental care or other facility or institution which provides extended health care to resident patients.

(f) The term "prescription" means an order for medication which is dispensed to or for an ultimate user but does not include an order for medication which is dispensed for immediate administration to the ultimate user. (E.g., an order to dispense a drug to a bed patient for immediate administration in a hospital is not a prescription.)

(g) The terms "register" and "registered" refer to registration required and permitted by section 303 of the Act (21 U.S.C. 823).

§ 1306.03   Persons entitled to issue prescriptions.

(a) A prescription for a controlled substance may be issued only by an individual practitioner who is:

(1) authorized to prescribe controlled substances by the jurisdiction in which he is licensed to practice his profession and

(2) either registered or exempted from registration pursuant to §§ 1301.24(c) and 1301.25 of this chapter.

(b) A prescription issued by an individual practitioner may be communicated to a pharmacist by an employee or agent of the individual practitioner.

§ 1306.04   Purpose of issue of prescription.

(a) A prescription for a controlled substance to be effective must be issued for a legitimate medical purpose by an individual practitioner acting in the usual course of his professional practice. The responsibility for the proper prescribing and dispensing of controlled substances is upon the prescribing practitioner, but a corresponding responsibility rests with the pharmacist who fills the prescription. An order purporting to be a prescription issued not in the usual course of professional treatment or in legitimate and authorized research is not a prescription within the meaning and intent of section 309 of the Act (21 U.S.C. 829) and the person knowingly filling such a purported prescription, as well as the person issuing it, shall be subject to the penalties provided for violations of the provisions of law relating to controlled substances.

(b) A prescription may not be issued in order for an individual practitioner to obtain controlled substances for supplying the individual practitioner for the purpose of general dispensing to patients.

(c) A prescription may not be issued for the dispensing of narcotic drugs listed in any schedule for "detoxification treatment" or "maintenance treatment" as defined in Section 102 of the Act (21 U.S.C. 802).

§ 1306.05   Manner of issuance of prescriptions.

(a) All prescriptions for controlled substances shall be dated as of, and signed on, the day when issued and shall bear the full name and address of the patient, the drug name, strength, dosage form, quantity prescribed, directions for use, and the name, address, and registration number of the practitioner. A practitioner may sign a prescription in the same manner as he would sign a check or legal document (e.g., J. H. Smith or John H. Smith). Where an oral order is not permitted, prescriptions shall be written with ink or indelible pencil or typewriter and shall be manually signed by the practitioner. The prescriptions may be prepared by a secretary or agent for the signature of a practitioner, but the prescribing practitioner is responsible in case the prescription does not conform in all essential respects to the law and regulations. A corresponding liability rests upon the pharmacist who fills a prescription not prepared in the form prescribed by these regulations.

(b) An intern, resident, or foreign-trained physician, or physician on the staff of a Veterans Administration facility, exempted from registration under § 1301.24(c) shall include on all prescriptions issued by him the registration number of the hospital or other institution and the special internal code number assigned to him by the hospital or other institution as provided

in § 1301.24(c), in lieu of the registration number of the practitioner required by this section. Each written prescription shall have the name of the physician stamped, typed, or handprinted on it, as well as the signature of the physician.

(c) An official exempted from registration under § 1301.25 shall include on all prescriptions issued by him his branch of service or agency (e.g., "U. S. Army" or "Public Health Service") and his service identification number, in lieu of the registration number of the practitioner required by this section. The service identification number for a Public Health Service employee is his Social Security identification number. Each prescription shall have the name of the officer stamped, typed, or handprinted on it, as well as the signature of the officer.

§ 1306.06   Persons entitled to fill prescriptions.

A prescription for controlled substances may only be filled by a pharmacist acting in the usual course of his professional practice and either registered individually or employed in a registered pharmacy or registered institutional practitioner.

§ 1306.07   Administering or dispensing of narcotic drugs.

(a) The administering or dispensing directly (but not prescribing) of narcotic drugs listed in any schedule to a narcotic drug dependent person for "detoxification treatment" or "maintenance treatment" as defined in section 102 of the Act (21 U.S.C. 802) shall be deemed to be within the meaning of the term "in the course of his professional practice or research" in section 308(e) and section 102(20) of the Act (21 U.S.C. 828(e)): *Provided*, That the practitioner is separately registered with the Attorney General as required by section 303(g) of the Act (21 U.S.C. 823(g)) and then thereafter complies with the regulatory standards imposed relative to treatment qualification, security, records and unsupervised use of drugs pursuant to such Act.

(b) Nothing in this section shall prohibit a physician who is not specifically registered to conduct a narcotic treatment program from administering (but not prescribing) narcotic drugs to a person for the purpose of relieving acute withdrawal symptoms when necessary while arrangements are being made for referral for treatment. Not more than one day's medication may be administered to the person or for the person's use at one time. Such emergency treatment may be carried out for not more than three days and may not be renewed or extended.

(c) This section is not intended to impose any limitations on a physician or authorized hospital staff to administer or dispense narcotic drugs in a hospital to maintain or detoxify a person as an incidental adjunct to medical or surgical treatment of conditions other than addiction, or to administer or dispense narcotic drugs to persons with intractable pain in which no relief or cure is possible or none has been found after reasonable efforts.

Controlled Substances Listed in Schedule II

§ 1306.11   Requirement of prescription.

(a) A pharmacist may dispense directly a controlled substance listed in Schedule II, which is a prescription drug as determined under the Federal Food, Drug, and Cosmetic Act, only pursuant to a written prescription signed by the prescribing individual practitioner, except as provided in paragraph (d) of this section.

(b) An individual practitioner may administer or dispense directly a controlled substance listed in Schedule II in the course of his professional practice without a prescription, subject to § 1306.07.

(c) An institutional practitioner may administer or dispense directly (but not prescribe) a controlled substance listed in Schedule II only pursuant to a written prescription signed by the prescribing individual practitioner or to an order for medication made by an individual practitioner which is dispensed for immediate administration to the ultimate user.

(d) In the case of an emergency situation, as defined by the Secretary in § 290.10 of this title, a pharmacist may dispense a controlled substance listed in Schedule II upon receiving oral authorization of a prescribing individual practitioner, provided that:

(1) The quantity prescribed and dispensed is limited to the amount adequate to treat the patient during the emergency period (dispensing beyond the emergency period must be pursuant to a written prescription signed by the prescribing individual practitioner);

(2) The prescription shall be immediately reduced to writing by the pharmacist and shall contain all information required in § 1306.05, except for the signature of the prescribing individual practitioner;

(3) If the prescribing individual practitioner is not known to the pharmacist, he must make a reasonable effort to determine that the oral authorization came from a registered individual practitioner, which may include a callback to the prescribing individual practitioner using his phone number as listed in the telephone directory and/or other good faith efforts to insure his identity; and

(4) Within 72 hours after authorizing an emergency oral prescription, the prescribing individual practitioner shall cause a written prescription for the emergency quantity prescribed to be delivered to the dispensing pharmacist. In addition to conforming to the requirements of § 1306.05, the prescription shall have written on its face "Authorization for Emergency Dispensing," and the date of the oral order. The written prescription may be delivered to the pharmacist in person or by mail, but if delivered by mail it must be postmarked within the 72-hour period. Upon receipt, the dispensing pharmacist shall attach this prescription to the oral emergency prescription which had earlier been reduced to writing. The pharmacist shall notify the nearest office of the Administration if the prescribing individual practitioner fails to deliver a written prescription to him; failure of the pharmacist to do so shall void the authority conferred by this paragraph to dispense without a written prescription of a prescribing individual practitioner.

§ 1306.12   Refilling prescriptions.

The refilling of a prescription for a controlled substance listed in Schedule II is prohibited.

§ 1306.13   Partial filling of prescriptions.

(a) The partial filling of a prescription for a controlled substance listed in Schedule II is permissible, if the pharmacist is unable to supply the full quantity called for in a written or emergency oral prescription and he makes a notation of the quantity supplied on the face of the written prescription (or written record of the emergency oral prescription). The remaining portion of the prescription may be filled within 72 hours of the first partial filling; however, if the remaining portion is not or cannot be filled within the 72-hour period, the pharmacist shall so notify the prescribing individual practitioner. No further quantity may be supplied beyond 72 hours without a new prescription.

(b) A prescription for a Schedule II controlled substance written for a patient in a Long Term Care Facility (LTCF) or for a patient with a medical diagnosis documenting a terminal illness may be filled in partial quantities to include individual dosage units. If there is any question whether a patient may be classified as having a terminal illness, the pharmacist must contact the practitioner prior to partially filling the prescription. Both the pharmacist and the prescribing practitioner have a corresponding responsibility to assure that the controlled substance is for a terminally ill patient. The pharmacist must record on the prescription whether the patient is "terminally ill" or an "LTCF patient." A prescription that is partially filled and does not contain the notation "terminally ill" or "LTCF patient" shall be deemed to have been filled in violation of the Act. For each

partial filling, the dispensing pharmacist shall record on the back of the prescription (or on another appropriate record, uniformly maintained, and readily retrievable) the date of the partial filling, quantity dispensed, remaining quantity authorized to be dispensed, and the identification of the dispensing pharmacist. Prior to any subsequent partial filling the pharmacist is to determine that the additional partial filling is necessary. The total quantity of Schedule II controlled substances dispensed in all partial fillings must not exceed the total quantity prescribed. Schedule II prescriptions for patients in a LTCF or patients with a medical diagnosis documenting a terminal illness shall be valid for a period not to exceed 60 days from the issue date unless sooner terminated by the discontinuance of medication.

(c) Information pertaining to current Schedule II prescriptions for patients in a LTCF or for patients with a medical diagnosis documenting a terminal illness may be maintained in a computerized system if this system has the capability to permit:

(1) Output (display or printout) of the original prescription number, date of issue, identification of prescribing individual practitioner, identification of patient, address of the LTCF or address of the hospital or residence of the patient, identification of medication authorized (to include dosage, form, strength, and quantity), listing of the partial fillings that have been dispensed under each prescription and the information required in § 1306.13(b).

(2) Immediate (real time) updating of the prescription record each time a partial filling of the prescription is conducted.

(3) Retrieval of partially filled Schedule II prescription information is the same as required by § 1306.22(b) (4) and (5) for Schedule III and IV prescription refill information.

§ 1306.14   Labeling of substances.

(a) The pharmacist filling a written or emergency oral prescription for a controlled substance listed in Schedule II shall affix to the package a label showing date of filling, the pharmacy name and address, the serial number of the prescription, the name of the patient, the name of the prescribing practitioner, and directions for use and cautionary statements, if any, contained in such prescription or required by law.

(b) The requirements of paragraph (a) of this section do not apply when a controlled substance listed in Schedule II is prescribed for administration to an ultimate user who is institutionalized: *Provided,* That:

(1) Not more than a 7-day supply of the controlled substance listed in Schedule II is dispensed at one time;

(2) The controlled substance listed in Schedule II is not in the possession of the ultimate user prior to the administration;

(3) The institution maintains appropriate safeguards and records regarding the proper administration, control, dispensing, and storage of the controlled substance listed in Schedule II; and

(4) The system employed by the pharmacist in filling a prescription is adequate to identify the supplier, the product, and the patient, and to set forth the directions for use and cautionary statements, if any, contained in the prescription or required by law.

§ 1306.15   Filing of prescriptions.

All written prescriptions and written records of emergency oral prescriptions shall be kept in accordance with requirements of § 1304.04(h) of this chapter.

Controlled Substances Listed in Schedules III and IV

§ 1306.21   Requirement of prescription.

(a) A pharmacist may dispense directly a controlled substance listed in Schedule III or IV, which is a prescription drug as determined under the Federal Food, Drug, and Cosmetic Act, only pursuant to either a written prescription signed by a prescribing individual practitioner or an oral prescription made by a prescribing individual practitioner and promptly reduced to writing by the pharmacist containing all information required in § 1306.05, except for the signature of the prescribing individual practitioner.

(b) An individual practitioner may administer or dispense directly a controlled substance listed in Schedule III or IV in the course of his professional practice without a prescription, subject to § 1306.07.

(c) An institutional practitioner may administer or dispense directly (but not prescribe) a controlled substance listed in Schedule III or IV pursuant to a written prescription signed by a prescribing individual practitioner, or pursuant to an oral prescription made by a prescribing individual practitioner and promptly reduced to writing by the pharmacist (containing all information required in § 1306.05 except for the signature of the prescribing individual practitioner), or pursuant to an order for medication made by an individual practitioner which is dispensed for immediate administration to the ultimate user, subject to § 1306.07.

§ 1306.22   Refilling of prescriptions.

(a) No prescription for a controlled substance listed in Schedule III or IV shall be filled or refilled more than 6 months after the date on which such prescription was issued and no such prescription authorized to be refilled may be refilled more than five times. Each refilling of a prescription shall be entered on the back of the prescription or on another appropriate document. If entered on another document, such as a medication record, the document must be uniformly maintained and readily retrievable. The following information must be retrievable by the prescription number consisting of the name and dosage form of the controlled substance, the date filled or refilled, the quantity dispensed, initials of the dispensing pharmacist for each refill, and the total number of refills for that prescription. If the pharmacist merely initials and dates the back of the prescription it shall be deemed that the full face amount of the prescription has been dispensed. The prescribing practitioner may authorize additional refills of Schedule III or IV controlled substances on the original prescription through an oral refill authorization transmitted to the pharmacist provided the following conditions are met:

(1) The total quantity authorized, including the amount of the original prescription, does not exceed five refills nor extend beyond six months from the date of issue of the original prescription.

(2) The pharmacist obtaining the oral authorization records on the reverse of the original prescription the date, quantity of refill, number of additional refills authorized, and initials the prescription showing who received the authorization from the prescribing practitioner who issued the original prescription.

(3) The quantity of each additional refill authorized is equal to or less than the quantity authorized for the initial filling of the original prescription.

(4) The prescribing practitioner must execute a new and separate prescription for any additional quantities beyond the five refill, six-month limitation.

(b) As an alternative to the procedures provided by subsection (a), an automated data processing system may be used for the storage and retrieval of refill information for prescription orders for controlled substances in Schedules III and IV, subject to the following conditions:

(1) Any such proposed computerized system must provide on-line retrieval (via CRT display or hard-copy printout) of original prescription order information for those prescription orders which are currently authorized for refilling. This shall include, but is not limited to, data such as the original prescription number, date of issuance of the original prescription order by the practitioner, full name and address of the patient, name, address, and DEA registration number of the practitioner, and the name, strength, dosage form, quantity of the controlled substance prescribed (and quantity dispensed if different from the quantity prescribed), and the total number of refills authorized by the prescribing practitioner.

(2) Any such proposed computerized system must also provide on-line retrieval (via CRT display or hard-copy printout) of the current refill history for Schedule III or IV controlled substance prescription orders (those authorized for refill during the past six months). This refill history shall include, but is not limited to, the name of the controlled substance, the date of refill, the quantity dispensed, the identification code, or name or initials of the dispensing pharmacist for each refill and the total number of refills dispensed to date for that prescription order.

(3) Documentation of the fact that the refill information entered into the computer each time a pharmacist refills an original prescription order for a Schedule III or IV controlled substance is correct must be provided by the individual pharmacist who makes use of such a system. If such a system provides a hard-copy printout of each day's controlled substance prescription order refill data, that printout shall be verified, dated, and signed by the individual pharmacist who refilled such a prescription order. The individual pharmacist must verify that the data indicated is correct and then sign this document in the same manner as he would sign a check or legal document (e.g., J. H. Smith, or John H. Smith). This document shall be maintained in a separate file at that pharmacy for a period of two years from the dispensing date. This printout of the day's controlled substance prescription order refill data must be provided to each pharmacy using such a computerized system within 72 hours of the date on which the refill was dispensed. It must be verified and signed by each pharmacist who is involved with such dispensing. In lieu of such a printout, the pharmacy shall maintain a bound log book, or separate file, in which each individual pharmacist involved in such dispensing shall sign a statement (in the manner previously described) each day, attesting to the fact that the refill information entered into the computer that day has been reviewed by him and is correct as shown. Such a book or file must be maintained at the pharmacy employing such a system for a period of two years after the date of dispensing the appropriately authorized refill.

(4) Any such computerized system shall have the capability of producing a printout of any refill data which the user pharmacy is responsible for maintaining under the Act and its implementing regulations. For example, this would include a refill-by-refill audit trail for any specified strength and dosage form of any controlled substance (by either brand or generic name or both). Such a printout must indicate name of the prescribing practitioner, name and address of the patient, quantity dispensed on each refill, date of dispensing for each refill, name or identification code of the dispensing pharmacist, and the number of the original prescription order. In any computerized system employed by a user pharmacy the central recordkeeping location must be capable of sending the printout to the pharmacy within 48 hours, and if a DEA Special Agent or Compliance Investigator requests a copy of such printout from the user pharmacy, it must, if requested to do so by the Agent or Investigator, verify the printout transmittal capability of its system by documentation (e.g., postmark).

(5) In the event that a pharmacy which employs such a computerized system experiences system down-time, the pharmacy must have an auxiliary procedure which will be used for documentation of refills of Schedule III and IV controlled substance prescription orders. This auxiliary procedure must insure that refills are authorized by the original prescription order, that the maximum number of refills has not been exceeded, and that all of the appropriate data are retained for on-line data entry as soon as the computer system is available for use again.

(c) When filing refill information for original prescription orders for Schedule III or IV controlled substances, a pharmacy may use only one of the two systems described in paragraph (a) or (b) of this section.

§ 1306.23 Partial filling of prescriptions.

The partial filling of a prescription for a controlled substance listed in Schedule III or IV is permissible, provided that:

(a) Each partial filling is recorded in the same manner as a refilling,

(b) The total quantity dispensed in all partial fillings does not exceed the total quantity prescribed, and

(c) No dispensing occurs after 6 months after the date on which the prescription was issued.

§ 1306.24 Labeling of substances.

(a) The pharmacist filling a prescription for a controlled substance listed in Schedule III or IV shall affix to the package a label showing the pharmacy name and address, the serial number and date of initial filling, the name of the patient, the name of the practitioner issuing the prescription, and directions for use and cautionary statements, if any, contained in such prescription as required by law.

(b) The requirements of paragraph (a) of this section do not apply when a controlled substance listed in Schedule III or IV is prescribed for administration to an ultimate user who is institutionalized: *Provided*, That:

(1) Not more than a 34-day supply or 100 dosage units, whichever is less, of the controlled substance listed in Schedule III or IV is dispensed at one time;

(2) The controlled substance listed in Schedule III or IV is not in the possession of the ultimate user prior to administration;

(3) The institution maintains appropriate safeguards and records the proper administration, control, dispensing, and storage of the controlled substance listed in Schedule III or IV; and

(4) The system employed by the pharmacist in filling a prescription is adequate to identify the supplier, the product and the patient, and to set forth the directions for use and cautionary statements, if any, contained in the prescription or required by law.

§ 1306.25 Filing prescriptions.

All prescriptions for controlled substances listed in Schedules III and IV shall be kept in accordance with § 1304.04(h) of this chapter.

§ 1306.26 Transfer between pharmacies of prescription information for Schedules III, IV, and V controlled substances for refill purposes.

(a) The transfer of original prescription information for a controlled substance listed in Schedules III, IV or V for the purpose of refill dispensing is permissible between pharmacies on a one time basis subject to the following requirements:

(1) The transfer is communicated directly between two licensed pharmacists and the transferring pharmacist records the following information:

(i) Write the word "VOID" on the face of the invalidated prescription.

(ii) Record on the reverse of the invalidated prescription the name, address and DEA registration number of the pharmacy to which it was transferred and the name of the pharmacist receiving the prescription information.

(iii) Record the date of the transfer and the name of the pharmacist transferring the information.

(b) The pharmacist receiving the transferred prescription information shall reduce to writing the following:

(1) Write the word "transfer" on the face of the transferred prescription.

(2) Provide all information required to be on a prescription pursuant to 21 CFR 1306.05 and include:

(i) Date of issuance of original prescription;

(ii) Original number of refills authorized on original prescription;

(iii) Date of original dispensing;

(iv) Number of valid refills remaining and date of last refill;

(v) Pharmacy's name, address, DEA registration number and original prescription number from which the prescription information was transferred;

(vi) Name of transferor pharmacist.

(3) Both the original and transferred prescription must be maintained for a period of two years from the date of last refill.

(c) Pharmacies electronically accessing the same prescription record must satisfy all information requirements of a manual mode for prescription transferral.

(d) The procedure allowing the transfer of prescription information for refill purposes is permissible only if allowable under existing state or other applicable law.

Controlled Substances Listed in Schedule V

§ 1306.31 Requirement of prescription.

(a) A pharmacist may dispense directly a controlled substance listed in Schedule V pursuant to a prescription as required for controlled substances listed in Schedules III and IV in § 1306.21. A prescription for a controlled substance listed in Schedule V may be refilled only as expressly authorized by the prescribing individual practitioner on the prescription; if no such authorization is given, the prescription may not be refilled. A pharmacist dispensing such substance pursuant to a prescription shall label the substance in accordance with § 1306.24 and file the prescription in accordance with § 1306.25.

(b) An individual practitioner may administer or dispense directly a controlled substance listed in Schedule V in the course of his professional practice without a prescription, subject to § 1306.07.

(c) An institutional practitioner may administer or dispense directly (but not prescribe) a controlled substance listed in Schedule V only pursuant to a written prescription signed by the prescribing individual practitioner, or pursuant to an oral prescription made by a prescribing individual practitioner and promptly reduced to writing by the pharmacist (containing all information required in § 1306.05 except for the signature of the prescribing individual practitioner), or pursuant to an order for medication made by an individual practitioner which is dispensed for immediate administration to the ultimate user, subject to § 1306.07.

§ 1306.32 Dispensing without prescription.

A controlled substance listed in Schedule V, and a controlled substance listed in Schedule II, III, or IV which is not a prescription drug as determined under the Federal Food, Drug, and Cosmetic Act, may be dispensed by a pharmacist without a prescription to a purchaser at retail, provided that:

(a) Such dispensing is made only by a pharmacist (as defined in § 1306.02(d)), and not by a nonpharmacist employee even if under the supervision of a pharmacist (although after the pharmacist has fulfilled his professional and legal responsibilities set forth in this section, the actual cash, credit transaction, or delivery, may be completed by a nonpharmacist);

(b) Not more than 240 cc. (8 ounces) of any such controlled substance containing opium, nor more than 120 cc. (4 ounces) of any other such controlled substance nor more than 48 dosage units of any such controlled substance containing opium, nor more than 24 dosage units of any other such controlled substance may be dispensed at retail to the same purchaser in any given 48-hour period;

(c) The purchaser is at least 18 years of age;

(d) The pharmacist requires every purchaser of a controlled substance under this section not known to him to furnish suitable identification (including proof of age where appropriate);

(e) A bound record book for dispensing of controlled substances under this section is maintained by the pharmacist, which book shall contain the name and address of the purchaser, the name and quantity of controlled substance purchased, the date of each purchase, and the name or initials of the pharmacist who dispensed the substance to the purchaser (the book shall be maintained in accordance with the recordkeeping requirement of § 1304.04 of this chapter); and

(f) A prescription is not required for distribution or dispensing of the substance pursuant to any other Federal, State or local law.

Miscellaneous

§ 1307.02   Application of State law and other Federal law.

Nothing in Parts 1301–1308, 1311, 1312, or 1316 of this chapter shall be construed as authorizing or permitting any person to do any act which such person is not authorized or permitted to do under other Federal laws or obligations under international treaties, conventions or protocols, or under the law of the State in which he desires to do such act nor shall compliance with such Parts be construed as compliance with other Federal or State laws unless expressly provided in such other laws.

§ 1307.03   Exceptions to regulations.

Any person may apply for an exception to the application of any provision of Parts 1301–1308, 1311, 1312, or 1316 of this chapter by filing a written request stating the reasons for such exception. Requests shall be filed with the Administrator, Drug Enforcement Administration, Department of Justice, Washington, D. C. 20537. The Administrator may grant an exception in his discretion, but in no case shall he be required to grant an exception to any person which is not otherwise required by law or the regulations cited in this section.

Special Exceptions for Manufacture and Distribution of Controlled Substances

§ 1307.11   Distribution by dispenser to another practitioner.

(a) A practitioner who is registered to dispense a controlled substance may distribute (without being registered to distribute) a quantity of such substance to another practitioner for the purpose of general dispensing by the practitioner to his or its patients: *Provided*, That:

(1) The practitioner to whom the controlled substance is to be distributed is registered under the Act to dispense that controlled substance;

(2) The distribution is recorded by the distributing practitioner in accordance with § 1304.24(e) of this chapter and by the receiving practitioner in accordance with § 1304.24(c) of this chapter;

(3) If the substance is listed in Schedule I or II, an order form is used as required in Part 1305 of this chapter;

(4) The total number of dosage units of all controlled substances distributed by the practitioner pursuant to this section and § 1301.28 of this chapter during each calendar year in which the practitioner is registered to dispense does not exceed 5 percent of the total number of dosage units of all controlled substances distributed and dispensed by the practitioner during the same calendar year.

(b) If, during any calendar year in which the practitioner is registered to dispense, the practitioner has reason to believe that the total number of dosage units of all controlled substances which will be distributed by him pursuant to this section and § 1301.28 of this chapter will exceed 5 percent of the total number of dosage units of all controlled substances distributed

and dispensed by him during that calendar year, the practitioner shall obtain a registration to distribute controlled substances.

§ 1307.12   Manufacture and distribution of narcotic solutions and compounds by a pharmacist.

As an incident to a distribution under § 1307.11, a pharmacist may manufacture (without being registered to manufacture) an aqueous or oleaginous solution or solid dosage form containing a narcotic controlled substance in a proportion not exceeding 20 percent of the complete solution, compound, or mixture.

§ 1307.13   Distribution to supplier.

Any person lawfully in possession of a controlled substance listed in any schedule may distribute (without being registered to distribute) that substance to the person from whom he obtained it or to the manufacturer of the substance, provided that a written record is maintained which indicates the date of the transaction, the name, form and quantity of the substance, the name, address, and registration number, if any, of the person making the distribution, and the name, address, and registration number, if known, of the supplier or manufacturer. In the case of returning a controlled substance listed in Schedule I or II, an order form shall be used in the manner prescribed in Part 1305 of this chapter and be maintained as the written record of the transaction. Any person not required to register pursuant to sections 302(c) or 1007(b) (1) of the Act (21 U.S.C. 823(c) or 957(b) (1)) shall be exempt from maintaining the records required by this section.

§ 1307.14   Distribution upon discontinuance or transfer of business.

(a) Any registrant desiring to discontinue business activities altogether or with respect to controlled substances (without transferring such business activities to another person) shall return for cancellation his certificate of registration, and any unexecuted order forms in his possession, to the Registration Unit, Drug Enforcement Administration, Department of Justice, Post Office Box 28083, Central Station, Washington, D. C. 20005. Any controlled substances in his possession may be disposed of in accordance with § 1307.21.

(b) Any registrant desiring to discontinue business activities altogether or with respect to controlled substances (by transferring such business activities to another person) shall submit in person or by registered or certified mail, return receipt requested, to the Special Agent in Charge in his area, at least 14 days in advance of the date of the proposed transfer (unless the Special Agent in Charge waives this time limitation in individual instances), the following information:

(1) The name, address, registration number, and authorized business activity of the registrant discontinuing the business (registrant-transferor);

(2) The name, address, registration number, and authorized business activity of the person acquiring the business (registrant-transferee);

(3) Whether the business activities will be continued at the location registered by the person discontinuing business, or moved to another location (if the latter, the address of the new location should be listed);

(4) Whether the registrant-transferor has a quota to manufacture or procure any controlled substance listed in Schedule I or II (if so, the basic class or class of the substance should be indicated); and

(5) The date on which the transfer of controlled substances will occur.

(c) Unless the registrant-transferor is informed by the Regional Administrator,[1] before the date on which the transfer was stated to occur, that the transfer may not occur, the registrant-transferor may distribute (without being registered to distribute) controlled substances in his possession to the registrant-transferee in accordance with the following:

(1) On the date of transfer of the controlled substances, a complete inventory of all controlled substances being transferred shall be taken in accordance with §§ 1304.11–1304.19 of this chapter. This inventory shall serve as the final inventory of the registrant-transferor and the initial inventory of the registrant-transferee, and a copy of the inventory shall be included in the records of each person. It shall not be necessary to file a copy of the inventory with the Administration unless requested by the Regional Administrator (Special Agent in Charge). Transfers of any substances listed in Schedule I or II shall require the use of order forms in accordance with Part 1305 of this chapter.

(2) On the date of transfer of the controlled substances, all records required to be kept by the registrant-transferor with reference to the controlled substances being transferred, under Part 1304 of this chapter, shall be transferred to the registrant-transferee. Responsibility for the accuracy of records prior to the date of transfer remains with the transferor, but responsibility for custody and maintenance shall be upon the transferee.

(3) In the case of registrants required to make reports pursuant to Part 1304 of this chapter, a report marked "Final" will be prepared and submitted by the registrant-transferor showing the disposition of all the controlled substances for which a report is required; no additional report will be required from him, if no further transactions involving controlled substances are consummated by him. The initial report of the registrant-transferee shall account for transactions beginning with the day next succeeding the date of discontinuance or transfer of business by the transferor-registrant and the substances transferred to him shall be reported as receipts in his initial report.

---

[1]Special Agent in Charge.

Disposal of Controlled Substances

§ 1307.21   Procedure for disposing of controlled substances.

(a) Any person in possession of any controlled substance and desiring or required to disposed of such substance may request the Special Agent in Charge of the Administration in the area in which the person is located for authority and instructions to dispose of such substance. The request should be made as follows:

(1) If the person is a registrant required to make reports pursuant to Part 1304 of this chapter, he shall list the controlled substance or substances which he desires to dispose of on the "b" subpart of the report normally filed by him, and submit three copies of that subpart to the Special Agent in Charge of the Administration in his area;

(2) If the person is a registrant not required to make reports pursuant to Part 1304 of this chapter, he shall list the controlled substance or substances which he desires to dispose of on DEA Form 41, and submit three copies of that form to the Special Agent in Charge in his area; and

(3) If the person is not a registrant, he shall submit to the Special Agent in Charge a letter stating:

(i) The name and address of the person;

(ii) The name and quantity of each controlled substance to be disposed of;

(iii) How the applicant obtained the substance, if known; and

(iv) The name, address, and registration number, if known, of the person who possessed the controlled substances prior to the applicant, if known.

(b) The Special Agent in Charge shall authorize and instruct the applicant to dispose of the controlled substance in one of the following manners:

(1) By transfer to person registered under the Act and authorized to possess the substance;

(2) By delivery to an agent of the Administration or to the nearest office of the Administration;

(3) By destruction in the presence of an agent of the Administration or other authorized person; or

(4) By such other means as the Special Agent in Charge may determine to assure that the substance does not become available to unauthorized persons.

(c) In the event that a registrant is required regularly to dispose of controlled substances, the Special Agent in Charge may authorize the registrant to dispose of such substances, in accordance with paragraph (b) of this section, without prior approval of the Administration in each instance, on the condition that the registrant keep records of such disposals and file periodic reports with the Special Agent in Charge summarizing the disposals made by the registrant. In granting such authority, the Special Agent in Charge may place such conditions as he deems proper on the disposal of controlled substances, including the method of disposal and the frequency and detail of reports.

(d) This section shall not be construed as affecting or altering in any way the disposal of controlled substances through procedures provided in laws and regulations adopted by any State.

Schedules of Controlled Substances

§ 1308.02   Definitions.

(b) The term *anabolic steroid* means any drug or hormonal substance, chemically and pharmacologically related to testosterone (other than estrogens, progestins, and corticosteroids) that promotes muscle growth, and includes:

(1) Boldenone;
(2) Chlorotestosterone (4-chlortestosterone);
(3) Clostebol;
(4) Dehydrochlormethyltestosterone;
(5) Dihydrotestosterone (4-dihydrotestosterone);
(6) Drostanolone;
(7) Ethylestrenol;
(8) Fluoxymesterone;
(9) Formebulone (formebolone);
(10) Mesterolone;
(11) Methandienone;
(12) Methandranone;
(13) Methandriol;
(14) Methandrostenolone;
(15) Methenolone;
(16) Methyltestosterone;
(17) Mibolerone;
(18) Nandrolone;
(19) Norethandrolone;
(20) Oxandrolone;
(21) Oxymesterone;
(22) Oxymetholone;
(23) Stanolone;

(24) Stanozolol;

(25) Testolactone;

(26) Testosterone;

(27) Trenbolone; and

(28) Any salt, ester, or isomer of a drug or substance described or listed in this paragraph, if that salt, ester, or isomer promotes muscle growth. Except such term does not include an anabolic steroid which is expressly intended for administration through implants to cattle or other non-human species and which has been approved by the Secretary of Health and Human Services for such administration. If any person prescribes, dispenses, or distributes such steroid for human use, such person shall be considered to have prescribed, dispensed, or distributed an anabolic steroid within the meaning of this paragraph.

(d) The term "isomer" means the optical isomer, except as used in § 1308.11(d) and § 1308.12(b)(4). As used in § 1308.11(d), the term "isomer" means the optical, positional, or geometric isomer. As used in § 1308.12(b)(4), the term "isomer" means the optical or geometric isomer.

(e) The term "interested person" means any person adversely affected or aggrieved by any rule or proposed rule issuable pursuant to section 201 of the Act.

(f) The term "narcotic drug" means any of the following whether produced directly or indirectly by extraction from substances of vegetable origin or independently by means of chemical synthesis or by a combination of extraction and chemical synthesis:

(1) Opium, opiates, derivatives of opium and opiates, including their isomers, esters, ethers, salts, and salts of isomers, esters, and ethers whenever the existence of such isomers, esters, ethers and salts is possible within the specific chemical designation. Such term does not include the isoquinoline alkaloids of opium.

(2) Poppy straw and concentrate of poppy straw.

(3) Coca leaves, except coco leaves and extracts of coca leaves from which cocaine, ecgonine and derivatives of ecgonine or their salts have been removed.

(4) Cocaine, its salts, optical and geometric isomers, and salts of isomers.

(5) Ecgonine, its derivatives, their salts, isomers and salts of isomers.

(6) Any compound, mixture, or preparation which contains any quantity of any of the substances referred to in subparagraphs (1) through (5).

§ 1308.11   Schedule I.

(a) Schedule I shall consist of the drugs and other substances, by whatever official name, common or usual name, chemical name, or brand name designated, listed in this section. Each drug or substance has been assigned the DEA Controlled Substances Code Number set forth opposite it.

(b) *Opiates.* Unless specifically excepted or unless listed in another schedule, any of the following opiates, including their isomers, esters, ethers, salts, and salts of isomers, esters and ethers, whenever the existence of such isomers, esters, ethers and salts is possible within the specific chemical designation (for purposes of paragraph (b)(34) only, the term isomer includes the optical and geometric isomers):

(1) Acetyl-alpha-methylfentanyl (N-[1-(1-methyl-2-phenethyl)-4-piperidinyl]-N-phenylacetamide)................. 9815

(2) Acetylmethadol 9601

(3) Allylprodine............................ 9602

(4) Alphacetylmethadol 9603

(5) Alphameprodine......................... 9604

(6) Alphamethadol.......................... 9605

(7) Alpha-methylfentanyl (N-[1-(alpha-methyl-beta-phenyl)ethyl-4-piperidyl] propion-anilide; 1-(1-methyl-2-phenylethyl)-4-(N-propanilido) piperidine)................. 9814

(8) Alpha-methylthiofentanyl (N-[1-methyl-2-(2-thienyl)ethyl-4-piperidinyl]-N-phenylpropanamide)................... 9832

(9) Benzethidine 9606

(10) Betacetylmethadol...................... 9607

(11) Beta-hydroxyfentanyl (N-[1-(2-hydroxy-2-phenethyl)-4-piperidinyl]-N-phenylpropanamide) 9830

(12) Beta-hydroxy-3-methylfentanyl (other name: N-[1-(2-hydroxy-2-phenethyl)-3-methyl-4-piperidinyl]-N-phenylpropanamide) 9831

(13) Betameprodine 9608

(14) Betamethadol 9609

(15) Betaprodine 9611

(16) Clonitazene 9612

(17) Dextromoramide 9613

(18) Diampromide 9615

(19) Diethylthiambutene 9616

(20) Difenoxin 9168

(21) Dimenoxadol 9617

(22) Dimepheptanol 9618

(23) Dimethylthiambutene.................. 9619

(24) Dioxaphetyl butyrate 9621

(25) Dipipanone 9622

(26) Ethylmethylthiambutene............... 9623

(27) Etonitazene 9624

(28) Etoxeridine 9625

(29) Furethidine 9626

(30) Hydroxypethidine 9627

(31) Ketobemidone......................... 9628

(32) Levomoramide 9629

(33) Levophenacylmorphan.................. 9631

(34) 3-Methylfentanyl(N-[3-methyl-1-(2-phenylethyl)-4-piperidyl]-N-phenylpropanamide)................... 9813

(35) 3-Methylthiofentanyl [(3-methyl-1-(2-thienyl)ethyl-4-piperidinyl]-N-phenylpropanamide).................. 9833

(36) Morpheridine 9632

(37) MPPP (1-methyl-4-phenyl-4-propionoxypiperidine) 9661

(38) Noracymethadol 9633

(39) Norlevorphanol....................... 9634

(40) Normethadone 9635

(41) Norpipanone 9636

(42) Para-fluorofentanyl (N-(4-fluorophenyl)-N-[1-(2-phenethyl)-4-piperidinyl]propanamide................ 9812

(43) Phenadoxone 9637

(44) PEPAP (1-(-2-phenethyl)-4-phenyl-4-acetoxypiperidine 9663

(45) Phenampromide 9638

(46) Phenomorphan 9647

(47) Phenoperidine........................ 9641

(48) Piritramide........................... 9642

(49) Proheptazine 9643

(50) Properidine.......................... 9644

(51) Propiram............................. 9649

(52) Racemoramide 9645

(53) Thiofentanyl (N-phenyl-N-[1-(2-thienyl)ethyl-4-piperidinyl]-propanamide....... 9835

(54) Tilidine.............................. 9750

(55)   Trimeperidine.............................   9646

(c) *Opium derivatives.* Unless specifically excepted or unless listed in another schedule, any of the following opium derivatives, its salts, isomers, and salts of isomers whenever the existence of such salts, isomers, and salts of isomers is possible within the specific chemical designation:

(1)	Acetorphine...........................	9319
(2)	Acetyldihydrocodeine.................	9051
(3)	Benzylmorphine......................	9052
(4)	Codeine methylbromide	9070
(5)	Codeine-N-Oxide.....................	9053
(6)	Cyprenorphine	9054
(7)	Desomorphine........................	9055
(8)	Dihydromorphine.....................	9145
(9)	Drotebanol	9335
(10)	Etorphine (except hydrochloride salt)	9056
(11)	Heroin	9200
(12)	Hydromorphinol......................	9301
(13)	Methyldesorphine....................	9302
(14)	Methyldihydromorphine	9304
(15)	Morphine methylbromide	9305
(16)	Morphine methylsulfonate	9306
(17)	Morphine-N-Oxide	9307
(18)	Myrophine	9308
(19)	Nicocodeine..........................	9309
(20)	Nicomorphine........................	9312
(21)	Normorphine.........................	9313
(22)	Pholcodine	9314
(23)	Thebacon	9315

(d) *Hallucinogenic substances.* Unless specifically excepted or unless listed in another schedule, any material, compound, mixture, or preparation, which contains any quantity of the following hallucinogenic substances, or which contains any of its salts, isomers, and salts of isomers whenever the existence of such salts, isomers, and salts of isomers is possible within the specific chemical designation (for purposes of this paragraph only, the term "isomer" includes the optical, position and geometric isomers):

(1)   4-bromo-2,5-dimethoxyamphetamine   7391
Some trade or other names: 4-bromo-2,5-dimethoxy-α-methylphenethylamine; 4-bromo-2,5-DMA.

(2)   2,5-dimethoxyamphetamine...............   7396
Some trade or other names: 2,5-dimethoxy-α-methylphenethylamine; 2,5-DMA.

(3)   4-methoxyamphetamine...................   7411
Some trade or other names: 4-methoxy-α-methylphenethylamine; paramethoxyamphetamine; PMA.

(4)   5-methoxy-3,4-methylenedioxyamphetamine.........   7401

(5)   4-methyl-2,5-dimethoxyamphetamine......   7395
Some trade and other names: 4-methyl-2,5-dimethoxy-α-methylphenethylamine; "DOM"; and "STP."

(6)   3,4-methylenedioxy amphetamine   7400

(7)   3,4-methylenedioxymethamphetamine (MDMA)..........................   7405

(8)   3,4-methylenedioxy-N-ethylamphetamine (also known as N-ethyl-alpha-methyl-3,4(methylenedioxy)phenethylamine, N-ethyl MDA, MDE, MDEA   7404

(9)   N-hydroxy-3,4-methylenedioxyamphetamine (also known as N-hydroxy-alpha-methyl-3,4(methylenedioxy)-phenethylamine, and N-hydroxy MDA   7402

(10)   3,4,5-trimethoxy amphetamine............   7390

(11)   Bufotenine..............................   7433

Some trade and other names: 3-(β-Dimethylaminoethyl)-5-hydroxyindole; 3-(2-dimethylaminoethyl)-5-indolol; N,N-dimethylserotonin; 5-hydroxy-N,N-dimethyltryptamine; mappine.

(12)   Diethyltryptamine.......................   7434
Some trade and other names: N,N-Diethyltryptamine; DET.

(13)   Dimethyltryptamine   7435
Some trade or other names: DMT.

(14)   Ibogaine   7260
Some trade and other names: 7-Ethyl-6,6β,7,8,9,10,12,13-octahydro-2-methoxy-6,9-methano-5H-pyrido [1′,2′:1,2]azepino [5,4-b] indole; tabernanthe iboga.

(15)   Lysergic acid diethylamide   7315

(16)   Marihuana...........................   7360

(17)   Mescaline.............................   7381

(18)   Parahexyl.............................   7374
Some trade or other names: 3-Hexyl-1-hydroxy-7,8,9,10-tetrahydro-6,6,9-trimethyl-6H-dibenzo[b,d]pyran; Synhexyl.

(19)   Peyote..................................   7415
Meaning all parts of the plant presently classified botanically as *Lophophora Williamsii Lemaire,* whether growing or not, the seeds thereof, any extract from any part of such plant, and every compound, manufacture, salt, derivative, mixture, or preparation of such plant, its seeds or extracts.

(Interprets 21 U.S.C. 812(c), Schedule I(c)(12))

(20)   N-ethyl-3-piperidyl benzilate.............   7482

(21)   N-methyl-3-piperidyl benzilate   7484

(22)   Psilocybin..............................   7437

(23)   Psilocyn................................   7438

(24)   Tetrahydrocannabinols...................   7370
Synthetic equivalents of the substances contained in the plant, or in the resinous extractives of Cannabis, sp. and/or synthetic substances, derivatives, and their isomers with similar chemical structure and pharmacological activity such as the following:
Δ1 cis or trans tetrahydrocannabinol, and their optical isomers.
Δ6 cis or trans tetrahydrocannabinol, and their optical isomers.
Δ3,4 cis or trans tetrahydrocannabinol, and its optical isomers.
(Since nomenclature of these substances is not internationally standardized, compounds of these structures, regardless of numerical designation of atomic positions covered.)

(25)   Ethylamine analog of phencyclidine.......   7455
Some trade or other names: N-ethyl-1-phenylcyclohexylamine, (1-phenylcyclohexyl)ethylamine, N-(1-phenylcyclohexyl) ethylamine, cyclohexamine, PCE.

(26)   Pyrrolidine analog of phencyclidine   7458
Some trade or other names: 1-(1-phenylcyclohexyl)pyrrolidine, PCPy, PHP.

(27)   Thiophene analog of phencyclidine........   7470
Some trade or other names: 1-[1-(2-thienyl)-cyclohexyl]-piperidine, 2-thienyl analog of phencyclidine, TPCP, TCP.

(28) 1-[1-(2-thienyl)cyclohexyl]pyrrolidine...... 7473
Some other names: TCPY

(e) *Depressants.* Unless specifically excepted or unless listed in another schedule, any material compound, mixture, or preparation which contains any quantity of the following substances having a depressant effect on the central nervous system, including its salts, isomers, and salts of isomers whenever the existence of such salts, isomers, and salts of isomers is possible within the specific chemical designation:

(1) Mecloqualone........................... 2572
(2) Methaqualone........................... 2565

(f) *Stimulants.* Unless specifically excepted or unless listed in another schedule, any material, compound, mixture, or preparation which contains any quantity of the following substances having a stimulant effect on the central nervous system, including its salts, isomers, and salts of isomers:

(1) Fenethylline............................ 1503
(2) (±)cis-4-methylaminorex[(±)cis-4,5-dihydro-4-methyl-5-phenyl-2-oxazolamine]..... 1590
(3) N-ethylamphetamine.................... 1475
(4) N,N-dimethylamphetamine (also known as N,N,alpha-trimethylbenzeneethanamine; N,N,alpha-trimethylphenethylamine)...... 1480

(g) Temporary listing of substances subject to emergency scheduling. Any material, compound, mixture or preparation which contains any quantity of the following substances:

(1) N-[1-benzyl-4-piperidyl]-N-phenylpropanamide (benzylfentanyl), its optical isomers, salts and salts of isomers........ 9818
(2) N-[1-(2-thienyl)methyl-4-piperidyl]-N-phenylpropanamide (thenylfentanyl), its optical isomers, salts and salts of isomers............................. 9834

§ 1308.12 Schedule II.

(a) Schedule II shall consist of the drugs and other substances, by whatever official name, common or usual name, chemical name, or brand name designated, listed in this section. Each drug or substance has been assigned the Controlled Substances Code Number set forth opposite it.

(b) *Substances, vegetable origin or chemical synthesis.* Unless specifically excepted or unless listed in another schedule, any of the following substances whether produced directly or indirectly by extraction from substances of vegetable origin, or independently by means of chemical synthesis, or by a combination of extraction and chemical synthesis:

(1) Opium and opiate, and any salt, compound, derivative, or preparation of opium or opiate, excluding apomorphine, dextrorphan, nalbuphine, nalmefene, naloxone, and naltrexone, and their respective salts, but including the following:

(1) Raw opium 9600
(2) Opium extracts 9610
(3) Opium fluid extracts 9620
(4) Powdered opium........................ 9639
(5) Granulated opium...................... 9640
(6) Tincture of opium..................... 9630
(7) Codeine............................... 9050
(8) Ethylmorphine......................... 9190
(9) Etorphine hydrochloride............... 9059
(10) Hydrocodone.......................... 9193
(11) Hydromorphone........................ 9150
(12) Metopon.............................. 9260
(13) Morphine............................. 9300
(14) Oxycodone............................ 9143

(15) Oxymorphone........................... 9652
(16) Thebaine.............................. 9333

(2) Any salt, compound, derivative, or preparation thereof which is chemically equivalent or identical with any of the substances referred to in paragraph (b) (1) of this section, except that these substances shall not include the isoquinoline alkaloids of opium.

(3) Opium poppy and poppy straw.

(4) Coca leaves (9040) and any salt, compound, derivative or preparation of coca leaves (including cocaine (9041) and ecgonine (9180) and their salts, isomers, derivatives and salts of isomers and derivatives), and any salt, compound, derivative, or preparation thereof which is chemically equivalent or identical with any of these substances, except that the substances shall not include decocainized coca leaves or extraction of coca leaves, which extractions do not contain cocaine or ecgonine.

(5) Concentrate of poppy straw (the crude extract of poppy straw in either liquid, solid or powder form which contains the phenanthrine alkaloids of the opium poppy), 9670.

(c) *Opiates.* Unless specifically excepted or unless in another schedule any of the following opiates, including its isomers, esters, ethers, salts and salts of isomers, esters and ethers whenever the existence of such isomers, esters, ethers, and salts is possible within the specific chemical designation, dextrorphan and levopropoxyphene excepted:

(1) Alfentanil............................. 9737
(2) Alphaprodine 9010
(3) Anileridine........................... 9020
(4) Benzitramide.......................... 9800
(5) Bulk Dextropropoxyphene (nondosage forms) 9273
(6) Carfentanil........................... 9743
(7) Dihydrocodeine 9120
(8) Diphenoxylate......................... 9170
(9) Fentanyl 9801
(10) Isomethadone......................... 9226
(11) Levomethorphan 9210
(12) Levorphanol......................... 9220
(13) Metazocine 9240
(14) Methadone........................... 9250
(15) Methadone-Intermediate, 4-cyano-2-dimethylamino-4,4-diphenyl butane... 9254
(16) Moramide-Intermediate, 2-methyl-3-morpholino-1,1-diphenylpropane-carboxylic acid 9802
(17) Pethidine (meperidine) 9230
(18) Pethidine-Intermediate-A, 4-cyano-1-methyl-4-phenylpiperidine.................... 9232
(19) Pethidine-Intermediate-B, ethyl-4-phenylpiperidine-4-carboxylate 9233
(20) Pethidine-Intermediate-C, 1-methyl-4-phenylpiperidine-4-carboxylic acid 9234
(21) Phenazocine.......................... 9715
(22) Piminodine........................... 9730
(23) Racemethorphan 9732
(24) Racemorphan 9733
(25) Sufentanil........................... 9740

(d) *Stimulants.* Unless specifically excepted or unless listed in another schedule, any material, compound, mixture, or preparation which contains any quantity of the following substances having a stimulant effect on the central nervous system:

(1) Amphetamine, its salts, optical isomers, and salts of its optical isomers 1100
(2) Methamphetamine, its salts, isomers, and salts of its isomers 1105
(3) Phenmetrazine and its salts.............. 1631
(4) Methylphenidate 1724

(e) *Depressants.* Unless specifically excepted or unless listed in another schedule, any material, compound, mixture, or preparation which contains any quantity of the following substances having a depressant effect on the central nervous system, including its salts, isomers, and salts of isomers whenever the existence of such salts, isomers, and salts of isomers is possible within the specific chemical designation:

(1)	Amobarbital	2125
(2)	Glutethimide	2550
(3)	Pentobarbital	2270
(4)	Phencyclidine	7471
(5)	Secobarbital	2315

(f) *Hallucinogenic substances.*

(1) Dronabinol (synthetic) in sesame oil and encapsulated in a soft gelatin capsule in a U.S. Food and Drug Administration approved drug product[1] ... 7369

[Some other names for dronabinol: (6a*R*-*trans*)-6a,7,8,10a-tetrahydro-6,6,9-trimethyl-3-pentyl-6H-dibenzo[b,d]pyran-1-ol, or (−)-delta-9-(trans)-tetrahydrocannabinol]

(2) Nabilone ... 7379

[Another name for nabilone: (±)-*trans*-3-(1,1-dimethylheptyl)-6,6a,7,8,10,10a-hexahydro-1-hydroxy-6,6-dimethyl-9H-dibenzo[b,d]pyran-9-one].

[1]*DEA Statement of Policy: Any person registered by DEA to distribute, prescribe, administer or dispense controlled substances in Schedule II who engages in the distribution or dispensing of dronabinol for medical indications outside the approved use associated with cancer treatment, except within the confines of a structured and recognized research program, may subject his or her controlled substances registration to review under the provisions of 21 U.S.C. 823(f) and 824(a)(4) as being inconsistent with the public interest. DEA will take action to revoke that such distribution or dispensing constitutes a threat to the public health and safety, and in addition will pursue any criminal sanctions which may be warranted under 21 U.S.C. 841(a)(1). See United States v. Moore, 423 U.S. 122 (1975).*

(g) *Immediate precursors.* Unless specifically excepted or unless listed in another schedule, any material, compound, mixture, or preparation which contains any quantity of the following substances:

(1) Immediate precursor to amphetamine and methamphetamine:

    (i) Phenylacetone ... 8501

    Some trade or other names: phenyl-2-propanone; P2P; benzyl methyl ketone; methyl benzyl ketone;

(2) Immediate precursors to phencyclidine (PCP):

    (i) 1-phenylcyclohexylamine ... 7460
    (ii) 1-piperidinocyclohexanecarbonitrile (PCC) ... 8603

§ 1308.13 Schedule III.

(a) Schedule III shall consist of the drugs and other substances, by whatever official name, common or usual name, chemical name, or brand name designated, listed in this section. Each drug or substance has been assigned the DEA Controlled Substances Code Number set forth opposite it.

(b) *Stimulants.* Unless specifically excepted or unless listed in another schedule, any material, compound, mixture, or preparation which contains any quantity of the following substances having a stimulant effect on the central nervous system, including its salts, isomers (whether optical, position, or geometric), and salts of such isomers whenever the existence of such

salts, isomers, and salts of isomers is possible within the specific chemical designation:

(1) Those compounds, mixtures, or preparations in dosage unit form containing any stimulant substances listed in Schedule II which compounds, mixtures, or preparations were listed on August 25, 1971, as excepted compounds under § 308.32, and any other drug of the quantitative composition shown in that list for those drugs or which is the same except that it contains a lesser quantity of controlled substances ... 1405

(2)	Benzphetamine	1228
(3)	Chlorphentermine	1645
(4)	Clortermine	1647
(5)	Phendimetrazine	1615

(c) *Depressants.* Unless specifically excepted or unless listed in another schedule, any material, compound, mixture, or preparation which contains any quantity of the following substances having a depressant effect on the central nervous system:

(1) Any compound, mixture or preparation containing:

(i) Amobarbital	2128
(ii) Secobarbital	2316
(iii) Pentobarbital	2271

    or any salt thereof and one or more other active medicinal ingredients which are not listed in any schedule.

(2) Any suppository dosage form containing:

(i) Amobarbital	2126
(ii) Secobarbital	2316
(iii) Pentobarbital	2271

    or any salt of any of these drugs and approved by the Food and Drug Administration for marketing only as a suppository.

(3) Any substance which contains any quantity of a derivative of barbituric acid or any salt thereof ... 2100

(4)	Chlorhexadol	2510
(5)	Lysergic acid	7300
(6)	Lysergic acid amide	7310
(7)	Methyprylon	2575
(8)	Sulfondiethylmethane	2600
(9)	Sulfonethylmethane	2605
(10)	Sulfonmethane	2610
(11)	Tiletamine and zolazepam or any salt thereof	7295

    Some trade or other names for a tiletamine-zolazepam combination product: Telazol.

    Some trade or other names for tiletamine: 2-(ethylamino)-2-(2-thienyl)-cyclohexanone.

    Some trade or other names for zolazepam: 4-(2-fluorophenyl)-6,8-dihydro-1,3,8-trimethylpyrazolo-[3,4-e][1,4]-diazepin-7(1H)-one, flupyrazapon.

Nalorphine ... 9400

(e) *Narcotics drugs.* Unless specifically excepted or unless listed in another schedule, any material, compound, mixture, or preparation containing any of the following narcotic drugs, or their salts calculated as the free anhydrous base or alkaloid, in limited quantities as set forth below:

(1) Not more than 1.8 grams of codeine per 100 milliliters or not more than 90 milligrams per dosage unit, with an equal or greater quantity of an isoquinoline alkaloid of opium 9803

(2) Not more than 1.8 grams of codeine per 100 milliliters or not more than 90 milligrams per dosage unit, with one or more active, nonnarcotic ingredients in recognized therapeutic amounts 9804

(3) Not more than 300 milligrams of dihydro-codeinone (hydrocodone) per 100 milliliters or not more than 15 milligrams per dosage unit, with a fourfold or greater quantity of an isoquinoline alkaloid of opium 9805

(4) Not more than 300 milligrams of dihydro-codeinone (hydrocodone) per 100 milliliters or not more than 15 milligrams per dosage unit, with one or more active non-narcotic ingredients in recognized therapeutic amounts 9806

(5) Not more than 1.8 grams of dihydrocodeine per 100 milliliters or not more than 90 milligrams per dosage unit, with one or more active nonnarcotic ingredients in recognized therapeutic amounts 9807

(6) Not more than 300 milligrams of ethylmorphine per 100 milliliters or not more than 15 milligrams per dosage unit, with one or more active, nonnarcotic ingredients in recognized therapeutic amounts 9808

(7) Not more than 500 milligrams of opium per 100 milliliters or per 100 grams or not more than 25 milligrams per dosage unit, with one or more active, nonnarcotic ingredients in recognized therapeutic amounts 9809

(8) Not more than 50 milligrams of morphine per 100 milliliters or per 100 grams, with one or more active, nonnarcotic ingredients in recognized therapeutic amounts... 9810

(f) *Anabolic steroids.* Unless specifically excepted or unless listed in another schedule, any material, compound, mixture, or preparation containing any quantity of the following substances, including its salts, isomers, and salts of isomers whenever the existence of such salts of isomers is possible within the specific chemical designation:

(1) Anabolic Steroids 4000

§ 1308.14   Schedule IV.

(a) Schedule IV shall consist of the drugs and other substances, by whatever official name, common or usual name, chemical name, or brand name designated, listed in this section. Each drug or substance has been assigned the DEA Controlled Substances Code Number set forth opposite it.

(b) *Narcotic drugs.* Unless specifically excepted or unless listed in another schedule, any material, compound, mixture, or preparation containing any of the following narcotic drugs, or their salts calculated as the free anhydrous base or alkaloid, in limited quantities as set forth below:

(1) Not more than 1 milligram of difenoxin (DEA Drug Code No. 9618) and not less than 25 micrograms of atropine sulfate per dosage unit.

(2) Dextropropoxyphene (alpha-(+)-4-dimethyl-amino-1,2-diphenyl-3-methyl-2-propionoxybutane)...................... 9273

(c) *Depressants.* Unless specifically excepted or unless listed in another schedule, any material, compound, mixture, or preparation which contains any quantity of the following substances, including its salts, isomers, and salts of isomers whenever the existence of such salts, isomers, and salts of isomers is possible within the specific chemical designation:

(1) Alprazolam 2882
(2) Barbital................................. 2145
(3) Bromazepam.............................. 2748
(4) Camazepam............................... 2749
(5) Chloral betaine.......................... 2460
(6) Chloral hydrate.......................... 2465
(7) Chlordiazepoxide........................ 2744
(8) Clobazam................................ 2751
(9) Clonazepam............................. 2737
(10) Clorazepate............................ 2768
(11) Clotiazepam............................ 2752
(12) Cloxazolam............................. 2753
(13) Delorazepam............................ 2754
(14) Diazepam............................... 2765
(15) Estazolam.............................. 2756
(16) Ethchlorvynol.......................... 2540
(17) Ethinamate............................. 2545
(18) Ethyl loflazepate....................... 2758
(19) Fludiazepam............................ 2759
(20) Flunitrazepam.......................... 2763
(21) Flurazepam............................. 2767
(22) Halazepam.............................. 2762
(23) Haloxazolam............................ 2771
(24) Ketazolam.............................. 2772
(25) Loprazolam............................. 2773
(26) Lorazepam............................. 2885
(27) Lormetazepam.......................... 2774
(28) Mebutamate............................ 2800
(29) Medazepam............................. 2836
(30) Meprobamate........................... 2820
(31) Methohexital........................... 2264
(32) Methylphenobarbital (mephobarbital) 2250
(33) Midazolam............................. 2884
(34) Nimetazepam........................... 2837
(35) Nitrazepam............................ 2834
(36) Nordiazepam........................... 2838
(37) Oxazepam.............................. 2835
(38) Oxazolam.............................. 2839
(39) Paraldehyde............................ 2585
(40) Petrichloral........................... 2591
(41) Phenobarbital.......................... 2285
(42) Pinazepam............................. 2883
(43) Prazepam.............................. 2764
(44) Quazepam.............................. 2881
(45) Temazepam............................. 2925
(46) Tetrazepam............................ 2886
(47) Triazolam............................. 2887

(d) *Fenfluramine.* Any material, compound, mixture, or preparation which contains any quantity of the following substances, including its salts, isomers (whether optical, position, or geometric), and salts of such isomers whenever the existence of such salts, isomers, and salts of isomers is possible:

(1) Fenfluramine............................. 1670

(e) *Stimulants.* Unless specifically excepted or unless listed in another schedule, any material, compound, mixture, or preparation which contains any quantity of the following substances having a stimulant effect on the central nervous system, including its salts, isomers and salts of isomers:

(1) Cathine [(+)-norpseudoephedrine]......... 1230
(2) Diethylpropion 1610
(3) Fencamfamin 1760

(4) Fenproporex 1575
(5) Mazindol 1605
(6) Mefenorex 1580
(7) Pemoline (including organometallic complexes and chelates thereof) 1530
(8) Phentermine 1640
(9) Pipradrol..................................... 1750
(10) SPA ((−)-1-dimethylamino-1,2-diphenylethane) 1635

(f) *Other substances*. Unless specifically excepted or unless listed in another schedule, any material, compound, mixture or preparation which contains any quantity of the following substances, including its salts:

(1) Pentazocine 9709

§ 1308.15   Schedule V.

(a) Schedule V shall consist of the drugs and other substances, by whatever official name, common or usual name, chemical name, or brand name designated, listed in this section.

(b) *Narcotic drugs*. Unless specifically excepted or unless listed in another schedule, any material, compound, mixture, or preparation containing any of the following narcotic drugs and their salts, as set forth below:

(1) Buprenorphine 9064

(c) Narcotic drugs containing nonnarcotic active medicinal ingredients. Any compound, mixture, or preparation containing any of the following narcotic drugs, or their salts calculated as the free anhydrous base or alkaloid, in limited quantities as set forth below, which shall include one or more nonnarcotic active medicinal ingredients in sufficient proportion to confer upon the compound, mixture, or preparation valuable medicinal qualities other than those possessed by narcotic drugs alone:

(1) Not more than 200 milligrams of codeine per 100 milliliters or per 100 grams.

(2) Not more than 100 milligrams of dihydrocodeine per 100 milliliters or per 100 grams.

(3) Not more than 100 milligrams of ethylmorphine per 100 milliliters or per 100 grams.

(4) Not more than 2.5 milligrams of diphenoxylate and not less than 25 micrograms of atropine sulfate per dosage unit.

(5) Not more than 100 milligrams of opium per 100 milliliters or per 100 grams.

(6) Not more than 0.5 milligram of difenoxin (DEA Drug Code No. 9618) and not less than 25 micrograms of atropine sulfate per dosage unit.

(d) *Stimulants*. Unless specifically exempted or excluded or unless listed in another schedule, any material, compound, mixture, or preparation which contains any quantity of the following substances having a stimulant effect on the central nervous system, including its salts, isomers and salts of isomers:

(1) Pyrovalerone 1485

Inspections

§ 1316.02   Definitions.

As used in this Subpart, the following terms shall have the meanings specified:

(c) The term "controlled premises" means—(1) Places where original or other records or documents required under the Act are kept or required to be kept, and

(2) Places, including factories, warehouses, or other establishments, and conveyances, where persons registered under the Act or exempted from registration under the Act may lawfully hold, manufacture, or distribute, dispense, administer, or otherwise dispose of controlled substances.

(e) The term "inspector" means an officer or employee of the Administration authorized by the Administrator to make inspections under the Act.

(f) The term "register" and "registration" refer to registration required and permitted by sections 303 and 1008 of the Act (21 U.S.C. 823 and 958).

§ 1316.03   Authority to make inspections.

In carrying out his functions under the Act, the Administrator, through his inspectors, is authorized in accordance with sections 510 and 1015 of the Act (21 U.S.C. 880 and 965) to enter controlled premises and conduct administrative inspections thereof, for the purpose of:

(a) Inspecting, copying, and verifying the correctness of records, reports, or other documents required to be kept or made under the Act and regulations promulgated under the Act, including, but not limited to, inventory and other records required to be kept pursuant to Part 1304 of this chapter, order form records required to be kept pursuant to Part 1305 of this chapter, prescription and distribution records required to be kept pursuant to Part 1306 of this chapter, tableting machines, and encapsulating machines required to be kept pursuant to part 1310 of this chapter, import/export records of listed chemicals required to be kept pursuant to part 1313 of this chapter, shipping records identifying the name of each carrier used and the date and quantity of each shipment, and storage records identifying the name of each warehouse used and the date and quantity of each storage;

(b) Inspecting within reasonable limits and in a reasonable manner all pertinent equipment, finished and unfinished controlled substances and other substances or materials, containers, and labeling found at the controlled premises relating to this Act;

(c) Making a physical inventory of all controlled substances on-hand at the premises;

(d) Collecting samples of controlled substances or precursors (in the event any samples are collected during an inspection, the inspector shall issue a receipt for such samples on DEA Form 84 to the owner, operator, or agent in charge of the premises);

(e) Checking of records and information on distribution of controlled substances by the registrant as they relate to total distribution of the registrant (i.e., has the distribution in controlled substances increased markedly within the past year, and if so why); and

(f) Except as provided in § 1316.04, all other things therein (including records, files, papers, processes, controls and facilities) appropriate for verification of the records, reports, documents referred to above or otherwise bearing on the provisions of the Act and the regulations thereunder.

§ 1316.04   Exclusion from inspection.

(a) Unless the owner, operator or agent in charge of the controlled premises so consents in writing, no inspection authorized by these regulations shall extend to:

(1) Financial data;

(2) Sales data other than shipping data; or

(3) Pricing data.

§ 1316.05   Entry.

An inspection shall be carried out by an inspector. Any such inspector, upon (a) stating his purpose and (b) presenting to the owner, operator or agent in charge of the premises to be inspected (1) appropriate credentials, and (2) written notice of his inspection authority under § 1314.06 of this chapter, and (c) receiving informed consent under § 1316.08 or through the use of administrative warrant issued under §§ 1316.09–1316.14, shall have the right to enter such premises and conduct inspections at reasonable times and in a reasonable manner.

§ 1316.06   Notice of inspection.

The notice of inspection (DEA (or DNB) Form 82) shall contain:

(a) The name and title of the owner, operator, or agent in charge of the controlled premises;

(b) The controlled premises name;

(c) The address of the controlled premises to be inspected;

(d) The date and time of the inspection;

(e) A statement that a notice of inspection is given pursuant to section 510 of the Act (21 U.S.C. 880);

(f) A reproduction of the pertinent parts of section 510 of the Act; and

(g) The signature of the inspector.

§ 1316.07 Requirement for administrative inspection warrant; exceptions.

In all cases where an inspection is contemplated, an administrative inspection warrant is required pursuant to section 510 of the Act (21 U.S.C. 880), except that such warrant shall not be required for establishments applying for initial registration under the Act, for the inspection of books and records pursuant to an administrative subpoena issued in accordance with section 506 of the Act (21 U.S.C. 876) nor for entries in administrative inspections (including seizures of property):

(a) With the consent of the owner, operator, or agent in charge of the controlled premises as set forth in § 1316.08;

(b) In situations presenting imminent danger to health or safety;

(c) In situations involving inspection of conveyances where there is reasonable cause to obtain a warrant;

(d) In any other exceptional or emergency circumstance or time or opportunity to apply for a warrant is lacking; or

(e) In any other situations where a warrant is not constitutionally required.

§ 1316.08 Consent to inspection.

(a) An administrative inspection warrant shall not be required if informed consent is obtained from the owner, operator, or agent in charge of the controlled premises to be inspected;

(b) Wherever possible, informed consent shall consist of a written statement signed by the owner, operator, or agent in charge of the premises to be inspected and witnessed by two persons. The written consent shall contain the following information:

(1) That he (the owner, operator, or agent in charge of the premises) has been informed of his constitutional right not to have an administrative inspection made without an administrative inspection warrant;

(2) That he has right to refuse to consent to such an inspection;

(3) That anything of an incriminating nature which may be found may be seized and used against him in a criminal prosecution;

(4) That he has been presented with a notice of inspection as set forth in § 1316.06;

(5) That the consent given by him is voluntary and without threats of any kind; and

(6) That he may withdraw his consent at any time during the course of inspection.

(c) The written consent shall be produced in duplicate and be distributed as follows:

(1) The original will be retained by the inspector; and

(2) The duplicate will be given to the person inspected.

§ 1316.11 Execution of warrants.

An administrative inspection warrant shall be executed and returned as required by, and any inventory or seizure made shall comply with the requirements of, section 510(d) (3) of the Act (21 U.S.C. 880(d) (3)). The inspection shall begin as soon as is practicable after the issuance of the administrative inspection warrant and shall be completed with reasonable promptness. The inspection shall be conducted during regular business hours and shall be completed in a reasonable manner.

§ 1316.12 Refusal to allow inspection with an administrative warrant.

If a registrant or any person subject to the Act refuses to permit execution of an administrative warrant or impedes the inspector in the execution of that warrant, he shall be advised that such refusal or action constitutes a violation of section 402(a) (6) of the Act (21 U.S.C. (a) (6)). If he persists and the circumstances warrant, he shall be arrested and the inspection shall commence or continue.

§ 1316.13 Frequency of administrative inspections.

Except where circumstances otherwise dictate, it is the intent of the Administration to inspect all manufacturers of controlled substances listed in Schedules I and II and distributors of controlled substances listed in Schedule I once each year; and to inspect all distributors of controlled substances listed in Schedules II through V and manufacturers of controlled substances listed in Schedules III through V once every 3 years.

⟨1076⟩ FEDERAL FOOD, DRUG, AND COSMETIC ACT REQUIREMENTS RELATING TO DRUGS FOR HUMAN USE

Selected portions of the Federal Food, Drug, and Cosmetic Act as it relates to the regulation of drugs for human use are presented here as a service to practitioners and students of pharmacy and medicine. The complete text of the Act can be found in Title 21 of the United States Code. The corresponding section number of the code appear in brackets after the section number of the Act.

In addition to federal requirements, statutes governing drugs and their quality have been enacted by various states. In many cases, state requirements parallel those of the federal law. However, this should not be assumed to be the case and individual state laws and requirements should be consulted also.

Publication of these sections in the United States Pharmacopeia is for purposes of information and does not impart to them any legal effect.

Inquiries regarding these requirements should be directed to the U. S. Food and Drug Administration, 5600 Fishers Lane, Rockville, Md.   20857.

INDEX TO SELECTED PORTIONS OF THE FEDERAL FOOD, DRUG, AND COSMETIC ACT RELATED TO DRUGS FOR HUMAN USE PRESENTED HEREIN
§ 1   Title
§ 201   Definitions

(e)	person
(g) (1)	drug
(g) (2)	counterfeit drug
(j)	official compendium
(k)	label
(l)	immediate container
(m)	labeling
(n)	misleading labeling or advertising
(o)	antiseptic
(p)	new drug
(t) (1)	color additive
(u)	safe

§ 301   Prohibited Acts Regarding Adulterated and Misbranded Drugs

(a)	introduction into interstate commerce
(b)	in interstate commerce
(c)	receipt and delivery
(d)	introduction into interstate commerce in violation of new drug requirements
(e)	failure to permit access or copying or to make reports
(f)	refusal to permit inspection
(g)	manufacture

(h)   giving a false guarantee
(i)   forging, counterfeiting
(k)   while held for sale
(o)   failure to provide to practitioners required labeling
(p)   failure to register
(t)   importation or marketing of samples and coupons

§ 303   Penalties

(a)   fine or imprisonment: repeat offenders or violation with intent to defraud or mislead
(b) (1) fines and imprisonment for importing or marketing samples or coupons
(b) (2) fines or imprisonment; employees
(b) (3) failure to report
(b) (4) limits on manufacturer or distributor responsibility
(b) (5) informant rewards
(c)   defenses
(d)   food and drug guarantee

§ 501   Adulterated Drugs

(a)   filthy, putrid, decomposed substances insanitary conditions failure to conform to good manufacturing practices poisonous or deleterious container unsafe color additive
(b)   failure to comply with compendial standards
(c)   failure to comply with purported strength, quality, or purity
(d)   other substance mixed with or substituted therefor

§ 502   Misbranded Drugs

(a)   false and misleading labeling
(b)   name and place of manufacturer, packer, or distributor quantity statement
(c)   conspicuousness of statements
(d)   label statement for certain narcotic and hypnotic substances
(e)   established name and quantity requirements
(f)   directions for use and adequate warnings
(g)   compendial packaging and labeling requirements
(h)   packaging requirements for drugs subject to deterioration
(i)   misleading containers and imitations
(j)   dangerous to health as labeled
(k)   uncertified insulin
(l)   uncertified antibiotic
(m)   nonconforming color additive
(n)   advertising requirements
(o)   unregistered establishment or failure to bear identification symbol
(p)   failure to comply with Poison Prevention Packaging Act

§ 503   Exemptions from Labeling and Packaging Requirements; Sales Restrictions of Drug Samples

(a)   exemptions for repacking
(b) (1) prescription drug classification
(b) (2) dispensed prescription drug labeling requirements
(b) (4) federal caution statement required
(c) (1) drug sample marketing prohibited
(c) (2) coupon marketing prohibited
(c) (3) hospital or charity resale restrictions
(d) (1) restrictions on distribution of drug samples
(d) (2) requirements for sampling by mail
(d) (3) other distribution requirements
(e) (1) wholesale distributor restrictions
(e) (2) state licensure requirements
(e) (3) distributor and wholesale distribution definitions

§ 505   New Drugs

§ 506   Certification of Drugs Containing Insulin

§ 507   Certification of Antibiotics

§ 508   Authority to Designate Official Names

§ 510   Registration Requirements

(g)   nonapplicability to pharmacies and practitioners

§ 525   Recommendations for Investigations of Drugs for Rare Diseases or Conditions

§ 526   Designation of Drugs for Rare Diseases or Conditions

§ 527   Protection of Unpatented Drugs for Rare Diseases or Conditions

§ 528   Open Protocols for Investigations of Drugs for Rare Diseases or Conditions

§ 703   Records of Interstate Shipment

§ 704   Inspections

§ 707   Cooperation in Revision of USP and Development of Analytical Methods

Short Title

§ 1   This Act may be cited as the Federal Food, Drug, and Cosmetic Act.

Definitions

§ 201 [321]   For the purposes of this Act—

(e) The term "person" includes individual, partnership, corporation, and association.

(g) (1) The term "drug" means (A) articles recognized in the official United States Pharmacopeia, official Homeopathic Pharmacopeia of the United States, or official National Formulary, or any supplement to any of them; and (B) articles intended for use in the diagnosis, cure, mitigation, treatment, or prevention of disease in man or other animals; and (C) articles (other than food) intended to affect the structure or any function of the body of man or other animals; and (D) articles intended for use as a component of any articles specified in clause (A), (B), or (C); but does not include devices or their components, parts, or accessories.

(2) The term "counterfeit drug" means a drug which, or the container or labeling of which, without authorization, bears the trademark, trade name, or other identifying mark, imprint, or device, or any likeness thereof, of a drug manufacturer, processor, packer, or distributor other than the person or persons who in fact manufactured, processed, packed, or distributed such drug and which thereby falsely purports or is represented to be the product of, or to have been packed or distributed by, such other drug manufacturer, processor, packer, or distributor.

(j) The term "official compendium" means the official United States Pharmacopeia, official Homeopathic Pharmacopeia of the United States, official National Formulary, or any supplement to any of them.

(k) The term "label" means a display of written, printed, or graphic matter upon the immediate container of any article; and a requirement made by or under authority of this Act that any word, statement, or other information appear on the label shall not be considered to be complied with unless such word, statement, or other information also appears on the outside container or wrapper, if any there be, of the retail package of such article, or is easily legible through the outside container or wrapper.

(l) The term "immediate container" does not include package liners.

(m) The term "labeling" means all labels and other written, printed, or graphic matter (1) upon any article or any of its containers or wrappers, or (2) accompanying such article.

(n) If an article is alleged to be misbranded because the labeling or advertising is misleading, then in determining whether the labeling or advertising is misleading there shall be taken into account (among other things) not only representations made or suggested by statement, word, design, device, or any combination thereof, but also the extent to which the labeling or advertising fails to reveal facts material in the light of such representations or material with respect to consequences which may result from the use of the article to which the labeling or advertising relates under the conditions of use prescribed in the labeling or advertising thereof or under such conditions of use as are customary or usual.

(o) The representation of a drug, in its labeling, as an antiseptic shall be considered to be a representation that it is a germicide, except in the case of a drug purporting to be, or represented as, an antiseptic for inhibitory use as a wet dressing, ointment, dusting powder, or such other use as involves prolonged contact with the body.

(p) The term "new drug" means—

(1) Any drug (except a new animal drug or an animal feed bearing or containing a new animal drug) the composition of which is such that such drug is not generally recognized, among experts qualified by scientific training and experience to evaluate the safety and effectiveness of drugs, as safe and effective for use under the conditions prescribed, recommended, or suggested in the labeling thereof, except that such a drug not so recognized shall not be deemed to be a "new drug" if at any time prior to the enactment of this Act it was subject to the Food and Drugs Act of June 30, 1906, as amended, and if at such time its labeling contained the same representations concerning the conditions of its use; or

(2) Any drug (except a new animal drug or an animal feed bearing or containing a new animal drug) the composition of which is such that such drug, as a result of investigations to determine its safety and effectiveness for use under such conditions, has become so recognized, but which has not, otherwise than in such investigations, been used to a material extent or for a material time under such conditions.

(t) (1) The term "color additive" means a material which—

(A) is a dye, pigment, or other substance made by a process of synthesis or similar artifice, or extracted, isolated, or otherwise derived, with or without intermediate or final change of identity, from a vegetable, animal, mineral, or other source, and

(B) when added or applied to a food, drug, or cosmetic, or to the human body or any part thereof, is capable (alone or through reaction with other substance) of imparting color thereto:

except that such term does not include any material which the Secretary, by regulation, determines is used (or intended to be used) solely for a purpose or purposes other than coloring.

(2) The term "color" includes black, white, and intermediate grays.

(u) The term "safe," as used in paragraph(s) of this section and in sections 409, 512, and 706, has reference to the health of man or animal.

Prohibited Acts

§ 301 [331] The following acts and the causing thereof are hereby prohibited:

(a) The introduction or delivery for introduction into interstate commerce of any food, drug, device, or cosmetic that is adulterated or misbranded.

(b) The adulteration or misbranding of any food, drug, device, or cosmetic in interstate commerce.

(c) The receipt in interstate commerce of any food, drug, device, or cosmetic that is adulterated or misbranded, and the delivery or proffered delivery thereof for pay or otherwise.

(d) The introduction or delivery for introduction into interstate commerce of any article in violation of section 404 or 505.

(e) The refusal to permit access to or copying of any record as required by section 703; or the failure to establish or maintain any record, or make any report, required under section 505 (i) or (j), 507 (d) or (g), 512 (j), (l) or (m), 515 (f) or 519, or the

refusal to permit access to or verification or copying of any such required record.

(f) The refusal to permit entry or inspection as authorized by section 704.

(g) The manufacture within any Territory of any food, drug, device, or cosmetic that is adulterated or misbranded.

(h) The giving of a guaranty or undertaking referred to in section 303 (c) (2), which guaranty or undertaking is false, except by a person who relied upon a guaranty or undertaking to the same effect signed by, and containing the name and address of, the person residing in the United States from whom he received in good faith the food, drug, device, or cosmetic; or the giving of a guaranty or undertaking referred to in section 303 (c) (3), which guaranty or undertaking is false.

(i) (1) Forging, counterfeiting, simulating, or falsely representing, or without proper authority using any mark, stamp, tag, label, or other identification device authorized or required by regulations promulgated under the provisions of section 404, 506, 507, or 706.

(2) Making, selling, disposing of, or keeping in possession, control, or custody, or concealing any punch, die, plate, stone, or other thing designed to print, imprint, or reproduce the trademark, trade name, or other identifying mark, imprint, or device of another or any likeness of any of the foregoing upon any drug or container or labeling thereof so as to render such drug a counterfeit drug.

(3) The doing of any act which causes a drug to be a counterfeit drug, or the sale or dispensing, or the holding for sale or dispensing, of a counterfeit drug.

(k) The alteration, mutilation, destruction, obliteration, or removal of the whole or any part of the labeling of, or the doing of any other act with respect to, a food, drug, device, or cosmetic, if such act is done while such article is held for sale (whether or not the first sale) after shipment in interstate commerce and results in such article being adulterated or misbranded.

(l) The using, on the labeling of any drug or device or in any advertising relating to such drug or device, of any representation or suggestion that approval of an application with respect to such drug or device is in effect under section 505, 515, or 520 (g), as the case may be, or that such drug or device complies with the provisions of such action.

(n) The using, in labeling, advertising or other sales promotion of any reference to any report or analysis furnished in compliance with section 704.

(p) The failure to register in accordance with section 510, the failure to provide any information required by section 510 (j) or 510 (k), or the failure to provide a notice required by section 510 (j) (2).

(t) The importation of a drug in violation of section 801 (d) (1), the sale, purchase, or trade of a drug or drug sample or the offer to sell, purchase, or trade a drug or drug sample in violation of section 503 (c), the sale, purchase, or trade of a coupon, the offer to sell, purchase, or trade such a coupon, or the counterfeiting of such a coupon in violation of section 503 (c) (2), the distribution of a drug sample in violation of section 530 (d) of the failure to otherwise comply with the requirements of section 503 (d), or the distribution of drugs in violation of section 503 (e) or the failure to otherwise comply with the requirements of section 503 (e).

Penalties

§ 303 [333]   (a) (1) Any person who violates a provision of section 301 shall be imprisoned for not more than one year or fined not more than $1,000, or both.

(2) Notwithstanding the provisions of paragraph (1) of this section, if any person commits such a violation after a conviction of him under this section has become final, or commits such a violation with the intent to defraud or mislead, such person shall

be imprisoned for not more than three years or fined not more than $10,000 or both.

(b) (1) Notwithstanding subsection (a), any person who violates section 301 (t) because of an importation of a drug in violation of section 801 (d) (1), because of a sale, purchase, or trade of a drug or drug sample or the offer to sell, purchase, or trade a drug or drug sample in violation of section 503 (c), because of the sale, purchase, or trade of a coupon, the offer to sell, purchase, or trade such a coupon, or the counterfeiting of such a coupon in violation of section 503 (c) (2), or the distribution of drugs in violation of section 503 (e) (2) (A) shall be imprisoned for not more than 10 years or fined not more than $250,000, or both.

(2) Any manufacturer or distributor who distributes drug samples by means other than the mail or common carrier whose representative, during the course of the representative's employment or association with the manufacturer or distributor, violated section 301 (t) because of a violation of section 503 (c) (1) or violated any State law prohibiting the sale, purchase, or trade of a drug sample subject to section 503 (b) or the offer to sell, purchase, or trade such a drug sample shall, upon conviction of the representative for such violation, be subject to the following civil penalties:

(A) A civil penalty of not more than $50,000 for each of the first two such violations resulting in a conviction of any representative of the manufacturer or distributor in any 10-year period.

(B) A civil penalty of not more than $1,000,000 for each violation resulting in a conviction of any representative after the second conviction in any 10-year period.
For the purposes of this paragraph, multiple convictions of one or more persons arising out of the same event or transaction, or a related series of events or transactions, shall be considered as one violation.

(3) Any manufacturer or distributor who violates section 301 (t) because of a failure to make a report required by section 503 (d) (3) (E) shall be subject to a civil penalty of not more than $100,000.

(4) (A) If a manufacturer or distributor or any representative of such manufacturer or distributor provides information leading to the arrest and conviction of any representative of that manufacturer or distributor for a violation of section 301 (t) because of a sale, purchase, or trade or offer to purchase, sell, or trade a drug sample in violation of section 503 (c) (1) or for a violation of State law prohibiting the sale, purchase, or trade or offer to sell, purchase, or trade a drug sample, the conviction of such representative shall not be considered as a violation for purposes of paragraph (2).

(B) If, in an action brought under paragraph (2) against a manufacturer or distributor relating to the conviction of a representative of such manufacturer or distributor for the sale, purchase, or trade of a drug or the offer to sell, purchase, or trade a drug, it is shown, by clear and convincing evidence—

(i) that the manufacturer or distributor conducted, before the arrest of such representative for the violation which resulted in such conviction, an investigation of events or transactions which would have led to the reporting of information leading to the arrest and conviction of such representative for such purchase, sale, or trade or offer to purchase, sell, or trade, or

(ii) that, except in the case of the conviction of a representative employed in a supervisory function, despite diligent implementation by the manufacturer or distributor of an independent audit and security system designed to detect such a violation, the manufacturer or distributor could not reasonably have been expected to have detected such violation, the conviction of such representative shall not be considered as a conviction for purpose of paragraph (2).

(5) If a person provides information leading to the arrest and conviction of a person for a violation of section 301 (t) because of the sale, purchase, or trade of a drug sample or the offer to sell, purchase, or trade a drug sample in violation of section 503 (c) (1), such person shall be entitled to one-half of the criminal fine imposed and collected for such violation but not more than $125,000.

(c) No person shall be subject to the penalties of subsection (a) of this section, (1) for having received in interstate commerce any article and delivered it or proffered delivery of it, if such delivery or proffer was made in good faith, unless he refuses to furnish on request of an officer or employee duly designated by the Secretary the name and address of the person from whom he purchased or received such article and copies of all documents, if any there be, pertaining to the delivery of the article to him; or (2) for having violated section 301 (a) or (d), if he establishes a guaranty or undertaking signed by, and containing the name and address of, the person residing in the United States from whom he received in good faith the article, to the effect, in case of an alleged violation of section 301 (a), that such article is not adulterated or misbranded, within the meaning of this Act, designating this Act, or to the effect, in case of an alleged violation of section 301 (d), that such article is not an article which may not, under the provisions of section 404 or 505, be introduced into interstate commerce; or (3) for having violated section 301 (a), where the violation exists because the article is adulterated by reason of containing a color additive not from a batch certified in accordance with regulations promulgated by the Secretary under this Act, if such person establishes a guaranty or undertaking signed by, and containing the name and address of, the manufacturer of the color additive, to the effect that such color additive was from a batch certified in accordance with the applicable regulations promulgated by the Secretary under this Act; or (4) for having violated section 301 (b), (c), or (k) by failure to comply with section 502 (f) in respect to an article received in interstate commerce to which neither section 503 (a) nor section 503 (b) (1) is applicable if the delivery or proffered delivery was made in good faith and the labeling at the time thereof contained the same directions for use and warning statements as were contained in the labeling at the time of such receipt of such article; or (5) for having violated section 301 (i) (2) if such person acted in good faith and had no reason to believe that use of the punch, die, plate, stone, or other thing involved would result in a drug being a counterfeit drug, or for having violated section 301 (i) (3) if the person doing the act or causing it to be done acted in good faith and had no reason to believe that the drug was a counterfeit drug.

Adulterated Drugs

§ 501 [351] A drug or device shall be deemed to be adulterated—

(a) (1) if it consists in whole or in part of any filthy, putrid, or decomposed substance; or (2) (A) if it has been prepared, packed, or held under insanitary conditions whereby it may have been contaminated with filth, or whereby it may have been rendered injurious to health; or (B) if it is a drug and the methods used in, or the facilities or controls used for, its manufacture, processing, packing, or holding do not conform to or are not operated or administered in conformity with current good manufacturing practice to assure that such drug meets the requirements of this Act as to safety and has the identity and strength, and meets the quality and purity characteristics, which it purports or is represented to possess; or (3) if its container is composed, in whole or in part, of any poisonous or deleterious substance which may render the contents injurious to health; or (4) if (A) it bears or contains, for purposes of coloring only, a color additive which is unsafe within the meaning of section 706 (a), or (B) it is a color additive the intended use of which in or on drugs or devices is for purposes of coloring only and is unsafe within the meaning of section 706 (a);

(b) If it purports to be or is represented as a drug the name of which is recognized in an official compendium, and its strength differs from, or its quality or purity falls below, the standards set forth in such compendium. Such determination as to strength, quality, or purity shall be made in accordance with the tests or methods of assay set forth in such compendium, except that whenever tests or methods of assays have not been prescribed in such compendium, or such tests or methods of assay as are prescribed are, in the judgment of the Secretary, insufficient for the making of such determination, the Secretary shall bring such fact to the attention of the appropriate body charged with the revision of such compendium, and if such body fails within a reasonable time to prescribe tests or methods of assay which, in the judgment of the Secretary, are sufficient for purposes of this paragraph, then the Secretary shall promulgate regulations prescribing appropriate tests or methods of assay in accordance with which such determination as to strength, quality, or purity shall be made. No drug defined in an official compendium shall be deemed to be adulterated under this paragraph because it differs from the standard of strength, quality, or purity therefor set forth in such compendium, if its difference in strength, quality, or purity from such standards is plainly stated on its label. Whenever a drug is recognized in both the United States Pharmacopeia and the Homeopathic Pharmacopeia of the United States it shall be subject to the requirements of the United States Pharmacopeia unless it is labeled and offered for sale as a homeopathic drug, in which case it shall be subject to the provisions of the Homeopathic Pharmacopeia of the United States and not to those of the United States Pharmacopeia.

(c) If it is not subject to the provisions of paragraph (b) of this section and its strength differs from, or its purity or quality falls below, that which it purports or is represented to possess.

(d) If it is a drug and any substance has been (1) mixed or packed therewith so as to reduce its quality or strength or (2) substituted wholly or in part therefor.

Misbranded Drugs

§ 502 [352] A drug or device shall be deemed to be misbranded—

(a) If its labeling is false or misleading in any particular.

(b) If in a package form unless it bears a label containing (1) the name and place of business of the manufacturer, packer, or distributor; and (2) an accurate statement of the quantity of the contents in terms of weight, measure, or numerical count: *Provided*, That under clause (2) of this paragraph reasonable variations shall be permitted, and exemptions as to small packages shall be established, by regulations prescribed by the Secretary.

(c) If any word, statement, or other information required by or under authority of this Act to appear cn the label or labeling is not prominently placed thereon with such conspicuousness (as compared with other words, statements, designs, or devices, in the labeling) and in such terms as to render it likely to be read and understood by the ordinary individual under customary conditions of purchase and use.

(d) If it is for use by man and contains any quantity of the narcotic or hypnotic substance alpha-eucaine, barbituric acid, beta-eucaine, bromal, cannabis, carbromal, chloral, coca, cocaine, codeine, heroin, marijuana, morphine, opium, paraldehyde, peyote, or sulfonmethane; or any chemical derivative of such substance, which derivative has been by the Secretary, after investigation, found to be, and by regulations designated as, habit forming; unless its label bears the name, and quantity or proportion of such substance or derivative and in juxtaposition therewith the statement "Warning—May be habit forming."

(e) (1) If it is a drug, unless (A) its label bears, to the exclusion of any other nonproprietary name (except the applicable systematic chemical name or the chemical formula), (i) the established name (as defined in subparagraph (3)) of the drug, if such there be, and (ii) in case it is fabricated from two or more ingredients, the established name and quantity of each active ingredient, including the quantity, kind, and proportion of any alcohol, and also including whether active or not, the established name and quantity or proportion of any bromides, ether, chloroform, acetanilide, acetophenetidin, amidopyrine, antipyrine, atropine, hyoscine, hyoscyamine, arsenic, digitalis, digitalis glucosides, mercury, ouabain, strophanthin, strychnine, thyroid, or any derivative or preparation of any such substances, contained therein: *Provided*, That the requirement for stating the quantity of the active ingredients, other than the quantity of those specifically named in this paragraph, shall apply only to prescription drugs; and (B) for any prescription drug the established name of such drug or ingredient, as the case may be, on such label (and on any labeling on which a name for such drug or ingredient is used) is printed prominently and in type at least half as large as that used thereon for any proprietary name or designation for such drug or ingredient: and *Provided*, That to the extent that compliance with the requirements of clause (A) (ii) or clause (B) of this subparagraph is impracticable, exemptions shall be established by regulations promulgated by the Secretary.

(3) As used in paragraph (l) the term "established name," with respect to a drug or ingredient thereof, means (A) the applicable official name designated pursuant to section 508, or (B) if there is no such name and such drug, or such ingredient, is an article recognized in an official compendium, then the official title thereof in such compendium or (C) if neither clause (A) nor clause (B) of this subparagraph applies, then the common or usual name, if any, of such drug or of such ingredient: *Provided further*, That where clause (B) of this subparagraph applies to an article recognized in the United States Pharmacopeia and in the Homeopathic Pharmacopeia under different official titles, the official title used in the United States Pharmacopeia shall apply unless it is labeled and offered for sale as a homeopathic drug, in which case the official title used in the Homeopathic Pharmacopeia shall apply.

(f) Unless its labeling bears (1) adequate directions for use; and (2) such adequate warnings against use in those pathological conditions or by children where its use may be dangerous to health, or against unsafe dosage or methods or duration of administration or application, in such manner and form, as are necessary for the protection of users: *Provided,* That where any requirement of clause (1) of this paragraph, as applied to any drug or device, is not necessary for the protection of the public health, the Secretary shall promulgate regulations exempting such drug or device from such requirement.

(g) If it purports to be a drug the name of which is recognized in an official compendium, unless it is packaged and labeled as prescribed therein: *Provided*, That the method of packing may be modified with the consent of the Secretary. Whenever a drug is recognized in both the United States Pharmacopeia and the Homeopathic Pharmacopeia of the United States, it shall be subject to the requirements of the United States Pharmacopeia with respect to packaging, and labeling unless it is labeled and offered for sale as a homeopathic drug, in which case it shall be subject to the provisions of the Homeopathic Pharmacopeia of the United States, and not to those of the United States Pharmacopeia: *Provided further*, That, in the event of inconsistency between the requirements of this paragraph and those of paragraph (e) as to the name by which the drug or its ingredients shall be designated, the requirements of paragraph (e) shall prevail.

(h) If it has been found by the Secretary to be a drug liable to deterioration, unless it is packaged in such form and manner, and its label bears a statement of such precautions, as the Secretary shall by regulations require as necessary for the protection of the public health. No such regulation shall be established for any drug recognized in an official compendium until the Secretary shall have informed the appropriate body charged with the revision of such compendium of the need for such packaging or labeling requirements and such body shall have failed within a reasonable time to prescribe such requirements.

(i) (1) If it is a drug and its container is so made, formed, or filled as to be misleading; or (2) if it is an imitation of another drug; or (3) if it is offered for sale under the name of another drug.

(j) If it is dangerous to health when used in the dosage or manner, or with the frequency or duration prescribed, recommended, or suggested in the labeling thereof.

(k) If it is, or purports to be, or is represented as a drug composed wholly or partly of insulin, unless (1) it is from a batch with respect to which a certificate or release has been issued pursuant to section 506, and (2) such certificate or release is in effect with respect to such drug.

(l) If it is, or purports to be, or is represented as a drug (except a drug for use in animals other than man) composed wholly or partly of any kind of penicillin, streptomycin, chlortetracycline, chloramphenicol, bacitracin, or any other antibiotic drug, or any derivative thereof, unless (1) it is from a batch with respect to which a certificate or release has been issued pursuant to section 507, and (2) such certificate or release is in effect with respect to such drug; *Provided,* That this paragraph shall not apply to any drug or class of drugs exempted by regulations promulgated under section 507 (c) or (d).

(m) If it is a color additive the intended use of which is for the purpose of coloring only, unless its packaging and labeling are in conformity with such packaging and labeling requirements applicable to such color additive, as may be contained in regulations issued under section 706.

(n) In the case of any prescription drug distributed or offered for sale in any State, unless the manufacturer, packer, or distributor thereof includes in all advertisements and other descriptive printed matter issued or caused to be issued by the manufacturer, packer, or distributor with respect to that drug a true statement of (1) the established name as defined in section 502 (e), printed prominently and in type at least half as large as that used for any trade or brand name thereof, (2) the formula showing quantitatively each ingredient of such drug to the extent required for labels under section 502 (e), and (3) such other information in brief summary relating to side effects, contraindications, and effectiveness as shall be required in regulations which shall be issued by the Secretary in accordance with the procedure specified in section 701 (e) of this Act: *Provided,* That (A) except in extraordinary circumstances, no regulation issued under this paragraph shall require prior approval by the Secretary of the content of any advertisement, and (B) no advertisement of a prescription drug, published after the effective date of regulations issued under this paragraph applicable to advertisements of prescription drugs, shall, with respect to the matters specified in this paragraph or covered by such regulations, be subject to the provisions of sections 12 through 17 of the Federal Trade Commission Act, as amended (15 U.S.C. 52–57). This paragraph (n) shall not be applicable to any printed matter which the Secretary determines to be labeling as defined in section 201 (m) of this Act. Nothing in the Convention on Psychotropic Substances, signed at Vienna, Austria, on February 21, 1971, shall be construed to prevent drug price communications to consumers.

(o) If it was manufactured, prepared, propagated, compounded, or processed in an establishment in any State not duly registered under section 510, if it was not included in a list required by section 510 (j), if a notice or other information respecting it was not provided as required by such section or

section 510 (k), or if it does not bear such symbols from the uniform system for identification of devices prescribed under section 510 (e) as the Secretary by regulation requires.

(p) If it is a drug and its packaging or labeling is in violation of an applicable regulation issued pursuant to section 3 or 4 of the Poison Prevention Packing Act of 1970.

Exemptions in Case of Drugs

§ **503** [353]   (a) The Secretary is hereby directed to promulgate regulations exempting from any labeling or packaging requirement of this Act drugs and devices which are, in accordance with the practice of the trade, to be processed, labeled, or repacked in substantial quantities at establishments other than those where originally processed or packed, on condition that such drugs and devices are not adulterated or misbranded under the provisions of this Act upon removal from such processing, labeling, or repacking establishment.

(b) (1) A drug intended for use by man which—

(A) is a habit-forming drug to which section 502 (d) applies; or

(B) because of its toxicity or other potentiality for harmful effect, or the method of its use, or the collateral measures necessary to its use, is not safe for use except under the supervision of a practitioner licensed by law to administer such drug; or

(C) is limited by an approved application under section 505 to use under the professional supervision of a practitioner licensed by law to administer such drug;

shall be dispensed only (i) upon a written prescription of a practitioner licensed by law to administer such drug, or (ii) upon an oral prescription of such practitioner which is reduced promptly to writing and filed by the pharmacist, or (iii) by refilling any such written or oral prescription if such refilling is authorized by the prescriber either in the original prescription or by oral order which is reduced promptly to writing and filed by the pharmacist. The act of dispensing a drug contrary to the provisions of this paragraph shall be deemed to be an act which results in the drug being misbranded while held for sale.

(2) Any drug dispensed by filling or refilling a written or oral prescription of a practitioner licensed by law to administer such drug shall be exempt from the requirements of section 502, except paragraphs (a), (i) (2) and (3), (k), and (l), and the packaging requirements of paragraphs (g), (h), and (p), if the drug bears a label containing the name and address of the dispenser, the serial number and date of the prescription or of its filling, the name of the prescriber, and, if stated in the prescription, the name of the patient, and the directions for use and cautionary statements, if any, contained in such prescription. This exemption shall not apply to any drug dispensed in the course of the conduct of a business of dispensing drugs pursuant to diagnosis by mail, or to a drug dispensed in violation of paragraph (1) of this subsection.

(3) The Secretary may by regulation remove drugs subject to section 502 (d) and section 505 from the requirements of paragraph (1) of this subsection when such requirements are not necessary for the protection of the public health.

(4) A drug which is subject to paragraph (1) of this subsection shall be deemed to be misbranded if at any time prior to dispensing its label fails to bear the statement "Caution: Federal law prohibits dispensing without prescription." A drug to which paragraph (1) of this subsection does not apply shall be deemed to be misbranded if at any time prior to dispensing its label bears the caution statement quoted in the preceding sentence.

(5) Nothing in this subsection shall be construed to relieve any person from any requirement prescribed by or under authority of law with respect to drugs now included or which may hereafter be included within the classifications stated in section 3220 of the Internal Revenue Code (26 U.S.C. 3220), or to

marijuana as defined in section 3238 (b) of the Internal Revenue Code (26 U.S.C. 3238 (b)).

(c) (1) No person may sell, purchase, or trade or offer to sell, purchase, or trade any drug sample. For purposes of this paragraph and subsection (d), the term 'drug sample' means a unit of a drug, subject ot subsection (b), which is not intended to be sold and is intended to promote the sale of the drug. Nothing in this paragraph shall subject an officer or executive of a drug manufacturer or distributor to criminal liability solely because of a sale, purchase, trade, or offer to sell, purchase, or trade in violation of this paragraph by other employees of the manufacturer or distributor.

(2) No person may sell, purchase, or trade, offer to sell, purchase, or trade, or counterfeit any coupon. For purposes of this paragraph, the term 'coupon' means a form which may be redeemed, at no cost or at a reduced cost, for a drug which is prescribed in accordance with section 503 (b).

(3) (A) No person may sell, purchase, or trade, or offer to sell, purchase, or trade, any drug—

(i) which is subject to subsection (b), and

(ii) (I) which was purchased by a public or private hospital or other health care entity, or

(II) which was donated or supplied at a reduced price to a charitable organization described in section 501 (c) (3) of the Internal Revenue Code of 1954.

(B) Subparagraph (A) does not apply to—

(i) the purchase or other acquisition by a hospital or other health care entity which is a member of a group purchasing organization of a drug for its own use from the group purchasing organization or from other hospitals or health care entities which are members of such organization,

(ii) the sale, purchase, or trade of a drug or an offer to sell, purchase, or trade a drug by an organization described in subparagraph (A) (ii) (II) to a nonprofit affiliate of the organization to the extent otherwise permitted by law,

(iii) a sale, purchase, or trade of a drug or an offer to sell, purchase, or trade a drug among hospitals or other health care entities which are under common control,

(iv) a sale, purchase, or trade of a drug or an offer to sell, purchase, or trade a drug for emergency medical reasons, or

(v) a sale, purchase, or trade of a drug, an offer to sell, purchase, or trade a drug, or the dispensing of a drug pursuant to a prescription executed in accordance with section 503 (b).

For purposes of this paragraph, the term 'entity' does not include a wholesale distributor of drugs or a retail pharmacy licensed under State law and the term 'emergency medical reasons' includes transfers of a drug between health care entities or from a health care entity to a retail pharmacy undertaken to alleviate temporary shortages of the drug arising from delays in or interruptions of regular distribution schedules.

(d) (1) Except as provided in paragraphs (2) and (3), no representative of drug manufacturer or distributor may distribute any drug sample.

(2) (A) The manufacturer or distributor of a drug subject to subsection (b) may, in accordance with this paragraph, distribute drug samples by mail or common carrier to practitioners licensed to prescribe such drugs, or, at the request of a licensed practitioner, to pharmacies of hospitals or other health care entities. Such a distribution of drug samples may only be made—

(i) in response to a written request for drug samples made on a form which meets the requirements of subparagraph (B), and

(ii) under a system which requires the recipient of the drug sample to execute a written receipt for the drug sample upon its delivery and the return of the receipt to the manufacturer or distributor.

(B) A written request for a drug sample required by subparagraph (A) (i) shall contain—

(i) the name, address, professional designation, and signature of the practitioner making the request,

(ii) the identity of the drug sample requested and the quantity requested,

(iii) the name of the manufacturer of the drug sample requested, and

(iv) the date of the request.

(C) Each drug manufacturer or distributor which makes distributions by mail or common carrier under this paragraph shall maintain, for a period of 3 years, the request forms submitted for such distributions and shall maintain a record of distributions of drug samples which identifies the drugs distributed and the recipients of the distributions. Forms, receipts, and records required to be maintained under this subparagraph shall be made available by the drug manufacturer or distributor to Federal and State officials engaged in the regulation of drugs and in the enforcement of laws applicable to drugs.

(3) The manufacturer or distributor of a drug subject to subsection (b) may, by means other than mail or common carrier, distribute drug samples only if the manufacturer or distributor makes the distributions in accordance with subparagraph (A) and carries out the activities described in subparagraphs (B) through (F) as follows:

(A) Drug samples may only be distributed—

(i) to practitioners licensed to prescribe such drugs if they make a written request for the drug samples, or

(ii) at the written request of such a licensed practitioner, to pharmacies of hospitals or other health care entities. A written request for drug samples shall be made on a form which contains the practitioner's name, address, and professional designation, the identity of the drug sample requested, the quantity of drug samples requested, the name of the manufacturer or distributor of the drug sample, the date of the request and signature of the practitioner making the request.

(B) Drug manufacturers or distributors shall store drug samples under conditions that will maintain their stability, integrity, and effectiveness and will assure that the drug samples will be free of contamination, deterioration, and adulteration.

(C) Drug manufacturers or distributors shall conduct, at least annually, a complete and accurate inventory of all drug samples in the possession of representatives of the manufacturer or distributor. Drug manufacturers or distributors shall maintain lists of the names and addresses of each of their representatives who distribute drug samples and of the sites where drug samples are stored. Drug manufacturers or distributors shall maintain records for at least 3 years of all drug samples distributed, destroyed, or returned to the manufacturer or distributor, of all inventories maintained under this subparagraph, of all thefts or significant losses of drug samples, and of all requests made under subparagraph (A) for drug samples. Records and lists maintained under this subparagraph shall be made available by the drug manufacturer or distributor to the Secretary upon request.

(D) Drug manufacturers or distributors shall notify the Secretary of any significant loss of drug samples and any known theft of drug samples.

(E) Drug manufacturers or distributors shall report to the Secretary any conviction of their representatives for violations of section 503 (c) (1) or a State law because of the sale, purchase, or trade of a drug sample or the offer to sell, purchase, or trade a drug sample.

(F) Drug manufacturers or distributors shall provide to the Secretary the name and telephone number of the individual responsible for responding to a request for information respecting drug samples.

(e) (1) Each person who is engaged in the wholesale distribution of drugs subject to subsection (b) and who is not an authorized distributor of record of such drugs shall provide to each wholesale distributor of such drugs a statement identifying each sale of the drug (including the date of the sale) before the sale to such wholesale distributor. Each manufacturer shall maintain at its corporate offices a curent list of such authorized distributors.

(2) (A) No person may engage in the wholesale distribution in interstate commerce of drugs subject to subsection (b) in a State unless such person is licensed by the State in accordance with the guidelines issued under subparagraph (B).

(B) The Secretary shall by regulation issue guidelines establishing minimum standards, terms, and conditions for the licensing of persons to make wholesale distributions in interstate commerce of drugs subject to subsection (b). Such guidelines shall prescribe requirements for the storage and handling of such drugs and for the establishment and maintenance of records of the distributions of such drugs.

(3) For the purposes of this subsection—

(A) the term 'authorized distributors of record' means those distributors with whom a manufacturer has established an ongoing relationship to distribute such manufacturer's products, and

(B) the term 'wholesale distribution' means distribution of drugs subject to subsection (b) to other than the consumer or patient but does not include intracompany sales and does not include distributions of drugs described in subsection (c) (3) (B).

New Drugs

§ 505 [355] (a) No person shall introduce or deliver for introduction into interstate commerce any new drug, unless an approval of an application filed pursuant to subsection (b) or (j) is effective with respect to such drug.

(b) (1) Any person may file with the Secretary an application with respect to any drug subject to the provisions of subsection (a). Such persons shall submit to the Secretary as a part of the application (A) full reports of investigations which have been made to show whether or not such drug is safe for use and whether such drug is effective in use; (B) a full list of the articles used as components of such drug; (C) a full statement of the composition of such drug; (D) a full description of the methods used in, and the facilities and controls used for, the manufacture, processing, and packing of such drug; (E) such samples of such drug and of the articles used as components thereof as the Secretary may require; and (F) specimens of the labeling proposed to be used for such drug. The applicant shall file with the application the patent number and the expiration date of any patent which claims the drug for which the applicant submitted the application or which claims a method of using such drug and with respect to which a claim of patent infringement could reasonably be asserted if a person not licensed by the owner engaged in the manufacture, use, or sale of the drug. If an application is filed under this subsection for a drug and a patent which claims such drug or a method of using such drug is issued after the filing date but before approval of the application, the applicant shall amend the application to include the information required by the preceding sentence. Upon approval of the application, the Secretary shall publish information submitted under the two preceding sentences.

(2) An application submitted under paragraph (1) for a drug for which the investigations described in clause (A) of such paragraph and relied upon by the applicant for approval of the application were not conducted by or for the applicant and for which the applicant has not obtained a right of reference or use from the person by or for whom the investigations were conducted shall also include—

(A) a certification, in the opinion of the applicant and to the best of his knowledge, with respect to each patent which claims the drug for which such investigations were conducted

or which claims a use for such drug for which the applicant is seeking approval under this subsection and for which information is required to be filed under paragraph (1) or subsection (c)—

(i) that such patent information has not been filed,

(ii) that such patent has expired,

(iii) of the date on which such patent will expire, or

(iv) that such patent is invalid or will not be infringed by the manufacture, use, or sale of the new drug for which the application is submitted; and

(B) if with respect to the drug for which investigations described in paragraph (1) (A) were conducted information was filed under paragraph (1) or subsection (c) for a method of use patent which does not claim a use for which the applicant is seeking approval under this subsection, a statement that the method of use patent does not claim such a use.

(3) (A) An applicant who makes a certification described in paragraph (2) (A) (iv) shall include in the application a statement that the applicant will give the notice required by subparagraph (B) to—

(i) each owner of the patent which is the subject of the certification or the representative of such owner designated to receive such notice, and

(ii) the holder of the approved application under subsection (b) for the drug which is claimed by the patent or a use of which is claimed by the patent or the representative of such holder designated to receive such notice.

(B) The notice referred to in subparagraph (A) shall state that an application has been submitted under this subsection for the drug with respect to which the certification is made to obtain approval to engage in the commercial manufacture, use, or sale of the drug before the expiration of the patent referred to in the certification. Such notice shall include a detailed statement of the factual and legal basis of the applicant's opinion that the patent is not valid or will not be infringed.

(C) If an application is amended to include a certification described in paragraph (2) (A) (iv), the notice required by subparagraph (B) shall be given when the amended application is submitted.

(c) (1) Within one hundred and eighty days after the filing of an application under subsection (b), or such additional period as may be agreed upon by the Secretary and the applicant, the Secretary shall either—

(A) approve the application if he then finds that none of the grounds for denying approval specified in subsection (d) applies, or

(B) give the applicant notice of an opportunity for a hearing before the Secretary under subsection (d) on the question whether such application is approvable. If the applicant elects to accept the opportunity for hearing by written request within thirty days after such notice, such hearing shall commence not more than ninety days after the expiration of such thirty days unless the Secretary and the applicant otherwise agree. Any such hearing shall thereafter be conducted on an expedited basis and the Secretary's order thereon shall be issued within ninety days after the date fixed by the Secretary for filing final briefs.

(2) If the patent information described in subsection (b) could not be filed with the submission of an application under subsection (b) because the application was filed before the patent information was required under subsection (b) or a patent was issued after the application was approved under such subsection, the holder of an approved application shall file with the Secretary the patent number and the expiration date of any patent which claims the drug for which the application was submitted or which claims a method of using such drug and with respect to which a claim of patent infringement could reasonably be asserted if a person not licensed by the owner engaged in the

manufacture, use, or sale of the drug. If the holder of an approved application could not file patent information under subsection (b) because it was not required at the time the application was approved, the holder shall file such information under this subsection not later than thirty days after the date of the enactment of this sentence, and if the holder of an approved application could not file patent information under subsection (b) because no patent had been issued when an application was filed or approved, the holder shall file such information under this subsection not later than thirty days after the date the patent involved is issued. Upon the submission of patent information under this subsection, the Secretary shall publish it.

(3) The approval of an application filed under subsection (b) which contains a certification required by paragraph (2) of such subsection shall be made effective on the last applicable date determined under the following:

(A) If the applicant only made a certification described in clause (i) or (ii) of subsection (b) (2) (A) or in both such clauses, the approval may be made effective immediately.

(B) If the applicant made a certification described in clause (iii) of subsection (b) (2) (A), the approval may be made effective on the date certified under clause (iii).

(C) If the applicant made a certification described in clause (iv) of subsection (b) (2) (A), the approval shall be made effective immediately unless an action is brought for infringement of a patent which is the subject of the certification before the expiration of forty-five days from the date the notice provided under paragraph (3) (B) is received. If such an action is brought before the expiration of such days, the approval may be made effective upon the expiration of the thirty-month period beginning on the date of the receipt of the notice provided under paragraph (3) (B) or such shorter or longer period as the court may order because either party to the action failed to reasonably cooperate in expediting the action, except that—

(i) if before the expiration of such period the court decides that such patent is invalid or not infringed, the approval may be made effective on the date of the court decision,

(ii) if before the expiration of such period the court decides that such patent has been infringed, the approval may be made effective on such date as the court orders under section 271 (e) (4) (A) of title 35, United States Code, or

(iii) if before the expiration of such period the court grants a preliminary injunction prohibiting the applicant from engaging in the commercial manufacture or sale of the drug until the court decides the issues of patent validity and infringement and if the court decides that such patent is invalid or not infringed, the approval shall be made effective on the date of such court decision.

In such an action, each of the parties shall reasonably cooperate in expediting the action. Until the expiration of forty-five days from the date the notice made under paragraph (3) (B) is received, no action may be brought under section 2201 of title 28, United States Code, for a declaratory judgment with respect to the patent. Any action brought under such section 2201 shall be brought in the judicial district where the defendant has its principal place of business or a regular and established place of business.

(D) (i) If an application (other than an abbreviated new drug application) submitted under subsection (b) for a drug, no active ingredient (including any ester or salt of the active ingredient) of which has been approved in any other application under subsection (b), was approved during the period beginning January 1, 1982, and ending on the date of the enactment of this subsection, the Secretary may not make the approval of another application for a drug for which the investigations described in clause (A) of subsection (b) (1) and relied upon by the applicant for approval of the application were not conducted by or for the applicant and for which the applicant has not obtained a right of reference or use from the person by or for

whom the investigations were conducted effective before the expiration of ten years from the date of the approval of the application previously approved under subsection (b).

(ii) If an application submitted under subsection (b) for a drug, no active ingredient (including any ester or salt of the active ingredient) of which has been approved in any other application under subsection (b), is approved after the date of the enactment of this clause, no application which refers to the drug for which the subsection (b) application was submitted and for which the investigations described in clause (A) of subsection (b) (1) and relied upon by the applicant for approval of the application were not conducted by or for the applicant and for which the applicant has not obtained a right of reference or use from the person by or for whom the investigations were conducted may be submitted under subsection (b) before the expiration of five years from the date of the approval of the application under subsection (b), except that such an application may be submitted under subsection (b) after the expiration of four years from the date of the approval of the subsection (b) application if it contains a certification of patent invalidity or noninfringement described in clause (iv) of subsection (b) (2) (A). The approval of such an application shall be made effective in accordance with this paragraph except that, if an action for patent infringement is commenced during the one-year period beginning forty-eight months after the date of the approval of the subsection (b) application, the thirty-month period referred to in subparagraph (C) shall be extended by such amount of time (if any) which is required for seven and one-half years to have elapsed from the date of approval of the subsection (b) application.

(iii) If an application submitted under subsection (b) for a drug, which includes an active ingredient (including any ester or salt of the active ingredient) that has been approved in another application approved under subsection (b), is approved after the date of the enactment of this clause and if such application contains reports of new clinical investigations (other than bioavailability studies) essential to the approval of the application and conducted or sponsored by the applicant, the Secretary may not make the approval of an application submitted under subsection (b) for the conditions of approval of such drug in the approved subsection (b) application effective before the expiration of three years from the date of the approval of the application under subsection (b) if the investigations described in clause (A) of subsection (b) (1) and relied upon by the applicant for approval of the application were not conducted by or for the applicant and if the applicant has not obtained a right of reference or use from the person by or for whom the investigations were conducted.

(iv) If a supplement to an application approved under subsection (b) is approved after the date of enactment of this clause and the supplement contains reports of new clinical investigations (other than bioavailability studies) essential to the approval of the supplement and conducted or sponsored by the person submitting the supplement, the Secretary may not make the approval of an application submitted under subsection (b) for a change approved in the supplement effective before the expiration of three years from the date of the approval of the supplement under subsection (b) if the investigations described in clause (A) of subsection (b) (1) and relied upon by the applicant for approval of the application were not conducted by or for the applicant and if the applicant has not obtained a right of reference or use from the person by or for whom the investigations were conducted.

(v) If an application (or supplement to an application) submitted under subsection (b) for a drug, which includes an active ingredient (including any ester or salt of the active ingredient) that has been approved in another application under subsection (b), was approved during the period beginning January 1, 1982, and ending on the date of the enactment of this clause, the

Secretary may not make the approval of an application submitted under this subsection and for which the investigations described in clause (A) of subsection (b) (1) and relied upon by the applicant for approval of the application were not conducted by or for the applicant and for which the applicant has not obtained a right of reference or use from the person by or for whom the investigations were conducted and which refers to the drug for which the subsection (b) application was submitted effective before the expiration of two years from the date of enactment of this clause.

(d) If the Secretary finds, after due notice to the applicant in accordance with subsection (c) and giving him an opportunity for a hearing, in accordance with said subsection, that (1) the investigations, reports of which are required to be submitted to the Secretary pursuant to subsection (b), do not include adequate tests by all methods reasonably applicable to show whether or not such drug is safe for use under the conditions prescribed, recommended, or suggested in the proposed labeling thereof; (2) the results of such tests show that such drug is unsafe for use under such conditions or do not show that such drug is safe for use under such conditions; (3) the methods used in, and the facilities and controls used for, the manufacture, processing, and packing of such drug are inadequate to preserve its identity, strength, quality, and purity; (4) upon the basis of the information submitted to him as part of the application, or upon the basis of any other information before him with respect to such drug, he has insufficient information to determine whether such drug is safe for use under such conditions; or (5) evaluated on the basis of the information submitted to him as part of the application and any other information before him with respect to such drug, there is a lack of substantial evidence that the drug will have the effect it purports or is represented to have under the conditions of use prescribed, recommended, or suggested in the proposed labeling thereof; or

(6) the application failed to contain the patent information prescribed by subsection (b); or

(7) based on a fair evaluation of all material facts, such labeling is false or misleading in any particular; he shall issue an order refusing to approve the application. If, after such notice and opportunity for hearing, the Secretary finds that clauses (1) through (6) do not apply, he shall issue an order approving the application. As used in this subsection and subsection (e), the term "substantial evidence" means evidence consisting of adequate and well-controlled investigations, including clinical investigations, by experts qualified by scientific training and experience to evaluate the effectiveness of the drug involved, on the basis of which it could fairly and responsibly be concluded by such experts that the drug will have the effect it purports or is represented to have under the conditions of use prescribed, recommended, or suggested in the labeling or proposed labeling thereof.

(e) The Secretary shall, after due notice and opportunity for hearing to the applicant, withdraw approval of an application with respect to any drug under this section if the Secretary finds (1) that clinical or other experience, tests, or other scientific data show that such drug is unsafe for use under the conditions of use upon the basis of which the application was approved; (2) that new evidence of clinical experience, not contained in such application or not available to the Secretary until after such application was approved, or tests by new methods, or tests by methods not deemed reasonably applicable when such application was approved, evaluated together with the evidence available to the Secretary when the application was approved, shows that such drug is not shown to be safe for use under the conditions of use upon the basis of which the application was approved; or (3) on the basis of new information before him with respect to such drug, evaluated together with the evidence available to him when the application was approved, that there is a lack of substantial evidence that the drug

will have the effect it purports or is represented to have under the conditions of use prescribed, recommended, or suggested in the labeling thereof; or

(4) the patent information prescribed by subsection (c) was not filed within thirty days after the receipt of written notice from the Secretary specifying the failure to file such information; or

(5) that the application contains any untrue statement of a material fact: *Provided*, That if the Secretary (or in his absence the officer acting as Secretary) finds that there is an imminent hazard to the public health, he may suspend the approval of such application immediately, and give the applicant prompt notice of his action and afford the applicant the opportunity for an expedited hearing under this subsection; but the authority conferred by this proviso to suspend the approval of an application shall not be delegated. The Secretary may also, after due notice and opportunity for hearing to the applicant, withdraw the approval of an application submitted under subsection (b) or (j) with respect to any drug under this section if the Secretary finds (1) that the applicant has failed to establish a system for maintaining required records, or has repeatedly or deliberately failed to maintain such records or to make required reports, in accordance with a regulation or order under subsection (k) or to comply with the notice requirements of section 510 (k) (2), or the applicant has refused to permit access to, or copying or verification of, such records as required by paragraph (2) of such subsection; or (2) that on the basis of new information before him, evaluated together with the evidence before him when the application was approved, the methods used in, or the facilities and controls used for, the manufacture, processing, and packing of such drug are inadequate to assure and preserve its identity, strength, quality, and purity and were not made adequate within a reasonable time after receipt of written notice from the Secretary specifying the matter complained of; or (3) that on the basis of new information before him, evaluated together with the evidence before him when the application was approved, the labeling of such drug, based on a fair evaluation of all material facts, is false or misleading in any particular and was not corrected within a reasonable time after receipt of written notice from the Secretary specifying the matter complained of. Any order under this subsection shall state the findings upon which it is based.

(f) Whenever the Secretary finds that the facts so require, he shall revoke any previous order under subsection (d) or (e) refusing, withdrawing, or suspending approval of an application and shall approve such application or reinstate such approval, as may be appropriate.

(g) Orders of the Secretary issued under this section shall be served (1) in person by any officer or employee of the Department designated by the Secretary or (2) by mailing the order by registered mail or by certified mail addressed to the applicant or respondent at his last-known address in the records of the Secretary

(h) An appeal may be taken by the applicant from an order of the Secretary refusing or withdrawing approval of an application under this section. Such appeal shall be taken by filing in the United States court of appeals for the circuit wherein such applicant resides or has his principal place of business, or in the United States Court of Appeals for the District of Columbia Circuit, within sixty days after the entry of such order, a written petition praying that the order of the Secretary be set aside. A copy of such petition shall be forthwith transmitted by the clerk of the court to the Secretary, or any officer designated by him for that purpose, and thereupon the Secretary shall certify and file in the court the record upon which the order complained of was entered, as provided in section 2112 of title 28, United States Code. Upon the filing of such petition such court shall have exclusive jurisdiction to affirm or set aside such order, except that until the filing of the record the Secretary may modify or set aside his order. No objection to the order of the Secretary shall be considered by the court unless such objection shall have been urged before the Secretary or unless there were reasonable grounds for failure so to do. The finding of the Secretary as to the facts, if supported by substantial evidence, shall be conclusive. If any person shall apply to the court for leave to adduce additional evidence, and shall show to the satisfaction of the court that such additional evidence is material and that there were reasonable grounds for failure to adduce such evidence in the proceeding before the Secretary, the court may order such additional evidence to be taken before the Secretary and to be adduced upon the hearing in such manner and upon such terms and conditions as to the court may seem proper. The Secretary may modify his findings as to the facts by reason of the additional evidence so taken, and he shall file with the court such modified findings which, if supported by substantial evidence, shall be conclusive, and his recommendation, if any, for the setting aside of the original order. The judgment of the court affirming or setting aside any such order of the Secretary shall be final, subject to review by the Supreme Court of the United States upon certiorari or certification as provided in section 1254 of title 28 of the United States Code. The commencement of proceedings under this subsection shall not, unless specifically ordered by the court to the contrary, operate as a stay of the Secretary's order.

(i) The Secretary shall promulgate regulations for exempting from the operation of the foregoing subsections of this section drugs intended solely for investigational use by experts qualified by scientific training and experience to investigate the safety and effectiveness of drugs. Such regulations may, within the discretion of the Secretary, among other conditions relating to the protection of the public health, provide for conditioning such exemption upon—

(1) the submission to the Secretary, before any clinical testing of a new drug is undertaken, of reports, by the manufacturer or the sponsor of the investigation of such drug, or preclinical tests (including tests on animals) of such drug adequate to justify the proposed clinical testing;

(2) the manufacturer or the sponsor of the investigation of a new drug proposed to be distributed to investigators for clinical testing obtaining a signed agreement from each of such investigators that patients to whom the drug is administered will be under his personal supervision, or under the supervision of investigators responsible to him, and that he will not supply such drug to any other investigator, or to clinics, for administration to human beings; and

(3) the establishment and maintenance of such records, and the making of such reports to the Secretary, by the manufacturer or the sponsor of the investigation of such drug, of data (including but not limited to analytical reports by investigators) obtained as the result of such investigational use of such drug, as the Secretary finds will enable him to evaluate the safety and effectiveness of such drug in the event of the filing of an application pursuant to subsection (b).

Such regulations shall provide that such exemption shall be conditioned upon the manufacturer, or the sponsor of the investigation, requiring that experts using such drugs for investigational purposes certify to such manufacturer or sponsor that they will inform any human beings to whom such drugs, or any controls used in connection therewith, are being administered, or their representatives, that such drugs are being used for investigational purposes and will obtain the consent of such human beings or their representatives, except where they deem it not feasible or, in their professional judgment, contrary to the best interests of such human beings. Nothing in this subsection shall be construed to require any clinical investigator to submit directly to the Secretary reports on the investigational use of drugs.

(j) (1) Any person may file with the Secretary an abbreviated application for the approval of a new drug.

(2) (A) An abbreviated application for a new drug shall contain—

(i) information to show that the conditions of use prescribed, recommended, or suggested in the labeling proposed for the new drug have been previously approved for a drug listed under paragraph (6) (hereinafter in this subsection referred to as a listed drug);

(ii) (I) if the listed drug referred to in clause (i) has only one active ingredient, information to show that the active ingredient of the new drug is the same as that of the listed drug;

(II) if the listed drug referred to in clause (i) has more than one active ingredient, information to show that the active ingredients of the new drug are the same as those of the listed drug, or

(III) if the listed drug referred to in clause (i) has more than one active ingredient and if one of the active ingredients of the new drug is different and the application is filed pursuant to the approval of a petition filed under subparagraph (C), information to show that the other active ingredients of the new drug are the same as the active ingredients of the listed drug, information to show that the different active ingredient is an active ingredient of a listed drug or of a drug which does not meet the requirements of section 201 (p), and such other information respecting the different active ingredient with respect to which the petition was filed as the Secretary may require;

(iii) information to show that the route of administration, the dosage form, and the strength of the new drug are the same as those of the listed drug referred to in clause (i) or, if the route of administration, the dosage form, or the strength of the new drug is different and the application is filed pursuant to the approval of a petition filed under subparagraph (C), such information respecting the route of administration, dosage form, or strength with respect to which the petition was filed as the Secretary may require;

(iv) information to show that the new drug is bioequivalent to the listed drug referred to in clause (i), except that if the application is filed pursuant to the approval of a petition filed under subparagraph (C), information to show that the active ingredients of the new drug are of the same pharmacological or therapeutic class as those of the listed drug referred to in clause (i) and the new drug can be expected to have the same therapeutic effect as the listed drug when administered to patients for a condition of use referred to in clause (i);

(v) information to show that the labeling proposed for the new drug is the same as the labeling approved for the listed drug referred to in clause (i) except for changes required because of differences approved under a petition filed under subparagraph (C) or because the new drug and the listed drug are produced or distributed by different manufacturers;

(vi) the items specified in clauses (B) through (F) of subsection (b) (1);

(vii) a certification, in the opinion of the applicant and to the best of his knowledge, with respect to each patent which claims the listed drug referred to in clause (i) or which claims a use for such listed drug for which the applicant is seeking approval under this subsection and for which information is required to be filed under subsection (b) or (c)—

(I) that such patent information has not been filed,

(II) that such patent has expired,

(III) of the date on which such patent will expire, or

(IV) that such patent is invalid or will not be infringed by the manufacture, use, or sale of the new drug for which the application is submitted; and

(viii) if with respect to the listed drug referred to in clause (i) information was filed under subsection (b) or (c) for a method of use patent which does not claim a use for which the applicant is seeking approval under this subsection, a statement that the method of use patent does not claim such a use.

The Secretary may not require that an abbreviated application contain information in addition to that required by clauses (i) through (viii).

(B) (i) An applicant who makes a certification described in subparagraph (A) (vii) (IV) shall include in the application a statement that the applicant will give the notice required by clause (ii) to—

(I) each owner of the patent which is the subject of the certification or the representative of such owner designated to receive such notice, and

(II) the holder of the approved application under subsection (b) for the drug which is claimed by the patent or a use of which is claimed by the patent or the representative of such holder designated to receive such notice.

(ii) The notice referred to in clause (i) shall state that an application, which contains data from bioavailability or bioequivalence studies, has been submitted under this subsection for the drug with respect to which the certification is made to obtain approval to engage in the commercial manufacture, use, or sale of such drug before the expiration of the patent referred to in the certification. Such notice shall include a detailed statement of the factual and legal basis of the applicant's opinion that the patent is not valid or will not be infringed.

(iii) If an application is amended to include a certification described in subparagraph (A) (vii) (IV), the notice required by clause (ii) shall be given when the amended application is submitted.

(C) If a person wants to submit an abbreviated application for a new drug which has a different active ingredient or whose route of administration, dosage form, or strength differ from that of a listed drug, such person shall submit a petition to the Secretary seeking permission to file such an application. The Secretary shall approve or disapprove a petition submitted under this subparagraph within ninety days of the date the petition is submitted. The Secretary shall approve such a petition unless the Secretary finds—

(i) that investigations must be conducted to show the safety and effectiveness of the drug or of any of its active ingredients, the route of administration, the dosage form, or strength which differ from the listed drug; or

(ii) that any drug with a different active ingredient may not be adequately evaluated for approval as safe and effective on the basis of the information required to be submitted in an abbreviated application.

(3) Subject to paragraph (4), the Secretary shall approve an application for a drug unless the Secretary finds—

(A) the methods used in, or the facilities and controls used for, the manufacture, processing, and packing of the drug are inadequate to assure and preserve its identity, strength, quality, and purity;

(B) information submitted with the application is insufficient to show that each of the proposed conditions of use have been previously approved for the listed drug referred to in the application;

(C) (i) if the listed drug has only one active ingredient, information submitted with the application is insufficient to show that the active ingredient is the same as that of the listed drug;

(ii) if the listed drug has more than one active ingredient, information submitted with the application is insufficient to show that the active ingredients are the same as the active ingredients of the listed drug, or

(iii) if the listed drug has more than one active ingredient and if the application is for a drug which has an active ingredient different from the listed drug, information submitted with the application is insufficient to show—

(I) that the other active ingredients are the same as the active ingredients of the listed drug, or

(II) that the different active ingredient is an active ingredient of a listed drug or a drug which does not meet the requirements of section 201 (p),
or no petition to file an application for the drug with the different ingredient was approved under paragraph (2) (C);

(D) (i) if the application is for a drug whose route of administration, dosage form, or strength of the drug is the same as the route of administration, dosage form, or strength of the listed drug referred to in the application, information submitted in the application is insufficient to show that the route of administration, dosage form, or strength is the same as that of the listed drug, or

(ii) if the application is for a drug whose route of administration, dosage form, or strength of the drug is different from that of the listed drug referred to in the application, no petition to file an application for the drug with the different route of administration, dosage form, or strength was approved under paragraph (2) (C);

(E) if the application was filed pursuant to the approval of a petition under paragraph (2) (C), the application did not contain the information required by the Secretary respecting the active ingredient, route of administration, dosage form, or strength which is not the same;

(F) information submitted in the application is insufficient to show that the drug is bioequivalent to the listed drug referred to in the application or, if the application was filed pursuant to a petition approved under paragraph (2) (C), information submitted in the application is insufficient to show that the active ingredients of the new drug are of the same pharmacological or therapeutic class as those of the listed drug referred to in paragraph (2) (A) (i) and that the new drug can be expected to have the same therapeutic effect as the listed drug when administered to patients for a condition of use referred to in such paragraph;

(G) information submitted in the application is insufficient to show that the labeling proposed for the drug is the same as the labeling approved for the listed drug referred to in the application except for changes required because of differences approved under a petition filed under paragraph (2) (C) or because the drug and the listed drug are produced or distributed by different manufacturers;

(H) information submitted in the application or any other information available to the Secretary shows that (i) the inactive ingredients of the drug are unsafe for use under the conditions prescribed, recommended, or suggested in the labeling proposed for the drug, or (ii) the composition of the drug is unsafe under such conditions because of the type or quantity of inactive ingredients included or the manner in which the inactive ingredients are included;

(I) the approval under subsection (c) of the listed drug referred to in the application under this subsection has been withdrawn or suspended for grounds described in the first sentence of subsection (e), the Secretary has published a notice of opportunity for hearing to withdraw approval of the listed drug under subsection (c) for grounds described in the first sentence of subsection (e), the approval under this subsection of the listed drug referred to in the application under this subsection has been withdrawn or suspended under paragraph (5), or the Secretary has determined that the listed drug has been withdrawn from sale for safety or effectiveness reasons;

(J) the application does not meet any other requirement of paragraph (2) (A); or

(K) the application contains an untrue statement of material fact.

(4) (A) Within one hundred and eighty days of the initial receipt of an application under paragraph (2) or within such additional period as may be agreed upon by the Secretary and the applicant, the Secretary shall approve or disapprove the application.

(B) The approval of an application submitted under paragraph (2) shall be made effective on the last applicable date determined under the following:

(i) If the applicant only made a certification described in subclause (I) or (II) of paragraph (2) (A) (vii) or in both such subclauses, the approval may be made effective immediately.

(ii) If the applicant made a certification described in subclause (III) of paragraph (2) (A) (vii), the approval may be made effective on the date certified under subclause (III).

(iii) If the applicant made a certification described in subclause (IV) of paragraph (2) (A) (vii), the approval shall be made effective immediately unless an action is brought for infringement of a patent which is the subject of the certification before the expiration of forty-five days from the date the notice provided under paragraph (2) (B) (i) is received. If such an action is brought before the expiration of such days, the approval shall be made effective upon the expiration of the thirty-month period beginning on the date of the receipt of the notice provided under paragraph (2) (B) (i) or such shorter or longer period as the court may order because either party to the action failed to reasonably cooperate in expediting the action, except that—

(I) if before the expiration of such period the court decides that such patent is invalid or not infringed, the approval shall be made effective on the date of the court decision,

(II) if before the expiration of such period the court decides that such patent has been infringed, the approval shall be made effective on such date as the court orders under section 271 (e) (4) (A) of title 35, United States Code, or

(III) if before the expiration of such period the court grants a preliminary injunction prohibiting the applicant from engaging in the commercial manufacture or sale of the drug until the court decides the issues of patent validity and infringement and if the court decides that such patent is invalid or not infringed, the approval shall be made effective on the date of such court decision.

In such an action, each of the parties shall reasonably cooperate in expediting the action. Until the expiration of forty-five days from the date the notice made under paragraph (2) (B) (i) is received, no action may be brought under section 2201 of title 28, United States Code, for a declaratory judgment with respect to the patent. Any action brought under section 2201 shall be brought in the judicial district where the defendant has its principal place of business or a regular and established place of business.

(iv) If the application contains a certification described in subclause (IV) of paragraph (2) (A) (vii) and is for a drug for which a previous application has been submitted under this subsection continuing such a certification, the application shall be made effective not earlier than one hundred and eighty days after—

(I) the date the Secretary receives notice from the applicant under the previous application of the first commercial marketing of the drug under the previous application, or

(II) the date of a decision of a court in an action described in clause (iii) holding the patent which is the subject of the certification to be invalid or not infringed, whichever is earlier.

(C) If the Secretary decides to disapprove an application, the Secretary shall give the applicant notice of an opportunity for a hearing before the Secretary on the question of whether such application is approvable. If the applicant elects to accept the opportunity for hearing by written request within thirty days after such notice, such hearing shall commence not more than ninety days after the expiration of such thirty days unless the Secretary and the applicant otherwise agree. Any such hearing shall thereafter be conducted on an expedited basis and the Secretary's order thereon shall be issued within ninety days after the date fixed by the Secretary for filing final briefs.

(D) (i) If an application (other than an abbreviated new drug application) submitted under subsection (b) for a drug, no active ingredient (including any ester or salt of the active ingredient) of which has been approved in any other application under subsection (b), was approved during the period beginning January 1, 1982, and ending on the date of the enactment of this subsection, the Secretary may not make the approval of an application submitted under this subsection which refers to the drug for which the subsection (b) application was submitted effective before the expiration of ten years from the date of the approval of the application under subsection (b).

(ii) If an application submitted under subsection (b) for a drug, no active ingredient (including any ester or salt of the active ingredient) of which has been approved in any other application under subsection (b), is approved after the date of the enactment of this subsection, no application may be submitted under this subsection which refers to the drug for which the subsection (b) application was submitted before the expiration of five years from the date of the approval of the application under subsection (b), except that such an application may be submitted under this subsection after the expiration of four years from the date of the approval of the subsection (b) application if it contains a certification of patent invalidity or noninfringement described in subclause (IV) of paragraph (2) (A) (vii). The approval of such an application shall be made effective in accordance with subparagraph (B) except that, if an action for patent infringement is commenced during the one-year period beginning forty-eight months after the date of the approval of the subsection (b) application, the thirty-month period referred to in subparagraph (B) (iii) shall be extended by such amount of time (if any) which is required for seven and one-half years to have elapsed from the date of approval of the subsection (b) application.

(iii) If an application submitted under subsection (b) for a drug, which includes an active ingredient (including any ester or salt of the active ingredient) that has been approved in another application approved under subsection (b), is approved after the date of enactment of this subsection and if such application contains reports of new clinical investigations (other than bioavailability studies) essential to the approval of the application and conducted or sponsored by the applicant, the Secretary may not make the approval of an application submitted under this subsection for the conditions of approval of such drug in the subsection (b) application effective before the expiration of three years from the date of the approval of the application under subsection (b) for such drug.

(iv) If a supplement to an application approved under subsection (b) is approved after the date of enactment of this subsection and the supplement contains reports of new clinical investigations (other than bioavailability studies) essential to the approval of the supplement and conducted or sponsored by the person submitting the supplement, the Secretary may not make the approval of an application submitted under this subsection for a change approved in the supplement effective before the expiration of three years from the date of the approval of the supplement under subsection (b).

(v) If an application (or supplement to an application) submitted under subsection (b) for a drug, which includes an active ingredient (including any ester or salt of the active ingredient) that has been approved in another application under subsection (b), was approved during the period beginning January 1, 1982, and ending on the date of the enactment of this subsection, the Secretary may not make the approval of an application submitted under this subsection which refers to the drug for which the subsection (b) application was submitted or which refers to a change approved in a supplement to the subsection (b) application effective before the expiration of two years from the date of enactment of this subsection.

(5) If a drug approved under this subsection refers in its approved application to a drug the approval of which was withdrawn or suspended for grounds described in the first sentence of subsection (e) or was withdrawn or suspended under this paragraph or which, as determined by the Secretary, has been withdrawn from sale for safety or effectiveness reasons, the approval of the drug under this subsection shall be withdrawn or suspended—

(A) for the same period as the withdrawal or suspension under subsection (e) or this paragraph, or

(B) if the listed drug has been withdrawn from sale, for the period of withdrawal from sale or, if earlier, the period ending on the date the Secretary determines that the withdrawal from sale is not for safety or effectiveness reasons.

(6) (A) (i) Within sixty days of the date of the enactment of this subsection, the Secretary shall publish and make available to the public—

(I) a list in alphabetical order of the official and proprietary name of each drug which has been approved for safety and effectiveness under subsection (c) before the date of the enactment of this subsection;

(II) the date of approval if the drug is approved after 1981 and the number of the application which was approved; and

(III) whether in vitro or in vivo bioequivalence studies, or both such studies, are required for applications filed under this subsection which will refer to the drug published.

(ii) Every thirty days after the publication of the first list under clause (i) the Secretary shall revise the list to include each drug which has been approved for safety and effectiveness under subsection (c) or approved under this subsection during the thirty-day period.

(iii) When patent information submitted under subsection (b) or (c) respecting a drug included on the list is to be published by the Secretary the Secretary shall, in revisions made under clause (ii), include such information for such drug.

(B) A drug approved for safety and effectiveness under subsection (c) or approved under this subsection shall, for purposes of this subsection, be considered to have been published under subparagraph (A) on the date of its approval or the date of enactment, whichever is later.

(C) If the approval of a drug was withdrawn or suspended for grounds described in the first sentence of subsection (e) or was withdrawn or suspended under paragraph (5) or if the Secretary determines that a drug has been withdrawn from sale for safety or effectiveness reasons, it may not be published in the list under subparagraph (A) or, if the withdrawal or suspension occurred after its publication in such list, it shall be immediately removed from such list—

(i) for the same period as the withdrawal or suspension under subsection (e) or paragraph (5), or

(ii) if the listed drug has been withdrawn from sale, for the period of withdrawal from sale or, if earlier, the period ending on the date the Secretary determines that the withdrawal from sale is not for safety or effectiveness reasons.

A notice of the removal shall be published in the Federal Register.

(7) For purposes of this subsection:

(A) The term 'bioavailability' means the rate and extent to which the active ingredient or therapeutic ingredient is absorbed from a drug and becomes available at the site of drug action.

(B) A drug shall be considered to be bioequivalent to a listed drug if—

(i) the rate and extent of absorption of the drug do not show a significant difference from the rate and extent of absorption of the listed drug when administered at the same molar dose of the therapeutic ingredient under similar experimental conditions in either a single dose or multiple doses; or

(ii) the extent of absorption of the drug does not show a significant difference from the extent of absorption of the listed drug when administered at the same molar dose of the therapeutic ingredient under similar experimental conditions in either a single dose or multiple doses and the difference from the listed drug in the rate of absorption of the drug is intentional, is reflected in its proposed labeling, is not essential to the attainment of effective body drug concentrations on chronic use, and is considered medically insignificant for the drug.

(k) (1) In the case of any drug for which an approval of an application filed under subsection (b) or (j) is in effect, the applicant shall establish and maintain such records, and make such reports to the Secretary, of data relating to clinical experience and other data or information, received or otherwise obtained by such applicant with respect to such drug, as the Secretary may by general regulation, or by order with respect to such application, prescribe on the basis of a finding that such records and reports are necessary in order to enable the Secretary to determine, or facilitate a determination, whether there is or may be ground for invoking subsection (e) of this section: *Provided, however,* That regulations and orders issued under subsection and under subsection (i) shall have due regard for the professional ethics of the medical profession and the interests of patients and shall provide, where the Secretary deems it to be appropriate, for the examination, upon request, by the persons to whom such regulations or orders are applicable, of similar information received or otherwise obtained by the Secretary.

(2) Every person required under this section to maintain records, and every person in charge or custody thereof, shall, upon request of an officer or employee designated by the Secretary, permit such officer or employee at all reasonable times to have access to and copy and verify such records.

(l) Safety and effectiveness data and information which has been submitted in an application under subsection (b) for a drug and which has not previously been disclosed to the public shall be made available to the public, upon request, unless extraordinary circumstances are shown—

(1) if no work is being or will be undertaken to have the application approved,

(2) if the Secretary has determined that the application is not approvable and all legal appeals have been exhausted,

(3) if approval of the application under subsection (c) is withdrawn and all legal appeals have been exhausted,

(4) if the Secretary has determined that such drug is not a new drug, or

(5) upon the effective date of the approval of the first application under subsection (j) which refers to such drug or upon the date upon which the approval of an application under subsection (j) which refers to such drug could be made effective if such an application had been submitted.

(m) For purposes of this section, the term 'patent' means a patent issued by the Patent and Trademark Office of the Department of Commerce.

Certification of Drugs Containing Insulin

§ 506 [356] (a) The Secretary, pursuant to regulations promulgated by him, shall provide for the certification of batches of drugs composed wholly or partly of insulin. A batch of any such drug shall be certified if such drug has such characteristics of identity and such batch has such characteristics of strength, quality, and purity, as the Secretary prescribes in such regulations as necessary to adequately insure safety and efficacy of use, but shall not otherwise be certified. Prior to the effective date of such regulations the Secretary, in lieu of certification, shall issue a release for any batch which, in his judgment, may be released without risk as to the safety and efficacy of its use. Such release shall prescribe the date of its expiration and other conditions under which it shall cease to be effective as to such batch and as to portions thereof.

(b) Regulations providing for such certification shall contain such provisions as are necessary to carry out the purposes of this section, including provisions prescribing (1) standards of identity and of strength, quality, and purity; (2) tests and methods of assay to determine compliance with such standards; (3) effective periods for certificates, and other conditions under which they shall cease to be effective as to certified batches and as to portions thereof; (4) administration and procedure; and (5) such fees, specified in such regulations, as are necessary to provide, equip, and maintain an adequate certification service. Such regulations shall prescribe no standard of identity or of strength, quality, or purity for any drug different from the standard of identity, strength, quality, or purity set forth for such drug in an official compendium.

(c) Such regulations, insofar as they prescribe tests or methods of assay to determine strength, quality, or purity of any drug, different from the tests or methods of assay set forth for such drug in an official compendium, shall be prescribed, after notice and opportunity for revision of such compendium, in the manner provided in the second sentence of section 501 (b). The provisions of subsections (e), (f), and (g) of section 701 shall be applicable to such portion of any regulation as prescribes any such different test or method, but shall not be applicable to any other portion of any such regulation.

Certification of Antibiotics

§ **507** [357] (a) The Secretary, pursuant to regulations promulgated by him, shall provide for the certification of batches of drugs (except drugs for use in animals other than man) composed wholly or partly of any kind of penicillin, streptomycin, chlortetracycline, chloramphenicol, bacitracin, or any other antibiotic drug, or any derivative thereof. A batch of any such drug shall be certified if such drug has such characteristics of identity and such batch has such characteristics of strength, quality, and purity, as the Secretary prescribes in such regulations as necessary to adequately insure safety and efficacy of use, but shall not otherwise be certified. Prior to the effective date of such regulations the Secretary, in lieu of certification, shall issue a release for any batch which, in his judgment, may be released without risk as to the safety and efficacy of its use. Such release shall prescribe the date of its expiration and other conditions under which it shall cease to be effective as to such batch and as to portions thereof. For purposes of this section and of section 502 (l), the term "antibiotic drug" means any drug intended for use by man containing any quantity of any chemical substance which is produced by a microorganism and which has the capacity to inhibit or destroy microorganisms in dilute solution (including the chemically synthesized equivalent of any such substance).

(b) Regulations providing for such certification shall contain such provisions as are necessary to carry out the purposes of this section, including provisions prescribing (1) standards of identity and of strength, quality, and purity; (2) tests and methods of assay to determine compliance with such standards; (3) effective periods for certificates, and other conditions under which they shall cease to be effective as to certified batches and as to portions thereof; (4) administration and procedure; and (5) such fees, specified in such regulations, as are necessary to provide, equip, and maintain an adequate certification service. Such regulations shall prescribe only such tests and methods

of assay as will provide for certification or rejection within the shortest time consistent with the purposes of this section.

(c) Whenever in the judgment of the Secretary, the requirements of this section and of section 502 (l) with respect to any drug or class of drugs are not necessary to insure safety and efficacy of use, the Secretary shall promulgate regulations exempting such drug or class of drugs from such requirements. In deciding whether an antibiotic drug, or class of antibiotic drugs, is to be exempted from the requirement of certification the Secretary shall give consideration, among other relevant factors, to—

(1) whether such drug or class of drugs is manufactured by a person who has, or hereafter shall have, produced fifty consecutive batches of such drug or class of drugs in compliance with the regulations for the certification thereof within a period of not more than eighteen calendar months, upon the application by such person to the Secretary; or

(2) whether such drug or class of drugs is manufactured by any person who has otherwise demonstrated such consistency in the production of such drug or class of drugs, in compliance with the regulations for the certification thereof, as in the judgment of the Secretary is adequate to insure the safety and efficacy of use thereof. When an antibiotic drug or a drug manufacturer has been exempted from the requirement of certification, the manufacturer may still obtain certification of a batch or batches of that drug if he applies for and meets the requirements for certification. Nothing in this Act shall be deemed to prevent a manufacturer or distributor of an antibiotic drug from making a truthful statement in labeling or advertising of the product as to whether it has been certified or exempted from the requirement of certification.

(d) The Secretary shall promulgate regulations exempting from any requirement of this section and of section 502 (l), (1) drugs which are to be stored, processed, labeled, or repacked at establishments other than those where manufactured, on condition that such drugs comply with all such requirements upon removal from such establishments; (2) drugs which conform to applicable standards of identity, strength, quality, and purity prescribed by these regulations and are intended for use in manufacturing other drugs; and (3) drugs which are intended solely for investigational use by experts qualified by scientific training and experience to investigate the safety and efficacy of drugs. Such regulations may, within the discretion of the Secretary, among other conditions relating to the protection of the public health, provide for conditioning the exemption under clause (3) upon—

(1) the submission to the Secretary, before any clinical testing of a new drug is undertaken, of reports, by the manufacturer or the sponsor of the investigation of such drug, of preclinical tests (including tests on animals) of such drug adequate to justify the proposed clinical testing;

(2) the manufacturer or the sponsor of the investigation of a new drug proposed to be distributed to investigators for clinical testing obtaining a signed agreement from each of such investigators that patients to whom the drug is administered will be under his personal supervision, or under the supervision of investigators responsible to him, and that he will not apply such drug to any other investigator, or to clinics, for administration to human beings; and

(3) the establishment and maintenance of such records, and the making of such reports to the Secretary, by the manufacturer or the sponsor of the investigation of such drug, of data (including but not limited to analytical reports by investigators) obtained as the result of such investigational use of such drug, as the Secretary finds will enable him to evaluate the safety and effectiveness of such drug in the event of the filing of an application for certification or release pursuant to subsection (a).

Such regulations shall provide that such exemption shall be conditioned upon the manufacturer, or the sponsor of the investigation, requiring that experts using such drugs for investigational purposes certify to such manufacturer or sponsor that they will inform any human beings to whom such drugs, or any controls used in connection therewith, are being administered, or their representatives, that such drugs are being used for investigational purposes and will obtain the consent of such human beings or their representatives, except where they deem it not feasible or, in their professional judgment, contrary to the best interests of such human beings. Nothing in this subsection shall be construed to require any clinical investigator to submit directly to the Secretary reports on the investigational use of drugs.

(e) No drug which is subject to section 507 shall be deemed to be subject to any provision of section 505 except a new drug exempted from the requirements of this section and of section 502 (l) pursuant to regulations promulgated by the Secretary: *Provided*, That, for purposes of section 505, the initial request for certification, as thereafter duly amended, pursuant to section 507, of a new drug so exempted shall be considered a part of the application filed pursuant to section 505 (b) with respect to the person filing such request and to such drug as of the date of the exemption. Compliance of any drug subject to section 502 (l) or 507 with section 501 (b) and 502 (g) shall be determined by the application of the standards of strength, quality, and purity, the tests and methods of assay, and the requirements of packaging, and labeling, respectively, prescribed by regulations promulgated under section 507.

(f) Any interested person may file with the Secretary a petition proposing the issuance, amendment, or repeal of any regulation contemplated by this section. The petition shall set forth the proposal in general terms and shall state reasonable grounds therefor. The Secretary shall give public notice of the proposal and an opportunity for all interested persons to present their views thereon, orally or in writing, and as soon as practicable thereafter shall make public his action upon such proposal. At any time prior to the thirtieth day after such action is made public any interested person may file objections to such action, specifying with particularity the changes desired, stating reasonable grounds therefor, and requesting a public hearing upon such objections. The Secretary shall thereupon, after due notice, hold such public hearing. As soon as practicable after completion of the hearing, the Secretary shall by order make public his action on such objections. The Secretary shall base his order only on substantial evidence of record at the hearing and shall set forth as part of the order detailed findings of fact on which the order is based. The order shall be subject to the provision of section 701 (f) and (g).

(g) (1) Every person engaged in manufacturing, compounding, or processing any drug within the purview of this section with respect to which a certificate or release has been issued pursuant to this section shall establish and maintain such records, and make such reports to the Secretary, of data relating to clinical experience and other data or information, received or otherwise obtained by such person with respect to such drug, as the Secretary may by general regulation, or by order with respect to such certification or release, prescribe on the basis of a finding that such records and reports are necessary in order to enable the Secretary to make, or to facilitate, a determination as to whether such certification or release should be rescinded or whether any regulation issued under this section should be amended or repealed: *Provided, however*, That regulations and orders issued under this subsection and under clause (3) of subsection (d) shall have due regard for the professional ethics of the medical profession and the interests of patients and shall provide, where the Secretary deems it to be appropriate, for the examination, upon request, by the persons to whom such

regulations or orders are applicable, of similar information received or otherwise obtained by the Secretary.

(2) Every person required under this section to maintain records, and every person having charge or custody thereof, shall, upon request of an officer or employee designated by the Secretary, permit such officer or employee at all reasonable times to have access to and copy and verify such records.

(h) In the case of a drug for which, on the day immediately preceding the effective date of this subsection, a prior approval of an application under section 505 had not been withdrawn under section 505 (e), the initial issuance of regulations providing for certification or exemption of such drug under this section 507 shall, with respect to the conditions of use prescribed, recommended, or suggested in the labeling covered by such application, not be conditioned upon an affirmative finding of the efficacy of such drug. Any subsequent amendment or repeal of such regulations so as no longer to provide for such certification or exemption on the ground of a lack of efficacy of such drug for use under such conditions of use may be effected only on or after that effective date of clause (3) of the first sentence of section 505 (e) which would be applicable to such drug under such conditions of use if such drug were subject to section 505 (e), and then only if (1) such amendment or repeal is made in accordance with the procedure specified in subsection (f) of this section (except that such amendment or repeal may be initiated either by a proposal of the Secretary or by a petition of any interested person) and (2) the Secretary finds, on the basis of new information with respect to such drug evaluated together with the information before him when the application under section 505 became effective or was approved, that there is a lack of substantial evidence (as defined in section 505 (d)) that the drug has the effect it purports or is represented to have under such conditions of use.

Authority to Designate Official Names

§ 508 [358] (a) The Secretary may designate an official name for any drug or device if he determines that such action is necessary or desirable in the interest of usefulness and simplicity. Any official name designated under this section for any drug or device shall be the only official name of that drug or device used in any official compendium published after such name has been prescribed or for any other purpose of this Act. In no event, however, shall the Secretary establish an official name so as to infringe a valid trademark.

(b) Within a reasonable time after the effective date of this section, and at such other times as he may deem necessary, the Secretary shall cause a review to be made of the official names by which drugs are identified in the official United States Pharmacopeia, the official Homeopathic Pharmacopeia of the United States, and the official National Formulary, and all supplements thereto and at such times as he may deem necessary shall cause a review to be made of the official names by which devices are identified in any official compendium (and all supplements thereto), to determine whether revision of any of those names is necessary or desirable in the interest of usefulness and simplicity.

(c) Whenever he determines after any such review that (1) any such official name is unduly complex or is not useful for any other reason, (2) two or more official names have been applied to a single drug or device, or to two or more drugs which are identical in chemical structure and pharmacological action and which are substantially identical in strength, quality, and purity or to two or more devices which are substantially equivalent in design and purpose, or (3) no official name has been applied to a medically useful drug or device, he shall transmit in writing to the compiler of each official compendium in which that drug or drugs or device are identified and recognized his request for the recommendation of a single official name for such drug or drugs or device which will have usefulness and simplicity. Whenever such a single official name has not been recommended within one hundred and eighty days after such request, or the Secretary determines that any name so recommended is not useful for any reason, he shall designate a single official name for such drug or drugs or device. Whenever he determines that the name so recommended is useful, he shall designate that name as the official name of such drug or drugs or device. Such designation shall be made as a regulation upon public notice and in accordance with the procedure set forth in section 4 of the Administrative Procedure Act (5 U.S.C. 1003).

(d) After each such review, and at such other times as the Secretary may determine to be necessary or desirable, the Secretary shall cause to be compiled, published, and publicly distributed a list which shall list all revised official names of drugs or devices designated under this section and shall contain such descriptive and explanatory matter as the Secretary may determine to be required for the effective use of those names.

(e) Upon a request in writing by any compiler of an official compendium that the Secretary exercise the authority granted to him under section 508 (a), he shall upon public notice and in accordance with the procedure set forth in section 4 of the Administrative Procedure Act (5 U.S.C. 1003) designate the official name of the drug or device for which the request is made.

Registration Requirements

§ 510 [360] (a) As used in this section—

(1) the term "manufacture, preparation, propagation, compounding, or processing" shall include repackaging or otherwise changing the container, wrapper, or labeling of any drug package or device package in furtherance of the distribution of the drug or device from the original place of manufacture to the person who makes final delivery or sale to the ultimate consumer or user; and

(2) the term "name" shall include in the case of a partnership the name of each partner and, in the case of a corporation, the name of each corporate officer and director, and the State of incorporation.

(b) On or before December 31 of each year every person who owns or operates any establishment in any State engaged in the manufacture, preparation, propagation, compounding, or processing of a drug or drugs or a device or devices shall register with the Secretary his name, places of business, and all such establishments.

(c) Every person upon first engaging in the manufacture, preparation, propagation, compounding, or processing of a drug or drugs or a device or devices in any establishment which he owns or operates in any State shall immediately register with the Secretary his name, place of business, and such establishment.

(d) Every person duly registered in accordance with the foregoing subsections of this section shall immediately register with the Secretary any additional establishment which he owns or operates in any State and in which he begins the manufacture, preparation, propagation, compounding, or processing of a drug or drugs or a device or devices.

(e) The Secretary may assign a registration number to any person or any establishment registered in accordance with this section. The Secretary may also assign a listing number to each drug or class of drugs listed under subsection (j). Any number assigned pursuant to the preceding sentence shall be the same as that assigned pursuant to the National Drug Code. The Secretary may by regulation prescribe a uniform system for the identification of devices intended for human use and may require that persons who are required to list such devices pursuant to subsection (j) shall list such devices in accordance with such system.

(f) The Secretary shall make available for inspection, to any person so requesting, any registration filed pursuant to this section, except that any list submitted pursuant to paragraph (3) of subsection (j) and the information accompanying any list or notice filed under paragraph (1) or (2) of that subsection shall be exempt from such inspection unless the Secretary finds that such an exemption would be inconsistent with protection of the public health.

(g) The foregoing subsections of this section shall not apply to—

(1) pharmacies which maintain establishments in conformance with any applicable local laws regulating the practice of pharmacy and medicine and which are regularly engaged in dispensing prescription drugs or devices, upon prescriptions of practitioners licensed to administer such drugs or devices to patients under the care of such practitioners in the course of their professional practice, and which do not manufacture, prepare, propagate, compound, or process drugs or devices for sale other than in the regular course of their business of dispensing or selling drugs or devices at retail;

(2) practitioners licensed by law to prescribe or administer drugs or devices and who manufacture, prepare, propagate, compound, or process drugs or devices solely for use in the course of their professional practice;

(3) persons who manufacture, prepare, propagate, compound, or process drugs or devices solely for use in research, teaching, or chemical analysis and not for sale;

(4) such other classes of persons as the Secretary may by regulation exempt from the application of this section upon a finding that registration by such classes of persons in accordance with this section is not necessary for the protection of the public health.

(h) Every establishment in any State registered with the Secretary pursuant to this section shall be subject to inspection pursuant to section 704 and every such establishment engaged in the manufacture, propagation, compounding, or processing of a drug or drugs or of a device or devices classified in class II or III shall be so inspected by one or more officers or employees duly designated by the Secretary at least once in the two-year period beginning with the date of registration of such establishment pursuant to this section and at least once in every successive two-year period thereafter.

(i) Any establishment within any foreign country engaged in the manufacture, preparation, propagation, compounding, or processing of a drug or drugs or a device or devices shall be permitted to register under this section pursuant to regulations promulgated by the Secretary. Such regulations shall require such establishment to provide the information required by subsection (j) and shall require such establishment to provide the information required by subsection (j) in the case of a device or devices and shall include provisions for registration of any such establishment upon condition that adequate and effective means are available, by arrangement with the government of such foreign country or otherwise, to enable the Secretary to determine from time to time whether drugs or devices manufactured, prepared, propagated, compounded or processed in such establishment, if imported or offered for import into the United States, shall be refused admission on any of the grounds set forth in section 801 (a) of this Act.

(j) (1) Every person who registers with the Secretary under subsection (b), (c), or (d) shall, at the time of registration under any such subsection, file with the Secretary a list of all drugs and a list of all devices and a brief statement of the basis for believing that each device included in the list is a device rather than a drug (with each drug and device in each list listed by its established name as defined in section 502 (e) and by any proprietary name) which is being manufactured, prepared, propagated, compounded, or processed by him for commercial distribution and which he has not included in any list of drugs or devices filed by him with the Secretary under this paragraph or paragraph (2) before such time of registration. Such list shall be prepared in such form and manner as the Secretary may prescribe and shall be accompanied by—

(A) in the case of a drug contained in the applicable list and subject to section 505, 506, 507, or 523, or a device intended for human use contained in the applicable list with respect to which a performance standard has been established under section 514 or which is subject to section 515, a reference to the authority for the marketing of such drug or device and a copy of all labeling for such drug or device;

(B) in the case of any other drug or device contained in an applicable list—

(i) which drug is subject to section 503 (b) (1), or which device is a restricted device, a copy of all labeling for such drug or device, a representative sampling of advertisements for such drug or device, and, upon request made by the Secretary for good cause, a copy of all advertisements for a particular drug product or device, or

(ii) which drug is not subject to section 503 (b) (1) or which device is not a restricted device, the label and package insert for such drug or device and a representative sampling of any other labeling for such drug or device;

(C) in the case of any drug contained in an applicable list which is described in subparagraph (B), a quantitative listing of its active ingredient or ingredients, except that with respect to a particular drug product the Secretary may require the submission of a quantitative listing of all ingredients if he finds that such submission is necessary to carry out the purposes of this Act; and

(D) if the registrant filing a list has determined that a particular drug product or device contained in such list is not subject to section 505, 506, 507, or 512, or the particular device contained in such list is not subject to a performance standard established under section 514 or to section 515 or is not a restricted device, a brief statement of the basis on which the registrant made such determination if the Secretary requests such a statement with respect to that particular drug product or device.

(2) Each person who registers with the Secretary under this subsection shall report to the Secretary once during the month of June of each year and once during the month of December of each year the following information:

(A) A list of each drug or device introduced by the registrant for commercial distribution which has not been included in any list previously filed by him with the Secretary under this subparagraph or paragraph (1) of this subsection. A list under this subparagraph shall list a drug or device by its established name (as defined in section 502 (e)) and by any proprietary name it may have and shall be accompanied by the other information required by paragraph (1).

(B) If since the date the registrant last made a report under this paragraph (or if he has not made a report under this paragraph, since the effective date of this subsection) he has discontinued the manufacture, preparation, propagation, compounding, or processing for commercial distribution of a drug or device included in a list filed by him under subparagraph (A) or paragraph (1); notice of such discontinuance, the date of such discontinuance, and the identity (by established name as defined in section 502 (e) and by any proprietary name) of such drug or device.

(C) If since the date the registrant reported pursuant to subparagraph (B) a notice of discontinuance he has resumed the manufacture, preparation, propagation, compounding, or processing for commercial distribution of the drug or device with respect to which such notice of discontinuance was reported; notice of such resumption, the date of such resumption, the identity of such drug or device (each by established name (as defined in section 502 (e)) and by any proprietary name),

and the other information required by paragraph (1), unless the registrant has previously reported such resumption to the Secretary pursuant to this subparagraph.

(D) Any material change in any information previously submitted pursuant to this paragraph or paragraph (1).

(3) The Secretary may also require each registrant under this section to submit a list of each drug product which (A) the registrant is manufacturing, preparing, propagating, compounding, or processing for commercial distribution, and (B) contains a particular ingredient. The Secretary may not require the submission of such a list unless he has made a finding that the submission of such a list is necessary to carry out the purposes of this Act.

Drugs for Rare Diseases or Conditions

RECOMMENDATIONS FOR INVESTIGATIONS OF DRUGS FOR RARE DISEASES OR CONDITIONS

§ 525 [360aa] (a) The sponsor of a drug for a disease or condition which is rare in the States may request the Secretary to provide written recommendations for the non-clinical and clinical investigations which must be conducted with the drug before—

(1) it may be approved for such disease or condition under section 505, or

(2) if the drug is a biological product, before it may be licensed for such disease or condition under section 351 of the Public Health Service Act.

If the Secretary has reason to believe that a drug for which a request is made under this section is a drug for a disease or condition which is rare in the States, the Secretary shall provide the person making the request written recommendations for the non-clinical and clinical investigations which the Secretary believes, on the basis of information available to the Secretary at the time of the request under this section, would be necessary for approval of such drug for such disease or condition under section 505 or licensing under section 351 of the Public Health Service Act for such disease or condition.

(b) The Secretary shall by regulation promulgate procedures for the implementation of subsection (a).

DESIGNATION OF DRUGS FOR RARE DISEASES OR CONDITIONS

§ 526 [360bb] (a) (1) The manufacturer or the sponsor of a drug may request the Secretary to designate the drug as a drug for a rare disease or condition. If the Secretary finds that a drug for which a request is submitted under this subsection is being or will be investigated for a rare disease or condition and—

(A) if an application for such drug is approved under section 505, or

(B) if the drug is a biological product, a license is issued under section 351 of the Public Health Service Act,

the approval or license would be for use for such disease or condition, the Secretary shall designate the drug as a drug for such disease or condition. A request for a designation of a drug under this subsection shall contain the consent of the applicant to notice being given by the Secretary under subsection (b) respecting the designation of the drug.

(2) For purposes of paragraph (1), the term 'rare disease or condition' means any disease or condition *which (A) affects less than 200,000 persons in the U.S. or (B) affects more than 200,000 persons in the U.S. and for which* there is no reasonable expectation that the cost of developing and making available in the United States a drug for such disease or condition will be recovered from sales in the United States of such drug. Determinations under the preceding sentence with respect to any drug shall be made on the basis of the facts and circumstances as of the date the request for designation of the drug under this subsection is made.

(b) Notice respecting the designation of a drug under subsection (a) shall be made available to the public.

(c) The Secretary shall by regulation promulgate procedures for the implementation of subsection (a).

PROTECTION FOR UNPATENTED DRUGS FOR RARE DISEASES OR CONDITIONS

§ **527** [360cc] (a) Except as provided in subsection (b), if the Secretary—

(1) approves an application filed pursuant to section 505 (b), or

(2) issues a license under section 351 of the Public Health Service Act for a drug designated under section 526 for a rare disease or condition and for which a United States Letter of Patent may not be issued, the Secretary may not approve another application under section 505 (b) or issue another license under section 351 of the Public Health Service Act for such drug for such disease or condition for a person who is not the holder of such approved application or of such license until the expiration of seven years from the date of the approval of the approved application or the issuance of the license. Section 505 (c) (2) does not apply to the refusal to approve an application under the preceding sentence.

(b) If an application filed pursuant to section 505 (b) is approved for a drug designated under section 526 for a rare disease or condition or a license is issued under section 351 of the Public Health Service Act for such a drug and if a United States Letter of Patent may not be issued for the drug, the Secretary may, during the seven-year period beginning on the date of the application approval or of the issuance of the license, approve another application under section 505 (b), or, if the drug is a biological product, issue a license under section 351 of the Public Health Service Act, for such drug for such disease or condition for a person who is not the holder of such approved application or of such license if—

(1) The Secretary finds, after providing the holder notice and opportunity for the submission of views, that in such period the holder of the approved application or of the license cannot assure the availability of sufficient quantities of the drug to meet the needs of persons with the disease or condition for which the drug was designated; or

(2) such holder provides the Secretary in writing the consent of such holder for the approval of other applications or the issuance of other licenses before the expiration of such seven-year period.

OPEN PROTOCOLS FOR INVESTIGATIONS OF DRUGS FOR RARE DISEASES OR CONDITIONS

§ **528** [360dd] If a drug is designated under section 526 as a drug for a rare disease or condition and if notice of a claimed exemption under section 505 (i) or regulations issued thereunder is filed for such drug, the Secretary shall encourage the sponsor of such drug to design protocols for clinical investigations of the drug which may be conducted under the exemption to permit the addition to the investigations of persons with the disease or condition who need the drug to treat the disease or condition and who cannot be satisfactorily treated by available alternative drugs.

Records of Interstate Shipment

§ **703** [373] For the purpose of enforcing the provisions of this Act, carriers engaged in interstate commerce, and persons receiving foods, drugs, devices, or cosmetics in interstate commerce or holding such articles so received, shall, upon the request of an officer or employee duly designated by the Secretary, permit such officer or employee, at reasonable times, to have access to and to copy all records showing the movement in interstate commerce of any food, drug, device, or cosmetic, or

the holding thereof during or after such movement, and the quantity, shipper, and consignee thereof; and it shall be unlawful for any such carrier or person to fail to permit such access to and copying of any such record so requested when such request is accompanied by a statement in writing specifying the nature or kind of food, drug, device, or cosmetic to which such request relates: *Provided,* That evidence obtained under this section, or any evidence which is directly or indirectly derived from such evidence, shall not be used in a criminal prosecution of the person from whom obtained: *Provided further,* That carriers shall not be subject to the other provisions of this Act by reason of their receipt, carriage, holding, or delivery of food, drugs, devices, or cosmetics in the usual course of business as carriers.

Inspections

§ **704** [374] (a) (1) For purposes of enforcement of this Chapter, officers or employees duly designated by the Secretary, upon presenting appropriate credentials and a written notice to the owner, operator, or agent in charge, are authorized (A) to enter, at reasonable times, any factory, warehouse, or establishment in which food, drugs, devices, or cosmetics are manufactured, processed, packed, or held, for introduction into interstate commerce or after such introduction, or to enter any vehicle being used to transport or hold such food, drugs, devices or cosmetics in interstate commerce; and (B) to inspect, at reasonable times and within reasonable limits and in a reasonable manner, such factory, warehouse, establishment, or vehicle and all pertinent equipment, finished and unfinished materials, containers, and labeling therein. In the case of any factory, warehouse, establishment, or consulting laboratory in which prescription drugs or restricted devices are manufactured, processed, packed, or held, the inspection shall extend to all things therein (including records, files, papers, processes, controls, and facilities) bearing on whether prescription drugs or restricted devices which are adulterated or misbranded within the meaning of this Chapter, or which may not be manufactured, introduced into interstate commerce, or sold, or offered for sale by reason of any provision of this Chapter, have been or are being manufactured, processed, packed, transported, or held in any such place, or otherwise bearing on violation of this Chapter. No inspection authorized by the preceding sentence or by paragraph (3) shall extend to financial data, sales data other than shipment data, pricing data, personnel data (other than data as to qualifications of technical and professional personnel performing functions subject to this Chapter, and research data (other than data relating to new drugs, antibiotic drugs, and devices and subject to reporting and inspection under regulations lawfully issued pursuant to section 505 (i) or (j), section 507 (d) or (g), section 519, or 520 (g), and data relating to other drugs or devices which in the case of a new drug would be subject to reporting or inspection under lawful regulations issued pursuant to section 505 (j) of the title). A separate notice shall be given for each such inspection, but a notice shall not be given for each such inspection, but a notice shall not be required for each entry made during the period covered by the inspection. Each such inspection shall be commenced and completed with reasonable promptness.

(2) The provisions of the second sentence of this subsection shall not apply to—

(A) pharmacies which maintain establishments in conformance with any applicable local laws regulating the practice of pharmacy and medicine and which are regularly engaged in dispensing prescription drugs, or devices upon prescriptions of practitioners licensed to administer such drugs or devices to patients under the care of such practitioners in the course of their professional practice, and which do not, either through a subsidiary or otherwise, manufacture, prepare, propagate, compound, or process drugs or devices for sale other than in the regular course of their business of dispensing or selling drugs or devices at retail;

(B) practitioners licensed by law to prescribe or administer drugs or prescribe or use devices, as the case may be, and who manufacture, prepare, propagate, compound, or process drugs or manufacture or process devices solely for use in the course of their professional practice;

(C) persons who manufacture, prepare, propagate, compound, or process drugs or manufacture or process devices solely for use in research, teaching, or chemical analysis and not for sale;

(D) such other classes of persons as the Secretary may by regulation exempt from the application of this section upon a finding that inspection as applied to such classes of persons in accordance with this section is not necessary for the protection of the public health.

(b) Upon completion of any such inspection of a factory, warehouse, consulting laboratory, or other establishment, and prior to leaving the premises, the officer or employee making the inspection shall give to the owner, operator, or agent in charge a report in writing setting forth any conditions or practices observed by him which, in his judgment, indicate that any food, drug, device, or cosmetic in such establishment (1) consists in whole or in part of any filthy, putrid, or decomposed substance, or (2) has been prepared, packed, or held under insanitary conditions whereby it may have become contaminated with filth, or whereby it may have been rendered injurious to health. A copy of such report shall be sent promptly to the Secretary.

(c) If the officer or employee making any such inspection of a factory, warehouse, or other establishment has obtained any sample in the course of the inspection, upon completion of the inspection and prior to leaving the premises he shall give to the owner, operator, or agent in charge a receipt describing the samples obtained.

Revision of United States Pharmacopeia; Development of Analysis and Mechanical and Physical Tests

§ 707 [377] The Secretary, in carrying into effect the provisions of this chapter, is authorized hereafter to cooperate with associations and scientific societies in the revision of the United States Pharmacopeia and in the development of methods of analysis and mechanical and physical tests necessary to carry out the work of the Food and Drug Administration.

⟨1077⟩ GOOD MANUFACTURING PRACTICE FOR FINISHED PHARMACEUTICALS

As is indicated in the General Notices, tolerances stated in the United States Pharmacopeia and in the National Formulary are based upon the consideration that the article is produced under recognized principles of good manufacturing practice. In the United States, a drug not produced in accordance with current good manufacturing practices may be considered to be adulterated. The U. S. Food and Drug Administration has published regulations setting forth minimum current good manufacturing practices for the preparation of drug products. While the regulations are directed primarily to drug manufacturers, the principles embodied therein may be helpful to those engaged in the practice of pharmacy and it is for this reason that these regulations are reproduced here.

Publication of these regulations in this Pharmacopeia is for purposes of information and does not impart to them any legal effect under the Federal Food, Drug, and Cosmetic Act.

Part 210—Current Good Manufacturing Practices in Manufacturing, Processing, Packing, or Holding of Drugs: General

§ 210.1 Status of current good manufacturing practice regulations.

(a) The regulations set forth in this part and in Parts 211 through 229 of this chapter contain the minimum current good manufacturing practice for methods to be used in, and the facilities or controls to be used for, the manufacture, processing, packing, or holding of a drug to assure that such drug meets the requirements of the act as to safety, and has the identity and strength and meets the quality and purity characteristics that it purports or is represented to possess.

(b) The failure to comply with any regulation set forth in this part and in Parts 211 through 229 of this chapter in the manufacture, processing, packing, or holding of a drug shall render such drug to be adulterated under section 501(a)(2)(B) of the act and such drug, as well as the person who is responsible for the failure to comply, shall be subject to regulatory action.

§ 210.2 Applicability of current good manufacturing practice regulations.

(a) The regulations in this part and in Parts 211 through 229 of this chapter as they may pertain to a drug and in Parts 600 through 680 of this chapter as they may pertain to a biological product for human use, shall be considered to supplement, not supersede, each other, unless the regulations explicitly provide otherwise. In the event that it is impossible to comply with all applicable regulations in these parts, the regulations specifically applicable to the drug in question shall supersede the more general.

(b) If a person engages in only some operations subject to the regulations in this part and in Parts 211 through 229 and Parts 600 through 680 of this chapter, and not in others, that person need only comply with those regulations applicable to the operations in which he or she is engaged.

§ 210.3 Definitions.

(a) The definitions and interpretations contained in section 201 of the act shall be applicable to such terms when used in this part and in Parts 211 through 229 of this chapter.

(b) The following definitions of terms apply to this part and to Parts 211 through 229 of this chapter.

(1) "Act" means the Federal Food, Drug, and Cosmetic Act, as amended (21 U.S.C. 301 et seq.).

(2) "Batch" means a specific quantity of a drug or other material that is intended to have uniform character and quality, within specified limits, and is produced according to a single manufacturing order during the same cycle of manufacture.

(3) "Component" means any ingredient intended for use in the manufacture of a drug product, including those that may not appear in such drug product.

(4) "Drug product" means a finished dosage form, for example, tablet, capsule, solution, etc., that contains an active drug ingredient generally, but not necessarily, in association with inactive ingredients. The term also includes a finished dosage form that does not contain an active ingredient but is intended to be used as a placebo.

(5) "Fiber" means any particulate contaminant with a length at least three times greater than its width.

(6) "Non-fiber-releasing filter" means any filter, which after any appropriate pretreatment such as washing or flushing, will not release fibers into the component or drug product that is being filtered. All filters composed of asbestos are deemed to be fiber-releasing filters.

(7) "Active ingredient" means any component that is intended to furnish pharmacological activity or other direct effect in the diagnosis, cure, mitigation, treatment, or prevention of disease, or to affect the structure of any function of the body of man or other animals. The term includes those components that may undergo chemical change in the manufacture of the

drug product and be present in the drug product in a modified form intended to furnish the specified activity or effect.

(8) "Inactive ingredient" means any component other than an "active ingredient."

(9) "In-process material" means any material fabricated, compounded, blended, or derived by chemical reaction that is produced for, and used in the preparation of the drug product.

(10) "Lot" means a batch, or a specific identified portion of a batch, having uniform character and quality within specified limits; or, in the case of a drug product produced by continuous process, it is a specific identified amount produced in a unit of time or quantity in a manner that assures its having uniform character and quality within specified limits.

(11) "Lot number, control number, or batch number" means any distinctive combination of letters, numbers, or symbols, or any combination of them, from which the complete history of the manufacture, processing, packing, holding, and distribution of a batch or lot of drug product or other material can be determined.

(12) "Manufacture, processing, packing, or holding of a drug product" includes packaging and labeling operations, testing, and quality control of drug products.

(15) "Quality control unit" means any person or organizational element designated by the firm to be responsible for the duties relating to quality control.

(16) "Strength" means:

(i) The concentration of the drug substance (for example, weight/weight, weight/volume, or unit dose/volume basis), and/or

(ii) The potency, that is, the therapeutic activity of the drug product as indicated by appropriate laboratory tests or by adequately developed and controlled clinical data (expressed, for example, in terms of units by reference to a standard).

(17) "Theoretical yield" means the quantity that would be produced at any appropriate phase of manufacture, processing, or packing of a particular drug product, based upon the quantity of components to be used, in the absence of any loss or error in actual production.

(18) "Actual yield" means the quantity that is actually produced at any appropriate phase of manufacture, processing, or packing of a particular drug product.

(19) "Percentage of theoretical yield" means the ratio of the actual yield (at any appropriate phase of manufacture, processing, or packing of a particular drug product) to the theoretical yield (at the same phase), stated as a percentage.

(20) "Acceptance criteria" means the product specifications and acceptance/rejection criteria, such as acceptable quality level and unacceptable quality level, with an associated sampling plan, that are necessary for making a decision to accept or reject a lot or batch (or any other convenient subgroups of manufactured units).

(21) "Representative sample" means a sample that consists of a number of units that are drawn based on rational criteria such as random sampling and intended to assure that the sample accurately portrays the material being sampled.

Part 211—Current Good Manufacturing Practice for Finished Pharmaceuticals

Subpart A—General Provisions

§ 211.1   Scope.
§ 211.3   Definitions.

Subpart B—Organization and Personnel

§ 211.22   Responsibilities of quality control unit.
§ 211.25   Personnel qualifications.
§ 211.28   Personnel responsibilities.
§ 211.34   Consultants.

Subpart C—Buildings and Facilities

§ 211.42   Design and construction features.
§ 211.44   Lighting.
§ 211.46   Ventilation, air filtration, air heating and cooling.
§ 211.48   Plumbing.
§ 211.50   Sewage and refuse.
§ 211.52   Washing and toilet facilities.
§ 211.56   Sanitation.
§ 211.58   Maintenance.

Subpart D—Equipment

§ 211.63   Equipment design, size, and location.
§ 211.65   Equipment construction.
§ 211.67   Equipment cleaning and maintenance.
§ 211.68   Automatic, mechanical, and electronic equipment.
§ 211.72   Filters.

Subpart E—Control of Components and Drug Product Containers and Closures

§ 211.80   General requirements.
§ 211.82   Receipt and storage of untested components, drug product containers, and closures.
§ 211.84   Testing and approval or rejection of components, drug product containers, and closures.
§ 211.86   Use of approved components, drug product containers, and closures.
§ 211.87   Retesting of approved components, drug product containers, and closures.
§ 211.89   Rejected components, drug product containers, and closures.
§ 211.94   Drug product containers and closures.

Subpart F—Production and Process Controls

§ 211.100   Written procedures; deviations.
§ 211.101   Charge-in of components.
§ 211.103   Calculation of yield.
§ 211.105   Equipment identification.
§ 211.110   Sampling and testing of in-process materials and drug products.
§ 211.111   Time limitations on production.
§ 211.113   Control of microbiological contamination.
§ 211.115   Reprocessing.

Subpart G—Packaging and Labeling Control

§ 211.122   Materials examination and usage criteria.
§ 211.125   Labeling issuance.
§ 211.130   Packaging and labeling operations.
§ 211.132   Tamper-resistant packaging requirements for over-the-counter human drug products.
§ 211.134   Drug product inspection.
§ 211.137   Expiration dating.

Subpart H—Holding and Distribution

§ 211.142   Warehousing procedures.
§ 211.150   Distribution procedures.

Subpart I—Laboratory Controls

§ 211.160   General requirements.
§ 211.165   Testing and release for distribution.
§ 211.166   Stability testing.
§ 211.167   Special testing requirements.
§ 211.170   Reserve samples.
§ 211.173   Laboratory animals.
§ 211.176   Penicillin contamination.

Subpart J—Records and Reports

§ 211.180   General requirements.
§ 211.182   Equipment cleaning and use log.
§ 211.184   Component, drug product container, closure, and labeling records.
§ 211.186   Master production and control records.
§ 211.188   Batch production and control records.
§ 211.192   Production record review.
§ 211.194   Laboratory records.
§ 211.196   Distribution records.
§ 211.198   Complaint files.

Subpart K—Returned and Salvaged Drug Products

§ 211.204   Returned drug products.
§ 211.208   Drug product salvaging.

Subpart A—General Provisions

§ 211.1 Scope.

(a) The regulations in this part contain the minimum current good manufacturing practice for preparation of drug products for administration to humans or animals.

(b) The current good manufacturing practice regulations in this chapter, as they pertain to drug products, and in Parts 600 through 680 of this chapter, as they pertain to biological products for human use, shall be considered to supplement, not supersede, the regulations in this part unless the regulations explicitly provide otherwise. In the event it is impossible to comply with applicable regulations both in this part and in other parts of this chapter or in Parts 600 through 680 of this chapter, the regulation specifically applicable to the drug product in question shall supersede the regulation in this part.

Subpart B—Organization and Personnel

§ 211.22 Responsibilities of quality control unit.

(a) There shall be a quality control unit that shall have the responsibility and authority to approve or reject all components, drug product containers, closures, in-process materials, packaging material, labeling, and drug products, and the authority to review production records to assure that no errors have occurred or, if errors have occurred, that they have been fully investigated. The quality control unit shall be responsible for approving or rejecting drug products manufactured, processed, packed, or held under contract by another company.

(b) Adequate laboratory facilities for the testing and approval (or rejection) of components, drug product containers, closures, packaging materials, in-process materials, and drug products shall be available to the quality control unit.

(c) The quality control unit shall have the responsibility for approving or rejecting all procedures or specifications impacting on the identity, strength, quality, and purity of the drug product.

(d) The responsibilities and procedures applicable to the quality control unit shall be in writing; such written procedures shall be followed.

§ 211.25 Personnel qualifications.

(a) Each person engaged in the manufacture, processing, packing, or holding of a drug product shall have education, training, and experience, or any combination thereof, to enable that person to perform the assigned functions. Training shall be in the particular operations that the employee performs and in current good manufacturing practice (including the current good manufacturing practice regulations in this chapter and written procedures required by these regulations) as they relate to the employee's functions. Training in current good manufacturing practice shall be conducted by qualified individuals on a continuing basis and with sufficient frequency to assure that employees remain familiar with CGMP requirements applicable to them.

(b) Each person responsible for supervising the manufacture, processing, packing, or holding of a drug product shall have the education, training, and experience, or any combination thereof, to perform assigned functions in such a manner as to provide assurance that the drug product has the safety, identity, strength, quality, and purity that it purports or is represented to possess.

(c) There shall be an adequate number of qualified personnel to perform and supervise the manufacture, processing, packing, or holding of each drug product.

§ 211.28 Personnel responsibilities.

(a) Personnel engaged in the manufacture, processing, packing, or holding of a drug product shall wear clean clothing appropriate for the duties they perform. Protective apparel, such as head, face, hand, and arm coverings, shall be worn as necessary to protect drug products from contamination.

(b) Personnel shall practice good sanitation and health habits.

(c) Only personnel authorized by supervisory personnel shall enter those areas of the buildings and facilities designated as limited-access areas.

(d) Any person shown at any time (either by medical examination or supervisory observation) to have an apparent illness or open lesions that may adversely affect the safety or quality of drug products shall be excluded from direct contact with components, drug product containers, closures, in-process materials, and drug products until the condition is corrected or determined by competent medical personnel not to jeopardize the safety or quality of drug products. All personnel shall be instructed to report to supervisory personnel any health conditions that may have an adverse effect on drug products.

§ 211.34 Consultants.

Consultants advising on the manufacture, processing, packing, or holding of drug products shall have sufficient education, training, and experience, or any combination thereof, to advise on the subject for which they are retained. Records shall be maintained stating the name, address, and qualifications of any consultants and the type of service they provide.

Subpart C—Buildings and Facilities

§ 211.42 Design and construction features.

(a) Any building or buildings used in the manufacture, processing, packing, or holding of a drug product shall be of suitable size, construction and location to facilitate cleaning, maintenance, and proper operations.

(b) Any such building shall have adequate space for the orderly placement of equipment and materials to prevent mixups between different components, drug product containers, closures, labeling, in-process materials, or drug products, and to prevent contamination. The flow of components, drug product containers, closures, labeling, in-process materials, and drug products through the building or buildings shall be designed to prevent contamination.

(c) Operations shall be performed within specifically defined areas of adequate size. There shall be separate or defined areas for the firm's operations to prevent contamination or mixups as follows:

(1) Receipt, identification, storage, and withholding from use of components, drug product containers, closures, and labeling, pending the appropriate sampling, testing, or examination by the quality control unit before release for manufacturing or packaging;

(2) Holding rejected components, drug product containers, closures, and labeling before disposition;

(3) Storage of released components, drug product containers, closures, and labeling;

(4) Storage of in-process materials;

(5) Manufacturing and processing operations;

(6) Packaging and labeling operations;

(7) Quarantine storage before release of drug products;

(8) Storage of drug products after release;

(9) Control and laboratory operations;

(10) Aseptic processing, which includes as appropriate:

(i) Floors, walls, and ceilings of smooth, hard surfaces that are easily cleanable;

(ii) Temperature and humidity controls;

(iii) An air supply filtered through high-efficiency particulate air filters under positive pressure, regardless of whether flow is laminar or nonlaminar;

(iv) A system for monitoring environmental conditions;

(v) A system for cleaning and disinfecting the room and equipment to produce aseptic conditions;

(vi) A system for maintaining any equipment used to control the aseptic conditions.

(d) Operations relating to the manufacture, processing, and packing of penicillin shall be performed in facilities separate from those used for other drug products for human use.

§ 211.44   Lighting.

Adequate lighting shall be provided in all areas.

§ 211.46   Ventilation, air filtration, air heating and cooling.

(a) Adequate ventilation shall be provided.

(b) Equipment for adequate control over air pressure, microorganisms, dust, humidity, and temperature shall be provided when appropriate for the manufacture, processing, packing, or holding of a drug product.

(c) Air filtration systems, including prefilters and particulate matter air filters, shall be used when appropriate on air supplies to production areas. If air is recirculated to production areas, measures shall be taken to control recirculation of dust from production. In areas where air contamination occurs during production, there shall be adequate exhaust systems or other systems adequate to control contaminants.

(d) Air-handling systems for the manufacture, processing, and packing of penicillin shall be completely separate from those for other drug products for human use.

§ 211.48   Plumbing.

(a) Potable water shall be supplied under continuous positive pressure in a plumbing system free of defects that could contribute contamination to any drug product. Potable water shall meet the standards prescribed in the Environmental Protection Agency's Primary Drinking Water Regulations set forth in 40 CFR Part 141. Water not meeting such standards shall not be permitted in the potable water system.

(b) Drains shall be of adequate size and, where connected directly to a sewer, shall be provided with an air break or other mechanical device to prevent back-siphonage.

§ 211.50   Sewage and refuse.

Sewage, trash, and other refuse in and from the building and immediate premises shall be disposed of in a safe and sanitary manner.

§ 211.52   Washing and toilet facilities.

Adequate washing facilities shall be provided, including hot and cold water, soap or detergent, air driers or single-service towels, and clean toilet facilities easily accessible to working areas.

§ 211.56   Sanitation.

(a) Any building used in the manufacture, processing, packing, or holding of a drug product shall be maintained in a clean and sanitary condition. Any such building shall be free of infestation by rodents, birds, insects, and other vermin (other than laboratory animals). Trash and organic waste matter shall be held and disposed of in a timely and sanitary manner.

(b) There shall be written procedures assigning responsibility for sanitation and describing in sufficient detail the cleaning schedules, methods, equipment, and materials to be used in cleaning the buildings and facilities; such written procedures shall be followed.

(c) There shall be written procedures for use of suitable rodenticides, insecticides, fungicides, fumigating agents, and cleaning and sanitizing agents. Such written procedures shall be designed to prevent the contamination of equipment, components, drug product containers, closures, packaging, labeling materials, or drug products and shall be followed. Rodenticides, insecticides, and fungicides shall not be used unless registered and used in accordance with the Federal Insecticide, Fungicide, and Rodenticide Act (7 U.S.C. 135).

(d) Sanitation procedures shall apply to work performed by contractors or temporary employees as well as work performed by full-time employees during the ordinary course of operations.

§ 211.58   Maintenance.

Any building used in the manufacture, processing, packing, or holding of a drug product shall be maintained in a good state of repair.

Subpart D—Equipment

§ 211.63   Equipment design, size, and location.

Equipment used in the manufacture, processing, packing, or holding of a drug product shall be of appropriate design, adequate size, and suitably located to facilitate operations for its intended use and for its cleaning and maintenance.

§ 211.65   Equipment construction.

(a) Equipment shall be constructed so that surfaces that contact components, in-process materials, or drug products shall not be reactive, additive, or absorptive so as to alter the safety, identity, strength, quality, or purity of the drug product beyond the official or other established requirements.

(b) Any substances required for operation, such as lubricants or coolants, shall not come into contact with components, drug product containers, closures, in-process materials, or drug products so as to alter the safety, identity, strength, quality, or purity of the drug product beyond the official or other established requirements.

§ 211.67   Equipment cleaning and maintenance.

(a) Equipment and utensils shall be cleaned, maintained, and sanitized at appropriate intervals to prevent malfunctions or contamination that would alter the safety, identity, strength, quality, or purity of the drug product beyond the official or other established requirements.

(b) Written procedures shall be established and followed for cleaning and maintenance of equipment, including utensils, used in the manufacture, processing, packing, or holding of a drug product. These procedures shall include, but are not necessarily limited to, the following:

(1) Assignment of responsibility for cleaning and maintaining equipment;

(2) Maintenance and cleaning schedules, including, where appropriate, sanitizing schedules;

(3) A description in sufficient detail of the methods, equipment, and materials used in cleaning and maintenance operations, and the methods of disassembling and reassembling equipment as necessary to assure proper cleaning and maintenance;

(4) Removal or obliteration of previous batch identification;

(5) Protection of clean equipment from contamination prior to use;

(6) Inspection of equipment for cleanliness immediately before use.

(c) Records shall be kept of maintenance, cleaning, sanitizing, and inspection as specified in §§211.180 and 211.182.

§ 211.68 Automatic, mechanical, and electronic equipment.

(a) Automatic, mechanical, or electronic equipment or other types of equipment, including computers, or related systems that will perform a function satisfactorily, may be used in the manufacture, processing, packing, and holding of a drug product. If such equipment is so used, it shall be routinely calibrated, inspected, or checked according to a written program designed to assure proper performance. Written records of those calibration checks and inspections shall be maintained.

(b) Appropriate controls shall be exercised over computer or related systems to assure that changes in master production and control records or other records are instituted only by authorized personnel. Input to and output from the computer or related system of formulas or other records or data shall be checked for accuracy. A backup file of data entered into the computer or related system shall be maintained except where certain data, such as calculations performed in connection with laboratory analysis, are eliminated by computerization or other automated processes. In such instances a written record of the program shall be maintained along with appropriate validation data. Hard copy or alternative systems, such as duplicates, tapes, or microfilm, designed to assure that backup data are exact and complete and that it is secure from alteration, inadvertent erasures, or loss shall be maintained.

§ 211.72 Filters.

Filters for liquid filtration used in the manufacture, processing, or packing of injectable drug products intended for human use shall not release fibers into such products. Fiber-releasing filters may not be used in the manufacture, processing, or packing of these injectable drug products unless it is not possible to manufacture such drug products without the use of such filters. If use of a fiber-releasing filter is necessary, an additional non-fiber-releasing filter of 0.22 micron maximum mean porosity (0.45 micron if the manufacturing conditions so dictate) shall subsequently be used to reduce the content of particles in the injectable drug product. Use of an asbestos-containing filter, with or without subsequent use of a specific non-fiber-releasing filter, is permissible only upon submission of proof to the appropriate bureau of the Food and Drug Administration that use of a non-fiber-releasing filter will, or is likely to, compromise the safety or effectiveness of the injectable drug product.

Subpart E—Control of Components and Drug Product Containers and Closures

§ 211.80 General requirements.

(a) There shall be written procedures describing in sufficient detail the receipt, identification, storage, handling, sampling, testing, and approval or rejection of components and drug product containers and closures; such written procedures shall be followed.

(b) Components and drug product containers and closures shall at all times be handled and stored in a manner to prevent contamination.

(c) Bagged or boxed components of drug product containers, or closures shall be stored off the floor and suitably spaced to permit cleaning and inspection.

(d) Each container or grouping of containers for components or drug product containers, or closures shall be identified with a distinctive code for each lot in each shipment received. This code shall be used in recording the disposition of each lot. Each lot shall be appropriately identified as to its status (i.e., quarantined, approved, or rejected).

§ 211.82 Receipt and storage of untested components, drug product containers, and closures.

(a) Upon receipt and before acceptance, each container or grouping of containers of components, drug product containers, and closures shall be examined visually for appropriate labeling as to contents, container damage or broken seals, and contamination.

(b) Components, drug product containers, and closures shall be stored under quarantine until they have been tested or examined, as appropriate, and released. Storage within the area shall conform to the requirements of §211.80.

§ 211.84 Testing and approval or rejection of components, drug product containers, and closures.

(a) Each lot of components, drug product containers, and closures shall be withheld from use until the lot has been sampled, tested, or examined, as appropriate, and released for use by the quality control unit.

(b) Representative samples of each shipment of each lot shall be collected for testing or examination. The number of containers to be sampled, and the amount of material to be taken from each container, shall be based upon appropriate criteria such as statistical criteria for component variability, confidence levels, and degree of precision desired, the past quality history of the supplier, and the quantity needed for analysis and reserve where required by §211.170.

(c) Samples shall be collected in accordance with the following procedures:

(1) The containers of components selected shall be cleaned where necessary, by appropriate means.

(2) The containers shall be opened, sampled, and resealed in a manner designed to prevent contamination of their contents and contamination of other components, drug product containers, or closures.

(3) Sterile equipment and aseptic sampling techniques shall be used when necessary.

(4) If it is necessary to sample a component from the top, middle, and bottom of its container, such sample subdivisions shall not be composited for testing.

(5) Sample containers shall be identified so that the following information can be determined: name of the material sampled, the lot number, the container from which the sample was taken, the data on which the sample was taken, and the name of the person who collected the sample.

(6) Containers from which samples have been taken shall be marked to show that samples have been removed from them.

(d) Samples shall be examined and tested as follows:

(1) At least one test shall be conducted to verify the identity of each component of a drug product. Specific identity tests, if they exist, shall be used.

(2) Each component shall be tested for conformity with all appropriate written specifications for purity, strength, and quality. In lieu of such testing by the manufacturer, a report of analysis may be accepted from the supplier of a component, provided that at least one specific identity test is conducted on such component by the manufacturer, and provided that the manufacturer establishes the reliability of the supplier's analyses through appropriate validation of the supplier's test results at appropriate intervals.

(3) Containers and closures shall be tested for conformance with all appropriate written procedures. In lieu of such testing by the manufacturer, a certificate of testing may be accepted from the supplier, provided that at least a visual identification is conducted on such containers/closures by the manufacturer and provided that the manufacturer establishes the reliability of the supplier's test results through appropriate validation of the supplier's test results at appropriate intervals.

(4) When appropriate, components shall be microscopically examined.

(5) Each lot of a component, drug product container, or closure that is liable to contamination with filth, insect infestation, or other extraneous adulterant shall be examined against established specifications for such contamination.

(6) Each lot of a component, drug product container, or closure that is liable to microbiological contamination that is objectionable in view of its intended use shall be subjected to microbiological tests before use.

(e) Any lot of components, drug product containers, or closures that meets the appropriate written specifications of identity, strength, quality, and purity and related tests under paragraph (d) of this section may be approved and released for use. Any lot of such material that does not meet such specifications shall be rejected.

§ 211.86 Use of approved components, drug product containers, and closures.

Components, drug product containers, and closures approved for use shall be rotated so that the oldest approved stock is used first. Deviation from this requirement is permitted if such deviation is temporary and appropriate.

§ 211.87 Retesting of approved components, drug product containers, and closures.

Components, drug product containers, and closures shall be retested or reexamined, as appropriate, for identity, strength, quality, and purity and approved or rejected by the quality control unit in accordance with §211.84 as necessary, e.g., after storage for long periods or after exposure to air, heat or other conditions that might adversely affect the component, drug product container, or closure.

§ 211.89 Rejected components, drug product containers, and closures.

Rejected components, drug product containers, and closures shall be identified and controlled under a quarantine system designed to prevent their use in manufacturing or processing operations for which they are unsuitable.

§ 211.94 Drug product containers and closures.

(a) Drug product containers and closures shall not be reactive, additive, or absorptive so as to alter the safety, identity, strength, quality, or purity of the drug beyond the official or established requirements.

(b) Container closure systems shall provide adequate protection against foreseeable external factors in storage and use that can cause deterioration or contamination of the drug product.

(c) Drug product containers and closures shall be clean and, where indicated by the nature of the drug, sterilized and processed to remove pyrogenic properties to assure that they are suitable for their intended use.

(d) Standards or specifications, methods of testing, and, where indicated, methods of cleaning, sterilizing, and processing to remove pyrogenic properties shall be written and followed for drug product containers and closures.

Subpart F—Production and Process Controls

§ 211.100 Written procedures; deviations.

(a) There shall be written procedures for production and process control designed to assure that the drug products have the identity, strength, quality, and purity they purport or are represented to possess. Such procedures shall include all requirements in this subpart. These written procedures, including any changes, shall be drafted, reviewed, and approved by the appropriate organizational units and reviewed and approved by the quality control unit.

(b) Written production and process control procedures shall be followed in the execution of the various production and process control functions and shall be documented at the time of performance. Any deviation from the written procedures shall be recorded and justified.

§ 211.101 Charge-in of components.

Written production and control procedures shall include the following, which are designed to assure that the drug products produced have the identity, strength, quality, and purity they purport or are represented to possess:

(a) The batch shall be formulated with the intent to provide not less than 100 percent of the labeled or established amount of active ingredient.

(b) Components for drug product manufacturing shall be weighed, measured, or subdivided as appropriate. If a component is removed from the original container to another, the new container shall be identified with the following information:

(1) Component name or item code;

(2) Receiving or control number;

(3) Weight or measure in new container;

(4) Batch for which component was dispensed, including its product name, strength, and lot number.

(c) Weighing, measuring, or subdividing operations for components shall be adequately supervised. Each container of component dispensed to manufacturing shall be examined by a second person to assure that:

(1) The component was released by the quality control unit;

(2) The weight or measure is correct as stated in the batch production records;

(3) The containers are properly identified.

(d) Each component shall be added to the batch by one person and verified by a second person.

§ 211.103 Calculation of yield.

Actual yields and percentages of theoretical yield shall be determined at the conclusion of each appropriate phase of manufacturing, processing, packaging, or holding of the drug product. Such calculations shall be performed by one person and independently verified by a second person.

§ 211.105 Equipment identification.

(a) All compounding and storage containers, processing lines, and major equipment used using the production of a batch of a drug product shall be properly identified at all times to indicate their contents and, when necessary, the phase of processing of the batch.

(b) Major equipment shall be identified by a distinctive identification number or code that shall be recorded in the batch production record to show the specific equipment used in the manufacture of each batch of a drug product. In cases where only one of a particular type of equipment exists in a manufacturing facility, the name of the equipment may be used in lieu of a distinctive identification number or code.

§ 211.110 Sampling and testing of in-process materials and drug products.

(a) To assure batch uniformity and integrity of drug products, written procedures shall be established and followed that describe the in-process controls, and tests, or examinations to be conducted on appropriate samples of in-process materials of each batch. Such control procedures shall be established to monitor the output and to validate the performance of those manufacturing processes that may be responsible for causing variability in the characteristics of in-process material and the drug product. Such control procedures shall include, but are not limited to, the following, where appropriate:

(1) Tablet or capsule weight variation;

(2) Disintegration time;

(3) Adequacy of mixing to assure uniformity and homogeneity;

(4) Dissolution time and rate;

(5) Clarity, completeness, or pH of solutions.

(b) Valid in-process specifications for such characteristics shall be consistent with drug product final specifications and shall be derived from previous acceptable process average and process variability estimates where possible and determined by the application of suitable statistical procedures where appropriate. Examination and testing of samples shall assure that the drug product and in-process material conform to specifications.

(c) In-process materials shall be tested for identity, strength, quality, and purity as appropriate, and approved or rejected by the quality control unit, during the production process, e.g., at commencement or completion of significant phases or after storage for long periods.

(d) Rejected in-process materials shall be identified and controlled under a quarantine system designed to prevent their use in manufacturing or processing operations for which they are unsuitable.

§ 211.111 Time limitations on production.

When appropriate, time limits for the completion of each phase of production shall be established to assure the quality of the drug product. Deviation from established time limits may be acceptable if such deviation does not compromise the quality of the drug product.Such deviation shall be justified and documented.

§ 211.113 Control of microbiological contamination.

(a) Appropriate written procedures, designed to prevent objectionable microorganisms in drug products not required to be sterile, shall be established and followed.

(b) Appropriate written procedures, designed to prevent microbiological contamination of drug products purporting to be sterile, shall be established and followed. Such procedures shall include validation of any sterilization process.

§ 211.115 Reprocessing.

(a) Written procedures shall be established and followed prescribing a system for reprocessing batches that do not conform to standards or specifications and the steps to be taken to insure that the reprocessed batches will conform with all established standards, specifications, and characteristics.

(b) Reprocessing shall not be performed without the review and approval of the quality control unit.

Subpart G—Packaging and Labeling Control

§ 211.122 Materials examination and usage criteria.

(a) There shall be written procedures describing in sufficient detail the receipt, identification, storage, handling, sampling, examination, and/or testing of labeling and packaging materials; such written procedures shall be followed. Labeling and packaging materials shall be representatively sampled, and examined or tested upon receipt and before use in packaging or labeling of a drug product.

(b) Any labeling or packaging materials meeting appropriate written specifications may be approved and released for use. Any labeling or packaging materials that do not meet such specifications shall be rejected to prevent their use in operations for which they are unsuitable.

(c) Records shall be maintained for each shipment received of each different labeling and packaging material indicating receipt, examination or testing, and whether accepted or rejected.

(d) Labels and other labeling materials for each different drug product, strength, dosage form, or quantity of contents shall be stored separately with suitable identification. Access to the storage area shall be limited to authorized personnel.

(e) Obsolete and outdated labels, labeling, and other packaging materials shall be destroyed.

(f) Gang printing of labeling to be used for different drug products or different strengths of the same drug product (or labeling of the same size and identical or similar format and/or color schemes) shall be minimized. If gang printing is employed, packaging and labeling operations shall provide for special control procedures, taking into consideration sheet layout, stacking, cutting, and handling during and after printing.

(g) Printing devices on, or associated with, manufacturing lines used to imprint labeling upon the drug product unit label or case shall be monitored to assure that all imprinting conforms to the print specified in the batch production record.

§ 211.125 Labeling issuance.

(a) Strict control shall be exercised over labeling issued for use in drug product labeling operations.

(b) Labeling materials issued for a batch shall be carefully examined for identity and conformity to the labeling specified in the master or batch production records.

(c) Procedures shall be utilized to reconcile the quantities of labeling issued, used, and returned, and shall require evaluation of discrepancies found between the quantity of drug product finished and the quantity of labeling issued when such discrepancies are outside narrow preset limits based on historical operating data. Such discrepancies shall be investigated in accordance with §211.192.

(d) All excess labeling bearing lot or control numbers shall be destroyed.

(e) Returned labeling shall be maintained and stored in a manner to prevent mixups and provide proper identification.

(f) Procedures shall be written describing in sufficient detail the control procedures employed for the issuance of labeling; such written procedures shall be followed.

§ 211.130 Packaging and labeling operations.

There shall be written procedures designed to assure that correct labels, labeling, and packaging materials are used for drug products; such written procedures shall be followed. These procedures shall incorporate the following features:

(a) Prevention of mixups and cross-contamination by physical or spatial separation from operations on other drug products.

(b) Identification of the drug product with a lot or control number that permits determination of the history of the manufacture and control of the batch.

(c) Examination of packaging and labeling materials for suitability and correctness before packaging operations, and documentation of such examination in the batch production record.

(d) Inspection of the packaging and labeling facilities immediately before use to assure that all drug products have been removed from previous operations. Inspection shall also be made to assure that packaging and labeling materials not suitable for subsequent operations have been removed. Results of inspection shall be documented in the batch production records.

§ 211.132 Tamper-resistant packaging requirements for over-the-counter human drug products.

(a) *General.* Because most over-the-counter (OTC) human drug products are not now packaged in tamper-resistant retail packages, there is the opportunity for the malicious adulteration of OTC drug products with health risks to individuals who unknowingly purchase adulterated products and with loss of consumer confidence in the security of OTC drug product packages. The Food and Drug Administration has the authority and responsibility under the Federal Food, Drug, and Cosmetic Act (the act) to establish a uniform national requirement for tamper-resistant packaging of OTC drug products that will improve the security of OTC drug packaging and help assure the safety and effectiveness of OTC drug products. An OTC drug product (except a dermatological, dentifrice, insulin, or lozenge product) for retail sale that is not packaged in a tamper-resistant package or that is not properly labeled under this section is adulterated under section 501 of the act or misbranded under section 502 of the act, or both.

(b) *Requirement for tamper-resistant package.* Each manufacturer and packer who packages an OTC drug product (except a dermatological, dentifrice, insulin, or lozenge product) for retail sale, shall package the product in a tamper-resistant package, if this product is accessible to the public while held for sale. A tamper-resistant package is one having an indicator or barrier to entry which, if breached or missing, can reasonably be expected to provide visible evidence to consumers that tampering has occurred. To reduce the likelihood of substitution of a tamper-resistant feature after tampering, the indicator or barrier to entry is required to be distinctive by design (e.g., an aerosol product container) or by the use of an identifying characteristic (e.g., a pattern, name, registered trademark, logo, or picture). For purposes of this section, the term "distinctive by design" means the packaging cannot be duplicated with commonly available materials or through commonly available processes. For purposes of this section, the term "aerosol product" means a product which depends upon the power of a liquified or compressed gas to expel the contents from the container. A tamper-resistant package may involve an immediate-container and closure system or secondary-container or carton system or any combination of systems intended to provide a visual indication of package integrity. The tamper-resistant feature shall be designed to and shall remain intact when handled in a reasonable manner during manufacture, distribution, and retail display.

(c) *Labeling.* Each retail package of an OTC drug product covered by this section, except ammonia inhalant in crushable glass ampules, aerosol products as defined in paragraph (b) of this section, or containers of compressed medical oxygen, is required to bear a statement that is prominently placed so that consumers are alerted to the specific tamper-resistant feature of the package. The labeling statement is also required to be so placed that it will be unaffected if the tamper-resistant feature of the package is breached or missing. If the tamper-resistant feature chosen to meet the requirement in paragraph (b) of this section is one that uses an identifying characteristic, that characteristic is required to be referred to in the labeling statement. For example, the labeling statement on a bottle with a shrink band could say "For your protection, this bottle has an imprinted seal around the neck."

(d) *Requests for exemptions from packaging and labeling requirements.* A manufacturer or packer may request an exemption from the packaging and labeling requirements of this section. A request for an exemption is required to be submitted in the form of a citizen petition under §10.30 of this chapter and should be clearly identified on the envelope as a "Request for Exemption from Tamper-resistant Rule." The petition is required to contain the following:

(1) The name of the drug product or, if the petition seeks an exemption for a drug class, the name of the drug class, and a list of products within that class.

(2) The reasons that the drug product's compliance with the tamper-resistant packaging or labeling requirements of this section is unnecessary or cannot be achieved.

(3) A description of alternative steps that are available, or that the petitioner has already taken, to reduce the likelihood that the product or drug class will be the subject of malicious adulteration.

(4) Other information justifying an exemption.

This information collection requirement has been approved by the Office of Management and Budget under number 0910–0149.

(e) *OTC drug products subject to approved new drug applications.* Holders of approved new drug applications for OTC drug products are required under §314.8 (a) (4) (vi), (5) (xi), or (d) (5) of this chapter to provide for changes in packaging, and under §314.8 (a) (5) (xii) to provide for changes in labeling to comply with the requirements of this section.

(f) *Poison Prevention Packaging Act of 1970.* This section does not affect any requirements for "special packaging" as defined under §310.3 (1) of this chapter and required under the Poison Prevention Packaging Act of 1970.

(g) *Effective date.* OTC drug products, except dermatological, dentifrice, insulin, and lozenge products, are required to comply with the requirements of this section on the dates listed below except to the extent that a product's manufacturer or packer has obtained an exemption from a packaging or labeling requirement.

(1) *Initial effective date for packaging requirements.*

(i) The packaging requirement in paragraph (b) of this section is effective on February 7, 1983 for each affected OTC drug product (except oral and vaginal tablets, vaginal and rectal suppositories, and one-piece soft gelatin capsules) packaged for retail sale on or after that date, except for the requirement in paragraph (b) of this section for a distinctive indicator or barrier to entry.

(ii) The packaging requirements in paragraph (b) of this section is effective on May 5, 1983 for each OTC drug product that is an oral or vaginal tablet, a vaginal or rectal suppository, or one-piece soft gelatin capsules packaged for retail sale on or after that date.

(2) *Initial effective date for labeling requirements.* The requirement in paragraph (b) of this section that the indicator or barrier to entry be distinctive by design and the requirement in paragraph (c) of this section for a labeling statement are effective on May 5, 1983 for each affected OTC drug product packaged on or after that date.

(3) *Retail level effective date.* The tamper-resistant packaging requirement of paragraph (b) of this section is effective on February 6, 1984 for each affected OTC drug product held for sale on or after that date that was packaged for retail sale before May 5, 1983. This does not include the requirement in paragraph (b) of this section that the indicator or barrier to entry be distinctive by design. Products packaged for retail sale after May 5, 1983, are required to be in compliance with all aspects of the regulations without regard to the retail level effective date.

§ 211.134   Drug product inspection.

(a) Packaged and labeled products shall be examined during finishing operations to provide assurance that containers and packages in the lot have the correct label.

(b) A representative sample of units shall be collected at the completion of finishing operations and shall be visually examined for correct labeling.

(c) Results of these examinations shall be recorded in the batch production or control records.

§ 211.137   Expiration dating.

(a) To assure that a drug product meets applicable standards of identity, strength, quality, and purity at the time of use, it shall bear an expiration date determined by appropriate stability testing described in §211.166.

(b) Expiration dates shall be related to any storage conditions stated on the labeling, as determined by stability studies described in §211.166.

(c) If the drug product is to be reconstituted at the time of dispensing, its labeling shall bear expiration information for both the reconstituted and unreconstituted drug products.

(d) Expiration dates shall appear on labeling in accordance with the requirements of §201.17 of this chapter.

(e) Homeopathic drug products shall be exempt from the requirements of this section.

(f) Allergenic extracts that are labeled "No U.S. Standard of Potency" are exempt from the requirements of this section.

(g) Pending consideration of a proposed exemption, published in the FEDERAL REGISTER of September 29, 1978, the requirements in this section shall not be enforced for human OTC drug products if their labeling does not bear dosage limitations and they are stable for at least 3 years as supported by appropriate stability data.

Subpart H—Holding and Distribution

§ 211.142 Warehousing procedures.

Written procedures describing the warehousing of drug products shall be established and followed. They shall include:

(a) Quarantine of drug products before release by the quality control unit.

(b) Storage of drug products under appropriate conditions of temperature, humidity, and light so that the identity, strength, quality, and purity of the drug products are not affected.

§ 211.150 Distribution procedures.

Written procedures shall be established, and followed, describing the distribution of drug products. They shall include:

(a) A procedure whereby the oldest approved stock of a drug product is distributed first. Deviation from this requirement is permitted if such deviation is temporary and appropriate.

(b) A system by which the distribution of each lot of drug product can be readily determined to facilitate its recall if necessary.

Subpart I—Laboratory Controls

§ 211.160 General requirements.

(a) The establishment of any specifications, standards, sampling plans, test procedures, or other laboratory control mechanisms required by this subpart, including any change in such specifications, standards, sampling plans, test procedures, or other laboratory control mechanisms, shall be drafted by the appropriate organizational unit and reviewed and approved by the quality control unit. The requirements in this subpart shall be followed and shall be documented at the time of performance. Any deviation from the written specifications, standards, sampling plans, test procedures, or other laboratory control mechanisms shall be recorded and justified.

(b) Laboratory controls shall include the establishment of scientifically sound and appropriate specifications, standards, sampling plans, and test procedures designed to assure that components, drug product containers, closures, in-process materials, labeling, and drug products conform to appropriate standards of identity, strength, quality, and purity. Laboratory controls shall include:

(1) Determination of conformance to appropriate written specifications for the acceptance of each lot within each shipment of components, drug product containers, closures, and labeling used in the manufacture, processing, packing, or holding of drug products. The specifications shall include a description of the sampling and testing procedures used. Samples shall be representative and adequately identified. Such procedures shall also require appropriate retesting of any component, drug product container, or closure that is subject to deterioration.

(2) Determination of conformance to written specifications and a description of sampling and testing procedures for in-process materials. Such samples shall be representative and properly identified.

(3) Determination of conformance to written descriptions of sampling procedures and appropriate specifications for drug products. Such samples shall be representative and properly identified.

(4) The calibration of instruments, apparatus, gauges, and recording devices at suitable intervals in accordance with an established written program containing specific directions, schedules, limits for accuracy and precision, and provisions for remedial action in the event accuracy and/or precision limits are not met. Instruments, apparatus, gauges, and recording devices not meeting established specifications shall not be used.

§ 211.165 Testing and release for distribution.

(a) For each batch of drug product, there shall be appropriate laboratory determination of satisfactory conformance to final specifications for the drug product, including the identity and strength of each active ingredient, prior to release. Where sterility and/or pyrogen testing are conducted on specific batches of short-lived radiopharmaceuticals, such batches may be released prior to completion of sterility and/or pyrogen testing, provided such testing is completed as soon as possible.

(b) There shall be appropriate laboratory testing, as necessary, of each batch of drug product required to be free of objectionable microorganisms.

(c) Any sampling and testing plans shall be described in written procedures that shall include the method of sampling and the number of units per batch to be tested; such written procedure shall be followed.

(d) Acceptance criteria for the sampling and testing conducted by the quality control unit shall be adequate to assure that batches of drug products meet each appropriate specification and appropriate statistical quality control criteria as a condition for their approval and release. The statistical quality control criteria shall include appropriate acceptance levels and/or appropriate rejection levels.

(e) The accuracy, sensitivity, specificity, and reproducibility of test methods employed by the firm shall be established and documented. Such validation and documentation may be accomplished in accordance with §211.194 (a) (2).

(f) Drug products failing to meet established standards or specifications and any other relevant quality control criteria shall be rejected. Reprocessing may be performed. Prior to acceptance and use, reprocessed material must meet appropriate standards, specifications, and any other relevant criteria.

§ 211.166 Stability testing.

(a) There shall be a written testing program designed to assess the stability characteristics of drug products. The results of such stability testing shall be used in determining appropriate storage conditions and expiration dates. The written program shall be followed and shall include:

(1) Sample size and test intervals based on statistical criteria for each attribute examined to assure valid estimates of stability;

(2) Storage conditions for samples retained for testing;

(3) Reliable, meaningful, and specific test methods;

(4) Testing of the drug product in the same container-closure system as that in which the drug product is marketed;

(5) Testing of drug products for reconstitution at the time of dispensing (as directed in the labeling) as well as after they are reconstituted.

(b) An adequate number of batches of each drug product shall be tested to determine an appropriate expiration date and a record of such data shall be maintained. Accelerated studies, combined with basic stability information on the components, drug products, and container-closure system, may be used to support tentative expiration dates provided full shelf life studies are not available and are being conducted. Where data from accelerated studies are used to project a tentative expiration date that is beyond a date supported by actual shelf life studies, there must be stability studies conducted, including drug product testing at appropriate intervals, until the tentative expiration date is verified or the appropriate expiration date determined.

(c) For homeopathic drug products, the requirements of this section are as follows:

(1) There shall be a written assessment of stability based at least on testing or examination of the drug product for compatibility of the ingredients, and based on marketing experience with the drug product to indicate that there is no degradation of the product for the normal or expected period of use.

(2) Evaluation of stability shall be based on the same container-closure system in which the drug product is being marketed.

(d) Allergenic extracts that are labeled "No U.S. Standard of Potency" are exempt from the requirements of this section.

§ 211.167 Special testing requirements.

(a) For each batch of drug product purporting to be sterile and/or pyrogen-free, there shall be appropriate laboratory testing to determine conformance to such requirements. The test procedures shall be in writing and shall be followed.

(b) For each batch of ophthalmic ointment, there shall be appropriate testing to determine conformance to specifications regarding the presence of foreign particles and harsh or abrasive substances. The test procedures shall be in writing and shall be followed.

(c) For each batch of controlled-release dosage form, there shall be appropriate laboratory testing to determine conformance to the specifications for the rate of release of each active ingredient. The test procedures shall be in writing and shall be followed.

§ 211.170 Reserve samples.

(a) An appropriately identified reserve sample that is representative of each lot in each shipment of each active ingredient shall be retained. The reserve sample consists of at least twice the quantity necessary for all tests required to determine whether the active ingredient meets its established specifications, except for sterility and pyrogen testing. The retention time is as follows:

(1) For an active ingredient in a drug product other than those described in paragraphs (a) (2) and (3) of this section, the reserve sample shall be retained for 1 year after the expiration date of the last lot of the drug product containing the active ingredient.

(2) For an active ingredient in a radioactive drug product, except for nonradioactive reagent kits, the reserve sample shall be retained for:

(i) Three months after the expiration date of the last lot of the drug product containing the active ingredient if the expiration dating period of the drug product is 30 days or less; or

(ii) Six months after the expiration date of the last lot of the drug product containing the active ingredient if the expiration dating period of the drug product is more than 30 days.

(3) For an active ingredient in an OTC drug product that is exempt from bearing an expiration date under §211.137, the reserve sample shall be retained for 3 years after distribution of the last lot of the drug product containing the active ingredient.

(b) An appropriately identified reserve sample that is representative of each lot or batch of drug product shall be retained and stored under conditions consistent with product labeling. The reserve sample shall be stored in the same immediate container-closure system in which the drug product is marketed or in one that has essentially the same characteristics. The reserve sample consists of at least twice the quantity necessary to perform all the required tests, except those for sterility and pyrogens. Reserve samples, except those drug products described in paragraph (b) (2), shall be examined visually at least once a year for evidence of deterioration unless visual examination would affect the integrity of the reserve samples. Any evidence of reserve sample deterioration shall be investigated in accordance with §211.192. The results of the examination shall be

recorded and maintained with other stability data on the drug product. Reserve samples of compressed medical gases need not be retained. The retention time is as follows:

(1) For a drug product other than those described in paragraphs (b) (2) and (3) of this section, the reserve sample shall be retained for 1 year after the expiration date of the drug product.

(2) For a radioactive drug product, except for nonradioactive reagent kits, the reserve sample shall be retained for:

(i) Three months after the expiration date of the drug product if the expiration dating period of the drug product is 30 days or less; or

(ii) Six months after the expiration date of the drug product if the expiration dating period of the drug product is more than 30 days.

(3) For an OTC drug product that is exempt from bearing an expiration date under § 211.137, the reserve sample must be retained for 3 years after the lot or batch of drug product is distributed.

§ 211.173 Laboratory animals.

Animals used in testing components, in-process materials, or drug products for compliance with established specifications shall be maintained and controlled in a manner that assures their suitability for their intended use. They shall be identified, and adequate records shall be maintained showing the history of their use.

§ 211.176 Penicillin contamination.

If a reasonable possibility exists that a non-penicillin drug product has been exposed to cross-contamination with penicillin, the non-penicillin drug product shall be tested for the presence of penicillin. Such drug product shall not be marketed if detectable levels are found when tested according to procedures specified in 'Procedures for Detecting and Measuring Penicillin Contamination in Drugs,' which is incorporated by reference. Copies are available from the Bureau of Drugs (HFD-430), Food and Drug Administration, 200 C St., SW., Washington, D. C. 20204, or available for inspection at the Office of the Federal Register, 1100 L St. NW., Washington, D. C. 20408. [ED. NOTE—The Bureau of Drugs (HFD-430) is now designated as National Center for Drugs and Biologics (HFN-416).]

Subpart J—Records and Reports

§ 211.180 General requirements.

(a) Any production, control, or distribution record that is required to be maintained in compliance with this part and is specifically associated with a batch of a drug product shall be retained for at least 1 year after the expiration date of the batch or, in the case of certain OTC drug products lacking expiration dating because they meet the criteria for exemption under §211.137, 3 years after distribution of the batch.

(b) Records shall be maintained for all components, drug product containers, closures, and labeling for at least 1 year after the expiration date or, in the case of certain OTC drug products lacking expiration dating because they meet the criteria for exemption under §211.137, 3 years after distribution of the last lot of drug product incorporating the component or using the container, closure, or labeling.

(c) All records required under this part, or copies of such records, shall be readily available for authorized inspection during the retention period at the establishment where the activities described in such records occurred. These records or copies thereof shall be subject to photocopying or other means of reproduction as part of such inspection. Records that can be immediately retrieved from another location by computer or other electronic means shall be considered as meeting the requirements of this paragraph.

(d) Records required under this part may be retained either as original records or as true copies such as photocopies, microfilm, microfiche, or other accurate reproductions of the original records. Where reduction techniques, such as microfilming, are used, suitable reader and photocopying equipment shall be readily available.

(e) Written records required by this part shall be maintained so that data therein can be used for evaluating, at least annually, the quality standards of each drug product to determine the need for changes in drug product specifications or manufacturing or control procedures. Written procedures shall be established and followed for such evaluations and shall include provisions for:

(1) A review of every batch, whether approved or rejected, and, where applicable, records associated with the batch.

(2) A review of complaints, recalls, returned or salvaged drug products, and investigations conducted under §211.192 for each drug product.

(f) Procedures shall be established to assure that the responsible officials of the firm, if they are not personally involved in or immediately aware of such actions, are notified in writing of any investigations conducted under §§211.198, 211.204, or 211.208 of these regulations, any recalls, reports of inspectional observations issued by the Food and Drug Administration, or any regulatory actions relating to good manufacturing practices brought by the Food and Drug Administration.

§ 211.182   Equipment cleaning and use log.

A written record of major equipment cleaning, maintenance (except routine maintenance such as lubrication and adjustments), and use shall be included in individual equipment logs that show the date, time, product, and lot number of each batch processed. If equipment is dedicated to manufacture of one product, then individual equipment logs are not required, provided that lots or batches of such product follow in numerical order and are manufactured in numerical sequence. In cases where dedicated equipment is employed, the records of cleaning, maintenance, and use shall be part of the batch record. The persons performing and double-checking the cleaning and maintenance shall date and sign or initial the log indicating that the work was performed. Entries in the log shall be in chronological order.

§ 211.184   Component, drug product container, closure, and labeling records.

These records shall include the following:

(a) The identity and quantity of each shipment of each lot of components, drug product containers, closures, and labeling; the name of the supplier; the supplier's lot number(s) if known; the receiving code as specified in §211.80; and the date of receipt. The name and location of the prime manufacturer, if different from the supplier, shall be listed if known.

(b) The results of any test or examination performed (including those performed as required by §211.82 (a), §211.84 (d), or §211.122 (a)) and the conclusions derived therefrom.

(c) An individual inventory record of each component, drug product container, and closure and, for each component, a reconciliation of the use of each lot of such component. The inventory record shall contain sufficient information to allow determination of any batch or lot of drug product associated with the use of each component, drug product container, and closure.

(d) Documentation of the examination and review of labels and labeling for conformity with established specifications in accord with §§211.122 (c) and 211.130 (c).

(e) The disposition of rejected components, drug product containers, closure, and labeling.

§ 211.186   Master production and control records.

(a) To assure uniformity from batch to batch, master production and control records for each drug product, including each batch size thereof, shall be prepared, dated, and signed (full signature, handwritten) by one person and independently checked, dated, and signed by a second person. The preparation of master production and control records shall be described in a written procedure and such written procedure shall be followed.

(b) Master production and control records shall include:

(1) The name and strength of the product and a description of the dosage form;

(2) The name and weight or measure of each active ingredient per dosage unit or per unit of weight or measure of the drug product, and a statement of the total weight or measure of any dosage unit;

(3) A complete list of components designated by names or codes sufficiently specific to indicate any special quality characteristic;

(4) An accurate statement of the weight or measure of each component, using the same weight system (metric, avoirdupois, or apothecary) for each component. Reasonable variations may be permitted, however, in the amount of components necessary for the preparation in the dosage form, provided they are justified in the master production and control records;

(5) A statement concerning any calculated excess of component;

(6) A statement of theoretical weight or measure at appropriate phases of processing;

(7) A statement of theoretical yield, including the maximum and minimum percentages of theoretical yield beyond which investigation according to §211.192 is required;

(8) A description of the drug product containers, closures, and packaging materials, including a specimen or copy of each label and all other labeling signed and dated by the person or persons responsible for approval of such labeling;

(9) Complete manufacturing and control instructions, sampling and testing procedures, specifications, special notations, and precautions to be followed.

§ 211.188   Batch production and control records.

Batch production and control records shall be prepared for each batch of drug product produced and shall include complete information relating to the production and control of each batch. These records shall include:

(a) An accurate reproduction of the appropriate master production or control record, checked for accuracy, dated, and signed;

(b) Documentation that each significant step in the manufacture, processing, packing, or holding of the batch was accomplished, including:

(1) Dates;

(2) Identity of individual major equipment and lines used;

(3) Specific identification of each batch of component or in-process material used;

(4) Weights and measures of components used in the course of processing;

(5) In-process and laboratory control results;

(6) Inspection of the packaging and labeling area before and after use;

(7) A statement of the actual yield and a statement of the percentage of theoretical yield at appropriate phases of processing;

(8) Complete labeling control records, including specimens or copies of all labeling used;

(9) Description of drug product containers and closures;

(10) Any sampling performed;

(11) Identification of the persons performing and directly supervising or checking each significant step in the operation;

(12) Any investigation made according to §211.192;

(13) Results of examinations made in accordance with §211.134.

§ 211.192 Production record review.

All drug product production and control records, including those for packaging and labeling, shall be reviewed and approved by the quality control unit to determine compliance with all established, approved written procedures before a batch is released or distributed. Any unexplained discrepancy (including a percentage of theoretical yield exceeding the maximum or minimum percentages established in master production and control records) or the failure of a batch or any of its components to meet any of its specifications shall be thoroughly investigated, whether or not the batch has already been distributed. The investigation shall extend to other batches of the same drug product and other drug products that may have been associated with the specific failure or discrepancy. A written record of the investigation shall be made and shall include the conclusions and followup.

§ 211.194 Laboratory records.

(a) Laboratory records shall include complete data derived from all tests necessary to assure compliance with established specifications and standards, including examinations and assays, as follows:

(1) A description of the sample received for testing with identification of source (that is, location from where sample was obtained), quantity, lot number or other distinctive code, date sample was taken, and date sample was received for testing.

(2) A statement of each method used in the testing of the sample. The statement shall indicate the location of data that establish that the methods used in the testing of the sample meet proper standards of accuracy and reliability as applied to the product tested. (If the method employed is in the current revision of the United States Pharmacopeia, National Formulary, Association of Official Analytical Chemists, Book of Methods,* or in other recognized standard references, or is detailed in an approved new drug application and the referenced method is not modified, a statement indicating the method and reference will suffice). The suitability of all testing methods used shall be verified under actual conditions of use.

(3) A statement of the weight or measure of sample used for each test, where appropriate.

(4) A complete record of all data secured in the course of each test, including all graphs, charts, and spectra from laboratory instrumentation, properly identified to show the specific component, drug product container, closure, in-process material, or drug product, and lot tested.

(5) A record of all calculations performed in connection with the test, including units of measure, conversion factors, and equivalency factors.

(6) A statement of the results of tests and how the results compare with established standards of identity, strength, quality, and purity for the component, drug product container, closure, in-process material, or drug product tested.

(7) The initials or signature of the person who performs each test and the date(s) the tests were performed.

(8) The initials or signature of a second person showing that the original records have been reviewed for accuracy, completeness, and compliance with established standards.

(b) Complete records shall be maintained of any modification of an established method employed in testing. Such records shall include the reason for the modification and data to verify that the modification produced results that are at least as accurate and reliable for the material being tested as the established method.

(c) Complete records shall be maintained of any testing and standardization of laboratory reference standards, reagents, and standard solutions.

(d) Complete records shall be maintained of the periodic calibration of laboratory instruments, apparatus, gauges, and recording devices required by §211.160 (b) (4).

(e) Complete records shall be maintained of all stability testing performed in accordance with §211.166.

---

*Copies may be obtained from: Association of Official Analytical Chemists, P.O. Box 540, Benjamin Franklin Station, Washington, DC 20204.

---

§ 211.196 Distribution records.

Distribution records shall contain the name and strength of the product and a description of the dosage form, name and address of the consignee, date and quantity shipped, and lot or control number of the drug product.

§ 211.198 Complaint files.

(a) Written procedures describing the handling of all written and oral complaints regarding a drug product shall be established and followed. Such procedures shall include provisions for review by the quality control unit, of any complaint involving the possible failure of a drug product to meet any of its specifications and, for such drug products, a determination as to the need for an investigation in accordance with §211.192.

(b) A written record of each complaint shall be maintained in a file designated for drug product complaints. The file regarding such drug product complaints shall be maintained at the establishment where the drug product involved was manufactured, processed, or packed, or such file may be maintained at another facility if the written records in such files are readily available for inspection at that other facility. Written records involving a drug product shall be maintained until at least 1 year after the expiration date of the drug product, or 1 year after the date that the complaint was received, whichever is longer. In the case of certain OTC drug products lacking expiration dating because they meet the criteria for exemption under §211.137, such written records shall be maintained for 3 years after distribution of the drug product.

(1) The written record shall include the following information, where known: the name and strength of the drug product, lot number, name of complainant, nature of complaint, and reply to complainant.

(2) Where an investigation under §211.192 is conducted, the written record shall include the findings of the investigation and followup. The record or copy of the record of the investigation shall be maintained at the establishment where the investigation occurred in accordance with §211.180 (c).

(3) Where an investigation under §211.192 is not conducted, the written record shall include the reason that an investigation was found not to be necessary and the name of the responsible person making such a determination.

Subpart K—Returned and Salvaged Drug Products

§ 211.204 Returned drug products.

Returned drug products shall be identified as such and held. If the conditions under which returned drug products have been held, stored, or shipped before or during their return, or if the condition of the drug product, its container, carton, or labeling, as a result of storage or shipping, casts doubt on the safety, identity, strength, quality or purity of the drug product, the returned drug product shall be destroyed unless examination, testing, or other investigations prove the drug product meets appropriate standards of safety, identity, strength, quality, or purity. A drug product may be reprocessed provided the subsequent drug product meets appropriate standards, specifications, and characteristics. Records of returned drug products shall be maintained and shall include the name and label potency of the drug product dosage form, lot number (or control number or batch number), reason for the return, quantity returned, date of disposition, and ultimate disposition of the returned drug product. If the reason for a drug product being returned implicates associated batches, an appropriate investigation shall be conducted in accordance with the requirements of §211.192. Procedures for the holding, testing, and reprocessing of returned drug products shall be in writing and shall be followed.

§ 211.208 Drug product salvaging.

Drug products that have been subjected to improper storage conditions including extremes in temperature, humidity, smoke, fumes, pressure, age, or radiation due to natural disasters, fires, accidents, or equipment failures shall not be salvaged and returned to the marketplace. Whenever there is a question whether drug products have been subjected to such conditions, salvaging operations may be conducted only if there is (a) evidence from laboratory tests and assays (including animal feeding studies where applicable) that the drug products meet all applicable standards of identity, strength, quality, and purity and (b) evidence from inspection of the premises that the drug products and their associated packaging were not subjected to improper storage conditions as a result of the disaster or accident. Organoleptic examinations shall be acceptable only as supplemental evidence that the drug products meet appropriate standards of identity, strength, quality, and purity. Records including name, lot number, and disposition shall be maintained for drug products subject to this section.

⟨1141⟩ PACKAGING—CHILD-SAFETY

The Poison Prevention Packaging Act is administered and enforced by the Consumer Product Safety Commission of the federal government. The purpose of the law is to decrease the chance that children may obtain access to poisons. The act applies not only to drugs, but also to other household substances. The Commission is authorized to promulgate regulations providing standards for special packaging of any household substance where that special packaging will help to protect children from serious injury or illness resulting from the handling, using, or ingesting of such substance. Special packaging of this type is not necessarily packaging that all children under 5 years of age cannot open, but is packaging that makes it difficult for most children under the age of 5 to open the package or to obtain a harmful amount of the contents. On the other hand, the packaging should not be difficult for normal adults to open.

Not all hazardous household substances are subject to special packaging requirements. However, once a special packaging requirement is published, special packaging becomes the rule, and conventional packaging the exception. There are basically four ways by which exceptions are allowed for drugs:

(1) The substance is specifically exempted by regulation;

(2) If the drug is dispensed on prescription, the prescriber directs in the prescription order that it be dispensed in a non-complying package;

(3) The purchaser of a prescription drug so requests;

(4) The manufacturer (or packer) of a drug for sale without prescription may provide a single-size, noncomplying package provided it bears conspicuous labeling stating, "This package for households without young children," or, if the package is small, stating, "Package not child-resistant," and provided the manufacturer also supplies the substance in complying packages.

The Commission has taken the view that in the case of prescription drugs, the manufacturer has the primary responsibility to provide special packaging where the manufacturer places the drug in a container clearly intended to be utilized in dispensing the drug for use in the home. If the pharmacist transfers a drug from the manufacturer's container to a dispensing container, the responsibility shifts to him. The fact that a manufacturer fails to provide suitable dispensing packaging does not relieve the pharmacist of this responsibility. It should be noted also that there is no special exemption for single-unit or unit-dose packages in the Act. Therefore, in order to comply, such unit packages, if they do not meet child-resistant standards, are to be placed in an outer package that does comply. Drugs placed in containers having dual-purpose closures must be dispensed in the child-resistant mode unless the physician has specified, or the patient has requested, the conventional mode.

Although special packaging should not be difficult for normal adults to open, it is recognized that some individuals having physical limitations, e.g., some elderly persons or arthritics, may have difficulties. Where pharmacists are aware of such infirmities, the proper procedure is to make the patient aware that non-complying packages are available for his or her prescription medication and that the choice is his or hers, with regard to the need for taking into account the likelihood of young children's gaining access to the medication.

Failure to dispense a drug in a child-resistant container where such is required may be a violation of the Federal Food, Drug, and Cosmetic Act (misbranding). Where a question may arise with regard to whether or not a particular container meets the requirements of the Poison Prevention Packaging Act, the manufacturer or the supplier should be consulted.

A child-resistant container that meets the requirements of the Poison Prevention Packaging Act is required to meet also the requirements of the Federal Food, Drug, and Cosmetic Act, and, if it is used to contain an official drug, the requirements of the official compendia. Because safety closures may lose their effectiveness through repeated opening and closing, replacement of the container and/or the cap should be made if the prescription is refilled.

There is no prohibition against utilizing safety packaging in those instances where the Consumer Product Safety Commission does not require it.

Where a non-complying container is dispensed upon the request of a patient, written documentation is advisable. Although there is no statutory requirement that this be done, such documentation might be important in the event that a subsequent question arises, such as in a negligence suit. A blanket waiver is permissible, but this option is limited to the purchaser.

Problems or defects with child-safety containers may be reported through the Drug Product Problem Reporting Program. Reports received through this program are forwarded to the Consumer Product Safety Commission by the Food and Drug Administration. Questions concerning compliance with the law should be directed to the Consumer Product Safety Commission, Washington, D. C. 20207.

Following are the standards and protocol for testing special packaging. (See also first paragraph under *The Poison Prevention Packaging Act and Regulations*.)

§ 1700.15 Poison prevention packaging standards.

To protect children from serious personal injury or serious illness resulting from handling, using, or ingesting household substances, the Commission has determined that packaging designed and constructed to meet the following standards shall be regarded as "special packaging" within the meaning of section 2(4) of the act. Specific application of these standards to substances requiring special packaging is in accordance with § 1700.14.

(a) *General requirements.* The special packaging must continue to function with the effectiveness specifications set forth in paragraph (b) of this section when in actual contact with the substance contained therein. This requirement may be satisfied by appropriate scientific evaluation of the compatibility of the substance with the special packaging to determine that the chemical and physical characteristics of the substance will not compromise or interfere with the proper functioning of the special packaging. The special packaging must also continue to function with the effectiveness specifications set forth in paragraph (b) of this section for the number of openings and closings customary for its size and contents. This requirement may be satisfied by appropriate technical evaluation based on physical wear and stress factors, force required for activation, and other such relevant factors which establish that, for the duration of normal use, the effectiveness specifications of the packaging would not be expected to lessen.

(b) *Effectiveness specifications.* Special packaging, tested by the method described in § 1700.20, shall meet the following specifications:

(1) Child-resistant effectiveness of not less than 85 percent without a demonstration and not less than 80 percent after a demonstration of the proper means of opening such special packaging. In the case of unit packaging, child-resistant effectiveness of not less than 80 percent.

(2) Adult-use effectiveness of not less than 90 percent.

(c) *Reuse of special packaging.* Special packaging for substances subject to the provisions of this paragraph shall not be reused.

(d) *Restricted flow.* Special packaging subject to the provisions of this paragraph shall be special packaging from which the flow of liquid is so restricted that not more than 2 milliliters of the contents can be obtained when the inverted, opened container is shaken or squeezed once or when the container is otherwise activated once.

§ 1700.20   Testing procedure for special packaging.

(a) The protocol for testing "special packaging" as defined in section 2(4) of the act shall be as follows:

(1) Use 200 children between the ages of 42 and 51 months inclusive, evenly distributed by age and sex, to test the ability of the special packaging to resist opening by children. The even age distribution shall be determined by having 20 children (plus or minus 10 percent) whose nearest age is 42 months, 20 whose nearest age is 43 months, 20 at 44 months, etc., up to and including 20 at 51 months of age. There should be no more than a 10 percent preponderance of either sex in each age group. The children selected should be healthy and normal and should have no obvious or overt physical or mental handicap.

(2) The children shall be divided into groups of two each. The testing shall be done in a location that is familiar to the children; for example, their customary nursery school or regular kindergarten. No child shall test more than two special packages, and each package shall be of a different type. For each test, the paired children shall receive the same special packaging simultaneously. When more than one special packaging is being tested, they shall be presented to the paired children in random order, and this order shall be recorded. The special packaging, each test unit of which, if appropriate, has previously been opened and properly resecured by the tester, shall be given to each of the two children with a request for them to open it. (In the case of unit packaging, it shall be presented exposed so that the individual units are immediately available to the child.) Each child shall be allowed up to 5 minutes to open the special packaging. For those children unable to open the special packaging after the first 5 minutes, a single visual demonstration, without verbal explanation, shall be given by the demonstrator. A second 5 minutes shall then be allowed for opening the special packaging. (In the case of unit packaging, a single visual demonstration, without verbal explanation, will be provided at the end of the first 5 minutes only for those test subjects who have not opened at least one unit package, and a second 5 minutes

allowed for all subjects.) If a child fails to use his teeth to open the special packaging during the first 5 minutes, the demonstrator shall instruct him, before the start of the second 5-minute period, that he is permitted to use his teeth if he wishes.

(3) Records shall be kept on the number of children who were and were not able to open the special packaging, with and without demonstration. (In the case of unit packaging, records shall be kept on the number of individual units opened or gained access to by each child.) The percent of child-resistant effectiveness shall be the number of children tested, less the test failures, divided by two. A test failure shall be any child who opens the special packaging or gains access to its contents. In the case of unit packaging, however, a test failure shall be any child who opens or gains access to the number of individual units which constitute the amount that may produce serious personal injury or serious illness, or a child who opens or gains access to more than 8 individual units, whichever number is lower, during the full 10 minutes of testing. The determination of the amount of a substance that may produce serious personal injury or serious illness shall be based on a 25-pound child. Manufacturers or packagers intending to use unit packaging for a substance requiring special packaging are requested to submit such toxicological data to the Commission.

(4) One hundred adults, age 18 to 45 years inclusive, with no overt physical or mental handicaps, and 70 percent of whom are female, shall comprise the test panel for normal adults. The adults shall be tested individually, rather than in groups of two or more. The adults shall receive only such printed instructions on how to open and properly resecure the special packaging as will appear on the package as it is delivered to the consumer. Five minutes shall be allowed to complete the opening and, if appropriate, the resecuring process.

(5) Records shall be kept on the number of adults unable to open and the number of the other adults tested who fail to properly resecure the special packaging. The number of adults who successfully open the special packaging and then properly resecure the special packaging (if resecuring is appropriate) is the percent of adult-use effectiveness of the special packaging. In the case of unit packaging, the percent of adult-use effectiveness shall be the number of adults who successfully open a single package.

(b) The standards published as regulations issued for the purpose of designating particular substances as being subject to the requirements for special packaging under the act will stipulate the percent of child-resistant effectiveness and adult-use effectiveness required for each and, where appropriate, will include any other conditions deemed necessary and provided for in the act.

(c) It is recommended that manufacturers of special packaging, or producers of substances subject to regulations issued pursuant to the act, submit to the Commission summaries of data resulting from tests conducted in accordance with this protocol.

THE POISON PREVENTION PACKAGING ACT AND REGULATIONS

Selective portions of the Poison Prevention Packaging Act and Regulations promulgated thereunder that are believed to be of most interest to practitioners and students of pharmacy and medicine are presented here as a service to the professions and with the cooperation of the Consumer Product Safety Commission. The publication of these sections in The United States Pharmacopeia is for purposes of information and does not impart to them any legal effect.

SEC. 2. For the purpose of this Act—

(2) The term "household substance" means any substance which is customarily produced or distributed for sale for consumption or use, or customarily stored, by individuals in or about the household and which is—

(A) a hazardous substance as that term is defined in section 2(f) of the Federal Hazardous Substances Act (15 U.S.C. 1261(f));

(B) an economic poison as that term is defined in section 2a of the Federal Insecticide, Fungicide, and Rodenticide Act (7 U.S.C. 135(a));

(C) a food, drug, or cosmetic as those terms are defined in section 201 of the Federal Food, Drug, and Cosmetic Act (21 U.S.C. 321); or

(D) a substance intended for use as fuel when stored in a portable container and used in the heating, cooking, or refrigeration system of a house.

(3) The term "package" means the immediate container or wrapping in which any household substance is contained for consumption, use, or storage by individuals in or about the household, and, for purposes of section 4(a)(2) of this Act, also means any outer container or wrapping used in the retail display of any such substances to consumers. Such term does not include—

(A) any shipping container or wrapping used solely for the transportation of any household substance in bulk or in quantity to manufacturers, packers, or processors, or to wholesale or retail distributors thereof, or

(B) any shipping container or outer wrapping used by retailers to ship or deliver any household substance to consumers unless it is the only such container or wrapping.

(4) The term "special packaging" means packaging that is designed or constructed to be significantly difficult for children under five years of age to open or obtain a toxic or harmful amount of the substance contained therein within a reasonable time and not difficult for normal adults to use properly, but does not mean packaging which all such children cannot open or obtain a toxic or harmful amount within a reasonable time.

(5) The term "labeling" means all labels and other written, printed, or graphic matter (A) upon any household substance or its package, or (B) accompanying such substance.

SEC. 3. (a) The Secretary, after consultation with the technical advisory committee provided for in section 6 of this Act, may establish in accordance with the provisions of this Act, by regulation, standards for the special packaging of any household substance if he finds that—

(1) the degree or nature of the hazard to children in the availability of such substance, by reason of its packaging, is such that special packaging is required to protect children from serious personal injury or serious illness resulting from handling, using, or ingesting such substance; and

(2) the special packaging to be required by such standard is technically feasible, practicable, and appropriate for such substance.

(b) In establishing a standard under this section, the Secretary shall consider—

(1) the reasonableness of such standard;

(2) available scientific, medical, and engineering data concerning special packaging and concerning childhood accidental ingestions, illness, and injury caused by household substances;

(3) the manufacturing practices of industries affected by this Act; and

(4) the nature and use of the household substance.

(c) In carrying out this Act, the Secretary shall publish his findings, his reasons therefor, and citation of the sections of statutes which authorize his action.

(d) Nothing in this Act shall authorize the Secretary to prescribe specific packaging designs, product content, package quantity, or, with the exception of authority granted in section 4(a) (2) of this Act, labeling. In the case of a household substance for which special packaging is required pursuant to a regulation under this section, the Secretary may in such regulation prohibit the packaging of such substance in packages which he determines are unnecessarily attractive to children.

SEC. 4. (a) For the purpose of making any household substance which is subject to a standard established under section 3 readily available to elderly or handicapped persons unable to use such substance when packaged in compliance with such standard, the manufacturer or packer, as the case may be, may package any household substance, subject to such a standard, in packaging of a single size which does not comply with such standard if—

(1) the manufacturer (or packer) also supplies such substance in packages which comply with such standard; and

(2) the packages of such substances which do not meet such standard bear conspicuous labeling stating: "This package for households without young children"; except that the Secretary may by regulation prescribe a substitute statement to the same effect for packaging too small to accommodate such labeling.

(b) In the case of a household substance which is subject to such a standard and which is dispensed pursuant to an order of a physician, dentist, or other licensed medical practitioner authorized to prescribe, such substance may be dispensed in noncomplying packages only when directed in such order or when requested by the purchaser.

(c) In the case of a household substance subject to such a standard which is packaged under subsection (a) in a noncomplying package, if the Secretary determines that such substance is not also being supplied by a manufacturer (or packer) in popular size packages which comply with such standard, he may, after giving the manufacturer (or packer) an opportunity to comply with the purposes of this Act, by order require such substance to be packaged by such manufacturer (or packer) exclusively in special packaging complying with such standard if he finds, after opportunity for hearing, that such exclusive use of special packaging is necessary to accomplish the purposes of this Act.

SEC. 502 [352]. A drug or device shall be deemed to be misbranded—

"(p) If it is a drug and its packaging or labeling is in violation of an applicable regulation issued pursuant to section 3 or 4 of the Poison Prevention Packaging Act of 1970."

Poison Prevention Packaging Act of 1970 Regulations

§ 1700.14 Substances requiring special packaging.

(a) *Substances.* The Commission has determined that the degree or nature of the hazard to children in the availability of the following substances, by reason of their packaging, is such that special packaging is required to protect children from serious personal injury or serious illness resulting from handling, using, or ingesting such substances, and that the special packaging herein required is technically feasible, practicable, and appropriate for these substances:

(1) *Aspirin.* Any aspirin-containing preparation for human use in a dosage form intended for oral administration shall be packaged in accordance with the provisions of § 1700.15(a), (b), and (c), except the following:

(i) Effervescent tablets containing aspirin, other than those intended for pediatric use, provided the dry tablet contains not more than 15 percent aspirin and has an oral LD-50 in rats of 5 grams or more per kilogram of body weight.

(ii) Unflavored aspirin-containing preparations in powder form (other than those intended for pediatric use) that are packaged in unit doses providing not more than 15.4 grains of aspirin per unit dose and that contain no other substance subject to the provisions of this section.

(3) *Methyl salicylate.* Liquid preparations containing more than 5 percent by weight of methyl salicylate, other than those packaged in pressurized spray containers, shall be packaged in accordance with the provisions of § 1700.15(a), (b), and (c).

(4) *Controlled drugs.* Any preparation for human use that consists in whole or in part of any substance subject to control under the Comprehensive Drug Abuse Prevention and Control Act of 1970 (21 U.S.C. 801 et seq.) and that is in a dosage form intended for oral administration shall be packaged in accordance with the provisions of § 1700.15(a), (b), and (c).

(6) *Turpentine.* Household substances in liquid form containing 10 percent or more by weight of turpentine shall be packaged in accordance with the provisions of § 1700.15(a) and (b).

(10) *Prescription drugs.* Any drug for human use that is in a dosage form intended for oral administration and that is required by Federal law to be dispensed only by or upon an oral or written prescription of a practitioner licensed by law to administer such drug shall be packaged in accordance with the provisions of § 1700.15(a), (b), and (c), except for the following:

(i) Sublingual dosage forms of nitroglycerin.

(ii) Sublingual and chewable forms of isosorbide dinitrate in dosage strengths of 10 milligrams or less.

(iii) Erythromycin ethylsuccinate granules for oral suspension and oral suspensions in packages containing not more than 8 grams of the equivalent of erythromycin.

(iv) Cyclically administered oral contraceptives in manufacturers' mnemonic (memory-aid) dispenser packages that rely solely upon the activity of one or more progestogen or estrogen substances.

(v) Anhydrous cholestyramine in powder form.

(vi) All unit-dose forms of potassium supplements, including individually wrapped effervescent tablets, unit-dose vials of liquid potassium, and powdered potassium in unit-dose packets, containing not more than 50 milliequivalents of potassium per unit dose.

(vii) Sodium fluoride drug preparations, including liquid and tablet forms, containing no more than 264 milligrams of sodium fluoride per package and containing no other substances subject to this § 1700.14(a)(10).

(viii) Betamethasone tablets packaged in manufacturers' dispenser packages, containing no more than 12.6 milligrams betamethasone.

(ix) Pancrelipase preparations in tablet, capsule, or powder form and containing no other substances subject to this § 1700.14(a)(10).

(x) Prednisone in tablet form, when dispensed in packages containing no more than 105 mg of the drug, and containing no other substances subject to this §1700.14(a)(10).

(xiii) Mebendazole in tablet form in packages containing not more than 600 mg of the drug, and containing no other substance subject to the provisions of this section.

(xiv) Methylprednisolone in tablet form in packages containing not more than 84 mg of the drug and containing no other substance subject to the provisions of this section.

(xv) Colestipol in powder form in packages containing not more than 5 grams of the drug and containing no other substance subject to the provisions of this section.

(xvi) Erythromycin ethylsuccinate tablets in packages containing no more than the equivalent of 16 grams erythromycin.

(xvii) Conjugated Estrogen Tablets, USP, when dispensed in mnemonic packages containing not more than 32 mg of the drug and containing no other substances subject to this § 1700.14(a)(10).

(xviii) Norethindrone Acetate Tablets, USP, when dispensed in mnemonic packages containing not more than 50 mg of the drug and containing no other substances subject to this § 1700.14(a)(10).

(xix) Medroxyprogesterone acetate tablets.

(12) *Iron-containing drugs.* With the exception of: (i) Animal feeds used as vehicles for the administration of drugs, and (ii) those preparations in which iron is present solely as a colorant, noninjectable animal and human drugs providing iron for therapeutic or prophylactic purposes, and containing a total amount of elemental iron, from any source, in a single package, equivalent to 250 mg or more elemental iron in a concentration of 0.025 percent or more on a weight to volume basis for liquids and 0.05 percent or more on a weight-to-weight basis for nonliquids (e.g., powders, granules, tablets, capsules, wafers, gels, viscous products, such as pastes and ointments, etc.) shall be packaged in accordance with the provisions of § 1700.15(a), (b), and (c).

(13) *Dietary supplements containing iron.* With the exception of those preparations in which iron is present solely as a colorant, dietary supplements, as defined in § 1700.1(a)(3), that contain an equivalent of 250 mg or more of elemental iron, from any source, in a single package in concentrations of 0.025 percent or more on a weight to volume basis for liquids and 0.05 percent or more on a weight-to-weight basis for nonliquids (e.g., powders, granules, tablets, capsules, wafers, gels, viscous products, such as pastes and ointments, etc.) shall be packaged in accordance with the provisions of § 1700.15(a), (b), and (c).

(16) *Acetaminophen.* Preparations for human use in a dosage form intended for oral administration and containing in a single package a total of more than one gram acetaminophen shall be packaged in accordance with the provisions of § 1700.15(a), (b), and (c), except the following—

(i) Effervescent tablets or granules containing acetaminophen, provided the dry tablet or granules contain less than 15 percent acetaminophen, the tablet or granules have an oral LD-50 of 5 grams or greater per kilogram of body weight, and the tablet or granules contain no other substance subject to the provisions of this section.

(ii) Unflavored acetaminophen-containing preparations in powder form (other than those intended for pediatric use) that are packaged in unit doses providing not more than 13 grains of acetaminophen per unit dose and that contain no other substance subject to this § 1700.14(a).

(17) *Diphenhydramine.* Preparations for human use in a dosage form intended for oral administration and containing more than the equivalent of 66 mg diphenhydramine base in a single package shall be packaged in accordance with the provisions of § 1700.15(a), (b), and (c), if packaged on or after February 11, 1985.

Guide to General Chapters

General Tests and Assays

General Requirements for Tests and Assays

⟨ 1⟩ Injections
⟨ 11⟩ USP Reference Standards

Apparatus for Tests and Assays

⟨ 16⟩ Automated Methods of Analysis
⟨ 21⟩ Thermometers
⟨ 31⟩ Volumetric Apparatus
⟨ 41⟩ Weights and Balances

Microbiological Tests

⟨ 51⟩ Antimicrobial Preservatives—Effectiveness
⟨ 61⟩ Microbial Limit Tests
⟨ 71⟩ Sterility Tests

Biological Tests and Assays

⟨ 81⟩ Antibiotics—Microbial Assays
⟨ 85⟩ Bacterial Endotoxins Test
⟨ 87⟩ Biological Reactivity Tests, In-vitro
⟨ 88⟩ Biological Reactivity Tests, In-vivo
⟨ 91⟩ Calcium Pantothenate Assay
⟨101⟩ Depressor Substances Test
⟨111⟩ Design and Analysis of Biological Assays
⟨115⟩ Dexpanthenol Assay
⟨121⟩ Insulin Assay
⟨141⟩ Protein—Biological Adequacy Test
⟨151⟩ Pyrogen Test
⟨161⟩ Transfusion and Infusion Assemblies
⟨171⟩ Vitamin B$_{12}$ Activity Assay

Chemical Tests and Assays

IDENTIFICATION TESTS

⟨181⟩ Identification—Organic Nitrogenous Bases
⟨191⟩ Identification Tests—General
⟨193⟩ Identification—Tetracyclines
⟨201⟩ Thin-layer Chromatographic Identification Test

LIMIT TESTS

⟨211⟩ Arsenic
⟨216⟩ Calcium, Potassium, and Sodium
⟨221⟩ Chloride and Sulfate
⟨224⟩ Dioxane
⟨226⟩ 4-Epianhydrotetracycline
⟨231⟩ Heavy Metals
⟨241⟩ Iron
⟨251⟩ Lead
⟨261⟩ Mercury
⟨271⟩ Readily Carbonizable Substances Test
⟨281⟩ Residue on Ignition
⟨291⟩ Selenium

OTHER TESTS AND ASSAYS

⟨301⟩ Acid-neutralizing Capacity
⟨311⟩ Alginates Assay
⟨321⟩ Alkaloidal Drug Assays; Proximate Assays
⟨331⟩ Amphetamine Assay
⟨341⟩ Antimicrobial Agents—Content
⟨351⟩ Assay for Steroids
⟨361⟩ Barbiturate Assay
⟨371⟩ Cobalamin Radiotracer Assay
⟨381⟩ Elastomeric Closures for Injections
⟨391⟩ Epinephrine Assay
⟨401⟩ Fats and Fixed Oils
⟨411⟩ Folic Acid Assay
⟨421⟩ Hydroxypropoxy Determination
⟨425⟩ Iodometric Assay—Antibiotics
⟨431⟩ Methoxy Determination
⟨441⟩ Niacin or Niacinamide Assay
⟨451⟩ Nitrite Titration
⟨461⟩ Nitrogen Determination
⟨466⟩ Ordinary Impurities
⟨468⟩ Oxygen Determination
⟨471⟩ Oxygen Flask Combustion
⟨475⟩ Penicillin G Determination
⟨481⟩ Riboflavin Assay
⟨501⟩ Salts of Organic Nitrogenous Bases
⟨511⟩ Single-steroid Assay
⟨521⟩ Sulfonamides
⟨531⟩ Thiamine Assay
⟨541⟩ Titrimetry
⟨551⟩ Alpha Tocopherol Assay

⟨561⟩ Vegetable Drugs—Sampling and Methods of Analysis
⟨571⟩ Vitamin A Assay
⟨581⟩ Vitamin D Assay
⟨591⟩ Zinc Determination

Physical Tests and Determinations

⟨601⟩ Aerosols
⟨611⟩ Alcohol Determination
⟨621⟩ Chromatography
⟨631⟩ Color and Achromicity
⟨641⟩ Completeness of Solution
⟨651⟩ Congealing Temperature
⟨661⟩ Containers
⟨671⟩ Containers—Permeation
⟨691⟩ Cotton
⟨695⟩ Crystallinity
⟨701⟩ Disintegration
⟨711⟩ Dissolution
⟨721⟩ Distilling Range
⟨724⟩ Drug Release
⟨726⟩ Electrophoresis
⟨731⟩ Loss on Drying
⟨733⟩ Loss on Ignition
⟨736⟩ Mass Spectrometry
⟨741⟩ Melting Range or Temperature
⟨751⟩ Metal Particles in Ophthalmic Ointments
⟨755⟩ Minimum Fill
⟨761⟩ Nuclear Magnetic Resonance
⟨771⟩ Ophthalmic Ointments
⟨781⟩ Optical Rotation
⟨785⟩ Osmolarity
⟨788⟩ Particulate Matter in Injections
⟨791⟩ pH
⟨801⟩ Polarography
⟨811⟩ Powder Fineness
⟨821⟩ Radioactivity
⟨831⟩ Refractive Index
⟨841⟩ Specific Gravity
⟨851⟩ Spectrophotometry and Light-scattering
⟨861⟩ Sutures—Diameter
⟨871⟩ Sutures—Needle Attachment
⟨881⟩ Tensile Strength
⟨891⟩ Thermal Analysis
⟨901⟩ Ultraviolet Absorbance of Citrus Oils
⟨905⟩ Uniformity of Dosage Units
⟨911⟩ Viscosity
⟨921⟩ Water Determination
⟨941⟩ X-ray Diffraction

General Information

⟨1001⟩ Antacid Effectiveness
⟨1035⟩ Biological Indicators
⟨1041⟩ Biologics
⟨1051⟩ Cleaning Glass Apparatus
⟨1061⟩ Color—Instrumental Measurement
⟨1071⟩ Controlled Substances Act Regulations
⟨1076⟩ Federal Food, Drug and Cosmetic Act Requirements Relating to Drugs for Human Use
⟨1077⟩ Good Manufacturing Practice for Finished Pharmaceuticals
⟨1081⟩ Gel Strength of Gelatin
⟨1086⟩ Impurities in Official Articles
⟨1091⟩ Labeling of Inactive Ingredients
⟨1101⟩ Medicine Dropper
⟨1111⟩ Microbiological Attributes of Nonsterile Pharmaceutical Products
⟨1121⟩ Nomenclature
⟨1141⟩ Packaging—Child-safety

⟨1151⟩ Pharmaceutical Dosage Forms
⟨1171⟩ Phase-solubility Analysis
⟨1176⟩ Prescription Balances and Volumetric Apparatus
⟨1181⟩ Scanning Electron Microscopy
⟨1191⟩ Stability Considerations in Dispensing Practice

⟨1211⟩ Sterilization and Sterility Assurance of Compendial
       Articles
⟨1221⟩ Teaspoon
⟨1225⟩ Validation of Compendial Methods
⟨1231⟩ Water for Pharmaceutical Purposes
⟨1241⟩ Water-solid Interactions in Pharmaceutical Systems

III

Section III

CHEMISTRY AND COMPENDIAL REQUIREMENTS

ACACIA

Description: Acacia NF—Practically odorless.

NF category: Emulsifying and/or solubilizing agent; suspending and/or viscosity-increasing agent; tablet binder.

Solubility: Acacia NF—Insoluble in alcohol. One gram dissolves in 2 mL of water; the resulting solution flows readily and is acid to litmus.

NF requirements: Acacia NF—Preserve in tight containers. Acacia is the dried gummy exudate from the stems and branches of *Acacia senegal* (Linné) Willdenow or of other related African species of *Acacia* (Fam. Leguminosae). Meets the requirements for Botanic characteristics, Identification, Microbial limit, Specific rotation ($-25°$ to $-35°$, calculated on the anhydrous basis, determined on a 1.0% w/v solution), Water (not more than 15.0%), Total ash (not more than 4.0%), Acid-insoluble ash (not more than 0.5%), Insoluble residue (not more than 50 mg), Arsenic (3 ppm), Lead (0.001%), Heavy metals (0.004%), Starch or dextrin, Tannin-bearing gums, and Organic volatile impurities.

ACEBUTOLOL

Chemical name: Acebutolol hydrochloride—Butanamide, N-[3-acetyl-4-[2-hydroxy-3-[(1-methylethyl)amino]propoxy]-phenyl]-, ($\pm$)-, monohydrochloride.

Molecular formula: Acebutolol hydrochloride—$C_{18}H_{28}N_2O_4 \cdot HCl$.

Molecular weight: Acebutolol hydrochloride—372.9.

Description: Acebutolol hydrochloride—White or slightly off-white powder. The melting point is 141–145 °C.

pKa: 9.20.

Solubility: Freely soluble in water; less soluble in alcohol.

Other characteristics: Lipid solubility—Low.

USP requirements:
Acebutolol Hydrochloride Capsules—Not in USP.
Acebutolol Hydrochloride Tablets—Not in USP.

ACETAMINOPHEN

Chemical name: Acetamide, N-(4-hydroxyphenyl)-.

Molecular formula: $C_8H_9NO_2$.

Molecular weight: 151.16.

Description: Acetaminophen USP—White, odorless, crystalline powder.

Solubility: Acetaminophen USP—Soluble in boiling water and in 1 N sodium hydroxide; freely soluble in alcohol.

USP requirements:
Acetaminophen USP—Preserve in tight, light-resistant containers. Contains not less than 98.0% and not more than 101.0% of acetaminophen, calculated on the anhydrous basis. Meets the requirements for Identification, Melting range (168–172 °C), Water (not more than 0.5%), Residue on ignition (not more than 0.1%), Chloride (not more than 0.014%), Sulfate (not more than 0.02%), Sulfide, Heavy metals (not more than 0.001%), Readily carbonizable substances, Free *p*-aminophenol (not more than 0.005%), *p*-Chloroacetanilide (not more than 0.001%), and Organic volatile impurities.

Acetaminophen Capsules USP—Preserve in tight containers. Contain the labeled amount, within ± 10%. Meet the requirements for Identification, Dissolution (75% in 45 minutes in water in Apparatus 2 at 50 rpm), and Uniformity of dosage units.

Acetaminophen Oral Solution USP—Preserve in tight containers. Contains the labeled amount, within ± 10%. Meets the requirements for Identification, pH (3.8–6.1), and Alcohol content, if present (the labeled amount, within −10% to +15%).

Acetaminophen Suppositories USP—Preserve in well-closed containers, in a cool place. Contain the labeled amount, within ± 10%. Meet the requirement for Identification.

Acetaminophen Oral Suspension USP—Preserve in tight containers. A suspension of acetaminophen in a suitable aqueous vehicle. Contains the labeled amount, within ± 10%. Meets the requirements for Identification and pH (4.5–6.9).

Acetaminophen Tablets USP—Preserve in tight containers. Label Tablets that must be chewed to indicate that they are to be chewed before swallowing. Contain the labeled amount, within ± 10%. Meet the requirements for Identification, Dissolution (80% in 30 minutes in pH 5.8 phosphate buffer in Apparatus 2 at 50 rpm), and Uniformity of dosage units.

Acetaminophen Wafers—Not in USP.

ACETAMINOPHEN AND ASPIRIN

For *Acetaminophen* and *Aspirin*—See individual listings for chemistry information.

USP requirements: Acetaminophen and Aspirin Tablets USP—Preserve in tight containers. Contain the labeled amounts of acetaminophen and aspirin, within ± 10%. Meet the requirements for Identification, Dissolution (75% of each ingredient in 45 minutes in water in Apparatus 2 at 50 rpm), Uniformity of dosage units, and Salicylic acid (not more than 3.0%).

ACETAMINOPHEN, ASPIRIN, AND CAFFEINE

For *Acetaminophen*, *Aspirin*, and *Caffeine*—See individual listings for chemistry information.

USP requirements:
Acetaminophen, Aspirin, and Caffeine Capsules USP—Preserve in tight containers. Contain the labeled amounts of

III

acetaminophen, aspirin, and caffeine, within ±10%. Meet the requirements for Identification, Dissolution (75% of each ingredient in 45 minutes in water in Apparatus 1 at 100 rpm), Uniformity of dosage units, and Salicylic acid (not more than 3.0%).

Acetaminophen, Aspirin, and Caffeine Oral Powders—Not in USP.

Acetaminophen, Aspirin, and Caffeine Tablets USP—Preserve in well-closed containers. Contain the labeled amounts of acetaminophen, aspirin, and caffeine, within ±10%. Meet the requirements for Identification, Dissolution (75% of each ingredient in 60 minutes in water in Apparatus 2 at 100 rpm), Uniformity of dosage units, and Salicylic acid (not more than 3.0%).

Buffered Acetaminophen, Aspirin, and Caffeine Tablets—Not in USP.

ACETAMINOPHEN, ASPIRIN, CODEINE, MAGNESIUM HYDROXIDE, AND ALUMINUM HYDROXIDE

For *Acetaminophen, Aspirin, Codeine, Magnesia* (Magnesium Hydroxide), and *Alumina* (Aluminum Hydroxide)—See individual listings for chemistry information.

USP requirements: Buffered Acetaminophen, Aspirin, and Codeine Phosphate Tablets—Not in USP.

ACETAMINOPHEN, ASPIRIN, AND SALICYLAMIDE

For *Acetaminophen, Aspirin*, and *Salicylamide*—See individual listings for chemistry information.

USP requirements: Buffered Acetaminophen, Aspirin, and Salicylamide Tablets—Not in USP.

ACETAMINOPHEN, ASPIRIN, SALICYLAMIDE, AND CAFFEINE

For *Acetaminophen, Aspirin, Salicylamide*, and *Caffeine*—See individual listings for chemistry information.

USP requirements: Acetaminophen, Aspirin, Salicylamide, and Caffeine Tablets—Not in USP.

ACETAMINOPHEN, ASPIRIN, SALICYLAMIDE, CODEINE, AND CAFFEINE

For *Acetaminophen, Aspirin, Salicylamide, Codeine*, and *Caffeine*—See individual listings for chemistry information.

USP requirements: Acetaminophen, Aspirin, Salicylamide, Codeine Phosphate, and Caffeine Tablets—Not in USP.

ACETAMINOPHEN AND CAFFEINE

For *Acetaminophen* and *Caffeine*—See individual listings for chemistry information.

USP requirements:

Acetaminophen and Caffeine Capsules USP—Preserve in tight containers. Contain the labeled amounts of acetaminophen and caffeine (anhydrous), within ±10%. Meet the requirements for Identification, Dissolution (75% of the labeled amounts of acetaminophen and caffeine in 45 minutes in water in Apparatus 1 at 100 rpm), and Uniformity of dosage units.

Acetaminophen and Caffeine Tablets USP—Preserve in tight containers. Contain the labeled amounts of acetaminophen and caffeine (anhydrous), within ±10%. Meet the requirements for Identification, Dissolution (75% of the labeled amounts of acetaminophen and caffeine in 60 minutes in water in Apparatus 2 at 100 rpm), and Uniformity of dosage units.

ACETAMINOPHEN, CALCIUM CARBONATE, POTASSIUM AND SODIUM BICARBONATES, AND CITRIC ACID

For *Acetaminophen, Calcium Carbonate, Potassium Bicarbonate, Sodium Bicarbonate*, and *Citric Acid*—See individual listings for chemistry information.

USP requirements: Acetaminophen Effervescent Tablets for Oral Solution—Not in USP.

ACETAMINOPHEN AND CODEINE

For *Acetaminophen* and *Codeine*—See individual listings for chemistry information.

USP requirements:

Acetaminophen and Codeine Phosphate Capsules USP—Preserve in tight, light-resistant containers. Contain the labeled amounts of acetaminophen and of codeine phosphate, within ±10%. Meet the requirements for Identification, Dissolution (75% of each ingredient in 30 minutes in 0.1 N hydrochloric acid in Apparatus 2 at 50 rpm), and Uniformity of dosage units.

Acetaminophen and Codeine Phosphate Elixir USP—Preserve in tight, light-resistant containers. Contains the labeled amounts of acetaminophen and codeine phosphate, within ±10%. Meets the requirements for Identification, pH (4.0–6.1), and Alcohol content (6.0–8.5%).

Acetaminophen and Codeine Phosphate Oral Suspension—Not in USP.

Acetaminophen and Codeine Phosphate Tablets USP—Preserve in tight, light-resistant containers. Contain the labeled amounts of acetaminophen and of codeine phosphate, within ±10%. Meet the requirements for Identification, Dissolution (75% of each ingredient in 45 minutes in 0.1 N hydrochloric acid in Apparatus 2 at 50 rpm), and Uniformity of dosage units.

ACETAMINOPHEN, CODEINE, AND CAFFEINE

For *Acetaminophen, Codeine*, and *Caffeine*—See individual listings for chemistry information.

USP requirements:

Acetaminophen, Codeine Phosphate, and Caffeine Capsules—Not in USP.

Acetaminophen, Codeine Phosphate, and Caffeine Tablets—Not in USP.

ACETAMINOPHEN AND DIPHENHYDRAMINE

For *Acetaminophen* and *Diphenhydramine*—See individual listings for chemistry information.

USP requirements: Acetaminophen and Diphenhydramine Citrate Tablets USP—Preserve in tight containers. Contain the labeled amounts of acetaminophen and diphenhydramine citrate, within ±10%. Meet the requirements for Identification, Dissolution (75% in 45 minutes in water in Apparatus 2 at 50 rpm), and Uniformity of dosage units.

ACETAMINOPHEN AND SALICYLAMIDE

For *Acetaminophen* and *Salicylamide*—See individual listings for chemistry information.

USP requirements:

Acetaminophen and Salicylamide Capsules—Not in USP.

Acetaminophen and Salicylamide Tablets—Not in USP.

ACETAMINOPHEN, SALICYLAMIDE, AND CAFFEINE

For *Acetaminophen*, *Salicylamide*, and *Caffeine*—See individual listings for chemistry information.

USP requirements:

Acetaminophen, Salicylamide, and Caffeine Capsules—Not in USP.
Acetaminophen, Salicylamide, and Caffeine Tablets—Not in USP.

ACETAMINOPHEN, SODIUM BICARBONATE, AND CITRIC ACID

For *Acetaminophen*, *Sodium Bicarbonate*, and *Citric Acid*—See individual listings for chemistry information.

USP requirements: Acetaminophen for Effervescent Oral Solution USP—Preserve in tight containers. Contains not less than 5.63 grams and not more than 6.88 grams of acetaminophen in each 100 grams. Meets the requirements for Identification and Minimum fill (when packaged in multiple-unit containers) or Uniformity of dosage units (when packaged in single-unit containers).

ACETAZOLAMIDE

Chemical name:

Acetazolamide—Acetamide, *N*-[5-(aminosulfonyl)-1,3,4-thiadiazol-2-yl]-.
Acetazolamide sodium [sterile]—Acetamide, *N*-[5-(aminosulfonyl)-1,3,4-thiadiazol-2-yl]-, monosodium salt.

Molecular formula:

Acetazolamide—$C_4H_6N_4O_3S_2$.
Acetazolamide sodium [sterile]—$C_4H_5N_4NaO_3S_2$.

Molecular weight:

Acetazolamide—222.24.
Acetazolamide sodium [sterile]—244.22.

Description:

Acetazolamide USP—White to faintly yellowish white, crystalline, odorless powder.
Sterile Acetazolamide Sodium USP—White solid, having the characteristic appearance of freeze-dried products.

Solubility: Acetazolamide USP—Very slightly soluble in water; sparingly soluble in practically boiling water; slightly soluble in alcohol.

USP requirements:

Acetazolamide USP—Preserve in well-closed containers. Contains not less than 98.0% and not more than 102.0% of acetazolamide, calculated on the anhydrous basis. Meets the requirements for Identification, Water (not more than 0.5%), Residue on ignition (not more than 0.1%), Chloride (0.014%), Sulfate (0.04%), Selenium (0.003%, a 200-mg specimen being used), Heavy metals (not more than 0.002%), Silver-reducing substances (not less than 4.8 mL of 0.1 *N* ammonium thiocyanate is required), Ordinary impurities, and Organic volatile impurities.
Acetazolamide Extended-release Capsules—Not in USP.
Acetazolamide Tablets USP—Preserve in well-closed containers. Contain the labeled amount, within ±5%. Meet the requirements for Identification, Dissolution (not less than 75% in 60 minutes in 0.1 *N* hydrochloric acid in Apparatus 1 at 100 rpm), and Uniformity of dosage units.
Sterile Acetazolamide Sodium USP—Preserve in Containers for Sterile Solids, preferably of Type III glass. It is prepared from Acetazolamide with the aid of Sodium Hydroxide. It is suitable for parenteral use. The contents of each container, when constituted as directed in the labeling, yields a solution containing an amount of acetazolamide sodium equivalent to the labeled amount of acetazolamide, within −5% to +10%. Meets the requirements for Completeness of solution, Constituted solution, Identification, Bacterial endotoxins, pH (9.0–10.0, in a freshly prepared solution [1 in 10]), Sterility tests, Uniformity of dosage units, and Labeling under Injections.

ACETIC ACID

Chemical name:

Acetic acid—Acetic acid.
Acetic acid, glacial—Acetic acid.

Molecular formula: Acetic acid, glacial—$C_2H_4O_2$.

Molecular weight: Acetic acid, glacial—60.05.

Description:

Acetic Acid NF—Clear, colorless liquid, having a strong, characteristic odor. Specific gravity is about 1.045.
NF category: Acidifying agent; buffering agent.
Glacial Acetic Acid USP—Clear, colorless liquid, having a pungent, characteristic odor. Boils at about 118 °C. Specific gravity is about 1.05.
NF category: Acidifying agent.

Solubility:

Acetic Acid NF—Miscible with water, with alcohol, and with glycerin.
Glacial Acetic Acid USP—Miscible with water, with alcohol, and with glycerin.

USP requirements:

Acetic Acid Irrigation USP—Preserve in single-dose containers, preferably of Type I or Type II glass. It may be packaged in suitable plastic containers. A sterile solution of Glacial Acetic Acid in Water for Injection. Contains, in each 100 mL, not less than 237.5 mg and not more than 262.5 mg of glacial acetic acid. Meets the requirements for Identification, Bacterial endotoxins, pH (2.8–3.4), and Injections, except that the container in which it is packaged may be designed to empty rapidly and may exceed 1000 mL in capacity.
Acetic Acid Otic Solution USP—Preserve in tight containers. A solution of Glacial Acetic Acid in a suitable nonaqueous solvent. Contains an amount of glacial acetic acid equivalent to the labeled amount, within −15% to +30%. Meets the requirements for Identification and pH (2.0–4.0, when diluted with an equal volume of water).
Glacial Acetic Acid USP—Preserve in tight containers. Contains not less than 99.5% and not more than 100.5%, by weight, of glacial acetic acid. Meets the requirements for Identification, Congealing temperature (not lower than 15.6 °C), Nonvolatile residue (not more than 1.0 mg), Chloride, Sulfate, Heavy metals (not more than 5 ppm), and Readily oxidizable substances.

NF requirements: Acetic Acid NF—Preserve in tight containers. A solution. Contains not less than 36.0% and not more than 37.0%, by weight, of acetic acid. Meets the requirements for Identification, Nonvolatile residue (not more than 1.0 mg [0.005%]), Chloride, Sulfate, Heavy metals (not more than 0.001%), Readily oxidizable substances, and Organic volatile impurities.

ACETOHEXAMIDE

Chemical group: Sulfonylurea.

Chemical name: Benzenesulfonamide, 4-acetyl-*N*-[[cyclohexylamino]carbonyl]-.

Molecular formula: $C_{15}H_{20}N_2O_4S$.

Molecular weight: 324.39.

Description: Acetohexamide USP—White, crystalline, practically odorless powder.

Solubility: Acetohexamide USP—Practically insoluble in water and in ether; soluble in pyridine and in dilute solutions of alkali hydroxides; slightly soluble in alcohol and in chloroform.

USP requirements:
Acetohexamide USP—Preserve in well-closed containers. Contains not less than 97.0% and not more than 101.0% of acetohexamide, calculated on the dried basis. Meets the requirements for Identification, Melting range (182.5–187 °C), Loss on drying (not more than 1.0%), Selenium (0.003%, a 200-mg specimen mixed with 200 mg of magnesium oxide being used), Residue on ignition (not more than 0.1%), Heavy metals (not more than 0.002%), and Organic volatile impurities.
Acetohexamide Tablets USP—Preserve in well-closed containers. Contain the labeled amount, within ± 7%. Meet the requirements for Identification, Dissolution (50% in 60 minutes in pH 7.6 phosphate buffer in Apparatus 1 at 100 rpm), and Uniformity of dosage units.

ACETOHYDROXAMIC ACID

Chemical name: Acetamide, N-hydroxy-.

Molecular formula: $C_2H_5NO_2$.

Molecular weight: 75.07.

Description: Acetohydroxamic Acid USP—White, slightly hygroscopic, crystalline powder. Melts, after drying at about 80 °C for 2 to 4 hours, at about 88 °C.

pKa: 9.32.

Solubility: Acetohydroxamic Acid USP—Freely soluble in water and in alcohol; very slightly soluble in chloroform.

Other characteristics: Chelates metals, especially iron.

USP requirements:
Acetohydroxamic Acid USP—Preserve in tight containers, and store in a cool, dry place. Acetohydroxamic Acid is dried over phosphorus pentoxide for 16 hours. Contains not less than 98.0% and not more than 101.0% of acetohydroxamic acid. Meets the requirements for Completeness of solution, Color of solution (absorbance not greater than 0.050), Identification, Loss on drying (not more than 1.0%), Residue on ignition (not more than 0.1%), Heavy metals (not more than 0.002%), Hydroxylamine (not more than 0.5%), and Organic volatile impurities.
Acetohydroxamic Acid Tablets USP—Preserve in tight containers. Contain the labeled amount, within ± 10%. Meet the requirements for Identification, Dissolution (85% in 30 minutes in water in Apparatus 1 at 100 rpm), Uniformity of dosage units, and Hydroxylamine (not more than 0.5%).

ACETONE

Chemical name: 2-Propanone.

Molecular formula: C_3H_6O.

Molecular weight: 58.08.

Description: Acetone NF—Transparent, colorless, mobile, volatile liquid, having a characteristic odor. A solution (1 in 2) is neutral to litmus.
NF category: Solvent.

Solubility: Acetone NF—Miscible with water, with alcohol, with ether, with chloroform, and with most volatile oils.

NF requirements: Acetone NF—Preserve in tight containers, remote from fire. Contains not less than 99.0% of acetone, calculated on the anhydrous basis. Meets the requirements for Identification, Specific gravity (not more than 0.789), Water (0.5%), Nonvolatile residue (not more than 0.004%), Readily oxidizable substances, and Organic volatile impurities.
Caution: Acetone is very flammable. Do not use where it may be ignited.

ACETOPHENAZINE

Chemical group: Piperazine phenothiazine.

Chemical name: Acetophenazine maleate—Ethanone, 1-[10-[3-[4-(2-hydroxyethyl)-1-piperazinyl]propyl]-10H-phenothiazin-2-yl]-, (Z) 2-butenedioate (1:2) (salt).

Molecular formula: Acetophenazine maleate—$C_{23}H_{29}N_3O_2S \cdot 2C_4H_4O_4$.

Molecular weight: Acetophenazine maleate—643.71.

Description: Acetophenazine Maleate USP—Fine, yellow powder. Melts at about 165 °C, with decomposition.

Solubility: Acetophenazine Maleate USP—Soluble in water; slightly soluble in acetone and in alcohol.

USP requirements:
Acetophenazine Maleate USP—Preserve in tight, light-resistant containers. Acetophenazine Maleate is dried at 65 °C for 4 hours. Contains not less than 97.0% and not more than 103.0% of acetophenazine maleate. Meets the requirements for Identification, Loss on drying (not more than 0.5%), Residue on ignition (not more than 0.1%), Ordinary impurities, and Organic volatile impurities.
Acetophenazine Maleate Tablets USP—Preserve in tight, light-resistant containers. Contain the labeled amount, within ± 10%. Meet the requirements for Identification, Dissolution (75% in 45 minutes in 0.1 N hydrochloric acid in Apparatus 2 at 50 rpm), and Uniformity of dosage units.

ACETYLCHOLINE

Chemical name: Acetylcholine chloride—Ethanaminium, 2-(acetyloxy)-N,N,N-trimethyl-, chloride.

Molecular formula: Acetylcholine chloride—$C_7H_{16}ClNO_2$.

Molecular weight: Acetylcholine chloride—181.66.

Description: Acetylcholine Chloride USP—White or off-white crystals or crystalline powder.

Solubility: Acetylcholine Chloride USP—Very soluble in water; freely soluble in alcohol; insoluble in ether. Is decomposed by hot water and by alkalies.

USP requirements:
Acetylcholine Chloride USP—Preserve in tight containers. Contains not less than 98.0% and not more than 102.0% of acetylcholine chloride, calculated on the dried basis. Meets the requirements for Identification, Melting range (149–152 °C), Acidity, Loss on drying (not more than

1.0%), Residue on ignition (not more than 0.2%), Chloride content (19.3–19.8%, calculated on dried basis), and Organic volatile impurities.

Acetylcholine Chloride for Ophthalmic Solution USP—Preserve in Containers for Sterile Solids. A sterile mixture of Acetylcholine Chloride with Mannitol or other suitable diluent, prepared by freeze-drying. Contains the labeled amount, within −10% to +15%. Meets the requirements for Constituted solution, Identification, Acidity, Water (not more than 1.0%), Sterility tests, and Uniformity of dosage units.

ACETYLCYSTEINE

Source: The N-acetyl derivative of the naturally occurring amino acid, L-cysteine.

Chemical name: L-Cysteine, *N*-acetyl-.

Molecular formula: $C_5H_9NO_3S$.

Molecular weight: 163.19.

Description: Acetylcysteine USP—White, crystalline powder, having a slight acetic odor.

Solubility: Acetylcysteine USP—Freely soluble in water and in alcohol; practically insoluble in chloroform and in ether.

USP requirements:

Acetylcysteine USP—Preserve in tight containers. Contains not less than 98.0% and not more than 102.0% of acetylcysteine, calculated on the dried basis. Meets the requirements for Identification, Melting range (104–110 °C), Specific rotation (+21° to +27°), pH (2.0–2.8, in a solution [1 in 100]), Loss on drying (not more than 1.0%), Residue on ignition (not more than 0.5%), Heavy metals (not more than 0.001%), and Organic volatile impurities.

Acetylcysteine Injection—Not in USP.

Acetylcysteine Solution USP—Preserve in single-unit or in multiple-unit tight containers that effectively exclude oxygen. A sterile solution of Acetylcysteine in water, prepared with the aid of Sodium Hydroxide. Contains the labeled amount, within ±10%. Meets the requirements for Identification, Sterility, and pH (6.0–7.5).

ACETYLCYSTEINE AND ISOPROTERENOL

For *Acetylcysteine* and *Isoproterenol*—See individual listings for chemistry information.

USP requirements: Acetylcysteine and Isoproterenol Hydrochloride Inhalation Solution USP—Preserve in single-dose or in multiple-dose containers, preferably of Type I glass, tightly closed with a glass or polyethylene closure. A sterile solution of Acetylcysteine and Isoproterenol Hydrochloride in water. The label indicates that the Inhalation Solution is not to be used if its color is pinkish or darker than slightly yellow or if it contains a precipitate. Contains the labeled amounts of acetylcysteine, within ±10%, and isoproterenol hydrochloride, within −10% to +15%. Meets the requirements for Color and clarity, Identification, Sterility, and pH (6.0–7.0).

ACRISORCIN

Chemical name: 1,3-Benzenediol, 4-hexyl-, compd. with 9-acridinamine (1:1).

Molecular formula: $C_{12}H_{18}O_2 \cdot C_{13}H_{10}N_2$.

Molecular weight: 388.51

Description: Acrisorcin USP—Yellow, odorless powder. Melts at about 190 °C, with decomposition.

Solubility: Acrisorcin USP—Very slightly soluble in water and in ether; soluble in alcohol; slightly soluble in chloroform.

USP requirements:

Acrisorcin USP—Preserve in well-closed containers. Contains not less than 97.0% and not more than 101.0% of acrisorcin, calculated on the dried basis. Meets the requirements for Identification, Loss on drying (not more than 1.0%), and Residue on ignition (not more than 0.2%).

Acrisorcin Cream USP—Preserve in collapsible tubes or in tight containers. It is Acrisorcin in a suitable water-miscible base. Contains the labeled amount, within ±10%. Meets the requirements for Identification and Minimum fill.

ACYCLOVIR

Chemical group: Synthetic acyclic purine nucleoside analog.

Chemical name:

Acyclovir—6*H*-Purin-6-one, 2-amino-1,9-dihydro-9-[(2-hydroxyethoxy)methyl]-.

Acyclovir sodium—6*H*-Purin-6-one, 2-amino-1,9-dihydro-9-[(2-hydroxyethoxy)methyl]-, monosodium salt.

Molecular formula:

Acyclovir—$C_8H_{11}N_5O_3$.

Acyclovir sodium—$C_8H_{10}N_5NaO_3$.

Molecular weight:

Acyclovir—225.21.

Acyclovir sodium—247.19.

Description: Acyclovir USP—White to off-white crystalline powder. Melts at temperatures higher than 250 °C, with decomposition.

Solubility: Acyclovir USP—Soluble in 0.1 N hydrochloric acid; sparingly soluble in water; insoluble in alcohol.

USP requirements:

Acyclovir USP—Preserve in tight containers. Contains not less than 98.0% and not more than 101.0% of acyclovir, calculated on the anhydrous basis. Meets the requirements for Identification, Water (not more than 6.0%), Ordinary impurities, and Organic volatile impurities.

Acyclovir Capsules—Not in USP.

Acyclovir Ointment—Not in USP.

Acyclovir Oral Suspension—Not in USP.

Acyclovir Tablets—Not in USP.

Sterile Acyclovir Sodium—Not in USP.

ADENINE

Chemical name: 1*H*-Purin-6-amine.

Molecular formula: $C_5H_5N_5$.

Molecular weight: 135.13.

Description: Adenine USP—White crystals or crystalline powder. Is odorless.

Solubility: Adenine USP—Very slightly soluble in water; sparingly soluble in boiling water; slightly soluble in alcohol; practically insoluble in ether and in chloroform.

USP requirements: Adenine USP—Preserve in well-closed containers. Contains not less than 98.0% and not more than 102.0% of adenine, calculated on the dried basis. Meets the requirements for Identification, Loss on drying (not more than 1.0%), Residue on ignition (not more than 0.1%), Heavy metals (0.001%), Organic impurities, Nitrogen content (50.2–53.4%, calculated on the dried basis), and Organic volatile impurities.

ADENOSINE

Chemical name: Adenosine.

Molecular formula: $C_{10}H_{13}N_5O_4$.

Molecular weight: 267.24.

Description: White crystalline powder.

Solubility: Soluble in water; practically insoluble in alcohol.

USP requirements: Adenosine Injection—Not in USP.

AGAR

Description: Agar NF—Odorless or has a slight odor.
  NF category: Suspending and/or viscosity-increasing agent.

Solubility: Agar NF—Insoluble in cold water; soluble in boiling water.

NF requirements: Agar NF—Agar is the dried, hydrophilic, colloidal substance extracted from *Gelidium cartilagineum,* (Linné) Gaillon (Fam. Gelidiaceae), *Gracilaria confervoides,* (Linné) Greville (Fam. Sphaerococcaceae), and related red algae (Class Rhodophyceae). Meets the requirements for Botanic characteristics, Identification, Microbial limit, Water (not more than 20.0%), Total ash (not more than 6.5%, on a dry-weight basis), Acid-insoluble ash (not more than 0.5%, on a dry-weight basis), Foreign organic matter (not more than 1.0%), Foreign insoluble matter (not more than 1.0%), Arsenic (not more than 3 ppm), Lead (not more than 0.001%), Heavy metals (not more than 0.004%), Foreign starch, Gelatin, and Water absorption.

MEDICAL AIR

USP requirements: Medical Air USP—Preserve in cylinders or in a low pressure collecting tank. Containers used for Medical Air are not to be treated with any toxic, sleep-inducing, or narcosis-producing compounds, and are not to be treated with any compound that would be irritating to the respiratory tract when the Medical Air is used. [Note—Reduce the container pressure by means of a regulator. Measure the gases with a gas volume meter downstream from the detector tube in order to minimize contamination or change of the specimens.] It is a natural or synthetic mixture of gases consisting largely of nitrogen and oxygen. Where it is piped directly from the collecting tank to the point of use, label each outlet "Medical Air." Contains not less than 19.5% and not more than 23.5%, by volume, of oxygen. Meets the requirements for Water and oil, Odor, Carbon dioxide (not more than 0.05%), Carbon monoxide (not more than 0.001%), Nitric oxide and nitrogen dioxide (not more than 2.5 ppm), and Sulfur dioxide (not more than 5 ppm).

ALANINE

Chemical name: L-Alanine.

Molecular formula: $C_3H_7NO_2$.

Molecular weight: 89.09.

Description: Alanine USP—White, odorless crystals or crystalline powder.

Solubility: Alanine USP—Freely soluble in water; slightly soluble in 80% alcohol; insoluble in ether.

USP requirements: Alanine USP—Preserve in well-closed containers. Contains not less than 98.5% and not more than 101.5% of alanine, as L-alanine, calculated on the dried basis. Meets the requirements for Identification, Specific rotation ($+13.7°$ to $+15.1°$, calculated on the dried basis), pH (5.5–7.0 in a solution [1 in 20]), Loss on drying (not more than 0.2%), Residue on ignition (not more than 0.15%), Chloride (0.05%), Sulfate (0.03%), Arsenic (1.5 ppm), Iron (0.003%), Heavy metals (not more than 0.0015%), and Organic volatile impurities.

ALBENDAZOLE

Chemical name: Carbamic acid, [5-(propylthio)-1*H*-benzimidazol-2-yl]-, methyl ester.

Molecular formula: $C_{12}H_{15}N_3O_2S$.

Molecular weight: 265.33.

Description: Colorless crystals with a melting point of 208–210 °C.

USP requirements: Albendazole USP—Preserve in well-closed containers. Contains not less than 98.0% and not more than 102.0% of albendazole, calculated on the dried basis. Meets the requirements for Identification, Loss on drying (not more than 0.5%), Residue on ignition (not more than 0.2%), and Chromatographic purity.

ALBUMIN HUMAN

Description: Albumin Human USP—Practically odorless, moderately viscous, clear, brownish fluid.

USP requirements: Albumin Human USP—Preserve at the temperature indicated on the label. A sterile, non-pyrogenic preparation of serum albumin obtained by fractionating material (source blood, plasma, serum, or placentas) from healthy human donors, the source material being tested for the absence of hepatitis B surface antigen. It is made by a process that yields a product that is safe for intravenous use. Label it to state that it is not to be used if it is turbid and that it is to be used within 4 hours after the container is entered. Label it also to state the osmotic equivalent in terms of plasma, the sodium content, and the type of source material (venous plasma, placental plasma, or both) from which it was prepared. Label it also to indicate that additional fluids are needed when the 20-grams-per-100-mL or 25-grams-per-100-mL product is administered to a markedly dehydrated patient. Not less than 96% of its total protein is albumin. It is a solution containing, in each 100 mL, either 25 grams of serum albumin osmotically equivalent to 500 mL of normal human plasma, or 20 grams equivalent to 400 mL, or 5 grams equivalent to 100 mL, or 4 grams equivalent to 80 mL thereof, and contains not less than 93.75% and not more than 106.25% of the labeled amount in the case of the solution containing 4 grams in each 100 mL, and not less than 94.0% and not more than 106.0% of the labeled amount in the other cases. Contains no added antimicrobial agent, but may contain sodium acetyltryptophanate with or without sodium caprylate as a stabilizing agent. It has a sodium content of not less than 130 mEq per liter and not more than 160 mEq per liter. It has a heme content such that the absorbance of a solution, diluted to contain 1% of protein, in a 1-cm holding cell, measured at a wavelength of 403 nanometers, is not more than 0.25. Meets the requirements of the tests for heat stability and for pH, and for Expiration date (the expiration date is not later than 5 years after issue from manufacturer's cold storage [5 °C, 3 years] if labeling recommends storage between 2 and 10 °C; not later than 3 years after issue from manufacturer's cold storage [5 °C, 3 years] if labeling recommends storage at temperatures not higher than 37 °C; and not later than 10 years after date of manufacture if in a hermetically sealed metal container and labeling recommends storage between 2 and 10 °C). Conforms to the regulations of the U.S. Food and Drug Administration concerning biologics.

ALBUTEROL

Chemical name:
Albuterol—1,3-Benzenedimethanol, alpha¹-[[(1,1-dimethylethyl)amino]methyl]-4-hydroxy-.
Albuterol sulfate—1,3-Benzenedimethanol, alpha¹-[[(1,1-dimethylethyl)amino]methyl]-4-hydroxy-, sulfate (2:1) (salt).

Molecular formula:
Albuterol—$C_{13}H_{21}NO_3$.
Albuterol sulfate—$(C_{13}H_{21}NO_3)_2 \cdot H_2SO_4$.

Molecular weight:
Albuterol—239.31.
Albuterol sulfate—576.70.

Description:
Albuterol USP—White, crystalline powder. Melts at about 156 °C.
Albuterol Sulfate USP—White or practically white powder.

Solubility:
Albuterol USP—Sparingly soluble in water; soluble in alcohol.
Albuterol Sulfate USP—Freely soluble in water; slightly soluble in alcohol, in chloroform, and in ether.

USP requirements:
Albuterol USP—Preserve in well-closed, light-resistant containers. Contains not less than 98.5% and not more than 101.0% of albuterol, calculated on the anhydrous basis. Meets the requirements for Identification, Water (not more than 0.5%), Residue on ignition (not more than 0.1%), and Chromatographic purity (total impurities not greater than 2.0%).
Albuterol Inhalation Aerosol—Not in USP.
Albuterol Tablets USP—Preserve in well-closed, light-resistant containers. Label Tablets to state both the content of the active moiety and the content of the salt used in formulating the article. Contain an amount of albuterol sulfate equivalent to the labeled amount of albuterol, within ±10%. Meet the requirements for Identification, Dissolution (80% in 30 minutes in water in Apparatus 2 at 50 rpm), Uniformity of dosage units, and Related substances (not more than 3.5%).
Albuterol Sulfate USP—Preserve in well-closed, light-resistant containers. Contains not less than 98.5% and not more than 101.0% of albuterol sulfate, calculated on the anhydrous basis. Meets the requirements for Identification, Water (not more than 0.5%), Residue on ignition (not more than 0.1%), Chromatographic purity, and Organic volatile impurities.
Albuterol Sulfate for Inhalation—Not in USP.
Albuterol Sulfate Injection—Not in USP.
Albuterol Sulfate Inhalation Solution—Not in USP.
Albuterol Sulfate Oral Solution—Not in USP.
Albuterol Sulfate Syrup—Not in USP.
Albuterol Sulfate Extended-release Tablets—Not in USP.

ALCLOMETASONE

Chemical name: Alclometasone dipropionate—Pregna-1,4-diene-3,20-dione, 7-chloro-11-hydroxy-16-methyl-17,21-bis(1-oxopropoxy)-, (7 alpha,11 beta,16 alpha)-.

Molecular formula: Alclometasone dipropionate—$C_{28}H_{37}ClO_7$.

Molecular weight: Alclometasone dipropionate—521.05.

Description: Alclometasone dipropionate—White powder.

Solubility: Alclometasone dipropionate—Insoluble in water; slightly soluble in propylene glycol; moderately soluble in hexylene glycol.

USP requirements:
Alclometasone Dipropionate USP—Preserve in tight containers. Contains not less than 97.0% and not more than 102.0% of alclometasone dipropionate, calculated on the dried basis. Meets the requirements for Identification, Specific rotation (+21° to +25°, calculated on the dried basis, determined in a solution in dioxane containing 30 mg per mL), Loss on drying (not more than 0.5%), Residue on ignition (not more than 0.1%), Heavy metals (0.003%), and Chromatographic purity (not more than 3.0% of related compounds).
Alclometasone Dipropionate Cream USP—Preserve in collapsible tubes or in tight containers. Contains the labeled amount, within ±10%, in a suitable cream base. Meets the requirements for Identification, Microbial limits, and Minimum fill.
Alclometasone Dipropionate Ointment USP—Preserve in collapsible tubes or in tight containers. Contains the labeled amount, within ±10%, in a suitable ointment base. Meets the requirements for Identification, Microbial limits, and Minimum fill.

ALCOHOL

Chemical name: Ethanol.

Molecular formula: C_2H_6O.

Molecular weight: 46.07.

Description: Alcohol USP—Clear, colorless, mobile, volatile liquid. Has a characteristic odor. Is readily volatilized even at low temperatures, and boils at about 78 °C. Is flammable. NF category: Solvent.

Solubility: Alcohol USP—Miscible with water and with practically all organic solvents.

USP requirements: Alcohol USP—Preserve in tight containers, remote from fire. Contains not less than 92.3% and not more than 93.8%, by weight, corresponding to not less than 94.9% and not more than 96.0%, by volume, at 15.56 °C, of alcohol. Meets the requirements for Identification, Specific gravity (0.812–0.816 at 15.56 °C, indicating between 92.3% and 93.8%, by weight, or between 94.9 and 96.0%, by volume, of alcohol), Acidity (not more than 0.90 mL of 0.020 N sodium hydroxide is required for neutralization), Nonvolatile residue, Water-insoluble substances, Aldehydes and other foreign organic substances, Amyl alcohol and nonvolatile, carbonizable substances, etc., Fusel oil constituents, Acetone and isopropyl alcohol, and Methanol.

DEHYDRATED ALCOHOL

Chemical name: Ethanol.

Molecular formula: C_2H_6O.

Molecular weight: 46.07.

Description: Dehydrated Alcohol USP—Clear, colorless, mobile, volatile liquid. Has a characteristic odor. Is readily volatilized even at low temperatures, and boils at about 78 °C. Is flammable.

Solubility: Dehydrated Alcohol USP— Miscible with water and with practically all organic solvents.

USP requirements:

Dehydrated Alcohol USP—Preserve in tight containers, remote from fire. Contains not less than 99.2%, by weight, corresponding to not less than 99.5%, by volume, of alcohol at 15.56 °C. Meets the requirements for Identification, Specific gravity (not more than 0.7964 at 15.56 °C, indicating not less than 99.2% of alcohol by weight), Acidity (not more than 0.90 mL of 0.020 N sodium hydroxide required for neutralization), Nonvolatile residue, Water-insoluble substances, Aldehydes and other foreign organic substances, Amyl alcohol and nonvolatile, carbonizable substances, Ultraviolet absorbance (absorbance is not more than 0.30 at 220 nanometers, 0.18 at 230 nanometers, 0.08 at 240 nanometers, and 0.02 at 270 nanometers to 350 nanometers, the curve drawn through these points is smooth), Fusel oil constituents, Acetone and isopropyl alcohol, and Methanol.

Dehydrated Alcohol Injection USP—Preserve in single-dose containers, preferably of Type I glass. The container may contain an inert gas in the headspace. It is Dehydrated Alcohol suitable for parenteral use. Meets the requirements for Specific gravity (not more than 0.8035 at 15.56 °C, indicating not less than 96.8%, by weight, of alcohol) and Acidity (not more than 10.0 mL of 0.020 N sodium hydroxide is required for neutralization), for Identification, Nonvolatile residue, Water-insoluble substances, Aldehydes and other foreign organic substances, Amyl alcohol and nonvolatile, carbonizable substances, Ultraviolet absorbance, Fusel oil constituents, Acetone and isopropyl alcohol, and Methanol under Dehydrated Alcohol, and for Injections.

DILUTED ALCOHOL

Description: Diluted Alcohol NF—Clear, colorless, mobile liquid, having a characteristic odor.

NF category: Solvent.

NF requirements: Diluted Alcohol NF—Preserve in tight containers, remote from fire. A mixture of Alcohol and water. Contains not less than 41.0% and not more than 42.0%, by weight, corresponding to not less than 48.4% and not more than 49.5%, by volume, at 15.56 °C, of alcohol.

Prepare Diluted Alcohol as follows: 500 mL of Alcohol and 500 mL of Purified Water. Measure the Alcohol and the Purified Water separately at the same temperature, and mix. If the water and the Alcohol and the resulting mixture are measured at 25 °C, the volume of the mixture will be about 970 mL.

Meets the requirements for Specific gravity (0.935–0.937 at 15.56 °C, indicating 41.0–42.0%, by weight, or 48.4–49.5%, by volume, of alcohol), and for the tests under Alcohol, allowance being made for the difference in alcohol concentration.

RUBBING ALCOHOL

Description: Rubbing Alcohol USP—Transparent, colorless, or colored as desired, mobile, volatile liquid. Has, in the absence of added odorous constituents, a characteristic odor. Is flammable.

USP requirements: Rubbing Alcohol USP—Preserve in tight containers, remote from fire. Rubbing Alcohol and all preparations under the classification of Rubbing Alcohols are manufactured in accordance with the requirements of the U.S. Treasury Department, Bureau of Alcohol, Tobacco, and

Firearms, Formula 23-H (8 parts by volume of acetone, 1.5 parts by volume of methyl isobutyl ketone, and 100 parts by volume of ethyl alcohol) being used. Label it to indicate that it is flammable. Contains not less than 68.5% and not more than 71.5% by volume of dehydrated alcohol, the remainder consisting of water and the denaturants, with or without color additives, and perfume oils. Contains, in each 100 mL, not less than 355 mg of sucrose octaacetate or not less than 1.40 mg of denatonium benzoate. Meets the requirements for Specific gravity (0.8691–0.8771 at 15.56 °C), Nonvolatile residue (where the denaturant is sucrose octaacetate, not less than 89 mg; where the denaturant is denatonium benzoate, not less than 2.8 mg), and Methanol. Complies with the requirements of the Bureau of Alcohol, Tobacco, and Firearms of the U.S. Treasury Department.

Note: Rubbing Alcohol is packaged, labeled, and sold in accordance with the regulations issued by the U.S. Treasury Department, Bureau of Alcohol, Tobacco, and Firearms.

ALCOHOL AND ACETONE

For *Alcohol* and *Acetone*—See individual listings for chemistry information.

USP requirements:

Alcohol and Acetone Detergent Lotion—Not in USP.
Alcohol and Acetone Pledgets—Not in USP.

ALCOHOL AND DEXTROSE

For *Alcohol* and *Dextrose*—See individual listings for chemistry information.

USP requirements: Alcohol in Dextrose Injection USP—Preserve in single-dose containers, preferably of Type I or Type II glass. A sterile solution of Alcohol and Dextrose in Water for Injection. The label states the total osmolarity of the solution expressed in mOsmol per liter. Contains the labeled amounts of alcohol, within ±10%, and dextrose, within ±5%. Meets the requirements for Identification, Bacterial endotoxins, pH (3.5–6.5), Heavy metals (0.0005C%, in which C is the labeled amount, in grams, of Dextrose per mL of Injection), 5-Hydroxymethylfurfural and related substances (absorbance not more than 0.25), and Injections.

ALCOHOL AND SULFUR

Chemical name:

Alcohol—Ethanol.
Sulfur, precipitated—Sulfur.
Sulfur, sublimed—Sulfur.

Molecular formula:

Alcohol—C_2H_6O.
Sulfur, precipitated—S.
Sulfur, sublimed—S.

Molecular weight:

Alcohol—46.07.
Sulfur, precipitated—32.06.
Sulfur, sublimed—32.06.

Description:

Alcohol USP—Clear, colorless, mobile, volatile liquid. Has a characteristic odor. Is readily volatilized even at low temperatures, and boils at about 78 °C. Is flammable.

NF category: Solvent.

Precipitated Sulfur USP—Very fine, pale yellow, amorphous or microcrystalline powder. Is odorless.

Sublimed Sulfur USP—Fine, yellow, crystalline powder, having a faint odor.

Solubility:
Alcohol USP—Miscible with water and with practically all organic solvents.
Precipitated Sulfur USP—Practically insoluble in water; very soluble in carbon disulfide; slightly soluble in olive oil; very slightly soluble in alcohol.
Sublimed Sulfur USP—Practically insoluble in water; sparingly soluble in olive oil; practically insoluble in alcohol.

USP requirements:
Alcohol and Sulfur Gel—Not in USP.
Alcohol and Sulfur Lotion—Not in USP.

ALFENTANIL

Chemical group: Fentanyl derivatives are anilinopiperidine-derivative opioid analgesics and are chemically related to anileridine and meperidine.

Chemical name: Alfentanil hydrochloride—Propanamide, *N*-[1-[2-(4-ethyl-4,5-dihydro-5-oxo-1*H*-tetrazol-1-yl)ethyl]-4-(methoxymethyl)-4-piperidinyl]-*N*-phenyl, monohydrochloride, monohydrate.

Molecular formula: Alfentanil hydrochloride—$C_{21}H_{32}N_6O_3 \cdot HCl \cdot H_2O$.

Molecular weight: Alfentanil hydrochloride—471.00.

Solubility: Alfentanil hydrochloride—Soluble in water.

pKa: 6.5.

Other characteristics: Partition coefficient (octanol:water)—Alfentanil hydrochloride: At pH 7.4—130.

USP requirements: Alfentanil Hydrochloride Injection—Not in USP.

ALGINIC ACID

Description: Alginic Acid NF—White to yellowish white, fibrous powder. Odorless, or practically odorless.
NF category: Suspending and/or viscosity-increasing agent; tablet binder; tablet disintegrant.

Solubility: Alginic Acid NF—Insoluble in water and in organic solvents; soluble in alkaline solutions.

NF requirements: Alginic Acid NF—Preserve in well-closed containers. It is a hydrophilic colloidal carbohydrate extracted with dilute alkali from various species of brown seaweeds (Phaeophyceae). Meets the requirements for Identification, Microbial limits, pH (1.5–3.5, in a 3 in 100 dispersion in water), Loss on drying (not more than 15.0%), Ash (not more than 4.0%), Arsenic (3 ppm), Lead, Heavy metals (0.004%), and Acid value (not less than 230, calculated on the dried basis).

ALLOPURINOL

Chemical group: A structural analogue of hypoxanthine.

Chemical name: 4*H*-Pyrazolo[3,4-*d*]pyrimidin-4-one, 1,5-dihydro-.

Molecular formula: $C_5H_4N_4O$.

Molecular weight: 136.11.

Description: Allopurinol USP—Fluffy white to off-white powder, having only a slight odor.

pKa: 10.2.

Solubility: Allopurinol USP—Very slightly soluble in water and in alcohol; soluble in solutions of potassium and sodium hydroxides; practically insoluble in chloroform and in ether.

USP requirements:
Allopurinol USP—Preserve in well-closed containers. Contains not less than 98.0% and not more than 101.0% of allopurinol, calculated on the dried basis. Meets the requirements for Identification, Loss on drying (not more than 0.5%), Chromatographic impurities (0.2%), and Organic volatile impurities.
Allopurinol Tablets USP—Preserve in well-closed containers. Contain the labeled amount, within ±7%. Meet the requirements for Identification, Dissolution (75% in 45 minutes in 0.1 *N* hydrochloric acid in Apparatus 2 at 75 rpm), and Uniformity of dosage units.

ALMOND OIL

Description: Almond Oil NF—Clear, pale straw-colored or colorless, oily liquid. Remains clear at –10 °C, and does not congeal until cooled to almost –20 °C.
NF category: Flavors and perfumes; oleaginous vehicle.

Solubility: Almond Oil NF—Slightly soluble in alcohol; miscible with ether, with chloroform, and with solvent hexane.

NF requirements: Almond Oil NF—Preserve in tight containers. It is the fixed oil obtained by expression from the kernels of varieties of *Prunus amygdalus* Batsch (Fam. Rosaceae). Meets the requirements for Specific gravity (0.910–0.915), Foreign kernel oils, Cottonseed oil, Sesame oil, Mineral oil and foreign fatty oils, Foreign oils, Free fatty acids (not more than 5.0 mL of 0.10 *N* sodium hydroxide), Iodine value (95–105), and Saponification value (190–200).

ALOE

Description: Aloe USP—Has a characteristic, somewhat sour and disagreeable, odor.

USP requirements: Aloe USP—It is the dried latex of the leaves of *Aloe barbadensis* Miller (*Aloe vera* Linné), known in commerce as Curaçao Aloe, or of *Aloe ferox* Miller and hybrids of this species with *Aloe africana* Miller and *Aloe spicata* Baker, known in commerce as Cape Aloe (Fam. Liliaceae). Aloe yields not less than 50.0% of water-soluble extractive. Meets the requirements for Botanic characteristics, Identification, Water (not more than 12.0%, determined by drying at 105 °C for 5 hours), Total ash (not more than 4.0%), and Alcohol-insoluble substances (not more than 10.0% of weight of Aloe taken).

ALPHA₁-PROTEINASE INHIBITOR, HUMAN

Source: Prepared from pooled human plasma of normal donors by modification and refinements of the cold ethanol method of Cohn.

Other characteristics: When alpha₁-PI is reconstituted, it has a pH of 6.6 to 7.4.

USP requirements: Alpha₁-proteinase Inhibitor, Human, for Injection—Not in USP.

ALPRAZOLAM

Chemical name: 4*H*-[1,2,4]Triazolo[4,3-*a*][1,4]benzodiazepine, 8-chloro-1-methyl-6-phenyl-.

Molecular formula: $C_{17}H_{13}ClN_4$.

Molecular weight: 308.77.

Description: Alprazolam USP—A white to off-white crystalline powder. Melts at about 225 °C.

Solubility: Alprazolam USP—Insoluble in water; slightly soluble in ethyl acetate; sparingly soluble in acetone; soluble in alcohol; freely soluble in chloroform.

USP requirements:
Alprazolam USP—Preserve in well-closed containers. Contains not less than 98.0% and not more than 102.0% of alprazolam. Meets the requirements for Identification, Loss on drying (not more than 0.5%), Residue on ignition (not more than 0.5%), Heavy metals (0.002%), and Chromatographic purity.
Caution: Care should be taken to prevent inhaling particles of Alprazolam and exposing the skin to it.
Alprazolam Tablets USP—Preserve in tight, light-resistant containers. Contain the labeled amount, within ±10%. Meet the requirements for Identification, Dissolution (80% in 30 minutes in Working buffer solution in Apparatus 1 at 100 rpm), and Uniformity of dosage units.

ALPROSTADIL

Chemical name: Prost-13-en-1-oic acid, 11,15-dihydroxy-9-oxo-, (11 alpha,13E,15S)-.

Molecular formula: $C_{20}H_{34}O_5$.

Molecular weight: 354.49.

Description: Alprostadil USP—A white to off-white, crystalline powder. Melts at about 110 °C.

pKa: 6.3 in 60% ethanol in water.

Solubility: Alprostadil USP—Soluble in water; freely soluble in alcohol; soluble in acetone; slightly soluble in ethyl acetate; very slightly soluble in chloroform and in ether.

USP requirements:
Alprostadil USP—Preserve in tight containers, in a refrigerator. Contains not less than 95.0% and not more than 105.0% of alprostadil, calculated on the anhydrous basis. Meets the requirements for Identification, Water (not more than 0.5%, using 0.5 grams), Residue on ignition (not more than 0.5%, using 0.3 grams), Prostaglandin A_1, prostaglandin B_1, and 13,14-dihydroprostaglandin E_1 (total not more than 0.5%), and Foreign prostaglandins (not more than 3.0% total and no single foreign prostaglandin greater than 2.0%).
Caution: Great care should be taken to prevent inhaling particles of Alprostadil and exposing the skin to it.
Alprostadil Injection USP—Preserve in single-dose containers, preferably of Type I glass. Store in a refrigerator. A sterile solution of Alprostadil in Dehydrated Alcohol. Contains the labeled amount, within −10% to +15%. Meets the requirements for Identification, Bacterial endotoxins (not more than 5 USP Endotoxin units per 100 mcg of alprostadil), Sterility, Water (not more than 0.4%), and Injections.

ALSEROXYLON

Chemical source: An extract of *Rauwolfia serpentina* standardized so that it contains 7.5 to 10% of the reserpine-rescinnamine group alkaloids, calculated as reserpine.
Solubility: Slightly soluble in water; freely soluble in alcohol.

USP requirements: Alseroxylon Tablets—Not in USP.

ALTEPLASE

Source: An enzymatic glycoprotein composed of 527 amino acids. It is produced by recombinant DNA technology using the complementary DNA for natural human tissue-type plasminogen activator obtained from a human melanoma cell line.

Molecular weight: About 68,000 daltons.

Description: A white to off-white lyophilized powder.

USP requirements: Alteplase, Recombinant, for Injection—Not in USP.

ALTRETAMINE

Source: Synthetic s-triazine derivative.

Chemical name: 1,3,5-Triazine-2,4,6-triamine, N,N,N',N',N'',N''-hexamethyl-

Molecular formula: $C_9H_{18}N_6$.

Molecular weight: 210.28.

Description: White, crystalline powder, with a melting point of 172 °C ± 1 °C.

Solubility: Practically insoluble in water, but increasingly soluble at pH 3 and below.

USP requirements: Altretamine Capsules—Not in USP.

ALUM

Chemical name:
Ammonium alum—Sulfuric acid, aluminum ammonium salt (2:1:1), dodecahydrate.
Potassium alum—Sulfuric acid, aluminum potassium salt (2:1:1), dodecahydrate.

Molecular formula:
Ammonium alum—$AlNH_4(SO_4)_2 \cdot 12H_2O$.
Potassium alum—$AlK(SO_4)_2 \cdot 12H_2O$.

Molecular weight:
Ammonium alum—453.32.
Potassium alum—474.38.

Description:
Ammonium Alum USP—Large, colorless crystals, crystalline fragments, or white powder. Is odorless. Its solutions are acid to litmus.
Potassium Alum USP—Large, colorless crystals, crystalline fragments, or white powder. Is odorless. Its solutions are acid to litmus.

Solubility:
Ammonium Alum USP—Freely soluble in water; very soluble in boiling water; freely but slowly soluble in glycerin; insoluble in alcohol.
Potassium Alum USP—Freely soluble in water; very soluble in boiling water; freely but slowly soluble in glycerin; insoluble in alcohol.

USP requirements:
Ammonium Alum USP—Contains not less than 99.0% and not more than 100.5% of ammonium alum, calculated on the dried basis. Meets the requirements for Identification, Loss on drying (45.0–48.0%), Alkalies and alkaline earths (not more than 0.5%), Arsenic (3 ppm), Heavy metals (not more than 0.002%), and Iron.
Potassium Alum USP—Preserve in well-closed containers. Contains not less than 99.0% and not more than 100.5%

of potassium alum, calculated on the dried basis. Meets the requirements for Identification, Loss on drying (43.0–46.0%), Arsenic (3 ppm), Heavy metals (not more than 0.002%), and Iron.

ALUMINA AND MAGNESIA

For *Alumina* (Aluminum Hydroxide) and *Magnesia* (Magnesium Hydroxide)—See individual listings for chemistry information.

USP requirements:

Alumina and Magnesia Oral Suspension USP—Preserve in tight containers, and avoid freezing. A mixture containing Aluminum Hydroxide and Magnesium Hydroxide. Oral Suspension may be labeled to state the aluminum hydroxide content in terms of the equivalent amount of dried aluminum hydroxide gel, on the basis that each mg of dried gel is equivalent to 0.765 mg of aluminum hydroxide. Contains the equivalent of the labeled amounts of aluminum hydroxide and magnesium hydroxide, within ±10%. Meets the requirements for Identification, Microbial limits, Acid-neutralizing capacity, pH (7.3–8.5), Chloride (0.14%), and Sulfate (0.1%), and for Arsenic and Heavy metals under Aluminum Hydroxide Gel.

Alumina and Magnesia Tablets USP—Preserve in well-closed containers. Tablets prepared with the use of Dried Aluminum Hydroxide Gel may be labeled to state the aluminum hydroxide content in terms of the equivalent amount of dried aluminum hydroxide gel, on the basis that each mg of dried gel is equivalent to 0.765 mg of aluminum hydroxide. Contain the equivalent of the labeled amounts of aluminum hydroxide and magnesium hydroxide, within ±10%. Meet the requirements for Identification, Disintegration (10 minutes, in simulated gastric fluid TS), Uniformity of dosage units, and Acid-neutralizing capacity.

ALUMINA, MAGNESIA, AND CALCIUM CARBONATE

For *Alumina* (Aluminum Hydroxide), *Magnesia* (Magnesium Hydroxide), and *Calcium Carbonate*—See individual listings for chemistry information.

USP requirements:

Alumina, Magnesia, and Calcium Carbonate Oral Suspension USP—Preserve in tight containers, and avoid freezing. Oral Suspension may be labeled to state the aluminum hydroxide content in terms of the equivalent amount of dried aluminum hydroxide gel, on the basis that each mg of dried gel is equivalent to 0.765 mg of aluminum hydroxide. Contains the labeled amounts of aluminum hydroxide, magnesium hydroxide, and calcium carbonate, within ±10%. Meets the requirements for Identification, Microbial limits, pH (7.5–8.5), Chloride (0.14%), Sulfate (0.1%), and Acid-neutralizing capacity, and for Arsenic and Heavy metals under Aluminum Hydroxide Gel.

Alumina, Magnesia, and Calcium Carbonate Tablets USP—Preserve in well-closed containers. Label the Tablets to indicate that they are to be chewed before being swallowed. Tablets prepared with the use of Dried Aluminum Hydroxide Gel may be labeled to state the aluminum hydroxide content in terms of the equivalent amount of dried aluminum hydroxide gel, on the basis that each mg of dried gel is equivalent to 0.765 mg of aluminum hydroxide. Contain the labeled amounts of aluminum hydroxide, magnesium hydroxide, and calcium carbonate, within ±10%. Meet the requirements for Identification, Disintegration (45 minutes), Uniformity of dosage units, and Acid-neutralizing capacity.

ALUMINA, MAGNESIA, CALCIUM CARBONATE, AND SIMETHICONE

For *Alumina* (Aluminum Hydroxide), *Magnesia* (Magnesium Hydroxide), *Calcium Carbonate,* and *Simethicone*—See individual listings for chemistry information.

USP requirements: Alumina, Magnesia, Calcium Carbonate, and Simethicone Tablets USP—Preserve in well-closed containers. The labeling indicates that Tablets are to be chewed before swallowing. Label Tablets to state the sodium content, if it is greater than 5 mg per Tablet. Contain the equivalent of the labeled amounts of aluminum hydroxide and magnesium hydroxide, within ±10%, the labeled amount of calcium carbonate, within ±10%, and an amount of polydimethylsiloxane equivalent to the labeled amount of simethicone, within ±15%. Meet the requirements for Identification, Uniformity of dosage units, Acid-neutralizing capacity, Defoaming activity, Microbial limits, and Sodium content.

ALUMINA, MAGNESIA, AND SIMETHICONE

For *Alumina* (Aluminum Hydroxide), *Magnesia* (Magnesium Hydroxide), and *Simethicone*—See individual listings for chemistry information.

USP requirements:

Alumina, Magnesia, and Simethicone Oral Suspension USP—Preserve in tight containers, and avoid freezing. Oral Suspension may be labeled to state the aluminum hydroxide content in terms of the equivalent amount of dried aluminum hydroxide gel, on the basis that each mg of dried gel is equivalent to 0.765 mg of aluminum hydroxide. Label it to state the sodium content if it is greater than 1 mg per mL. Contains the equivalent of the labeled amounts of aluminum hydroxide and magnesium hydroxide, within −10% to +15%. Contains an amount of polydimethylsiloxane equivalent to the labeled amount of simethicone, within ±15%. Meets the requirements for Identification, Microbial limits, Acid-neutralizing capacity, pH (7.0–8.6), Defoaming activity (not more than 45 seconds), and Sodium.

Alumina, Magnesia, and Simethicone Tablets USP—Preserve in well-closed containers. Label Tablets to indicate that they are to be chewed before being swallowed. Label Tablets to state the sodium content if it is greater than 5 mg per Tablet. Tablets may be labeled to state the aluminum hydroxide content in terms of the equivalent amount of dried aluminum hydroxide gel, on the basis that each mg of dried gel is equivalent to 0.765 mg of aluminum hydroxide. Contain the equivalent of the labeled amounts of aluminum hydroxide and magnesium hydroxide, within −10% to +15%. Contain an amount of polydimethylsiloxane equivalent to the labeled amount of simethicone, within ±15%. Meet the requirements for Identification, Uniformity of dosage units, Acid-neutralizing capacity, Defoaming activity, and Sodium.

ALUMINA AND MAGNESIUM CARBONATE

For *Alumina* (Aluminum Hydroxide) and *Magnesium Carbonate*—See individual listings for chemistry information.

USP requirements:

Alumina and Magnesium Carbonate Oral Suspension USP—Preserve in tight containers, and avoid freezing. Contains the equivalent of the labeled amounts of aluminum hydroxide and magnesium carbonate, within ±10%. Meets the requirements for Identification, Microbial limits, pH (7.5–9.5), and Acid-neutralizing capacity.

Alumina and Magnesium Carbonate Tablets USP—Preserve in tight containers. Contain the equivalent of the labeled amounts of aluminum hydroxide and magnesium carbonate, within ±10%. Meet the requirements for Identification, Disintegration (10 minutes, in simulated gastric fluid TS), Uniformity of dosage units, and Acid-neutralizing capacity (not less than 5 mEq of acid is consumed by the minimum single dose recommended in the labeling).

ALUMINA, MAGNESIUM CARBONATE, AND MAGNESIUM OXIDE

For *Alumina* (Aluminum Hydroxide), *Magnesium Carbonate,* and *Magnesium Oxide*—See individual listings for chemistry information.

USP requirements: Alumina, Magnesium Carbonate, and Magnesium Oxide Tablets USP—Preserve in tight containers. Contain the equivalent of the labeled amounts of aluminum hydroxide and magnesium carbonate, within ±10%. Contain the labeled amount of magnesium oxide, within ±15%. Meet the requirements for Identification, Disintegration (10 minutes, in simulated gastric fluid TS), Uniformity of dosage units, and Acid-neutralizing capacity (not less than 5 mEq of acid is consumed by the minimum single dose recommended in the labeling).

ALUMINA AND MAGNESIUM TRISILICATE

For *Alumina* (Aluminum Hydroxide) and *Magnesium Trisilicate*—See individual listings for chemistry information.

USP requirements:

Alumina and Magnesium Trisilicate Oral Suspension USP—Preserve in tight containers. Contains the equivalent of the labeled amount of aluminum hydroxide, within ±10%, and the labeled amount of magnesium trisilicate, within ±10%. Meets the requirements for Identification, Acid-neutralizing capacity (not less than 5 mEq of acid is consumed by the minimum single dose recommended in the labeling), and pH (7.5–8.5).

Alumina and Magnesium Trisilicate Tablets USP—Preserve in well-closed containers. Tablets prepared with the use of Dried Aluminum Hydroxide Gel may be labeled to state the aluminum hydroxide content in terms of the equivalent amount of dried aluminum hydroxide gel, on the basis that each mg of dried gel is equivalent to 0.765 mg of aluminum hydroxide. Tablets intended for the temporary relief of heartburn (acid indigestion) due to acid reflux are so labeled. Tablets that must be chewed before swallowing are so labeled. Contain the equivalent of the labeled amount of aluminum hydroxide, within ±10%, and the labeled amount of magnesium trisilicate, within ±10%. Meet the requirements for Identification, Disintegration (10 minutes, in simulated gastric fluid TS [Note: Tablets that must be chewed before swallowing are exempt from this requirement]), Uniformity of dosage units, and Acid-neutralizing capacity (not less than 5 mEq of acid is consumed by the minimum single dose recommended in the labeling [Note: Tablets labeled for the temporary relief of heartburn (acid indigestion) due to acid reflux are exempt from this requirement]).

ALUMINA, MAGNESIUM TRISILICATE, AND SODIUM BICARBONATE

For *Alumina* (Aluminum Hydroxide), *Magnesium Trisilicate* and *Sodium Bicarbonate*—See individual listings for chemistry information.

USP requirements: Alumina, Magnesium Trisilicate, and Sodium Bicarbonate Chewable Tablets—Not in USP.

ALUMINUM ACETATE

Chemical name: Acetic acid, aluminum salt.

Molecular formula: $C_6H_9AlO_6$.

Molecular weight: 204.12.

Description: Aluminum Acetate Topical Solution USP—Clear, colorless liquid having a faint odor of acetic acid. Specific gravity is about 1.02.

USP requirements: Aluminum Acetate Topical Solution USP—Preserve in tight containers. Yields, from each 100 mL, not less than 1.20 grams and not more than 1.45 grams of aluminum oxide, and not less than 4.24 grams and not more than 5.12 grams of acetic acid, corresponding to not less than 4.8 grams and not more than 5.8 grams of aluminum acetate. May be stabilized by the addition of not more than 0.6% of Boric Acid.

Prepare Aluminum Acetate Topical Solution as follows: 545 mL of Aluminum Subacetate Topical Solution, 15 mL of Glacial Acetic Acid, and a sufficient quantity of Purified Water to make 1000 mL. Add the Glacial Acetic Acid to the Aluminum Subacetate Topical Solution and sufficient Water to make 1000 mL. Mix, and filter, if necessary.

Meets the requirements for Identification, pH (3.6–4.4), Limit of boric acid, and Heavy metals (not more than 0.001%).

Note: Dispense only clear Aluminum Acetate Topical Solution.

ALUMINUM CARBONATE, BASIC

Source: Aluminum carbonate—An aluminum oxycarbonate of indefinite composition.

Solubility: Insoluble in water and in alcohol; soluble in dilute mineral acids and in solutions of fixed alkali hydroxides.

USP requirements:

Basic Aluminum Carbonate Gel USP—Preserve in tight containers, and avoid freezing. Contains an amount of aluminum carbonate equivalent to the labeled amount of aluminum hydroxide, within ±10%. Meets the requirements for Identification, Microbial limits, pH (5.5–8.0), Chloride (0.37%), Sulfate (0.06%), Arsenic (not more than 0.8 ppm), and Heavy metals (not more than 6.7 ppm).

Dried Basic Aluminum Carbonate Gel Capsules USP—Preserve in well-closed containers. Capsules may be labeled to state the aluminum hydroxide content in terms of the equivalent amount of dried aluminum hydroxide gel, on the basis that each mg of dried aluminum hydroxide gel is equivalent to 0.765 mg of aluminum hydroxide. Contain an amount of aluminum carbonate equivalent to the labeled amount of aluminum hydroxide, within ±10%. Meet the requirements for Identification, Disintegration (10 minutes, in simulated gastric fluid TS), Uniformity of dosage units, and Acid-neutralizing capacity (0.0385 mEq per mg of aluminum hydroxide).

Dried Basic Aluminum Carbonate Gel Tablets USP—Preserve in well-closed containers. Tablets may be labeled to state the aluminum hydroxide content in terms of the equivalent amount of dried aluminum hydroxide gel, on the basis that each mg of dried aluminum hydroxide gel is equivalent to 0.765 mg of aluminum hydroxide. Contain an amount of aluminum carbonate equivalent to the labeled amount of aluminum hydroxide, within ±10%. Meet the requirements for Identification, Disintegration (10 minutes, in simulated gastric fluid TS), Uniformity of dosage units, and Acid-neutralizing capacity (0.0385 mEq per mg of aluminum hydroxide).

ALUMINUM CHLORIDE

Chemical name: Aluminum chloride, hexahydrate.

Molecular formula: $AlCl_3 \cdot 6H_2O$.

Molecular weight: 241.43.

Description: Aluminum Chloride USP—White, or yellowish white, deliquescent, crystalline powder. Is practically odorless. Its solutions are acid to litmus.

Solubility: Aluminum Chloride USP—Very soluble in water; freely soluble in alcohol; soluble in glycerin.

USP requirements: Aluminum Chloride USP—Preserve in tight containers. Contains not less than 95.0% and not more than 102.0% of aluminum chloride, calculated on the anhydrous basis. Meets the requirements for Identification, Water (42.0–48.0%), Sulfate, Alkalies and alkaline earths (not more than 0.5%), Arsenic (8 ppm), Heavy metals (not more than 0.002%), and Iron (not more than 0.001%).

ALUMINUM HYDROXIDE

Source: An amorphous form of aluminum hydroxide in which there is a partial substitution of carbonate for hydroxide.

Chemical name: Aluminum hydroxide.

Molecular formula: $Al(OH)_3$.

Molecular weight: 78.00.

Description:
Aluminum Hydroxide Gel USP—White, viscous suspension, from which small amounts of clear liquid may separate on standing.
Dried Aluminum Hydroxide Gel USP—White, odorless, amorphous powder.

Solubility: Dried Aluminum Hydroxide Gel USP—Insoluble in water and in alcohol; soluble in dilute mineral acids and in solutions of fixed alkali hydroxides.

USP requirements:
Aluminum Hydroxide Gel USP—Preserve in tight containers, and avoid freezing. A suspension, each 100 grams of which contains the equivalent of not less than 5.5 grams and not more than 6.7 grams of aluminum hydroxide, in the form of amorphous aluminum hydroxide in which there is a partial substitution of carbonate for hydroxide. Meets the requirements for Identification, Microbial limits, Acid-neutralizing capacity (not less than 65% of the expected mEq value; each mg of aluminum hydroxide has an expected acid-neutralizing capacity value of 0.0385 mEq), pH (5.5–8.0), Chloride (not more than 0.28%), Sulfate (not more than 0.05%), Arsenic (not more than 0.6 ppm), and Heavy metals (not more than 5 ppm).
Dried Aluminum Hydroxide Gel USP—Preserve in tight containers. An amorphous form of aluminum hydroxide in which there is a partial substitution of carbonate for hydroxide. Where the quantity of dried aluminum hydroxide gel equivalent is stated in the labeling of any preparation, this shall be understood to be on the basis that each mg of dried gel is equivalent to 0.765 mg of aluminum hydroxide. Contains the equivalent of not less than 76.5% of aluminum hydroxide, and may contain varying quantities of basic aluminum carbonate and bicarbonate. Meets the requirements for Identification, Acid-neutralizing capacity (not less than 25.0 mEq per gram), pH (not more than 10.0, in an aqueous dispersion [1 in 25]), Chloride (not more than 0.85%), Sulfate (not more than 0.6%), Arsenic (not more than 8 ppm), and Heavy metals (not more than 0.006%).

Dried Aluminum Hydroxide Gel Capsules USP—Preserve in well-closed containers. Capsules may be labeled to state the aluminum hydroxide content in terms of the equivalent amount of dried aluminum hydroxide gel, on the basis that each mg of dried gel is equivalent to 0.765 mg of aluminum hydroxide. Contain the labeled amount, within ±10%. Meet the requirements for Identification, Disintegration (10 minutes, in simulated gastric fluid TS), Uniformity of dosage units, and Acid-neutralizing capacity (not less than 5 mEq of acid consumed by the minimum single dose recommended in the labeling, and not less than 55.0% of the expected mEq value, calculated from the labeled quantity of aluminum hydroxide; each mg of aluminum hydroxide has an expected acid-neutralizing capacity value of 0.0385 mEq).
Dried Aluminum Hydroxide Gel Tablets USP—Preserve in well-closed containers. Tablets may be labeled to state the aluminum hydroxide content in terms of the equivalent amount of dried aluminum hydroxide gel, on the basis that each mg of dried gel is equivalent to 0.765 mg of aluminum hydroxide. Contain the labeled amount, within ±10%. Meet the requirements for Identification, Disintegration (10 minutes, in simulated gastric fluid TS), Uniformity of dosage units, and Acid-neutralizing capacity (not less than 5 mEq of acid consumed by the minimun single dose recommended in the labeling, and not less than 55.0% of the expected mEq value, calculated from the labeled quantity of aluminum hydroxide; each mg of aluminum hydroxide has an expected acid-neutralizing capacity value of 0.0385 mEq).

ALUMINUM MONOSTEARATE

Chemical name: Aluminum, dihydroxy(octadecanoato-*O*-)

Molecular formula: $C_{18}H_{37}AlO_4$.

Molecular weight: 344.47.

Description: Aluminum Monostearate NF—Fine, white to yellowish white bulky powder, having a faint, characteristic odor.
NF category: Suspending and/or viscosity-increasing agent.

Solubility: Aluminum Monostearate NF—Insoluble in water, in alcohol, and in ether.

NF requirements: Aluminum Monostearate NF—Preserve in well-closed containers. A compound of aluminum with a mixture of solid organic acids obtained from fats, and consists chiefly of variable proportions of aluminum monostearate and aluminum monopalmitate. Contains the equivalent of not less than 14.5% and not more than 16.5% of aluminum oxide. Meets the requirements for Identification, Loss on drying (not more than 2.0%), Arsenic (not more than 4 ppm), and Heavy metals (not more than 0.005%).

ALUMINUM PHOSPHATE

Chemical name: Phosphoric acid, aluminum salt (1:1).

Molecular formula: $AlPO_4$.

Molecular weight: 121.95.

Description: Aluminum Phosphate Gel USP—White, viscous suspension from which small amounts of water separate on standing.

USP requirements: Aluminum Phosphate Gel USP—Preserve in tight containers. A water suspension. Contains not less than 4.0% and not more than 5.0% (w/w) of aluminum phosphate. Meets the requirements for Identification, pH (6.0–7.2), Chloride (not more than 0.16%), Soluble phosphate (not more than 0.30%), Sulfate (0.05%), Arsenic (not more than 0.6 ppm), and Heavy metals (not more than 5 ppm).

ALUMINUM SUBACETATE

Chemical name: Aluminum, bis(acetato-*O*)hydroxy-.

Molecular formula: $C_4H_7AlO_5$.

Molecular weight: 162.08.

Description: Aluminum Subacetate Topical Solution USP— Clear, colorless or faintly yellow liquid, having an odor of acetic acid and an acid reaction to litmus. Gradually becomes turbid on standing, through separation of a more basic salt.

USP requirements: Aluminum Subacetate Topical Solution USP—Preserve in tight containers. Yields, from each 100 mL, not less than 2.30 grams and not more than 2.60 grams of aluminum oxide, and not less than 5.43 grams and not more than 6.13 grams of acetic acid. May be stabilized by the addition of not more than 0.9% of boric acid.

Aluminum Subacetate Topical Solution may be prepared as follows: 145 grams of Aluminum Sulfate, 160 mL of Acetic Acid, 70 grams of Precipitated Calcium Carbonate, and a sufficient quantity of Purified Water to make 1000 mL. Dissolve the Aluminum Sulfate in 600 mL of cold water, filter the solution, and add the Precipitated Calcium Carbonate gradually, in several portions, with constant stirring. Then slowly add the Acetic Acid, mix, and set the mixture aside for 24 hours. Filter the product with the aid of vacuum if necessary, returning the first portion of the filtrate to the funnel. Wash the magma on the filter with small portions of cold water, until the total filtrate measures 1000 mL.

Meets the requirements for Identification, pH (3.8–4.6), and Limit of boric acid.

ALUMINUM SULFATE

Chemical name: Sulfuric acid, aluminum salt (3:2), hydrate.

Molecular formula: $Al_2(SO_4)_3 \cdot xH_2O$.

Molecular weight: 342.14 (anhydrous).

Description: Aluminum Sulfate USP—White, crystalline powder, shining plates, or crystalline fragments. Is stable in air. Is odorless.

Solubility: Aluminum Sulfate USP—Freely soluble in water; insoluble in alcohol.

USP requirements: Aluminum Sulfate USP—Preserve in well-closed containers. Contains not less than 54.0% and not more than 59.0% of anhydrous aluminum sulfate. Contains a varying amount of water of crystallization. Meets the requirements for Identification, pH (not less than 2.9, in a solution [1 in 20]), Water (41.0–46.0%), Alkalies and alkaline earths (not more than 0.4%), Ammonium salts, Arsenic (3 ppm), Heavy metals (not more than 0.004%), and Iron.

AMANTADINE

Chemical name: Amantadine hydrochloride—Tricyclo[3.3.1.1³,⁷]decan-1-amine, hydrochloride.

Molecular formula: Amantadine hydrochloride—$C_{10}H_{17}N \cdot HCl$.

Molecular weight: Amantadine hydrochloride—187.71.

Description: Amantadine Hydrochloride USP—White or practically white, crystalline powder.

Solubility: Amantadine Hydrochloride USP—Freely soluble in water; soluble in alcohol and in chloroform.

USP requirements:
Amantadine Hydrochloride USP—Preserve in well-closed containers. Contains not less than 98.5% and not more than 101.5% of amantadine hydrochloride. Meets the requirements for Clarity and color of solution, Identification, pH (3.0–5.5, in a solution [1 in 5]), Heavy metals (not more than 0.001%), and Organic volatile impurities.
Amantadine Hydrochloride Capsules USP—Preserve in tight containers. Contain the labeled amount, within ±5%. Meet the requirements for Identification, Dissolution (75% in 45 minutes in water in Apparatus 1 at 100 rpm), and Uniformity of dosage units.
Amantadine Hydrochloride Syrup USP—Preserve in tight containers. Contains the labeled amount, within ±5%. Meets the requirement for Identification.

AMBENONIUM

Source: Synthetic quaternary ammonium compound.

Chemical name: Ambenonium chloride—Benzenemethanaminium, *N,N'*-[(1,2-dioxo-1,2-ethanediyl)bis(imino-2,1-ethanediyl)]bis[2-chloro-*N,N*-diethyl-, dichloride.

Molecular formula: Ambenonium chloride—$C_{28}H_{42}Cl_4N_4O_2$.

Molecular weight: Ambenonium chloride—608.48.

Description: Ambenonium chloride—White, odorless powder; melting point 196–199 °C.

Solubility: Ambenonium chloride—Soluble in water and in alcohol; slightly soluble in chloroform; practically insoluble in acetone and in ether.

USP requirements: Ambenonium Chloride Tablets—Not in USP.

AMCINONIDE

Chemical name: Pregna-1,4-diene-3,20-dione, 21-(acetyloxy)-16,17-[cyclopentylidenebis(oxy)]-9-fluoro-11-hydroxy-, (11 beta,16 alpha)-.

Molecular formula: $C_{28}H_{35}FO_7$.

Molecular weight: 502.58.

Description: White to cream colored crystalline powder, having not more than a slight odor. Its melting point range is 248–252 °C.

USP requirements:
Amcinonide USP—Preserve in well-closed containers. Contains not less than 97.0% and not more than 102.0% of amcinonide, calculated on the dried basis. Meets the requirements for Identification, Specific rotation (+89.4° to +94.0°, calculated on the dried basis, determined in a solution in chloroform containing 100 mg in each 10 mL), Loss on drying (not more than 1.0%), and Heavy metals (0.002%).
Amcinonide Cream USP—Preserve in tight containers. It is Amcinonide in a suitable cream base. Contains the labeled amount, within −10% to +15%. Meets the requirements for Identification, Microbial limits, Minimum fill, and pH (3.5–5.2).
Amcinonide Lotion—Not in USP.
Amcinonide Ointment USP—Preserve in tight containers. It is Amcinonide in a suitable ointment base. Contains the labeled amount, within −10% to +15%. Meets the requirements for Identification, Microbial limits, and Minimum fill.

AMDINOCILLIN

Chemical name: 4-Thia-1-azabicyclo[3.2.0]heptane-2-carboxylic acid, 6-[[(hexahydro-1*H*-azepin-1-yl)methylene]amino]-3,3-dimethyl-7-oxo-, [2*S*-(2 alpha,5 alpha,6 beta)]-.

Molecular formula: $C_{15}H_{23}N_3O_3S$.

Molecular weight: 325.43.

Description: Sterile Amdinocillin USP—White to off-white crystalline powder. Melts at 141–143 °C, with decomposition.

Solubility: Sterile Amdinocillin USP—Freely soluble in water and in methanol.

USP requirements: Sterile Amdinocillin USP—Preserve in Containers for Sterile Solids. It is amdinocillin suitable for parenteral use. Contains not less than 950 mcg and not more than 1050 mcg per mg (anhydrous) and, where packaged for dispensing, contains the labeled amount, within −10% to +20%. Meets the requirements for Constituted solution, Identification, Crystallinity, Bacterial endotoxins, Sterility, pH (4.0–6.2, in a solution [1 in 10]), Water (not more than 0.5%), Particulate matter, and Hexamethyleneimine (not more than 2.0%), for Uniformity of dosage units, and for Labeling under Injections.

AMIKACIN

Source: Semi-synthetic; derived from kanamycin.

Chemical group: Aminoglycoside.

Chemical name:

Amikacin—D-Streptamine, *O*-3-amino-3-deoxy-alpha-D-glucopyranosyl-(1→6)-*O*-[6-amino-6-deoxy-alpha-D-glucopyranosyl-(1→4)]-*N*¹-(4-amino-2-hydroxy-1-oxobutyl)-2-deoxy-, (*S*)-.

Amikacin sulfate—D-Streptamine, *O*-3-amino-3-deoxy-alpha-D-glucopyranosyl-(1→6)-*O*-[6-amino-6-deoxy-alpha-D-glucopyranosyl-(1→4)]-*N*¹-(4-amino-2-hydroxy-1-oxobutyl)-2-deoxy-, (*S*)-, sulfate (1:2 or 1:1.8) (salt).

Molecular formula:

Amikacin—$C_{22}H_{43}N_5O_{13}$.

Amikacin sulfate—$C_{22}H_{43}N_5O_{13} \cdot 2H_2SO_4$ or $C_{22}H_{43}N_5O_{13} \cdot 1.8\ H_2SO_4$.

Molecular weight:

Amikacin—585.61.

Amikacin sulfate 2 H₂O—781.75.

Amikacin sulfate 1.8 H₂O—762.14.

Description:

Amikacin USP—White, crystalline powder.

Amikacin sulfate—White, crystalline powder.

Amikacin sulfate injection—Sterile, colorless to light straw colored solution. It has a pH adjusted to 4.5 with sulfuric acid.

Solubility:

Amikacin USP—Sparingly soluble in water.

Amikacin sulfate—Freely soluble in water.

USP requirements:

Amikacin USP—Preserve in tight containers. Has a potency of not less than 900 mcg of amikacin per mg, calculated on the anhydrous basis. Meets the requirements for Identification, Specific rotation (+97° to +105°, calculated on the anhydrous basis, determined in a solution containing 20 mg per mL), Crystallinity, pH (9.5–11.5, in a solution containing 10 mg per mL), Water (not more than 8.5%), and Residue on ignition (not more than 1.0%).

Amikacin Sulfate USP—Preserve in tight containers. Label it to indicate whether its molar ratio of amikacin to hydrogen sulfate is 1:2 or 1:1.8. Amikacin Sulfate having a molar ratio of amikacin to hydrogen sulfate of 1:2 contains an amount of amikacin sulfate equivalent to not less than 674 mcg and not more than 786 mcg of amikacin per mg, calculated on the dried basis. Amikacin Sulfate having a molar ratio of amikacin to hydrogen sulfate of 1:1.8 contains an amount of amikacin sulfate equivalent to not less than 691 mcg and not more than 806 mcg of amikacin per mg, calculated on the dried basis. Meets the requirements for Identification, Specific rotation (+76° to +84°, calculated on the dried basis, determined in a solution containing 20 mg per mL), Crystallinity, pH (2.0–4.0 [1:2 salt], or 6.0–7.3 [1:1.8 salt], in a solution containing 10 mg per mL), Loss on drying (not more than 13.0%), and Residue on ignition (not more than 1.0%).

Amikacin Sulfate Injection USP—Preserve in single-dose or in multiple-dose containers, preferably of Type I or Type III glass. A sterile solution of Amikacin Sulfate in Water for Injection, or of Amikacin in Water for Injection prepared with the aid of Sulfuric Acid. Contains an amount of amikacin sulfate equivalent to the labeled amount of amikacin, within −10% to +20%. Meets the requirements for Identification, Bacterial endotoxins, pH (3.5–5.5), Particulate matter, and Injections.

AMILORIDE

Chemical name: Amiloride hydrochloride—Pyrazinecarboxamide, 3,5-diamino-*N*-(aminoiminomethyl)-6-chloro-, monohydrochloride dihydrate.

Molecular formula: Amiloride hydrochloride—$C_6H_8ClN_7O \cdot HCl \cdot 2H_2O$.

Molecular weight: Amiloride hydrochloride—302.12.

Description: Amiloride Hydrochloride USP—Yellow to greenish yellow, odorless or practically odorless powder.

pKa: Amiloride—8.7.

Solubility: Amiloride Hydrochloride USP—Slightly soluble in water; insoluble in ether, in ethyl acetate, in acetone, and in chloroform; freely soluble in dimethylsulfoxide; sparingly soluble in methanol.

USP requirements:

Amiloride Hydrochloride USP—Preserve in well-closed containers. Contains not less than 98.0% and not more than 101.0% of amiloride hydrochloride, calculated on the dried basis. Meets the requirements for Identification, Acidity, Loss on drying (11.0–13.0%), Residue on ignition (not more than 0.1%), Heavy metals (not more than 0.002%), Chromatographic purity, and Organic volatile impurities.

Amiloride Hydrochloride Tablets USP—Preserve in well-closed containers. Contain the labeled amount, within ±10%. Meet the requirements for Identification, Dissolution (80% in 30 minutes in 0.1 *N* hydrochloric acid in Apparatus 2 at 50 rpm), and Uniformity of dosage units.

AMILORIDE AND HYDROCHLOROTHIAZIDE

For *Amiloride* and *Hydrochlorothiazide*—See individual listings for chemistry information.

USP requirements: Amiloride Hydrochloride and Hydrochlorothiazide Tablets USP—Preserve in well-closed containers. Contain the labeled amounts of amiloride hydrochloride and hydrochlorothiazide, within ±10%. Meet the requirements for Identification, Dissolution (80% of amiloride hydrochloride and 75% of hydrochlorothiazide in 30 minutes in 0.1 *N* hydrochloric acid in Apparatus 2 at 50 rpm), 4-Amino-6-chloro-1,3-benzenedisulfonamide (not more than 1.0%), and Uniformity of dosage units.

AMINOBENZOATE POTASSIUM

Molecular formula: $C_7H_6KNO_2$.

Molecular weight: 175.23.

Solubility: Very freely soluble in water; less soluble in alcohol; practically insoluble in ether.

Other characteristics: pH is approximately 7 in a 1% solution; slightly alkaline to litmus.

USP requirements:
Aminobenzoate Potassium USP—Preserve in well-closed containers. Contains not less than 98.5% and not more than 101.0% of aminobenzoate potassium, calculated on the dried basis. Meets the requirements for Identification, pH (8.0–9.0, in a solution [1 in 20]), Loss on drying (not more than 1.0%), Chloride (not more than 0.02%), Sulfate (not more than 0.02%), Heavy metals (not more than 0.002%), and Volatile diazotizable substances (not more than 0.002%, as *p*-toluidine).
Aminobenzoate Potassium Capsules USP—Preserve in well-closed containers. Contain the labeled amount, within ±10%. Meet the requirements for Identification, Dissolution (75% in 45 minutes in water in Apparatus 1 at 100 rpm), and Uniformity of dosage units.
Aminobenzoate Potassium for Oral Solution USP—Preserve in tight containers. Contains the labeled amount, within ±10%. Meets the requirements for Identification, pH (7.0–9.0, in a solution [1 in 10]), Minimum fill (multiple-unit containers), and Uniformity of dosage units (single-unit containers).
Aminobenzoate Potassium Tablets USP—Preserve in well-closed containers. Contain the labeled amount, within ±10%. Meet the requirements for Identification, Dissolution (75% in 45 minutes in water in Apparatus 1 at 100 rpm), and Uniformity of dosage units.

AMINOBENZOATE SODIUM

Molecular formula: $C_7H_6NNaO_2$.

Molecular weight: 159.12.

USP requirements: Aminobenzoate Sodium USP—Preserve in well-closed containers. Contains not less than 98.5% and not more than 101.0% of aminobenzoate sodium, calculated on the dried basis. Meets the requirements for Identification, pH (8.0–9.0, in a solution [1 in 20]), Loss on drying (not more than 1.0%), Chloride (0.02%), Sulfate (0.02%), Heavy metals (0.002%), and Volatile diazotizable substances (not more than 0.002%, as *p*-toluidine).

AMINOBENZOIC ACID

Chemical name: Benzoic acid, 4-amino.

Molecular formula: $C_7H_7NO_2$.

Molecular weight: 137.14.

Description:
Aminobenzoic Acid USP—White or slightly yellow, odorless crystals or crystalline powder. Discolors on exposure to air or light.

Aminobenzoic Acid Topical Solution USP—Straw-colored solution having the odor of alcohol.

Solubility: Aminobenzoic Acid USP—Slightly soluble in water and in chloroform; freely soluble in alcohol and in solutions of alkali hydroxides and carbonates; sparingly soluble in ether.

USP requirements:
Aminobenzoic Acid USP—Preserve in tight, light-resistant containers. Contains not less than 98.5% and not more than 101.5% of aminobenzoic acid, calculated on the dried basis. Meets the requirements for Identification, Melting range (186–189 °C), Loss on drying (not more than 0.2%), Residue on ignition (not more than 0.1%), Heavy metals (0.002%), Volatile diazotizable substances (not more than 0.002%, as *p*-toluidine), and Ordinary impurities.
Aminobenzoic Acid Gel USP—Preserve in tight, light-resistant containers. Contains the labeled amount, within ±10%. Meets the requirements for Identification, Minimum fill, pH (4.0–6.0), and Alcohol content (42.3–54.0% [w/w]).
Aminobenzoic Acid Topical Solution USP—Preserve in tight, light-resistant containers. Contains, in each mL, not less than 45 mg and not more than 55 mg of aminobenzoic acid. Meets the requirements for Identification, Specific gravity (0.895–0.905), and Alcohol content (65–75%).

AMINOCAPROIC ACID

Chemical name: Hexanoic acid, 6-amino-.

Molecular formula: $C_6H_{13}NO_2$.

Molecular weight: 131.17.

Description: Aminocaproic Acid USP—Fine, white, crystalline powder. Is odorless, or practically odorless. Its solutions are neutral to litmus. Melts at about 205 °C.

Solubility: Aminocaproic Acid USP—Freely soluble in water, in acids, and in alkalies; slightly soluble in methanol and in alcohol; practically insoluble in chloroform and in ether.

USP requirements:
Aminocaproic Acid USP—Preserve in tight containers. Contains not less than 98.5% and not more than 100.5% of aminocaproic acid, calculated on the anhydrous basis. Meets the requirements for Identification, Water (not more than 0.5%), Residue on ignition (not more than 0.1%), and Heavy metals (0.002%).
Aminocaproic Acid Injection USP—Preserve in single-dose or in multiple-dose containers, preferably of Type I glass. A sterile solution of Aminocaproic Acid in Water for Injection. Contains the labeled amount, within −5% to +7.5%. Meets the requirements for Identification, Pyrogen, pH (6.0–7.6), and Injections.
Aminocaproic Acid Syrup USP—Preserve in tight containers. Contains the labeled amount, within −5% to +15%. Meets the requirements for Identification and pH (6.1–6.6).
Aminocaproic Acid Tablets USP—Preserve in tight containers. Contain the labeled amount, within ±5%. Meet the requirements for Identification, Dissolution (75% in 45 minutes in water in Apparatus 1 at 100 rpm), and Uniformity of dosage units.

AMINOGLUTETHIMIDE

Chemical name: 2,6-Piperidinedione, 3-(4-aminophenyl)-3-ethyl-.

Molecular formula: $C_{13}H_{16}N_2O_2$.

Molecular weight: 232.28.

Description: Aminoglutethimide USP—Fine, white, or creamy white, crystalline powder.

Solubility: Aminoglutethimide USP—Very slightly soluble in water; readily soluble in most organic solvents. Forms water-soluble salts with strong acids.

USP requirements:

Aminoglutethimide USP—Preserve in well-closed containers. Contains not less than 98.0% and not more than 102.0% of aminoglutethimide, calculated on the dried basis. Meets the requirements for Identification, pH (6.2–7.3, in a 1 in 1000 solution in dilute methanol [1 in 20]), Loss on drying (not more than 0.5%), Residue on ignition (not more than 0.1%), Heavy metals (not more than 0.001%), Sulfate, Chromatographic purity and limit of *m*-aminoglutethimide (not more than 1.0% total impurities, other than *m*-aminoglutethimide), Azo-aminoglutethimide (not more than 0.03%), and Organic volatile impurities.

Aminoglutethimide Tablets USP—Preserve in tight, light-resistant containers. Contain the labeled amount, within ±10%. Meet the requirements for Identification, Dissolution (70% in 30 minutes in dilute hydrochloric acid [7 in 1000] in Apparatus 1 at 100 rpm), Uniformity of dosage units, and Chromatographic purity (not more than 2.0% total impurities, other than *m*-aminoglutethimide).

AMINOHIPPURATE SODIUM

Chemical name: Glycine, *N*-(4-aminobenzoyl)-, monosodium salt.

Molecular formula: $C_9H_9N_2NaO_3$.

Molecular weight: 216.17.

USP requirements: Aminohippurate Sodium Injection USP—Preserve in single-dose or in multiple-dose containers, preferably of Type I glass. A sterile solution of Aminohippuric Acid in Water for Injection prepared with the aid of Sodium Hydroxide. Contains the labeled amount, within ±5%. Meets the requirements for Identification, Bacterial endotoxins, pH (6.7–7.6), and Injections.

AMINOHIPPURIC ACID

Chemical name: Glycine, *N*-(4-aminobenzoyl)-.

Molecular formula: $C_9H_{10}N_2O_3$.

Molecular weight: 194.19.

Description: Aminohippuric Acid USP—White, crystalline powder. Discolors on exposure to light. Melts at about 195 °C, with decomposition.

Solubility: Aminohippuric Acid USP—Sparingly soluble in water and in alcohol; freely soluble in alkaline solutions, with some decomposition, and in diluted hydrochloric acid; very slightly soluble in carbon tetrachloride, in chloroform, and in ether.

USP requirements: Aminohippuric Acid USP—Preserve in tight, light-resistant containers. Contains not less than 98.0% and not more than 100.5% of aminohippuric acid, calculated on the dried basis. Meets the requirements for Identification, Loss on drying (not more than 0.25%), Residue on ignition (not more than 0.25%), and Heavy metals (0.001%).

AMINOPHYLLINE

Source: The ethylenediamine salt of theophylline.

Chemical name: 1*H*-Purine-2,6-dione, 3,7-dihydro-1,3-dimethyl-, compd. with 1,2-ethanediamine (2:1).

Molecular formula: $C_{16}H_{24}N_{10}O_4$.

Molecular weight: 420.43.

Description:

Aminophylline USP—White or slightly yellowish granules or powder, having a slight ammoniacal odor. Upon exposure to air, it gradually loses ethylenediamine and absorbs carbon dioxide with the liberation of free theophylline. Its solutions are alkaline to litmus.

Aminophylline Tablets USP—May have a faint ammoniacal odor.

Solubility: Aminophylline USP—One gram dissolves in 25 mL of water to give a clear solution; one gram dissolved in 5 mL of water crystallizes upon standing, but redissolves when a small amount of ethylenediamine is added. Insoluble in alcohol and in ether.

USP requirements:

Aminophylline USP—Preserve in tight containers. It is anhydrous or contains not more than two molecules of water of hydration. Label it to indicate whether it is anhydrous or hydrous, and also to state the content of anhydrous theophylline. Contains not less than 84.0% and not more than 87.4% of anhydrous theophylline, calculated on the anhydrous basis. Meets the requirements for Identification, Water (not more than 0.75% [anhydrous form] and not more than 7.9% [hydrous form]), Residue on ignition (not more than 0.15%), Ethylenediamine content (157–175 mg per gram of theophylline), and Organic volatile impurities.

Aminophylline Enema USP—Preserve in single-dose or in multiple-dose containers. An aqueous solution of Aminophylline, prepared with the aid of Ethylenediamine. Label the Enema to state the content of anhydrous theophylline. Contains an amount of aminophylline equivalent to the labeled amount of anhydrous theophylline, within ±10%. Aminophylline Enema may contain an excess of ethylenediamine, but no other substance may be added for the purpose of pH adjustment. Meets the requirements for Identification, pH (9.0–9.5), and Ethylenediamine content (218–267 mg per gram of anhydrous theophylline).

Aminophylline Injection USP—Preserve in single-dose containers from which carbon dioxide has been excluded, preferably of Type I glass, protected from light. A sterile solution of Aminophylline in Water for Injection, or a sterile solution of Theophylline in Water for Injection prepared with the aid of Ethylenediamine. Label the Injection to state the content of anhydrous theophylline. Contains, in each mL, an amount of aminophylline equivalent to the labeled amount of anhydrous theophylline, within ±7%. Aminophylline Injection may contain an excess of Ethylenediamine, but no other substance may be added for the purpose of pH adjustment. Meets the requirements for Identification, pH (8.6–9.0), Particulate matter, Injections, and Ethylenediamine content (166–192 mg per gram of anhydrous theophylline).

Note: Do not use the Injection if crystals have separated.

Aminophylline Oral Solution USP—Preserve in tight containers. An aqueous solution of Aminophylline, prepared with the aid of Ethylenediamine. Label the Oral Solution to state the content of anhydrous theophylline. Contains an amount of aminophylline equivalent to the labeled amount of anhydrous theophylline, within ±10%. Aminophylline Oral Solution may contain an excess of ethylenediamine, but no other substance may be added for the purpose of pH adjustment. Meets the requirements for Identification, pH (8.5–9.7), and Ethylenediamine content (176–283 mg per gram of anhydrous theophylline).

Aminophylline Suppositories USP—Preserve in well-closed containers, in a cold place. Label the Suppositories to state the content of anhydrous theophylline. Contain an amount of aminophylline equivalent to the labeled amount of anhydrous theophylline, within ± 10%. Meet the requirements for Identification and Ethylenediamine content (152–190 mg per gram of anhydrous theophylline).

Aminophylline Tablets USP—Preserve in tight containers. Label the Tablets to state the content of anhydrous theophylline. Contain an amount of aminophylline equivalent to the labeled amount of anhydrous theophylline, within ± 7%. Meet the requirements for Identification, Disintegration (30 minutes, for enteric-coated tablets), Dissolution (75% in 45 minutes in water in Apparatus 2 at 50 rpm, for uncoated or plain coated tablets), Uniformity of dosage units, and Ethylenediamine content (152–178 mg per gram of anhydrous theophylline).

Note: The ammoniacal odor present in the vapor space above Aminophylline Tablets is often quite strong, especially when bottles having suitably tight closures are newly opened. This is due to ethylenediamine vapor pressure build-up, a natural condition in the case of aminophylline.

Aminophylline Extended-release Tablets—Not in USP.

AMINOPHYLLINE AND SODIUM CHLORIDE

For *Aminophylline* and *Sodium Chloride*—See individual listings for chemistry information.

USP requirements: Aminophylline and Sodium Chloride Injection—Not in USP.

AMINOSALICYLATE SODIUM

Chemical name: Benzoic acid, 4-amino-2-hydroxy-, monosodium salt, dihydrate.

Molecular formula: $C_7H_6NNaO_3 \cdot 2H_2O$.

Molecular weight: 211.15.

Description: Aminosalicylate Sodium USP—White to cream-colored, crystalline powder. Is practically odorless. Its solutions decompose slowly and darken in color.

Solubility: Aminosalicylate Sodium USP—Freely soluble in water; sparingly soluble in alcohol; very slightly soluble in ether and in chloroform.

USP requirements:

Aminosalicylate Sodium USP—Preserve in tight, light-resistant containers, protected from excessive heat. Contains not less than 98.0% and not more than 101.0% of aminosalicylate sodium, calculated on the anhydrous basis. Meets the requirements for Clarity and color of solution, Identification, pH (6.5–8.5, in a solution [1 in 50]), Water (16.0–18.0%), Chloride (not more than 0.042%), Heavy metals (not more than 0.003%), m-Aminophenol (not more than 0.25%), Hydrogen sulfide, sulfur dioxide, and amyl alcohol, and Organic volatile impurities.

Note: Prepare solutions of Aminosalicylate Sodium within 24 hours of administration. Under no circumstances use a solution if its color is darker than that of a freshly prepared solution.

Aminosalicylate Sodium Tablets USP—Preserve in tight, light-resistant containers, protected from excessive heat. Contain the labeled amount, within ± 5%. Meet the requirements for Identification, Dissolution (75% in 45 minutes in water in Apparatus 1 at 100 rpm), Uniformity of dosage units, and m-Aminophenol (not more than 1.0%).

AMINOSALICYLIC ACID

Chemical name: Benzoic acid, 4-amino-2-hydroxy-.

Molecular formula: $C_7H_7NO_3$.

Molecular weight: 153.14.

Description: Aminosalicylic Acid USP—White or practically white, bulky powder, that darkens on exposure to light and to air. Is odorless, or has a slight acetous odor.

Solubility: Aminosalicylic Acid USP—Slightly soluble in water and in ether; soluble in alcohol.

USP requirements:

Aminosalicylic Acid USP—Preserve in tight, light-resistant containers, at a temperature not exceeding 30 °C. Contains not less than 98.5% and not more than 100.5% of aminosalicylic acid, calculated on the anhydrous basis. Meets the requirements for Clarity and color of solution, Identification, pH (3.0–3.7, in a saturated solution), Water (not more than 0.5%), Residue on ignition (not more than 0.2%), Chloride (0.042%), Heavy metals (0.003%), m-Aminophenol (not more than 0.25%), and Hydrogen sulfide, sulfur dioxide, and amyl alcohol.

Note: Under no circumstances use a solution prepared from Aminosalicylic Acid if its color is darker than that of a freshly prepared solution.

Aminosalicylic Acid Tablets USP—Preserve in tight, light-resistant containers, at a temperature not exceeding 30 °C. Contain the labeled amount, within ± 5%. Meet the requirements for Identification, Dissolution (75% in 45 minutes in pH 7.5 phosphate buffer in Apparatus 1 at 100 rpm), Uniformity of dosage units, and m-Aminophenol (not more than 1.0%).

AMIODARONE

Chemical group: Benzofuran derivative.

Chemical name: Amiodarone hydrochloride—2-Butyl-3-benzofuranyl 4-[2-(diethylamino)-ethoxy]-3-5-diiodophenyl ketone, hydrochloride.

Molecular formula: Amiodarone hydrochloride—$C_{25}H_{29}I_2NO_3 \cdot HCl$.

Molecular weight: Amiodarone hydrochloride—681.8.

Description: Amiodarone hydrochloride—White to cream-colored crystalline powder.

pKa: 5.6.

Solubility: Amiodarone hydrochloride—Slightly soluble in water; soluble in alcohol; freely soluble in chloroform.

Other characteristics: Amiodarone hydrochloride—Contains 37.3% iodine by weight; highly lipophilic.

USP requirements: Amiodarone Hydrochloride Tablets—Not in USP.

AMITRIPTYLINE

Chemical group: Dibenzocycloheptadiene derivative.

Chemical name: Amitriptyline hydrochloride—1-Propanamine, 3-(10,11-dihydro-5H-dibenzo[a,d]cyclohepten-5-ylidene)-N,N-dimethyl-, hydrochloride.

Molecular formula: Amitriptyline hydrochloride—$C_{20}H_{23}N \cdot HCl$.

Molecular weight: Amitriptyline hydrochloride—313.87.

Description: Amitriptyline Hydrochloride USP—White or practically white, odorless or practically odorless, crystalline powder or small crystals.

pKa: Amitriptyline—9.4.

Solubility: Amitriptyline Hydrochloride USP—Freely soluble in water, in alcohol, in chloroform, and in methanol; insoluble in ether.

Other characteristics: Tertiary amine.

USP requirements:

Amitriptyline Hydrochloride USP—Preserve in well-closed containers. Contains not less than 99.0% and not more than 100.5% of amitriptyline hydrochloride, calculated on the dried basis. Meets the requirements for Identification, Melting range (195–199 °C), pH (5.0–6.0, in a solution [1 in 100]), Loss on drying (not more than 0.5%), Residue on ignition (not more than 0.1%), Heavy metals (0.001%), Chromatographic purity, and Organic volatile impurities.

Amitriptyline Hydrochloride Injection USP—Preserve in single-dose or in multiple-dose containers, preferably of Type I glass. A sterile solution of Amitriptyline Hydrochloride in Water for Injection. Contains the labeled amount, within ± 10%. Meets the requirements for Identification, Pyrogen, pH (4.0–6.0), and Injections.

Amitriptyline Hydrochloride Tablets USP—Preserve in well-closed containers. Contain the labeled amount, within ± 10%. Meet the requirements for Identification, Dissolution (75% in 45 minutes in 0.1 N hydrochloric acid in Apparatus 1 at 100 rpm), and Uniformity of dosage units.

Amitriptyline Pamoate Syrup—Not in USP.

AMMONIA N 13

Source: Different methods are being used in the various clinical facilities for the on-site production of $^{13}NH_3$. It can be produced by irradiation of ^{16}O-water with protons and subsequent reduction using De Varda's alloy or titanium (III) salts. The resultant $^{13}NH_3$ is collected as the ammonium ion in saline solution.

Chemical name: Ammonia-^{13}N.

Molecular formula: $H_3{}^{13}N$.

Molecular weight: 16.00.

USP requirements: Ammonia N 13 Injection USP—Preserve in single-dose or in multiple-dose containers that are adequately shielded. A sterile, aqueous solution, suitable for intravenous administration, of $^{13}NH_3$ in which a portion of the molecules are labeled with radioactive ^{13}N. Label it to include the following, in addition to the information specified for Labeling under Injections: the time and date of calibration; the amount of ^{13}N as ammonia expressed as total megabecquerels (or millicuries) per mL, at time of calibration; the expiration time and date; the name and quantity of any added preservative or stabilizer; and the statement "Caution—Radioactive Material." The labeling indicates that in making dosage calculations correction is to be made for radioactive decay and also indicates that the radioactive half-life of ^{13}N is 9.96 minutes. The label indicates "Do not use if cloudy or if it contains particulate matter." Contains the labeled amount of ^{13}N expressed in megabecquerels (or millicuries) per mL, within ± 10%, at the time indicated in the labeling. Meets the requirements for Specific activity (not less than 37×10^5 megabecquerels [100 curies] per mmol), Radionuclide identification, Bacterial endotoxins, pH (4.5–8.5), Radiochemical purity, Radionuclidic purity, Chemical

purity, and Injections (except that the Injection may be distributed or dispensed prior to completion of the test for Sterility, the latter test being started on the day following final manufacture, and except that it is not subject to the recommendation in Volume in Container).

STRONG AMMONIA SOLUTION

Chemical name: Ammonia.

Molecular formula: NH_3.

Molecular weight: 17.03.

Description: Strong Ammonia Solution NF—Clear, colorless liquid, having an exceedingly pungent, characteristic odor. Specific gravity is about 0.90.

NF category: Alkalizing agent.

NF requirements: Strong Ammonia Solution NF—Preserve in tight containers at a temperature not above 25 °C. A solution of ammonia containing not less than 27.0% and not more than 31.0% (w/w) of ammonia. On exposure to air it loses ammonia rapidly. Meets the requirements for Identification, Nonvolatile residue (not more than 0.05%), Heavy metals (not more than 0.0013%), and Readily oxidizable substances.

Caution: Use care in handling Strong Ammonia Solution because of the caustic nature of the Solution and the irritating properties of its vapor. Cool the container well before opening, and cover the closure with a cloth or similar material while opening. Do not taste Strong Ammonia Solution, and avoid inhalation of its vapor.

AROMATIC AMMONIA SPIRIT

Description: Aromatic Ammonia Spirit USP—Practically colorless liquid when recently prepared, but gradually acquiring a yellow color on standing. Has an aromatic and pungent odor, and is affected by light. Specific gravity is about 0.90.

USP requirements: Aromatic Ammonia Spirit USP—Preserve in tight, light-resistant containers, at a temperature not exceeding 30 °C. A hydroalcoholic solution that contains, in each 100 mL, not less than 1.7 grams and not more than 2.1 grams of total ammonia, and Ammonium Carbonate corresponding to not less than 3.5 grams and not more than 4.5 grams. Meets the requirement for Alcohol content (62.0–68.0%).

AMMONIO METHACRYLATE COPOLYMER

Description: Ammonio Methacrylate Copolymer NF—Colorless, clear to white-opaque granules with a faint amine-like odor.

NF category: Coating agent.

Solubility: Ammonio Methacrylate Copolymer NF—Soluble to freely soluble in methanol, in alcohol, and in isopropyl alcohol, each of which contains small amounts of water; soluble to freely soluble in acetone, in ethyl acetate, and in methylene chloride. The solutions are clear to slightly cloudy. Insoluble in petroleum ether and in water.

NF requirements: Ammonio Methacrylate Copolymer NF—Preserve in tight containers at a temperature not exceeding 30 °C. A fully polymerized copolymer of acrylic and methacrylic acid esters with a low content of quaternary ammonium groups. It is available in 2 types, which differ in content of ammonio methacrylate units. Label it to state whether it is Type A or B. Meets the requirements for Identification, Viscosity, Loss on drying (not more than 3.0%),

Residue on ignition (not more than 0.1%), Arsenic (2 ppm), Heavy metals (0.002%), and Monomers.

AMMONIUM CARBONATE

Chemical name: Carbonic acid, monoammonium salt, mixt. with ammonium carbamate.

Description: Ammonium Carbonate NF—White powder, or hard, white or translucent masses, having a strong odor of ammonia without empyreuma. Its solutions are alkaline to litmus. On exposure to air, it loses ammonia and carbon dioxide, becoming opaque, and is finally converted to friable porous lumps or a white powder of ammonium bicarbonate.
NF category: Alkalizing agent; buffering agent.

Solubility: Ammonium Carbonate NF—Freely soluble in water, but decomposed by hot water.

NF requirements: Ammonium Carbonate NF—Preserve in tight, light-resistant containers, at a temperature not above 30 °C. Consists of ammonium bicarbonate and ammonium carbamate in varying proportions. It yields not less than 30.0% and not more than 34.0% of ammonia. Meets the requirements for Identification, Residue on ignition (not more than 0.1%), Chloride (not more than 0.0035%), Sulfate (not more than 0.005%), and Heavy metals (not more than 0.001%).

AMMONIUM CHLORIDE

Chemical name: Ammonium chloride.

Molecular formula: NH_4Cl.

Molecular weight: 53.49.

Description: Ammonium Chloride USP—Colorless crystals or white, fine or coarse, crystalline powder. Is somewhat hygroscopic.

Solubility: Ammonium Chloride USP—Freely soluble in water and in glycerin, and even more so in boiling water; sparingly soluble in alcohol.

USP requirements:
Ammonium Chloride USP—Preserve in tight containers. Contains not less than 99.5% and not more than 100.5% of ammonium chloride, calculated on the dried basis. Meets the requirements for Identification, pH (4.6–6.0, in a solution [1 in 20]), Loss on drying (not more than 0.5%), Residue on ignition (not more than 0.1%), Thiocyanate, and Heavy metals (not more than 0.001%).
Ammonium Chloride Injection USP—Preserve in single-dose or in multiple-dose containers, preferably of Type I or Type II glass. A sterile solution of Ammonium Chloride in Water for Injection. The label states the content of ammonium chloride in terms of weight and of milliequivalents in a given volume. The label states also the total osmolar concentration in mOsmol per liter or per mL. The label states that the Injection is not for direct injection but is to be diluted with Sodium Chloride Injection to the appropriate strength before use. Contains the labeled amount, within ±5%. Hydrochloric acid may be added to adjust the pH. Meets the requirements for Identification, Pyrogen, pH (4.0–6.0, in a concentration of not more than 100 mg of ammonium chloride per mL), Particulate matter, Chloride content (63.0–70.3%), and Injections.
Ammonium Chloride Delayed-release Tablets USP—Preserve in tight containers. Contain the labeled amount, within ±6%. Ammonium Chloride Delayed-release Tablets are enteric-coated. Meet the requirements for Identification, Disintegration (2 hours, determined as directed for Enteric-coated Tablets), and Thiocyanate.

AMMONIUM MOLYBDATE

Chemical name: Molybdate ($Mo_7O_{24}{}^{6-}$), hexaammonium, tetrahydrate.

Molecular formula: $(NH_4)_6Mo_7O_{24} \cdot 4H_2O$.

Molecular weight: 1235.86.

Description: Colorless or slightly greenish or yellowish crystals.

Solubility: Soluble in 2.3 parts water; practically insoluble in alcohol.

USP requirements:
Ammonium Molybdate USP—Preserve in tight containers. Contains not less than 99.3% and not more than 101.8% of ammonium molybdate. Meets the requirements for Identification, Insoluble substances (not more than 0.005%), Chloride (not more than 0.002%), Nitrate, Sulfate (not more than 0.02%), Arsenate, phosphate, and silicate, Phosphate (not more than 5 ppm), Magnesium and alkali salts (not more than 0.02%), and Heavy metals (not more than 0.001%).
Ammonium Molybdate Injection USP—Preserve in single-dose or in multiple-dose containers, preferably of Type I or Type II glass. A sterile solution of Ammonium Molybdate in Water for Injection. Label the Injection to indicate that it is to be diluted to the appropriate strength with Sterile Water for Injection or other suitable fluid prior to administration. Contains an amount of ammonium molybdate equivalent to the labeled amount of molybdenum, within ±15%. Meets the requirements for Identification, Pyrogen, pH (3.0–6.0), Particulate matter, and Injections.

AMMONIUM PHOSPHATE

Chemical name: Phosphoric acid, diammonium salt.

Molecular formula: $(NH_4)_2HPO_4$.

Molecular weight: 132.06.

Description: Ammonium Phosphate NF—Colorless or white granules or powder.
NF category: Buffering agent.

Solubility: Ammonium Phosphate NF—Freely soluble in water; practically insoluble in acetone and in alcohol.

NF requirements: Ammonium Phosphate NF—Preserve in tight containers. Contains not less than 96.0% and not more than 102.0% of ammonium phosphate. Meets the requirements for Identification, pH (7.6–8.2, in a solution [1 in 100]), Chloride (not more than 0.03%), Sulfate (not more than 0.15%), Arsenic (not more than 3 ppm), and Heavy metals (not more than 0.001%).

AMOBARBITAL

Chemical name:
Amobarbital—2,4,6(1*H*,3*H*,5*H*)-Pyrimidinetrione, 5-ethyl-5-(3-methylbutyl)-.
Amobarbital sodium—2,4,6(1*H*,3*H*,5*H*)-Pyrimidinetrione, 5-ethyl-5-(3-methylbutyl)-, monosodium salt.

Molecular formula:
Amobarbital—$C_{11}H_{18}N_2O_3$.
Amobarbital sodium—$C_{11}H_{17}N_2NaO_3$.

Molecular weight:
Amobarbital—226.27.
Amobarbital sodium—248.26.

Description:
Amobarbital USP—White, odorless, crystalline powder. Its saturated solution has a pH of about 5.6, determined potentiometrically.

Amobarbital Sodium USP—White, friable, granular powder. Is odorless and hygroscopic. Its solutions decompose on standing, heat accelerating the decomposition.

Solubility:
Amobarbital USP—Very slightly soluble in water; freely soluble in alcohol and in ether; soluble in chloroform and in solutions of fixed alkali hydroxides and carbonates.

Amobarbital Sodium USP—Very soluble in water; soluble in alcohol; practically insoluble in ether and in chloroform.

USP requirements:
Amobarbital USP—Preserve in well-closed containers. Contains not less than 98.5% and not more than 101.0% of amobarbital, calculated on the dried basis. Meets the requirements for Identification, Melting range (156–161 °C, but the range between beginning and end of melting does not exceed 3 °C), Loss on drying (not more than 1.0%), Residue on ignition (not more than 0.1%), and Organic volatile impurities.

Amobarbital Tablets USP—Preserve in well-closed containers. Contain the labeled amount, within ± 10%. Meet the requirements for Identification, Dissolution (70% in 30 minutes in pH 7.6 phosphate buffer in Apparatus 1 at 100 rpm), and Uniformity of dosage units.

Amobarbital Sodium USP—Preserve in tight containers. Contains not less than 98.5% and not more than 100.5% of amobarbital sodium, calculated on the dried basis. Meets the requirements for Completeness of solution, Identification, pH (9.6–10.4), Loss on drying (not more than 2.0%), Heavy metals (not more than 0.003%), and Organic volatile impurities.

Amobarbital Sodium Capsules USP—Preserve in tight containers. Contain the labeled amount, within ± 10%. Meet the requirements for Identification, Dissolution (75% in 60 minutes in water in Apparatus 1 at 100 rpm), and Uniformity of dosage units.

Sterile Amobarbital Sodium USP—Preserve in Containers for Sterile Solids. It is Amobarbital Sodium suitable for parenteral use. Meets the requirements for Constituted solution, Loss on drying (not more than 1.0%), and Identification tests, for Completeness of solution, Bacterial endotoxins, pH, and Heavy metals under Amobarbital Sodium, and for Sterility tests, Uniformity of dosage units, and Labeling under Injections.

AMODIAQUINE

Chemical name:
Amodiaquine—Phenol, 4-[(7-chloro-4-quinolinyl)amino]-2-[(diethylamino)methyl]-.

Amodiaquine hydrochloride—Phenol, 4-[(7-chloro-4-quinolinyl)amino]-2-[(diethylamino)methyl]-, dihydrochloride, dihydrate.

Molecular formula:
Amodiaquine—$C_{20}H_{22}ClN_3O$.

Amodiaquine hydrochloride—$C_{20}H_{22}ClN_3O \cdot 2HCl \cdot 2H_2O$.

Molecular weight:
Amodiaquine—355.87.

Amodiaquine hydrochloride—464.82.

Description:
Amodiaquine USP—Very pale yellow to light tan-yellow, odorless powder.

Amodiaquine Hydrochloride USP—Yellow, crystalline powder. Is odorless.

Solubility:
Amodiaquine USP—Practically insoluble in water; sparingly soluble in 1.0 N hydrochloric acid; slightly soluble in alcohol.

Amodiaquine Hydrochoride USP—Soluble in water; sparingly soluble in alcohol; very slightly soluble in chloroform and in ether.

USP requirements:
Amodiaquine USP—Preserve in tight containers. Contains not less than 97.0% and not more than 103.0% of amodiaquine, calculated on the anhydrous basis. Meets the requirements for Identification, Water (not more than 0.5%), Residue on ignition (not more than 0.2%), Chromatographic purity, and Organic volatile impurities.

Amodiaquine Hydrochloride USP—Preserve in tight containers. Contains not less than 97.0% and not more than 103.0% of amodiaquine hydrochloride, calculated on the anhydrous basis. Meets the requirements for Completeness of solution, Identification, Water (7.0–9.0%), Residue on ignition (not more than 0.2%), Chromatographic purity, and Organic volatile impurities.

Amodiaquine Hydrochloride Tablets USP—Preserve in tight containers. Contain an amount of amodiaquine hydrochloride equivalent to the labeled amount of amodiaquine, within ± 7%. Meet the requirements for Identification, Dissolution (75% in 30 minutes in water in Apparatus 2 at 50 rpm), and Uniformity of dosage units.

AMOXAPINE

Chemical group: Dibenzoxazepine.

Chemical name: Dibenz[b,f][1,4]oxazepine, 2-chloro-11-(1-piperazinyl)-.

Molecular formula: $C_{17}H_{16}ClN_3O$.

Molecular weight: 313.79.

Description: Amoxapine USP—White to yellowish crystalline powder.

pKa: 7.6.

Solubility: Amoxapine USP—Freely soluble in chloroform; soluble in tetrahydrofuran; sparingly soluble in methanol and in toluene; slightly soluble in acetone; practically insoluble in water.

Other characteristics: Secondary amine.

USP requirements:
Amoxapine USP—Preserve in tight containers. Contains not less than 98.5% and not more than 101.0% of amoxapine, calculated on the dried basis. Meets the requirements for Identification, Melting range (177–181 °C), Loss on drying (not more than 0.5%), Residue on ignition (not more than 0.1%), and Chromatographic purity.

Amoxapine Tablets USP—Preserve in well-closed containers. Contain the labeled amount, within ± 10%. Meet the requirements for Identification and Uniformity of dosage units.

AMOXICILLIN

Source: Semisynthetic derivative of ampicillin.

Chemical group: Semisynthetic penicillin.

Chemical name: 4-Thia-1-azabicyclo[3.2.0]heptane-2-carboxylic acid, 6-[[amino(4-hydroxyphenyl)acetyl]amino]-3,3-dimethyl-7-oxo-, trihydrate[2S-[2 alpha,5 alpha,6 beta(S*)]]-.

Molecular formula: $C_{16}H_{19}N_3O_5S \cdot 3H_2O$.

Molecular weight: 419.45.

Description: Amoxicillin USP—White, practically odorless, crystalline powder.

Solubility: Amoxicillin USP—Slightly soluble in water and in methanol; insoluble in carbon tetrachloride and in chloroform.

USP requirements:

Amoxicillin USP—Preserve in tight containers, at controlled room temperature. Label it to indicate that it is to be used in the manufacture of nonparenteral drugs only. Contains not less than 90.0% of amoxicillin, calculated on the anhydrous basis. It has a potency equivalent to not less than 900 mcg and not more than 1050 mcg of amoxicillin per mg, calculated on the anhydrous basis. Meets the requirements for Identification, Crystallinity, pH (3.5–6.0, in a solution containing 2 mg per mL), Water (11.5–14.5%), and Dimethylaniline (not more than 0.002%).

Amoxicillin Capsules USP—Preserve in tight containers, at controlled room temperature. Contain the labeled amount, within −10% to +20%. Meet the requirements for Identification, Dissolution (80% in 90 minutes in water in Apparatus 1 at 100 rpm), Uniformity of dosage units, and Water (not more than 14.5%).

Amoxicillin Intramammary Infusion USP—Preserve in well-closed disposable syringes. A suspension of Amoxicillin in a suitable vegetable oil vehicle. Label it to indicate that it is intended for veterinary use only. Contains the labeled amount, within −10% to +20%. Contains a suitable dispersing agent and preservative. Meets the requirements for Identification and Water (not more than 1.0%).

Sterile Amoxicillin USP—Preserve in Containers for Sterile Solids. It is Amoxicillin suitable for parenteral use. Label it to indicate that it is intended for veterinary use only. It has a potency equivalent to not less than 900 mcg and not more than 1050 mcg of amoxicillin per mg, calculated on the anhydrous basis. Meets the requirements for Bacterial endotoxins and Sterility, and for Identification test, Crystallinity, pH, Water, and Dimethylaniline under Amoxicillin.

Sterile Amoxicillin for Suspension USP—Preserve in Containers for Sterile Solids. A sterile mixture of Amoxicillin and one or more suitable buffers, preservatives, stabilizers, and suspending agents. Label it to indicate that it is for veterinary use only. Contains the labeled amount, within −10% to +20%. Meets the requirements for Identification, Bacterial endotoxins, Sterility, pH (5.0–7.0, in the suspension constituted as directed in the labeling), and Water (11.0–14.0%).

Amoxicillin Oral Suspension USP—Preserve in multiple-dose containers equipped with a suitable dosing pump. A suspension of Amoxicillin in Soybean Oil. Label it to indicate that it is for veterinary use only. Contains the labeled amount, within −10% to +20%. Meets the requirements for Identification and Water (not more than 2.0%).

Amoxicillin for Oral Suspension USP—Preserve in tight containers, at controlled room temperature. Contains the labeled amount, within −10% to +20%. Contains one or more suitable buffers, colors, flavors, preservatives, stabilizers, sweeteners, and suspending agents. Meets the requirements for Identification, pH (5.0–7.5 [constituted as directed in the labeling]), Water (not more than 3.0%), Deliverable volume (multiple-unit containers), and Uniformity of dosage units (single-unit containers).

Amoxicillin Tablets USP—Preserve in tight containers, at controlled room temperature. Label chewable Tablets to indicate that they are to be chewed before swallowing. Label film-coated Tablets or Tablets having a diameter of greater than 15 mm to indicate that they are intended for veterinary use only. Contain the labeled amount, within −10% to +20%. Meet the requirements for Identification, Disintegration (30 minutes, in simulated gastric fluid TS [chewable Tablets and Tablets having a diameter of greater than 15 mm are exempt]), and Water (not more than 6.0%, not more than 7.0% for film-coated Tablets, not more than 7.5% for Tablets having a diameter greater than 15 mm).

AMOXICILLIN AND CLAVULANATE

Source:

Amoxicillin—Semisynthetic penicillin.

Clavulanic acid—Fermentation product of the mold *Streptomyces clavuligerus*.

Chemical group:

Amoxicillin—Semisynthetic analog of ampicillin.

Clavulanic acid—A naturally occurring beta-lactam, structurally related to the penicillin nucleus.

Chemical name:

Amoxicillin—4-Thia-1-azabicyclo[3.2.0]heptane-2-carboxylic acid, 6-[[amino(4-hydroxyphenyl)acetyl]amino]-3,3-dimethyl-7-oxo-, trihydrate[2S-[2 alpha,5 alpha,6 beta(S*)]]-.

Clavulanate potassium—4-Oxa-1-azabicyclo[3.2.0]heptane-2-carboxylic acid, 3-(2-hydroxyethylidene)-7-oxo-, monopotassium salt, [2R-(2 alpha,3Z,5 alpha)]-.

Clavulanic acid—(Z)-(2R,5R)-3-(2-Hydroxyethylidene)-7-oxo-4-oxa-1-azabicyclo[3.2.0]heptane-2-carboxylic acid.

Molecular formula:

Amoxicillin—$C_{16}H_{19}N_3O_5S \cdot 3H_2O$.

Clavulanate potassium—$C_8H_8KNO_5$.

Clavulanic acid—$C_8H_9NO_5$.

Molecular weight:

Amoxicillin—419.45.

Clavulanate potassium—237.25.

Clavulanic acid—199.16.

Description:

Amoxicillin USP—White, practically odorless, crystalline powder.

Clavulanate Potassium USP—White to off-white powder. Is moisture-sensitive.

pKa: Clavulanic acid—2.7.

Solubility:

Amoxicillin USP—Slightly soluble in water and in methanol; insoluble in carbon tetrachloride and in chloroform.

Clavulanate Potassium USP—Freely soluble in water, but stability in aqueous solution is not good, optimum stability at a pH of 6.0–6.3; soluble in methanol, with decomposition.

Other characteristics: Clavulanate potassium—Stable at neutral pH.

USP requirements:

Amoxicillin and Clavulanate Potassium for Oral Suspension USP—Preserve in tight containers, at controlled room temperature. Contains the labeled amount of amoxicillin, within −10% to +20%, and an amount of clavulanate potassium equivalent to the labeled amount of clavulanic acid, within −10% to +25%. Contains one or more suitable buffers, colors, flavors, preservatives, stabilizers, sweeteners, and suspending agents. Meets the requirements for Identification, pH (4.8–6.6 [constituted as directed in the labeling]), and Water (not more than 7.5% [25 mg of amoxicillin per mL]; not more than 8.5% [50 mg of amoxicillin per mL]).

Amoxicillin and Clavulanate Potassium Tablets USP—Preserve in tight containers. Label chewable Tablets to include the word "chewable" in juxtaposition to the official name. The labeling indicates that chewable Tablets may be chewed before being swallowed or may be swallowed whole. Tablets intended for veterinary use only are so labeled. Contain the labeled amount of amoxicillin, within −10% to +20%, and an amount of clavulanate potassium equivalent to the labeled amount of clavulanic acid, within −10% to +20%. Meet the requirements for Identification, Disintegration (30 minutes, in simulated gastric fluid TS [veterinary use only]), Dissolution (85% in 30 minutes in water in Apparatus 2 at 75 rpm [veterinary use exempt]), Uniformity of dosage units, and Water (not more than 6.0% where the Tablets are labeled as being chewable; not more than 7.0% [250 mg of amoxicillin or less]; not more than 10.0% [greater than 250 mg of amoxicillin]).

AMPHETAMINE

Chemical name: Amphetamine sulfate—Benzeneethanamine, alpha-methyl-, sulfate (2:1), (±)-.

Molecular formula: Amphetamine sulfate—$(C_9H_{13}N)_2 \cdot H_2SO_4$.

Molecular weight: Amphetamine sulfate—368.49.

Description: Amphetamine Sulfate USP—White, odorless, crystalline powder. Its solutions are acid to litmus, having a pH of 5 to 6.

Solubility: Amphetamine Sulfate USP—Freely soluble in water; slightly soluble in alcohol; practically insoluble in ether.

USP requirements:
Amphetamine Sulfate USP—Preserve in well-closed containers. Amphetamine Sulfate is dried at 105 °C for 2 hours. Contains not less than 98.0% and not more than 100.5% of amphetamine sulfate. Meets the requirements for Identification, Loss on drying (not more than 1.0%), Residue on ignition (not more than 0.2%), Dextroamphetamine, Ordinary impurities, and Organic volatile impurities.

Amphetamine Sulfate Tablets USP—Preserve in well-closed containers. Contain the labeled amount, within ±7%. Meet the requirements for Identification, Dissolution (75% in 45 minutes in water in Apparatus 1 at 100 rpm), and Uniformity of dosage units.

AMPHOTERICIN B

Source: Antifungal antibiotic derived from a strain of *Streptomyces nodosus*.

Chemical name: Amphotericin B.

Molecular formula: $C_{47}H_{73}NO_{17}$.

Molecular weight: 924.09.

Description: Amphotericin B USP—Yellow to orange powder; odorless or practically so.

Solubility:
Amphotericin B USP—Insoluble in water, in anhydrous alcohol, in ether, and in toluene; soluble in dimethylformamide, in dimethyl sulfoxide, and in propylene glycol; slightly soluble in methanol.

Amphotericin B for Injection USP—It yields a colloidal dispersion in water.

Other characteristics: Solubilized by the addition of sodium desoxycholate, which yields a colloidal dispersion in water after reconstitution.

USP requirements:
Amphotericin B USP—Preserve in tight, light-resistant containers, in a cold place. Label it to state whether it is intended for use in preparing dermatological and oral dosage forms or parenteral dosage forms. Has a potency of not less than 750 mcg of amphotericin B per mg, calculated on the dried basis. Meets the requirements for Identification, Loss on drying (not more than 5.0%), Residue on ignition (not more than 0.5% [Note—Amphotericin B intended for use in preparing dermatological creams, lotions, and ointments, and oral suspensions and capsules, yields not more than 3.0%]), and Amphotericin A (not more than 5.0%, calculated on the dried basis [Note—Amphotericin B intended for use in preparing dermatological creams, lotions, and ointments, and oral suspensions and capsules, contains not more than 15% of amphotericin A, calculated on the dried basis]).

Amphotericin B Cream USP—Preserve in collapsible tubes, or in other well-closed containers. Contains the labeled amount, within −10% to +25%. Meets the requirement for Minimum fill.

Amphotericin B for Injection USP—Preserve in Containers for Sterile Solids, in a refrigerator and protected from light. A sterile complex of amphotericin B and deoxycholate sodium and one or more suitable buffers. Label it to indicate that it is intended for use by intravenous infusion to hospitalized patients only, and that the solution should be protected from light during administration. Contains the labeled amount, within −10% to +20%. Meets the requirements for Pyrogen, Sterility, pH (7.2–8.0 [10 mg per mL]), and Loss on drying (not more than 8.0%), and for Uniformity of dosage units and Labeling under Injections.

Amphotericin B Lotion USP—Preserve in well-closed containers. Contains the labeled amount, within −10% to +25%. Meets the requirements for Minimum fill and pH (5.0–7.0).

Amphotericin B Ointment USP—Preserve in collapsible tubes, or in other well-closed containers. It is Amphotericin B in a suitable ointment base. Contains the labeled amount, within −10% to +25%. Meets the requirements for Minimum fill and Water (not more than 1.0%).

AMPICILLIN

Source: Semisynthetic penicillin

Chemical name:
Ampicillin—4-Thia-1-azabicyclo[3.2.0]heptane-2-carboxylic acid, 6-[(aminophenylacetyl)amino]-3,3-dimethyl-7-oxo-, [2S-[2 alpha,5 alpha,6 beta(S*)]]-.
Ampicillin sodium—4-Thia-1-azabicyclo[3.2.0]heptane-2-carboxylic acid, 6-[(aminophenylacetyl)amino]-3,3-dimethyl-7-oxo-, monosodium salt, [2S-[2 alpha,5 alpha,6 beta(S*)]]-.

Molecular formula:
Ampicillin—$C_{16}H_{19}N_3O_4S$.
Ampicillin sodium—$C_{16}H_{18}N_3NaO_4S$.

Molecular weight:
Ampicillin—349.40.
Ampicillin sodium—371.39.

Description:
Ampicillin USP—White, practically odorless, crystalline powder.

Sterile Ampicillin Sodium USP—White to off-white, odorless or practically odorless, crystalline powder. Is hygroscopic.

Solubility:

Ampicillin USP—Slightly soluble in water and in methanol; insoluble in carbon tetrachloride and in chloroform.

Sterile Ampicillin Sodium USP—Very soluble in water and in isotonic sodium chloride and dextrose solutions.

USP requirements:

Ampicillin USP—Preserve in tight containers. It is anhydrous or contains three molecules of water of hydration. Label it to indicate whether it is anhydrous or is the trihydrate. Where the quantity of ampicillin is indicated in the labeling of any preparation containing Ampicillin, this shall be understood to be in terms of anhydrous ampicillin. Contains not less than 900 mcg and not more than 1050 mcg of ampicillin per mg, calculated on the anhydrous basis. Meets the requirements for Identification, Crystallinity, pH (3.5–6.0, in a solution containing 10 mg per mL), Loss on drying (not more than 2.0% for anhydrous; 12.0–15.0% for trihydrate), and Dimethylaniline (not more than 0.002%).

Ampicillin Boluses USP—Preserve in tight containers. Label Boluses to indicate that they are for veterinary use only. Contain an amount of ampicillin (as the trihydrate) equivalent to the labeled amount of ampicillin, within −10% to +20%. Meet the requirements for Identification, Uniformity of dosage units, and Loss on drying (not more than 5.0%).

Ampicillin Capsules USP—Preserve in tight containers. Label Capsules to indicate whether the ampicillin therein is in the anhydrous form or is the trihydrate. Contain an amount of ampicillin (anhydrous or as the trihydrate) equivalent to the labeled amount of ampicillin, within −10% to +20%. Meet the requirements for Identification, Dissolution (75% in 45 minutes in water in Apparatus 1 at 100 rpm), Uniformity of dosage units, and Loss on drying (not more than 4.0% [anhydrous]; and 10.0–15.0% [trihydrate]).

Ampicillin Soluble Powder USP—Preserve in tight containers. A dry mixture of Ampicillin (as the trihydrate) and one or more suitable diluents and stabilizing agents. Label it to indicate that it is for veterinary use only. Contains an amount of ampicillin (as the trihydrate) equivalent to the labeled amount of ampicillin, within −10% to +20%. Meets the requirements for Identification, pH (3.5–6.0, in an aqueous solution containing the equivalent of 20 mg of ampicillin per mL), and Water (not more than 5.0%).

Sterile Ampicillin USP—Preserve in Containers for Sterile Solids. It is the trihydrate form of Ampicillin suitable for parenteral use. Label it to indicate that it is the trihydrate. Where the quantity of ampicillin is indicated in the labeling of any preparation containing Sterile Ampicillin, this shall be understood to be in terms of anhydrous ampicillin. Contains not less than 900 mcg and not more than 1050 mcg of ampicillin per mg, calculated on the dried basis. Meets the requirements for Bacterial endotoxins, Sterility, and Loss on drying (12.0–15.0%), for Identification test, and for pH, Dimethylaniline, and Crystallinity under Ampicillin.

Sterile Ampicillin Suspension USP—Preserve in single-dose or in multiple-dose containers, preferably of Type I glass. A sterile suspension of Ampicillin in a suitable oil vehicle. Label it to indicate that it is for veterinary use only. Contains an amount of ampicillin (as the trihydrate) equivalent to the labeled amount of ampicillin, within −10% to +20%. Meets the requirements for Identification, Sterility, and Water (not more than 4.0%).

Sterile Ampicillin for Suspension USP—Preserve in Containers for Sterile Solids. A dry mixture of Ampicillin (as the trihydrate) and one or more suitable buffers, preservatives, stabilizers, and suspending agents. Contains an amount of ampicillin (as the trihydrate) equivalent to the labeled amount of ampicillin, within −10% to +20%. Meets the requirements for Identification, Bacterial endotoxins, pH (5.0–7.0 [constituted as directed in the labeling]), Loss on drying (11.4–14.0%), Sterility under Sterile Ampicillin Suspension, Uniformity of dosage units, and Labeling under Injections.

Ampicillin for Oral Suspension USP—Preserve in tight containers. Label it to indicate whether the ampicillin therein is in the anhydrous form or is the trihydrate. Contains an amount of ampicillin (anhydrous or as the trihydrate) equivalent to the labeled amount of ampicillin, within −10% to +20%, when constituted as directed. Contains one or more suitable buffers, colors, flavors, preservatives, and sweetening ingredients. Meets the requirements for Identification, pH (5.0–7.5 [constituted as directed in the labeling]), Water (not more than 2.5%, not more than 5.0% [trihydrate and 100 mg per mL]), Deliverable volume (multiple-unit containers), and Uniformity of dosage units (single-unit containers).

Ampicillin Tablets USP—Preserve in tight containers. Label Tablets to indicate whether the ampicillin therein is in the anhydrous form or is the trihydrate. Label chewable Tablets to indicate that they are to be chewed before being swallowed. Tablets intended for veterinary use only are so labeled. Contain an amount of Ampicillin (anhydrous form or trihydrate form) equivalent to the labeled amount of ampicillin, within −10% to +20%. Meet the requirements for Identification, Dissolution (75% in 45 minutes in water in Apparatus 1 at 100 rpm), Uniformity of dosage units, Loss on drying (where the Tablets contain anhydrous ampicillin, not more than 4.0% for powder from nonchewable Tablets and not more than 3.0% for powder from chewable Tablets; where the Tablets contain ampicillin as the trihydrate, not more than 13.0% for powder from Tablets for veterinary use), and Water (where chewable Tablets contain ampicillin trihydrate, not more than 5.0%; where nonchewable Tablets contain ampicillin trihydrate, 9.5–12.0%).

Sterile Ampicillin Sodium USP—Preserve in Containers for Sterile Solids. Protect the constituted solution from freezing. Contains an amount of ampicillin sodium equivalent to not less than 845 mcg and not more than 988 mcg of ampicillin per mg (anhydrous) and, where packaged for dispensing, contains an amount of ampicillin sodium equivalent to the labeled amount of ampicillin within −10% to +15%. Meets the requirements for Constituted solution, Identification, Crystallinity (Note—Sterile Ampicillin Sodium in the freeze-dried form is exempt from this requirement), Bacterial endotoxins, pH (8.0–10.0 in a solution containing 10.0 mg of ampicillin per mg), Water (not more than 2.0%), Particulate matter, and Dimethylaniline (not more than 0.002%), and Methylene chloride (not more than 0.2%), and for Sterility tests, Uniformity of dosage units, and Labeling under Injections.

AMPICILLIN AND PROBENECID

For *Ampicillin* and *Probenecid*—See individual listings for chemistry information.

USP requirements:

Ampicillin and Probenecid Capsules USP—Preserve in tight containers. Contain an amount of ampicillin (as the trihydrate) equivalent to the labeled amount of ampicillin, within −10% to +20%, and the labeled amount of probenecid, within ±10%. Meet the requirements for Loss on drying (8.5–13.0%) and Uniformity of dosage units.

Ampicillin and Probenecid for Oral Suspension USP—Preserve in tight, unit-dose containers. Contains an amount of ampicillin (as the trihydrate) equivalent to the labeled amount of ampicillin, within −10% to +20%, and the labeled amount of probenecid, within ±10%. Contains one or more suitable colors, flavors, and suspending agents. Meets the requirements for pH (5.0–7.5, in the suspension constituted as directed in the labeling), Water (not more than 5.0%), Deliverable volume (for solid packaged in multiple-unit containers), and Uniformity of dosage units (for solid packaged in single-unit containers).

AMPICILLIN AND SULBACTAM

For *Ampicillin* and *Sulbactam*—See individual listings for chemistry information.

USP requirements: Sterile Ampicillin Sodium and Sulbactam Sodium USP—Preserve in Containers for Sterile Solids. A sterile, dry mixture of Sterile Ampicillin Sodium and Sterile Sulbactam Sodium. Contains amounts of ampicillin sodium and sulbactam sodium equivalent to the labeled amounts of ampicillin and sulbactam, within −10% to +15%, the labeled amounts representing proportions of ampicillin to sulbactam of 2:1. Contains an amount of ampicillin sodium equivalent to not less than 563 mcg of ampicillin and an amount of sulbactam sodium equivalent to not less than 280 mcg of sulbactam per mg, calculated on the anhydrous basis. Meets the requirements for Constituted solution, Identification, Bacterial endotoxins, Sterility, pH (8.0–10.0, in a solution containing 10 mg of ampicillin and 5 mg of sulbactam per mL), Water (not more than 2.0%), and Particulate matter, and for Uniformity of dosage units and Labeling under Injections.

AMPROLIUM

Chemical group: Vitamin B_1 or thiamine structural analog.

Chemical name: 1-[(4-Amino-2-propyl-5-pyrimidinyl)methyl]-2-methylpyridinium chloride monohydrochloride.

Molecular formula: $C_{14}H_{19}ClN_4 \cdot HCl$.

Molecular weight: 315.25.

Description: Amprolium USP—White to light yellow powder.

Solubility: Amprolium USP—Freely soluble in water, in methanol, in alcohol, and in dimethylformamide; sparingly soluble in dehydrated alcohol; practically insoluble in isopropyl alcohol, in butyl alcohol, and in acetone.

USP requirements:
Amprolium USP—Preserve in well-closed containers. Label it to indicate that it is for veterinary use only. Contains not less than 97.0% and not more than 101.0% of amprolium, calculated on the dried basis. Meets the requirements for Identification and Loss on drying (not more than 1.0%).
Amprolium Soluble Powder USP—Preserve in tight containers. Label it to indicate that it is for veterinary use only. Contains the labeled amount, within ±5%. Meets the requirement for Identification.
Amprolium Oral Solution USP—Preserve in tight containers. Label it to indicate that it is for veterinary use only. Contains the labeled amount, within ±7%. Meets the requirements for Identification and pH (2.5–3.0).

AMRINONE

Chemical name: Amrinone lactate—5-Amino[3,4′-bipyridin]-6(1*H*)-one 2-hydroxypropanate.

Molecular formula: $C_{10}H_9N_3O$.

Molecular weight: 187.20.

Description: Pale yellow crystalline compound.

Solubility: Solubilities in water at pH 4.1, 6.0, and 8.0 are 25, 0.9, and 0.7 mg per mL, respectively.

USP requirements: Amrinone Lactate Injection—Not in USP.

AMYL NITRITE

Chemical group: Mixture of nitrous acid, 2-methylbutyl ester, and nitrous acid, 3-methylbutyl ester.

Molecular formula: $C_5H_{11}NO_2$.

Molecular weight: 117.15.

Description: Amyl Nitrite USP—Clear, yellowish liquid, having a peculiar, ethereal, fruity odor. Is volatile even at low temperatures, and is flammable. Boils at about 96 °C.

Solubility: Amyl Nitrite USP—Practically insoluble in water. Miscible with alcohol and with ether.

USP requirements:
Amyl Nitrite USP—Preserve in tight containers, and store in a cool place, protected from light. A mixture of the nitrite esters of 3-methyl-1-butanol and 2-methyl-1-butanol. Contains not less than 85.0% and not more than 103.0% of amyl nitrite. Meets the requirements for Identification, Specific gravity (0.870–0.876), Acidity, Nonvolatile residue (0.02%), Total nitrites (not less than 97.0%), and Organic volatile impurities.
Caution: Amyl Nitrite is very flammable. Do not use where it may be ignited.
Amyl Nitrite Inhalant USP—Preserve in tight, unit-dose glass containers, wrapped loosely in gauze or other suitable material, and store in a cool place, protected from light. Contains a mixture of the nitrite esters of 3-methyl-1-butanol and 2-methyl-1-butanol. Contains the labeled amount, within −20% to +5%. Contains a suitable stabilizer. Meets the requirements for Specific gravity (0.870–0.880), Total nitrites (not less than 95.0%), for Identification tests, and for Acidity under Amyl Nitrite.
Caution: Amyl Nitrite Inhalant is very flammable. Do not use where it may be ignited.

AMYLENE HYDRATE

Chemical name: 2-Butanol, 2-methyl-.

Molecular formula: $C_5H_{12}O$.

Molecular weight: 88.15.

Description: Amylene Hydrate NF—Clear, colorless liquid, having a camphoraceous odor. Its solutions are neutral to litmus.
NF category: Solvent.

Solubility: Amylene Hydrate NF—Freely soluble in water; miscible with alcohol, with chloroform, with ether, and with glycerin.

NF requirements: Amylene Hydrate NF—Preserve in tight containers. Contains not less than 99.0% and not more than 100.0% of amylene hydrate. Meets the requirements for Identification, Specific gravity (0.803–0.807), Distilling range (97–103 °C), Water (not more than 0.5%), Nonvolatile residue (not more than 0.02%), Heavy metals (not more than 0.0005%), Readily oxidizable substances, Aldehyde, and Organic volatile impurities.

ANETHOLE

Chemical name: Benzene, 1-methoxy-4-(1-propenyl)-, (E)-.

Molecular formula: $C_{10}H_{12}O$.

Molecular weight: 148.20.

Description: Anethole NF—Colorless or faintly yellow liquid at or above 23 °C. Has the aromatic odor of anise. Affected by light.
  NF category: Flavors and perfumes.

Solubility: Anethole NF—Very slightly soluble in water; freely soluble in alcohol; readily miscible with ether and with chloroform.

NF requirements: Anethole NF—Preserve in tight, light-resistant containers. It is obtained from Anise Oil and other sources, or is prepared synthetically. Label it to indicate whether it is obtained from natural sources or is prepared synthetically. Meets the requirements for Specific gravity (0.983–0.988), Congealing temperature (not less than 20 °C), Distilling range (231–237 °C), Angular rotation (−0.15° to +0.15°), Refractive index (1.557–1.561), Heavy metals (not more than 0.004%), Aldehydes and ketones, Phenols, and Organic volatile impurities.

ANILERIDINE

Chemical name:
  Anileridine—4-Piperidinecarboxylic acid, 1-[2-(4-amino-phenyl)ethyl]-4-phenyl-, ethyl ester.
  Anileridine hydrochloride—4-Piperidinecarboxylic acid, 1-[2-(4-aminophenyl)ethyl]-4-phenyl-, ethyl ester, dihydrochloride.

Molecular formula:
  Anileridine—$C_{22}H_{28}N_2O_2$.
  Anileridine hydrochloride—$C_{22}H_{28}N_2O_2 \cdot 2HCl$.

Molecular weight:
  Anileridine—352.48.
  Anileridine hydrochloride—425.40.

Description:
  Anileridine USP—White to yellowish white, odorless to practically odorless, crystalline powder. Is oxidized on exposure to air and light, becoming darker in color. It exhibits polymorphism, and of two crystalline forms observed, one melts at about 80 °C and the other at about 89 °C.
  Anileridine Hydrochloride USP—White or nearly white, odorless, crystalline powder. Is stable in air. Melts at about 270 °C, with decomposition.

Solubility:
  Anileridine USP—Very slightly soluble in water; freely soluble in alcohol and in chloroform; soluble in ether although it may show turbidity.
  Anileridine Hydrochloride USP—Freely soluble in water; sparingly soluble in alcohol; practically insoluble in ether and in chloroform.

USP requirements:
  Anileridine USP—Preserve in tight, light-resistant containers. Contains not less than 98.5% and not more than 101.0% of anileridine, calculated on the anhydrous basis. Meets the requirements for Identification, Water (not more than 1.0%), Residue on ignition (not more than 0.1%), and Chloride (0.040%).
  Anileridine Injection USP—Preserve in single-dose or in multiple-dose containers, preferably of Type I glass, protected from light. A sterile solution of Anileridine in Water

for Injection, prepared with the aid of Phosphoric Acid. Contains the labeled amount, as the phosphate, within −10% to +15%. Meets the requirements for Identification, Bacterial endotoxins, pH (4.5–5.0), and Injections.
  Anileridine Hydrochloride USP—Preserve in tight, light-resistant containers. Contains not less than 96.0% and not more than 102.0% of anileridine hydrochloride, calculated on the dried basis. Meets the requirements for Identification, pH (2.5–3.0, in a solution [1 in 20]), Loss on drying (not more than 1.0%), Residue on ignition (not more than 0.1%), and Chloride content (16.0–17.2%).
  Anileridine Hydrochloride Tablets USP—Preserve in tight, light-resistant containers. Contain an amount of anileridine hydrochloride equivalent to the labeled amount of anileridine, within ±5%. Meet the requirements for Identification, Dissolution (65% in 45 minutes in 0.1 N hydrochloric acid in Apparatus 1 at 100 rpm), and Uniformity of dosage units.

ANISINDIONE

Chemical group: Indandione derivative.

Chemical name: 2-(p-Methoxyphenyl)indane-1,3-dione.

Molecular formula: $C_{16}H_{12}O_3$.

Molecular weight: 252.27.

Description: White or off-white, crystalline powder.

Solubility: Practically insoluble in water.

USP requirements: Anisindione Tablets—Not in USP.

ANISOTROPINE

Source: Synthetic amine compound.

Chemical group: Quaternary ammonium salt.

Chemical name: Anisotropine methylbromide—8-Azoniabicyclo[3.2.1]octane, 8,8-dimethyl-3-[(1-oxo-2-propylpentyl)oxy]-, bromide, endo-.

Molecular formula: Anisotropine methylbromide—$C_{17}H_{32}BrNO_2$.

Molecular weight: Anisotropine methylbromide—362.35.

Solubility: Anisotropine methylbromide—Soluble in water; sparingly soluble in alcohol.

USP requirements: Anisotropine Methylbromide Tablets—Not in USP.

ANISTREPLASE

Source: Prepared in vitro by acylating human plasma–derived, purified, heat-treated lys-plasminogen and purified streptokinase from group C beta-hemolytic streptococci.

Chemical name: Anistreplase.

Molecular weight: 131,000 daltons.

Description: White to off-white powder.

USP requirements: Anistreplase for Injection—Not in USP.

ANTAZOLINE

Chemical name: Antazoline phosphate—1H-Imidazole-2-methanamine, 4,5-dihydro-N-phenyl-N-(phenylmethyl)-, phosphate (1:1).

Molecular formula: Antazoline phosphate—$C_{17}H_{19}N_3 \cdot H_3PO_4$.

Molecular weight: Antazoline phosphate—363.35.

Description: Antazoline Phosphate USP—White to off-white, crystalline powder.

Solubility: Antazoline Phosphate USP—Soluble in water; sparingly soluble in methanol; practically insoluble in ether.

USP requirements: Antazoline Phosphate USP—Preserve in tight containers. Contains not less than 98.0% and not more than 101.0% of antazoline phosphate, calculated on the dried basis. Meets the requirements for Identification, Melting range (194–198 °C, with decomposition), pH (4.0–5.0, in a solution [1 in 50]), Loss on drying (not more than 0.5%), and Chromatographic purity.

ANTHRALIN

Chemical name: 9(10H)-Anthracenone, 1,8-dihydroxy-.

Molecular formula: $C_{14}H_{10}O_3$.

Molecular weight: 226.23.

Description: Anthralin USP—Yellowish brown, crystalline powder. Is odorless.

Solubility: Anthralin USP—Insoluble in water; soluble in chloroform, in acetone, and in solutions of alkali hydroxides; slightly soluble in alcohol, in ether, and in glacial acetic acid.

USP requirements:
Anthralin USP—Preserve in tight containers in a cool place. Protect from light. Contains not less than 97.0% and not more than 102.0% of anthralin, calculated on the dried basis. Meets the requirements for Identification, Melting range (178–181 °C), Acidity or alkalinity, Loss on drying (not more than 0.5%), Residue on ignition (not more than 0.1%), Chloride, and Sulfate.

Anthralin Cream USP—Preserve in tight containers, in a cool place. Protect from light. It is Anthralin in an aqueous (oil-in-water) or oily (water-in-oil) cream vehicle. Label it to indicate whether the cream vehicle is aqueous or oily. If labeled to contain more than 0.1% of anthralin, contains the labeled amount, within −10% to +15%; if labeled to contain 0.1% or less of anthralin, contains the labeled amount, within −10% to +30%.

Anthralin Ointment USP—Preserve in tight containers, in a cool place. Protect from light. It is Anthralin in a petrolatum or other oleaginous vehicle. If labeled to contain more than 0.1% of anthralin, contains the labeled amount, within −10% to +15%; if labeled to contain 0.1% or less of anthralin, contains the labeled amount, within −10% to +30%.

ANTICOAGULANT CITRATE DEXTROSE

Description: Anticoagulant Citrate Dextrose Solution USP—Clear, colorless, odorless liquid. Is dextrorotatory.

USP requirements: Anticoagulant Citrate Dextrose Solution USP—Preserve in single-dose containers, of colorless, transparent, Type I or Type II glass, or of a suitable plastic material. A sterile solution of Citric Acid, Sodium Citrate, and Dextrose in Water for Injection. Label it to indicate the number of mL of Solution required per 100 mL of whole blood or the number of mL of Solution required per volume of whole blood to be collected. Contains in each 1000 mL of Solution A, not less than 20.59 grams and not more than 22.75 grams of Total Citrate, expressed as citric acid, anhydrous, and not less than 23.28 grams and not more than 25.73 grams of Dextrose, and not less than 4.90 grams and not more than 5.42 grams of Sodium. Contains in each 1000 mL of Solution B, not less than 12.37 grams and not more than 13.67 grams of Total Citrate, expressed as citric acid, anhydrous, and not less than 13.96 grams and not more than 15.44 grams of Dextrose, and not less than 2.94 grams and not more than 3.25 grams of Sodium. Contains no antimicrobial agents.

Prepare Anticoagulant Citrate Dextrose Solution as follows: Solution A—7.3 grams of Citric Acid (anhydrous), 22.0 grams of Sodium Citrate (dihydrate), 24.5 grams of Dextrose (monohydrate), and a sufficient quantity of Water for Injection, to make 1000 mL. Solution B—4.4 grams of Citric Acid (anhydrous), 13.2 grams of Sodium Citrate (dihydrate), 14.7 grams of Dextrose (monohydrate), and a sufficient quantity of Water for Injection, to make 1000 mL. Dissolve the ingredients, and mix. Filter the solution until clear, place immediately in suitable containers, and sterilize. If desired, 8 grams and 4.8 grams of monohydrated citric acid may be used instead of the indicated, respective amounts of anhydrous citric acid; 19.3 grams and 11.6 grams of anhydrous sodium citrate may be used instead of the indicated, respective amounts of dihydrated sodium citrate; and 22.3 grams and 13.4 grams of anhydrous dextrose may be used instead of the indicated, respective amounts of monohydrated dextrose.

Meets the requirements for Identification, Bacterial endotoxins, pH (4.5–5.5), Chloride (0.0035%), and Injections.

ANTICOAGULANT CITRATE PHOSPHATE DEXTROSE

Description: Anticoagulant Citrate Phosphate Dextrose Solution USP—Clear, colorless to slightly yellow, odorless liquid. Is dextrorotatory.

USP requirements: Anticoagulant Citrate Phosphate Dextrose Solution USP—Preserve in single-dose containers, of colorless, transparent, Type I or Type II glass, or of a suitable plastic material. A sterile solution of Citric Acid, Sodium Citrate, Monobasic Sodium Phosphate, and Dextrose in Water for Injection. Label it to indicate the number of mL of Solution required per 100 mL of whole blood or the number of mL of Solution required per volume of whole blood to be collected. Contains, in each 1000 mL, not less than 2.11 grams and not more than 2.33 grams of monobasic sodium phosphate; not less than 24.22 grams and not more than 26.78 grams of dextrose; not less than 19.16 grams and not more than 21.18 grams of total citrate, expressed as citric acid, anhydrous; and not less than 6.21 grams and not more than 6.86 grams of Sodium. Contains no antimicrobial agents.

Prepare Anticoagulant Citrate Phosphate Dextrose Solution as follows: 2.99 grams of Citric Acid (anhydrous), 26.3 grams of Sodium Citrate (dihydrate), 2.22 grams of Monobasic Sodium Phosphate (monohydrate), 25.5 grams of Dextrose (monohydrate), and a sufficient quantity of Water for Injection, to make 1000 mL. Dissolve the ingredients, and mix. Filter the solution until clear, place immediately in suitable containers, and sterilize. If desired, 3.27 grams of monohydrated citric acid may be used instead of the indicated amount of anhydrous citric acid; 23.06 grams of anhydrous sodium citrate may be used instead of the indicated amount of dihydrated sodium citrate; 1.93 grams of anhydrous monobasic sodium phosphate may be used instead of the indicated amount of monohydrated monobasic sodium phosphate; and 23.2 grams of anhydrous dextrose may be used instead of the indicated amount of monohydrated dextrose.

Meets the requirements for Identification, Bacterial endotoxins, pH (5.0–6.0), Chloride (0.0035%), and Injections.

ANTICOAGULANT CITRATE PHOSPHATE DEXTROSE ADENINE

USP requirements: Anticoagulant Citrate Phosphate Dextrose Adenine Solution USP—Preserve in single-dose containers, of colorless, transparent, Type I or Type II glass, or of a suitable plastic material. A sterile solution of Citric Acid, Sodium Citrate, Monobasic Sodium Phosphate, Dextrose, and Adenine in Water for Injection. Label it to indicate the number of mL of solution required per 100 mL of whole blood or the number of mL of solution required per volume of whole blood to be collected. Contains, in each 1000 mL, not less than 2.11 grams and not more than 2.33 grams of monobasic sodium phosphate; not less than 30.30 grams and not more than 33.50 grams of dextrose; not less than 19.16 grams and not more than 21.18 grams of total citrate, expressed as citric acid, anhydrous; not less than 6.21 grams and not more than 6.86 grams of sodium; and not less than 0.247 grams and not more than 0.303 grams of adenine. Contains no antimicrobial agents.

Prepare Anticoagulant Citrate Phosphate Dextrose Adenine Solution as follows: 2.99 grams of Citric Acid (anhydrous), 26.3 grams of Sodium Citrate (dihydrate), 2.22 grams of Monobasic Sodium Phosphate (monohydrate), 31.9 grams of Dextrose (monohydrate), 0.275 grams of Adenine, and a sufficient quantity of Water for Injection, to make 1000 mL. Dissolve the ingredients, and mix. Filter the solution until clear, place immediately in suitable containers, and sterilize. If desired, 3.27 grams of monohydrated citric acid may be used instead of the indicated amount of anhydrous citric acid; 23.06 grams of anhydrous sodium citrate may be used instead of the indicated amount of dihydrated sodium citrate; 1.93 grams of anhydrous monobasic sodium phosphate may be used instead of the indicated amount of monohydrated monobasic sodium phosphate; and 29.0 grams of anhydrous dextrose may be used instead of the indicated amount of monohydrated dextrose.

Meets the requirements for Bacterial endotoxins, pH (5.0–6.0), Chloride (0.0035%), and Injections.

ANTICOAGULANT HEPARIN

USP requirements: Anticoagulant Heparin Solution USP—Preserve in single-dose containers, of colorless, transparent, Type I or Type II glass, or of a suitable plastic material. A sterile solution of Heparin Sodium in Sodium Chloride Injection. Its potency is within ±10% of the potency stated on the label in terms of USP Heparin Units. Label it in terms of USP Heparin Units, and to indicate the number of mL of Solution required per 100 mL of whole blood. Contains not less than 0.85% and not more than 0.95% of sodium chloride. May be buffered. Contains no antimicrobial agents.

Prepare Anticoagulant Heparin Solution as follows: 75,000 Units of Heparin Sodium and a sufficient quantity of Sodium Chloride Injection to make 1000 mL. Add the Heparin Sodium, in solid form or in solution, to the Sodium Chloride Injection, mix, filter if necessary, and sterilize.

Meets the requirements for Bacterial endotoxins, pH (5.0–7.5), and Injections.

ANTICOAGULANT SODIUM CITRATE

Description: Anticoagulant Sodium Citrate Solution USP—Clear and colorless liquid.

USP requirements: Anticoagulant Sodium Citrate Solution USP—Preserve in single-dose containers, preferably of Type I or Type II glass. A sterile solution of Sodium Citrate in Water for Injection. Contains, in each 100 mL, not less than 3.80 grams and not more than 4.20 grams of sodium citrate,

dihydrate. Contains no antimicrobial agents.

Prepare Anticoagulant Sodium Citrate Solution as follows: 40 grams of Sodium Citrate (dihydrate) and a sufficient quantity of Water for Injection, to make 1000 mL. Dissolve the Sodium Citrate in sufficient Water for Injection to make 1000 mL, and filter until clear. Place the solution in suitable containers, and sterilize.

Note: Anhydrous sodium citrate (35.1 grams) may be used instead of the dihydrate.

Meets the requirements for Identification, pH (6.4–7.5), Bacterial endotoxins, and Injections.

ANTIHEMOPHILIC FACTOR

Description: Antihemophilic Factor USP—White or yellowish powder. On constitution is opalescent with a slight blue tinge or is a yellowish liquid.

USP requirements: Antihemophilic Factor USP—Preserve in hermetic containers, in a refrigerator, unless otherwise indicated. A sterile, freeze-dried powder containing the Factor VIII fraction prepared from units of human venous plasma that have been tested for the absence of hepatitis B surface antigen, obtained from whole-blood donors and pooled. May contain Heparin Sodium or Sodium Citrate. Label it to state that it is to be used within 4 hours after constitution, that it is for intravenous administration, and that a filter is to be used in the administration equipment. Meets the requirements of the test for potency, by comparison with the U.S. Standard Antihemophilic Factor (Factor VIII) or with a working reference that has been calibrated with it, in containing ±20% of the potency stated on the label, the stated potency being not less than 100 Antihemophilic Factor Units per gram of protein. Meets the requirements of the test for Pyrogen, the test dose being 10 Antihemophilic Factor Units per kg, and for Expiration date (not later than 2 years from date of manufacture, within which time it may be stored at room temperature and used within 6 months of the time of such storage. Conforms to the regulations of the U.S. Food and Drug Administration concerning biologics.

CRYOPRECIPITATED ANTIHEMOPHILIC FACTOR

Description: Cryoprecipitated Antihemophilic Factor USP—Yellowish frozen solid. On thawing becomes a very viscous, yellow, gummy liquid.

USP requirements: Cryoprecipitated Antihemophilic Factor USP—Preserve in hermetic containers at a temperature of −18 °C or lower. A sterile, frozen concentrate of human antihemophilic factor prepared from the Factor VIII–rich cryoprotein fraction of human venous plasma obtained from suitable whole-blood donors from a single unit of plasma derived from whole blood or by plasmapheresis, collected and processed in a closed system. Contains no preservative. Label it to indicate the ABO blood group designation and the identification number of the donor from whom the source material was obtained. Label it also with the type and result of a serologic test for syphilis, or to indicate that it was nonreactive in such test; with the type and result of a test for hepatitis B surface antigen, or to indicate that it was nonreactive in such test; with a warning not to use it if there is evidence of breakage or thawing; with instructions to thaw it before use to a temperature between 20 and 37 °C, after which it is to be stored at room temperature and used as soon as possible but within 6 hours after thawing; to state that it is to be used within 4 hours after the container is entered; and to state that it is for intravenous administration, and that a filter is to be used in the administration equipment. Meets the requirements of the test for potency by comparison with the U.S. Standard Antihemophilic Factor (Factor VIII) or with a working reference that has been calibrated with it, in having an average potency of not less than 80 Antihemophilic Factor Units per container, made at intervals of not more than 1 month during the dating period. Meets the requirement for Expiration date (not later than 1 year from the date of collection of source material). Conforms to the regulations of the U.S. Food and Drug Administration concerning biologics.

ANTIMONY POTASSIUM TARTRATE

Chemical name: Antimonate(2-), bis[mu-[2,3-dihydroxybutane-dioato(4-)-O^1,O^2:O^3,O^4]]-di-, dipotassium, trihydrate, stereoisomer.

Molecular formula: $C_8H_4K_2O_{12}Sb_2 \cdot 3H_2O$.

Molecular weight: 667.85.

Description: Antimony Potassium Tartrate USP—Colorless, odorless, transparent crystals, or white powder. The crystals effloresce upon exposure to air and do not readily rehydrate even on exposure to high humidity. Its solutions are acid to litmus.

Solubility: Antimony Potassium Tartrate USP—Freely soluble in boiling water; soluble in water and in glycerin; insoluble in alcohol.

USP requirements: Antimony Potassium Tartrate USP—Preserve in well-closed containers. Contains not less than 99.0% and not more than 103.0% of antimony potassium tartrate. Meets the requirements for Completeness of solution, Identification, Lead (not more than 0.002%), Acidity or alkalinity, Loss on drying (not more than 2.7%), and Arsenic (0.015%).

ANTIMONY SODIUM TARTRATE

Chemical name: Antimonate(2-), bis[mu-[2,3-dihydroxybutane-dioato(4-)-O^1,O^2:O^3,O^4]]di-, disodium, stereoisomer.

Molecular formula: $C_8H_4Na_2O_{12}Sb_2$.

Molecular weight: 581.59.

Description: Antimony Sodium Tartrate USP—Colorless, odorless, transparent crystals, or white powder. The crystals effloresce upon exposure to air.

Solubility: Antimony Sodium Tartrate USP—Freely soluble in water; insoluble in alcohol.

USP requirements: Antimony Sodium Tartrate USP—Preserve in well-closed containers. Contains not less than 98.0% and not more than 101.0% of antimony sodium tartrate, calculated on the dried basis. Meets the requirements for Identification, Acidity or alkalinity, Loss on drying (not more than 6.0%), Arsenic (8 ppm), and Lead (not more than 0.002%).

ANTIPYRINE

Chemical name: 1,2-Dihydro-1,5-dimethyl-2-phenyl-3H-pyrazol-3-one.

Molecular formula: $C_{11}H_{12}N_2O$.

Molecular weight: 188.23.

Description: Antipyrine USP—Colorless crystals, or white, crystalline powder. Is odorless. Its solutions are neutral to litmus.

Solubility: Antipyrine USP—Very soluble in water; freely soluble in alcohol and in chloroform; sparingly soluble in ether.

USP requirements: Antipyrine USP—Preserve in tight containers. Contains not less than 99.0% and not more than 100.5% of antipyrine, calculated on the dried basis. Meets the requirements for Completeness and color of solution, Identification, Melting range (110–112.5 °C), Loss on drying (not more than 1.0%), Residue on ignition (not more than 0.15%), Heavy metals (not more than 0.002%), and Ordinary impurities.

ANTIPYRINE AND BENZOCAINE

For *Antipyrine* and *Benzocaine*—See individual listings for chemistry information.

USP requirements: Antipyrine and Benzocaine Otic Solution USP—Preserve in tight, light-resistant containers. A solution of Antipyrine and Benzocaine in Glycerin. Contains the labeled amounts of antipyrine and benzocaine, within ± 10%. Meets the requirements for Identification and Water (not more than 1.0%).

Note: In the preparation of this Otic Solution, use Glycerin that has a low water content, in order that the Otic Solution may comply with the *Water* limit. This may be ensured by using Glycerin having a specific gravity of not less than 1.2607, corresponding to a concentration of 99.5%.

ANTIPYRINE, BENZOCAINE, AND PHENYLEPHRINE

For *Antipyrine, Benzocaine* and *Phenylephrine*—See individual listings for chemistry information.

USP requirements: Antipyrine, Benzocaine, and Phenylephrine Hydrochloride Otic Solution USP—Preserve in tight, light-resistant containers. A solution of Antipyrine, Benzocaine, and Phenylephrine Hydrochloride in a suitable nonaqueous solvent. Contains the labeled amounts, within ± 10%. Meets the requirement for Identification.

ANTIRABIES SERUM

Description: Antirabies Serum USP—Transparent or slightly opalescent liquid, faint brownish, yellowish, or greenish in color, and practically odorless or having a slight odor because of the antimicrobial agent.

USP requirements: Antirabies Serum USP—Preserve at a temperature between 2 and 8 °C. A sterile, non-pyrogenic solution containing antiviral substances obtained from the blood serum or plasma of a healthy animal, usually the horse, that has been immunized against rabies by means of vaccine. Its potency is determined in mice using the Serum Neutralization Test (SNT) or, in cell culture using the Rapid Fluorescent Focus Inhibition Test (RFFIT) in comparison with the U.S. Standard Rabies Immune Globulin. The CVS strain of rabies virus (mouse-adapted or cell culture adapted) is used as the challenge strain. Label it to indicate the species of animal in which it was prepared. Contains a suitable antimicrobial agent. Meets the requirement for Expiration date (not later than 2 years after date of issue from manufacturer's cold storage [5 °C, 1 year; or 0 °C, 2 years]). Conforms to the regulations of the U.S. Food and Drug Administration concerning biologics.

ANTITHROMBIN III (HUMAN)

Chemical group: A glycoprotein.

Molecular weight: 58,000.

Description: Sterile, white powder.

Other characteristics: Antithrombin III (Human) for Injection—Has a pH of 6.5–7.5 after reconstitution.

USP requirements: Antithrombin III (Human) for Injection—Not in USP.

ANTIVENIN (CROTALIDAE) POLYVALENT

Description: Antivenin (Crotalidae) Polyvalent USP—Solid exhibiting the characteristic structure of a freeze-dried solid; light cream in color.

USP requirements: Antivenin (Crotalidae) Polyvalent USP—Preserve in single-dose containers, and avoid exposure to excessive heat. A sterile, non-pyrogenic preparation derived by drying a frozen solution of specific venom-neutralizing globulins obtained from the serum of healthy horses immunized against venoms of four species of pit vipers, *Crotalus atrox, Crotalus adamanteus, Crotalus durissus terrificus,* and *Bothrops atrox* (Fam. Crotalidae). It is standardized by biological assay on mice, in terms of one dose of antivenin neutralizing the venoms in not less than the number of mouse LD_{50} stated, of *Crotalus atrox* (Western diamondback), 180; *Crotalus durissus terrificus* (South American rattlesnake), 1320; and *Bothrops atrox* (South American fer de lance), 780. Label it to indicate the species of snakes against which the Antivenin is to be used, and to state that it was prepared from horse serum. When constituted as specified in the labeling, it is opalescent and contains not more than 20.0% of solids, determined by drying 1 mL at 105 °C to constant weight (± 1 mg). Meets the requirements for general safety and Expiration date (for Antivenin containing a 10% excess of potency, not more than 5 years after date of issue from manufacturer's cold storage [5 °C, 1 year; or 0 °C, 2 years]). Conforms to the regulations of the U.S. Food and Drug Administration concerning biologics.

ANTIVENIN (LATRODECTUS MACTANS)

USP requirements: Antivenin (Latrodectus mactans) USP—Preserve in single-dose containers, and avoid exposure to excessive heat. It is the sterile, non-pyrogenic preparation derived by drying a frozen solution of specific venom-neutralizing globulins obtained from the serum of healthy horses immunized against venom of black widow spiders (*Latrodectus mactans*). It is standardized by biological assay on mice, in terms of one dose of antivenin neutralizing the venom of *Latrodectus mactans* in not less than 6000 mouse LD_{50}. Label it to indicate the species of spider against which the Antivenin is to be used, that it is not intended to protect against bites from other spider species, and to state that it was prepared in the horse. Thimerosal 1:10,000 is added as a preservative. When constituted as specified in the labeling, it is opalescent and contains not more than 20.0% of solids. Meets the requirement for Expiration date (for Antivenin containing a 10% excess of potency, not more than 5 years after date of issue from manufacturer's cold storage [5 °C, 1 year; or 0 °C, 2 years]). Conforms to the regulations of the U.S. Food and Drug Administration concerning biologics.

ANTIVENIN (MICRURUS FULVIUS)

Description: Antivenin (Micrurus Fulvius) USP—Solid exhibiting the characteristic structure of a freeze-dried solid; light cream in color.

USP requirements: Antivenin (Micrurus Fulvius) USP—Preserve in single-dose containers, and avoid exposure to excessive heat. It is the sterile, non-pyrogenic preparation derived by drying a frozen solution of specific venom-neutralizing globulins obtained from the serum of healthy horses immunized against venom of the Eastern Coral snake (*Micrurus fulvius*). It is standardized by biological assay on mice, in terms of one dose of antivenin neutralizing the venom of *Micrurus fulvius* in not less than 250 mouse LD_{50}. Label it to indicate the species of snake against which the Antivenin is to be used, and to state that it was prepared in the horse. When constituted as specified in the labeling, it is opalescent and contains not more than 20.0% of solids, determined by drying 1 mL at 105 °C to constant weight (± 1 mg). Meets the requirements for general safety and Expiration date (for Antivenin containing a 10% excess of potency, not more than 5 years after date of issue from manufacturer's cold storage [5 °C, 1 year; or 0 °C, 2 years]). Conforms to the regulations of the U.S. Food and Drug Administration concerning biologics.

APOMORPHINE

Chemical name: Apomorphine hydrochloride—$4H$-Dibenzo-[*de,g*]quinoline-10,11-diol, 5,6,6a,7-tetrahydro-6-methyl-, hydrochloride, hemihydrate, (*R*)-.

Molecular formula: Apomorphine hydrochloride—$C_{17}H_{17}NO_2 \cdot HCl \cdot \frac{1}{2}H_2O$.

Molecular weight: Apomorphine hydrochloride—312.80.

Description: Apomorphine Hydrochloride USP—Minute, white or grayish white, glistening crystals or white powder. Is odorless. It gradually acquires a green color on exposure to light and to air. Its solutions are neutral to litmus.

Solubility: Apomorphine Hydrochloride USP—Sparingly soluble in water and in alcohol; soluble in water at 80 °C; very slightly soluble in chloroform and in ether.

USP requirements:
  Apomorphine Hydrochloride USP—Preserve in small, tight, light-resistant containers. Containers from which Apomorphine Hydrochloride is to be taken for immediate use in compounding prescriptions contain not more than 350 mg. Contains not less than 98.5% and not more than 100.5% of apomorphine hydrochloride, calculated on the dried basis. Meets the requirements for Color of solution, Identification, Specific rotation (−60.5° to −63.0°, calculated on the dried basis), Loss on drying (2.0–3.5%), Residue on ignition (not more than 0.1%), Decomposition products, and Ordinary impurities.
  Apomorphine Hydrochloride Tablets USP—Preserve in tight, light-resistant containers. Contain the labeled amount, within ± 10%. Meet the requirements for Color of solution, Identification, Disintegration (15 minutes), and Uniformity of dosage units.

APRACLONIDINE

Chemical name: Apraclonidine hydrochloride—1,4-Benzenediamine, 2,6-dichloro-N^1-2-imidazolidinylidene-, monohydrochloride.

Molecular formula: Apraclonidine hydrochloride—$C_9H_{10}Cl_2N_4 \cdot HCl$.

Molecular weight: Apraclonidine hydrochloride—281.57.

Description: Apraclonidine Hydrochloride USP—White to off-white, odorless to practically odorless powder.

pKa: 9.22.

Solubility: Apraclonidine Hydrochloride USP—Soluble in methanol; sparingly soluble in water and in alcohol; insoluble in chloroform, in ethyl acetate, and in hexanes.

USP requirements:

Apraclonidine Hydrochloride USP—Preserve in tight, light-resistant containers. Contains not less than 98.0% and not more than 102.0% of apraclonidine hydrochloride, calculated on the dried basis. Meets the requirements for Identification, pH (4.9–5.9, in a solution [1 in 100]), Loss on drying (not more than 1.0%), Residue on ignition (not more than 0.1%), Heavy metals (not more than 0.002%), and Chromatographic purity (not more than 1.0% for any individual impurity and not more than 2.0% total impurities).

Apraclonidine Ophthalmic Solution USP—Preserve in tight, light-resistant containers. A sterile, aqueous solution of Apraclonidine Hydrochloride. Contains an amount of apraclonidine hydrochloride equivalent to the labeled amount of apraclonidine, within −10% to +15%. Meets the requirements for Identification, Sterility, and pH (4.4–7.8).

APROBARBITAL

Chemical name: 5-Allyl-5-isopropylbarbituric acid.

Molecular formula: $C_{10}H_{14}N_2O_3$.

Molecular weight: 210.23.

Description: White crystalline powder.

Solubility: Slightly soluble in water; soluble in alcohol.

USP requirements: Aprobarbital Elixir—Not in USP.

ARGININE

Chemical name:

Arginine—L-Arginine.

Arginine hydrochloride—L-Arginine monohydrochloride.

Molecular formula:

Arginine—$C_6H_{14}N_4O_2$.

Arginine hydrochloride—$C_6H_{14}N_4O_2 \cdot HCl$.

Molecular weight:

Arginine—174.20.

Arginine hydrochloride—210.66.

Description:

Arginine USP—White, practically odorless crystals.

Arginine Hydrochloride USP—White crystals or crystalline powder, practically odorless.

Solubility:

Arginine USP—Freely soluble in water; sparingly soluble in alcohol; insoluble in ether.

Arginine Hydrochloride USP—Freely soluble in water.

USP requirements:

Arginine USP—Preserve in well-closed containers. Contains not less than 98.5% and not more than 101.5% of arginine, as L-arginine, calculated on the dried basis. Meets the requirements for Identification, Specific rotation (+26.2° to +27.6°, calculated on the dried basis), Loss on drying (not more than 0.5%), Residue on ignition (not more than 0.3%), Chloride (0.05%), Sulfate (0.03%), Arsenic (not more than 1.5 ppm), Iron (0.003%), Heavy metals (not more than 0.0015%), and Organic volatile impurities.

Arginine Hydrochloride USP—Preserve in well-closed containers. Contains not less than 98.5% and not more than

101.5% of arginine hydrochloride, calculated on the dried basis. Meets the requirements for Identification, Specific rotation (+21.4° to +23.6°, calculated on the dried basis), Loss on drying (not more than 0.2%), Residue on ignition (not more than 0.1%), Sulfate (0.03%), Arsenic (not more than 1.5 ppm), Chloride content (16.5–17.1%), Heavy metals (not more than 0.002%), and Organic volatile impurities.

Arginine Hydrochloride Injection USP—Preserve in single-dose containers, preferably of Type II glass. A sterile solution of Arginine Hydrochloride in Water for Injection. The label states the total osmolar concentration in mOsmol per liter. Where the contents are less than 100 mL, or where the label states that the Injection is not for direct injection but is to be diluted before use, the label alternatively may state the total osmolar concentration in mOsmol per mL. Contains not less than 9.5% and not more than 10.5% of arginine hydrochloride. Contains no antimicrobial agents. Meets the requirements for Identification, Bacterial endotoxins, pH (5.0–6.5), and Injections.

Note: The chloride ion content of Arginine Hydrochloride Injection is approximately 475 mEq per liter.

AROMATIC ELIXIR

Description: Aromatic Elixir NF—NF category: Flavored and/or sweetened vehicle.

NF requirements: Aromatic Elixir NF—Preserve in tight containers.

Prepare Aromatic Elixir as follows: Suitable essential oil(s), 375 mL of Syrup, 30 grams of Talc, and a sufficient quantity of Alcohol and Purified Water to make 1000 mL. Dissolve the oil(s) in Alcohol to make 250 mL. To this solution add the Syrup in several portions, agitating vigorously after each addition, and afterwards add, in the same manner, the required quantity of Purified Water. Mix the Talc with the liquid, and filter through a filter wetted with Diluted Alcohol, returning the filtrate until a clear liquid is obtained.

Meets the requirements for Alcohol content (21.0–23.0%) and Organic volatile impurities.

ASCORBIC ACID

Chemical name: L-Ascorbic acid.

Molecular formula: $C_6H_8O_6$.

Molecular weight: 176.13.

Description: Ascorbic Acid USP—White or slightly yellow crystals or powder. On exposure to light it gradually darkens. In the dry state, is reasonably stable in air, but in solution rapidly oxidizes. Melts at about 190 °C.

NF category: Antioxidant.

pKa: 4.2 and 11.6.

Solubility: Ascorbic Acid USP—Freely soluble in water; sparingly soluble in alcohol; insoluble in chloroform and in ether.

USP requirements:

Ascorbic Acid USP—Preserve in tight, light-resistant containers. Contains not less than 99.0% and not more than 100.5% of ascorbic acid. Meets the requirements for Identification, Specific rotation (+20.5° to +21.5°), Residue on ignition (not more than 0.1%), and Heavy metals (not more than 0.002%).

Ascorbic Acid Extended-release Capsules—Not in USP.

Ascorbic Acid Injection USP—Preserve in light-resistant, single-dose containers, preferably of Type I or Type II glass. A sterile solution, in Water for Injection, of Ascorbic Acid prepared with the aid of Sodium Hydroxide, Sodium Carbonate, or Sodium Bicarbonate. In addition to meeting the requirements for Labeling under Injections, fused-seal containers of the Injection in concentrations of 250 mg per mL and greater are labeled to indicate that since pressure may develop on long storage, precautions should be taken to wrap the container in a protective covering while it is being opened. Contains the labeled amount, within ± 10%. Meets the requirements for Identification, Bacterial endotoxins, pH (5.5–7.0), Oxalate, and Injections.

Ascorbic Acid Oral Solution USP—Preserve in tight, light-resistant containers. A solution of Ascorbic Acid in a hydroxylic organic solvent or an aqueous mixture thereof. Label Oral Solution that contains alcohol to state the alcohol content. Contains the labeled amount, within ± 10%. Meets requirements for Identification and Alcohol content (90–110%).

Ascorbic Acid Syrup—Not in USP.

Ascorbic Acid Tablets USP—Preserve in tight, light-resistant containers. Contain the labeled amount, within ± 10%. Meet requirements for Identification, Disintegration (30 minutes), and Uniformity of dosage units.

Ascorbic Acid Extended-release Tablets—Not in USP.

ASCORBYL PALMITATE

Chemical name: L-Ascorbic acid, 6-hexadecanoate.

Molecular formula: $C_{22}H_{38}O_7$.

Molecular weight: 414.54.

Description: Ascorbyl Palmitate NF—White to yellowish white powder, having a characteristic odor.

NF category: Antioxidant.

Solubility: Ascorbyl Palmitate NF—Very slightly soluble in water and in vegetable oils; soluble in alcohol.

NF requirements: Ascorbyl Palmitate NF—Preserve in tight containers, in a cool, dry place. Contains not less than 95.0% and not more than 100.5% of ascorbyl palmitate, calculated on the dried basis. Meets the requirements for Identification, Melting range (107–117 °C), Specific rotation (+21° to +24°, calculated on the dried basis), Loss on drying (not more than 2.0%), Residue on ignition (not more than 0.1%), and Heavy metals (0.001%).

ASPARAGINASE

Source: Asparaginase is a high molecular weight enzyme obtained commercially from *Escherichia coli.*

Chemical name: Asparaginase.

Description: White, crystalline powder.

Solubility: Freely soluble in water; practically insoluble in methanol, in acetone, and in chloroform.

Other characteristics: Slightly hygroscopic; active at pH 6.5 to 8.0.

USP requirements: Asparaginase for Injection—Not in USP.

ASPARTAME

Chemical Name: L-Phenylalanine, *N*-L-alpha-aspartyl-, 1-methyl ester.

Molecular formula: $C_{14}H_{18}N_2O_5$.

Molecular weight: 294.31.

Description: Aspartame NF—White, odorless, crystalline powder. Melts at about 246 °C. The pH of an 8 in 1000 solution is about 5.

NF category: Sweetening agent.

Solubility: Aspartame NF—Sparingly soluble in water; slightly soluble in alcohol.

NF requirements: Aspartame NF—Preserve in well-closed containers. Contains not less than 98.0% and not more than 102.0% of aspartame, calculated on the dried basis. Meets the requirements for Identification, Transmittance, Specific rotation (+14.5° to +16.5°, calculated on the dried basis), Loss on drying (not more than 4.5%), Residue on ignition (not more than 0.2%), Arsenic (not more than 3 ppm), Heavy metals (not more than 0.001%), Other related substances, 5-Benzyl-3,6-dioxo-2-piperazineacetic acid, and Organic volatile impurities.

ASPIRIN

Chemical name: Benzoic acid, 2-(acetyloxy)-.

Molecular formula: $C_9H_8O_4$.

Molecular weight: 180.16.

Description: Aspirin USP—White crystals, commonly tabular or needle-like, or white, crystalline powder. Is odorless or has a faint odor. Is stable in dry air; in moist air it gradually hydrolyzes to salicylic and acetic acids.

pKa: 3.5.

Solubility: Aspirin USP—Slightly soluble in water; freely soluble in alcohol; soluble in chloroform and in ether; sparingly soluble in absolute ether.

USP requirements:

Aspirin USP—Preserve in tight containers. Contains not less than 99.5% and not more than 100.5% of aspirin, calculated on the dried basis. Meets the requirements for Identification, Loss on drying (not more than 0.5%), Residue on ignition (not more than 0.05%), Chloride (not more than 0.014%), Sulfate (not more than 0.04%), Nonaspirin salicylates (not more than 0.1%), Heavy metals (not more than 0.001%), Readily carbonizable substances, Substances insoluble in sodium carbonate TS, and Organic volatile impurities.

Aspirin Capsules USP—Preserve in tight containers. Contain the labeled amount, within ± 7%. Meet the requirements for Identification, Dissolution (80% in 30 minutes in 0.05 *M* acetate buffer [pH 4.5 ± 0.05] in Apparatus 1 at 100 rpm), Uniformity of dosage units, and Free salicylic acid (not more than 0.75%, calculated on the labeled aspirin content).

Note: Capsules that are enteric-coated or the contents of which are enteric-coated meet the requirements for Aspirin Delayed-release Capsules USP.

Aspirin Delayed-release Capsules USP—Preserve in tight containers. The label indicates that Aspirin Delayed-release Capsules or the contents thereof are enteric-coated. Contain the labeled amount, within ± 7%. Meet the requirements for Identification, Drug release, Uniformity of dosage units, and Free salicylic acid (not more than 3.0%).

Aspirin Suppositories USP—Preserve in well-closed containers, in a cool place. Contain the labeled amount, within ± 10%. Meet the requirements for Identification and Nonaspirin salicylates (not more than 3.0%).

Aspirin Tablets USP—Preserve in tight containers. Preserve flavored or sweetened Tablets of 81-mg size or smaller in containers holding not more than 36 Tablets each. Contain the labeled amount, within ±10%. Tablets of larger than 81-mg size contain no sweeteners or other flavors. Meet the requirements for Identification, Dissolution (80% in 30 minutes in 0.05 *M* acetate buffer [pH 4.5 ±0.05] in Apparatus 1 at 50 rpm), Uniformity of dosage units, and Free salicylic acid (not more than 0.3% [uncoated tablets] or 3.0% [coated tablets]).

Note: Tablets that are enteric-coated meet the requirements for Aspirin Delayed-release Tablets USP.

Aspirin Chewing Gum Tablets—Not in USP.

Aspirin Delayed-release Tablets USP—Preserve in tight containers. The label indicates that Aspirin Delayed-release Tablets are enteric-coated. Contain the labeled amount, within ±5%. Meet the requirements for Identification, Drug release, Uniformity of dosage units, and Free salicylic acid (not more than 3.0%).

Aspirin Extended-release Tablets USP—Preserve in tight containers. Label to indicate the Drug release test with which the product complies. Contain the labeled amount, within ±5%. Meet the requirements for Identification, Drug release, Uniformity of dosage units, and Free salicylic acid (not more than 3.0%).

BUFFERED ASPIRIN

Chemical name: Aspirin—Benzoic acid, 2-(acetyloxy)-.

Molecular formula: Aspirin—$C_9H_8O_4$.

Molecular weight: Aspirin—180.16.

Description: Aspirin USP—White crystals, commonly tabular or needle-like, or white, crystalline powder. Is odorless or has a faint odor. Is stable in dry air; in moist air it gradually hydrolyzes to salicylic and acetic acids.

pKa: Aspirin—3.5.

Solubility: Aspirin USP—Slightly soluble in water; freely soluble in alcohol; soluble in chloroform and in ether; sparingly soluble in absolute ether.

USP requirements: Buffered Aspirin Tablets USP—Preserve in tight containers. Contain Aspirin and suitable buffering agents. Contain the labeled amount of aspirin, within ±10%. Meet the requirements for Identification, Dissolution (80% in 30 minutes in 0.05 *M* acetate buffer [pH 4.5 ± 0.05] in Apparatus 2 at 75 rpm), Uniformity of dosage units, Acid-neutralizing capacity (not less than 1.9 mEq of acid is consumed for each 325 mg of aspirin in the Tablets), and Free salicylic acid limit (not more than 3%).

ASPIRIN, ALUMINA, AND MAGNESIA

For *Aspirin, Alumina* (Aluminum Hydroxide), and *Magnesia* (Magnesium Hydroxide)—See individual listings for chemistry information.

USP requirements: Aspirin, Alumina, and Magnesia Tablets USP—Preserve in tight containers. Contain the labeled amount of aspirin, within ±10%, and amounts of alumina and magnesia equivalent to the labeled amounts of aluminum hydroxide and magnesium hydroxide, within ±10%. Meet the requirements for Identification, Dissolution (75% in 45 minutes in 0.05 *M* acetate buffer [pH 4.5 ± 0.05] in Apparatus 2 at 75 rpm), Uniformity of dosage units, Acid-neutralizing capacity (not less than 1.9 mEq of acid is consumed for each 325 mg of aspirin in the Tablets), and Free salicylic acid limit (not more than 3.0%).

ASPIRIN, ALUMINA, AND MAGNESIUM OXIDE

For *Aspirin, Alumina* (Aluminum Hydroxide), and *Magnesium Oxide*—See individual listings for chemistry information.

USP requirements: Aspirin, Alumina, and Magnesium Oxide Tablets USP—Preserve in tight containers. Contain the labeled amounts of aspirin and magnesium oxide, within ±10%, and an amount of alumina equivalent to the labeled amount of aluminum hydroxide, within ±10%. Meet the requirements for Identification, Dissolution (75% in 45 minutes in 0.05 *M* acetate buffer [pH 4.5 ±0.05] in Apparatus 2 at 75 rpm), Uniformity of dosage units, Acid-neutralizing capacity (not less than 1.9 mEq of acid is consumed for each 325 mg of aspirin in the Tablets), and Free salicylic acid limit (not more than 3%).

ASPIRIN AND CAFFEINE

For *Aspirin* and *Caffeine*—See individual listings for chemistry information.

USP requirements:
Aspirin and Caffeine Capsules—Not in USP.
Aspirin and Caffeine Tablets—Not in USP.

BUFFERED ASPIRIN AND CAFFEINE

Source: Caffeine—Coffee, tea, cola, and cocoa or chocolate. May also be synthesized from urea or dimethylurea.

Chemical group: Caffeine—Methylated xanthine.

Chemical name:
Aspirin—Benzoic acid, 2-(acetyloxy)-.
Caffeine—1*H*-Purine-2,6-dione, 3,7-dihydro-1,3,7-trimethyl-.

Molecular formula:
Aspirin—$C_9H_8O_4$.
Caffeine—$C_8H_{10}N_4O_2$ (anhydrous); $C_8H_{10}N_4O_2 \cdot H_2O$ (monohydrate).

Molecular weight:
Aspirin—180.16.
Caffeine—194.19 (anhydrous); 212.21 (monohydrate).

Description:
Aspirin USP—White crystals, commonly tabular or needle-like, or white, crystalline powder. Is odorless or has a faint odor. Is stable in dry air; in moist air it gradually hydrolyzes to salicylic and acetic acids.
Caffeine USP—White powder or white, glistening needles, usually matted together. Is odorless. Its solutions are neutral to litmus. The hydrate is efflorescent in air.

pKa: Aspirin—3.5.

Solubility:
Aspirin USP—Slightly soluble in water; freely soluble in alcohol; soluble in chloroform and in ether; sparingly soluble in absolute ether.
Caffeine USP—Sparingly soluble in water and in alcohol; freely soluble in chloroform; slightly soluble in ether.
The aqueous solubility of caffeine is increased by organic acids or their alkali salts, such as citrates, benzoates, salicylates, or cinnamates, which dissociate to yield caffeine when dissolved in biological fluids.

USP requirements: Buffered Aspirin and Caffeine Tablets—Not in USP.

ASPIRIN, CAFFEINE, AND DIHYDROCODEINE

For *Aspirin, Caffeine,* and *Dihydrocodeine*—See individual listings for chemistry information.

USP requirements: Aspirin, Caffeine, and Dihydrocodeine Capsules USP—Preserve in tight containers. Label Capsules to state both the content of the dihydrocodeine active moiety and the content of the dihydrocodeine bitartrate salt used in formulating the article. Contain the labeled amounts of aspirin and caffeine and an amount of dihydrocodeine equivalent to the labeled amount of dihydrocodeine bitartrate, within ±10%. Meet the requirements for Identification, Dissolution (75% in 45 minutes in 0.05 *M* acetate buffer [pH 4.50 ± 0.05] in Apparatus 1 at 50 rpm), Uniformity of dosage units, and Salicylic acid limit (not more than 3.0%).

ASPIRIN AND CODEINE

For *Aspirin* and *Codeine*—See individual listings for chemistry information.

USP requirements: Aspirin and Codeine Phosphate Tablets USP—Preserve in well-closed, light-resistant containers. Contain the labeled amounts of aspirin and codeine phosphate hemihydrate, within ±10%. Meet the requirements for Identification, Dissolution (75% of each ingredient in 30 minutes in 0.05 *M* acetate buffer [pH 4.5 ± 0.05] in Apparatus 2 at 75 rpm), Uniformity of dosage units, and Free salicylic acid (not more than 3.0%).

ASPIRIN, CODEINE, AND CAFFEINE

For *Aspirin, Codeine,* and *Caffeine*—See individual listings for chemistry information.

USP requirements:
Aspirin, Codeine Phosphate, and Caffeine Capsules USP—Preserve in well-closed, light-resistant containers. Contain the labeled amounts of aspirin, codeine phosphate hemihydrate, and caffeine, within ±10%. Meet the requirements for Identification, Uniformity of dosage units, and Salicylic acid (not more than 3.0%).
Aspirin, Codeine Phosphate, and Caffeine Tablets USP—Preserve in well-closed, light-resistant containers. Contain the labeled amounts of aspirin, codeine phosphate hemihydrate, and caffeine, within ±10%. Meet the requirements for Identification, Uniformity of dosage units, and Salicylic acid (not more than 3.0%).

ASPIRIN, CODEINE, CAFFEINE, ALUMINA, AND MAGNESIA

For *Aspirin, Codeine, Caffeine, Alumina* (Aluminum Hydroxide), and *Magnesia* (Magnesium Hydroxide)—See individual listings for chemistry information.

USP requirements: Aspirin, Codeine Phosphate, Caffeine, Alumina, and Magnesia Tablets—Not in USP.

ASPIRIN, SODIUM BICARBONATE, AND CITRIC ACID

For *Aspirin, Sodium Bicarbonate,* and *Citric Acid*—See individual listings for chemistry information.

USP requirements: Aspirin Effervescent Tablets for Oral Solution USP—Preserve in tight containers. Contain Aspirin and an effervescent mixture of a suitable organic acid and an alkali metal bicarbonate and/or carbonate. Contain the labeled amount of aspirin, within ±10%. Meet the requirements for Identification, Solution time (within 5 minutes in water at 17.5 ± 2.5 °C), Uniformity of dosage units, Acid-neutralizing capacity (not less than 5.0 mEq of acid is consumed by one Tablet), and Free salicylate (not more than 8%).

ASTEMIZOLE

Chemical name: 1*H*-Benzimidazol-2-amine, 1-[(4-fluoro-phenyl)methyl]-*N*-[1-[2-(4-methoxyphenyl)ethyl]-4-piperi-dinyl]-.

Molecular formula: $C_{28}H_{31}FN_4O$.

Molecular weight: 458.58.

Description: White to almost white powder. It has a melting point of 173–177 °C.

Solubility: Insoluble in water; soluble in chloroform and in methanol; slightly soluble in ethanol.

USP requirements:
Astemizole Oral Suspension—Not in USP.
Astemizole Tablets—Not in USP.

ATENOLOL

Chemical name: Benzeneacetamide, 4-[2-hydroxy-3-[(1-methyl-ethyl)amino]propoxy]-.

Molecular formula: $C_{14}H_{22}N_2O_3$.

Molecular weight: 266.34.

Description: White or almost white, odorless or almost odorless powder.

Solubility: Sparingly soluble in water; soluble in absolute alcohol; practically insoluble in ether.

Other characteristics: Lipid solubility—Very low (log partition coefficient for octanol/water is 0.23).

USP requirements:
Atenolol Injection—Not in USP.
Atenolol Tablets—Not in USP.

ATENOLOL AND CHLORTHALIDONE

For *Atenolol* and *Chlorthalidone*—See individual listings for chemistry information.

USP requirements: Atenolol and Chlorthalidone Tablets—Not in USP.

ATRACURIUM

Chemical name: Atracurium besylate—Isoquinolinium, 2,2'-[1,5-pentanediylbis[oxy(3-oxo-3,1-propanediyl)]]bis[1-[(3,4-dimethoxyphenyl)methyl]-1,2,3,4-tetrahydro-6,7-dimethoxy-2-methyl-, dibenzenesulfonate.

Molecular formula: Atracurium besylate—$C_{65}H_{82}N_2O_{18}S_2$.

Molecular weight: Atracurium besylate—1243.49.

Description: Atracurium besylate injection—Sterile, non-pyrogenic aqueous solution. The pH is adjusted to 3.25–3.65 with benzenesulfonic acid.

USP requirements: Atracurium Besylate Injection—Not in USP.

ATROPINE

Source: Naturally occurring alkaloid—The naturally occurring belladonna alkaloids are found in various solanaceous plants, including *Atropa belladonna, Datura stamonium,* and *Duboisia myoporoides.* The active alkaloids of belladonna include hyoscyamine (which racemizes to atropine on extraction) and scopolamine (hyoscine). Hyoscyamine, the levo-isomer of atropine, is the major active alkaloid of belladonna.

Chemical group: Tertiary amine, natural; an aminoalcohol ester.

Chemical name:
Atropine—Benzeneacetic acid, alpha-(hydroxymethyl)-8-methyl-8-azabicyclo[3.2.1]oct-3-yl ester, *endo*-(±)-.

Atropine Sulfate—Benzeneacetic acid, alpha-(hydroxy-methyl)-, 8-methyl-8-azabicyclo[3.2.1]oct-3-yl ester, *endo*-(±)-, sulfate (2:1) (salt), monohydrate.

Molecular formula:
Atropine—$C_{17}H_{23}NO_3$.
Atropine Sulfate—$(C_{17}H_{23}NO_3)_2 \cdot H_2SO_4 \cdot H_2O$.

Molecular weight:
Atropine—289.37.
Atropine Sulfate—694.84.

Description:
Atropine USP—White crystals, usually needle-like, or white, crystalline powder. Its saturated solution is alkaline to phenolphthalein TS. Is optically inactive, but usually contains some levorotatory hyoscyamine.
Atropine Sulfate USP—Colorless crystals, or white, crystalline powder. Odorless; effloresces in dry air; is slowly affected by light.

Solubility:
Atropine USP—Slightly soluble in water, and sparingly soluble in water at 80 °C; freely soluble in alcohol and in chloroform; soluble in glycerin and in ether.
Atropine Sulfate USP—Very soluble in water; freely soluble in alcohol and even more so in boiling alcohol; freely soluble in glycerin.

USP requirements:
Atropine USP—Preserve in tight, light-resistant containers. Contains not less than 99.0% and not more than 100.5% of atropine, calculated on the anhydrous basis. Meets the requirements for Identification, Melting range (114–118 °C), Optical rotation (−0.70° to +0.05° [limit of hyoscyamine]), Water (not more than 0.2%), Residue on ignition (not more than 0.1%), Readily carbonizable substances, Foreign alkaloids and other impurities (0.2%), and Organic volatile impurities.
  Caution: Handle Atropine with exceptional care, since it is highly potent.
Atropine Sulfate USP—Preserve in tight containers. Contains not less than 98.5% and not more than 101.0% of atropine sulfate, calculated on the anhydrous basis. Meets the requirements for Identification, Melting temperature (not lower than 187 °C, determined after drying at 120 °C for 4 hours), Optical rotation (−0.60° to +0.05° [limit of hyoscyamine]), Acidity, Water (not more than 4.0%), Residue on ignition (not more than 0.2%), Other alkaloids, and Organic volatile impurities.
  Caution: Handle Atropine Sulfate with exceptional care, since it is highly potent.
Atropine Sulfate Injection USP—Preserve in single-dose or in multiple-dose containers, preferably of Type I glass. A sterile solution of Atropine Sulfate in Water for Injection. Contains the labeled amount, within ±7%. Meets the requirements for Identification, Bacterial endotoxins, pH (3.0–6.5), and Injections.
Atropine Sulfate Ophthalmic Ointment USP—Preserve in collapsible ophthalmic ointment tubes. It is Atropine Sulfate in a suitable ophthalmic ointment base. Contains the labeled amount, within ±10%. It is sterile. Meets the requirements for Identification, Sterility, and Metal particles.
Atropine Sulfate Ophthalmic Solution USP—Preserve in tight containers. A sterile, aqueous solution of Atropine Sulfate. Contains the labeled amount, within ±7%. May contain suitable stabilizers and antimicrobial agents. Meets the requirements for Identification, Sterility, and pH (3.5–6.0).
Atropine Sulfate Tablets USP—Preserve in well-closed containers. Contain the labeled amount, within ±10%. Meet the requirements for Identification, Disintegration (15 minutes), and Uniformity of dosage units.
Atropine Sulfate Soluble Tablets—Not in USP.

ATROPINE, HYOSCYAMINE, METHENAMINE, METHYLENE BLUE, PHENYL SALICYLATE, AND BENZOIC ACID

Chemical name:
Atropine sulfate—Benzeneacetic acid, alpha-(hydroxy-methyl)-, 8-methyl-8-azabicyclo[3.2.1]oct-3-yl ester, *endo*-(±)-, sulfate (2:1) (salt), monohydrate.
Hyoscyamine—Benzeneacetic acid, alpha-(hydroxymethyl)-, 8-methyl-8-azabicyclo[3.2.1]oct-3-yl ester, [3(*S*)-*endo*]-.
Methenamine—1,3,5,7-Tetraazatricyclo[3.3.1.1³,⁷]decane.
Methylene blue—Phenothiazin-5-ium, 3,7-bis(dimethyl-amino)-, chloride, trihydrate.
Benzoic acid—Benzoic acid.

Molecular formula:
Atropine sulfate—$(C_{17}H_{23}NO_3)_2 \cdot H_2SO_4 \cdot H_2O$.
Hyoscyamine—$C_{17}H_{23}NO_3$.
Methenamine—$C_6H_{12}N_4$.
Methylene blue—$C_{16}H_{18}ClN_3S \cdot 3H_2O$.
Benzoic acid—$C_7H_6O_2$.

Molecular weight:
Atropine sulfate—694.84.
Hyoscyamine—289.37.
Methenamine—140.19.
Methylene blue—373.90.
Benzoic acid—122.12.

Description:
Atropine Sulfate USP—Colorless crystals, or white, crystalline powder. Odorless; effloresces in dry air; is slowly affected by light.
Hyoscyamine USP—White, crystalline powder. Is affected by light. Its solutions are alkaline to litmus.
Methenamine USP—Colorless, lustrous crystals or white, crystalline powder. Is practically odorless. When brought into contact with fire, it readily ignites, burning with a smokeless flame. It sublimes at about 260 °C, without melting. Its solutions are alkaline to litmus.
Methylene Blue USP—Dark green crystals or crystalline powder having a bronze-like luster. Is odorless or practically so, and is stable in air. Its solutions in water and in alcohol are deep blue in color.
Benzoic Acid USP—White crystals, scales, or needles. Has a slight odor, usually suggesting benzaldehyde or benzoin. Somewhat volatile at moderately warm temperatures. Freely volatile in steam.

NF category: Antimicrobial preservative.

Solubility:
Atropine Sulfate USP—Very soluble in water; freely soluble in alcohol and even more so in boiling alcohol; freely soluble in glycerin.
Hyoscyamine USP—Slightly soluble in water; freely soluble in alcohol, in chloroform, and in dilute acids; sparingly soluble in ether.
Methenamine USP—Freely soluble in water; soluble in alcohol and in chloroform.
Methylene Blue USP—Soluble in water and in chloroform; sparingly soluble in alcohol.
Benzoic Acid USP—Slightly soluble in water; freely soluble in alcohol, in chloroform, and in ether.

USP requirements: Atropine Sulfate, Hyoscyamine, Methenamine, Methylene Blue, Phenyl Salicylate, and Benzoic Acid Tablets—Not in USP.

ATROPINE, HYOSCYAMINE, SCOPOLAMINE, AND PHENOBARBITAL

For *Atropine*, *Hyoscyamine*, *Scopolamine*, and *Phenobarbital*—See individual listings for chemistry information.

USP requirements:
   Atropine Sulfate, Hyoscyamine Sulfate (or Hyoscyamine Hydrobromide), Scopolamine Hydrobromide, and Phenobarbital Capsules—Not in USP.
   Atropine Sulfate, Hyoscyamine Sulfate (or Hyoscyamine Hydrobromide), Scopolamine Hydrobromide, and Phenobarbital Elixir—Not in USP.
   Atropine Sulfate, Hyoscyamine Sulfate (or Hyoscyamine Hydrobromide), Scopolamine Hydrobromide, and Phenobarbital Tablets—Not in USP.
   Atropine Sulfate, Hyoscyamine Sulfate, Scopolamine Hydrobromide, and Phenobarbital Extended-release Tablets—Not in USP.

ATROPINE AND PHENOBARBITAL

For *Atropine* and *Phenobarbital*—See individual listings for chemistry information.

USP requirements:
   Atropine Sulfate and Phenobarbital Capsules—Not in USP.
   Atropine Sulfate and Phenobarbital Elixir—Not in USP.
   Atropine Sulfate and Phenobarbital Tablets—Not in USP.

ATTAPULGITE

Description:
   Activated Attapulgite USP—Cream-colored, micronized, non-swelling powder, free from gritty particles. The high heat treatment used in its preparation causes it to yield only moderately viscous aqueous suspensions, its dispersion consisting mainly of particle groups.
   Colloidal Activated Attapulgite USP—Cream-colored, micronized, non-swelling powder, free from gritty particles. Yields viscous aqueous suspensions, as a result of dispersion into its constituent ultimate particles.

Solubility:
   Activated Attapulgite USP—Insoluble in water.
   Colloidal Activated Attapulgite USP—Insoluble in water.

USP requirements:
   Activated Attapulgite USP—Preserve in well-closed containers. A highly heat-treated, processed, native magnesium aluminum silicate. Meets the requirements for Identification, Loss on drying (not more than 4.0%), Volatile matter (3.0–7.5%, on the dried basis), Loss on ignition (4.0–12.0%), Acid-soluble matter (not more than 25%), and Powder fineness, and for tests for Microbial limit, pH, Carbonate, Arsenic and Lead, and Adsorptive capacity, under Colloidal Activated Attapulgite.
   Colloidal Activated Attapulgite USP—Preserve in well-closed containers. A purified native magnesium aluminum silicate. Meets the requirements for Identification, Microbial limit, pH (7.0–9.5), Loss on drying (5.0–17.0%), Volatile matter (7.5–12.5%, on the dried basis), Loss on ignition (17.0–27.0%), Acid-soluble matter (not more than 15%), Carbonate, Arsenic and Lead, Powder fineness, and Adsorptive capacity.
   Attapulgite Oral Suspension—Not in USP.
   Attapulgite Tablets—Not in USP.

AURANOFIN

Chemical name: Gold, (2,3,4,6-tetra-*O*-acetyl-1-thio-beta-D-glucopyranosato-*S*)(triethylphosphine)-.

Molecular formula: $C_{20}H_{34}AuO_9PS$.

Molecular weight: 678.48.

Description: White, odorless, crystalline powder.

USP requirements: Auranofin Capsules—Not in USP.

AUROTHIOGLUCOSE

Chemical name: Gold, (1-thio-D-glucopyranosato)-.

Molecular formula: $C_6H_{11}AuO_5S$.

Molecular weight: 392.18.

Description: Aurothioglucose USP—Yellow, odorless or practically odorless powder. Is stable in air. An aqueous solution is unstable on long standing. The pH of its 1 in 100 solution is about 6.3.

Solubility: Aurothioglucose USP—Freely soluble in water; practically insoluble in acetone, in alcohol, in chloroform, and in ether.

USP requirements:
   Aurothioglucose USP—Preserve in tight, light-resistant containers. Contains not less than 95.0% and not more than 105.0% of aurothioglucose, calculated on the dried basis. It is stabilized by the addition of a small amount of Sodium Acetate. Meets the requirements for Identification, Specific rotation (+65° to +75°, calculated on the dried basis, determined in a solution containing 100 mg in each 10 mL), and Loss on drying (not more than 1.0%).
   Sterile Aurothioglucose Suspension USP—Preserve in single-dose or in multiple-dose containers, preferably of Type I glass. Protect from light. A sterile suspension of Aurothioglucose in a suitable vegetable oil. Contains the labeled amount, within ±10%. Meets the requirements for Identification and Injections.

AZAPERONE

Chemical name: 1-Butanone, 1-(4-fluorophenyl)-4-[4-(2-pyridinyl)-1-piperazinyl]-.

Molecular formula: $C_{19}H_{22}FN_3O$.

Molecular weight: 327.40.

Description: White to yellowish-white microcrystalline powder. Melting point 90–95 °C.

Solubility: Practically insoluble in water; soluble 1 in 29 of alcohol, 1 in 4 of chloroform, and 1 in 31 of ether.

USP requirements:
   Azaperone USP—Preserve in well-closed containers, protected from light. Label it to indicate that it is for veterinary use only. Contains not less than 98.0% and not more than 102.0% of azaperone, calculated on the dried basis. Meets the requirements for Identification, Melting range (92–95 °C), Loss on drying (not more than 0.5%), Residue on ignition (not more than 0.1%), and Chromatographic purity.
   Azaperone Injection USP—Preserve in single-dose or in multiple-dose containers, preferably of Type I glass, protected from light. A sterile solution of Azaperone in Water for Injection, prepared with the aid of Tartaric Acid. Label it to indicate that it is for veterinary use only. Contains the labeled amount, within ±10%. Meets the requirements for Identification, pH (4.0–5.6), and Injections.

AZATADINE

Chemical group: Piperidine derivative.

Chemical name: Azatadine maleate—5*H*-Benzo[5,6]cyclohepta-[1,2-*b*]pyridine, 6,11-dihydro-11-(1-methyl-4-piperidinylidene)-, (*Z*)-2-butenedioate (1:2).

Molecular formula: Azatadine maleate—$C_{20}H_{22}N_2 \cdot 2C_4H_4O_4$.

Molecular weight: Azatadine maleate—522.55.

Description: Azatadine Maleate USP—White to light cream-colored, odorless powder. Melts at about 153 °C.

pKa: Azatadine maleate—9.3.

Solubility: Azatadine Maleate USP—Freely soluble in water, in alcohol, in chloroform, and in methanol; practically insoluble in ether.

USP requirements:

Azatadine Maleate USP—Preserve in well-closed containers. Contains not less than 98.0% and not more than 102.0% of azatadine maleate, calculated on the dried basis. Meets the requirements for Identification, Loss on drying (not more than 1.0%), Residue on ignition (not more than 0.1%), and Chromatographic purity (not less than 98.0%).

Azatadine Maleate Tablets USP—Preserve in well-closed containers. Contain the labeled amount, within ±10%. Meet the requirements for Identification, Dissolution (80% in 30 minutes in 0.1 N hydrochloric acid in Apparatus 2 at 50 rpm), and Uniformity of dosage units.

AZATADINE AND PSEUDOEPHEDRINE

For *Azatadine* and *Pseudoephedrine*—See individual listings for chemistry information.

USP requirements: Azatadine Maleate and Pseudoephedrine Sulfate Extended-release Tablets—Not in USP.

AZATHIOPRINE

Chemical name: 1*H*-Purine, 6-[(1-methyl-4-nitro-1*H*-imidazol-5-yl)thio]-.

Molecular formula: $C_9H_7N_7O_2S$.

Molecular weight: 277.26.

Description:

Azathioprine USP—Pale yellow, odorless powder.

Azathioprine Sodium for Injection USP—Bright yellow, hygroscopic, amorphous mass or cake.

Solubility: Azathioprine USP—Insoluble in water; soluble in dilute solutions of alkali hydroxides; sparingly soluble in dilute mineral acids; very slightly soluble in alcohol and in chloroform.

USP requirements:

Azathioprine USP—Preserve in tight, light-resistant containers. Contains not less than 98.0% and not more than 101.5% of azathioprine, calculated on the dried basis. Meets the requirements for Identification, Acidity or alkalinity, Loss on drying (not more than 1.0%), Residue on ignition (not more than 0.1%), Limit of mercaptopurine (1.0%), and Organic volatile impurities.

Azathioprine Tablets USP—Protect from light. Contain the labeled amount, within ±7%. Meet the requirements for Identification, Dissolution (65% in 45 minutes in water in Apparatus 2 at 50 rpm), and Uniformity of dosage units.

Azathioprine Sodium for Injection USP—Preserve in Containers for Sterile Solids, at controlled room temperature. A sterile solid prepared by the freeze-drying of an aqueous solution of Azathioprine and Sodium Hydroxide. Contains the labeled amount, within ±7%. Meets the requirements for Completeness of solution, Identification, Bacterial endotoxins, pH (9.8–11.0), Water (not more

than 7.0%), and Limit of mercaptopurine (3.0%), and for Injections and Uniformity of dosage units.

AZLOCILLIN

Chemical name: Azlocillin sodium—4-Thia-1-azabicyclo-[3.2.0]heptane-2-carboxylic acid, 3,3-dimethyl-7-oxo-6-[[[[(2-oxo-1-imidazolidinyl)carbonyl]amino]phenylacetyl]amino]-, monosodium salt, [2*S*-[2 alpha,5 alpha,6 beta(*S**)]]-.

Molecular formula: Azlocillin sodium—$C_{20}H_{22}N_5NaO_6S$.

Molecular weight: Azlocillin sodium—483.47.

Description: Sterile Azlocillin Sodium USP—White to pale yellow powder.

Solubility: Sterile Azlocillin Sodium USP—Freely soluble in water; soluble in methanol and in dimethylformamide; slightly soluble in alcohol and in isopropyl alcohol.

USP requirements: Sterile Azlocillin Sodium USP—Preserve in Containers for Sterile Solids. It is azlocillin sodium suitable for parenteral use. It has a potency equivalent to not less than 859 mcg and not more than 1000 mcg of azlocillin per mg, calculated on the anhydrous basis, and, where packaged for dispensing, contains an amount of azlocillin sodium equivalent to the labeled amount of azlocillin, within −10% to +15%. Meets the requirements for Constituted solution, Identification, Specific rotation (+170° to +200° determined in a solution containing 10 mg per mL), Bacterial endotoxins, Sterility, pH (6.0–8.0 in a solution containing the equivalent of 100 mg of azlocillin per mL]), Water (not more than 2.5%), and Particulate matter, and for Uniformity of dosage units and for Labeling under Injections.

AZTREONAM

Chemical group: Monobactams (*mono*cyclic *bac*terially produced beta-lac*tams*).

Chemical name: Propanoic acid, 2-[[[1-(2-amino-4-thiazolyl)-2-[(2-methyl-4-oxo-1-sulfo-3-azetidinyl)amino]-2-oxoethylidene]amino]oxy]-2-methyl-, [2*S*-[2 alpha,3 beta(*Z*)]]-.

Molecular formula: $C_{13}H_{17}N_5O_8S_2$.

Molecular weight: 435.43.

Description: White crystalline, odorless powder.

Solubility: Very slightly soluble in ethanol; slightly soluble in methanol; soluble in dimethylformamide and in dimethylsulfoxide; practically insoluble in toluene, in chloroform, and in ethyl acetate.

Other characteristics: pH of aqueous solutions—4.5 to 7.5.

USP requirements:

Aztreonam USP—Preserve in tight containers. Contains not less than 90.0% and not more than 105.0% of aztreonam. Meets the requirements for Identification, Water (not more than 2.0%), Residue on ignition (not more than 0.1%), and Heavy metals (not more than 0.003%).

Aztreonam Injection USP—Preserve in Containers for Sterile Solids. Maintain in the frozen state. A sterile solution of Aztreonam and Arginine and a suitable osmolality adjusting substance in Water for Injection. It meets the requirements for Labeling under Injections. The label states that it is to be thawed just prior to use, describes conditions for proper storage of the resultant solution, and directs that the solution is not to be refrozen. Contains the labeled amount of aztreonam, within −10% to +20%. Meets the requirements for Identification, Pyrogen, Sterility, pH (4.5–7.5), and Particulate matter.

Aztreonam for Injection USP—Preserve in Containers for Sterile Solids. A dry mixture of Sterile Aztreonam and Arginine. Contains not less than 90.0% and not more than 105.0% of aztreonam, calculated on the anhydrous and arginine-free basis. Each container contains the labeled amount, within −10% to +20%. Meets the requirements for Constituted solution, Identification, Bacterial endotoxins, Sterility, pH (4.5–7.5 [100 mg per mL]), Water (not more than 2.0%), Particulate matter, and Content of arginine, and for Uniformity of dosage units and Labeling under Injections.

Sterile Aztreonam USP—Preserve in Containers for Sterile Solids. It is Aztreonam suitable for parenteral use. Contains the labeled amount, within −10% to +5%. Meets the requirements for Bacterial endotoxins and Sterility, and for Identification test, Water, Residue on ignition, and Heavy metals under Aztreonam.

BACAMPICILLIN

Chemical group: A semi-synthetic penicillin, an analogue of ampicillin.

Chemical name: Bacampicillin hydrochloride—4-Thia-1-azabicyclo[3.2.0]heptane-2-carboxylic acid, 6-[(aminophenylacetyl)amino]-3,3-dimethyl-7-oxo-, 1-[(ethoxycarbonyl)oxy]ethyl ester, monohydrochloride, [2S-[2 alpha,5 alpha,6 beta-(S*)]]-.

Molecular formula: Bacampicillin hydrochloride—$C_{21}H_{27}N_3O_7S \cdot HCl$.

Molecular weight: Bacampicillin hydrochloride—501.98.

Description: Bacampicillin Hydrochloride USP—White or practically white powder. Is hygroscopic.

Solubility: Bacampicillin Hydrochloride USP—Soluble in methylene chloride and in water; freely soluble in alcohol and in chloroform; very slightly soluble in ether.

USP requirements:
Bacampicillin Hydrochloride USP—Preserve in tight containers. It has a potency of not less than 623 mcg and not more than 727 mcg of ampicillin per mg. Meets the requirements for Identification, pH (3.0–4.5, in a solution containing 20 mg per mL), and Water (not more than 1.0%).
Bacampicillin Hydrochloride for Oral Suspension USP—Preserve in tight containers. Contains an amount of bacampicillin hydrochloride equivalent to the labeled amount of ampicillin, when constituted as directed, within −10% to +25%. Contains one or more suitable buffers, colors, flavors, suspending agents, and sweetening ingredients. Meets the requirements for Identification, pH (6.5–8.0, in the suspension constituted as directed in the labeling), Loss on drying (not more than 2.0%), Uniformity of dosage units (single-unit containers), and Deliverable volume (multiple-unit containers).
Bacampicillin Hydrochloride Tablets USP—Preserve in tight containers. Contain an amount of bacampicillin hydrochloride equivalent to the labeled amount of ampicillin, within −10% to +25%. Meet the requirements for Identification, Dissolution (85% in 30 minutes in water in Apparatus 2 at 75 rpm), Uniformity of dosage units, and Water (not more than 2.5%).

BACILLUS CALMETTE-GUÉRIN (BCG) VACCINE

Source: Obtained from a live culture of the bacillus Calmette-Guérin strain of *Mycobacterium tuberculosis* var. *bovis*. Commercially available strains (which are substrains of the

Pasteur Institute strain) include the Armand-Frappier, Connaught, Glaxo, and Tice substrains.

Description: BCG Vaccine USP—White to creamy white, dried mass, having the characteristic texture of material dried in the frozen state.

USP requirements:
BCG Live (Connaught Strain)—Not USP.
BCG Vaccine USP (Tice Strain)—Preserve in hermetic containers, preferably of Type I glass, at a temperature between 2 and 8 °C. A dried, living culture of the bacillus Calmette-Guérin strain of *Mycobacterium tuberculosis* var. *bovis,* grown in a suitable medium from a seed strain of known history that has been maintained to preserve its capacity for conferring immunity. Contains an amount of viable bacteria such that inoculation, in the recommended dose, of tuberculin-negative persons results in an acceptable tuberculin conversion rate. It is free from other organisms, and contains a suitable stabilizer. Contains no antimicrobial agent. Meets the requirements for expiration date (not later than 6 months after date of issue, or not later than 1 year after date of issue if stored at a temperature below 5° C). Conforms to the regulations of the U.S. Food and Drug Administration concerning biologics.
Note: Use the Vaccine immediately after its constitution, and discard any unused portion after 2 hours.

BACITRACIN

Chemical name:
Bacitracin—Bacitracin.
Bacitracin zinc—Bacitracins, zinc complex.

Description:
Bacitracin USP—White to pale buff powder, odorless or having a slight odor. Is hygroscopic. Its solutions deteriorate rapidly at room temperature. Is precipitated from its solutions and is inactivated by salts of many of the heavy metals.
Sterile Bacitracin USP—White to pale buff powder, odorless or having a slight odor. Is hygroscopic. Its solutions deteriorate rapidly at room temperature. May be amorphous when prepared by freeze-drying. Is precipitated from its solutions and is inactivated by salts of many of the heavy metals.
Bacitracin Zinc USP—White to pale tan powder, odorless or having a slight odor. Is hygroscopic.

Solubility:
Bacitracin USP—Freely soluble in water; soluble in alcohol, in methanol, and in glacial acetic acid, the solution in the organic solvents usually showing some insoluble residue; insoluble in acetone, in chloroform, and in ether.
Sterile Bacitracin USP—Freely soluble in water; soluble in alcohol, in methanol, and in glacial acetic acid, the solution in the organic solvents usually showing some insoluble residue; insoluble in acetone, in chloroform, and in ether.
Bacitracin Zinc USP—Sparingly soluble in water.

USP requirements:
Bacitracin USP—Preserve in tight containers, and store in a cool place. A polypeptide produced by the growth of an organism of the *licheniformis* group of *Bacillus subtilis* (Fam. Bacillaceae). Where it is packaged for prescription compounding, label it to indicate that it is not sterile and that the potency cannot be assured for longer than 60 days after opening, and to state the number of Bacitracin Units per milligram. Has a potency of not less than 40 Bacitracin Units per mg. Meets the requirements

for Identification, pH (5.5–7.5, in a solution containing 10,000 Bacitracin Units per mL), and Loss on drying (not more than 5.0%).

Bacitracin Ointment USP—Preserve in well-closed containers containing not more than 60 grams, unless labeled solely for hospital use, preferably at controlled room temperature. It is Bacitracin in an anhydrous ointment base. Contains the labeled amount, within −10% to +40%. Meets the requirements for Identification, Minimum fill, and Water (not more than 0.5%).

Bacitracin Ophthalmic Ointment USP—Preserve in collapsible ophthalmic ointment tubes. A sterile preparation of Bacitracin in an anhydrous ointment base. Contains the labeled amount, within −10% to +40%. Meets the requirements for Identification, Sterility, Water (not more than 0.5%), and Metal particles.

Sterile Bacitracin USP—Preserve in Containers for Sterile Solids, and store in a cool place. Has a potency of not less than 50 Bacitracin Units per mg. In addition, where packaged for dispensing, contains the labeled amount, within −10% to +15%. Meets the requirements for Constituted solution, Bacterial endotoxins, Sterility, Residue on ignition (not more than 3.0%), and Heavy metals (not more than 0.003%), for Identification test, and for tests for pH, and for Loss on drying under Bacitracin. Where packaged for dispensing, meets the requirements for Injections and Uniformity of dosage units. Where intended for use in preparing sterile ophthalmic dosage forms, it is exempt from the requirements for Pyrogen, Residue on ignition, and Heavy metals.

Soluble Bacitracin Methylene Disalicylate USP—Preserve in well-closed containers. A mixture of bacitracin methylene disalicylate and Sodium Bicarbonate. Label it to indicate that it is for veterinary use only. Has a potency of not less than 8 Bacitracin Units per mg, calculated on the dried basis. Meets the requirements for Loss on drying (not more than 8.5%) and pH (8.0–9.5, in a solution containing 25 mg of specimen per mL).

Bacitracin Methylene Disalicylate Soluble Powder USP—Preserve in tight containers. Label it to indicate that it is for veterinary use only. Label it to state the content of bacitracin in terms of grams per pound, each gram of bacitracin being equivalent to 42,000 Bacitracin Units. Contains an amount of bacitracin methylene disalicylate equivalent to the labeled amount of Bacitracin, within −10% to +20%. Meets the requirements for Loss on drying (not more than 8.5%) and pH (8.0–9.5, in a solution containing 50 mg of specimen per mL).

Bacitracin Zinc USP—Preserve in tight containers, and store in a cool place. It is the zinc salt of a kind of bacitracin or a mixture of two or more such salts. Label it to indicate that it is to be used in the manufacture of nonparenteral drugs only. Where it is packaged for prescription compounding, label it to indicate that it is not sterile and that the potency cannot be assured for longer than 60 days after opening, and to state the number of Bacitracin Units per mg. Has a potency of not less than 40 Bacitracin Units per mg. Contains not less than 2.0% and not more than 10.0% of zinc, calculated on the dried basis. Meets the requirements for Identification, pH (6.0–7.5, in a [saturated] solution containing approximately 100 mg per mL), Loss on drying (not more than 5.0%), and Zinc content.

Bacitracin Zinc Ointment USP—Preserve in well-closed containers containing not more than 60 grams, unless labeled solely for hospital use, preferably at controlled room temperature. It is Bacitracin Zinc in an anhydrous ointment base. Contains an amount of bacitracin zinc equivalent to the labeled amount of bacitracin, within −10% to +40%. Meets the requirements for Identification, Minimum fill, and Water (not more than 0.5%).

Bacitracin Zinc Soluble Powder USP—Preserve in tight containers. A mixture of bacitracin zinc and zinc proteinates. Label it to indicate that it is for veterinary use only. Label it to state the content of bacitracin in terms of grams per pound, each gram of bacitracin being equivalent to 42,000 Bacitracin Units. Contains an amount of bacitracin zinc equivalent to the labeled amount of bacitracin, within −10% to +20%. Meets the requirements for Loss on drying (not more than 5.0%) and Zinc content (not more than 2.0 grams of Zinc for each 42,000 Bacitracin Units).

Sterile Bacitracin Zinc USP—Preserve in Containers for Sterile Solids. It is Bacitracin Zinc suitable for use in the manufacture of sterile topical dosage forms. Label it to indicate that it is to be used in the manufacture of topical drugs only. Has a potency of not less than 40 Bacitracin Units per mg. Meets the requirements for Sterility, and for Identification test, pH, Loss on drying, and Zinc content under Bacitracin Zinc.

BACITRACIN AND POLYMYXIN B

For *Bacitracin* and *Polymyxin B*—See individual listings for chemistry information.

USP requirements:

Bacitracin and Polymyxin B Sulfate Topical Aerosol USP—Preserve in pressurized containers, and avoid exposure to excessive heat. A suspension of Bacitracin and Polymyxin B Sulfate in a suitable vehicle, packaged in a pressurized container with a suitable inert propellant. Contains the labeled amount of bacitracin, within −10% to +30%, and an amount of polymyxin B sulfate equivalent to the labeled amount of polymyxin B, within −10% to +30%. Meets the requirements for Identification and Water (not more than 0.5%), and for Leak testing and Pressure testing under Aerosols.

Bacitracin Zinc and Polymyxin B Sulfate Ointment USP—Preserve in well-closed, light-resistant containers. Contains amounts of bacitracin zinc and polymyxin B sulfate equivalent to the labeled amounts of bacitracin and polymyxin B, within −10% to +30%. Meets the requirements for Identification, Minimum fill, and Water (not more than 0.5%).

Bacitracin Zinc and Polymyxin B Sulfate Ophthalmic Ointment USP—Preserve in collapsible ophthalmic ointment tubes. Contains amounts of bacitracin zinc and polymyxin B sulfate equivalent to the labeled amounts of bacitracin and polymyxin B, within −10% to +30%. Meets the requirements for Identification, Sterility, Minimum fill, Water (not more than 0.5%), and Metal particles.

BACLOFEN

Chemical name: Butanoic acid, 4-amino-3-(4-chlorophenyl)-.

Molecular formula: $C_{10}H_{12}ClNO_2$.

Molecular weight: 213.66.

Description: Baclofen USP—White to off-white, crystalline powder. Is odorless or practically so.

Solubility: Baclofen USP—Slightly soluble in water; very slightly soluble in methanol; insoluble in chloroform.

USP requirements:

Baclofen USP—Preserve in tight containers. Contains not less than 99.0% and not more than 101.0% of baclofen, calculated on the anhydrous basis. Meets the requirements for Identification, Water (not more than 3.0%), Residue on ignition (not more than 0.3%), Heavy metals (0.001%), and Related substances.

Baclofen Tablets USP—Preserve in well-closed containers. Contain the labeled amount, within ±10%. Meet the requirements for Identification, Dissolution (75% in 30 minutes in 0.1 N hydrochloric acid in Apparatus 2 at 50 rpm), Limit of 4-(4-Chlorophenyl)-2-pyrrolidinone (not more than 4.0%), and Uniformity of dosage units.

ADHESIVE BANDAGE

Description: Adhesive Bandage USP—The compress of Adhesive Bandage is substantially free from loose threads or ravelings. The adhesive strip may be perforated, and the back may be coated with a water-repellent film.

USP requirements: Adhesive Bandage USP—Package Adhesive Bandage that does not exceed 15 cm (6 inches) in width individually in such manner that sterility is maintained until the individual package is opened. Package individual packages in a second protective container. Adhesive Bandage consists of a compress of four layers of Type I Absorbent Gauze, or other suitable material, affixed to a film or fabric coated with a pressure-sensitive adhesive substance. It is sterile. The adhesive surface is protected by a suitable removable covering. The label of the second protective container bears a statement that the contents may not be sterile if the individual package has been damaged or previously opened, and it bears the names of any added antimicrobial agents. Each individual package is labeled to indicate the dimensions of the compress and the name of the manufacturer, packer, or distributor, and each protective container indicates also the address of the manufacturer, packer, or distributor. Meets the requirement for Sterility.

GAUZE BANDAGE

Description: Gauze Bandage USP—One continuous piece, tightly rolled, in various widths and lengths and substantially free from loose threads and ravelings.

USP requirements: Gauze Bandage USP—Gauze Bandage that has been rendered sterile is so packaged that the sterility of the contents of the package is maintained until the package is opened for use. It is Type I Absorbent Gauze. Its length is not less than 98.0% of that declared on the label, and its average width is not more than 1.6 mm less than the declared width. Contains no dye or other additives. The width and length of the Bandage and the number of pieces contained, and the name of the manufacturer, packer, or distributor, are stated on the package. The designation "non-sterilized" or "not sterilized" appears prominently on the package unless the Gauze Bandage has been rendered sterile, in which case it may be labeled to indicate that it is sterile and that the contents may not be sterile if the package bears evidence of damage or if the package has been previously opened.

Note: Before determining the thread count, dimensions, and weight, hold the Bandage, unrolled for not less than 4 hours in a standard atmosphere of 65 ± 2% relative humidity at 21 ± 1.1 °C (70 ± 2 °F).

Meets the requirements for Thread count (not more than 3 threads per inch allowed in either warp or filling, provided that the combined variations do not exceed 5 threads per square inch), Width (average of 5 measurements not more than 1.6 mm [1/16 inch] less than labeled width), Length (not less than 98.0% of labeled length), Weight (calculated weight in grams per 0.894 square meter is not less than 39.2 grams), Absorbency (complete submersion of entire bandage roll takes place in not more than 30 seconds), and Sterility, and of the tests for Ignited residue, Acid or alkali, and Dextrin or starch, in water extract, Residue on ignition, Fatty matter, and Alcohol-soluble dyes under Absorbent Gauze.

BARIUM HYDROXIDE LIME

Description: Barium Hydroxide Lime USP—White or grayish white granules. May have a color if an indicator has been added.

NF category: Sorbent, carbon dioxide.

USP requirements: Barium Hydroxide Lime USP—Preserve in tight containers. A mixture of barium hydroxide octahydrate and Calcium Hydroxide. May contain also Potassium Hydroxide and may contain an indicator that is inert toward anesthetic gases such as Ether, Cyclopropane, and Nitrous Oxide, and that changes color when the Barium Hydroxide Lime no longer can absorb carbon dioxide. If an indicator has been added, the name and color change of such indicator are stated on the container label. The container label indicates also the mesh size in terms of standard mesh sieve sizes. Meets the requirements for Identification, Size of granules, Loss on drying (11.0 to 16.0%), Hardness, and Carbon dioxide absorbency (not less than 19.0%).

Caution: Since Barium Hydroxide Lime contains a soluble form of barium, it is toxic if swallowed.

BARIUM SULFATE

Chemical name: Sulfuric acid, barium salt (1:1).

Molecular formula: $BaSO_4$.

Molecular weight: 233.39.

Description:
Barium Sulfate USP—Fine, white, odorless, bulky powder, free from grittiness.
Barium Sulfate for Suspension USP—White or colored, bulky or granular powder.

Solubility: Barium Sulfate USP—Practically insoluble in water, in organic solvents, and in solutions of acids and of alkalies.

USP requirements:
Barium Sulfate USP—Preserve in well-closed containers. Contains not less than 97.5% and not more than 100.5% of barium sulfate. Meets the requirements for Identification, Bulkiness, Acidity or alkalinity, Sulfide (0.5 ppm), Acid-soluble substances (not more than 0.3%), Soluble barium salts, Arsenic (not more than 0.8 ppm), and Heavy metals (not more than 0.001%).
Barium Sulfate for Suspension USP—Preserve in well-closed containers. A dry mixture of Barium Sulfate and one or more suitable dispersing and/or suspending agents. Contains the labeled amount, within −10%. Meets the requirements for Identification, pH (4.0–10.0, in a 60% [w/w] aqueous suspension), Loss on drying (not more than 1.0%), and Heavy metals (not more than 0.001%), and for tests for Sulfide and Arsenic under Barium Sulfate.

BECLOMETHASONE

Chemical name:
Beclomethasone dipropionate—Pregna-1,4-diene-3,20-dione, 9-chloro-11-hydroxy-16-methyl-17,21-bis(1-oxopropoxy)-, (11 beta,16 beta)-.
Beclomethasone dipropionate, monohydrate—9-Chloro-11 beta, 17,21-trihydroxy-16 beta-methylpregna-1, 4-diene-3, 20-dione 17,21-dipropionate, monohydrate.

Molecular formula:
Beclomethasone dipropionate—$C_{28}H_{37}ClO_7$.
Beclomethasone dipropionate monohydrate—$C_{28}H_{37}ClO_7 \cdot H_2O$.

Molecular weight:
Beclomethasone dipropionate—521.05.
Beclomethasone dipropionate monohydrate—539.06.

Description:
Beclomethasone Dipropionate USP—White to cream white, odorless powder.
Beclomethasone dipropionate monohydrate—White to creamy white, odorless powder.

Solubility:
Beclomethasone Dipropionate USP—Very slightly soluble in water; very soluble in chloroform; freely soluble in acetone and in alcohol.
Beclomethasone dipropionate monohydrate—Very slightly soluble in water; very soluble in chloroform; freely soluble in acetone and in alcohol.

USP requirements:
Beclomethasone Dipropionate USP—Preserve in well-closed containers. It is anhydrous or contains one molecule of water of hydration. Contains not less than 97.0% and not more than 103.0% of beclomethasone dipropionate, calculated on the dried basis. Meets the requirements for Identification, Specific rotation (+88° to +94°, calculated on the dried basis, determined in a solution in dioxane containing 100 mg in each 10 mL), Loss on drying (not more than 0.5% [anhydrous], 2.8–3.8% [monohydrate]), and Residue on ignition (not more than 0.1%).
Beclomethasone Dipropionate Inhalation Aerosol—Not in USP.
Beclomethasone Dipropionate Nasal Aerosol—Not in USP.
Beclomethasone Dipropionate Cream—Not in USP.
Beclomethasone Dipropionate for Inhalation—Not in USP.
Beclomethasone Dipropionate Lotion—Not in USP.
Beclomethasone Dipropionate Ointment—Not in USP.
Beclomethasone Dipropionate Monohydrate Nasal Spray—Not in USP.

BELLADONNA

Source: Naturally occurring alkaloid—The naturally occurring belladonna alkaloids are found in various solanaceous plants, including *Atropa belladonna, Datura stamonium,* and *Duboisia myoporoides.* The active alkaloids of belladonna include hyoscyamine (which racemizes to atropine on extraction) and scopolamine (hyoscine). Hyoscyamine, the levo-isomer of atropine, is the major active alkaloid of belladonna.

Description: Belladonna Leaf USP—When moistened, its odor is slight, somewhat tobacco-like.

USP requirements:
Belladonna Extract USP—Preserve in tight containers, at a temperature not exceeding 30 °C. Contains in each 100 grams, not less than 1.15 grams and not more than 1.35 grams of the alkaloids of belladonna leaf.
Belladonna Extract Tablets USP—Preserve in tight, light-resistant containers. Contain the labeled amount of the alkaloids of belladonna leaf, within ± 10%. Meet the requirements for Identification, Disintegration (30 minutes), and Uniformity of dosage units.
Belladonna Leaf USP—Preserve in well-closed containers and avoid long exposure to direct sunlight. Preserve powdered Belladonna Leaf in light-resistant containers. Consists of the dried leaf and flowering or fruiting top of *Atropa belladonna* Linné or of its variety *acuminata* Royle ex Lindley (Fam. Solanaceae). Belladonna Leaf yields not less than 0.35% of the alkaloids of belladonna leaf. Meets the requirements for Botanic characteristics, Acid-insoluble ash (not more than 3.0%), and Belladonna stems (proportion of belladonna stems over 10 mm in diameter not more than 3.0%).
Belladonna Tincture USP—Preserve in tight, light-resistant containers, and avoid exposure to direct sunlight and to excessive heat. Contains, per 100 mL, not less than 27 mg and not more than 33 mg of the alkaloids of the belladonna leaf. Meets the requirement for Alcohol content (65.0–70.0%).

BELLADONNA AND BUTABARBITAL

For *Belladonna* and *Butabarbital*—See individual listings for chemistry information.

USP requirements:
Belladonna Extract and Butabarbital Sodium Elixir—Not in USP.
Belladonna Extract and Butabarbital Sodium Tablets—Not in USP.

BELLADONNA AND PHENOBARBITAL

For *Belladonna* and *Phenobarbital*—See individual listings for chemistry information.

USP requirements: Belladonna Extract and Phenobarbital Tablets—Not in USP.

BENDROFLUMETHIAZIDE

Chemical name: 2*H*-1,2,4-Benzothiadiazine-7-sulfonamide, 3,4-dihydro-3-(phenylmethyl)-6-(trifluoromethyl)-, 1,1-dioxide-.

Molecular formula: $C_{15}H_{14}F_3N_3O_4S_2$.

Molecular weight: 421.41.

Description: Bendroflumethiazide USP—White to cream-colored, finely divided, crystalline powder. Is odorless or has a slight odor. Melts at about 220 °C.

pKa: 8.5.

Solubility: Bendroflumethiazide USP—Practically insoluble in water; freely soluble in alcohol and in acetone.

USP requirements:
Bendroflumethiazide USP—Preserve in tight containers. Contains not less than 98.0% and not more than 102.0% of bendroflumethiazide, calculated on the anhydrous basis. Meets the requirements for Identification, Water (not more than 0.5%), Residue on ignition (not more than 0.2%), Heavy metals (not more than 0.002%), Selenium (0.003%), Limit of 2,4-disulfamyl-5-trifluoromethylaniline (not more than 1.5%), and Organic volatile impurities.
Bendroflumethiazide Tablets USP—Preserve in tight containers. Contain the labeled amount, within ± 10%. Meet the requirements for Identification, Dissolution (75% in 45 minutes in 0.1 *N* hydrochloric acid in Apparatus 2 at 50 rpm), and Uniformity of dosage units.

BENOXINATE

Chemical name: Benoxinate hydrochloride—Benzoic acid, 4-amino-3-butoxy-, 2-(diethylamino)ethyl ester, monohydrochloride.

Molecular formula: Benoxinate hydrochloride—$C_{17}H_{28}N_2O_3 \cdot$ HCl.

Molecular weight: Benoxinate hydrochloride—344.88.

Description: Benoxinate Hydrochloride USP—White, or slightly off-white, crystals or crystalline powder. Is odorless, or has a slight characteristic odor. Its solutions are neutral to litmus, and it melts at about 158 °C.

Solubility: Benoxinate Hydrochloride USP—Very soluble in water; freely soluble in chloroform and in alcohol; insoluble in ether.

USP requirements:
Benoxinate Hydrochloride USP—Preserve in well-closed containers. Contains not less than 98.5% and not more than 101.5% of benoxinate hydrochloride, calculated on the dried basis. Meets the requirements for Identification, pH (5.0–6.0, in a solution [1 in 100]), Loss on drying (not more than 1.0%), Residue on ignition (not more than 0.2%), and Ordinary impurities.
Benoxinate Hydrochloride Ophthalmic Solution USP—Preserve in tight containers. A sterile solution of Benoxinate Hydrochloride in water. Contains the labeled amount, within ±5%. Meets the requirements for Identification, Sterility, and pH (3.0–6.0).

BENTIROMIDE

Chemical group: Synthetic peptide attached to para-aminobenzoic acid (PABA) by a chymotrypsin-labile bond.

Chemical name: Benzoic acid, 4-[[2-(benzoylamino)-3-(4-hydroxyphenyl)-1-oxopropyl]amino]-, (S)-.

Molecular formula: $C_{23}H_{20}N_2O_5$.

Molecular weight: 404.42.

Description: White crystals. Melting point is about 240 °C.

pKa: 5.4.

Solubility: Practically insoluble in water, dilute acid, and ether; sparingly soluble in ethanol; freely soluble in dilute alkali.

USP requirements: Bentiromide Oral Solution—Not in USP.

BENTONITE

Chemical name: Bentonite.

Description:
Bentonite NF—Very fine, odorless, pale buff or cream-colored to grayish powder, free from grit. It is hygroscopic.
NF category: Suspending and/or viscosity-increasing agent.
Purified Bentonite NF—Odorless, fine (micronized) powder or small flakes that are creamy when viewed on their flat surfaces and tan to brown when viewed on their edges.
NF category: Suspending and/or viscosity-increasing agent.
Bentonite Magma NF—NF category: Suspending and/or viscosity-increasing agent.

Solubility:
Bentonite NF—Insoluble in water, but swells to approximately twelve times its volume when added to water. Insoluble in, and does not swell in, organic solvents.
Purified Bentonite NF—Insoluble in water and in alcohol. Swells when added to water or glycerin.

NF requirements:
Bentonite NF—Preserve in tight containers. A native, colloidal, hydrated aluminum silicate. Label it to indicate that absorption of atmospheric moisture should be avoided following the opening of the original package, preferably by storage of the remainder of the contents in a tight container. Meets the requirements for Identification, Microbial limit, pH (9.5–10.5), Loss on drying (5.0–8.0%),

Arsenic (not more than 5 ppm), Lead (0.004%), Gel formation, Swelling power, and Fineness of powder.
Purified Bentonite NF—Preserve in tight containers. A colloidal montmorillonite that has been processed to remove grit and non-swellable ore components. Meets the requirements for Identification, Viscosity (40–200 centipoises), Microbial limits, pH (9.0–10.0, in a suspension [5 in 100] in water), Acid demand (pH not more than 4.0), Loss on drying (not more than 8.0%), Arsenic (not more than 3 ppm), and Lead (0.0015%).
Bentonite Magma NF—Preserve in tight containers.
Prepare Bentonite Magma as follows: 50 grams of Bentonite and a sufficient quantity of Purified Water to make 1000 grams. Sprinkle the Bentonite, in portions, upon 800 grams of hot purified water, allowing each portion to become thoroughly wetted without stirring. Allow it to stand with occasional stirring for 24 hours. Stir until a uniform magma is obtained, add Purified Water to make 1000 grams, and mix. The Magma may be prepared also by mechanical means such as by use of a blender, as follows: Place about 500 grams of Purified Water in the blender, and while the machine is running, add the Bentonite. Add Purified Water to make up to about 1000 grams or up to the operating capacity of the blender. Blend the mixture for 5 to 10 minutes, add Purified Water to make 1000 grams, and mix.
Meets the requirement for Microbial limit.

BENZALDEHYDE

Chemical name: Benzaldehyde.

Molecular formula: C_7H_6O.

Molecular weight: 106.12.

Description:
Benzaldehyde NF—Colorless, strongly refractive liquid, having an odor resembling that of bitter almond oil. Is affected by light.
NF category: Flavors and perfumes.
Compound Benzaldehyde Elixir NF—NF category: Flavored and/or sweetened vehicle.

Solubility: Benzaldehyde NF—Slightly soluble in water; miscible with alcohol, with ether, and with fixed and volatile oils.

NF requirements:
Benzaldehyde NF—Preserve in well-filled, tight, light-resistant containers. Contains not less than 98.0% and not more than 100.5% of benzaldehyde. Meets the requirements for Specific gravity (1.041–1.046 at 25 °C), Refractive index (1.544–1.546 at 20 °C), Hydrocyanic acid, Chlorinated compounds, Nitrobenzene, and Organic volatile impurities.
Compound Benzaldehyde Elixir NF—Preserve in tight, light-resistant containers. Contains 0.05% Benzaldehyde in a suitably flavored and sweetened hydroalcoholic vehicle. Meets the requirements for Alcohol content (3.0–5.0%) and Organic volatile impurities.

BENZALKONIUM CHLORIDE

Chemical name: Ammonium, alkyldimethyl(phenylmethyl)-, chloride.

Description:
Benzalkonium Chloride NF—White or yellowish white, thick gel or gelatinous pieces. Usually has a mild, aromatic

odor. Its aqueous solution foams strongly when shaken, and usually is slightly alkaline.

NF category: Antimicrobial preservative; wetting and/or solubilizing agent.

Benzalkonium Chloride Solution NF—Clear liquid; colorless or slightly yellow unless a color has been added. It has an aromatic odor.

NF category: Antimicrobial preservative.

Solubility: Benzalkonium Chloride NF—Very soluble in water and in alcohol. Anhydrous form slightly soluble in ether.

USP requirements: Benzalkonium Chloride Vaginal Suppositories—Not in USP.

NF requirements:

Benzalkonium Chloride NF—Preserve in tight containers. A mixture of alkylbenzyldimethylammonium chlorides, the composition of which is restricted within certain limits. Meets the requirements for Identification, Water (not more than 15.0%), Residue on ignition (not more than 2.0%), Water-insoluble matter, Foreign amines, and Ratio of alkyl components.

Benzalkonium Chloride Solution NF—Preserve in tight containers, and prevent contact with metals. Contains the labeled amount, within ±5%, in concentrations of 1.0% or more; and contains the labeled amount, within ±7%, in concentrations of less than 1.0%. May contain a suitable coloring agent and may contain not more than 10% of alcohol. Meets the requirements for Identification, Microbial limit, Alcohol (if present, 95.0–105.0% of labeled amount), and Foreign amines.

Caution: Mixing Benzalkonium Chloride Solution with ordinary soaps and with anionic detergents may decrease or destroy the bacteriostatic activity of the Solution.

BENZETHONIUM

Chemical name: Benzethonium chloride—Benzenemethanaminium, *N,N*-dimethyl-*N*-[2-[2-[4-(1,1,3,3-tetramethylbutyl)phenoxy]ethoxy]ethyl]-, chloride.

Molecular formula: Benzethonium chloride—$C_{27}H_{42}ClNO_2$.

Molecular weight: Benzethonium chloride—448.09.

Description:

Benzethonium Chloride USP—White crystals, having a mild odor. Its solution (1 in 100) is slightly alkaline to litmus.

NF category: Antimicrobial preservative; wetting and/or solubilizing agent.

Benzethonium Chloride Solution USP—Odorless, clear liquid, slightly alkaline to litmus.

Benzethonium Chloride Tincture USP—Clear liquid, having the characteristic odor of acetone and of alcohol.

Solubility: Benzethonium Chloride USP—Soluble in water, in alcohol, and in chloroform; slightly soluble in ether.

USP requirements:

Benzethonium Chloride USP—Preserve in tight, light-resistant containers. Contains not less than 97.0% and not more than 103.0% of benzethonium chloride, calculated on the dried basis. Meets the requirements for Identification, Melting range (158–163 °C), Loss on drying (not more than 5.0%), Residue on ignition (not more than 0.1%), and Ammonium compounds.

Benzethonium Chloride Topical Solution USP—Preserve in tight, light-resistant containers. Contains the labeled amount, within ±5%. Meets the requirements for Identification, Oxidizing substances, and Nitrites.

Benzethonium Chloride Tincture USP—Preserve in tight, light-resistant containers. Contains in each 100 mL, not less than 190 mg and not more than 210 mg of benzethonium chloride.

Prepare Benzethonium Chloride Tincture as follows: 2 grams of Benzethonium Chloride, 685 mL of Alcohol, 100 mL of Acetone, and a sufficient quantity of Purified Water to make 1000 mL. Dissolve the Benzethonium Chloride in a mixture of the Alcohol and the Acetone. Add sufficient Purified Water to make 1000 mL.

Meets the requirements for Identification, Specific gravity (0.868–0.876), and Alcohol and acetone content (62.0–68.0% of alcohol, and 9.0–11.0% of acetone).

Note: Benzethonium Chloride Tincture may be colored by the addition of any suitable color or combination of colors certified by the FDA for use in drugs.

BENZOCAINE

Chemical group: Ester, aminobenzoic acid (PABA)–derivative.

Chemical name: Benzoic acid, 4-amino-, ethyl ester.

Molecular formula: $C_9H_{11}NO_2$.

Molecular weight: 165.19.

Description: Benzocaine USP—Small, white crystals or white, crystalline powder. Is odorless and is stable in air.

Solubility: Benzocaine USP—Very slightly soluble in water; freely soluble in alcohol, in chloroform, and in ether; sparingly soluble in almond oil and in olive oil; dissolves in dilute acids.

USP requirements:

Benzocaine USP—Preserve in well-closed containers. Benzocaine is dried over phosphorus pentoxide for 3 hours. Contains not less than 98.0% and not more than 101.0% of benzocaine. Meets the requirements for Identification, Melting range (88–92 °C, but the range between beginning and end of melting is not more than 2 °C), Reaction, Loss on drying (not more than 1.0%), Residue on ignition (not more than 0.1%), Chloride, Heavy metals (not more than 0.001%), Readily carbonizable substances, and Ordinary impurities (not more than 1%).

Benzocaine Topical Aerosol USP (Solution)—Preserve in pressurized containers, and avoid exposure to excessive heat. A solution of Benzocaine in a pressurized container. Contains the labeled amount, within ±10%. Meets the requirements for Identification and for Leak testing under Aerosols.

Benzocaine Cream USP—Preserve in tight containers, protected from light, and avoid prolonged exposure to temperatures exceeding 30 °C. It is Benzocaine in a suitable cream base. Contains the labeled amount, within ±10%. Meets the requirements for Identification, Microbial limits, and Minimum fill.

Benzocaine Gel—Not in USP.

Benzocaine Jelly—Not in USP.

Benzocaine Lozenges—Not in USP.

Benzocaine Ointment USP—Preserve in tight containers, protected from light, and avoid prolonged exposure to temperatures exceeding 30 °C. It is Benzocaine in a suitable ointment base. Contains the labeled amount, within ±10%. Meets the requirements for Identification, Microbial limits, and Minimum fill.

Benzocaine Dental Paste—Not in USP.

Benzocaine Otic Solution USP—Preserve in tight, light-resistant containers. Contains the labeled amount, within ±10%. Meets the requirements for Identification and Microbial limits.

Benzocaine Topical Solution USP—Preserve in tight containers, protected from light, and avoid prolonged exposure to temperatures exceeding 30 °C. A solution of Benzocaine in a suitable solvent. Contains the labeled amount, within ± 10%. Contains a suitable antimicrobial agent. Meets the requirements for Identification and Microbial limits.

BENZOCAINE, BUTAMBEN, AND TETRACAINE

For *Benzocaine, Butamben,* and *Tetracaine*—See individual listings for chemistry information.

USP requirements:
Benzocaine, Butamben, and Tetracaine Hydrochloride Topical Aerosol Solution—Not in USP.
Benzocaine, Butamben, and Tetracaine Hydrochloride Gel—Not in USP.
Benzocaine, Butamben, and Tetracaine Hydrochloride Ointment—Not in USP.
Benzocaine, Butamben, and Tetracaine Hydrochloride Topical Solution—Not in USP.

BENZOCAINE AND MENTHOL

For *Benzocaine* and *Menthol*—See individual listings for chemistry information.

USP requirements:
Benzocaine and Menthol Lotion—Not in USP.
Benzocaine and Menthol Topical Aerosol Solution—Not in USP.

BENZOIC ACID

Chemical name: Benzoic acid.

Molecular formula: $C_7H_6O_2$.

Molecular weight: 122.12.

Description: Benzoic Acid USP—White crystals, scales, or needles. Has a slight odor, usually suggesting benzaldehyde or benzoin. Somewhat volatile at moderately warm temperatures. Freely volatile in steam.
NF category: Antimicrobial preservative.

Solubility: Benzoic Acid USP—Slightly soluble in water; freely soluble in alcohol, in chloroform, and in ether.

USP requirements: Benzoic Acid USP—Preserve in well-closed containers. Contains not less than 99.5% and not more than 100.5% of benzoic acid, calculated on the anhydrous basis. Meets the requirements for Identification, Congealing range (121–123 °C), Water (not more than 0.7%, a 1 in 2 solution of methanol in pyridine being used as the solvent), Residue on ignition (not more than 0.05%), Arsenic (not more than 3 ppm), Heavy metals (not more than 0.001%), Readily carbonizable substances, and Readily oxidizable substances.

BENZOIC AND SALICYLIC ACIDS

For *Benzoic Acid* and *Salicylic Acid*—See individual listings for chemistry information.

USP requirements: Benzoic and Salicylic Acids Ointment USP—Preserve in well-closed containers, and avoid exposure to temperatures exceeding 30 °C. It is Benzoic Acid and Salicylic Acid, present in a ratio of about 2 to 1, in a suitable ointment base. Label Ointment to indicate the concentrations of Benzoic Acid and Salicylic Acid and to indicate whether the ointment base is water-soluble or water-insoluble. Contains the labeled amounts, within ± 10%. Meets the requirements for Identification and Minimum fill.

BENZOIN

Description: Benzoin USP—Sumatra Benzoin has an aromatic and balsamic odor. When heated it does not emit a pinaceous odor. When Sumatra Benzoin is digested with boiling water, the odor suggests cinnamates or storax. Siam Benzoin has an agreeable, balsamic, vanilla-like odor.

USP requirements:
Benzoin USP—Preserve in well-closed containers. It is the balsamic resin obtained from *Styrax benzoin* Dryander or *Styrax paralleloneurus* Perkins, known in commerce as Sumatra Benzoin, or from *Styrax tonkinensis* (Pièrre) Craib ex Hartwich, or other species of the Section *Anthostyrax* of the genus *Styrax*, known in commerce as Siam Benzoin (Fam. Styraceae). Label it to indicate whether it is Sumatra Benzoin or Siam Benzoin. Sumatra Benzoin yields not less than 75.0% of alcohol-soluble extractive, and Siam Benzoin yields not less than 90.0% of alcohol-soluble extractive. Meets the requirements for Botanic characteristics, Identification, Benzoic acid (not less than 6.0% for Sumatra Benzoin; not less than 12.0% for Siam Benzoin), Acid-insoluble ash (not more than 1.0% for Sumatra Benzoin; not more than 0.5% for Siam Benzoin), and Foreign organic matter (not more than 1.0% for Siam Benzoin).
Compound Benzoin Tincture USP—Preserve in tight, light-resistant containers, and avoid exposure to direct sunlight and to excessive heat. Label it to indicate that it is flammable.
Prepare Compound Benzoin Tincture as follows: 100 grams of Benzoin, in moderately coarse powder, 20 grams of Aloe, in moderately coarse powder, 80 grams of Storax, and 40 grams of Tolu Balsam to make 1000 mL. Prepare a Tincture by Process M, using alcohol as the menstruum.
Meets the requirements for Specific gravity (0.870–0.885), Alcohol content (74.0–80.0%, the dilution to approximately 2% alcohol being made with methanol instead of with water), and Nonvolatile residue (525–675 mg).

BENZONATATE

Chemical name: Benzoic acid, 4-(butylamino)-, 2,5,8,11,-14,17,20,23,26-nonaoxaoctacos-28-yl ester.

Molecular formula: $C_{30}H_{53}NO_{11}$ (Average).

Molecular weight: 603.00 (Average).

Description: Benzonatate USP—Clear, pale yellow, viscous liquid, having a faint, characteristic odor.

Solubility: Benzonatate USP—Miscible with water in all proportions. Freely soluble in chloroform and in alcohol.

USP requirements:
Benzonatate USP—Preserve in tight, light-resistant containers. Contains not less than 95.0% and not more than 105.0% of benzonatate. Meets the requirements for Identification, Refractive index (1.509–1.511 at 20 °C), Water (not more than 0.3%), Residue on ignition (not more than 0.1%), Arsenic (1.5 ppm), Chloride (0.0035%), Sulfate (0.04%), Heavy metals (0.001%), and Organic volatile impurities.
Benzonatate Capsules USP—Preserve in tight, light-resistant containers. Contain the labeled amount, within ± 10%. Meet the requirements for Identification and Uniformity of dosage units.

BENZOYL PEROXIDE

Chemical name: Dibenzoyl peroxide.

Molecular formula: $C_{14}H_{10}O_4$ (anhydrous).

Molecular weight: 242.23 (anhydrous).

Description:

Hydrous Benzoyl Peroxide USP—White, granular powder, having a characteristic odor.

Benzoyl Peroxide Gel USP—A soft, white gel, having a characteristic odor.

Benzoyl Peroxide Lotion USP—White, viscous, creamy lotion, having a characteristic odor.

Solubility: Hydrous Benzoyl Peroxide USP—Sparingly soluble in water and in alcohol; soluble in acetone, in chloroform, and in ether.

USP requirements:

Hydrous Benzoyl Peroxide USP—Store in the original container, at room temperature. [Note—Do not transfer Hydrous Benzoyl Peroxide to metal or glass containers fitted with friction tops. Do not return unused material to its original container, but destroy it by treatment with sodium hydroxide solution (1 in 10) until addition of a crystal of potassium iodide results in no release of free iodine.] Contains not less than 65.0% and not more than 82.0% of anhydrous benzoyl peroxide. Contains about 26% of water for the purpose of reducing flammability and shock sensitivity. Meets the requirements for Identification and Chromatographic purity.

Caution: Hydrous Benzoyl Peroxide may explode at temperatures higher than 60 °C or cause fires in the presence of reducing substances. Store it in the original container, treated to reduce static charges.

Benzoyl Peroxide Cleansing Bar—Not in USP.

Benzoyl Peroxide Cream—Not in USP.

Benzoyl Peroxide Gel USP—Preserve in tight containers. It is benzoyl peroxide in a suitable gel base. Contains the labeled amount, within −10% to +25%. Meets the requirements for Identification, pH (3.5–6.0), and Related substances.

Benzoyl Peroxide Lotion USP—Preserve in tight containers. It is benzoyl peroxide in a suitable lotion base. Contains the labeled amount, within ±10%. Meets the requirements for Identification, pH (2.8–6.6), and Related substances.

Benzoyl Peroxide Cleansing Lotion—Not in USP.

Benzoyl Peroxide Facial Mask—Not in USP.

Benzoyl Peroxide Stick—Not in USP.

BENZPHETAMINE

Chemical group: Phenethylamine (amphetamine-like).

Chemical name: Benzphetamine hydrochloride—(+)-N-Benzyl-N,alpha-dimethylphenethylamine hydrochloride.

Molecular formula: Benzphetamine hydrochloride—$C_{17}H_{21}N \cdot HCl$.

Molecular weight: Benzphetamine hydrochloride—275.82.

Description: Benzphetamine hydrochloride—White crystalline powder.

Solubility: Benzphetamine hydrochloride—Readily soluble in water and in 95% ethanol.

USP requirements: Benzphetamine Hydrochloride Tablets—Not in USP.

BENZTHIAZIDE

Chemical name: 2H-1,2,4-Benzothiadiazine-7-sulfonamide, 6-chloro-3-[[(phenylmethyl)thio]methyl]-, 1,1-dioxide.

Molecular formula: $C_{15}H_{14}ClN_3O_4S_3$.

Molecular weight: 431.93.

Description: Benzthiazide USP—White, crystalline powder, having a characteristic odor. Melts at about 240 °C.

Solubility: Benzthiazide USP—Practically insoluble in water; freely soluble in dimethylformamide and in solutions of fixed alkali hydroxides; slightly soluble in acetone; practically insoluble in ether and in chloroform.

USP requirements:

Benzthiazide USP—Preserve in tight containers. Contains not less than 98.0% and not more than 101.5% of benzthiazide, calculated on the dried basis. Meets the requirements for Identification, Loss on drying (not more than 1.0%), Residue on ignition (not more than 0.2%), Selenium (0.003%), Heavy metals (not more than 0.0025%), Diazotizable substances, and Organic volatile impurities.

Benzthiazide Tablets USP—Preserve in tight containers. Contain the labeled amount, within ±10%. Meet the requirements for Identification, Disintegration (15 minutes), and Uniformity of dosage units.

BENZTROPINE

Chemical group: Synthetic tertiary amine.

Chemical name: Benztropine mesylate—8-Azabicyclo[3.2.1]-octane, 3-(diphenylmethoxy)-, *endo*, methanesulfonate.

Molecular formula: Benztropine mesylate—$C_{21}H_{25}NO \cdot CH_4O_3S$.

Molecular weight: Benztropine mesylate—403.54.

Description: Benztropine Mesylate USP—White, slightly hygroscopic, crystalline powder.

Solubility: Benztropine Mesylate USP—Very soluble in water; freely soluble in alcohol; very slightly soluble in ether.

USP requirements:

Benztropine Mesylate USP—Preserve in tight containers. Contains not less than 98.0% and not more than 100.5% of benztropine mesylate, calculated on the dried basis. Meets the requirements for Identification, Melting range (141–145 °C), Loss on drying (not more than 5.0%), Residue on ignition (not more than 0.1%), and Organic volatile impurities.

Benztropine Mesylate Injection USP—Preserve in single-dose or in multiple-dose containers, preferably of Type I glass. A sterile solution of Benztropine Mesylate in Water for Injection. Contains the labeled amount, within ±10%. Meets the requirements for Identification, Bacterial endotoxins, pH (5.0–8.0), and Injections.

Benztropine Mesylate Tablets USP—Preserve in well-closed containers. Contain the labeled amount, within ±10%. Meet the requirements for Identification, Dissolution (80% in 30 minutes in 0.1 N hydrochloric acid in Apparatus 2 at 50 rpm), and Uniformity of dosage units.

BENZYL ALCOHOL

Chemical name: Benzenemethanol.

Molecular formula: C_7H_8O.

Molecular weight: 108.14.

Description: Benzyl Alcohol NF—Colorless liquid, having a faint, aromatic odor. Boils at about 206 °C, without decomposition. It is neutral to litmus.

NF category: Antimicrobial preservative.

Solubility: Benzyl Alcohol NF—Sparingly soluble in water; freely soluble in 50% alcohol. Miscible with alcohol, with ether, and with chloroform.

NF requirements: Benzyl Alcohol NF—Preserve in tight containers, and prevent exposure to light. Contains not less than 97.0% and not more than 100.5% of benzyl alcohol. Meets the requirements for Identification, Specific gravity (1.042–1.047), Refractive index (1.539–1.541 at 20 °C), Residue on ignition (not more than 0.005%), Acidity, Nonvolatile residue, Halogenated compounds and halides (0.03% as chlorine), Benzaldehyde (not more than 0.20%), and Organic volatile impurities.

BENZYL BENZOATE

Chemical name: Benzoic acid, phenylmethyl ester.

Molecular formula: $C_{14}H_{12}O_2$.

Molecular weight: 212.25.

Description: Benzyl Benzoate USP—Clear, colorless, oily liquid having a slight aromatic odor.

NF category: Solvent.

Solubility: Benzyl Benzoate USP—Practically insoluble in water and in glycerin; miscible with alcohol, with ether, and with chloroform.

USP requirements:
Benzyl Benzoate USP—Preserve in tight, well-filled, light-resistant containers, and avoid exposure to excessive heat. Contains not less than 99.0% and not more than 100.5% of benzyl benzoate. Meets the requirements for Identification, Specific gravity (1.116–1.120), Congealing temperature (not lower than 18.0 °C), Refractive index (1.568–1.570 at 20 °C), Aldehyde, Acidity, and Organic volatile impurities.
Benzyl Benzoate Lotion USP—Preserve in tight containers. Contains not less than 26.0% and not more than 30.0% (w/w) of benzyl benzoate.
Prepare Benzyl Benzoate Lotion as follows: 250 mL of Benzyl Benzoate, 5 grams of Triethanolamine, 20 grams of Oleic Acid, and 750 mL of Purified Water to make about 1000 mL. Mix the Triethanolamine with the Oleic Acid, add the Benzyl Benzoate, and mix. Transfer the mixture to a suitable container of about 2000-mL capacity, add 250 mL of Purified Water, and shake the mixture thoroughly. Finally add the remaining Purified Water, and again shake thoroughly.
Meets the requirement for pH (8.5–9.2).

BENZYLPENICILLOYL POLYLYSINE

USP requirements:
Benzylpenicilloyl Polylysine Concentrate USP—Preserve in tight containers. It has a molar concentration of benzylpenicilloyl moiety of not less than 0.0125 *M* and not more than 0.020 *M*. Contains one or more suitable buffers. Meets the requirements for pH (6.5–8.5, the undiluted Concentrate being used), Penicillenate (not more than 0.00020 *M*) and penamaldate (not more than 0.00060 *M*), and Benzylpenicilloyl substitution (50–70%).
Benzylpenicilloyl Polylysine Injection USP—Preserve in single-dose or in multiple-dose containers, preferably of Type I glass, in a refrigerator. It has a molar concentration of benzylpenicilloyl moiety of not less than 5.4×10^{-5} *M* and not more than 7.0×10^{-5} *M*. Contains one or more suitable buffers. Meets the requirements for Pyrogen, Sterility, and pH (6.5–8.5).

BEPRIDIL

Chemical name: Bepridil hydrochloride—1-Pyrrolideneethanamine, beta-[(2-methylpropoxy)methyl]-*N*-phenyl-*N*-(phenylmethyl)-, monohydrochloride, monohydrate.

Molecular formula: Bepridil hydrochloride—$C_{24}H_{34}N_2O\cdot$ $HCl\cdot H_2O$.

Molecular weight: Bepridil hydrochloride—421.02.

Description: Bepridil hydrochloride—White to off-white, crystalline powder.

Solubility: Bepridil hydrochloride—Slightly soluble in water; very soluble in ethanol, in methanol, and in chloroform; freely soluble in acetone.

USP requirements: Bepridil Hydrochloride Tablets—Not in USP.

BETA CAROTENE

Chemical name: Beta,beta-Carotene.

Molecular formula: $C_{40}H_{56}$.

Molecular weight: 536.88.

Description: Beta Carotene USP—Red or reddish brown to violet-brown crystals or crystalline powder.

Solubility: Beta Carotene USP—Insoluble in water and in acids and alkalies; soluble in carbon disulfide, and in chloroform; sparingly soluble in ether, in solvent hexane, and in vegetable oils; practically insoluble in methanol and in alcohol.

USP requirements:
Beta Carotene USP—Preserve in tight, light-resistant containers. Contains not less than 96.0% and not more than 101.0% of beta carotene. Meets the requirements for Identification, Melting range (176–182 °C, with decomposition), Loss on drying (not more than 0.2%), Residue on ignition (not more than 0.2%, 2 grams of specimen being used), Heavy metals (0.001%), and Arsenic (3 ppm).
Beta Carotene Capsules USP—Preserve in tight, light-resistant containers. Contain the labeled amount, within −10% to +25%. Meet the requirements for Identification and Uniformity of dosage units.
Beta Carotene Tablets—Not in USP.

BETAINE

Chemical name: Betaine hydrochloride—Methanaminium, 1-carboxy-*N*,*N*,*N*-trimethyl-, chloride.

Molecular formula: Betaine hydrochloride—$C_5H_{11}NO_2\cdot HCl$.

Molecular weight: Betaine hydrochloride—153.61.

USP requirements: Betaine Hydrochloride USP—Preserve in well-closed containers. Contains not less than 98.0% and not more than 100.5% of betaine hydrochloride, calculated on the anhydrous basis. Meets the requirements for Identification, pH (0.8–1.2, in a solution [1 in 4]), Water (not more than 0.5%), Residue on ignition (not more than 0.1%), Arsenic (2 ppm), and Heavy metals (0.001%).

BETAMETHASONE

Chemical name:
Betamethasone—Pregna-1,4-diene-3,20-dione, 9-fluoro-11,17,21-trihydroxy-16-methyl-, (11 beta,16 beta)-.

Betamethasone acetate—Pregna-1,4-diene-3,20-dione, 9-fluoro-11,17-dihydroxy-16-methyl-21-(acetyloxy)-, (11 beta,16 beta)-.

Betamethasone benzoate—Pregna-1,4-diene-3,20-dione, 17-(benzoyloxy)-9-fluoro-11,21-dihydroxy-16-methyl-, (11 beta,16 beta)-.

Betamethasone dipropionate—Pregna-1,4-diene-3,20-dione, 9-fluoro-11-hydroxy-16-methyl-17,21-bis(1-oxopropoxy)-, (11 beta,16 beta).

Betamethasone sodium phosphate—Pregna-1,4-diene-3,20-dione, 9-fluoro-11,17-dihydroxy-16-methyl-21-(phosphonooxy)-, disodium salt, (11 beta,16 beta)-.

Betamethasone valerate—Pregna-1,4-diene-3,20-dione, 9-fluoro-11,21-dihydroxy-16-methyl-17-[(1-oxopentyl)oxy]-fluoro-11,21-dihydroxy-16-methyl-17-[(1-oxopentyl)oxy]-, (11 beta,16 beta)-.

Molecular formula:

Betamethasone—$C_{22}H_{29}FO_5$.

Betamethasone acetate—$C_{24}H_{31}FO_6$.

Betamethasone benzoate—$C_{29}H_{33}FO_6$.

Betamethasone dipropionate—$C_{28}H_{37}FO_7$.

Betamethasone sodium phosphate—$C_{22}H_{28}FNa_2O_8P$.

Betamethasone valerate—$C_{27}H_{37}FO_6$.

Molecular weight:

Betamethasone—392.47.

Betamethasone acetate—434.50.

Betamethasone benzoate—496.57.

Betamethasone dipropionate—504.59.

Betamethasone sodium phosphate—516.41.

Betamethasone valerate—476.58.

Description:

Betamethasone USP—White to practically white, odorless, crystalline powder. Melts at about 240 °C, with some decomposition.

Betamethasone Acetate USP—White to creamy white, odorless powder. Sinters and resolidifies at about 165 °C, and remelts at about 200 or 220 °C, with decomposition.

Betamethasone Benzoate USP—White to practically white, practically odorless powder. Melts at about 220 °C, with decomposition.

Betamethasone Dipropionate USP—White to cream-white, odorless powder.

Betamethasone Sodium Phosphate USP—White to practically white, odorless powder. Is hygroscopic.

Betamethasone Valerate USP—White to practically white, odorless powder. Melts at about 190 °C, with decomposition.

Solubility:

Betamethasone USP—Insoluble in water; sparingly soluble in acetone, in alcohol, in dioxane, and in methanol; very slightly soluble in chloroform and in ether.

Betamethasone Acetate USP—Practically insoluble in water; freely soluble in acetone; soluble in alcohol and in chloroform.

Betamethasone Benzoate USP—Insoluble in water; soluble in alcohol, in methanol, and in chloroform.

Betamethasone Dipropionate USP—Insoluble in water; freely soluble in acetone and in chloroform; sparingly soluble in alcohol.

Betamethasone Sodium Phosphate USP—Freely soluble in water and in methanol; practically insoluble in acetone and in chloroform.

Betamethasone Valerate USP—Practically insoluble in water; freely soluble in acetone and in chloroform; soluble in alcohol; slightly soluble in ether.

USP requirements:

Betamethasone USP—Preserve in well-closed containers. Contains not less than 97.0% and not more than 103.0% of betamethasone, calculated on the dried basis. Meets the requirements for Identification, Specific rotation (+112° to +120°, calculated on the dried basis), Loss on drying (not more than 1.0%), Residue on ignition (not more than 0.2%), Ordinary impurities, and Organic volatile impurities.

Betamethasone Cream USP—Preserve in collapsible tubes or in tight containers. Contains the labeled amount, within −10% to +15%, in a suitable cream base. Meets the requirements for Identification, Microbial limits, and Minimum fill.

Betamethasone Syrup USP—Preserve in well-closed containers. Contains the labeled amount, within −10% to +15%. Meets the requirement for Identification.

Betamethasone Tablets USP—Preserve in well-closed containers. Contain the labeled amount, within ±10%. Meet the requirements for Identification, Dissolution (75% in 45 minutes in water in Apparatus 2 at 50 rpm), and Uniformity of dosage units.

Betamethasone Effervescent Tablets—Not in USP.

Betamethasone Acetate USP—Preserve in tight containers. Contains not less than 97.0% and not more than 103.0% of betamethasone acetate, calculated on the anhydrous basis. Meets the requirements for Identification, Specific rotation (+120° to +128°, calculated on the anhydrous basis), Water (not more than 4.0%), Residue on ignition (not more than 0.2%), and Ordinary impurities.

Betamethasone Benzoate USP—Preserve in tight containers. Contains not less than 98.0% and not more than 102.0% of betamethasone benzoate, calculated on the dried basis. Meets the requirements for Identification, Specific rotation (+60° to +66°, calculated on the dried basis), Loss on drying (not more than 0.5%), and Related steroids.

Betamethasone Benzoate Cream—Not in USP.

Betamethasone Benzoate Gel USP—Preserve in collapsible tubes or tight containers. Contains an amount of betamethasone benzoate equivalent to the labeled amount of betamethasone, within ±10%. Meets the requirements for Identification, Microbial limits, and Minimum fill.

Betamethasone Benzoate Lotion—Not in USP.

Betamethasone Dipropionate USP—Preserve in well-closed containers. Contains not less than 97.0% and not more than 103.0% of betamethasone dipropionate, calculated on the dried basis. Meets the requirements for Identification, Specific rotation (+63° to +70°, calculated on the dried basis), Loss on drying (not more than 1.0%), Residue on ignition (not more than 0.2%), and Ordinary impurities.

Betamethasone Dipropionate Topical Aerosol USP—Preserve in tight, pressurized containers, and avoid exposure to excessive heat. A solution, in suitable propellants in a pressurized container. Contains an amount of betamethasone dipropionate equivalent to the labeled amount of betamethasone, within ±10%. Meets the requirements for Identification, and for Leak testing and Pressure testing under Aerosols.

Betamethasone Dipropionate Cream USP—Preserve in collapsible tubes or in tight containers. Contains an amount of betamethasone dipropionate equivalent to the labeled amount of betamethasone, within ±10%, in a suitable cream base. Meets the requirements for Identification and Minimum fill.

Betamethasone Dipropionate Gel—Not in USP.

Betamethasone Dipropionate Lotion USP—Preserve in tight containers. Contains an amount of betamethasone dipropionate equivalent to the labeled amount of betamethasone, within ±10%, in a suitable lotion base. Meets the requirements for Identification and Minimum fill.

Betamethasone Dipropionate Ointment USP—Preserve in collapsible tubes or in well-closed containers. Contains an amount of betamethasone dipropionate equivalent to the labeled amount of betamethasone, within ±10%, in a suitable ointment base. Meets the requirements for Identification and Minimum fill.

Betamethasone Disodium Phosphate Enema—Not in USP.

Betamethasone Disodium Phosphate Dental Pellets—Not in USP.

Betamethasone Sodium Phosphate USP—Preserve in tight containers. Contains not less than 97.0% and not more than 103.0% of betamethasone sodium phosphate, calculated on the anhydrous basis. Meets the requirements for Identification, Specific rotation (+99° to +105°, calculated on the anhydrous basis), Water (not more than 10.0%), Phosphate ions (not more than 1.0%), and Free betamethasone (not more than 1.0%).

Betamethasone Sodium Phosphate Injection USP—Preserve in single-dose or in multiple-dose containers, preferably of Type I glass. A sterile solution of Betamethasone Sodium Phosphate in Water for Injection. Contains an amount of betamethasone sodium phosphate equivalent to the labeled amount of betamethasone, within ±10%. Meets the requirements for Identification, Bacterial endotoxins, pH (8.0–9.0), Particulate matter, and Injections.

Betamethasone Sodium Phosphate Ophthalmic/Otic Solution—Not in USP.

Betamethasone Sodium Phosphate Extended-release Tablets—Not in USP.

Sterile Betamethasone Sodium Phosphate and Betamethasone Acetate Suspension USP—Preserve in multiple-dose containers, preferably of Type I glass. A sterile preparation of Betamethasone Sodium Phosphate in solution and Betamethasone Acetate in suspension in Water for Injection. Contains an amount of betamethasone sodium phosphate equivalent to the labeled amount of betamethasone, within −10% to +15%, and the labeled amount of betamethasone acetate, within −10% to +15%. Meets the requirements for Identification, Bacterial endotoxins, pH (6.8–7.2), and Injections.

Betamethasone Valerate USP—Preserve in tight containers. Contains not less than 97.0% and not more than 103.0% of betamethasone valerate, calculated on the dried basis. Meets the requirements for Identification, Specific rotation (+75° to +82°, calculated on the dried basis), Loss on drying (not more than 0.5%), and Residue on ignition (not more than 0.2%).

Betamethasone Valerate Cream USP—Preserve in collapsible tubes or in tight containers. Contains an amount of betamethasone valerate equivalent to the labeled amount of betamethasone, within ±10%, in a suitable cream base. Meets the requirements for Identification, Microbial limits, and Minimum fill.

Betamethasone Valerate Lotion USP—Preserve in tight, light-resistant containers, and store at controlled room temperature. Contains an amount of betamethasone valerate equivalent to the labeled amount of betamethasone, within −5% to +15%. Meets the requirements for Identification, Microbial limits, pH (4.0–6.0), and Minimum fill.

Betamethasone Valerate Ointment USP—Preserve in collapsible tubes or in tight containers, and avoid exposure to excessive heat. Contains an amount of betamethasone valerate equivalent to the labeled amount of betamethasone, within ±10%, in a suitable ointment base. Meets the requirements for Identification, Microbial limits, and Minimum fill.

BETAXOLOL

Chemical name: Betaxolol hydrochloride—2-Propanol, 1-[4-[2-(cyclopropylmethoxy)ethyl]phenoxy]-3-[(1-methylethyl)-amino]-, hydrochloride, (±)-.

Molecular formula: Betaxolol hydrochloride—$C_{18}H_{29}NO_3 \cdot HCl$.

Molecular weight: Betaxolol hydrochloride—343.89.

Description: Betaxolol Hydrochloride USP—White, crystalline powder.

pKa: 9.4.

Solubility: Betaxolol Hydrochloride USP—Freely soluble in water, in alcohol, in chloroform, and in methanol.

USP requirements:

Betaxolol Ophthalmic Solution USP—Preserve in tight containers. A sterile, aqueous, isotonic solution of Betaxolol Hydrochloride. Label Ophthalmic Solution to state both the content of the betaxolol active moiety and the content of the salt used in formulating the article. Contains a suitable antimicrobial preservative. Contains an amount of betaxolol hydrochloride equivalent to the labeled amount of betaxolol, within ±10%. Meets the requirements for Identification, Sterility, and pH (4.0–8.0).

Betaxolol Hydrochloride USP—Preserve in tight containers. Contains not less than 98.5% and not more than 101.5% of betaxolol hydrochloride, calculated on the dried basis. Meets the requirements for Identification, Melting range (113–117 °C), pH (4.5–6.5, in a solution [1 in 50]), Loss on drying (not more than 1.0%), Residue on ignition (not more than 0.1%), Heavy metals (not more than 0.002%), and Chromatographic purity.

Betaxolol Hydrochloride Ophthalmic Suspension—Not in USP.

Betaxolol Hydrochloride Tablets—Not in USP.

BETHANECHOL

Chemical group: Synthetic ester, structurally related to acetylcholine.

Chemical name: Bethanechol chloride—1-Propanaminium, 2-[(aminocarbonyl)oxy]-*N,N,N*-trimethyl-, chloride.

Molecular formula: Bethanechol chloride—$C_7H_{17}ClN_2O_2$.

Molecular weight: Bethanechol chloride—196.68.

Description: Bethanechol Chloride USP—Colorless or white crystals or white, crystalline powder, usually having a slight, amine-like odor. Is hygroscopic. Exhibits polymorphism, and of two crystalline forms observed, one melts at about 211 °C and the other melts at about 219 °C.

Solubility: Bethanechol Chloride USP—Freely soluble in water and in alcohol; insoluble in chloroform and in ether.

USP requirements:

Bethanechol Chloride USP—Preserve in tight containers. Contains not less than 98.0% and not more than 101.5% of bethanechol chloride, calculated on the dried basis. Meets the requirements for Identification, pH (5.5–6.5, in a solution [1 in 100]), Loss on drying (not more than 1.0%), Residue on ignition (not more than 0.1%), Chloride content (17.7–18.3%), Heavy metals (not more than 0.003%), and Organic volatile impurities.

Bethanechol Chloride Injection USP—Preserve in single-dose containers, preferably of Type I glass. A sterile solution of Bethanechol Chloride in Water for Injection. Contains the labeled amount, within ±5%. Meets the requirements for Identification, Bacterial endotoxins, pH (5.5–7.5), and Injections.

Bethanechol Chloride Tablets USP—Preserve in tight containers. Contain the labeled amount, within ±10%. Meet the requirements for Identification, Dissolution (80% in

30 minutes in 0.1 N hydrochloric acid in Apparatus 2 at 50 rpm), and Uniformity of dosage units.

BIOLOGICAL INDICATOR FOR DRY-HEAT STERILIZATION, PAPER STRIP

USP requirements: Biological Indicator for Dry-heat Sterilization, Paper Strip USP—Preserve in the original package under the conditions recommended on the label, and protect from light, toxic substances, excessive heat, and moisture. A preparation of viable spores made from a culture derived from a specified strain of *Bacillus subtilis* subspecies *niger*, on a suitable grade of paper carrier, individually packaged in a suitable container readily penetrable by dry heat, and characterized for predictable resistance to dry-heat sterilization. Label it to state that it is a Biological Indicator for Dry-heat Sterilization on a paper carrier, to indicate its D value, the method used to determine such D value, i.e., by spore count or fraction negative procedure after graded exposures to the sterilization conditions, survival time and kill time under the sterilization conditions stated on the label, its particular viable spore count, with a statement that such count has been determined after preliminary heat treatment, and its recommended storage conditions. State in the labeling the size of the paper carrier, the strain and ATCC number from which the spores were derived, and instructions for spore recovery and for its safe disposal. Indicate in the labeling that the stated D value is reproducible only under the exact conditions under which it was determined, that the user would not necessarily obtain the same result, and that the user would need to determine its suitability for the particular use. The packaged Biological Indicator for Dry-heat Sterilization, Paper Strip, has a particular labeled spore count per carrier of not less than 10^4 and not more than 10^9 spores. When labeled for and subjected to dry-heat sterilization conditions at a particular temperature, it has a survival time and kill time appropriate to the labeled spore count and to the decimal reduction value (D value, in minutes) of the preparation, specified by: Survival time (in minutes) = not less than (labeled D value) $\times$ ($\log_{10}$ labeled spore count per carrier $-$ 2); and Kill time (in minutes) = not more than (labeled D value) $\times$ ($\log_{10}$ labeled spore count per carrier $+$ 4). Meets the requirements for Expiration date (not less than 18 months from the date of manufacture, the date of manufacture being the date on which the first determination of the total viable population was made), Identification, Resistance performance tests, Purity, and Stability.

Note: See Biological Indicators in *USP* for directives on selection of suitable indicators and on their applicability for different sterilization cycles, and for the characteristics of the basic or prototype article.

BIOLOGICAL INDICATOR FOR ETHYLENE OXIDE STERILIZATION, PAPER STRIP

USP requirements: Biological Indicator for Ethylene Oxide Sterilization, Paper Strip USP.—Preserve in the original package under the conditions recommended on the label, and protect it from light, toxic substances, excessive heat, and moisture. A preparation of viable spores made from a culture derived from a specified strain of *Bacillus subtilis* subspecies *niger*, on a suitable grade of paper carrier, individually packaged in a suitable container readily penetrable by ethylene oxide sterilizing gas mixture, and characterized for predictable resistance to sterilization with such gas. Label it to state that it is a Biological Indicator for Ethylene Oxide Sterilization on a paper carrier, to indicate its D value, the method used to determine such D value, i.e., by spore count or fraction negative procedure after graded exposures to the sterilization conditions, survival time and kill time under the

sterilization conditions stated on the label, its particular viable spore count, with a statement that such count has been determined after preliminary heat treatment, and its recommended storage conditions. State in the labeling the size of the paper carrier, the strain and ATCC number from which the spores were derived, and instructions for spore recovery and for its safe disposal. Indicate in the labeling that the stated D value is reproducible only under the exact conditions under which it was determined, that the user would not necessarily obtain the same result and that the user would need to determine its suitability for the particular use. The packaged Biological Indicator for Ethylene Oxide Sterilization, Paper Strip, has a particular labeled spore count per carrier of not less than 10^4 and not more than 10^9 spores. Where labeled for and subjected to particular ethylene oxide sterilization conditions of a gaseous mixture, temperature, and relative humidity, it has a survival time and kill time appropriate to the labeled spore count and to the decimal reduction value (D value, in minutes) of the preparation, specified by: Survival time (in minutes) = not less than (labeled D value) $\times$ ($\log_{10}$ labeled spore count per carrier $-$ 2); and Kill time (in minutes) = not more than (labeled D value) $\times$ ($\log_{10}$ labeled spore count per carrier $+$ 4). Meets the requirements for Expiration date (not less than 18 months from the date of manufacture, the date of manufacture being the date on which the first determination of the total viable population was made), Identification, Resistance performance tests, Purity, and Stability.

Note: See Biological Indicators in *USP* for directives on selection of suitable indicators and on their applicability for different sterilization cycles, and for the characteristics of the basic or prototype article.

BIOLOGICAL INDICATOR FOR STEAM STERILIZATION, PAPER STRIP

USP requirements: Biological Indicator for Steam Sterilization, Paper Strip USP—Preserve in the original package under the conditions recommended on the label, and protect it from light, toxic substances, excessive heat, and moisture. A preparation of viable spores made from a culture derived from a specified strain of *Bacillus stearothermophilus*, on a suitable grade of paper carrier, individually packaged in a suitable container readily penetrable by steam, and characterized for predictable resistance to steam sterilization. Label it to state that it is a Biological Indicator for Steam Sterilization on a paper carrier, to indicate its D value, the method used to determine such D value, i.e., by spore count or fraction negative procedure after graded exposures to the sterilization conditions, survival time and kill time under the sterilization conditions stated on the label, its particular viable spore count, with a statement that such count has been determined after preliminary heat treatment, and its recommended storage conditions. State in the labeling the size of the paper carrier, the strain and ATCC number from which the spores were derived, and instructions for spore recovery and for its safe disposal. Indicate in the labeling that the stated D value is reproducible only under the exact conditions under which it was determined, that the user would not necessarily obtain the same result, and that the user would need to determine its suitability for the particular use. The packaged Biological Indicator for Steam Sterilization, Paper Strip, has a particular labeled spore count per carrier of not less than 10^4 and not more than 10^9 spores. When labeled for and subjected to steam sterilization conditions at a particular temperature, it has a survival time and kill time appropriate to the labeled spore count and to the decimal reduction value (D value, in minutes) of the preparation, specified by: Survival time (in minutes) = not less than (labeled D value) $\times$ ($\log_{10}$ labeled spore count per carrier

— 2); and Kill time (in minutes) = not more than (labeled D value) × (log₁₀ labeled spore count per carrier + 4). Meets the requirements for Expiration date (not less than 18 months from the date of manufacture, the date of manufacture being the date on which the first determination of the total viable population was made), Identification, Resistance performance tests, Purity, and Stability.

Note: See Biological Indicators in *USP* for directives on selection of suitable indicators and on their applicability for different sterilization cycles, and for the characteristics of the basic or prototype article.

BIOTIN

Chemical name: 1*H*-Thieno[3,4-*d*]imidazole-4-pentanoic acid, hexahydro-2-oxo-, [3a*S*-(3a alpha,4 beta,6a alpha)]-.

Molecular formula: $C_{10}H_{16}N_2O_3S$.

Molecular weight: 244.31.

Description: Biotin USP—Practically white, crystalline powder.

Solubility: Biotin USP—Very slightly soluble in water and in alcohol; insoluble in other common organic solvents.

USP requirements:
Biotin USP—Store in tight containers. Contains not less than 97.5% and not more than 100.5% of biotin. Meets the requirements for Identification, Specific rotation (+89° to +93°), and Organic volatile impurities.
Biotin Capsules—Not in USP.
Biotin Tablets—Not in USP.

BIPERIDEN

Chemical group: Synthetic tertiary amine.

Chemical name:
Biperiden—1-Piperidinepropanol, alpha-bicyclo[2.2.1]hept-5-en-2-yl-alpha-phenyl-.
Biperiden hydrochloride—1-Piperidinepropanol, alpha-bicyclo[2.2.1]hept-5-en-2-yl-alpha-phenyl-, hydrochloride.
Biperiden lactate—1-Piperidinepropanol, alpha-bicyclo-[2.2.1]hept-5-en-2-yl-alpha-phenyl-, compounded with 2-hydroxypropanoic acid (1:1).

Molecular formula:
Biperiden—$C_{21}H_{29}NO$.
Biperiden hydrochloride—$C_{21}H_{29}NO \cdot HCl$.
Biperiden lactate—$C_{21}H_{29}NO \cdot C_3H_6O_3$.

Molecular weight:
Biperiden—311.47.
Biperiden hydrochloride—347.93.
Biperiden lactate—401.54.

Description:
Biperiden USP—White, practically odorless, crystalline powder.
Biperiden Hydrochloride USP—White, practically odorless, crystalline powder. Melts at about 275 °C, with decomposition. Is optically inactive.

Solubility:
Biperiden USP—Practically insoluble in water; freely soluble in chloroform; sparingly soluble in alcohol.
Biperiden Hydrochloride USP—Slightly soluble in water, in ether, in alcohol, and in chloroform; sparingly soluble in methanol.

USP requirements:
Biperiden USP—Preserve in well-closed, light-resistant containers. Contains not less than 98.0% and not more than

101.0% of biperiden, calculated on the dried basis. Meets the requirements for Identification, Melting range (112–116 °C), Loss on drying (not more than 1.0%), Residue on ignition (not more than 0.1%), and Ordinary impurities.
Biperiden Hydrochloride USP—Preserve in well-closed, light-resistant containers. Contains not less than 98.0% and not more than 101.0% of biperiden hydrochloride, calculated on the dried basis. Meets the requirements for Identification, Loss on drying (not more than 0.5%), and Ordinary impurities.
Biperiden Hydrochloride Tablets USP—Preserve in tight containers. Contain the labeled amount, within ±7%. Meet the requirements for Identification, Dissolution (75% in 45 minutes in 0.1 *N* hydrochloric acid in Apparatus 2 at 50 rpm), and Uniformity of dosage units.
Biperiden Lactate Injection USP—Preserve in single-dose containers, preferably of Type I glass, protected from light. A sterile solution of biperiden lactate in Water for Injection, prepared from Biperiden with the aid of Lactic Acid. Contains the labeled amount, within ±5%. Meets the requirements for Identification, Bacterial endotoxins, pH (4.8–5.8), and Injections.

BISACODYL

Chemical group: Diphenylmethane derivatives.

Chemical name: Phenol, 4,4′-(2-pyridinylmethylene)bis-, diacetate (ester).

Molecular formula: $C_{22}H_{19}NO_4$.

Molecular weight: 361.40.

Description: Bisacodyl USP—White to off-white, crystalline powder, in which the number of particles having a longest diameter smaller than 50 micrometers predominate.

Solubility: Bisacodyl USP—Practically insoluble in water; soluble in chloroform; sparingly soluble in alcohol and in methanol; slightly soluble in ether.

USP requirements:
Bisacodyl USP—Preserve in well-closed containers. Contains not less than 98.0% and not more than 101.0% of bisacodyl, calculated on the dried basis. Meets the requirements for Identification, Melting range (131–135 °C), Loss on drying (not more than 0.5%), Residue on ignition (not more than 0.1%), and Heavy metals (0.001%).
Caution: Avoid inhalation and contact with the eyes, skin, and mucous membranes.
Bisacodyl Rectal Solution—Not in USP.
Bisacodyl Suppositories USP—Preserve in well-closed containers at a temperature not exceeding 30 °C. Contain the labeled amount, within ±10%. Meet the requirement for Identification.
Bisacodyl Tablets USP—Preserve in well-closed containers at a temperature not exceeding 30 °C. Label Tablets to indicate that they are enteric-coated. Contain the labeled amount, within ±10%. Bisacodyl Tablets are enteric-coated. Meet the requirements for Identification, Disintegration (tablets do not disintegrate after 1 hour of agitation in simulated gastric fluid TS, but then disintegrate within 45 minutes in simulated intestinal fluid TS), and Uniformity of dosage units.
Bisacodyl Tannex Powder for Rectal Solution—Not in USP.

BISACODYL AND DOCUSATE

For *Bisacodyl* and *Docusate*—See individual listings for chemistry information.

USP requirements: Bisacodyl and Docusate Sodium Tablets—Not in USP.

BISMUTH

Chemical name:
Bismuth subgallate—Gallic acid bismuth basic salt.
Bismuth subnitrate—Bismuth hydroxide nitrate oxide $(Bi_5O(OH)_9(NO_3)_4)$.
Bismuth subsalicylate—(2-Hydroxybenzoato-O^1)-oxobismuth.

Molecular formula:
Bismuth subgallate—$C_7H_5BiO_6$.
Bismuth subnitrate—$Bi_5O(OH)_9(NO_3)_4$.
Bismuth subsalicylate—$C_7H_5BiO_4$.

Molecular weight:
Bismuth subgallate—394.09.
Bismuth subnitrate—1461.99.
Bismuth subsalicylate—362.09.

Description:
Bismuth Subgallate USP—Amorphous, bright yellow powder. Odorless. Stable in air, but affected by light.
Bismuth Subnitrate USP—White, slightly hygroscopic powder.

Solubility:
Bismuth Subgallate USP—Dissolves readily with decomposition in warm, moderately dilute hydrochloric, nitric, or sulfuric acid; readily dissolved by solutions of alkali hydroxides, forming a clear, yellow liquid, which rapidly assumes a deep red color. Practically insoluble in water, in alcohol, in chloroform, and in ether; insoluble in very dilute mineral acids.
Bismuth Subnitrate USP—Practically insoluble in water and in alcohol; readily dissolved by hydrochloric acid or by nitric acid.
Bismuth subsalicylate—Practically insoluble in water or in alcohol; soluble in alkali; decomposed by hot water.

USP requirements:
Bismuth Subgallate USP—Preserve in tight, light-resistant containers. A basic salt. When dried at 105 °C for 3 hours, contains an amount of bismuth subgallate equivalent to not less than 52.0% and not more than 57.0% of bismuth trioxide. Meets the requirements for Identification, Loss on drying (not more than 7.0%), Nitrate, Alkalies and alkaline earths (not more than 0.5%), Arsenic (not more than 7.5 ppm), Copper, Lead, and Silver, and Free gallic acid (not more than 0.5%).
Bismuth Subnitrate USP—Preserve in well-closed containers. A basic salt. Contains an amount of bismuth subnitrate equivalent to not less than 79.0% of bismuth trioxide, calculated on the dried basis. Meets the requirements for Identification, Loss on drying (not more than 3.0%), Carbonate, Chloride (not more than 0.035%), Sulfate, Alkalies and alkaline earths (not more than 0.5%), Ammonium salts, Arsenic (not more than 8 ppm), Copper, Lead, and Silver.
Bismuth Subsalicylate Oral Suspension—Not in USP.
Bismuth Subsalicylate Chewable Tablets—Not in USP.

MILK OF BISMUTH

Description: Milk of Bismuth USP—Thick, white, opaque suspension that separates on standing. Is odorless.

Solubility: Milk of Bismuth USP—Miscible with water and with alcohol.

USP requirements: Milk of Bismuth USP—Preserve in tight containers, and protect from freezing. Contains bismuth hydroxide and bismuth subcarbonate in suspension in water, and yields not less than 5.2% and not more than 5.8% (w/w) of bismuth trioxide.

Prepare Milk of Bismuth as follows: 80 grams of Bismuth Subnitrate, 120 mL of Nitric Acid, 10 grams of Ammonium Carbonate, and a sufficient amount of, each, Strong Ammonia Solution and Purified Water, to make 1000 mL. Mix the Bismuth Subnitrate with 60 mL of Purified Water and 60 mL of the Nitric Acid in a suitable container, and agitate, warming gently until solution is effected. Pour this solution, with constant stirring, into 5000 mL of Purified Water containing 60 mL of the Nitric Acid. Dilute 160 mL of Strong Ammonia Solution with 4300 mL of Purified Water in a glazed or glass vessel of at least 12,000-mL capacity. Dissolve the Ammonium Carbonate in this solution, and then pour the bismuth solution quickly into it with constant stirring. Add sufficient 6 N ammonium hydroxide, if necessary, to render the mixture distinctly alkaline, allow to stand until the precipitate has settled, then pour or siphon off the supernatant liquid, and wash the precipitate twice with Purified Water, by decantation. Transfer the magma to a strainer of close texture, so as to provide continuous washing with Purified Water, the outlet tube being elevated to prevent the surface of the magma from becoming dry. When the washings no longer yield a pink color with phenolphthalein TS, drain the moist preparation, transfer to a graduated vessel, add sufficient Purified Water to make 1000 mL, and mix.

Note: This method of preparation may be varied, provided the product meets the requirements.

Meets the requirements for Identification, Microbial limits, Water-soluble substances (not more than 0.1%), Alkalies and alkaline earths (not more than 0.3%), Arsenic (not more than 0.8 ppm), and Lead.

BITOLTEROL

Chemical name: Bitolterol mesylate—Benzoic acid, 4-methyl-, 4-[2-[(1,1-dimethylethyl)amino]-1-hydroxyethyl]-1,2-phenylene ester methanesulfonate (salt).

Molecular formula: Bitolterol mesylate—$C_{28}H_{31}NO_5 \cdot CH_4O_3S$.

Molecular weight: Bitolterol mesylate—557.66.

Description: Bitolterol mesylate—White to off-white, crystalline powder.

Solubility: Bitolterol mesylate—Sparingly soluble to soluble in water; freely soluble in alcohol.

USP requirements: Bitolterol Mesylate Inhalation Aerosol—Not in USP.

BLEOMYCIN

Source: Bleomycin is a mixture of glycopeptide antibiotics isolated from a strain of *Streptomyces verticillus* and converted into sulfates.

Chemical name: Bleomycin sulfate—Bleomycin sulfate (salt).

Description: Sterile Bleomycin Sulfate USP—Cream-colored, amorphous powder.

Solubility: Sterile Bleomycin Sulfate USP—Very soluble in water.

Other characteristics: Hygroscopic; inactivated in vitro by agents containing sulfhydryl groups, hydrogen peroxide, and ascorbic acid.

USP requirements: Sterile Bleomycin Sulfate USP—Preserve in Containers for Sterile Solids. It is the sulfate salt of bleomycin, a mixture of basic cytotoxic glycopeptides produced by the growth of *Streptomyces verticillus*, or produced by other means. Contains not less than 1.5 Bleomycin Units and not more than 2.0 Bleomycin Units per mg and, where packaged for dispensing, contains an amount of bleomycin sulfate equivalent to the labeled amount of bleomycin, within −10% to +20%. Meets the requirements for Constituted solution, Identification, Depressor substances, Bacterial endotoxins, Sterility, pH (4.5–6.0, in a solution containing 10 Bleomycin Units per mL), Loss on drying (not more than 6.0%), Content of bleomycins, and Copper (not more than 0.02%), and, where packaged for dispensing, for Uniformity of dosage units and Labeling under Injections.

ANTI-A BLOOD GROUPING SERUM

Description: Anti-A Blood Grouping Serum USP—Liquid Serum is a clear or slightly opalescent fluid unless artificially colored blue. Dried Serum is light yellow to deep cream color, unless artificially colored as indicated for liquid Serum. The liquid Serum may develop slight turbidity on storage. The dried Serum may show slight turbidity upon reconstitution for use.

USP requirements: Anti-A Blood Grouping Serum USP—Preserve at a temperature between 2 and 8 °C. A sterile, liquid or dried preparation containing the particular blood group antibodies derived from high-titered blood plasma or serum of human subjects, with or without stimulation by the injection of Blood Group Specific Substance A (or AB). Agglutinates human red cells containing A-antigens, i.e., blood groups A and AB (including subgroups A_1, A_2, A_1B, and A_2B but not necessarily weaker subgroups). Contains a suitable antimicrobial preservative. Label it to state that the source material was not reactive for hepatitis B surface antigen, but that no known test method offers assurance that products derived from human blood will not transmit hepatitis. Label it also to state that it is for in-vitro diagnostic use. [Note: The labeling is in black lettering imprinted on paper that is white or is colored completely or in part to match the specified blue color standard.] Meets the requirements of the tests for potency, specificity, and avidity. All fresh or frozen red blood cell suspensions used for these tests are prepared under specified conditions and meet specified criteria. Meets the requirement for Expiration date (for liquid Serum, not later than 1 year, and for dried Serum, not later than 5 years after date of issue from manufacturer's cold storage [5 °C, 1 year; or 0 °C, 2 years], provided that the expiration date for dried Serum is not later than 1 year after constitution). Conforms to the regulations of the U.S. Food and Drug Administration concerning biologics.

ANTI-B BLOOD GROUPING SERUM

Description: Anti-B Blood Grouping Serum USP—Liquid Serum is a clear or slightly opalescent fluid unless artificially colored yellow. Dried Serum is light yellow to deep cream color, unless artificially colored as indicated for liquid Serum. The liquid Serum may develop a slight turbidity on storage. The dried Serum may show slight turbidity upon reconstitution for use.

USP requirements: Anti-B Blood Grouping Serum USP—Preserve at a temperature between 2 and 8 °C. A sterile, liquid or dried preparation containing the particular blood group antibodies derived from high-titered blood plasma or serum of human subjects, with or without stimulation by the injection of Blood Group Specific Substance B (or AB). Agglutinates human red cells containing B-antigens, i.e., blood groups B and AB (including subgroups A_1B and A_2B). Contains a suitable antimicrobial preservative. Label it to state

that the source material was not reactive for hepatitis B surface antigen, but that no known test method offers assurance that products derived from human blood will not transmit hepatitis. Label it also to state that it is for in-vitro diagnostic use. [Note: The labeling is in black lettering imprinted on paper that is white or is colored completely or in part to match the specified yellow color standard.] Meets the requirements of the tests for potency, specificity, and avidity. All fresh or frozen red blood cell suspensions used for these tests are prepared under specified conditions and meet specified criteria. Meets the requirement for Expiration date (for liquid Serum, not later than 1 year, and for dried Serum, not later than 5 years after date of issue from manufacturer's cold storage [5 °C, 1 year; or 0 °C, 2 years], provided that the expiration date for dried Serum is not later than 1 year after constitution). Conforms to the regulations of the U.S. Food and Drug Administration concerning biologics.

BLOOD GROUPING SERUMS

USP requirements: Blood Grouping Serums USP—Preserve at a temperature between 2 and 8 °C. Each serum is a sterile, liquid or dried preparation containing one or more of the particular blood group antibodies derived from high-titered blood plasma or serum of human subjects, with or without stimulation by the injection of red cells or other substances, or of animals after stimulation by substances that cause such antibody production. Causes either directly, or indirectly by the antiglobulin test, the visible agglutination of human red cells containing the particular antigen(s) for which it is specific. Contains a suitable antimicrobial preservative. Label each to state the source of the product if other than human and, if of human origin, to state that the source material was not reactive for hepatitis B surface antigen, but that no known test method offers assurance that products derived from human blood will not transmit hepatitis. Label each also to state that it is for in-vitro diagnostic use. Meets the requirements of the tests for potency, specificity, and avidity. All fresh or frozen red blood cell suspensions used for these tests are prepared under specified conditions and meet specified criteria. Meets the requirement for Expiration date (for liquid Serum, not later than 1 year, and for dried Serum, not later than 5 years after date of issue from manufacturer's cold storage [5 °C, 1 year; or 0 °C, 2 years], provided that the expiration date for dried Serum is not later than 1 year after constitution). Blood Grouping Serums conform to the regulations of the U.S. Food and Drug Administration concerning biologics.

Note: This monograph deals with those Blood Grouping Serums for which there are no individual monographs and which are not routinely used or required for the testing of blood or blood products for transfusion.

BLOOD GROUPING SERUMS ANTI-D, ANTI-C, ANTI-E, ANTI-c, ANTI-e

Description: Blood Grouping Serums Anti-D, Anti-C, Anti-E, Anti-c, Anti-e USP—The liquid Serums are clear, slightly yellowish fluids, that may develop slight turbidity on storage. The dried Serums are light yellow to deep cream color.

USP requirements: Blood Grouping Serums Anti-D, Anti-C, Anti-E, Anti-c, Anti-e USP—Preserve at a temperature between 2 and 8 °C. They are sterile, liquid or dried preparations derived from the blood plasma or serum of human subjects who have developed specific Rh antibodies. They are free from agglutinins for the A or B antigens and from alloantibodies other than those for which claims are made in the labeling. Contain a suitable antimicrobial preservative. Liquid serums are not artificially colored. Label each to state that the source material was not reactive for hepatitis B surface antigen, but that no known test method offers assurance that products derived from human blood will not transmit hepatitis. Label each to state that it is for in-vitro diagnostic use. Meet the requirements of the tests for potency, avidity, and specificity. All fresh or frozen red blood cell suspensions used for these tests are prepared under specified conditions and meet specified criteria. Meet the requirement for Expiration date (for liquid Serums, not later than 1 year, and for dried Serums, not later than 5 years, after date of issue from manufacturer's cold storage [5 °C, 1 year; or 0 °C, 2 years], provided that the expiration date for dried Serum is not later than 1 year after constitution). Conform to the regulations of the U.S. Food and Drug Administration concerning biologics.

BLOOD GROUP SPECIFIC SUBSTANCES A, B, AND AB

Description: Blood Group Specific Substances A, B, and AB USP—Clear solution that may have a slight odor because of the preservative.

USP requirements: Blood Group Specific Substances A, B, and AB USP—Preserve in single-dose containers, each containing a volume of not more than 1 mL consisting of a solution containing not more than 1.25 mg of Blood Group Specific Substance powder, at a temperature between 2 and 8 °C. Dispense it in the unopened container in which it was placed by the manufacturer. A sterile, pyrogen-free, nonanaphylactic isotonic solution of the polysaccharide-amino acid complexes that are capable of neutralizing the anti-A and the anti-B isoagglutinins of group O blood, and are used in the immunization of plasma donors for the production of in-vitro diagnostic reagents. Contains no added preservative. Blood Group Specific Substance A is prepared from hog stomach (gastric mucin), and Blood Group Specific Substances B and AB are prepared from horse stomach (gastric mucosa). It has a total nitrogen content of not more than 8%, calculated on the moisture- and ash-free basis. Label it to state that it was derived from porcine or equine stomachs, whichever is applicable, and that it contains a single dose consisting of the stated content of dry weight of powder dissolved in the stated volume of product. Label it also to state the route of administration, and to state that it is not to be administered intravenously nor to fertile women. Label Blood Group Specific Substance B with a warning that it may contain immunogenic A activity. Meets the requirements of the test for potency (including identity). Meets the requirements for Expiration date (not more than 2 years after date of issue from manufacturer's cold storage [5 °C, 1 year; or 0 °C, 2 years]), pH (6.0–6.8), and of the tests for safety and for anaphylaxis. Conforms to the regulations of the U.S. Food and Drug Administration concerning biologics.

RED BLOOD CELLS

Description: Red Blood Cells USP—Dark red in color when packed. May show a slight creamy layer on the surface and a small supernatant layer of yellow or opalescent plasma. Also supplied in deep-frozen form with added cryophylactic substance to extend storage time.

USP requirements: Red Blood Cells USP—Preserve in a hermetic container, which is of colorless, transparent, sterile, pyrogen-free Type I or Type II glass, or of a suitable plastic material in which it was placed by the processor. Store if unfrozen at a temperature between 1 and 6 °C, held constant within a 2 °C range except during shipment when the temperature may be between 1 and 10 °C, and store if for extended manufacturers' storage in frozen form at −65 °C

or colder. The container of Red Blood Cells is accompanied by a securely attached smaller container holding an original pilot sample of blood taken from the donor at the same time as the whole human blood, or a pilot sample of Red Blood Cells removed at the time of its preparation. It is the remaining red blood cells of whole human blood that have been collected from suitable whole blood donors, and from which plasma has been removed. Red Blood Cells may be prepared at any time during the dating period of the whole blood from which it is derived, by centrifuging or undisturbed sedimentation for the separation of plasma and cells, not later than 21 days after the blood has been drawn, except that when acid citrate dextrose adenine solution has been used as the anticoagulant, such preparation may be made within 35 days therefrom. Contains a portion of the plasma sufficient to ensure optional cell preservation or contains a cryophylactic substance if it is for extended manufacturers' storage at −65 °C or colder. In addition to labeling requirements of Whole Blood applicable to this product, label it to indicate the approved variation to which it conforms, such as "Frozen," or "Deglycerolized." Label it also with the instruction to use a filter in the administration equipment. Meets the requirement for Expiration date (for unfrozen Red Blood Cells, not later than that of the whole human blood from which it is derived if plasma has not been removed, except that if the hermetic seal of the container is broken during preparation, the expiration date is not later than 24 hours after the seal is broken; for frozen Red Blood Cells, not later than 3 years after the date of collection of the source blood when stored at −65 °C or colder and not later than 24 hours after removal from −65 °C storage provided it is then stored at the temperature for unfrozen Red Blood Cells). Conforms to the regulations of the U.S. Food and Drug Administration concerning biologics.

WHOLE BLOOD

Description: Whole Blood USP—Deep red, opaque liquid from which the corpuscles readily settle upon standing for 24 to 48 hours, leaving a clear, yellowish or pinkish supernatant layer of plasma.

USP requirements: Whole Blood USP—Preserve in the container into which it was originally drawn. Use pyrogen-free, sterile containers of colorless, transparent, Type I or Type II glass, or of a suitable plastic material. The container is provided with a hermetic contamination-proof closure. Accessory equipment supplied with the blood is sterile and pyrogen-free. Store at a temperature between 1 and 6 °C held constant within a 2 °C range, except during shipment, when the temperature may be between 1 and 10 °C. The container of Whole Blood is accompanied by at least one securely attached smaller container holding an original pilot sample of blood, for test purposes, taken at the same time from the same donor, with the same anticoagulant. Both containers bear the donor's identification symbol or number. It is blood that has been collected from suitable whole blood human donors under rigid aseptic precautions, for transfusion to human recipients. Contains citrate ion (acid citrate dextrose or citrate phosphate dextrose or citrate phosphate dextrose with adenine) or Heparin Sodium as an anticoagulant. May consist of blood from which the antihemophilic factor has been removed, in which case it is termed "Modified." Label it to indicate the donor classification, quantity and kind of anticoagulant used and the corresponding volume of blood, the designation of ABO blood group and Rh factors, and in the case of Group O blood, whether or not isoagglutinin titers or other tests for exclusion of specified Group O bloods were performed and to indicate any group classification of the blood resulting therefrom. If an ABO blood group color scheme is used, the labeling color used shall be: Group A (yellow), Group B (pink), Group O (blue), and Group AB (white). Label it also with the type and result of a serologic test for syphilis, or to indicate that it was non-reactive in such test; and with the type and result of a test for hepatitis B surface antigen, or to indicate that it was non-reactive in such test. If it has been issued prior to determination of test results, label it also with a warning not to use it until the test results have been received and to specify that a cross-match be performed. Where applicable, label it as "Modified," and indicate that antihemophilic factor has been removed and that it should not be used for patients requiring that factor. Meets the requirements of tests made on a pilot sample in non-reacting in a serologic test for syphilis; for ABO blood group designation; and for classification in regard to Rh type, including those tests specified for variants and other related factors. Containers of Whole Blood shall not be entered for sterility testing prior to use of the blood for transfusion. [Note: Whole Blood may be issued prior to the results of testing, under the specified provisions.] Meets the requirement for Expiridation date (not later than 21 days after the date of bleeding the donor, if it contains anticoagulant citrate dextrose solution or anticoagulant citrate phosphate dextrose solution, as the anticoagulant; or not later than 35 days if it contains anticoagulant citrate phosphate dextrose adenine solution as the anticoagulant; or not later than 48 hours after date of bleeding the donor, if it contains heparin ion as the anticoagulant). Conforms to the regulations of the U.S. Food and Drug Administration concerning biologics.

BORIC ACID

Chemical name: Boric acid (H_3BO_3).

Molecular formula: H_3BO_3.

Molecular weight: 61.83.

Description: Boric Acid NF—Colorless, odorless scales of a somewhat pearly luster, or crystals, or white powder that is slightly unctuous to the touch. Stable in air.
   NF category: Buffering agent.

Solubility: Boric Acid NF—Soluble in water and in alcohol; freely soluble in glycerin, in boiling water, and in boiling alcohol.

NF requirements: Boric Acid NF—Preserve in well-closed containers. Label the container with a warning that it is not for internal use. Contains not less than 99.5% and not more than 100.5% of boric acid, calculated on the dried basis. Meets the requirements for Solubility in alcohol, Completeness of solution, Identification, Loss on drying (not more than 0.5%), Arsenic (8 ppm), and Heavy metals (not more than 0.002%).

BOTULISM ANTITOXIN

Description: Botulism Antitoxin USP—Transparent or slightly opalescent liquid, practically colorless, and practically odorless or having an odor because of the antimicrobial agent.

USP requirements: Botulism Antitoxin USP—Preserve in single-dose containers only, at a temperature between 2 and 8 °C. A sterile, non-pyrogenic solution of the refined and concentrated antitoxic antibodies, chiefly globulins, obtained from the blood of healthy horses that have been immunized against the toxins produced by the type A and type B and/or type E strains of *Clostridium botulinum*. Label it to state that it was prepared from horse blood. Its potency is determined with the U.S. Standard Botulism Antitoxin of the relevant type, tested by neutralizing activity in mice of the

corresponding U.S. Control Botulism Test Toxin. Contains not more than 20% of solids, and contains a suitable antimicrobial agent. Meets the requirement for Expiration date (for Antitoxin containing a 20% excess of potency, not later than 5 years after date of issue from manufacturer's cold storage [5 °C, 1 year; or 0 °C, 2 years]). Conforms to the regulations of the U.S. Food and Drug Administration concerning biologics.

BRETYLIUM

Chemical group: Bretylium is a bromobenzyl quaternary ammonium compound.

Chemical name: Bretylium tosylate—Benzenemethanaminium, 2-bromo-*N*-ethyl-*N*,*N*-dimethyl-, salt with 4-methylbenzenesulfonic acid (1:1).

Molecular formula: Bretylium tosylate—$C_{18}H_{24}BrNO_3S$.

Molecular weight: Bretylium tosylate—414.36.

Description: Bretylium tosylate—White, crystalline powder.

Solubility: Bretylium tosylate—Freely soluble in water and in alcohol.

USP requirements:
   Bretylium Tosylate Injection—Not in USP.
   Bretylium Tosylate in 5% Dextrose Injection—Not in USP.

BROMAZEPAM

Chemical name: 2*H*-1,4-Benzodiazepin-2-one, 7-bromo-1,3-dihydro-5-(2-pyridinyl)-.

Molecular formula: $C_{14}H_{10}BrN_3O$.

Molecular weight: 316.16.

USP requirements: Bromazepam Tablets—Not in USP.

BROMOCRIPTINE

Source: Bromocriptine is an ergot derivative.

Chemical name: Bromocriptine mesylate—Ergotaman-3′,6′,18-trione, 2-bromo-12′-hydroxy-2′-(1-methylethyl)-5′-(2-methylpropyl)-, monomethanesulfonate (salt), (5′alpha)-.

Molecular formula: Bromocriptine mesylate—$C_{32}H_{40}BrN_5O_5 \cdot CH_4SO_3$.

Molecular weight: Bromocriptine mesylate—750.70.

Description: Bromocriptine Mesylate USP—White or slightly colored, fine crystalline powder; odorless or having a weak, characteristic odor.

Solubility: Bromocriptine mesylate—Practically insoluble in water; sparingly soluble in dehydrated alcohol; soluble in alcohol; very slightly soluble in chloroform; freely soluble in methyl alcohol.

USP requirements:
   Bromocriptine Mesylate USP—Preserve in tight, light-resistant containers, in a cold place. Contains not less than 98.0% and not more than 102.0% of bromocriptine mesylate, calculated on the dried basis. Meets the requirements for Identification, Color of solution, Specific rotation (+95° to +105°, calculated on the dried basis), Loss on drying (not more than 4.0%), Residue on ignition (not more than 0.1%), Heavy metals (not more than 0.002%), Related substances (not more than 1.0%), Methanesulfonic acid content (12.5–13.4%, calculated on the dried basis), and Organic volatile impurities.

Bromocriptine Mesylate Capsules—Not in USP.

Bromocriptine Mesylate Tablets USP—Preserve in tight, light-resistant containers. Contain an amount of bromocriptine mesylate equivalent to the labeled amount of bromocriptine, within ± 10%. Meet the requirements for Identification, Related substances (not more than 5.0%), Dissolution (80% in 60 minutes in 0.1 N hydrochloric acid in Apparatus 1 at 120 rpm), and Uniformity of dosage units.

BROMODIPHENHYDRAMINE

Chemical name: Bromodiphenhydramine hydrochloride—Ethanamine, 2-[(4-bromophenyl)phenylmethoxy]-*N*,*N*-dimethyl-, hydrochloride.

Molecular formula: Bromodiphenhydramine hydrochloride—$C_{17}H_{20}BrNO \cdot HCl$.

Molecular weight: Bromodiphenhydramine hydrochloride—370.72.

Description: Bromodiphenhydramine Hydrochloride USP—White to pale buff, crystalline powder, having no more than a faint odor.

Solubility: Bromodiphenhydramine Hydrochloride USP—Freely soluble in water and in alcohol; soluble in isopropyl alcohol; insoluble in ether and in solvent hexane.

USP requirements:

Bromodiphenhydramine Hydrochloride USP—Preserve in tight containers. Contains not less than 98.0% and not more than 101.0%, calculated on the dried basis. Meets the requirements for Identification, Melting range (148–152 °C), Loss on drying (not more than 0.5%), and Organic volatile impurities.

Bromodiphenhydramine Hydrochloride Capsules USP—Preserve in tight containers. Contain the labeled amount, within ± 7%. Meet the requirements for Identification, Dissolution (75% in 45 minutes in water in Apparatus 1 at 100 rpm), and Uniformity of dosage units.

Bromodiphenhydramine Hydrochloride Elixir USP—Preserve in tight, light-resistant containers. Contains the labeled amount, within ± 7%. Meets the requirements for Identification and Alcohol content (12.0–15.0%).

BROMODIPHENHYDRAMINE AND CODEINE

For *Bromodiphenhydramine* and *Codeine*—See individual listings for chemistry information.

USP requirements: Bromodiphenhydramine Hydrochloride and Codeine Phosphate Syrup—Not in USP.

BROMODIPHENHYDRAMINE, DIPHENHYDRAMINE, CODEINE, AMMONIUM CHLORIDE, AND POTASSIUM GUAIACOLSULFONATE

Chemical group: Bromodiphenhydramine; Diphenhydramine—Ethanolamine derivatives.

Chemical name:

Bromodiphenhydramine hydrochloride—Ethanamine, 2-[(4-bromophenyl)phenylmethoxy]-*N*,*N*-dimethyl-, hydrochloride.

Diphenhydramine hydrochloride—Ethanamine, 2-(diphenylmethoxy)-*N*,*N*-dimethyl-, hydrochloride.

Codeine phosphate—Morphinan-6-ol, 7,8-didehydro-4,5-epoxy-3-methoxy-17-methyl-, (5 alpha,6 alpha)-, phosphate (1:1) (salt), hemihydrate.

Ammonium chloride—Ammonium chloride.

Potassium guaiacolsulfonate—Benzenesulfonic acid, hydroxymethoxy-, monopotassium salt, hemihydrate.

Molecular formula:

Bromodiphenhydramine hydrochloride—$C_{17}H_{20}BrNO \cdot HCl$.

Diphenhydramine hydrochloride—$C_{17}H_{21}NO \cdot HCl$.

Codeine phosphate—$C_{18}H_{21}NO_3 \cdot H_3PO_4 \cdot \frac{1}{2}H_2O$ (hemihydrate); $C_{18}H_{21}NO_3 \cdot H_3PO_4$ (anhydrous).

Ammonium chloride—NH_4Cl.

Potassium guaiacolsulfonate—$C_7H_7KO_5S \cdot \frac{1}{2}H_2O$.

Molecular weight:

Bromodiphenhydramine hydrochloride—370.72.

Diphenhydramine hydrochloride—291.82.

Codeine phosphate—406.37 (hemihydrate); 397.36 (anhydrous).

Ammonium chloride—53.49.

Potassium guaiacolsulfonate—251.29.

Description:

Bromodiphenhydramine Hydrochloride USP—White to pale buff, crystalline powder, having no more than a faint odor.

Diphenhydramine Hydrochloride USP—White, odorless, crystalline powder. Slowly darkens on exposure to light. Its solutions are practically neutral to litmus.

Codeine Phosphate USP—Fine, white, needle-shaped crystals, or white, crystalline powder. Is odorless, and is affected by light. Its solutions are acid to litmus.

Ammonium Chloride USP—Colorless crystals or white, fine or coarse, crystalline powder. Is somewhat hygroscopic.

pKa: Diphenhydramine hydrochloride—9.

Solubility:

Bromodiphenhydramine Hydrochloride USP—Freely soluble in water and in alcohol; soluble in isopropyl alcohol; insoluble in ether and in solvent hexane.

Diphenhydramine Hydrochloride USP—Freely soluble in water, in alcohol, and in chloroform; sparingly soluble in acetone; very slightly soluble in ether.

Codeine Phosphate USP—Freely soluble in water; very soluble in hot water; slightly soluble in alcohol but more so in boiling alcohol.

Ammonium Chloride USP—Freely soluble in water and in glycerin, and even more so in boiling water; sparingly soluble in alcohol.

USP requirements: Bromodiphenhydramine Hydrochloride, Diphenhydramine Hydrochloride, Codeine Phosphate, Ammonium Chloride, and Potassium Guaiacolsulfonate Oral Solution—Not in USP.

BROMPHENIRAMINE

Chemical group: Propylamine derivative (alkylamine).

Chemical name: Brompheniramine maleate—2-Pyridinepropanamine, gamma-(4-bromophenyl)-*N*,*N*-dimethyl-, (*Z*)-butenedioate (1:1).

Molecular formula: Brompheniramine maleate—$C_{16}H_{19}BrN_2 \cdot C_4H_4O_4$.

Molecular weight: Brompheniramine maleate—435.32.

Description: Brompheniramine Maleate USP—White, odorless, crystalline powder.

pKa: Brompheniramine maleate—3.59 and 9.12.

Solubility: Brompheniramine Maleate USP—Freely soluble in water; soluble in alcohol and in chloroform; slightly soluble in ether.

USP requirements:

Brompheniramine Maleate USP—Preserve in tight, light-resistant containers. It is dried at 105 °C for 3 hours. Contains not less than 98.0% and not more than 100.5% of brompheniramine maleate. Meets the requirements for Identification, Melting range (130–135 °C), pH (4.0–5.0, in a solution [1 in 100]), Loss on drying (not more than 0.5%), Residue on ignition (not more than 0.2%), Related compounds, and Organic volatile impurities.

Brompheniramine Maleate Elixir USP—Preserve in well-closed, light-resistant containers. Contains the labeled amount, within ±5%. Meets the requirements for Identification, pH (2.5–3.5), and Alcohol content (2.7–3.3%).

Brompheniramine Maleate Injection USP—Preserve in single-dose or in multiple-dose containers, preferably of Type I glass, protected from light. A sterile solution of Brompheniramine Maleate in Water for Injection. Contains the labeled amount, within ±10%. Meets the requirements for Identification, pH (6.3–7.3), and Injections.

Brompheniramine Maleate Tablets USP—Preserve in tight containers. Contain the labeled amount, within ±5%. Meet the requirements for Identification, Dissolution (75% in 45 minutes in water in Apparatus 1 at 100 rpm), and Uniformity of dosage units.

Brompheniramine Maleate Extended-release Tablets—Not in USP.

BROMPHENIRAMINE AND PHENYLEPHRINE

For *Brompheniramine* and *Phenylephrine*—See individual listings for chemistry information.

USP requirements:

Brompheniramine Maleate and Phenylephrine Hydrochloride Elixir—Not in USP.

Brompheniramine Maleate and Phenylephrine Hydrochloride Tablets—Not in USP.

BROMPHENIRAMINE, PHENYLEPHRINE, AND PHENYLPROPANOLAMINE

For *Brompheniramine*, *Phenylephrine*, and *Phenylpropanolamine*—See individual listings for chemistry information.

USP requirements:

Brompheniramine Maleate, Phenylephrine Hydrochloride, and Phenylpropanolamine Hydrochloride Elixir—Not in USP.

Brompheniramine Maleate, Phenylephrine Hydrochloride, and Phenylpropanolamine Hydrochloride Oral Solution—Not in USP.

Brompheniramine Maleate, Phenylephrine Hydrochloride, and Phenylpropanolamine Hydrochloride Tablets—Not in USP.

Brompheniramine Maleate, Phenylephrine Hydrochloride, and Phenylpropanolamine Hydrochloride Extended-release Tablets—Not in USP.

BROMPHENIRAMINE, PHENYLEPHRINE, PHENYLPROPANOLAMINE, AND ACETAMINOPHEN

For *Brompheniramine*, *Phenylephrine*, *Phenylpropanolamine*, and *Acetaminophen*—See individual listings for chemistry information.

USP requirements:

Brompheniramine Maleate, Phenylephrine Hydrochloride, Phenylpropanolamine Hydrochloride, and Acetaminophen Oral Solution—Not in USP.

Brompheniramine Maleate, Phenylephrine Hydrochloride, Phenylpropanolamine Hydrochloride, and Acetaminophen Tablets—Not in USP.

BROMPHENIRAMINE, PHENYLEPHRINE, PHENYLPROPANOLAMINE, AND CODEINE

For *Brompheniramine*, *Phenylephrine*, *Phenylpropanolamine*, and *Codeine*—See individual listings for chemistry information.

USP requirements: Brompheniramine Maleate, Phenylephrine Hydrochloride, Phenylpropanolamine Hydrochloride, and Codeine Phosphate Tablets—Not in USP.

BROMPHENIRAMINE, PHENYLEPHRINE, PHENYLPROPANOLAMINE, CODEINE, AND GUAIFENESIN

For *Brompheniramine*, *Phenylephrine*, *Phenylpropanolamine*, *Codeine*, and *Guaifenesin*—See individual listings for chemistry information.

USP requirements: Brompheniramine Maleate, Phenylephrine Hydrochloride, Phenylpropanolamine Hydrochloride, Codeine Phosphate, and Guaifenesin Syrup—Not in USP.

BROMPHENIRAMINE, PHENYLEPHRINE, PHENYLPROPANOLAMINE, AND DEXTROMETHORPHAN

For *Brompheniramine*, *Phenylephrine*, *Phenylpropanolamine*, and *Dextromethorphan*—See individual listings for chemistry information.

USP requirements:

Brompheniramine Maleate, Phenylephrine Hydrochloride, Phenylpropanolamine Hydrochloride, and Dextromethorphan Hydrobromide Elixir—Not in USP.

Brompheniramine Maleate, Phenylephrine Hydrochloride, Phenylpropanolamine Hydrochloride, and Dextromethorphan Hydrobromide Tablets—Not in USP.

BROMPHENIRAMINE, PHENYLEPHRINE, PHENYLPROPANOLAMINE, AND GUAIFENESIN

For *Brompheniramine*, *Phenylephrine*, *Phenylpropanolamine*, and *Guaifenesin*—See individual listings for chemistry information.

USP requirements: Brompheniramine Maleate, Phenylephrine Hydrochloride, Phenylpropanolamine Hydrochloride, and Guaifenesin Syrup—Not in USP.

BROMPHENIRAMINE, PHENYLEPHRINE, PHENYLPROPANOLAMINE, HYDROCODONE, AND GUAIFENESIN

For *Brompheniramine*, *Phenylephrine*, *Phenylpropanolamine*, *Hydrocodone*, and *Guaifenesin*—See individual listings for chemistry information.

USP requirements: Brompheniramine Maleate, Phenylephrine Hydrochloride, Phenylpropanolamine Hydrochloride, Hydrocodone Bitartrate, and Guaifenesin Oral Solution—Not in USP.

BROMPHENIRAMINE AND PHENYLPROPANOLAMINE

For *Brompheniramine* and *Phenylpropanolamine*—See individual listings for chemistry information.

USP requirements:

Brompheniramine Maleate and Phenylpropanolamine Hydrochloride Elixir—Not in USP.

Brompheniramine Maleate and Phenylpropanolamine Hydrochloride Tablets—Not in USP.

Brompheniramine Maleate and Phenylpropanolamine Hydrochloride Extended-release Tablets—Not in USP.

BROMPHENIRAMINE, PHENYLPROPANOLAMINE, AND ASPIRIN

For *Brompheniramine, Phenylpropanolamine*, and *Aspirin*—See individual listings for chemistry information.

USP requirements: Brompheniramine Maleate, Phenylpropanolamine Bitartrate, and Aspirin Tablets for Oral Solution—Not in USP.

BROMPHENIRAMINE, PHENYLPROPANOLAMINE, AND CODEINE

For *Brompheniramine, Phenylpropanolamine*, and *Codeine*—See individual listings for chemistry information.

USP requirements: Brompheniramine Maleate, Phenylpropanolamine Hydrochloride, and Codeine Phosphate Syrup—Not in USP.

BROMPHENIRAMINE, PHENYLPROPANOLAMINE, AND DEXTROMETHORPHAN

For *Brompheniramine, Phenylpropanolamine*, and *Dextromethorphan*—See individual listings for chemistry information.

USP requirements: Brompheniramine Maleate, Phenylpropanolamine Hydrochloride, and Dextromethorphan Hydrobromide Syrup—Not in USP.

BROMPHENIRAMINE, PHENYLTOLOXAMINE, AND PHENYLEPHRINE

Chemical group:
Brompheniramine—Propylamine derivative (alkylamine).
Phenyltoloxamine citrate—Ethanolamine derivative.

Chemical name:
Brompheniramine maleate—2-Pyridinepropanamine, gamma-(4-bromophenyl)-*N,N*-dimethyl-, (*Z*)-butenedioate (1:1).
Phenyltoloxamine citrate—2-(2-Benzylphenoxy)-*N,N*-dimethylethylamine dihydrogen citrate.
Phenylephrine hydrochloride—Benzenemethanol, 3-hydroxy-alpha-[(methylamino)methyl]-, hydrochloride.

Molecular formula:
Brompheniramine maleate—$C_{16}H_{19}BrN_2 \cdot C_4H_4O_4$.
Phenyltoloxamine citrate—$C_{17}H_{21}NO \cdot C_6H_8O_7$.
Phenylephrine hydrochloride—$C_9H_{13}NO_2 \cdot HCl$.

Molecular weight:
Brompheniramine maleate—435.32.
Phenyltoloxamine citrate—447.5.
Phenylephrine hydrochloride—203.67.

Description:
Brompheniramine Maleate USP—White, odorless, crystalline powder.
Phenyltoloxamine citrate—It has a melting point of 138–140 °C.
Phenylephrine Hydrochloride USP—White or practically white, odorless crystals.

pKa: Brompheniramine maleate—3.59 and 9.12.

Solubility:
Brompheniramine Maleate USP—Freely soluble in water; soluble in alcohol and in chloroform; slightly soluble in ether.
Phenyltoloxamine citrate—Soluble in water.
Phenylephrine Hydrochloride USP—Freely soluble in water and in alcohol.

USP requirements: Brompheniramine Maleate, Phenyltoloxamine Citrate, and Phenylephrine Hydrochloride Extended-release Capsules—Not in USP.

BROMPHENIRAMINE AND PSEUDOEPHEDRINE

For *Brompheniramine* and *Pseudoephedrine*—See individual listings for chemistry information.

USP Requirements:
Brompheniramine Maleate and Pseudoephedrine Hydrochloride Extended-release Capsules—Not in USP.
Brompheniramine Maleate and Pseudoephedrine Hydrochloride Syrup—Not in USP.
Brompheniramine Maleate and Pseudoephedrine Hydrochloride Tablets—Not in USP.
Brompheniramine Maleate and Pseudoephedrine Sulfate Syrup USP—Contains the labeled amounts of brompheniramine maleate and pseudoephedrine sulfate, within ± 10%. Meets the requirement for Identification.

BROMPHENIRAMINE, PSEUDOEPHEDRINE, AND DEXTROMETHORPHAN

For *Brompheniramine, Pseudoephedrine*, and *Dextromethorphan*—See individual listings for chemistry information.

USP requirements: Brompheniramine Maleate, Pseudoephedrine Hydrochloride, and Dextromethorphan Hydrobromide Syrup—Not in USP.

BUCLIZINE

Chemical group: Piperazine-derivative antihistamine.

Chemical name: Buclizine hydrochloride—Piperazine, 1-[(4-chlorophenyl)phenylmethyl]-4-[[4-(1,1-dimethylethyl)-phenyl]methyl]-, dihydrochloride.

Molecular formula: Buclizine hydrochloride—$C_{28}H_{33}ClN_2 \cdot 2HCl$.

Molecular weight: Buclizine hydrochloride—505.96.

Description: Buclizine hydrochloride—White, crystalline powder.

Solubility: Buclizine hydrochloride—Slightly soluble in water; insoluble in the usual organic solvents.

USP requirements: Buclizine Hydrochloride Chewable Tablets—Not in USP.

BUMETANIDE

Chemical name: Benzoic acid, 3-(aminosulfonyl)-5-(butylamino)-4-phenoxy-.

Molecular formula: $C_{17}H_{20}N_2O_5S$.

Molecular weight: 364.42.

Description: Bumetanide USP—Practically white powder.

Solubility: Bumetanide USP—Slightly soluble in water; soluble in alkaline solutions.

USP requirements:
Bumetanide USP—Preserve in tight, light-resistant containers. Contains not less than 98.0% and not more than 102.0% of bumetanide, calculated on the dried basis. Meets the requirements for Identification, Loss on drying (not more than 0.5%), Residue on ignition (not more than 0.1%), Heavy metals (0.002%), and Chromatographic purity.
Bumetanide Injection USP—Preserve in single-dose or in multiple-dose containers, preferably of Type I glass, protected from light. A sterile solution of Bumetanide in Water for Injection. Contains the labeled amount, within

±10%. Meets the requirements for Identification, Bacterial endotoxins, pH (6.8–7.8), Chromatographic purity, and Injections.

Bumetanide Tablets USP—Preserve in tight, light-resistant containers. Contain the labeled amount, within ±10%. Meet the requirements for Identification, Dissolution (85% in 30 minutes in water in Apparatus 2 at 50 rpm), Chromatographic purity, and Uniformity of dosage units.

BUPIVACAINE

Chemical group: Amide.

Chemical name: Bupivacaine hydrochloride—2-Piperidinecarboxamide, 1-butyl-*N*-(2,6-dimethylphenyl)-, monohydrochloride, monohydrate.

Molecular formula:
Bupivacaine hydrochloride—$C_{18}H_{28}N_2O \cdot HCl$ (anhydrous).
Bupivacaine hydrochloride—$C_{18}H_{28}N_2O \cdot HCl \cdot H_2O$ (monohydrate).

Molecular weight:
Bupivacaine hydrochloride—324.89 (anhydrous).
Bupivacaine hydrochloride—342.91 (monohydrate).

Description:
Bupivacaine Hydrochloride USP—White, odorless, crystalline powder. Melts at about 248 °C, with decomposition.
Bupivacaine Hydrochloride Injection USP—Clear, colorless solution.

pKa: 8.1.

Solubility: Bupivacaine Hydrochloride USP—Freely soluble in water and in alcohol; slightly soluble in chloroform and in acetone.

USP requirements:
Bupivacaine Hydrochloride USP—Preserve in well-closed containers. Contains not less than 98.5% and not more than 101.5% of bupivacaine hydrochloride, calculated on the anhydrous basis. Meets the requirements for Identification, pH (4.5–6.0, in a solution [1 in 100]), Water (4.0–6.0%), Residue on ignition (not more than 0.1%), Heavy metals (not more than 0.001%), Residual solvents (not more than 2.0%), and Chromatographic purity.
Bupivacaine Hydrochloride Injection USP—Preserve in single-dose or in multiple-dose containers, preferably of Type I glass. Injection labeled to contain 0.5% or less of bupivacaine hydrochloride may be packaged in 50-mL multiple-dose containers. A sterile solution of Bupivacaine Hydrochloride in Water for Injection. Contains the labeled amount, within ±7%. Meets the requirements for Identification, Bacterial endotoxins, pH (4.0–6.5), and Injections.

BUPIVACAINE AND DEXTROSE

For *Bupivacaine* and *Dextrose*—See individual listings for chemistry information.

USP requirements: Bupivacaine in Dextrose Injection USP—Preserve in single-dose containers, preferably of Type I glass. A sterile solution of Bupivacaine Hydrochloride and Dextrose in Water for Injection. Contains an amount of bupivacaine equivalent to the labeled amount of anhydrous bupivacaine hydrochloride and the labeled amount of dextrose, within ±7%. It contains no preservative. Meets the requirements for Identification, Bacterial endotoxins, and Injections.

BUPIVACAINE AND EPINEPHRINE

For *Bupivacaine* and *Epinephrine*—See individual listings for chemistry information.

USP requirements: Bupivacaine and Epinephrine Injection USP—Preserve in single-dose or in multiple-dose containers, preferably of Type I glass, protected from light. Injection labeled to contain 0.5% or less of bupivacaine hydrochloride may be packaged in 50-mL multiple-dose containers. A sterile solution of Bupivacaine Hydrochloride and Epinephrine or Epinephrine Bitartrate in Water for Injection. The content of epinephrine does not exceed 0.001% (1 in 100,000). The label indicates that the Injection is not to be used if its color is pinkish or darker than slightly yellow or if it contains a precipitate. Contains an amount of bupivacaine equivalent to the labeled amount of bupivacaine hydrochloride, within ±7%, and the equivalent of the labeled amount of epinephrine, within −10% to +15%. Meets the requirements for Identification, Color and clarity, Bacterial endotoxins, pH (3.3–5.5), and Injections.

BUPRENORPHINE

Chemical group: Buprenorphine is a thebaine derivative.

Chemical name: Buprenorphine hydrochloride—6,14-Ethenomorphinan-7-methanol, 17-(cyclopropylmethyl)-alpha-(1,1-dimethylethyl)-4,5-epoxy-18,19-dihydro-3-hydroxy-6-methoxy-alpha-methyl-, hydrochloride, [5 alpha,7 alpha (*S*)]-.

Molecular formula: Buprenorphine hydrochloride—$C_{29}H_{41}NO_4 \cdot HCl$.

Molecular weight: Buprenorphine hydrochloride—504.11.

Description: Buprenorphine hydrochloride—White powder.

pKa: 8.42 and 9.92.

Solubility: Buprenorphine hydrochloride—Limited solubility in water.

Other characteristics: Weakly acidic; highly lipophilic.

USP requirements: Buprenorphine Hydrochloride Injection—Not in USP.

BUPROPION

Chemical group: Phenylaminoketone.
Note: Chemically *unrelated* to tricyclic, tetracyclic, or other antidepressants. Structure closely resembles diethylpropion. Related to phenylethylamines.

Chemical name: Bupropion hydrochloride—1-Propanone, 1-(3-chlorophenyl)-2-[(1,1-dimethylethyl)amino]-, hydrochloride, (±)-.

Molecular formula: Bupropion hydrochloride—$C_{13}H_{18}ClNO \cdot HCl$.

Molecular weight: Bupropion hydrochloride—276.21.

Description: White crystalline powder.

Solubility: Highly soluble in water.

USP requirements: Bupropion Hydrochloride Tablets—Not in USP.

BUSERELIN

Chemical name: Buserelin acetate—Luteinizing hormone-releasing factor (pig), 6-[*O*-(1,1-dimethylethyl)-D-serine]-9-(*N*-ethyl-L-prolinamide)-10-deglycinamide-, monoacetate (salt).

Molecular formula: Buserelin acetate—$C_{60}H_{86}N_{16}O_{13} \cdot C_2H_4O_2$.

Molecular weight: Buserelin acetate—1299.49.

Description: Buserelin acetate—Amorphous, white substance.

Solubility: Buserelin acetate—Freely soluble in water and in dilute acids.

Other characteristics: Buserelin acetate—Weak base.

USP requirements:
Buserelin Acetate Injection—Not in USP.
Buserelin Acetate Nasal Solution—Not in USP.

BUSPIRONE

Chemical group: Azaspirodecanedione, a nonbenzodiazepine.

Chemical name: Buspirone hydrochloride—8-Azaspiro[4,5]-decane-7,9-dione, 8-[4-[4-(2-pyrimidinyl)-1-piperazinyl]-butyl]-, monohydrochloride.

Molecular formula: Buspirone hydrochloride—$C_{21}H_{31}N_5O_2 \cdot$ HCl.

Molecular weight: Buspirone hydrochloride—421.97.

Description: Buspirone hydrochloride—White, crystalline compound.

Solubility: Buspirone hydrochloride—Soluble in water.

Other characteristics: A fat-soluble, dibasic heterocyclic compound. Not chemically related to benzodiazepines, barbiturates, or other sedative/antianxiety agents.

USP requirements: Buspirone Hydrochloride Tablets—Not in USP.

BUSULFAN

Chemical name: 1,4-Butanediol, dimethanesulfonate.

Molecular formula: $C_6H_{14}O_6S_2$.

Molecular weight: 246.29.

Description: Busulfan USP—White, crystalline powder.

Solubility: Busulfan USP—Very slightly soluble in water; sparingly soluble in acetone; slightly soluble in alcohol.

USP requirements:
Busulfan USP—Preserve in tight containers. The label bears a warning that great care should be taken to prevent inhaling particles of Busulfan and exposing the skin to it. Contains not less than 98.0% and not more than 100.5% of busulfan, calculated on the dried basis. Meets the requirements for Identification, Melting range (115–118 °C), Loss on drying (not more than 2.0%), Residue on ignition (not more than 0.1%), and Organic volatile impurities.
Busulfan Tablets USP—Preserve in well-closed containers. Contain the labeled amount, within ± 7%. Meet the requirements for Identification, Disintegration (30 minutes, the use of disks being omitted), and Uniformity of dosage units.

BUTABARBITAL

Chemical name:
Butabarbital—2,4,6(1H,3H,5H)-Pyrimidinetrione, 5-ethyl-5-(1-methylpropyl)-.
Butabarbital sodium—2,4,6(1H,3H,5H)-Pyrimidinetrione, 5-ethyl-5-(1-methylpropyl)-, monosodium salt.

Molecular formula:
Butabarbital—$C_{10}H_{16}N_2O_3$.
Butabarbital sodium—$C_{10}H_{15}N_2NaO_3$.

Molecular weight:
Butabarbital—212.25.
Butabarbital sodium—234.23.

Description:
Butabarbital USP—White, odorless, crystalline powder.
Butabarbital Sodium USP—White powder.

Solubility:
Butabarbital USP—Very slightly soluble in water; soluble in alcohol, in chloroform, in ether, and in solutions of alkali hydroxides and carbonates.
Butabarbital Sodium USP—Freely soluble in water and in alcohol; practically insoluble in absolute ether.

USP requirements:
Butabarbital USP—Preserve in tight containers. Contains not less than 98.5% and not more than 101.0% of butabarbital, calculated on the dried basis. Meets the requirements for Identification, Melting range (164–167 °C), Loss on drying (not more than 1.0%), Residue on ignition (not more than 0.1%), Chromatographic purity, and Organic volatile impurities.
Butabarbital Sodium USP—Preserve in tight containers. Contains not less than 98.2% and not more than 100.5% of butabarbital sodium, calculated on the dried basis. Meets the requirements for Completeness of solution, Identification, pH (10.0–11.2), Loss on drying (not more than 5.0%), Heavy metals (not more than 0.003%), Chromatographic purity, and Organic volatile impurities.
Butabarbital Sodium Capsules USP—Preserve in well-closed containers. Contain the labeled amount, within ± 10%. Meet the requirements for Identification, Dissolution (75% in 45 minutes in water in Apparatus 1 at 100 rpm), and Uniformity of dosage units.
Butabarbital Sodium Elixir USP—Preserve in tight containers. Contains the labeled amount, within ± 10%. Meets the requirements for Identification and Alcohol content (95.0–115.0% of labeled amount).
Butabarbital Sodium Tablets USP—Preserve in well-closed containers. Contain the labeled amount, within ± 10%. Meet the requirements for Identification, Dissolution (75% in 45 minutes in water in Apparatus 1 at 100 rpm), and Uniformity of dosage units.

BUTACAINE

Chemical group: Ester, aminobenzoic acid (PABA)–derivative.

Chemical name: 3-(Dibutylamino)-1-propanol, 4-aminobenzoate.

Molecular formula: $C_{18}H_{30}N_2O_2$.

Molecular weight: 306.44.

USP requirements: Butacaine Dental Ointment—Not in USP.

BUTALBITAL

Chemical name: 2,4,6(1H,3H,5H)-Pyrimidinetrione, 5-(2-methylpropyl)-5-(2-propenyl)-.

Molecular formula: $C_{11}H_{16}N_2O_3$.

Molecular weight: 224.26.

Description: Butalbital USP—White, crystalline, odorless powder. Is stable in air. Its saturated solution is acid to litmus.

Solubility: Butalbital USP—Freely soluble in alcohol, in ether, and in chloroform; slightly soluble in cold water; soluble in boiling water, and in solutions of fixed alkalies and alkali carbonates.

USP requirements: Butalbital USP—Preserve in well-closed containers. Contains not less than 98.0% and not more than 102.0% of butalbital, calculated on the dried basis. Meets the requirements for Identification, Melting range (138–141 °C), Loss on drying (not more than 0.2%), Residue on ignition (not more than 0.1%), Heavy metals (not more than 0.002%), Chromatographic purity, and Organic volatile impurities.

BUTALBITAL AND ACETAMINOPHEN

For *Butalbital* and *Acetaminophen*—See individual listings for chemistry information.

USP requirements:
Butalbital and Acetaminophen Capsules—Not in USP.
Butalbital and Acetaminophen Tablets—Not in USP.

BUTALBITAL, ACETAMINOPHEN, AND CAFFEINE

For *Butalbital, Acetaminophen*, and *Caffeine*—See individual listings for chemistry information.

USP requirements:
Butalbital, Acetaminophen, and Caffeine Capsules—Not in USP.
Butalbital, Acetaminophen, and Caffeine Tablets USP—Preserve in tight containers. Contain the labeled amounts of each ingredient, within ± 10%. Meet the requirements for Identification, Dissolution (80% in 30 minutes in water in Apparatus 2 at 50 rpm), and Uniformity of dosage units.

BUTALBITAL AND ASPIRIN

For *Butalbital* and *Aspirin*—See individual listings for chemistry information.

USP requirements: Butalbital and Aspirin Tablets USP—Preserve in tight containers. Contain the labeled amounts of butalbital and aspirin, within ± 10%. Meet the requirements for Identification, Dissolution (75% of each ingredient in 60 minutes in water in Apparatus 1 at 100 rpm), Uniformity of dosage units, and Limit of free salicylic acid (not more than 3%).

BUTALBITAL, ASPIRIN, AND CAFFEINE

For *Butalbital, Aspirin*, and *Caffeine*—See individual listings for chemistry information.

USP requirements:
Butalbital, Aspirin, and Caffeine Capsules—Not in USP.
Butalbital, Aspirin, and Caffeine Tablets—Not in USP.

BUTALBITAL, ASPIRIN, CODEINE, AND CAFFEINE

For *Butalbital, Aspirin, Codeine*, and *Caffeine*—See individual listings for chemistry information.

USP requirements:
Butalbital, Aspirin, Codeine Phosphate, and Caffeine Capsules—Not in USP.
Butalbital, Aspirin, Codeine Phosphate, and Caffeine Tablets—Not in USP.

BUTAMBEN

Chemical group: Ester, aminobenzoic acid (PABA)–derivative.

Chemical name:
Butamben—Benzoic acid, 4-amino-, butyl ester.
Butamben picrate—Benzoic acid, 4-amino-, butyl ester, compound with 2,4,6-trinitrophenol (2:1).

Molecular formula:
Butamben—$C_{11}H_{15}NO_2$.
Butamben picrate—$(C_{11}H_{15}NO_2)_2 \cdot C_6H_3N_3O_7$.

Molecular weight:
Butamben—193.25.
Butamben picrate—615.60.

Description: Butamben USP—White, crystalline powder. Is odorless.

Solubility: Butamben USP—Very slightly soluble in water; soluble in dilute acids, in alcohol, in chloroform, in ether, and in fixed oils. Is slowly hydrolyzed when boiled with water.

USP requirements:
Butamben USP—Preserve in well-closed containers. Butamben is dried over phosphorus pentoxide for 3 hours. Contains not less than 98.0% and not more than 101.0% of butamben. Meets the requirements for Completeness and color of solution, Identification, Melting range (57–59 °C), Reaction, Loss on drying (not more than 1.0%), Residue on ignition (not more than 0.2%), Chloride, and Heavy metals (not more than 0.001%).
Butamben Picrate Ointment—Not in USP.

BUTANE

Molecular formula: C_4H_{10}.

Molecular weight: 58.12.

Description: Butane NF—Colorless, flammable gas (boiling temperature is about –0.5 °C). Vapor pressure at 21 °C is about 1620 mm of mercury (17 psig).
NF category: Aerosol propellant.

Solubility: Butane NF—One volume of water dissolves 0.15 volume, and 1 volume of alcohol dissolves 18 volumes at 17 °C and 770 mm; 1 volume of ether or chloroform at 17 °C dissolves 25 or 30 volumes, respectively.

NF requirements: Butane NF—Preserve in tight cylinders, and prevent exposure to excessive heat. Contains not less than 97.0% of *n*-butane. Meets the requirements for Identification, Water (not more than 0.001%), High-boiling residues (not more than 5 ppm), Acidity of residue, and Sulfur compounds.
Caution: Butane is highly flammable and explosive.

BUTOCONAZOLE

Chemical name: Butoconazole nitrate—1*H*-Imidazole, 1-[4-(4-chlorophenyl)-2-[(2,6-dichlorophenyl)thio]butyl]-, mononitrate, (±)-.

Molecular formula: Butoconazole nitrate—$C_{19}H_{17}Cl_3N_2S \cdot HNO_3$.

Molecular weight: Butoconazole nitrate—474.79.

Description: Butoconazole Nitrate USP—White to off-white, crystalline powder. Melts at about 160 °C.

Solubility: Butoconazole Nitrate USP—Practically insoluble in water; very slightly soluble in ethyl acetate; slightly soluble in acetonitrile, in acetone, in dichloromethane, and in tetrahydrofuran; sparingly soluble in methanol.

USP requirements:
Butoconazole Nitrate USP—Preserve in well-closed, light-resistant containers. Contains not less than 98.0% and not more than 102.0% of butoconazole, calculated on the dried basis. Meets the requirements for Identification, Loss on drying (not more than 1.0%), Residue on ignition (not more than 0.1%), and Ordinary impurities.
Butoconazole Nitrate Cream USP—Preserve in collapsible tubes or in tight containers. Avoid excessive heat and avoid freezing. It is Butoconazole Nitrate in a suitable cream base. Cream that is intended for use as a vaginal preparation may be labeled Butoconazole Nitrate Vaginal Cream. Contains the labeled amount, within ± 10%. Meets the requirements for Identification and Minimum fill.

BUTORPHANOL

Chemical name: Butorphanol tartrate—Morphinan-3,14-diol, 17-(cyclobutylmethyl)-, (−)-, [S-(R*,R*)]-2,3-dihydroxy-butanedioate (1:1) (salt).

Molecular formula: Butorphanol tartrate—$C_{21}H_{29}NO_2 \cdot C_4H_6O_6$.

Molecular weight: Butorphanol tartrate—477.55.

Description: Butorphanol Tartrate USP—White powder. Its solutions are slightly acidic. Melts between 217 °C and 219 °C, with decomposition.

Solubility: Butorphanol Tartrate USP—Sparingly soluble in water; slightly soluble in methanol; insoluble in alcohol, in chloroform, in ethyl acetate, in ethyl ether, and in hexane; soluble in dilute acids.

USP requirements:
Butorphanol Tartrate USP—Preserve in tight containers. Contains not less than 98.0% and not more than 102.0% of butorphanol tartrate, calculated on the anhydrous basis. Meets the requirements for Identification, Specific rotation (−60° to −66°, calculated on the anhydrous basis), Water (not more than 2.0%), Residue on ignition (not more than 0.1%), Heavy metals (not more than 0.003%), and Chromatographic purity (not more than 2.0%).
Butorphanol Tartrate Injection USP—Preserve in single-dose or in multiple-dose containers, preferably of Type I glass, protected from light. A sterile solution of Butorphanol Tartrate in Water for Injection. Contains the labeled amount, within ± 10%. Meets the requirements for Identification, Bacterial endotoxins, pH (3.0–5.5), and Injections.

BUTYL ALCOHOL

Molecular formula: $C_4H_{10}O$.

Molecular weight: 74.12.

Description: Butyl Alcohol NF—Clear, colorless, mobile liquid, having a characteristic, penetrating vinous odor.
NF category: Solvent.

Solubility: Butyl Alcohol NF—Soluble in water. Miscible with alcohol, with ether, and with many other organic solvents.

NF requirements: Butyl Alcohol NF—Preserve in tight containers, and prevent exposure to excessive heat. It is *n*-butyl alcohol. Meets the requirements for Specific gravity (0.807–0.809), Distilling range (distils within a range of 1.5 °C, including 117.7 °C), Acidity, Water (not more than 0.1%),

Nonvolatile residue (not more than 0.004%), Aldehydes, and Butyl ether (not more than 0.2%).

BUTYLATED HYDROXYANISOLE

Chemical name: Phenol, (1,1-dimethylethyl)-4-methoxy.

Molecular formula: $C_{11}H_{16}O_2$.

Molecular weight: 180.25.

Description: Butylated Hydroxyanisole NF—White or slightly yellow, waxy solid, having a faint, characteristic odor.
NF category: Antioxidant.

Solubility: Butylated Hydroxyanisole NF—Insoluble in water; freely soluble in alcohol, in propylene glycol, in chloroform, and in ether.

NF requirements: Butylated Hydroxyanisole NF—Preserve in well-closed containers. Contains not less than 98.5% of butylated hydroxyanisole. Meets the requirements for Identification, Residue on ignition (not more than 0.01%, determined on a 10-gram specimen), Arsenic (not more than 3 ppm), Heavy metals (not more than 0.001%), and Organic volatile impurities.

BUTYLATED HYDROXYTOLUENE

Chemical name: Phenol, 2,6-bis(1,1-dimethylethyl)-4-methyl-.

Molecular formula: $C_{15}H_{24}O$.

Molecular weight: 220.35.

Description: Butylated Hydroxytoluene NF—White, crystalline solid, having a faint characteristic odor.
NF category: Antioxidant.

Solubility: Butylated Hydroxytoluene NF—Insoluble in water and in propylene glycol; freely soluble in alcohol, in chloroform, and in ether.

NF requirements: Butylated Hydroxytoluene NF—Preserve in well-closed containers. Contains not less than 99.0% of butylated hydroxytoluene. Meets the requirements for Identification, Congealing temperature (not less than 69.2 °C, corresponding to not less than 99.0% of butylated hydroxytoluene), Residue on ignition (not more than 0.002%), Arsenic (not more than 3 ppm), and Heavy metals (not more than 0.001%).

BUTYLPARABEN

Chemical name: Benzoic acid, 4-hydroxy-, butyl ester.

Molecular formula: $C_{11}H_{14}O_3$.

Molecular weight: 194.23.

Description: Butylparaben NF—Small, colorless crystals or white powder.
NF category: Antimicrobial preservative.

Solubility: Butylparaben NF—Very slightly soluble in water and in glycerin; freely soluble in acetone, in alcohol, in ether, and in propylene glycol.

NF requirements: Butylparaben NF—Preserve in well-closed containers. Contains not less than 99.0% and not more than 100.5% of butylparaben, calculated on the dried basis. Meets the requirements for Identification, Melting range (68–72 °C), Acidity, Loss on drying (not more than 0.5%), and Residue on ignition (not more than 0.05%).

CAFFEINE

Source: Coffee, tea, cola, and cocoa or chocolate. May also be synthesized from urea or dimethylurea.

Chemical group: Methylated xanthine.

Chemical name: 1*H*-Purine-2,6-dione, 3,7-dihydro-1,3,7-trimethyl-.

Molecular formula:
Caffeine (anhydrous)—$C_8H_{10}N_4O_2$.
Caffeine (monohydrate)—$C_8H_{10}N_4O_2 \cdot H_2O$.

Molecular weight:
Caffeine (anhydrous)—194.19.
Caffeine (monohydrate)—212.21.

Description: Caffeine USP—White powder or white, glistening needles, usually matted together. Is odorless. Its solutions are neutral to litmus. The hydrate is efflorescent in air.

Solubility: Caffeine USP—Sparingly soluble in water and in alcohol; freely soluble in chloroform; slightly soluble in ether.

The aqueous solubility of caffeine is increased by organic acids or their alkali salts, such as citrates, benzoates, salicylates, or cinnamates, which dissociate to yield caffeine when dissolved in biological fluids.

USP requirements:
Caffeine USP—Preserve hydrous Caffeine in tight containers. Preserve anhydrous Caffeine in well-closed containers. It is anhydrous or contains one molecule of water of hydration. Label it to indicate whether it is anhydrous or hydrous. Contains not less than 98.5% and not more than 101.0% of caffeine, calculated on the anhydrous basis. Meets the requirements for Identification, Melting range (235–237.5 °C, determined after drying at 80 °C for 4 hours), Water (not more than 0.5% [anhydrous], not more than 8.5% [hydrous]), Residue on ignition (not more than 0.1%), Arsenic (3 ppm), Heavy metals (0.001%), Readily carbonizable substances, Other alkaloids, and Organic volatile impurities.
Caffeine Extended-release Capsules—Not in USP.
Caffeine Tablets—Not in USP.

CITRATED CAFFEINE

Source: Caffeine—Coffee, tea, cola, and cocoa or chocolate. May also be synthesized from urea or dimethylurea.

Chemical group: Caffeine—Methylated xanthine.

Chemical name:
Caffeine—1*H*-Purine-2,6-dione, 3,7-dihydro-1,3,7-trimethyl-.
Citric acid—1,2,3-Propanetricarboxylic acid, 2-hydroxy-.

Molecular formula:
Caffeine—$C_8H_{10}N_4O_2$ (anhydrous); $C_8H_{10}N_4O_2 \cdot H_2O$ (monohydrate).
Citric acid—$C_6H_8O_7$ (anhydrous); $C_6H_8O_7 \cdot H_2O$ (monohydrate).

Molecular weight:
Caffeine—194.19 (anhydrous); 212.21 (monohydrate).
Citric acid—192.12 (anhydrous); 210.14 (monohydrate).

Description:
Caffeine USP—White powder or white, glistening needles, usually matted together. Is odorless. Its solutions are neutral to litmus. The hydrate is efflorescent in air.
Citric Acid USP—Colorless, translucent crystals, or white, granular to fine crystalline powder. Odorless or practically odorless. The hydrous form is efflorescent in dry air.
NF category: Acidifying agent; buffering agent.

Solubility:
Caffeine USP—Sparingly soluble in water and in alcohol; freely soluble in chloroform; slightly soluble in ether.

The aqueous solubility of caffeine is increased by organic acids or their alkali salts, such as citrates, benzoates, salicylates, or cinnamates, which dissociate to yield caffeine when dissolved in biological fluids.

Citric Acid USP—Very soluble in water; freely soluble in alcohol; sparingly soluble in ether.

USP requirements:
Citrated Caffeine Injection—Not in USP.
Citrated Caffeine Solution—Not in USP.
Citrated Caffeine Tablets—Not in USP.

CAFFEINE AND SODIUM BENZOATE

For *Caffeine* and *Sodium Benzoate*—See individual listings for chemistry information.

USP requirements: Caffeine and Sodium Benzoate Injection USP—Preserve in single-dose containers, preferably of Type I glass. A sterile solution of Caffeine and Sodium Benzoate in Water for Injection. Contains an amount of anhydrous caffeine equivalent to 45–52.0%, and an amount of sodium benzoate equivalent to 47.55–55.5%, of the labeled amounts of caffeine and sodium benzoate. Meets the requirements for Identification, Bacterial endotoxins, pH (6.5–8.5), and Injections.

CALAMINE

Chemical name: Iron oxide (Fe_2O_3), mixture with zinc oxide.

Description: Calamine USP—Pink, odorless, fine powder.

Solubility: Calamine USP—Insoluble in water; practically completely soluble in mineral acids.

USP requirements:
Calamine USP—Preserve in well-closed containers. It is Zinc Oxide with a small proportion of ferric oxide. Contains, after ignition, not less than 98.0% and not more than 100.5% of zinc oxide. Meets the requirements for Identification, Microbial limits, Loss on ignition (not more than 2.0%), Acid-insoluble substances (not more than 2.0%), Alkaline substances, Arsenic (not more than 8 ppm), Calcium, Calcium or magnesium, and Lead.
Calamine Lotion USP—Preserve in tight containers.

Prepare Calamine Lotion as follows: 80 grams of Calamine, 80 grams of Zinc Oxide, 20 mL of Glycerin, 250 mL of Bentonite Magma, and a sufficient quantity of Calcium Hydroxide Topical Solution to make 1000 mL. Dilute the Bentonite Magma with an equal volume of Calcium Hydroxide Topical Solution. Mix the powders intimately with the Glycerin and about 100 mL of the diluted magma, triturating until a smooth, uniform paste is formed. Gradually incorporate the remainder of the diluted magma. Finally add enough Calcium Hydroxide Solution to make 1000 mL, and shake well. If a more viscous consistency in the Lotion is desired, the quantity of Bentonite Magma may be increased to not more than 400 mL.

Meets the requirement for Microbial limits.

Note: Shake Calamine Lotion well before dispensing.

PHENOLATED CALAMINE

Chemical name:
Calamine—Iron oxide (Fe_2O_3), mixture with zinc oxide.
Phenol—Phenol.

Molecular formula: Phenol—C₆H₆O.

Molecular weight: Phenol—94.11.

Description:
Calamine USP—Pink, odorless, fine powder.
Phenol USP—Colorless to light pink, interlaced or separate, needleshaped crystals, or white to light pink, crystalline mass. It has a characteristic odor. Liquefied by warming, and by the addition of 10% of water. Boils at about 182 °C, and its vapor is flammable. Gradually darkens on exposure to light and air.
NF category: Antimicrobial preservative.

Solubility:
Calamine USP—Insoluble in water; practically completely soluble in mineral acids.
Phenol USP—Soluble in water; very soluble in alcohol, in glycerin, in chloroform, in ether, and in fixed and volatile oils; sparingly soluble in mineral oil.

USP requirements: Phenolated Calamine Lotion USP—Preserve in tight containers.
Prepare Phenolated Calamine Lotion as follows: 10 mL of Liquefied Phenol and 990 mL of Calamine Lotion, to make 1000 mL. Mix the ingredients.
Note: Shake Phenolated Calamine Lotion well before dispensing.

CALCIFEDIOL

Chemical name: 9,10-Secocholesta-5,7,10(19)-triene-3,25-diol monohydrate, (3 beta,5Z,7E)-.

Molecular formula: C₂₇H₄₄O₂·H₂O.

Molecular weight: 418.66.

Description: A white powder. It has a melting point of about 105 °C.

Solubility: Practically insoluble in water; soluble in organic solvents.

USP requirements:
Calcifediol USP—Preserve in tight, light-resistant containers at controlled room temperature. Contains not less than 97.0% and not more than 103.0% of calcifediol. Meets the requirements for Identification, Water (3.8–5.0%, determined on a 0.2-gram specimen), and Organic volatile impurities.
Calcifediol Capsules USP—Preserve in tight, light-resistant containers. Contain the labeled amount, within −10% to +20%. Meet the requirements for Identification, Disintegration (30 minutes), and Uniformity of dosage units.

CALCITONIN

Source:
Calcitonin-human—A synthetic polypeptide hormone of 32 amino acids in the same linear sequence found in naturally occurring human calcitonin and differing from salmon calcitonin at 16 of the amino acid sites.
Calcitonin-salmon—A synthetic polypeptide hormone of 32 amino acids in the same linear sequence found in calcitonin of salmon origin.

Molecular formula:
Calcitonin-human—C₁₅₁H₂₂₆N₄₀O₄₅S₃·3HCl.
Calcitonin-salmon—C₁₄₅H₂₄₀N₄₄O₄₈S₂.

Molecular weight:
Calcitonin-human—3527.20.
Calcitonin-salmon—3431.88.

Description:
Calcitonin-human—White to off-white amorphous powder.
Calcitonin-salmon—White or almost white, light powder.

Solubility:
Calcitonin-human—Soluble in water, in physiological salt solution, in dilute acid, and in dilute base; sparingly soluble in methanol; practically insoluble in chloroform.
Calcitonin-salmon—Freely soluble in water.

USP requirements:
Calcitonin-Human for Injection—Not in USP.
Calcitonin-Salmon Injection—Not in USP.

CALCITRIOL

Chemical name: 9,10-Secocholesta-5,7,10(19)-triene-1,3,25-triol, (1 alpha,3 beta,5Z,7E)-.

Molecular formula: C₂₇H₄₄O₃.

Molecular weight: 416.64.

Description: A practically white crystalline compound with a melting range of 111–115 °C.

Solubility: Insoluble in water; soluble in organic solvents.

USP requirements:
Calcitriol Capsules—Not in USP.
Calcitriol Injection—Not in USP.

CALCIUM ACETATE

Chemical name: Acetic acid, calcium salt.

Molecular formula: C₄H₆CaO₄.

Molecular weight: 158.17.

Description: White, odorless, or almost odorless, hygroscopic powder.

Solubility: Soluble 1 in 3 of water; slightly soluble in alcohol.

USP requirements:
Calcium Acetate USP—Preserve in tight containers. Where Calcium Acetate is intended for use in hemodialysis or peritoneal dialysis it is so labeled. Contains not less than 99.0% and not more than 100.5% of calcium acetate, calculated on the anhydrous basis. Meets the requirements for Identification, pH (6.3–9.6, in a solution [1 in 20]), Water (not more than 7.0%), Fluoride (not more than 0.005%), Arsenic (not more than 3 ppm), Heavy metals (not more than 0.0025%), Lead (not more than 0.001%), Chloride (not more than 0.05%), Sulfate (not more than 0.06%), Nitrate, Readily oxidizable substances, Aluminum (not more than 2 ppm), Barium (not more than 0.005%), Magnesium (not more than 0.05%), Potassium (not more than 0.05%), Sodium (not more than 0.5%), Strontium (not more than 0.05%), and Organic volatile impurities.
Calcium Acetate Tablets—Not in USP.

CALCIUM CARBONATE

Chemical name: Carbonic acid, calcium salt (1:1).

Molecular formula: CaCO₃.

Molecular weight: 100.09.

Description: Calcium Carbonate USP—Fine, white, odorless, microcrystalline powder. Is stable in air.
NF category: Tablet and/or capsule diluent.

Solubility: Calcium Carbonate USP—Practically insoluble in water. Its solubility in water is increased by the presence of any ammonium salt or of carbon dioxide. The presence of any alkali hydroxide reduces its solubility. Insoluble in alcohol. Dissolves with effervescence in 1 *N* acetic acid, in 3 *N* hydrochloric acid, and 2 *N* nitric acid.

USP requirements:
Calcium Carbonate USP—Preserve in well-closed containers. When dried at 200 °C for 4 hours, contains an amount of calcium equivalent to not less than 98.0% and not more than 100.5% of calcium carbonate. Meets the requirements for Identification, Loss on drying (not more than 2.0%), Acid-insoluble substances (not more than 0.2%), Fluoride (not more than 0.005%), Arsenic (not more than 3 ppm), Barium, Lead (not more than 3 ppm), Iron (0.1%), Mercury (not more than 0.5 ppm), Heavy metals (not more than 0.002%), and Magnesium and alkali salts (not more than 1.0%).
Calcium Carbonate Capsules—Not in USP.
Calcium Carbonate Chewing Gum—Not in USP.
Calcium Carbonate Oral Suspension USP—Preserve in tight containers, and avoid freezing. Contains the labeled amount, within ± 10%. Meets the requirements for Identification, Microbial limits, pH (7.5–8.7), and of the tests for Fluoride, Arsenic, Lead, and Heavy metals under Calcium Carbonate.
Calcium Carbonate Tablets USP—Preserve in well-closed containers. Contain the labeled amount, within ± 7.5%. Meet the requirements for Identification, Disintegration (10 minutes, where Tablets are labeled solely for antacid use), Dissolution (75% in 30 minutes in 0.1 *N* hydrochloric acid in Apparatus 2 at 75 rpm, for Tablets labeled for any indication other than, or in addition to, antacid use), Uniformity of dosage units, and Acid-neutralizing capacity.
Calcium Carbonate (Oyster-shell derived) Tablets—Not in USP.
Calcium Carbonate (Oyster-shell derived) Chewable Tablets—Not in USP.

CALCIUM CARBONATE AND MAGNESIA

For *Calcium Carbonate* and *Magnesia* (Magnesium Hydroxide)—See individual listings for chemistry information.

USP requirements: Calcium Carbonate and Magnesia Tablets USP—Preserve in well-closed containers. Label the Tablets to indicate that they are to be chewed before being swallowed. Contain the labeled amount of calcium carbonate, within ± 10%, and an amount of magnesia equivalent to the labeled amount of magnesium hydroxide, within ± 10%. Meet the requirements for Identification, Disintegration (30 minutes, with simulated gastric fluid TS being used as the test medium), Uniformity of dosage units, and Acid-neutralizing capacity.

CALCIUM CARBONATE, MAGNESIA, AND SIMETHICONE

For *Calcium Carbonate*, *Magnesia* (Magnesium Hydroxide), and *Simethicone*—See individual listings for chemistry information.

USP requirements: Calcium Carbonate, Magnesia, and Simethicone Tablets USP—Preserve in well-closed containers. Label it to indicate that Tablets are to be chewed before swallowing. Label Tablets to state the sodium content, in mg per Tablet, if it is greater than 5 mg per Tablet. Contain the labeled amount of calcium carbonate, within ± 10%, an amount of magnesia equivalent to the labeled amount of magnesium hydroxide, within ± 10%, and an amount of polydimethylsiloxane equivalent to the labeled amount of simethicone, within ± 15%. Meet the requirements for Identification, Uniformity of dosage units, Acid-neutralizing capacity (not less than 5 mEq of acid is consumed by the minimum single dose recommended in the labeling), Defoaming activity (not more than 45 seconds), and Sodium content (if so labeled, each tablet contains not more than the number of mg of sodium stated on the label).

CALCIUM AND MAGNESIUM CARBONATES

For *Calcium Carbonate* and *Magnesium Carbonate*—See individual listings for chemistry information.

USP requirements:
Calcium and Magnesium Carbonates Oral Suspension—Not in USP.
Calcium and Magnesium Carbonates Tablets USP—Preserve in well-closed containers. Contain the labeled amount of calcium carbonate, within ± 10%, and the labeled amount of magnesium carbonate, within ± 15%. Meet the requirements for Identification, Disintegration (10 minutes in simulated gastric fluid TS), Uniformity of dosage units, and Acid-neutralizing capacity.

CALCIUM AND MAGNESIUM CARBONATES AND MAGNESIUM OXIDE

For *Calcium Carbonate*, *Magnesium Carbonate*, and *Magnesium Oxide*—See individual listings for chemistry information.

USP requirements: Calcium and Magnesium Carbonates and Magnesium Oxide Tablets—Not in USP.

CALCIUM CARBONATE AND SIMETHICONE

For *Calcium Carbonate* and *Simethicone*—See individual listings for chemistry information.

USP requirements:
Calcium Carbonate and Simethicone Oral Suspension—Not in USP.
Calcium Carbonate and Simethicone Chewable Tablets—Not in USP.

CALCIUM CHLORIDE

Chemical name: Calcium chloride, dihydrate.

Molecular formula: $CaCl_2 \cdot 2H_2O$.

Molecular weight: 147.02.

Description: Calcium Chloride USP—White, hard, odorless fragments or granules; deliquescent.
NF category: Desiccant.

Solubility: Calcium Chloride USP—Freely soluble in water, in alcohol, and in boiling alcohol; very soluble in boiling water.

USP requirements:
Calcium Chloride USP—Preserve in tight containers. Where Calcium Chloride is intended for use in hemodialysis, it is so labeled. Contains an amount of calcium chloride equivalent to the labeled amount of calcium chloride dihydrate, within −1% to +7%. Meets the requirements for Identification, pH (4.5–9.2, in a solution [1 in 20]), Arsenic (3 ppm), Heavy metals (not more than 0.001%), Iron, aluminum, and phosphate, Magnesium and alkali salts (not more than 1.0%), Aluminum (where it is labeled for use in hemodialysis, not more than 1 ppm), and Organic volatile impurities.

Calcium Chloride Injection USP—Preserve in single-dose containers, preferably of Type I glass. A sterile solution of Calcium Chloride in Water for Injection. The label states the total osmolar concentration in mOsmol per liter. Where the contents are less than 100 mL, or where the label states that the Injection is not for direct injection but is to be diluted before use, the label alternatively may state the total osmolar concentration in mOsmol per mL. Contains the labeled amount, within ±5%. Meets the requirements for Identification, Bacterial endotoxins, pH (5.5–7.5 in the undiluted Injection), Particulate matter, and Injections.

CALCIUM CITRATE

Chemical name: 1,2,3-Propanetricarboxylic acid, 2-hydroxy-, calcium salt (2:3), tetrahydrate.

Molecular formula: $C_{12}H_{10}Ca_3O_{14} \cdot 4H_2O$.

Molecular weight: 570.50.

Description: Calcium Citrate USP—White, odorless, crystalline powder.

Solubility: Calcium Citrate USP—Slightly soluble in water; freely soluble in diluted 3 *N* hydrochloric acid and in diluted 2 *N* nitric acid; insoluble in alcohol.

USP requirements:
Calcium Citrate USP—Preserve in well-closed containers. Contains four molecules of water of hydration. When dried at 150 °C to constant weight, contains not less than 97.5% and not more than 100.5% of anhydrous calcium citrate. Meets the requirements for Identification, Loss on drying (10.0–13.3%), Arsenic (not more than 3 ppm), Fluoride (not more than 0.003%), Acid-insoluble substances (not more than 0.2%), Lead (not more than 0.001%), and Heavy metals (not more than 0.002%).
Calcium Citrate Tablets—Not in USP.
Calcium Citrate Effervescent Tablets—Not in USP.

CALCIUM GLUBIONATE

Chemical name: Calcium, (4-*O*-beta-D-galactopyranosyl-D-gluconato-O¹)(D-gluconato-O¹)-, monohydrate.

Molecular formula: $C_{18}H_{32}CaO_{19} \cdot H_2O$.

Molecular weight: 610.53.

USP requirements: Calcium Glubionate Syrup USP—Preserve in tight containers, at a temperature not exceeding 30 °C, and avoid freezing. A solution containing equimolar amounts of Calcium Gluconate and Calcium Lactobionate or with Calcium Lactobionate predominating. Contains an amount of calcium glubionate equivalent to the labeled amount of calcium, within ±5%. Meets the requirements for Identification and pH (3.4–4.5).

CALCIUM GLUCEPTATE

Chemical name: Glucoheptonic acid, calcium salt (2:1).

Molecular formula: $C_{14}H_{26}CaO_{16}$.

Molecular weight: 490.43.

Description: Calcium Gluceptate USP—White to faintly yellow, amorphous powder. Is stable in air, but the hydrous forms may lose part of their water of hydration on standing.

Solubility: Calcium Gluceptate USP—Freely soluble in water; insoluble in alcohol and in many other organic solvents.

USP requirements:
Calcium Gluceptate USP—Preserve in well-closed containers. It is anhydrous or contains varying amounts of water of hydration. Consists of the calcium salt of the alpha epimer of glucoheptonic acid or of a mixture of the alpha and beta epimers of glucoheptonic acid. Label it to indicate whether it is hydrous or anhydrous; if hydrous, label it to indicate also the degree of hydration. Contains not less than 95.0% and not more than 102.0% of calcium gluceptate, calculated on the dried basis. Meets the requirements for Identification, pH (6.0–8.0, in a solution [1 in 10]), Loss on drying (not more than 1.0% [anhydrous], not more than 6.9% [2H₂O], and not more than 11.4% [3½H₂O]), Chloride (not more than 0.07%), Sulfate (not more than 0.05%), Arsenic (not more than 1 ppm), Heavy metals (not more than 0.002%), Reducing sugars, and Organic volatile impurities.
Calcium Gluceptate Injection USP—Preserve in tight, single-dose containers, preferably of Type I or Type II glass. A sterile solution of Calcium Gluceptate in Water for Injection. The label states the total osmolar concentration in mOsmol per liter. Where the contents are less than 100 mL, or where the label states that the Injection is not for direct injection but is to be diluted before use, the label alternatively may state the total osmolar concentration in mOsm per mL. Contains an amount of calcium gluceptate equivalent to the labeled amount of calcium, within ±5%. Meets the requirements for Identification, Bacterial endotoxins, pH (5.6–7.0), Particulate matter, and Injections.

CALCIUM GLUCONATE

Chemical name: D-Gluconic acid, calcium salt (2:1).

Molecular formula: $C_{12}H_{22}CaO_{14}$.

Molecular weight: 430.38.

Description: Calcium Gluconate USP—White, crystalline, odorless granules or powder. Is stable in air. Its solutions are neutral to litmus.

Solubility: Calcium Gluconate USP—Sparingly (and slowly) soluble in water; freely soluble in boiling water; insoluble in alcohol.

USP requirements:
Calcium Gluconate USP—Preserve in well-closed containers. It is anhydrous or contains one molecule of water of hydration. Label it to indicate whether it is anhydrous or is the monohydrate. Where the quantity of calcium gluconate is indicated in the labeling of any preparation containing Calcium Gluconate, this shall be understood to be in terms of anhydrous calcium gluconate. Calcium Gluconate intended for use in preparing injectable dosage forms is so labeled. Calcium Gluconate not intended for use in preparing injectable dosage forms is so labeled; in addition, it may be labeled also as intended for use in preparing oral dosage forms. The anhydrous form contains not less than 98.0% and not more than 102.0% of calcium gluconate, calculated on the dried basis. The monohydrate form contains not less than 99.0% and not more than 101.0% of calcium gluconate (monohydrate) where labeled as intended for use in preparing injectable dosage forms, and not less than 98.5% and not more than 102.0% of calcium gluconate (monohydrate) where labeled as not intended for use in preparing injectable dosage forms. Meets the requirements for Identification, Loss on drying (for the anhydrous, not more than 3.0%; for the monohydrate, where labeled as intended for use in preparing injectable dosage forms, not more than 1.0%

and where labeled as not intended for use in preparing injectable dosage forms, not more than 2.0%), Chloride (not more than 0.005%, and where labeled as not intended for use in preparation of injectable dosage forms, not more than 0.07%), Sulfate (not more than 0.005%, and where labeled as not intended for use in preparation of injectable dosage forms, not more than 0.05%), Arsenic (not more than 3 ppm), Heavy metals (not more than 0.001% [Note: Where Calcium Gluconate is labeled as not intended for use in preparation of injectable dosage forms, not more than 0.002%]), Reducing substances (not more than 1.0%), Magnesium and alkali metals (not more than 0.4% [Note: Calcium Gluconate labeled as not intended for use in preparing injectable dosage forms is exempt from this requirement]), Iron (not more than 5 ppm [Note: Calcium Gluconate labeled as not intended for use in preparation of injectable dosage forms is exempt from this requirement]), Phosphate (0.01% [Note: Calcium Gluconate labeled as not intended for use in preparation of injectable dosage forms is exempt from this requirement]), Oxalate (not more than 0.01% [Note: Calcium Gluconate labeled as not intended for use in preparation of injectable dosage forms is exempt from this requirement]), and Organic volatile impurities.

Calcium Gluconate Injection USP—Preserve in single-dose containers, preferably of Type I glass. A sterile solution of Calcium Gluconate in Water for Injection. Label the Injection to indicate its content, if any, of added calcium salts, calculated as percentage of calcium in the Injection. The label states the total osmolar concentration in mOsmol per liter. Where the contents are less than 100 mL, or where the label states that the Injection is not for direct injection but is to be diluted before use, the label alternatively may state the total osmolar concentration in mOsmol per mL. Contains an amount of calcium gluconate equivalent to the labeled amount of calcium, within ± 5%. The calcium is in the form of calcium gluconate, except that a small amount may be replaced with an equal amount of calcium in the form of Calcium Saccharate, or other suitable calcium salts, for the purpose of stabilization. It may require warming before use if crystallization has occurred. Meets the requirements for Identification, Bacterial endotoxins, pH (6.0–8.2), Particulate matter, and Injections.

Note: If crystallization has occurred, warming may dissolve the precipitate. The Injection must be clear at the time of use.

Calcium Gluconate Tablets USP—Preserve in well-closed containers. Contain the labeled amount, within ± 5%. Meet the requirements for Identification, Dissolution (75% in 45 minutes in water in Apparatus 2 at 50 rpm), and Uniformity of dosage units.

CALCIUM GLYCEROPHOSPHATE AND CALCIUM LACTATE

Chemical name:
Calcium glycerophosphate—1,2,3-Propanetriol, mono-(dihydrogen phosphate) calcium salt (1:1).
Calcium lactate—Propanoic acid, 2-hydroxy-, calcium salt (2:1), hydrate.

Molecular formula:
Calcium glycerophosphate—$C_3H_7CaO_6P$.
Calcium lactate—$C_6H_{10}CaO_6 \cdot xH_2O$.

Molecular weight:
Calcium glycerophosphate—210.15.
Calcium lactate—218.22 (anhydrous).

Description:
Calcium glycerophosphate—Fine, odorless, slightly hygroscopic powder.
Calcium Lactate USP—White, practically odorless granules or powder. The pentahydrate is somewhat efflorescent and at 120 °C becomes anhydrous.

Solubility:
Calcium glycerophosphate—Soluble in about 50 parts of water; almost insoluble in alcohol and in boiling water.
Calcium Lactate USP—The pentahydrate is soluble in water; practically insoluble in alcohol.

USP requirements: Calcium Glycerophosphate and Calcium Lactate Injection—Not in USP.

CALCIUM HYDROXIDE

Chemical name: Calcium hydroxide.

Molecular formula: $Ca(OH)_2$.

Molecular weight: 74.09.

Description:
Calcium Hydroxide USP—White powder.
Calcium Hydroxide Solution USP—Clear, colorless liquid. Is alkaline to litmus.

Solubility: Calcium Hydroxide USP—Slightly soluble in water; soluble in glycerin and in syrup; very slightly soluble in boiling water; insoluble in alcohol.

USP requirements:
Calcium Hydroxide USP—Preserve in tight containers. Contains not less than 95.0% and not more than 100.5% of calcium hydroxide. Meets the requirements for Identification, Acid-insoluble substances (not more than 0.5%), Carbonate, Arsenic (not more than 3 ppm), Heavy metals (not more than 0.004%), and Magnesium and alkali salts (not more than 4.8%).

Calcium Hydroxide Topical Solution USP—Preserve in well-filled, tight containers, at a temperature not exceeding 25 °C. A solution containing, in each 100 mL, not less than 140 mg of Calcium Hydroxide.

Prepare Calcium Hydroxide Topical Solution as follows: 3 grams of Calcium Hydroxide and 1000 mL of Purified Water. Add the Calcium Hydroxide to 1000 mL of cool Purified Water, and agitate the mixture vigorously and repeatedly during 1 hour. Allow the excess calcium hydroxide to settle. Dispense only the clear, supernatant liquid.

Meets the requirements for Identification and Alkalies and their carbonates.

Note: The solubility of calcium hydroxide varies with the temperature at which the solution is stored, being about 170 mg per 100 mL at 15 °C, and less at a higher temperature. The official concentration is based upon a temperature of 25 °C. The undissolved portion of the mixture is not suitable for preparing additional quantities of Calcium Hydroxide Topical Solution.

CALCIUM LACTATE

Chemical name: Propanoic acid, 2-hydroxy-, calcium salt (2:1), hydrate.

Molecular formula: $C_6H_{10}CaO_6 \cdot xH_2O$.

Molecular weight: 218.22 (anhydrous).

Description: Calcium Lactate USP—White, practically odorless granules or powder. The pentahydrate is somewhat efflorescent and at 120 °C becomes anhydrous.

Solubility: Calcium Lactate USP—The pentahydrate is soluble in water; practically insoluble in alcohol.

USP requirements:

Calcium Lactate USP—Preserve in tight containers. The label indicates whether it is the dried form or is hydrous; if the latter, the label indicates the degree of hydration. Where the quantity of Calcium Lactate is indicated in the labeling of any preparation containing Calcium Lactate, this shall be understood to be in terms of calcium lactate pentahydrate. Contains not less than 98.0% and not more than 101.0% of calcium lactate, calculated on the dried basis. Meets the requirements for Identification, Acidity, Loss on drying (22.0–27.0% [pentahydrate], 15.0–20.0% [trihydrate], 5.0–8.0% [monohydrate], and not more than 3.0% [dried form]), Heavy metals (not more than 0.002%), Magnesium and alkali salts (not more than 1.0%), Volatile fatty acid, and Organic volatile impurities.

Calcium Lactate Tablets USP—Preserve in tight containers. The quantity of calcium lactate stated in the labeling is in terms of calcium lactate pentahydrate. Contain the labeled amount, within ±6%. Meet the requirements for Identification, Dissolution (75% in 45 minutes in water in Apparatus 1 at 100 rpm), and Uniformity of dosage units.

Note: An equivalent amount of Calcium Lactate with less water of hydration may be used in place of calcium lactate pentahydrate in preparing Calcium Lactate Tablets.

CALCIUM LACTOBIONATE

Chemical name: D-Gluconic acid, 4-O-beta-D-galactopyranosyl-, calcium salt (2:1), dihydrate.

Molecular formula: $C_{24}H_{42}CaO_{24} \cdot 2H_2O$.

Molecular weight: 790.69.

USP requirements: Calcium Lactobionate USP—Preserve in well-closed containers. Contains not less than 96.0% and not more than 102.0% of calcium lactobionate. Meets the requirements for Identification, Specific rotation (+22.0° to +26.5°, determined in a solution containing 1 gram in each 10 mL), pH (5.4–7.4, in a solution [1 in 20]), Halides (0.04%), Sulfate (0.05%), Arsenic (not more than 3 ppm), Heavy metals (not more than 0.002%), Reducing substances (not more than 1.0%), and Organic volatile impurities.

CALCIUM LEVULINATE

Chemical name: Pentanoic acid, 4-oxo-, calcium salt (2:1), dihydrate.

Molecular formula: $C_{10}H_{14}CaO_6 \cdot 2H_2O$.

Molecular weight: 306.33.

Description: Calcium Levulinate USP—White, crystalline or amorphous, powder, having a faint odor suggestive of burnt sugar.

Solubility: Calcium Levulinate USP—Freely soluble in water; slightly soluble in alcohol; insoluble in ether and in chloroform.

USP requirements:

Calcium Levulinate USP—Preserve in well-closed containers. Contains not less than 97.5% and not more than 100.5% of calcium levulinate, calculated on the dried basis. Meets the requirements for Identification, Melting range (119–125 °C), pH 7.0–8.5, in a solution [1 in 10]),

Loss on drying (10.5–12.0%), Chloride (0.07%), Sulfate (0.05%), Arsenic (not more than 3 ppm), Heavy metals (not more than 0.002%), Reducing sugars, and Organic volatile impurities.

Calcium Levulinate Injection USP—Preserve in single-dose containers, preferably of Type I glass. A sterile solution of Calcium Levulinate in Water for Injection. The label states the total osmolar concentration in mOsmol per liter. Where the contents are less than 100 mL, or where the label states that the Injection is not for direct injection but is to be diluted before use, the label alternatively may state the total osmolar concentration in mOsmol per mL. Contains the labeled amount, within ±5%. Meets the requirements for Identification, Bacterial endotoxins, pH (6.0–8.0), Particulate matter, and Injections.

CALCIUM PANTOTHENATE

Chemical name: Beta-alanine, N-(2,4-dihydroxy-3,3-dimethyl-1-oxobutyl)-, calcium salt (2:1), (R)-.

Molecular formula: $C_{18}H_{32}CaN_2O_{10}$.

Molecular weight: 476.54.

Description: Calcium Pantothenate USP—Slightly hygroscopic, white powder. Odorless.

Solubility: Calcium Pantothenate USP—Freely soluble in water; soluble in glycerin; practically insoluble in alcohol, in chloroform, and in ether.

USP requirements:

Calcium Pantothenate USP—Preserve in tight containers. It is the calcium salt of the dextrorotatory isomer of pantothenic acid. Contains not less than 5.7% and not more than 6.0% of nitrogen, and not less than 8.2% and not more than 8.6% of calcium, both calculated on the dried basis. Meets the requirements for Identification, Specific rotation (+25.0° to +27.5°, calculated on the dried basis, determined in a solution containing 500 mg in each 10 mL), Alkalinity, Loss on drying (not more than 5.0%), Heavy metals (not more than 0.002%), Ordinary impurities (not more than 1.0%), Nitrogen content, Calcium content, and Organic volatile impurities.

Calcium Pantothenate Tablets USP—Preserve in tight containers. Label Tablets to indicate the content of dextrorotatory calcium pantothenate. Contain the labeled amount of the dextrorotatory isomer of Calcium Pantothenate, within −5% to +15%. Meet the requirements for Identification, Disintegration (30 minutes), Uniformity of dosage units, and Calcium content.

RACEMIC CALCIUM PANTOTHENATE

Chemical name: Beta-alanine, N-(2,4-dihydroxy-3,3-dimethyl-1-oxobutyl)-, calcium salt (2:1), (±)-.

Molecular formula: $C_{18}H_{32}CaN_2O_{10}$.

Molecular weight: 476.54.

Description: Racemic Calcium Pantothenate USP—White, slightly hygroscopic powder, having a faint, characteristic odor. Is stable in air. Its solutions are neutral or alkaline to litmus. Is optically inactive.

Solubility: Racemic Calcium Pantothenate USP—Freely soluble in water; soluble in glycerin; practically insoluble in alcohol, in chloroform, and in ether.

USP requirements: Racemic Calcium Pantothenate USP—Preserve in tight containers. A mixture of the calcium salts of the dextrorotatory and levorotatory isomers of pantothenic acid. Label preparations containing it in terms of the equivalent amount of dextrorotatory calcium pantothenate. Contains not less than 5.7% and not more than 6.0% of nitrogen, and not less than 8.2% and not more than 8.6% of calcium, both calculated on the dried basis. Meets the requirements for Specific rotation ($-0.05°$ to $+0.05°$, calculated on the dried basis, determined in a solution containing 500 mg in each 10 mL), Alkalinity, and Organic volatile impurities, and for Identification tests, Loss on drying, Heavy metals, Nitrogen content, and Calcium content under Calcium Pantothenate.

Note: The physiological activity of Racemic Calcium Pantothenate is approximately one-half that of Calcium Pantothenate.

DIBASIC CALCIUM PHOSPHATE

Chemical name: Phosphoric acid, calcium salt (1:1).

Molecular formula: $CaHPO_4$.

Molecular weight: 136.06.

Description: Dibasic Calcium Phosphate USP—White, odorless powder; stable in air.

NF category: Tablet and/or capsule diluent.

Solubility: Dibasic Calcium Phosphate USP—Practically insoluble in water; soluble in 3 N hydrochloric acid and in 2 N nitric acid; insoluble in alcohol.

USP requirements:

Dibasic Calcium Phosphate USP—Preserve in well-closed containers. It is anhydrous or contains two molecules of water of hydration. Label it to indicate whether it is anhydrous or the dihydrate. Contains not less than 98.0% and not more than 105.0% of anhydrous calcium phosphate, or of dibasic calcium phosphate dihydrate. Meets the requirements for Identification, Loss on ignition (6.6–8.5% [anhydrous Dibasic Calcium Phosphate], 24.5–26.5% [dihydrate form of Dibasic Calcium Phosphate]), Acid-insoluble substances (not more than 0.2%), Carbonate, Chloride (not more than 0.25%), Fluoride (not more than 0.005%), Sulfate (not more than 0.5%), Arsenic (not more than 3 ppm), Barium, and Heavy metals (not more than 0.003%).

Dibasic Calcium Phosphate Tablets USP—Preserve in well-closed containers. The quantity of dibasic calcium phosphate stated in the labeling is in terms of Dibasic Calcium Phosphate dihydrate. Contain the labeled amount, within ±7.5%. Meet the requirements for Identification, Disintegration (30 minutes), and Uniformity of dosage units.

Note: An equivalent amount of Dibasic Calcium Phosphate with less water of hydration may be used in place of Dibasic Calcium Phosphate dihydrate in preparing Dibasic Calcium Phosphate Tablets.

TRIBASIC CALCIUM PHOSPHATE

Chemical name: Calcium hydroxide phosphate.

Molecular formula: $Ca_5(OH)(PO_4)_3$.

Molecular weight: 502.32.

Description: Tribasic Calcium Phosphate NF—White, odorless, powder. Is stable in air.

NF category: Tablet and/or capsule diluent.

Solubility: Tribasic Calcium Phosphate NF—Practically insoluble in water; readily soluble in 3 N hydrochloric acid and in 2 N nitric acid; insoluble in alcohol.

USP requirements: Tribasic Calcium Phosphate Tablets—Not in USP.

NF requirements: Tribasic Calcium Phosphate NF—Preserve in well-closed containers. A variable mixture of calcium phosphates having the approximate composition $10CaO \cdot 3P_2O_5 \cdot H_2O$. Contains an amount of tribasic calcium phosphate equivalent to not less than 34.0% and not more than 40.0% of calcium. Meets the requirements for Identification, Loss on ignition (not more than 8.0%), Water-soluble substances (not more than 0.5%), Acid-insoluble substances (not more than 0.2%), Carbonate, Chloride (not more than 0.14%), Fluoride (not more than 0.0075%), Nitrate, Sulfate (not more than 0.8%), Arsenic (not more than 3 ppm), Barium, Dibasic salt and calcium oxide, and Heavy metals (not more than 0.003%).

CALCIUM POLYCARBOPHIL

Chemical name: Calcium polycarbophil.

Description: Calcium Polycarbophil USP—White to creamy white powder.

Solubility: Calcium Polycarbophil USP—Insoluble in water, in dilute acids, in dilute alkalies, and in common organic solvents.

USP requirements:

Calcium Polycarbophil USP—Preserve in tight containers. It is the calcium salt of polyacrylic acid cross-linked with divinyl glycol. Meets the requirements for Identification, Loss on drying (not more than 10.0%), Absorbing power, and Calcium content (18.0–22.0%, calculated on the dried basis).

Calcium Polycarbophil Tablets—Not in USP.
Calcium Polycarbophil Chewable Tablets—Not in USP.

CALCIUM SACCHARATE

Chemical name: D-Glucaric acid, calcium salt (1:1) tetrahydrate.

Molecular formula: $C_6H_8CaO_8 \cdot 4H_2O$.

Molecular weight: 320.27.

Description: Calcium Saccharate USP—White, odorless, crystalline powder.

Solubility: Calcium Saccharate USP—Very slightly soluble in cold water; slightly soluble in boiling water; very slightly soluble in alcohol; practically insoluble in ether and in chloroform; soluble in dilute mineral acids and in solutions of calcium gluconate.

USP requirements: Calcium Saccharate USP—Preserve in well-closed containers. It is the calcium salt of D-saccharic acid. Contains not less than 98.5% and not more than 102.0% of calcium saccharate. Meets the requirements for Identification, Specific rotation ($+18.5°$ to $+22.5°$, determined in a solution in 4.8 N hydrochloric acid containing 600 mg in each 10 mL that has been allowed to stand for 1 hour), Arsenic (not more than 3 ppm), Chloride (0.07%), Sulfate (0.12%), Heavy metals (0.002%), and Sucrose and reducing sugars.

CALCIUM SILICATE

Molecular formula:

Calcium metasilicate—$CaSiO_3$.
Calcium diorthosilicate—Ca_2SiO_4.
Calcium trisilicate—Ca_3SiO_5.

Molecular weight:
 Calcium metasilicate—116.2
 Calcium diorthosilicate—172.2
 Calcium trisilicate—228.3

Description: Calcium Silicate NF—White to off-white, free-flowing powder that remains so after absorbing relatively large amounts of water or other liquids.
 NF category: Glidant and/or anticaking agent.

Solubility: Calcium Silicate NF—Insoluble in water. Forms a gel with mineral acids.

NF requirements: Calcium Silicate NF—Preserve in well-closed containers. A compound of calcium oxide and silicon dioxide. Contains not less than 25.0% of calcium oxide and not less than 45.0% of silicon dioxide. Meets the requirements for Identification, pH (8.4–10.2, determined in a well-mixed aqueous suspension [1 in 20]), Loss on ignition (not more than 20.0%), Fluoride (10 ppm), Arsenic (3 ppm), Lead (not more than 0.001%), Heavy metals (not more than 0.004%), Ratio of calcium oxide to silicon dioxide (1.65–2.65), and Sum of calcium oxide, silicon dioxide, and Loss on ignition (not less than 90.0%).

CALCIUM STEARATE

Chemical name: Octadecanoic acid, calcium salt.

Molecular formula: $C_{36}H_{70}CaO_4$.

Molecular weight: 607.00.

Description: Calcium Stearate NF—Fine, white to yellowish white, bulky powder having a slight, characteristic odor. Is unctuous, and is free from grittiness.
 NF category: Tablet and/or capsule lubricant.

Solubility: Calcium Stearate NF—Insoluble in water, in alcohol, and in ether.

NF requirements: Calcium Stearate NF—Preserve in well-closed containers. A compound of calcium with a mixture of solid organic acids obtained from fats, and consists chiefly of variable proportions of calcium stearate and calcium palmitate. Contains the equivalent of not less than 9.0% and not more than 10.5% of calcium oxide. Meets the requirements for Identification, Loss on drying (not more than 4.0%), Arsenic (not more than 3 ppm), and Heavy metals (not more than 0.001%).

CALCIUM SULFATE

Chemical name: Sulfuric acid, calcium salt (1:1).

Molecular formula: $CaSO_4$.

Molecular weight: 136.14.

Description: Calcium Sulfate NF—Fine, white to slightly yellow-white, odorless powder.
 NF category: Desiccant; tablet and/or capsule diluent.

Solubility: Calcium Sulfate NF—Slightly soluble in water; soluble in 3 *N* hydrochloric acid.

NF requirements: Calcium Sulfate NF—Preserve in well-closed containers. It is anhydrous or contains two molecules of water of hydration. Label it to indicate whether it is anhydrous or the dihydrate. Contains not less than 98.0% and not more than 101.0% of calcium sulfate, calculated on the dried basis. Meets the requirements for Identification, Loss on drying (not more than 1.5% [anhydrous], 19.0–23.0% [dihydrate]),

Iron (not more than 0.01%), and Heavy metals (not more than 0.001%).

CAMPHOR

Chemical name: Bicyclo[2.2.1]heptane-2-one, 1,7,7-trimethyl-.

Molecular formula: $C_{10}H_{16}O$.

Molecular weight: 152.24.

Description: Camphor USP—Colorless or white crystals, granules, or crystalline masses; or colorless to white, translucent, tough masses. Has a penetrating, characteristic odor. Specific gravity is about 0.99. Slowly volatilizes at ordinary temperatures.

Solubility: Camphor USP—Slightly soluble in water; very soluble in alcohol, in chloroform, and in ether; freely soluble in carbon disulfide, in solvent hexane, and in fixed and volatile oils.

USP requirements:
 Camphor USP—Preserve in tight containers, and avoid exposure to excessive heat. A ketone obtained from *Cinnamomum camphora* (Linné) Nees et Ebermaier (Fam. Lauraceae) (Natural Camphor) or produced synthetically (Synthetic Camphor). Label it to indicate whether it is obtained from natural sources or is prepared synthetically. Meets the requirements for Melting range (174–179 °C), Specific rotation (+41° to +43° for natural Camphor), Water, Nonvolatile residue (not more than 0.05%), and Halogens (not more than 0.035%).
 Camphor Spirit USP—Preserve in tight containers. An alcohol solution containing, in each 100 mL, not less than 9.0 grams and not more than 11.0 grams of camphor.
 Prepare Camphor Spirit as follows: 100 grams of Camphor and a sufficient quantity of alcohol to make 1000 mL. Dissolve the camphor in about 800 mL of the alcohol, and add alcohol to make 1000 mL. Filter, if necessary.
 Meets the requirement for Alcohol content (80.0–87.0%, the dilution to approximately 2% alcohol being made with methanol instead of with water).

CANDICIDIN

Chemical name: Candicidin.

Description: Candicidin USP—Yellow to brown powder.

Solubility: Candicidin USP—Sparingly soluble in water; very slightly soluble in alcohol, in acetone, and in butyl alcohol.

USP requirements:
 Candicidin USP—Preserve in tight containers, in a refrigerator. A substance produced by the growth of *Streptomyces griseus* Waksman et Henrici (Fam. Streptomycetaceae). It has a potency of not less than 1000 mcg per mg, calculated on the dried basis. Meets the requirements for Identification, pH (8.0–10.0, in an aqueous suspension containing 10 mg per mL), and Loss on drying (not more than 4.0%).
 Candicidin Ointment USP—Preserve in well-closed containers, in a refrigerator. Contains the labeled amount, within −10% to +40%. Meets the requirements for Minimum fill and Water (not more than 0.1%).
 Candicidin Vaginal Tablets USP—Preserve in tight containers, in a refrigerator. Contain the labeled amount, within −10% to +50%. Meet the requirements for Disintegration (30 minutes) and Loss on drying (not more than 1.0%).

CAPREOMYCIN

Source: A complex of four microbiologically active components derived from *Streptomyces capreolus*.

Chemical group: Polypeptide antibiotic.

Chemical name: Capreomycin sulfate.

Description: Sterile Capreomycin Sulfate USP—White to practically white, amorphous powder.

Solubility: Sterile Capreomycin Sulfate USP—Freely soluble in water; practically insoluble in most organic solvents.

USP requirements: Sterile Capreomycin Sulfate USP—Preserve in Containers for Sterile Solids. The constituted solution may be stored for 48 hours at room temperature, and up to 14 days in a refrigerator. It is the disulfate salt of capreomycin, a polypeptide mixture produced by the growth of *Streptomyces capreolus*, suitable for parenteral use. Contains an amount of capreomycin sulfate equivalent to not less than 700 mcg and not more than 1050 mcg of capreomycin per mg and, where packaged for dispensing, contains an amount of capreomycin sulfate equivalent to the labeled amount of capreomycin, within −10% to +15%. Meets the requirements for Constituted solution, Identification, Depressor substances, Bacterial endotoxins, pH (4.5–7.5, in a solution containing 30 mg per mL [or, where packaged for dispensing, in the solution constituted as directed in the labeling]), Loss on drying (not more than 10.0%), Residue on ignition (not more than 3.0%), Heavy metals (not more than 0.003%), Capreomycin I content (not less than 90.0%), and Injections.

CAPSAICIN

Source: Naturally occurring substance derived from plants of the Solanaceae family.

Chemical name: Trans-8-methyl-*N*-vanillyl-6-nonenamide.

Molecular formula: $C_{18}H_{27}NO_3$.

Molecular weight: 305.4.

Description: White, crystalline powder.

Solubility: Practically insoluble in water; very soluble in alcohol, in ether, and in chloroform.

USP requirements: Capsaicin Cream—Not in USP.

CAPTOPRIL

Chemical name: L-Proline, 1-[(2*S*)-3-mercapto-2-methyl-1-oxopropyl]-.

Molecular formula: $C_9H_{15}NO_3S$.

Molecular weight: 217.28.

Description: Captopril USP—White to off-white, crystalline powder, which may have a characteristic, sulfide-like odor. Melts in the range of 104 to 110 °C.

pKa: 3.7 and 9.8 (apparent).

Solubility: Captopril USP—Freely soluble in water, in methanol, in alcohol, and in chloroform.

USP requirements:
Captopril USP—Preserve in tight containers. Contains not less than 97.5% and not more than 102.0% of captopril, calculated on the dried basis. Meets the requirements for Identification, Specific rotation (−125° to −134°, calculated on the dried basis, determined in a solution in

absolute alcohol containing 10 mg per mL), Loss on drying (not more than 1.0%), Residue on ignition (not more than 0.2%), Heavy metals (not more than 0.003%), Related substances (not more than 0.1%), and Organic volatile impurities.
Captopril Tablets USP—Preserve in tight containers. Contain the labeled amount, within ± 10%. Meet the requirements for Identification, Dissolution (80% in 20 minutes in 0.1 *N* hydrochloric acid in Apparatus 1 at 50 rpm), Related substance (not more than 3.0%), and Uniformity of dosage units.

CAPTOPRIL AND HYDROCHLOROTHIAZIDE

For *Captopril* and *Hydrochlorothiazide*—See individual listings for chemistry information.

USP requirements: Captopril and Hydrochlorothiazide Tablets—Not in USP.

CARAMEL

Description: Caramel NF—Thick, dark brown liquid having the characteristic odor of burnt sugar. One part dissolved in 1000 parts of water yields a clear solution having a distinct yellowish orange color. The color of the solution is not changed and no precipitate is formed after exposure to sunlight for 6 hours. When spread in a thin layer on a glass plate, it appears homogeneous, reddish brown, and transparent.
NF category: Color.

Solubility: Caramel NF—Miscible with water. Soluble in dilute alcohol up to 55% (v/v). Immiscible with ether, with chloroform, with acetone, and with solvent hexane.

NF requirements: Caramel NF—Preserve in tight containers. A concentrated solution of the product obtained by heating sugar or glucose until the sweet taste is destroyed and a uniform dark brown mass results, a small amount of alkali or of alkaline carbonate or a trace of mineral acid being added while heating. Meets the requirements for Specific gravity (not less than 1.30), Purity, Microbial limits, Ash (not more than 8.0%), Arsenic (3 ppm), and Lead (10 ppm).
Note: Where included in articles for coloring purposes, Caramel complies with the regulations of the U.S. Food and Drug Administration concerning color additives.

CARBACHOL

Chemical name: Ethanaminium, 2-[(aminocarbonyl)oxy]-*N,N,N*-trimethyl-, chloride.

Molecular formula: $C_6H_{15}ClN_2O_2$.

Molecular weight: 182.65.

Description: White or faintly yellow hygroscopic crystals or crystalline powder; odorless or with a faint amine-like odor. Its solutions in water are neutral to litmus.

Solubility: Soluble 1 in 1 of water and 1 in 50 of alcohol; practically insoluble in chloroform and in ether.

USP requirements:
Carbachol USP—Preserve in tight containers. Contains not less than 99.0% and not more than 101.0% of carbachol, calculated on the dried basis. Meets the requirements for Identification, Melting range (200–204 °C, with some decomposition), Loss on drying (not more than 2.0%), Residue on ignition (not more than 0.1%), and Ordinary impurities.
Carbachol Intraocular Solution USP—Preserve in tight containers, at controlled room temperature, and protect from

freezing. A sterile solution of Carbachol in an aqueous medium. Label it to indicate that it is for single-dose intraocular use only, and that the unused portion is to be discarded. Contains the labeled amount, within −10% to +15%. Contains no preservatives or antimicrobial agents. Meets the requirements for Identification, Sterility, and pH (5.0–7.5).

Carbachol Ophthalmic Solution USP—Preserve in tight containers. A sterile solution of Carbachol in an isotonic, aqueous medium. Contains the labeled amount, within ±5%. Meets the requirements for Identification, Sterility, and pH (5.0–7.0).

CARBAMAZEPINE

Chemical group: Tricyclic iminostilbene derivative. Structurally resembles the psychoactive agents imipramine, chlorpromazine, and maprotiline; shares some structural features with the anticonvulsant agents phenytoin, clonazepam, and phenobarbital.

Chemical name: 5*H*-Dibenz[*b,f*]azepine-5-carboxamide.

Molecular formula: $C_{15}H_{12}N_2O$.

Molecular weight: 236.27.

Description: Carbamazepine USP—White to off-white powder.

pKa: 7.

Solubility: Carbamazepine USP—Practically insoluble in water; soluble in alcohol and in acetone.

USP requirements:
Carbamazepine USP—Preserve in tight containers. Contains not less than 98.0% and not more than 102.0% of carbamazepine, calculated on the dried basis. Meets the requirements for Identification, X-ray diffraction, Acidity (not more than 1.0 mL of 0.010 N sodium hydroxide required for each 1.0 gram of Carbamazepine), Alkalinity (not more than 1.0 mL of 0.010 N hydrochloric acid required for each 1.0 gram of Carbamazepine), Loss on drying (not more than 0.5%), Residue on ignition (not more than 0.1%), Chloride (not more than 0.014%), Heavy metals (not more than 0.001%), Chromatographic purity (not more than 0.2% for any single impurity and not more than 0.5% total impurities), and Organic volatile impurities.

Carbamazepine Oral Suspension USP—Preserve in tight, light-resistant containers, protected from freezing and from excessive heat. Contains the labeled amount, within ±10%. Meets the requirements for Identification and Microbial limits.

Carbamazepine Tablets USP—Preserve in tight containers, preferably of glass. Dispense Carbamazepine Tablets in a container labeled "Store in a dry place. Protect from moisture." Contain the labeled amount, within ±8%. Meet the requirements for Identification, Dissolution (75% in 60 minutes in water containing 1% sodium lauryl sulfate in Apparatus 2 at 75 rpm), Water (not more than 5.0%), and Uniformity of dosage units.

Carbamazepine Extended-release Tablets—Not in USP.

CARBAMIDE PEROXIDE

Chemical name: Urea, compd. with hydrogen peroxide (1:1).

Molecular formula: $CH_6N_2O_3$.

Molecular weight: 94.07.

Description: Carbamide Peroxide Topical Solution USP—Clear, colorless, viscous liquid, having a characteristic odor.

USP requirements:
Carbamide Peroxide USP—Preserve in tight, light-resistant containers, and avoid exposure to excessive heat. Contains not less than 96.0% and not more than 102.0% of carbamide peroxide. Meets the requirements for Identification and Organic volatile impurities.

Carbamide Peroxide Topical Solution USP—Preserve in tight, light-resistant containers, and avoid exposure to excessive heat. A solution in anhydrous glycerin of Carbamide Peroxide or of carbamide peroxide prepared from hydrogen peroxide and Urea. Contains the labeled amount, by weight, within −22% to +10%. Meets the requirements for Identification, Specific gravity (1.245–1.272), and pH (4.0–7.5).

CARBENICILLIN

Chemical name:
Carbenicillin disodium—4-Thia-1-azabicyclo[3.2.0]heptane-2-carboxylic acid, 6-[(carboxyphenylacetyl)amino]-3,3-dimethyl-7-oxo, disodium salt, [6S-(2 alpha,5 alpha,6 beta)]-.
Carbenicillin indanyl sodium—4-Thia-1-azabicyclo[3.2.0]-heptane-2-carboxylic acid, 6-[[3-[(2,3-dihydro-1H-inden-5-yl)-oxy]-1,3-dioxo-2-phenylpropyl]amino]-3,3-dimethyl-7-oxo-, monosodium salt, [2S-(2 alpha,5 alpha,6 beta)]-.

Molecular formula:
Carbenicillin disodium—$C_{17}H_{16}N_2Na_2O_6S$.
Carbenicillin indanyl sodium—$C_{26}H_{25}N_2NaO_6S$.

Molecular weight:
Carbenicillin disodium—422.36.
Carbenicillin indanyl sodium—516.54.

Description:
Sterile Carbenicillin Disodium USP—White to off-white, crystalline powder.
Carbenicillin Indanyl Sodium USP—White to off-white powder.

Solubility:
Sterile Carbenicillin Disodium USP—Freely soluble in water; soluble in alcohol; practically insoluble in chloroform and in ether.
Carbenicillin Indanyl Sodium USP—Soluble in water and in alcohol.

USP requirements:
Sterile Carbenicillin Disodium USP—Preserve in Containers for Sterile Solids. Contains an amount of carbenicillin disodium equivalent to not less than 770 mcg of carbenicillin per mg, calculated on the anhydrous basis and, where packaged for dispensing, contains an amount of carbenicillin disodium equivalent to the labeled amount of carbenicillin, within −10% to +20%. Meets the requirements for Constituted solution, Identification, Bacterial endotoxins, Sterility, pH (6.5–8.0, in a solution containing 10 mg of carbenicillin per mL [or, where packaged for dispensing, in the solution constituted as directed in the labeling]), Water (not more than 6.0%), and Particulate matter, for Uniformity of dosage units, and for Constituted solutions and Labeling under Injections.

Carbenicillin Indanyl Sodium USP—Preserve in tight containers. For periods up to 18 months, store at controlled room temperature. It has a potency equivalent to not less than 630 mcg and not more then 769 mcg of carbenicillin per mg, calculated on the anhydrous basis. Meets the requirements for Identification, pH (5.0–8.0, in a solution containing 100 mg per mL), and Water (not more than 2.0%).

Carbenicillin Indanyl Sodium Tablets USP—Preserve in tight containers. Contain an amount of carbenicillin indanyl sodium equivalent to the labeled amount of carbenicillin, within −10% to +20%. Meet the requirements for Identification, Dissolution (75% in 45 minutes in water in Apparatus 1 at 100 rpm), Uniformity of dosage units, and Water (not more than 2.0%).

CARBIDOPA

Chemical group: Hydrazine analog of levodopa; inhibitor of L-aromatic amino acid decarboxylase.

Chemical name: Benzenepropanoic acid, alpha-hydrazino-3,4-dihydroxy-alpha-methyl-, monohydrate, (*S*).

Molecular formula: $C_{10}H_{14}N_2O_4 \cdot H_2O$.

Molecular weight: 244.25.

Description: Carbidopa USP—White to creamy white, odorless or practically odorless, powder.

Solubility: Carbidopa USP—Slightly soluble in water; freely soluble in 3 *N* hydrochloric acid; slightly soluble in methanol; practically insoluble in alcohol, in acetone, in chloroform, and in ether.

USP requirements: Carbidopa USP—Preserve in well-closed, light-resistant containers. Contains not less than 98.0% and not more than 101.0% of carbidopa. Meets the requirements for Identification, Specific rotation (−21.0° to −23.5°, calculated as the monohydrate), Loss on drying (6.9–7.9%), Residue on ignition (not more than 0.1%), Heavy metals (not more than 0.001%), and Methyldopa and 3-*O*-methylcarbidopa (not more than 0.5%).

CARBIDOPA AND LEVODOPA

For *Carbidopa* and *Levodopa*—See individual listings for chemistry information.

USP requirements:
Carbidopa and Levodopa Tablets USP—Preserve in well-closed, light-resistant containers. Contain the labeled amounts of carbidopa and levodopa, within ±10%. Meet the requirements for Identification, Dissolution (80% of each ingredient in 30 minutes in 0.1 *N* hydrochloric acid in Apparatus 1 at 50 rpm), and Uniformity of dosage units.
Carbidopa and Levodopa Extended-release Tablets—Not in USP.

CARBINOXAMINE

Chemical group: Ethanolamine derivative.

Chemical name: Carbinoxamine maleate—Ethanamine, 2-[(4-chlorophenyl)-2-pyridinylmethoxy]-*N*,*N*-dimethyl-, (*Z*)-2-butenedioate (1:1).

Molecular formula: Carbinoxamine maleate—$C_{16}H_{19}ClN_2O \cdot C_4H_4O_4$.

Molecular weight: Carbinoxamine maleate—406.87.

Description: Carbinoxamine Maleate USP—White, odorless, crystalline powder.

pKa: Carbinoxamine maleate—8.1.

Solubility: Carbinoxamine Maleate USP—Very soluble in water; freely soluble in alcohol and in chloroform; very slightly soluble in ether.

USP requirements:
Carbinoxamine Maleate USP—Preserve in tight, light-resistant containers. It is dried at 105 °C for 2 hours. Contains not less than 98.0% and not more than 102.0% of carbinoxamine maleate. Meets the requirements for Identification, Melting range (116–121 °C, determined after drying), pH (4.6–5.1, in a solution [1 in 100]), Loss on drying (not more than 0.5%), Residue on ignition (not more than 0.1%), Ordinary impurities, and Organic volatile impurities
Carbinoxamine Maleate Tablets USP—Preserve in tight, light-resistant containers. Contain the labeled amount, within ±7%. Meet the requirements for Identification, Dissolution (75% in 45 minutes in water in Apparatus 2 at 50 rpm), and Uniformity of dosage units.

CARBINOXAMINE AND PSEUDOEPHEDRINE

For *Carbinoxamine* and *Pseudoephedrine*—See individual listings for chemistry information.

USP requirements:
Carbinoxamine Maleate and Pseudoephedrine Hydrochloride Oral Solution—Not in USP.
Carbinoxamine Maleate and Pseudoephedrine Hydrochloride Syrup—Not in USP.
Carbinoxamine Maleate and Pseudoephedrine Hydrochloride Tablets—Not in USP.
Carbinoxamine Maleate and Pseudoephedrine Hydrochloride Extended-release Tablets—Not in USP.

CARBINOXAMINE, PSEUDOEPHEDRINE, AND DEXTROMETHORPHAN

For *Carbinoxamine*, *Pseudoephedrine*, and *Dextromethorphan*—See individual listings for chemistry information.

USP requirements:
Carbinoxamine Maleate, Pseudoephedrine Hydrochloride, and Dextromethorphan Hydrobromide Oral Solution—Not in USP.
Carbinoxamine Maleate, Pseudoephedrine Hydrochloride, and Dextromethorphan Hydrobromide Syrup—Not in USP.

CARBINOXAMINE, PSEUDOEPHEDRINE, AND GUAIFENESIN

For *Carbinoxamine*, *Pseudoephedrine*, and *Guaifenesin*—See individual listings for chemistry information.

USP requirements:
Carbinoxamine Maleate, Pseudoephedrine Hydrochloride, and Guaifenesin Capsules—Not in USP.
Carbinoxamine Maleate, Pseudoephedrine Hydrochloride, and Guaifenesin Oral Solution—Not in USP.

CARBOL-FUCHSIN

Chemical name:
Basic fuchsin—Benzenamine, 4-[(4-aminophenyl)(4-imino-2,5-cyclohexadien-1-ylidene)methyl]-2-methyl-, monohydrochloride.
Phenol—Phenol.
Resorcinol—1,3-Benzenediol.
Acetone—2-Propanone.
Alcohol—Ethanol.

Molecular formula:
Phenol—C_6H_6O.
Resorcinol—$C_6H_6O_2$.
Acetone—C_3H_6O.
Alcohol—C_2H_6O.

Molecular weight:
Phenol—94.11.
Resorcinol—110.11.
Acetone—58.08.
Alcohol—46.07.

Description:
Basic Fuchsin USP—Dark green powder or greenish glistening crystalline fragments, having a bronze-like luster and not more than a faint odor.

Phenol USP—Colorless to light pink, interlaced or separate, needle-shaped crystals, or white to light pink, crystalline mass. Has a characteristic odor. Is liquefied by warming and by the addition of 10% of water. Boils at about 182 °C, and its vapor is flammable. Gradually darkens on exposure to light and air.

NF category: Antimicrobial preservative.

Resorcinol USP—White, or practically white, needle-shaped crystals or powder. Has a faint, characteristic odor. Acquires a pink tint on exposure to light and air. Its solution (1 in 20) is neutral or acid to litmus.

Acetone USP—Transparent, colorless, mobile, volatile liquid, having a characteristic odor. A solution (1 in 2) is neutral to litmus.

NF category: Solvent.

Alcohol USP—Clear, colorless, mobile, volatile liquid. Has a characteristic odor. Is readily volatilized even at low temperatures, and boils at about 78 °C. Is flammable.

NF category: Solvent.

Carbol-Fuchsin Topical Solution USP—Dark purple liquid, which appears purplish red when spread in a thin film.

Solubility:
Basic Fuchsin USP—Soluble in water, in alcohol, and in amyl alcohol; insoluble in ether.

Phenol USP—Soluble in water; very soluble in alcohol, in glycerin, in chloroform, in ether, and in fixed and volatile oils; sparingly soluble in mineral oil.

Resorcinol USP—Freely soluble in water, in alcohol, in glycerin, and in ether; slightly soluble in chloroform.

Acetone USP—Miscible with water, with alcohol, with ether, with chloroform, and with most volatile oils.

Alcohol USP—Miscible with water and with practically all organic solvents.

USP requirements: Carbol-Fuchsin Topical Solution USP—Preserve in tight, light-resistant containers.

Prepare Carbol-Fuchsin Topical Solution as follows: 3 grams of Basic Fuchsin, 45 grams of Phenol, 100 grams of Resorcinol, 50 mL of Acetone, 100 mL of Alcohol, and a sufficient quantity of Purified Water, to make 1000 mL. Dissolve the Basic Fuchsin in a mixture of the Acetone and Alcohol, and add to this solution the Phenol and Resorcinol previously dissolved in 725 mL of Purified Water. Then add sufficient Purified Water to make the product measure 1000 mL, and mix.

Meets the requirements for Specific gravity (0.990–1.050) and Alcohol content (7.0–10.0%).

CARBOMER

Chemical name:
Carbomer 910—Polymer of 2-propenoic acid, cross-linked with allyl ethers of pentaerythritol.

Carbomer 934—Polymer of 2-propenoic acid, cross-linked with allyl ethers of sucrose.

Carbomer 934P—Polymer of 2-propenoic acid, cross-linked with allyl ethers of sucrose or pentaerythritol.

Carbomer 940—Polymer of 2-propenoic acid, cross-linked with allyl ethers of pentaerythritol.

Carbomer 941—Polymer of 2-propenoic acid, cross-linked with allyl ethers of pentaerythritol.

Description: Carbomer 910 NF; Carbomer 934 NF; Carbomer 934P NF; Carbomer 940 NF; Carbomer 941 NF; Carbomer 1342 NF—White, fluffy powder, having a slight, characteristic odor. Hygroscopic. The pH of a 1 in 100 dispersion is about 3.

NF category: Suspending and/or viscosity-increasing agent.

Solubility: Carbomer 910 NF; Carbomer 934 NF; Carbomer 934P NF; Carbomer 940 NF; Carbomer 941 NF; Carbomer 1342 NF—When neutralized with alkali hydroxides or with amines, it dissolves in water, in alcohol, and in glycerin.

NF requirements:
Carbomer 910 NF—Preserve in tight containers. A high molecular weight polymer of acrylic acid cross-linked with allyl ethers of pentaerythritol. Label it to indicate that it is not intended for internal use. Previously dried in vacuum at 80 °C for 1 hour, contains not less than 56.0% and not more than 68.0% of carboxylic acid groups. Meets the requirements for Viscosity (3000–7000 centipoises for neutralized 1.0% aqueous dispersion) and Benzene (not more than 0.5%), and for Identification, Loss on drying, and Heavy metals under Carbomer 934P.

Carbomer 934 NF—Preserve in tight containers. A high molecular weight polymer of acrylic acid cross-linked with allyl ethers of sucrose. Label it to indicate that it is not intended for internal use. Previously dried in vacuum at 80 °C for 1 hour, contains not less than 56.0% and not more than 68.0% of carboxylic acid groups. Meets the requirements for Viscosity (30,500–39,400 centipoises for neutralized 0.5% aqueous dispersion) and Benzene (not more than 0.5%), and for Identification, Loss on drying, and Heavy metals under Carbomer 934P.

Carbomer 934P NF—Preserve in tight containers. A high molecular weight polymer of acrylic acid cross-linked with allyl ethers of sucrose or pentaerythritol. Previously dried in vacuum at 80 °C for 1 hour, contains not less than 56.0% and not more than 68.0% of carboxylic acid groups. Meets the requirements for Identification, Viscosity (29,400–39,400 centipoises for neutralized 0.5% aqueous dispersion), Loss on drying (not more than 2.0%), Heavy metals (not more than 0.002%), and Benzene (not more than 0.01%).

Carbomer 940 NF—Preserve in tight containers. A high molecular weight polymer of acrylic acid cross-linked with allyl ethers of pentaerythritol. Label it to indicate that it is not intended for internal use. Previously dried in vacuum at 80 °C for 1 hour, contains not less than 56.0% and not more than 68.0% of carboxylic acid groups. Meets the requirements for Viscosity (40,000–60,000 centipoises for neutralized 0.5% aqueous dispersion) and Benzene (not more than 0.5%), and for Identification, Loss on drying, and Heavy metals under Carbomer 934P.

Carbomer 941 NF—Preserve in tight containers. A high molecular weight polymer of acrylic acid cross-linked with allyl ethers of pentaerythritol. Label it to indicate that it is not intended for internal use. Previously dried in vacuum at 80 °C for 1 hour, contains not less than 56.0% and not more than 68.0% of carboxylic acid groups. Meets the requirements for Viscosity (4,000–11,000 centipoises for neutralized 0.5% aqueous dispersion) and Benzene (not more than 0.5%), and for Identification, Loss on drying, and Heavy metals under Carbomer 934P.

Carbomer 1342 NF—Preserve in tight containers. A high molecular weight copolymer of acrylic acid and a long chain alkyl methacrylate cross-linked with allyl ethers of pentaerythritol. Label it to indicate that it is not intended for internal use. Previously dried in vacuum at 80 °C for

1 hour, contains not less than 52.0% and not more than 62.0% of carboxylic acid groups. Meets the requirements for Identification, Viscosity (9,500–26,500 centipoises for neutralized 1.0% aqueous dispersion), Carboxylic acid content, and Benzene (not more than 0.2%), and for Loss on drying and Heavy metals under Carbomer 934P.

CARBON DIOXIDE

Chemical name: Carbon dioxide.

Molecular formula: CO_2.

Molecular weight: 44.01.

Description: Carbon Dioxide USP—Odorless, colorless gas. Its solutions are acid to litmus. One liter at 0 °C and at a pressure of 760 mm of mercury weighs 1.977 grams.
NF category: Air displacement.

Solubility: Carbon Dioxide USP—One volume dissolves in about 1 volume of water.

USP requirements: Carbon Dioxide USP—Preserve in cylinders. Contains not less than 99.0%, by volume, of carbon dioxide. Meets the requirements for Identification, Carbon monoxide (not more than 0.001%), Hydrogen sulfide (not more than 1 ppm), Nitric oxide (not more than 2.5 ppm), Nitrogen dioxide (not more than 2.5 ppm), Ammonia (not more than 0.0025%), Sulfur dioxide (not more than 5 ppm), and Water (not more than 150 mg per cubic meter).

CARBON TETRACHLORIDE

Chemical name: Methane, tetrachloro-.

Molecular formula: CCl_4.

Molecular weight: 153.82.

Description: Carbon Tetrachloride NF—Clear, colorless, mobile liquid, having a characteristic ethereal odor resembling that of chloroform.
NF category: Solvent.

Solubility: Carbon Tetrachloride NF—Practically insoluble in water. Miscible with alcohol, with ether, with chloroform, with solvent hexane, and with fixed and volatile oils.

NF requirements: Carbon Tetrachloride NF—Preserve in tight, light-resistant containers, at a temperature not exceeding 30 °C. Contains not less than 99.0% and not more than 100.5% of carbon tetrachloride. Meets the requirements for Specific gravity (1.588–1.590, indicating 99.0–100.5% of carbon tetrachloride), Distilling range (76.0–78.0 °C), Acidity, Nonvolatile residue (not more than 0.002%), Chloride and free chlorine, Readily carbonizable substances, and Carbon disulfide.

Caution: Avoid contact; vapor and liquid are poisonous. Care should be taken not to vaporize Carbon Tetrachloride in the presence of a flame because of the production of harmful gases (mainly phosgene).

CARBOPLATIN

Chemical group: A metal coordination complex.

Chemical name: Platinum, diammine[1,1-cyclobutanedicarboxylato(2-)O,O']-, (SP-4-2).

Molecular formula: $C_6H_{12}N_2O_4Pt$.

Molecular weight: 371.25.

Description: White to off-white crystalline powder.

Solubility: Soluble in water at a rate of approximately 14 mg per mL; virtually insoluble in ethanol, in acetone, and in dimethylacetamide.

Other characteristics: pH of a 1% solution is 5–7.

USP requirements:
Carboplatin Injection—Not in USP.
Carboplatin for Injection—Not in USP.

CARBOPROST

Source: Carboprost tromethamine—the tromethamine salt of the (15S)-15 methyl analogue of naturally occurring prostaglandin $F_{2\text{-alpha}}$.

Chemical name: Carboprost tromethamine—Prosta-5,13-dien-1-oic acid, 9,11,15-trihydroxy-15-methyl-, (5Z,9 alpha,11 alpha,13E,15S)-, compound with 2-amino-2-(hydroxymethyl)-1,3-propanediol (1:1).

Molecular formula: Carboprost tromethamine—$C_{21}H_{36}O_5 \cdot C_4H_{11}NO_3$.

Molecular weight: Carboprost tromethamine—489.65.

Description: Carboprost tromethamine—White to slightly off-white crystalline powder. It has a melting point between 95 and 105 °C, depending on the rate of heating.

Solubility: Carboprost tromethamine—Dissolves readily in water at room temperature at a concentration greater than 75 mg per mL.

USP requirements:
Carboprost Tromethamine USP—Preserve in well-closed containers, in a freezer. Contains not less than 95.0% and not more than 105.0% of carboprost tromethamine, calculated on the dried basis. Meets the requirements for Identification, Specific rotation (+18° to +24°, calculated on the dried basis, determined in an alcohol solution containing 10 mg per mL), Loss on drying (not more than 1.0%), Residue on ignition (not more than 0.5%), and Limit of 15R-epimer and 5-trans isomer (not more than 3.0%).

Caution: Great care should be taken to prevent inhaling particles of Carboprost Tromethamine and exposing the skin to it.

Carboprost Tromethamine Injection USP—Preserve in single-dose or in multiple-dose containers, preferably of Type I glass, in a refrigerator. A sterile solution of Carboprost Tromethamine in aqueous solution, which may contain also benzyl alcohol, sodium chloride, and tromethamine. Contains an amount of carboprost tromethamine equivalent to the labeled amount of carboprost, within ±10%. Meets the requirements for Identification, Bacterial endotoxins, pH (7.0–8.0), and Injections.

CARBOXYMETHYLCELLULOSE

Chemical group: Semisynthetic hydrophilic derivative of cellulose.

Chemical name:
Carboxymethylcellulose calcium—Cellulose, carboxymethyl ether, calcium salt.
Carboxymethylcellulose sodium (carmellose)—Cellulose, carboxymethyl ether, sodium salt.

Description:
Carboxymethylcellulose Calcium NF—White to yellowish white powder. Is hygroscopic. The pH of the suspension, obtained by shaking 1 gram with 100 mL of water, is between 4.5 and 6.0.
  NF category: Suspending and/or viscosity-increasing agent.
Carboxymethylcellulose Sodium USP—White to cream-colored powder or granules. The powder is hygroscopic.
  NF category: Coating agent; suspending and/or viscosity-increasing agent; tablet binder.
Carboxymethylcellulose Sodium 12 NF—White to cream-colored powder or granules. The powder is hygroscopic.
  NF category: Suspending and/or viscosity-increasing agent.

Solubility:
Carboxymethylcellulose Calcium NF—Practically insoluble in alcohol, in acetone, in ether, and in chloroform. It swells with water to form a suspension.
Carboxymethylcellulose Sodium USP—Is easily dispersed in water to form colloidal solutions. Insoluble in alcohol, in ether, and in most other organic solvents.
Carboxymethylcellulose Sodium 12 NF—Is easily dispersed in water to form colloidal solutions. Insoluble in alcohol, in ether, and in most other organic solvents.

USP requirements:
Carboxymethylcellulose Sodium USP—Preserve in tight containers. It is the sodium salt of a polycarboxymethyl ether of cellulose. Label it to indicate the viscosity in solutions of stated concentrations of either 1% (w/w) or 2% (w/w). Contains not less than 6.5% and not more than 9.5% of sodium, calculated on the dried basis. Meets the requirements for Identification, pH (6.5–8.5 in a solution [1 in 100]), Viscosity, Loss on drying (not more than 10.0%), and Heavy metals (not more than 0.004%).
Carboxymethylcellulose Sodium Paste USP—Preserve in well-closed containers, and avoid prolonged exposure to temperatures exceeding 30 °C. Contains not less than 16.0% and not more than 17.0% of carboxymethylcellulose sodium. Meets the requirements for Identification, Microbial limits, Loss on drying (not more than 2.0%), Heavy metals (not more than 0.005%), and Consistency.
Carboxymethylcellulose Sodium Tablets USP—Preserve in tight containers. Contain an amount of sodium equivalent to not less than 6.5% and not more than 9.5% of the labeled amount of carboxymethylcellulose sodium. Meet the requirements for Identification, Disintegration (2 hours), and Uniformity of dosage units.

NF requirements:
Carboxymethylcellulose Calcium NF—Preserve in tight containers. It is the calcium salt of a polycarboxymethyl ether of cellulose. Meets the requirements for Identification, Alkalinity, Loss on drying (not more than 10.0%), Residue on ignition (10.0–20.0%), Chloride (not more than 0.36%), Silicate (not more than 1.5%), Sulfate (not more than 0.96%), Arsenic (not more than 0.001%), Heavy metals (not more than 0.002%), and Starch.
Carboxymethylcellulose Sodium 12 NF—Preserve in tight containers. It is the sodium salt of a polycarboxymethyl ether of cellulose. Label it to indicate the viscosity in solutions of stated concentrations of either 1% (w/w) or 2% (w/w). Its degree of substitution is not less than 1.15 and not more than 1.45, corresponding to a sodium content of not less than 10.5% and not more than 12.0%, calculated on the dried basis. Meets the requirements for Identification, Viscosity, pH (6.5–8.5, in a solution [1 in 100]), Loss on drying (not more than 10.0%), Heavy metals (not more than 0.004%), Sodium chloride and Sodium

glycolate (not more than 0.5%), and Degree of substitution.

CARBOXYMETHYLCELLULOSE, CASANTHRANOL, AND DOCUSATE

For *Carboxymethylcellulose, Casanthranol,* and *Docusate*—See individual listings for chemistry information.

USP requirements: Carboxymethylcellulose Sodium, Casanthranol, and Docusate Sodium Capsules—Not in USP.

CARBOXYMETHYLCELLULOSE AND DOCUSATE

For *Carboxymethylcellulose* and *Docusate*—See individual listings for chemistry information.

USP requirements: Carboxymethylcellulose Sodium and Docusate Sodium Capsules—Not in USP.

CARISOPRODOL

Chemical name: 2-Methyl-2-propyl-1,3-propanediol carbamate isopropylcarbamate.

Molecular formula: $C_{12}H_{24}N_2O_4$.

Molecular weight: 260.33.

Description: Carisoprodol USP—White, crystalline powder, having a mild, characteristic odor.

Solubility: Carisoprodol USP—Very slightly soluble in water; freely soluble in alcohol, in chloroform, and in acetone.

USP requirements:
Carisoprodol USP—Preserve in tight containers. Contains not less than 98.0% and not more than 102.0% of carisoprodol, calculated on the dried basis. Meets the requirements for Identification, Melting range (91–94 °C), Loss on drying (not more than 0.5%), Heavy metals (not more than 0.001%), Meprobamate (not more than 0.5%), and Organic volatile impurities.
Carisoprodol Tablets USP—Preserve in well-closed containers. Contain the labeled amount, within ±10%. Meet the requirements for Identification, Dissolution (80% in 60 minutes in 0.05 *M* phosphate buffer [pH 6.9] containing 5 units of alpha-amylase per mL in Apparatus 2 at 75 rpm), and Uniformity of dosage units.

CARISOPRODOL AND ASPIRIN

For *Carisoprodol* and *Aspirin*—See individual listings for chemistry information.

USP requirements: Carisoprodol and Aspirin Tablets USP—Preserve in well-closed containers. Contain the labeled amounts, within ±10%. Meet the requirements for Identification, Dissolution (75% of each active ingredient in 45 minutes in water in Apparatus 2 at 75 rpm), Uniformity of dosage units, and Limit of free salicylic acid (not more than 3.0%).

CARISOPRODOL, ASPIRIN, AND CODEINE

For *Carisoprodol, Aspirin,* and *Codeine*—See individual listings for chemistry information.

USP requirements: Carisoprodol, Aspirin, and Codeine Phosphate Tablets USP—Preserve in well-closed containers. Contain the labeled amounts, within ±10%. Meet the requirements for Identification, Dissolution (75% of each active ingredient in 45 minutes in water in Apparatus 2 at 75 rpm),

Uniformity of dosage units, and Limit of free salicylic acid (not more than 3.0%).

CARMUSTINE

Chemical name: Urea, *N,N'*-bis(2-chloroethyl)-*N*-nitroso-.

Molecular formula: $C_5H_9Cl_2N_3O_2$.

Molecular weight: 214.05.

Description: Lyophilized pale yellow flakes or congealed mass.

Solubility: Highly soluble in alcohol and lipids; poorly soluble in water.

USP requirements: Carmustine for Injection—Not in USP.

CARPHENAZINE

Chemical name: Carphenazine maleate—1-Propanone, 1-[10-[3-[4-(2-hydroxyethyl)-1-piperazinyl]propyl]-10*H*-phenothiazin-2-yl]-, (*Z*)-2-butenedioate (1:2).

Molecular formula: Carphenazine maleate—$C_{24}H_{31}N_3O_2S \cdot 2C_4H_4O_4$.

Molecular weight: Carphenazine maleate—657.73.

Description: Carphenazine Maleate USP—Yellow, finely divided powder. Is odorless, or has a slight odor.

Solubility: Carphenazine Maleate USP—Slightly soluble in water and in alcohol; practically insoluble in ether.

USP requirements:
Carphenazine Maleate USP—Preserve in tight, light-resistant containers. Contains not less than 98.0% and not more than 102.0% of carphenazine maleate, calculated on the anhydrous basis. Meets the requirements for Identification, Melting range (176–185 °C, with decomposition, but the range between beginning and end of melting is not more than 3 °C), pH (2.5–3.5, in a suspension [1 in 100]), Water (not more than 1.0%), Residue on ignition (not more than 0.2%), Heavy metals (not more than 0.0025%), and Ordinary impurities.
Carphenazine Maleate Oral Solution USP—Preserve in tight, light-resistant containers. Contains the labeled amount, within −5% to +10%. Meets the requirements for Identification and pH (5.8–6.8).

CARRAGEENAN

Chemical name: Carrageenan.

Description: Carrageenan NF—Yellowish or tan to white, coarse to fine powder. Practically odorless.
NF category: Suspending and/or viscosity-increasing agent.

Solubility: Carrageenan NF—Soluble in water at a temperature of about 80 °C, forming a viscous, clear or slightly opalescent solution that flows readily. Disperses in water more readily if first moistened with alcohol, glycerin, or a saturated solution of sucrose in water.

NF requirements: Carrageenan NF—Preserve in tight containers, preferably in a cool place. It is the hydrocolloid obtained by extraction with water or aqueous alkali from some members of the class *Rhodophyceae* (red seaweeds). It consists chiefly of potassium, sodium, calcium, magnesium, and ammonium sulfate esters of galactose and 3,6-anhydrogalactose copolymers, which are subclassified by slight structural differences. The ester sulfate content for Carrageenan is 18 to 40%. In addition, contains inorganic

salts that originate from the seaweed and from the process of recovery from the extract. Meets the requirements for Identification, Solubility in water (not more than 30 mL of water required to dissolve 1 gram at 80 °C), Viscosity (not less than 5 centipoises at 75 °C), Microbial limits, Loss on drying (not more than 12.5%), Acid-insoluble matter (not more than 2.0% of Carrageenan taken), Total ash (not more than 35.0%), Arsenic (not more than 3 ppm), Lead (not more than 0.001%), and Heavy metals (not more than 0.004%).

CARTEOLOL

Chemical name: Carteolol hydrochloride—2(1*H*)-Quinolinone, 5-[3-[(1,1-dimethylethyl)amino]-2-hydroxypropoxy]-3,4-dihydro-, monohydrochloride.

Molecular formula: Carteolol hydrochloride—$C_{16}H_{24}N_2O_3 \cdot HCL$.

Molecular weight: Carteolol hydrochloride—328.84.

Description: Carteolol hydrochloride—White crystalline powder.

pKa: 9.74.

Solubility: Carteolol hydrochloride—Soluble in water; slightly soluble in ethanol.

Other characteristics: Lipid solubility—Low.

USP requirements: Carteolol Hydrochloride Tablets—Not in USP.

CASANTHRANOL

Source: A purified mixture of the anthranol glycosides derived from *Cascara sagrada*.

Chemical group: Anthraquinones.

Description: Casanthranol USP—Light tan to brown, amorphous, hygroscopic powder.

Solubility: Casanthranol USP—Freely soluble in water, with some residue; partially soluble in methanol and in hot isopropyl alcohol; practically insoluble in acetone.

USP requirements:
Casanthranol USP—Preserve in tight, light-resistant containers, at a temperature not exceeding 30 °C. It is obtained from Cascara Sagrada. Contains in each 100 grams not less than 20.0 grams of total hydroxyanthracene derivatives, calculated on the dried basis, calculated as cascaroside A. Not less than 80.0% of the total hydroxyanthracene derivatives consists of cascarosides, calculated as cascaroside A. Meets the requirements for Loss on drying (not more than 10.0%), Residue on ignition (not more than 4.0%), and Heavy metals (not more than 0.0025%).
Casanthranol Syrup—Not in USP.

CASANTHRANOL AND DOCUSATE

For *Casanthranol* and *Docusate*—See individual listings for chemistry information.

USP requirements:
Casanthranol and Docusate Potassium Capsules—Not in USP.
Casanthranol and Docusate Sodium Capsules—Not in USP.
Casanthranol and Docusate Sodium Syrup—Not in USP.
Casanthranol and Docusate Sodium Tablets—Not in USP.

CASCARA SAGRADA

Source: Dried bark of *Rhamnus purshiana* (buckthorn tree); main active principles are cascarosides A and B (glycosides of barbaloin) and cascarosides C and D (glycosides of chrysaloin).

Chemical group: Anthraquinones.

Description: Cascara Sagrada USP—Has a distinct odor.

USP requirements:

Cascara Sagrada USP—The dried bark of *Rhamnus purshiana* De Candolle (Fam. Rhamnaceae). Yields not less than 7.0% of total hydroxyanthracene derivatives, calculated as cascaroside A, and calculated on the dried basis. Not less than 60% of the total hydroxyanthracene derivatives consists of cascarosides, calculated as cascaroside A. Meets the requirements for Botanic characteristics, Identification, Water (not more than 12.0%), and Foreign organic matter (not more than 4.0%).

Note: Collect Cascara Sagrada not less than one year prior to use.

Cascara Sagrada Extract USP—Preserve in tight, light-resistant containers, at a temperature not exceeding 30 °C. Contains, in each 100 grams, not less than 10.0 grams and not more than 12.0 grams of hydroxyanthracene derivatives, of which not less than 50.0% consists of cascarosides, both calculated as cascaroside A.

Prepare Cascara Sagrada Extract as follow: Mix 900 grams of Cascara Sagrada, in coarse powder, with 4000 mL of boiling water, and macerate the mixture for 3 hours. Then transfer it to a percolator, allow it to drain, exhaust it by percolation, using boiling water as the menstruum, and collect about 5000 mL of percolate. Evaporate the percolate to dryness, reduce the extract to a fine powder, and, after assaying, add sufficient starch, dried at 100 °C, or other inert, non-toxic diluents to make the product contain, in each 100 grams, 11 grams of hydroxyanthracene derivatives. Mix the powders, and pass the Extract through a number 60 sieve.

Cascara Tablets USP—Preserve in tight containers; if the Tablets are coated, well-closed containers may be used. They are prepared from Cascara Sagrada Extract. Contain an amount of hydroxyanthracene derivatives, calculated as cascaroside A, not less than 9.35% and not more than 12.65% of the labeled amount of Cascara Sagrada Extract. Not less than 50% of the hydroxyanthracene derivatives are cascarosides, calculated as cascaroside A. Meet the requirements for Disintegration (60 minutes) and Uniformity of dosage units.

Cascara Sagrada Fluidextract USP—Preserve in tight, light-resistant containers, and avoid exposure to direct sunlight and to excessive heat.

Prepare Cascara Sagrada Fluidextract as follows: To 1000 grams of coarsely ground Cascara Sagrada add 3000 mL of boiling water, mix, and allow to macerate in a suitable percolator for 2 hours. Allow the percolation to proceed at a moderate rate, gradually adding boiling water until the drug is practically exhausted of its active principles. Evaporate the percolate on a water bath or in a vacuum still to not more than 800 mL, cool, add 200 mL of alcohol and, if necessary, add sufficient water to make the product measure 1000 mL. Mix.

Meets the requirement for Alcohol content (18.0–20.0%).

Aromatic Cascara Fluidextract USP—Preserve in tight, light-resistant containers and avoid exposure to direct sunlight and to excessive heat.

Prepare Aromatic Cascara Fluidextract as follows: 1000 grams of Cascara Sagrada, in very coarse powder, 120 grams of Magnesium Oxide, Suitable sweetening agent(s), Suitable essential oils(s), Suitable flavoring agent(s), 200 mL of Alcohol, and a sufficient quantity of Purified Water, to make 1000 mL. Mix the Cascara Sagrada with the Magnesium Oxide, moisten it uniformly with 2000 mL of boiling water, and set it aside in a shallow container for 48 hours, stirring it occasionally. Pack it in a percolator, and percolate with boiling water until the drug is exhausted. Evaporate the percolate, at a temperature not exceeding 100 °C, to 750 mL, and at once dissolve in it the flavoring agent(s). When the liquid has cooled, add the Alcohol, in which the sweetening agent(s) and oils have been dissolved, add sufficient water to make the Aromatic Fluidextract measure 1000 mL, and mix.

Meets the requirement for Alcohol content (18.0–20.0%).

CASCARA SAGRADA AND ALOE

For *Cascara Sagrada* and *Aloe*—See individual listings for chemistry information.

USP requirements: Cascara Sagrada and Aloe Tablets—Not in USP.

CASCARA SAGRADA AND PHENOLPHTHALEIN

For *Cascara Sagrada* and *Phenolphthalein*—See individual listings for chemistry information.

USP requirements: Cascara Sagrada Extract and Phenolphthalein Tablets—Not in USP.

CASTOR OIL

Source: Fixed oil obtained from the seeds of *Ricinus communis*.

Chemical group: Glycerides.

Description:

Castor Oil USP—Pale yellowish or almost colorless, transparent, viscid liquid. It has a faint, mild odor; it is free from foreign and rancid odor.

NF category: Plasticizer.

Hydrogenated Castor Oil NF—White, crystalline wax.

NF category: Stiffening agent.

Solubility:

Castor Oil USP—Soluble in alcohol; miscible with dehydrated alcohol, with glacial acetic acid, with chloroform, and with ether.

Hydrogenated Castor Oil NF—Insoluble in water and in most common organic solvents.

USP requirements:

Castor Oil USP—Preserve in tight containers, and avoid exposure to excessive heat. The fixed oil obtained from the seed of *Ricinus communis* Linné (Fam. Euphorbiaceae). Contains no added substances. Meets the requirements for Specific gravity (0.957–0.961), Distinction from most other fixed oils, Heavy metals (not more than 0.001%), Free fatty acids (not more than 3.5 mL of 0.10 N sodium hydroxide to neutralize 10 grams), Hydroxyl value (160–168), Iodine value (83–88), and Saponification value (176–182).

Aromatic Castor Oil USP—Preserve in tight containers. It is Castor Oil containing suitable flavoring agents. Contains the labeled amount, within −5%. Meets the requirement for Alcohol content (not more than 4.0%).

Castor Oil Capsules USP—Preserve in tight containers, preferably at controlled room temperature. Contain the labeled amount, within ±10%, calculated from the tests for Weight variation and Specific gravity. Meet the requirements for Identification and Uniformity of dosage units, and for Specific gravity, Hydroxyl value, Iodine value, and Saponification value under Castor Oil.

Castor Oil Emulsion USP—Preserve in tight containers. Contains the labeled amount, within −10% to +20%. Meets the requirement for Identification.

NF requirements: Hydrogenated Castor Oil NF—Preserve in tight containers, and avoid exposure to excessive heat. It is refined, bleached, hydrogenated, and deodorized Castor Oil, consisting mainly of the triglyceride of hydroxystearic acid. Meets the requirements for Melting range (85–88 °C), Heavy metals (not more than 0.001%), Free fatty acids (not more than 11.0 mL of 0.1 N sodium hydroxide), Hydroxyl value (154–162), Iodine value (not more than 5), and Saponification value (176–182).

CEFACLOR

Source: Semisynthetic cephalosporin.

Chemical name: 5-Thia-1-azabicyclo[4.2.0]oct-2-ene-2-carboxylic acid, 7-[(aminophenylacetyl)amino]-3-chloro-8-oxo-, monohydrate, [6R-[6 alpha,7 beta(R*)]]-.

Molecular formula: $C_{15}H_{14}ClN_3O_4S \cdot H_2O$.

Molecular weight: 385.82.

Description: White, crystalline solid.

Solubility: Soluble in water (1 in 100); practically insoluble in most organic solvents.

Other characteristics: A 2.5% aqueous suspension has a pH of 3.0–4.5.

USP requirements:
Cefaclor USP—Preserve in tight containers. It has a potency of not less than 860 mcg and not more than 1050 mcg of anhydrous cefaclor per mg. Meets the requirements for Identification, Crystallinity, pH (3.0–4.5, in an aqueous suspension containing 25 mg per mL), and Water (3.0–8.0%).

Cefaclor Capsules USP—Preserve in tight containers. Contain an amount of cefaclor equivalent to the labeled amount of anhydrous cefaclor, within −10% to +20%. Meet the requirements for Identification, Uniformity of dosage units, and Water (not more than 8.0%).

Cefaclor for Oral Suspension USP—Preserve in tight containers. A dry mixture of Cefaclor and one or more suitable buffers, colors, diluents, and flavors. Contains an amount of cefaclor equivalent to the labeled amount of anhydrous cefaclor, within −10% to +20%. Meets the requirements for Identification, pH (2.5–5.0, in the suspension constituted as directed in the labeling), Uniformity of dosage units (solid packaged in single-unit containers), Deliverable volume (solid packaged in multiple-unit containers), and Water (not more than 2.0%).

CEFADROXIL

Source: Semisynthetic cephalosporin.

Chemical name: 5-Thia-1-azabicyclo[4.2.0]oct-2-ene-2-carboxylic acid, 7-[[amino(4-hydroxyphenyl)acetyl]amino]-3-methyl-8-oxo-, monohydrate, [6R-[6 alpha,7 beta(R*)]]-.

Molecular formula: $C_{16}H_{17}N_3O_5S \cdot H_2O$.

Molecular weight: 381.40.

Description: Cefadroxil USP—White to off-white, crystalline powder.

Solubility: Cefadroxil USP—Slightly soluble in water; practically insoluble in alcohol, in chloroform, and in ether.

Other characteristics: Acid-stable.

USP requirements:
Cefadroxil USP—Preserve in tight containers. It has a potency equivalent to not less than 900 mcg and not more than 1050 mcg of cefadroxil per mg, calculated on the anhydrous basis. Meets the requirements for Identification, Crystallinity, pH (4.0–6.0, in a suspension containing 50 mg per mL), and Water (4.2–6.0%).

Cefadroxil Capsules USP—Preserve in tight containers. Contain an amount of cefadroxil equivalent to the labeled amount of anhydrous cefadroxil, within −10% to +20%. Meet the requirements for Identification, Dissolution (75% in 45 minutes in water in Apparatus 1 at 100 rpm), Uniformity of dosage units, and Water (not more than 7.0%).

Cefadroxil for Oral Suspension USP—Preserve in tight containers. A dry mixture of Cefadroxil and one or more suitable buffers, colors, diluents, and flavors. Contains an amount of cefadroxil equivalent to the labeled amount of anhydrous cefadroxil, within −10% to +20%. Meets the requirements for Identification, pH (4.5–6.0, in the suspension constituted as directed in the labeling), Uniformity of dosage units (solid packaged in single-unit containers), Deliverable volume (solid packaged in multiple-unit containers), and Water (not more than 2.0%).

Cefadroxil Tablets USP—Preserve in tight containers. Contain an amount of cefadroxil equivalent to the labeled amount of anhydrous cefadroxil, within −10% to +20%. Meet the requirements for Identification, Dissolution (75% in 30 minutes in water in Apparatus 2 at 50 rpm), Uniformity of dosage units, and Water (not more than 8.0%).

CEFAMANDOLE

Source: Semisynthetic cephalosporin.

Chemical name:
Cefamandole nafate—5-Thia-1-azabicyclo[4.2.0]oct-2-ene-2-carboxylic acid, 7-[[(formyloxy)phenylacetyl]amino]-3-[[(1-methyl-1H-tetrazol-5-yl)thio]methyl]-8-oxo-, monosodium salt, [6R-[6 alpha,7 beta(R*)]].

Cefamandole sodium—5-Thia-1-azabicyclo[4.2.0]oct-2-ene-2-carboxylic acid, 7-[(hydroxyphenylacetyl)amino]-3-[[(1-methyl-1H-tetrazol-5-yl)thio]methyl]-8-oxo-, [6R-[6 alpha,7 beta(R*)]]-, monosodium salt.

Molecular formula:
Cefamandole nafate—$C_{19}H_{17}N_6NaO_6S_2$.
Cefamandole sodium—$C_{18}H_{17}N_6NaO_5S_2$.

Molecular weight:
Cefamandole nafate—512.49.
Cefamandole sodium—484.48.

Description:
Sterile Cefamandole Nafate USP—White, odorless, crystalline solid.

Cefamandole nafate for injection—After addition of diluent, cefamandole nafate rapidly hydrolyzes to cefamandole. Solutions of cefamandole nafate range from light yellow to amber, depending on concentration and diluent used.

Cefamandole Sodium USP—White to light yellowish-white, odorless crystalline powder.

Solubility:
Sterile Cefamandole Nafate USP—Soluble in water and in methanol; practically insoluble in ether, in chloroform, and in cyclohexane.

Cefamandole Sodium USP—Freely soluble in water and in dimethylformamide; soluble in methanol; slightly soluble in dehydrated alcohol; very slightly soluble in acetone.

Other characteristics: Cefamandole nafate—The pH of freshly reconstituted solutions usually ranges from 6.0 to 8.5.

USP requirements:

Cefamandole Nafate for Injection USP—Preserve in Containers for Sterile Solids. A sterile mixture of Sterile Cefamandole Nafate or cefamandole nafate and one or more suitable buffers. It has a potency equivalent to not less than 810 mcg and not more than 1000 mcg of cefamandole per mg, calculated on the anhydrous and sodium carbonate-free basis. Contains an amount of cefamandole nafate equivalent to the labeled amount of cefamandole, within −10% to +15%. Meets the requirements for Constituted solution, Identification, Bacterial endotoxins, Sterility, pH (6.0–8.0 [100 mg per mL after 30 minutes]), Water (not more than 3.0%), and Particulate matter, and for Uniformity of dosage units and Injections.

Sterile Cefamandole Nafate USP—Preserve in Containers for Sterile Solids. It is Cefamandole Nafate suitable for parenteral use. Contains an amount of cefamandole nafate equivalent to not less than 810 mcg and not more than 1000 mcg of cefamandole per mg, calculated on the anhydrous basis. Meets the requirements for Identification, Bacterial endotoxins, Sterility, pH (3.5–7.0, in a solution containing 100 mg per mL), and Water (not more than 2.0%).

Cefamandole Sodium for Injection USP—Preserve in Containers for Sterile Solids. A sterile mixture of Sterile Cefamandole Sodium and one or more suitable buffers. Contains an amount of cefamandole sodium equivalent to the labeled amount of cefamandole, within −10% to +15%. Meets the requirements for Constituted solution, Identification, Bacterial endotoxins, Sterility, pH (6.0–8.5, in a solution containing 100 mg of cefamandole per mL), Water (not more than 3.0%), and Particulate matter, and for Uniformity of dosage units and Labeling under Injections.

Sterile Cefamandole Sodium USP—Preserve in Containers for Sterile Solids. It has a potency equivalent to not less than 860 mcg and not more than 1000 mcg of cefamandole per mg, calculated on the anhydrous basis. Meets the requirements for Identification, Bacterial endotoxins, Sterility, pH (3.5–7.0, in a solution [1 in 10]), Water (not more than 3.0%), and Particulate matter.

CEFAZOLIN

Source: Semisynthetic cephalosporin.

Chemical name:

Cefazolin—5-Thia-1-azabicyclo[4.2.0]oct-2-ene-2-carboxylic acid, 3-[[(5-methyl-1,3,4-thiadiazol-2-yl)thio]methyl]-8-oxo-7-[[1*H*-tetrazol-1-yl)acetyl]amino]-(6*R-trans*).

Cefazolin sodium—5-Thia-1-azabicyclo[4.2.0]oct-2-ene-2-carboxylic acid, 3-[[(5-methyl-1,3,4-thiadiazol-2-yl)thio]methyl]-8-oxo-7-[[(1*H*-tetrazol-1-yl)acetyl]amino]-, monosodium salt (6*R-trans*)-.

Molecular formula:

Cefazolin—$C_{14}H_{14}N_8O_4S_3$.

Cefazolin sodium—$C_{14}H_{13}N_8NaO_4S_3$.

Molecular weight:

Cefazolin—454.50.

Cefazolin sodium—476.48.

Description:

Cefazolin—Melting point 198–200 °C.

Cefazolin sodium—White to off-white, almost odorless, crystalline powder.

Sterile Cefazolin Sodium USP—White to off-white, practically odorless, crystalline powder, or white to off-white solid having the characteristic appearance of products prepared by freeze-drying.

Solubility:

Cefazolin—Easily soluble in dimethylformamide, and in pyridine; soluble in aqueous acetone, in aqueous dioxane, and in aqueous ethanol; slightly soluble in methanol; practically insoluble in chloroform and in ether.

Cefazolin sodium—Freely soluble in water, in 0.9% sodium chloride solution, and in glucose solutions; very slightly soluble in alcohol; practically insoluble in ether and in chloroform.

Sterile Cefazolin Sodium USP—Freely soluble in water, in saline TS, and in dextrose solutions; very slightly soluble in alcohol; practically insoluble in chloroform and in ether.

Other characteristics: A 10% solution in water has a pH of 4.5 to 6.0.

USP requirements:

Cefazolin USP—Preserve in tight containers. Contains not less than 950 mcg and not more than 1030 mcg of cefazolin per mg, calculated on the anhydrous basis. Meets the requirements for Identification, Water (not more than 2.0%), and Heavy metals (not more than 0.002%).

Cefazolin Sodium Injection USP—Preserve in Containers for Injections. Maintain in the frozen state. A sterile solution of Cefazolin and Sodium Bicarbonate diluted with a suitable isoosmotic diluent. It meets the requirements for Labeling under Injections. The label states that it is to be thawed just prior to use, describes conditions for proper storage of the resultant solution, and directs that the solution is not to be refrozen. Contains an amount of cefazolin sodium equivalent to the labeled amount of cefazolin, within −10% to +15%. Meets the requirements for Identification, Bacterial endotoxins, Sterility, pH (4.5–7.0), and Particulate matter.

Sterile Cefazolin Sodium USP—Preserve in Containers for Sterile Solids. Contains an amount of cefazolin sodium equivalent to not less than 850 mcg and not more than 1050 mcg of cefazolin per mg, calculated on the anhydrous basis, and, where packaged for dispensing, contains an amount of cefazolin sodium equivalent to the labeled amount of cefazolin, within −10% to +15%. Meets the requirements for Constituted solution, Identification, Specific rotation (−24° to −10°), Bacterial endotoxins, Sterility, pH (4.5–6.0 in a solution containing 100 mg of cefazolin per mL), Water (not more than 6.0%), and Particulate matter, and for Uniformity of dosage units and Labeling under Injections.

CEFIXIME

Chemical name: 5-Thia-1-azabicyclo[4.2.0]oct-2-ene-2-carboxylic acid, 7-[[(2-amino-4-thiazolyl)[(carboxymethoxy)imino]acetyl]amino]-3-ethenyl-8-oxo-, trihydrate, [6*R*-[6 alpha, 7 beta(*Z*)]]-.

Molecular formula: $C_{16}H_{15}N_5O_7S_2 \cdot 3H_2O$.

Molecular weight: 507.49.

Description: Cefixime USP—White to light yellow, crystalline powder.

Solubility: Cefixime USP—Very soluble in water, in alcohol, in glycerin, and in propylene glycol; freely soluble in 70% sorbitol and in octanol.

USP requirements:

Cefixime USP—Preserve in tight containers. Label to indicate that it is the trihydrate form. Where the quantity of cefixime is indicated in the labeling of any preparation containing Cefixime, this shall be understood to be in terms of anhydrous cefixime. Contains the equivalent of not less than 950 mcg and not more than 1030 mcg of cefixime per mg, calculated on the anhydrous basis. Meets the requirements for Identification, Specific rotation (−75° to −88°, calculated on the anhydrous basis), Crystallinity, pH (2.6–4.1, in a solution containing the equivalent of 0.7 mg of cefixime per mL), and Water (9.0–12.0%).

Cefixime for Oral Suspension USP—Preserve in tight containers. A dry mixture of Cefixime and one or more suitable diluents, flavors, preservatives, and suspending agents. Label it to indicate that the cefixime contained therein is in the trihydrate form. Contains the labeled amount of anhydrous cefixime, within −10% to +20%, per mL when constituted as directed in the labeling. Meets the requirements for Identification, Uniformity of dosage units (solid packaged in single-unit containers), Deliverable volume (solid packaged in multiple-unit containers), pH (2.5–4.5, in the suspension constituted as directed in the labeling), and Water (not more than 2.0%).

Cefixime Tablets USP—Preserve in tight containers. Label Tablets to indicate that the cefixime contained therein is in the trihydrate form. Contain the labeled amount of anhydrous cefixime, within ±10%. Meet the requirements for Identification, Dissolution (75% in 45 minutes in 0.05 *M* potassium phosphate buffer [pH 7.2] in Apparatus 1 at 100 rpm), Uniformity of dosage units, and Water (not more than 10.0%).

CEFMENOXIME

Chemical name: Cefmenoxime hydrochloride—5-Thia-1-azabicyclo[4.2.0]oct-2-ene-2-carboxylic acid, 7-[[[(2-amino-4-thiazolyl)(methoxyimino)acetyl]amino]-3-[[[(1-methyl-1*H*-tetrazol-5-yl)thio]methyl]-8-oxo-, hydrochloride (2:1), [6*R*-[6 alpha,7 beta(*Z*)]]-.

Molecular formula: Cefmenoxime hydrochloride—$(C_{16}H_{17}N_9O_5S_3)_2 \cdot HCl$.

Molecular weight: Cefmenoxime hydrochloride—1059.56.

USP requirements:

Cefmenoxime for Injection USP—Preserve in Containers for Sterile Solids. A sterile mixture of Sterile Cefmenoxime Hydrochloride and Sodium Carbonate. Contains not less than 869 mcg and not more than 1015 mcg of cefmenoxime per mg, calculated on the dried and sodium carbonate-free basis, and the labeled amount of cefmenoxime, within −10% to +15%. Meets the requirements for Identification, Pyrogen, Sterility, pH (6.4–7.9, in a solution containing the equivalent of 100 mg of cefmenoxime per mL), Loss on drying (not more than 1.5%), Particulate matter, and Sodium carbonate content.

Sterile Cefmenoxime Hydrochloride USP—Preserve in Containers for Sterile Solids. It is Cefmenoxime Hydrochloride suitable for parenteral use. Contains an amount of cefmenoxime hydrochloride equivalent to not less than 869 mcg and not more than 1015 mcg of cefmenoxime per mg, calculated on the anhydrous basis. Meets the requirements for Identification, Crystallinity, Pyrogen, Sterility, and Water (not more than 1.5%).

CEFMETAZOLE

Chemical name: Cefmetazole sodium—5-Thia-1-azabicyclo[4.2.0]oct-2-ene-2-carboxylic acid, 7-[[[(cyanomethyl)thio]acetyl]amino]-7-methoxy-3-[[(1-methyl-1*H*-tetrazol-5-yl)thio]methyl]-8-oxo-, monosodium salt, (6*R-cis*)-.

Molecular formula: Cefmetazole sodium—$C_{15}H_{16}N_7NaO_5S_3$.

Molecular weight: Cefmetazole sodium—493.51.

Description: Sterile Cefmetazole Sodium USP—White solid having the characteristic appearance of products prepared by freeze-drying.

Solubility: Sterile Cefmetazole Sodium USP—Very soluble in water and in methanol; soluble in acetone; practically insoluble in chloroform.

USP requirements:

Sterile Cefmetazole Sodium USP—Preserve in Containers for Sterile Solids. Contains the equivalent of not less than 860 mcg and not more than 1003 mcg of cefmetazole per mg, calculated on the anhydrous basis. In addition, where packaged for dispensing, contains an amount of cefmetazole sodium equivalent to the labeled amount of cefmetazole, within −10% to +20%. Meets the requirements for Identification, Bacterial endotoxins, Sterility, pH (4.2–6.2, in a solution [1 in 10]), Water (not more than 0.5%), and Particulate matter, and for Uniformity of dosage units, and for Labeling under Injections.

Cefmetazole Sodium for Injection—Not in USP.

CEFONICID

Source: Semisynthetic cephalosporin.

Chemical name: Cefonicid sodium—5-Thia-1-azabicyclo[4.2.0]oct-2-ene-2-carboxylic acid, 7-[(hydroxyphenylacetyl)amino]-8-oxo-3-[[[1-(sulfomethyl)-1*H*-tetrazol-5-yl]thio]methyl]disodium salt, [6*R*-[6 alpha,7 beta(*R**)]].

Molecular formula: Cefonicid sodium—$C_{18}H_{16}N_6Na_2O_8S_3$.

Molecular weight: Cefonicid sodium—586.52.

Description: Sterile Cefonicid Sodium USP—White to off-white solid having the characteristic appearance of products prepared by freeze-drying.

Solubility: Sterile Cefonicid Sodium USP—Freely soluble in water, in 0.9% sodium chloride solution, and in 5% dextrose solution; soluble in methanol; very slightly soluble in dehydrated alcohol.

USP requirements: Sterile Cefonicid Sodium USP—Preserve in Containers for Sterile Solids. It is cefonicid sodium suitable for parenteral use. Contains an amount of cefonicid sodium equivalent to not less than 832 mcg and not more than 970 mcg of cefonicid per mg, calculated on the anhydrous basis, and, where packaged for dispensing, contains an amount of cefonicid sodium equivalent to the labeled amount of cefonicid, within −10% to +20%. Meets the requirements for Constituted solution, Identification, Bacterial endotoxins, Sterility, Specific rotation (−37° to −47°, calculated on the anhydrous basis), pH (3.5–6.5, in a solution [1 in 20]), Water (not more than 5.0%), and Particulate matter, and for Uniformity of dosage units and for Labeling under Injections.

CEFOPERAZONE

Source: Semisynthetic cephalosporin.

Chemical name: Cefoperazone sodium—5-Thia-1-azabicyclo[4.2.0]oct-2-ene-2-carboxylic acid, 7-[[[[(4-ethyl-2,3-dioxo-1-piperazinyl)carbonyl]amino](4-hydroxyphenyl)acetyl]amino]-3-[[(1-methyl-1*H*-tetrazol-5-yl)thio]methyl]-8-oxo, monosodium salt, [6*R*-[6 alpha,7 beta(*R**)]]-.

Molecular formula: Cefoperazone sodium—$C_{25}H_{26}N_9NaO_8S_2$.

Molecular weight: Cefoperazone sodium—667.65.

Description:
Cefoperazone Sodium USP—White to pale buff crystalline powder.

Sterile Cefoperazone Sodium USP—White to pale buff, crystalline powder or white to pale buff solid having the characteristic appearance of products prepared by freeze-drying.

Solubility:
Cefoperazone Sodium USP—Freely soluble in water and in methanol; slightly soluble in dehydrated alcohol; insoluble in acetone, in ethyl acetate, and in ether.

Sterile Cefoperazone Sodium USP—Freely soluble in water, in sodium chloride solution, and in dextrose solution.

USP requirements:
Cefoperazone Sodium USP—Preserve in tight containers. Contains the equivalent of not less than 870 mcg and not more than 1015 mcg of cefoperazone per mg, calculated on the anhydrous basis. Meets the requirements for Identification, Crystallinity (Note: Cefoperazone Sodium in the freeze-dried form is exempt from this requirement), pH (4.5–6.5, in a solution [1 in 4]), and Water (not more than 5.0%, except that where it is in the freeze-dried form, the limit is not more than 2.0%).

Cefoperazone Sodium Injection USP—Preserve in Containers for Injections. Maintain in the frozen state. A sterile solution of Cefoperazone Sodium and a suitable osmolality-adjusting substance in Water for Injection. Meets the requirements for Labeling under Injections. The label states that it is to be thawed just prior to use, describes conditions for proper storage of the resultant solution, and directs that the solution is not to be refrozen. Contains an amount of cefoperazone sodium equivalent to the labeled amount of cefoperazone, within −10% to +20%. Meets the requirements for Identification, Pyrogen, Sterility, pH (4.5–6.5), and Particulate matter.

Sterile Cefoperazone Sodium USP—Preserve in Containers for Sterile Solids. It is Cefoperazone Sodium suitable for parenteral use. Contains an amount of cefoperazone sodium equivalent to not less than 870 mcg and not more than 1015 mcg of cefoperazone per mg, calculated on the anhydrous basis, and where packaged for dispensing, contains an amount of cefoperazone sodium equivalent to the labeled amount of cefoperazone, within −10% to +20%. Meets the requirements for Constituted solution, Identification, Crystallinity (Note: Sterile Cefoperazone Sodium packaged for dispensing in the freeze-dried form is exempt from this requirement), Bacterial endotoxins, Sterility, pH (4.5–6.5 in a solution [1 in 4]), Water (not more than 5.0%; where packaged for dispensing in the freeze-dried form, not more than 2.0%), and Particulate matter, and for Uniformity of dosage units and for Labeling under Injections.

CEFORANIDE

Source: Semisynthetic cephalosporin.

Chemical name: 5-Thia-1-azabicyclo[4.2.0]oct-2-ene-2-carboxylic acid, 7-[[[2-(aminomethyl)phenyl]acetyl]amino]-3-[[[1-(carboxymethyl)-1*H*-tetrazol-5-yl]thio]methyl]-8-oxo-, (6*R*-trans)-.

Molecular formula: $C_{20}H_{21}N_7O_6S_2$.

Molecular weight: 519.55.

Description:
Ceforanide for injection—Solutions of ceforanide range in color from light yellow to amber depending on the concentration and diluent used.

Sterile Ceforanide USP—White to off-white powder.

Solubility: Sterile Ceforanide USP—Practically insoluble in water, in methanol, in chloroform, and in ether; very soluble in 1 *N* sodium hydroxide.

Other characteristics: Ceforanide for injection—The pH of the solution ranges from 5.5 to 8.5.

USP requirements:
Ceforanide for Injection USP—Preserve in Containers for Sterile Solids. A sterile mixture of Sterile Ceforanide and L-Lysine. Contains not less than 900 mcg and not more than 1050 mcg of ceforanide per mg on the L-Lysine-free basis, and the labeled amount, within −10% to +15%. Meets the requirements for Identification, Bacterial endotoxins, Sterility, pH (5.5–8.5, constituted as directed in the labeling), Water (not more than 3.0%), Particulate matter, and L-Lysine content, and for Uniformity of dosage units and for Labeling under Injections.

Sterile Ceforanide USP—Preserve in Containers for Sterile Solids. It is ceforanide suitable for parenteral use. Contains not less than 900 mcg and not more than 1050 mcg of ceforanide per mg. Meets the requirements for Identification, Bacterial endotoxins, Sterility, pH (2.5–4.5, in a suspension containing 50 mg per mL), and Water (not more than 5.0%).

CEFOTAXIME

Source: Semisynthetic cephalosporin.

Chemical name: Cefotaxime sodium—5-Thia-1-azabicyclo[4.2.0]oct-2-ene-2-carboxylic acid, 3-[(acetyloxy)methyl]-7-[[(2-amino-4-thiazolyl)(methoxyimino)acetyl]amino]-8-oxo-, monosodium salt, [6*R*-[6 alpha,7 beta(*Z*)]]-.

Molecular formula: Cefotaxime sodium—$C_{16}H_{16}N_5NaO_7S_2$.

Molecular weight: Cefotaxime sodium—477.44.

Description:
Cefotaxime Sodium USP—Off-white to pale yellow crystalline powder.

Cefotaxime sodium injection—Solutions of cefotaxime sodium range from very pale yellow to light amber depending on the concentration and the diluent used.

Solubility: Cefotaxime Sodium USP—Freely soluble in water; practically insoluble in organic solvents.

Other characteristics: Cefotaxime sodium injection—Has a pH of 5.0–7.5.

USP requirements:
Cefotaxime Sodium USP—Preserve in tight containers. Contains an amount of cefotaxime sodium equivalent to not less than 855 mcg and not more than 1002 mcg of cefotaxime per mg, calculated on the anhydrous basis. Meets the requirements for Identification, pH (4.5–6.5, in a solution [1 in 10]), and Water (not more than 6.0%).

Cefotaxime Sodium Injection USP—Preserve in single-dose containers. Maintain in the frozen state. A sterile solution of Cefotaxime Sodium in Water for Injection. Contains one or more suitable buffers. Meets the requirements for Labeling under Injections. The label states that it is to be thawed just prior to use, describes conditions for proper storage of the resultant solution, and directs that the solution is not to be refrozen. Contains an amount of cefotaxime sodium equivalent to the labeled amount of cefotaxime, within ±10%. Meets the requirements for Identification, Bacterial endotoxins, Sterility, pH (5.0–7.5), and Particulate matter.

Sterile Cefotaxime Sodium USP—Preserve in Containers for Sterile Solids. It is Cefotaxime Sodium suitable for parenteral use. Contains an amount of cefotaxime sodium equivalent to not less than 855 mcg and not more than 1002 mcg of cefotaxime per mg, calculated on the anhydrous basis and, where packaged for dispensing, contains an amount of cefotaxime sodium equivalent to the labeled amount of cefotaxime, within ± 10%. Meets the requirements for Constituted solution, Bacterial endotoxins, Sterility, and Particulate matter, and for Identification tests, pH, and Water under Cefotaxime Sodium. In addition, where packaged for dispensing, it meets the requirements for Uniformity of dosage units and for Labeling under Injections.

CEFOTETAN

Source: Semisynthetic cephamycin.

Chemical name: Cefotetan disodium—5-Thia-1-azabicyclo[4.2.0]-oct-2-ene-2-carboxylic acid, 7-[[[4-(2-amino-1-carboxy-2-oxoethylidene)-1,3-dithietan-2-yl]carbonyl]amino]-7-methoxy-3-[[(1-methyl-1H-tetrazol-5-yl)thio]methyl]-8-oxo-, disodium salt, [6R-(6 alpha,7 alpha)]-.

Molecular formula: Cefotetan disodium—$C_{17}H_{15}N_7Na_2O_8S_4$.

Molecular weight: Cefotetan disodium—619.57.

Description:
Cefotetan disodium—White to pale yellow powder.
Cefotetan disodium injection—Solution varies from colorless to yellow, depending on the concentration.

Solubility: Cefotetan disodium—Very soluble in water.

Other characteristics: Cefotetan disodium—The pH of freshly reconstituted solutions is usually between 4.5 and 6.5.

USP requirements: Sterile Cefotetan Disodium USP—Preserve in Containers for Sterile Solids. It is Cefotetan Disodium suitable for parenteral use. Contains an amount of cefotetan disodium equivalent to not less than 830 mcg and not more than 970 mcg of cefotetan per mg, calculated on the anhydrous basis, and, where packaged for dispensing, contains an amount of cefotetan disodium equivalent to the labeled amount of cefotetan, within −10% to +20%. Meets the requirements for Constituted solution, Identification, Bacterial endotoxins, Sterility, pH (4.0–6.5, in a solution [1 in 10]), Water (not more than 1.5%), and Particulate matter, and for Uniformity of dosage units, and for Labeling under Injections.

CEFOTIAM

Chemical name: Cefotiam hydrochloride—5-Thia-1-azabicyclo[4.2.0]oct-2-ene-2-carboxylic acid, 7-[[(2-amino-4-thiazolyl)acetyl]-amino]-3-[[[1-[2-(dimethylamino)ethyl]-1H-tetrazol-5-yl]thio]methyl]-8-oxo, hydrochloride, (6R-trans)-.

Molecular formula: Cefotiam hydrochloride—$C_{18}H_{23}N_9O_4S_3\cdot$2HCl.

Molecular weight: Cefotiam hydrochloride—598.54.

Description: Cefotiam hydrochloride—White to light yellow crystals.

Solubility: Cefotiam hydrochloride—Soluble in methanol; slightly soluble in ethanol.

USP requirements:
Cefotiam for Injection USP—Preserve in Containers for Sterile Solids. A sterile mixture of Sterile Cefotiam Hydrochloride and Sodium Carbonate. Contains not less than

790 mcg and not more than 925 mcg of cefotiam per mg, calculated on the dried and sodium carbonate-free basis, and the labeled amount of cefotiam, within −10% to +20%. Meets the requirements for Identification, Pyrogen, Sterility, pH (5.7–7.2, in a solution containing the equivalent of 100 mg of cefotiam per mL), Loss on drying (not more than 6.0%), Particulate matter, and Sodium carbonate content.
Sterile Cefotiam Hydrochloride USP—Preserve in Containers for Sterile Solids. It is cefotiam hydrochloride suitable for parenteral use. Contains the equivalent of not less than 790 mcg and not more than 925 mcg of cefotiam per mg, calculated on the anhydrous basis. Meets the requirements for Identification, Crystallinity, Pyrogen, Sterility, and Water (not more than 7.0%).

CEFOXITIN

Source: Cefoxitin sodium—Semisynthetic cephamycin derived from cephamycin C, produced by *Streptomyces lactamdurans.*

Chemical name: Cefoxitin sodium—5-Thia-1-azabicyclo[4.2.0]-oct-2-ene-2-carboxylic acid, 3-[[(aminocarbonyl)oxy]methyl]-7-methoxy-8-oxo-7-[(2-thienylacetyl)amino]-, sodium salt, (6R-cis)-.

Molecular formula: Cefoxitin sodium—$C_{16}H_{16}N_3NaO_7S_2$.

Molecular weight: Cefoxitin sodium—449.43.

Description: Sterile Cefoxitin Sodium USP—White to off-white, granules or powder, having a slight characteristic odor. Is somewhat hygroscopic.

Solubility: Sterile Cefoxitin Sodium USP—Very soluble in water; soluble in methanol; sparingly soluble in dimethylformamide; slightly soluble in acetone; insoluble in ether and in chloroform.

USP requirements:
Cefoxitin Sodium USP—Preserve in tight containers. Contains an amount of cefoxitin sodium equivalent to not less than 927 mcg and not more than 970 mcg of cefoxitin per mg, corresponding to not less than 97.5% and not more than 102.0% of cefoxitin sodium, calculated on the anhydrous and acetone- and methanol-free basis. Meets the requirements for Identification, Specific rotation (+206° to +214°, calculated on the anhydrous and acetone- and methanol-free basis), Crystallinity, pH (4.2–7.0, in a solution containing 100 mg per mL), Water (not more than 1.0%), Heavy metals (not more than 0.002%), and Acetone and methanol (not more than 0.7% of acetone and 0.1% of methanol).
Cefoxitin Sodium Injection USP—Preserve in Containers for Injections. Maintain in the frozen state. A sterile solution of Cefoxitin Sodium and one or more suitable buffer substances in Water for Injection. Contains Dextrose or Sodium Chloride as a tonicity-adjusting agent. Meets the requirements for Labeling under Injections. The label states that it is to be thawed just prior to use, describes conditions for proper storage of the resultant solution, and directs that the solution is not to be refrozen. Contains an amount of cefoxitin sodium equivalent to the labeled amount of cefoxitin, within −10% to +20%. Meets the requirements for Identification, Bacterial endotoxins, Sterility, pH (4.5–8.0), and Particulate matter.
Sterile Cefoxitin Sodium USP—Preserve in Containers for Sterile Solids. Contains an amount of cefoxitin sodium equivalent to not less than 927 mcg and not more than 970 mcg of cefoxitin per mg, corresponding to not less than 97.5% and not more than 102.0% of cefoxitin sodium, calculated on the anhydrous and acetone- and

methanol-free basis and, where packaged for dispensing, contains an amount of cefoxitin sodium equivalent to the labeled amount of cefoxitin, within -10% to $+20\%$. Meets the requirements for Constituted solution, Bacterial endotoxins, Sterility, and Particulate matter, and for Identification tests, Specific rotation, Crystallinity, pH, Water, Heavy metals, and Acetone and methanol under Cefoxitin Sodium. In addition, where packaged for dispensing, meets the requirements for Uniformity of dosage units and for Labeling under Injections.

CEFPIRAMIDE

Chemical name: 5-Thia-1-azabicyclo[4.2.0]oct-2-ene-2-carboxylic acid, 7-[[[[(4-hydroxy-6-methyl-3-pyridinyl)-carbonyl]amino](4-hydroxyphenyl)acetyl]amino]-3-[[(1-methyl-1*H*-tetrazol-5-yl)thio]methyl]-8-oxo-, [6*R*-[6 alpha,7 beta(*R**)]]-.

Molecular formula: $C_{25}H_{24}N_8O_7S_2$.

Molecular weight: 612.63.

Description: Yellow crystals. Melting point is 213–215 °C.

USP requirements:
Cefpiramide USP—Preserve in tight containers. Contains the equivalent of not less than 974 mcg and not more than 1026 mcg of cefpiramide per mg, calculated on the anhydrous basis. Meets the requirements for Identification, Specific rotation ($-100°$ to $-112°$, calculated on the anhydrous basis), Crystallinity, pH (3.0–5.0, in a suspension [1 in 200]), Water (not more than 9.0%), and Related substances (not more than 2.0%).
Cefpiramide for Injection USP—Preserve in Containers for Sterile Solids. A sterile mixture of Cefpiramide, Sodium Benzoate, and other buffers and preservatives. Contains not less than 754 mcg and not more than 924 mcg of cefpiramide per mg, calculated on the anhydrous basis, and where packaged for dispensing contains the labeled amount, within -10% to $+20\%$. Meets the requirements for Identification, Pyrogen, Sterility, pH (6.0–8.0, in a solution containing the equivalent of 100 mg of cefpiramide per mL), Water (not more than 3.0%), and Particulate matter.

CEFPROZIL

Source: Semisynthetic cephalosporin.

Chemical name: 5-Thia-1-azabicyclo[4.2.0]oct-2-ene-2-carboxylic acid, 7-[[amino(4-hydroxyphenyl)acetyl]amino]-8-oxo-3-(1-propenyl)-, [6*R*-[6 alpha,7 beta(*R**)]]-.

Molecular formula: $C_{18}H_{19}N_3O_5S$.

Molecular weight: 389.43.

Description: White to yellowish powder.

USP requirements:
Cefprozil Oral Suspension—Not in USP.
Cefprozil Tablets—Not in USP.

CEFTAZIDIME

Source: Semisynthetic cephalosporin.

Chemical name: Pyridinium, 1-[[7-[[(2-amino-4-thiazolyl)[(1-carboxy-1-methylethoxy)imino]acetyl]amino]-2-carboxy-8-oxo-5-thia-1-azabicyclo[4.2.0]oct-2-en-3-yl]methyl]-, hydroxide, inner salt, pentahydrate, [6*R*-[6 alpha,7 beta(*Z*)]]-.

Molecular formula: $C_{22}H_{22}N_6O_7S_2 \cdot 5H_2O$.

Molecular weight: 636.65.

Description: Ceftazidime for injection—Solutions of ceftazidime range in color from light yellow to amber, depending upon the diluent and volume used.

Other characteristics: Ceftazidime for injection—The pH of freshly constituted solutions usually ranges from 5 to 8.

USP requirements:
Ceftazidime USP—Preserve in tight containers. Contains not less than 95.0% and not more than 102.0% of ceftazidime, calculated on the dried basis. Meets the requirements for Identification, Crystallinity, pH (3.0–4.0, in a solution containing 5 mg per mL), Loss on drying (13.0–15.0%), and High molecular weight ceftazidime polymer (not more than 0.05%).
Ceftazidime Injection USP—Preserve in Containers for Injections. Maintain in the frozen state. A sterile isoosmotic solution of Ceftazidime in Water for Injection. Meets the requirements for Labeling under Injections. The label states that it is to be thawed just prior to use, describes conditions for proper storage of the resultant solution, and directs that the solution is not to be refrozen. Contains one or more suitable buffers and a tonicity-adjusting agent. Contains an amount equivalent to the labeled amount of anhydrous ceftazidime, within -10% to $+20\%$. Meets the requirements for Identification, Pyrogen, Sterility, pH (5.0–7.5), and Particulate matter.
Ceftazidime for Injection USP—Preserve in Containers for Sterile Solids, protected from light. A sterile mixture of Sterile Ceftazidime and Sodium Carbonate. Contains not less than 90.0% and not more than 105.0% of ceftazidime, on the dried and sodium carbonate-free basis, and contains an amount equivalent to the labeled amount of anhydrous ceftazidine, within -10% to $+20\%$. Meets the requirements for Identification, Bacterial endotoxins, Sterility, pH (5.0–7.5 [100 mg per mL constituted in the sealed container, taking care to relieve the pressure inside the container during constitution]), Loss on drying (not more than 13.5%), Particulate matter, Sodium carbonate, and High molecular weight ceftazidime polymer (not more than 0.4%), and for Uniformity of dosage units and Labeling under Injections.
Sterile Ceftazidime USP—Preserve in Containers for Sterile Solids, protected from light. It is ceftazidime pentahydrate suitable for parenteral use. Contains the labeled amount of ceftazidime, within -5% to $+2\%$, calculated on the dried basis. Meets the requirements for Bacterial endotoxins and Sterility, and for Identification test, Crystallinity, pH, Loss on drying, and High molecular weight ceftazidime polymer under Ceftazidime. In addition, where packaged for dispensing, meets the requirements for Uniformity of dosage units and for Labeling under Injections.

CEFTIZOXIME

Source: Semisynthetic cephalosporin.

Chemical name: Ceftizoxime sodium—5-Thia-1-azabicyclo[4.2.0]oct-2-ene-2-carboxylic acid, 7-[[(2,3-dihydro-2-imino-4-thiazolyl)(methoxyimino)acetyl]amino]-8-oxomono-sodium salt, [6*R*-[6 alpha,7 beta(*Z*)]]-.

Molecular formula: Ceftizoxime sodium—$C_{13}H_{12}N_5NaO_5S_2$.

Molecular weight: Ceftizoxime sodium—405.38.

Description:
Ceftizoxime Sodium USP—White to pale yellow crystalline powder.

Sterile ceftizoxime sodium—White to pale yellow crystalline powder.

Solubility: Ceftizoxime Sodium USP—Freely soluble in water.

Other characteristics: Ceftizoxime sodium—A 10% solution in water has a pH of 6 to 8. The USP injection has a pH of 5.5 to 8.0.

USP requirements:
Ceftizoxime Sodium USP—Preserve in tight containers. Contains an amount of ceftizoxime sodium equivalent to not less than 850 mcg and not more than 995 mcg of ceftizoxime per mg, calculated on the anhydrous basis. Meets the requirements for Identification, Crystallinity, pH (6.0–8.0, in a solution [1 in 10]), and Water (not more than 8.5%).

Ceftizoxime Sodium Injection USP—Preserve in Containers for Injections. Maintain in the frozen state. A sterile solution of Ceftizoxime Sodium in a suitable isoosmotic diluent. It meets the requirements for Labeling under Injections. The label states that it is to be thawed just prior to use, describes conditions for proper storage of the resultant solution, and directs that the solution is not to be refrozen. Contains an amount of ceftizoxime sodium equivalent to the labeled amount of ceftizoxime, within −10% to +15%. Meets the requirements for Identification, Bacterial endotoxins, Sterility, pH (5.5–8.0), and Particulate matter.

Sterile Ceftizoxime Sodium USP—Preserve in Containers for Sterile Solids. It is ceftizoxime sodium suitable for parenteral use. Contains an amount of ceftizoxime sodium equivalent to not less than 850 mcg and not more than 995 mcg of ceftizoxime per mg, calculated on the anhydrous basis and, where packaged for dispensing, contains an amount of ceftizoxime sodium equivalent to the labeled amount of ceftizoxime, within −10% to +15%. Meets the requirements for Constituted solution, Identification, Crystallinity, Bacterial endotoxins, Sterility, pH (6.0–8.0 in a solution [1 in 10]), Water (not more than 8.5%), and Particulate matter, and for Uniformity of dosage units and Labeling under Injections.

CEFTRIAXONE

Source: Semisynthetic cephalosporin.

Chemical name: Ceftriaxone sodium—5-Thia-1-azabicyclo[4.2.0]oct-2-ene-2-carboxylic acid, 7-[[(2-amino-4-thiazolyl)(methoxyimino)acetyl]amino]-8-oxo-3-[[(1,2,5,6-tetrahydro-2-methyl-5,6-dioxo-1,2,4-triazin-3-yl)thio]methyl]-, disodium salt, [6R-[6 alpha,7 beta(Z)]]-, hydrate (2:7).

Molecular formula: Ceftriaxone sodium—$C_{18}H_{16}N_8Na_2O_7S_3$ (anhydrous).

Molecular weight: Ceftriaxone sodium—598.53 (anhydrous).

Description:
Ceftriaxone sodium—White to yellowish-orange crystalline powder.

Ceftriaxone injection—The color of ceftriaxone sodium solution ranges from light yellow to amber, depending on the length of storage and the concentration and diluent used.

Sterile Ceftriaxone Sodium USP—White to yellowish-orange crystalline powder.

Solubility:
Ceftriaxone sodium—Readily soluble in water; sparingly soluble in methanol; very slightly soluble in alcohol.

Sterile Ceftriaxone Sodium USP—Freely soluble in water; sparingly soluble in methanol; very slightly soluble in alcohol.

USP requirements:
Ceftriaxone Sodium USP—Preserve in tight containers. Contains an amount of ceftriaxone sodium equivalent to not less than 795 mcg of ceftriaxone per mg, calculated on the anhydrous basis. Meets the requirements for Identification, Crystallinity, pH (6.0–8.0 in a solution [1 in 10]), and Water (8.0–11.0%).

Ceftriaxone Sodium Injection USP—Preserve in Containers for Injections. Maintain in the frozen state. A sterile solution of Ceftriaxone Sodium in a suitable isoosmotic diluent. It meets the requirements for Labeling under Injections. The label states that it is to be thawed just prior to use, describes conditions for proper storage of the resultant solution, and directs that the solution is not to be refrozen. Contains an amount of ceftriaxone sodium equivalent to the labeled amount of ceftriaxone, within −10% to +15%. Meets the requirements for Identification, Pyrogen, Sterility, pH (6.0–8.0), and Particulate matter.

Sterile Ceftriaxone Sodium USP—Preserve in Containers for Sterile Solids. It is Ceftriaxone Sodium suitable for parenteral use. Where it is not packaged for dispensing, it contains an amount of ceftriaxone sodium equivalent to not less than 795 mcg of ceftriaxone per mg, calculated on the anhydrous basis. Where it is packaged for dispensing, it contains an amount of ceftriaxone sodium equivalent to not less than 776 mcg of ceftriaxone per mg, calculated on the anhydrous basis and contains an amount of ceftriaxone sodium equivalent to the labeled amount of ceftriaxone, within −10% to +15%. Meets the requirements for Constituted solution, Bacterial endotoxins, Sterility, and Particulate matter, and for Identification tests, Crystallinity, pH, and Water under Ceftriaxone Sodium. In addition, where packaged for dispensing, meets the requirements for Uniformity of dosage units and for Labeling under Injections.

CEFUROXIME

Source: Semisynthetic cephalosporin.

Chemical name:
Cefuroxime axetil—5-Thia-1-azabicyclo[4.2.0]oct-2-ene-2-carboxylic acid, 3-[[(aminocarbonyl)oxy]methyl]-7-[[2-furanyl(methoxyimino)acetyl]amino]-8-oxo-, 1-(acetyloxy)ethyl ester, [6R-[6 alpha,7 beta(Z)]]-.

Cefuroxime sodium—5-Thia-1-azabicyclo[4.2.0]oct-2-ene-2-carboxylic acid, 3-[[(aminocarbonyl)oxy]methyl]-7-[[2-furanyl(methoxyimino)acetyl]amino]-8-oxo-, monosodium salt [6R-[6 alpha,7 beta(Z)]]-.

Molecular formula:
Cefuroxime axetil—$C_{20}H_{22}N_4O_{10}S$.
Cefuroxime sodium—$C_{16}H_{15}N_4NaO_8S$.

Molecular weight:
Cefuroxime axetil—510.48.
Cefuroxime sodium—446.37.

Description:
Cefuroxime sodium—White to faintly yellow crystalline powder.

Sterile Cefuroxime Sodium USP—White or faintly yellow powder.

Sterile cefuroxime sodium for injection—Solutions range from light yellow to amber, depending on the concentration and the diluent used.

Solubility:
Cefuroxime sodium—Soluble in water; sparingly soluble in ethanol; insoluble in chloroform, in toluene, in ether, in ethyl acetate, and in acetone.

Sterile Cefuroxime Sodium USP—Soluble in water; sparingly soluble in alcohol; insoluble in chloroform, in toluene, in ether, in ethyl acetate, and in acetone.

Other characteristics: Sterile cefuroxime sodium for injection— The pH of freshly reconstituted solutions usually ranges from 6.0 to 8.5.

USP requirements:

Cefuroxime Axetil USP—Preserve in tight containers. A mixture of the amorphous diastereoisomers of cefuroxime axetil. Contains an amount of cefuroxime axetil equivalent to not less than 745 mcg and not more than 875 mcg of cefuroxime per mg, calculated on the anhydrous basis. Meets the requirements for Identification, Crystallinity, Water (not more than 1.5%), and Diastereoisomer ratio (0.48–0.55).

Cefuroxime Axetil Tablets USP—Preserve in well-closed containers. Contain an amount of cefuroxime axetil equivalent to the labeled amount of cefuroxime, within ±10%. Meet the requirements for Identification, Dissolution (60% in 15 minutes, 75% in 45 minutes in 0.07 N hydrochloric acid in Apparatus 2 at 55 rpm), Uniformity of dosage units, and Water (not more than 6.0%).

Cefuroxime Sodium USP—Preserve in tight containers. Contains an amount of cefuroxime sodium equivalent to not less than 855 mcg and not more than 1000 mcg of cefuroxime, calculated on the anhydrous basis. Meets the requirements for Identification, pH (6.0–8.5, in a solution [1 in 10]), and Water (not more than 3.5%).

Cefuroxime Sodium Injection USP—Preserve in Containers for Injections. Maintain in the frozen state. A sterile isoosmotic solution of Cefuroxime Sodium in Water for Injection. Contains one or more suitable buffers and a tonicity-adjusting agent. It meets the requirements for Labeling under Injections. The label states that it is to be thawed just prior to use, describes conditions for proper storage of the resultant solution, and directs that the solution is not to be refrozen. Contains an amount of cefuroxime sodium equivalent to the labeled amount of cefuroxime, within −10% to +20%. Meets the requirements for Identification, Pyrogen, Sterility, pH (5.0–7.5), and Particulate matter, and for Uniformity of dosage units and Labeling under Injections.

Sterile Cefuroxime Sodium USP—Preserve in Containers for Sterile Solids. It is Cefuroxime Sodium suitable for parenteral use. Contains an amount of cefuroxime sodium equivalent to not less than 855 mcg and not more than 1000 mcg of cefuroxime per mg, calculated on the anhydrous basis and, where packaged for dispensing, contains an amount of cefuroxime sodium equivalent to the labeled amount of cefuroxime, within −10% to +20%. Meets the requirements for Constituted solution, Bacterial endotoxins, Sterility, and Particulate matter, and for Identification tests, pH, and Water under Cefuroxime Sodium. In addition, where packaged for dispensing, meets the requirements for Uniformity of dosage units and for Labeling under Injections.

CELLULOSE ACETATE

Chemical name: Cellulose acetate.

Description: Cellulose Acetate NF—Fine, white powder or free-flowing pellets. Available in a range of viscosities and acetyl contents.

NF category: Coating agent; polymer membrane, insoluble.

Solubility: Cellulose Acetate NF—High viscosity, which reflects high molecular weight, decreases solubility slightly. High acetyl content cellulose acetates generally have more

limited solubility in commonly used organic solvents than low acetyl content cellulose acetates, but are more soluble in methylene chloride. All acetyl content cellulose acetates are insoluble in alcohol and in water; soluble in dioxane and in dimethylformamide.

NF requirements: Cellulose Acetate NF—Preserve in well-closed containers. It is partially or completely acetylated cellulose. Label it to indicate the percentage content of acetyl. Contains not less than 29.0% and not more than 44.8%, by weight, of acetyl groups. Its acetyl content is not less than 90.0% and not more than 110.0% of that indicated on the label. Meets the requirements for Identification, Loss on drying (not more than 5.0%), Residue on ignition (not more than 0.1%), Heavy metals (not more than 0.001%), Free acid (not more than 0.1%, on the dried basis), and Acetyl content.

CELLULOSE ACETATE PHTHALATE

Chemical name: Cellulose, acetate, 1,2-benzenedicarboxylate.

Description: Cellulose Acetate Phthalate NF—Free-flowing, white powder. It may have a slight odor of acetic acid.

NF category: Coating agent.

Solubility: Cellulose Acetate Phthalate NF—Insoluble in water and in alcohol; soluble in acetone and in dioxane.

NF requirements: Cellulose Acetate Phthalate NF—Preserve in tight containers. A reaction product of phthalic anhydride and a partial acetate ester of cellulose. Contains not less than 21.5% and not more than 26.0% of acetyl groups and not less than 30.0% and not more than 36.0% of phthalyl groups, calculated on the anhydrous, acid-free basis. Meets the requirements for Identification, Viscosity (45–90 centipoises), Water (not more than 5.0%), Residue on ignition (not more than 0.1%), Free acid (not more than 6.0%), Phthalyl content, and Acetyl content.

MICROCRYSTALLINE CELLULOSE

Chemical name: Cellulose.

Description: Microcrystalline Cellulose NF—Fine, white, odorless, crystalline powder. It consists of free-flowing, nonfibrous particles that may be compressed into self-binding tablets which disintegrate rapidly in water.

NF category: Tablet binder; tablet disintegrant; tablet and/ or capsule diluent.

Solubility: Microcrystalline Cellulose NF—Insoluble in water, in dilute acids, and in most organic solvents; practically insoluble in sodium hydroxide solution (1 in 20).

NF requirements: Microcrystalline Cellulose NF—Preserve in tight containers. A purified, partially depolymerized cellulose prepared by treating alpha cellulose, obtained as a pulp from fibrous plant material, with mineral acids. Contains an amount of microcrystalline cellulose equivalent to not less than 97.0% and not more than 102.0% of cellulose, calculated on the dried basis. Meets the requirements for Identification, pH (5.5–7.0 for the grades of Microcrystalline Cellulose that have a sieve fraction greater than 5% retained on the 37-mcg screen, and 5.0–7.0 for the grades with less than 5% retained on the 37-mcg screen), Loss on drying (not more than 5.0%), Residue on ignition (not more than 0.05%), Water-soluble substances (not more than 0.16% of residue obtained for the grades that have a sieve fraction more than 5% retention on the 37-mcg screen; not more than 0.24% of residue obtained for the grades that have a sieve fraction not more than 5% retention on the 37-mcg screen), Heavy metals (not more than 0.001%), and Starch.

MICROCRYSTALLINE CELLULOSE AND CARBOXYMETHYLCELLULOSE SODIUM

Chemical name:
Microcrystalline cellulose—Cellulose.
Carboxymethylcellulose sodium—Cellulose, carboxymethyl ether, sodium salt.

Description: Microcrystalline Cellulose and Carboxymethylcellulose Sodium NF—Odorless, white to off-white, coarse to fine powder.
NF category: Suspending and/or viscosity-increasing agent.

Solubility: Microcrystalline Cellulose and Carboxymethylcellulose Sodium NF—Swells in water, producing, when dispersed, a white, opaque dispersion or gel. Insoluble in organic solvents and in dilute acids.

NF requirements: Microcrystalline Cellulose and Carboxymethylcellulose Sodium NF—Preserve in tight containers. Store in a dry place, and avoid exposure to excessive heat. A colloid-forming, attrited mixture of Microcrystalline Cellulose and Carboxymethylcellulose Sodium. Label it to indicate the percentage content of carboxymethylcellulose sodium and the viscosity of the dispersion in water of the designated weight percentage composition. Contains not less than 75.0% and not more than 125.0% of the labeled amount of carboxymethylcellulose sodium, calculated on the dried basis. The viscosity of its aqueous dispersion of percent by weight stated on the label is 60.0 to 140.0% of that stated on the label in centipoises. Meets the requirements for Identification, Viscosity, pH (6.0–8.0), Loss on drying (not more than 8.0%), Residue on ignition (not more than 5.0%), and Heavy metals (not more than 0.001%).

OXIDIZED CELLULOSE

Description: Oxidized Cellulose USP—In the form of gauze or lint. Is slightly off-white in color, and has a slight, charred odor.

Solubility: Oxidized Cellulose USP—Insoluble in water and in acids; soluble in dilute alkalies.

USP requirements: Oxidized Cellulose USP—Preserve in Containers for Sterile Solids, protected from direct sunlight. Store in a cold place. The package bears a statement to the effect that the sterility of Oxidized Cellulose cannot be guaranteed if the package bears evidence of damage, or if the package has been previously opened. Oxidized Cellulose meets the requirements for Labeling under Injections. Contains not less than 16.0% and not more than 24.0% of carboxyl groups, calculated on the dried basis. It is sterile. Meets the requirements for Identification, Sterility, Loss on drying (not more than 15.0%), Residue on ignition (not more than 0.15%), Nitrogen as nitrate or nitrite (not more than 0.5%), and Formaldehyde (0.5%).

OXIDIZED REGENERATED CELLULOSE

Description: Oxidized Regenerated Cellulose USP—A knit fabric, usually in the form of sterile strips. Slightly off-white, having a slight odor.

Solubility: Oxidized Regenerated Cellulose USP—Insoluble in water and in dilute acids; soluble in dilute alkalies.

USP requirements: Oxidized Regenerated Cellulose USP—Preserve in Containers for Sterile Solids, protected from direct sunlight. Store at controlled room temperature. The package bears a statement to the effect that the sterility of Oxidized Regenerated Cellulose cannot be guaranteed if the package bears evidence of damage, or if the package has been previously opened. Oxidized Regenerated Cellulose meets the requirements for Labeling under Injections. Contains not less than 18.0% and not more than 24.0% of carboxyl groups, calculated on the dried basis. It is sterile. Meets the requirements for Identification, Sterility, Loss on drying (not more than 15%), Residue on ignition (not more than 0.15%), Nitrogen content (not more than 0.5%), and Formaldehyde (absorbance not more than 0.5%).

POWDERED CELLULOSE

Description: Powdered Cellulose NF—White, odorless substance, consisting of fibrous particles. Exhibits degrees of fineness ranging from a free-flowing dense powder to a coarse, fluffy, non-flowing material.
NF category: Filtering aid sorbent; tablet and/or capsule diluent.

Solubility: Powdered Cellulose NF—Insoluble in water, in dilute acids, and in nearly all organic solvents; slightly soluble in sodium hydroxide solution (1 in 20).

NF requirements: Powdered Cellulose NF—Preserve in well-closed containers. A purified, mechanically disintegrated cellulose prepared by processing alpha cellulose obtained as a pulp from fibrous plant materials. Contains not less than 97.0% and not more than 102.0% of cellulose, calculated on the dried basis. Meets the requirements for Identification, pH (5.0–7.5), Loss on drying (not more than 7.0%), Residue on ignition (not more than 0.3%, calculated on the dried basis, the addition of sulfuric acid being omitted from the procedure), Water-soluble substances (not more than 1.5%), Heavy metals (not more than 0.001%), and Starch.

CELLULOSE SODIUM PHOSPHATE

Source: An insoluble, nonabsorbable ion-exchange resin made by phosphorylation of cellulose.

Chemical name: Cellulose, dihydrogen phosphate, disodium salt.

Description: Cellulose Sodium Phosphate USP—Free-flowing cream-colored, odorless powder.

Solubility: Cellulose Sodium Phosphate USP—Insoluble in water, in dilute acids, and in most organic solvents.

Other characteristics: Exchanges sodium for calcium and other polyvalent cations. Inorganic phosphate content is approximately 34%; sodium content is approximately 11%.

USP requirements: Cellulose Sodium Phosphate USP (For Oral Suspension)—Preserve in well-closed containers. It is prepared by phosphorylation of alpha cellulose. Has an inorganic bound phosphate content of not less than 31.0% and not more than 36.0%, calculated on the dried basis. Meets the requirements for pH (6.0–9.0, for the filtrate), Loss on drying (not more than 10.0%), Nitrogen (not more than 1.0%), Heavy metals (not more than 0.004%), Calcium binding capacity (not less than 1.8 mmol per gram), Sodium content (9.5–13.0%), Free phosphate (not more than 3.5%, calculated on the dried basis), and Inorganic bound phosphate.

CEPHALEXIN

Source: Semisynthetic cephalosporin.

Chemical name:
Cephalexin—5-Thia-1-azabicyclo[4.2.0]oct-2-ene-2-carboxylic acid, 7-[(aminophenylacetyl)amino]-3-methyl-8-oxo-, monohydrate [6R-[6 alpha,7 beta(R*)]]-.

Cephalexin hydrochloride—5-Thia-1-azabicyclo[4.2.0]oct-2-ene-2-carboxylic acid, 7-[(aminophenylacetyl)amino]-3-methyl-8-oxo-, monohydrochloride, monohydrate, [6R-[6 alpha,7 beta(R*)]]-.

Molecular formula:
Cephalexin—$C_{16}H_{17}N_3O_4S \cdot H_2O$.
Cephalexin hydrochloride—$C_{16}H_{17}N_3O_4S \cdot HCl \cdot H_2O$.

Molecular weight:
Cephalexin—365.40.
Cephalexin hydrochloride—401.86.

Description:
Cephalexin USP—White to off-white, crystalline powder.
Cephalexin Hydrochloride USP—White to off-white crystalline powder.

Solubility:
Cephalexin USP—Slightly soluble in water; practically insoluble in alcohol, in chloroform, and in ether.
Cephalexin Hydrochloride USP—Soluble to the extent of 10 mg per mL in water, in acetone, in acetonitrile, in alcohol, in dimethylformamide, and in methanol; practically insoluble in chloroform, in ether, in ethyl acetate, and in isopropyl alcohol.

Other characteristics: A zwitterion (contains both a basic and an acidic group); isoelectric point of cephalexin in water is approximately 4.5 to 5.

USP requirements:
Cephalexin USP—Preserve in tight containers. It has a potency of not less than 900 mcg of cephalexin per mg, calculated on the anhydrous basis. Meets the requirements for Identification, Crystallinity, pH (3.0–5.5, in an aqueous suspension containing 50 mg per mL), Water (4.0–8.0%), and Related substances (not more than 5.0%).
Cephalexin Capsules USP—Preserve in tight containers. Contain an amount of cephalexin equivalent to the labeled amount of anhydrous cephalexin, within −10% to +20%. Meet the requirements for Identification, Dissolution (75% in 45 minutes in water in Apparatus 1 at 100 rpm), Uniformity of dosage units, and Water (not more than 10.0%).
Cephalexin for Oral Suspension USP—Preserve in tight containers. A dry mixture of Cephalexin and one or more suitable buffers, colors, diluents, and flavors. Contains an amount of cephalexin equivalent to the labeled amount of anhydrous cephalexin per mL when constituted as directed in the labeling, within −10% to +20%. Meets the requirements for Identification, Uniformity of dosage units (solid packaged in single-unit containers), pH (3.0–6.0, in the suspension constituted as directed in the labeling), Water (not more than 2.0%), and Deliverable volume (solid packaged in multiple-unit containers).
Cephalexin Tablets USP—Preserve in tight containers. They are prepared from Cephalexin or Cephalexin Hydrochloride. The label states whether the Tablets contain Cephalexin or Cephalexin Hydrochloride. Contain an amount of cephalexin equivalent to the labeled amount of anhydrous cephalexin, within −10% to +20%. Meet the requirements for Identification, Dissolution (75% in 45 minutes in water in Apparatus 1 at 150 rpm), Uniformity of dosage units, and Water (not more than 9.0% where Tablets contain Cephalexin; not more than 8.0% where Tablets contain Cephalexin Hydrochloride).
Cephalexin Hydrochloride USP—Preserve in tight containers. Contains an amount of cephalexin hydrochloride equivalent to not less than 800 mcg and not more than 880 mcg of anhydrous cephalexin per mg. Meets the requirements for Identification, Crystallinity, pH (1.5–3.0, in a solution containing 10 mg per mL), Water (3.0–6.5%), and Related substances (not more than 5.0%).

CEPHALOTHIN

Source: Semisynthetic cephalosporin; cephalosporanic acid nucleus derived from cephalosporin C, produced by the fungus *Cephalosporium*.

Chemical name: Cephalothin sodium—5-Thia-1-azabicyclo[4.2.0]oct-2-ene-2-carboxylic acid, 3-[(acetyloxy)methyl]-8-oxo-7-[(2-thienylacetyl)amino]-, monosodium salt, (6R-trans)-.

Molecular formula: Cephalothin sodium—$C_{16}H_{15}N_2NaO_6S_2$.

Molecular weight: Cephalothin sodium—418.41.

Description: Sterile Cephalothin Sodium USP—White to off-white, practically odorless, crystalline powder.

Solubility: Sterile Cephalothin Sodium USP—Freely soluble in water, in saline TS, and in dextrose solutions; insoluble in most organic solvents.

Other characteristics: Cephalothin sodium for injection—Contains 30 mg of sodium bicarbonate per gram of cephalothin sodium. Since free cephalothin acid does not form within the pH range produced by the addition of sodium bicarbonate, solubility and freezability are thereby enhanced.

USP requirements:
Cephalothin Sodium USP—Preserve in tight containers. Contains an amount of cephalothin sodium equivalent to not less than 850 mcg of cephalothin per mg, calculated on the dried basis. Meets the requirements for Identification, Specific rotation (+124° to +134°, calculated on the dried basis), Crystallinity, Pyrogen, pH (4.5–7.0, in a solution containing 250 mg per mL, or, where packaged for dispensing, in the solution constituted as directed in the labeling), and Loss on drying (not more than 1.5%).
Cephalothin Sodium Injection USP—Preserve in Containers for Injections. Maintain in the frozen state. A sterile solution of Cephalothin Sodium, or Sterile Cephalothin Sodium, in Water for Injection. Meets the requirements for Labeling under Injections. The label states that it is to be thawed just prior to use, describes conditions for proper storage of the resultant solution, and directs that the solution is not to be refrozen. Contains an amount of cephalothin sodium equivalent to the labeled amount of cephalothin, within −10% to +15%. Meets the requirements for pH (6.0–8.5) and Particulate matter, for Identification test A under Cephalothin Sodium, and for Pyrogen and Sterility under Sterile Cephalothin Sodium.
Cephalothin Sodium for Injection USP—Preserve in Containers for Sterile Solids. A sterile mixture of Sterile Cephalothin Sodium or cephalothin sodium and one or more suitable buffers. Contains an amount of cephalothin sodium equivalent to not less than 850 mcg of cephalothin per mg, calculated on the dried and sodium bicarbonate-free basis, and, where packaged for dispensing, contains an amount of cephalothin sodium equivalent to the labeled amount of cephalothin, within −10% to +15%. Meets the requirements for Constituted solution, Specific rotation (+124° to +134°, in a solution containing a known amount of specimen, equivalent to about 50 mg of cephalothin, per mL, calculated on the dried and sodium bicarbonate-free basis), Bacterial endotoxins, pH (6.0–8.5, in the solution constituted as directed in the labeling), and Particulate matter, for Identification test A and Loss on drying under Cephalothin Sodium, for Sterility under Sterile Cephalothin Sodium, and for Uniformity of dosage units and Labeling under Injections.

Sterile Cephalothin Sodium USP—Preserve in Containers for Sterile Solids. It is cephalothin sodium suitable for parenteral use. Contains an amount of cephalothin sodium equivalent to not less than 850 mcg of cephalothin per mg, calculated on the dried basis. In addition, where packaged for dispensing, contains an amount of cephalothin sodium equivalent to the labeled amount of cephalothin, within −10% to +15%. Meets the requirements for Constituted solution, Bacterial endotoxins, Sterility, pH (4.5–7.0, in a solution containing 250 mg per mL, or, where packaged for dispensing, in the solution constituted as directed in the labeling), and Particulate matter, and for Identification tests, Specific rotation, Crystallinity, and Loss on drying under Cephalothin Sodium. In addition, where packaged for dispensing, meets the requirements for Injections and for Uniformity of dosage units.

CEPHAPIRIN

Source: Semisynthetic cephalosporin.

Chemical name: Cephapirin sodium—5-Thia-1-azabicyclo[4.2.0]oct-2-ene-2-carboxylic acid, 3-[(acetyloxy)methyl]-8-oxo-7-[[(4-pyridylthio)acetyl]amino]-, monosodium salt, [6R-trans]-.

Molecular formula: Cephapirin sodium—$C_{17}H_{16}N_3NaO_6S_2$.

Molecular weight: Cephapirin sodium—445.44.

Description: Sterile Cephapirin Sodium USP—White to off-white crystalline powder, odorless or having a slight odor.

Solubility: Sterile Cephapirin Sodium USP—Very soluble in water; insoluble in most organic solvents.

USP requirements: Sterile Cephapirin Sodium USP—Preserve in Containers for Sterile Solids. Contains an amount of cephapirin sodium equivalent to not less than 855 mcg and not more than 1000 mcg of cephapirin per mg and, where packaged for dispensing, contains an amount of cephapirin sodium equivalent to the labeled amount of cephapirin, within −10% to +15%. Meets the requirements for Constituted solution, Identification, Crystallinity, Bacterial endotoxins, Sterility, pH (6.5–8.5, in a solution containing 10 mg of cephapirin per mL), Water (not more than 2.0%), Particulate matter, and for Uniformity of dosage units and Labeling under Injections.

CEPHRADINE

Source: Semisynthetic cephalosporin.

Chemical name: 5-Thia-1-azabicyclo[4.2.0]oct-2-ene-2-carboxylic acid, 7-[(amino-1,4-cyclohexadien-1-ylacetyl)amino]-3-methyl-8-oxo-, [6R-[6 alpha,7 beta(R*)]]-.

Molecular formula: $C_{16}H_{19}N_3O_4S$.

Molecular weight: 349.40.

Description: Cephradine USP—White to off-white, crystalline powder.

Solubility: Cephradine USP—Sparingly soluble in water; very slightly soluble in alcohol and in chloroform; practically insoluble in ether.

USP requirements:
Cephradine USP—Preserve in tight containers. Where it is the dihydrate form, the label so indicates. Where the quantity of cephradine is indicated in the labeling of any preparation containing Cephradine, this shall be understood to be in terms of anhydrous cephradine. Has a potency of not less than 900 mcg and not more than 1050

mcg of cephradine per mg, calculated on the anhydrous basis. Meets the requirements for Identification, Crystallinity, pH (3.5–6.0, in a solution containing 10 mg per mL), Water (not more than 6.0%, except that if it is the dihydrate form, the limit is 8.5–10.5%), and Cephalexin (not more than 5.0%, calculated on the anhydrous basis).
Cephradine Capsules USP—Preserve in tight containers. The quantity of cephradine stated in the labeling is in terms of anhydrous cephradine. Contain the labeled amount, within −10% to +20%. Meet the requirements for Identification, Dissolution (75% in 45 minutes in 0.12 N hydrochloric acid in Apparatus 1 at 100 rpm), Uniformity of dosage units, and Loss on drying (not more than 7.0%).
Cephradine for Injection USP—Preserve in Containers for Sterile Solids. A dry mixture of Cephradine and one or more suitable buffers and solubilizers. Contains the labeled amount, within −10% to +15%. Meets the requirements for Identification, Bacterial endotoxins, pH (8.0–9.6, in a solution containing 10 mg per mL), Loss on drying (not more than 5.0%), and Particulate matter, for Sterility under Sterile Cephradine, and for Uniformity of dosage units and Labeling under Injections.
Cephradine for Oral Suspension USP—Preserve in tight containers. A dry mixture of Cephradine and one or more suitable buffers, colors, diluents, and flavors. Contains the labeled amount, within −10% to +25%. Meets the requirements for Identification, Uniformity of dosage units (solid packaged in single-unit containers), pH (3.5–6.0, in the suspension constituted as directed in the labeling), Water (not more than 1.5%), and Deliverable volume (solid packaged in multiple-unit containers).
Sterile Cephradine USP—Preserve in Containers for Sterile Solids. Contains not less than 900 mcg and not more than 1050 mcg of cephradine per mg, calculated on the anhydrous basis, and, where packaged for dispensing, contains the labeled amount, within −10% to +15%. Meets the requirements for Constituted solution, Bacterial endotoxins, and Sterility, for Identification test, pH, Water, Crystallinity, and Cephalexin under Cephradine, and for Uniformity of dosage units and Labeling under Injections.
Cephradine Tablets USP—Preserve in tight containers. Contain the labeled amount, within −10% to +20%. Meet the requirements for Identification, Dissolution (85% in 60 minutes in 0.12 N hydrochloric acid in Apparatus 2 at 75 rpm), Uniformity of dosage units, and Water (not more than 6.0%).

CETOSTEARYL ALCOHOL

Description: Cetostearyl Alcohol NF—Unctuous, white flakes or granules having a faint, characteristic odor.

NF category: Stiffening agent.

Solubility: Cetostearyl Alcohol NF—Insoluble in water; soluble in alcohol and in ether.

NF requirements: Cetostearyl Alcohol NF—Preserve in well-closed containers. Contains not less than 40.0% of stearyl alcohol, and the sum of the stearyl alcohol content and the cetyl alcohol content is not less than 90.0%. Meets the requirements for Identification, Melting range (48–55 °C), Acid value (not more than 2), Iodine value (not more than 4), and Hydroxyl value (208–228).

CETYL ALCOHOL

Chemical name: 1-Hexadecanol.

Molecular formula: $C_{16}H_{34}O$.

Molecular weight: 242.44.

Description: Cetyl Alcohol NF—Unctuous, white flakes, granules, cubes, or castings. Has a faint characteristic odor. Usually melts in the range between 45–50 °C.
NF category: Stiffening agent.

Solubility: Cetyl Alcohol NF—Insoluble in water; soluble in alcohol and in ether, the solubility increasing with an increase in temperature.

NF requirements: Cetyl Alcohol NF—Preserve in well-closed containers. Contains not less than 90.0% of cetyl alcohol, the remainder consisting chiefly of related alcohols. Meets the requirements for Identification, Acid value (not more than 2), Iodine value (not more than 5), and Hydroxyl value (218–238).

CETYL ESTERS WAX

Description: Cetyl Esters Wax NF—White to off-white, somewhat translucent flakes, having a crystalline structure and a pearly luster when caked. It has a faint odor and has a specific gravity of about 0.83 at 50 °C.
NF category: Stiffening agent.

Solubility: Cetyl Esters Wax NF—Insoluble in water; soluble in boiling alcohol, in ether, in chloroform, and in fixed and volatile oils; slightly soluble in cold solvent hexane; practically insoluble in cold alcohol.

NF requirements: Cetyl Esters Wax NF—Preserve in well-closed containers in a dry place, and prevent exposure to excessive heat. A mixture consisting primarily of esters of saturated fatty alcohols and saturated fatty acids. Meets the requirements for Melting range (43–47 °C), Acid value (not more than 5), Iodine value (not more than 1), Saponification value (109–120), and Paraffin and free acids.

CETYLPYRIDINIUM

Chemical name: Cetylpyridinium chloride—Pyridinium, 1-hexadecyl-, chloride, monohydrate.

Molecular formula: Cetylpyridinium chloride—$C_{21}H_{38}ClN \cdot H_2O$.

Molecular weight: Cetylpyridinium chloride—358.01.

Description:
Cetylpyridinium Chloride USP—White powder, having a slight, characteristic odor.
NF category: Antimicrobial preservative; wetting and/or solubilizing agent.
Cetylpyridinium Chloride Topical Solution USP—Clear liquid. Is colorless unless a color has been added; has an aromatic odor.

Solubility: Cetylpyridinium Chloride USP—Very soluble in water, in alcohol, and in chloroform; slightly soluble in ether.

USP requirements:
Cetylpyridinium Chloride USP—Preserve in well-closed containers. Contains not less than 99.0% and not more than 102.0% of cetylpyridinium chloride, calculated on the anhydrous basis. Meets the requirements for Identification, Melting range (80–84 °C), Acidity, Water (4.5–5.5%), Residue on ignition (not more than 0.2%, calculated on the anhydrous basis), Heavy metals (not more than 0.002%), Pyridine, and Organic volatile impurities.
Cetylpyridinium Chloride Lozenges USP—Preserve in well-closed containers. Contain the labeled amount, within −10% to +25%, in a suitable molded base. Meet the requirement for Identification.

Cetylpyridinium Chloride Topical Solution USP—Preserve in tight containers. Contains the labeled amount, within ±5%. Meets the requirement for Identification.

ACTIVATED CHARCOAL

Source: Carbon residue derived from heating organic material in the absence of oxygen.

Description: Activated Charcoal USP—Fine, black, odorless powder, free from gritty matter.
NF category: Sorbent.

Solubility: Activated charcoal—Practically insoluble in all usual solvents.

USP requirements:
Activated Charcoal USP—Preserve in well-closed containers. It is the residue from the destructive distillation of various organic materials, treated to increase its adsorptive power. Meets the requirements for Microbial limits, Reaction (neutral to litmus), Loss on drying (not more than 15.0%), Residue on ignition (not more than 4.0%), Acid-soluble substances (not more than 3.5%), Chloride (not more than 0.2%), Sulfate (not more than 0.2%), Sulfide, Cyanogen compounds, Heavy metals (not more than 0.005%), Uncarbonized constituents, and Adsorptive power.
Activated Charcoal Capsules—Not in USP.
Activated Charcoal Oral Suspension—Not in USP.
Activated Charcoal Tablets—Not in USP.

ACTIVATED CHARCOAL AND SORBITOL

For *Activated Charcoal* and *Sorbitol*—See individual listings for chemistry information.

USP requirements: Activated Charcoal and Sorbitol Oral Suspension—Not in USP.

CHENODIOL

Source: Chenodeoxycholic acid, a naturally occurring human bile acid.

Chemical name: Cholan-24-oic acid, 3,7-dihydroxy-, (3 alpha,- 5 beta,7 alpha)-.

Molecular formula: $C_{24}H_{40}O_4$.

Molecular weight: 392.58.

Description: White powder consisting of crystalline and amorphous particles.

Solubility: Practically insoluble in water; freely soluble in methanol, in acetone, and in acetic acid.

USP requirements: Chenodiol Tablets—Not in USP.

CHLOPHEDIANOL

Chemical name: Chlophedianol hydrochloride—Benzenemethanol, 2-chloro-alpha-[2-(dimethylamino)ethyl]-alpha-phenyl-, hydrochloride.

Molecular formula: Chlophedianol hydrochloride—$C_{17}H_{20}ClNO \cdot HCl$.

Molecular weight: Chlophedianol hydrochloride—326.26.

Description: Chlophedianol hydrochloride—White, crystalline powder. Melting point 190–191 °C.

Solubility: Chlophedianol hydrochloride—Freely soluble in water, in methanol, and in ethanol. Sparingly soluble in ether and in ethyl acetate.

USP requirements: Chlophedianol Hydrochloride Syrup—Not in USP.

CHLORAL HYDRATE

Chemical name: 1,1-Ethanediol, 2,2,2-trichloro-.

Molecular formula: $C_2H_3Cl_3O_2$.

Molecular weight: 165.40.

Description: Chloral Hydrate USP—Colorless, transparent, or white crystals having an aromatic, penetrating, and slightly acrid odor. Melts at about 55 °C, and slowly volatilizes when exposed to air.

Solubility: Chloral Hydrate USP—Very soluble in water and in olive oil; freely soluble in alcohol, in chloroform, and in ether.

USP requirements:
Chloral Hydrate USP—Preserve in tight containers. Contains not less than 99.5% and not more than 102.5% of chloral hydrate. Meets the requirements for Identification, Acidity, Residue on ignition (not more than 0.1%), Chloride (not more than 0.007%), Readily carbonizable substances, and Organic volatile impurities.
Chloral Hydrate Capsules USP—Preserve in tight containers, preferably at controlled room temperature. Contain the labeled amount, within −5% to +10%. Meet the requirements for Identification and Uniformity of dosage units.
Chloral Hydrate Suppositories—Not in USP.
Chloral Hydrate Syrup USP—Preserve in tight, light-resistant containers. Contains the labeled amount, within −5% to +10%. Meets the requirement for Identification.

CHLORAMBUCIL

Chemical name: Benzenebutanoic acid, 4-[bis(2-chloroethyl)amino]-.

Molecular formula: $C_{14}H_{19}Cl_2NO_2$.

Molecular weight: 304.22.

Description: Chlorambucil USP—Off-white, slightly granular powder.

pKa: 1.3 and 5.8.

Solubility: Chlorambucil USP—Very slightly soluble in water; freely soluble in acetone; soluble in dilute alkali.

USP requirements:
Chlorambucil USP—Preserve in tight, light-resistant containers. Contains not less than 98.0% and not more than 101.0% of chlorambucil, calculated on the anhydrous basis. Meets the requirements for Identification, Melting range (65–69 °C), Water (not more than 0.5%), and Organic volatile impurities.
　　Caution: Great care should be taken to prevent inhaling particles of Chlorambucil and exposing the skin to it.
Chlorambucil Tablets USP—Preserve coated Tablets in well-closed containers; preserve uncoated Tablets in well-closed, light-resistant containers. Contain the labeled amount, within −15% to +10%. Meet the requirements for Identification, Disintegration (15 minutes, the use of disks being omitted), and Uniformity of dosage units.

CHLORAMPHENICOL

Source: Originally derived from *Streptomyces venezuelae*.

Chemical name:
Chloramphenicol—Acetamide, 2,2-dichloro-*N*-[2-hydroxy-1-(hydroxymethyl)-2-(4-nitrophenyl)ethyl]-, [*R*-(*R**,*R**)]-.
Chloramphenicol palmitate—Hexadecanoic acid, 2-[(2,2-dichloroacetyl)amino]-3-hydroxy-3-(4-nitrophenyl) propyl ester, [*R*-(*R**,*R**)]-.

Molecular formula:
Chloramphenicol—$C_{11}H_{12}Cl_2N_2O_5$.
Chloramphenicol palmitate—$C_{27}H_{42}Cl_2N_2O_6$.
Chloramphenicol sodium succinate—$C_{15}H_{15}Cl_2N_2NaO_8$.

Molecular weight:
Chloramphenicol—323.13.
Chloramphenicol palmitate—561.54.
Chloramphenicol sodium succinate—445.19.

Description:
Chloramphenicol USP—Fine, white to grayish white or yellowish white, needle-like crystals or elongated plates. Its solutions are practically neutral to litmus. Is reasonably stable in neutral or moderately acid solutions. Its alcohol solution is dextrorotatory and its ethyl acetate solution is levorotatory.
Chloramphenicol Palmitate USP—Fine, white, unctuous, crystalline powder, having a faint odor.
Sterile Chloramphenicol Sodium Succinate USP—Light yellow powder.

Solubility:
Chloramphenicol USP—Slightly soluble in water; freely soluble in alcohol, in propylene glycol, in acetone, and in ethyl acetate.
Chloramphenicol Palmitate USP—Insoluble in water; freely soluble in acetone and in chloroform; soluble in ether; sparingly soluble in alcohol; very slightly soluble in solvent hexane.
Sterile Chloramphenicol Sodium Succinate USP—Freely soluble in water and in alcohol.

USP requirements:
Chloramphenicol USP—Preserve in tight containers. Contains not less than 97.0% and not more than 103.0% of chloramphenicol. Meets the requirements for Identification, Melting range (149–153 °C), Specific rotation (+17.0° to +20.0°), Crystallinity, pH (4.5–7.5, in an aqueous suspension containing 25 mg per mL), and Chromatographic purity (not more than 2.0%).
Chloramphenicol Capsules USP—Preserve in tight containers. Contain the labeled amount, within −10% to +20%. Meet the requirements for Identification, Dissolution (85% in 30 minutes in 0.1 *N* hydrochloric acid in Apparatus 1 at 100 rpm), and Uniformity of dosage units.
Chloramphenicol Cream USP—Preserve in collapsible tubes or in tight containers. Contains the labeled amount, within −10% to +30%. Meets the requirements for Identification and Minimum fill.
Chloramphenicol Injection USP—Preserve in single-dose or in multiple-dose containers. A sterile solution of Chloramphenicol in one or more suitable solvents. Label it to indicate that it is for veterinary use only. Contains the labeled amount, within −10% to +15%. Meets the requirements for Identification, Bacterial endotoxins, Sterility, pH (5.0–8.0, in a solution diluted with water [1:1]), and Injections.
Chloramphenicol Ophthalmic Ointment USP—Preserve in collapsible ophthalmic ointment tubes. Contains the labeled amount, within −10% to +30%. Meets the requirements for Identification, Sterility, Minimum fill, and Metal particles.

Chloramphenicol Ophthalmic Solution USP—Preserve in tight containers, and store in a refrigerator until dispensed. The containers or individual cartons are sealed and tamper-proof so that sterility is assured at time of first use. A sterile solution of Chloramphenicol. The labeling states that there is a 21-day beyond-use period after dispensing. Contains the labeled amount, within −10% to +30%. Meets the requirements for Identification, Sterility, and pH (7.0–7.5, except that in the case of Ophthalmic Solution that is unbuffered or is labeled for veterinary use it is 3.0–6.0).

Chloramphenicol for Ophthalmic Solution USP—Preserve in tight containers. A sterile, dry mixture of Chloramphenicol with or without one or more suitable buffers, diluents, and preservatives. If packaged in combination with a container of solvent, label it with a warning that it is not for injection. Contains the labeled amount, within −10% to +30%, when constituted as directed. Meets the requirements for Identification, Sterility, and pH (7.1–7.5, in an aqueous solution containing 5 mg of chloramphenicol per mL).

Chloramphenicol Oral Solution USP—Preserve in tight containers. A solution of Chloramphenicol in a suitable solvent. Label it to indicate that it is for veterinary use only and that it is not to be used in animals raised for food production. Contains the labeled amount, within −10% to +20%. Contains one or more suitable buffers and preservatives. Meets the requirements for Identification and pH (5.0–8.5, when diluted with an equal volume of water).

Chloramphenicol Otic Solution USP—Preserve in tight containers. A sterile solution of Chloramphenicol in a suitable solvent. Contains the labeled amount, within −10% to +30%. Meets the requirements for Identification, Sterility, pH (4.0–8.0, when diluted with an equal volume of water), and Water (not more than 2.0%).

Sterile Chloramphenicol USP—Preserve in Containers for Sterile Solids. It is Chloramphenicol suitable for parenteral use. Contains not less than 97.0% and not more than 103.0% of chloramphenicol. Meets the requirements for Bacterial endotoxins and Sterility, and for Identification test, Melting range, Specific rotation, pH, and Crystallinity under Chloramphenicol.

Chloramphenicol Tablets USP—Preserve in tight containers. Label Tablets to indicate that they are for veterinary use only and are not to be used in animals raised for food production. Contain the labeled amount, within −10% to +20%. Meet the requirements for Identification, Disintegration (60 minutes), and Uniformity of dosage units.

Chloramphenicol Palmitate USP—Preserve in tight containers. It has a potency equivalent to not less than 555 mcg and not more than 595 mcg of chloramphenicol per mg. Meets the requirements for Identification, Melting range (87–95 °C), Specific rotation (+21° to +25°), Crystallinity, Loss on drying (not more than 0.5%), Acidity, and Free chloramphenicol (absorbance not more than 0.045%).

Chloramphenicol Palmitate Oral Suspension USP—Preserve in tight, light-resistant containers. Contains an amount of chloramphenicol palmitate equivalent to the labeled amount of chloramphenicol, within −10% to +20%. Contains one or more suitable buffers, colors, flavors, preservatives, and suspending agents. Meets the requirements for Identification, Uniformity of dosage units (suspension packaged in single-unit containers), pH (4.5–7.0), Polymorph A, and Deliverable volume (suspension packaged in multiple-unit containers).

Sterile Chloramphenicol Sodium Succinate USP—Preserve in Containers for Sterile Solids. Contains an amount of chloramphenicol sodium succinate equivalent to not less than 650 mcg and not more than 765 mcg of chloramphenicol per mg and, where packaged for dispensing and constituted as directed in the labeling, contains an amount of chloramphenicol sodium succinate equivalent to the labeled amount of chloramphenicol, within −10% to +15%. Meets the requirements for Identification, Specific rotation (+5.0° to +8.0°, calculated on the anhydrous basis, determined in a solution containing 50 mg per mL), Bacterial endotoxins, Sterility, pH (6.4–7.0, in a solution containing the equivalent of 250 mg of chloramphenicol per mL), Water (not more than 5.0%), Particulate matter, and Free chloramphenicol (not more than 2.0%).

CHLORAMPHENICOL AND HYDROCORTISONE

For *Chloramphenicol* and *Hydrocortisone*—See individual listings for chemistry information.

USP requirements: Chloramphenicol and Hydrocortisone Acetate for Ophthalmic Suspension USP—A sterile, dry mixture of Chloramphenicol and Hydrocortisone Acetate with or without one or more suitable buffers, diluents, and preservatives. If packaged in combination with a container of solvent, label it with a warning that it is not for injection. Contains the labeled amounts of chloramphenicol, within −10% to +30%, and hydrocortisone acetate, within −10% to +15%, when constituted as directed. Meets the requirements for Identification, Sterility, and pH (7.1–7.5, in an aqueous suspension containing 5 mg of chloramphenicol per mL).

CHLORAMPHENICOL AND POLYMYXIN B

For *Chloramphenicol* and *Polymyxin B*—See individual listings for chemistry information.

USP requirements: Chloramphenicol and Polymyxin B Sulfate Ophthalmic Ointment USP—Preserve in collapsible ophthalmic ointment tubes. Contains the labeled amount of chloramphenicol, within −10% to +20%, and an amount of polymyxin B sulfate equivalent to the labeled amount of polymyxin B, within −10% to +25%. Meets the requirements for Identification, Sterility, and Metal particles.

CHLORAMPHENICOL, POLYMYXIN B, AND HYDROCORTISONE

For *Chloramphenicol*, *Polymyxin B*, and *Hydrocortisone*—See individual listings for chemistry information.

USP requirements: Chloramphenicol, Polymyxin B Sulfate, and Hydrocortisone Acetate Ophthalmic Ointment USP—Preserve in collapsible ophthalmic ointment tubes. Contains the labeled amount of chloramphenicol, within −10% to +20%, an amount of polymyxin B sulfate equivalent to the labeled amount of polymyxin B, within −10% to +25%, and the labeled amount of hydrocortisone acetate, within −10% to +15%. Meets the requirements for Identification, Sterility, Minimum fill, and Metal particles.

CHLORAMPHENICOL AND PREDNISOLONE

For *Chloramphenicol* and *Prednisolone*—See individual listings for chemistry information.

USP requirements: Chloramphenicol and Prednisolone Ophthalmic Ointment USP—Preserve in collapsible ophthalmic ointment tubes. Contains the labeled amounts of chloramphenicol, within −10% to +30%, and prednisolone, within −10% to +15%. Meets the requirements for Identification, Sterility, Minimum fill, and Metal particles.

CHLORDIAZEPOXIDE

Chemical name:

Chlordiazepoxide—3H-1,4-Benzodiazepin-2-amine, 7-chloro-N-methyl-5-phenyl, 4-oxide.

Chlordiazepoxide hydrochloride—3H-1,4-Benzodiazepin-2-amine, 7-chloro-N-methyl-5-phenyl-, 4-oxide, monohydrochloride.

Molecular formula:

Chlordiazepoxide—$C_{16}H_{14}ClN_3O$.

Chlordiazepoxide hydrochloride—$C_{16}H_{14}ClN_3O \cdot HCl$.

Molecular weight:

Chlordiazepoxide—299.76.

Chlordiazepoxide hydrochloride—336.22.

Description:

Chlordiazepoxide USP—Yellow, practically odorless, crystalline powder. Is sensitive to sunlight. Melts at about 240 °C.

Chlordiazepoxide Hydrochloride USP—White or practically white, odorless, crystalline powder. Is affected by sunlight.

Sterile Chlordiazepoxide Hydrochloride USP—White or practically white, odorless, crystalline powder. Is affected by sunlight.

Solubility:

Chlordiazepoxide USP—Insoluble in water; sparingly soluble in chloroform and in alcohol.

Chlordiazepoxide Hydrochloride USP—Soluble in water and in alcohol; insoluble in solvent hexane.

Sterile Chlordiazepoxide Hydrochloride USP—Soluble in water and in alcohol; insoluble in solvent hexane.

USP requirements:

Chlordiazepoxide USP—Preserve in tight, light-resistant containers. Contains not less than 98.0% and not more than 102.0% of chlordiazepoxide, calculated on the dried basis. Meets the requirements for Identification, Loss on drying (not more than 0.3%), Residue on ignition (not more than 0.1%), Heavy metals (not more than 0.002%), and Related compounds.

Chlordiazepoxide Tablets USP—Preserve in tight, light-resistant containers. Contain the labeled amount, within ±10%. Meet the requirements for Identification, Dissolution (85% in 30 minutes in simulated gastric fluid TS, prepared without pepsin, in Apparatus 1 at 100 rpm), Uniformity of dosage units, and Related compounds.

Chlordiazepoxide Hydrochloride USP—Preserve in tight, light-resistant containers. Contains not less than 98.0% and not more than 102.0% of chlordiazepoxide hydrochloride, calculated on the dried basis. Meets the requirements for Identification, Melting range (212–218 °C, with decomposition), Loss on drying (not more than 0.5%), Residue on ignition (not more than 0.1%), Heavy metals (not more than 0.002%), Related compounds, and Organic volatile impurities.

Chlordiazepoxide Hydrochloride Capsules USP—Preserve in tight, light-resistant containers. Contain the labeled amount, within ±10%. Meet the requirements for Identification, Dissolution (85% in 30 minutes in water in Apparatus 1 at 100 rpm), Uniformity of dosage units, and Related compounds.

Sterile Chlordiazepoxide Hydrochloride USP—Preserve in Containers for Sterile Solids, protected from light. It is Chlordiazepoxide Hydrochloride suitable for parenteral use. Meets the requirements for Completeness of solution, Constituted solution, Bacterial endotoxins, pH (2.5–3.5, in a solution [1 in 100]), for Identification tests, Loss on

drying and Heavy metals under Chlordiazepoxide Hydrochloride, for Related compounds under Chlordiazepoxide, and for Sterility tests, Uniformity of dosage units, and Labeling under Injections.

CHLORDIAZEPOXIDE AND AMITRIPTYLINE

For *Chlordiazepoxide* and *Amitriptyline*—See individual listings for chemistry information.

USP requirements: Chlordiazepoxide and Amitriptyline Hydrochloride Tablets USP—Preserve in tight, light-resistant containers. Contain the labeled amount of chlordiazepoxide, within ±10%, and an amount of amitriptyline hydrochloride equivalent to the labeled amount of amitriptyline, within ±10%. Meet the requirements for Identification, Dissolution (85% of chlordiazepoxide and an amount of amitriptyline hydrochloride equivalent to not less than 85% of amitriptyline in 30 minutes in simulated gastric fluid TS, prepared without pepsin, in Apparatus 1 at 100 rpm), Uniformity of dosage units, and Related compounds.

CHLORDIAZEPOXIDE AND CLIDINIUM

For *Chlordiazepoxide* and *Clidinium*—See individual listings for chemistry information.

USP requirements: Chlordiazepoxide Hydrochloride and Clidinium Bromide Capsules USP—Preserve in tight, light-resistant containers. Contain the labeled amounts of chlordiazepoxide hydrochloride and clidinium bromide, within ± 10%. Meet the requirements for Identification, Dissolution (75% of each active ingredient in 30 minutes in water in Apparatus 1 at 100 rpm), Uniformity of dosage units, and Related compounds.

CHLORHEXIDINE

Chemical group: Chlorhexidine gluconate is a bis-biguanide.

Chemical name: Chlorhexidine gluconate—2,4,11,13-Tetraazatetradecanediimidamide, N,N''-bis(4-chlorophenyl)-3,12-diimino-, di-D-gluconate.

Molecular formula: Chlorhexidine gluconate—$C_{22}H_{30}Cl_2N_{10} \cdot 2C_6H_{12}O_7$.

Molecular weight: Chlorhexidine gluconate—897.77.

Other characteristics: Chlorhexidine gluconate—A 5% v/v aqueous solution has a pH of 5.5 to 7.

USP requirements: Chlorhexidine Gluconate Oral Rinse—Not in USP.

CHLORMEZANONE

Chemical group: A substituted metathiazanone compound.

Chemical name: 2-(p-Chlorophenyl)tetrahydro-3-methyl-4H-1,3-thiazin-4-one 1,1-dioxide.

Molecular formula: $C_{11}H_{12}ClNO_3S$.

Molecular weight: 273.73.

Description: A white, crystalline powder with a faint characteristic odor.

Solubility: Soluble in water (less than 0.25% w/v) and in alcohol.

USP requirements: Chlormezanone Tablets—Not in USP.

CHLOROBUTANOL

Chemical name: 2-Propanol, 1,1,1-trichloro-2-methyl-.

Molecular formula: $C_4H_7Cl_3O$ (anhydrous).

Molecular weight: 177.46 (anhydrous).

Description: Chlorobutanol NF—Colorless to white crystals, having a characteristic, somewhat camphoraceous, odor. The anhydrous form melts at about 95 °C, and the hydrous form melts at about 76 °C.
  NF category: Antimicrobial preservative.

Solubility: Chlorobutanol NF—Slightly soluble in water; freely soluble in alcohol, in ether, in chloroform, and in volatile oils; soluble in glycerin.

NF requirements: Chlorobutanol NF—Preserve in tight containers. It is anhydrous or contains not more than ½ molecule of water of hydration. Label it to indicate whether it is anhydrous or hydrous. Contains not less than 98.0% and not more than 100.5% of chlorobutanol, calculated on the anhydrous basis. Meets the requirements for Identification, Reaction, Water (for anhydrous, not more than 1.0%; for hydrous, not more than 6.0%), and Chloride (not more than 0.07%).

CHLOROCRESOL

Chemical name: Phenol, 4-chloro-3-methyl-.

Molecular formula: C_7H_7ClO.

Molecular weight: 142.58.

Description: Chlorocresol NF—Colorless or practically colorless crystals or crystalline powder, having a characteristic, nontarry odor. Volatile in steam.
  NF category: Antimicrobial preservative.

Solubility: Chlorocresol NF—Slightly soluble in water and more soluble in hot water; very soluble in alcohol; soluble in ether, in terpenes, in fixed oils, and in solutions of alkali hydroxides.

NF requirements: Chlorocresol NF—Preserve in tight, light-resistant containers. Contains not less than 99.0% and not more than 101.0% of chlorocresol. Meets the requirements for Completeness of solution, Identification, Melting range (63–66 °C), and Nonvolatile residue (not more than 0.1%).

CHLOROFORM

Chemical name: Methane, trichloro-.

Molecular formula: $CHCl_3$.

Molecular weight: 119.38.

Description: Chloroform NF—Clear, colorless, mobile liquid, having a characteristic, ethereal odor. It is not flammable, but its heated vapor burns with a green flame. Boils at about 61 °C. Affected by light.
  NF category: Solvent.

Solubility: Chloroform NF—Slightly soluble in water. Miscible with alcohol, with ether, with solvent hexane, and with fixed and volatile oils.

NF requirements: Chloroform NF—Preserve in tight, light-resistant containers, at a temperature not exceeding 30 °C. Contains not less than 99.0% and not more than 99.5% of chloroform, the remainder consisting of alcohol. Meets the requirements for Specific gravity (1.476–1.480), Nonvolatile residue (not more than 0.002%), Free chlorine, Readily carbonizable substances, Chlorinated decomposition products and chloride, Acid and phosgene, and Aldehyde and ketone.
  Caution: Care should be taken not to vaporize Chloroform in the presence of a flame, because of the production of harmful gases.

CHLOROPROCAINE

Chemical group: Ester, aminobenzoic acid (PABA)-derivative.

Chemical name: Chloroprocaine hydrochloride—Benzoic acid, 4-amino-2-chloro-, 2-(diethylamino)ethyl ester, monohydrochloride.

Molecular formula: Chloroprocaine hydrochloride—$C_{13}H_{19}ClN_2O_2 \cdot HCl$.

Molecular weight: Chloroprocaine hydrochloride—307.22.

Description: Chloroprocaine Hydrochloride USP—White, crystalline powder. Is odorless, and is stable in air. Its solutions are acid to litmus.

pKa: 9.0.

Solubility: Chloroprocaine Hydrochloride USP—Soluble in water; slightly soluble in alcohol; very slightly soluble in chloroform; practically insoluble in ether.

USP requirements:
  Chloroprocaine Hydrochloride USP—Preserve in well-closed containers. Contains not less than 98.0% and not more than 102.0% of chloroprocaine hydrochloride, calculated on the dried basis. Meets the requirements for Identification, Melting range (173–176 °C), Acidity, Loss on drying (not more than 1.0%), Residue on ignition (not more than 0.2%), and Related substances (not more than 0.625%).
  Chloroprocaine Hydrochloride Injection USP—Preserve in single-dose or in multiple-dose containers, preferably of Type I glass. A sterile solution of Chloroprocaine Hydrochloride in Water for Injection. Contains the labeled amount, within ± 5%. Meets the requirements for Identification, pH (2.7–4.0), Related substances (not more than 3.0%), and Injections.

CHLOROQUINE

Chemical name:
  Chloroquine—1,4-Pentanediamine, N^4-(7-chloro-4-quinolinyl)-N^1,N^1-diethyl.
  Chloroquine hydrochloride—1,4-Pentanediamine, N^4-(7-chloro-4-quinolinyl)-N^1,N^1-diethyl-, dihydrochloride.
  Chloroquine phosphate—1,4-Pentanediamine, N^4-(7-chloro-4-quinolinyl)-N^1,N^1-diethyl-, phosphate (1:2).

Molecular formula:
  Chloroquine—$C_{18}H_{26}ClN_3$.
  Chloroquine hydrochloride—$C_{18}H_{26}ClN_3 \cdot 2HCl$.
  Chloroquine phosphate—$C_{18}H_{26}ClN_3 \cdot 2H_3PO_4$.

Molecular weight:
  Chloroquine—319.88.
  Chloroquine hydrochloride—392.80.
  Chloroquine phosphate—515.87.

Description:
  Chloroquine USP—White or slightly yellow, crystalline powder. Is odorless.
  Chloroquine Hydrochloride Injection USP—Colorless liquid.
  Chloroquine Phosphate USP—White, crystalline powder. Is odorless and is discolored slowly on exposure to light. Its

solutions have a pH of about 4.5. Exists in two polymorphic forms, one melting between 193 °C and 195 °C and the other between 210 °C and 215 °C; mixture of the forms melts between 193 °C and 215 °C.

Solubility:
Chloroquine USP—Very slightly soluble in water; soluble in dilute acids, in chloroform, and in ether.
Chloroquine Phosphate USP—Freely soluble in water; practically insoluble in alcohol, in chloroform, and in ether.

USP requirements:
Chloroquine USP—Preserve in well-closed containers. Contains not less than 98.0% and not more than 102.0% of chloroquine, calculated on the dried basis. Meets the requirements for Identification, Melting range (87–92 °C), Loss on drying (not more than 2.0%), Residue on ignition (not more than 0.2%), and Organic volatile impurities.
Chloroquine Hydrochloride Injection USP—Preserve in single-dose containers, preferably of Type I glass. A sterile solution of Chloroquine in Water for Injection prepared with the aid of Hydrochloric Acid. Contains, in each mL, not less than 47.5 mg and not more than 52.5 mg of chloroquine hydrochloride. Meets the requirements for Identification, Bacterial endotoxins, pH (5.5–6.5), and Injections.
Chloroquine Phosphate USP—Preserve in well-closed containers. Contains not less than 98.0% and not more than 102.0% of chloroquine phosphate, calculated on the dried basis. Meets the requirements for Identification, Loss on drying (not more than 2.0%), and Organic volatile impurities.
Chloroquine Phosphate Tablets USP—Preserve in well-closed containers. Contain the labeled amount, within ±7%. Meet the requirements for Identification, Dissolution (75% in 45 minutes in water in Apparatus 2 at 100 rpm), and Uniformity of dosage units.

CHLOROTHIAZIDE

Chemical name:
Chlorothiazide—2H-1,2,4-Benzothiadiazine-7-sulfonamide, 6-chloro-, 1,1-dioxide.
Chlorothiazide sodium—2H-1,2,4-Benzothiadiazine-7-sulfonamide, 6-chloro-, 1,1-dioxide, monosodium salt.

Molecular formula:
Chlorothiazide—$C_7H_6ClN_3O_4S_2$.
Chlorothiazide sodium—$C_7H_5ClN_3NaO_4S_2$.

Molecular weight:
Chlorothiazide—295.72.
Chlorothiazide sodium—317.70.

Description: Chlorothiazide USP—White or practically white, crystalline, odorless powder. Melts at about 340 °C, with decomposition.

pKa: 6.7 and 9.5.

Solubility: Chlorothiazide USP—Very slightly soluble in water; freely soluble in dimethylformamide and in dimethyl sulfoxide; slightly soluble in methanol and in pyridine; practically insoluble in ether and in chloroform.

USP requirements:
Chlorothiazide USP—Preserve in well-closed containers. Contains not less than 98.0% and not more than 102.0% of chlorothiazide, calculated on the dried basis. Meets the requirements for Identification, Loss on drying (not more than 1.0%), Residue on ignition (not more than 0.1%), Chloride (not more than 0.05%), Selenium

(0.003%), Heavy metals (not more than 0.001%), 4-Amino-6-chloro-1,3-benzenedisulfonamide (not more than 1.0%), and Organic volatile impurities.
Chlorothiazide Oral Suspension USP—Preserve in tight containers. Contains the labeled amount, within ±10%. Meets the requirements for Identification and pH (3.2–4.0).
Chlorothiazide Tablets USP—Preserve in well-closed containers. Contain the labeled amount, within ±10%. Meet the requirements for Identification, Dissolution (75% in 60 minutes in 0.05 M phosphate buffer [pH 8.0] in Apparatus 2 at 75 rpm), and Uniformity of dosage units.
Chlorothiazide Sodium for Injection USP—Preserve in Containers for Sterile Solids. A sterile, freeze-dried mixture of Chlorothiazide Sodium (prepared by the neutralization of Chlorothiazide with the aid of Sodium Hydroxide) and Mannitol. Contains an amount of chlorothiazide sodium equivalent to the labeled amount of chlorothiazide, within ±7%. Meets the requirements for Constituted solution, Identification, Bacterial endotoxins, pH (9.2–10.0, in a solution prepared as directed in the labeling), Uniformity of dosage units, and Injections.

CHLOROTRIANISENE

Source: Synthetic compound.

Chemical name: Benzene, 1,1',1''-(1-chloro-1-ethenyl-2-ylidene)-tris[4-methoxy]-.

Molecular formula: $C_{23}H_{21}ClO_3$.

Molecular weight: 380.87.

Description: Small, white crystals or crystalline powder. It is odorless.

Solubility: Very slightly soluble in water; slightly soluble in alcohol.

USP requirements:
Chlorotrianisene USP—Preserve in tight containers. It is dried in vacuum at 60 °C for 6 hours. Contains not less than 97.0% and not more than 103.0% of chlorotrianisene. Meets the requirements for Identification, Loss on drying (not more than 1.0%), Residue on ignition (not more than 1.0%), Heavy metals (not more than 0.002%), Volatile related compounds (not more than 1.0%), and Organic volatile impurities.
Chlorotrianisene Capsules USP—Preserve in well-closed containers, protected from excessive heat, cold, and moisture. Label Chlorotrianisene Capsules to indicate the vehicle used in the Capsules. Contain the labeled amount, within ±7%. Meet the requirements for Identification and Uniformity of dosage units.

CHLOROXINE

Chemical name: 8-Quinolinol, 5,7-dichloro-.

Molecular formula: $C_9H_5Cl_2NO$.

Molecular weight: 214.05.

Description: Melting point 179–180 °C.

Solubility: Soluble in acetone; slightly soluble in cold alcohol and in acetic acid; readily soluble in sodium and potassium hydroxides and in acids, forming yellow solutions.

USP requirements: Chloroxine Lotion Shampoo—Not in USP.

CHLOROXYLENOL

Chemical name: Phenol, 4-chloro-3,5-dimethyl-.

Molecular formula: C_8H_9ClO.

Molecular weight: 156.61.

Description: Chloroxylenol USP—White crystals or crystalline powder, having a characteristic odor. Volatile in steam.

Solubility: Chloroxylenol USP—Very slightly soluble in water; freely soluble in alcohol, in ether, in terpenes, in fixed oils, and in solutions of alkali hydroxides.

USP requirements: Chloroxylenol USP—Preserve in well-closed containers. Contains not less than 98.5% of chloroxylenol. Meets the requirements for Identification, Melting range (114–116 °C), Residue on ignition (not more than 0.1%), Iron (not more than 0.01%), Water (not more than 0.5%), and Chromatographic purity.

CHLORPHENESIN

Chemical name: Chlorphenesin carbamate—1,2-Propanediol, 3-(4-chlorophenoxy)-, 1-carbamate.

Molecular formula: Chlorphenesin carbamate—$C_{10}H_{12}ClNO_4$.

Molecular weight: Chlorphenesin carbamate—245.66.

Description: Chlorphenesin carbamate—White to off-white crystalline solid.

Solubility: Chlorphenesin carbamate—Almost insoluble in cold water or in cyclohexane; fairly readily soluble in dioxane; readily soluble in ethyl acetate, in 95.0% ethanol, and in acetone.

USP requirements: Chlorphenesin Carbamate Tablets—Not in USP.

CHLORPHENIRAMINE

Chemical group: Propylamine derivative (alkylamine).

Chemical name:
Chlorpheniramine maleate—2-Pyridinepropanamine, gamma-(4-chlorophenyl)-*N,N*-dimethyl-, (*Z*)-2-butenedioate (1:1).
Chlorpheniramine polistirex—Benzene, diethenyl-, polymer with ethenylbenzene, sulfonated, complex with gamma-(4-chlorophenyl)-*N,N*-dimethyl-2-pyridinepropanamine.

Molecular formula: Chlorpheniramine maleate—$C_{16}H_{19}ClN_2 \cdot C_4H_4O_4$.

Molecular weight: Chlorpheniramine maleate—390.87.

Description: Chlorpheniramine Maleate USP—White, odorless, crystalline powder. Its solutions have a pH between 4 and 5.

pKa: Chlorpheniramine maleate—9.2.

Solubility: Chlorpheniramine Maleate USP—Freely soluble in water; soluble in alcohol and in chloroform; slightly soluble in ether.

USP requirements:
Chlorpheniramine Maleate USP—Preserve in tight, light-resistant containers. Contains not less than 98.0% and not more than 100.5% of chlorpheniramine maleate, calculated on the dried basis. Meets the requirements for Identification, Melting range (130–135 °C), Loss on drying (not more than 0.5%), Residue on ignition (not more than

0.2%), Related compounds (not more than 2.0%), and Organic volatile impurities.
Chlorpheniramine Maleate Extended-release Capsules USP—Preserve in tight containers. Contain the labeled amount, within ± 10%. Meet the requirements for Identification and Uniformity of dosage units.
Chlorpheniramine Maleate Injection USP—Preserve in single-dose or in multiple-dose containers, preferably of Type I glass, protected from light. A sterile solution of Chlorpheniramine Maleate in Water for Injection. Contains the labeled amount, within ± 10%. Meets the requirements for Identification, Bacterial endotoxins, pH (4.0–5.2), and Injections.
Chlorpheniramine Maleate Oral Solution—Not in USP.
Chlorpheniramine Maleate Syrup USP—Preserve in tight, light-resistant containers. Contains the labeled amount, within ± 10%. Meets the requirements for Identification and Alcohol content (6.0–8.0%).
Chlorpheniramine Maleate Tablets USP—Preserve in tight containers. Contain the labeled amount, within ± 7%. Meet the requirements for Identification, Dissolution (75% in 45 minutes in water in Apparatus 2 at 50 rpm), and Uniformity of dosage units.
Chlorpheniramine Maleate Extended-release Tablets—Not in USP.

CHLORPHENIRAMINE, CODEINE, ASPIRIN, AND CAFFEINE

For *Chlorpheniramine*, *Codeine*, *Aspirin*, and *Caffeine*—See individual listings for chemistry information.

USP requirements: Chlorpheniramine Maleate, Codeine Phosphate, Aspirin, and Caffeine Tablets—Not in USP.

CHLORPHENIRAMINE, CODEINE, AND GUAIFENESIN

For *Chlorpheniramine*, *Codeine*, and *Guaifenesin*—See individual listings for chemistry information.

USP requirements: Chlorpheniramine Maleate, Codeine Phosphate, and Guaifenesin Syrup—Not in USP.

CHLORPHENIRAMINE AND DEXTROMETHORPHAN

For *Chlorpheniramine* and *Dextromethorphan*—See individual listings for chemistry information.

USP requirements: Chlorpheniramine Maleate and Dextromethorphan Hydrobromide Oral Solution—Not in USP.

CHLORPHENIRAMINE, DEXTROMETHORPHAN, AND ACETAMINOPHEN

For *Chlorpheniramine*, *Dextromethorphan*, and *Acetaminophen*—See individual listings for chemistry information.

USP requirements: Chlorpheniramine Maleate, Dextromethorphan Hydrobromide, and Acetaminophen Capsules—Not in USP.

CHLORPHENIRAMINE, EPHEDRINE, AND GUAIFENESIN

For *Chlorpheniramine*, *Ephedrine*, and *Guaifenesin*—See individual listings for chemistry information.

USP requirements: Chlorpheniramine Maleate, Ephedrine Sulfate, and Guaifenesin Oral Solution—Not in USP.

CHLORPHENIRAMINE, EPHEDRINE, PHENYLEPHRINE, AND CARBETAPENTANE

Chemical group: Chlorpheniramine—Propylamine derivative (alkylamine).

USP requirements:
  Chlorpheniramine Tannate, Ephedrine Tannate, Phenylephrine Tannate, and Carbetapentane Tannate Oral Suspension—Not in USP.
  Chlorpheniramine Tannate, Ephedrine Tannate, Phenylephrine Tannate, and Carbetapentane Tannate Tablets—Not in USP.

CHLORPHENIRAMINE, EPHEDRINE, PHENYLEPHRINE, DEXTROMETHORPHAN, AMMONIUM CHLORIDE, AND IPECAC

For *Chlorpheniramine, Ephedrine, Phenylephrine, Dextromethorphan, Ammonium Chloride,* and *Ipecac*—See individual listings for chemistry information.

USP requirements: Chlorpheniramine Maleate, Ephedrine Hydrochloride, Phenylephrine Hydrochloride, Dextromethorphan Hydrobromide, Ammonium Chloride, and Ipecac Fluidextract Syrup—Not in USP.

CHLORPHENIRAMINE, PHENINDAMINE, PHENYLEPHRINE, DEXTROMETHORPHAN, ACETAMINOPHEN, SALICYLAMIDE, CAFFEINE, AND ASCORBIC ACID

For *Chlorpheniramine, Phenindamine, Phenylephrine, Dextromethorphan, Acetaminophen, Salicylamide, Caffeine,* and *Ascorbic Acid*—See individual listings for chemistry information.

USP requirements: Chlorpheniramine Maleate, Phenindamine Tartrate, Phenylephrine Hydrochloride, Dextromethorphan Hydrobromide, Acetaminophen, Salicylamide, Caffeine, and Ascorbic Acid Tablets—Not in USP.

CHLORPHENIRAMINE, PHENINDAMINE, AND PHENYLPROPANOLAMINE

For *Chlorpheniramine, Phenindamine,* and *Phenylpropanolamine*—See individual listings for chemistry information.

USP requirements: Chlorpheniramine Maleate, Phenindamine Tartrate, and Phenylpropanolamine Hydrochloride Extended-release Tablets—Not in USP.

CHLORPHENIRAMINE, PHENINDAMINE, PYRILAMINE, PHENYLEPHRINE, HYDROCODONE, AND AMMONIUM CHLORIDE

For *Chlorpheniramine, Phenindamine, Pyrilamine, Phenylephrine, Hydrocodone,* and *Ammonium Chloride*—See individual listings for chemistry information.

USP requirements: Chlorpheniramine Maleate, Phenindamine Tartrate, Pyrilamine Maleate, Phenylephrine Hydrochloride, Hydrocodone Bitartrate, and Ammonium Chloride Syrup—Not in USP.

CHLORPHENIRAMINE, PHENIRAMINE, PYRILAMINE, PHENYLEPHRINE, HYDROCODONE, SALICYLAMIDE, CAFFEINE, AND ASCORBIC ACID

Source: Caffeine—Coffee, tea, cola, and cocoa or chocolate. May also be synthesized from urea or dimethylurea.

Chemical group:
  Chlorpheniramine; Pheniramine—Propylamine derivatives (alkylamines).
  Pyrilamine—Ethylenediamine derivative.

Caffeine—Methylated xanthine.

Chemical name:
  Chlorpheniramine maleate—2-Pyridinepropanamine, gamma-(4-chlorophenyl)-*N*,N-dimethyl-, (*Z*)-2-butenedioate (1:1).
  Pheniramine maleate—2-[alpha-[2-Dimethylaminoethyl]-benzyl]pyridine bimaleate.
  Pyrilamine maleate—1,2-Ethanediamine, *N*-[(4-methoxyphenyl)methyl]-*N'*,*N'*-dimethyl-*N*-2-pyridinyl-, (*Z*)-2-butenedioate (1:1).
  Phenylephrine hydrochloride—Benzenemethanol, 3-hydroxy-alpha-[(methylamino)methyl]-, hydrochloride.
  Hydrocodone bitartrate—Morphinan-6-one, 4,5-epoxy-3-methoxy-17-methyl-, (5 alpha)-, [*R*-(*R**,*R**)]-2,3-dihydroxybutanedioate (1:1), hydrate (2:5).
  Salicylamide—Benzamide, 2-hydroxy-.
  Caffeine—1*H*-Purine-2,6-dione, 3,7-dihydro-1,3,7-trimethyl-.
  Ascorbic acid—L-Ascorbic acid.

Molecular formula:
  Chlorpheniramine maleate—$C_{16}H_{19}ClN_2 \cdot C_4H_4O_4$.
  Pheniramine maleate—$C_{16}H_{20}N_2 \cdot C_4H_4O_4$.
  Pyrilamine maleate—$C_{17}H_{23}N_3O \cdot C_4H_4O_4$.
  Phenylephrine hydrochloride—$C_9H_{13}NO_2 \cdot HCl$.
  Hydrocodone bitartrate—$C_{18}H_{21}NO_3 \cdot C_4H_6O_6 \cdot 2\frac{1}{2}H_2O$ (hydrate); $C_{18}H_{21}NO_3 \cdot C_4H_6O_6$ (anhydrous).
  Salicylamide—$C_7H_7NO_2$.
  Caffeine (anhydrous)—$C_8H_{10}N_4O_2$.
  Ascorbic acid—$C_6H_8O_6$.

Molecular weight:
  Chlorpheniramine maleate—390.87.
  Pheniramine maleate—356.43.
  Pyrilamine maleate—401.46.
  Phenylephrine hydrochloride—203.67.
  Hydrocodone bitartrate—494.50 (hydrate); 449.46 (anhydrous).
  Salicylamide—137.14.
  Caffeine (anhydrous)—194.19.
  Ascorbic acid—176.13.

Description:
  Chlorpheniramine Maleate USP—White, odorless, crystalline powder. Its solutions have a pH between 4 and 5.
  Pheniramine maleate—A white or almost white crystalline powder, odorless or with a slight odor.
  Pyrilamine Maleate USP—White, crystalline powder, usually having a faint odor. Its solutions are acid to litmus.
  Phenylephrine Hydrochloride USP—White or practically white, odorless crystals.
  Hydrocodone Bitartrate USP—Fine, white crystals or a crystalline powder. Is affected by light.
  Salicylamide USP—White, practically odorless, crystalline powder.
  Caffeine USP—White powder, or white, glistening needles, usually matted together. Is odorless. Its solutions are neutral to litmus. The hydrate is efflorescent in air.
  Ascorbic Acid USP—White or slightly yellow crystals or powder. On exposure to light it gradually darkens. In the dry state, is reasonably stable in air, but in solution rapidly oxidizes. Melts at about 190 °C.

  NF category: Antioxidant.

pKa:
  Chlorpheniramine maleate—9.2.
  Ascorbic acid—4.2 and 11.6.

Solubility:
  Chlorpheniramine Maleate USP—Freely soluble in water; soluble in alcohol and in chloroform; slightly soluble in ether.

Pheniramine maleate—Soluble in water, in alcohol, and in chloroform; very slightly soluble in ether.

Pyrilamine Maleate USP—Very soluble in water; freely soluble in alcohol and in chloroform; slightly soluble in ether.

Phenylephrine Hydrochloride USP—Freely soluble in water and in alcohol.

Hydrocodone Bitartrate USP—Soluble in water; slightly soluble in alcohol; insoluble in ether and in chloroform.

Salicylamide USP—Slightly soluble in water and in chloroform; soluble in alcohol and in propylene glycol; freely soluble in ether and in solutions of alkalies.

Caffeine USP—Sparingly soluble in water and in alcohol; freely soluble in chloroform; slightly soluble in ether.

The aqueous solubility of caffeine is increased by organic acids or their alkali salts, such as citrates, benzoates, salicylates, or cinnamates, which dissociate to yield caffeine when dissolved in biological fluids.

Ascorbic Acid USP—Freely soluble in water; sparingly soluble in alcohol; insoluble in chloroform and in ether.

USP requirements: Chlorpheniramine Maleate, Pheniramine Maleate, Pyrilamine Maleate, Phenylephrine Hydrochloride, Hydrocodone Bitartrate, Salicylamide, Caffeine, and Ascorbic Acid Capsules—Not in USP.

CHLORPHENIRAMINE AND PHENYLEPHRINE

For *Chlorpheniramine* and *Phenylephrine*—See individual listings for chemistry information.

USP requirements:

Chlorpheniramine Maleate and Phenylephrine Hydrochloride Extended-release Capsules—Not in USP.

Chlorpheniramine Maleate and Phenylephrine Hydrochloride Elixir—Not in USP.

Chlorpheniramine Maleate and Phenylephrine Hydrochloride Syrup—Not in USP.

Chlorpheniramine Maleate and Phenylephrine Hydrochloride Tablets—Not in USP.

Chlorpheniramine Maleate and Phenylephrine Hydrochloride Chewable Tablets—Not in USP.

CHLORPHENIRAMINE, PHENYLEPHRINE, AND ACETAMINOPHEN

For *Chlorpheniramine, Phenylephrine,* and *Acetaminophen*—See individual listings for chemistry information.

USP requirements: Chlorpheniramine Maleate, Phenylephrine Hydrochloride, and Acetaminophen Tablets—Not in USP.

CHLORPHENIRAMINE, PHENYLEPHRINE, ACETAMINOPHEN, AND CAFFEINE

For *Chlorpheniramine, Phenylephrine, Acetaminophen,* and *Caffeine*—See individual listings for chemistry information.

USP requirements: Chlorpheniramine Maleate, Phenylephrine Hydrochloride, Acetaminophen, and Caffeine Tablets—Not in USP.

CHLORPHENIRAMINE, PHENYLEPHRINE, ACETAMINOPHEN, AND SALICYLAMIDE

For *Chlorpheniramine, Phenylephrine, Acetaminophen,* and *Salicylamide*—See individual listings for chemistry information.

USP requirements:

Chlorpheniramine Maleate, Phenylephrine Hydrochloride, Acetaminophen, and Salicylamide Capsules—Not in USP.

Chlorpheniramine Maleate, Phenylephrine Hydrochloride, Acetaminophen, and Salicylamide Tablets—Not in USP.

CHLORPHENIRAMINE, PHENYLEPHRINE, ACETAMINOPHEN, SALICYLAMIDE, AND CAFFEINE

For *Chlorpheniramine, Phenylephrine, Acetaminophen, Salicylamide,* and *Caffeine*—See individual listings for chemistry information.

USP requirements: Chlorpheniramine Maleate, Phenylephrine Hydrochloride, Acetaminophen, Salicylamide, and Caffeine Capsules—Not in USP.

CHLORPHENIRAMINE, PHENYLEPHRINE, CODEINE, AMMONIUM CHLORIDE, POTASSIUM GUAIACOLSULFONATE, AND SODIUM CITRATE

Chemical group: Chlorpheniramine—Propylamine derivative (alkylamine).

Chemical name:

Chlorpheniramine maleate—2-Pyridinepropanamine, gamma-(4-chlorophenyl)-*N*,*N*-dimethyl-, (*Z*)-2-butenedioate (1:1).

Phenylephrine hydrochloride—Benzenemethanol, 3-hydroxy-alpha-[(methylamino)methyl]-, hydrochloride.

Codeine phosphate—Morphinan-6-ol, 7,8-didehydro-4,5-epoxy-3-methoxy-17-methyl-, (5 alpha,6 alpha)-, phosphate (1:1) (salt), hemihydrate.

Ammonium chloride—Ammonium chloride.

Potassium guaiacolsulfonate—Benzenesulfonic acid, hydroxymethoxy-, monopotassium salt, hemihydrate.

Sodium citrate—1,2,3-Propanetricarboxylic acid, 2-hydroxy-, trisodium salt.

Molecular formula:

Chlorpheniramine maleate—$C_{16}H_{19}ClN_2 \cdot C_4H_4O_4$.

Phenylephrine hydrochloride—$C_9H_{13}NO_2 \cdot HCl$.

Codeine phosphate—$C_{18}H_{21}NO_3 \cdot H_3PO_4 \cdot \frac{1}{2}H_2O$ (hemihydrate); $C_{18}H_{21}NO_3 \cdot H_3PO_4$ (anhydrous).

Ammonium chloride—NH_4Cl.

Potassium guaiacolsulfonate—$C_7H_7KO_5S \cdot \frac{1}{2}H_2O$.

Sodium citrate—$C_6H_5Na_3O_7$.

Molecular weight:

Chlorpheniramine maleate—390.87.

Phenylephrine hydrochloride—203.67.

Codeine phosphate—406.37 (hemihydrate); 397.36 (anhydrous).

Ammonium chloride—53.49.

Potassium guaiacolsulfonate—251.29.

Sodium citrate—258.07 (anhydrous).

Description:

Chlorpheniramine Maleate USP—White, odorless, crystalline powder. Its solutions have a pH between 4 and 5.

Phenylephrine Hydrochloride USP—White or practically white, odorless crystals.

Codeine Phosphate USP—Fine, white, needle-shaped crystals, or white, crystalline powder. Odorless. Is affected by light. Its solutions are acid to litmus.

Ammonium Chloride USP—Colorless crystals or white, fine or coarse, crystalline powder. Is somewhat hygroscopic.

Sodium Citrate USP—Colorless crystals or white, crystalline powder.

NF category: Buffering agent.

pKa: Chlorpheniramine maleate—9.2.

Solubility:

Chlorpheniramine Maleate USP—Freely soluble in water; soluble in alcohol and in chloroform; slightly soluble in ether.

Phenylephrine Hydrochloride USP—Freely soluble in water and in alcohol.

Codeine Phosphate USP—Freely soluble in water; very soluble in hot water; slightly soluble in alcohol but more so in boiling alcohol.

Ammonium Chloride USP—Freely soluble in water and in glycerin, and even more so in boiling water; sparingly soluble in alcohol.

Sodium Citrate USP—Hydrous form freely soluble in water and very soluble in boiling water. Insoluble in alcohol.

USP requirements: Chlorpheniramine Maleate, Phenylephrine Hydrochloride, Codeine Phosphate, Ammonium Chloride, Potassium Guaiacolsulfonate, and Sodium Citrate Oral Solution—Not in USP.

CHLORPHENIRAMINE, PHENYLEPHRINE, CODEINE, AND POTASSIUM IODIDE

For *Chlorpheniramine*, *Phenylephrine*, *Codeine*, and *Potassium Iodide*—See individual listings for chemistry information.

USP requirements: Chlorpheniramine Maleate, Phenylephrine Hydrochloride, Codeine Phosphate, and Potassium Iodide Syrup—Not in USP.

CHLORPHENIRAMINE, PHENYLEPHRINE, AND DEXTROMETHORPHAN

For *Chlorpheniramine*, *Phenylephrine*, and *Dextromethorphan*—See individual listings for chemistry information.

USP requirements:
Chlorpheniramine Maleate, Phenylephrine Hydrochloride, and Dextromethorphan Hydrobromide Oral Solution—Not in USP.
Chlorpheniramine Maleate, Phenylephrine Hydrochloride, and Dextromethorphan Hydrobromide Tablets—Not in USP.

CHLORPHENIRAMINE, PHENYLEPHRINE, DEXTROMETHORPHAN, ACETAMINOPHEN, AND SALICYLAMIDE

For *Chlorpheniramine*, *Phenylephrine*, *Dextromethorphan*, *Acetaminophen*, and *Salicylamide*—See individual listings for chemistry information.

USP requirements: Chlorpheniramine Maleate, Phenylephrine Hydrochloride, Dextromethorphan Hydrobromide, Acetaminophen, and Salicylamide Tablets—Not in USP.

CHLORPHENIRAMINE, PHENYLEPHRINE, DEXTROMETHORPHAN, AND GUAIFENESIN

For *Chlorpheniramine*, *Phenylephrine*, *Dextromethorphan*, and *Guaifenesin*—See individual listings for chemistry information.

USP requirements: Chlorpheniramine Maleate, Phenylephrine Hydrochloride, Dextromethorphan Hydrobromide, and Guaifenesin Syrup—Not in USP.

CHLORPHENIRAMINE, PHENYLEPHRINE, DEXTROMETHORPHAN, GUAIFENESIN, AND AMMONIUM CHLORIDE

For *Chlorpheniramine*, *Phenylephrine*, *Dextromethorphan*, *Guaifenesin*, and *Ammonium Chloride*—See individual listings for chemistry information.

USP requirements: Chlorpheniramine Maleate, Phenylephrine Hydrochloride, Dextromethorphan Hydrobromide, Guaifenesin, and Ammonium Chloride Oral Solution—Not in USP.

CHLORPHENIRAMINE, PHENYLEPHRINE, AND GUAIFENESIN

For *Chlorpheniramine*, *Phenylephrine*, and *Guaifenesin*—See individual listings for chemistry information.

USP requirements: Chlorpheniramine Maleate, Phenylephrine Hydrochloride, and Guaifenesin Oral Solution—Not in USP.

CHLORPHENIRAMINE, PHENYLEPHRINE, AND HYDROCODONE

For *Chlorpheniramine*, *Phenylephrine*, and *Hydrocodone*—See individual listings for chemistry information.

USP requirements:
Chlorpheniramine Maleate, Phenylephrine Hydrochloride, and Hydrocodone Bitartrate Oral Solution—Not in USP.
Chlorpheniramine Maleate, Phenylephrine Hydrochloride, and Hydrocodone Bitartrate Syrup—Not in USP.

CHLORPHENIRAMINE, PHENYLEPHRINE, HYDROCODONE, ACETAMINOPHEN, AND CAFFEINE

For *Chlorpheniramine*, *Phenylephrine*, *Hydrocodone*, *Acetaminophen*, and *Caffeine*—See individual listings for chemistry information.

USP requirements: Chlorpheniramine Maleate, Phenylephrine Hydrochloride, Hydrocodone Bitartrate, Acetaminophen, and Caffeine Tablets—Not in USP.

CHLORPHENIRAMINE, PHENYLEPHRINE, AND PHENYLPROPANOLAMINE

For *Chlorpheniramine*, *Phenylephrine*, and *Phenylpropanolamine*—See individual listings for chemistry information.

USP requirements:
Chlorpheniramine Maleate, Phenylephrine Hydrochloride, and Phenylpropanolamine Hydrochloride Extended-release Capsules—Not in USP.
Chlorpheniramine Maleate, Phenylephrine Hydrochloride, and Phenylpropanolamine Hydrochloride Tablets—Not in USP.

CHLORPHENIRAMINE, PHENYLEPHRINE, PHENYLPROPANOLAMINE, CARBETAPENTANE, AND POTASSIUM GUAIACOLSULFONATE

Chemical group:
Chlorpheniramine—Propylamine derivative (alkylamine).
Phenylpropanolamine—A synthetic phenylisopropanolamine.

Chemical name:
Chlorpheniramine maleate—2-Pyridinepropanamine, gamma-(4-chlorophenyl)-*N,N*-dimethyl-, (*Z*)-2-butenedioate (1:1).
Phenylephrine hydrochloride—Benzenemethanol, 3-hydroxy-alpha-[(methylamino)methyl]-, hydrochloride.
Phenylpropanolamine hydrochloride—Benzenemethanol, alpha-(1-aminoethyl)-, hydrochloride, (*R**,*S**)-, (±).
Carbetapentane citrate—2-[2-(Diethylamino)ethoxy]ethyl 1-phenylcyclopentanecarboxylate citrate (1:1).
Potassium guaiacolsulfonate—Benzenesulfonic acid, hydroxymethoxy-, monopotassium salt, hemihydrate.

Molecular formula:
Chlorpheniramine maleate—$C_{16}H_{19}ClN_2\cdot C_4H_4O_4$.
Phenylephrine hydrochloride—$C_9H_{13}NO_2\cdot HCl$.
Phenylpropanolamine hydrochloride—$C_9H_{13}NO\cdot HCl$.
Carbetapentane citrate—$C_{20}H_{31}NO_3\cdot C_6H_8O_7$.
Potassium guaiacolsulfonate—$C_7H_7KO_5S\cdot\frac{1}{2}H_2O$.

Molecular weight:
   Chlorpheniramine maleate—390.87.
   Phenylephrine hydrochloride—203.67.
   Phenylpropanolamine hydrochloride—187.67.
   Carbetapentane citrate—525.60.
   Potassium guaiacolsulfonate—251.29.

Description:
   Chlorpheniramine Maleate USP—White, odorless, crystalline powder. Its solutions have a pH between 4 and 5.
   Phenylephrine Hydrochloride USP—White or practically white, odorless crystals.
   Phenylpropanolamine Hydrochloride USP—White, crystalline powder, having a slight aromatic odor. Is affected by light.

pKa:
   Chlorpheniramine maleate—9.2.
   Phenylpropanolamine—9.

Solubility:
   Chlorpheniramine Maleate USP—Freely soluble in water; soluble in alcohol and in chloroform; slightly soluble in ether.
   Phenylephrine Hydrochloride USP—Freely soluble in water and in alcohol.
   Phenylpropanolamine Hydrochloride USP—Freely soluble in water and in alcohol; insoluble in ether.

Other characteristics: Phenylpropanolamine—Similar in structure and action to ephedrine and amphetamine but with less central nervous system (CNS) stimulation.

USP requirements:
   Chlorpheniramine Maleate, Phenylephrine Hydrochloride, Phenylpropanolamine Hydrochloride, Carbetapentane Citrate, and Potassium Guaiacolsulfonate Capsules—Not in USP.
   Chlorpheniramine Maleate, Phenylephrine Hydrochloride, Phenylpropanolamine Hydrochloride, Carbetapentane Citrate, and Potassium Guaiacolsulfonate Syrup—Not in USP.

CHLORPHENIRAMINE, PHENYLEPHRINE, PHENYLPROPANOLAMINE, AND CODEINE

For *Chlorpheniramine, Phenylephrine, Phenylpropanolamine*, and *Codeine*—See individual listings for chemistry information.

USP requirements: Chlorpheniramine Maleate, Phenylephrine Hydrochloride, Phenylpropanolamine Hydrochloride, and Codeine Phosphate Syrup—Not in USP.

CHLORPHENIRAMINE, PHENYLEPHRINE, PHENYLPROPANOLAMINE, AND DEXTROMETHORPHAN

For *Chlorpheniramine, Phenylephrine, Phenylpropanolamine*, and *Dextromethorphan*—See individual listings for chemistry information.

USP requirements: Chlorpheniramine Maleate, Phenylephrine Hydrochloride, Phenylpropanolamine Hydrochloride, and Dextromethorphan Hydrobromide Syrup—Not in USP.

CHLORPHENIRAMINE, PHENYLEPHRINE, PHENYLPROPANOLAMINE, DEXTROMETHORPHAN, GUAIFENESIN, AND ACETAMINOPHEN

For *Chlorpheniramine, Phenylephrine, Phenylpropanolamine, Dextromethorphan, Guaifenesin*, and *Acetaminophen*—See individual listings for chemistry information.

USP requirements:
   Chlorpheniramine Maleate, Phenylephrine Hydrochloride, Phenylpropanolamine Hydrochloride, Dextromethorphan Hydrobromide, Guaifenesin, and Acetaminophen Syrup—Not in USP.
   Chlorpheniramine Maleate, Phenylephrine Hydrochloride, Phenylpropanolamine Hydrochloride, Dextromethorphan Hydrobromide, Guaifenesin, and Acetaminophen Tablets—Not in USP.

CHLORPHENIRAMINE, PHENYLEPHRINE, PHENYLPROPANOLAMINE, AND DIHYDROCODEINE

For *Chlorpheniramine, Phenylephrine, Phenylpropanolamine* and *Dihydrocodeine*—See individual listings for chemistry information.

USP requirements: Chlorpheniramine Maleate, Phenylephrine Hydrochloride, Phenylpropanolamine Hydrochloride, and Dihydrocodeine Bitartrate Syrup—Not in USP.

CHLORPHENIRAMINE AND PHENYLPROPANOLAMINE

For *Chlorpheniramine* and *Phenylpropanolamine*—See individual listings for chemistry information.

USP requirements:
   Chlorpheniramine Maleate and Phenylpropanolamine Hydrochloride Extended-release Capsules—Not in USP.
   Chlorpheniramine Maleate and Phenylpropanolamine Hydrochloride Granules—Not in USP.
   Chlorpheniramine Maleate and Phenylpropanolamine Hydrochloride Oral Solution—Not in USP.
   Chlorpheniramine Maleate and Phenylpropanolamine Hydrochloride Syrup—Not in USP.
   Chlorpheniramine Maleate and Phenylpropanolamine Hydrochloride Tablets—Not in USP.
   Chlorpheniramine Maleate and Phenylpropanolamine Hydrochloride Chewable Tablets—Not in USP.
   Chlorpheniramine Maleate and Phenylpropanolamine Hydrochloride Extended-release Tablets—Not in USP.
   Chlorpheniramine and Phenylpropanolamine Polistirexes Extended-release Oral Suspension—Not in USP.

CHLORPHENIRAMINE, PHENYLPROPANOLAMINE, AND ACETAMINOPHEN

For *Chlorpheniramine, Phenylpropanolamine*, and *Acetaminophen*—See individual listings for chemistry information.

USP requirements:
   Chlorpheniramine Maleate, Phenylpropanolamine Hydrochloride, and Acetaminophen Capsules—Not in USP.
   Chlorpheniramine Maleate, Phenylpropanolamine Hydrochloride, and Acetaminophen Tablets—Not in USP.
   Chlorpheniramine Maleate, Phenylpropanolamine Hydrochloride, and Acetaminophen Chewable Tablets—Not in USP.
   Chlorpheniramine Maleate, Phenylpropanolamine Hydrochloride, and Acetaminophen Effervescent Tablets—Not in USP.
   Chlorpheniramine Maleate, Phenylpropanolamine Hydrochloride, and Acetaminophen Extended-release Tablets—Not in USP.

CHLORPHENIRAMINE, PHENYLPROPANOLAMINE, ACETAMINOPHEN, AND CAFFEINE

For *Chlorpheniramine, Phenylpropanolamine, Acetaminophen*, and *Caffeine*—See individual listings for chemistry information.

USP requirements: Chlorpheniramine Maleate, Phenylpropanolamine Hydrochloride, Acetaminophen, and Caffeine Tablets—Not in USP.

CHLORPHENIRAMINE, PHENYLPROPANOLAMINE, ACETAMINOPHEN, AND SALICYLAMIDE

For *Chlorpheniramine, Phenylpropanolamine, Acetaminophen,* and *Salicylamide*—See individual listings for chemistry information.

USP requirements: Chlorpheniramine Maleate, Phenylpropanolamine Hydrochloride, Acetaminophen, and Salicylamide Extended-release Tablets—Not in USP.

CHLORPHENIRAMINE, PHENYLPROPANOLAMINE, AND ASPIRIN

For *Chlorpheniramine, Phenylpropanolamine,* and *Aspirin*—See individual listings for chemistry information.

USP requirements:
Chlorpheniramine Maleate, Phenylpropanolamine Bitartrate, and Aspirin for Oral Solution—Not in USP.
Chlorpheniramine Maleate, Phenylpropanolamine Hydrochloride, and Aspirin for Oral Solution—Not in USP.
Chlorpheniramine Maleate, Phenylpropanolamine Hydrochloride, and Aspirin Tablets—Not in USP.

CHLORPHENIRAMINE, PHENYLPROPANOLAMINE, ASPIRIN, AND CAFFEINE

For *Chlorpheniramine, Phenylpropanolamine, Aspirin,* and *Caffeine*—See individual listings for chemistry information.

USP requirements:
Chlorpheniramine Maleate, Phenylpropanolamine Hydrochloride, Aspirin, and Caffeine Capsules—Not in USP.
Chlorpheniramine Maleate, Phenylpropanolamine Hydrochloride, Aspirin, and Caffeine Tablets—Not in USP.

CHLORPHENIRAMINE, PHENYLPROPANOLAMINE, AND CARAMIPHEN

Chemical group:
Chlorpheniramine—Propylamine derivative (alkylamine).
Phenylpropanolamine—A synthetic phenylisopropanolamine.

Chemical name:
Chlorpheniramine maleate—2-Pyridinepropanamine, gamma-(4-chlorophenyl)-*N,N*-dimethyl-, (*Z*)-2-butenedioate (1:1).
Phenylpropanolamine hydrochloride—Benzenemethanol, alpha-(1-aminoethyl)-, hydrochloride, (*R*,S**)-, (±).
Caramiphen edisylate—1-Phenylcyclopentane-1-carboxylic acid, 2-diethylaminoethyl ester, 1,2-ethanedisulfonate (2:1).

Molecular formula:
Chlorpheniramine maleate—$C_{16}H_{19}ClN_2 \cdot C_4H_4O_4$.
Phenylpropanolamine hydrochloride—$C_9H_{13}NO \cdot HCl$.
Caramiphen edisylate—$(C_{18}H_{27}NO_2)_2 \cdot C_2H_6O_6S_2$.

Molecular weight:
Chlorpheniramine maleate—390.87.
Phenylpropanolamine hydrochloride—187.67.
Caramiphen edisylate—769.03.

Description:
Chlorpheniramine Maleate USP—White, odorless, crystalline powder. Its solutions have a pH between 4 and 5.
Phenylpropanolamine Hydrochloride USP—White, crystalline powder, having a slight aromatic odor. Is affected by light.
Caramiphen edisylate—Off-white crystals. Melting point 115–116 °C.

pKa:
Chlorpheniramine maleate—9.2.
Phenylpropanolamine—9.

Solubility:
Chlorpheniramine Maleate USP—Freely soluble in water; soluble in alcohol and in chloroform; slightly soluble in ether.
Phenylpropanolamine Hydrochloride USP—Freely soluble in water and in alcohol; insoluble in ether.
Caramiphen edisylate—One gram dissolves in about 2 mL of water; soluble in alcohol.

Other characteristics: Phenylpropanolamine—Similar in structure and action to ephedrine and amphetamine but with less central nervous system (CNS) stimulation.

USP requirements: Chlorpheniramine Maleate, Phenylpropanolamine Hydrochloride, and Caramiphen Edisylate Extended-release Capsules—Not in USP.

CHLORPHENIRAMINE, PHENYLPROPANOLAMINE, CODEINE, GUAIFENESIN, AND ACETAMINOPHEN

For *Chlorpheniramine, Phenylpropanolamine, Codeine, Guaifenesin,* and *Acetaminophen*—See individual listings for chemistry information.

USP requirements:
Chlorpheniramine Maleate, Phenylpropanolamine Hydrochloride, Codeine Phosphate, Guaifenesin, and Acetaminophen Syrup—Not in USP.
Chlorpheniramine Maleate, Phenylpropanolamine Hydrochloride, Codeine Phosphate, Guaifenesin, and Acetaminophen Tablets—Not in USP.

CHLORPHENIRAMINE, PHENYLPROPANOLAMINE, AND DEXTROMETHORPHAN

For *Chlorpheniramine, Phenylpropanolamine,* and *Dextromethorphan*—See individual listings for chemistry information.

USP requirements:
Chlorpheniramine Maleate, Phenylpropanolamine Hydrochloride, and Dextromethorphan Hydrobromide Oral Gel—Not in USP.
Chlorpheniramine Maleate, Phenylpropanolamine Hydrochloride, and Dextromethorphan Hydrobromide Granules—Not in USP.
Chlorpheniramine Maleate, Phenylpropanolamine Hydrochloride, and Dextromethorphan Hydrobromide Oral Solution—Not in USP.
Chlorpheniramine Maleate, Phenylpropanolamine Hydrochloride, and Dextromethorphan Hydrobromide Syrup—Not in USP.
Chlorpheniramine Maleate, Phenylpropanolamine Hydrochloride, and Dextromethorphan Hydrobromide Tablets—Not in USP.

CHLORPHENIRAMINE, PHENYLPROPANOLAMINE, DEXTROMETHORPHAN, AND ACETAMINOPHEN

For *Chlorpheniramine, Phenylpropanolamine, Dextromethorphan,* and *Acetaminophen*—See individual listings for chemistry information.

USP requirements:
Chlorpheniramine Maleate, Phenylpropanolamine Hydrochloride, Dextromethorphan Hydrobromide, and Acetaminophen Capsules—Not in USP.
Chlorpheniramine Maleate, Phenylpropanolamine Hydrochloride, Dextromethorphan Hydrobromide, and Acetaminophen Oral Solution—Not in USP.
Chlorpheniramine Maleate, Phenylpropanolamine Hydrochloride, Dextromethorphan Hydrobromide, and Acetaminophen Tablets—Not in USP.

CHLORPHENIRAMINE, PHENYLPROPANOLAMINE, DEXTROMETHORPHAN, ACETAMINOPHEN, AND CAFFEINE

For *Chlorpheniramine, Phenylpropanolamine, Dextromethorphan, Acetaminophen,* and *Caffeine*—See individual listings for chemistry information.

USP requirements: Chlorpheniramine Maleate, Phenylpropanolamine Hydrochloride, Dextromethorphan Hydrobromide, Acetaminophen, and Caffeine Capsules—Not in USP.

CHLORPHENIRAMINE, PHENYLPROPANOLAMINE, DEXTROMETHORPHAN, AND AMMONIUM CHLORIDE

For *Chlorpheniramine, Phenylpropanolamine, Dextromethorphan,* and *Ammonium Chloride*—See individual listings for chemistry information.

USP requirements: Chlorpheniramine Maleate, Phenylpropanolamine Hydrochloride, Dextromethorphan Hydrobromide, and Ammonium Chloride Syrup—Not in USP.

CHLORPHENIRAMINE, PHENYLPROPANOLAMINE, AND GUAIFENESIN

For *Chlorpheniramine, Phenylpropanolamine,* and *Guaifenesin*—See individual listings for chemistry information.

USP requirements: Chlorpheniramine Maleate, Phenylpropanolamine Hydrochloride, and Guaifenesin Oral Solution—Not in USP.

CHLORPHENIRAMINE, PHENYLPROPANOLAMINE, GUAIFENESIN, SODIUM CITRATE, AND CITRIC ACID

For *Chlorpheniramine, Phenylpropanolamine, Guaifenesin, Sodium Citrate* and *Citric Acid*—See individual listings for chemistry information.

USP requirements: Chlorpheniramine Maleate, Phenylpropanolamine Hydrochloride, Guaifenesin, Sodium Citrate, and Citric Acid Oral Solution—Not in USP.

CHLORPHENIRAMINE, PHENYLPROPANOLAMINE, HYDROCODONE, GUAIFENESIN, AND SALICYLAMIDE

For *Chlorpheniramine, Phenylpropanolamine, Hydrocodone, Guaifenesin,* and *Salicylamide*—See individual listings for chemistry information.

USP requirements: Chlorpheniramine Maleate, Phenylpropanolamine Hydrochloride, Hydrocodone Bitartrate, Guaifenesin, and Salicylamide Tablets—Not in USP.

CHLORPHENIRAMINE, PHENYLTOLOXAMINE, EPHEDRINE, CODEINE, AND GUAIACOL

Chemical group: Chlorpheniramine—Propylamine derivative (alkylamine).

Chemical name: Guaiacol carbonate—Carbonic acid bis(2-methoxyphenyl) ester; guaiacol carbonic acid neutral ester; carbonic acid guaiacol ether.

Molecular formula: Guaiacol carbonate—$C_{15}H_{14}O_5$.

Molecular weight: Guaiacol carbonate—274.26.

Description: Guaiacol carbonate—Odorless needles from ethanol. It has a melting point of 88.1 °C.

Solubility: Guaiacol carbonate—Practically insoluble in water; soluble in ethanol, in chloroform, and in ether; slightly soluble in liquid fatty acids.

USP requirements: Chlorpheniramine Resin Complex, Phenyltoloxamine Resin Complex, Ephedrine Resin Complex, Codeine Resin Complex, and Guaiacol Carbonate Oral Suspension—Not in USP.

CHLORPHENIRAMINE, PHENYLTOLOXAMINE, AND PHENYLEPHRINE

Chemical group:
Chlorpheniramine—Propylamine derivative (alkylamine).
Phenyltoloxamine citrate—Ethanolamine derivative.

Chemical name:
Chlorpheniramine maleate—2-Pyridinepropanamine, gamma-(4-chlorophenyl)-*N,N*-dimethyl-, (*Z*)-2-butenedioate (1:1).
Phenyltoloxamine citrate—2-(2-Benzylphenoxy)-*NN*-dimethylethylamine dihydrogen citrate.
Phenylephrine hydrochloride—Benzenemethanol, 3-hydroxy-alpha-[(methylamino)methyl]-, hydrochloride.

Molecular formula:
Chlorpheniramine maleate—$C_{16}H_{19}ClN_2 \cdot C_4H_4O_4$.
Phenyltoloxamine citrate—$C_{17}H_{21}NO \cdot C_6H_8O_7$.
Phenylephrine hydrochloride—$C_9H_{13}NO_2 \cdot HCl$.

Molecular weight:
Chlorpheniramine maleate—390.87.
Phenyltoloxamine citrate—447.5.
Phenylephrine hydrochloride—203.67.

Description:
Chlorpheniramine Maleate USP—White, odorless, crystalline powder. Its solutions have a pH between 4 and 5.
Phenylephrine Hydrochloride USP—White or practically white, odorless crystals.

pKa: Chlorpheniramine maleate—9.2.

Solubility:
Chlorpheniramine Maleate USP—Freely soluble in water; soluble in alcohol and in chloroform; slightly soluble in ether.
Phenylephrine Hydrochloride USP—Freely soluble in water and in alcohol.

USP requirements:
Chlorpheniramine Maleate, Phenyltoloxamine Citrate, and Phenylephrine Hydrochloride Extended-release Capsules—Not in USP.
Chlorpheniramine Maleate, Phenyltoloxamine Citrate, and Phenylephrine Hydrochloride Tablets—Not in USP.

CHLORPHENIRAMINE, PHENYLTOLOXAMINE, PHENYLEPHRINE, AND PHENYLPROPANOLAMINE

Chemical group:
Chlorpheniramine—Propylamine derivative (alkylamine).
Phenyltoloxamine citrate—Ethanolamine derivative.
Phenylpropanolamine—A synthetic phenylisopropanolamine.

Chemical name:
Chlorpheniramine maleate—2-Pyridinepropanamine, gamma-(4-chlorophenyl)-*N,N*-dimethyl-, (*Z*)-2-butenedioate (1:1).
Phenyltoloxamine citrate—2-(2-Benzylphenoxy)-*NN*-dimethylethylamine dihydrogen citrate.
Phenylephrine hydrochloride—Benzenemethanol, 3-hydroxy-alpha-[(methylamino)methyl]-, hydrochloride.
Phenylpropanolamine hydrochloride—Benzenemethanol, alpha-(1-aminoethyl)-, hydrochloride, (*R*,S**)-, (±).

Molecular formula:
Chlorpheniramine maleate—$C_{16}H_{19}ClN_2 \cdot C_4H_4O_4$.

Phenyltoloxamine citrate—$C_{17}H_{21}NO \cdot C_6H_8O_7$.
Phenylephrine hydrochloride—$C_9H_{13}NO_2 \cdot HCl$.
Phenylpropanolamine hydrochloride—$C_9H_{13}NO \cdot HCl$.

Molecular weight:
Chlorpheniramine maleate—390.87.
Phenyltoloxamine citrate—447.5.
Phenylephrine hydrochloride—203.67.
Phenylpropanolamine hydrochloride—187.67.

Description:
Chlorpheniramine Maleate USP—White, odorless, crystalline powder. Its solutions have a pH between 4 and 5.
Phenylephrine Hydrochloride USP—White or practically white, odorless crystals.
Phenylpropanolamine Hydrochloride USP—White, crystalline powder, having a slight aromatic odor. Is affected by light.

pKa:
Chlorpheniramine maleate—9.2.
Phenylpropanolamine hydrochloride—9.

Solubility:
Chlorpheniramine Maleate USP—Freely soluble in water; soluble in alcohol and in chloroform; slightly soluble in ether.
Phenylephrine Hydrochloride USP—Freely soluble in water and in alcohol.
Phenylpropanolamine Hydrochloride USP—Freely soluble in water and in alcohol; insoluble in ether.

Other characteristics: Phenylpropanolamine—Similar in structure and action to ephedrine and amphetamine but with less central nervous system (CNS) stimulation.

USP requirements:
Chlorpheniramine Maleate, Phenyltoloxamine Citrate, Phenylephrine Hydrochloride, and Phenylpropanolamine Hydrochloride Extended-release Capsules—Not in USP.
Chlorpheniramine Maleate, Phenyltoloxamine Citrate, Phenylephrine Hydrochloride, and Phenylpropanolamine Hydrochloride Oral Solution—Not in USP.
Chlorpheniramine Maleate, Phenyltoloxamine Citrate, Phenylephrine Hydrochloride, and Phenylpropanolamine Hydrochloride Syrup—Not in USP.
Chlorpheniramine Maleate, Phenyltoloxamine Citrate, Phenylephrine Hydrochloride, and Phenylpropanolamine Hydrochloride Extended-release Tablets—Not in USP.

CHLORPHENIRAMINE, PHENYLTOLOXAMINE, PHENYLPROPANOLAMINE, AND ACETAMINOPHEN

Chemical group:
Chlorpheniramine—Propylamine derivative (alkylamine).
Phenylpropanolamine—A synthetic phenylisopropanolamine.

Chemical name:
Chlorpheniramine maleate—2-Pyridinepropanamine, gamma-(4-chlorophenyl)-N,N-dimethyl-, (Z)-2-butenedioate (1:1).
Phenyltoloxamine dihydrogen citrate—2-(2-Benzylphenoxy)-NN-dimethylethylamine dihydrogen citrate.
Phenylpropanolamine hydrochloride—Benzenemethanol, alpha-(1-aminoethyl)-, hydrochloride, (R*,S*)-, (±).
Acetaminophen—Acetamide, N-(4-hydroxyphenyl)-.

Molecular formula:
Chlorpheniramine maleate—$C_{16}H_{19}ClN_2 \cdot C_4H_4O_4$.
Phenyltoloxamine dihydrogen citrate—$C_{17}H_{21}NO \cdot C_6H_8O_7$.
Phenylpropanolamine hydrochloride—$C_9H_{13}NO \cdot HCl$.
Acetaminophen—$C_8H_9NO_2$.

Molecular weight:
Chlorpheniramine maleate—390.87.
Phenyltoloxamine dihydrogen citrate—447.5.
Phenylpropanolamine hydrochloride—187.67.
Acetaminophen—151.16.

Description:
Chlorpheniramine Maleate USP—White, odorless, crystalline powder. Its solutions have a pH between 4 and 5.
Phenyltoloxamine dihydrogen citrate—It has a melting point of 138–140 °C.
Phenylpropanolamine Hydrochloride USP—White, crystalline powder, having a slight aromatic odor. Is affected by light.
Acetaminophen USP—White, odorless, crystalline powder.

pKa:
Chlorpheniramine maleate—9.2.
Phenylpropanolamine hydrochloride—9.

Solubility:
Chlorpheniramine Maleate USP—Freely soluble in water; soluble in alcohol and in chloroform; slightly soluble in ether.
Phenyltoloxamine dihydrogen citrate—Soluble in water.
Phenylpropanolamine Hydrochloride USP—Freely soluble in water and in alcohol; insoluble in ether.
Acetaminophen USP—Soluble in boiling water and in 1 N sodium hydroxide; freely soluble in alcohol.

Other characteristics: Phenylpropanolamine—Similar in structure and action to ephedrine and amphetamine but with less central nervous system (CNS) stimulation.

USP requirements: Chlorpheniramine Maleate, Phenyltoloxamine Dihydrogen Citrate, Phenylpropanolamine Hydrochloride, and Acetaminophen Capsules—Not in USP.

CHLORPHENIRAMINE, PHENYLTOLOXAMINE, PHENYLPROPANOLAMINE, DEXTROMETHORPHAN, AND GUAIFENESIN

Source: Dextromethorphan—Methylated dextroisomer of levorphanol.

Chemical group:
Chlorpheniramine—Propylamine derivative (alkylamine).
Phenylpropanolamine—A synthetic phenylisopropanolamine.
Dextromethorphan—Nonopioid, morphinan-derivative.

Chemical name:
Chlorpheniramine maleate—2-Pyridinepropanamine, gamma-(4-chlorophenyl)-N,N-dimethyl-, (Z)-2-butenedioate (1:1).
Phenyltoloxamine citrate—2-(2-Benzylphenoxy)-NN-dimethylethylamine dihydrogen citrate.
Phenylpropanolamine hydrochloride—Benzenemethanol, alpha-(1-aminoethyl)-, hydrochloride, (R*,S*)-, (±).
Dextromethorphan hydrobromide—Morphinan, 3-methoxy-17-methyl-, (9 alpha,13 alpha,14 alpha)-, hydrobromide, monohydrate.
Guaifenesin—1,2-Propanediol, 3-(2-methoxyphenoxy)-.

Molecular formula:
Chlorpheniramine maleate—$C_{16}H_{19}ClN_2 \cdot C_4H_4O_4$.
Phenyltoloxamine citrate—$C_{17}H_{21}NO \cdot C_6H_8O_7$.
Phenylpropanolamine hydrochloride—$C_9H_{13}NO \cdot HCl$.
Dextromethorphan hydrobromide—$C_{18}H_{25}NO \cdot HBr \cdot H_2O$.
Guaifenesin—$C_{10}H_{14}O_4$.

Molecular weight:
Chlorpheniramine maleate—390.87.

Phenyltoloxamine citrate—447.5.
Phenylpropanolamine hydrochloride—187.67.
Dextromethorphan hydrobromide—370.33.
Guaifenesin—198.22.

Description:
Chlorpheniramine Maleate USP—White, odorless, crystalline powder. Its solutions have a pH between 4 and 5.
Phenylpropanolamine Hydrochloride USP—White, crystalline powder, having a slight aromatic odor. Is affected by light.
Dextromethorphan Hydrobromide USP—Practically white crystals or crystalline powder, having a faint odor. Melts at about 126 °C, with decomposition.
Guaifenesin USP—White to slightly gray, crystalline powder. May have a slight characteristic odor.

pKa:
Chlorpheniramine maleate—9.2.
Phenylpropanolamine hydrochloride—9.

Solubility:
Chlorpheniramine Maleate USP—Freely soluble in water; soluble in alcohol and in chloroform; slightly soluble in ether.
Phenylpropanolamine Hydrochloride USP—Freely soluble in water and in alcohol; insoluble in ether.
Dextromethorphan Hydrobromide USP—Sparingly soluble in water; freely soluble in alcohol and in chloroform; insoluble in ether.
Guaifenesin USP—Soluble in water, in alcohol, in chloroform, in glycerin, and in propylene glycol.

Other characteristics: Phenylpropanolamine—Similar in structure and action to ephedrine and amphetamine but with less central nervous system (CNS) stimulation.

USP requirements: Chlorpheniramine Maleate, Phenyltoloxamine Citrate, Phenylpropanolamine Hydrochloride, Dextromethorphan Hydrobromide, and Guaifenesin Syrup—Not in USP.

CHLORPHENIRAMINE AND PSEUDOEPHEDRINE

For *Chlorpheniramine* and *Pseudoephedrine*—See individual listings for chemistry information.

USP requirements:
Chlorpheniramine Maleate and Pseudoephedrine Hydrochloride Capsules—Not in USP.
Chlorpheniramine Maleate and Pseudoephedrine Hydrochloride Extended-release Capsules—Not in USP.
Chlorpheniramine Maleate and Pseudoephedrine Hydrochloride Oral Solution—Not in USP.
Chlorpheniramine Maleate and Pseudoephedrine Hydrochloride Syrup—Not in USP.
Chlorpheniramine Maleate and Pseudoephedrine Hydrochloride Tablets—Not in USP.
Chlorpheniramine Maleate and Pseudoephedrine Sulfate Tablets—Not in USP.
Chlorpheniramine Maleate and Pseudoephedrine Sulfate Extended-release Tablets—Not in USP.

CHLORPHENIRAMINE, PSEUDOEPHEDRINE, AND ACETAMINOPHEN

For *Chlorpheniramine*, *Pseudoephedrine*, and *Acetaminophen*—See individual listings for chemistry information.

USP requirements:
Chlorpheniramine Maleate, Pseudoephedrine Hydrochloride, and Acetaminophen Capsules—Not in USP.
Chlorpheniramine Maleate, Pseudoephedrine Hydrochloride, and Acetaminophen Oral Solution—Not in USP.
Chlorpheniramine Maleate, Pseudoephedrine Hydrochloride, and Acetaminophen for Oral Solution—Not in USP.
Chlorpheniramine Maleate, Pseudoephedrine Hydrochloride, and Acetaminophen Tablets—Not in USP.

CHLORPHENIRAMINE, PSEUDOEPHEDRINE, AND CODEINE

For *Chlorpheniramine*, *Pseudoephedrine*, and *Codeine*—See individual listings for chemistry information.

USP requirements:
Chlorpheniramine Maleate, Pseudoephedrine Hydrochloride, and Codeine Phosphate Elixir—Not in USP.
Chlorpheniramine Maleate, Pseudoephedrine Hydrochloride, and Codeine Phosphate Oral Solution—Not in USP.

CHLORPHENIRAMINE, PSEUDOEPHEDRINE, AND DEXTROMETHORPHAN

For *Chlorpheniramine*, *Pseudoephedrine*, and *Dextromethorphan*—See individual listings for chemistry information.

USP requirements:
Chlorpheniramine Maleate, Pseudoephedrine Hydrochloride, and Dextromethorphan Hydrobromide Oral Solution—Not in USP.
Chlorpheniramine Maleate, Pseudoephedrine Hydrochloride, and Dextromethorphan Hydrobromide Syrup—Not in USP.
Chlorpheniramine Maleate, Pseudoephedrine Hydrochloride, and Dextromethorphan Hydrobromide Chewable Tablets—Not in USP.

CHLORPHENIRAMINE, PSEUDOEPHEDRINE, DEXTROMETHORPHAN, AND ACETAMINOPHEN

For *Chlorpheniramine*, *Pseudoephedrine*, *Dextromethorphan*, and *Acetaminophen*—See individual listings for chemistry information.

USP requirements:
Chlorpheniramine Maleate, Pseudoephedrine Hydrochloride, Dextromethorphan Hydrobromide, and Acetaminophen Capsules—Not in USP.
Chlorpheniramine Maleate, Pseudoephedrine Hydrochloride, Dextromethorphan Hydrobromide, and Acetaminophen Oral Solution—Not in USP.
Chlorpheniramine Maleate, Pseudoephedrine Hydrochloride, Dextromethorphan Hydrobromide, and Acetaminophen for Oral Solution—Not in USP.
Chlorpheniramine Maleate, Pseudoephedrine Hydrochloride, Dextromethorphan Hydrobromide, and Acetaminophen Tablets—Not in USP.

CHLORPHENIRAMINE, PSEUDOEPHEDRINE, DEXTROMETHORPHAN, GUAIFENESIN, AND ASPIRIN

For *Chlorpheniramine*, *Pseudoephedrine*, *Dextromethorphan*, *Guaifenesin*, and *Aspirin*—See individual listings for chemistry information.

USP requirements: Chlorpheniramine Maleate, Pseudoephedrine Hydrochloride, Dextromethorphan Hydrobromide, Guaifenesin, and Aspirin Tablets—Not in USP.

CHLORPHENIRAMINE, PSEUDOEPHEDRINE, AND GUAIFENESIN

For *Chlorpheniramine*, *Pseudoephedrine*, and *Guaifenesin*—See individual listings for chemistry information.

USP requirements: Chlorpheniramine Maleate, Pseudoephedrine Hydrochloride, and Guaifenesin Extended-release Tablets—Not in USP.

CHLORPHENIRAMINE, PSEUDOEPHEDRINE, AND HYDROCODONE

For *Chlorpheniramine*, *Pseudoephedrine*, and *Hydrocodone*—See individual listings for chemistry information.

USP requirements: Chlorpheniramine Maleate, Pseudoephedrine Hydrochloride, and Hydrocodone Bitartrate Oral Solution—Not in USP.

CHLORPHENIRAMINE, PYRILAMINE, AND PHENYLEPHRINE

For *Chlorpheniramine*, *Pyrilamine*, and *Phenylephrine*—See individual listings for chemistry information.

USP requirements:
Chlorpheniramine Tannate, Pyrilamine Tannate, and Phenylephrine Tannate Oral Suspension—Not in USP.
Chlorpheniramine Tannate, Pyrilamine Tannate, and Phenylephrine Tannate Tablets—Not in USP.
Chlorpheniramine Tannate, Pyrilamine Tannate, and Phenylephrine Tannate Extended-release Tablets—Not in USP.

CHLORPHENIRAMINE, PYRILAMINE, PHENYLEPHRINE, AND ACETAMINOPHEN

For *Chlorpheniramine*, *Pyrilamine*, *Phenylephrine*, and *Acetaminophen*—See individual listings for chemistry information.

USP requirements: Chlorpheniramine Maleate, Pyrilamine Maleate, Phenylephrine Hydrochloride, and Acetaminophen Tablets—Not in USP.

CHLORPHENIRAMINE, PYRILAMINE, PHENYLEPHRINE, AND PHENYLPROPANOLAMINE

For *Chlorpheniramine*, *Pyrilamine*, *Phenylephrine*, and *Phenylpropanolamine*—See individual listings for chemistry information.

USP requirements: Chlorpheniramine Maleate, Pyrilamine Maleate, Phenylephrine Hydrochloride, and Phenylpropanolamine Hydrochloride Tablets—Not in USP.

CHLORPHENIRAMINE, PYRILAMINE, PHENYLEPHRINE, PHENYLPROPANOLAMINE, AND ACETAMINOPHEN

For *Chlorpheniramine*, *Pyrilamine*, *Phenylephrine*, *Phenylpropanolamine*, and *Acetaminophen*—See individual listings for chemistry information.

USP requirements: Chlorpheniramine Maleate, Pyrilamine Maleate, Phenylephrine Hydrochloride, Phenylpropanolamine Hydrochloride, and Acetaminophen Tablets—Not in USP.

CHLORPROMAZINE

Chemical group: Aliphatic phenothiazine.

Chemical name:
Chlorpromazine—10*H*-Phenothiazine-10-propanamine, 2-chloro-*N,N*-dimethyl-.
Chlorpromazine hydrochloride—10*H*-Phenothiazine-10-propanamine, 2-chloro-*N,N*-dimethyl-, monohydrochloride.

Molecular formula:
Chlorpromazine—$C_{17}H_{19}ClN_2S$.
Chlorpromazine hydrochloride—$C_{17}H_{19}ClN_2S \cdot HCl$.

Molecular weight:
Chlorpromazine—318.86.
Chlorpromazine hydrochloride—355.32.

Description:
Chlorpromazine USP—White, crystalline solid, having an amine-like odor. Darkens on prolonged exposure to light. Melts at about 60 °C.
Chlorpromazine Hydrochloride USP—White or slightly creamy white, odorless, crystalline powder. Darkens on prolonged exposure to light.

Solubility:
Chlorpromazine USP—Practically insoluble in water and in dilute alkali hydroxides; freely soluble in alcohol, in chloroform, in ether, and in dilute mineral acids.
Chlorpromazine Hydrochloride USP—Very soluble in water; freely soluble in alcohol and in chloroform; insoluble in ether.

USP requirements:
Chlorpromazine USP—Preserve in tight, light-resistant containers. Contains not less than 98.0% and not more than 101.0% of chlorpromazine, calculated on the dried basis. Meets the requirements for Identification, Loss on drying (not more than 1.0%), Other alkylated phenothiazines, and Organic volatile impurities.
Chlorpromazine Suppositories USP—Preserve in well-closed, light-resistant containers, at controlled room temperature. Contain the labeled amount, within ±10%. Meet the requirements for Identification and Other alkylated phenothiazines.
Chlorpromazine Hydrochloride USP—Preserve in tight, light-resistant containers. Contains not less than 98.0% and not more than 101.5% of chlorpromazine hydrochloride, calculated on the dried basis. Meets the requirements for Identification, Melting range (195–198 °C), Loss on drying (not more than 0.5%), Residue on ignition (not more than 0.1%), Other alkylated phenothiazines, and Organic volatile impurities.
Chlorpromazine Hydrochloride Extended-release Capsules—Not in USP.
Chlorpromazine Hydrochloride Oral Concentrate USP—Preserve in tight, light-resistant containers. Label it to indicate that it must be diluted prior to administration. Contains the labeled amount, within ±10%. Meets the requirements for Identification, Microbial limits, pH (2.3–4.1), and Chlorpromazine sulfoxide.
Chlorpromazine Hydrochloride Injection USP—Preserve in single-dose or in multiple-dose containers, preferably of Type I glass, protected from light. A sterile solution of Chlorpromazine Hydrochloride in Water for Injection. Contains, in each mL, not less than 23.75 mg and not more than 26.25 mg of chlorpromazine hydrochloride. Meets the requirements for Identification, Bacterial endotoxins, pH (3.4–5.4), Injections, and Chlorpromazine sulfoxide.
Chlorpromazine Hydrochloride Syrup USP—Preserve in tight, light-resistant containers. Contains, in each 100 mL, not less than 190 mg and not more than 210 mg of chlorpromazine hydrochloride. Meets the requirement for Identification and Chlorpromazine sulfoxide.
Chlorpromazine Hydrochloride Tablets USP—Preserve in well-closed, light-resistant containers. Contain the labeled amount, within ±5%. Meet the requirements for Identification, Dissolution (80% in 30 minutes in 0.1 *N* hydrochloric acid in Apparatus 1 at 50 rpm), Uniformity of dosage units, and Other alkylated phenothiazines.

CHLORPROPAMIDE

Chemical group: Sulfonylurea.

Chemical name: Benzenesulfonamide, 4-chloro-*N*-[(propylamino)carbonyl]-.

Molecular formula: $C_{10}H_{13}ClN_2O_3S$.

Molecular weight: 276.74.

Description: Chlorpropamide USP—White, crystalline powder, having a slight odor.

pKa: 4.8.

Solubility: Chlorpropamide USP—Practically insoluble in water; soluble in alcohol; sparingly soluble in chloroform.

USP requirements:
Chlorpropamide USP—Preserve in well-closed containers. Contains not less than 97.0% and not more than 103.0% of chlorpropamide, calculated on the dried basis. Meets the requirements for Identification, Melting range (126–129 °C), Loss on drying (not more than 1.0%), Selenium (0.003%), Heavy metals (not more than 0.003%), and Residue on ignition (not more than 0.4%).
Chlorpropamide Tablets USP—Preserve in well-closed containers. Contain the labeled amount, within ± 10%. Meet the requirements for Identification, Dissolution (75% in 60 minutes in water in Apparatus 2 at 50 rpm), and Uniformity of dosage units.

CHLORPROTHIXENE

Chemical group: Thioxanthene.

Chemical name: 1-Propanamine, 3-(2-chloro-9*H*-thioxanthen-9-ylidene)-*N,N*-dimethyl-, (*Z*)-.

Molecular formula: $C_{18}H_{18}ClNS$.

Molecular weight: 315.86.

Description: Chlorprothixene USP—Yellow, crystalline powder, having a slight amine-like odor.

Solubility: Chlorprothixene USP—Practically insoluble in water; soluble in alcohol and in ether; freely soluble in chloroform.

Other characteristics: Structurally and pharmacologically similar to the piperazine phenothiazines, which are acetophenazine, fluphenazine, perphenazine, prochlorperazine, and trifluoperazine.

USP requirements:
Chlorprothixene USP—Preserve in tight, light-resistant containers. Contains not less than 99.0% and not more than 101.0% of chlorprothixene, calculated on the dried basis. Meets the requirements for Identification, Melting range (96.5–101.5 °C), Loss on drying (not more than 0.1%), Residue on ignition (not more than 0.1%), Heavy metals (not more than 0.002%), Limit of (*E*)-chlorprothixene [(*E*)-2-chloro-*N,N*-dimethylthioxanthene-Delta$^{9,\,gamma}$-propylamine (not more than 3.0%), and Organic volatile impurities.
Chlorprothixene Injection USP—Preserve in single-dose, low-actinic containers, protected from light. A sterile solution of Chlorprothixene in Water for Injection, prepared with the aid of Hydrochloric Acid. Contains the labeled amount, within ± 5%. Meets the requirements for Identification, Bacterial endotoxins, pH (3.0–4.0), and Injections.
Chlorprothixene Oral Suspension USP—Preserve in tight, light-resistant containers. Contains the labeled amount, within ± 10%. Meets the requirements for Identification and pH (3.5–4.5).
Chlorprothixene Tablets USP—Preserve in well-closed, light-resistant containers. Contain the labeled amount, within ± 7%. Meet the requirements for Identification, Dissolution (75% in 30 minutes in 0.1 *N* hydrochloric acid in Apparatus 1 at 100 rpm), and Uniformity of dosage units.

CHLORTETRACYCLINE

Chemical name: Chlortetracycline hydrochloride—2-Naphthacenecarboxamide, 7-chloro-4-(dimethylamino)-1,4,4a,5,5a,-6,11,12a-octahydro-3,6,10,12,12a-pentahydroxy-6-methyl-1,11-dioxo-, monohydrochloride [4*S*-(4 alpha,4a alpha,5a alpha,6 beta,12a alpha)]-.

Molecular formula: Chlortetracycline hydrochloride—$C_{22}H_{23}$-$ClN_2O_8 \cdot HCl$.

Molecular weight: Chlortetracycline hydrochloride—515.35.

Description: Chlortetracycline Hydrochloride USP—Yellow, crystalline powder. Is odorless. Is stable in air, but is slowly affected by light.

Solubility: Chlortetracycline Hydrochloride USP—Sparingly soluble in water; soluble in solutions of alkali hydroxides and carbonates; slightly soluble in alcohol; practically insoluble in acetone, in chloroform, in dioxane, and in ether.

USP requirements:
Chlortetracycline Bisulfate USP—Preserve in tight, light-resistant containers. Label it to indicate that it is intended for veterinary use only. It has a potency equivalent to not less than 760 mcg of chlortetracycline hydrochloride per mg, calculated on the dried and butyl alcohol-free basis. Meets the requirements for Identification, Crystallinity, Safety, Loss on drying (not more than 2.0%), Sulfate content (not less than 15.0%, calculated on the dried and butyl alcohol-free basis), and Butyl alcohol (not more than 15.0%).
Chlortetracycline Hydrochloride USP—Preserve in tight, light-resistant containers. It has a potency of not less than 900 mcg of chlortetracycline hydrochloride per mg. Meets the requirements for Identification, Specific rotation (−235° to −250°, calculated on the dried basis), Crystallinity, pH (2.3–3.3, in a solution containing 10 mg per mL), and Loss on drying (not more than 2.0%).
Note: Chlortetracycline Hydrochloride labeled solely for use in preparing oral veterinary dosage forms has a potency of not less than 820 mcg of chlortetracycline hydrochloride per mg.
Chlortetracycline Hydrochloride Capsules USP—Preserve in tight, light-resistant containers. Contain the labeled amount, within −10% to +20%. Meet the requirements for Identification, Dissolution (75% in 45 minutes in water in Apparatus 2 at 75 rpm), Uniformity of dosage units, and Loss on drying (not more than 1.0%).
Chlortetracycline Hydrochloride Ointment USP—Preserve in collapsible tubes or in well-closed, light-resistant containers. Contains the labeled amount, within −10% to +25%, in a suitable ointment base. Meets the requirements for Water (not more than 0.5%) and Minimum fill.
Chlortetracycline Hydrochloride Ophthalmic Ointment USP—Preserve in collapsible ophthalmic ointment tubes. Contains the labeled amount, within −10% to +25%. Meets the requirements for Sterility, Minimum fill, Water (not more than 0.5%), and Metal particles.
Chlortetracycline Hydrochloride Soluble Powder USP—Preserve in tight containers, protected from light. Label it to indicate that it is intended for oral veterinary use only. Contains the labeled amount, within −10% to +25%. Meets the requirement for Loss on drying (not more than 2.0%).
Sterile Chlortetracycline Hydrochloride USP—Preserve in Containers for Sterile Solids. It is Chlortetracycline Hydrochloride suitable for parenteral use. It has a potency of not less than 900 mcg of chlortetracycline hydrochloride per mg. Meets the requirements for Depressor substances, Bacterial endotoxins, Sterility, and for Identification tests, pH, Specific rotation, Loss on drying, and Crystallinity under Chlortetracycline Hydrochloride.

Chlortetracycline Hydrochloride Tablets USP—Preserve in tight containers, protected from light. Label Tablets to indicate that they are intended for veterinary use only. Contain the labeled amount, within −10% to +20%. Meet the requirements for Identification, Disintegration (1 hour, with simulated gastric fluid TS being used as the test medium instead of water), Uniformity of dosage units, and Water (not more than 3.0%, or where the Tablets have a diameter of greater than 15 mm, not more than 6.0%).

CHLORTETRACYCLINE AND SULFAMETHAZINE

USP requirements: Chlortetracycline and Sulfamethazine Bisulfates Soluble Powder USP—Preserve in tight, light-resistant containers. A dry mixture of Chlortetracycline Bisulfate and Sulfamethazine Bisulfate and one or more suitable buffers and diluents. Label it to indicate that it is intended for veterinary use only. Contains amounts of chlortetracycline and sulfamethazine bisulfates equivalent to the labeled amounts of chlortetracycline hydrochloride and sulfamethazine, within −15% to +25%. Meets the requirement for Loss on drying (not more than 2.0%).

CHLORTHALIDONE

Chemical name: Benzenesulfonamide, 2-chloro-5-(2,3-dihydro-1-hydroxy-3-oxo-1*H*-isoindol-1-yl)-.

Molecular formula: $C_{14}H_{11}ClN_2O_4S$.

Molecular weight: 338.76.

Description: Chlorthalidone USP—White to yellowish white, crystalline powder. Melts at a temperature above 215 °C, with decomposition.

pKa: 9.4.

Solubility: Chlorthalidone USP—Practically insoluble in water, in ether, and in chloroform; soluble in methanol; slightly soluble in alcohol.

USP requirements:
Chlorthalidone USP—Preserve in well-closed containers. Contains not less than 98.0% and not more than 102.0% of chlorthalidone, calculated on the dried basis. Meets the requirements for Identification, Loss on drying (not more than 0.4%), Residue on ignition (not more than 0.1%), Chloride (not more than 0.035%), Heavy metals (not more than 0.001%), and Limit of 4′-chloro-3′-sulfamoyl-2-benzophenone carboxylic acid (CCA) (not more than 1.0%).
Chlorthalidone Tablets USP—Preserve in well-closed containers. Contain the labeled amount, within ± 8%. Meet the requirements for Identification, Dissolution (50% in 60 minutes in water in Apparatus 2 at 100 rpm), and Uniformity of dosage units.

CHLORZOXAZONE

Chemical name: 2(3*H*)-Benzoxazolone, 5-chloro-.

Molecular formula: $C_7H_4ClNO_2$.

Molecular weight: 169.57.

Description: Chlorzoxazone USP—White or practically white, practically odorless, crystalline powder.

Solubility: Chlorzoxazone USP—Slightly soluble in water; sparingly soluble in alcohol, in isopropyl alcohol, and in methanol; soluble in solutions of alkali hydroxides and ammonia.

USP requirements:
Chlorzoxazone USP—Preserve in tight containers. Contains not less than 98.0% and not more than 102.0% of chlorzoxazone, calculated on the dried basis. Meets the requirements for Identification, Melting range (189–194 °C), Loss on drying (not more than 0.5%), Heavy metals (not more than 0.002%), Residue on ignition (not more than 0.15%), Chromatographic impurities, Chlorine content (20.6–21.2%, calculated on the dried basis), and Organic volatile impurities.
Chlorzoxazone Tablets USP—Preserve in tight containers. Contain the labeled amount, within ± 10%. Meet the requirements for Identification, Dissolution (75% in 60 minutes in phosphate buffer [pH 8.0] in Apparatus 2 at 75 rpm), and Uniformity of dosage units.

CHLORZOXAZONE AND ACETAMINOPHEN

For *Chlorzoxazone* and *Acetaminophen*—See individual listings for chemistry information.

USP requirements:
Chlorzoxazone and Acetaminophen Capsules—Not in USP.
Chlorzoxazone and Acetaminophen Tablets —Not in USP.

CHOLECALCIFEROL

Chemical name: 9,10-Secocholesta-5,7,10(19)-trien-3-ol, (3 beta,5*Z*,7*E*)-.

Molecular formula: $C_{27}H_{44}O$.

Molecular weight: 384.64.

Description: Cholecalciferol USP—White, odorless crystals. Is affected by air and by light. Melts at about 85 °C.

Solubility: Cholecalciferol USP—Insoluble in water; soluble in alcohol, in chloroform, and in fatty oils.

USP requirements: Cholecalciferol USP—Preserve in hermetically sealed containers under nitrogen, in a cool place and protected from light. Contains not less than 97.0% and not more than 103.0% of cholecalciferol. Meets the requirements for Identification and Specific rotation (+105° to +112°, determined in a solution in alcohol containing 50 mg in each 10 mL).

CHOLERA VACCINE

Description: Cholera Vaccine USP—Practically water-clear liquid to milky suspension, nearly odorless or having a faint odor because of the antimicrobial agent.

USP requirements: Cholera Vaccine USP—Preserve at a temperature between 2 and 8 °C. A sterile suspension, in Sodium Chloride Injection or other suitable diluent, of killed cholera vibrios (*Vibrio cholerae*) of a strain or strains selected for high antigenic efficiency, shown to yield a vaccine not less potent than vaccines prepared from Inaba strain 35A3 and Ogawa strain 41. It is prepared from equal portions of suspensions of cholera vibrios of the Inaba and Ogawa strains. Label it to state that it is to be well shaken before use and that it is not to be frozen. It has a labeled potency of 8 units per serotype per mL. Its potency, determined by the specific mouse potency test based on the U.S. Standard Cholera Vaccines for the respective serotypes, is not less than 4.4 units per serotype per mL. Contains a suitable antimicrobial agent. Meets the requirements of the specific mouse toxicity test and of the test for nitrogen content, and for Expiration date (not later than 18 months after date of issue from manufacturer's cold storage [5 °C, 1 year]). Conforms to the regulations of the U.S. Food and Drug Administration concerning biologics.

CHOLESTEROL

Chemical name: Cholest-5-en-3-ol, (3 beta)-.

Molecular formula: $C_{27}H_{46}O$.

Molecular weight: 386.66.

Description: Cholesterol NF—White or faintly yellow, practically odorless, pearly leaflets, needles, powder, or granules. Acquires a yellow to pale tan color on prolonged exposure to light.
NF category: Emulsifying and/or solubilizing agent.

Solubility: Cholesterol NF—Insoluble in water; soluble in acetone, in chloroform, in dioxane, in ether, in ethyl acetate, in solvent hexane, and in vegetable oils; sparingly soluble in dehydrated alcohol; slightly (and slowly) soluble in alcohol.

NF requirements: Cholesterol NF—Preserve in well-closed, light-resistant containers. A steroid alcohol used as an emulsifying agent. Meets the requirements for Solubility in alcohol, Identification, Melting range (147–150 °C), Specific rotation (−34° to −38°), Acidity, Loss on drying (not more than 0.3%), and Residue on ignition (not more than 0.1%).

CHOLESTYRAMINE

Chemical group: Cholestyramine is an anion-exchange resin.

Chemical name: Cholestyramine resin—Cholestyramine.

Description: Cholestyramine Resin USP—White to buff-colored, hygroscopic, fine powder. Is odorless or has not more than a slight amine-like odor.

Solubility: Cholestyramine Resin USP—Insoluble in water, in alcohol, in chloroform, and in ether.

USP requirements:
Cholestyramine Resin USP—Preserve in tight containers. A strongly basic anion-exchange resin in the chloride form, consisting of styrene-divinylbenzene copolymer with quaternary ammonium functional groups. Each gram exchanges not less than 1.8 grams and not more than 2.2 grams of sodium glycocholate, calculated on the dried basis. Meets the requirements for Identification, pH (4.0–6.0, in a slurry [1 in 100]), Loss on drying (not more than 12.0%), Residue on ignition (not more than 0.1%), Heavy metals (not more than 0.002%), Dialyzable quaternary amines (absorbance not more than 0.05% as benzyltrimethylammonium chloride), Chloride content (13.0–17.0%, calculated on the dried basis), and Exchange capacity.
Cholestyramine Chewable Bar—Not in USP.
Cholestyramine for Oral Suspension USP—Preserve in tight containers. A mixture of Cholestyramine Resin with suitable excipients and coloring and flavoring agents. Contains the labeled amount of dried cholestyramine resin, within ±15%. Meets the requirements for Identification, Uniformity of dosage units, and Loss on drying (not more than 12.0%).

CHOLINE SALICYLATE

Chemical name: (2-Hydroxyethyl)trimethylammonium salicylate.

Molecular formula: $C_{12}H_{19}NO_4$.

Molecular weight: 241.29.

Description: White, hygroscopic solid with a melting point of about 50 °C.

Solubility: Freely soluble in water; soluble in most hydrophilic solvents; insoluble in organic solvents.

USP requirements: Choline Salicylate Oral Solution—Not in USP.

CHOLINE AND MAGNESIUM SALICYLATES

Chemical name:
Choline salicylate—(2-Hydroxyethyl)trimethylammonium salicylate.
Magnesium salicylate—Magnesium, bis(2-hydroxybenzoato-O^1,O^2)-, tetrahydrate.

Molecular formula:
Choline salicylate—$C_{12}H_{19}NO_4$.
Magnesium salicylate—$C_{14}H_{10}MgO_6 \cdot 4H_2O$ (tetrahydrate); $C_{14}H_{10}MgO_6$ (anhydrous).

Molecular weight:
Choline salicylate—241.29.
Magnesium salicylate—370.60 (tetrahydrate); 298.53 (anhydrous).

Description: Magnesium salicylate—White to slightly pink, free-flowing crystalline powder; odorless or has a faint characteristic odor. Its aqueous solution is acid to litmus.

Solubility: Magnesium salicylate—1 gram dissolves in 13 mL of water; soluble in alcohol.

USP requirements:
Choline and Magnesium Salicylates Oral Solution—Not in USP.
Choline and Magnesium Salicylates Tablets—Not in USP.

CHROMIC CHLORIDE

Chemical name: Chromium chloride ($CrCl_3$) hexahydrate.

Molecular formula: $CrCl_3 \cdot 6H_2O$.

Molecular weight: 266.48.

Description: Chromic Chloride USP—Dark green, odorless, slightly deliquescent crystals.

Solubility: Chromic Chloride USP—Soluble in water and in alcohol; slightly soluble in acetone; practically insoluble in ether.

USP requirements:
Chromic Chloride USP—Preserve in tight containers. Contains not less than 98.0% and not more than 101.0% of chromic chloride. Meets the requirements for Identification, Insoluble matter (not more than 0.01%), Substances not precipitated by ammonium hydroxide (not more than 0.20% as sulfate), Sulfate (not more than 0.01%), and Iron (not more than 0.01%).
Chromic Chloride Injection USP—Preserve in single-dose or in multiple-dose containers, preferably of Type I or Type II glass. A sterile solution of Chromic Chloride in Water for Injection. Label the Injection to indicate that it is to be diluted to the appropriate strength with Sterile Water for Injection or other suitable fluid prior to administration. Contains an amount of chromic chloride equivalent to the labeled amount of chromium, within ±10%. Meets the requirements for Identification, Bacterial endotoxins, pH (1.5–2.5), and Injections.

CHYMOPAPAIN

Source: A proteolytic enzyme isolated from the crude latex of *Carica papaya*, differing from papain in electrophoretic mobility, solubility, and substrate specificity.

Chemical name: Chymopapain.

Molecular weight: Approximately 27,000.

USP requirements: Chymopapain for Injection—Not in USP.

CHYMOTRYPSIN

Chemical name: Chymotrypsin.

Description: Chymotrypsin USP—White to yellowish white, crystalline or amorphous, odorless, powder.

Solubility: Chymotrypsin USP—An amount equivalent to 100,000 USP Units is soluble in 10 mL of water and in 10 mL of saline TS.

USP requirements:
Chymotrypsin USP—Preserve in tight containers, and avoid exposure to excessive heat. A proteolytic enzyme crystallized from an extract of the pancreas gland of the ox, *Bos taurus* Linné (Fam. Bovidae). Contains not less than 1000 USP Chymotrypsin Units in each mg, calculated on the dried basis, and not less than 90.0% and not more than 110.0% of the labeled potency, as determined by the *Assay*. Meets the requirements for Microbial limits, Loss on drying (not more than 5.0%), Residue on ignition (not more than 2.5%), and Trypsin (not more than 1.0%).
Chymotrypsin for Ophthalmic Solution USP—Preserve in single-dose containers, preferably of Type I glass, and avoid exposure to excessive heat. It is sterile Chymotrypsin. When constituted as directed in the labeling, yields a solution containing the labeled potency, within ± 20%. Meets the requirements for Completeness of solution, Identification, pH (4.3–8.7, in the solution constituted as directed in the labeling), and Uniformity of dosage units, for the test for Trypsin under Chymotrypsin, and for Sterility tests.

CICLOPIROX

Chemical group: Synthetic pyridinone derivative; chemically unrelated to the imidazole.

Chemical name: Ciclopirox olamine—2(1*H*)-Pyridinone, 6-cyclohexyl-1-hydroxy-4-methyl-, compd. with 2-aminoethanol (1:1).

Molecular formula: Ciclopirox olamine—$C_{12}H_{17}NO_2 \cdot C_2H_7NO$.

Molecular weight: Ciclopirox olamine—268.36.

Description: Ciclopirox olamine—White to pale yellow crystalline powder.

Solubility: Ciclopirox olamine—Soluble in methanol.

Other characteristics: Ciclopirox olamine—1% cream has a pH of 7.

USP requirements:
Ciclopirox Olamine USP—Preserve in well-closed containers. Contains an amount of ciclopirox olamine equivalent to not less than 75.7% and not more than 78.0% of ciclopirox, calculated on the dried basis. Meets the requirements for Identification, Loss on drying (not more than 1.5%), Residue on ignition (not more than 0.1%), Heavy metals (not more than 0.002%), pH (8.0–9.0, in a solution [1 in 100]), and Monoethanolamine content

(289–298 mg per gram of ciclopirox, calculated on the anhydrous basis).
Ciclopirox Olamine Cream USP—Preserve in collapsible tubes, at controlled room temperature. Contains the labeled amount, within ± 10%. Meets the requirements for Identification, Minimum fill, pH (5.0–8.0), and Benzyl alcohol content (90.0–110.0% of labeled amount).
Ciclopirox Olamine Lotion—Not in USP.

CILASTATIN

Chemical name: Cilastatin sodium—2-Heptenoic acid, 7-[(2-amino-2-carboxyethyl)thio]-2-[[[(2,2-dimethylcyclopropyl)carbonyl]amino]-, monosodium salt, [R-[R*,S*(Z)]]-.

Molecular formula: Cilastatin sodium—$C_{16}H_{25}N_2NaO_5S$.

Molecular weight: Cilastatin sodium—380.43.

Description: Cilastatin Sodium USP—White to tan-colored powder.

Solubility: Cilastatin Sodium USP—Soluble in water and in methanol.

USP requirements: Sterile Cilastatin Sodium USP—Preserve in Containers for Sterile Solids, and store in a cold place. It is cilastatin sodium suitable for parenteral use. Contains not less than 98.0% and not more than 101.5% of cilastatin sodium, calculated on the anhydrous and solvent-free basis. Meets the requirements for Identification, Bacterial endotoxins, Sterility, pH (6.5–7.5, in a solution [1 in 100]), Specific rotation (+41.5° to +44.5°, calculated on the anhydrous and solvent-free basis), Water (not more than 2.0%), Heavy metals (not more than 0.002%), Solvents (not more than 1.0% of acetone, 0.5% of methanol, and 0.4% of mesityl oxide), and Chromatographic purity (not more than 0.5%).

CIMETIDINE

Chemical group: Imidazole derivative of histamine.

Chemical name:
Cimetidine—Guanidine, *N''*-cyano-*N*-methyl-*N'*-[2-[[(5-methyl-1*H*-imidazol-4-yl)methyl]thio]ethyl]-.
Cimetidine hydrochloride—Guanidine, *N''*-cyano-*N*-methyl-*N'*-[2-[[(5-methyl-1*H*-imidazol-4-yl)methyl]thio]ethyl]-, monohydrochloride.

Molecular formula:
Cimetidine—$C_{10}H_{16}N_6S$.
Cimetidine hydrochloride—$C_{10}H_{16}N_6S \cdot HCl$.

Molecular weight:
Cimetidine—252.34.
Cimetidine hydrochloride—288.80.

Description: Cimetidine USP—White to off-white, crystalline powder; odorless, or having a slight mercaptan odor.

pKa:
Cimetidine—7.09.
Cimetidine hydrochloride—7.11.

Solubility:
Cimetidine USP—Soluble in alcohol and in polyethylene glycol 400; freely soluble in methanol; sparingly soluble in isopropyl alcohol; slightly soluble in water and in chloroform; practically insoluble in ether.
Cimetidine hydrochloride—Freely soluble in water; soluble in alcohol; very slightly soluble in chloroform; and practically insoluble in ether.

USP requirements:
Cimetidine USP—Preserve in tight, light-resistant containers, at controlled room temperature. Contains not less than 98.0% and not more than 102.0% of cimetidine, calculated on the dried basis. Meets the requirements for Identification, Selenium (0.002%), Melting range (139–144 °C), Loss on drying (not more than 1.0%), Residue on ignition (not more than 0.2%), Heavy metals (not more than 0.002%), and Chromatographic purity.
Cimetidine Tablets USP—Preserve in tight, light-resistant containers, at controlled room temperature. Contain the labeled amount, within ±10%. Meet the requirements for Identification, Dissolution (75% in 15 minutes in water in Apparatus 1 at 100 rpm), and Uniformity of dosage units.
Cimetidine Hydrochloride Injection—Not in USP.
Cimetidine Hydrochloride Oral Solution—Not in USP.

CINOXACIN

Chemical group: Similar in chemical structure to nalidixic acid and oxolinic acid.

Chemical name: [1,3]Dioxolo[4,5-g]cinnoline-3-carboxylic acid, l-ethyl-1,4-dihydro-4-oxo-.

Molecular formula: $C_{12}H_{10}N_2O_5$.

Molecular weight: 262.22.

Description: Cinoxacin USP—White to yellowish white, crystalline solid. Is odorless.

Solubility: Cinoxacin USP—Insoluble in water and in most common organic solvents; soluble in alkaline solution.

USP requirements:
Cinoxacin USP—Preserve in tight containers. Contains not less than 97.0% and not more than 102.0% of cinoxacin, calculated on the dried basis. Meets the requirements for Identification, Loss on drying (not more than 1.0%), and Related substances (not more than 1.0%).
Cinoxacin Capsules USP—Preserve in well-closed containers. Contain the labeled amount, within ±10%. Meet the requirements for Identification, Dissolution (60% in 30 minutes in phosphate buffer [pH 6.5] in Apparatus 1 at 100 rpm), and Uniformity of dosage units.

CINOXATE

Chemical name: Propenoic acid, 3-(4-methoxyphenyl)-, 2-ethoxyethyl ester.

Molecular formula: $C_{14}H_{18}O_4$.

Molecular weight: 250.29.

Description: Cinoxate USP—Slightly yellow, practically odorless, viscous liquid.

Solubility: Cinoxate USP—Very slightly soluble in water; slightly soluble in glycerin; soluble in propylene glycol. Miscible with alcohol and with vegetable oils.

USP requirements:
Cinoxate USP—Preserve in tight, light-resistant containers. Contains not less than 98.0% and not more than 101.0% of cinoxate. Meets the requirements for Identification, Specific gravity (1.100–1.105), Refractive index (1.564–1.569), and Acidity.
Cinoxate Lotion USP—Preserve in tight, light-resistant containers. It is Cinoxate in a suitable hydroalcoholic vehicle. Contains the labeled amount, within ±10%. Meets the

requirements for Identification, pH (5.4–6.4), and Alcohol content (47–57%).

CIPROFLOXACIN

Chemical group: Fluoroquinolone derivative; structurally related to cinoxacin, nalidixic acid, norfloxacin, and other quinolones.

Chemical name:
Ciprofloxacin—3-Quinolinecarboxylic acid, 1-cyclopropyl-6-fluoro-1,4-dihydro-4-oxo-7-(1-piperazinyl)-.
Ciprofloxacin hydrochloride—3-Quinolinecarboxylic acid, 1-cyclopropyl-6-fluoro-1,4-dihydro-4-oxo-7-(1-piperazinyl)-, monohydrochloride, monohydrate.

Molecular formula:
Ciprofloxacin—$C_{17}H_{18}FN_3O_3$.
Ciprofloxacin hydrochloride—$C_{17}H_{18}FN_3O_3 \cdot HCl \cdot H_2O$.

Molecular weight:
Ciprofloxacin—331.35.
Ciprofloxacin hydrochloride—385.82.

Description: Ciprofloxacin Hydrochloride USP—Faintly yellowish to light yellow crystals.

Solubility: Ciprofloxacin Hydrochloride USP—Sparingly soluble in water; slightly soluble in acetic acid and in methanol; very slightly soluble in dehydrated alcohol; practically insoluble in acetone, in acetonitrile, in ethyl acetate, in hexane, and in methylene chloride.

USP requirements:
Ciprofloxacin Injection—Not in USP.
Ciprofloxacin for Injection—Not in USP.
Ciprofloxacin Tablets USP—Preserve in well-closed containers. Contain an amount of ciprofloxacin hydrochloride equivalent to the labeled amount of ciprofloxacin, within ±10%. Meet the requirements for Identification, Dissolution (80% in 30 minutes in water in Apparatus 2 at 50 rpm), and Uniformity of dosage units.
Ciprofloxacin Hydrochloride USP—Preserve in tight, light-resistant containers. Contains not less than 98.0% and not more than 102.0% of ciprofloxacin hydrochloride, calculated on the anhydrous basis. Meets the requirements for Identification, pH (3.0–4.5, in a solution [1 in 40]), Water (4.7–6.7%), Residue on ignition (not more than 0.1%), Sulfate (not more than 0.04%), Heavy metals (not more than 0.002%), Fluoroquinolonic acid (not more than 0.2%), and Chromatographic purity (not more than 0.7%).

CISPLATIN

Chemical group: A heavy metal complex.

Chemical name: Platinum, diamminedichloro-, (SP-4-2)-.

Molecular formula: $Cl_2H_6N_2Pt$.

Molecular weight: 300.06.

Description: White lyophilized powder. It has a melting point of 207 °C.

Solubility: Soluble in water or saline at 1 mg per mL and in dimethylformamide at 24 mg per mL.

USP requirements:
Cisplatin USP—Preserve in tight containers. Protect from light. Contains not less than 98.0% and not more than 102.0% of cisplatin, calculated on the anhydrous basis. Meets the requirements for Identification, Crystallinity, Water (not more than 1.0%), UV purity ratio (ratio of

absorbance at the maximum near 301 nanometers to that at the minimum near 246 nanometers is not less than 4.5), Platinum content (64.42–65.22%, on the anhydrous basis), Trichloroammineplatinate (not more than 1.0%), and Transplatin (not more than 2.0%).

Caution: Cisplatin is potentially cytotoxic. Great care should be taken to prevent inhaling particles and exposing the skin to it.

Cisplatin Injection—Not in USP.

Cisplatin for Injection USP—Preserve in Containers for Sterile Solids. Protect from light. A sterile, lyophilized mixture of Cisplatin, Mannitol, and Sodium Chloride. Contains the labeled amount, within ±10%. Meets the requirements for Identification, Constituted solution, Pyrogen, Sterility, pH (3.5–6.2, in the solution constituted as directed in the labeling, using Sterile Water for Injection), Water (not more than 2.0%), Uniformity of dosage units, Trichloroammineplatinate (not more than 1.0%), and Transplatin (not more than 2.0%), and for Labeling under Injections.

Caution: Cisplatin is potentially cytotoxic. Great care should be taken in handling the powder and preparing solutions.

CITRIC ACID

Chemical name: 1,2,3-Propanetricarboxylic acid, 2-hydroxy-.

Molecular formula: $C_6H_8O_7$ (anhydrous); $C_6H_8O_7 \cdot H_2O$ (monohydrate).

Molecular weight: 192.12 (anhydrous); 210.14 (monohydrate).

Description: Citric Acid USP—Colorless, translucent crystals, or white, granular to fine crystalline powder. Odorless or practically odorless. The hydrous form is efflorescent in dry air.
NF category: Acidifying agent; buffering agent.

Solubility: Citric Acid USP—Very soluble in water; freely soluble in alcohol; sparingly soluble in ether.

USP requirements: Citric Acid USP—Preserve in tight containers. It is anhydrous or contains one molecule of water of hydration. Label it to indicate whether it is anhydrous or hydrous. Contains not less than 99.5% and not more than 100.5% of citric acid, calculated on the anhydrous basis. Meets the requirements for Identification, Water (not more than 0.5% for anhydrous form and not more than 8.8% for hydrous form), Residue on ignition (not more than 0.05%), Oxalate, Sulfate, Arsenic (not more than 3 ppm), Heavy metals (not more than 0.001%), and Readily carbonizable substances.

CITRIC ACID AND D-GLUCONIC ACID

Chemical name: Citric acid—1,2,3-Propanetricarboxylic acid, 2-hydroxy-.

Molecular formula:
Citric acid—$C_6H_8O_7$ (anhydrous); $C_6H_8O_7 \cdot H_2O$ (monohydrate).
D-Gluconic acid—$C_6H_{12}O_7$.

Molecular weight:
Citric acid—192.12 (anhydrous); 210.14 (monohydrate).
D-Gluconic acid—196.16.

Description:
Citric Acid USP—Colorless, translucent crystals, or white, granular to fine crystalline powder. Odorless or practically odorless. The hydrous form is efflorescent in dry air.
NF category: Acidifying agent; buffering agent.
D-Gluconic acid—Melting point 131 °C.

Solubility:
Citric Acid USP—Very soluble in water; freely soluble in alcohol; sparingly soluble in ether.
D-Gluconic acid—Freely soluble in water; slightly soluble in alcohol; insoluble in ether and most other organic solvents.

USP requirements: Citric Acid and D-Gluconic Acid for Topical Solution—Not in USP.

CITRIC ACID, MAGNESIUM OXIDE, AND SODIUM CARBONATE

For *Citric Acid, Magnesium Oxide,* and *Sodium Carbonate*—See individual listings for chemistry information.

USP requirements: Citric Acid, Magnesium Oxide, and Sodium Carbonate Irrigation USP—Preserve in single-dose containers, preferably of Type I or Type II glass. A sterile solution of Citric Acid, Magnesium Oxide, and Sodium Carbonate in Water for Injection. Contains an amount of citric acid equivalent to the labeled amount of citric acid (as the monohydrate), within ±5%, and the labeled amounts of magnesium oxide and sodium carbonate, within ±5%. Meets the requirements for Identification, Bacterial endotoxins, pH (3.8–4.2), and Injections (except that the container may be designed to empty rapidly, and may exceed 1000 mL in capacity).

CLARITHROMYCIN

Chemical name: Erythromycin, 6-*O*-methyl-.

Molecular formula: $C_{38}H_{69}NO_{13}$.

Molecular weight: 747.96.

Description: White to off-white crystalline powder.

Solubility: Soluble in acetone; slightly soluble in methanol, in ethanol, and in acetonitrile; practically insoluble in water.

USP requirements: Clarithromycin Tablets—Not in USP.

CLAVULANATE

Chemical name:
Clavulanate potassium—4-Oxa-1-azabicyclo[3.2.0]heptane-2-carboxylic acid, 3-(2-hydroxyethylidene)-7-oxo-, monopotassium salt, [2R-(2 alpha,3Z,5 alpha)]-.
Clavulanic acid—(Z)-(2R,5R)-3-(2-Hydroxyethylidene)-7-oxo-4-oxa-1-azabicyclo[3.2.0]heptane-2-carboxylic acid.

Molecular formula:
Clavulanate potassium—$C_8H_8KNO_5$.
Clavulanic acid—$C_8H_9NO_5$.

Molecular weight:
Clavulanate potassium—237.25.
Clavulanic acid—199.16.

Description: Clavulanate Potassium USP—White to off-white powder. Is moisture-sensitive.

Solubility: Clavulanate Potassium USP—Freely soluble in water, but stability in aqueous solution is not good, optimum stability at a pH of 6.0 to 6.3; soluble in methanol, with decomposition.

USP requirements:
Clavulanate Potassium USP—Preserve in tight containers. Contains an amount of clavulanate potassium equivalent

to not less than 75.5% and not more than 92.0% of clavulanic acid, calculated on the anhydrous basis. Meets the requirements for Identification, pH (5.5–8.0, in a solution [1 in 100]), Water (not more than 1.5%), and Clavam-2-carboxylate potassium (not more than 0.01%).

Sterile Clavulanate Potassium USP—Preserve in Containers for Sterile Solids. It is clavulanate potassium suitable for parenteral use. Contains an amount of clavulanate potassium equivalent to not less than 75.5% and not more than 92.0% of clavulanic acid, calculated on the anhydrous basis. Meets the requirements for Pyrogen and Sterility, and for Identification tests, pH, Water, and Clavam-2-carboxylate potassium under Clavulanate Potassium.

CLEMASTINE

Chemical group: Ethanolamine derivative.

Chemical name: Clemastine fumarate—Pyrrolidine, 2-[2-[1-(4-chlorophenyl)-1-phenylethoxy]ethyl]-1-methyl-, [R-(R*,R*)]-, (E)-2-butenedioate (1:1).

Molecular formula: Clemastine fumarate—$C_{21}H_{26}ClNO \cdot C_4H_4O_4$.

Molecular weight: Clemastine fumarate—459.97.

Description: Clemastine Fumarate USP—Colorless to faintly yellow, odorless, crystalline powder. Its solutions are acid to litmus.

Solubility: Clemastine Fumarate USP—Very slightly soluble in water; slightly soluble in methanol; very slightly soluble in chloroform.

USP requirements:
Clemastine Fumarate USP—Preserve in tight, light-resistant containers, at a temperature not exceeding 25 °C. Contains not less than 98.0% and not more than 102.0% of clemastine fumarate, calculated on the dried basis. Meets the requirements for Clarity and color of solution, Identification, Specific rotation (+15.0° to 18.0°, calculated on the dried basis), pH (3.2–4.2, in a suspension [1 in 10]), Loss on drying (not more than 0.5%), Heavy metals (not more than 0.002%), and Chromatographic purity.
Clemastine Fumarate Syrup—Not in USP.
Clemastine Fumarate Tablets USP—Preserve in well-closed containers. Contain the labeled amount, within ±10%. Meet the requirements for Identification, Dissolution (75% in 30 minutes in citrate buffer [pH 4.0] in Apparatus 2 at 50 rpm), and Uniformity of dosage units.

CLEMASTINE AND PHENYLPROPANOLAMINE

For *Clemastine* and *Phenylpropanolamine*—See individual listings for chemistry information.

USP requirements: Clemastine Fumarate and Phenylpropanolamine Hydrochloride Extended-release Tablets—Not in USP.

CLIDINIUM

Source: Synthetic amine compound; an aminoalcohol.

Chemical group: Quaternary ammonium compound, synthetic.

Chemical name: Clidinium bromide—1-Azoniabicyclo[2.2.2]-octane, 3-[(hydroxydiphenylacetyl)oxy]-1-methyl-, bromide.

Molecular formula: Clidinium bromide—$C_{22}H_{26}BrNO_3$.

Molecular weight: Clidinium bromide—432.36.

Description: Clidinium Bromide USP—White to nearly white, practically odorless, crystalline powder. Is optically inactive. Melts at about 242 °C.

Solubility: Clidinium Bromide USP—Soluble in water and in alcohol; slightly soluble in ether.

USP requirements:
Clidinium Bromide USP—Preserve in tight, light-resistant containers. Contains not less than 99.0% and not more than 100.5% of clidinium bromide, calculated on the dried basis. Meets the requirements for Identification, Loss on drying (not more than 0.5%), Residue on ignition (not more than 0.1%), Heavy metals (not more than 0.002%), Related compounds, and Organic volatile impurities.
Clidinium Bromide Capsules USP—Preserve in tight, light-resistant containers. Contain the labeled amount, within ±10%. Meet the requirements for Identification, Dissolution (80% in 15 minutes in 0.1 N hydrochloric acid in Apparatus 1 at 100 rpm), Uniformity of dosage units, and Related compounds.

CLINDAMYCIN

Source: Semi-synthetic; 7(S)-chloro derivative of lincomycin.

Chemical group: Lincomycins.

Chemical name:
Clindamycin hydrochloride—L-*threo*-alpha-D-*galacto*-Octopyranoside, methyl 7-chloro-6,7,8-trideoxy-6-[[(1-methyl-4-propyl-2-pyrrolidinyl)carbonyl]amino]-1-thio-, (2S-*trans*)-, monohydrochloride.
Clindamycin palmitate hydrochloride—L-*threo*-alpha-D-*galacto*-Octopyranoside, methyl 7-chloro-6,7,8-trideoxy-6-[[(1-methyl-4-propyl-2-pyrrolidinyl)carbonyl]amino]-1-thio-2-hexadecanoate, monohydrochloride, (2S-*trans*)-.
Clindamycin phosphate—L-*threo*-alpha-D-*galacto*-Octopyranoside, methyl 7-chloro-6,7,8-trideoxy-6-[[(1-methyl-4-propyl-2-pyrrolidinyl)carbonyl]amino]-1-thio-, 2-(dihydrogen phosphate), (2S-*trans*)-.

Molecular formula:
Clindamycin hydrochloride—$C_{18}H_{33}ClN_2O_5S \cdot HCl$.
Clindamycin palmitate hydrochloride—$C_{34}H_{63}ClN_2O_6S \cdot HCl$.
Clindamycin phosphate—$C_{18}H_{34}ClN_2O_8PS$.

Molecular weight:
Clindamycin hydrochloride—461.44.
Clindamycin palmitate hydrochloride—699.86.
Clindamycin phosphate—504.96.

Description:
Clindamycin Hydrochloride USP—White or practically white, crystalline powder. Is odorless or has a faint mercaptan-like odor. Is stable in the presence of air and light. Its solutions are acidic and are dextrorotatory.
Clindamycin Palmitate Hydrochloride USP—White to off-white amorphous powder, having a characteristic odor.
Clindamycin Phosphate USP—White to off-white, hygroscopic, crystalline powder. Is odorless or practically odorless.

Solubility:
Clindamycin Hydrochloride USP—Freely soluble in water, in dimethylformamide, and in methanol; soluble in alcohol; practically insoluble in acetone.
Clindamycin Palmitate Hydrochloride USP—Very soluble in ethyl acetate and in dimethylformamide; freely soluble in water, in ether, in chloroform, and in alcohol.

Clindamycin Phosphate USP—Freely soluble in water; slightly soluble in dehydrated alcohol; very slightly soluble in acetone; practically insoluble in chloroform and in ether.

USP requirements:

Clindamycin Hydrochloride USP—Preserve in tight containers. It is the hydrated hydrochloride salt of clindamycin, a substance produced by the chlorination of lincomycin. Has a potency equivalent to not less than 800 mcg of clindamycin per mg. Meets the requirements for Identification, Crystallinity, pH (3.0–5.5, in a solution containing 100 mg per mL), and Water (3.0–6.0%).

Clindamycin Hydrochloride Capsules USP—Preserve in tight containers. Contain an amount of clindamycin hydrochloride equivalent to the labeled amount of clindamycin, within −10% to +20%. Meet the requirements for Identification, Dissolution (80% in 30 minutes in water in Apparatus 1 at 100 rpm), Uniformity of dosage units, and Water (not more than 7.0%).

Clindamycin Palmitate Hydrochloride USP—Preserve in tight containers. Has a potency equivalent to not less than 540 mcg of clindamycin per mg. Meets the requirements for Identification, pH (2.8–3.8, in a solution containing 10 mg per mL), Water (not more than 3.0%), and Residue on ignition (not more than 0.5%).

Clindamycin Palmitate Hydrochloride for Oral Solution USP—Preserve in tight containers. A dry mixture of Clindamycin Palmitate Hydrochloride and one or more suitable buffers, colors, diluents, flavors, and preservatives. Contains an amount of clindamycin palmitate hydrochloride equivalent to the labeled amount of clindamycin (15 mg per mL when constituted as directed in the labeling), within −10% to +20%. Meets the requirements for Uniformity of dosage units (solid packaged in single-unit containers), pH (2.5–5.0, in the solution constituted as directed in the labeling), Water (not more than 3.0%), and Deliverable volume (solid packaged in multiple-unit containers).

Clindamycin Phosphate USP—Preserve in tight containers. Has a potency equivalent to not less than 758 mcg of clindamycin per mg, calculated on the anhydrous basis. Meets the requirements for Identification, Crystallinity, Bacterial endotoxins, pH (3.5–4.5, in a solution containing 10 mg per mL), and Water (not more than 6.0%), and for Depressor substances under Sterile Clindamycin Phosphate (for Clindamycin Phosphate intended for use in making Clindamycin Phosphate Injection).

Clindamycin Phosphate Gel USP—Preserve in tight containers. Contains an amount of clindamycin phosphate equivalent to the labeled amount of clindamycin, within ±10%. Meets the requirements for Identification, Minimum fill, and pH (4.5–6.5).

Clindamycin Phosphate Injection USP—Preserve in single-dose or in multiple-dose containers, preferably of Type I glass, or in suitable plastic containers. A sterile solution of Sterile Clindamycin Phosphate or Clindamycin Phosphate in Water for Injection with one or more suitable preservatives, sequestering agents, or tonicity-adjusting agents. It meets the requirement for Labeling under Injections. Where it is maintained in the frozen state, the label states that it is to be thawed just prior to use, describes the conditions for proper storage of the resultant solution, and directs that the solution is not to be refrozen. Contains an amount of clindamycin phosphate equivalent to the labeled amount of clindamycin, within −10% to +20%. Meets the requirements for Identification, Bacterial endotoxins, pH (5.5–7.0), Particulate matter, and Injections.

Clindamycin Phosphate Topical Solution USP—Preserve in tight containers. Contains an amount of clindamycin phosphate equivalent to the labeled amount of clindamycin, within ±10%. Meets the requirements for Identification and pH (4.0–7.0).

Clindamycin Phosphate Topical Suspension USP—Preserve in tight containers. Contains an amount of clindamycin phosphate equivalent to the labeled amount of clindamycin, within ±10%. Meets the requirements for Identification, Minimum fill, and pH (4.5–6.5).

Sterile Clindamycin Phosphate USP—Preserve in Containers for Sterile Solids. It is Clindamycin Phosphate suitable for parenteral use. Has a potency equivalent to not less than 758 mcg of clindamycin per mg, calculated on the anhydrous basis. Meets the requirements for Depressor substances, Bacterial endotoxins, and Sterility, and for Identification test, pH, Water, and Crystallinity under Clindamycin Phosphate.

CLIOQUINOL

Chemical name: 8-Quinolinol, 5-chloro-7-iodo-.

Molecular formula: C_9H_5ClINO.

Molecular weight: 305.50.

Description: Clioquinol USP—Voluminous, spongy, yellowish white to brownish yellow powder, having a slight, characteristic odor. Darkens on exposure to light. Melts at about 180 °C, with decomposition.

Solubility: Clioquinol USP—Practically insoluble in water and in alcohol; soluble in hot ethyl acetate and in hot glacial acetic acid.

USP requirements:

Clioquinol USP—Preserve in tight, light-resistant containers. It is dried over phosphorus pentoxide for 5 hours. Contains not less than 93.0% and not more than 100.5% of clioquinol (the 5-chloro-7-iodo-8-quinolinol isomer). Meets the requirements for Identification, Loss on drying (not more than 0.5%), Residue on ignition (not more than 0.5%), and Free iodine and iodide.

Clioquinol Cream USP—Preserve in collapsible tubes or tight, light-resistant containers. Contains the labeled amount, within ±10%, in a suitable cream base. Meets the requirement for Identification.

Clioquinol Ointment USP—Preserve in collapsible tubes or tight, light-resistant containers. Contains the labeled amount, within ±10%, in a suitable ointment base. Meets the requirement for Identification.

Compound Clioquinol Powder USP—Preserve in well-closed, light-resistant containers. Contains not less than 22.5% and not more than 27.5% of clioquinol.

Prepare Compound Clioquinol Powder as follows: 250 grams of Clioquinol, 25 grams of Lactic Acid, 200 grams of Zinc Stearate, and 525 grams of Lactose to make 1000 grams. Mix the Lactic Acid with the Lactose, then add the Clioquinol and the Zinc Stearate, and mix.

Meets the requirement for Identification.

CLIOQUINOL AND FLUMETHASONE

For *Clioquinol* and *Flumethasone*—See individual listings for chemistry information.

USP requirements:

Clioquinol and Flumethasone Pivalate Cream—Not in USP.

Clioquinol and Flumethasone Pivalate Ointment—Not in USP.

Clioquinol and Flumethasone Pivalate Otic Solution—Not in USP.

CLIOQUINOL AND HYDROCORTISONE

For *Clioquinol* and *Hydrocortisone*—See individual listings for chemistry information.

USP requirements:

Clioquinol and Hydrocortisone Cream USP—Preserve in collapsible tubes or in tight, light-resistant containers. Contains the labeled amounts of clioquinol and hydrocortisone, within ± 10%, in a suitable cream base. Meets the requirements for Identification and Minimum fill.

Clioquinol and Hydrocortisone Lotion—Not in USP.

Clioquinol and Hydrocortisone Ointment USP—Preserve in collapsible tubes or in tight, light-resistant containers. Contains the labeled amounts of clioquinol and hydrocortisone, within ± 10%, in a suitable ointment base. Meets the requirements for Identification and Minimum fill.

CLOBETASOL

Chemical name: Clobetasol propionate—Pregna-1,4-diene-3,20-dione, 21-chloro-9-fluoro-11-hydroxy-16-methyl-17-(1-oxopropoxy)-, (11 beta,16 beta)-.

Molecular formula: Clobetasol propionate—$C_{25}H_{32}ClFO_5$.

Molecular weight: Clobetasol propionate—466.99.

Description: Clobetasol propionate—White to cream-colored crystalline powder.

Solubility: Clobetasol propionate—Insoluble in water.

USP requirements:

Clobetasol Propionate Cream—Not in USP.
Clobetasol Propionate Ointment—Not in USP.
Clobetasol Propionate Solution—Not in USP.

CLOBETASONE

Chemical name: Clobetasone butyrate—Pregna-1,4-diene-3,11,20-trione, 21-chloro-9-fluoro-16-methyl-17-(1-oxobutoxy)-, (16 beta)-.

Molecular formula: Clobetasone butyrate—$C_{26}H_{32}ClFO_5$.

Molecular weight: Clobetasone butyrate—479.00.

Description: Clobetasone butyrate—White to cream-colored crystalline powder.

USP requirements:

Clobetasone Butyrate Cream—Not in USP.
Clobetasone Butyrate Ointment—Not in USP.

CLOCORTOLONE

Chemical name: Clocortolone pivalate—Pregna-1,4-diene-3,20-dione, 9-chloro-21-(2,2-dimethyl-1-oxopropoxy)-6-fluoro-11-hydroxy-16-methyl-, (6 alpha,11 beta,16 alpha)-.

Molecular formula: Clocortolone pivalate—$C_{27}H_{36}ClFO_5$.

Molecular weight: Clocortolone pivalate—495.03.

Description: Clocortolone Pivalate USP—White to yellowish white, odorless powder. Melts at about 230 °C, with decomposition.

Solubility: Clocortolone Pivalate USP—Freely soluble in chloroform and in dioxane; soluble in acetone; sparingly soluble in alcohol; slightly soluble in ether.

USP requirements:

Clocortolone USP—Preserve in tight, light-resistant containers. Contains not less than 97.0% and not more than 103.0% of clocortolone pivalate, calculated on the dried basis. Meets the requirements for Color and clarity of solution, Identification, Specific rotation (+125° to +135°, calculated on the dried basis), Loss on drying (not more than 1.0%), Residue on ignition (not more than 0.2%), and Chromatographic impurities (not more than 3.0%).

Clocortolone Pivalate Cream USP—Preserve in collapsible tubes or in tight, light-resistant containers. Contains the labeled amount, within ± 10%, in a suitable cream base. Meets the requirements for Identification, Minimum fill, pH (5.0–7.0, in a 1 in 10 aqueous dispersion), and Particle size determination (no particle more than 50 microns when measured in the longitudinal axis).

CLOFAZIMINE

Chemical group: Substituted iminophenazine dye.

Chemical name: 2-Phenazinamine, *N*,5-bis(4-chlorophenyl)-3,5-dihydro-3-[(1-methylethyl)imino]-.

Molecular formula: $C_{27}H_{22}Cl_2N_4$.

Molecular weight: 473.40.

Description: Reddish-brown powder.

Solubility: Soluble in chloroform; poorly soluble in acetone and in ethyl acetate; sparingly soluble in methanol and in ethanol; virtually insoluble in water.

Other characteristics: Highly lipophilic.

USP requirements:

Clofazimine USP—Preserve in tight, light-resistant containers, at room temperature. Contains not less than 98.5% and not more than 101.5% of clofazimine, calculated on the dried basis. Meets the requirements for Identification, Loss on drying (not more than 0.5%), Residue on ignition (not more than 0.1%), and Chromatographic purity.

Clofazimine Capsules USP—Preserve in well-closed containers. Contain the labeled amount, within ± 10%. Meet the requirements for Identification, Disintegration (15 minutes, in simulated gastric fluid TS), Uniformity of dosage units, and Chromatographic purity.

CLOFIBRATE

Chemical name: Propanoic acid, 2-(4-chlorophenoxy)-2-methyl-, ethyl ester.

Molecular formula: $C_{12}H_{15}ClO_3$.

Molecular weight: 242.70.

Description: Clofibrate USP—Colorless to pale yellow liquid having a characteristic odor.

Solubility: Clofibrate USP—Insoluble in water; soluble in acetone, in alcohol, and in chloroform.

USP requirements:

Clofibrate USP—Preserve in tight, light-resistant containers. Contains not less than 97.0% and not more than 103.0% of clofibrate, calculated on the anhydrous basis. Meets the requirements for Identification, Refractive index (1.500–1.505, at 20 °C), Acidity, Water (not more than 0.2%), Chromatographic impurities (not more than 0.12%), *p*-Chlorophenol (not more than 0.003%), and Organic volatile impurities.

Clofibrate Capsules USP—Preserve in well-closed, light-resistant containers. Contain the labeled amount, within ± 10%. Meet the requirements for Identification, Dissolution (75% in 180 minutes in sodium lauryl sulfate solution [5 in 100] in Apparatus 2 at 75 rpm), and Uniformity of dosage units.

CLOMIPHENE

Chemical name: Clomiphene citrate—Ethanamine, 2-[4-(2-chloro-1,2-diphenylethenyl)phenoxy]-N,N-diethyl-, 2-hydroxy-1,2,3-propanetricarboxylate (1:1).

Molecular formula: Clomiphene citrate—$C_{26}H_{28}ClNO \cdot C_6H_8O_7$.

Molecular weight: Clomiphene citrate—598.09.

Description: Clomiphene Citrate USP—White to pale yellow, essentially odorless powder.

Solubility: Clomiphene Citrate USP—Slightly soluble in water and in chloroform; freely soluble in methanol; sparingly soluble in alcohol; insoluble in ether.

USP requirements:
Clomiphene Citrate USP—Preserve in well-closed containers. Contains not less than 98.0% and not more than 101.0% of a mixture of the (E)- and (Z)- geometric isomers of clomiphene citrate, calculated on the anhydrous basis. Contains not less than 30.0% and not more than 50.0% of the Z-isomer, [(Z)-2-[4-(2-chloro-1,2-diphenylethenyl)phenoxy]-N,N-diethylethanamine 2-hydroxy-1,2,3-propanetricarboxylate (1:1). Meets the requirements for Identification, Water (not more than 1.0%), Heavy metals (not more than 0.002%), Z-isomer (30.0–50.0%), Limit of related compounds (not more than 1.0% of any single extraneous volatile substance and not more than 2.0% of total extraneous volatile substances), and Organic volatile impurities.
Clomiphene Citrate Tablets USP—Preserve in well-closed containers, protected from light. Contain the labeled amount, within ±7%. Meet the requirements for Identification, Dissolution (75% in 60 minutes in water in Apparatus 1 at 100 rpm), and Uniformity of dosage units.

CLOMIPRAMINE

Chemical group: Dibenzazepine.

Chemical name: Clomipramine hydrochloride—5H-Dibenz[b,f]azepine-5-propanamine, 3-chloro-10,11-dihydro-N,N-dimethyl-, monohydrochloride.

Molecular formula: Clomipramine hydrochloride—$C_{19}H_{23}ClN_2 \cdot HCl$.

Molecular weight: Clomipramine hydrochloride—351.32.

Description: Clomipramine hydrochloride—White to off-white crystalline powder.

Solubility: Clomipramine hydrochloride—Freely soluble in water, in methanol, and in methylene chloride; insoluble in ethyl ether and in hexane.

Other characteristics: Clomipramine hydrochloride—A 10% solution has a pH of 3.5–5.0.

USP requirements:
Clomipramine Hydrochloride Capsules—Not in USP.
Clomipramine Hydrochloride Tablets—Not in USP.

CLONAZEPAM

Chemical name: 2H-1,4-Benzodiazepin-2-one, 5-(2-chlorophenyl)-1,3-dihydro-7-nitro-.

Molecular formula: $C_{15}H_{10}ClN_3O_3$.

Molecular weight: 315.72.

Description: Clonazepam USP—Light yellow powder, having a faint odor. Melts at about 239 °C.

Solubility: Clonazepam USP—Insoluble in water; sparingly soluble in acetone and in chloroform; slightly soluble in alcohol and in ether.

USP requirements:
Clonazepam USP—Preserve in tight, light-resistant containers, at room temperature. Contains not less than 99.0% and not more than 101.0% of clonazepam, calculated on the dried basis. Meets the requirements for Identification, Loss on drying (not more than 0.5%), Residue on ignition (not more than 0.1%), Heavy metals (not more than 0.002%), Related compounds (not more than 0.5% of 3-amino-4-(2-chlorophenyl)-6-nitrocarbostyril and not more than 0.5% of 2-amino-2'-chloro-5-nitrobenzophenone), and Organic volatile impurities.
Clonazepam Tablets USP—Preserve in tight, light-resistant containers, at room temperature. Contain the labeled amount, within ±10%. Meet the requirements for Identification, Dissolution (80% in 60 minutes in degassed water in Apparatus 2 at 100 rpm), Uniformity of dosage units, and Related compounds (not more than 1.0% of 3-Amino-4-(2-chlorophenyl)-6-nitrocarbostyril and not more than 1.0% of 2-Amino-2'-chloro-5-nitrobenzophenone).

CLONIDINE

Chemical name:
Clonidine—Benzenamine, 2,6-dichloro-N-2-imidazolidinylidene-.
Clonidine hydrochloride—Benzenamine, 2,6-dichloro-N-2-imidazolidinylidene-, monohydrochloride.

Molecular formula:
Clonidine—$C_9H_9Cl_2N_3$.
Clonidine hydrochloride—$C_9H_9Cl_2N_3 \cdot HCl$.

Molecular weight:
Clonidine—230.10.
Clonidine hydrochloride—266.56.

Description: Clonidine hydrochloride—Odorless, white, crystalline substance.

Solubility: Clonidine hydrochloride—Soluble in water and in alcohol; practically insoluble in chloroform and in ether.

Other characteristics: Clonidine hydrochloride—The pH of a 10% aqueous solution is between 3 and 5.

USP requirements:
Clonidine Transdermal System—Not in USP.
Clonidine Hydrochloride USP—Preserve in tight containers. Contains not less than 98.5% and not more than 101.0% of clonidine hydrochloride, calculated on the dried basis. Meets the requirements for Identification, pH (3.5–5.5, in a solution [1 in 20]), Loss on drying (not more than 0.5%), Residue on ignition (not more than 0.1%), and Chromatographic purity.
Clonidine Hydrochloride Tablets USP—Preserve in well-closed containers. Contain the labeled amount, within ±10%. Meet the requirements for Identification, Dissolution (75% in 30 minutes in water in Apparatus 2 at 50 rpm), and Uniformity of dosage units.

CLONIDINE AND CHLORTHALIDONE

For *Clonidine* and *Chlorthalidone*—See individual listings for chemistry information.

USP requirements: Clonidine Hydrochloride and Chlorthalidone Tablets USP—Preserve in well-closed containers. Contain the labeled amounts of clonidine hydrochloride and chlorthalidone, within ±10%. Meet the requirements for Identification, Dissolution (80% of clonidine hydrochloride and 50% of chlorthalidone in 60 minutes in water in Apparatus 2 at 100 rpm), and Uniformity of dosage units.

CLORAZEPATE

Chemical name: Clorazepate dipotassium—1*H*-1,4-Benzodiazepine-3-carboxylic acid, 7-chloro-2,3-dihydro-2-oxo-5-phenyl-, potassium salt compd. with potassium hydroxide (1:1).

Molecular formula: Clorazepate dipotassium—$C_{16}H_{11}ClK_2N_2O_4$.

Molecular weight: Clorazepate dipotassium—408.92.

Description: Clorazepate Dipotassium USP—Light yellow, crystalline powder. Darkens on exposure to light.

Solubility: Clorazepate Dipotassium USP—Soluble in water but, upon standing, may precipitate from the solution; slightly soluble in alcohol and in isopropyl alcohol; practically insoluble in acetone, in chloroform, in ether, and in methylene chloride.

USP requirements:
Clorazepate Dipotassium USP—Preserve under nitrogen in tight, light-resistant containers. Contains not less than 98.5% and not more than 101.5% of clorazepate dipotassium, calculated on the dried basis. Meets the requirements for Identification, Loss on drying (not more than 0.5%), Heavy metals (not more than 0.002%), Related compounds (not more than 1.0%), and Organic volatile impurities.
Clorazepate Dipotassium Capsules—Not in USP.
Clorazepate Dipotassium Tablets—Not in USP.

CLOTRIMAZOLE

Chemical name: 1*H*-Imidazole, 1-[(2-chlorophenyl)diphenylmethyl]-.

Molecular formula: $C_{22}H_{17}ClN_2$.

Molecular weight: 344.84.

Description: Clotrimazole USP—White to pale yellow, crystalline powder. Melts at about 142 °C, with decomposition.

Solubility: Clotrimazole USP—Practically insoluble in water; freely soluble in methanol, in acetone, in chloroform, and in alcohol.

USP requirements:
Clotrimazole USP—Preserve in tight containers. Contains not less than 98.0% and not more than 102.0% of clotrimazole, calculated on the dried basis. Meets the requirements for Identification, Loss on drying (not more than 0.5%), Residue on ignition (not more than 0.1%), Heavy metals (not more than 0.001%), Imidazole (not more than 0.5%), and (*o*-Chlorophenyl)diphenylmethanol (not more than 0.5%).
Clotrimazole Cream USP—Preserve in collapsible tubes or in tight containers, at a temperature between 2 and 30 °C. Cream that is intended for use as a vaginal preparation may be labeled Clotrimazole Vaginal Cream. Contains the labeled amount, within ±10%. Meets the requirement for Identification.
Clotrimazole Lotion USP—Preserve in tight containers, at a temperature between 2 and 30 °C. Contains the labeled amount, within ±10%. Meets the requirements for Identification, pH (5.0–7.0), Microbial limits, and (*o*-Chlorophenyl)diphenylmethanol (not more than 5%).
Clotrimazole Lozenges—Not in USP.
Clotrimazole Topical Solution USP—Preserve in tight containers, at a temperature between 2 and 30 °C. A solution of Clotrimazole in a suitable nonaqueous, hydrophilic solvent. Contains the labeled amount, within −10% to +15%. Meets the requirement for Identification.
Clotrimazole Vaginal Tablets USP—Preserve in well-closed containers. Contain the labeled amount, within ±10%. Meet the requirements for Identification, Disintegration (20 minutes), and Uniformity of dosage units.

CLOTRIMAZOLE AND BETAMETHASONE

For *Clotrimazole* and *Betamethasone*—See individual listings for chemistry information.

USP requirements: Clotrimazole and Betamethasone Dipropionate Cream USP—Preserve in collapsible tubes or in tight containers. Contains the labeled amount of clotrimazole, within ±10%, and an amount of betamethasone dipropionate equivalent to the labeled amount of betamethasone, within ±10%, in a suitable cream base. Meets the requirements for Identification, Microbial limits, and Minimum fill.

CLOXACILLIN

Chemical name:
Cloxacillin benzathine—4-Thia-1-azabicyclo[3.2.0]heptane-2-carboxylic acid, 6-[[[3-(2-chlorophenyl)-5-methyl-4-isoxazolyl]carbonyl]amino]-3,3-dimethyl-7-oxo-, [2*S*-(2 alpha,5 alpha,6 beta)]-, compd. with *N,N'*bis(phenylmethyl)-1,2-ethanediamine (2:1).
Cloxacillin sodium—4-Thia-1-azabicyclo[3.2.0]heptane-2-carboxylic acid, 6-[[[3-(2-chlorophenyl)-5-methyl-4-isoxazolyl]carbonyl]amino]-3,3-dimethyl-7-oxo-, monosodium salt, monohydrate, [2*S*-(2 alpha,5 alpha,6 beta)]-.

Molecular formula:
Cloxacillin benzathine—$(C_{19}H_{18}ClN_3O_5S)_2 \cdot C_{16}H_{20}N_2$.
Cloxacillin sodium—$C_{19}H_{17}ClN_3NaO_5S \cdot H_2O$.

Molecular weight:
Cloxacillin benzathine—1112.11.
Cloxacillin sodium—475.88.

Description:
Cloxacillin Benzathine USP—White or almost white, almost odorless, crystals or crystalline powder.
Cloxacillin Sodium USP—White, odorless, crystalline powder.

Solubility:
Cloxacillin Benzathine USP—Slightly soluble in water, in alcohol, and in isopropyl alcohol; soluble in chloroform and in methanol; sparingly soluble in acetone.
Cloxacillin Sodium USP—Freely soluble in water; soluble in alcohol; slightly soluble in chloroform.

USP requirements:
Cloxacillin Benzathine USP—Preserve in tight containers. Label it to indicate that it is for veterinary use only. Has a potency equivalent to not less than 704 mcg and not more than 821 mcg of cloxacillin per mg, calculated on the anhydrous basis. Meets the requirements for Identification, Crystallinity, pH (3.0–6.5, in a suspension containing 10 mg per mL), and Water (not more than 5.0%).
Cloxacillin Benzathine Intramammary Infusion USP—Preserve in disposable syringes that are well-closed containers, except that where the Infusion is labeled as sterile, the individual syringes or cartons are sealed and tamperproof so that sterility is assured at time of use. A suspension of Cloxacillin Benzathine or Sterile Cloxacillin Benzathine in a suitable oil vehicle. Label it to indicate that it is for veterinary use only. Infusion that is sterile may be so labeled. Contains an amount of cloxacillin benzathine equivalent to the labeled amount of cloxacillin, within −10% to +20%. Meets the requirements for Identification, Sterility (where labeled as being sterile), and Water (not more than 1.0%).
Sterile Cloxacillin Benzathine USP—Preserve in tight containers. Label it to indicate that it is for veterinary use only. Has a potency equivalent to not less than 704 mcg and not more than 821 mcg of cloxacillin per mg, calculated on the anhydrous basis. Meets the requirements for Sterility and for Identification, Crystallinity, pH, and Water under Cloxacillin Benzathine.

Cloxacillin Sodium USP—Preserve in tight containers, at a temperature not exceeding 25 °C. Contains the equivalent of not less than 825 mcg of cloxacillin per mg. Meets the requirements for Identification, Crystallinity, pH (4.5–7.5, in a solution containing 10 mg per mL), Water (3.0–5.0%), and Dimethylaniline.

Cloxacillin Sodium Capsules USP—Preserve in tight containers. Contain an amount of cloxacillin sodium equivalent to the labeled amount of cloxacillin, within −10% to +20%. Meet the requirements for Dissolution (75% in 45 minutes in water in Apparatus 1 at 100 rpm), Uniformity of dosage units, and Water (not more than 5.0%).

Cloxacillin Sodium Intramammary Infusion USP—Preserve in disposable syringes that are well-closed containers, except that where the Infusion is labeled as sterile, the individual syringes or cartons are sealed and tamperproof so that sterility is assured at time of use. A suspension of Sterile Cloxacillin Sodium in a suitable natural or chemically modified vegetable oil vehicle with a suitable dispersing agent. Label it to indicate that it is for veterinary use only. Infusion that is sterile may be so labeled. Contains an amount of cloxacillin sodium equivalent to the labeled amount of cloxacillin, within −10% to +20%. Meets the requirements for Identification, Sterility, and Water (not more than 1.0%).

Cloxacillin Sodium Injection—Not in USP.

Cloxacillin Sodium for Oral Solution USP—Preserve in tight containers. A dry mixture of Cloxacillin Sodium and one or more suitable buffers, colors, flavors, and preservatives. Contains an amount of cloxacillin sodium equivalent to the labeled amount of cloxacillin, within −10% to +20%. Meets the requirements for pH (5.0–7.5, in the solution constituted as directed in the labeling), Water (not more than 1.0%), Uniformity of dosage units (solid packaged in single-unit containers), and Deliverable volume (multiple-unit containers).

Sterile Cloxacillin Sodium USP—Preserve in tight containers. Label it to indicate that it is for veterinary use only. Contains an amount of cloxacillin sodium equivalent to not less than 825 mcg of cloxacillin per mg. Meets the requirements for Bacterial endotoxins and Sterility, and for Identification tests, Crystallinity, pH, Water, and Dimethylaniline under Cloxacillin Sodium.

COAL TAR

Description: Coal Tar USP—Nearly black, viscous liquid, heavier than water, having a characteristic, naphthalene-like odor.

Solubility: Coal Tar USP—Slightly soluble in water, to which it imparts its characteristic odor and a faintly alkaline reaction. Partially soluble in acetone, in alcohol, in carbon disulfide, in chloroform, in ether, in methanol, and in solvent hexane.

USP requirements:

Coal Tar USP—Preserve in tight containers. It is the tar obtained as a by-product during the destructive distillation of bituminous coal at temperatures in the range of 900 to 1100 °C. It may be processed further either by extraction with alcohol and suitable dispersing agents and maceration times or by fractional distillation with or without the use of suitable solvents. Meets the requirement for Residue on ignition (not more than 2.0%, from 100 mg).

Coal Tar Cleansing Bar—Not in USP.
Coal Tar Cream—Not in USP.
Coal Tar Gel—Not in USP.
Coal Tar Lotion—Not in USP.
Coal Tar Ointment USP—Preserve in tight containers.

Prepare Coal Tar Ointment as follows: 10 grams of Coal Tar, 5 grams of Polysorbate 80, and 985 grams of Zinc Oxide Paste to make 1000 grams. Blend the Coal Tar with the Polysorbate 80, and incorporate the mixture with the Zinc Oxide Paste.

Coal Tar Shampoo—Not in USP.
Coal Tar Topical Solution USP—Preserve in tight containers.

Prepare Coal Tar Topical Solution as follows: 200 grams of Coal Tar, 50 grams of Polysorbate 80, and a sufficient quantity of Alcohol, to make 1000 mL. Mix the Coal Tar with 500 grams of washed sand, and add the Polysorbate 80 and 700 mL of Alcohol. Macerate the mixture for 7 days in a closed vessel with frequent agitation. Filter, and rinse the vessel and the filter with sufficient Alcohol to make the product measure 1000 mL.

Meets the requirement for Alcohol content (81.0–86.0%).

Coal Tar Topical Suspension—Not in USP.

COCAINE

Source: An alkaloid obtained from the leaves of *Erythroxylum coca* and other species of *Erythroxylum*.

Chemical name:
Cocaine—8-Azabicyclo[3.2.1]octane-2-carboxylic acid, 3-(benzoyloxy)-8-methyl-, methyl ester, [1*R*-(*exo,exo*)]-.
Cocaine hydrochloride—8-Azabicyclo[3.2.1]octane-2-carboxylic acid, 3-(benzoyloxy)-8-methyl-, methyl ester, hydrochloride, [1*R*-(*exo,exo*)]-.

Molecular formula:
Cocaine—$C_{17}H_{21}NO_4$.
Cocaine hydrochloride—$C_{17}H_{21}NO_4 \cdot HCl$.

Molecular weight:
Cocaine—303.36.
Cocaine hydrochloride—339.82.

Description:
Cocaine USP—Colorless to white crystals or white, crystalline powder. Is levorotatory in 3 *N* hydrochloric acid solution. Its saturated solution is alkaline to litmus.
Cocaine Hydrochloride USP—Colorless crystals or white, crystalline powder.

Solubility:
Cocaine USP—Slightly soluble in water; very soluble in warm alcohol; freely soluble in alcohol, in chloroform, and in ether; soluble in olive oil; sparingly soluble in mineral oil.
Cocaine Hydrochloride USP—Very soluble in water; freely soluble in alcohol; soluble in chloroform and in glycerin; insoluble in ether.

USP requirements:
Cocaine USP—Preserve in well-closed, light-resistant containers. Dried over phosphorus pentoxide for 3 hours, contains not less than 99.0% and not more than 101.0% of cocaine. Meets the requirements for Identification, Melting range (96–98 °C), Loss on drying (not more than 1.0%), Residue on ignition (not more than 0.1%), Readily carbonizable substances, Cinnamyl-cocaine and other reducing substances, and Isoatropyl-cocaine.
Cocaine Hydrochloride USP—Preserve in well-closed, light-resistant containers. Contains not less than 99.0% and not more than 101.0% of cocaine hydrochloride, calculated on the dried basis. Meets the requirements for Identification, Specific rotation (−71° to −73°, determined in a solution containing the equivalent of 200 mg in each 10 mL, the test specimen previously having been dried over silica gel for 3 hours), Acidity, Loss on drying (not more than 1.0%), Residue on ignition (not more than 0.1%), Readily carbonizable substances, Cinnamyl-cocaine and other reducing substances, and Isoatropyl-cocaine.

Cocaine Hydrochloride Topical Solution—Not in USP.
Cocaine Hydrochloride Viscous Topical Solution—Not in USP.
Cocaine Hydrochloride Tablets for Topical Solution USP—Preserve in well-closed, light-resistant containers. Contain the labeled amount, within ±9%. Meet the requirements for Identification, Disintegration (15 minutes), and Uniformity of dosage units.

COCCIDIOIDIN

Description: Coccidioidin USP—Clear, practically colorless or amber-colored liquid.

USP requirements: Coccidioidin USP—Preserve at a temperature between 2 and 8 °C. A sterile solution containing the antigens obtained from the by-products of mycelial growth or from the spherules of the fungus *Coccidioides immitis*. Contains a suitable antimicrobial agent. Label it to state that any dilutions made of the product should be stored in a refrigerator and used within 24 hours. Label it also to state that a separate syringe and needle shall be used for each individual injection. Has a potency such that the 1:100 dilution is bioequivalent to the U.S. Reference Coccidioidin 1:100. Meets the requirement for Expiration date (not later than 3 years after date of issue from manufacturer's cold storage [5 °C, 1 year] for the mycelial product and not later than 18 months after date of issue from manufacturer's cold storage [5 °C, 18 months] for the spherule-derived product). Conforms to the regulations of the U.S. Food and Drug Administration concerning biologics.

COCOA BUTTER

Description: Cocoa Butter NF—Yellowish white solid, having a faint, agreeable odor. Usually brittle at temperatures below 25 °C.

NF category: Suppository base.

Solubility: Cocoa Butter NF—Freely soluble in ether and in chloroform; soluble in boiling dehydrated alcohol; slightly soluble in alcohol.

NF requirements: Cocoa Butter NF—Preserve in well-closed containers. It is the fat obtained from the seed of *Theobroma cacao* Linné (Fam. Sterculiaceae). Meets the requirements for Refractive index (1.454–1.459 at 40 °C), Wax, stearin, and tallow, Solidification range of the fatty acids (45–50 °C), Free fatty acids, Iodine value (33–42), and Saponification value (188–198).

CODEINE

Chemical name:
Codeine—Morphinan-6-ol, 7,8-didehydro-4,5-epoxy-3-methoxy-17-methyl-, monohydrate, (5 alpha,6 alpha)-.
Codeine phosphate—Morphinan-6-ol, 7,8-didehydro-4,5-epoxy-3-methoxy-17-methyl-, (5 alpha,6 alpha)-, phosphate (1:1) (salt), hemihydrate.
Codeine polistirex—Benzene, diethenyl-, polymer with ethenylbenzene, sulfonated, complex with (5 alpha,6 alpha)-7,8-didehydro-4,5-epoxy-3-methoxy-17-methylmorphinan-6-ol.
Codeine sulfate—Morphinan-6-ol, 7,8-didehydro-4,5-epoxy-3-methoxy-17-methyl-, (5 alpha,6 alpha)-, sulfate (2:1) (salt), trihydrate.

Molecular formula:
Codeine—$C_{18}H_{21}NO_3 \cdot H_2O$ (monohydrate); $C_{18}H_{21}NO_3$ (anhydrous).
Codeine phosphate—$C_{18}H_{21}NO_3 \cdot H_3PO_4 \cdot \frac{1}{2}H_2O$ (hemihydrate); $C_{18}H_{21}NO_3 \cdot H_3PO_4$ (anhydrous).
Codeine sulfate—$(C_{18}H_{21}NO_3)_2 \cdot H_2SO_4 \cdot 3H_2O$ (trihydrate); $(C_{18}H_{21}NO_3)_2 \cdot H_2SO_4$ (anhydrous).

Molecular weight:
Codeine—317.38 (monohydrate); 299.37 (anhydrous).
Codeine phosphate—406.37 (hemihydrate); 397.36 (anhydrous).
Codeine sulfate—750.86 (trihydrate); 696.81 (anhydrous).

Description:
Codeine USP—Colorless or white crystals or white, crystalline powder. Effloresces slowly in dry air, and is affected by light. In acid or alcohol solutions it is levorotatory. Its saturated solution is alkaline to litmus.
Codeine Phosphate USP—Fine, white, needle-shaped crystals, or white, crystalline powder. Odorless. Is affected by light. Its solutions are acid to litmus.
Codeine Sulfate USP—White crystals, usually needle-like, or white, crystalline powder. Is affected by light.

Solubility:
Codeine USP—Slightly soluble in water; very soluble in chloroform; freely soluble in alcohol; sparingly soluble in ether. When heated in an amount of water insufficient for complete solution, it melts to oily drops which crystallize on cooling.
Codeine Phosphate USP—Freely soluble in water; very soluble in hot water; slightly soluble in alcohol but more so in boiling alcohol.
Codeine Sulfate USP—Soluble in water; freely soluble in water at 80 °C; very slightly soluble in alcohol; insoluble in chloroform and in ether.

USP requirements:
Codeine USP—Preserve in tight, light-resistant containers. Dried at 80 °C for 4 hours, contains not less than 98.5% and not more than 100.5% of anhydrous codeine. Meets the requirements for Identification, Melting range (154–158 °C, the range between beginning and end of melting not more than 2 °C), Loss on drying (not more than 6.0%), Residue on ignition (not more than 0.1%), Readily carbonizable substances, Chromatographic purity, and Morphine.
Codeine Phosphate USP—Preserve in tight, light-resistant containers. Contains not less than 99.0% and not more than 101.5% of codeine phosphate, calculated on the anhydrous basis. Meets the requirements for Identification, Acidity, Water (not more than 3.0%), Chloride, Sulfate, Morphine, and Chromatographic purity.
Codeine Phosphate Injection USP—Preserve in single-dose or in multiple-dose containers, preferably of Type I glass, protected from light. A sterile solution of Codeine Phosphate in Water for Injection. Contains the labeled amount of codeine phosphate (as the hemihydrate), within ±7%. Meets the requirements for Identification, Bacterial endotoxins, pH (3.0–6.0), Morphine, and Injections.

Note: Do not use the Injection if it is more than slightly discolored or contains a precipitate.

Codeine Phosphate Oral Solution—Not in USP.
Codeine Phosphate Tablets USP—Preserve in well-closed, light-resistant containers. Contain the labeled amount of codeine phosphate (as the hemihydrate), within ±7%. Meet the requirements for Identification, Dissolution (75% in 45 minutes in water in Apparatus 2 at 50 rpm), Uniformity of dosage units, and Morphine.
Codeine Phosphate Soluble Tablets—Not in USP.
Codeine Sulfate USP—Preserve in tight, light-resistant containers. Dried at 105 °C for 3 hours, contains not less than 98.5% and not more than 100.5% of anhydrous codeine sulfate. Meets the requirements for Identification, Specific rotation (−112.5° to −115.0°, calculated on the dried basis), Acidity, Water (6.0–7.5%), Residue on ignition (not more than 0.1%), Readily carbonizable substances, Chromatographic purity, and Morphine.

Codeine Sulfate Tablets USP—Preserve in well-closed containers. Contain the labeled amount of codeine sulfate (as the trihydrate), within ±7%. Meet the requirements for Identification, Dissolution (75% in 45 minutes in water in Apparatus 1 at 100 rpm), and Uniformity of dosage units.

Codeine Sulfate Soluble Tablets—Not in USP.

CODEINE AND CALCIUM IODIDE

Chemical name: Codeine—Morphinan-6-ol, 7,8-didehydro-4,5-epoxy-3-methoxy-17-methyl-, monohydrate, (5 alpha,6 alpha)-.

Molecular formula:
Codeine—$C_{18}H_{21}NO_3 \cdot H_2O$.
Calcium iodide—CaI_2.

Molecular weight:
Codeine—317.38.
Calcium iodide—293.9.

Description:
Codeine USP—Colorless or white crystals or white, crystalline powder. It effloresces slowly in dry air, and is affected by light. In acid or alcohol solutions it is levorotatory. Its saturated solution is alkaline to litmus.
Calcium iodide—Very hygroscopic. Aqueous solution is neutral or slightly alkaline.

Solubility:
Codeine USP—Slightly soluble in water; very soluble in chloroform; freely soluble in alcohol; sparingly soluble in ether. When heated in an amount of water insufficient for complete solution, it melts to oily drops which crystallize on cooling.
Calcium iodide—Very soluble in water, in methanol, in ethanol, and in acetone; practically insoluble in ether and in dioxane.

USP requirements: Codeine and Calcium Iodide Syrup—Not in USP.

CODEINE AND IODINATED GLYCEROL

For *Codeine* and *Iodinated Glycerol*—See individual listings for chemistry information.

USP requirements: Codeine Phosphate and Iodinated Glycerol Oral Solution—Not in USP.

COD LIVER OIL

Description: Cod Liver Oil USP—Thin, oily liquid, having a characteristic, slightly fishy but not rancid odor.

Solubility: Cod Liver Oil USP—Slightly soluble in alcohol; freely soluble in ether, in chloroform, in carbon disulfide, and in ethyl acetate.

USP requirements: Cod Liver Oil USP—Preserve in tight containers. It may be bottled or otherwise packaged in containers from which air has been expelled by the production of a vacuum or by an inert gas. It is the partially destearinated fixed oil obtained from fresh livers of *Gadus morrhua* Linné and other species of Fam. Gadidae. The vitamin A potency and vitamin D potency, when designated on the label, are expressed in USP Units per gram of oil. The potencies may be expressed also in metric units, on the basis that 1 USP Vitamin A Unit = 0.3 mcg and 40 USP Vitamin D Units = 1 mcg. Contains, in each gram, not less than 255 mcg (850 USP Units) of vitamin A and not less than 2.125 mcg (85 USP Units) of vitamin D. Meets the requirements for Identification for vitamin A, Specific gravity (0.918–0.927), Color, Nondestearinated cod liver oil, Unsaponifiable matter (not more than 1.30%), Acid value (not more than 1.0 mL of 0.10 sodium hydroxide required), Iodine value (145–180), and Saponification value (180–192).

COLCHICINE

Source: An alkaloid derived from various species of *Colchicum*.

Chemical name: Acetamide, *N*-(5,6,7,9-tetrahydro-1,2,3,10-tetramethoxy-9-oxobenzo[*a*]heptalen-7-yl)-, (*S*)-.

Molecular formula: $C_{22}H_{25}NO_6$.

Molecular weight: 399.44.

Description: Colchicine USP—Pale yellow to pale greenish yellow, amorphous scales, or powder or crystalline powder. Is odorless or nearly so, and darkens on exposure to light.

pKa: 1.7 and 12.4.

Solubility: Colchicine USP—Soluble in water; freely soluble in alcohol and in chloroform; slightly soluble in ether.

USP requirements:
Colchicine USP—Preserve in tight, light-resistant containers. An alkaloid obtained from various species of *Colchicum*. Contains not less than 94.0% and not more than 101.0% of colchicine, calculated on the anhydrous, solvent-free basis. Meets the requirements for Identification, Specific rotation (−240° to −250°, calculated on the anhydrous and solvent-free basis), Water (not more than 3.0%), Colchiceine, Chloroform and ethyl acetate, Chromatographic purity, and Organic volatile impurities.
Colchicine Injection USP—Preserve in single-dose containers, preferably of Type I glass, protected from light. A sterile solution of Colchicine in Water for Injection, prepared from Colchicine with the aid of Sodium Hydroxide. Contains the labeled amount, within ±10%. Meets the requirements for Identification, Bacterial endotoxins, pH (6.0–7.2, in a solution of Injection containing 1.0 mg of potassium chloride in each mL), and Injections.
Caution: Colchicine is extremely poisonous.
Colchicine Tablets USP—Preserve in well-closed, light-resistant containers. Contain the labeled amount, within ±10%. Meet the requirements for Identification, Dissolution (75% in 30 minutes in water in Apparatus 1 at 100 rpm), and Uniformity of dosage units.

COLESTIPOL

Chemical group: An anion-exchange resin.

Chemical name: Colestipol hydrochloride—Colestipol hydrochloride. Copolymer of diethylenetriamine and 1-chloro-2,3-epoxypropane, hydrochloride (with approximately 1 out of 5 amine nitrogens protonated).

Description: Colestipol Hydrochloride USP—Yellow to orange beads.

Solubility: Colestipol Hydrochloride USP—Swells but does not dissolve in water or dilute aqueous solutions of acid or alkali. Insoluble in the common organic solvents.

USP requirements:
Colestipol Hydrochloride USP—Preserve in tight containers. An insoluble, high molecular weight basic anion-exchange copolymer of diethylenetriamine and 1-chloro-2,3-epoxypropane with approximately one out of five amino

nitrogens protonated. Each gram binds not less than 1.1 mEq and not more than 1.6 mEq of sodium cholate, calculated as cholate binding capacity. Meets the requirements for Identification, pH (6.0–7.5), Loss on drying (not more than 1.0%), Residue on ignition (not more than 0.3%), Heavy metals (not more than 0.002%), Chloride content (6.5–9.0%, calculated on the dried basis), Water absorption (3.3–5.3 grams of water per gram), Cholate binding capacity (1.1–1.6 mEq per gram), Water-soluble substances (not more than 0.5%), and Colestipol exchange capacity (9.0–11.0 mEq of sodium hydroxide per gram).

Colestipol Hydrochloride for Oral Suspension USP—Preserve in tight, single-dose or multiple-dose containers. A mixture of Colestipol Hydrochloride with a suitable flow-promoting agent. Each gram binds not less than 1.1 mEq and not more than 1.6 mEq of sodium cholate, calculated as the cholate binding capacity. Meets the requirements for Minimum fill and Water-soluble substances (not more than 0.5%), and for Cholate binding capacity, Identification, Water absorption, and pH under Colestipol Hydrochloride.

COLISTIMETHATE

Chemical name: Colistimethate sodium—Colistimethate sodium.

Molecular formula: $C_{58}H_{105}N_{16}Na_5O_{28}S_5$ (colistin A component); $C_{57}H_{103}N_{16}Na_5O_{28}S_5$ (colistin B component).

Molecular weight: 1749.81 (colistin A component); 1735.78 (colistin B component).

Description: Sterile Colistimethate Sodium USP—White to slightly yellow, odorless, fine powder.

Solubility: Sterile Colistimethate Sodium USP—Freely soluble in water; soluble in methanol; insoluble in acetone and in ether.

USP requirements: Sterile Colistimethate Sodium USP—Preserve in Containers for Sterile Solids. It is colistimethate sodium suitable for parenteral use. Contains an amount of colistimethate sodium equivalent to not less than 390 mcg of colistin per mg and, where packaged for dispensing, contains an amount of colistimethate sodium equivalent to the labeled amount of colistin, within −10% to +20%. Meets the requirements for Constituted solution, Identification, Bacterial endotoxins, Sterility, pH (6.5–8.5, in a solution containing 10 mg per mL), Loss on drying (not more than 7.0%), Heavy metals (not more than 0.003%), and Free colistin. Where packaged for dispensing, meets the requirements for Uniformity of dosage units and for Constituted solutions and Labeling under Injections.

COLISTIN

Chemical name: Colistin sulfate—Colistin, sulfate.

Molecular formula:
Sulfate, Colistin A component—$C_{53}H_{100}N_{16}O_{13}\cdot2\frac{1}{2}H_2SO_4$.
Sulfate, Colistin B component—$C_{52}H_{98}N_{16}O_{13}\cdot2\frac{1}{2}H_2SO_4$.

Molecular weight:
Sulfate, Colistin A component—1414.65.
Sulfate, Colistin B component—1400.63.

Description: Colistin Sulfate USP—White to slightly yellow, odorless, fine powder.

Solubility: Colistin Sulfate USP—Freely soluble in water; slightly soluble in methanol; insoluble in acetone and in ether.

USP requirements:
Colistin Sulfate USP—Preserve in tight containers. It is the sulfate salt of an antibacterial substance produced by the growth of *Bacillus polymyxa* var. *colistinus*. Has a potency equivalent to not less than 500 mcg of colistin per mg. Meets the requirements for Identification, pH (4.0–7.0, in a solution containing 10 mg per mL), and Loss on drying (not more than 7.0%).

Colistin Sulfate for Oral Suspension USP—Preserve in tight containers, protected from light. A dry mixture of Colistin Sulfate with or without one or more suitable buffers, colors, diluents, dispersants, and flavors. Contains an amount of colistin sulfate equivalent to the labeled amount of colistin, within −10% to +20%. Meets the requirements for Uniformity of dosage units (solid packaged in single-unit containers), Deliverable volume (solid packaged in multiple-unit containers), pH (5.0–6.0, in the suspension constituted as directed in the labeling), and Loss on drying (not more than 3.0%).

COLISTIN, NEOMYCIN, AND HYDROCORTISONE

For *Colistin*, *Neomycin*, and *Hydrocortisone*—See individual listings for chemistry information.

USP requirements: Colistin and Neomycin Sulfates and Hydrocortisone Acetate Otic Suspension USP—Preserve in tight containers. A sterile suspension. Contains an amount of colistin sulfate equivalent to the labeled amount of colistin, within −10% to +35%, an amount of neomycin sulfate equivalent to the labeled amount of neomycin, within −10% to +25%, and the labeled amount of hydrocortisone acetate, within ±10%. Contains one or more suitable buffers, detergents, dispersants, and preservatives. Meets the requirements for Sterility and pH (4.8–5.2).

Note: Where Colistin and Neomycin Sulfates and Hydrocortisone Acetate Otic Suspension is prescribed, without reference to the quantity of colistin, neomycin, or hydrocortisone acetate contained therein, a product containing 3.0 mg of colistin, 3.3 mg of neomycin, and 10 mg of hydrocortisone acetate per mL shall be dispensed.

COLLODION

Description: Flexible Collodion USP—Clear, or slightly opalescent, viscous liquid. Is colorless or slightly yellow, and has the odor of ether. The strong odor of camphor becomes noticeable as the ether evaporates.

USP requirements:
Collodion USP—Preserve in tight containers, at a temperature not exceeding 30 °C, remote from fire. The label bears a caution statement to the effect that Collodion is highly flammable. Contains not less than 5.0%, by weight, of pyroxylin.

Prepare Collodion as follows: 40 grams of Pyroxylin, 750 mL of Ether, and 250 mL of Alcohol to make about 1000 mL. Add the Alcohol and Ether to the Pyroxylin contained in a suitable container, and insert the stopper into the container well. Shake the mixture occasionally until the Pyroxylin is dissolved.

Meets the requirements for Identification, Specific gravity (0.765–0.775), Acidity, and Alcohol content (22.0–26.0%).

Caution: Collodion is highly flammable.

Flexible Collodion USP—Preserve in tight containers, at a temperature not exceeding 30 °C, remote from fire. The label bears a caution statement to the effect that Flexible Collodion is highly flammable.

Prepare Flexible Collodion as follows: 20 grams of Camphor, 30 grams of Castor Oil, and a sufficient quantity of Collodion, to make 1000 grams. Weigh the ingredients, successively, into a dry, tared bottle, insert the stopper in the bottle, and shake the mixture until the camphor is dissolved.

Meets the requirements for Identification, Specific gravity (0.770–0.790), and Alcohol content (21.0–25.0%).

COPPER

Chemical name: Copper gluconate—Copper, bis (D-gluconato-O^1,O^2)-.

Molecular formula: Copper gluconate—$C_{12}H_{22}CuO_{14}$.

Molecular weight: Copper gluconate—453.84.

USP requirements:
Copper Gluconate USP—Preserve in well-closed containers. Contains not less than 98.0% and not more than 102.0% of copper gluconate. Meets the requirements for Identification, Chloride (not more than 0.07%), Sulfate (not more than 0.05%), Arsenic (not more than 3 ppm), Lead (not more than 0.0025%), and Reducing substances (not more than 1.0%).
Copper Gluconate Tablets—Not in USP.

CORN OIL

Description: Corn Oil NF—Clear, light yellow oily liquid, having a faint, characteristic odor.
NF category: Solvent; oleaginous vehicle.

Solubility: Corn Oil NF—Slightly soluble in alcohol; miscible with ether, with chloroform, and with solvent hexane.

NF requirements: Corn Oil NF—Preserve in tight, light-resistant containers, and avoid exposure to excessive heat. It is the refined fixed oil obtained from the embryo of *Zea mays* Linné (Fam. Gramineae). Meets the requirements for Specific gravity (0.914–0.921), Heavy metals (not more than 0.001%), Cottonseed oil, Fatty acid composition, Free fatty acids, Iodine value (102–130), Saponification value (187–193), and Unsaponifiable matter (not more than 1.5%).

CORTICOTROPIN

Chemical name:
Corticotropin—Corticotropin.
Corticotropin, repository—Corticotropin.
Corticotropin zinc hydroxide—Corticotropin zinc hydroxide.

Description:
Corticotropin Injection USP—Colorless or light straw-colored liquid.
Corticotropin for Injection USP—White or practically white, soluble, amorphous solid having the characteristic appearance of substances prepared by freeze-drying.
Repository Corticotropin Injection USP—Colorless or light straw-colored liquid, which may be quite viscid at room temperature. Is odorless or has an odor of an antimicrobial agent.
Sterile Corticotropin Zinc Hydroxide Suspension USP—Flocculent, white, aqueous suspension, free from large particles following moderate shaking.

USP requirements:
Corticotropin Injection USP—Preserve in single-dose or in multiple-dose containers, preferably of Type I glass. Store in a cold place. A sterile solution, in a suitable diluent,

of the material containing the polypeptide hormone having the property of increasing the rate of secretion of adrenal corticosteroids, which is obtained from the anterior lobe of the pituitary of mammals used for food by man. If the labeling of Corticotropin Injection recommends intravenous administration, include specific information on dosage. Its potency is within −20% to +25% of the potency stated on the label in USP Corticotropin Units. Meets the requirements for Vasopressin activity, Bacterial endotoxins, pH (3.0–7.0), Particulate matter, and Injections.
Corticotropin for Injection USP—Preserve in Containers for Sterile Solids. A sterile, dry material containing the polypeptide hormone having the property of increasing the rate of secretion of adrenal corticosteroids, which is obtained from the anterior lobe of the pituitary of mammals used for food by man. If the labeling of Corticotropin for Injection recommends intravenous administration, include specific information on dosage. Its potency is within −20% to +25% of the potency stated on the label in USP Corticotropin Units. Meets the requirements for Vasopressin activity, Bacterial endotoxins, pH (2.5–6.0, in a solution constituted as directed in the labeling supplied by the manufacturer), and Particulate matter, and for Sterility tests, Uniformity of dosage units, Constituted solutions and Labeling under Injections.
Repository Corticotropin Injection USP—Preserve in single-dose or in multiple-dose containers, preferably of Type I glass. It is corticotropin in a solution of partially hydrolyzed gelatin. Its potency is within −20% to +25% of the potency stated on the label in USP Corticotropin Units. Meets the requirements for Bacterial endotoxins, for Vasopressin activity and pH under Corticotropin Injection, and for Injections.
Sterile Corticotropin Zinc Hydroxide Suspension USP—Preserve in single-dose or in multiple-dose containers, preferably of Type I glass. Store at controlled room temperature. A sterile suspension of corticotropin adsorbed on zinc hydroxide. Label it to indicate that it is not recommended for intravenous use and that the suspension is to be well shaken before use. The container label and the package label state the potency in USP Corticotropin Units in each mL. Its potency is within −20% to +25% of the potency stated on the label in USP Corticotropin Units. Contains not less than 1800 mcg and not more than 2200 mcg of zinc, and not less than 604 mcg and not more than 776 mcg of anhydrous dibasic sodium phosphate, for each 40 USP Corticotropin Units. Meets the requirements for Bacterial endotoxins, pH (7.5–8.5), Zinc, Anhydrous dibasic sodium phosphate, and Injections.

CORTISONE

Chemical name: Cortisone acetate—Pregn-4-ene-3,11,20-trione, 21-(acetyloxy)-17-hydroxy-.

Molecular formula: Cortisone acetate—$C_{23}H_{30}O_6$.

Molecular weight: Cortisone acetate—402.49.

Description: Cortisone Acetate USP—White or practically white, odorless, crystalline powder. Is stable in air. Melts at about 240 °C, with some decomposition.

Solubility: Cortisone Acetate USP—Insoluble in water; freely soluble in chloroform; soluble in dioxane; sparingly soluble in acetone; slightly soluble in alcohol.

USP requirements:
Cortisone Acetate USP—Preserve in well-closed containers. Contains not less than 97.0% and not more than 102.0% of cortisone acetate, calculated on the dried basis. Meets

the requirements for Identification, Specific rotation (+208° to +217°, calculated on the dried basis), Loss on drying (not more than 1.0%), Residue on ignition (negligible), and Ordinary impurities.

Sterile Cortisone Acetate Suspension USP—Preserve in single-dose or in multiple-dose containers, preferably of Type I glass. A sterile suspension of Cortisone Acetate in a suitable aqueous medium. Contains the labeled amount, within ±10%. Meets the requirements for Identification, pH (5.0–7.0), and Injections.

Cortisone Acetate Tablets USP—Preserve in well-closed containers. Contain the labeled amount, within ±10%. Meet the requirements for Identification, Dissolution (60% in 30 minutes in a mixture of isopropyl alcohol and dilute hydrochloric acid [1 in 100] in Apparatus 1 at 100 rpm), and Uniformity of dosage units.

COSYNTROPIN

Source: Synthetic polypeptide identical to the first 24 of the 39 amino acids of corticotropin.

Chemical name: Alpha$^{1-24}$-Corticotropin.

Molecular formula: $C_{136}H_{210}N_{40}O_{31}S$.

Molecular weight: 2933.46.

Description: White to off-white lyophilized mixture.

Solubility: Soluble in water.

USP requirements: Cosyntropin for Injection—Not in USP.

PURIFIED COTTON

Description: Purified Cotton USP—White, soft, fine filament-like hairs appearing under the microscope as hollow, flattened and twisted bands, striate and slightly thickened at the edges. Is practically odorless.

Solubility: Purified Cotton USP—Insoluble in ordinary solvents; soluble in ammoniated cupric oxide TS.

USP requirements: Purified Cotton USP—Package it in rolls of not more than 500 grams of a continuous lap, with a light-weight paper running under the entire lap, the paper being of such width that it may be folded over the edges of the lap to a distance of at least 25 millimeters, the two together being tightly and evenly rolled, and enclosed and sealed in a well-closed container. It may be packaged also in other types of containers if these are so constructed that the sterility of the product is maintained. It is the hair of the seed of cultivated varieties of *Gossypium hirsutum* Linné, or of other species of *Gossypium* (Fam. Malvaceae), freed from adhering impurities, deprived of fatty matter, bleached, and sterilized in its final container. Its label bears a statement to the effect that the sterility cannot be guaranteed if the package bears evidence of damage or if the package has been opened previously. Meets the requirements for Alkalinity or acidity, Residue on ignition (not more than 0.20%), Water-soluble substances (not more than 0.35%), Fatty matter (not more than 0.7%), Dyes, Other foreign matter, Fiber length and Absorbency (not less than 60% of fibers, by weight, are 12.5 millimeters or greater in length and not more than 10% of fibers, by weight, are 6.25 millimeters or less in length; retains not less than 24 times its weight of water), and Sterility.

COTTONSEED OIL

Description: Cottonseed Oil NF—Pale yellow, oily liquid. It is odorless or nearly so. At temperatures below 10 °C particles of solid fat may separate from the Oil, and at about 0 to −5 °C, the oil becomes a solid or nearly so.

NF category: Solvent; oleaginous vehicle.

Solubility: Cottonseed Oil NF—Slightly soluble in alcohol. Miscible with ether, with chloroform, with solvent hexane, and with carbon disulfide.

NF requirements: Cottonseed Oil NF—Preserve in tight, light-resistant containers, and avoid exposure to excessive heat. It is the refined fixed oil obtained from the seed of cultivated plants of various varieties of *Gossypium hirsutum* Linné or of other species of *Gossypium* (Fam. Malvaceae). Meets the requirements for Identification, Specific gravity (0.915–0.921), Heavy metals (not more than 0.001%), Trichloroethylene, Solidification range of the fatty acids (31–35 °C), Free fatty acids, Iodine value (109–120), and Saponification value (190–198).

CREATININE

Molecular formula: $C_4H_7N_3O$.

Molecular weight: 113.12.

Description: Creatinine NF—White crystals or crystalline powder. Is odorless.

NF category: Bulking agent for freeze-drying.

Solubility: Creatinine NF—Soluble in water; slightly soluble in alcohol; practically insoluble in acetone, in ether, and in chloroform.

NF requirements: Creatinine NF—Preserve in well-closed containers. Contains not less than 98.5% and not more than 102.0% of creatinine, as Creatinine, calculated on the dried basis. Meets the requirements for Identification, Loss on drying (not more than 3.0%), Residue on ignition (not more than 0.2%), and Heavy metals (not more than 0.001%).

CRESOL

Chemical name: Phenol, methyl-.

Molecular formula: C_7H_8O.

Molecular weight: 108.14.

Description: Cresol NF—Colorless, or yellowish to brownish yellow, or pinkish, highly refractive liquid, becoming darker with age and on exposure to light. It has a phenol-like, sometimes empyreumatic odor. A saturated solution of it is neutral or only slightly acid to litmus.

NF category: Antimicrobial preservative.

Solubility: Cresol NF—Sparingly soluble in water, usually forming a cloudy solution; dissolves in solutions of fixed alkali hydroxides. Miscible with alcohol, with ether, and with glycerin.

NF requirements: Cresol NF—Preserve in tight, light-resistant containers. A mixture of isomeric cresols obtained from coal tar or from petroleum. Meets the requirements for Identification, Specific gravity (1.030–1.038), Distilling range (195–205 °C, not less than 90.0% distils), Hydrocarbons, and Phenol (not more than 5.0%).

CROMOLYN

Chemical name: Cromolyn sodium—4H-1-Benzopyran-2-carboxylic acid, 5,5′-[(2-hydroxy-1,3-propanediyl)bis(oxy)]bis-[4-oxo-, disodium salt].

Molecular formula: Cromolyn sodium—$C_{23}H_{14}Na_2O_{11}$.

Molecular weight: Cromolyn sodium—512.34.

Description:
Cromolyn Sodium USP—White, odorless, crystalline powder. Is hygroscopic.
Cromolyn Sodium for Inhalation USP—White to creamy white, odorless, hygroscopic, and very finely divided powder.

Solubility: Cromolyn Sodium USP—Soluble in water; insoluble in alcohol and in chloroform.

USP requirements:
Cromolyn Sodium USP—Preserve in tight containers. Contains not less than 98.0% and not more than 101.0% of cromolyn sodium, calculated on the dried basis. Meets the requirements for Identification, Acidity or alkalinity, Loss on drying (not more than 10.0%), Related compounds, Oxalate, and Organic volatile impurities.
Cromolyn Sodium Capsules—Not in USP.
Cromolyn Sodium Inhalation USP (Solution)—Preserve in single-unit, double-ended glass ampuls or in low-density polyethylene ampuls. A sterile, aqueous solution of Cromolyn Sodium. The label indicates that the Inhalation is not to be used if it contains a precipitate. Contains the labeled amount, within ±10%. Meets the requirements for Identification, Related compounds, pH (4.0–7.0), Sterility, and Uniformity of dosage units.
Cromolyn Sodium Inhalation Aerosol—Not in USP.
Cromolyn Sodium for Inhalation USP (Capsules)—Preserve in tight, light-resistant containers. Avoid excessive heat. A mixture of equal parts of Lactose and Cromolyn Sodium contained in a hard gelatin capsule. Contains the labeled amount, within −5% to +25%. Meets the requirements for Identification and Uniformity of dosage units.
Cromolyn Sodium for Nasal Insufflation—Not in USP.
Cromolyn Sodium Nasal Solution USP—Preserve in tight, light-resistant containers. An aqueous solution of Cromolyn Sodium. Contains the labeled amount, within ±10%. Meets the requirements for Identification, pH (4.0–7.0), and Related compounds.
Cromolyn Sodium Ophthalmic Solution USP—Preserve in tight, light-resistant, single-dose or multiple-dose containers. Ophthalmic Solution that is packaged in multiple-dose containers contains a suitable antimicrobial agent. A sterile, aqueous solution of Cromolyn Sodium. Contains the labeled amount, within ±10%. Meets the requirements for Identification, Sterility, pH (4.0–7.0), and Related compounds.

CROSCARMELLOSE SODIUM

Description: Croscarmellose Sodium NF—White, free-flowing powder.
NF category: Tablet disintegrant.

Solubility: Croscarmellose Sodium NF—Partially soluble in water; insoluble in alcohol, in ether, and in other organic solvents.

NF requirements: Croscarmellose Sodium NF—Preserve in tight containers. A cross-linked polymer of carboxymethylcellulose sodium. Meets the requirements for Identification, pH (5.0—7.0), Loss on drying (not more than 10.0%), Heavy metals (not more than 0.001%), Sodium chloride and sodium glycolate (not more than 0.5%), Degree of substitution (0.60–0.85, calculated on the dried basis), Content of water-soluble material (1.0–10.0%), and Settling volume (10.0–30.0 mL).

CROSPOVIDONE

Chemical name: 1-Ethenyl-2-pyrrolidinone homopolymer.

Molecular formula: $(C_6H_9NO)_n$.

Description: Crospovidone NF—White to creamy-white, hygroscopic powder, having a faint odor.
NF category: Tablet disintegrant.

Solubility: Crospovidone NF—Insoluble in water and in ordinary organic solvents.

NF requirements: Crospovidone NF—Preserve in tight containers. A water-insoluble synthetic, cross-linked homopolymer of N-vinyl-2-pyrrolidinone. Contains not less than 11.0% and not more than 12.8% of nitrogen, calculated on the anhydrous basis. Meets the requirements for Identification, pH (5.0–8.0, in an aqueous suspension [1 in 100]), Water (not more than 5.0%), Residue on ignition (not more than 0.4%), Water-soluble substances (not more than 1.5%), Heavy metals (not more than 0.001%), Vinylpyrrolidinone (not more than 0.1%), and Nitrogen content.

CROTAMITON

Chemical name: 2-Butenamide, N-ethyl-N-(2-methylphenyl)-.

Molecular formula: $C_{13}H_{17}NO$.

Molecular weight: 203.28.

Description: Crotamiton USP—Colorless to slightly yellowish oil, having a faint amine-like odor.

Solubility: Crotamiton USP—Soluble in alcohol and in methanol.

USP requirements:
Crotamiton USP—Preserve in tight, light-resistant containers. A mixture of cis and trans isomers containing not less than 97.0% and not more than 103.0% of crotamiton. Meets the requirements for Identification, Specific gravity (1.008–1.011 at 20 °C), Refractive index (1.540–1.543 at 20 °C), Residue on ignition (not more than 0.1%), and Bound halogen.
Crotamiton Cream USP—Preserve in collapsible tubes or in tight, light-resistant containers. Contains the labeled amount, within ±7%. Meets the requirements for Identification and Minimum fill.
Crotamiton Lotion—Not in USP.

CUPRIC CHLORIDE

Chemical name: Copper chloride ($CuCl_2$) dihydrate.

Molecular formula: $CuCl_2 \cdot 2H_2O$.

Molecular weight: 170.48.

Description: Cupric Chloride USP—Bluish green, deliquescent crystals.

Solubility: Cupric Chloride USP—Freely soluble in water; soluble in alcohol; slightly soluble in ether.

USP requirements:
Cupric Chloride USP—Preserve in tight containers. Contains not less than 99.0% and not more than 100.5% of cupric chloride, calculated on the dried basis. Meets the requirements for Identification, Loss on drying (20.9–21.4%), Insoluble matter (not more than 0.01%), Sulfate (not more than 0.005%), Substances not precipitated by hydrogen sulfide (not more than 0.1%), Iron, Other metals, and Organic volatile impurities.

Cupric Chloride Injection USP—Preserve in single-dose or in multiple-dose containers, preferably of Type I or Type II glass. A sterile solution of Cupric Chloride in Water for Injection. Label the Injection to indicate that it is to be diluted to the appropriate strength with Sterile Water for Injection or other suitable fluid prior to administration. Contains an amount of cupric chloride equivalent to the labeled amount of copper, within ±5%. Meets the requirements for Identification, Bacterial endotoxins, pH (1.5–2.5), Particulate matter, and Injections.

CUPRIC SULFATE

Chemical name: Sulfuric acid, copper(2+) salt (1:1), pentahydrate.

Molecular formula: $CuSO_4 \cdot 5H_2O$.

Molecular weight: 249.68.

Description: Cupric Sulfate USP—Deep blue, triclinic crystals or blue, crystalline granules or powder. It effloresces slowly in dry air. Its solutions are acid to litmus.

Solubility: Cupric Sulfate USP—Freely soluble in water and in glycerin; very soluble in boiling water; slightly soluble in alcohol.

USP requirements:
Cupric Sulfate USP—Preserve in tight containers. Dried at 250 °C to constant weight, contains not less than 98.5% and not more than 100.5% of cupric sulfate. Meets the requirements for Identification, Loss on drying (33.0–36.5%), Alkalies and alkaline earths (not more than 0.3%), and Substances not precipitated by hydrogen sulfide (not more than 0.3%).

Cupric Sulfate Injection USP—Preserve in single-dose or in multiple-dose containers, preferably of Type I or Type II glass. A sterile solution of Cupric Sulfate in Water for Injection. Label the Injection to indicate that it is to be diluted to the appropriate strength with Sterile Water for Injection or other suitable fluid prior to administration. Contains an amount of cupric sulfate equivalent to the labeled amount of copper, within ±5%. Meets the requirements for Identification, Bacterial endotoxins, pH (2.0–3.5), Particulate matter, and Injections.

CYANOCOBALAMIN

Source: Synthetic form of vitamin B_{12}.

Chemical name: Vitamin B_{12}.

Molecular formula: $C_{63}H_{88}CoN_{14}O_{14}P$.

Molecular weight: 1324.46.

Description: Cyanocobalamin USP—Dark red crystals or amorphous or crystalline red powder. In the anhydrous form, it is very hygroscopic and when exposed to air it may absorb about 12% of water.

Solubility: Cyanocobalamin USP—Sparingly soluble in water; soluble in alcohol; insoluble in acetone, in chloroform, and in ether.

USP requirements:
Cyanocobalamin USP—Preserve in tight, light-resistant containers. Contains not less than 96.0% and not more than 100.5% of cyanocobalamin, calculated on the dried basis. Meets the requirements for Identification, Loss on drying (not more than 12.0%), and Pseudo cyanocobalamin.

Cyanocobalamin Injection USP—Preserve in light-resistant, single-dose or multiple-dose containers, preferably of Type I glass. A sterile solution of Cyanocobalamin in Water for Injection, or in Water for Injection rendered isotonic by the addition of Sodium Chloride. Contains the labeled amount of anhydrous cyanocobalamin, within −5% to +15%. Meets the requirements for Identification, Bacterial endotoxins, pH (4.5–7.0), and Injections.

Cyanocobalamin Tablets—Not in USP.

CYANOCOBALAMIN Co 57

Chemical name: Vitamin B_{12}-^{57}Co.

Molecular formula: $C_{63}H_{88}{}^{57}CoN_{14}O_{14}P$.

Description:
Cyanocobalamin Co 57 Capsules USP—May contain a small amount of solid or solids, or may appear empty.
Cyanocobalamin Co 57 Oral Solution USP—Clear, colorless to pink solution.

USP requirements:
Cyanocobalamin Co 57 Capsules USP—Preserve in well-closed, light-resistant containers. Contain Cyanocobalamin in which a portion of the molecules contain radioactive cobalt (^{57}Co) in the molecular structure. Label Capsules to include the following: the date of calibration; the amount of cyanocobalamin expressed in micrograms per Capsule; the amount of ^{57}Co as cyanocobalamin expressed in megabecquerels (or microcuries) per Capsule at the time of calibration; the expiration date; and the statement, "Caution—Radioactive Material." The labeling indicates that in making dosage calculations, correction is to be made for radioactive decay, and also indicates that the radioactive half-life of ^{57}Co is 270.9 days. Contain the labeled amount of ^{57}Co, within ±10%, as cyanocobalamin expressed in megabecquerels (or microcuries) at the time indicated in the labeling. Contain the labeled amount of cyanocobalamin, within ±10%. The specific activity is not less than 0.02 megabecquerel (0.5 microcurie) per mcg of cyanocobalamin. Meet the requirements for Radionuclide identification, Uniformity of dosage units, Radiochemical purity, and Cyanocobalamin content.

Cyanocobalamin Co 57 Oral Solution USP—Preserve in tight containers, and protect from light. A solution suitable for oral administration, containing Cyanocobalamin in which a portion of the molecules contain radioactive cobalt (^{57}Co) in the molecular structure. Label it to include the following: the date of calibration; the amount of ^{57}Co as cyanocobalamin expressed as total megabecquerels (or microcuries) and as megabecquerels (or microcuries) per mL at the time of calibration; the amount of cyanocobalamin expressed in mcg per mL; the name and quantity of the added preservative; the expiration date; and the statement, "Caution—Radioactive Material." The labeling indicates that in making dosage calculations, correction is to be made for radioactive decay, and also indicates that the radioactive half-life of ^{57}Co is 270.9 days, and directs that the Oral Solution be protected from light. Contains the labeled amount of ^{57}Co, within ±10%, as cyanocobalamin expressed in megabecquerels (or microcuries) per mL at the time indicated in the labeling. Contains the labeled amount of cyanocobalamin, within ±10%. The specific activity is not less than 0.02 megabecquerel (0.5 microcurie) per mcg of cyanocobalamin. Contains a suitable antimicrobial agent. Meets the requirements for Radionuclide identification, pH (4.0–5.5), Radiochemical purity (not less than 95.0%), and Cyanocobalamin content.

CYANOCOBALAMIN Co 60

Chemical name: Vitamin B_{12}-^{60}Co.

Molecular formula: $C_{63}H_{88}{}^{60}CoN_{14}O_{14}P$.

Description:
Cyanocobalamin Co 60 Capsules USP—Capsules may contain a small, rectangular solid, or may appear empty.
Cyanocobalamin Co 60 Oral Solution USP—Clear, colorless to pink solution.

USP requirements:
Cyanocobalamin Co 60 Capsules USP—Preserve in well-closed, light-resistant containers. Contain Cyanocobalamin in which a portion of the molecules contain radioactive cobalt (^{60}Co) in the molecular structure. Label Capsules to include the following: the date of calibration; the amount of cyanocobalamin expressed in mcg per Capsule; the amount of ^{60}Co as cyanocobalamin expressed in megabecquerels (or microcuries) per Capsule on the date of calibration; the expiration date; and the statement, "Caution—Radioactive Material." The labeling indicates that in making dosage calculations, correction is to be made for radioactive decay, and also indicates that the radioactive half-life of ^{60}Co is 5.27 years. Contain the labeled amount of ^{60}Co, within ±10%, as cyanocobalamin expressed in megabecquerels (or microcuries) on the date indicated in the labeling. Contain the labeled amount of cyanocobalamin, within ±10%. The specific activity is not less than 0.02 megabecquerel (0.5 microcurie) per mcg of cyanocobalamin. Meet the requirements for Radionuclide identification, Uniformity of dosage units, and Cyanocobalamin content.
Cyanocobalamin Co 60 Oral Solution USP—Preserve in single-dose or in multiple-dose containers, protected from light. A solution suitable for oral administration, containing Cyanocobalamin in which a portion of the molecules contain radioactive cobalt (^{60}Co) in the molecular structure. Label it to include the following: the date of calibration; the amount of ^{60}Co as cyanocobalamin expressed as total megabecquerels (or microcuries) and as megabecquerels (or microcuries) per mL on the date of calibration; the amount of cyanocobalamin expressed in mcg per mL; the name and quantity of the added preservative; the expiration date; and the statement, "Caution—Radioactive Material." The labeling indicates that in making dosage calculations, correction is to be made for radioactive decay, and also indicates that the radioactive half-life of ^{60}Co is 5.27 years. Contains the labeled amount of ^{60}Co, within ±10%, as cyanocobalamin expressed in megabecquerels (or microcuries) per mL on the date indicated in the labeling. Contains the labeled amount of cyanocobalamin per mL, within ±10%. The amount of cobalt 60 as cyanocobalamin is not more than 0.04 megabecquerel (1 microcurie) per mL. The specific activity is not less than 0.02 megabecquerel (0.5 microcurie) per mcg of cyanocobalamin. Contains a suitable antimicrobial agent. Meets the requirements for Radionuclide identification, pH (4.0–5.5), Radiochemical purity, and Cyanocobalamin content.

CYCLACILLIN

Chemical name: 4-Thia-1-azabicyclo[3.2.0]heptane-2-carboxylic acid, 6-[[(1-aminocyclohexyl)carbonyl]amino]-3,3-dimethyl-7-oxo-, [2S-(2 alpha,5 alpha,6 beta)]-.

Molecular formula: $C_{15}H_{23}N_3O_4S$.

Molecular weight: 341.42.

Description: White, crystalline, anhydrous powder.

Solubility: Sparingly soluble in water.

USP requirements:
Cyclacillin USP—Preserve in tight containers. Contains not less than 90.0% of cyclacillin, calculated on the anhydrous basis. Has a potency of not less than 900 mcg and not more than 1050 mcg of cyclacillin per mg. Meets the requirements for Identification, Crystallinity, pH (4.0–6.5, in a solution containing 10 mg per mL), Water (not more than 1.0%), Concordance (not more than 6.0%), and Content of cyclacillin.
Cyclacillin for Oral Suspension USP—Preserve in tight containers. A dry mixture of Cyclacillin with one or more suitable buffers, colors, flavors, preservatives, sweeteners, and suspending agents. Contains the labeled amount, within −10% to +20%. Meets the requirements for Identification, Uniformity of dosage units (solid packaged in single-unit containers), Deliverable volume (multiple-unit containers), pH (4.5–6.5, in the suspension constituted as directed in the labeling), and Water (not more than 1.5%).
Cyclacillin Tablets USP—Preserve in tight containers. Contain the labeled amount, within −10% to +20%. Meet the requirements for Identification, Dissolution (75% in 45 minutes in water in Apparatus 2 at 50 rpm), and Water (not more than 5.0%).

CYCLANDELATE

Chemical name: 3,3,5-Trimethylcyclohexanol alpha-phenyl-alpha-hydroxyacetate.

Molecular formula: $C_{17}H_{24}O_3$.

Molecular weight: 276.37.

Description: White, amorphous powder having a faint menthol-like odor.

Solubility: Slightly soluble in water; highly soluble in ethyl alcohol and organic solvents.

USP requirements:
Cyclandelate Capsules—Not in USP.
Cyclandelate Tablets—Not in USP.

CYCLIZINE

Chemical group: Piperazine-derivative antihistamine.

Chemical name:
Cyclizine—Piperazine, 1-(diphenylmethyl)-4-methyl-.
Cyclizine hydrochloride—Piperazine, 1-(diphenylmethyl)-4-methyl-, monohydrochloride.
Cyclizine lactate—Piperazine, 1-(diphenylmethyl)-4-methyl-, mono(2-hydroxypropanoate).

Molecular formula:
Cyclizine—$C_{18}H_{22}N_2$.
Cyclizine hydrochloride—$C_{18}H_{22}N_2 \cdot HCl$.
Cyclizine lactate—$C_{18}H_{22}N_2 \cdot C_3H_6O_3$.

Molecular weight:
Cyclizine—266.39.
Cyclizine hydrochloride—302.85.
Cyclizine lactate—356.46.

Description:
Cyclizine USP—White, or creamy white, crystalline, practically odorless powder.
Cyclizine Hydrochloride USP—White, crystalline powder or small, colorless crystals. Is odorless or nearly so. Melts indistinctly at about 285 °C, with decomposition.

pka: 7.7.

Solubility:

Cyclizine USP—Slightly soluble in water; soluble in alcohol and in chloroform.

Cyclizine Hydrochloride USP—Slightly soluble in water and in alcohol; sparingly soluble in chloroform; insoluble in ether.

USP requirements:

Cyclizine USP—Preserve in tight, light-resistant containers. Contains not less than 98.0% and not more than 100.5% of cyclizine, calculated on the anhydrous basis. Meets the requirements for Clarity and color of solution, Identification, Melting range (106–109 °C), pH (7.6–8.6, in a saturated solution), Water (not more than 1.0%), Residue on ignition (not more than 0.1%), Chloride (not more than 0.014%), Ordinary impurities, and Organic volatile impurities.

Cyclizine Hydrochloride USP—Preserve in tight, light-resistant containers. Contains not less than 98.0% and not more than 100.5% of cyclizine hydrochloride, calculated on the dried basis. Meets the requirements for Identification, pH (4.5–5.5, determined potentiometrically in a 1 in 50 solution), Loss on drying (not more than 1.0%), Residue on ignition (not more than 0.2%), and Ordinary impurities.

Cyclizine Hydrochloride Tablets USP—Preserve in tight, light-resistant containers. Contain the labeled amount, within ±7%. Meet the requirements for Identification, Dissolution (75% in 45 minutes in water in Apparatus 2 at 50 rpm), and Uniformity of dosage units.

Cyclizine Lactate Injection USP—Preserve in single-dose containers, preferably of Type I glass, protected from light. A sterile solution of cyclizine lactate in Water for Injection, prepared from Cyclizine with the aid of Lactic Acid. Contains the labeled amount, within ±5%. Meets the requirements for Identification, pH (3.2–4.7), and Injections.

CYCLOBENZAPRINE

Chemical name: Cyclobenzaprine hydrochloride—1-Propanamine, 3-(5H-dibenzo[a,d]cyclohepten-5-ylidene)-N,N-dimethyl-, hydrochloride.

Molecular formula: Cyclobenzaprine hydrochloride—$C_{20}H_{21}N \cdot HCl$.

Molecular weight: Cyclobenzaprine hydrochloride—311.85.

Description: Cyclobenzaprine Hydrochloride USP—White to off-white, odorless, crystalline powder.

pKa: 8.47 (25 °C).

Solubility: Cyclobenzaprine Hydrochloride USP—Freely soluble in water, in alcohol, and in methanol; sparingly soluble in isopropanol; slightly soluble in chloroform and in methylene chloride; insoluble in hydrocarbons.

USP requirements:

Cyclobenzaprine Hydrochloride USP—Preserve in well-closed containers. Contains not less than 99.0% and not more than 101.0% of cyclobenzaprine hydrochloride, calculated on the dried basis. Meets the requirements for Identification, Melting range (215–219 °C, not more than 2 °C range between beginning and end of melting), Loss on drying (not more than 1.0%), Residue on ignition (not more than 0.1%), Heavy metals (not more than 0.001%), and Chromatographic purity.

Cyclobenzaprine Hydrochloride Tablets USP—Preserve in well-closed containers. Contain the labeled amount, within ±10%. Meet the requirements for Identification, Dissolution (75% in 30 minutes in 0.1 N hydrochloric acid

in Apparatus 1 at 50 rpm), and Uniformity of dosage units.

CYCLOMETHICONE

Chemical name: Cyclopolydimethylsiloxane.

Molecular formula: $(C_2H_6OSi)_n$.

Description: Cyclomethicone NF—NF category: Water repelling agent.

NF requirements: Cyclomethicone NF—Preserve in tight containers. A fully methylated cyclic siloxane containing repeating units of the formula $[-(CH_3)_2SiO-]_n$, in which n is 4, 5, or 6, or a mixture of them. Label it to state, as part of the official title, the n-value of the Cyclomethicone. Where it is a mixture of 2 or 3 such cyclic siloxanes, the label states the n-value and percentage of each in the mixture. Contains not less than 98.0% of cyclomethicone, calculated as the sum of cyclomethicone 4, cyclomethicone 5, and cyclomethicone 6, and not less than 95.0% and not more than 105.0% of the labeled amount of any one or more of the individual cyclomethicone components. Meets the requirements for Identification and Nonvolatile residue (not more than 0.15% [w/w]).

CYCLOPENTOLATE

Chemical name: Cyclopentolate hydrochloride—Benzeneacetic acid, alpha-(1-hydroxycyclopentyl)-, 2-(dimethylamino)ethyl ester, hydrochloride.

Molecular formula: Cyclopentolate hydrochloride—$C_{17}H_{25}NO_3 \cdot HCl$.

Molecular weight: Cyclopentolate hydrochloride—327.85.

Description: Cyclopentolate Hydrochloride USP—White, crystalline powder, which upon standing develops a characteristic odor. Its solutions are acid to litmus. Melts at about 138 °C, the melt appearing opaque.

Solubility: Cyclopentolate Hydrochloride USP—Very soluble in water; freely soluble in alcohol; insoluble in ether.

USP requirements:

Cyclopentolate Hydrochloride USP—Preserve in tight containers, and store in a cold place. Contains not less than 98.0% and not more than 100.5% of cyclopentolate hydrochloride, calculated on the dried basis. Meets the requirements for Identification, pH (4.5–5.5, in a solution [1 in 100]), Loss on drying (not more than 0.5%), Residue on ignition (not more than 0.05%), and Chromatographic purity.

Cyclopentolate Hydrochloride Ophthalmic Solution USP—Preserve in tight containers, and store at controlled room temperature. A sterile, aqueous solution of Cyclopentolate Hydrochloride. Contains the labeled amount, within ±10%. Meets the requirements for Identification, Sterility, and pH (3.0–5.5).

CYCLOPHOSPHAMIDE

Chemical name: 2H-1,3,2-Oxazaphosphorin-2-amine, N,N-bis(2-chloroethyl)tetrahydro-, 2-oxide, monohydrate.

Molecular formula: $C_7H_{15}Cl_2N_2O_2P \cdot H_2O$.

Molecular weight: 279.10.

Description: Cyclophosphamide USP—White, crystalline powder. Liquefies upon loss of its water of crystallization.

Solubility: Cyclophosphamide USP—Soluble in water and in alcohol.

USP requirements:

Cyclophosphamide USP—Preserve in tight containers, at a temperature between 2 and 30 °C. Contains not less than 97.0% and not more than 103.0% of cyclophosphamide, calculated on the anhydrous basis. Meets the requirements for Identification, pH (3.9–7.1, in a solution [1 in 100]), Water (5.7–6.8%), and Heavy metals (not more than 0.002%).

Caution: Great care should be taken in handling Cyclophosphamide, as it is a potent cytotoxic agent.

Cyclophosphamide for Injection USP—Preserve in Containers for Sterile Solids. Storage at a temperature not exceeding 25 °C is recommended. It will withstand brief exposure to temperatures up to 30 °C, but is to be protected from temperatures above 30 °C. A sterile mixture of Cyclophosphamide with or without a suitable diluent. Contains an amount of cyclophosphamide equivalent to the labeled amount of anhydrous cyclophosphamide, within ±10%. Meets the requirements for Constituted solution, Identification, Bacterial endotoxins, and pH (3.0–7.5), and for Sterility tests, Uniformity of dosage units, and Labeling under Injections.

Cyclophosphamide Oral Solution—Not in USP.

Cyclophosphamide Tablets USP—Preserve in tight containers. Storage at a temperature not exceeding 25 °C is recommended. Tablets will withstand brief exposure to temperatures up to 30 °C, but are to be protected from temperatures above 30 °C. Contain an amount of cyclophosphamide equivalent to the labeled amount of anhydrous cyclophosphamide, within ±10%. Meet the requirements for Identification, Disintegration (30 minutes, determined as directed under Uncoated Tablets), and Uniformity of dosage units.

CYCLOPROPANE

Chemical name: Cyclopropane.

Molecular formula: C_3H_6.

Molecular weight: 42.08.

Description: Cyclopropane USP—Colorless gas having a characteristic odor. One liter at a pressure of 760 millimeters and a temperature of 0 °C weighs about 1.88 grams.

Solubility: Cyclopropane USP—One volume dissolves in about 2.7 volumes of water at 15 °C. Freely soluble in alcohol; soluble in fixed oils.

USP requirements: Cyclopropane USP—Preserve in cylinders. The label bears a warning that cyclopropane is highly flammable and is not to be used where it may be ignited. Contains not less than 99.0%, by volume, of cyclopropane. Meets the requirements for Acidity or alkalinity, Carbon dioxide (not more than 0.03%), Halogens (not more than 0.02% as chloride), and Propylene, allene, and other unsaturated hydrocarbons.

Caution: Cyclopropane is highly flammable. Do not use where it may be ignited.

CYCLOSERINE

Source: Produced by a strain of *Streptomyces orchidaceus*; has also been synthesized.

Chemical name: 3-Isoxazolidinone, 4-amino-, (R)-.

Molecular formula: $C_3H_6N_2O_2$.

Molecular weight: 102.09.

Description: Cycloserine USP—White to pale yellow, crystalline powder. Is odorless or has a faint odor. Is hygroscopic and deteriorates upon absorbing water. Its solutions are dextrorotatory.

Solubility: Cycloserine USP—Freely soluble in water.

Other characteristics: Stable in alkaline solution, but rapidly destroyed at neutral or acid pH.

USP requirements:

Cycloserine USP—Preserve in tight containers. Has a potency of not less than 900 mcg of cycloserine per mg. Meets the requirements for Identification, Crystallinity, pH (5.5–6.5, in a solution [1 in 10]), Loss on drying (not more than 1.0%), Residue on ignition (not more than 0.5%), and Condensation products (not more than 0.80).

Cycloserine Capsules USP—Preserve in tight containers. Contain the labeled amount, within −10% to +20%. Meet the requirements for Identification, Dissolution (75% in 45 minutes in water in Apparatus 1 at 100 rpm), Uniformity of dosage units, and Loss on drying (not more than 1.0%).

CYCLOSPORINE

Chemical name: Cyclosporin A.

Molecular formula: $C_{62}H_{111}N_{11}O_{12}$.

Molecular weight: 1202.63.

Description: White or off-white finely crystalline powder with a weak characteristic odor.

Solubility: Soluble in methanol, in ethanol, in acetone, in ether, and in chloroform; slightly soluble in water and in saturated hydrocarbons.

Other characteristics: Lipophilic; hydrophobic.

USP requirements:

Cyclosporine USP—Preserve in tight, light-resistant containers. Contains not less than 975 mcg and not more than 1020 mcg of cyclosporine per mg, calculated on the dried basis. Meets the requirements for Identification, Loss on drying (not more than 2.0%), and Heavy metals (not more than 0.002%).

Cyclosporine Capsules—Not in USP.

Cyclosporine Concentrate for Injection USP—Preserve in single-dose or in multiple-dose containers. A sterile solution of Cyclosporine in a suitable vehicle. Label it to indicate that it is to be diluted with a suitable parenteral vehicle prior to intravenous infusion. Contains the labeled amount, within ±10%. Meets the requirements for Identification, Bacterial endotoxins, Sterility, and Alcohol content (where present, the labeled amount, within ±20%).

Cyclosporine Oral Solution USP—Preserve in tight containers. A solution of Cyclosporine in a suitable vehicle. Contains the labeled amount, within ±10%. Meets the requirements for Identification and Alcohol content (where present, the labeled amount, within ±20%).

CYCLOTHIAZIDE

Chemical name: 2H-1,2,4-Benzothiadiazine-7-sulfonamide, 3-bicyclo[2.2.1]hept-5-en-2-yl-6-chloro-3,4-dihydro-, 1,1-dioxide.

Molecular formula: $C_{14}H_{16}ClN_3O_4S_2$.

Molecular weight: 389.87.

Description: White, crystalline solid. It has a melting point of approximately 220 °C.

pKa: 10.7 in water.

Solubility: Moderately soluble in hot ethyl alcohol and in hot dilute alcohol; very soluble in cold ethyl acetate (an ethyl acetate solvate is formed); relatively insoluble in ether and in chloroform.

USP requirements:
Cyclothiazide USP—Preserve in well-closed containers. Contains not less than 98.0% and not more than 102.0% of cyclothiazide, calculated on the anhydrous basis. Meets the requirements for Identification, Melting range (217–225 °C, not more than 4 °C range between beginning and end of melting), Water (not more than 1.0%), Residue on ignition (not more than 0.2%), Selenium (0.003%), Diazotizable substances (not more than 1.0%), and Organic volatile substances.

Cyclothiazide Tablets USP—Preserve in well-closed containers. Contain the labeled amount, within ± 10%. Meet the requirements for Identification, Dissolution (70% in 60 minutes in water in Apparatus 2 at 50 rpm), and Uniformity of dosage units.

CYPROHEPTADINE

Chemical group: Piperidine derivative.

Chemical name: Cyproheptadine hydrochloride—Piperidine,4-(5H-dibenzo[a,d]-cyclohepten-5-ylidene)-1-methyl-, hydrochloride, sesquihydrate.

Molecular formula: Cyproheptadine hydrochloride—$C_{21}H_{21}N \cdot HCl \cdot 1\frac{1}{2}H_2O$.

Molecular weight: Cyproheptadine hydrochloride—350.89.

Description: Cyproheptadine Hydrochloride USP—White to slightly yellow, odorless or practically odorless, crystalline powder.

pKa: Cyproheptadine hydrochloride—9.3.

Solubility: Cyproheptadine Hydrochloride USP—Slightly soluble in water; freely soluble in methanol; soluble in chloroform; sparingly soluble in alcohol; practically insoluble in ether.

USP requirements:
Cyproheptadine Hydrochloride USP—Preserve in well-closed containers. Previously dried, contains not less than 98.5% and not more than 100.5% of cyproheptadine hydrochloride. Meets the requirements for Identification, Acidity, Loss on drying (7.0–9.0%), Residue on ignition (not more than 0.1%), Heavy metals (not more than 0.003%), and Organic volatile impurities.

Cyproheptadine Hydrochloride Syrup USP—Preserve in tight containers. Contains the labeled amount, within ± 10%. Meets the requirements for Identification and pH (3.5–4.5).

Cyproheptadine Hydrochloride Tablets USP—Preserve in well-closed containers. Contain the labeled amount, within ± 10%. Meet the requirements for Identification, Dissolution (80% in 30 minutes in 0.1 N hydrochloric acid in Apparatus 2 at 50 rpm), and Uniformity of dosage units.

CYSTEINE

Chemical name: Cysteine hydrochloride—L-Cysteine hydrochloride monohydrate.

Molecular formula: Cysteine hydrochloride—$C_3H_7NO_2S \cdot HCl \cdot H_2O$.

Molecular weight: Cysteine hydrochloride—175.63.

Description: Cysteine Hydrochloride USP—White crystals or crystalline powder.

Solubility: Cysteine Hydrochloride USP—Soluble in water, in alcohol, and in acetone.

USP requirements:
Cysteine Hydrochloride USP—Preserve in well-closed containers. Contains not less than 98.5% and not more than 101.5% of cysteine hydrochloride, as L-cysteine hydrochloride, calculated on the dried basis. Meets the requirements for Identification, Specific rotation (+5.7° to +6.8°, calculated on the dried basis), Loss on drying (8.0–12.0%), Residue on ignition (not more than 0.4%), Sulfate (not more than 0.03%), Arsenic (not more than 1.5 ppm), Iron (0.003%), Heavy metals (not more than 0.0015%), Chloride content (19.8–20.8%), and Organic volatile impurities.

Cysteine Hydrochloride Injection USP—Preserve in single-dose or in multiple-dose containers, preferably of Type I glass. A sterile solution of Cysteine Hydrochloride in Water for Injection. Contains the labeled amount, within ± 15%. Meets the requirements for Identification, Bacterial endotoxins, pH (1.0–2.5), Heavy metals (not more than 2 ppm), and Injections.

CYTARABINE

Chemical name: 2(1H)-Pyrimidinone, 4-amino-1-beta-D-arabinofuranosyl-.

Molecular formula: $C_9H_{13}N_3O_5$.

Molecular weight: 243.22.

Description: Cytarabine USP—Odorless, white to off-white, crystalline powder.

pKa: 4.35 in 60% aqueous ethanol.

Solubility: Cytarabine USP—Freely soluble in water; slightly soluble in alcohol and in chloroform.

USP requirements:
Cytarabine USP—Preserve in well-closed, light-resistant containers. Contains not less than 95.0% and not more than 105.0% of cytarabine, calculated on the dried basis. Meets the requirements for Identification, Specific rotation (+154° to +160°, calculated on the dried basis), Loss on drying (not more than 1.0%), Residue on ignition (not more than 0.5%), Heavy metals (not more than 0.001%), and Related substances (not more than 0.5%).

Sterile Cytarabine USP—Preserve in Containers for Sterile Solids. It is Cytarabine suitable for parenteral use. Contains the labeled amount, within ± 10%. Meets the requirements for Constituted solution, Identification, pH (4.0–6.0, in a solution containing the equivalent of 10 mg of cytarabine per mL), Water (not more than 3.0%), and Bacterial endotoxins, and for Sterility tests, Uniformity of dosage units, and Labeling under Injections. The drug substance in the vial meets the requirements for Cytarabine.

DACARBAZINE

Chemical name: 1H-Imidazole-4-carboxamide, 5-(3,3-dimethyl-1-triazenyl)-.

Molecular formula: $C_6H_{10}N_6O$.

Molecular weight: 182.18.

Description: Colorless to ivory colored solid which is light sensitive.

pKa: 4.42.

Solubility: Slightly soluble in water and in alcohol.

USP requirements:
Dacarbazine USP—Preserve in tight, light-resistant containers, in a refrigerator. Contains not less than 97.0% and not more than 102.0% of dacarbazine. Meets the requirements for Identification, Residue on ignition (not more than 0.1%), and Related compounds.

Caution: Great care should be taken in handling Dacarbazine, as it is a potent cytotoxic agent.

Dacarbazine for Injection USP—Preserve in single-dose or multiple-dose Containers for Sterile Solids, preferably of Type I glass, protected from light. A sterile, freeze-dried mixture of Dacarbazine and suitable buffers or diluents. Contains the labeled amount, within ± 10%. Meets the requirements for Completeness of solution, Constituted solution, Identification, Pyrogen, pH (3.0–4.0), Water (not more than 1.5%), and 2-Azahypoxanthine (not more than 1.0%), and for Sterility tests, Uniformity of dosage units, and Labeling under Injections.

Caution: Great care should be taken to prevent inhaling particles of Dacarbazine for Injection and exposing the skin to it.

DACTINOMYCIN

Source: An actinomycin derived from a mixture of actinomycins produced by *Streptomyces parvullus*.

Chemical name: Actinomycin D. Specific stereoisomer of N,N′-[(2-amino-4,6-dimethyl-3-oxo-3H-phenoxazine-1,9-diyl)bis-[carbonylimino(2-hydroxypropylidene)carbonyliminoisobutylidenecarbonyl-1,2-pyrrolidinediylcarbonyl(methylimino)methylenecarbonyl]]bis[N-methyl-L-valine] dilactone.

Molecular formula: $C_{62}H_{86}N_{12}O_{16}$.

Molecular weight: 1255.43.

Description: Dactinomycin USP—Bright red, crystalline powder. Is somewhat hygroscopic and is affected by light and heat.

Solubility: Dactinomycin USP—Soluble in water at 10 °C and slightly soluble in water at 37 °C; freely soluble in alcohol; very slightly soluble in ether.

USP requirements:
Dactinomycin USP—Preserve in tight containers, protected from light and excessive heat. Contains not less than 950 mcg and not more than 1030 mcg of dactinomycin per mg, calculated on the dried basis. Meets the requirements for Identification, Specific rotation (−292° to −317°, calculated on the dried basis), Crystallinity, Bacterial endotoxins, and Loss on drying (not more than 5.0%).

Caution: Great care should be taken to prevent inhaling particles of Dactinomycin and exposing the skin to it.

Dactinomycin for Injection USP—Preserve in light-resistant Containers for Sterile Solids. A sterile mixture of Dactinomycin and Mannitol. Label it to include the statement, "Protect from light." Contains the labeled amount, within −10% to +20%, the labeled amount being 0.5 mg in each container. Meets the requirements for Constituted solution, Identification, Bacterial endotoxins, Sterility, pH (5.5–7.5, in the solution constituted as directed in the labeling), Loss on drying (not more than 4.0%), and Injections.

Caution: Great care should be taken to prevent inhaling particles of Dactinomycin and exposing the skin to it.

DANAZOL

Chemical name: Pregna-2,4-dien-20-yno[2,3-d]isoxazol-17-ol,(17 alpha)-.

Molecular formula: $C_{22}H_{27}NO_2$.

Molecular weight: 337.46.

Description: Danazol USP—White to pale yellow, crystalline powder. Melts at about 225 °C, with some decomposition.

Solubility: Danazol USP—Practically insoluble or insoluble in water and in hexane; freely soluble in chloroform; soluble in acetone; sparingly soluble in alcohol; slightly soluble in ether.

USP requirements:
Danazol USP—Preserve in tight, light-resistant containers. Contains not less than 97.0% and not more than 102.0% of danazol, calculated on the dried basis. Meets the requirements for Identification, Specific rotation (+21° to +27°, calculated on the dried basis), Loss on drying (not more than 2.0%), Chromatogrpahic impurities, and Organic volatile impurities.

Danazol Capsules USP—Preserve in well-closed containers. Contain the labeled amount, within ± 10%. Meet the requirements for Identification, Dissolution (65% in 30 minutes in isopropyl alcohol in 0.1 N hydrochloric acid [4 in 10] in Apparatus 2 at 80 rpm), and Uniformity of dosage units.

DANTHRON AND DOCUSATE

Chemical group:
Danthron—Anthraquinones.
Docusate—Surfactants, anionic.

Chemical name:
Danthron—9,10-Anthracenedione, 1,8-dihydroxy-.
Docusate sodium—Butanedioic acid, sulfo-, 1,4-bis(2-ethylhexyl) ester, sodium salt.

Molecular formula:
Danthron—$C_{14}H_8O_4$.
Docusate sodium—$C_{20}H_{37}NaO_7S$.

Molecular weight:
Danthron—240.21.
Docusate sodium—444.56.

Description:
Danthron—Orange, odorless or almost odorless, crystalline powder.
Docusate Sodium USP—White, wax-like, plastic solid, having a characteristic odor suggestive of octyl alcohol, but no odor of other solvents.

NF category: Wetting and/or solubilizing agent.

Solubility:
Danthron—Practically insoluble in water; very slightly soluble in alcohol; soluble in chloroform and in hot glacial acetic acid; slightly soluble in ether; dissolves in solutions of alkali hydroxides.
Docusate Sodium USP—Sparingly soluble in water; very soluble in solvent hexane; freely soluble in alcohol and in glycerin.

USP requirements:
Danthron and Docusate Sodium Capsules—Not in USP.
Danthron and Docusate Sodium Tablets—Not in USP.

DANTROLENE

Chemical name: Dantrolene sodium—2,4-Imidazolidinedione, 1-[[[5-(4-nitrophenyl)-2-furanyl]methylene]amino]-, sodium salt, hydrate (2:7).

Molecular formula: Dantrolene sodium—$C_{14}H_9N_4NaO_5 \cdot 3\frac{1}{2}$-$H_2O$.

Molecular weight: Dantrolene sodium—399.29.

Description: Dantrolene sodium—Orange powder.

Solubility: Dantrolene sodium—Slightly soluble in water, but due to its slightly acidic nature the solubility increases somewhat in alkaline solution.

USP requirements:
Dantrolene Sodium Capsules—Not in USP.
Dantrolene Sodium for Injection—Not in USP.

DAPIPRAZOLE

Chemical name: Dapiprazole hydrochloride—1,2,4-Triazolo[4,3-*a*]pyridine, 5,6,7,8-tetrahydro-3-[2-[4-(2-methylphenyl)-1-piperazinyl]ethyl]-, monohydrochloride.

Molecular formula: Dapiprazole hydrochloride—$C_{19}H_{27}N_5 \cdot HCl$.

Molecular weight: Dapiprazole hydrochloride—361.92.

Description: Dapiprazole hydrochloride—Sterile, white, lyophilized powder.

Solubility: Dapiprazole hydrochloride—Soluble in water.

USP requirements: Dapiprazole Hydrochloride Powder for Topical Solution—Not in USP.

DAPSONE

Chemical group: Sulfone.

Chemical name: Benzenamine, 4,4′-sulfonylbis-.

Molecular formula: $C_{12}H_{12}N_2O_2S$.

Molecular weight: 248.30.

Description: Dapsone USP—White or creamy white, crystalline powder. Is odorless.

Solubility: Dapsone USP—Very slightly soluble in water; freely soluble in alcohol; soluble in acetone and in dilute mineral acids.

USP requirements:
Dapsone USP—Preserve in well-closed, light-resistant containers. Contains not less than 99.0% and not more than 101.0% of dapsone, calculated on the dried basis. Meets the requirements for Identification, Melting range (175–181 °C), Loss on drying (not more than 1.5%), Residue on ignition (not more than 0.1%), Selenium (0.003%), Chromatographic purity, and Organic volatile impurities.
Dapsone Tablets USP—Preserve in well-closed, light-resistant containers. Contain the labeled amount, within ±7.5%. Meet the requirements for Identification, Dissolution (75% in 60 minutes in dilute hydrochloric acid [2 in 100] in Apparatus 1 at 100 rpm), and Uniformity of dosage units.

DAUNORUBICIN

Source: An anthracycline glycoside obtained from *Streptomyces peucetius*.

Chemical name: Daunorubicin hydrochloride—5,12-Naphthacenedione, 8-acetyl-10-[(3-amino-2,3,6-trideoxy-alpha-L-*lyxo*-hexopyranosyl)]oxy]-7,8,9,10-tetrahydro-6,8,11-trihydroxy-1-methoxy-, (8*S-cis*)-, hydrochloride.

Molecular formula: Daunorubicin hydrochloride—$C_{27}H_{29}$-$NO_{10} \cdot HCl$.

Molecular weight: Daunorubicin hydrochloride—563.99.

Description: Daunorubicin Hydrochloride USP—Orange-red, crystalline, hygroscopic powder.

pKa: 10.3.

Solubility: Daunorubicin Hydrochloride USP—Freely soluble in water and in methanol; slightly soluble in alcohol; very slightly soluble in chloroform; practically insoluble in acetone.

USP requirements:
Daunorubicin Hydrochloride USP—Preserve in tight containers, protected from light and excessive heat. Has a potency equivalent to not less than 842 mcg and not more than 1030 mcg of daunorubicin per mg. Meets the requirements for Identification, Crystallinity, pH (4.5–6.5, in a solution containing 5 mg per mL), and Water (not more than 3.0%).
  Caution: Great care should be taken to prevent inhaling particles of daunorubicin hydrochloride and exposing the skin to it.
Daunorubicin Hydrochloride for Injection USP—Preserve in light-resistant Containers for Sterile Solids. A sterile mixture of Daunorubicin Hydrochloride and Mannitol. Contains an amount of daunorubicin hydrochloride equivalent to the labeled amount of daunorubicin, within −10% to +15%. Meets the requirements for Constituted solution, Identification, Depressor substances, Pyrogen, pH (4.5–6.5, in the solution constituted as directed in the labeling), Water (not more than 3.0%), and Injections.

DEFEROXAMINE

Source: Isolated as the iron chelate from *Streptomyces pilosus* and treated chemically to obtain the metal-free ligand.

Chemical name: Deferoxamine mesylate—Butanediamide, *N′*-[5-[[4-[[5-(acetylhydroxyamino)pentyl]amino]-1,4-dioxobutyl]-hydroxyamino]pentyl]-*N*-(5-aminopentyl)-*N*-hydroxy-, monomethanesulfonate.

Molecular formula: Deferoxamine mesylate—$C_{25}H_{48}N_6O_8 \cdot CH_4O_3S$.

Molecular weight: Deferoxamine mesylate—656.79.

Description: Deferoxamine Mesylate USP—White to off-white powder.

Solubility: Deferoxamine Mesylate USP—Freely soluble in water; slightly soluble in methanol.

USP requirements:
Deferoxamine Mesylate USP—Preserve in tight containers. Contains not less than 98.0% and not more than 102.0% of deferoxamine mesylate, calculated on the anhydrous basis. Meets the requirements for Identification, pH (4.0–6.0, in a solution [1 in 100]), Water (not more than 2.0%), Residue on ignition (not more than 0.1%), Chloride (not more than 0.012%), Sulfate (not more than 0.04%), and Heavy metals (not more than 0.001%).
Sterile Deferoxamine Mesylate USP—Preserve in single-dose or in multiple-dose containers, preferably of Type I glass. It is Deferoxamine Mesylate suitable for parenteral use. Contains the labeled amount, within ±10%. Meets the requirements for Constituted solution, Identification, pH (4.0–6.0, in a solution [1 in 100]), Bacterial endotoxins, Water (not more than 1.5%), Injections, and Uniformity of dosage units.

DEHYDROACETIC ACID

Chemical name: 2*H*-Pyran-2,4(3*H*)-dione, 3-acetyl-6-methyl-.

Molecular formula: $C_8H_8O_4$.

Molecular weight: 168.15.

Description: Dehydroacetic Acid NF—White or nearly white, crystalline powder. Odorless or practically odorless.
  NF category: Antimicrobial preservative.

Solubility: Dehydroacetic Acid NF—Very slightly soluble in water, freely soluble in acetone; soluble in aqueous solutions of fixed alkalies; sparingly soluble in alcohol.

NF requirements: Dehydroacetic Acid NF—Preserve in well-closed containers. Contains not less than 98.0% and not more than 100.5% of dehydroacetic acid, calculated on the anhydrous basis. Meets the requirements for Identification, Melting range (109–111 °C), Water (not more than 1.0%), Residue on ignition (not more than 0.1%), Arsenic (not more than 3 ppm), Heavy metals (not more than 0.001%), and Organic volatile impurities.

DEHYDROCHOLIC ACID

Source: Oxidized bile acid produced from the main constituent of ox bile, cholic acid.

Chemical name: Cholan-24-oic acid, 3,7,12-trioxo-, (5 beta)-.

Molecular formula: $C_{24}H_{34}O_5$.

Molecular weight: 402.53.

Description: Dehydrocholic Acid USP—White, fluffy, odorless powder.

Solubility: Dehydrocholic Acid USP—Practically insoluble in water; soluble in glacial acetic acid and in solutions of alkali hydroxides and carbonates; slightly soluble in alcohol and in ether; sparingly soluble in chloroform (the solutions in alcohol and in chloroform usually are slightly turbid).

USP requirements:
  Dehydrocholic Acid USP—Preserve in well-closed containers. Contains not less than 98.5% and not more than 101.0% of dehydrocholic acid, calculated on the dried basis. Dehydrocholic Acid for parenteral use melts between 237 and 242 °C. Meets the requirements for Identification, Melting range (231–242 °C, not more than 3 °C between beginning and end of melting), Specific rotation (+29.0° to +32.5°, calculated on the dried basis), Microbial limit, Loss on drying (not more than 1.0%), Residue on ignition (not more than 0.3%), Odor on boiling, Barium, Heavy metals (not more than 0.002%), and Organic volatile impurities.
  Dehydrocholic Acid Tablets USP—Preserve in well-closed containers. Contain the labeled amount, within ±6%. Meet the requirements for Identification, Microbial limit, Disintegration (30 minutes), and Uniformity of dosage units.

DEHYDROCHOLIC ACID AND DOCUSATE

For *Dehydrocholic Acid* and *Docusate*—See individual listings for chemistry information.

USP requirements:
  Dehydrocholic Acid and Docusate Sodium Capsules—Not in USP.

Dehydrocholic Acid and Docusate Sodium Tablets—Not in USP.

DEHYDROCHOLIC ACID, DOCUSATE, AND PHENOLPHTHALEIN

For *Dehydrocholic Acid, Docusate,* and *Phenolphthalein*—See individual listings for chemistry information.

USP requirements: Dehydrocholic Acid, Docusate Sodium, and Phenolphthalein Capsules—Not in USP.

DEMECARIUM

Chemical name: Demecarium bromide—Benzenaminium, 3,3′-[1,10-decanediylbis[(methylimino)carbonyloxy]]bis[*N,N,N*-trimethyl-, dibromide.

Molecular formula: Demecarium bromide—$C_{32}H_{52}Br_2N_4O_4$.

Molecular weight: Demecarium bromide—716.60.

Description: Demecarium Bromide USP—White or slightly yellow, slightly hygroscopic, crystalline powder.

Solubility: Demecarium Bromide USP—Freely soluble in water and in alcohol; soluble in ether; sparingly soluble in acetone.

USP requirements:
  Demecarium Bromide USP—Preserve in tight, light-resistant containers. Contains not less than 95.0% and not more than 100.5% of demecarium bromide, calculated on the anhydrous basis. Meets the requirements for Identification, pH (5.0–7.0, in a solution [1 in 100]), Water (not more than 2.0%), Residue on ignition (not more than 0.1%), Heavy metals (not more than 0.002%), and *m*-Trimethylammoniophenol bromide.
  Demecarium Bromide Ophthalmic Solution USP—Preserve in tight, light-resistant containers. A sterile, aqueous solution of Demecarium Bromide. Contains the labeled amount, within ±8%. Contains a suitable antimicrobial agent. Meets the requirements for Identification and Sterility.

DEMECLOCYCLINE

Chemical name:
  Demeclocycline—2-Naphthacenecarboxamide, 7-chloro-4-(dimethylamino)-1,4,4a,5,5a,6,11,12a-octahydro-3,6,10,12,12a-pentahydroxy-1,11-dioxo-, [4*S*-(4 alpha,4a alpha,5a alpha,6 beta,12a alpha)]-.
  Demeclocycline hydrochloride—2-Naphthacenecarboxamide, 7-chloro-4-(dimethylamino)-1,4,4a,5,5a,6,11,12a-octahydro-3,6,10,12,12a-pentahydroxy-1,11-dioxo-, monohydrochloride, [4*S*-(4 alpha,4a alpha,5a alpha,6 beta,12a alpha)]-.

Molecular formula:
  Demeclocycline—$C_{21}H_{21}ClN_2O_8$.
  Demeclocycline hydrochloride—$C_{21}H_{21}ClN_2O_8 \cdot HCl$.

Molecular weight:
  Demeclocycline—464.86.
  Demeclocycline hydrochloride—501.32.

Description:
  Demeclocycline USP—Yellow, crystalline odorless powder.
  Demeclocycline Hydrochloride USP—Yellow, crystalline, odorless powder.

Solubility:
  Demeclocycline USP—Sparingly soluble in water; soluble in alcohol. Dissolves readily in 3 *N* hydrochloric acid and in alkaline solutions.

Demeclocycline Hydrochloride USP—Sparingly soluble in water and in solutions of alkali hydroxides and carbonates; slightly soluble in alcohol; practically insoluble in acetone and in chloroform.

USP requirements:

Demeclocycline USP—Preserve in tight, light-resistant containers. Has a potency equivalent to not less than 970 mcg of demeclocycline hydrochloride per mg, calculated on the anhydrous basis. Meets the requirements for Identification, Crystallinity, pH (4.0–5.5, in a solution containing 10 mg per mL), and Water (4.3–6.7%).

Demeclocycline Oral Suspension USP—Preserve in tight containers, protected from light. Contains an amount of demeclocycline equivalent to the labeled amount of demeclocycline hydrochloride, within −10% to +25%. Meets the requirement for pH (4.0–5.8).

Demeclocycline Hydrochloride USP—Preserve in tight, light-resistant containers. Has a potency of not less than 900 mcg of demeclocycline hydrochloride per mg, calculated on the dried basis. Meets the requirements for Identification, Crystallinity, pH (2.0–3.0, in a solution containing 10 mg per mL), and Loss on drying (not more than 2.0%).

Demeclocycline Hydrochloride Capsules USP—Preserve in tight, light-resistant containers. Contain the labeled amount, within −10% to +25%. Meet the requirements for Dissolution (75% in 45 minutes in water in Apparatus 2 at 75 rpm), Uniformity of dosage units, and Loss on drying (not more than 2.0%; not more than 8.0% if the Capsules contain starch).

Demeclocycline Hydrochloride Tablets USP—Preserve in tight, light-resistant containers. Contain the labeled amount, within −10% to +25%. Meet the requirements for Dissolution (75% in 45 minutes in water in Apparatus 2 at 75 rpm), Uniformity of dosage units, and Loss on drying (not more than 2.0%).

DEMECLOCYCLINE AND NYSTATIN

For *Demeclocycline* and *Nystatin*—See individual listings for chemistry information.

USP requirements:

Demeclocycline Hydrochloride and Nystatin Capsules USP—Preserve in tight, light-resistant containers. Contain the labeled amounts of demeclocycline hydrochloride, within −10% to +25%, and USP Nystatin Units, within −10% to +35%. Meet the requirements for Identification, Dissolution (75% of the labeled amount of demeclocycline hydrochloride in 45 minutes in water in Apparatus 2 at 75 rpm), and Loss on drying (not more than 5.0%).

Demeclocycline Hydrochloride and Nystatin Tablets USP—Preserve in tight, light-resistant containers. Contain the labeled amounts of demeclocycline hydrochloride, within −10% to +25%, and USP Nystatin Units, within −10% to +35%. Meet the requirements for Identification, Dissolution (75% of the labeled amount of demeclocycline hydrochloride in 45 minutes in water in Apparatus 2 at 75 rpm), and Loss on drying (not more than 4.0%).

DENATONIUM BENZOATE

Chemical name: Benzenemethanaminium, *N*-[2-[(2,6-dimethylphenyl)amino]-2-oxoethyl]-*N*,*N*-diethyl-, benzoate, monohydrate.

Molecular formula: $C_{28}H_{34}N_2O_3 \cdot H_2O$ (hydrous).

Molecular weight: 464.60 (hydrous); 446.59 (anhydrous).

Description: Denatonium Benzoate NF—NF category: Alcohol denaturant.

Solubility: Denatonium Benzoate NF—Freely soluble in water and in alcohol; very soluble in chloroform and in methanol; very slightly soluble in ether.

NF requirements: Denatonium Benzoate NF—Preserve in tight containers. Dried at 105 °C for 2 hours, contains one molecule of water of hydration, or is anhydrous. Label it to indicate whether it is hydrous or anhydrous. When dried at 105 °C for 2 hours, contains not less than 99.5% and not more than 101.0% of denatonium benzoate. Meets the requirements for Identification, Melting range (163–170 °C), pH (6.5–7.5, in a solution [3 in 100]), Loss on drying (not more than 1.0%), Residue on ignition (not more than 0.1%), and Chloride (not more than 0.2%).

DENTAL-TYPE SILICA

Description: Dental-Type Silica NF—Fine, white, hygroscopic, odorless, amorphous powder, in which the diameter of the average particle ranges between 0.5 micrometer and 40 micrometers.

NF category: Glidant and/or anticaking agent; suspending and/or viscosity-increasing agent.

Solubility: Dental-Type Silica NF—Insoluble in water, in alcohol, and in acid (except hydrofluoric acid); soluble in hot solutions of alkali hydroxides.

NF requirements: Dental-Type Silica NF—Preserve in tight containers. It is obtained from sodium silicate solution by destabilizing with acid in such a way as to yield very fine particles. The sum of the Assay value and the Sodium Sulfate content is not less than 98.0%. Label it to indicate the maximum percentage of Loss on drying. Meets the requirements for pH (4.0–8.5 in a slurry [1 in 20]), Loss on drying, and Sodium sulfate (not more than 4.0%), and for Loss on ignition, Chloride, Arsenic, and Heavy metals under Silicon Dioxide.

DESERPIDINE

Source: A pure alkaloid obtained from *Rauwolfia serpentina*.

Chemical name: Methyl 17 alpha-methoxy-18 beta-[(3,4,5-trimethoxybenzoyl)oxy]-3 beta,20 alpha-yohimban-16 beta-carboxylate.

Molecular formula: $C_{32}H_{38}N_2O_8$.

Molecular weight: 578.66.

Description: White to light yellow, crystalline powder.

pKa: 5.67.

Solubility: Insoluble in water; slightly soluble in alcohol.

USP requirements: Deserpidine Tablets—Not in USP.

DESERPIDINE AND HYDROCHLOROTHIAZIDE

For *Deserpidine* and *Hydrochlorothiazide*—See individual listings for chemistry information.

USP requirements: Deserpidine and Hydrochlorothiazide Tablets—Not in USP.

DESERPIDINE AND METHYCLOTHIAZIDE

For *Deserpidine* and *Methyclothiazide*—See individual listings for chemistry information.

USP requirements: Deserpidine and Methyclothiazide Tablets—Not in USP.

DESIPRAMINE

Chemical group: Dibenzazepine.

Chemical name: Desipramine hydrochloride—5*H*-Dibenz[*b*,*f*]-azepine-5-propanamine, 10,11-dihydro-*N*-methyl-, mono-hydrochloride.

Molecular formula: Desipramine hydrochloride—$C_{18}H_{22}N_2 \cdot$ HCl.

Molecular weight: Desipramine hydrochloride—302.85.

Description: Desipramine Hydrochloride USP—White to off-white, crystalline powder. Melts at about 213 °C.

pKa: 1.5 and 10.2.

Solubility: Desipramine Hydrochloride USP—Soluble in water and in alcohol; freely soluble in methanol and in chloroform; insoluble in ether.

Other characteristics: Secondary amine.

USP requirements:
Desipramine Hydrochloride USP—Preserve in tight containers. Dried in a vacuum at 105 °C for 2 hours, contains not less than 98.0% and not more than 100.5% of desipramine hydrochloride. Meets the requirements for Identification, Loss on drying (not more than 0.5%), Residue on ignition (not more than 0.1%), Heavy metals (not more than 0.001%), Iminodibenzyl, and Organic volatile impurities.
Desipramine Hydrochloride Capsules USP—Preserve in tight containers. Contain the labeled amount, within ±8%. Meet the requirements for Identification, Dissolution (75% in 45 minutes in water in Apparatus 1 at 100 rpm), and Uniformity of dosage units.
Desipramine Hydrochloride Tablets USP—Preserve in tight containers. Contain the labeled amount, within ±5%. Meet the requirements for Identification, Dissolution (75% in 60 minutes in 0.1 N hydrochloric acid in Apparatus 2 at 50 rpm), and Uniformity of dosage units.

DESLANOSIDE

Source: Obtained naturally from *Digitalis lanata* or may be produced synthetically.

Chemical name: Card-20(22)-enolide, 3-[(*O*-beta-D-glucopyra-nosyl-(1→4)-*O*-2,6-dideoxy-beta-D-*ribo*-hexopyranosyl-(1→4)-*O*-2,6-dideoxy-beta-D-*ribo*-hexopyranosyl-(1→4)-2,6-dideoxy-beta-D-*ribo*-hexopyranosyl)oxy]-12,14-dihydroxy-, (3 beta, 5 beta, 12 beta)-.

Molecular formula: $C_{47}H_{74}O_{19}$.

Molecular weight: 943.09.

Description: Odorless, hygroscopic, white crystals or crystalline powder.

Solubility: Practically insoluble in water, in chloroform, and in ether; very slightly soluble in alcohol and in methyl alcohol.

USP requirements:
Deslanoside USP—Preserve in tight, light-resistant containers. Contains not less than 95.0% and not more than 103.0% of deslanoside, calculated on the dried basis. Meets the requirements for Identification, Specific rotation (+7.0° to +8.5°, calculated on the dried basis), Loss on drying (not more than 5.0%), and Residue on ignition (not more than 0.2%).
Deslanoside Injection USP—Preserve in single-dose containers, preferably of Type I glass. A sterile solution of Deslanoside in a suitable solvent. Contains the labeled

amount, within ±10%. Meets the requirements for Identification, pH (5.5–7.0), and Injections.

DESMOPRESSIN

Source: Synthetic polypeptide structurally related to the posterior pituitary hormone arginine vasopressin (antidiuretic hormone).

Chemical name: Desmopressin acetate—Vasopressin, 1-(3-mercaptopropanoic acid)-8-D-arginine-, monoacetate (salt), trihydrate.

Molecular formula: Desmopressin acetate—$C_{48}H_{68}N_{14}O_{14}\text{-}S_2 \cdot 3H_2O$.

Molecular weight: Desmopressin acetate—1183.32.

USP requirements:
Desmopressin Acetate Injection—Not in USP.
Desmopressin Acetate Nasal Solution—Not in USP.

DESONIDE

Chemical name: Pregna-1,4-diene-3,20-dione, 11,21-dihydroxy-16,17-[(1-methylethylidene)bis(oxy)]-, (11 beta, 16 alpha)-.

Molecular formula: $C_{24}H_{32}O_6$.

Molecular weight: 416.51.

Description: Small plates of white to off-white, odorless powder.

USP requirements:
Desonide Cream—Not in USP.
Desonide Ointment—Not in USP.

DESONIDE AND ACETIC ACID

For *Desonide* and *Acetic Acid*—See individual listings for chemistry information.

USP requirements: Desonide and Acetic Acid Otic Solution—Not in USP.

DESOXIMETASONE

Chemical name: Pregna-1,4-diene-3,20-dione, 9-fluoro-11,21-dihydroxy-16-methyl-, (11 beta,16 alpha)-.

Molecular formula: $C_{22}H_{29}FO_4$.

Molecular weight: 376.47.

Description: Desoximetasone USP—White to practically white, odorless, crystalline powder.

Solubility: Desoximetasone USP—Insoluble in water; freely soluble in alcohol, in acetone, and in chloroform.

USP requirements:
Desoximetasone USP—Preserve in well-closed containers. Contains not less than 97.0% and not more than 103.0% of desoximetasone, calculated on the dried basis. Meets the requirements for Identification, Melting range (206–218 °C, not more than 4 °C between beginning and end of melting), Specific rotation (+107° to +112 °, calculated on the dried basis), Loss on drying (not more than 1.0%), Residue on ignition (not more than 0.2%), and Heavy metals (not more than 0.002%).
Desoximetasone Cream USP—Preserve in collapsible tubes, at controlled room temperature. It is Desoximetasone in an emollient cream base. Contains the labeled amount, within ±10%. Meets the requirements for Identification, Minimum fill, and pH (4.0–8.0).

Desoximetasone Gel USP—Preserve in collapsible tubes, at controlled room temperature. Contains the labeled amount, within ± 10%. Meets the requirements for Identification, Minimum fill, and Alcohol content (18.0–24.0% [w/w]).

Desoximetasone Ointment USP—Preserve in collapsible tubes, at controlled room temperature. Contains the labeled amount, within ± 10%. Meets the requirements for Identification and Minimum fill.

DESOXYCORTICOSTERONE

Chemical name:
Desoxycorticosterone acetate—Pregn-4-ene-3,20-dione, 21-(acetyloxy)-.
Desoxycorticosterone pivalate—Pregn-4-ene-3,20-dione, 21-(2,2-dimethyl-1-oxopropoxy)-.

Molecular formula:
Desoxycorticosterone acetate—$C_{23}H_{32}O_4$.
Desoxycorticosterone pivalate—$C_{26}H_{38}O_4$.

Molecular weight:
Desoxycorticosterone acetate—372.50.
Desoxycorticosterone pivalate—414.58.

Description:
Desoxycorticosterone Acetate USP—White or creamy white, crystalline powder. Is odorless, and is stable in air.
Desoxycorticosterone Pivalate USP—White or creamy white, crystalline powder. Is odorless, and is stable in air.

Solubility:
Desoxycorticosterone Acetate USP—Practically insoluble in water; sparingly soluble in alcohol, in acetone, and in dioxane; slightly soluble in vegetable oils.
Desoxycorticosterone Pivalate USP—Practically insoluble in water; soluble in dioxane; sparingly soluble in acetone; slightly soluble in alcohol, in methanol, in ether, and in vegetable oils.

USP requirements:
Desoxycorticosterone Acetate USP—Preserve in well-closed, light-resistant containers. Contains not less than 97.0% and not more than 103.0% of desoxycorticosterone acetate, calculated on the dried basis. Meets the requirements for Identification, Melting range (155–161 °C), Specific rotation (+171° to +179°, determined in a solution in dioxane containing 100 mg in each 10 mL), and Loss on drying (not more than 0.5%).
Desoxycorticosterone Acetate Injection USP—Preserve in single-dose or in multiple-dose containers, preferably of Type I or Type III glass, protected from light. A sterile solution of Desoxycorticosterone Acetate in vegetable oil. Contains the labeled amount, within −10% to +15%. Meets the requirements for Identification, Bacterial endotoxins, and Injections.
Desoxycorticosterone Acetate Pellets USP—Preserve in tight containers suitable for maintaining sterile contents, holding one pellet each. Desoxycorticosterone Acetate Pellets are sterile pellets composed of Desoxycorticosterone Acetate in compressed form, without the presence of any binder, diluent, or excipient. Contain the labeled amount, within ± 3%. Meet the requirements for Identification, Solubility in alcohol, Melting range (155–161 °C), Specific rotation (+171° to +179°, determined in a solution in dioxane containing 100 mg in each 10 mL), Sterility, and Weight variation (average weight of 5 Pellets 95–105% of labeled weight; each Pellet weighs 90–110% of labeled weight).
Desoxycorticosterone Pivalate USP—Preserve in well-closed, light-resistant containers. Contains not less than 97.0%

and not more than 103.0% of desoxycorticosterone pivalate, calculated on the dried basis. Meets the requirements for Identification, Melting range (200–206 °C), Specific rotation (+155° to +163°, calculated on the dried basis), and Loss on drying (not more than 0.5%).
Sterile Desoxycorticosterone Pivalate Suspension USP—Preserve in single-dose or in multiple-dose containers, preferably of Type I glass, protected from light. A sterile suspension of Desoxycorticosterone Pivalate in an aqueous medium. Contains the labeled amount, within ± 10%. Meets the requirements for Identification, Bacterial endotoxins, pH (5.0–7.0), and Injections.

DEXAMETHASONE

Chemical name:
Dexamethasone—Pregna-1,4-diene-3,20-dione, 9-fluoro-11,17,21-trihydroxy-16-methyl-, (11 beta,16 alpha)-.
Dexamethasone acetate—Pregna-1,4-diene-3,20-dione, 21-(acetyloxy)-9-fluoro-11,17-dihydroxy-16-methyl, monohydrate, (11 beta,16 alpha)-.
Dexamethasone sodium phosphate—Pregna-1,4-diene-3,20-dione, 9-fluoro-11,17-dihydroxy-16-methyl-21-(phosphonooxy)-, disodium salt, (11 beta,16 alpha)-.

Molecular formula:
Dexamethasone—$C_{22}H_{29}FO_5$.
Dexamethasone acetate (anhydrous)—$C_{24}H_{31}FO_6$.
Dexamethasone acetate (monohydrate)—$C_{24}H_{31}FO_6 \cdot H_2O$.
Dexamethasone sodium phosphate—$C_{22}H_{28}FNa_2O_8P$.

Molecular weight:
Dexamethasone—392.47.
Dexamethasone acetate (anhydrous)—434.50.
Dexamethasone acetate (monohydrate)—452.52.
Dexamethasone sodium phosphate—516.41.

Description:
Dexamethasone USP—White to practically white, odorless, crystalline powder. Is stable in air. Melts at about 250 °C, with some decomposition.
Dexamethasone Acetate USP—Clear, white to off-white, odorless powder.
Dexamethasone Sodium Phosphate USP— White or slightly yellow, crystalline powder. Is odorless or has a slight odor of alcohol, and is exceedingly hygroscopic.

Solubility:
Dexamethasone USP—Practically insoluble in water; sparingly soluble in acetone, in alcohol, in dioxane, and in methanol; slightly soluble in chloroform; very slightly soluble in ether.
Dexamethasone Acetate USP—Practically insoluble in water; freely soluble in methanol, in acetone, and in dioxane.
Dexamethasone Sodium Phosphate USP—Freely soluble in water; slightly soluble in alcohol; very slightly soluble in dioxane; insoluble in chloroform and in ether.

USP requirements:
Dexamethasone USP—Preserve in well-closed containers. Contains not less than 97.0% and not more than 102.0% of dexamethasone, calculated on the dried basis. Meets the requirements for Identification, Specific rotation (+72° to +80°, calculated on the dried basis), Loss on drying (not more than 0.5%), Residue on ignition (not more than 0.2% from 250 mg), and Ordinary impurities.
Dexamethasone Topical Aerosol USP—Preserve in pressurized containers, and avoid exposure to excessive heat. It is Dexamethasone in a suitable lotion base mixed with suitable propellants in a pressurized container. Delivers the labeled amount, within −10% to +20%. Meets the

requirements for Identification and Microbial limits, and for Leak testing and Pressure testing under Aerosols.

Dexamethasone Elixir USP—Preserve in tight containers. Contains the labeled amount, within ±10%. Meets the requirements for Identification and Alcohol content (3.8–5.7%, *n*-propyl alcohol being used as the internal standard).

Dexamethasone Gel USP—Preserve in collapsible tubes. Keep tightly closed. Avoid exposure to temperatures exceeding 30 °C. Contains the labeled amount, within ±10%. Meets the requirements for Identification and Minimum fill.

Dexamethasone Ophthalmic Ointment—Not in USP.

Dexamethasone Oral Solution—Not in USP.

Dexamethasone Ophthalmic Suspension USP—Preserve in tight containers. A sterile, aqueous suspension of dexamethasone containing a suitable antimicrobial preservative. Contains the labeled amount, within ±10%. Meets the requirements for Identification, Sterility, and pH (5.0–6.0).

Dexamethasone Tablets USP—Preserve in well-closed containers. Contain the labeled amount, within ±10%. Meet the requirements for Identification, Dissolution (70% in 45 minutes in dilute hydrochloric acid [1 in 100] in Apparatus 1 at 100 rpm), and Uniformity of dosage units.

Dexamethasone Acetate USP—Preserve in well-closed containers. Contains one molecule of water of hydration or is anhydrous. Label it to indicate whether it is hydrous or anhydrous. Contains not less than 97.0% and not more than 102.0% of dexamethasone acetate, calculated on the dried basis. Meets the requirements for Identification, Specific rotation (+82° to +88°, calculated on the dried basis), Loss on drying (3.5–4.5% for the hydrous, not more than 0.4% for the anhydrous), Residue on ignition (not more than 0.1%), Heavy metals (not more than 0.002%), and Organic volatile impurities.

Sterile Dexamethasone Acetate Suspension USP—Preserve in single-dose or in multiple-dose containers, preferably of Type I glass. A sterile suspension of Dexamethasone Acetate in Water for Injection. Contains an amount of dexamethasone acetate monohydrate equivalent to the labeled amount of anhydrous dexamethasone, within ±10%. Meets the requirements for Identification, Bacterial endotoxins, pH (5.0–7.5), and Injections.

Dexamethasone Sodium Phosphate USP—Preserve in tight containers. Contains not less than 97.0% and not more than 102.0% of dexamethasone sodium phosphate, calculated on the water-free and alcohol-free basis. Meets the requirements for Identification, Specific rotation (+74° to +82°, calculated on the water-free and alcohol-free basis), pH (7.5–10.5, in a solution [1 in 100]), Water (sum of percentages of water content and of alcohol content not more than 16.0%), Alcohol (not more than 8.0%), Phosphate ions (not more than 1.0%), and Free dexamethasone (not more than 1.0%).

Dexamethasone Sodium Phosphate Inhalation Aerosol USP—Preserve in tight, pressurized containers, and avoid exposure to excessive heat. A suspension, in suitable propellants and alcohol, in a pressurized container, of dexamethasone sodium phosphate. Contains an amount of dexamethasone sodium phosphate equivalent to the labeled amount of dexamethasone phosphate, within ±10%. Delivers the labeled dose of dexamethasone phosphate, within ±20% per metered spray. Meets the requirements for Identification and Alcohol content (1.7–2.3%), for Leak testing and Pressure testing under Aerosols, and for Unit spray content (not less than 80.0% and not more than 120.0% of the labeled amount of dexamethasone phosphate is delivered per spray).

Dexamethasone Sodium Phosphate Nasal Aerosol—Not in USP.

Dexamethasone Sodium Phosphate Cream USP—Preserve in collapsible tubes or in tight containers. Contains an amount of dexamethasone sodium phosphate equivalent to the labeled amount of dexamethasone phosphate, within −10% to +15%. Meets the requirements for Identification, Microbial limits, and Minimum fill.

Dexamethasone Sodium Phosphate Injection USP—Preserve in single-dose or in multiple-dose containers, preferably of Type I glass, protected from light. A sterile solution of Dexamethasone Sodium Phosphate in Water for Injection. Contains an amount of dexamethasone sodium phosphate equivalent to the labeled amount of dexamethasone phosphate, within −10% to +15%, present as the disodium salt. Meets the requirements for Identification, Bacterial endotoxins, pH (7.0–8.5), and Injections.

Dexamethasone Sodium Phosphate Ophthalmic Ointment USP—Preserve in collapsible ophthalmic ointment tubes. A sterile ointment. Contains an amount of dexamethasone sodium phosphate equivalent to the labeled amount of dexamethasone phosphate, within −10% to +15%. Meets the requirements for Identification, Minimum fill, Sterility, and Metal particles.

Dexamethasone Sodium Phosphate Ophthalmic Solution USP—Preserve in tight, light-resistant containers. A sterile, aqueous solution of Dexamethasone Sodium Phosphate. Contains an amount of dexamethasone sodium phosphate equivalent to the labeled amount of dexamethasone phosphate, within −10% to +15%. Meets the requirements for Identification, pH (6.6–7.8), and Sterility.

DEXBROMPHENIRAMINE

Chemical group: Propylamine derivative (alkylamine).

Chemical name: Dexbrompheniramine maleate—2-Pyridinepropanamine, gamma-(4-bromophenyl)-*N,N*-dimethyl-, (*S*)-, (*Z*)-2-butenedioate (1:1).

Molecular formula: Dexbrompheniramine maleate—$C_{16}H_{19}BrN_2 \cdot C_4H_4O_4$.

Molecular weight: Dexbrompheniramine maleate—435.32.

Description: Dexbrompheniramine Maleate USP—White, odorless, crystalline powder. Exists in two polymorphic forms, one melting between 106 and 107 °C and the other between 112 and 113 °C. Mixtures of the forms may melt between 105 and 113 °C. The pH of a solution (1 in 100) is about 5.

Solubility: Dexbrompheniramine Maleate USP—Freely soluble in water; soluble in alcohol and in chloroform.

USP requirements: Dexbrompheniramine Maleate USP—Preserve in tight, light-resistant containers. Contains not less than 98.0% and not more than 100.5% of dexbrompheniramine maleate, calculated on the dried basis. Meets the requirements for Identification, Specific rotation (+35.0° to +38.5°, calculated on the dried basis), Loss on drying (not more than 0.5%), Residue on ignition (not more than 0.2%), Related compounds (not more than 2.0%), and Organic volatile impurities.

DEXBROMPHENIRAMINE AND PSEUDOEPHEDRINE

For *Dexbrompheniramine* and *Pseudoephedrine*—See individual listings for chemistry information.

USP requirements:

Dexbrompheniramine Maleate and Pseudoephedrine Sulfate Extended-release Capsules—Not in USP.

Dexbrompheniramine Maleate and Pseudoephedrine Sulfate Syrup—Not in USP.
Dexbrompheniramine Maleate and Pseudoephedrine Sulfate Tablets—Not in USP.
Dexbrompheniramine Maleate and Pseudoephedrine Sulfate Extended-release Tablets—Not in USP.

DEXBROMPHENIRAMINE, PSEUDOEPHEDRINE, AND ACETAMINOPHEN

For *Dexbrompheniramine, Pseudoephedrine,* and *Acetaminophen*—See individual listings for chemistry information.

USP requirements: Dexbrompheniramine Maleate, Pseudoephedrine Hydrochloride, and Acetaminophen Extended-release Tablets—Not in USP.

DEXCHLORPHENIRAMINE

Chemical group: Propylamine derivative (alkylamine).

Chemical name: Dexchlorpheniramine maleate—2-Pyridinepropanamine, gamma-(4-chlorophenyl)-*N,N*-dimethyl-, (*S*)-, (*Z*)-2-butenedioate (1:1).

Molecular formula: Dexchlorpheniramine maleate—$C_{16}H_{19}Cl$-$N_2 \cdot C_4H_4O_4$.

Molecular weight: Dexchlorpheniramine maleate—390.87.

Description: Dexchlorpheniramine Maleate USP—White, odorless, crystalline powder.

Solubility: Dexchlorpheniramine Maleate USP—Freely soluble in water; soluble in alcohol and in chloroform; slightly soluble in ether.

USP requirements:
Dexchlorpheniramine Maleate USP—Preserve in tight, light-resistant containers. Dried at 65 °C for 4 hours, contains not less than 98.0% and not more than 100.5% of dexchlorpheniramine maleate. Meets the requirements for Identification, Melting range (110–115 °C), Specific rotation (+39.5° to +43.0°, calculated on the dried basis), pH (4.0–5.0, in a solution [1 in 100]), Loss on drying (not more than 0.5%), Residue on ignition (not more than 0.2%), Related compounds (not more than 2.0%), and Organic volatile impurities.
Dexchlorpheniramine Maleate Syrup USP—Preserve in tight, light-resistant containers. Contains the labeled amount, within ±10%. Meets the requirements for Identification and Alcohol content (5.0–7.0%).
Dexchlorpheniramine Maleate Tablets USP—Preserve in tight containers. Contain the labeled amount, within ±10%. Meet the requirements for Identification, Dissolution (75% in 45 minutes in water in Apparatus 2 at 50 rpm), and Uniformity of dosage units.
Dexchlorpheniramine Maleate Extended-release Tablets—Not in USP.

DEXCHLORPHENIRAMINE, PSEUDOEPHEDRINE, AND GUAIFENESIN

For *Dexchlorpheniramine, Pseudoephedrine,* and *Guaifenesin*—See individual listings for chemistry information.

USP requirements: Dexchlorpheniramine Maleate, Pseudoephedrine Sulfate, and Guaifenesin Oral Solution—Not in USP.

DEXPANTHENOL

Chemical name: Butanamide, 2,4-dihydroxy-*N*-(3-hydroxypropyl)-3,3-dimethyl-, (*R*)-.

Molecular formula: $C_9H_{19}NO_4$.

Molecular weight: 205.25

Description: Dexpanthenol USP—Clear, viscous, somewhat hygroscopic liquid, having a slight, characteristic odor. Some crystallization may occur on standing.

Solubility: Dexpanthenol USP—Freely soluble in water, in alcohol, in methanol, and in propylene glycol; soluble in chloroform and in ether; slightly soluble in glycerin.

USP requirements:
Dexpanthenol USP—Preserve in tight containers. Contains not less than 98.0% and not more than 102.0% of dexpanthenol, calculated on the anhydrous basis. Meets the requirements for Identification, Specific rotation (+29.0° to +31.5°, calculated on the anhydrous basis), Refractive index (1.495–1.502 at 20 °C), Water (not more than 1.0%), Residue on ignition (not more than 0.1%), and Aminopropanol (not more than 1.0%).
Dexpanthenol Preparation USP—Preserve in tight containers. Contains not less than 94.5% and not more than 98.5% of dexpanthenol, and not less than 2.7% and not more than 4.2% of pantolactone, both calculated on the anhydrous basis. Meets the requirements for Identification, Specific rotation (+27.5° to +30.0°, calculated on the anhydrous basis), and Pantolactone, and for Refractive index, Water, Residue on ignition, and Aminopropanol under Dexpanthenol.

DEXTRATES

Description: Dextrates NF—Free-flowing, porous, white, odorless, spherical granules consisting of aggregates of microcrystals. May be compressed directly into self-binding tablets.
NF category: Sweetening agent; tablet and/or capsule diluent.

Solubility: Dextrates NF—Freely soluble in water; heating increases its solubility in water; soluble in dilute acids and alkalies and in basic organic solvents such as pyridine; insoluble in the common organic solvents.

NF requirements: Dextrates NF—Preserve in well-closed containers in a cool, dry place. A purified mixture of saccharides resulting from the controlled enzymatic hydrolysis of starch. Label it to state whether it is anhydrous or hydrated. Contains dextrose equivalent to not less than 93.0% and not more than 99.0%, calculated on the dried basis. Meets the requirements for pH (3.8–5.8, determined in a 1 in 5 solution in carbon dioxide-free water), Loss on drying (for the anhydrous not more than 2.0%, for the hydrated form 7.8–9.2%), Residue on ignition (not more than 0.1%), Heavy metals (not more than 5 ppm), Dextrose equivalent, and Organic volatile impurities.

DEXTRIN

Description: Dextrin NF—Free-flowing, white, yellow, or brown powder.
NF category: Suspending and/or viscosity-increasing agent; tablet binder; tablet and/or capsule diluent.

Solubility: Dextrin NF—Its solubility in water varies; it is usually very soluble, but often contains an insoluble portion.

NF requirements: Dextrin NF—Preserve in well-closed containers. It is starch or partially hydrolyzed starch, modified by heating in a dry state, with or without acids, alkalies, or pH control agents. Meets the requirements for Botanic characteristics, Identification, Loss on drying (not more than 13.0%), Acidity, Residue on ignition (not more than 0.5%),

Chloride (not more than 0.2%), Arsenic (not more than 3 ppm), Heavy metals (not more than 0.004%), Protein, Reducing sugars, and Organic volatile impurities.

DEXTROAMPHETAMINE

Chemical name: Dextroamphetamine sulfate—Benzeneethanamine, alpha-methyl-, (*S*)-, sulfate (2:1).

Molecular formula: Dextroamphetamine sulfate—$(C_9H_{13}N)_2 \cdot H_2SO_4$.

Molecular weight: Dextroamphetamine sulfate—368.49.

Description: Dextroamphetamine Sulfate USP—White, odorless, crystalline powder.

Solubility: Dextroamphetamine Sulfate USP—Soluble in water; slightly soluble in alcohol; insoluble in ether.

USP requirements:
Dextroamphetamine Sulfate USP—Preserve in well-closed containers. It is the dextrorotatory isomer of amphetamine sulfate. Contains not less than 98.0% and not more than 101.0% of amphetamine sulfate, calculated on the dried basis. Meets the requirements for Identification, Specific rotation (+20° to +23.5°, calculated on the dried basis), pH (5.0–6.0, in a solution [1 in 20]), Loss on drying (not more than 1.0%), Residue on ignition (not more than 0.1%), Ordinary impurities, and Organic volatile impurities.

Dextroamphetamine Sulfate Capsules USP—Preserve in tight containers. Contain the labeled amount, within ±10%. Meet the requirements for Identification, Dissolution (75% in 45 minutes in water in Apparatus 1 at 100 rpm) and Uniformity of dosage units.

Dextroamphetamine Sulfate Extended-release Capsules—Not in USP.

Dextroamphetamine Sulfate Elixir USP—Preserve in tight, light-resistant containers. Contains, in each 100 mL, not less than 90.0 mg and not more than 110.0 mg of dextroamphetamine sulfate. Meets the requirements for Identification, Alcohol content (9.0–11.0%), and Isomeric purity.

Dextroamphetamine Sulfate Tablets USP—Preserve in well-closed containers. Contain the labeled amount, within ±7%. Meet the requirements for Identification, Dissolution (75% in 45 minutes in water in Apparatus 1 at 100 rpm), Uniformity of dosage units, and Isomeric purity.

DEXTROMETHORPHAN

Source: Methylated dextroisomer of levorphanol.

Chemical group: Synthetic derivative of morphine.

Chemical name:
Dextromethorphan—Morphinan, 3-methoxy-17-methyl-, (9 alpha,13 alpha,14 alpha)-.

Dextromethorphan hydrobromide—Morphinan, 3-methoxy-17-methyl-, (9 alpha,13 alpha,14 alpha)-, hydrobromide, monohydrate.

Dextromethorphan polistirex—Benzene, diethenyl-, polymer with ethenylbenzene, sulfonated, complex with (9 alpha,13 alpha,14 alpha)-3-methoxy-17-methylmorphinan.

Molecular formula:
Dextromethorphan—$C_{18}H_{25}NO$.
Dextromethorphan hydrobromide—$C_{18}H_{25}NO \cdot HBr \cdot H_2O$.

Molecular weight:
Dextromethorphan—271.40.
Dextromethorphan hydrobromide—370.33.

Description:
Dextromethorphan USP—Practically white to slightly yellow, odorless, crystalline powder. Eleven mg of Dextromethorphan is equivalent to 15 mg of dextromethorphan hydrobromide monohydrate.

Dextromethorphan Hydrobromide USP—Practically white crystals or crystalline powder, having a faint odor. Melts at about 126 °C, with decomposition.

Solubility:
Dextromethorphan USP—Practically insoluble in water; freely soluble in chloroform.

Dextromethorphan Hydrobromide USP—Sparingly soluble in water; freely soluble in alcohol and in chloroform; insoluble in ether.

USP requirements:
Dextromethorphan USP—Preserve in tight containers. Contains not less than 98.0% and not more than 101.0% of dextromethorphan, calculated on the anhydrous basis. Meets the requirements for Identification, Melting range (109.5–112.5 °C), Specific rotation, Water (not more than 0.5%), Residue on ignition (not more than 0.1%), Heavy metals (not more than 0.002%), Dimethylaniline (not more than 0.001%), and Phenolic compounds.

Dextromethorphan Hydrobromide USP—Preserve in tight containers. Contains not less than 98.0% and not more than 102.0% of dextromethorphan hydrobromide, calculated on the anhydrous basis. Meets the requirements for Identification, Specific rotation, pH (5.2–6.5, in a solution [1 in 100]), Water (3.5–5.5%), Residue on ignition (not more than 0.1%), *N,N*-Dimethylaniline (not more than 0.001%), and Phenolic compounds.

Dextromethorphan Hydrobromide Capsules—Not in USP.

Dextromethorphan Hydrobromide Lozenges—Not in USP.

Dextromethorphan Hydrobromide Syrup USP—Preserve in tight, light-resistant containers. Contains the labeled amount, within ±5%. Meets the requirement for Identification.

Dextromethorphan Hydrobromide Chewable Tablets—Not in USP.

Dextromethorphan Polistirex Extended-release Oral Suspension—Not in USP.

DEXTROMETHORPHAN AND GUAIFENESIN

For *Dextromethorphan* and *Guaifenesin*—See individual listings for chemistry information.

USP requirements:
Dextromethorphan Hydrobromide and Guaifenesin Capsules—Not in USP.

Dextromethorphan Hydrobromide and Guaifenesin Oral Gel—Not in USP.

Dextromethorphan Hydrobromide and Guaifenesin Oral Solution—Not in USP.

Dextromethorphan Hydrobromide and Guaifenesin Syrup—Not in USP.

Dextromethorphan Hydrobromide and Guaifenesin Tablets—Not in USP.

DEXTROMETHORPHAN, GUAIFENESIN, POTASSIUM CITRATE, AND CITRIC ACID

For *Dextromethorphan, Guaifenesin, Potassium Citrate,* and *Citric Acid*—See individual listings for chemistry information.

USP requirements: Dextromethorphan Hydrobromide, Guaifenesin, Potassium Citrate, and Citric Acid Syrup—Not in USP.

DEXTROMETHORPHAN AND IODINATED GLYCEROL

For *Dextromethorphan* and *Iodinated Glycerol*—See individual listings for chemistry information.

USP requirements: Dextromethorphan Hydrobromide and Iodinated Glycerol Oral Solution—Not in USP.

DEXTROSE

Chemical name: D-Glucose, monohydrate.

Molecular formula: $C_6H_{12}O_6 \cdot H_2O$ (monohydrate); $C_6H_{12}O_6$ (anhydrous).

Molecular weight: 198.17 (monohydrate); 180.16 (anhydrous).

Description: Dextrose USP—Colorless crystals or white, crystalline or granular powder. Is odorless.

NF category: Sweetening agent; tonicity agent.

Solubility: Dextrose USP—Freely soluble in water; very soluble in boiling water; soluble in boiling alcohol; slightly soluble in alcohol.

USP requirements:

Dextrose USP—Preserve in well-closed containers. A sugar usually obtained by the hydrolysis of Starch. Contains one molecule of water of hydration or is anhydrous. Label it to indicate whether it is hydrous or anhydrous. Meets the requirements for Identification, Color of solution, Specific rotation ($+52.6°$ to $+53.2°$, calculated on anhydrous basis), Acidity, Water (hydrous form loses 7.5–9.5%; anhydrous form loses not more than 0.5%), Residue on ignition (not more than 0.1%), Chloride (not more than 0.018%), Sulfate (not more than 0.025%), Arsenic (not more than 1 ppm), Heavy metals (not more than 5 ppm), Dextrin, and Soluble starch, sulfites.

Dextrose Injection USP—Preserve in single-dose glass or plastic containers. Glass containers are preferably of Type I or Type II glass. A sterile solution of Dextrose in Water for Injection. The label states the total osmolar concentration in mOsmol per liter. Where the contents are less than 100 mL, or where the label states that the Injection is not for direct injection but is to be diluted before use, the label alternatively may state the total osmolar concentration in mOsmol per mL. Contains the labeled amount of dextrose monohydrate, within ±5%. Contains no antimicrobial agents. Meets the requirements for Identification, Pyrogen, pH (3.5–6.5), Particulate matter, Heavy metals (not more than $0.0005C$%), 5-Hydroxymethylfurfural and related substances (absorbance not more than 0.25), and Injections.

DEXTROSE AND ELECTROLYTES

For *Calcium Chloride, Citric Acid, Dextrose, Dibasic Sodium Phosphate, Magnesium Chloride, Potassium Chloride, Potassium Citrate, Sodium Bicarbonate, Sodium Chloride,* and *Sodium Citrate*—See individual listings for chemistry information.

USP requirements:

Dextrose and Electrolytes Solution—Not in USP.

Oral Rehydration Salts USP (For Oral Solution)—Preserve in tight containers, and avoid exposure to temperatures in excess of 30 °C. The Sodium Bicarbonate or Sodium Citrate component may be omitted from the mixture and packaged in a separate, accompanying container. A dry mixture of Sodium Chloride, Potassium Chloride, Sodium Bicarbonate, and Dextrose (anhydrous). Alternatively, it may contain Sodium Citrate (anhydrous or dihydrate) instead of Sodium Bicarbonate. It may contain Dextrose (monohydrate) instead of Dextrose (anhydrous),

provided that the Sodium Bicarbonate or Sodium Citrate is packaged in a separate, accompanying container. Contains the equivalent of the amounts of sodium, potassium, chloride, and bicarbonate or citrate, calculated from the labeled amounts of sodium chloride, potassium chloride, and sodium bicarbonate [or sodium citrate (anhydrous or dihydrate)], within ±10%. Contains the labeled amounts of anhydrous dextrose or dextrose monohydrate, within ±10%. The label indicates prominently whether Sodium Bicarbonate or Sodium Citrate is a component by the placement of the word "Bicarbonate" or "Citrate," as appropriate, in juxtaposition to the official title. The label states the name and quantity, in grams, of each component in each unit-dose container, or in a stated quantity, in grams, of Salts in a multiple-unit container. The label states the net weight in each container, and provides directions for constitution. Where packaged in individual unit-dose pouches, the label instructs the user not to open until the time of use. The label states also that any solution that remains unused 24 hours after constitution is to be discarded. Meets the requirements for Identification, Loss on drying (not more than 1.0%), Minimum fill, and pH (7.0–8.8, in the solution constituted as directed in labeling).

DEXTROSE EXCIPIENT

Description: Dextrose Excipient NF—Colorless crystals or white, crystalline or granular powder. Is odorless.

NF category: Sweetening agent; tablet and/or capsule diluent.

Solubility: Dextrose Excipient NF—Freely soluble in water; very soluble in boiling water; sparingly soluble in boiling alcohol; slightly soluble in alcohol.

NF requirements: Dextrose Excipient NF—Preserve in well-closed containers. A sugar usually obtained by hydrolysis of starch. Contains one molecule of water of hydration. Label it to indicate that it is not intended for parenteral use. Meets the requirements for Specific rotation ($+52.5°$ to $+53.5°$, calculated on anhydrous basis), Water (7.5–9.5%), and Organic volatile impurities, and for Identification test, Color of solution, Acidity, Residue on ignition, Chloride, Sulfate, Arsenic, Heavy metals, Dextrin, and Soluble starch, sulfites under Dextrose.

DEXTROSE AND SODIUM CHLORIDE

For *Dextrose* and *Sodium Chloride*—See individual listings for chemistry information.

USP requirements: Dextrose and Sodium Chloride Injection USP—Preserve in single-dose glass or plastic containers. Glass containers are preferably of Type I or Type II glass. A sterile solution of Dextrose and Sodium Chloride in Water for Injection. The label states the total osmolar concentration in mOsmol per liter. Where the contents are less than 100 mL, or where the label states that the Injection is not for direct injection but is to be diluted before use, the label alternatively may state the total osmolar concentration in mOsmol per mL. Contains the labeled amounts, within ±5%. Contains no antimicrobial agents. Meets the requirements for Identification, Pyrogen, pH (3.5–6.5, determined on a portion diluted with water, if necessary, to a concentration of not more than 5% of dextrose), 5-Hydroxymethylfurfural and related substances (absorbance not more than 0.25), and Injections.

DEXTROTHYROXINE

Chemical name: Dextrothyroxine sodium—D-Tyrosine, O-(4-hydroxy-3,5-diiodophenyl)-3,5-diiodo-, monosodium salt hydrate.

Molecular formula: Dextrothyroxine sodium—$C_{15}H_{10}I_4NNaO_4 \cdot xH_2O$.

Molecular weight: Dextrothyroxine sodium—798.86 (anhydrous).

Description: Dextrothyroxine sodium—Light yellow to buff-colored, odorless powder which may assume a slight pink color on exposure to light.

Solubility: Dextrothyroxine sodium—Soluble 1 in 700 of water and 1 in 300 of alcohol; soluble in solutions of alkali hydroxides and in hot solutions of alkali carbonates; practically insoluble in acetone, in chloroform, and in ether.

USP requirements: Dextrothyroxine Sodium Tablets—Not in USP.

DEZOCINE

Chemical group: An opioid agonist/antagonist analgesic of the aminotetralin series.

Chemical name: 5,11-Methanobenzocyclodecen-3-ol, 13-amino-5,6,7,8,9,10,11,12-octahydro-5-methyl-, (5 alpha,11 alpha,13S*)-, (–)-.

Molecular formula: $C_{16}H_{23}NO$.

Molecular weight: 245.36.

Other characteristics: *n*-Octanol:Water partition coefficient—1.7.

USP requirements: Dezocine Injection—Not in USP.

DIACETYLATED MONOGLYCERIDES

Description: Diacetylated Monoglycerides NF—Clear liquid. NF category: Plasticizer.

Solubility: Diacetylated Monoglycerides NF—Very soluble in 80% (w/w) aqueous alcohol, in vegetable oils, and in mineral oils; sparingly soluble in 70% alcohol.

NF requirements: Diacetylated Monoglycerides NF—Preserve in tight, light-resistant containers. It is glycerin esterified with edible fat-forming fatty acids and acetic acid. It may be prepared by the interesterification of edible oils with triacetin in the presence of catalytic agents, followed by molecular distillation, or by the direct acetylation of edible monoglycerides with acetic anhydride without the use of catalyst or molecular distillation. Meets the requirements for Identification, Residue on ignition (not more than 0.1%), Arsenic (not more than 3 ppm), Heavy metals (not more than 0.001%), Acid value (not more than 3), Hydroxyl value (not more than 15), and Saponification value (365–385).

DIATRIZOATE AND IODIPAMIDE

For *Diatrizoate* and *Iodipamide*—See individual listings for chemistry information.

USP requirements: Diatrizoate Meglumine and Iodipamide Meglumine Injection—Not in USP.

DIATRIZOATES

Chemical group: Ionic, monomeric, triiodinated benzoic acid derivative.

Chemical name:
Diatrizoate meglumine—Benzoic acid, 3,5-bis(acetylamino)-2,4,6-triiodo-, compd. with 1-deoxy-1-(methylamino)-D-glucitol (1:1).

Diatrizoate sodium—Benzoic acid, 3,5-bis(acetylamino)-2,4,6-triiodo-, monosodium salt.

Molecular formula:
Diatrizoate meglumine—$C_{11}H_9I_3N_2O_4 \cdot C_7H_{17}NO_5$.
Diatrizoate sodium—$C_{11}H_8I_3N_2NaO_4$.

Molecular weight:
Diatrizoate meglumine—809.13.
Diatrizoate sodium—635.90.

Description:
Diatrizoate Meglumine USP—White, odorless powder.
Diatrizoate Meglumine Injection USP—Clear, colorless to pale yellow, slightly viscous liquid.
Diatrizoate Meglumine and Diatrizoate Sodium Injection USP—Clear, colorless to pale yellow, slightly viscous liquid. May crystallize at room temperature or below.
Diatrizoate Sodium USP—White, odorless powder.
Diatrizoate Sodium Injection USP—Clear, colorless to pale yellow, slightly viscous liquid.
Diatrizoate Sodium Solution USP—Clear, pale yellow to light brown liquid.

Solubility:
Diatrizoate Meglumine USP—Freely soluble in water.
Diatrizoate Sodium USP—Soluble in water; slightly soluble in alcohol; practically insoluble in acetone and in ether.

Other characteristics: High osmolality.

USP requirements:
Diatrizoate Meglumine USP—Preserve in well-closed containers. Contains not less than 98.0% and not more than 102.0% of diatrizoate meglumine, calculated on the dried basis. Meets the requirements for Identification, Specific rotation (−5.65° to −6.37°, calculated on the dried basis), Loss on drying (not more than 1.0%), Residue on ignition (not more than 0.1%), Free aromatic amine (absorbance not more than 0.05%), Iodine and iodide (0.02% iodide), and Heavy metals (not more than 0.002%).
Diatrizoate Meglumine Injection USP—Preserve Injection intended for intravascular injection either in single-dose containers, preferably of Type I or Type III glass, protected from light or, where intended for administration with a pressure injector through a suitable transfer connection, in similar glass 500-mL or 1000-mL bottles, protected from light. Injection packaged for other than intravascular use may be packaged in 100-mL multiple-dose containers, preferably of Type I or Type III glass, protected from light. A sterile solution of Diatrizoate Meglumine in Water for Injection, or a sterile solution of Diatrizoic Acid in Water for Injection prepared with the aid of Meglumine. Label containers of Injection intended for intravascular injection, where packaged in single-dose containers, to direct the user to discard any unused portion remaining in the container or, where packaged in bulk bottles to state, "Bulk Container—only for sterile filling of pressure injectors," to state that it contains no antimicrobial preservatives, and to direct the user to discard any unused portion remaining in the container after 6 hours. Indicate also in the labeling of bulk bottles that a pressure injector is to be charged with a dose just prior to administration of the Injection. Label containers of Injection intended for other than intravascular injection to show that the contents are not intended for intravascular injection. Contains the labeled amount, within ±5%. Diatrizoate Meglumine Injection intended for intravascular use contains no antimicrobial agents. Meets the requirements for Identification, Pyrogen, pH (6.0–7.7), Free aromatic amine, Iodine and iodide (0.02% iodide), Heavy metals (not more than 0.002%), Meglumine content (22.9–25.3% of the labeled amount of diatrizoate meglumine), and Injections.

Diatrizoate Meglumine and Diatrizoate Sodium Injection USP—Preserve either in single-dose containers, preferably of Type I or Type III glass, protected from light or, where intended for administration with a pressure injector through a suitable transfer connection, in similar glass 500-mL or 1000-mL bottles, protected from light. A sterile solution of Diatrizoate Meglumine and Diatrizoate Sodium in Water for Injection, or a sterile solution of Diatrizoic Acid in Water for Injection prepared with the aid of Sodium Hydroxide and Meglumine. Label containers of Injection intended for intravascular injection, where packaged in single-dose containers, to direct the user to discard any unused portion remaining in the container or, where packaged in bulk bottles to state, "Bulk Container—only for sterile filling of pressure injectors," to state that it contains no antimicrobial preservatives, and to direct the user to discard any unused portion remaining in the container after 6 hours. Indicate also in the labeling of bulk bottles that a pressure injector is to be charged with a dose just prior to administration of the Injection. Label containers of Injection intended for other than intravascular injection to show that the contents are not intended for intravascular injection. Contains the labeled amounts of diatrizoate meglumine and iodine, within ±5%. Diatrizoate Meglumine and Diatrizoate Sodium Injection intended for intravascular use contains no antimicrobial agents. Meets the requirements for Identification, Pyrogen, pH (6.0–7.7), Free aromatic amine, Iodine and iodide (0.02% iodide), Heavy metals (not more than 0.002%), and Injections.

Diatrizoate Meglumine and Diatrizoate Sodium Solution USP—Preserve in tight, light-resistant containers. A solution of Diatrizoic Acid in Purified Water prepared with the aid of Meglumine and Sodium Hydroxide. Label the container to indicate that the contents are not intended for parenteral use. Contains the labeled amounts of diatrizoate meglumine and iodine, within ±5%. Meets the requirements for Identification, pH (6.0–7.6), and Iodine and iodide (0.02% iodide).

Diatrizoate Sodium USP—Preserve in well-closed containers. Contains not less than 98.0% and not more than 102.0% of diatrizoate sodium, calculated on the anhydrous basis. Meets the requirements for Identification, Water (not more than 10.0%), Free aromatic amine, Iodine and iodide (0.02% iodide), and Heavy metals (not more than 0.002%).

Diatrizoate Sodium Injection USP—Preserve Injection intended for intravascular injection in single-dose containers, preferably of Type I or Type III glass, protected from light. Injection intended for other than intravascular use may be packaged in 100-mL multiple-dose containers, preferably of Type I or Type III glass, protected from light. A sterile solution of Diatrizoate Sodium in Water for Injection, or a sterile solution of Diatrizoic Acid in Water for Injection prepared with the aid of Sodium Hydroxide. Label containers of Injection intended for intravascular injection to direct the user to discard any unused portion remaining in the container. Label containers of Injection intended for other than intravascular injection to show that the contents are not intended for intravascular injection. Contains the labeled amount, within ±5%. Diatrizoate Sodium Injection intended for intravascular use contains no antimicrobial agents. Meets the requirements for Identification, Pyrogen, pH (6.0–7.7), Free aromatic amine, Iodine and iodide (0.02% iodide), Heavy metals (not more than 0.002%), and Injections.

Diatrizoate Sodium Solution USP—Preserve in tight, light-resistant containers. A solution of Diatrizoate Sodium in Purified Water, or a solution of Diatrizoic Acid in Purified Water prepared with the aid of Sodium Hydroxide. Label the container to indicate that the contents are not intended for parenteral use. Contains the labeled amount, within ±5%. Meets the requirements for Identification, pH (4.5–7.5), and Iodine and iodide (0.02% iodide).

Diatrizoate Sodium for Solution—Not in USP.

DIATRIZOIC ACID

Chemical name: Benzoic acid, 3,5-bis(acetylamino)-2,4,6-triiodo-.

Molecular formula: $C_{11}H_9I_3N_2O_4$.

Molecular weight: 613.92.

Description: Diatrizoic Acid USP—White, odorless powder.

Solubility: Diatrizoic Acid USP—Very slightly soluble in water and in alcohol; soluble in dimethylformamide and in alkali hydroxide solutions.

USP requirements: Diatrizoic Acid USP—Preserve in well-closed containers. It is anhydrous or contains two molecules of water of hydration. Label it to indicate whether it is anhydrous or hydrous. Contains not less than 98.0% and not more than 102.0% of diatrizoic acid, calculated on the anhydrous basis. Meets the requirements for Identification, Water (for anhydrous not more than 1.0%, for hydrous 4.5–7.0%), Residue on ignition (not more than 0.1%), Free aromatic amine (absorbance not more than 0.05%), Iodine and iodide (0.02% iodide), and Heavy metals (not more than 0.002%).

DIAZEPAM

Chemical name: 2H-1,4-Benzodiazepin-2-one, 7-chloro-1,3-dihydro-1-methyl-5-phenyl-.

Molecular formula: $C_{16}H_{13}ClN_2O$.

Molecular weight: 284.75.

Description: Diazepam USP—Off-white to yellow, practically odorless, crystalline powder.

Solubility: Diazepam USP—Practically insoluble in water; freely soluble in chloroform; soluble in alcohol.

USP requirements:

Diazepam USP—Preserve in tight, light-resistant containers. Contains not less than 98.5% and not more than 101.0% of diazepam, calculated on the dried basis. Meets the requirements for Identification, Melting range (131–135 °C), Loss on drying (not more than 0.5%), Residue on ignition (not more than 0.1%), Heavy metals (not more than 0.002%), Related compounds, and Organic volatile impurities.

Diazepam Capsules USP—Preserve in tight, light-resistant containers. Contain the labeled amount, within ±10%. Meet the requirements for Identification, Dissolution (85% in 45 minutes in 0.1 N hydrochloric acid in Apparatus 1 at 100 rpm), and Uniformity of dosage units.

Diazepam Extended-release Capsules USP—Preserve in tight, light-resistant containers. Contain the labeled amount, within ±10%. Meet the requirements for Identification, Drug release (15–27% in 0.042D hours, 49–66% in 0.167D hours, 76–96% in 0.333D hours, and 85–115% in 0.500D hours in simulated gastric fluid TS, prepared without enzymes, in Apparatus 1 at 100 rpm), and Uniformity of dosage units.

Sterile Diazepam Emulsion—Not in USP.

Diazepam Injection USP—Preserve in single-dose or in multiple-dose containers, preferably of Type I glass, protected from light. A sterile solution of Diazepam in a suitable medium. Contains the labeled amount, within ±10%.

Meets the requirements for Identification, Bacterial endotoxins, pH (6.2–6.9), and Injections.

Diazepam Oral Solution—Not in USP.

Diazepam Tablets USP—Preserve in tight, light-resistant containers. Contain the labeled amount, within ±10%. Meet the requirements for Identification, Dissolution (85% in 30 minutes in 0.1 N hydrochloric acid in Apparatus 1 at 100 rpm), and Uniformity of dosage units.

DIAZOXIDE

Chemical group: A nondiuretic benzothiadiazine derivative.

Chemical name: 2H-1,2,4-Benzothiadiazine, 7-chloro-3-methyl-, 1,1-dioxide.

Molecular formula: $C_8H_7ClN_2O_2S$.

Molecular weight: 230.67.

Description: Diazoxide USP—White or cream-white crystals or crystalline powder.

pKa: 8.5.

Solubility: Diazoxide USP—Practically insoluble to sparingly soluble in water and in most organic solvents; very soluble in strong alkaline solutions; freely soluble in dimethylformamide.

USP requirements:
Diazoxide USP—Preserve in well-closed containers. Contains not less than 97.0% and not more than 102.0% of diazoxide, calculated on the dried basis. Meets the requirements for Identification, Loss on drying (not more than 0.5%), and Residue on ignition (not more than 0.1%).

Diazoxide Capsules USP—Preserve in well-closed containers. Contain the labeled amount, within ±10%. Meet the requirements for Identification, Dissolution (75% in 45 minutes in phosphate buffer [pH 7.6] in Apparatus 1 at 100 rpm), and Uniformity of dosage units.

Diazoxide Injection USP—Preserve in single-dose containers, preferably of Type I glass, protected from light. A sterile solution of Diazoxide in Water for Injection, prepared with the aid of Sodium Hydroxide. Contains the labeled amount, within ±10%. Meets the requirements for Identification, pH (11.2–11.9), Bacterial endotoxins, and Injections.

Diazoxide Oral Suspension USP—Preserve in tight, light-resistant containers. Contains the labeled amount, within ±10%. Meets the requirements for Identification.

DIBUCAINE

Chemical group: Amide.

Chemical name:
Dibucaine—4-Quinolinecarboxamide, 2-butoxy-N-[2-(diethylamino)ethyl]-.
Dibucaine hydrochloride—4-Quinolinecarboxamide, 2-butoxy-N-[2-(diethylamino)ethyl]-, monohydrochloride.

Molecular formula:
Dibucaine—$C_{20}H_{29}N_3O_2$.
Dibucaine hydrochloride—$C_{20}H_{29}N_3O_2 \cdot HCl$.

Molecular weight:
Dibucaine—343.47.
Dibucaine hydrochloride—379.93.

Description:
Dibucaine USP—White to off-white powder, having a slight, characteristic odor. Darkens on exposure to light.

Dibucaine Hydrochloride USP—Colorless or white to off-white crystals or white to off-white, crystalline powder. Is odorless, is somewhat hygroscopic, and darkens on exposure to light. Its solutions have a pH of about 5.5.

pKa: 8.8.

Solubility:
Dibucaine USP—Slightly soluble in water; soluble in 1 N hydrochloric acid and in ether.
Dibucaine Hydrochloride USP—Freely soluble in water, in alcohol, in acetone, and in chloroform.

USP requirements:
Dibucaine USP—Preserve in tight, light-resistant containers. Contains not less than 97.0% and not more than 100.5% of dibucaine, calculated on the dried basis. Meets the requirements for Identification, Melting range (62.5–66.0 °C, determined after drying), Loss on drying (not more than 1.0%), Residue on ignition (not more than 0.2%), and Chromatographic purity.

Dibucaine Cream USP—Preserve in collapsible tubes or in tight, light-resistant containers. Contains the labeled amount, within ±10%, in a suitable cream base. Meets the requirements for Identification, Microbial limits, and Minimum fill.

Dibucaine Ointment USP—Preserve in collapsible tubes or in tight, light-resistant containers. Contains the labeled amount, within ±10%, in a suitable ointment base. Meets the requirements for Identification, Microbial limits, and Minimum fill.

Dibucaine Hydrochloride USP—Preserve in tight, light-resistant containers. Contains not less than 97.0% and not more than 100.5% of dibucaine hydrochloride, calculated on the dried basis. Meets the requirements for Identification, Loss on drying (not more than 2.0%), Residue on ignition (not more than 0.1%), and Chromatographic purity.

Dibucaine Hydrochloride Injection—Preserve in single-dose or in multiple-dose containers, preferably of Type I glass, and protect from light. A sterile solution of Dibucaine Hydrochloride in Water for Injection. Contains the labeled amount, within ±5%. Meets the requirements for Identification, Bacterial endotoxins, pH (4.5–7.0), Particulate matter, and Injections.

DIBUTYL SEBACATE

Description: Dibutyl Sebacate NF—Colorless, oily liquid of very mild odor.

NF category: Plasticizer.

Solubility: Dibutyl Sebacate NF—Soluble in alcohol, in isopropyl alcohol, and in mineral oil; very slightly soluble in propylene glycol; practically insoluble in water and in glycerin.

NF requirements: Dibutyl Sebacate NF—Preserve in tight containers. Consists of esters of n-butyl alcohol and saturated dibasic acids, principally sebacic acid. Contains not less than 92.0% of dibutyl sebacate. Meets the requirements for Specific gravity (0.935–0.939 at 20 °C), Refractive index (1.429–1.441), Acid value (not more than 0.1), and Saponification value (352–357).

DICHLORODIFLUOROMETHANE

Chemical name: Methane, dichlorodifluoro-.

Molecular formula: CCl_2F_2.

Molecular weight: 120.91.

Description: Dichlorodifluoromethane NF—Clear, colorless gas having a faint ethereal odor. Its vapor pressure at 25 °C is about 4880 mm of mercury (80 psig).

NF category: Aerosol propellant.

NF requirements: Dichlorodifluoromethane NF—Preserve in tight cylinders, and avoid exposure to excessive heat. Meets the requirements for Identification, Boiling temperature (approximately −30 °C), Water (not more than 0.001%), High-boiling residues (not more than 0.01%), and Inorganic chlorides.

DICHLOROTETRAFLUOROETHANE

Chemical name: Ethane, 1,2-dichloro-1,1,2,2-tetrafluoro-.

Molecular formula: $C_2Cl_2F_4$.

Molecular weight: 170.92.

Description: Dichlorotetrafluoroethane NF—Clear, colorless gas having a faint ethereal odor. Its vapor pressure at 25 °C is about 1620 mm of mercury (17 psig). Usually contains between 6% and 10% of its isomer, 1,1-dichloro-1,2,2,2-tetrafluoro ethane.

NF category: Aerosol propellant.

NF requirements: Dichlorotetrafluoroethane NF—Preserve in tight cylinders and avoid exposure to excessive heat. Meets the requirements for Identification, Boiling temperature (approximately 4 °C), Water (not more than 0.001%), High-boiling residues (not more than 0.01%), and Inorganic chlorides.

DICHLORPHENAMIDE

Chemical name: 1,3-Benzenedisulfonamide, 4,5-dichloro-.

Molecular formula: $C_6H_6Cl_2N_2O_4S_2$.

Molecular weight: 305.15.

Description: White or practically white, crystalline compound.

Solubility: Very slightly soluble in water; soluble in dilute solutions of sodium carbonate and sodium hydroxide

USP requirements:
Dichlorphenamide USP—Preserve in well-closed containers. Contains not less than 98.0% and not more than 101.0% of dichlorphenamide, calculated on the dried basis. Meets the requirements for Identification, Melting range (236.5–240 °C), Loss on drying (not more than 1.0%), Residue on ignition (not more than 0.2%), Chloride (not more than 0.20%), Selenium (0.003%), Heavy metals (not more than 0.001%), and Organic volatile impurities.
Dichlorphenamide Tablets USP—Preserve in well-closed containers. Contain the labeled amount, within ±8%. Meet the requirements for Identification, Dissolution (80% in 60 minutes in 0.1 M phosphate buffer [pH 8.0] in Apparatus 2 at 75 rpm), and Uniformity of dosage units.

DICLOFENAC

Chemical group: Phenylacetic acid derivative.

Chemical name: Diclofenac sodium—Benzeneacetic acid, 2-[(2,6-dichlorophenyl)amino]-, monosodium salt.

Molecular formula: Diclofenac sodium—$C_{14}H_{10}Cl_2NNaO_2$.

Molecular weight: Diclofenac sodium—318.13.

Description: Diclofenac sodium—Faintly yellow-white to light beige, virtually odorless, slightly hygroscopic, crystalline powder.

Solubility: Diclofenac sodium—Freely soluble in methanol; sparingly soluble in water; very slightly soluble in acetonitrile; insoluble in chloroform and in 0.1 N hydrochloric acid.

USP requirements:
Diclofenac Delayed-release Tablets—Not in USP.
Diclofenac Sodium Ophthalmic Solution—Not in USP.
Diclofenac Sodium Suppositories—Not in USP.
Diclofenac Sodium Delayed-release Tablets—Not in USP.
Diclofenac Sodium Extended-release Tablets—Not in USP.

DICLOXACILLIN

Chemical name: Dicloxacillin sodium—4-Thia-1-azabicyclo[3.2.0]heptane-2-carboxylic acid, 6-[[[3-(2,6-dichlorophenyl)-5-methyl-4-isoxazolyl]carbonyl]amino]-3,3-dimethyl-7-oxo-, monosodium salt, monohydrate, [2S-(2 alpha,5 alpha,6 beta)]-.

Molecular formula: Dicloxacillin sodium—$C_{19}H_{16}Cl_2N_3NaO_5S \cdot H_2O$.

Molecular weight: Dicloxacillin sodium—510.32.

Description: Dicloxacillin Sodium USP—White to off-white, crystalline powder.

Solubility: Dicloxacillin Sodium USP—Freely soluble in water.

USP requirements:
Dicloxacillin Sodium USP—Preserve in tight containers. Contains an amount of dicloxacillin sodium equivalent to not less than 850 mcg of dicloxacillin per mg. Meets the requirements for Identification, Crystallinity, pH (4.5–7.5, in a solution containing 10 mg per mL), Water (3.0–5.0%), and Dimethylaniline.
Dicloxacillin Sodium Capsules USP—Preserve in tight containers. Contain an amount of dicloxacillin sodium equivalent to the labeled amount of dicloxacillin, within −10% to +20%. Meet the requirements for Identification, Dissolution (75% in 45 minutes in water in Apparatus 1 at 100 rpm), Uniformity of dosage units, and Water (not more than 5.0%).
Sterile Dicloxacillin Sodium USP—Preserve in Containers for Sterile Solids. It is Dicloxacillin Sodium suitable for parenteral use. Contains an amount of dicloxacillin sodium equivalent to not less than 850 mcg of dicloxacillin per mg and, where packaged for dispensing, contains an amount of dicloxacillin sodium equivalent to the labeled amount of dicloxacillin, within −10% to +20%. Meets the requirements for Constituted solution, Bacterial endotoxins, Sterility, pH (4.5–7.5, in a solution containing 10 mg per mL or, where packaged for dispensing, in the solution constituted as directed in the labeling), and Particulate matter, for Identification tests, Water, Dimethylaniline, and Crystallinity under Dicloxacillin Sodium, and for Uniformity of dosage units and Labeling under Injections.
Dicloxacillin Sodium for Oral Suspension USP—Preserve in tight containers. A dry mixture of Dicloxacillin Sodium and one or more suitable buffers, colors, flavors, and preservatives. Contains an amount of dicloxacillin sodium equivalent to the labeled amount of dicloxacillin, within −10% to +20%. Meets the requirements for Identification, pH (4.5–7.5, in the suspension constituted as directed in the labeling]), Water (not more than 2.0%), Uniformity of dosage units (solid packaged in single-unit containers), and Deliverable volume (solid packaged in multiple-unit containers).

DICUMAROL

Chemical group: Coumarin derivative.

Chemical name: 2*H*-1-Benzopyran-2-one], 3,3′-Methylenebis[4-hydroxy-.

Molecular formula: $C_{19}H_{12}O_6$.

Molecular weight: 336.30.

Description: Dicumarol USP—White or creamy white, crystalline powder, having a faint, pleasant odor. Melts at about 290 °C.

Solubility: Dicumarol USP—Practically insoluble in water, in alcohol, and in ether; readily soluble in solutions of fixed alkali hydroxides; slightly soluble in chloroform.

USP requirements:
  Dicumarol USP—Preserve in well-closed containers. Contains not less than 98.5% and not more than 101.0% of dicumarol, calculated on the dried basis. Meets the requirements for Identification, Acidity, Loss on drying (not more than 0.5%), Residue on ignition (not more than 0.25%), and Ordinary impurities.
  Dicumarol Tablets USP—Preserve in well-closed containers. Label Tablets to state that Dicumarol Tablets may not be interchangeable with Dicumarol Capsules without retitration of the patient. Contain the labeled amount, within ±10%. Meet the requirements for Identification, Dissolution (60% in 30 minutes in 0.1 *M* tris buffer in Apparatus 1 at 100 rpm), and Uniformity of dosage units.

DICYCLOMINE

Source: Synthetic amine compound.

Chemical group: Tertiary amine, synthetic.

Chemical name: Dicyclomine hydrochloride—[Bicyclohexyl]-1-carboxylic acid, 2-(diethylamino)ethyl ester, hydrochloride.

Molecular formula: Dicyclomine hydrochloride—$C_{19}H_{35}NO_2 \cdot$ HCl.

Molecular weight: Dicyclomine hydrochloride—345.95.

Description:
  Dicyclomine Hydrochloride USP—Fine, white, crystalline powder. Is practically odorless.
  Dicyclomine Hydrochloride Injection USP—Colorless solution, which may have the odor of a preservative.

pKa: 9.0.

Solubility: Dicyclomine Hydrochloride USP—Soluble in water; freely soluble in alcohol and in chloroform; very slightly soluble in ether.

USP requirements:
  Dicyclomine Hydrochloride USP—Preserve in well-closed containers. Contains not less than 99.0% and not more than 102.0% of dicyclomine hydrochloride, calculated on the dried basis. Meets the requirements for Identification, Melting range (169–174 °C), pH (5.0–5.5, in a solution [1 in 100]), Readily carbonizable substances, and Organic volatile impurities.
  Dicyclomine Hydrochloride Capsules USP—Preserve in well-closed containers. Contain the labeled amount, within ±7%. Meet the requirements for Identification, Dissolution (75% in 45 minutes in 0.01 *N* hydrochloric acid in Apparatus 2 at 50 rpm), and Uniformity of dosage units.
  Dicyclomine Hydrochloride Injection USP—Preserve in single-dose or in multiple-dose containers, preferably of Type

I glass. A sterile, isotonic solution of Dicyclomine Hydrochloride in Water for Injection. Contains the labeled amount, within ±7%. Meets the requirements for Identification, Bacterial endotoxins, and Injections.
  Dicyclomine Hydrochloride Syrup USP—Preserve in tight containers. Contains the labeled amount, within ±5%. Meets the requirement for Identification.
  Dicyclomine Hydrochloride Tablets USP—Preserve in well-closed containers. Contain the labeled amount, within ±7%. Meet the requirements for Identification, Dissolution (75% in 45 minutes in 0.01 *N* hydrochloric acid in Apparatus 2 at 50 rpm), and Uniformity of dosage units.

DIDANOSINE

Chemical name: Inosine, 2′,3′-dideoxy-.

Molecular formula: $C_{10}H_{12}N_4O_3$.

Molecular weight: 236.23.

Description: White, crystalline powder. Unstable in acidic solutions.

Solubility: Aqueous solubility at 25 °C and pH of approximately 6 is 27.3 mg per mL.

USP requirements:
  Didanosine for Oral Solution—Not in USP.
  Buffered Didanosine for Oral Solution—Not in USP.
  Didanosine Chewable/Dispersible Tablets—Not in USP.

DIENESTROL

Chemical name: Phenol, 4,4′-(1,2-diethylidene-1,2-ethanediyl)bis-, (*E,E*)-.

Molecular formula: $C_{18}H_{18}O_2$.

Molecular weight: 266.34.

Description: Dienestrol USP—Colorless, white or practically white, needle-like crystals, or white or practically white, crystalline powder. Is odorless.

Solubility: Dienestrol USP—Practically insoluble in water; soluble in alcohol, in acetone, in ether, in methanol, in propylene glycol, and in solutions of alkali hydroxides; slightly soluble in chloroform and in fatty oils.

USP requirements:
  Dienestrol USP—Preserve in well-closed containers. Contains not less than 98.0% and not more than 100.5% of dienestrol, calculated on the dried basis. Meets the requirements for Identification, Melting range (227–234 °C, not more than 3 °C between beginning and end of melting), Loss on drying (not more than 0.5%), and Residue on ignition (not more than 0.2%).
  Dienestrol Cream USP—Preserve in collapsible tubes or in tight containers. It is Dienestrol in a suitable water-miscible base. Contains the labeled amount, within ±10%. Meets the requirements for Identification and Minimum fill.

DIETHANOLAMINE

Chemical name: Ethanol, 2,2′-iminobis-.

Molecular formula: $C_4H_{11}NO_2$.

Molecular weight: 105.14.

Description: Diethanolamine NF—White or clear, colorless crystals, deliquescing in moist air; or colorless liquid.

NF category: Alkalizing agent; emulsifying and/or solubilizing agent.

Solubility: Diethanolamine NF—Miscible with water, with alcohol, with acetone, with chloroform, and with glycerin. Slightly soluble to insoluble in ether and in petroleum ether.

NF requirements: Diethanolamine NF—Preserve in tight, light-resistant containers. A mixture of ethanolamines, consisting largely of diethanolamine. Contains not less than 98.5% and not more than 101.0% of ethanolamines, calculated on the anhydrous basis as diethanolamine. Meets the requirements for Identification, Refractive index (1.473–1.476, at 30 °C), Water (not more than 0.15%), and Triethanolamine (not more than 1.0%).

DIETHYLCARBAMAZINE

Chemical group: Piperazine derivative.

Chemical name: Diethylcarbamazine citrate—1-Piperazinecarboxamide, N,N-diethyl-4-methyl-, 2-hydroxy-1,2,3-propanetricarboxylate.

Molecular formula: Diethylcarbamazine citrate—$C_{10}H_{21}N_3O \cdot C_6H_8O_7$.

Molecular weight: Diethylcarbamazine citrate—391.42.

Description: Diethylcarbamazine Citrate USP—White, crystalline powder. Melts at about 136 °C, with decomposition. Is odorless or has a slight odor; is slightly hygroscopic.

Solubility: Diethylcarbamazine Citrate USP—Very soluble in water; sparingly soluble in alcohol; practically insoluble in acetone, in chloroform, and in ether.

USP requirements:

Diethylcarbamazine Citrate USP—Preserve in tight containers. Contains not less than 98.0% and not more than 100.5% of diethylcarbamazine citrate, calculated on the anhydrous basis. Meets the requirements for Identification, Water (not more than 0.5%), Residue on ignition (not more than 0.1%), Heavy metals (not more than 0.002%), and Ordinary impurities.

Diethylcarbamazine Citrate Tablets USP—Preserve in tight containers. Contain the labeled amount, within ± 5%. Meet the requirements for Identification, Disintegration (for Tablets labeled solely for veterinary use: 30 minutes), Dissolution (75% in 45 minutes in water in Apparatus 2 at 50 rpm), and Uniformity of dosage units.

Note: Diethylcarbamazine Citrate Tablets labeled solely for veterinary use are exempt from the requirements of the test for *Dissolution*.

DIETHYL PHTHALATE

Chemical name: 1,2-Benzenedicarboxylic acid, diethyl ester.

Molecular formula: $C_{12}H_{14}O_4$.

Molecular weight: 222.24.

Description: Diethyl Phthalate NF—Colorless, practically odorless, oily liquid.

NF category: Plasticizer.

Solubility: Diethyl Phthalate NF—Insoluble in water. Miscible with alcohol, with ether, and with other usual organic solvents.

NF requirements: Diethyl Phthalate NF—Preserve in tight containers. Contains not less than 98.0% and not more than 102.0% of diethyl phthalate, calculated on the anhydrous

basis. Meets the requirements for Identification, Specific gravity (1.118–1.122, at 20 °C), Refractive index (1.500–1.505, at 20 °C), Acidity, Water (not more than 0.2%), and Residue on ignition (not more than 0.02%).

Caution: Avoid contact.

DIETHYLPROPION

Chemical group: Phenethylamine.

Chemical name: Diethylpropion hydrochloride—1-Propanone, 2-(diethylamino)-1-phenyl-, hydrochloride.

Molecular formula: Diethylpropion hydrochloride—$C_{13}H_{19}NO \cdot HCl$.

Molecular weight: Diethylpropion hydrochloride—241.76.

Description: Diethylpropion Hydrochloride USP—White to off-white, fine crystalline powder. Is odorless, or has a slight characteristic odor. It melts at about 175 °C, with decomposition.

Solubility: Diethylpropion Hydrochloride USP—Freely soluble in water, in chloroform, and in alcohol; practically insoluble in ether.

USP requirements:

Diethylpropion Hydrochloride USP—Preserve in well-closed, light-resistant containers. The label indicates whether it contains tartaric acid as a stabilizer. Contains not less than 97.0% and not more than 103.0% of diethylpropion hydrochloride, calculated on the anhydrous basis. Meets the requirements for Identification, Water (not more than 0.5%), Secondary amines (not more than 0.5%), Free bromine, Hydrobromic acid and bromide, Chromatographic purity, and Organic volatile impurities.

Diethylpropion Hydrochloride Extended-release Capsules—Not in USP.

Diethylpropion Hydrochloride Tablets USP—Preserve in well-closed containers. Contain the labeled amount, within ± 10%. Meet the requirements for Identification, Dissolution (75% in 45 minutes in water in Apparatus 2 at 50 rpm), and Uniformity of dosage units.

Diethylpropion Hydrochloride Extended-release Tablets—Not in USP.

DIETHYLSTILBESTROL

Chemical name:

Diethylstilbestrol—Phenol 4,4′-(1,2-diethyl-1,2-ethenediyl)bis-, (E)-.

Diethylstilbestrol diphosphate—Phenol, 4,4′-(1,2-diethyl-1,2-ethenediyl)bis-, bis(dihydrogen phosphate), (E)-.

Molecular formula:

Diethylstilbestrol—$C_{18}H_{20}O_2$.

Diethylstilbestrol diphosphate—$C_{18}H_{22}O_8P_2$.

Molecular weight:

Diethylstilbestrol—268.35.

Diethylstilbestrol diphosphate—428.31.

Description:

Diethylstilbestrol USP—White, odorless, crystalline powder.

Diethylstilbestrol Diphosphate USP—Off-white, odorless, crystalline powder.

Diethylstilbestrol Diphosphate Injection USP—Colorless to light, straw-colored liquid.

Solubility:

Diethylstilbestrol USP—Practically insoluble in water; soluble in alcohol, in chloroform, in ether, in fatty oils, and in dilute alkali hydroxides.

Diethylstilbestrol Diphosphate USP—Sparingly soluble in water; soluble in alcohol and in dilute alkali.

USP requirements:

Diethylstilbestrol USP—Preserve in tight, light-resistant containers. Contains not less than 97.0% and not more than 100.5% of diethylstilbestrol, calculated on the dried basis. Meets the requirements for Identification, Melting range (169–175 °C, not more than 4 °C between beginning and end of melting), Acidity and alkalinity, Loss on drying (not more than 0.5%), Residue on ignition (not more than 0.05%), and Organic volatile impurities.

Diethylstilbestrol Injection USP—Preserve in light-resistant, single-dose or multiple-dose containers, preferably of Type I glass. A sterile solution of Diethylstilbestrol in a suitable vegetable oil. Contains the labeled amount, within ± 10%. Meets the requirements for Identification, Bacterial endotoxins, and Injections.

Diethylstilbestrol Tablets USP—Preserve in well-closed containers. Contain the labeled amount, within ± 10%. Meet the requirements for Identification, Disintegration (30 minutes), and Uniformity of dosage units.

Diethylstilbestrol Diphosphate USP—Preserve in tight containers, at a temperature not exceeding 21 °C. Contains not less than 95.0% and not more than 101.0% of diethylstilbestrol diphosphate, calculated on the dried basis. Meets the requirements for Identification, Loss on drying (not more than 1.0%), Chloride (not more than 1.5%), Free diethylstilbestrol (not more than 0.15%), Diethylstilbestrol monophosphate (not more than 1.5%), Pyridine (absorbance not more than 0.5%), and Organic volatile impurities.

Diethylstilbestrol Diphosphate Injection USP—Preserve in single-dose or in multiple-dose containers. A sterile, buffered solution of Diethylstilbestrol Diphosphate. Contains not less than 45.0 mg and not more than 55.0 mg of diethylstilbestrol diphosphate in each mL. Meets the requirements for Identification, Bacterial endotoxins, pH (9.0–10.5), Free diethylstilbestrol (not more than 0.2 mg per mL of Injection), Diethylstilbestrol monophosphate (not more than 2.0 mg per mL of Injection), and Injections.

Diethylstilbestrol Diphosphate Tablets—Not in USP.

DIETHYLSTILBESTROL AND METHYLTESTOSTERONE

For *Diethylstilbestrol* and *Methyltestosterone*—See individual listings for chemistry information.

USP requirements: Diethylstilbestrol and Methyltestosterone Tablets—Not in USP.

DIETHYLTOLUAMIDE

Chemical name: Benzamide, *N,N*-diethyl-3-methyl-.

Molecular formula: $C_{12}H_{17}NO$.

Molecular weight: 191.27.

Description: Diethyltoluamide USP—Colorless liquid, having a faint, pleasant odor. Boils at about 111 °C under a pressure of 1 mm of mercury.

Solubility: Diethyltoluamide USP—Practically insoluble in water and in glycerin. Miscible with alcohol, with isopropyl alcohol, with ether, with chloroform, and with carbon disulfide.

USP requirements:

Diethyltoluamide USP—Preserve in tight containers. Contains not less than 95.0% and not more than 103.0% of the *meta*-isomer of diethyltoluamide, calculated on the

anhydrous basis. Meets the requirements for Identification, Specific gravity (0.996–1.002), Refractive index (1.520–1.524), Acidity, and Water (not more than 0.5%).

Diethyltoluamide Topical Solution USP—Preserve in tight containers. A solution of Diethyltoluamide in Alcohol or Isopropyl Alcohol. Contains the labeled amount of the meta isomer of diethyltoluamide, within ± 8%. If it contains Alcohol, contains the labeled amount of alcohol, within ± 5%. Meets the requirements for Identification and Alcohol content (if present, 29.0–89.0%).

DIFENOXIN AND ATROPINE

Source: Atropine—Naturally occurring alkaloid. The naturally occurring belladonna alkaloids are found in various solanaceous plants, including *Atropa belladonna, Datura stamonium,* and *Duboisia myoporoides.* The active alkaloids of belladonna include hyoscyamine (which racemizes to atropine on extraction) and scopolamine (hyoscine). Hyoscyamine, the levoisomer of atropine, is the major active alkaloid of belladonna.

Chemical group:

Atropine—Natural tertiary amine; an aminoalcohol ester.
Difenoxin—Diphenoxylic acid, principal active metabolite of diphenoxylate.

Chemical name:

Atropine sulfate—Benzeneacetic acid, alpha-(hydroxymethyl)-, 8-methyl-8-azabicyclo[3.2.1]oct-3-yl ester, *endo*-(±)-, sulfate (2:1) (salt), monohydrate.
Difenoxin hydrochloride—1-(3-Cyano-3,3-diphenylpropyl)-4-phenyl-4-piperidinecarboxylic acid monohydrochloride.

Molecular formula:

Atropine sulfate—$(C_{17}H_{23}NO_3)_2 \cdot H_2SO_4 \cdot H_2O$.
Difenoxin hydrochloride—$C_{28}H_{28}N_2O_2 \cdot HCl$.

Molecular weight:

Atropine sulfate—694.84.
Difenoxin hydrochloride—461.0.

Description:

Atropine Sulfate USP—Colorless crystals, or white, crystalline powder. Odorless; effloresces in dry air; is slowly affected by light.
Difenoxin hydrochloride—White amorphous powder. It has a melting point of 290 °C.

Solubility:

Atropine Sulfate USP—Very soluble in water; freely soluble in alcohol and even more so in boiling alcohol; freely soluble in glycerin.
Difenoxin hydrochloride—Very slightly soluble in water; sparingly soluble in chloroform, in tetrahydrofuran, in dimethylacetamide, and in dimethyl sulfoxide.

USP requirements: Difenoxin Hydrochloride and Atropine Sulfate Tablets—Not in USP.

DIFLORASONE

Chemical name: Diflorasone diacetate—Pregna-1,4-diene-3,20-dione, 17,21-bis(acetyloxy)-6,9-difluoro-11-hydroxy-16-methyl-, (6 alpha,11 beta,16 beta)-.

Molecular formula: Diflorasone diacetate—$C_{26}H_{32}F_2O_7$.

Molecular weight: Diflorasone diacetate—494.53.

Description: Diflorasone Diacetate USP—White to pale yellow, crystalline powder.

Solubility: Diflorasone Diacetate USP—Insoluble in water; soluble in methanol and in acetone; sparingly soluble in ethyl acetate; slightly soluble in toluene; very slightly soluble in ether.

USP requirements:

Diflorasone Diacetate USP—Preserve in tight containers. Contains not less than 97.0% and not more than 103.0% of diflorasone diacetate, calculated on the dried basis. Meets the requirements for Identification, Specific rotation (+58° to +68°), Loss on drying (not more than 0.5%), and Residue on ignition (not more than 0.5%).

Diflorasone Diacetate Cream USP—Preserve in collapsible tubes, preferably at controlled room temperature. Contains the labeled amount, within ±10%. Meets the requirements for Identification, Microbial limits, and Minimum fill.

Diflorasone Diacetate Ointment USP—Preserve in collapsible tubes, preferably at controlled room temperature. Contains the labeled amount, within ±10%. Meets the requirements for Identification, Microbial limits, and Minimum fill.

DIFLUCORTOLONE

Chemical name: Diflucortolone valerate—6 alpha,9 alpha-Difluoro-11 beta,21-dihydroxy-16 alpha-methylpregna-1,4-diene-3,20-dione 21-valerate.

Molecular formula: Diflucortolone valerate—$C_{27}H_{36}F_2O_5$.

Molecular weight: Diflucortolone valerate—478.6.

Description: Diflucortolone valerate—Melting point 200–205 °C.

Solubility: Diflucortolone valerate—Soluble in chloroform; slightly soluble in methyl alcohol; practically insoluble in ether.

USP requirements:

Diflucortolone Valerate Cream—Not in USP.
Diflucortolone Valerate Ointment—Not in USP.

DIFLUNISAL

Chemical group: Salicylic acid derivative. However, diflunisal is not metabolized to salicylic acid in vivo.

Chemical name: [1,1'-Biphenyl]-3-carboxylic acid, 2',4'-difluoro-4-hydroxy-.

Molecular formula: $C_{13}H_8F_2O_3$.

Molecular weight: 250.20.

Description: Diflunisal USP—White to off-white, practically odorless powder.

pKa: 3.3.

Solubility: Diflunisal USP—Freely soluble in alcohol and in methanol; soluble in acetone and in ethyl acetate; slightly soluble in chloroform, in carbon tetrachloride, and in methylene chloride; insoluble in hexane and in water.

USP requirements:

Diflunisal USP—Preserve in well-closed containers. Contains not less than 98.0% and not more than 101.5% of diflunisal, calculated on the dried basis. Meets the requirements for Identification, Loss on drying (not more than 0.3%), Residue on ignition (not more than 0.1%), Heavy metals (not more than 0.001%), Chromatographic purity, and Organic volatile impurities.

Diflunisal Tablets USP—Preserve in well-closed containers. Contain the labeled amount, within ±10%. Meet the requirements for Identification, Dissolution (80% in 30 minutes in 0.1 *M* Tris buffer [pH 7.2] in Apparatus 2 at 50 rpm), and Uniformity of dosage units.

DIGITALIS

USP requirements:

Digitalis USP—Preserve in containers that protect it from absorbing moisture. Digitalis labeled to indicate that it is to be used only in the manufacture of glycosides is exempt from the moisture and storage requirements. It is the dried leaf of *Digitalis purpurea* Linné (Fam Scrophulariaceae). The potency of Digitalis is such that, when assayed as directed, 100 mg is equivalent to not less than 1 USP Digitalis Unit. (One Digitalis Unit represents the potency of 100 mg of USP Digitalis RS.) Meets the requirements for Botanic characteristics, Acid-insoluble ash (not more than 5.0%), Foreign organic matter (not more than 2.0%), and Water (not more than 6.0%).

Note: When Digitalis is prescribed, Powdered Digitalis is to be dispensed.

Powdered Digitalis USP—Preserve in tight, light-resistant containers. A package of suitable desiccant may be enclosed in the container. It is Digitalis dried at a temperature not exceeding 60 °C, reduced to a fine or a very fine powder, and adjusted, if necessary to conform to the official potency by admixture with sufficient Lactose, Starch or exhausted marc of digitalis, or with Powdered Digitalis having either a lower or a higher potency. The potency of Powdered Digitalis is such that, when assayed as directed, 100 mg is equivalent to 1 USP Digitalis Unit. (One Digitalis Unit represents the potency of 100 mg of USP Digitalis RS.) Meets the requirements for Identification, Microbial limit, Acid-insoluble ash (not more than 5.0%), and Water (not more than 5.0%).

Digitalis Capsules USP—Preserve in tight containers. Contain an amount of Powdered Digitalis equivalent to the labeled potency, within −15% to +20%. Meet the requirements for Microbial limit and Uniformity of dosage units.

Digitalis Tablets USP—Preserve in tight containers. Contain an amount of Powdered Digitalis equivalent to the labeled potency, within −15% to +20%. Meet the requirements for Disintegration (30 minutes), Microbial limit, and Uniformity of dosage units.

DIGITOXIN

Source: Obtained naturally from *Digitalis purpurea* (digitoxin, digitalis) and *Digitalis lanata* (digoxin, digitoxin, deslanoside) or may be produced synthetically.

Chemical name: Card-20(22)-enolide, 3-[(*O*-2,6-dideoxy-beta-D-*ribo*-hexopyranosyl-(1→4)-*O*-2,6-dideoxy-beta-D-*ribo*-hexopyranosyl-(1→4)-2,6-dideoxy-beta-D-*ribo*-hexopyranosyl)-oxy]-14-hydroxy, (3 beta,5 beta)-.

Molecular formula: $C_{41}H_{64}O_{13}$.

Molecular weight: 764.95.

Description: Digitoxin USP—White or pale buff, odorless, microcrystalline powder.

Solubility: Digitoxin USP—Practically insoluble in water; sparingly soluble in chloroform; slightly soluble in alcohol; very slightly soluble in ether.

USP requirements:

Digitoxin USP—Preserve in tight containers. A cardiotonic glycoside obtained from *Digitalis purpurea* Linné, *Digitalis lanata* Ehrhart (Fam. Scrophulariaceae), and other suitable species of *Digitalis*. Contains not less than 92.0% and not more than 103.0% of digitoxin, calculated on the dried basis. Meets the requirements for Identification, Loss on drying (not more than 1.5%), and Residue on ignition.

Caution: Handle Digitoxin with exceptional care since it is highly potent.

Digitoxin Capsules—Not in USP.

Digitoxin Injection USP—Preserve in single-dose or in multiple-dose containers, preferably of Type I glass, protected from light. A sterile solution of Digitoxin in 5 to 50% (v/v) of alcohol, and may contain Glycerin or other suitable solubilizing agents. Contains the labeled amount, within ±10%. Meets the requirements for Identification, Bacterial endotoxins, Alcohol content (90.0–110.0% of labeled percentage of alcohol), and Injections.

Digitoxin Tablets USP—Preserve in well-closed containers. Contain the labeled amount, within ±10%. Meet the requirements for Identification, Dissolution (60% dissolved in 30 minutes and 85% dissolved in 60 minutes in dilute hydrochloric acid [3 in 500] in Apparatus 1 at 120 ± 5 rpm), and Uniformity of dosage units.

Note: Avoid the use of strongly adsorbing substances, such as bentonite, in the manufacture of Digitoxin Tablets.

DIGOXIN

Source: Obtained naturally from *Digitalis lanata* or may be produced synthetically.

Chemical name: Card-20(22)-enolide, 3-[(O-2,6-dideoxy-beta-D-ribo-hexopyranosyl-(1→4)-O-2,6-dideoxy-beta-D-ribo-hexopyranosyl-(1→4)-2,6-dideoxy-beta-D-ribo-hexopyranosyl)oxy]-12,14-dihydroxy-, (3 beta,5 beta,12 beta)-.

Molecular formula: $C_{41}H_{64}O_{14}$.

Molecular weight: 780.95.

Description: Digoxin USP—Clear to white, odorless crystals or white, odorless crystalline powder.

Solubility: Digoxin USP—Practically insoluble in water and in ether; freely soluble in pyridine; slightly soluble in diluted alcohol and in chloroform.

USP requirements:

Digoxin USP—Preserve in tight containers. A cardiotonic glycoside obtained from the leaves of *Digitalis lanata* Ehrhart (Fam. Scrophulariaceae). Contains not less than 95.0% and not more than 101.0% of digoxin, calculated on the dried basis. Meets the requirements for Identification, Loss on drying (not more than 1.0%), Residue on ignition (not more than 0.5%), and Related glycosides (not more than 3.0%).

Caution: Handle Digoxin with exceptional care, since it is extremely poisonous.

Digoxin Capsules—Not in USP.

Digoxin Elixir USP—Preserve in tight containers, and avoid exposure to excessive heat. Contains, in each 100 mL, not less than 4.50 mg and not more than 5.25 mg of digoxin. Meets the requirements for Identification and Alcohol content (9.0–11.5%).

Digoxin Injection USP—Preserve in single-dose containers, preferably of Type I glass. Avoid exposure to excessive heat. A sterile solution of Digoxin in Water for Injection and Alcohol or other suitable solvents. Contains the labeled amount, within −10% to +5%. Meets the requirements for Identification, Bacterial endotoxins, Alcohol content (9.0–11.0%), and Injections.

Digoxin Tablets USP—Preserve in tight containers. Contain the labeled amount, within −10% to +5%. Meet the requirements for Identification, Dissolution (65% for not fewer than eleven-twelfths of the Tablets tested, and 55% for any individual Tablet, in 60 minutes in 0.1 N hydrochloric acid in Apparatus 1 at 120 rpm), and Uniformity of dosage units.

DIGOXIN IMMUNE FAB (OVINE)

Source: Produced by a process involving immunization of sheep with digoxin that has been coupled as a hapten to human serum albumin, to stimulate production of digoxin-specific antibodies. After papain digestion of the antibody, digoxin-specific antigen binding (Fab) fragments (molecular weight 50,000 daltons) are isolated and purified by affinity chromatography.

Molecular weight: 50,000.

Description: Sterile, lyophilized powder.

USP requirements: Digoxin Immune Fab (Ovine) for Injection—Not in USP.

DIHYDROCODEINE

Chemical name: Dihydrocodeine bitartrate—Morphinan-6-ol, 4,5-epoxy-3-methoxy-17-methyl-, (5 alpha,6 alpha)-2,3-dihydroxybutanedioate (1:1) (salt).

Molecular formula: Dihydrocodeine bitartrate—$C_{18}H_{23}NO_3\cdot C_4H_6O_6$.

Molecular weight: Dihydrocodeine bitartrate—451.47.

Description: Dihydrocodeine bitartrate—Odorless, or almost odorless, colorless crystals or white crystalline powder.

Solubility: Dihydrocodeine bitartrate—Soluble in water; sparingly soluble in alcohol; practically insoluble in ether.

Other characteristics: Dihydrocodeine bitartrate—A 10% solution in water has a pH of 3.2–4.2.

USP requirements: Dihydrocodeine Bitartrate USP—Preserve in tight containers. Contains not less than 98.5% and not more than 100.5% of dihydrocodeine bitartrate, calculated on the dried basis. Meets the requirements for Identification, Melting range (186–190 °C, not more than 2.5 °C between beginning and end of melting), Specific rotation (−72° to −75°, calculated on the dried basis), pH (3.0–3.5, in a solution [1 in 20]), Loss on drying (not more than 0.5%), Residue on ignition (not more than 0.1%), Ammonium salts, and Ordinary impurities.

DIHYDROCODEINE, ACETAMINOPHEN, AND CAFFEINE

For *Dihydrocodeine, Acetaminophen,* and *Caffeine*—See individual listings for chemistry information.

USP requirements: Dihydrocodeine Bitartrate, Acetaminophen, and Caffeine Capsules—Not in USP.

DIHYDROERGOTAMINE

Chemical name: Dihydroergotamine mesylate—Ergotaman-3′,6′,18-trione,9,10-dihydro-12′-hydroxy-2′-methyl-5′-(phenylmethyl)-, (5′ alpha)-, monomethanesulfonate (salt).

Molecular formula: Dihydroergotamine mesylate—$C_{33}H_{37}N_5$-$O_5 \cdot CH_4O_3S$.

Molecular weight: Dihydroergotamine mesylate—679.79.

Description: Dihydroergotamine Mesylate USP—White to slightly yellowish powder, or off-white to faintly red powder, having a faint odor.

pKa: 6.75.

Solubility: Dihydroergotamine Mesylate USP—Slightly soluble in water and in chloroform; soluble in alcohol.

USP requirements: Dihydroergotamine Mesylate Injection USP—Preserve in single-dose containers, preferably of Type I glass, protected from light. A sterile solution of Dihydroergotamine Mesylate in Water for Injection. Contains the labeled amount, within ±10%. Meets the requirements for Identification, pH (3.2–4.0), and Injections.

DIHYDROERGOTAMINE, HEPARIN, AND LIDOCAINE

For *Dihydroergotamine*, *Heparin*, and *Lidocaine*—See individual listings for chemistry information.

USP requirements: Dihydroergotamine Mesylate, Heparin Sodium, and Lidocaine Hydrochloride Injection USP—Preserve in single-dose or in multiple-dose containers, preferably of Type I glass. A sterile solution of Dihydroergotamine Mesylate, Heparin Sodium, and Lidocaine Hydrochloride in Water for Injection. Contains the labeled amounts of dihydroergotamine mesylate and lidocaine hydrochloride, within ±10%, and exhibits the labeled potency of heparin, within ±10%, stated on the label in terms of USP Heparin Units. Meets the requirements for Identification, Bacterial endotoxins, pH (5.0–6.5, determined on a portion diluted with an equal volume of potassium nitrate solution [1 in 100]), and Injections.

Note: Heparin Units are consistently established on the basis of the Assay set forth in *USP*, independently of International Units, and the respective units are not equivalent.

DIHYDROSTREPTOMYCIN

Chemical name: Dihydrostreptomycin sulfate—Dihydrostreptomycinium sulfate(2:3)(salt).

Molecular formula: Dihydrostreptomycin sulfate—$(C_{21}H_{41}N_7O_{12})_2 \cdot 3H_2SO_4$.

Molecular weight: Dihydrostreptomycin sulfate—1461.41.

Description: Dihydrostreptomycin Sulfate USP—White or almost white, amorphous or crystalline powder. Amorphous form is hygroscopic.

Solubility: Dihydrostreptomycin Sulfate USP—Freely soluble in water; practically insoluble in acetone, in chloroform, and in methanol.

USP requirements:
Dihydrostreptomycin Sulfate Boluses USP—Preserve in tight containers. Label Boluses to indicate that they are intended for veterinary use only. Contain an amount of dihydrostreptomycin sulfate equivalent to the labeled amount of dihydrostreptomycin, within −15% to +20%. Meet the requirement for Loss on drying (not more than 10.0%).
Dihydrostreptomycin Sulfate Injection USP—Preserve in single-dose or in multiple-dose containers. Label it to indicate that it is intended for veterinary use only. Contains an amount of dihydrostreptomycin sulfate equivalent to the labeled amount of dihydrostreptomycin, within −10%

to +20%. Contains one or more suitable preservatives. Meets the requirements for Identification, Depressor substances, Bacterial endotoxins, Sterility, and pH (5.0–8.0).
Sterile Dihydrostreptomycin Sulfate USP—Preserve in containers for Sterile Solids. It is Dihydrostreptomycin Sulfate suitable for parenteral use. Label it to indicate that it is intended for veterinary use only. If it is crystalline, it may be so labeled. Contains an amount of dihydrostreptomycin sulfate equivalent to not less than 650 mcg of dihydrostreptomycin per mg, except that if it is labeled as being crystalline contains an amount of dihydrostreptomycin sulfate equivalent to not less than 725 mcg of dihydrostreptomycin per mg. Meets the requirements for Depressor substances, Bacterial endotoxins, and Sterility, and for Identification tests, Crystallinity, pH (4.5–7.0), Loss on drying (not more than 14.0%), and Streptomycin (not more than 5.0%) under Dihydrostreptomycin Sulfate.

DIHYDROTACHYSTEROL

Chemical name: 9,10-Secoergosta-5,7,22-trien-3-ol, (3 beta,-5E,7E,10 alpha,22E)-.

Molecular formula: $C_{28}H_{46}O$.

Molecular weight: 398.67.

Description: Dihydrotachysterol USP—Colorless or white, odorless crystals, or white, odorless, crystalline powder.

Solubility: Dihydrotachysterol USP—Practically insoluble in water; soluble in alcohol; freely soluble in ether and in chloroform; sparingly soluble in vegetable oils.

USP requirements:
Dihydrotachysterol Capsules USP—Preserve in well-closed, light-resistant containers. Contain a solution of Dihydrotachysterol in a suitable vegetable oil. Contain the labeled amount, within ±10%. Meet the requirements for Identification and Uniformity of dosage units.
Dihydrotachysterol Oral Solution USP—Preserve in tight, light-resistant glass containers. Contains the labeled amount, within ±10%. Meets the requirement for Identification.
Dihydrotachysterol Tablets USP—Preserve in well-closed, light-resistant containers. Contain the labeled amount, within ±10%. Meet the requirements for Identification, Disintegration (10 minutes), and Uniformity of dosage units.

DIHYDROXYALUMINUM AMINOACETATE

Source: A basic salt of aluminum and glycine.

Chemical name: Aluminum, (glycinato-N,O)dihydroxy-, hydrate.

Molecular formula: $C_2H_6AlNO_4 \cdot xH_2O$.

Molecular weight: 135.06 (anhydrous).

Description:
Dihydroxyaluminum Aminoacetate USP—White, odorless powder.
Dihydroxyaluminum Aminoacetate Magma USP—White, viscous suspension, from which small amounts of water may separate on standing.

Solubility: Dihydroxyaluminum Aminoacetate USP—Insoluble in water and in organic solvents; soluble in dilute mineral acids and in solutions of fixed alkalies.

USP requirements:

Dihydroxyaluminum Aminoacetate Capsules USP—Preserve in well-closed containers. Contain the labeled amount, within ±10%. Meet the requirements for Identification, Disintegration (10 minutes, in simulated gastric fluid TS), Uniformity of dosage units, Acid-neutralizing capacity (not less than 5 mEq of acid consumed by minimum single dose recommended in labeling), and pH (6.5–7.5, in a suspension of Capsule powder equivalent to about 1 gram of dihydroxyaluminum aminoacetate in 25 mL of water).

Dihydroxyaluminum Aminoacetate Magma USP—Preserve in tight containers, and protect from freezing. A suspension that contains the labeled amount, within ±10%. Meets the requirements for Identification, Microbial limits, Acid-neutralizing capacity, and pH (6.5–7.5, in a dilution in water, equivalent to about 1 gram of dihydroxyaluminum aminoacetate in 25 mL).

Dihydroxyaluminum Aminoacetate Tablets USP—Preserve in well-closed containers. Contain the labeled amount, within ±10%. Meet the requirements for Identification, Disintegration (10 minutes in simulated gastric fluid TS), Acid-neutralizing capacity, pH (6.5–7.5, in a suspension of ground Tablet powder in water, equivalent to about 1 gram of dihydroxyaluminum aminoacetate in 25 mL of water), and Uniformity of dosage units.

DIHYDROXYALUMINUM SODIUM CARBONATE

Chemical name: Aluminum, [carbonato(1-)-O]dihydroxy-, monosodium salt.

Molecular formula: $NaAl(OH)_2CO_3$.

Molecular weight: 144.00.

Description: Dihydroxyaluminum Sodium Carbonate USP—Fine, white, odorless powder.

Solubility: Dihydroxyaluminum Sodium Carbonate USP—Practically insoluble in water and in organic solvents; soluble in dilute mineral acids with the evolution of carbon dioxide.

USP requirements: Dihydroxyaluminum Sodium Carbonate Tablets USP—Preserve in well-closed containers. Label the Tablets to indicate that they are to be chewed before swallowing. Contain the labeled amount, within ±10%. Meet the requirements for Identification, Acid-neutralizing capacity, and Uniformity of dosage units.

DIISOPROPANOLAMINE

Chemical name: 2-Propanol, 1,1′-iminobis-.

Molecular formula: $C_6H_{15}NO_2$.

Molecular weight: 133.19.

Description: Diisopropanolamine NF—NF category: Alkalizing agent.

NF requirements: Diisopropanolamine NF—Preserve in tight, light-resistant containers. A mixture of isopropanolamines, consisting largely of diisopropanolamine. Contains not less than 98.0% and not more than 102.0% of isopropanolamines, calculated on the anhydrous basis. Meets the requirements for Identification, Water (not more than 0.50%), Triisopropanolamine (not more than 1.0%), and Organic volatile impurities.

DILTIAZEM

Chemical name: Diltiazem hydrochloride—1,5-Benzothiazepin-4(5H)one, 3-(acetyloxy)-5-[2-(dimethylamino)ethyl]-2,3-dihydro-2-(4-methoxyphenyl)-, monohydrochloride, (+)-cis-.

Molecular formula: Diltiazem hydrochloride—$C_{22}H_{26}N_2O_4S \cdot HCl$.

Molecular weight: Diltiazem hydrochloride—450.98.

Description: Diltiazem Hydrochloride USP— White, odorless, crystalline powder or small crystals. Melts at about 210 °C, with decompostion.

Solubility: Diltiazem Hydrochloride USP—Freely soluble in chloroform, in formic acid, in methanol, and in water; sparingly soluble in dehydrated alcohol; insoluble in ether.

USP requirements:

Diltiazem Extended-release Capsules USP—Preserve in tight containers. Label Extended-release Capsules to state both the content of the active moiety and the content of the diltiazem salt used in formulating the article. Contain the labeled amount of Diltiazem Hydrochloride, within ±10%. Meet the requirements for Identification and Uniformity of dosage units.

Diltiazem Injection—Not in USP.

Diltiazem Tablets USP—Preserve in tight, light-resistant containers. Label Tablets to state both the content of the active moiety and the content of the diltiazem salt used in formulating the article. Contain the labeled amount of diltiazem hydrochloride, within ±10%. Meet the requirements for Identification and Uniformity of dosage units.

DIMENHYDRINATE

Chemical group: Ethanolamine derivative.

Chemical name: 1H-Purine-2,6-dione, 8-chloro-3,7-dihydro-1,3-dimethyl-, compd. with 2-(diphenylmethoxy)-N,N-dimethylethanamine (1:1).

Molecular formula: $C_{17}H_{21}NO \cdot C_7H_7ClN_4O_2$.

Molecular weight: 469.97.

Description: Dimenhydrinate USP—White, crystalline, odorless powder.

Solubility: Dimenhydrinate USP—Slightly soluble in water; freely soluble in alcohol and in chloroform; sparingly soluble in ether.

USP requirements:

Dimenhydrinate Capsules—Not in USP.

Dimenhydrinate Extended-release Capsules—Not in USP.

Dimenhydrinate Elixir—Not in USP.

Dimenhydrinate Injection USP—Preserve in single-dose or in multiple-dose containers, preferably of Type I or Type III glass. A solution of Dimenhydrinate in a mixture of Propylene Glycol and water. Contains the labeled amount, within ±5%. Meets the requirements for Identification, pH (6.4–7.2), 8-Chlorotheophylline content, and Injections.

Dimenhydrinate Suppositories—Not in USP.

Dimenhydrinate Syrup USP—Preserve in tight containers. Contains the labeled amount, within ±6%. Meets the requirements for Identification, Alcohol content (4.0–6.0%), and 8-Chlorotheophylline content.

Dimenhydrinate Tablets USP—Preserve in well-closed containers. Contain the labeled amount, within ±5%. Meet the requirements for Identification, Dissolution (75% in 45 minutes in water in Apparatus 2 at 50 rpm), Uniformity of dosage units, and 8-Chlorotheophylline content.

DIMERCAPROL

Chemical group: Dithiol.

Chemical name: 1-Propanol, 2,3-dimercapto.

Molecular formula: $C_3H_8OS_2$.

Molecular weight: 124.22.

Description:

Dimercaprol USP—Colorless or practically colorless liquid, having a disagreeable, mercaptan-like odor.

Dimercaprol Injection USP—Yellow, viscous solution having a pungent, disagreeable odor. Specific gravity is about 0.978.

Solubility: Dimercaprol USP—Soluble in water, in alcohol, in benzyl benzoate, and in methanol.

USP requirements: Dimercaprol Injection USP—Preserve in single-dose or in multiple-dose containers, preferably of Type I or Type III glass. A sterile solution of Dimercaprol in a mixture of Benzyl Benzoate and vegetable oil. Contains, in each 100 grams, not less than 9.0 grams and not more than 11.0 grams of dimercaprol. Meets the requirements for 1,2,3-Trimercaptopropane and related impurities and Injections, except that at times it may be turbid or contain small amounts of flocculent material.

DIMETHICONE

Chemical name: Dimethicone.

Description: Dimethicone NF—Clear, colorless, odorless liquid. NF category: Antifoaming agent; water repelling agent.

Solubility: Dimethicone NF—Insoluble in water, in methanol, in alcohol, and in acetone; very slightly soluble in isopropyl alcohol; soluble in chlorinated hydrocarbons, in toluene, in xylene, in *n*-hexane, in petroleum spirits, in ether, and in amyl acetate.

NF requirements: Dimethicone NF—Preserve in tight containers. A mixture of fully methylated linear siloxane polymers containing repeating units of the formula $[-(CH_3)_2SiO-]_n$, stabilized with trimethylsiloxy endblocking units of the formula $[(CH_3)_3SiO-]$, wherein *n* has an average value such that the corresponding nominal viscosity is in a discrete range between 20 and 12,500 centistokes. Label it to indicate its nominal viscosity value. Dimethicone intended for use in coating containers that come in contact with articles for parenteral use is so labeled. Contains not less than 97.0% and not more than 103.0% of polydimethylsiloxane. The requirements for viscosity, specific gravity, refractive index, and loss on heating differ for the several types of Dimethicone. Meets the requirements for Identification, Specific gravity, Viscosity, Refractive index, Acidity, Loss on heating, and Heavy metals (not more than 0.001%). Additionally, Dimethicone intended for use in coating containers that come in contact with articles for parenteral use meets the requirements for Pyrogen and Biological suitability.

DIMETHYL SULFOXIDE

Chemical name: Methane, sulfinylbis-.

Molecular formula: C_2H_6OS.

Molecular weight: 78.13.

Description: Dimethyl Sulfoxide USP—Clear, colorless, odorless, hygroscopic liquid. Melts at about 18.4 °C. Boils at about 189 °C.

Solubility: Dimethyl Sulfoxide USP—Soluble in water; practically insoluble in acetone, in alcohol, in chloroform, and in ether.

USP requirements:

Dimethyl Sulfoxide Irrigation USP—Preserve in single-dose containers, and store at controlled room temperature, protected from strong light. A sterile solution of Dimethyl Sulfoxide in Water for Injection. Label it to indicate prominently that it is not intended for injection. Contains the labeled amount, within ± 5%. Meets the requirements for Identification, Bacterial endotoxins, Sterility, and pH (5.0–7.0, when diluted with water to obtain a solution containing 50 mg of dimethyl sulfoxide per mL).

Dimethyl Sulfoxide Gel—Not in USP.

Dimethyl Sulfoxide Solution—Not in USP.

DINOPROST

Source: Dinoprost tromethamine is the tromethamine salt of naturally occurring prostaglandin $F_{2\text{-alpha}}$.

Chemical name: Dinoprost tromethamine—Prosta-5,13-dien-1-oic acid, 9,11,15-trihydroxy-, (5*Z*,9 alpha,11 alpha,13*E*,-15*S*)-, compd. with 2-amino-2-(hydroxymethyl)-1,3-propanediol (1:1).

Molecular formula: Dinoprost tromethamine—$C_{20}H_{34}O_5 \cdot C_4H_{11}NO_3$.

Molecular weight: Dinoprost tromethamine—475.62.

Description: Dinoprost Tromethamine USP—White to off-white, crystalline powder.

Solubility: Dinoprost Tromethamine USP—Very soluble in water; freely soluble in dimethylformamide; soluble in methanol; slightly soluble in chloroform.

USP requirements: Dinoprost Tromethamine Injection USP—Preserve in single-dose or in multiple-dose containers, preferably of Type I glass. A sterile solution of Dinoprost Tromethamine in Water for Injection. Contains an amount of dinoprost tromethamine equivalent to the labeled amount of dinoprost, within ± 10%. Meets the requirements for Identification, Bacterial endotoxins, pH (7.0–9.0), and Injections, and for Sterility tests.

DINOPROSTONE

Source: Dinoprostone is the naturally occurring prostaglandin E_2.

Chemical name: Prosta-5,13-dien-1-oic acid, 11,15-dihydroxy-9-oxo-, (5*Z*,11 alpha,13*E*,15*S*)-.

Molecular formula: $C_{20}H_{32}O_5$.

Molecular weight: 352.47.

Description: White crystalline powder. Melting point 64–71 °C.

Solubility: Soluble in ethanol and in 25% ethanol in water; soluble in water to the extent of 130 mg/100 mL.

USP requirements:

Dinoprostone Cervical Gel—Not in USP.

Dinoprostone Vaginal Suppositories—Not in USP.

DIOXYBENZONE AND OXYBENZONE

Chemical name:

Dioxybenzone—Methanone, (2-hydroxy-4-methoxyphenyl)(2-hydroxyphenyl)-.

Oxybenzone—Methanone, (2-hydroxy-4-methoxyphenyl)phenyl-.

Molecular formula:
Dioxybenzone—$C_{14}H_{12}O_4$.
Oxybenzone—$C_{14}H_{12}O_3$.

Molecular weight:
Dioxybenzone—244.25.
Oxybenzone—228.25.

Description:
Dioxybenzone USP—Yellow powder.
Oxybenzone USP—Pale yellow powder.

Solubility:
Dioxybenzone USP—Practically insoluble in water; freely soluble in alcohol and in toluene.
Oxybenzone USP—Practically insoluble in water; freely soluble in alcohol and in toluene.

USP requirements: Dioxybenzone and Oxybenzone Cream USP—Preserve in tight containers. A mixture of approximately equal parts of Dioxybenzone and Oxybenzone in a suitable cream base. Contains, in each 100 grams, not less than 2.7 grams and not more than 3.3 grams each of dioxybenzone and oxybenzone. Meets the requirements for Identification and Minimum fill.

DIPERODON

Chemical name: 1,2-Propanediol, 3-(1-piperidinyl)-, bis(phenylcarbamate) (ester), monohydrate.

Molecular formula: $C_{22}H_{27}N_3O_4 \cdot H_2O$.

Molecular weight: 415.49.

Description: Diperodon USP—White to cream-colored powder having a characteristic odor.

Solubility: Diperodon USP—Insoluble in water.

USP requirements: Diperodon Ointment USP—Preserve in collapsible tubes or in tight containers. Contains an amount of diperodon equivalent to the labeled amount of anhydrous diperodon, within ±10%, in a suitable ointment base. Meets the requirements for Identification and Minimum fill.

DIPHEMANIL

Chemical name: Diphemanil methylsulfate—Piperidinium, 4-(diphenylmethylene)-1,1-dimethyl-, methyl sulfate.

Molecular formula: Diphemanil methylsulfate—$C_{21}H_{27}NO_4S$.

Molecular weight Diphemanil methylsulfate—389.51.

Description: Diphemanil Methylsulfate USP—White or nearly white, crystalline solid, having a a faint characteristic odor. Is stable to heat and to light, and is somewhat hygroscopic.

Solubility: Diphemanil Methylsulfate USP—Sparingly soluble in water, in alcohol, and in chloroform.

USP requirements: Diphemanil Methylsulfate Tablets USP—Preserve in tight containers. Contain the labeled amount, within ±7.5%. Meet the requirements for Identification, Dissolution (80% in 30 minutes in water in Apparatus 1 at 100 rpm), and Uniformity of dosage units.

DIPHENHYDRAMINE

Chemical group: Ethanolamine derivative.

Chemical name:
Diphenhydramine citrate—Ethanamine, 2-(diphenylmethoxy)-*N,N*-dimethyl-, 2-hydroxy-1,2,3-propanetricarboxylate (1:1).

Diphenhydramine hydrochloride—Ethanamine, 2-(diphenylmethoxy)-*N,N*-dimethyl-, hydrochloride.

Molecular formula:
Diphenhydramine citrate—$C_{17}H_{21}NO \cdot C_6H_8O_7$.
Diphenhydramine hydrochloride—$C_{17}H_{21}NO \cdot HCl$.

Molecular weight:
Diphenhydramine citrate—447.49.
Diphenhydramine hydrochloride—291.82.

Description: Diphenhydramine Hydrochloride USP—White, odorless, crystalline powder. Slowly darkens on exposure to light. Its solutions are practically neutral to litmus.

pKa: Diphenhydramine hydrochloride—9.

Solubility: Diphenhydramine Hydrochloride USP—Freely soluble in water, in alcohol, and in chloroform; sparingly soluble in acetone; very slightly soluble in ether.

USP requirements:
Diphenhydramine Hydrochloride Capsules USP—Preserve in tight containers. Contain the labeled amount, within ±10%. Meet the requirements for Identification, Dissolution (75% in 45 minutes in water in Apparatus 1 at 100 rpm), and Uniformity of dosage units.
Diphenhydramine Hydrochloride Elixir USP—Preserve in tight, light-resistant containers. Contains the labeled amount, within ±10%. Meets the requirements for Identification and Alcohol content (12.0–15.0%).
Diphenhydramine Hydrochloride Injection USP—Preserve in single-dose or in multiple-dose containers, preferably of Type I glass, protected from light. A sterile solution of Diphenhydramine Hydrochloride in Water for Injection. Contains the labeled amount, within ±10%. Meets the requirements for Identification, Bacterial endotoxins, pH (4.0–6.5), and Injections.
Diphenhydramine Hydrochloride Syrup—Not in USP.
Diphenyhydramine Hydrochloride Tablets—Not in USP.

DIPHENHYDRAMINE, CODEINE, AND AMMONIUM CHLORIDE

For *Diphenhydramine*, *Codeine*, and *Ammonium Chloride*—See individual listings for chemistry information.

USP requirements: Diphenhydramine Hydrochloride, Codeine Phosphate, and Ammonium Chloride Syrup—Not in USP.

DIPHENHYDRAMINE, DEXTROMETHORPHAN, AND AMMONIUM CHLORIDE

For *Diphenhydramine*, *Dextromethorphan*, and *Ammonium Chloride*—See individual listings for chemistry information.

USP requirements: Diphenhydramine Hydrochloride, Dextromethorphan Hydrobromide, and Ammonium Chloride Syrup—Not in USP.

DIPHENHYDRAMINE, PHENYLPROPANOLAMINE, AND ASPIRIN

For *Diphenhydramine*, *Phenylpropanolamine*, and *Aspirin*—See individual listings for chemistry information.

USP requirements: Diphenhydramine Citrate, Phenylpropanolamine Bitartrate, and Aspirin Tablets for Oral Solution—Not in USP.

DIPHENHYDRAMINE AND PSEUDOEPHEDRINE

For *Diphenhydramine* and *Pseudoephedrine*—See individual listings for chemistry information.

USP requirements:
Diphenhydramine and Pseudoephedrine Capsules USP—Preserve in tight containers. Contain the labeled amounts

of diphenhydramine hydrochloride and pseudoephedrine hydrochloride, within ± 10%. Label Capsules to state both the contents of the active moieties and the contents of the salts used in formulating the article. Meet the requirements for Identification, Dissolution (75% of each active ingredient in 30 minutes in water in Apparatus 1 at 100 rpm), Uniformity of dosage units, and Related compounds (sum of amounts of benzhydrol and benzophenone not more than 2% [w/w] of diphenhydramine hydrochloride).

Diphenhydramine and Pseudoephedrine Hydrochlorides Oral Solution—Not in USP.

Diphenhydramine and Pseudoephedrine Hydrochlorides Tablets—Not in USP.

DIPHENHYDRAMINE, PSEUDOEPHEDRINE, AND ACETAMINOPHEN

For *Diphenhydramine*, *Pseudoephedrine*, and *Acetaminophen*—See individual listings for chemistry information.

USP requirements:

Diphenhydramine Hydrochloride, Pseudoephedrine Hydrochloride, and Acetaminophen Oral Solution—Not in USP.

Diphenhydramine Hydrochloride, Pseudoephedrine Hydrochloride, and Acetaminophen Tablets—Not in USP.

DIPHENHYDRAMINE, PSEUDOEPHEDRINE, DEXTROMETHORPHAN, AND ACETAMINOPHEN

For *Diphenhydramine*, *Pseudoephedrine*, *Dextromethorphan*, and *Acetaminophen*—See individual listings for chemistry information.

USP requirements: Diphenhydramine Hydrochloride, Pseudoephedrine Hydrochloride, Dextromethorphan Hydrobromide, and Acetaminophen Oral Solution—Not in USP.

DIPHENIDOL

Chemical name: Diphenidol hydrochloride—1-Piperidinebutanol, alpha,alpha-diphenyl, hydrochloride.

Molecular formula: Diphenidol hydrochloride—$C_{21}H_{27}NO \cdot HCl$.

Molecular weight: Diphenidol hydrochloride—345.91.

Description: Diphenidol hydrochloride—Melting point 212–214 °C.

Solubility: Diphenidol hydrochloride—Freely soluble in methanol; soluble in water and in chloroform; practically insoluble in ether.

USP requirements: Diphenidol Hydrochloride Tablets—Not in USP.

DIPHENOXYLATE AND ATROPINE

Chemical group:

Diphenoxylate hydrochloride—Similar in structure to meperidine.

Atropine—Natural tertiary amine; an aminoalcohol ester.

Chemical name:

Diphenoxylate hydrochloride—4-Piperidinecarboxylic acid, 1-(3-cyano-3,3-diphenylpropyl)-4-phenyl-, ethyl ester, monohydrochloride.

Atropine sulfate—Benzeneacetic acid, alpha-(hydroxymethyl)-, 8-methyl-8-azabicyclo[3.2.1]oct-3-yl ester, *endo*-(±)-, sulfate (2:1) (salt), monohydrate.

Molecular formula:

Diphenoxylate hydrochloride—$C_{30}H_{32}N_2O_2 \cdot HCl$.

Atropine sulfate—$(C_{17}H_{23}NO_3)_2 \cdot H_2SO_4 \cdot H_2O$.

Molecular weight:

Diphenoxylate hydrochloride—489.06.

Atropine sulfate—694.84.

Description:

Diphenoxylate Hydrochloride USP—White, odorless, crystalline powder. Its saturated solution has a pH of about 3.3.

Atropine Sulfate USP—Colorless crystals, or white, crystalline powder. Odorless; effloresces in dry air; is slowly affected by light.

Solubility:

Diphenoxylate Hydrochloride USP—Slightly soluble in water and in isopropanol; freely soluble in chloroform; soluble in methanol; sparingly soluble in alcohol and in acetone; practically insoluble in ether and in solvent hexane.

Atropine Sulfate USP—Very soluble in water; freely soluble in alcohol and even more so in boiling alcohol; freely soluble in glycerin.

USP requirements:

Diphenoxylate Hydrochloride and Atropine Sulfate Oral Solution USP—Preserve in tight, light-resistant containers. Contains the labeled amount of diphenoxylate hydrochloride, within ± 7%, and the labeled amount of atropine sulfate, within ± 20%. Meets the requirements for Identification, pH (3.0–4.3, determined in a dilution of the Oral Solution with an equal volume of water), and Alcohol content (13.5–16.5%).

Diphenoxylate Hydrochloride and Atropine Sulfate Tablets USP—Preserve in well-closed, light-resistant containers. Contain the labeled amount of diphenoxylate hydrochloride, within ± 5%, and the labeled amount of atropine sulfate, within ± 20%. Meet the requirements for Identification, Dissolution (75% of the labeled amount of diphenoxylate hydrochloride in 45 minutes in 0.2 *M* acetic acid in Apparatus 1 at 150 rpm), and Uniformity of dosage units.

DIPHENYLPYRALINE

Chemical group: Piperidine derivative.

Chemical name: Diphenylpyraline hydrochloride—Piperidine, 4-(diphenylmethoxy)-1-methyl-, hydrochloride.

Molecular formula: Diphenylpyraline hydrochloride—$C_{19}H_{23}NO \cdot HCl$.

Molecular weight: Diphenylpyraline hydrochloride—317.86.

Description: Diphenylpyraline hydrochloride—White or almost white, odorless or almost odorless, crystalline powder.

Solubility: Diphenylpyraline hydrochloride—Soluble 1 in 1 of water, 1 in 3 of alcohol, and 1 in 2 of chloroform; practically insoluble in ether.

USP requirements: Diphenylpyraline Hydrochloride Extended-release Capsules—Not in USP.

DIPHENYLPYRALINE, PHENYLEPHRINE, AND CODEINE

For *Diphenylpyraline*, *Phenylephrine*, and *Codeine*—See individual listings for chemistry information.

USP requirements: Diphenylpyraline Hydrochloride, Phenylephrine Hydrochloride, and Codeine Phosphate Oral Solution—Not in USP.

DIPHENYLPYRALINE, PHENYLEPHRINE, AND DEXTROMETHORPHAN

For *Diphenylpyraline*, *Phenylephrine*, and *Dextromethorphan*—See individual listings for chemistry information.

USP requirements: Diphenylpyraline Hydrochloride, Phenylephrine Hydrochloride, and Dextromethorphan Hydrobromide Syrup—Not in USP.

DIPHENYLPYRALINE, PHENYLEPHRINE, AND HYDROCODONE

For *Diphenylpyraline*, *Phenylephrine*, and *Hydrocodone*—See individual listings for chemistry information.

USP requirements:
Diphenylpyraline Hydrochloride, Phenylephrine Hydrochloride, and Hydrocodone Bitartrate Oral Solution—Not in USP.
Diphenylpyraline Hydrochloride, Phenylephrine Hydrochloride, and Hydrocodone Bitartrate Syrup—Not in USP.

DIPHENYLPYRALINE, PHENYLEPHRINE, HYDROCODONE, AND GUAIFENESIN

For *Diphenylpyraline*, *Phenylephrine*, *Hydrocodone*, and *Guaifenesin*—See individual listings for chemistry information.

USP requirements: Diphenylpyraline Hydrochloride, Phenylephrine Hydrochloride, Hydrocodone Bitartrate, and Guaifenesin Oral Solution—Not in USP.

DIPHTHERIA ANTITOXIN

Description: Diphtheria Antitoxin USP—Transparent or slightly opalescent liquid, practically colorless, and practically odorless or having an odor because of the preservative.

USP requirements: Diphtheria Antitoxin USP—Preserve at a temperature between 2 and 8 °C. A sterile, non-pyrogenic solution of the refined and concentrated proteins, chiefly globulins, containing antitoxic antibodies obtained from the blood serum or plasma of healthy horses that have been immunized against diphtheria toxin or toxoid. Label it to state that it was prepared from horse serum or plasma. Has a potency of not less than 500 antitoxin units per mL based on the U.S. Standard Diphtheria Antitoxin, and a diphtheria test toxin, tested in guinea pigs. Contains not more than 20.0% of solids. Meets the requirement for Expiration date (for Antitoxin containing a 20% excess of potency, not later than 5 years after date of issue from manufacturer's cold storage). Conforms to the regulations of the U.S. Food and Drug Administration concerning biologics.

DIPHTHERIA TOXIN FOR SCHICK TEST

Description: Diphtheria Toxin for Schick Test USP—Transparent liquid.

USP requirements: Diphtheria Toxin for Schick Test USP—Preserve at a temperature between 2 and 8 °C. A sterile solution of the diluted, standardized toxic products of growth of the diphtheria bacillus (*Corynebacterium diphtheriae*) of which the parent toxin contains not less than 400 MLD (minimum lethal doses) per mL or 400,000 MRD (minimum skin reaction doses) per mL in guinea pigs. Potency is determined in terms of the U.S. Standard Diphtheria Toxin for Schick Test, tested in guinea pigs. Meets the requirement for Expiration date (not later than 1 year after date of issue from manufacturer's cold storage [5 °C, 1 year]). Conforms to the regulations of the U.S. Food and Drug Administration concerning biologics.

DIPHTHERIA TOXOID

Description: Diphtheria Toxoid USP—Clear, brownish yellow, or slightly turbid liquid, free from evident clumps or particles, having a faint, characteristic odor.

USP requirements: Diphtheria Toxoid USP—Preserve at a temperature between 2 and 8 °C. A sterile solution of the formaldehyde-treated products of growth of the diphtheria bacillus (*Corynebacterium diphtheriae*). Label it to state that it is not to be frozen. Meets the requirements of the specific guinea pig potency and detoxification tests. Contains not more than 0.02% of residual free formaldehyde. Contains a preservative other than a phenoloid compound. Meets the requirement for Expiration date (not later than 2 years after date of issue from manufacturer's cold storage [5 °C, 1 year]). Conforms to the regulations of the U.S. Food and Drug Administration concerning biologics.

DIPHTHERIA TOXOID ADSORBED

Description: Diphtheria Toxoid Adsorbed USP—White, slightly gray, or slightly pink suspension, free from evident clumps after shaking.

USP requirements: Diphtheria Toxoid Adsorbed USP—Preserve at a temperature between 2 and 8 °C. A sterile preparation of plain diphtheria toxoid that meets all of the requirements for that product with the exception of those for antigenicity, and that has been precipitated or adsorbed by alum, aluminum hydroxide, or aluminum phosphate adjuvants. Label it to state that it is to be well shaken before use and that it is not to be frozen. Meets the requirements of the specific guinea pig antigenicity test in the production of not less than 2 units of antitoxin per mL based on the U.S. Standard Diphtheria Antitoxin and a diphtheria test toxin. Meets the requirements of the specific guinea pig detoxification test. Meets the requirements for Expiration date (not later than 2 years after date of issue from manufacturer's cold storage [5 °C, 1 year]) and Aluminum content (not more than 0.85 mg per single injection, determined by analysis, or not more than 1.14 mg calculated on the basis of the amount of aluminum compound added). Conforms to the regulations of the U.S. Food and Drug Administration concerning biologics.

DIPHTHERIA AND TETANUS TOXOIDS

Description: Diphtheria and Tetanus Toxoids USP—Clear, colorless to brownish yellow or very slightly turbid liquid, free from evident clumps or particles, having a characteristic odor.

USP requirements: Diphtheria and Tetanus Toxoids USP—Preserve at a temperature between 2 and 8 °C. A sterile solution prepared by mixing suitable quantities of fluid diphtheria toxoid and fluid tetanus toxoid. Label it to state that it is not to be frozen. The antigenicity or potency and the proportions of the toxoids are such as to provide an immunizing dose of each toxoid in the total dosage prescribed in the labeling, and each component meets the requirements for those products. Contains not more than 0.02% of residual free formaldehyde. Meets the requirement for Expiration date (not later than 2 years after date of issue from manufacturer's cold storage [5 °C, 1 year]). Conforms to the regulations of the U.S. Food and Drug Administration concerning biologics.

DIPHTHERIA AND TETANUS TOXOIDS ADSORBED

Description: Diphtheria and Tetanus Toxoids Adsorbed USP—Turbid, and white, slightly gray, or slightly pink suspension, free from evident clumps after shaking.

USP requirements: Diphtheria and Tetanus Toxoids Adsorbed USP—Preserve at a temperature between 2 and 8 °C. A sterile suspension prepared by mixing suitable quantities of plain or adsorbed diphtheria toxoid and plain or adsorbed tetanus toxoid, and an aluminum adsorbing agent if plain toxoids are used. Label it to state that it is to be well shaken before use and that it is not to be frozen. The antigenicity or potency and the proportions of the toxoids are such as to provide an immunizing dose of each toxoid in the total dosage prescribed in the labeling, and each component meets the requirements for those products. Contains not more than 0.02% of residual free formaldehyde. Meets the requirement for Expiration date (not later than 2 years after date of issue from manufacturer's cold storage [5 °C, 1 year]). Conforms to the regulations of the U.S. Food and Drug Administration concerning biologics.

DIPHTHERIA AND TETANUS TOXOIDS AND PERTUSSIS VACCINE

Description: Diphtheria and Tetanus Toxoids and Pertussis Vaccine USP—More or less turbid, whitish to light yellowish or brownish liquid, free from evident clumps after shaking, having a faint odor because of the toxoid components, the antimicrobial agent, or both.

USP requirements: Diphtheria and Tetanus Toxoids and Pertussis Vaccine USP—Preserve at a temperature between 2 and 8 °C. A sterile suspension prepared by mixing suitable quantities of pertussis vaccine component of killed pertussis bacilli (*Bordetella pertussis*), or a fraction of this organism, fluid diphtheria toxoid, and fluid tetanus toxoid. Label it to state that it is to be well shaken before use and that it is not to be frozen. The antigenicity or potency and the proportions of the components are such as to provide an immunizing dose of each product in the total dosage prescribed in the labeling, and each component meets the requirements for those products. Meets the requirement for Expiration date (not later than 18 months after date of issue from manufacturer's cold storage [5 °C, 1 year]). Conforms to the regulations of the U.S. Food and Drug Administration concerning biologics.

DIPHTHERIA AND TETANUS TOXOIDS AND PERTUSSIS VACCINE ADSORBED

Source: Diphtheria, tetanus toxoids, and pertussis vaccine consists of a mixture of the detoxified toxins (toxoids) of diphtheria and tetanus and inactivated *B. pertussis* bacteria that have been adsorbed onto an aluminum salt.

Description: Diphtheria and Tetanus Toxoids and Pertussis Vaccine Adsorbed USP—Markedly turbid, whitish liquid, free from evident clumps after shaking; nearly odorless or having a faint odor because of the preservative.

USP requirements: Diphtheria and Tetanus Toxoids and Pertussis Vaccine Adsorbed USP—Preserve at a temperature between 2 and 8 °C. A sterile suspension prepared by mixing suitable quantities of plain or adsorbed diphtheria toxoid, plain or adsorbed tetanus toxoid, plain or adsorbed pertussis vaccine, and an aluminum adsorbing agent if plain antigen components are used. Label it to state that it is to be well shaken before use and that it is not to be frozen. The antigenicity or potency and the proportions of the components are such as to provide an immunizing dose of each product in the total dosage prescribed in the labeling, and each component meets the requirements for those products. Meets the requirement for Expiration date (not later than 18 months after date of issue from manufacturer's cold storage [5 °C, 1 year]). Conforms to the regulations of the U.S. Food and Drug Administration concerning biologics.

DIPIVEFRIN

Source: Formed by the diesterification of epinephrine and pivalic acid.

Chemical name: Dipivefrin hydrochloride—Propanoic acid, 2,2-dimethyl-, 4-[1-hydroxy-2-(methylamino)ethyl]-1,2-phenylene ester, hydrochloride, (±)-.

Molecular formula: Dipivefrin hydrochloride—$C_{19}H_{29}NO_5 \cdot HCl$.

Molecular weight: Dipivefrin hydrochloride—387.90.

Description: Dipivefrin Hydrochloride USP—White, crystalline powder or small crystals, having a faint odor.

Solubility: Dipivefrin Hydrochloride USP—Very soluble in water.

USP requirements: Dipivefrin Hydrochloride Ophthalmic Solution USP—Preserve in tight, light-resistant containers. A sterile, aqueous solution of Dipivefrin Hydrochloride. Contains the labeled amount, within −10% to +15%. Contains a suitable antimicrobial agent. Meets the requirements for Identification, Sterility, and pH (2.5–3.5).

DIPYRIDAMOLE

Chemical name: Ethanol, 2,2′,2″,2‴-[(4,8-di-1-piperidinylpyrimido[5,4-*d*]pyrimidine-2,6-diyl)dinitrilo]tetrakis-.

Molecular formula: $C_{24}H_{40}N_8O_4$.

Molecular weight: 504.63.

Description: Dipyridamole USP—Intensely yellow, crystalline powder or needles.

Solubility: Dipyridamole USP—Very soluble in methanol, in alcohol, and in chloroform; slightly soluble in water; very slightly soluble in acetone and in ethyl acetate.

USP requirements:
Dipyridamole Injection—Not in USP.
Dipyridamole Tablets USP—Preserve in tight, light-resistant containers. Contain the labeled amount, within ±10%. Meet the requirements for Identification, Dissolution (70% in 30 minutes in 0.1 *N* hydrochloric acid in Apparatus 2 at 50 rpm), and Uniformity of dosage units.

DISOPYRAMIDE

Chemical name:
Disopyramide—2-Pyridineacetamide, alpha-[2-[bis(1-methylethyl)amino]ethyl]-alpha-phenyl-.
Disopyramide phosphate—2-Pyridineacetamide, alpha-[2-[bis(1-methylethyl)amino]ethyl]-alpha-phenyl-, phosphate (1:1).

Molecular formula:
Disopyramide—$C_{21}H_{29}N_3O$.
Disopyramide phosphate—$C_{21}H_{29}N_3O \cdot H_3PO_4$.

Molecular weight:
Disopyramide—339.48.
Disopyramide phosphate—437.47.

Description:
Disopyramide—White, odorless or almost odorless powder.
Disopyramide Phosphate USP—White or practically white, odorless powder. Melts at about 205 °C, with decomposition.

pKa: 8.4.

Solubility:

Disopyramide—Slightly soluble in water; soluble 1 in 10 of alcohol, 1 in 5 of chloroform, and 1 in 5 of ether.

Disopyramide Phosphate USP—Freely soluble in water; slightly soluble in alcohol; practically insoluble in chloroform and in ether.

Other characteristics: Partition coefficient—3.1 at pH 7.2 (chloroform : water, of the free base).

USP requirements:

Disopyramide Capsules—Not in USP.

Disopyramide Phosphate Capsules USP—Preserve in well-closed containers. Contain an amount of Disopyramide Phosphate equivalent to the labeled amount of disopyramide, within ±10%. Meet the requirements for Identification, Dissolution (80% in 20 minutes in water in Apparatus 2 at 50 rpm), and Uniformity of dosage units.

Disopyramide Phosphate Extended-release Capsules USP—Preserve in well-closed containers. Contain an amount of Disopyramide Phosphate equivalent to the labeled amount of disopyramide, within ±10%. Meet the requirements for Identification, Drug release (5–25% in 0.083 D hours, 17–43% in 0.167 D hours, 50–80% in 0.417 D hours, and not less than 85% in 1.000 D hours in pH 2.5, 0.1 M phosphate buffer in Apparatus 1 at 100 rpm), and Uniformity of dosage units.

Disopyramide Phosphate Extended-release Tablets—Not in USP.

DISULFIRAM

Chemical name: Thioperoxydicarbonic diamide [(H₂N)C(S)]₂S₂, tetraethyl-.

Molecular formula: $C_{10}H_{20}N_2S_4$.

Molecular weight: 296.52.

Description: Disulfiram USP—White to off-white, odorless, crystalline powder.

Solubility: Disulfiram USP—Very slightly soluble in water; soluble in acetone, in alcohol, in carbon disulfide, and in chloroform.

USP requirements: Disulfiram Tablets USP—Preserve in tight, light-resistant containers. Contain the labeled amount, within ±10%. Meet the requirements for Identification, Disintegration (15 minutes, the use of disks being omitted), and Uniformity of dosage units.

DIVALPROEX SODIUM

Chemical name: Pentanoic acid, 2-propyl-, sodium salt (2:1).

Molecular formula: $C_{16}H_{31}NaO_4$.

Molecular weight: 310.41.

Description: White powder, having a characteristic odor.

Solubility: Insoluble in water; very soluble in alcohol.

USP requirements:

Divalproex Sodium Delayed-release Capsules—Not in USP.

Divalproex Sodium Delayed-release Tablets—Not in USP.

DOBUTAMINE

Chemical group: A synthetic catecholamine.

Chemical name: Dobutamine hydrochloride—1,2-Benzenediol, 4-[2-[[3-(4-hydroxyphenyl)-1-methylpropyl]amino]ethyl]-, hydrochloride, (±)-.

Molecular formula: Dobutamine hydrochloride—$C_{18}H_{23}NO_3\cdot$HCl.

Molecular weight: Dobutamine hydrochloride—337.85.

Description: Dobutamine Hydrochloride USP—White to practically white, crystalline powder.

pKa: 9.4.

Solubility: Dobutamine Hydrochloride USP—Sparingly soluble in water and in methanol; soluble in alcohol and in pyridine.

USP requirements:

Dobutamine Hydrochloride Injection—Not in USP.

Dobutamine Hydrochloride for Injection USP—Preserve in Containers for Sterile Solids, at controlled room temperature. A sterile mixture of Dobutamine Hydrochloride with suitable diluents. Contains an amount of dobutamine hydrochloride equivalent to the labeled amount of dobutamine, within ± 10%. Meets the requirements for Constituted solution, Identification, Pyrogen, Uniformity of dosage units, pH (2.5–5.5), Particulate matter, and Injections.

Caution: Great care should be taken to prevent inhaling particles of Dobutamine Hydrochloride for Injection and exposing the skin to it. Protect the eyes.

DOCUSATE

Chemical group: Anionic surfactants.

Chemical name:

Docusate calcium—Butanedioic acid, sulfo-, 1,4-bis(2-ethylhexyl) ester, calcium salt.

Docusate potassium—Butanedioic acid, sulfo-, 1,4-bis(2-ethylhexyl) ester, potassium salt.

Docusate sodium—Butanedioic acid, sulfo-, 1,4-bis(2-ethylhexyl) ester, sodium salt.

Molecular formula:

Docusate calcium—$C_{40}H_{74}CaO_{14}S_2$.

Docusate potassium—$C_{20}H_{37}KO_7S$.

Docusate sodium—$C_{20}H_{37}NaO_7S$.

Molecular weight:

Docusate calcium—883.22.

Docusate potassium—460.67.

Docusate sodium—444.56.

Description:

Docusate Calcium USP—White, amorphous solid, having the characteristic odor of octyl alcohol. It is free of the odor of other solvents.

Docusate Potassium USP—White, amorphous solid, having a characteristic odor suggestive of octyl alcohol.

Docusate Sodium USP—White, wax-like, plastic solid, having a characteristic odor suggestive of octyl alcohol, but no odor of other solvents.

NF category: Wetting and/or solubilizing agent.

Solubility:

Docusate Calcium USP—Very slightly soluble in water; very soluble in alcohol, in polyethylene glycol 400, and in corn oil.

Docusate Potassium USP—Sparingly soluble in water; very soluble in solvent hexane; soluble in alcohol and in glycerin.

Docusate Sodium USP—Sparingly soluble in water; very soluble in solvent hexane; freely soluble in alcohol and in glycerin.

USP requirements:

Docusate Calcium Capsules USP—Preserve in tight containers, and store at controlled room temperature in a dry place. Contain the labeled amount, within ±15%. Meet the requirements for Identification and Uniformity of dosage units.

Docusate Potassium Capsules USP—Preserve in tight containers, and store at controlled room temperature. Contain the labeled amount, within ±10%. Meet the requirements for Identification and Uniformity of dosage units.

Docusate Sodium USP—Preserve in well-closed containers. Contains not less than 99.0% and not more than 100.5% of docusate sodium, calculated on the anhydrous basis. Meets the requirements for Clarity of solution, Identification, Water (not more than 2%), Residue on ignition (15.5–16.5%, calculated on anhydrous basis), Arsenic (not more than 3 ppm), Heavy metals (not more than 0.001%), and Bis(2-ethylhexyl) maleate (not more than 0.4%).

Docusate Sodium Capsules USP—Preserve in tight containers, and store at controlled room temperature. Contain the labeled amount, within ±10%. Meet the requirements for Identification and Uniformity of dosage units.

Docusate Sodium Solution USP (Oral)—Preserve in tight containers. Contains the labeled amount, within ±10%. Meets the requirements for Identification and pH (4.5–6.9).

Docusate Sodium Rectal Solution—Not in USP.

Docusate Sodium Syrup USP—Preserve in tight, light-resistant containers. Contains the labeled amount, within ±10%. Meets the requirements for Identification and pH (5.5–6.5).

Docusate Sodium Tablets USP—Preserve in well-closed containers. Contain the labeled amount, within ±10%. Meet the requirements for Identification, Disintegration (1 hour, simulated gastric fluid TS being substituted for water in the test for Uncoated Tablets), and Uniformity of dosage units.

DOCUSATE AND PHENOLPHTHALEIN

For *Docusate* and *Phenolphthalein*—See individual listings for chemistry information.

USP requirements:

Docusate Calcium and Phenolphthalein Capsules—Not in USP.

Docusate Sodium and Phenolphthalein Capsules—Not in USP.

Docusate Sodium and Phenolphthalein Tablets—Not in USP.

Docusate Sodium and Phenolphthalein Chewable Tablets—Not in USP.

DOPAMINE

Chemical group: A naturally occurring biochemical catecholamine precursor of norepinephrine.

Chemical name: Dopamine hydrochloride—1,2-Benzenediol, 4-(2-aminoethyl)-, hydrochloride.

Molecular formula: Dopamine hydrochloride—$C_8H_{11}NO_2 \cdot HCl$.

Molecular weight: Dopamine hydrochloride—189.64.

Description: Dopamine Hydrochloride USP—White to off-white, crystalline powder. May have a slight odor of hydrochloric acid. Melts at about 240 °C, with decomposition.

Solubility: Dopamine Hydrochloride USP—Freely soluble in water, in methanol, and in aqueous solutions of alkali hydroxides; insoluble in ether and in chloroform.

USP requirements: Dopamine Hydrochloride Injection USP—Preserve in single-dose containers of Type I glass. A sterile solution of Dopamine Hydrochloride in Water for Injection. It may contain a suitable antioxidant. Label it to indicate

that the Injection is to be diluted with a suitable parenteral vehicle prior to intravenous infusion. Contains the labeled amount, within ±5%. Meets the requirements for Identification, Bacterial endotoxins, pH (2.5–5.0), Particulate matter, and Injections.

Note: Do not use the Injection if it is darker than slightly yellow or discolored in any other way.

DOPAMINE AND DEXTROSE

For *Dopamine* and *Dextrose*—See individual listings for chemistry information.

USP requirements: Dopamine Hydrochloride and Dextrose Injection USP—Preserve in single-dose glass or plastic containers. Glass containers are preferably of Type I or Type II glass. A sterile solution of Dopamine Hydrochloride and Dextrose in Water for Injection. The label states the total osmolar concentration in mOsmol per liter. Where the contents are less than 100 mL, or where the label states that the Injection is not for direct injection but is to be diluted before use, the label alternatively may state the total osmolar concentration in mOsm per mL. Contains the labeled amounts, within ±5%. Meets the requirements for Identification, Bacterial endotoxins, pH (2.5–4.5), Particulate matter, and Injections.

Note: Do not use the Injection if it is darker than slightly yellow or discolored in any other way.

DOXACURIUM

Chemical name: Doxacurium chloride—Isoquinolinium, 2,2′-[(1,4-dioxo-1,4-butanediyl)bis(oxy-3,1-propanediyl)]-bis[1,2,3,4-tetrahydro-6,7,8-trimethoxy-2-methyl-1-[(3,4,5-trimethoxyphenyl)-methyl]-, dichloride, [1 alpha,2 beta(1′S*,2′R*)]-, mixture with (±)-[1 alpha,2 beta(1′R*,2′S*)]-2,2′-[(1,4-dioxo-1,4-butanediyl)bis(oxy-3,1-propanediyl)]bis-[1,2,3,4-tetrahydro-6,7,8-trimethoxy-2-methyl-1-[(3,4,5-trimethoxyphenyl)methyl]isoquinolinium] dichloride.

Molecular formula: Doxacurium chloride—$C_{56}H_{78}Cl_2N_2O_{16}$.

Molecular weight: Doxacurium chloride—1106.15.

Description: Doxacurium chloride injection—Sterile, nonpyrogenic aqueous solution.

Other characteristics:

Doxacurium chloride—N-octanol:water partition coefficient 0.

Doxacurium chloride injection—pH 3.9–5.0.

USP requirements: Doxacurium Chloride Injection—Not in USP.

DOXAPRAM

Chemical name: Doxapram hydrochloride—2-Pyrrolidinone, 1-ethyl-4-[2-(4-morpholinyl)ethyl]-3,3-diphenyl-, monohydrochloride, monohydrate.

Molecular formula: Doxapram hydrochloride—$C_{24}H_{30}N_2O_2 \cdot HCl \cdot H_2O$.

Molecular weight: Doxapram hydrochloride—432.99.

Description: Doxapram Hydrochloride USP—White to off-white, odorless, crystalline powder. Melts at about 220 °C.

Solubility: Doxapram Hydrochloride USP—Soluble in water and in chloroform; sparingly soluble in alcohol; practically insoluble in ether.

USP requirements: Doxapram Hydrochloride Injection USP—Preserve in single-dose or in multiple-dose containers, preferably of Type I glass. A sterile solution of Doxapram Hydrochloride in Water for Injection. Contains the labeled amount, within ±10%. Meets the requirements for Identification, Bacterial endotoxins, pH (3.5–5.0), and Injections.

DOXEPIN

Chemical group: Doxepin hydrochloride—Dibenzoxepin derivative.

Chemical name: Doxepin hydrochloride—1-Propanamine, 3-dibenz[b,e]oxepin-11(6H)ylidene-N,N-dimethyl-, hydrochloride.

Molecular formula: Doxepin hydrochloride—$C_{19}H_{21}NO \cdot HCl$.

Molecular weight: Doxepin hydrochloride—315.84.

Description: Doxepin hydrochloride—White, crystalline solid.

pKa: 9.0.

Solubility: Doxepin hydrochloride—Readily soluble in water, in lower alcohols, and in chloroform.

Other characteristics: Tertiary amine.

USP requirements:
Doxepin Hydrochloride Capsules USP—Preserve in well-closed containers. Contain an amount of doxepin hydrochloride equivalent to the labeled amount of doxepin, within ±10%. Meet the requirements for Identification, Dissolution (80% in 30 minutes in water in Apparatus 1 at 50 rpm), Uniformity of dosage units, and Water (not more than 9.0%).

Doxepin Hydrochloride Oral Solution USP—Preserve in tight, light-resistant containers. Label it to indicate that it is to be diluted with water or other suitable fluid to approximately 120 mL, just prior to administration. Contains an amount of doxepin hydrochloride equivalent to the labeled amount of doxepin, within ±10%. Meets the requirements for Identification and pH (4.0–7.0).

DOXORUBICIN

Source: An anthracycline glycoside obtained from *Streptomyces peucetius* var. *caesius*.

Chemical name: Doxorubicin hydrochloride—5,12-Naphthacenedione, 10-[(3-amino-2,3,6-trideoxy-alpha-L-*lyxo*-hexopyranosyl)oxy]-7,8,9,10-tetrahydro-6,8,11-trihydroxy-8-(hydroxyacetyl)-1-methoxy-, hydrochloride (8S-*cis*)-.

Molecular formula: Doxorubicin hydrochloride—$C_{27}H_{29}NO_{11} \cdot HCl$.

Molecular weight: Doxorubicin hydrochloride—579.99.

Description: Doxorubicin Hydrochloride USP—Red-orange, hygroscopic, crystalline powder.

Solubility: Doxorubicin Hydrochloride USP—Soluble in water, in isotonic sodium chloride solution, and in methanol; practically insoluble in chloroform, in ether, and in other organic solvents.

Other characteristics: Unstable in solutions with a pH less than 3 or greater than 7.

USP requirements:
Doxorubicin Hydrochloride Injection USP—Preserve in single-dose or in multiple-dose containers, preferably of Type I glass, protected from light. Store in a refrigerator. Injection may be packaged in multiple-dose containers not exceeding 100 mL in volume. A sterile solution of Doxorubicin Hydrochloride in Sterile Water for Injection made isoosmotic with Sodium Chloride, Dextrose, or other suitable added substances. Contains the labeled amount, within −10% to +15%. Meets the requirements for Identification, Bacterial endotoxins, Sterility, pH (2.5–4.5), and Injections.

Doxorubicin Hydrochloride for Injection USP—Preserve in Containers for Sterile Solids, except that multiple-dose containers may provide for the withdrawal of not more than 100 mL when constituted as directed in the labeling. A sterile mixture of Doxorubicin Hydrochloride and Lactose. Contains the labeled amount, within −10% to +15%. Meets the requirements for Constituted solution, Bacterial endotoxins, Sterility, pH (4.5–6.5, in the solution constituted as directed in the labeling, except that water is used as the diluent), Water (not more than 4.0%), for Identification under Doxorubicin Hydrochloride, and for Uniformity of dosage units and Labeling under Injections.

Caution: Great care should be taken to prevent inhaling particles of Doxorubicin Hydrochloride and exposing the skin to it.

DOXYCYCLINE

Chemical name:
Doxycycline—2-Naphthacenecarboxamide, 4-(dimethylamino) - 1,4,4a,5,5a,6,11,12a - octahydro - 3,5,10,12,12a - pentahydroxy-6-methyl-1,11-dioxo-, [4S-(4 alpha,4a alpha,-5 alpha,5a alpha,6 alpha,12a alpha)]-, monohydrate.
Doxycycline hyclate—2-Naphthacenecarboxamide, 4-(dimethylamino)-1,4,4a,5,5a,6,11,12a-octahydro-3,5,10,12,12a-pentahydroxy-6-methyl-1,11-dioxo-, monohydrochloride, compd. with ethanol (2:1), monohydrate, [4S-(4 alpha,4a alpha,5 alpha,5a alpha,6 alpha,12a alpha)]-.

Molecular formula:
Doxycycline—$C_{22}H_{24}N_2O_8 \cdot H_2O$.
Doxycycline hyclate—$(C_{22}H_{24}N_2O_8 \cdot HCl)_2 \cdot C_2H_6O \cdot H_2O$.

Molecular weight:
Doxycycline—462.46.
Doxycycline hyclate—1025.89.

Description:
Doxycycline USP—Yellow, crystalline powder.
Doxycycline Hyclate USP—Yellow, crystalline powder.

Solubility:
Doxycycline USP—Very slightly soluble in water; freely soluble in dilute acid and in alkali hydroxide solutions; sparingly soluble in alcohol; practically insoluble in chloroform and in ether.
Doxycycline Hyclate USP—Soluble in water and in solutions of alkali hydroxides and carbonates; slightly soluble in alcohol; practically insoluble in chloroform and in ether.

USP requirements:
Doxycycline for Oral Suspension USP—Preserve in tight, light-resistant containers. It contains one or more suitable buffers, colors, diluents, flavors, and preservatives. Contains the labeled amount, within −10% to +25% when constituted as directed. Meets the requirements for Identification, pH (5.0–6.5, in the suspension constituted as directed in the labeling), Deliverable volume, Water (not more than 3.0%), and Uniformity of dosage units (single-unit containers).

Doxycycline Calcium Oral Suspension USP—Preserve in tight, light-resistant containers. Prepared from Doxycycline Hyclate, and contains one or more suitable buffers, colors, diluents, flavors, and preservatives. Contains an amount of doxycycline calcium equivalent to the labeled amount of doxycycline, within −10% to +25%. Meets the requirements for Identification, pH (6.5–8.0), Deliverable volume, and Uniformity of dosage units (single-unit containers).

Doxycycline Hyclate Capsules USP—Preserve in tight, light-resistant containers. Contain an amount of doxycycline hyclate equivalent to the labeled amount of doxycycline, within −10% to +20%. Meet the requirements for Identification, Dissolution (80% in 30 minutes in water in Apparatus 2 at 75 rpm), Uniformity of dosage units, and Water (not more than 5.0%).

Doxycycline Hyclate Delayed-release Capsules USP—Preserve in tight, light-resistant containers. The label indicates that the contents of the Delayed-release Capsules are enteric-coated. Contain an amount of doxycycline hyclate equivalent to the labeled amount of doxycycline, within −10% to +20%. Meet the requirements for Identification, Drug release (Acid stage—50% [Level 1 and Level 2] in 20 minutes in 0.06 N hydrochloric acid in Apparatus 1 at 50 rpm; Buffer stage—85% in 30 minutes in neutralized phthalate buffer [pH 5.5] in Apparatus 1 at 50 rpm), Uniformity of dosage units, and Water (not more than 5.0%).

Doxycycline Hyclate for Injection USP—Preserve in Containers for Sterile Solids, protected from light. A sterile, dry mixture of Doxycycline Hyclate and a suitable buffer or a sterile-filtered and lyophilized mixture of Doxycycline Hyclate and a suitable buffer. Contains an amount of doxycycline hyclate equivalent to the labeled amount of doxycycline, within −10% to +20%. Meets the requirements for Constituted solution, Identification, Depressor substances, Bacterial endotoxins, Sterility, pH (1.8–3.3, in the solution constituted as directed in the labeling), Loss on drying (not more than 2.0%), and Particulate matter.

Sterile Doxycycline Hyclate USP—Preserve in Containers for Sterile Solids, protected from light. It is Doxycycline Hyclate suitable for parenteral use. It has a potency equivalent to not less than 800 mcg and not more than 920 mcg of doxycycline per mg. Meets the requirements for Depressor substances, Bacterial endotoxins, and Sterility, and for Identification test, pH, Water, and Crystallinity under Doxycycline Hyclate.

Doxycycline Hyclate Tablets USP—Preserve in tight, light-resistant containers. Contain an amount of doxycycline hyclate equivalent to the labeled amount of doxycycline, within −10% to +20%. Meet the requirements for Identification, Dissolution (85% in 90 minutes in water in Apparatus 2 at 75 rpm), Uniformity of dosage units, and Water (not more than 5.0%).

DOXYLAMINE

Chemical group: Doxylamine succinate—Ethanolamine derivative.

Chemical name: Doxylamine succinate—Ethanamine, N,N-dimethyl-2-[1-phenyl-1-(2-pyridinyl)ethoxy]-, butanedioate (1:1).

Molecular formula: Doxylamine succinate—$C_{17}H_{22}N_2O \cdot C_4H_6O_4$.

Molecular weight: Doxylamine succinate—388.46.

Description: Doxylamine Succinate USP—White or creamy white powder, having a characteristic odor.

pKa: Doxylamine succinate—5.8 and 9.3.

Solubility: Doxylamine Succinate USP—Very soluble in water and in alcohol; freely soluble in chloroform; very slightly soluble in ether.

USP requirements:
Doxylamine Succinate Syrup USP—Preserve in tight, light-resistant containers. Contains the labeled amount, within ±8%. Meets the requirement for Identification.

Doxylamine Succinate Tablets USP—Preserve in well-closed, light-resistant containers. Contain the labeled amount, within ±8%. Meet the requirements for Identification, Dissolution (80% in 30 minutes in 0.1 N hydrochloric acid in Apparatus 2 at 50 rpm), and Uniformity of dosage units.

DOXYLAMINE, PSEUDOEPHEDRINE, DEXTROMETHORPHAN, AND ACETAMINOPHEN

For *Doxylamine, Pseudoephedrine, Dextromethorphan,* and *Acetaminophen*—See individual listings for chemistry information.

USP requirements: Doxylamine Succinate, Pseudoephedrine Hydrochloride, Dextromethorphan Hydrobromide, and Acetaminophen Oral Solution—Not in USP.

DRONABINOL

Chemical group: A cannabinoid; synthetic form of one of the major active substances in *Cannabis sativa* L. (marijuana).

Chemical name: 6H-Dibenzo[b,d]pyran-1-ol, 6a,7,8,10a-tetrahydro-6,6,9-trimethyl-3-pentyl-, (6aR-trans)-.

Molecular formula: $C_{21}H_{30}O_2$.

Molecular weight: 314.47.

Description: Viscous, oily liquid.

Solubility: Insoluble in water; soluble in 1 part of alcohol or acetone, 3 parts of glycerol; soluble in fixed oils.

USP requirements: Dronabinol Capsules USP—Preserve in well-closed, light-resistant containers, in a cool place. Contain dronabinol in sesame oil. Contain the labeled amount, within ±10%. Meet the requirements for Identification and Uniformity of dosage units.

DROPERIDOL

Chemical name: 2H-Benzimidazol-2-one, 1-[1-[4-(4-fluorophenyl)-4-oxobutyl]-1,2,3,6-tetrahydro-4-pyridinyl]-1,3-dihydro-.

Molecular formula: $C_{22}H_{22}FN_3O_2$.

Molecular weight: 379.43.

Description: Droperidol USP—White to light tan, amorphous or microcrystalline powder.

Solubility: Droperidol USP—Practically insoluble in water; freely soluble in chloroform; slightly soluble in alcohol and in ether.

USP requirements: Droperidol Injection USP—Preserve in single-dose or in multiple-dose containers, preferably of Type I glass, protected from light. A sterile solution of Droperidol in Water for Injection, prepared with the aid of Lactic Acid. Contains the labeled amount of droperidol, as the lactate, within ±10%. Meets the requirements for Identification, Bacterial endotoxins, pH (3.0–3.8), Related substances, and Injections.

ABSORBABLE DUSTING POWDER

Description: Absorbable Dusting Powder USP—White, odorless powder.

USP requirements: Absorbable Dusting Powder USP—Preserve in well-closed containers. It may be preserved in sealed paper packets. An absorbable powder prepared by processing cornstarch and intended for use as a lubricant for surgical gloves. Contains not more than 2.0% of magnesium oxide. Meets the requirements for Identification, Stability to autoclaving, Sedimentation, pH (10.0–10.8, in a 1 in 10 suspension), Loss on drying (not more than 12%), Residue on ignition (not more than 3.0%), and Heavy metals (not more than 0.001%).

DYCLONINE

Chemical name: Dyclonine hydrochloride—1-Propanone, 1-(4-butoxyphenyl)-3-(1-piperidinyl)-, hydrochloride.

Molecular formula: Dyclonine hydrochloride—$C_{18}H_{27}NO_2 \cdot HCl$.

Molecular weight: Dyclonine hydrochloride—325.88.

Description: Dyclonine Hydrochloride USP—White crystals or white crystalline powder, which may have a slight odor.

Solubility: Dyclonine Hydrochloride USP—Soluble in water, in acetone, in alcohol, and in chloroform.

USP requirements:
Dyclonine Hydrochloride Gel USP—Preserve in collapsible, opaque plastic tubes or in tight, light-resistant glass containers. [Note: Do not use aluminum or tin tubes.] Contains the labeled amount, within ±10%. Meets the requirements for Identification and pH (2.0–4.0).
Dyclonine Hydrochloride Lozenges—Not in USP.
Dyclonine Hydrochloride Oral Topical Solution—Not in USP.
Dyclonine Hydrochloride Topical Solution USP—Preserve in tight, light-resistant containers. A sterile, aqueous solution of Dyclonine Hydrochloride. Contains the labeled amount, within ±8%. Meets the requirements for Identification, Sterility, and pH (3.0–5.0).

DYDROGESTERONE

Chemical name: Pregna-4,6-diene-3,20-dione, (9 beta, 10 alpha)-.

Molecular formula: $C_{21}H_{28}O_2$.

Molecular weight: 312.45.

Description: Dydrogesterone USP—White to pale yellow, crystalline powder.

Solubility: Dydrogesterone USP—Practically insoluble in water; sparingly soluble in alcohol.

USP requirements: Dydrogesterone Tablets USP—Preserve in well-closed containers. Contain the labeled amount, within ±10%. Meet the requirements for Identification, Dissolution (75% in 45 minutes in water : isopropyl alcohol [89:11] in Apparatus 2 at 100 rpm), and Uniformity of dosage units.

DYPHYLLINE

Source: A chemical derivative of theophylline, but not a theophylline salt as are the other agents.

Chemical name: 1*H*-Purine-2,6-dione, 7-(2,3-dihydroxypropyl)-3,7-dihydro-1,3-dimethyl-.

Molecular formula: $C_{10}H_{14}N_4O_4$.

Molecular weight: 254.25.

Description: Dyphylline USP—White, odorless, amorphous or crystalline solid.

Solubility: Dyphylline USP—Freely soluble in water; sparingly soluble in alcohol and in chloroform; practically insoluble in ether.

USP requirements:
Dyphylline Elixir USP—Preserve in tight containers. Contains the labeled amount, within ±10%. Meets the requirements for Identification and Alcohol content (±10% of labeled amount).
Dyphylline Injection USP—Preserve in single-dose or in multiple-dose containers, preferably of Type I glass, protected from light. To avoid precipitation, store at a temperature of not below 15 °C, but avoid excessive heat. Label it to indicate that the Injection is not to be used if crystals have separated. Contains the labeled amount, within ±10%. Meets the requirements for Identification, Bacterial endotoxins, pH (5.0–8.0), and Injections.
Dyphylline Oral Solution—Not in USP.
Dyphylline Tablets USP—Preserve in tight containers. Contain the labeled amount, within ±10%. Meet the requirements for Identification, Dissolution (75% in 45 minutes in water in Apparatus 1 at 100 rpm), and Uniformity of dosage units.

DYPHYLLINE AND GUAIFENESIN

For *Dyphylline* and *Guaifenesin*—See individual listings for chemistry information.

USP requirements:
Dyphylline and Guaifenesin Elixir USP—Preserve in tight containers. Contains the labeled amounts of dyphylline and guaifenesin, within ±10%. Meets the requirements for Identification, pH (5.0–7.0), and Alcohol content (labeled amount, within ±10%).
Dyphylline and Guaifenesin Tablets USP—Preserve in tight containers. Contain the labeled amounts of dyphylline and guaifenesin, within ±10%. Meet the requirements for Identification, Dissolution (75% of each active ingredient in 45 minutes in water in Apparatus 1 at 100 rpm), and Uniformity of dosage units.

ECHOTHIOPHATE

Chemical name: Echothiophate iodide—Ethanaminium, 2-[(diethoxyphosphinyl)thio]-*N*,*N*,*N*-trimethyl-, iodide.

Molecular formula: Echothiophate iodide—$C_9H_{23}INO_3PS$.

Molecular weight: Echothiophate iodide—383.22.

Description:
Echothiophate Iodide USP—White, crystalline, hygroscopic solid having a slight mercaptan-like odor. Its solutions have a pH of about 4.
Echothiophate Iodide for Ophthalmic Solution USP—White, amorphous powder.

Solubility: Echothiophate Iodide USP—Freely soluble in water and in methanol; soluble in dehydrated alcohol; practically insoluble in other organic solvents.

USP requirements: Echothiophate Iodide for Ophthalmic Solution USP—Preserve in tight containers, preferably of Type I glass, at controlled room temperature. It is sterile Echothiophate Iodide. Contains the labeled amount, within −5% to +15%. Meets the requirements for Completeness of solution, Identification, Sterility, and Water (not more than 2.0%).

ECONAZOLE

Chemical group: Synthetic imidazole derivative, structurally related to miconazole.

Chemical name: Econazole nitrate—1*H*-Imidazole, 1-[2-[(4-chlorophenyl)methoxy]-2-(2,4-dichlorophenyl)ethyl]-, mononitrate, (±)-.

Molecular formula: Econazole nitrate—$C_{18}H_{15}Cl_3N_2O \cdot HNO_3$.

Molecular weight: Econazole nitrate—444.70.

Description: Econazole Nitrate USP—White or practically white, crystalline powder, having not more than a slight odor.

Solubility: Econazole Nitrate USP—Very slightly soluble in water and in ether; slightly soluble in alcohol; sparingly soluble in chloroform; soluble in methanol.

USP requirements:
Econazole Nitrate Cream—Not in USP.
Econazole Nitrate Vaginal Suppositories—Not in USP.

EDETATE CALCIUM DISODIUM

Chemical group: A mixture of the dihydrate (predominantly) and trihydrate of calcium disodium ethylenediaminetetraacetate.

Chemical name: Calciate(2-), [[*N*,*N'*-1,2-ethanediylbis[*N*-(carboxymethyl)glycinato]](4-)-*N*,*N'*,*O*,*O'*,*O^N*,*O^{N'}*], disodium, hydrate, (*OC*-6-21)-.

Molecular formula: $C_{10}H_{12}CaN_2Na_2O_8 \cdot xH_2O$.

Molecular weight: 374.27 (anhydrous).

Description: Edetate Calcium Disodium USP—White, crystalline granules or white, crystalline powder; odorless; slightly hygroscopic; stable in air.

Solubility: Edetate Calcium Disodium USP—Freely soluble in water.

USP requirements: Edetate Calcium Disodium Injection USP—Preserve in single-dose containers, preferably of Type I glass. A sterile solution of Edetate Calcium Disodium in Water for Injection. Contains, in each mL, not less than 180 mg and not more than 220 mg of edetate calcium disodium. Meets the requirements for Identification, Bacterial endotoxins, pH (6.5–8.0), Particulate matter, and Injections.

EDETATE DISODIUM

Chemical group: The disodium salt of ethylenediamine tetraacetic acid (EDTA).

Chemical name: Glycine, *N*,*N'*-1,2-ethanediylbis[*N*-(carboxymethyl)-, disodium salt, dihydrate.

Molecular formula: $C_{10}H_{14}N_2Na_2O_8 \cdot 2H_2O$.

Molecular weight: 372.24.

Description: Edetate Disodium USP—White, crystalline powder.
NF category: Chelating agent; complexing agent.

Solubility: Edetate Disodium USP—Soluble in water.

USP requirements:
Edetate Disodium USP—Preserve in well-closed containers. Contains not less than 99.0% and not more than 101.0% of edetate disodium, calculated on the dried basis. Meets the requirements for Identification, pH (4.0–6.0, in a solution [1 in 20]), Loss on drying (8.7–11.4%), Calcium,

Heavy metals (not more than 0.005%), and Nitrilotriacetic acid (0.1%).
Edetate Disodium Injection USP—Preserve in single-dose containers, preferably of Type I glass. A sterile solution of Edetate Disodium in Water for Injection, which as a result of pH adjustment, contains varying amounts of the disodium and trisodium salts. Contains the labeled amount, within ±10%. Meets requirements for Identification, Pyrogen, pH (6.5–7.5), and Injections.
Edetate Disodium Ophthalmic Solution—Not in USP.

EDETIC ACID

Chemical name: Glycine, *N*,*N'*-1,2-ethanediylbis[*N*-(carboxymethyl)-.

Molecular formula: $C_{10}H_{16}N_2O_8$.

Molecular weight: 292.24.

Description: Edetic Acid NF—White, crystalline powder. Melts above 220 °C, with decomposition.
NF category: Chelating agent; complexing agent.

Solubility: Edetic Acid NF—Very slightly soluble in water; soluble in solutions of alkali hydroxides.

NF requirements: Edetic Acid NF—Preserve in well-closed containers. Contains not less than 98.0% and not more than 100.5% of edetic acid. Meets the requirements for Identification, Residue on ignition (not more than 0.2%), Heavy metals (not more than 0.003%), Nitrilotriacetic acid (0.3%), and Iron (0.005%).

EDROPHONIUM

Chemical group: Synthetic quaternary ammonium compound.

Chemical name: Edrophonium chloride—Benzenaminium, *N*-ethyl-3-hydroxy-*N*,*N*-dimethyl-, chloride.

Molecular formula: Edrophonium chloride—$C_{10}H_{16}ClNO$.

Molecular weight: Edrophonium chloride—201.70.

Description: Edrophonium Chloride USP—White, odorless, crystalline powder. Its solution (1 in 10) is practically colorless.

Solubility: Edrophonium Chloride USP—Very soluble in water; freely soluble in alcohol; insoluble in chloroform and in ether.

USP requirements: Edrophonium Chloride Injection USP—Preserve in single-dose or multiple-dose containers, preferably of Type I glass. A sterile solution of Edrophonium Chloride in Water for Injection. Label Injection in multiple-dose containers to indicate an expiration date of not later than 3 years after date of manufacture, and label Injection in single-dose containers to indicate an expiration date of not later than 4 years after the date of manufacture. Contains the labeled amount, within ±5%. Meets the requirements for Identification, Bacterial endotoxins, pH (5.0–5.8), and Injections.

EDROPHONIUM AND ATROPINE

For *Edrophonium* and *Atropine*—See individual listings for chemistry information.

USP requirements: Edrophonium Chloride and Atropine Sulfate Injection—Not in USP.

EFLORNITHINE

Chemical name: Eflornithine hydrochloride—DL-Ornithine, 2-(difluoromethyl)-, monohydrochloride, monohydrate.

Molecular formula: Eflornithine hydrochloride—$C_6H_{12}F_2N_2O_2 \cdot HCl \cdot H_2O$.

Molecular weight: Eflornithine hydrochloride—236.65.

Description: Eflornithine hydrochloride—White to off-white, odorless, crystalline powder.

Solubility: Eflornithine hydrochloride—Freely soluble in water and sparingly soluble in ethanol.

USP requirements: Eflornithine Hydrochloride for Injection Concentrate—Not in USP.

TRACE ELEMENTS

USP requirements: Trace Elements Injection USP—Preserve in single-dose or in multiple-dose containers, preferably of Type I or Type II glass. A sterile solution in Water for Injection of two or more of the following: Zinc Chloride or Zinc Sulfate, Cupric Chloride or Cupric Sulfate, Chromic Chloride, Manganese Chloride or Manganese Sulfate, Selenious Acid, Sodium Iodide, and Ammonium Molybdate. Label the Injection to specify that it is to be diluted to the appropriate strength with Sterile Water for Injection or other suitable fluid prior to administration. The label shows by an appropriate number juxtaposed to the official name, the number of trace elements contained in the Injection according to the following: zinc and copper (2), and then cumulatively, chromium (3), manganese (4), selenium (5), iodine (6), and molybdenum (7). Other combinations are indicated separately by citing the number of trace elements contained in each followed by an asterisk that is repeated with the list of labeled ingredients. Label the Injection for its contents of zinc chloride ($ZnCl_2$), zinc sulfate ($ZnSO_4 \cdot 7H_2O$), cupric chloride ($CuCl_2$), cupric sulfate ($CuSO_4$), chromic chloride ($CrCl_2$), manganese chloride ($MnCl_2$), manganese sulfate ($MnSO_4$), selenious acid (H_2SeO_3), sodium iodide (NaI), and ammonium molybdate [$(NH_4)Mo_7 \cdot 4H_2O$], and for elemental zinc (Zn), copper (Cu), chromium (Cr), manganese (Mn), selenium (Se), iodine (I), and molybdenum (Mo), as appropriate in relation to the ingredients claimed to be present. Contains the labeled amounts of zinc (Zn), copper (Cu), chromium (Cr), manganese (Mn), selenium (Se), iodine (I), and molybdenum (Mo), within ±10%. Meets the requirements for Identification, Pyrogen, pH (1.5–3.5), Particulate matter, and Injection.

EMETINE

Chemical name: Emetine hydrochloride—Emetan, 6′,7′,10,11-tetramethoxy-, dihydrochloride.

Molecular formula: Emetine hydrochloride—$C_{29}H_{40}N_2O_4 \cdot 2HCl$.

Molecular weight: Emetine hydrochloride—553.57.

Description: Emetine Hydrochloride USP—White or very slightly yellowish, odorless, crystalline powder. Affected by light.

Solubility: Emetine Hydrochloride USP—Freely soluble in water and in alcohol.

USP requirements: Emetine Hydrochloride Injection USP—Preserve in single-dose, light-resistant containers, preferably of Type I glass. A sterile solution of Emetine Hydrochloride in Water for Injection. Contains an amount of anhydrous emetine hydrochloride equivalent to the labeled amount of emetine hydrochloride, within −16% to −6%. Meets the requirements for Identification, Bacterial endotoxins, pH (3.0–5.0), Cephaeline, and Injections.

ENALAPRIL

Chemical name: Enalapril maleate—L-Proline, 1-[N-[1-(ethoxycarbonyl)-3-phenylpropyl]-L-alanyl]-, (S)-, (Z)-2-butenedioate (1:1).

Molecular formula: Enalapril maleate—$C_{20}H_{28}N_2O_5 \cdot C_4H_4O_4$.

Molecular weight: Enalapril maleate—492.52.

Description: Enalapril Maleate USP—Off-white, crystalline powder. Melts at about 144 °C.

Solubility: Enalapril Maleate USP—Practically insoluble in nonpolar organic solvents; slightly soluble in semipolar organic solvents; sparingly soluble in water; soluble in alcohol; freely soluble in methanol and in dimethylformamide.

USP requirements: Enalapril Maleate Tablets USP—Preserve in well-closed containers. Contain the labeled amount, within ±10%. Meet the requirements for Identification, Dissolution (80% in 30 minutes in water in Apparatus 2 at 50 rpm), Uniformity of dosage units, and Related compounds.

ENALAPRIL AND HYDROCHLOROTHIAZIDE

For *Enalapril* and *Hydrochlorothiazide*—See individual listings for chemistry information.

USP requirements: Enalapril Maleate and Hydrochlorothiazide Tablets—Not in USP.

ENALAPRILAT

Chemical name: L-Proline, 1-[N-(1-carboxy-3-phenylpropyl)-L-alanyl]-, dihydrate, (S)-.

Molecular formula: $C_{18}H_{24}N_2O_5 \cdot 2H_2O$.

Molecular weight: 384.43.

Description: Enalaprilat USP—White to nearly white, hygroscopic, crystalline powder.

Solubility: Enalaprilat USP—Sparingly soluble in methanol and in dimethylformamide; slightly soluble in water and in isopropyl alcohol; very slightly soluble in acetone, in alcohol, and in hexane; practically insoluble in acetonitrile and in chloroform.

USP requirements: Enalaprilat Injection—Not in USP.

ENCAINIDE

Chemical name: Encainide hydrochloride—Benzamide, 4-methoxy-N-[2-[2-(1-methyl-2-piperidinyl)ethyl]phenyl]-, monohydrochloride, (±)-.

Molecular formula: Encainide hydrochloride—$C_{22}H_{28}N_2O_2 \cdot HCl$.

Molecular weight: Encainide hydrochloride—388.94.

Description: White solid.

Solubility: Freely soluble in water; slightly soluble in ethanol; insoluble in heptane.

USP requirements: Encainide Hydrochloride Capsules—Not in USP.

ENFLURANE

Chemical name: Ethane, 2-chloro-1-(difluoromethoxy)-1,1,2-trifluoro-.

Molecular formula: $C_3H_2ClF_5O$.

Molecular weight: 184.49.

Description: Enflurane USP—Clear, colorless, stable, volatile liquid, having a mild, sweet odor. Is non-flammable.

Solubility: Enflurane USP—Slightly soluble in water; miscible with organic solvents, fats, and oils.

Other characteristics:
Blood-to-Gas partition coefficient—1.91 at 37 °C.
Oil-to-Gas partition coefficient—98.5 at 37 °C.

USP requirements: Enflurane USP—Preserve in tight, light-resistant containers, and avoid exposure to excessive heat. Contains not less than 99.0% and not more than 100.0% of enflurane, calculated on the anhydrous basis. Meets the requirements for Identification, Specific gravity (1.516–1.519), Distilling range (55.5–57.5 °C, a correction factor of 0.041 °C per mm being applied as necessary), Refractive index (1.3020–1.3038 at 20 °C), Acidity or alkalinity, Water (not more than 0.14%), Nonvolatile residue, Chloride, and Fluoride ions (not more than 10 mcg per mL).

EPHEDRINE

Chemical name:
Ephedrine hydrochloride—Benzenemethanol, alpha-[1-(methylamino)ethyl]-, hydrochloride, [R-(R*,S*)]-.
Ephedrine sulfate—Benzenemethanol, alpha-[1-(methylamino)ethyl]-, [R-(R*,S*)]-, sulfate (2:1) (salt).

Molecular formula:
Ephedrine hydrochloride—$C_{10}H_{15}NO \cdot HCl$.
Ephedrine sulfate—$(C_{10}H_{15}NO)_2 \cdot H_2SO_4$.

Molecular weight:
Ephedrine hydrochloride—201.70.
Ephedrine sulfate—428.54.

Description:
Ephedrine Hydrochloride USP—Fine, white, odorless crystals or powder. Is affected by light.
Ephedrine Sulfate USP—Fine, white, odorless crystals or powder. Darkens on exposure to light.
Ephedrine Sulfate Nasal Solution USP—Clear, colorless solution. Is neutral or slightly acid to litmus.

Solubility:
Ephedrine Hydrochloride USP—Freely soluble in water; soluble in alcohol; insoluble in ether.
Ephedrine Sulfate USP—Freely soluble in water; sparingly soluble in alcohol.

USP requirements:
Ephedrine Sulfate Capsules USP—Preserve in tight, light-resistant containers. Contain the labeled amount, within ±8%. Meet the requirements for Identification, Dissolution (80% in 30 minutes in water in Apparatus 1 at 100 rpm), and Uniformity of dosage units.
Ephedrine Sulfate Injection USP—Preserve in single-dose or in multiple-dose, light-resistant containers, preferably of Type I glass. A sterile solution of Ephedrine Sulfate in Water for Injection. Contains the labeled amount, within ±5%. Meets the requirements for Identification, Bacterial endotoxins, pH (4.5–7.0), and Injections.
Ephedrine Sulfate Nasal Solution USP—Preserve in tight, light-resistant containers. Contains the labeled amount,

within ±7%. Meets the requirements for Identification and Microbial limits.
Ephedrine Sulfate Syrup USP—Preserve in tight, light-resistant containers, and avoid exposure to excessive heat. Contains, in each 100 mL, not less than 360 mg and not more than 440 mg of ephedrine sulfate. Meets the requirements for Identification and Alcohol content (2.0–4.0%).
Ephedrine Sulfate Tablets USP—Preserve in well-closed containers. Contain the labeled amount, within ±7%. Meet the requirements for Identification, Dissolution (75% in 45 minutes in water in Apparatus 2 at 50 rpm), and Uniformity of dosage units.

EPHEDRINE AND GUAIFENESIN

For *Ephedrine* and *Guaifenesin*—See individual listings for chemistry information.

USP requirements:
Ephedrine Hydrochloride and Guaifenesin Capsules—Not in USP.
Ephedrine Hydrochloride and Guaifenesin Syrup—Not in USP.

EPHEDRINE AND PHENOBARBITAL

For *Ephedrine* and *Phenobarbital*—See individual listings for chemistry information.

USP requirements: Ephedrine Sulfate and Phenobarbital Capsules USP—Preserve in well-closed containers. Contain the labeled amounts of ephedrine sulfate and phenobarbital, within ±9%. Meet the requirements for Identification, Dissolution (75% of each active ingredient in 45 minutes in water in Apparatus 1 at 100 rpm), and Uniformity of dosage units.

EPHEDRINE AND POTASSIUM IODIDE

For *Ephedrine* and *Potassium Iodide*—See individual listings for chemistry information.

USP requirements: Ephedrine Hydrochloride and Potassium Iodide Syrup—Not in USP.

EPINEPHRINE

Chemical name:
Epinephrine—1,2-Benzenediol, 4-[1-hydroxy-2-(methylamino)ethyl]-, (R)-.
Epinephrine bitartrate—1,2-Benzenediol, 4-[1-hydroxy-2-(methylamino)ethyl]-, (R)-, [R-(R*,R*)]-2,3-dihydroxybutanedioate (1:1) (salt).

Molecular formula:
Epinephrine—$C_9H_{13}NO_3$.
Epinephrine bitartrate—$C_9H_{13}NO_3 \cdot C_4H_6O_6$.

Molecular weight:
Epinephrine—183.21.
Epinephrine bitartrate—333.29.

Description:
Epinephrine USP—White to practically white, odorless, microcrystalline powder or granules, gradually darkening on exposure to light and air. With acids, it forms salts that are readily soluble in water, and the base may be recovered by the addition of ammonia water or alkali carbonates. Its solutions are alkaline to litmus.
Epinephrine Injection USP—Practically colorless, slightly acid liquid. Gradually turns dark on exposure to light and to air.

Epinephrine Inhalation Solution USP—Practically colorless, slightly acid liquid. Gradually turns dark on exposure to light and air.

Epinephrine Nasal Solution USP—Nearly colorless, slightly acid liquid. Gradually turns dark on exposure to light and air.

Epinephrine Ophthalmic Solution USP—Colorless to faint yellow solution. Gradually turns dark on exposure to light and air.

Epinephrine Bitartrate USP—White, or grayish white or light brownish gray, odorless, crystalline powder. Slowly darkens on exposure to air and light. Its solutions are acid to litmus, having a pH of about 3.5.

Epinephrine Bitartrate for Ophthalmic Solution USP—White to off-white solid.

Solubility:

Epinephrine USP—Very slightly soluble in water and in alcohol; insoluble in ether, in chloroform, and in fixed and volatile oils.

Epinephrine Bitartrate USP—Freely soluble in water; slightly soluble in alcohol; practically insoluble in chloroform and in ether.

USP requirements:

Epinephrine Inhalation Aerosol USP—Preserve in small, nonreactive, light-resistant aerosol containers equipped with metered-dose valves and provided with oral inhalation actuators. A solution of Epinephrine in propellants and Alcohol prepared with the aid of mineral acid in a pressurized container. Contains the labeled amount within −10% to +15%, and delivers the labeled dose per inhalation, within ±25%, through an oral inhalation actuator. Meets the requirements for Identification and Unit spray content, and for Leak testing under Aerosols.

Epinephrine Injection USP—Preserve in single-dose or in multiple-dose, light-resistant containers, preferably of Type I glass. A sterile solution of Epinephrine in Water for Injection prepared with the aid of Hydrochloric acid. The label indicates that the Injection is not to be used if its color is pinkish or darker than slightly yellow or if it contains a precipitate. Contains the labeled amount, within −10% to +15%. Meets the requirements for Color and clarity, Identification, Bacterial endotoxins, pH (2.2–5.0), Total acidity, and Injections.

Epinephrine Inhalation Solution USP—Preserve in small, well-filled, tight, light-resistant containers. A solution of Epinephrine in Purified Water prepared with the aid of Hydrochloric Acid. The label indicates that the Inhalation Solution is not to be used if its color is pinkish or darker than slightly yellow or if it contains a precipitate. Contains, in each 100 mL, not less than 0.9 grams and not more than 1.15 grams of epinephrine. Meets the requirements for Color and clarity and Identification.

Epinephrine Nasal Solution USP—Preserve in small, well-filled, tight, light-resistant containers. A solution of Epinephrine in Purified Water prepared with the aid of Hydrochloric Acid. The label indicates that the Nasal Solution is not to be used if its color is pinkish or darker than slightly yellow or if it contains a precipitate. Contains, in each 100 mL, not less than 90 mg and not more than 115 mg of epinephrine. Meets the requirements for Color and clarity and Identification.

Epinephrine Ophthalmic Solution USP—Preserve in tight, light-resistant containers. A sterile, aqueous solution of Epinephrine prepared with the aid of Hydrochloric Acid. The label indicates that the Ophthalmic Solution is not to be used if its color is pinkish or darker than slightly yellow or if it contains a precipitate. Contains the labeled amount, within −10% to +15%. It contains a suitable antibacterial agent. Meets the requirements for Color and clarity, Identification, Sterility, and pH (2.2–4.5).

Sterile Epinephrine Suspension—Not in USP.

Sterile Epinephrine Oil Suspension USP—Preserve in single-dose, light-resistant containers, preferably of Type I or Type III glass. A sterile suspension of Epinephrine in a suitable vegetable oil. Contains, in each mL, not less than 1.8 mg and not more than 2.4 mg of epinephrine. Meets the requirement for Injections.

Epinephrine Bitartrate Inhalation Aerosol USP—Preserve in small, nonreactive, light-resistant aerosol containers equipped with metered-dose valves and provided with oral inhalation actuators. A suspension of microfine Epinephrine Bitartrate in propellants in a pressurized container. Contains the labeled amount, within ±10%, and delivers the labeled dose per inhalation, within ±25%, through an oral inhalation actuator. Meets the requirements for Identification, Unit spray content, and Particle size, and for Leak testing under Aerosols.

Epinephrine Bitartrate Ophthalmic Solution USP—Preserve in small, well-filled, tight, light-resistant containers. A sterile, buffered, aqueous solution of Epinephrine Bitartrate. The label indicates that the Ophthalmic Solution is not to be used if its color is pinkish or darker than slightly yellow or if it contains a precipitate. Contains an amount of epinephrine bitartrate equivalent to the labeled amount of epinephrine, within −10% to +15%. It contains a suitable antibacterial agent. Meets the requirements for Color and clarity and pH (3.0–3.8), and for Identification test for Epinephrine Nasal Solution and Sterility tests.

Epinephrine Bitartrate for Ophthalmic Solution USP—Preserve in Containers for Sterile Solids. A sterile, dry mixture of Epinephrine Bitartrate and suitable antioxidants, prepared by freeze-drying. Contains an amount of epinephrine bitartrate equivalent to the labeled amount of epinephrine, within ±10%. Meets the requirements for Completeness of solution and Constituted solution, and for Identification test under Epinephrine Nasal Solution, Sterility tests, and Uniformity of dosage units.

EPINEPHRYL BORATE

Chemical name: 1,3,2-Benzodioxaborole-5-methanol, 2-hydroxy-alpha-[(methylamino)methyl]-, (R)-.

Molecular formula: $C_9H_{12}BNO_4$.

Molecular weight: 209.01.

Description: Epinephryl Borate Ophthalmic Solution USP—Clear, pale yellow liquid, gradually darkening on exposure to light and to air.

USP requirements: Epinephryl Borate Ophthalmic Solution USP—Preserve in small, well-filled, tight, light-resistant containers. A sterile solution in water of Epinephrine as a borate complex. The label indicates that the Ophthalmic Solution is not to be used if its color is pinkish or darker than slightly yellow or if it contains a precipitate. Contains an amount of epinephryl borate equivalent to the labeled amount of epinephrine, within −10% to +15%. Contains a suitable antibacterial agent and one or more suitable preservatives and buffering agents. Meets the requirements for Color and clarity, Identification, Sterility, and pH (5.5–7.6).

EPOETIN ALFA

Chemical name: 1-165-Erythropoietin (human clone lambda-HEPOFL13 protein moiety).

Molecular formula: $C_{809}H_{1301}N_{229}O_{240}S_5$ (amino acid sequence).

Molecular weight: 30,400.00 ± 400.

USP requirements: Epoetin Alfa, Recombinant, Injection—Not in USP.

ERGOCALCIFEROL

Chemical name: 9,10-Secoergosta-5,7,10(19),22-tetraen-3-ol, (3 beta,5Z,7E,22E)-.

Molecular formula: $C_{28}H_{44}O$.

Molecular weight: 396.65.

Description:
Ergocalciferol USP—White, odorless crystals. Is affected by air and by light.
Ergocalciferol Oral Solution USP—Clear liquid having the characteristics of the solvent used in preparing the Solution.

Solubility: Ergocalciferol USP—Insoluble in water; soluble in alcohol, in chloroform, in ether, and in fatty oils.

USP requirements:
Ergocalciferol Capsules USP—Preserve in tight, light-resistant containers. Usually consist of an edible vegetable oil solution of Ergocalciferol, encapsulated with Gelatin. Label the Capsules to indicate the content of ergocalciferol in mg. The activity may be expressed also in terms of USP Units, on the basis that 40 USP Vitamin D Units = 1 mcg. Contain not less than 100.0% and not more than 120.0% of the labeled amount. Meet the requirements for Uniformity of dosage units.
Ergocalciferol Injection—Not in USP.
Ergocalciferol Oral Solution USP—Preserve in tight, light-resistant containers. A solution of Ergocalciferol in an edible vegetable oil, in Polysorbate 80, or in Propylene Glycol. Label the Oral Solution to indicate the concentration of ergocalciferol in mg. The activity may be expressed also in terms of USP Units, on the basis that 40 USP Vitamin D Units = 1 mcg. Contains not less than 100.0% and not more than 120.0% of the labeled amount.
Ergocalciferol Tablets USP—Preserve in tight, light-resistant containers. Label the Tablets to indicate the content of ergocalciferol in mg. The activity may be expressed also in terms of USP Units, on the basis that 40 USP Vitamin D Units = 1 mcg. Contain not less than 100.0% and not more than 120.0% of the labeled amount. Meet the requirements for Identification, Disintegration (30 minutes), and Uniformity of dosage units.

ERGOLOID MESYLATES

Chemical name: Ergotaman-3′,6′,18-trione, 9,10-dihydro-12′-hydroxy-2′,5′-bis(1-methylethyl)-, (5′ alpha,10 alpha)-, monomethanesulfonate (salt) mixture with 9,10 alpha-dihydro-12′-hydroxy-2′-(1-methylethyl)-5′alpha-(phenylmethyl)ergotaman-3′,6′,18-trione monomethanesulfonate (salt), 9,10 alpha-dihydro-12′-hydroxy-2′-(1-methylethyl)-5′alpha-(2-methylpropyl)ergotaman-3′,6′,18-trione monomethanesulfonate (salt), and 9,10 alpha-dihydro-12′-hydroxy-2′-(1-methylethyl)-5′alpha-(1-methylpropyl)ergotaman-3′,6′,18-trione monomethanesulfonate (salt).

Molecular formula:
Dihydroergocornine mesylate—$C_{31}H_{41}N_5O_5 \cdot CH_4O_3S$.
Dihydroergocristine mesylate—$C_{35}H_{41}N_5O_5 \cdot CH_4O_3S$.
Dihydro-alpha-ergocryptine mesylate—$C_{32}H_{43}N_5O_5 \cdot CH_4O_3S$.
Dihydro-beta-ergocryptine mesylate—$C_{32}H_{43}N_5O_5 \cdot CH_4O_3S$.

Molecular weight:
Dihydroergocornine mesylate—659.80.

Dihydroergocristine mesylate—707.84.
Dihydro-alpha-ergocryptine mesylate—673.82.
Dihydro-beta-ergocryptine mesylate—673.82.

Description: Ergoloid Mesylates USP—White to off-white, microcrystalline or amorphous, practically odorless powder.

Solubility: Ergoloid Mesylates USP—Slightly soluble in water; soluble in methanol and in alcohol; sparingly soluble in acetone.

USP requirements:
Ergoloid Mesylates Capsules—Not in USP.
Ergoloid Mesylates Oral Solution USP—Preserve in tight, light-resistant containers at a temperature not exceeding 30 °C. Contains the labeled amount, within ± 10%, consisting of not less than 30.3% and not more than 36.3% of the methanesulfonate salt of each of the individual alkaloids (dihydroergocristine, dihydroergocornine, and dihydroergocryptine); the ratio of alpha- to beta-dihydroergocryptine mesylate is not less than 1.5:1.0 and not more than 2.5:1.0. Meets the requirements for Identification and Alcohol content (the labeled amount of ethanol, within ± 10%).
Ergoloid Mesylates Tablets USP—Preserve in tight, light-resistant containers. Label Tablets to indicate whether they are intended for sublingual administration or for swallowing. Contain the labeled amount, within ± 10%, consisting of not less than 30.3% and not more than 36.3% of the methanesulfonate salt of each of the individual alkaloids (dihydroergocristine, dihydroergocornine, and dihydroergocryptine); the ratio of alpha- to beta-dihydroergocryptine mesylate is not less than 1.5:1.0 and not more than 2.5:1.0. Meet the requirements for Identification, Disintegration (15 minutes, for Tablets intended for sublingual use), Dissolution (75% in 30 minutes in water in Apparatus 2 at 50 rpm, for Tablets intended to be swallowed), and Uniformity of dosage units.

ERGONOVINE

Chemical group: Ergot alkaloid.

Chemical name: Ergonovine maleate—Ergoline-8-carboxamide, 9,10-didehydro-N-(2-hydroxy-1-methylethyl)-6-methyl-, [8 beta(S)]-, (Z)-2-butenedioate (1:1) (salt).

Molecular formula: Ergonovine maleate—$C_{19}H_{23}N_3O_2 \cdot C_4H_4O_4$.

Molecular weight: Ergonovine maleate—441.48.

Description: Ergonovine Maleate USP—White to grayish white or faintly yellow, odorless, microcrystalline powder. Darkens with age and on exposure to light.

Solubility: Ergonovine Maleate USP—Sparingly soluble in water; slightly soluble in alcohol; insoluble in ether and in chloroform.

USP requirements:
Ergonovine Maleate Injection USP—Preserve in single-dose, light-resistant containers, preferably of Type I glass, and store in a cold place. A sterile solution of Ergonovine Maleate in Water for Injection. Contains the labeled amount, within ± 10%. Meets the requirements for Identification, pH (2.7–3.5), Related alkaloids, and Injections.
Ergonovine Maleate Tablets USP—Preserve in well-closed containers. Contain the labeled amount, within ± 10%. Meet the requirements for Identification, Dissolution (75% in 45 minutes in water in Apparatus 1 at 100 rpm), Uniformity of dosage units, and Related alkaloids.

ERGOTAMINE

Chemical name: Ergotamine tartrate—Ergotaman-3′,6′,18-trione, 12′-hydroxy-2′-methyl-5′-(phenylmethyl)-, (5′alpha)-, [R-(R*,R*)]-2,3-dihydroxybutanedioate (2:1) (salt).

Molecular formula: Ergotamine tartrate—$(C_{33}H_{35}N_5O_5)_2 \cdot C_4H_6O_6$.

Molecular weight: Ergotamine tartrate—1313.43.

Description: Ergotamine Tartrate USP—Colorless crystals or white to yellowish white, crystalline powder. Is odorless. Melts at about 180 °C, with decomposition.

Solubility: Ergotamine Tartrate USP—One gram dissolves in about 3200 mL of water; in the presence of a slight excess of tartaric acid, 1 gram dissolves in about 500 mL of water. Slightly soluble in alcohol.

USP requirements:

Ergotamine Tartrate Inhalation Aerosol USP—Preserve in small, non-reactive, light-resistant aerosol containers equipped with metered-dose valves and provided with oral inhalation actuators. A suspension of microfine Ergotamine Tartrate in propellants in a pressurized container. Contains the labeled amount, within ±10%, and delivers within ±25% of the labeled amount per inhalation, through an oral inhalation actuator. Meets the requirements for Identification, Unit spray content, and Particle size, and for Leak testing under Aerosols.

Ergotamine Tartrate Injection USP—Preserve in single-dose, light-resistant containers, preferably of Type I glass. A sterile solution of Ergotamine Tartrate and the tartrates of its epimer, ergotaminine, and of other related alkaloids, in Water for Injection to which Tartaric Acid or suitable stabilizers have been added. The total alkaloid content, in each mL, is not less than 450 mcg and not more than 550 mcg. The content of ergotamine tartrate is not less than 52.0% and not more than 74.0% of the content of total alkaloid; the content of ergotaminine tartrate is not more than 45.0% of the content of total alkaloid. Meets the requirements for Bacterial endotoxins, pH (3.5–4.0) and Injections.

Ergotamine Tartrate Tablets USP—Preserve in well-closed, light-resistant containers. Label Tablets to indicate whether they are intended for sublingual administration or for swallowing. Contain the labeled amount, within ±10%. Meet the requirements for Identification, Disintegration (5 minutes, for Tablets intended for sublingual use), Dissolution (75% in 30 minutes in tartaric acid solution [1 in 100] in Apparatus 2 at 75 rpm, for Tablets intended to be swallowed), and Uniformity of dosage units.

ERGOTAMINE, BELLADONNA ALKALOIDS, AND PHENOBARBITAL

For *Ergotamine*, *Belladonna Alkaloids* (Atropine, Belladonna, Hyoscyamine, and Scopolamine), and *Phenobarbital*—See individual listings for chemistry information.

USP requirements:

Ergotamine Tartrate, Belladonna Alkaloids, and Phenobarbital Sodium Tablets—Not in USP.

Ergotamine Tartrate, Belladonna Alkaloids, and Phenobarbital Sodium Extended-release Tablets—Not in USP.

ERGOTAMINE AND CAFFEINE

For *Ergotamine* and *Caffeine*—See individual listings for chemistry information.

USP requirements:

Ergotamine Tartrate and Caffeine Suppositories USP—Preserve in tight containers at a temperature not above 25 °C. Do not expose unwrapped Suppositories to sunlight. Contain the labeled amounts of ergotamine tartrate and caffeine, within ±10%. Meet the requirements for Identification.

Ergotamine Tartrate and Caffeine Tablets USP—Preserve in well-closed, light-resistant containers. Contain the labeled amounts of ergotamine tartrate and caffeine, within ±10%. Meet the requirements for Identification, Dissolution (70% of ergotamine tartrate and 75% of caffeine in 30 minutes in tartaric acid solution [1 in 100] in Apparatus 2 at 75 rpm), and Uniformity of dosage units.

ERGOTAMINE, CAFFEINE, BELLADONNA ALKALOIDS, AND PENTOBARBITAL

For *Ergotamine*, *Caffeine*, *Belladonna Alkaloids* (Anisotropine, Atropine, Belladonna, Hyoscyamine, Methscopolamine, and Scopolamine), and *Pentobarbital*—See individual listings for chemistry information.

USP requirements:

Ergotamine Tartrate, Caffeine, Belladonna Alkaloids, and Pentobarbital Suppositories—Not in USP.

Ergotamine Tartrate, Caffeine, Belladonna Alkaloids, and Pentobarbital Sodium Tablets—Not in USP.

ERGOTAMINE, CAFFEINE, AND CYCLIZINE

For *Ergotamine*, *Caffeine*, and *Cyclizine*—See individual listings for chemistry information.

USP requirements: Ergotamine Tartrate, Caffeine Hydrate, and Cyclizine Hydrochloride Tablets—Not in USP.

ERGOTAMINE, CAFFEINE, AND DIMENHYDRINATE

For *Ergotamine*, *Caffeine*, and *Dimenhydrinate*—See individual listings for chemistry information.

USP requirements: Ergotamine Tartrate, Caffeine, and Dimenhydrinate Capsules—Not in USP.

ERGOTAMINE, CAFFEINE, AND DIPHENHYDRAMINE

For *Ergotamine*, *Citrated Caffeine*, and *Diphenhydramine*—See individual listings for chemistry information.

USP requirements: Ergotamine Tartrate, Caffeine Citrate, and Diphenhydramine Hydrochloride Capsules—Not in USP.

ERYTHRITYL TETRANITRATE

Chemical name: 1,2,3,4-Butanetetrol, tetranitrate, (R*, S*)-.

Molecular formula: $C_4H_6N_4O_{12}$.

Molecular weight: 302.11.

Description: Diluted Erythrityl Tetranitrate USP—White powder, having a slight odor of nitric oxides.

Solubility: Undiluted erythrityl tetranitrate—Practically insoluble in water; soluble in acetone, in acetonitrile, and in alcohol.

USP requirements: Erythrityl Tetranitrate Tablets USP—Preserve in tight containers, and avoid exposure to excessive heat. Erythrityl Tetranitrate Tablets are prepared from Diluted Erythrityl Tetranitrate. Contain the labeled amount of diluted erythrityl tetranitrate, within ±10%. Meet the requirements for Identification, Disintegration (10 minutes), and Uniformity of dosage units.

Caution—Undiluted erythrityl tetranitrate is a powerful explosive, and proper precautions must be taken in handling. It can be exploded by percussion or by excessive heat. Only extremely small amounts should be isolated.

ERYTHROMYCIN

Source: Produced from a strain of *Streptomyces erythraeus*.

Chemical group: Macrolide group of antibiotics.

Chemical name:

Erythromycin—Erythromycin.

Erythromycin estolate—Erythromycin, 2'-propanoate, dodecyl sulfate (salt).

Erythromycin ethylsuccinate—Erythromycin 2'-(ethyl butanedioate).

Erythromycin gluceptate—Erythromycin monoglucoheptonate (salt).

Erythromycin lactobionate—Erythromycin mono(4-O-beta-D-galactopyranosyl-D-gluconate) (salt).

Erythromycin stearate—Erythromycin octadecanoate (salt).

Molecular formula:

Erythromycin—$C_{37}H_{67}NO_{13}$.

Erythromycin estolate—$C_{40}H_{71}NO_{14} \cdot C_{12}H_{26}O_4S$.

Erythromycin ethylsuccinate—$C_{43}H_{75}NO_{16}$.

Erythromycin gluceptate—$C_{37}H_{67}NO_{13} \cdot C_7H_{14}O_8$.

Erythromycin lactobionate—$C_{37}H_{67}NO_{13} \cdot C_{12}H_{22}O_{12}$.

Erythromycin stearate—$C_{37}H_{67}NO_{13} \cdot C_{18}H_{36}O_2$.

Molecular weight:

Erythromycin—733.94.

Erythromycin estolate—1056.39.

Erythromycin ethylsuccinate—862.06.

Erythromycin gluceptate—960.12.

Erythromycin lactobionate—1092.23.

Erythromycin stearate—1018.42.

Description:

Erythromycin USP—White or slightly yellow, crystalline powder. Is odorless or practically odorless.

Erythromycin Estolate USP—White, crystalline powder. Is odorless or practically odorless.

Erythromycin Ethylsuccinate USP—White or slightly yellow crystalline powder. Is odorless or practically odorless.

Sterile Erythromycin Gluceptate USP—White powder. Is odorless or practically odorless, and is slightly hygroscopic. Its solution (1 in 20) is neutral or slightly acid.

Erythromycin Lactobionate for Injection USP—White or slightly yellow crystals or powder, having a faint odor. Its solution (1 in 20) is neutral or slightly alkaline.

Erythromycin Stearate USP—White or slightly yellow crystals or powder. Is odorless or may have a slight, earthy odor.

Solubility:

Erythromycin USP—Slightly soluble in water; soluble in alcohol, in chloroform, and in ether.

Erythromycin Estolate USP—Soluble in alcohol, in acetone, and in chloroform; practically insoluble in water.

Erythromycin Ethylsuccinate USP—Very slightly soluble in water; freely soluble in alcohol, in chloroform, and in polyethylene glycol 400.

Sterile Erythromycin Gluceptate USP—Freely soluble in water, in alcohol, and in methanol; slightly soluble in acetone and in chloroform; practically insoluble in ether.

Erythromycin Lactobionate for Injection USP—Freely soluble in water, in alcohol, and in methanol; slightly soluble in acetone and in chloroform; practically insoluble in ether.

Erythromycin Stearate USP—Practically insoluble in water; soluble in alcohol, in chloroform, in methanol, and in ether.

USP requirements:

Erythromycin Delayed-release Capsules USP—Preserve in tight containers. Contain the labeled amount, within −10% to +15%. Meet the requirements for Identification, Drug release (Method B—80% in 60 minutes for Acid stage and 60 minutes for Buffer stage in Apparatus 1 at 50 rpm), and Water (not more than 7.5%).

Erythromycin Topical Gel USP—Preserve in tight containers. It is Erythromycin in a suitable gel vehicle. Contains the labeled amount, within −10% to +25%. Meets the requirements for Identification and Minimum fill.

Erythromycin Ointment USP—Preserve in collapsible tubes or in other tight containers, preferably at controlled room temperature. It is Erythromycin in a suitable ointment base. Contains the labeled amount, within −10% to +25%. Meets the requirements for Identification, Minimum fill, and Water (not more than 1.0%).

Erythromycin Ophthalmic Ointment USP—Preserve in collapsible ophthalmic ointment tubes. A sterile preparation of Erythromycin in a suitable ointment base. Contains the labeled amount, within −10% to +20%. Meets the requirements for Identification, Sterility, Minimum fill, and Metal particles, and for Water under Erythromycin Ointment.

Erythromycin Pledgets USP—Preserve in tight containers. Suitable absorbent pads impregnated with Erythromycin Topical Solution. Label Pledgets to indicate that each Pledget is to be used once and then discarded. Label Pledgets also to indicate the volume, in mL, of Erythromycin Topical Solution contained in each Pledget, and the concentration, in mg of erythromycin per mL, of the Erythromycin Topical Solution. Contain not less than 90% of the labeled volume of Erythromycin Topical Solution. The Erythromycin Topical Solution expressed from Erythromycin Pledgets meets the requirements for Identification, Water, and Alcohol content under Erythromycin Topical Solution.

Erythromycin Topical Solution USP—Preserve in tight containers. A solution of Erythromycin in a suitable vehicle. Contains the labeled amount, within −10% to +25%. Meets the requirements for Identification, Water (not more than 8.0% [20 mg per mL]; not more than 5.0% [15 mg per mL]; or not more than 2.0% [acetone-containing solutions]), and Alcohol content (the labeled amount, within ±7.5%).

Erythromycin Tablets USP—Preserve in tight containers. Contain the labeled amount, within −10% to +20%. Meet the requirements for Identification, Dissolution (70% in 60 minutes in 0.05 M phosphate buffer [pH 6.8] in Apparatus 2 at 50 rpm), Uniformity of dosage units, and Loss on drying (not more than 5.0%).

Note: Tablets that are enteric-coated meet the requirements for Erythromycin Delayed-release Tablets.

Erythromycin Delayed-release Tablets USP—Preserve in tight containers. The label indicates that Erythromycin Delayed-release Tablets are enteric-coated. Contain the labeled amount, within −10% to +20%. Meet the requirements for Identification, Drug Release (Method B—75% in 60 minutes for Acid stage and 60 minutes for Buffer stage in Apparatus 1 at 100 rpm), Uniformity of dosage units, and Water (not more than 6.0%).

Erythromycin Estolate Capsules USP—Preserve in tight containers. Contain an amount of erythromycin estolate equivalent to the labeled amount of erythromycin, within −10% to +15%. Meet the requirements for Identification, Uniformity of dosage units, and Water (not more than 5.0%).

Erythromycin Estolate Oral Suspension USP—Preserve in tight containers, in a cold place. Contains one or more suitable buffers, colors, diluents, dispersants, and flavors.

Contains an amount of erythromycin estolate equivalent to the labeled amount of erythromycin, within −10% to +15%. Meets the requirements for Identification, Deliverable volume, pH (3.5–6.5), and Uniformity of dosage units (single-unit containers).

Erythromycin Estolate for Oral Suspension USP—Preserve in tight containers. A dry mixture of Erythromycin Estolate with one or more suitable buffers, colors, diluents, dispersants, and flavors. Contains an amount of erythromycin estolate equivalent to the labeled amount of erythromycin, within −10% to +15%. Meets the requirements for Identification, pH (5.0–7.0 [if pediatric drops, between 5.0 and 5.5], in the suspension constituted as directed in the labeling), Deliverable volume, Uniformity of dosage units, and Water (not more than 2.0%).

Erythromycin Estolate Tablets USP—Preserve in tight containers. Label Tablets to indicate whether they are to be chewed before swallowing. Contain an amount of erythromycin estolate equivalent to the labeled amount of erythromycin, within −10% to +20% (+15%, if chewable). Meet the requirements for Identification, Disintegration (30 minutes [Note: Chewable tablets are exempt from this requirement]), Uniformity of dosage units, and Water (not more than 5.0%; if chewable, not more than 4.0%).

Erythromycin Ethylsuccinate Injection USP—Preserve in single-dose or in multiple-dose containers, preferably of Type I glass. A sterile solution of Erythromycin Ethylsuccinate in Polyethylene Glycol 400, and contains 2% of butylaminobenzoate and a suitable preservative. Contains an amount of erythromycin ethylsuccinate equivalent to the labeled amount of erythromycin, within −10% to +15%. Meets the requirements for Sterility, Water (not more than 1.5%), and Injections.

Erythromycin Ethylsuccinate Oral Suspension USP—Preserve in tight containers, and store in a cold place. A suspension of Erythromycin Ethylsuccinate containing one or more suitable buffers, colors, dispersants, flavors, and preservatives. Contains an amount of erythromycin ethylsuccinate equivalent to the labeled amount of erythromycin, within −10% to +20%. Meets the requirements for Identification, pH (6.5–8.5), Deliverable volume, and Uniformity of dosage units (single-unit containers).

Erythromycin Ethylsuccinate for Oral Suspension USP—Preserve in tight containers. A dry mixture of Erythromycin Ethylsuccinate with one or more suitable buffers, colors, diluents, dispersants, and flavors. Contains an amount of erythromycin ethylsuccinate equivalent to the labeled amount of erythromycin, within −10% to +20%. Meets the requirements for Identification, pH (7.0–9.0, in the suspension constituted as directed in the labeling), Loss on drying (not more than 1.0%), Deliverable volume, and Uniformity of dosage units (single-unit containers).

Erythromycin Ethylsuccinate Tablets USP—Preserve in tight containers. Label chewable Tablets to indicate that they are to be chewed before swallowing. Contain an amount of erythromycin ethylsuccinate equivalent to the labeled amount of erythromycin, within −10% to +20%. Meet the requirements for Identification, Dissolution (75% in 45 minutes in 0.1 N hydrochloric acid in Apparatus 2 at 50 rpm), Uniformity of dosage units, Loss on drying (not more than 4.0% [Note: Chewable Tablets are exempt from this requirement]), and Water (Chewable Tablets only, not more than 5.0%).

Sterile Erythromycin Gluceptate USP—Preserve in Containers for Sterile Solids. It is Erythromycin Gluceptate suitable for parenteral use. Has a potency equivalent to not less than 600 mcg of erythromycin per mg, calculated on the anhydrous basis. In addition, where packaged for dispensing, contains an amount of erythromycin gluceptate equivalent to the labeled amount of erythromycin,

within −10% to +15%. Meets the requirements for Identification, Bacterial endotoxins, Sterility, pH (6.0–8.0, in a solution containing 25 mg per mL), Water (not more than 5.0%), Particulate matter, and, where packaged for dispensing, Uniformity of dosage units, and Constituted solutions and for Labeling under Injections.

Erythromycin Lactobionate for Injection USP—Preserve in Containers for Sterile Solids. A sterile, dry mixture of erythromycin lactobionate and a suitable preservative. Contains an amount of erythromycin lactobionate equivalent to the labeled amount of erythromycin, within −10% to +20%. Meets the requirements for Constituted solution, Identification, Bacterial endotoxins, pH (6.5–7.5, in a solution containing the equivalent of 50 mg of erythromycin per mL), Water (not more than 5.0%), Particulate matter, and Heavy metals (not more than 0.005%), and for Injections.

Erythromycin Stearate Oral Suspension—Not in USP.

Erythromycin Stearate for Oral Suspension USP—Preserve in tight containers. A dry mixture of Erythromycin Stearate with one or more suitable buffers, colors, diluents, dispersants, and flavors. Contains an amount of erythromycin stearate equivalent to the labeled amount of erythromycin, within −10% to +20%. Meets the requirements for Identification, pH (6.0–9.0, in the suspension constituted as directed in the labeling), Water (not more than 2.0%), Deliverable volume, and Uniformity of dosage units.

Erythromycin Stearate Tablets USP—Preserve in tight containers. Contain an amount of erythromycin stearate equivalent to the labeled amount of erythromycin, within −10% to +20%. Meet the requirements for Identification, Dissolution (75% in 120 minutes in monobasic sodium phosphate buffer in Apparatus 2 at 100 rpm), Uniformity of dosage units, and Loss on drying (not more than 5.0%).

ERYTHROMYCIN AND BENZOYL PEROXIDE

For *Erythromycin* and *Benzoyl Peroxide*—See individual listings for chemistry information.

USP requirements: Erythromycin and Benzoyl Peroxide Topical Gel USP—Before mixing, preserve the Erythromycin and the vehicle containing benzoyl peroxide in separate, tight containers. After mixing, preserve the mixture in tight containers. A mixture of Erythromycin in a suitable gel vehicle containing benzoyl peroxide and one or more suitable dispersants, stabilizers, and wetting agents. Contains the labeled amounts, within −10% to +25%. Meets the requirements for Identification, Benzoyl peroxide related substances, and Minimum fill.

ERYTHROMYCIN AND SULFISOXAZOLE

For *Erythromycin* and *Sulfisoxazole*—See individual listings for chemistry information.

USP requirements:

Erythromycin Estolate and Sulfisoxazole Acetyl Oral Suspension USP—Preserve in tight containers. Contains an amount of erythromycin estolate equivalent to the labeled amount of erythromycin, within −10% to +20%, and an amount of sulfisoxazole acetyl equivalent to the labeled amount of sulfisoxazole, within −10% to +15%. Contains one or more suitable buffers, colors, diluents, emulsifiers, flavors, preservatives, and suspending agents. Meets the requirements for Identification, Uniformity of dosage units (single-unit containers), Deliverable volume, and pH (3.5–6.5).

Erythromycin Ethylsuccinate and Sulfisoxazole Acetyl for Oral Suspension USP—Preserve in tight containers. A dry mixture of Erythromycin Ethylsuccinate and Sulfi-soxazole Acetyl with one or more suitable buffers, colors, flavors, surfactants, and suspending agents. Contains an amount of erythromycin ethylsuccinate equivalent to the labeled amount of erythromycin, within −10% to +20%, and an amount of sulfisoxazole acetyl equivalent to the labeled amount of sulfisoxazole, within −10% to +15%. Meets the requirements for Identification, pH (5.0–7.0, in the suspension constituted as directed in the labeling), Loss on drying (not more than 1.0%), Deliverable volume, and Uniformity of dosage units (single-unit containers).

Note: Where Erythromycin Ethylsuccinate and Sulfisox-azole Acetyl for Oral Suspension is prescribed, with-out reference to the quantity of erythromycin or sul-fisoxazole contained therein, a product containing 40 mg of erythromycin and 120 mg of sulfisoxazole per mL when constituted as directed in the labeling shall be dispensed.

ERYTHROSINE

Chemical name: Erythrosine sodium—Spiro[isobenzofuran-1(3H),9′-[9H]-xanthen]-3-one, 3′,6′-dihydroxy-2′,4′,5′,7′-te-traiodo-, disodium salt, monohydrate.

Molecular formula: Erythrosine sodium—$C_{20}H_6I_4Na_2O_5 \cdot H_2O$.

Molecular weight: Erythrosine sodium—897.88.

Description: Erythrosine Sodium USP—Red or brownish red, odorless powder. Dissolves in water to form a bluish red solution that shows no fluorescence in ordinary light. Hy-groscopic.

Solubility: Erythrosine Sodium USP—Soluble in water, in glyc-erin, and in propylene glycol; sparingly soluble in alcohol; insoluble in fats and in oils.

USP requirements:
Erythrosine Sodium Topical Solution USP—Preserve in tight, light-resistant containers. A solution of Erythrosine So-dium in Purified Water. Contains the labeled amount, within ±10%, calculated as hydrous erythrosine sodium. Contains one or more suitable flavoring and preservative agents. Meets the requirements for Identification and pH (6.8–8.0).
Erythrosine Sodium Soluble Tablets USP—Preserve in tight, moisture-resistant, light-resistant containers. Contain the labeled amount, within ±10%, calculated as hydrous erythrosine sodium. Meet the requirements for Identifi-cation and Uniformity of dosage units.

ESMOLOL

Chemical name: Esmolol hydrochloride—Benzenepropanoic acid, 4-[2-hydroxy-3-[(1-methylethyl)amino]propoxy]-, methyl es-ter, hydrochloride, (±)-.

Molecular formula: Esmolol hydrochloride—$C_{16}H_{25}NO_4 \cdot HCl$.

Molecular weight: Esmolol hydrochloride—331.84.

Description: Esmolol hydrochloride—White to off-white crys-talline powder; injection is clear, colorless to light yellow.

Solubility: Esmolol hydrochloride—Very soluble in water; freely soluble in alcohol.

Other characteristics: Partition coefficient—Esmolol hydro-chloride: Octanol/water at pH 7.0—0.42.

USP requirements: Esmolol Hydrochloride Injection—Not in USP.

ESTAZOLAM

Chemical group: A triazolobenzodiazepine derivative.

Chemical name: 4H-[1,2,4]Triazolo[4,3-a][1,4]benzodiazepine, 8-chloro-6-phenyl-.

Molecular formula: $C_{16}H_{11}ClN_4$.

Molecular weight: 294.74.

Description: Fine, white, odorless powder.

Solubility: Soluble in alcohol; practically insoluble in water.

USP requirements: Estazolam Tablets—Not in USP.

ESTRADIOL

Source:
Estradiol—Naturally occurring compound.
Estradiol cypionate; Estradiol valerate—Semi-synthetic compound.

Chemical name:
Estradiol—Estra-1,3,5(10)-triene-3,17-diol, (17 beta)-.
Estradiol cypionate—Estra-1,3,5(10)-triene-3,17-diol, (17 beta)-, 17-cyclopentanepropanoate.
Estradiol valerate—Estra-1,3,5(10)-triene-3,17-diol(17 beta)-, 17-pentanoate.

Molecular formula:
Estradiol—$C_{18}H_{24}O_2$.
Estradiol cypionate—$C_{26}H_{36}O_3$.
Estradiol valerate—$C_{23}H_{32}O_3$.

Molecular weight:
Estradiol—272.39.
Estradiol cypionate—396.57.
Estradiol valerate—356.50.

Description:
Estradiol USP—White or creamy white, small crystals or crystalline powder. Is odorless, and is stable in air. Is hygroscopic.
Estradiol Cypionate USP—White to practically white, crys-talline powder. Is odorless or has a slight odor.
Estradiol Valerate USP—White, crystalline powder. Is usu-ally odorless but may have a faint, fatty odor.

Solubility:
Estradiol USP—Practically insoluble in water; soluble in alcohol, in acetone, in dioxane, in chloroform, and in so-lutions of fixed alkali hydroxides; sparingly soluble in vegetable oils.
Estradiol Cypionate USP—Insoluble in water; soluble in al-cohol, in acetone, in chloroform, and in dioxane; sparingly soluble in vegetable oils.
Estradiol Valerate USP—Practically insoluble in water; sol-uble in castor oil, in methanol, in benzyl benzoate, and in dioxane; sparingly soluble in sesame oil and in peanut oil.

USP requirements:
Estradiol Vaginal Cream USP—Preserve in collapsible tubes or in tight containers. Contains the labeled amount, within ±10% in a suitable cream base. Meets the requirements for Identification, Microbial limits, Minimum fill, and pH (3.5–6.5).
Estradiol Pellets USP—Preserve in tight containers, suitable for maintaining sterile contents, that hold 1 Pellet each. Sterile pellets composed of Estradiol in compressed form, without the presence of any binder, diluent, or excipient. Contain the labeled amount, within ±3%. Meet the re-quirements for Solubility in chloroform, Identification,

Melting range (173–179 °C), Specific rotation (+76 ° to +83 °, calculated on the anhydrous basis), Water (not more than 3.5%), and Weight variation (for 5 pellets, average weight within ±5% of labeled weight; for each pellet, within ±10% of labeled weight), and the requirements under Sterility tests.

Sterile Estradiol Suspension USP—Preserve in single-dose or in multiple-dose containers, preferably of Type I glass. A sterile suspension of Estradiol in Water for Injection. Contains the labeled amount, within ±10%. Meets the requirements for Identification, Bacterial endotoxins, Uniformity of dosage units, and Injections.

Estradiol Tablets USP—Preserve in tight, light-resistant containers. Contain the labeled amount, within −10% to +15%. Meet the requirements for Identification, Dissolution (75% in 60 minutes in 0.3% sodium lauryl sulfate in water in Apparatus 2 at 100 rpm), and Uniformity of dosage units.

Estradiol Transdermal System—Not in USP.

Estradiol Cypionate Injection USP—Preserve in single-dose or in multiple-dose, light-resistant containers, preferably of Type I glass. A sterile solution of Estradiol Cypionate in a suitable oil. Contains the labeled amount, within ±10%. Meets the requirements for Identification and Injections.

Estradiol Valerate Injection USP—Preserve in single-dose or in multiple-dose, light-resistant containers, preferably of Type I or Type III glass. A sterile solution of Estradiol Valerate in a suitable vegetable oil. Contains the labeled amount, within −10% to +15%. Meets the requirements for Identification, Limit of estradiol (not more than 3.0%), and Injections.

ESTRAMUSTINE

Chemical name: Estramustine phosphate sodium—Estra-1,3,5(10)-triene-3,17-diol (17 beta)-, 3-[bis(2-chloroethyl)carbamate] 17-(dihydrogen phosphate), disodium salt.

Molecular formula: Estramustine phosphate sodium—$C_{23}H_{30}Cl_2NNa_2O_6P$.

Molecular weight: Estramustine phosphate sodium—564.35.

Description: Estramustine phosphate sodium—Off-white powder.

Solubility: Estramustine phosphate sodium—Readily soluble in water.

USP requirements: Estramustine Phosphate Sodium Capsules—Not in USP.

ESTROGENS, CONJUGATED

Source: Naturally occurring compound.

Description: Estrogens, Conjugated USP—Conjugated estrogens obtained from natural sources is a buff-colored, amorphous powder, odorless or having a slight, characteristic odor. The synthetic form is a white to light buff, crystalline or amorphous powder, odorless or having a slight odor.

USP requirements:
Conjugated Estrogens Vaginal Cream—Not in USP.
Conjugated Estrogens for Injection—Not in USP.
Conjugated Estrogens Tablets USP—Preserve in well-closed containers. Contain the labeled amount of conjugated estrogens as the total of sodium estrone sulfate and sodium equilin sulfate, within −27% to −5%. The ratio of sodium equilin sulfate to sodium estrone sulfate is not less than 0.35 and not more than 0.65. Meet the requirements

for Identification, Dissolution (75% in 1 hour in simulated gastric fluid TS, without pepsin, in a modified Disintegration basket assembly), and Uniformity of dosage units.

ESTROGENS, CONJUGATED, AND METHYLTESTOSTERONE

For *Estrogens, Conjugated*, and *Methyltestosterone*—See individual listings for chemistry information.

USP requirements: Conjugated Estrogens and Methyltestosterone Tablets—Not in USP.

ESTROGENS, ESTERIFIED

Source: Naturally occurring compound.

Description: Estrogens, Esterified USP—White or buff-colored, amorphous powder, odorless or having a slight, characteristic odor.

USP requirements: Esterified Estrogens Tablets USP—Preserve in well-closed containers. Contain the labeled amount of esterified estrogens as the total of sodium estrone sulfate and sodium equilin sulfate, within −10% to +15%. The ratio of sodium equilin sulfate to sodium estrone sulfate is not less than 0.071 and not more than 0.20. Meet the requirements for Identification, Disintegration (60 minutes), and Uniformity of dosage units.

ESTROGENS, ESTERIFIED, AND METHYLTESTOSTERONE

For *Estrogens, Esterified*, and *Methyltestosterone*—See individual listings for chemistry information.

USP requirements: Esterified Estrogens and Methyltestosterone Tablets—Not in USP.

ESTRONE

Source: Naturally occurring compound.

Chemical name: Estra-1,3,5(10)-trien-17-one, 3-hydroxy-.

Molecular formula: $C_{18}H_{22}O_2$.

Molecular weight: 270.37.

Description: Estrone USP—Small, white crystals or white to creamy white, crystalline powder. Is odorless, and is stable in air. Melts at about 260 °C.

Solubility: Estrone USP—Practically insoluble in water; soluble in alcohol, in acetone, in dioxane, and in vegetable oils; slightly soluble in solutions of fixed alkali hydroxides.

USP requirements:
Estrone Vaginal Cream—Not in USP.
Estrone Injection USP—Preserve in single-dose or in multiple-dose containers, preferably of Type I glass. A sterile solution of Estrone in a suitable oil. Contains the labeled amount, within −10% to +15%. Meets the requirements for Identification and Injections.
Estrone Vaginal Suppositories—Not in USP.
Sterile Estrone Suspension USP—Preserve in single-dose or in multiple-dose containers, preferably of Type I glass. A sterile suspension of Estrone in Water for Injection. Contains the labeled amount, within −10% to +15%. Meets the requirements for Identification, Bacterial endotoxins, Uniformity of dosage units, and Injections.

ESTROPIPATE

Source: Semi-synthetic compound.

Chemical name: Estra-1,3,5(10)-trien-17-one, 3-(sulfooxy)-, compd. with piperazine (1:1).

Molecular formula: $C_{18}H_{22}O_5S \cdot C_4H_{10}N_2$.

Molecular weight: 436.56.

Description: Estropipate USP—White to yellowish white, fine crystalline powder. Is odorless, or may have a slight odor. Melts at about 190 °C to a light brown, viscous liquid which solidifies, on further heating, and finally melts at about 245 °C, with decomposition.

Solubility: Estropipate USP—Very slightly soluble in water, in alcohol, in chloroform, and in ether; soluble in warm water.

USP requirements:
Estropipate Vaginal Cream USP—Preserve in collapsible tubes. Contains the labeled amount, within −10% to +20%, in a suitable cream base. Meets the requirements for Identification and Minimum fill.
Estropipate Tablets USP—Preserve in well-closed containers. Contain the labeled amount, within ± 10%. Meet the requirements for Identification, Dissolution (75% in 60 minutes in water in Apparatus 2 at 75 rpm), and Uniformity of dosage units.

ETHACRYNATE SODIUM

Chemical name: Acetic acid, [2,3-dichloro-4-(2-methylene-1-oxobutyl)phenoxy]-, sodium salt.

Molecular formula: $C_{13}H_{11}Cl_2NaO_4$.

Molecular weight: 325.12.

Description: Ethacrynate sodium for injection—White, crystalline powder.

Solubility: Ethacrynate sodium for injection—Solubility of about 70 mg/mL in water at 25 °C.

USP requirements: Ethacrynate Sodium for Injection USP—Preserve in Containers for Sterile Solids. It is a sterile, freeze-dried powder prepared by the neutralization of Ethacrynic Acid with the aid of Sodium Hydroxide. Label it to indicate that it was prepared by freeze-drying, having been filled into its container in the form of a true solution. Contains an amount of ethacrynate sodium equivalent to the labeled amount of ethacrynic acid, within ± 10%. Meets the requirements for Constituted solution, Identification, Bacterial endotoxins, pH (6.3–7.7), and for Sterility tests, Uniformity of dosage units, and Labeling under Injections.

ETHACRYNIC ACID

Chemical name: Acetic acid, [2,3-dichloro-4-(2-methylene-1-oxobutyl)phenoxy]-.

Molecular formula: $C_{13}H_{12}Cl_2O_4$.

Molecular weight: 303.14.

Description: Ethacrynic Acid USP—White or practically white, odorless or practically odorless, crystalline powder.

pKa: 3.5.

Solubility: Ethacrynic Acid USP—Very slightly soluble in water; freely soluble in alcohol, in chloroform, and in ether.

USP requirements:
Ethacrynic Acid Oral Solution—Not in USP.

Ethacrynic Acid Tablets USP—Preserve in well-closed containers. Contain the labeled amount, within ± 10%. Meet the requirements for Identification, Dissolution (75% in 45 minutes in 0.1 *M* phosphate buffer [pH 8.0] in Apparatus 2 at 50 rpm), and Uniformity of dosage units.

ETHAMBUTOL

Chemical name: Ethambutol hydrochloride—1-Butanol, 2,2′-(1,2-ethanediyldiimino)bis-, dihydrochloride, [*S*-(*R**,*R**)]-.

Molecular formula: Ethambutol hydrochloride—$C_{10}H_{24}N_2O_2 \cdot 2HCl$.

Molecular weight: Ethambutol hydrochloride—277.23.

Description: Ethambutol Hydrochloride USP—White, crystalline powder.

Solubility: Ethambutol Hydrochloride USP—Freely soluble in water; soluble in alcohol and in methanol; slightly soluble in ether and in chloroform.

USP requirements: Ethambutol Hydrochloride Tablets USP—Preserve in well-closed containers. Contain the labeled amount, within ± 5%. Meet the requirements for Identification, Dissolution (75% in 45 minutes in water in Apparatus 1 at 100 rpm), Uniformity of dosage units, and Aminobutanol (not more than 1.0%).

ETHCHLORVYNOL

Chemical name: 1-Penten-4-yn-3-ol, 1-chloro-3-ethyl-.

Molecular formula: C_7H_9ClO.

Molecular weight: 144.60.

Description: Ethchlorvynol USP—Colorless to yellow, slightly viscous liquid, having a characteristic pungent odor. Darkens on exposure to light and to air.

Solubility: Ethchlorvynol USP—Immiscible with water; miscible with most organic solvents.

USP requirements: Ethchlorvynol Capsules USP—Preserve in tight, light-resistant containers. Contain the labeled amount of *E*-ethchlorvynol, within ± 10%. Meet the requirements for Identification and Uniformity of dosage units.

ETHER

Chemical name: Ethane, 1,1′-oxybis-.

Molecular formula: $C_4H_{10}O$.

Molecular weight: 74.12.

Description: Ether USP—Colorless, mobile, volatile liquid, having a characteristic odor. Is slowly oxidized by the action of air and light, with the formation of peroxides. Boils at about 35 °C.

Solubility: Ether USP—Soluble in water. Miscible with alcohol, with chloroform, with solvent hexane, and with fixed and volatile oils.

USP requirements: Ether USP—Preserve in partly filled, tight, light-resistant containers, at a temperature not exceeding 30 °C, remote from fire. Contains not less than 96.0% and not more than 98.0% of ether, the remainder consisting of alcohol and water. Meets the requirements for Specific gravity (0.713–0.716 [indicating 96.0–98.0% of ether]), Acidity, Water (not more than 0.2%), Nonvolatile residue (not more than 0.003%), Foreign odor, Aldehyde, Peroxide (not more than 0.3 ppm), and Low-boiling hydrocarbons.

ETHINAMATE

Chemical name: Cyclohexanol, 1-ethynyl-, carbamate.

Molecular formula: $C_9H_{13}NO_2$.

Molecular weight: 167.21.

Description: Ethinamate USP—White, essentially odorless powder. Its saturated aqueous solution has a pH of about 6.5.

Solubility: Ethinamate USP—Slightly soluble in water; freely soluble in alcohol, in chloroform, and in ether.

USP requirements: Ethinamate Capsules USP—Preserve in tight containers. Contain the labeled amount, within ± 10%. Meet the requirements for Identification, Dissolution (75% in 45 minutes in water in Apparatus 2 at 50 rpm), and Uniformity of dosage units.

ETHINYL ESTRADIOL

Source: Semi-synthetic compound.

Chemical name: 19-Norpregna-1,3,5(10)-trien-20-yne-3,17-diol, (17 alpha)-.

Molecular formula: $C_{20}H_{24}O_2$.

Molecular weight: 296.41.

Description: Ethinyl Estradiol USP—White to creamy white, odorless, crystalline powder.

Solubility: Ethinyl Estradiol USP—Insoluble in water; soluble in alcohol, in chloroform, in ether, in vegetable oils, and in solutions of fixed alkali hydroxides.

USP requirements: Ethinyl Estradiol Tablets USP—Preserve in well-closed containers. Contain the labeled amount, within −10% to +15%. Meet the requirements for Identification, Disintegration (30 minutes), and Uniformity of dosage units.

ETHIODIZED OIL

Description: Ethiodized Oil Injection USP—Straw-colored to amber-colored, oily liquid. May possess an alliaceous odor.

Solubility: Ethiodized Oil Injection USP—Insoluble in water; soluble in acetone, in chloroform, in ether, and in solvent hexane.

USP requirements: Ethiodized Oil Injection USP—Preserve in well-filled, light-resistant, single-dose or multiple-dose containers. An iodine addition product of the ethyl ester of the fatty acids of poppyseed oil, containing not less than 35.2% and not more than 38.9% of organically combined iodine. It is sterile. Meets the requirements for Identification, Specific gravity (1.280–1.293, at 15 °C), Viscosity (50–100 centipoises, at 15 °C), Sterility, Acidity, and Free iodine.

ETHIONAMIDE

Chemical group: Synthetic derivative of isonicotinic acid.

Chemical name: 4-Pyridinecarbothioamide, 2-ethyl-.

Molecular formula: $C_8H_{10}N_2S$.

Molecular weight: 166.24.

Description: Ethionamide USP—Bright yellow powder, having a faint to moderate sulfide-like odor.

Solubility: Ethionamide USP—Slightly soluble in water, in chloroform, and in ether; soluble in methanol; sparingly soluble in alcohol and in propylene glycol.

USP requirements: Ethionamide Tablets USP—Preserve in tight containers. Contain the labeled amount, within −5% to +10%. Meet the requirements for Identification, Disintegration (15 minutes, the use of disks being omitted), and Uniformity of dosage units.

ETHOPROPAZINE

Chemical group: Phenothiazine derivative.

Chemical name: Ethopropazine hydrochloride—10H-Phenothiazine-10-ethanamine, N,N-diethyl-alpha-methyl-, monohydrochloride.

Molecular formula: Ethopropazine hydrochloride—$C_{19}H_{24}N_2S \cdot$ HCl.

Molecular weight: Ethopropazine hydrochloride—348.93.

Description: Ethopropazine Hydrochloride USP—White or slightly off-white, odorless, crystalline powder. Melts at about 210 °C, with decomposition.

Solubility: Ethopropazine Hydrochloride USP—Soluble in water at 40 °C; slightly soluble in water at 20 °C; soluble in alcohol and in chloroform; sparingly soluble in acetone; insoluble in ether.

USP requirements: Ethopropazine Hydrochloride Tablets USP—Preserve in well-closed containers, protected from light. Contain the labeled amount, within ± 10%. Meet the requirements for Identification, Dissolution (75% in 45 minutes in 0.1 N hydrochloric acid in Apparatus 1 at 100 rpm), Uniformity of dosage units, and Other alkylated phenothiazines.

ETHOSUXIMIDE

Chemical name: 2,5-Pyrrolidinedione, 3-ethyl-3-methyl-.

Molecular formula: $C_7H_{11}NO_2$.

Molecular weight: 141.17.

Description: Ethosuximide USP—White to off-white, crystalline powder or waxy solid, having a characteristic odor.

Solubility: Ethosuximide USP—Freely soluble in water and in chloroform; very soluble in alcohol and in ether; very slightly soluble in solvent hexane.

USP requirements:
Ethosuximide Capsules USP—Preserve in tight containers. Contain the labeled amount, within ± 7%, as a solution in Polyethylene Glycol 400 or other suitable solvent. Meet the requirements for Identification and Uniformity of dosage units.
Ethosuximide Syrup—Not in USP.

ETHOTOIN

Chemical group: Related to the barbiturates in chemical structure, but having a five-membered ring.

Chemical name: 3-Ethyl-5-phenylimidazolidin-2,4-dione.

Molecular formula: $C_{11}H_{12}N_2O_2$.

Molecular weight: 204.23.

Description: Ethotoin USP—White, crystalline powder.

Solubility: Ethotoin USP—Insoluble in water; freely soluble in dehydrated alcohol and in chloroform; soluble in ether.

USP requirements: Ethotoin Tablets USP—Preserve in tight containers. Contain the labeled amount, within ±10%. Meet the requirements for Identification, Dissolution (80% in 60 minutes in 0.1 N hydrochloric acid in Apparatus 2 at 100 rpm), and Uniformity of dosage units.

ETHYL ACETATE

Chemical name: Acetic acid, ethyl ester.

Molecular formula: $C_4H_8O_2$.

Molecular weight: 88.11.

Description: Ethyl Acetate NF—Transparent, colorless liquid, having a fragrant, refreshing, slightly acetous odor.
NF category: Flavors and perfumes; solvent.

Solubility: Ethyl Acetate NF—Soluble in water; miscible with alcohol, with ether, with fixed oils, and with volatile oils.

NF requirements: Ethyl Acetate NF—Preserve in tight containers, and avoid exposure to excessive heat. Contains not less than 99.0% and not more than 100.5% of ethyl acetate. Meets the requirements for Identification, Specific gravity (0.894–0.898), Acidity, Nonvolatile residue (not more than 0.02%), Readily carbonizable substances, Methyl compounds, Chromatographic purity, and Organic volatile impurities.

ETHYLCELLULOSE

Chemical name: Cellulose, ethyl ester.

Description: Ethylcellulose NF—Free-flowing, white to light tan powder. It forms films that have a refractive index of about 1.47. Its aqueous suspensions are neutral to litmus.
NF category: Coating agent; tablet binder.

Solubility: Ethylcellulose NF—Insoluble in water, in glycerin, and in propylene glycol. Ethylcellulose containing less than 46.5% of ethoxy groups is freely soluble in tetrahydrofuran, in methyl acetate, in chloroform, and in mixtures of aromatic hydrocarbons with alcohol. Ethylcellulose containing not less than 46.5% of ethoxy groups is freely soluble in alcohol, in methanol, in toluene, in chloroform, and in ethyl acetate.

NF requirements:
Ethylcellulose NF—Preserve in well-closed containers. An ethyl ether of cellulose. Label it to indicate its viscosity (under the conditions specified herein), and its ethoxy content. When dried at 105 °C for 2 hours, contains not less than 44.0% and not more than 51.0% of ethoxy ($-OC_2H_5$) groups. Meets the requirements for Identification, Viscosity, Loss on drying (not more than 3.0%), Residue on ignition (not more than 0.4%), Arsenic (not more than 3 ppm), Lead (not more than 10 ppm), and Heavy metals (not more than 40 ppm).
Ethylcellulose Aqueous Dispersion NF—Preserve in tight containers, and protect from freezing. A colloidal dispersion of Ethylcellulose in water. The labeling states the ethoxy content of the Ethylcellulose and the percentage of Ethylcellulose. Contains the labeled amount of Ethylcellulose, within ±10%. Contains suitable amounts of Cetyl Alcohol and Sodium Lauryl Sulfate, which assist in the formation and stabilization of the dispersion. Meets the requirements for Identification, Viscosity (not more than 150 centipoises), pH (4.0–7.0), Loss on drying (not more than 71.0%), Heavy metals (not more than 0.001%), and Organic volatile impurities.

ETHYLNOREPINEPHRINE

Chemical name: Ethylnorepinephrine hydrochloride—1,2-Benzenediol, 4-(2-amino-1-hydroxybutyl)-, hydrochloride.

Molecular formula: Ethylnorepinephrine hydrochloride—$C_{10}H_{15}NO_3 \cdot HCl$.

Molecular weight: Ethylnorepinephrine hydrochloride—233.69.

Description: Ethylnorepinephrine Hydrochloride USP—White to practically white, crystalline powder, which gradually darkens on exposure to light. Melts at about 190 °C, with decomposition.

Solubility: Ethylnorepinephrine Hydrochloride USP—Soluble in water and in alcohol; practically insoluble in ether.

USP requirements: Ethylnorepinephrine Hydrochloride Injection USP—Preserve in single-dose or in multiple-dose, light-resistant containers, preferably of Type I glass. A sterile solution of Ethylnorepinephrine Hydrochloride in Water for Injection. Contains the labeled amount, within −10% to +15%. Meets the requirements for Identification, Bacterial endotoxins, pH (2.5–5.0), and Injections.
Note: Do not use the Injection if it is brown or contains a precipitate.

ETHYL OLEATE

Chemical name: 9-Octadecenoic acid, (Z)-, ethyl ester.

Molecular formula: $C_{20}H_{38}O_2$.

Molecular weight: 310.52.

Description: Ethyl Oleate NF—Mobile, practically colorless liquid.
NF category: Vehicle (oleaginous).

Solubility: Ethyl Oleate NF—Insoluble in water; miscible with vegetable oils, with mineral oil, with alcohol, and with most organic solvents.

NF requirements: Ethyl Oleate NF—Preserve in tight, light-resistant containers. Consists of esters of ethyl alcohol and high molecular weight fatty acids, principally oleic acid. Meets the requirements for Specific gravity, (0.866–0.874 at 20 °C), Viscosity (not less than 5.15 centipoises), Refractive index (1.443–1.450), Acid value (not more than 0.5), Iodine value (75–85), and Saponification value (177–188).

ETHYLPARABEN

Chemical name: Benzoic acid, 4-hydroxy-, ethyl ester.

Molecular formula: $C_9H_{10}O_3$.

Molecular weight: 166.18.

Description: Ethylparaben NF—Small, colorless crystals or white powder.
NF category: Antimicrobial preservative.

Solubility: Ethylparaben NF—Slightly soluble in water and in glycerin; freely soluble in acetone, in alcohol, in ether, and in propylene glycol.

NF requirements: Ethylparaben NF—Preserve in well-closed containers. Contains not less than 99.0% and not more than 100.5% of ethylparaben, calculated on the dried basis. Meets the requirements for Identification and Melting range (115–118 °C), and for Acidity, Loss on drying, and Residue on ignition under Butylparaben.

ETHYL VANILLIN

Chemical name: Benzaldehyde, 3-ethoxy-4-hydroxy-.

Molecular formula: $C_9H_{10}O_3$.

Molecular weight: 166.18.

Description: Ethyl Vanillin NF—Fine, white or slightly yellowish crystals. Its odor is similar to the odor of vanillin. It is affected by light. Its solutions are acid to litmus.
NF category: Flavors and perfumes.

Solubility: Ethyl Vanillin NF—Sparingly soluble in water at 50 °C; freely soluble in alcohol, in chloroform, in ether, and in solutions of alkali hydroxides.

NF requirements: Ethyl Vanillin NF—Preserve in tight, light-resistant containers. Dried over phosphorus pentoxide for 4 hours, contains not less than 98.0% and not more than 101.0% of ethyl vanillin. Meets the requirements for Identification, Melting range (76–78 °C), Loss on drying (not more than 1.0%), and Residue on ignition (not more than 0.1%).

ETHYNODIOL DIACETATE AND ETHINYL ESTRADIOL

Chemical name:
Ethynodiol diacetate—19-Norpregn-4-en-20-yne-3,17-diol, diacetate, (3 beta,17 alpha)-.
Ethinyl estradiol—19-Norpregna-1,3,5(10)-trien-20-yne-3,17-diol, (17 alpha)-.

Molecular formula:
Ethynodiol diacetate—$C_{24}H_{32}O_4$.
Ethinyl estradiol—$C_{20}H_{24}O_2$.

Molecular weight:
Ethynodiol diacetate—384.51.
Ethinyl estradiol—296.41.

Description:
Ethynodiol Diacetate USP—White, odorless, crystalline powder. Is stable in air.
Ethinyl Estradiol USP—White to creamy white, odorless, crystalline powder.

Solubility:
Ethynodiol Diacetate USP—Insoluble in water; very soluble in chloroform; freely soluble in ether; soluble in alcohol; sparingly soluble in fixed oils.
Ethinyl Estradiol USP—Insoluble in water; soluble in alcohol, in chloroform, in ether, in vegetable oils, and in solutions of fixed alkali hydroxides.

USP requirements: Ethynodiol Diacetate and Ethinyl Estradiol Tablets USP—Preserve in well-closed containers. Contain the labeled amount of ethynodiol diacetate, within ±7%, and the labeled amount of ethinyl estradiol, within ±10%. Meet the requirements for Identification, Disintegration (15 minutes, the use of disks being omitted), and Uniformity of dosage units.

ETHYNODIOL DIACETATE AND MESTRANOL

Chemical name:
Ethynodiol diacetate—19-Norpregn-4-en-20-yne-3,17-diol, diacetate, (3 beta,17 alpha)-.
Mestranol—19-Norpregna-1,3,5(10)-trien-20-yn-17-ol, 3-methoxy-, (17 alpha)-.

Molecular formula:
Ethynodiol diacetate—$C_{24}H_{32}O_4$.
Mestranol—$C_{21}H_{26}O_2$.

Molecular weight:
Ethynodiol diacetate—384.51.
Mestranol—310.44.

Description:
Ethynodiol Diacetate USP—White, odorless, crystalline powder. Is stable in air.
Mestranol USP—White to creamy white, odorless, crystalline powder.

Solubility:
Ethynodiol Diacetate USP—Insoluble in water; very soluble in chloroform; freely soluble in ether; soluble in alcohol; sparingly soluble in fixed oils.
Mestranol USP—Insoluble in water; freely soluble in chloroform; soluble in dioxane; sparingly soluble in dehydrated alcohol; slightly soluble in methanol.

USP requirements: Ethynodiol Diacetate and Mestranol Tablets USP—Preserve in well-closed containers. Contain the labeled amounts of ethynodiol diacetate and mestranol, within ±10%. Meet the requirements for Identification, Disintegration (15 minutes, the use of disks being omitted), and Uniformity of dosage units.

ETIDOCAINE

Chemical group: Amide.

Chemical name: Etidocaine hydrochloride—Butanamide, *N*-(2,6-dimethylphenyl)-2-(ethylpropylamine)-, monohydrochloride.

Molecular formula: Etidocaine hydrochloride—$C_{17}H_{28}N_2O \cdot HCl$.

Molecular weight: Etidocaine hydrochloride—312.88.

Description: Etidocaine hydrochloride—White, crystalline powder.

pKa: 7.74.

Solubility: Etidocaine hydrochloride—Soluble in water; freely soluble in alcohol.

USP requirements: Etidocaine Hydrochloride Injection—Not in USP.

ETIDOCAINE AND EPINEPHRINE

For *Etidocaine* and *Epinephrine*—See individual listings for chemistry information.

USP requirements: Etidocaine Hydrochloride and Epinephrine Injection—Not in USP.

ETIDRONATE

Source: Synthetic analogue of inorganic pyrophosphate.

Chemical group: Diphosphonate.

Chemical name: Etidronate disodium—Phosphonic acid, (1-hydroxyethylidene)bis-, disodium salt.

Molecular formula: Etidronate disodium—$C_2H_6Na_2O_7P_2$.

Molecular weight: Etidronate disodium—249.99.

Description: Etidronate disodium—White powder.

Solubility: Etidronate disodium—Highly soluble in water.

USP requirements:
Etidronate Disodium Injection—Not in USP.

Etidronate Disodium Tablets USP—Preserve in tight containers. Contain the labeled amount, within ±10%. Meet the requirements for Identification, Dissolution (70% in 30 minutes in water in Apparatus 1 at 100 rpm), and Uniformity of dosage units.

ETODOLAC

Chemical name: Pyrano[3,4-*b*]indole-1-acetic acid, 1,8-diethyl-1,3,4,9-tetrahydro-.

Molecular formula: $C_{17}H_{21}NO_3$.

Molecular weight: 287.36.

Description: White, crystalline compound.

pKa: 4.65.

Solubility: Insoluble in water; soluble in alcohols, in chloroform, in dimethyl sulfoxide, and in aqueous polyethylene glycol.

Other characteristics: N-octanol:water partition coefficient 11.4 at pH 7.4.

USP requirements: Etodolac Capsules—Not in USP.

ETOMIDATE

Chemical name: 1*H*-Imidazole-5-carboxylic acid, 1-(1-phenylethyl)-, ethyl ester, (+)-.

Molecular formula: $C_{14}H_{16}N_2O_2$.

Molecular weight: 244.29.

Description: A white or yellowish crystalline or amorphous powder. Melting point about 67 °C.

Solubility: Soluble in water at 25 °C (0.0045 mg/100 mL), in chloroform, in methanol, in ethanol, in propylene glycol, and in acetone.

USP requirements: Etomidate Injection—Not in USP.

ETOPOSIDE

Source: Etoposide (also known as VP-16 or VP-16-213) is a semisynthetic podophyllotoxin of the mandrake plant.

Chemical name: Furo[3′,4′:6,7]naphtho[2,3-*d*]-1,3-dioxol-6(5a*H*)-one-, 9-[(4,6-*O*-ethylidene-beta-D-glucopyranosyl)oxy]-5,8,8a,9-tetrahydro-5-(4-hydroxy-3,5-dimethoxyphenyl), [5*R*-[5 alpha,5a beta,8a alpha,9 beta(*R**)]]-.

Molecular formula: $C_{29}H_{32}O_{13}$.

Molecular weight: 588.56.

Description: White to yellow-brown powder. Melts at about 221 °C.

Solubility: Very soluble in methanol and in chloroform; slightly soluble in ethanol; sparingly soluble in water and in ether; made more miscible with water by means of organic solvents.

Other characteristics: Lipophilic.

USP requirements:
Etoposide Capsules—Not in USP.
Etoposide Injection—Not in USP.

ETRETINATE

Source: Ethyl ester of an aromatic analog of retinoic acid.

Chemical group: Related to both retinoic acid and retinol (vitamin A).

Chemical name: 2,4,6,8-Nonatetraenoic acid, 9-(4-methoxy-2,3,6-trimethylphenyl)-, ethyl ester, (*all-E*-).

Molecular formula: $C_{23}H_{30}O_3$.

Molecular weight: 354.49.

Description: Greenish-yellow to yellow powder.

Solubility: Insoluble in water.

Other characteristics: Both etretinate and its pharmacologically active metabolite, acetretin (etretin), have an all-*trans* structure.

USP requirements: Etretinate Capsules—Not in USP.

EUCATROPINE

Chemical name: Eucatropine hydrochloride—Benzeneacetic acid, alpha-hydroxy-, 1,2,2,6-tetramethyl-4-piperidinyl ester hydrochloride.

Molecular formula: Eucatropine hydrochloride—$C_{17}H_{25}NO_3 \cdot$ HCl.

Molecular weight: Eucatropine hydrochloride—327.85.

Description: Eucatropine Hydrochloride USP—White, granular, odorless powder. Its solutions are neutral to litmus.

Solubility: Eucatropine Hydrochloride USP—Very soluble in water; freely soluble in alcohol and in chloroform; insoluble in ether.

USP requirements: Eucatropine Hydrochloride Ophthalmic Solution USP—Preserve in tight containers. A sterile, isotonic, aqueous solution of Eucatropine Hydrochloride. Contains the labeled amount, within ±5%. Meets the requirements for Identification, Sterility, and pH (4.0–5.0).

EUGENOL

Chemical name: Phenol, 2-methoxy-4-(2-propenyl)-.

Molecular formula: $C_{10}H_{12}O_2$.

Molecular weight: 164.20.

Description: Eugenol USP—Colorless or pale yellow liquid, having a strongly aromatic odor of clove. Upon exposure to air, it darkens and thickens. Is optically inactive.

Solubility: Eugenol USP—Slightly soluble in water. Miscible with alcohol, with chloroform, with ether, and with fixed oils.

USP requirements: Eugenol USP—Preserve in tight, light-resistant containers. It is obtained from Clove Oil and from other sources. Meets the requirements for Solubility in 70% alcohol (1 volume dissolves in 2 volumes of 70% alcohol), Specific gravity (1.064–1.070), Distilling range (not less than 95% at 250–255 °C), Refractive index (1.540–1.542 at 20 °C), Heavy metals (not more than 0.004%), Hydrocarbons, and Phenol.

EVANS BLUE

Chemical name: 1,3-Naphthalenedisulfonic acid, 6,6′-[(3,3′-dimethyl[1,1′-biphenyl]-4,4′-diyl)bis(azo)]bis[4-amino-5-hydroxy]-, tetrasodium salt.

Molecular formula: $C_{34}H_{24}N_6Na_4O_{14}S_4$.

Molecular weight: 960.79.

Description: Evans Blue USP—Green, bluish green, or brown, odorless powder.

Solubility: Evans Blue USP—Very soluble in water; very slightly soluble in alcohol; practically insoluble in carbon tetrachloride, in chloroform, and in ether.

USP requirements: Evans Blue Injection USP—Preserve in single-dose containers, preferably of Type I glass. A sterile solution of Evans Blue in Water for Injection. Contains, in each mL, not less than 4.30 mg and not more than 4.75 mg of Evans Blue. Meets the requirements for Identification, Bacterial endotoxins, pH (5.5–7.5), and Injections.

FACTOR IX COMPLEX

USP requirements: Factor IX Complex USP—Preserve in hermetic containers in a refrigerator. A sterile, freeze-dried powder consisting of partially purified Factor IX fraction, as well as concentrated Factors II, VII, and X fractions, of venous plasma obtained from healthy human donors. Contains no preservative. Label it with a warning that it is to be used within 4 hours after constitution, and to state that it is for intravenous administration and that a filter is to be used in the administration equipment. Meets the requirements of the test for potency in having within ±20% of the potency stated on the label in Factor IX Units by comparison with the U.S. Factor IX Standard or with a working reference that has been calibrated with it. Meets the requirement for Expiration date (not later than 2 years from the date of manufacture). Conforms to the regulations of the U.S. Food and Drug Administration concerning biologics.

FAMOTIDINE

Chemical group: Thiazole derivative of histamine.

Chemical name: Propanimidamide, N'-(aminosulfonyl)-3-[[[2-[(diaminomethylene)amino]-4-thiazolyl]methyl]thio]-.

Molecular formula: $C_8H_{15}N_7O_2S_3$.

Molecular weight: 337.43.

Description: Famotidine USP—White to pale yellowish-white crystalline powder. Sensitive to light.

Solubility: Famotidine USP—Freely soluble in dimethylformamide and in glacial acetic acid; slightly soluble in methanol; very slightly soluble in water; practically insoluble in acetone, in alcohol, in chloroform, in ether, and in ethyl acetate.

USP requirements:
Famotidine Injection—Not in USP.
Famotidine for Oral Suspension—Not in USP.
Famotidine Tablets USP—Preserve in well-closed, light-resistant containers. Contain the labeled amount, within ±10%. Meet the requirements for Identification, Dissolution (75% in 30 minutes in 0.1 M phosphate buffer [pH 4.5] in Apparatus 2 at 50 rpm), and Uniformity of dosage units.

HARD FAT

Description: Hard Fat NF—White mass; almost odorless and free from rancid odor; greasy to the touch. On warming, melts to give a colorless or slightly yellowish liquid. When the molten material is shaken with an equal quantity of hot water, a white emulsion is formed.

NF category: Stiffening agent; suppository base.

Solubility: Hard Fat NF—Practically insoluble in water; freely soluble in ether; slightly soluble in alcohol.

NF requirements: Hard Fat NF—Preserve in tight containers at a temperature that is 5 °C or more below the melting range stated in the labeling. A mixture of glycerides of saturated fatty acids. The labeling includes a melting range, which is not greater than 4 °C and which is between 27 and 44 °C. Meets the requirements for Melting range, Residue on ignition (not more than 0.05%), Acid value (not more than 1.0), Iodine value (not more than 7.0), Saponification value (215–255), Hydroxyl value (not more than 70), Unsaponifiable matter (not more than 3.0%), and Alkaline impurities.

FAT EMULSIONS

Source:
Egg phosphatides—A mixture of naturally occurring phospholipids which are isolated from the egg yolk.
Safflower oil—Refined fixed oil obtained from seeds of the safflower, or false (bastard) saffron, *Carthamus tinctorius* (Compositae).
Soybean oil—Obtained from soybeans by solvent extraction using petroleum hydrocarbons or, to a lesser extent, by expression using continuous screw press operations.

Chemical name:
Glycerin—1,2,3-Propanetriol.
Linoleic acid—(Z,Z)-9,12-Octadecadienoic acid.
Linolenic acid—(Z,Z,Z)-9,12,15-Octadecatrienoic acid.
Oleic acid—9-Octadecenoic acid, (Z)-.
Palmitic acid—Hexadecanoic acid.
Stearic acid—Octadecanoic acid.

Molecular formula:
Glycerin—$C_3H_8O_3$.
Linoleic acid—$C_{18}H_{32}O_2$.
Linolenic acid—$C_{18}H_{30}O_2$.
Oleic acid—$C_{18}H_{34}O_2$.
Palmitic acid—$C_{16}H_{32}O_2$.
Stearic acid—$C_{18}H_{36}O_2$.

Molecular weight:
Glycerin—92.09.
Linoleic acid—280.44.
Linolenic acid—278.42.
Oleic acid—282.47.
Palmitic acid—256.42.
Stearic acid—284.47.

Description:
Glycerin USP—Clear, colorless, syrupy liquid. Has not more than a slight characteristic odor, which is neither harsh nor disagreeable. Is hygroscopic. Its solutions are neutral to litmus.
NF category: Humectant; plasticizer; solvent; tonicity agent.
Linoleic acid—Colorless oil; easily oxidized by air; cannot be distilled without decomposition.
Linolenic acid—Colorless liquid.
Oleic Acid NF—Colorless to pale yellow, oily liquid when freshly prepared, but on exposure to air it gradually absorbs oxygen and darkens. It has a characteristic, lard-like odor. When strongly heated in air, it is decomposed with the production of acrid vapors.
NF category: Emulsifying and/or solubilizing agent.
Palmitic acid—White crystalline scales. Melting point 63–64 °C.
Safflower oil—Thickens and becomes rancid on prolonged exposure to air.
Soybean Oil USP—Clear, pale yellow, oily liquid having a characteristic odor.
NF category: Oleaginous vehicle.

Stearic Acid NF—Hard, white or faintly yellowish, somewhat glossy and crystalline solid, or white or yellowish white powder. Slight odor, suggesting tallow.

NF category: Emulsifying and/or solubilizing agent; tablet and/or capsule lubricant.

Solubility:

Glycerin USP—Miscible with water and with alcohol. Insoluble in chloroform, in ether, and in fixed and volatile oils.

Linoleic acid—Freely soluble in ether; soluble in absolute alcohol. One mL dissolves in 10 mL petroleum ether. Miscible with dimethylformamide, with fat solvents, and with oils.

Linolenic acid—Insoluble in water; soluble in organic solvents.

Oleic Acid NF—Practically insoluble in water. Miscible with alcohol, with chloroform, with ether, and with fixed and volatile oils.

Palmitic acid—Insoluble in water; sparingly soluble in cold alcohol or in petroleum ether; freely soluble in hot alcohol, in ether, in propyl alcohol, and in chloroform.

Safflower oil—Soluble in the usual oil and fat solvents.

Soybean Oil USP—Insoluble in water; miscible with ether and with chloroform.

Stearic Acid NF—Practically insoluble in water; freely soluble in chloroform and in ether; soluble in alcohol.

USP requirements: Fat Emulsions Injection—Not in USP.

FELODIPINE

Chemical group: Dihydropyridine derivative.

Chemical name: 3,5-Pyridinedicarboxylic acid, 4-(2,3-dichlorophenyl)-1,4-dihydro-2,6-dimethyl-, ethyl methyl ester.

Molecular formula: $C_{18}H_{19}Cl_2NO_4$.

Molecular weight: 384.26.

Description: Slightly yellowish, crystalline powder.

Solubility: Insoluble in water; freely soluble in dichloromethane and in ethanol.

USP requirements: Felodipine Extended-release Tablets—Not in USP.

FENFLURAMINE

Chemical group: Phenethylamine.

Chemical name: Fenfluramine hydrochloride—Benzeneethanamine, N-ethyl-alpha-methyl-3-(trifluoromethyl)-, hydrochloride.

Molecular formula: Fenfluramine hydrochloride—$C_{12}H_{16}F_3N\cdot HCl$.

Molecular weight: Fenfluramine hydrochloride—267.72.

Description: Fenfluramine hydrochloride—White, odorless, or almost odorless, crystalline powder.

Solubility: Fenfluramine hydrochloride—Soluble 1 in 20 of water, 1 in 10 of alcohol, and in chloroform; practically insoluble in ether.

USP requirements:

Fenfluramine Hydrochloride Extended-release Capsules—Not in USP.

Fenfluramine Hydrochloride Tablets—Not in USP.

Fenfluramine Hydrochloride Extended-release Tablets—Not in USP.

FENOPROFEN

Chemical group: Phenylpropionic acid derivative nonsteroidal anti-inflammatory.

Chemical name: Fenoprofen calcium—Benzeneacetic acid, alpha-methyl-3-phenoxy-, calcium salt dihydrate, (±)-.

Molecular formula: Fenoprofen calcium—$C_{30}H_{26}CaO_6\cdot2H_2O$.

Molecular weight: Fenoprofen calcium—558.64.

Description: Fenoprofen Calcium USP—White, crystalline powder.

pKa: Fenoprofen calcium—4.5 (25 °C).

Solubility: Fenoprofen Calcium USP—Slightly soluble in n-hexanol, in methanol, and in water; practically insoluble in chloroform.

USP requirements:

Fenoprofen Calcium Capsules USP—Preserve in well-closed containers. Contain an amount of fenoprofen calcium equivalent to the labeled amount of fenoprofen, within ±10%. Meet the requirements for Identification, Dissolution (75% in 60 minutes in phosphate buffer [pH 7.0] in Apparatus 1 [10-mesh basket] at 100 rpm), and Uniformity of dosage units.

Fenoprofen Calcium Tablets USP—Preserve in well-closed containers. Contain an amount of fenoprofen calcium equivalent to the labeled amount of fenoprofen, within ±10%. Meet the requirements for Identification, Dissolution (75% in 60 minutes in phosphate buffer [pH 7.0] in Apparatus 1 [10-mesh basket] at 100 rpm), and Uniformity of dosage units.

FENOTEROL

Chemical name: Fenoterol hydrobromide—1,3-Benzenediol, 5-[1-hydroxy-2-[[2-(4-hydroxyphenyl)-1-methylethyl]amino]ethyl]-, hydrobromide.

Molecular formula: Fenoterol hydrobromide—$C_{17}H_{21}NO_4\cdot HBr$.

Molecular weight: Fenoterol hydrobromide—384.28.

Description: Fenoterol hydrobromide—White, odorless, crystalline powder. Melting point approximately 230 °C.

Solubility: Fenoterol hydrobromide—Soluble in water and in alcohol; practically insoluble in chloroform.

USP requirements:

Fenoterol Hydrobromide Inhalation Aerosol—Not in USP.

Fenoterol Hydrobromide Inhalation Solution—Not in USP.

Fenoterol Hydrobromide Tablets—Not in USP.

FENTANYL

Chemical group: Fentanyl derivatives are anilinopiperidine-derivative opioid analgesics and are chemically related to anileridine and meperidine.

Chemical name: Fentanyl citrate—Propanamide, N-phenyl-N-[1-(2-phenylethyl)-4-piperidinyl]-, 2-hydroxy-1,2,3-propanetricarboxylate (1:1).

Molecular formula: Fentanyl citrate—$C_{22}H_{28}N_2O\cdot C_6H_8O_7$.

Molecular weight: Fentanyl citrate—528.60.

Description: Fentanyl Citrate USP—White, crystalline powder or white, glistening crystals. Melts at about 150 °C, with decomposition.

pKa: 8.4.

Solubility: Fentanyl Citrate USP—Sparingly soluble in water; soluble in methanol; slightly soluble in chloroform.

Other characteristics: Partition coefficient (octanol:water)—Fentanyl citrate: At pH 7.4—816.

USP requirements:
Fentanyl Citrate Injection USP—Preserve in single-dose containers, preferably of Type I glass, protected from light. A sterile solution of Fentanyl Citrate in Water for Injection. Contains an amount of fentanyl citrate equivalent to the labeled amount of fentanyl, present as the citrate, within ±10%. Meets the requirements for Identification, Bacterial endotoxins, pH (4.0–7.5), and Injections.
Fentanyl Transdermal Systems—Not in USP.

FERRIC OXIDE

Molecular formula: Fe_2O_3.

Molecular weight: 159.69.

Description: Ferric Oxide NF—Powder exhibiting two basic colors (red and yellow) or other shades produced on blending the basic colors.
NF category: Color.

Solubility: Ferric Oxide NF—Insoluble in water and in organic solvents; dissolves in hydrochloric acid upon warming, a small amount of insoluble residue usually remaining.

NF requirements: Ferric Oxide NF—Preserve in well-closed containers. Contains not less than 97.0% and not more than 100.5% of ferric oxide, calculated on the ignited basis. [Note: The U.S. Food and Drug Administration requires that not more than 3 ppm arsenic, not more than 10 ppm lead, and not more than 3 ppm mercury be present (21 CFR 73.1200).] Meets the requirements for Identification, Water-soluble substances (not more than 1.0%), Acid-insoluble substances (not more than 0.1%), and Organic colors and lakes.

FERROUS CITRATE Fe 59

Chemical name: 1,2,3-Propanetricarboxylic acid, 2-hydroxy-, iron(2+)-^{59}Fe salt.

Molecular formula: $C_{12}H_{10}{}^{59}Fe_3O_{14}$.

USP requirements: Ferrous Citrate Fe 59 Injection USP—Preserve in single-dose or in multiple-dose containers. A sterile solution of radioactive iron (^{59}Fe) in the ferrous state and complexed with citrate ion in Water for Injection. Iron 59 is produced by the neutron bombardment of iron 58. Label it to include the following, in addition to the information specified for Labeling under Injections: the date of calibration; the amount of ^{59}Fe as ferrous citrate expressed as total megabecquerels (or millicuries) and concentration as megabecquerels (or millicuries) per mL on the date of calibration; the expiration date; and the statement, "Caution—Radioactive Material." The labeling indicates that correction is to be made for radioactive decay, and also indicates that the radioactive half-life of ^{59}Fe is 44.6 days. Contains the labeled amount of ^{59}Fe, within ±10%, expressed in megabecquerels (or microcuries or millicuries) per mL at the time indicated in the labeling. Its specific activity is not less than 185 megabecquerels (5 millicuries) per mg of ferrous citrate on the date of manufacture. Meets the requirements for Radionuclide identification, Bacterial endotoxins, pH (5.0–7.0), and Injections (not subject to the recommendation on Volume in Container).

FERROUS FUMARATE

Chemical name: 2-Butenedioic acid, (*E*)-, iron(2+) salt.

Molecular formula: $C_4H_2FeO_4$.

Molecular weight: 169.90.

Description: Ferrous Fumarate USP—Reddish orange to red-brown, odorless powder. May contain soft lumps that produce a yellow streak when crushed.

Solubility: Ferrous Fumarate USP—Slightly soluble in water; very slightly soluble in alcohol. Its solubility in dilute hydrochloric acid is limited by the separation of fumaric acid.

USP requirements:
Ferrous Fumarate Capsules—Not in USP.
Ferrous Fumarate Extended-release Capsules—Not in USP.
Ferrous Fumarate Oral Solution—Not in USP.
Ferrous Fumarate Oral Suspension—Not in USP.
Ferrous Fumarate Tablets USP—Preserve in tight containers. Label Tablets in terms of ferrous fumarate and in terms of elemental iron. Contain the labeled amount, within −5% to +10%. Meet the requirements for Identification, Disintegration (30 minutes), and Uniformity of dosage units.

FERROUS FUMARATE AND DOCUSATE

For *Ferrous Fumarate* and *Docusate*—See individual listings for chemistry information.

USP requirements: Ferrous Fumarate and Docusate Sodium Extended-release Tablets USP—Preserve in well-closed containers. Label Tablets in terms of the content of ferrous fumarate and in terms of the content of elemental iron. Contain the labeled amount of ferrous fumarate, within ±10%, and the labeled amount of docusate sodium, within −10% to +15%. Meet the requirement for Uniformity of dosage units.

FERROUS GLUCONATE

Chemical name: D-Gluconic acid, iron(2+) salt (2:1), dihydrate.

Molecular formula: $C_{12}H_{22}FeO_{14} \cdot 2H_2O$.

Molecular weight: 482.17.

Description: Ferrous Gluconate USP—Yellowish gray or pale greenish yellow, fine powder or granules, having a slight odor resembling that of burned sugar. Its solution (1 in 20) is acid to litmus.

Solubility: Ferrous Gluconate USP—Soluble in water, with slight heating; practically insoluble in alcohol.

USP requirements:
Ferrous Gluconate Capsules USP—Preserve in tight containers. Label Capsules in terms of the content of ferrous gluconate and in terms of the content of elemental iron. Contain the labeled amount, within ±7%. Meet the requirements for Identification, Dissolution (75% in 45 minutes in 0.1 N hydrochloric acid in Apparatus 1 at 100 rpm), and Uniformity of dosage units.
Ferrous Gluconate Elixir USP—Preserve in tight, light-resistant containers. Label Elixir in terms of the content of ferrous gluconate and in terms of the content of elemental iron. Contains the labeled amount, within ±6%. Meets the requirements for Identification, pH (3.4–3.8), and Alcohol content (6.3–7.7%).
Ferrous Gluconate Syrup—Not in USP.
Ferrous Gluconate Tablets USP—Preserve in tight containers. Label Tablets in terms of the content of ferrous

gluconate and in terms of the content of elemental iron. Contain the labeled amount, within ±7%. Meet the requirements for Identification, Dissolution (80% in 80 minutes in simulated gastric fluid TS in Apparatus 2 at 150 rpm), and Uniformity of dosage units.

FERROUS SULFATE

Chemical name:

Ferrous sulfate—Sulfuric acid, iron(2+) salt (1:1), heptahydrate.

Ferrous sulfate, dried—Sulfuric acid, iron(2+) salt (1:1), hydrate.

Molecular formula:

Ferrous sulfate—$FeSO_4 \cdot 7H_2O$.

Ferrous sulfate, dried—$FeSO_4 \cdot xH_2O$.

Molecular weight:

Ferrous sulfate—278.01.

Ferrous sulfate, dried—151.90.

Description:

Ferrous Sulfate USP—Pale, bluish green crystals or granules. Is odorless and efflorescent in dry air. Oxidizes readily in moist air to form brownish yellow basic ferric sulfate. Its solution (1 in 10) is acid to litmus, having a pH of about 3.7.

Ferrous Sulfate, Dried USP—Grayish white to buff-colored powder, consisting primarily of $FeSO_4 \cdot H_2O$ with varying amounts of $FeSO_4 \cdot 4H_2O$.

Solubility:

Ferrous Sulfate USP—Freely soluble in water; very soluble in boiling water; insoluble in alcohol.

Ferrous Sulfate, Dried USP—Slowly soluble in water; insoluble in alcohol.

USP requirements:

Ferrous Sulfate (Dried) Capsules—Not in USP.

Ferrous Sulfate Extended-release Capsules—Not in USP.

Ferrous Sulfate Elixir—Not in USP.

Ferrous Sulfate Oral Solution USP—Preserve in tight, light-resistant containers. Label Oral Solution in terms of the content of ferrous sulfate and in terms of the content of elemental iron. Contains the labeled amount, within ±6%. Meets the requirements for Identification and pH (1.8–5.3).

Ferrous Sulfate Syrup USP—Preserve in tight containers. Label Syrup in terms of the content of ferrous sulfate and in terms of the content of elemental iron. Contains, in each 100 mL, not less than 3.75 grams and not more than 4.25 grams of Ferrous Sulfate, equivalent to not less than 0.75 grams and not more than 0.85 grams of elemental iron.

Prepare Ferrous Sulfate Syrup as follows: 40 grams of Ferrous Sulfate, 2.1 grams of Citric Acid, hydrous, 2 mL of Peppermint Spirit, 825 grams of Sucrose, and a sufficient quantity of Purified Water, to make 1000 mL. Dissolve the Ferrous Sulfate, the Citric Acid, the Peppermint Spirit, and 200 grams of the Sucrose in 450 mL of Purified Water, and filter the solution until clear. Dissolve the remainder of the Sucrose in the clear filtrate, and add Purified Water to make 1000 mL. Mix, and filter, if necessary, through a pledget of cotton.

Meets the requirement for Identification.

Ferrous Sulfate Tablets USP—Preserve in tight containers. Label Tablets in terms of ferrous sulfate and in terms of elemental iron. Contain the labeled amount, within −5% to +10%. Meet the requirements for Identification, Disintegration (30 minutes), and Uniformity of dosage units.

Note: An equivalent amount of Dried Ferrous Sulfate may be used in place of ferrous sulfate heptahydrate in preparing Ferrous Sulfate Tablets.

Ferrous Sulfate Enteric-coated Tablets—Not in USP.

Ferrous Sulfate Extended-release Tablets—Not in USP.

Ferrous Sulfate (Dried) Extended-release Tablets—Not in USP.

FILGRASTIM

Chemical name: Colony-stimulating factor (human clone 1034), *N*-L-methionyl-.

Molecular formula: $C_{845}H_{1339}N_{223}O_{243}S_9$.

Molecular weight: 18,800.00 daltons.

USP requirements: Filgrastim Injection—Not in USP.

FLAVOXATE

Chemical name: Flavoxate hydrochloride—4*H*-1-Benzopyran-8-carboxylic acid, 3-methyl-4-oxo-2-phenyl-, 2-(1-piperidinyl)ethyl ester, hydrochloride.

Molecular formula: Flavoxate hydrochloride—$C_{24}H_{25}NO_4 \cdot HCl$.

Molecular weight: Flavoxate hydrochloride—427.93.

Description: Flavoxate hydrochloride—Off-white, crystalline powder. Melts at about 230 °C, with decomposition.

Solubility: Flavoxate hydrochloride—One gram dissolves in 6 mL water or in 500 mL alcohol.

USP requirements: Flavoxate Hydrochloride Tablets—Not in USP.

FLECAINIDE

Chemical name: Flecainide acetate—Benzamide, *N*-(2-piperidinylmethyl)-2,5-bis(2,2,2-trifluoroethoxy)-, monoacetate.

Molecular formula: Flecainide acetate—$C_{17}H_{20}F_6N_2O_3 \cdot C_2H_4O_2$.

Molecular weight: Flecainide acetate—474.40.

Description: Flecainide acetate—White crystalline substance.

pKa: Flecainide acetate—9.3.

Solubility: Flecainide acetate—Aqueous: 48.4 mg per mL at 37 °C.

USP requirements: Flecainide Acetate Tablets—Not in USP.

FLOCTAFENINE

Chemical name: Benzoic acid, 2-[[8-(trifluoromethyl)-4-quinolinyl]amino]-, 2,3-dihydroxypropyl ester.

Molecular formula: $C_{20}H_{17}F_3N_2O_4$.

Molecular weight: 406.36.

Description: Melting point 179–180 °C.

Solubility: Soluble in alcohol and in acetone; very slightly soluble in ether, in chloroform, and in methylene chloride; insoluble in water.

USP requirements: Floctafenine Tablets—Not in USP.

FLOXURIDINE

Chemical group: A fluorinated pyrimidine derivative.

Chemical name: Uridine, 2'-deoxy-5-fluoro-.

Molecular formula: $C_9H_{11}FN_2O_5$.

Molecular weight: 246.19.

Description: White to off-white odorless solid.

Solubility: Freely soluble in water; soluble in alcohol.

Other characteristics: Hydrophilic.

USP requirements: Sterile Floxuridine USP—Preserve in Containers for Sterile Solids, as described under Injections, protected from light. Store containers of constituted Sterile Floxuridine under refrigeration for not more than 2 weeks. It is lyophilized Floxuridine suitable for intraarterial infusion. Contains the labeled amount, within ±10%. Meets the requirements for Constituted solution, Identification, Pyrogen, Uniformity of dosage units, pH (4.0–5.5 in a solution [1 in 50]), and Injections (Sterile Solids).

FLUCONAZOLE

Chemical group: Bis-triazole antifungal.

Chemical name: 1 *H*-1,2,4-Triazole-1-ethanol, alpha-(2,4-difluorophenyl)-alpha-(1*H*-1,2,4-triazol-1-ylmethyl)-.

Molecular formula: $C_{13}H_{12}F_2N_6O$.

Molecular weight: 306.27.

Description: White crystalline solid.

Solubility: Slightly soluble in water and in saline.

USP requirements:
  Fluconazole Injection—Not in USP.
  Fluconazole Tablets—Not in USP.

FLUCYTOSINE

Chemical group: Fluorinated pyrimidine derivative; chemically related to fluorouracil and floxuridine.

Chemical name: Cytosine, 5-fluoro-.

Molecular formula: $C_4H_4FN_3O$.

Molecular weight: 129.09.

Description: Flucytosine USP—White to off-white, crystalline powder. Is odorless or has a slight odor.

Solubility: Flucytosine USP—Sparingly soluble in water; slightly soluble in alcohol; practically insoluble in chloroform and in ether.

USP requirements: Flucytosine Capsules USP—Preserve in tight, light-resistant containers. Contain the labeled amount, within ±10%. Meet the requirements for Identification, Dissolution (75% in 45 minutes in water in Apparatus 2 at 100 rpm), and Uniformity of dosage units.

FLUDEOXYGLUCOSE F 18

Source: Different methods are being used in the various clinical facilities for the on-site production of FDG injection. It can be prepared either by the electrophilic reaction of ^{18}F-enriched fluorine gas with 3,4,6-tri-O-acetyl-D-glucal or by the nucleophilic reaction of ^{18}F-labeled acetylhypofluorite with suitably protected D-mannopyranose. The fluorinated product is hydrolyzed with acid to give a mixture of 2-fluoro-2-deoxy-D-glucose and 2-fluoro-2-deoxy-D-mannose. Subsequently, it is purified by column chromatography and dissolved in an appropriate solvent, most commonly 0.9% saline.

Chemical group: D-glucose analog.

Chemical name: Alpha-D-glucopyranose, 2-deoxy-2-(fluoro-^{18}F)-.

Molecular formula: $C_6H_{11}{}^{18}FO_5$.

Molecular weight: 182.

pKa: None between pH 1–13.

Solubility: Very soluble in water.

Other characteristics: Partition coefficient—Hydrocarbon:water (<0.001).

USP requirements: Fludeoxyglucose F 18 Injection USP—Preserve in single-dose or in multiple-dose containers that are adequately shielded. A sterile, isotonic aqueous solution, suitable for intravenous administration, of 2-deoxy-2-[^{18}F]fluoro-D-glucose in which a portion of the molecules are labeled with radioactive ^{18}F. Label it to include the following, in addition to the information specified for Labeling under Injection: the time and date of calibration; the amount of ^{18}F as fludeoxyglucose expressed as total MBq (or millicurie) per mL, at the time of calibration; the expiration date; the name and quantity of any added preservative or stabilizer; and the statement, "Caution, Radioactive Material." The labeling indicates that in making dosage calculations, correction is to be made for radioactive decay. The radioactive half-life of ^{18}F is 110 minutes. The label indicates "Do not use if cloudy or if it contains particulate matter." Contains the labeled amount of ^{18}F, within ±10%, expressed in MBq (or millicurie) per mL at the time indicated in the labeling. It has a Specific activity of not less than 37×10^3 MBq (1 curie) per mmol. Meets the requirements for Radionuclide identification, Bacterial endotoxins, pH (4.5–8.5), Radiochemical purity, Isomeric purity, Radionuclidic purity, Chemical purity, and Injections, except that the Injection may be distributed or dispensed prior to completion of the test for Sterility, the latter test being started on the day following final manufacture, and except that it is not subject to the recommendation on Volume in Container.

FLUDROCORTISONE

Chemical name: Fludrocortisone acetate—Pregn-4-ene-3,20-dione, 21-(acetyloxy)-9-fluoro-11,17-dihydroxy-, (11 beta)-.

Molecular formula: Fludrocortisone acetate—$C_{23}H_{31}FO_6$.

Molecular weight: Fludrocortisone acetate—422.49.

Description: Fludrocortisone Acetate USP—White to pale yellow crystals or crystalline powder. Is odorless or practically odorless. Is hygroscopic.

Solubility: Fludrocortisone Acetate USP—Insoluble in water; slightly soluble in ether; sparingly soluble in alcohol and in chloroform.

USP requirements: Fludrocortisone Acetate Tablets USP—Preserve in well-closed containers. Contain the labeled amount, within ±10%. Meet the requirements for Identification, Disintegration (30 minutes), and Uniformity of dosage units.

FLUMAZENIL

Chemical name: 4*H*-Imidazo[1,5-alpha][1,4]benzodiazepine-3-carboxylic acid, 8-fluoro-5,6-dihydro-5-methyl-6-oxo-, ethyl ester.

Molecular formula: $C_{15}H_{14}FN_3O_3$.

Molecular weight: 303.29.

Description: White to off-white crystalline compound.

Solubility: Insoluble in water; slightly soluble in acidic aqueous solutions.

Other characteristics: Octanol:buffer partition coefficient—14 to 1 at pH 7.4.

USP requirements: Flumazenil Injection—Not in USP.

FLUMETHASONE

Chemical name: Flumethasone pivalate—Pregna-1,4-diene-3,20-dione, 21-(2,2-dimethyl-1-oxopropoxy)-6,9-difluoro-11,17-di-hydroxy-16-methyl-, (6 alpha, 11 beta, 16 alpha)-.

Molecular formula: Flumethasone pivalate—$C_{27}H_{36}F_2O_6$.

Molecular weight: Flumethasone pivalate—494.57.

Description: Flumethasone Pivalate USP—White to off-white, crystalline powder.

Solubility: Flumethasone Pivalate USP—Insoluble in water; slightly soluble in methanol; very slightly soluble in chloroform and in methylene chloride.

USP requirements:
Flumethasone Pivalate Cream USP—Preserve in collapsible tubes. Contains the labeled amount, within ±10%, in a suitable cream base. Meets the requirements for Identification, Microbial limits, and Minimum fill.
Flumethasone Pivalate Ointment—Not in USP.

FLUNARIZINE

Chemical name: Flunarizine hydrochloride—Piperazine, 1-[bis(4-fluorophenyl)methyl]-4-(3-phenyl-2-propenyl)-, dihydrochloride, (E)-.

Molecular formula: Flunarizine hydrochloride—$C_{26}H_{26}F_2N_2 \cdot$ 2HCl.

Molecular weight: Flunarizine hydrochloride—477.42.

Description: White to pale cream colored powder.

Solubility: Soluble in dimethylsulfoxide, in polyethylene glycol (PEG) 400, in propylene glycol, in N,N-dimethylformamide, and in methanol; poorly soluble in water and in ethanol (0.1–1.0%).

USP requirements: Flunarizine Hydrochloride Capsules—Not in USP.

FLUNISOLIDE

Chemical name: Pregna-1,4-diene-3,20-dione, 6-fluoro-11,21-dihydroxy-16,17-[(1-methylethylidene)bis(oxy)]-, hemihy-drate, (6 alpha, 11 beta, 16 alpha)-.

Molecular formula: $C_{24}H_{31}FO_6 \cdot \frac{1}{2}H_2O$.

Molecular weight: 443.51.

Description: Flunisolide USP—White to creamy-white, crystalline powder. Melts at about 245 °C, with decomposition.

Solubility: Flunisolide USP—Practically insoluble in water; soluble in acetone; sparingly soluble in chloroform; slightly soluble in methanol.

USP requirements:
Flunisolide Inhalation Aerosol—Not in USP.
Flunisolide Nasal Solution USP—Preserve in tight containers, protected from light, at controlled room temperature. An aqueous, buffered solution of Flunisolide. It is supplied in a form suitable for nasal administration. Contains the labeled amount, within ±10%. Meets the requirements for Identification, pH (4.5–6.0), and Quantity delivered per spray (17–33 mcg).

FLUOCINOLONE

Chemical name: Fluocinolone acetonide—Pregna-1,4-diene-3,20-dione, 6,9-difluoro-11,21-dihydroxy-16,17-[(1-methylethyli-dene)bis(oxy)]-, (6 alpha,11 beta,16 alpha)-.

Molecular formula:
Fluocinolone acetonide (anhydrous)—$C_{24}H_{30}F_2O_6$.
Fluocinolone acetonide (dihydrate)—$C_{24}H_{30}F_2O_6 \cdot 2H_2O$.

Molecular weight:
Fluocinolone acetonide (anhydrous)—452.50.
Fluocinolone acetonide (dihydrate)—488.53.

Description: Fluocinolone Acetonide USP—White or practically white, odorless, crystalline powder. Is stable in air. Melts at about 270 °C, with decomposition.

Solubility: Fluocinolone Acetonide USP—Insoluble in water; soluble in methanol; slightly soluble in ether and in chloroform.

USP requirements:
Fluocinolone Acetonide Cream USP—Preserve in collapsible tubes or in tight containers. Contains the labeled amount, within ±10%. Meets the requirements for Identification, Microbial limits, and Minimum fill.
Fluocinolone Acetonide Ointment USP—Preserve in collapsible tubes or in tight containers. Contains the labeled amount, within ±10%. Meets the requirements for Identification, Microbial limits, and Minimum fill.
Fluocinolone Acetonide Topical Solution USP—Preserve in tight containers. Contains the labeled amount, within ±10%. Meets the requirements for Identification and Microbial limits.

FLUOCINONIDE

Chemical name: Pregna-1,4-diene-3,20-dione, 21-(acetyloxy)-6,9-difluoro-11-hydroxy-16,17-[(1-methylethylidene)bis(oxy)]-, (6 alpha,11 beta,16 alpha)-.

Molecular formula: $C_{26}H_{32}F_2O_7$.

Molecular weight: 494.53.

Description: Fluocinonide USP—White to cream-colored, crystalline powder, having not more than a slight odor.

Solubility: Fluocinonide USP—Practically insoluble in water; sparingly soluble in acetone and in chloroform; slightly soluble in alcohol, in methanol, and in dioxane; very slightly soluble in ether.

USP requirements:
Fluocinonide Cream USP—Preserve in collapsible tubes or in tight containers. Contains the labeled amount, within ±10%. Meets the requirements for Identification, Microbial limits, and Minimum fill.
Fluocinonide Gel USP—Preserve in collapsible tubes or in tight containers. Contains the labeled amount, within ±10%. Meets the requirements for Identification and Minimum fill.

Fluocinonide Ointment USP—Preserve in collapsible tubes or in tight containers. Contains the labeled amount, within ±10%. Meets the requirements for Identification and Minimum fill.

Fluocinonide Topical Solution USP—Preserve in tight containers. Contains the labeled amount, within ±10%. Meets the requirements for Identification, Alcohol content (28.4–39.0%), and Minimum fill.

FLUORESCEIN

Chemical name:
Fluorescein—Spiro[isobenzofuran-1(3H),9′-[9H]xanthen]-3-one,3′6′-dihydroxy-.
Fluorescein sodium—Spiro[isobenzofuran-1(3H),9′-[9H]-xanthene]-3-one, 3′6′-dihydroxy, disodium salt.

Molecular formula:
Fluorescein—$C_{20}H_{12}O_5$.
Fluorescein sodium—$C_{20}H_{10}Na_2O_5$.

Molecular weight:
Fluorescein—332.31.
Fluorescein sodium—376.28.

Description:
Fluorescein USP—Yellowish red to red, odorless powder.
Fluorescein Sodium USP—Orange-red, hygroscopic, odorless powder.
Fluorescein Sodium Ophthalmic Strip USP—Each Strip is a dry, white piece of paper, one end of which is rounded and is uniformly orange-red in color because of the fluorescein sodium impregnated in the paper.

Solubility:
Fluorescein USP—Insoluble in water; soluble in dilute alkali hydroxides.
Fluorescein Sodium USP—Freely soluble in water; sparingly soluble in alcohol.

USP requirements:
Fluorescein Injection USP—Preserve in single-dose containers, preferably of Type I glass. A sterile solution, in Water for Injection, of Fluorescein prepared with the aid of Sodium Hydroxide. Contains an amount of fluorescein equivalent to the labeled amount of fluorescein sodium, within ±10%. Meets the requirements for Identification, Pyrogen, pH (8.0–9.8), and Injections.
Fluorescein Sodium Ophthalmic Strips USP—Package not more than 2 Strips in a single-unit container in such manner as to maintain sterility until the package is opened. Package individual packages in a second protective container. The label of the second protective container bears a statement that the contents may not be sterile if the individual package has been damaged or previously opened. The label states the amount of fluorescein sodium in each Strip. Contain the labeled amount, within +60%. Meet the requirements for Identification, Sterility, and Content uniformity (85.0–175.0% of labeled amount).

FLUORESCEIN AND BENOXINATE

For *Fluorescein* and *Benoxinate*—See individual listings for chemistry information.

USP requirements: Fluorescein Sodium and Benoxinate Hydrochloride Ophthalmic Solution USP—Preserve in tight, light-resistant containers. A sterile aqueous solution of Fluorescein Sodium and Benoxinate Hydrochloride. Contains the labeled amounts, within −10% to +20%. Contains a suitable preservative. Meets the requirements for Identification, Sterility, and pH (4.3–5.3).

FLUORESCEIN AND PROPARACAINE

For *Fluorescein* and *Proparacaine*—See individual listings for chemistry information.

USP requirements: Fluorescein Sodium and Proparacaine Hydrochloride Ophthalmic Solution USP—Preserve in tight, light-resistant containers, preferably of Type I amber glass, and store in a refrigerator. A sterile aqueous solution of Fluorescein Sodium and Proparacaine Hydrochloride. Label it to state that it is to be stored in a refrigerator before and after the container is opened. Contains the labeled amounts, within ±10%. Contains a suitable preservative. Meets the requirements for Identification, Sterility, and pH (4.0–5.2).

FLUORODOPA F 18

Chemical name: L-Tyrosine, 2-(fluoro-^{18}F)-5-hydroxy-.

Molecular formula: $C_9H_{10}{}^{18}FNO_4$.

Molecular weight: 214.19.

USP requirements: Fluorodopa F 18 Injection USP—Preserve in single-dose or in multiple-dose containers that are adequately shielded. A sterile, isotonic aqueous solution, suitable for intravenous administration of 6-[^{18}F]fluorolevodopa in which a portion of the molecules are labeled with radioactive ^{18}F. Label it to include the following, in addition to the information specified for Labeling under Injections: the time and date of calibration; the amount of ^{18}F as fluorodopa expressed as total megabecquerels (MBq or millicuries) per mL, at time of calibration; the expiration date; the name and quantity of any added preservative or stabilizer; and the statement "Caution—Radioactive Material." The labeling indicates that in making dosage calculations correction is to be made for radioactive decay. The radioactive half-life of ^{18}F is 110 minutes. The label indicates "Do not use if cloudy or if it contains particulate matter." Contains the labeled amount of ^{18}F expressed in megabecquerels (MBq or millicuries) per mL at the time indicated in the labeling, within ±10%. Meets the requirements for Specific activity (not less than 3.7×10^3 MBq [100 millicuries] per mmol), Radionuclide identification, Bacterial endotoxins, pH (4.0–5.0), Radiochemical purity, Radionuclidic purity, Chemical purity, Enantiomeric purity, and Injections (except that the Injection may be distributed or dispensed prior to completion of the test for Sterility, the latter test being started on the day following final manufacture, and except that it is not subject to the recommendation of Volume in Container).

FLUOROMETHOLONE

Chemical name:
Fluorometholone—Pregna-1,4-diene-3,20-dione, 9-fluoro-11,17-dihydroxy-6-methyl-, (6 alpha,11 beta)-.
Fluorometholone acetate—Pregna-1,4-diene-3,20-dione, 17-(acetyloxy)-9-fluoro-11-hydroxy-6-methyl-, (6 alpha,11 beta)-.

Molecular formula:
Fluorometholone—$C_{22}H_{29}FO_4$.
Fluorometholone acetate—$C_{24}H_{31}FO_5$.

Molecular weight:
Fluorometholone—376.47.
Fluorometholone acetate—418.51.

Description: Fluorometholone USP—White to yellowish white, odorless, crystalline powder. Melts at about 280 °C, with some decomposition.

Solubility: Fluorometholone USP—Practically insoluble in water; slightly soluble in alcohol; very slightly soluble in chloroform and in ether.

USP requirements:

Fluorometholone Cream USP—Preserve in collapsible tubes. Contains the labeled amount, within ±10%. Meets the requirements for Identification, Microbial limits, and Minimum fill.

Fluorometholone Ophthalmic Ointment—Not in USP.

Fluorometholone Ophthalmic Suspension USP—Preserve in tight containers. A sterile suspension of Fluorometholone in a suitable aqueous medium. Contains the labeled amount, within ±10%. Meets the requirements for Identification, Sterility, and pH (6.0–7.5).

Fluorometholone Acetate Ophthalmic Suspension—Not in USP.

FLUOROURACIL

Chemical name: 2,4(1H,3H)-Pyrimidinedione, 5-fluoro-.

Molecular formula: $C_4H_3FN_2O_2$.

Molecular weight: 130.08.

Description: Fluorouracil USP—White to practically white, practically odorless, crystalline powder. Decomposes at about 282 °C.

pKa: 8.0 and 13.0.

Solubility: Fluorouracil USP—Sparingly soluble in water; slightly soluble in alcohol; practically insoluble in chloroform and in ether.

USP requirements:

Fluorouracil Cream USP—Preserve in tight containers, at controlled room temperature. Contains the labeled amount, within ±10%. Meets the requirements for Identification, Microbial limits, and Minimum fill.

Fluorouracil Injection USP—Preserve in single-dose containers, preferably of Type I glass, at controlled room temperature. Avoid freezing and exposure to light. A sterile solution of Fluorouracil in Water for Injection, prepared with the aid of Sodium Hydroxide. Label it to indicate the expiration date, which is not more than 24 months after date of manufacture. Contains, in each mL, not less than 45 mg and not more than 55 mg of fluorouracil. Meets the requirements for Identification, Pyrogen, pH (8.6–9.4), and Injections.

Note: If a precipitate is formed as a result of exposure to low temperatures, redissolve it by heating to 60 °C with vigorous shaking, and allow to cool to body temperature prior to use.

Fluorouracil Topical Solution USP—Preserve in tight containers, at controlled room temperature. Contains the labeled amount, within ±10%. Meets the requirements for Identification and Microbial limits.

FLUOXETINE

Chemical group: Cyclic, propylamine-derivative. Chemically unrelated to tricyclic, tetracyclic, or other available antidepressants.

Chemical name:

Fluoxetine—Benzenepropanamine, N-methyl-gamma-[4-(trifluoromethyl)phenoxy]-, (±)-.

Fluoxetine hydrochloride—Benzenepropanamine, N-methyl-gamma-[4-(trifluoromethyl)phenoxy]-, hydrochloride, (±)-.

Molecular formula:

Fluoxetine—$C_{17}H_{18}F_3NO$.

Fluoxetine hydrochloride—$C_{17}H_{18}F_3NO \cdot HCl$.

Molecular weight:

Fluoxetine—309.33.

Fluoxetine hydrochloride—345.79.

Description: Fluoxetine hydrochloride—White to off-white crystalline solid.

Solubility: Fluoxetine hydrochloride—Soluble in water.

USP requirements:

Fluoxetine Oral Solution—Not in USP.

Fluoxetine Hydrochloride Capsules—Not in USP.

FLUOXYMESTERONE

Chemical group: Synthetic androgen; halogenated derivative of 17-alpha-methyltestosterone.

Chemical name: Androst-4-en-3-one, 9-fluoro-11,17-dihydroxy-17-methyl-, (11 beta,17 beta)-.

Molecular formula: $C_{20}H_{29}FO_3$.

Molecular weight: 336.45.

Description: Fluoxymesterone USP—White or practically white, odorless, crystalline powder. Melts at about 240 °C, with some decomposition.

Solubility: Fluoxymesterone USP—Practically insoluble in water; sparingly soluble in alcohol; slightly soluble in chloroform.

USP requirements: Fluoxymesterone Tablets USP—Preserve in well-closed containers, protected from light. Contain the labeled amount, within ±10%. Meet the requirements for Identification, Dissolution (70% in 60 minutes in 0.1 N hydrochloric acid in Apparatus 2 at 75 rpm), and Uniformity of dosage units.

FLUOXYMESTERONE AND ETHINYL ESTRADIOL

For *Fluoxymesterone* and *Ethinyl Estradiol*—See individual listings for chemistry information.

USP requirements: Fluoxymesterone and Ethinyl Estradiol Tablets—Not in USP.

FLUPENTHIXOL

Chemical group: Thioxanthene.

Chemical name:

Flupenthixol decanoate—Cis-2-trifluoromethyl-9-(3-(4-(2-hydroxyethyl)-1-piperazinyl)-propylidene)-thioxanthene decanoate acid ester.

Flupenthixol dihydrochloride—2-Trifluoromethyl-9-(3-(4-(2-hydroxyethyl)-1-piperazinyl)-propylidene)-thioxanthene dihydrochloride.

Molecular formula:

Flupenthixol decanoate—$C_{33}H_{43}F_3N_2O_2S$.

Flupenthixol dihydrochloride—$C_{23}H_{25}F_3N_2OS \cdot 2HCl$.

Molecular weight:

Flupenthixol decanoate—588.8.

Flupenthixol dihydrochloride—507.4.

Description:

Flupenthixol decanoate—Yellow oil with a slight odor.

Flupenthixol dihydrochloride—White or yellowish white powder.

Solubility:

Flupenthixol decanoate—Very slightly soluble in water; soluble in alcohol; freely soluble in chloroform and in ether.

Flupenthixol dihydrochloride—Soluble in water and in alcohol.

Other characteristics: Structurally and pharmacologically similar to the piperazine phenothiazines, which are acetophenazine, fluphenazine, perphenazine, prochlorperazine, and trifluoperazine.

USP requirements:
Flupenthixol Decanoate Injection—Not in USP.
Flupenthixol Dihydrochloride Tablets—Not in USP.

FLUPHENAZINE

Chemical group: Piperazine.

Chemical name:
Fluphenazine decanoate—2-{4-[3-(2-Trifluoromethylphenothiazin-10-yl)propyl]-piperazin-1-yl}ethyl decanoate.
Fluphenazine enanthate—Heptanoic acid, 2-[4-[3-[2-(trifluoromethyl)-10H-phenothiazin-10-yl]propyl]-1-piperazinyl]ethyl ester.
Fluphenazine hydrochloride—1-Piperazineethanol, 4-[3-[2-(trifluoromethyl)-10H-phenothiazin-10-yl]propyl]-, dihydrochloride.

Molecular formula:
Fluphenazine decanoate—$C_{32}H_{44}F_3N_3O_2S$.
Fluphenazine enanthate—$C_{29}H_{38}F_3N_3O_2S$.
Fluphenazine hydrochloride—$C_{22}H_{26}F_3N_3OS \cdot 2HCl$.

Molecular weight:
Fluphenazine decanoate—591.8.
Fluphenazine enanthate—549.69.
Fluphenazine hydrochloride—510.44.

Description:
Fluphenazine decanoate—Pale yellow viscous liquid or a yellow crystalline oily solid with a faint ester-like odor.
Fluphenazine Enanthate USP—Pale yellow to yellow-orange, clear to slightly turbid, viscous liquid, having a characteristic odor; unstable in strong light, but stable to air at room temperature.
Fluphenazine Hydrochloride USP—White or nearly white, odorless, crystalline powder; melts, within a range of 5°, at a temperature above 225 °C.

Solubility:
Fluphenazine decanoate—Practically insoluble in water; miscible with dehydrated alcohol, with chloroform, and with ether; soluble in fixed oils.
Fluphenazine Enanthate USP—Insoluble in water; freely soluble in alcohol, in chloroform, and in ether.
Fluphenazine Hydrochloride USP—Freely soluble in water; slightly soluble in acetone, in alcohol, and in chloroform; practically insoluble in ether.

USP requirements:
Fluphenazine Decanoate Injection—Not in USP.
Fluphenazine Enanthate Injection USP—Preserve in single-dose or in multiple-dose containers, preferably of Type I or Type III glass, protected from light. A sterile solution of Fluphenazine Enanthate in a suitable vegetable oil. Contains the labeled amount, within ±10%. Meets the requirements for Identification and Injections.
Fluphenazine Hydrochloride Elixir USP—Preserve in tight containers, protected from light. Contains the labeled amount, within ±10%. Meets the requirements for Identification, pH (5.3–5.8), and Alcohol content (13.5–15.0%).
Fluphenazine Hydrochloride Injection USP—Preserve in single-dose or in multiple-dose containers, preferably of Type I glass, protected from light. A sterile solution of

Fluphenazine Hydrochloride in Water for Injection. Contains the labeled amount, within −5% to +10%. Meets the requirements for Identification, pH (4.8–5.2), and Injections.
Fluphenazine Hydrochloride Oral Solution USP—Preserve in tight containers, protected from light. An aqueous solution of Fluphenazine Hydrochloride. Contains the labeled amount, within ±10%. Label it to indicate that it is to be diluted to appropriate strength with water or other suitable fluid prior to administration. Meets the requirements for Identification, pH (4.0–5.0), and Alcohol content (90.0–110.0% of the labeled amount, the labeled amount being not more than 15.0%).
Fluphenazine Hydrochloride Tablets USP—Preserve in tight, light-resistant containers. Contain the labeled amount, within ±10%. Meet the requirements for Identification, Dissolution (75% in 45 minutes in 0.1 N hydrochloric acid in Apparatus 1 at 100 rpm), and Uniformity of dosage units.

FLURANDRENOLIDE

Chemical name: Pregn-4-ene-3,20-dione, 6-fluoro-11,21-dihydroxy-16,17-[(1-methylethylidene)bis(oxy)]-, (6 alpha,11 beta,16 alpha)-.

Molecular formula: $C_{24}H_{33}FO_6$.

Molecular weight: 436.52.

Description: Flurandrenolide USP—White to off-white, fluffy, crystalline powder. Is odorless.

Solubility: Flurandrenolide USP—Practically insoluble in water and in ether; freely soluble in chloroform; soluble in methanol; sparingly soluble in alcohol.

USP requirements:
Flurandrenolide Cream USP—Preserve in tight containers, protected from light. Contains the labeled amount, within ±10%. Meets the requirements for Identification, Microbial limits, and Minimum fill.
Flurandrenolide Lotion USP—Preserve in tight containers, protected from heat, light, and freezing. Contains the labeled amount, within ±10%. Meets the requirements for Identification, Microbial limits, pH (3.5–6.0), and Minimum fill.
Flurandrenolide Ointment USP—Preserve in tight containers, protected from light. Contains the labeled amount, within ±10%. Meets the requirements for Identification, Microbial limits, and Minimum fill.
Flurandrenolide Tape USP—Preserve at controlled room temperature. A non-porous, pliable, adhesive-type tape having Flurandrenolide impregnated in the adhesive material, the adhesive material on one side being transported on a removable, protective slit-paper liner. Contains the labeled amount, within −20% to +25%. Meets the requirements for Identification and Microbial limits.

FLURAZEPAM

Chemical name:
Flurazepam hydrochloride—2H-1,4-Benzodiazepin-2-one, 7-chloro-1-[2-(diethylamino)ethyl]-5-(2-fluorophenyl)-1,3-dihydro-, dihydrochloride.
Flurazepam monohydrochloride—7-Chloro-1-(2-diethylaminoethyl)-5-(2-fluorophenyl)-1,3-dihydro-1,4-benzodiazepin-2-one hydrochloride.

Molecular formula:
Flurazepam hydrochloride—$C_{21}H_{23}ClFN_3O \cdot 2HCl$.
Flurazepam monohydrochloride—$C_{21}H_{23}ClFN_3O \cdot HCl$.

Molecular weight:
Flurazepam hydrochloride—460.81.
Flurazepam monohydrochloride—424.4.

Description: Flurazepam Hydrochloride USP—Off-white to yellow, crystalline powder. Is odorless, or has a slight odor, and its solutions are acid to litmus. Melts at about 212 °C, with decomposition.

Solubility: Flurazepam Hydrochloride USP—Freely soluble in water and in alcohol; slightly soluble in isopropyl alcohol and in chloroform.

USP requirements:
Flurazepam Hydrochloride Capsules USP—Preserve in tight, light-resistant containers. Contain the labeled amount, within ±10%. Meet the requirements for Identification, Dissolution (75% in 20 minutes in 0.1 N hydrochloric acid in Apparatus 1 at 100 rpm), and Uniformity of dosage units.
Flurazepam Monohydrochloride Tablets—Not in USP.

FLURBIPROFEN

Chemical group: A phenylalkanoic acid–derivative nonsteroidal anti-inflammatory agent chemically related to fenoprofen, ibuprofen, ketoprofen, naproxen, and tiaprofenic acid.

Chemical name:
Flurbiprofen—[1,1′-Biphenyl]-4-acetic acid, 2-fluoro-alpha-methyl-, (±)-.
Flurbiprofen sodium—[1,1′-Biphenyl]-4-acetic acid, 2-fluoro-alpha-methyl, sodium salt dihydrate, (±)-.

Molecular formula:
Flurbiprofen—$C_{15}H_{13}FO_2$.
Flurbiprofen sodium—$C_{15}H_{12}FNaO_2 \cdot 2H_2O$.

Molecular weight:
Flurbiprofen—244.26.
Flurbiprofen sodium—302.28.

Description: White or slightly yellow crystalline powder.

pKa: 4.22.

Solubility: Slightly soluble in water at pH 7.0; readily soluble in most polar solvents.

Other characteristics: Acidic.

USP requirements:
Flurbiprofen Extended-release Capsules—Not in USP.
Flurbiprofen Tablets—Not in USP.
Flurbiprofen Sodium Ophthalmic Solution USP—Preserve in tight containers. Contains the labeled amount, within ±10%. Meets the requirements for Identification, pH (6.0–7.0), Antimicrobial preservatives—Effectiveness, and Sterility.

FLUTAMIDE

Chemical name: Propanamide, 2-methyl-N-[4-nitro-3-(trifluoromethyl)phenyl]-.

Molecular formula: $C_{11}H_{11}F_3N_2O_3$.

Molecular weight: 276.21.

Description: Buff to yellow powder.

Solubility: Practically insoluble in water.

USP requirements:
Flutamide Capsules—Not in USP.
Flutamide Tablets—Not in USP.

FOLIC ACID

Chemical name: L-Glutamic acid, N-[4-[[(2-amino-1,4-dihydro-4-oxo-6-pteridinyl)methyl]amino]benzoyl]-.

Molecular formula: $C_{19}H_{19}N_7O_6$.

Molecular weight: 441.40.

Description:
Folic Acid USP—Yellow, yellow-brownish, or yellowish orange, odorless, crystalline powder.
Folic Acid Injection USP—Clear, yellow to orange-yellow, alkaline liquid.

Solubility: Folic Acid USP—Very slightly soluble in water; insoluble in alcohol, in acetone, in chloroform, and in ether; readily dissolves in dilute solutions of alkali hydroxides and carbonates, and is soluble in hot, 3 N hydrochloric acid and in hot, 2 N sulfuric acid. Soluble in hydrochloric acid and in sulfuric acid, yielding very pale yellow solutions.

USP requirements:
Folic Acid Injection USP—Preserve in single-dose or in multiple-dose containers, preferably of Type I glass, protected from light. A sterile solution of Folic Acid in Water for Injection prepared with the aid of Sodium Hydroxide or Sodium Carbonate. Contains the labeled amount, within −5% to +10%. Meets the requirements for Identification, Bacterial endotoxins, pH (8.0–11.0), and Injections.
Folic Acid Tablets USP—Preserve in well-closed containers. Contain the labeled amount, within −10% to +15%. Meet the requirements for Identification, Disintegration (30 minutes), and Uniformity of dosage units.

FORMALDEHYDE

Chemical name: Formaldehyde solution—Formaldehyde.

Molecular formula: Formaldehyde solution—CH_2O.

Molecular weight: Formaldehyde solution—30.03.

Description: Formaldehyde Solution USP—Clear, colorless or practically colorless liquid, having a pungent odor. The vapor from it irritates the mucous membrane of the throat and nose. On long standing, especially in the cold, it may become cloudy because of the separation of paraformaldehyde. This cloudiness disappears when the solution is warmed.

Solubility: Formaldehyde Solution USP—Miscible with water and with alcohol.

USP requirements: Formaldehyde Solution USP—Preserve in tight containers, preferably at a temperature not below 15 °C. The label of bulk containers of Formaldehyde Solution directs the drug repackager to demonstrate compliance with the USP *Assay* limit for formaldehyde of not less than 37.0%, by weight, immediately prior to repackaging. In bulk containers, contains not less than 37.0%, by weight, of formaldehyde, with methanol added to prevent polymerization. In small containers (4 liters or less), contains not less than 36.5%, by weight, of formaldehyde, with methanol present to prevent polymerization. Meets the requirements for Identification and Acidity (20.0 mL of Formaldehyde Solution consumes not more than 10.0 mL of 0.1 N sodium hydroxide).

FOSCARNET

Chemical group: Pyrophosphate analog.

Chemical name: Foscarnet sodium—Phosphinecarboxylic acid, dihydroxy-, oxide, trisodium salt.

Molecular formula:
Foscarnet sodium—CNa_3O_5P.
Foscarnet sodium hexahydrate—$Na_3CO_5P·6H_2O$.

Molecular weight:
Foscarnet sodium—191.95.
Foscarnet sodium hexahydrate—300.1.

Description:
Foscarnet sodium—White, crystalline powder.
Foscarnet sodium injection—Clear and colorless solution.
Foscarnet sodium—Soluble in water at pH 7 and 25 °C (about 5% w/w).

Other characteristics: Foscarnet sodium injection—pH is 7.4.

USP requirements: Foscarnet Sodium Injection—Not in USP.

FRUCTOSE

Chemical name: D-Fructose.

Molecular formula: $C_6H_{12}O_6$.

Molecular weight: 180.16.

Description: Fructose USP—Colorless crystals or white crystalline powder. Odorless.
NF category: Sweetening agent; tablet and/or capsule diluent.

Solubility: Fructose USP—Freely soluble in water; soluble in alcohol and in methanol.

USP requirements:
Fructose USP—Preserve in well-closed containers. Dried in vacuum at 70 °C for 4 hours, contains not less than 98.0% and not more than 102.0% of fructose. Meets the requirements for Identification, Color of solution, Acidity, Loss on drying (not more than 0.5%), Residue on ignition (not more than 0.5%), Chloride (not more than 0.018%), Sulfate (not more than 0.025%), Arsenic (not more than 1 ppm), Calcium and magnesium (as calcium) (not more than 0.005% calcium), Heavy metals (not more than 5 ppm), and Hydroxymethylfurfural.
Fructose Injection USP—Preserve in single-dose containers, preferably of Type I or Type II glass. A sterile solution of Fructose in Water for Injection. The label states the total osmolar concentration in mOsmol per liter. Where the contents are less than 100 mL, or where the label states that the Injection is not for direct injection but is to be diluted before use, the label alternatively may state the total osmolar concentration in mOsmol per mL. Contains the labeled amount, within ±5%. Contains no antimicrobial agents. Meets the requirements for Identification, Bacterial endotoxins, pH (3.0–6.0), Heavy metals (not more than 5 ppm), Hydroxymethylfurfural, and Injections.

FRUCTOSE, DEXTROSE, AND PHOSPHORIC ACID

For *Fructose, Dextrose,* and *Phosphoric Acid*—See individual listings for chemistry information.

USP requirements: Fructose, Dextrose, and Phosphoric Acid Oral Solution—Not in USP.

FRUCTOSE AND SODIUM CHLORIDE

For *Fructose* and *Sodium Chloride*—See individual listings for chemistry information.

USP requirements: Fructose and Sodium Chloride Injection USP—Preserve in single-dose containers, preferably of Type I or Type II glass. A sterile solution of Fructose and Sodium Chloride in Water for Injection. The label states the total osmolar concentration in mOsmol per liter. Where the contents are less than 100 mL, or where the label states that the Injection is not for direct injection but is to be diluted before use, the label alternatively may state the total osmolar concentration in mOsmol per mL. Contains the labeled amounts of fructose and sodium chloride, within ±5%. Contains no antimicrobial agents. Meets the requirements for Identification, Bacterial endotoxins, pH (3.0–6.0), Heavy metals (not more than 5 ppm), Hydroxymethylfurfural, and Injections.

FUMARIC ACID

Chemical name: 2-Butenedioic acid, [*E*]-.

Molecular formula: $C_4H_4O_4$.

Molecular weight: 116.07.

Description: Fumaric Acid NF—White, odorless granules or crystalline powder.
NF category: Acidifying agent.

Solubility: Fumaric Acid NF—Soluble in alcohol; slightly soluble in water and in ether; very slightly soluble in chloroform.

NF requirements: Fumaric Acid NF—Preserve in well-closed containers. Contains not less than 99.5% and not more than 100.5% of fumaric acid, calculated on the anhydrous basis. Meets the requirements for Identification, Water (0.5%), Residue on ignition (not more than 0.1%), Heavy metals (not more than 0.001%), Maleic acid (not more than 0.1%), and Organic volatile impurities.

FURAZOLIDONE

Chemical group: Nitrofuran.

Chemical name: 2-Oxazolidinone, 3-[[(5-nitro-2-furanyl)methylene]amino]-.

Molecular formula: $C_8H_7N_3O_5$.

Molecular weight: 225.16.

Description: Furazolidone USP—Yellow, odorless, crystalline powder.

Solubility: Furazolidone USP—Practically insoluble in water, in alcohol, and in carbon tetrachloride.

USP requirements:
Furazolidone Oral Suspension USP—Preserve in tight, light-resistant containers, and avoid exposure to excessive heat. A suspension of Furazolidone in a suitable aqueous vehicle. Contains the labeled amount, within ±10%. Meets the requirements for Identification and pH (6.0–8.5).
Furazolidone Tablets USP—Preserve in tight, light-resistant containers, and avoid exposure to excessive heat. Contain the labeled amount, within ±10%. Meet the requirements for Identification and Uniformity of dosage units.

FUROSEMIDE

Chemical name: Benzoic acid, 5-(aminosulfonyl)-4-chloro-2-[(2-furanylmethyl)amino]-.

Molecular formula: $C_{12}H_{11}ClN_2O_5S$.

Molecular weight: 330.74.

Description:
Furosemide USP—White to slightly yellow, odorless, crystalline powder.

Furosemide Injection USP—Clear, colorless solution.

pKa: 3.9.

Solubility: Furosemide USP—Practically insoluble in water; freely soluble in acetone, in dimethylformamide, and in solutions of alkali hydroxides; soluble in methanol; sparingly soluble in alcohol; slightly soluble in ether; very slightly soluble in chloroform.

USP requirements:
Furosemide Bolus—Not in USP.
Furosemide Injection USP—Store in single-dose or in multiple-dose, light-resistant containers, of Type I glass. A sterile solution of Furosemide in Water for Injection prepared with the aid of Sodium Hydroxide. Contains the labeled amount, within ±10%. Meets the requirements for Identification, Bacterial endotoxins, pH (8.0–9.3), Particulate matter, 4-Chloro-5-sulfamoylanthranilic acid (not more than 1.0%), and Injections.
Furosemide Oral Solution—Not in USP.
Furosemide Syrup—Not in USP.
Furosemide Tablets USP—Preserve in well-closed, light-resistant containers. Contain the labeled amount, within ±10%. Meet the requirements for Identification, Dissolution (80.0% in 60 minutes in phosphate buffer [pH 5.8] in Apparatus 2 at 50 rpm), Uniformity of dosage units, and 4-Chloro-5-sulfamoylanthranilic acid (not more than 0.8%).

GADOPENTETATE

Chemical name: Gadopentetate dimeglumine—Gadolinate(2−), [*N*,*N*-bis[2-[bis(carboxymethyl)amino]ethyl]glycinato(5−)]-, dihydrogen, compound with 1-deoxy-1-(methylamino)-D-glucitol (1:2).

Molecular formula: Gadopentetate dimeglumine—$C_{14}H_{20}GdN_3O_{10} \cdot 2C_7H_{17}NO_5$.

Molecular weight: Gadopentetate dimeglumine—938.01.

Description: Gadopentetate dimeglumine injection—Clear, colorless to slightly yellow aqueous solution, with a pH of 6.5–8.0.

Solubility: Gadopentetate dimeglumine—Freely soluble in water.

USP requirements: Gadopentetate Dimeglumine Injection—Not in USP.

GALLAMINE

Chemical name: Gallamine triethiodide—Ethanaminium, 2,2′,2″-[1,2,3-benzenetriyltris(oxy)]tris[*N*,*N*,*N*-triethyl]-, triiodide.

Molecular formula: Gallamine triethiodide—$C_{30}H_{60}I_3N_3O_3$.

Molecular weight: Gallamine triethiodide—891.54.

Description: Gallamine Triethiodide USP—White, odorless, amorphous powder. Is hygroscopic.

Solubility: Gallamine Triethiodide USP—Very soluble in water; sparingly soluble in alcohol; very slightly soluble in chloroform.

USP requirements: Gallamine Triethiodide Injection USP—Preserve in single-dose or in multiple-dose containers, preferably of Type I glass, protected from light. A sterile solution of Gallamine Triethiodide in Water for Injection. Contains the labeled amount, within ±5%. Meets the requirements for Identification, Bacterial endotoxins, pH (6.5–7.5), and Injections.

GALLIUM CITRATE Ga 67

Chemical name: 1,2,3-Propanetricarboxylic acid, 2-hydroxy-, gallium-^{67}Ga (1:1) salt.

Molecular formula: $C_6H_5{}^{67}GaO_7$.

USP requirements: Gallium Citrate Ga 67 Injection USP—Preserve in single-dose or in multiple-dose containers. A sterile aqueous solution of radioactive, essentially carrier-free, gallium citrate Ga 67 suitable for intravenous administration. Label it to include the following, in addition to the information specified for Labeling under Injections: the time and date of calibration; the amount of ^{67}Ga as labeled gallium citrate expressed as total megabecquerels (or microcuries or millicuries) and concentration as megabecquerels (or microcuries or millicuries) per mL at the time of calibration; the expiration date and time; and the statement, "Caution—Radioactive Material." The labeling indicates that in making dosage calculations, correction is to be made for radioactive decay, and also indicates that the radioactive half-life of ^{67}Ga is 78.26 hours. Contains the labeled amount of ^{67}Ga as citrate, within ±10%, expressed in megabecquerels (or microcuries or millicuries) per mL at the time indicated in the labeling. Meets the requirements for Bacterial endotoxins, pH (4.5–8.0), Radiochemical purity, Radionuclide identification, Radionuclidic purity, and Injections (except that the Injection may be distributed or dispensed prior to completion of the test for Sterility, the latter test being started on the day of manufacture, and except that it is not subject to the recommendation of Volume in Container).

GALLIUM NITRATE

Molecular formula: $Ga(NO_3)_3 \cdot 9(H_2O)$.

Molecular weight: 417.87 (nonahydrate).

Description:
Gallium nitrate—White, slightly hygroscopic, crystalline powder (nonahydrate).
Gallium nitrate injection—Clear, colorless, odorless, sterile solution.

USP requirements: Gallium Nitrate Injection—Not in USP.

GANCICLOVIR

Chemical name: Ganciclovir sodium—6*H*-Purin-6-one, 2-amino-1,9-dihydro-9-[[2-hydroxy-1-(hydroxymethyl)ethoxy]methyl]-, monosodium salt.

Molecular formula: Ganciclovir sodium—$C_9H_{12}N_5NaO_4$.

Molecular weight: Ganciclovir sodium—277.22.

Description: White to off-white solid.

pKa: 2.2 and 9.4.

Solubility: Soluble in water at 25 °C—4.3 mg/mL at pH 7.

USP requirements: Sterile Ganciclovir Sodium—Not in USP.

ABSORBENT GAUZE

USP requirements: Absorbent Gauze USP—Preserve in well-closed containers. Absorbent Gauze that has been rendered sterile is so packaged that the sterility of the contents of the package is maintained until the package is opened for use. It is cotton, or a mixture of cotton and not more than 53.0%, by weight, of rayon, and is in the form of a plain woven cloth conforming to the standards set forth in *USP*. Absorbent

Gauze that has been rendered sterile is packaged to protect it from contamination. Its type or thread count, length, and width, and the number of pieces contained, are stated on the container, and the designation "non-sterilized" or "not sterilized" appears prominently thereon unless the Gauze has been rendered sterile, in which case it may be labeled to indicate that it is sterile. The package label of sterile Gauze indicates that the contents may not be sterile if the package bears evidence of damage or has been previously opened. The name of the manufacturer, packer, or distributor is stated on the package. Meets the requirements for General characteristics, Thread count, Length (not less than 98.0% of that stated on label), Width (average of three measurements is within 1.6 mm of width stated on label), Weight, Absorbency (complete submersion takes place in not more than 30 seconds), Sterility, Dried and ignited residue, Acid or alkali, and Dextrin or starch, in water extract, Residue on ignition, Fatty matter, Alcohol-soluble dyes, and Cotton and rayon content.

Note: Condition all Absorbent Gauze for not less than 4 hours in a standard atmosphere of 65 ± 2% relative humidity at 21 ± 1.1 °C (70 ± 2 °F), before determining the weight, thread count, and absorbency. Remove the Absorbent Gauze from its wrappings before placing it in the conditioning atmosphere, and if it is in the form of bolts or rolls, cut the quantity necessary for the various tests from the piece, excluding the first two and the last two meters when the total quantity of Gauze available so permits.

PETROLATUM GAUZE

USP requirements: Petrolatum Gauze USP—Each Petrolatum Gauze unit is so packaged individually that the sterility of the unit is maintained until the package is opened for use. It is Absorbent Gauze saturated with White Petrolatum. The package label bears a statement to the effect that the sterility of the Petrolatum Gauze cannot be guaranteed if the package bears evidence of damage or has been opened previously. The package label states the width, length, and type or thread count of the Gauze. The weight of the petrolatum in the gauze is not less than 70.0% and not more than 80.0% of the weight of petrolatum gauze. Petrolatum Gauze is sterile. May be prepared by adding, under aseptic conditions, molten, sterile, White Petrolatum to dry, sterile, Absorbent Gauze, previously cut to size, in the ratio of 60 grams of petrolatum to each 20 grams of gauze. Meets the requirements for Sterility, of tests under White Petrolatum, and of tests for Thread count, Length, Width, and Weight under Absorbent Gauze.

GELATIN

Description: Gelatin NF—Sheets, flakes, or shreds, or coarse to fine powder. Faintly yellow or amber in color, the color varying in depth according to the particle size. It has a slight, characteristic, bouillon-like odor in solution. Stable in air when dry, but subject to microbic decomposition when moist or in solution. Gelatin has any suitable strength that is designated by Bloom Gelometer number. Type A Gelatin exhibits an isoelectric point between pH 7 and pH 9, and Type B Gelatin exhibits an isoelectric point between pH 4.7 and pH 5.2.

NF category: Coating agent; suspending and/or viscosity-increasing agent; tablet binder.

Solubility: Gelatin NF—Insoluble in cold water, but swells and softens when immersed in it, gradually absorbing from 5 to 10 times its own weight of water. Soluble in hot water, in 6 N acetic acid, and in a hot mixture of glycerin and water.

Insoluble in alcohol, in chloroform, in ether, and in fixed and volatile oils.

NF requirements: Gelatin NF—Preserve in well-closed containers in a dry place. A product obtained by the partial hydrolysis of collagen derived from the skin, white connective tissue, and bones of animals. Gelatin derived from an acid-treated precursor is known as Type A, and Gelatin derived from an alkali-treated precursor is known as Type B. Gelatin, where being used in the manufacture of capsules, or for the coating of tablets, may be colored with a certified color, may contain not more than 0.15% of sulfur dioxide, and may contain a suitable concentration of sodium lauryl sulfate and suitable antimicrobial agents. Meets the requirements for Identification, Microbial limits, Residue on ignition (not more than 2.0%), Odor and water-insoluble substances, Sulfur dioxide, Arsenic (not more than 0.8 ppm), and Heavy metals (not more than 0.005%).

ABSORBABLE GELATIN

Description:
Absorbable Gelatin Film USP—Light amber, transparent, pliable film which becomes rubbery when moistened.
Absorbable Gelatin Sponge USP—Light, nearly white, nonelastic, tough, porous, hydrophilic solid.

Solubility:
Absorbable Gelatin Film USP—Insoluble in water.
Absorbable Gelatin Sponge USP—Insoluble in water.

USP requirements:
Absorbable Gelatin Film USP—Preserve in hermetically sealed or other suitable container in such manner that the sterility of the product is maintained until the container is opened for use. It is Gelatin in the form of a sterile, absorbable, water-insoluble film. The package bears a statement to the effect that the sterility of Absorbable Gelatin Film cannot be guaranteed if the package bears evidence of damage, or if the package has been previously opened. Meets the requirements for Sterility, Residue on ignition (not more than 2.0%), and Proteolytic digest (average time of 3 proteolytic digest determinations, 4–8 hours). {R-2}
Absorbable Gelatin Sponge USP—Preserve in a hermetically sealed or other suitable container in such manner that the sterility of the product is maintained until the container is opened for use. It is Gelatin in the form of a sterile, absorbable, water-insoluble sponge. The package bears a statement to the effect that the sterility of Absorbable Gelatin Sponge cannot be guaranteed if the package bears evidence of damage, or if the package has been previously opened. Meets the requirements for Sterility, Residue on ignition (not more than 2.0%), Digestibility (average digestion time of 3 determinations not more than 75 minutes), and Water absorption (not less than 35 times its weight of water).

GEMFIBROZIL

Chemical name: Pentanoic acid, 5-(2,5-dimethylphenoxy)-2,2-dimethyl-.

Molecular formula: $C_{15}H_{22}O_3$.

Molecular weight: 250.34.

Description: Gemfibrozil USP—White, waxy, crystalline solid.

Solubility: Gemfibrozil USP—Practically insoluble in water; soluble in alcohol, in methanol, and in chloroform.

USP requirements:

Gemfibrozil Capsules USP—Preserve in tight containers. Contain the labeled amount, within ±10%. Meet the requirements for Identification, Dissolution (80% in 45 minutes in 0.2 *M* phosphate buffer [pH 7.5] in Apparatus 2 at 50 rpm), and Uniformity of dosage units.

Gemfibrozil Tablets—Not in USP.

GENTAMICIN

Source: Derived from the actinomycete *Micromonospora purpurea.*

Chemical group: Aminoglycosides.

Chemical name: Gentamicin sulfate—Gentamicin sulfate (salt).

Description:

Gentamicin Sulfate USP—White to buff powder.

Gentamicin Sulfate Injection USP—Clear, slightly yellow solution, having a faint odor.

Solubility: Gentamicin Sulfate USP—Freely soluble in water; insoluble in alcohol, in acetone, in chloroform, and in ether.

USP requirements:

Gentamicin Sulfate Cream USP—Preserve in collapsible tubes or in other tight containers, and avoid exposure to excessive heat. Contains an amount of gentamicin sulfate equivalent to the labeled amount of gentamicin, within −10% to +35%. Meets the requirements for Identification and Minimum fill.

Gentamicin Sulfate Uterine Infusion—Not in USP.

Gentamicin Sulfate Injection USP—Preserve in single-dose or in multiple-dose containers, preferably of Type I glass. A sterile solution of Gentamicin Sulfate in Water for Injection. It may contain suitable buffers, preservatives, and sequestering agents, unless it is intended for intrathecal use, in which case it contains only suitable tonicity agents. Contains an amount of gentamicin sulfate equivalent to the labeled amount of gentamicin, within −10% to +25%. Meets the requirements for Identification, Bacterial endotoxins, pH (3.0–5.5), Particulate matter, and Injections.

Gentamicin Sulfate Ointment USP—Preserve in collapsible tubes or in other tight containers, and avoid exposure to excessive heat. Contains an amount of gentamicin sulfate equivalent to the labeled amount of gentamicin, within −10% to +35%. Meets the requirements for Identification, Minimum fill, and Water (not more than 1.0%).

Gentamicin Sulfate Ophthalmic Ointment USP—Preserve in collapsible ophthalmic ointment tubes, and avoid exposure to excessive heat. Contains an amount of gentamicin sulfate equivalent to the labeled amount of gentamicin, within −10% to +35%. Meets the requirements for Identification, Sterility, Minimum fill, and Metal particles, and for Water under Gentamicin Sulfate Ointment.

Gentamicin Sulfate Soluble Powder—Not in USP.

Gentamicin Sulfate Ophthalmic Solution USP—Preserve in tight containers, and avoid exposure to excessive heat. A sterile, buffered solution of Gentamicin Sulfate with preservatives. Contains an amount of gentamicin sulfate equivalent to the labeled amount of gentamicin, within −10% to +35%. Meets the requirements for pH (6.5–7.5) and for Identification test under Gentamicin Sulfate Injection and Sterility tests.

Gentamicin Sulfate Oral Solution—Not in USP.

Gentamicin Sulfate Otic Solution—Not in USP.

Sterile Gentamicin Sulfate USP—Preserve in Containers for Sterile Solids. It is Gentamicin Sulfate suitable for parenteral use. It has a potency equivalent to not less than 590 mcg of gentamicin per mg, calculated on the dried basis. Meets the requirements for Pyrogen and Sterility, and for Identification tests, Specific rotation (+107° to +121°, calculated on the dried basis), pH (3.5–5.5, in a solution [1 in 25]), Loss on drying (not more than 18.0%), Methanol, and Content of gentamicins under Gentamicin Sulfate.

GENTAMICIN AND PREDNISOLONE

For *Gentamicin* and *Prednisolone*—See individual listings for chemistry information.

USP requirements:

Gentamicin and Prednisolone Acetate Ophthalmic Ointment USP—Preserve in collapsible ophthalmic ointment tubes, and avoid exposure to excessive heat. Contains the equivalent of the labeled amount of gentamicin, within −10% to +20%, and the labeled amount of prednisolone acetate, within ±10%. Meets the requirements for Identification, Sterility, Minimum fill, Water (not more than 2.0%), and Metal particles.

Gentamicin and Prednisolone Acetate Ophthalmic Suspension USP—Preserve in tight containers. A sterile aqueous suspension containing Gentamicin Sulfate and Prednisolone Acetate. Contains an amount of gentamicin sulfate equivalent to the labeled amount of gentamicin, within −10% to +30%, and the labeled amount of prednisolone acetate, within ±10%. Meets the requirements for Identification, Sterility, and pH (5.4–6.6).

GENTAMICIN AND SODIUM CHLORIDE

For *Gentamicin* and *Sodium Chloride*—See individual listings for chemistry information.

USP requirements: Gentamicin Sulfate in Sodium Chloride Injection—Not in USP.

GENTIAN VIOLET

Chemical name: Methanaminium, *N*-[4-[bis[4-(dimethylamino)phenyl]methylene]-2,5-cyclohexadien-1-ylidene]-*N*-methyl-, chloride; also known as methylrosaniline chloride and basic violet 3.

Molecular formula: $C_{25}H_{30}ClN_3$.

Molecular weight: 407.99.

Description:

Gentian Violet USP—Dark green powder or greenish, glistening pieces having a metallic luster, and having not more than a faint odor.

Gentian Violet Cream USP—Dark purple, water-washable cream.

Gentian Violet Topical Solution USP—Purple liquid, having a slight odor of alcohol. A dilution (1 in 100), viewed downward through 1 cm of depth, is deep purple in color.

Solubility: Gentian Violet USP—Sparingly soluble in water; soluble in alcohol, in glycerin, and in chloroform; insoluble in ether.

USP requirements:

Gentian Violet Cream USP—Preserve in collapsible tubes, or in other tight containers, and avoid exposure to excessive heat. It is Gentian Violet in a suitable cream base. Contains, in each 100 grams, not less than 1.20 grams and not more than 1.60 grams of gentian violet, calculated as hexamethylpararosaniline chloride. Meets the requirements for Identification and Minimum fill.

Gentian Violet Topical Solution USP—Preserve in tight containers. Contains, in each 100 mL, not less than 0.95 gram and not more than 1.05 grams of gentian violet, calculated as hexamethylpararosaniline chloride. Meets the requirements for Identification, Solution of residue in alcohol, and Alcohol content (8.0–10.0%).

Gentian Violet Vaginal Tampons—Not in USP.

GENTISIC ACID ETHANOLAMIDE

Molecular formula: $C_9H_{11}NO_4$.

Molecular weight: 197.19.

Description: Gentisic Acid Ethanolamide NF—White to tan powder. Melts at about 149 °C.

NF category: Complexing agent.

Solubility: Gentisic Acid Ethanolamide NF—Sparingly soluble in water; freely soluble in acetone, in methanol, and in alcohol; very slightly soluble in ether; practically insoluble in chloroform.

NF requirements: Gentisic Acid Ethanolamide NF—Preserve in well-closed containers. Contains not less than 99.0% and not more than 100.5% of gentisic acid ethanolamide, calculated on the dried basis. Meets the requirements for Identification, Loss on drying (not more than 0.5%), Residue on ignition (not more than 0.1%), Chloride, Sulfate (not more than 0.02%), Heavy metals (not more than 0.001%), Chromatographic impurities, and Organic volatile impurities.

PHARMACEUTICAL GLAZE

Description: Pharmaceutical Glaze NF—NF category: Coating agent.

NF requirements: Pharmaceutical Glaze NF—Preserve in tight, lined metal or plastic containers, protected from excessive heat, preferably at a temperature below 25 °C. A specially denatured alcoholic solution of Shellac containing between 20.0 and 57.0% of anhydrous shellac, and is made with either anhydrous alcohol or alcohol containing 5% of water by volume. The solvent is a specially denatured alcohol approved for glaze manufacturing by the Internal Revenue Service. Label it to indicate the shellac type and concentration, the composition of the solvent, and the quantity of titanium dioxide, if present. Where titanium dioxide or waxes are present, the label states that the Glaze requires mixing before use. Meets the requirements for Identification, Arsenic, Heavy metals, and Rosin under Shellac, Acid value under Shellac, and Wax under Shellac.

GLIPIZIDE

Chemical group: Sulfonylurea.

Chemical name: Pyrazinecarboxamide, N-[2-[4-[[[(cyclohexylamino)carbonyl]amino]sulfonyl]phenyl]ethyl]-5-methyl-.

Molecular formula: $C_{21}H_{27}N_5O_4S$.

Molecular weight: 445.54.

Description: Whitish, odorless powder.

pKa: 5.9.

Solubility: Insoluble in water and in alcohols; soluble in 0.1 N sodium hydroxide; freely soluble in dimethylformamide.

USP requirements: Glipizide Tablets—Not in USP.

ANTI-HUMAN GLOBULIN SERUM

USP requirements: Anti-Human Globulin Serum USP—Preserve at a temperature between 2 and 8 °C. A sterile, liquid preparation of serum produced by immunizing lower animals such as rabbits or goats with human serum or plasma, or with selected human plasma proteins. It is free from agglutinins and from hemolysins to non-sensitized human red cells of all blood groups. Contains a suitable antimicrobial preservative. Label it to state the animal source of the product. Label it also to state the specific antibody activities present; to state the application for which the reagent is intended; to include a cautionary statement that it does not contain antibodies to immunoglobulins or that it does not contain antibodies to complement components, wherever and whichever is applicable; and to state that it is for in-vitro diagnostic use. [Note: The lettering on the label of the general-purpose polyspecific reagent is black on a white background. The label of all other Anti-Human Globulin Serum containers is in white lettering on a black background.] Anti-Human Globulin Serums containing Anti-IgG meet the requirements of the test for potency, in parallel with the U.S. Reference Anti-Human Globulin (Anti-IgG) Serum (at a 1:4 dilution) when tested with red cells suspended in isotonic saline sensitized with decreasing amounts of non-agglutinating Anti-D (Anti-Rh$_o$) serum, and with cells sensitized in the same manner with an immunoglobulin IgG Anti-Fy^a serum of similar potency. Anti-Human Globulin Serum containing one or more Anti-complement components meets the requirements of the tests for potency in giving a 2+ agglutination reaction (i.e., agglutinated cells dislodged into many small clumps of equal size) by the low-ionic sucrose or sucrose-trypsin procedures when tested as recommended in the labeling. Anti-Human Globulin Serum containing Anti-3Cd activity meets the requirements for stability, by potency testing of representative lots every 3 months during the dating period. Meets the requirement for Expiration date (not later than 1 year after the date of issue from manufacturer's cold storage [5 °C, 1 year; or 0 °C, 2 years]). Conforms to the regulations of the U.S. Food and Drug Administration concerning biologics.

IMMUNE GLOBULIN

Description: Immune Globulin USP—Transparent or slightly opalescent liquid, either colorless or of a brownish color due to denatured hemoglobin. Practically odorless. May develop a slight, granular deposit during storage.

USP requirements: Immune Globulin USP—Preserve at a temperature between 2 and 8 °C. A sterile, non-pyrogenic solution of globulins that contains many antibodies normally present in adult human blood, prepared by pooling approximately equal amounts of material (source blood, plasma, serum, or placentas) from not less than 1000 donors. Label it to state that passive immunization with Immune Globulin modifies hepatitis A, prevents or modifies measles, and provides replacement therapy in persons having hypo- or agammaglobulinemia, that it is not standardized with respect to antibody titers against hepatitis B surface antigen and that it should be used for prophylaxis of viral hepatitis type B only when the specific Immune Globulin is not available, that it may be of benefit in women who have been exposed to rubella in the first trimester of pregnancy but who would not consider a therapeutic abortion, and that it may be used in immunosuppressed patients for passive immunization against varicella if the specific Immune Globulin is not available. Label it also to state that it is not indicated for routine prophylaxis or treatment of rubella, poliomyelitis or mumps, or for allergy or asthma in patients who have normal levels of immunoglobulin, that the plasma units from which it has been derived have been tested and found non-reactive for hepatitis B surface antigen, and that it should not be administered intravenously but be given intramuscularly, preferably in the gluteal region. Contains not less than 15 grams and not more than 18 grams of protein per 100 mL, not less than 90.0% of which is gamma globulin. Contains 0.3 M glycine as a stabilizing agent and contains a suitable preservative. It has a potency of component antibodies of diphtheria antitoxin based on the U.S. Standard Diphtheria Antitoxin and a diphtheria test toxin, tested in guinea pigs (not less than 2 antitoxin units per mL), and antibodies for measles and poliovirus. Meets the requirements of the tests for heat stability in absence of gelation on heating, and for pH. Meets the requirement for Expiration date (not later than 3 years after date of issue from manufacturer's cold storage [5 °C, 3 years]. Conforms to the regulations of the U.S. Food and Drug Administration concerning biologics.

RH₀ (D) IMMUNE GLOBULIN

Description: RH₀ (D) Immune Globulin USP—Transparent or slightly opalescent liquid. Practically colorless and practically odorless. May develop a slight, granular deposit during storage.

USP requirements: RH₀ (D) Immune Globulin USP—Preserve at a temperature between 2 and 8 °C. A sterile, non-pyrogenic solution of globulins derived from human blood plasma containing antibody to the erythrocyte factor Rh₀ (D). Contains not less than 10 grams and not more than 18 grams of protein per 100 mL, not less than 90.0% of which is gamma globulin. It has a potency, determined by a suitable method, not less than that of the U.S. Reference Rh₀ (D) Immune Globulin. Contains 0.3 M glycine as a stabilizing agent and contains a suitable preservative. Meets the requirement for Expiration date (not later than 6 months from the date of issue from manufacturer's cold storage, or not later than 1 year from the date of manufacture, as indicated on the label). Conforms to the regulations of the U.S. Food and Drug Administration concerning biologics.

GLUCAGON

Source: Extracted from beef or porcine pancreas.

Chemical name: Glucagon (pig).

Molecular formula: $C_{153}H_{225}N_{43}O_{49}S$.

Molecular weight: 3482.78.

Description:
Glucagon USP—Fine, white or faintly colored, crystalline powder. Is practically odorless.
Glucagon for Injection USP—White, odorless powder.

Solubility: Glucagon USP—Soluble in dilute alkali and acid solutions; insoluble in most organic solvents.

Other characteristics: A single-chain polypeptide containing 29 amino acid residues. Chemically unrelated to insulin. One USP Unit of glucagon is equivalent to 1 International Unit of glucagon and also to about 1 mg of glucagon.

USP requirements: Glucagon for Injection USP—Preserve in Containers for Sterile Solids. Preserve the accompanying solvent in single-dose or in multiple-dose containers, preferably of Type I glass. A mixture of the hydrochloride of Glucagon with one or more suitable, dry diluents. Contains the labeled amount, within −20% to +25%. Meets the requirements for Constituted solution, pH (2.5–3.0), Clarity of solution, Sterility tests, Labeling, and Uniformity of dosage units.

GLUCOSE ENZYMATIC TEST STRIP

USP requirements: Glucose Enzymatic Test Strip USP—Preserve in the original container, in a dry place, at controlled room temperature. Consists of the enzymes glucose oxidase and horseradish peroxidase, a suitable substrate for the reaction of hydrogen peroxide catalyzed by peroxidase, and other inactive ingredients impregnated and dried on filter paper. When tested in human urine containing known glucose concentrations, it reacts in the specified times to produce colors corresponding to the color chart provided. Meets the requirements for Identification and Calibration.

LIQUID GLUCOSE

Description: Liquid Glucose NF—Colorless or yellowish, thick, syrupy liquid. Odorless or nearly odorless.
NF category: Tablet binder.

Solubility: Liquid Glucose NF—Miscible with water; sparingly soluble in alcohol.

NF requirements: Liquid Glucose NF—Preserve in tight containers. A product obtained by the incomplete hydrolysis of starch. Consists chiefly of dextrose, dextrins, maltose, and water. Meets the requirements for Identification, Acidity, Water (not more than 21.0%), Residue on ignition (not more than 0.5%), Sulfite, Arsenic (not more than 1 ppm), Heavy metals (not more than 0.001%), Starch, and Organic volatile impurities.

GLUTARAL

Chemical name: Pentanedial.

Molecular formula: $C_5H_8O_2$.

Molecular weight: 100.12.

Description: Glutaral Concentrate USP—Clear, colorless or faintly yellow liquid, having a characteristic, irritating odor.

USP requirements: Glutaral Concentrate USP—Preserve in tight containers, protected from light, and avoid exposure to excessive heat. A solution of glutaraldehyde in Purified Water. Contains the labeled amount, within +4%, the labeled amount being 50.0 grams of glutaral per 100.0 grams of Concentrate. Meets the requirements for Clarity of solution, Identification, Specific gravity (1.128 to 1.135 at 20 °C/20 °C), Acidity (not more than 0.4% of acid (w/w), calculated as acetic acid), pH (3.7–4.5), and Heavy metals (not more than 0.001%).

NF requirements: Glutaral Disinfectant Solution NF—Preserve in tight, light-resistant containers, and avoid exposure to excessive heat. Contains, by weight, the labeled amount of glutaral, within +10%. Meets the requirements for Identification and pH (2.7–3.7).

GLUTETHIMIDE

Chemical name: 2,6-Piperidinedione, 3-ethyl-3-phenyl-.

Molecular formula: $C_{13}H_{15}NO_2$.

Molecular weight: 217.27.

Description: Glutethimide USP—White, crystalline powder. Its saturated solution is acid to litmus.

Solubility: Glutethimide USP—Practically insoluble in water; freely soluble in ethyl acetate, in acetone, in ether, and in chloroform; soluble in alcohol and in methanol.

USP requirements:

Glutethimide Capsules USP—Preserve in well-closed containers. Contain the labeled amount, within ±5%. Meet the requirements for Identification, Dissolution (75% in 45 minutes in water in Apparatus 1 at 100 rpm), and Uniformity of dosage units.

Glutethimide Tablets USP—Preserve in well-closed containers. Contain the labeled amount, within ±10%. Meet the requirements for Identification, Dissolution (70% in 60 minutes in water in Apparatus 2 at 50 rpm), and Uniformity of dosage units.

GLYBURIDE

Chemical group: Sulfonylurea.

Chemical name: Benzamide, 5-chloro-*N*-[2-[4-[[[(cyclohexylamino)carbonyl]amino]sulfonyl]phenyl]ethyl]-2-methoxy-.

Molecular formula: $C_{23}H_{28}ClN_3O_5S$.

Molecular weight: 494.00.

Description: White, crystalline compound.

pKa: 5.3.

Solubility: Practically insoluble in water and in ether; soluble 1 in 330 of alcohol, 1 in 36 of chloroform, and 1 in 250 of methyl alcohol.

USP requirements: Glyburide Tablets—Not in USP.

GLYCERIN

Chemical name: 1,2,3-Propanetriol.

Molecular formula: $C_3H_8O_3$.

Molecular weight: 92.09.

Description: Glycerin USP—Clear, colorless, syrupy liquid. Has not more than a slight characteristic odor, which is neither harsh nor disagreeable. Is hygroscopic. Its solutions are neutral to litmus.

NF category: Humectant; plasticizer; solvent; tonicity agent.

Solubility: Glycerin USP—Miscible with water and with alcohol. Insoluble in chloroform, in ether, and in fixed and volatile oils.

USP requirements:

Glycerin USP—Preserve in tight containers. Contains not less than 95.0% and not more than 101.0% of glycerin. Meets the requirements for Identification, Specific gravity (not less than 1.249), Color, Residue on ignition (not more than 0.01%), Chloride (not more than 0.001%), Sulfate (not more than 0.002%), Arsenic (not more than 1.5 ppm), Heavy metals (not more than 5 ppm), Chlorinated compounds (not more than 0.003% of chlorine), and Fatty acids and esters.

Glycerin Ophthalmic Solution USP—Preserve in tight containers of glass or plastic, containing not more than 15 mL, protected from light. The container or individual carton is sealed and tamper-proof so that sterility is assured at time of first use. A sterile, anhydrous solution of Glycerin, containing the labeled amount, within −1.5%. [Note: In the preparation of this Ophthalmic Solution, use Glycerin that has a low water content, in order that the Ophthalmic Solution may comply with the Water limit. This may be ensured by using Glycerin having a specific gravity of not less than 1.2607, corresponding to a concentration of 99.5%.] Meets the requirements for

Identification, Sterility, pH (4.5–7.5), and Water (not more than 1.0%).

Note: Do not use the Ophthalmic Solution if it contains crystals, or if it is cloudy or discolored or contains a precipitate.

Glycerin Oral Solution USP—Preserve in tight containers. Contains the labeled amount, within ±5%. Meets the requirements for Identification and pH (5.5–7.5).

Glycerin Rectal Solution—Not in USP.

Glycerin Suppositories USP—Preserve in well-closed containers. Contain Glycerin solidified with Sodium Stearate. Contain the labeled amount, by weight, of glycerin, within −25% to −10%. Meet the requirements for Identification and Water (not more than 15.0%).

GLYCERYL BEHENATE

Description: Glyceryl Behenate NF—Fine powder, having a faint odor. Melts at about 70 °C.

NF category: Tablet and/or capsule lubricant.

Solubility: Glyceryl Behenate NF—Practically insoluble in water and in alcohol; soluble in chloroform.

NF requirements: Glyceryl Behenate NF—Preserve in tight containers, at a temperature not higher than 35 °C. A mixture of glycerides of fatty acids, mainly behenic acid. Meets the requirements for Identification, Residue on ignition (not more than 0.1%), Heavy metals (not more than 0.001%), Acid value (not more than 4), Iodine value (not more than 3), Saponification value (145–165), 1-Monoglycerides (12.0–18.0%), and Free glycerin (not more than 1.0%).

GLYCERYL MONOSTEARATE

Chemical name: Octadecanoic acid, monoester with 1,2,3-propanetriol.

Molecular formula: $C_{21}H_{42}O_4$.

Molecular weight: 358.56.

Description: Glyceryl Monostearate NF—White, wax-like solid, or white, wax-like beads or flakes. Slight agreeable fatty odor. Affected by light.

NF category: Emulsifying and/or solubilizing agent.

Solubility: Glyceryl Monostearate NF—Dissolves in hot organic solvents such as alcohol, mineral or fixed oils, ether, and acetone. Insoluble in water, but it may be dispersed in hot water with the aid of a small amount of soap or other suitable surface-active agent.

NF requirements: Glyceryl Monostearate NF—Preserve in tight, light-resistant containers. Contains not less than 90.0% of monoglycerides of saturated fatty acids, chiefly glyceryl monostearate and glyceryl monopalmitate. Meets the requirements for Melting range (not less than 55 °C), Residue on ignition (not more than 0.5%), Arsenic (not more than 3 ppm), Heavy metals (not more than 0.001%), Acid value (not more than 6), Iodine value (not more than 3), Saponification value (155–165), Hydroxyl value (300–330), and Free glycerin (not more than 1.2%).

GLYCINE

Chemical name: Glycine.

Molecular formula: $C_2H_5NO_2$.

Molecular weight: 75.07.

Description: Glycine USP—White, odorless, crystalline powder. Its solutions are acid to litmus.

Solubility: Glycine USP—Freely soluble in water; very slightly soluble in alcohol and in ether.

USP requirements: Glycine Irrigation USP—Preserve in single-dose containers, preferably of Type I or Type II glass. A sterile solution of Glycine in Water for Injection. Contains the labeled amount, within ±5%. Meets the requirements for Identification, Bacterial endotoxins, pH (4.5–6.5), and Injections (except the container in which the solution is packaged may be designed to empty rapidly and may exceed 1000 mL in capacity).

GLYCOPYRROLATE

Source: An aminoalcohol ester.

Chemical group: Quaternary ammonium compound.

Chemical name: Pyrrolidinium, 3-[(cyclopentylhydroxyphenyl-acetyl)oxy]-1,1-dimethyl-, bromide.

Molecular formula: $C_{19}H_{28}BrNO_3$.

Molecular weight: 398.34.

Description: Glycopyrrolate USP—White, odorless, crystalline powder.

Solubility: Glycopyrrolate USP—Soluble in water and in alcohol; practically insoluble in chloroform and in ether.

USP requirements:
Glycopyrrolate Injection USP—Preserve in single-dose or in multiple-dose containers, preferably of Type I glass. A sterile solution of Glycopyrrolate in Water for Injection. Contains the labeled amount, within ±7%. Meets the requirements for Identification, Bacterial endotoxins, pH (2.0–3.0), and Injections.
Glycopyrrolate Tablets USP—Preserve in tight containers. Contain the labeled amount, within ±7%. Meet the requirements for Identification, Dissolution (75% in 45 minutes in water in Apparatus 1 at 100 rpm), and Uniformity of dosage units.

GOLD SODIUM THIOMALATE

Chemical name: Butanedioic acid, mercapto-, monogold(1+) sodium salt.

Molecular formula: $C_4H_3AuNa_2O_4S + C_4H_4AuNaO_4S$.

Molecular weight: 758.16.

Description: Gold sodium thiomalate—White to yellowish white, odorless or practically odorless, lumpy solid.

Solubility: Gold sodium thiomalate—Very soluble in water; insoluble in alcohol, in ether, and in most organic solvents.

USP requirements: Gold Sodium Thiomalate Injection USP—Preserve in single-dose or in multiple-dose containers, preferably of Type I glass, protected from light. A sterile solution of Gold Sodium Thiomalate in Water for Injection. Contains the labeled amount, within ±5%. Meets the requirements for Identification, pH (5.8–6.5), and Injections.

GONADORELIN

Source: Gonadorelin is a gonad stimulating principle (luteinizing hormone-releasing factor). Source of this compound may be sheep, pig, or other species, or it could be synthetic.

Chemical name:
Gonadorelin acetate—5-Oxo-L-prolyl-L-histidyl-L-tryptophyl-L-seryl-L-tyrosylglycyl-L-leucyl-L-arginyl-L-prolyl-glycinamide acetate (salt) hydrate.
Gonadorelin hydrochloride—5-Oxo-L-prolyl-L-histidyl-L-tryptophyl-L-seryl-L-tyrosyl-glycyl-L-leucyl-L-prolylglycinamide hydrochloride.

Molecular formula:
Gonadorelin acetate—$C_{55}H_{75}N_{17}O_{13} \cdot xC_2H_4O_2 \cdot yH_2O$.
Gonadorelin hydrochloride—$C_{55}H_{75}N_{17}O_{13} \cdot xHCl$.
Note: Gonadorelin hydrochloride is $C_{55}H_{75}N_{17}O_{13}$ as the monohydrochloride or the dihydrochloride or as a mixture of these.

Molecular weight: 1182.33.

Description: White powder. Hygroscopic and moisture-sensitive.

Solubility: Soluble in alcohol and in water.

USP requirements:
Gonadorelin Acetate for Injection—Not in USP.
Gonadorelin Hydrochloride for Injection—Not in USP.

CHORIONIC GONADOTROPIN

Source: Extracted from urine of pregnant women (produced by the placenta).

Description:
Chorionic Gonadotropin USP—White or practically white, amorphous powder.
Chorionic Gonadotropin for Injection USP—White or practically white, amorphous solid having the characteristic appearance of substances prepared by freeze-drying.

Solubility: Chorionic Gonadotropin USP—Freely soluble in water.

USP requirements: Chorionic Gonadotropin for Injection USP—Preserve in Containers for Sterile Solids. A sterile, dry mixture of Chorionic Gonadotropin with suitable diluents and buffers. Label it to indicate the expiration date. Contains the labeled amount in USP Chorionic Gonadotropin Units, within −20% to +25%. Meets the requirements for Constituted solution, Bacterial endotoxins, pH (6.0–8.0), Estrogenic activity, and Uniformity of dosage units, and for Sterility tests and Labeling under Injections.

GOSERELIN

Source: Goserelin acetate—Synthetic decapeptide analog of luteinizing hormone-releasing hormone (LHRH).

Chemical name: Goserelin acetate—L-pyroglutamyl-L-histidyl-L-tryptophyl-L-seryl-L-tyrosyl-D-(0-tert-butyl)seryl-L-leucyl-L-arginyl-L-prolyl-azaglycine amide acetate.

Molecular formula: Goserelin acetate—$C_{61}H_{87}N_{18}O_{16}$.

Molecular weight: Goserelin acetate—1328.

Description: Goserelin acetate—Off-white powder.

Solubility: Goserelin acetate—Freely soluble in glacial acetic acid; soluble in water, in 0.1 M hydrochloric acid, in 0.1 M sodium hydroxide, in dimethylformamide, and in dimethyl sulfoxide; practically insoluble in acetone, in chloroform, and in ether.

USP requirements:
Goserelin Acetate Implants—Not in USP.
Goserelin Acetate Injection—Not in USP.

GRAMICIDIN

Chemical name: Gramicidin.

Description: Gramicidin USP—White or practically white, odorless, crystalline powder.

Solubility: Gramicidin USP—Insoluble in water; soluble in alcohol.

USP requirements: Gramicidin USP—Preserve in tight containers. An antibacterial substance produced by the growth of *Bacillus brevis* Dubos (Fam. Bacillaceae). May be obtained from tyrothricin. Has a potency of not less than 900 mcg of gramicidin per mg, calculated on the dried basis. Meets the requirements for Identification, Melting temperature (not less than 229 °C, determined after drying), Crystallinity, Loss on drying (not more than 3.0%), and Residue on ignition (not more than 1.0%).

GREEN SOAP

Description: Green Soap USP—Soft, unctuous, yellowish white to brownish or greenish yellow, transparent to translucent mass. Has a slight, characteristic odor, often suggesting the oil from which it was prepared. Its solution (1 in 20) is alkaline to bromothymol blue TS.

USP requirements:
Green Soap USP—Preserve in well-closed containers. A potassium soap made by the saponification of suitable vegetable oils, excluding coconut oil and palm kernel oil, without the removal of glycerin.

Green Soap may be prepared as follows: 380 grams of the Vegetable Oil, 20 grams of Oleic Acid, 91.7 grams of Potassium Hydroxide (total alkali 85%), 50 mL of Glycerin, and a sufficient quantity of Purified Water to make about 1000 grams. Mix the oil and the Oleic Acid, and heat the mixture to about 80 °C. Dissolve the Potassium Hydroxide in a mixture of the Glycerin and 100 mL of Purified Water, and add the solution, while it is still hot, to the hot oil. Stir the mixture vigorously until emulsified, then heat while continuing the stirring, until the mixture is homogeneous and a test portion will dissolve to give a clear solution in hot water. Add hot purified water to make the product weigh 1000 grams, continuing the stirring until the Soap is homogeneous.

Meets the requirements for Water (not more than 52.0%), Alcohol-insoluble substances (not more than 3.0%), Free alkali hydroxides (not more than 0.25% of potassium hydroxide), Alkali carbonates (0.35%, as potassium carbonate), Unsaponified matter, and Characteristics of the liberated fatty acids.
Green Soap Tincture USP—Preserve in tight containers.
Prepare Green Soap Tincture as follows: 650 grams of Green Soap, Suitable essential oil(s), 316 mL of Alcohol, and a sufficient quantity of Purified Water to make 1000 mL. Mix the oil(s) and Alcohol, dissolve in this the Green Soap by stirring or by agitation, set the solution aside for 24 hours, filter through paper, and add water to make 1000 mL.

Meets the requirements for Identification, pH (9.5–11.5), and Alcohol content (28.0–32.0%).

GRISEOFULVIN

Source: Antifungal antibiotic derived from a species of *Penicillium*.

Chemical name: Spiro[benzofuran-2(3*H*),1'-[2]cyclohexene]-3,4'-dione, 7-chloro-2',4,6-trimethoxy-6'-methyl-, (1'*S-trans*)-.

Molecular formula: $C_{17}H_{17}ClO_6$.

Molecular weight: 352.77.

Description: Griseofulvin USP—White to creamy white, odorless powder, in which particles of the order of 4 micrometers in diameter predominate.

Solubility: Griseofulvin USP—Very slightly soluble in water; soluble in acetone, in dimethylformamide, and in chloroform; sparingly soluble in alcohol.

USP requirements:
Griseofulvin Capsules USP (Microsize)—Preserve in tight containers. The label indicates that the griseofulvin contained is known as griseofulvin (microsize). Contain the labeled amount, within −10% to +15%. Meet the requirements for Identification, Dissolution (80% in 30 minutes in water containing 5.4 mg of sodium lauryl sulfate per mL in Apparatus 2 at 100 rpm), Uniformity of dosage units, and Loss on drying (not more than 1.0%).
Griseofulvin Oral Suspension USP (Microsize)—Preserve in tight containers. Contains one or more suitable colors, diluents, flavors, preservatives, and wetting agents. The label indicates that the griseofulvin contained is known as griseofulvin (microsize). Contains the labeled amount, within −10% to +15%. Meets the requirements for Identification, pH (5.5–7.5), Deliverable volume (multiple-unit containers), and Uniformity of dosage units (single-unit containers).
Griseofulvin Tablets USP (Microsize)—Preserve in tight containers. The label indicates that the griseofulvin contained is known as griseofulvin (microsize). Contain the labeled amount, within −10% to +15%. Meet the requirements for Identification, Dissolution (70% in 60 minutes in water containing 40.0 mg of sodium lauryl sulfate per mL in Apparatus 2 at 100 rpm), Uniformity of dosage units, and Loss on drying (not more than 5.0%).
Ultramicrosize Griseofulvin Tablets USP—Preserve in well-closed containers. Composed of ultramicrosize crystals of Griseofulvin dispersed in Polyethylene Glycol 6000 or dispersed by other suitable means. Contain the labeled amount, within −10% to +15%. Meet the requirements for Identification, Dissolution (85% in 60 minutes in water containing 5.4 mg of sodium lauryl sulfate per mL in Apparatus 2 at 100 rpm), Uniformity of dosage units, and Loss on drying (not more than 5.0%).

GUAIFENESIN

Chemical name: 1,2-Propanediol, 3-(2-methoxyphenoxy)-.

Molecular formula: $C_{10}H_{14}O_4$.

Molecular weight: 198.22.

Description: Guaifenesin USP—White to slightly gray, crystalline powder. May have a slight characteristic odor.

Solubility: Guaifenesin USP—Soluble in water, in alcohol, in chloroform, in glycerin, and in propylene glycol.

USP requirements:
Guaifenesin Capsules USP—Preserve in tight containers. Contain the labeled amount, within ±10%. Meet the requirements for Identification, Dissolution (75% in 45 minutes in water in Apparatus 1 at 100 rpm), and Uniformity of dosage units.
Guaifenesin Extended-release Capsules—Not in USP.
Guaifenesin Oral Solution—Not in USP.
Guaifenesin Syrup USP—Preserve in tight containers. Contains the labeled amount, within ±5%. Meets the requirements for Identification, pH (2.3–3.0), and Alcohol content (if present, 90.0–115.0% of labeled amount).

Guaifenesin Tablets USP—Preserve in tight containers. Contain the labeled amount, within ±10%. Meet the requirements for Identification, Dissolution (75% in 45 minutes in water in Apparatus 2 at 50 rpm), and Uniformity of dosage units.

Guaifenesin Extended-release Tablets—Not in USP.

GUAIFENESIN AND CODEINE

For *Guaifenesin* and *Codeine*—See individual listings for chemistry information.

USP requirements:

Guaifenesin and Codeine Phosphate Oral Solution—Not in USP.

Guaifenesin and Codeine Phosphate Syrup USP—Preserve in tight, light-resistant containers, at controlled room temperature. Contains the labeled amounts, within ±10%. Meets the requirements for Identification, pH (2.3–3.0), and Alcohol content (3.5–4.4%).

GUANABENZ

Chemical name: Guanabenz acetate—Hydrazinecarboximidamide, 2-[(2,6-dichlorophenyl)methylene]-, monoacetate.

Molecular formula: Guanabenz acetate—$C_8H_8Cl_2N_4 \cdot C_2H_4O_2$.

Molecular weight: Guanabenz acetate—291.14.

Description: Guanabenz Acetate USP—White or almost white powder having not more than a slight odor.

Solubility: Guanabenz Acetate USP—Sparingly soluble in water and in 0.1 N hydrochloric acid; soluble in alcohol and in propylene glycol.

USP requirements: Guanabenz Acetate Tablets USP—Preserve in tight, light-resistant containers. Contain an amount of guanabenz acetate equivalent to the labeled amount of guanabenz, within ±10%. Meet the requirements for Identification, Dissolution (75% in 60 minutes in water in Apparatus 2 at 50 rpm), Uniformity of dosage units, and Chromatographic purity.

GUANADREL

Chemical name: Guanadrel sulfate—Guanidine (1,4-dioxaspiro[4.5]dec-2-ylmethyl)-, sulfate (2:1).

Molecular formula: Guanadrel sulfate—$(C_{10}H_{19}N_3O_2)_2 \cdot H_2SO_4$.

Molecular weight: Guanadrel sulfate—524.63.

Description: Guanadrel Sulfate USP—White to off-white, crystalline powder. Melts at about 235 °C, with decomposition.

Solubility: Guanadrel Sulfate USP—Soluble in water; sparingly soluble in methanol; slightly soluble in alcohol and in acetone.

USP requirements: Guanadrel Sulfate Tablets USP—Preserve in tight, light-resistant containers. Contain the labeled amount, within ±10%. Meet the requirements for Identification, Dissolution (70% in 20 minutes in Working buffer solution in Apparatus 2 at 50 rpm), and Uniformity of dosage units.

GUANETHIDINE

Chemical name:

Guanethidine monosulfate—Guanidine, [2-(hexahydro-1(2*H*)-azocinyl)ethyl]-, sulfate (1:1).

Guanethidine sulfate—Guanidine, [2-(hexahydro-1(2*H*)-azocinyl)ethyl]-, sulfate (2:1).

Molecular formula:

Guanethidine monosulfate—$C_{10}H_{22}N_4 \cdot H_2SO_4$.

Guanethidine sulfate—$(C_{10}H_{22}N_4)_2 \cdot H_2SO_4$.

Molecular weight:

Guanethidine monosulfate—296.38.

Guanethidine sulfate—494.69.

Description: Guanethidine Monosulfate USP—White to off-white, crystalline powder.

pKa: 9.0 and 12.0.

Solubility: Guanethidine Monosulfate USP—Very soluble in water; sparingly soluble in alcohol; practically insoluble in chloroform.

USP requirements: Guanethidine Monosulfate Tablets USP—Preserve in well-closed containers. Contain an amount of guanethidine monosulfate equivalent to the labeled amount of guanethidine sulfate, within ±10%. Meet the requirements for Identification, Dissolution (75% in 45 minutes in water in Apparatus 1 at 100 rpm), and Uniformity of dosage units.

GUANETHIDINE AND HYDROCHLOROTHIAZIDE

For *Guanethidine* and *Hydrochlorothiazide*—See individual listings for chemistry information.

USP requirements: Guanethidine Monosulfate and Hydrochlorothiazide Tablets—Not in USP.

GUANFACINE

Chemical name: Guanfacine hydrochloride—Benzeneacetamide, *N*-(aminoiminomethyl)-2,6-dichloro-, monohydrochloride.

Molecular formula: Guanfacine hydrochloride—$C_9H_9Cl_2N_3O \cdot HCl$.

Molecular weight: Guanfacine hydrochloride—282.56.

Description: Guanfacine hydrochloride—White to off-white powder.

Solubility: Guanfacine hydrochloride—Sparingly soluble in water and in alcohol; slightly soluble in acetone.

USP requirements: Guanfacine Hydrochloride Tablets—Not in USP.

GUAR GUM

Description: Guar Gum NF—White to yellowish white, practically odorless powder.

NF category: Suspending and/or viscosity-increasing agent; tablet binder.

Solubility: Guar Gum NF—Dispersible in hot or cold water, forming a colloidal solution.

NF requirements: Guar Gum NF—Preserve in well-closed containers. A gum obtained from the ground endosperms of *Cyamopsis tetragonolobus* (Linné) Taub. (Fam. Leguminosae). Consists chiefly of a high molecular weight hydrocolloidal polysaccharide composed of galactan and mannan units combined through glycosidic linkages, which may be described chemically as a galactomannan. Meets the requirements for Identification, Loss on drying (not more than 15.0%), Ash (not more than 1.5%), Acid-insoluble matter (not more than 7.0%), Arsenic (not more than 3 ppm), Lead (not more than 0.001%), Heavy metals (not more than

0.002%), Protein (not more than 10.0%), Starch, and Galactomannans (not less than 66.0%).

GUTTA PERCHA

Source: *Trans* isomer of rubber prepared from the exudate of various trees of the genus *Palaquium*, Fam. *Sapotaceae*.

Description: Gutta Percha USP—Lumps or blocks of variable size; externally brown or grayish brown to grayish white in color; internally reddish yellow or reddish gray and having a laminated or fibrous appearance. Is flexible but only slightly elastic. Has a slight, characteristic odor.

Solubility: Gutta Percha USP—Insoluble in water; about 90% soluble in chloroform; partly soluble in carbon disulfide and in turpentine oil.

USP requirements: Gutta Percha USP—Preserve under water in well-closed containers, protected from light. It is the coagulated, dried, purified latex of the trees of the genera *Palaquium* and *Payena* and most commonly *Palaquium gutta* (Hooker) Baillon (Fam. Sapotaceae). Meets the requirement for Residue on ignition (not more than 1.7%).

HAEMOPHILUS B CONJUGATE VACCINE

Source: Purified capsular polysaccharide, a polymer of ribose, ribitol, and phosphate (PRP), from the bacterium *Haemophilus influenzae* type b (Hib), strain Eagen. The polysaccharide has been conjugated to the diphtheria toxoid via a linker 6-carbon molecule, the oligosaccharide has been derived from the polysaccharide and has been bound directly to CRM_{197} (a nontoxic variant of diphtheria toxin) by reductive amination, or the polysaccharide has been covalently bound to an outer membrane protein complex (OMPC) of the B11 strain of *Neisseria meningitidis* serogroup B. Hib is an encapsulated gram-negative coccobacillus that is the most common cause of bacterial meningitis and a leading cause of serious, systemic bacterial disease in young children in the U.S.

Description: The conjugate vaccine is a clear, colorless solution.

USP requirements: Haemophilus b Conjugate Vaccine Injection—Not in USP.

HAEMOPHILUS B POLYSACCHARIDE VACCINE

Source: Purified capsular polysaccharide, a polymer of ribose, ribitol, and phosphate (PRP), from the bacterium *Haemophilus influenzae* type b (Hib). Hib is an encapsulated gram-negative coccobacillus that is the most common cause of bacterial meningitis and a leading cause of serious, systemic bacterial disease in young children in the U.S.

Description: When reconstituted, the polysaccharide vaccine is a clear, colorless liquid.

Other characteristics: The pH is 6.6 to 7.1.

USP requirements: Haemophilus b Polysaccharide Vaccine for Injection—Not in USP.

HALAZEPAM

Chemical name: 2*H*-1,4-Benzodiazepin-2-one, 7-chloro-1,3-dihydro-5-phenyl-1-(2,2,2-trifluoroethyl)-.

Molecular formula: $C_{17}H_{12}ClF_3N_2O$.

Molecular weight: 352.74.

Description: Halazepam USP—Fine, white to light cream-colored powder. Melts at about 165 °C.

Solubility: Halazepam USP—Freely soluble in chloroform; soluble in methanol; very slightly soluble in water.

USP requirements: Halazepam Tablets USP—Preserve in well-closed containers. Contain the labeled amount, within ± 10%. Meet the requirements for Identification, Dissolution (75% in 30 minutes in 0.1 *N* hydrochloric acid in Apparatus 1 at 100 rpm), and Uniformity of dosage units.

HALAZONE

Chemical name: Benzoic acid, 4-[(dichloroamino)sulfonyl]-.

Molecular formula: $C_7H_5Cl_2NO_4S$.

Molecular weight: 270.09.

Description: Halazone USP—White, crystalline powder, having a characteristic chlorine-like odor. Affected by light. Melts at about 194 °C, with decomposition.

Solubility:
Halazone USP—Very slightly soluble in water and in chloroform; soluble in glacial acetic acid. Dissolves in solutions of alkali hydroxides and carbonates with the formation of a salt.
Halazone Tablets for Solution USP—Soluble in water.

USP requirements: Halazone Tablets for Solution USP—Preserve in tight, light-resistant containers. Label Tablets to indicate that they are not intended to be swallowed. Contain the labeled amount, within −10% to +35%. Meet the requirements for Identification, Disintegration (10 minutes), Uniformity of dosage units, and pH (not less than 7.0, in a solution of 1 Tablet, containing 4 mg of halazone, in 200 mL of water).

HALCINONIDE

Chemical name: Pregn-4-ene-3,20-dione, 21-chloro-9-fluoro-11-hydroxy-16,17-[(1-methylethylidene)bis(oxy)]-, (11 beta, 16 alpha)-.

Molecular formula: $C_{24}H_{32}ClFO_5$.

Molecular weight: 454.97.

Description: Halcinonide USP—White to off-white, odorless, crystalline powder.

Solubility: Halcinonide USP—Soluble in acetone and in chloroform; slightly soluble in alcohol and in ethyl ether; insoluble in water and in hexanes.

USP requirements:
Halcinonide Cream USP—Preserve in well-closed containers. It is Halcinonide in a suitable cream base. Contains the labeled amount, within ± 10%. Meets the requirements for Identification, Microbial limits, and Minimum fill.
Halcinonide Ointment USP—Preserve in well-closed containers. It is Halcinonide in a suitable ointment base. Contains the labeled amount, within ± 10%. Meets the requirements for Identification, Microbial limits, and Minimum fill.
Halcinonide Topical Solution USP—Preserve in well-closed containers. It is Halcinonide in a suitable aqueous vehicle. Contains the labeled amount, within ± 10%. Meets the requirements for Identification and Microbial limits.

HALOPERIDOL

Chemical group: A butyrophenone derivative.

Chemical name:
Haloperidol—1-Butanone, 4-[4-(4-chlorophenyl)-4-hydroxy-1-piperidinyl]-1-(4-fluorophenyl)-.
Haloperidol decanoate—Decanoic acid, 4-(4-chlorophenyl)-1-[4-(4-fluorophenyl)-4-oxobutyl]-4-piperidinyl ester.

Molecular formula:
Haloperidol—$C_{21}H_{23}ClFNO_2$.
Haloperidol decanoate—$C_{31}H_{41}ClFNO_3$.

Molecular weight:
Haloperidol—375.87.
Haloperidol decanoate—530.12.

Description: Haloperidol USP—White to faintly yellowish, amorphous or microcrystalline powder. Its saturated solution is neutral to litmus.

Solubility:
Haloperidol USP—Practically insoluble in water; soluble in chloroform; sparingly soluble in alcohol; slightly soluble in ether.
Haloperidol decanoate—Practically insoluble in water; soluble in most organic solvents.

USP requirements:
Haloperidol Injection USP—Preserve in single-dose or in multiple-dose containers, preferably of Type I glass, protected from light. A sterile solution of Haloperidol in Water for Injection, prepared with the aid of Lactic Acid. Contains the labeled amount, within ±10%. Meets the requirements for Identification, Bacterial endotoxins, pH (3.0–3.8), and Injections.
Haloperidol Oral Solution USP—Preserve in tight, light-resistant containers. A solution of Haloperidol in Water, prepared with the aid of Lactic Acid. Contains the labeled amount, within ±10%. Meets the requirements for Identification and pH (2.75–3.75).
Haloperidol Tablets USP—Preserve in tight, light-resistant containers. Contain the labeled amount, within ±10%. Meet the requirements for Identification, Dissolution (80% in 60 minutes in simulated gastric fluid TS, without the enzyme, in Apparatus 1 at 100 rpm), and Uniformity of dosage units.
Haloperidol Decanoate Injection—Not in USP.

HALOPROGIN

Chemical name: Benzene, 1,2,4-trichloro-5-[(3-iodo-2-propynyl)oxy]-.

Molecular formula: $C_9H_4Cl_3IO$.

Molecular weight: 361.39.

Description: White or pale yellow crystals. Melting point is about 113–114 °C.

Solubility: Very slightly soluble in water; easily soluble in methanol and in ethanol.

USP requirements:
Haloprogin Cream USP—Preserve in tight, light-resistant containers, at controlled room temperature. Contains the labeled amount, within ±10%. Meets the requirements for Identification, Microbial limits, Minimum fill, and Water (not more than 3.0%).
Haloprogin Topical Solution USP—Preserve in tight, light-resistant containers, at controlled room temperature. Contains the labeled amount, within ±10%. Meets the requirements for Identification, Specific gravity (0.838–0.852), and Alcohol (the labeled amount, within ±5%).

HALOTHANE

Chemical name: Ethane, 2-bromo-2-chloro-1,1,1-trifluoro-.

Molecular formula: $C_2HBrClF_3$.

Molecular weight: 197.38.

Description: Halothane USP—Colorless, mobile, nonflammable, heavy liquid, having a characteristic odor resembling that of chloroform.

Solubility: Halothane USP—Slightly soluble in water; miscible with alcohol, with chloroform, with ether, and with fixed oils.

Other characteristics:
Blood-to-Gas partition coefficient—2.5 at 37 °C.
Olive oil-to-water partition coefficient—220 at 37 °C.

USP requirements: Halothane USP—Preserve in tight, light-resistant containers, preferably of Type NP glass, and avoid exposure to excessive heat. Dispense it only in the original container. Contains 0.008% to 0.012% of thymol, by weight, as a stabilizer. Meets the requirements for Identification, Specific gravity (1.872–1.877 at 20 °C), Distilling range (not less than 95% within a 1° range between 49 and 51 °C; not less than 100% between 49 and 51 °C, a correction factor of 0.040 °C per mm being applied as necessary), Refractive index (1.369–1.371 at 20 °C), Acidity or alkalinity, Water (not more than 0.03%), Nonvolatile residue (not more than 1 mg per 50 mL), Chloride and bromide, Thymol content, and Chromatographic purity.

HELIUM

Chemical name: Helium.

Molecular formula: He.

Molecular weight: 4.00.

Description: Helium USP—Colorless, odorless gas, which is not combustible and does not support combustion. At 0 °C and at a pressure of 760 mm of mercury, 1000 mL of the gas weighs about 180 mg.

Solubility: Helium USP—Very slightly soluble in water.

USP requirements: Helium USP—Preserve in cylinders. Contains not less than 99.0%, by volume, of helium. Meets the requirements for Identification, Odor, Carbon monoxide (not more than 0.001%), and Air (not more than 1.0%).

HEPARIN

Source:
Heparin is present in mammalian tissues and is usually obtained from the intestinal mucosa or other suitable tissues of domestic mammals used for food by man.
Heparin calcium is the calcium salt, and heparin sodium is the sodium salt, of a sulfated glycosaminoglycan of mixed mucopolysaccharides varying in molecular weights. Heparin is composed of polymers of alternating derivatives of D-glycosamine (N-sulfated or N-acetylated) and uronic acid (L-iduronic acid or D-glucuronic acid) joined by glycosidic linkages, the components being liberated in varying proportions on complete hydrolysis. It is a mixture of active principles.

Description:
Heparin calcium—White or almost white, moderately hygroscopic powder.
Heparin Sodium USP—White or pale-colored, amorphous powder. Is odorless or practically so, and is hygroscopic.

Solubility:

Heparin calcium—Soluble 1 in less than 5 of water.
Heparin Sodium USP—Soluble in water.

Other characteristics: Highly acidic.

USP requirements:

Heparin Lock Flush Solution USP—Preserve in single-dose pre-filled syringes or containers, or in multiple-dose containers, preferably of Type I glass. A sterile preparation of Heparin Sodium Injection with sufficient Sodium Chloride to make it isotonic with blood. Label it to indicate the volume of the total contents, and to indicate the potency in terms of USP Heparin Units only per mL, except that single unit-dose containers may be labeled additionally to indicate the single unit-dose volume and the total number of USP Heparin Units in the contents. Where it is labeled with total content, the label states clearly that the entire contents are to be used or, if not, any remaining portion is to be discarded. Label it to indicate the organ and species from which the heparin sodium is derived. The label states also that the Solution is intended for maintenance of patency of intravenous injection devices only, and that it is not to be used for anticoagulant therapy. The label states also that in the case of Solution having a concentration of 10 USP Heparin Units per mL, it may alter, and that in the case of higher concentrations it will alter, the results of blood coagulation tests. Exhibits the labeled potency, within −10% to +20%, stated in terms of USP Heparin Units. Contains not more than 1.00% of sodium chloride. Meets the requirements for pH (5.0–7.5), Particulate matter, Pyrogen test, and Injections.

Heparin Calcium Injection USP—Preserve in single-dose or in multiple-dose containers, preferably of Type I glass. A sterile solution of Heparin Calcium in Water for Injection. Label it to indicate the volume of the total contents and the potency in terms of USP Heparin Units only per mL, except that single unit-dose containers may be labeled additionally to indicate the single unit-dose volume and the total number of USP Heparin Units in the contents. Where it is labeled with total content, the label states also that the entire contents are to be used or, if not, any remaining portion is to be discarded. Label it to indicate also the organ and species from which it is derived. Exhibits the labeled potency, within ±10%, stated in terms of USP Heparin Units. Meets the requirements for Pyrogen, pH (5.0–7.5), Particulate matter, Injections, and Anti-factor X_a activity.

Note: USP Heparin Units are consistently established on the basis of the Assay set forth in *USP*, independently of International Units, and the respective units are not equivalent. The USP Units for Anti-factor X_a activity are defined by the USP Heparin Sodium Reference Standard.

Heparin Sodium Injection USP—Preserve in single-dose or in multiple-dose containers, preferably of Type I glass. A sterile solution of Heparin Sodium in Water for Injection. Label it to indicate the volume of the total contents and the potency in terms of USP Heparin Units only per mL, except that single unit-dose containers may be labeled additionally to indicate the single unit-dose volume and the total number of USP Heparin Units in the contents. Where it is labeled with total content, the label states also that the entire contents are to be used or, if not, any remaining portion is to be discarded. Label it to indicate also the organ and species from which it is derived. Exhibits the labeled potency, within ±10%, stated in terms of USP Heparin Units. Meets the requirements for Pyrogen, pH (5.0–7.5), Particulate matter, Anti-factor X_a activity, and Injections.

Note: USP Heparin Units are consistently established on the basis of the Assay set forth in *USP*, independently of International Units, and the respective units are not equivalent. The USP Units for Anti-factor X_a activity are defined by the USP Heparin Sodium Reference Standard.

HEPARIN AND DEXTROSE

For *Heparin* and *Dextrose*—See individual listings for chemistry information.

USP requirements: Heparin Sodium in Dextrose Injection—Not in USP.

HEPARIN AND SODIUM CHLORIDE

For *Heparin* and *Sodium Chloride*—See individual listings for chemistry information.

USP requirements: Heparin Sodium in Sodium Chloride Injection—Not in USP.

HEPATITIS B IMMUNE GLOBULIN

USP requirements: Hepatitis B Immune Globulin USP—Preserve at a temperature between 2 and 8 °C. A sterile, non-pyrogenic solution free from turbidity, consisting of globulins derived from the blood plasma of human donors who have high titers of antibodies against hepatitis B surface antigen. Label it to state that it is not for intravenous injection. Contains not less than 10.0 grams and not more than 18.0 grams of protein per 100 mL, of which not less than 80% is monomeric immunoglobulin G, having no ultracentrifugally detectable fragments, nor aggregates having a sedimentation coefficient greater than 12S. Contains 0.3 *M* glycine as a stabilizing agent, and contains a suitable preservative. Has a potency per mL not less than that of the U.S. Reference Hepatitis B Immune Globulin tested by an approved radioimmunoassay for the detection and measurement of antibody to hepatitis B surface antigen. Has a pH between 6.4 and 7.2, measured in a solution diluted to contain 1% of protein with 0.15 *M* sodium chloride. Meets the requirements of the test for heat stability and for Expiration date (not later than 1 year after the date of manufacture, such date being that of the first valid potency test of the product). Conforms to the regulations of the U.S. Food and Drug Administration concerning biologics.

HEPATITIS B VACCINE RECOMBINANT

Source:

A non-infectious subunit viral vaccine derived from hepatitis B surface antigen (HBsAg) produced in yeast cells. A portion of the hepatitis B virus gene, coding for HBsAg, is cloned into yeast, and the vaccine for hepatitis B is produced from cultures of this recombinant yeast strain according to methods developed in the Merck Sharp and Dohme Research Laboratories.

The antigen is harvested and purified from fermentation cultures of a recombinant strain of the teast *Saccharomyces cerevisiae* containing the gene for the *adw* subtype of HBsAg.

USP requirements: Hepatitis B Vaccine Recombinant Sterile Suspension—Not in USP.

HEPATITIS B VIRUS VACCINE INACTIVATED

USP requirements: Hepatitis B Virus Vaccine Inactivated USP—Preserve at a temperature between 2 and 8 °C. A sterile preparation consisting of a suspension of particles of Hepatitis B surface antigen (HBsAg) isolated from the plasma of HBsAg carriers; treated with pepsin at pH 2, 8 *M* urea, and 1:4000 formalin so as to inactivate any hepatitis B virus and any representative viruses from all known virus groups that may be present; purified by ultracentrifugation and biochemical procedures and standardized to a concentration of 35 mcg to 55 mcg of Lowry (HBsAg) protein per mL. The preparation is adsorbed on aluminum hydroxide and diluted to a concentration of 20 mcg Lowry protein per mL or other appropriate concentration, depending on the intended use. Label it to state the content of HBsAg protein per recommended dose. Label it also to state that it is to be shaken before use and that it is not to be frozen. Contains not more than 0.62 mg of aluminum per mL and not more than 0.02% of residual free formaldehyde. Contains thimerosal as a preservative. Meets the requirements for potency in animal tests using mice and by a quantitative parallel line radioimmunoassay, of tests for pyrogen, for general safety, and for Expiration date (not later than 3 years from the date of manufacture, the date of manufacture being the date on which the last valid potency test was initiated).

HETACILLIN

Chemical name:
Hetacillin—4-Thia-1-azabicyclo[3.2.0]heptane-2-carboxylic acid, 6-(2,2-dimethyl-5-oxo-4-phenyl-1-imidazolidinyl)-3,3-dimethyl-7-oxo-, [2*S*-[2 alpha,5 alpha,6 beta(*S**)]]-.
Hetacillin potassium—4-Thia-1-azabicyclo[3.2.0]heptane-2-carboxylic acid, 6-(2,2-dimethyl-5-oxo-4-phenyl-1-imidazolidinyl)-3,3-dimethyl-7-oxo-, monopotassium salt, [2*S*-[2 alpha,5 alpha,6 beta(*S**)]]-.

Molecular formula:
Hetacillin—$C_{19}H_{23}N_3O_4S$.
Hetacillin potassium—$C_{19}H_{22}KN_3O_4S$.

Molecular weight:
Hetacillin—389.47.
Hetacillin potassium—427.56.

Description:
Hetacillin USP—White to off-white, crystalline powder.
Hetacillin Potassium USP—White to light buff, crystalline powder.

Solubility:
Hetacillin USP—Practically insoluble in water and in most organic solvents; soluble in dilute sodium hydroxide solution and in methanol.
Hetacillin Potassium USP—Freely soluble in water; soluble in alcohol.

USP requirements:
Hetacillin for Oral Suspension USP—Preserve in tight containers. Contains an amount of hetacillin equivalent to the labeled amount of ampicillin, within −10% to +20%. Contains one or more suitable colors, flavors, preservatives, sweeteners, and suspending agents. Meets the requirements for Identification, pH (2.0–5.0, in the suspension constituted as directed in the labeling), Water (not more than 2.0%), Deliverable volume, and Uniformity of dosage units (for solid packaged in single-unit containers).
Hetacillin Tablets USP—Preserve in tight containers. Label Tablets to indicate that they are to be chewed before swallowing. Contain an amount of hetacillin equivalent to the labeled amount of ampicillin, within −10% to +20%. Meet the requirements for Identification, Dissolution (75% in 45 minutes in 0.05 *M* phosphate buffer [pH 7.6] in Apparatus 2 at 50 rpm), Uniformity of dosage units, and Water (not more than 2.0%).

Hetacillin Potassium Capsules USP—Preserve in tight containers. Contain an amount of hetacillin potassium equivalent to the labeled amount of ampicillin, within −10% to +20%. Meet the requirements for Identification, Dissolution (75% in 45 minutes in water in Apparatus 1 at 100 rpm), Uniformity of dosage units, and Water (not more than 3.0%).
Hetacillin Potassium Intramammary Infusion USP—Preserve in suitable, well-closed, disposable syringes. A suspension of Hetacillin Potassium in a Peanut Oil vehicle with a suitable dispersing agent. Label it to indicate that it is for veterinary use only. Contains an amount of hetacillin potassium equivalent to the labeled amount of ampicillin, within −10% to +20%. Meets the requirements for Identification and Water (not more than 1.0%).
Sterile Hetacillin Potassium USP—Preserve in Containers for Sterile Solids. It is Hetacillin Potassium suitable for parenteral use. Contains an amount of hetacillin potassium equivalent to the labeled amount of ampicillin, within −10% to +20%. Meets the requirements for Bacterial endotoxins, Sterility, pH (7.0–9.0, in the solution constituted as directed in the labeling), for Identification tests, pH, Water, Crystallinity, and Hetacillin content under Hetacillin Potassium, and for Uniformity of dosage units and Labeling under Injections.
Hetacillin Potassium Oral Suspension USP—Preserve in tight containers. It is Hetacillin Potassium suspended in a suitable nonaqueous vehicle. Label it to indicate that it is for veterinary use only. Contains an amount of hetacillin potassium equivalent to the labeled amount of ampicillin, within −10% to +20%. Contains one or more suitable colors, flavors, and gelling agents. Meets the requirements for Identification, Deliverable volume, Uniformity of dosage units (for suspension packaged in single-unit containers), pH (7.0–9.0), and Water (not more than 1.0%).
Hetacillin Potassium Tablets USP—Preserve in tight containers. Label Tablets to indicate that they are for veterinary use only. Contain an amount of hetacillin potassium equivalent to the labeled amount of ampicillin, within −10% to +20%. Meet the requirements for Identification, Disintegration (30 minutes), and Water (not more than 5.0%).

HEXACHLOROPHENE

Chemical name: Phenol, 2,2′-methylenebis[3,4,6-trichloro-.

Molecular formula: $C_{13}H_6Cl_6O_2$.

Molecular weight: 406.91.

Description:
Hexachlorophene USP—White to light tan, crystalline powder. Odorless, or has only a slight, phenolic odor.
Hexachlorophene Liquid Soap USP—Clear, amber-colored liquid, having a slight, characteristic odor. Its solution (1 in 20) is clear and has an alkaline reaction.

Solubility: Hexachlorophene USP—Insoluble in water; freely soluble in acetone, in alcohol, and in ether; soluble in chloroform and in dilute solutions of fixed alkali hydroxides.

USP requirements:
Hexachlorophene Cleansing Emulsion USP—Preserve in tight, light-resistant, non-metallic containers. It is Hexachlorophene in a suitable aqueous vehicle. Contains the labeled amount, within ±10%. Contains no coloring agents. Meets the requirements for Identification, Microbial limits, and pH (5.0–6.0).
Hexachlorophene Liquid Soap USP—Preserve in tight, light-resistant containers. A solution of Hexachlorophene in a

10.0 to 13.0% solution of a potassium soap. Solutions of higher concentrations of hexachlorophene and potassium soap, in which the ratios of these components are consistent with the official limits, may be labeled "For the preparation of Hexachlorophene Liquid Soap, USP," provided that the label indicates also that the soap is a concentrate, and provided that directions are given for dilution to the official strength. Contains, in each 100 grams, not less than 225 mg and not more than 260 mg of hexachlorophene. Meets the requirements for Identification, Microbial limits, Water (86.5–90.0% by weight of the portion of Soap taken), Alcohol-insoluble substances (not more than 3.0%), Free alkali hydroxides (not more than 0.05% of potassium hydroxide), and Alkali carbonates (not more than 0.35% of potassium carbonate).

Note: The inclusion of non-ionic detergents in Hexachlorophene Liquid Soap in amounts greater than 8% on a total weight basis may decrease the bacteriostatic activity of the Soap.

HEXYLCAINE

Chemical name: Hexylcaine hydrochloride—2-Propanol, 1-(cyclohexylamino)-, benzoate (ester), hydrochloride.

Molecular formula: Hexylcaine hydrochloride—$C_{16}H_{23}NO_2 \cdot$ HCl.

Molecular weight: Hexylcaine hydrochloride—297.82.

Description:
Hexylcaine Hydrochloride USP—White powder, having not more than a slight, aromatic odor.
Hexylcaine Hydrochloride Topical Solution USP—Clear, colorless solution of Hexylcaine Hydrochloride in water.

Solubility: Hexylcaine Hydrochloride USP—Soluble in water; freely soluble in alcohol and in chloroform; practically insoluble in ether.

USP requirements: Hexylcaine Hydrochloride Topical Solution USP—Preserve in tight containers. Contains the labeled amount, within ±7%. Meets the requirements for Identification and pH (3.0–5.0).

HEXYLENE GLYCOL

Chemical name: 2,4-Pentanediol, 2-methyl-.

Molecular formula: $C_6H_{14}O_2$.

Molecular weight: 118.17.

Description: Hexylene Glycol NF—Clear, colorless, viscous liquid. Absorbs moisture when exposed to moist air.
NF category: Humectant; solvent.

Solubility: Hexylene Glycol NF—Miscible with water and with many organic solvents, including alcohol, ether, chloroform, acetone, and hexanes.

NF requirements: Hexylene Glycol NF—Preserve in tight containers. Hexylene Glycol is 2-methyl-2,4-pentanediol. Meets the requirements for Identification, Specific gravity (0.917–0.923), Refractive index (1.424–1.430), Acidity, and Water (not more than 0.5%).

HEXYLRESORCINOL

Chemical name: 1,3-Benzenediol, 4-hexyl-.

Molecular formula: $C_{12}H_{18}O_2$.

Molecular weight: 194.27

Description: White or yellowish-white, acicular crystals, crystalline plates, or crystalline powder with a pungent odor. Acquires a brownish-pink tint on exposure to light and air. Melting point 62–68 °C.

Solubility: Soluble 1 in 2000 of water; freely soluble in alcohol, in chloroform, in ether, in glycerol, in methyl alcohol, and in fixed oils; very slightly soluble in petroleum spirit.

USP requirements: Hexylresorcinol Lozenges USP—Preserve in well-closed containers. Contain the labeled amount, within ±10%. Meet the requirements for Identification and Uniformity of dosage units.

HISTAMINE

Chemical group: Low molecular weight–amine.

Chemical name: Histamine phosphate—1*H*-Imidazole-4-ethanamine, phosphate (1:2).

Molecular formula: Histamine phosphate—$C_5H_9N_3 \cdot 2H_3PO_4$.

Molecular weight: Histamine phosphate—307.14.

Description: Histamine Phosphate USP—Colorless, odorless, long prismatic crystals. Is stable in air but is affected by light. Its solutions are acid to litmus.

Solubility: Histamine Phosphate USP—Freely soluble in water.

USP requirements: Histamine Phosphate Injection USP—Preserve in single-dose or in multiple-dose containers, preferably of Type I glass, protected from light. A sterile solution of Histamine Phosphate in Water for Injection. Contains the labeled amount, within ±10%. Meets the requirements for Identification, Bacterial endotoxins, pH (3.0–6.0), and Injections.

HISTOPLASMIN

Description: Histoplasmin USP—Clear, red liquid.

Solubility: Histoplasmin USP—Miscible with water.

USP requirements: Histoplasmin USP—Preserve at a temperature between 2 and 8 °C. A clear, colorless, sterile solution containing standardized culture filtrates of *Histoplasma capsulatum* grown on liquid synthetic medium. Label it to state that only the diluent supplied is to be used for making dilutions, and that it is not to be injected other than intradermally. Label it also to state that a separate syringe and needle shall be used for each individual injection. It has a potency of the 1:100 dilution equivalent to and determined in terms of the Histoplasmin Reference diluted 1:100 tested in guinea pigs. Meets the requirement for Expiration date (not later than 2 years after date of issue from manufacturer's cold storage [5 °C, 1 year]). Conforms to the regulations of the U.S. Food and Drug Administration concerning biologics.

HOMATROPINE

Source: A semisynthetic tertiary amine derivative of mandelic acid and tropine. Homatropine methylbromide and methscopolamine bromide are quaternary ammonium derivatives of homatropine and scopolamine, respectively.

Chemical group: Quaternary ammonium compound, semisynthetic.

Chemical name:
Homatropine hydrobromide—Benzeneacetic acid, alpha-hydroxy-, 8-methyl-8-azabicyclo[3.2.1]oct-3-yl ester, hydrobromide, *endo*-(±)-.

Homatropine methylbromide—8-Azoniabicyclo[3.2.1]octane, 3-[(hydroxyphenylacetyl)oxy]-8,8-dimethyl-, bromide, *endo-*.

Molecular formula:
Homatropine hydrobromide—$C_{16}H_{21}NO_3 \cdot HBr$.
Homatropine methylbromide—$C_{17}H_{24}BrNO_3$.

Molecular weight:
Homatropine hydrobromide—356.26.
Homatropine methylbromide—370.29.

Description:
Homatropine Hydrobromide USP—White crystals, or white, crystalline powder. Is affected by light.
Homatropine Methylbromide USP—White, odorless powder. Slowly darkens on exposure to light. Melts at about 190 °C.

Solubility:
Homatropine Hydrobromide USP—Freely soluble in water; sparingly soluble in alcohol; slightly soluble in chloroform; insoluble in ether.
Homatropine Methylbromide USP—Very soluble in water; freely soluble in alcohol and in acetone containing about 20% of water; practically insoluble in ether and in acetone.

USP requirements:
Homatropine Hydrobromide Ophthalmic Solution USP—Preserve in tight containers. A sterile, buffered, aqueous solution of Homatropine Hydrobromide. Contains the labeled amount, within ± 5%. Meets the requirements for Identification, Sterility, and pH (2.5–5.0).
Homatropine Methylbromide Tablets USP—Preserve in tight, light-resistant containers. Contain the labeled amount, within ± 10%. Meet the requirements for Identification, Dissolution (75% in 45 minutes in water in Apparatus 2 at 50 rpm), and Uniformity of dosage units.

HYALURONIDASE

Description: White or yellowish-white powder.

Solubility: Very soluble in water; practically insoluble in alcohol, in acetone, and in ether.

USP requirements:
Hyaluronidase Injection USP—Preserve in single-dose or in multiple-dose containers, preferably of Type I glass, in a refrigerator. A sterile solution of dry, soluble enzyme product, prepared from mammalian testes and capable of hydrolyzing mucopolysaccharides of the type of hyaluronic acid, in Water for Injection. Contains the labeled amount of USP Hyaluronidase Units, within − 10%. Contains not more than 0.25 mcg of tyrosine for each USP Hyaluronidase Unit. Meets the requirements for Tyrosine (not more than 0.25 mcg for each USP Hyaluronidase Unit), Bacterial endotoxins, pH (6.4–7.4), and Injections.
Hyaluronidase for Injection USP—Preserve in Containers for Sterile Solids, preferably of Type I or Type III glass, at controlled room temperature. A sterile, dry, soluble, enzyme product prepared from mammalian testes and capable of hydrolyzing mucopolysaccharides of the type of hyaluronic acid. Its potency, in USP Hyaluronidase Units, is not less than the labeled potency. Contains not more than 0.25 mcg of tyrosine for each USP Hyaluronidase Unit. Meets the requirements for Tyrosine (not more than 0.25 mcg for each USP Hyaluronidase Unit), Bacterial endotoxins, and Sterility.

HYDRALAZINE

Chemical name: Hydralazine hydrochloride—Phthalazine, 1-hydrazino-, monohydrochloride.

Molecular formula: Hydralazine hydrochloride—$C_8H_8N_4 \cdot HCl$.

Molecular weight: Hydralazine hydrochloride—196.64.

Description: Hydralazine Hydrochloride USP—White to off-white, odorless, crystalline powder. Melts at about 275 °C, with decomposition.

pKa: 7.3.

Solubility: Hydralazine Hydrochloride USP—Soluble in water; slightly soluble in alcohol; very slightly soluble in ether.

USP requirements:
Hydralazine Hydrochloride Injection USP—Preserve in single-dose or in multiple-dose containers, preferably of Type I glass. A sterile solution of Hydralazine Hydrochloride in Water for Injection. Contains the labeled amount, within ± 5%. Meets the requirements for Identification, Bacterial endotoxins, pH (3.4–4.4), Particulate matter, and Injections.
Hydralazine Hydrochloride Tablets USP—Preserve in tight, light-resistant containers. Contain the labeled amount, within ± 10%. Meet the requirements for Identification, Dissolution (60% in 30 minutes in 0.1 N hydrochloric acid in Apparatus 1 at 100 rpm), and Uniformity of dosage units.

HYDRALAZINE AND HYDROCHLOROTHIAZIDE

For *Hydralazine* and *Hydrochlorothiazide*—See individual listings for chemistry information.

USP requirements:
Hydralazine Hydrochloride and Hydrochlorothiazide Capsules—Not in USP.
Hydralazine Hydrochloride and Hydrochlorothiazide Tablets—Not in USP.

HYDROCHLORIC ACID

Chemical name: Hydrochloric acid.

Molecular formula: HCl.

Molecular weight: 36.46.

Description: Hydrochloric Acid NF—Colorless, fuming liquid, having a pungent odor. It ceases to fume when it is diluted with 2 volumes of water. Specific gravity is about 1.18.
NF category: Acidifying agent.

NF requirements: Hydrochloric Acid NF—Preserve in tight containers. Contains not less than 36.5% and not more than 38.0%, by weight, of hydrochloric acid. Meets the requirements for Identification, Residue on ignition (not more than 0.008%), Bromide or iodide, Free bromine or chlorine, Sulfate, and Sulfite, Arsenic (not more than 1 ppm), and Heavy metals (not more than 5 ppm).

DILUTED HYDROCHLORIC ACID

Description: Diluted Hydrochloric Acid NF—Colorless, odorless liquid. Specific gravity is about 1.05.
NF category: Acidifying agent.

NF requirements: Diluted Hydrochloric Acid NF—Preserve in tight containers. Contains, in each 100 mL, not less than 9.5 grams and not more than 10.5 grams of hydrochloric acid.

Diluted Hydrochloric Acid may be prepared as follows: 226 mL of Hydrochloric Acid and a sufficient quantity of Purified Water to make 1000 mL. Mix the ingredients.

Meets the requirements for Identification, Residue on ignition, Sulfite, Sulfate, Arsenic (not more than 0.6 ppm), Heavy metals (not more than 5 ppm), and Free bromine or chlorine.

HYDROCHLOROTHIAZIDE

Chemical name: 2H-1,2,4-Benzothiadiazine-7-sulfonamide, 6-chloro-3,4-dihydro-, 1,1-dioxide.

Molecular formula: $C_7H_8ClN_3O_4S_2$.

Molecular weight: 297.73.

Description: Hydrochlorothiazide USP—White or practically white, practically odorless, crystalline powder.

pKa: 7.9 and 9.2.

Solubility: Hydrochlorothiazide USP—Slightly soluble in water; freely soluble in sodium hydroxide solution, in *n*-butylamine, and in dimethylformamide; sparingly soluble in methanol; insoluble in ether, in chloroform, and in dilute mineral acids.

USP requirements:
Hydrochlorothiazide Oral Solution—Not in USP.
Hydrochlorothiazide Tablets USP—Preserve in well-closed containers. Contain the labeled amount, within ± 10%. Meet the requirements for Identification, Dissolution (60% in 60 minutes in 0.1 *N* hydrochloric acid in Apparatus 1 at 100 rpm), Uniformity of dosage units, and 4-Amino-6-chloro-1,3-benzenedisulfonamide.

HYDROCODONE

Chemical name: Hydrocodone bitartrate—Morphinan-6-one, 4,5-epoxy-3-methoxy-17-methyl-, (5 alpha)-, [*R*-(*R**,*R**)]-2,3-dihydroxybutanedioate (1:1), hydrate (2:5).

Molecular formula: Hydrocodone bitartrate—$C_{18}H_{21}NO_3 \cdot C_4H_6O_6 \cdot 2\frac{1}{2}H_2O$ (hydrate); $C_{18}H_{21}NO_3 \cdot C_4H_6O_6$ (anhydrous).

Molecular weight: Hydrocodone bitartrate—494.50 (hydrate); 449.46 (anhydrous).

Description: Hydrocodone Bitartrate USP—Fine, white crystals or a crystalline powder. Is affected by light.

Solubility: Hydrocodone Bitartrate USP—Soluble in water; slightly soluble in alcohol; insoluble in ether and in chloroform.

USP requirements:
Hydrocodone Bitartrate Syrup—Not in USP.
Hydrocodone Bitartrate Tablets USP—Preserve in tight, light-resistant containers. Contain the labeled amount, within ± 10%. Meet the requirements for Identification, Dissolution (75% in 45 minutes in water in Apparatus 2 at 50 rpm), and Uniformity of dosage units.

HYDROCODONE AND ACETAMINOPHEN

For *Hydrocodone* and *Acetaminophen*—See individual listings for chemistry information.

USP requirements:
Hydrocodone Bitartrate and Acetaminophen Capsules—Not in USP.
Hydrocodone Bitartrate and Acetaminophen Oral Solution—Not in USP.

Hydrocodone Bitartrate and Acetaminophen Tablets—Not in USP.

HYDROCODONE AND ASPIRIN

For *Hydrocodone* and *Aspirin*—See individual listings for chemistry information.

USP requirements: Hydrocodone Bitartrate and Aspirin Tablets—Not in USP.

HYDROCODONE, ASPIRIN, AND CAFFEINE

For *Hydrocodone*, *Aspirin*, and *Caffeine*—See individual listings for chemistry information.

USP requirements: Hydrocodone Bitartrate, Aspirin, and Caffeine Tablets—Not in USP.

HYDROCODONE AND GUAIFENESIN

For *Hydrocodone* and *Guaifenesin*—See individual listings for chemistry information.

USP requirements:
Hydrocodone Bitartrate and Guaifenesin Oral Solution—Not in USP.
Hydrocodone Bitartrate and Guaifenesin Syrup—Not in USP.
Hydrocodone Bitartrate and Guaifenesin Tablets—Not in USP.

HYDROCODONE AND HOMATROPINE

For *Hydrocodone* and *Homatropine*—See individual listings for chemistry information.

USP requirements:
Hydrocodone Bitartrate and Homatropine Methylbromide Syrup—Not in USP.
Hydrocodone Bitartrate and Homatropine Methylbromide Tablets—Not in USP.

HYDROCODONE AND POTASSIUM GUAIACOLSULFONATE

Chemical name:
Hydrocodone bitartrate—Morphinan-6-one, 4,5-epoxy-3-methoxy-17-methyl-, (5 alpha)-, [*R*-(*R**,*R**)]-2,3-dihydroxybutanedioate (1:1), hydrate (2:5).
Potassium guaiacolsulfonate—Benzenesulfonic acid, hydroxymethoxy-, monopotassium salt, hemihydrate.

Molecular formula:
Hydrocodone bitartrate—$C_{18}H_{21}NO_3 \cdot C_4H_6O_6 \cdot 2\frac{1}{2}H_2O$ (hydrate); $C_{18}H_{21}NO_3 \cdot C_4H_6O_6$ (anhydrous).
Potassium guaiacolsulfonate—$C_7H_7KO_5S \cdot \frac{1}{2}H_2O$.

Molecular weight:
Hydrocodone bitartrate—494.50 (hydrate); 449.46 (anhydrous).
Potassium guaiacolsulfonate—251.29.

Description: Hydrocodone Bitartrate USP—Fine, white crystals or a crystalline powder. Is affected by light.

Solubility: Hydrocodone Bitartrate USP—Soluble in water; slightly soluble in alcohol; insoluble in ether and in chloroform.

USP requirements: Hydrocodone Bitartrate and Potassium Guaiacolsulfonate Syrup—Not in USP.

HYDROCORTISONE

Chemical name:
Hydrocortisone—Pregn-4-ene-3,20-dione, 11,17,21,trihydroxy-, (11 beta)-.

Hydrocortisone acetate—Pregn-4-ene-3,20-dione, 21-(acetyloxy)-11,17-dihydroxy-, (11 beta)-.

Hydrocortisone butyrate—Pregn-4-ene-3,20-dione, 11,21-dihydroxy-17-(1-oxobutoxy)-, (11 beta)-.

Hydrocortisone cypionate—Pregn-4-ene-3,20-dione, 21-(3-cyclopentyl-1-oxopropoxy)-11,17-dihydroxy-, (11 beta)-.

Hydrocortisone sodium phosphate—Pregn-4-ene-3,20-dione, 11,17-dihydroxy-21-(phosphonooxy)-, disodium salt, (11 beta)-.

Hydrocortisone sodium succinate—Pregn-4-ene-3,20-dione, 21-(3-carboxy-1-oxopropoxy)-11,17-dihydroxy-, monosodium salt, (11 beta)-.

Hydrocortisone valerate—Pregn-4-ene-3,20-dione, 11,21-dihydroxy-17-[(1-oxopentyl)oxy]-, (11 beta)-.

Molecular formula:
Hydrocortisone—$C_{21}H_{30}O_5$.
Hydrocortisone acetate—$C_{23}H_{32}O_6$.
Hydrocortisone butyrate—$C_{25}H_{36}O_6$.
Hydrocortisone cypionate—$C_{29}H_{42}O_6$.
Hydrocortisone sodium phosphate—$C_{21}H_{29}Na_2O_8P$.
Hydrocortisone sodium succinate—$C_{25}H_{33}NaO_8$.
Hydrocortisone valerate—$C_{26}H_{38}O_6$.

Molecular weight:
Hydrocortisone—362.47.
Hydrocortisone acetate—404.50.
Hydrocortisone butyrate—432.56.
Hydrocortisone cypionate—486.65.
Hydrocortisone sodium phosphate—486.41.
Hydrocortisone sodium succinate—484.52.
Hydrocortisone valerate—446.58.

Description:
Hydrocortisone USP—White to practically white, odorless, crystalline powder. Melts at about 215 °C, with decomposition.

Hydrocortisone Acetate USP—White to practically white, odorless, crystalline powder. Melts at about 200 °C, with decomposition.

Hydrocortisone Butyrate USP—White to practically white, practically odorless, crystalline powder.

Hydrocortisone Cypionate USP—White to practically white crystalline powder. Is odorless, or has a slight odor.

Hydrocortisone Sodium Phosphate USP—White to light yellow, odorless or practically odorless, powder. Is exceedingly hygroscopic.

Hydrocortisone Sodium Succinate USP—White or nearly white, odorless, hygroscopic, amorphous solid.

Solubility:
Hydrocortisone USP—Very slightly soluble in water and in ether; sparingly soluble in acetone and in alcohol; slightly soluble in chloroform.

Hydrocortisone Acetate USP—Insoluble in water; slightly soluble in alcohol and in chloroform.

Hydrocortisone Butyrate USP—Practically insoluble in water; slightly soluble in ether; soluble in methanol, in alcohol, and in acetone; freely soluble in chloroform.

Hydrocortisone Cypionate USP—Insoluble in water; very soluble in chloroform; soluble in alcohol; slightly soluble in ether.

Hydrocortisone Sodium Phosphate USP—Freely soluble in water; slightly soluble in alcohol; practically insoluble in chloroform, in dioxane, and in ether.

Hydrocortisone Sodium Succinate USP—Very soluble in water and in alcohol; very slightly soluble in acetone; insoluble in chloroform.

USP requirements:
Hydrocortisone Cream USP—Preserve in tight containers. It is Hydrocortisone in a suitable cream base. Contains the labeled amount, within ±10%. Meets the requirements for Identification, Microbial limits, and Minimum fill.

Hydrocortisone Enema USP—Preserve in tight containers. Contains the labeled amount, within ±10%. Meets the requirements for Identification and pH (5.5–7.0).

Hydrocortisone Gel USP—Preserve in tight containers. It is Hydrocortisone in a suitable hydroalcoholic gel base. Contains the labeled amount, within ±10%. Meets the requirements for Identification and Minimum fill.

Hydrocortisone Lotion USP—Preserve in tight containers. It is Hydrocortisone in a suitable aqueous vehicle. Contains the labeled amount, within ±10%. Meets the requirements for Identification, Microbial limits, and Minimum fill.

Hydrocortisone Ointment USP—Preserve in well-closed containers. It is Hydrocortisone in a suitable ointment base. Contains the labeled amount, within ±10%. Meets the requirements for Identification, Microbial limits, and Minimum fill.

Hydrocortisone Rectal Ointment—Not in USP.
Hydrocortisone Topical Solution—Not in USP.
Hydrocortisone Topical Aerosol Solution—Not in USP.
Hydrocortisone Topical Spray Solution—Not in USP.
Hydrocortisone Suppositories—Not in USP.

Sterile Hydrocortisone Suspension USP—Preserve in single-dose or in multiple-dose containers, preferably of Type I glass. A sterile suspension of Hydrocortisone in Water for Injection. Contains the labeled amount, within ±10%. Meets the requirements for Identification, Bacterial endotoxins, pH (5.0–7.0), and Injections.

Hydrocortisone Tablets USP—Preserve in well-closed containers. Contain the labeled amount, within ±10%. Meet the requirements for Identification, Dissolution (70% in 30 minutes in water in Apparatus 2 at 50 rpm), and Uniformity of dosage units.

Hydrocortisone Acetate Rectal Aerosol (Foam)—Not in USP.
Hydrocortisone Acetate Topical Aerosol (Foam)—Not in USP.

Hydrocortisone Acetate Cream USP—Preserve in well-closed containers. It is Hydrocortisone Acetate in a suitable cream base. Contains the labeled amount, within ±10%. Meets the requirements for Identification, Microbial limits, and Minimum fill.

Hydrocortisone Acetate Lotion USP—Preserve in tight containers. It is Hydrocortisone Acetate in a suitable aqueous vehicle. Contains the labeled amount, within ±10%. Meets the requirements for Identification and Minimum fill.

Hydrocortisone Acetate Ointment USP—Preserve in well-closed containers. It is Hydrocortisone Acetate in a suitable ointment base. Contains the labeled amount, within ±10%. Meets the requirements for Identification, Microbial limits, and Minimum fill.

Hydrocortisone Acetate Ophthalmic Ointment USP—Preserve in collapsible ophthalmic ointment tubes. It is Hydrocortisone Acetate in a suitable ophthalmic ointment base. It is sterile. Contains the labeled amount of total steroids, calculated as hydrocortisone acetate, within ±10%. Meets the requirements for Identification, Sterility, Minimum fill, and Particulate matter.

Hydrocortisone Acetate Dental Paste—Not in USP.
Hydrocortisone Acetate Suppositories—Not in USP.

Hydrocortisone Acetate Ophthalmic Suspension USP—Preserve in tight containers. A sterile suspension of Hydrocortisone Acetate in an aqueous medium containing a suitable antimicrobial agent. Contains the labeled amount of total steroids, calculated as Hydrocortisone Acetate, within ± 10%. Meets the requirements for Identification, Sterility, and pH (6.0–8.0).

Sterile Hydrocortisone Acetate Suspension USP—Preserve in single-dose or in multiple-dose containers, preferably of Type I glass. A sterile suspension of Hydrocortisone Acetate in a suitable aqueous medium. Contains the labeled amount of total steroids, calculated as hydrocortisone acetate, within ± 10%. Meets the requirements for Identification, pH (5.0–7.0), and Injections.

Hydrocortisone Butyrate Cream USP—Preserve in well-closed containers. It is Hydrocortisone Butyrate in a suitable cream base. Contains the labeled amount, within ± 10%. Meets the requirements for Identification, pH (3.5–4.5), Microbial limits, and Minimum fill.

Hydrocortisone Butyrate Ointment—Not in USP.

Hydrocortisone Cypionate Oral Suspension USP—Preserve in tight, light-resistant containers. Contains an amount of hydrocortisone cypionate equivalent to the labeled amount of hydrocortisone, within ± 10%. Meets the requirements for Identification and pH (2.8–3.2).

Hydrocortisone Sodium Phosphate Injection USP—Preserve in single-dose or in multiple-dose containers, preferably of Type I glass. A sterile, buffered solution of Hydrocortisone Sodium Phosphate in Water for Injection. Contains an amount of hydrocortisone sodium phosphate equivalent to the labeled amount of hydrocortisone, within −10% to +15%. Meets the requirements for Identification, Bacterial endotoxins, pH (7.5–8.5), Particulate matter, and Injections.

Hydrocortisone Sodium Succinate for Injection USP—Preserve in Containers for Sterile Solids. A sterile mixture of Hydrocortisone Sodium Succinate and suitable buffers. It may be prepared from Hydrocortisone Sodium Succinate, or from Hydrocortisone Hemisuccinate with the aid of Sodium Hydroxide or Sodium Carbonate. Label it to indicate that the constituted solution prepared from Hydrocortisone Sodium Succinate for Injection is suitable for use only if it is clear, and that the solution is to be discarded after 3 days. Label it to indicate that it was prepared by freeze-drying, having been filled into its container in the form of a true solution. Contains an amount of hydrocortisone sodium succinate equivalent to the labeled amount of hydrocortisone, within ± 10%, in single-compartment containers, or in the volume of solution designated on the label of containers that are constructed to hold in separate compartments the Hydrocortisone Sodium Succinate for Injection and a solvent. Meets the requirements for Constituted solution, Identification, Bacterial endotoxins, pH (7.0–8.0 in a solution containing the equivalent of 50 mg of hydrocortisone per mL), Loss on drying (not more than 2.0%), Particulate matter, and Free hydrocortisone (not more than 6.7%), and for Sterility tests, Uniformity of dosage units, and Labeling under Injections.

Hydrocortisone Valerate Cream USP—Preserve in well-closed containers. It is Hydrocortisone Valerate in a suitable cream base. Contains the labeled amount, within ± 10%. Meets the requirements for Identification and Minimum fill.

Hydrocortisone Valerate Ointment—Not in USP.

HYDROCORTISONE AND ACETIC ACID

For *Hydrocortisone* and *Acetic Acid*—See individual listings for chemistry information.

USP requirements: Hydrocortisone and Acetic Acid Otic Solution USP—Preserve in tight, light-resistant containers. A solution of Hydrocortisone and Glacial Acetic Acid in a suitable nonaqueous solvent. Contains the labeled amount of hydrocortisone, within −10% to +20%, and the labeled

amount of acetic acid, within −15% to +30%. Meets the requirements for Identification and pH (2.0–4.0, when diluted with an equal volume of water).

HYDROCORTISONE AND UREA

For *Hydrocortisone* and *Urea*—See individual listings for chemistry information.

USP requirements: Hydrocortisone and Urea Cream—Not in USP.

HYDROFLUMETHIAZIDE

Chemical name: 2*H*-1,2,4-Benzothiadiazine-7-sulfonamide, 3,4-dihydro-6-(trifluoromethyl)-, 1,1-dioxide.

Molecular formula: $C_8H_8F_3N_3O_4S_2$.

Molecular weight: 331.28.

Description: Hydroflumethiazide USP—White to cream-colored, finely divided, odorless, crystalline powder.

pKa: 8.9 and 10.7.

Solubility: Hydroflumethiazide USP—Very slightly soluble in water; freely soluble in acetone; soluble in alcohol.

USP requirements: Hydroflumethiazide Tablets USP—Preserve in tight containers. Contain the labeled amount, within ± 5%. Meet the requirements for Identification, Dissolution (80% in 60 minutes in dilute hydrochloric acid [1 in 100] in Apparatus 2 at 50 rpm), and Uniformity of dosage units.

HYDROGEN PEROXIDE

Chemical name: Hydrogen peroxide.

Molecular formula: H_2O_2.

Molecular weight: 34.01.

Description:

Hydrogen Peroxide Concentrate USP—Clear, colorless liquid. Acid to litmus. Slowly decomposes, and is affected by light.

Hydrogen Peroxide Solution USP—Clear, colorless liquid, odorless or having an odor resembling that of ozone. Acid to litmus. Rapidly decomposes when in contact with many oxidizing as well as reducing substances. When rapidly heated, it may decompose suddenly. Affected by light. Specific gravity is about 1.01.

USP requirements:

Hydrogen Peroxide Concentrate USP—Preserve in partially-filled containers having a small vent in the closure, and store in a cool place. Label it to indicate the name and amount of any added preservative. Contains not less than 29.0% and not more than 32.0%, by weight, of hydrogen peroxide. Contains not more than 0.05% of a suitable preservative or preservatives. Meets the requirements for Acidity and Chloride (not more than 0.005%), and for Identification test, Nonvolatile residue, Heavy metals, and Limit of preservative under Hydrogen Peroxide Topical Solution.

Caution: Hydrogen Peroxide Concentrate is a strong oxidant.

Hydrogen Peroxide Topical Solution USP—Preserve in tight, light-resistant containers, at controlled room temperature. Contains, in each 100 mL, not less than 2.5 grams and not more than 3.5 grams of Hydrogen Peroxide. Contains not more than 0.05% of a suitable preservative or preservatives. Meets the requirements for Identification, Acidity, Nonvolatile residue, Barium, Heavy metals (not more than 5 ppm), and Limit of preservative (not more than 0.05%).

HYDROMORPHONE

Chemical name: Hydromorphone hydrochloride—Morphinan-6-one, 4,5-epoxy-3-hydroxy-17-methyl-, hydrochloride, (5 alpha)-.

Molecular formula: Hydromorphone hydrochloride—$C_{17}H_{19}NO_3 \cdot HCl$.

Molecular weight: Hydromorphone hydrochloride—321.80.

Description: Hydromorphone Hydrochloride USP—Fine, white or practically white, odorless, crystalline powder. Is affected by light.

Solubility: Hydromorphone Hydrochloride USP—Freely soluble in water; sparingly soluble in alcohol; practically insoluble in ether.

USP requirements:
Hydromorphone Hydrochloride Injection USP—Preserve in single-dose or in multiple-dose containers, preferably of Type I glass, protected from light. A sterile solution of Hydromorphone Hydrochloride in Water for Injection. Contains the labeled amount, within ±5%. Meets the requirements for Identification, Bacterial endotoxins, pH (3.5–5.5), and Injections.
Hydromorphone Hydrochloride Suppositories—Not in USP.
Hydromorphone Hydrochloride Tablets USP—Preserve in tight, light-resistant containers. Contain the labeled amount, within ±10%. Meet the requirements for Identification, Dissolution (75% in 45 minutes in water in Apparatus 2 at 50 rpm), and Uniformity of dosage units.

HYDROMORPHONE AND GUAIFENESIN

For *Hydromorphone* and *Guaifenesin*—See individual listings for chemistry information.

USP requirements: Hydromorphone Hydrochloride and Guaifenesin Syrup—Not in USP.

HYDROQUINONE

Chemical name: 1,4-Benzenediol.

Molecular formula: $C_6H_6O_2$.

Molecular weight: 110.11.

Description: Hydroquinone USP—Fine white needles. Darkens upon exposure to light and to air.

Solubility: Hydroquinone USP—Freely soluble in water, in alcohol, and in ether.

USP requirements:
Hydroquinone Cream USP—Preserve in well-closed, light-resistant containers. Contains the labeled amount, within ±6%. Meets the requirements for Identification and Minimum fill.
Hydroquinone Topical Solution USP—Preserve in tight, light-resistant containers. Contains the labeled amount, within −5% to +10%. Meets the requirements for Identification and pH (3.0–4.2).

HYDROXOCOBALAMIN

Source: Synthetic form of vitamin B_{12}.

Chemical name: Cobinamide, dihydroxide, dihydrogen phosphate (ester), mono(inner salt), 3'-ester with 5,6-dimethyl-1-alpha-D-ribofuranosyl-1H-benzimidazole.

Molecular formula: $C_{62}H_{89}CoN_{13}O_{15}P$.

Molecular weight: 1346.37.

Description: Hydroxocobalamin USP—Dark red crystals or red crystalline powder. Is odorless, or has not more than a slight acetone odor. The anhydrous form is very hygroscopic.

Solubility: Hydroxocobalamin USP—Sparingly soluble in water, in alcohol, and in methanol; practically insoluble in acetone, in ether, and in chloroform.

USP requirements: Hydroxocobalamin Injection USP—Preserve in single-dose or in multiple-dose containers, preferably of Type I glass, protected from light. A sterile solution of Hydroxocobalamin in Water for Injection. Contains the labeled amount, within −5% to +15%. Meets the requirements for Identification, Bacterial endotoxins, pH (3.5–5.0), and Injections.

HYDROXYAMPHETAMINE

Chemical name: Hydroxyamphetamine hydrobromide—Phenol, 4-(2-aminopropyl)-, hydrobromide.

Molecular formula: Hydroxyamphetamine hydrobromide—$C_9H_{13}NO \cdot HBr$.

Molecular weight: Hydroxyamphetamine hydrobromide—232.12.

Description: Hydroxyamphetamine Hydrobromide USP—White, crystalline powder. Its solutions are slightly acid to litmus, having a pH of about 5.

Solubility: Hydroxyamphetamine Hydrobromide USP—Freely soluble in water and in alcohol; slightly soluble in chloroform; practically insoluble in ether.

USP requirements: Hydroxyamphetamine Hydrobromide Ophthalmic Solution USP—Preserve in tight, light-resistant containers. A sterile, buffered, aqueous solution of Hydroxyamphetamine Hydrobromide. Contains the labeled amount, within ±5%. Contains a suitable antimicrobial agent. Meets the requirements for Identification, Sterility, and pH (4.2–6.0).

HYDROXYCHLOROQUINE

Chemical name: Hydroxychloroquine sulfate—Ethanol, 2-[[4-[(7-chloro-4-quinolinyl)amino]pentyl]ethylamino]-, sulfate (1:1) salt.

Molecular formula: Hydroxychloroquine sulfate—$C_{18}H_{26}ClN_3O \cdot H_2SO_4$.

Molecular weight: Hydroxychloroquine sulfate—433.95.

Description: Hydroxychloroquine Sulfate USP—White or practically white, crystalline powder. Is odorless. Its solutions have a pH of about 4.5. Exists in two forms, the usual form melting at about 240 °C and the other form melting at about 198 °C.

Solubility: Hydroxychloroquine Sulfate USP—Freely soluble in water; practically insoluble in alcohol, in chloroform, and in ether.

USP requirements: Hydroxychloroquine Sulfate Tablets USP—
Preserve in tight, light-resistant containers. Contain the labeled amount, within ±7%. Meet the requirements for Identification, Dissolution (70% in 60 minutes in water in Apparatus 2 at 100 rpm), and Uniformity of dosage units.

HYDROXYETHYL CELLULOSE

Chemical name: Cellulose, 2-hydroxyethyl ether.

Description: Hydroxyethyl Cellulose NF—White to light tan, practically odorless, hygroscopic powder.
NF category: Suspending and/or viscosity-increasing agent.

Solubility: Hydroxyethyl Cellulose NF—Soluble in hot water and in cold water, giving a colloidal solution; practically insoluble in alcohol and in most organic solvents.

NF requirements: Hydroxyethyl Cellulose NF—Preserve in well-closed containers. A partially substituted poly(hydroxyethyl) ether of cellulose. It is available in several grades, varying in viscosity and degree of substitution, and some grades are modified to improve their dispersion in water. The labeling indicates its viscosity, under specified conditions, in aqueous solution. The indicated viscosity may be in the form of a range encompassing 50% to 150% of the average value. Meets the requirements for Identification, Viscosity (not less than 50% and not more than 150%, where stated as a single value, or it is between the maximum and minimum values, where stated as a range of viscosities), pH (6.0–8.5, in a solution [1 in 100]), Loss on drying (not more than 10.0%), Residue on ignition (not more than 5.0%), Lead (not more than 0.001%), Arsenic (not more than 3 ppm), Heavy metals (not more than 0.004%), and Organic volatile impurities.

HYDROXYPROGESTERONE

Chemical name: Hydroxyprogesterone caproate—Pregn-4-ene-3,20-dione, 17-[(1-oxohexyl)oxy]-.

Molecular formula: Hydroxyprogesterone caproate—$C_{27}H_{40}O_4$.

Molecular weight: Hydroxyprogesterone caproate—428.61.

Description: Hydroxyprogesterone Caproate USP—White or creamy white, crystalline powder. Is odorless or has a slight odor.

Solubility: Hydroxyprogesterone Caproate USP—Insoluble in water; soluble in ether.

USP requirements: Hydroxyprogesterone Caproate Injection USP—Preserve in single-dose or in multiple-dose containers, preferably of Type I or Type III glass. A sterile solution of Hydroxyprogesterone Caproate in a suitable vegetable oil. Contains the labeled amount, within ±10%. Meets the requirements for Identification, Water (not more than 0.2%), and Injections.

HYDROXYPROPYL CELLULOSE

Chemical name: Cellulose, 2-hydroxypropyl ether.

Description: Hydroxypropyl Cellulose NF—White to cream-colored, practically odorless, granular solid or powder. Is hygroscopic after drying.
NF category: Coating agent; suspending and/or viscosity-increasing agent.

Solubility: Hydroxypropyl Cellulose NF—Soluble in cold water, in alcohol, in chloroform, and in propylene glycol, giving a colloidal solution; insoluble in hot water.

USP requirements: Hydroxypropyl Cellulose Ocular System USP—Preserve in single-dose containers, at a temperature not exceeding 30 °C. Contains the labeled amount, within ±15%. Contains no other substance. It is sterile. Meets the requirements for Identification, Sterility, and Weight variation.

NF requirements: Hydroxypropyl Cellulose NF—Store in well-closed containers. A partially substituted poly(hydroxypropyl) ether of cellulose. Label it to indicate the viscosity in an aqueous solution of stated concentration and temperature. The indicated viscosity may be in the form of a range encompassing 50% to 150% of the average value. When dried at 105 °C for 3 hours, contains not more than 80.5% of hydroxypropoxy groups. Meets the requirements for Identification, Apparent viscosity, pH (5.0–8.0, in a solution [1 in 100]), Loss on drying (not more than 5.0%), Residue on ignition (except for silica, not more than 0.2%), Arsenic (not more than 3 ppm), Lead (not more than 0.001%), Heavy metals (not more than 0.004%), and Organic volatile impurities.

LOW-SUBSTITUTED HYDROXYPROPYL CELLULOSE

Description: Low-Substituted Hydroxypropyl Cellulose NF—White to yellowish white, practically odorless, fibrous or granular powder. Is hygroscopic. The pH of the suspension, obtained by shaking 1.0 gram with 100 mL of water, is between 5.0 and 7.5.
NF category: Tablet disintegrant and/or tablet binder.

Solubility: Low-Substituted Hydroxypropyl Cellulose NF—Practically insoluble in ethanol and in ether. Dissolves in a solution of sodium hydroxide (1 in 10), and produces a viscous solution. Swells in water, in sodium carbonate TS, and in 2 N hydrochloric acid.

NF requirements: Low-Substituted Hydroxypropyl Cellulose NF—Preserve in tight containers. A low-substituted hydroxypropyl ether of cellulose. When dried at 105 °C for 1 hour, contains not less than 5.0% and not more than 16.0% of hydroxypropoxy groups ($-OCH_2CHOHCH_3$). Meets the requirements for Identification, Loss on drying (not more than 5.0%), Residue on ignition (not more than 0.5%), Chloride (not more than 0.36%), Arsenic (not more than 2 ppm), and Heavy metals (not more than 0.001%).

HYDROXYPROPYL METHYLCELLULOSE

Chemical name: Cellulose, 2-hydroxypropyl methyl ether.

Description: Hydroxypropyl Methylcellulose USP—White to slightly off-white, fibrous or granular powder. Swells in water and produces a clear to opalescent, viscous, colloidal mixture.
NF category: Coating agent; suspending and/or viscosity-increasing agent; tablet binder.

Solubility: Hydroxypropyl Methylcellulose USP—Insoluble in dehydrated alcohol, in ether, and in chloroform.

USP requirements:
Hydroxypropyl Methylcellulose USP—Preserve in well-closed containers. A propylene glycol ether of methylcellulose. Label it to indicate its substitution type and its viscosity type [viscosity of a solution (1 in 50)]. When dried at 105 °C for 2 hours, contains methoxy and hydroxypropoxy groups conforming to the limits for the 4 substitution types for methoxy and hydroxypropoxy contents. Meets the requirements for Identification, Apparent viscosity, Loss on drying (not more than 5.0%), Residue on ignition (not more than 1.5% for labeled viscosity of greater than 50 centipoises, 3% for labeled viscosity of 50 centipoises

or less, or 5% of all labeled viscosities.), Arsenic (not more than 3 ppm), and Heavy metals (not more than 0.001%).
Hydroxypropyl Methylcellulose Ophthalmic Solution USP—Preserve in tight containers. A sterile solution of Hydroxypropyl Methylcellulose. Contains the labeled amount, within ±15%. Meets the requirements for Identification, Sterility, and pH (6.0–7.8).

HYDROXYPROPYL METHYLCELLULOSE PHTHALATE

Description: Hydroxypropyl Methylcellulose Phthalate NF—White powder or granules. Is odorless.
NF category: Coating agent.

Solubility: Hydroxypropyl Methylcellulose Phthalate NF—Practically insoluble in water, in dehydrated alcohol, and in hexane. Produces a viscous solution in a mixture of methanol and dichloromethane (1:1), or in a mixture of dehydrated alcohol and acetone (1:1). Dissolves in 1 *N* sodium hydroxide.

NF requirements: Hydroxypropyl Methylcellulose Phthalate NF—Preserve in well-closed containers. A monophthalic acid ester of hydroxypropyl methylcellulose. Label it to indicate its substitution type and its viscosity. When dried at 105 °C for 1 hour, contains methoxy, hydroxypropoxy, and phthalyl groups conforming to the limits for the 2 substitution types for methoxy, hydroxypropxy, and phthalyl. Meets the requirements for Clarity and color of solution, Identification, Viscosity (80–120% of that indicated by the label), Loss on drying (not more than 5.0%), Residue on ignition (not more than 0.20%), Chloride (not more than 0.07%), Arsenic (not more than 2 ppm), Heavy metals (not more than 0.001%), Free phthalic acid (not more than 1.0%), Phthalyl content, and Methoxy and hydroxypropoxy contents.

HYDROXYSTILBAMIDINE

Chemical name: Hydroxystilbamidine isethionate—Benzenecarboximidamide, 4-[2-[4-(aminoiminomethyl)phenyl]ethenyl]-3-hydroxy-, bis(2-hydroxyethanesulfonate) (salt).

Molecular formula: Hydroxystilbamidine isethionate—$C_{16}H_{16}N_4O\cdot2C_2H_6O_4S$.

Molecular weight: Hydroxystilbamidine isethionate—532.58.

Description:
Hydroxystilbamidine Isethionate USP—Yellow, fine, odorless, crystalline powder. Is stable in air but decomposes upon exposure to light. Melts at about 280 °C.
Sterile Hydroxystilbamidine Isethionate USP—Yellow, fine, odorless, crystalline powder. Is stable in air, but decomposes upon exposure to light. Melts at about 280 °C.

Solubility:
Hydroxystilbamidine Isethionate USP—Soluble in water; slightly soluble in alcohol; insoluble in ether.
Sterile Hydroxystilbamidine Isethionate USP—Soluble in water; slightly soluble in alcohol; insoluble in ether.

USP requirements:
Hydroxystilbamidine Isethionate USP—Preserve in tight, light-resistant containers. Contains not less than 95.0% and not more than 105.0% of hydroxystilbamidine isethionate, calculated on the dried basis. Meets the requirements for Identification, pH (4.0–5.5, in a solution [1 in 100]), Loss on drying (not more than 1.0%), Residue on ignition (not more than 0.1%), Selenium (0.003%), and Heavy metals (not more than 0.001%).
Sterile Hydroxystilbamidine Isethionate USP—Preserve in light-resistant Containers for Sterile Solids. It is Hydroxystilbamidine Isethionate suitable for parenteral use.

Meets the requirements for Completeness of solution, Constituted solution, and Bacterial endotoxins, for Identification tests, pH, Loss on drying, Residue on ignition, Selenium, and Heavy metals under Hydroxystilbamidine Isethionate, and for Sterility tests, Uniformity of dosage units, and Labeling under Injections.

HYDROXYUREA

Chemical name: Urea, hydroxy-.

Molecular formula: $CH_4N_2O_2$.

Molecular weight: 76.05.

Description: Hydroxyurea USP—White to off-white powder. Is somewhat hygroscopic, decomposing in the presence of moisture. Melts at a temperature exceeding 133 °C, with decomposition.

Solubility: Hydroxyurea USP—Freely soluble in water and in hot alcohol.

USP requirements: Hydroxyurea Capsules USP—Preserve in tight containers, in a dry atmosphere. Contain the labeled amount, within ±10%. Meet the requirements for Identification and Uniformity of dosage units.

HYDROXYZINE

Chemical group: Piperazine derivative.

Chemical name:
Hydroxyzine hydrochloride—Ethanol, 2-[2-[4-[(4-chlorophenyl)phenylmethyl]-1-piperazinyl]ethoxy]-, dihydrochloride.
Hydroxyzine pamoate—Ethanol, 2-[2-[4-[(4-chlorophenyl)phenylmethyl]-1-piperazinyl]ethoxy]-, compd. with 4,4′-methylenebis[3-hydroxy-2-naphthalenecarboxylic acid] (1:1).

Molecular formula:
Hydroxyzine hydrochloride—$C_{21}H_{27}ClN_2O_2\cdot2HCl$.
Hydroxyzine pamoate—$C_{21}H_{27}ClN_2O_2\cdot C_{23}H_{16}O_6$.

Molecular weight:
Hydroxyzine hydrochloride—447.83.
Hydroxyzine pamoate—763.29.

Description:
Hydroxyzine Hydrochloride USP—White, odorless powder. Melts at about 200 °C, with decomposition.
Hydroxyzine Pamoate USP—Light yellow, practically odorless powder.

pKa: Hydroxyzine hydrochloride—2.6 and 7.

Solubility:
Hydroxyzine Hydrochloride USP—Very soluble in water; soluble in chloroform; slightly soluble in acetone; practically insoluble in ether.
Hydroxyzine Pamoate USP—Practically insoluble in water and in methanol; freely soluble in dimethylformamide.

USP requirements:
Hydroxyzine Hydrochloride Capsules—Not in USP.
Hydroxyzine Hydrochloride Injection USP—Preserve in single-dose or multiple-dose containers, protected from light. A sterile solution of Hydroxyzine Hydrochloride in Water for Injection. Contains the labeled amount, within ±10%. Meets the requirements for Identification, Bacterial endotoxins, pH (3.5–6.0), Limit of 4-chlorobenzophenone (not more than 0.2%), and Injections.

Hydroxyzine Hydrochloride Syrup USP—Preserve in tight, light-resistant containers. Contains the labeled amount, within ± 10%. Meets the requirement for Identification.

Hydroxyzine Hydrochloride Tablets USP—Preserve in tight containers. Contain the labeled amount, within ± 10%. Meet the requirements for Identification, Dissolution (75% in 45 minutes in water in a modified basket-rack assembly as directed for Uncoated tablets under Disintegration), and Uniformity of dosage units.

Hydroxyzine Pamoate Capsules USP—Preserve in well-closed containers. Contain an amount of hydroxyzine pamoate equivalent to the labeled amount of hydroxyzine hydrochloride, within ± 10%. Meet the requirements for Identification, Dissolution (75% in 60 minutes in 0.1 N hydrochloric acid in Apparatus 2 at 50 rpm), and Uniformity of dosage units.

Hydroxyzine Pamoate Oral Suspension USP—Preserve in tight, light-resistant containers. Contains an amount of hydroxyzine pamoate equivalent to the labeled amount of hydroxyzine hydrochloride, within ± 10%. Meets the requirements for Identification and pH (4.5–7.0).

HYOSCYAMINE

Source: The levo-isomer of atropine; the major active alkaloid of belladonna.

Chemical group: Natural tertiary amine.

Chemical name:
Hyoscyamine—Benzeneacetic acid, alpha-(hydroxymethyl)-, 8-methyl-8-azabicyclo[3.2.1]oct-3-yl ester, [3(S)-endo]-.
Hyoscyamine sulfate—Benzeneacetic acid, alpha-(hydroxymethyl)-, 8-methyl-8-azabicyclo[3.2.1]oct-3-yl ester, [3(S)-endo]-, sulfate (2:1), dihydrate.

Molecular formula:
Hyoscyamine—$C_{17}H_{23}NO_3$.
Hyoscyamine sulfate—$(C_{17}H_{23}NO_3)_2 \cdot H_2SO_4 \cdot 2H_2O$.

Molecular weight:
Hyoscyamine—289.37.
Hyoscyamine sulfate—712.85.

Description:
Hyoscyamine USP—White, crystalline powder. Is affected by light. Its solutions are alkaline to litmus.
Hyoscyamine Sulfate USP—White, odorless crystals or crystalline powder. Is deliquescent and is affected by light. The pH of a solution (1 in 100) is about 5.3.

Solubility:
Hyoscyamine USP—Slightly soluble in water; freely soluble in alcohol, in chloroform, and in dilute acids; sparingly soluble in ether.
Hyoscyamine Sulfate USP—Very soluble in water; freely soluble in alcohol; practically insoluble in ether.

USP requirements:
Hyoscyamine Tablets USP—Preserve in well-closed, light-resistant containers. Contain the labeled amount, within ± 10%. Meet the requirements for Identification, Disintegration (30 minutes, the use of disks being omitted), and Uniformity of dosage units.
Hyoscyamine Sulfate Extended-release Capsules—Not in USP.
Hyoscyamine Sulfate Elixir USP—Preserve in tight, light-resistant containers, at controlled room temperature. Contains the labeled amount, within ± 10%. Meets the requirements for Identification, pH (3.0–6.5), and Alcohol content (90.0–110.0% of labeled amount).
Hyoscyamine Sulfate Injection USP—Preserve in single-dose or in multiple-dose containers, preferably of Type I glass,

at controlled room temperature. A sterile solution of Hyoscyamine Sulfate in Water for Injection. Contains the labeled amount, within ± 7%. Meets the requirements for Identification, Bacterial endotoxins, pH (3.0–6.5), and Injections.
Hyoscyamine Sulfate Oral Solution USP—Preserve in tight, light-resistant containers, at controlled room temperature. Contains the labeled amount, within ± 10%. Meets the requirements for Identification and pH (3.0–6.5).
Hyoscyamine Sulfate Tablets USP—Preserve in tight, light-resistant containers. Contain the labeled amount, within ± 10%. Meet the requirements for Identification, Disintegration (15 minutes), and Uniformity of dosage units.

HYOSCYAMINE AND PHENOBARBITAL

For *Hyoscyamine* and *Phenobarbital*—See individual listings for chemistry information.

USP requirements:
Hyoscyamine Sulfate and Phenobarbital Elixir—Not in USP.
Hyoscyamine Sulfate and Phenobarbital Oral Solution—Not in USP.
Hyoscyamine Sulfate and Phenobarbital Tablets—Not in USP.

HYPOPHOSPHOROUS ACID

Chemical name: Phosphinic acid.

Molecular formula: H_3PO_2.

Molecular weight: 66.00.

Description: Hypophosphorous Acid NF—Colorless or slightly yellow, odorless liquid. Specific gravity is about 1.13.
NF category: Antioxidant.

NF requirements: Hypophosphorous Acid NF—Preserve in tight containers. Contains not less than 30.0% and not more than 32.0% of hypophosphorous acid. Meets the requirements for Identification, Arsenic, Barium, and Oxalate (not more than 1.5 ppm arsenic), and Heavy metals (not more than 0.002%).

IBUPROFEN

Chemical group: Propionic acid derivative.

Chemical name: Benzeneacetic acid, alpha-methyl-4-(2-methylpropyl), (±)-.

Molecular formula: $C_{13}H_{18}O_2$.

Molecular weight: 206.28.

Description: Ibuprofen USP—White to off-white, crystalline powder, having a slight, characteristic odor.

pKa: 4.43.

Solubility: Ibuprofen USP—Practically insoluble in water; very soluble in alcohol, in methanol, in acetone, and in chloroform; slightly soluble in ethyl acetate.

USP requirements:
Ibuprofen USP—Preserve in tight containers. Contains not less than 97.0% and not more than 103.0% of ibuprofen, calculated on the anhydrous basis. Meets the requirements for Identification, Water (not more than 1.0%), Residue on ignition (not more than 0.5%), Heavy metals (not more than 0.002%), Chromatographic purity, and Organic volatile impurities.
Ibuprofen Capsules—Not in USP.
Ibuprofen Oral Suspension—Not in USP.

Ibuprofen Tablets USP—Preserve in well-closed containers. Contain the labeled amount, within ± 10%. Meet the requirements for Identification, Dissolution (70% in 30 minutes in pH 7.2 phosphate buffer in Apparatus 1 at 150 rpm), Uniformity of dosage units, and Water (not more than 5.0%).

ICHTHAMMOL

Chemical name: Ichthammol.

Description: Ichthammol USP—Reddish brown to brownish black, viscous fluid, having a strong, characteristic, empyreumatic odor.

Solubility: Ichthammol USP—Miscible with water, with glycerin, and with fixed oils and fats. Partially soluble in alcohol and in ether.

USP requirements:

Ichthammol USP—Preserve in well-closed containers. It is obtained by the destructive distillation of certain bituminous schists, sulfonation of the distillate, and neutralization of the product with ammonia. Yields not less than 2.5% of ammonia and not less than 10.0% of total sulfur. Meets the requirements for Identification, Loss on drying (not more than 50.0%), Residue on ignition (not more than 0.5%), and Limit for ammonium sulfate (not more than 8.0%).

Ichthammol Ointment USP—Preserve in collapsible tubes or in tight containers, and avoid prolonged exposure to temperatures exceeding 30 °C. Contains an amount of Ichthammol equivalent to not less than 0.25% of ammonia.

Prepare Ichthammol Ointment as follows: 100 grams of Ichthammol, 100 grams of Anhydrous Lanolin, 800 grams of Petrolatum, to make 1000 grams. Thoroughly incorporate the Ichthammol with the Anhydrous Lanolin, and combine this mixture with the Petrolatum.

IDARUBICIN

Chemical name: Idarubicin hydrochloride—5,12-Naphthacenedione, 9-acetyl-7-[(3-amino-2,3,6-trideoxy-alpha-L-lyxo-hexopyranosyl)oxy]-7,8,9,10-tetrahydro-6,9,11-trihydroxy-hydrochloride, (7S-cis)-.

Molecular formula: Idarubicin hydrochloride—$C_{26}H_{27}NO_9 \cdot HCl$.

Molecular weight: Idarubicin hydrochloride—533.96.

USP requirements: Idarubicin Hydrochloride for Injection—Not in USP.

IDOXURIDINE

Chemical group: An antimetabolite of thymidine.

Chemical name: Uridine, 2'-deoxy-5-iodo-.

Molecular formula: $C_9H_{11}IN_2O_5$.

Molecular weight: 354.10.

Description: Idoxuridine USP—White, crystalline, practically odorless powder.

Solubility: Idoxuridine USP—Slightly soluble in water and in alcohol; practically insoluble in chloroform and in ether.

USP requirements:

Idoxuridine USP—Preserve in tight, light-resistant containers. Contains not less than 98.0% and not more than 101.0% of idoxuridine, calculated on the dried basis. Meets

the requirements for Identification and Loss on drying (not more than 1.0%).

Idoxuridine Ophthalmic Ointment USP—Preserve in collapsible ophthalmic ointment tubes in a cool place. It is Idoxuridine in a Petrolatum base. It is sterile. Contains 0.45% to 0.55% of idoxuridine. Meets the requirements for Identification, Sterility, and Metal particles.

Idoxuridine Ophthalmic Solution USP—Preserve in tight, light-resistant containers in a cold place. A sterile, aqueous solution of Idoxuridine. Contains 0.09% to 0.11% of idoxuridine. Meets the requirements for Identification, Sterility, and pH (4.5–7.0).

IFOSFAMIDE

Chemical name: 2H-1,3,2-Oxazaphosphorin-2-amine, N,3-bis(2-chloroethyl)tetrahydro-, 2-oxide.

Molecular formula: $C_7H_{15}Cl_2N_2O_2P$.

Molecular weight: 261.09.

Description: Ifosfamide USP—White, crystalline powder. Melts at about 40 °C.

Solubility: Ifosfamide USP—Freely soluble in water; very soluble in alcohol, in ethyl acetate, in isopropyl alcohol, in methanol, and in methylene chloride; very slightly soluble in hexanes.

USP requirements:

Ifosfamide USP—Preserve in tight containers at a temperature not exceeding 25 °C. Contains not less than 98.0% and not more than 102.0% of ifosfamide. Meets the requirements for Identification, pH (4.0–7.0 in a solution [1 in 10]), Water (not more than 0.3%), Heavy metals (not more than 0.002%), Ionic chloride (not more than 0.018%), Chloroform-insoluble phosphorus (not more than 0.0415%), and Limit of 2-chloroethylamine hydrochloride (not more than 0.25%).

Caution: Great care should be taken in handling Ifosfamide, as it is a potent cytotoxic agent and suspected carcinogen.

Ifosfamide for Injection—Not in USP.

Sterile Ifosfamide USP—Preserve in Containers for Sterile Solids, at controlled room temperature. It is Ifosfamide suitable for parenteral use. Contains the labeled amount, within ± 10%. Meets the requirements for Identification, Bacterial endotoxins, pH (4.0–7.0), Water (not more than 0.3%), and for Sterility tests, Uniformity of dosage units, and Labeling under Injections.

Caution: Great care should be taken in handling Ifosfamide, as it is a potent cytotoxic agent and suspected carcinogen.

IMIDUREA

Chemical name: N,N''-Methylenebis [N'-[3-(hydroxymethyl)-2,5-dioxo-4-imidazolidinyl]urea].

Molecular formula: $C_{11}H_{16}N_8O_8$.

Molecular weight: 388.30.

Description: Imidurea NF—White, odorless powder.

Solubility: Imidurea NF—Soluble in water and in glycerin; sparingly soluble in propylene glycol; insoluble in most organic solvents.

NF requirements: Imidurea NF—Preserve in tight containers. Contains not less than 26.0% and not more than 28.0% of nitrogen, calculated on the dried basis. Meets the requirements for Color and clarity of solution, Identification, pH (6.0–7.5, in a solution [1 in 100]), Loss on drying (not more than 3.0%), Residue on ignition (not more than 3.0%), Heavy metals (not more than 0.001%), Nitrogen content, and Organic volatile impurities.

IMIPENEM

Source: Derivative of thienamycin, produced by the soil organism *Streptomyces cattleya*.

Chemical group: A carbapenem, which is a subclass of the beta-lactams.

Chemical name: 1-Azabicyclo[3.2.0]hept-2-ene-2-carboxylic acid, 6-(1-hydroxyethyl)-3-[[2-[(iminomethyl)amino]ethyl]thio]-7-oxo-, monohydrate, [5*R*-[5 alpha,6 alpha(*R**)]]-.

Molecular formula: $C_{12}H_{17}N_3O_4S\cdot H_2O$.

Molecular weight: 317.36.

Description: Imipenem USP—White to tan-colored crystalline powder.

Solubility: Imipenem USP—Sparingly soluble in water; slightly soluble in methanol.

USP requirements: Sterile Imipenem USP—Preserve in Containers for Sterile Solids, and store in a cold place. It is imipenem suitable for parenteral use. Contains the equivalent of not less than 98.0% and not more than 101.0% of imipenem monohydrate. Meets the requirements for Identification, Specific rotation (+84° to +89°, calculated on the dried basis), Crystallinity, Bacterial endotoxins, Sterility, Loss on drying (5.0–8.0%), Residue on ignition (not more than 0.2%), Heavy metals (not more than 0.002%), and Solvents (not more than 0.25%).

IMIPENEM AND CILASTATIN

For *Imipenem* and *Cilastatin*—See individual listings for chemistry information.

USP requirements:
Imipenem and Cilastatin Sodium for Injection—Not in USP.
Imipenem and Cilastatin Sodium for Suspension—Not in USP.

IMIPRAMINE

Chemical group: Dibenzazepine.

Chemical name:
Imipramine hydrochloride—5*H*-Dibenz[*b,f*]azepine-5-propanamine, 10,11-dihydro-*N,N*-dimethyl-, monohydrochloride.
Imipramine pamoate—5-(3-[Dimethylamino)propyl]-10,11-dihydro-5*H*-dibenz[*b,f*]azepine 4,4′-methylenebis-(3-hydroxy-2-naphthoate)(2:1).

Molecular formula:
Imipramine hydrochloride—$C_{19}H_{24}N_2\cdot HCl$.
Imipramine pamoate—$(C_{19}H_{24}N_2)_2\cdot C_{23}H_{16}O_6$.

Molecular weight:
Imipramine hydrochloride—316.87.
Imipramine pamoate—949.21.

Description:
Imipramine Hydrochloride USP—White to off-white, odorless or practically odorless, crystalline powder.
Imipramine pamoate—Fine, yellow, odorless powder.

pKa: 9.5.

Solubility:
Imipramine Hydrochloride USP—Freely soluble in water and in alcohol; soluble in acetone; insoluble in ether.
Imipramine pamoate—Soluble in ethanol, in acetone, in ether, in chloroform, and in carbon tetrachloride. Insoluble in water.

USP requirements:
Imipramine Hydrochloride USP— Preserve in tight containers. Contains not less than 98.0% and not more than 102.0% of imipramine hydrochloride, calculated on the dried basis. Meets the requirements for Identification, Melting range (170–174 °C), Loss on drying (not more than 0.5%), Residue on ignition (not more than 0.1%), Heavy metals (not more than 0.001%), Iminodibenzyl (absorbance not more than 0.1%), and Organic volatile impurities.
Imipramine Hydrochloride Injection USP—Preserve in single-dose containers, preferably of Type I glass. A sterile solution of Imipramine Hydrochloride in Water for Injection. Contains, in each mL, not less than 11.5 mg and not more than 13.5 mg of imipramine hydrochloride. Meets the requirements for Identification, Bacterial endotoxins, pH (4.0–5.0), and Injections.
Imipramine Hydrochloride Tablets USP—Preserve in tight containers. Contain the labeled amount, within ±7%. Meet the requirements for Identification, Dissolution (75% in 45 minutes in 0.1 N hydrochloric acid in Apparatus 1 at 100 rpm), and Uniformity of dosage units.
Imipramine Pamoate Capsules—Not in USP.

INDAPAMIDE

Chemical name: Benzamide, 3-(aminosulfonyl)-4-chloro-*N*-(2,3-dihydro-2-methyl-1*H*-indol-1-yl)-.

Molecular formula: $C_{16}H_{16}ClN_3O_3S$.

Molecular weight: 365.83.

Description: Indapamide USP—White to off-white crystalline powder. Melts between 167 and 170 °C.

Solubility: Indapamide USP—Soluble in methanol, in alcohol, in acetonitrile, in glacial acetic acid, and in ethyl acetate; very slightly soluble in ether and in chloroform; practically insoluble in water.

USP requirements:
Indapamide USP—Preserve in well-closed containers. Contains not less than 98.0% and not more than 101.0% of indapamide, calculated on the dried basis. Meets the requirements for Identification, Loss on drying (not more than 3.0%), Residue on ignition (not more than 0.1%), and Chromatographic purity.
Indapamide Tablets USP—Preserve in well-closed containers. Contain the labeled amount, within ±10%. Meet the requirements for Identification, Dissolution (75% in 60 minutes in simulated gastric fluid TS [without enzyme] in Apparatus 1 at 100 rpm), and Uniformity of dosage units.

INDECAINIDE

Chemical name: Indecainide hydrochloride—9*H*-Fluorene-9-carboxamide, 9-[3-[(1-methylethyl)amino]propyl]-, monohydrochloride.

Molecular formula: Indecainide hydrochloride—$C_{20}H_{24}N_2O\cdot HCl$.

Molecular weight: Indecainide hydrochloride—344.88.

Description: Indecainide hydrochloride—White crystalline solid.

pKa: Indecainide hydrochloride—10.2 in 66% N,N-dimethyl-formamide; 10.6 in water.

Solubility: Indecainide hydrochloride—Freely soluble in water, and in methanol; slightly soluble in chloroform; practically insoluble in diethyl ether, in ethyl acetate, and in toluene.

Other characteristics: Indecainide hydrochloride—The octanol/water partition coefficient is 0.76.

USP requirements: Indecainide Hydrochloride Extended-release Tablets—Not in USP.

INDIGOTINDISULFONATE

Chemical name: Indigotindisulfonate sodium—1*H*-Indole-5-sulfonic acid, 2-(1,3-dihydro-3-oxo-5-sulfo-2*H*-indol-2-ylidene)-2,3-dihydro-3-oxo-, disodium salt.

Molecular formula: Indigotindisulfonate sodium—$C_{16}H_8N_2Na_2O_8S_2$.

Molecular weight: Indigotindisulfonate sodium—466.35.

Description: Indigotindisulfonate Sodium USP—Dusky, purplish blue powder, or blue granules having a coppery luster. Affected by light. Its solutions have a blue or bluish purple color.

Solubility: Indigotindisulfonate Sodium USP—Slightly soluble in water and in alcohol; practically insoluble in most other organic solvents.

USP requirements:
Indigotindisulfonate Sodium USP—Preserve in tight, light-resistant containers. Contains not less than 96.0% and not more than 102.0% of sodium indigotinsulfonates, calculated on the dried basis as indigotindisulfonate sodium. Meets the requirements for Identification, Loss on drying (not more than 5.0%), Water-insoluble substances, Arsenic (not more than 8 ppm), Lead (not more than 0.001%), and Sulfur content (13.0–14.0%, calculated on the dried basis).
Indigotindisulfonate Sodium Injection USP—Preserve in single-dose, light-resistant containers, preferably of Type I glass. A sterile solution of Indigotindisulfonate Sodium in Water for Injection. Contains the labeled amount, within −10% to +5%. Meets the requirements for Identification, Bacterial endotoxins, pH (3.0–6.5), and Injections.

INDIUM In 111 OXYQUINOLINE

Source: Saturated (1:3) complex of indium and oxyquinoline (oxine), a chelating agent.

Chemical name: Indium-¹¹¹*In*, tris(8-quinolinolato-*N*¹,*O*⁸)-.

Molecular formula: $C_{27}H_{18}{}^{111}InN_3O_3$.

Molecular weight: 543.46.

USP requirements: Indium In 111 Oxyquinoline Solution USP—Preserve in single-unit containers at a temperature between 15 and 25 °C. A sterile, nonpyrogenic, isotonic aqueous solution suitable for the radiolabeling of blood cells, especially leukocytes and platelets, containing radioactive indium (¹¹¹In) in the form of a complex with 8-hydroxyquinoline, the latter being present in excess. Label it to contain the following, in addition to the information specified for Labeling under Injections: the time and date of calibration; the amount of ¹¹¹In as the 8-hydroxyquinoline complex expressed as total megabecquerels (or millicuries) and concentration as megabecquerels (or millicuries) per mL on the date and time of calibration; the expiration date; the statement, "Not for direct administration. Use only for radiolabeling of leucocytes in vitro. Administer radiolabeled cells subsequently by intravenous injection;" and the statement, "Caution—Radioactive Material." The labeling indicates that in making dosage calculations, correction is to be made for radioactive decay, and also indicates that the radioactive half-life of ¹¹¹In is 67.9 hours. Contains the labeled amount of ¹¹¹In, within ±10%, as the 8-hydroxyquinoline complex expressed as megabecquerels (or millicuries) per mL at the time indicated in the labeling. Other chemical forms of radioactivity do not exceed 10.0% of the total radioactivity. Meets the requirements for Specific activity (not less than 1.85 gigabecquerels [50 millicuries] per mcg of indium), Pyrogen, pH (6.5–7.5), Radionuclide identification, Radiochemical purity, and Radionuclidic purity.

INDIUM In 111 PENTETATE

USP requirements: Indium In 111 Pentetate Injection USP—Preserve in single-dose containers. A sterile, isotonic solution suitable for intrathecal administration, containing radioactive indium (¹¹¹In) in the form of a chelate of pentetic acid. Label it to include the following, in addition to the information specified for Labeling under Injections: the time and date of calibration; the amount of ¹¹¹In as labeled pentetic acid complex expressed as total megabecquerels (or millicuries or microcuries) and concentration as megabecquerels (or microcuries or millicuries) per mL on the date and time of calibration; the expiration date; and the statement, "Caution—Radioactive Material." The labeling indicates that in making dosage calculations, correction is to be made for radioactive decay, and also indicates that the radioactive half-life of ¹¹¹In is 2.83 days. Contains the labeled amount of ¹¹¹In, within ±10%, as pentetic acid complex expressed in megabecquerels (or microcuries or millicuries) per mL at the time indicated in the labeling. Other chemical forms of radioactivity do not exceed 10.0% of the total radioactivity. Meets the requirements for Bacterial endotoxins, pH (7.0–8.0), Radionuclide identification, Radiochemical purity (not less than 90.0%), Radionuclidic purity, and Injections (except that the Injection may be distributed or dispensed prior to completion of the test for Sterility, the latter test being started on the day of final manufacture, and except that it is not subject to the recommendation on Volume in Container).

INDOCYANINE GREEN

Chemical name: 1*H*-Benz[*e*]indolium, 2-[7-[1,3-dihydro-1,1-dimethyl-3-(4-sulfobutyl)-2*H*-benz[*e*]indol-2-ylidene]-1,3,5-heptatrienyl]-1,1-dimethyl-3-(4-sulfobutyl)-, hydroxide, inner salt, sodium salt.

Molecular formula: $C_{43}H_{47}N_2NaO_6S_2$.

Molecular weight: 774.96.

Description:
Indocyanine Green USP—Olive-brown, dark green, blue-green, dark blue, or black powder. Odorless, or has a slight odor. Its solutions are deep emerald-green in color. The pH of a solution (1 in 200) is about 6. Its aqueous solutions are stable for about 8 hours.
Sterile Indocyanine Green USP—Olive-brown, dark green, blue-green, dark blue, or black powder. Odorless, or has a slight odor. Its solutions are deep emerald-green in color. The pH of a solution (1 in 200) is about 6. Its aqueous solutions are stable for about 8 hours.

Solubility: Indocyanine Green USP—Soluble in water and in methanol; practically insoluble in most other organic solvents.

USP requirements: Sterile Indocyanine Green USP—Preserve in Containers for Sterile Solids. It is Indocyanine Green suitable for parenteral use. Contains the labeled amount, within ±10%. Meets the requirements for Constituted solution, Bacterial endotoxins, pH (5.5–6.5, in a solution [1 in 200]), and Content variation, and for Identification tests, Arsenic (not more than 8 ppm), Lead (not more than 0.001%), and Sodium iodide (not more than 5.0%) under Indocyanine Green, and for Sterility tests and Labeling under Injections.

INDOMETHACIN

Chemical group: An indoleacetic acid derivative nonsteroidal anti-inflammatory agent structurally related to the pyrrole-acetic acid derivative sulindac.

Chemical name:
Indomethacin—1H-Indole-3-acetic acid, 1-(4-chloroben-zoyl)-5-methoxy-2-methyl-.
Indomethacin sodium—1H-Indole-3-acetic acid, 1-(4-chlo-robenzoyl)-5-methoxy-2-methyl-, sodium salt, trihydrate.

Molecular formula:
Indomethacin—$C_{19}H_{16}ClNO_4$.
Indomethacin sodium (trihydrate)—$C_{19}H_{15}ClNNaO_4 \cdot 3H_2O$.

Molecular weight:
Indomethacin—357.79.
Indomethacin sodium (trihydrate)—433.82.

Description: Indomethacin USP—Pale yellow to yellow-tan, crystalline powder, having not more than a slight odor. Is sensitive to light. Melts at about 162 °C. Exhibits polymorphism.

pKa: 4.5.

Solubility: Indomethacin USP—Practically insoluble in water; sparingly soluble in alcohol, in chloroform, and in ether.

USP requirements:
Indomethacin Capsules USP—Preserve in well-closed containers. Contain the labeled amount, within ±10%. Meet the requirements for Identification, Dissolution (80% in 20 minutes in 1 volume of phosphate buffer [pH 7.2] mixed with 4 volumes of water in Apparatus 1 at 100 rpm), and Uniformity of dosage units.
Indomethacin Extended-release Capsules USP—Preserve in well-closed containers. Label it to indicate the Drug Release test with which the product complies. Contain the labeled amount, within ±10%. Meet the requirements for Identification, Drug release, Uniformity of dosage units, and Limit of 4-Chlorobenzoic acid (not more than 0.44%).
Indomethacin Suppositories USP—Preserve in well-closed containers, at controlled room temperature. Contain the labeled amount, within ±10%. Meet the requirements for Identification, Dissolution (75% in 60 minutes in 0.1 M phosphate buffer [pH 7.2] in Apparatus 2 at 50 rpm), and Uniformity of dosage units.
Indomethacin Ophthalmic Suspension—Not in USP
Indomethacin Oral Suspension USP—Preserve in tight, light-resistant containers. Contains the labeled amount, within ±10%. Meets the requirements for Identification, Dissolution (80% in 20 minutes in 0.01 M phosphate buffer [pH 7.2] in Apparatus 2 at 50 rpm), pH (3.0–5.0), 4-Chlorobenzoic acid (not more than 0.44%), and Sorbic acid content (where present, 80.0–120.0% of labeled amount).
Sterile Indomethacin Sodium USP—Preserve in Containers for Sterile Solids. Contains the labeled amount, within ±10%. Meets the requirements for Constituted solution, Identification, Pyrogen, pH (6.0–7.5, in a 1 in 2000 solution), Particulate matter, and Chromatographic purity, and for Sterility tests, Uniformity of dosage units, and Labeling under Injections.

INFLUENZA VIRUS VACCINE

Source: Influenza vaccine is available as either a whole-virus or split-virus preparation. The vaccine is prepared from highly purified, egg-grown influenza viruses that have been inactivated to yield a whole-virus preparation. The split-virus vaccine is produced by chemically treating a whole-virus preparation to cause inactivation and disruption of a significant proportion of the virus into smaller subunit particles called subvirions. The preparation is then refined to remove the unwanted substances.

Description: Slightly turbid liquid or suspension, which may have a slightly yellow or reddish tinge and may have an odor because of the preservative.

Note: The Canadian product is more likely to be bluish.

Other characteristics: The viral antigen content of both the whole-virus vaccine and the split-virus vaccine has been standardized by immunodiffusion tests, according to current U.S. Public Health Service requirements. Each 0.5 mL dose contains the proportions and not less than the microgram amounts of hemagglutinin antigens (mcg HA) representative of the specific components recommended for the present year's vaccine.

USP requirements: Influenza Virus Vaccine USP—Preserve at a temperature between 2 and 8 °C. A sterile, aqueous suspension of suitably inactivated influenza virus types A and B, either individually or combined, or virus sub-units prepared from the extra-embryonic fluid of influenza virus–infected chicken embryo. Label it to state that it is to be shaken before use and that it is not to be frozen. Label it also to state that it was prepared in embryonated chicken eggs. The strains of influenza virus used in the preparation of this Vaccine are those designated by the U.S. Government's Expert Committee on Influenza and recommended by the Surgeon General of the U.S. Public Health Service. Influenza Virus Vaccine has a composition of such strains and a content of virus antigen of each, designated for the particular season, of not less than the specified weight (in micrograms) of influenza virus hemagglutinin determined in specific radial-immunodiffusion tests relative to the U.S. Reference Influenza Virus Vaccine. If formalin is used for inactivation, it contains not more than 0.02% of residual free formaldehyde. Meets the requirements for Expiration date (not later than 18 months after date of issue from manufacturer's cold storage [5 °C, 1 year]). Conforms to the regulations of the U.S. Food and Drug Administration concerning biologics.

INSULIN

Chemical name: Insulin (ox), 8A-L-threonine-10A-L-isoleucine-.

Molecular formula:
Insulin—$C_{256}H_{381}N_{65}O_{76}S_6$ (pork); $C_{254}H_{377}N_{65}O_{75}S_6$ (beef).
Insulin Human—$C_{257}H_{383}N_{65}O_{77}S_6$.

Molecular weight:
Insulin—5777.59 (pork); 5733.54 (beef).
Insulin Human—5807.62.

Description:

Insulin USP—White or practically white crystals.

Insulin Injection USP—The Injection containing, in each mL, not more than 100 USP Units is a clear, colorless or almost colorless liquid; the Injection containing, in each mL, 500 Units may be straw-colored. Contains between 0.1% and 0.25% (w/v) of either phenol or cresol. Contains between 1.4% and 1.8% (w/v) of glycerin.

Insulin Zinc Suspension USP—Practically colorless suspension of a mixture of characteristic crystals predominantly between 10 micrometers and 40 micrometers in maximum dimension and many particles that have no uniform shape and do not exceed 2 micrometers in maximum dimension. Contains between 0.15% and 0.17% (w/v) of sodium acetate, between 0.65% and 0.75% (w/v) of sodium chloride, and between 0.09% and 0.11% (w/v) of methylparaben.

Isophane Insulin Suspension USP—White suspension of rod-shaped crystals, free from large aggregates of crystals following moderate agitation. Contains either (1) between 1.4% and 1.8% (w/v) of glycerin, between 0.15% and 0.17% (w/v) of metacresol, and between 0.06% and 0.07% (w/v) of phenol, or (2) between 1.4% and 1.8% (w/v) of glycerin and between 0.20% and 0.25% (w/v) of phenol. Contains between 0.15% and 0.25% (w/v) of dibasic sodium phosphate. When examined microscopically, the insoluble matter in the Suspension is crystalline, and contains not more than traces of amorphous material.

Extended Insulin Zinc Suspension USP—Practically colorless suspension of a mixture of characteristic crystals the maximum dimension of which is predominantly between 10 micrometers and 40 micrometers. Contains between 0.15% and 0.17% (w/v) of sodium acetate, between 0.65% and 0.75% (w/v) of sodium chloride, and between 0.09% and 0.11% (w/v) of methylparaben.

Prompt Insulin Zinc Suspension USP—Practically colorless suspension of particles that have no uniform shape and the maximum dimension of which does not exceed 2 micrometers. Contains between 0.15% and 0.17% (w/v) of sodium acetate, between 0.65% and 0.75% (w/v) of sodium chloride, and between 0.09% and 0.11% (w/v) of methylparaben.

Protamine Zinc Insulin Suspension USP—White or practically white suspension, free from large particles following moderate agitation. Contains between 1.4% and 1.8% (w/v) of glycerin, and either between 0.18% and 0.22% (w/v) of cresol or between 0.22% and 0.28% (w/v) of phenol. Contains between 0.15% and 0.25% (w/v) of dibasic sodium phosphate, and between 1.0 mg and 1.5 mg of protamine for each 100 USP Insulin Units.

Solubility:
Insulin USP—Soluble in solutions of dilute acids and alkalies.

USP requirements:

Insulin Injection USP—Preserve in a refrigerator. Avoid freezing. Dispense it in the unopened, multiple-dose container in which it was placed by the manufacturer. The container for Insulin Injection, up to 100 USP Units in each mL, is of approximately 10-mL capacity and contains not less than 10 mL of the Injection, and the container for Insulin Injection, 500 USP Units per mL, is of approximately 20-mL capacity and contains not less than 20 mL of the Injection. A sterile, acidified or neutral solution of Insulin. The Injection container label and package label state the potency in USP Insulin Units in each mL, based on the results of *Assay A*, and the expiration date, which is not later than 24 months after the immediate container was filled. If the Injection is prepared from neutral solution, the word "neutral" appears on the label. Label it to indicate the one or more animal

species to which it is related, as porcine, as bovine, or as a mixture of porcine and bovine. Where it is highly purified, label it as such. Label it to state that it is to be stored in a refrigerator and that freezing is to be avoided. It has a biological potency, determined by *Assay A,* of ±5% of the potency stated on the label, expressed in USP Insulin Units, the potency being 40, 100, or 500 USP Insulin Units in each mL. Meets the requirements for Identification, Bacterial endotoxins, Sterility, pH (2.5–3.5 for acidified and 7.0–7.8 for neutral), Particulate matter, Residue on ignition, Nitrogen content (not more than 0.7 mg for each 100 USP Insulin Units), Zinc content (10–40 mcg for each 100 USP Insulin Units), and Injections, and, where highly purified, for Proinsulin content and High molecular weight protein.

Insulin Human Injection USP—Preserve in a refrigerator and avoid freezing. The container for Insulin Human Injection, 40 or 100 USP Units in each mL, is of approximately 10-mL capacity and contains not less than 10 mL of the Injection, and the container for Insulin Human Injection, 500 USP Units per mL, is of approximately 20-mL capacity and contains not less than 20 mL of the Injection. A sterile solution of Insulin Human in Water for Injection. The Injection container label and package label state the potency in USP Insulin Human Units in each mL on the basis of the results of the *Assay*, and the expiration date, which is not later than 24 months after the immediate container was filled. The labeling states also that it has been prepared either with Insulin Human derived by enzyme modification of pork pancreas Insulin or with Insulin Human obtained from microbial synthesis, whichever is applicable. Label it to state that it is to be stored in a refrigerator and that freezing is to be avoided. It has a potency, determined chromatographically, of ±5% of the potency stated on the label, expressed in USP Insulin Human Units in each mL. Meets the requirements for Identification, Bacterial endotoxins, Sterility, Biological potency (labeled potency ±5%), pH (7.0–7.8), Particulate matter, Nitrogen content (not more than 0.7 mg for each 100 USP Insulin Human Units), Zinc content (10–40 mcg for each 100 USP Insulin Human Units), and Injections, and for High molecular weight protein, and, where derived from pork pancreas insulin, for Proinsulin content, and Pancreatic polypeptide content under Insulin Human.

Buffered Insulin Human Injection—Not in USP.

Insulin Injection and Isophane Insulin, Human Semisynthetic Injection—Not in USP.

Isophane Insulin Suspension USP—Preserve in a refrigerator. Avoid freezing. Dispense it in the unopened, multiple-dose container in which it was placed by the manufacturer. The container is of approximately 10-mL capacity and contains not less than 10 mL of the Suspension. A sterile suspension of zinc-insulin crystals and Protamine Sulfate in buffered Water for Injection, combined in a manner such that the solid phase of the suspension consists of crystals composed of insulin, protamine, and zinc. The Protamine Sulfate is prepared from the sperm or from the mature testes of fish belonging to the genus *Oncorhynchus* Suckley, or *Salmo* Linné (Fam. Salmonidae). Label it to indicate the one or more animal species to which it is related, as porcine, as bovine, or as a mixture of porcine and bovine. Where it is highly purified, label it as such. The Suspension container label states that the Suspension is to be shaken carefully before use. The container label and the package label state the potency in USP Insulin Units in each mL, and the expiration date, which is not later than 24 months after the immediate container was filled. Label it to state that it is to be stored in a refrigerator and that freezing is to be avoided. Each mL of Isophane Insulin Suspension is prepared from sufficient insulin to provide 40, 80, or 100 USP Insulin Units of insulin activity. Meets the requirements for Identification, Sterility, pH (7.0–7.8), Nitrogen content (not more than 0.85 mg for each 100 USP Insulin Units), Zinc content (0.01–0.04 mg for each 100 USP Insulin Units), and Biological activity of the supernatant liquid.

Isophane Insulin, Human, Suspension—Not in USP.

Isophane Insulin Suspension and Insulin Injection—Not in USP.

Isophane Insulin, Human, Suspension and Insulin Human Injection—Not in USP.

Insulin Zinc Suspension USP—Preserve in a refrigerator. Avoid freezing. Dispense it in the unopened, multiple-dose container in which it was placed by the manufacturer. The container is of approximately 10-mL capacity and contains not less than 10 mL of the Suspension. A sterile suspension of Insulin in buffered Water for Injection, modified by the addition of Zinc Chloride in a manner such that the solid phase of the suspension consists of a mixture of crystalline and amorphous insulin in a ratio of approximately 7 parts of crystals to 3 parts of amorphous material. Label it to indicate the one or more animal species to which it is related, as porcine, as bovine, or as a mixture of porcine and bovine. Where it is highly purified, label it as such. The Suspension container label states that the Suspension is to be shaken carefully before use. The container label and the package label state the potency in USP Insulin Units in each mL, and the expiration date, which is not later than 24 months after the immediate container was filled. Label it to state that it is to be stored in a refrigerator and that freezing is to be avoided. Each mL of Insulin Zinc Suspension is prepared from sufficient insulin to provide 40, 80, or 100 USP Insulin Units of insulin activity. Meets the requirements for Identification, Sterility, pH (7.0–7.8), Nitrogen content (not more than 0.70 mg for each 100 USP Insulin Units), Zinc content (0.12–0.25 mg for each 100 USP Insulin Units), Zinc in the supernatant liquid, and Insulin not extracted by buffered acetone solution.

Insulin Zinc, Human, Suspension—Not in USP.

Extended Insulin Zinc Suspension USP—Preserve in a refrigerator. Avoid freezing. Dispense it in the unopened multiple-dose container in which it was placed by the manufacturer. The container is of approximately 10-mL capacity and contains not less than 10 mL of the Suspension. A sterile suspension of Insulin in buffered Water for Injection, modified by the addition of Zinc Chloride in a manner such that the solid phase of the suspension is predominantly crystalline. Label it to indicate the one or more animal species to which it is related, as porcine, as bovine, or as a mixture of porcine and bovine. Its container label states that the Suspension is to be shaken carefully before use. Its container label and its package label state the potency in USP Insulin Units in each mL, and the expiration date, which is not later than 24 months after the immediate container was filled. Label it to state that it is to be stored in a refrigerator and that freezing is to be avoided. In its preparation, sufficient insulin is used to provide 40, 80, or 100 USP Insulin Units for each mL of the Suspension. Meets the requirements for Identification, Sterility, pH (7.0–7.8), Nitrogen content (not more than 0.70 mg for each 100 USP Insulin Units), Zinc content (0.12–0.25 mg for each 100 USP Insulin Units), Zinc in the supernatant liquid, and Insulin not extracted by buffered acetone solution.

Extended Insulin Zinc, Human, Suspension—Not in USP.

Prompt Insulin Zinc Suspension USP—Preserve in a refrigerator. Avoid freezing. Dispense it in the unopened, multiple-dose container in which it was placed by the manufacturer. The container is of approximately 10-mL capacity

and contains not less than 10 mL of the Suspension. A sterile suspension of Insulin in buffered Water for Injection, modified by the addition of Zinc Chloride in a manner such that the solid phase of the suspension is amorphous. Label it to indicate the one or more animal species to which it is related, as porcine, as bovine, or as a mixture of porcine and bovine. Its container label states that the Suspension is to be shaken carefully before use. Its container label and its package label state the potency in USP Insulin Units in each mL, and the expiration date, which is not later than 24 months after the immediate container was filled. Label it to state that it is to be stored in a refrigerator and that freezing is to be avoided. In its preparation, sufficient insulin is used to provide 40, 80, or 100 USP Insulin Units for each mL of the Suspension. Meets the requirements for Identification, Sterility, pH (7.0–7.8), Nitrogen content (not more than 0.70 mg for each 100 USP Insulin Units), Zinc content (0.12–0.25 mg for each 100 USP Insulin Units), Zinc in the supernatant liquid, and Insulin not extracted by buffered acetone solution.

Protamine Zinc Insulin Suspension USP—Preserve in a refrigerator. Avoid freezing. Dispense it in the unopened, multiple-dose container in which it was placed by the manufacturer. The container is of approximately 10-mL capacity and contains not less than 10 mL of the Suspension. A sterile suspension of Insulin in buffered Water for Injection modified by the addition of Zinc Chloride and Protamine Sulfate. The Protamine Sulfate is prepared from the sperm or from the mature testes of fish belonging to the genus *Oncorhynchus* Suckley, or *Salmo* Linné (Fam. Salmonidae), and conforms to the regulations of the U.S. Food and Drug Administration. Label it to indicate the one or more animal species to which it is related, as porcine, as bovine, or as a mixture of porcine and bovine. Where it is highly purified, label it as such. The Suspension container label states that the Suspension is to be shaken carefully before use. The container label and package label state the potency in USP Insulin Units in each mL, and the expiration date, which is not later than 24 months after the immediate container was filled. Label it to state that it is to be stored in a refrigerator and that freezing is to be avoided. In the preparation of Protamine Zinc Insulin Suspension, the amount of insulin used is sufficient to provide 40, 80, or 100 USP Insulin Units for each mL of the Suspension. Meets the requirements for Identification, Sterility, pH (7.1–7.4), Nitrogen content (not more than 1.25 mg for each 100 USP Insulin Units), Zinc content (0.15–0.25 mg for each 100 USP Insulin Units), and Biological reaction.

INTERFERON ALFA

Source:

Interferon Alfa-2a, recombinant—Synthetic. A protein chain of 165 amino acids produced by a recombinant DNA process involving genetically engineered *Escherichia coli*. Recombinant interferon alfa-2a has a lysine group at position 23. Purification procedure for recombinant interferon alfa-2a includes affinity chromatography using a murine monoclonal antibody.

Interferon Alfa-2b, recombinant—Synthetic. A protein chain of 165 amino acids produced by a recombinant DNA process involving genetically engineered *Escherichia coli*. Recombinant interferon alfa-2b has an arginine group at position 23. Purification of recombinant interferon alfa-2b is done by proprietary methods.

Interferon Alfa-n1 (lns)—A highly purified blend of natural human alpha interferons, obtained from human lymphoblastoid cells following induction with Sendai virus.

Interferon Alfa-n3—A protein chain of approximately 166 amino acids. Manufactured from pooled units of human leukocytes that have been induced by incomplete infection with an avian virus (Sendai virus) to produce interferon alfa-n3. The manufacturing process includes immunoaffinity chromatography with a murine monoclonal antibody, acidification (pH 2) for 5 days at 4 °C, and gel filtration chromatography.

Chemical group: Related to naturally occurring alfa interferons. Interferons are produced and secreted by cells in response to viral infections or various synthetic and biologic inducers; alfa interferons are produced mainly by leukocytes.

Chemical name:
Interferon Alfa-2a—Interferon alphaA (human leukocyte protein moiety reduced).
Interferon Alfa-2b—Interferon alpha2b (human leukocyte clone Hif-SN206 protein moiety reduced).
Interferon Alfa-n1—alpha-Interferons.
Interferon Alfa-n3—Interferons, alpha-.

Molecular formula:
Interferon Alfa-2a—$C_{860}H_{1353}N_{227}O_{255}S_9$.
Interferon Alfa-2b—$C_{860}H_{1353}N_{229}O_{255}S_9$.

Molecular weight:
Interferon Alfa-2a—19,241.11.
Interferon Alfa-2b—19,269.12.

Solubility: Water-soluble.

USP requirements:
Interferon Alfa-2a, Recombinant, Injection—Not in USP.
Interferon Alfa-2a, Recombinant, for Injection—Not in USP.
Interferon Alfa-2b, Recombinant, for Injection—Not in USP.
Interferon Alfa-n1 (lns) Injection—Not in USP.
Interferon Alfa-n3 Injection—Not in USP.

INTERFERON GAMMA

Chemical name: Interferon gamma-1b—1-139-Interferon gamma (human lymphocyte protein moiety reduced), N^2-L-methionyl-.

Molecular formula: Interferon gamma-1b—$C_{734}H_{1166}N_{204}O_{216}S_5$.

Molecular weight: Interferon gamma-1b—16,464.87.

Description: Interferon gamma-1b injection—Sterile, clear, colorless solution.

USP requirements: Interferon Gamma-1b Injection—Not in USP.

INULIN

Source: A polysaccharide obtained from the tubers of *Dahlia variabilis, Helianthus tuberosus,* and other genera of the family Compositae.

Chemical name: Inulin.

Molecular formula: $C_6H_{11}O_5(C_6H_{10}O_5)_nOH$.

Description: Inulin USP—White, friable, chalk-like, amorphous, odorless powder.

Solubility: Inulin USP—Soluble in hot water; slightly soluble in cold water and in organic solvents.

Other characteristics: Hygroscopic.

USP requirements: Inulin Injection—Not in USP.

INULIN AND SODIUM CHLORIDE

For *Inulin* and *Sodium Chloride*—See individual listings for chemistry information.

USP requirements: Inulin in Sodium Chloride Injection USP—Preserve in single-dose containers, preferably of Type I or Type II glass. A sterile solution, which may be supersaturated, of Inulin and Sodium Chloride in Water for Injection. May require heating before use if crystallization has occurred. Contains the labeled amounts of inulin, within ± 10%, and sodium chloride, within ± 5%. Contains no antimicrobial agents. Meets the requirements for Clarity, Bacterial endotoxins, pH (5.0–7.0), Free fructose (2.2 mg per mL), and Injections.

IOCETAMIC ACID

Chemical group: Ionic, triiodinated benzoic acid derivative.

Chemical name: Propanoic acid, 3-[acetyl(3-amino-2,4,6-triiodophenyl)amino]-2-methyl-.

Molecular formula: $C_{12}H_{13}I_3N_2O_3$.

Molecular weight: 613.96.

Description: White to light cream-colored powder. Melting point 224–225 °C.

pKa: 4.1 and 4.25.

Solubility: Practically insoluble in water; very slightly soluble in ether and in ethanol; slightly soluble in acetone and in chloroform.

USP requirements: Iocetamic Acid Tablets USP—Preserve in tight containers. Contain the labeled amount, within ± 10%. Meet the requirements for Identification, Dissolution (35% in 30 minutes and 50% in 60 minutes in simulated intestinal fluid TS, prepared without pancreatin, in Apparatus 1 at 150 rpm), and Uniformity of dosage units.

IODINATED GLYCEROL

Chemical group: An isomeric mixture formed by the interaction of iodine and glycerol, the active ingredient thought to be iodopropylidene glycerol; contains about 50% of organically bound iodine.

Chemical name: 1,3-Dioxolane-4-methanol, 2-(1-iodoethyl)-.

Molecular formula: $C_6H_{11}IO_3$.

Molecular weight: 258.06.

Description: Viscous, amber liquid stable in acid media, including gastric juice, which contains virtually no inorganic iodide and no free iodine.

Solubility: Miscible with water, with alcohol, and with glycerin; soluble in ether, in chloroform, in isobutyl alcohol, in methyl acetate, in ethyl acetate, in methyl formate, and in tetrahydrofuran.

USP requirements:
Iodinated Glycerol Elixir—Not in USP.
Iodinated Glycerol Oral Solution—Not in USP.
Iodinated Glycerol Tablets—Not in USP.

IODINATED I 125 ALBUMIN

Description: Iodinated I 125 Albumin Injection USP—Clear, colorless to slightly yellow solution. Upon standing, both the Albumin and the glass container may darken as a result of the effects of the radiation.

USP requirements: Iodinated I 125 Albumin Injection USP—Preserve in single-dose or multiple-dose containers, at a temperature between 2 and 8 °C. A sterile, buffered, isotonic solution containing normal human albumin adjusted to provide not more than 37 MBq (or 1 millicurie) of radioactivity per mL. Derived by mild iodination of normal human albumin with the use of radioactive iodine (^{125}I) to introduce not more than one gram-atom of iodine for each gram-molecule (60,000 grams) of albumin. Label it to include the following, in addition to the information specified for Labeling under Injections: the date of calibration; the amount of ^{125}I as iodinated albumin, expressed as total megabecquerels (or microcuries or millicuries), and concentration as megabecquerels (or microcuries or millicuries) per mL on the date of calibration; the expiration date; and the statement, "Caution—Radioactive Material." The labeling indicates that in making dosage calculations, correction is to be made for radioactive decay, and also indicates that the radioactive half-life of ^{125}I is 60 days. Contains the labeled amount of ^{125}I, within ±5%, as iodinated albumin, expressed in megabecquerels (or microcuries or in millicuries) per mL at the time indicated in the labeling. Other forms of radioactivity do not exceed 3% of the total radioactivity. Its production and distribution are subject to federal regulations. Meets the requirements for Radionuclide identification, Bacterial endotoxins, pH (7.0–8.5), Radiochemical purity (not less than 97.0%), and for Biologics and Injections (except that it is not subject to the recommendation on Volume in Container and meets all other applicable requirements of the U.S. Food and Drug Administration).

IODINATED I 131 ALBUMIN

Description:

Iodinated I 131 Albumin Injection USP—Clear, colorless to slightly yellow solution. Upon standing, both the albumin and the glass container may darken as a result of the effects of the radiation.

Iodinated I 131 Albumin Aggregated Injection USP—Dilute suspension of white to faintly yellow particles, which may settle on standing. The glass container may darken on standing, as a result of the effects of the radiation.

USP requirements:

Iodinated I 131 Albumin Injection USP—A sterile, buffered, isotonic solution containing normal human albumin adjusted to provide not more than 37 MBq (1 millicurie) of radioactivity per mL. Derived by mild iodination of normal human albumin with the use of radioactive iodine (^{131}I) to introduce not more than one gram-atom of iodine for each gram-molecule (60,000 grams) of albumin. Label it to include the following, in addition to the information specified for Labeling under Injections: the date of calibration; the amount of ^{131}I as iodinated albumin expressed as total megabecquerels (or millicuries or microcuries), and concentration as megabecquerels (or millicuries or microcuries) per mL on the date of calibration; the expiration date; and the statement, "Caution—Radioactive Material." The labeling indicates that in making dosage calculations, correction is to be made for radioactive decay, and also indicates that the radioactive half-life of ^{131}I is 8.08 days. Contains the labeled amount of ^{131}I, within ±5%, as iodinated albumin, expressed in megabecquerels (or millicuries or microcuries) per mL at the time indicated in the labeling. Other forms of radioactivity do not exceed 3% of the total radioactivity. Its production and distribution are subject to federal regulations. Meets the requirements for Radionuclide identification, for Packaging and storage, Bacterial endotoxins, pH (7.0–8.5), and Radiochemical purity under

Iodinated I 125 Albumin Injection USP, and for Biologics and Injections (except that it is not subject to the recommendation on Volume in Container and meets all other applicable requirements of the U.S. Food and Drug Administration.

Iodinated I 131 Albumin Aggregated Injection USP—Preserve in single-dose or in multiple-dose containers, at a temperature between 2 and 8 °C. A sterile aqueous suspension of Albumin Human that has been iodinated with ^{131}I and denatured to produce aggregates of controlled particle size. Label it to include the following, in addition to the information specified for Labeling under Injections: the time and date of calibration; the amount of ^{131}I as aggregated albumin expressed as total megabecquerels (or microcuries or millicuries) and as aggregated albumin in mg per mL on the date of calibration; the expiration date; and the statement, "Caution—Radioactive Material." The labeling indicates that in making dosage calculations, correction is to be made for radioactive decay, and also indicates that the radioactive half-life of ^{131}I is 8.08 days; in addition, the labeling states that it is not to be used if clumping of the albumin is observed and directs that the container be agitated before the contents are withdrawn into a syringe. Each mL of the suspension contains not less than 300 mcg and not more than 3.0 mg of aggregated albumin with a specific activity of not less than 7.4 megabecquerels (200 microcuries) per mg and not more than 44.4 megabecquerels (1.2 millicuries) per mg of aggregated albumin. Contains the labeled amount of ^{131}I, within ±5%, as aggregated albumin, expressed in megabecquerels (or microcuries) per mL or megabecquerels (or millicuries) per mL at the time indicated in the labeling. Other chemical forms of radioactivity do not exceed 6% of the total radioactivity. Its production and distribution are subject to federal regulations. Meets the requirements for Radionuclide identification and pH (5.0–6.0), for Biologics and Injections (except that it is not subject to the recommendation on Volume in Container), and for Particle size, Bacterial endotoxins, and Radiochemical purity under Technetium Tc 99m Albumin Aggregated Injection (except that in the test for Radiochemical purity, not more than 6% of the radioactivity is found in the supernatant liquid following centrifugation).

IODINE

Chemical name: Iodine.

Molecular formula: I.

Molecular weight: 126.90.

Description:

Iodine USP—Heavy, grayish black plates or granules, having a metallic luster and a characteristic odor.

Iodine Topical Solution USP—Transparent, reddish brown liquid, having the odor of iodine.

Iodine Tincture USP—Transparent liquid having a reddish brown color and the odor of iodine and of alcohol.

Solubility: Iodine USP—Very slightly soluble in water; freely soluble in carbon disulfide, in chloroform, in carbon tetrachloride, and in ether; soluble in alcohol and in solutions of iodides; sparingly soluble in glycerin.

USP requirements:

Iodine Topical Solution USP—Preserve in tight, light-resistant containers, at a temperature not exceeding 35 °C. Contains, in each 100 mL, not less than 1.8 grams and not more than 2.2 grams of iodine, and not less than 2.1 grams and not more than 2.6 grams of sodium iodide.

Prepare Iodine Topical Solution as follows: 20 grams of Iodine, 24 grams of Sodium Iodide, and a sufficient quantity of Purified Water to make 1000 mL. Dissolve the Iodine and the Sodium Iodide in 50 mL of Purified Water, then add Purified Water to make 1000 mL.

Meets the requirement for Identification.

Iodine Tincture USP—Preserve in tight containers. Contains, in each 100 mL, not less than 1.8 grams and not more than 2.2 grams of iodine, and not less than 2.1 grams and not more than 2.6 grams of sodium iodide.

Iodine Tincture may be prepared by dissolving 20 grams of iodine and 24 grams of Sodium Iodide in 500 mL of Alcohol and then adding Purified Water to make the product measure 1000 mL.

Meets the requirements for Identification and Alcohol content (44.0–50.0%).

STRONG IODINE

Chemical group: Iodine and inorganic iodides.

Chemical name:
Iodine—Iodine.
Potassium iodide—Potassium iodide.

Molecular formula:
Iodine—I.
Potassium Iodide—KI.

Molecular weight:
Iodine—126.90.
Potassium Iodide—166.00.

Description:
Iodine USP—Heavy, grayish black plates or granules, having a metallic luster and a characteristic odor.
Strong Iodine Solution USP—Transparent liquid having a deep brown color and having the odor of iodine.
Potassium Iodide USP—Hexahedral crystals, either transparent and colorless or somewhat opaque and white, or a white, granular powder. Is slightly hygroscopic. Its solutions are neutral or alkaline to litmus.

Solubility:
Iodine USP—Very slightly soluble in water; freely soluble in carbon disulfide, in chloroform, in carbon tetrachloride, and in ether; soluble in alcohol and in solutions of iodides; sparingly soluble in glycerin.
Potassium Iodide USP—Very soluble in water and even more soluble in boiling water; freely soluble in glycerin; soluble in alcohol.

USP requirements:
Strong Iodine Solution USP—Preserve in tight containers, preferably at a temperature not exceeding 35 °C. Contains, in each 100 mL, not less than 4.5 grams and not more than 5.5 grams of iodine, and not less than 9.5 grams and not more than 10.5 grams of potassium iodide.
Strong Iodine Solution may be prepared by dissolving 50 grams of Iodine and 100 grams of Potassium Iodide in 100 mL of Purified Water, then adding Purified Water to make the product measure 1000 mL.

Meets the requirement for Identification.

Strong Iodine Tincture USP—Preserve in tight, light-resistant containers. Contains, in each 100 mL, not less than 6.8 grams and not more than 7.5 grams of iodine, and not less than 4.7 grams and not more than 5.5 grams of potassium iodide.

Strong Iodine Tincture may be prepared by dissolving 50 grams of Potassium Iodide in 50 mL of Purified Water,

adding 70 grams of Iodine, and agitating until solution is effected, and then adding Alcohol to make the product measure 1000 mL.

Meets the requirements for Identification and Alcohol content (82.5–88.5%).

IODIPAMIDE

Chemical group: Ionic, dimeric, triiodinated benzoic acid derivative.

Chemical name: Iodipamide meglumine—Benzoic acid, 3,3′-[(1,6-dioxo-1,6-hexanediyl)diimino]bis[2,4,6-triiodo-, compd. with 1-deoxy-1-(methylamino)-D-glucitol (1:2).

Molecular formula: Iodipamide meglumine—$C_{20}H_{14}I_6N_2O_6 \cdot 2C_7H_{17}NO_5$.

Molecular weight: Iodipamide meglumine—1530.20.

Description:
Iodipamide USP—White, practically odorless, crystalline powder.
Iodipamide Meglumine Injection USP—Clear, colorless to pale yellow, slightly viscous liquid.

Solubility: Iodipamide USP—Very slightly soluble in water, in chloroform, and in ether; slightly soluble in alcohol.

USP requirements: Iodipamide Meglumine Injection USP—Preserve in single-dose containers, preferably of Type I or Type III glass, protected from light. A sterile solution of Iodipamide in Water for Injection, prepared with the aid of Meglumine. Label containers of Injection intended for intravascular injection to direct the user to discard any unused portion remaining in the container. Label containers of Injection intended for other than intravascular injection to show that the contents are not intended for intravascular injection. Contains the labeled amount, within ± 5%. Iodipamide Meglumine Injection intended for intravascular use contains no antimicrobial agents. Meets the requirements for Identification, Bacterial endotoxins, pH (6.5–7.7), Free aromatic amine, and Meglumine content (24.2–26.8% of the labeled amount of iodipamide meglumine), for the tests for Iodine and iodide and Heavy metals under Diatrizoate Meglumine Injection, and for Injections.

IODOHIPPURATE SODIUM I 123

Chemical name: Glycine, N-[2-(iodo-^{123}I)benzoyl]-, monosodium salt.

Molecular formula: $C_9H_7{}^{123}INNaO_3$.

USP requirements: Iodohippurate Sodium I 123 Injection USP—Preserve in single-dose or in multiple-dose containers that are adequately shielded. A sterile, aqueous solution containing o-iodohippurate sodium in which a portion of the molecules contain radioactive iodine (^{123}I) in the molecular structure. Label it to include the following, in addition to the information specified for Labeling under Injections: the time and date of calibration; the amount of I 123 as iodohippurate sodium expressed as total megabecquerels (or microcuries or millicuries) per mL at the time of calibration; the name and quantity of any added preservative or stabilizer; the expiration time; and the statement, "Caution—Radioactive Material." The labeling indicates that in making dosage calculations, correction is to be made for radioactive decay, and also indicates that the radioactive half-life of I 123 is 13.2 hours. Contains the labeled amount of I 123, within ± 10%, as iodohippurate sodium expressed in megabecquerels (or microcuries or millicuries) per mL at the time indicated in the labeling. Contains the labeled amount of *o*-iodohippuric acid, within ±10%. Other chemical forms of radioactivity do not exceed 3.0% of total radioactivity. Meets the requirements for Radionuclide identification, Bacterial endotoxins, pH (7.0–8.5), Radionuclidic purity (not less than 85%), Radiochemical purity, Biological distribution, and Injections (except that the Injection may be distributed or dispensed prior to completion of the test for Sterility, the latter test being started on the day of final manufacture, and except that it is not subject to the recommendation on Volume in Container).

IODOHIPPURATE SODIUM I 131

Chemical name: Glycine, *N*-[2-(iodo-^{131}*I*)benzoyl]-, monosodium salt.

Molecular formula: $C_9H_7^{131}INNaO_3$.

Description: Iodohippurate Sodium 131 USP—Clear, colorless solution. Upon standing, both the Injection and the glass container may darken as a result of the effects of the radiation.

USP requirements: Iodohippurate Sodium I 131 Injection USP— Preserve in single-dose or in multiple-dose containers. A sterile solution containing *o*-iodohippurate sodium in which a portion of the molecules contain radioactive iodine (^{131}I) in the molecular structure. Label it to include the following, in addition to the information specified for Labeling under Injections: the time and date of calibration; the amount of ^{131}I as iodohippurate sodium expressed as total megabecquerels (or microcuries or millicuries) and as megabecquerels (or microcuries or millicuries) per mL at the time of calibration; the expiration date; and the statement, "Caution—Radioactive Material." The labeling indicates that in making dosage calculations, correction is to be made for radioactive decay, and also indicates that the radioactive half-life of ^{131}I is 8.08 days. Contains the labeled amount of ^{131}I, within ±10%, as iodohippurate sodium expressed in megabecquerels (or microcuries or millicuries) per mL at the time indicated in the labeling. Other chemical forms of radioactivity do not exceed 3.0% of the total radioactivity. Meets the requirements for Radionuclide identification, Bacterial endotoxins, pH (7.0–8.5), Radiochemical purity, and Injections (except that the Injection may be distributed or dispensed prior to the completion of the test for Sterility, the latter test being started on the day of final manufacture and except that it is not subject to the recommendation on Volume in Container).

IODOQUINOL

Chemical group: Halogenated 8-hydroxyquinoline.

Chemical name: 8-Quinolinol, 5,7-diiodo-.

Molecular formula: $C_9H_5I_2NO$.

Molecular weight: 396.95.

Description: Iodoquinol USP—Light yellowish to tan, microcrystalline powder not readily wetted by water. Is odorless or has a faint odor; is stable in air. Melts with decomposition.

Solubility: Iodoquinol USP—Practically insoluble in water; sparingly soluble in alcohol and in ether.

USP requirements: Iodoquinol Tablets USP—Preserve in well-closed containers. Contain the labeled amount, within ±5%. Meet the requirements for Identification, Disintegration (1 hour), Uniformity of dosage units, and Soluble iodides.

IOFETAMINE I 123

Chemical name: Iofetamine hydrochloride I 123—Benzeneethanamine, 4-(iodo-^{123}*I*)-alpha-methyl-*N*-(1-methylethyl)-, hydrochloride, (±)-.

Molecular formula: Iofetamine hydrochloride I 123—$C_{12}H_{18}$-^{123}IN·HCl.

Molecular weight: Iofetamine hydrochloride I 123—335.74.

Description: Iofetamine hydrochloride I 123—Melting point 156–158 °C.

USP requirements: Iofetamine Hydrochloride I 123 Injection— Not in USP.

IOHEXOL

Chemical group: Non-ionic, monomeric, triiodinated benzoic acid derivative.

Chemical name: 1,3-Benzenedicarboxamide, 5-[acetyl(2,3-dihydroxypropyl)amino]-*N,N'*-bis(2,3-dihydroxypropyl)-2,4,6-triiodo.

Molecular formula: $C_{19}H_{26}I_3N_3O_9$.

Molecular weight: 821.14.

Description: Iohexol injection—Colorless to pale yellow solution.

Solubility: Soluble in water.

Other characteristics: Low osmolality. The osmolality of iohexol injection with iodine concentrations of 180, 240, 300, and 350 mg per mL is 408, 520, 672, and 844 mOsmol per kg of water, respectively.

USP requirements: Iohexol Injection—Not in USP.

IOPAMIDOL

Chemical group: A nonionic contrast medium.

Chemical name: 1,3-Benzenedicarboxamide, *N,N'*-bis[2-hydroxy-1-(hydroxymethyl)ethyl]-5-[(2-hydroxy-1-oxopropyl)amino]-2,4,6-triiodo-, (*S*)-.

Molecular formula: $C_{17}H_{22}I_3N_3O_8$.

Molecular weight: 777.09.

Description:
Iopamidol USP—Practically odorless, white to off-white powder.
Iopamidol injection—Clear, colorless to pale yellow.

Solubility: Iopamidol USP—Very soluble in water; sparingly soluble in methanol; practically insoluble in alcohol and in chloroform.

Other characteristics: Low osmolality. The osmolality of iopamidol injection with iodine concentrations of 200, 300, and 370 mg per mL is 413, 616, and 796 mOsmol per kg of water, respectively.

USP requirements: Iopamidol Injection USP—Preserve Injection intended for intravascular or intrathecal use in single-dose containers, preferably of Type I glass, and protected from light. A sterile solution of Iopamidol in Water for Injection. Label containers of Injection to direct the user to discard any unused portion remaining in the container and to check for the presence of particulate matter before using. Contains the labeled amount, within ±5%. Iopamidol Injection intended for intravascular or intrathecal use contains no antimicrobial agents. Meets the requirements for Identification, Bacterial endotoxins, pH (6.5–7.5), Free aromatic amine, Free iodine, Free iodide (not more than 0.04 mg of iodide per mL), and Injections.

IOPANOIC ACID

Chemical group: Ionic, triiodinated benzoic acid derivative.

Chemical name: Benzenepropanoic acid, 3-amino-alpha-ethyl-2,4,6-triiodo-.

Molecular formula: $C_{11}H_{12}I_3NO_2$.

Molecular weight: 570.93.

Description: Iopanoic Acid USP—Cream-colored powder. Has a faint, characteristic odor. Affected by light.

pKa: 4.8.

Solubility: Iopanoic Acid USP—Insoluble in water; soluble in alcohol, in chloroform, and in ether; soluble in solutions of alkali hydroxides and carbonates.

USP requirements: Iopanoic Acid Tablets USP—Preserve in tight, light-resistant containers. Contain the labeled amount, within ±5%. Meet the requirements for Identification, Disintegration (30 minutes), Uniformity of dosage units, and Halide ions.

IOPHENDYLATE

Chemical group: Ionic organic iodine compound.

Chemical name: Benzenedecanoic acid, iodo-iota-methyl-, ethyl ester.

Molecular formula: $C_{19}H_{29}IO_2$.

Molecular weight: 416.34.

Description:
Iophendylate USP—Colorless to pale yellow, viscous liquid, the color darkening on long exposure to air. Is odorless or has a faint ethereal odor.
Iophendylate Injection USP—Colorless to pale yellow, viscous liquid, the color darkening on long exposure to air. Is odorless or has a faintly ethereal odor.

Solubility:
Iophendylate USP—Very slightly soluble in water; freely soluble in alcohol, in chloroform, and in ether.
Iophendylate Injection USP—Very slightly soluble in water; freely soluble in alcohol, in chloroform, and in ether.

Other characteristics: Iophendylate injection—Immiscible with CSF; high specific gravity in relation to that of CSF.

USP requirements: Iophendylate Injection USP—Preserve in single-dose containers, preferably of Type I glass, protected from light. It is sterile Iophendylate. Contains the labeled amount, within ±2%. Meets the requirements for Bacterial endotoxins, for Identification, Specific gravity (1.248–1.257), Refractive index (1.524–1.526), Residue on ignition (not more than 0.1%), Free acids (not more than 0.3% as iodophenylundecanoic acid), Free iodine (absorbance not more than 7.5 ppm), and Saponification value (132–142) under Iophendylate, and for Injections.

IOTHALAMATE

Chemical group: Ionic, monomeric, triiodinated benzoic acid derivative.

Chemical name:
Iothalamate meglumine—Benzoic acid, 3-(acetylamino)-2,4,6-triiodo-5-[(methylamino)carbonyl]-, compd. with 1-deoxy-1-(methylamino)-D-glucitol (1:1).

Iothalamate sodium—Benzoic acid, 3-(acetylamino)-2,4,6-triiodo-5-[(methylamino)carbonyl]-, monosodium salt.

Molecular formula:
Iothalamate meglumine—$C_{11}H_9I_3N_2O_4 \cdot C_7H_{17}NO_5$.
Iothalamate sodium—$C_{11}H_8I_3N_2NaO_4$.

Molecular weight:
Iothalamate meglumine—809.13.
Iothalamate sodium—635.90.

Description:
Iothalamate Meglumine Injection USP—Clear, colorless to pale yellow, slightly viscous liquid.
Iothalamate Meglumine and Iothalamate Sodium Injection USP—Clear, colorless to pale yellow, slightly viscous liquid.
Iothalamate Sodium Injection USP—Clear, colorless to pale yellow, slightly viscous liquid.

USP requirements:
Iothalamate Meglumine Injection USP—Preserve in single-dose containers, preferably of Type I glass, protected from light. A sterile solution of Iothalamic Acid in Water for Injection, prepared with the aid of Meglumine. Label containers of Injection intended for intravascular injection to direct the user to discard any unused portion remaining in the container. Label containers of Injection intended for other than intravascular injection to show that the contents are not intended for intravascular injection. Contains the labeled amount, within ±5%. Iothalamate Meglumine Injection intended for intravascular use contains no antimicrobial agents. Meets the requirements for Identification, Bacterial endotoxins, pH (6.5–7.7), Free aromatic amine, Iodine and iodide, Heavy metals (not more than 0.002%), Meglumine content (22.9% to 25.3% of the labeled amount of iothalamate meglumine), and Injections.
Iothalamate Meglumine and Iothalamate Sodium Injection USP—Preserve in single-dose containers, preferably of Type I glass, protected from light. A sterile solution of Iothalamic Acid in Water for Injection, prepared with the aid of Meglumine and Sodium Hydroxide. Label containers of Injection intended for intravascular injection to direct the user to discard any unused portion remaining in the container. Label containers of Injection intended for other than intravascular injection to show that the contents are not intended for intravascular injection. Contains the labeled amounts of iothalamate meglumine and iothalamate sodium, within ±5%. Iothalamate Meglumine and Iothalamate Sodium Injection intended for intravascular use contains no antimicrobial agents. Meets the requirements for Identification, Bacterial endotoxins, pH (6.5–7.7), Free aromatic amine, Iodine and iodide (not more than 0.02% iodide), Heavy metals (not more than 0.002%), and Injections.
Iothalamate Sodium Injection USP—Preserve in single-dose containers, preferably of Type I glass, protected from light. A sterile solution of Iothalamic Acid in Water for Injection prepared with the aid of Sodium Hydroxide. Label containers of the Injection intended for intravascular injection to direct the user to discard any unused portion remaining in the container. Label containers of the Injection intended for other than intravascular injection to show that the contents are not intended for intravascular injection. Contains the labeled amount, within ±5%. Iothalamate Sodium Injection intended for intravascular use contains no antimicrobial agents. Meets the requirements for Identification, Bacterial endotoxins, pH (6.5–7.7), Free aromatic amine, Iodine and iodide (not more than 0.02% of iodide), Heavy metals (not more than 0.002%), and Injections.

IOVERSOL

Chemical name: 1,3-Benzenedicarboxamide, *N,N'*-bis(2,3-dihydroxypropyl)-5-[(hydroxyacetyl)(2-hydroxyethyl)amino]-2,4,6-triiodo-.

Molecular formula: $C_{18}H_{24}I_3N_3O_9$.

Molecular weight: 807.12.

USP requirements: Ioversol Injection—Not in USP.

IOXAGLATE

Chemical group: Ionic, dimeric, contrast agent; benzoic acid salt.

Chemical name:
Ioxaglate meglumine—Benzoic acid, 3-[[[[3-(acetylmethylamino)-2,4,6-triiodo-5-[(methylamino)carbonyl]benzoyl]amino]acetyl]amino]-5-[[(2-hydroxyethyl)amino]carbonyl]-2,4,6-triiodo-, compound with 1-deoxy-1-(methylamino)-D-glucitol (1:1).
Ioxaglate sodium—Benzoic acid, 3-[[[[3-(acetylmethylamino)-2,4,6-triiodo-5-[(methylamino)carbonyl]benzoyl]amino]acetyl]amino]-5-[[(2-hydroxyethyl)amino]carbonyl]-2,4,6-triiodo-, sodium salt.

Molecular formula:
Ioxaglate meglumine—$C_{24}H_{21}I_6N_5O_8 \cdot C_7H_{17}NO_5$.
Ioxaglate sodium—$C_{24}H_{20}I_6N_5NaO_8$.

Molecular weight:
Ioxaglate meglumine—1464.10.
Ioxaglate sodium—1290.87.

Solubility: Soluble in water.

USP requirements: Ioxaglate Meglumine and Ioxaglate Sodium Injection—Not in USP.

IPECAC

Description: Powdered Ipecac USP—Pale brown, weak yellow, or light olive-gray powder.

USP requirements: Ipecac Syrup USP—Preserve in tight containers, preferably at a temperature not exceeding 25 °C. Containers intended for sale to the public without prescription contain not more than 30 mL of Ipecac Syrup USP. Contains, in each 100 mL, not less than 123 mg and not more than 157 mg of the total ether-soluble alkaloids of ipecac. The content of emetine and cephaeline together is not less than 90.0% of the amount of the total ether-soluble alkaloids. The content of cephaeline varies from an amount equal to, to an amount not more than 2.5 times, the content of emetine.

Prepare Ipecac Syrup as follows: 70 grams of Powdered Ipecac, 100 mL of Glycerin, and a sufficient quantity of Syrup to make 1000 mL. Exhaust the powdered Ipecac by percolation, using a mixture of 3 volumes of alcohol and 1 volume of water as the menstruum, macerating for 72 hours, and percolating slowly. Reduce the entire percolate to a volume of 70 mL by evaporation at a temperature not exceeding 60 °C and preferably in vacuum, and add 140 mL of water. Allow the mixture to stand overnight, filter, and wash the residue on the filter with water. Evaporate the filtrate and washings to 40 mL, and to this add 2.5 mL of hydrochloric acid and 20 mL of alcohol, mix, and filter. Wash the filter with a mixture of 30 volumes of alcohol, 3.5 volumes of hydrochloric acid, and 66.5 volumes of water, using a volume sufficient to produce 70 mL of the filtrate. Add 100 mL of Glycerin and enough Syrup to make the product measure 1000 mL, and mix.

Meets the requirements for Microbial limits and Alcohol content (1.0–2.5%).

IPODATE

Chemical group: Triiodinated benzoic acid derivative.

Chemical name:
Ipodate calcium—Benzenepropanoic acid, 3-[[(dimethylamino)methylene]amino]-2,4,6-triiodo-, calcium salt.
Ipodate sodium—Benzenepropanoic acid, 3-[[(dimethylamino)methylene]amino]-2,4,6-triiodo-, sodium salt.

Molecular formula:
Ipodate calcium—$C_{24}H_{24}CaI_6N_4O_4$.
Ipodate sodium—$C_{12}H_{12}I_3N_2NaO_2$.

Molecular weight:
Ipodate calcium—1233.99.
Ipodate sodium—619.94.

Description:
Ipodate Calcium USP—White to off-white, odorless, fine, crystalline powder.
Ipodate Sodium USP—White to off-white, odorless, fine, crystalline powder.

Solubility:
Ipodate Calcium USP—Slightly soluble in water, in alcohol, in chloroform, and in methanol.
Ipodate Sodium USP—Freely soluble in water, in alcohol, and in methanol; very slightly soluble in chloroform.

USP requirements:
Ipodate Calcium for Oral Suspension USP—Preserve in well-closed containers. A dry mixture of Ipodate Calcium and one or more suitable suspending, dispersing, and flavoring agents. Contains the labeled amount, within ± 15%. Meets the requirements for Identification and Minimum fill.
Ipodate Sodium Capsules USP—Preserve in tight containers. Contain the labeled amount, within ± 10%. Meet the requirements for Identification and Uniformity of dosage units.

IPRATROPIUM

Source: A synthetic quaternary ammonium derivative of atropine.

Chemical name: Ipratropium bromide—8-Azoniabicyclo[3.2.1]octane, 3-(3-hydroxy-1-oxo-2-phenylpropoxy)-8-methyl-8-(1-methylethyl)-, bromide, monohydrate(*endo,-syn*)-, (±)-.

Molecular formula: Ipratropium bromide—$C_{20}H_{30}BrNO_3 \cdot H_2O$.

Molecular weight: Ipratropium bromide—430.38.

Description: Ipratropium bromide—A white, crystalline substance.

Solubility: Ipratropium bromide—Freely soluble in water and in lower alcohols; insoluble in lipophilic solvents such as chloroform, ether, and fluorocarbons. Has a low lipid solubility.

Other characteristics: Ipratropium bromide—Fairly stable in neutral solutions and in acid solutions; rapidly hydrolyzed in alkaline solutions.

USP requirements:
Ipratropium Bromide Inhalation Aerosol—Not in USP.
Ipratropium Bromide Nasal Inhalation—Not in USP.
Ipratropium Bromide Inhalation Solution—Not in USP.

IRON DEXTRAN

Chemical name: A complex of ferric oxyhydroxide and a low-molecular weight dextran derivative.

Description: Iron Dextran Injection USP—Dark brown, slightly viscous liquid.

USP requirements: Iron Dextran Injection USP—Preserve in single-dose or in multiple-dose containers, preferably of Type I or Type II glass. A sterile, colloidal solution of ferric hydroxide in complex with partially hydrolyzed Dextran of low molecular weight, in Water for Injection. Contains the labeled amount of iron, within ±5%. Meets the requirements for Identification, Pyrogen, Acute toxicity, Absorption from injection site, pH (5.2–6.5), Nonvolatile residue, Chloride content, Phenol content (not more than 0.5% as a preservative), and Injections.

IRON-POLYSACCHARIDE

Source: A complex of ferric iron and a low-molecular weight polysaccharide.

Description: An amorphous brown powder.

Solubility: Very soluble in water; insoluble in alcohol.

USP requirements:
Iron-Polysaccharide Capsules—Not in USP.
Iron-Polysaccharide Elixir—Not in USP.
Iron-Polysaccharide Tablets—Not in USP.

IRON SORBITEX

Description: Iron Sorbitex Injection USP—Clear liquid, having a dark brown color.

USP requirements: Iron Sorbitex Injection USP—Preserve in single-dose containers, preferably of Type I glass. A sterile solution of a complex of iron, Sorbitol, and Citric Acid that is stabilized with the aid of Dextrin and an excess of Sorbitol. Label it to indicate its expiration date, which is not more than 24 months after date of manufacture. Contains an amount of iron sorbitex equivalent to the labeled amount of iron, within −6% to +4%. Meets the requirements for Identification, Specific gravity (1.17–1.19 at 20 °C), Viscosity (8–13 centipoises, determined at 20 °C with a capillary tube viscometer), Bacterial endotoxins, pH (7.2–7.9), Ferrous iron (not more than 8.5 mg per mL), and Injections.

ISOBUTANE

Molecular formula: C_4H_{10}.

Molecular weight: 58.12.

Description: Isobutane NF—Colorless, flammable gas (boiling temperature is about −11 °C). Vapor pressure at 21 °C is about 2950 mm of mercury (31 psig).
NF category: Aerosol propellant.

NF requirements: Isobutane NF—Preserve in tight cylinders and prevent exposure to excessive heat. Contains not less than 95.0% of isobutane. Meets the requirements for Identification, Water (not more than 0.001%), High-boiling residues (not more than 5 ppm), Acidity of residue, and Sulfur compounds.
Caution: Isobutane is highly flammable and explosive.

ISOCARBOXAZID

Chemical group: Hydrazine derivative, structurally similar to amphetamine.

Chemical name: 3-Isoxazolecarboxylic acid, 5-methyl-, 2-(phenylmethyl)hydrazide.

Molecular formula: $C_{12}H_{13}N_3O_2$.

Molecular weight: 231.25.

Description: Isocarboxazid USP—White, or practically white, crystalline powder, having a slight characteristic odor.

Solubility: Isocarboxazid USP—Slightly soluble in water; very soluble in chloroform; soluble in alcohol.

USP requirements: Isocarboxazid Tablets USP—Preserve in well-closed, light-resistant containers. Contain the labeled amount, within ±5%. Meet the requirements for Identification, Dissolution (80% in 45 minutes in 0.1 N hydrochloric acid in Apparatus 2 at 50 rpm), and Uniformity of dosage units.

ISOETHARINE

Chemical name:
Isoetharine hydrochloride—1,2-Benzenediol, 4-[1-hydroxy-2-[(1-methylethyl)amino]butyl]-, hydrochloride.
Isoetharine mesylate—1,2-Benzenediol, 4-[1-hydroxy-2-[(1-methylethyl)amino]butyl]-, methanesulfonate (salt).

Molecular formula:
Isoetharine hydrochloride—$C_{13}H_{21}NO_3 \cdot HCl$.
Isoetharine mesylate—$C_{13}H_{21}NO_3 \cdot CH_4O_3S$.

Molecular weight:
Isoetharine hydrochloride—275.77.
Isoetharine mesylate—335.41.

Description:
Isoetharine Inhalation Solution USP—Colorless or slightly yellow, slightly acid liquid, gradually turning dark on exposure to air and light.
Isoetharine Hydrochloride USP—White to off-white, odorless, crystalline solid. Melts between 196 and 208 °C, with decomposition.
Isoetharine Mesylate USP—White or practically white, odorless crystals.

Solubility:
Isoetharine Hydrochloride USP—Soluble in water; sparingly soluble in alcohol; practically insoluble in ether.
Isoetharine Mesylate USP—Freely soluble in water; soluble in alcohol; practically insoluble in acetone and in ether.

USP requirements:
Isoetharine Inhalation Solution USP—Preserve in small, well-filled, tight containers, protected from light. A solution of Isoetharine Hydrochloride in Purified Water. The label indicates that the Inhalation Solution is not to be used if its color is pinkish or darker than slightly yellow or if it contains a precipitate. Contains the labeled amount of isoetharine hydrochloride, within ±8%. Meets the requirements for Color and clarity, Identification and pH (2.5–5.5).
Isoetharine Mesylate Inhalation Aerosol USP—Preserve in small, nonreactive, light-resistant, aerosol containers equipped with metered-dose valves and provided with oral inhalation actuators. A solution of Isoetharine Mesylate in Alcohol in an inert propellant base. Contains the labeled amount within ±10%, and delivers the labeled dose per inhalation, within ±25%, through an oral inhalation

actuator. Meets the requirements for Identification, Alcohol content (25.9–35.0% [w/w]), and Unit spray content, and for Leak testing under Aerosols.

ISOFLURANE

Chemical name: Ethane, 2-chloro-2-(difluoromethoxy)-1,1,1-trifluoro-.

Molecular formula: $C_3H_2ClF_5O$.

Molecular weight: 184.49.

Description: Isoflurane USP—Clear, colorless, volatile liquid, having a slight odor. Boils at about 49 °C.

Solubility: Isoflurane USP—Insoluble in water; miscible with common organic solvents and with fats and oils.

Other characteristics:
Blood-to-Gas partition coefficient at 37 °C—1.43.
Oil-to-Gas partition coefficient at 37 °C—90.8.

USP requirements: Isoflurane USP—Preserve in tight, light-resistant containers. Contains not less than 99.0% and not more than 101.0% of isoflurane, calculated on the anhydrous basis. Meets the requirements for Identification, Refractive index (1.2990–1.3005 at 20 °C), Water (not more than 0.14%), Chloride (not more than 0.001%), Nonvolatile residue (not more than 0.02%), and Fluoride (not more than 0.001%).

ISOFLUROPHATE

Chemical name: Phosphorofluoridic acid, bis(1-methylethyl) ester.

Molecular formula: $C_6H_{14}FO_3P$.

Molecular weight: 184.15.

Description: Isoflurophate USP—Clear, colorless or faintly yellow, liquid. Its vapor is extremely irritating to the eye and mucous membranes. Is decomposed by moisture, with the formation of hydrogen fluoride. Specific gravity is about 1.05.

Solubility: Isoflurophate USP—Sparingly soluble in water; soluble in alcohol and in vegetable oils.

USP requirements: Isoflurophate Ophthalmic Ointment USP—Preserve in collapsible ophthalmic ointment tubes. Label it to indicate the expiration date, which is not later than 2 years after date of manufacture. Contains not less than 0.0225% and not more than 0.0275% of isoflurophate, in a suitable anhydrous ointment base. It is sterile. Meets the requirements for Identification, Irritation, Sterility, Minimum fill, Water (not more than 0.03%), and Metal particles.

ISOMETHEPTENE, DICHLORALPHENAZONE, AND ACETAMINOPHEN

Chemical name:
Isometheptene—N,1,5-Trimethyl-4-hexenylamine.
Dichloralphenazone—1,2-Dihydro-1,5-dimethyl-2-phenyl-3H-pyrazol-3-one compd. with 2,2,2-trichloro-1,1-ethanediol(1:2).
Acetaminophen—Acetamide, N-(4-hydroxyphenyl)-.

Molecular formula:
Isometheptene mucate—$(C_9H_{19}N)_2 \cdot C_6H_{10}O_8$.
Dichloralphenazone—$C_{15}H_{18}Cl_6N_2O_5$.
Acetaminophen—$C_8H_9NO_2$.

Molecular weight:
Isometheptene mucate—492.7.
Dichloralphenazone—519.04.
Acetaminophen—151.16.

Description:
Isometheptene mucate—White crystalline powder having a characteristic aromatic odor.
Dichloralphenazone—White, microcrystalline powder, with a slight odor characteristic of chloral hydrate. Melting point 64–67 °C.
Acetaminophen USP—White, odorless, crystalline powder.

Solubility:
Isometheptene mucate—Freely soluble in water; solubility in alcohol about 5 grams/100 mL; almost insoluble in ether and in chloroform.
Dichloralphenazone—Soluble 1 in 10 of water, 1 in 1 of alcohol, and 1 in 2 of chloroform; soluble in dilute acids.
Acetaminophen USP—Soluble in boiling water and in 1 N sodium hydroxide; freely soluble in alcohol.

USP requirements: Isometheptene Mucate, Dichloralphenazone, and Acetaminophen Capsules—Not in USP.

ISONIAZID

Chemical group: Hydrazide derivative of isonicotinic acid.

Chemical name: 4-Pyridinecarboxylic acid, hydrazide.

Molecular formula: $C_6H_7N_3O$.

Molecular weight: 137.14.

Description:
Isoniazid USP—Colorless or white crystals or white, crystalline powder. Is odorless and is slowly affected by exposure to air and to light.
Isoniazid Injection USP—Clear, colorless to faintly greenish yellow liquid. Gradually darkens on exposure to air and to light. Tends to crystallize at low temperatures.

Solubility: Isoniazid USP—Freely soluble in water; sparingly soluble in alcohol; slightly soluble in chloroform and in ether.

USP requirements:
Isoniazid Injection USP—Preserve in single-dose or in multiple-dose containers, preferably of Type I glass, protected from light. A sterile solution of Isoniazid in Water for Injection. Its package label states that if crystallization has occurred, the Injection should be warmed to redissolve the crystals prior to use. Contains the labeled amount, within ± 10%. Meets the requirements for Identification, Bacterial endotoxins, pH (6.0–7.0), and for Injections.
Isoniazid Syrup USP—Preserve in tight, light-resistant containers. Contains, in each 100 mL, not less than 0.93 gram and not more than 1.10 grams of isoniazid. Meets the requirement for Identification.
Isoniazid Tablets USP—Preserve in well-closed, light-resistant containers. Contain the labeled amount, within ± 10%. Meet the requirements for Identification, Dissolution (80% in 45 minutes in 0.1 N hydrochloric acid in Apparatus 1 at 100 rpm), and Uniformity of dosage units.

ISOPROPAMIDE

Source: Synthetic amine compound.

Chemical group: Quaternary ammonium compound, synthetic.

Chemical name: Isopropamide iodide—Benzenepropanaminium, gamma-(aminocarbonyl)-N-methyl-N,N-bis(1-methylethyl)-gamma-phenyl-, iodide.

Molecular formula: Isopropamide iodide—$C_{23}H_{33}IN_2O$.

Molecular weight: Isopropamide iodide—480.43.

Description: Isopropamide Iodide USP—White to pale yellow, crystalline powder.

Solubility: Isopropamide Iodide USP—Sparingly soluble in water; freely soluble in chloroform and in alcohol; very slightly soluble in ether.

USP requirements: Isopropamide Iodide Tablets USP—Preserve in well-closed containers. Contain an amount of isopropamide iodide equivalent to the labeled amount of isopropamide, within ±7%. Meet the requirements for Identification, Dissolution (70% in 60 minutes in water in Apparatus 2 at 100 rpm), and Uniformity of dosage units.

ISOPROPYL ALCOHOL

Chemical name: 2-Propanol.

Molecular formula: C_3H_8O.

Molecular weight: 60.10.

Description: Isopropyl Alcohol USP—Transparent, colorless, mobile, volatile liquid, having a characteristic odor. Is flammable.
NF category: Solvent.

Solubility: Isopropyl Alcohol USP—Miscible with water, with alcohol, with ether, and with chloroform.

USP requirements: Isopropyl Alcohol USP—Preserve in tight containers, remote from heat. Contains not less than 99.0% of isopropyl alcohol. Meets the requirements for Identification, Specific gravity (0.783–0.787), Refractive index (1.376–1.378 at 20 °C), Acidity, and Nonvolatile residue (not more than 0.005%).

AZEOTROPIC ISOPROPYL ALCOHOL

Description: Azeotropic Isopropyl Alcohol USP—Transparent, colorless, mobile, volatile liquid, having a characteristic odor. Is flammable.

Solubility: Azeotropic Isopropyl Alcohol USP—Miscible with water, with alcohol, with ether, and with chloroform.

USP requirements: Azeotropic Isopropyl Alcohol USP—Preserve in tight containers, remote from heat. Contains not less than 91.0% and not more than 93.0% of isopropyl alcohol, by volume, the remainder consisting of water. Meets the requirements for Identification, Specific gravity (0.815–0.810, indicating 91.0–93.0% by volume of isopropyl alcohol), Refractive index (1.376–1.378 at 20 °C), Acidity, Nonvolatile residue (not more than 0.005%), and Volatile impurities.

ISOPROPYL MYRISTATE

Chemical name: Tetradecanoic acid, 1-methylethyl ester.

Molecular formula: $C_{17}H_{34}O_2$.

Molecular weight: 270.45.

Description: Isopropyl Myristate NF—Clear, practically colorless, oily liquid. It is practically odorless and congeals at about 5 °C.
NF category: Oleaginous vehicle.

Solubility: Isopropyl Myristate NF—Insoluble in water, in glycerin, and in propylene glycol; freely soluble in 90% alcohol; miscible with most organic solvents and with fixed oils.

NF requirements: Isopropyl Myristate NF—Preserve in tight, light-resistant containers. Consists of esters of isopropyl alcohol and saturated high molecular weight fatty acids, principally myristic acid. Contains not less than 90.0% of isopropyl myristate. Meets the requirements for Identification, Specific gravity (0.846–0.854), Refractive index (1.432–1.436 at 20 °C), Residue on ignition (not more than 0.1%), Acid value (not more than 1), Saponification value (202–212), and Iodine value (not more than 1).

ISOPROPYL PALMITATE

Chemical name: Hexadecanoic acid, 1-methylethyl ester.

Molecular formula: $C_{19}H_{38}O_2$.

Molecular weight: 298.51.

Description: Isopropyl Palmitate NF—Colorless, mobile liquid having a very slight odor.
NF category: Oleaginous vehicle.

Solubility: Isopropyl Palmitate NF—Soluble in acetone, in castor oil, in chloroform, in cottonseed oil, in ethyl acetate, in alcohol, and in mineral oil; insoluble in water, in glycerin, and in propylene glycol.

NF requirements: Isopropyl Palmitate NF—Preserve in tight, light-resistant containers. Consists of esters of isopropyl alcohol and saturated high molecular weight fatty acids. Contains not less than 90.0% of isopropyl palmitate. Meets the requirements for Identification, Specific gravity (0.850–0.855), Refractive index (1.435–1.438), Residue on ignition (not more than 0.1%), Acid value (not more than 1), Iodine value (not more than 1), and Saponification value (183–193).

ISOPROPYL RUBBING ALCOHOL

USP requirements: Isopropyl Rubbing Alcohol USP—Preserve in tight containers, remote from heat. Label it to indicate that it is flammable. Contains not less than 68.0% and not more than 72.0% of isopropyl alcohol, by volume, the remainder consisting of water, with or without suitable stabilizers, perfume oils, and color additives certified by the U.S. Food and Drug Administration for use in drugs. Meets the requirements for Specific gravity (0.872–0.883 at 20 °C), Acidity, and Nonvolatile residue (not more than 0.01%).

ISOPROTERENOL

Chemical name:
Isoproterenol hydrochloride—1,2-Benzenediol, 4-[1-hydroxy-2-[(1-methylethyl)amino]ethyl]-, hydrochloride.
Isoproterenol sulfate—1,2-Benzenediol, 4-[1-hydroxy-2-[(methylethyl)amino]ethyl]-, sulfate (2:1) (salt), dihydrate.

Molecular formula:
Isoproterenol hydrochloride—$C_{11}H_{17}NO_3 \cdot HCl$.
Isoproterenol sulfate—$(C_{11}H_{17}NO_3)_2 \cdot H_2SO_4 \cdot 2H_2O$.

Molecular weight:
Isoproterenol hydrochloride—247.72.
Isoproterenol sulfate—556.62.

Description:
Isoproterenol Inhalation Solution USP—Colorless or practically colorless, slightly acid liquid, gradually turning dark on exposure to air and to light.
Isoproterenol Hydrochloride USP—White to practically white, odorless, crystalline powder. Gradually darkens on exposure to air and to light. Its solutions become pink to

brownish pink on standing exposed to air, and almost immediately so when rendered alkaline. Its solution (1 in 100) has a pH of about 5.

Isoproterenol Hydrochloride Injection USP—Colorless or practically colorless liquid, gradually turning dark on exposure to air and to light.

Isoproterenol Sulfate USP—White to practically white, odorless, crystalline powder. It gradually darkens on exposure to air and to light. Its solutions become pink to brownish pink on standing exposed to air, doing so almost immediately when rendered alkaline. A solution (1 in 100) has a pH of about 5.

Solubility:

Isoproterenol Hydrochloride USP—Freely soluble in water; sparingly soluble in alcohol and less soluble in dehydrated alcohol; insoluble in chloroform and in ether.

Isoproterenol Sulfate USP—Freely soluble in water; very slightly soluble in alcohol and in ether.

USP requirements:

Isoproterenol Inhalation Solution USP—Preserve in small, well-filled, tight containers, protected from light. Label it to indicate that the Inhalation Solution is not to be used if its color is pinkish or darker than slightly yellow or if it contains a precipitate. A solution of Isoproterenol Hydrochloride in Purified Water. It may contain Sodium Chloride. Contains the labeled amount of isoproterenol hydrochloride, within −10% to +15%. Meets the requirements for Color and clarity, Identification and pH (2.5–5.5).

Isoproterenol Hydrochloride Inhalation Aerosol USP—Preserve in small, nonreactive, light-resistant aerosol containers equipped with metered-dose valves and provided with oral inhalation actuators. A solution of Isoproterenol Hydrochloride in Alcohol in an inert propellant base. Contains the labeled amount within −10% to +15%, and delivers the labeled dose per inhalation, within ±25%, through an oral inhalation actuator. Meets the requirements for Identification, Alcohol content (28.5–38.5% [w/w]), and Unit spray content, and for Leak testing under Aerosols.

Isoproterenol Hydrochloride Injection USP—Preserve in single-dose containers, preferably of Type I glass, protected from light. Label it to indicate that the Injection is not to be used if its color is pinkish or darker than slightly yellow or if it contains a precipitate. A sterile solution of Isoproterenol Hydrochloride in Water for Injection. Contains the labeled amount, within −10% to +15%. Meets the requirements for Color and clarity, Identification, pH (2.5–4.5), Particulate matter, and Injections.

Isoproterenol Hydrochloride Tablets USP—Preserve in well-closed, light-resistant containers. Contain the labeled amount, within ±7%. Meet the requirements for Identification, Dissolution (75% in 45 minutes in water in Apparatus 2 at 50 rpm), and Uniformity of dosage units.

Isoproterenol Sulfate Inhalation Aerosol USP—Preserve in small, nonreactive, light-resistant aerosol containers equipped with metered-dose valves and provided with oral inhalation actuators. A suspension of microfine Isoproterenol Sulfate in fluorochlorohydrocarbon propellants in a pressurized container. Contains the labeled amount within ±10%, and delivers the labeled dose per inhalation, within ±25%, through an oral inhalation actuator. Meets the requirements for Identification, Microbial limits, Unit spray content, and Particle size, and for Leak testing under Aerosols.

Isoproterenol Sulfate Inhalation Solution USP—Store in small, well-filled, tight containers, protected from light. A solution of Isoproterenol Sulfate in Purified Water.

Label it to indicate that the Inhalation Solution is not to be used if its color is pinkish or darker than slightly yellow or if it contains a precipitate. Contains the labeled amount, within −10% to +15%. Meets the requirements for Color and clarity and Identification.

ISOPROTERENOL AND PHENYLEPHRINE

Chemical name:

Isoproterenol hydrochloride—1,2-Benzenediol, 4-[1-hydroxy-2-[(1-methylethyl)amino]ethyl]-, hydrochloride.

Phenylephrine hydrochloride—Benzenemethanol, 3-hydroxy-alpha-[(methylamino)methyl]-, hydrochloride.

Molecular formula:

Isoproterenol hydrochloride—$C_{11}H_{17}NO_3 \cdot HCl$.

Phenylephrine bitartrate—$C_9H_{13}NO_2 \cdot C_4H_6O_6$.

Phenylephrine hydrochloride—$C_9H_{13}NO_2 \cdot HCl$.

Molecular weight:

Isoproterenol hydrochloride—247.72.

Phenylephrine bitartrate—317.29.

Phenylephrine hydrochloride—203.67.

Description:

Isoproterenol Hydrochloride USP—White to practically white, odorless, crystalline powder. Gradually darkens on exposure to air and to light. Its solutions become pink to brownish pink on standing exposed to air, and almost immediately so when rendered alkaline. Its solution (1 in 100) has a pH of about 5.

Phenylephrine bitartrate—White, crystalline powder.

Phenylephrine Hydrochloride USP—White or practically white, odorless crystals.

Solubility:

Isoproterenol Hydrochloride USP—Freely soluble in water; sparingly soluble in alcohol and less soluble in dehydrated alcohol; insoluble in chloroform and in ether.

Phenylephrine bitartrate—Soluble in water; insoluble in alcohol.

Phenylephrine Hydrochloride USP—Freely soluble in water and in alcohol.

USP requirements:

Isoproterenol Hydrochloride and Phenylephrine Bitartrate Inhalation Aerosol USP—Preserve in small, non-reactive, light-resistant aerosol containers equipped with metered-dose valves and provided with oral inhalation actuators. A suspension of microfine Isoproterenol Hydrochloride and Phenylephrine Bitartrate in suitable propellants in a pressurized container. Contains the labeled amounts of isoproterenol hydrochloride and phenylephrine bitartrate within ±10%, and delivers the labeled dose per inhalation, within ±25%, through an oral inhalation actuator. Meets the requirements for Identification, Unit spray content, and Particle size, and for Leak testing under Aerosols.

Isoproterenol Hydrochloride and Phenylephrine Hydrochloride Inhalation Aerosol—Not in USP.

ISOSORBIDE

Chemical name:

Isosorbide—D-Glucitol, 1,4:3,6-dianhydro.

Isosorbide dinitrate—D-Glucitol, 1,4:3,6-dianhydro-, dinitrate.

Isosorbide mononitrate—D-Glucitol, 1,4:3,6-dianhydro-, 5-nitrate.

Molecular formula:

Isosorbide—$C_6H_{10}O_4$.

Isosorbide dinitrate—$C_6H_8N_2O_8$.
Isosorbide mononitrate—$C_6H_9NO_6$.

Molecular weight:
Isosorbide—146.14.
Isosorbide dinitrate—236.14.
Isosorbide mononitrate—191.14.

Description:
Isosorbide Concentrate USP—Colorless to slightly yellow liquid.
Diluted Isosorbide Dinitrate USP—Ivory-white, odorless powder. (Note: Undiluted isosorbide dinitrate occurs as white, crystalline rosettes.)

Solubility:
Isosorbide Concentrate USP—Soluble in water and in alcohol.
Undiluted isosorbide dinitrate—Very slightly soluble in water; very soluble in acetone; freely soluble in chloroform; sparingly soluble in alcohol.

USP requirements:
Isosorbide Oral Solution USP—Preserve in tight containers. Contains the labeled amount, within ±10%. Meets the requirements for Identification and pH (3.2–3.8).
Isosorbide Dinitrate Capsules—Not in USP.
Isosorbide Dinitrate Extended-release Capsules USP—Preserve in well-closed containers. Contain the labeled amount, within ±10%. Meet the requirements for Identification and Uniformity of dosage units.
Isosorbide Dinitrate Tablets USP—Preserve in well-closed containers. Contain the labeled amount, within ±10%. Meet the requirements for Identification, Dissolution (70% in 45 minutes in water in Apparatus 2 at 75 rpm), and Uniformity of dosage units.
Isosorbide Dinitrate Chewable Tablets USP—Preserve in well-closed containers. Contain the labeled amount, within ±10%. Meet the requirements for Identification and Uniformity of dosage units.
Isosorbide Dinitrate Extended-release Tablets USP—Preserve in well-closed containers. Contain the labeled amount, within ±10%. Meet the requirements for Identification and Uniformity of dosage units.
Isosorbide Dinitrate Sublingual Tablets USP—Preserve in well-closed containers. Contain the labeled amount, within ±10%. Meet the requirements for Identification, Disintegration (2 minutes), Dissolution (50% in 15 minutes and 70% in 30 minutes in water in Apparatus 2 at 50 rpm), and Uniformity of dosage units.
Isosorbide Mononitrate Tablets—Not in USP.

ISOTRETINOIN

Chemical group: Vitamin A derivative (retinoid).

Chemical name: Retinoic acid, 13-*cis*-.

Molecular formula: $C_{20}H_{28}O_2$.

Molecular weight: 300.44.

Description: Isotretinoin USP—Yellow crystals.

Solubility: Isotretinoin USP—Practically insoluble in water; soluble in chloroform; sparingly soluble in alcohol, in isopropyl alcohol, and in polyethylene glycol 400.

USP requirements: Isotretinoin Capsules—Not in USP.

ISOXSUPRINE

Chemical name: Isoxsuprine hydrochloride—Benzenemethanol, 4-hydroxy-alpha-[1-[(1-methyl-2-phenoxyethyl)amino]-ethyl]-, hydrochloride, stereoisomer.

Molecular formula: Isoxsuprine hydrochloride—$C_{18}H_{23}NO_3 \cdot$ HCl.

Molecular weight: Isoxsuprine hydrochloride—337.85.

Description: Isoxsuprine Hydrochloride USP—White, odorless, crystalline powder. Melts, with decomposition, at about 200 °C.

Solubility: Isoxsuprine Hydrochloride USP—Slightly soluble in water; sparingly soluble in alcohol.

USP requirements:
Isoxsuprine Hydrochloride Injection USP—Preserve in single-dose or in multiple-dose containers, preferably of Type I glass. A sterile solution of Isoxsuprine Hydrochloride in Water for Injection. Contains the labeled amount, within ±5%. Meets the requirements for Identification, Bacterial endotoxins, pH (4.9–6.0), and Injections.
Isoxsuprine Hydrochloride Tablets USP—Preserve in tight containers. Contain the labeled amount, within ±7%. Meet the requirements for Identification, Dissolution (75% in 45 minutes in water in Apparatus 1 at 100 rpm), and Uniformity of dosage units.

ISRADIPINE

Chemical name: 3,5-Pyridinedicarboxylic acid, 4-(4-benzofurazanyl)-1,4-dihydro-2,6-dimethyl-, methyl 1-methylethyl ester, (±)-.

Molecular formula: $C_{19}H_{21}N_3O_5$.

Molecular weight: 371.39.

Description: Yellow, fine crystalline powder. Is odorless or has a faint characteristic odor.

Solubility: Practically insoluble in water; soluble in ethanol; freely soluble in acetone, in chloroform, and in methylene chloride.

USP requirements: Isradipine Capsules—Not in USP.

IVERMECTIN

Source: Semisynthetic macrocyclic lactone produced by the actinomycete *Streptomyces avermitilis*.

Chemical group: Avermectins.

Other characteristics: A mixture of Ivermectin component B_{1a} and Ivermectin component B_{1b}.

USP requirements:
Ivermectin for Injection—Not in USP.
Ivermectin Paste—Not in USP.
Ivermectin Oral Solution—Not in USP.
Ivermectin Tablets—Not in USP.
Ivermectin Chewable Tablets—Not in USP.

JUNIPER TAR

Description: Juniper Tar USP—Dark brown, clear, thick liquid, having a tarry odor.

Solubility: Juniper Tar USP—Very slightly soluble in water; partially soluble in solvent hexane. One volume dissolves in 9 volumes of alcohol. Dissolves in 3 volumes of ether, leaving only a slight, flocculent residue. Miscible with amyl alcohol, with chloroform, and with glacial acetic acid.

USP requirements: Juniper Tar USP—Preserve in tight, light-resistant containers, and avoid exposure to excessive heat. It is the empyreumatic volatile oil obtained from the woody portions of *Juniperus oxycedrus* Linné (Fam. Pinaceae).

Meets the requirements for Identification, Specific gravity (0.950–1.055), Reaction, and Rosin or rosin oils.

KANAMYCIN

Source: Derived from *Streptomyces kanamyceticus*.

Chemical group: Aminoglycosides.

Chemical name: Kanamycin sulfate—D-Streptamine, *O*-3-amino-3-deoxy-alpha-D-glucopyranosyl(1→6)-*O*-[6-amino-6-deoxy-alpha-D-glucopyranosyl(1→4)]-2-deoxy-, sulfate (1:1) (salt).

Molecular formula: Kanamycin sulfate—$C_{18}H_{36}N_4O_{11} \cdot H_2SO_4$.

Molecular weight: Kanamycin sulfate—582.58.

Description: Kanamycin Sulfate USP—White, odorless, crystalline powder.

Solubility: Kanamycin Sulfate USP—Freely soluble in water; insoluble in acetone and in ethyl acetate.

USP requirements:
Kanamycin Sulfate Capsules USP—Preserve in tight containers. Contain an amount of kanamycin sulfate equivalent to the labeled amount of kanamycin, within −10% to +15%. Meet the requirements for Identification, Dissolution (75% in 45 minutes in 0.1 N hydrochloric acid in Apparatus 1 at 100 rpm), and Loss on drying (not more than 4.0%).

Kanamycin Sulfate Injection USP—Preserve in single-dose or in multiple-dose containers preferably of Type I or Type III glass. Contains suitable buffers and preservatives. Contains an amount of kanamycin sulfate equivalent to the labeled amount of kanamycin, within −10% to +15%. Meets the requirements for Identification, Bacterial endotoxins, Sterility, pH (3.5–5.0), and Particulate matter.

Sterile Kanamycin Sulfate USP—Preserve in Containers for Sterile Solids. It is Kanamycin Sulfate suitable for parenteral use. Has a potency equivalent to not less than 750 mcg of kanamycin per mg, calculated on the dried basis. Meets the requirements for Bacterial endotoxins and Sterility and for Identification tests, pH, Loss on drying, Residue on ignition, Crystallinity, and Chromatographic purity under Kanamycin Sulfate.

KAOLIN

Description: Kaolin USP—Soft, white or yellowish white powder or lumps. When moistened with water, it assumes a darker color and develops a marked clay-like odor.

NF category: Tablet and/or capsule diluent.

Solubility: Kaolin USP—Insoluble in water, in cold, dilute acids, and in solutions of alkali hydroxides.

USP requirements: Kaolin USP—Preserve in well-closed containers. It is a native hydrated aluminum silicate, powdered and freed from gritty particles by elutriation. Meets the requirements for Identification, Microbial limits, Loss on ignition (not more than 15.0%), Acid-soluble substances (not more than 2.0%), Carbonate, Iron, and Lead (not more than 0.001%).

KAOLIN AND PECTIN

For *Kaolin* and *Pectin*—See individual listings for chemistry information.

USP requirements: Kaolin and Pectin Oral Suspension—Not in USP.

KAOLIN, PECTIN, BELLADONNA ALKALOIDS, AND OPIUM

For *Kaolin, Pectin, Hyoscyamine, Atropine, Scopolamine,* and *Opium*—See individual listings for chemistry information.

USP requirements: Kaolin, Pectin, Hyoscyamine Sulfate, Atropine Sulfate, Scopolamine Hydrobromide, and Opium Oral Suspension—Not in USP.

KAOLIN, PECTIN, AND PAREGORIC

For *Kaolin, Pectin,* and *Paregoric*—See individual listings for chemistry information.

USP requirements: Kaolin, Pectin, and Paregoric Oral Suspension—Not in USP.

KETAMINE

Chemical name: Ketamine hydrochloride—Cyclohexanone, 2-(2-chlorophenyl)-2-(methylamino)-, hydrochloride.

Molecular formula: Ketamine hydrochloride—$C_{13}H_{16}ClNO \cdot HCl$.

Molecular weight: Ketamine hydrochloride—274.19.

Description: Ketamine Hydrochloride USP—White, crystalline powder, having a slight, characteristic odor.

Solubility: Ketamine Hydrochloride USP—Freely soluble in water and in methanol; soluble in alcohol; sparingly soluble in chloroform.

USP requirements: Ketamine Hydrochloride Injection USP—Preserve in single-dose or in multiple-dose containers, preferably of Type I glass, protected from light and heat. A sterile solution of Ketamine Hydrochloride in Water for Injection. Contains an amount of ketamine hydrochloride equivalent to the labeled amount of ketamine, within ±5%. Meets the requirements for Identification, Bacterial endotoxins, pH (3.0–5.0), and Injections.

KETAZOLAM

Chemical name: 4*H*-[1,3]-Oxazino[3,2-*d*]-[1,4]benzodiazepine-4,7(6*H*)-dione, 11-chloro-8,12b-dihydro-2,8-dimethyl-.

Molecular formula: $C_{20}H_{17}ClN_2O_3$.

Molecular weight: 368.82.

Description: Melting point 182–183.5 °C.

USP requirements: Ketazolam Capsules—Not in USP.

KETOCONAZOLE

Chemical group: Imidazoles.

Chemical name: Piperazine, 1-acetyl-4-[4-[[2-(2,4-dichlorophenyl)-2-(1*H*-imidazol-1-ylmethyl)-1,3-dioxolan-4-yl]methoxy]phenyl]-, *cis*-.

Molecular formula: $C_{26}H_{28}Cl_2N_4O_4$.

Molecular weight: 531.44.

Description: Almost white to slightly beige powder.

Solubility: Freely soluble in chloroform, in methanol, and in diluted hydrochloric acid; sparingly soluble in isopropyl alcohol and in acetone; practically insoluble in water.

Other characteristics: Weakly dibasic; requires acidity for dissolution and absorption.

USP requirements:
Ketoconazole Cream—Not in USP.
Ketoconazole Shampoo—Not in USP.
Ketoconazole Oral Suspension—Not in USP.
Ketoconazole Tablets USP—Preserve in well-closed containers. Contain the labeled amount, within ±10%. Meet the requirements for Identification, Disintegration (10 minutes), and Uniformity of dosage units.

KETOPROFEN

Chemical group: Propionic acid derivative.

Chemical name: Benzeneacetic acid, 3-benzoyl-alpha-methyl-.

Molecular formula: $C_{16}H_{14}O_3$.

Molecular weight: 254.28.

Description: White or off-white, odorless, nonhygroscopic, fine to granular powder. Melts at about 95 °C.

Solubility: Freely soluble in ethanol, in chloroform, in acetone, and in ether; soluble in strong alkali; practically insoluble in water at 20 °C.

Other characteristics: Highly lipophilic.

USP requirements:
Ketoprofen Capsules—Not in USP.
Ketoprofen Delayed-release Capsules—Not in USP.
Ketoprofen Suppositories—Not in USP.
Ketoprofen Delayed-release Tablets—Not in USP.
Ketoprofen Extended-release Tablets—Not in USP.

KETOROLAC

Chemical name: Ketorolac tromethamine—1*H*-Pyrrolizine-1-carboxylic acid, 5-benzoyl-2,3-dihydro, (±)-, compound with 2-amino-2-(hydroxymethyl)-1,3-propanediol (1:1).

Molecular formula: Ketorolac tromethamine—$C_{19}H_{24}N_2O_6$.

Molecular weight: Ketorolac tromethamine—376.41.

Description: Ketorolac tromethamine injection—Clear and slightly yellow in color.

pKa: Ketorolac tromethamine—3.54.

Solubility: Ketorolac tromethamine—Soluble in water.

Other characteristics: Ketorolac tromethamine—*n*-Octanol: water partition coefficient—0.26.

USP requirements:
Ketorolac Tromethamine Injection—Not in USP.
Ketorolac Tromethamine Tablets—Not in USP.

KRYPTON Kr 81m

Chemical name: Krypton, isotope of mass 81 (metastable).

Molecular formula: Kr 81m.

USP requirements: Krypton Kr 81m USP—The generator column is enclosed in a lead container. The unit is stored at room temperature. A gas suitable only for inhalation in diagnostic studies, and is obtained from a generator that contains rubidium 81 adsorbed on an immobilized suitable column support. Rubidium 81 decays with a half-life of 4.58 hours and forms its radioactive daughter ^{81m}Kr, which is eluted from the generator by passage of humidified oxygen or air through the column. Rubidium 81 is produced in an accelerator by proton bombardment of Kr 82. Other radio-isotopes of rubidium are produced and are present on the generator column. These other radioisotopes do not decay to ^{81m}Kr. The labeling indicates the name and address of the manufacturer, the name of the generator, the quantity of ^{81}Rb at the date and time of calibration, and the statement, "Caution—Radioactive Material." The labeling indicates that in making dosage calculations, correction is to be made for radioactive decay, and also indicates that the radioactive half-life of ^{81m}Kr is 13.1 seconds. The column contains the labeled amount of Rb 81, within ±10%, at the date and time indicated in the labeling, and on elution yields not less than 80.0% of ^{81m}Kr. Meets the requirements for Radionuclide identification and Radionuclidic purity.

LABETALOL

Chemical name: Labetalol hydrochloride—Benzamide, 2-hydroxy-5-[1-hydroxy-2-[(1-methyl-3-phenylpropyl)amino]ethyl]-, monohydrochloride.

Molecular formula: Labetalol hydrochloride—$C_{19}H_{24}N_2O_3 \cdot HCl$.

Molecular weight: Labetalol hydrochloride—364.87.

Description: Labetalol Hydrochloride USP—White to off-white powder. Melts at about 180 °C, with decomposition.

pKa: 9.45.

Solubility: Labetalol Hydrochloride USP—Soluble in water and in alcohol; insoluble in ether and in chloroform.

Other characteristics: Lipid solubility—Low.

USP requirements:
Labetalol Hydrochloride Injection USP—Preserve in single-dose containers, or in multiple-dose containers not exceeding 60 mL in volume, preferably of Type I glass, at a temperature between 2 and 30 °C. Avoid freezing and exposure to light. A sterile solution of Labetalol Hydrochloride in Water for Injection. Contains the labeled amount, within ±10%. Meets the requirements for Identification, Bacterial endotoxins, pH (3.0–4.5), and Injections.
Labetalol Hydrochloride Tablets USP—Preserve in tight, light-resistant containers, at a temperature between 2 and 30 °C. Contain the labeled amount, within ±10%. Meet the requirements for Identification, Dissolution (80% in 45 minutes in water in Apparatus 2 at 50 rpm), and Uniformity of dosage units.

LABETALOL AND HYDROCHLOROTHIAZIDE

For *Labetalol* and *Hydrochlorothiazide*—See individual listings for chemistry information.

USP requirements: Labetalol Hydrochloride and Hydrochlorothiazide Tablets—Not in USP.

LACTIC ACID

Chemical name: Propanoic acid, 2-hydroxy-.

Molecular formula: $C_3H_6O_3$.

Molecular weight: 90.08.

Description: Lactic Acid USP—Colorless or yellowish, practically odorless, syrupy liquid. Is hygroscopic. When it is concentrated by boiling, lactic acid lactate is formed. Specific gravity is about 1.20.

NF category: Buffering agent.

Solubility: Lactic Acid USP—Miscible with water, with alcohol, and with ether. Insoluble in chloroform.

USP requirements: Lactic Acid USP—Preserve in tight containers. A mixture of lactic acid and lactic acid lactate equivalent to a total of not less than 85.0% and not more than 90.0%, by weight, of lactic acid. It is obtained by the lactic fermentation of sugars or prepared synthetically. Lactic Acid obtained by fermentation of sugars is levorotatory, while that prepared synthetically is racemic. [Note: Lactic Acid prepared by fermentation becomes dextrorotatory on dilution, which hydrolyzes L(−) lactic acid lactate to L(+) lactic acid.] Label it to indicate whether it is levorotatory or racemic. Meets the requirements for Identification, Specific rotation (−0.05° to +0.05°, for racemic Lactic Acid), Residue on ignition (not more than 0.05%), Sugars, Chloride, Citric, oxalic, phosphoric, or tartaric acid, Sulfate, Heavy metals (not more than 0.001%), and Readily carbonizable substances.

LACTOSE

Chemical name: D-Glucose, 4-O-beta-D-galactopyranosyl-.

Molecular formula: $C_{12}H_{22}O_{11}$.

Molecular weight: 342.30 (anhydrous).

Description: Lactose NF—White or creamy white, hard, crystalline masses or powder. It is odorless. Stable in air, but readily absorbs odors.
NF category: Tablet and/or capsule diluent.

Solubility: Lactose NF—Freely (and slowly) soluble in water, and even more soluble in boiling water; very slightly soluble in alcohol; insoluble in chloroform and in ether.

NF requirements: Lactose NF—Preserve in well-closed containers. A sugar obtained from milk. It is anhydrous or contains one molecule of water of hydration. Label it to indicate whether it is anhydrous or hydrous. If it has been prepared by a spray-dried process, the label so indicates. Meets the requirements for Clarity and color of solution, Identification, Specific rotation (+54.8° to +55.5°, calculated on the anhydrous basis), Microbial limits, Acidity or alkalinity, Water (not more than 1.0% for anhydrous, not more than 5.5% for hydrous), Residue on ignition (not more than 0.1%), Alcohol-soluble residue, and Heavy metals (not more than 5 ppm).

LACTULOSE

Chemical name: D-Fructose, 4-O-beta-D-galactopyranosyl-.

Molecular formula: $C_{12}H_{22}O_{11}$.

Molecular weight: 342.30.

Description: Lactulose Concentrate USP—Colorless to amber syrupy liquid, which may exhibit some precipitation and darkening upon standing.

Solubility: Lactulose Concentrate USP—Miscible with water.

USP requirements:
Lactulose Concentrate USP—Preserve in tight containers, preferably at a temperature between 2 and 30 °C. Avoid subfreezing temperatures. A solution of sugars prepared from Lactose. Consists principally of lactulose together with minor quantities of lactose and galactose, and traces of other related sugars and water. Contains the labeled amount, within ±5%. Contains no added substances. Meets the requirements for Identification, Refractive index (not less than 1.451, at 20 °C), Residue on ignition (not more than 0.1%), and Limit of related substances.
Lactulose Solution USP—Preserve in tight containers, preferably at a temperature between 2 and 30 °C. Avoid

subfreezing temperatures. A solution in water prepared from Lactulose Concentrate. Contains the labeled amount, within ±10%. Meets the requirements for Microbial limits and pH (3.0–7.0, after 15 minutes of contact with the electrodes), and for Identification tests and Limit of related substances under Lactulose Concentrate.

LANOLIN

Description: Lanolin USP—Yellow, tenacious, unctuous mass, having a slight characteristic odor.
NF category: Ointment base.

Solubility: Lanolin USP—Insoluble in water, but mixes without separation with about twice its weight of water. Sparingly soluble in cold alcohol; more soluble in hot alcohol; freely soluble in ether and in chloroform.

USP requirements: Lanolin USP—Preserve in well-closed containers, preferably at controlled room temperature. It is the purified, wax-like substance from the wool of sheep, *Ovis aries* Linné (Fam. Bovidae), that has been cleaned, decolorized, and deodorized. The label states that it is not to be used undiluted. Contains not more than 0.25% of water. Meets the requirements for Melting range (38–44 °C), Acidity, Alkalinity, Water (not more than 0.25%), Residue on ignition (not more than 0.1%), Water-soluble acids and alkalies, Water-soluble oxidizable substances, Chloride (not more than 0.035%), Ammonia, Iodine value (18–36), Petrolatum, and Foreign substances (not more than 40 ppm).

LANOLIN ALCOHOLS

Description: Lanolin Alcohols NF—Hard, waxy, amber solid, having a characteristic odor.
NF category: Emulsifying and/or solubilizing agent.

Solubility: Lanolin Alcohols NF—Insoluble in water; slightly soluble in alcohol; freely soluble in chloroform, in ether, and in petroleum ether.

NF requirements: Lanolin Alcohols NF—Preserve in well-closed, light-resistant containers, preferably at controlled room temperature. A mixture of aliphatic alcohols, triterpenoid alcohols, and sterols, obtained by the hydrolysis of Lanolin. Contains not less than 30.0% of cholesterol. Meets the requirements for Identification, Melting range (not below 56 °C), Acidity and alkalinity, Loss on drying (not more than 0.5%), Residue on ignition (not more than 0.15%), Copper (5 ppm), Acid value (not more than 2), and Saponifaction value (not more than 12).

MODIFIED LANOLIN

USP requirements: Modified Lanolin USP—Preserve in tight, preferably rust-proof containers, preferably at controlled room temperature. It is the purified wax-like substance from the wool of sheep, *Ovis aries* Linné (Fam. Bovidae), that has been processed to reduce the contents of free lanolin alcohols and detergent and pesticide residues. Contains not more than 0.25% of water. Meets the requirements for Acidity, Alkalinity, Water (not more than 0.25%), Water-soluble acids and alkalies, Ammonia, Related substances (not more than 6%), Foreign substances (not more than 3 ppm for total pesticides and not more than 1 ppm for individual pesticide), and Petrolatum.

LECITHIN

Description: Lecithin NF—The consistency of both natural grades and refined grades of lecithin may vary from plastic to fluid, depending upon free fatty acid and oil content, and upon the presence or absence of other diluents. Its color varies from light yellow to brown, depending on the source, on crop variations, and on whether it is bleached or unbleached. Odorless, or has a characteristic, slight, nutlike odor.

NF category: Emulsifying and/or solubilizing agent.

Solubility: Lecithin NF—Partially soluble in water, but it readily hydrates to form emulsions. The oil-free phosphatides are soluble in fatty acids, but are practically insoluble in fixed oils. When all phosphatide fractions are present, lecithin is partially soluble in alcohol and practically insoluble in acetone.

NF requirements: Lecithin NF—Preserve in well-closed containers. A complex mixture of acetone-insoluble phosphatides, which consist chiefly of phosphatidyl choline, phosphatidyl ethanolamine, phosphatidyl serine, and phosphatidyl inositol, combined with various amounts of other substances such as triglycerides, fatty acids, and carbohydrates, as separated from the crude vegetable oil source. Contains not less than 50.0% of Acetone-insoluble matter. Meets the requirements for Water (not more than 1.5%), Arsenic (not more than 3 ppm), Lead (not more than 0.001%), Heavy metals (not more than 0.004%), Acid value (not more than 36), Hexane-insoluble matter (not more than 0.3%), and Acetone-insoluble matter.

LEUCOVORIN

Chemical name: Leucovorin calcium—L-Glutamic acid, *N*-[4-[[(2-amino-5-formyl-1,4,5,6,7,8-hexahydro-4-oxo-6-pteridinyl)methyl]amino]benzoyl]-, calcium salt (1:1).

Molecular formula: Leucovorin calcium—$C_{20}H_{21}CaN_7O_7$.

Molecular weight: Leucovorin calcium—511.51.

Description:
Leucovorin Calcium USP—Yellowish white or yellow, odorless powder.
Leucovorin Calcium Injection USP—Clear, yellowish solution.

pKa: 3.1, 4.8, and 10.4.

Solubility: Leucovorin Calcium USP—Very soluble in water; practically insoluble in alcohol.

USP requirements:
Leucovorin Calcium Injection USP—Preserve in single-dose, light-resistant containers, preferably of Type I glass. A sterile solution of Leucovorin Calcium in Water for Injection. Contains an amount of leucovorin calcium equivalent to the labeled amount of leucovorin, within −10% to +20%. Meets the requirements for Identification, pH (6.5–8.5), and Injections.
Leucovorin Calcium for Injection—Not in USP.
Leucovorin Calcium for Oral Solution—Not in USP.
Leucovorin Calcium Tablets—Not in USP.

LEUKOCYTE TYPING SERUM

USP requirements: Leukocyte Typing Serum USP—Preserve at the temperature recommended by the manufacturer. A dried or liquid preparation of serum derived from plasma or blood obtained from animals or from human donors containing an antibody or antibodies for identification of leukocyte antigens. Label it to state the source of the product if other than human and, if of human origin, to state either that the source material was found reactive for hepatitis B surface antigen and that the product may transmit hepatitis, or that the source material was not reactive for hepatitis B

surface antigen but that no known test method offers assurance that products derived from human blood will not transmit hepatitis. Label it also to include the name of the specific antibody or antibodies present and the requirements for potency in relation to the antigen(s) of the corresponding specificity with which it complies; the permissible limits of error for specificity reactions with which it complies; the name of the test method or methods recommended for the product; and a statement that it is for in-vitro diagnostic use. Provide with the package enclosure the following: adequate directions for performing the tests, including a description of all recommended test methods; descriptions of all supplementary reagents, including one of a suitable complement source; description of precautions in use, including a warning against exposure of the product to carbon dioxide; a caution statement to the effect that more than one antiserum is to be used for each specificity, that the antiserum is not to be diluted, and that cross-reacting antigens exist; and directions for constitution of the product, including instructions for the use, storage, and labeling of the constituted product. Meets the requirements of the test for potency and for specificity. Meets the requirement for Expiration date (for dried Serum, not later than 2 years after date of issue from manufacturer's cold storage [5 °C, 1 year; or 0 °C, 2 years] and for liquid Serum not later than 1 year after such issue [5 °C, 1 year]). Conforms to the regulations of the U.S. Food and Drug Administration concerning biologics.

LEUPROLIDE

Source: Luteinizing hormone–releasing hormone analog.

Chemical name: Leuprolide acetate—Luteinizing hormone–releasing factor (pig), 6-D-leucine-9-(*N*-ethyl-L-prolinamide)-10-deglycinamide-, monoacetate (salt).

Molecular formula: Leuprolide acetate—$C_{59}H_{84}N_{16}O_{12} \cdot C_2H_4O_2$.

Molecular weight: Leuprolide acetate—1269.47.

Description: Leuprolide acetate—White to off-white powder.

Solubility: Leuprolide acetate—Solubility greater than 250 mg/mL in water and greater than 1 g/mL in alcohol at 25 °C.

USP requirements:
Leuprolide Acetate Injection—Not in USP.
Leuprolide Acetate for Injection—Not in USP.

LEVAMISOLE

Chemical name: Levamisole hydrochloride—Imidazo[2,1-*b*]thiazole, 2,3,5,6-tetrahydro-6-phenyl-, monohydrochloride, (*S*)-.

Molecular formula: Levamisole hydrochloride—$C_{11}H_{12}N_2S \cdot$ HCl.

Molecular weight: Levamisole hydrochloride—240.75.

Description: Levamisole Hydrochloride USP—White or almost white crystalline powder.

Solubility: Levamisole Hydrochloride USP—Freely soluble in water; soluble in alcohol; slightly soluble in methylene chloride; practically insoluble in ether.

USP requirements:
Levamisole Hydrochloride Bolus—Not in USP.
Levamisole Hydrochloride Paste—Not in USP.
Levamisole Hydrochloride Soluble Powder—Not in USP.
Levamisole Hydrochloride Soluble Powder for Drench—Not in USP.
Levamisole Hydrochloride Tablets—Not in USP.

LEVOBUNOLOL

Chemical name: Levobunolol hydrochloride—1(2*H*)-Naphthalenone, 5-[3-[(1,1-dimethylethyl)amino]-2-hydroxypropoxy]-3,4-dihydro-, hydrochloride, (−)-.

Molecular formula: Levobunolol hydrochloride—$C_{17}H_{25}NO_3 \cdot$ HCl.

Molecular weight: Levobunolol hydrochloride—327.85.

Description: Levobunolol hydrochloride—White, crystalline, odorless powder.

pKa: Levobunolol hydrochloride—9.4.

Solubility: Levobunolol hydrochloride—Solubility of 300 mg/mL in water and 24 mg/mL in alcohol at 25 °C.

USP requirements: Levobunolol Hydrochloride Ophthalmic Solution USP—Preserve in tight containers. Contains the labeled amount, within ±10%. Meets the requirements for Identification, pH (5.5–7.5), Antimicrobial preservatives—Effectiveness, and Sterility.

LEVOCARNITINE

Source: Naturally occurring amino acid derivative.

Chemical name: 1-Propanaminium, 3-carboxy-2-hydroxy-*N,N,N*-trimethyl-, hydroxide, inner salt, (*R*)-.

Molecular formula: $C_7H_{15}NO_3$.

Molecular weight: 161.20.

Description: Levocarnitine USP—White, odorless crystals or crystalline powder. Hygroscopic.

Solubility: Levocarnitine USP—Freely soluble in water and in hot alcohol; practically insoluble in acetone and in ether.

USP requirements:
Levocarnitine Capsules—Not in USP.
Levocarnitine Oral Solution USP—Preserve in tight containers. A solution of Levocarnitine in water. Contains suitable antimicrobial agents. Contains the labeled amount, within ±10%. Meets the requirements for Identification and pH (4.0–6.0).
Levocarnitine Tablets—Not in USP.

LEVODOPA

Chemical group: L-dihydroxyphenylalanine; precursor of dopamine.

Chemical name: L-Tyrosine, 3-hydroxy-.

Molecular formula: $C_9H_{11}NO_4$.

Molecular weight: 197.19.

Description: Levodopa USP—White to off-white, odorless, crystalline powder. In the presence of moisture, is rapidly oxidized by atmospheric oxygen and darkens.

Solubility: Levodopa USP—Slightly soluble in water; freely soluble in 3 *N* hydrochloric acid; insoluble in alcohol.

USP requirements:
Levodopa Capsules USP—Preserve in tight, light-resistant containers, in a dry place, and prevent exposure to excessive heat. Contain the labeled amount, within ±10%. Meet the requirements for Identification, Dissolution (75% in 30 minutes in 0.1 *N* hydrochloric acid in Apparatus 1 at 100 rpm), Related compounds, and Uniformity of dosage units.

Levodopa Tablets USP—Preserve in tight, light-resistant containers, in a dry place, and prevent exposure to excessive heat. Contain the labeled amount, within ±10%. Meet the requirements for Identification, Dissolution (75% in 30 minutes in 0.1 *N* hydrochloric acid in Apparatus 1 at 100 rpm), Related compounds, and Uniformity of dosage units.

LEVONORGESTREL

Chemical name: 18,19-Dinorpregn-4-en-20-yn-3-one, 13-ethyl-17-hydroxy-, (17 alpha)-(−)-.

Molecular formula: $C_{21}H_{28}O_2$.

Molecular weight: 312.45.

Description: Levonorgestrel USP—White or practically white, odorless powder.

Solubility: Levonorgestrel USP—Practically insoluble in water; soluble in chloroform; slightly soluble in alcohol.

USP requirements: Levonorgestrel Implants—Not in USP.

LEVONORGESTREL AND ETHINYL ESTRADIOL

For *Levonorgestrel and Ethinyl Estradiol*—See individual listings for chemistry information.

USP requirements: Levonorgestrel and Ethinyl Estradiol Tablets USP—Preserve in well-closed containers. Contain the labeled amounts of levonorgestrel and ethinyl estradiol, within ±10%. Meet the requirements for Identification, Dissolution (for uncoated tablets, 60% of levonorgestrel in 30 minutes and 75% of ethinyl estradiol in 60 minutes; for sugar-coated tablets, 60% of levonorgestrel in 60 minutes and 60% of ethinyl estradiol in 60 minutes; both, in polysorbate 80 [5 ppm] in Water in Apparatus 2 at 75 rpm), and Uniformity of dosage units.

LEVOPROPOXYPHENE

Chemical name: Levopropoxyphene napsylate—Benzeneethanol, alpha-[2-(dimethylamino)-1-methylethyl]-alpha-phenyl-, propanoate (ester), [*R*-(*R*,S**)]-, compd. with 2-naphthalenesulfonic acid (1:1), monohydrate.

Molecular formula: Levopropoxyphene napsylate—$C_{22}H_{29}NO_2 \cdot C_{10}H_8O_3S \cdot H_2O$.

Molecular weight: Levopropoxyphene napsylate—565.72.

Description: Levopropoxyphene Napsylate USP—White powder, having essentially no odor.

Solubility: Levopropoxyphene Napsylate USP—Very slightly soluble in water; soluble in methanol, in alcohol, in chloroform, and in acetone.

USP requirements:
Levopropoxyphene Napsylate Capsules USP—Preserve in tight containers. Contain an amount of levopropoxyphene napsylate equivalent to the labeled amount of levopropoxyphene, within ±10%. Meet the requirements for Identification, Dissolution (75% in 60 minutes in acetate buffer [pH 4.5] in Apparatus 1 at 100 rpm) and Uniformity of dosage units.
Levopropoxyphene Napsylate Oral Suspension USP—Preserve in tight containers, protected from light. Avoid freezing. Contains an amount of levopropoxyphene napsylate equivalent to the labeled amount of levopropoxyphene, within ±10%. Meets the requirements for Identification and Alcohol content (0.5–1.5%).

LEVORPHANOL

Chemical name: Levorphanol tartrate—Morphinan-3-ol, 17-methyl-, [R-(R*,R*)]-2,3-dihydroxybutanedioate (1:1) (salt), dihydrate.

Molecular formula: Levorphanol tartrate—$C_{17}H_{23}NO \cdot C_4H_6O_6 \cdot 2H_2O$ (dihydrate); $C_{17}H_{23}NO \cdot C_4H_6O_6$ (anhydrous).

Molecular weight: Levorphanol tartrate—443.49 (dihydrate); 407.46 (anhydrous).

Description: Levorphanol Tartrate USP—Practically white, odorless, crystalline powder. Melts, in a sealed tube, at about 110 °C, with decomposition.

Solubility: Levorphanol Tartrate USP—Sparingly soluble in water; slightly soluble in alcohol; insoluble in chloroform and in ether.

USP requirements:
Levorphanol Tartrate Injection USP—Preserve in single-dose or in multiple-dose containers, preferably of Type I glass. A sterile solution of Levorphanol Tartrate in Water for Injection. Contains the labeled amount, within ±7%. Meets the requirements for Identification, Bacterial endotoxins, pH (4.1–4.5), and Injections.
Levorphanol Tartrate Tablets USP—Preserve in well-closed containers. Contain the labeled amount, within ±7%. Meet the requirements for Identification, Dissolution (75% in 30 minutes in water in Apparatus 2 at 50 rpm), and Uniformity of dosage units.

LEVOTHYROXINE

Chemical name: Levothyroxine sodium—L-Tyrosine, O-(4-hydroxy-3,5-diiodophenyl)-3,5-diiodo-, monosodium salt, hydrate.

Molecular formula: Levothyroxine sodium—$C_{15}H_{10}I_4NNaO_4 \cdot xH_2O$.

Molecular weight: Levothyroxine sodium—798.86 (anhydrous).

Description: Levothyroxine Sodium USP—Light yellow to buff-colored, odorless, hygroscopic powder. Is stable in dry air but may assume a slight pink color upon exposure to light. The pH of a saturated solution is about 8.9.

Solubility: Levothyroxine Sodium USP—Very slightly soluble in water; soluble in solutions of alkali hydroxides and in hot solutions of alkali carbonates; slightly soluble in alcohol; insoluble in acetone, in chloroform, and in ether.

USP requirements:
Levothyroxine Sodium Injection—Not in USP.
Levothyroxine Sodium for Injection—Not in USP.
Levothyroxine Sodium Powder—Not in USP.
Levothyroxine Sodium Tablets USP—Preserve in tight, light-resistant containers. Contain the labeled amount, within ±10%. Meet the requirements for Identification, Dissolution (55% in 80 minutes in 0.05 M phosphate buffer [pH 7.4] in Apparatus 2 at 100 rpm), Uniformity of dosage units, Soluble halides (not more than 7.1%), and Liothyronine sodium (not more than 2.0%).

LIDOCAINE

Chemical group: Amide.

Chemical name:
Lidocaine—Acetamide, 2-(diethylamino)-N-(2,6-dimethylphenyl)-.

Lidocaine hydrochloride—Acetamide, 2-(diethylamino)-N-(2,6-dimethylphenyl)-, monohydrochloride, monohydrate.

Molecular formula:
Lidocaine—$C_{14}H_{22}N_2O$.
Lidocaine hydrochloride—$C_{14}H_{22}N_2O \cdot HCl \cdot H_2O$.

Molecular weight:
Lidocaine—234.34.
Lidocaine hydrochloride—288.82.

Description:
Lidocaine USP—White or slightly yellow, crystalline powder. Has a characteristic odor and is stable in air.
Lidocaine Hydrochloride USP—White, odorless, crystalline powder.

pKa:
Lidocaine—7.9.
Lidocaine hydrochloride—7.86.

Solubility:
Lidocaine USP—Practically insoluble in water; very soluble in alcohol and in chloroform; freely soluble in ether; dissolves in oils.
Lidocaine Hydrochloride USP—Very soluble in water and in alcohol; soluble in chloroform; insoluble in ether.

USP requirements:
Lidocaine Topical Aerosol USP (Solution)—Preserve in non-reactive aerosol containers equipped with metered-dose valves. A solution of Lidocaine in a suitable flavored vehicle with suitable propellants in a pressurized container equipped with a metering valve. Contains the labeled amount, within ±10%, and delivers within ±15% of the labeled amount per actuation. Meets the requirements for Identification and Microbial limits and for Leak Testing under Aerosols.
Lidocaine Ointment USP—Preserve in tight containers. It is Lidocaine in a suitable hydrophilic ointment base. Contains the labeled amount, within ±5%. Meets the requirements for Identification, Microbial limits, and Minimum fill.
Lidocaine Oral Topical Solution USP—Preserve in tight containers. Contains the labeled amount, within ±5%. Contains a suitable flavor. Meets the requirement for Identification.
Lidocaine Hydrochloride Injection USP—Preserve in single-dose or in multiple-dose containers, preferably of Type I glass. A sterile solution of Lidocaine Hydrochloride in Water for Injection, or a sterile solution prepared from Lidocaine with the aid of Hydrochloric Acid in Water for Injection. Injection may be packaged in 50-mL multiple-dose containers. Injections that are of such concentration that they are not intended for direct injection into tissues are labeled to indicate that they are to be diluted prior to administration. Contains the labeled amount, within ±5%. Meets the requirements for Identification, Bacterial endotoxins, pH (5.0–7.0), Particulate matter, and Injections.
Lidocaine Hydrochloride Jelly USP—Preserve in tight containers. It is Lidocaine Hydrochloride in a suitable, water-soluble, sterile, viscous base. Contains the labeled amount, within ±5%. Meets the requirements for Identification, Sterility, Minimum fill, and pH (6.0–7.0).
Lidocaine Hydrochloride Ointment—Not in USP.
Lidocaine Hydrochloride Topical Solution USP—Preserve in tight containers. Contains the labeled amount, within ±5%. Meets the requirements for Identification and pH (5.0–7.0).
Lidocaine Hydrochloride Oral Topical Solution USP—Preserve in tight containers. Contains the labeled amount,

within ±5%. Contains a suitable flavor and/or sweetening agent. Meets the requirements for Identification and pH (5.0–7.0).

Sterile Lidocaine Hydrochloride USP—Preserve in Containers for Sterile Solids. It is Lidocaine Hydrochloride suitable for parenteral use. Contains the labeled amount, within ±5%. Meets the requirements for Bacterial endotoxins, for Identification test, Melting range, Water, Residue on ignition, Sulfate, and Heavy metals under Lidocaine Hydrochloride, for Sterility tests, Uniformity of dosage units, and Constituted solutions, and for Labeling under Injections.

LIDOCAINE AND DEXTROSE

For *Lidocaine* and *Dextrose*—See individual listings for chemistry information.

USP requirements: Lidocaine Hydrochloride and Dextrose Injection USP—Preserve in single-dose containers of Type I or Type II glass, or of a suitable plastic material. A sterile solution of Lidocaine Hydrochloride and Dextrose in Water for Injection. Contains the labeled amounts of lidocaine hydrochloride and dextrose, within ±5%. Meets the requirements for Identification, Bacterial endotoxins, pH (3.0–7.0), and Injections.

LIDOCAINE AND EPINEPHRINE

For *Lidocaine* and *Epinephrine*—See individual listings for chemistry information.

USP requirements: Lidocaine and Epinephrine Injection USP—Preserve in single-dose or in multiple-dose, light-resistant containers, preferably of Type I glass. A sterile solution prepared from Lidocaine Hydrochloride and Epinephrine with the aid of Hydrochloric Acid in Water for Injection, or a sterile solution prepared from Lidocaine and Epinephrine with the aid of Hydrochloric Acid in Water for Injection, or a sterile solution of Lidocaine Hydrochloride and Epinephrine Bitartrate in Water for Injection. The content of epinephrine does not exceed 0.002% (1 in 50,000). The label indicates that the Injection is not to be used if its color is pinkish or darker than slightly yellow or if it contains a precipitate. Contains the equivalent of the labeled amount of lidocaine hydrochloride, within ±5%, and the equivalent of the labeled amount of epinephrine, within −10% to +15%. Meets the requirements for Color and clarity, Bacterial endotoxins, and pH (3.3–5.5), for Identification test under Lidocaine Hydrochloride Injection, and for Injections.

LIDOCAINE AND PRILOCAINE

For *Lidocaine* and *Prilocaine*—See individual listings for chemistry information.

USP requirements: Lidocaine and Prilocaine Cream—Not in USP.

LIME

Chemical name: Calcium oxide.

Molecular formula: CaO.

Molecular weight: 56.08.

Description: Lime USP—Hard, white or grayish white masses or granules, or white or grayish white powder. Is odorless.

Solubility: Lime USP—Slightly soluble in water; very slightly soluble in boiling water.

USP requirements: Lime USP—Preserve in tight containers. When freshly ignited to constant weight, contains not less than 95.0% of lime. Meets the requirements for Identification, Loss on ignition (not more than 10.0%), Insoluble substances (not more than 1.0%), Carbonate, and Magnesium and alkali salts.

LINCOMYCIN

Source: Produced by the growth of *Streptomyces lincolnensis var. lincolnensis.*

Chemical name: Lincomycin hydrochloride—D-*erythro*-alpha-D-*galacto*-Octopyranoside, methyl 6,8-dideoxy-6-[[(1-methyl-4-propyl-2-pyrrolidinyl)carbonyl]amino]-1-thio-, monohydrochloride, monohydrate, (2S-*trans*)-.

Molecular formula: Lincomycin hydrochloride—$C_{18}H_{34}N_2O_6S \cdot HCl \cdot H_2O$.

Molecular weight: Lincomycin hydrochloride—461.01.

Description:
Lincomycin Hydrochloride USP—White or practically white, crystalline powder. Is odorless or has a faint odor. Is stable in the presence of air and light. Its solutions are acid and are dextrorotatory.
Lincomycin Hydrochloride Injection USP—Clear, colorless to slightly yellow solution, having a slight odor.

Solubility: Lincomycin Hydrochloride USP—Freely soluble in water; soluble in dimethylformamide; very slightly soluble in acetone.

USP requirements:
Lincomycin Hydrochloride Capsules USP—Preserve in tight containers. Contain an amount of lincomycin hydrochloride equivalent to the labeled amount of lincomycin, within −10% to +20%. Meet the requirements for Dissolution (75% in 45 minutes in water in Apparatus 1 at 100 rpm), Uniformity of dosage units, and Water (not more than 7.0%).
Lincomycin Hydrochloride Injection USP—Preserve in single-dose or in multiple-dose containers, preferably of Type I glass. A sterile solution of Lincomycin Hydrochloride in Water for Injection. It contains benzyl alcohol as a preservative. Contains an amount of lincomycin hydrochloride equivalent to the labeled amount of lincomycin, within −10% to +20%. Meets the requirements for Sterility, Bacterial endotoxins, pH (3.0–5.5), Particulate matter, and Injections.
Sterile Lincomycin Hydrochloride USP—Preserve in Containers for Sterile Solids. It is Lincomycin Hydrochloride suitable for parenteral use. It has a potency equivalent to not less than 790 mcg of lincomycin per mg. Meets the requirements for Depressor substances, Bacterial endotoxins, and Sterility, and for Identification test, Specific rotation (+135° to +150°, calculated on the anhydrous basis), pH (3.0–5.5, in a solution [1 in 10]), Water (3.0–6.0%), Crystallinity, and Lincomycin B (not more than 5.0%) under Lincomycin Hydrochloride.
Lincomycin Hydrochloride Syrup USP—Preserve in tight containers. Contains an amount of Lincomycin Hydrochloride equivalent to the labeled amount of lincomycin, within −10% to +20%, and one or more suitable colors, flavors, preservatives, and sweeteners in water. Meets the requirements for pH (3–5.5), Deliverable volume (for syrup packaged in multiple-unit containers), and Uniformity of dosage units (for syrup packaged in single-unit containers).

LINDANE

Chemical name: Cyclohexane, 1,2,3,4,5,6-hexachloro-, (1 alpha,2 alpha,3 beta,4 alpha,5 alpha,6 beta)-.

Molecular formula: $C_6H_6Cl_6$.

Molecular weight: 290.83.

Description: Lindane USP—White, crystalline powder, having a slight, musty odor.

Solubility: Lindane USP—Practically insoluble in water; freely soluble in chloroform; soluble in dehydrated alcohol; sparingly soluble in ether; slightly soluble in ethylene glycol.

USP requirements:
Lindane Cream USP—Preserve in tight containers. It is Lindane in a suitable cream base. Contains the labeled amount, within ± 10%. Meets the requirements for Identification and pH (8.0–9.0, in a 1 in 5 dilution).
Lindane Lotion USP—Preserve in tight containers. It is Lindane in a suitable aqueous vehicle. Contains the labeled amount, within ± 10%. Meets the requirements for Identification and pH (6.5–8.5).
Lindane Shampoo USP—Preserve in tight containers. It is Lindane in a suitable vehicle. Contains the labeled amount, within ± 10%. Meets the requirements for Identification and pH (6.2–7.0).

LIOTHYRONINE

Chemical name: Liothyronine sodium—L-Tyrosine, *O*-(4-hydroxy-3-iodophenyl)-3,5-diiodo-, monosodium salt.

Molecular formula: Liothyronine sodium—$C_{15}H_{11}I_3NNaO_4$.

Molecular weight: Liothyronine sodium—672.96.

Description: Liothyronine Sodium USP—Light tan, odorless, crystalline powder.

Solubility: Liothyronine Sodium USP—Very slightly soluble in water; slightly soluble in alcohol; practically insoluble in most other organic solvents.

USP requirements:
Liothyronine Sodium Injection—Not in USP.
Liothyronine Sodium Tablets USP—Preserve in tight containers. Contain an amount of liothyronine sodium equivalent to the labeled amount of liothyronine, within ± 10%. Meet the requirements for Identification, Disintegration (30 minutes), and Uniformity of dosage units.

LIOTRIX

Source: A mixture of liothyronine sodium and levothyroxine sodium, in a ratio of 1:1 in terms of biological activity, or in a ratio of 1:4 in terms of weight.

Chemical name: L-Tyrosine, *O*-(4-hydroxy-3,5-diiodophenyl)-3,5-diiodo-, monosodium salt, hydrate, mixt. with *O*-(4-hydroxy-3-iodophenyl)-3,5-diiodo-L-tyrosine monosodium salt.

USP requirements: Liotrix Tablets USP—Preserve in tight containers. Contain the labeled amounts of levothyroxine sodium and liothyronine sodium, within ± 10%. Meet the requirements for Identification, Disintegration (30 minutes), and Uniformity of dosage units.

LISINOPRIL

Chemical name: L-Proline, 1-[*N*²-(1-carboxy-3-phenylpropyl)-L-lysyl]-, dihydrate, (*S*)-.

Molecular formula: $C_{21}H_{31}N_3O_5 \cdot 2H_2O$.

Molecular weight: 441.52.

Description: Lisinopril USP—White, crystalline powder. Melts at about 160 °C, with decomposition.

Solubility: Lisinopril USP—Soluble in water; sparingly soluble in methanol; practically insoluble in alcohol, in acetone, in acetonitrile, and in chloroform.

USP requirements: Lisinopril Tablets USP—Preserve in tight containers. Contain the labeled amount, within ± 10%. Meet the requirements for Identification, Dissolution (80% in 30 minutes in 0.1 *N* hydrochloric acid in Apparatus 2 at 50 rpm), Uniformity of dosage units, and Related compounds.

LISINOPRIL AND HYDROCHLOROTHIAZIDE

For *Lisinopril* and *Hydrochlorothiazide*—See individual listings for chemistry information.

USP requirements: Lisinopril and Hydrochlorothiazide Tablets—Not in USP.

LITHIUM

Chemical name:
Lithium carbonate—Carbonic acid, dilithium salt.
Lithium citrate—1,2,3-Propanetricarboxylic acid, 2-hydroxy-trilithium salt tetrahydrate.

Molecular formula:
Lithium carbonate—Li_2CO_3.
Lithium citrate—$C_6H_5Li_3O_7 \cdot 4H_2O$.

Molecular weight:
Lithium carbonate—73.89.
Lithium citrate—282.00.

Description:
Lithium Carbonate USP—White, granular, odorless powder.
Lithium Citrate USP—White, odorless, deliquescent powder or granules.

Solubility:
Lithium Carbonate USP—Sparingly soluble in water; very slightly soluble in alcohol. Dissolves, with effervescence, in dilute mineral acids.
Lithium Citrate USP—Freely soluble in water; slightly soluble in alcohol.

Other characteristics: A monovalent cation; salts share some chemical characteristics with salts of sodium and potassium.

USP requirements:
Lithium Carbonate Capsules USP—Preserve in well-closed containers. Contain the labeled amount, within ± 5%. Meet the requirements for Identification, Dissolution (60% in 30 minutes in water in Apparatus 1 at 100 rpm), and Uniformity of dosage units.
Lithium Carbonate Slow-release Capsules—Not in USP.
Lithium Carbonate Tablets USP—Preserve in well-closed containers. Contain the labeled amount, within ± 5%. Meet the requirements for Identification, Dissolution (60% in 30 minutes in water in Apparatus 1 at 100 rpm), and Uniformity of dosage units.
Lithium Carbonate Extended-release Tablets USP—Preserve in well-closed containers. Contain the labeled amount, within ± 10%. Meet the requirements for Identification and Uniformity of dosage units.
Lithium Citrate Syrup USP—Preserve in tight containers. It is prepared from Lithium Citrate or Lithium Hydroxide to which an excess of Citric Acid has been added. Contains an amount of lithium citrate equivalent to the

labeled amount of lithium, within ±10%. Meets the requirements for Identification and pH (4.0–5.0).

LOMUSTINE

Chemical name: Urea, N-(2-chloroethyl)-N′-cyclohexyl-N-nitroso-.

Molecular formula: $C_9H_{16}ClN_3O_2$.

Molecular weight: 233.70.

Description: Yellow powder.

Solubility: Soluble in 10% ethanol and in absolute alcohol; relatively insoluble in water; highly soluble in lipids.

USP requirements: Lomustine Capsules—Not in USP.

LOPERAMIDE

Source: Synthetic piperidine derivative.

Chemical group: Opiate agonist.

Chemical name: Loperamide hydrochloride—1-Piperidinebutanamide, 4-(4-chlorophenyl)-4-hydroxy-N,N-dimethyl-alpha, alpha-diphenyl-, monohydrochloride.

Molecular formula: Loperamide hydrochloride—$C_{29}H_{33}ClN_2O_2 \cdot HCl$.

Molecular weight: Loperamide hydrochloride—513.51.

Description: Loperamide Hydrochloride USP—White to slightly yellow powder. Melts at about 225 °C, with some decomposition.

pKa: 8.6.

Solubility: Loperamide Hydrochloride USP—Freely soluble in methanol, in isopropyl alcohol, and in chloroform; slightly soluble in water and in dilute acids.

USP requirements:
Loperamide Hydrochloride Capsules USP—Preserve in well-closed containers. Contain the labeled amount, within ±10%. Meet the requirements for Identification, Dissolution (70% in 30 minutes in pH 4.7 acetate buffer in Apparatus 1 at 100 rpm), and Uniformity of dosage units.
Loperamide Hydrochloride Oral Solution—Not in USP.
Loperamide Hydrochloride Tablets—Not in USP.

LORATADINE

Chemical name: 1-Piperidinecarboxylic acid, 4-(8-chloro-5,6-dihydro-11H-benzo[5,6]cyclohepta[1,2-b]pyridin-11-ylidene)-, ethyl ester.

Molecular formula: $C_{22}H_{23}ClN_2O_2$.

Molecular weight: 382.89.

Description: Melting point 134–136 °C.

USP requirements: Loratadine Tablets—Not in USP.

LORAZEPAM

Chemical name: 2H-1,4-Benzodiazepin-2-one, 7-chloro-5-(2-chlorophenyl)-1,3-dihydro-3-hydroxy-.

Molecular formula: $C_{15}H_{10}Cl_2N_2O_2$.

Molecular weight: 321.16.

Description: Lorazepam USP—White or practically white, practically odorless powder.

Solubility: Lorazepam USP—Insoluble in water; sparingly soluble in alcohol; slightly soluble in chloroform.

USP requirements:
Lorazepam Injection USP—Preserve in a single-dose or in multiple-dose containers, preferably of Type I glass, protected from light. A sterile solution of Lorazepam in a suitable medium. Contains the labeled amount, within ±10%. Meets the requirements for Identification, Bacterial endotoxins, Related compounds, and Injections.
Lorazepam Concentrated Oral Solution—Not in USP.
Lorazepam Tablets USP—Preserve in tight, light-resistant containers. Contain the labeled amount, within ±10%. Meet the requirements for Identification, Dissolution (60% in 30 minutes and 80% in 60 minutes in water in Apparatus 1 at 100 rpm), Uniformity of dosage units, and Related compounds.
Lorazepam Sublingual Tablets—Not in USP.

LOVASTATIN

Source: Isolated from a strain of *Aspergillus terreus*.

Chemical name: Butanoic acid, 2-methyl-, 1,2,3,7,8,8a-hexahydro-3,7-dimethyl-8-[2-(tetrahydro-4-hydroxy-6-oxo-2H-pyran-2-yl)ethyl]-1-naphthalenyl ester, [1S-[1 alpha(R*), 3 alpha,7 beta,8 beta(2S*,4S*)]8a beta]]-.

Molecular formula: $C_{24}H_{36}O_5$.

Molecular weight: 404.55.

Description: White, nonhygroscopic crystalline powder.

Solubility: Insoluble in water; sparingly soluble in ethanol, in methanol, and in acetonitrile.

USP requirements: Lovastatin Tablets—Not in USP.

LOXAPINE

Chemical group: A tricyclic dibenzoxazepine derivative.

Chemical name:
Loxapine—Dibenz[b,f][1,4]oxazepine, 2-chloro-11-(4-methyl-1-piperazinyl)-.
Loxapine succinate—Butanedioic acid, compd. with 2-chloro-11-(4-methyl-1-piperazinyl)dibenz[b,f][1,4]oxazepine (1:1).

Molecular formula:
Loxapine—$C_{18}H_{18}ClN_3O$.
Loxapine hydrochloride—$C_{18}H_{18}ClN_3O \cdot HCl$.
Loxapine succinate—$C_{18}H_{18}ClN_3O \cdot C_4H_6O_4$.

Molecular weight:
Loxapine—327.81.
Loxapine hydrochloride—364.3.
Loxapine succinate—445.90.

Description: Loxapine Succinate USP—White to yellowish, crystalline powder. Is odorless.

pKa: 6.6.

Solubility: Loxapine succinate—Slightly soluble in water and in alcohol.

USP requirements:
Loxapine Capsules USP—Preserve in tight containers. Contain an amount of loxapine succinate equivalent to the

labeled amount of loxapine, within ±10%. Label Capsules to state both the content of the active moiety and the content of the salt used in formulating the article. Meet the requirements for Identification, Dissolution (75% in 45 minutes in water in Apparatus 1 at 100 rpm), and Uniformity of dosage units.
Loxapine Hydrochloride Injection—Not in USP.
Loxapine Hydrochloride Oral Solution—Not in USP.
Loxapine Succinate Capsules—Not in USP.
Loxapine Succinate Tablets—Not in USP.

LYPRESSIN

Source: A synthetic vasopressin analog.

Chemical name: Vasopressin, 8-L-lysine-.

Molecular formula: $C_{46}H_{65}N_{13}O_{12}S_2$.

Molecular weight: 1056.22.

Description: Hygroscopic, crystalline powder.

Solubility: Freely soluble in water.

USP requirements: Lypressin Nasal Solution USP—Preserve in containers suitable for administering the contents by spraying into the nasal cavities in a controlled individualized dosage. A solution, in a suitable diluent, of the polypeptide hormone, prepared synthetically and free from foreign proteins, which has the properties of causing the contraction of vascular and other smooth muscle and of producing antidiuresis, and which is present in the posterior lobe of the pituitary of healthy pigs. Contains suitable preservatives, and is packaged in a form suitable for nasal administration so that the required dose can be controlled as required. Label it to indicate that it is for intranasal administration only. Label it also to state that the package insert should be consulted for instructions to regulate the dosage according to symptoms. Each mL possesses a pressor activity of the labeled activity of USP Posterior Pituitary Units, within −15% to +20%. Meets the requirements for Oxytocic activity and pH (3.0–4.3).

MAFENIDE

Chemical group: Methylated sulfonamide.

Chemical name: Mafenide acetate—Benzenesulfonamide, 4-(aminomethyl)-, monoacetate.

Molecular formula: Mafenide acetate—$C_7H_{10}N_2O_2S·C_2H_4O_2$.

Molecular weight: Mafenide acetate—246.28.

Description: Mafenide Acetate USP—White, crystalline powder.

Solubility: Mafenide Acetate USP—Freely soluble in water.

Other characteristics: Sulfonamides have certain chemical similarities to some goitrogens, diuretics (acetazolamide and thiazides), and oral antidiabetic agents.

USP requirements:
Mafenide Acetate Cream USP—Preserve in tight, light-resistant containers, and avoid exposure to excessive heat. It is Mafenide Acetate in a water-miscible, oil-in-water cream base, containing suitable preservatives. Contains an amount of mafenide acetate equivalent to the labeled amount of mafenide, within ±10%. Meets the requirement for Identification.
Mafenide Acetate Solution—Not in USP.

MAGALDRATE

Source: A combination of aluminum and magnesium hydroxides and sulfate.

Chemical name: Aluminum magnesium hydroxide sulfate.

Molecular formula: $Al_5Mg_{10}(OH)_{31}(SO_4)_2·xH_2O$.

Molecular weight: 1097.38 (anhydrous approx.).

Description: Magaldrate USP—White, odorless, crystalline powder.

Solubility: Magaldrate USP—Insoluble in water and in alcohol; soluble in dilute solutions of mineral acids.

USP requirements:
Magaldrate Oral Suspension USP—Preserve in tight containers. Contains the labeled amount of magaldrate, within ±10%. Meets the requirements for Identification, Microbial limits, Acid-neutralizing capacity, Magnesium hydroxide content (492–666 mg per gram of labeled amount of magaldrate), and Aluminum hydroxide content (321–459 mg per gram of labeled amount of magaldrate), and for Arsenic and Heavy metals under Magaldrate.
Magaldrate Tablets USP—Preserve in well-closed containers. Label Tablets to indicate whether they are to be swallowed or to be chewed. Contain the labeled amount of magaldrate, within ±10%. Meet the requirements for Identification, Microbial limit, Disintegration (2 minutes, for Magaldrate Tablets labeled to be swallowed), Uniformity of dosage units, Acid-neutralizing capacity, Magnesium hydroxide content (492–666 mg per gram of labeled amount of magaldrate), and Aluminum hydroxide content (321–459 mg per gram of labeled amount of magaldrate).

MAGALDRATE AND SIMETHICONE

For *Magaldrate* and *Simethicone*—See individual listings for chemistry information.

USP requirements:
Magaldrate and Simethicone Oral Suspension USP—Preserve in tight containers, and keep from freezing. Contains the labeled amount of magaldrate, within ±10%. Contains an amount of polydimethylsiloxane equivalent to the labeled amount of simethicone, within ±15%. Meets the requirements for Identification, Acid-neutralizing capacity, Defoaming activity, Microbial limits, Magnesium hydroxide content (492–666 mg per gram of labeled amount of magaldrate), and Aluminum hydroxide content (321–459 mg per gram of labeled amount of magaldrate), and for Arsenic and Heavy metals under Magaldrate.
Magaldrate and Simethicone Tablets USP (Chewable)—Preserve in well-closed containers. Label Tablets to indicate that they are to be chewed before being swallowed. Contain the labeled amount of magaldrate, within ±10%. Contain an amount of polydimethylsiloxane equivalent to the labeled amount of simethicone, within ±15%. Meet the requirements for Identification, Microbial limit, Uniformity of dosage units, Acid-neutralizing capacity, Magnesium hydroxide content (492–666 mg per gram of labeled amount of magaldrate), and Aluminum hydroxide content (321–459 mg per gram of labeled amount of magaldrate).

MAGNESIUM ALUMINUM SILICATE

Description: Magnesium Aluminum Silicate NF—Odorless, fine (micronized) powder or small flakes that are creamy when viewed on their flat surfaces and tan to brown when viewed on their edges.

NF category: Suspending and/or viscosity-increasing agent.

Solubility: Magnesium Aluminum Silicate NF—Insoluble in water and in alcohol. Swells when added to water or glycerin.

NF requirements: Magnesium Aluminum Silicate NF—Preserve in tight containers. A blend of colloidal montmorillonite and saponite that has been processed to remove grit and non-swellable ore components. It is available in 4 types that differ in requirements for viscosity and ratio of aluminum content to magnesium content. Label it to indicate its type. Meets the requirements for Identification, Viscosity, Microbial limits, pH (9.0–10.0, in a suspension [5 in 100] in water), Acid demand (pH not more than 4.0), Loss on drying (not more than 8.0%), Arsenic (not more than 3 ppm), and Lead.

MAGNESIUM CARBONATE

Chemical name: Carbonic acid, magnesium salt, basic; or, Carbonic acid, magnesium salt (1:1), hydrate.

Molecular formula:
Magnesium carbonate—$MgCO_3 \cdot H_2O$.
Magnesium carbonate, basic (approx.)—$(MgCO_3)_4 \cdot Mg(OH)_2 \cdot 5H_2O$.

Molecular weight:
Magnesium carbonate—102.33.
Magnesium carbonate, basic (approx.)—485.65.

Description: Magnesium Carbonate USP—Light, white, friable masses or bulky, white powder. Is odorless, and is stable in air.

Solubility: Magnesium Carbonate USP—Practically insoluble in water; to which, however, it imparts a slightly alkaline reaction; insoluble in alcohol, but is dissolved by dilute acids with effervescence.

USP requirements: Magnesium Carbonate USP—Preserve in well-closed containers. A basic hydrated magnesium carbonate or a normal hydrated magnesium carbonate. Contains the equivalent of not less than 40.0% and not more than 43.5% of magnesium oxide. Meets the requirements for Identification, Microbial limit, Soluble salts (not more than 1.0%), Acid-insoluble substances (not more than 0.05%), Arsenic (not more than 4 ppm), Calcium (not more than 0.45%), Heavy metals (not more than 0.003%), and Iron (not more than 0.02%).

MAGNESIUM CARBONATE AND SODIUM BICARBONATE

For *Magnesium Carbonate* and *Sodium Bicarbonate*—See individual listings for chemistry information.

USP requirements: Magnesium Carbonate and Sodium Bicarbonate for Oral Suspension USP—Preserve in tight containers. Contains the labeled amounts of magnesium carbonate and sodium bicarbonate, within ±10%. Meets the requirements for Identification, Acid-neutralizing capacity, and Minimum fill.

MAGNESIUM CHLORIDE

Chemical name: Magnesium chloride, hexahydrate.

Molecular formula: $MgCl_2 \cdot 6H_2O$.

Molecular weight: 203.30.

Description: Magnesium Chloride USP—Colorless, odorless, deliquescent flakes or crystals, which lose water when heated to 100 °C and lose hydrochloric acid when heated to 110 °C.

Solubility: Magnesium Chloride USP—Very soluble in water; freely soluble in alcohol.

USP requirements: Magnesium Chloride USP—Preserve in tight containers. Where Magnesium Chloride is intended for use in hemodialysis, it is so labeled. Contains not less than 98.0% and not more than 101.0% of magnesium chloride. Meets the requirements for Identification, pH (4.5–7.0, in a 1 in 20 solution in carbon dioxide-free water), Insoluble matter (not more than 0.005%), Sulfate (not more than 0.005%), Arsenic (not more than 3 ppm), Aluminum (where it is labeled as intended for use in hemodialysis, not more than 1 ppm), Barium, Calcium (not more than 0.01%), Potassium, Heavy metals (not more than 0.001%), and Organic volatile impurities.

MAGNESIUM CITRATE

Chemical name: 1,2,3-Propanetricarboxylic acid, hydroxy-, magnesium salt (2:3).

Molecular formula: $C_{12}H_{10}Mg_3O_{14}$.

Molecular weight: 451.12.

Description: Magnesium Citrate Oral Solution USP—Colorless to slightly yellow, clear, effervescent liquid.

USP requirements: Magnesium Citrate Oral Solution USP—Preserve at controlled room temperature or in a cool place, in bottles containing not less than 200 mL. A sterilized or pasteurized solution. Contains, in each 100 mL, not less than 7.59 grams of anhydrous citric acid and an amount of magnesium citrate equivalent to not less than 1.55 grams and not more than 1.9 grams of magnesium oxide.

Prepare Magnesium Citrate Oral Solution as follows: 15 grams of Magnesium Carbonate, 27.4 grams of Anhydrous Citric Acid, 60 mL of Syrup, 5 grams of Talc, 0.1 mL of Lemon Oil, 2.5 grams of Potassium Bicarbonate, and a sufficient quantity of Purified Water to make 350 mL. Dissolve the anhydrous Citric Acid in 150 mL of hot Purified Water in a suitable dish, slowly add the Magnesium Carbonate, previously mixed with 100 mL of Purified Water, and stir until it is dissolved. Then add the Syrup, heat the mixed liquids to the boiling point, immediately add the Lemon Oil, previously triturated with the Talc, and filter the mixture, while hot, into a strong bottle (previously rinsed with boiling Purified Water) of suitable capacity. Add boiled Purified Water to make the product measure 350 mL. Use Purified Cotton as a stopper for the bottle, allow to cool, add the Potassium Bicarbonate, and immediately insert the stopper in the bottle securely. Finally, shake the solution occasionally until the Potassium Bicarbonate is dissolved, cap the bottle, and sterilize or pasteurize the solution.

Note: An amount (30 grams) of citric acid containing 1 molecule of water of hydration, equivalent to 27.4 grams of anhydrous citric acid, may be used in the foregoing formula. In this process the 2.5 grams of potassium bicarbonate may be replaced by 2.1 grams of sodium bicarbonate, preferably in tablet form. The Oral Solution may be further carbonated by the use of carbon dioxide under pressure.

Meets the requirements for Identification, Chloride (not more than 0.01%), Sulfate (not more than 0.015%), and Tartaric acid.

MAGNESIUM GLUCONATE

Chemical name: D-Gluconic acid, magnesium salt (2:1), hydrate.

Molecular formula: $C_{12}H_{22}MgO_{14} \cdot xH_2O$.

Molecular weight: 450.63 (dihydrate).

Description: Magnesium Gluconate USP—Colorless crystals or white powder or granules. Odorless.

Solubility: Magnesium Gluconate USP—Freely soluble in water; very slightly soluble in alcohol; insoluble in ether.

USP requirements: Magnesium Gluconate Tablets USP—Preserve in well-closed containers. Contain the labeled amount, within ±5%. Meet the requirements for Identification, Dissolution (80% in 30 minutes in water in Apparatus 2 at 50 rpm), and Uniformity of dosage units.

MAGNESIUM HYDROXIDE

Chemical name: Magnesium hydroxide.

Molecular formula: $Mg(OH)_2$.

Molecular weight: 58.32.

Description: Magnesium Hydroxide USP—Bulky, white powder.

Solubility: Magnesium Hydroxide USP—Practically insoluble in water and in alcohol; soluble in dilute acids.

USP requirements:
   Magnesia Tablets USP—Preserve in well-closed containers. Contain an amount of magnesia equivalent to the labeled amount of magnesium hydroxide, within ±7%. Meet the requirements for Identification, Disintegration (10 minutes, simulated gastric fluid TS), Acid-neutralizing capacity, and Uniformity of dosage units.
   Milk of Magnesia USP—Preserve in tight containers, preferably at a temperature not exceeding 35 °C. Avoid freezing. A suspension of Magnesium Hydroxide. Double- or Triple-strength Milk of Magnesia is so labeled, or may be labeled as 2X or 3X Concentrated Milk of Magnesia, respectively. Milk of Magnesia, Double-strength Milk of Magnesia, and Triple-strength Milk of Magnesia contain an amount of magnesia equivalent to the labeled amount of magnesium hydroxide, within −10% to +15%, the labeled amount being 80, 160, and 240 mg of magnesium hydroxide per mL, respectively. Meets the requirements for Identification, Acid-neutralizing capacity, Microbial limits, Soluble alkalies, Soluble salts, Carbonate and acid-insoluble matter, Arsenic (not more than $2/W$ ppm, W being the weight, in grams, of specimen taken), Calcium (not more than 0.07%), and Heavy metals (not more than $20/W$ ppm, the W being the weight, in grams, of specimen taken).
   Magnesium Hydroxide Paste USP—Preserve in tight containers. An aqueous paste of magnesium hydroxide, each 100 grams of which contains not less than 29.0 grams and not more than 33.0 grams of magnesium hydroxide. Meets the requirements for Identification, Microbial limits, Soluble alkalies, Soluble salts (not more than 12 mg from 1.67 grams of Paste), Carbonate and acid-insoluble matter, Arsenic (not more than 0.6 ppm, based on amount of diluted Paste taken), Calcium (not more than 0.7% based on the magnesium hydroxide content), and Heavy metals (not more than 5 ppm, based on amount of diluted Paste taken).

MAGNESIUM HYDROXIDE AND MINERAL OIL

For *Magnesium Hydroxide* and *Mineral Oil*—See individual listings for chemistry information.

USP requirements: Milk of Magnesia and Mineral Oil Emulsion—Not in USP.

MAGNESIUM HYDROXIDE, MINERAL OIL, AND GLYCERIN

For *Magnesium Hydroxide, Mineral Oil,* and *Glycerin*—See individual listings for chemistry information.

USP requirements: Milk of Magnesia, Mineral Oil, and Glycerin Emulsion—Not in USP.

MAGNESIUM OXIDE

Chemical name: Magnesium oxide.

Molecular formula: MgO.

Molecular weight: 40.30.

Description: Magnesium Oxide USP—Very bulky, white powder known as Light Magnesium Oxide or relatively dense, white powder known as Heavy Magnesium Oxide. Five grams of Light Magnesium Oxide occupies a volume of approximately 40 to 50 mL, while 5 grams of Heavy Magnesium Oxide occupies a volume of approximately 10 to 20 mL.

Solubility: Magnesium Oxide USP—Practically insoluble in water; soluble in dilute acids; insoluble in alcohol.

USP requirements:
   Magnesium Oxide Capsules USP—Preserve in well-closed containers. Contain the labeled amount, within ±10%. Meet the requirements for Identification, Disintegration (10 minutes in simulated gastric fluid TS), Acid-neutralizing capacity, and Uniformity of dosage units.
   Magnesium Oxide Tablets USP—Preserve in well-closed containers. Contain the labeled amount, within ±10%. Meet the requirements for Disintegration (10 minutes in simulated gastric fluid TS), Acid-neutralizing capacity, and Uniformity of dosage units, and for Identification tests under Magnesium Oxide Capsules.

MAGNESIUM PHOSPHATE

Chemical name: Phosphoric acid, magnesium salt (2:3), pentahydrate.

Molecular formula: $Mg_3(PO_4)_2 \cdot 5H_2O$.

Molecular weight: 352.93.

Description: Magnesium Phosphate USP—White, odorless powder.

Solubility: Magnesium Phosphate USP—Almost insoluble in water; readily soluble in diluted mineral acids.

USP requirements: Magnesium Phosphate USP—Preserve in well-closed containers. Ignited at 425 °C to constant weight, contains not less than 98.0% and not more than 101.5% of magnesium phosphate. Meets the requirements for Identification, Microbial limit, Loss on ignition (20.0–27.0%), Acid-insoluble substances (not more than 0.2%), Soluble substances (not more than 1.5%), Carbonate, Chloride (not more than 0.14%), Nitrate, Sulfate (not more than 0.6%), Arsenic (not more than 3 ppm), Barium, Calcium, Heavy metals (not more than 0.003%), Dibasic salt and magnesium oxide, and Lead (not more than 5 ppm).

MAGNESIUM SALICYLATE

Chemical name: Magnesium, bis(2-hydroxybenzoato-O^1,O^2)-, tetrahydrate.

Molecular formula: $C_{14}H_{10}MgO_6 \cdot 4H_2O$ (tetrahydrate); $C_{14}H_{10}MgO_6$ (anhydrous).

Molecular weight: 370.60 (tetrahydrate); 298.53 (anhydrous).

Description: White, odorless, efflorescent, crystalline powder.

Solubility: Soluble in 13 parts water; soluble in alcohol.

USP requirements: Magnesium Salicylate Tablets USP—Preserve in tight containers. Contain an amount of magnesium salicylate tetrahydrate equivalent to the labeled amount of anhydrous magnesium salicylate, within ±5%. Meet the requirements for Identification, Dissolution (80% in 120 minutes in water in Apparatus 2 at 50 rpm), and Uniformity of dosage units.

MAGNESIUM SILICATE

Description: Magnesium Silicate NF—Fine, white, odorless powder, free from grittiness.
NF category: Glidant and/or anticaking agent.

Solubility: Magnesium Silicate NF—Insoluble in water and in alcohol. Readily decomposed by mineral acids.

NF requirements: Magnesium Silicate NF—Preserve in well-closed containers. A compound of magnesium oxide and silicon dioxide. Contains not less than 15.0% of magnesium oxide and not less than 67.0% of silicon dioxide, calculated on the ignited basis. Meets the requirements for Identification, pH (7.0–10.8, determined in a well-mixed aqueous suspension [1 in 10]), Loss on drying (not more than 15.0%), Loss on ignition (not more than 15%), Soluble salts (not more than 3.0%), Fluoride (not more than 10 ppm), Free alkali, Arsenic (not more than 3 ppm), Lead (not more than 0.001%), Ratio of silicon dioxide to magnesium oxide (2.50–4.50), and Heavy metals (not more than 0.004%).

MAGNESIUM STEARATE

Chemical name: Octadecanoic acid, magnesium salt.

Molecular formula: $C_{36}H_{70}MgO_4$.

Molecular weight: 591.25.

Description: Magnesium Stearate NF—Fine, white, bulky powder, having a faint, characteristic odor. It is unctuous, adheres readily to the skin, and is free from grittiness.
NF category: Tablet and/or capsule lubricant.

Solubility: Magnesium Stearate NF—Insoluble in water, in alcohol, and in ether.

NF requirements: Magnesium Stearate NF—Preserve in well-closed containers. A compound of magnesium with a mixture of solid organic acids obtained from fats, consisting chiefly of variable proportions of magnesium stearate and magnesium palmitate. Contains the equivalent of not less than 6.8% and not more than 8.3% of magnesium oxide. Meets the requirements for Identification, Microbial limits, Loss on drying (not more than 4.0%), and Lead (not more than 0.001%).

MAGNESIUM SULFATE

Chemical name: Sulfuric acid magnesium salt (1:1), heptahydrate.

Molecular formula: $MgSO_4 \cdot 7H_2O$.

Molecular weight: 246.47.

Description: Magnesium Sulfate USP—Small, colorless crystals, usually needle-like. It effloresces in warm, dry air.

Solubility: Magnesium Sulfate USP—Freely soluble in water; freely (and slowly) soluble in glycerin; very soluble in boiling water; sparingly soluble in alcohol.

USP requirements:
Magnesium Sulfate USP (Crystals)—Preserve in well-closed containers. The label states whether it is the monohydrate, the dried form, or the heptahydrate. Magnesium Sulfate intended for use in preparing parenteral dosage forms is so labeled. Magnesium Sulfate not intended for use in preparing parenteral dosage forms is so labeled; in addition, it may be labeled also as intended for use in preparing nonparenteral dosage forms. When rendered anhydrous by ignition, contains not less than 99.0% and not more than 100.5% of magnesium sulfate. Meets the requirements for Identification, pH (5.0–9.2, in a solution [1 in 20]), Loss on ignition (monohydrate, 13.0–16.0%; dried form, 22.0–28.0%; heptahydrate, 40.0–52.0%), Chloride (not more than 0.014%), Arsenic (not more than 3 ppm), Heavy metals (not more than 0.001%), Selenium (not more than 0.003%), Iron (not more than 0.002%, when intended for use in preparing nonparenteral dosage forms; not more than 0.5 ppm, when intended for use in preparing parenteral dosage forms), and Organic volatile impurities.
Magnesium Sulfate Injection USP—Preserve in single-dose or in multiple-dose containers, preferably of Type I glass. A sterile solution of Magnesium Sulfate in Water for Injection. The label states the total osmolar concentration in mOsmol per liter. Where the contents are less than 100 mL, or where the label states that the Injection is not for direct injection but is to be diluted before use, the label alternatively may state the total osmolar concentration in mOsmol per mL. Contains the labeled amount, within ±7%. Meets the requirements for Identification, Bacterial endotoxins, pH (5.5–7.0 in a 5% solution), Particulate matter, and Injections.
Magnesium Sulfate Tablets—Not in USP.

MAGNESIUM TRISILICATE

Chemical name: Silicic acid ($H_4Si_3O_8$), magnesium salt (1:2), hydrate.

Molecular formula: $2MgO \cdot 3SiO_2 \cdot xH_2O$.

Molecular weight: 260.86 (anhydrous).

Description: Magnesium Trisilicate USP—Fine, white, odorless powder, free from grittiness.

Solubility: Magnesium Trisilicate USP—Insoluble in water and in alcohol. Is readily decomposed by mineral acids.

USP requirements: Magnesium Trisilicate Tablets USP—Preserve in well-closed containers. Contain the labeled amount, within ±10%. Meet the requirements for Identification, Disintegration (10 minutes, in simulated gastric fluid TS), Acid-neutralizing capacity (not less than 5 mEq of acid is consumed by the minimum single dose recommended in the labeling), and Uniformity of dosage units.

MAGNESIUM TRISILICATE, ALUMINA, AND MAGNESIA

For *Magnesium Trisilicate, Alumina* (Aluminum Hydroxide), and *Magnesia* (Magnesium Hydroxide)—See individual listings for chemistry information.

USP requirements:
Magnesium Trisilicate, Alumina, and Magnesia Oral Suspension—Not in USP.

Magnesium Trisilicate, Alumina, and Magnesia Chewable Tablets—Not in USP.

MALATHION

Chemical name: Butanedioic acid, [(dimethoxyphosphino-thioyl)-thio]-, diethyl ester.

Molecular formula: $C_{10}H_{19}O_6PS_2$.

Molecular weight: 330.35.

Description: Malathion USP—Yellow to deep brown liquid, having a characteristic odor. Congeals at about 2.9 °C.

Solubility: Malathion USP—Slightly soluble in water. Miscible with alcohols, with esters, with ketones, with ethers, with aromatic and alkylated aromatic hydrocarbons, and with vegetable oils.

USP requirements: Malathion Lotion USP—Preserve in tight, glass containers. It is Malathion in a suitable isopropyl alcohol vehicle. The labeling states the percentage (v/v) of isopropyl alcohol in the Lotion. Contains the labeled amount, within ± 10%. Meets the requirements for Identification and Isopropyl alcohol content (90–110% of labeled amount).

MALIC ACID

Chemical name: Hydroxybutanedioic acid.

Molecular formula: $C_4H_6O_5$.

Molecular weight: 134.09.

Description: Malic Acid NF—White, or practically white, crystalline powder or granules. Melts at about 130 °C.
NF category: Acidifying agent.

Solubility: Malic Acid NF—Very soluble in water; freely soluble in alcohol.

NF requirements: Malic Acid NF—Preserve in well-closed containers. Contains not less than 99.0% and not more than 100.5% of malic acid. Meets the requirements for Identification, Specific rotation (−0.10° to +0.10°), Residue on ignition (not more than 0.1%), Water-insoluble substances (not more than 0.1%), Heavy metals (not more than 0.002%), Fumaric and maleic acids (not more than 1.0% of fumaric acid; not more than 0.05% of maleic acid), and Organic volatile impurities.

MALTODEXTRIN

Description: Maltodextrin NF—White, hygroscopic powder or granules.
NF category: Tablet and/or capsule diluent; coating agent; tablet binder; viscosity-increasing agent.

Solubility: Maltodextrin NF—Freely soluble or readily dispersible in water; slightly soluble to insoluble in anhydrous alcohol.

NF requirements: Maltodextrin NF—Preserve in tight containers, or in well-closed containers at a temperature not exceeding 30 °C and a relative humidity not exceeding 50%. A nonsweet, nutritive saccharide mixture of polymers that consist of D-glucose units, with a Dextrose Equivalent less than 20. Prepared by the partial hydrolysis of a food grade starch with suitable acids and/or enzymes. May be physically modified to improve its physical and functional characteristics. Meets the requirements for Microbial limits, pH (4.0–7.0, in a 1 in 5 solution in carbon dioxide-free water), Loss on drying (not more than 6.0%), Residue on ignition

(not more than 0.5%), Heavy metals (not more than 5 ppm), Protein (not more than 0.1%), Sulfur dioxide (not more than 0.004%), and Dextrose equivalent (not more than 20).

MALT SOUP EXTRACT

Source: Obtained from the grain of one or more varieties of barley; contains 73% maltose, 12% other polymeric carbohydrates, 7% protein, 1.5% potassium, and small amounts of calcium, magnesium, phosphorus, and vitamins.

USP requirements:
Malt Soup Extract Powder—Not in USP.
Malt Soup Extract Oral Solution—Not in USP.
Malt Soup Extract Tablets—Not in USP.

MALT SOUP EXTRACT AND PSYLLIUM

For *Malt Soup Extract* and *Psyllium*—See individual listings for chemistry information.

USP requirements: Malt Soup Extract and Psyllium Powder—Not in USP.

MANGANESE

Chemical name:
Manganese chloride—Manganese chloride ($MnCl_2$) tetrahydrate.
Manganese sulfate—Sulfuric acid, manganese(2+) salt (1:1) monohydrate.

Molecular formula:
Manganese chloride—$MnCl_2 \cdot 4H_2O$.
Manganese sulfate—$MnSO_4 \cdot H_2O$.

Molecular weight:
Manganese chloride—197.91.
Manganese sulfate—169.01.

Description:
Manganese Chloride USP—Large, irregular, pink, odorless, translucent crystals.
Manganese Sulfate USP—Pale red, slightly efflorescent crystals, or purple, odorless powder.

Solubility:
Manganese Chloride USP—Soluble in water and in alcohol; insoluble in ether.
Manganese Sulfate USP—Soluble in water; insoluble in alcohol.

USP requirements:
Manganese Chloride Injection USP—Preserve in single-dose or in multiple-dose containers, preferably of Type I or Type II glass. A sterile solution of Manganese Chloride in Water for Injection. Label the Injection to indicate that it is to be diluted to the appropriate strength with Sterile Water for Injection or other suitable fluid prior to administration. Contains an amount of manganese chloride equivalent to the labeled amount of manganese, within ± 5%. Meets the requirements for Identification, Bacterial endotoxins, pH (1.5–2.5), Particulate matter, and Injections.
Manganese Sulfate Injection USP—Preserve in single-dose or in multiple-dose containers, preferably of Type I or Type II glass. A sterile solution of Manganese Sulfate in Water for Injection. Label the Injection to indicate that it is to be diluted to the appropriate strength with Sterile Water for Injection or other suitable fluid prior to administration. Contains an amount of manganese sulfate equivalent to the labeled amount of manganese, within

±5%. Meets the requirements for Identification, Bacterial endotoxins, pH (2.0–3.5), Particulate matter, and Injections.

MANNITOL

Chemical name: D-Mannitol.

Molecular formula: $C_6H_{14}O_6$.

Molecular weight: 182.17.

Description: Mannitol USP—White, crystalline powder or free-flowing granules. Is odorless.
NF category: Sweetening agent; tablet and/or capsule diluent; tonicity agent; bulking agent for freeze-drying.

Solubility: Mannitol USP—Freely soluble in water; soluble in alkaline solutions; slightly soluble in pyridine; very slightly soluble in alcohol; practically insoluble in ether.

USP requirements:
Mannitol USP—Preserve in well-closed containers. Contains not less than 96.0% and not more than 101.5% of mannitol, calculated on the dried basis. Meets the requirements for Identification, Melting range (165–169 °C), Specific rotation (+137° to +145°), Acidity, Loss on drying (not more than 0.3%), Chloride (not more than 0.007%), Sulfate (not more than 0.01%), Arsenic (not more than 1 ppm), and Reducing sugars.
Mannitol Injection USP—Preserve in single-dose glass or plastic containers. Glass containers are preferably of Type I or Type II glass. A sterile solution, which may be supersaturated, of Mannitol in Water for Injection. Contains no antimicrobial agents. May require warming or autoclaving before use if crystallization has occurred. The label states the total osmolar concentration in mOsmol per liter. Where the contents are less than 100 mL, or where the label states that the Injection is not for direct injection but is to be diluted before use, the label alternatively may state the total osmolar concentration in mOsmol per mL. Contains the labeled amount, within ±5%. Meets the requirements for Identification, Specific rotation, Pyrogen, pH (4.5–7.0), Particulate matter, and Injections.

MANNITOL AND SODIUM CHLORIDE

For *Mannitol* and *Sodium Chloride*—See individual listings for chemistry information.

USP requirements: Mannitol in Sodium Chloride Injection USP—A sterile solution of Mannitol and Sodium Chloride in Water for Injection. The label states the total osmolar concentration in mOsmol per liter. Where the contents are less than 100 mL, or where the label states that the Injection is not for direct injection but is to be diluted before use, the label alternatively may state the total osmolar concentration in mOsmol per mL. Contains the labeled amounts of mannitol and sodium chloride, within ±5%. Contains no antimicrobial agents. Meets the requirements for Identification, Bacterial endotoxins, and pH (4.5–7.0), for Packaging and storage under Mannitol Injection, and for Injections.

MAPROTILINE

Chemical group: Dibenzo-bicyclo-octadiene.

Chemical name: Maprotiline hydrochloride—9,10-Ethano-anthracene-9(10H)-propanamine, N-methyl-, hydrochloride.

Molecular formula: Maprotiline hydrochloride—$C_{20}H_{23}N \cdot HCl$.

Molecular weight: Maprotiline hydrochloride—313.87.

Description: Maprotiline Hydrochloride USP—Fine, white to off-white, crystalline powder. Is practically odorless.

Solubility: Maprotiline Hydrochloride USP—Freely soluble in methanol and in chloroform; slightly soluble in water; practically insoluble in isooctane.

USP requirements: Maprotiline Hydrochloride Tablets USP—Preserve in well-closed containers. Contain the labeled amount, within ±10%. Meet the requirements for Identification, Dissolution (75% in 60 minutes in dilute hydrochloric acid [7 in 1000] in Apparatus 2 at 50 rpm), and Uniformity of dosage units.

MAZINDOL

Chemical group: Imidazoisoindole.

Chemical name: 3H-Imidazo[2,1-a]isoindol-5-ol, 5-(4-chlorophenyl)-2,5-dihydro-.

Molecular formula: $C_{16}H_{13}ClN_2O$.

Molecular weight: 284.74.

Description: Mazindol USP—White to off-white, crystalline powder, having not more than a faint odor.

Solubility: Mazindol USP—Insoluble in water; slightly soluble in methanol and in chloroform.

USP requirements: Mazindol Tablets USP—Preserve in tight containers, at a temperature not exceeding 25 °C. Contain the labeled amount, within ±10%. Meet the requirements for Identification, Dissolution (60% in 60 minutes in 0.1 N hydrochloric acid in Apparatus 2 at 50 rpm), and Uniformity of dosage units.

MEASLES AND MUMPS VIRUS VACCINE LIVE

Description: Measles and Mumps Virus Vaccine Live USP—Solid having the characteristic appearance of substances dried from the frozen state. The Vaccine is to be constituted with a suitable diluent just prior to use. Constituted vaccine undergoes loss of potency on exposure to sunlight.

USP requirements: Measles and Mumps Virus Vaccine Live USP—Preserve in single-dose containers, or in light-resistant, multiple-dose containers, at a temperature between 2 and 8 °C. Multiple-dose containers for 50 doses are adapted for use only in jet injectors, and those for 10 doses for use by jet or syringe injection. A bacterially sterile preparation of a combination of live measles virus and live mumps virus such that each component is prepared in conformity with and meets the requirements for Measles Virus Vaccine Live and for Mumps Virus Vaccine Live, whichever is applicable. Each component provides an immunizing dose and meets the requirements of the corresponding Virus Vaccine in the total dosage prescribed in the labeling. Label the Vaccine in multiple-dose containers to indicate that the contents are intended solely for use by jet injector or for use by either jet or syringe injection, whichever is applicable. Label the Vaccine in single-dose containers, if such containers are not light-resistant, to state that it should be protected from sunlight. Label it also to state that constituted Vaccine should be discarded if not used within 8 hours. Meets the requirement for Expiration date (1 to 2 years, depending on the manufacturer's data, after date of issue from manufacturer's cold storage [−20 °C, 1 year]). Conforms to the regulations of the U.S. Food and Drug Administration concerning biologics.

MEASLES, MUMPS, AND RUBELLA VIRUS VACCINE LIVE

Description: Measles, Mumps, and Rubella Virus Vaccine Live USP—Solid having the characteristic appearance of substances dried from the frozen state. The Vaccine is to be constituted with a suitable diluent just prior to use. Constituted vaccine undergoes loss of potency on exposure to sunlight.

USP requirements: Measles, Mumps, and Rubella Virus Vaccine Live USP—Preserve in single-dose containers, or in light-resistant, multiple-dose containers, at a temperature between 2 and 8 °C. Multiple-dose containers for 50 doses are adapted for use only in jet injectors, and those for 10 doses for use by jet or syringe injection. A bacterially sterile preparation of a combination of live measles virus, live mumps virus, and live rubella virus such that each component is prepared in conformity with and meets the requirements for Measles Virus Vaccine Live, for Mumps Virus Vaccine Live, and for Rubella Virus Vaccine Live, whichever is applicable. Each component provides an immunizing dose and meets the requirements of the corresponding Virus Vaccine in the total dosage prescribed in the labeling. Label the Vaccine in multiple-dose containers to indicate that the contents are intended solely for use by jet injector or for use by either jet or syringe injection, whichever is applicable. Label the Vaccine in single-dose containers, if such containers are not light-resistant, to state that it should be protected from sunlight. Label it also to state that constituted Vaccine should be discarded if not used within 8 hours. Meets the requirement for Expiration date (1 to 2 years, depending on the manufacturer's data, after date of issue from manufacturer's cold storage [−20 °C, 1 year]). Conforms to the regulations of the U.S. Food and Drug Administration concerning biologics.

MEASLES AND RUBELLA VIRUS VACCINE LIVE

Description: Measles and Rubella Virus Vaccine Live USP— Solid having the characteristic appearance of substances dried from the frozen state. The Vaccine is to be constituted with a suitable diluent just prior to use. Constituted vaccine undergoes loss of potency on exposure to sunlight.

USP requirements: Measles and Rubella Virus Vaccine Live USP—Preserve in single-dose containers, or in light-resistant, multiple-dose containers, at a temperature between 2 and 8 °C. Multiple-dose containers for 50 doses are adapted for use only in jet injectors, and those for 10 doses for use by jet or syringe injection. A bacterially sterile preparation of a combination of live measles virus and live rubella virus such that each component is prepared in conformity with and meets the requirements for Measles Virus Vaccine Live and for Rubella Virus Vaccine Live, whichever is applicable. Each component provides an immunizing dose and meets the requirements of the corresponding Virus Vaccine in the total dosage prescribed in the labeling. Label the Vaccine in multiple-dose containers to indicate that the contents are intended solely for use by jet injector or for use by either jet or syringe injection, whichever is applicable. Label the Vaccine in single-dose containers, if such containers are not light-resistant, to state that it should be protected from sunlight. Label it also to state that constituted Vaccine should be discarded if not used within 8 hours. Meets the requirement for Expiration date (1 to 2 years, depending on the manufacturer's data, after date of issue from manufacturer's cold storage [−20 °C, 1 year]). Conforms to the regulations of the U.S. Food and Drug Administration concerning biologics.

MEASLES VIRUS VACCINE LIVE

Source: The currently available vaccine in the U.S. (*Attenuvax*, MSD) contains a lyophilized preparation of a more attenuated line of live measles virus derived from Enders' attenuated Edmonston strain. Further modification of the virus was achieved by multiple passage of Edmonston virus in cell cultures of chick embryo at low temperature. *Attenuvax*, Morson (UK) and Measles Virus Vaccine, Live Attenuated (Dried), Connaught (Canada) brands of live measles virus vaccine, also contain the Enders' attenuated Edmonston strain.

Description: Measles Virus Vaccine Live USP—Solid having the characteristic appearance of substances dried from the frozen state. Undergoes loss of potency on exposure to sunlight. The Vaccine is to be constituted with a suitable diluent just prior to use.

Other characteristics: Slightly acidic, pH 6.2 to 6.6.

USP requirements: Measles Virus Vaccine Live USP—Preserve in single-dose containers, or in light-resistant, multiple-dose containers, at a temperature between 2 and 8 °C. Multiple-dose containers for 50 doses are adapted for use only in jet injectors, and those for 10 doses for use by jet or syringe injection. A bacterially sterile preparation of live virus derived from a strain of measles virus tested for neurovirulence in monkeys, for safety, and for immunogenicity, free from all demonstrable viable microbial agents except unavoidable bacteriophage, and found suitable for human immunization. The strain is grown for purposes of vaccine production on chicken embryo primary cell tissue cultures derived from pathogen-free flocks, meets the requirements of the specific safety tests in adult and suckling mice; the requirements of the tests in monkey kidney, chicken embryo and human tissue cell cultures and embryonated eggs; and the requirements of the tests for absence of *Mycobacterium tuberculosis* and of avian leucosis, unless the production cultures were derived from certified avian leucosis-free sources and the control fluids were tested for avian leucosis. The strain cultures are treated to remove all intact tissue cells. The Vaccine meets the requirements of the specific tissue culture test for live virus titer, in a single immunizing dose, of not less than the equivalent of 1000 $TCID_{50}$ (quantity of virus estimated to infect 50% of inoculated cultures × 1000) when tested in parallel with the U.S. Reference Measles Virus, Live Attenuated. Label the Vaccine in multiple-dose containers to indicate that the contents are intended solely for use by jet injector or for use by either jet or syringe injection, whichever is applicable. Label the Vaccine in single-dose containers, if such containers are not light-resistant, to state that it should be protected from sunlight. Label it also to state that constituted Vaccine should be discarded if not used within 8 hours. Meets the requirement for Expiration date (1 to 2 years, depending on the manufacturer's data, after date of issue from manufacturer's cold storage [−20 °C, 1 year]). Conforms to the regulations of the U.S. Food and Drug Administration concerning biologics.

MEBENDAZOLE

Chemical group: Benzimidazole carbamate derivative; structurally related to thiabendazole.

Chemical name: Carbamic acid, (5-benzoyl-1*H*-benzimidazol-2-yl)-, methyl ester.

Molecular formula: $C_{16}H_{13}N_3O_3$.

Molecular weight: 295.30.

Description: Mebendazole USP—White to slightly yellow powder. Is almost odorless. Melts at about 290 °C.

Solubility: Mebendazole USP—Practically insoluble in water, in dilute solutions of mineral acids, in alcohol, in ether, and in chloroform; freely soluble in formic acid.

USP requirements: Mebendazole Tablets USP—Preserve in well-closed containers. Contain the labeled amount, within ±10%. Meet the requirements for Identification, Disintegration (10 minutes), and Uniformity of dosage units.

MECAMYLAMINE

Chemical name: Mecamylamine hydrochloride—Bicyclo-[2.2.1]heptan-2-amine, N,2,3,3-tetramethyl-, hydrochloride.

Molecular formula: Mecamylamine hydrochloride—$C_{11}H_{21}N \cdot HCl$.

Molecular weight: Mecamylamine hydrochloride—203.75.

Description: Mecamylamine hydrochloride—White, odorless or practically odorless, crystalline powder. Melts at about 245 °C, with decomposition.

pKa: 11.2.

Solubility: Mecamylamine hydrochloride—Freely soluble in water and in chloroform; soluble in isopropyl alcohol; practically insoluble in ether.

USP requirements: Mecamylamine Hydrochloride Tablets USP—Preserve in well-closed containers. Contain the labeled amount, within ±10%. Meet the requirements for Identification, Dissolution (75% in 30 minutes in water in Apparatus 2 at 50 rpm), and Uniformity of dosage units.

MECHLORETHAMINE

Chemical name: Mechlorethamine hydrochloride—Ethanamine, 2-chloro-N-(2-chloroethyl)-N-methyl-, hydrochloride.

Molecular formula: Mechlorethamine hydrochloride—$C_5H_{11}Cl_2N \cdot HCl$.

Molecular weight: Mechlorethamine hydrochloride—192.52.

Description: Mechlorethamine Hydrochloride USP—White, crystalline powder. Is hygroscopic.

pKa: 6.1.

Solubility: Mechlorethamine hydrochloride—Very soluble in water; soluble in alcohol.

USP requirements:
Mechlorethamine Hydrochloride for Injection USP—Preserve in Containers for Sterile Solids. A sterile mixture of Mechlorethamine Hydrochloride with Sodium Chloride or other suitable diluent. The label bears a warning that great care should be taken to prevent inhaling particles of Mechlorethamine Hydrochloride for Injection and exposing the skin to it. Contains the labeled amount, within ±10%. Meets the requirements for Labeling under Injections, Completeness of solution, Constituted solution, Identification, Bacterial endotoxins, pH (3.0–5.0, in a solution [1 in 50]), Water (not more than 1.0%), and Particulate matter, and for Sterility tests and Uniformity of dosage units.
Mechlorethamine Hydrochloride Ointment—Not in USP.
Mechlorethamine Hydrochloride Topical Solution—Not in USP.

MECLIZINE

Chemical group: Piperazine derivative.

Chemical name: Meclizine hydrochloride—Piperazine, 1-[(4-chlorophenyl)phenylmethyl]-4-[(3-methylphenyl)methyl]-, dihydrochloride, monohydrate.

Molecular formula: Meclizine hydrochloride—$C_{25}H_{27}ClN_2 \cdot 2HCl \cdot H_2O$.

Molecular weight: Meclizine hydrochloride—481.89.

Description: Meclizine Hydrochloride USP—White or slightly yellowish, crystalline powder. Has a slight odor.

Solubility: Meclizine Hydrochloride USP—Practically insoluble in water and in ether; freely soluble in chloroform, in pyridine, and in acid-alcohol-water mixtures; slightly soluble in dilute acids and in alcohol.

USP requirements:
Meclizine Hydrochloride Capsules—Not in USP.
Meclizine Hydrochloride Tablets USP—Preserve in well-closed containers. Contain the labeled amount, within −5% to +10%. Meet the requirements for Identification, Dissolution (75% in 45 minutes in 0.1 N hydrochloric acid in Apparatus 1 at 100 rpm), and Uniformity of dosage units.

MECLOCYCLINE

Chemical name: Meclocycline sulfosalicylate—2-Naphthacenecarboxamide, 7-chloro-4-(dimethylamino)-1,4,4a,5,5a,6,-11,12a-octahydro-3,5,10,12,12a-pentahydroxy-6-methylene-1,11-dioxo-, [4S-(4 alpha,4a alpha,5 alpha,5a alpha,12a alpha)]-, mono(2-hydroxy-5-sulfobenzoate) (salt).

Molecular formula: Meclocycline sulfosalicylate—$C_{22}H_{21}ClN_2O_8 \cdot C_7H_6O_6S$.

Molecular weight: Meclocycline sulfosalicylate—695.05.

Description: Meclocycline sulfosalicylate—Yellow, crystalline powder.

USP requirements: Meclocycline Sulfosalicylate Cream USP—Preserve in tight containers, protected from light. Contains an amount of meclocycline sulfosalicylate equivalent to the labeled amount of meclocycline, within −10% to +25%. Meets the requirement for Minimum fill.

MECLOFENAMATE

Chemical group: Fenamate derivative.

Chemical name: Meclofenamate sodium—Benzoic acid, 2-[(2,6-dichloro-3-methylphenyl)amino]-, monosodium salt, monohydrate.

Molecular formula: Meclofenamate sodium—$C_{14}H_{10}Cl_2NNaO_2 \cdot H_2O$.

Molecular weight: Meclofenamate sodium—336.15.

Description: Meclofenamate Sodium USP—White to creamy white, odorless to almost odorless, crystalline powder.

Solubility: Meclofenamate Sodium USP—Soluble in methanol; slightly soluble in chloroform; practically insoluble in ether. Freely soluble in water, the solution sometimes being somewhat turbid due to partial hydrolysis and absorption of carbon dioxide; the solution is clear above pH 11.5.

USP requirements: Meclofenamate Sodium Capsules USP—Preserve in tight, light-resistant containers. Contain an amount of meclofenamate sodium equivalent to the labeled amount of meclofenamic acid, within ±10%. Meet the requirements for Identification, Dissolution (75% in 45 minutes in 0.05 M phosphate buffer [pH 8.0] in Apparatus 2 at 50 rpm), and Uniformity of dosage units.

MEDROXYPROGESTERONE

Chemical name: Medroxyprogesterone acetate—Pregn-4-ene-3,20-dione, 17-(acetyloxy)-6-methyl-, (6 alpha)-.

Molecular formula: Medroxyprogesterone acetate—$C_{24}H_{34}O_4$.

Molecular weight: Medroxyprogesterone acetate—386.53.

Description: Medroxyprogesterone Acetate USP—White to off-white, odorless, crystalline powder. Melts at about 205 °C. Is stable in air.

Solubility: Medroxyprogesterone Acetate USP—Insoluble in water; freely soluble in chloroform; soluble in acetone and in dioxane; sparingly soluble in alcohol and in methanol; slightly soluble in ether.

USP requirements:
Sterile Medroxyprogesterone Acetate Suspension USP—Preserve in single-dose or in multiple-dose containers, preferably of Type I glass. A sterile suspension of Medroxyprogesterone Acetate in a suitable aqueous medium. Contains the labeled amount, within ± 10%. Meets the requirements for Identification, pH (3.0–7.0), and Injections.
Medroxyprogesterone Acetate Tablets USP—Preserve in well-closed containers. Contain the labeled amount, within ± 7%. Meet the requirements for Identification, Dissolution (50% in 45 minutes in 0.5% sodium lauryl sulfate in Apparatus 2 at 50 rpm), and Uniformity of dosage units.

MEDRYSONE

Chemical name: Pregn-4-ene-3,20-dione, 11-hydroxy-6-methyl-, (6 alpha,11 beta)-.

Molecular formula: $C_{22}H_{32}O_3$.

Molecular weight: 344.49.

Description: Medrysone USP—White to off-white, crystalline powder. Is odorless or may have a slight odor. Melts at about 158 °C, with decomposition.

Solubility: Medrysone USP—Sparingly soluble in water; soluble in methylene chloride and in chloroform.

USP requirements: Medrysone Ophthalmic Suspension USP—Preserve in tight, light-resistant containers. A sterile suspension of Medrysone in a buffered aqueous medium containing a suitable antimicrobial agent and preservative. Contains the labeled amount, within −10% to +15%. Meets the requirements for Identification, Sterility, and pH (6.2–7.5).

MEFENAMIC ACID

Chemical group: Fenamate derivative.

Chemical name: Benzoic acid, 2-[(2,3-dimethylphenyl)amino]-.

Molecular formula: $C_{15}H_{15}NO_2$.

Molecular weight: 241.29.

Description: Mefenamic Acid USP—White to off-white, crystalline powder. Melts at about 230 °C, with decomposition.

pKa: 4.2.

Solubility: Mefenamic Acid USP—Soluble in solutions of alkali hydroxides; sparingly soluble in chloroform; slightly soluble in alcohol and in methanol; practically insoluble in water.

USP requirements: Mefenamic Acid Capsules USP—Preserve in tight containers. Contain the labeled amount, within ± 10%.

Meet the requirements for Identification and Uniformity of dosage units.

MEFLOQUINE

Chemical name: Mefloquine hydrochloride—4-Quinolinemethanol, alpha-2-piperidinyl-2,8-bis(trifluoromethyl)-, monohydrochloride, ($R*,S*$)- (±)-.

Molecular formula: Mefloquine hydrochloride—$C_{17}H_{16}F_6N_2O$·HCl.

Molecular weight: Mefloquine hydrochloride—414.78.

Description: Mefloquine hydrochloride—White to almost white crystalline compound.

Solubility: Mefloquine hydrochloride—Slightly soluble in water.

USP requirements: Mefloquine Hydrochloride Tablets—Not in USP.

MEGESTROL

Chemical name: Megestrol acetate—Pregna-4,6-diene-3,20-dione, 17-(acetyloxy)-6-methyl-.

Molecular formula: Megestrol acetate—$C_{24}H_{32}O_4$.

Molecular weight: Megestrol acetate—384.51.

Description: Megestrol Acetate USP—White to creamy white, essentially odorless, crystalline powder. Is unstable under aqueous conditions at pH 7 or above.

Solubility: Megestrol Acetate USP—Insoluble in water; sparingly soluble in alcohol; slightly soluble in ether and in fixed oils; soluble in acetone; very soluble in chloroform.

USP requirements: Megestrol Acetate Tablets USP—Preserve in well-closed containers. Contain the labeled amount, within ± 7%. Meet the requirements for Identification, Dissolution (75% in 60 minutes in 1% sodium lauryl sulfate in Apparatus 2 at 100 rpm), and Uniformity of dosage units.

MELPHALAN

Chemical name: L-Phenylalanine, 4-[bis(2-chloroethyl)amino]-.

Molecular formula: $C_{13}H_{18}Cl_2N_2O_2$.

Molecular weight: 305.20.

Description: Melphalan USP—Off-white to buff powder, having a faint odor. Melts at about 180 °C, with decomposition.

Solubility: Melphalan USP—Practically insoluble in water, in chloroform, and in ether; soluble in dilute mineral acids; slightly soluble in alcohol and in methanol.

USP requirements: Melphalan Tablets USP—Preserve in well-closed, light-resistant, glass containers. Contain the labeled amount, within ± 10%. Meet the requirements for Identification, Disintegration (15 minutes), and Uniformity of dosage units.

MENADIOL

Chemical name: Menadiol sodium diphosphate—1,4-Naphthalenediol, 2-methyl-, bis(dihydrogen phosphate), tetrasodium salt, hexahydrate.

Molecular formula: Menadiol sodium diphosphate—$C_{11}H_8Na_4O_8P_2$·$6H_2O$.

Molecular weight: Menadiol sodium diphosphate—530.18.

Description: Menadiol Sodium Diphosphate USP—White to pink powder, having a characteristic odor. Is hygroscopic. Its solutions are neutral or slightly alkaline to litmus, having a pH of about 8.

Solubility: Menadiol Sodium Diphosphate USP—Very soluble in water; insoluble in alcohol.

USP requirements:

Menadiol Sodium Diphosphate Injection USP—Preserve in single-dose, light-resistant containers, preferably of Type I glass. A sterile solution of Menadiol Sodium Diphosphate in Water for Injection. Contains the labeled amount, within −5% to +10%. Meets the requirements for Identification, Bacterial endotoxins, pH (7.5–8.5), and Injections.

Menadiol Sodium Diphosphate Tablets USP—Preserve in well-closed, light-resistant containers. Contain the labeled amount, within −5% to +10%. Meet the requirements for Identification, Dissolution (75% in 30 minutes in 0.1 N hydrochloric acid in Apparatus 1 at 100 rpm), and Uniformity of dosage units.

MENADIONE

Chemical name: 1,4-Naphthalenedione, 2-methyl.

Molecular formula: $C_{11}H_8O_2$.

Molecular weight: 172.18.

Description: Menadione USP—Bright yellow, crystalline, practically odorless powder. Affected by sunlight.

Solubility: Menadione USP—Practically insoluble in water; soluble in vegetable oils; sparingly soluble in chloroform and in alcohol.

USP requirements: Menadione Injection USP—Preserve in single-dose or in multiple-dose containers, preferably of Type I glass. A sterile solution of Menadione in oil. Contains the labeled amount, within −10% to +20%. Meets the requirements for Bacterial endotoxins and Injections.

MENINGOCOCCAL POLYSACCHARIDE VACCINE

Source: The vaccine currently available in the U.S. and Canada contains a freeze-dried preparation of the group-specific polysaccharide antigens from *Neisseria meningitidis*, Group A, Group C, Group Y, and Group W-135.

USP requirements:

Meningococcal Polysaccharide Vaccine for Injection—Not in USP.

Meningococcal Polysaccharide Vaccine Group A USP—Preserve in multiple-dose containers for subcutaneous or jet injection at a temperature between 2 and 8 °C. (Note: Use the constituted vaccine immediately after its constitution, or if stored in a refrigerator within 8 hours after constitution.) A sterile preparation of the group-specific polysaccharide antigen from *Neisseria meningitidis*, Group A, consisting of a polymer of *N*-acetyl mannosamine phosphate. Contains 50 mcg of isolated product and 2.5 to 5 mg of lactose as a stabilizer per 0.5-mL dose, when constituted as directed. The constituting fluid is Bacteriostatic Sodium Chloride Injection in which the antimicrobial agent is Thimerosal in a suitable concentration. Meets the requirements of the tests for potency, and for Expiration date (not later than 18 months after date of issue from manufacturer's cold storage [−20 °C, 6 months]). Conforms to the regulations of the U.S. Food and Drug Administration concerning biologics.

Meningococcal Polysaccharide Vaccine Groups A and C Combined USP—Preserve in multiple-dose containers for subcutaneous or jet injection at a temperature between 2 and 8 °C. (Note: Use the constituted vaccine immediately after its constitution, or if stored in a refrigerator within 8 hours after constitution.) A sterile preparation consisting of Meningococcal Polysaccharide Group A and C specific antigens. Contains 50 mcg of each isolated product and 2.5 to 5 mg of lactose as a stabilizer per 0.5-mL dose, when constituted as directed. The constituting fluid is Bacteriostatic Sodium Chloride Injection in which the antimicrobial agent is Thimerosal in a suitable concentration. Each component meets the requirements for antigenicity or potency, and for Expiration date (not later than 18 months after date of issue from manufacturer's cold storage [−20 °C, 6 months]). Conforms to the regulations of the U.S. Food and Drug Administration concerning biologics.

Meningococcal Polysaccharide Vaccine Group C USP—Preserve in multiple-dose containers for subcutaneous or jet injection at a temperature between 2 and 8 °C. (Note: Use the constituted vaccine immediately after its constitution, or if stored in a refrigerator within 8 hours after constitution.) A sterile preparation of the group-specific polysaccharide antigen from *Neisseria meningitidis*, Group C, consisting of a polymer of sialic acid. Contains 50 mcg of isolated product and 2.5 to 5 mg of lactose as a stabilizer per 0.5-mL dose, when constituted as directed. The constituting fluid is Bacteriostatic Sodium Chloride Injection in which the antimicrobial agent is Thimerosal in a suitable concentration. Meets the requirements of the tests for potency, and for Expiration date (not later than 18 months after date of issue from manufacturer's cold storage [−20 °C, 6 months]). Conforms to the regulations of the U.S. Food and Drug Administration concerning biologics.

MENOTROPINS

Source: Extracted from urine of postmenopausal women.

Chemical name: Follicle stimulating hormone.

USP requirements: Menotropins for Injection USP—Preserve in Containers for Sterile Solids. A sterile, freeze-dried mixture of menotropins and suitable excipients. Contains labeled potencies of Follicle-stimulating Hormone and Luteinizing Hormone, within −20% to +25%. Meets the requirements for Constituted solution, Bacterial endotoxins, and pH (6.0–7.0, in the solution constituted as directed in the labeling), and for Sterility tests, Uniformity of dosage units, and Labeling under Injections.

MENTHOL

Chemical name: Cyclohexanol, 5-methyl-2-(1-methylethyl)-.

Molecular formula: $C_{10}H_{20}O$.

Molecular weight: 156.27.

Description: Menthol USP—Colorless, hexagonal crystals, usually needle-like, or in fused masses, or crystalline powder. It has a pleasant, peppermint-like odor.

NF category: Flavors and perfumes.

Solubility: Menthol USP—Slightly soluble in water; very soluble in alcohol, in chloroform, in ether, and in solvent hexane; freely soluble in glacial acetic acid, in mineral oil, and in fixed and volatile oils.

USP requirements: Menthol USP—Preserve in tight containers, preferably at controlled room temperature. An alcohol obtained from diverse mint oils or prepared synthetically. Menthol may be levorotatory (*l*-Menthol), from natural or synthetic sources, or racemic (*dl*-Menthol). Label it to indicate whether it is levorotatory or racemic. Meets the requirements for Identification, Melting range of *l*-Menthol (41–44 °C), Congealing range of *dl*-Menthol, Specific rotation (−45° to −51° for *l*-Menthol; −2° to +2° for *dl*-Menthol), Nonvolatile residue (not more than 0.05%), Readily oxidizable substances in *dl*-Menthol, Chromatographic purity, and Organic volatile impurities.

MEPENZOLATE

Chemical group: Synthetic quaternary ammonium compound.

Chemical name: Mepenzolate bromide—Piperidinium, 3-[(hydroxydiphenylacetyl)oxy]-1,1-dimethyl-, bromide.

Molecular formula: Mepenzolate bromide—$C_{21}H_{26}BrNO_3$.

Molecular weight: Mepenzolate bromide—420.35.

Description: Mepenzolate bromide—White or light cream-colored powder.

Solubility: Mepenzolate bromide—Slightly soluble in water and in chloroform; freely soluble in methanol; practically insoluble in ether.

USP requirements:
Mepenzolate Bromide Syrup USP—Preserve in tight, light-resistant containers. Contains the labeled amount, within ±7%. Meets the requirement for Identification.
Mepenzolate Bromide Tablets USP—Preserve in well-closed containers. Contain the labeled amount, within ±7%. Meet the requirements for Identification, Disintegration (30 minutes), and Uniformity of dosage units.

MEPERIDINE

Chemical name: Meperidine hydrochloride—4-Piperidinecarboxylic acid, 1-methyl-4-phenyl-, ethyl ester, hydrochloride.

Molecular formula: Meperidine hydrochloride—$C_{15}H_{21}NO_2 \cdot$ HCl.

Molecular weight: Meperidine hydrochloride—283.80.

Description: Meperidine Hydrochloride USP—Fine, white, crystalline, odorless powder. The pH of a solution (1 in 20) is about 5.

Solubility: Meperidine Hydrochloride USP—Very soluble in water; soluble in alcohol; sparingly soluble in ether.

USP requirements:
Meperidine Hydrochloride Injection USP—Preserve in single-dose or in multiple-dose containers, preferably of Type I glass. A sterile solution of Meperidine Hydrochloride in Water for Injection. Contains the labeled amount, within ±5%. Meets the requirements for Identification, Bacterial endotoxins, pH (3.5–6.0), and Injections.
Meperidine Hydrochloride Syrup USP—Preserve in tight, light-resistant containers. Contains the labeled amount, within ±5%. Meets the requirements for Identification and pH (3.5–4.1).
Meperidine Hydrochloride Tablets USP—Preserve in well-closed, light-resistant containers. Contain the labeled amount, within ±5%. Meet the requirements for Identification, Dissolution (75% in 45 minutes in water in Apparatus 1 at 100 rpm), and Uniformity of dosage units.

MEPERIDINE AND ACETAMINOPHEN

For *Meperidine* and *Acetaminophen*—See individual listings for chemistry information.

USP requirements: Meperidine Hydrochloride and Acetaminophen Tablets—Not in USP.

MEPHENTERMINE

Chemical group: Structurally similar to methamphetamine.

Chemical name: Mephentermine sulfate—Benzeneethanamine, *N*,alpha,alpha-trimethyl-, sulfate (2:1).

Molecular formula: Mephentermine sulfate—$(C_{11}H_{17}N)_2 \cdot$ H_2SO_4.

Molecular weight: Mephentermine sulfate—424.60.

Description: Mephentermine Sulfate USP—White, odorless crystals or crystalline powder. Its solutions are slightly acid to litmus, having a pH of about 6.

pKa: 10.11.

Solubility: Mephentermine Sulfate USP—Soluble in water; slightly soluble in alcohol; insoluble in chloroform.

USP requirements: Mephentermine Sulfate Injection USP—Preserve in single-dose or in multiple-dose containers, preferably of Type I glass. A sterile solution of Mephentermine Sulfate in Water for Injection. Contains an amount of mephentermine sulfate equivalent to the labeled amount of mephentermine, within ±5%. Meets the requirements for Identification, Bacterial endotoxins, pH (4.0–6.5), Particulate matter, and Injections.

MEPHENYTOIN

Chemical group: Related to the barbiturates in chemical structure, but having a five-membered ring.

Chemical name: 2,4-Imidazolidinedione, 5-ethyl-3-methyl-5-phenyl-.

Molecular formula: $C_{12}H_{14}N_2O_2$.

Molecular weight: 218.25.

Description: Mephenytoin USP—White, crystalline powder.

Solubility: Mephenytoin USP—Very slightly soluble in water; freely soluble in chloroform; soluble in alcohol and in aqueous solutions of alkali hydroxides; sparingly soluble in ether.

USP requirements: Mephenytoin Tablets USP—Preserve in well-closed containers. Contain the labeled amount, within ±10%. Meet the requirements for Dissolution (70% in 60 minutes in water in Apparatus 2 at 75 rpm), and Uniformity of dosage units.

MEPHOBARBITAL

Chemical name: 2,4,6(1*H*,3*H*,5*H*)-Pyrimidinetrione, 5-ethyl-1-methyl-5-phenyl-.

Molecular formula: $C_{13}H_{14}N_2O_3$.

Molecular weight: 246.27.

Description: Mephobarbital USP—White, odorless, crystalline powder. Its saturated solution is acid to litmus.

Solubility: Mephobarbital USP—Slightly soluble in water, in alcohol, and in ether; soluble in chloroform and in solutions of fixed alkali hydroxides and carbonates.

USP requirements: Mephobarbital Tablets USP—Preserve in well-closed containers. Contain the labeled amount, within −5% to +10%. Meet the requirements for Identification, Dissolution (70% in 75 minutes in alkaline borate buffer [pH 10.0] in Apparatus 2 at 75 rpm), and Uniformity of dosage units.

MEPIVACAINE

Chemical group: Amide.

Chemical name: Mepivacaine hydrochloride—2-Piperidinecarboxamide, N-(2,6-dimethylphenyl)-1-methyl-, monohydrochloride.

Molecular formula: Mepivacaine hydrochloride—$C_{15}H_{22}N_2O \cdot HCl$.

Molecular weight: Mepivacaine hydrochloride—282.81.

Description: Mepivacaine Hydrochloride USP—White, odorless, crystalline solid. The pH of a solution (1 in 50) is about 4.5.

pKa: Mepivacaine hydrochloride—7.6 and 7.8.

Solubility: Mepivacaine Hydrochloride USP—Freely soluble in water and in methanol; very slightly soluble in chloroform; practically insoluble in ether.

USP requirements: Mepivacaine Hydrochloride Injection USP—Preserve in single-dose or in multiple-dose containers, preferably of Type I glass. Injection labeled to contain 2% or less of mepivacaine hydrochloride may be packaged in 50-mL multiple-dose containers. A sterile solution of Mepivacaine Hydrochloride in Water for Injection. Contains the labeled amount, within ±5%. Meets the requirements for Identification, Bacterial endotoxins, pH (4.5–6.8), and Injections.

MEPIVACAINE AND LEVONORDEFRIN

Chemical group: Mepivacaine—Amide.

Chemical name:
Mepivacaine hydrochloride—2-Piperidinecarboxamide, N-(2,6-dimethylphenyl)-1-methyl-, monohydrochloride.
Levonordefrin—1,2-Benzenediol, 4-(2-amino-1-hydroxypropyl)-, [R-(R*,S*)]-.

Molecular formula:
Mepivacaine hydrochloride—$C_{15}H_{22}N_2O \cdot HCl$.
Levonordefrin—$C_9H_{13}NO_3$.

Molecular weight:
Mepivacaine hydrochloride—282.81.
Levonordefrin—183.21.

Description:
Mepivacaine Hydrochloride USP—White, odorless, crystalline solid. The pH of a solution (1 in 50) is about 4.5.
Levonordefrin USP—White to buff-colored, odorless, crystalline solid. Melts at about 210 °C.

pKa: Mepivacaine hydrochloride—7.6 and 7.8.

Solubility:
Mepivacaine Hydrochloride USP—Freely soluble in water and in methanol; very slightly soluble in chloroform; practically insoluble in ether.
Levonordefrin USP—Practically insoluble in water; freely soluble in aqueous solutions of mineral acids; slightly soluble in acetone, in chloroform, in alcohol, and in ether.

USP requirements: Mepivacaine Hydrochloride and Levonordefrin Injection USP—Preserve in single-dose or in multiple-dose containers, preferably of Type I glass. A sterile solution of Mepivacaine Hydrochloride and Levonordefrin in Water for Injection. The label indicates that the Injection is not to be used if its color is pinkish or darker than slightly yellow or if it contains a precipitate. Contains the labeled amount of mepivacaine hydrochloride, within ±5%, and the labeled amount of levonordefrin, within ±10%. Meets the requirements for Color and clarity, Identification, Bacterial endotoxins, pH (3.3–5.5), and Injections.

MEPROBAMATE

Chemical group: A carbamate derivative.

Chemical name: 1,3-Propanediol, 2-methyl-2-propyl-, dicarbamate.

Molecular formula: $C_9H_{18}N_2O_4$.

Molecular weight: 218.25.

Description: Meprobamate USP—White powder, having a characteristic odor.

Solubility: Meprobamate USP—Slightly soluble in water; freely soluble in acetone and in alcohol; sparingly soluble in ether.

USP requirements:
Meprobamate Extended-release Capsules—Not in USP.
Meprobamate Oral Suspension USP—Preserve in tight containers. Contains the labeled amount, within −5% to +10%. Meets the requirement for Identification.
Meprobamate Tablets USP—Preserve in well-closed containers. Contain the labeled amount, within ±10%. Meet the requirements for Identification, Dissolution (60% in 30 minutes in deaerated water in Apparatus 1 at 100 rpm), and Uniformity of dosage units.

MEPROBAMATE AND ASPIRIN

For *Meprobamate* and *Aspirin*—See individual listings for chemistry information.

USP requirements: Meprobamate and Aspirin Tablets—Not in USP.

MEPRYLCAINE AND EPINEPHRINE

Chemical name:
Meprylcaine hydrochloride—1-Propanol-2-methyl-2-(propylamino)-, benzoate (ester), hydrochloride.
Epinephrine—1,2-Benzenediol, 4-[1-hydroxy-2-(methylamino)ethyl]-, (R)-.

Molecular formula:
Meprylcaine hydrochloride—$C_{14}H_{21}NO_2 \cdot HCl$.
Epinephrine—$C_9H_{13}NO_3$.

Molecular weight:
Meprylcaine hydrochloride—271.79.
Epinephrine—183.21.

Description:
Meprylcaine Hydrochloride USP—White, odorless, crystalline solid. The pH of a solution (1 in 50) is about 5.7.
Epinephrine USP—White to practically white, odorless, microcrystalline powder or granules, gradually darkening on exposure to light and air. With acids it forms salts that are readily soluble in water, and the base may be recovered by the addition of ammonia water or alkali carbonates. Its solutions are alkaline to litmus.

Solubility:

Meprylcaine Hydrochloride USP—Freely soluble in water, in alcohol, and in chloroform; slightly soluble in acetone.

Epinephrine USP—Very slightly soluble in water and in alcohol; insoluble in ether, in chloroform, and in fixed and volatile oils.

USP requirements: Meprylcaine Hydrochloride and Epinephrine Injection USP—Preserve in single-dose containers, preferably of Type I glass, protected from light. A sterile solution of Meprylcaine Hydrochloride and Epinephrine in Water for Injection. The label indicates that the Injection is not to be used if its color is pinkish or darker than slightly yellow or if it contains a precipitate. Contains the labeled amounts of meprylcaine hydrochloride, within ±10%, and epinephrine, within −5% to +10%. Meets the requirements for Color and clarity, Identification, Bacterial endotoxins, and Injections.

MERCAPTOPURINE

Chemical name: 6*H*-Purine-6-thione, 1,7-dihydro-, monohydrate.

Molecular formula: $C_5H_4N_4S \cdot H_2O$.

Molecular weight: 170.19.

Description: Mercaptopurine USP—Yellow, odorless or practically odorless, crystalline powder. Melts at a temperature exceeding 308 °C, with decomposition.

pKa: 7.6.

Solubility: Mercaptopurine USP—Insoluble in water, in acetone, and in ether; soluble in hot alcohol and in dilute alkali solutions; slightly soluble in 2 *N* sulfuric acid.

USP requirements: Mercaptopurine Tablets USP—Preserve in well-closed containers. Contain the labeled amount, within −7% to +10%. Meet the requirements for Identification, Disintegration (30 minutes), and Uniformity of dosage units.

AMMONIATED MERCURY

Chemical name: Mercury amide chloride.

Molecular formula: $Hg(NH_2)Cl$.

Molecular weight: 252.07.

Description: Ammoniated Mercury USP—White, pulverulent pieces or white, amorphous powder. Is odorless, and is stable in air, but darkens on exposure to light.

Solubility: Ammoniated Mercury USP—Insoluble in water, and in alcohol; readily soluble in warm hydrochloric, nitric, and acetic acids.

USP requirements:

Ammoniated Mercury Ointment USP—Preserve in collapsible tubes or in well-closed, light-resistant containers. Contains the labeled amount, within ±10%, in a suitable oleaginous ointment base. Meets the requirements for Identification and Minimum fill.

Ammoniated Mercury Ophthalmic Ointment USP—Preserve in collapsible ophthalmic ointment tubes. A sterile ointment. Contains the labeled amount, within ±10%, in a suitable oleaginous ointment base. Meets the requirements for Sterility, Metal particles, and Identification tests, and for Minimum fill under Ammoniated Mercury Ointment.

MESALAMINE

Chemical group: The active moiety of the prodrug sulfasalazine, which belongs to the salicylate and sulfonamide groups.

Chemical name: Benzoic acid, 5-amino-2-hydroxy-.

Molecular formula: $C_7H_7NO_3$.

Molecular weight: 153.14.

Description: Mesalamine USP—Light tan to pink colored needle-shaped crystals. Color may darken on exposure to air. Odorless or may have a slight characteristic odor.

Solubility: Mesalamine USP—Slightly soluble in water; very slightly soluble in methanol, in dehydrated alcohol, and in acetone; practically insoluble in *n*-butyl alcohol, in chloroform, in ether, in ethyl acetate, in *n*-hexane, in methylene chloride, and in *n*-propyl alcohol; soluble in dilute hydrochloric acid and in dilute alkali hydroxides.

USP requirements:

Mesalamine Delayed-release Tablets—Not in USP.

Mesalamine Suppositories—Not in USP.

Mesalamine Rectal Suspension—Not in USP.

MESNA

Chemical name: Ethanesulfonic acid, 2-mercapto-, monosodium salt.

Molecular formula: $C_2H_5NaO_3S_2$.

Molecular weight: 164.17.

Description: Mesna injection—Clear and colorless solution, with a pH of 6.5–8.5.

USP requirements: Mesna Injection—Not in USP.

MESORIDAZINE

Chemical group: Mesoridazine besylate—Salt of a metabolite of thioridazine, a phenothiazine derivative.

Chemical name: Mesoridazine besylate—10*H*-Phenothiazine, 10-[2-(1-methyl-2-piperidinyl)ethyl]-2-(methylsulfinyl)-, monobenzenesulfonate.

Molecular formula: Mesoridazine besylate—$C_{21}H_{26}N_2OS_2 \cdot C_6H_6O_3S$.

Molecular weight: Mesoridazine besylate—544.74.

Description: Mesoridazine Besylate USP—White to pale yellowish powder, having not more than a faint odor. Melts at about 178 °C, with decomposition.

Solubility: Mesoridazine Besylate USP—Freely soluble in water, in chloroform, and in methanol.

USP requirements:

Mesoridazine Besylate Injection USP—Preserve in single-dose containers, preferably of Type I glass, protected from light. A sterile solution of Mesoridazine Besylate in Water for Injection. Contains an amount of mesoridazine besylate equivalent to the labeled amount of mesoridazine, within ±10%. Meets the requirements for Identification, Bacterial endotoxins, pH (4.0–5.0), and Injections.

Mesoridazine Besylate Oral Solution USP—Preserve in tight, light-resistant containers, at a temperature not exceeding 25 °C. Contains an amount of mesoridazine besylate equivalent to the labeled amount of mesoridazine, within ±10%. Label it to indicate that it is to be diluted to the appropriate strength with water or other suitable fluid prior to administration. Meets the requirements for Identification and Alcohol content (0.25–1.0%).

Mesoridazine Besylate Tablets USP—Preserve in well-closed, light-resistant containers. Preserve Tablets having an opaque coating in well-closed containers. Contain an amount of mesoridazine besylate equivalent to the labeled amount of mesoridazine, within ±10%. Meet the requirements for Identification, Dissolution (80% in 60 minutes in 0.1 N hydrochloric acid in Apparatus 2 at 100 rpm), and Uniformity of dosage units.

METAPROTERENOL

Chemical name: Metaproterenol sulfate—1,3-Benzenediol, 5-[1-hydroxy-2-[(1-methylethyl)amino]ethyl]-, sulfate (2:1) (salt).

Molecular formula: Metaproterenol sulfate—$(C_{11}H_{17}NO_3)_2\cdot H_2SO_4$.

Molecular weight: Metaproterenol sulfate—520.59.

Description: Metaproterenol Sulfate USP—White to off-white, crystalline powder.

Solubility: Metaproterenol Sulfate USP—Freely soluble in water.

USP requirements:

Metaproterenol Sulfate Inhalation Aerosol USP—Preserve in small, nonreactive, light-resistant aerosol containers equipped with metered-dose valves and provided with oral inhalation actuators. A suspension of microfine Metaproterenol Sulfate in fluorochlorohydrocarbon propellants in a pressurized container. Contains the labeled amount within ±10%, and delivers the labeled dose per inhalation, within ±25%, through an oral inhalation actuator. Meets the requirements for Identification, Unit spray content, Particle size, and Water (not more than 0.075%), and for Leak testing under Aerosols.

Metaproterenol Sulfate Inhalation Solution USP—Store in small, well-filled, tight containers, protected from light. A solution of Metaproterenol Sulfate in Purified Water. Label it to indicate that the Inhalation Solution is not to be used if its color is pinkish or darker than slightly yellow or if it contains a precipitate. Contains the labeled amount, within ±10%. Meets the requirements for Color and clarity, Identification, and pH (2.8–4.0).

Metaproterenol Sulfate Syrup USP—Preserve in tight, light-resistant containers. Contains the labeled amount, within ±10%. Meets the requirements for Identification and pH (2.5–4.0, in a solution obtained by mixing 1 volume of Syrup and 4 volumes of water).

Metaproterenol Sulfate Tablets USP—Preserve in well-closed, light-resistant containers. Contain the labeled amount, within ±8%. Meet the requirements for Identification, Dissolution (70% in 30 minutes in water in Apparatus 2 at 50 rpm), and Uniformity of dosage units.

METARAMINOL

Chemical name: Metaraminol bitartrate—Benzenemethanol, alpha-(1-aminoethyl)-3-hydroxy-, [R-(R*,S*)]-, [R-(R*,R*)]-2,3-dihydroxybutanedioate (1:1) (salt).

Molecular formula: Metaraminol bitartrate—$C_9H_{13}NO_2\cdot C_4H_6O_6$.

Molecular weight: Metaraminol bitartrate—317.29.

Description: Metaraminol bitartrate—White, practically odorless, crystalline powder.

Solubility: Metaraminol bitartrate—Freely soluble in water; slightly soluble in alcohol; practically insoluble in chloroform and in ether.

USP requirements: Metaraminol Bitartrate Injection USP—Preserve in single-dose or in multiple-dose containers, preferably of Type I glass, protected from light. A sterile solution of Metaraminol Bitartrate in Water for Injection. Contains, in each mL, an amount of metaraminol bitartrate equivalent to not less than 9.0 mg and not more than 11.0 mg of metaraminol. Meets the requirements for Identification, Bacterial endotoxins, pH (3.2–4.5), Particulate matter, and Injections.

METAXALONE

Chemical name: 2-Oxazolidinone, 5-[(3,5-dimethylphenoxy)methyl]-.

Molecular formula: $C_{12}H_{15}NO_3$.

Molecular weight: 221.26.

Description: White, crystalline powder. Melts at about 123 °C.

Solubility: Very slightly soluble in water; soluble in alcohol; freely soluble in chloroform.

USP requirements: Metaxalone Tablets—Not in USP.

METHACHOLINE

Chemical name: Methacholine chloride—1-Propanaminium, 2-(acetyloxy)-N,N,N-trimethyl-, chloride.

Molecular formula: Methacholine chloride—$C_8H_{18}ClNO_2$.

Molecular weight: Methacholine chloride—195.69.

Description: Methacholine Chloride USP—Colorless or white crystals, or white, crystalline powder. Is odorless or has a slight odor, and is very hygroscopic. Its solutions are neutral to litmus.

Solubility: Methacholine Chloride USP—Very soluble in water; freely soluble in alcohol and in chloroform.

USP requirements: Methacholine Chloride for Inhalation—Not in USP.

METHACRYLIC ACID COPOLYMER

Description: Methacrylic Acid Copolymer NF—White powder, having a faint characteristic odor.

NF category: Coating agent.

Solubility: Methacrylic Acid Copolymer NF—The polymer is insoluble in water, in diluted acids, in simulated gastric fluid TS, and in buffer solutions of up to pH 5; soluble in diluted alkali, in simulated intestinal fluid TS, and in buffer solutions of pH 7 and above. The solubility between pH 5.5 and pH 7 depends on the content of methacrylic acid units in the copolymer. Soluble to freely soluble in methanol, in alcohol, in isopropyl alcohol, and in acetone, each of which contains not less than 3% of water.

NF requirements: Methacrylic Acid Copolymer NF—Preserve in tight containers. A fully polymerized copolymer of methacrylic acid and an acrylic or methacrylic ester. It is available in 3 types, which differ in content of methacrylic acid units and viscosity. Label it to state whether it is Type A, B, or C. Meets the requirements for Identification, Viscosity, Loss on drying (not more than 5.0%), Residue on ignition (not more than 0.1% for Types A and B; not more than 0.4% for Type C), Arsenic (not more than 2 ppm), Heavy metals (not more than 0.002%), Monomers (not more than 0.3%), and Organic volatile impurities.

METHACYCLINE

Chemical name: Methacycline hydrochloride—2-Naphthacene-carboxamide, 4-(dimethylamino)-1,4,4a,5,5a,6,11,12a-octahydro-3,5,10,12,12a-pentahydroxy-6-methylene-1,11-dioxo-, monohydrochloride, [4S-(4 alpha,4a alpha,5 alpha,5a alpha,12a alpha)]-.

Molecular formula: Methacycline hydrochloride—$C_{22}H_{22}N_2O_8 \cdot HCl$.

Molecular weight: Methacycline hydrochloride—478.89.

Description: Methacycline Hydrochloride USP—Yellow to dark yellow, crystalline powder.

Solubility: Methacycline Hydrochloride USP—Soluble in water.

USP requirements:
Methacycline Hydrochloride Capsules USP—Preserve in tight, light-resistant containers. Contain an amount of methacycline hydrochloride equivalent to the labeled amount of methacycline, within −10% to +20%. Meet the requirements for Dissolution (70% in 60 minutes in water in Apparatus 1 at 100 rpm), Uniformity of dosage units, and Water (not more than 7.5%).
Methacycline Hydrochloride Oral Suspension USP—Preserve in tight, light-resistant containers. Contains an amount of methacycline hydrochloride equivalent to the labeled amount of methacycline, within −10% to +25%. Contains one or more suitable and harmless buffers, colors, diluents, dispersants, flavors, and preservatives. Meets the requirements for pH (6.5–8.0), Deliverable volume (for Suspension packaged in multiple-unit containers), and Uniformity of dosage units (for Suspension packaged in single-unit containers).

METHADONE

Chemical name: Methadone hydrochloride—3-Heptanone, 6-(dimethylamino)-4,4-diphenyl-, hydrochloride.

Molecular formula: Methadone hydrochloride—$C_{21}H_{27}NO \cdot HCl$.

Molecular weight: Methadone hydrochloride—345.91.

Description:
Methadone Hydrochloride USP—Colorless crystals or white, crystalline, odorless powder.
Methadone Hydrochloride Oral Concentrate USP—Clear to slightly hazy, syrupy liquid.

Solubility: Methadone Hydrochloride USP—Soluble in water; freely soluble in alcohol and in chloroform; practically insoluble in ether and in glycerin.

USP requirements:
Methadone Hydrochloride Oral Concentrate USP—Preserve in tight containers, protected from light, at controlled room temperature. Label it to indicate that it is to be diluted with water or other liquid to 30 mL or more prior to administration. Contains, in each mL, not less than 9.0 mg and not more than 11.0 mg of methadone hydrochloride. Contains a suitable preservative. Meets the requirements for Identification and pH (1.0–6.0).
Methadone Hydrochloride Injection USP—Preserve in single-dose or in multiple-dose, light-resistant containers, preferably of Type I glass. A sterile solution of Methadone Hydrochloride in Water for Injection. Contains, in each mL, not less than 9.5 mg and not more than 10.5 mg of methadone hydrochloride. Meets the requirements for Identification, Bacterial endotoxins, pH (3.0–6.5), and Injections.
Methadone Hydrochloride Oral Solution USP—Preserve in tight containers, protected from light, at controlled room

temperature. Contains the labeled amount, within ± 10%. Meets the requirements for Identification, pH (1.0–4.0), and Alcohol content (7.0–9.0%).
Methadone Hydrochloride Tablets USP—Preserve in well-closed containers. Label Tablets that are not intended for oral administration as intact Tablets to state that they are dispersible tablets or to indicate that they are intended for dispersion in a liquid prior to oral administration of the prescribed dose. Contain the labeled amount, within ± 7%. Meet the requirements for Identification, Disintegration (for dispersible Tablets, 15 minutes, the use of disks being omitted), Dissolution (for Tablets intended to be swallowed, 75% in 45 minutes in water in Apparatus 1 at 100 rpm), and Uniformity of dosage units.

METHAMPHETAMINE

Chemical name: Methamphetamine hydrochloride—(+)-N,alpha-Dimethylphenethylamine hydrochloride.

Molecular formula: Methamphetamine hydrochloride—$C_{10}H_{15}N \cdot HCl$.

Molecular weight: Methamphetamine hydrochloride—185.70.

Description: Methamphetamine Hydrochloride USP—White crystals or white, crystalline powder. Is odorless or practically so. Its solutions have a pH of about 6.

Solubility: Methamphetamine Hydrochloride USP—Freely soluble in water, in alcohol, and in chloroform; very slightly soluble in absolute ether.

USP requirements:
Methamphetamine Tablets USP—Preserve in tight, light-resistant containers. Label Tablets to state both the content of the active moiety and the content of the salt used in formulating the article. Contain the labeled amount of methamphetamine hydrochloride, within ± 10%. Meet the requirements for Identification, Dissolution (75% in 45 minutes in water in Apparatus 2 at 50 rpm), and Uniformity of dosage units.
Methamphetamine Hydrochloride Extended-release Tablets—Not in USP.

METHANTHELINE

Source: Synthetic amine compound.

Chemical group: Quaternary ammonium compound.

Chemical name: Methantheline bromide—Ethanaminium, N,N-diethyl-N-methyl-2-[(9H-xanthen-9-ylcarbonyl)oxy]-, bromide.

Molecular formula: Methantheline bromide—$C_{21}H_{26}BrNO_3$.

Molecular weight: Methantheline bromide—420.35.

Description:
Methantheline Bromide USP—White or nearly white, practically odorless powder. Its solutions have a pH of about 5.
Sterile Methantheline Bromide USP—White or nearly white, practically odorless powder. Its solutions have a pH of about 5.

Solubility:
Methantheline Bromide USP—Very soluble in water; freely soluble in alcohol and in chloroform; practically insoluble in ether. Its water solution decomposes on standing.
Sterile Methantheline Bromide USP—Very soluble in water; freely soluble in alcohol and in chloroform; practically

insoluble in ether. Its water solution decomposes on standing.

USP requirements:

Methantheline Bromide Tablets USP—Preserve in well-closed containers. Contain the labeled amount, within ±5%. Meet the requirements for Identification, Dissolution (75% in 45 minutes in water in Apparatus 2 at 50 rpm), and Uniformity of dosage units.

Sterile Methantheline Bromide USP—Preserve in Containers for Sterile Solids. Contains the labeled amount, within ±2%, calculated on the dried basis. Meets the requirements for Completeness of solution, Constituted solution, Pyrogen, and Uniformity of dosage units, for Identification tests, Melting range, Loss on drying, and Residue on ignition under Methantheline Bromide, and for Sterility tests and Labeling under Injections.

METHARBITAL

Chemical name: 2,4,6(1H,3H,5H)-Pyrimidinetrione, 5,5-diethyl-1-methyl-.

Molecular formula: $C_9H_{14}N_2O_3$.

Molecular weight: 198.22.

Description: Metharbital USP—White to nearly white, crystalline powder, having a faint aromatic odor. The pH of a saturated solution is about 6.

Solubility: Metharbital USP—Slightly soluble in water; soluble in alcohol; sparingly soluble in ether.

USP requirements: Metharbital Tablets USP—Preserve in tight containers. Contain the labeled amount, within ±5%. Meet the requirements for Identification, Dissolution (75% in 45 minutes in water in Apparatus 1 at 100 rpm), and Uniformity of dosage units.

METHAZOLAMIDE

Chemical name: Acetamide, N-[5-(aminosulfonyl)-3-methyl-1,3,-4-thiadiazol-2(3H)-ylidene]-.

Molecular formula: $C_5H_8N_4O_3S_2$.

Molecular weight: 236.26.

Description: Methazolamide USP—White or faintly yellow, crystalline powder having a slight odor. Melts at about 213 °C.

Solubility: Methazolamide USP—Very slightly soluble in water and in alcohol; soluble in dimethylformamide; slightly soluble in acetone.

USP requirements: Methazolamide Tablets USP—Preserve in well-closed containers. Contain the labeled amount, within ±5%. Meet the requirements for Identification, Dissolution (75% in 45 minutes in acetate buffer [pH 4.5] in Apparatus 2 at 100 rpm), and Uniformity of dosage units.

METHDILAZINE

Chemical name:

Methdilazine—10H-Phenothiazine, 10-[(1-methyl-3-pyrrolidinyl)methyl]-.

Methdilazine hydrochloride—10H-Phenothiazine, 10-[(1-methyl-3-pyrrolidinyl)methyl]-, monohydrochloride.

Molecular formula:

Methdilazine—$C_{18}H_{20}N_2S$.

Methdilazine hydrochloride—$C_{18}H_{20}N_2S \cdot HCl$.

Molecular weight:

Methdilazine—296.43.

Methdilazine hydrochloride—332.89.

Description:

Methdilazine USP—Light tan, crystalline powder, having a characteristic odor.

Methdilazine Hydrochloride USP—Light tan, crystalline powder, having a slight, characteristic odor.

Solubility:

Methdilazine USP—Practically insoluble in water; freely soluble in 3 N hydrochloric acid; soluble in alcohol and in chloroform.

Methdilazine Hydrochloride USP—Freely soluble in water, in alcohol, and in chloroform.

USP requirements:

Methdilazine Tablets USP—Preserve in tight, light-resistant containers. Contains the labeled amount, within ±7%. Meets the requirements for Identification, Disintegration (30 minutes), and Uniformity of dosage units.

Methdilazine Hydrochloride Syrup USP—Preserve in tight, light-resistant containers. Contains the labeled amount, within ±7%. Meets the requirements for Identification, pH (3.3–4.1), and Alcohol content (6.5–7.5%).

Methdilazine Hydrochloride Tablets USP—Preserve in tight, light-resistant containers. Contain the labeled amount, within ±7%. Meet the requirements for Identification, Dissolution (75% in 45 minutes in water in Apparatus 1 at 100 rpm), and Uniformity of dosage units.

METHENAMINE

Chemical name:

Methenamine—1,3,5,7-Tetraazatricyclo[3.3.1.1^{3,7}]decane.

Methenamine hippurate—Glycine, N-benzoyl, compd. with 1,3,5,7-tetraazatricyclo[3.3.1.1^{3,7}]decane (1:1).

Methenamine mandelate—Benzeneacetic acid, alpha-hydroxy-, compd. with 1,3,5,7-tetraazatricyclo[3.3.-1.1^{3,7}]decane (1:1).

Molecular formula:

Methenamine—$C_6H_{12}N_4$.

Methenamine hippurate—$C_6H_{12}N_4 \cdot C_9H_9NO_3$.

Methenamine mandelate—$C_6H_{12}N_4 \cdot C_8H_8O_3$.

Molecular weight:

Methenamine—140.19.

Methenamine hippurate—319.36.

Methenamine mandelate—292.34.

Description:

Methenamine USP—Colorless, lustrous crystals or white, crystalline powder. Is practically odorless. When brought into contact with fire, it readily ignites, burning with a smokeless flame. It sublimes at about 260 °C, without melting. Its solutions are alkaline to litmus.

Methenamine hippurate—White crystalline powder.

Methenamine Mandelate USP—White crystalline powder. Is practically odorless. Its solutions have a pH of about 4. Melts at about 127 °C, with decomposition.

Solubility:

Methenamine USP—Freely soluble in water; soluble in alcohol and in chloroform.

Methenamine hippurate—Freely soluble in water and in alcohol.

Methenamine Mandelate USP—Very soluble in water; soluble in alcohol and in chloroform; slightly soluble in ether.

USP requirements:

Methenamine Elixir USP—Preserve in tight containers. Contains the labeled amount, within ±10%. Meets the requirements for Identification and Alcohol content (19.0–21.0%).

Methenamine Tablets USP—Preserve in well-closed containers. Contain the labeled amount, within ±5%. Meet the requirements for Identification, Dissolution (75% in 45 minutes in water in Apparatus 1 at 100 rpm), and Uniformity of dosage units.

Methenamine Hippurate Tablets USP—Preserve in well-closed containers. Contain the labeled amount, within ±5%. Meet the requirements for Identification, Disintegration (30 minutes), and Uniformity of dosage units.

Methenamine Mandelate for Oral Solution USP—Preserve in well-closed containers. Label Methenamine Mandelate for Oral Solution that contains insoluble ingredients to indicate that the aqueous constituted Oral Solution contains dissolved methenamine mandelate but may remain turbid because of the presence of added substances. Contains the labeled amount, within ±10%. Meets the requirements for Identification, pH (4.0–4.5 in a mixture of 1 gram with 30 mL of water), and Water (not more than 0.5%).

Methenamine Mandelate Oral Suspension USP—Preserve in tight containers. It is Methenamine Mandelate suspended in vegetable oil. Contains the labeled amount, within ±10%. Meets the requirements for Identification and Water (not more than 0.1%).

Methenamine Mandelate Tablets USP—Preserve in well-closed containers. Contain the labeled amount, within ±5%. Meet the requirements for Identification, Disintegration (for enteric-coated Tablets, 2 hours and 30 minutes), Dissolution (for uncoated or plain coated Tablets, 75% in 45 minutes in water in Apparatus 1 at 100 rpm), and Uniformity of dosage units.

METHENAMINE AND SODIUM PHOSPHATE

For *Methenamine* and *Sodium Phosphate*—See individual listings for chemistry information.

USP requirements: Methenamine and Monobasic Sodium Phosphate Tablets USP—Preserve in tight containers. Contain the labeled amounts of methenamine and monobasic sodium phosphate, within ±7.5%. Meet the requirements for Identification, Dissolution (75% in 45 minutes in water in Apparatus 1 at 100 rpm), Uniformity of dosage units, and Ammonium salts.

METHICILLIN

Chemical name: Methicillin sodium—4-Thia-1-azabicyclo-[3.2.0]heptane-2-carboxylic acid, 6-[(2,6-dimethoxybenzoyl)amino]-3,3-dimethyl-7-oxo-, monosodium salt, monohydrate, [2S-(2 alpha,5 alpha,6 beta)]-.

Molecular formula: Methicillin sodium—$C_{17}H_{19}N_2NaO_6S \cdot H_2O$.

Molecular weight: Methicillin sodium—420.41.

Description:
Methicillin Sodium for Injection USP—Fine, white, crystalline powder, odorless or having a slight odor.
Sterile Methicillin Sodium USP—Fine, white, crystalline powder, odorless or having a slight odor.

Solubility:
Methicillin Sodium for Injection USP—Freely soluble in water, in methanol, and in pyridine; slightly soluble in propyl and amyl alcohols, in chloroform, and in ethylene chloride; insoluble in acetone and in ether.
Sterile Methicillin Sodium USP—Freely soluble in water, in methanol, and in pyridine; slightly soluble in propyl and amyl alcohols, in chloroform, and in ethylene chloride; insoluble in acetone and in ether.

USP requirements:
Methicillin Sodium for Injection USP—Preserve in Containers for Sterile Solids, at controlled room temperature. A sterile mixture of Sterile Methicillin Sodium and Sodium Citrate. Contains an amount of methicillin sodium equivalent to the labeled amount of methicillin, within −10% to +15%. Meets the requirements for Constituted solution, Identification, Bacterial endotoxins, Sterility, pH (6.0–8.5, in a solution containing 10 mg per mL), Water (not more than 6.0%), and Particulate matter, and for Uniformity of dosage units and Labeling under Injections.
Sterile Methicillin Sodium USP—Preserve in Containers for Sterile Solids, at controlled room temperature. It is Methicillin Sodium for parenteral use. It has a potency equivalent to not less than 815 mcg of methicillin per mg. Meets the requirements for Identification, Crystallinity, Bacterial endotoxins, Sterility, pH (5.0–7.5, in a solution containing 10 mg per mL), and Water (3.0–6.0%).

METHIMAZOLE

Chemical group: Thioamide derivative.

Chemical name: 2H-Imidazole-2-thione, 1,3-dihydro-1-methyl-.

Molecular formula: $C_4H_6N_2S$.

Molecular weight: 114.16.

Description: Methimazole USP—White to pale buff, crystalline powder, having a faint, characteristic odor. It solutions are practically neutral to litmus.

Solubility: Methimazole USP—Freely soluble in water, in alcohol, and in chloroform; slightly soluble in ether.

USP requirements: Methimazole Tablets USP—Preserve in well-closed, light-resistant containers. Contain the labeled amount, within ±6%. Meet the requirements for Identification, Dissolution (80% in 30 minutes in water in Apparatus 1 at 100 rpm), and Uniformity of dosage units.

METHOCARBAMOL

Chemical name: 1,2-Propanediol, 3-(2-methoxyphenoxy)-, 1-carbamate.

Molecular formula: $C_{11}H_{15}NO_5$.

Molecular weight: 241.24.

Description: Methocarbamol USP—White powder, odorless, or having a slight characteristic odor. Melts at about 94 °C, or, if previously ground to a fine powder, melts at about 90 °C.

Solubility: Methocarbamol USP—Sparingly soluble in water and in chloroform; soluble in alcohol only with heating; insoluble in n-hexane.

USP requirements:
Methocarbamol Injection USP—Preserve in single-dose containers, preferably of Type I glass. A sterile solution of Methocarbamol in an aqueous solution of Polyethylene Glycol 300. Contains the labeled amount, within ±5%. Meets the requirements for Identification, Bacterial endotoxins, pH (3.5–6.0), Particulate matter under Small-volume Injections, Aldehydes (not more than 0.01%, as formaldehyde), and Injections.

Methocarbamol Tablets USP—Preserve in tight containers. Contain the labeled amount, within ±5%. Meet the requirements for Identification, Dissolution (75% in 45 minutes in water in Apparatus 2 at 50 rpm), and Uniformity of dosage units.

METHOHEXITAL

Chemical group: Methohexital sodium—A methylated oxybarbiturate; differs chemically from the established barbiturate anesthetics in that it contains no sulfur.

Chemical name:
Methohexital—2,4,6(1H,3H,5H)-Pyrimidinetrione, 1-methyl-5-(1-methyl-2-pentynyl)-5-(2-propenyl)-, (±)-.
Methohexital sodium—2,4,6(1H,3H,5H)-Pyrimidinetrione, 1-methyl-5-(1-methyl-2-pentynyl)-5-(2-propenyl)-, (±)-, monosodium salt.

Molecular formula:
Methohexital—$C_{14}H_{18}N_2O_3$.
Methohexital sodium—$C_{14}H_{17}N_2NaO_3$.

Molecular weight:
Methohexital—262.31.
Methohexital sodium—284.29.

Description:
Methohexital USP—White to faintly yellowish white, crystalline odorless powder.
Methohexital Sodium for Injection USP—White to off-white hygroscopic powder. Is essentially odorless.

Solubility:
Methohexital USP—Very slightly soluble in water; slightly soluble in alcohol, in chloroform, and in dilute alkalies.
Methohexital sodium—Freely soluble in water.

Other characteristics:
Methohexital sodium—75% un-ionized at pH 7.4.
A 1% methohexital sodium solution in sterile water for injection has a pH of 10 to 11; a 0.2% methohexital sodium solution in 5% dextrose injection has a pH of 9.5 to 10.5.

USP requirements:
Methohexital Sodium for Injection USP—Preserve in Containers for Sterile Solids. A freeze-dried, sterile mixture of methohexital sodium and anhydrous Sodium Carbonate as a buffer, prepared from an aqueous solution of Methohexital, Sodium Hydroxide, and Sodium Carbonate. Contains the labeled amount, within ±10%. Meets the requirements for Completeness of solution, Constituted solution, Identification, Uniformity of dosage units, Bacterial endotoxins, pH (10.6–11.6), Loss on drying (not more than 2.0%), Heavy metals (not more than 0.001%), and Injections.
Methohexital Sodium for Rectal Solution—Not in USP.

METHOTREXATE

Chemical name: L-Glutamic acid, N-[4-[[(2,4-diamino-6-pteridinyl)methyl]methylamino]benzoyl]-.

Molecular formula: $C_{20}H_{22}N_8O_5$.

Molecular weight: 454.44.

Description: Methotrexate USP—Orange-brown, or yellow, crystalline powder.

Solubility: Methotrexate USP—Practically insoluble in water, in alcohol, in chloroform, and in ether; freely soluble in dilute solutions of alkali hydroxides and carbonates; slightly soluble in 6 N hydrochloric acid.

USP requirements:
Methotrexate Tablets USP—Preserve in well-closed containers. Contain the labeled amount, within ±10%. Meet the requirements for Identification, Dissolution (75% in 45 minutes in 0.1 N hydrochloric acid in Apparatus 2 at 50 rpm), and Uniformity of dosage units.
Methotrexate Sodium Injection USP—Preserve in single-dose or in multiple-dose containers, preferably of Type I glass, protected from light. A sterile solution of Methotrexate in Water for Injection prepared with the aid of Sodium Hydroxide. Contains the labeled amount of methotrexate, within −5% to +15%. Meets the requirements for Identification, Pyrogen, pH (7.0–9.0), and Injections.
Methotrexate Sodium for Injection USP—Preserve in Containers for Sterile Solids, protected from light. A sterile, freeze-dried preparation of methotrexate sodium with or without suitable added substances, buffers, and/or diluents. Contains an amount of methotrexate sodium equivalent to the labeled amount of methotrexate, within −5% to +15%. Meets the requirements for Constituted solution, Identification, Bacterial endotoxins, and pH (7.0–9.0 in a solution constituted as directed in the labeling, except that water is used as the diluent), and for Labeling under Injections, for Sterility tests and for Uniformity of dosage units.

Caution: Great care should be taken to prevent inhaling particles of methotrexate sodium and exposing the skin to it.

METHOTRIMEPRAZINE

Chemical group: Phenothiazine derivative.

Chemical name: 10H-Phenothiazine-10-propanamine, 2-methoxy-N,N,beta-trimethyl-, (−)-.

Molecular formula:
Methotrimeprazine—$C_{19}H_{24}N_2OS$.
Methotrimeprazine hydrochloride—$C_{19}H_{24}N_2OS \cdot HCl$.
Methotrimeprazine maleate—$C_{19}H_{24}N_2OS \cdot C_4H_4O_4$.

Molecular weight:
Methotrimeprazine—328.47.
Methotrimeprazine hydrochloride—364.9.
Methotrimeprazine maleate—444.5.

Description:
Methotrimeprazine USP—Fine, white, practically odorless, crystalline powder. Melts at about 126 °C.
Methotrimeprazine hydrochloride—White or slightly yellow, slightly hygroscopic crystalline powder. It deteriorates on exposure to air and light.

Solubility:
Methotrimeprazine USP—Practically insoluble in water; freely soluble in chloroform and in ether; sparingly soluble in methanol; sparingly soluble in alcohol at 25 °C; freely soluble in boiling alcohol.
Methotrimeprazine hydrochloride—Freely soluble in water, in alcohol, and in chloroform; practically insoluble in ether.
Methotrimeprazine maleate—Sparingly soluble in water and in ethanol.

USP requirements:
Methotrimeprazine Injection USP—Preserve in single-dose or in multiple-dose containers, preferably of Type I glass, protected from light. A sterile solution of Methotrimeprazine in Water for Injection, prepared with the aid of hydrochloric acid. Contains the labeled amount, as the hydrochloride, within ±10%. Meets the requirements for Identification, Bacterial endotoxins, pH (3.0–5.0), and Injections.

Methotrimeprazine Hydrochloride Oral Solution—Not in USP.
Methotrimeprazine Hydrochloride Syrup—Not in USP.
Methotrimeprazine Maleate Tablets—Not in USP.

METHOXAMINE

Chemical name: Methoxamine hydrochloride—Benzene-methanol, alpha-(1-aminoethyl)-2,5-dimethoxy-, hydrochloride.

Molecular formula: Methoxamine hydrochloride—$C_{11}H_{17}NO_3 \cdot HCl$.

Molecular weight: Methoxamine hydrochloride—247.72.

Description: Methoxamine Hydrochloride USP—Colorless or white, plate-like crystals or white, crystalline powder. Is odorless or has only a slight odor. Its solutions have a pH of about 5.

Solubility: Methoxamine Hydrochloride USP—Freely soluble in water; soluble in alcohol; practically insoluble in chloroform and in ether.

USP requirements: Methoxamine Hydrochloride Injection USP—Preserve in single-dose or in multiple-dose containers, preferably of Type I glass, and protect from light. Contains the labeled amount, within ± 7%. Meets the requirements for Identification, Bacterial endotoxins, pH (3.0–5.0), and Injections.

METHOXSALEN

Chemical name: 7H-Furo[3,2-g][1]benzopyran-7-one, 9-methoxy-.

Molecular formula: $C_{12}H_8O_4$.

Molecular weight: 216.19.

Description:
Methoxsalen USP—White to cream-colored, fluffy, needle-like crystals. Is odorless.
Methoxsalen Topical Solution USP—Clear, colorless liquid.

Solubility: Methoxsalen USP—Practically insoluble in water; freely soluble in chloroform; soluble in boiling alcohol, in acetone, in acetic acid, and in propylene glycol; sparingly soluble in boiling water and in ether.

USP requirements:
Methoxsalen Capsules USP—Preserve in tight, light-resistant containers. Contain the labeled amount, within ± 10%. Meet the requirements for Identification, Dissolution (75% in 45 minutes in water in Apparatus 2 at 50 rpm), and Uniformity of dosage units.
Methoxsalen Topical Solution USP—Store in tight, light-resistant containers. A solution of Methoxsalen in a suitable vehicle. Contains not less than 9.2 mg and not more than 10.8 mg of methoxsalen per mL. Meets the requirements for Identification and Alcohol content (66.5–77.0% ethanol).

METHOXYFLURANE

Chemical name: Ethane, 2,2-dichloro-1,1-difluoro-1-methoxy-.

Molecular formula: $C_3H_4Cl_2F_2O$.

Molecular weight: 164.97.

Description: Methoxyflurane USP—Clear, practically colorless, mobile liquid, having a characteristic odor. Boils at about 105 °C.

Solubility: Methoxyflurane USP—Miscible with alcohol, with acetone, with chloroform, with ether, and with fixed oils.

Other characteristics:
Blood-to-Gas (mean range) partition coefficient at 37 °C—10.20–14.06.
Oil-to-Gas partition coefficient at 37 °C—825.

USP requirements: Methoxyflurane USP—Preserve in tight, light-resistant containers, and avoid exposure to excessive heat. Contains not less than 99.9% and not more than 100.0% of methoxyflurane, calculated on the anhydrous basis. Meets the requirements for Identification, Specific gravity (1.420–1.425), Nonvolatile residue (not more than 1 mg per 50 mL), Acidity, Water (not more than 0.1%), and Foreign odor.

METHSCOPOLAMINE

Source: Quaternary ammonium derivative of scopolamine.

Chemical name: Methscopolamine bromide—3-Oxa-9-azoniatricyclo[3.3.1.0²,⁴]nonane, 7-(3-hydroxy-1-oxo-2-phenyl-propoxy)-9,9-dimethyl-, bromide, [7(S)-(1 alpha,2 beta,4 beta,5 alpha,7 beta)]-.

Molecular formula: Methscopolamine bromide—$C_{18}H_{24}BrNO_4$.

Molecular weight: Methscopolamine bromide—398.30.

Description: Methscopolamine Bromide USP—White crystals or white, odorless, crystalline powder. Melts at about 225 °C, with decomposition.

Solubility: Methscopolamine Bromide USP—Freely soluble in water; slightly soluble in alcohol; insoluble in acetone and in chloroform.

USP requirements: Methscopolamine Bromide Tablets USP—Preserve in tight containers. Contain the labeled amount, within ± 7%. Meet the requirements for Identification, Disintegration (15 minutes), and Uniformity of dosage units.

METHSUXIMIDE

Chemical name: 2,5-Pyrrolidinedione, 1,3-dimethyl-3-phenyl-.

Molecular formula: $C_{12}H_{13}NO_2$.

Molecular weight: 203.24.

Description: Methsuximide USP—White to grayish white, crystalline powder. Is odorless, or has not more than a slight odor.

Solubility: Methsuximide USP—Slightly soluble in hot water; very soluble in chloroform; freely soluble in alcohol and in ether.

USP requirements: Methsuximide Capsules USP—Preserve in tight containers, and avoid exposure to excessive heat. Contain the labeled amount, within ± 8%. Meet the requirements for Identification, Dissolution (75% in 120 minutes in water in Apparatus 1 at 100 rpm), and Uniformity of dosage units.

METHYCLOTHIAZIDE

Chemical name: 2H-1,2,4-Benzothiadiazine-7-sulfonamide, 6-chloro-3-(chloromethyl)-3,4-dihydro-2-methyl-, 1,1-dioxide.

Molecular formula: $C_9H_{11}Cl_2N_3O_4S_2$.

Molecular weight: 360.23.

Description: Methyclothiazide USP—White or practically white, crystalline powder. Is odorless, or has a slight odor.

pKa: 9.4.

Solubility: Methyclothiazide USP—Very slightly soluble in water and in chloroform; freely soluble in acetone and in pyridine; sparingly soluble in methanol; slightly soluble in alcohol.

USP requirements: Methyclothiazide Tablets USP—Preserve in well-closed containers. Contain the labeled amount, within ± 10%. Meet the requirements for Identification, Dissolution (70% in 60 minutes in 0.1 N hydrochloric acid in Apparatus 2 at 50 rpm), and Uniformity of dosage units.

METHYL ALCOHOL

Chemical name: Methanol.

Molecular formula: CH_4O.

Molecular weight: 32.04.

Description: Methyl Alcohol NF—Clear, colorless liquid, having a characteristic odor. Is flammable.
NF category: Solvent.

Solubility: Methyl Alcohol NF—Miscible with water, with alcohol, with ether, and with most other organic solvents.

NF requirements: Methyl Alcohol NF—Preserve in tight containers, remote from heat, sparks, and open flames. Contains not less than 99.5% of methyl alcohol. Meets the requirements for Identification, Acidity, Alkalinity (as ammonia, not more than 3 ppm), Water (not more than 0.1%), Nonvolatile residue (not more than 0.001% [w/w]), Readily carbonizable substances, Readily oxidizable substances, Acetone and aldehydes (as acetone, not more than 0.003%), and Organic volatile impurities.
Caution: Methyl Alcohol is poisonous.

METHYLBENZETHONIUM

Chemical name: Methylbenzethonium chloride—Benzenemethanaminium, N,N-dimethyl-N-[2-[2-[methyl-4-(1,1,3,3-tetramethylbutyl)phenoxy]ethoxy]ethyl]-, chloride, monohydrate.

Molecular formula: Methylbenzethonium chloride—$C_{28}H_{44}ClNO_2 \cdot H_2O$.

Molecular weight: Methylbenzethonium chloride—480.13.

Description: Methylbenzethonium Chloride USP—White, hygroscopic crystals, having a mild odor. Its solutions are neutral or slightly alkaline to litmus.

Solubility: Methylbenzethonium Chloride USP—Very soluble in water, in alcohol, and in ether; practically insoluble in chloroform.

USP requirements:
Methylbenzethonium Chloride Lotion USP—Preserve in tight containers. An emulsion containing the labeled amount, within ± 10%. Meets the requirements for Identification and pH (5.2–6.0).
Methylbenzethonium Chloride Ointment USP—Preserve in collapsible tubes or in tight containers. Contains the labeled amount, within ± 10%. Meets the requirements for Identification and pH (5.0–7.0, in a dispersion of it in carbon dioxide-free water [1 in 100]).
Methylbenzethonium Chloride Powder USP—Preserve in well-closed containers. Contains the labeled amount, within ± 15%, in a suitable fine powder base, free from grittiness. Meets the requirements for Identification, pH (9.0–10.5, in a dispersion of it in carbon dioxide-free water [1 in 100]), and Powder fineness (not less than 99% of it passes through a No. 200 sieve).

METHYLCELLULOSE

Chemical group: Semisynthetic hydrophilic derivative of cellulose.

Chemical name: Cellulose, methyl ether.

Description: Methylcellulose USP—White, fibrous powder or granules. Its aqueous suspensions are neutral to litmus. It swells in water and produces a clear to opalescent, viscous colloidal suspension.
NF category: Coating agent; suspending and/or viscosity-increasing agent; tablet binder.

Solubility: Methylcellulose USP—Insoluble in alcohol, in ether, and in chloroform; soluble in glacial acetic acid and in a mixture of equal volumes of alcohol and chloroform.

USP requirements:
Methylcellulose Capsules—Not in USP.
Methylcellulose USP (Granules or Powder)—Preserve in well-closed containers. A methyl ether of cellulose. When dried at 105 °C for 2 hours, contains not less than 27.5% and not more than 31.5% of methoxy (OCH_3) groups. Label it to indicate its viscosity type (viscosity of a solution [1 in 50]). Meets the requirements for Identification, Apparent viscosity (within ± 20% of labeled viscosity when 100 centipoises or less, within −25% to +40% of labeled viscosity when greater than 100 centipoises), Loss on drying (not more than 5.0%), Residue on ignition (not more than 1.5%), Arsenic (not more than 3 ppm), and Heavy metals (not more than 0.001%).
Methylcellulose Ophthalmic Solution USP—Preserve in tight containers. A sterile solution of Methylcellulose. Contains the labeled amount, within ± 15%. Meets the requirements for Identification, Sterility, and pH (6.0–7.8).
Methylcellulose Oral Solution USP—Preserve in tight, light-resistant containers, and avoid exposure to direct sunlight and to excessive heat. Avoid freezing. A flavored solution of Methylcellulose. Contains the labeled amount, within ± 15%. Meets the requirements for Identification, Microbial limits, and Alcohol content (3.5–6.5%).
Methylcellulose Tablets USP—Preserve in well-closed containers. Contain the labeled amount, within ± 10%. Meet the requirements for Identification, Disintegration (30 minutes), and Uniformity of dosage units.

METHYLDOPA

Chemical name:
Methyldopa—L-Tyrosine, 3-hydroxy-alpha-methyl-, sesquihydrate.
Methyldopate hydrochloride—L-Tyrosine, 3-hydroxy-alpha-methyl-, ethyl ester, hydrochloride.

Molecular formula:
Methyldopa—$C_{10}H_{13}NO_4 \cdot 1\frac{1}{2}H_2O$.
Methyldopate hydrochloride—$C_{12}H_{17}NO_4 \cdot HCl$.

Molecular weight:
Methyldopa—238.24.
Methyldopate hydrochloride—275.73.

Description:
Methyldopa USP—White to yellowish white, odorless, fine powder, which may contain friable lumps.
Methyldopate Hydrochloride USP—White or practically white, odorless or practically odorless, crystalline powder.

Solubility:

Methyldopa USP—Sparingly soluble in water; very soluble in 3 *N* hydrochloric acid; slightly soluble in alcohol; practically insoluble in ether.

Methyldopate Hydrochloride USP—Freely soluble in water, in alcohol, and in methanol; slightly soluble in chloroform; practically insoluble in ether.

USP requirements:

Methyldopa Oral Suspension USP—Preserve in tight, light-resistant containers, at a temperature not exceeding 26 °C. An aqueous suspension of Methyldopa. Contains one or more suitable flavors, wetting agents, and preservatives. Contains the labeled amount, within ± 10%. Meets the requirements for Identification, pH (3.0–5.0; 3.2–3.8 if sucrose is present), and Limit of methyldopa-glucose reaction product (if sucrose is present).

Methyldopa Tablets USP—Preserve in well-closed containers. Contain the labeled amount, within ± 10%. Meet the requirements for Identification, Dissolution (80% in 20 minutes in 0.1 *N* hydrochloric acid in Apparatus 2 at 50 rpm), and Uniformity of dosage units.

Methyldopate Hydrochloride Injection USP—Preserve in single-dose containers, preferably of Type I glass. A sterile solution of Methyldopate Hydrochloride in Water for Injection. Contains the labeled amount, within ± 10%. Meets the requirements for Identification, Bacterial endotoxins, pH (3.0–4.2), Particulate matter, and Injections.

METHYLDOPA AND CHLOROTHIAZIDE

For *Methyldopa* and *Chlorothiazide*—See individual listings for chemistry information.

USP requirements: Methyldopa and Chlorothiazide Tablets USP—Preserve in well-closed containers. Contain the labeled amounts, within ± 10%. Meet the requirements for Identification, Dissolution (80% of methyldopa in 30 minutes in 0.1 *N* hydrochloric acid in Apparatus 2 at 75 rpm; and 75% of chlorothiazide in 60 minutes in 0.05 *M* phosphate buffer [pH 8.0] in Apparatus 2 at 75 rpm), and Uniformity of dosage units.

METHYLDOPA AND HYDROCHLOROTHIAZIDE

For *Methyldopa* and *Hydrochlorothiazide*—See individual listings for chemistry information.

USP requirements: Methyldopa and Hydrochlorothiazide Tablets USP—Preserve in well-closed containers. Contain the labeled amounts, within ± 10%. Meet the requirements for Identification, Dissolution (80% of methyldopa in 30 minutes and 80% of hydrochlorothiazide in 60 minutes in 0.1 *N* hydrochloric acid in Apparatus 2 at 50 rpm), and Uniformity of dosage units.

METHYLENE BLUE

Chemical name: Phenothiazin-5-ium, 3,7-bis(dimethylamino)-, chloride, trihydrate.

Molecular formula: $C_{16}H_{18}ClN_3S \cdot 3H_2O$.

Molecular weight: 373.90.

Description: Methylene Blue USP—Dark green crystals or crystalline powder having a bronze-like luster. Odorless or practically so. Stable in air. Its solutions in water and in alcohol are deep blue in color.

Solubility: Methylene Blue USP—Soluble in water and in chloroform; sparingly soluble in alcohol.

USP requirements: Methylene Blue Injection USP—Preserve in single-dose containers, preferably of Type I glass. A sterile solution of Methylene Blue in Water for Injection. Contains, in each mL, not less than 9.5 mg and not more than 10.5 mg of methylene blue. Meets the requirements for Identification, Bacterial endotoxins, pH (3.0–4.5), and Injections.

METHYLENE CHLORIDE

Chemical name: Methane, dichloro-.

Molecular formula: CH_2Cl_2.

Molecular weight: 84.93.

Description: Methylene Chloride NF—Clear, colorless, mobile liquid, having an odor resembling that of chloroform.
NF category: Solvent.

Solubility: Methylene Chloride NF—Miscible with alcohol, with ether, and with fixed and volatile oils.

NF requirements: Methylene Chloride NF—Preserve in tight containers. Contains not less than 99.0% of methylene chloride. Meets the requirements for Identification, Specific gravity (1.318–1.322), Distilling range (39.5–40.5 °C), Water (not more than 0.02%), Hydrogen chloride, Nonvolatile residue (not more than 0.002%), Heavy metals (not more than 1 ppm), and Free chlorine.

Caution: Perform all steps involving evaporation of methylene chloride in a well-ventilated fume hood.

METHYLERGONOVINE

Chemical group: Semi-synthetic ergot alkaloid.

Chemical name: Methylergonovine maleate—Ergoline-8-carboxamide, 9,10-didehydro-*N*-[1-(hydroxymethyl)propyl]-6-methyl-, [8 beta(*S*)]-, (*Z*)-2-butenedioate (1:1) (salt).

Molecular formula: Methylergonovine maleate—$C_{20}H_{25}N_3O_2 \cdot C_4H_4O_4$.

Molecular weight: Methylergonovine maleate—455.51.

Description: Methylergonovine Maleate USP—White to pinkish tan, microcrystalline powder. Is odorless.

Solubility: Methylergonovine Maleate USP—Slightly soluble in water and in alcohol; very slightly soluble in chloroform and in ether.

USP requirements:

Methylergonovine Maleate Injection USP—Preserve in single-dose, light-resistant containers, preferably of Type I glass. A sterile solution of Methylergonovine Maleate in Water for Injection. Contains, in each mL, the labeled amount, within ± 10%. Meets the requirements for Identification, Bacterial endotoxins, pH (2.7–3.5), Related alkaloids, and Injections.

Methylergonovine Maleate Tablets USP—Preserve in tight, light-resistant containers. Contain the labeled amount, within ± 10%. Meet the requirements for Identification, Dissolution (70% in 30 minutes in tartaric acid solution [1 in 200] in Apparatus 2 at 100 rpm), Uniformity of dosage units, and Related alkaloids.

METHYL ISOBUTYL KETONE

Chemical name: 2-Pentanone, 4-methyl-.

Molecular formula: $C_6H_{12}O$.

Molecular weight: 100.16.

Description: Methyl Isobutyl Ketone NF—Transparent, colorless, mobile, volatile liquid, having a faint ketonic and camphoraceous odor.

NF category: Alcohol denaturant; solvent.

Solubility: Methyl Isobutyl Ketone NF—Slightly soluble in water; miscible with alcohol and with ether.

NF requirements: Methyl Isobutyl Ketone NF—Preserve in tight containers. Contains not less than 99.0% of methyl isobutyl ketone. Meets the requirements for Identification, Specific gravity (not more than 0.799), Distilling range (114–117 °C), Acidity, and Nonvolatile residue (not more than 0.008%).

METHYLPARABEN

Chemical name:
Methylparaben—Benzoic acid, 4-hydroxy-, methyl ester.
Methylparaben sodium—Benzoic acid, 4-hydroxy-, methyl ester, sodium salt.

Molecular formula:
Methylparaben—$C_8H_8O_3$.
Methylparaben sodium—$C_8H_7NaO_3$.

Molecular weight:
Methylparaben—152.15.
Methylparaben sodium—174.13.

Description:
Methylparaben NF—Small, colorless crystals, or white, crystalline powder. It is odorless, or has a faint, characteristic odor.
NF category: Antimicrobial preservative.
Methylparaben Sodium NF—White, hygroscopic powder.
NF category: Antimicrobial preservative.

Solubility:
Methylparaben NF—Slightly soluble in water and in carbon tetrachloride; freely soluble in alcohol and in ether.
Methylparaben Sodium NF—Freely soluble in water; sparingly soluble in alcohol; insoluble in fixed oils.

NF requirements:
Methylparaben NF—Preserve in well-closed containers. Contains not less than 99.0% and not more than 100.5% of methylparaben, calculated on the dried basis. Meets the requirements for Identification and Melting range (125–128 °C), and for Acidity, Loss on drying, and Residue on ignition under Butylparaben.
Methylparaben Sodium NF—Preserve in tight containers. Contains not less than 98.5% and not more than 101.5% of methylparaben sodium. Meets the requirements for Completeness of solution, Identification, pH (9.5–10.5, in a solution [1 in 1000]), Water (not more than 5.0%), Chloride (not more than 0.035%), Sulfate (not more than 0.12%), and Organic volatile impurities.

METHYLPHENIDATE

Chemical name: Methylphenidate hydrochloride—2-Piperidineacetic acid, alpha-phenyl-, methyl ester, hydrochloride, $(R*,R*)$-($\pm$)-.

Molecular formula: Methylphenidate hydrochloride—$C_{14}H_{19}NO_2\cdot HCl$.

Molecular weight: Methylphenidate hydrochloride—269.77.

Description: Methylphenidate Hydrochloride USP—White, odorless, fine, crystalline powder. Its solutions are acid to litmus.

Solubility: Methylphenidate Hydrochloride USP—Freely soluble in water and in methanol; soluble in alcohol; slightly soluble in chloroform and in acetone.

USP requirements:
Methylphenidate Hydrochloride Tablets USP—Preserve in tight containers. Contain the labeled amount, within ± 7%. Meet the requirements for Identification, Dissolution (75% in 45 minutes in water in Apparatus 1 at 100 rpm), and Uniformity of dosage units.
Methylphenidate Hydrochloride Extended-release Tablets USP—Preserve in tight containers. Contain the labeled amount, within ± 10%. Meet the requirements for Identification, Drug release (20 to 50% in 0.125D hours, 35 to 70% in 0.250D hours, 53 to 83% in 0.438D hours, 70 to 95% in 0.625D hours, not less than 80% in 0.875D hours, in water in Apparatus 2 at 50 rpm), and Uniformity of dosage units.

METHYLPREDNISOLONE

Chemical name:
Methylprednisolone—Pregna-1,4-diene-3,20-dione, 11,17,21-trihydroxy-6-methyl-, (6 alpha,11 beta)-.
Methylprednisolone acetate—Pregna-1,4-diene-3,20-dione, 21-(acetyloxy)-11,17-dihydroxy-6-methyl-, (6 alpha,11 beta)-.
Methylprednisolone hemisuccinate—Pregna-1,4-diene-3,20-dione, 21-(3-carboxy-1-oxopropoxy)-11,17-dihydroxy-6-methyl-, (6 alpha,11 beta)-.
Methylprednisolone sodium succinate—Pregna-1,4-diene-3,20-dione, 21-(3-carboxy-1-oxopropoxy)-11,17-dihydroxy-6-methyl-, monosodium salt, (6 alpha,11 beta)-.

Molecular formula:
Methylprednisolone—$C_{22}H_{30}O_5$.
Methylprednisolone acetate—$C_{24}H_{32}O_6$.
Methylprednisolone hemisuccinate—$C_{26}H_{34}O_8$.
Methylprednisolone sodium succinate—$C_{26}H_{33}NaO_8$.

Molecular weight:
Methylprednisolone—374.48.
Methylprednisolone acetate—416.51.
Methylprednisolone hemisuccinate—474.55.
Methylprednisolone sodium succinate—496.53.

Description:
Methylprednisolone USP—White to practically white, odorless, crystalline powder. Melts at about 240 °C, with some decomposition.
Methylprednisolone Acetate USP—White or practically white, odorless, crystalline powder. Melts at about 225 °C, with some decomposition.
Methylprednisolone Hemisuccinate USP—White or nearly white, odorless or nearly odorless, hygroscopic solid.
Methylprednisolone Sodium Succinate USP—White or nearly white, odorless, hygroscopic, amorphous solid.

Solubility:
Methylprednisolone USP—Practically insoluble in water; sparingly soluble in alcohol, in dioxane, and in methanol; slightly soluble in acetone and in chloroform; very slightly soluble in ether.
Methylprednisolone Acetate USP—Practically insoluble in water; soluble in dioxane; sparingly soluble in acetone, in alcohol, in chloroform, and in methanol; slightly soluble in ether.
Methylprednisolone Hemisuccinate USP—Very slightly soluble in water; freely soluble in alcohol; soluble in acetone.
Methylprednisolone Sodium Succinate USP—Very soluble in water and in alcohol; very slightly soluble in acetone; insoluble in chloroform.

USP requirements:

Methylprednisolone Tablets USP—Preserve in tight containers. Contain the labeled amount, within ±7.5%. Meet the requirements for Identification, Dissolution (50% in 30 minutes in water in Apparatus 1 at 100 rpm), and Uniformity of dosage units.

Methylprednisolone Acetate Cream USP—Preserve in collapsible tubes or in tight containers, protected from light. Contains the labeled amount, within ±10%. Meets the requirements for Identification and Minimum fill.

Methylprednisolone Acetate for Enema USP—Preserve in well-closed containers. A dry mixture of Methylprednisolone Acetate with one or more suitable excipients. Contains the labeled amount, within ±10%. Meets the requirements for Identification and Uniformity of dosage units.

Methylprednisolone Acetate Ointment—Not in USP.

Sterile Methylprednisolone Acetate Suspension USP—Preserve in single-dose or in multiple-dose containers, preferably of Type I glass. A sterile suspension of Methylprednisolone Acetate in a suitable aqueous medium. Contains the labeled amount, within ±10%. Meets the requirements for Identification, Uniformity of dosage units, pH (3.5–7.0), Particle size (minimum 99% are <20 micrometers in length [measured on longest axis] and minimum 75% are <10 micrometers in length, using 400x magnification), and Injections.

Methylprednisolone Sodium Succinate for Injection USP—Preserve in Containers for Sterile Solids. A sterile mixture of Methylprednisolone Sodium Succinate with suitable buffers. May be prepared from Methylprednisolone Sodium Succinate or from Methylprednisolone Hemisuccinate with the aid of Sodium Hydroxide or Sodium Carbonate. Contains an amount of methylprednisolone sodium succinate equivalent to the labeled amount of methylprednisolone, within ±10%, in the volume of constituted solution designated on the label. Meets the requirements for Constituted solution, Identification, Bacterial endotoxins, pH (7.0–8.0, in a solution containing about 50 mg of methylprednisolone sodium succinate per mL), Loss on drying (not more than 2.0%), Particulate matter, and Free methylprednisolone (not more than 6.6%), and for Sterility tests, Uniformity of dosage units, and Labeling under Injections.

METHYL SALICYLATE

Chemical name: Benzoic acid, 2-hydroxy-, methyl ester.

Molecular formula: $C_8H_8O_3$.

Molecular weight: 152.15.

Description: Methyl Salicylate NF—Colorless, yellowish, or reddish liquid, having the characteristic odor of wintergreen. It boils between 219 and 224 °C, with some decomposition. NF category: Flavors and perfumes.

Solubility: Methyl Salicylate NF—Slightly soluble in water; soluble in alcohol and in glacial acetic acid.

NF requirements: Methyl Salicylate NF—Preserve in tight containers. It is produced synthetically or is obtained by maceration and subsequent distillation with steam from the leaves of *Gaultheria procumbens* Linné (Fam. Ericaceae) or from the bark of *Betula lenta* Linné (Fam. Betulaceae). Label it to indicate whether it was made synthetically or distilled from either of the plants mentioned above. Contains not less than 98.0% and not more than 100.5% of methyl salicylate. Meets the requirements for Solubility in 70% alcohol (if it is synthetic, one volume dissolves in 7 volumes of 70% alcohol; if it is natural, one volume dissolves in 7 volumes of 70% alcohol, the solution having not more than a slight cloudiness), Identification, Specific gravity (for the synthetic, 1.180–1.185; for the natural, 1.176–1.182), Angular rotation, Refractive index (1.535–1.538 at 20 °C), and Heavy metals (not more than 0.004%).

METHYLTESTOSTERONE

Chemical group: Synthetic androgen; oral methylated androgen (17-alpha-alkylated androgen).

Chemical name: Androst-4-en-3-one, 17-hydroxy-17-methyl-, (17 beta)-.

Molecular formula: $C_{20}H_{30}O_2$.

Molecular weight: 302.46.

Description: Methyltestosterone USP—White or creamy white crystals or crystalline powder. Is odorless and is stable in air, but is slightly hygroscopic. Is affected by light.

Solubility: Methyltestosterone USP—Practically insoluble in water; soluble in alcohol, in methanol, in ether, and in other organic solvents; sparingly soluble in vegetable oils.

USP requirements:

Methyltestosterone Capsules USP—Preserve in well-closed containers. Contain the labeled amount, within ±10%. Meet the requirements for Identification, Dissolution (60% in 30 minutes in water in Apparatus 1 at 100 rpm), and Uniformity of dosage units.

Methyltestosterone Tablets USP—Preserve in well-closed containers. Contain the labeled amount, within ±10%. Meet the requirements for Identification, Disintegration (30 minutes. Tablets intended for buccal administration meet the requirements for Buccal Tablets), and Uniformity of dosage units.

METHYPRYLON

Chemical name: 2,4-Piperidinedione, 3,3-diethyl-5-methyl-.

Molecular formula: $C_{10}H_{17}NO_2$.

Molecular weight: 183.25.

Description: Methyprylon USP—White, or practically white, crystalline powder, having a slight, characteristic odor.

Solubility: Methyprylon USP—Soluble in water; freely soluble in alcohol, in chloroform, and in ether.

USP requirements:

Methyprylon Capsules USP—Preserve in tight, light-resistant containers. Contain the labeled amount, within ±10%. Meet the requirements for Identification, Dissolution (75% in 45 minutes in water in Apparatus 1 at 100 rpm), and Uniformity of dosage units.

Methyprylon Tablets USP—Preserve in tight, light-resistant containers. Contain the labeled amount, within ±5%. Meet the requirements for Identification, Dissolution (75% in 45 minutes in water in Apparatus 1 at 100 rpm), and Uniformity of dosage units.

METHYSERGIDE

Chemical name: Methysergide maleate—Ergoline-8-carboxamide, 9,10-didehydro-*N*-[1-(hydroxymethyl)propyl]-1,6-dimethyl-, (8 beta)-, (*Z*)-2-butenedioate (1:1) (salt).

Molecular formula: Methysergide maleate—$C_{21}H_{27}N_3O_2 \cdot C_4H_4O_4$.

Molecular weight: Methysergide maleate—469.54.

Description: Methysergide Maleate USP—White to yellowish white or reddish white, crystalline powder. Is odorless or has not more than a slight odor.

Solubility: Methysergide Maleate USP—Slightly soluble in water and in alcohol; very slightly soluble in chloroform; practically insoluble in ether.

USP requirements: Methysergide Maleate Tablets USP—Preserve in tight containers. Contain the labeled amount, within ±10%. Meet the requirements for Identification, Dissolution (70% in 30 minutes in tartaric acid solution [1 in 200] in Apparatus 2 at 100 rpm), and Uniformity of dosage units.

METIPRANOLOL

Chemical name: Phenol, 4-[2-hydroxy-3-[(1-methylethyl)amino]propoxy]-2,3,6-trimethyl-, (±)-, 1-acetate.

Molecular formula: $C_{17}H_{27}NO_4$.

Molecular weight: 309.40.

Description: White, odorless, crystalline powder.

Solubility: Metipranolol hydrochloride—Soluble in water.

USP requirements: Metipranolol Hydrochloride Ophthalmic Solution—Not in USP.

METOCLOPRAMIDE

Source: *p*-Aminobenzoic acid derivative, structurally related to procainamide.

Chemical name: Metoclopramide hydrochloride—Benzamide, 4-amino-5-chloro-*N*-[2-(diethylamino)ethyl]-2-methoxy-monohydrochloride, monohydrate.

Molecular formula: Metoclopramide hydrochloride—$C_{14}H_{22}ClN_3O_2 \cdot HCl \cdot H_2O$.

Molecular weight: Metoclopramide hydrochloride—354.28.

Description: Metoclopramide Hydrochloride USP—White or practically white, crystalline, odorless or practically odorless powder.

pKa: Metoclopramide hydrochloride—0.6 and 9.3.

Solubility: Metoclopramide Hydrochloride USP—Very soluble in water; freely soluble in alcohol; sparingly soluble in chloroform; practically insoluble in ether.

USP requirements:
Metoclopramide Injection USP—Preserve in single-dose or in multiple-dose containers, preferably of Type I glass, protected from light. (Note: Injection containing an antioxidant agent does not require protection from light.) A sterile solution of Metoclopramide Hydrochloride in Water for Injection. Contains the labeled amount, within ±10%. Meets the requirements for Identification, Bacterial endotoxins, pH (2.5–6.5), Particulate matter, and Injections.
Metoclopramide Oral Solution USP—Store in tight, light-resistant containers in a cool place. Protect from freezing. Contains an amount of Metoclopramide Hydrochloride equivalent to the labeled amount of metoclopramide, within ±10%. Meets the requirements for Identification and pH (2.0–5.5).
Metoclopramide Tablets USP—Preserve in tight, light-resistant containers. Contain an amount of metoclopramide

hydrochloride equivalent to the labeled amount of metoclopramide, within ±10%. Meet the requirements for Identification, Dissolution (75% in 30 minutes in water in Apparatus 1 at 50 rpm), and Uniformity of dosage units.
Metoclopramide Hydrochloride Syrup—Not in USP.

METOCURINE

Chemical name: Metocurine iodide—Tubocuraranium, 6,6',7',12'-tetramethoxy-2,2,2',2'-tetramethyl-, diiodide.

Molecular formula: Metocurine iodide—$C_{40}H_{48}I_2N_2O_6$.

Molecular weight: Metocurine iodide—906.64.

Description: Metocurine Iodide USP—White or pale yellow, crystalline powder.

Solubility: Metocurine Iodide USP—Slightly soluble in water, in 3 *N* hydrochloric acid, and in dilute solutions of sodium hydroxide; very slightly soluble in alcohol; practically insoluble in chloroform and in ether.

USP requirements: Metocurine Iodide Injection USP—Preserve in single-dose or in multiple-dose containers, preferably of Type I glass. Phenol, 0.5%, or some other suitable bacteriostatic substance, is added to the Injection in multiple-dose containers. A sterile solution of Metocurine Iodide in isotonic sodium chloride solution. Contains the labeled amount, within ±7%. Meets the requirements for Identification, Bacterial endotoxins, and Injections.

METOLAZONE

Chemical name: 6-Quinazolinesulfonamide, 7-chloro-1,2,3,4-tetrahydro-2-methyl-3-(2-methylphenyl)-4-oxo.

Molecular formula: $C_{16}H_{16}ClN_3O_3S$.

Molecular weight: 365.83.

Description: Colorless, odorless crystalline powder; is light-sensitive.

pKa: 9.72.

Solubility: Sparingly soluble in water; more soluble in plasma, in blood, in alkali, and in organic solvents.

USP requirements: Metolazone Tablets USP—Preserve in tight, light-resistant containers. Contain the labeled amount, within ±10%. Meet the requirements for Identification and Uniformity of dosage units.

METOPROLOL

Chemical name:
Metoprolol tartrate—2-Propanol, 1-[4-(2-methoxyethyl)phenoxy]-3-[(1-methylethyl)amino]-, (±)-, [R-(R*,R*)]-2,3-dihydroxybutanedioate (2:1) (salt).
Metoprolol succinate—(±)1-(isopropylamino)-3-[p-(2-methoxyethyl)phenoxy]-2-propanol succinate (2:1) (salt).

Molecular formula: Metoprolol tartrate—$(C_{15}H_{25}NO_3)_2 \cdot C_4H_6O_6$.

Molecular weight:
Metoprolol tartrate—684.82.
Metoprolol succinate—652.8.

Description:
Metoprolol Tartrate USP—White, crystalline powder.
Metoprolol succinate—White, crystalline powder.

pKa: Metoprolol tartrate—9.68.

Solubility:

Metoprolol Tartrate USP—Very soluble in water; freely soluble in methylene chloride, in chloroform, and in alcohol; slightly soluble in acetone; insoluble in ether.

Metoprolol succinate—Freely soluble in water; soluble in methanol; sparingly soluble in ethanol; slightly soluble in dichloromethane and in 2-propanol; practically insoluble in ethyl-acetate, in acetone, in diethylether, and in heptane.

Other characteristics: Lipid solubility—Moderate.

USP requirements:

Metoprolol Succinate Extended-release Tablets—Not in USP.

Metoprolol Tartrate Injection USP—Preserve in single-dose, light-resistant containers, preferably of Type I or Type II glass. A sterile solution of Metoprolol Tartrate in Water for Injection. Contains Sodium Chloride as a tonicity-adjusting agent. Contains the labeled amount, within ±10%. Meets the requirements for Identification, Bacterial endotoxins, pH (5.0–8.0), Sterility, and Injections.

Metoprolol Tartrate Tablets USP—Preserve in tight, light-resistant containers. Contain the labeled amount, within ±10%. Meet the requirements for Identification, Dissolution (75% in 30 minutes in simulated gastric fluid TS [without enzyme] in Apparatus 1 at 100 rpm), and Uniformity of dosage units.

Metoprolol Tartrate Extended-release Tablets—Not in USP.

METOPROLOL AND HYDROCHLOROTHIAZIDE

For *Metoprolol* and *Hydrochlorothiazide*—See individual listings for chemistry information.

USP requirements: Metoprolol Tartrate and Hydrochlorothiazide Tablets USP—Preserve in tight, light-resistant containers. Contain the labeled amounts, within ±10%. Meet the requirements for Identification, Dissolution (75% of metoprolol tartrate and 75% of hydrochlorothiazide in 30 minutes in simulated gastric fluid TS [without enzyme] in Apparatus 1 at 100 rpm), Uniformity of dosage units, and Diazotizable substances (not more than 1.0%).

METRIZAMIDE

Chemical group: Non-ionic, monomeric, triiodinated benzoic acid derivative.

Chemical name: D-Glucose, 2-[[3-(acetylamino)-5-(acetylmethylamino)-2,4,6-triiodobenzoyl]amino]-2-deoxy-.

Molecular formula: $C_{18}H_{22}I_3N_3O_8$.

Molecular weight: 789.10.

Description: White crystals.

Solubility: Very soluble in water (50% w/v) at room temperature.

Other characteristics: Low osmolality. The osmolality of metrizamide injection with iodine concentrations of 200 and 300 mg per mL is 340 and 484 mOsmol per kg of water, respectively.

USP requirements: Metrizamide for Injection—Not in USP.

METRONIDAZOLE

Chemical group: Nitroimidazoles.

Chemical name:

Metronidazole—1*H*-Imidazole-1-ethanol, 2-methyl-5-nitro-.

Metronidazole hydrochloride—1*H*-Imidazole-1-ethanol, 2-methyl-5-nitro-, hydrochloride.

Molecular formula:

Metronidazole—$C_6H_9N_3O_3$.

Metronidazole hydrochloride—$C_6H_9N_3O_3 \cdot HCl$.

Molecular weight:

Metronidazole—171.16.

Metronidazole hydrochloride—207.62.

Description: Metronidazole USP—White to pale yellow, odorless crystals or crystalline powder. Is stable in air, but darkens on exposure to light.

Solubility: Metronidazole USP—Sparingly soluble in water and in alcohol; slightly soluble in ether and in chloroform.

USP requirements:

Metronidazole Capsules—Not in USP.

Metronidazole Vaginal Cream—Not in USP.

Metronidazole Gel USP—Preserve in laminated collapsible tubes at controlled room temperature. Contains the labeled amount, within ±10%. Meets the requirements for Identification, pH (4.0–6.5), and Minimum fill.

Metronidazole Injection USP—Preserve in single-dose containers of Type I or Type II glass, or in suitable plastic containers, protected from light. A sterile, isotonic, buffered solution of Metronidazole in Water for Injection. Contains the labeled amount, within ±10%. Meets the requirements for Identification, Bacterial endotoxins, pH (4.5–7.0), Particulate matter, and Injections.

Metronidazole Vaginal Suppositories—Not in USP.

Metronidazole Tablets USP—Preserve in well-closed, light-resistant containers. Contain the labeled amount, within ±10%. Meet the requirements for Identification, Dissolution (85% in 60 minutes in 0.1 N hydrochloric acid in Apparatus 1 at 100 rpm), and Uniformity of dosage units.

Metronidazole Hydrochloride for Injection—Not in USP.

METRONIDAZOLE AND NYSTATIN

For *Metronidazole* and *Nystatin*—See individual listings for chemistry information.

USP requirements:

Metronidazole and Nystatin Vaginal Cream—Not in USP.

Metronidazole and Nystatin Vaginal Suppositories—Not in USP.

Metronidazole and Nystatin Vaginal Tablets—Not in USP.

METYRAPONE

Chemical name: 1-Propanone, 2-methyl-1,2-di-3-pyridinyl-.

Molecular formula: $C_{14}H_{14}N_2O$.

Molecular weight: 226.28.

Description: Metyrapone USP—White to light amber, fine, crystalline powder, having a characteristic odor. Darkens on exposure to light.

Solubility: Metyrapone USP—Sparingly soluble in water; soluble in methanol and in chloroform. It forms water-soluble salts with acids.

USP requirements: Metyrapone Tablets USP—Preserve in tight, light-resistant containers, and avoid exposure to excessive heat. Contain the labeled amount, within ±5%. Meet the requirements for Identification, Dissolution (60% in 45 minutes in 0.1 N hydrochloric acid in Apparatus 1 at 100 rpm), and Uniformity of dosage units.

METYROSINE

Chemical name: L-Tyrosine, alpha-methyl-, (–)-.

Molecular formula: $C_{10}H_{13}NO_3$.

Molecular weight: 195.22.

Description: White, crystalline compound.

pKa: 2.7 and 10.1.

Solubility: Very slightly soluble in water, in acetone, and in methanol; soluble in acidic aqueous solutions; soluble in alkaline aqueous solutions, but is subject to oxidative degradation in them; insoluble in chloroform.

USP requirements: Metyrosine Capsules USP—Preserve in well-closed containers. Contain the labeled amount, within ± 10%. Meet the requirements for Identification, Dissolution (75% in 60 minutes in 0.1 N hydrochloric acid in Apparatus 1 at 100 rpm), and Uniformity of dosage units.

MEXILETINE

Chemical name: Mexiletine hydrochloride—2-Propanamine, 1-(2,6-dimethylphenoxy)-, hydrochloride.

Molecular formula: Mexiletine hydrochloride—$C_{11}H_{17}NO \cdot HCl$.

Molecular weight: Mexiletine hydrochloride—215.72.

Description: Mexiletine hydrochloride—White to off-white crystalline powder.

pKa: 9.2.

Solubility: Mexiletine hydrochloride—Freely soluble in water and in alcohol.

USP requirements: Mexiletine Hydrochloride Capsules USP—Preserve in tight containers. Contain the labeled amount, within ± 10%. Meet the requirements for Identification, Dissolution (80% in 30 minutes in water in Apparatus 2 at 50 rpm), Uniformity of dosage units, and Related impurities (not more than 1.5%).

MEZLOCILLIN

Chemical name: Mezlocillin sodium—4-Thia-1-azabicyclo[3.2.0]heptane-2-carboxylic acid, 3,3-dimethyl-6-[[[[3-(methylsulfonyl)-2-oxo-1-imidazolidinyl]carbonyl]amino]phenylacetyl]amino]-7-oxo-, monosodium salt, [2S-[2 alpha,5 alpha,6 beta(S*)]].

Molecular formula: Mezlocillin sodium—$C_{21}H_{24}NaN_5O_8S_2$.

Molecular weight: Mezlocillin sodium—561.56.

Description: Mezlocillin sodium—White to pale yellow crystalline powder.

Solubility: Mezlocillin sodium—Freely soluble in water.

USP requirements: Sterile Mezlocillin Sodium USP—Preserve in Containers for Sterile Solids. It is mezlocillin sodium suitable for parenteral use. Contains an amount of mezlocillin sodium equivalent to not less than 838 mcg and not more than 978 mcg of mezlocillin per mg, calculated on the anhydrous basis and, where packaged for dispensing, contains an amount of mezlocillin sodium equivalent to the labeled amount of mezlocillin within −10% to +15%. Meets the requirements for Constituted solution, Identification, Specific rotation (+175° to +195°, calculated on the anhydrous basis), Bacterial endotoxins, Sterility, pH (4.5–8.0 in a solution [1 in 10]), Water (not more than 6.0%), and Particulate matter, and for Uniformity of dosage units and Labeling under Injections.

MICONAZOLE

Chemical group: Imidazoles.

Chemical name:
Miconazole—1H-Imidazole, 1-[2-(2,4-dichlorophenyl)-2-[(2,4-dichlorophenyl)methoxy]ethyl]-.
Miconazole nitrate—1H-Imidazole, 1-[2-(2,4-dichlorophenyl)-2-[(2,4-dichlorophenyl)methoxy]ethyl]-, mononitrate.

Molecular formula:
Miconazole—$C_{18}H_{14}Cl_4N_2O$.
Miconazole nitrate—$C_{18}H_{14}Cl_4N_2O \cdot HNO_3$.

Molecular weight:
Miconazole—416.14.
Miconazole nitrate—479.15.

Description:
Miconazole USP—White to pale cream powder. Melts in the range of 83 °C to 87 °C.
Miconazole Nitrate USP—White or practically white, crystalline powder, having not more than a slight odor. Melts in the range of 178 °C to 183 °C, with decomposition.

Solubility:
Miconazole USP—Insoluble in water; soluble in ether; freely soluble in alcohol, in methanol, in isopropyl alcohol, in acetone, in propylene glycol, in chloroform, and in dimethylformamide.
Miconazole Nitrate USP—Insoluble in ether; very slightly soluble in water and in isopropyl alcohol; slightly soluble in alcohol, in chloroform, and in propylene glycol; sparingly soluble in methanol; soluble in dimethylformamide; freely soluble in dimethylsulfoxide.

USP requirements:
Miconazole Injection USP—Preserve in single-dose containers, preferably of Type I glass, at controlled room temperature. A sterile solution of Miconazole in Water for Injection. Contains the labeled amount, within ± 10%. Meets the requirements for Identification, Bacterial endotoxins, pH (3.7–5.7), Particulate matter, and Injections.
Miconazole Nitrate Topical Aerosol Powder—Not in USP.
Miconazole Nitrate Topical Aerosol Solution—Not in USP.
Miconazole Nitrate Cream USP—Preserve in collapsible tubes or in tight containers. Contains the labeled amount, within ± 10%. Meets the requirements for Identification and Minimum fill.
Miconazole Nitrate Vaginal Cream—Not in USP.
Miconazole Nitrate Lotion—Not in USP.
Miconazole Nitrate Topical Powder USP—Preserve in well-closed containers. Contains the labeled amount, within ± 10%. Meets the requirements for Identification, Microbial limits, and Minimum fill.
Miconazole Nitrate Vaginal Suppositories USP—Preserve in tight containers, at controlled room temperature. Contain the labeled amount, within ± 10%. Meet the requirement for Identification.
Miconazole Nitrate Vaginal Tampons—Not in USP.

MIDAZOLAM

Source: 1,4 benzodiazepine derivative.

Chemical group: Benzodiazepine.

Chemical name: Midazolam hydrochloride—4H-Imidazo[1,5-a][1,4]benzodiazepine, 8-chloro-6-(2-fluorophenyl)-1-methyl-, monohydrochloride.

Molecular formula: Midazolam hydrochloride—C$_{18}$H$_{13}$ClFN$_3$·HCl.

Molecular weight: Midazolam hydrochloride—362.23.

Description: White to light yellow crystalline compound.

pKa: 6.0.

Solubility: Midazolam hydrochloride—Soluble in aqueous solutions. At physiologic pH, midazolam becomes highly lipophilic, and is one of the most lipid soluble of the benzodiazepines.

Other characteristics: Midazolam injection—An aqueous solution with an acidic pH of approximately 3.

USP requirements: Midazolam Hydrohcloride Injection—Not in USP.

MINERAL OIL

Source: Complex mixture of hydrocarbons derived from crude petroleum; aromatic amines and unsaturated hydrocarbons are removed when refined for human use, leaving various saturated hydrocarbons behind.

Description: Mineral Oil USP—Colorless, transparent, oily liquid, free, or practically free from fluorescence. Is odorless when cold, and develops not more than a faint odor of petroleum when heated.

NF category: Solvent; vehicle (oleaginous).

Solubility: Mineral Oil USP—Insoluble in water and in alcohol; soluble in volatile oils. Miscible with most fixed oils, but not with castor oil.

USP requirements:
Mineral Oil USP—Preserve in tight containers. A mixture of liquid hydrocarbons obtained from petroleum. Label it to indicate the name of any substance added as a stabilizer. Meets the requirements for Specific gravity (0.845–0.905), Viscosity (not less than 34.5 centistokes at 40.0 °C), Neutrality, Readily carbonizable substances, Limit of polynuclear compounds, and Solid paraffin.
Mineral Oil Emulsion USP—Preserve in tight containers.

Prepare Mineral Oil Emulsion as follows: 500 mL of Mineral Oil, 125 grams of Acacia in very fine powder, 100 mL of Syrup, 40 mg of Vanillin, 60 mL of Alcohol, and a sufficient quantity of Purified Water to make 1000 mL. Mix the Mineral Oil with the Powdered Acacia in a dry mortar, add 250 mL of Purified Water all at once, and emulsify the mixture. Then add, in divided portions, triturating after each addition, a mixture of the Syrup, 50 mL of Purified Water, and the Vanillin dissolved in the alcohol. Finally add Purified Water to make the product measure 1000 mL, and mix. The Vanillin may be replaced by not more than 1% of any other official flavoring substance or any mixture of official flavoring substances. Sixty mL of sweet orange peel tincture or 2 grams of benzoic acid may be used as a preservative in place of Alcohol.

Meets the requirement for Alcohol content (4.0–6.0%).
Mineral Oil Enema USP—Preserve in tight, single-unit containers. It is Mineral Oil that has been suitably packaged. Meets the requirements for Specific gravity (0.845–0.905), Viscosity (not less than 34.5 centistokes at 40.0 °C), and Neutrality.
Mineral Oil Gel—Not in USP.
Mineral Oil Oral Suspension—Not in USP.

LIGHT MINERAL OIL

Description: Light Mineral Oil NF—Colorless, transparent, oily liquid, free, or practically free, from fluorescence. Odorless when cold, and develops not more than a faint odor of petroleum when heated.

NF category: Tablet and/or capsule lubricant; vehicle (oleaginous).

Solubility: Light Mineral Oil NF—Insoluble in water and in alcohol; soluble in volatile oils. Miscible with most fixed oils, but not with castor oil.

USP requirements: Topical Light Mineral Oil USP—Preserve in tight containers. It is Light Mineral Oil that has been suitably packaged. Label it to indicate the name of any substance added as a stabilizer, and label packages intended for direct use by the public to indicate that it is not intended for internal use. Meets the requirements for Specific gravity (0.818–0.880) and Viscosity (not more than 33.5 centistokes at 40 °C), and for Neutrality and Solid paraffin under Mineral Oil.

NF requirements: Light Mineral Oil NF—Preserve in tight containers. A mixture of liquid hydrocarbons obtained from petroleum. Label it to indicate the name of any substance added as a stabilizer, and label packages intended for direct use by the public to indicate that it is not intended for internal use. Meets the requirements for Specific gravity (0.818–0.880) and Viscosity (not more than 33.5 centistokes at 40 °C), and for Neutrality, Readily carbonizable substances, Limit of polynuclear compounds, and Solid paraffin under Mineral Oil.

MINERAL OIL AND CASCARA SAGRADA

For *Mineral Oil* and *Cascara Sagrada*—See individual listings for chemistry information.

USP requirements: Mineral Oil and Cascara Sagrada Extract Emulsion—Not in USP.

MINERAL OIL, GLYCERIN, AND PHENOLPHTHALEIN

For *Mineral Oil, Glycerin,* and *Phenolphthalein*—See individual listings for chemistry information.

USP requirements: Mineral Oil, Glycerin, and Phenolphthalein Emulsion—Not in USP.

MINERAL OIL AND PHENOLPHTHALEIN

For *Mineral Oil* and *Phenolphthalein*—See individual listings for chemistry information.

USP requirements:
Mineral Oil and Phenolphthalein Emulsion—Not in USP.
Mineral Oil and Phenolphthalein Oral Suspension—Not in USP.

MINOCYCLINE

Chemical name: Minocycline hydrochloride—2-Naphthacenecarboxamide, 4,7-bis(dimethylamino)-1,4,4a,5,5a,6,11,12a-octahydro-3,10,12,12a-tetrahydroxy-1,11-dioxo-, monohydrochloride, [4S-(4 alpha,4a alpha,5a alpha,12a alpha)]-.

Molecular formula: Minocycline hydrochloride—C$_{23}$H$_{27}$N$_3$O$_7$·HCl.

Molecular weight: Minocycline hydrochloride—493.94.

Description: Minocycline Hydrochloride USP—Yellow, crystalline powder.

Solubility: Minocycline Hydrochloride USP—Soluble in water and in solutions of alkali hydroxides and carbonates; slightly soluble in alcohol; practically insoluble in chloroform and in ether.

USP requirements:
  Minocycline Hydrochloride Capsules USP—Preserve in tight, light-resistant containers. Contain an amount of minocycline hydrochloride equivalent to the labeled amount of minocycline, within −10% to +15%. Meet the requirements for Identification, Dissolution (75% in 45 minutes in water in Apparatus 2 at 50 rpm), Uniformity of dosage units, and Water (not more than 12.0%).
  Sterile Minocycline Hydrochloride USP—Preserve in Containers for Sterile Solids, protected from light. It is sterile, freeze-dried Minocycline Hydrochloride suitable for parenteral use. Contains an amount of minocycline hydrochloride equivalent to the labeled amount of minocycline, within −10% to +20%. Meets the requirements for Constituted solution, Identification, Depressor substances, Bacterial endotoxins, pH (2.0–3.5, in a solution containing the equivalent of 10 mg of minocycline per mL), Water (not more than 3.0%), Particulate matter, and Epiminocycline (not more than 6.0%), and for Sterility tests, Uniformity of dosage units, and Labeling under Injections.
  Minocycline Hydrochloride Oral Suspension USP—Preserve in tight, light-resistant containers. Contains one or more suitable diluents, flavors, preservatives, and wetting agents in an aqueous vehicle. Contains an amount of minocycline hydrochloride equivalent to the labeled amount of minocycline, within −10% to +30%. Meets the requirements for Identification, pH (7.0–9.0), Deliverable volume (multiple-unit containers), and Uniformity of dosage units (single-unit containers).
  Minocycline Hydrochloride Tablets USP—Preserve in tight, light-resistant containers. Contain an amount of minocycline hydrochloride equivalent to the labeled amount of minocycline, within −10% to +15%. Meet the requirements for Identification, Dissolution (75% in 45 minutes in water in Apparatus 2 at 50 rpm), Uniformity of dosage units, and Water (not more than 12.0%).

MINOXIDIL

Chemical name: 2,4-Pyrimidinediamine, 6-(1-piperidinyl)-, 3-oxide.

Molecular formula: $C_9H_{15}N_5O$.

Molecular weight: 209.25.

Description:
  Minoxidil USP—White to off-white, crystalline powder. Melts in the approximate range of between 248 and 268 °C, with decomposition.
  Minoxidil topical solution—Clear, colorless to slightly yellow solution.

pKa: 4.61.

Solubility: Minoxidil USP—Soluble in alcohol and in propylene glycol; sparingly soluble in methanol; slightly soluble in water; practically insoluble in chloroform, in acetone, in ethyl acetate, and in hexane.

USP requirements:
  Minoxidil Topical Solution—Not in USP.
  Minoxidil Tablets USP—Preserve in tight containers. Contain the labeled amount, within ±10%. Meet the requirements for Identification, Dissolution (50% in 15 minutes in phosphate buffer [pH 7.2] in Apparatus 1 at 75 rpm), and Uniformity of dosage units.

MISOPROSTOL

Chemical group: Synthetic prostaglandin E_1 analog.

Chemical name: Prost-13-en-1-oic acid, 11,16-dihydroxy-16-methyl-9-oxo-, methyl ester, (11 alpha,13E)-(±).

Molecular formula: $C_{22}H_{38}O_5$.

Molecular weight: 382.54.

Description: Light yellow, viscous liquid with a musty odor.

USP requirements: Misoprostol Tablets—Not in USP.

MITOMYCIN

Source: Isolated from the broth of *Streptomyces caespitosus*.

Chemical name: Azirino[2′,3′:3,4]pyrrolo[1,2-a]indole-4,7-dione, 6-amino-8-[[(aminocarbonyl)oxy]methyl]-1,1a,2,8,8a,8b-hexahydro-8a-methoxy-5-methyl-, [1aR-(1a alpha,8 beta,8a alpha,8b alpha)]-.

Molecular formula: $C_{15}H_{18}N_4O_5$.

Molecular weight: 334.33.

Description: Mitomycin USP—Blue-violet, crystalline powder.

Solubility: Mitomycin USP—Slightly soluble in water; soluble in acetone, in methanol, in butyl acetate, and in cyclohexanone.

USP requirements: Mitomycin for Injection USP—Preserve in Containers for Sterile Solids, protected from light. A dry mixture of Mitomycin and Mannitol. Contains the labeled amount, within −10% to +20%. Meets the requirements for Constituted solution, Identification, Depressor substances, Bacterial endotoxins, Sterility, pH (6.0–8.0, in the solution constituted as directed in the labeling), Water (not more than 5.0%), and Injections.

MITOTANE

Chemical name: Benzene, 1-chloro-2-[2,2-dichloro-1-(4-chlorophenyl)ethyl]-.

Molecular formula: $C_{14}H_{10}Cl_4$.

Molecular weight: 320.05.

Description: Mitotane USP—White, crystalline powder, having a slight aromatic odor.

Solubility: Mitotane USP—Practically insoluble in water; soluble in alcohol, in ether, in solvent hexane, and in fixed oils and fats.

USP requirements: Mitotane Tablets USP—Preserve in tight, light-resistant containers. Contain the labeled amount, within ±10%. Meet the requirements for Identification, Disintegration (15 minutes, the use of disks being omitted), and Uniformity of dosage units.

MITOXANTRONE

Chemical group: Synthetic anthracenedione.

Chemical name: Mitoxantrone hydrochloride—9,10-Anthracenedione, 1,4-dihydroxy-5,8-bis-[[2-[(2-hydroxyethyl)amino]ethyl]amino]-, dihydrochloride.

Molecular formula: Mitoxantrone hydrochloride—$C_{22}H_{28}N_4O_6 \cdot 2HCl$.

Molecular weight: Mitoxantrone hydrochloride—517.41.

Description:
Mitoxantrone Hydrochloride USP—Dark blue powder.
Mitoxantrone hydrochloride concentrate for injection—Dark blue aqueous solution.

Solubility: Mitoxantrone Hydrochloride USP—Sparingly soluble in water; slightly soluble in methanol; practically insoluble in acetone, in acetonitrile, and in chloroform.

USP requirements: Mitoxantrone for Injection Concentrate USP—Preserve in single-dose containers, preferably of Type I glass. A sterile solution of Mitoxantrone Hydrochloride in Water for Injection. Label Mitoxantrone for Injection Concentrate to state both the content of the active moiety and the name of the salt used in formulating the article. Label Mitoxantrone for Injection Concentrate to indicate that it is to be diluted to appropriate strength with water or other suitable fluid prior to administration. Contains the equivalent of the labeled amount of mitoxantrone, within −10% to +5%. Meets the requirements for Identification, Bacterial endotoxins, Sterility, pH (3.0–4.5), Related substances (not more than 3.0%), and Injections.

MOLINDONE

Chemical group: Dihydroindolone.

Chemical name: Molindone hydrochloride—4*H*-Indol-4-one, 3-ethyl-1,5,6,7-tetrahydro-2-methyl-5-(4-morpholinylmethyl)-, monohydrochloride.

Molecular formula: Molindone hydrochloride—$C_{16}H_{24}N_2O_2 \cdot$ HCl.

Molecular weight: Molindone hydrochloride—312.84.

Description: Molindone hydrochloride—White, crystalline powder.

pKa: 6.94.

Solubility: Molindone hydrochloride—Freely soluble in water and in alcohol.

USP requirements:
Molindone Hydrochloride Oral Solution—Not in USP.
Molindone Hydrochloride Tablets—Not in USP.

MOMETASONE

Chemical name: Mometasone furoate—Pregna-1,4-diene-3,20-dione, 9,21-dichloro-17-[(2-furanylcarbonyl)oxy]-11-hydroxy-16-methyl-, (11 beta,16 alpha)-.

Molecular formula: Mometasone furoate—$C_{27}H_{30}Cl_2O_6$.

Molecular weight: Mometasone furoate—521.44.

Description: Mometasone furoate—White to off-white powder.

Solubility: Mometasone furoate—Practically insoluble in water; slightly soluble in octanol; moderately soluble in ethyl alcohol.

USP requirements:
Mometasone Furoate Cream—Not in USP.
Mometasone Furoate Lotion—Not in USP.
Mometasone Furoate Ointment—Not in USP.

MONOBENZONE

Chemical name: Phenol, 4-(phenylmethoxy)-.

Molecular formula: $C_{13}H_{12}O_2$.

Molecular weight: 200.24.

Description: Monobenzone USP—White, odorless, crystalline powder.

Solubility:
Monobenzone USP—Practically insoluble in water; soluble in alcohol, in chloroform, in ether, and in acetone.
Monobenzone Ointment USP—Dispersible with, but not soluble in, water.

USP requirements: Monobenzone Cream USP—Preserve in tight containers, and avoid exposure to temperatures above 30 °C. Contains the labeled amount, within ±6%. Meets the requirement for Identification.

MONO- AND DI-ACETYLATED MONOGLYCERIDES

Description: Mono- and Di-acetylated Monoglycerides NF—White to pale yellow waxy solid, melting at about 45 °C.
NF category: Plasticizer.

Solubility: Mono- and Di-acetylated Monoglycerides NF—Soluble in ether and in chloroform; slightly soluble in carbon disulfide; insoluble in water.

NF requirements: Mono- and Di-acetylated Monoglycerides NF—Preserve in tight, light-resistant containers. It is glycerin esterified with edible fat-forming fatty acids and acetic acid. It may be prepared by the inter-esterification of edible oils with triacetin or a mixture of triacetin and glycerin, in the presence of catalytic agents, followed by molecular distillation, or by direct acetylation of edible monoglycerides and diglycerides with acetic anhydride with or without the use of catalysts or molecular distillation. Meets the requirements for Identification, Residue on ignition (not more than 0.5%), Arsenic (not more than 3 ppm), Heavy metals (not more than 0.001%), Acid value (not more than 3), Hydroxyl value (133–152), Saponification value (279–292), Free glycerin (not more than 1.5%), and Organic volatile impurities.

MONO- AND DI-GLYCERIDES

Description: Mono- and Di-glycerides NF—Varies in consistency from yellow liquids through ivory-colored plastics to hard ivory-colored solids having a bland odor.
NF category: Emulsifying and/or solubilizing agent.

Solubility: Mono- and Di-glycerides NF—Insoluble in water; soluble in alcohol, in ethyl acetate, in chloroform, and in other chlorinated hydrocarbons.

NF requirements: Mono- and Di-glycerides NF—Preserve in tight, light-resistant containers. A mixture of glycerol mono- and di-esters, with minor amounts of tri-esters, of fatty acids from edible oils. Contains not less than 40.0% of monoglycerides. The labeling indicates the monoglyceride content, hydroxyl value, iodine value, saponification value, and the name and quantity of any stabilizers. The monoglyceride content is within ±10% of the value indicated in the labeling. Meets the requirements for Residue on ignition (not more than 0.1%), Arsenic (not more than 3 ppm), Heavy metals (not more than 0.001%), Acid value (not more than 4), Hydroxyl value (90.0–110.0% of the value indicated in the labeling), Iodine value (90.0–110.0% of the value indicated in the labeling), Saponification value (90.0–110.0% of the value indicated in the labeling), Free glycerin (not more than 7.0%), and Organic volatile impurities.

MONOETHANOLAMINE

Chemical name: Ethanol, 2-amino-.

Molecular formula: C_2H_7NO.

Molecular weight: 61.08.

Description: Monoethanolamine NF—Clear, colorless, moderately viscous liquid, having a distinctly ammoniacal odor.

NF category: Emulsifying and/or solubilizing agent (adjunct).

Solubility: Monoethanolamine NF—Miscible with water, with acetone, with alcohol, with glycerin, and with chloroform. Immiscible with ether, with solvent hexane, and with fixed oils, although it dissolves in many essential oils.

NF requirements: Monoethanolamine NF—Preserve in tight, light-resistant containers. Contains not less than 98.0% and not more than 100.5%, by weight, of monoethanolamine. Meets the requirements for Specific gravity (1.013–1.016), Distilling range (not less than 95% distils at 167–173 °C), Residue on ignition (not more than 0.1%), and Organic volatile impurities.

MONOOCTANOIN

Source: A mixture of glycerol esters, principally Glyceryl Monooctanoate.

Chemical group: Mono- and diglycerides of medium chain length fatty acids.

Chemical name: Glyceryl-l-monooctanoate.

Molecular formula: $C_{11}H_{22}O_4$.

Molecular weight: 218.29.

Description: Melting point 39.5–40.5 °C.

USP requirements: Monooctanoin Irrigation—Not in USP.

MONOSODIUM GLUTAMATE

Molecular formula: $C_5H_8NNaO_4 \cdot H_2O$.

Molecular weight: 187.13.

Description: Monosodium Glutamate NF—White, practically odorless, free-flowing crystals or crystalline powder.

NF category: Flavors and perfumes.

Solubility: Monosodium Glutamate NF—Freely soluble in water; sparingly soluble in alcohol.

NF requirements: Monosodium Glutamate NF—Preserve in tight containers. Contains not less than 99.0% and not more than 100.5% of monosodium glutamate. Meets the requirements for Clarity and color of solution, Identification, Specific rotation (+24.8° to +25.3° at 20 °C), pH (6.7–7.2, in a solution [1 in 20]), Loss on drying (not more than 0.5%), Chloride (not more than 0.25%), Arsenic (not more than 3 ppm), Lead (not more than 10 ppm), Heavy metals (not more than 0.002%), and Organic volatile impurities.

MONOTHIOGLYCEROL

Chemical name: 1,2-Propanediol, 3-mercapto-.

Molecular formula: $C_3H_8O_2S$.

Molecular weight: 108.15.

Description: Monothioglycerol NF—Colorless or pale yellow viscous liquid, having a slight sulfidic odor. Hygroscopic.

NF category: Antioxidant.

Solubility: Monothioglycerol NF—Miscible with alcohol. Freely soluble in water; insoluble in ether.

NF requirements: Monothioglycerol NF—Preserve in tight containers. Contains not less than 97.0% and not more than 101.0% of monothioglycerol, calculated on the anhydrous basis. Meets the requirements for Specific gravity (1.241–1.250), Refractive index (1.521–1.526), pH (3.5–7.0, in a solution [1 in 10]), Water (not more than 5.0%), Residue on ignition (not more than 0.1%), Selenium (0.003%), Heavy metals (not more than 0.002%), and Organic volatile impurities.

MORICIZINE

Chemical name: Moricizine hydrochloride—10-(3-morpholinopropionyl) phenothiazine-2-carbamic acid ethyl ester hydrochloride.

Molecular formula: Moricizine hydrochloride—$C_{22}H_{25}N_3O_4S \cdot HCl$.

Molecular weight: Moricizine hydrochloride—464.

Description: Moricizine hydrochloride—White to tan crystalline powder.

pKa: Moricizine hydrochloride—6.4 (weak base).

Solubility: Moricizine hydrochloride—Freely soluble in water.

USP requirements: Moricizine Hydrochloride Tablets—Not in USP.

MORPHINE

Chemical name:

Morphine hydrochloride—Morphinan-3,6-diol, 7,8-didehydro-4,5-epoxy-17-methyl, (5 alpha,6 alpha)-, hydrochloride (1:1) (salt), trihydrate.

Morphine sulfate—Morphinan-3,6-diol, 7,8-didehydro-4,5-epoxy-17-methyl, (5 alpha,6 alpha)-, sulfate (2:1) (salt), pentahydrate.

Molecular formula:

Morphine hydrochloride—$C_{17}H_{19}NO_3 \cdot HCl \cdot 3H_2O$.

Morphine sulfate, pentahydrate—$(C_{17}H_{19}NO_3)_2 \cdot H_2SO_4 \cdot 5H_2O$.

Morphine sulfate, anhydrous—$(C_{17}H_{19}NO_3)_2 \cdot H_2SO_4$.

Molecular weight:

Morphine hydrochloride—375.8.

Morphine sulfate, pentahydrate—758.83.

Morphine sulfate, anhydrous—668.76.

Description:

Morphine hydrochloride—Colorless, silky crystals, cubical masses or a white or almost white, crystalline powder.

Morphine Sulfate USP—White, feathery, silky crystals, cubical masses of crystals, or white, crystalline powder. Is odorless, and when exposed to air it gradually loses water of hydration. Darkens on prolonged exposure to light.

Solubility:

Morphine hydrochloride—Freely soluble in boiling alcohol; soluble in water; sparingly soluble in alcohol; practically insoluble in chloroform and in ether.

Morphine Sulfate USP—Soluble in water; freely soluble in hot water; slightly soluble in alcohol but more so in hot alcohol; insoluble in chloroform and in ether.

USP requirements:

Morphine Hydrochloride Suppositories—Not in USP.

Morphine Hydrochloride Syrup—Not in USP.

Morphine Hydrochloride Tablets—Not in USP.

Morphine Hydrochloride Extended-release Tablets—Not in USP.

Morphine Sulfate Injection USP—Preserve in single-dose or in multiple-dose containers, preferably of Type I glass, protected from light. Preserve Injection labeled "Preservative-free" in single-dose containers. A sterile solution of Morphine Sulfate in Water for Injection. Label it to state that the Injection is not to be used if it is darker than pale yellow, if it is discolored in any other way, or if it contains a precipitate. Injection containing no antioxidant or antimicrobial agents prominently bears on its label the words "Preservative-free" and includes, in its labeling, its routes of administration and the statement that it is not to be heat-sterilized. Injection containing antioxidant or antimicrobial agents includes in its labeling its routes of administration and the statement that it is not for intrathecal or epidural use. Contains the labeled amount, within ±10%. Injection intended for intramuscular or intravenous administration may contain sodium chloride as a tonicity-adjusting agent, and suitable antioxidants and antimicrobial agents. Injection intended for intrathecal or epidural use may contain sodium chloride as a tonicity-adjusting agent, but contains no other added substances. Meets the requirements for Identification, Bacterial endotoxins, pH (2.5–6.5), Particulate matter, Injections, and Labeling under Injections.

Morphine Sulfate Oral Solution—Not in USP.
Morphine Sulfate Sterile Solution (Preservative-free)—Not in USP.
Morphine Sulfate Suppositories—Not in USP.
Morphine Sulfate Syrup—Not in USP.
Morphine Sulfate Tablets—Not in USP.
Morphine Sulfate Extended-release Tablets—Not in USP.
Morphine Sulfate Soluble Tablets—Not in USP.

MORRHUATE SODIUM

Description: Pale-yellowish, granular powder with a slight fishy odor.

Solubility: Soluble in water and in alcohol.

USP requirements: Morrhuate Sodium Injection USP—Preserve in single-dose or in multiple-dose containers, preferably of Type I glass. May be packaged in 50-mL multiple-dose containers. A sterile solution of the sodium salts of the fatty acids of Cod Liver Oil. Contains, in each mL, not less than 46.5 mg and not more than 53.5 mg of morrhuate sodium. Meets the requirements for Identification, Bacterial endotoxins, Acidity and alkalinity, Iodine value of the fatty acids (not less than 130), and Injections (except that at times it may show a slight turbidity or precipitate).

Note: Morrhuate Sodium Injection may show a separation of solid matter on standing. Do not use the material if such solid does not dissolve completely upon warming.

MOXALACTAM

Source: Semisynthetic 1-oxa-beta-lactam antibiotic structurally related to cephalosporins, cephamycins, and penicillins.

Chemical name: Moxalactam disodium—5-Oxa-1-azabicyclo[4.2.0]oct-2-ene-2-carboxylic acid, 7-[[carboxy(4-hydroxyphenyl)acetyl]amino]-7-methoxy-3-[[(1-methyl-1H-tetrazol-5-yl)thio]methyl]-8-oxo-, disodium salt.

Molecular formula: Moxalactam disodium—$C_{20}H_{18}N_6Na_2O_9S$.

Molecular weight: Moxalactam disodium—564.44.

Description: Moxalactam disodium—White to off-white powder with a faint characteristic odor.

Solubility: Moxalactam disodium—Very soluble in water.

USP requirements: Moxalactam Disodium for Injection USP—Preserve in Containers for Sterile Solids. A sterile mixture of moxalactam disodium and Mannitol. The mixture has a potency equivalent to not less than 722 mcg of moxalactam per mg. Contains an amount of moxalactam disodium equivalent to the labeled amount of moxalactam, within −10% to +20%. Meets the requirements for Constituted solution, Identification, Bacterial endotoxins, Sterility, pH (4.5–7.0 in a solution [1 in 10]), Water (not more than 3.0%), Particulate matter, and Isomer ratio (response ratio of R-isomer to S-isomer 0.8–1.4), and for Uniformity of dosage units and Labeling under Injections.

MUMPS SKIN TEST ANTIGEN

Description: Mumps Skin Test Antigen USP—Slightly turbid liquid.

USP requirements: Mumps Skin Test Antigen USP—Preserve at a temperature between 2 and 8 °C. A sterile suspension of formaldehyde-inactivated mumps virus prepared from the extra-embryonic fluids of the mumps virus–infected chicken embryo, concentrated and purified by differential centrifugation, and diluted with isotonic sodium chloride solution. Label it to state that it was prepared in embryonated chicken eggs and that a separate syringe and needle are to be used for each individual injection. Contains not less than 20 complement-fixing units in each mL. Contains approximately 0.006 M glycine as a stabilizing agent, and it contains a preservative. Meets the requirement for Expiration date (not later than 18 months after date of manufacture or date of issue from manufacturer's cold storage [5 °C, 1 year]). Conforms to the regulations of the U.S. Food and Drug Administration concerning biologics.

MUMPS VIRUS VACCINE LIVE

Source: The vaccine currently available in the U.S. (*Mumpsvax*, MSD) contains a lyophilized preparation of the Jeryl Lynn (B level) strain of mumps virus. This virus was adapted to and propagated in cell cultures of chick embryo free of avian leukosis virus and other adventitious agents. *Mumpsvax*, MSD (Canada) and Morson (U.K.) brands of mumps virus vaccine live, also contain the Jeryl Lynn strain of mumps virus.

Description: Mumps Virus Vaccine Live USP—Solid having the characteristic appearance of substances dried from the frozen state. The vaccine is to be constituted with a suitable diluent just prior to use. Constituted vaccine undergoes loss of potency on exposure to sunlight.

USP requirements: Mumps Virus Vaccine Live USP—Preserve in single-dose containers, or in light-resistant, multiple-dose containers, at a temperature between 2 and 8 °C. Multiple-dose containers for 50 doses are adapted for use only in jet injectors, and those for 10 doses for use by jet or syringe injection. A bacterially sterile preparation of live virus derived from a strain of mumps virus tested for neurovirulence in monkeys, and for immunogenicity, free from all demonstrable viable microbial agents except unavoidable bacteriophage, and found suitable for human immunization. The strain is grown for the purpose of vaccine production on chicken embryo primary cell tissue cultures derived from pathogen-free flocks, meets the requirements of the specific safety tests in adult and suckling mice; the requirements of the tests in monkey kidney, chicken embryo and human tissue cell cultures and embryonated eggs; and the requirements of the tests for absence of *Mycobacterium tuberculosis* and of avian leucosis, unless the production cultures were derived from certified avian leucosis-free sources and the control fluids were tested for avian leucosis. The strain cultures are treated to remove all intact tissue cells. The

Vaccine meets the requirements of the specific tissue culture test for live virus titer, in a single immunizing dose, of not less than the equivalent of 5000 $TCID_{50}$ (quantity of virus estimated to infect 50% of inoculated cultures $\times$ 5000) when tested in parallel with the U.S. Reference Mumps Virus, Live. Label the Vaccine in multiple-dose containers to indicate that the contents are intended solely for use by jet injector or for use by either jet or syringe injection, whichever is applicable. Label the Vaccine in single-dose containers, if such containers are not light-resistant, to state that it should be protected from sunlight. Label it also to state that constituted Vaccine should be discarded if not used within 8 hours. Meets the requirement for Expiration date (1 to 2 years, depending on the manufacturer's data, after date of issue from manufacturer's cold storage [−20 °C, 1 year]). Conforms to the regulations of the U.S. Food and Drug Administration concerning biologics.

MUPIROCIN

Source: Produced by fermentation of *Pseudomonas fluorescens*.

Chemical group: Structurally unrelated to other systemic or topical antibacterials.

Chemical name: Nonanoic acid, 9-[[3-methyl-1-oxo-4-[tetrahydro-3,4-dihydroxy-5-[[3-(2-hydroxy-1-methylpropyl)oxiranyl]methyl]2H-pyran-2-yl]-2-butenyl]oxy]-, [2S-[2 alpha(E), 3 beta,4 beta,5 alpha[2R*,3R*(1R*,2R*)]]]-.

Molecular formula: $C_{26}H_{44}O_9$.

Molecular weight: 500.63.

Description: White to off-white solid.

USP requirements: Mupirocin Ointment—Not in USP.

MUROMONAB-CD3

Source: Produced by a process involving fusion of mouse myeloma cells to lymphocytes from immunized animals to produce a hybridoma which secretes antigen-specific antibodies (murine monoclonal antibodies). Muromonab-CD3 is a biochemically purified $IgG_{2\ alpha}$ immunoglobulin with a heavy chain of approximately 50,000 daltons and a light chain of approximately 25,000 daltons.

USP requirements: Muromonab-CD3 Injection—Not in USP.

MYRISTYL ALCOHOL

Molecular formula: $C_{14}H_{30}O$.

Molecular weight: 214.39.

Description: Myristyl Alcohol NF—White wax-like mass. NF category: Oleaginous vehicle.

Solubility: Myristyl Alcohol NF—Soluble in ether; slightly soluble in alcohol; insoluble in water.

NF requirements: Myristyl Alcohol NF—Preserve in well-closed containers. Contains not less than 90.0% of myristyl alcohol, the remainder consisting chiefly of related alcohols. Meets the requirements for Identification, Melting range (36–40 °C), Acid value (not more than 2), Iodine value (not more than 1), Hydroxyl value (250–267), and Organic volatile impurities.

NABILONE

Chemical group: Synthetic cannabinoid. Resembles the cannabinols but is not a tetrahydrocannabinol.

Chemical name: 9H-Dibenzo[b,d]pyran-9-one, 3-(1,1-dimethylheptyl)-6,6a,7,8,10,10a-hexahydro-1-hydroxy-6,6-dimethyl-, trans-, (±)-.

Molecular formula: $C_{24}H_{36}O_3$.

Molecular weight: 372.55.

Description: White, polymorphic crystalline powder.

Solubility: In aqueous media, solubility less than 0.5 mg/L.

USP requirements: Nabilone Capsules—Not in USP.

NABUMETONE

Chemical name: 2-Butanone, 4-(6-methoxy-2-naphthalenyl)-.

Molecular formula: $C_{15}H_{16}O_2$.

Molecular weight: 228.29.

Description: White to off-white crystalline substance.

Solubility: Practically insoluble in water; soluble in alcohol and in most organic solvents.

Other characteristics: n-octanol:phosphate buffer partition coefficient—2400 at pH 7.4.

USP requirements: Nabumetone Tablets—Not in USP.

NADOLOL

Chemical name: 2,3-Naphthalenediol, 5-[3-[(1,1-dimethylethyl)amino]-2-hydroxypropoxy]-1,2,3,4-tetrahydro-, cis-.

Molecular formula: $C_{17}H_{27}NO_4$.

Molecular weight: 309.41.

Description: Nadolol USP—White to off-white, practically odorless, crystalline powder.

pKa: 9.67.

Solubility: Nadolol USP—Freely soluble in alcohol and in methanol; slightly soluble in chloroform, in methylene chloride, in isopropyl alcohol, and in water; insoluble in acetone, in ether, in hexane, and in trichloroethane.

Other characteristics: Lipid solubility—Low.

USP requirements: Nadolol Tablets USP—Preserve in tight containers. Contain the labeled amount, within ±10%. Meet the requirements for Identification, Dissolution (80% in 50 minutes in 0.1 N hydrochloric acid in Apparatus 1 at 100 rpm), and Uniformity of dosage units.

NADOLOL AND BENDROFLUMETHIAZIDE

For *Nadolol* and *Bendroflumethiazide*—See individual listings for chemistry information.

USP requirements: Nadolol and Bendroflumethiazide Tablets USP—Preserve in tight containers. Contain the labeled amounts, within ±10%. Meet the requirements for Identification, Dissolution (80% of each active ingredient in 30 minutes in 0.1 N hydrochloric acid in Apparatus 2 at 50 rpm), and Uniformity of dosage units.

NAFCILLIN

Chemical name: Nafcillin sodium—4-Thia-1-azabicyclo[3.2.0]heptane-2-carboxylic acid, 6-[[(2-ethoxy-1-naphthalenyl)carbonyl]amino]-3,3-dimethyl-7-oxo-, monosodium salt, monohydrate, [2S-(2 alpha,5 alpha,6 beta)].

Molecular formula: Nafcillin sodium—$C_{21}H_{21}N_2NaO_5S \cdot H_2O$.

Molecular weight: Nafcillin sodium—454.47.

Description:

Nafcillin Sodium USP—White to yellowish white powder, having not more than a slight characteristic odor.

Nafcillin Sodium for Injection USP—White to yellowish white powder, having not more than a slight characteristic odor.

Solubility:

Nafcillin Sodium USP—Freely soluble in water and in chloroform; soluble in alcohol.

Nafcillin Sodium for Injection USP—Freely soluble in water and in chloroform; soluble in alcohol.

USP requirements:

Nafcillin Sodium Capsules USP—Preserve in tight containers. Contain an amount of nafcillin sodium equivalent to the labeled amount of nafcillin, within −10% to +20%. Meet the requirements for Dissolution (75% in 45 minutes in water in Apparatus 1 at 100 rpm), Uniformity of dosage units, and Water (not more than 5.0%).

Nafcillin Sodium Injection USP—Preserve in Containers for Injections. Maintain in the frozen state. A sterile isoosmotic solution of Nafcillin Sodium and one or more buffer substances in Water for Injection. Contains dextrose as a tonicity-adjusting agent. The label states that it is to be thawed just prior to use, describes conditions for proper storage of the resultant solution, and directs that the solution is not to be refrozen. Contains an amount of nafcillin sodium equivalent to the labeled amount of nafcillin, within −10% to +20%. Contains no antimicrobial preservatives. Meets the requirements for Identification, Pyrogen, Sterility, pH (6.0–8.5), Particulate matter, and Labeling under Injections.

Nafcillin Sodium for Injection USP—Preserve in Containers for Sterile Solids. A sterile, dry mixture of Nafcillin Sodium and a suitable buffer. Contains an amount of nafcillin sodium equivalent to the labeled amount of nafcillin, within −10% to +20%. Meets the requirements for Constituted solution, Identification, Bacterial endotoxins, Sterility, pH (6.0–8.5, in the solution constituted as directed in the labeling), Water (3.5–5.3%), and Particulate matter, and for Uniformity of dosage units and Labeling under Injections.

Nafcillin Sodium for Oral Solution USP—Preserve in tight containers. Contains an amount of nafcillin sodium equivalent to the labeled amount of nafcillin, within −10% to +20%. Contains one or more suitable buffers, colors, diluents, dispersants, flavors, and preservatives. Meets the requirements for pH (5.5–7.5, in the solution constituted as directed in the labeling), Water (not more than 5.0%), Uniformity of dosage units (single-unit containers), and Deliverable volume (multiple-unit containers).

Sterile Nafcillin Sodium USP—Preserve in Containers for Sterile Solids. It is Nafcillin Sodium suitable for parenteral use. It has a potency equivalent to not less than 820 mcg of nafcillin per mg. Meets the requirements for Bacterial endotoxins and Sterility, and for Identification tests, pH, Water, and Crystallinity under Nafcillin Sodium.

Nafcillin Sodium Tablets USP—Preserve in tight, light-resistant containers. Contain an amount of nafcillin sodium equivalent to the labeled amount of nafcillin, within −10% to +20%. Meet the requirements for Dissolution (75% in 45 minutes in pH 4.0 buffer in Apparatus 2 at 50 rpm), Uniformity of dosage units, and Water (not more than 5.0%).

NAFTIFINE

Chemical group: Allylamine derivative.

Chemical name: Naftifine hydrochloride—1-Naphthalenemethanamine, *N*-methyl-*N*-(3-phenyl-2-propenyl)-, hydrochloride, (*E*)-.

Molecular formula: Naftifine hydrochloride—$C_{21}H_{21}N \cdot HCl$.

Molecular weight: Naftifine hydrochloride—323.86.

Description: Naftifine hydrochloride—White to yellow, fine, crystalline powder.

Solubility: Naftifine hydrochloride—0.68 mg/mL in water and 3.4 mg/mL in alcohol at 25 °C.

USP requirements:

Naftifine Hydrochloride Cream—Not in USP.

Naftifine Hydrochloride Gel—Not in USP.

NALBUPHINE

Chemical name: Nalbuphine hydrochloride—Morphinan-3,6,14-triol, 17-(cyclobutylmethyl)-4,5-epoxy-, hydrochloride, (5 alpha,6 alpha)-.

Molecular formula: Nalbuphine hydrochloride—$C_{21}H_{27}NO_4 \cdot HCl$.

Molecular weight: Nalbuphine hydrochloride—393.91.

Description: Nalbuphine hydrochloride—White to slightly off-white powder.

Solubility: Nalbuphine hydrochloride—Soluble in water; slightly soluble in alcohol.

USP requirements: Nalbuphine Hydrochloride Injection—Not in USP.

NALIDIXIC ACID

Chemical group: Closely related chemically to cinoxacin.

Chemical name: 1,8-Naphthyridine-3-carboxylic acid, 1-ethyl-1,4-dihydro-7-methyl-4-oxo-.

Molecular formula: $C_{12}H_{12}N_2O_3$.

Molecular weight: 232.24.

Description: Nalidixic Acid USP—White to very pale yellow, odorless, crystalline powder.

Solubility: Nalidixic Acid USP—Soluble in chloroform, in methylene chloride, and in solutions of fixed alkali hydroxides and carbonates; slightly soluble in acetone, in alcohol, in methanol, and in toluene; very slightly soluble in ether and in water.

USP requirements:

Nalidixic Acid Oral Suspension USP—Preserve in tight containers. Contains the labeled amount, within ±5%, in a suitable aqueous vehicle. Meets the requirement for Identification.

Nalidixic Acid Tablets USP—Preserve in tight containers. Contain the labeled amount, within ±7%. Meet the requirements for Identification, Dissolution (80% in 30 minutes in pH 8.60 buffer in Apparatus 2 at 60 rpm), and Uniformity of dosage units.

NALORPHINE

Chemical name: Nalorphine hydrochloride—Morphinan-3,6-diol, 7,8-didehydro-4,5-epoxy-17-(2-propenyl)-(5 alpha,6 alpha)-, hydrochloride.

Molecular formula: Nalorphine hydrochloride—$C_{19}H_{21}NO_3 \cdot HCl$.

Molecular weight: Nalorphine hydrochloride—347.84.

Description: Nalorphine hydrochloride—White or practically white, odorless, crystalline powder, slowly darkening on exposure to air and light. Melting point about 261 °C.

Solubility: Nalorphine hydrochloride—1 gram in about 8 mL of water or about 35 mL of alcohol; insoluble in chloroform or in ether; soluble in diluted alkali hydroxide solution.

USP requirements: Nalorphine Hydrochloride Injection USP—Preserve in single-dose or in multiple-dose containers, preferably of Type I glass. A suitably buffered, sterile solution of Nalorphine Hydrochloride in Water for Injection. Contains the labeled amount, within ±10%. Meets the requirements for Identification, Bacterial endotoxins, pH (6.0–7.5), and Injections.

NALOXONE

Chemical name: Naloxone hydrochloride—Morphinan-6-one, 4,5-epoxy-3,14-dihydroxy-17-(2-propenyl)-, hydrochloride, (5 alpha)-.

Molecular formula: Naloxone hydrochloride—$C_{19}H_{21}NO_4 \cdot HCl$.

Molecular weight: Naloxone hydrochloride—363.84.

Description:
Naloxone Hydrochloride USP—White to slightly off-white powder. Its aqueous solution is acidic.
Naloxone Hydrochloride Injection USP—Clear, colorless liquid.

Solubility: Naloxone Hydrochloride USP—Soluble in water, in dilute acids, and in strong alkali; slightly soluble in alcohol; practically insoluble in ether and in chloroform.

USP requirements: Naloxone Hydrochloride Injection USP—Preserve in single-dose or in multiple-dose containers of Type I glass, protected from light. A sterile, isotonic solution of Naloxone Hydrochloride in Water for Injection. Contains the labeled amount, within ±10%. Meets the requirements for Identification, Bacterial endotoxins, pH (3.0–4.5), and Injections.

NALTREXONE

Chemical group: A synthetic congener of oxymorphone; technically a thebaine derivative; also chemically related to the opioid antagonist naloxone.

Chemical name: Naltrexone hydrochloride—Morphinan-6-one, 17-(cyclopropylmethyl)-4,5-epoxy-3,14-dihydroxy-, hydrochloride, (5 alpha)-.

Molecular formula: Naltrexone hydrochloride—$C_{20}H_{23}NO_4 \cdot HCl$.

Molecular weight: Naltrexone hydrochloride—377.87.

Description: Naltrexone hydrochloride—White, crystalline compound.

Solubility: Naltrexone hydrochloride—Soluble in water to the extent of about 100 mg per mL.

USP requirements: Naltrexone Hydrochloride Tablets—Not in USP.

NANDROLONE

Chemical name:
Nandrolone decanoate—Estr-4-en-3-one, 17-[(1-oxodecyl)oxy]-, (17 beta)-.
Nandrolone phenpropionate—Estr-4-en-3-one, 17-(1-oxo-3-phenylpropoxy)-, (17 beta)-.

Molecular formula:
Nandrolone decanoate—$C_{28}H_{44}O_3$.
Nandrolone phenpropionate—$C_{27}H_{34}O_3$.

Molecular weight:
Nandrolone decanoate—428.65.
Nandrolone phenpropionate—406.56.

Description:
Nandrolone Decanoate USP—Fine, white to creamy white, crystalline powder. Is odorless, or may have a slight odor.
Nandrolone phenpropionate—Fine, white to creamy white, crystalline powder, having a slight, characteristic odor.

Solubility:
Nandrolone Decanoate USP—Practically insoluble in water; soluble in chloroform, in alcohol, in acetone, and in vegetable oils.
Nandrolone phenpropionate—Practically insoluble in water; soluble in alcohol, in chloroform, in dioxane, and in vegetable oils.

USP requirements:
Nandrolone Decanoate Injection USP—Preserve in single-dose or in multiple-dose containers, preferably of Type I glass, protected from light. A sterile solution of Nandrolone Decanoate in Sesame Oil, with a suitable preservative. Contains the labeled amount, within ±10%. Meets the requirements for Identification, Nandrolone (not more than 1.0%), and Injections.
Nandrolone Phenpropionate Injection USP—Preserve in single-dose or in multiple-dose containers, preferably of Type I glass, protected from light. A sterile solution of Nandrolone Phenpropionate in a suitable oil. Contains the labeled amount, within ±10%. Meets the requirements for Identification, Nandrolone, and Injections.

NAPHAZOLINE

Chemical name: Naphazoline hydrochloride—1*H*-Imidazole, 4,5-dihydro-2-(1-naphthalenylmethyl)-, monohydrochloride.

Molecular formula: Naphazoline hydrochloride—$C_{14}H_{14}N_2 \cdot HCl$.

Molecular weight: Naphazoline hydrochloride—246.74.

Description: Naphazoline Hydrochloride USP—White, crystalline powder. Is odorless. Melts at a temperature of about 255 °C, with decomposition.

Solubility: Naphazoline Hydrochloride USP—Freely soluble in water and in alcohol; very slightly soluble in chloroform; practically insoluble in ether.

USP requirements:
Naphazoline Hydrochloride Nasal Solution USP—Preserve in tight, light-resistant containers. A solution of Naphazoline Hydrochloride in water adjusted to a suitable pH and tonicity. Contains the labeled amount, within ±10%. Meets the requirement for Identification.
Naphazoline Hydrochloride Ophthalmic Solution USP—Preserve in tight containers. A sterile, buffered solution of Naphazoline Hydrochloride in water adjusted to a suitable tonicity. Contains the labeled amount, within −10% to +15%. Contains a suitable preservative. Meets the requirements for Identification, Sterility, and pH (5.5–7.0).

NAPROXEN

Chemical group: Propionic acid derivative.

Chemical name:
Naproxen—2-Naphthaleneacetic acid, 6-methoxy-alpha-methyl-, (+)-.

Naproxen sodium—2-Naphthaleneacetic acid, 6-methoxy-alpha-methyl-, sodium salt, (−)-.

Molecular formula:
Naproxen—$C_{14}H_{14}O_3$.
Naproxen sodium—$C_{14}H_{13}NaO_3$.

Molecular weight:
Naproxen—230.26.
Naproxen sodium—252.24.

Description:
Naproxen USP—White to off-white, practically odorless, crystalline powder.
Naproxen Sodium USP—White to creamy crystalline powder. Melts at about 255 °C, with decomposition.

pKa: 4.15 (apparent).

Solubility:
Naproxen USP—Practically insoluble in water; freely soluble in chloroform and in dehydrated alcohol; soluble in alcohol; sparingly soluble in ether.
Naproxen Sodium USP—Soluble in water and in methanol; sparingly soluble in alcohol; very slightly soluble in acetone; practically insoluble in chloroform and in toluene.

USP requirements:
Naproxen Suppositories—Not in USP.
Naproxen Oral Suspension—Not in USP.
Naproxen Tablets USP—Preserve in well-closed containers. Contain the labeled amount, within ±10%. Meet the requirements for Identification, Dissolution (70% in 45 minutes in 0.1 M phosphate buffer [pH 7.4] in Apparatus 2 at 50 rpm), and Uniformity of dosage units.
Naproxen Extended-release Tablets—Not in USP.
Naproxen Sodium Tablets USP—Preserve in well-closed containers. Contain the labeled amount, within ±10%. Meet the requirements for Identification, Dissolution (70% in 45 minutes in 0.1 M phosphate buffer [pH 7.4] in Apparatus 2 at 50 rpm), and Uniformity of dosage units.

NATAMYCIN

Source: Derived from *Streptomyces natalensis*.

Chemical group: Tetraene polyene antifungal.

Chemical name: Pimaricin.

Molecular formula: $C_{33}H_{47}NO_{13}$.

Molecular weight: 665.73.

Description: Natamycin USP—Off-white to cream-colored powder, which may contain up to 3 moles of water.

Solubility: Natamycin USP—Practically insoluble in water; slightly soluble in methanol; soluble in glacial acetic acid and in dimethylformamide.

USP requirements: Natamycin Ophthalmic Suspension USP—Preserve in tight, light-resistant containers. The containers or individual cartons are sealed and tamper-proof so that sterility is assured at time of first use. A sterile suspension of Natamycin in a suitable aqueous vehicle. Contains one or more suitable preservatives. Contains the labeled amount, within −10% to +25%. Meets the requirements for Identification, Sterility, and pH (5.0–7.5).

NEOMYCIN

Source: Derived from *Streptomyces fradiae*.

Chemical group: Aminoglycosides.

Chemical name: Neomycin sulfate.

Description: Neomycin Sulfate USP—White to slightly yellow powder, or cryodesiccated solid. Is odorless or practically so and is hygroscopic. Its solutions are dextrorotatory.

Solubility: Neomycin Sulfate USP—Freely soluble in water; very slightly soluble in alcohol; insoluble in acetone, in chloroform, and in ether.

USP requirements:
Neomycin Sulfate Cream USP—Preserve in well-closed containers, preferably at controlled room temperature. Contains an amount of neomycin sulfate equivalent to the labeled amount of neomycin, within −10% to +35%. Meets the requirements for Identification and Minimum fill.
Neomycin Sulfate Ointment USP—Preserve in well-closed containers, preferably at controlled room temperature. Contains an amount of neomycin sulfate equivalent to the labeled amount of neomycin, within −10% to +35%. Meets the requirements for Identification, Minimum fill, and Water (not more than 1.0%).
Neomycin Sulfate Ophthalmic Ointment USP—Preserve in collapsible ophthalmic ointment tubes. A sterile preparation of Neomycin Sulfate in a suitable ointment base. Contains an amount of neomycin sulfate equivalent to the labeled amount of neomycin, within −10% to +35%. Meets the requirements for Identification, Sterility, Minimum fill, Water (not more than 1.0%), and Metal particles.
Neomycin Sulfate Oral Solution USP—Preserve in tight, light-resistant containers, preferably at controlled room temperature. Contains an amount of neomycin sulfate equivalent to the labeled amount of neomycin, within −10% to +25%. Meets the requirements for Identification and pH (5.0–7.5).
Sterile Neomycin Sulfate USP—Preserve in Containers for Sterile Solids. It is Neomycin Sulfate suitable for parenteral use. Contains an amount of neomycin sulfate equivalent to not less than 600 mcg of neomycin per mg, calculated on the dried basis and, where packaged for dispensing, contains an amount of neomycin sulfate equivalent to the labeled amount of neomycin within −10% to +20%. Meets the requirements for Bacterial endotoxins and Sterility, and for Identification tests, pH, and Loss on drying under Neomycin Sulfate. Where packaged for dispensing, it meets also the requirements for Uniformity of dosage units and Labeling under Injections. Where intended for use in preparing sterile ophthalmic dosage forms, it is exempt from the requirements for Bacterial endotoxins.
Neomycin Sulfate Tablets USP—Preserve in tight containers. Contain an amount of neomycin sulfate equivalent to the labeled amount of neomycin, within −10% to +25%. Meet the requirements for Identification, Disintegration (60 minutes), Uniformity of dosage units, and Loss on drying (not more than 10.0%).

NEOMYCIN AND BACITRACIN

For *Neomycin* and *Bacitracin*—See individual listings for chemistry information.

USP requirements:
Neomycin Sulfate and Bacitracin Ointment USP—Preserve in tight, light-resistant containers, preferably at controlled room temperature. Contains amounts of neomycin sulfate and bacitracin equivalent to the labeled amounts of neomycin and bacitracin, within −10% to +30%. Meets the requirements for Identification, Minimum fill, and Water (not more than 0.5%).
Neomycin Sulfate and Bacitracin Zinc Ointment USP—Preserve in collapsible tubes or in well-closed containers.

Contains amounts of neomycin sulfate and bacitracin zinc equivalent to the labeled amounts of neomycin and bacitracin, within −10% to +30%. Meets the requirements for Identification, Minimum fill, and Water (not more than 0.5%).

NEOMYCIN AND DEXAMETHASONE

For *Neomycin* and *Dexamethasone*—See individual listings for chemistry information.

USP requirements:

Neomycin Sulfate and Dexamethasone Sodium Phosphate Cream USP—Preserve in collapsible tubes or in tight containers. Contains an amount of neomycin sulfate equivalent to the labeled amount of neomycin, within −10% to +35%, and an amount of dexamethasone sodium phosphate equivalent to the labeled amount of dexamethasone phosphate, within ±10%. Meets the requirements for Identification and Minimum fill.

Neomycin Sulfate and Dexamethasone Sodium Phosphate Ophthalmic Ointment USP—Preserve in collapsible ophthalmic ointment tubes. A sterile ointment containing Neomycin Sulfate and Dexamethasone Sodium Phosphate. Contains an amount of neomycin sulfate equivalent to the labeled amount of neomycin, within −10% to +35%, and an amount of dexamethasone sodium phosphate equivalent to the labeled amount of dexamethasone phosphate, within ±10%. Meets the requirements for Identification, Sterility, Minimum fill, Water (not more than 1.0%), and Metal particles.

Note: Where Neomycin Sulfate and Dexamethasone Sodium Phosphate Ophthalmic Ointment is prescribed without reference to the quantity of neomycin or dexamethasone phosphate contained therein, a product containing 3.5 mg of neomycin and 0.5 mg of dexamethasone phosphate per gram shall be dispensed.

Neomycin Sulfate and Dexamethasone Sodium Phosphate Ophthalmic Solution USP—Preserve in tight, light-resistant containers, and avoid exposure to excessive heat. A sterile, aqueous solution of Neomycin Sulfate and Dexamethasone Sodium Phosphate. Contains an amount of neomycin sulfate equivalent to the labeled amount of neomycin, within −10% to +30%, and an amount of dexamethasone sodium phosphate equivalent to the labeled amount of dexamethasone phosphate, within −10% to +15%. Meets the requirements for Identification, Sterility, and pH (6.0–8.0).

Note: Where Neomycin Sulfate and Dexamethasone Sodium Phosphate Ophthalmic Solution is prescribed, without reference to the amount of neomycin or dexamethasone phosphate contained therein, a product containing 3.5 mg of neomycin and 1.0 mg of dexamethasone phosphate per mL shall be dispensed.

NEOMYCIN AND FLUOCINOLONE

For *Neomycin* and *Fluocinolone*—See individual listings for chemistry information.

USP requirements: Neomycin Sulfate and Fluocinolone Acetonide Cream USP—Preserve in collapsible tubes or in tight containers. Contains an amount of neomycin sulfate equivalent to the labeled amount of neomycin, within −10% to +35%, and the labeled amount of fluocinolone acetonide, within ±10%. Meets the requirements for Identification and Minimum fill.

NEOMYCIN AND FLUOROMETHOLONE

For *Neomycin* and *Fluorometholone*—See individual listings for chemistry information.

USP requirements: Neomycin Sulfate and Fluorometholone Ointment USP—Preserve in collapsible tubes or in well-closed

containers. Contains an amount of neomycin sulfate equivalent to the labeled amount of neomycin, within −10% to +35%, and the labeled amount of fluorometholone, within ±10%. Meets the requirements for Identification, Minimum fill, and Water (not more than 1.0%).

NEOMYCIN AND FLURANDRENOLIDE

For *Neomycin* and *Flurandrenolide*—See individual listings for chemistry information.

USP requirements:

Neomycin Sulfate and Flurandrenolide Cream USP—Preserve in collapsible tubes or in tight containers, protected from light. Contains an amount of neomycin sulfate equivalent to the labeled amount of neomycin, within −10% to +35%, and the labeled amount of flurandrenolide, within ±10%. Meets the requirements for Identification and Minimum fill.

Neomycin Sulfate and Flurandrenolide Lotion USP—Preserve in tight containers, protected from light. Contains an amount of neomycin sulfate equivalent to the labeled amount of neomycin, within −10% to +30%, and the labeled amount of flurandrenolide, within ±10%. Meets the requirements for Identification, Microbial limits, and Minimum fill.

Neomycin Sulfate and Flurandrenolide Ointment USP—Preserve in collapsible tubes or in tight containers, protected from light. Contains an amount of neomycin sulfate equivalent to the labeled amount of neomycin, within −10% to +35%, and the labeled amount of flurandrenolide, within ±10%. Meets the requirements for Identification, Minimum fill, and Water (not more than 1.0%).

NEOMYCIN AND GRAMICIDIN

For *Neomycin* and *Gramicidin*—See individual listings for chemistry information.

USP requirements: Neomycin Sulfate and Gramicidin Ointment USP—Preserve in collapsible tubes or in well-closed containers. Contains amounts of neomycin sulfate and gramicidin equivalent to the labeled amounts of neomycin and gramicidin, within −10% to +40%. Meets the requirements for Identification, Minimum fill, and Water (not more than 1.0%).

NEOMYCIN AND HYDROCORTISONE

For *Neomycin* and *Hydrocortisone*—See individual listings for chemistry information.

USP requirements:

Neomycin Sulfate and Hydrocortisone Cream USP—Preserve in collapsible tubes or in well-closed containers. Contains an amount of neomycin sulfate equivalent to the labeled amount of neomycin, within −10% to +35%, and the labeled amount of hydrocortisone, within ±10%. Meets the requirements for Identification and Minimum fill.

Neomycin Sulfate and Hydrocortisone Ointment USP—Preserve in collapsible tubes or in well-closed containers. Contains an amount of neomycin sulfate equivalent to the labeled amount of neomycin, within −10% to +35%, and the labeled amount of hydrocortisone, within ±10%. Meets the requirements for Identification, Minimum fill, and Water (not more than 1.0%).

Neomycin Sulfate and Hydrocortisone Otic Suspension USP—Preserve in tight, light-resistant containers. A sterile suspension. Contains an amount of neomycin sulfate equivalent to the labeled amount of neomycin, within

−10% to +30%, and the labeled amount of hydrocortisone, within ±10%. Contains Acetic Acid. Meets the requirements for Sterility and pH (4.5–6.0).

> Note: Where Neomycin Sulfate and Hydrocortisone Otic Suspension is prescribed, without reference to the quantity of neomycin or hydrocortisone contained therein, a product containing 3.5 mg of neomycin and 10 mg of hydrocortisone per mL shall be dispensed.

Neomycin Sulfate and Hydrocortisone Acetate Cream USP—Preserve in well-closed containers. Contains an amount of neomycin sulfate equivalent to the labeled amount of neomycin, within −10% to +35%, and the labeled amount of hydrocortisone acetate, within ±10%. Meets the requirements for Identification and Minimum fill.

Neomycin Sulfate and Hydrocortisone Acetate Lotion USP—Preserve in well-closed containers. Contains an amount of neomycin sulfate equivalent to the labeled amount of neomycin, within −10% to +30%, and the labeled amount of hydrocortisone acetate, within ±10%. Meets the requirements for Identification and Minimum fill.

Neomycin Sulfate and Hydrocortisone Acetate Ointment USP—Preserve in collapsible tubes or in well-closed containers. Contains an amount of neomycin sulfate equivalent to the labeled amount of neomycin, within −10% to +35%, and the labeled amount of hydrocortisone acetate, within ±10%. Meets the requirements for Identification, Minimum fill, and Water (not more than 1.0%).

Neomycin Sulfate and Hydrocortisone Acetate Ophthalmic Ointment USP—Preserve in collapsible ophthalmic ointment tubes. Contains an amount of neomycin sulfate equivalent to the labeled amount of neomycin, within −10% to +35%, and the labeled amount of hydrocortisone acetate, within ±10%. Meets the requirements for Identification, Sterility, Minimum fill, Water (not more than 1.0%), and Metal particles.

Neomycin Sulfate and Hydrocortisone Acetate Ophthalmic Suspension USP—Preserve in tight containers. The containers or individual cartons are sealed and tamper-proof so that sterility is assured at time of first use. A sterile, aqueous suspension. Contains an amount of neomycin sulfate equivalent to the labeled amount of neomycin, within −10% to +30%, and the labeled amount of hydrocortisone acetate, within ±10%. Meets the requirements for Identification, Sterility, and pH (5.5–7.5).

NEOMYCIN AND METHYLPREDNISOLONE

For *Neomycin* and *Methylprednisolone*—See individual listings for chemistry information.

USP requirements: Neomycin Sulfate and Methylprednisolone Acetate Cream USP—Preserve in collapsible tubes or in tight containers, protected from light. Contains an amount of neomycin sulfate equivalent to the labeled amount of neomycin, within −10% to +35%, and the labeled amount of methylprednisone acetate, within ±10%. Meets the requirements for Identification and Minimum fill.

NEOMYCIN AND POLYMYXIN B

For *Neomycin* and *Polymyxin B*—See individual listings for chemistry information.

USP requirements:

Neomycin and Polymyxin B Sulfates Cream USP—Preserve in well-closed containers, preferably at controlled room temperature. Contains amounts of neomycin sulfate and polymyxin B sulfate equivalent to the labeled amounts of neomycin and polymyxin B, within −10% to +30%. Meets the requirements for Identification and Minimum fill.

Neomycin and Polymyxin B Sulfates Ophthalmic Ointment USP—Preserve in collapsible ophthalmic ointment tubes. A sterile ointment containing Neomycin Sulfate and Polymyxin B Sulfate. Contains amounts of neomycin sulfate and polymyxin B sulfate equivalent to the labeled amounts of neomycin and polymyxin B, within −10% to +30%. Meets the requirements for Identification, Sterility, Minimum fill, Water (not more than 0.5%), and Metal particles.

Neomycin and Polymyxin B Sulfates Solution for Irrigation USP—Preserve in tight containers. A sterile, aqueous solution. Label it to indicate that it is to be diluted for use in a urinary bladder irrigation and is not intended for injection. Contains amounts of neomycin sulfate and polymyxin B sulfate equivalent to the labeled amounts of neomycin and polymyxin B, within −10% to +30%. Meets the requirements for Identification, Sterility, and pH (4.5–6.0).

Neomycin and Polymyxin B Sulfates Ophthalmic Solution USP—Preserve in tight containers, and avoid exposure to excessive heat. Contains amounts of neomycin sulfate and polymyxin B sulfate equivalent to the labeled amounts of neomycin and polymyxin B, within −10% to +30%. Meets the requirements for Identification, Sterility, and pH (5.0–7.0).

NEOMYCIN, POLYMYXIN B, AND BACITRACIN

For *Neomycin, Polymyxin B,* and *Bacitracin*—See individual listings for chemistry information.

USP requirements:

Neomycin and Polymyxin B Sulfates and Bacitracin Ointment USP—Preserve in tight, light-resistant containers, preferably at controlled room temperature. Contains amounts of neomycin sulfate, polymyxin B sulfate, and bacitracin equivalent to the labeled amounts of neomycin, polymyxin B, and bacitracin, within −10% to +30%. Meets the requirements for Identification, Minimum fill, and Water (not more than 0.5%).

Neomycin and Polymyxin B Sulfates and Bacitracin Ophthalmic Ointment USP—Preserve in collapsible ophthalmic ointment tubes. A sterile ointment containing Neomycin Sulfate, Polymyxin B Sulfate, and Bacitracin. Contains amounts of neomycin sulfate, polymyxin B sulfate, and bacitracin equivalent to the labeled amounts of neomycin, polymyxin B, and bacitracin, within −10% to +40%. Meets the requirements for Identification, Sterility, Minimum fill, Water (not more than 0.5%), and Metal particles.

Neomycin and Polymyxin B Sulfates and Bacitracin Zinc Ointment USP—Preserve in well-closed containers, preferably at controlled room temperature. Contains amounts of neomycin sulfate, polymyxin B sulfate, and bacitracin zinc equivalent to the labeled amounts of neomycin, polymyxin B, and bacitracin, within −10% to +30%. Meets the requirements for Identification, Minimum fill, and Water (not more than 0.5%).

Neomycin and Polymyxin B Sulfates and Bacitracin Zinc Ophthalmic Ointment USP—Preserve in collapsible ophthalmic ointment tubes. Contains amounts of neomycin sulfate, polymyxin B sulfate, and bacitracin zinc equivalent to the labeled amounts of neomycin, polymyxin B, and bacitracin, within −10% to +40%. Meets the requirements for Identification, Sterility, Minimum fill, Water (not more than 0.5%), and Metal particles.

NEOMYCIN, POLYMYXIN B, BACITRACIN, AND HYDROCORTISONE

For *Neomycin, Polymyxin B, Bacitracin,* and *Hydrocortisone*—See individual listings for chemistry information.

USP requirements:

Neomycin and Polymyxin B Sulfates, Bacitracin, and Hydrocortisone Acetate Ointment USP—Preserve in collapsible tubes or in well-closed containers. Contains amounts of neomycin sulfate, polymyxin B sulfate, and bacitracin equivalent to the labeled amounts of neomycin, polymyxin B, and bacitracin, within −10% to +30%, and the labeled amount of hydrocortisone acetate, within ±10%, in a suitable ointment base. Meets the requirements for Identification, Minimum fill, and Water (not more than 0.5%).

Neomycin and Polymyxin B Sulfates, Bacitracin, and Hydrocortisone Acetate Ophthalmic Ointment USP—Preserve in collapsible ophthalmic ointment tubes. Contains amounts of neomycin sulfate, polymyxin B sulfate, and bacitracin equivalent to the labeled amounts of neomycin, polymyxin B, and bacitracin, within −10% to +40%, and the labeled amount of hydrocortisone acetate, within ±10%, in a suitable ointment base. Meets the requirements for Identification, Sterility, Minimum fill, Water (not more than 0.5%), and Metal particles.

Neomycin and Polymyxin B Sulfates, Bacitracin Zinc, and Hydrocortisone Ointment USP—Preserve in well-closed containers, preferably at controlled room temperature. Contains amounts of neomycin sulfate, polymyxin B sulfate, and bacitracin zinc equivalent to the labeled amounts of neomycin, polymyxin B, and bacitracin, within −10% to +30%, and the labeled amount of hydrocortisone, within ±10%. Meets the requirements for Identification, Minimum fill, and Water (not more than 0.5%).

Neomycin and Polymyxin B Sulfates, Bacitracin Zinc, and Hydrocortisone Ophthalmic Ointment USP—Preserve in collapsible ophthalmic ointment tubes. A sterile ointment containing Neomycin Sulfate, Polymyxin B Sulfate, Bacitracin Zinc, and Hydrocortisone. Contains amounts of neomycin sulfate, polymyxin B sulfate, and bacitracin zinc equivalent to the labeled amounts of neomycin, polymyxin B, and bacitracin, within −10% to +40%, and the labeled amount of hydrocortisone, within ±10%. Meets the requirements for Identification, Sterility, Minimum fill, Water (not more than 0.5%), and Metal particles.

Neomycin and Polymyxin B Sulfates, Bacitracin Zinc, and Hydrocortisone Acetate Ophthalmic Ointment USP—Preserve in collapsible ophthalmic ointment tubes. A sterile ointment containing Neomycin Sulfate, Polymyxin B Sulfate, Bacitracin Zinc, and Hydrocortisone Acetate. Contains amounts of neomycin sulfate, polymyxin B sulfate, and bacitracin zinc equivalent to the labeled amounts of neomycin, polymyxin B, and bacitracin, within −10% to +40%, and the labeled amount of hydrocortisone acetate, within ±10%. Meets the requirements for Identification, Sterility, Minimum fill, Water (not more than 0.5%), and Metal particles.

NEOMYCIN, POLYMYXIN B, BACITRACIN, AND LIDOCAINE

For *Neomycin, Polymyxin B, Bacitracin,* and *Lidocaine*—See individual listings for chemistry information.

USP requirements: Neomycin and Polymyxin B Sulfates, Bacitracin, and Lidocaine Ointment USP—Preserve in well-closed containers, preferably at controlled room temperature. Contains amounts of neomycin sulfate, polymyxin B sulfate, and bacitracin equivalent to the labeled amounts of

neomycin, polymyxin B, and bacitracin, within −10% to +30%, and the labeled amount of lidocaine, within ±10%. Meets the requirements for Identification, Minimum fill, and Water (not more than 0.5%).

NEOMYCIN, POLYMYXIN B, AND DEXAMETHASONE

For *Neomycin, Polymyxin B,* and *Dexamethasone*—See individual listings for chemistry information.

USP requirements:

Neomycin and Polymyxin B Sulfates and Dexamethasone Ophthalmic Ointment USP—Preserve in collapsible ophthalmic ointment tubes. Contains amounts of neomycin sulfate and polymyxin B sulfate equivalent to the labeled amounts of neomycin and polymyxin B, within −10% to +30%, and the labeled amount of dexamethasone, within ±10%. Meets the requirements for Identification, Sterility, Minimum fill, Water (not more than 0.5%), and Metal particles.

Neomycin and Polymyxin B Sulfates and Dexamethasone Ophthalmic Suspension USP—Preserve in tight, light-resistant containers in a cool place or at controlled room temperature. The containers or individual cartons are sealed and tamper-proof so that sterility is assured at time of first use. Contains amounts of neomycin sulfate and polymyxin B sulfate equivalent to the labeled amounts of neomycin and polymyxin B, within −10% to +30%, and the labeled amount of dexamethasone, within ±10%. Meets the requirements for Identification, Sterility, and pH (3.5–6.0).

NEOMYCIN, POLYMYXIN B, AND GRAMICIDIN

For *Neomycin, Polymyxin B,* and *Gramicidin*—See individual listings for chemistry information.

USP requirements:

Neomycin and Polymyxin B Sulfates and Gramicidin Cream USP—Preserve in collapsible tubes or in well-closed containers. Contains amounts of neomycin sulfate, polymyxin B sulfate, and gramicidin equivalent to the labeled amounts of neomycin, polymyxin B, and gramicidin, within −10% to +30%. Meets the requirement for Minimum fill.

Neomycin and Polymyxin B Sulfates and Gramicidin Ophthalmic Solution USP—Preserve in tight containers. The containers or individual cartons are sealed and tamper-proof so that sterility is assured at time of first use. A sterile, isotonic aqueous solution of Neomycin Sulfate, Polymyxin B Sulfate, and Gramicidin. Contains amounts of neomycin sulfate, polymyxin B sulfate, and gramicidin equivalent to the labeled amounts of neomycin, polymyxin B, and gramicidin, within −10% to +30%. Meets the requirements for Identification, Sterility, and pH (4.7–6.0).

NEOMYCIN, POLYMYXIN B, GRAMICIDIN, AND HYDROCORTISONE

For *Neomycin, Polymyxin B, Gramicidin,* and *Hydrocortisone*—See individual listings for chemistry information.

USP requirements: Neomycin and Polymyxin B Sulfates, Gramicidin, and Hydrocortisone Acetate Cream USP—Preserve in well-closed containers. Contains amounts of neomycin sulfate, polymyxin B sulfate, and gramicidin equivalent to the labeled amounts of neomycin, polymyxin B, and gramicidin, within −10% to +30%, and the labeled amount of hydrocortisone acetate, within ±10%. Meets the requirement for Minimum fill.

NEOMYCIN, POLYMYXIN B, AND HYDROCORTISONE

For *Neomycin, Polymyxin B,* and *Hydrocortisone*—See individual listings for chemistry information.

USP requirements:

Neomycin and Polymyxin B Sulfates and Hydrocortisone Otic Solution USP—Preserve in tight, light-resistant containers. The containers or individual cartons are sealed and tamper-proof so that sterility is assured at time of first use. A sterile solution containing Neomycin Sulfate, Polymyxin B Sulfate, and Hydrocortisone. Contains amounts of neomycin sulfate and polymyxin B sulfate equivalent to the labeled amounts of neomycin and polymyxin B, within −10% to +30%. Contains the labeled amount of hydrocortisone, within ±10%. Meets the requirements for Sterility and pH (2.0–4.5).

Neomycin and Polymyxin B Sulfates and Hydrocortisone Ophthalmic Suspension USP—Preserve in tight containers. The containers or individual cartons are sealed and tamper-proof so that sterility is assured at time of first use. A sterile, aqueous suspension of Neomycin Sulfate, Polymyxin B Sulfate, and Hydrocortisone. Contains amounts of neomycin sulfate and polymyxin B sulfate equivalent to the labeled amounts of neomycin and polymyxin B, within −10% to +30%. Contains the labeled amount of hydrocortisone, within ±10%. Meets the requirements for Identification, Sterility, and pH (4.1–7.0).

Neomycin and Polymyxin B Sulfates and Hydrocortisone Otic Suspension USP—Preserve in tight, light-resistant containers. The containers or individual cartons are sealed and tamper-proof so that sterility is assured at time of first use. A sterile suspension containing Neomycin Sulfate, Polymyxin B Sulfate, and Hydrocortisone. Contains amounts of neomycin sulfate and polymyxin B sulfate equivalent to the labeled amounts of neomycin and polymyxin B, within −10% to +30%. Contains the labeled amount of hydrocortisone, within ±10%. Meets the requirements for Identification, Sterility, and pH (3.0–7.0).

Neomycin and Polymyxin B Sulfates and Hydrocortisone Acetate Cream USP—Preserve in well-closed containers. Contains amounts of neomycin sulfate and polymyxin B sulfate equivalent to the labeled amounts of neomycin and polymyxin B, within −10% to +30%. Contains the labeled amount of hydrocortisone acetate, within ±10%. Meets the requirements for Identification and Minimum fill.

Neomycin and Polymyxin B Sulfates and Hydrocortisone Acetate Ophthalmic Suspension USP—Preserve in tight containers. The containers or individual cartons are sealed and tamper-proof so that sterility is assured at time of first use. A sterile suspension of Hydrocortisone Acetate in an aqueous solution of Neomycin Sulfate and Polymyxin B Sulfate. Contains amounts of neomycin sulfate and polymyxin B sulfate equivalent to the labeled amounts of neomycin and polymyxin B, within −10% to +25%. Contains the labeled amount of hydrocortisone acetate, within ±10%. Meets the requirements for Sterility and pH (5.0–7.0).

NEOMYCIN, POLYMYXIN B, AND PREDNISOLONE

For *Neomycin, Polymyxin B,* and *Prednisolone*—See individual listings for chemistry information.

USP requirements: Neomycin and Polymyxin B Sulfates and Prednisolone Acetate Ophthalmic Suspension USP—Preserve in tight containers. The containers or individual cartons are sealed and tamper-proof so that sterility is assured at time of first use. A sterile suspension of Prednisolone Acetate in an aqueous solution of Neomycin Sulfate and Polymyxin

B Sulfate. Contains amounts of neomycin sulfate and polymyxin B sulfate equivalent to the labeled amounts of neomycin and polymyxin B, within −10% to +25%, and the labeled amount of prednisolone acetate, within ±10%. Meets the requirements for Identification, Sterility, and pH (5.0–7.0).

NEOMYCIN AND PREDNISOLONE

For *Neomycin* and *Prednisolone*—See individual listings for chemistry information.

USP requirements:

Neomycin Sulfate and Prednisolone Acetate Ointment USP—Preserve in collapsible tubes or in tight containers, protected from light. Contains an amount of neomycin sulfate equivalent to the labeled amount of neomycin, within −10% to +35%, and the labeled amount of prednisolone acetate, within ±10%. Meets the requirements for Identification, Minimum fill, and Water (not more than 1.0%).

Neomycin Sulfate and Prednisolone Acetate Ophthalmic Ointment USP—Preserve in collapsible ophthalmic ointment tubes. A sterile ointment containing Neomycin Sulfate and Prednisolone Acetate. Contains an amount of neomycin sulfate equivalent to the labeled amount of neomycin, within −10% to +35%, and the labeled amount of prednisolone acetate, within ±10%. Meets the requirements for Identification, Sterility, Minimum fill, Water (not more than 1.0%), and Metal particles.

Neomycin Sulfate and Prednisolone Acetate Ophthalmic Suspension USP—Preserve in tight containers. The containers or individual cartons are sealed and tamper-proof so that sterility is assured at time of first use. Contains an amount of neomycin sulfate equivalent to the labeled amount of neomycin, within −10% to +30%, and the labeled amount of prednisolone acetate, within ±10%. Meets the requirements for Identification, Sterility, and pH (5.5–7.5).

Neomycin Sulfate and Prednisolone Sodium Phosphate Ophthalmic Ointment USP—Preserve in collapsible ophthalmic ointment tubes. A sterile ointment containing Neomycin Sulfate and Prednisolone Sodium Phosphate. Contains amounts of neomycin sulfate and prednisolone sodium phosphate equivalent to the labeled amounts of neomycin, within −10% to +35%, and prednisolone phosphate, within −10% to +15%. Meets the requirements for Identification, Sterility, Minimum fill, Water (not more than 1.0%), and Metal particles.

Note: Where Neomycin Sulfate and Prednisolone Sodium Phosphate Ophthalmic Ointment is prescribed without reference to the quantity of neomycin or prednisolone phosphate contained therein, a product containing 3.5 mg of neomycin and 2.5 mg of prednisolone phosphate per gram shall be dispensed.

NEOMYCIN, SULFACETAMIDE, AND PREDNISOLONE

For *Neomycin, Sulfacetamide,* and *Prednisolone*—See individual listings for chemistry information.

USP requirements: Neomycin Sulfate, Sulfacetamide Sodium, and Prednisolone Acetate Ophthalmic Ointment USP—Preserve in collapsible ophthalmic ointment tubes. Contains an amount of neomycin sulfate equivalent to the labeled amount of neomycin, within −10% to +35%, and the labeled amounts of sulfacetamide sodium and prednisolone acetate, within ±10%. Meets the requirements for Identification, Sterility, Minimum fill, and Metal particles.

NEOMYCIN AND TRIAMCINOLONE

For *Neomycin* and *Triamcinolone*—See individual listings for chemistry information.

USP requirements:

Neomycin Sulfate and Triamcinolone Acetonide Cream USP—Preserve in collapsible tubes or in tight containers. Contains an amount of neomycin sulfate equivalent to the labeled amount of neomycin, within −10% to +35%, and the labeled amount of triamcinolone acetonide, within ±10%. Meets the requirements for Identification and Minimum fill.

Neomycin Sulfate and Triamcinolone Acetonide Ophthalmic Ointment USP—Preserve in collapsible ophthalmic ointment tubes. Contains an amount of neomycin sulfate equivalent to the labeled amount of neomycin, within −10% to +35%, and the labeled amount of triamcinolone acetonide, within ±10%. Meets the requirements for Identification, Sterility, Minimum fill, Water (not more than 1.0%), and Metal particles.

NEOSTIGMINE

Source: Quaternary ammonium compound.

Chemical name:

Neostigmine bromide—Benzenaminium, 3-[[(dimethylamino)carbonyl]oxy]-*N,N,N*-trimethyl-, bromide.

Neostigmine methylsulfate—Benzenaminium, 3-[[(dimethylamino)carbonyl]oxy]-*N,N,N*-trimethyl-, methyl sulfate.

Molecular formula:

Neostigmine bromide—$C_{12}H_{19}BrN_2O_2$.

Neostigmine methylsulfate—$C_{13}H_{22}N_2O_6S$.

Molecular weight:

Neostigmine bromide—303.20.

Neostigmine methylsulfate—334.39.

Description:

Neostigmine bromide—White, crystalline powder. Odorless. Its solutions are neutral to litmus.

Neostigmine methylsulfate—White, crystalline powder. Odorless. Its solutions are neutral to litmus.

Solubility

Neostigmine bromide—Very soluble in water; soluble in alcohol; practically insoluble in ether.

Neostigmine methylsulfate—Very soluble in water; soluble in alcohol.

USP requirements:

Neostigmine Bromide Tablets USP—Preserve in tight containers. Contain the labeled amount, within ±7%. Meet the requirements for Identification, Dissolution (75% in 45 minutes in water in Apparatus 2 at 50 rpm), and Uniformity of dosage units.

Neostigmine Methylsulfate Injection USP—Preserve in single-dose or in multiple-dose containers, protected from light. A sterile solution of Neostigmine Methylsulfate in Water for Injection. Contains the labeled amount, within ±10%. Meets the requirements for Identification, pH (5.0–6.5), and Injections.

NETILMICIN

Source: Semi-synthetic derivative of sisomicin.

Chemical name: Netilmicin sulfate—D-Streptamine, *O*-3-deoxy-4-*C*-methyl-3-(methylamino)-beta-L-arabinopyranosyl-(1→6)-*O*-[2,6-diamino-2,3,4,6-tetradeoxy-alpha-D-*glycero*-hex-4-enopyranosyl-(1→4)]-2-deoxy-*N*¹-ethyl-, sulfate (2:5) (salt).

Molecular formula: Netilmicin sulfate—$(C_{21}H_{41}N_5O_7)_2 \cdot 5H_2SO_4$.

Molecular weight: Netilmicin sulfate—1441.54.

Description: Netilmicin sulfate—White- to buff-colored powder.

Solubility: Netilmicin sulfate—Readily soluble in water.

USP requirements: Netilmicin Sulfate Injection USP—Preserve in single-dose or in multiple-dose containers, preferably of Type I glass. A sterile solution of Netilmicin Sulfate in Water for Injection. Contains an amount of netilmicin sulfate equivalent to the labeled amount of netilmicin, within −10% to +15%. Meets the requirements for Identification, Bacterial endotoxins, Sterility, pH (3.5–6.0), Particulate matter, and Injections.

NIACIN

Chemical name: 3-Pyridinecarboxylic acid.

Molecular formula: $C_6H_5NO_2$.

Molecular weight: 123.11.

Description: Niacin USP—White crystals or crystalline powder. Is odorless, or has a slight odor. Melts at about 235 °C.

pKa: 4.85.

Solubility: Niacin USP—Sparingly soluble in water; freely soluble in boiling water, in boiling alcohol, and in solutions of alkali hydroxides and carbonates; practically insoluble in ether.

USP requirements:

Niacin Extended-release Capsules—Not in USP.

Niacin Injection USP—Preserve in single-dose or in multiple-dose containers, preferably of Type I glass. A sterile solution of Niacin and niacin sodium in Water for Injection, made with the aid of Sodium Carbonate or Sodium Hydroxide. Contains the labeled amount, within −5% to +10%. Meets the requirements for Identification, Bacterial endotoxins, pH (4.0–6.0), and Injections.

Niacin Oral Solution—Not in USP.

Niacin Tablets USP—Preserve in well-closed containers. Contain the labeled amount, within ±10%. Meet the requirements for Identification, Disintegration (30 minutes), and Uniformity of dosage units.

Niacin Extended-release Tablets—Not in USP.

NIACINAMIDE

Chemical name: 3-Pyridinecarboxamide.

Molecular formula: $C_6H_6N_2O$.

Molecular weight: 122.13.

Description: Niacinamide USP—White, crystalline powder. Is odorless or practically so. Its solutions are neutral to litmus.

pKa: 0.5 and 3.35.

Solubility: Niacinamide USP—Freely soluble in water and in alcohol; soluble in glycerin.

USP requirements:

Niacinamide Capsules—Not in USP.

Niacinamide Gel—Not in USP.

Niacinamide Injection USP—Preserve in single-dose or in multiple-dose containers, preferably of Type I glass. A sterile solution of Niacinamide in Water for Injection. Contains the labeled amount, within −5% to +10%.

Meets the requirements for Identification, Bacterial endotoxins, pH (5.0–7.0), and Injections.
Niacinamide Tablets USP—Preserve in tight containers. Contain the labeled amount, within ±10%. Meet the requirements for Identification, Disintegration (30 minutes), and Uniformity of dosage units.

NICARDIPINE

Chemical name: Nicardipine hydrochloride—3,5-Pyridinedicarboxylic acid, 1,4-dihydro-2,6-dimethyl-4-(3-nitrophenyl)-, methyl 2-[methyl(phenylmethyl)amino]ethyl ester, monohydrochloride.

Molecular formula: Nicardipine hydrochloride—$C_{26}H_{29}N_3O_6 \cdot$ HCl.

Molecular weight: Nicardipine hydrochloride—515.99.

Description: Nicardipine hydrochloride—Greenish-yellow, odorless, crystalline powder. Melts at about 169 °C.

Solubility: Nicardipine hydrochloride—Freely soluble in chloroform, in methanol, and in glacial acetic acid; sparingly soluble in anhydrous ethanol; slightly soluble in n-butanol, in water, in acetone, and in dioxane; very slightly soluble in ethyl acetate; practically insoluble in ether and in hexane.

USP requirements: Nicardipine Hydrochloride Capsules —Not in USP.

NICLOSAMIDE

Chemical group: Derivative of salicylanilide.

Chemical name: Benzamide, 5-chloro-*N*-(2-chloro-4-nitrophenyl)-2-hydroxy-.

Molecular formula: $C_{13}H_8Cl_2N_2O_4$.

Molecular weight: 327.12.

Description: Pale yellow crystals with a melting point of 225–230 °C.

Solubility: Practically insoluble in water; sparingly soluble in ethanol, in chloroform, and in ether.

USP requirements: Niclosamide Chewable Tablets—Not in USP.

NICOTINE

Chemical name:
Nicotine—(*S*)-3-(1-methyl-2-pyrrolidinyl)pyridine.
Nicotine polacrilex—2-Propenoic acid, 2-methyl-, polymer with diethenylbenzene, complex with (*S*)-3-(1-methyl-2-pyrrolidinyl)pyridine.

Molecular formula:
Nicotine—$C_{10}H_{14}N_2$.
Nicotine polacrilex—$[(C_4H_6O_2)_x(C_{10}H_{10})_y](C_{10}H_{14}N_2)$.

Molecular weight: 162.23.

Description: Colorless to pale yellow, strongly alkaline, oily, volatile, hygroscopic liquid; has a characteristic pungent odor; turns brown on exposure to air or light.

Solubility: Freely soluble in water.

USP requirements:
Nicotine Transdermal Systems—Not in USP.
Nicotine Polacrilex Chewing Gum Tablets—Not in USP.

NICOTINYL ALCOHOL

Chemical name:
Nicotinyl alcohol—3-Pyridinemethanol.
Nicotinyl tartrate—3-Pyridinemethanol tartrate (1:1) (salt).

Molecular formula:
Nicotinyl alcohol—C_6H_7NO.
Nicotinyl alcohol tartrate—$C_6H_7NO \cdot C_4H_6O_6$.

Molecular weight:
Nicotinyl alcohol—109.13.
Nicotinyl alcohol tartrate—259.2.

Description:
Nicotinyl alcohol—Very hygroscopic liquid.
Nicotinyl alcohol tartrate—White or almost white, odorless or almost odorless, crystalline powder.

Solubility:
Nicotinyl alcohol—Freely soluble in water and in ether; sparingly soluble in petroleum ether.
Nicotinyl alcohol tartrate—Freely soluble in water; slightly soluble in alcohol; practically insoluble in chloroform and in ether.

USP requirements: Nicotinyl Alcohol Tartrate Extended-release Tablets—Not in USP.

NIFEDIPINE

Chemical name: 3,5-Pyridinedicarboxylic acid, 1,4-dihydro-2,6-dimethyl-4-(2-nitrophenyl)-, dimethyl ester.

Molecular formula: $C_{17}H_{18}N_2O_6$.

Molecular weight: 346.34.

Description: Nifedipine USP—Yellow powder; affected by exposure to light.

Solubility: Nifedipine USP—Practically insoluble in water; freely soluble in acetone.

USP requirements:
Nifedipine Capsules USP—Preserve in tight, light-resistant containers at a temperature between 15 and 25 °C. Contain the labeled amount, within ±10%. Meet the requirements for Identification, Dissolution (80% in 20 minutes in simulated gastric fluid TS [without pepsin] in Apparatus 2 at 50 rpm), Uniformity of dosage units, and Related compounds.
Nifedipine Tablets—Not in USP.
Nifedipine Extended-release Tablets—Not in USP.

NIMODIPINE

Chemical name: 3,5-Pyridinedicarboxylic acid, 1,4-dihydro-2,6-dimethyl-4-(3-nitrophenyl)-, 2-methoxyethyl 1-methylethyl ester.

Molecular formula: $C_{21}H_{26}N_2O_7$.

Molecular weight: 418.45.

Description: Yellow crystalline substance.

Solubility: Practically insoluble in water.

USP requirements: Nimodipine Capsules—Not in USP.

NITRAZEPAM

Chemical name: 2*H*-1,4-Benzodiazepin-2-one, 1,3-dihydro-7-nitro-5-phenyl-.

Molecular formula: $C_{15}H_{11}N_3O_3$.

Molecular weight: 281.27.

Description: Yellow, crystalline powder.

Solubility: Practically insoluble in water; slightly soluble in alcohol and in ether; sparingly soluble in chloroform.

USP requirements: Nitrazepam Tablets—Not in USP.

NITRIC ACID

Chemical name: Nitric acid.

Molecular formula: HNO_3.

Molecular weight: 63.01.

Description: Nitric Acid NF—Highly corrosive, fuming liquid, having a characteristic, highly irritating odor. Stains animal tissue yellow. Boils at about 120 °C. Specific gravity is about 1.41.
NF category: Acidifying agent.

NF requirements: Nitric Acid NF—Preserve in tight containers. Contains not less than 69.0% and not more than 71.0%, by weight, of nitric acid. Meets the requirements for Clarity and color, Identification, Residue on ignition (not more than 5 ppm), Chloride (not more than 0.5 ppm), Sulfate (not more than 1 ppm), Arsenic (not more than 0.01 ppm), Iron (not more than 0.2 ppm), and Heavy metals (not more than 0.2 ppm).
Caution: Avoid contact since Nitric Acid rapidly destroys tissues.

NITROFURANTOIN

Chemical group: Nitrofuran derivative.

Chemical name: 2,4-Imidazolidinedione, 1-[[(5-nitro-2-furanyl)-methylene]amino]-.

Molecular formula: $C_8H_6N_4O_5$.

Molecular weight: 238.16.

Description: Nitrofurantoin USP—Lemon-yellow, odorless crystals or fine powder.

Solubility: Nitrofurantoin USP—Very slightly soluble in water and in alcohol; soluble in dimethylformamide.

USP requirements:
Nitrofurantoin Capsules USP—Preserve in tight, light-resistant containers. Contain the labeled amount, within ±10%. Meet the requirements for Identification, Uniformity of dosage units, and Nitrofurazone (not more than 0.01%).
Nitrofurantoin Oral Suspension USP—Preserve in tight, light-resistant containers. A suspension of Nitrofurantoin in a suitable, aqueous vehicle. Contains, in each 100 mL, not less than 460 mg and not more than 540 mg of nitrofurantoin. Meets the requirements for Identification, pH (4.5–6.5), and Limit of N-(aminocarbonyl)-N-[[(5-nitro-2-furanyl]methylene)amino]glycine.
Nitrofurantoin Tablets USP—Preserve in tight, light-resistant containers. Contain the labeled amount, within ±10%. Meet the requirements for Identification, Dissolution (25% in 60 minutes and 85% in 120 minutes in phosphate buffer [pH 7.2] in Apparatus 1 at 100 rpm), Uniformity of dosage units, and Nitrofurazone (not more than 0.01%).

NITROFURAZONE

Chemical name: Hydrazinecarboxamide, 2-[(5-nitro-2-furanyl)-methylene]-.

Molecular formula: $C_6H_6N_4O_4$.

Molecular weight: 198.14.

Description:
Nitrofurazone USP—Lemon yellow, odorless, crystalline powder. Darkens slowly on exposure to light. Melts at about 236 °C, with decomposition.
Nitrofurazone Cream USP—Yellow, opaque cream.
Nitrofurazone Ointment USP—Yellow, opaque, and has ointment-like consistency.
Nitrofurazone Topical Solution USP—Light yellow, clear, somewhat viscous liquid, having a faint, characteristic odor.

Solubility:
Nitrofurazone USP—Very slightly soluble in alcohol and in water; soluble in dimethylformamide; slightly soluble in propylene glycol and in polyethylene glycol mixtures; practically insoluble in chloroform and in ether.
Nitrofurazone Cream USP—Miscible with water.
Nitrofurazone Ointment USP—Miscible with water.
Nitrofurazone Topical Solution USP—Miscible with water.

USP requirements:
Nitrofurazone Cream USP—Preserve in tight, light-resistant containers. Avoid exposure to direct sunlight, strong fluorescent lighting, and excessive heat. It is Nitrofurazone in a suitable, emulsified water-miscible base. Contains the labeled amount, within ±10%. Meets the requirements for Identification and Minimum fill.
Note: Avoid exposure at all times to direct sunlight, excessive heat, strong fluorescent lighting, and alkaline materials.
Nitrofurazone Ointment USP—Preserve in tight, light-resistant containers. Avoid exposure to direct sunlight, strong fluorescent lighting, and excessive heat. It is Nitrofurazone in a suitable water-miscible base. Contains the labeled amount, within ±10%. Meets the requirements for Completeness of solution and Identification.
Nitrofurazone Topical Solution USP—Preserve in tight, light-resistant containers. Avoid exposure to direct sunlight and excessive heat. Contains the labeled amount, within ±5% (w/w). Meets the requirement for Identification.
Note: Avoid exposure at all times to direct sunlight, excessive heat, and alkaline materials.

NITROGEN

Chemical name: Nitrogen.

Molecular formula: N_2.

Molecular weight: 28.01.

Description: Nitrogen NF—Colorless, odorless gas. It is non-flammable and does not support combustion. One liter at 0 °C and at a pressure of 760 mm of mercury weighs about 1.251 grams.
NF category: Air displacement.

Solubility: Nitrogen NF—One volume dissolves in about 65 volumes of water and in about 9 volumes of alcohol at 20 °C and at a pressure of 760 mm of mercury.

NF requirements: Nitrogen NF—Preserve in cylinders. Contains not less than 99.0%, by volume, of nitrogen. Meets the requirements for Identification, Odor, Carbon monoxide (not more than 0.001%), and Oxygen (not more than 1.0%).

NITROGEN 97 PERCENT

NF requirements: Nitrogen 97 Percent NF—Preserve in cylinders or in a low-pressure collecting tank. It is Nitrogen produced from air by physical separation methods. Where it is piped directly from the collecting tank to the point of use, label each outlet "Nitrogen 97 Percent." Contains not less than 97.0%, by volume, of nitrogen. Meets the requirements for Identification, Odor, Carbon dioxide (not more than 0.03%), Carbon monoxide (not more than 0.001%), Nitric oxide and nitrogen dioxide (not more than 2.5 ppm), Sulfur dioxide (not more than 5 ppm), and Oxygen (not more than 3.0%).

NITROGLYCERIN

Chemical name: 1,2,3-Propanetriol, trinitrate.

Molecular formula: $C_3H_5N_3O_9$.

Molecular weight: 227.09.

Description: Diluted Nitroglycerin USP—White, odorless powder, when diluted with lactose. When diluted with propylene glycol or alcohol, it is a clear, colorless, or pale yellow liquid. (Note: Undiluted nitroglycerin is a white to pale yellow, thick, flammable, explosive liquid.)

Solubility: Undiluted nitroglycerin—Slightly soluble in water; soluble in methanol, in alcohol, in carbon disulfide, in acetone, in ethyl ether, in ethyl acetate, in glacial acetic acid, in toluene, in phenol, in chloroform, and in methylene chloride.

USP requirements:
Nitroglycerin Lingual Aerosol—Not in USP.
Nitroglycerin Extended-release Capsules—Not in USP.
Nitroglycerin Injection USP—Preserve in single-dose or in multiple-dose containers, preferably of Type I or Type II glass. A sterile solution prepared from Diluted Nitroglycerin; the solvent may contain Alcohol, Propylene Glycol, and Water for Injection. Where necessary, label it to indicate that it is to be diluted before use. Contains the labeled amount, within ±10%. Meets the requirements for Identification, Bacterial endotoxins, pH (3.0–6.5), Alcohol content (labeled amount, within ±10%), Particulate matter, and Injections.
Nitroglycerin Ointment USP—Preserve in tight containers. It is Diluted Nitroglycerin in a suitable ointment base. Label multiple-dose containers with a direction to close tightly, immediately after each use. Contains the labeled amount, within −10% to +15%. Meets the requirements for Identification, Minimum fill, and Homogeneity (within ±10% of mean value).
Nitroglycerin Transdermal Systems—Not in USP.
Nitroglycerin Tablets USP (Sublingual)—Preserve in tight containers, preferably of glass, at controlled room temperature. Each container holds not more than 100 Tablets. The labeling indicates that the Tablets are for sublingual use, and the label directs that the Tablets be dispensed in the original, unopened container, labeled with the following statement directed to the patient. "Warning: to prevent loss of potency, keep these tablets in the original container or in a supplemental Nitroglycerin container specifically labeled as being suitable for Nitroglycerin Tablets. Close tightly immediately after each use." Contain the labeled amount, within ±10%. Meet the requirements for Identification, Disintegration (2 minutes), and Uniformity of dosage units.
Nitroglycerin Extended-release Tablets—Not in USP.
Nitroglycerin Extended-release Buccal Tablets—Not in USP.

NITROMERSOL

Chemical name: 7-Oxa-8-mercurabicyclo[4.2.0]octa-1,3,5-triene, 5-methyl-2-nitro-.

Molecular formula: $C_7H_5HgNO_3$.

Molecular weight: 351.71.

Description:
Nitromersol USP—Brownish yellow to yellow granules or brownish yellow to yellow powder. Odorless. Affected by light.
Nitromersol Topical Solution USP—Clear, reddish orange solution. Affected by light.

Solubility: Nitromersol USP—Very slightly soluble in water, in alcohol, in acetone, and in ether; soluble in solutions of alkalies and of ammonia by opening of the anhydride ring and the formation of a salt.

USP requirements: Nitromersol Topical Solution USP—Preserve in tight, light-resistant containers. Yields, from each 100 mL, not less than 180.0 mg and not more than 220.0 mg of Nitromersol.
Prepare Nitromersol Topical Solution as follows: 2 grams of Nitromersol, 0.4 gram of Sodium Hydroxide, 4.25 grams of Sodium Carbonate, monohydrate, and a sufficient quantity of Purified Water to make 1000 mL. Dissolve the Sodium Hydroxide and the monohydrated Sodium Carbonate in 50 mL of Purified Water, add the Nitromersol, and stir until dissolved. Gradually add Purified Water to make 1000 mL.
Meets the requirements for Identification, Specific gravity (1.005–1.010), and Mercury ions.
Note: Prepare dilutions of Nitromersol Topical Solution as needed, since they tend to precipitate on standing.

NITROUS OXIDE

Chemical name: Nitrogen oxide (N_2O).

Molecular formula: N_2O.

Molecular weight: 44.01.

Description: Nitrous Oxide USP—Colorless gas, without appreciable odor. One liter at 0 °C and at a pressure of 760 mm of mercury weighs about 1.97 grams.

Solubility: Nitrous Oxide USP—One volume dissolves in about 1.4 volumes of water at 20 °C and at a pressure of 760 mm of mercury; freely soluble in alcohol; soluble in ether and in oils.

Other characteristics:
Blood-to-Gas partition coefficient at 37 °C—0.47.
Oil-to-Gas partition coefficient at 37 °C—1.4.

USP requirements: Nitrous Oxide USP—Preserve in cylinders. Contains not less than 99%, by volume, of nitrous oxide. Meets the requirements for Identification, Carbon monoxide (not more than 0.001%), Nitric oxide (not more than 1 ppm), Nitrogen dioxide (not more than 1 ppm), Halogens (not more than 1 ppm), Carbon dioxide (not more than 0.03%), Ammonia (not more than 0.0025%), Water (not more than 150 mg per cubic meter), and Air (not more than 1.0%).

NIZATIDINE

Chemical name: 1,1-Ethenediamine, N-[2-[[[2-[(dimethylamino)-methyl]-4-thiazolyl]methyl]thio]ethyl]-N'-methyl-2-nitro-.

Molecular formula: $C_{12}H_{21}N_5O_2S_2$.

Molecular weight: 331.45.

Description: Off-white to buff crystalline solid.

Solubility: Soluble in water.

USP requirements: Nizatidine Capsules USP—Preserve in tight, light-resistant containers. Store at controlled room temperature. Contain the labeled amount, within ± 10%. Meet the requirements for Identification, Dissolution (75% in 30 minutes in water in Apparatus 2 at 50 rpm), Uniformity of dosage units, and Related substances.

NONOXYNOL 9

Chemical name: Poly(oxy-1,2-ethanediyl), alpha-(4-nonylphenyl)-omega-hydroxy-.

Molecular formula: $C_{15}H_{24}O(C_2H_4O)_n$ (n = approximately 9).

Description: Nonoxynol 9 USP—Clear, colorless to light yellow viscous liquid.
  NF category: Wetting and/or solubilizing agent.

Solubility: Nonoxynol 9 USP—Soluble in water, in alcohol, and in corn oil.

USP requirements:
  Nonoxynol 9 USP—Preserve in tight containers. An anhydrous liquid mixture consisting chiefly of mononononylphenyl ethers of polyethylene glycols corresponding to the formula $C_9H_{19}C_6H_4(OCH_2CH_2)_nOH$, in which the average value of n is about 9. Contains not less than 90.0% and not more than 110.0% of nonoxynol 9. Meets the requirements for Identification, Acid value (not more than 0.2), Water (not more than 0.5%), Polyethylene glycol (not more than 1.6%), Cloud point (52–56 °C), Free ethylene oxide (not more than 5 ppm), Dioxane, and Organic volatile impurities.
  Nonoxynol 9 Vaginal Cream—Not in USP.
  Nonoxynol 9 Vaginal Film—Not in USP.
  Nonoxynol 9 Vaginal Foam—Not in USP.
  Nonoxynol 9 Vaginal Gel—Not in USP.
  Nonoxynol 9 Vaginal Jelly—Not in USP.
  Nonoxynol 9 Vaginal Sponge—Not in USP.
  Nonoxynol 9 Vaginal Suppositories—Not in USP.

NONOXYNOL 10

Chemical name: Poly(oxy-1,2-ethanediyl), alpha-(4-nonylphenyl)-omega-hydroxy-.

Description: Nonoxynol 10 NF—Colorless to light amber viscous liquid, having an aromatic odor.
  NF category: Wetting and/or solubilizing agent.

Solubility: Nonoxynol 10 NF—Soluble in polar organic solvents and in water.

NF requirements: Nonoxynol 10 NF—Preserve in tight containers. An anhydrous liquid mixture consisting chiefly of mononononylphenyl ethers of polyethylene glycols corresponding to the formula $C_9H_{19}C_6H_4(OCH_2CH_2)_nOH$, in which the average value of n is about 10. The labeling includes a cloud point range which is not greater than 6 °C and which is between 52 ° and 67 °C. Meets the requirements for Identification, Water (not more than 0.5%), Residue on ignition (not more than 0.4%), Arsenic (not more than 2 ppm), Heavy metals (not more than 0.002%), Hydroxyl value (81–97), Cloud point, and Organic volatile impurities.

NOREPINEPHRINE

Chemical group: A primary amine, differing from epinephrine by the absence of a methyl group on the nitrogen atom.

Chemical name: Norepinephrine bitartrate—1,2-Benzenediol, 4-(2-amino-1-hydroxyethyl)-, (R)-[R-(R*,R*)]-2,3-dihydroxybutanedioate (1:1) (salt), monohydrate.

Molecular formula: Norepinephrine bitartrate—$C_8H_{11}NO_3 \cdot C_4H_6O_6 \cdot H_2O$.

Molecular weight: Norepinephrine bitartrate—337.28.

Description:
  Norepinephrine Bitartrate USP—White or faintly gray, odorless, crystalline powder. Slowly darkens on exposure to air and light. Its solutions are acid to litmus, having a pH of about 3.5. Melts between 98 and 104 °C, without previous drying of the specimen, the melt being turbid.
  Norepinephrine Bitartrate Injection USP— Colorless or practically colorless liquid, gradually turning dark on exposure to air and light.

Solubility: Norepinephrine Bitartrate USP—Freely soluble in water; slightly soluble in alcohol; practically insoluble in chloroform and in ether.

USP requirements: Norepinephrine Bitartrate Injection USP—Preserve in single-dose, light-resistant containers, preferably of Type I glass. A sterile solution of Norepinephrine Bitartrate in Water for Injection. Label the Injection in terms of mg of norepinephrine per mL, and, where necessary, label it to indicate that it must be diluted prior to use. The label indicates that the Injection is not to be used if its color is pinkish or darker than slightly yellow or if it contains a precipitate. Contains an amount of norepinephrine bitartrate equivalent to the labeled amount of norepinephrine, within −10% to +15%. Meets the requirements for Color and clarity, Identification, Bacterial endotoxins, pH (3.0–4.5), Particulate matter, and Injections.

NORETHINDRONE

Chemical name:
  Norethindrone—19-Norpregn-4-en-20-yn-3-one, 17-hydroxy-, (17 alpha)-.
  Norethindrone acetate—19-Norpregn-4-en-20-yn-3-one, 17-(acetyloxy)-, (17 alpha).

Molecular formula:
  Norethindrone—$C_{20}H_{26}O_2$.
  Norethindrone acetate—$C_{22}H_{28}O_3$.

Molecular weight:
  Norethindrone—298.42.
  Norethindrone acetate—340.46.

Description:
  Norethindrone USP—White to creamy white, odorless, crystalline powder. Is stable in air.
  Norethindrone Acetate USP—White to creamy white, odorless, crystalline powder.

Solubility:
  Norethindrone USP—Practically insoluble in water; soluble in chloroform and in dioxane; sparingly soluble in alcohol; slightly soluble in ether.
  Norethindrone Acetate USP—Practically insoluble in water; very soluble in chloroform; freely soluble in dioxane; soluble in ether and in alcohol.

USP requirements:
  Norethindrone Tablets USP—Preserve in well-closed containers. Contain the labeled amount, within ± 10%. Meet

the requirements for Identification, Disintegration (15 minutes, the use of disks being omitted), and Uniformity of dosage units.

Norethindrone Acetate Tablets USP— Preserve in well-closed containers. Contain the labeled amount, within ±10%. Meet the requirements for Identification, Dissolution (70% in 60 minutes in dilute hydrochloric acid [1 in 100] containing 0.02% of sodium lauryl sulfate in Apparatus 1 at 100 rpm), and Uniformity of dosage units.

NORETHINDRONE AND ETHINYL ESTRADIOL

For *Norethindrone* and *Ethinyl Estradiol*—See individual listings for chemistry information.

USP requirements:

Norethindrone and Ethinyl Estradiol Tablets USP—Preserve in well-closed containers. Contain the labeled amounts of norethindrone and ethinyl estradiol, within ±10%. Meet the requirements for Identification, Dissolution (75% of each active ingredient in 60 minutes in 0.09% sodium lauryl sulfate in 0.1 N hydrochloric acid in Apparatus 2 at 75 rpm), and Uniformity of dosage units.

Norethindrone Acetate and Ethinyl Estradiol Tablets USP— Preserve in well-closed containers. Contain the labeled amount of norethindrone acetate, within ±10%, and the labeled amount of ethinyl estradiol, within ±12%. Meet the requirements for Identification, Disintegration (20 minutes, the use of disks being omitted), and Uniformity of dosage units.

NORETHINDRONE AND MESTRANOL

Chemical name:

Norethindrone—19-Norpregn-4-en-20-yn-3-one, 17-hydroxy-, (17 alpha)-.

Mestranol—19-Norpregna-1,3,5(10)-trien-20-yn-17-ol, 3-methoxy-, (17 alpha)-.

Molecular formula:

Norethindrone—$C_{20}H_{26}O_2$.

Mestranol—$C_{21}H_{26}O_2$.

Molecular weight:

Norethindrone—298.42.

Mestranol—310.44.

Description:

Norethindrone USP—White to creamy white, odorless, crystalline powder. Is stable in air.

Mestranol USP—White to creamy white, odorless, crystalline powder.

Solubility:

Norethindrone USP—Practically insoluble in water; soluble in chloroform and in dioxane; sparingly soluble in alcohol; slightly soluble in ether.

Mestranol USP—Insoluble in water; freely soluble in chloroform; soluble in dioxane; sparingly soluble in dehydrated alcohol; slightly soluble in methanol.

USP requirements: Norethindrone and Mestranol Tablets USP— Preserve in well-closed containers. Contain the labeled amounts of norethindrone and mestranol, within ±10%. Meet the requirements for Identification, Dissolution (75% of each active ingredient in 60 minutes in 0.09% sodium lauryl sulfate in 0.1 N hydrochloric acid in Apparatus 2 at 75 rpm), and Uniformity of dosage units.

NORETHYNODREL AND MESTRANOL

Chemical name:

Norethynodrel—19-Norpregn-5(10)-en-20-yn-3-one, 17-hydroxy-, (17 alpha)-.

Mestranol—19-Norpregna-1,3,5(10)-trien-20-yn-17-ol, 3-methoxy-, (17 alpha)-.

Molecular formula:

Norethynodrel—$C_{20}H_{26}O_2$.

Mestranol—$C_{21}H_{26}O_2$.

Molecular weight:

Norethynodrel—298.42.

Mestranol—310.44.

Description:

Norethynodrel USP—White or practically white, odorless, crystalline powder. Melts at about 175 °C, over a range of about 3°. Is stable in air.

Mestranol USP—White to creamy white, odorless, crystalline powder.

Solubility:

Norethynodrel USP—Very slightly soluble in water and in solvent hexane; freely soluble in chloroform; soluble in acetone; sparingly soluble in alcohol.

Mestranol USP—Insoluble in water; freely soluble in chloroform; soluble in dioxane; sparingly soluble in dehydrated alcohol; slightly soluble in methanol.

USP requirements: Norethynodrel and Mestranol Tablets—Not in USP.

NORFLOXACIN

Chemical group: Fluoroquinolone derivative; structurally related to cinoxacin, ciprofloxacin, nalidixic acid, and other quinolones.

Chemical name: 3-Quinolinecarboxylic acid, 1-ethyl-6-fluoro-1,4-dihydro-4-oxo-7-(1-piperazinyl)-.

Molecular formula: $C_{16}H_{18}FN_3O_3$.

Molecular weight: 319.34.

Description: Norfloxacin USP—White to pale yellow crystalline powder. Sensitive to light and moisture.

Solubility: Norfloxacin USP—Slightly soluble in acetone, in water, and in alcohol; freely soluble in acetic acid; sparingly soluble in chloroform; very slightly soluble in methanol and in ethyl acetate; insoluble in ether.

USP requirements:

Norfloxacin Ophthalmic Solution—Not in USP.

Norfloxacin Tablets USP—Preserve in well-closed containers. Contain the labeled amount, within ±10%. Meet the requirements for Identification, Dissolution (80% in 30 minutes in pH 4.0 buffer in Apparatus 2 at 50 rpm), and Uniformity of dosage units.

NORGESTREL

Chemical name: 18,19-Dinorpregn-4-en-20-yn-3-one, 13-ethyl-17-hydroxy-, (17 alpha)-(±)-.

Molecular formula: $C_{21}H_{28}O_2$.

Molecular weight: 312.45.

Description: Norgestrel USP—White or practically white, practically odorless, crystalline powder.

Solubility: Norgestrel USP—Insoluble in water; freely soluble in chloroform; sparingly soluble in alcohol.

USP requirements: Norgestrel Tablets USP—Preserve in well-closed containers. Contain the labeled amount, within ±10%. Meet the requirements for Identification, Disintegration (15 minutes, the use of disks being omitted), and Uniformity of dosage units.

NORGESTREL AND ETHINYL ESTRADIOL

For *Norgestrel* and *Ethinyl Estradiol*—See individual listings for chemistry information.

USP requirements: Norgestrel and Ethinyl Estradiol Tablets USP—Preserve in well-closed containers. Contain the labeled amounts of norgestrel and ethinyl estradiol, within ±10%. Meet the requirements for Identification, Disintegration (15 minutes, the use of disks being omitted), and Uniformity of dosage units.

NORTRIPTYLINE

Chemical group: Dibenzocycloheptadiene.

Chemical name: Nortriptyline hydrochloride—1-Propanamine, 3-(10,11-dihydro-5*H*-dibenzo[*a,d*]cyclohepten-5-ylidene)-*N*-methyl-, hydrochloride.

Molecular formula: Nortriptyline hydrochloride—$C_{19}H_{21}N \cdot HCl$.

Molecular weight: Nortriptyline hydrochloride—299.84.

Description: Nortriptyline Hydrochloride USP—White to off-white powder, having a slight, characteristic odor. Its solution (1 in 100) has a pH of about 5.

pKa: Nortriptyline hydrochloride—9.73.

Solubility: Nortriptyline Hydrochloride USP—Soluble in water and in chloroform; sparingly soluble in methanol; practically insoluble in ether and in most other organic solvents.

Other characteristics: Secondary amine.

USP requirements:
Nortriptyline Hydrochloride Capsules USP—Preserve in tight containers. Contain an amount of nortriptyline hydrochloride equivalent to the labeled amount of nortriptyline, within ±10%. Meet the requirements for Identification, Dissolution (70% in 30 minutes in water in Apparatus 1 at 100 rpm), and Uniformity of dosage units.
Nortriptyline Hydrochloride Oral Solution USP—Preserve in tight, light-resistant containers. Contains an amount of nortriptyline hydrochloride equivalent to the labeled amount of nortriptyline, within ±10%. Meets the requirements for Identification, pH (2.5–4.0), and Alcohol content (3.0–5.0%).

NOVOBIOCIN

Chemical name:
Novobiocin calcium—Benzamide, *N*-[7-[[3-*O*-(aminocarbonyl)-6-deoxy-5-*C*-methyl-4-*O*-methyl-beta-L-*lyxo*-hexopyranosyl]oxy]-4-hydroxy-8-methyl-2-oxo-2*H*-1-benzopyran-3-yl]-4-hydroxy-3-(3-methyl-2-butenyl)-, calcium salt (2:1).
Novobiocin sodium—Benzamide, *N*-[7-[[3-*O*-(aminocarbonyl)-6-deoxy-5-*C*-methyl-4-*O*-methyl beta-L-*lyxo*-hexopyranosyl]oxy]-4-hydroxy-8-methyl-2-oxo-2*H*-1-benzopyran-3-yl]-4-hydroxy-3-(3-methyl-2-butenyl)-, monosodium salt.

Molecular formula:
Novobiocin calcium—$C_{62}H_{70}CaN_4O_{22}$.
Novobiocin sodium—$C_{31}H_{35}N_2NaO_{11}$.

Molecular weight:
Novobiocin calcium—1263.33.
Novobiocin sodium—634.62.

Description:
Novobiocin Calcium USP—White or yellowish-white, odorless, crystalline powder.
Novobiocin Sodium USP—White or yellowish-white, odorless, hygroscopic crystalline powder.

Solubility:
Novobiocin Calcium USP—Slightly soluble in water and in ether; freely soluble in alcohol and in methanol; sparingly soluble in acetone and in butyl acetate; very slightly soluble in chloroform.
Novobiocin Sodium USP—Freely soluble in water, in alcohol, in methanol, in glycerin, and in propylene glycol; slightly soluble in butyl acetate; practically insoluble in acetone, in chloroform, and in ether.

USP requirements:
Novobiocin Calcium Oral Suspension USP—Preserve in tight, light-resistant containers. It is prepared from Novobiocin Calcium or Novobiocin Sodium reacted with a suitable calcium salt, and it contains one or more suitable buffers, colors, diluents, flavors, and preservatives. Contains an amount of novobiocin calcium or novobiocin sodium equivalent to the labeled amount of novobiocin, within −10% to +20%. Meets the requirements for Identification, pH (6.0–7.5), Deliverable volume (multiple-unit containers), and Uniformity of dosage units (single-unit containers).
Novobiocin Sodium Capsules USP—Preserve in tight, light-resistant containers. Contain an amount of novobiocin sodium equivalent to the labeled amount of novobiocin, within −10% to +20%. Meet the requirements for Identification and Loss on drying (not more than 6.0%).

NYLIDRIN

Chemical name: Nylidrin hydrochloride—Benzeneethanol, 4-hydroxy-alpha-[1-[(1-methyl-3-phenylpropyl)amino]ethyl]-, hydrochloride.

Molecular formula: Nylidrin hydrochloride—$C_{19}H_{25}NO_2 \cdot HCl$.

Molecular weight: Nylidrin hydrochloride—335.87.

Description: Nylidrin Hydrochloride USP—White, odorless, crystalline powder.

Solubility: Nylidrin Hydrochloride USP—Sparingly soluble in water and in alcohol; slightly soluble in chloroform and in ether.

USP requirements:
Nylidrin Hydrochloride Injection USP—Preserve in single-dose or in multiple-dose containers, preferably of Type I glass. A sterile solution of Nylidrin Hydrochloride in Water for Injection. Contains the labeled amount, within ±5%. Meets the requirements for Identification and Injections.
Nylidrin Hydrochloride Tablets USP—Preserve in tight containers. Contain the labeled amount, within ±7%. Meet the requirements for Identification, Dissolution (75% in 30 minutes in water in Apparatus 1 at 100 rpm), and Uniformity of dosage units.

NYSTATIN

Source: Derived from *Streptomyces noursei*.

Chemical group: Polyene antifungal.

Chemical name: Nystatin.

Description: Nystatin USP—Yellow to light tan powder, having an odor suggestive of cereals. Is hygroscopic, and is affected by long exposure to light, heat, and air.

Solubility: Nystatin USP—Very slightly soluble in water; slightly to sparingly soluble in alcohol, in methanol, in *n*-propyl alcohol, and in *n*-butyl alcohol; insoluble in chloroform and in ether.

USP requirements:

Nystatin Cream USP—Preserve in collapsible tubes, or in other tight containers, and avoid exposure to excessive heat. Contains the labeled amount of USP Nystatin Units, within −10% to +30%. Meets the requirement for Minimum fill.

Nystatin Vaginal Cream—Not in USP.

Nystatin Lotion USP—Preserve in tight containers, at controlled room temperature. Contains the labeled amount of USP Nystatin Units, within −10% to +40%. Meets the requirement for pH (5.5–7.5).

Nystatin Lozenges USP—Preserve in tight, light-resistant containers. Contain the labeled amount of USP Nystatin Units, within −10% to +25%. Meet the requirements for Disintegration (90 minutes, determined as set forth under Uncoated Tablets) and pH (5.0–7.5).

Nystatin Ointment USP—Preserve in well-closed containers, preferably at controlled room temperature. Contains the labeled amount of USP Nystatin Units, within −10% to +30%. Meets the requirements for Minimum fill and Water (not more than 0.5%).

Nystatin Topical Powder USP—Preserve in well-closed containers. A dry powder composed of Nystatin and Talc. Contains the labeled amount of USP Nystatin Units, within −10% to +30%. Meets the requirement for Loss on drying (not more than 2.0%).

Nystatin Vaginal Suppositories USP—Preserve in tight, light-resistant containers, at controlled room temperature. Contain the labeled amount of USP Nystatin Units, within −10% to +30%. Meet the requirement for Water (not more than 1.5%).

Nystatin Oral Suspension USP—Preserve in tight, light-resistant containers. Contains suitable dispersants, flavors, preservatives, and suspending agents. Contains the labeled amount of USP Nystatin Units, within −10% to +30%. Meets the requirements for pH (4.5–6.0; or 5.3–7.5 if it contains glycerin), Uniformity of dosage units (single-unit containers), and Deliverable volume (multiple-dose units).

Nystatin for Oral Suspension USP—Preserve in tight containers. A dry mixture of Nystatin with one or more suitable colors, diluents, suspending agents, flavors, and preservatives. Contains the labeled amount of USP Nystatin Units, within −10% to +40%. Meets the requirements for pH (4.9–5.5, in the suspension constituted as directed in the labeling) and Water (not more than 7.0%).

Nystatin Tablets USP—Preserve in tight, light-resistant containers. Label the Tablets to indicate that they are intended for oral use only (as distinguished from Vaginal Tablets). Contain the labeled amount of USP Nystatin Units, within −10% to +30%. Meet the requirements for Disintegration (120 minutes for plain-coated) and Loss on drying (not more than 5.0% for plain-coated; not more than 8.0% for film-coated).

Nystatin Vaginal Tablets USP—Preserve in tight, light-resistant containers and, where so specified in the labeling, in a refrigerator. Tablets composed of Nystatin with suitable binders, diluents and lubricants. Contain the labeled amount of USP Nystatin Units, within −10% to +40%. Meet the requirements for Disintegration (60 minutes) and Loss on drying (not more than 5.0%).

NYSTATIN AND CLIOQUINOL

For *Nystatin* and *Clioquinol*—See individual listings for chemistry information.

USP requirements: Nystatin and Clioquinol Ointment USP—Preserve in collapsible tubes or in tight, light-resistant containers, at controlled room temperature. Contains the labeled amount of USP Nystatin Units, within −10% to +40%, and the labeled amount of clioquinol, within ±10%. Meets the requirements for Identification, Minimum fill, and Water (not more than 0.5%).

NYSTATIN, NEOMYCIN, GRAMICIDIN, AND TRIAMCINOLONE

For *Nystatin, Neomycin, Gramicidin,* and *Triamcinolone*—See individual listings for chemistry information.

USP requirements:

Nystatin, Neomycin Sulfate, Gramicidin, and Triamcinolone Acetonide Cream USP—Preserve in tight containers. Contains amounts of nystatin, neomycin sulfate, and gramicidin equivalent to the labeled amounts of nystatin, neomycin, and gramicidin, within −10% to +40%, and the labeled amount of triamcinolone acetonide, within ±10%. Meets the requirements for Identification and Minimum fill.

Nystatin, Neomycin Sulfate, Gramicidin, and Triamcinolone Acetonide Ointment USP—Preserve in tight containers. Contains amounts of nystatin, neomycin sulfate, and gramicidin equivalent to the labeled amounts of nystatin, neomycin, and gramicidin, within −10% to +40%, and the labeled amount of triamcinolone acetonide, within ±10%. Meets the requirements for Identification, Water (not more than 0.5%), and Minimum fill.

NYSTATIN AND TRIAMCINOLONE

For *Nystatin* and *Triamcinolone*—See individual listings for chemistry information.

USP requirements:

Nystatin and Triamcinolone Acetonide Cream USP—Preserve in tight containers. Contains the labeled amount of USP Nystatin Units, within −10% to +40%, and the labeled amount of triamcinolone acetonide, within ±10%. Meets the requirements for Identification and Minimum fill.

Nystatin and Triamcinolone Acetonide Ointment USP—Preserve in tight containers. Contains the labeled amount of USP Nystatin Units, within −10% to +40%, and the labeled amount of triamcinolone acetonide, within ±10%. Meets the requirements for Identification, Minimum fill, and Water (not more than 0.5%).

OCTOXYNOL 9

Chemical name: Poly(oxy-1,2-ethanediyl), alpha-(octylphenyl)-omega-hydroxy-.

Molecular formula: $C_{34}H_{62}O_{11}$ (average).

Molecular weight: 647.00 (average).

Description: Octoxynol 9 NF—Clear, pale yellow, viscous liquid, having a faint odor.

NF category: Wetting and/or solubilizing agent.

Solubility: Octoxynol 9 NF—Miscible with water, with alcohol, and with acetone; soluble in toluene; practically insoluble in solvent hexane.

USP requirements:

Octoxynol 9 Vaginal Cream—Not in USP.

Octoxynol 9 Vaginal Jelly—Not in USP.

NF requirements: Octoxynol 9 NF—Preserve in tight containers. An anhydrous liquid mixture consisting chiefly of monooctylphenyl ethers of polyethylene glycols, corresponding to the formula $C_8H_{17}C_6H_4(OCH_2CH_2)_nOH$, in which the average value of *n* is 9. Meets the requirements for Identification, Water (not more than 0.5%), Residue on ignition (not more than 0.4%), Arsenic (not more than 2 ppm), Heavy metals (not more than 0.002%), Hydroxyl value (85–101), Cloud point (63–69 °C), Free ethylene oxide (not more than 5 ppm), and Dioxane.

OCTREOTIDE

Source: Synthetic octapeptide analog of somatostatin.

Chemical name:
  Octreotide—L-Cysteinamide, D-phenylalanyl-L-cysteinyl-L-phenylalanyl-D-tryptophyl-L-lysyl-L-threonyl-*N*-[2-hydroxy-1-(hydroxymethyl)propyl]-, cyclic (2→7)-disulfide, [*R*-(*R**,*R**)]-.
  Octreotide acetate—L-Cysteinamide, D-phenylalanyl-L-cysteinyl-L-phenylalanyl-D-tryptophyl-L-lysyl-L-threonyl-*N*-[2-hydroxy-1-(hydroxymethyl)propyl]-, cyclic (2→7)-disulfide, [*R*-(*R**,*R**)]-, acetate (salt).

Molecular formula:
  Octreotide—$C_{49}H_{66}N_{10}O_{10}S_2$.
  Octreotide acetate—$C_{49}H_{66}N_{10}O_{10}S_2 \cdot xC_2H_4O_2$.

Molecular weight: 1019.24.

Description: Octreotide acetate injection—Clear sterile solution.

USP requirements: Octreotide Acetate Injection—Not in USP.

OCTYLDODECANOL

Molecular formula: $C_{20}H_{42}O$.

Molecular weight: 298.55.

Description: Octyldodecanol NF—Clear, water-white, free-flowing liquid.
  NF category: Oleaginous vehicle.

Solubility: Octyldodecanol NF—Insoluble in water; soluble in alcohol and in ether.

NF requirements: Octyldodecanol NF—Preserve in tight containers. Contains not less than 90.0% of 2-octyldodecanol, the remainder consisting chiefly of related alcohols. Meets the requirements for Identification, Acid value (not more than 0.5), Iodine value (not more than 8), Hydroxyl value (175–190), Saponification value (not more than 5), and Organic volatile impurities.

OFLOXACIN

Chemical name: 7*H*-Pyrido[1,2,3-*de*]-1,4-benzoxazine-6-carboxylic acid, 9-fluoro-2,3-dihydro-3-methyl-10-(4-methyl-1-piperazinyl)-7-oxo-, (±)-.

Molecular formula: $C_{18}H_{20}FN_3O_4$.

Molecular weight: 361.37.

Description: Cream to pale yellow crystalline powder.

Solubility: At room temperature, aqueous solubility 60 mg/mL at pH 2–5, 4 mg/mL at pH 7, and 303 mg/mL at pH 9.8.

USP requirements: Ofloxacin Tablets—Not in USP.

HYDROPHILIC OINTMENT

Description: Hydrophilic Ointment USP—NF category: Ointment base.

USP requirements: Hydrophilic Ointment USP—Preserve in tight containers.
  Prepare Hydrophilic Ointment as follows: 0.25 gram of Methylparaben, 0.15 gram of Propylparaben, 10 grams of Sodium Lauryl Sulfate, 120 grams of Propylene Glycol, 250 grams of Stearyl Alcohol, 250 grams of White Petrolatum, and 370 grams of Purified Water, to make about 1000 grams. Melt the Stearyl Alcohol and the White Petrolatum on a steam bath, and warm to about 75 °C. Add the other ingredients, previously dissolved in the water and warmed to 75 °C, and stir the mixture until it congeals.

WHITE OINTMENT

Description: White Ointment USP—NF category: Ointment base.

USP requirements: White Ointment USP—Preserve in well-closed containers.
  Prepare White Ointment as follows: 50 grams of White Wax and 950 grams of White Petrolatum, to make 1000 grams. Melt the White Wax in a suitable dish on a water bath, add the White Petrolatum, warm until liquefied, then discontinue the heating, and stir the mixture until it begins to congeal.

YELLOW OINTMENT

Description: Yellow Ointment USP—NF category: Ointment base.

USP requirements: Yellow Ointment USP—Preserve in well-closed containers.
  Prepare Yellow Ointment as follows: 50 grams of Yellow Wax and 950 grams of Petrolatum, to make 1000 grams. Melt the Yellow Wax in a suitable dish on a steam bath, add the Petrolatum, warm until liquefied, then discontinue the heating, and stir the mixture until it begins to congeal.

OLEIC ACID

Chemical name: 9-Octadecenoic acid, (*Z*)-.

Molecular formula: $C_{18}H_{34}O_2$.

Molecular weight: 282.47.

Description: Oleic Acid NF—Colorless to pale yellow, oily liquid when freshly prepared, but on exposure to air it gradually absorbs oxygen and darkens. It has a characteristic, lard-like odor. When strongly heated in air, it is decomposed with the production of acrid vapors.
  NF category: Emulsifying and/or solubilizing agent.

Solubility: Oleic Acid NF—Practically insoluble in water. Miscible with alcohol, with chloroform, with ether, and with fixed and volatile oils.

NF requirements: Oleic Acid NF—Preserve in tight containers. It is manufactured from fats and oils derived from edible sources, and consists chiefly of (*Z*)-9-octadecenoic acid [$CH_3(CH_2)_7CH{:}CH(CH_2)_7COOH$]. If it is for external use only, the labeling so indicates. Meets the requirements for Specific gravity (0.889–0.895), Congealing temperature (not above 10 °C), Residue on ignition (not more than 0.01% [about]), Mineral acids, Neutral fat or mineral oil, Acid value (196–204), and Iodine value (85–95).

Note: Oleic Acid labeled solely for external use is exempt from the requirement that it be prepared from edible sources.

OLEOVITAMIN A AND D

Description: Oleovitamin A and D USP—Yellow to red, oily liquid, practically odorless or having a fish-like odor, and having no rancid odor. It is a clear liquid at temperatures exceeding 65 °C, and may crystallize on cooling. Unstable in air and in light.

Solubility: Oleovitamin A and D USP—Insoluble in water and in glycerin; very soluble in ether and in chloroform; soluble in dehydrated alcohol and in vegetable oils.

USP requirements: Oleovitamin A and D Capsules USP—Preserve in tight, light-resistant containers. Store in a dry place. Label the Capsules to indicate the content, in mg, of vitamin A in each capsule. The vitamin A content in each capsule may be expressed also in USP Vitamin A Units. Label the Capsules to show whether they contain ergocalciferol, cholecalciferol, or vitamin D from a natural source. Label the Capsules to indicate also the vitamin D content, in mcg, in each capsule. The vitamin D content may be expressed also in USP Vitamin D Units in each capsule. Contain the labeled amounts of vitamins A and D, within −10%. The oil in Oleovitamin A and D Capsules conforms to the definition for Oleovitamin A and D.

OLEYL ALCOHOL

Chemical name: 9-Octadecen-1-ol, (Z)-.

Molecular formula: $C_{18}H_{36}O$.

Molecular weight: 268.48.

Description: Oleyl Alcohol NF—Clear, colorless to light yellow, oily liquid. Has a faint characteristic odor.
   NF category: Emulsifying and/or solubilizing agent (stabilizer).

Solubility: Oleyl Alcohol NF—Insoluble in water; soluble in alcohol, in ether, in isopropyl alcohol, and in light mineral oil.

NF requirements: Oleyl Alcohol NF—Preserve in well-filled, tight containers, and store at controlled room temperature. A mixture of unsaturated and saturated high molecular weight fatty alcohols consisting chiefly of oleyl alcohol. Meets the requirements for Cloud point (not above 10 °C), Refractive index (1.458–1.460), Acid value (not more than 1), Hydroxyl value (205–215), and Iodine value (85–95).

OLIVE OIL

Description: Olive Oil NF—Pale yellow, or light greenish yellow, oily liquid, having a slight characteristic odor.
   NF category: Oleaginous vehicle.

Solubility: Olive Oil NF—Slightly soluble in alcohol. Miscible with ether, with chloroform, and with carbon disulfide.

NF requirements: Olive Oil NF—Preserve in tight containers and prevent exposure to excessive heat. The fixed oil obtained from the ripe fruit of *Olea europaea* Linné (Fam. Oleaceae). Meets the requirements for Specific gravity (0.910–0.915), Heavy metals (not more than 0.001%), Cottonseed oil, Peanut oil, Sesame oil, Teaseed oil, Solidification range of fatty acids (17–26 °C), Free fatty acids, Iodine value (79–88), and Saponification value (190–195).

OLSALAZINE

Chemical name: Olsalazine sodium—Benzoic acid, 3,3′-azobis[6-hydroxy-, disodium salt.

Molecular formula: Olsalazine sodium—$C_{14}H_8N_2Na_2O_6$.

Molecular weight: Olsalazine sodium—346.21.

Description: Olsalazine sodium—Yellow crystalline powder; melts with decomposition at 240 °C.

Solubility: Olsalazine sodium—Soluble in water and in dimethyl sulfoxide; practically insoluble in ethanol, in chloroform, and in ether.

USP requirements: Olsalazine Sodium Capsules—Not in USP.

OMEPRAZOLE

Chemical group: Substituted benzimidazole.

Chemical name: 1H-Benzimidazole, 5-methoxy-2-[[(4-methoxy-3,5-dimethyl-2-pyridinyl) methyl]sulfinyl]-.

Molecular formula: $C_{17}H_{19}N_3O_3S$.

Molecular weight: 345.42.

Description: White to off-white crystalline powder.

pKa: 4 and 8.8.

Solubility: Freely soluble in ethanol and in methanol; slightly soluble in acetone and in isopropanol; very slightly soluble in water.

Other characteristics: The stability of omeprazole is a function of pH; omeprazole is rapidly degraded in acid media, but has acceptable stability under alkaline conditions.

USP requirements: Omeprazole Delayed-release Capsules—Not in USP.

ONDANSETRON

Chemical name: Ondansetron hydrochloride—4H-Carbazol-4-one, 1,2,3,9-tetrahydro-9-methyl-3-[(2-methyl-1H-imidazol-1-yl)methyl]-, monohydrochloride, (±)-, dihydrate.

Molecular formula: Ondansetron hydrochloride—$C_{18}H_{19}N_3O \cdot HCl \cdot 2H_2O$.

Molecular weight: Ondansetron hydrochloride—365.86.

Description: Ondansetron hydrochloride—White to off-white powder.

Solubility: Ondansetron hydrochloride—Soluble in water and in normal saline.

USP requirements:
   Ondansetron Hydrochloride Injection—Not in USP.
   Ondansetron Hydrochloride Dihydrate Injection—Not in USP.
   Ondansetron Hydrochloride Dihydrate Tablets—Not in USP.

OPIUM

Source: The air-dried milky exudate obtained by incising the unripe capsules of *Papaver somniferum* Linné or its variety *album* De Candolle (Fam. Papaveraceae).

Description:
   Opium USP—Has a very characteristic odor.
   Powdered Opium USP—Light brown or moderately yellowish brown powder.

USP requirements:

Powdered Opium USP—Preserve in well-closed containers. It is Opium dried at a temperature not exceeding 70 °C, and reduced to a very fine powder. Yields not less than 10.0% and not more than 10.5% of anhydrous morphine. Meets the requirement for Botanic characteristics.

Opium Tincture USP (Laudanum)—Preserve in tight, light-resistant containers, and avoid exposure to direct sunlight and to excessive heat. Contains, in each 100 mL, not less than 0.90 gram and not more than 1.10 grams of anhydrous morphine.

Opium Tincture may be prepared as follows: Place 100 grams of granulated or sliced Opium in a suitable vessel. (Note: Do not use Powdered Opium.) Add 500 mL of boiling water, and allow to stand, with frequent stirring, for 24 hours. Transfer the mixture to a percolator, allow it to drain, percolate with water as the menstruum to complete extraction, and evaporate the percolate to a volume of 400 mL. Boil actively for not less than 15 minutes, and allow to stand overnight. Heat the mixture to 80 °C, add 50 grams of paraffin, and heat until the paraffin is melted. Beat the mixture thoroughly, and cool. Remove the paraffin, and filter the concentrate, washing the paraffin and the filter with sufficient water to make the filtrate measure 750 mL. Add 188 mL of alcohol to the filtrate, mix, and assay a 10-mL portion of the resulting solution as directed. Dilute the remaining solution with a mixture of 1 volume of alcohol and 4 volumes of water to obtain a Tincture containing 1 gram of anhydrous morphine in each 100 mL. Mix.

Meets the requirement for Alcohol content (17.0–21.0%).

Opium Alkaloids Hydrochlorides Injection—Not in USP.

ORANGE FLOWER OIL

Description: Orange Flower Oil NF—Pale yellow, slightly fluorescent liquid, which becomes reddish brown on exposure to light and air. Has a distinctive, fragrant odor, similar to that of orange blossoms. May become turbid or solid at low temperatures. Neutral to litmus.

NF category: Flavors and perfumes.

NF requirements: Orange Flower Oil NF—Preserve in tight, light-resistant containers. The volatile oil distilled from the fresh flowers of *Citrus aurantium* Linné (Fam. Rutaceae). Meets the requirements for Solubility in alcohol (miscible with an equal volume of alcohol and with about 2 volumes of 80% alcohol, the solution becoming cloudy on the further addition of 80% alcohol), Identification, Specific gravity (0.863–0.880), Angular rotation (+1.5° to +9.1°, in a 100-mm tube), and Heavy metals (not more than 0.004%).

ORPHENADRINE

Chemical name:

Orphenadrine citrate—Ethanamine, *N,N*-dimethyl-2-[(2-methylphenyl)phenylmethoxy]-, 2-hydroxy-1,2,3-propanetricarboxylate (1:1).

Orphenadrine hydrochloride—2-Dimethylaminoethyl 2-methylbenzhydryl ether hydrochloride.

Molecular formula:

Orphenadrine citrate—$C_{18}H_{23}NO \cdot C_6H_8O_7$.

Orphenadrine hydrochloride—$C_{18}H_{23}NO \cdot HCl$.

Molecular weight:

Orphenadrine citrate—461.51.

Orphenadrine hydrochloride—305.83.

Description:

Orphenadrine Citrate USP—White, practically odorless, crystalline powder.

Orphenadrine hydrochloride—White or almost white, odorless or almost odorless, crystalline powder.

Solubility:

Orphenadrine Citrate USP—Sparingly soluble in water; slightly soluble in alcohol; insoluble in chloroform and in ether.

Orphenadrine hydrochloride—Soluble 1 in 1 of water and of alcohol and 1 in 2 of chloroform; practically insoluble in ether.

USP requirements:

Orphenadrine Citrate Injection USP—Preserve in single-dose or in multiple-dose containers, preferably of Type I glass, protected from light. A sterile solution of Orphenadrine Citrate in Water for Injection, prepared with the aid of Sodium Hydroxide. Contains the labeled amount, within ±7%. Meets the requirements for Identification, Bacterial endotoxins, pH (5.0–6.0), and Injections.

Orphenadrine Citrate Extended-release Tablets—Not in USP.

Orphenadrine Hydrochloride Tablets—Not in USP.

ORPHENADRINE, ASPIRIN, AND CAFFEINE

For *Orphenadrine, Aspirin,* and *Caffeine*—See individual listings for chemistry information.

USP requirements: Orphenadrine Citrate, Aspirin, and Caffeine Tablets—Not in USP.

OXACILLIN

Chemical name: Oxacillin sodium—4-Thia-1-azabicyclo[3.2.0]heptane-2-carboxylic acid, 3,3-dimethyl-6-[[(5-methyl-3-phenyl-4-isoxazolyl)carbonyl]amino]-7-oxo-, monosodium salt, monohydrate, [2S-(2 alpha,5 alpha,6 beta)]-.

Molecular formula: Oxacillin sodium—$C_{19}H_{18}N_3NaO_5S \cdot H_2O$.

Molecular weight: Oxacillin sodium—441.43.

Description:

Oxacillin Sodium USP—Fine, white, crystalline powder, odorless or having a slight odor.

Oxacillin Sodium for Injection USP—Fine, white, crystalline powder, odorless or having a slight odor.

Solubility:

Oxacillin Sodium USP—Freely soluble in water, in methanol, and in dimethylsulfoxide; slightly soluble in absolute alcohol, in chloroform, in pyridine, and in methyl acetate; insoluble in ethyl acetate, in ether, and in ethylene chloride.

Oxacillin Sodium for Injection USP—Freely soluble in water, in methanol, and in dimethylsulfoxide; slightly soluble in absolute alcohol, in chloroform, in pyridine, and in methyl acetate; insoluble in ethyl acetate, in ether, and in ethylene chloride.

USP requirements:

Oxacillin Sodium Capsules USP—Preserve in tight containers, at controlled room temperature. Contain an amount of oxacillin sodium equivalent to the labeled amount of oxacillin, within −10% to +20%. Meet the requirements for Identification, Dissolution (75% in 45 minutes in water in Apparatus 1 at 100 rpm), Uniformity of dosage units, and Water (not more than 6.0%).

Oxacillin Sodium Injection USP—Preserve in Containers for Injections. Maintain in the frozen state. A sterile isoosmotic solution of Oxacillin Sodium in Water for Injection. Contains dextrose as a tonicity-adjusting agent and one or more suitable buffer substances. Contains no preservatives. The label states that it is to be thawed just prior to use, describes conditions for proper storage of the resultant solution, and directs that the solution is not to be refrozen. Contains an amount of oxacillin sodium equivalent to the labeled amount of oxacillin, within −10% to +15%. Meets the requirements for Identification, Pyrogen, Sterility, pH (6.0–8.5), Particulate matter, and Labeling under Injections.

Oxacillin Sodium for Injection USP—Preserve in Containers for Sterile Solids, at controlled room temperature. A sterile, dry mixture of Oxacillin Sodium and one or more suitable buffers. Contains an amount of oxacillin sodium equivalent to the labeled amount of oxacillin, within −10% to +15%. Meets the requirements for Constituted solution, Identification, Bacterial endotoxins, Sterility, Uniformity of dosage units, pH (6.0–8.5, in a solution containing 30 mg per mL), Water (not more than 6.0%), and Particulate matter.

Oxacillin Sodium for Oral Solution USP—Preserve in tight containers, at controlled room temperature. Contains one or more suitable buffers, colors, flavors, preservatives, and stabilizers. Contains an amount of oxacillin sodium equivalent to the labeled amount of oxacillin, within −10% to +20%. Meets the requirements for Identification, pH (5.0–7.5, in the solution constituted as directed in the labeling), Water (not more than 1.0%), Uniformity of dosage units (single-unit containers), and Deliverable volume (multiple-unit containers).

Sterile Oxacillin Sodium USP—Preserve in Containers for Sterile Solids. It is Oxacillin Sodium suitable for parenteral use. Contains an amount of oxacillin sodium equivalent to not less than 815 mcg and not more than 950 mcg of oxacillin per mg. Meets the requirements for Bacterial endotoxins and Sterility, and for Identification tests, pH (4.5–7.5, in a solution containing 30 mg per mL), Water (3.5–5.0%), and Crystallinity under Oxacillin Sodium.

OXAMNIQUINE

Chemical group: Tetrahydroquinoline derivative.

Chemical name: 6-Quinolinemethanol, 1,2,3,4-tetrahydro-2-[[(1-methylethyl)amino]methyl]-7-nitro-.

Molecular formula: $C_{14}H_{21}N_3O_3$.

Molecular weight: 279.34.

Description: Oxamniquine USP—Yellow-orange crystalline solid.

Solubility: Oxamniquine USP—Sparingly soluble in water; soluble in methanol, in chloroform, and in acetone.

USP requirements: Oxamniquine Capsules USP—Preserve in tight containers. Contain the labeled amount, within ±10%. Meet the requirements for Identification, Dissolution (70% in 60 minutes in 0.1 N hydrochloric acid in Apparatus 2 at 50 rpm), and Uniformity of dosage units.

OXANDROLONE

Chemical group: 17-alpha alkylated anabolic steroid.

Chemical name: 2-Oxaandrostan-3-one, 17-hydroxy-17-methyl-, (5 alpha,17 beta)-.

Molecular formula: $C_{19}H_{30}O_3$.

Molecular weight: 306.44.

Description: Oxandrolone USP—White, odorless, crystalline powder. Is stable in air, but darkens on exposure to light. Melts at about 225 °C.

Solubility: Oxandrolone USP—Practically insoluble in water; freely soluble in chloroform; sparingly soluble in alcohol and in acetone.

USP requirements: Oxandrolone Tablets USP—Preserve in tight, light-resistant containers. Contain the labeled amount, within ±8%. Meet the requirements for Identification, Disintegration (15 minutes), and Uniformity of dosage units.

OXAZEPAM

Chemical name: 2H-1,4-Benzodiazepin-2-one, 7-chloro-1,3-dihydro-3-hydroxy-5-phenyl-.

Molecular formula: $C_{15}H_{11}ClN_2O_2$.

Molecular weight: 286.72.

Description: Oxazepam USP—Creamy white to pale yellow powder. Is practically odorless.

Solubility: Oxazepam USP—Practically insoluble in water; slightly soluble in alcohol and in chloroform; very slightly soluble in ether.

USP requirements:
Oxazepam Capsules USP—Preserve in well-closed containers. Contain the labeled amount, within ±10%. Meet the requirements for Identification, Dissolution (75% in 60 minutes in 0.1 N hydrochloric acid in Apparatus 2 at 75 rpm), and Uniformity of dosage units.
Oxazepam Tablets USP—Preserve in well-closed containers. Contain the labeled amount, within ±10%. Meet the requirements for Identification, Dissolution (80% in 60 minutes in 0.1 N hydrochloric acid in Apparatus 2 at 50 rpm), and Uniformity of dosage units.

OXPRENOLOL

Chemical name: Oxprenolol hydrochloride—2-Propanol, 1-(o-allyloxyphenoxy)-3-isopropylamino-, hydrochloride.

Molecular formula: Oxprenolol hydrochloride—$C_{15}H_{23}NO_3$·HCl.

Molecular weight: Oxprenolol hydrochloride—301.81.

Description: Oxprenolol Hydrochloride USP—White, crystalline powder.

Solubility: Oxprenolol Hydrochloride USP—Freely soluble in alcohol, in chloroform, and in water; sparingly soluble in acetone; practically insoluble in ether.

Other characteristics: Lipid solubility—Moderate.

USP requirements:
Oxprenolol Tablets USP—Preserve in well-closed, light-resistant containers. Label Tablets to state both the content of the active moiety and the content of the salt used in formulating the article. Contain the labeled amount of oxprenolol hydrochloride, within ±10%. Meet the requirements for Identification, Dissolution (80% in 30 minutes in 0.1 N hydrochloric acid in Apparatus 1 at 100 rpm), and Uniformity of dosage units.
Oxprenolol Extended-release Tablets USP—Preserve in well-closed, light-resistant containers. Label Tablets to state both the content of the active moiety and the content of the salt used in formulating the article. Contain the labeled amount of oxprenolol hydrochloride, within ±10%. Meet the requirements for Identification, Drug release (15–45% in 1 hour in 0.1 N hydrochloric acid, 30–60% in 1 hour in Dissolution medium, 50–80% in 3 hours in Dissolution medium, and not less than 75% in 7 hours in

Dissolution medium, in Apparatus 1 at 100 rpm, the Dissolution medium being simulated intestinal fluid TS without enzyme), and Uniformity of dosage units.

OXTRIPHYLLINE

Source: The choline salt of theophylline.

Chemical name: Ethanaminium, 2-hydroxy-*N,N,N*-trimethyl-, salt with 3,7-dihydro-1,3-dimethyl-1*H*-purine-2,6-dione.

Molecular formula: $C_{12}H_{21}N_5O_3$.

Molecular weight: 283.33.

Description: Oxtriphylline USP—White, crystalline powder, having an amine-like odor. A solution (1 in 100) has a pH of about 10.3.

Solubility: Oxtriphylline USP—Freely soluble in water and in alcohol; very slightly soluble in chloroform.

USP requirements:
Oxtriphylline Oral Solution USP—Preserve in tight containers. Label Oral Solution to state both the content of oxtriphylline and the content of anhydrous theophylline. Contains an amount of oxtriphylline equivalent to the labeled amount of anhydrous theophylline, within ± 10%. Meets the requirements for Identification, pH (6.4–9.0), and Alcohol content (if present, 90–115% of labeled amount, the labeled amount being not more than 20.0%).
Oxtriphylline Syrup—Not in USP.
Oxtriphylline Tablets—Not in USP.
Oxtriphylline Delayed-release Tablets USP—Preserve in tight containers. Label Delayed-release Tablets to state both the content of oxtriphylline and the content of anhydrous theophylline. The label indicates that Oxtriphylline Delayed-release Tablets are enteric-coated. Contain an amount of oxtriphylline equivalent to the labeled amount of anhydrous theophylline, within ± 10%. Meet the requirements for Identification, Disintegration, and Uniformity of dosage units.
Oxtriphylline Extended-release Tablets USP—Preserve in tight containers. Label Extended-release Tablets to state both the content of oxtriphylline and the content of anhydrous theophylline. Contain an amount of oxtriphylline equivalent to the labeled amount of anhydrous theophylline, within ± 10%. Meet the requirements for Identification and Uniformity of dosage units.

OXTRIPHYLLINE AND GUAIFENESIN

For *Oxtriphylline* and *Guaifenesin*—See individual listings for chemistry information.

USP requirements:
Oxtriphylline and Guaifenesin Elixir—Not in USP.
Oxtriphylline and Guaifenesin Tablets—Not in USP.

OXYBUTYNIN

Chemical group: Synthetic tertiary amine.

Chemical name: Oxybutynin chloride—Benzeneacetic acid, alpha-cyclohexyl-alpha-hydroxy-, 4-(diethylamino)-2-butynyl ester hydrochloride.

Molecular formula: Oxybutynin chloride—$C_{22}H_{31}NO_3 \cdot HCl$.

Molecular weight: Oxybutynin chloride—393.95.

Description: Oxybutynin Chloride USP—White, crystalline, practically odorless powder.

pKa: Oxybutynin chloride—6.96.

Solubility: Oxybutynin Chloride USP—Freely soluble in water and in alcohol; very soluble in methanol and in chloroform; soluble in acetone; slightly soluble in ether; very slightly soluble in hexane.

USP requirements:
Oxybutynin Chloride Syrup USP—Preserve in tight, light-resistant containers. Contains the labeled amount, within ± 10%. Meets the requirement for Identification.
Oxybutynin Chloride Tablets USP—Preserve in tight, light-resistant containers. Contain the labeled amount, within ± 10%. Meet the requirements for Identification, Dissolution (80% in 30 minutes in water in Apparatus 2 at 50 rpm), and Uniformity of dosage units.

OXYCODONE

Chemical name:
Oxycodone—Morphinan-6-one, 4,5-epoxy-14-hydroxy-3-methoxy-17-methyl-, (5 alpha)-.
Oxycodone hydrochloride—Morphinan-6-one, 4,5-epoxy-14-hydroxy-3-methoxy-17-methyl-, hydrochloride, (5 alpha)-.

Molecular formula:
Oxycodone—$C_{18}H_{21}NO_4$.
Oxycodone hydrochloride—$C_{18}H_{21}NO_4 \cdot HCl$.

Molecular weight:
Oxycodone—315.37.
Oxycodone hydrochloride—351.83.

Description: Oxycodone Hydrochloride USP—White to off-white, hygroscopic crystals or powder. Is odorless.

Solubility: Oxycodone Hydrochloride USP—Soluble in water; slightly soluble in alcohol.

USP requirements:
Oxycodone Tablets USP—Preserve in tight, light-resistant containers. Label Tablets to state both the content of the active moiety and the content of the salt used in formulating the tablets. Contain the labeled amount of oxycodone hydrochloride, within ± 10%. Meet the requirements for Identification, Dissolution (70% in 45 minutes in water in Apparatus 2 at 50 rpm), and Uniformity of dosage units.
Oxycodone Hydrochloride Oral Solution USP—Preserve in tight, light-resistant containers. Contains the labeled amount, within ± 10%. Meets the requirements for Identification, pH (1.4–4.0), and Alcohol content (7.0–9.0%).
Oxycodone Hydrochloride Suppositories—Not in USP.

OXYCODONE AND ACETAMINOPHEN

For *Oxycodone* and *Acetaminophen*—See individual listings for chemistry information.

USP requirements:
Oxycodone and Acetaminophen Capsules USP—Preserve in tight, light-resistant containers. Contain Oxycodone Hydrochloride and Acetaminophen, or Oxycodone Hydrochloride, Oxycodone Terephthalate, and Acetaminophen. Label Capsules to indicate whether they contain Oxycodone Hydrochloride or Oxycodone Hydrochloride and Oxycodone Terephthalate. Capsules may be labeled to indicate the total content of oxycodone equivalent. Each mg of oxycodone hydrochloride or oxycodone terephthalate is equivalent to 0.8963 mg or 0.7915 mg of oxycodone, respectively. Contain the labeled amounts of oxycodone hydrochloride or oxycodone hydrochloride and oxycodone terephthalate, calculated as total oxycodone, and the labeled amount of acetaminophen, within ± 10%. Meet the requirements for Identification, Dissolution (75% of each

active ingredient in 45 minutes in 0.1 N hydrochloric acid in Apparatus 2 at 50 rpm), and Uniformity of dosage units.

Oxycodone and Acetaminophen Oral Solution—Not in USP.

Oxycodone and Acetaminophen Tablets USP—Preserve in tight, light-resistant containers. Contain Oxycodone Hydrochloride and Acetaminophen. Tablets may be labeled to indicate the content of oxycodone hydrochloride equivalent. Each mg of oxycodone is equivalent to 1.116 mg of oxycodone hydrochloride. Contain the labeled amounts of oxycodone and acetaminophen, within ±10%. Meet the requirements for Identification, Dissolution (75% of each active ingredient in 45 minutes in 0.1 N hydrochloric acid in Apparatus 2 at 50 rpm), and Uniformity of dosage units.

OXYCODONE AND ASPIRIN

For Oxycodone and Aspirin—See individual listings for chemistry information.

USP requirements: Oxycodone and Aspirin Tablets USP—Preserve in tight, light-resistant containers. Contain Oxycodone Hydrochloride and Aspirin, or Oxycodone Hydrochloride, Oxycodone Terephthalate, and Aspirin. Label Tablets to state both the content of the oxycodone active moiety and the content or contents of the salt or salts of oxycodone used in formulating the article. Contain the labeled amount of oxycodone, within ±7%, and the labeled amount of aspirin, within ±10%. Meet the requirements for Identification, Dissolution (80% of oxycodone and 75% of aspirin in 30 minutes in 0.05 M acetate buffer [pH 4.50] in Apparatus 1 at 50 rpm), Uniformity of dosage units, and Salicylic acid (not more than 3.0%).

OXYGEN

Chemical name: Oxygen.

Molecular formula: O_2.

Molecular weight: 32.00.

Description: Oxygen USP—Colorless, odorless gas, which supports combustion more energetically than does air. One liter at 0 °C and at a pressure of 760 mm of mercury weighs about 1.429 grams.

Solubility: Oxygen USP—One volume dissolves in about 32 volumes of water and in about 7 volumes of alcohol at 20 °C and at a pressure of 760 mm of mercury.

USP requirements: Oxygen USP—Preserve in cylinders or in a pressurized storage tank. Containers used for Oxygen must not be treated with any toxic, sleep-inducing, or narcosis-producing compounds, and must not be treated with any compound that will be irritating to the respiratory tract when the Oxygen is used. Label it to indicate whether or not it has been produced by the air-liquefaction process. Where it is piped directly from the cylinder or storage tank to the point of use, label each outlet "Oxygen." Contains not less than 99.0%, by volume, of oxygen. (Note: Oxygen that is produced by the air-liquefaction process is exempt from the requirements of the tests for Carbon dioxide and Carbon monoxide.) Meets the requirements for Identification, Odor, Carbon dioxide (not more than 0.03%), and Carbon monoxide (not more than 0.001%).

OXYGEN 93 PERCENT

USP requirements: Oxygen 93 Percent USP—Preserve in cylinders or in a low pressure collecting tank. Containers used for Oxygen 93 Percent must not be treated with any toxic,

sleep-inducing, or narcosis-producing compounds, and must not be treated with any compound that will be irritating to the respiratory tract when the Oxygen 93 Percent is used. It is Oxygen produced from air by the molecular sieve process. Where it is piped directly from the collecting tank to the point of use, label each outlet "Oxygen 93 Percent." Contains not less than 90.0% and not more than 96.0%, by volume, of oxygen, the remainder consisting mostly of argon and nitrogen. Meets the requirements for Identification, Odor, Carbon dioxide (not more than 0.03%), and Carbon monoxide (not more than 0.001%).

OXYMETAZOLINE

Source: Prepared from (4-tert-butyl-2,6-dimethyl-3-hydroxyphenyl)acetonitrile and ethylenediamine.

Chemical name: Oxymetazoline hydrochloride—Phenol, 3-[(4,5-dihydro-1H-imidazol-2-yl)methyl]-6-(1,1-dimethylethyl)-2,4-dimethyl-, monohydrochloride.

Molecular formula: Oxymetazoline hydrochloride—$C_{16}H_{24}N_2O \cdot HCl$.

Molecular weight: Oxymetazoline hydrochloride—296.84.

Description: Oxymetazoline Hydrochloride USP—White to practically white, fine crystalline powder. Is hygroscopic. Melts at about 300 °C, with decomposition.

Solubility: Oxymetazoline Hydrochloride USP—Soluble in water and in alcohol; practically insoluble in chloroform and in ether.

USP requirements:

Oxymetazoline Hydrochloride Nasal Solution USP—Preserve in tight containers. A solution of Oxymetazoline Hydrochloride in water adjusted to a suitable tonicity. Contains the labeled amount, within ±10%. Meets the requirements for Identification and pH (4.0–6.5).

Oxymetazoline Hydrochloride Ophthalmic Solution USP—Preserve in tight containers. A sterile, buffered solution of Oxymetazoline Hydrochloride in water adjusted to a suitable tonicity. Contains the labeled amount, within ±10%. Contains a suitable preservative. Meets the requirements for Identification, Sterility, and pH (5.8–6.8).

OXYMETHOLONE

Chemical group: 17-alpha alkylated anabolic steroid.

Chemical name: Androstan-3-one, 17-hydroxy-2-(hydroxymethylene)-17-methyl-, (5 alpha,17 beta)-.

Molecular formula: $C_{21}H_{32}O_3$.

Molecular weight: 332.48.

Description: Oxymetholone USP—White to creamy white, crystalline powder. Is odorless, and is stable in air.

Solubility: Oxymetholone USP—Practically insoluble in water; freely soluble in chloroform; soluble in dioxane; sparingly soluble in alcohol; slightly soluble in ether.

USP requirements: Oxymetholone Tablets USP—Preserve in well-closed containers. Contain the labeled amount, within ±10%. Meet the requirements for Identification, Dissolution (75% in 45 minutes in 0.05 M alkaline borate buffer [pH 8.5] in Apparatus 1 at 100 rpm), and Uniformity of dosage units.

OXYMORPHONE

Chemical name: Oxymorphone hydrochloride—Morphinan-6-one, 4,5-epoxy-3,14-dihydroxy-17-methyl-, hydrochloride, (5 alpha)-.

Molecular formula: Oxymorphone hydrochloride—$C_{17}H_{19}NO_4 \cdot HCl$.

Molecular weight: Oxymorphone hydrochloride—337.80.

Description: Oxymorphone Hydrochloride USP—White or slightly off-white, odorless powder. Darkens on exposure to light. Its aqueous solutions are slightly acidic.

Solubility: Oxymorphone Hydrochloride USP—Freely soluble in water; sparingly soluble in alcohol and in ether.

USP requirements:
Oxymorphone Hydrochloride Injection USP—Preserve in single-dose or in multiple-dose containers of Type I glass, protected from light. A sterile solution of Oxymorphone Hydrochloride in Water for Injection. Contains the labeled amount, within ±7%. Meets the requirements for Identification, Bacterial endotoxins, pH (2.7–4.5), and Injections.
Oxymorphone Hydrochloride Suppositories USP—Preserve in well-closed containers, and store in a refrigerator. Contain the labeled amount, within ±7%. Meet the requirement for Identification.

OXYPHENBUTAZONE

Chemical name: 3,5-Pyrazolidinedione, 4-butyl-1-(4-hydroxyphenyl)-2-phenyl-, monohydrate.

Molecular formula: $C_{19}H_{20}N_2O_3 \cdot H_2O$.

Molecular weight: 342.39.

Description: Oxyphenbutazone USP—White to yellowish white, odorless, crystalline powder. Melts over a wide range between about 85 and 100 °C.

Solubility: Oxyphenbutazone USP—Very slightly soluble in water; soluble in alcohol; freely soluble in acetone and in ether.

USP requirements: Oxyphenbutazone Tablets USP—Preserve in tight containers. Contain the labeled amount, within ±6%. Meet the requirements for Identification, Dissolution (60% in 30 minutes in phosphate buffer [pH 7.5] in Apparatus 1 at 100 rpm), and Uniformity of dosage units.

OXYPHENCYCLIMINE

Source: Synthetic amine compound.

Chemical group: Tertiary amine.

Chemical name: Oxyphencyclimine hydrochloride—Benzeneacetic acid, alpha-cyclohexyl-alpha-hydroxy-, (1,4,5,6-tetrahydro-1-methyl-2-pyrimidinyl)methyl ester monohydrochloride.

Molecular formula: Oxyphencyclimine hydrochloride—$C_{20}H_{28}N_2O_3 \cdot HCl$.

Molecular weight: Oxyphencyclimine hydrochloride—380.91.

Description: Oxyphencyclimine Hydrochloride USP—White, odorless, crystalline powder. Melts at about 234 °C.

Solubility: Oxyphencyclimine Hydrochloride USP—Sparingly soluble in water; soluble in methanol; slightly soluble in chloroform.

USP requirements: Oxyphencyclimine Hydrochloride Tablets USP—Preserve in tight containers. Contain the labeled amount, within ±10%. Meet the requirements for Identification, Dissolution (75% in 45 minutes in water in Apparatus 1 at 100 rpm), and Uniformity of dosage units.

OXYQUINOLINE SULFATE

Chemical name: 8-Quinolinol sulfate (2:1) (salt).

Molecular formula: $(C_9H_7NO)_2 \cdot H_2SO_4$.

Molecular weight: 388.39.

Description: Oxyquinoline Sulfate NF—Yellow powder. Melts at about 185 °C.
NF category: Complexing agent.

Solubility: Oxyquinoline Sulfate NF—Very soluble in water; freely soluble in methanol; slightly soluble in alcohol; practically insoluble in acetone and in ether.

NF requirements: Oxyquinoline Sulfate NF—Preserve in well-closed containers. It is 8-hydroxyquinoline sulfate. Contains not less than 97.0% and not more than 101.0% of oxyquinoline sulfate, calculated on the anhydrous basis. Meets the requirements for Identification, Water (4.0–6.0%), Residue on ignition (not more than 0.3%), Arsenic (not more than 3 ppm), Heavy metals (not more than 0.004%), and Organic volatile impurities.

OXYTETRACYCLINE

Chemical name:
Oxytetracycline—2-Naphthacenecarboxamide, 4-(dimethylamino)-1,4,4a,5,5a,6,11,12a-octahydro-3,5,6,10,12,-12a-hexahydroxy-6-methyl-1,11-dioxo-, [4S-(4 alpha,4a alpha,5 alpha,5a alpha,6 beta,12a alpha)]-, dihydrate.
Oxytetracycline calcium—2-Naphthacenecarboxamide, 4-(dimethylamino)-1,4,4a,5,5a,6,11,12a-octahydro-3,5,6,10,-12,12a-hexahydroxy-6-methyl-1,11-dioxo-, calcium salt, [4S-(4 alpha,4a alpha,5 alpha,5a alpha,6 beta,12a alpha)]-.
Oxytetracycline hydrochloride—2-Naphthacenecarboxamide, 4-(dimethylamino)-1,4,4a,5,5a,6,11,12a-octahydro-3,5,6,10,12,12a-hexahydroxy-6-methyl-1,11-dioxo-, monohydrochloride, [4S-(4 alpha,4a alpha,5 alpha,5a alpha,6 beta,12a alpha)]-.

Molecular formula:
Oxytetracycline—$C_{22}H_{24}N_2O_9 \cdot 2H_2O$.
Oxytetracycline calcium—$C_{44}H_{46}CaN_4O_{18}$.
Oxytetracycline hydrochloride—$C_{22}H_{24}N_2O_9 \cdot HCl$.

Molecular weight:
Oxytetracycline—496.47.
Oxytetracycline calcium—958.95.
Oxytetracycline hydrochloride—496.90.

Description:
Oxytetracycline USP—Pale yellow to tan, odorless, crystalline powder. Is stable in air, but exposure to strong sunlight causes it to darken. It loses potency in solutions of pH below 2, and is rapidly destroyed by alkali hydroxide solutions.
Oxytetracycline Calcium USP—Yellow to light brown, crystalline powder.
Oxytetracycline Hydrochloride USP—Yellow, odorless, crystalline powder. Is hygroscopic. Decomposes at a temperature exceeding 180 °C, and exposure to strong sunlight or to temperatures exceeding 90 °C in moist air causes it to darken. Its potency is diminished in solutions

having a pH below 2, and is rapidly destroyed by alkali hydroxide solutions.

Solubility:
Oxytetracycline USP—Very slightly soluble in water; freely soluble in 3 *N* hydrochloric acid and in alkaline solutions; sparingly soluble in alcohol.
Oxytetracycline Calcium USP—Insoluble in water.
Oxytetracycline Hydrochloride USP—Freely soluble in water, but crystals of oxytetracycline base separate as a result of partial hydrolysis of the hydrochloride. Sparingly soluble in alcohol and in methanol, and even less soluble in dehydrated alcohol; insoluble in chloroform and in ether.

USP requirements:
Oxytetracycline Injection USP—Preserve in single-dose or in multiple-dose containers, protected from light. A sterile solution of Oxytetracycline with or without one or more suitable anesthetics, antioxidants, buffers, complexing agents, preservatives, and solvents. Contains the labeled amount, within −10% to +20%, the labeled amount being 50 or 125 mg per mL. Meets the requirements for Depressor substances, Bacterial endotoxins, Sterility, and pH (8.0–9.0).
Sterile Oxytetracycline USP—Preserve in Containers for Sterile Solids, protected from light. It is Oxytetracycline suitable for parenteral use. It has a potency of not less than 832 mcg of oxytetracycline per mg. Meets the requirements for Depressor substances, Bacterial endotoxins, and Sterility, and for Identification tests, pH, Water, and Crystallinity under Oxytetracycline.
Oxytetracycline Tablets USP—Preserve in tight, light-resistant containers. Contain the labeled amount, within −10% to +20%. Meet the requirements for Dissolution (75% in 45 minutes in 0.1 *N* hydrochloric acid in Apparatus 1 at 100 rpm), Uniformity of dosage units, and Water (not more than 7.5%).
Oxytetracycline Calcium Oral Suspension USP—Preserve in tight, light-resistant containers. Contains an amount of oxytetracycline calcium equivalent to the labeled amount of oxytetracycline, within −10% to +20%. Contains one or more suitable buffers, colors, flavors, preservatives, stabilizers, and suspending agents. Meets the requirements for Identification, pH (5.0–8.0), Deliverable volume (for Suspension packaged in multiple-unit containers), and Uniformity of dosage units (for Suspension packaged in single-unit containers).
Oxytetracycline Hydrochloride Capsules USP—Preserve in tight, light-resistant containers. Contain an amount of oxytetracycline hydrochloride equivalent to the labeled amount of oxytetracycline, within −10% to +20%. Meet the requirements for Identification, Dissolution (80% in 60 minutes in water in Apparatus 2 at 75 rpm), Uniformity of dosage units, and Loss on drying (not more than 5.0%).
Oxytetracycline Hydrochloride for Injection USP—Preserve in Containers for Sterile Solids, protected from light. A sterile dry mixture of Sterile Oxytetracycline Hydrochloride and a suitable buffer. Contains an amount of oxytetracycline hydrochloride equivalent to the labeled amount of oxytetracycline, within −10% to +15%. Meets the requirements for Constituted solution, Bacterial endotoxins, pH (1.8–2.8, in a solution containing 25 mg per mL), Loss on drying (not more than 3.0%), and Particulate matter, for Identification test B under Oxytetracycline Hydrochloride, for Depressor substances and Sterility under Sterile Oxytetracycline Hydrochloride, and for Uniformity of dosage units and Labeling under Injections.
Sterile Oxytetracycline Hydrochloride USP—Preserve in Containers for Sterile Solids, protected from light. It is

Oxytetracycline Hydrochloride suitable for parenteral use. It has a potency equivalent to not less than 835 mcg of oxytetracycline per mg, calculated on the dried basis. Meets the requirements for Depressor substances, Bacterial endotoxins, and Sterility, and for Identification tests, pH, Loss on drying, and Crystallinity under Oxytetracycline Hydrochloride.

OXYTETRACYCLINE AND HYDROCORTISONE

For *Oxytetracycline* and *Hydrocortisone*—See individual listings for chemistry information.

USP requirements:
Oxytetracycline Hydrochloride and Hydrocortisone Ointment USP—Preserve in collapsible tubes or in well-closed, light-resistant containers. Contains an amount of oxytetracycline hydrochloride equivalent to the labeled amount of oxytetracycline, within −10% to +15%, and the labeled amount of hydrocortisone, within ±10%. Meets the requirements for Minimum fill and Water (not more than 1.0%).
Oxytetracycline Hydrochloride and Hydrocortisone Acetate Ophthalmic Suspension USP—Preserve in tight, light-resistant containers. The containers are sealed and tamper-proof so that sterility is assured at time of first use. A sterile suspension of Oxytetracycline Hydrochloride and Hydrocortisone Acetate in a suitable oil vehicle with one or more suitable suspending agents. Contains an amount of oxytetracycline hydrochloride equivalent to the labeled amount of oxytetracycline, within −10% to +15%, and the labeled amount of hydrocortisone acetate, within ±10%. Meets the requirements for Sterility and Water (not more than 1.0%).

OXYTETRACYCLINE AND NYSTATIN

For *Oxytetracycline* and *Nystatin*—See individual listings for chemistry information.

USP requirements:
Oxytetracycline and Nystatin Capsules USP—Preserve in tight, light-resistant containers. Contain the labeled amount of oxytetracycline, within −10% to +20%, and the labeled amount of USP Nystatin Units, within −10% to +35%. Meet the requirements for Identification, Dissolution (75% in 45 minutes in 0.1 *N* hydrochloric acid in Apparatus 1 at 100 rpm), Uniformity of dosage units, and Water (not more than 7.5%).
Oxytetracycline and Nystatin for Oral Suspension USP—Preserve in tight, light-resistant containers, at controlled room temperature. A dry mixture of Oxytetracycline and Nystatin with one or more suitable buffers, colors, diluents, flavors, suspending agents, and preservatives. When constituted as directed in the labeling, contains the labeled amount of oxytetracycline, within −10% to +20%, and the labeled amount of USP Nystatin Units, within −10% to +35%. Meets the requirements for pH (4.5–7.5, in the suspension constituted as directed in the labeling), Water (not more than 2.0%), Deliverable volume (for solid packaged in multiple-unit containers), and Uniformity of dosage units (for solid packaged in single-unit containers).

OXYTETRACYCLINE, PHENAZOPYRIDINE, AND SULFAMETHIZOLE

For *Oxytetracycline, Phenazopyridine,* and *Sulfamethizole*—See individual listings for chemistry information.

USP requirements: Oxytetracycline and Phenazopyridine Hydrochlorides and Sulfamethizole Capsules USP—Preserve in tight, light-resistant containers. Contain an amount of oxytetracycline hydrochloride equivalent to the labeled amount of oxytetracycline, within −10% to +20%, and the labeled amounts of phenazopyridine hydrochloride, within −10% to +15%, and sulfamethizole, within ±10%. Meet the requirements for Uniformity of dosage units and Loss on drying (not more than 5.0%).

OXYTETRACYCLINE AND POLYMYXIN B

For *Oxytetracycline* and *Polymyxin B*—See individual listings for chemistry information.

USP requirements:
Oxytetracycline Hydrochloride and Polymyxin B Sulfate Ointment USP—Preserve in collapsible tubes or in well-closed, light-resistant containers. Contains amounts of oxytetracycline hydrochloride and polymyxin B sulfate equivalent to the labeled amounts of oxytetracycline, within −10% to +20%, and polymyxin B, within −10% to +25%. Meets the requirements for Minimum fill and Water (not more than 1.0%).

Oxytetracycline Hydrochloride and Polymyxin B Sulfate Ophthalmic Ointment USP—Preserve in collapsible ophthalmic ointment tubes. A sterile ointment containing Oxytetracycline Hydrochloride and Polymyxin B Sulfate. Contains amounts of oxytetracycline hydrochloride and polymyxin B sulfate equivalent to the labeled amounts of oxytetracycline, within −10% to +20%, and polymyxin B, within −10% to +25%. Meets the requirements for Sterility, Minimum fill, Water (not more than 1.0%), and Metal particles.

Oxytetracycline Hydrochloride and Polymyxin B Sulfate Topical Powder USP—Preserve in well-closed containers. Contains amounts of oxytetracycline hydrochloride and polymyxin B sulfate equivalent to the labeled amounts of oxytetracycline and polymyxin B, within −10% to +20%, in a suitable fine powder base. Meets the requirements for Minimum fill and Loss on drying (not more than 2.0%).

Oxytetracycline Hydrochloride and Polymyxin B Sulfate Vaginal Tablets USP—Preserve in well-closed containers. Contain amounts of oxytetracycline hydrochloride and polymyxin B sulfate equivalent to the labeled amounts of oxytetracycline and polymyxin B, within −10% to +20%. Meet the requirement for Loss on drying (not more than 3.0%).

OXYTOCIN

Chemical name: Oxytocin.

Molecular formula: $C_{43}H_{66}N_{12}O_{12}S_2$.

Molecular weight: 1007.19.

Description: White powder.

Solubility: Soluble in water.

USP requirements:
Oxytocin Injection USP—Preserve in single-dose or in multiple-dose containers, preferably of Type I glass. Do not freeze. A sterile solution, in a suitable diluent, of material containing the polypeptide hormone having the property of causing the contraction of uterine, vascular, and other smooth muscle, which is prepared by synthesis or obtained from the posterior lobe of the pituitary of healthy, domestic animals used for food by man. Each mL of Oxytocin Injection possesses an oxytocic activity of that stated on the label in USP Posterior Pituitary Units, within −15% to +20%. Meets the requirements for pH (2.5–4.5), Particulate matter, Pressor activity, and Injections.

Oxytocin Nasal Solution USP—Preserve in containers suitable for administering the contents by spraying into the nasal cavities with the patient in the upright position, or for instillation in drop form. A solution, in a suitable diluent, of the polypeptide hormone, prepared synthetically, which has the property of causing the contraction of uterine, vascular, and other smooth muscle, and which is present in the posterior lobe of the pituitary of healthy, domestic animals used for food by man. Label it to indicate that it is for intranasal administration only. Contains suitable preservatives, and is packaged in a form suitable for nasal administration. Each mL of Oxytocin Nasal Solution possesses an oxytocic activity of that stated on the label in USP Posterior Pituitary Units, within −15% to +20%. Meets the requirements for pH (3.7–4.3) and Pressor activity.

PADIMATE O

Chemical name: Benzoic acid, 4-(dimethylamino)-, 2-ethylhexyl ester.

Molecular formula: $C_{17}H_{27}NO_2$.

Molecular weight: 277.41.

Description: Padimate O USP—Light yellow, mobile liquid having a faint, aromatic odor.

Solubility: Padimate O USP—Practically insoluble in water; soluble in alcohol, in isopropyl alcohol, and in mineral oil; practically insoluble in glycerin and in propylene glycol.

USP requirements: Padimate O Lotion USP—Preserve in tight, light-resistant containers. Contains the labeled amount, within ±10%. Meets the requirement for Identification.

PANCREATIN

Chemical name: Pancreatin.

Description: Pancreatin USP—Cream-colored, amorphous powder, having a faint, characteristic, but not offensive odor. It hydrolyzes fats to glycerol and fatty acids, changes protein into proteoses and derived substances, and converts starch into dextrins and sugars. Its greatest activities are in neutral or faintly alkaline media; more than traces of mineral acids or large amounts of alkali hydroxides make it inert. An excess of alkali carbonate also inhibits its action.

USP requirements:
Pancreatin Capsules USP—Preserve in tight containers, preferably at a temperature not exceeding 30 °C. Label Capsules to indicate minimum pancreatin fat digestive power; i.e., single strength, double strength, triple strength. Contain the labeled amount, within −10%. Meet the requirement for Microbial limit.

Pancreatin Tablets USP—Preserve in tight containers, preferably at a temperature not exceeding 30 °C. Label Tablets to indicate minimum pancreatin fat digestive power; i.e., single strength, double strength, triple strength. Contain the labeled amount, within −10%. Meet the requirements for Microbial limit and Disintegration (60 minutes).

PANCREATIN, PEPSIN, BILE SALTS, HYOSCYAMINE, ATROPINE, SCOPOLAMINE, AND PHENOBARBITAL

Source:
Pancreatin—Obtained from pancreas of the hog, *Sus scrofa* Linné var. *domesticus* Gray (Fam. Suidae) or of the ox, *Bos taurus* Linné (Fam. Bovidae).

Naturally occurring belladonna alkaloids—Found in various solanaceous plants, including *Atropa belladonna, Datura stramonium,* and *Duboisia myoporoides.* The active alkaloids of belladonna include hyoscyamine (which racemizes to atropine on extraction) and scopolamine (hyoscine). Hyoscyamine, the levo-isomer of atropine, is the major active alkaloid of belladonna.

Chemical name:

Hyoscyamine sulfate—Benzeneacetic acid, alpha-(hydroxymethyl)-, 8-methyl-8-azabicyclo[3.2.1]oct-3-yl ester, [3(*S*)-endo]-, sulfate (2:1), dihydrate.

Atropine sulfate—Benzeneacetic acid, alpha-(hydroxymethyl)-, 8-methyl-8-azabicyclo[3.2.1]oct-3-yl ester, *endo*-(±)-, sulfate (2:1) (salt), monohydrate.

Scopolamine hydrobromide—Benzeneacetic acid, alpha-(hydroxymethyl)-, 9-methyl-3-oxa-9-azatricyclo[3.3.-1.0^{2,4}]non-7-yl ester, hydrobromide, trihydrate, [7(*S*)-(1 alpha,2 beta,4 beta,5 alpha,7 beta)]-.

Phenobarbital—2,4,6(1*H*,3*H*,5*H*)-Pyrimidinetrione, 5-ethyl-5-phenyl-.

Molecular formula:

Hyoscyamine sulfate—$(C_{17}H_{23}NO_3)_2 \cdot H_2SO_4 \cdot 2H_2O$.

Atropine sulfate—$(C_{17}H_{23}NO_3)_2 \cdot H_2SO_4 \cdot H_2O$.

Scopolamine hydrobromide—$C_{17}H_{21}NO_4 \cdot HBr \cdot 3H_2O$.

Phenobarbital—$C_{12}H_{12}N_2O_3$.

Molecular weight:

Hyoscyamine sulfate—712.85.

Atropine sulfate—694.84.

Scopolamine hydrobromide—438.31.

Phenobarbital—232.24.

Description:

Pancreatin USP—Cream-colored, amorphous powder, having a faint, characteristic, but not offensive odor. It hydrolyzes fats to glycerol and fatty acids, changes protein into proteoses and derived substances, and converts starch into dextrins and sugars. Its greatest activities are in neutral or faintly alkaline media; more than traces of mineral acids or large amounts of alkali hydroxides make it inert. An excess of alkali carbonate also inhibits its action.

Hyoscyamine Sulfate USP—White, odorless crystals or crystalline powder. Is deliquescent and is affected by light. The pH of a solution (1 in 100) is about 5.3.

Atropine Sulfate USP—Colorless crystals, or white, crystalline powder. Odorless; effloresces in dry air; is slowly affected by light.

Scopolamine Hydrobromide USP—Colorless or white crystals or white, granular powder. Is odorless, and slightly efflorescent in dry air.

Phenobarbital USP—White, odorless, glistening, small crystals, or white, crystalline powder, which may exhibit polymorphism. Is stable in air. Its saturated solution has a pH of about 5.

pKa:

Atropine—9.8.

Scopolamine—7.55–7.81.

Solubility:

Hyoscyamine Sulfate USP—Very soluble in water; freely soluble in alcohol; practically insoluble in ether.

Atropine Sulfate USP—Very soluble in water; freely soluble in alcohol and even more so in boiling alcohol; freely soluble in glycerin.

Scopolamine Hydrobromide USP—Freely soluble in water; soluble in alcohol; slightly soluble in chloroform; insoluble in ether.

Phenobarbital USP—Very slightly soluble in water; soluble in alcohol, in ether, and in solutions of fixed alkali hydroxides and carbonates; sparingly soluble in chloroform.

USP requirements: Pancreatin, Pepsin, Bile Salts, Hyoscyamine Sulfate, Atropine Sulfate, Scopolamine Hydrobromide, and Phenobarbital Tablets—Not in USP.

PANCRELIPASE

Source: Obtained from pancreas of the hog, *Sus scrofa* Linné var. *domesticus* Gray (Fam. Suidae).

Chemical name: Lipase, triacylglycerol.

Description:

Pancrelipase USP—Cream-colored, amorphous powder, having a faint, characteristic, but not offensive odor. It hydrolyzes fats to glycerol and fatty acids, changes protein into proteoses and derived substances, and converts starch into dextrins and sugars. Its greatest activities are in neutral or faintly alkaline media; more than traces of mineral acids or large amounts of alkali hydroxides make it inert. An excess of alkali carbonate also inhibits its action.

Pancrelipase Capsules USP—The contents of the Capsules conform to the Description under Pancrelipase, except that the odor may vary with the flavoring agent used.

USP requirements:

Pancrelipase Capsules USP—Preserve in tight containers, preferably with a desiccant, at a temperature not exceeding 25 °C. Label Capsules to indicate lipase activity in USP Units. Contain an amount of pancrelipase equivalent to the labeled lipase activity, within −10% to +25%, expressed in USP Units, the labeled activity being not less than 8000 USP Units per capsule. They contain, in each capsule, the pancrelipase equivalent of not less than 30,000 USP Units of amylase activity, and not less than 30,000 USP Units of protease activity. Meet the requirements for Microbial limits and Loss on drying (not more than 5.0%).

Pancrelipase Delayed-release Capsules—Not in USP.

Pancrelipase Powder—Not in USP.

Pancrelipase Tablets USP—Preserve in tight containers, preferably with a desiccant, at a temperature not exceeding 25 °C. Label Tablets to indicate the lipase activity in USP Units. Contain an amount of pancrelipase equivalent to the labeled lipase activity, within −10% to +25%, expressed in USP Units, the labeled activity being not less than 8000 USP Units per Tablet. They contain, in each Tablet, the pancrelipase equivalent of not less than 30,000 USP Units of amylase activity, and not less than 30,000 USP Units of protease activity. Meet the requirements for Microbial limits, Disintegration (75 minutes), and Loss on drying (not more than 5.0%).

Pancrelipase Delayed-release Tablets—Not in USP.

PANCURONIUM

Chemical name: Pancuronium bromide—Piperidinium, 1,1′-[(2 beta,3 alpha,5 alpha,16 beta,17 beta)-3,17-bis(acetyloxy)-androstane-2,16-diyl]bis[1-methyl]-, dibromide.

Molecular formula: Pancuronium bromide—$C_{35}H_{60}Br_2N_2O_4$.

Molecular weight: Pancuronium bromide—732.68.

Description: Pancuronium bromide—White or almost white, odorless, hygroscopic crystals or crystalline powder.

Solubility: Pancuronium bromide—Soluble 1 in 1 of water, 1 in 5 of alcohol and of chloroform, 1 in 4 of dichloromethane, and 1 in 1 of methyl alcohol; practically insoluble in ether.

USP requirements: Pancuronium Bromide Injection—Not in USP.

PANTOTHENIC ACID

Chemical name: (+)-(*R*)-3-(2,4-Dihydroxy-3,3-dimethylbutyramido)propionic acid.

Molecular formula: $C_9H_{17}NO_5$.

Molecular weight: 219.2.

Description: Unstable, viscous oil. Extremely hygroscopic.

Solubility: Freely soluble in water, in ethyl acetate, in dioxane, and in glacial acetic acid; moderately soluble in ether and in amyl alcohol; practically insoluble in chloroform.

USP requirements: Pantothenic Acid Tablets—Not in USP.

PAPAIN

Source: A purified proteolytic substance derived from *Carica papaya* Linné (Fam. Caricaceae).

Description: Papain USP—White to light tan, amorphous powder.

Solubility: Papain USP—Soluble in water, the solution being colorless to light yellow and more or less opalescent; practically insoluble in alcohol, in chloroform, and in ether.

USP requirements: Papain Tablets for Topical Solution USP—Preserve in tight, light-resistant containers in a cool place. Contain not less than 100.0% of the labeled potency. Meet the requirements for Completeness of solution, Microbial limits, Disintegration (not more than 15 minutes at 23 ± 2 °C), and pH (6.9–8.0, determined in a solution of 1 Tablet in 10 mL).

PAPAVERINE

Chemical name: Papaverine hydrochloride—Isoquinoline, 1-[(3,4-dimethoxyphenyl)methyl]-6,7-dimethoxy-, hydrochloride.

Molecular formula: Papaverine hydrochloride—$C_{20}H_{21}NO_4 \cdot$ HCl.

Molecular weight: Papaverine hydrochloride—375.85.

Description: Papaverine Hydrochloride USP—White crystals or white, crystalline powder. Odorless. Optically inactive. Its solutions are acid to litmus. Melts at about 220 °C, with decomposition.

Solubility: Papaverine Hydrochloride USP—Soluble in water and in chloroform; slightly soluble in alcohol; practically insoluble in ether.

USP requirements:
Papaverine Hydrochloride Extended-release Capsules—Not in USP.
Papaverine Hydrochloride Injection USP—Preserve in single-dose or in multiple-dose containers, preferably of Type I glass. A sterile solution of Papaverine Hydrochloride in Water for Injection. Contains the labeled amount, within ±5%. Meets the requirements for Identification, Bacterial endotoxins, pH (not less than 3.0), and Injections.
Papaverine Hydrochloride Tablets USP—Preserve in tight containers. Contain the labeled amount, within ±7%. Meet the requirements for Identification, Dissolution (80% in 30 minutes in water in Apparatus 1 at 100 rpm), and Uniformity of dosage units.

CAMPHORATED PARACHLOROPHENOL

Chemical name:
Camphor—Bicyclo[2.2.1]heptane-2-one, 1,7,7-trimethyl-.
Parachlorophenol—Phenol, 4-chloro-.

Molecular formula:
Camphor—$C_{10}H_{16}O$.
Parachlorophenol—C_6H_5ClO.

Molecular weight:
Camphor—152.24.
Parachlorophenol—128.56.

Description:
Camphor USP—Colorless or white crystals, granules, or crystalline masses; or colorless to white, translucent, tough masses. Has a penetrating, characteristic odor. Specific gravity is about 0.99. Slowly volatilizes at ordinary temperatures.
Parachlorophenol USP—White or pink crystals having a characteristic phenolic odor. When undiluted, it whitens and cauterizes the skin and mucous membranes. Melts at about 42 °C.

Solubility:
Camphor USP—Slightly soluble in water; very soluble in alcohol, in chloroform, and in ether; freely soluble in carbon disulfide, in solvent hexane, and in fixed and volatile oils.
Parachlorophenol USP—Sparingly soluble in water and in liquid petrolatum; very soluble in alcohol, in glycerin, in chloroform, in ether, and in fixed and volatile oils; soluble in petrolatum.

USP requirements: Camphorated Parachlorophenol USP—Preserve in tight, light-resistant containers. A triturated mixture. Contains not less than 33.0% and not more than 37.0% of parachlorophenol and not less than 63.0% and not more than 67.0% of camphor. The sum of the percentages of parachlorophenol and camphor is not less than 97.0% and not more than 103.0%.

PARAFFIN

Description: Paraffin NF—Colorless or white, more or less translucent mass showing a crystalline structure. Odorless. Slightly greasy to the touch.
NF category: Stiffening agent.

Solubility: Paraffin NF—Insoluble in water and in alcohol; freely soluble in chloroform, in ether, in volatile oils, and in most warm fixed oils; slightly soluble in dehydrated alcohol.

NF requirements: Paraffin NF—Preserve in well-closed containers, and avoid exposure to excessive heat. A purified mixture of solid hydrocarbons obtained from petroleum. Meets the requirements for Identification, Congealing range (47–65 °C), Reaction, and Readily carbonizable substances.

SYNTHETIC PARAFFIN

Description: Synthetic Paraffin NF—Very hard, white, practically odorless wax. Contains mostly long-chain, unbranched, saturated hydrocarbons, with a small amount of branched hydrocarbons. Is represented by the formula C_nH_{2n+2}, in which *n* may range from 20 to about 100. The average molecular weight may range from 400 to 1400.

Solubility: Synthetic Paraffin NF—Insoluble in water; very slightly soluble in aliphatic, oxygenated, and halogenated hydrocarbon solvents; slightly soluble in aromatic and normal paraffinic solvents.

NF requirements: Synthetic Paraffin NF—Preserve in well-closed containers. Synthesized by the Fischer-Tropsch process from carbon monoxide and hydrogen, which are catalytically converted to a mixture of paraffin hydrocarbons; the lower molecular weight fractions are removed by distillation, and the residue is hydrogenated and further treated by percolation through activated charcoal. This mixture may be fractionated into its components by a solvent separation method, using a suitable synthetic isoparaffinic petroleum hydrocarbon solvent. The labeling indicates its congealing temperature, viscosity, and needle penetration range under specified conditions. Meets the requirements for Identification, Absorptivity (not more than 0.01), Heavy metals (not more than 0.002%), and Oil content (not more than 0.5%).

PARALDEHYDE

Chemical name: 1,3,5-Trioxane, 2,4,6-trimethyl-.

Molecular formula: $C_6H_{12}O_3$.

Molecular weight: 132.16.

Description: Paraldehyde USP—Colorless, transparent liquid. Has a strong, characteristic but not unpleasant or pungent odor. Specific gravity is about 0.99.

Solubility: Paraldehyde USP—Soluble in water, but less soluble in boiling water. Miscible with alcohol, with chloroform, with ether, and with volatile oils.

USP requirements:
Paraldehyde USP—Preserve in well-filled, tight, light-resistant containers, preferably of Type I or Type II glass, holding not more than 30 mL, at a temperature not exceeding 25 °C. Paraldehyde may be shipped in bulk containers holding a minimum of 22.5 kg (50 lb) to commercial drug repackagers only. The label of all containers of Paraldehyde, including those dispensed by the pharmacist, includes a statement directing the user to discard the unused contents of any container that has been opened for more than 24 hours. (Note: The label of bulk containers of Paraldehyde directs the commercial drug repackager to demonstrate compliance with the USP purity tests for Paraldehyde immediately prior to repackaging, and not to repackage from a container that has been opened longer than 24 hours.) Meets the requirements for Identification, Congealing temperature (not lower than 11 °C), Distilling range (120–126 °C), Acidity (not more than 0.5% as acetic acid), Nonvolatile residue (not more than 0.06%), Chloride, Sulfate, and Acetaldehyde (not more than 0.4%).
Note: Paraldehyde is subject to oxidation to form acetic acid. It may contain a suitable stabilizer.
Sterile Paraldehyde—Not in USP.

PARAMETHADIONE

Chemical group: Oxazolidinedione.

Chemical name: 2,4-Oxazolidinedione, 5-ethyl-3,5-dimethyl-.

Molecular formula: $C_7H_{11}NO_3$.

Molecular weight: 157.17.

Description: Paramethadione USP—Clear, colorless liquid. May have an aromatic odor. A solution (1 in 40) has a pH of about 6.

Solubility: Paramethadione USP—Sparingly soluble in water; freely soluble in alcohol, in chloroform, and in ether.

USP requirements:
Paramethadione Capsules USP—Preserve in tight containers. Contain the labeled amount, within ±10%. Meet the requirements for Identification and Uniformity of dosage units.

Paramethadione Oral Solution USP—Preserve in tight, light-resistant containers. A solution of Paramethadione in dilute Alcohol. Contains, in each mL, not less than 282 mg and not more than 318 mg of paramethadione. Meets the requirements for Identification and Alcohol content (62.0–68.0%).

PARAMETHASONE

Chemical name: Paramethasone acetate—Pregna-1,4-diene-3,20-dione, 21-(acetyloxy)-6-fluoro-11,17-dihydroxy-16-methyl-, (6 alpha,11 beta,16 alpha)-.

Molecular formula: Paramethasone acetate—$C_{24}H_{31}FO_6$.

Molecular weight: Paramethasone acetate—434.50.

Description: Paramethasone Acetate USP—Fluffy, white to creamy white, odorless, crystalline powder. Melts at about 240 °C, with decomposition.

Solubility: Paramethasone Acetate USP—Insoluble in water; soluble in chloroform, in ether, and in methanol.

USP requirements: Paramethasone Acetate Tablets USP—Preserve in well-closed containers. Contain the labeled amount, within ±15%. Meet the requirements for Identification, Disintegration (15 minutes, the use of disks being omitted), and Uniformity of dosage units.

PAREGORIC

USP requirements: Paregoric USP—Preserve in tight, light-resistant containers, and avoid exposure to direct sunlight and to excessive heat. Yields, from each 100 mL, not less than 35 mg and not more than 45 mg of anhydrous morphine.

Paregoric may be prepared as follows: 4.3 grams of Powdered Opium, Suitable essential oil(s), 3.8 grams of Benzoic Acid, 900 mL of Diluted Alcohol, and 38 mL of Glycerin to make about 950 mL. Macerate for 5 days the Powdered Opium, Benzoic Acid, and essential oil(s), with occasional agitation, in a mixture of 900 mL of Diluted Alcohol and 38 mL of Glycerin. Then filter, and pass enough Diluted Alcohol through the filter to obtain 950 mL of total filtrate. Assay a portion of this filtrate as directed, and dilute the remainder with a sufficient quantity of Diluted Alcohol containing, in each 100 mL, 400 mg of Benzoic Acid, 4 mL of Glycerin, and sufficient essential oil(s) to yield a solution containing, in each 100 mL, 40 mg of anhydrous morphine.

Meets the requirement for Alcohol content (43.0–47.0%).

Note: Paregoric may be prepared also by using Opium or Opium Tincture instead of Powdered Opium, the anhydrous morphine content being adjusted to 40 mg in each 100 mL and the alcohol content being adjusted to 45%.

PARGYLINE

Chemical name: Pargyline hydrochloride—Benzenemethanamine, N-methyl-N-2-propynyl-, hydrochloride.

Molecular formula: Pargyline hydrochloride—$C_{11}H_{13}N \cdot HCl$.

Molecular weight: Pargyline hydrochloride—195.69.

Description: Pargyline Hydrochloride USP—White or practically white, crystalline powder, having a slight odor. Sublimes slowly at elevated temperatures.

Solubility: Pargyline Hydrochloride USP—Very soluble in water; freely soluble in alcohol and in chloroform; very slightly soluble in acetone.

USP requirements: Pargyline Hydrochloride Tablets USP—Preserve in well-closed containers. Contain the labeled amount, within ±10%. Meet the requirements for Identification, Dissolution (70% in 60 minutes in phosphate buffer [pH 6.0] in Apparatus 2 at 100 rpm), and Uniformity of dosage units.

PARGYLINE AND METHYCLOTHIAZIDE

For *Pargyline* and *Methyclothiazide*—See individual listings for chemistry information.

USP requirements: Pargyline Hydrochloride and Methyclothiazide Tablets—Not in USP.

PAROMOMYCIN

Chemical name: Paromomycin sulfate—D-Streptamine, O-2-amino-2-deoxy-alpha-D-glucopyranosyl-(1→4)-O-[O-2,6-di-amino-2,6-dideoxy-beta-L-idopyranosyl-(1→3)-beta-D-ribo-furanosyl-(1→5)]-2-deoxy-, sulfate (salt).

Molecular formula: Paromomycin sulfate—$C_{23}H_{45}N_5O_{14} \cdot xH_2SO_4$.

Molecular weight: Paromomycin (base)—615.63.

Description: Paromomycin Sulfate USP—Creamy white to light yellow powder. Odorless or practically so. Very hygroscopic.

Solubility: Paromomycin Sulfate USP—Very soluble in water; insoluble in alcohol, in chloroform, and in ether.

USP requirements:
Paromomycin Sulfate Capsules USP—Preserve in tight containers. Contain an amount of paromomycin sulfate equivalent to the labeled amount of paromomycin, within −10% to +25%. Meet the requirements for Identification, Disintegration (15 minutes, the use of disks being omitted), Uniformity of dosage units, and Loss on drying (not more than 7.0%).
Paromomycin Sulfate Syrup USP—Preserve in tight containers. Contains an amount of paromomycin sulfate equivalent to the labeled amount of paromomycin, within −10% to +30%. Meets the requirements for pH (7.5–8.5), Deliverable volume (multiple-unit containers), and Uniformity of dosage units (single-unit containers).

PEANUT OIL

Description: Peanut Oil NF—Colorless or pale yellow oily liquid. May have a characteristic, nutty odor.

NF category: Solvent; vehicle (oleaginous).

Solubility: Peanut Oil NF—Very slightly soluble in alcohol. Miscible with ether, with chloroform, and with carbon disulfide.

NF requirements: Peanut Oil NF—Preserve in tight, light-resistant containers, and prevent exposure to excessive heat. It is the refined fixed oil obtained from the seed kernels of one or more of the cultivated varieties of *Arachis hypogaea* Linné (Fam. Leguminosae). Meets the requirements for Identification, Specific gravity (0.912–0.920), Refractive index (1.462–1.464 at 40 °C), Heavy metals (not more than 0.001%), Cottonseed oil, Rancidity, Solidification range of fatty acids (26–33 °C), Free fatty acids, Iodine value (84–100), Saponification value (185–195), and Unsaponifiable matter (not more than 1.5%).

PECTIN

Chemical name: Pectin.

Description: Pectin USP—Coarse or fine powder, yellowish white in color, almost odorless.
NF category: Suspending and/or viscosity-increasing agent.

Solubility: Pectin USP—Almost completely soluble in 20 parts of water, forming a viscous, opalescent, colloidal solution that flows readily and is acid to litmus. Is practically insoluble in alcohol or in diluted alcohol and in other organic solvents. Pectin dissolves in water more readily if first moistened with alcohol, glycerin, or simple syrup, or if first mixed with 3 or more parts of sucrose.

USP requirements: Pectin USP—Preserve in tight containers. A purified carbohydrate product obtained from the dilute acid extract of the inner portion of the rind of citrus fruits or from apple pomace. Consists chiefly of partially methoxylated polygalacturonic acids. Label it to indicate whether it is of apple or of citrus origin. Pectin yields not less than 6.7% of methoxy groups and not less than 74.0% of galacturonic acid, calculated on the dried basis. Meets the requirements for Identification, Microbial limit, Loss on drying (not more than 10.0%), Arsenic (not more than 3 ppm), Lead, and Sugars and organic acids.

Note: Commercial pectin for the production of jellied food products is standardized to the convenient "150 jelly grade" by addition of dextrose or other sugars, and sometimes contains sodium citrate or other buffer salts. This monograph refers to the pure pectin to which no such additions have been made.

PEG 3350 AND ELECTROLYTES

For *Polyethylene Glycol, Sodium Bicarbonate, Sodium Chloride, Sodium Sulfate,* and *Potassium Chloride*—See individual listings for chemistry information.

USP requirements: PEG 3350 and Electrolytes for Oral Solution USP—Preserve in tight containers. A mixture of Polyethylene Glycol 3350, Sodium Bicarbonate, Sodium Chloride, Sodium Sulfate (anhydrous), and Potassium Chloride. When constituted as directed in the labeling it contains the labeled amounts of polyethylene glycol 3350, potassium, sodium, bicarbonate, chloride, and sulfate, within ±10%, the labeled amounts per liter being 10 mmol (10 mEq) of potassium, 125 mmol (125 mEq) of sodium, 20 mmol (20 mEq) of bicarbonate, 35 mmol (35 mEq) of chloride, and 40 mmol (80 mEq) of sulfate. Meets the requirements for Completeness of solution, Identification, pH (7.5–9.5, in the solution prepared as directed in the labeling), Uniformity of dosage units, and Osmolarity (235–304 mOsmol, in the solution prepared as directed in the labeling).

PEGADEMASE

Source: Pegademase bovine—A conjugate of numerous strands of monomethoxypolyethylene glycol (PEG), covalently attached to the enzyme adenosine deaminase (ADA); ADA used in the manufacture of pegademase bovine is derived from bovine intestine.

Chemical name: Pegademase bovine—Deaminase, adenosine, cattle, reaction product with succinic anhydride, esters with polyethylene glycol, mono-Me ether.

Molecular weight: Pegademase bovine—5,000.

Description: Pegademase bovine injection—Clear, colorless solution; pH 7.2–7.4.

USP requirements: Pegademase Bovine Injection—Not in USP.

PEMOLINE

Chemical group: Oxazolidine.

Chemical name: 4(5*H*)-Oxazolone, 2-amino-5-phenyl-.

Molecular formula: $C_9H_8N_2O_2$.

Molecular weight: 176.17.

Description: White, odorless powder.

Solubility: Relatively insoluble (less than 1 mg/mL) in water, in chloroform, in ether, and in acetone; solubility in 95% ethyl alcohol 2.2 mg/mL.

USP requirements:
Pemoline Tablets—Not in USP.
Pemoline Chewable Tablets—Not in USP.

PENBUTOLOL

Chemical name: Penbutolol sulfate—2-Propanol, 1-(2-cyclopentylphenoxy)-3-[(1,1-dimethylethyl)amino]-, (*S*)-, sulfate (2:1) (salt).

Molecular formula: Penbutolol sulfate—$(C_{18}H_{29}NO_2)_2 \cdot H_2SO_4$.

Molecular weight: Penbutolol sulfate—680.94.

Description: White, odorless, crystalline powder.

pKa: 9.3.

Solubility: Soluble in methanol, in ethanol, and in chloroform.

Other characteristics: Lipid solubility—Moderate.

USP requirements: Penbutolol Sulfate Tablets—Not in USP.

PENICILLAMINE

Chemical name: D-Valine, 3-mercapto-.

Molecular formula: $C_5H_{11}NO_2S$.

Molecular weight: 149.21.

Description: Penicillamine USP—White or practically white, crystalline powder, having a slight, characteristic odor.

Solubility: Penicillamine USP—Freely soluble in water; slightly soluble in alcohol; insoluble in chloroform and in ether.

USP requirements:
Penicillamine Capsules USP—Preserve in tight containers. Contain the labeled amount, within ±10%. Meet the requirements for Identification, Dissolution (80% in 30 minutes in 0.1 *N* hydrochloric acid in Apparatus 1 at 100 rpm), Uniformity of dosage units, and Water (not more than 7.5%).
Penicillamine Tablets USP—Preserve in tight containers. Contain the labeled amount, within ±10%. Meet the requirements for Identification, Dissolution (60% in 60 minutes in 0.5% disodium EDTA in Apparatus 1 at 150 rpm), Uniformity of dosage units, and Loss on drying (not more than 3.0%).

PENICILLIN G

Chemical name:
Penicillin G—4-Thia-1-azabicyclo[3.2.0]heptane-2-carboxylic acid, 3,3-dimethyl-7-oxo-6-[(phenylacetyl)amino]-, [2*S*-(2 alpha,5 alpha,6 beta)]-.
Penicillin G benzathine—4-Thia-1-azabicyclo[3.2.0]heptane-2-carboxylic acid, 3,3-dimethyl-7-oxo-6-[(phenylacetyl)-amino]-, [2*S*-(2 alpha,5 alpha,6 beta)]-, compd. with

N,N′-bis(phenylmethyl)-1,2-ethanediamine (2:1), tetrahydrate.
Penicillin G potassium—4-Thia-1-azabicyclo[3.2.0]heptane-2-carboxylic acid, 3,3-dimethyl-7-oxo-6-[(phenylacetyl)amino]-, monopotassium salt, [2*S*-(2 alpha,5 alpha,6 beta)]-.
Penicillin G procaine—4-Thia-1-azabicyclo[3.2.0]heptane-2-carboxylic acid, 3,3-dimethyl-7-oxo-6-[(phenylacetyl)amino]-, [2*S*-(2 alpha,5 alpha,6 beta)]-, compd. with 2-(diethylamino)ethyl 4-aminobenzoate (1:1) monohydrate.
Penicillin G sodium (sterile)—4-Thia-1-azabicyclo-[3.2.0]heptane-2-carboxylic acid, 3,3-dimethyl-7-oxo-6-[(phenylacetyl)amino]-, [2*S*-(2 alpha,5 alpha,6 beta)]-, monosodium salt.

Molecular formula:
Penicillin G benzathine—$(C_{16}H_{18}N_2O_4S)_2 \cdot C_{16}H_{20}N_2 \cdot 4H_2O$.
Penicillin G potassium—$C_{16}H_{17}KN_2O_4S$.
Penicillin G procaine—$C_{16}H_{18}N_2O_4S \cdot C_{13}H_{20}N_2O_2 \cdot H_2O$.
Penicillin G sodium—$C_{16}H_{17}N_2NaO_4S$.

Molecular weight:
Penicillin G benzathine—981.19.
Penicillin G potassium—372.48.
Penicillin G procaine—588.72.
Penicillin G sodium—356.37.

Description:
Penicillin G Benzathine USP—White, odorless, crystalline powder.
Sterile Penicillin G Potassium USP—Colorless or white crystals, or white, crystalline powder. Is odorless or practically so, and is moderately hygroscopic. Its solutions are dextrorotatory. Its solutions retain substantially full potency for several days at temperatures below 15 °C, but are rapidly inactivated by acids, alkali hydroxides, glycerin, and oxidizing agents.
Sterile Penicillin G Procaine USP—White crystals or white, very fine, microcrystalline powder. Is odorless or practically odorless, and is relatively stable in air. Its solutions are dextrorotatory. Is rapidly inactivated by acids, by alkali hydroxides, and by oxidizing agents.
Sterile Penicillin G Sodium USP—Colorless or white crystals or white to slightly yellow, crystalline powder. Is odorless or practically odorless, and is moderately hygroscopic. Its solutions are dextrorotatory. Is relatively stable in air, but is inactivated by prolonged heating at about 100 °C, especially in the presence of moisture. Its solutions lose potency fairly rapidly at room temperature, but retain substantially full potency for several days at temperatures below 15 °C. Its solutions are rapidly inactivated by acids, alkali hydroxides, oxidizing agents, and penicillinase.

Solubility:
Penicillin G Benzathine USP—Very slightly soluble in water; sparingly soluble in alcohol.
Sterile Penicillin G Potassium USP—Very soluble in water, in saline TS, and in dextrose solutions; sparingly soluble in alcohol.
Sterile Penicillin G Procaine USP—Slightly soluble in water; soluble in alcohol and in chloroform.

USP requirements:
Sterile Penicillin G Benzathine USP—Preserve in Containers for Sterile Solids. It is Penicillin G Benzathine suitable for parenteral use. Has a potency of not less than 1090 and not more than 1272 Penicillin G Units per mg. Meets the requirements for Bacterial endotoxins and Sterility, and for Identification test, pH, Water, Crystallinity, Penicillin G content, and Benzathine content under Penicillin G Benzathine.

Penicillin G Benzathine Oral Suspension USP—Preserve in tight containers. Contains an amount of penicillin G benzathine equivalent to the labeled amount of penicillin G, within −10% to +20%. Contains one or more suitable buffers, colors, dispersants, flavors, and preservatives. Meets the requirements for Identification, pH (6.0–7.0), Uniformity of dosage units (single-unit containers), and Deliverable volume (multiple-unit containers).

Sterile Penicillin G Benzathine Suspension USP—Preserve in single-dose or in multiple-dose containers, preferably of Type I or Type II glass, in a refrigerator. A sterile suspension of Sterile Penicillin G Benzathine in Water for Injection with one or more suitable buffers, dispersants, preservatives, and suspending agents. Contains an amount of penicillin G benzathine equivalent to the labeled amount of penicillin G, within −10% to +15%. Meets the requirements for Identification, Bacterial endotoxins, Sterility, pH (5.0–7.5), and Injections.

Penicillin G Benzathine Tablets USP—Preserve in tight containers. Contain an amount of penicillin G benzathine equivalent to the labeled amount of penicillin G, within −10% to +20%. Meet the requirements for Identification, Disintegration (60 minutes in simulated gastric fluid TS), Uniformity of dosage units, and Water (not more than 8.0%).

Sterile Penicillin G Benzathine and Penicillin G Procaine Suspension USP—Preserve in single-dose or in multiple-dose containers, preferably of Type I or Type III glass. A sterile suspension of Sterile Penicillin G Benzathine and Sterile Penicillin G Procaine in Water for Injection. Contains the labeled amounts, within −10% to +15%. Meets the requirements for Identification and pH (5.0–7.5), for Pyrogen and Sterility under Sterile Penicillin G Procaine Suspension, and for Injections.

Penicillin G Potassium Capsules USP—Preserve in tight containers. Contain the labeled number of Penicillin G Units, within −10% to +20%. Meet the requirements for Identification, Dissolution (75% in 45 minutes in phosphate buffer [pH 6.0] in Apparatus 1 at 100 rpm), Uniformity of dosage units, and Loss on drying (not more than 1.5%).

Penicillin G Potassium Injection USP—Preserve in single-dose containers. Maintain in the frozen state. A sterile isoosmotic solution of Penicillin G Potassium in Water for Injection. Contains one or more suitable buffers and a tonicity-adjusting agent. The label states that it is to be thawed just prior to use, describes conditions for proper storage of the resultant solution, and directs that the solution is not to be refrozen. Contains the labeled number of Penicillin G Units, within −10% to +15%. Meets the requirements for Identification, Bacterial endotoxins, Sterility, pH (5.5–8.0), Particulate matter, and Labeling under Injections.

Penicillin G Potassium for Injection USP—Preserve in Containers for Sterile Solids. A sterile, dry mixture of Penicillin G Potassium with not less than 4.0% and not more than 5.0% of Sodium Citrate, of which not more than 0.15% may be replaced by Citric Acid. It has a potency of not less than 1355 and not more than 1595 Penicillin G Units per mg and, where packaged for dispensing, contains the labeled number of Penicillin G Units within −10% to +20%. Meets the requirements for Constituted solution, Identification, Crystallinity, Bacterial endotoxins, Sterility, pH (6.0–8.5, in a solution containing 60 mg per mL or, where packaged for dispensing, in the solution constituted as directed in the labeling), Loss on drying (not more than 1.5%), Particulate matter, and Penicillin G content (76.3–89.8%), and for Uniformity of dosage units, and Labeling under Injections.

Penicillin G Potassium for Oral Solution USP—Preserve in tight containers. A dry mixture of Penicillin G Potassium and one or more suitable buffers, colors, diluents, flavors, and preservatives. Contains the labeled number of Penicillin G Units when constituted as directed in the labeling, within −10% to +30%. Meets the requirements for Identification, pH (5.5–7.5, in the solution constituted as directed in the labeling), Water (not more than 1.0%), Uniformity of dosage units (single-unit containers), and Deliverable volume (multiple-unit containers).

Sterile Penicillin G Potassium USP—Preserve in Containers for Sterile Solids. It is Penicillin G Potassium suitable for parenteral use. It has a potency of not less than 1440 Penicillin G Units and not more than 1680 Penicillin G Units per mg and, where packaged for dispensing, contains the labeled number of Penicillin G Units, within −10% to +15%. Meets the requirements for Constituted solution, Bacterial endotoxins, Sterility, and Particulate matter, for Identification tests, pH (5.0–7.5, in a solution containing 60 mg per mL), Loss on drying (not more than 1.5%), Crystallinity, and Penicillin G content (80.8–94.3%) under Penicillin G Potassium, and for Uniformity of dosage units and Labeling under Injections.

Penicillin G Potassium Tablets USP—Preserve in tight containers. Contain the labeled number of Penicillin G Units, within −10% to +20%. Meet the requirements for Identification, Dissolution (70% in 60 minutes in phosphate buffer [pH 6.0] in Apparatus 2 at 75 rpm), Uniformity of dosage units, and Loss on drying (not more than 1.0%).

Penicillin G Potassium Tablets for Oral Solution USP—Preserve in tight containers. Contain the labeled number of Penicillin G Units, within −10% to +20%. Meet the requirements for Identification and Loss on drying (not more than 1.0%), and for Uniformity of dosage units under Penicillin G Potassium Tablets.

Penicillin G Procaine Intramammary Infusion USP—Preserve in well-closed disposable syringes. A suspension of Penicillin G Procaine in a suitable vegetable oil vehicle. Label it to indicate that it is for veterinary use only. Contains an amount of penicillin G procaine equivalent to the labeled amount of penicillin G, within −10% to +15%. Meets the requirements for Identification and Water (not more than 1.4%).

Sterile Penicillin G Procaine USP—Preserve in Containers for Sterile Solids. It is penicillin G procaine suitable for parenteral use. Has a potency of not less than 900 Penicillin G Units and not more than 1050 Penicillin G Units per mg. Meets the requirements for Identification, Crystallinity, Bacterial endotoxins, Sterility, pH (5.0–7.5, in a [saturated] solution containing about 300 mg per mL), Water (2.8–4.2%), and Penicillin G and procaine contents (37.5–43.0%).

Sterile Penicillin G Procaine Suspension USP—Preserve in single-dose or in multiple-dose containers, preferably of Type I or Type III glass, in a refrigerator. A sterile suspension of Sterile Penicillin G Procaine in Water for Injection and contains one or more suitable buffers, dispersants, or suspending agents, and a suitable preservative. It may contain procaine hydrochloride in a concentration not exceeding 2.0%. Contains an amount of penicillin G procaine equivalent to the labeled amount of penicillin G, within −10% to +15%, the labeled amount being not less than 300,000 Penicillin G Units per mL or per container. Meets the requirements for Identification, Pyrogen, Sterility, pH (5.0–7.5), and for Injections.

Sterile Penicillin G Procaine for Suspension USP—Preserve in single-dose or in multiple-dose containers, preferably of Type I or Type III glass. A sterile mixture of Sterile Penicillin G Procaine and one or more suitable buffers, dispersants, or suspending agents, and preservatives. Contains an amount of penicillin G procaine equivalent to the labeled amount of penicillin G, within −10% to +15%, the labeled amount being not less than 300,000 Penicillin G Units per container or per mL of constituted Suspension. Meets the requirements for Identification, pH (5.0–7.5, when constituted as directed in the labeling), and Water (2.8–4.2%), for Pyrogen and Sterility under Sterile Penicillin G Procaine Suspension, and for Injections and Uniformity of dosage units.

Penicillin G Sodium for Injection USP—Preserve in Containers for Sterile Solids. A sterile mixture of penicillin G sodium with not less than 4.0% and not more than 5.0% of Sodium Citrate, of which not more than 0.15% may be replaced by Citric Acid. It has a potency of not less than 1420 Penicillin G Units and not more than 1667 Penicillin G Units per mg and, where packaged for dispensing, contains an amount of penicillin G sodium equivalent to the labeled amount of penicillin G, within −10% to +20%. Meets the requirements for Constituted solution, Identification, Crystallinity, Bacterial endotoxins, pH (6.0–7.5, in a solution containing 60 mg per mL), Loss on drying (not more than 1.5%), Particulate matter, and Penicillin G content (80.0–93.8%), for Sterility under Sterile Penicillin G Sodium, and for Uniformity of dosage units and Labeling under Injections.

Note: It contains 2.0 mEq of sodium per million Penicillin G Units.

Sterile Penicillin G Sodium USP—Preserve in containers for Sterile Solids. It is penicillin G sodium suitable for parenteral use. It has a potency of not less than 1500 Penicillin G Units and not more than 1750 Penicillin G Units per mg. In addition, where packaged for dispensing, contains an amount of penicillin G sodium equivalent to the labeled amount of penicillin G, within −10% to +15%. Meets the requirements for Constituted solution, Identification, Crystallinity, Bacterial endotoxins, Sterility, pH (5.0–7.5, in a solution containing 60 mg per mL), Loss on drying (not more than 1.5%), Particulate matter, and Penicillin G content (84.5–98.5%), and for Uniformity of dosage units and Labeling under Injections.

PENICILLIN G PROCAINE AND ALUMINUM STEARATE

Chemical name:
Penicillin G procaine—4-Thia-1-azabicyclo[3.2.0]heptane-2-carboxylic acid, 3,3-dimethyl-7-oxo-6-[(phenylacetyl)-amino]-,[2S-(2alpha,5alpha,6beta]-,compd.with2-(diethyl-amino)ethyl 4-aminobenzoate (1:1) monohydrate.
Aluminum stearate—Octadecanoic acid aluminum salt.

Molecular formula:
Penicillin G procaine—$C_{16}H_{18}N_2O_4S \cdot C_{13}H_{20}N_2O_2 \cdot H_2O$.
Aluminum stearate—$C_{54}H_{105}AlO_6$.

Molecular weight:
Penicillin G procaine—588.72.
Aluminum stearate—877.35.

Description: Aluminum stearate—Melting point 117–120 °C.

Solubility: Aluminum stearate—Practically insoluble in water; when freshly made, soluble in alcohol, in oil turpentine, and in mineral oils.

USP requirements: Sterile Penicillin G Procaine with Aluminum Stearate Suspension USP—Preserve in single-dose or in multiple-dose containers, preferably of Type I or Type III glass. A sterile suspension of Sterile Penicillin G Procaine in a refined vegetable oil with one or more suitable dispersants and hardening agents. Contains an amount of penicillin G procaine equivalent to the labeled amount of penicillin G, within −10% to +15%. Meets the requirements for Bacterial endotoxins, Sterility, Water (not more than 1.4%), and Injections.

PENICILLIN G PROCAINE AND DIHYDROSTREPTOMYCIN

For *Penicillin G Procaine* and *Dihydrostreptomycin*—See individual listings for chemistry information.

USP requirements:
Penicillin G Procaine and Dihydrostreptomycin Sulfate Intramammary Infusion USP—Preserve in well-closed, disposable syringes. A suspension of Penicillin G Procaine and Dihydrostreptomycin Sulfate in a suitable vegetable oil vehicle. Label it to indicate that it is intended for veterinary use only. Contains amounts of penicillin G procaine and dihydrostreptomycin sulfate equivalent to the labeled amounts of Penicillin G Units and dihydrostreptomycin, within −10% to +20%. Meets the requirements for Identification and Water (not more than 1.4%).

Sterile Penicillin G Procaine and Dihydrostreptomycin Sulfate Suspension USP—Preserve in single-dose or in multiple-dose, tight containers. A sterile suspension of Sterile Penicillin G Procaine in a solution of Dihydrostreptomycin Sulfate in Water for Injection, and contains one or more suitable buffers, preservatives, and dispersing or suspending agents. May contain Procaine Hydrochloride in a concentration not exceeding 2.0%. Label it to indicate that it is intended for veterinary use only. Contains amounts of penicillin G procaine and dihydrostreptomycin sulfate equivalent to the labeled amounts of Penicillin G Units and dihydrostreptomycin, within −10% to +15%. Meets the requirements for Pyrogen, Sterility, and pH (5.0–8.0).

PENICILLIN G PROCAINE, DIHYDROSTREPTOMYCIN, CHLORPHENIRAMINE, AND DEXAMETHASONE

For *Penicillin G Procaine, Dihydrostreptomycin, Chlorpheniramine,* and *Dexamethasone*—See individual listings for chemistry information.

USP requirements: Sterile Penicillin G Procaine, Dihydrostreptomycin Sulfate, Chlorpheniramine Maleate, and Dexamethasone Suspension USP—Preserve in single-dose or in multiple-dose, tight containers, in a cool place. A sterile suspension of Sterile Penicillin G Procaine and Dexamethasone in a solution of Sterile Dihydrostreptomycin Sulfate and Chlorpheniramine Maleate in Water for Injection. Label it to indicate that it is intended for veterinary use only. Contains one or more suitable buffers, preservatives, and dispersing or suspending agents. May contain Procaine Hydrochloride in a concentration not exceeding 2.0%. Contains amounts of penicillin G procaine and dihydrostreptomycin sulfate equivalent to the labeled amounts of Penicillin G Units and dihydrostreptomycin, within −10% to +15%. Contains the labeled amounts of chlorpheniramine maleate and dexamethasone, within ±10%. Meets the requirements for Identification, Bacterial endotoxins, and pH (5.0–6.0), for Sterility under Sterile Penicillin G Procaine and Dihydrostreptomycin Sulfate Suspension, and for Injections.

PENICILLIN G PROCAINE, DIHYDROSTREPTOMYCIN, AND PREDNISOLONE

For *Penicillin G Procaine, Dihydrostreptomycin,* and *Prednisolone*—See individual listings for chemistry information.

USP requirements: Sterile Penicillin G Procaine, Dihydrostreptomycin Sulfate, and Prednisolone Suspension USP—Preserve in single-dose or in multiple-dose, tight containers. A sterile suspension of Sterile Penicillin G Procaine and Prednisolone in a solution of Sterile Dihydrostreptomycin Sulfate in Water for Injection. Contains one or more suitable buffers, dispersants, preservatives, and suspending agents. Label it to indicate that it is intended for veterinary use only, and is not to be used in animals to be slaughtered for human consumption. Contains amounts of penicillin G procaine and dihydrostreptomycin sulfate equivalent to the labeled number of Penicillin G Units, within −10% to +15%, and the labeled amount of dihydrostreptomycin, within −10% to +15%. Contains the labeled amount of prednisolone, within ±10%. Meets the requirements for Bacterial endotoxins, and for Sterility and pH under Sterile Penicillin G Procaine and Dihydrostreptomycin Sulfate Suspension.

PENICILLIN G PROCAINE, NEOMYCIN, POLYMYXIN B, AND HYDROCORTISONE

For *Penicillin G Procaine, Neomycin, Polymyxin B,* and *Hydrocortisone*—See individual listings for chemistry information.

USP requirements: Penicillin G Procaine, Neomycin and Polymyxin B Sulfates, and Hydrocortisone Acetate Topical Suspension USP—Preserve in well-closed containers. A suspension of Penicillin G Procaine, Neomycin Sulfate, Polymyxin B Sulfate, and Hydrocortisone Acetate in Peanut Oil or Sesame Oil. Label it to indicate that it is intended for veterinary use only. Contains amounts of penicillin G procaine, neomycin sulfate, and polymyxin B sulfate equivalent to the labeled amounts of Penicillin G Units, neomycin, and polymyxin B Units, within −10% to +40%. Contains the labeled amount of hydrocortisone acetate, within ±10%. Meets the requirement for Water (not more than 1.0%).

PENICILLIN G PROCAINE AND NOVOBIOCIN

For *Penicillin G Procaine* and *Novobiocin*—See individual listings for chemistry information.

USP requirements: Penicillin G Procaine and Novobiocin Sodium Intramammary Infusion USP—Preserve in disposable syringes that are well-closed containers. A suspension of Penicillin G Procaine and Novobiocin Sodium in a suitable vegetable oil vehicle. Contains a suitable preservative and suspending agent. Label it to indicate that it is for veterinary use only. Contains amounts of penicillin G procaine and novobiocin sodium equivalent to the labeled amounts of Penicillin G Units and novobiocin, within −10% to +25%. Meets the requirement for Water (not more than 1.0%).

PENICILLIN V

Chemical name:
Penicillin V—4-Thia-1-azabicyclo[3.2.0]heptane-2-carboxylic acid, 3,3-dimethyl-7-oxo-6-[(phenoxyacetyl)amino]-, [2S-(2 alpha,5 alpha,6 beta)]-.
Penicillin V benzathine—4-Thia-1-azabicyclo[3.2.0]heptane-2-carboxylic acid, 3,3-dimethyl-7-oxo-6-[(phenoxyacetyl)amino]-, [2S-(2 alpha,5 alpha,6 beta)]-, compd. with N,N'-bis(phenylmethyl)-1,2-ethanediamine (2:1).
Penicillin V potassium—4-Thia-1-azabicyclo[3.2.0]heptane-2-carboxylic acid, 3,3-dimethyl-7-oxo-6-[(phenoxyacetyl)amino]-, monopotassium salt, [2S-(2 alpha,5 alpha,6 beta)]-.

Molecular formula:
Penicillin V—$C_{16}H_{18}N_2O_5S$.
Penicillin V benzathine—$(C_{16}H_{18}N_2O_5S)_2 \cdot C_{16}H_{20}N_2$.
Penicillin V potassium—$C_{16}H_{17}KN_2O_5S$.

Molecular weight:
Penicillin V—350.39.
Penicillin V benzathine—941.12.
Penicillin V potassium—388.48.

Description:
Penicillin V USP—White, odorless, crystalline powder.

Penicillin V Benzathine USP—Practically white powder, having a characteristic odor.
Penicillin V Potassium USP—White, odorless, crystalline powder.

Solubility:
Penicillin V USP—Very slightly soluble in water; freely soluble in alcohol and in acetone; insoluble in fixed oils.
Penicillin V Benzathine USP—Very slightly soluble in water; slightly soluble in alcohol and in ether; sparingly soluble in chloroform.
Penicillin V Potassium USP—Very soluble in water; slightly soluble in alcohol; insoluble in acetone.

USP requirements:
Penicillin V for Oral Suspension USP—Preserve in tight containers. A dry mixture of Penicillin V with or without one or more suitable buffers, colors, flavors, and suspending agents. It may be labeled in terms of the weight of penicillin V contained therein, in addition to or instead of Units, on the basis that 1600 Penicillin V Units are equivalent to 1 mg of penicillin V. Contains the labeled number of Penicillin V Units, within −10% to +20%, when constituted as directed. Meets the requirements for Identification, Uniformity of dosage units (single-unit containers), Deliverable volume (multiple-unit containers), pH (2.0–4.0, in the suspension constituted as directed in the labeling), and Water (not more than 1.0%).

Penicillin V Tablets USP—Preserve in tight containers. Tablets may be labeled in terms of the weight of penicillin V contained therein, in addition to or instead of Units, on the basis that 1600 Penicillin V Units are equivalent to 1 mg of penicillin V. Contain the labeled number of Penicillin V Units, within −10% to +20%. Meet the requirements for Identification, Dissolution (75% in 45 minutes in water in Apparatus 2 at 50 rpm), Uniformity of dosage units, and Water (not more than 3.0%).

Penicillin V Benzathine Oral Suspension USP—Preserve in tight containers, and store in a refrigerator. It may be labeled in terms of the weight of penicillin V contained therein, in addition to or instead of Units, on the basis that 1600 Penicillin V Units are equivalent to 1 mg of penicillin V. Contains the labeled number of Penicillin V Units, within −10% to +20%. It contains one or more suitable buffers, colors, dispersants, flavors, and preservatives. Meets the requirements for Uniformity of dosage units (single-unit containers), Deliverable volume (multiple-unit containers), and pH (6.0–7.0).

Penicillin V Potassium for Oral Solution USP—Preserve in tight containers. A dry mixture of Penicillin V Potassium with or without one or more suitable buffers, colors, flavors, preservatives, and suspending agents. It may be labeled in terms of the weight of penicillin V contained therein, in addition to or instead of Units, on the basis that 1600 Penicillin V Units are equivalent to 1 mg of penicillin V. Contains the labeled number of Penicillin V Units, within −10% to +35%, when constituted as directed. Meets the requirements for Identification, pH (5.0–7.5, when constituted as directed in the labeling), Water (not more than 1.0%), Uniformity of dosage units (single-unit containers), and Deliverable volume (multiple-unit containers).

Penicillin V Potassium Tablets USP—Preserve in tight containers. Label chewable Tablets to indicate that they are to be chewed before swallowing. Tablets may be labeled in terms of the weight of penicillin V contained therein, in addition to or instead of Units, on the basis that 1600 Penicillin V Units are equivalent to 1 mg of penicillin V. Contain the labeled number of Penicillin V Units, within −10% to +20%. Meet the requirements for Identification, Dissolution (75% in 45 minutes in phosphate buffer [pH 6.0] in Apparatus 2 at 50 rpm), Uniformity of dosage units, and Loss on drying (not more than 1.5%).

PENTAERYTHRITOL TETRANITRATE

Chemical name: 1,3-Propanediol, 2,2-bis[(nitrooxy) methyl]-, dinitrate (ester).

Molecular formula: $C_5H_8N_4O_{12}$.

Molecular weight: 316.14.

Description: Diluted Pentaerythritol Tetranitrate USP—White to ivory-colored powder, having a faint, mild odor.

Solubility: Undiluted pentaerythritol tetranitrate—Soluble in acetone; slightly soluble in alcohol and in ether; practically insoluble in water.

USP requirements:
Pentaerythritol Tetranitrate Extended-release Capsules—Not in USP.
Pentaerythritol Tetranitrate Tablets USP—Preserve in tight containers. Prepared from Diluted Pentaerythritol Tetranitrate. Contain the labeled amount of Diluted Pentaerythritol Tetranitrate, within ±7%. Meet the requirements for Identification, Disintegration (10 minutes), and Uniformity of dosage units.
  Caution: Undiluted pentaerythritol tetranitrate is a powerful explosive; take proper precautions in handling. It can be exploded by percussion or by excessive heat. Only exceedingly small amounts should be isolated.
Pentaerythritol Tetranitrate Extended-release Tablets—Not in USP.

PENTAGASTRIN

Chemical name: L-Phenylalaninamide, *N*-[(1,1-dimethylethoxy)carbonyl]-beta-alanyl-L-tryptophyl-L-methionyl-L-alpha-aspartyl-.

Molecular formula: $C_{37}H_{49}N_7O_9S$.

Molecular weight: 767.90.

Description: Colorless crystalline solid.

Solubility: Soluble in dimethylformamide and in dimethylsulfoxide; almost insoluble in water, in ethanol, in ether, in chloroform, and in ethyl acetate.

USP requirements: Pentagastrin Injection—Not in USP.

PENTAMIDINE

Chemical group: Diamidine derivative, related to hydroxystilbamidine.

Chemical name: Pentamidine isethionate—4,4′-diamidinodiphenoxypentane di-(beta-hydroxyethanesulfonate).

Molecular formula: Pentamidine isethionate—$C_{19}H_{24}N_4O_2 \cdot 2C_2H_6O_4S$.

Molecular weight: Pentamidine isethionate—592.68.

Description: Pentamidine isethionate—White crystalline powder.

Solubility: Pentamidine isethionate—Soluble in water and in glycerin; insoluble in acetone, in chloroform, and in ether.

USP requirements:
Pentamidine Isethionate for Inhalation Solution—Not in USP.

Sterile Pentamidine Isethionate—Not in USP.

PENTAZOCINE

Chemical name:
Pentazocine hydrochloride—2,6-Methano-3-benzazocin-8-ol, 1,2,3,4,5,6-hexahydro-6,11-dimethyl-3-(3-methyl-2-butenyl)-, hydrochloride, (2 alpha,6 alpha,11*R**)-.
Pentazocine lactate—2,6-Methano-3-benzazocin-8-ol, 1,2,3,4,5,6-hexahydro-6,11-dimethyl-3-(3-methyl-2-butenyl)-, (2 alpha,6 alpha,11*R**)-, compd. with 2-hydroxypropanoic acid (1:1).

Molecular formula:
Pentazocine hydrochloride—$C_{19}H_{27}NO \cdot HCl$.
Pentazocine lactate—$C_{19}H_{27}NO \cdot C_3H_6O_3$.

Molecular weight:
Pentazocine hydrochloride—321.89.
Pentazocine lactate—375.51.

Description:
Pentazocine Hydrochloride USP—White, crystalline powder. It exhibits polymorphism, one form melting at about 254 °C and the other at about 218 °C.
Pentazocine lactate—White, crystalline substance.

Solubility:
Pentazocine Hydrochloride USP—Freely soluble in chloroform; soluble in alcohol; sparingly soluble in water; very slightly soluble in acetone and in ether.
Pentazocine lactate—Soluble in acidic aqueous solutions.

USP requirements:
Pentazocine Hydrochloride Tablets USP—Preserve in tight, light-resistant containers. Contain an amount of pentazocine hydrochloride equivalent to the labeled amount of pentazocine, within ±10%. Meet the requirements for Identification, Dissolution (75% in 45 minutes in water in Apparatus 2 at 50 rpm), and Uniformity of dosage units.
Pentazocine Lactate Injection USP—Preserve in single-dose or in multiple-dose containers, preferably of Type I glass. A sterile solution of pentazocine lactate in Water for Injection, prepared from Pentazocine with the aid of Lactic Acid. Contains an amount of pentazocine lactate equivalent to the labeled amount of pentazocine, within ±5%. Meets the requirements for Identification, Bacterial endotoxins, pH (4.0–5.0), and Injections.

PENTAZOCINE AND ACETAMINOPHEN

For *Pentazocine* and *Acetaminophen*—See individual listings for chemistry information.

USP requirements: Pentazocine Hydrochloride and Acetaminophen Tablets—Not in USP.

PENTAZOCINE AND ASPIRIN

For *Pentazocine* and *Aspirin*—See individual listings for chemistry information.

USP requirements: Pentazocine Hydrochloride and Aspirin Tablets USP—Preserve in tight, light-resistant containers. Contain an amount of pentazocine hydrochloride equivalent to the labeled amount of pentazocine, within ±10%, and the labeled amount of aspirin, within ±10%. Meet the requirements for Identification, Non-aspirin salicylates (not more than 3.0%), Dissolution (80% of pentazocine and 70% of aspirin in 30 minutes in water in Apparatus 1 at 80 rpm), and Uniformity of dosage units.

PENTAZOCINE AND NALOXONE

For *Pentazocine* and *Naloxone*—See individual listings for chemistry information.

USP requirements: Pentazocine and Naloxone Hydrochlorides Tablets USP—Preserve in tight, light-resistant containers. Contain amounts of pentazocine hydrochloride and naloxone hydrochloride equivalent to the labeled amounts of pentazocine and naloxone, within ± 10%. Meet the requirements for Identification, Dissolution (75% of pentazocine in 45 minutes in water in Apparatus 2 at 50 rpm), and Uniformity of dosage units.

PENTETIC ACID

Chemical name: Glycine, *N,N*-bis[2-[bis(carboxymethyl)amino]-ethyl]-.

Molecular formula: $C_{14}H_{23}N_3O_{10}$.

Molecular weight: 393.35.

USP requirements: Pentetic Acid USP—Preserve in well-closed containers. Contains not less than 98.0% and not more than 100.5% of pentetic acid. Meets the requirements for Identification, Melting range (215–225 °C), Residue on ignition (not more than 0.2%), Heavy metals (not more than 0.005%), Nitrilotriacetic acid, and Iron (not more than 0.01%).

PENTOBARBITAL

Chemical name:
Pentobarbital—2,4,6(1*H*,3*H*,5*H*)-Pyrimidinetrione, 5-ethyl-5-(1-methylbutyl)-.
Pentobarbital sodium—2,4,6(1*H*,3*H*,5*H*)-Pyrimidinetrione, 5-ethyl-5-(1-methylbutyl), monosodium salt.

Molecular formula:
Pentobarbital—$C_{11}H_{18}N_2O_3$.
Pentobarbital sodium—$C_{11}H_{17}N_2NaO_3$.

Molecular weight:
Pentobarbital—226.27.
Pentobarbital sodium—248.26.

Description:
Pentobarbital USP—White to practically white, fine, practically odorless powder. May occur in a polymorphic form that melts at about 116 °C. This form gradually reverts to the more stable higher-melting form upon being heated at about 110 °C.
Pentobarbital Sodium USP—White, crystalline granules or white powder. Is odorless or has a slight characteristic odor. Its solutions decompose on standing, heat accelerating the decomposition.

Solubility:
Pentobarbital USP—Very slightly soluble in water and in carbon tetrachloride; very soluble in alcohol, in methanol, in ether, in chloroform, and in acetone.
Pentobarbital Sodium USP—Very soluble in water; freely soluble in alcohol; practically insoluble in ether.

USP requirements:
Pentobarbital Elixir USP—Preserve in tight containers. Contains the labeled amount, within ± 7.5%. Meets the requirements for Identification and Alcohol content (16.0–20.0%).
Pentobarbital Sodium Capsules USP—Preserve in tight containers. Contain the labeled amount, within ± 7.5%. Meet the requirements for Identification, Dissolution (75% in 45 minutes in water in Apparatus 1 at 100 rpm), and Uniformity of dosage units.

Pentobarbital Sodium Injection USP—Preserve in single-dose or in multiple-dose containers, preferably of Type I glass. The Injection may be packaged in 50-mL containers. A sterile solution of Pentobarbital Sodium in a suitable solvent. Pentobarbital may be substituted for the equivalent amount of Pentobarbital Sodium, for adjustment of the pH. The label indicates that the Injection is not to be used if it contains a precipitate. Contains the equivalent of the labeled amount, within ± 8%. Meets the requirements for Identification, Bacterial endotoxins, pH (9.0–10.5), and Injections.
Pentobarbital Sodium Suppositories—Not in USP.

PENTOSTATIN

Chemical name: Imidazo[4,5-*d*][1,3]diazepin-8-ol, 3-(2-deoxy-beta-D-*erythro*-pentofuranosyl)-3,6,7,8-tetrahydro-, (*R*)-.

Molecular formula: $C_{11}H_{16}N_4O_4$.

Molecular weight: 268.27.

Description: White to off-white solid.

Solubility: Freely soluble in distilled water.

USP requirements: Pentostatin for Injection—Not in USP.

PENTOXIFYLLINE

Chemical group: A trisubstituted xanthine derivative.

Chemical name: 1*H*-purine-2,6-dione, 3,7-dihydro-3,7-dimethyl-1-(5-oxohexyl)-.

Molecular formula: $C_{13}H_{18}N_4O_3$.

Molecular weight: 278.31.

Description: Odorless, colorless, crystalline powder. Melts at 101–106 °C.

Solubility: Soluble in water and in ethanol; sparingly soluble in toluene.

USP requirements: Pentoxifylline Extended-release Tablets—Not in USP.

PEPPERMINT

Description: Peppermint NF—It has an aromatic odor.
NF category: Flavors and perfumes.

NF requirements: Peppermint NF—Consists of the dried leaf and flowering top of *Mentha piperita* Linné (Fam. Labiatae). Meets the requirements for Stems and other foreign organic matter and Botanic characteristics.

PEPPERMINT OIL

Description: Peppermint Oil NF—Colorless or pale yellow liquid, having a strong, penetrating, characteristic odor.
NF category: Flavors and perfumes.

NF requirements: Peppermint Oil NF—Preserve in tight containers, and prevent exposure to excessive heat. It is the volatile oil distilled with steam from the fresh overground parts of the flowering plant of *Mentha piperita* Linné (Fam. Labiatae), rectified by distillation and neither partially nor wholly dementholized. Yields not less than 5.0% of esters, calculated as menthyl acetate, and not less than 50.0% of total menthol, free and as esters. Meets the requirements for Solubility in 70% alcohol (one volume dissolves in 3 volumes of 70% alcohol, with not more than a slight opalescence),

Identification, Specific gravity (0.896–0.908), Angular rotation (−18° to −32° in a 100-mm tube), Refractive index (1.459–1.465 at 20 °C), Heavy metals (not more than 0.004%), and Dimethyl sulfide.

PEPPERMINT SPIRIT

Description: Peppermint Spirit USP—NF category: Flavors and perfumes.

USP requirements: Peppermint Spirit USP—Preserve in tight containers, protected from light. Contains, in each 100 mL, not less than 9.0 mL and not more than 11.0 mL of peppermint oil.

Prepare Peppermint Spirit as follows: 100 mL of Peppermint Oil, 10 grams of Peppermint, in coarse powder, and a sufficient quantity of Alcohol to make 1000 mL. Macerate the peppermint leaves, freed as much as possible from stems and coarsely powdered, for 1 hour in 500 mL of purified water, and then strongly express them. Add the moist, macerated leaves to 900 mL of alcohol, and allow the mixture to stand for 6 hours with frequent agitation. Filter, and to the filtrate add the oil and add alcohol to make the product measure 1000 mL.

Meets the requirement for Alcohol content (79.0–85.0%).

PEPPERMINT WATER

Description: Peppermint Water NF—NF category: Flavored and/or sweetened vehicle.

NF requirements: Peppermint Water NF—Preserve in tight containers. A clear, saturated solution of Peppermint Oil in Purified Water, prepared by one of the processes described under *Aromatic Waters*. Meets the requirement for Organic volatile impurities.

PERFLUOROCHEMICAL EMULSION

Molecular formula:
Perfluorodecalin—$C_{10}F_{18}$.
Perfluorotri-n-propylamine—$C_9F_{21}N$.

Description: Stable emulsion of synthetic perfluorochemicals (perfluorodecalin, perfluorotri-n-propylamine) in Water for Injection. Also contains Poloxamer 188 (a nonionic surfactant which is a polyoxyethylene [160]-polyoxypropylene [30] glycol block copolymer), glycerin, egg yolk phospholipids (a mixture of naturally occurring phospholipids isolated from egg yolk), dextrose (a naturally occurring sugar), and the potassium salt of oleic acid (a naturally occurring fatty acid), plus electrolytes in physiologic concentrations.

Other characteristics:
Osmolarity—Approximately 410 mOsmol per liter.
Mean particle diameter—Less than 270 nanometers as determined by laser light scattering spectrophotometry. The content of particles greater than 400 nanometers is less than 10%.
pH—After preparation for administration: 7.3.
Solubility of oxygen—At 37 °C and at partial pressure of oxygen (pO_2) of 760 mm Hg: 7 volume %. Increases with decreasing temperature; at 10 °C and pO_2 of 760 mm Hg, is 9 volume %.
Solubility of carbon dioxide—At 37 °C and at partial pressure of carbon dioxide (pCO_2) of 760 mm Hg: 66 volume %.
Viscosity—Less viscous than whole blood at 37 °C and physiological shear rates.

USP requirements: Perfluorochemical Emulsion for Injection—Not in USP.

PERGOLIDE

Source: Ergot derivative.

Chemical name: Pergolide mesylate—Ergoline, 8-[(methylthio)methyl]-6-propyl-, monomethanesulfonate, (8 beta)-.

Molecular formula: Pergolide mesylate—$C_{19}H_{26}N_2S \cdot CH_4O_3S$.

Molecular weight: Pergolide mesylate—410.59.

Description: Pergolide mesylate—Off-white crystals; melting point about 225 °C.

USP requirements: Pergolide Mesylate Tablets—Not in USP.

PERICYAZINE

Chemical group: Piperidine.

Chemical name: 10-[3-(4-Hydroxypiperidino)propyl]phenothiazine-2-carbonitrile.

Molecular formula: $C_{21}H_{23}N_3OS$.

Molecular weight: 365.19.

Description: A yellow almost odorless powder. Melts at 115 °C.

Solubility: Practically insoluble in water; soluble in alcohol and in acetone; freely soluble in chloroform; slightly soluble in ether.

USP requirements:
Pericyazine Capsules—Not in USP.
Pericyazine Oral Solution—Not in USP.

PERMETHRIN

Source: A mixture of the *cis* and *trans* isomers of a synthetic pyrethroid. Permethrin is the first pyrethroid formulated for human use.

Chemical name: Cyclopropanecarboxylic acid, 3-(2,2-dichloroethenyl)-2,2-dimethyl-, (3-phenoxyphenyl)methyl ester.

Molecular formula: $C_{21}H_{20}Cl_2O_3$.

Molecular weight: 391.29.

Description: A yellow to light orange-brown, low-melting solid or viscous liquid.

Solubility: Practically insoluble in water; soluble in nonpolar organic solvents.

USP requirements: Permethrin Lotion—Not in USP.

PERPHENAZINE

Chemical group: Piperazinyl phenothiazine.

Chemical name: Piperazineethanol, 4-[3-(2-chloro-10H-phenothiazin-10-yl)propyl]-.

Molecular formula: $C_{21}H_{26}ClN_3OS$.

Molecular weight: 403.97.

Description: Perphenazine USP—White to creamy white, odorless powder.

Solubility: Perphenazine USP—Practically insoluble in water; freely soluble in alcohol and in chloroform; soluble in acetone.

USP requirements:
Perphenazine Injection USP—Preserve in single-dose or in multiple-dose containers, preferably of Type I glass, protected from light. A sterile solution of Perphenazine in

Water for Injection, prepared with the aid of Citric Acid. Contains the labeled amount, as the citrate, within ±10%. Meets the requirements for Identification, Bacterial endotoxins, pH (4.2–5.6), and Injections.

Perphenazine Oral Solution USP—Preserve in well-closed, light-resistant containers. Contains the labeled amount, within ±10%. Meets the requirements for Identification and Perphenazine sulfoxide (not more than 5.0%).

Perphenazine Syrup USP—Preserve in well-closed, light-resistant containers. Contains the labeled amount, within ±10%. Meets the requirement for Identification.

Perphenazine Tablets USP—Preserve in tight, light-resistant containers. Contain the labeled amount, within ±10%. Meet the requirements for Identification, Dissolution (75% in 45 minutes in 0.1 N hydrochloric acid in Apparatus 2 at 50 rpm), and Uniformity of dosage units.

PERPHENAZINE AND AMITRIPTYLINE

For *Perphenazine* and *Amitriptyline*—See individual listings for chemistry information.

USP requirements: Perphenazine and Amitriptyline Hydrochloride Tablets USP—Preserve in well-closed containers. Contain the labeled amounts, within ±10%. Meet the requirements for Identification, Dissolution (75% of each active ingredient in 60 minutes in 0.1 N hydrochloric acid in Apparatus 2 at 50 rpm), and Uniformity of dosage units.

PERSIC OIL

Description: Persic Oil NF—Clear, pale straw-colored or colorless oily liquid. It is almost odorless. Not turbid at temperatures exceeding 15 °C.

NF category: Vehicle (oleaginous).

Solubility: Persic Oil NF—Slightly soluble in alcohol. Miscible with ether, with chloroform, and with solvent hexane.

NF requirements: Persic Oil NF—Preserve in tight containers. It is the oil expressed from the kernels of varieties of *Prunus armeniaca* Linné (Apricot Kernel Oil), or from the kernels of varieties of *Prunus persica* Sieb. et Zucc. (Peach Kernel Oil) (Fam. Rosaceae). Label it to indicate whether it was derived from apricot kernels or from peach kernels. Meets the requirements for Specific gravity (0.910–0.923), Heavy metals (not more than 0.004%), Mineral oil, Cottonseed oil, Sesame oil, Free fatty acids, Iodine value (90–108), and Saponification value (185–195).

PERTUSSIS IMMUNE GLOBULIN

Description: Pertussis Immune Globulin USP—Transparent or slightly opalescent liquid, practically colorless, free from turbidity or particles, and practically odorless. May develop a slight, granular deposit during storage. Is standardized for agglutinating activity with the U.S. Standard Antipertussis Serum.

USP requirements: Pertussis Immune Globulin USP—Preserve at a temperature between 2 and 8 °C. A sterile, non-pyrogenic solution of globulins derived from the blood plasma of adult human donors who have been immunized with pertussis vaccine such that each 1.25 mL contains not less than the amount of immune globulin to be equivalent to 25 mL of human hyperimmune serum. Contains a suitable preservative. Label it to state that it is not intended for intravenous injection. Meets the requirement for Expiration date (not later than 3 years after date of issue from manufacturer's cold storage [5 °C, 3 years]). Conforms to the regulations of the U.S. Food and Drug Administration concerning biologics.

PERTUSSIS VACCINE

Description: Pertussis Vaccine USP—More or less turbid, whitish liquid. Practically odorless, or having a faint odor because of the antimicrobial agent.

USP requirements: Pertussis Vaccine USP—Preserve at a temperature between 2 and 8 °C. A sterile bacterial fraction or suspension of killed pertussis bacilli (*Bordetella pertussis*) of a strain or strains selected for high antigenic efficiency. Label it to state that it is to be well shaken before use and that it is not to be frozen. It has a potency determined by the specific mouse potency test based on the U.S. Standard Pertussis Vaccine, and a pertussis challenge, of 12 protective units per total immunizing dose, and, in the case of whole bacterial vaccine, such dose contains not more than 60 opacity units. Contains a preservative. Meets the requirements of the specific mouse toxicity test and for Expiration date (not later than 18 months after date of issue from manufacturer's cold storage [5 °C, 1 year]). Conforms to the regulations of the U.S. Food and Drug Administration concerning biologics.

PERTUSSIS VACCINE ADSORBED

Description: Pertussis Vaccine Adsorbed USP—Markedly turbid, whitish liquid. Substantially odorless, or has a faint odor because of the antimicrobial agent.

USP requirements: Pertussis Vaccine Adsorbed USP—Preserve at a temperature between 2 and 8 °C, and avoid freezing. A sterile bacterial fraction or suspension, in a suitable diluent, of killed pertussis bacilli (*Bordetella pertussis*) of a strain or strains selected for high antigenic efficiency precipitated or adsorbed by the addition of aluminum hydroxide or aluminum phosphate, and re-suspended. Label it to state that it is to be well shaken before use and that it is not to be frozen. It has a potency determined by the specific mouse potency test based on the U.S. Standard Pertussis Vaccine, and a pertussis challenge, of 12 protective units per total immunizing dose, and, in the case of whole bacterial vaccine, such dose contains not more than 48 opacity units. Contains a preservative. Meets the requirements of the specific mouse toxicity test and for Expiration date (not later than 18 months after date of issue from manufacturer's cold storage [5 °C, 1 year]). Conforms to the regulations of the U.S. Food and Drug Administration concerning biologics.

PETROLATUM

Description: Petrolatum USP—Unctuous, yellowish to light amber mass, having not more than a slight fluorescence, even after being melted. It is transparent in thin layers. Free or practically free from odor.

NF category: Ointment base.

Solubility: Petrolatum USP—Insoluble in water; freely soluble in carbon disulfide, in chloroform, and in turpentine oil; soluble in ether, in solvent hexane, and in most fixed and volatile oils; practically insoluble in cold alcohol and hot alcohol and in cold dehydrated alcohol.

USP requirements: Petrolatum USP—Preserve in well-closed containers. A purified mixture of semisolid hydrocarbons obtained from petroleum. Label it to indicate the name and proportion of any added stabilizer. Meets the requirements for Specific gravity (0.815–0.880 at 60 °C), Melting range (38–60 °C), Consistency (value of 100–300), Alkalinity, Acidity, Residue on ignition (not more than 0.1%), Organic acids, Fixed oils, fats, and rosin, and Color.

HYDROPHILIC PETROLATUM

Description: Hydrophilic Petrolatum USP—NF category: Ointment base.

USP requirements: Hydrophilic Petrolatum USP—Prepare Hydrophilic Petrolatum as follows: 30 grams of Cholesterol, 30 grams of Stearyl Alcohol, 80 grams of White Wax, and 860 grams of White Petrolatum to make 1000 grams. Melt the Stearyl Alcohol and White Wax together on a steam bath, then add the Cholesterol, and stir until completely dissolved. Add the White Petrolatum, and mix. Remove from the bath, and stir until the mixture congeals.

WHITE PETROLATUM

Description: White Petrolatum USP—White or faintly yellowish, unctuous mass, transparent in thin layers even after cooling to 0 °C.
NF category: Ointment base.

Solubility: White Petrolatum USP—Insoluble in water; slightly soluble in cold or hot alcohol, and in cold dehydrated alcohol; freely soluble in carbon disulfide and in chloroform; soluble in ether, in solvent hexane, and in most fixed and volatile oils.

USP requirements: White Petrolatum USP—Preserve in well-closed containers. A purified mixture of semisolid hydrocarbons obtained from petroleum, and wholly or nearly decolorized. Label it to indicate the name and proportion of any added stabilizer. Meets the requirements for Residue on ignition (not more than 0.05%) and Color, and for Specific gravity, Melting range, Consistency, Alkalinity, Acidity, Organic acids, and Fixed oils, fats, and rosin under Petrolatum.

PHENACEMIDE

Chemical group: Acetylurea.

Chemical name: Benzeneacetamide, *N*-(aminocarbonyl)-.

Molecular formula: $C_9H_{10}N_2O_2$.

Molecular weight: 178.19.

Description: Phenacemide USP—White to practically white, fine crystalline powder. Is odorless, or practically odorless, and melts at about 213 °C.

Solubility: Phenacemide USP—Very slightly soluble in water, in alcohol, in chloroform, and in ether; slightly soluble in acetone and in methanol.

USP requirements: Phenacemide Tablets USP—Preserve in well-closed containers. Contain the labeled amount, within ±5%. Meet the requirements for Identification, Dissolution (35% in 60 minutes in 0.1 *N* hydrochloric acid in Apparatus 2 at 100 rpm), and Uniformity of dosage units.

PHENAZOPYRIDINE

Chemical name: Phenazopyridine hydrochloride—2,6-Pyridinediamine, 3-(phenylazo)-, monohydrochloride.

Molecular formula: Phenazopyridine hydrochloride—$C_{11}H_{11}N_5 \cdot HCl$.

Molecular weight: Phenazopyridine hydrochloride—249.70.

Description: Phenazopyridine Hydrochloride USP—Light or dark red to dark violet, crystalline powder. Is odorless, or has a slight odor. Melts at about 235 °C, with decomposition.

Solubility: Phenazopyridine Hydrochloride USP—Slightly soluble in water, in alcohol, and in chloroform.

USP requirements: Phenazopyridine Hydrochloride Tablets USP—Preserve in tight containers. Contain the labeled amount, within ±5%. Meet the requirements for Identification, Dissolution (75% in 45 minutes in water in Apparatus 2 at 50 rpm), and Uniformity of dosage units.

PHENDIMETRAZINE

Chemical group: Morpholine.

Chemical name: Phendimetrazine tartrate—Morpholine, 3,4-dimethyl-2-phenyl-, (2*S-trans*)-, [*R*-(*R**,*R**)]-2,3-dihydroxybutanedioate (1:1).

Molecular formula: Phendimetrazine tartrate—$C_{12}H_{17}NO \cdot C_4H_6O_6$.

Molecular weight: Phendimetrazine tartrate—341.36.

Description: Phendimetrazine Tartrate USP—White, odorless, crystalline powder.

Solubility: Phendimetrazine Tartrate USP—Freely soluble in water; sparingly soluble in warm alcohol; insoluble in chloroform, in acetone, and in ether. Phendimetrazine base is extracted by organic solvents from alkaline solution.

USP requirements:
Phendimetrazine Tartrate Capsules USP—Preserve in tight containers. Contain the labeled amount, within ±5%. Meet the requirements for Identification and Uniformity of dosage units.
Phendimetrazine Tartrate Extended-release Capsules—Not in USP.
Phendimetrazine Tartrate Tablets USP—Preserve in well-closed containers. Contain the labeled amount, within ±10%. Meet the requirements for Identification, Dissolution (60% in 45 minutes in water in Apparatus 1 at 100 rpm), and Uniformity of dosage units.
Phendimetrazine Tartrate Extended-release Tablets—Not in USP.

PHENELZINE

Chemical group: Hydrazine derivative.

Chemical name: Phenelzine sulfate—Hydrazine, (2-phenylethyl)-, sulfate (1:1).

Molecular formula: Phenelzine sulfate—$C_8H_{12}N_2 \cdot H_2SO_4$.

Molecular weight: Phenelzine sulfate—234.27.

Description: Phenelzine Sulfate USP—White to yellowish white powder, having a characteristic odor.

Solubility: Phenelzine Sulfate USP—Freely soluble in water; practically insoluble in alcohol, in chloroform, and in ether.

USP requirements: Phenelzine Sulfate Tablets USP—Preserve in tight containers, protected from heat and light. Contain an amount of phenelzine sulfate equivalent to the labeled amount of phenelzine, within ±5%. Meet the requirements for Identification, Disintegration (1 hour), and Uniformity of dosage units.

PHENINDAMINE

Chemical group: Piperidine derivative.

Chemical name: Phenindamine tartrate—2,3,4,9-Tetrahydro-2-methyl-9-phenyl-1*H*-indeno[2,1-*c*]pyridine.

Molecular formula: Phenindamine tartrate—$C_{19}H_{19}N \cdot C_4H_6O_6$.

Molecular weight: Phenindamine tartrate—411.45.

Description: Phenindamine tartrate—White or almost white, almost odorless, voluminous powder. A 1% solution in water has a pH of 3.4 to 3.9.

Solubility: Phenindamine tartrate—Soluble 1 in 70 of water; slightly soluble in alcohol; practically insoluble in chloroform and in ether.

USP requirements: Phenindamime Tartrate Tablets—Not in USP.

PHENINDAMINE, HYDROCODONE, AND GUAIFENESIN

For *Phenindamine*, *Hydrocodone*, and *Guaifenesin*—See individual listings for chemistry information.

USP requirements: Phenindamine Tartrate, Hydrocodone Bitartrate, and Guaifenesin Tablets—Not in USP.

PHENINDIONE

Chemical name: 1*H*-Indene-1,3(2*H*)-dione, 2-phenyl-.

Molecular formula: $C_{15}H_{10}O_2$.

Molecular weight: 222.24.

Description: Phenindione USP—Creamy white to pale yellow, almost odorless crystals or crystalline powder.

Solubility: Phenindione USP—Very slightly soluble in water; freely soluble in chloroform; slightly soluble in alcohol and in ether.

USP requirements: Phenindione Tablets USP—Preserve in well-closed containers. Contain the labeled amount, within ± 10%. Meet the requirements for Identification, Dissolution (85% in 45 minutes in phosphate buffer [pH 8.0] in Apparatus 1 at 100 rpm), and Uniformity of dosage units.

PHENIRAMINE, CODEINE, AND GUAIFENESIN

Chemical group: Pheniramine—Alkylamine derivative.

Chemical name:
Pheniramine maleate—2-[alpha-[2-Dimethylaminoethyl]-benzyl]pyridine bimaleate.
Codeine phosphate—Morphinan-6-ol, 7,8-didehydro-4,5-epoxy-3-methoxy-17-methyl-, (5 alpha,6 alpha)-, phosphate (1:1) (salt), hemihydrate.
Guaifenesin—1,2-Propanediol, 3-(2-methoxyphenoxy)-.

Molecular formula:
Pheniramine maleate—$C_{16}H_{20}N_2 \cdot C_4H_4O_4$.
Codeine phosphate—$C_{18}H_{21}NO_3 \cdot H_3PO_4 \cdot \frac{1}{2}H_2O$ (hemihydrate); $C_{18}H_{21}NO_3 \cdot H_3PO_4$ (anhydrous).
Guaifenesin—$C_{10}H_{14}O_4$.

Molecular weight:
Pheniramine maleate—356.43.
Codeine phosphate—406.37 (hemihydrate); 397.36 (anhydrous).
Guaifenesin—198.22.

Description:
Pheniramine maleate—White or almost white, crystalline powder, odorless or with a slight odor.
Codeine Phosphate USP—Fine, white, needle-shaped crystals, or white, crystalline powder. Is odorless, and is affected by light. Its solutions are acid to litmus.

Guaifenesin USP—White to slightly gray, crystalline powder. May have a slight characteristic odor.

Solubility:
Pheniramine maleate—Soluble 1 in 0.3 of water, 1 in 2.5 of alcohol, and 1 in 1.5 of chloroform; very slightly soluble in ether.
Codeine Phosphate USP—Freely soluble in water; very soluble in hot water; slightly soluble in alcohol but more so in boiling alcohol.
Guaifenesin USP—Soluble in water, in alcohol, in chloroform, in glycerin, and in propylene glycol.

USP requirements: Pheniramine Maleate, Codeine Phosphate, and Guaifenesin Syrup—Not in USP.

PHENIRAMINE, PHENYLEPHRINE, CODEINE, SODIUM CITRATE, SODIUM SALICYLATE, AND CAFFEINE

Source: Caffeine—Coffee, tea, cola, and cocoa or chocolate. May also be synthesized from urea or dimethylurea.

Chemical group:
Pheniramine—Alkylamine derivative.
Caffeine—Methylated xanthine.

Chemical name:
Pheniramine maleate—2-[alpha-[2-Dimethylaminoethyl]-benzyl]pyridine bimaleate.
Phenylephrine hydrochloride—Benzenemethanol, 3-hydroxy-alpha-[(methylamino)methyl]-, hydrochloride.
Codeine phosphate—Morphinan-6-ol, 7,8-didehydro-4,5-epoxy-3-methoxy-17-methyl-, (5 alpha,6 alpha)-, phosphate (1:1) (salt), hemihydrate.
Sodium citrate—1,2,3-Propanetricarboxylic acid, 2-hydroxy-, trisodium salt.
Sodium salicylate—Benzoic acid, 2-hydroxy-, monosodium salt.
Caffeine—1*H*-Purine-2,6-dione, 3,7-dihydro-1,3,7-trimethyl-.
Citric Acid—1,2,3-Propanetricarboxylic acid, 2-hydroxy-.

Molecular formula:
Pheniramine maleate—$C_{16}H_{20}N_2 \cdot C_4H_4O_4$.
Phenylephrine hydrochloride—$C_9H_{13}NO_2 \cdot HCl$.
Codeine phosphate—$C_{18}H_{21}NO_3 \cdot H_3PO_4 \cdot \frac{1}{2}H_2O$ (hemihydrate); $C_{18}H_{21}NO_3 \cdot H_3PO_4$ (anhydrous).
Sodium citrate—$C_6H_5Na_3O_7$.
Sodium salicylate—$C_7H_5NaO_3$.
Caffeine—$C_8H_{10}N_4O_2$ (anhydrous); $C_8H_{10}N_4O_2 \cdot H_2O$ (monohydrate).
Citric acid—$C_6H_8O_7$ (anhydrous); $C_6H_8O_7 \cdot H_2O$ (monohydrate).

Molecular weight:
Pheniramine maleate—356.43.
Phenylephrine hydrochloride—203.67.
Codeine phosphate—406.37 (hemihydrate); 397.36 (anhydrous).
Sodium citrate—258.07 (anhydrous).
Sodium salicylate—160.10.
Caffeine—194.19 (anhydrous); 212.21 (monohydrate).
Citric acid—192.12 (anhydrous); 210.14 (monohydrate).

Description:
Pheniramine maleate—White or almost white, crystalline powder, odorless or with a slight odor.
Phenylephrine Hydrochloride USP—White or practically white, odorless crystals.
Codeine Phosphate USP—Fine, white, needle-shaped crystals, or white, crystalline powder. Is odorless, and is affected by light. Its solutions are acid to litmus.

Sodium Citrate USP—Colorless crystals or white, crystalline powder.

NF category: Buffering agent.

Sodium Salicylate USP—Amorphous or microcrystalline powder or scales. Is colorless, or has not more than a faint, pink tinge. Is odorless, or has a faint, characteristic odor, and is affected by light. A freshly made solution (1 in 10) is neutral or acid to litmus.

Caffeine USP—White powder or white, glistening needles, usually matted together. Is odorless. Its solutions are neutral to litmus. The hydrate is efflorescent in air.

Citric Acid USP—Colorless, translucent crystals, or white, granular to fine crystalline powder. Odorless or practically odorless. The hydrous form is efflorescent in dry air.

NF category: Acidifying agent; buffering agent.

Solubility:

Pheniramine maleate—Soluble 1 in 0.3 of water, 1 in 2.5 of alcohol, and 1 in 1.5 of chloroform; very slightly soluble in ether.

Phenylephrine Hydrochloride USP—Freely soluble in water and in alcohol.

Codeine Phosphate USP—Freely soluble in water; very soluble in hot water; slightly soluble in alcohol but more so in boiling alcohol.

Sodium Citrate USP—Hydrous form freely soluble in water and very soluble in boiling water; insoluble in alcohol.

Sodium Salicylate USP—Freely (and slowly) soluble in water and in glycerin; very soluble in boiling water and in boiling alcohol; slowly soluble in alcohol.

Caffeine USP—Sparingly soluble in water and in alcohol; freely soluble in chloroform; slightly soluble in ether.

The aqueous solubility of caffeine is increased by organic acids or their alkali salts, such as citrates, benzoates, salicylates, or cinnamates, which dissociate to yield caffeine when dissolved in biological fluids.

Citric Acid USP—Very soluble in water; freely soluble in alcohol; sparingly soluble in ether.

USP requirements: Pheniramine Maleate, Phenylephrine Hydrochloride, Codeine Phosphate, Sodium Citrate, Sodium Salicylate, and Caffeine Citrate Syrup—Not in USP.

PHENIRAMINE, PHENYLEPHRINE, SODIUM SALICYLATE, AND CAFFEINE

Source: Caffeine—Coffee, tea, cola, and cocoa or chocolate. May also be synthesized from urea or dimethylurea.

Chemical group:

Pheniramine—Alkylamine derivative.

Caffeine—Methylated xanthine.

Chemical name:

Pheniramine maleate—2-[alpha-[2-Dimethylaminoethyl]-benzyl]pyridine bimaleate.

Phenylephrine hydrochloride—Benzenemethanol, 3-hydroxy-alpha-[(methylamino)methyl]-, hydrochloride.

Sodium salicylate—Benzoic acid, 2-hydroxy-, monosodium salt.

Caffeine—1*H*-Purine-2,6-dione, 3,7-dihydro-1,3,7-trimethyl-.

Molecular formula:

Pheniramine maleate—$C_{16}H_{20}N_2 \cdot C_4H_4O_4$.

Phenylephrine hydrochloride—$C_9H_{13}NO_2 \cdot HCl$.

Sodium salicylate—$C_7H_5NaO_3$.

Caffeine—$C_8H_{10}N_4O_2$ (anhydrous); $C_8H_{10}N_4O_2 \cdot H_2O$ (monohydrate).

Molecular weight:

Pheniramine maleate—356.43.

Phenylephrine hydrochloride—203.67.

Sodium salicylate—160.10.

Caffeine—194.19 (anhydrous); 212.21 (monohydrate).

Description:

Pheniramine maleate—White or almost white, crystalline powder, odorless or with a slight odor.

Phenylephrine Hydrochloride USP—White or practically white, odorless crystals.

Sodium Salicylate USP—Amorphous or microcrystalline powder or scales. Is colorless, or has not more than a faint, pink tinge. Is odorless, or has a faint, characteristic odor, and is affected by light. A freshly made solution (1 in 10) is neutral or acid to litmus.

Caffeine USP—White powder or white, glistening needles, usually matted together. Is odorless. Its solutions are neutral to litmus. The hydrate is efflorescent in air.

Solubility:

Pheniramine maleate—Soluble 1 in 0.3 of water, 1 in 2.5 of alcohol, and 1 in 1.5 of chloroform; very slightly soluble in ether.

Phenylephrine Hydrochloride USP—Freely soluble in water and in alcohol.

Sodium Salicylate USP—Freely (and slowly) soluble in water and in glycerin; very soluble in boiling water and in boiling alcohol; slowly soluble in alcohol.

Caffeine USP—Sparingly soluble in water and in alcohol; freely soluble in chloroform; slightly soluble in ether.

The aqueous solubility of caffeine is increased by organic acids or their alkali salts, such as citrates, benzoates, salicylates, or cinnamates, which dissociate to yield caffeine when dissolved in biological fluids.

USP requirements: Pheniramine, Maleate, Phenylephrine Hydrochloride, Sodium Salicylate, and Caffeine Oral Solution—Not in USP.

PHENIRAMINE, PHENYLTOLOXAMINE, PYRILAMINE, AND PHENYLPROPANOLAMINE

Chemical group:

Pheniramine—Alkylamine derivative.

Phenyltoloxamine citrate—Ethanolamine derivative.

Pyrilamine—Ethylenediamine derivative.

Chemical name:

Pheniramine maleate—2-[alpha-[2-Dimethylaminoethyl]-benzyl]pyridine bimaleate.

Phenyltoloxamine citrate—2-(2-Benzylphenoxy)-*N,N*-dimethylethylamine dihydrogen citrate.

Pyrilamine maleate—1,2-Ethanediamine, *N*-[(4-methoxyphenyl)methyl]-*N',N'*-dimethyl-*N*-2-pyridinyl-, (*Z*)-2-butenedioate (1:1).

Phenylpropanolamine hydrochloride—Benzenemethanol, alpha-(1-aminoethyl)-, hydrochloride, (*R*,S**)-, (±).

Molecular formula:

Pheniramine maleate—$C_{16}H_{20}N_2 \cdot C_4H_4O_4$.

Phenyltoloxamine citrate—$C_{17}H_{21}NO \cdot C_6H_8O_7$.

Pyrilamine maleate—$C_{17}H_{23}N_3O \cdot C_4H_4O_4$.

Phenylpropanolamine hydrochloride—$C_9H_{13}NO \cdot HCl$.

Molecular weight:

Pheniramine maleate—356.43.

Phenyltoloxamine citrate—447.5.

Pyrilamine maleate—401.46.

Phenylpropanolamine hydrochloride—187.67.

Description:

Pheniramine maleate—White or almost white, crystalline powder, odorless or with a slight odor.

Pyrilamine Maleate USP—White, crystalline powder, usually having a faint odor. Its solutions are acid to litmus.

Phenyltoloxamine citrate—It has a melting point of 138–140 °C.

Phenylpropanolamine Hydrochloride USP—White, crystalline powder, having a slight aromatic odor. Affected by light.

pKa: Phenylpropanolamine hydrochloride—9.

Solubility:

Pheniramine maleate—Soluble 1 in 0.3 of water, 1 in 2.5 of alcohol, and 1 in 1.5 of chloroform; very slightly soluble in ether.

Pyrilamine Maleate USP—Very soluble in water; freely soluble in alcohol and in chloroform; slightly soluble in ether.

Phenyltoloxamine citrate—Soluble in water.

Phenylpropanolamine Hydrochloride USP—Freely soluble in water and in alcohol; insoluble in ether.

USP requirements:

Pheniramine Maleate, Phenyltoloxamine Citrate, Pyrilamine Maleate, and Phenylpropanolamine Hydrochloride Extended-release Capsules—Not in USP.

Pheniramine Maleate, Phenyltoloxamine Citrate, Pyrilamine Maleate, and Phenylpropanolamine Hydrochloride Elixir—Not in USP.

PHENIRAMINE, PYRILAMINE, HYDROCODONE, POTASSIUM CITRATE, AND ASCORBIC ACID

Chemical group:

Pheniramine—Alkylamine derivative.

Pyrilamine—Ethylenediamine derivative.

Chemical name:

Pheniramine maleate—2-[alpha-[2-Dimethylaminoethyl]-benzyl]pyridine bimaleate.

Pyrilamine maleate—1,2-Ethanediamine, *N*-[(4-methoxy-phenyl) methyl]-*N'*,*N'*-dimethyl-*N*-2-pyridinyl-, (*Z*)-2-butenedioate (1:1).

Hydrocodone bitartrate—Morphinan-6-one, 4,5-epoxy-3-methoxy-17-methyl-, (5 alpha)-, [*R*-(*R**,*R**)]-2,3-dihydroxybutanedioate (1:1), hydrate (2:5).

Potassium citrate—1,2,3-Propanetricarboxylic acid, 2-hydroxy-, tripotassium salt, monohydrate.

Ascorbic acid—L-Ascorbic acid.

Molecular formula:

Pheniramine maleate—$C_{16}H_{20}N_2 \cdot C_4H_4O_4$.

Pyrilamine maleate—$C_{17}H_{23}N_3O \cdot C_4H_4O_4$.

Hydrocodone bitartrate—$C_{18}H_{21}NO_3 \cdot C_4H_6O_6 \cdot 2\frac{1}{2}H_2O$ (hydrate); $C_{18}H_{21}NO_3 \cdot C_4H_6O_6$ (anhydrous).

Potassium citrate—$C_6H_5K_3O_7 \cdot H_2O$.

Ascorbic acid—$C_6H_8O_6$.

Molecular weight:

Pheniramine maleate—356.43.

Pyrilamine maleate—401.46.

Hydrocodone bitartrate—494.50 (hydrate); 449.46 (anhydrous).

Potassium citrate—324.41.

Ascorbic acid—176.13.

Description:

Pheniramine maleate—White or almost white, crystalline powder, odorless or with a slight odor.

Pyrilamine Maleate USP—White, crystalline powder, usually having a faint odor. Its solutions are acid to litmus.

Hydrocodone Bitartrate USP—Fine, white crystals or a crystalline powder. Is affected by light.

Potassium Citrate USP—Transparent crystals or white, granular powder. Is odorless and is deliquescent when exposed to moist air.

Ascorbic Acid USP—White or slightly yellow crystals or powder. On exposure to light it gradually darkens. In the dry state, is reasonably stable in air, but in solution rapidly oxidizes. Melts at about 190 °C.

NF category: Antioxidant.

Solubility:

Pheniramine maleate—Soluble 1 in 0.3 of water, 1 in 2.5 of alcohol, and 1 in 1.5 of chloroform; very slightly soluble in ether.

Pyrilamine Maleate USP—Very soluble in water; freely soluble in alcohol and in chloroform; slightly soluble in ether.

Hydrocodone Bitartrate USP—Soluble in water; slightly soluble in alcohol; insoluble in ether and in chloroform.

Potassium Citrate USP—Freely soluble in water; almost insoluble in alcohol.

Ascorbic Acid USP—Freely soluble in water; sparingly soluble in alcohol; insoluble in chloroform and in ether.

USP requirements: Pheniramine Maleate, Pyrilamine Maleate, Hydrocodone Bitartrate, Potassium Citrate, and Ascorbic Acid Syrup—Not in USP.

PHENIRAMINE, PYRILAMINE, PHENYLEPHRINE, PHENYLPROPANOLAMINE, AND HYDROCODONE

Chemical group:

Pheniramine—Alkylamine derivative.

Pyrilamine—Ethylenediamine derivative.

Chemical name:

Pheniramine maleate—2-[alpha-[2-Dimethylaminoethyl]-benzyl]pyridine bimaleate.

Pyrilamine maleate—1,2-Ethanediamine, *N*-[(4-methoxy-phenyl)methyl]-*N'*,*N'*-dimethyl-*N*-2-pyridinyl-, (*Z*)-2-butenedioate (1:1).

Phenylephrine hydrochloride—Benzenemethanol, 3-hydroxy-alpha-[(methylamino)methyl]-, hydrochloride.

Phenylpropanolamine hydrochloride—Benzenemethanol, alpha-(1-aminoethyl)-, hydrochloride, (*R**,*S**)-, (±).

Hydrocodone bitartrate—Morphinan-6-one, 4,5-epoxy-3-methoxy-17-methyl-, (5 alpha)-, [*R*-(*R**,*R**)]-2,3-dihydroxybutanedioate (1:1), hydrate (2:5).

Molecular formula:

Pheniramine maleate—$C_{16}H_{20}N_2 \cdot C_4H_4O_4$.

Pyrilamine maleate—$C_{17}H_{23}N_3O \cdot C_4H_4O_4$.

Phenylephrine hydrochloride—$C_9H_{13}NO_2 \cdot HCl$.

Phenylpropanolamine hydrochloride—$C_9H_{13}NO \cdot HCl$.

Hydrocodone bitartrate—$C_{18}H_{21}NO_3 \cdot C_4H_6O_6 \cdot 2\frac{1}{2}H_2O$ (hydrate); $C_{18}H_{21}NO_3 \cdot C_4H_6O_6$ (anhydrous).

Molecular weight:

Pheniramine maleate—356.43.

Pyrilamine maleate—401.46.

Phenylephrine hydrochloride—203.67.

Phenylpropanolamine hydrochloride—187.67.

Hydrocodone bitartrate—494.50 (hydrate); 449.46 (anhydrous).

Description:

Pheniramine maleate—White or almost white, crystalline powder, odorless or with a slight odor.

Pyrilamine Maleate USP—White, crystalline powder, usually having a faint odor. Its solutions are acid to litmus.

Phenylephrine Hydrochloride USP—White or practically white, odorless crystals.

Phenylpropanolamine Hydrochloride USP—White, crystalline powder, having a slight aromatic odor. Is affected by light.

Hydrocodone Bitartrate USP—Fine, white crystals or a crystalline powder. Is affected by light.

pKa: Phenylpropanolamine hydrochloride—9.

Solubility:

Pheniramine maleate—Soluble 1 in 0.3 of water, 1 in 2.5 of alcohol, and 1 in 1.5 of chloroform; very slightly soluble in ether.

Pyrilamine Maleate USP—Very soluble in water; freely soluble in alcohol and in chloroform; slightly soluble in ether.

Phenylephrine Hydrochloride USP—Freely soluble in water and in alcohol.

Phenylpropanolamine Hydrochloride USP—Freely soluble in water and in alcohol; insoluble in ether.

Hydrocodone Bitartrate USP—Soluble in water; slightly soluble in alcohol; insoluble in ether and in chloroform.

USP requirements: Pheniramine Maleate, Pyrilamine Maleate, Phenylephrine Hydrochloride, Phenylpropanolamine Hydrochloride, and Hydrocodone Bitartrate Oral Solution—Not in USP.

PHENIRAMINE, PYRILAMINE, AND PHENYLPROPANOLAMINE

Chemical group:

Pheniramine—Alkylamine derivative.

Pyrilamine—Ethylenediamine derivative.

Chemical name:

Pheniramine maleate—2-[alpha-[2-Dimethylaminoethyl]-benzyl]pyridine bimaleate.

Pyrilamine maleate—1,2-Ethanediamine, N-[(4-methoxyphenyl)methyl]-N',N'-dimethyl-N-2-pyridinyl-, (Z)-2-butenedioate (1:1).

Phenylpropanolamine hydrochloride—Benzenemethanol, alpha-(1-aminoethyl)-, hydrochloride, ($R*$,$S*$)-, (±).

Molecular formula:

Pheniramine maleate—$C_{16}H_{20}N_2 \cdot C_4H_4O_4$.

Pyrilamine maleate—$C_{17}H_{23}N_3O \cdot C_4H_4O_4$.

Phenylpropanolamine hydrochloride—$C_9H_{13}NO \cdot HCl$.

Molecular weight:

Pheniramine maleate—356.43.

Pyrilamine maleate—401.46.

Phenylpropanolamine hydrochloride—187.67.

Description:

Pheniramine maleate—White or almost white, crystalline powder, odorless or with a slight odor.

Pyrilamine Maleate USP—White, crystalline powder, usually having a faint odor. Its solutions are acid to litmus.

Phenylpropanolamine Hydrochloride USP—White, crystalline powder, having a slight aromatic odor. Affected by light.

pKa: Phenylpropanolamine hydrochloride—9.

Solubility:

Pheniramine maleate—Soluble 1 in 0.3 of water, 1 in 2.5 of alcohol, and 1 in 1.5 of chloroform; very slightly soluble in ether.

Pyrilamine Maleate USP—Very soluble in water; freely soluble in alcohol and in chloroform; slightly soluble in ether.

Phenylpropanolamine Hydrochloride USP—Freely soluble in water and in alcohol; insoluble in ether.

USP requirements:

Pheniramine Maleate, Pyrilamine Maleate, and Phenylpropanolamine Hydrochloride Oral Solution—Not in USP.

Pheniramine Maleate, Pyrilamine Maleate, and Phenylpropanolamine Hydrochloride Extended-release Tablets—Not in USP.

PHENIRAMINE, PYRILAMINE, PHENYLPROPANOLAMINE, AND ASPIRIN

Chemical group:

Pheniramine—Alkylamine derivative.

Pyrilamine—Ethylenediamine derivative.

Chemical name:

Pheniramine maleate—2-[alpha-[2-Dimethylaminoethyl]-benzyl]pyridine bimaleate.

Pyrilamine maleate—1,2-Ethanediamine, N-[(4-methoxyphenyl)methyl]-N',N'-dimethyl-N-2-pyridinyl-, (Z)-2-butenedioate (1:1).

Phenylpropanolamine hydrochloride—Benzenemethanol, alpha-(1-aminoethyl)-, hydrochloride, ($R*$,$S*$)-, (±).

Aspirin—Benzoic acid, 2-(acetyloxy)-.

Molecular formula:

Pheniramine maleate—$C_{16}H_{20}N_2 \cdot C_4H_4O_4$.

Pyrilamine maleate—$C_{17}H_{23}N_3O \cdot C_4H_4O_4$.

Phenylpropanolamine hydrochloride—$C_9H_{13}NO \cdot HCl$.

Aspirin—$C_9H_8O_4$.

Molecular weight:

Pheniramine maleate—356.43.

Pyrilamine maleate—401.46.

Phenylpropanolamine hydrochloride—187.67.

Aspirin—180.16.

Description:

Pheniramine maleate—White or almost white, crystalline powder, odorless or with a slight odor.

Pyrilamine Maleate USP—White, crystalline powder, usually having a faint odor. Its solutions are acid to litmus.

Phenylpropanolamine Hydrochloride USP—White, crystalline powder, having a slight aromatic odor. Affected by light.

Aspirin USP—White crystals, commonly tabular or needle-like, or white, crystalline powder. Is odorless or has a faint odor. Is stable in dry air; in moist air it gradually hydrolyzes to salicylic and acetic acids.

pKa:

Phenylpropanolamine hydrochloride—9.

Aspirin—3.5.

Solubility:

Pheniramine maleate—Soluble 1 in 0.3 of water, 1 in 2.5 of alcohol, and 1 in 1.5 of chloroform; very slightly soluble in ether.

Pyrilamine Maleate USP—Very soluble in water; freely soluble in alcohol and in chloroform; slightly soluble in ether.

Phenylpropanolamine Hydrochloride USP—Freely soluble in water and in alcohol; insoluble in ether.

Aspirin USP—Slightly soluble in water; freely soluble in alcohol; soluble in chloroform and in ether; sparingly soluble in absolute ether.

USP requirements: Pheniramine Maleate, Pyrilamine Maleate, Phenylpropanolamine Hydrochloride, and Aspirin Tablets—Not in USP.

PHENIRAMINE, PYRILAMINE, PHENYLPROPANOLAMINE, AND CODEINE

Chemical group:

Pheniramine—Alkylamine derivative.

Pyrilamine—Ethylenediamine derivative.

Chemical name:

Pheniramine maleate—2-[alpha-[2-Dimethylaminoethyl]-benzyl]pyridine bimaleate.

Pyrilamine maleate—1,2-Ethanediamine, *N*-[(4-methoxy-phenyl)methyl]-*N′,N′*-dimethyl-*N*-2-pyridinyl-, (*Z*)-2-butenedioate (1:1).
Phenylpropanolamine hydrochloride—Benzenemethanol, alpha-(1-aminoethyl)-, hydrochloride, (*R**,*S**)-, (±).
Codeine phosphate—Morphinan-6-ol, 7,8-didehydro-4,5-epoxy-3-methoxy-17-methyl-, (5 alpha,6 alpha)-, phosphate (1:1) (salt), hemihydrate.

Molecular formula:
Pheniramine maleate—$C_{16}H_{20}N_2 \cdot C_4H_4O_4$.
Pyrilamine maleate—$C_{17}H_{23}N_3O \cdot C_4H_4O_4$.
Phenylpropanolamine hydrochloride—$C_9H_{13}NO \cdot HCl$.
Codeine phosphate—$C_{18}H_{21}NO_3 \cdot H_3PO_4 \cdot \frac{1}{2}H_2O$ (hemihydrate); $C_{18}H_{21}NO_3 \cdot H_3PO_4$ (anhydrous).

Molecular weight:
Pheniramine maleate—356.43.
Pyrilamine maleate—401.46.
Phenylpropanolamine hydrochloride—187.67.
Codeine phosphate—406.37 (hemihydrate); 397.36 (anhydrous).

Description:
Pheniramine maleate—White or almost white, crystalline powder, odorless or with a slight odor.
Pyrilamine Maleate USP—White, crystalline powder, usually having a faint odor. Its solutions are acid to litmus.
Phenylpropanolamine Hydrochloride USP—White, crystalline powder, having a slight aromatic odor. Affected by light.
Codeine Phosphate USP—Fine, white, needle-shaped crystals, or white, crystalline powder. Is odorless, and is affected by light. Its solutions are acid to litmus.

pKa: Phenylpropanolamine hydrochloride—9.

Solubility:
Pheniramine maleate—Soluble 1 in 0.3 of water, 1 in 2.5 of alcohol, and 1 in 1.5 of chloroform; very slightly soluble in ether.
Pyrilamine Maleate USP—Very soluble in water; freely soluble in alcohol and in chloroform; slightly soluble in ether.
Phenylpropanolamine Hydrochloride USP—Freely soluble in water and in alcohol; insoluble in ether.
Codeine Phosphate USP—Freely soluble in water; very soluble in hot water; slightly soluble in alcohol but more so in boiling alcohol.

USP requirements: Pheniramine Maleate, Pyrilamine Maleate, Phenylpropanolamine Hydrochloride and Codeine Phosphate Syrup—Not in USP.

PHENIRAMINE, PYRILAMINE, PHENYLPROPANOLAMINE, CODEINE, ACETAMINOPHEN, AND CAFFEINE

Source: Caffeine—Coffee, tea, cola, and cocoa or chocolate. May also be synthesized from urea or dimethylurea.

Chemical group:
Pheniramine—Alkylamine derivative.
Pyrilamine—Ethylenediamine derivative.
Caffeine—Methylated xanthine.

Chemical name:
Pheniramine maleate—2-[alpha-[2-Dimethylaminoethyl]-benzyl]pyridine bimaleate.
Pyrilamine maleate—1,2-Ethanediamine, *N*-[(4-methoxy-phenyl)methyl]-*N′,N′*-dimethyl-*N*-2-pyridinyl-, (*Z*)-2-butenedioate (1:1).

Phenylpropanolamine hydrochloride—Benzenemethanol, alpha-(1-aminoethyl)-, hydrochloride, (*R**,*S**)-, (±).
Codeine phosphate—Morphinan-6-ol, 7,8-didehydro-4,5-epoxy-3-methoxy-17-methyl-, (5 alpha,6 alpha)-, phosphate (1:1) (salt), hemihydrate.
Acetaminophen—Acetamide, *N*-(4-hydroxyphenyl)-.
Caffeine—1*H*-Purine-2,6-dione, 3,7-dihydro-1,3,7-trimethyl-.

Molecular formula:
Pheniramine maleate—$C_{16}H_{20}N_2 \cdot C_4H_4O_4$.
Pyrilamine maleate—$C_{17}H_{23}N_3O \cdot C_4H_4O_4$.
Phenylpropanolamine hydrochloride—$C_9H_{13}NO \cdot HCl$.
Codeine phosphate—$C_{18}H_{21}NO_3 \cdot H_3PO_4 \cdot \frac{1}{2}H_2O$ (hemihydrate); $C_{18}H_{21}NO_3 \cdot H_3PO_4$ (anhydrous).
Acetaminophen—$C_8H_9NO_2$.
Caffeine—$C_8H_{10}N_4O_2$ (anhydrous); $C_8H_{10}N_4O_2 \cdot H_2O$ (monohydrate).

Molecular weight:
Pheniramine maleate—356.43.
Pyrilamine maleate—401.46.
Phenylpropanolamine hydrochloride—187.67.
Codeine phosphate—406.37 (hemihydrate); 397.36 (anhydrous).
Acetaminophen—151.16.
Caffeine—194.19 (anhydrous); 212.21 (monohydrate).

Description:
Pheniramine maleate—White or almost white, crystalline powder, odorless or with a slight odor.
Pyrilamine Maleate USP—White, crystalline powder, usually having a faint odor. Its solutions are acid to litmus.
Phenylpropanolamine Hydrochloride USP—White, crystalline powder, having a slight aromatic odor. Is affected by light.
Codeine Phosphate USP—Fine, white, needle-shaped crystals, or white, crystalline powder. Is odorless, and is affected by light. Its solutions are acid to litmus.
Acetaminophen USP—White, odorless, crystalline powder.
Caffeine USP—White powder, or white, glistening needles, usually matted together. Is odorless. Its solutions are neutral to litmus. The hydrate is efflorescent in air.

pKa: Phenylpropanolamine hydrochloride—9.

Solubility:
Pheniramine maleate—Soluble 1 in 0.3 of water, 1 in 2.5 of alcohol, and 1 in 1.5 of chloroform; very slightly soluble in ether.
Pyrilamine Maleate USP—Very soluble in water; freely soluble in alcohol and in chloroform; slightly soluble in ether.
Phenylpropanolamine Hydrochloride USP—Freely soluble in water and in alcohol; insoluble in ether.
Codeine Phosphate USP—Freely soluble in water; very soluble in hot water; slightly soluble in alcohol but more so in boiling alcohol.
Acetaminophen USP—Soluble in boiling water and in 1 *N* sodium hydroxide; freely soluble in alcohol.
Caffeine USP—Sparingly soluble in water and in alcohol; freely soluble in chloroform; slightly soluble in ether.

The aqueous solubility of caffeine is increased by organic acids or their alkali salts, such as citrates, benzoates, salicylates, or cinnamates, which dissociate to yield caffeine when dissolved in biological fluids.

USP requirements: Pheniramine Maleate, Pyrilamine Maleate, Phenylpropanolamine Hydrochloride, Codeine Phosphate, Acetaminophen, and Caffeine Tablets—Not in USP.

PHENIRAMINE, PYRILAMINE, PHENYLPROPANOLAMINE, AND DEXTROMETHORPHAN

Source: Dextromethorphan—Methylated dextroisomer of levorphanol.

Chemical group:
Pheniramine—Alkylamine derivative.
Pyrilamine—Ethylenediamine derivative.
Dextromethorphan—Synthetic derivative of morphine.

Chemical name:
Pheniramine maleate—2-[alpha-[2-Dimethylaminoethyl]-benzyl]pyridine bimaleate.
Pyrilamine maleate—1,2-Ethanediamine, *N*-[(4-methoxy-phenyl)methyl]-*N',N'*-dimethyl-*N*-2-pyridinyl-, (*Z*)-2-butenedioate (1:1).
Phenylpropanolamine hydrochloride—Benzenemethanol, alpha-(1-aminoethyl)-, hydrochloride, (*R*,S**)-, (±).
Dextromethorphan hydrobromide—Morphinan, 3-methoxy-17-methyl-, (9 alpha,13 alpha,14 alpha)-, hydrobromide, monohydrate.

Molecular formula:
Pheniramine maleate—$C_{16}H_{20}N_2 \cdot C_4H_4O_4$.
Pyrilamine maleate—$C_{17}H_{23}N_3O \cdot C_4H_4O_4$.
Phenylpropanolamine hydrochloride—$C_9H_{13}NO \cdot HCl$.
Dextromethorphan hydrobromide—$C_{18}H_{25}NO \cdot HBr \cdot H_2O$.

Molecular weight:
Pheniramine maleate—356.43.
Pyrilamine maleate—401.46.
Phenylpropanolamine hydrochloride—187.67.
Dextromethorphan hydrobromide—370.33.

Description:
Pheniramine maleate—White or almost white, crystalline powder, odorless or with a slight odor.
Pyrilamine Maleate USP—White, crystalline powder, usually having a faint odor. Its solutions are acid to litmus.
Phenylpropanolamine Hydrochloride USP—White, crystalline powder, having a slight aromatic odor. Is affected by light.
Dextromethorphan Hydrobromide USP—Practically white crystals or crystalline powder, having a faint odor. Melts at about 126 °C, with decomposition.

pKa: Phenylpropanolamine hydrochloride—9.

Solubility:
Pheniramine maleate—Soluble 1 in 0.3 of water, 1 in 2.5 of alcohol, and 1 in 1.5 of chloroform; very slightly soluble in ether.
Pyrilamine Maleate USP—Very soluble in water; freely soluble in alcohol and in chloroform; slightly soluble in ether.
Phenylpropanolamine Hydrochloride USP—Freely soluble in water and in alcohol; insoluble in ether.
Dextromethorphan Hydrobromide USP—Sparingly soluble in water; freely soluble in alcohol and in chloroform; insoluble in ether.

USP requirements: Pheniramine Maleate, Pyrilamine Maleate, Phenylpropanolamine Hydrochloride, and Dextromethorphan Hydrobromide Syrup—Not in USP.

PHENIRAMINE, PYRILAMINE, PHENYLPROPANOLAMINE, DEXTROMETHORPHAN, AND AMMONIUM CHLORIDE

Source: Dextromethorphan—Methylated dextroisomer of levorphanol.

Chemical group:
Pheniramine—Alkylamine derivative.
Pyrilamine—Ethylenediamine derivative.
Dextromethorphan—Synthetic derivative of morphine.

Chemical name:
Pheniramine maleate—2-[alpha-[2-Dimethylaminoethyl]-benzyl]pyridine bimaleate.
Pyrilamine maleate—1,2-Ethanediamine, *N*-[(4-methoxy-phenyl)methyl]-*N',N'*-dimethyl-*N*-2-pyridinyl-, (*Z*)-2-butenedioate (1:1).
Phenylpropanolamine hydrochloride—Benzenemethanol, alpha-(1-aminoethyl)-, hydrochloride, (*R*,S**)-, (±).
Dextromethorphan hydrobromide—Morphinan, 3-methoxy-17-methyl-, (9 alpha,13 alpha,14 alpha)-, hydrobromide, monohydrate.
Ammonium chloride—Ammonium chloride.

Molecular formula:
Pheniramine maleate—$C_{16}H_{20}N_2 \cdot C_4H_4O_4$.
Pyrilamine maleate—$C_{17}H_{23}N_3O \cdot C_4H_4O_4$.
Phenylpropanolamine hydrochloride—$C_9H_{13}NO \cdot HCl$.
Dextromethorphan hydrobromide—$C_{18}H_{25}NO \cdot HBr \cdot H_2O$.
Ammonium chloride—NH_4Cl.

Molecular weight:
Pheniramine maleate—356.43.
Pyrilamine maleate—401.46.
Phenylpropanolamine hydrochloride—187.67.
Dextromethorphan hydrobromide—370.33.
Ammonium chloride—53.49.

Description:
Pheniramine maleate—White or almost white, crystalline powder, odorless or with a slight odor.
Pyrilamine Maleate USP—White, crystalline powder, usually having a faint odor. Its solutions are acid to litmus.
Phenylpropanolamine Hydrochloride USP—White, crystalline powder, having a slight aromatic odor. Is affected by light.
Dextromethorphan Hydrobromide USP—Practically white crystals or crystalline powder, having a faint odor. Melts at about 126 °C, with decomposition.
Ammonium Chloride USP—Colorless crystals or white, fine or coarse, crystalline powder. Is somewhat hygroscopic.

pKa: Phenylpropanolamine hydrochloride—9.

Solubility:
Pheniramine maleate—Soluble 1 in 0.3 of water, 1 in 2.5 of alcohol, and 1 in 1.5 of chloroform; very slightly soluble in ether.
Pyrilamine Maleate USP—Very soluble in water; freely soluble in alcohol and in chloroform; slightly soluble in ether.
Phenylpropanolamine Hydrochloride USP—Freely soluble in water and in alcohol; insoluble in ether.
Dextromethorphan Hydrobromide USP—Sparingly soluble in water; freely soluble in alcohol and in chloroform; insoluble in ether.
Ammonium Chloride USP—Freely soluble in water and in glycerin, and even more so in boiling water; sparingly soluble in alcohol.

USP requirements: Pheniramine Maleate, Pyrilamine Maleate, Phenylpropanolamine Hydrochloride, Dextromethorphan Hydrobromide, and Ammonium Chloride Syrup—Not in USP.

PHENIRAMINE, PYRILAMINE, PHENYLPROPANOLAMINE, DEXTROMETHORPHAN, AND GUAIFENESIN

Source: Dextromethorphan—Methylated dextroisomer of levorphanol.

Chemical group:
Pheniramine—Alkylamine derivative.

Pyrilamine—Ethylenediamine derivative.
Dextromethorphan—Synthetic derivative of morphine.

Chemical name:
Pheniramine maleate—2-[alpha-[2-Dimethylaminoethyl]-benzyl]pyridine bimaleate.
Pyrilamine maleate—1,2-Ethanediamine, N-[(4-methoxyphenyl)methyl]-N',N'-dimethyl-N-2-pyridinyl-, (Z)-2-butenedioate (1:1).
Phenylpropanolamine hydrochloride—Benzenemethanol, alpha-(1-aminoethyl)-, hydrochloride, (R*,S*)-, (±).
Dextromethorphan hydrobromide—Morphinan, 3-methoxy-17-methyl-, (9 alpha,13 alpha,14 alpha)-, hydrobromide, monohydrate.
Guaifenesin—1,2-Propanediol, 3-(2-methoxyphenoxy)-.

Molecular formula:
Pheniramine maleate—$C_{16}H_{20}N_2 \cdot C_4H_4O_4$.
Pyrilamine maleate—$C_{17}H_{23}N_3O \cdot C_4H_4O_4$.
Phenylpropanolamine hydrochloride—$C_9H_{13}NO \cdot HCl$.
Dextromethorphan hydrobromide—$C_{18}H_{25}NO \cdot HBr \cdot H_2O$.
Guaifenesin—$C_{10}H_{14}O_4$.

Molecular weight:
Pheniramine maleate—356.43.
Pyrilamine maleate—401.46.
Phenylpropanolamine hydrochloride—187.67.
Dextromethorphan hydrobromide—370.33.
Guaifenesin—198.22.

Description:
Pheniramine maleate—White or almost white, crystalline powder, odorless or with a slight odor.
Pyrilamine Maleate USP—White, crystalline powder, usually having a faint odor. Its solutions are acid to litmus.
Phenylpropanolamine Hydrochloride USP—White, crystalline powder, having a slight aromatic odor. Is affected by light.
Dextromethorphan Hydrobromide USP—Practically white crystals or crystalline powder, having a faint odor. Melts at about 126 °C, with decomposition.
Guaifenesin USP—White to slightly gray, crystalline powder. May have a slight characteristic odor.

pKa: Phenylpropanolamine hydrochloride—9.

Solubility:
Pheniramine maleate—Soluble 1 in 0.3 of water, 1 in 2.5 of alcohol, and 1 in 1.5 of chloroform; very slightly soluble in ether.
Pyrilamine Maleate USP—Very soluble in water; freely soluble in alcohol and in chloroform; slightly soluble in ether.
Phenylpropanolamine Hydrochloride USP—Freely soluble in water and in alcohol; insoluble in ether.
Dextromethorphan Hydrobromide USP—Sparingly soluble in water; freely soluble in alcohol and in chloroform; insoluble in ether.
Guaifenesin USP—Soluble in water, in alcohol, in chloroform, in glycerin, and in propylene glycol.

USP requirements: Pheniramine Maleate, Pyrilamine Maleate, Phenylpropanolamine Hydrochloride, Dextromethorphan Hydrobromide, and Guaifenesin Oral Solution—Not in USP.

PHENIRAMINE, PYRILAMINE, PHENYLPROPANOLAMINE, AND GUAIFENESIN

Chemical group:
Pheniramine—Alkylamine derivative.
Pyrilamine—Ethylenediamine derivative.

Chemical name:
Pheniramine maleate—2-[alpha-[2-Dimethylaminoethyl]-benzyl]pyridine bimaleate.

Pyrilamine maleate—1,2-Ethanediamine, N-[(4-methoxyphenyl)methyl]-N',N'-dimethyl-N-2-pyridinyl-, (Z)-2-butenedioate (1:1).
Phenylpropanolamine hydrochloride—Benzenemethanol, alpha-(1-aminoethyl)-, hydrochloride, (R*,S*)-, (±).
Guaifenesin—1,2-Propanediol, 3-(2-methoxyphenoxy)-.

Molecular formula:
Pheniramine maleate—$C_{16}H_{20}N_2 \cdot C_4H_4O_4$.
Pyrilamine maleate—$C_{17}H_{23}N_3O \cdot C_4H_4O_4$.
Phenylpropanolamine hydrochloride—$C_9H_{13}NO \cdot HCl$.
Guaifenesin—$C_{10}H_{14}O_4$.

Molecular weight:
Pheniramine maleate—356.43.
Pyrilamine maleate—401.46.
Phenylpropanolamine hydrochloride—187.67.
Guaifenesin—198.22.

Description:
Pheniramine maleate—White or almost white, crystalline powder, odorless or with a slight odor.
Pyrilamine Maleate USP—White, crystalline powder, usually having a faint odor. Its solutions are acid to litmus.
Phenylpropanolamine Hydrochloride USP—White, crystalline powder, having a slight aromatic odor. Is affected by light.
Guaifenesin USP—White to slightly gray, crystalline powder. May have a slight characteristic odor.

pKa: Phenylpropanolamine hydrochloride—9.

Solubility:
Pheniramine maleate—Soluble 1 in 0.3 of water, 1 in 2.5 of alcohol, and 1 in 1.5 of chloroform; very slightly soluble in ether.
Pyrilamine Maleate USP—Very soluble in water; freely soluble in alcohol and in chloroform; slightly soluble in ether.
Phenylpropanolamine Hydrochloride USP—Freely soluble in water and in alcohol; insoluble in ether.
Guaifenesin USP—Soluble in water, in alcohol, in chloroform, in glycerin, and in propylene glycol.

USP requirements: Pheniramine Maleate, Pyrilamine Maleate, Phenylpropanolamine Hydrochloride, and Guaifenesin Oral Solution—Not in USP.

PHENIRAMINE, PYRILAMINE, PHENYLPROPANOLAMINE, AND HYDROCODONE

Chemical group:
Pheniramine—Alkylamine derivative.
Pyrilamine—Ethylenediamine derivative.

Chemical name:
Pheniramine maleate—2-[alpha-[2-Dimethylaminoethyl]-benzyl]pyridine bimaleate.
Pyrilamine maleate—1,2-Ethanediamine, N-[(4-methoxyphenyl)methyl]-N',N'-dimethyl-N-2-pyridinyl-, (Z)-2-butenedioate (1:1).
Phenylpropanolamine hydrochloride—Benzenemethanol, alpha-(1-aminoethyl)-, hydrochloride, (R*,S*)-, (±).
Hydrocodone bitartrate—Morphinan-6-one, 4,5-epoxy-3-methoxy-17-methyl-, (5 alpha)-, [R-(R*,R*)]-2,3-dihydroxybutanedioate (1:1), hydrate (2:5).

Molecular formula:
Pheniramine maleate—$C_{16}H_{20}N_2 \cdot C_4H_4O_4$.
Pyrilamine maleate—$C_{17}H_{23}N_3O \cdot C_4H_4O_4$.
Phenylpropanolamine hydrochloride—$C_9H_{13}NO \cdot HCl$.
Hydrocodone bitartrate—$C_{18}H_{21}NO_3 \cdot C_4H_6O_6 \cdot 2\frac{1}{2}H_2O$ (hydrate); $C_{18}H_{21}NO_3 \cdot C_4H_6O_6$ (anhydrous).

Molecular weight:
Pheniramine maleate—356.43.
Pyrilamine maleate—401.46.
Phenylpropanolamine hydrochloride—187.67.
Hydrocodone bitartrate—494.50 (hydrate); 449.46 (anhydrous).

Description:
Pheniramine maleate—White or almost white, crystalline powder, odorless or with a slight odor.
Pyrilamine Maleate USP—White, crystalline powder, usually having a faint odor. Its solutions are acid to litmus.
Phenylpropanolamine Hydrochloride USP—White, crystalline powder, having a slight aromatic odor. Is affected by light.
Hydrocodone Bitartrate USP—Fine, white crystals or a crystalline powder. Is affected by light.

pKa: Phenylpropanolamine hydrochloride—9.

Solubility:
Pheniramine maleate—Soluble 1 in 0.3 of water, 1 in 2.5 of alcohol, and 1 in 1.5 of chloroform; very slightly soluble in ether.
Pyrilamine Maleate USP—Very soluble in water; freely soluble in alcohol and in chloroform; slightly soluble in ether.
Phenylpropanolamine Hydrochloride USP—Freely soluble in water and in alcohol; insoluble in ether.
Hydrocodone Bitartrate USP—Soluble in water; slightly soluble in alcohol; insoluble in ether and in chloroform.

USP requirements: Pheniramine Maleate, Pyrilamine Maleate, Phenylpropanolamine Hydrochloride, and Hydrocodone Bitartrate Oral Solution—Not in USP.

PHENIRAMINE, PYRILAMINE, PHENYLPROPANOLAMINE, HYDROCODONE, AND GUAIFENESIN

Chemical group:
Pheniramine—Alkylamine derivative.
Pyrilamine—Ethylenediamine derivative.

Chemical name:
Pheniramine maleate—2-[alpha-[2-Dimethylaminoethyl]-benzyl]pyridine bimaleate.
Pyrilamine maleate—1,2-Ethanediamine, N-[(4-methoxyphenyl)methyl]-N',N'-dimethyl-N-2-pyridinyl-, (Z)-2-butenedioate (1:1).
Phenylpropanolamine hydrochloride—Benzenemethanol, alpha-(1-aminoethyl)-, hydrochloride, ($R*,S*$)-, ($\pm$).
Hydrocodone bitartrate—Morphinan-6-one, 4,5-epoxy-3-methoxy-17-methyl-, (5 alpha)-, [R-($R*,R*$)]-2,3-dihydroxybutanedioate (1:1), hydrate (2:5).
Guaifenesin—1,2-Propanediol, 3-(2-methoxyphenoxy)-.

Molecular formula:
Pheniramine maleate—$C_{16}H_{20}N_2 \cdot C_4H_4O_4$.
Pyrilamine maleate—$C_{17}H_{23}N_3O \cdot C_4H_4O_4$.
Phenylpropanolamine hydrochloride—$C_9H_{13}NO \cdot HCl$.
Hydrocodone bitartrate—$C_{18}H_{21}NO_3 \cdot C_4H_6O_6 \cdot 2\frac{1}{2}H_2O$ (hydrate); $C_{18}H_{21}NO_3 \cdot C_4H_6O_6$ (anhydrous).
Guaifenesin—$C_{10}H_{14}O_4$.

Molecular weight:
Pheniramine maleate—356.43.
Pyrilamine maleate—401.46.
Phenylpropanolamine hydrochloride—187.67.
Hydrocodone bitartrate—494.50 (hydrate); 449.46 (anhydrous).
Guaifenesin—198.22.

Description:
Pheniramine maleate—White or almost white, crystalline powder, odorless or with a slight odor.
Pyrilamine Maleate USP—White, crystalline powder, usually having a faint odor. Its solutions are acid to litmus.
Phenylpropanolamine Hydrochloride USP—White, crystalline powder, having a slight aromatic odor. Is affected by light.
Hydrocodone Bitartrate USP—Fine, white crystals or a crystalline powder. Is affected by light.
Guaifenesin USP—White to slightly gray, crystalline powder. May have a slight characteristic odor.

pKa: Phenylpropanolamine hydrochloride—9.

Solubility:
Pheniramine maleate—Soluble 1 in 0.3 of water, 1 in 2.5 of alcohol, and 1 in 1.5 of chloroform; very slightly soluble in ether.
Pyrilamine Maleate USP—Very soluble in water; freely soluble in alcohol and in chloroform; slightly soluble in ether.
Phenylpropanolamine Hydrochloride USP—Freely soluble in water and in alcohol; insoluble in ether.
Hydrocodone Bitartrate USP—Soluble in water; slightly soluble in alcohol; insoluble in ether and in chloroform.
Guaifenesin USP—Soluble in water, in alcohol, in chloroform, in glycerin, and in propylene glycol.

USP requirements: Pheniramine Maleate, Pyrilamine Maleate, Phenylpropanolamine Hydrochloride, Hydrocodone Bitartrate, and Guaifenesin Oral Solution—Not in USP.

PHENMETRAZINE

Chemical group: Morpholine.

Chemical name: Phenmetrazine hydrochloride—Morpholine, 3-methyl-2-phenyl-, hydrochloride.

Molecular formula: Phenmetrazine hydrochloride—$C_{11}H_{15}NO \cdot HCl$.

Molecular weight: Phenmetrazine hydrochloride—213.71.

Description: Phenmetrazine Hydrochloride USP—White to off-white, crystalline powder.

Solubility: Phenmetrazine Hydrochloride USP—Very soluble in water; freely soluble in alcohol and in chloroform.

USP requirements: Phenmetrazine Hydrochloride Tablets USP—Preserve in tight containers. Contain the labeled amount, within $\pm 7\%$. Meet the requirements for Identification, Dissolution (75% in 45 minutes in water in Apparatus 2 at 50 rpm), and Uniformity of dosage units.

PHENOBARBITAL

Chemical name:
Phenobarbital—2,4,6(1H,3H,5H)-Pyrimidinetrione, 5-ethyl-5-phenyl-.
Phenobarbital sodium—2,4,6(1H,3H,5H)-Pyrimidinetrione, 5-ethyl-5-phenyl-, monosodium salt.

Molecular formula:
Phenobarbital—$C_{12}H_{12}N_2O_3$.
Phenobarbital sodium—$C_{12}H_{11}N_2NaO_3$.

Molecular weight:
Phenobarbital—232.24.
Phenobarbital sodium—254.22.

Description:

Phenobarbital USP—White, odorless, glistening, small crystals, or white, crystalline powder, which may exhibit polymorphism. Is stable in air. Its saturated solution has a pH of about 5.

Phenobarbital Sodium USP—Flaky crystals, or white, crystalline granules, or white powder. Is odorless and is hygroscopic. Its solutions are alkaline to phenolphthalein TS, and decompose on standing.

Solubility:

Phenobarbital USP—Very slightly soluble in water; soluble in alcohol, in ether, and in solutions of fixed alkali hydroxides and carbonates; sparingly soluble in chloroform.

Phenobarbital Sodium USP—Very soluble in water; soluble in alcohol; practically insoluble in ether and in chloroform.

USP requirements:

Phenobarbital Capsules—Not in USP.

Phenobarbital Elixir USP—Preserve in tight, light-resistant containers. Contains the labeled amount, within ±10%. Meets the requirements for Identification and Alcohol content (12.0–15.0%).

Phenobarbital Tablets USP—Preserve in well-closed containers. Contain the labeled amount, within ±10%. Meet the requirements for Identification, Dissolution (75% in 45 minutes in water in Apparatus 2 at 50 rpm), and Uniformity of dosage units.

Phenobarbital Sodium Injection USP—Preserve in single-dose or in multiple-dose containers, preferably of Type I glass. A sterile solution of Phenobarbital Sodium in a suitable solvent. Phenobarbital may be substituted for the equivalent amount of Phenobarbital Sodium, for adjustment of the pH. The label indicates that the Injection is not to be used if it contains a precipitate. Contains the labeled amount, within −10% to +5%. Meets the requirements for Identification, Bacterial endotoxins, pH (9.2–10.2), and Injections.

Sterile Phenobarbital Sodium USP—Preserve in Containers for Sterile Solids. It is Phenobarbital Sodium suitable for parenteral use. Meets the requirements for Constituted solution and Bacterial endotoxins, for Identification tests, Completeness of solution, pH (9.2–10.2), Loss on drying (not more than 7.0%), and Heavy metals (not more than 0.003%) under Phenobarbital Sodium, and for Sterility tests, Uniformity of dosage units, and Labeling under Injections.

PHENOL

Chemical name: Phenol.

Molecular formula: C_6H_6O.

Molecular weight: 94.11.

Description: Phenol USP—Colorless to light pink, interlaced or separate, needleshaped crystals, or white to light pink, crystalline mass. It has a characteristic odor. Liquefied by warming, and by the addition of 10% of water. Boils at about 182 °C, and its vapor is flammable. Gradually darkens on exposure to light and air.

NF category: Antimicrobial preservative.

Solubility: Phenol USP—Soluble in water. Very soluble in alcohol, in glycerin, in chloroform, in ether, and in fixed and volatile oils; sparingly soluble in mineral oil.

USP requirements: Phenol USP—Preserve in tight, light-resistant containers. Label it to indicate the name and amount of any substance added as a stabilizer. Contains not less than

99.0% and not more than 100.5% of phenol, calculated on the anhydrous basis. Meets the requirements for Clarity of solution and reaction, Identification, Congealing temperature (not lower than 39 °C), Water (not more than 0.5%), Nonvolatile residue (not more than 0.05%), and Organic volatile impurities.

Caution: Avoid contact with skin, since serious burns may result.

LIQUEFIED PHENOL

Description: Liquefied Phenol USP—Colorless to pink liquid, which may develop a red tint upon exposure to air or light. Has a characteristic, somewhat aromatic odor. It whitens and cauterizes the skin and mucous membranes. Specific gravity is about 1.065.

Solubility: Liquefied Phenol USP—Miscible with alcohol, with ether, and with glycerin. A mixture of equal volumes of Liquefied Phenol and glycerin is miscible with water.

USP requirements: Liquefied Phenol USP—Preserve in tight, light-resistant containers. It is Phenol maintained in a liquid condition by the presence of about 10% of water. Label it to indicate the name and amount of any substance added as a stabilizer. Contains not less than 89.0% by weight of phenol. Meets the requirements for Distilling range (not higher than 182.5 °C) and Organic volatile impurities, and for Identifications tests, Clarity of solution and reaction, and Nonvolatile residue under Phenol.

Caution: Avoid contact with skin, since serious burns may result.

Note: When phenol is to be mixed with a fixed oil, mineral oil, or white petrolatum, use crystalline Phenol, not Liquefied Phenol.

PHENOLPHTHALEIN

Chemical group: Diphenylmethane derivative.

Chemical name: 1(3H)-Isobenzofuranone, 3,3-bis(4-hydroxyphenyl)-.

Molecular formula: $C_{20}H_{14}O_4$.

Molecular weight: 318.33.

Description: Phenolphthalein USP—White or faintly yellowish white, crystalline powder. Is odorless, and is stable in air.

Solubility: Phenolphthalein USP—Practically insoluble in water; soluble in alcohol; sparingly soluble in ether.

USP requirements:

Phenolphthalein Chewing Gum—Not in USP.

Phenolphthalein Tablets USP—Preserve in tight containers. Where Tablets contain Yellow Phenolphthalein, the labeling so indicates. Contain the labeled amount, within ±10%. Meet the requirements for Identification, Disintegration (30 minutes), and Uniformity of dosage units.

Phenolphthalein Wafers—Not in USP.

PHENOLSULFONPHTHALEIN

Chemical name: Phenol, 4,4′-(3H-2,1-benzoxathiol-3-ylidene)bis-, (S,S-dioxide).

Molecular formula: $C_{19}H_{14}O_5S$.

Molecular weight: 354.38.

Description: Bright to dark red, odorless, crystalline powder.

pKa: 7.9.

Solubility: Very slightly soluble in water; slightly soluble in alcohol; freely soluble in solutions of alkali hydroxides and carbonates; practically insoluble in chloroform and in ether.

USP requirements: Phenolsulfonphthalein Injection—Not in USP.

PHENOXYBENZAMINE

Chemical name: Phenoxybenzamine hydrochloride—Benzenemethanamine, *N*-(2-chloroethyl)-*N*-(1-methyl-2-phenoxyethyl)-, hydrochloride.

Molecular formula: Phenoxybenzamine hydrochloride—$C_{18}H_{22}ClNO \cdot HCl$.

Molecular weight: Phenoxybenzamine hydrochloride—340.29.

Description: Phenoxybenzamine hydrochloride—Colorless, crystalline powder. Melting point is 136 to 141 °C.

pKa: Phenoxybenzamine hydrochloride—4.4.

Solubility: Phenoxybenzamine hydrochloride—Soluble in water, in alcohol, and in chloroform; insoluble in ether.

USP requirements: Phenoxybenzamine Hydrochloride Capsules USP—Preserve in well-closed containers. Contain the labeled amount, within ±10%. Meet the requirements for Identification, Dissolution (75% in 45 minutes in 0.1 *N* hydrochloric acid in Apparatus 1 at 100 rpm), and Uniformity of dosage units.

PHENPROCOUMON

Chemical name: 2*H*-1-Benzopyran-2-one, 4-hydroxy-3-(1-phenylpropyl)-.

Molecular formula: $C_{18}H_{16}O_3$.

Molecular weight: 280.32.

Description: Phenprocoumon USP—Fine, white, crystalline powder. Odorless, or has a slight odor.

Solubility: Phenprocoumon USP—Practically insoluble in water; soluble in chloroform, in methanol, and in solutions of alkali hydroxides.

USP requirements: Phenprocoumon Tablets USP—Preserve in well-closed containers. Contain the labeled amount, within ±10%. Meet the requirements for Identification, Dissolution (75% in 45 minutes in water in Apparatus 2 at 50 rpm), and Uniformity of dosage units.

PHENSUXIMIDE

Chemical name: 2,5-Pyrrolidinedione, 1-methyl-3-phenyl-.

Molecular formula: $C_{11}H_{11}NO_2$.

Molecular weight: 189.21.

Description: Phensuximide USP—White to off-white crystalline powder. Is odorless, or has not more than a slight odor.

Solubility: Phensuximide USP—Slightly soluble in water; very soluble in chloroform; soluble in alcohol.

USP requirements: Phensuximide Capsules USP—Preserve in tight containers. Contain the labeled amount, within ±7%. Meet the requirements for Identification, Dissolution (75% in 120 minutes in water in Apparatus 1 at 100 rpm), and Uniformity of dosage units.

PHENTERMINE

Chemical group: Phenethylamine.

Chemical name:
Phentermine—Benzeneethanamine, alpha,alpha-dimethyl-.
Phentermine hydrochloride—Benzeneethanamine, alpha,alpha-dimethyl-, hydrochloride.

Molecular formula:
Phentermine—$C_{10}H_{15}N$.
Phentermine hydrochloride—$C_{10}H_{15}N \cdot HCl$.

Molecular weight:
Phentermine—149.24.
Phentermine hydrochloride—185.70.

Description: Phentermine Hydrochloride USP—White, odorless, hygroscopic, crystalline powder.

Solubility: Phentermine Hydrochloride USP—Soluble in water and in the lower alcohols; slightly soluble in chloroform; insoluble in ether.

USP requirements:
Phentermine Hydrochloride Capsules USP—Preserve in tight containers. Contain the labeled amount, within ±10%. Meet the requirements for Identification, Dissolution (75% in 45 minutes in water in Apparatus 2 at 50 rpm), and Uniformity of dosage units.
Phentermine Hydrochloride Tablets USP—Preserve in tight containers. Contain the labeled amount, within ±10%. Meet the requirements for Identification, Dissolution (75% in 45 minutes in water in Apparatus 2 at 50 rpm), and Uniformity of dosage units.
Phentermine Resin Capsules—Not in USP.

PHENTOLAMINE

Chemical name: Phentolamine mesylate—Phenol, 3-[[(4,5-dihydro-1*H*-imidazol-2-yl)methyl](4-methylphenyl)amino]-, monomethanesulfonate (salt).

Molecular formula: Phentolamine mesylate—$C_{17}H_{19}N_3O \cdot CH_4O_3S$.

Molecular weight: Phentolamine mesylate—377.46.

Description: Phentolamine Mesylate USP—White or off-white, odorless, crystalline powder. Its solutions are acid to litmus, having a pH of about 5, and slowly deteriorate. Melts at about 178 °C.

Solubility: Phentolamine Mesylate USP—Freely soluble in water and in alcohol; slightly soluble in chloroform.

USP requirements: Phentolamine Mesylate for Injection USP—Preserve in Containers for Sterile Solids. It is sterile Phentolamine Mesylate or a sterile mixture of Phentolamine Mesylate with a suitable buffer or suitable diluents. Contains the labeled amount, within ±10%. Meets the requirements for Constituted solution, Identification, Uniformity of dosage units, Bacterial endotoxins, and pH (4.5–6.5 in a freshly prepared solution of 1 in 100), and for Sterility tests and Labeling under Injections.

PHENYLBUTAZONE

Chemical group: Pyrazole derivative.

Chemical name: 3,5-Pyrazolidinedione, 4-butyl-1,2-diphenyl-.

Molecular formula: $C_{19}H_{20}N_2O_2$.

Molecular weight: 308.38.

Description: Phenylbutazone USP—White to off-white, odorless, crystalline powder.

Solubility: Phenylbutazone USP—Very slightly soluble in water; freely soluble in acetone and in ether; soluble in alcohol.

USP requirements:
Phenylbutazone Bolus—Not in USP.
Phenylbutazone Capsules USP—Preserve in tight containers. Contain the labeled amount, within ±10%. Meet the requirements for Identification, Dissolution (60% in 30 minutes in phosphate buffer [pH 7.5] in Apparatus 1 at 100 rpm), and Uniformity of dosage units.
Phenylbutazone Granules—Not in USP.
Phenylbutazone Injection—Not in USP.
Phenylbutazone Paste—Not in USP.
Phenylbutazone Tablets USP—Preserve in tight containers. Contain the labeled amount, within ±7%. Meet the requirements for Identification, Dissolution (60% in 30 minutes in simulated intestinal fluid TS [without the enzyme] in Apparatus 1 at 100 rpm), and Uniformity of dosage units.
Phenylbutazone Tablets, Buffered—Not in USP.
Phenylbutazone Delayed-release Tablets—Not in USP.

PHENYLEPHRINE

Chemical name: Phenylephrine hydrochloride—Benzenemethanol, 3-hydroxy-alpha-[(methylamino)methyl]-, hydrochloride.

Molecular formula: Phenylephrine hydrochloride—$C_9H_{13}NO_2 \cdot HCl$.

Molecular weight: Phenylephrine hydrochloride—203.67.

Description:
Phenylephrine Hydrochloride USP—White or practically white, odorless crystals.
Phenylephrine Hydrochloride Nasal Solution USP—Clear, colorless or slightly yellow, odorless liquid. Is neutral or acid to litmus.
Phenylephrine Hydrochloride Ophthalmic Solution USP—Clear, colorless or slightly yellow liquid, depending on the concentration.

Solubility: Phenylephrine Hydrochloride USP—Freely soluble in water and in alcohol.

USP requirements:
Phenylephrine Hydrochloride Injection USP—Preserve in single-dose or in multiple-dose containers, preferably of Type I glass, protected from light. A sterile solution of Phenylephrine Hydrochloride in Water for Injection. Contains the labeled amount, within −10% to +15%. Meets the requirements for Identification, Bacterial endotoxins, pH (3.0–6.5), and Injections.
Phenylephrine Hydrochloride Nasal Jelly USP—Preserve in tight containers. Contains the labeled amount, within ±10%. Meets the requirements for Identification and Minimum fill.
Phenylephrine Hydrochloride Nasal Solution USP—Preserve in tight, light-resistant containers. Contains the labeled amount, within −10% to +15%. Meets the requirement for Identification.
Phenylephrine Hydrochloride Ophthalmic Solution USP—Preserve in tight, light-resistant containers of not more than 15-mL size. A sterile, aqueous solution of Phenylephrine Hydrochloride. Contains the labeled amount, within −10% to +15%. Meets the requirements for Identification, Sterility, and pH (4.0–7.5 for buffered Ophthalmic Solution; 3.0–4.5 for unbuffered Ophthalmic Solution).

PHENYLEPHRINE AND ACETAMINOPHEN

For *Phenylephrine* and *Acetaminophen*—See individual listings for chemistry information.

USP requirements:
Phenylephrine Hydrochloride and Acetaminophen for Oral Solution—Not in USP.
Phenylephrine Hydrochloride and Acetaminophen Chewable Tablets—Not in USP.

PHENYLEPHRINE AND DEXTROMETHORPHAN

For *Phenylephrine* and *Dextromethorphan*—See individual listings for chemistry information.

USP requirements: Phenylephrine Hydrochloride and Dextromethorphan Hydrobromide Oral Suspension—Not in USP.

PHENYLEPHRINE, DEXTROMETHORPHAN, AND GUAIFENESIN

For *Phenylephrine, Dextromethorphan,* and *Guaifenesin*—See individual listings for chemistry information.

USP requirements: Phenylephrine Hydrochloride, Dextromethorphan Hydrobromide, and Guaifenesin Syrup—Not in USP.

PHENYLEPHRINE, DEXTROMETHORPHAN, GUAIFENESIN, AND ACETAMINOPHEN

For *Phenylephrine, Dextromethorphan, Guaifenesin,* and *Acetaminophen*—See individual listings for chemistry information.

USP requirements: Phenylephrine Hydrochloride, Dextromethorphan Hydrobromide, Guaifenesin, and Acetaminophen Tablets—Not in USP.

PHENYLEPHRINE, GUAIFENESIN, ACETAMINOPHEN, SALICYLAMIDE, AND CAFFEINE

For *Phenylephrine, Guaifenesin, Acetaminophen, Salicylamide,* and *Caffeine*—See individual listings for chemistry information.

USP requirements: Phenylephrine Hydrochloride, Guaifenesin, Acetaminophen, Salicylamide, and Caffeine Tablets—Not in USP.

PHENYLEPHRINE, HYDROCODONE, AND GUAIFENESIN

For *Phenylephrine, Hydrocodone,* and *Guaifenesin*—See individual listings for chemistry information.

USP requirements: Phenylephrine Hydrochloride, Hydrocodone Bitartrate, and Guaifenesin Syrup—Not in USP.

PHENYLEPHRINE, PHENYLPROPANOLAMINE, AND GUAIFENESIN

For *Phenylephrine, Phenylpropanolamine,* and *Guaifenesin*—See individual listings for chemistry information.

USP requirements:
Phenylephrine Hydrochloride, Phenylpropanolamine Hydrochloride, and Guaifenesin Capsules—Not in USP.
Phenylephrine Hydrochloride, Phenylpropanolamine Hydrochloride, and Guaifenesin Oral Solution—Not in USP.
Phenylephrine Hydrochloride, Phenylpropanolamine Hydrochloride, and Guaifenesin Tablets—Not in USP.

PHENYLETHYL ALCOHOL

Chemical name: Benzeneethanol.

Molecular formula: $C_8H_{10}O$.

Molecular weight: 122.17.

Description: Phenylethyl Alcohol USP—Colorless liquid, having a rose-like odor.

NF category: Antimicrobial preservative.

Solubility: Phenylethyl Alcohol USP—Sparingly soluble in water; very soluble in alcohol, in fixed oils, in glycerin, and in propylene glycol; slightly soluble in mineral oil.

USP requirements: Phenylethyl Alcohol USP—Preserve in tight, light-resistant containers, and store in a cool, dry place. Meets the requirements for Identification, Specific gravity (1.017–1.020), Refractive index (1.531–1.534 at 20 °C), Residue on ignition (not more than 0.005%), Chlorinated compounds, and Aldehyde.

PHENYLMERCURIC ACETATE

Chemical name: Mercury, (acetato-O)phenyl-.

Molecular formula: $C_8H_8HgO_2$.

Molecular weight: 336.74.

Description: Phenylmercuric Acetate NF—White to creamy white crystalline powder, or small, white prisms or leaflets. Odorless.

NF category: Antimicrobial preservative.

Solubility: Phenylmercuric Acetate NF—Slightly soluble in water; soluble in alcohol and in acetone.

NF requirements: Phenylmercuric Acetate NF—Preserve in tight, light-resistant containers. Contains not less than 98.0% and not more than 100.5% of phenylmercuric acetate. Meets the requirements for Identification, Melting range (149–153 °C), Residue on ignition (not more than 0.2%), Mercuric salts and heavy metals, and Polymercurated benzene compounds (not more than 1.5%).

PHENYLMERCURIC NITRATE

Chemical name: Mercury, (nitrato-O)phenyl-.

Molecular formula: $C_6H_5HgNo_3$.

Molecular weight: 339.70.

Description: Phenylmercuric Nitrate NF—White, crystalline powder. Affected by light. Its saturated solution is acid to litmus.

NF category: Antimicrobial preservative.

Solubility: Phenylmercuric Nitrate NF—Very slightly soluble in water; slightly soluble in alcohol and in glycerin. It is more soluble in the presence of either nitric acid or alkali hydroxides.

NF requirements: Phenylmercuric Nitrate NF—Preserve in tight, light-resistant containers. A mixture of phenylmercuric nitrate and phenylmercuric hydroxide containing not less than 87.0% and not more than 87.9% of phenylmercuric ion, and not less than 62.75% and not more than 63.50% of mercury. Meets the requirements for Identification, Residue on ignition (not more than 0.1%), and Mercury ions.

PHENYLPROPANOLAMINE

Chemical group: A synthetic phenylisopropanolamine.

Chemical name:
Phenylpropanolamine hydrochloride—Benzenemethanol, alpha-(1-aminoethyl)-, hydrochloride, (R^*,S^*)-, ($\pm$).

Phenylpropanolamine polistirex—Benzene, diethenyl-, polymer with ethenylbenzene, sulfonated, complex with ($\pm$)-(R^*,S^*)-alpha-(1-aminoethyl)benzenemethanol.

Molecular formula: Phenylpropanolamine hydrochloride—$C_9H_{13}NO \cdot HCl$.

Molecular weight: Phenylpropanolamine hydrochloride—187.67.

Description: Phenylpropanolamine Hydrochloride USP—White, crystalline powder, having a slight aromatic odor. Is affected by light.

pKa: Phenylpropanolamine hydrochloride—9.

Solubility: Phenylpropanolamine Hydrochloride USP—Freely soluble in water and in alcohol; insoluble in ether.

Other characteristics: Similar in structure and action to ephedrine but with less central nervous system (CNS) stimulation.

USP requirements:
Phenylpropanolamine Hydrochloride Capsules—Not in USP.
Phenylpropanolamine Hydrochloride Extended-release Capsules USP—Preserve in tight, light-resistant containers. Label Capsules to indicate the Drug Release Test with which the product complies. Contain the labeled amount, within ±10%. Meet the requirements for Identification, Drug release (15–45% in 3 hours, 40–70% in 6 hours, and not less than 70% in 12 hours in water in Apparatus 1 at 100 rpm for Drug Release Test 1; 5–30% in 1 hour, 30–65% in 3 hours, and not less than 70% in 6 hours in 0.1 N hydrochloric acid for 1 hour and in phosphate buffer [pH 6.8 ±0.05] for 1 hour in Apparatus 1 at 200 rpm for Drug Release Test 2), and Uniformity of dosage units.
Phenylpropanolamine Hydrochloride Tablets—Not in USP.
Phenylpropanolamine Hydrochloride Extended-release Tablets USP—Preserve in tight, light-resistant containers. The labeling states the in-vitro Drug release test conditions of times and tolerances, as directed under Drug release. Contain the labeled amount, within ±10%. Meet the requirements for Identification, Drug release, and Uniformity of dosage units.

PHENYLPROPANOLAMINE AND ACETAMINOPHEN

For *Phenylpropanolamine* and *Acetaminophen*—See individual listings for chemistry information.

USP requirements:
Phenylpropanolamine Hydrochloride and Acetaminophen Capsules—Not in USP.
Phenylpropanolamine Hydrochloride and Acetaminophen Oral Solution—Not in USP.
Phenylpropanolamine Hydrochloride and Acetaminophen Tablets—Not in USP.
Phenylpropanolamine Hydrochloride and Acetaminophen Chewable Tablets—Not in USP.

PHENYLPROPANOLAMINE, ACETAMINOPHEN, AND ASPIRIN

For *Phenylpropanolamine, Acetaminophen,* and *Aspirin*—See individual listings for chemistry information.

USP requirements: Phenylpropanolamine Hydrochloride, Acetaminophen, and Aspirin Capsules—Not in USP.

PHENYLPROPANOLAMINE, ACETAMINOPHEN, ASPIRIN, AND CAFFEINE

For *Phenylpropanolamine, Acetaminophen, Aspirin,* and *Caffeine*—See individual listings for chemistry information.

USP requirements: Phenylpropanolamine Hydrochloride, Acetaminophen, Aspirin, and Caffeine Capsules—Not in USP.

PHENYLPROPANOLAMINE, ACETAMINOPHEN, AND CAFFEINE

For *Phenylpropanolamine, Acetaminophen,* and *Caffeine*—See individual listings for chemistry information.

USP requirements: Phenylpropanolamine Hydrochloride, Acetaminophen, and Caffeine Tablets—Not in USP.

PHENYLPROPANOLAMINE, ACETAMINOPHEN, SALICYLAMIDE, AND CAFFEINE

For *Phenylpropanolamine, Acetaminophen, Salicylamide,* and *Caffeine*—See individual listings for chemistry information.

USP requirements: Phenylpropanolamine Hydrochloride, Acetaminophen, Salicylamide, and Caffeine Capsules—Not in USP.

PHENYLPROPANOLAMINE AND CARAMIPHEN

Chemical name:
Phenylpropanolamine hydrochloride—Benzenemethanol, alpha-(1-aminoethyl)-, hydrochloride, (R^*,S^*)-, $(\pm)$.
Caramiphen edisylate—1-Phenylcyclopentane-1-carboxylic acid, 2-diethylaminoethyl ester, 1,2-ethanedisulfonate (2:1).

Molecular formula:
Phenylpropanolamine hydrochloride—$C_9H_{13}NO \cdot HCl$.
Caramiphen edisylate—$(C_{18}H_{27}NO_2)_2 \cdot C_2H_6O_6S_2$.

Molecular weight:
Phenylpropanolamine hydrochloride—187.67.
Caramiphen edisylate—769.03.

Description:
Phenylpropanolamine Hydrochloride USP—White, crystalline powder, having a slight aromatic odor. Is affected by light.
Caramiphen edisylate—Off-white crystals with a melting point of 115–116 °C.

pKa: Phenylpropanolamine hydrochloride—9.

Solubility:
Phenylpropanolamine Hydrochloride USP—Freely soluble in water and in alcohol; insoluble in ether.
Caramiphen edisylate—1 gram dissolves in about 2 mL of water; soluble in alcohol.

USP requirements:
Phenylpropanolamine Hydrochloride and Caramiphen Edisylate Extended-release Capsules—Not in USP.
Phenylpropanolamine Hydrochloride and Caramiphen Edisylate Oral Solution—Not in USP.

PHENYLPROPANOLAMINE, CODEINE, AND GUAIFENESIN

For *Phenylpropanolamine, Codeine,* and *Guaifenesin*—See individual listings for chemistry information.

USP requirements:
Phenylpropanolamine Hydrochloride, Codeine Phosphate, and Guaifenesin Oral Solution—Not in USP.
Phenylpropanolamine Hydrochloride, Codeine Phosphate, and Guaifenesin Oral Suspension—Not in USP.
Phenylpropanolamine Hydrochloride, Codeine Phosphate, and Guaifenesin Syrup—Not in USP.

PHENYLPROPANOLAMINE AND DEXTROMETHORPHAN

For *Phenylpropanolamine* and *Dextromethorphan*—See individual listings for chemistry information.

USP requirements:
Phenylpropanolamine Hydrochloride and Dextromethorphan Hydrobromide Oral Gel—Not in USP.

Phenylpropanolamine Hydrochloride and Dextromethorphan Hydrobromide Granules—Not in USP.
Phenylpropanolamine Hydrochloride and Dextromethorphan Hydrobromide Lozenges—Not in USP.
Phenylpropanolamine Hydrochloride and Dextromethorphan Hydrobromide Oral Solution—Not in USP.
Phenylpropanolamine Hydrochloride and Dextromethorphan Hydrobromide Syrup—Not in USP.

PHENYLPROPANOLAMINE, DEXTROMETHORPHAN, AND ACETAMINOPHEN

For *Phenylpropanolamine, Dextromethorphan,* and *Acetaminophen*—See individual listings for chemistry information.

USP requirements:
Phenylpropanolamine Hydrochloride, Dextromethorphan Hydrobromide, and Acetaminophen Oral Solution—Not in USP.
Phenylpropanolamine Hydrochloride, Dextromethorphan Hydrobromide, and Acetaminophen Tablets—Not in USP.

PHENYLPROPANOLAMINE, DEXTROMETHORPHAN, AND GUAIFENESIN

For *Pheylpropanolanine, Dextromethorphan,* and *Guaifenesin*—See individual listings for chemistry information.

USP requirements:
Phenylpropanolamine Hydrochloride, Dextromethorphan Hydrobromide, and Guaifenesin Oral Solution—Not in USP.
Phenylpropanolamine Hydrochloride, Dextromethorphan Hydrobromide, and Guaifenesin Syrup—Not in USP.

PHENYLPROPANOLAMINE AND GUAIFENESIN

For *Phenylpropanolamine* and *Guaifenesin*—See individual listings for chemistry information.

USP requirements:
Phenylpropanolamine Hydrochloride and Guaifenesin Extended-release Capsules—Not in USP.
Phenylpropanolamine Hydrochloride and Guaifenesin Granules—Not in USP.
Phenylpropanolamine Hydrochloride and Guaifenesin Oral Solution—Not in USP.
Phenylpropanolamine Hydrochloride and Guaifenesin Syrup—Not in USP.
Phenylpropanolamine Hydrochloride and Guaifenesin Extended-release Tablets—Not in USP.

PHENYLPROPANOLAMINE AND HYDROCODONE

For *Phenylpropanolamine* and *Hydrocodone*—See individual listings for chemistry information.

USP requirements:
Phenylpropanolamine Hydrochloride and Hydrocodone Bitartrate Oral Solution—Not in USP.
Phenylpropanolamine Hydrochloride and Hydrocodone Bitartrate Syrup—Not in USP.

PHENYLTOLOXAMINE AND HYDROCODONE

Chemical name: Hydrocodone polistirex—Benzene, diethenyl-, polymer with ethenylbenzene, sulfonated, complex with (5 alpha)-4,5-epoxy-3-methoxy-17-methylmorphinan-6-one.

USP requirements:
Phenyltoloxamine Polistirex and Hydrocodone Polistirex Capsules—Not in USP.

Phenyltoloxamine Polistirex and Hydrocodone Polistirex Oral Suspension—Not in USP.

PHENYLTOLOXAMINE, PHENYLPROPANOLAMINE, AND ACETAMINOPHEN

Chemical name:
Phenyltoloxamine citrate—2-(2-Benzylphenoxy)-*N,N*-dimethylethylamine dihydrogen citrate.
Phenylpropanolamine hydrochloride—Benzenemethanol, alpha-(1-aminoethyl)-, hydrochloride, (*R**,*S**)-, (±).
Acetaminophen—Acetamide, *N*-(4-hydroxyphenyl)-.

Molecular formula:
Phenyltoloxamine citrate—$C_{17}H_{21}NO \cdot C_6H_8O_7$.
Phenylpropanolamine hydrochloride—$C_9H_{13}NO \cdot HCl$.
Acetaminophen—$C_8H_9NO_2$.

Molecular weight:
Phenyltoloxamine citrate—447.5.
Phenylpropanolamine hydrochloride—187.67.
Acetaminophen—151.16.

Description:
Phenyltoloxamine citrate—It has a melting point of 138–140 °C.
Phenylpropanolamine Hydrochloride USP—White, crystalline powder, having a slight aromatic odor. Affected by light.
Acetaminophen USP—White, odorless, crystalline powder.

pKa: Phenylpropanolamine hydrochloride—9.

Solubility:
Phenyltoloxamine citrate—Soluble in water.
Phenylpropanolamine Hydrochloride USP—Freely soluble in water and in alcohol; insoluble in ether.
Acetaminophen USP—Soluble in boiling water and in 1 *N* sodium hydroxide; freely soluble in alcohol.

USP requirements: Phenyltoloxamine Citrate, Phenylpropanolamine Hydrochloride, and Acetaminophen Extended-release Tablets—Not in USP.

PHENYTOIN

Chemical group: Related to the barbiturates in chemical structure, but has a five-membered ring.

Chemical name:
Phenytoin—2,4-Imidazolidinedione, 5,5-diphenyl-.
Phenytoin sodium—2,4-Imidazolidinedione, 5,5-diphenyl-, monosodium salt.

Molecular formula:
Phenytoin—$C_{15}H_{12}N_2O_2$.
Phenytoin sodium—$C_{15}H_{11}N_2NaO_2$.

Molecular weight:
Phenytoin—252.27.
Phenytoin sodium—274.25.

Description:
Phenytoin USP—White, odorless powder. Melts at about 295 °C.
Phenytoin Sodium USP—White, odorless powder. Is somewhat hygroscopic and on exposure to air gradually absorbs carbon dioxide.

pKa: 8.06–8.33 (apparent).

Solubility:
Phenytoin USP—Practically insoluble in water; soluble in hot alcohol; slightly soluble in cold alcohol, in chloroform, and in ether.

Phenytoin Sodium USP—Freely soluble in water, the solution usually being somewhat turbid due to partial hydrolysis and absorption of carbon dioxide. Soluble in alcohol; practically insoluble in ether and in chloroform.

USP requirements:
Phenytoin Oral Suspension USP—Preserve in tight containers. Avoid freezing. It is Phenytoin suspended in a suitable medium. Contains the labeled amount, within ±10%. Meets the requirement for Identification.
Phenytoin Tablets USP—Preserve in well-closed containers. Label the Tablets to indicate that they are to be chewed. Contain the labeled amount, within ±7%. Meet the requirements for Identification and Uniformity of dosage units.
Extended Phenytoin Sodium Capsules USP—Preserve in tight containers. Contain the labeled amount, within ±7%. Meet the requirements for Identification, Dissolution (not more than 40% in 30 minutes, 55% in 60 minutes, and not less than 70% in 120 minutes in water in Apparatus 1 at 50 rpm), and Uniformity of dosage units.
Prompt Phenytoin Sodium Capsules USP—Preserve in tight containers. Label Prompt Phenytoin Sodium Capsules with the statement, "Not for once-a-day dosing," printed immediately under the official name, in a bold and contrasting color and/or enclosed within a box. Contain the labeled amount, within ±7%. Meet the requirements for Identification, Dissolution (85% in 30 minutes in water in Apparatus 1 at 50 rpm), and Uniformity of dosage units.
Phenytoin Sodium Injection USP—Preserve in single-dose or in multiple-dose containers, preferably of Type I glass, at controlled room temperature. A sterile solution of Phenytoin Sodium with Propylene Glycol and Alcohol in Water for Injection. Contains the labeled amount, within ±10%. Meets the requirements for Identification, Bacterial endotoxins, pH (10.0–12.3), Alcohol and propylene glycol content (9–11% alcohol; 37–43% propylene glycol), Particulate matter, and Injections.
Note: Do not use the Injection if it is hazy or contains a precipitate.

CHROMIC PHOSPHATE P 32

Chemical name: Phosphoric-^{32}P acid, chromium(3+) salt (1:1).

Molecular formula: $Cr^{32}PO_4$.

Description: Grayish-green to brownish-green suspension.

USP requirements: Chromic Phosphate P 32 Suspension USP—Preserve in single-dose or in multiple-dose containers. A sterile, aqueous suspension of radioactive chromic phosphate P 32 in a 30% Dextrose solution suitable for intraperitoneal, intrapleural, or interstitial administration. Label it to include the following, in addition to the information specified for Labeling under Injections: the time and date of calibration; the amount of ^{32}P as labeled chromic phosphate expressed as total megabecquerels (or millicuries) and concentration as megabecquerels (or millicuries) per mL at the time of calibration; the expiration date; and the statements, "Caution—Radioactive Material," and "For intracavitary use only." The labeling indicates that in making dosage calculations, correction is to be made for radioactive decay, and also indicates that the radioactive half-life of ^{32}P is 14.3 days. Contains the labeled amount, within ±10%, of ^{32}P as chromic phosphate expressed in megabecquerels (or millicuries) per mL at the time indicated in the labeling. Other chemical forms of radioactivity do not exceed 5.0% of the total radioactivity. Meets the requirements for Radionuclide identification, Bacterial endotoxins, pH (3.0–5.0), Radiochemical purity, and Injections (except that the Suspension may be distributed or dispensed prior to the completion of the test for Sterility, the latter test being started on the day of final manufacture, and except that it is not subject to the recommendations on Volume in Container).

SODIUM PHOSPHATE P 32

Chemical name: Phosphoric-^{32}P acid, disodium salt.

Description: Sodium Phosphate P 32 Solution USP—Clear, colorless solution. Upon standing, both the solution and the glass container may darken as a result of the effects of the radiation.

USP requirements: Sodium Phosphate P 32 Solution USP—Preserve in single-dose or in multiple-dose containers that previously have been treated to prevent adsorption. A solution suitable for either oral or intravenous administration, containing radioactive phosphorus processed in the form of Dibasic Sodium Phosphate from the neutron bombardment of elemental sulfur. Label it to include the following: the time and date of calibration; the amount of ^{32}P as phosphate expressed in total megabecquerels (or microcuries or millicuries) and in megabecquerels (or microcuries or in millicuries) per mL at the time of calibration; the name and quantity of any added preservative or stabilizer; a statement of the intended use, whether oral or intravenous; a statement of whether the contents are intended for diagnostic or therapeutic use; the expiration date; and the statements, "Caution—Radioactive Material" and "Not for intracavitary use." The labeling indicates that in making dosage calculations, correction is to be made for radioactive decay, and also indicates that the radioactive half-life of ^{32}P is 14.3 days. Contains the labeled amount of ^{32}P, within ±10%, as phosphate expressed in megabecquerels (or microcuries or millicuries) per mL at the time indicated in the labeling. Other chemical forms of radioactivity are absent. Meets the requirements for Radionuclide identification, Bacterial endotoxins, pH (5.0–6.0), Radiochemical purity, and Injections (if for intravenous use, except that the Solution may be distributed or dispensed prior to completion of the test for Sterility, the latter test being started on the day of final manufacture, and except that it is not subject to the recommendation on Volume in Container).

PHOSPHORIC ACID

Chemical name: Phosphoric acid.

Molecular formula: H_3PO_4.

Molecular weight: 98.00.

Description: Phosphoric Acid NF—Colorless, odorless liquid of syrupy consistency. Specific gravity is about 1.71.
NF category: Acidifying agent; buffering agent.

Solubility: Phosphoric Acid NF—Miscible with water and with alcohol.

NF requirements: Phosphoric Acid NF—Preserve in tight containers. Contains not less than 85.0% and not more than 88.0%, by weight, of phosphoric acid. Meets the requirements for Identification, Nitrate, Phosphorous or hypophosphorous acid, Sulfate, Arsenic (not more than 3 ppm), Alkali phosphates, and Heavy metals (not more than 0.001%).
Caution: Avoid contact, as Phosphoric Acid rapidly destroys tissues.

DILUTED PHOSPHORIC ACID

Description: Diluted Phosphoric Acid NF—Clear, colorless, odorless liquid. Specific gravity is about 1.057.
NF category: Acidifying agent.

NF requirements: Diluted Phosphoric Acid NF—Preserve in tight containers. Contains, in each 100 mL, not less than 9.5 grams and not more than 10.5 grams of phosphoric acid.
Prepare Diluted Phosphoric Acid as follows: 69 mL of Phosphoric Acid and a sufficient quantity of Purified Water to make 1000 mL. Mix the ingredients.
Meets the requirements for Alkali phosphates, Arsenic (not more than 1.5 ppm), and Heavy metals (not more than 5 ppm), and for Identification test, Nitrate, Phosphorous or hypophosphorous acid, and Sulfate under Phosphoric Acid.

PHYSOSTIGMINE

Source: Derivative of Calabar bean. An alkaloid usually obtained from the dried ripe seeds of *Physostigma venenosum*.

Chemical name:
Physostigmine salicylate—Pyrrolo[2,3-*b*]indol-5-ol, 1,2,3,3a,8,8a-hexahydro-1,3a,8-trimethyl-, methylcarbamate (ester), (3a*S-cis*)-, mono(2-hydroxybenzoate).
Physostigmine sulfate—Pyrrolo[2,3-*b*]indol-5-ol, 1,2,3,3a,8,8a-hexahydro-1,3a,8-trimethyl-, methylcarbamate (ester), (3a*S-cis*)-, sulfate (2:1).

Molecular formula:
Physostigmine salicylate—$C_{15}H_{21}N_3O_2 \cdot C_7H_6O_3$.
Physostigmine sulfate—$(C_{15}H_{21}N_3O_2)_2 \cdot H_2SO_4$.

Molecular weight:
Physostigmine salicylate—413.47.
Physostigmine sulfate—648.77.

Description:
Physostigmine Salicylate USP—White, shining, odorless crystals or white powder. Acquires a red tint when exposed to heat, light, air, or contact with traces of metals for long periods. Melts at about 184 °C.
Physostigmine Sulfate USP—White, odorless, microcrystalline powder. Is deliquescent in moist air and acquires a red tint when exposed to heat, light, air, or contact with traces of metals for long periods. Melts at about 143 °C.

Solubility:
Physostigmine Salicylate USP—Sparingly soluble in water; freely soluble in chloroform; soluble in alcohol; slightly soluble in ether.
Physostigmine Sulfate USP—Freely soluble in water; very soluble in alcohol; very slightly soluble in ether.

USP requirements:
Physostigmine Salicylate Injection USP—Preserve in single-dose containers, preferably of Type I glass, protected from light. A sterile solution of Physostigmine Salicylate in Water for Injection. Contains the labeled amount, within ±10%. Meets the requirements for Identification, Bacterial endotoxins, pH (3.5–5.0), and Injections.
Note: Do not use the Injection if it is more than slightly discolored.
Physostigmine Salicylate Ophthalmic Solution USP—Preserve in tight, light-resistant containers. A sterile aqueous solution of Physostigmine Salicylate. Contains the labeled amount, within ±10%. Meets the requirements for Identification, Sterility, and pH (2.0–4.0).
Physostigmine Sulfate Ophthalmic Ointment USP—Preserve in collapsible ophthalmic ointment tubes. Contains the labeled amount, within ±10%. It is sterile. Meets the requirements for Identification, Sterility, and Metal particles.

PHYTONADIONE

Chemical name: 1,4-Naphthalenedione, 2-methyl-3-(3,7,11,15-tetramethyl-2-hexadecenyl)-, [R-[R*,R*-(E)]]-.

Molecular formula: $C_{31}H_{46}O_2$.

Molecular weight: 450.70.

Description: Phytonadione USP—Clear, yellow to amber, very viscous, odorless or practically odorless liquid, having a specific gravity of about 0.967. Is stable in air, but decomposes on exposure to sunlight.

Solubility: Phytonadione USP—Insoluble in water; soluble in dehydrated alcohol, in chloroform, in ether, and in vegetable oils; slightly soluble in alcohol.

USP requirements:
Phytonadione Injection USP—Preserve in single-dose or in multiple-dose containers, preferably of Type I glass, protected from light. A sterile, aqueous dispersion of Phytonadione. Contains the labeled amount, within ±10%. It contains suitable solubilizing and/or dispersing agents. Meets the requirements for Identification, Bacterial endotoxins, pH (3.5–7.0), and Injections.
Phytonadione Tablets USP—Preserve in well-closed, light-resistant containers. Contain the labeled amount, within ±10%. Meet the requirements for Identification, Disintegration (30 minutes), and Uniformity of dosage units.

PILOCARPINE

Chemical name:
Pilocarpine—2(3H)-Furanone, 3-ethyldihydro-4-[(1-methyl-1H-imidazol-5-yl)methyl]-, (3S-cis)-.
Pilocarpine hydrochloride—2(3H)-Furanone, 3-ethyldihydro-4-[(1-methyl-1H-imidazol-5-yl)methyl]-, monohydrochloride, (3S-cis)-.
Pilocarpine nitrate—2(3H)-Furanone, 3-ethyldihydro-4-[(1-methyl-1H-imidazol-5-yl)methyl]-, (3S-cis)-, mononitrate.

Molecular formula:
Pilocarpine—$C_{11}H_{16}N_2O_2$.
Pilocarpine hydrochloride—$C_{11}H_{16}N_2O_2 \cdot HCl$.
Pilocarpine nitrate—$C_{11}H_{16}N_2O_2 \cdot HNO_3$.

Molecular weight:
Pilocarpine—208.26.
Pilocarpine hydrochloride—244.72.
Pilocarpine nitrate—271.27.

Description:
Pilocarpine USP—A viscous, oily liquid, or crystals melting at about 34 °C. Exceedingly hygroscopic.
Pilocarpine Hydrochloride USP—Colorless, translucent, odorless crystals. Is hygroscopic and is affected by light. Its solutions are acid to litmus.
Pilocarpine Nitrate USP—Shining, white crystals. Is stable in air but is affected by light. Its solutions are acid to litmus.

Solubility:
Pilocarpine USP—Soluble in water, in alcohol, and in chloroform; practically insoluble in petroleum ether; sparingly soluble in ether.
Pilocarpine Hydrochloride USP—Very soluble in water; freely soluble in alcohol; slightly soluble in chloroform; insoluble in ether.
Pilocarpine Nitrate USP—Freely soluble in water; sparingly soluble in alcohol; insoluble in chloroform and in ether.

USP requirements:
Pilocarpine Ocular System USP—Preserve in single-dose containers, in a cold place. It is sterile. Contains the labeled amount, within ±15%. Meets the requirements for Identification, Sterility, Uniformity of dosage units (for capsules), and Drug release pattern.

Pilocarpine Hydrochloride Ophthalmic Gel—Not in USP.
Pilocarpine Hydrochloride Ophthalmic Solution USP—Preserve in tight containers. A sterile, buffered, aqueous solution of Pilocarpine Hydrochloride. Contains the labeled amount, within ±10%. Meets the requirements for Identification, Sterility, and pH (3.5–5.5).
Pilocarpine Nitrate Ophthalmic Solution USP—Preserve in tight, light-resistant containers. A sterile, buffered aqueous solution of Pilocarpine Nitrate. Contains the labeled amount, within ±10%. Meets the requirements for Identification, Sterility, and pH (4.0–5.5).

PIMOZIDE

Chemical group: A diphenylbutylpiperidine derivative.

Chemical name: 2H-Benzimidazol-2-one, 1-[1-[4,4-bis(4-fluorophenyl)butyl]-4-piperidinyl]-1,3-dihydro-.

Molecular formula: $C_{28}H_{29}F_2N_3O$.

Molecular weight: 461.55.

Description: Pimozide USP—White, crystalline powder.

Solubility: Pimozide USP—Insoluble in water; slightly soluble in ether and in alcohol; freely soluble in chloroform.

USP requirements: Pimozide Tablets USP—Preserve in tight, light-resistant containers. Contain the labeled amount, within ±10%. Meet the requirements for Identification, Dissolution (80% in 45 minutes in 0.1 N hydrochloric acid in Apparatus 2 at 50 rpm), and Uniformity of dosage units.

PINDOLOL

Chemical name: 2-Propanol, 1-(1H-indol-4-yloxy)-3-[(1-methylethyl)amino]-.

Molecular formula: $C_{14}H_{20}N_2O_2$.

Molecular weight: 248.32.

Description: Pindolol USP—White to off-white, crystalline powder, having a faint odor.

Solubility: Pindolol USP—Practically insoluble in water; slightly soluble in methanol; very slightly soluble in chloroform.

Other characteristics: Lipid solubility—Moderate.

USP requirements: Pindolol Tablets USP—Preserve in well-closed containers, protected from light. Contain the labeled amount, within ±10%. Meet the requirements for Identification, Dissolution (80% in 15 minutes in 0.1 N hydrochloric acid in Apparatus 2 at 50 rpm), Uniformity of dosage units, and Chromatographic purity.

PINDOLOL AND HYDROCHLOROTHIAZIDE

For *Pindolol* and *Hydrochlorothiazide*—See individual listings for chemistry information.

USP requirements: Pindolol and Hydrochlorothiazide Tablets—Not in USP.

PIPECURONIUM

Chemical name: Pipecuronium bromide—Piperazinium, 4,4'-[(2 beta,3 alpha,5 alpha,16 beta,17 beta)-3,17-bis(acetyloxy)androstane-2,16-diyl]bis[1,1-dimethyl-, dibromide, dihydrate.

Molecular formula: Pipecuronium bromide—$C_{35}H_{62}Br_2N_4O_4 \cdot 2H_2O$.

Molecular weight: Pipecuronium bromide—798.74.

Description: Pipecuronium bromide—Melting point 262–264 °C.

USP requirements: Pipecuronium Bromide for Injection—Not in USP.

PIPERACETAZINE

Chemical name: Ethanone, 1-[10-[3-[4-(2-hydroxyethyl)-1-piperidinyl]propyl]-10*H*-phenothiazin-2-yl]-.

Molecular formula: $C_{24}H_{30}N_2O_2S$.

Molecular weight: 410.57.

Description: Piperacetazine USP—Yellow, granular powder.

Solubility: Piperacetazine USP—Practically insoluble in water; freely soluble in chloroform; soluble in alcohol and in dilute hydrochloric acid.

USP requirements: Piperacetazine Tablets USP—Preserve in well-closed, light-resistant containers. Contain the labeled amount, within ±7%. Meet the requirements for Identification, Dissolution (75% in 45 minutes in 0.1 N hydrochloric acid in Apparatus 1 at 100 rpm), and Uniformity of dosage units.

PIPERACILLIN

Chemical name: Piperacillin sodium—4-Thia-1-azabicyclo[3.2.0]heptane-2-carboxylic acid, 6-[[[[(4-ethyl-2,3-dioxo-1-piperazinyl)carbonyl]amino]phenylacetyl]amino]-3,-3-dimethyl-7-oxo-, monosodium salt, [2*S*-[2 alpha,-5 alpha,6 beta(*S**)]].

Molecular formula: Piperacillin sodium—$C_{23}H_{26}N_5NaO_7S$.

Molecular weight: Piperacillin sodium—539.54.

Description: Sterile Piperacillin Sodium USP—White to off-white solid having the characteristic appearance of products prepared by freeze-drying.

Solubility: Sterile Piperacillin Sodium USP—Freely soluble in water and in alcohol.

USP requirements: Sterile Piperacillin Sodium USP—Preserve in Containers for Sterile Solids. It is piperacillin sodium suitable for parenteral use. It has a potency equivalent to not less than 863 mcg and not more than 1007 mcg of piperacillin per mg, calculated on the anhydrous basis and, where packaged for dispensing, contains an amount of piperacillin sodium equivalent to the labeled amount of piperacillin within −10% to +20%. Meets the requirements for Constituted solution, Identification, Bacterial endotoxins, Sterility, pH (5.5–7.5, in a solution containing 400 mg per mL), Water (not more than 1.0%), and Particulate matter, and for Uniformity of dosage units and Labeling under Injections.

PIPERAZINE

Chemical name:
Piperazine—Piperazine.
Piperazine adipate—Hexanedioic acid compd. with piperazine (1:1).
Piperazine citrate—Piperazine, 2-hydroxy-1,2,3-propanetricarboxylate (3:2), hydrate.
Piperazine phosphate—Piperazine phosphate (1:1), monohydrate.

Molecular formula:
Piperazine—$C_4H_{10}N_2$.

Piperazine adipate—$C_4H_{10}N_2 \cdot C_6H_{10}O_4$.
Piperazine citrate—$(C_4H_{10}N_2)_3 \cdot 2C_6H_8O_7 \cdot xH_2O$.
Piperazine phosphate—$C_4H_{10}N_2 \cdot H_3PO_4 \cdot H_2O$.

Molecular weight:
Piperazine—86.14.
Piperazine adipate—232.3.
Piperazine citrate (anhydrous)—642.66.
Piperazine phosphate—202.15.

Description:
Piperazine USP—White to slightly off-white lumps or flakes, having an ammoniacal odor.
Piperazine adipate—White, crystalline powder.
Piperazine Citrate USP—White, crystalline powder, having not more than a slight odor. Its solution (1 in 10) has a pH of about 5.
Piperazine phosphate—White odorless, or almost odorless, crystalline powder. A 1% solution in water has a pH of 6.0–6.5.

Solubility:
Piperazine USP—Soluble in water and in alcohol; insoluble in ether.
Piperazine adipate—Soluble 1 in 18 of water; practically insoluble in alcohol.
Piperazine Citrate USP—Soluble in water; insoluble in alcohol and in ether.
Piperazine phosphate—Soluble 1 in 60 of water; practically insoluble in alcohol.

USP requirements:
Piperazine Adipate Capsules—Not in USP.
Piperazine Adipate Oral Suspension—Not in USP.
Piperazine Adipate for Oral Suspension—Not in USP.
Piperazine Citrate Capsules—Not in USP.
Piperazine Citrate Syrup USP—Preserve in tight containers. Prepared from Piperazine Citrate or from Piperazine to which an equivalent amount of Citric Acid is added. Contains an amount of piperazine citrate equivalent to the labeled amount of piperazine hexahydrate, within ±7%. Meets the requirement for Identification.
Piperazine Citrate Tablets USP—Preserve in tight containers. Contain an amount of piperazine citrate equivalent to the labeled amount of piperazine hexahydrate, within ±7%. Meet the requirements for Identification, Dissolution (75% in 45 minutes in water in Apparatus 2 at 50 rpm), and Uniformity of dosage units.
Piperazine Dihydrochloride Soluble Powder for Solution—Not in USP.
Piperazine Phosphate Monohydrate Oral Solution—Not in USP.

PIPOBROMAN

Chemical name: Piperazine, 1,4-bis(3-bromo-1-oxopropyl)-.

Molecular formula: $C_{10}H_{16}Br_2N_2O_2$.

Molecular weight: 356.06.

Description: Pipobroman USP—White, or practically white, crystalline powder, having a slightly sharp, fruity odor.

Solubility: Pipobroman USP—Slightly soluble in water; freely soluble in chloroform; soluble in acetone; sparingly soluble in alcohol; very slightly soluble in ether.

USP requirements: Pipobroman Tablets USP—Preserve in well-closed containers. Contain the labeled amount, within ±10%. Meet the requirements for Identification, Disintegration (45 minutes, the use of disks being omitted), and Uniformity of dosage units.

PIPOTIAZINE

Chemical group: Piperidine phenothiazine.

Chemical name: Pipotiazine palmitate—Hexadecanoic acid, 2-[1-[3-[2-[(dimethylamino)sulfonyl]-10H-phenothiazin-10-yl]propyl]-4-piperidinyl]ethyl ester.

Molecular formula: Pipotiazine palmitate—$C_{40}H_{63}N_3O_4S_2$.

Molecular weight: Pipotiazine palmitate—714.08.

USP requirements: Pipotiazine Palmitate Injection—Not in USP.

PIRBUTEROL

Chemical name: Pirbuterol acetate—2,6-Pyridinedimethanol, alpha^6-[[(1,1-dimethylethyl)amino]methyl]-3-hydroxy-, monoacetate (salt).

Molecular formula: Pirbuterol acetate—$C_{12}H_{20}N_2O_3 \cdot C_2H_4O_2$.

Molecular weight: Pirbuterol acetate—300.35.

Description: Pirbuterol acetate—A white, crystalline powder.

Solubility: Pirbuterol acetate—Freely soluble in water.

USP requirements: Pirbuterol Acetate Inhalation Aerosol—Not in USP.

PIRENZEPINE

Source: Synthetic amine compound.

Chemical group: Tertiary amine, synthetic.

Chemical name: Pirenzepine hydrochloride—6H-Pyrido[2,3-b][1,4]benzodiazepin-6-one, 5,11-dihydro-11-[(4-methyl-1-piperazinyl)acetyl]-, dihydrochloride.

Molecular formula: Pirenzepine hydrochloride—$C_{19}H_{21}N_5O_2 \cdot 2HCl$.

Molecular weight: Pirenzepine hydrochloride—424.33.

Solubility: Pirenzepine hydrochloride—Soluble in water; slightly soluble in methanol; practically insoluble in ether.

USP requirements: Pirenzepine Hydrochloride Tablets—Not in USP.

PIROXICAM

Chemical group: Oxicam derivative.

Chemical name: 2H-1,2-Benzothiazine-3-carboxamide, 4-hydroxy-2-methyl-N-2-pyridinyl-, 1,1-dioxide.

Molecular formula: $C_{15}H_{13}N_3O_4S$.

Molecular weight: 331.35.

Description: Piroxicam USP—Off-white to light tan or light yellow, odorless powder. Forms a monohydrate that is yellow.

pKa: 1.8 and 5.1.

Solubility: Piroxicam USP—Very slightly soluble in water, in dilute acids, and in most organic solvents; slightly soluble in alcohol and in aqueous alkaline solutions.

USP requirements:
Piroxicam Capsules USP—Preserve in tight, light-resistant containers. Contain the labeled amount, within ±7.5%. Meet the requirements for Identification, Dissolution (75% in 45 minutes in simulated gastric fluid TS, prepared without pepsin, in Apparatus 1 at 50 rpm), Uniformity of dosage units, and Water (not more than 8.0%).
Piroxicam Suppositories—Not in USP.

POSTERIOR PITUITARY

USP requirements: Posterior Pituitary Injection USP—Preserve in single-dose or in multiple-dose containers, preferably of Type I glass. Do not freeze. A sterile solution, in a suitable diluent, of material containing the polypeptide hormones having the property of causing the contraction of uterine, vascular, and other smooth muscle, which is prepared from the posterior lobe of the pituitary body of healthy, domestic animals used for food by man. Each mL of Posterior Pituitary Injection possesses oxytocic and pressor activities of not less than 85.0% and not more than 120.0% of those stated on the label in USP Posterior Pituitary Units. Meets the requirements for Bacterial endotoxins, pH (2.5–4.5), and Injections.

PLAGUE VACCINE

Description: Plague Vaccine USP—Turbid, whitish liquid, practically odorless, or having a faint odor because of the preservative.

USP requirements: Plague Vaccine USP—Preserve at a temperature between 2 and 8 °C. A sterile suspension of plague bacilli (*Yersinia pestis*) of the 195/P strain grown on E medium, harvested and killed by the addition of formaldehyde. Its potency is determined with the specific mouse protection test on the basis of the U.S. Reference Plague Vaccine. Label it to state that it is to be well shaken before use and that it is not to be frozen. Meets the requirements of the specific mouse test for inactivation and for Expiration date (not later than 18 months after date of issue from manufacturer's cold storage [5 °C, 1 year]) and Potency test. Conforms to the regulations of the U.S. Food and Drug Administration concerning biologics.

PLANTAGO SEED

Description: Plantago Seed USP—All varieties are practically odorless.

USP requirements: Plantago Seed USP—Preserve in well-closed containers, secure against insect attack. It is the cleaned, dried, ripe seed of *Plantago psyllium* Linné, or of *Plantago indica* Linné (*Plantago arenaria* Waldstein et Kitaibel), known in commerce as Spanish or French Psyllium Seed; or of *Plantago ovata* Forskal, known in commerce as Blond Psyllium or Indian Plantago Seed (Fam. Plantaginaceae). Meets the requirements for Botanic characteristics, Water absorption, Total ash (not more than 4.0%), Acid-insoluble ash (not more than 1.0%), and Foreign organic matter (not more than 0.50%).

PLASMA PROTEIN FRACTION

USP requirements: Plasma Protein Fraction USP—Preserve at the temperature indicated on the label. A sterile preparation of serum albumin and globulin obtained by fractionating material (source blood, plasma, or serum) from healthy human donors, the source material being tested for the absence of hepatitis B surface antigen. It is made by a process that yields a product having protein components of approved composition and sedimentation coefficient content. Label it to state that it is not to be used if it is turbid and that it is to be used within 4 hours after the container is entered. Label it also to state the osmotic equivalent in terms of plasma and the sodium content. Not less than 83% of its total protein is albumin and not more than 17% of its total protein consists of alpha and beta globulins. Not more than 1% of its total protein has the electrophoretic properties of gamma globulin. A solution containing, in each 100 mL, 5 grams of protein, and contains the labeled amount, within ±6%. Contains no added antimicrobial agent, but contains sodium acetyltryptophanate with or without sodium caprylate as a stabilizing agent. Has a sodium content of not less than 130 mEq per liter and not more than 160 mEq per liter and a potassium content of not more than 2 mEq per liter. Has a pH between 6.7 and 7.3, measured in a solution diluted to contain 1% of protein with 0.15 M sodium chloride. Meets the requirements of the test for heat stability and for Expiration date (minimum date not later than 5 years after issue from manufacturer's cold storage [5 °C, 1 year] if labeling recommends storage between 2 and 10 °C; not later than 3 years after issue from manufacturer's cold storage [5 °C, 1 year] if labeling recommends storage at temperatures not higher than 30 °C). Conforms to the regulations of the U.S. Food and Drug Administration concerning biologics.

PLATELET CONCENTRATE

USP requirements: Platelet Concentrate USP—Preserve in hermetic containers of colorless, transparent, sterile, pyrogen-free Type I or Type II glass, or of a suitable plastic material. Preserve at the temperature relevant to the volume of resuspension plasma, either between 20 and 24 °C or between 1 and 6 °C, the latter except during shipment, when the temperature may be between 1 and 10 °C. In addition to the labeling requirements of Whole Blood applicable to this product, label it to state the volume of original plasma present, the kind and volume of anticoagulant solution present in the original plasma, the blood group designation of the source blood, and the hour of expiration on the stated expiration date. Where labeled for storage at 20 to 24 °C, label it also to state that a continuous gentle agitation shall be maintained, or where labeled for storage at 1 to 6 °C, to state that such agitation is optional. Label it also with the type and result of a serologic test for syphilis, or to indicate that it was nonreactive in such test; with the type and result of a test for hepatitis B surface antigen, or to indicate that it was nonreactive in such test; with a warning that it is to be used as soon as possible but not more than 4 hours after entering the container; to state that a filter is to be used in the administration equipment; and to state that the instruction circular provided is to be consulted for directions for use. Contains the platelets taken from plasma obtained by whole blood collection, by plasmapheresis, or by platelet-pheresis, from a single suitable human donor of whole blood; or from a plasmapheresis donor; or from a plateletpheresis donor who meets the criteria described in the product license application (in which case the collection procedure is as described therein), except where a licensed physician has determined that the recipient is to be transfused with the platelets from a specific donor (in which case the plateletpheresis procedure is performed under the supervision of a licensed physician who is aware of the health status of the donor and has certified that the donor's health permits such procedure). In all cases, the collection of source material is made by a single, uninterrupted venipuncture with minimal damage to and manipulation of the donor's tissue. Concentrate consists of such platelets suspended in a specified volume of the original plasma, the separation of plasma and resuspension of the platelets being done in a closed system, within 4 hours of collection of the whole blood or plasma. The separation of platelets is by a procedure shown to yield an unclumped product without visible hemolysis, with a content of not less than 5.5×10^{10} platelets per unit in not less than 75% of

the units tested, and the volume of original plasma used for resuspension of the separated platelets is such that the product has a pH of not less than 6 during the storage period when kept at the selected storage temperature, the selected storage temperature and corresponding volume of resuspension plasma being either 30 to 50 mL of plasma for storage at 20 to 24 °C, or 20 to 30 mL of plasma for storage at 1 to 6 °C. Meets the aforementioned requirements for platelet count, pH, and actual plasma volume, when tested 72 hours after preparation, and for Expiration date (not more than 72 hours from the time of collection of the source material). Conforms to the regulations of the U.S. Food and Drug Administration concerning biologics.

PLICAMYCIN

Source: Antibiotic produced by *Streptomyces argillaceus, Streptomyces tanashiensis,* and *Streptomyces plicatus.*

Chemical name: Plicamycin.

Molecular formula: $C_{52}H_{76}O_{24}$.

Molecular weight: 1085.16.

Description: Plicamycin USP—Yellow, odorless, hygroscopic, crystalline powder.

Solubility: Plicamycin USP—Slightly soluble in water and in methanol; very slightly soluble in alcohol; freely soluble in ethyl acetate.

USP requirements: Plicamycin for Injection USP—Preserve in light-resistant Containers for Sterile Solids, at a temperature between 2 and 8 °C. A sterile, dry mixture of Plicamycin and Mannitol. Label it with the mandatory instruction to consult the professional information for dosage and warnings, and with the warning that it is intended for hospital use only, under the direct supervision of a physician. Contains the labeled amount, within ±10%. Meets the requirements for Constituted solution, Identification, Depressor substances, Bacterial endotoxins, Sterility, pH (5.0–7.5), and Water (not more than 2.0%).

PNEUMOCOCCAL VACCINE POLYVALENT

Source:
The currently available vaccines in the U.S. (*Pneumovax 23*, MSD, and *Pnu-Imune 23*, Lederle) contain a mixture of purified capsular polysaccharides from the 23 most prevalent pneumococcal types responsible for approximately 90% of serious pneumococcal disease. Each of the pneumococcal polysaccharide types is produced separately. The resultant 23 polysaccharides are separated from the cells, purified, and combined to give 25 mcg of each type per 0.5-mL dose of the final vaccine.
Pneumovax 23, MSD (Canada) brand of pneumococcal vaccine polyvalent, also contains 23 polysaccharides.

Other characteristics:
The U.S. nomenclature for these 23 types is: 1, 2, 3, 4, 5, 26, 51, 8, 9, 68, 34, 43, 12, 14, 54, 17, 56, 57, 19, 20, 22, 23, 70.
The Danish nomenclature for these 23 types is: 1, 2, 3, 4, 5, 6B, 7F, 8, 9N, 9V, 10A, 11A, 12F, 14, 15B, 17F, 18C, 19A, 19F, 20, 22F, 23F, 33F.

USP requirements: Pneumococcal Vaccine Polyvalent Injection—Not in USP.

PODOPHYLLUM

Source: Podophyllum resin—Dried resin from the roots and rhizomes of *Podophyllum peltatum* (mandrake or May apple plant), the North American variety; active constituents are lignans including podophyllotoxin (20%), alpha-peltatin (10%), and beta-peltatin (5%).

Description: Podophyllum Resin USP—Amorphous powder, varying in color from light brown to greenish yellow, turning darker when subjected to a temperature exceeding 25 °C or when exposed to light. Its alcohol solution is acid to moistened litmus paper.

Solubility: Podophyllum Resin USP—Soluble in alcohol with a slight opalescence; partially soluble in ether and in chloroform.

The major active constituent of podophyllum, podophyllotoxin, is lipid soluble.

USP requirements: Podophyllum Resin Topical Solution USP—Preserve in tight, light-resistant containers. A solution in Alcohol consisting of Podophyllum Resin and an alcoholic extract of Benzoin. Contains, in each 100 mL, not less than 10 grams and not more than 13 grams of hexane-insoluble matter. Meets requirements for Identification and Alcohol content (69.0–72.0%).

Caution: Podophyllum Resin Topical Solution is highly irritating to the eye and to mucous membranes in general.

POLACRILIN POTASSIUM

Chemical name: 2-Propenoic acid, 2-methyl-, polymer with divinylbenzene, potassium salt.

Description: Polacrilin Potassium NF—White to off-white, free-flowing powder. It has a faint odor or is odorless.

NF category: Tablet disintegrant.

Solubility: Polacrilin Potassium NF—Insoluble in water and in most liquids.

NF requirements: Polacrilin Potassium NF—Preserve in well-closed containers. It is the potassium salt of a unifunctional low-cross-linked carboxylic cation-exchange resin prepared from methacrylic acid and divinylbenzene. When previously dried at 105 °C for 6 hours, contains not less than 20.6% and not more than 25.1% of potassium. Meets the requirements for Identification, Loss on drying (not more than 10.0%), Powder fineness, Arsenic (not more than 3 ppm), Iron (not more than 0.01%), Sodium (not more than 0.20%), and Heavy metals (not more than 0.002%).

POLIOVIRUS VACCINE

Source:

Poliovirus vaccine inactivated (IPV)—Produced from a mixture of three types of attenuated polioviruses that have been propagated in monkey kidney cell culture. The polioviruses are then inactivated with formaldehyde.

Poliovirus vaccine inactivated enhanced potency (enhanced-potency IPV)—Produced in human diploid cells and the resultant polioviruses have been inactivated.

Poliovirus vaccine live oral (OPV)—Produced from a mixture of three types of attenuated polioviruses that have been propagated in monkey kidney cell culture. OPV contains the live, attenuated polioviruses.

Description:

Poliovirus Vaccine Inactivated USP—Clear, reddish-tinged or yellowish liquid, that may have a slight odor because of the preservative.

Poliovirus vaccine inactivated enhanced-potency—Clear, colorless liquid.

Poliovirus Vaccine Live Oral USP—Generally frozen but, in liquid form, is clear and colorless, or may have a yellow or red tinge.

USP requirements:

Poliovirus Vaccine Inactivated USP (Injection)—Preserve at a temperature between 2 and 8 °C. A sterile aqueous suspension of inactivated poliomyelitis virus of Types 1, 2, and 3. Label it to state that it is to be well shaken before use. Label it also to state that it was prepared in monkey tissue cultures. The virus strains are grown separately in primary cell cultures of monkey kidney tissue, and from a virus suspension with a virus titer of not less than $10^{6.5}$ TCID$_{50}$ measured in comparison with the U.S. Reference Poliovirus of the corresponding type, are inactivated so as to reduce the virus titer by a factor of 10^{-8}, and after inactivation are combined in suitable proportions. No extraneous protein, capable of producing allergenic effects upon injection into human subjects, is added to the final virus production medium. If animal serum is used at any stage, its calculated concentration in the final medium does not exceed 1 part per million. Suitable antimicrobial agents may be used during the production. Meets the requirements of the specific monkey potency test by virus neutralizing antibody production, based on the U.S. Reference Poliovirus Antiserum, such that the ratio of the geometric mean titer of the group of monkey serums representing the vaccine to the mean titer value of the reference serum is not less than 1.29 for Type 1, 1.13 for Type 2, and 0.72 for Type 3. Meets the requirement for Expiration date (not later than 1 year after date of issue from manufacturer's cold storage [5 °C, 1 year]). Conforms to the regulations of the U.S. Food and Drug Administration concerning biologics.

Poliovirus Vaccine Inactivated Enhanced Potency (Injection)—Not in USP.

Poliovirus Vaccine Live Oral USP (Oral Solution)—Preserve in single-dose or in multiple-dose containers at a temperature that will maintain ice continuously in a solid state. Preserve thawed Vaccine at a temperature between 2 and 8 °C. A preparation of a combination of the three types of live, attenuated polioviruses derived from strains of virus tested for neurovirulence in monkeys in comparison with the U.S. Reference Attenuated Poliovirus, Type 1, for such tests, and for immunogenicity, free from all demonstrable viable microbial agents except unavoidable bacteriophage, and found suitable for human immunization. The strains are grown, for purposes of vaccine production, separately in primary cell cultures of monkey renal tissue. Label the Vaccine to state that it may be thawed and refrozen not more than 10 times, provided that the thawed material is kept refrigerated and the total cumulative duration of the thaw is not more than 24 hours. Label the Vaccine to state the type of tissue in which it was prepared and to state that it is not for injection. Meets the requirements of the specific monkey neurovirulence test in comparison with the Reference Attenuated Poliovirus, and the requirements of the specific in-vitro marker tests. The Vaccine meets the requirements of the specific tissue culture tests for live virus titer, in a single immunizing dose, of not less than $10^{5.4}$ to $10^{6.4}$ for Type 1, $10^{4.5}$ to $10^{5.5}$ for Type 2, and $10^{5.2}$ to $10^{6.2}$ for Type 3, using the U.S. Reference Poliovirus, Live, Attenuated of the corresponding type for correlation of such titers. The Vaccine is filtered to prevent possible inclusion of bacteria in the final product. Meets the requirement for Expiration date (not later than 1 year after date of issue from manufacturer's cold storage [−10 °C, 1 year]). Conforms to the regulations of the U.S. Food and Drug Administration concerning biologics.

POLOXAMER

Chemical group: Surfactants, nonionic.

Chemical name: Oxirane, methyl-, polymer with oxirane.

Molecular formula: $HO(C_2H_4O)_a(C_3H_6O)_b(C_2H_4O)_aH$.

Molecular weight: Average—
Poloxamer 124: 2090–2360.
Poloxamer 188: 7680–9510.
Poloxamer 237: 6840–8830.
Poloxamer 338: 12700–17400.
Poloxamer 407: 9840–14600.

Description: Poloxamer NF—Poloxamer 124 is a colorless liquid, having a mild odor. When solidified, it melts at about 16 °C. Poloxamer 188 (melting at about 52 °C), Poloxamer 237 (melting at about 49 °C), Poloxamer 338 (melting at about 57 °C), and Poloxamer 407 (melting at about 56 °C), are white, prilled or cast solids, odorless, or having a very mild odor.

NF category: Emulsifying and/or solubilizing agent.

Solubility: Poloxamer NF—Poloxamer 124 is freely soluble in water, in alcohol, in isopropyl alcohol, in propylene glycol, and in xylene. Poloxamer 188 is freely soluble in water and in alcohol. Poloxamer 237 is freely soluble in water and in alcohol; sparingly soluble in isopropyl alcohol and in xylene. Poloxamer 338 is freely soluble in water and in alcohol; sparingly soluble in propylene glycol. Poloxamer 407 is freely soluble in water, in alcohol, and in isopropyl alcohol.

USP requirements: Poloxamer 188 Capsules—Not in USP.

NF requirements: Poloxamer NF—Preserve in tight containers. A synthetic block copolymer of ethylene oxide and propylene oxide. It is available in several types. Label it to state, as part of the official title, the Poloxamer number. Meets the requirements for Average molecular weight, Weight percent oxyethylene, pH (5.0–7.5, in a solution [1 in 40]), Unsaturation, Heavy metals (not more than 0.002%), Organic volatile impurities, and Free ethylene oxide, propylene oxide, and 1, 4-dioxane (not more than 5 ppm of each).

POLYETHYLENE EXCIPIENT

Description: Polyethylene Excipient NF—White, translucent, partially crystalline and partially amorphous resin. Available in various grades and types, differing from one another in molecular weight, molecular weight distribution, degree of chain branching, and extent of crystallinity.

NF category: Stiffening agent.

Solubility: Polyethylene Excipient NF—Insoluble in water.

NF requirements: Polyethylene Excipient NF—Preserve in well-closed containers. A homopolymer produced by the direct polymerization of ethylene. Meets the requirements for Identification, Intrinsic viscosity in 1,2,3,4-tetrahydronaphthalene (not less than 0.126), Heavy metals (not more than 0.004%), and Volatile substances (not more than 0.5%).

POLYETHYLENE GLYCOL

Chemical name: Poly(oxy-1,2-ethanediyl, alpha-hydro-omega-hydroxy-.

Molecular formula: $H(OCH_2CH_2)_nOH$.

Description: Polyethylene Glycol NF—Polyethylene Glycol is usually designated by a number that corresponds approximately to its average molecular weight. As the average molecular weight increases, the water solubility, vapor pressure, hygroscopicity, and solubility in organic solvents decrease, while congealing temperature, specific gravity, flash point, and viscosity increase. Liquid grades occur as clear to slightly hazy, colorless or practically colorless, slightly hygroscopic, viscous liquids, having a slight, characteristic odor, and a specific gravity at 25 °C of about 1.12. Solid grades occur

as practically odorless white, waxy, plastic material having a consistency similar to beeswax, or as creamy white flakes, beads, or powders. The accompanying table states the approximate congealing temperatures that are characteristic of commonly available grades.

Nominal Molecular Weight Polyethylene Glycol	Approximate Congealing Temperature (°C)
300	−11
400	6
600	20
900	34
1000	38
1450	44
3350	56
4500	58
8000	60

NF category: Coating agent; plasticizer; solvent; suppository base; tablet and/or capsule lubricant.

Solubility: Polyethylene Glycol NF—Liquid grades are miscible with water; solid grades are freely soluble in water; and all are soluble in acetone, in alcohol, in chloroform, in ethylene glycol monoethyl ether, in ethyl acetate, and in toluene; all are insoluble in ether and in hexane.

NF requirements: Polyethylene Glycol NF—Preserve in tight containers. An addition polymer of ethylene oxide and water, represented by the formula $H(OCH_2CH_2)_nOH$, in which *n* represents the average number of of oxyethylene groups. The average molecular weight is not less than 95.0% and not more than 105.0% of the labeled nominal value if the labeled nominal value is below 1000; it is not less than 90.0% and not more than 110.0% of the labeled nominal value if the labeled nominal value is between 1000 and 7000; it is not less than 87.5% and not more than 112.5% of the labeled nominal value if the labeled nominal value is above 7000. Label it to state, as part of the official title, the average nominal molecular weight of the Polyethylene Glycol. Meets the requirements for Completeness and color of solution, Viscosity, Average molecular weight, pH (4.5–7.5), Residue on ignition (not more than 0.1%), Arsenic (not more than 3 ppm), Free ethylene oxide and 1, 4-dioxane (not more than 10 ppm of each), Limit of ethylene glycol and diethylene glycol (not more than 0.25%), and Heavy metals (not more than 5 ppm).

POLYETHYLENE GLYCOL MONOMETHYL ETHER

Chemical name: Poly(oxy-1,2-ethanediyl), alpha-methyl-omega-hydroxy-.

Description: Polyethylene Glycol Monomethyl Ether NF—Polyethylene Glycol Monomethyl Ether is usually designated by a number that corresponds approximately to its average molecular weight. As the average molecular weight increases, the water solubility, vapor pressure, hygroscopicity, and solubility in organic solvents decrease, while congealing temperature, specific gravity, flash point, and viscosity increase. Liquid grades occur as clear to slightly hazy, colorless or practically colorless, slightly hygroscopic, viscous liquids, having a slight, characteristic odor, and a specific gravity at 25 °C of about 1.09–1.10. Solid grades occur as practically odorless, white, waxy, plastic material having a consistency similar to beeswax, or as creamy white flakes, beads, or powders. The accompanying table states the approximate congealing temperatures that are characteristic of commonly available grades.

Nominal Molecular Weight Polyethylene Glycol Monomethyl Ether	Approximate Congealing Temperature (°C)
350	−7
550	17
750	28
1000	35
2000	51
5000	59
8000	60
10000	61

NF category: Ointment base; solvent; plasticizer.

Solubility: Polyethylene Glycol Monomethyl Ether NF—Liquid grades are miscible with water; solid grades are freely soluble in water; and all are soluble in acetone, in alcohol, in chloroform, in ethylene glycol monoethyl ether, in ethyl acetate, and in toluene; all are insoluble in ether and in hexane.

NF requirements: Polyethylene Glycol Monomethyl Ether NF—Preserve in tight containers. An addition polymer of ethylene oxide and methanol, represented by the formula $CH_3(OCH_2CH_2)_nOH$, in which n represents the average number of oxyethylene groups. The average molecular weight is not less than 95.0% and not more than 105.0% of the labeled nominal value if the labeled nominal value is below 1000; it is not less than 90.0% and not more than 110.0% of the labeled nominal value if the labeled nominal value is between 1000 and 4750; it is not less than 87.5% and not more than 112.5% of the labeled nominal value if the labeled nominal value is above 4750. Label it to state, as part of the official title, the average nominal molecular weight of the Polyethylene Glycol Monomethyl Ether. Meets the requirements for Completeness and color of solution, Viscosity, Average molecular weight, pH (4.5–7.5), Residue on ignition (not more than 0.1%), Arsenic (not more than 3 ppm), Limit of ethylene glycol and diethylene glycol (not more than 0.25%), Heavy metals (not more than 5 ppm), Free ethylene oxide and 1,4-dioxane (not more than 10 ppm of each), and 2-Methoxyethanol (not more than 10 ppm).

POLYETHYLENE GLYCOL OINTMENT

Description: Polyethylene Glycol Ointment NF—NF category: Ointment base.

NF requirements: Polyethylene Glycol Ointment NF—Preserve in well-closed containers.

Prepare Polyethylene Glycol Oinment as follows: 400 grams of Polyethylene Glycol 3350 and 600 grams of Polyethylene Glycol 400 to make 1000 grams. Heat the two ingredients on a water bath to 65 °C. Allow to cool, and stir until congealed. If a firmer preparation is desired, replace up to 100 grams of the polyethylene glycol 400 with an equal amount of polyethylene glycol 3350.

Note: If 6% to 25% of an aqueous solution is to be incorporated in Polyethylene Glycol Ointment, replace 50 grams of the polyethylene glycol 3350 with an equal amount of stearyl alcohol.

POLYETHYLENE OXIDE

Description: Polyethylene Oxide NF—Polyethylene oxide resins are high molecular weight polymers having the common structure $(-O-CH_2CH_2-)_n$, in which n, the degree of polymerization, varies from about 2000 to over 100,000. Polyethylene oxide, being a polyether, strongly hydrogen, bonds with water. It is nonionic and undergoes salting-out effects associated with neutral molecules in solutions of high dielectric media. Salting-out effects manifest themselves in depressing the upper temperature limit of solubility, and in reducing the viscosity of both dilute and concentrated solutions of the polymers. All molecular weight grades are powdered or granular solids.

NF category: Suspending and/or viscosity-increasing agent; tablet binder.

Solubility: Polyethylene Oxide NF—Soluble in water, but, because of the high solution viscosities obtained (see table), solutions over 1% in water may be difficult to prepare.

Approximate Molecular Weight	Typical Solution Viscosity (cps), 25 °C	
	5% Solution	1% Solution
100,000	40	
200,000	100	
300,000	800	
400,000	3000	
600,000	6000	
900,000	15000	
4,000,000		3500
5,000,000		5500

The water solubility, hygroscopicity, solubility in organic solvents, and melting point do not vary in the specified molecular weight range. At room temperature polyethylene oxide is miscible with water in all proportions. At concentrations of about 20% polymer in water the solutions are nontacky, reversible, elastic gels. At higher concentrations, the solutions are tough, elastic materials with the water acting as a plasticizer. Polyethylene oxide is also freely soluble in acetonitrile, in ethylene dichloride, in trichloroethylene, and in methylene chloride. Heating may be required to obtain solutions in many other organic solvents. It is insoluble in aliphatic hydrocarbons, in ethylene glycol, in diethylene glycol, and in glycerol.

NF requirements: Polyethylene Oxide NF—Preserve in tight, light-resistant containers. A nonionic homopolymer of ethylene oxide, represented by the formula $(OCH_2CH_2)_n$, in which n represents the average number of oxyethylene groups. It is a white powder obtainable in several grades, varying in viscosity profile when dissolved in water. May contain not more than 3.0% of silicon dioxide. The labeling indicates its viscosity profile in aqueous solution. Meets the requirements for Identification, Loss on drying (not more than 1.0%), Silicon dioxide and Non–silicon dioxide residue on ignition (not more than 2.0%), Arsenic (not more than 3 ppm), Heavy metals (not more than 0.001%), and Free ethylene oxide (not more than 0.001%).

POLYMYXIN B

Source: Derived from polymyxin B_1 and polymyxin B_2, which are produced by the growth of *Bacillus polymyxa*.

Chemical group: Polypeptide.

Chemical name: Polymyxin B, sulfate.

Description: Polymyxin B Sulfate USP—White to buff-colored powder. Odorless or has a faint odor.

Solubility: Polymyxin B Sulfate USP—Freely soluble in water; slightly soluble in alcohol.

USP requirements: Sterile Polymyxin B Sulfate USP—Preserve in Containers for Sterile Solids, protected from light. It is Polymyxin B Sulfate suitable for parenteral use. Label it to indicate that where it is administered intramuscularly and/or intrathecally, it is to be given only to patients hospitalized so as to provide constant supervision by a physician. It has a potency of not less than 6000 Polymyxin B Units per mg, calculated on the dried basis. Contains, where packaged for dispensing, an amount of polymyxin B sulfate equivalent to the labeled amount of polymyxin B, within −10% to +20%. Meets the requirements for Constituted solution, Pyrogen, Sterility, Particulate matter, Residue on ignition (not more than 5.0%), and Heavy metals (not more than 0.01%), for Identification tests, pH, and Loss on drying under Polymyxin B Sulfate, and where packaged for dispensing, for Uniformity of dosage units and Labeling under Injections. Where intended for use in preparing sterile ophthalmic dosage forms, it is exempt from requirements for Pyrogen, Particulate matter, and Heavy metals.

POLYMYXIN B AND BACITRACIN

For *Polymyxin B* and *Bacitracin*—See individual listings for chemistry information.

USP requirements:
Polymyxin B Sulfate and Bacitracin Zinc Topical Aerosol USP—Preserve in pressurized containers, and avoid exposure to excessive heat. Contains amounts of polymyxin B sulfate and bacitracin zinc equivalent to the labeled amounts of polymyxin B and bacitracin, within −10% to +30%. Meets the requirements for Identification, Microbial limits, and Water (not more than 0.5%), and for Leak testing and Pressure testing under Aerosols.
Polymyxin B Sulfate and Bacitracin Zinc Topical Powder USP—Preserve in well-closed containers. Contains amounts of polymyxin B sulfate and bacitracin zinc equivalent to the labeled amounts of polymyxin B and bacitracin, within −10% to +30%. Meets the requirements for Microbial limits and Water (not more than 7.0%).

POLYMYXIN B AND HYDROCORTISONE

For *Polymyxin B* and *Hydrocortisone*—See individual listings for chemistry information.

USP requirements: Polymyxin B Sulfate and Hydrocortisone Otic Solution USP—Preserve in tight, light-resistant containers. A sterile solution. Contains an amount of polymyxin B sulfate equivalent to the labeled amount of polymyxin B, within −10% to +30%, and the labeled amount of hydrocortisone, within ±10%. Meets the requirements for Sterility and pH (3.0–5.0).
Note: Where Polymyxin B Sulfate and Hydrocortisone Otic Solution is prescribed, without reference to the quantity of polymyxin B or hydrocortisone contained therein, a product containing 10,000 Polymyxin B Units and 5 mg of hydrocortisone per mL shall be dispensed.

POLYOXYL 10 OLEYL ETHER

Chemical name: Polyoxy-1,2-ethanediyl, alpha-[(Z)-9-octade-cenyl-omega-hydroxy-.

Description: Polyoxyl 10 Oleyl Ether NF—White, soft semi-solid, or pale yellow liquid, having a bland odor.
NF category: Emulsifying and/or solubilizing agent; wetting and or solubilizing agent.

Solubility: Polyoxyl 10 Oleyl Ether NF—Soluble in water and in alcohol; dispersible in mineral oil and in propylene glycol, with possible separation on standing.

NF requirements: Polyoxyl 10 Oleyl Ether NF—Preserve in tight containers, in a cool place. A mixture of the monooleyl ethers of mixed polyoxyethylene diols, the average polymer length being equivalent to not less than 8.6 and not more than 10.4 oxyethylene units. Label it to indicate the names

and proportions of any added stabilizers. Meets the requirements for Identification, Water (not more than 3.0%), Residue on ignition (not more than 0.4%), Arsenic (not more than 2 ppm), Heavy metals (not more than 0.002%), Acid value (not more than 1.0), Hydroxyl value (75–95), Iodine value (23–40), Saponification value (not more than 3), Free polyethylene glycols (not more than 7.5%), Free ethylene oxide (not more than 0.01%), Average polymer length, and Organic volatile impurities.

POLYOXYL 20 CETOSTEARYL ETHER

Description: Polyoxyl 20 Cetostearyl Ether NF—Cream-colored, waxy, unctuous mass, melting, when heated, to a clear, brownish yellow liquid.
NF category: Emulsifying and/or solubilizing agent; wetting and/or solubilizing agent.

Solubility: Polyoxyl 20 Cetostearyl Ether NF—Soluble in water, in alcohol, and in acetone; insoluble in solvent hexane.

NF requirements: Polyoxyl 20 Cetostearyl Ether NF—Preserve in tight containers in a cool place. A mixture of monoceto-stearyl (mixed hexadecyl and octadecyl) ethers of mixed polyoxyethylene diols, the average polymer length being equivalent to not less than 17.2 and not more than 25.0 oxyethylene units. Meets the requirements for Identification, pH (4.5–7.5, determined in a solution [1 in 10]), Water (not more than 1.0%), Residue on ignition (not more than 0.4%), Arsenic (not more than 2 ppm), Heavy metals (not more than 0.002%), Acid value (not more than 0.5%), Hydroxyl value (42–60), Saponification value (not more than 2), Free polyethylene glycols (not more than 7.5%), Free ethylene oxide (not more than 0.01%), Average polymer length, and Organic volatile impurities.

POLYOXYL 35 CASTOR OIL

Description: Polyoxyl 35 Castor Oil NF—Yellow, oily liquid, having a faint, characteristic odor.
NF category: Emulsifying and/or solubilizing agent; wetting and/or solubilizing agent.

Solubility: Polyoxyl 35 Castor Oil NF—Very soluble in water, producing a practically odorless and colorless solution; soluble in alcohol and in ethyl acetate; insoluble in mineral oils.

NF requirements: Polyoxyl 35 Castor Oil NF—Preserve in tight containers. Contains mainly the tri-ricinoleate ester of ethoxylated glycerol, with smaller amounts of polyethylene glycol ricinoleate and the corresponding free glycols. Results from the reaction of glycerol ricinoleate with about 35 moles of ethylene oxide. Meets the requirements for Identification, Specific gravity (1.05–1.06), Viscosity (650–850 centipoises at 25 °C), Water (not more than 3.0%), Residue on ignition (not more than 0.3%), Heavy metals (not more than 0.001%), Acid value (not more than 2.0), Hydroxyl value (65–80), Iodine value (25–35), Saponification value (60–75), and Organic volatile impurities.

POLYOXYL 40 HYDROGENATED CASTOR OIL

Description: Polyoxyl 40 Hydrogenated Castor Oil NF—White to yellowish paste or pasty liquid, having a faint odor.
NF category: Emulsifying and/or solubilizing agent; wetting and/or solubilizing agent.

Solubility: Polyoxyl 40 Hydrogenated Castor Oil NF—Very soluble in water, producing a practically odorless and colorless solution; soluble in alcohol and in ethyl acetate; insoluble in mineral oils.

NF requirements: Polyoxyl 40 Hydrogenated Castor Oil NF—Preserve in tight containers. Contains mainly the tri-hydroxy-stearate ester of ethoxylated glycerol, with smaller amounts of polyethylene glycol tri-hydroxystearate and of the corresponding free glycols. Results from the reaction of glycerol tri-hydroxystearate with about 40 to 45 moles of ethylene oxide. Meets the requirements for Identification, Congealing temperature (20–30 °C), Water (not more than 3.0%), Residue on ignition (not more than 0.3%), Heavy metals (not more than 0.001%), Acid value (not more than 2.0), Hydroxyl value (60–80), Iodine value (not more than 2.0), Saponification value (45–69), and Organic volatile impurities.

POLYOXYL 40 STEARATE

Chemical name: Poly(oxy-1,2-ethanediyl), alpha-hydro-omega-hydroxy-, octadecanoate.

Description: Polyoxyl 40 Stearate NF—Waxy, white to light tan solid. It is odorless or has a faint fat-like odor.
   NF category: Emulsifying and/or solubilizing agent; wetting and/or solubilizing agent.

Solubility: Polyoxyl 40 Stearate NF—Soluble in water, in alcohol, in ether, and in acetone; insoluble in mineral oil and in vegetable oils.

NF requirements: Polyoxyl 40 Stearate NF—Preserve in tight containers. A mixture of the monoesters and diesters of Stearic Acid or Purified Stearic Acid with mixed polyoxyethylene diols, the average polymer length being about 40 oxyethylene units. Meets the requirements for Identification, Congealing temperature (37–47 °C), Water (not more than 3.0%), Arsenic (not more than 3 ppm), Heavy metals (not more than 0.001%), Acid value (not more than 2), Hydroxyl value (25–40), Saponification value (25–35), Free polyethylene glycols (17–27%), and Organic volatile impurities.

POLYOXYL 50 STEARATE

Chemical name: Poly(oxy-1,2-ethanediyl), alpha-(1-oxooctade-cyl)-omega-hydroxy-.

Description: Polyoxyl 50 Stearate NF—Soft, cream-colored, waxy solid, having a faint, fat-like odor. Melts at about 45 °C.
   NF category: Wetting and/or solubilizing agent.

Solubility: Polyoxyl 50 Stearate NF—Soluble in water and in isopropyl alcohol.

NF requirements: Polyoxyl 50 Stearate NF—Preserve in tight containers. A mixture of the monostearate and distearate esters of mixed polyoxyethylene diols and the corresponding free diols. The average polymer length is about 50 oxyethylene units. Meets the requirements for Identification, Free polyethylene glycols (17–27%), Acid value (not more than 2), Hydroxyl value (23–35), Saponification value (20–28), and Organic volatile impurities, and for Water, Arsenic, and Heavy metals under Polyoxyl 40 Stearate.

POLYSORBATE 20

Chemical name: Sorbitan, monododecanoate, poly(oxy-1,2-ethanediyl) derivs.

Molecular formula: $C_{58}H_{114}O_{26}$ (approximate).

Description: Polysorbate 20 NF—Lemon to amber liquid, having a faint characteristic odor.
   NF category: Emulsifying and/or solubilizing agent; wetting and/or solubilizing agent.

Solubility: Polysorbate 20 NF—Soluble in water, in alcohol, in ethyl acetate, in methanol, and in dioxane; insoluble in mineral oil.

NF requirements: Polysorbate 20 NF—Preserve in tight containers. A laurate ester of sorbitol and its anhydrides copolymerized with approximately 20 moles of ethylene oxide for each mole of sorbitol and sorbitol anhydrides. Meets the requirements for Identification, Hydroxyl value (96–108), and Saponification value (40–50), and for Water, Residue on ignition, Arsenic, Heavy metals, and Acid value under Polysorbate 80.

POLYSORBATE 40

Chemical name: Sorbitan, monohexadecanoate, poly(oxy-1,2-ethanediyl) derivs.

Molecular formula: $C_{62}H_{122}O_{26}$ (approximate).

Description: Polysorbate 40 NF—Yellow liquid, having a faint, characteristic odor.
   NF category: Emulsifying and/or solubilizing agent; wetting and/or solubilizing agent.

Solubility: Polysorbate 40 NF—Soluble in water and in alcohol; insoluble in mineral oil and in vegetable oils.

NF requirements: Polysorbate 40 NF—Preserve in tight containers. A palmitate ester of sorbitol and its anhydrides copolymerized with approximately 20 moles of ethylene oxide for each mole of sorbitol and sorbitol anhydrides. Meets the requirements for Identification, Hydroxyl value (89–105), and Saponification value (41–52), and for Water, Residue on ignition, Arsenic, Heavy metals, and Acid value under Polysorbate 80.

POLYSORBATE 60

Chemical name: Sorbitan, monooctadecanoate, poly(oxy-1,2-ethanediyl) derivs.

Molecular formula: $C_{64}H_{126}O_{26}$ (approximate).

Description: Polysorbate 60 NF—Lemon- to orange-colored, oily liquid or semi-gel, having a faint, characteristic odor.
   NF category: Emulsifying and/or solubilizing agent; wetting and/or solubilizing agent.

Solubility: Polysorbate 60 NF—Soluble in water, in ethyl acetate, and in toluene; insoluble in mineral oil and in vegetable oils.

NF requirements: Polysorbate 60 NF—Preserve in tight containers. A mixture of stearate and palmitate esters of sorbitol and its anhydrides copolymerized with approximately 20 moles of ethylene oxide for each mole of sorbitol and sorbitol anhydrides. Meets the requirements for Identification, Hydroxyl value (81–96), and Saponification value (45–55), and for Water, Residue on ignition, Arsenic, Heavy metals, and Acid value under Polysorbate 80.

POLYSORBATE 80

Chemical name: Sorbitan, mono-9-octadecenoate, poly(oxy-1,2-ethanediyl) derivs., (Z)-.

Description: Polysorbate 80 NF—Lemon- to amber-colored, oily liquid, having a faint, characteristic odor.
   NF category: Emulsifying and/or solubilizing agent; wetting and/or solubilizing agent.

Solubility: Polysorbate 80 NF—Very soluble in water, producing an odorless and practically colorless solution; soluble in alcohol and in ethyl acetate; insoluble in mineral oil.

NF requirements: Polysorbate 80 NF—Preserve in tight containers. An oleate ester of sorbitol and its anhydrides copolymerized with approximately 20 moles of ethylene oxide for each mole of sorbitol and sorbitol anhydrides. Meets the requirements for Identification, Specific gravity (1.06–1.09), Viscosity (300–500 centistokes when determined at 25 °C), Water (not more than 3.0%), Residue on ignition (not more than 0.25%), Arsenic (not more than 1 ppm), Heavy metals (not more than 0.001%), Acid value (2.2), Hydroxyl value (65–80), and Saponification value (45–55).

POLYTHIAZIDE

Chemical name: 2*H*-1,2,4-Benzothiadiazine-7-sulfonamide, 6-chloro-3,4-dihydro-2-methyl-3-[[(2,2,2-trifluoroethyl)thio]-methyl]-, 1,1-dioxide.

Molecular formula: $C_{11}H_{13}ClF_3N_3O_4S_3$.

Molecular weight: 439.87.

Description: Polythiazide USP—White, crystalline powder, having a characteristic odor.

Solubility: Polythiazide USP—Practically insoluble in water and in chloroform; soluble in methanol and in acetone.

USP requirements: Polythiazide Tablets USP—Preserve in tight, light-resistant containers. Contain the labeled amount, within ± 10%. Meet the requirements for Identification, Dissolution (50% in 90 minutes in dilute hydrochloric acid [1 in 100] in Apparatus 2 at 50 rpm), and Uniformity of dosage units.

POLYVINYL ACETATE PHTHALATE

Description: Polyvinyl Acetate Phthalate NF—Free-flowing, white powder. May have a slight odor of acetic acid.
  NF category: Coating agent.

Solubility: Polyvinyl Acetate Phthalate NF—Insoluble in water, in methylene chloride, and in chloroform. Soluble in methanol and in alcohol.

NF requirements: Polyvinyl Acetate Phthalate NF—Preserve in tight containers. A reaction product of phthalic anhydride and partially hydrolyzed polyvinyl acetate. Contains not less than 55.0% and not more than 62.0% of phthalyl (*o*-carboxybenzoyl, $C_8H_5O_3$) groups, calculated on an anhydrous acid-free basis. Meets the requirements for Identification, Viscosity (7–11 centipoises, determined at 25 °C ± 0.2 °C [apparent]), Water (not more than 5.0%), Residue on ignition (not more than 1.0%), Free phthalic acid (not more than 0.6%, on the anhydrous basis), Free acid other than phthalic (not more than 0.6%, on the anhydrous basis), and Phthalyl content.

POLYVINYL ALCOHOL

Chemical name: Ethenol, homopolymer.

Molecular formula: $(C_2H_4O)_n$.

Description: Polyvinyl Alcohol USP—White to cream-colored granules, or white to cream-colored powder. Is odorless..
  NF category: Suspending and/or viscosity-increasing agent.

Solubility: Polyvinyl Alcohol USP—Freely soluble in water at room temperature. Solution may be effected more rapidly at somewhat higher temperatures.

USP requirements: Polyvinyl Alcohol USP—Preserve in well-closed containers. A water-soluble synthetic resin, represented by the formula: $(C_2H_4O)_n$, in which the average value of *n* lies between 500 and 5000. Prepared by 85 to 89% hydrolysis of polyvinyl acetate. The apparent viscosity, in centipoises, at 20 °C, of a solution containing 4 grams of Polyvinyl Alcohol in each 100 grams, is within ±15% of that stated on the label. Meets the requirements for Viscosity, pH (5.0–8.0, in a solution [1 in 25]), Loss on drying (not more than 5.0%), Residue on ignition (not more than 2.0%), Water-insoluble substances (not more than 0.1%), Degree of hydrolysis (85–89%), and Organic volatile impurities.

SULFURATED POTASH

Chemical name: Thiosulfuric acid, dipotassium salt, mixt. with potassium sulfide (K_2S_x).

Description: Sulfurated Potash USP—Irregular, liver-brown pieces when freshly made, changing to a greenish-yellow. Has an odor of hydrogen sulfide and decomposes on exposure to air. A solution (1 in 10) is light brown in color and is alkaline to litmus.

Solubility: Sulfurated Potash USP—Freely soluble in water, usually leaving a slight residue. Alcohol dissolves only the sulfides.

USP requirements: Sulfurated Potash USP—Preserve in tight containers. Containers from which it is to be taken for immediate use in compounding prescriptions contain not more than 120 grams. A mixture composed chiefly of potassium polysulfides and potassium thiosulfate. Contains not less than 12.8% of sulfur in combination as sulfide. Meets the requirement for Identification.

POTASSIUM ACETATE

Chemical name: Acetic acid, potassium salt.

Molecular formula: $C_2H_3KO_2$.

Molecular weight: 98.14.

Description: Potassium Acetate USP—Colorless, monoclinic crystals or white, crystalline powder. Is odorless, or has a faint acetous odor. Deliquesces on exposure to moist air.

Solubility: Potassium Acetate USP—Very soluble in water; freely soluble in alcohol.

USP requirements: Potassium Acetate Injection USP—Preserve in single-dose or in multiple-dose containers, preferably of Type I or Type II glass. A sterile solution of Potassium Acetate in Water for Injection. The label states the potassium acetate content in terms of weight and of milliequivalents in a given volume. Label the Injection to indicate that it is to be diluted to appropriate strength with water or other suitable fluid prior to administration. The label states also the total osmolar concentration in mOsmol per liter. Where the contents are less than 100 mL, or where the label states that the Injection is not for direct injection but is to be diluted before use, the label alternatively may state the total osmolar concentration in mOsmol per mL. Contains the labeled amount, within ±5%. Meets the requirements for Identification, Bacterial endotoxins, pH (5.5–8.0, when diluted with water to 1.0% of potassium acetate), Particulate matter, and Injections.

POTASSIUM BENZOATE

Chemical name: Benzoic acid, potassium salt.

Molecular formula: $C_7H_5KO_2$.

Molecular weight: 160.21.

Description: Potassium Benzoate NF—White, odorless, or practically odorless, granular or crystalline powder. Stable in air. NF category: Antimicrobial preservative.

Solubility: Potassium Benzoate NF—Freely soluble in water; sparingly soluble in alcohol and somewhat more soluble in 90% alcohol.

NF requirements: Potassium Benzoate NF—Preserve in well-closed containers. Contains not less than 99.0% and not more than 100.5% of potassium benzoate, calculated on the anhydrous basis. Meets the requirements for Identification, Alkalinity, Water (not more than 1.5%), Arsenic (not more than 3 ppm), Heavy metals (not more than 0.001%), and Organic volatile impurities.

POTASSIUM BICARBONATE

Chemical name: Carbonic acid, monopotassium salt.

Molecular formula: $KHCO_3$.

Molecular weight: 100.12.

Description: Potassium Bicarbonate USP—Colorless, transparent, monoclinic prisms or as a white, granular powder. Is odorless, and is stable in air. Its solutions are neutral or alkaline to phenolphthalein TS.

Solubility: Potassium Bicarbonate USP—Freely soluble in water; practically insoluble in alcohol.

USP requirements: Potassium Bicarbonate Effervescent Tablets for Oral Solution USP—Preserve in tight containers, protected from excessive heat. The label states the potassium content in terms of weight and in terms of milliequivalents. Where Tablets are packaged in individual pouches, the label instructs the user not to open until the time of use. Contain an amount of potassium bicarbonate equivalent to the labeled amount of potassium, within ±10%. Meet the requirements for Identification and Uniformity of dosage units.

POTASSIUM BICARBONATE AND POTASSIUM CHLORIDE

For *Potassium Bicarbonate* and *Potassium Chloride*—See individual listings for chemistry information.

USP requirements:

Potassium Bicarbonate and Potassium Chloride for Effervescent Oral Solution USP—Preserve in tight containers, protected from excessive heat. The label states the potassium and chloride contents in terms of weight and in terms of milliequivalents. Where packaged in individual pouches, the label instructs the user not to open until the time of use. Contains amounts of potassium bicarbonate and potassium chloride equivalent to the labeled amounts of potassium and chloride, within ±10%. Meets the requirements for Identification, Uniformity of dosage units (single-unit containers), and Minimum fill (multiple-unit containers).

Potassium Bicarbonate and Potassium Chloride Effervescent Tablets for Oral Solution USP—Preserve in tight containers, protected from excessive heat. The label states the potassium and chloride contents in terms of weight and in terms of milliequivalents. Where Tablets are packaged in individual pouches, the label instructs the user not to open until the time of use. Contain amounts of potassium bicarbonate and potassium chloride equivalent to the labeled amounts of potassium and chloride, within ±10%. Meet the requirements for Identification and Uniformity of dosage units.

POTASSIUM BICARBONATE AND POTASSIUM CITRATE

For *Potassium Bicarbonate* and *Potassium Citrate*—See individual listings for chemistry information.

USP requirements: Potassium Bicarbonate and Potassium Citrate Effervescent Tablets for Oral Solution—Not in USP.

POTASSIUM AND SODIUM BICARBONATES AND CITRIC ACID

For *Potassium Bicarbonate, Sodium Bicarbonate,* and *Citric Acid*—See individual listings for chemistry information.

USP requirements: Potassium and Sodium Bicarbonates and Citric Acid Effervescent Tablets for Oral Solution USP—Preserve in tight containers. Label it to state the sodium content. The label states also that Tablets are to be dissolved in water before being taken. Contain the labeled amounts of potassium bicarbonate, sodium bicarbonate, and anhydrous citric acid, within ±10%. Meet the requirements for Identification and Acid-neutralizing capacity (not less than 5 mEq of acid consumed per single dose).

POTASSIUM BITARTRATE AND SODIUM BICARBONATE

Chemical name:
Potassium bitartrate—Potassium acid tartrate.
Sodium bicarbonate—Carbonic acid monosodium salt.

Molecular formula:
Potassium bitartrate—$C_4H_5KO_6$.
Sodium bicarbonate—$NaHCO_3$.

Molecular weight:
Potassium bitartrate—188.18.
Sodium bicarbonate 84.01.

Description:
Potassium bitartrate—Odorless, or almost odorless, crystals or white crystalline powder.
Sodium Bicarbonate USP—White, crystalline powder. Is stable in dry air, but slowly decomposes in moist air. Its solutions, when freshly prepared with cold water, without shaking, are alkaline to litmus. The alkalinity increases as the solutions stand, as they are agitated, or as they are heated.
NF category: Alkalizing agent.

Solubility:
Potassium bitartrate—Soluble 1 in 90 of water and 1 in 16 of boiling water; practically insoluble in alcohol.
Sodium Bicarbonate USP—Soluble in water; insoluble in alcohol.

USP requirements: Potassium Bitartrate and Sodium Bicarbonate Suppositories—Not in USP.

POTASSIUM CARBONATE

Chemical name: Carbonic acid, dipotassium salt.

Molecular formula: K_2CO_3.

Molecular weight: 138.21.

Description: Hygroscopic, odorless granules or granular powder.

Solubility: Soluble in 1 part cold, 0.7 part boiling water; practically insoluble in alcohol.

USP requirements: Potassium Carbonate USP—Preserve in well-closed containers. Contains not less than 99.5% and not more than 100.5% of potassium carbonate, calculated on the dried basis. Meets the requirements for Identification, Loss on drying (not more than 0.5%), Insoluble substances, Arsenic (not more than 2 ppm), Heavy metals (not more than 0.0005%), and Organic volatile impurities.

POTASSIUM CHLORIDE

Chemical name: Potassium chloride.

Molecular formula: KCl.

Molecular weight: 74.55.

Description: Potassium Chloride USP—Colorless, elongated, prismatic, or cubical crystals, or white, granular powder. Is odorless and is stable in air. Its solutions are neutral to litmus. NF category: Tonicity agent.

Solubility: Potassium Chloride USP—Freely soluble in water and even more soluble in boiling water; insoluble in alcohol.

USP requirements:
Potassium Chloride USP—Preserve in well-closed containers. Where Potassium Chloride is intended for use in hemodialysis, it is so labeled. Contains not less than 99.0% and not more than 100.5% of potassium chloride, calculated on the dried basis. Meets the requirements for Identification, Acidity or alkalinity, Loss on drying (not more than 1.0%), Iodide or bromide, Arsenic (not more than 3 ppm), Calcium and magnesium, Heavy metals (not more than 0.001%), Sodium, Aluminum (not more than 1 ppm), and Organic volatile impurities.

Potassium Chloride Extended-release Capsules USP—Preserve in tight containers at a temperature not exceeding 30 °C. Contain the labeled amount, within ±10%. Meet the requirements for Identification, Dissolution (not more than 35% in 2 hours in water in Apparatus 1 at 100 rpm), and Uniformity of dosage units.

Potassium Chloride for Injection Concentrate USP—Preserve in single-dose or in multiple-dose containers, preferably of Type I or Type II glass. A sterile solution of Potassium Chloride in Water for Injection. The label states the potassium chloride content in terms of weight and of milliequivalents in a given volume. Label Potassium Chloride for Injection Concentrate to indicate that it is to be diluted to appropriate strength with water or other suitable fluid prior to administration. Immediately following the name, the label bears the boxed warning (in large letters): **Concentrate Must be Diluted Before Use.** The cap of the container and the overseal of the cap must be black and both bear the words: "Must be Diluted" in readily legible type, in a color that stands out from its background. Ampuls shall be identified by a black band or a series of black bands above the constriction. The label states also the total osmolar concentration in mOsmol per liter. Contains the labeled amount, within ±5%. Meets the requirements for Identification, Pyrogen, pH (4.0–8.0), Particulate matter, and Injections.

Potassium Chloride Oral Solution USP—Preserve in tight containers. Contains the labeled amount, within ±5%. May contain alcohol. Meets the requirements for Identification and Alcohol content (90.0–115.0% of the labeled amount which is not more than 7.5%).

Potassium Chloride for Oral Solution USP—Preserve in tight containers. A dry mixture of Potassium Chloride and one or more suitable colors, diluents, and flavors. The label states the Potassium Chloride content in terms of weight and in terms of milliequivalents. Contains the labeled amount, within ±10%. Meets the requirements for Identification, Uniformity of dosage units (single-unit containers), and Minimum fill (multiple-unit containers).

Potassium Chloride for Oral Suspension—Not in USP.

Potassium Chloride Extended-release Tablets USP—Preserve in tight containers at a temperature not exceeding 30 °C. Contain the labeled amount, within ±10%. Meet the requirements for Identification, Dissolution (not more than 35% in 2 hours in water in Apparatus 2 at 50 rpm), and Uniformity of dosage units.

POTASSIUM CHLORIDE AND DEXTROSE

For *Potassium Chloride* and *Dextrose*—See individual listings for chemistry information.

USP requirements: Potassium Chloride in Dextrose Injection USP—Preserve in single-dose glass or plastic containers. Glass containers are preferably of Type I or Type II glass. A sterile solution of Potassium Chloride and Dextrose in Water for Injection. The label states the total osmolar concentration in mOsmol per liter. Where the contents are less than 100 mL, or where the label states that the Injection is not for direct injection but is to be diluted before use, the label alternatively may state the total osmolar concentration in mOsmol per mL. The content of potassium, in milliequivalents, is prominently displayed on the label. Contains the labeled amounts of potassium chloride, within −5% to +10%, and dextrose, within ±5%. Contains no antimicrobial agents. Meets the requirements for Identification, Pyrogen, pH (3.5–6.5, determined on a portion diluted with water, if necessary, to a concentration of not more than 5% of dextrose), 5-Hydroxymethylfurfural and related substances, and Injections, and for Heavy metals under Dextrose Injection.

POTASSIUM CHLORIDE, DEXTROSE, AND SODIUM CHLORIDE

For *Potassium Chloride, Dextrose,* and *Sodium Chloride*—See individual listings for chemistry information.

USP requirements: Potassium Chloride in Dextrose and Sodium Chloride Injection USP—Preserve in single-dose containers, preferably of Type I or Type II glass, or of a suitable plastic. A sterile solution of Potassium Chloride, Dextrose, and Sodium Chloride in Water for Injection. The label states the potassium, sodium, and chloride contents in terms of milliequivalents in a given volume. The label states also the total osmolar concentration in mOsmol per liter. Where the contents are less than 100 mL, the label alternatively may state the total osmolar concentration in mOsmol per mL. Contains the equivalent of the labeled amounts of potassium and chloride, within −5% to +10%, and the equivalent of the labeled amounts of dextrose and sodium, within ±5%. Contains no antimicrobial agents. Meets the requirements for Identification, Pyrogen, pH (3.5–6.5), Heavy metals, 5-Hydroxymethylfurfural and related substances, and Injections.

POTASSIUM CHLORIDE, LACTATED RINGER'S, AND DEXTROSE

For *Potassium Chloride, Calcium Chloride, Sodium Chloride, Sodium Lactate,* and *Dextrose*—See individual listings for chemistry information.

USP requirements: Potassium Chloride in Lactated Ringer's and Dextrose Injection USP—Preserve in single-dose glass or plastic containers. Glass containers are preferably of Type I or Type II glass. A sterile solution of Calcium Chloride, Potassium Chloride, Sodium Chloride, and Sodium Lactate in Water for Injection. The label states the total osmolar concentration in mOsmol per liter. Where the contents are less than 100 mL, the label alternatively may state the total osmolar concentration in mOsmol per mL. The label includes also the warning: "Not for use in the treatment of lactic acidosis." Contains, in each 100 mL, not less than 285.0 mg and not more than 315.0 mg of sodium (as sodium chloride and sodium lactate), not less than 4.90 mg and not more than 6.00 mg of calcium (calcium, equivalent to not less than 18.0 mg and not more than 22.0 mg of hydrous calcium chloride), and not less than 231.0 mg and not more than 261.0 mg of lactate (lactate, equivalent to not less than 290.0 mg and not more than 330.0 mg of sodium lactate). Contains the labeled amounts of Potassium Chloride and dextrose, within ±5%, and the equivalent of the labeled amount of chloride (chloride, as sodium chloride, potassium chloride, and hydrous calcium chloride), within ±10%. Contains no antimicrobial agents. Meets the requirements for Identification, Bacterial endotoxins, pH (3.5–6.5), Heavy metals, 5-Hydroxymethylfurfural and related substances (absorbance not more than 0.25), and Injections.

POTASSIUM CHLORIDE, POTASSIUM BICARBONATE, AND POTASSIUM CITRATE

For *Potassium Chloride, Potassium Bicarbonate,* and *Potassium Citrate*—See individual listings for chemistry information.

USP requirements: Potassium Chloride, Potassium Bicarbonate, and Potassium Citrate Effervescent Tablets for Oral Solution USP—Preserve in tight containers, protected from excessive heat. The label states the potassium and chloride contents in terms of weight and in terms of milliequivalents. Where Tablets are packaged in individual pouches, the label instructs the user not to open until the time of use. Contain the equivalent of the labeled amounts of potassium and chloride, within ±10%. Meet the requirements for Identification and Uniformity of dosage units.

POTASSIUM CHLORIDE AND SODIUM CHLORIDE

For *Potassium Chloride* and *Sodium Chloride*—See individual listings for chemistry information.

USP requirements: Potassium Chloride in Sodium Chloride Injection USP—Preserve in single-dose containers, preferably of Type I or Type II glass, or of a suitable plastic. A sterile solution of Potassium Chloride and Sodium Chloride in Water for Injection. The label states the potassium, sodium, and chloride contents in terms of milliequivalents in a given volume. The label states also the total osmolar concentration in mOsmol per liter. Where the contents are less than 100 mL, the label may alternatively state the total osmolar concentration in mOsmol per mL. Contains the equivalent of the labeled amounts of potassium and chloride, within −5% to +10%, and the equivalent of the labeled amount of sodium, within ±5%. Contains no antimicrobial agents. Meets the requirements for Identification, Pyrogen, pH (3.5–6.5), Heavy metals, and Injections.

POTASSIUM CITRATE

Chemical name: 1,2,3-Propanetricarboxylic acid, 2-hydroxy-, tripotassium salt, monohydrate.

Molecular formula: $C_6H_5K_3O_7 \cdot H_2O$.

Molecular weight: 324.41.

Description: Potassium Citrate USP—Transparent crystals or white, granular powder. Is odorless and is deliquescent when exposed to moist air.

NF category: Buffering agent.

Solubility: Potassium Citrate USP—Freely soluble in water; almost insoluble in alcohol.

USP requirements:
Potassium Citrate USP—Preserve in tight containers. Contains not less than 99.0% and not more than 100.5% of potassium citrate, calculated on the dried basis. Meets the requirements for Identification, Alkalinity, Loss on drying (3.0–6.0%), Tartrate, Heavy metals (not more than 0.001%), and Organic volatile impurities.
Potassium Citrate Tablets—Not in USP.
Potassium Citrate Extended-release Tablets USP—Preserve in tight containers. Contain the labeled amount, within ±10%. Meet the requirements for Identification, Dissolution (not more than 45% in 30 minutes, not more than 60% in 1 hour, and not less than 80% in 3 hours, in water in Apparatus 2 at 50 rpm), Uniformity of dosage units, and Potassium content (38.4–40.2%).

POTASSIUM CITRATE AND CITRIC ACID

For *Potassium Citrate* and *Citric Acid*—See individual listings for chemistry information.

USP requirements:
Potassium Citrate and Citric Acid Oral Solution USP—Preserve in tight containers. A solution of Potassium Citrate and Citric Acid in a suitable aqueous medium. Contains, in each 100 mL, not less than 7.55 grams and not more than 8.35 grams of potassium; not less than 12.18 grams and not more than 13.46 grams of citrate, equivalent to not less than 20.9 grams and not more than 23.1 grams of potassium citrate monohydrate; and not less than 6.34 grams and not more than 7.02 grams of citric acid monohydrate. Meets the requirements for Identification and pH (4.9–5.4).
Note: The potassium ion content of Potassium Citrate and Citric Acid Oral Solution is approximately 2 mEq per mL.
Potassium Citrate and Citric Acid for Oral Solution—Not in USP.

POTASSIUM CITRATE AND SODIUM CITRATE

For *Potassium Citrate* and *Sodium Citrate*—See individual listings for chemistry information.

USP requirements: Potassium Citrate and Sodium Citrate Tablets—Not in USP.

POTASSIUM GLUCONATE

Chemical name: D-Gluconic acid, monopotassium salt.

Molecular formula: $C_6H_{11}KO_7$.

Molecular weight: 234.25.

Description: Potassium Gluconate USP—White to yellowish white, crystalline powder or granules. Is odorless and is stable in air. Its solutions are slightly alkaline to litmus.

Solubility: Potassium Gluconate USP—Freely soluble in water; practically insoluble in dehydrated alcohol, in ether, and in chloroform.

USP requirements:
Potassium Gluconate Elixir USP—Preserve in tight, light-resistant containers. Contains the labeled amount, within ±5%. Meets the requirements for Identification and Alcohol content (4.5–5.5%).
Potassium Gluconate Tablets USP—Preserve in tight containers. Contain the labeled amount, within ±5%. Meet the requirements for Identification, Dissolution (75% in 45 minutes in water in Apparatus 2 at 100 rpm), and Uniformity of dosage units.

POTASSIUM GLUCONATE AND POTASSIUM CHLORIDE

For *Potassium Gluconate* and *Potassium Chloride*—See individual listings for chemistry information.

USP requirements:
Potassium Gluconate and Potassium Chloride Oral Solution USP—Preserve in tight containers. A solution of Potassium Gluconate and Potassium Chloride in a suitable aqueous medium. Label it to state the potassium and chloride contents in terms of milliequivalents of each in a given volume of Oral Solution. Contains the equivalent of the labeled amounts of potassium and chloride, within ±10%. Meets the requirement for Identification.

Potassium Gluconate and Potassium Chloride for Oral Solution USP—Preserve in tight containers. A dry mixture of Potassium Gluconate and Potassium Chloride and one or more suitable colors, diluents, and flavors. Label it to state the potassium and chloride contents in terms of milliequivalents. Where packaged in unit-dose pouches, the label instructs the user not to open until the time of use. Contains the equivalent of the labeled amounts of potassium and chloride, within ±10%. Meets the requirements for Identification and Minimum fill.

POTASSIUM GLUCONATE AND POTASSIUM CITRATE

For *Potassium Gluconate* and *Potassium Citrate*—See individual listings for chemistry information.

USP requirements: Potassium Gluconate and Potassium Citrate Oral Solution USP—Preserve in tight containers. A solution of Potassium Gluconate and Potassium Citrate in a suitable aqueous medium. Label it to state the potassium content in terms of milliequivalents in a given volume of Oral Solution. Contains the equivalent of the labeled amount of potassium, within ±10%. Meets the requirement for Identification.

POTASSIUM GLUCONATE, POTASSIUM CITRATE, AND AMMONIUM CHLORIDE

For *Potassium Gluconate*, *Potassium Citrate*, and *Ammonium Chloride*—See individual listings for chemistry information.

USP requirements: Potassium Gluconate, Potassium Citrate, and Ammonium Chloride Oral Solution USP—Preserve in tight containers. A solution of Potassium Gluconate, Potassium Citrate, and Ammonium Chloride in a suitable aqueous medium. Label it to state the potassium and chloride contents in terms of milliequivalents of each in a given volume of Oral Solution. Contains the equivalent of the labeled amounts of potassium and chloride, within ±10%. Meets the requirement for Identification.

POTASSIUM GUAIACOLSULFONATE

Chemical name: Benzenesulfonic acid, hydroxymethoxy-, monopotassium salt, hemihydrate.

Molecular formula: $C_7H_7KO_5S \cdot \frac{1}{2}H_2O$.

Molecular weight: 251.29 (hemihydrate); 242.29 (anhydrous).

Description: White, odorless crystals or crystalline powder. Gradually turns pink on exposure to air and light.

Solubility: Soluble in 7.5 parts water; almost insoluble in alcohol; insoluble in ether.

USP requirements: Potassium Guaiacolsulfonate USP—Preserve in well-closed, light-resistant containers. Contains not less than 98.0% and not more than 102.0% of potassium guaiacolsulfonate, calculated on the anhydrous basis. Meets

the requirements for Identification, Water (3.0–6.0%), Selenium (not more than 0.003%), Sulfate, and Heavy metals (not more than 0.002%).

POTASSIUM HYDROXIDE

Chemical name: Potassium hydroxide.

Molecular formula: KOH.

Molecular weight: 56.11.

Description: Potassium Hydroxide NF—White or practically white fused masses, or small pellets, or flakes, or sticks, or other forms. It is hard and brittle and shows a crystalline fracture. Exposed to air, it rapidly absorbs carbon dioxide and moisture, and deliquesces.

NF category: Alkalizing agent.

Solubility: Potassium Hydroxide NF—Freely soluble in water, in alcohol, and in glycerin; very soluble in boiling alcohol.

NF requirements: Potassium Hydroxide NF—Preserve in tight containers. Contains not less than 85.0% of total alkali, calculated as potassium hydroxide, including not more than 3.5% of anhydrous potassium carbonate. Meets the requirements for Identification, Insoluble substances, and Heavy metals (not more than 0.003%).

Caution: Exercise great care in handling Potassium Hydroxide, as it rapidly destroys tissues.

POTASSIUM IODIDE

Chemical group: Inorganic iodides.

Chemical name: Potassium iodide.

Molecular formula: KI.

Molecular weight: 166.00.

Description:
Potassium Iodide USP—Hexahedral crystals, either transparent and colorless or somewhat opaque and white, or a white, granular powder. Is slightly hygroscopic. Its solutions are neutral or alkaline to litmus.

Potassium Iodide Oral Solution USP—Clear, colorless, odorless liquid. Is neutral or alkaline to litmus. Specific gravity is about 1.70.

Solubility: Potassium Iodide USP—Very soluble in water and even more soluble in boiling water; freely soluble in glycerin; soluble in alcohol.

USP requirements:
Potassium Iodide Oral Solution USP—Preserve in tight, light-resistant containers. Contains the labeled amount, within ±6%. Meets the requirement for Identification.

Note: If Potassium Iodide Oral Solution is not to be used within a short time, add 0.5 mg of sodium thiosulfate for each gram of potassium iodide. Crystals of potassium iodide may form in Potassium Iodide Oral Solution under normal conditions of storage, especially if refrigerated.

Potassium Iodide Syrup—Not in USP.

Potassium Iodide Tablets USP—Preserve in tight containers. Contain the labeled amount, within ±6% for Tablets of 300 mg or more; within ±7.5% for Tablets of less than 300 mg. Meet the requirements for Identification, Disintegration (for Enteric-coated Tablets, the tablets do not disintegrate after 1 hour of agitation in simulated gastric fluid TS, but they disintegrate within 90 minutes in simulated intestinal fluid TS), Dissolution (for uncoated Tablets, 75% in 15 minutes in water in Apparatus 2 at 50 rpm), and Uniformity of dosage units.

POTASSIUM METABISULFITE

Chemical name: Disulfurous acid, dipotassium salt.

Molecular formula: $K_2S_2O_5$.

Molecular weight: 222.31.

Description: Potassium Metabisulfite NF—White or colorless, free-flowing crystals, crystalline powder, or granules, usually having an odor of sulfur dioxide. Gradually oxidizes in air to the sulfate. Its solutions are acid to litmus.
NF category: Antioxidant.

Solubility: Potassium Metabisulfite NF—Soluble in water; insoluble in alcohol.

NF requirements: Potassium Metabisulfite NF—Preserve in well-fitted, tight containers, and avoid exposure to excessive heat. Contains an amount of potassium metabisulfite equivalent to not less than 51.8% and not more than 57.6% of sulfur dioxide. Meets the requirements for Identification, Arsenic (not more than 3 ppm), Iron (not more than 0.001%), Heavy metals (not more than 0.001%), and Organic volatile impurities.

POTASSIUM METAPHOSPHATE

Chemical name: Metaphosphoric acid (HPO_3), potassium salt.

Molecular formula: KPO_3.

Molecular weight: 118.07.

Description: Potassium Metaphosphate NF—White, odorless powder.
NF category: Buffering agent.

Solubility: Potassium Metaphosphate NF—Insoluble in water; soluble in dilute solutions of sodium salts.

NF requirements: Potassium Metaphosphate NF—Preserve in well-closed containers. A straight-chain polyphosphate, having a high degree of polymerization. Contains the equivalent of not less than 59.0% and not more than 61.0% of phosphorus pentoxide. Meets the requirements for Identification, Viscosity (6.5–15 centipoises), Fluoride (not more than 0.001%), Arsenic (not more than 3 ppm), Lead (not more than 5 ppm), and Heavy metals (not more than 0.002%).

POTASSIUM PERMANGANATE

Chemical name: Permanganic acid ($HMnO_4$), potassium salt.

Molecular formula: $KMnO_4$.

Molecular weight: 158.03.

Description: Potassium Permanganate USP—Dark purple crystals, almost opaque by transmitted light and of a blue metallic luster by reflected light. Its color is sometimes modified by a dark bronze-like appearance. Is stable in air.

Solubility: Potassium Permanganate USP—Soluble in water; freely soluble in boiling water.

USP requirements: Potassium Permanganate USP—Preserve in well-closed containers. Contains not less than 99.0% and not more than 100.5% of potassium permanganate, calculated on the dried basis. Meets the requirements for Identification,

Loss on drying (not more than 0.5%), and Insoluble substances (not more than 0.2%).
Caution: Observe great care in handling Potassium Permanganate, as dangerous explosions may occur if it is brought into contact with organic or other readily oxidizable substances, either in solution or in the dry state.

DIBASIC POTASSIUM PHOSPHATE

Chemical name: Phosphoric acid, dipotassium salt.

Molecular formula: K_2HPO_4.

Molecular weight: 174.18.

Description: Dibasic Potassium Phosphate USP—Colorless or white, somewhat hygroscopic, granular powder. The pH of a solution (1 in 20) is about 8.5 to 9.6.
NF category: Buffering agent.

Solubility: Dibasic Potassium Phosphate USP—Freely soluble in water; very slightly soluble in alcohol.

USP requirements: Dibasic Potassium Phosphate USP—Preserve in well-closed containers. Contains not less than 98.0% and not more than 100.5% of dibasic potassium phosphate, calculated on the dried basis. Meets the requirements for Identification, pH (8.5–9.6, in a solution [1 in 20]), Loss on drying (not more than 1.0%), Insoluble substances (not more than 0.2%), Carbonate, Chloride (not more than 0.03%), Sulfate (not more than 0.1%), Fluoride (not more than 0.001%), Arsenic (not more than 3 ppm), Iron (not more than 0.003%), Sodium, Heavy metals (not more than 0.001%), and Monobasic or tribasic salt.

MONOBASIC POTASSIUM PHOSPHATE

Chemical name: Phosphoric acid, monopotassium salt.

Molecular formula: KH_2PO_4.

Molecular weight: 136.09.

Description: Monobasic Potassium Phosphate NF—Colorless crystals or white, granular or crystalline powder. Is odorless, and is stable in air. The pH of a solution (1 in 100) is about 4.5.
NF category: Buffering agent.

Solubility: Monobasic Potassium Phosphate NF—Freely soluble in water; practically insoluble in alcohol.

USP requirements: Monobasic Potassium Phosphate Tablets for Oral Solution—Not in USP.

NF requirements: Monobasic Potassium Phosphate NF—Preserve in tight containers. Dried at 105 °C for 4 hours, contains not less than 98.0% and not more than 100.5% of monobasic potassium phosphate. Meets the requirements for Identification, Loss on drying (not more than 1.0%), Insoluble substances (not more than 0.2%), Fluoride (not more than 0.001%), Arsenic (not more than 3 ppm), Heavy metals (not more than 0.002%), Lead (not more than 5 ppm), and Organic volatile impurities.

POTASSIUM PHOSPHATES

For *Monobasic Potassium Phosphate* and *Dibasic Potassium Phosphate*—See individual listings for chemistry information.

USP requirements:
Potassium Phosphates Capsules for Oral Solution—Not in USP.

Potassium Phosphates Injection USP—Preserve in single-dose containers, preferably of Type I glass. A sterile solution of Monobasic Potassium Phosphate and Dibasic Potassium Phosphate in Water for Injection. The label states the potassium content in terms of milliequivalents in a given volume, and states also the elemental phosphorus content in terms of millimoles in a given volume. Label the Injection to indicate that it is to be diluted to appropriate strength with water or other suitable fluid prior to administration, and that once opened any unused portion is to be discarded. The label states also the total osmolar concentration in mOsmol per liter. Where the contents are less than 100 mL, or where the label states that the Injection is not for direct injection but is to be diluted before use, the label alternatively may state the total osmolar concentration in mOsmol per mL. Contains the labeled amounts of monobasic potassium phosphate and dibasic potassium phosphate, within ±5%. Contains no bacteriostat or other preservative. Meets the requirements for Identification, Bacterial endotoxins, Particulate matter, and Injections.

Potassium Phosphates for Oral Solution—Not in USP.

POTASSIUM AND SODIUM PHOSPHATES

For *Dibasic Potassium Phosphate, Dibasic Sodium Phosphate, Monobasic Potassium Phosphate,* and *Monobasic Sodium Phosphate*—See individual listings for chemistry information.

USP requirements:

Potassium and Sodium Phosphates Capsules for Oral Solution—Not in USP.

Potassium and Sodium Phosphates for Oral Solution—Not in USP.

Potassium and Sodium Phosphates Tablets for Oral Solution—Not in USP.

MONOBASIC POTASSIUM AND SODIUM PHOSPHATES

For *Monobasic Potassium Phosphate* and *Monobasic Sodium Phosphate*—See individual listings for chemistry information.

USP requirements: Monobasic Potassium and Sodium Phosphates Tablets for Oral Solution—Not in USP.

POTASSIUM SODIUM TARTRATE

Chemical name: Butanedioic acid, 2,3-dihydroxy-, [R-(R*,R*)]-, monopotassium monosodium salt, tetrahydrate.

Molecular formula: $C_4H_4KNaO_6 \cdot 4H_2O$.

Molecular weight: 282.22 (tetrahydrate); 210.16 (anhydrous).

Description: Potassium Sodium Tartrate USP—Colorless crystals or white, crystalline powder. As it effloresces slightly in warm, dry air, the crystals are often coated with a white powder.

Solubility: Potassium Sodium Tartrate USP—Freely soluble in water; practically insoluble in alcohol.

USP requirements: Potassium Sodium Tartrate USP—Preserve in tight containers. Contains not less than 99.0% and not more than 102.0% of potassium sodium tartrate, calculated on the anhydrous basis. Meets the requirements for Identification, Alkalinity, Water (21.0–27.0%), Ammonia, and Heavy metals (not more than 0.001%).

POTASSIUM SORBATE

Chemical name: 2,4-Hexadienoic acid, (E,E')- potassium salt.

Molecular formula: $C_6H_7KO_2$.

Molecular weight: 150.22.

Description: Potassium Sorbate NF—White crystals or powder, having a characteristic odor. Melts at about 270 °C, with decomposition.

NF category: Antimicrobial preservative.

Solubility: Potassium Sorbate NF—Freely soluble in water; soluble in alcohol.

NF requirements: Potassium Sorbate NF—Preserve in tight containers, protected from light, and avoid exposure to excessive heat. Contains not less than 98.0% and not more than 101.0% of potassium sorbate, calculated on the dried basis. Meets the requirements for Identification, Acidity or alkalinity, Loss on drying (not more than 1.0%), Heavy metals (not more than 0.001%), and Organic volatile impurities.

POVIDONE

Chemical name: 2-Pyrrolidinone, 1-ethenyl-, homopolymer.

Molecular formula: $(C_6H_9NO)_n$.

Description: Povidone USP—White to creamy white powder, having a faint odor. Is hygroscopic.

NF category: Suspending and/or viscosity-increasing agent; tablet binder.

Solubility: Povidone USP—Soluble in water, in alcohol, and in chloroform; insoluble in ether.

USP requirements: Povidone USP—Preserve in tight containers. A synthetic polymer consisting essentially of linear 1-vinyl-2-pyrrolidinone groups, the degree of polymerization of which results in polymers of various molecular weights. It is characterized by its viscosity in aqueous solution, relative to that of water, expressed as a K-value, ranging from 10 to 120. Label it to state, as part of the official title, the K-value or K-value range of the Povidone. The K-value of Povidone having a nominal K-value of 15 or less is not less than 85.0% and not more than 115.0% of the nominal K-value, and the K-value of Povidone having a nominal K-value or nominal K-value range with an average of more than 15 is not less than 90.0% and not more than 108.0% of the nominal K-value or average of the nominal K-value range. Meets the requirements for Identification, pH (3.0–7.0, in a solution [1 in 20]), Water (not more than 5.0%), Residue on ignition (not more than 0.1%), Lead (not more than 10 ppm), Aldehydes (not more than 0.20%), Hydrazine (not more than 1 ppm), Vinylpyrrolidinone (not more than 0.2%), K-value, and Nitrogen content (11.5–12.8%, on the anhydrous basis).

POVIDONE-IODINE

Chemical name: 2-Pyrrolidinone, 1-ethenyl-, homopolymer, compd. with iodine.

Molecular formula: $(C_6H_9NO)_n \cdot xI$.

Description:

Povidone-Iodine USP—Yellowish brown, amorphous powder, having a slight characteristic odor. Its solution is acid to litmus.

Povidone-Iodine Topical Aerosol Solution USP—The liquid obtained from Povidone-Iodine Topical Aerosol Solution is transparent, having a reddish-brown color.

Solubility: Povidone-Iodine USP—Soluble in water and in alcohol; practically insoluble in chloroform, in carbon tetrachloride, in ether, in solvent hexane, and in acetone.

USP requirements:

Povidone-Iodine Ointment USP—Preserve in tight containers. An emulsion, solution, or suspension of Povidone-Iodine in a suitable water-soluble ointment base. Contains an amount of povidone-iodine equivalent to the labeled amount of iodine, within −15% to +20%. Meets the requirements for Identification, Minimum fill, and pH (1.5–6.5, determined in a solution [1 in 20]).

Povidone-Iodine Topical Aerosol Solution USP—Preserve in pressurized containers, and avoid exposure to excessive heat. A solution of Povidone-Iodine under nitrogen in a pressurized container. Contains an amount of povidone-iodine equivalent to the labeled amount of iodine, within −15% to +20%. Meets the requirements for Identification and pH (not more than 6.0), and for Leak testing and Pressure testing under Aerosols.

Povidone-Iodine Cleansing Solution USP—Preserve in tight containers. A solution of Povidone-Iodine with one or more suitable surface-active agents. Contains an amount of povidone-iodine equivalent to the labeled amount of iodine, within −15% to +20%. Meets the requirements for Identification, pH (1.5–6.5), and Alcohol content (if present, within ±10% of labeled amount).

PRALIDOXIME

Chemical name: Pralidoxime chloride—Pyridinium, 2-[(hydroxyimino)methyl]-1-methyl-, chloride.

Molecular formula: Pralidoxime chloride—$C_7H_9ClN_2O$.

Molecular weight: Pralidoxime chloride—172.61.

Description:

Pralidoxime Chloride USP—White to pale-yellow, crystalline powder. Odorless and stable in air.

Sterile Pralidoxime Chloride USP—White to pale-yellow, crystalline powder. Odorless and stable in air.

Solubility:

Pralidoxime Chloride USP—Freely soluble in water.

Sterile Pralidoxime Chloride USP—Freely soluble in water.

USP requirements:

Sterile Pralidoxime Chloride USP—Preserve in Containers for Sterile Solids. It is Pralidoxime Chloride suitable for parenteral use. Contains the labeled amount, within ±10%. Meets the requirements for Completeness of solution, Constituted solution, Bacterial endotoxins, and pH (3.5–4.5, in a solution [1 in 20]), for Identification tests, Loss on drying (not more than 2.0%) and Heavy metals (not more than 0.002%) under Pralidoxime Chloride, and for Sterility tests, Uniformity of dosage units, and Labeling under Injections.

Pralidoxime Chloride Tablets USP—Preserve in well-closed containers. Contain the labeled amount, within ±5%. Meet the requirements for Identification, Dissolution (55% in 60 minutes in water in Apparatus 1 at 100 rpm), and Uniformity of dosage units.

PRAMOXINE

Chemical name:

Pramoxine—4-[3-(4-Butoxyphenoxy)propyl]morpholine.

Pramoxine hydrochloride—Morpholine, 4-[3-(4-butoxyphenoxy)propyl]-, hydrochloride.

Molecular formula:

Pramoxine—$C_{17}H_{27}NO_3$.

Pramoxine hydrochloride—$C_{17}H_{27}NO_3 \cdot HCl$.

Molecular weight:

Pramoxine—293.41.

Pramoxine hydrochloride—329.87.

Description: Pramoxine Hydrochloride USP—White to practically white, crystalline powder. May have a slight aromatic odor. The pH of a solution (1 in 100) is about 4.5.

Solubility: Pramoxine Hydrochloride USP—Freely soluble in water and in alcohol; soluble in chloroform; very slightly soluble in ether.

USP requirements:

Pramoxine Hydrochloride Cream USP—Preserve in tight containers. Contains the labeled amount, within ±10%, in a suitable water-miscible base. Meets the requirements for Identification, Microbial limits, and Minimum fill.

Pramoxine Hydrochloride Aerosol Foam—Not in USP.

Pramoxine Hydrochloride Jelly USP—Preserve in tight containers, preferably in collapsible tubes. Contains the labeled amount, within ±6%. Meets the requirements for Identification and Microbial limits.

Pramoxine Hydrochloride Lotion—Not in USP.

Pramoxine Hydrochloride Ointment—Not in USP.

Pramoxine and Pramoxine Hydrochloride Suppositories—Not in USP.

PRAVASTATIN

Chemical name: Pravastatin sodium—1-Naphthalene-heptanoic acid, 1,2,6,7,8,8a-hexahydro-beta,delta,6-trihydroxy-2-methyl-8-(2-methyl-1-oxobutoxy)-, monosodium salt, [1S-[1 alpha(betaS*,deltaS*),2 alpha,6 alpha,8 beta(R*),8a alpha]]-.

Molecular formula: Pravastatin sodium—$C_{23}H_{35}NaO_7$.

Molecular weight: Pravastatin sodium—446.52.

Description: Pravastatin sodium—Odorless, white to off-white, fine or crystalline powder.

Solubility: Pravastatin sodium—Soluble in methanol and in water; slightly soluble in isopropanol; practically insoluble in acetone, in acetonitrile, in chloroform, and in ether.

Other characteristics: Pravastatin sodium—Partition coefficient (octanol/water) 0.59 at pH 7.0.

USP requirements: Pravastatin Sodium Tablets—Not in USP.

PRAZEPAM

Chemical name: 2H-1,4-Benzodiazepin-2-one, 7-chloro-1-(cyclopropylmethyl)-1,3-dihydro-5-phenyl-.

Molecular formula: $C_{19}H_{17}ClN_2O$.

Molecular weight: 324.81.

Description: Prazepam USP—White to off-white crystalline powder.

Solubility: Prazepam USP—Freely soluble in acetone; soluble in dilute mineral acids, in alcohol, and in chloroform.

USP requirements:

Prazepam Capsules USP—Preserve in tight, light-resistant containers. Contain the labeled amount, within ±10%. Meet the requirements for Identification, Dissolution (80% in 60 minutes in 0.1 N hydrochloric acid in Apparatus 1 at 50 rpm), and Uniformity of dosage units.

Prazepam Tablets USP—Preserve in tight, light-resistant containers. Contain the labeled amount, within ±10%. Meet the requirements for Identification, Dissolution (80% in 60 minutes in 0.1 N hydrochloric acid in Apparatus 1 at 50 rpm), and Uniformity of dosage units.

PRAZIQUANTEL

Chemical group: An acylated isoquinoline-pyrazine derivative.

Chemical name: 4H-Pyrazino[2,1-a]isoquinolin-4-one, 2-(cyclohexylcarbonyl)-1,2,3,6,7,11b-hexahydro-.

Molecular formula: $C_{19}H_{24}N_2O_2$.

Molecular weight: 312.41.

Description: Praziquantel USP—White or practically white, crystalline powder; odorless or having a faint characteristic odor.

Solubility: Praziquantel USP—Very slightly soluble in water; freely soluble in alcohol and in chloroform.

Other characteristics: Hygroscopic.

USP requirements:
Praziquantel Injection—Not in USP.
Praziquantel Tablets USP—Preserve in tight containers. Contain the labeled amount, within ±10%. Meet the requirements for Identification, Dissolution (75% in 60 minutes in 0.1 N hydrochloric acid containing 2.0 mg of sodium lauryl sulfate per mL in Apparatus 2 at 50 rpm), and Uniformity of dosage units.

PRAZOSIN

Chemical name: Prazosin hydrochloride—Piperazine, 1-(4-amino-6,7-dimethoxy-2-quinazolinyl)-4-(2-furanylcarbonyl)-, monohydrochloride.

Molecular formula: Prazosin hydrochloride—$C_{19}H_{21}N_5O_4 \cdot HCl$.

Molecular weight: Prazosin hydrochloride—419.87.

Description: Prazosin Hydrochloride USP—White to tan powder.

pKa: 6.5 in 1:1 water and ethanol solution.

Solubility: Prazosin Hydrochloride USP—Slightly soluble in water, in methanol, in dimethylformamide, and in dimethylacetamide; very slightly soluble in alcohol; practically insoluble in chloroform and in acetone.

USP requirements:
Prazosin Hydrochloride Capsules USP—Preserve in well-closed, light-resistant containers. Contain an amount of prazosin hydrochloride equivalent to the labeled amount of prazosin, within ±10%. Meet the requirements for Identification, Dissolution (75% in 60 minutes in 0.1 N hydrochloric acid containing 3% sodium lauryl sulfate in Apparatus 1 at 100 rpm), and Uniformity of dosage units.
Caution: Care should be taken to prevent inhaling particles of Prazosin Hydrochloride and to prevent its contacting any part of the body.
Prazosin Hydrochloride Tablets—Not in USP.

PRAZOSIN AND POLYTHIAZIDE

For *Prazosin* and *Polythiazide*—See individual listings for chemistry information.

USP requirements: Prazosin Hydrochloride and Polythiazide Capsules—Not in USP.

PREDNISOLONE

Chemical name:
Prednisolone—Pregna-1,4-diene-3,20-dione, 11,17,21-trihydroxy-, (11 beta)-.
Prednisolone acetate—Pregna-1,4-diene-3,20-dione, 21-(acetyloxy)-11,17-dihydroxy-, (11 beta)-.
Prednisolone hemisuccinate—Pregna-1,4-diene-3,20-dione, 21-(3-carboxy-1-oxopropoxy)-11,17-dihydroxy-, (11 beta)-.
Prednisolone sodium phosphate—Pregna-1,4-diene-3,20-dione, 11,17-dihydroxy-21-(phosphonooxy)-, disodium salt, (11 beta)-.
Prednisolone tebutate—Pregna-1,4-diene-3,20-dione, 11,17-dihydroxy-21-[(3,3-dimethyl-1-oxobutyl)oxy]-, (11 beta)-.

Molecular formula:
Prednisolone—$C_{21}H_{28}O_5$ (anhydrous).
Prednisolone acetate—$C_{23}H_{30}O_6$.
Prednisolone hemisuccinate—$C_{25}H_{32}O_8$.
Prednisolone sodium phosphate—$C_{21}H_{27}Na_2O_8P$.
Prednisolone tebutate—$C_{27}H_{38}O_6$.

Molecular weight:
Prednisolone—360.45 (anhydrous).
Prednisolone acetate—402.49.
Prednisolone hemisuccinate—460.52.
Prednisolone sodium phosphate—484.39.
Prednisolone tebutate—458.59.

Description:
Prednisolone USP—White to practically white, odorless, crystalline powder. Melts at about 235 °C, with some decomposition.
Prednisolone Acetate USP—White to practically white, odorless, crystalline powder. Melts at about 235 °C, with some decomposition.
Prednisolone Hemisuccinate USP—Fine, creamy white powder with friable lumps; practically odorless. Melts at about 205 °C, with decomposition.
Prednisolone Sodium Phosphate USP—White or slightly yellow, friable granules or powder. Is odorless or has a slight odor. Is slightly hygroscopic.
Prednisolone Sodium Succinate for Injection USP—Creamy white powder with friable lumps, having a slight odor.
Prednisolone Tebutate USP—White to slightly yellow, free-flowing powder, which may show some soft lumps. Is odorless or has not more than a moderate, characteristic odor. Is hygroscopic.

Solubility:
Prednisolone USP—Very slightly soluble in water; soluble in methanol and in dioxane; sparingly soluble in acetone and in alcohol; slightly soluble in chloroform.
Prednisolone Acetate USP—Practically insoluble in water; slightly soluble in acetone, in alcohol, and in chloroform.
Prednisolone Hemisuccinate USP—Very slightly soluble in water; freely soluble in alcohol; soluble in acetone.
Prednisolone Sodium Phosphate USP—Freely soluble in water; soluble in methanol; slightly soluble in alcohol and in chloroform; very slightly soluble in acetone and in dioxane.
Prednisolone Tebutate USP—Very slightly soluble in water; freely soluble in chloroform and in dioxane; soluble in acetone; sparingly soluble in alcohol and in methanol.

USP requirements:
Prednisolone Cream USP—Preserve in collapsible tubes or in tight containers. Contains the labeled amount, within ±10%, in a suitable cream base. Meets the requirements for Identification and Minimum fill.
Prednisolone Syrup USP—Preserve in tight, light-resistant containers. Contains the labeled amount, within ±10%. Prednisolone Syrup may contain alcohol. Meets the requirements for Identification, pH (3.0–4.5), and Alcohol content (if present, 2.0–5.0%).
Prednisolone Tablets USP—Preserve in well-closed containers. Contain the labeled amount, within ±10%. Meet

the requirements for Identification, Dissolution (70% in 30 minutes in water in Apparatus 2 at 50 rpm), and Uniformity of dosage units.

Prednisolone Acetate Ophthalmic Suspension USP—Preserve in tight containers. A sterile, aqueous suspension of prednisolone acetate containing a suitable antimicrobial preservative. Contains the labeled amount, within −10% to +15%. Meets the requirements for Identification, Sterility, and pH (5.0–6.0).

Sterile Prednisolone Acetate Suspension USP—Preserve in single-dose or in multiple-dose containers, preferably of Type I glass. A sterile suspension of Prednisolone Acetate in a suitable aqueous medium. Contains the labeled amount, within ±10%. Meets the requirements for Identification, pH (5.0–7.5), and Injections.

Sterile Prednisolone Acetate and Prednisolone Sodium Phosphate Suspension—Not in USP.

Prednisolone Sodium Phosphate Injection USP—Preserve in single-dose or in multiple-dose containers, preferably of Type I glass, protected from light. A sterile solution of Prednisolone Sodium Phosphate in Water for Injection. Contains an amount of prednisolone sodium phosphate equivalent to the labeled amount of prednisolone phosphate, present as the disodium salt, within ±10%. Meets the requirements for Identification, Bacterial endotoxins, pH (7.0–8.0), Particulate matter, and Injections.

Prednisolone Sodium Phosphate Ophthalmic Solution USP—Preserve in tight, light-resistant containers. A sterile solution of Prednisolone Sodium Phosphate in a buffered, aqueous medium. Contains an amount of prednisolone sodium phosphate equivalent to the labeled amount of prednisolone phosphate, present as the disodium salt, within −10% to +15%. Meets the requirements for Identification, Sterility, and pH (6.2–8.2).

Prednisolone Sodium Phosphate Oral Solution—Not in USP.

Prednisolone Sodium Succinate for Injection USP—Preserve in Containers for Sterile Solids. It is sterile prednisolone sodium succinate prepared from Prednisolone Hemisuccinate with the aid of Sodium Hydroxide or Sodium Carbonate. Contains an amount of prednisolone sodium succinate equivalent to the labeled amount of prednisolone, within ±10%. Contains suitable buffers. Meets the requirements for Constituted solution, Identification, Bacterial endotoxins, pH (6.7–8.0, determined in the solution constituted as directed in the labeling), Loss on drying (not more than 2.0%), and Particulate matter, and for Sterility tests, Uniformity of dosage units, and Labeling under Injections.

Sterile Prednisolone Tebutate Suspension USP—Preserve in single-dose or in multiple-dose containers, preferably of Type I glass. A sterile suspension of Prednisolone Tebutate in a suitable aqueous medium. Contains the labeled amount, within ±10%. Meets the requirements for Identification, Bacterial endotoxins, pH (6.0–8.0), and Injections.

PREDNISONE

Chemical name: Pregna-1,4-diene-3,11,20-trione, 17,21-dihydroxy-.

Molecular formula: $C_{21}H_{26}O_5$.

Molecular weight: 358.43.

Description: Prednisone USP—White to practically white, odorless, crystalline powder. Melts at about 230 °C, with some decomposition.

Solubility: Prednisone USP—Very slightly soluble in water; slightly soluble in alcohol, in chloroform, in dioxane, and in methanol.

USP requirements:

Prednisone Oral Solution USP—Preserve in tight containers. Contains the labeled amount, within ±10%. Meets the requirements for Identification, pH (2.6–4.0), and Alcohol content (4.0–6.0%).

Prednisone Syrup USP—Preserve in tight containers. Contains the labeled amount, within ±10%. Meets the requirements for Identification, Specific gravity (1.220–1.280 at 25 °C), pH (3.0–4.5), and Alcohol content (2.0–5.0%).

Prednisone Tablets USP—Preserve in well-closed containers. Contain the labeled amount, within ±10%. Meet the requirements for Identification, Dissolution (80% in 30 minutes in water in Apparatus 2 at 50 rpm), and Uniformity of dosage units.

PRILOCAINE

Chemical group: Amide.

Chemical name: Prilocaine hydrochloride—Propanamide, N-(2-methylphenyl)-2-(propylamino)-, monohydrochloride.

Molecular formula: Prilocaine hydrochloride—$C_{13}H_{20}N_2O\cdot HCl$.

Molecular weight: Prilocaine hydrochloride—256.77.

Description: Prilocaine Hydrochloride USP—White, odorless, crystalline powder.

pKa: 7.9.

Solubility: Prilocaine Hydrochloride USP—Freely soluble in water and in alcohol; slightly soluble in chloroform; very slightly soluble in acetone; practically insoluble in ether.

USP requirements: Prilocaine Hydrochloride Injection USP—Preserve in single-dose or in multiple-dose containers, preferably of Type I glass. A sterile solution of Prilocaine Hydrochloride in Water for Injection. Contains the labeled amount, ±5%. Meets the requirements for Identification, Bacterial endotoxins, pH (6.0–7.0), and Injections.

PRILOCAINE AND EPINEPHRINE

For Prilocaine and Epinephrine—See individual listings for chemistry information.

USP requirements: Prilocaine and Epinephrine Injection USP—Preserve in single-dose or in multiple-dose, light-resistant containers, preferably of Type I glass. A sterile solution prepared from Prilocaine Hydrochloride and Epinephrine with the aid of Hydrochloric Acid in Water for Injection, or a sterile solution of Prilocaine Hydrochloride and Epinephrine Bitartrate in Water for Injection. The content of epinephrine does not exceed 0.002% (1 in 50,000). The label indicates that the Injection is not to be used if its color is pinkish or darker than slightly yellow or if it contains a precipitate. Contains the labeled amount of prilocaine hydrochloride, within ±5%, and the labeled amount of epinephrine, within −10% to +15%. Meets the requirements for Color and clarity, Identification, Bacterial endotoxins, pH (3.3–5.5), and Injections.

PRIMAQUINE

Chemical group: 8-Aminoquinolines.

Chemical name: Primaquine phosphate—1,4-Pentanediamine, N^4-(6-methoxy-8-quinolinyl)-, phosphate (1:2).

Molecular formula: Primaquine phosphate—$C_{15}H_{21}N_3O\cdot 2H_3PO_4$.

Molecular weight: Primaquine phosphate—455.34.

Description: Primaquine Phosphate USP—Orange-red, crystalline powder. Is odorless. Its solutions are acid to litmus. Melts at about 200 °C.

Solubility: Primaquine Phosphate USP—Soluble in water; insoluble in chloroform and in ether.

USP requirements: Primaquine Phosphate Tablets USP—Preserve in well-closed, light-resistant containers. Contain the labeled amount, within ±7%. Meet the requirements for Identification, Dissolution (75% in 60 minutes in simulated gastric fluid TS in Apparatus 2 at 100 rpm), and Uniformity of dosage units.

PRIMIDONE

Chemical group: A congener of phenobarbital in which the carbonyl oxygen of the urea moiety is replaced by two hydrogen atoms.

Chemical name: 4,6(1H,5H)-Pyrimidinedione, 5-ethyldihydro-5-phenyl-.

Molecular formula: $C_{12}H_{14}N_2O_2$.

Molecular weight: 218.25.

Description: Primidone USP—White, crystalline powder. Is odorless.

Solubility: Primidone USP—Very slightly soluble in water and in most organic solvents; slightly soluble in alcohol.

Other characteristics: Highly stable compound; no acidic properties, in contrast to its barbiturate analog.

USP requirements:
Primidone Oral Suspension USP—Preserve in tight, light-resistant containers. A suspension of Primidone in a suitable aqueous vehicle. Contains, in each 100 mL, not less than 4.5 grams and not more than 5.5 grams of primidone. Meets the requirements for Identification and pH (5.5–8.5).
Primidone Tablets USP—Preserve in well-closed containers. Contain the labeled amount, within ±5%. Meet the requirements for Identification, Dissolution (75% in 60 minutes in water in Apparatus 2 at 50 rpm), and Uniformity of dosage units.

PROBENECID

Chemical name: Benzoic acid, 4-[(dipropylamino)sulfonyl]-.

Molecular formula: $C_{13}H_{19}NO_4S$.

Molecular weight: 285.36.

Description: Probenecid USP—White or practically white, fine, crystalline powder. Is practically odorless.

pKa: 3.4.

Solubility: Probenecid USP—Practically insoluble in water and in dilute acids; soluble in dilute alkali, in chloroform, in alcohol, and in acetone.

USP requirements: Probenecid Tablets USP—Preserve in well-closed containers. Contain the labeled amount, within ±7%. Meet the requirements for Identification, Dissolution (80% in 30 minutes in simulated intestinal fluid TS [pH 7.5 ± 0.1], prepared without pancreatin, in Apparatus 2 at 50 rpm), and Uniformity of dosage units.

PROBENECID AND COLCHICINE

For *Probenecid* and *Colchicine*—See individual listings for chemistry information.

USP requirements: Probenecid and Colchicine Tablets USP—Preserve in well-closed, light-resistant containers. Contain the labeled amount of colchicine, within −10% to +15%, and the labeled amount of probenecid, within ±10%. Meet the requirements for Identification, Dissolution (80% of each active ingredient in 30 minutes in 0.05 M phosphate buffer [pH 7.5] in Apparatus 2 at 50 rpm), and Uniformity of dosage units.

PROBUCOL

Chemical name: Phenol, 4,4'-[(1-methylethylidene)bis(thio)]-bis[2,6-bis(1,1-dimethylethyl)-.

Molecular formula: $C_{31}H_{48}O_2S_2$.

Molecular weight: 516.84.

Description: Probucol USP—White to off-white, crystalline powder.

Solubility: Probucol USP—Insoluble in water; freely soluble in chloroform and in n-propyl alcohol; soluble in alcohol and in solvent hexane.

USP requirements: Probucol Tablets—Not in USP.

PROCAINAMIDE

Chemical name: Procainamide hydrochloride—Benzamide, 4-amino-N-[2-(diethylamino)ethyl]-, monohydrochloride.

Molecular formula: Procainamide hydrochloride—$C_{13}H_{21}N_3O \cdot HCl$.

Molecular weight: Procainamide hydrochloride—271.79.

Description:
Procainamide Hydrochloride USP—White to tan, crystalline powder. Is odorless. Its solution (1 in 10) has a pH of 5.0–6.5.
Procainamide Hydrochloride Injection USP—Colorless, or having not more than a slight yellow color.

pKa: 9.23.

Solubility: Procainamide Hydrochloride USP—Very soluble in water; soluble in alcohol; slightly soluble in chloroform; very slightly soluble in ether.

USP requirements:
Procainamide Hydrochloride Capsules USP—Preserve in tight containers. Contain the labeled amount, within ±5%. Meet the requirements for Identification, Dissolution (75% in 90 minutes in 0.1 N hydrochloric acid in Apparatus 2 at 50 rpm), and Uniformity of dosage units.
Procainamide Hydrochloride Injection USP—Preserve in single-dose or in multiple-dose containers, preferably of Type I glass. A sterile solution of Procainamide Hydrochloride in Water for Injection. Label it to indicate that the Injection is not to be used if it is darker than slightly yellow, or is discolored in any other way. Contains the labeled amount, within ±5%. Meets the requirements for Identification, Bacterial endotoxins, pH (4.0–6.0), Particulate matter, and Injections.
Procainamide Hydrochloride Tablets USP—Preserve in tight containers. Contain the labeled amount, within ±5%. Meet the requirements for Identification, Dissolution (80% in 75 minutes in 0.1 N hydrochloric acid in Apparatus 1 at 100 rpm), and Uniformity of dosage units.

Procainamide Hydrochloride Extended-release Tablets USP—Preserve in tight containers. Contain the labeled amount, within ±7%. Meet the requirements for Identification and Uniformity of dosage units.

PROCAINE

Chemical group: Ester.

Chemical name: Procaine hydrochloride—Benzoic acid, 4-amino-, 2-(diethylamino)ethyl ester, monohydrochloride.

Molecular formula: Procaine hydrochloride—$C_{13}H_{20}N_2O_2 \cdot HCl$.

Molecular weight: Procaine hydrochloride—272.77.

Description:
Procaine Hydrochloride USP—Small, white crystals or white, crystalline powder. Is odorless.
Procaine Hydrochloride Injection USP—Clear, colorless liquid.
Sterile Procaine Hydrochloride USP—Small, white crystals or white, crystalline powder. Is odorless.

pKa: 8.9.

Solubility:
Procaine Hydrochloride USP—Freely soluble in water; soluble in alcohol; slightly soluble in chloroform; practically insoluble in ether.
Sterile Procaine Hydrochloride USP—Freely soluble in water; soluble in alcohol; slightly soluble in chloroform; practically insoluble in ether.

USP requirements:
Procaine Hydrochloride Injection USP—Preserve in single-dose or in multiple-dose containers, preferably of Type I or Type II glass. The Injection may be packaged in 100-mL multiple-dose containers. A sterile solution of Procaine Hydrochloride in Water for Injection. Contains the labeled amount, within ±5%. Meets the requirements for Identification, Bacterial endotoxins, pH (3.0–5.5), Particulate matter, and Injections.
Sterile Procaine Hydrochloride USP—Preserve in Containers for Sterile Solids. Each package contains not more than 1 gram, and the container may be of such size as to permit solution within the container. It is Procaine Hydrochloride suitable for parenteral use. Meets the requirements for Completeness of solution, Constituted solution, Bacterial endotoxins, and Particulate matter, for Identification tests, Melting range (153–158 °C), Acidity, and Loss on drying (not more than 1.0%) under Procaine Hydrochloride, and for Sterility tests, Uniformity of dosage units, and Labeling under Injections.

PROCAINE AND EPINEPHRINE

For *Procaine* and *Epinephrine*—See individual listings for chemistry information.

USP requirements: Procaine Hydrochloride and Epinephrine Injection USP—Preserve in single-dose or in multiple-dose, light-resistant containers, preferably of Type I or Type II glass. A sterile solution of Procaine Hydrochloride and epinephrine hydrochloride in Water for Injection. The content of epinephrine does not exceed 0.002% (1 in 50,000). The label indicates that the Injection is not to be used if its color is pinkish or darker than slightly yellow or if it contains a precipitate. Contains the labeled amounts of procaine hydrochloride, within ±5%, and epinephrine, within −10% to +15%. Meets the requirements for Color and clarity, Identification, Bacterial endotoxins, pH (3.0–5.5), Content of epinephrine, and Injections.

PROCAINE AND PHENYLEPHRINE

For *Procaine* and *Phenylephrine*—See individual listings for chemistry information.

USP requirements: Procaine and Phenylephrine Hydrochlorides Injection USP—Preserve in single-dose or in multiple-dose containers, preferably of Type I glass. A sterile solution of Procaine Hydrochloride and Phenylephrine Hydrochloride in Water for Injection. Contains the labeled amounts of procaine hydrochloride, within ±5%, and phenylephrine hydrochloride, within ±10%. Meets the requirements for Identification, Bacterial endotoxins, pH (3.0–5.5), and Injections.

PROCAINE, TETRACAINE, AND LEVONORDEFRIN

Chemical name:
Procaine hydrochloride—Benzoic acid, 4-amino-, 2-(diethylamino)ethyl ester, monohydrochloride.
Tetracaine hydrochloride—Benzoic acid, 4-(butylamino)-, 2-(dimethylamino)ethyl ester, monohydrochloride.
Levonordefrin—1,2-Benzenediol, 4-(2-amino-1-hydroxypropyl)-, [R-(R*,S*)]-.

Molecular formula:
Procaine hydrochloride—$C_{13}H_{20}N_2O_2 \cdot HCl$.
Tetracaine hydrochloride—$C_{15}H_{24}N_2O_2 \cdot HCl$.
Levonordefrin—$C_9H_{13}NO_3$.

Molecular weight:
Procaine hydrochloride—272.77.
Tetracaine hydrochloride—300.83.
Levonordefrin—183.21.

Description:
Procaine Hydrochloride USP—Small, white crystals, or white, crystalline powder. Odorless.
Tetracaine Hydrochloride USP—Fine, white, crystalline, odorless powder. Its solutions are neutral to litmus. Melts at about 148 °C, or may occur in either of two other polymorphic modifications that melt at about 134 °C and 139 °C, respectively. Mixtures of the forms may melt within the range of 134–147 °C. Hygroscopic.
Levonordefrin USP—White to buff-colored, odorless, crystalline solid. Melts at about 210 °C.

Solubility:
Procaine Hydrochloride USP—Freely soluble in water; soluble in alcohol; slightly soluble in chloroform; practically insoluble in ether.
Tetracaine Hydrochloride USP—Very soluble in water; soluble in alcohol; insoluble in ether.
Levonordefrin USP—Practically insoluble in water; freely soluble in aqueous solutions of mineral acids; slightly soluble in acetone, in chloroform, in alcohol, and in ether.

USP requirements: Procaine and Tetracaine Hydrochlorides and Levonordefrin Injection USP—Preserve in single-dose or in multiple-dose containers, preferably of Type I glass. A sterile solution of Procaine Hydrochloride, Tetracaine Hydrochloride, and Levonordefrin in Water for Injection. The label indicates that the Injection is not to be used if its color is pinkish or darker than slightly yellow or if it contains a precipitate. Contains the labeled amounts of procaine hydrochloride and tetracaine hydrochloride, within ±5%, and levonordefrin, within ±10%. Meets the requirements for Color and clarity, Identification, Bacterial endotoxins, pH (3.5–5.0), and Injections.

PROCARBAZINE

Chemical name: Procarbazine hydrochloride—Benzamide, *N*-(1-methylethyl)-4-[(2-methylhydrazino)methyl]-, monohydrochloride.

Molecular formula: Procarbazine hydrochloride—$C_{12}H_{19}N_3O \cdot HCl$.

Molecular weight: Procarbazine hydrochloride—257.76.

Description: Procarbazine hydrochloride—White to pale yellow, crystalline powder.

Solubility: Procarbazine hydrochloride—Soluble but unstable in water or in aqueous solutions.

USP requirements: Procarbazine Hydrochloride Capsules USP—Preserve in tight, light-resistant containers. Contain the labeled amount, within ±10%. Meet the requirements for Identification, Dissolution (75% in 45 minutes in water in Apparatus 2 at 50 rpm), and Uniformity of dosage units.

PROCATEROL

Chemical name: Procaterol hydrochloride hemihydrate—8-hydroxy-5-[1-hydroxy-2[(1-methylethyl)amino]butyl]-2-(1H)quinolone, monohydrochloride, hemihydrate, racemic mixture of (±) (R*,S*) isomers.

Molecular formula: Procaterol hydrochloride hemihydrate—$C_{16}H_{22}N_2O_3 \cdot HCl \cdot \frac{1}{2}H_2O$.

Molecular weight: Procaterol hydrochloride hemihydrate—335.83.

Description: Procaterol hydrochloride hemihydrate—White to off-white powder, unstable to light.

Solubility: Procaterol hydrochloride hemihydrate—Soluble in water and in methanol; slightly soluble in ethanol; practically insoluble in acetone, in ether, in ethyl acetate, and in chloroform.

USP requirements: Procaterol Hydrochloride Hemihydrate Inhalation Aerosol—Not in USP.

PROCHLORPERAZINE

Chemical group: Phenothiazine derivative of piperazine group.

Chemical name:
Prochlorperazine—10H-Phenothiazine, 2-chloro-10-[3-(4-methyl-1-piperazinyl)propyl]-.
Prochlorperazine edisylate—10H-Phenothiazine, 2-chloro-10-[3-(4-methyl-1-piperazinyl)propyl]-, 1,2-ethanedisulfonate (1:1).
Prochlorperazine maleate—10H-Phenothiazine, 2-chloro-10-[3-(4-methyl-1-piperazinyl)propyl]-, (Z)-2-butenedioate (1:2).
Prochlorperazine mesylate—10H-Phenothiazine, 2-chloro-10-[3-(4-methyl-1-piperazinyl)propyl]-, dimethanesulphonate.

Molecular formula:
Prochlorperazine—$C_{20}H_{24}ClN_3S$.
Prochlorperazine edisylate—$C_{20}H_{24}ClN_3S \cdot C_2H_6O_6S_2$.
Prochlorperazine maleate—$C_{20}H_{24}ClN_3S \cdot 2C_4H_4O_4$.
Prochlorperazine mesylate—$C_{20}H_{24}ClN_3S \cdot 2CH_3SO_3H$.

Molecular weight:
Prochlorperazine—373.94.
Prochlorperazine edisylate—564.13.
Prochlorperazine maleate—606.09.
Prochlorperazine mesylate—566.1.

Description:
Prochlorperazine USP—Clear, pale yellow, viscous liquid. Is sensitive to light.
Prochlorperazine Edisylate USP—White to very light yellow, odorless, crystalline powder. Its solutions are acid to litmus.
Prochlorperazine Maleate USP—White or pale yellow, practically odorless, crystalline powder. Its saturated solution is acid to litmus.
Prochlorperazine mesylate—White or almost white odorless powder.

Solubility:
Prochlorperazine USP—Very slightly soluble in water; freely soluble in alcohol, in chloroform, and in ether.
Prochlorperazine Edisylate USP—Freely soluble in water; very slightly soluble in alcohol; insoluble in ether and in chloroform.
Prochlorperazine Maleate USP—Practically insoluble in water and in alcohol; slightly soluble in warm chloroform.
Prochlorperazine mesylate—Soluble 1 in less than 0.5 of water and 1 in 40 of alcohol; slightly soluble in chloroform; practically insoluble in ether.

USP requirements:
Prochlorperazine Suppositories USP—Preserve in tight containers at a temperature below 37 °C. Do not expose the unwrapped Suppositories to sunlight. Contain the labeled amount, within ±10%. Meet the requirement for Identification.
Prochlorperazine Edisylate Injection USP—Preserve in single-dose or in multiple-dose containers, preferably of Type I glass, protected from light. A sterile solution of Prochlorperazine Edisylate in Water for Injection. Contains an amount of prochlorperazine edisylate equivalent to the labeled amount of prochlorperazine, within ±10%. Meets the requirements for Identification, Bacterial endotoxins, pH (4.2–6.2), and Injections.
Prochlorperazine Edisylate Oral Solution USP—Preserve in tight, light-resistant containers. Label it to indicate that it is to be diluted to appropriate strength with water or other suitable fluid prior to administration. Contains an amount of prochlorperazine edisylate equivalent to the labeled amount of prochlorperazine, within ±8%. Meets the requirement for Identification.
Prochlorperazine Edisylate Syrup USP—Preserve in tight, light-resistant containers. Contains, in each 100 mL, an amount of prochlorperazine edisylate equivalent to not less than 92.0 mg and not more than 108.0 mg of prochlorperazine. Meets the requirement for Identification.
Prochlorperazine Maleate Extended-release Capsules—Not in USP.
Prochlorperazine Maleate Tablets USP—Preserve in well-closed containers, protected from light. Contain the labeled amount, within ±5%. Meet the requirements for Identification, Dissolution (75% in 60 minutes in 0.1 N hydrochloric acid in Apparatus 2 at 75 rpm), and Uniformity of dosage units.
Prochlorperazine Mesylate Injection—Not in USP.
Prochlorperazine Mesylate Syrup—Not in USP.

PROCYCLIDINE

Chemical group: Synthetic tertiary amine.

Chemical name: Procyclidine hydrochloride—1-Pyrrolidinepropanol, alpha-cyclohexyl-alpha-phenyl-, hydrochloride.

Molecular formula: Procyclidine hydrochloride—$C_{19}H_{29}NO \cdot HCl$.

Molecular weight: Procyclidine hydrochloride—323.91.

Description: Procyclidine Hydrochloride USP—White, crystalline powder, having a moderate, characteristic odor. Melts at about 225 °C, with decomposition.

Solubility: Procyclidine Hydrochloride USP—Soluble in water and in alcohol; insoluble in ether and in acetone.

USP requirements:

Procyclidine Hydrochloride Elixir—Not in USP.

Procyclidine Hydrochloride Tablets USP—Preserve in tight containers, and store in dry place. Contain the labeled amount, within ±7%. Meet the requirements for Identification, Dissolution (75% in 45 minutes in water in Apparatus 2 at 50 rpm), Related compounds, and Uniformity of dosage units.

PROGESTERONE

Chemical name: Pregn-4-ene-3,20-dione.

Molecular formula: $C_{21}H_{30}O_2$.

Molecular weight: 314.47.

Description: Progesterone USP—White or creamy white, odorless, crystalline powder. Is stable in air.

Solubility: Progesterone USP—Practically insoluble in water; soluble in alcohol, in acetone, and in dioxane; sparingly soluble in vegetable oils.

USP requirements:

Progesterone Injection USP—Preserve in single-dose or in multiple-dose containers, preferably of Type I or Type III glass. A sterile solution of Progesterone in a suitable solvent. Contains the labeled amount, within ±10%. Meets the requirements for Identification and Injections.

Progesterone Rectal Suppositories—Not in USP.

Progesterone Vaginal Suppositories—Not in USP.

Sterile Progesterone Suspension USP—Preserve in single-dose or in multiple-dose containers, preferably of Type I glass. A sterile suspension of Progesterone in Water for Injection. Contains the labeled amount, within ±7%. Meets the requirements for Identification, pH (4.0–7.5), and Injections.

Progesterone Intrauterine Contraceptive System USP—Preserve in sealed, single-unit containers. Contains the labeled amount, within ±10%. It is sterile. Meets the requirements for Identification, Sterility, Uniformity of dosage units, Chromatographic impurities (not more than 3% total), and Drug-release pattern.

PROMAZINE

Chemical group: Aliphatic phenothiazine.

Chemical name: Promazine hydrochloride—10*H*-Phenothiazine-10-propanamine, *N,N*-dimethyl-, monohydrochloride.

Molecular formula: Promazine hydrochloride—$C_{17}H_{20}N_2S \cdot$ HCl.

Molecular weight: Promazine hydrochloride—320.88.

Description: Promazine Hydrochloride USP—White to slightly yellow, practically odorless, crystalline powder. It oxidizes upon prolonged exposure to air and acquires a blue or pink color.

Solubility: Promazine Hydrochloride USP—Freely soluble in water and in chloroform.

USP requirements:

Promazine Hydrochloride Injection USP—Preserve in single-dose or in multiple-dose containers, preferably of Type I glass, protected from light. A sterile solution of Promazine Hydrochloride in Water for Injection. Contains the labeled amount, within −5% to +10%. Meets the requirements for Identification, Bacterial endotoxins, pH (4.0–5.5), and Injections.

Promazine Hydrochloride Oral Solution USP—Preserve in tight, light-resistant containers. Contains the labeled amount, within −5% to +10%. Meets the requirements for Identification and pH (5.0–5.5).

Promazine Hydrochloride Syrup USP—Preserve in tight, light-resistant containers. Contains the labeled amount, within −5% to +10%. Meets the requirement for Identification.

Promazine Hydrochloride Tablets USP—Preserve in tight, light-resistant containers. Contain the labeled amount, within −5% to +10%. Meet the requirements for Identification, Disintegration (30 minutes), and Uniformity of dosage units.

PROMETHAZINE

Chemical group: Phenothiazine derivative.

Chemical name: Promethazine hydrochloride—10*H*-Phenothiazine-10-ethanamine, *N,N*,alpha-trimethyl-, monohydrochloride.

Molecular formula: Promethazine hydrochloride—$C_{17}H_{20}N_2$-S·HCl.

Molecular weight: Promethazine hydrochloride—320.88.

Description: Promethazine Hydrochloride USP—White to faint yellow, practically odorless, crystalline powder. Slowly oxidizes, and acquires a blue color, on prolonged exposure to air.

pKa: 9.1.

Solubility: Promethazine Hydrochloride USP—Very soluble in water, in hot dehydrated alcohol, and in chloroform; practically insoluble in ether, in acetone, and in ethyl acetate.

USP requirements:

Promethazine Hydrochloride Injection USP—Preserve in single-dose or in multiple-dose containers, preferably of Type I glass, protected from light. A sterile solution of Promethazine Hydrochloride in Water for Injection. Contains the labeled amount, within −5% to +10%. Meets the requirements for Identification, pH (4.0–5.5), and Injections.

Promethazine Hydrochloride Suppositories USP—Preserve in tight, light-resistant containers, and store in a cold place. Contain the labeled amount, within −5% to +10%. Meet the requirement for Identification.

Promethazine Hydrochloride Syrup USP—Preserve in tight, light-resistant containers. Contains the labeled amount, within ±10%. Meets the requirement for Identification.

Promethazine Hydrochloride Tablets USP—Preserve in tight, light-resistant containers. Contain the labeled amount, within −5% to +10%. Meet the requirements for Identification, Dissolution (75% in 45 minutes in 0.1 *N* hydrochloric acid in Apparatus 1 at 100 rpm), and Uniformity of dosage units.

PROMETHAZINE AND CODEINE

For *Promethazine* and *Codeine*—See individual listings for chemistry information.

USP requirements: Promethazine Hydrochloride and Codeine Phosphate Syrup—Not in USP.

PROMETHAZINE AND DEXTROMETHORPHAN

For *Promethazine* and *Dextromethorphan*—See individual listings for chemistry information.

USP requirements: Promethazine Hydrochloride and Dextromethorphan Hydrobromide Syrup—Not in USP.

PROMETHAZINE AND PHENYLEPHRINE

For *Promethazine* and *Phenylephrine*—See individual listings for chemistry information.

USP requirements: Promethazine Hydrochloride and Phenylephrine Hydrochloride Syrup—Not in USP.

PROMETHAZINE, PHENYLEPHRINE, AND CODEINE

For *Promethazine*, *Phenylephrine*, and *Codeine*—See individual listings for chemistry information.

USP requirements: Promethazine Hydrochloride, Phenylephrine Hydrochloride, and Codeine Phosphate Syrup—Not in USP.

PROMETHAZINE AND PSEUDOEPHEDRINE

For *Promethazine* and *Pseudoephedrine*—See individual listings for chemistry information.

USP requirements: Promethazine Hydrochloride and Pseudoephedrine Hydrochloride Tablets—Not in USP.

PROPAFENONE

Chemical name: Propafenone hydrochloride—1-Propanone, 1-[2-[2-hydroxy-3-(propylamino)propoxy]phenyl]-3-phenyl-, hydrochloride.

Molecular formula: Propafenone hydrochloride—$C_{21}H_{27}NO_3 \cdot HCl$.

Molecular weight: Propafenone hydrochloride—377.91.

Description: Propafenone hydrochloride—Colorless crystals or white crystalline powder.

Solubility: Propafenone hydrochloride—Slightly soluble in water (20 °C), in chloroform, and in ethanol.

USP requirements: Propafenone Hydrochloride Tablets—Not in USP.

PROPANE

Molecular formula: C_3H_8.

Molecular weight: 44.10.

Description: Propane NF—Colorless, flammable gas (boiling temperature is about −42 °C). Vapor pressure at 21 °C is about 10290 mm of mercury (108 psig).

NF category: Aerosol propellant.

Solubility: Propane NF—One hundred volumes of water dissolves 6.5 volumes at 17.8 °C and 753 mm pressure; 100 volumes of anhydrous alcohol dissolves 790 volumes at 16.6 °C and 754 mm pressure; 100 volumes of ether dissolves 926 volumes at 16.6 °C and 757 mm pressure; 100 volumes of chloroform dissolves 1299 volumes at 21.6 °C and 757 mm pressure.

NF requirements: Propane NF—Preserve in tight cylinders, and prevent exposure to excessive heat. Contains not less than 98.0% of propane. Meets the requirements for Identification, Water (not more than 0.001%), High-boiling residues (not more than 5 ppm), Acidity of residue, and Sulfur compounds.

Caution: Propane is highly flammable and explosive.

PROPANTHELINE

Source: Synthetic amine compound.

Chemical group: Quaternary ammonium compound, synthetic.

Chemical name: Propantheline bromide—2-Propanaminium, *N*-methyl-*N*-(1-methylethyl)-*N*-[2-[(9*H*-xanthen-9-ylcarbonyl)oxy]ethyl]-, bromide.

Molecular formula: Propantheline bromide—$C_{23}H_{30}BrNO_3$.

Molecular weight: Propantheline bromide—448.40.

Description:
Propantheline Bromide USP—White or practically white crystals. Is odorless. Melts at about 160 °C, with decomposition.
Sterile Propantheline Bromide USP—White or practically white crystals. Is odorless.

Solubility:
Propantheline Bromide USP—Very soluble in water, in alcohol, and in chloroform; practically insoluble in ether.
Sterile Propantheline Bromide USP—Very soluble in water, in alcohol, and in chloroform; practically insoluble in ether.

USP requirements:
Sterile Propantheline Bromide USP—Preserve in Containers for Sterile Solids. It is Propantheline Bromide suitable for parenteral use. Meets the requirements for Completeness of solution, Constituted solution, and Bacterial endotoxins, for Identification tests, Loss on drying, Residue on ignition, Related compounds, and Bromide content under Propantheline Bromide, and for Sterility tests, Uniformity of dosage units, and Labeling under Injections.
Propantheline Bromide Tablets USP—Preserve in well-closed containers. Contain the labeled amount, within ±10%. Meet the requirements for Identification, Dissolution (75% in 45 minutes in Acetate buffer [pH 4.5 +0.05] in Apparatus 2 at 50 rpm), Related compounds, and Uniformity of dosage units.

PROPARACAINE

Chemical name: Proparacaine hydrochloride—Benzoic acid, 3-amino-4-propoxy, 2-(diethylamino)ethyl ester, monohydrochloride.

Molecular formula: Proparacaine hydrochloride—$C_{16}H_{26}N_2O_3 \cdot HCl$.

Molecular weight: Proparacaine hydrochloride—330.85.

Description:
Proparacaine Hydrochloride USP—White to off-white, or faintly buff-colored, odorless, crystalline powder. Its solutions are neutral to litmus.
Proparacaine Hydrochloride Ophthalmic Solution USP—Colorless or faint yellow solution.

Solubility: Proparacaine Hydrochloride USP—Soluble in water, in warm alcohol, and in methanol; insoluble in ether.

USP requirements: Proparacaine Hydrochloride Ophthalmic Solution USP—Preserve in tight, light-resistant containers. A sterile, aqueous solution of Proparacaine Hydrochloride. Label it to indicate that it is to be stored in a refrigerator after the container is opened. Contains the labeled amount, within −5% to +10%. Meets the requirements for Identification, Sterility, and pH (3.5–6.0).

PROPIOMAZINE

Chemical name: Propiomazine hydrochloride—1-Propanone, 1-[10-[2-(dimethylamino)propyl]-10*H*-phenothiazin-2-yl]-, monohydrochloride.

Molecular formula: Propiomazine hydrochloride—$C_{20}H_{24}N_2OS \cdot HCl$.

Molecular weight: Propiomazine hydrochloride—376.94.

Description: Propiomazine Hydrochloride USP—Yellow, practically odorless powder.

Solubility: Propiomazine Hydrochloride USP—Very soluble in water; freely soluble in alcohol.

USP requirements: Propiomazine Hydrochloride Injection USP—Preserve in single-dose containers, preferably of Type I glass, at controlled room temperature, protected from light. A sterile solution of Propiomazine Hydrochloride in Water for Injection. Contains the labeled amount, within −5% to +10%. Meets the requirements for Identification, Bacterial endotoxins, pH (4.7–5.3), and Injections.

Note: Do not use the Injection if it is cloudy or contains a precipitate.

PROPIONIC ACID

Molecular formula: $C_3H_6O_2$.

Molecular weight: 74.08.

Description: Propionic Acid NF—Oily liquid, having a slight, pungent, rancid odor.

Solubility: Propionic Acid NF—Miscible with water and with alcohol and with various other organic solvents.

NF requirements: Propionic Acid NF—Preserve in tight containers. Contains not less than 99.5% and not more than 100.5%, by weight, of propionic acid. Meets the requirements for Specific gravity (0.988–0.993), Distilling range (138.5–142.5 °C), Nonvolatile residue, Arsenic (not more than 3 ppm), Heavy metals (not more than 0.001%), Readily oxidizable substances, Aldehydes, and Organic volatile impurities.

PROPOFOL

Chemical group: Alkyl phenol.

Chemical name: Phenol, 2,6-bis(1-methylethyl).

Molecular formula: $C_{12}H_{18}O$.

Molecular weight: 178.27.

Description: Propofol exists as an oil at room temperature. Propofol injection is formulated as a white, oil-in-water emulsion and has a pH of 7–8.5.

Solubility: Propofol—Very slightly soluble in water.

USP requirements: Propofol Injection—Not in USP.

PROPOXYCAINE, PROCAINE, AND LEVONORDEFRIN

Chemical group: Propoxycaine; Procaine—Esters.

Chemical name:

Propoxycaine hydrochloride—Benzoic acid, 4-amino-2-propoxy-, 2-(diethylamino)ethyl ester, monohydrochloride.

Procaine hydrochloride—Benzoic acid, 4-amino-, 2-(diethylamino)ethyl ester, monohydrochloride.

Levonordefrin—1,2-Benzenediol, 4-(2-amino-1-hydroxypropyl)-, [R-(R*,S*)]-.

Molecular formula:

Propoxycaine hydrochloride—$C_{16}H_{26}N_2O_3 \cdot HCl$.

Procaine hydrochloride—$C_{13}H_{20}N_2O_2 \cdot HCl$.

Levonordefrin—$C_9H_{13}NO_3$.

Molecular weight:

Propoxycaine hydrochloride—330.85.

Procaine hydrochloride—272.77.

Levonordefrin—183.21.

Description:

Propoxycaine Hydrochloride USP—White, odorless, crystalline solid which discolors on prolonged exposure to light and to air. The pH of a solution (1 in 50) is about 5.4.

Procaine Hydrochloride USP—Small, white crystals or white, crystalline powder. Is odorless.

Levonordefrin USP—White to buff-colored, odorless, crystalline solid. Melts at about 210 °C.

Solubility:

Propoxycaine Hydrochloride USP—Freely soluble in water; soluble in alcohol; sparingly soluble in ether; practically insoluble in acetone and in chloroform.

Procaine Hydrochloride USP—Freely soluble in water; soluble in alcohol; slightly soluble in chloroform; practically insoluble in ether.

Levonordefrin USP—Practically insoluble in water; freely soluble in aqueous solutions of mineral acids; slightly soluble in acetone, in chloroform, in alcohol, and in ether.

USP requirements: Propoxycaine and Procaine Hydrochlorides and Levonordefrin Injection USP—Preserve in single-dose containers, preferably of Type I glass. A sterile solution of Propoxycaine Hydrochloride, Procaine Hydrochloride, and Levonordefrin in Water for Injection. The label indicates that the Injection is not to be used if its color is pinkish or darker than slightly yellow or if it contains a precipitate. Contains the labeled amounts of propoxycaine hydrochloride and procaine hydrochloride, within ±5%, and the labeled amount of levonordefrin, within ±10%. Meets the requirements for Color and clarity, Identification, Bacterial endotoxins, pH (3.5–5.0), and Injections.

PROPOXYCAINE, PROCAINE, AND NOREPINEPHRINE

Chemical group:

Propoxycaine; Procaine—Esters.

Norepinephrine—A primary amine, differing from epinephrine by the absence of a methyl group on the nitrogen atom.

Chemical name:

Propoxycaine hydrochloride—Benzoic acid, 4-amino-2-propoxy-, 2-(diethylamino)ethyl ester, monohydrochloride.

Procaine hydrochloride—Benzoic acid, 4-amino-, 2-(diethylamino)ethyl ester, monohydrochloride.

Norepinephrine bitartrate—1,2-Benzenediol, 4-(2-amino-1-hydroxyethyl)-, (R)-[R-(R*,R*)]-2,3-dihydroxybutanedioate (1:1) (salt), monohydrate.

Molecular formula:

Propoxycaine hydrochloride—$C_{16}H_{26}N_2O_3 \cdot HCl$.

Procaine hydrochloride—$C_{13}H_{20}N_2O_2 \cdot HCl$.

Norepinephrine Bitartrate—$C_8H_{11}NO_3 \cdot C_4H_6O_6 \cdot H_2O$.

Molecular weight:

Propoxycaine hydrochloride—330.85.

Procaine hydrochloride—272.77.

Norepinephrine bitartrate—337.28.

Description:
Propoxycaine Hydrochloride USP—White, odorless, crystalline solid which discolors on prolonged exposure to light and to air. The pH of a solution (1 in 50) is about 5.4.
Procaine Hydrochloride USP—Small, white crystals or white, crystalline powder. Is odorless.
Norepinephrine Bitartrate USP—White or faintly gray, odorless, crystalline powder. Slowly darkens on exposure to air and light. Its solutions are acid to litmus, having a pH of about 3.5. Melts between 98° and 104 °C, without previous drying of the specimen, the melt being turbid.

Solubility:
Propoxycaine Hydrochloride USP—Freely soluble in water; soluble in alcohol; sparingly soluble in ether; practically insoluble in acetone and in chloroform.
Procaine Hydrochloride USP—Freely soluble in water; soluble in alcohol; slightly soluble in chloroform; practically insoluble in ether.
Norepinephrine Bitartrate USP—Freely soluble in water; slightly soluble in alcohol; practically insoluble in chloroform and in ether.

USP requirements: Propoxycaine and Procaine Hydrochlorides and Norepinephrine Bitartrate Injection USP—Preserve in single-dose or in multiple-dose containers, preferably of Type I glass. A sterile solution of Propoxycaine Hydrochloride, Procaine Hydrochloride, and Norepinephrine Bitartrate in Water for Injection. The label indicates that the Injection is not to be used if its color is pinkish or darker than slightly yellow or if it contains a precipitate. Contains the labeled amounts of propoxycaine hydrochloride and procaine hydrochloride, within ±5%, and an amount of norepinephrine bitartrate equivalent to the labeled amount of norepinephrine, within ±10%. Meets the requirements for Color and clarity, Identification, Bacterial endotoxins, pH (3.5–5.0), and Injections.

PROPOXYPHENE
Chemical name:
Propoxyphene hydrochloride—Benzeneethanol, alpha-[2-(dimethylamino)-1-methylethyl]-alpha-phenyl-, propanoate (ester), hydrochloride, [S-(R*,S*)]-.
Propoxyphene napsylate—Benzeneethanol, alpha-[2-(dimethylamino)-1-methylethyl]-alpha-phenyl-, propanoate (ester), [S-(R*,S*)]-, compound with 2-naphthalenesulfonic acid (1:1), monohydrate.

Molecular formula:
Propoxyphene hydrochloride—$C_{22}H_{29}NO_2 \cdot HCl$.
Propoxyphene napsylate—$C_{22}H_{29}NO_2 \cdot C_{10}H_8O_3S \cdot H_2O$ (monohydrate); $C_{22}H_{29}NO_2 \cdot C_{10}H_8O_3S$ (anhydrous).

Molecular weight:
Propoxyphene hydrochloride—375.94.
Propoxyphene napsylate—565.72 (monohydrate); 547.71 (anhydrous).

Description:
Propoxyphene Hydrochloride USP—White, crystalline powder. Is odorless.
Propoxyphene Napsylate USP—White powder, having essentially no odor.

Solubility:
Propoxyphene Hydrochloride USP—Freely soluble in water; soluble in alcohol, in chloroform, and in acetone; practically insoluble in ether.
Propoxyphene Napsylate USP—Very slightly soluble in water; soluble in methanol, in alcohol, in chloroform, and in acetone.

USP requirements:
Propoxyphene Hydrochloride Capsules USP—Preserve in tight containers. Contain the labeled amount, within ±7.5%. Meet the requirements for Identification, Dissolution (85% in 60 minutes in acetate buffer [pH 4.5] in Apparatus 1 at 100 rpm), and Uniformity of dosage units.
Propoxyphene Hydrochloride Tablets—Not in USP.
Propoxyphene Napsylate Capsules—Not in USP.
Propoxyphene Napsylate Oral Suspension USP—Preserve in tight containers, protected from light. Avoid freezing. Contains the labeled amount, within ±10%. Meets the requirements for Identification and Alcohol content (0.5–1.5%).
Propoxyphene Napsylate Tablets USP—Preserve in tight containers. Contain the labeled amount, within ±10%. Meet the requirements for Identification, Dissolution (75% in 60 minutes in acetate buffer [pH 4.5] in Apparatus 1 at 100 rpm), and Uniformity of dosage units.

PROPOXYPHENE AND ACETAMINOPHEN
For *Propoxyphene* and *Acetaminophen*—See individual listings for chemistry information.

USP requirements:
Propoxyphene Hydrochloride and Acetaminophen Capsules—Not in USP.
Propoxyphene Hydrochloride and Acetaminophen Tablets USP—Preserve in tight containers. Contain the labeled amounts of propoxyphene hydrochloride and acetaminophen, within ±10%. Meet the requirements for Identification, Dissolution (75% of propoxyphene hydrochloride in 30 minutes in acetate buffer [pH 4.5] in Apparatus 2 at 50 rpm), and Uniformity of dosage units (with respect to propoxyphene hydrochloride).
Propoxyphene Napsylate and Acetaminophen Tablets USP—Preserve in tight containers, at controlled room temperature. Contain the labeled amounts of propoxyphene napsylate and acetaminophen, within ±10%. Meet the requirements for Identification, Dissolution (75% of each active ingredient in 60 minutes in acetate buffer [pH 4.5] in Apparatus 1 at 100 rpm), and Uniformity of dosage units (with respect to propoxyphene napsylate and acetaminophen).

PROPOXYPHENE AND ASPIRIN
For *Propoxyphene* and *Aspirin*—See individual listings for chemistry information.

USP requirements:
Propoxyphene Hydrochloride and Aspirin Capsules—Not in USP.
Propoxyphene Napsylate and Aspirin Capsules—Not in USP.
Propoxyphene Napsylate and Aspirin Tablets USP—Preserve in tight containers, at controlled room temperature. Contain the labeled amounts of propoxyphene napsylate and aspirin, within ±10%. Meet the requirements for Identification, Dissolution (75% of each active ingredient in 60 minutes in acetate buffer [pH 4.5] in Apparatus 1 at 100 rpm), Uniformity of dosage units (with respect to propoxyphene napsylate), and Free salicylic acid (not more than 3.0% of labeled amount of aspirin).

PROPOXYPHENE, ASPIRIN, AND CAFFEINE
For *Propoxyphene, Aspirin,* and *Caffeine*—See individual listings for chemistry information.

USP requirements:
Propoxyphene Hydrochloride, Aspirin, and Caffeine Capsules USP—Preserve in tight containers at controlled room

temperature. Contain the labeled amounts of propoxyphene hydrochloride, aspirin, and caffeine, within ±10%. Meet the requirements for Identification, Dissolution (75% of the aspirin and 85% of the propoxyphene hydrochloride in 60 minutes in acetate buffer [pH 4.5] in Apparatus 1 at 100 rpm), Free salicylic acid (not more than 3.0% of labeled amount of aspirin), and Uniformity of dosage units (with respect to propoxyphene hydrochloride and caffeine).

Note: Where Propoxyphene Hydrochloride, Aspirin, and Caffeine Capsules are prescribed, the quantity of propoxyphene hydrochloride is to be specified. Where the Capsules are prescribed without reference to the quantity of aspirin or caffeine contained therein, a product containing 389 mg of aspirin and 32.4 mg of caffeine shall be dispensed.

Propoxyphene Hydrochloride, Aspirin, and Caffeine Tablets—Not in USP.

Propoxyphene Napsylate, Aspirin, and Caffeine Capsules—Not in USP.

PROPRANOLOL

Chemical name: Propranolol hydrochloride—2-Propanol, 1-[(1-methylethyl)amino]-3-(1-naphthalenyloxy)-, hydrochloride.

Molecular formula: Propranolol hydrochloride—$C_{16}H_{21}NO_2\cdot$HCl.

Molecular weight: Propranolol hydrochloride—295.81.

Description: Propranolol Hydrochloride USP—White to off-white, crystalline powder. Is odorless. Melts at about 164 °C.

Solubility: Propranolol Hydrochloride USP—Soluble in water and in alcohol; slightly soluble in chloroform; practically insoluble in ether.

Other characteristics: Lipid solubility—High.

USP requirements:
Propranolol Hydrochloride Extended-release Capsules USP—Preserve in well-closed containers. The labeling states the Drug Release Test with which the product complies. Contain the labeled amount, within ±10%. Meet the requirements for Identification, Drug release (for Test 1: not more than 30% in 1.5 hours in buffer solution [pH 1.2 for the Acid stage], and 35–60% in 4 hours, 55–80% in 8 hours, 70–95% in 14 hours, and 81–110% in 24 hours in buffer solution [pH 6.8 for the Buffer stage] in Apparatus 1 at 100 rpm; for Test 2: not more than 20% in 1 hour in buffer solution [pH 1.2 for the Acid stage], and 20–45% in 3 hours, 45–80% in 6 hours, and not less than 80% in 12 hours in buffer solution [pH 7.5 for the Buffer stage] in Apparatus 1 at 50 rpm), and Uniformity of dosage units.

Propranolol Hydrochloride Injection USP—Preserve in single-dose, light-resistant containers, preferably of Type I glass. A sterile solution of Propranolol Hydrochloride in Water for Injection. Contains the labeled amount, within ±10%. Meets the requirements for Identification, Bacterial endotoxins, pH (2.8–4.0), and Injections.

Propranolol Hydrochloride Oral Solution—Not in USP.

Propranolol Hydrochloride Tablets USP—Preserve in well-closed, light-resistant containers. Contain the labeled amount, within ±10%. Meet the requirements for Identification, Dissolution (75% in 30 minutes in dilute hydrochloric acid [1 in 100] in Apparatus 1 at 100 rpm), and Uniformity of dosage units.

PROPRANOLOL AND HYDROCHLOROTHIAZIDE

For *Propranolol* and *Hydrochlorothiazide*—See individual listings for chemistry information.

USP requirements:
Propranolol Hydrochloride and Hydrochlorothiazide Extended-release Capsules USP—Preserve in well-closed containers. Contain the labeled amounts, within ±10%. Meet the requirements for Identification, Drug release (propranolol hydrochloride: not more than 30% in 0.0625 *D* hours in buffer solution [pH 1.5 for the Acid stage], 35–60% in 0.167 *D* hours, 55–80% in 0.333 *D* hours, 70–95% in 0.583 *D* hours, and 83–108% in 1.00 *D* hours in buffer solution [pH 6.8 for the Buffer stage]; hydrochlorothiazide: not less than 80% in 30 minutes in buffer solution [pH 1.5], in Apparatus 1 at 100 rpm), Related substance (not more than 1.0%), and Uniformity of dosage units.

Propranolol Hydrochloride and Hydrochlorothiazide Tablets USP—Preserve in well-closed containers. Contain the labeled amounts, within ±10%. Meet the requirements for Identification, Dissolution (80% of each active ingredient in 30 minutes in 0.1 *N* hydrochloric acid in Apparatus 1 at 100 rpm), and Uniformity of dosage units.

PROPYLENE CARBONATE

Chemical name: 4-Methyl-1,3-dioxolan-2-one.

Molecular formula: $C_4H_6O_3$.

Molecular weight: 102.09.

Description: Propylene Carbonate NF—Clear, colorless, mobile liquid.
NF category: Solvent.

Solubility: Propylene Carbonate NF—Freely soluble in water; insoluble in hexane; miscible with alcohol and with chloroform.

NF requirements: Propylene Carbonate NF—Preserve in tight containers. Contains not less than 99.0% and not more than 100.5% of propylene carbonate. Meets the requirements for Identification, Specific gravity (1.203–1.210 at 20 °C), pH (6.0–7.5), Residue on ignition (not more than 0.01%), and Organic volatile impurities.

PROPYLENE GLYCOL

Chemical name: 1,2-Propanediol.

Molecular formula: $C_3H_8O_2$.

Molecular weight: 76.10.

Description: Propylene Glycol USP—Clear, colorless, viscous liquid. It is practically odorless. It absorbs moisture when exposed to moist air.
NF category: Humectant; plasticizer; solvent.

Solubility: Propylene Glycol USP—Miscible with water, with acetone, and with chloroform. Soluble in ether and will dissolve many essential oils, but is immiscible with fixed oils.

USP requirements: Propylene Glycol USP—Preserve in tight containers. Contains not less than 99.5% of propylene glycol. Meets the requirements for Identification, Specific gravity (1.035–1.037), Acidity, Water (not more than 0.2%), Residue on ignition, Chloride (not more than 0.007%), Sulfate (not more than 0.006%), Arsenic (not more than 3 ppm), and Heavy metals (not more than 5 ppm).

PROPYLENE GLYCOL ALGINATE

Description: Propylene Glycol Alginate NF—White to yellowish fibrous or granular powder. Practically odorless.

NF category: Suspending and/or viscosity-increasing agent.

Solubility: Propylene Glycol Alginate NF—Soluble in water, in solutions of dilute organic acids, and, depending on the degree of esterification, in hydroalcoholic mixtures containing up to 60% by weight of alcohol to form stable, viscous colloidal solutions at a pH of 3.

NF requirements: Propylene Glycol Alginate NF—Preserve in well-closed containers. A propylene glycol ester of alginic acid. Each gram yields not less than 0.16 and not more than 0.20 gram of carbon dioxide, calculated on the dried basis. Meets the requirements for Identification, Microbial limits, Loss on drying (not more than 20.0%), Ash (not more than 10.0%, calculated on the dried basis), Arsenic (not more than 3 ppm), Lead (not more than 0.001%), Heavy metals (not more than 0.004%), Free carboxyl groups, and Esterified carboxyl groups.

PROPYLENE GLYCOL DIACETATE

Molecular formula: $C_7H_{12}O_4$.

Molecular weight: 160.17.

Description: Propylene Glycol Diacetate NF—Clear, colorless liquid, having a mild, fruity odor.

NF category: Emulsifying and/or solubilizing agent.

Solubility: Propylene Glycol Diacetate NF—Soluble in water.

NF requirements: Propylene Glycol Diacetate NF—Preserve in tight containers, and avoid contact with metal. Contains not less than 98.0% and not more than 102.0% of propylene glycol diacetate. Meets the requirements for Identification, Specific gravity (1.040–1.060), Refractive index (1.4130–1.4150 at 20 °C), pH (4.0–6.0, in a solution [1 in 20]), Acetic acid (not more than 0.2%), Chromatographic purity, and Organic volatile impurities.

PROPYLENE GLYCOL MONOSTEARATE

Chemical name: Octadecanoic acid, monoester with 1,2-propanediol.

Molecular formula: $C_{21}H_{42}O_3$.

Molecular weight: 342.56.

Description: Propylene Glycol Monostearate NF—White, wax-like solid, or white, wax-like beads or flakes. It has a slight, agreeable, fatty odor.

NF category: Emulsifying and/or solubilizing agent.

Solubility: Propylene Glycol Monostearate NF—Insoluble in water, but may be dispersed in hot water with the aid of a small amount of soap or other suitable surface-active agent; soluble in organic solvents, such as alcohol, mineral or fixed oils, ether, and acetone.

NF requirements: Propylene Glycol Monostearate NF—Preserve in well-closed containers. A mixture of the propylene glycol mono- and di-esters of stearic and palmitic acids. Contains not less than 90.0% of monoesters of saturated fatty acids, chiefly propylene glycol monostearate and propylene glycol monopalmitate. Meets the requirements for Congealing temperature (not lower than 45 °C), Residue on ignition (not more than 0.5%), Acid value (not more than 4), Saponification value (155–165), Hydroxyl value (160–175), Iodine value (not more than 3), Free glycerin and propylene glycol, and Propylene glycol monoesters.

PROPYL GALLATE

Chemical name: Benzoic acid, 3,4,5-trihydroxy-, propyl ester.

Molecular formula: $C_{10}H_{12}O_5$.

Molecular weight: 212.20.

Description: Propyl Gallate NF—White, crystalline powder, having a very slight, characteristic odor.

NF category: Antioxidant.

Solubility: Propyl Gallate NF—Slightly soluble in water; freely soluble in alcohol.

NF requirements: Propyl Gallate NF—Preserve in tight containers, protected from light, and avoid contact with metals. Contains not less than 98.0% and not more than 102.0% of propyl gallate, calculated on the dried basis. Meets the requirements for Identification, Melting range (146–150 °C), Loss on drying (not more than 0.5%), Residue on ignition (not more than 0.1%), and Heavy metals (not more than 0.001%).

PROPYLHEXEDRINE

Chemical name: Cyclohexaneethanamine, N,alpha-dimethyl-, (±).

Molecular weight: $C_{10}H_{21}N$.

Molecular weight: 155.28.

Description: Propylhexedrine USP—Clear, colorless liquid, having a characteristic, amine-like odor. Volatilizes slowly at room temperature. Absorbs carbon dioxide from the air, and its solutions are alkaline to litmus. Boils at about 205 °C.

Solubility: Propylhexedrine USP—Very slightly soluble in water. Miscible with alcohol, with chloroform, and with ether.

USP requirements: Propylhexedrine Inhalant USP—Preserve in tight containers (inhalers), and avoid exposure to excessive heat. Consists of cylindrical rolls of suitable fibrous material impregnated with Propylhexedrine, usually aromatized, and contained in a suitable inhaler. Inhaler contains the labeled amount, within −10% to +25%. Meets the requirement for Identification.

PROPYLIODONE

Chemical name: 1(4H)-Pyridineacetic acid, 3,5-diiodo-4-oxo-, propyl ester.

Molecular formula: $C_{10}H_{11}I_2NO_3$.

Molecular weight: 447.01.

Description: Propyliodone USP—White or almost white, crystalline powder. Odorless or has a faint odor.

Solubility: Propyliodone USP—Practically insoluble in water; soluble in acetone, in alcohol, and in ether.

USP requirements: Sterile Propyliodone Oil Suspension USP—Preserve in single-dose, light-resistant containers. A sterile suspension of Propyliodone in Peanut Oil. Contains not less than 57.0% and not more than 63.0% of propyliodone. Meets the requirements for Identification, Weight per mL (1.236–1.276 grams), Iodine and iodide, and Injections.

PROPYLPARABEN

Chemical name: Benzoic acid, 4-hydroxy-, propyl ester.

Molecular formula: $C_{10}H_{12}O_3$.

Molecular weight: 180.20.

Description: Propylparaben NF—Small, colorless crystals or white powder.
NF category: Antimicrobial preservative.

Solubility: Propylparaben NF—Very slightly soluble in water; freely soluble in alcohol and in ether; slightly soluble in boiling water.

NF requirements: Propylparaben NF—Preserve in well-closed containers. Contains not less than 99.0% and not more than 100.5% of propylparaben, calculated on the dried basis. Meets the requirements for Identification, Melting range (95–98 °C), and Organic volatile impurities, and for Acidity, Loss on drying, and Residue on ignition under Butylparaben.

PROPYLPARABEN SODIUM

Chemical name: Benzoic acid, 4-hydroxy-, propyl ester, sodium salt.

Molecular formula: $C_{10}H_{11}NaO_3$.

Molecular weight: 202.19.

Description: Propylparaben Sodium NF—White powder. It is odorless and hygroscopic.
NF category: Antimicrobial preservative.

Solubility: Propylparaben Sodium NF—Freely soluble in water; sparingly soluble in alcohol; insoluble in fixed oils.

NF requirements: Propylparaben Sodium NF—Preserve in tight containers. Contains not less than 98.5% and not more than 101.5% of propylparaben sodium, calculated on the anhydrous basis. Meets the requirements for Completeness of solution, Identification, pH (9.5–10.5, in a solution [1 in 1000]), Water (not more than 5.0%), Chloride (not more than 0.035%), Sulfate (not more than 0.12%), and Organic volatile impurities.

PROPYLTHIOURACIL

Chemical group: Thioamide derivative.

Chemical name: 4(1*H*)-Pyrimidinone, 2,3-dihydro-6-propyl-2-thioxo-.

Molecular formula: $C_7H_{10}N_2OS$.

Molecular weight: 170.23.

Description: Propylthiouracil USP—White, powdery, crystalline substance; starch-like in appearance and to the touch.

Solubility: Propylthiouracil USP—Slightly soluble in water; sparingly soluble in alcohol; slightly soluble in chloroform and in ether; soluble in ammonium hydroxide and in alkali hydroxides.

USP requirements: Propylthiouracil Tablets USP—Preserve in well-closed containers. Contain the labeled amount, within ±7%. Meet the requirements for Identification, Dissolution (85% in 30 minutes in water in Apparatus 1 at 100 rpm), and Uniformity of dosage units.

PROTAMINE

Source: Protamine sulfate—A purified mixture of simple protein principles obtained from the sperm or testes of suitable species of fish.

Description:
Protamine Sulfate Injection USP—Colorless solution, which may have the odor of a preservative.
Protamine Sulfate for Injection USP—White, odorless powder, having the characteristic appearance of solids dried from the frozen state.

USP requirements:
Protamine Sulfate Injection USP—Preserve in single-dose containers, preferably of Type I glass. Store in a refrigerator. A sterile, isotonic solution of Protamine Sulfate. Label it to indicate the approximate neutralization capacity in USP Heparin Units. Contains the labeled amount, within −10% to +20%. Meets the requirements for Identification (tests for Sulfate), Bacterial endotoxins, and Injections.
Protamine Sulfate for Injection USP—Preserve in Containers for Sterile Solids. Preserve the accompanying solvent in single-dose or in multiple-dose containers, preferably of Type I glass. A sterile mixture of Protamine Sulfate with one or more suitable, dry diluents. Label it to indicate the approximate neutralization capacity in USP Heparin Units. Contains the labeled amount, within −10% to +20%. Meets the requirements for Constituted solution (under Injections at time of use), Pyrogen, pH and clarity of solution (6.5–7.5, and the solution is clear), and Uniformity of dosage units, and both the medication and the accompanying solvent meet the requirements for Sterility tests and Labeling under Injections.

PROTEIN HYDROLYSATE

Description: Protein Hydrolysate Injection USP—Yellowish to reddish amber, transparent liquid.

USP requirements: Protein Hydrolysate Injection USP—Preserve in single-dose containers, preferably of Type I or Type II glass, and avoid excessive heat. A sterile solution of amino acids and short-chain peptides which represent the approximate nutritive equivalent of the casein, lactalbumin, plasma, fibrin, or other suitable protein from which it is derived by acid, enzymatic, or other method of hydrolysis. It may be modified by partial removal and restoration or addition of one or more amino acids. It may contain alcohol, dextrose, or other carbohydrate suitable for intravenous infusion. Not less than 50.0% of the total nitrogen present is in the form of alpha-amino nitrogen. The label of the immediate container bears in a subtitle the name of the protein from which the hydrolysate has been derived and the word "modified" if one or more of the "essential" amino acids has been partially removed, restored, or added. The label bears a statement of the pH range; the name and percentage of any added other nutritive ingredient; the method of hydrolysis; the nature of the modification, if any, in amino acid content after hydrolysis; the percentage of each essential amino acid or its equivalent; the approximate protein equivalent, in grams per liter; the approximate number of calories per liter; the percentage of the total nitrogen in the form of alpha-amino nitrogen; and the quantity of the sodium and of the potassium ions present in each 100 mL of the Injection. Injection that contains not more than 30 mg of sodium per 100 mL may be labeled "Protein Hydrolysate Injection, Low Sodium," or by a similar title the approximate equivalent thereof. The label states the total osmolar concentration in mOsmol per liter. Where the contents are less than 100 mL, or where the

III/346   **Chemistry and Compendial Requirements**

label states that the Injection is not for direct injection but is to be diluted before use, the label may alternatively state the total osmolar concentration in mOsmol per mL. Meets the requirements for Non-antigenicity, Bacterial endotoxins, Biological adequacy (for Protein), pH (4.0–7.0, determined potentiometrically, but the variation from the pH range stated on the label is not greater than ± 0.5 pH unit), Nitrogen content, alpha-Amino nitrogen, Potassium content, Sodium content, and Injections.

PROTIRELIN

Source: A synthetic tripeptide thought to be structurally identical to the naturally occurring thyrotropin-releasing hormone produced by the hypothalamus.

Chemical name: L-Prolinamide, 5-oxo-L-prolyl-L-histidyl-.

Molecular formula: $C_{16}H_{22}N_6O_4$.

Molecular weight: 362.39.

Description: Slightly yellowish hygroscopic powder.

Solubility: Very soluble in water and in methanol; soluble in isopropanol.

USP requirements: Protirelin Injection—Not in USP.

PROTRIPTYLINE

Chemical group: Dibenzocycloheptadiene.

Chemical name: Protriptyline hydrochloride—5H-Dibenzo-[a,d]cycloheptene-5-propanamine, N-methyl-, hydrochloride.

Molecular formula: Protriptyline hydrochloride—$C_{19}H_{21}N \cdot HCl$.

Molecular weight: Protriptyline hydrochloride—299.84.

Description: Protriptyline Hydrochloride USP—White to yellowish powder. Is odorless, or has not more than a slight odor. Melts at about 168 °C.

Solubility: Protriptyline Hydrochloride USP—Freely soluble in water, in alcohol, and in chloroform; practically insoluble in ether.

Other characteristics: Secondary amine.

USP requirements: Protriptyline Hydrochloride Tablets USP—Preserve in tight containers. Contain the labeled amount, within ± 10%. Meet the requirements for Identification, Dissolution (75% in 45 minutes in water in Apparatus 1 at 100 rpm), and Uniformity of dosage units.

PSEUDOEPHEDRINE

Chemical name:
Pseudoephedrine hydrochloride—Benzenemethanol, alpha-[1-(methylamino)ethyl]-, [S-(R*,R*)]-, hydrochloride.
Pseudoephedrine sulfate—Benzenemethanol, alpha-[1-(methylamino)ethyl]-, [S-(R*,R*)]-, sulfate (2:1) (salt).

Molecular formula:
Pseudoephedrine hydrochloride—$C_{10}H_{15}NO \cdot HCl$.
Pseudoephedrine sulfate—$(C_{10}H_{15}NO)_2 \cdot H_2SO_4$.

Molecular weight:
Pseudoephedrine hydrochloride—201.70.
Pseudoephedrine sulfate—428.54.

Description:
Pseudoephedrine Hydrochloride USP—Fine, white to off-white crystals or powder, having a faint characteristic odor.
Pseudoephedrine Sulfate USP—White crystals or crystalline powder. Is odorless.

Solubility:
Pseudoephedrine Hydrochloride USP—Very soluble in water; freely soluble in alcohol; sparingly soluble in chloroform.
Pseudoephedrine Sulfate USP—Freely soluble in alcohol.

USP requirements:
Pseudoephedrine Hydrochloride Capsules—Not in USP.
Pseudoephedrine Hydrochloride Extended-release Capsules—Not in USP.
Pseudoephedrine Hydrochloride Oral Solution—Not in USP.
Pseudoephedrine Hydrochloride Syrup USP—Preserve in tight, light-resistant containers. Contains the labeled amount, within ± 10%. Meets the requirements for Identification and Reaction (acid to litmus).
Pseudoephedrine Hydrochloride Tablets USP—Preserve in tight containers. Contain the labeled amount, within ± 7%. Meet the requirements for Identification, Dissolution (75% in 45 minutes in water in Apparatus 2 at 50 rpm), and Uniformity of dosage units.
Pseudoephedrine Sulfate Tablets—Not in USP.
Pseudoephedrine Sulfate Extended-release Tablets—Not in USP.

PSEUDOEPHEDRINE AND ACETAMINOPHEN

For *Pseudoephedrine* and *Acetaminophen*—See individual listings for chemistry information.

USP requirements:
Pseudoephedrine Hydrochloride and Acetaminophen Capsules—Not in USP.
Pseudoephedrine Hydrochloride and Acetaminophen Tablets—Not in USP.

PSEUDOEPHEDRINE, ACETAMINOPHEN, AND CAFFEINE

For *Pseudoephedrine, Acetaminophen,* and *Caffeine*—See individual listings for chemistry information.

USP requirements: Pseudoephedrine Hydrochloride, Acetaminophen, and Caffeine Capsules—Not in USP.

PSEUDOEPHEDRINE AND ASPIRIN

For *Pseudoephedrine* and *Aspirin*—See individual listings for chemistry information.

USP requirements: Pseudoephedrine Hydrochloride and Aspirin Tablets—Not in USP.

PSEUDOEPHEDRINE, ASPIRIN, AND CAFFEINE

For *Pseudoephedrine, Aspirin,* and *Caffeine*—See individual listings for chemistry information.

USP requirements: Pseudoephedrine Hydrochloride, Aspirin, and Caffeine Capsules—Not in USP.

PSEUDOEPHEDRINE AND CODEINE

For *Pseudoephedrine* and *Codeine*—See individual listings for chemistry information.

USP requirements:
Pseudoephedrine Hydrochloride and Codeine Phosphate Capsules—Not in USP.

Pseudoephedrine Hydrochloride and Codeine Phosphate Syrup—Not in USP.

PSEUDOEPHEDRINE, CODEINE, AND GUAIFENESIN

For *Pseudoephedrine, Codeine,* and *Guaifenesin*—See individual listings for chemistry information.

USP requirements:
Pseudoephedrine Hydrochloride, Codeine Phosphate, and Guaifenesin Oral Solution—Not in USP.
Pseudoephedrine Hydrochloride, Codeine Phosphate, and Guaifenesin Syrup—Not in USP.

PSEUDOEPHEDRINE AND DEXTROMETHORPHAN

For *Pseudoephedrine* and *Dextromethorphan*—See individual listings for chemistry information.

USP requirements:
Pseudoephedrine Hydrochloride and Dextromethorphan Hydrobromide Oral Solution—Not in USP.
Pseudoephedrine Hydrochloride and Dextromethorphan Hydrobromide Chewable Tablets—Not in USP.

PSEUDOEPHEDRINE, DEXTROMETHORPHAN, AND ACETAMINOPHEN

For *Pseudoephedrine, Dextromethorphan,* and *Acetaminophen*—See individual listings for chemistry information.

USP requirements:
Pseudoephedrine Hydrochloride, Dextromethorphan Hydrobromide, and Acetaminophen Oral Solution—Not in USP.
Pseudoephedrine Hydrochloride, Dextromethorphan Hydrobromide, and Acetaminophen Tablets—Not in USP.

PSEUDOEPHEDRINE, DEXTROMETHORPHAN, AND GUAIFENESIN

For *Pseudoephedrine, Dextromethorphan,* and *Guaifenesin*—See individual listings for chemistry information.

USP requirements:
Pseudoephedrine Hydrochloride, Dextromethorphan Hydrobromide, and Guaifenesin Capsules—Not in USP.
Pseudoephedrine Hydrochloride, Dextromethorphan Hydrobromide, and Guaifenesin Oral Solution—Not in USP.
Pseudoephedrine Hydrochloride, Dextromethorphan Hydrobromide, and Guaifenesin Syrup—Not in USP.

PSEUDOEPHEDRINE, DEXTROMETHORPHAN, GUAIFENESIN, AND ACETAMINOPHEN

For *Pseudoephedrine, Dextromethorphan, Guaifenesin,* and *Acetaminophen*—See individual listings for chemistry information.

USP requirements:
Pseudoephedrine Hydrochloride, Dextromethorphan Hydrobromide, Guaifenesin, and Acetaminophen Oral Solution—Not in USP.
Pseudoephedrine Hydrochloride, Dextromethorphan Hydrobromide, Guaifenesin, and Acetaminophen Tablets—Not in USP.

PSEUDOEPHEDRINE AND GUAIFENESIN

For *Pseudoephedrine* and *Guaifenesin*—See individual listings for chemistry information.

USP requirements:
Pseudoephedrine Hydrochloride and Guaifenesin Extended-release Capsules—Not in USP.

Pseudoephedrine Hydrochloride and Guaifenesin Oral Solution—Not in USP.
Pseudoephedrine Hydrochloride and Guaifenesin Syrup—Not in USP.
Pseudoephedrine Hydrochloride and Guaifenesin Tablets—Not in USP.
Pseudoephedrine Hydrochloride and Guaifenesin Extended-release Tablets—Not in USP.

PSEUDOEPHEDRINE AND HYDROCODONE

For *Pseudoephedrine* and *Hydrocodone*—See individual listings for chemistry information.

USP requirements:
Pseudoephedrine Hydrochloride and Hydrocodone Bitartrate Oral Solution—Not in USP.
Pseudoephedrine Hydrochloride and Hydrocodone Bitartrate Syrup—Not in USP.

PSEUDOEPHEDRINE, HYDROCODONE, AND GUAIFENESIN

For *Pseudoephedrine, Hydrocodone,* and *Guaifenesin*—See individual listings for chemistry information.

USP requirements:
Pseudoephedrine Hydrochloride, Hydrocodone Bitartrate, and Guaifenesin Oral Solution—Not in USP.
Pseudoephedrine Hydrochloride, Hydrocodone Bitartrate, and Guaifenesin Syrup—Not in USP.
Pseudoephedrine Hydrochloride, Hydrocodone Bitartrate, and Guaifenesin Tablets—Not in USP.

PSEUDOEPHEDRINE AND IBUPROFEN

For *Pseudoephedrine* and *Ibuprofen*—See individual listings for chemistry information.

USP requirements: Pseudoephedrine Hydrochloride and Ibuprofen Tablets—Not in USP.

PSYLLIUM

Source: Psyllium seed—Cleaned, dried, ripe seed of *Plantago psyllium* and related species having a high content of hemicellulose mucilages.

USP requirements:
Psyllium Caramels—Not in USP.
Psyllium Granules—Not in USP.
Psyllium Powder—Not in USP.

PSYLLIUM HUSK

USP requirements: Psyllium Husk USP—Preserve in well-closed containers, secured against insect attack. It is the cleaned, dried seed coat (epidermis) separated by winnowing and thrashing from the seeds of *Plantago ovata* Forskal, known in commerce as Blond Psyllium or Indian Psyllium or Ispaghula, or from *Plantago psyllium* Linné or from *Plantago indica* Linné (*Plantago arenaria* Waldstein et Kitaibel) known in commerce as Spanish or French Psyllium (Fam. Plantaginaceae), in whole or in powdered form. Meets the requirements for Botanic characteristics, Identification, Microbial limits, Total ash (not more than 4.0%), Acid-insoluble ash (not more than 1.0%), Water (not more than 12.0%), Light extraneous matter (not more than 15%), Heavy extraneous matter (not more than 1.1%), Insect infestation, and Swell volume.

PSYLLIUM HYDROPHILIC MUCILLOID

Source: Obtained from the coating of *Plantago ovata*; contains about 50% hemicellulose.

Description: White to cream-colored, slightly granular powder with little or no odor.

USP requirements:
Psyllium Hydrophilic Mucilloid Granules—Not in USP.
Psyllium Hydrophilic Mucilloid Powder—Not in USP.
Psyllium Hydrophilic Mucilloid Effervescent Powder—Not in USP.
Psyllium Hydrophilic Mucilloid for Oral Suspension USP—Preserve in tight containers. A dry mixture of Psyllium Husk with suitable additives. Meets the requirements for Identification, Microbial limits, and Swell volume.
Psyllium Hydrophilic Mucilloid Wafers—Not in USP.

PSYLLIUM HYDROPHILIC MUCILLOID AND CARBOXYMETHYLCELLULOSE

For *Psyllium Hydrophilic Mucilloid* and *Carboxymethylcellulose*—See individual listings for chemistry information.

USP requirements: Psyllium Hydrophilic Mucilloid and Carboxymethylcellulose Sodium Granules—Not in USP.

PSYLLIUM HYDROPHILIC MUCILLOID AND SENNA

For *Psyllium Hydrophilic Mucilloid* and *Senna*—See individual listings for chemistry information.

USP requirements: Psyllium Hydrophilic Mucilloid and Senna Granules—Not in USP.

PSYLLIUM HYDROPHILIC MUCILLOID AND SENNOSIDES

For *Psyllium Hydrophilic Mucilloid* and *Sennosides*—See individual listings for chemistry information.

USP requirements: Psyllium Hydrophilic Mucilloid and Sennosides Powder—Not in USP.

PSYLLIUM AND SENNA

For *Psyllium* and *Senna*—See individual listings for chemistry information.

USP requirements: Psyllium and Senna Granules—Not in USP.

PUMICE

Description: Pumice USP—Very light, hard, rough, porous, grayish masses or gritty, grayish powder. Is odorless and stable in air.

Solubility: Pumice USP—Practically insoluble in water; is not attacked by acids.

USP requirements: Pumice USP—Preserve in well-closed containers. A substance of volcanic origin, consisting chiefly of complex silicates of aluminum, potassium, and sodium. Label powdered Pumice to indicate, in descriptive terms, the fineness of the powder. Powdered Pumice meets requirements for several sizes (Pumice Flour or Superfine Pumice, Fine Pumice, and Coarse Pumice). Meets the requirements for Water-soluble substances (not more than 0.20%), Acid-soluble substances (not more than 6.0%), and Iron.

PYRANTEL

Chemical name: Pyrantel pamoate—Pyrimidine, 1,4,5,6-tetra-hydro-1-methyl-2-[2-(2-thienyl)ethenyl]-, (*E*)-, compd. with 4,4′-methylenebis[3-hydroxy-2-naphthalenecarboxylic acid] (1:1).

Molecular formula: Pyrantel pamoate—$C_{11}H_{14}N_2S \cdot C_{23}H_{16}O_6$.

Molecular weight: Pyrantel pamoate—594.68.

Description: Pyrantel Pamoate USP—Yellow to tan solid.

Solubility: Pyrantel Pamoate USP—Practically insoluble in water and in methanol; soluble in dimethylsulfoxide; slightly soluble in dimethylformamide.

USP requirements:
Pyrantel Pamoate Oral Suspension USP—Preserve in tight, light-resistant containers. A suspension of Pyrantel Pamoate in a suitable aqueous vehicle. Contains an amount of pyrantel pamoate equivalent to the labeled amount of pyrantel, within ± 10%. Meets the requirements for Identification and pH (4.5–6.0).
Pyrantel Pamoate Tablets—Not in USP.

PYRAZINAMIDE

Source: Pyrazine derivative of nicotinamide.

Chemical name: Pyrazinecarboxamide.

Molecular formula: $C_5H_5N_3O$.

Molecular weight: 123.11.

Description: Pyrazinamide USP—White to practically white, odorless or practically odorless, crystalline powder.

Solubility: Pyrazinamide USP—Sparingly soluble in water; slightly soluble in alcohol, in ether, and in chloroform.

USP requirements: Pyrazinamide Tablets USP—Preserve in well-closed containers. Contain the labeled amount, within ± 7%. Meet the requirements for Identification, Dissolution (75% in 45 minutes in water in Apparatus 2 at 50 rpm), and Uniformity of dosage units.

PYRETHRINS AND PIPERONYL BUTOXIDE

Source:
Pyrethrins—Obtained from flowers of the pyrethrum plant, *Chrysanthemum cincerariaefolium*, which is related to the ragweed plant; esters formed by the combination of chrysanthenic and pyrethric acids and pyrethrolone, cinerolone, and jasmolone alcohols.
Piperonyl butoxide—A synthetic piperic acid derivative.

Chemical name: Piperonyl butoxide—5-[2-(2-Butoxyethoxy)ethoxymethyl]-6-propyl-1,3-benzodioxole.

Molecular formula: Piperonyl butoxide—$C_{19}H_{30}O_5$.

Molecular weight: Piperonyl butoxide—338.44.

Description:
Pyrethrins—Viscous liquid.
Piperonyl butoxide—Yellow or pale brown oily liquid with a faint characteristic odor.

Solubility:
Pyrethrins—Practically insoluble in water; soluble in alcohol, in petroleum ether, in kerosene, in carbon tetrachloride, in ethylene dichloride, and in nitromethane.
Piperonyl butoxide—Very slightly soluble in water; miscible with alcohol, with chloroform, with ether, with petroleum oils, and with liquefied aerosol propellants.

USP requirements:
Pyrethrins and Piperonyl Butoxide Gel—Not in USP.
Pyrethrins and Piperonyl Butoxide Solution Shampoo—Not in USP.
Pyrethrins and Piperonyl Butoxide Topical Solution—Not in USP.

PYRIDOSTIGMINE

Source: Synthetic quaternary ammonium compound.

Chemical name: Pyridostigmine bromide—Pyridinium, 3-[[(dimethylamino)carbonyl]oxy]-1-methyl-, bromide.

Molecular formula: Pyridostigmine bromide—$C_9H_{13}BrN_2O_2$.

Molecular weight: Pyridostigmine bromide—261.12.

Description: Pyridostigmine Bromide USP—White or practically white, crystalline powder, having an agreeable, characteristic odor. Hygroscopic.

Solubility: Pyridostigmine Bromide USP—Freely soluble in water, in alcohol, and in chloroform; slightly soluble in solvent hexane; practically insoluble in ether.

USP requirements:
Pyridostigmine Bromide Injection USP—Preserve in single-dose containers, preferably of Type I glass, protected from light. A sterile solution of Pyridostigmine Bromide in a suitable medium. Contains the labeled amount, within ±10%. Meets the requirements for Identification, Bacterial endotoxins, pH (4.5–5.5), and Injections.
Pyridostigmine Bromide Syrup USP—Preserve in tight, light-resistant containers. Contains, in each 100 mL, not less than 1.08 grams and not more than 1.32 grams of pyridostigmine bromide. Meets the requirement for Identification.
Pyridostigmine Bromide Tablets USP—Preserve in tight containers. Contain the labeled amount, within ±5%. Meet the requirements for Identification, Dissolution (75% in 45 minutes in water in Apparatus 2 at 50 rpm), and Uniformity of dosage units.
Pyridostigmine Bromide Extended-release Tablets—Not in USP.

PYRIDOXINE

Chemical name: Pyridoxine hydrochloride—3,4-Pyridinedimethanol, 5-hydroxy-6-methyl-, hydrochloride.

Molecular formula: Pyridoxine hydrochloride—$C_8H_{11}NO_3 \cdot HCl$.

Molecular weight: Pyridoxine hydrochloride—205.64.

Description: Pyridoxine Hydrochloride USP—White to practically white crystals or crystalline powder. Is stable in air, and is slowly affected by sunlight. Its solutions have a pH of about 3.

Solubility: Pyridoxine Hydrochloride USP—Freely soluble in water; slightly soluble in alcohol; insoluble in ether.

USP requirements:
Pyridoxine Hydrochloride Extended-release Capsules—Not in USP.
Pyridoxine Hydrochloride Injection USP—Preserve in single-dose or in multiple-dose containers, preferably of Type I glass, protected from light. A sterile solution of Pyridoxine Hydrochloride in Water for Injection. Contains the labeled amount, within −5% to +15%. Meets the requirements for Identification, Bacterial endotoxins, pH (2.0–3.8), and Injections.

Pyridoxine Hydrochloride Tablets USP—Preserve in well-closed containers, protected from light. Contain the labeled amount, within −5% to +15%. Meet the requirements for Identification, Disintegration (30 minutes), and Uniformity of dosage units.

PYRILAMINE

Chemical group: Ethylenediamine derivative.

Chemical name: Pyrilamine maleate—1,2-Ethanediamine, *N*-[(4-methoxyphenyl)methyl]-*N′,N′*-dimethyl-*N*-2-pyridinyl-, (*Z*)-2-butenedioate (1:1).

Molecular formula: Pyrilamine maleate—$C_{17}H_{23}N_3O \cdot C_4H_4O_4$.

Molecular weight: Pyrilamine maleate—401.46.

Description: Pyrilamine Maleate USP—White, crystalline powder, usually having a faint odor. Its solutions are acid to litmus.

Solubility: Pyrilamine Maleate USP—Very soluble in water; freely soluble in alcohol and in chloroform; slightly soluble in ether.

USP requirements: Pyrilamine Maleate Tablets USP—Preserve in well-closed containers. Contain the labeled amount, within ±7%. Meet the requirements for Identification, Dissolution (75% in 45 minutes in water in Apparatus 2 at 50 rpm), and Uniformity of dosage units.

PYRILAMINE, CODEINE, AND TERPIN HYDRATE

For *Pyrilamine, Codeine,* and *Terpin Hydrate*—See individual listings for chemistry information.

USP requirements: Pyrilamine Maleate, Codeine Phosphate, and Terpin Hydrate Syrup—Not in USP.

PYRILAMINE, PHENYLEPHRINE, ASPIRIN, AND CAFFEINE

For *Pyrilamine, Phenylephrine, Aspirin,* and *Caffeine*—See individual listings for chemistry information.

USP requirements: Pyrilamine Maleate, Phenylephrine Hydrochloride, Aspirin, and Caffeine Tablets—Not in USP.

PYRILAMINE, PHENYLEPHRINE, AND CODEINE

For *Pyrilamine, Phenylephrine,* and *Codeine*—See individual listings for chemistry information.

USP requirements: Pyrilamine Maleate, Phenylephrine Hydrochloride, and Codeine Phosphate Syrup—Not in USP.

PYRILAMINE, PHENYLEPHRINE, AND DEXTROMETHORPHAN

For *Pyrilamine, Phenylephrine,* and *Dextromethorphan*—See individual listings for chemistry information.

USP requirements: Pyrilamine Maleate, Phenylephrine Hydrochloride, and Dextromethorphan Hydrobromide Oral Solution—Not in USP.

PYRILAMINE, PHENYLEPHRINE, DEXTROMETHORPHAN, AND ACETAMINOPHEN

For *Pyrilamine, Phenylephrine, Dextromethorphan,* and *Acetaminophen*—See individual listings for chemistry information.

USP requirements: Pyrilamine Maleate, Phenylephrine Hydrochloride, Dextromethorphan Hydrobromide, and Acetaminophen Oral Solution—Not in USP.

PYRILAMINE, PHENYLEPHRINE, AND HYDROCODONE

For *Pyrilamine, Phenylephrine,* and *Hydrocodone*—See individual listings for chemistry information.

USP requirements: Pyrilamine Maleate, Phenylephrine Hydrochloride, and Hydrocodone Bitartrate Syrup—Not in USP.

PYRILAMINE, PHENYLEPHRINE, HYDROCODONE, AND AMMONIUM CHLORIDE

For *Pyrilamine, Phenylephrine, Hydrocodone,* and *Ammonium Chloride*—See individual listings for chemistry information.

USP requirements: Pyrilamine Maleate, Phenylephrine Hydrochloride, Hydrocodone Bitartrate, and Ammonium Chloride Syrup—Not in USP.

PYRILAMINE, PHENYLPROPANOLAMINE, ACETAMINOPHEN, AND CAFFEINE

For *Pyrilamine, Phenylpropanolamine, Acetaminophen,* and *Caffeine*—See individual listings for chemistry information.

USP requirements: Pyrilamine Maleate, Phenylpropanolamine Hydrochloride, Acetaminophen, and Caffeine Tablets—Not in USP.

PYRILAMINE, PHENYLPROPANOLAMINE, DEXTROMETHORPHAN, GUAIFENESIN, POTASSIUM CITRATE, AND CITRIC ACID

For *Pyrilamine, Phenylpropanolamine, Dextromethorphan, Guaifenesin, Potassium Citrate,* and *Citric Acid*—See individual listings for chemistry information.

USP requirements: Pyrilamine Maleate, Phenylpropanolamine Hydrochloride, Dextromethorphan Hydrobromide, Guaifenesin, Potassium Citrate, and Citric Acid Syrup—Not in USP.

PYRILAMINE, PHENYLPROPANOLAMINE, DEXTROMETHORPHAN, AND SODIUM SALICYLATE

For *Pyrilamine, Phenylpropanolamine, Dextromethorphan,* and *Sodium Salicylate*—See individual listings for chemistry information.

USP requirements: Pyrilamine Maleate, Phenylpropanolamine Hydrochloride, Dextromethorphan Hydrobromide, and Sodium Salicylate Oral Solution—Not in USP.

PYRIMETHAMINE

Chemical group: Structurally related to trimethoprim.

Chemical name: 2,4-Pyrimidinediamine, 5-(4-chlorophenyl)-6-ethyl-.

Molecular formula: $C_{12}H_{13}ClN_4$.

Molecular weight: 248.71.

Description: Pyrimethamine USP—White, odorless, crystalline powder.

Solubility: Pyrimethamine USP—Practically insoluble in water; slightly soluble in acetone, in alcohol, and in chloroform.

USP requirements: Pyrimethamine Tablets USP—Preserve in tight, light-resistant containers. Contain the labeled amount, within ±7%. Meet the requirements for Identification, Dissolution (75% in 45 minutes in 0.1 N hydrochloric acid in Apparatus 2 at 50 rpm), and Uniformity of dosage units.

PYRITHIONE

Chemical name: Pyrithione zinc—Zinc, bis(1-hydroxy-2(1H)-pyridinethionato-O,S)-(T-4)-.

Molecular formula: Pyrithione zinc—$C_{10}H_8N_2O_2S_2Zn$.

Molecular weight: Pyrithione zinc—317.69.

Description: Pyrithione zinc—Off-white to gray colored powder with not more than a mild characteristic odor.

Solubility: Pyrithione zinc—Soluble in dimethylsulfoxide; practically insoluble in acetone, in alcohol, and in water.

USP requirements:
Pyrithione Zinc Bar Shampoo—Not in USP.
Pyrithione Zinc Cream Shampoo—Not in USP.
Pyrithione Zinc Lotion Shampoo—Not in USP.

PYRVINIUM

Chemical group: Cyanine dye.

Chemical name: Pyrvinium pamoate—Quinolinium, 6-(dimethylamino)-2-[2-(2,5-dimethyl-1-phenyl-1H-pyrrol-3-yl)ethenyl]-1-methyl-, salt with 4,4′-methylenebis[3-hydroxy-2-naphthalenecarboxylic acid] (2:1).

Molecular formula: Pyrvinium pamoate—$C_{75}H_{70}N_6O_6$.

Molecular weight: Pyrvinium pamoate—1151.41.

Description:
Pyrvinium Pamoate USP—Bright orange or orange-red to practically black, crystalline powder.
Pyrvinium Pamoate Oral Suspension USP—Dark red, opaque suspension of essentially very fine, amorphous particles or aggregates, usually less than 10 micrometers in size. Larger particles, some of which may be crystals, up to 100 micrometers in size also may be present.

Solubility: Pyrvinium Pamoate USP—Practically insoluble in water and in ether; freely soluble in glacial acetic acid; slightly soluble in chloroform and in methoxyethanol; very slightly soluble in methanol.

USP requirements:
Pyrvinium Pamoate Oral Suspension USP—Preserve in tight, light-resistant containers. Contains, in each 100 mL, an amount of pyrvinium pamoate equivalent to not less than 0.90 gram and not more than 1.10 grams of pyrvinium. Meets the requirements for Identification and pH (6.0–8.0).
Pyrvinium Pamoate Tablets USP—Preserve in tight, light-resistant containers. Contain an amount of pyrvinium pamoate equivalent to the labeled amount of pyrvinium, within ±8%. Meet the requirements for Identification, Disintegration (30 minutes), and Uniformity of dosage units.

QUAZEPAM

Chemical name: 2H-1,4-Benzodiazepine-2-thione, 7-chloro-5-(2-fluorophenyl)-1,3-dihydro-1-(2,2,2-trifluoroethyl)-.

Molecular formula: $C_{17}H_{11}ClF_4N_2S$.

Molecular weight: 386.79.

Description: White, crystalline compound.

Solubility: Soluble in ethanol; insoluble in water.

USP requirements: Quazepam Tablets—Not in USP.

QUINACRINE

Chemical group: Acridine derivative.

Chemical name: Quinacrine hydrochloride—1,4-Pentanedi-amine, N^4-(6-chloro-2-methoxy-9-acridinyl)-N^1,N^1-diethyl-, dihydrochloride, dihydrate.

Molecular formula: Quinacrine hydrochloride—$C_{23}H_{30}ClN_3O \cdot 2HCl \cdot 2H_2O$.

Molecular weight: Quinacrine hydrochloride—508.91.

Description: Quinacrine Hydrochloride USP—Bright yellow, crystalline powder. Is odorless. Its solution (1 in 100) has a pH of about 4.5. Melts at about 250 °C, with decomposition.

Solubility: Quinacrine Hydrochloride USP—Sparingly soluble in water; soluble in alcohol.

USP requirements: Quinacrine Hydrochloride Tablets USP—Preserve in tight containers. Contain the labeled amount, within ±7%. Meet the requirements for Identification, Dissolution (75% in 45 minutes in water in Apparatus 2 at 50 rpm), and Uniformity of dosage units.

QUINAPRIL

Chemical name: Quinapril hydrochloride—3-Isoquinolinecar-boxylic acid, 2-[2-[[1-(ethoxycarbonyl)-3-phenylpropyl]-amino]-1-oxopropyl]-1,2,3,4-tetrahydro-, monohydrochlo-ride, [3S-[2[R*(R*)],3R*]].

Molecular formula: Quinapril hydrochloride—$C_{25}H_{30}N_2O_5 \cdot HCl$.

Molecular weight: Quinapril hydrochloride—474.98.

Description: Quinapril hydrochloride—White to off-white amorphous powder.

Solubility: Quinapril hydrochloride—Freely soluble in aqueous solvents.

USP requirements: Quinapril Hydrochloride Tablets—Not in USP.

QUINESTROL

Chemical name: 19-Norpregna-1,3,5(10)-trien-20-yn-17-ol, 3-(cyclopentyloxy)-, (17 alpha)-.

Molecular formula: $C_{25}H_{32}O_2$.

Molecular weight: 364.53.

Description: Quinestrol USP—White, practically odorless powder.

Solubility: Quinestrol USP—Insoluble in water; soluble in alcohol, in chloroform, and in ether.

USP requirements: Quinestrol Tablets USP—Preserve in well-closed containers. Contain the labeled amount, within ±10%. Meet the requirements for Identification, Dissolution (80% in 30 minutes in 0.29% sodium lauryl sulfate in Apparatus 2 at 50 rpm), and Uniformity of dosage units.

QUINETHAZONE

Chemical name: 6-Quinazolinesulfonamide, 7-chloro-2-ethyl-1,2,3,4-tetrahydro-4-oxo-.

Molecular formula: $C_{10}H_{12}ClN_3O_3S$.

Molecular weight: 289.74.

Description: Quinethazone USP—White to yellowish white, crystalline powder.

pKa: 9.3 and 10.7.

Solubility: Quinethazone USP—Very slightly soluble in water; freely soluble in solutions of alkali hydroxides and carbon-ates; sparingly soluble in pyridine; slightly soluble in alcohol.

USP requirements: Quinethazone Tablets USP—Preserve in tight containers. Contain the labeled amount, within ±7.5%. Meet the requirements for Identification, Disintegration (30 minutes), and Uniformity of dosage units.

QUINIDINE

Source: Quinidine polygalacturonate—A polymer of quinidine and polygalacturonic acid.

Chemical name:

Quinidine gluconate—Cinchonan-9-ol, 6'-methoxy-, (9S)-, mono-D-gluconate (salt).

Quinidine sulfate—Cinchonan-9-ol, 6'-methoxy-, (9S)-, sul-fate (2:1) (salt), dihydrate.

Molecular formula:

Quinidine gluconate—$C_{20}H_{24}N_2O_2 \cdot C_6H_{12}O_7$.

Quinidine polygalacturonate—$(C_{20}H_{24}N_2O_2 \cdot C_6H_{10}O_7 \cdot H_2O)_x$.

Quinidine sulfate—$(C_{20}H_{24}N_2O_2)_2 \cdot H_2SO_4 \cdot 2H_2O$.

Molecular weight:

Quinidine gluconate—520.58.

Quinidine sulfate—782.95.

Description:

Quinidine Gluconate USP—White powder. Odorless.

Quinidine polygalacturonate—Creamy white, amorphous powder.

Quinidine Sulfate USP—Fine, needle-like, white crystals, frequently cohering in masses, or fine, white powder. Is odorless, and darkens on exposure to light. Its solutions are neutral or alkaline to litmus.

Solubility:

Quinidine Gluconate USP—Freely soluble in water; slightly soluble in alcohol.

Quinidine polygalacturonate—Sparingly soluble in water; freely soluble in hot 40% alcohol.

Quinidine Sulfate USP—Slightly soluble in water; soluble in alcohol and in chloroform; insoluble in ether.

USP requirements:

Quinidine Gluconate Injection USP—Preserve in single-dose or in multiple-dose containers, preferably of Type I glass. A sterile solution of Quinidine Gluconate in Water for Injection. Contains, in each mL, amounts of quinidine gluconate and dihydroquinidine gluconate totaling not less than 76 mg and not more than 84 mg of quinidine glu-conate, calculated as quinidine gluconate. Meets the re-quirements for Identification, Bacterial endotoxins, Chro-matographic purity, and Injections.

Quinidine Gluconate Tablets—Not in USP.

Quinidine Gluconate Extended-release Tablets USP—Pre-serve in well-closed, light-resistant containers. Contain amounts of quinidine gluconate and dihydroquinidine glu-conate totaling the labeled amount of quinidine gluco-nate, calculated as quinidine gluconate, within ±10%. Meet the requirements for Identification, Chromato-graphic purity, and Uniformity of dosage units.

Quinidine Polygalacturonate Tablets—Not in USP.

Quinidine Sulfate Capsules USP—Preserve in tight, light-resistant containers. Contain amounts of quinidine sulfate and dihydroquinidine sulfate totaling the labeled amount of quinidine sulfate, calculated as quinidine sulfate, within ±10%. Meet the requirements for Identification, Dissolution (85% in 30 minutes in 0.1 N hydrochloric acid in Apparatus 1 at 100 rpm), Uniformity of dosage units, and Chromatographic purity.

Quinidine Sulfate Injection—Not in USP.

Quinidine Sulfate Tablets USP—Preserve in well-closed, light-resistant containers. Contain amounts of quinidine sulfate and dihydroquinidine sulfate totaling the labeled amount of quinidine sulfate, calculated as quinidine sulfate, within ±10%. Meet the requirements for Identification, Dissolution (85% in 30 minutes in 0.1 N hydrochloric acid in Apparatus 1 at 100 rpm), Uniformity of dosage units, and Chromatographic purity.

Quinidine Sulfate Extended-release Tablets USP—Preserve in well-closed, light-resistant containers. Contain amounts of quinidine sulfate and dihydroquinidine sulfate totaling the labeled amount of quinidine sulfate, calculated as quinidine sulfate, within ±10%. Meet the requirements for Identification, Drug release (20–50% in 0.125D hours, 43–73% in 0.500D hours, and not less than 70% in 1.50D hours in 0.1 N hydrochloric acid in Apparatus 1 at 100 rpm), Uniformity of dosage units, and Chromatographic purity.

QUININE

Chemical name: Quinine sulfate—Cinchonan-9-ol, 6'-methoxy-, (8 alpha,9R)-, sulfate (2:1) (salt), dihydrate.

Molecular formula: Quinine sulfate—$(C_{20}H_{24}N_2O_2)_2 \cdot H_2SO_4 \cdot 2H_2O$.

Molecular weight: Quinine sulfate—782.95.

Description: Quinine Sulfate USP—White, fine, needle-like crystals, usually lusterless, making a light and readily compressible mass. Is odorless. It darkens on exposure to light. Its saturated solution is neutral or alkaline to litmus.

Solubility: Quinine Sulfate USP—Slightly soluble in water, in alcohol, in chloroform, and in ether; freely soluble in alcohol at 80 °C, and in a mixture of 2 volumes of chloroform and 1 volume of dehydrated alcohol; sparingly soluble in water at 100 °C.

USP requirements:

Quinine Sulfate Capsules USP—Preserve in tight containers. Contain amounts of quinine sulfate and dihydroquinine sulfate totaling the labeled amount of quinine sulfate, calculated as quinine sulfate dihydrate, within ±10%. Meet the requirements for Identification, Dissolution (75% in 45 minutes in 0.1 N hydrochloric acid in Apparatus 1 at 100 rpm), Uniformity of dosage units, and Chromatographic purity.

Quinine Sulfate Tablets USP—Preserve in well-closed containers. Contain amounts of quinine sulfate and dihydroquinine sulfate totaling the labeled amount of quinine sulfate, calculated as quinine sulfate dihydrate, within ±10%. Meet the requirements for Identification, Dissolution (75% in 45 minutes in 0.1 N hydrochloric acid in Apparatus 1 at 100 rpm), Uniformity of dosage units, and Chromatographic purity.

RABIES IMMUNE GLOBULIN

Description: Rabies Immune Globulin USP—Transparent or slightly opalescent liquid, practically colorless and practically odorless. May develop a slight, granular deposit during storage.

USP requirements: Rabies Immune Globulin USP—Preserve at a temperature between 2 and 8 °C. A sterile, non-pyrogenic, slightly opalescent solution consisting of globulins derived from blood plasma or serum that has been tested for the absence of hepatitis B surface antigen, derived from selected adult human donors who have been immunized with rabies vaccine and have developed high titers of rabies antibody. Label it to state that it is not for intravenous injection. Has a potency such that when labeled as 150 International Units (IU) per mL, it has a geometric mean lower limit (95% confidence) potency value of not less than 110 IU per mL, and proportionate lower limit potency values for other labeled potencies, based on the U.S. Standard Rabies Immune Globulin and using the CVS Virus challenge, by neutralization test in mice or tissue culture. Contains not less than 10 grams and not more than 18 grams of protein per 100 mL, of which not less than 80% is monomeric immunoglobilin G, having a sedimentation coefficient in the range of 6.0 to 7.5S, with no fragments having a sedimentation coefficient less than 6S and no aggregates having a sedimentation coefficient greater than 12S. Contains 0.3 M glycine as a stabilizing agent, and it contains a suitable preservative. Has a pH of 6.4–7.2, measured in a solution diluted to contain 1% of protein with 0.15 M sodium chloride. Meets the requirements of the test for heat stability and for Expiration date (not later than 1 year after date of issue from manufacturer's cold storage [5 °C, 1 year]). Conforms to the regulations of the U.S. Food and Drug Administration concerning biologics.

RABIES VACCINE

Description: Rabies Vaccine USP—White to straw-colored, amorphous pellet, which may or may not become fragmented when shaken.

USP requirements: Rabies Vaccine USP—Preserve at a temperature between 2 and 8 °C. A sterile preparation, in dried or liquid form, of inactivated rabies virus harvested from inoculated diploid cell cultures. Label it to state that it contains rabies antigen equivalent to not less than 2.5 IU per dose and that it is intended for intramuscular injection only. The cell cultures are shown to consist of diploid cells by tests of karyology, to be non-tumorigenic by tests in hamsters treated with anti-lymphocytic serum (ALS), and to be free from extraneous agents by tests in animals or cell-culture systems. The harvested virus meets the requirements for identity by serological tests, for absence of infectivity by tests in mice or cell-culture systems, and for absence of extraneous agents by tests in animals or cell-culture systems. The Vaccine meets the requirements for absence of live virus by tests using a suitable virus amplification system involving inoculation and incubation of sensitive cell cultures for not less than 14 days followed by inoculation of the cell-culture fluid thereafter into not less than 20 adult mice. Has a potency of rabies antigen equivalent to not less than 2.5 International Units for Rabies Vaccine, per dose, determined with the specific mouse protection test using the U.S. Standard Rabies Vaccine. Meets the requirements for general safety and Expiration date (not later than 2 years after date of issue from manufacturer's cold storage [5 °C, 1 year]). Conforms to the regulations of the U.S. Food and Drug Administration concerning biologics.

RACEPINEPHRINE

Chemical name: 1,2-Benzenediol, 4-[1-hydroxy-2-(methylamino)ethyl]-, (±)-.

Molecular formula:
Racepinephrine—$C_9H_{13}NO_3$.
Racepinephrine hydrochloride—$C_9H_{13}NO_3 \cdot HCl$.

Molecular weight:
Racepinephrine—183.21.
Racepinephrine hydrochloride—219.67.

Description:
Racepinephrine USP—White to nearly white, crystalline, odorless powder, gradually darkening on exposure to light and air. With acids, it forms salts that are readily soluble in water, and the base may be recovered by the addition of ammonium hydroxide.
Racepinephrine Hydrochloride USP—Fine, white, odorless powder. Darkens on exposure to light and air. Its solutions are acid to litmus.

Solubility:
Racepinephrine USP—Very slightly soluble in water and in alcohol; insoluble in ether, in chloroform, and in fixed and volatile oils.
Racepinephrine Hydrochloride USP—Freely soluble in water; sparingly soluble in alcohol.

USP requirements: Racepinephrine Inhalation Solution USP—Preserve in tight, light-resistant containers. Do not freeze. A solution of Racepinephrine in Purified Water prepared with the aid of Hydrochloric Acid or of Racepinephrine Hydrochloride in Purified Water. The label indicates that the Inhalation Solution is not to be used if its color is pinkish or darker than slightly yellow or if it contains a precipitate. Contains the labeled amount, within ±10%. Meets the requirements for Color and clarity, Identification, and pH (2.0–3.5).

RANITIDINE

Chemical group: Amino-alkyl furan derivative of histamine.

Chemical name:
Ranitidine—1,1-Ethenediamine, N-[2-[[[5-[(dimethyl-amino)methyl]-2-furanyl]methyl]thio]ethyl]-N'-methyl-2-nitro-.
Ranitidine hydrochloride—1,1-Ethenediamine, N-[2-[[[5-[(dimethylamino)methyl]-2-furanyl]methyl]thio]ethyl]-N'-methyl-2-nitro-, monohydrochloride.

Molecular formula:
Ranitidine—$C_{13}H_{22}N_4O_3S$.
Ranitidine hydrochloride—$C_{13}H_{22}N_4O_3S \cdot HCl$.

Molecular weight:
Ranitidine—314.40.
Ranitidine hydrochloride—350.87.

Description: Ranitidine Hydrochloride USP—White to pale yellow, crystalline, practically odorless powder. Is sensitive to light and moisture. Melts at about 140 °C, with decomposition.

pKa: 8.2 and 2.7.

Solubility: Ranitidine Hydrochloride USP—Very soluble in water; moderately soluble in alcohol; and sparingly soluble in chloroform.

USP requirements:
Ranitidine Capsules—Not in USP.
Ranitidine Injection USP—Preserve in single-dose or in multiple-dose containers of Type I glass, protected from light. Store below 30 °C (86 °F). Do not freeze. A sterile solution of Ranitidine Hydrochloride in Water for Injection. Label Injection to state both the content of the active moiety and the content of the salt used in formulating the article. Contain the labeled amount, within ±10%. Meets the requirements for Identification, Bacterial endotoxins, pH (6.7–7.3), Particulate matter, Chromatographic purity, and Injections.
Ranitidine Oral Solution USP—Preserve in tight, light-resistant containers. Store below 25 °C. Do not freeze. A solution of Ranitidine Hydrochloride in water. Label Oral Solution to state both the content of the active moiety and the content of the ranitidine salt used in formulating the article. Contains the equivalent of the labeled amount of ranitidine, within ±10%. Meets the requirements for Identification, Antimicrobial preservatives—effectiveness, Microbial limits, pH (6.7–7.5), and Chromatographic purity.
Ranitidine Tablets USP—Preserve in tight, light-resistant containers. Label Tablets to state both the content of the active moiety and the content of the salt used in formulating the article. Contain the labeled amount, within ±10%. Meet the requirements for Identification, Dissolution (80% in 45 minutes in water in Apparatus 2 at 50 rpm), Chromatographic purity, and Uniformity of dosage units.
Ranitidine Hydrochloride Syrup—Not in USP.

RANITIDINE AND SODIUM CHLORIDE

For *Ranitidine* and *Sodium Chloride*—See individual listings for chemistry information.

USP requirements: Ranitidine in Sodium Chloride Injection USP—Preserve in intact flexible containers meeting the general requirements in Containers, protected from light. Store at room temperature. Do not freeze. A sterile solution of Ranitidine Hydrochloride and Sodium Chloride in Water for Injection. Label Ranitidine in Sodium Chloride Injection to state both the content of the active moiety and the content of the ranitidine salt used in formulating the article. Contains the labeled amounts of both ranitidine and sodium chloride, within ±10%. Meets the requirements for Identification, Bacterial endotoxins, pH (6.7–7.3), Chromatographic purity, and Injections.

RAUWOLFIA SERPENTINA

Source: Powdered *Rauwolfia serpentina* standardized so that it contains 0.15 to 0.20% of the reserpine-rescinnamine group alkaloids, calculated as reserpine.

Description: Powdered rauwolfia serpentina—Light tan to light brown powder.

Solubility: Powdered rauwolfia serpentina—Slightly soluble in water; sparingly soluble in alcohol.

USP requirements: Rauwolfia Serpentina Tablets USP—Preserve in tight, light-resistant containers. Contain an amount of reserpine-rescinnamine group alkaloids, calculated as reserpine, equivalent to not less than 0.15% and not more than 0.20% of the labeled amount of powdered rauwolfia serpentina. Meet the requirements for Identification, Microbial limit, Disintegration (30 minutes), and Uniformity of dosage units.

RAUWOLFIA SERPENTINA AND BENDROFLUMETHIAZIDE

For *Rauwolfia Serpentina* and *Bendroflumethiazide*—See individual listings for chemistry information.

USP requirements: Rauwolfia Serpentina and Bendroflumethiazide Tablets—Not in USP.

PURIFIED RAYON

Description: Purified Rayon USP—White, lustrous or dull, fine, soft, filamentous fibers, appearing under the microscope as round, oval, or slightly flattened translucent rods, straight or crimped, striate and with serrate cross-sectional edges. Is practically odorless.

Solubility: Purified Rayon USP—Very soluble in ammoniated cupric oxide TS and in dilute sulfuric acid (3 in 5); insoluble in ordinary solvents.

USP requirements: Purified Rayon USP—A fibrous form of bleached, regenerated cellulose. May contain not more than 1.25% of titanium dioxide. Meets the requirements for Alkalinity or acidity, Residue on ignition (not more than 1.50%, from 5.0 grams), Acid-insoluble ash (not more than 1.25%), Water-soluble substances (not more than 1.0%), and Fiber length and absorbency, and for Dyes and Other foreign matter under Purified Cotton.

RESERPINE

Chemical source: A pure crystalline alkaloid obtained from *Rauwolfia serpentina*.

Chemical name: Yohimban-16-carboxylic acid, 11,17-dimethoxy-18-[(3,4,5-trimethoxybenzoyl)oxy]-, methyl ester, (3 beta,16 beta,17 alpha,18 beta,20 alpha)-.

Molecular formula: $C_{33}H_{40}N_2O_9$.

Molecular weight: 608.69.

Description: Reserpine USP—White or pale buff to slightly yellowish, odorless, crystalline powder. Darkens slowly on exposure to light, but more rapidly when in solution.

pKa: 6.6.

Solubility: Reserpine USP—Insoluble in water; freely soluble in acetic acid and in chloroform; very slightly soluble in alcohol and in ether.

USP requirements:
Reserpine Elixir USP—Preserve in tight, light-resistant containers. Contains the labeled amount, within ± 10%. Meets the requirements for Identification and Alcohol content (11.0–13.0%).

Reserpine Injection USP—Preserve in single-dose (or, if stabilizers are present, in multiple-dose), light-resistant containers, preferably of Type I glass. A sterile solution of Reserpine in Water for Injection, prepared with the aid of a suitable acid. Contains the labeled amount, within ± 10%. Contains suitable antioxidants. Meets the requirements for Identification, Bacterial endotoxins, pH (3.0–4.0), Other alkaloids, and Injections.

Reserpine Tablets USP—Preserve in tight, light-resistant containers. Contain the labeled amount, within ± 10%. Meet the requirements for Identification, Other alkaloids, Dissolution (75% in 45 minutes in 0.1 N acetic acid in Apparatus 1 at 100 rpm), and Uniformity of dosage units.

RESERPINE AND CHLOROTHIAZIDE

For *Reserpine* and *Chlorothiazide*—See individual listings for chemistry information.

USP requirements: Reserpine and Chlorothiazide Tablets USP—Preserve in tight, light-resistant containers. Contain the labeled amount of reserpine, within ± 10%, and the labeled amount of chlorothiazide, within ± 7%. Meet the requirements for Identification, Dissolution (75% of each active ingredient in 60 minutes in mixture of phosphate buffer [pH

8.0] and *n*-propyl alcohol [3:2] in Apparatus 2 at 75 rpm), and Uniformity of dosage units.

RESERPINE AND CHLORTHALIDONE

For *Reserpine* and *Chlorthalidone*—See individual listings for chemistry information.

USP requirements: Reserpine and Chlorthalidone Tablets—Not in USP.

RESERPINE AND HYDRALAZINE

For *Reserpine* and *Hydralazine*—See individual listings for chemistry information.

USP requirements: Reserpine and Hydralazine Hydrochloride Tablets—Not in USP.

RESERPINE, HYDRALAZINE, AND HYDROCHLOROTHIAZIDE

For *Reserpine, Hydralazine,* and *Hydrochlorothiazide*—See individual listings for chemistry information.

USP requirements: Reserpine, Hydralazine Hydrochloride, and Hydrochlorothiazide Tablets USP—Preserve in tight, light-resistant containers. Contain the labeled amount of reserpine, within ± 10%, and the labeled amounts of hydralazine hydrochloride and hydrochlorothiazide, within ± 7%. Meet the requirements for Identification, Disintegration (30 minutes), Uniformity of dosage units, and Diazotizable substances.

Note: Where Reserpine, Hydralazine Hydrochloride, and Hydrochlorothiazide Tablets are prescribed, without reference to the quantity of reserpine, hydralazine hydrochloride, or hydrochlorothiazide contained therein, a product containing 0.1 mg of reserpine, 25 mg of hydralazine hydrochloride, and 15 mg of hydrochlorothiazide shall be dispensed.

RESERPINE AND HYDROCHLOROTHIAZIDE

For *Reserpine* and *Hydrochlorothiazide*—See individual listings for chemistry information.

USP requirements: Reserpine and Hydrochlorothiazide Tablets USP—Preserve in tight, light-resistant containers. Contain the labeled amount of reserpine, within ± 10%, and the labeled amount of hydrochlorothiazide, within ± 7%. Meet the requirements for Identification, Dissolution (80% of reserpine in 45 minutes and 80% of hydrochlorothiazide in 60 minutes in mixture of 0.1 N hydrochloric acid and *n*-propyl alcohol [3:2] in Apparatus 2 at 50 rpm), Diazotizable substances, and Uniformity of dosage units.

RESERPINE AND HYDROFLUMETHIAZIDE

For *Reserpine* and *Hydroflumethiazide*—See individual listings for chemistry information.

USP requirements: Reserpine and Hydroflumethiazide Tablets—Not in USP.

RESERPINE AND METHYCLOTHIAZIDE

For *Reserpine* and *Methyclothiazide*—See individual listings for chemistry information.

USP requirements: Reserpine and Methyclothiazide Tablets—Not in USP.

RESERPINE AND POLYTHIAZIDE

For *Reserpine* and *Polythiazide*—See individual listings for chemistry information.

USP requirements: Reserpine and Polythiazide Tablets—Not in USP.

RESERPINE AND QUINETHAZONE

For *Reserpine* and *Quinethazone*—See individual listings for chemistry information.

USP requirements: Reserpine and Quinethazone Tablets—Not in USP.

RESERPINE AND TRICHLORMETHIAZIDE

For *Reserpine* and *Trichlormethiazide*—See individual listings for chemistry information.

USP requirements: Reserpine and Trichlormethiazide Tablets—Not in USP.

RESORCINOL

Chemical name: 1,3-Benzenediol.

Molecular formula: $C_6H_6O_2$.

Molecular weight: 110.11.

Description: Resorcinol USP—White, or practically white, needle-shaped crystals or powder. Has a faint, characteristic odor. Acquires a pink tint on exposure to light and air. Its solution (1 in 20) is neutral or acid to litmus.

Solubility: Resorcinol USP—Freely soluble in water, in alcohol, in glycerin, and in ether; slightly soluble in chloroform.

USP requirements:
Resorcinol Lotion—Not in USP.
Resorcinol Ointment—Not in USP.
Compound Resorcinol Ointment USP—Preserve in tight containers and avoid prolonged exposure to temperatures exceeding 30 °C.
   Prepare Compound Resorcinol Ointment as follows: 60 grams of Resorcinol, 60 grams of Zinc Oxide, 60 grams of Bismuth Subnitrate, 20 grams of Juniper Tar, 100 grams of Yellow Wax, 290 grams of Petrolatum, 280 grams of Anhydrous Lanolin, and 130 grams of Glycerin, to make 1000 grams of Compound Resorcinol Ointment. Melt the Yellow Wax and the Anhydrous Lanolin in a dish on a steam bath. Triturate the Zinc Oxide and the Bismuth Subnitrate with the Petrolatum until smooth, and add it to the melted mixture. Dissolve the Resorcinol in the Glycerin, incorporate the solution with the warm mixture just prepared, then add the Juniper Tar, and stir the Ointment until it congeals.

RESORCINOL AND SULFUR

For *Resorcinol* and *Sulfur*—See individual listings for chemistry information.

USP requirements:
Resorcinol and Sulfur Cake—Not in USP.
Resorcinol and Sulfur Cream—Not in USP.
Resorcinol and Sulfur Gel—Not in USP.
Resorcinol and Sulfur Lotion USP—Preserve in tight containers. It is Resorcinol and Sulfur in a suitable hydroalcoholic vehicle. Contains the labeled amount of resorcinol, within ± 10%, and the labeled amount of sulfur, within −5% to +10%. Meets the requirements for Identification and Alcohol content (90.0–110.0%).
Resorcinol and Sulfur Stick—Not in USP.

RIBAVIRIN

Chemical group: A synthetic nucleoside; structurally related to inosine, guanosine, and xanthosine.

Chemical name: 1*H*-1,2,4-Triazole-3-carboxamide, 1-beta-D-ribofuranosyl-.

Molecular formula: $C_8H_{12}N_4O_5$.

Molecular weight: 244.21.

Description: Ribavirin USP—White, crystalline powder.

Solubility: Ribavirin USP—Freely soluble in water; slightly soluble in dehydrated alcohol.

USP requirements: Ribavirin for Inhalation Solution USP—Preserve in tight containers, in a dry place at controlled room temperature. A sterile, freeze-dried, form of ribavirin. The labeling indicates that Ribavirin for Inhalation Solution must be constituted with a measured volume of Sterile Water for Injection or with Sterile Water for Inhalation containing no preservatives, and that the constituted solution is to be administered only by a small-particle aerosol generator. When constituted as directed in the labeling, the inhalation solution so obtained contains the labeled amount, within ± 5%. Meets the requirements for Identification, Sterility, pH (5.0–6.9, in the solution constituted as directed in the labeling), and Chromatographic purity, and for Specific rotation (−34.9° to −37.1°, calculated on the dried basis, in a solution containing 1 gram in each 10 mL), Loss on drying (not more than 0.5%), Residue on ignition (not more than 0.25%), and Heavy metals (not more than 0.001%) under Ribavirin.

RIBOFLAVIN

Chemical name: Riboflavine.

Molecular formula: $C_{17}H_{20}N_4O_6$.

Molecular weight: 376.37.

Description: Riboflavin USP—Yellow to orange-yellow, crystalline powder having a slight odor. Melts at about 280 °C. Its saturated solution is neutral to litmus. When dry, it is not appreciably affected by diffused light, but when in solution, light induces quite rapid deterioration, especially in the presence of alkalies.

pKa: 10.2.

Solubility: Riboflavin USP—Very slightly soluble in water, in alcohol, and in isotonic sodium chloride solution; very soluble in dilute solutions of alkalies; insoluble in ether and in chloroform.

USP requirements:
Riboflavin Injection USP—Preserve in light-resistant, single-dose or multiple-dose containers, preferably of Type I glass. A sterile solution of Riboflavin in Water for Injection. Contains the labeled amount, within −5% to +20%. Meets the requirements for Identification, Bacterial endotoxins, pH (4.5–7.0), and Injections.
Riboflavin Tablets USP—Preserve in tight, light-resistant containers. Contain the labeled amount, within −5% to +15%. Meet the requirements for Disintegration (30 minutes) and Uniformity of dosage units.

RICE SYRUP SOLIDS AND ELECTROLYTES

Chemical name:
Sodium chloride—Sodium chloride.
Potassium citrate—1,2,3-Propanetricarboxylic acid, 2-hydroxy-, tripotassium salt, monohydrate.

Sodium citrate—1,2,3-Propanetricarboxylic acid, 2-hydroxy-, trisodium salt.

Citric acid—1,2,3-Propanetricarboxylic acid, 2-hydroxy-.

Molecular formula:
Sodium chloride—NaCl.
Potassium citrate—$C_6H_5K_3O_7 \cdot H_2O$.
Sodium citrate—$C_6H_5Na_3O_7$.
Citric acid—$C_6H_8O_7$ (anhydrous); $C_6H_8O_7 \cdot H_2O$ (monohydrate).

Molecular weight:
Sodium chloride—58.44.
Potassium citrate—324.41.
Sodium citrate—258.07 (anhydrous).
Citric acid—192.12 (anhydrous); 210.14 (monohydrate).

Description:
Sodium Chloride USP—Colorless, cubic crystals or white crystalline powder.
  NF category: Tonicity agent.
Potassium Citrate USP—Transparent crystals or white, granular powder. Is odorless and is deliquescent when exposed to moist air.
  NF category: Buffering agent.
Sodium Citrate USP—Colorless crystals or white, crystalline powder.
  NF category: Buffering agent.
Citric Acid USP—Colorless, translucent crystals, or white, granular to fine crystalline powder. Odorless or practically odorless. The hydrous form is efflorescent in dry air.
  NF category: Acidifying agent; buffering agent.

Solubility:
Sodium Chloride USP—Freely soluble in water; and slightly more soluble in boiling water; soluble in glycerin; slightly soluble in alcohol.
Potassium Citrate USP—Freely soluble in water; almost insoluble in alcohol.
Sodium Citrate USP—Hydrous form freely soluble in water and very soluble in boiling water. Insoluble in alcohol.
Citric Acid USP—Very soluble in water; freely soluble in alcohol; sparingly soluble in ether.

USP requirements: Rice Syrup Solids and Electrolytes Solution—Not in USP.

RIFAMPIN

Source: Semisynthetic derivative of rifamycin B.

Chemical name: Rifamycin, 3-[[(4-methyl-1-piperazinyl)-imino]methyl]-.

Molecular formula: $C_{43}H_{58}N_4O_{12}$.

Molecular weight: 822.95.

Description: Rifampin USP—Red-brown, crystalline powder.

Solubility: Rifampin USP—Very slightly soluble in water; freely soluble in chloroform; soluble in ethyl acetate and in methanol.

USP requirements:
Rifampin Capsules USP—Preserve in tight, light-resistant containers, protected from excessive heat. Contain the labeled amount, within ±10%. Meet the requirements for Identification, Uniformity of dosage units, Dissolution (75% in 45 minutes in 0.1 *N* hydrochloric acid in Apparatus 1 at 50 rpm), and Loss on drying (not more than 3.0%).

Rifampin for Injection USP—Preserve in Containers for Sterile Solids. Contains the labeled amount, within −10% to +15%. Meets the requirements for Identification, Bacterial endotoxins, Sterility, pH (7.8–8.8, in a solution containing 60 mg of rifampin per mL), Water (not more than 3.0%), and Particulate matter.

RIFAMPIN AND ISONIAZID

For *Rifampin* and *Isoniazid*—See individual listings for chemistry information.

USP requirements: Rifampin and Isoniazid Capsules USP—Preserve in tight, light-resistant containers, and avoid exposure to excessive heat. Contain the labeled amount of rifampin, within −10% to +30%, and the labeled amount of isoniazid, within ±10%. Meet the requirement for Loss on drying (not more than 3.0%).

Note: Where Rifampin and Isoniazid Capsules are prescribed without reference to the quantity of rifampin or isoniazid contained therein, a product containing 300 mg of rifampin and 150 mg of isoniazid shall be dispensed.

RINGER'S

For *Sodium Chloride, Potassium Chloride,* and *Calcium Chloride*—See individual listings for chemistry information.

USP requirements:
Ringer's Injection USP—Preserve in single-dose glass or plastic containers. Glass containers are preferably of Type I or Type II glass. A sterile solution of Sodium Chloride, Potassium Chloride, and Calcium Chloride in Water for Injection. The label states the total osmolar concentration in mOsmol per liter. Where the contents are less than 100 mL, the label alternatively may state the total osmolar concentration in mOsmol per mL. Contains, in each 100 mL, not less than 323.0 mg and not more than 354.0 mg of sodium (equivalent to not less than 820.0 mg and not more than 900.0 mg of sodium chloride); not less than 14.9 mg and not more than 16.5 mg of potassium (equivalent to not less than 28.5 mg and not more than 31.5 mg of potassium chloride); not less than 8.20 mg and not more than 9.80 mg of calcium (equivalent to not less than 30.0 mg and not more than 36.0 mg of calcium chloride dihydrate); and not less than 523.0 mg and not more than 580.0 mg of chloride (as sodium chloride, potassium chloride, and calcium chloride dihydrate). Contains no antimicrobial agents.

Prepare Ringer's Injection as follows: Combine 8.6 grams of Sodium Chloride, 0.3 grams of Potassium Chloride, 0.33 grams of Calcium Chloride, and a sufficient quantity of Water for Injection, to make 1000 mL. Dissolve the three salts in the Water for Injection, filter until clear, place in suitable containers, and sterilize.

Meets the requirements for Identification, Bacterial endotoxins, pH (5.0–7.5), Heavy metals (not more than 0.3 ppm), and Injections.

Note: The calcium, chloride, potassium, and sodium ion contents of Ringer's Injection are approximately 4.5, 156, 4, and 147.5 milliequivalents per liter, respectively.

Ringer's Irrigation USP—Preserve in single-dose glass or plastic containers. Glass containers are preferably of Type I or Type II glass. The container may be designed to empty rapidly and may contain a volume of more than 1 liter. It is Ringer's Injection that has been suitably packaged, and it contains no antimicrobial agents. The designation "not for injection" appears prominently on the label. Meets the requirements for Sterility and for Identification tests, pH, and Heavy metals under Ringer's Injection.

LACTATED RINGER'S

For *Calcium Chloride, Potassium Chloride, Sodium Chloride* and *Sodium Lactate*—See individual listings for chemistry information.

USP requirements: Lactated Ringer's Injection USP—Preserve in single-dose glass or plastic containers. Glass containers are preferably of Type I or Type II glass. A sterile solution of Calcium Chloride, Potassium Chloride, Sodium Chloride, and Sodium Lactate in Water for Injection. The label states the total osmolar concentration in mOsmol per liter. Where the contents are less than 100 mL, the label alternatively may state the total osmolar concentration in mOsmol per mL. The label includes also the warning: "Not for use in the treatment of lactic acidosis." Contains, in each 100 mL, not less than 285.0 mg and not more than 315.0 mg of sodium (as sodium chloride and sodium lactate), not less than 14.1 mg and not more than 17.3 mg of potassium (equivalent to not less than 27.0 mg and not more than 33.0 mg of potassium chloride), not less than 4.90 mg and not more than 6.00 mg of calcium (equivalent to not less than 18.0 mg and not more than 22.0 mg of calcium chloride dihydrate), not less than 368.0 mg and not more than 408.0 mg of chloride (as sodium chloride, potassium chloride, and calcium chloride dihydrate), and not less than 231.0 mg and not more than 261.0 mg of lactate (equivalent to not less than 290.0 mg and not more than 330.0 mg of sodium lactate). Contains no antimicrobial agents. Meets the requirements for Identification, Bacterial endotoxins, pH (6.0–7.5), Heavy metals (not more than 0.3 ppm), and Injections.

Note: The calcium, potassium, and sodium contents of Lactated Ringer's Injection are approximately 2.7, 4, and 130 milliequivalents per liter, respectively.

RITODRINE

Chemical name: Ritodrine hydrochloride—Benzenemethanol, 4-hydroxy-alpha-[1-[[2-(4-hydroxyphenyl)ethyl]amino]ethyl]-, hydrochloride, ($R*$, $S*$)-.

Molecular formula: Ritodrine hydrochloride—$C_{17}H_{21}NO_3 \cdot HCl$.

Molecular weight: Ritodrine hydrochloride—323.82.

Description: Ritodrine Hydrochloride USP—White to nearly white, odorless or practically odorless, crystalline powder. Melts at about 200 °C.

Solubility: Ritodrine Hydrochloride USP—Freely soluble in water and in alcohol; soluble in *n*-propyl alcohol; practically insoluble in ether.

USP requirements:
Ritodrine Hydrochloride Injection USP—Preserve in single-dose containers, preferably of Type I glass. Store at room temperature, preferably below 30 °C. A sterile solution of Ritodrine Hydrochloride in Water for Injection. Contains the labeled amount, within ±10%. Meets the requirements for Identification, Bacterial endotoxins, pH (4.8–5.5), and Injections.
Ritodrine Hydrochloride Tablets USP—Preserve in tight containers. Store at room temperature, preferably below 30 °C. Contain the labeled amount, within ±10%. Meet the requirements for Identification, Dissolution (80% in 30 minutes in 0.1 *N* hydrochloric acid in Apparatus 2 at 50 rpm), and Uniformity of dosage units.

ROLITETRACYCLINE

Chemical name: 2-Naphthacenecarboxamide, 4-(dimethylamino)-1,4,4a,5,5a,6,11,12a-octahydro-3,6,10,12,12a-pentahydroxy-6-methyl-1,11-dioxo-*N*-(1-pyrrolidinylmethyl)-, [4S-(4 alpha,4a alpha,5a alpha,6 beta,12a alpha)]-.

Molecular formula: $C_{27}H_{33}N_3O_8$.

Molecular weight: 527.57.

Description: Sterile Rolitetracycline USP—Light yellow, crystalline powder, having a characteristic, musty, amine-like odor.

Solubility: Sterile Rolitetracycline USP—Soluble in water and in acetone; slightly soluble in dehydrated alcohol; very slightly soluble in ether.

USP requirements:
Rolitetracycline for Injection USP—Preserve in Containers for Sterile Solids, protected from light. A sterile dry mixture of Sterile Rolitetracycline and one or more suitable buffers, and if intended for intramuscular use, one or more suitable anesthetics. Contains the labeled amount, within −10% to +15%. Meets the requirements for Constituted solution, Depressor substances (exempt from this requirement when intended for intramuscular use only), Bacterial endotoxins, Sterility, pH (3.0–4.5, in the solution constituted as directed in the labeling), and Loss on drying (not more than 5.0%).
Sterile Rolitetracycline USP—Preserve in Containers for Sterile Solids, protected from light. It is rolitetracycline suitable for parenteral use. It has a potency of not less than 900 mcg of rolitetracycline per mg, calculated on the anhydrous basis. Meets the requirements for Identification, Crystallinity, Depressor substances, Bacterial endotoxins, Sterility, pH (7–9, in a solution containing 10 mg per mL), and Water (not more than 3.0%).

ROSE BENGAL SODIUM I 131

Chemical name: Spiro[isobenzofuran-1(3H),9'-[9H]-xanthene]-3-one, 4,5,6,7-tetrachloro-3',6'-dihydroxy-2',4',5',7'-tetraiodo-, disodium salt, labeled with iodine-131.

Molecular formula: $C_{20}H_2Cl_4{}^{131}I_4Na_2O_5$.

Description: Sodium Rose Bengal I 131 Injection USP—Clear, deep-red solution.

USP requirements: Rose Bengal Sodium I 131 Injection USP—Preserve in single-dose or in multiple-dose containers. A sterile solution containing rose bengal sodium in which a portion of the molecules contain radioactive iodine (^{131}I) in the molecular structure. Label it to include the following, in addition to the information specified for Labeling under Injections: the time and date of calibration; the amount of ^{131}I as rose bengal sodium expressed as total megabecquerels (or microcuries or millicuries) and as megabecquerels (or microcuries or millicuries) per mL on the date of calibration; the expiration date; and the statement, "Caution—Radioactive Material." The labeling indicates that in making dosage calculations, correction is to be made for radioactive decay, and also indicates that the radioactive half-life of ^{131}I is 8.08 days. Contains the labeled amount of ^{131}I, within ±10%, as rose bengal sodium expressed in megabecquerels (or microcuries or millicuries) per mL at the time indicated in the labeling. Contains the labeled amount of rose bengal sodium, within ±10%. Other chemical forms of radioactivity do not exceed 10% of the total radioactivity. Meets the requirements for Radionuclide identification, Bacterial endotoxins, pH (7.0–8.5), Radiochemical purity, and Injections (except that the Injection may be distributed or dispensed prior to the completion of the test for Sterility, the latter test being started on the day of final manufacture, and except that it is not subject to the recommendation on Volume in Container).

ROSE OIL

Description: Rose Oil NF—Colorless or yellow liquid, having the characteristic odor of rose. At 25 °C it is a viscous liquid. Upon gradual cooling, it changes to a translucent, crystalline mass, easily liquefied by warming.

NF category: Flavors and perfumes.

NF requirements: Rose Oil NF—Preserve in well-filled, tight containers. A volatile oil distilled with steam from the fresh flowers of *Rosa gallica* Linné, *Rosa damascena* Miller, *Rosa alba* Linné, *Rosa centifolia* Linné, and varieties of these species (Fam. Rosaceae). Meets the requirements for Solubility test (1 mL is miscible with 1 mL of chloroform without turbidity. Add 20 mL of 90% alcohol to this mixture: the resulting liquid is neutral or acid to moistened litmus paper and, upon standing at 20 °C, deposits crystals within 5 minutes), Specific gravity (0.848–0.863 at 30 °C compared with water at 15 °C), Angular rotation ($-1°$ to $-4°$ when determined in a 100-mm tube), and Refractive index (1.457–1.463 at 30 °C).

ROSE WATER

Description: Rose Water Ointment USP—NF category: Ointment base.

USP requirements: Rose Water Ointment USP—Preserve in tight, light-resistant containers.

Prepare Rose Water Ointment as follows: 125 grams of Cetyl Esters Wax, 120 grams of White Wax, 560 grams of Almond Oil, 5 grams of Sodium Borate, 25 mL of Stronger Rose Water, 165 mL of Purified Water, and 200 microliters of Rose Oil, to make about 1000 grams of Rose Water Ointment. Reduce the cetyl esters wax and the white wax to small pieces, melt them on a steam bath, add the almond oil, and continue heating until the temperature of the mixture reaches 70 °C. Dissolve the sodium borate in the purified water and the stronger rose water, warmed to 70 °C, and gradually add the warm aqueous phase to the melted oil phase, stirring rapidly and continuously until it has cooled to about 45 °C. Then incorporate the rose oil.

Note: Rose Water Ointment is free from rancidity. If the Ointment has been chilled, warm it slightly before attempting to incorporate other ingredients.

STRONGER ROSE WATER

Description: Stronger Rose Water NF—Practically colorless and clear, having the pleasant odor of fresh rose blossoms. It is free from empyreuma, mustiness, and fungal growths.

NF category: Flavors and perfumes.

NF requirements: Stronger Rose Water NF—The odor of Stronger Rose Water is best preserved by allowing a limited access of fresh air to the container. A saturated solution of the odoriferous principles of the flowers of *Rosa centifolia* Linné (Fam. Rosaceae) prepared by distilling the fresh flowers with water and separating the excess volatile oil from the clear, water portion of the distillate. Meets the requirements for Reaction (neutral or acid to litmus), Residue on evaporation (not more than 0.015%), Heavy metals (not more than 2 ppm), and Organic volatile impurities.

Note: Stronger Rose Water, diluted with an equal volume of purified water, may be supplied when "Rose Water" is required.

RUBELLA AND MUMPS VIRUS VACCINE LIVE

Description: Rubella and Mumps Virus Vaccine Live USP— Solid having the characteristic appearance of substances dried from the frozen state. The Vaccine is to be constituted with a suitable diluent just prior to use. Constituted vaccine undergoes loss of potency on exposure to sunlight.

USP requirements: Rubella and Mumps Virus Vaccine Live USP—Preserve in single-dose containers, or in light-resistant, multiple-dose containers, at a temperature between 2 and 8 °C. Multiple-dose containers for 50 doses are adapted for use only in jet injectors, and those for 10 doses for use by jet or syringe injection. A bacterially sterile preparation of a combination of live rubella virus and live mumps virus such that each component is prepared in conformity with and meets the requirements for Rubella Virus Vaccine Live, and for Mumps Virus Vaccine Live, whichever is applicable. Label the Vaccine in multiple-dose containers to indicate that the contents are intended solely for use by jet injector or for use by either jet or syringe injection, whichever is applicable. Label the Vaccine in single-dose containers, if such containers are not light-resistant, to state that it should be protected from sunlight. Label it also to state that constituted Vaccine should be discarded if not used within 8 hours. Meets the requirement for Expiration date (1 to 2 years, depending on the manufacturer's data, after date of issue from manufacturer's cold storage [-20 °C, 1 year]). Conforms to the regulations of the U.S. Food and Drug Administration concerning biologics.

RUBELLA VIRUS VACCINE LIVE

Source:
The vaccine currently available in the U.S. contains a sterile, lyophilized preparation of live, attenuated Wistar Institute RA 27/3 strain of rubella virus. The virus is propagated in human diploid (WI-38) cell culture.
The vaccines currently available in Canada also contain the RA 27/3 strain of rubella virus.

Description: Rubella Virus Vaccine Live USP—Solid having the characteristic appearance of substances dried from the frozen state. Undergoes loss of potency on exposure to sunlight. The vaccine is to be constituted with a suitable diluent just prior to use.

Other characteristics: Slightly acidic, pH 6.2 to 6.6.

USP requirements: Rubella Virus Vaccine Live USP—Preserve in single-dose containers, or in light-resistant, multiple-dose containers, at a temperature between 2 and 8 °C. Multiple-dose containers for 50 doses are adapted for use only in jet injectors, and those for 10 doses for use by jet or syringe injection. A bacterially sterile preparation of live virus derived from a strain of rubella virus that has been tested for neurovirulence in monkeys, and for immunogenicity, that is free from all demonstrable viable microbial agents except unavoidable bacteriophage, and that has been found suitable for human immunization. The strain is grown, for purposes of vaccine production, on primary cell cultures of duck embryo tissue, derived from pathogen-free flocks, or on primary cell cultures of a designated strain of human tissue, provided that the same cell culture system is used as that in which the strain was tested. The strain meets the requirements of the specific safety tests in adult and suckling mice; and the requirements of the tests in monkey kidney, chicken embryo, and human tissue cell cultures and embryonated eggs. In the case of virus grown in duck embryo cell cultures, the strain meets the requirements of the test by inoculation of embryonated duck eggs, and of the tests for absence of *Mycobacterium tuberculosis* and of avian leucosis. In the case of virus grown in rabbit kidney cell cultures, the strain meets the requirements of the tests by inoculation of rabbits and guinea pigs, and of the tests for absence of *Mycobacterium tuberculosis* and of known adventitious agents of rabbits. In the case of virus grown in human tissue cell cultures, the strain meets the requirements of the specific safety tests and tests for absence of *Mycobacterium tuberculosis* or other adventitious agents tests by inoculation of rabbits and guinea pigs and the requirements for karyology and of the tests for absence of adventitious and other infective agents, including hemadsorption viruses and *Mycoplasma,* in human diploid cell cultures. The strain cultures are treated to remove all intact tissue cells. The Vaccine meets the requirements of the specific tissue culture test for live virus titer, in a single immunizing dose, of not less than the equivalent of 1000 TCID$_{50}$ (quantity of virus estimated to infect 50% of inoculated cultures $\times$ 1000) when tested in parallel with the U.S. Reference Rubella Virus, Live. Label the Vaccine in multiple-dose containers to indicate that the contents are intended solely for use by jet injector or for use by either jet or syringe injection, whichever is applicable. Label the Vaccine in single-dose containers, if such containers are not light-resistant, to state that it should be protected from sunlight. Label it also to state that constituted Vaccine should be discarded if not used within 8 hours. Meets the requirement for Expiration date (1 to 2 years, depending on the manufacturer's data, after date of issue from manufacturer's cold storage [$-20\,°C$, 1 year]). Conforms to the regulations of the U.S. Food and Drug Administration concerning biologics.

RUBIDIUM RB 82

Molecular formula: ^{82}RbCl.

USP requirements: Rubidium Rb 82 Injection—Not in USP.

SACCHARIN

Chemical name:
Saccharin—1,2-Benzisothiazol-3(2*H*)-one, 1,1-dioxide.
Saccharin calcium—1,2-Benzisothiazol-3(2*H*)-one, 1,1-dioxide, calcium salt, hydrate (2:7).
Saccharin sodium—1,2-Benzisothiazol-3(2*H*)-one, 1,1-dioxide, sodium salt, dihydrate.

Molecular formula:
Saccharin—$C_7H_5NO_3S$.
Saccharin calcium—$C_{14}H_8CaN_2O_6S_2 \cdot 3\frac{1}{2}H_2O$.
Saccharin sodium—$C_7H_4NNaO_3S \cdot 2H_2O$.

Molecular weight:
Saccharin—183.18.
Saccharin calcium—467.48.
Saccharin sodium—241.19.

Description:
Saccharin NF—White crystals or white crystalline powder. Odorless or has a faint, aromatic odor. Its solutions are acid to litmus.
   NF category: Sweetening agent.
Saccharin Calcium USP—White crystals or white, crystalline powder. Odorless or has a faint aromatic odor.
   NF category: Sweetening agent.
Saccharin Sodium USP—White crystals or white crystalline powder. Odorless or has a faint aromatic odor. When in powdered form it usually contains about ⅓ the theoretical amount of water of hydration as a result of efflorescence.
   NF category: Sweetening agent.

Solubility:
Saccharin NF—Slightly soluble in water, in chloroform, and in ether; soluble in boiling water; sparingly soluble in alcohol. Readily dissolved by dilute solutions of ammonia,

by solutions of alkali hydroxides, and by solutions of alkali carbonates with the evolution of carbon dioxide.
Saccharin Calcium USP—Freely soluble in water.
Saccharin Sodium USP—Freely soluble in water; sparingly soluble in alcohol.

USP requirements:
Saccharin Calcium USP—Preserve in well-closed containers. Where the quantity of saccharin calcium is indicated in the labeling of any preparation containing Saccharin Calcium, this shall be expressed in terms of saccharin. Contains not less than 98.0% and not more than 101.0% of saccharin calcium, calculated on the anhydrous basis. Meets the requirements for Identification, Water (not more than 15.0%), Benzoate and salicylate, Arsenic (not more than 3 ppm), Selenium (not more than 0.003%), Toluenesulfonamides (not more than 0.0025%), Heavy metals (not more than 0.001%), Readily carbonizable substances, and Organic volatile impurities.
Saccharin Sodium USP—Preserve in well-closed containers. Where the quantity of saccharin sodium is indicated in the labeling of any preparation containing Saccharin Sodium, this shall be expressed in terms of saccharin. Contains not less than 98.0% and not more than 101.0% of saccharin sodium, calculated on the anhydrous basis. Meets the requirements for Identification, Alkalinity, Toluenesulfonamides (not more than 0.0025%), and Heavy metals (not more than 0.001%), and for Identification tests, Water, Benzoate and salicylate, Arsenic, Selenium, and Readily carbonizable substances under Saccharin Calcium.
Saccharin Sodium Oral Solution USP—Preserve in tight containers. Contains an amount of saccharin sodium equivalent to the labeled amount of saccharin, within ±5%. Meets the requirements for Identification and pH (3.0–5.0).
Saccharin Sodium Tablets USP—Preserve in well-closed containers. Contain an amount of saccharin sodium equivalent to the labeled amount of saccharin, within −5% to +10%. Meet the requirements for Completeness of solution, Identification, and Ammonium salts.

NF requirements: Saccharin NF—Preserve in well-closed containers. Contains not less than 98.0% and not more than 101.0% of saccharin, calculated on the dried basis. Meets the requirements for Identification, Melting range (226–230 °C), Loss on drying (not more than 1.0%), Residue on ignition (not more than 0.2%), Toluenesulfonamides (not more than 0.0025%), Arsenic (not more than 3 ppm), Selenium (not more than 0.003%), Heavy metals (not more than 0.001%), Readily carbonizable substances, Benzoic and salicylic acids, and Organic volatile impurities.

SAFFLOWER OIL

Description: Safflower Oil USP—Light yellow oil. Thickens and becomes rancid on prolonged exposure to air.
   NF category: Vehicle (oleaginous).

Solubility: Safflower Oil USP—Insoluble in water. Miscible with ether and with chloroform.

USP requirements: Safflower Oil USP—Preserve in tight, light-resistant containers. It is the refined fixed oil obtained from the seed of *Carthamus tinctorius* Linné (Fam. Compositae). Meets the requirements for Fatty acid composition, Free fatty acids, Iodine value (135–150), Heavy metals (not more than 0.001%), Unsaponifiable matter (not more than 1.5%), and Peroxide (not more than 10.0).

SALICYLAMIDE

Chemical name: Benzamide, 2-hydroxy-.

Molecular formula: $C_7H_7NO_2$.

Molecular weight: 137.14.

Description: Salicylamide USP—White, practically odorless, crystalline powder.

Solubility: Salicylamide USP—Slightly soluble in water and in chloroform; soluble in alcohol and in propylene glycol; freely soluble in ether and in solutions of alkalies.

USP requirements: Salicylamide USP—Preserve in well-closed containers. Contains not less than 98.0% and not more than 102.0% of salicylamide, calculated on the anhydrous basis. Meets the requirements for Identification, Melting range (139–142 °C), Water (not more than 0.5%), Residue on ignition (not more than 0.1%), Heavy metals (not more than 0.001%), Chromatographic purity, and Organic volatile impurities.

SALICYLIC ACID

Chemical name: Benzoic acid, 2-hydroxy-.

Molecular formula: $C_7H_6O_3$.

Molecular weight: 138.12.

Description: Salicylic Acid USP—White crystals, usually in fine needles, or fluffy, white, crystalline powder. Is stable in air. The synthetic form is white and odorless. When prepared from natural methyl salicylate, it may have a slightly yellow or pink tint, and a faint, mint-like odor.

Solubility: Salicylic Acid USP—Slightly soluble in water; freely soluble in alcohol and in ether; soluble in boiling water; sparingly soluble in chloroform.

USP requirements:
Salicylic Acid Collodion USP—Preserve in tight containers at controlled room temperature, remote from fire. Contains not less than 9.5% and not more than 11.5% of salicylic acid.

Prepare Salicylic Acid Collodion as follows: 100 grams of Salicylic Acid and a sufficient quantity of Flexible Collodion to make 1000 mL. Dissolve the Salicylic Acid in about 750 mL of Flexible Collodion, add sufficient of the latter to make the product measure 1000 mL, and mix.

Salicylic Acid Cream—Not in USP.
Salicylic Acid Topical Foam USP—Preserve in tight containers. Contains the labeled amount, within ± 10%. Meets the requirements for Identification and pH (5.0–6.0).
Salicylic Acid Gel USP—Preserve in collapsible tubes or in tight containers, preferably at controlled room temperature. It is Salicylic Acid in a suitable viscous hydrophilic vehicle. Contains the labeled amount, within ± 10%. Meets the requirements for Identification, Water (not more than 15.0%), and Alcohol content (if present, 90.0–110.0%).
Salicylic Acid Lotion—Not in USP.
Salicylic Acid Ointment—Not in USP.
Salicylic Acid Pads—Not in USP.
Salicylic Acid Plaster USP—Preserve in well-closed containers, preferably at controlled room temperature. A uniform mixture of Salicylic Acid in a suitable base, spread on paper, cotton cloth, or other suitable backing material. The plaster mass contains the labeled amount, within ± 10%.
Salicylic Acid Shampoo—Not in USP.
Salicylic Acid Soap—Not in USP.
Salicylic Acid Topical Solution—Not in USP.

SALICYLIC ACID AND SULFUR

For *Salicylic Acid* and *Sulfur*—See individual listings for chemistry information.

USP requirements:
Salicylic Acid and Sulfur Cream—Not in USP.
Salicylic Acid and Sulfur Cleansing Cream—Not in USP.
Salicylic Acid and Sulfur Lotion—Not in USP.
Salicylic Acid and Sulfur Cleansing Lotion—Not in USP.
Salicylic Acid and Sulfur Cream Shampoo—Not in USP.
Salicylic Acid and Sulfur Lotion Shampoo—Not in USP.
Salicylic Acid and Sulfur Suspension Shampoo—Not in USP.
Salicylic Acid and Sulfur Bar Soap—Not in USP.
Salicylic Acid and Sulfur Cleansing Suspension—Not in USP.
Salicylic Acid and Sulfur Topical Suspension—Not in USP.

SALICYLIC ACID, SULFUR, AND COAL TAR

For *Salicylic Acid, Sulfur,* and *Coal Tar*—See individual listings for chemistry information.

USP requirements:
Salicylic Acid, Sulfur, and Coal Tar Cream Shampoo—Not in USP.
Salicylic Acid, Sulfur, and Coal Tar Lotion Shampoo—Not in USP.

SALSALATE

Chemical name: Benzoic acid, 2-hydroxy-, 2-carboxyphenyl ester.

Molecular formula: $C_{14}H_{10}O_5$.

Molecular weight: 258.23.

Description: Odorless or almost odorless, white or almost white powder.

Solubility: Very slightly soluble in water; soluble 1 in 6 of alcohol, 1 in 8 of chloroform, and 1 in 12 of ether.

USP requirements:
Salsalate Capsules USP—Preserve in tight containers. Contain the labeled amount, within ± 10%. Meet the requirements for Identification, Disintegration (30 minutes, simulated gastric fluid TS [without pepsin] being used), Uniformity of dosage units, and Salicylic acid (not more than 1.5%).
Salsalate Tablets—Not in USP.

SARGRAMOSTIM

Source: A single chain, glycosylated polypeptide of 127 amino acid residues expressed from *Saccharomyces cerevisiae*.

Chemical name: Colony-stimulating factor 2 (human clone pHG$_{25}$ protein moiety), 23-L-leucine-.

Molecular formula: $C_{639}H_{1002}N_{168}O_{196}S_8$ (protein moiety).

Molecular weight: 15,500–19,500 daltons.

Description: White, crystalline powder.

Solubility: In water, 500 mcg per mL.

USP requirements: Sargramostim for Injection—Not in USP.

SCHICK TEST CONTROL

Description: Schick Test Control USP—Transparent liquid.

USP requirements: Schick Test Control USP—Preserve at a temperature between 2 and 8 °C. It is Diphtheria Toxin for Schick Test that has been inactivated by heat for use as control for the Schick Test. Meets the requirements of the specific guinea pig test for detoxification by injection of not less than 2.0 mL into each of at least four guinea pigs. The animals are observed daily for 30 days and during this period show no evidence of diphtheria toxin poisoning (extensive necrosis, paralysis, or specific lethality). Meets the requirement for Expiration date (not later than 1 year after date of issue from manufacturer's cold storage [5 °C, 1 year]). Conforms to the regulations of the U.S. Food and Drug Administration concerning biologics.

SCOPOLAMINE

Source: Naturally occurring alkaloid.

Chemical group: Tertiary amine, natural.

Chemical name:
Scopolamine butylbromide—(1S,3s,5R,6R,7S)-8-Butyl-6,7-epoxy-3-[(S)-tropoyloxy]tropanium bromide.
Scopolamine hydrobromide—Benzeneacetic acid, alpha-(hydroxymethyl)-, 9-methyl-3-oxa-9-azatricyclo-[3.3.1.0^{2,4}]-non-7-yl ester, hydrobromide, trihydrate, [7(S)-(1 alpha,2 beta,4 beta,5 alpha,7 beta)]-.

Molecular formula:
Scopolamine butylbromide—$C_{21}H_{30}BrNO_4$.
Scopolamine hydrobromide—$C_{17}H_{21}NO_4 \cdot HBr \cdot 3H_2O$.

Molecular weight:
Scopolamine butylbromide—440.4.
Scopolamine hydrobromide—438.31.

Description:
Scopolamine butylbromide—White or almost white, odorless or almost odorless, crystalline powder.
Scopolamine Hydrobromide USP—Colorless or white crystals or white, granular powder. Is odorless, and slightly efflorescent in dry air.

pKa: 7.55 (23 °C)–7.81 (25 °C).

Solubility:
Scopolamine butylbromide—Soluble 1 in 1 of water, 1 in 50 of alcohol, and 1 in 5 of chloroform.
Scopolamine Hydrobromide USP—Freely soluble in water; soluble in alcohol; slightly soluble in chloroform; insoluble in ether.

USP requirements:
Scopolamine Transdermal System—Not in USP.
Scopolamine Butylbromide Injection—Not in USP.
Scopolamine Butylbromide Suppositories—Not in USP.
Scopolamine Butylbromide Tablets—Not in USP.
Scopolamine Hydrobromide Injection USP—Preserve in light-resistant, single-dose or multiple-dose containers, preferably of Type I glass. A sterile solution of Scopolamine Hydrobromide in Water for Injection. Contains the labeled amount, within ± 10%. Meets the requirements for Identification, Bacterial endotoxins, pH (3.5–6.5), and Injections.
Scopolamine Hydrobromide Ophthalmic Ointment USP—Preserve in collapsible ophthalmic ointment tubes. It is Scopolamine Hydrobromide in a suitable ophthalmic ointment base. It is sterile. Contains the labeled amount, within ± 10%. Meets the requirements for Identification, Sterility, and Metal particles.
Scopolamine Hydrobromide Ophthalmic Solution USP—Preserve in tight containers. A sterile, buffered, aqueous solution of Scopolamine Hydrobromide. Contains the labeled amount, within ± 10%. Meets the requirements for Identification, Sterility, and pH (4.0–6.0).
Scopolamine Hydrobromide Tablets USP—Preserve in tight, light-resistant containers. Contain the labeled amount of scopolamine hydrobromide, within ± 10%. Meet the requirements for Identification, Disintegration (15 minutes, the use of disks being omitted), and Uniformity of dosage units.

SECOBARBITAL

Chemical name:
Secobarbital—2,4,6(1H,3H,5H)-Pyrimidinetrione, 5-(1-methylbutyl)-5-(2-propenyl)-.
Secobarbital sodium—2,4,6(1H,3H,5H)-Pyrimidinetrione, 5-(1-methylbutyl)-5-(2-propenyl)-, monosodium salt.

Molecular formula:
Secobarbital—$C_{12}H_{18}N_2O_3$.
Secobarbital sodium—$C_{12}H_{17}N_2NaO_3$.

Molecular weight:
Secobarbital—238.29.
Secobarbital sodium—260.27.

Description:
Secobarbital USP—White, amorphous or crystalline, odorless powder. Its saturated solution has a pH of about 5.6.
Secobarbital Sodium USP—White powder. Is odorless and is hygroscopic. Its solutions decompose on standing, heat accelerating the decomposition.

Solubility:
Secobarbital USP—Very slightly soluble in water; freely soluble in alcohol, in ether, and in solutions of fixed alkali hydroxides and carbonates; soluble in chloroform.
Secobarbital Sodium USP—Very soluble in water; soluble in alcohol; practically insoluble in ether.

USP requirements:
Secobarbital Elixir USP—Preserve in tight containers. Contains, in each 100 mL, not less than 417 mg and not more than 461 mg of secobarbital, in a suitable, flavored vehicle. Meets the requirements for Identification and Alcohol content (10.0–14.0%).
Secobarbital Sodium Capsules USP—Preserve in tight containers. Contain the labeled amount, within ± 7.5%. Meet the requirements for Identification, Dissolution (75% in 60 minutes in water in Apparatus 1 at 100 rpm), and Uniformity of dosage units.
Secobarbital Sodium Injection USP—Preserve in single-dose or in multiple-dose containers, preferably of Type I glass, protected from light, in a refrigerator. A sterile solution of Secobarbital Sodium in a suitable solvent. The label indicates that the Injection is not to be used if it contains a precipitate. Contains the labeled amount, within ± 10%. Meets the requirements for Identification, Bacterial endotoxins, pH (9.0–10.5), and Injections.
Sterile Secobarbital Sodium USP—Preserve in Containers for Sterile Solids. It is Secobarbital Sodium suitable for parenteral use. Contains the labeled amount, within ± 10%. Meets the requirements for Constituted solution and Bacterial endotoxins, for Identification tests, pH, Completeness of solution, Loss on drying, and Heavy metals under Secobarbital Sodium, and for Sterility tests, Uniformity of dosage units, and Labeling under Injections.

SECOBARBITAL AND AMOBARBITAL

For *Secobarbital* and *Amobarbital*—See individual listings for chemistry information.

USP requirements: Secobarbital Sodium and Amobarbital Sodium Capsules USP—Preserve in well-closed containers. Contain the labeled amounts of secobarbital sodium and amobarbital sodium, within ± 10%. Meet the requirements for Identification, Dissolution (60% of each active ingredient in 60 minutes in water in Apparatus 1 at 100 rpm), and Uniformity of dosage units.

SELEGILINE

Chemical name: Selegiline hydrochloride—(R)-$(-)$-N,2-Dimethyl-N-2-propynylphenethylamine hydrochloride.

Molecular formula: Selegiline hydrochloride—$C_{13}H_{17}N \cdot HCl$.

Molecular weight: Selegiline hydrochloride—223.75.

Description: Selegiline hydrochloride—White to near white, crystalline powder.

Solubility: Selegiline hydrochloride—Freely soluble in water, in chloroform, and in methanol.

USP requirements: Selegiline Hydrochloride Tablets—Not in USP.

SELENIOUS ACID

Chemical name: Selenium dioxide, monohydrated.

Molecular formula: H_2SeO_3.

Molecular weight: 128.97.

USP requirements: Selenious Acid Injection USP—Preserve in single-dose or in multiple-dose containers, preferably of Type I or Type II glass. A sterile solution in Water for Injection of Selenious Acid or of selenium dissolved in nitric acid. Label the Injection to indicate that it is to be diluted to the appropriate strength with Sterile Water for Injection or other suitable fluid prior to administration. Contains an amount of selenious acid equivalent to the labeled amount of selenium, within ± 5%. Meets the requirements for Identification, Bacterial endotoxins, pH (1.8–2.4), Particulate matter, and Injections.

SELENIUM SULFIDE

Chemical name: Selenium sulfide (SeS_2).

Molecular formula: SeS_2.

Molecular weight: 143.08.

Description: Selenium Sulfide USP—Reddish brown to bright orange powder, having not more than a faint odor.

Solubility: Selenium Sulfide USP—Practically insoluble in water and in organic solvents.

USP requirements: Selenium Sulfide Lotion USP—Preserve in tight containers. An aqueous, stabilized suspension of Selenium Sulfide. Contains the labeled amount, within ± 10%. Contains suitable buffering and dispersing agents. Meets the requirements for Identification and pH (2.0–6.0).

Note: Where labeled for use as a shampoo, it contains a detergent. Where labeled for other uses, it may contain a detergent.

SELENOMETHIONINE SE 75

Chemical name: Butanoic acid, 2-amino-4-(methylseleno-^{75}Se)-, (S)-.

Molecular formula: $C_5H_{11}NO_2{}^{75}Se$.

Description: Selenomethionine Se 75 Injection USP—Clear, colorless to pale yellow liquid.

USP requirements: Selenomethionine Se 75 Injection USP—Preserve in single-dose or in multiple-dose containers, at a temperature between 2 and 8 °C, unless otherwise specified by the manufacturer. A sterile, aqueous solution of radioactive L-selenomethionine which is the analog of the essential amino acid, methionine, in which the sulfur atom is replaced by a selenium atom. Label it to include the following, in addition to the information specified for Labeling under Injections: the date of calibration; the amount of ^{75}Se as selenomethionine expressed as total megabecquerels (or microcuries or millicuries), and concentration as megabecquerels (or microcuries or millicuries) per mL at the time of calibration; the expiration date; and the statement, "Caution—Radioactive Material." The labeling indicates that in making dosage calculations, correction is to be made for radioactive decay, and also indicates that the radioactive half-life of ^{75}Se is 120 days. Contains the labeled amount of ^{75}Se, within ± 10%, expressed in megabecquerels (or microcuries or millicuries) per mL at the time indicated in the labeling. Its specific activity is not less than 37.0 MBq (1.0 millicurie) per mg of selenium at the time of manufacture. Meets the requirements for Radionuclide identification, Bacterial endotoxins, pH (3.5–8.0), Radiochemical purity, and Injections (except that it is not subject to the recommendation on Volume in Container).

SENNA

Source: Dried leaflet of *Cassia acutifolia* or *Cassia angustifolia*; main active cathartic principles are sennosides A and B.
   Standardized senna concentrate—Standardized powder from deseeded, ground senna pod.
   Standardized extract of senna fruit—Hydroalcoholic extract of senna pod.

Chemical group: Anthraquinones.

USP requirements:
   Senna Fluidextract USP—Preserve in tight, light-resistant containers, and avoid exposure to direct sunlight and excessive heat.

   Prepare Senna Fluidextract as follows: Mix 1000 grams of Senna, in coarse powder, with a sufficient quantity (600 mL to 800 mL) of menstruum consisting of a mixture of 1 volume of alcohol and 2 volumes of water to make it evenly and distinctly damp. After 15 minutes, pack the mixture firmly into a suitable percolator, and cover the drug with additional menstruum. Macerate for 24 hours, then percolate at a moderate rate, adding fresh menstruum, until the drug is practically exhausted of its active principles. Reserve the first 800 mL of percolate, and use it to dissolve the residue from the additional percolate that has been concentrated to a soft extract at a temperature not to exceed 60 °C. Add water and alcohol to make the product measure 1000 mL, and mix.

   Meets the requirement for Alcohol content (23.0–27.0%).

   Senna Granules—Not in USP.
   Senna Oral Solution—Not in USP.
   Senna Suppositories—Not in USP.
   Senna Syrup USP—Preserve in tight containers, at a temperature not exceeding 25 °C.

Prepare Senna Syrup as follows: 250 mL of Senna Fluidextract, Suitable essential oil(s), 635 grams of Sucrose, and a sufficient quantity of Purified Water to make 1000 mL. Mix the oil(s) with the Senna Fluidextract, and gradually add 330 mL of Purified Water. Allow the mixture to stand for 24 hours in a cool place, with occasional agitation, then filter, and pass enough Purified Water through the filter to obtain 580 mL of filtrate. Dissolve the Sucrose in this liquid, and add sufficient Purified Water to make the product measure 1000 mL. Mix, and strain.

Meets the requirement for Alcohol content (5.0–7.0%).

Senna Tablets—Not in USP.

SENNA AND DOCUSATE

For *Senna* and *Docusate*—See individual listings for chemistry information.

USP requirements: Senna and Docusate Sodium Tablets—Not in USP.

SENNOSIDES

Chemical group: Anthraquinones.

Description: Brownish powder.

USP requirements: Sennosides Tablets USP—Preserve in well-closed containers. Contain the labeled amount, within ±10%. Meet the requirements for Identification, Dissolution (75% in 120 minutes in water in Apparatus 1 at 100 rpm), and Uniformity of dosage units.

SESAME OIL

Description: Sesame Oil NF—Pale yellow, oily liquid. Practically odorless.

NF category: Solvent; vehicle (oleaginous).

Solubility: Sesame Oil NF—Slightly soluble in alcohol. Miscible with ether, with chloroform, with solvent hexane, and with carbon disulfide.

NF requirements: Sesame Oil NF—Preserve in tight, light-resistant containers, and prevent exposure to excessive heat. It is the refined fixed oil obtained from the seed of one or more cultivated varieties of *Sesamum indicum* Linné (Fam. Pedaliaceae). Meets the requirements for Identification, Specific gravity (0.916–0.921), Heavy metals (not more than 0.001%), Cottonseed oil, Solidification range of fatty acids (20–25 °C), Free fatty acids, Iodine value (103–116), Saponification value (188–195), and Unsaponifiable matter (not more than 1.5%).

SHELLAC

Description: Shellac NF—
Orange Shellac: Thin, hard, brittle, transparent, pale lemon-yellow to brownish orange flakes, having little or no odor.
Bleached Shellac: Opaque, amorphous cream to yellow granules or coarse powder, having little or no odor.
NF category: Coating agent.

Solubility: Shellac NF—Insoluble in water; very slowly soluble in alcohol, 85 to 95% (w/w); in ether, 13 to 15%; in petroleum ether, 2 to 6%; soluble in aqueous solutions of ethanolamines, alkalies, and borax; sparingly soluble in oil of turpentine.

NF requirements: Shellac NF—Preserve in well-closed containers, preferably in a cold place. It is obtained by the

purification of Lac, the resinous secretion of the insect *Laccifer Lacca Kerr* (Fam. Coccidae). Orange Shellac is produced either by a process of filtration in the molten state, or by hot solvent process, or both. Orange Shellac may retain most of its wax or be dewaxed, and may contain lesser amounts of the natural color than originally present. Bleached (White) Shellac is prepared by dissolving the Lac in aqueous sodium carbonate, bleaching the solution with sodium hypochlorite and precipitating the Bleached Shellac with 2 N sulfuric acid. Removal of the wax, by filtration, during the process results in Refined Bleached Shellac. Label it to indicate whether it is bleached or is orange, and whether it is dewaxed or wax-containing. Meets the requirements for Identification, Loss on drying, Arsenic (not more than 1.5 ppm), Heavy metals (not more than 0.001%), Acid value, Wax, and Rosin. Shellac conforms to the specifications in the accompanying table.

	Acid value (on dried basis)	Loss on drying	Wax
Orange Shellac	between 68 and 76	not more than 2.0%	not more than 5.5%
Dewaxed Orange Shellac	between 71 and 79	not more than 2.0%	not more than 0.2%
Regular Bleached Shellac	between 73 and 89	not more than 6.0%	not more than 5.5%
Refined Bleached Shellac	between 75 and 91	not more than 6.0%	not more than 0.2%

PURIFIED SILICEOUS EARTH

Description: Purified Siliceous Earth NF—Very fine, white, light gray, or pale buff mixture of amorphous powder and lesser amounts of crystalline polymorphs, including quartz and cristobalite. It is gritty, readily absorbs moisture, and retains about 4 times its weight of water without becoming fluid.

NF category: Filtering aid; sorbent.

Solubility: Purified Siliceous Earth NF—Insoluble in water, in acids, and in dilute solutions of alkali hydroxides.

NF requirements: Purified Siliceous Earth NF—Preserve in well-closed containers. A form of silica (SiO_2) consisting of the frustules and fragments of diatoms, purified by calcining. Meets the requirements for Loss on drying (not more than 0.5%), Loss on ignition (not more than 2.0%), Acid-soluble substances (not more than 2.0%), Water-soluble substances (not more than 0.2%), Leachable arsenic (not more than 0.001%), Leachable lead (not more than 0.001%), and Non-siliceous substances.

SILICON DIOXIDE

Molecular formula: $SiO_2 xH_2O$.

Molecular weight: 60.08 (anhydrous).

Description: Silicon Dioxide NF—Fine, white, hygroscopic, odorless, amorphous powder, in which the diameter of the average particles ranges between 2 and 10 micrometers.

NF category: Desiccant; suspending and/or viscosity-increasing agent.

Solubility: Silicon Dioxide NF—Insoluble in water, in alcohol, and in other organic solvents; soluble in hot solutions of alkali hydroxides.

NF requirements: Silicon Dioxide NF—Preserve in tight containers, protected from moisture. It is obtained by insolubilizing the dissolved silica in sodium silicate solution. Where obtained by addition of sodium silicate to a mineral acid, the product is termed silica gel; where obtained by the destabilization of a solution of sodium silicate in such manner as to yield very fine particles, the product is termed precipitated silica. Label it to state whether it is silica gel or precipitated silica. After ignition at 1000 °C for not less than 1 hour, contains not less than 99.0% of anhydrous silicon dioxide. Meets the requirements for Identification, pH (4–8, in a slurry [1 in 20]), Loss on drying (not more than 5.0%), Loss on ignition (not more than 8.5%), Chloride (not more than 0.1%), Sulfate (not more than 0.5%), Arsenic (not more than 3 ppm), and Heavy metals (not more than 0.003%).

COLLOIDAL SILICON DIOXIDE

Chemical name: Silica.

Molecular formula: SiO_2.

Molecular weight: 60.08.

Description: Colloidal Silicon Dioxide NF—Light, white, nongritty powder of extremely fine particle size (about 15 nm).
   NF category: Glidant and/or anticaking agent; suspending and/or viscosity-increasing agent.

Solubility: Colloidal Silicon Dioxide NF—Insoluble in water and in acid (except hydrofluoric); soluble in hot solutions of alkali hydroxides.

NF requirements: Colloidal Silicon Dioxide NF—Preserve in well-closed containers. A submicroscopic fumed silica prepared by the vapor-phase hydrolysis of a silicon compound. When ignited at 1000 °C for 2 hours, contains not less than 99.0% and not more than 100.5% of silicon dioxide. Meets the requirements for Identification, pH (3.5–4.4, in a 1 in 25 dispersion), Loss on drying (not more than 2.5%), Loss on ignition (not more than 2.0%), and Arsenic (not more than 8 ppm).

SILVER NITRATE

Chemical name: Nitric acid silver(1+) salt.

Molecular formula: $AgNO_3$.

Molecular weight: 169.87.

Description: Silver Nitrate USP—Colorless or white crystals. The pH of its solutions is about 5.5. On exposure to light in the presence of organic matter, it becomes gray or grayish black.

Solubility: Silver Nitrate USP—Very soluble in water and even more so in boiling water; sparingly soluble in alcohol; freely soluble in boiling alcohol; slightly soluble in ether.

USP requirements: Silver Nitrate Ophthalmic Solution USP—Preserve it protected from light, in inert, collapsible capsules or in other suitable single-dose containers. A solution of Silver Nitrate in a water medium. The solution may be buffered by the addition of Sodium Acetate. Contains the labeled amount, within ±5%. Meets the requirements for Clarity and color of solution, Identification, Sterility, and pH (4.5–6.0).

SILVER SULFADIAZINE

Chemical group: Metal sulfanilamide derivative.

Chemical name: Benzenesulfonamide, 4-amino-*N*-2-pyrimidinyl-, monosilver(1+) salt.

Molecular formula: $C_{10}H_9AgN_4O_2S$.

Molecular weight: 357.13.

Description: Silver Sulfadiazine USP—White to creamy-white, crystalline powder, odorless to having a slight odor. Is stable in air, but turns yellow on exposure to light.

Solubility: Silver Sulfadiazine USP—Slightly soluble in acetone; practically insoluble in alcohol, in chloroform, and in ether; freely soluble in 30% ammonium solution; decomposes in moderately strong mineral acids.

Other characteristics: Sulfonamides have certain chemical similarities to some goitrogens, diuretics (acetazolamide and thiazides), and oral antidiabetic agents.

USP requirements: Silver Sulfadiazine Cream USP—Preserve in collapsible tubes or in tight, light-resistant containers. Contains the labeled amount, within ±10%. Meets the requirements for Identification, Microbial limits, Minimum fill, and pH (4.0–7.0, determined in the supernatant liquid obtained from a 1 in 20 mixture of the Cream in water).

SIMETHICONE

Chemical name: Simethicone.

Description: Simethicone USP—Translucent, gray, viscous fluid.
   NF category: Antifoaming agent; water-repelling agent.

Solubility: Simethicone USP—Insoluble in water and in alcohol. The liquid phase is soluble in chloroform and in ether, but silicon dioxide remains as a residue in these solvents.

USP requirements:
   Simethicone USP—Preserve in tight containers. A mixture of fully methylated linear siloxane polymers containing repeating units of the formula $[-(CH_3)_2SiO-]_n$, stabilized with trimethylsiloxy end-blocking units of the formula $[(CH_3)_3SiO-]$, and silicon dioxide. Contains not less than 90.5% and not more than 99.0% of polydimethylsiloxane, and not less than 4.0% and not more than 7.0% of silicon dioxide. Meets the requirements for Identification, Loss on heating (not more than 18.0%), Heavy metals (not more than 0.001%), Defoaming activity (not more than 15 seconds), and Silicon dioxide content.
   Simethicone Capsules USP—Preserve in well-closed containers. Contain an amount of polydimethylsiloxane equivalent to the labeled amount of simethicone, within ±15%. Meet the requirements for Identification, Disintegration (30 minutes), Uniformity of dosage units, and Defoaming activity.
   Simethicone Emulsion USP—Preserve in tight containers. A water-dispersible form of Simethicone composed of Simethicone, suitable emulsifiers, preservatives, and water. Contains an amount of polydimethylsiloxane equivalent to the labeled amount of simethicone, within −15% to +10%. Meets the requirements for Identification, Microbial limit (total aerobic microbial count not more than 100 per gram), Heavy metals (not more than 0.001%), and Defoaming activity (not more than 15 seconds).
   Simethicone Oral Suspension USP—Preserve in tight, light-resistant containers. A suspension of Simethicone in Water. Contains an amount of polydimethylsiloxane equivalent to the labeled amount of simethicone, within ±15%. Meets the requirements for Identification, pH (4.4–4.6), and Defoaming activity (not more than 45 seconds).
   Simethicone Tablets USP—Preserve in well-closed containers. Contain an amount of polydimethylsiloxane equivalent to the labeled amount of simethicone, within ±15%. Meet the requirements for Identification, Disintegration (30 minutes), Defoaming activity, and Uniformity of dosage units.

SIMETHICONE, ALUMINA, CALCIUM CARBONATE, AND MAGNESIA

For *Simethicone, Alumina* (Aluminum Hydroxide), *Calcium Carbonate,* and *Magnesia* (Magnesium Hydroxide)—See individual listings for chemistry information.

USP requirements: Simethicone, Alumina, Calcium Carbonate, and Magnesia Chewable Tablets—Not in USP.

SIMETHICONE, ALUMINA, MAGNESIUM CARBONATE, AND MAGNESIA

For *Simethicone, Alumina* (Aluminum Hydroxide), *Magnesium Carbonate,* and *Magnesia* (Magnesium Hydroxide)—See individual listings for chemistry information.

USP requirements: Simethicone, Alumina, Magnesium Carbonate, and Magnesia Chewable Tablets—Not in USP.

SIMVASTATIN

Chemical name: Butanoic acid, 2,2-dimethyl-, 1,2,3,7,8,8a-hexahydro-3,7-dimethyl-8-[2-(tetrahydro-4-hydroxy-6-oxo-2*H*-pyran-2-yl)ethyl]-1-naphthalenyl ester, [1*S*-[1 alpha,3 alpha,7 beta,8 beta(2*S**,4*S**),8a beta]]-.

Molecular formula: $C_{25}H_{38}O_5$.

Molecular weight: 418.57.

Description: White, crystalline powder.

Solubility: Soluble in chloroform (610 mg/mL), in methanol (200 mg/mL), in ethanol (160 mg/mL), and in water (0.03 mg/mL).

USP requirements: Simvastatin Tablets—Not in USP.

SISOMICIN

Chemical name: Sisomicin sulfate—D-Streptamine, (2*S-cis*)-4-*O*-[3-amino-6-(aminomethyl)-3,4-dihydro-2*H*-pyran-2-yl]-2-deoxy-6-*O*-[3-deoxy-4-*C*-methyl-3-(methylamino)-beta-L-arabinopyranosyl]-, sulfate (2:5) (salt).

Molecular formula: Sisomicin sulfate—$(C_{19}H_{37}N_5O_7)_2 \cdot 5H_2SO_4$.

Molecular weight: Sisomicin sulfate—1385.43.

USP requirements: Sisomicin Sulfate Injection USP—Preserve in single-dose or in multiple-dose containers, preferably of Type I glass. A sterile solution of Sisomicin Sulfate in Water for Injection. Contains an amount of sisomicin sulfate equivalent to the labeled amount of sisomicin, within −10% to +20%. Meets the requirements for Identification, Bacterial endotoxins, pH (2.5–5.5), and Injections.

SMALLPOX VACCINE

Description: Smallpox Vaccine USP—Liquid vaccine is a turbid, whitish to greenish suspension, which may have a slight odor due to the antimicrobial agent. Dried vaccine is a yellow to grayish pellet, which may or may not become fragmented when shaken.

USP requirements: Smallpox Vaccine USP—Preserve and dispense in the containers in which it was placed by the manufacturer. Keep liquid Vaccine during storage and in shipment at a temperature below 0 °C. Keep dried Vaccine at a temperature between 2 and 8 °C. A suspension or solid containing the living virus of vaccinia of a strain of approved origin and manipulation, that has been grown in the skin of a vaccinated bovine calf. Label it to state that it contains not more than 200 microorganisms per mL in the case of

Vaccine intended for multiple-puncture administration, or that it contains not more than 1 microorganism per 100 doses in the case of Vaccine intended for jet injection, unless it meets the requirements for sterility. In the case of Vaccine intended for jet injection, so state on the label. In the case of dried Vaccine, label it to state that after constitution it is to be well shaken before use. Label it also to state that it was prepared in the bovine calf. Meets the requirements of the specific potency test using embryonated chicken eggs in comparison with the U.S. Reference Smallpox Vaccine in the case of Vaccine intended for multiple-puncture administration or with such Reference Vaccine diluted (1:30) in the case of Vaccine intended for jet injection, and the requirements for the tests for absence of specific microorganisms. Meets the requirement for Expiration date (for liquid Vaccine, not later than 3 months after date of issue from manufacturer's cold storage [−10° C, 9 months as glycerinated or equivalent preparation]; for dried Vaccine, not later than 18 months after date of issue from manufacturer's cold storage [5 °C, 6 months]). Conforms to the regulations of the U.S. Food and Drug Administration concerning biologics.

SODA LIME

Description: Soda Lime NF—White or grayish white granules. It may have a color if an indicator has been added.

NF category: Sorbent, carbon dioxide.

NF requirements: Soda Lime NF—A mixture of Calcium Hydroxide and Sodium or Potassium Hydroxide or both. May contain an indicator that is inert toward anesthetic gases such as Ether, Cyclopropane, and Nitrous Oxide, and that changes color when the Soda Lime no longer can absorb Carbon Dioxide. Meets the requirements for Identification, Loss on drying (12.0 to 19.0%), Moisture absorption (increase in weight not more than 7.5%), Hardness, and Carbon dioxide absorbency (not less than 19.0%), and for Packaging and storage, Labeling, and Size of granules under Barium Hydroxide Lime.

SODIUM ACETATE

Chemical name: Acetic acid, sodium salt, trihydrate.

Molecular formula: $C_2H_3NaO_2 \cdot 3H_2O$ (hydrate); $C_2H_3NaO_2$ (anhydrous).

Molecular weight: 136.08 (hydrate); 82.03 (anhydrous).

Description: Sodium Acetate USP—Colorless, transparent crystals, or white, granular crystalline powder, or white flakes. It is odorless, or has a faint, acetous odor. Efflorescent in warm, dry air.

NF category: Buffering agent.

Solubility: Sodium Acetate USP—Very soluble in water; soluble in alcohol.

USP requirements:
Sodium Acetate USP—Preserve in tight containers. Contains 3 molecules of water of hydration, or is anhydrous. Contains not less than 99.0% and not more than 101.0% of sodium acetate, calculated on the dried basis. Label it to indicate whether it is the trihydrate or is anhydrous. Where Sodium Acetate is intended for use in hemodialysis, it is so labeled. Meets the requirements for Identification, pH (7.5–9.2, in a solution in carbon dioxide–free water containing the equivalent of 30 mg of anhydrous sodium acetate per mL), Loss on drying (38.0–41.0% for the hydrous, not more than 1.0% for the anhydrous), Insoluble matter (not more than 0.05%), Chloride (not more than 0.035%), Sulfate (not more than

0.005%), Arsenic (not more than 3 ppm), Calcium and magnesium, Potassium, Heavy metals (not more than 0.001%), and Aluminum (not more than 0.2 ppm).

Sodium Acetate Injection USP—Preserve in single-dose containers, preferably of Type I glass. A sterile solution of Sodium Acetate in Water for Injection. The label states the sodium acetate content in terms of weight and of milliequivalents in a given volume. Label the Injection to indicate that it is to be diluted to appropriate strength with water or other suitable fluid prior to administration. The label states also the total osmolar concentration in mOsmol per liter. Where the contents are less than 100 mL, or where the label states that the Injection is not for direct injection but is to be diluted before use, the label alternatively may state the total osmolar concentration in mOsmol per mL. Contains the labeled amount, within ±5%. Meets the requirements for Identification, Bacterial endotoxins, pH (6.0–7.0), Particulate matter, and Injections.

Sodium Acetate Solution USP—Preserve in tight containers. An aqueous solution of Sodium Acetate. Contains the labeled amount, within ±3% (w/w). Meets the requirements for Identification, pH (7.5–9.2, when diluted with carbon dioxide–free water to contain 5% of solids), Insoluble matter (not more than 0.005%), Chloride (not more than 0.035%), Sulfate (not more than 0.005%), Arsenic (not more than 3 ppm), Calcium and magnesium, Potassium, and Heavy metals (not more than 0.001%).

SODIUM ALGINATE

Chemical name: Alginic acid, sodium salt.

Description: Sodium Alginate NF—Practically odorless, coarse or fine powder, yellowish white in color.

NF category: Suspending and/or viscosity-increasing agent.

Solubility: Sodium Alginate NF—Soluble in water, forming a viscous, colloidal solution; insoluble in alcohol and in hydroalcoholic solutions in which the alcohol content is greater than about 30% by weight; insoluble in chloroform, in ether, and in acids when the pH of the resulting solution becomes lower than about 3.

NF requirements: Sodium Alginate NF—Preserve in tight containers. It is the purified carbohydrate product extracted from brown seaweeds by the use of dilute alkali. Consists chiefly of the sodium salt of Alginic Acid, a polyuronic acid composed of beta-D-mannuronic acid residues linked so that the carboxyl group of each unit is free while the aldehyde group is shielded by a glycosidic linkage. Contains not less than 90.8% and not more than 106.0% of sodium alginate of average equivalent weight 222.00, calculated on the dried basis. Meets the requirements for Identification, Microbial limits, Loss on drying (not more than 15.0%), Ash (18.0–24.0%), Arsenic (not more than 1.5 ppm), Lead (not more than 0.001%), and Heavy metals (not more than 0.004%).

SODIUM ASCORBATE

Chemical name: L-Ascorbic acid, monosodium salt.

Molecular formula: $C_6H_7NaO_6$.

Molecular weight: 198.11.

Description: Sodium Ascorbate USP—White or very faintly yellow crystals or crystalline powder. Is odorless or practically odorless. Is relatively stable in air. On exposure to light it gradually darkens.

Solubility: Sodium Ascorbate USP—Freely soluble in water; very slightly soluble in alcohol; insoluble in chloroform and in ether.

USP requirements: Sodium Ascorbate Injection—Not in USP.

SODIUM BENZOATE

Chemical name: Benzoic acid, sodium salt.

Molecular formula: $C_7H_5NaO_2$.

Molecular weight: 144.11.

Description: Sodium Benzoate NF—White, odorless or practically odorless, granular or crystalline powder. It is stable in air.

NF category: Antimicrobial preservative.

Solubility: Sodium Benzoate NF—Freely soluble in water; sparingly soluble in alcohol, and somewhat more soluble in 90% alcohol.

NF requirements: Sodium Benzoate NF—Preserve in well-closed containers. Contains not less than 99.0% and not more than 100.5% of sodium benzoate. Meets the requirements for Identification, Alkalinity, Water (not more than 1.5%), Arsenic (not more than 3 ppm), and Heavy metals (not more than 0.001%).

SODIUM BENZOATE AND SODIUM PHENYLACETATE

Chemical name:
Sodium benzoate—Benzoic acid, sodium salt.
Sodium phenylacetate—Benzeneacetic acid, sodium salt.

Molecular formula:
Sodium benzoate—$C_7H_5NaO_2$.
Sodium phenylacetate—$C_8H_7NaO_2$.

Molecular weight:
Sodium benzoate—144.11.
Sodium phenylacetate—158.13.

Description: Sodium Benzoate NF—White, odorless or practically odorless, granular or crystalline powder. It is stable in air.

NF category: Antimicrobial preservative.

Solubility: Sodium Benzoate NF—Freely soluble in water; sparingly soluble in alcohol, and somewhat more soluble in 90% alcohol.

Other characteristics: The pH of the undiluted sodium benzoate and sodium phenylacetate combination solution is approximately 6.0.

USP requirements: Sodium Benzoate and Sodium Phenylacetate Oral Solution—Not in USP.

SODIUM BICARBONATE

Chemical name: Carbonic acid monosodium salt.

Molecular formula: $NaHCO_3$.

Molecular weight: 84.01.

Description: Sodium Bicarbonate USP—White, crystalline powder. Is stable in dry air, but slowly decomposes in moist air. Its solutions, when freshly prepared with cold water, without shaking, are alkaline to litmus. The alkalinity increases as the solutions stand, as they are agitated, or as they are heated.

NF category: Alkalizing agent.

Solubility: Sodium Bicarbonate USP—Soluble in water; insoluble in alcohol.

USP requirements:
Sodium Bicarbonate USP—Preserve in well-closed containers. Contains not less than 99.0% and not more than 100.5% of sodium bicarbonate, calculated on the dried basis. Meets the requirements for Identification, Loss on drying (not more than 0.25%), Insoluble substances, Carbonate (where it is labeled as intended for use in hemodialysis, not more than 0.23%), Normal carbonate, Chloride (not more than 0.015%), Sulfate (not more than 0.015%), Ammonia, Aluminum (where it is labeled as intended for use in hemodialysis, not more than 2 ppm), Arsenic (not more than 2 ppm), Calcium and magnesium (where it is labeled as intended for use in hemodialysis, not more than 0.01% for calcium, and not more than 0.004% for magnesium), Copper (where it is labeled as intended for use in hemodialysis, not more than 1 ppm), Iron (where it is labeled as intended for use in hemodialysis, not more than 5 ppm), Heavy metals (not more than 5 ppm), and Organics (where it is labeled as intended for use in hemodialysis, not more than 0.01%).
Effervescent Sodium Bicarbonate—Not in USP.
Sodium Bicarbonate Injection USP—Preserve in single-dose containers, of Type I glass. A sterile solution of Sodium Bicarbonate in Water for Injection, the pH of which may be adjusted by means of Carbon Dioxide. The label states the total osmolar concentration in mOsmol per liter. Where the contents are less than 100 mL, or where the label states that the Injection is not for direct injection, but is to be diluted before use, the label alternatively may state the total osmolar concentration in mOsmol per mL. Contains the labeled amount, within ±5%. Meets the requirements for Identification, Bacterial endotoxins, pH (7.0–8.5), Particulate matter, and Injections.
Note: Do not use the Injection if it contains a precipitate.
Sodium Bicarbonate Oral Powder USP—Preserve in well-closed containers. Contains Sodium Bicarbonate and suitable added substances. Label Oral Powder to indicate that it is for oral use only. Contains not less than 98.5% and not more than 100.5% of sodium bicarbonate, calculated on the dried basis. Meets the requirements for Identification and Loss on drying under Sodium Bicarbonate.
Sodium Bicarbonate Tablets USP—Preserve in well-closed containers. Contain the labeled amount, within ±5%. Meet the requirements for Identification, Disintegration (30 minutes, simulated gastric fluid TS being substituted for water in the test), and Uniformity of dosage units.

SODIUM BORATE

Chemical name: Borax.

Molecular formula: $Na_2B_4O_7 \cdot 10H_2O$.

Molecular weight: 381.37.

Description: Sodium Borate NF—Colorless, transparent crystals or white crystalline powder. It is odorless. Its solutions are alkaline to phenolphthalein TS. As it effloresces in warm, dry air, the crystals are often coated with white powder.
NF category: Alkalizing agent.

Solubility: Sodium Borate NF—Soluble in water; freely soluble in boiling water and in glycerin; insoluble in alcohol.

NF requirements: Sodium Borate NF—Preserve in tight containers. Contains an amount of anhydrous sodium borate equivalent to not less than 99.0% and not more than 105.0% of hydrous sodium borate. Meets the requirements for Identification, Carbonate and bicarbonate, Arsenic (not more than 8 ppm), Heavy metals (not more than 0.002%), and Organic volatile impurities.

SODIUM CARBONATE

Chemical name: Carbonic acid, disodium salt.

Molecular formula: Na_2CO_3 (anhydrous); $Na_2CO_3 \cdot H_2O$ (monohydrate).

Molecular weight: 105.99 (anhydrous); 124.00 (monohydrate).

Description: Sodium Carbonate NF—Colorless crystals, or white crystalline powder or granules. Stable in air under ordinary conditions. When exposed to air above 50 °C, the hydrous salt effloresces and, at 100 °C, becomes anhydrous.
NF category: Alkalizing agent.

Solubility: Sodium Carbonate NF—Freely soluble in water, but still more soluble in boiling water.

NF requirements: Sodium Carbonate NF—Preserve in well-closed containers. It is anhydrous or contains one molecule of water of hydration. Label it to indicate whether it is anhydrous or hydrous. Contains not less than 99.5% and not more than 100.5% of sodium carbonate, calculated on the anhydrous basis. Meets the requirements for Identification, Water (for the anhydrous form, not more than 0.5%; for the hydrous form, 12.0–15.0%), Arsenic (not more than 3 ppm), Heavy metals (not more than 0.001%), and Organic volatile impurities.

SODIUM CHLORIDE

Chemical name: Sodium chloride.

Molecular formula: NaCl.

Molecular weight: 58.44.

Description:
Sodium Chloride USP—Colorless, cubic crystals or white crystalline powder.
NF category: Tonicity agent.
Sodium Chloride Inhalation Solution USP—Clear, colorless solution.
Bacteriostatic Sodium Chloride Injection USP—Clear, colorless solution, odorless or having the odor of the bacteriostatic substance.
NF category: Vehicle (sterile).
Sodium Chloride Irrigation USP—Clear, colorless solution.

Solubility: Sodium Chloride USP—Freely soluble in water; and slightly more soluble in boiling water; soluble in glycerin; slightly soluble in alcohol.

USP requirements:
Sodium Chloride USP—Preserve in well-closed containers. Where Sodium Chloride is intended for use in hemodialysis, it is so labeled. Contains not less than 99.0% and not more than 101.0% of sodium chloride, calculated on the dried basis. Contains no added substance. Meets the requirements for Identification, Acidity or alkalinity, Loss on drying (not more than 0.5%), Arsenic (not more than 3 ppm), Barium, Iodide or bromide, Calcium and magnesium (not more than 0.005%), Iron (not more than 2 ppm), Sulfate (not more than 0.015%), Sodium ferrocyanide, Aluminum (where it is labeled as intended for use in hemodialysis, not more than 0.2 ppm), and Heavy metals (not more than 5 ppm).
Sodium Chloride Injection USP—Preserve in single-dose glass or plastic containers. Glass containers are preferably of Type I or Type II glass. A sterile solution of Sodium Chloride in Water for Injection. Contains no antimicrobial agents. The label states the total osmolar concentration in mOsmol per liter. Where the contents are less than

100 mL, or where the label states that the Injection is not for direct injection but is to be diluted before use, the label alternatively may state the total osmolar concentration in mOsmol per mL. Contains the labeled amount, within ±5%. Meets the requirements for Identification, Bacterial endotoxins, pH (4.5–7.0), Particulate matter, Iron (not more than 2 ppm), Heavy metals (not more than 0.001%, based on amount of sodium chloride), and Injections.

Bacteriostatic Sodium Chloride Injection USP—Preserve in single-dose or in multiple-dose containers, of not larger than 30-mL size, preferably of Type I or Type II glass. A sterile, isotonic solution of Sodium Chloride in Water for Injection, containing one or more suitable antimicrobial agents. Label it to indicate the name(s) and proportion(s) of the added antimicrobial agent(s). Label it also to include the statement, "NOT FOR USE IN NEWBORNS," in boldface capital letters, on the label immediately under the official name, printed in a contrasting color, preferably red. Alternatively, the statement may be placed prominently elsewhere on the label if the statement is enclosed within a box. Contains not less than 0.85% and not more than 0.95% of sodium chloride. Meets the requirements for Antimicrobial agent(s), Bacterial endotoxins, and Particulate matter, for Identification test, pH, Iron, and Heavy metals under Sodium Chloride Injection, and for Injections.

Note: Use Bacteriostatic Sodium Chloride Injection with due regard for the compatibility of the antimicrobial agent or agents it contains with the particular medicinal substance that is to be dissolved or diluted.

Sodium Chloride Irrigation USP—Preserve in single-dose glass or plastic containers. Glass containers are preferably of Type I or Type II glass. The container may be designed to empty rapidly and may contain a volume of more than 1 liter. It is Sodium Chloride Injection that has been suitably packaged, and it contains no antimicrobial agents. The designation "not for injection" appears prominently on the label. Contains the labeled amount, within ±5%. Meets the requirements for Identification, Bacterial endotoxins, and Sterility, and for pH, Iron, and Heavy metals under Sodium Chloride Injection.

Sodium Chloride Ophthalmic Ointment USP—Preserve in collapsible ophthalmic ointment tubes. It is Sodium Chloride in a suitable ophthalmic ointment base. Contains the labeled amount, within ±10%. Meets the requirements for Identification, Sterility, Minimum fill, and Particulate matter.

Sodium Chloride Inhalation Solution USP—Preserve in single-dose containers. A sterile solution of Sodium Chloride in water purified by distillation or by reverse osmosis and rendered sterile. Contains the labeled amount, within ±10%. Contains no antimicrobial agents or other added substances. Meets the requirements for Identification, Sterility, and pH (4.5–7.0).

Sodium Chloride Ophthalmic Solution USP—Preserve in tight containers. A sterile solution of Sodium Chloride. Contains the labeled amount, within ±10%. Contains a buffer. Meets the requirements for Identification, Sterility, and pH (6.0–8.0).

Sodium Chloride Tablets USP—Preserve in well-closed containers. Contain the labeled amount, within ±5%. Meet the requirements for Identification, Iodide or bromide, Barium, Calcium and magnesium, Disintegration (30 minutes), and Uniformity of dosage units.

Sodium Chloride Tablets for Solution USP—Composed of Sodium Chloride in compressed form, containing no added substance. Contain the labeled amount, within ±5%. Meet the requirements for Identification test, Packaging and storage, Iodide or bromide, Barium, Calcium and magnesium, Disintegration, and Uniformity of dosage units under Sodium Chloride Tablets.

SODIUM CHLORIDE AND DEXTROSE

For *Sodium Chloride* and *Dextrose*—See individual listings for chemistry information.

USP requirements: Sodium Chloride and Dextrose Tablets USP—Preserve in well-closed containers. Contain the labeled amounts, within ±7.5%. Meet the requirements for Identification, Disintegration (30 minutes), and Uniformity of dosage units.

SODIUM CHROMATE Cr 51

Chemical name: Chromic acid ($H_2{}^{51}CrO_4$), disodium salt.

Molecular formula: $Na_2{}^{51}CrO_4$.

Description: Sodium Chromate Cr 51 Injection USP—Clear, slightly yellow solution.

USP requirements: Sodium Chromate Cr 51 Injection USP—Preserve in single-dose or in multiple-dose containers. A sterile solution of radioactive chromium (^{51}Cr) processed in the form of sodium chromate in Water for Injection. For those uses where an isotonic solution is required, Sodium Chloride may be added in appropriate amounts. Chromium 51 is produced by the neutron bombardment of enriched chromium 50. Label it to include the following, in addition to the information specified for Labeling under Injections: the time and date of calibration; the amount of sodium chromate expressed in micrograms per mL; the amount of ^{51}Cr as sodium chromate expressed as total megabecquerels (or millicuries) and as megabecquerels (or millicuries) per mL at the time of calibration; a statement to indicate whether the contents are intended for diagnostic or therapeutic use; the expiration date; and the statement, "Caution—Radioactive Material." The labeling indicates that in making dosage calculations, correction is to be made for radioactive decay and the quantity of chromium, and also indicates that the radioactive half-life of ^{51}Cr is 27.8 days. Contains the labeled amount of ^{51}Cr, within ±10%, as sodium chromate expressed in megabecquerels (or millicuries) per mL at the time indicated in the labeling. The sodium chromate content is not less than 90.0% and not more than 110.0% of the labeled amount. The specific activity is not less than 370 megabecquerels (10 millicuries) per mg of sodium chromate at the end of the expiry period. Other chemical forms of radioactivity do not exceed 10.0% of the total radioactivity. Meets the requirements for Radionuclide identification, Bacterial endotoxins, pH (7.5–8.5), Radiochemical purity, and Injections (except that it is not subject to the recommendation on Volume in Container).

SODIUM CITRATE

Chemical name: 1,2,3-Propanetricarboxylic acid, 2-hydroxy-, trisodium salt.

Molecular formula: $C_6H_5Na_3O_7$ (anhydrous); $C_6H_5Na_3O_7\cdot2H_2O$ (hydrous).

Molecular weight: 258.07 (anhydrous); 294.10 (hydrous).

Description: Sodium Citrate USP—Colorless crystals or white, crystalline powder.
NF category: Buffering agent.

Solubility: Sodium Citrate USP—Hydrous form freely soluble in water and very soluble in boiling water. Insoluble in alcohol.

USP requirements: Sodium Citrate USP—Preserve in tight containers. It is anhydrous or contains 2 molecules of water of hydration. Label it to indicate whether it is anhydrous or hydrous. Contains not less than 99.0% and not more than 100.5% of sodium citrate, calculated on the anhydrous basis. Meets the requirements for Identification, Alkalinity, Water (10.0–13.0% for the hydrous form, not more than 1.0% for the anhydrous form), Tartrate, and Heavy metals (not more than 0.001%).

SODIUM CITRATE AND CITRIC ACID

For *Sodium Citrate* and *Citric Acid*—See individual listings for chemistry information.

Description: Sodium Citrate and Citric Acid Oral Solution USP—Clear solution having the color of any added preservative or flavoring agents.

USP requirements: Sodium Citrate and Citric Acid Oral Solution USP—Preserve in tight containers. A solution of Sodium Citrate and Citric Acid in a suitable aqueous medium. Contains, in each 100 mL, not less than 2.23 grams and not more than 2.46 grams of sodium, and not less than 6.11 grams and not more than 6.75 grams of citrate, equivalent to not less than 9.5 grams and not more than 10.5 grams of sodium citrate dihydrate; and not less than 6.34 grams and not more than 7.02 grams of citric acid monohydrate. Meets the requirements for Identification and pH (4.0–4.4).

SODIUM DEHYDROACETATE

Chemical name: 2*H*-Pyran-2,4(3*H*)-dione, 3-acetyl-6-methyl-, monosodium salt.

Molecular formula: $C_8H_7NaO_4$.

Molecular weight: 190.13.

Description: Sodium Dehydroacetate NF—White or practically white odorless powder.

NF category: Antimicrobial preservative.

Solubility: Sodium Dehydroacetate NF—Freely soluble in water, in propylene glycol, and in glycerin.

NF requirements: Sodium Dehydroacetate NF—Preserve in well-closed containers. Contains not less than 98.0% and not more than 100.5% of sodium dehydroacetate, calculated on the anhydrous basis. Meets the requirements for Identification, Water (8.5–10.0%), Arsenic (not more than 3 ppm), Heavy metals (not more than 0.001%), and Organic volatile impurities.

SODIUM FLUORIDE

Chemical name: Sodium fluoride.

Molecular formula: NaF.

Molecular weight: 41.99.

Description: Sodium Fluoride USP—White, odorless powder.

Solubility: Sodium Fluoride USP—Soluble in water; insoluble in alcohol.

USP requirements:
Sodium Fluoride Oral Solution USP—Preserve in tight containers, plastic containers being used for Oral Solution having a pH below 7.5. Label Oral Solution in terms of the content of sodium fluoride (NaF) and in terms of the content of fluoride ion. Contains the labeled amount, within ±10%. Meets the requirement for Identification.

Sodium Fluoride Tablets USP—Preserve in tight containers. Label Tablets in terms of the content of sodium fluoride (NaF) and in terms of the content of fluoride ion. Tablets that are to be chewed may be labeled as Sodium Fluoride Chewable Tablets. Contain the labeled amount, within ±10%. Meet the requirements for Identification, Disintegration (15 minutes), and Uniformity of dosage units.

SODIUM FLUORIDE AND PHOSPHORIC ACID

For *Sodium Fluoride* and *Phosphoric Acid*—See individual listings for chemistry information.

USP requirements:
Sodium Fluoride and Phosphoric Acid Gel USP—Preserve in tight, plastic containers. Label Gel in terms of the content of sodium fluoride (NaF) and in terms of the content of fluoride ion. Contains the labeled amount of fluoride ion, within ±10%, in an aqueous medium containing a suitable viscosity-inducing agent. Meets the requirements for Identification, Viscosity (7,000–20,000 centipoises), and pH (3.0–4.0).

Sodium Fluoride and Phosphoric Acid Topical Solution USP—Preserve in tight, plastic containers. Label Topical Solution in terms of the content of sodium fluoride (NaF) and in terms of the content of fluoride ion. Contains the labeled amount of fluoride ion, within ±10%. Meets the requirements for Identification tests and pH under Sodium Fluoride and Phosphoric Acid Gel.

SODIUM FORMALDEHYDE SULFOXYLATE

Chemical name: Methanesulfinic acid, hydroxy-, monosodium salt.

Molecular formula: CH_3NaO_3S.

Molecular weight: 118.08.

Description: Sodium Formaldehyde Sulfoxylate NF—White crystals or hard white masses, having the characteristic odor of garlic.

NF category: Antioxidant.

Solubility: Sodium Formaldehyde Sulfoxylate NF—Freely soluble in water; slightly soluble in alcohol, in ether, and in chloroform.

NF requirements: Sodium Formaldehyde Sulfoxylate NF—Preserve in well-closed, light-resistant containers, and store at controlled room temperature. Contains an amount of sodium formaldehyde sulfoxylate equivalent to not less than 45.5% and not more than 54.5% of sulfur dioxide, calculated on the dried basis. Meets the requirements for Clarity and color of solution, Identification, Alkalinity, pH (9.5–10.5, in a solution [1 in 50]), Loss on drying (not more than 27.0%), Sulfide, Iron (not more than 0.0025%), Sodium sulfite (not more than 5.0%, calculated on the dried basis), and Organic volatile impurities.

SODIUM HYDROXIDE

Chemical name: Sodium hydroxide.

Molecular formula: NaOH.

Molecular weight: 40.00.

Description: Sodium Hydroxide NF—White or practically white, fused masses, in small pellets, in flakes, or sticks, or in other forms. It is hard and brittle and shows a crystalline fracture. Exposed to the air, it rapidly absorbs carbon dioxide and moisture.

NF category: Alkalizing agent.

Solubility: Sodium Hydroxide NF—Freely soluble in water and in alcohol.

NF requirements: Sodium Hydroxide NF—Preserve in tight containers. Contains not less than 95.0% and not more than 100.5% of total alkali, calculated as sodium hydroxide, including not more than 3.0% of anhydrous sodium carbonate. Meets the requirements for Identification, Insoluble substances and organic matter, Potassium, and Heavy metals (not more than 0.003%).

Caution: Exercise great care in handling Sodium Hydroxide, as it rapidly destroys tissues.

SODIUM HYPOCHLORITE

Chemical name: Hypochlorous acid, sodium salt.

Molecular formula: NaClO.

Molecular weight: 74.44.

Description: Sodium Hypochlorite Solution USP—Clear, pale greenish yellow liquid, having the odor of chlorine. Affected by light.

USP requirements: Sodium Hypochlorite Solution USP—Preserve in tight, light-resistant containers, at a temperature not exceeding 25 °C. Contains not less than 4.0% and not more than 6.0%, by weight, of sodium hypochlorite. Meets the requirement for Identification.

Caution: This solution is not suitable for application to wounds.

SODIUM IODIDE

Chemical name: Sodium iodide.

Molecular formula: NaI.

Molecular weight: 149.89.

Description: Sodium Iodide USP—Colorless, odorless crystals, or white, crystalline powder. Is deliquescent in moist air, and develops a brown tint upon decomposition.

Solubility: Sodium Iodide USP—Very soluble in water; freely soluble in alcohol and in glycerin.

USP requirements: Sodium Iodide USP—Preserve in tight containers. Contains not less than 99.0% and not more than 101.5% of sodium iodide, calculated on the anhydrous basis. Meets the requirements for Identification, Alkalinity, Water (not more than 2.0%), Iodate, Nitrate, nitrite, and ammonia, Thiosulfate and barium, Potassium, Heavy metals (not more than 0.001%), and Organic volatile impurities.

SODIUM IODIDE I 123

Molecular formula: Na¹²³I.

Description:

Sodium Iodide I 123 Capsules USP—Capsules may contain a small amount of solid or solids, or may appear empty.

Sodium Iodide I 123 Solution USP—Clear, colorless solution. Upon standing, both the Solution and the glass container may darken as a result of the effects of the radiation.

USP requirements:

Sodium Iodide I 123 Capsules USP—Preserve in well-closed containers that are adequately shielded. Contain radioactive iodine (¹²³I) processed in the form of Sodium Iodide obtained from the bombardment of enriched tellurium 124 with protons or of enriched tellurium 122 with deuterons or by the decay of xenon 123 in such manner

that it is carrier-free. Label Capsules to include the following: the name of the Capsules; the name, address, and batch or lot number of the manufacturer; the time and date of calibration; the amount of ¹²³I as iodide expressed in megabecquerels (or microcuries or millicuries) per Capsule at the time of calibration; the name and quantity of any added preservative or stabilizer; a statement indicating that the Capsules are for oral use only; the expiration date and time; and the statement, "Caution—Radioactive Material." The labeling indicates that in making dosage calculations, correction is to be made for radioactive decay, and also indicates that the radioactive half-life of ¹²³I is 13.2 hours. Contain the labeled amount of ¹²³I, within ±10%, as iodide expressed in megabecquerels (or microcuries or millicuries) at the time indicated in the labeling. Other chemical forms of radioactivity do not exceed 5% of the total radioactivity. Meet the requirements for Radionuclide identification, Uniformity of dosage units, Radionuclidic purity (not less than 85.0%), and Radiochemical purity.

Sodium Iodide I 123 Solution USP—Preserve in single-dose or in multiple-dose containers that previously have been treated to prevent adsorption, if necessary. A solution, suitable for oral or for intravenous administration, containing radioactive iodine (¹²³I) processed in the form of Sodium Iodide, obtained from the bombardment of enriched tellurium 124 with protons or of enriched tellurium 122 with deuterons, or by the decay of xenon 123 in such manner that it is carrier-free. Label it to include the following: the time and date of calibration; the amount of ¹²³I as iodide expressed as total megabecquerels (or microcuries or millicuries) per mL at the time of calibration; the name and quantity of any added preservative or stabilizer; a statement indicating whether the contents are intended for oral or for intravenous use; the expiration date and time; and the statement, "Caution—Radioactive Material." The labeling indicates that in making dosage calculations, correction is to be made for radioactive decay, and also indicates that the radioactive half-life of ¹²³I is 13.2 hours. Contains the labeled amount of ¹²³I, within ±10%, as iodide expressed in megabecquerels (or microcuries or in millicuries) per mL at the time indicated in the labeling. Other chemical forms of radioactivity do not exceed 5% of the total radioactivity. Meets the requirements for Radionuclide identification, Radionuclidic purity (not less than 85.0%), Bacterial endotoxins, pH (7.5–9.0), Radiochemical purity, and Injections (if for intravenous use, except that it may be distributed or dispensed prior to completion of the test for Sterility, the latter test being started on the day of final manufacture, and except that it is not subject to the recommendation on Volume in Container).

SODIUM IODIDE I 125

Chemical name: Sodium iodide (Na¹²⁵I).

Molecular formula: Na¹²⁵I.

Description: Sodium Iodide I 125 Solution USP—Clear, colorless solution. Upon standing, both the Solution and the glass container may darken as a result of the effects of the radiation.

USP requirements:

Sodium Iodide I 125 Capsules USP—Preserve in well-closed containers that are adequately shielded. Contain radioactive iodine (¹²⁵I) processed in the form of Sodium Iodide in such manner that it is carrier-free. Label Capsules to include the following: the date of calibration; the amount of ¹²⁵I as iodide expressed as total megabecquerels (or microcuries or millicuries) at the time of calibration; the name and quantity of any added preservative or stabilizer; a statement indicating that the Capsules are for oral use only; the expiration date; and the statement, "Caution—Radioactive Material." The labeling indicates that in making dosage calculations, correction is to be made for radioactive decay, and also indicates that the radioactive half-life of ^{125}I is 60 days. Contain the labeled amount of ^{125}I, within $\pm 10\%$, as iodide expressed in megabecquerels (or microcuries or in millicuries) at the time indicated in the labeling. Other chemical forms of radioactivity do not exceed 5% of the total radioactivity. Meet the requirements for Radionuclide identification, Uniformity of dosage units, and Radiochemical purity.

Sodium Iodide I 125 Solution USP—Preserve in single-dose or in multiple-dose containers that previously have been treated to prevent adsorption. A solution suitable for either oral or intravenous administration, containing radioactive iodine (^{125}I) processed in the form of sodium iodide from the neutron bombardment of xenon gas in such a manner that it is essentially carrier-free. Label it to include the following: the name of the Solution; the name, address, and batch or lot number of the manufacturer; the date of calibration; the amount of ^{125}I as iodide expressed as total megabecquerels (or microcuries or millicuries) and as megabecquerels (or microcuries or millicuries) per mL at the time of calibration; the name and quantity of any added preservative or stabilizer; a statement of the intended use, whether oral or intravenous; a statement of whether diagnostic or therapeutic; the expiration date; and the statement, "Caution—Radioactive Material." The labeling indicates that in making dosage calculations, correction is to be made for radioactive decay, and also indicates that the radioactive half-life of ^{125}I is 60 days. Contains the labeled amount of ^{125}I, within $\pm 15\%$, as iodide expressed in megabecquerels (or microcuries or in millicuries) per mL at the time indicated in the labeling. Other chemical forms of radioactivity do not exceed 5% of the total radioactivity. Meets the requirements for Radionuclide identification, Bacterial endotoxins, pH (7.5–9.0), Radiochemical purity, and Injections (for solution intended for intravenous use, except that it is not subject to the recommendation on Volume in Container).

SODIUM IODIDE I 131

Chemical name: Sodium iodide ($Na^{131}I$).

Molecular formula: $Na^{131}I$.

Description:

Sodium Iodide I 131 Capsules USP—May contain a small amount of solid or solids, or may appear empty.

Sodium Iodide I 131 Solution USP—Clear, colorless solution. Upon standing, both the Solution and the glass container may darken as a result of the effects of the radiation.

USP requirements:

Sodium Iodide I 131 Capsules USP—Preserve in well-closed containers. Contain radioactive iodine (^{131}I) processed in the form of Sodium Iodide from products of uranium fission or the neutron bombardment of tellurium in such a manner that it is essentially carrier-free and contains only minute amounts of naturally occurring iodine 127. Label Capsules to include the following: the date of calibration; the amount of ^{131}I as iodide expressed in megabecquerels (or microcuries or in millicuries) per Capsule at the time of calibration; a statement of whether the contents are intended for diagnostic or therapeutic use; the expiration date; and the statement, "Caution—Radioactive Material." The labeling indicates that in

making dosage calculations, correction is to be made for radioactive decay, and also indicates that the radioactive half-life of ^{131}I is 8.08 days. Contain the labeled amount of ^{131}I, within $\pm 10\%$, as iodide expressed in megabecquerels (or microcuries or in millicuries) at the time indicated in the labeling. Other chemical forms of radioactivity do not exceed 5% of the total radioactivity. Meet the requirements for Radionuclide identification, Uniformity of dosage units, and Radiochemical purity.

Sodium Iodide I 131 Solution USP—Preserve in single-dose or in multiple-dose containers that previously have been treated to prevent adsorption. A solution suitable for either oral or intravenous administration, containing radioactive iodine (^{131}I) processed in the form of Sodium Iodide from the products of uranium fission or the neutron bombardment of tellurium in such a manner that it is essentially carrier-free and contains only minute amounts of naturally occurring iodine 127. Label it to include the following: the time and date of calibration; the amount of ^{131}I as iodide expressed as total megabecquerels (or microcuries or millicuries) and as megabecquerels (or microcuries or millicuries) per mL at the time of calibration; the name and quantity of any added preservative or stabilizer; a statement of the intended use, whether oral or intravenous; a statement of whether the contents are intended for diagnostic or therapeutic use; the expiration date; and the statement, "Caution—Radioactive Material." The labeling indicates that in making dosage calculations, correction is to be made for radioactive decay, and also indicates that the radioactive half-life of ^{131}I is 8.08 days. Contains the labeled amount of ^{131}I, within $\pm 10\%$, as iodide expressed in megabecquerels (or microcuries or in millicuries) per mL at the time indicated in the labeling. Other chemical forms of radioactivity do not exceed 5% of the total radioactivity. Meets the requirements for Radionuclide identification, Bacterial endotoxins (if intended for intravenous use), pH (7.5–9.0), Radiochemical purity, and Injections (if for intravenous use, except that the Solution may be distributed or dispensed prior to completion of the test for Sterility, the latter test being started on the day of final manufacture, and except that it is not subject to the recommendation on Volume in Container).

SODIUM LACTATE

Chemical name: Sodium lactate—Propanoic acid, 2-hydroxy-, monosodium salt.

Molecular formula: Sodium lactate—$C_3H_5NaO_3$.

Molecular weight: Sodium lactate—112.06.

Description: Sodium Lactate Solution USP—Clear, colorless or practically colorless, slightly viscous liquid, odorless, or having a slight, not unpleasant odor.

NF category: Buffering agent.

Solubility: Sodium Lactate Solution USP—Miscible with water.

USP requirements:

Sodium Lactate Injection USP—Preserve in single-dose glass or plastic containers. Glass containers are preferably of Type I or Type II glass. It is sterile Sodium Lactate Solution in Water for Injection, or a sterile solution of Lactic Acid in Water for Injection prepared with the aid of Sodium Hydroxide. The label states the total osmolar concentration in mOsmol per liter. Where the contents are less than 100 mL, or where the label states that the Injection is not for direct injection but is to be diluted before use, the label alternatively may state the total osmolar concentration in mOsmol per mL. The label includes also the warning: "Not for use in the treatment of lactic acidosis." Contains the labeled amount, within -5% to $+10\%$. Meets the requirements for Identification, Bacterial endotoxins, pH (6.0–7.3, the Injection being diluted with water, if necessary, to approximately 0.16 M [20 mg per mL]), Particulate matter, Heavy metals (not more than 0.001%), and Injections.

Sodium Lactate Solution USP—Preserve in tight containers. An aqueous solution containing not less than 50.0%, by weight, of monosodium lactate. Label it to indicate its content of sodium lactate. Contains the labeled amount, within ±2%. Meets the requirements for Identification, pH (5.0–9.0), Chloride (not more than 0.05%), Citrate, oxalate, phosphate, or tartrate, Sulfate, Heavy metals (not more than 0.001%), Sugars, and Methanol and methyl esters.

SODIUM LAURYL SULFATE

Chemical name: Sulfuric acid monododecyl ester sodium salt.

Molecular formula: $C_{12}H_{25}NaO_4S$.

Molecular weight: 288.38.

Description: Sodium Lauryl Sulfate NF—Small, white or light yellow crystals having a slight characteristic odor.

NF category: Emulsifying and/or solubilizing agent; wetting and/or solubilizing agent.

Solubility: Sodium Lauryl Sulfate NF—Freely soluble in water, forming an opalescent solution.

NF requirements: Sodium Lauryl Sulfate NF—Preserve in well-closed containers. A mixture of sodium alkyl sulfates consisting chiefly of sodium lauryl sulfate $[CH_3(CH_2)_{10}-CH_2OSO_3Na]$. The combined content of sodium chloride and sodium sulfate is not more than 8.0%. Meets the requirements for Identification, Alkalinity, Arsenic (not more than 3 ppm), Heavy metals (not more than 0.002%), Sodium chloride, Sodium sulfate, Unsulfated alcohols (not more than 4.0%), and Total alcohols (not less than 59.0%).

SODIUM METABISULFITE

Chemical name: Disulfurous acid, disodium salt.

Molecular formula: $Na_2S_2O_5$.

Molecular weight: 190.10.

Description: Sodium Metabisulfite NF—White crystals or white to yellowish crystalline powder, having the odor of sulfur dioxide.

NF category: Antioxidant.

Solubility: Sodium Metabisulfite NF—Freely soluble in water and in glycerin; slightly soluble in alcohol.

NF requirements: Sodium Metabisulfite NF—Preserve in well-filled, tight containers, and avoid exposure to excessive heat. Contains an amount of sodium metabisulfite equivalent to not less than 65.0% and not more than 67.4% of sulfur dioxide. Meets the requirements for Identification, Chloride (not more than 0.05%), Thiosulfate (not more than 0.05%), Arsenic (not more than 3 ppm), Iron (not more than 0.002%), and Heavy metals (not more than 0.002%).

SODIUM MONOFLUOROPHOSPHATE

Chemical name: Phosphorofluoridic acid, disodium salt.

Molecular formula: Na_2PFO_3.

Molecular weight: 143.95.

Description: Sodium Monofluorophosphate USP—White to slightly gray, odorless powder.

Solubility: Sodium Monofluorophosphate USP—Freely soluble in water.

USP requirements: Sodium Monofluorophosphate USP—Preserve in well-closed containers. Contains not less than 91.7% and not more than 100.5% of sodium monofluorophosphate, calculated on the dried basis. Meets the requirements for Identification, pH (6.5–8.0, in a solution [1 in 50]), Loss on drying (not more than 0.2%), Arsenic (not more than 3 ppm), Limit of fluoride ion (not more than 1.2%), Heavy metals (not more than 0.005%), and Organic volatile impurities.

SODIUM NITRITE

Chemical name: Nitrous acid, sodium salt.

Molecular formula: $NaNO_2$

Molecular weight: 69.00.

Description:
Sodium Nitrite USP—White to slightly yellow, granular powder, or white or practically white, opaque, fused masses or sticks. Deliquescent in air. Its solutions are alkaline to litmus.
Sodium Nitrite Injection USP—Clear, colorless liquid.

Solubility: Sodium Nitrite USP—Freely soluble in water; sparingly soluble in alcohol.

USP requirements: Sodium Nitrite Injection USP—Preserve in single-dose containers, of Type I glass. A sterile solution of Sodium Nitrite in Water for Injection. Contains the labeled amount, within ±5%. Meets the requirements for Identification, Pyrogen, pH (7.0–9.0), and Injections.

SODIUM NITROPRUSSIDE

Chemical name: Sodium nitroprusside—Ferrate(2-), pentakis(cyano-*C*)nitrosyl-, disodium, dihydrate, (*OC*-6-22)-.

Molecular formula: Sodium nitroprusside—$Na_2[Fe(CN)_5\cdot NO]\cdot 2H_2O$.

Molecular weight: Sodium nitroprusside—297.95.

Description:
Sodium Nitroprusside USP—Reddish brown, practically odorless, crystals or powder.
Sterile Sodium Nitroprusside USP—Reddish brown, practically odorless, crystals or powder.

Solubility:
Sodium Nitroprusside USP—Freely soluble in water; slightly soluble in alcohol; very slightly soluble in chloroform.
Sterile Sodium Nitroprusside USP—Freely soluble in water; slightly soluble in alcohol; very slightly soluble in chloroform.

USP requirements: Sterile Sodium Nitroprusside USP—Preserve protected from light in Containers for Sterile Solids. It is Sodium Nitroprusside suitable for parenteral use. Contains the labeled amount, within ±10%. Meets the requirements for Constituted solution, Identification, Pyrogen, and Water (not more than 15.0%), for Identification test under Sodium Nitroprusside, and for Sterility tests, Uniformity of dosage units, and Labeling under Injections.

SODIUM PERTECHNETATE Tc 99m

Chemical name: Pertechnetic acid ($H^{99m}TcO_4$), sodium salt.

Molecular formula: $Na^{99m}TcO_4$.

Description: Sodium Pertechnetate Tc 99m Injection USP—Clear, colorless solution.

USP requirements: Sodium Pertechnetate Tc 99m Injection USP—Preserve in single-dose or in multiple-dose containers. A sterile solution, suitable for intravenous or oral administration, containing radioactive technetium (^{99m}Tc) in the form of sodium pertechnetate and sufficient Sodium Chloride to make the solution isotonic. Technetium 99m is a radioactive nuclide formed by the radioactive decay of molybdenum 99. Molybdenum 99 is a radioactive isotope of molybdenum and may be formed by the neutron bombardment of molybdenum 98 or as a product of uranium fission. If intended for intravenous use, label it with the information specified for Labeling under Injections. Label it also to include the following: the time and date of calibration; the amount of ^{99m}Tc as sodium pertechnetate expressed as total megabecquerels (or millicuries) and as megabecquerels (or millicuries) per mL on the date and time of calibration; a statement of the intended use whether oral or intravenous; the expiration date; and the statement, "Caution—Radioactive Material." If the Injection has been prepared from molybdenum 99 produced from uranium fission, the label so states. The labeling indicates that in making dosage calculations, correction is to be made for radioactive decay, and also indicates that the radioactive half-life of ^{99m}Tc is 6.0 hours. Contains the labeled amount of ^{99m}Tc, within ±10%, at the date and hour stated on the label. Other chemical forms of ^{99m}Tc do not exceed 5% of the total radioactivity. Meets the requirements for Radionuclide identification, Bacterial endotoxins, pH (4.5–7.5), Radiochemical purity, Radionuclidic purity, Chemical purity, and Injections (except that the Injection may be distributed or dispensed prior to the completion of the test for Sterility, the latter test being started on the day of manufacture, and except that it is not subject to the recommendation on Volume in Container).

DIBASIC SODIUM PHOSPHATE

Chemical name: Phosphoric acid, disodium salt, heptahydrate.

Molecular formula: $Na_2HPO_4 \cdot 7H_2O$.

Molecular weight: 268.07.

Description:

Dibasic Sodium Phosphate USP (dried)—White powder that readily absorbs moisture.

    NF category: Buffering agent.

Dibasic Sodium Phosphate USP (heptahydrate)—Colorless or white, granular or caked salt. Effloresces in warm, dry air. Its solutions are alkaline to phenolphthalein TS, a 0.1 *M* solution having a pH of about 9.

    NF category: Buffering agent.

Solubility:

Dibasic Sodium Phosphate USP (dried)—Freely soluble in water; insoluble in alcohol.

Dibasic Sodium Phosphate USP (heptahydrate)—Freely soluble in water; very slightly soluble in alcohol.

USP requirements:

Dibasic Sodium Phosphate USP—Preserve in tight containers. It is dried or contains 7 molecules of water of hydration. Label it to indicate whether it is dried or is the heptahydrate. Contains not less than 98.0% and not more than 100.5% of dibasic sodium phosphate, calculated on the dried basis. Meets the requirements for Identification, Loss on drying (not more than 5.0% for the dried form and 43.0–50.0% for the heptahydrate), Insoluble substances (not more than 0.4%), Chloride (not more than 0.06%), Sulfate (not more than 0.2%), Arsenic (not more than 16 ppm), and Heavy metals (not more than 0.002%).

Effervescent Sodium Phosphate—Not in USP.

MONOBASIC SODIUM PHOSPHATE

Chemical name: Phosphoric acid, monosodium salt, monohydrate; phosphoric acid, monosodium salt, dihydrate.

Molecular formula: $NaH_2PO_4 \cdot xH_2O$.

Molecular weight: 137.99 (monohydrate); 119.98 (anhydrous); 156.01 (dihydrate).

Description: Monobasic Sodium Phosphate USP—Colorless crystals or white, crystalline powder. Odorless and slightly deliquescent. Its solutions are acid to litmus and effervesce with sodium carbonate.

    NF category: Buffering agent.

Solubility: Monobasic Sodium Phosphate USP—Freely soluble in water; practically insoluble in alcohol.

USP requirements: Monobasic Sodium Phosphate USP—Preserve in well-closed containers. Contains 1 or 2 molecules of water of hydration, or is anhydrous. Label it to indicate whether it is anhydrous or is the monohydrate or the dihydrate. Contains not less than 98.0% and not more than 103.0% of monobasic sodium phosphate, calculated on the anhydrous basis. Meets the requirements for Identification, pH (4.1–4.5, in a solution containing the equivalent of 1.0 gram of monobasic sodium phosphate [monohydrate] in 20 mL of water), Water (less than 2.0% for the anhydrous form, 10.0–15.0% for the monohydrate, 18.0–26.5% for the dihydrate), Insoluble substances (not more than 0.2%), Chloride (not more than 0.014%), Sulfate (not more than 0.15%), Aluminum, calcium, and related elements, Arsenic (not more than 8 ppm), Heavy metals (not more than 0.002%), and Organic volatile impurities.

SODIUM PHOSPHATES

For *Dibasic Sodium Phosphate* and *Monobasic Sodium Phosphate*—See individual listings for chemistry information.

USP requirements:

Sodium Phosphates Enema USP—Preserve in well-closed, single-unit containers. A solution of Dibasic Sodium Phosphate and Monobasic Sodium Phosphate, or Dibasic Sodium Phosphate and Phosphoric Acid, in Purified Water. Contains, in each 100 mL, not less than 5.7 grams and not more than 6.3 grams of dibasic sodium phosphate (heptahydrate), and not less than 15.2 grams and not more than 16.8 grams of monobasic sodium phosphate (monohydrate). Meets the requirements for Identification, Specific gravity (1.121–1.128), pH (5.0–5.8), Chloride (not more than 0.008%), Arsenic (not more than 2 ppm), and Heavy metals (not more than 0.001%).

Sodium Phosphates Injection USP—Preserve in single-dose containers, preferably of Type I glass. A sterile solution of Monobasic Sodium Phosphate and Dibasic Sodium Phosphate in Water for Injection. The label states the sodium content in terms of milliequivalents in a given volume, and states also the phosphorus content in terms of millimoles in a given volume. Label the Injection to indicate that it is to be diluted to appropriate strength with water or other suitable fluid prior to administration, and that once opened any unused portion is to be discarded. The label states also the total osmolar concentration in mOsmol per liter. Where the contents are less than 100 mL, or where the label states that the Injection is not for direct injection but is to be diluted before use, the label alternatively may state the total osmolar concentration in mOsmol per mL. Contains the labeled amounts of monobasic sodium phosphate and dibasic sodium phosphate, within ±5%. Contains no bacteriostat or other preservative. Meets the requirements for Identification, Bacterial endotoxins, Particulate matter, and Injections.

Sodium Phosphates Oral Solution USP—Preserve in tight containers. A solution of Dibasic Sodium Phosphate and Monobasic Sodium Phosphate, or Dibasic Sodium Phosphate and Phosphoric Acid, in Purified Water. Contains, in each 100 mL, not less than 17.1 grams and not more than 18.9 grams of dibasic sodium phosphate (heptahydrate), and not less than 45.6 grams and not more than 50.4 grams of monobasic sodium phosphate (monohydrate). Meets the requirements for Identification, pH (4.4–5.2), Chloride (not more than 0.01%), Arsenic (not more than 2 ppm), and Heavy metals (not more than 0.001%).

SODIUM POLYSTYRENE SULFONATE

Chemical name: Benzene, diethenyl-, polymer with ethenylbenzene, sulfonated, sodium salt.

Description: Sodium Polystyrene Sulfonate USP—Golden brown, fine powder. Is odorless.

Solubility: Sodium Polystyrene Sulfonate USP—Insoluble in water.

USP requirements:

Sodium Polystyrene Sulfonate USP (for Suspension)—Preserve in well-closed containers. A cation-exchange resin prepared in the sodium form. Sodium Polystyrene Sulfonate that is intended for preparing suspensions for oral or rectal administration may be labeled Sodium Polystyrene Sulfonate for Suspension. Each gram exchanges not less than 110 mg and not more than 135 mg of potassium, calculated on the anhydrous basis. Meets the requirements for Water (not more than 10.0%), Ammonia, Sodium content (9.4–11.0%, calculated on the anhydrous basis), and Potassium exchange capacity.

Sodium Polystyrene Sulfonate Suspension USP—Preserve in well-closed containers, protected from freezing and from excessive heat. A suspension of Sodium Polystyrene Sulfonate in an aqueous vehicle containing a suitable quantity of sorbitol. Label it to state the quantity of sorbitol in a given volume of Suspension. Contains the labeled amount of sorbitol, within ±10%. Each gram of the labeled amount of sodium polystyrene sulfonate exchanges not less than 110 mg and not more than 135 mg of potassium. Meets the requirements for Microbial limits, Sodium content (9.4–11.0%, based on the labeled amount) and Potassium exchange capacity.

SODIUM PROPIONATE

Chemical name: Propanoic acid, sodium salt, hydrate.

Molecular formula: $C_3H_5NaO_2 \cdot xH_2O$.

Molecular weight: 96.06 (anhydrous).

Description: Sodium Propionate NF—Colorless, transparent crystals or granular, crystalline powder. Odorless, or has a slight acetic-butyric odor. Deliquescent in moist air.

NF category: Antimicrobial preservative.

Solubility: Sodium Propionate NF—Very soluble in water; soluble in alcohol.

NF requirements: Sodium Propionate NF—Preserve in tight containers. Dried at 105 °C for 2 hours, contains not less than 99.0% and not more than 100.5% of anhydrous sodium propionate. Meets the requirements for Identification, Alkalinity, Water (not more than 1.0%), Arsenic (not more

than 3 ppm), Heavy metals (not more than 0.001%), and Organic volatile impurities.

SODIUM SALICYLATE

Chemical name: Benzoic acid, 2-hydroxy-, monosodium salt.

Molecular formula: $C_7H_5NaO_3$.

Molecular weight: 160.10.

Description: Sodium Salicylate USP—Amorphous or microcrystalline powder or scales. Is colorless, or has not more than a faint, pink tinge. Is odorless, or has a faint, characteristic odor, and is affected by light. A freshly made solution (1 in 10) is neutral or acid to litmus.

Solubility: Sodium Salicylate USP—Freely (and slowly) soluble in water and in glycerin; very soluble in boiling water and in boiling alcohol; slowly soluble in alcohol.

USP requirements:

Sodium Salicylate Tablets USP—Preserve in well-closed containers. Contain the labeled amount, within ±5%. Meet the requirements for Identification, Dissolution (75% in 45 minutes in water in Apparatus 1 at 100 rpm), and Uniformity of dosage units.

Sodium Salicylate Delayed-release Tablets—Not in USP.

SODIUM STARCH GLYCOLATE

Description: Sodium Starch Glycolate NF—White, odorless, relatively free-flowing powder; available in several different viscosity grades. A 2% (w/v) dispersion in cold water settles, on standing, in the form of a highly hydrated layer.

NF category: Tablet disintegrant.

NF requirements: Sodium Starch Glycolate NF—Preserve in well-closed containers, preferably protected from wide variations in temperature and humidity, which may cause caking. It is the sodium salt of a carboxymethyl ether of starch. The labeling indicates the pH range. Contains not less than 2.8% and not more than 4.2% of sodium on the dried, alcohol-washed basis. It may contain not more than 7.0% of Sodium Chloride. Meets the requirements for Identification, Microbial limits, pH (3.0–5.0 or 5.5–7.5), Loss on drying (not more than 10.0%), Iron (not more than 0.002%), Heavy metals (not more than 0.002%), and Sodium chloride.

SODIUM STEARATE

Chemical name: Octadecanoic acid, sodium salt.

Molecular formula: $C_{18}H_{35}NaO_2$.

Molecular weight: 306.46.

Description: Sodium Stearate NF—Fine, white powder, soapy to the touch, usually having a slight tallow-like odor. It is affected by light. Its solutions are alkaline to phenolphthalein TS.

NF category: Emulsifying and/or solubilizing agent.

Solubility: Sodium Stearate NF—Slowly soluble in cold water and in cold alcohol; readily soluble in hot water and in hot alcohol.

NF requirements: Sodium Stearate NF—Preserve in well-closed, light-resistant containers. A mixture of sodium stearate and sodium palmitate, which together constitute not less than 90.0% of the total content. The content of sodium stearate is not less than 40.0% of the total. Contains small amounts of the sodium salts of other fatty acids. Meets the requirements for Identification, Acidity, Loss on drying (not more than 5.0%), Alcohol-insoluble substances, Iodine value of fatty acids (not more than 4.0), Acid value of fatty acids (196–211), and Organic volatile impurities.

SODIUM STEARYL FUMARATE

Description: Sodium Stearyl Fumarate NF—Fine, white powder.

NF category: Tablet and/or capsule lubricant.

Solubility: Sodium Stearyl Fumarate NF—Slightly soluble in methanol; practically insoluble in water.

NF requirements: Sodium Stearyl Fumarate NF—Preserve in well-closed containers. Contains not less than 99.0% and not more than 101.5% of sodium stearyl fumarate. Meets the requirements for Identification, Water (not more than 5.0%), Arsenic (not more than 3 ppm), Lead (not more than 0.001%), Heavy metals (not more than 0.002%), Limit of sodium stearyl maleate and stearyl alcohol (not more than 0.25% of sodium stearyl maleate and not more than 0.5% of stearyl alcohol), and Saponification value (142.2–146.0, calculated on the anhydrous basis).

SODIUM SULFATE

Chemical name: Sulfuric acid disodium salt, decahydrate.

Molecular formula: $Na_2SO_4 \cdot 10H_2O$.

Molecular weight: 322.19.

Description: Sodium Sulfate USP—Large, colorless, odorless, transparent crystals, or granular powder. Effloresces rapidly in air, liquifies in its water of hydration at about 33 °C, and loses all of its water of hydration at about 100 °C.

Solubility: Sodium Sulfate USP—Freely soluble in water; soluble in glycerin; insoluble in alcohol.

USP requirements: Sodium Sulfate Injection USP—Preserve in single-dose containers, preferably of Type I glass. A sterile, concentrated solution of Sodium Sulfate in Water for Injection, which upon dilution is suitable for parenteral use. Label it to indicate that it is to be diluted before injection to render it isotonic (3.89% of sodium sulfate decahydrate). Contains the labeled amount, within ± 5%. Meets the requirements for Identification, Pyrogen, pH (5.0–6.5), and Injections.

SODIUM THIOSULFATE

Chemical name: Thiosulfuric acid, disodium salt, pentahydrate.

Molecular formula: $Na_2S_2O_3 \cdot 5H_2O$.

Molecular weight: 248.17.

Description: Sodium Thiosulfate USP—Large, colorless crystals or coarse, crystalline powder. It is deliquescent in moist air and effloresces in dry air at temperatures exceeding 33 °C. Its solutions are neutral or faintly alkaline to litmus.

NF category: Antioxidant.

Solubility: Sodium Thiosulfate USP—Very soluble in water; insoluble in alcohol.

USP requirements:
Sodium Thiosulfate USP—Preserve in tight containers. Contains not less than 99.0% and not more than 100.5% of sodium thiosulfate, calculated on the anhydrous basis.

Meets the requirements for Identification, Water (32.0–37.0%), Arsenic (not more than 3 ppm), Calcium, and Heavy metals (not more than 0.002%).
Sodium Thiosulfate Injection USP—Preserve in single-dose containers, of Type I glass. A sterile solution of Sodium Thiosulfate in freshly boiled Water for Injection. Contains the labeled amount, within ± 5%. Meets the requirements for Identification, Bacterial endotoxins, pH (6.0–9.5), and Injections.

SOMATREM

Source: Biosynthetic. A single polypeptide chain of 192 amino acids, one more (methionine) than naturally occurring human growth hormone, produced by a recombinant DNA process in *Escherichia coli*.

Chemical name: Somatotropin (human), *N*-L-methionyl-.

Molecular formula: $C_{995}H_{1537}N_{263}O_{301}S_8$.

Molecular weight: 22,256.21.

USP requirements: Somatrem for Injection—Not in USP.

SOMATROPIN

Source:
Somatropin, pituitary-derived—Obtained from the anterior lobe of the human pituitary gland. A single polypeptide chain of 191 amino acids.
Somatropin, recombinant—Biosynthetic, produced by a recombinant DNA process in *Escherichia coli*; same amino acid sequence as pituitary-derived somatropin. A single polypeptide chain of 191 amino acids.

Chemical name: Growth hormone (human).

Molecular formula: $C_{990}H_{1528}N_{262}O_{300}S_7$.

Molecular weight: 21,500.00.

USP requirements:
Somatropin, Pituitary-derived, for Injection—Not in USP.
Somatropin, Recombinant, for Injection—Not in USP.

SORBIC ACID

Chemical name: 2,4-Hexadienoic acid, (*E,E*)-.

Molecular formula: $C_6H_8O_2$.

Molecular weight: 112.13.

Description: Sorbic Acid NF—Free-flowing, white, crystalline powder, having a characteristic odor.
NF category: Antimicrobial preservative.

Solubility: Sorbic Acid NF—Slightly soluble in water; soluble in alcohol and in ether.

NF requirements: Sorbic Acid NF—Preserve in tight containers, protected from light, and avoid exposure to excessive heat. Contains not less than 99.0% and not more than 101.0% of sorbic acid, calculated on the anhydrous basis. Meets the requirements for Identification, Melting range (132–135 °C), Water (not more than 0.5%), Residue on ignition (not more than 0.2%), and Heavy metals (not more than 0.001%).

SORBITAN MONOLAURATE

Chemical name: Sorbitan, esters, monododecanoate.

Description: Sorbitan Monolaurate NF—Yellow to amber oily liquid, having a bland, characteristic odor.

NF category: Emulsifying and/or solubilizing agent; wetting and/or solubilizing agent.

Solubility: Sorbitan Monolaurate NF—Insoluble in water; soluble in mineral oil; slightly soluble in cottonseed oil and in ethyl acetate.

NF requirements: Sorbitan Monolaurate NF—Preserve in tight containers. A partial ester of lauric acid with Sorbitol and its mono- and dianhydrides. Yields, upon saponification, not less than 55.0% and not more than 63.0% of fatty acids, and not less than 39.0% and not more than 45.0% of polyols (w/w). Meets the requirements for Identification, Water (not more than 1.5%), Residue on ignition (not more than 0.5%), Heavy metals (not more than 0.001%), Acid value (not more than 8), Hydroxyl value (330–358), Saponification value (158–170), and Organic volatile impurities.

SORBITAN MONOOLEATE

Chemical name: Sorbitan esters, mono(Z)-9-octadecenoate.

Molecular formula: $C_{24}H_{44}O_6$ (approximate).

Description: Sorbitan Monooleate NF—Viscous, yellow to amber-colored, oily liquid, having a bland, characteristic odor.
  NF category: Emulsifying and/or solubilizing agent; wetting and/or solubilizing agent.

Solubility: Sorbitan Monooleate NF—Insoluble in water and in propylene glycol. Miscible with mineral and vegetable oils.

NF requirements: Sorbitan Monooleate NF—Preserve in tight containers. A partial oleate ester of Sorbitol and its mono- and dianhydrides. Yields, upon saponification, not less than 72.0% and not more than 78.0% of fatty acids, and not less than 25.0% and not more than 31.0% of polyols (w/w). Meets the requirements for Identification, Water (not more than 1.0%), Residue on ignition (not more than 0.5%), Heavy metals (not more than 0.001%), Acid value (not more than 8), Hydroxyl value (190–215), Iodine value (62–76), and Saponification value (145–160).

SORBITAN MONOPALMITATE

Chemical name: Sorbitan, esters, monohexadecanoate.

Molecular formula: $C_{22}H_{42}O_6$ (approximate).

Description: Sorbitan Monopalmitate NF—Cream-colored, waxy solid, having a faint fatty odor.
  NF category: Emulsifying and/or solubilizing agent; wetting and/or solubilizing agent.

Solubility: Sorbitan Monopalmitate NF—Insoluble in water; soluble in warm absolute alcohol; soluble, with haze, in warm peanut oil and in warm mineral oil.

NF requirements: Sorbitan Monopalmitate NF—Preserve in well-closed containers. A partial ester of palmitic acid with Sorbitol and its mono- and dianhydrides. Yields, upon saponification, not less than 63.0% and not more than 71.0% of fatty acids, and not less than 32.0% and not more than 38.0% of polyols (w/w). Meets the requirements for Identification, Water (not more than 1.5%), Residue on ignition (not more than 0.5%), Heavy metals (not more than 0.001%), Acid value (not more than 8), Hydroxyl value (275–305), and Saponification value (140–150).

SORBITAN MONOSTEARATE

Chemical name: Sorbitan, esters, monooctadecanoate.

Molecular formula: $C_{24}H_{46}O_6$ (approximate).

Description: Sorbitan Monostearate NF—Cream-colored to tan, hard, waxy solid, having a bland odor.

NF category: Emulsifying and/or solubilizing agent; wetting and/or solubilizing agent.

Solubility: Sorbitan Monostearate NF—Insoluble in cold water and in acetone; dispersible in warm water; soluble, with haze, above 50 °C in mineral oil and in ethyl acetate.

NF requirements: Sorbitan Monostearate NF—Preserve in well-closed containers. A partial ester of Stearic Acid with Sorbitol and its mono- and dianhydrides. Yields, upon saponification, not less than 68.0% and not more than 76.0% of fatty acids, and not less than 27.0% and not more than 34.0% of polyols (w/w). Meets the requirements for Identification, Water (not more than 1.5%), Residue on ignition (not more than 0.5%), Heavy metals (not more than 0.001%), Acid value (not more than 10), Hydroxyl value (235–260), and Saponification value (147–157).

SORBITOL

Chemical name: D-Glucitol.

Molecular formula: $C_6H_{14}O_6$.

Molecular weight: 182.17.

Description:
  Sorbitol NF—White, hygroscopic powder, granules, or flakes.
    NF category: Humectant; sweetening agent; tablet and/or capsule diluent.
  Sorbitol Solution USP—Clear, colorless, syrupy liquid. Neutral to litmus.
    NF category: Sweetening agent; vehicle (flavored and/or sweetened).

Solubility: Sorbitol NF—Very soluble in water; slightly soluble in alcohol, in methanol, and in acetic acid.

USP requirements: Sorbitol Solution USP—Preserve in tight containers. A water solution containing, in each 100.0 grams, not less than 64.0 grams of D–sorbitol. Meets the requirements for Identification, Specific gravity (not less than 1.285), Refractive index (1.455–1.465 at 20 °C), Water (28.5–31.5%), Residue on ignition (not more than 0.1%), Chloride (not more than 0.005%), Sulfate (not more than 0.010%), Arsenic (not more than 2.5 ppm), Heavy metals (not more than 0.001%), and Reducing sugars.

NF requirements: Sorbitol NF—Preserve in tight containers. Contains not less than 91.0% and not more than 100.5% of sorbitol, calculated on the anhydrous basis. May contain small amounts of other polyhydric alcohols. Meets the requirements for Identification, Water (not more than 1.0%), Residue on ignition (not more than 0.1%), Chloride (not more than 0.0050%), Sulfate (not more than 0.010%), Arsenic (not more than 3 ppm), Heavy metals (not more than 0.001%), Reducing sugars, and Total sugars.

SOTALOL

Chemical name: Sotalol hydrochloride—Methanesulfonamide, N-[4-[1-hydroxy-2-[(1-methylethyl)amino]ethyl]phenyl]-, monohydrochloride.

Molecular formula: Sotalol hydrochloride—$C_{12}H_{20}N_2O_3S \cdot HCl$.

Molecular weight: Sotalol hydrochloride—308.82.

Description: Sotalol hydrochloride—White, crystalline solid. Melting point 206.5–207 °C with decomposition.

Solubility: Sotalol hydrochloride—Freely soluble in water; slightly soluble in chloroform.

Other characteristics: Lipid solubility—Low.

USP requirements: Sotalol Hydrochloride Tablets—Not in USP.

SOYBEAN OIL

Description: Soybean Oil USP—Clear, pale yellow, oily liquid having a characteristic odor.
NF category: Vehicle (oleaginous).

Solubility: Soybean Oil USP—Insoluble in water. Miscible with ether and with chloroform.

USP requirements: Soybean Oil USP—Preserve in tight, light-resistant containers, and avoid exposure to excessive heat. It is the refined fixed oil obtained from the seeds of the soya plant *Glycine soja* (Fam. Leguminosae). Meets the requirements for Specific gravity (0.916–0.922), Refractive index (1.465–1.475), Heavy metals (not more than 0.001%), Free fatty acids, Fatty acid composition, Iodine value (120–141), Saponification value (180–200), Unsaponifiable matter (not more than 1.0%), Cottonseed oil, and Peroxide.

SPECTINOMYCIN

Source: Produced by a species of the soil microorganism *Streptomyces spectabilis*.

Chemical group: Aminocyclitol antibiotic.

Chemical name: Spectinomycin hydrochloride—$4H$-Pyrano[2,3-*b*][1,4]benzodioxin-4-one, decahydro-4a,7,9-trihydroxy-2-methyl-6,8-bis(methylamino)-, dihydrochloride, pentahydrate.

Molecular formula: Spectinomycin hydrochloride—$C_{14}H_{24}N_2O_7 \cdot 2HCl \cdot 5H_2O$.

Molecular weight: Spectinomycin hydrochloride—495.35.

Description: Sterile Spectinomycin Hydrochloride USP—White to pale-buff crystalline powder.

Solubility: Sterile Spectinomycin Hydrochloride USP—Freely soluble in water; practically insoluble in alcohol, in chloroform, and in ether.

USP requirements:
Sterile Spectinomycin Hydrochloride USP—Preserve in Containers for Sterile Solids. Has a potency equivalent to not less than 603 mcg of spectinomycin per mg. Meets the requirements for Identification, Crystallinity, Depressor substances, Bacterial endotoxins, Sterility, pH (3.8–5.6, in a solution containing 10 mg per mL [where packaged for dispensing, 4.0–7.0, in the solution constituted as directed in the labeling]), Water (16.0–20.0%), and Residue on ignition (not more than 1.0%).
Sterile Spectinomycin Hydrochloride for Suspension USP—Preserve in Containers for Sterile Solids. It is Sterile Spectinomycin Hydrochloride packaged for dispensing. Contains an amount of spectinomycin hydrochloride equivalent to the labeled amount of spectinomycin, within −10% to +20%. Conforms to the definition and meets the requirements for Identification test, Crystallinity, Pyrogen, Sterility, pH, Water, and Residue on ignition under Sterile Spectinomycin Hydrochloride, and for Uniformity of dosage units and Labeling under Injections.

SPIRONOLACTONE

Chemical name: Pregn-4-ene-21-carboxylic acid, 7-(acetylthio)-17-hydroxy-3-oxo-, gamma-lactone, (7 alpha,17 alpha)-.

Molecular formula: $C_{24}H_{32}O_4S$.

Molecular weight: 416.57.

Description: Spironolactone USP—Light cream-colored to light tan, crystalline powder. Has a faint to mild mercaptan-like odor; is stable in air.

Solubility: Spironolactone USP—Practically insoluble in water; freely soluble in chloroform; soluble in ethyl acetate and in alcohol; slightly soluble in methanol and in fixed oils.

USP requirements: Spironolactone Tablets USP—Preserve in tight, light-resistant containers. Contain the labeled amount, within ±5%. Meet the requirements for Identification, Dissolution (75% in 60 minutes in 0.1 N hydrochloric acid containing 0.1% of sodium lauryl sulfate in Apparatus 2 at 75 rpm), and Uniformity of dosage units.

SPIRONOLACTONE AND HYDROCHLOROTHIAZIDE

For *Spironolactone* and *Hydrochlorothiazide*—See individual listings for chemistry information.

USP requirements: Spironolactone and Hydrochlorothiazide Tablets USP—Preserve in tight, light-resistant containers. Contain the labeled amounts, within ±10%. Meet the requirements for Identification, Dissolution (75% of each active ingredient in 60 minutes in 0.1 N hydrochloric acid containing 0.1% sodium lauryl sulfate in Apparatus 2 at 75 rpm), and Uniformity of dosage units.

SQUALANE

Chemical name: Tetracosane, 2,6,10,15,19,23-hexamethyl-.

Molecular formula: $C_{30}H_{62}$.

Molecular weight: 422.82.

Description: Squalane NF—Colorless, practically odorless transparent oil.
NF category: Ointment base; vehicle (oleaginous).

Solubility: Squalane NF—Insoluble in water; very slightly soluble in absolute alcohol; slightly soluble in acetone. Miscible with ether and with chloroform.

NF requirements: Squalane NF—Preserve in tight containers. A saturated hydrocarbon obtained by hydrogenation of squalene, an aliphatic triterpene occurring in some fish oils. Meets the requirements for Identification, Specific gravity (0.807–0.810 at 20 °C), Refractive index (1.4510–1.4525 at 20 °C), Residue on ignition (not more than 0.5%), Acid value (not more than 0.2), Iodine value (not more than 4), Saponification value (not more than 2), and Chromatographic purity.

STANNOUS FLUORIDE

Chemical name: Tin fluoride (SnF_2).

Molecular formula: SnF_2.

Molecular weight: 156.69.

Description: Stannous Fluoride USP—White, crystalline powder. Melts at about 213 °C.

Solubility: Stannous Fluoride USP—Freely soluble in water; practically insoluble in alcohol, in ether, and in chloroform.

USP requirements: Stannous Fluoride Gel USP—Preserve in well-closed containers. Contains the labeled amount, within −5% to +15%, in a suitable medium containing a suitable viscosity-inducing agent. Meets the requirements for Identification, Viscosity (600–170,000 centipoises), pH (2.8–4.0, in a freshly prepared mixture with water [1:1]), and Stannous ion content (not less than 68.2% of the labeled amount of stannous fluoride).

Note: If Glycerin is used as the medium in preparation of this Gel, use Glycerin that has a low water content, that is, Glycerin having a specific gravity of not less than 1.2607, corresponding to a concentration of 99.5%.

STANOZOLOL

Chemical group: 17-alpha alkylated anabolic steroid.

Chemical name: 2'H-Androst-2-eno[3,2-c]pyrazol-17-ol, 17-methyl-, (5 alpha,17 beta)-.

Molecular formula: $C_{21}H_{32}N_2O$.

Molecular weight: 328.50.

Description: Stanozolol USP—Odorless, crystalline powder, occurring in two forms: as needles, melting at about 155 °C, and as prisms, melting at about 235 °C.

Solubility: Stanozolol USP—Insoluble in water; soluble in dimethylformamide; sparingly soluble in alcohol and in chloroform; slightly soluble in ethyl acetate and in acetone.

USP requirements: Stanozolol Tablets USP—Preserve in tight, light-resistant containers. Contain the labeled amount, within ± 10%. Meet the requirements for Identification, Dissolution (75% in 45 minutes in 0.1 N hydrochloric acid in Apparatus 2 at 50 rpm), and Uniformity of dosage units.

STARCH

Chemical name: Starch.

Description: Starch NF—Irregular, angular, white masses or fine powder. Odorless.
   NF category: Tablet and/or capsule diluent; tablet disintegrant.

Solubility: Starch NF—Insoluble in cold water and in alcohol.

NF requirements: Starch NF—Preserve in well-closed containers. Consists of the granules separated from the mature grain of corn (*Zea mays* Linné [Fam. Gramineae]) or of wheat (*Triticum aestivum* Linné [Fam. Gramineae]), or from tubers of the potato (*Solanum tuberosum* Linné [Fam. Solanaceae]) or of tapioca (*Manihot utilissima* Pehl [Fam. Euphorbi Aceae]). Label it to indicate the botanical source from which it was derived. Meets the requirements for Botanic characteristics, Identification, Microbial limits, pH (4.5–7.0 for Corn starch, Tapioca starch, and Wheat starch, and 5.0–8.0 for Potato starch), Loss on drying (not more than 14.0%), Residue on ignition (not more than 0.5%), Iron (not more than 0.002%), Oxidizing substances (not more than 0.002%), and Sulfur dioxide (not more than 0.008%).

Note: Starches obtained from different botanical sources may not have identical properties with respect to their use for specific pharmaceutical purposes, e.g., as a tablet-disintegrating agent. Therefore, types of starch should not be interchanged unless performance equivalency has been ascertained.

PREGELATINIZED STARCH

Description: Pregelatinized Starch NF—Moderately coarse to fine, white to off-white powder. Odorless.
   NF category: Tablet binder; tablet and/or capsule diluent; tablet disintegrant.

Solubility: Pregelatinized Starch NF—Slightly soluble to soluble in cold water; insoluble in alcohol.

NF requirements: Pregelatinized Starch NF—It is Starch that has been chemically and/or mechanically processed to rupture all or part of the granules in the presence of water and subsequently dried. Some types of Pregelatinized Starch may be modified to render them compressible and flowable in character. Meets the requirements for pH (4.5–7.0, determined potentiometrically), Iron (not more than 0.002%), Oxidizing substances, and Sulfur dioxide (not more than 0.008%), and for Identification test B, Packaging and storage, Labeling, Microbial limits, Loss on drying, and Residue on ignition under Starch.

TOPICAL STARCH

USP requirements: Topical Starch USP—Preserve in well-closed containers. Consists of granules separated from the mature grain of corn (*Zea mays* Linné [Fam. Gramineae]). Meets the requirements for Botanic characteristics, Identification, Microbial limits, pH (4.5–7.0, determined potentiometrically), Loss on drying (not more than 14.0%), Residue on ignition (not more than 0.5%), Iron (not more than 0.001%), Oxidizing substances (not more than 0.018%), and Sulfur dioxide (not more than 0.008%).

STEARIC ACID

Chemical name: Octadecanoic acid.

Molecular formula: $C_{18}H_{36}O_2$.

Molecular weight: 284.48.

Description: Stearic Acid NF—Hard, white or faintly yellowish, somewhat glossy and crystalline solid, or white or yellowish-white powder. Slight odor, suggesting tallow.
   NF category: Emulsifying and/or solubilizing agent; tablet and/or capsule lubricant.

Solubility: Stearic Acid NF—Practically insoluble in water; freely soluble in chloroform and in ether; soluble in alcohol.

NF requirements: Stearic Acid NF—Preserve in well-closed containers. It is manufactured from fats and oils derived from edible sources and is a mixture of Stearic Acid and palmitic acid. The content of Stearic Acid is not less than 40.0%, and the sum of the two is not less than 90.0%. If it is for external use only, the labeling so indicates. Meets the requirements for Congealing temperature (not lower than 54 °C), Residue on ignition (not more than 0.1%), Heavy metals (not more than 0.001%), Mineral acid, Neutral fat or paraffin, Iodine value (not more than 4), and Organic volatile impurities.

Note: Stearic Acid labeled solely for external use is exempt from the requirement that it be prepared from edible sources.

PURIFIED STEARIC ACID

Description: Purified Stearic Acid NF—Hard, white or faintly yellowish, somewhat glossy and crystalline solid, or white or yellowish-white powder. Its odor is slight, suggesting tallow.
   NF category: Tablet and/or capsule lubricant.

Solubility: Purified Stearic Acid NF—Practically insoluble in water; freely soluble in chloroform and in ether; soluble in alcohol.

NF requirements: Purified Stearic Acid NF—Preserve in well-closed containers. It is manufactured from fats and oils derived from edible sources and is a mixture of Stearic Acid and palmitic acid, which together constitute not less than 96.0% of the total content. The content of Stearic Acid is not less than 90.0% of the total. If it is for external use only, the labeling so indicates. Meets the requirements for Congealing temperature (66–69 °C), Acid value (195–200), Iodine value (not more than 1.5), and Organic volatile impurities, and for Residue on ignition, Heavy metals, Mineral acid, and Neutral fat or paraffin under Stearic Acid.

Note: Purified Stearic Acid labeled solely for external use is exempt from the requirement that it be prepared from edible sources.

STEARYL ALCOHOL

Chemical name: 1-Octadecanol.

Molecular formula: $C_{18}H_{38}O$.

Molecular weight: 270.50.

Description: Stearyl Alcohol NF—Unctuous, white flakes or granules. Has a faint, characteristic odor.
NF category: Stiffening agent.

Solubility: Stearyl Alcohol NF—Insoluble in water; soluble in alcohol and in ether.

NF requirements: Stearyl Alcohol NF—Preserve in well-closed containers. Contains not less than 90.0% of stearyl alcohol, the remainder consisting chiefly of related alcohols. Meets the requirements for Identification, Melting range (55–60 °C), Acid value (not more than 2), Iodine value (not more than 2), and Hydroxyl value (195–220).

STREPTOKINASE

Source: A protein obtained from culture filtrates of certain strains of *Streptococcus hemolyticus* group C.

Molecular weight: About 46,000 daltons.

Description: Hygroscopic white powder or friable solid.

Solubility: Freely soluble in water.

USP requirements: Streptokinase for Injection—Not in USP.

STREPTOMYCIN

Source: Derived from *Streptomyces griseus*.

Chemical name: Streptomycin sulfate—D-Streptamine, *O*-2-deoxy-2-(methylamino)-alpha-L-glucopyranosyl-(1→2)-*O*-5-deoxy-3-*C*-formyl-alpha-L-lyxofuranosyl-(1→4)-*N*,*N*′-bis(aminoiminomethyl)-, sulfate (2:3) (salt).

Molecular formula: Streptomycin sulfate—$(C_{21}H_{39}N_7O_{12})_2 \cdot 3H_2SO_4$.

Molecular weight: Streptomycin sulfate—1457.38.

Description:
Streptomycin Sulfate Injection USP—Clear, colorless to yellow, viscous liquid. Is odorless or has a slight odor.
Sterile Streptomycin Sulfate USP—White or practically white powder. Is odorless or has not more than a faint odor. Is hygroscopic, but is stable in air and on exposure to light. Its solutions are acid to practically neutral to litmus.

Solubility: Sterile Streptomycin Sulfate USP—Freely soluble in water; very slightly soluble in alcohol; practically insoluble in chloroform.

USP requirements:
Streptomycin Sulfate Injection USP—Preserve in single-dose or in multiple-dose containers, preferably of Type I glass. Contains an amount of streptomycin sulfate equivalent to the labeled amount of streptomycin, within −10% to +15%. Meets the requirements for Bacterial endotoxins and pH (5.0–8.0), for Identification test A, Depressor substances, and Sterility under Sterile Streptomycin Sulfate, and for Injections.
Sterile Streptomycin Sulfate USP—Preserve in Containers for Sterile Solids. Contains an amount of streptomycin sulfate equivalent to not less than 650 mcg and not more than 850 mcg of streptomycin per mg and, where packaged for dispensing, contains an amount of streptomycin sulfate equivalent to the labeled amount of streptomycin, within −10% to +15%. Meets the requirements for Constituted solution, Identification, Depressor substances, Bacterial endotoxins, Sterility, pH (4.5–7.0, in a solution containing 200 mg of streptomycin per mL), and Loss on drying (not more than 5.0%), and for Uniformity of dosage units and Labeling under Injections.

STREPTOZOCIN

Chemical name: D-Glucopyranose, 2-deoxy-2-[[(methylnitrosoamino)carbonyl]amino]-.

Molecular formula: $C_8H_{15}N_3O_7$.

Molecular weight: 265.22.

Description: Ivory-colored crystalline powder.

Solubility: Very soluble in water or in physiological saline; soluble in alcohol.

USP requirements: Streptozocin for Injection—Not in USP.

SUCCINYLCHOLINE

Chemical name: Succinylcholine chloride—Ethanaminium, 2,2′-[(1,4-dioxo-1,4-butanediyl)bis(oxy)]bis[*N*,*N*,*N*-trimethyl-], dichloride.

Molecular formula: Succinylcholine chloride—$C_{14}H_{30}Cl_2N_2O_4$.

Molecular weight: Succinylcholine chloride—361.31.

Description:
Succinylcholine Chloride USP—White, odorless, crystalline powder. Its solutions have a pH of about 4. The dihydrate form melts at about 160 °C; the anhydrous form melts at about 190 °C, and is hygroscopic.
Sterile Succinylcholine Chloride USP—White, odorless, crystalline powder. Its solutions have a pH of about 4. The dihydrate form melts at about 160 °C; the anhydrous form melts at about 190 °C, and is hygroscopic.

Solubility:
Succinylcholine Chloride USP—Freely soluble in water; slightly soluble in alcohol and in chloroform; practically insoluble in ether.
Sterile Succinylcholine Chloride USP—Freely soluble in water; slightly soluble in alcohol and in chloroform; practically insoluble in ether.

USP requirements:
Succinylcholine Chloride Injection USP—Preserve in single-dose or in multiple-dose containers, preferably of Type I or Type II glass, in a refrigerator. A sterile solution of Succinylcholine Chloride in a suitable aqueous vehicle. Label it to indicate, as its expiration date, the month and year not more than 2 years from the month during which

the Injection was last assayed and released by the manufacturer. Contains an amount of succinylcholine chloride equivalent to the labeled amount of anhydrous succinylcholine chloride, within ± 10%. Meets the requirements for Identification, Bacterial endotoxins, pH (3.0–4.5), and Injections.

Sterile Succinylcholine Chloride USP—Preserve in Containers for Sterile Solids. It is Succinylcholine Chloride suitable for parenteral use. Meets the requirements for Completeness of solution, Constituted solution, Bacterial endotoxins, and Chromatographic purity, for Identification, Water, Residue on ignition, Ammonium salts, and Chloride content under Succinylcholine Chloride, and for Sterility, Uniformity of dosage units, and Labeling under Injections.

SUCRALFATE

Chemical name: Alpha-D-glucopyranoside, beta-D-fructofuranosyl-, octakis(hydrogen sulfate), aluminum complex.

Molecular formula: $C_{12}H_mAl_{16}O_nS_8$.

Description: Whitish or white, odorless, amorphous powder.

Solubility: Soluble in dilute hydrochloric acid and in sodium hydroxide; practically insoluble in water, in boiling water, in ethanol, and in chloroform.

Other characteristics: Metal salt of a sulfated disaccharide.

USP requirements:
Sucralfate Oral Suspension–Not in USP.
Sucralfate Tablets—Not in USP.

SUCROSE

Chemical name: Alpha-D-glucopyranoside, beta-D-fructofuranosyl-.

Molecular formula: $C_{12}H_{22}O_{11}$.

Molecular weight: 342.30.

Description: Sucrose NF—Colorless or white crystals, crystalline masses or blocks, or white crystalline powder. Odorless and stable in air. Its solutions are neutral to litmus.
NF category: Coating agent; sweetening agent; tablet and/or capsule diluent.

Solubility: Sucrose NF—Very soluble in water, and even more soluble in boiling water; slightly soluble in alcohol; insoluble in chloroform and in ether.

NF requirements: Sucrose NF—Preserve in well-closed containers. A sugar obtained from *Saccharum officinarum* Linné (Fam. Gramineae), *Beta vulgaris* Linné (Fam. Chenopodiaceae), and other sources. Contains no added substances. Meets the requirements for Specific rotation (not less than +65.9°), Residue on ignition (not more than 0.05%), Chloride (not more than 0.0035%), Sulfate (not more than 0.006%), Calcium, Heavy metals (not more than 5 ppm), and Invert sugar.

SUCROSE OCTAACETATE

Chemical name: Alpha-D-glucopyranoside, 1,3,4,6-tetra-*O*-acetyl-beta-D-fructofuranosyl, tetraacetate.

Molecular formula: $C_{28}H_{38}O_{19}$.

Molecular weight: 678.60.

Description: Sucrose Octaacetate NF—White, practically odorless powder. Hygroscopic.
NF category: Alcohol denaturant.

Solubility: Sucrose Octaacetate NF—Very slightly soluble in water; very soluble in methanol and in chloroform; soluble in alcohol and in ether.

NF requirements: Sucrose Octaacetate NF—Preserve in tight containers. Contains not less than 98.0% and not more than 100.5% of sucrose octaacetate, calculated on the anhydrous basis. Meets the requirements for Melting temperature (not lower than 78 °C), Acidity, Water (not more than 1.0%), and Residue on ignition (not more than 0.1%).

SUFENTANIL

Chemical group: Fentanyl derivatives are anilinopiperidine-derivative opioid analgesics and are chemically related to anileridine and meperidine.

Chemical name: Sufentanil citrate—Propanamide, *N*-[4-(methoxymethyl)-1-[2-(thienyl)ethyl]-4-piperidinyl]-*N*-phenyl-, 2-hydroxy-1,2,3-propanetricarboxylate (1:1).

Molecular formula: Sufentanil citrate—$C_{22}H_{30}N_2O_2S \cdot C_6H_8O_7$.

Molecular weight: Sufentanil citrate—578.68.

Description: Sufentanil citrate—White to slightly yellowish powder melting at 133–140 °C.

pKa: Sufentanil citrate—8.01.

Solubility: Sufentanil citrate—Freely soluble in methanol; soluble in water; sparingly soluble in ethanol.

Other characteristics: Log partition coefficient (*n*-octanol/aqueous buffer solution at pH 10.8–3.95.

USP requirements: Sufentanil Citrate Injection—Not in USP.

COMPRESSIBLE SUGAR

Description: Compressible Sugar NF—Practically white, crystalline, odorless powder. Stable in air.
NF category: Sweetening agent; tablet and/or capsule diluent.

Solubility: Compressible Sugar NF—The sucrose portion of Compressible Sugar is very soluble in water.

NF requirements: Compressible Sugar NF—Preserve in well-closed containers. Previously dried at 105 °C for 4 hours, contains not less than 95.0% and not more than 98.0% of sucrose. Meets the requirements for Identification, Microbial limits, Loss on drying (0.25–1.0%), Residue on ignition (not more than 0.1%), Chloride, Sulfate, Calcium, and Heavy metals (not more than 0.014% for chloride, not more than 0.010% for sulfate, and not more than 5 ppm for heavy metals).

CONFECTIONER'S SUGAR

Description: Confectioner's Sugar NF—Fine, white, odorless powder. Stable in air.
NF category: Sweetening agent; tablet and/or capsule diluent.

Solubility: Confectioner's Sugar NF—The sucrose portion of Confectioner's Sugar is soluble in cold water. Freely soluble in boiling water.

NF requirements: Confectioner's Sugar NF—Preserve in well-closed containers. It is Sucrose ground together with corn starch to a fine powder. Contains not less than 95.0% of sucrose, calculated on the dried basis. Meets the requirements for Identification, Specific rotation, Chloride, Calcium, Sulfate, and Heavy metals (not less than +62.6°, calculated on the dried basis, for specific rotation, not more than 0.014% for chloride, not more than 0.006% for sulfate, and not more than 5 ppm for heavy metals), Microbial limits, Loss on drying (not more than 1.0%), and Residue on ignition (not more than 0.08%).

INVERT SUGAR

USP requirements: Invert Sugar Injection USP—Preserve in single-dose containers, preferably of Type I or Type II glass, or of a suitable plastic material. A sterile solution of a mixture of equal amounts of Dextrose and Fructose in Water for Injection, or an equivalent sterile solution produced by the hydrolysis of Sucrose, in Water for Injection. The label states the total osmolar concentration in mOsmol per liter. Contains the labeled amount of fructose, within ± 5%. Contains no antimicrobial agents. Meets the requirements for Identification, Bacterial endotoxins, pH (3.0–6.5), Chloride (not more than 0.012%), Heavy metals, 5-Hydroxymethyl-furfural and related substances (absorbance not more than 0.25), Completeness of inversion, and Injections.

Note: Invert Sugar Injection that is produced by mixing Dextrose and Fructose is exempt from the requirement of the test for Completeness of inversion.

SUGAR SPHERES

Description: Sugar Spheres NF—Hard, brittle, free-flowing, spherical masses ranging generally in size from 10- to 60-mesh. Usually white, but may be colored.

NF category: Vehicle (solid carrier).

Solubility: Sugar Spheres NF—Solubility in water varies according to the sugar-to-starch ratio.

NF requirements: Sugar Spheres NF—Preserve in well-closed containers. The label states the nominal particle size range. Contain not less than 62.5% and not more than 91.5% of sucrose, calculated on the dried basis, the remainder consisting chiefly of starch. Consist of approximately spherical particles of a labeled nominal size range. Meet the requirements for Identification and Specific rotation ($+41°$ to $+61°$, calculated on the dried basis, for specific rotation), Microbial limits, Loss on drying (not more than 4.0%), Residue on ignition (not more than 0.25%), Particle size, and Heavy metals (not more than 5 ppm).

SULBACTAM

Chemical name: Sulbactam sodium—4-Thia-1-azabicy-clo[3.2.0]heptane-2-carboxylic acid, 3,3-dimethyl-7-oxo-, 4,4-dioxide, sodium salt, (2S-*cis*)-.

Molecular formula: Sulbactam sodium—$C_8H_{10}NNaO_5S$.

Molecular weight: Sulbactam sodium—255.22.

USP requirements: Sterile Sulbactam Sodium USP—Preserve in tight containers. It is sulbactam sodium suitable for parenteral use. Contains not less than 886 mcg and not more than 941 mcg of sulbactam, calculated on the anhydrous basis. Meets the requirements for Identification, Crystallinity, Pyrogen, Sterility, and Water (not more than 1.0%).

TRIPLE SULFA

For *Sulfathiazole, Sulfacetamide,* and *Sulfabenzamide*—See individual listings for chemistry information.

USP requirements:

Triple Sulfa Vaginal Cream USP—Preserve in well-closed, light-resistant containers, or in collapsible tubes. Contains the labeled amounts of sulfathiazole, sulfacetamide, and sulfabenzamide, within ± 10%. Meets the requirements for Identification, Minimum fill, and pH (3.0–4.0).

Triple Sulfa Vaginal Tablets USP—Preserve in well-closed, light-resistant containers. Contain the labeled amounts of sulfathiazole, sulfacetamide, and sulfabenzamide, within ± 10%. Meet the requirements for Identification, Disintegration (30 minutes), and Uniformity of dosage units.

SULFABENZAMIDE

Chemical name: Benzamide, *N*-[(4-aminophenyl)sulfonyl]-.

Molecular formula: $C_{13}H_{12}N_2O_3S$.

Molecular weight: 276.31.

Description: Sulfabenzamide USP—Fine, white, practically odorless powder.

Solubility: Sulfabenzamide USP—Insoluble in water and in ether; soluble in alcohol, in acetone, and in sodium hydroxide TS.

USP requirements: Sulfabenzamide USP—Preserve in well-closed, light-resistant containers. Contains not less than 99.0% and not more than 100.5% of sulfabenzamide, calculated on the dried basis. Meets the requirements for Color and clarity of solution, Identification, Melting range (180–184 °C), Loss on drying (not more than 0.5%), Selenium (not more than 0.001%), Heavy metals (not more than 0.002%), and Ordinary impurities.

SULFACETAMIDE

Chemical name:

Sulfacetamide—Acetamide, *N*-[(4-aminophenyl)sulfonyl]-.

Sulfacetamide sodium—Acetamide, *N*-[(4-aminophenyl)-sulfonyl]-, monosodium salt, monohydrate.

Molecular formula:

Sulfacetamide—$C_8H_{10}N_2O_3S$.

Sulfacetamide sodium—$C_8H_9N_2NaO_3S \cdot H_2O$.

Molecular weight:

Sulfacetamide—214.24.

Sulfacetamide sodium—254.24.

Description:

Sulfacetamide USP—White, crystalline, odorless powder. Its aqueous solutions are sensitive to light, and are unstable when acidic or strongly alkaline.

Sulfacetamide Sodium USP—White, crystalline powder. Is odorless.

Solubility:

Sulfacetamide USP—Slightly soluble in water and in ether; freely soluble in dilute mineral acids and in solutions of potassium and sodium hydroxides; soluble in alcohol; very slightly soluble in chloroform.

Sulfacetamide Sodium USP—Freely soluble in water; sparingly soluble in alcohol; practically insoluble in chloroform and in ether.

USP requirements:

Sulfacetamide Sodium Ophthalmic Ointment USP— Preserve in collapsible ophthalmic ointment tubes. It is sterile. Contains the labeled amount, within ± 10%. Meets the requirements for Identification, Sterility, and Metal particles.

Sulfacetamide Sodium Ophthalmic Solution USP—Preserve in tight, light-resistant containers, in a cool place. A sterile solution. Contains the labeled amount, within + 10%. Meets the requirements for Identification and Sterility.

SULFACETAMIDE AND PREDNISOLONE

For *Sulfacetamide* and *Prednisolone*—See individual listings for chemistry information.

USP requirements:

Sulfacetamide Sodium and Prednisolone Acetate Ophthalmic Ointment USP—Preserve in collapsible ophthalmic ointment tubes that are tamper-proof so that sterility is assured at time of first use. A sterile ointment. Contains the labeled amounts, within ±10%. Meets the requirements for Identification, Minimum fill, Sterility, and Metal particles.

Sulfacetamide Sodium and Prednisolone Acetate Ophthalmic Suspension USP—Preserve in tight containers. The containers or individual cartons are sealed and tamper-proof so that sterility is assured at time of first use. A sterile, aqueous suspension. Contains the labeled amounts, within ±10%. Meets the requirements for Identification, Sterility, and pH (6.0–7.4).

SULFACYTINE

Chemical name: Benzenesulfonamide, 4-amino-N-(1-ethyl-1,2-dihydro-2-oxo-4-pyrimidinyl)-.

Molecular formula: $C_{12}H_{14}N_4O_3S$.

Molecular weight: 294.33.

Description: White to cream-colored crystalline powder. Melts at about 169 °C.

Solubility: Slightly soluble in water.

Other characteristics: Sulfonamides have certain chemical similarities to some goitrogens, diuretics (acetazolamide and thiazides), and oral antidiabetic agents.

USP requirements: Sulfacytine Tablets—Not in USP.

SULFADIAZINE

Chemical name:

Sulfadiazine—Benzenesulfonamide, 4-amino-N-2-pyrimidinyl-.

Sulfadiazine sodium—Benzenesulfonamide, 4-amino-N-2-pyrimidinyl-, monosodium salt.

Molecular formula:

Sulfadiazine—$C_{10}H_{10}N_4O_2S$.

Sulfadiazine sodium—$C_{10}H_9N_4NaO_2S$.

Molecular weight:

Sulfadiazine—250.27.

Sulfadiazine sodium—272.26.

Description

Sulfadiazine USP—White or slightly yellow powder. Odorless or nearly odorless and stable in air, but slowly darkens on exposure to light.

Sulfadiazine Sodium USP—White powder. On prolonged exposure to humid air it absorbs carbon dioxide with liberation of sulfadiazine and becomes incompletely soluble in water. Its solutions are alkaline to phenolphthalein. Affected by light.

Solubility:

Sulfadiazine USP—Practically insoluble in water; freely soluble in dilute mineral acids, in solutions of potassium and sodium hydroxides, and in ammonia TS; sparingly soluble in alcohol and in acetone; slightly soluble in human serum at 37 °C.

Sulfadiazine Sodium USP—Freely soluble in water; slightly soluble in alcohol.

USP requirements:

Sulfadiazine Tablets USP—Preserve in well-closed, light-resistant containers. Contain the labeled amount, within ±5%. Meet the requirements for Identification, Dissolution (70% in 90 minutes in 0.1 N hydrochloric acid in Apparatus 2 at 75 rpm), and Uniformity of dosage units.

Sulfadiazine Sodium Injection USP—Preserve in single-dose, light-resistant containers, of Type I glass. A sterile solution of Sulfadiazine Sodium in Water for Injection. Contains, in each mL, not less than 237.5 mg and not more than 262.5 mg of sulfadiazine sodium. Meets the requirements for Identification, Bacterial endotoxins, pH (8.5–10.5), Particulate matter, and Injections.

SULFADIAZINE AND TRIMETHOPRIM

For *Sulfadiazine* and *Trimethoprim*—See individual listings for chemistry information.

USP requirements:

Sulfadiazine and Trimethoprim Oral Suspension—Not in USP.

Sulfadiazine and Trimethoprim Tablets—Not in USP.

SULFADOXINE AND PYRIMETHAMINE

Chemical group:

Sulfadoxine—Sulfonamides (long-acting).

Pyrimethamine—Structurally related to trimethoprim.

Chemical name:

Sulfadoxine—Benzenesulfonamide, 4-amino-N-(5,6-dimethoxy-4-pyrimidinyl)-.

Pyrimethamine—2,4-Pyrimidinediamine, 5-(4-chlorophenyl)-6-ethyl-.

Molecular formula:

Sulfadoxine—$C_{12}H_{14}N_4O_4S$.

Pyrimethamine—$C_{12}H_{13}ClN_4$.

Molecular weight:

Sulfadoxine—310.33.

Pyrimethamine—248.71.

Description:

Sulfadoxine—White or creamy-white odorless, crystalline powder, melting at 197–200 °C.

Pyrimethamine USP—White, odorless, crystalline powder.

Solubility:

Sulfadoxine—Very slightly soluble in water; slightly soluble in alcohol and in methanol; practically insoluble in ether.

Pyrimethamine USP—Practically insoluble in water; slightly soluble in acetone, in alcohol, and in chloroform.

Other characteristics: Sulfadoxine—Sulfonamides have certain chemical similarities to some goitrogens, diuretics (acetazolamide and thiazides), and oral antidiabetic agents.

USP requirements: Sulfadoxine and Pyrimethamine Tablets USP—Preserve in well-closed, light-resistant containers. Contain the labeled amounts, within ±10%. Meet the requirements for Identification, Dissolution (60% of each active ingredient in 30 minutes in phosphate buffer [pH 6.8] in Apparatus 2 at 75 rpm), and Uniformity of dosage units.

SULFAMERAZINE

Chemical name: Benzenesulfonamide, 4-amino-*N*-(4-methyl-2-pyrimidinyl)-.

Molecular formula: $C_{11}H_{12}N_4O_2S$.

Molecular weight: 264.30.

Description: Sulfamerazine USP—White or faintly yellowish white crystals or powder. Odorless or practically odorless. Stable in air, but slowly darkens on exposure to light.

Solubility: Sulfamerazine USP—Very slightly soluble in water; sparingly soluble in acetone; slightly soluble in alcohol; very slightly soluble in ether and in chloroform.

USP requirements: Sulfamerazine Tablets USP—Preserve in well-closed containers. Contain the labeled amount, within ±5%. Meet the requirements for Identification, Dissolution (75% in 45 minutes in water in Apparatus 1 at 100 rpm), and Uniformity of dosage units.

SULFAMETHIZOLE

Chemical name: Benzenesulfonamide, 4-amino-*N*-(5-methyl-1,3,4-thiadiazol-2-yl)-.

Molecular formula: $C_9H_{10}N_4O_2S_2$.

Molecular weight: 270.32.

Description: Sulfamethizole USP—White crystals or powder. Practically odorless, and has no odor of hydrogen sulfide.

Solubility: Sulfamethizole USP—Very slightly soluble in water, in chloroform, and in ether; freely soluble in solutions of ammonium, potassium, and sodium hydroxides; soluble in dilute mineral acids and in acetone; sparingly soluble in alcohol.

USP requirements:
Sulfamethizole Oral Suspension USP—Preserve in tight, light-resistant containers. Contains the labeled amount, within ±10%, in a buffered aqueous suspension. Meets the requirement for Identification.
Sulfamethizole Tablets USP—Preserve in well-closed containers. Contain the labeled amount, within ±5%. Meet the requirements for Identification, Dissolution (75% in 30 minutes in 0.1 N hydrochloric acid in Apparatus 2 at 50 rpm), and Uniformity of dosage units.

SULFAMETHOXAZOLE

Chemical name: Benzenesulfonamide, 4-amino-*N*-(5-methyl-3-isoxazolyl)-.

Molecular formula: $C_{10}H_{11}N_3O_3S$.

Molecular weight: 253.28.

Description: Sulfamethoxazole USP—White to off-white, practically odorless, crystalline powder.

Solubility: Sulfamethoxazole USP—Practically insoluble in water, in ether, and in chloroform; freely soluble in acetone and in dilute solutions of sodium hydroxide; sparingly soluble in alcohol.

Other characteristics: Sulfonamides have certain chemical similarities to some goitrogens, diuretics (acetazolamide and thiazides), and oral antidiabetic agents.

USP requirements:
Sulfamethoxazole Oral Suspension USP—Preserve in tight, light-resistant containers. Contains the labeled amount,

within −5% to + 10%. Meets the requirement for Identification.
Sulfamethoxazole Tablets USP—Preserve in well-closed, light-resistant containers. Contain the labeled amount, within ±5%. Meet the requirements for Identification, Dissolution (50% in 20 minutes in dilute hydrochloric acid [7 in 100] in Apparatus 1 at 100 rpm), and Uniformity of dosage units.

SULFAMETHOXAZOLE AND PHENAZOPYRIDINE

For *Sulfamethoxazole* and *Phenazopyridine*—See individual listings for chemistry information.

USP requirements: Sulfamethoxazole and Phenazopyridine Hydrochloride Tablets—Not in USP.

SULFAMETHOXAZOLE AND TRIMETHOPRIM

For *Sulfamethoxazole* and *Trimethoprim*—See individual listings for chemistry information.

USP requirements:
Sulfamethoxazole and Trimethoprim for Injection Concentrate USP—Preserve in single-dose, light-resistant containers, preferably of Type I glass. Sulfamethoxazole and Trimethoprim for Injection Concentrate may be packaged in 50-mL multiple-dose containers. A sterile solution of Sulfamethoxazole and Trimethoprim in Water for Injection which, when diluted with Dextrose Injection, is suitable for intravenous infusion. Label it to indicate that it is to be diluted with 5% Dextrose Injection prior to administration. Contains the labeled amounts, within ±10%. Meets the requirements for Identification, Pyrogen, pH (9.5–10.5), Particulate matter, Related compounds (not more than 0.5% of trimethoprim degradation product, 0.5% of sulfanilamide, and 0.3% of sulfanilic acid), and Injections.
Sulfamethoxazole and Trimethoprim Oral Suspension USP—Preserve in tight, light-resistant containers. Contains the labeled amounts, within ±10%. Meets the requirements for Identification, pH (5.0–6.5), Alcohol content (not more than 0.5%), and Chromatographic purity (not more than 0.5% of trimethoprim degradation product, 0.5% of sulfanilamide, 0.3% of sulfanilic acid, and 3.0% of sulfamethoxazole N₄-glucoside).
Sulfamethoxazole and Trimethoprim Tablets USP—Preserve in well-closed, light-resistant containers. Contain the labeled amounts, within ±7%. Meet the requirements for Identification, Dissolution (70% of each active ingredient in 60 minutes in 0.1 N hydrochloric acid in Apparatus 2 at 75 rpm), and Uniformity of dosage units.

SULFANILAMIDE

Chemical name: *p*-Aminobenzenesulfonamide.

Molecular formula: $C_6H_8N_2O_2S$.

Molecular weight: 172.21.

Description: White, odorless, crystalline powder.

Solubility: Slightly soluble in water, in alcohol, in acetone, in glycerin, in propylene glycol, in hydrochloric acid, and in solutions of potassium and sodium hydroxide; practically insoluble in chloroform, in ether, and in petroleum ether.

USP requirements:
    Sulfanilamide Vaginal Cream—Not in USP.
    Sulfanilamide Vaginal Suppositories—Not in USP.

SULFANILAMIDE, AMINACRINE, AND ALLANTOIN

Chemical name:
    Sulfanilamide—p-Aminobenzenesulfonamide.
    Aminacrine hydrochloride—9-Acridinamine monohydrochloride.
    Allantoin—Urea, (2,5-dioxo-4-imidazolidinyl)-.

Molecular formula:
    Sulfanilamide—$C_6H_8N_2O_2S$.
    Aminacrine hydrochloride—$C_{13}H_{10}N_2 \cdot HCl$.
    Allantoin—$C_4H_6N_4O_3$.

Molecular weight:
    Sulfanilamide—172.21.
    Aminacrine hydrochloride—320.70.
    Allantoin—158.12.

Description:
    Sulfanilamide—White, odorless crystalline powder.
    Aminacrine hydrochloride—Pale yellow, crystalline powder; highly fluorescent.
    Allantoin—Colorless crystals, melting at 238 °C.

Solubility:
    Sulfanilamide—Slightly soluble in water, in alcohol, in acetone, in glycerin, in propylene glycol, in hydrochloric acid, and in solutions of potassium and sodium hydroxide; practically insoluble in chloroform, in ether, and in petroleum ether.
    Aminacrine hydrochloride—1 gram soluble in 300 mL of water and in 150 mL of alcohol; soluble in glycerin.
    Allantoin—1 gram dissolves in 190 mL of water or in 500 mL of alcohol; nearly insoluble in ether.

USP requirements:
    Sulfanilamide, Aminacrine Hydrochloride, and Allantoin Vaginal Cream—Not in USP.
    Sulfanilamide, Aminacrine Hydrochloride, and Allantoin Vaginal Suppositories—Not in USP.

SULFAPYRIDINE

Chemical group: Sulfonamide.

Chemical name: Benzenesulfonamide, 4-amino-N-2-pyridinyl-.

Molecular formula: $C_{11}H_{11}N_3O_2S$.

Molecular weight: 249.29.

Description: Sulfapyridine USP—White or faintly yellowish white crystals, granules, or powder. Is odorless or practically odorless, and is stable in air, but slowly darkens on exposure to light.

Solubility: Sulfapyridine USP—Very slightly soluble in water; freely soluble in dilute mineral acids and in solutions of potassium and sodium hydroxides; sparingly soluble in acetone; slightly soluble in alcohol.

Other characteristics: Sulfonamides have certain chemical similarities to some goitrogens, diuretics (acetazolamide and thiazides), and oral hypoglycemic agents.

USP requirements: Sulfapyridine Tablets USP—Preserve in well-closed, light-resistant containers. Contain the labeled amount, within ±5%. Meet the requirements for Identification, Dissolution (70% in 60 minutes in 0.1 N hydrochloric acid in Apparatus 2 at 50 rpm), and Uniformity of dosage units.

SULFASALAZINE

Source: Synthesized by the diazotization of sulfapyridine and the coupling of the diazonium salt with salicylic acid.

Chemical name: Benzoic acid, 2-hydroxy-5-[[4-[(2-pyridinylamino)sulfonyl]phenyl]azo]-.

Molecular formula: $C_{18}H_{14}N_4O_5S$.

Molecular weight: 398.39.

Description: Sulfasalazine USP—Bright yellow or brownish yellow, odorless, fine powder. Melts at about 255 °C, with decomposition.

Solubility: Sulfasalazine USP—Very slightly soluble in alcohol; practically insoluble in water, in ether, and in chloroform; soluble in aqueous solutions of alkali hydroxides.

USP requirements:
    Sulfasalazine Oral Suspension—Not in USP.
    Sulfasalazine Tablets USP—Preserve in well-closed containers. Contain the labeled amount, within ±5%. Meet the requirements for Identification, Disintegration (15 minutes, for Tablets that are enteric-coated), Dissolution (85% in 60 minutes in phosphate buffer [pH 7.5] in Apparatus 1 at 100 rpm), and Uniformity of dosage units.

SULFATHIAZOLE

Chemical name: Benzenesulfonamide, 4-amino-N-2-thiazolyl-.

Molecular formula: $C_9H_9N_3O_2S_2$.

Molecular weight: 255.31.

Description: Sulfathiazole USP—Fine, white or faintly yellowish white, practically odorless powder.

Solubility: Sulfathiazole USP—Very slightly soluble in water; soluble in acetone, in dilute mineral acids, in solutions of alkali hydroxides, and in 6 N ammonium hydroxide; slightly soluble in alcohol.

USP requirements: Sulfathiazole USP—Preserve in well-closed, light-resistant containers. Contains not less than 99.0% and not more than 100.5% of sulfathiazole, calculated on the dried basis. Meets the requirements for Identification, Melting range (200–204 °C), Acidity, Loss on drying (not more than 0.5%), Residue on ignition (not more than 0.1%), Chloride (not more than 0.014%), Sulfate (not more than 0.04%), Heavy metals (not more than 0.002%), and Ordinary impurities.

SULFINPYRAZONE

Chemical group: A pyrazole compound chemically related to phenylbutazone.

Chemical name: 3,5-Pyrazolidinedione, 1,2-diphenyl-4-[2-(phenylsulfinyl)ethyl]-.

Molecular formula: $C_{23}H_{20}N_2O_3S$.

Molecular weight: 404.48.

Description: Sulfinpyrazone USP—White to off-white powder.

pKa: 2.8.

Solubility: Sulfinpyrazone USP—Practically insoluble in water and in solvent hexane; soluble in alcohol and in acetone; sparingly soluble in dilute alkali.

USP requirements:
    Sulfinpyrazone Capsules USP—Preserve in well-closed containers. Contain the labeled amount, within ±7%. Meet

the requirements for Identification, Dissolution (75% in 45 minutes in phosphate buffer [pH 7.5] in Apparatus 1 at 100 rpm), and Uniformity of dosage units.

Sulfinpyrazone Tablets USP—Preserve in well-closed containers. Contain the labeled amount, within ±7%. Meet the requirements for Identification, Dissolution (75% in 45 minutes in phosphate buffer [pH 7.5] in Apparatus 1 at 100 rpm), and Uniformity of dosage units.

SULFISOXAZOLE

Chemical name:

Sulfisoxazole—Benzenesulfonamide, 4-amino-N-(3,4-dimethyl-5-isoxazolyl)-.

Sulfisoxazole acetyl—Acetamide, N-[(4-aminophenyl)-sulfonyl]-N-(3,4-dimethyl-5-isoxazolyl)-.

Sulfisoxazole diolamine—Benzenesulfonamide, 4-amino-N-(3,4-dimethyl-5-isoxazolyl)-, compd. with 2,2'-iminobis[ethanol] (1:1).

Molecular formula:

Sulfisoxazole—$C_{11}H_{13}N_3O_3S$.

Sulfisoxazole acetyl—$C_{13}H_{15}N_3O_4S$.

Sulfisoxazole diolamine—$C_{11}H_{13}N_3O_3S \cdot C_4H_{11}NO_2$.

Molecular weight:

Sulfisoxazole—267.30.

Sulfisoxazole acetyl—309.34.

Sulfisoxazole diolamine—372.44.

Description:

Sulfisoxazole USP—White to slightly yellowish, odorless, crystalline powder.

Sulfisoxazole Acetyl USP—White or slightly yellow, crystalline powder.

Sulfisoxazole Diolamine USP—White to off-white, fine crystalline, odorless powder.

Solubility:

Sulfisoxazole USP—Very slightly soluble in water; soluble in boiling alcohol and in 3 N hydrochloric acid.

Sulfisoxazole Acetyl USP—Practically insoluble in water; sparingly soluble in chloroform; slightly soluble in alcohol.

Sulfisoxazole Diolamine USP—Freely soluble in water; soluble in alcohol.

Other characteristics: Sulfonamides have certain chemical similarities to some goitrogens, diuretics (acetazolamide and thiazides), and oral antidiabetic agents.

USP requirements:

Sulfisoxazole Tablets USP—Preserve in well-closed, light-resistant containers. Contain the labeled amount, within ±5%. Meet the requirements for Identification, Dissolution (70% in 30 minutes in dilute hydrochloric acid [1 in 12.5] in Apparatus 1 at 100 rpm), and Uniformity of dosage units.

Sulfisoxazole Acetyl Oral Suspension USP—Preserve in tight, light-resistant containers. Contains an amount of sulfisoxazole acetyl equivalent to the labeled amount of sulfisoxazole, within ±7%. Meets the requirements for Identification and pH (5.0–5.5).

Sulfisoxazole Acetyl Oral Syrup—Not in USP.

Sulfisoxazole Diolamine Injection USP—Preserve in single-dose or in multiple-dose containers, preferably of Type I glass, protected from light. A sterile solution of Sulfisoxazole Diolamine in Water for Injection. Contains an amount of sulfisoxazole diolamine equivalent to the labeled amount of sulfisoxazole, within ±10%. Meets the requirements for Identification, Pyrogen, pH (7.0–8.5), Particulate matter, and Injections.

Sulfisoxazole Diolamine Ophthalmic Ointment USP—Preserve in collapsible ophthalmic ointment tubes. A sterile ointment. Contains an amount of sulfisoxazole diolamine equivalent to the labeled amount of sulfisoxazole, within ±10%. Meets the requirements for Identification, Sterility, Minimum fill, Leakage, and Metal particles.

Sulfisoxazole Diolamine Ophthalmic Solution USP—Preserve in tight, light-resistant containers. A sterile solution. Contains an amount of sulfisoxazole diolamine equivalent to the labeled amount of sulfisoxazole, within −10% to +15%. Meets the requirements for Identification, Sterility, and pH (7.2–8.2).

SULFISOXAZOLE, AMINACRINE, AND ALLANTOIN

Chemical name:

Sulfisoxazole—Benzenesulfonamide, 4-amino-N-(3,4-dimethyl-5-isoxazolyl)-.

Aminacrine hydrochloride—9-Acridinamine monohydrochloride.

Allantoin—Urea, (2,5-dioxo-4-imidazolidinyl)-.

Molecular formula:

Sulfisoxazole—$C_{11}H_{13}N_3O_3S$.

Aminacrine hydrochloride—$C_{13}H_{10}N_2 \cdot HCl$.

Allantoin—$C_4H_6N_4O_3$.

Molecular weight:

Sulfisoxazole—267.30.

Aminacrine hydrochloride—320.70.

Allantoin—158.12.

Description:

Sulfisoxazole USP—White to slightly yellowish, odorless, crystalline powder.

Aminacrine hydrochloride—Pale yellow, crystalline powder; highly fluorescent.

Allantoin—Colorless crystals, melting at 238 °C.

Solubility:

Sulfisoxazole USP—Very slightly soluble in water; soluble in boiling alcohol and in 3 N hydrochloric acid.

Aminacrine hydrochloride—1 gram soluble in 300 mL of water and in 150 mL of alcohol; soluble in glycerin.

Allantoin—1 gram dissolves in 190 mL of water or in 500 mL of alcohol; nearly insoluble in ether.

USP requirements: Sulfisoxazole, Aminacrine Hydrochloride, and Allantoin Vaginal Cream— Not in USP.

SULFISOXAZOLE AND PHENAZOPYRIDINE

For *Sulfisoxazole* and *Phenazopyridine*—See individual listings for chemistry information.

USP requirements: Sulfisoxazole and Phenazopyridine Hydrochloride Tablets—Not in USP.

SULFOBROMOPHTHALEIN

Chemical name: Sulfobromophthalein sodium—Benzenesulfonic acid, 3,3'-(4,5,6,7-tetrabromo-3-oxo-1(3H)-isobenzofuranylidine)bis[6-hydroxy-, disodium salt.

Molecular formula: Sulfobromophthalein sodium—$C_{20}H_8Br_4Na_2O_{10}S_2$.

Molecular weight: Sulfobromophthalein sodium—837.99.

Description: Sulfobromophthalein Sodium USP—White, crystalline powder. Odorless. Hygroscopic.

Solubility: Sulfobromophthalein Sodium USP—Soluble in water; insoluble in acetone and in alcohol.

USP requirements: Sulfobromophthalein Sodium Injection USP—Preserve in single-dose containers, preferably of Type I glass. A colorless, or almost colorless, sterile solution of Sulfobromophthalein Sodium in Water for Injection. Contains, in each mL, not less than 47 mg and not more than 53 mg of sulfobromophthalein sodium. Meets the requirements for Identification, Bacterial endotoxins, pH (5.0–6.5, a suitable agar-potassium nitrate salt bridge being used), and Injections.

SULFOXONE

Chemical name: Sulfoxone sodium—Methanesulfinic acid, [sulfonylbis(1,4-phenyleneimino)]bis-, disodium salt.

Molecular formula: Sulfoxone sodium—$C_{14}H_{14}N_2Na_2O_6S_3$.

Molecular weight: Sulfoxone sodium—448.43.

Description: Sulfoxone Sodium USP—White to pale yellow powder, having a characteristic odor.

Solubility: Sulfoxone Sodium USP—Soluble in water, yielding a clear to hazy, pale yellow solution; very slightly soluble in alcohol.

USP requirements: Sulfoxone Sodium Tablets USP—Preserve in tight, light-resistant containers. Contain the labeled amount, within ± 5%. Sulfoxone Sodium Tablets are enteric coated. Meet the requirements for Identification, Disintegration (not within 1 hour in simulated gastric fluid TS, but within 2 hours, in simulated intestinal TS, the procedure for *Enteric-coated Tablets* being used), Uniformity of dosage units, and Suitability test.

SULFUR

Chemical name: Precipitated sulfur—Sulfur.

Molecular formula: Precipitated sulfur—S.

Molecular weight: Precipitated sulfur—32.06.

Description: Precipitated Sulfur USP—Very fine, pale yellow, amorphous or microcrystalline powder. Is odorless.

Solubility: Precipitated Sulfur USP—Practically insoluble in water; very soluble in carbon disulfide; slightly soluble in olive oil; very slightly soluble in alcohol.

USP requirements:
Precipitated Sulfur USP—Preserve in well-closed containers. Contains not less than 99.5% and not more than 100.5% of sulfur, calculated on the anhydrous basis. Meets the requirements for Identification, Reaction, Water (not more than 0.5%), Residue on ignition (not more than 0.3%), and Other forms of sulfur.
Sulfur Cream—Not in USP.
Sulfur Lotion—Not in USP.
Sulfur Ointment USP—Preserve in well-closed containers, and avoid prolonged exposure to excessive heat. Contains not less than 9.5% and not more than 10.5% of Sulfur.
Prepare Sulfur Ointment as follows: 100 grams of Precipitated Sulfur, 100 grams of Mineral Oil, and 800 grams of White Ointment, to make 1000 grams. Levigate the sulfur with the Mineral Oil to a smooth paste, and then incorporate with the White Ointment.
Sulfur Bar Soap—Not in USP.

SUBLIMED SULFUR

Chemical name: Sulfur.

Molecular formula: S.

Molecular weight: 32.06.

Description: Sublimed Sulfur USP—Fine, yellow, crystalline powder, having a faint odor.

Solubility: Sublimed Sulfur USP—Practically insoluble in water and in alcohol; sparingly soluble in olive oil.

USP requirements: Sublimed Sulfur USP—Preserve in well-closed containers. Dried over phosphorus pentoxide for 4 hours, contains not less than 99.5% and not more than 100.5% of sulfur. Meets the requirements for Solubility in carbon disulfide, Identification, Residue on ignition (not more than 0.5%), and Arsenic (not more than 4 ppm).

SULFURATED LIME

Source: Mixture of sublimed sulfur, lime, and water resulting in formation of calcium pentasulfide and calcium thiosulfate.

Description: Sulfurated lime solution—Clear orange liquid with a slight odor of hydrogen sulfide.

USP requirements:
Sulfurated Lime Mask—Not in USP.
Sulfurated Lime Topical Solution—Not in USP.

SULFUR DIOXIDE

Chemical name: Sulfur dioxide.

Molecular formula: SO_2.

Molecular weight: 64.06.

Description: Sulfur Dioxide NF—Colorless, non-flammable gas, possessing a strong suffocating odor characteristic of burning sulfur. Under pressure, it condenses readily to a colorless liquid that boils at –10 °C, and has a density of approximately 1.5.
NF category: Antioxidant.

Solubility: Sulfur Dioxide NF—At 20 °C and at standard pressure, approximately 36 volumes dissolve in 1 volume of water, and approximately 114 volumes dissolve in 1 volume of alcohol. Soluble also in ether and in chloroform.

NF requirements: Sulfur Dioxide NF—Preserve in cylinders. Note: Sulfur Dioxide is used most in the form of a gas in pharmaceutical applications, and the monograph deals with it for such purposes. However, it is usually packaged under pressure; hence, the NF specifications are designed for testing it in liquid form. Contains not less than 97.0%, by volume, of sulfur dioxide. Meets the requirements for Water (not more than 2.0%), Nonvolatile residue (not more than 0.0025%), and Sulfuric acid (not more than 0.002%).
Caution: Sulfur Dioxide is poisonous.

SULFURIC ACID

Chemical name: Sulfuric acid.

Molecular formula: H_2SO_4.

Molecular weight: 98.07.

Description: Sulfuric Acid NF—Clear, colorless, oily liquid. Very caustic and corrosive. Specific gravity is about 1.84.
NF category: Acidifying agent.

Solubility: Sulfuric Acid NF—Miscible with water and with alcohol with the generation of much heat.

NF requirements: Sulfuric Acid NF—Preserve in tight containers. Contains not less than 95.0% and not more than 98.0%, by weight, of sulfuric acid. Meets the requirements for Identification, Residue on ignition (not more than 0.005%), Chloride (not more than 0.005%), Arsenic (not more than 1 ppm), Heavy metals (not more than 5 ppm), and Reducing substances.

Caution: When Sulfuric Acid is to be mixed with other liquids, always add it to the diluent, and exercise great caution.

SULINDAC

Chemical group: Pyrroleacetic acid derivative.

Chemical name: 1*H*-Indene-3-acetic acid, 5-fluoro-2-methyl-1-[[4-(methylsulfinyl)phenyl]methylene]-, (*Z*)-.

Molecular formula: $C_{20}H_{17}FO_3S$.

Molecular weight: 356.41.

Description: Sulindac USP—Yellow, crystalline powder, which is odorless or practically so.

Solubility: Sulindac USP—Slightly soluble in methanol, in alcohol, in acetone, and in chloroform; very slightly soluble in isopropanol and in ethyl acetate; practically insoluble in hexane and in water.

USP requirements: Sulindac Tablets USP—Preserve in well-closed containers. Contain the labeled amount, within ±10%. Meet the requirements for Identification, Dissolution (80% in 45 minutes in 0.1 *M* phosphate buffer [pH 7.2] in Apparatus 2 at 50 rpm), Uniformity of dosage units, and Related compounds (not more than 3.0%).

SUPROFEN

Chemical name: Benzeneacetic acid, alpha-methyl-4-(2-thienylcarbonyl)-.

Molecular formula: $C_{14}H_{12}O_3S$.

Molecular weight: 260.31.

Description: Suprofen USP—White to off-white powder, odorless to having a slight odor.

Solubility: Suprofen USP—Sparingly soluble in water.

USP requirements: Suprofen Ophthalmic Solution USP—Preserve in tight containers. A sterile, buffered, aqueous solution of Suprofen adjusted to a suitable tonicity. Contains a suitable antimicrobial preservative. Contains the labeled amount, within −10% to +15%. Meets the requirements for Identification, Sterility, and pH (6.5–8.0).

SUTILAINS

Source: Proteolytic enzymes derived from *Bacillus subtilis*.

Chemical name: Sutilains.

Description: Sutilains USP—Cream-colored powder.

USP requirements: Sutilains Ointment USP—Preserve in collapsible tubes or in tight containers, and store in a refrigerator. Contains the labeled potency of sutilains, within −15% to +25%, in a suitable ointment base. Meets the requirement for Sterility.

Note: One USP Casein Unit of proteolytic activity is contained in the amount of sutilains which, when incubated with 35 mg of denatured casein at 37 °C, produces in 1 minute a hydrolysate whose absorbance at 275 nanometers is equal to that of a tyrosine solution containing 1.5 mcg of USP Tyrosine Reference Standard per mL.

ABSORBABLE SURGICAL SUTURE

USP requirements: Absorbable Surgical Suture USP—Preserve dry or in fluid, in containers (packets) so designed that sterility is maintained until the container is opened. A number of such containers may be placed in a box. A sterile, flexible strand prepared from collagen derived from healthy mammals, or from a synthetic polymer. Suture prepared from synthetic polymer may be in either monofilament or multifilament form. It is capable of being absorbed by living mammalian tissue, but may be treated to modify its resistance to absorption. Its diameter and tensile strength correspond to the size designation indicated on the label, within the limits prescribed in *USP*. It may be modified with respect to body or texture. It may be impregnated or treated with a suitable coating, softening, or antimicrobial agent. It may be colored by a color additive approved by the U.S. Food and Drug Administration. The collagen suture is designated as either *Plain Suture* or *Chromic Suture*. Both types consist of processed strands of collagen, but *Chromic Suture* is processed by physical or chemical means so as to provide greater resistance to absorption in living mammalian tissue. The label of each individual container (packet) of Suture indicates the size, length, type of Suture, kind of needle (if a needle is included), number of sutures (if multiple), lot number, and name of the manufacturer or distributor. If removable needles are used, the labeling so indicates. Suture size is designated by the metric size (gauge number) and the corresponding USP size. The label of the box indicates also the address of the manufacturer, packer, or distributor, and the composition of any packaging fluids used. Note: If the Suture is packaged with a fluid, make the required measurements for the following tests within 2 minutes after removing it from the fluid—Length, Diameter, Tensile strength, and Needle attachment. Meets the requirements for Length (not less than 95.0% of length stated on label), Diameter, Tensile strength, Needle attachment, Sterility, Extractable color (if Suture is dyed), and Soluble chromium compounds.

NONABSORBABLE SURGICAL SUTURE

USP requirements: Nonabsorbable Surgical Suture USP—Preserve non-sterilized Suture in well-closed containers. Preserve sterile Suture dry or in fluid, in containers (packets) so designed that sterility is maintained until the container is opened. A number of such containers may be placed in a box. A flexible strand of material that is suitably resistant to the action of living mammalian tissue. It may be in either monofilament or multifilament form. If it is a multifilament strand, the individual filaments may be combined by spinning, twisting, braiding, or any combination thereof. It may be either sterile or nonsterile. Its diameter and tensile strength correspond to the size designation indicated on the label, within the limits prescribed in *USP*. It may be modified with respect to body or texture, or to reduce capillarity, and may be suitably bleached. It may be impregnated or treated with a suitable coating, softening, or antimicrobial agent. It may be colored by a color additive approved by the U.S. Food and Drug Administration. Nonabsorbable Surgical Suture is classed and typed as follows: *Class I* Suture is composed of silk or synthetic fibers of monofilament, twisted or braided construction where the coating, if any, does not significantly affect thickness (e.g., braided silk, polyester, or nylon; microfilament nylon, or polypropylene). *Class II* Suture is composed of cotton or linen fibers or coated natural or synthetic fibers where the coating significantly affects thickness but does not contribute significantly to strength (e.g., virgin silk sutures). *Class III* Suture is composed of monofilament or multifilament metal wire. The label of each individual container (packet) of Suture indicates the material from which the Suture is made, the size, construction, and length of the

Suture, whether it is sterile or non-sterile, kind of needle (if a needle is included), number of sutures (if multiple), lot number, and name of the manufacturer or distributor. If removable needles are used, the labeling so indicates. Suture size is designated by the metric size (gauge number) and the corresponding USP size. The label of the box indicates also the address of the manufacturer, packer, or distributor, and the composition of any packaging fluids used. Note: If the Suture is packaged with a fluid, make the required measurements for the following tests within 2 minutes after removing it from the fluid—Length, Diameter, Tensile strength, and Needle attachment. Meets the requirements for Length (not less than 95.0% of length stated on label), Diameter, Tensile strength, Needle attachment, Sterility, and Extractable color (if Suture is dyed).

SYRUP

Description: Syrup NF—NF category: Sweetening agent; tablet binder; flavored and/or sweetened vehicle.

NF requirements: Syrup NF—Preserve in tight containers, preferably in a cool place. A solution of Sucrose in Purified Water. Contains a preservative unless it is used when freshly prepared.
Prepare Syrup as follows: 850 grams of Sucrose and a sufficient quantity of Purified Water to make 1000 mL. It may be prepared by the use of boiling water or, preferably, without heat, by the following process. Place the Sucrose in a suitable percolator, the neck of which is nearly filled with loosely packed cotton, moistened, after packing, with a few drops of water. Pour carefully about 450 mL of Purified Water upon the Sucrose, and regulate the outflow to a steady drip of percolate. Return the percolate, if necessary, until all of the Sucrose has been dissolved. Then wash the inside of the percolator and the cotton with sufficient Purified Water to bring the volume of the percolate to 1000 mL, and mix.
Meets the requirements for Specific gravity (not less than 1.30) and Organic volatile impurities.

TALBUTAL

Chemical name: 2,4,6(1H,3H,5H)-Pyrimidinetrione, 5-(1-methylpropyl)-5-(2-propenyl)-.

Molecular formula: $C_{11}H_{16}N_2O_3$.

Molecular weight: 224.26.

Description: Talbutal USP—White, crystalline powder, which may have a slight odor of caramel. Melts at about 108 °C, or at about 111 °C in the polymorphic form.

Solubility: Talbutal USP—Slightly soluble in water; freely soluble in alcohol and in chloroform; soluble in glacial acetic acid and in aqueous solutions of sodium hydroxide and sodium carbonate; sparingly soluble in ether.

USP requirements: Talbutal Tablets USP—Preserve in tight containers. Contain the labeled amount, within ±10%. Meet the requirements for Identification, Dissolution (75% in 45 minutes in water in Apparatus 2 at 50 rpm), and Uniformity of dosage units.

TALC

Description: Talc USP—Very fine, white or grayish-white, crystalline powder. It is unctuous, adheres readily to the skin, and is free from grittiness.
  NF category: Glidant and/or anticaking agent; tablet and/or capsule lubricant.

USP requirements: Talc USP—Preserve in well-closed containers. A native, hydrous magnesium silicate, sometimes containing a small proportion of aluminum silicate. Meets the requirements for Identification, Microbial limit, Loss on ignition (not more than 6.5%), Acid-soluble substances (not more than 2.0%), Reaction and soluble substances (not more than 0.1%), Water-soluble iron, Arsenic, Heavy metals, and Lead (not more than 3 ppm for arsenic, not more than 0.004% for heavy metals, and not more than 0.001% for lead).

TAMOXIFEN

Chemical name: Tamoxifen citrate—Ethanamine, 2-[4-(1,2-diphenyl-1-butenyl)phenoxy]-N,N-dimethyl, (Z)-, 2-hydroxy-1,2,3-propanetricarboxylate (1:1).

Molecular formula: Tamoxifen citrate—$C_{26}H_{29}NO\cdot C_6H_8O_7$.

Molecular weight: Tamoxifen citrate—563.65.

Description: Tamoxifen Citrate USP—White, fine, crystalline powder. Melts at about 142 °C, with decomposition.

pKa: 8.85.

Solubility: Tamoxifen Citrate USP—Very slightly soluble in water, in acetone, in chloroform, and in alcohol; soluble in methanol.

USP requirements:
  Tamoxifen Citrate Tablets USP—Preserve in well-closed, light-resistant containers. Contain an amount of tamoxifen citrate equivalent to the labeled amount of tamoxifen, within ±10%. Meet the requirements for Identification, Dissolution (75% in 30 minutes in 0.02 N hydrochloric acid in Apparatus 1 at 100 rpm), and Uniformity of dosage units.
  Tamoxifen Citrate Enteric-coated Tablets—Not in USP.

TANNIC ACID

Chemical name: Tannin.

Description: Tannic Acid USP—Amorphous powder, glistening scales, or spongy masses, varying in color from yellowish-white to light brown. Is odorless or has a faint, characteristic odor.

Solubility: Tannic Acid USP—Very soluble in water, in acetone, and in alcohol; freely soluble in diluted alcohol, and only slightly soluble in dehydrated alcohol; practically insoluble in chloroform, in ether, and in solvent hexane; 1 gram dissolves in about 1 mL of warm glycerin.

USP requirements: Tannic Acid USP—Preserve in tight, light-resistant containers. A tannin usually obtained from nutgalls, the excrescences produced on the young twigs of *Quercus infectoria* Oliver, and allied species of *Quercus* Linné (Fam. Fagaceae), from the seed pods of Tara (*Caesalpinia spinosa*), or from the nutgalls or leaves of sumac (any of a genus *Rhus*). Meets the requirements for Identification, Loss on drying (not more than 12.0%), Residue on ignition (not more than 1.0%), Arsenic (not more than 3 ppm), Heavy metals (not more than 0.004%), Gum or dextrin, Resinous substances, and Organic volatile impurities.

ADHESIVE TAPE

USP requirements: Adhesive Tape USP—Preserve in well-closed containers, and prevent exposure to excessive heat and to sunlight. Adhesive Tape that has been rendered sterile is so packaged that the sterility of the contents of the package is maintained until the package is opened for use. Consists of fabric and/or film evenly coated on one side with a pressure-sensitive, adhesive mixture. Its length is not less than 98.0% of that declared on the label, and its average width is not less than 95.0% of the declared width. If Adhesive Tape has been rendered sterile, it is protected from contamination by appropriate packaging. The package label of Adhesive Tape that has been rendered sterile indicates that the contents may not be sterile if the package bears evidence of damage or previously has been opened. The package label indicates the length and width of the Tape, and the name of the manufacturer, packer, or distributor. Meets the requirements for Dimensions (length, not less than 98.0% of labeled length; width, average of 5 measurements not less than 95% of the labeled width of Tape), Tensile strength, Adhesive strength, and Sterility.

TARTARIC ACID

Chemical name: Butanedioic acid, 2,3-dihydroxy-; Butanedioic acid, 2,3-dihydroxy-, [R-(R*,R*)]-.

Molecular formula: $C_4H_6O_6$.

Molecular weight: 150.09.

Description: Tartaric Acid NF—Colorless or translucent crystals, or white, fine to granular, crystalline powder. Odorless. Stable in air.
NF category: Acidifying agent.

Solubility: Tartaric Acid NF—Very soluble in water; freely soluble in alcohol.

NF requirements: Tartaric Acid NF—Preserve in well-closed containers. Dried over phosphorus pentoxide for 3 hours, contains not less than 99.7% and not more than 100.5% of tartaric acid. Meets the requirements for Identification, Specific rotation (+12.0° to +13.0°, calculated on the dried basis), Loss on drying (not more than 0.5%), Residue on ignition (not more than 0.1%), Oxalate, Sulfate, Heavy metals (not more than 0.001%), and Organic volatile impurities.

TECHNETIUM Tc 99m ALBUMIN

USP requirements: Technetium Tc 99m Albumin Injection USP—Preserve in single-dose or in multiple-dose containers, at a temperature between 2 and 8 °C. A sterile, aqueous solution, suitable for intravenous administration, of Albumin Human that is labeled with ^{99m}Tc. Label it to include the following, in addition to the information specified for Labeling under Injections: the time and date of calibration; the amount of ^{99m}Tc as albumin expressed as total megabecquerels (or microcuries or millicuries) and concentration as megabecquerels (or microcuries or millicuries) per mL at the time of calibration; the expiration date; and the statement, "Caution—Radioactive Material." The labeling indicates that in making dosage calculations, correction is to be made for radioactive decay, and also indicates that the radioactive half-life of ^{99m}Tc is 6.0 hours. Contains the labeled amount of ^{99m}Tc, within ± 10%, as albumin expressed in megabecquerels (or microcuries or millicuries) per mL at the time indicated in the labeling. Other chemical forms of radioactivity do not exceed 10.0% of the total radioactivity. Its production and distribution are subject to U.S. regulations. Meets the requirements for Bacterial endotoxins, pH (2.5–5.0), Radiochemical purity, and Biological distribution, for Radionuclide identification and Radionuclidic purity under Sodium Pertechnetate Tc 99m Injection, and for Injections (except that it may be distributed or dispensed prior to completion of the test for Sterility, the latter test being started on the day of final manufacture, and except that it

is not subject to the recommendation on Volume in Container).

TECHNETIUM Tc 99m ALBUMIN AGGREGATED

Description: Technetium Tc 99m Aggregated Albumin Injection USP—Milky suspension, from which particles settle upon standing.

USP requirements: Technetium Tc 99m Albumin Aggregated Injection USP—Preserve in single-dose or in multiple-dose containers, at a temperature between 2 and 8 °C. A sterile, aqueous suspension of Albumin Human that has been denatured to produce aggregates of controlled particle size that are labeled with ^{99m}Tc. Suitable for intravenous administration. Label it to include the following, in addition to the information specified for Labeling under Injections: the time and date of calibration; the amount of ^{99m}Tc as aggregated albumin expressed as total megabecquerels (or millicuries or microcuries) and concentration as megabecquerels (or microcuries or millicuries) per mL at the time of calibration; the expiration date; and the statement, "Caution—Radioactive Material." The labeling indicates that in making dosage calculations, correction is to be made for radioactive decay, and also indicates that the radioactive half-life of ^{99m}Tc is 6.0 hours. In addition, the labeling states that it is not to be used if clumping of the albumin is observed and directs that the container be agitated before the contents are withdrawn into a syringe. Its production and distribution are subject to U.S. regulations. Contains the labeled amount of ^{99m}Tc, within ± 10%, as aggregated albumin expressed in megabecquerels (or microcuries or millicuries) per mL at the time indicated in the labeling. Other chemical forms of radioactivity do not exceed 10.0% of the total radioactivity. Meets the requirements for Particle size, Bacterial endotoxins, pH (3.8–8.0), Radiochemical purity, Protein concentration, and Biological distribution, for Radionuclide identification and Radionuclidic purity under Sodium Pertechnetate Tc 99m Injection, and for Injections (except that it may be distributed or dispensed prior to completion of the test for Sterility, the latter test being started on the day of final manufacture, and except that it is not subject to the recommendation on Volume in Container).

TECHNETIUM Tc 99m ALBUMIN COLLOID

USP requirements: Technetium Tc 99m Albumin Colloid Injection USP—Preserve in single-dose or in multiple-dose containers, at a temperature between 2 and 8 °C. A sterile, pyrogen-free, aqueous suspension of Albumin Human that has been denatured to produce colloids of controlled particle size and that are labeled with ^{99m}Tc. Label it to include the following, in addition to the information specified for Labeling under Injections: the time and date of calibration; the amount of ^{99m}Tc expressed as total megabecquerels (or millicuries) and concentration as megabecquerels (or millicuries) per mL at the time of calibration; the expiration date and time and a statement, "Caution—Radioactive Material." The labeling indicates that in making dosage calculations, correction is to be made for radioactive decay, and also indicates that the radioactive half-life of ^{99m}Tc is 6.0 hours. In addition, the labeling states that it is not to be used if clumping of the albumin is observed, and directs that the container be agitated before the contents are withdrawn into a syringe. Contains the labeled amount of ^{99m}Tc, within ± 10%, as albumin colloid complex, expressed in megabecquerels (or millicuries) per mL at the time indicated on the label. The vials are sealed under a suitable inert atmosphere. Its production and distribution are subject to U.S. regulations. Other chemical forms of radioactivity do not exceed

10.0% of the total radioactivity. Meets the requirements for Bacterial endotoxins, pH (7.5–8.5), Radiochemical purity, Particle size distribution, Biological distribution, and Albumin content, for Radionuclide identification and Radionuclidic purity under Sodium Pertechnetate Tc 99m Injection, and for Injections (except that it may be distributed or dispensed prior to completion of the test for Sterility, the latter test being started on the date of manufacture, and except that it is not subject to the recommendation on Volume in Container).

TECHNETIUM Tc 99m ANTIMONY TRISULFIDE COLLOID

USP requirements: Technetium Tc 99m Antimony Trisulfide Colloid Injection—Not in USP.

TECHNETIUM Tc 99m DISOFENIN

Chemical group: Disofenin—derivative of iminodiacetic acid (IDA).

Chemical name: Disofenin—Glycine, *N*-[2-[[2,6-bis(1-methylethyl)phenyl]amino]-2-ox-oethyl]-*N*-(carboxymethyl)-.

Molecular formula: Disofenin—$C_{18}H_{26}N_2O_5$.

Molecular weight: Disofenin—350.41.

USP requirements: Technetium Tc 99m Disofenin Injection USP—Preserve in single-dose or in multiple-dose containers sealed under a suitable inert atmosphere. A sterile, aqueous solution, suitable for intravenous administration, of disofenin that is labeled with ^{99m}Tc. Label it to include the following, in addition to the information specified for Labeling under Injections: the time and date of preparation; the amount of ^{99m}Tc expressed as total megabecquerels (or microcuries or millicuries) and concentration as megabecquerels (or microcuries or millicuries) per mL at the time of preparation; the expiration date and time; and a statement, "Caution—Radioactive Material." The labeling indicates that in making dosage calculations, correction is to be made for radioactive decay, and also indicates that the radioactive half-life of ^{99m}Tc is 6.0 hours. Contains the labeled amount of ^{99m}Tc, within ± 10%, as a disofenin complex, expressed in megabecquerels (or microcuries or millicuries) per mL at the time indicated on the labeling. Contains a suitable reducing agent. Meets the requirements for pH (4.0–5.0), Radiochemical purity, and Biological distribution, for Radionuclide identification, Radionuclidic purity, and Bacterial endotoxins under Sodium Pertechnetate Tc 99m Injection, and for Injections (except that it may be distributed or dispensed prior to completion of the test for Sterility, the latter test being started on the date of preparation, and except that it is not subject to the recommendation on Volume in Container).

TECHNETIUM Tc 99m ETIDRONATE

USP requirements: Technetium Tc 99m Etidronate Injection USP—Preserve in single-dose or in multiple-dose containers. A sterile, clear, colorless solution, suitable for intravenous administration, of radioactive technetium (^{99m}Tc) in the form of a chelate of etidronate sodium. Label it to include the following, in addition to the information specified for Labeling under Injections: the time and date of calibration; the amount of ^{99m}Tc as labeled etidronate expressed as total megabecquerels (or microcuries or millicuries) and concentration as megabecquerels (or microcuries or millicuries) per mL at the time of calibration; the expiration date and time; and the statement, "Caution—Radioactive Material." The labeling indicates that in making dosage calculations, correction is to be made for radioactive decay, and also indicates

that the radioactive half-life of ^{99m}Tc is 6.0 hours. Contains the labeled amount of ^{99m}Tc, within ± 10%, as chelate expressed in megabecquerels (or microcuries or millicuries) per mL at the time indicated in the labeling. Other chemical forms of radioactivity do not exceed 10.0% of the total radioactivity. Meets the requirements for pH (2.5–7.0), and for Bacterial endotoxins, Radiochemical purity, Biological distribution, and Other requirements under Technetium Tc 99m Pyrophosphate Injection.

TECHNETIUM Tc 99m EXAMETAZIME

Chemical name: Exametazime—2-Butanone, 3,3'-[(2,2-dimethyl-1,3-propanediyl)diimino]bis-, dioxime, [*R**,*R**-(*E*,*E*)]-(±)-.

Chemical formula: Exametazime—$C_{13}H_{28}N_4O_2$.

Molecular weight: Exametazime—272.39.

USP requirements: Technetium Tc 99m Exametazime Injection—Not in USP.

TECHNETIUM Tc 99m FERPENTETATE

Chemical name: Iron, ascorbic acid and *N*,*N*-bis[2-[bis(carboxymethyl)amino]ethyl]glycine complex, metastable technetium-99 labeled.

Description: Technetium Tc 99m Ferpentetate Injection USP—Clear, light brown to yellow solution.

USP requirements: Technetium Tc 99m Ferpentetate Injection USP—Preserve in single-dose or in multiple-dose containers, at a temperature between 2 and 8 °C. Protect from light. A sterile, aqueous solution of iron ascorbate pentetic acid that is complexed with ^{99m}Tc. It is suitable for intravenous administration. Label it to include the following, in addition to the information specified for Labeling under Injections: the time and date of calibration; the amount of ^{99m}Tc as labeled ferpentetate expressed as total megabecquerels (or microcuries or millicuries) and concentration as megabecquerels (or microcuries or millicuries) per mL at the time of calibration; the expiration date; and the statement, "Caution—Radioactive Material." The labeling indicates that in making dosage calculations, correction is to be made for radioactive decay, and also indicates that the radioactive half-life of ^{99m}Tc is 6.0 hours. Contains the labeled amount of ^{99m}Tc, within ± 10%, as the ferpentetate expressed in megabecquerels (or microcuries or millicuries) per mL at the time indicated in the labeling. Other chemical forms of radioactivity do not exceed 10.0% of the total radioactivity. Meets the requirements for Bacterial endotoxins, pH (4.0–5.5), Radiochemical purity, and Biological distribution, for Radionuclide identification and Radionuclidic purity under Sodium Pertechnetate Tc 99m Injection, and for Injections (except that it may be distributed or dispensed prior to completion of test for Sterility, the latter test being started on the day of manufacture, and except that it is not subject to the recommendation on Volume in Container).

TECHNETIUM Tc 99m GLUCEPTATE

Chemical name: D-*glycero*-D-*gulo*-Heptonic acid, technetium-^{99m}Tc complex.

USP requirements: Technetium Tc 99m Gluceptate Injection USP—Preserve in single-dose or in multiple-dose containers, at a temperature between 2 and 8 °C . A sterile, aqueous solution, suitable for intravenous administration, of sodium gluceptate and stannous chloride that is labeled with ^{99m}Tc.

Label it to include the following, in addition to the information specified for Labeling under Injections: the time and date of calibration; the amount of ^{99m}Tc as labeled stannous gluceptate expressed as total megabecquerels (or microcuries or millicuries) and concentration as megabecquerels (or microcuries or millicuries) per mL at the time of calibration; the expiration date and time; and the statement, "Caution—Radioactive Material." The labeling indicates that in making dosage calculations, correction is to be made for radioactive decay, and also indicates that the radioactive half-life of ^{99m}Tc is 6.0 hours. Contains the labeled amount of ^{99m}Tc, within ±10%, as stannous gluceptate complex expressed in megabecquerels (or microcuries or millicuries) per mL at the time indicated in the labeling. Other chemical forms of radioactivity do not exceed 10.0% of the total radioactivity. Meets the requirements for Bacterial endotoxins, pH (4.0–8.0), Radiochemical purity, and Biological distribution, for Radionuclide identification and Radionuclidic purity under Sodium Pertechnetate Tc 99m Injection, and for Injections (except that it may be distributed or dispensed prior to completion of the test for Sterility, the latter test being started on the date of manufacture, and except that it is not subject to the recommendation on Volume in Container).

TECHNETIUM Tc 99m LIDOFENIN

Chemical source: Lidofenin—Derivative of iminodiacetic acid (IDA).

Chemical name: Lidofenin—Glycine, N-(carboxymethyl)-N-[2-[(2,6-dimethylphenyl)amino]-2-oxoethyl]-.

Molecular formula: Lidofenin—$C_{14}H_{18}N_2O_5$.

Molecular weight: Lidofenin—294.31.

Description: Lidofenin—Possesses both a lipophilic component and a hydrophilic group; forms an anionic bis-complex with Tc 99m.

USP requirements: Technetium Tc 99m Lidofenin Injection USP—Preserve in single-dose or in multiple-dose containers at a temperature between 2 and 8 °C. A sterile, clear, colorless solution of lidofenin complexed to radioactive technetium (^{99m}Tc) in the form of a chelate. Label it to include the following, in addition to the information specified for Labeling under Injections: the time and date of calibration; the amount of ^{99m}Tc as labeled lidofenin expressed as total megabecquerels (or millicuries) per mL at the time of calibration; the expiration date and time; the storage temperature and the statement, "Caution—Radioactive Material." The labeling indicates that, in making dosage calculations, correction is to be made for radioactive decay, and also indicates that the radioactive half-life of ^{99m}Tc is 6.0 hours. Contains the labeled amount of ^{99m}Tc, within ±10%, as the lidofenin chelate, expressed in megabecquerels (or millicuries) per mL at the time indicated in the labeling. Other chemical forms of radioactivity do not exceed 10.0% of the total radioactivity. Meets the requirements for Bacterial endotoxins, pH (3.5–5.0), Radiochemical purity, and Biological distribution, for Radionuclide identification and Radionuclidic purity under Sodium Pertechnetate Tc 99m Injection, and for Injections (except that it may be distributed or dispensed prior to completion of the test for Sterility, the latter test being started on the day of manufacture, and except that it is not subject to the recommendation on Volume in Container).

TECHNETIUM Tc 99m MEBROFENIN

Chemical source: Mebrofenin—Derivative of iminodiacetic acid (IDA).

Chemical name: Mebrofenin—Glycine, N-[2-[(3-bromo-2,4,6-trimethylphenyl)amino]-2-oxoethyl]-N-(carboxymethyl)-.

Molecular formula: Mebrofenin—$C_{15}H_{19}BrN_2O_5$.

Molecular weight: Mebrofenin—387.23.

Description: Mebrofenin—Possesses both a lipophilic component and a hydrophilic group; forms an anionic bis-complex with Tc 99m.

USP requirements: Technetium Tc 99m Mebrofenin Injection—Not in USP.

TECHNETIUM Tc 99m MEDRONATE

Chemical group: Medronate is a phosphonate compound.

USP requirements: Technetium Tc 99m Medronate Injection USP—Preserve in single-dose or in multiple-dose containers at a temperature specified in the labeling. A sterile, aqueous solution, suitable for intravenous administration, of sodium medronate and stannous chloride or stannous fluoride that is labeled with radioactive Tc 99m. Contains the labeled amount of Tc 99m, within ±10%, as stannous medronate complex expressed in megabecquerels (or microcuries or millicuries) per mL at the date and time indicated in the labeling. Other chemical forms of radioactivity do not exceed 10.0% of the total radioactivity. Meets the requirements for Bacterial endotoxins, pH (4.0–7.8), and Radiochemical purity, for Radionuclide identification and Radionuclidic purity under Sodium Pertechnetate Tc 99m Injection, for Labeling and Biological distribution under Technetium Tc 99m Pyrophosphate Injection, and for Injections (except that it may be distributed or dispensed prior to completion of the test for Sterility, the latter test being started on the day of manufacture, and except that it is not subject to the recommendation on Volume in Container).

TECHNETIUM Tc 99m MERTIATIDE

Chemical name: Technetate(2–)-^{99m}TC, [N-[N-[N-(mercaptoacetyl)glycyl]glycyl]glycinato(5–)-N,N', N'',S]-oxo-, disodium, (SP-5-25)-.

Molecular formula: $C_8H_8N_3Na_2O_6S^{99m}Tc$.

USP requirements: Technetium Tc 99m Mertiatide Injection—Not in USP.

TECHNETIUM Tc 99m OXIDRONATE

Chemical group: Oxidronate is a phosphonate compound.

USP requirements: Technetium Tc 99m Oxidronate Injection USP—Preserve in single-dose or in multiple-dose containers. A sterile, clear, colorless solution, suitable for intravenous administration, of radioactive technetium (^{99m}Tc) in the form of a chelate of oxidronate sodium. Label it to include the following, in addition to the information specified for Labeling under Injections: the time and date of calibration; the amount of ^{99m}Tc as labeled oxidronate expressed as total megabecquerels (or microcuries or millicuries) and concentration as megabecquerels (or microcuries or millicuries) per mL at the time of calibration; the expiration date and time; and the statement, "Caution—Radioactive Material." The labeling indicates that in making dosage calculations, correction is to be made for radioactive decay, and also indicates that the radioactive half-life of ^{99m}Tc is 6.0 hours. Contains the labeled amount of ^{99m}Tc, within ±10%, as chelate expressed in megabecquerels (or microcuries or millicuries) per mL at the date and time indicated in the labeling. Other chemical forms of radioactivity do not exceed 10.0% of the total radioactivity. Meets the requirements for pH (2.5–7.0), and for Bacterial endotoxins, Radiochemical purity, Biological distribution, and Other requirements under Technetium Tc 99m Pyrophosphate Injection.

TECHNETIUM Tc 99m PENTETATE

Chemical name: Technetate(1-)^{99m}Tc, [*N,N*-bis[2-[bis(carboxymethyl)amino]ethyl]glycinato(5-)]-, sodium.

Molecular formula: $C_{14}H_{18}N_3NaO_{10}{}^{99m}Tc$.

Description: Technetium Tc 99m Pentetate Injection USP—Clear, colorless solution.

USP requirements: Technetium Tc 99m Pentetate Injection USP—Preserve in single-dose or in multiple-dose containers, at a temperature between 2 and 8 °C. A sterile solution of pentetic acid that is complexed with ^{99m}Tc in Sodium Chloride Injection. It is suitable for intravenous administration. Label it to include the following, in addition to the information specified for Labeling under Injections: the time and date of calibration; the amount of ^{99m}Tc as labeled pentetic acid complex expressed as total megabecquerels (or millicuries or microcuries) and concentration as megabecquerels (or microcuries or millicuries) per mL at the time of calibration; the expiration date; and the statement, "Caution—Radioactive Material." The labeling indicates that in making dosage calculations, correction is to be made for radioactive decay, and also indicates that the radioactive half-life of ^{99m}Tc is 6.0 hours. Contains the labeled amount of ^{99m}Tc, within ±10%, as the pentetic acid complex, expressed in megabecquerels (or microcuries or millicuries) per mL at the time indicated on the labeling. Other chemical forms of radioactivity do not exceed 10.0% of the total radioactivity. Meets the requirements for pH (3.8–7.5) and Radiochemical purity, for Radionuclide identification and Radionuclidic purity under Sodium Pertechnetate Tc 99m Injection, for Bacterial endotoxins and Biological distribution under Technetium Tc 99m Ferpentetate Injection, and for Injections (except that it may be distributed or dispensed prior to completion of the test for Sterility, the latter test being started on the day of manufacture, and except that it is not subject to the recommendation on Volume in Container).

TECHNETIUM Tc 99m PYROPHOSPHATE

Chemical name:
Sodium pyrophosphate—Diphosphoric acid, tetrasodium salt.
Stannous chloride—Tin chloride ($SnCl_2$) dihydrate.

Molecular formula:
Sodium pyrophosphate—$Na_4P_2O_7$.
Stannous chloride—$SnCl_2 \cdot 2H_2O$.

Molecular weight:
Sodium pyrophosphate—265.90.
Stannous chloride—225.63.

USP requirements: Technetium Tc 99m Pyrophosphate Injection USP—Preserve in single-dose or in multiple-dose containers, at a temperature between 2 and 8 °C. A sterile aqueous solution, suitable for intravenous administration, of pyrophosphate that is labeled with ^{99m}Tc. Label it to include the following, in addition to the information specified for Labeling under Injections: the time and date of calibration; the amount of ^{99m}Tc as labeled tetrasodium pyrophosphate expressed as total megabecquerels (or microcuries or millicuries) and concentration as megabecquerels (or microcuries or millicuries) per mL at the time of calibration; the expiration date and time; and the statement, "Caution—Radioactive Material." The labeling indicates that in making dosage calculations, correction is to be made for radioactive

decay, and also indicates that the radioactive half-life of ^{99m}Tc is 6.0 hours. Contains the labeled amount of ^{99m}Tc, within ±10%, as pyrophosphate expressed in megabecquerels (or microcuries or millicuries) per mL at the time indicated in the labeling. Other chemical forms of radioactivity do not exceed 10.0% of the total radioactivity. Meets the requirements for Bacterial endotoxins, pH (4.0–7.5), Radiochemical purity, and Biological distribution, for Radionuclide identification and Radionuclidic purity under Sodium Pertechnetate Tc 99m Injection, and for Injections (except that it may be distributed or dispensed prior to completion of the test for Sterility, the latter test being started on the day of final manufacture, and except that it is not subject to the recommendation on Volume in Container).

TECHNETIUM Tc 99m (PYRO- AND TRIMETA-) PHOSPHATES

Chemical name:
Sodium pyrophosphate—Diphosphoric acid, tetrasodium salt.
Sodium trimetaphosphate—Metaphosphoric acid ($H_3P_3O_9$), trisodium salt.
Stannous chloride—Tin chloride ($SnCl_2$) dihydrate.

Molecular formula:
Sodium pyrophosphate—$Na_4P_2O_7$.
Sodium trimetaphosphate—$Na_3P_3O_9$.
Stannous chloride—$SnCl_2 \cdot 2H_2O$.

Molecular weight:
Sodium pyrophosphate—265.90.
Sodium trimetaphosphate—305.89.
Stannous chloride—225.63.

Description: Technetium Tc 99m (Pyro- and Trimeta-) Phosphates Injection USP—Clear solution.

USP requirements: Technetium Tc 99m (Pyro- and trimeta-) Phosphates Injection USP—A sterile, aqueous solution, suitable for intravenous administration, composed of sodium pyrophosphate, sodium trimetaphosphate, and stannous chloride labeled with radioactive Tc 99m. Contains the labeled amount of ^{99m}Tc, within ±10%, as phosphate expressed in megabecquerels (or microcuries or millicuries) per mL at the time indicated in the labeling. Other chemical forms of radioactivity do not exceed 10.0% of the total radioactivity. Meets the requirements for pH (4.0–7.0) and Radiochemical purity, for Radionuclide identification and Radionuclidic purity under Sodium Pertechnetate Tc 99m Injection, for Packaging and storage, Labeling, Bacterial endotoxins, and Biological distribution under Technetium Tc 99m Pyrophosphate Injection, and for Injections (except that it may be distributed or dispensed prior to completion of the test for Sterility, the latter test being started on the day of final manufacture, and except that it is not subject to the recommendation on Volume in Container).

TECHNETIUM Tc 99m SESTAMIBI

Chemical name: Technetium(1+)-^{99m}Tc, hexakis(1-isocyano-2-methoxy-2-methylpropane)-, (*OC*-6-11)-.

Molecular formula: $C_{36}H_{66}N_6O_6{}^{99m}Tc$.

USP requirements: Technetium Tc 99m Sestamibi Injection—Not in USP.

TECHNETIUM Tc 99m SUCCIMER

Chemical name: meso-2,3-Dimercaptosuccinic acid, ^{99m}Tc complex.

Description: Clear, colorless aqueous solution.

USP requirements: Technetium Tc 99m Succimer Injection USP—Preserve in single-dose containers, at a temperature between 15 and 30 °C. Do not freeze or store above 30 °C. Protect from light. A sterile, clear, colorless, aqueous solution of succimer complexed with ^{99m}Tc. It is suitable for intravenous administration. Label it to include the following, in addition to the information specified for Labeling under Injections: the time and date of calibration; the amount of ^{99m}Tc as labeled succimer expressed as total megabecquerels (or microcuries or millicuries) and concentration as megabecquerels (or microcuries or millicuries) per mL at the time of calibration; the expiration date and time; and the statement, "Caution—Radioactive Material." The labeling indicates that in making dosage calculations, correction is to be made for radioactive decay, and also indicates that the radioactive half-life of ^{99m}Tc is 6.0 hours. In addition, the labeling states that it is not to be used if discoloration or particulate matter is observed. (Note: A beyond-use time of 30 minutes shall be stated on the label upon constitution with Sodium Pertechnetate Tc 99m Injection.) Contains not less than 85% of the labeled amount of ^{99m}Tc as the succimer complex expressed in megabecquerels (or microcuries or millicuries) per mL at the time indicated in the labeling. Other chemical forms of radioactivity do not exceed 15.0% of the total radioactivity. Meets the requirements for Bacterial endotoxins, pH (2.0–3.0), Radiochemical purity, and Biological distribution, for Radionuclide identification and Radionuclidic purity under Sodium Pertechnetate Tc 99m Injection, and for Injections (except that it may be distributed or dispensed prior to completion of the test for Sterility, the latter test being started on the day of final manufacture, and except that it is not subject to the recommendation on Volume in Container).

TECHNETIUM Tc 99m SULFUR COLLOID

Description: Technetium Tc 99m Sulfur Colloid Injection USP— Colloidal dispersion. Slightly opalescent, colorless to light tan liquid.

USP requirements: Technetium Tc 99m Sulfur Colloid Injection USP—Store in single-dose or in multiple-dose containers. A sterile, colloidal dispersion of sulfur labeled with radioactive ^{99m}Tc, suitable for intravenous administration. Label it to include the following, in addition to the information specified for Labeling under Injections: the time and date of calibration; the amount of ^{99m}Tc as sulfur colloid expressed as total megabecquerels (or microcuries or millicuries) and concentration as megabecquerels (or microcuries or millicuries) per mL at the time of calibration; the expiration date; and the statement, "Caution—Radioactive Material." The labeling indicates that in making dosage calculations, correction is to be made for radioactive decay, and also indicates that the radioactive half-life of ^{99m}Tc is 6.0 hours; in addition, the labeling states that it is not to be used if flocculent material is visible and directs that the container be agitated before the Injection is withdrawn into a syringe. Contains the labeled amount of ^{99m}Tc, within ± 10%, as sulfur colloid expressed in megabecquerels (or microcuries or millicuries) per mL at the time indicated in the labeling. Other chemical forms of radioactivity do not exceed 8% of the total radioactivity. Meets the requirements for Bacterial endotoxins, pH (4.5–7.5), Radionuclidic purity under Sodium Pertechnetate Tc 99m Injection, Radiochemical purity, Biological distribution, and Injections (except that the Injection may be distributed or dispensed prior to completion of the test for Sterility, the latter test being started on the day of final manufacture, and except that it is not subject to the recommendation on Volume in Container).

Note: Agitate the container before withdrawing the Injection into a syringe.

TECHNETIUM Tc 99m TEBOROXIME

Chemical name: Technetium-^{99m}Tc, [bis[(1,2-cyclohexanedione dioximato)(1-)-O][(1,2-cyclohexanedione dioximato)(2-)-O]methylborato(2-)-N,N',N'',N''',N'''',N''''']-chloro-, (TPS-7-1-232'4'54)-.

Molecular formula: $C_{19}H_{29}BClN_6O_6{}^{99m}Tc$.

USP requirements: Technetium Tc 99m Teboroxime Injection—Not in USP.

TEMAZEPAM

Chemical name: 2H-1,4-Benzodiazepin-2-one, 7-chloro-1,3-dihydro-3-hydroxy-1-methyl-5-phenyl-.

Molecular formula: $C_{16}H_{13}ClN_2O_2$.

Molecular weight: 300.74.

Description: White, crystalline substance.

Solubility: Very slightly soluble in water; sparingly soluble in alcohol.

USP requirements:
Temazepam Capsules—Not in USP.
Temazepam Tablets—Not in USP.

TERAZOSIN

Chemical group: Quinazoline derivative.

Chemical name: Terazosin hydrochloride—Piperazine, 1-(4-amino-6,7-dimethoxy-2-quinazolinyl)-4-[(tetrahydro-2-furanyl)carbonyl]-, monohydrochloride, dihydrate. Is a racemic mixture, both components of which are active.

Molecular formula: Terazosin hydrochloride—$C_{19}H_{25}N_5O_4\cdot$HCl$\cdot2H_2O$.

Molecular weight: Terazosin hydrochloride—459.93.

Description: Terazosin hydrochloride—White, crystalline substance.

pKa: 7.04.

Solubility: Terazosin hydrochloride—Freely soluble in water and in isotonic saline.

USP requirements: Terazosin Hydrochloride Tablets—Not in USP.

TERBUTALINE

Chemical name: Terbutaline sulfate—1,3-Benzenediol, 5-[2-[(1,1-dimethylethyl)amino]-1-hydroxyethyl]-, sulfate (2:1) (salt).

Molecular formula: Terbutaline sulfate—$(C_{12}H_{19}NO_3)_2\cdot H_2SO_4$.

Molecular weight: Terbutaline sulfate—548.65.

Description: Terbutaline Sulfate USP—White to gray-white, crystalline powder. Is odorless or has a faint odor of acetic acid.

Solubility: Terbutaline Sulfate USP—Soluble in water and in 0.1 N hydrochloric acid; slightly soluble in methanol; insoluble in chloroform.

USP requirements:
Terbutaline Sulfate Inhalation Aerosol—Not in USP.
Terbutaline Sulfate Injection USP—Preserve in single-dose containers, preferably of Type I glass, protected from light, at controlled room temperature. A sterile solution

of Terbutaline Sulfate in Water for Injection. Contains the labeled amount, within ±10%. Meets the requirements for Identification, Bacterial endotoxins, pH (3.0–5.0), and Injections.

Note: Do not use the Injection if it is discolored.

Terbutaline Sulfate Tablets USP—Preserve in tight containers, at controlled room temperature. Contain the labeled amount, within ±10%. Meet the requirements for Identification, Dissolution (75% in 45 minutes in water in Apparatus 1 at 100 rpm), and Uniformity of dosage units.

TERCONAZOLE

Chemical name: Piperazine, 1-[4-[[2-(2,4-dichlorophenyl)-2-(1*H*-1,2,4-triazol-1-ylmethyl)-1,3-dioxolan-4-yl]methoxy]phenyl]-4-(1-methylethyl)-, *cis*-.

Molecular formula: $C_{26}H_{31}Cl_2N_5O_3$.

Molecular weight: 532.47.

Description: White to almost white powder.

Solubility: Soluble in butanol; sparingly soluble in ethanol; insoluble in water.

USP requirements:
Terconazole Vaginal Cream—Not in USP.
Terconazole Vaginal Suppositories—Not in USP.

TERFENADINE

Chemical group: Butyrophenone derivative.

Chemical name: 1-Piperidinebutanol, alpha-[4-(1,1-dimethylethyl)phenyl]-4-(hydroxydiphenylmethyl)-.

Molecular formula: $C_{32}H_{41}NO_2$.

Molecular weight: 471.68.

Description: Terfenadine USP—White to off-white, crystalline powder.

Solubility: Terfenadine USP—Slightly soluble in water, in hexane, and in 0.1 *N* hydrochloric acid; freely soluble in chloroform; soluble in alcohol, in methanol, in octanol, and in toluene.

USP requirements: Terfenadine Tablets USP—Preserve in tight, light-resistant containers. Contain the labeled amount, within ±10%. Meet the requirements for Identification and Uniformity of dosage units.

TERFENADINE AND PSEUDOEPHEDRINE

For *Terfenadine* and *Pseudoephedrine*—See individual listings for chemistry information.

USP requirements: Terfenadine and Pseudoephedrine Hydrochloride Extended-release Tablets—Not in USP.

TERIPARATIDE

Source: Teriparatide acetate—A synthetic polypeptide hormone consisting of the 1–34 fragment of human parathyroid hormone, the biologically active N-terminal region of the 84-amino-acid native hormone.

Chemical name: Teriparatide acetate—L-Phenylalanine, L-seryl-L-valyl-L-seryl-L-alpha-glutamyl-L-isoleucyl-L-glutaminyl-L-leucyl-L-methionyl-L-histadyl-L-asparaginyl-L-leucylglycyl-L-lysyl-L-histidyl-L-leucyl-L-asparaginyl-L-seryl-L-methionyl-L-alpha-glutamyl-L-arginyl-L-valyl-L-alpha-glutamyl-L-tryptophyl-L-leucyl-L-arginyl-L-lysyl-L-lysyl-L-leucyl-L-glutaminyl-L-alpha-aspartyl-L-valyl-L-histidyl-L-asparaginyl-, acetate (salt) hydrate.

Molecular formula: Teriparatide acetate—$C_{181}H_{291}N_{55}O_{51}S_2 \cdot xH_2O \cdot yC_2H_4O_2$.

USP requirements: Teriparatide Acetate for Injection—Not in USP.

TERPIN HYDRATE

Chemical name: Cyclohexanemethanol, 4-hydroxy-alpha,alpha,4-trimethyl-, monohydrate.

Molecular formula: $C_{10}H_{20}O_2 \cdot H_2O$.

Molecular weight: 190.28.

Description: Terpin Hydrate USP—Colorless, lustrous crystals or white powder. Has a slight odor, and effloresces in dry air. A hot solution (1 in 100) is neutral to litmus. When dried in vacuum at 60 °C for 2 hours, it melts at about 103 °C.

Solubility: Terpin Hydrate USP—Slightly soluble in water, in chloroform, and in ether; very soluble in boiling alcohol; soluble in alcohol; sparingly soluble in boiling water.

USP requirements: Terpin Hydrate Elixir USP—Preserve in tight containers. Contains, in each 100 mL, not less than 1.53 grams and not more than 1.87 grams of terpin hydrate. Meets the requirement for Alcohol content (39.0–44.0%).

TERPIN HYDRATE AND CODEINE

For *Terpin Hydrate* and *Codeine*—See individual listings for chemistry information.

USP requirements:
Terpin Hydrate and Codeine Elixir USP—Preserve in tight containers. Contains, in each 100 mL, not less than 1.53 grams and not more than 1.87 grams of terpin hydrate, and not less than 180 mg and not more than 220 mg of codeine. Meets the requirements for Identification and Alcohol content (39.0–44.0%).
Terpin Hydrate and Codeine Sulfate Oral Solution—Not in USP.

TERPIN HYDRATE AND DEXTROMETHORPHAN

For *Terpin Hydrate* and *Dextromethorphan*—See individual listings for chemistry information.

USP requirements: Terpin Hydrate and Dextromethorphan Hydrobromide Elixir USP—Preserve in tight containers. Contains, in each 100 mL, not less than 1.53 grams and not more than 1.87 grams of terpin hydrate, and not less than 180 mg and not more than 220 mg of dextromethorphan hydrobromide. Meets the requirements for Identification and Alcohol content (39.0–44.0%).

TESTOLACTONE

Chemical name: D-Homo-17a-oxaandrosta-1,4-diene-3,17-dione.

Molecular formula: $C_{19}H_{24}O_3$.

Molecular weight: 300.40.

Description: Testolactone USP—White to off-white, practically odorless, crystalline powder. Melts at about 218 °C.

Solubility: Testolactone USP—Slightly soluble in water and in benzyl alcohol; soluble in alcohol and in chloroform; insoluble in ether and in solvent hexane.

USP requirements:

Sterile Testolactone Suspension USP—Preserve in single-dose or in multiple-dose containers, preferably of Type I glass. A sterile suspension of Testolactone in a suitable aqueous medium. Contains the labeled amount, within −10% to +20%. Meets the requirements for Identification, Uniformity of dosage units, Bacterial endotoxins, pH (5.0–7.5), and Injections.

Testolactone Tablets USP—Preserve in tight containers. Contain the labeled amount, within ±10%. Meet the requirements for Identification, Dissolution (80% in 120 minutes in 0.1 *N* hydrochloric acid in Apparatus 2 at 75 rpm), and Uniformity of dosage units.

TESTOSTERONE

Chemical group:

Testosterone—Naturally occurring androgen.

Testosterone cypionate, testosterone enanthate, and testosterone propionate—Semi-synthetic androgens.

Chemical name:

Testosterone—Androst-4-en-3-one, 17-hydroxy-, (17 beta)-.

Testosterone cypionate—Androst-4-en-3-one, 17-(3-cyclopentyl-1-oxopropoxy)-, (17 beta)-.

Testosterone enanthate—Androst-4-en-3-one, 17-[(1-oxoheptyl)oxy]-, (17 beta)-.

Testosterone propionate—Androst-4-en-3-one, 17-(1-oxopropoxy)-, (17 beta)-.

Molecular formula:

Testosterone—$C_{19}H_{28}O_2$.

Testosterone cypionate—$C_{27}H_{40}O_3$.

Testosterone enanthate—$C_{26}H_{40}O_3$.

Testosterone propionate—$C_{22}H_{32}O_3$.

Molecular weight:

Testosterone—288.43.

Testosterone cypionate—412.61.

Testosterone enanthate—400.60.

Testosterone propionate—344.49.

Description:

Testosterone USP—White or slightly creamy white crystals or crystalline powder. Is odorless, and is stable in air.

Testosterone Cypionate USP—White or creamy white, crystalline powder. Is odorless or has a slight odor, and is stable in air.

Testosterone Enanthate USP—White or creamy white, crystalline powder. Is odorless or has a faint odor characteristic of heptanoic acid.

Testosterone Propionate USP—White or creamy white crystals or crystalline powder. Is odorless and is stable in air.

Solubility:

Testosterone USP—Practically insoluble in water; freely soluble in dehydrated alcohol and in chloroform; soluble in dioxane and in vegetable oils; slightly soluble in ether.

Testosterone Cypionate USP—Insoluble in water; freely soluble in alcohol, in chloroform, in dioxane, and in ether; soluble in vegetable oils.

Testosterone Enanthate USP—Insoluble in water; very soluble in ether; soluble in vegetable oils.

Testosterone Propionate USP—Insoluble in water; freely soluble in alcohol, in dioxane, in ether, and in other organic solvents; soluble in vegetable oils.

USP requirements:

Testosterone Pellets USP—Preserve in tight containers holding one pellet each and suitable for maintaining sterile contents. They are sterile pellets composed of Testosterone in compressed form, without the presence of any binder, diluent, or excipient. Contain the labeled amount, within ±3%. Meet the requirements for Identification, Melting range, and Specific rotation under Testosterone, Solubility in chloroform, Sterility, and Weight variation (95.0–105.0% of labeled weight of testosterone for average weight of 5 Pellets, and 90.0–110.0% of labeled weight of testosterone for each Pellet).

Sterile Testosterone Suspension USP—Preserve in single-dose or in multiple-dose containers, preferably of Type I glass. A sterile suspension of Testosterone in an aqueous medium. Contains the labeled amount, within ±10%. Meets the requirements for Identification, Uniformity of dosage units, Bacterial endotoxins, pH (4.0–7.5), and Injections.

Testosterone Cypionate Injection USP—Preserve in single-dose or in multiple-dose containers, preferably of Type I glass, protected from light. A sterile solution of Testosterone Cypionate in a suitable vegetable oil. Contains the labeled amount, within ±10%. Meets the requirements for Identification and Injections.

Testosterone Enanthate Injection USP—Preserve in single-dose or in multiple-dose containers, preferably of Type I glass. A sterile solution of Testosterone Enanthate in a suitable vegetable oil. Contains the labeled amount, within ±10%. Meets the requirements for Identification and Injections.

Testosterone Propionate Injection USP—Preserve in single-dose or in multiple-dose containers, preferably of Type I glass. A sterile solution of Testosterone Propionate in a suitable vegetable oil. Contains the labeled amount, within ±12%. Meets the requirements for Identification and Injections.

TESTOSTERONE AND ESTRADIOL

Chemical name:

Testosterone cypionate—Androst-4-en-3-one, 17-(3-cyclopentyl-1-oxopropoxy)-, (17 beta)-.

Testosterone enanthate—Androst-4-en-3-one, 17-[(1-oxoheptyl)oxy]-, (17 beta)-.

Estradiol cypionate—Estra-1,3,5(10)-triene-3,17-diol, (17 beta)-, 17-cyclopentanepropanoate.

Estradiol valerate—Estra-1,3,5(10)-triene-3,17-diol(17 beta)-, 17-pentanoate.

Estradiol benzoate—Estra-1,3,5(10)-triene-3,17-diol, (17 beta)-, 3-benzoate.

Molecular formula:

Testosterone cypionate—$C_{27}H_{40}O_3$.

Testosterone enanthate—$C_{26}H_{40}O_3$.

Estradiol cypionate—$C_{26}H_{36}O_3$.

Estradiol valerate—$C_{23}H_{32}O_3$.

Estradiol benzoate—$C_{25}H_{28}O_3$.

Molecular weight:

Testosterone cypionate—412.61.

Testosterone enanthate—400.60.

Estradiol cypionate—396.57.

Estradiol valerate—356.50.

Estradiol benzoate—376.49.

Description:

Testosterone Cypionate USP—White or creamy white, crystalline powder. Is odorless or has a slight odor, and is stable in air.

Testosterone Enanthate USP—White or creamy white, crystalline powder. Is odorless or has a faint odor characteristic of heptanoic acid.

Estradiol Cypionate USP—White to practically white, crystalline powder. Is odorless or has a slight odor.

Estradiol Valerate USP—White, crystalline powder. Is usually odorless but may have a faint, fatty odor.

Estradiol benzoate—Colorless crystals or a white or almost white crystalline powder.

Solubility:
Testosterone Cypionate USP—Insoluble in water; freely soluble in alcohol, in chloroform, in dioxane, and in ether; soluble in vegetable oils.

Testosterone Enanthate USP—Insoluble in water; very soluble in ether; soluble in vegetable oils.

Estradiol Cypionate USP—Insoluble in water; soluble in alcohol, in acetone, in chloroform, and in dioxane; sparingly soluble in vegetable oils.

Estradiol Valerate USP—Practically insoluble in water; soluble in castor oil, in methanol, in benzyl benzoate, and in dioxane; sparingly soluble in sesame oil and in peanut oil.

Estradiol benzoate—Practically insoluble in water; slightly soluble in alcohol and in fixed oils; soluble 1 in 50 of acetone.

USP requirements:
Testosterone Cypionate and Estradiol Cypionate Injection—Not in USP.

Testosterone Enanthate and Estradiol Valerate Injection—Not in USP.

Testosterone Enanthate Benzilic Acid Hydrazone, Estradiol Dienanthate, and Estradiol Benzoate Injection—Not in USP.

TETANUS ANTITOXIN

Description: Tetanus Antitoxin USP—Transparent or slightly opalescent liquid, faint brownish, yellowish, or greenish in color and practically odorless or having an odor because of the antimicrobial agent.

USP requirements: Tetanus Antitoxin USP—Preserve at a temperature between 2 and 8 °C. A sterile, non-pyrogenic solution of the refined and concentrated proteins, chiefly globulins, containing antitoxic antibodies obtained from the blood serum or plasma of healthy horses that have been immunized against tetanus toxin or toxoid. It has a potency of not less than 400 antitoxin units per mL based on the U.S. Standard Tetanus Antitoxin and the U.S. Control Tetanus Test Toxin, tested in guinea pigs. Label it to state that it was prepared from horse serum or plasma. Meets the requirement for Expiration date (for Antitoxin containing a 20% excess of potency, not later than 5 years after date of issue from manufacturer's cold storage [5 °C, 1 year; or 0 °C, 2 years]). Conforms to the regulations of the U.S. Food and Drug Administration concerning biologics.

TETANUS IMMUNE GLOBULIN

Description: Tetanus Immune Globulin USP—Transparent or slightly opalescent liquid, practically colorless and practically odorless. May develop a slight granular deposit during storage.

USP requirements: Tetanus Immune Globulin USP—Preserve at a temperature between 2 and 8 °C. A sterile, non-pyrogenic solution of globulins derived from the blood plasma of adult human donors who have been immunized with tetanus toxoid. It has a potency of not less than 50 antitoxin units

per mL based on the U.S. Standard Tetanus Antitoxin and the U.S. Control Tetanus Test Toxin, tested in guinea pigs. Contains not less than 10 grams and not more than 18 grams of protein per 100 mL, of which not less than 90% is gamma globulin. Contains 0.3 M glycine as a stabilizing agent, and contains a suitable preservative. Label it to state that it is not for intravenous injection. Meets the requirement for Expiration date (for Tetanus Immune Globulin containing a 10% excess of potency, not later than 3 years after date of issue from manufacturer's cold storage [5 °C, 1 year]). Conforms to the regulations of the U.S. Food and Drug Administration concerning biologics.

TETANUS TOXOID

Source: Tetanus toxoid adsorbed and fluid are prepared by growing the tetanus bacilli *Clostridium tetani* on a protein-free, semi-synthetic medium. The tetanus toxin produced by these bacilli is detoxified using formaldehyde and forms the tetanus toxoid. Thimerosal is added as a preservative. In addition, for tetanus toxoid adsorbed, aluminum phosphate or aluminum potassium sulfate is used as a mineral adjuvant to adsorb the tetanus antigens. This prolongs and enhances the antigenic properties by retarding the rate of absorption of the injected toxoid into the body.

Description:
Tetanus Toxoid USP—Clear, colorless to brownish yellow, or slightly turbid liquid, free from evident clumps or particles, having a characteristic odor or an odor of formaldehyde.

Tetanus Toxoid Adsorbed USP—Turbid, white, slightly gray, or slightly pink suspension, free from evident clumps after shaking.

USP requirements:
Tetanus Toxoid USP—Preserve at a temperature between 2 and 8 °C. A sterile solution of the formaldehyde-treated products of growth of the tetanus bacillus (*Clostridium tetani*). Label it to state that it is not to be frozen. Meets the requirements of the specific guinea pig potency test of antitoxin production based on the U.S. Standard Tetanus Antitoxin and the U.S. Control Tetanus Test Toxin. Meets the requirements of the specific guinea pig detoxification test. Contains not more than 0.02% of residual free formaldehyde. Contains a preservative other than a phenoloid compound. Meets the requirement for Expiration date (not later than 2 years after date of issue from manufacturer's cold storage [5 °C, 1 year]). Conforms to the regulations of the U.S. Food and Drug Administration concerning biologics.

Tetanus Toxoid Adsorbed USP—Preserve at a temperature between 2 and 8 °C. A sterile preparation of plain tetanus toxoid that meets all of the requirements for that product with the exception of those for potency, and that has been precipitated or adsorbed by alum, aluminum hydroxide, or aluminum phosphate adjuvants. Label it to state that it is to be well shaken before use and that it is not to be frozen. Meets the requirements of the specific mouse or guinea pig potency test of antitoxin production based on the U.S. Standard Tetanus Antitoxin and the U.S. Control Test Tetanus Toxin. Meets the requirements of the specific guinea pig detoxification test. Meets the requirements for Expiration date (not later than 2 years after date of issue from manufacturer's cold storage [5 °C, 1 year]) and Aluminum content. Conforms to the regulations of the U.S. Food and Drug Administration concerning biologics.

TETANUS AND DIPHTHERIA TOXOIDS ADSORBED FOR ADULT USE

Description: Tetanus and Diphtheria Toxoids Adsorbed for Adult Use USP—Turbid, white, slightly gray, or cream-colored suspension, free from evident clumps after shaking.

USP requirements: Tetanus and Diphtheria Toxoids Adsorbed for Adult Use USP—Preserve at a temperature between 2 and 8 °C. A sterile suspension prepared by mixing suitable quantities of adsorbed diphtheria toxoid and adsorbed tetanus toxoid using the same precipitating or adsorbing agent for both toxoids. The antigenicity or potency and the proportions of the toxoids are such as to provide, in each dose prescribed in the labeling, an immunizing dose of Tetanus Toxoid Adsorbed as defined for that product, and one-tenth of the immunizing dose of Diphtheria Toxoid Adsorbed as defined for that product for children, such that in the specific guinea pig antigenicity test it meets the requirement of production of not less than 0.5 unit of diphtheria antitoxin per mL and each immunizing dose has an antigen content of not more than 2 Lf (flocculating units) value as measured with the U.S. Reference Diphtheria Antitoxin for Flocculation Test. Each component meets the other requirements for those products. Contains not more than 0.02% of residual free formaldehyde. Label it to state that it is to be well shaken before use and that it is not to be frozen. Meets the requirement for Expiration date (not later than 2 years after date of issue from manufacturer's cold storage [5 °C, 1 year]). Conforms to the regulations of the U.S. Food and Drug Administration concerning biologics.

TETRACAINE

Chemical group: Ester, aminobenzoic acid (PABA)–derivative.

Chemical name:
Tetracaine—Benzoic acid, 4-(butylamino)-, 2-(dimethylamino)ethyl ester.
Tetracaine hydrochloride—Benzoic acid, 4-(butylamino)-, 2-(dimethylamino)ethyl ester, monohydrochloride.

Molecular formula:
Tetracaine—$C_{15}H_{24}N_2O_2$.
Tetracaine hydrochloride—$C_{15}H_{24}N_2O_2 \cdot HCl$.

Molecular weight:
Tetracaine—264.37.
Tetracaine hydrochloride—300.83.

Description:
Tetracaine USP—White or light yellow, waxy solid.
Tetracaine Hydrochloride USP—Fine, white, crystalline, odorless powder. Its solutions are neutral to litmus. Melts at about 148 °C, or may occur in either of two other polymorphic modifications that melt at about 134 °C and 139 °C, respectively. Mixtures of the forms may melt within the range of 134 to 147 °C. Is hygroscopic.
Sterile Tetracaine Hydrochloride USP—Fine, white, crystalline, odorless powder. Its solutions are neutral to litmus. Melts at about 148 °C, or may occur in either of two other polymorphic modifications that melt at about 134 °C and 139 °C, respectively. Mixtures of the forms may melt within the range of 134 to 147 °C. Is hygroscopic.

pKa: 8.2.

Solubility:
Tetracaine USP—Very slightly soluble in water; soluble in alcohol, in ether, and in chloroform.
Tetracaine Hydrochloride USP—Very soluble in water; soluble in alcohol; insoluble in ether.

Sterile Tetracaine Hydrochloride USP—Very soluble in water; soluble in alcohol; insoluble in ether.

USP requirements:
Tetracaine Ointment USP—Preserve in collapsible ointment tubes. Contains the labeled amount, within ± 10%, in a suitable ointment base. Meets the requirements for Identification, Microbial limits, and Minimum fill.
Tetracaine Ophthalmic Ointment USP—Preserve in collapsible ophthalmic ointment tubes. A sterile ointment. Contains not less than 0.45% and not more than 0.55% of Tetracaine in White Petrolatum. Meets the requirements for Identification, Sterility, Minimum fill, and Metal particles.
Tetracaine Topical Aerosol Solution—Not in USP.
Tetracaine Hydrochloride Cream USP—Preserve in collapsible, lined metal tubes. Contains an amount of tetracaine hydrochloride equivalent to the labeled amount of tetracaine, within ±10%, in a suitable water-miscible base. Meets the requirements for Identification, Microbial limits, Minimum fill, and pH (3.2–3.8).
Tetracaine Hydrochloride Injection USP—Preserve in single-dose or in multiple-dose containers, preferably of Type I glass, under refrigeration and protected from light. It may be packaged in 100-mL multiple-dose containers. Injection supplied as a component of spinal anesthesia trays may be stored at room temperature for 12 months. A sterile solution of Tetracaine Hydrochloride in Water for Injection. Label it to indicate that the Injection is not to be used if it contains crystals, or if it is cloudy or discolored. Contains the labeled amount, within ±5%. Meets the requirements for Identification, Bacterial endotoxins, pH (3.2–6.0), Particulate matter, and Injections.
Tetracaine Hydrochloride Ophthalmic Solution USP—Preserve in tight, light-resistant containers. A sterile, aqueous solution of Tetracaine Hydrochloride. Label it to indicate that the Ophthalmic Solution is not to be used if it contains crystals, or if it is cloudy or discolored. Contains the labeled amount, within ±10%. Meets the requirements for Identification, Sterility, and pH (3.7–6.0).
Sterile Tetracaine Hydrochloride USP—Preserve in Containers for Sterile Solids, preferably of Type I glass. It is Tetracaine Hydrochloride suitable for parenteral use. Contains not less than 98.0% and not more than 101.0% of tetracaine hydrochloride, calculated on anhydrous basis. Meets the requirements for Completeness of solution, Constituted solution, Identification, Container content variation, Bacterial endotoxins, pH (5.0–6.0, in a solution [1 in 100]), Water (not more than 2.0%), Residue on ignition (not more than 0.1%), and Chromatographic purity, and for Sterility tests and Labeling under Injections.
Tetracaine Hydrochloride Topical Solution USP—Preserve in tight, light-resistant containers. An aqueous solution of Tetracaine Hydrochloride. Contains a suitable antimicrobial agent. Label it to indicate that the Topical Solution is not to be used if it contains crystals, or if it is cloudy or discolored. Contains the labeled amount, within ±5%. Meets the requirements for Identification and pH (4.5–6.0).

TETRACAINE AND DEXTROSE

For *Tetracaine* and *Dextrose*—See individual listings for chemistry information.

USP requirements: Tetracaine Hydrochloride in Dextrose Injection USP—Preserve in single-dose or in multiple-dose containers, preferably of Type I glass, under refrigeration and protected from light. It may be packaged in 100-mL multiple-dose containers. Injection supplied as a component of spinal anesthesia trays may be stored at room temperature for 12 months. A sterile solution of Tetracaine Hydrochloride and Dextrose in Water for Injection. Label it to indicate that the Injection is not to be used if it contains crystals, or if it is cloudy or discolored. Contains the labeled amounts, within ± 5%. Meets the requirements for Identification, Bacterial endotoxins, pH (3.5–6.0), Particulate matter under Small-volume injections, and Injections.

TETRACAINE AND MENTHOL

For *Tetracaine* and *Menthol*—See individual listings for chemistry information.

USP requirements: Tetracaine and Menthol Ointment USP—Preserve in collapsible ointment tubes. Contains the labeled amounts, within ± 10%, in a suitable ointment base. Meets the requirements for Identification and Minimum fill.

TETRACYCLINE

Chemical name:
   Tetracycline—2-Naphthacenecarboxamide, 4-(dimethyl-amino)-1,4,4a,5,5a,6,11,12a-octahydro-3,6,10,12,12a-pentahydroxy-6-methyl-1,11-dioxo-, [4S-(4 alpha,4a alpha,5a alpha,6 beta,12a alpha)]-.
   Tetracycline hydrochloride—2-Naphthacenecarboxamide, 4-(dimethylamino)-1,4,4a,5,5a,6,11,12a-octahydro-3,6,-10,12,12a-pentahydroxy-6-methyl-1,11-dioxo-, monohydrochloride, [4S-(4 alpha,4a alpha,5a alpha,6 beta,12a alpha)]-.
   Tetracycline phosphate complex—2-Naphthacenecarboxamide, 4-(dimethylamino)-1,4,4a,5,5a,6,11,12a-octahydro-3,6,10,12,12a-pentahydroxy-6-methyl-1,11-dioxo, [4S-(4 alpha,4a alpha,5a alpha,6 beta,12a alpha)]-, phosphate complex.

Molecular formula:
   Tetracycline—$C_{22}H_{24}N_2O_8$.
   Tetracycline hydrochloride—$C_{22}H_{24}N_2O_8 \cdot HCl$.

Molecular weight:
   Tetracycline—444.44.
   Tetracycline hydrochloride—480.90.

Description:
   Tetracycline USP—Yellow, odorless, crystalline powder. Is stable in air, but exposure to strong sunlight causes it to darken. It loses potency in solutions of pH below 2, and is rapidly destroyed by alkali hydroxide solutions.
   Tetracycline Hydrochloride USP—Yellow, odorless, crystalline powder. Is moderately hygroscopic. Is stable in air, but exposure to strong sunlight in moist air causes it to darken. It loses potency in solution at a pH below 2, and is rapidly destroyed by alkali hydroxide solutions.
   Tetracycline Phosphate Complex USP—Yellow, crystalline powder, having a faint, characteristic odor.

Solubility:
   Tetracycline USP—Very slightly soluble in water; freely soluble in dilute acid and in alkali hydroxide solutions; sparingly soluble in alcohol; practically insoluble in chloroform and in ether.
   Tetracycline Hydrochloride USP—Soluble in water and in solutions of alkali hydroxides and carbonates; slightly soluble in alcohol; practically insoluble in chloroform and in ether.
   Tetracycline Phosphate Complex USP—Sparingly soluble in water; slightly soluble in methanol; very slightly soluble in acetone.

USP requirements:
   Tetracycline Boluses USP—Preserve in tight containers. Label Boluses to indicate that they are intended for veterinary use only. Contain an amount of tetracycline equivalent to the labeled amount of tetracycline hydrochloride, within −10% to +20%. Meet the requirements for Identification, Uniformity of dosage units, and Loss on drying (not more than 3.0%; or for Boluses greater than 15 mm in diameter, not more than 6.0%).
   Tetracycline Oral Suspension USP—Preserve in tight, light-resistant containers. It is Tetracycline with or without one or more suitable buffers, preservatives, stabilizers, and suspending agents. Contains an amount of tetracycline equivalent to the labeled amount of tetracycline hydrochloride, within −10% to +25%. Meets the requirements for Identification, pH (3.5–6.0), 4-Epianhydrotetracycline (not more than 5.0%), Uniformity of dosage units (single-unit containers), and Deliverable volume.
   Tetracycline Hydrochloride Capsules USP—Preserve in tight, light-resistant containers. Contain the labeled amount, within −10% to +25%. Meet the requirements for Identification, Dissolution (70% in 60 minutes in water in Apparatus 2 at 75 rpm), Uniformity of dosage units, Loss on drying (not more than 4.0%), and 4-Epianhydrotetracycline (not more than 3.0%).
   Tetracycline Hydrochloride for Injection USP—Preserve in Containers for Sterile Solids, protected from light. A sterile, dry mixture of Sterile Tetracycline Hydrochloride, one form of which contains Magnesium Chloride or magnesium ascorbate and one or more suitable buffers, and the other form of which contains one or more suitable stabilizing agents. Label Tetracycline Hydrochloride for Injection that contains an anesthetic agent to indicate that it is intended for intramuscular administration only. Contains the labeled amount, within −10% to +15%. Meets the requirements for Constituted solution, Identification, Bacterial endotoxins, Sterility, pH (2.0–3.0, in a solution containing 10 mg per mL), Loss on drying (not more than 5.0%), Particulate matter, and 4-Epianhydrotetracycline (not more than 3.0%), and for Uniformity of dosage units and Labeling under Injections. Where it is labeled for intravenous use it meets the requirements for Depressor substances under Sterile Tetracycline Hydrochloride.
   Tetracycline Hydrochloride Ointment USP—Preserve in well-closed containers, preferably at controlled room temperature. Contains the labeled amount, within −10% to +25%. Meets the requirements for Identification, Minimum fill, and Water (not more than 1.0%).
   Tetracycline Hydrochloride Ophthalmic Ointment USP—Preserve in collapsible ophthalmic ointment tubes. Contains the labeled amount, within −10% to +25%. Meets the requirements for Sterility, Minimum fill, Water (not more than 0.5%), and Metal particles.
   Tetracycline Hydrochloride Soluble Powder USP—Preserve in tight containers. Label it to indicate that it is intended for veterinary use only. Contains the labeled amount, within −10% to +25%. Meets the requirements for Identification and Loss on drying (not more than 2.0%).
   Tetracycline Hydrochloride for Topical Solution USP—Preserve in tight, light-resistant containers. A dry mixture of Tetracycline Hydrochloride and Epitetracycline Hydrochloride with Sodium Metabisulfite packaged in conjunction with a suitable aqueous vehicle. Contains the labeled amount of tetracycline hydrochloride, within −10% to +30%, when constituted as directed. Meets the requirements for Identification, pH (1.9–3.5, in the solution constituted as directed in the labeling), Loss on drying (not more than 5.0%), and Epitetracycline hydrochloride content.

Sterile Tetracycline Hydrochloride USP—Preserve in Containers for Sterile Solids, protected from light. It is Tetracycline Hydrochloride suitable for parenteral use. Has a potency of not less than 900 mcg of tetracycline hydrochloride per mg and, where packaged for dispensing, contains the equivalent of the labeled amount of tetracycline hydrochloride, within −10% to +15%. Meets the requirements for Constituted solution, Depressor substances, Bacterial endotoxins, Sterility, and Particulate matter, for Identification tests, Crystallinity, pH, Loss on drying, and 4-Epianhydrotetracycline under Tetracycline Hydrochloride, and, where packaged for dispensing, for Uniformity of dosage units and Labeling under Injections.

Tetracycline Hydrochloride Ophthalmic Suspension USP—Preserve in tight, light-resistant containers of glass or plastic, containing not more than 15 mL. The containers or individual cartons are sealed and tamper-proof so that sterility is assured at time of first use. A sterile suspension of Sterile Tetracycline Hydrochloride in a suitable oil. Contains the labeled amount, within −10% to +25%. Meets the requirements for Identification, Sterility, and Water (not more than 0.5%).

Tetracycline Hydrochloride Tablets USP—Preserve in tight, light-resistant containers. Contain the labeled amount, within −10% to +25%. Meet the requirements for Identification, Dissolution (70% in 60 minutes in water in Apparatus 2 at 75 rpm), Uniformity of dosage units, Loss on drying (not more than 3.0%), and 4-Epianhydrotetracycline (not more than 3.0%).

Tetracycline Phosphate Complex Capsules USP—Preserve in tight, light-resistant containers. Contain an amount of tetracycline phosphate complex equivalent to the labeled amount of tetracycline hydrochloride, within −10% to +25%. Meet the requirements for Identification, Dissolution (75% in 30 minutes in 0.1 N hydrochloric acid in Apparatus 1 at 100 rpm), Uniformity of dosage units, Loss on drying (not more than 9.0%), and 4-Epianhydrotetracycline (not more than 3.0%).

Tetracycline Phosphate Complex for Injection USP—Preserve in Containers for Sterile Solids, protected from light. A sterile, dry mixture of Sterile Tetracycline Phosphate Complex and Magnesium Chloride or magnesium ascorbate, and one or more suitable buffers. Contains an amount of tetracycline phosphate complex equivalent to the labeled amount of tetracycline hydrochloride, within −10% to +15%. Meets the requirements for Constituted solution, Identification, Bacterial endotoxins, Sterility, pH (2.0–3.0, in a solution containing 10 mg per mL), Loss on drying (not more than 5.0%), Particulate matter, and 4-Epianhydrotetracycline (not more than 3.0%), and for Uniformity of dosage units and Labeling under Injections.

Sterile Tetracycline Phosphate Complex USP—Preserve in Containers for Sterile Solids, protected from light. It is Tetracycline Phosphate Complex suitable for parenteral use. Has a potency equivalent to not less than 750 mcg of tetracycline hydrochloride per mg, calculated on the anhydrous basis. Meets the requirements for Depressor substances and Sterility, and for Identification tests, pH, Water, Chloride, Crystallinity, Tetracycline, and 4-Epianhydrotetracycline under Tetracycline Phosphate Complex.

TETRACYCLINE AND NOVOBIOCIN

For *Tetracycline* and *Novobiocin*—See individual listings for chemistry information.

USP requirements:

Tetracycline Hydrochloride and Novobiocin Sodium Tablets USP—Preserve in tight containers. Label Tablets to indicate that they are intended for veterinary use only. Contain amounts of tetracycline hydrochloride and novobiocin sodium equivalent to the labeled amounts of

tetracycline hydrochloride and novobiocin, within −10% to +25%. Meet the requirements for Identification, Disintegration (60 minutes, simulated gastric fluid TS being substituted for water in the test), Uniformity of dosage units, Loss on drying (not more than 6.0%), and 4-Epianhydrotetracycline (not more than 2.0%).

Tetracycline Phosphate Complex and Novobiocin Sodium Capsules USP—Preserve in tight containers. Label Capsules to indicate that they are intended for veterinary use only. Contain amounts of tetracycline phosphate complex and novobiocin sodium equivalent to the labeled amounts of tetracycline hydrochloride and novobiocin, within −10% to +20%. Meet the requirements for Identification, Uniformity of dosage units, Loss on drying (not more than 9.0%), and 4-Epianhydrotetracycline (not more than 3.0%).

TETRACYCLINE, NOVOBIOCIN, AND PREDNISOLONE

For *Tetracycline, Novobiocin,* and *Prednisolone*—See individual listings for chemistry information.

USP requirements: Tetracycline Hydrochloride, Novobiocin Sodium, and Prednisolone Tablets USP—Preserve in tight containers. Label Tablets to indicate that they are intended for veterinary use only. Contain amounts of tetracycline hydrochloride and novobiocin sodium equivalent to the labeled amounts of tetracycline hydrochloride and novobiocin, within −10% to +25%, and the labeled amount of prednisolone, within ±10%. Meet the requirements for Disintegration (60 minutes, simulated gastric fluid TS being substituted for water in the test), Uniformity of dosage units, and 4-Epianhydrotetracycline (not more than 2.0%), and for Identification test and Loss on drying under Tetracycline Hydrochloride and Novobiocin Sodium Tablets.

TETRACYCLINE AND NYSTATIN

For *Tetracycline* and *Nystatin*—See individual listings for chemistry information.

USP requirements: Tetracycline Hydrochloride and Nystatin Capsules USP—Preserve in tight, light-resistant containers. Contain the labeled amount of tetracycline hydrochloride, within −10% to +25%, and the labeled amount of USP Nystatin Units, within −10% to +35%. Meet the requirements for Identification, Dissolution (70% in 60 minutes in water in Apparatus 2 at 75 rpm), Loss on drying (not more than 4.0%), and 4-Epianhydrotetracycline (not more than 3.0%).

TETRAHYDROZOLINE

Chemical name: Tetrahydrozoline hydrochloride—1H-Imidazole, 4,5-dihydro-2-(1,2,3,4-tetrahydro-1-naphthalenyl)-, monohydrochloride.

Molecular formula: Tetrahydrozoline hydrochloride—$C_{13}H_{16}N_2 \cdot HCl$.

Molecular weight: Tetrahydrozoline hydrochloride—236.74.

Description: Tetrahydrozoline Hydrochloride USP—White, odorless solid. Melts at about 256 °C, with decomposition.

Solubility: Tetrahydrozoline Hydrochloride USP—Freely soluble in water and in alcohol; very slightly soluble in chloroform; practically insoluble in ether.

USP requirements:

Tetrahydrozoline Hydrochloride Nasal Solution USP—Preserve in tight containers. A solution of Tetrahydrozoline Hydrochloride in water adjusted to a suitable tonicity.

Contains the labeled amount, within ±10%. Meets the requirements for Identification, Microbial limits, and pH (5.3–6.5).

Tetrahydrozoline Hydrochloride Ophthalmic Solution USP— Preserve in tight containers. A sterile, isotonic solution of Tetrahydrozoline Hydrochloride in water. Contains the labeled amount, within ±10%. Meets the requirements for Identification, Sterility, and pH (5.8–6.5).

THALLOUS CHLORIDE Tl 201

Chemical name: Thallium chloride ($^{201}TlCl$).

Molecular formula: $^{201}TlCl$.

USP requirements: Thallous Chloride Tl 201 Injection USP— Preserve in single-dose or in multiple-dose containers. A sterile, isotonic, aqueous solution of radioactive thallium (^{201}Tl) in the form of thallous chloride suitable for intravenous administration. Label it to include the following, in addition to the information specified for Labeling under Injections: the time and date of calibration; the amount of ^{201}Tl as labeled thallous chloride expressed as total megabecquerels (or microcuries or millicuries) and concentration as megabecquerels (or microcuries or millicuries) per mL at the time of calibration; the expiration date and time; and the statement, "Caution—Radioactive Material." The labeling indicates that in making dosage calculations, correction is to be made for radioactive decay, and also indicates that the radioactive half-life of ^{201}Tl is 73.1 hours. Contains the labeled amount of ^{201}Tl, within ±10%, as chloride, expressed in megabecquerels (or microcuries or millicuries) per mL, at the time indicated in the labeling. Other chemical forms of radioactivity do not exceed 5.0% of the total radioactivity. Meets the requirements for Radionuclide identification, Bacterial endotoxins, pH (4.5–7.5), Radiochemical purity, Radionuclidic purity, Thallium, Iron, Copper, and Injections (except that the Injection may be distributed or dispensed prior to completion of the test for Sterility, the latter test being started on the day of final manufacture, and except that it is not subject to the recommendation on Volume in Container).

THEOPHYLLINE

Source: Theophylline sodium glycinate—An equimolar mixture of theophylline sodium and aminoacetic acid (glycine).

Chemical name:

Theophylline—1*H*-Purine-2,6-dione, 3,7-dihydro-1,3-dimethyl-, monohydrate.

Theophylline sodium glycinate—Glycine, mixt. with 3,7-dihydro-1,3-dimethyl-1*H*-purine-2,6-dione, monosodium salt.

Molecular formula: $C_7H_8N_4O_2 \cdot H_2O$ (hydrous); $C_7H_8N_4O_2$ (anhydrous).

Molecular weight: 198.18 (hydrous); 180.17 (anhydrous).

Description:

Theophylline USP—White, odorless, crystalline powder. Is stable in air.

Theophylline Sodium Glycinate USP—White, crystalline powder having a slight ammoniacal odor.

Solubility:

Theophylline USP—Slightly soluble in water, but more soluble in hot water; freely soluble in solutions of alkali hydroxides and in ammonia; sparingly soluble in alcohol, in chloroform, and in ether.

Theophylline Sodium Glycinate USP—Freely soluble in water; very slightly soluble in alcohol; practically insoluble in chloroform.

USP requirements:

Theophylline Capsules USP—Preserve in well-closed containers. Contain the labeled amount of anhydrous theophylline, within ±10%. Meet the requirements for Identification, Dissolution (80% in 60 minutes in water in Apparatus 2 at 50 rpm), and Uniformity of dosage units.

Theophylline Extended-release Capsules USP—Preserve in well-closed containers. The labeling indicates whether the product is intended for dosing every 12 or 24 hours, and states with which in-vitro Drug release test the product complies. Contain the labeled amount of anhydrous theophylline, within ±10%. Meet the requirements for Identification, Drug release, and Uniformity of dosage units.

Theophylline Elixir—Not in USP.

Theophylline Oral Solution—Not in USP.

Theophylline Oral Suspension—Not in USP.

Theophylline Syrup—Not in USP.

Theophylline Tablets USP—Preserve in well-closed containers. Contain the labeled amount of anhydrous theophylline, within ±6%. Meet the requirements for Identification, Dissolution (80% in 45 minutes in water in Apparatus 2 at 50 rpm), and Uniformity of dosage units.

Theophylline Extended-release Tablets—Not in USP.

Theophylline Sodium Glycinate Elixir USP—Preserve in tight containers. Label Elixir to state both the content of theophylline sodium glycinate and the content of anhydrous theophylline. Contains an amount of theophylline sodium glycinate equivalent to the labeled amount of anhydrous theophylline, within ±7%. Meets the requirements for Identification, pH (8.3–9.1), and Alcohol content (17.0–23.0%).

Theophylline Sodium Glycinate Tablets USP—Preserve in well-closed containers. Label Tablets to state both the content of theophylline sodium glycinate and the content of anhydrous theophylline. Contain an amount of theophylline sodium glycinate equivalent to the labeled amount of anhydrous theophylline, within ±7%. Meet the requirements for Identification, Dissolution (75% in 45 minutes in water in Apparatus 1 at 100 rpm), and Uniformity of dosage units.

THEOPHYLLINE IN DEXTROSE

For *Theophylline* and *Dextrose*—See individual listings for chemistry information.

USP requirements: Theophylline in Dextrose Injection USP— Preserve in single-dose containers, preferably of Type I or Type II glass, or of a suitable plastic material. A sterile solution of Theophylline and Dextrose in Water for Injection. Contains the labeled amount of anhydrous theophylline, within ±7%, and the labeled amount of dextrose, within ±5%. Meets the requirements for Identification, Bacterial endotoxin, pH (3.5–6.5), 5-Hydroxymethylfurfural and related substances (absorbance not more than 0.25), and Injections.

THEOPHYLLINE, EPHEDRINE, GUAIFENESIN, AND BUTABARBITAL

For *Theophylline, Ephedrine, Guaifenesin,* and *Butabarbital*—See individual listings for chemistry information.

USP requirements:

Theophylline, Ephedrine Hydrochloride, Guaifenesin, and Butabarbital Capsules—Not in USP.

Theophylline, Ephedrine Hydrochloride, Guaifenesin, and Butabarbital Elixir—Not in USP.

THEOPHYLLINE, EPHEDRINE, GUAIFENESIN, AND PHENOBARBITAL

For *Theophylline, Ephedrine, Guaifenesin,* and *Phenobarbital*—See individual listings for chemistry information.

USP requirements:

Theophylline, Ephedrine Hydrochloride, Guaifenesin, and Phenobarbital Elixir—Not in USP.

Theophylline, Ephedrine Hydrochloride, Guaifenesin, and Phenobarbital Tablets—Not in USP.

Theophylline, Ephedrine Sulfate, Guaifenesin, and Phenobarbital Elixir—Not in USP.

Theophylline, Ephedrine Sulfate, Guaifenesin, and Phenobarbital Tablets—Not in USP.

THEOPHYLLINE, EPHEDRINE, AND HYDROXYZINE

For *Theophylline, Ephedrine,* and *Hydroxyzine*—See individual listings for chemistry information.

USP requirements:

Theophylline, Ephedrine Sulfate, and Hydroxyzine Hydrochloride Syrup—Not in USP.

Theophylline, Ephedrine Sulfate, and Hydroxyzine Hydrochloride Tablets—Not in USP.

THEOPHYLLINE, EPHEDRINE, AND PHENOBARBITAL

For *Theophylline, Ephedrine,* and *Phenobarbital*—See individual listings for chemistry information.

USP requirements:

Theophylline, Ephedrine Hydrochloride, and Phenobarbital Elixir—Not in USP.

Theophylline, Ephedrine Hydrochloride, and Phenobarbital Suspension—Not in USP.

Theophylline, Ephedrine Hydrochloride, and Phenobarbital Tablets USP—Preserve in tight containers. Contain the labeled amounts of anhydrous theophylline, ephedrine hydrochloride, and phenobarbital, within ±10%. Meet the requirements for Identification, Dissolution (75% of each active ingredient in 30 minutes in water in Apparatus 1 at 100 rpm), and Uniformity of dosage units.

Theophylline, Ephedrine Hydrochloride, and Phenobarbital Extended-release Tablets—Not in USP.

THEOPHYLLINE AND GUAIFENESIN

For *Theophylline* and *Guaifenesin*—See individual listings for chemistry information.

USP requirements:

Theophylline and Guaifenesin Capsules USP—Preserve in tight containers. Contain the labeled amounts of anhydrous theophylline and guaifenesin, within ±10%. Meet the requirements for Identification and Uniformity of dosage units.

Theophylline and Guaifenesin Elixir—Not in USP.

Theophylline and Guaifenesin Oral Solution USP—Preserve in tight containers. Contains the labeled amount of anhydrous theophylline, within ±10%, and the labeled amount of guaifenesin, within ±13.3%. Meets the requirements for Identification and Alcohol content (if present, 90.0–110.0% of labeled amount).

Theophylline and Guaifenesin Syrup—Not in USP.

Theophylline and Guaifenesin Tablets—Not in USP.

Theophylline Sodium Glycinate and Guaifenesin Elixir—Not in USP.

Theophylline Sodium Glycinate and Guaifenesin Syrup—Not in USP.

Theophylline Sodium Glycinate and Guaifenesin Tablets—Not in USP.

THIABENDAZOLE

Chemical group: Benzimidazole derivative; structurally related to mebendazole.

Chemical name: 1*H*-Benzimidazole, 2-(4-thiazolyl)-.

Molecular formula: $C_{10}H_7N_3S$.

Molecular weight: 201.25.

Description: Thiabendazole USP—White to practically white, odorless or practically odorless powder.

Solubility: Thiabendazole USP—Practically insoluble in water; slightly soluble in acetone and in alcohol; very slightly soluble in chloroform and in ether.

USP requirements:

Thiabendazole Oral Suspension USP—Preserve in tight containers. Contains the labeled amount, within ±10%. Meets the requirements for Identification and pH (3.4–4.2).

Thiabendazole Topical Suspension—Not in USP.

Thiabendazole Tablets USP—Preserve in tight containers. Label the Tablets to indicate that they are to be chewed before swallowing. Contain the labeled amount, within ±10%. Meet the requirements for Identification and Uniformity of dosage units.

THIAMINE

Chemical name:

Thiamine hydrochloride—Thiazolium, 3-[(4-amino-2-methyl-5-pyrimidinyl)methyl]-5-(2-hydroxyethyl)-4-methyl-, chloride, monohydrochloride.

Thiamine mononitrate—Thiazolium, 3-[(4-amino-2-methyl-5-pyrimidinyl)methyl]-5-(2-hydroxyethyl)-4-methyl-, nitrate (salt).

Molecular formula:

Thiamine hydrochloride—$C_{12}H_{17}ClN_4OS \cdot HCl$.

Thiamine mononitrate—$C_{12}H_{17}N_5O_4S$.

Molecular weight:

Thiamine hydrochloride—337.27.

Thiamine mononitrate—327.36.

Description:

Thiamine Hydrochloride USP—White crystals or crystalline powder, usually having a slight, characteristic odor. When exposed to air, the anhydrous product rapidly absorbs about 4% of water. Melts at about 248 °C, with some decomposition.

Thiamine Mononitrate USP—White crystals or crystalline powder, usually having a slight, characteristic odor.

pKa: Thiamine hydrochloride—4.8 and 9.0.

Solubility:

Thiamine Hydrochloride USP—Freely soluble in water; soluble in glycerin; slightly soluble in alcohol; insoluble in ether.

Thiamine Mononitrate USP—Sparingly soluble in water; slightly soluble in alcohol and in chloroform.

USP requirements:

Thiamine Hydrochloride Elixir USP—Preserve in tight, light-resistant containers. Contains the labeled amount, within −5% to +35%. Meets the requirements for Identification and Alcohol content (8.5–20.0%).

Thiamine Hydrochloride Injection USP—Preserve in single-dose or in multiple-dose containers, preferably of Type I glass, protected from light. A sterile solution of Thiamine Hydrochloride in Water for Injection. Contains the labeled amount, within ±10%. Meets the requirements for

Identification, Bacterial endotoxins, pH (2.5–4.5), and Injections.

Thiamine Hydrochloride Tablets USP—Preserve in tight, light-resistant containers. Contain the labeled amount, within ± 10%. Meet the requirements for Identification, Disintegration (30 minutes), and Uniformity of dosage units.

Thiamine Mononitrate Elixir USP—Preserve in tight, light-resistant containers. Contains the labeled amount, within −5% to +15%. Meets the requirements for Identification and Alcohol content (7.5–10.5%).

THIAMYLAL

Chemical group: Thiamylal sodium—A thiobarbiturate.

Chemical name: Thiamylal sodium—4,6-(1H,5H)-Pyrimidinedione, dihydro-5-(1-methylbutyl)-5-(2-propenyl)-2-thioxo-, monosodium salt.

Molecular formula: Thiamylal sodium—$C_{12}H_{17}N_2NaO_2S$.

Molecular weight: Thiamylal sodium—276.33.

Description: Thiamylal Sodium for Injection USP—Pale yellow, hygroscopic powder, having a disagreeable odor.

USP requirements:
Thiamylal Sodium for Injection USP—Preserve in Containers for Sterile Solids. A sterile mixture of thiamylal with anhydrous Sodium Carbonate as a buffer. Contains the labeled amount, within ± 7%. Meets the requirements for Labeling under injections, Completeness of solution, Constituted solution, Identification, Sterility, Uniformity of dosage units, Bacterial endotoxins, pH (10.7–11.5, in the solution prepared as directed in the test for Completeness of solution), Loss on drying (not more than 2.0%), and Heavy metals (not more than 0.003%).

Thiamylal Sodium for Rectal Solution—Not in USP.

THIETHYLPERAZINE

Chemical name:
Thiethylperazine malate—10H-Phenothiazine, 2-(ethylthio)-10-[3-(4-methyl-1-piperazinyl)propyl]-, 2-hydroxy-1,4-butanedioate (1:2).
Thiethylperazine maleate—10H-Phenothiazine, 2-(ethylthio)-10-[3-(4-methyl-1-piperazinyl)propyl]-, (Z)-2-butenedioate (1:2).

Molecular formula:
Thiethylperazine malate—$C_{22}H_{29}N_3S_2 \cdot 2C_4H_6O_5$.
Thiethylperazine maleate—$C_{22}H_{29}N_3S_2 \cdot 2C_4H_4O_4$.

Molecular weight:
Thiethylperazine malate—667.79.
Thiethylperazine maleate—631.76.

Description:
Thiethylperazine malate—White to faintly yellow crystalline powder with not more than a slight odor.
Thiethylperazine Maleate USP—Yellowish, granular powder. Odorless or has not more than a slight odor. Melts at about 183 °C, with decomposition.

Solubility:
Thiethylperazine malate—Soluble 1 in 40 of water, 1 in 90 of alcohol, 1 in 525 of chloroform, and 1 in 3400 of ether.
Thiethylperazine Maleate USP—Practically insoluble in water; slightly soluble in methanol; practically insoluble in chloroform.

USP requirements:
Thiethylperazine Malate Injection USP—Preserve in single-dose containers, preferably of Type I glass, protected from light. A sterile solution of Thiethylperazine Malate in Water for Injection. Contains the labeled amount, within ± 10%. Meets the requirements for Identification, Bacterial endotoxins, pH (3.0–4.0), and Injections.

Thiethylperazine Maleate Suppositories USP—Preserve in tight containers at temperatures below 25 °C. Do not expose unwrapped Suppositories to sunlight. Contain the labeled amount, within ± 10%. Meet the requirement for Identification.

Thiethylperazine Maleate Tablets USP—Preserve in tight, light-resistant containers. Contain the labeled amount, within ± 10%. Meet the requirements for Identification, Dissolution (75% in 30 minutes in 0.1 N hydrochloric acid in Apparatus 1 at 120 rpm), and Uniformity of dosage units.

THIMEROSAL

Chemical name: Mercury, ethyl (2-mercaptobenzoato-S)-, sodium salt.

Molecular formula: $C_9H_9HgNaO_2S$.

Molecular weight: 404.81.

Description:
Thimerosal USP—Light cream-colored, crystalline powder, having a slight characteristic odor. Affected by light. The pH of a solution (1 in 100) is about 6.7.
NF category: Antimicrobial preservative.
Thimerosal Topical Solution USP—Clear liquid, having a slight characteristic odor. Affected by light.
Thimerosal Tincture USP—Transparent, mobile liquid, having the characteristic odor of alcohol and acetone. Affected by light.

Solubility: Thimerosal USP—Freely soluble in water; soluble in alcohol; practically insoluble in ether.

USP requirements:
Thimerosal USP—Preserve in tight, light-resistant containers. Contains not less than 97.0% and not more than 101.0% of thimerosal, calculated on the dried basis. Meets the requirements for Identification, Loss on drying (not more than 0.5%), Ether-soluble substances (not more than 0.8%), Mercury ions (not more than 0.70%), and Readily carbonizable substances.

Thimerosal Topical Aerosol USP—Preserve in tight, light-resistant, pressurized containers, and avoid exposure to excessive heat. An alcoholic solution of Thimerosal mixed with suitable propellants in a pressurized container. Contains the labeled amount, within ± 15%. Meets the requirements for Identification and Alcohol content (18.7–25.3% [w/w]), and for Leak testing and Pressure testing under Aerosols.

Note: Thimerosal Topical Aerosol is sensitive to some metals.

Thimerosal Topical Solution USP—Preserve in tight, light-resistant containers, and avoid exposure to excessive heat. Contains, in each 100 mL, not less than 95 mg and not more than 105 mg of thimerosal. Meets the requirements for Identification and pH (9.6–10.2).

Note: Thimerosal Topical Solution is sensitive to some metals.

Thimerosal Tincture USP—Preserve in tight, light-resistant containers, and avoid exposure to excessive heat. Contains, in each 100 mL, not less than 90 mg and not more than 110 mg of thimerosal. Meets the requirements for Identification and Alcohol content (45.0–55.0%).

Note: Thimerosal Tincture is sensitive to some metals.

THIOGUANINE

Chemical name: 6*H*-Purine-6-thione, 2-amino-1,7-dihydro-.

Molecular formula: $C_5H_5N_5S \cdot xH_2O$.

Molecular weight: 167.19 (anhydrous).

Description: Thioguanine USP—Pale yellow, odorless or practically odorless, crystalline powder.

pKa: 8.1.

Solubility: Thioguanine USP—Insoluble in water, in alcohol, and in chloroform; freely soluble in dilute solutions of alkali hydroxides.

USP requirements: Thioguanine Tablets USP—Preserve in tight containers. Contain the labeled amount, within ±7%. Meet the requirements for Identification, Dissolution (75% in 45 minutes in water in Apparatus 2 at 50 rpm), and Uniformity of dosage units.

THIOPENTAL

Chemical group: A thiobarbiturate, the sulfur analog of pentobarbital sodium.

Chemical name: Thiopental sodium—4,6(1*H*,5*H*)-Pyrimidinedione, 5-ethyldihydro-5-(1-methylbutyl)-2-thioxo-, monosodium salt.

Molecular formula: Thiopental sodium—$C_{11}H_{17}N_2NaO_2S$.

Molecular weight: Thiopental sodium—264.32.

Description:
Thiopental Sodium USP—White to off-white, crystalline powder, or yellowish-white to pale greenish-yellow, hygroscopic powder. May have a disagreeable odor. Its solutions are alkaline to litmus. Its solutions decompose on standing, and on boiling precipitation occurs.
Thiopental Sodium for Injection USP—White to off-white, crystalline powder, or yellowish-white to pale greenish-yellow, hygroscopic powder. May have a disagreeable odor. Its solutions are alkaline to litmus. Its solutions decompose on standing, and on boiling precipitation occurs.

pKa: Thiopental sodium—7.4.

Solubility: Thiopental Sodium USP—Soluble in water and in alcohol; insoluble in absolute ether and in solvent hexane.

USP requirements:
Thiopental Sodium for Injection USP—Preserve in Containers for Sterile Solids, preferably of Type III glass. A sterile mixture of Thiopental Sodium and anhydrous Sodium Carbonate as a buffer. Contains the labeled amount, within ±7%. Meets the requirements for Completeness of solution, Constituted solution, Bacterial endotoxins, and pH (10.2–11.2), for Identification tests and Heavy metals under Thiopental Sodium, and for Sterility tests, Uniformity of dosage units, and Labeling under Injections.
Thiopental Sodium for Rectal Solution—Not in USP.
Thiopental Sodium Rectal Suspension—Not in USP.

THIOPROPAZATE

Chemical group: Piperazine phenothiazine derivative.

Chemical name: Thiopropazate hydrochloride—4-[3-(2-Chlorophenothiazin-10-yl)propyl]-1-piperazineethanol acetate dihydrochloride.

Molecular formula: Thiopropazate hydrochloride—$C_{23}H_{28}ClN_3O_2S \cdot 2HCl$.

Molecular weight: Thiopropazate hydrochloride—518.94.

Description: Thiopropazate hydrochloride—White or pale yellow crystalline powder with a faint odor.

Solubility: Thiopropazate hydrochloride—Soluble 1 in 4 of water, 1 in 130 of alcohol, and 1 in 65 of chloroform; practically insoluble in ether.

USP requirements: Thiopropazate Hydrochloride Tablets—Not in USP.

THIOPROPERAZINE

Chemical group: Phenothiazine.

Chemical name: Thioproperazine mesylate—*NN*-Dimethyl-10-[3-(4-methylpiperazin-1-yl)propyl]phenothiazine-2-sulphonamide dimethanesulphonate.

Molecular formula: Thioproperazine mesylate—$C_{22}H_{30}N_4O_2S_2 \cdot 2CH_4O_3S$.

Molecular weight: Thioproperazine mesylate—638.8.

Description: Thioproperazine mesylate—Slightly hygroscopic white powder with a yellowish tint.

Solubility: Thioproperazine mesylate—Readily soluble in water; slightly soluble in ethanol; practically insoluble in methanol and in dimethylformamide.

USP requirements: Thioproperazine Mesylate Tablets—Not in USP.

THIORIDAZINE

Chemical group: Piperidine.

Chemical name:
Thioridazine—10*H*-Phenothiazine, 10-[2-(1-methyl-2-piperidinyl)ethyl]-2-(methylthio)-.
Thioridazine hydrochloride—10*H*-Phenothiazine, 10-[2-(1-methyl-2-piperidinyl)ethyl]-2-(methylthio)-, monohydrochloride.

Molecular formula:
Thioridazine—$C_{21}H_{26}N_2S_2$.
Thioridazine hydrochloride—$C_{21}H_{26}N_2S_2 \cdot HCl$.

Molecular weight:
Thioridazine—370.57.
Thioridazine hydrochloride—407.03.

Description:
Thioridazine USP—White to slightly yellow, crystalline or micronized powder, odorless or having a faint odor.
Thioridazine Hydrochloride USP—White to slightly yellow, granular powder, having a faint odor.

Solubility:
Thioridazine USP—Practically insoluble in water; freely soluble in dehydrated alcohol and in ether; very soluble in chloroform.
Thioridazine Hydrochloride USP—Freely soluble in water, in methanol, and in chloroform; insoluble in ether.

USP requirements:
Thioridazine Oral Suspension USP—Preserve in tight, light-resistant containers, at a temperature not exceeding 30 °C. Contains the labeled amount, within ±10%. Meets the requirements for Identification, Specific gravity (1.180–1.310), and pH (8.0–10.0).
Thioridazine Hydrochloride Oral Solution USP—Preserve in tight, light-resistant containers, at controlled room temperature. Label it to indicate that it is to be diluted to

appropriate strength with water or other suitable fluid prior to administration. Contains the labeled amount, within ±10%. Meets the requirements for Identification and Alcohol content (not more than 4.75%).

Thioridazine Hydrochloride Tablets USP—Preserve in tight, light-resistant containers. Contain the labeled amount, within ±10%. Meet the requirements for Identification, Dissolution (75% in 60 minutes in 0.1 *N* hydrochloric acid in Apparatus 2 at 75 rpm), and Uniformity of dosage units.

THIOTEPA

Chemical name: Aziridine,1,1′,1″-phosphinothioylidynetris-.

Molecular formula: $C_6H_{12}N_3PS$.

Molecular weight: 189.21.

Description:
Thiotepa USP—Fine, white, crystalline flakes, having a faint odor.
Thiotepa for Injection USP—White powder.

Solubility: Thiotepa USP—Freely soluble in water, in alcohol, in chloroform, and in ether.

USP requirements: Thiotepa for Injection USP—Preserve in Containers for Sterile Solids, and store in a refrigerator, protected from light. It is Thiotepa, with or without added substances, that is suitable for parenteral use. Contains the labeled amount, within −5% to +10%. Meets the requirements for Completeness of solution, Identification, pH (7.0–8.6, in a solution, constituted as directed in the labeling, containing 10 mg of thiotepa per mL), Loss on drying (not more than 0.5%), and Bacterial endotoxins, and for Sterility tests, Uniformity of dosage units, and Labeling under Injections.

THIOTHIXENE

Chemical group: Thioxanthene derivative.

Chemical name:
Thiothixene—9*H*-Thioxanthene-2-sulfonamide, *N,N*-dimethyl-9-[3-(4-methyl-1-piperazinyl)propylidene]-, (*Z*)-.
Thiothixene hydrochloride—9*H*-Thioxanthene-2-sulfonamide, *N,N*-dimethyl-9-[3-(4-methyl-1-piperazinyl)propylidene]-, dihydrochloride, dihydrate (*Z*)-.

Molecular formula:
Thiothixene—$C_{23}H_{29}N_3O_2S_2$.
Thiothixene hydrochloride—$C_{23}H_{29}N_3O_2S_2 \cdot 2HCl \cdot 2H_2O$.

Molecular weight:
Thiothixene—443.62.
Thiothixene hydrochloride—552.57.

Description:
Thiothixene USP—White to tan, practically odorless crystals. Is affected by light.
Thiothixene Hydrochloride USP—White, or practically white, crystalline powder, having a slight odor. Is affected by light.

Solubility:
Thiothixene USP—Practically insoluble in water; very soluble in chloroform; slightly soluble in methanol and in acetone.
Thiothixene Hydrochloride USP—Soluble in water; slightly soluble in chloroform; practically insoluble in acetone and in ether.

Other characteristics: Structurally and pharmacologically similar to the piperazine phenothiazines.

USP requirements:
Thiothixene Capsules USP—Preserve in well-closed, light-resistant containers. Contain the labeled amount, within ±10%. Meet the requirements for Identification, Dissolution (75% in 15 minutes in solution of 2.0 grams of sodium chloride and 7 mL of hydrochloric acid in water to make 1000 mL in Apparatus 1 at 150 rpm), and Uniformity of dosage units.

Thiothixene Hydrochloride Injection USP—Preserve in single-dose containers, preferably of Type I glass, protected from light. A sterile solution of Thiothixene Hydrochloride in Water for Injection. Contains an amount of thiothixene hydrochloride equivalent to the labeled amount of thiothixene, within ±10%. Meets the requirements for Identification, Bacterial endotoxins, pH (2.5–3.5), and Injections.

Thiothixene Hydrochloride for Injection USP—Preserve in light-resistant Containers for Sterile Solids. A sterile, dry mixture of Thiothixene Hydrochloride and Mannitol. Contains an amount of thiothixene hydrochloride equivalent to the labeled amount of thiothixene, within ±10%. Meets the requirements for Identification, Bacterial endotoxins, pH (2.3–3.7, in the solution constituted as directed in the labeling), Water (not more than 4.0%), and Injections.

Thiothixene Hydrochloride Oral Solution USP—Preserve in tight, light-resistant containers. Contains an amount of thiothixene hydrochloride equivalent to the labeled amount of thiothixene, within ±10%. Meets the requirements for Identification, pH (2.0–3.0), and Alcohol content (if present, within ±10% of the labeled amount, the labeled amount being not more than 7.0%).

THONZONIUM BROMIDE

Chemical name: 1-Hexadecanaminium, *N*-[2-[[(4-methoxyphenyl)methyl]-2-pyrimidinylamino]ethyl]-*N,N*-dimethyl-, bromide.

Molecular formula: $C_{32}H_{55}BrN_4O$.

Molecular weight: 591.72.

USP requirements: Thonzonium Bromide USP—Preserve in tight containers. Contains not less than 97.0% and not more than 103.0% of thonzonium bromide, calculated on the anhydrous basis. Meets the requirements for Identification, Melting range (93–97 °C), Water (not more than 0.5%), Residue on ignition (not more than 0.2%), Ordinary impurities, and Organic volatile impurities.

THROMBIN

Description: Thrombin USP—White to grayish, amorphous substance dried from the frozen state.

USP requirements: Thrombin USP—Preserve at a temperature between 2 and 8 °C. Dispense it in the unopened container in which it was placed by the manufacturer. A sterile, freeze-dried powder derived from bovine plasma containing the protein substance prepared from prothrombin through interaction with added thromboplastin in the presence of calcium. It is capable, without the addition of other substances, of causing the clotting of whole blood, plasma, or a solution of fibrinogen. Its potency is determined in U.S. Units in terms of the U.S. Standard Thrombin in a test comparing clotting times of fibrinogen solution. Label it to indicate that solutions of Thrombin are to be used within a few hours after preparation, and are not to be injected into or otherwise allowed to enter large blood vessels. Meets the requirement for Expiration date (not more than 3 years after date of manufacture). Conforms to the regulations of the U.S. Food and Drug Administration concerning biologics.

THYMOL

Chemical name: Phenol, 5-methyl-2-(1-methylethyl)-.

Molecular formula: $C_{10}H_{14}O$.

Molecular weight: 150.22.

Description: Thymol NF—Colorless, often large, crystals, or white, crystalline powder, having an aromatic, thyme-like odor. Affected by light. Its alcohol solution is neutral to litmus.

NF category: Antimicrobial preservative; flavors and perfumes.

Solubility: Thymol NF—Very slightly soluble in water; freely soluble in alcohol, in chloroform, in ether, and in olive oil; soluble in glacial acetic acid and in fixed and volatile oils.

NF requirements: Thymol NF—Preserve in tight, light-resistant containers. Contains not less than 99.0% and not more than 101.0% of thymol. Meets the requirements for Identification, Melting range (48–51 °C, but when melted, Thymol remains liquid at a considerably lower temperature), and Nonvolatile residue (not more than 0.05%).

THYROGLOBULIN

Source: Substance obtained by the fractionation of thyroid glands from the hog, *Sus scrofa* Linné var. *domesticus* Gray (Fam. *Suidae*), containing not less than 0.7% of total iodine (I).

Chemical name: Thyroglobulin.

Description: Thyroglobulin USP—Cream to tan-colored, free-flowing powder, having a slight, characteristic odor.

Solubility: Thyroglobulin USP—Insoluble in water, in dimethylformamide, in alcohol, in hydrochloric acid, in chloroform, and in carbon tetrachloride.

USP requirements: Thyroglobulin Tablets USP—Preserve in tight containers. Contain the labeled amount of levothyroxine, within ± 15%, and the labeled amount of liothyronine, within ±10%, the labeled amounts being 36 mcg of levothyroxine and 12 mcg of liothyronine for each 65 mg (1 grain) of the labeled content of thyroglobulin. Meet the requirements for Identification, Microbial limits, Disintegration (15 minutes), and Uniformity of dosage units.

THYROID

Description: Thyroid USP—Yellowish to buff-colored, amorphous powder, having a slight, characteristic, meat-like odor.

USP requirements:
Thyroid Tablets USP—Preserve in tight containers. Contain the labeled amount of levothyroxine, within ±15%, and the labeled amount of liothyronine, within ±10%, the labeled amounts being 38 mcg of levothyroxine and 9 mcg of liothyronine for each 65 mg (1 grain) of the labeled content of thyroid. Meet the requirements for Microbial limit, Disintegration (15 minutes), Uniformity of dosage units, and Inorganic iodides (not more than 0.004%).
Thyroid Enteric-coated Tablets—Not in USP.

THYROTROPIN

Source: Thyroid stimulating hormone (TSH) isolated from bovine anterior pituitary.

Molecular weight: Range of 28,000–30,000.

Solubility: Dissolves readily in physiologic saline.

USP requirements: Thyrotropin for Injection—Not in USP.

TIAPROFENIC ACID

Chemical group: Propionic acid derivative.

Chemical name: 5-Benzoyl-alpha-methyl-2-thiopheneacetic acid.

Molecular formula: $C_{14}H_{12}O_3S$.

Molecular weight: 260.31.

Description: White, microcrystalline powder. Melts at about 95 °C.

pKa: 3.0.

Solubility: Readily soluble in alcohol, in chloroform, and in acetone; sparingly soluble in water.

USP requirements: Tiaprofenic Acid Tablets—Not in USP.

TICARCILLIN

Chemical name:
Ticarcillin disodium—4-Thia-1-azabicyclo[3.2.0]heptane-2-carboxylic acid, 6-[(carboxy-3-thienylacetyl)amino]-3,3-dimethyl-7-oxo-, disodium salt, [2S-[2 alpha,5 alpha,6 beta(S*)]]-.
Ticarcillin monosodium—4-Thia-1-azabicyclo[3.2.0]heptane-2-carboxylic acid, 6-[(carboxy-3-thienylacetyl)amino]-3,3-dimethyl-7-oxo, monosodium salt, [2S-[2 alpha,5 alpha,6 beta(S*)]]-, monohydrate.

Molecular formula:
Ticarcillin disodium—$C_{15}H_{14}N_2Na_2O_6S_2$.
Ticarcillin monosodium monohydrate—$C_{15}H_{15}N_2NaO_6S_2 \cdot H_2O$.

Molecular weight:
Ticarcillin disodium—428.38.
Ticarcillin monosodium monohydrate—424.42.

Description: Sterile Ticarcillin Disodium USP—White to pale yellow powder, or white to pale yellow solid having the characteristic appearance of products prepared by freeze-drying.

Solubility: Sterile Ticarcillin Disodium USP—Freely soluble in water.

USP requirements:
Sterile Ticarcillin Disodium USP—Preserve in Containers for Sterile Solids. It is ticarcillin disodium suitable for parenteral use. It has a potency equivalent to not less than 800 mcg of ticarcillin per mg, calculated on the anhydrous basis, and, where packaged for dispensing, contains an amount of ticarcillin disodium equivalent to the labeled amount of ticarcillin, within −10% to +15%. Meets the requirements for Constituted solution, Identification, Bacterial endotoxins, Sterility, pH (6.0–8.0, in a solution containing 10 mg of ticarcillin per mL [or in the solution constituted as directed in the labeling]), Water (not more than 6.0%), Particulate matter, and Ticarcillin content (80.0–94.0%, calculated on the anhydrous basis). Where packaged for dispensing, meets the requirements for Uniformity of dosage units and Labeling under Injections.

III/406   **Chemistry and Compendial Requirements**

Ticarcillin Monosodium USP—Preserve in tight containers. Contains the equivalent of not less than 890 mcg of ticarcillin per mg, calculated on the anhydrous basis. Meets the requirements for Identification, Crystallinity, pH (2.5–4.0, in a solution containing the equivalent of 10 mg of ticarcillin per mL), and Water (4.0–6.0%).

TICARCILLIN AND CLAVULANATE

For *Ticarcillin* and *Clavulanate*—See individual listings for chemistry information.

USP requirements:
Ticarcillin Disodium and Clavulanate Potassium Injection USP—Preserve in Containers for Injections. Maintain in the frozen state. A sterile isoosmotic solution of Ticarcillin Monosodium and Clavulanate Potassium in Water for Injection. Contains one or more suitable buffering agents and a tonicity-adjusting agent. The label states that it is to be thawed just prior to use, describes conditions for proper storage of the resultant solution, and directs that the solution is not to be refrozen. Contains an amount of ticarcillin disodium equivalent to the labeled amount of ticarcillin, within −10 to +15%, and an amount of clavulanate potassium equivalent to the labeled amount of clavulanic acid, within −15% to +20%. Meets the requirements for Identification, Pyrogen, Sterility, pH (5.5–7.5), and Particulate matter, for Uniformity of dosage units, and for Labeling under Injections.
Sterile Ticarcillin Disodium and Clavulanate Potassium USP—Preserve in Containers for Sterile Solids. A sterile, dry mixture of Sterile Ticarcillin Disodium and Sterile Clavulanate Potassium. Contains amounts of ticarcillin disodium and clavulanate potassium equivalent to the labeled amount of ticarcillin, within −10% to +15%, and clavulanic acid, within −15% to +20%, the labeled amounts representing proportions of ticarcillin to clavulanic acid of 15:1 or 30:1. Where the proportion is 15:1, contains not less than 733 mcg of ticarcillin per mg, calculated on the anhydrous basis. Where the proportion is 30:1, contains not less than 755 mcg of ticarcillin per mg, calculated on the anhydrous basis. Meets the requirements for Constituted solution, Identification, Bacterial endotoxins, Sterility, pH (5.5–7.5, in a solution [1 in 10]), Water (not more than 4.2%), and Particulate matter, for Uniformity of dosage units, and for Labeling under Injections.

TICLOPIDINE

Chemical name: Ticlopidine hydrochloride—Thieno[3,2-c]pyridine, 5-[(2-chlorophenyl)methyl]-4,5,6,7-tetrahydro-, hydrochloride.

Molecular formula: Ticlopidine hydrochloride—$C_{14}H_{14}ClNS \cdot HCl$.

Molecular weight: Ticlopidine hydrochloride—300.25.

Description: Ticlopidine hydrochloride—White crystalline solid.

Solubility: Ticlopidine hydrochloride—Freely soluble in water and in self buffers to a pH of 3.6, and in methanol; sparingly soluble in methylene chloride and in ethanol; slightly soluble in acetone; insoluble in a buffer solution of pH 6.3.

USP requirements: Ticlopidine Hydrochloride Tablets—Not in USP.

TIMOLOL

Chemical name: Timolol maleate—2-Propanol, 1-[(1,1-dimethylethyl)amino]-3-[[4-(4-morpholinyl)-1,2,5-thiadiazol-3-yl]oxy]-, (*S*)-, (*Z*)-2-butenedioate (1:1) (salt).

Molecular formula: Timolol maleate—$C_{13}H_{24}N_4O_3S \cdot C_4H_4O_4$.

Molecular weight: Timolol maleate—432.49.

Description: Timolol Maleate USP—White to practically white, odorless or practically odorless, powder.

pKa: Approximately 9 in water at 25 °C.

Solubility: Timolol Maleate USP—Freely soluble in water; soluble in alcohol and in methanol; sparingly soluble in chloroform and in propylene glycol; insoluble in ether and in cyclohexane.

Other characteristics: Lipid solubility—Moderate.

USP requirements:
Timolol Maleate Ophthalmic Solution USP—Preserve in tight, light-resistant containers. A sterile aqueous solution of Timolol Maleate. Contains an amount of timolol maleate equivalent to the labeled amount of timolol, within ±10%. Meets the requirements for Identification, Sterility, and pH (6.5–7.5).
Timolol Maleate Tablets USP—Preserve in well-closed containers. Contain the labeled amount, within ±10%. Meet the requirements for Identification, Dissolution (80% in 20 minutes in 0.1 N hydrochloric acid in Apparatus 1 at 100 rpm), and Uniformity of dosage units.

TIMOLOL AND HYDROCHLOROTHIAZIDE

For *Timolol* and *Hydrochlorothiazide*—See individual listings for chemistry information.

USP requirements: Timolol Maleate and Hydrochlorothiazide Tablets USP—Preserve in well-closed, light-resistant containers. Contain the labeled amounts, within ±10%. Meet the requirements for Identification, Dissolution (80% of each active ingredient in 20 minutes in 0.1 N hydrochloric acid in Apparatus 2 at 50 rpm), Limit of 4-amino-6-chloro-1,3-benzenedisulfonamide (not more than 1.0%), and Uniformity of dosage units.

TIOCONAZOLE

Chemical name: 1*H*-Imidazole, 1-[2-[(2-chloro-3-thienyl)methoxy]-2-(2,4-dichlorophenyl)ethyl]-.

Molecular formula: $C_{16}H_{13}Cl_3N_2OS$.

Molecular weight: 387.71.

Description: White to off-white crystalline solid.

Solubility: Moderately soluble in chloroform, in methanol, in ethanol, and in ethyl acetate; virtually insoluble in water.

USP requirements:
Tioconazole Cream USP—Preserve in tight containers. Contains the labeled amount, within ±10%, in a suitable cream base. Meets the requirements for Identification, Microbial limits, Minimum fill, and pH (3.0–6.0, in a 1:1 aqueous suspension of the Cream).
Tioconazole Vaginal Ointment—Not in USP.
Tioconazole Vaginal Suppositories—Not in USP.

TIOPRONIN

Chemical name: *N*-(2-Mercaptopropionyl)glycine.

Molecular formula: $C_5H_9NO_3S$.

Molecular weight: 163.19.

Description: A white, crystalline powder with a characteristic sulphurous odor.

Solubility: Soluble in water.

Other characteristics: Chemically similar to penicillamine.

USP requirements: Tiopronin Tablets—Not in USP.

TITANIUM DIOXIDE

Chemical name: Titanium oxide (TiO_2).

Molecular formula: TiO_2.

Molecular weight: 79.88.

Description: Titanium Dioxide USP—White, odorless powder. Its 1 in 10 suspension in water is neutral to litmus.
NF category: Coating agent.

Solubility: Titanium Dioxide USP—Insoluble in water, in hydrochloric acid, in nitric acid, and in 2 N sulfuric acid. Dissolves in hydrofluoric acid and in hot sulfuric acid. It is rendered soluble by fusion with potassium bisulfate or with alkali carbonates or hydroxides.

USP requirements: Titanium Dioxide USP—Preserve in well-closed containers. Contains not less than 99.0% and not more than 100.5% of titanium dioxide, calculated on the dried basis. Meets the requirements for Identification, Loss on drying (not more than 0.5%), Loss on ignition (not more than 0.5%), Water-soluble substances (not more than 0.25%), Acid-soluble substances (not more than 0.5%), and Arsenic (not more than 1ppm).
Note: The U.S. Food and Drug Administration requires the content of lead to be not more than 0.001%, that of antimony to be not more than 2 ppm, and that of mercury to be not more than 1 ppm.

TOBRAMYCIN

Source: Derived from *Streptomyces tenebrarius*.

Chemical group: Aminoglycoside.

Chemical name:
Tobramycin—D-Streptamine, *O*-3-amino-3-deoxy-alpha-D-glucopyranosyl-(1→6)-*O*-[2,6-diamino-2,3,6-trideoxy-alpha-D-*ribo*-hexopyranosyl-(1→4)]-2-deoxy-.
Tobramycin sulfate—D-Streptamine, *O*-3-amino-3-deoxy-alpha-D-glucopyranosyl-(1→6)-*O*-[2,6-diamino-2,3,6-trideoxy-alpha-D-*ribo*-hexopyranosyl-(1→4)]-2-deoxy-, sulfate (2:5) (salt).

Molecular formula:
Tobramycin—$C_{18}H_{37}N_5O_9$.
Tobramycin sulfate—$(C_{18}H_{37}N_5O_9)_2 \cdot 5H_2SO_4$.

Molecular weight:
Tobramycin—467.52.
Tobramycin sulfate—1425.39.

Description:
Tobramycin USP—White to off-white, hygroscopic powder.
Tobramycin Sulfate Injection USP—Clear, colorless solution.

Solubility: Tobramycin USP—Freely soluble in water; very slightly soluble in alcohol; practically insoluble in chloroform and in ether.

USP requirements:
Tobramycin Ophthalmic Ointment USP—Preserve in collapsible ophthalmic ointment tubes. Contains the labeled amount, within −10% to +20%. Meets the requirements for Identification, Sterility, Minimum fill, Water (not more than 1.0%), and Metal particles.

Tobramycin Ophthalmic Solution USP—Preserve in tight containers, and avoid exposure to excessive heat. Contains the labeled amount, within −10% to +20%. Meets the requirements for Identification, Sterility, and pH (7.0–8.0).

Tobramycin Sulfate Injection USP—Preserve in single-dose or in multiple-dose glass or plastic containers. Glass containers are preferably of Type I glass. A sterile solution of Tobramycin Sulfate or of Sterile Tobramycin Sulfate in Water for Injection, or of Tobramycin in Water for Injection prepared with the aid of Sulfuric Acid. Contains an amount of tobramycin sulfate equivalent to the labeled amount of tobramycin, within −10% to +20%. Meets the requirements for Identification, Bacterial endotoxins, Sterility, pH (3.0–6.5), Particulate matter, and Injections.

Sterile Tobramycin Sulfate USP—Preserve in Containers for Sterile Solids. It is tobramycin sulfate suitable for parenteral use. Has a potency of not less than 634 mcg and not more than 739 mcg of tobramycin per mg and, where packaged for dispensing, contains an amount of tobramycin sulfate equivalent to the labeled amount of tobramycin within −10% to +15%. Meets the requirements for Identification, Constituted solution, Bacterial endotoxins, Sterility, pH (6.0–8.0, in a solution containing 40 mg per mL [or, where packaged for dispensing, in the solution constituted as directed in the labeling]), Water (not more than 2.0%), and Particulate matter, for Residue on ignition and Heavy metals under Tobramycin, and for Uniformity of dosage units (where packaged for dispensing) and Labeling under Injections.

TOBRAMYCIN AND DEXAMETHASONE

For *Tobramycin* and *Dexamethasone*—See individual listings for chemistry information.

USP requirements:
Tobramycin and Dexamethasone Ophthalmic Ointment USP—Preserve in collapsible ophthalmic ointment tubes. Contains the labeled amount of tobramycin, within −10% to +20%, and the labeled amount of dexamethasone, within ±10%. Meets the requirements for Identification, Minimum fill, Water (not more than 1.0%), and Metal particles.

Tobramycin and Dexamethasone Ophthalmic Suspension USP—Preserve in tight containers. A sterile aqueous suspension containing Tobramycin and Dexamethasone. Contains the labeled amount of tobramycin, within −10% to +20%, and the labeled amount of dexamethasone, within ±10%. Meets the requirements for Identification, Sterility, and pH (5.0–6.0).

TOBRAMYCIN AND FLUOROMETHOLONE

For *Tobramycin* and *Fluorometholone*—See individual listings for chemistry information.

USP requirements: Tobramycin and Fluorometholone Acetate Ophthalmic Suspension USP—Preserve in tight containers. A sterile aqueous suspension of Tobramycin and Fluorometholone Acetate. Contains the labeled amount of tobramycin, within −10% to +20%, and the labeled amount of fluorometholone acetate, within −10% to +15%. Meets the requirements for Identification, Sterility, and pH (6.0–7.0).

TOCAINIDE

Chemical name: Tocainide hydrochloride—Propanamide, 2-amino-*N*-(2,6-dimethylphenyl)-, hydrochloride.

Molecular formula: Tocainide hydrochloride—$C_{11}H_{16}N_2O \cdot HCl$.

Molecular weight: Tocainide hydrochloride—228.72.

Description: Tocainide Hydrochloride USP—Fine, white, odorless powder.

pKa: 7.7.

Solubility: Tocainide Hydrochloride USP—Freely soluble in water and in alcohol; practically insoluble in chloroform and in ether.

USP requirements: Tocainide Hydrochloride Tablets USP—Preserve in well-closed containers. Contain the labeled amount, within ±5%. Meet the requirements for Identification, Dissolution (80% in 30 minutes in water in Apparatus 2 at 50 rpm), and Uniformity of dosage units.

TOCOPHEROLS EXCIPIENT

Description: Tocopherols Excipient NF—Brownish red to red, clear, viscous oil, having a mild, characteristic odor. May show a slight separation of waxlike constituents in microcrystalline form. Oxidizes and darkens slowly in air and on exposure to light, particularly in alkaline media.

NF category: Antioxidant.

Solubility: Tocopherols Excipient NF—Insoluble in water; soluble in alcohol; miscible with acetone, with chloroform, with ether, and with vegetable oils.

NF requirements: Tocopherols Excipient NF—Preserve in tight containers, protected from light. Protect with a blanket of an inert gas. A vegetable oil solution containing not less than 50.0% of total tocopherols, of which not less than 80.0% consists of varying amounts of beta, gamma, and delta tocopherols. Label it to indicate the content, in mg per gram, of total tocopherols, and of the sum of beta, gamma, and delta tocopherols. Meets the requirements for Identification and Acidity.

TOLAZAMIDE

Chemical group: Sulfonylurea.

Chemical name: Benzenesulfonamide, *N*-[[(hexahydro-1*H*-azepin-1-yl)amino]carbonyl]-4-methyl-.

Molecular formula: $C_{14}H_{21}N_3O_3S$.

Molecular weight: 311.40.

Description: Tolazamide USP—White to off-white, powder, odorless or having a slight odor. Melts with decomposition in the approximate range of 161 to 173 °C.

pKa: 3.5 and 5.7.

Solubility: Tolazamide USP—Very slightly soluble in water; freely soluble in chloroform; soluble in acetone; slightly soluble in alcohol.

USP requirements: Tolazamide Tablets USP—Preserve in tight containers. Contain the labeled amount, within ±5%. Meet the requirements for Identification, Dissolution (70% in 30 minutes in 0.05 *M* Tris(hydroxymethyl)aminomethane, adjusted, if necessary, with hydrochloric acid to a pH of 7.6, in Apparatus 2 at 75 rpm), and Uniformity of dosage units.

TOLAZOLINE

Chemical group: Imidazoline derivative, structurally related to phentolamine.

Chemical name: Tolazoline hydrochloride—1*H*-Imidazole, 4,5-dihydro-2-(phenylmethyl)-, monohydrochloride.

Molecular formula: Tolazoline hydrochloride—$C_{10}H_{12}N_2 \cdot HCl$.

Molecular weight: Tolazoline hydrochloride—196.68.

Description: Tolazoline Hydrochloride USP—White to off-white, crystalline powder. Its solutions are slightly acid to litmus.

pKa: 10.3.

Solubility: Tolazoline Hydrochloride USP—Freely soluble in water and in alcohol.

USP requirements:

Tolazoline Hydrochloride Injection USP—Preserve in single-dose or in multiple-dose containers, preferably of Type I glass. A sterile solution of Tolazoline Hydrochloride in Water for Injection. Contains the labeled amount, within ±5%. Meets the requirements for Identification, Bacterial endotoxins, pH (3.0–4.0), and Injections.

Tolazoline Hydrochloride Tablets USP—Preserve in well-closed containers. Contain the labeled amount, within ±5%. Meet the requirements for Identification, Dissolution (75% in 45 minutes in water in Apparatus 2 at 50 rpm), and Uniformity of dosage units.

TOLBUTAMIDE

Chemical group: Sulfonylurea.

Chemical name:

Tolbutamide—Benzenesulfonamide, *N*-[(butylamino)carbonyl]-4-methyl-.

Tolbutamide sodium—Benzenesulfonamide, *N*-[(butylamino)carbonyl]-4-methyl-, monosodium salt.

Molecular formula:

Tolbutamide—$C_{12}H_{18}N_2O_3S$.

Tolbutamide sodium—$C_{12}H_{17}N_2NaO_3S$.

Molecular weight:

Tolbutamide—270.35.

Tolbutamide sodium—292.33.

Description:

Tolbutamide USP—White, or practically white, crystalline powder. Is practically odorless.

Sterile Tolbutamide Sodium USP—White to off-white, practically odorless, crystalline powder.

pKa: 5.3.

Solubility:

Tolbutamide USP—Practically insoluble in water; soluble in alcohol and in chloroform.

Sterile Tolbutamide Sodium USP—Freely soluble in water; soluble in alcohol and in chloroform; very slightly soluble in ether.

USP requirements:

Tolbutamide Tablets USP—Preserve in well-closed containers. Contain the labeled amount, within ±10%. Meet the requirements for Identification, Dissolution (70% in 30 minutes in phosphate buffer [pH 7.4] in Apparatus 2 at 75 rpm), and Uniformity of dosage units.

Sterile Tolbutamide Sodium USP—Preserve in Containers for Sterile Solids. It is prepared from Tolbutamide with the aid of Sodium Hydroxide. It is suitable for parenteral use. Contains an amount of tolbutamide sodium equivalent to the labeled amount of tolbutamide, within ±5%. Meets the requirements for Constituted solution, Identification, Bacterial endotoxins, pH (8.0–9.8, in a solution containing 50 mg per mL), and Loss on drying (not more than 1.0%), and for Sterility, Uniformity of dosage units, and Labeling under Injections.

TOLMETIN

Chemical group: Pyrroleacetic acid derivative.

Chemical name: Tolmetin sodium—1*H*-Pyrrole-2-acetic acid, 1-methyl-5-(4-methylbenzoyl)-, sodium salt, dihydrate.

Molecular formula: Tolmetin sodium—$C_{15}H_{14}NNaO_3 \cdot 2H_2O$.

Molecular weight: Tolmetin sodium—315.30.

Description: Tolmetin Sodium USP—Light yellow to light orange, crystalline powder.

pKa: Tolmetin sodium—3.5.

Solubility: Tolmetin Sodium USP—Freely soluble in water and in methanol; slightly soluble in alcohol; very slightly soluble in chloroform.

USP requirements:

Tolmetin Sodium Capsules USP—Preserve in tight containers. Contain an amount of tolmetin sodium equivalent to the labeled amount of tolmetin, within ±7%. Meet the requirements for Identification, Dissolution (85% in 30 minutes in phosphate buffer [pH 4.5] in Apparatus 2 at 50 rpm), and Uniformity of dosage units.

Tolmetin Sodium Tablets USP—Preserve in well-closed containers. Contain an amount of tolmetin sodium equivalent to the labeled amount of tolmetin, within ±10%. Meet the requirements for Identification, Dissolution (75% in 30 minutes in phosphate buffer [pH 4.5] in Apparatus 2 at 50 rpm), and Uniformity of dosage units.

TOLNAFTATE

Chemical name: Carbamothioic acid, methyl(3-methylphenyl)-, *O*-2-naphthalenyl ester.

Molecular formula: $C_{19}H_{17}NOS$.

Molecular weight: 307.41.

Description: Tolnaftate USP—White to creamy white, fine powder, having a slight odor.

Solubility: Tolnaftate USP—Practically insoluble in water; freely soluble in acetone and in chloroform; sparingly soluble in ether; slightly soluble in alcohol.

USP requirements:

Tolnaftate Cream USP—Preserve in tight containers. Contains the labeled amount, within ±10%. Meets the requirements for Identification and Minimum fill.

Tolnaftate Gel USP—Preserve in tight containers. Contains the labeled amount, within ±10%. Meets the requirements for Identification and Minimum fill.

Tolnaftate Powder USP—Preserve in tight containers. Contains the labeled amount, within ±10%. Meets the requirements for Identification and Minimum fill.

Tolnaftate Topical Aerosol Powder USP—Preserve in tight, pressurized containers, and avoid exposure to excessive heat. A suspension of powder in suitable propellants in a pressurized container. Contains the labeled amount, within ±10%. Meets the requirements for Identification and for Leak testing and Pressure testing under Aerosols.

Tolnaftate Topical Solution USP—Preserve in tight containers. Contains the labeled amount, within −10% to +15%. Meets the requirement for Identification.

Tolnaftate Topical Aerosol Solution—Not in USP.

TOLU BALSAM

Description:

Tolu Balsam USP—Brown or yellowish-brown, plastic solid, transparent in thin layers and brittle when old, dried, or exposed to cold temperatures. Has a pleasant, aromatic odor resembling that of vanilla.

NF category: Flavors and perfumes.

Tolu Balsam Syrup NF—NF category: Flavored and/or sweetened vehicle.

Tolu Balsam Tincture NF—NF category: Flavors and perfumes.

Solubility: Tolu Balsam USP—Practically insoluble in water and in solvent hexane; soluble in alcohol, in chloroform, and in ether, sometimes with a slight residue or turbidity.

USP requirements: Tolu Balsam USP—Preserve in tight containers, and avoid exposure to excessive heat. A balsam obtained from *Myroxylon balsamum* (Linné) Harms (Fam. Leguminosae). Meets the requirements for Rosin, rosin oil, and copaiba, Acid value (112–168), and Saponification value (154–220).

NF requirements:

Tolu Balsam Syrup NF—Preserve in tight containers, at a temperature not above 25 °C.

Prepare Tolu Balsam Syrup as follows: 50 mL of Tolu Balsam Tincture, 10 grams of Magnesium Carbonate, 820 grams of Sucrose and a sufficient quantity of Purified Water to make 1000 mL. Add the tincture all at once to the Magnesium Carbonate and 60 grams of the Sucrose in a mortar, and mix. Gradually add 430 mL of Purified Water with trituration, and filter. Dissolve the remainder of the Sucrose in the clear filtrate with gentle heating, strain the syrup while warm, and add sufficient Purified Water through the strainer to make the product measure 1000 mL. Mix.

Meets the requirements for Alcohol content (3.0–5.0%) and Organic volatile impurities.

Note: Tolu Balsam Syrup may be prepared also as follows: Place 760 grams of the Sucrose in a suitable percolator, the neck of which is nearly filled with loosely-packed cotton, moistened after packing with a few drops of water. Pour the filtrate, obtained as directed in the preceding instructions, upon the Sucrose, and regulate the outflow to a steady drip of percolate. When all of the liquid has run through, return portions of the percolate, if necessary, to dissolve all the Sucrose. Then pass enough Purified Water through the cotton to make the product measure 1000 mL. Mix.

Tolu Balsam Tincture NF—Preserve in tight, light-resistant containers, and avoid exposure to direct sunlight and to excessive heat.

Prepare Tolu Balsam Tincture as follows: 200 grams of Tolu Balsam to make 1000 mL. Prepare a tincture by Process M, using alcohol as the menstruum.

Meets the requirements for Alcohol content (77.0–83.0%) and Organic volatile impurities.

TRAGACANTH

Description: Tragacanth NF—Odorless.

NF category: Suspending and/or viscosity-increasing agent.

NF requirements: Tragacanth NF—Preserve in well-closed containers. The dried gummy exudation from *Astragalus gummifer* Labillardière, or other Asiatic species of *Astragalus* (Fam. Leguminosae). Meets the requirements for Botanic characteristics, Identification, Microbial limits, Arsenic (not more than 3 ppm), Lead (not more than 0.001%), Heavy metals (not more than 0.004%), and Karaya gum.

TRANEXAMIC ACID

Chemical name: Cyclohexanecarboxylic acid, 4-(aminomethyl)-, *trans*-.

Molecular formula: $C_8H_{15}NO_2$.

Molecular weight: 157.21.

Description: White, crystalline powder.

Solubility: Freely soluble in water and in glacial acetic acid; practically insoluble in alcohol and in ether.

USP requirements:
Tranexamic Acid Injection—Not in USP.
Tranexamic Acid Tablets—Not in USP.

TRANYLCYPROMINE

Chemical group: Nonhydrazine derivative structurally similar to amphetamine, with the exception of a cyclopropyl rather than an isopropyl side chain.

Chemical name: Tranylcypromine sulfate—Cyclopropanamine, 2-phenyl-, *trans*-(±)-, sulfate (2:1).

Molecular formula: Tranylcypromine sulfate—$(C_9H_{11}N)_2 \cdot H_2SO_4$.

Molecular weight: Tranylcypromine sulfate—364.46.

Description: Tranylcypromine sulfate—White or almost white crystalline powder, odorless or having a faint, cinnamaldehyde-like odor.

Solubility: Tranylcypromine sulfate—Soluble 1 in 25 of water; very slightly soluble in alcohol and in ether; practically insoluble in chloroform.

USP requirements: Tranylcypromine Sulfate Tablets—Not in USP.

TRAZODONE

Chemical group: Triazolopyridine derivative.

Chemical name: Trazodone hydrochloride—1,2,4-Triazolo[4,3-*a*]pyridin-3(2*H*)-one, 2-[3-[4-(3-chlorophenyl)-1-piperazinyl]propyl]-, monohydrochloride.

Molecular formula: Trazodone hydrochloride—$C_{19}H_{22}ClN_5O \cdot HCl$.

Molecular weight: Trazodone hydrochloride—408.33.

Description: Trazodone Hydrochloride USP—White to off-white crystalline powder. Melts between 231 and 234 °C when the melting point determination is carried out in an evacuated capillary tube; otherwise melts with decomposition over a broad range below 230 °C.

Solubility: Trazodone Hydrochloride USP—Sparingly soluble in chloroform and in water.

Other characteristics: Not chemically related to tricyclic, tetracyclic, or other known antidepressants.

USP requirements: Trazodone Tablets USP—Preserve in tight, light-resistant containers. Contain the labeled amount of trazodone hydrochloride, within ±10%. Label Tablets to state both the content of the active moiety and the content of the salt used in formulating the article. Meet the requirements for Identification, Dissolution (80% in 60 minutes in 0.01 *N* hydrochloric acid in Apparatus 2 at 50 rpm), and Uniformity of dosage units.

TRETINOIN

Chemical name: Retinoic acid.

Molecular formula: $C_{20}H_{28}O_2$.

Molecular weight: 300.44.

Description: Tretinoin USP—Yellow to light-orange, crystalline powder.

Solubility: Tretinoin USP—Insoluble in water; slightly soluble in alcohol and in chloroform.

USP requirements:
Tretinoin Cream USP—Preserve in collapsible tubes or in tight, light-resistant containers. Contains the labeled amount, within −10% to +30%. Meets the requirements for Identification and Minimum fill.
Tretinoin Gel USP—Preserve in tight containers, protected from light. Contains the labeled amount, within −10% to +30%. Meets the requirements for Identification and Minimum fill.
Tretinoin Topical Solution USP—Preserve in tight, light-resistant containers. A solution of Tretinoin in a suitable nonaqueous, hydrophilic solvent. Contains the labeled amount (w/w), within −10% to +35%. Meets the requirements for Identification and Alcohol content (50.0–60.0%).

TRIACETIN

Chemical name: 1,2,3-Propanetriol triacetate.

Molecular formula: $C_9H_{14}O_6$.

Molecular weight: 218.21.

Description: Triacetin USP—Colorless, somewhat oily liquid having a slight fatty odor.
NF category: Plasticizer.

Solubility: Triacetin USP—Soluble in water; slightly soluble in carbon disulfide. Miscible with alcohol, with ether, and with chloroform.

USP requirements: Triacetin USP—Preserve in tight containers. Contains not less than 97.0% and not more than 100.5% of triacetin, calculated on the anhydrous basis. Meets the requirements for Identification, Specific gravity (1.152–1.158), Refractive index (1.429–1.430), Acidity, and Water (not more than 0.2%).

TRIAMCINOLONE

Chemical name:
Triamcinolone—Pregna-1,4-diene-3,20-dione, 9-fluoro-11,16,17,21-tetrahydroxy-, (11 beta,16 alpha).
Triamcinolone acetonide—Pregna-1,4-diene-3,20-dione, 9-fluoro-11,21-dihydroxy-16,17-[(1-methylethylidene)bis(oxy)]-, (11 beta,16 alpha)-.
Triamcinolone diacetate—Pregna-1,4-diene-3,20-dione, 16,21-bis(acetyloxy)-9-fluoro-11,17-dihydroxy-, (11 beta,16 alpha).
Triamcinolone hexacetonide—Pregna-1,4-diene-3,20-dione, 21-(3,3-dimethyl-1-oxobutoxy)-9-fluoro-11-hydroxy-16,17-[(1-methylethylidene)bis(oxy)]-, (11 beta,16 alpha)-.

Molecular formula:
Triamcinolone—$C_{21}H_{27}FO_6$.
Triamcinolone acetonide—$C_{24}H_{31}FO_6$.
Triamcinolone diacetate—$C_{25}H_{31}FO_8$.
Triamcinolone hexacetonide—$C_{30}H_{41}FO_7$.

Molecular weight:
  Triamcinolone—394.44.
  Triamcinolone acetonide—434.50.
  Triamcinolone diacetate—478.51.
  Triamcinolone hexacetonide—532.65.

Description:
  Triamcinolone USP—White or practically white, odorless, crystalline powder.
  Triamcinolone Acetonide USP—White to cream-colored, crystalline powder, having not more than a slight odor.
  Triamcinolone Diacetate USP—Fine, white to off-white, crystalline powder, having not more than a slight odor.
  Triamcinolone Hexacetonide USP—White to cream-colored powder.

Solubility:
  Triamcinolone USP—Very slightly soluble in water, in chloroform, and in ether; slightly soluble in alcohol and in methanol.
  Triamcinolone Acetonide USP—Practically insoluble in water; sparingly soluble in dehydrated alcohol, in chloroform, and in methanol.
  Triamcinolone Diacetate USP—Practically insoluble in water; soluble in chloroform; sparingly soluble in alcohol and in methanol; slightly soluble in ether.
  Triamcinolone Hexacetonide USP—Practically insoluble in water; soluble in chloroform; slightly soluble in methanol.

USP requirements:
  Triamcinolone Tablets USP—Preserve in well-closed containers. Contain the labeled amount, within ±10%. Meet the requirements for Identification, Dissolution (75% in 45 minutes in 0.1 N hydrochloric acid in Apparatus 1 at 100 rpm), and Uniformity of dosage units.
  Triamcinolone Acetonide Inhalation Aerosol—Not in USP.
  Triamcinolone Acetonide Nasal Aerosol—Not in USP.
  Triamcinolone Acetonide Topical Aerosol USP—Preserve in pressurized containers, and avoid exposure to excessive heat. A solution of Triamcinolone Acetonide in a suitable propellant in a pressurized container. Contains the labeled amount, within −10% to +15%. Meets the requirements for Identification and Microbial limits, and for Leak testing and Pressure testing under Aerosols.
  Triamcinolone Acetonide Cream USP—Preserve in tight containers. It is Triamcinolone Acetonide in a suitable cream base. Contains the labeled amount, within −10% to +15%. Meets the requirements for Identification, Microbial limits, and Minimum fill.
  Triamcinolone Acetonide Lotion USP—Preserve in tight containers. It is Triamcinolone Acetonide in a suitable lotion base. Contains the labeled amount, within ±10%. Meets the requirements for Identification, Microbial limits, and Minimum fill.
  Triamcinolone Acetonide Ointment USP—Preserve in well-closed containers. It is Triamcinolone Acetonide in a suitable ointment base. Contains the labeled amount, within −10% to +15%. Meets the requirements for Identification, Microbial limits, and Minimum fill.
  Triamcinolone Acetonide Dental Paste USP—Preserve in tight containers. It is Triamcinolone Acetonide in a suitable emollient paste. Contains the labeled amount, within −10% to +15%. Meets the requirements for Identification, Microbial limits, and Minimum fill.
  Sterile Triamcinolone Acetonide Suspension USP—Preserve in single-dose or in multiple-dose containers, preferably of Type I glass, protected from light. A sterile suspension of Triamcinolone Acetonide in a suitable aqueous medium. Contains the labeled amount, within −10% to +15%. Meets the requirements for Identification, Bacterial endotoxins, pH (5.0–7.5), and Injections.

  Sterile Triamcinolone Diacetate Suspension USP—Preserve in single-dose or in multiple-dose containers, preferably of Type I glass. A sterile suspension of Triamcinolone Diacetate in a suitable aqueous medium. Contains the labeled amount, within −10% to +15%. Meets the requirements for Identification, Uniformity of dosage units, Bacterial endotoxins, pH (4.5–7.5), and Injections.
  Triamcinolone Diacetate Syrup USP—Preserve in tight, light-resistant containers. Contains the labeled amount, within ±10%. Contains a suitable preservative. Meets the requirement for Identification.
  Sterile Triamcinolone Hexacetonide Suspension USP—Preserve in single-dose or in multiple-dose containers, preferably of Type I glass. A sterile suspension of Triamcinolone Hexacetonide in a suitable aqueous medium. Contains the labeled amount, within −10% to +15%. Meets the requirements for Identification, Bacterial endotoxins, pH (4.0–8.0), and Injections.

TRIAMTERENE

Chemical name: 2,4,7-Pteridinetriamine, 6-phenyl-.

Molecular formula: $C_{12}H_{11}N_7$.

Molecular weight: 253.27.

Description: Triamterene USP—Yellow, odorless, crystalline powder.

pKa: 6.2.

Solubility: Triamterene USP—Practically insoluble in water, in chloroform, in ether, and in dilute alkali hydroxides; soluble in formic acid; sparingly soluble in methoxyethanol; very slightly soluble in acetic acid, in alcohol, and in dilute mineral acids.

USP requirements:
  Triamterene Capsules USP—Preserve in tight, light-resistant containers. Contain the labeled amount, within ±7%. Meet the requirements for Identification and Uniformity of dosage units.
  Triamterene Tablets—Not in USP.

TRIAMTERENE AND HYDROCHLOROTHIAZIDE

For *Triamterene* and *Hydrochlorothiazide*—See individual listings for chemistry information.

USP requirements:
  Triamterene and Hydrochlorothiazide Capsules USP—Preserve in tight, light-resistant containers. Contain the labeled amounts, within ±10%. Meet the requirements for Identification, Related compounds (not more than 1.0%), and Uniformity of dosage units.
  Note: The Capsules and Tablets dosage forms should not be considered bioequivalent. If patients are to be transferred from one dosage form to the other, retitration and appropriate changes in dosage may be necessary.
  Triamterene and Hydrochlorothiazide Tablets USP—Preserve in tight, light-resistant containers. Contain the labeled amounts, within ±10%. Meet the requirements for Identification, Dissolution (80% of each active ingredient in 30 minutes in 0.1 N hydrochloric acid in Apparatus 2 at 75 rpm), Related compounds (not more than 1.0%), and Uniformity of dosage units.
  Note: The Capsules and Tablets dosage forms should not be considered bioequivalent. If patients are to be transferred from one dosage form to the other, retitration and appropriate changes in dosage may be necessary.

TRIAZOLAM

Chemical name: 4*H*-[1,2,4]Triazolo[4,3-*a*][1,4]benzodiazepine, 8-chloro-6-(2-chlorophenyl)-1-methyl-.

Molecular formula: $C_{17}H_{12}Cl_2N_4$.

Molecular weight: 343.21.

Description: Triazolam USP—White to off-white, practically odorless, crystalline powder.

Solubility: Triazolam USP—Soluble in chloroform; slightly soluble in alcohol; practically insoluble in ether and in water.

USP requirements: Triazolam Tablets USP—Preserve in tight, light-resistant containers. Contain the labeled amount, within ± 10%. Meet the requirements for Identification, Dissolution (70% in 30 minutes in water in Apparatus 2 at 50 rpm), and Uniformity of dosage units.

TRICHLORMETHIAZIDE

Chemical name: 2*H*-1,2,4-Benzothiadiazine-7-sulfonamide, 6-chloro-3-(dichloromethyl)-3,4-dihydro-, 1,1-dioxide.

Molecular formula: $C_8H_8Cl_3N_3O_4S_2$.

Molecular weight: 380.65.

Description: Trichlormethiazide USP—White or practically white, crystalline powder. Is odorless, or has a slight characteristic odor. Melts at about 274 °C, with decomposition.

pKa: 8.6.

Solubility: Trichlormethiazide USP—Very slightly soluble in water, in ether, and in chloroform; freely soluble in acetone; soluble in methanol; sparingly soluble in alcohol.

USP requirements: Trichlormethiazide Tablets USP—Preserve in tight containers. Contain the labeled amount, within ± 10%. Meet the requirements for Identification, Dissolution (65% in 60 minutes in water in Apparatus 2 at 50 rpm), and Uniformity of dosage units.

TRICHLOROMONOFLUOROMETHANE

Chemical name: Methane, trichlorofluoro-.

Molecular formula: CCl_3F.

Molecular weight: 137.37.

Description: Trichloromonofluoromethane NF—Clear, colorless gas, having a faint, ethereal odor. Its vapor pressure at 25 °C is about 796 mm of mercury (1 psig).

NF category: Aerosol propellant.

NF requirements: Trichloromonofluoromethane NF—Preserve in tight cylinders, and avoid exposure to excessive heat. Meets the requirements for Identification, Boiling temperature (approximately 24 °C), Water (not more than 0.001%), High-boiling residues (not more than 0.01%), and Inorganic chlorides.

TRICITRATES

For *Sodium Citrate, Potassium Citrate,* and *Citric Acid*—See individual listings for chemistry information.

USP requirements: Tricitrates Oral Solution USP—Preserve in tight containers. A solution of Sodium Citrate, Potassium Citrate, and Citric Acid in a suitable aqueous medium. Contains, in each 100 mL, not less than 2.23 grams and not more than 2.46 grams of sodium, equivalent to not less than 9.5

grams and not more than 10.5 grams of sodium citrate dihydrate; not less than 3.78 grams and not more than 4.18 grams of potassium, equivalent to not less than 10.45 grams and not more than 11.55 grams of potassium citrate monohydrate; not less than 12.20 grams and not more than 13.48 grams of citrate as sodium citrate and potassium citrate; and not less than 6.34 grams and not more than 7.02 grams of citric acid monohydrate. Meets the requirements for Identification and pH (4.9–5.4).

Note: The sodium and potassium ion contents of Tricitrates Oral Solution are each approximately 1 mEq per mL.

TRIDIHEXETHYL

Source: Synthetic amine compound.

Chemical group: Quaternary ammonium compound, synthetic.

Chemical name: Tridihexethyl chloride—Benzenepropanaminium, gamma-cyclohexyl-*N,N,N*-triethyl-gamma-hydroxy-, chloride.

Molecular formula: Tridihexethyl chloride—$C_{21}H_{36}ClNO$.

Molecular weight: Tridihexethyl chloride—353.97.

Description: Tridihexethyl Chloride USP—White, odorless, crystalline powder.

Solubility: Tridihexethyl Chloride USP—Freely soluble in water, in methanol, and in chloroform; practically insoluble in ether and in acetone.

USP requirements:
Tridihexethyl Chloride Injection USP—Preserve in single-dose containers, preferably of Type I glass. A sterile solution of Tridihexethyl Chloride in Water for Injection. Contains the labeled amount, within ± 10%. Meets the requirements for Identification, Bacterial endotoxins, pH (5.0–7.5), and Injections.
Tridihexethyl Chloride Tablets USP—Preserve in tight containers. Contain the labeled amount, within ± 10%. Meet the requirements for Identification, Dissolution (75% in 45 minutes in water in Apparatus 1 at 100 rpm), and Uniformity of dosage units.

TRIENTINE

Chemical name: Trientine hydrochloride—1,2-Ethanediamine, *N,N*'-bis(2-aminoethyl)-, dihydrochloride.

Molecular formula: Trientine hydrochloride—$C_6H_{18}N_4 \cdot 2HCl$.

Molecular weight: Trientine hydrochloride—219.16.

Description: Trientine Hydrochloride USP—White to pale yellow, crystalline powder. Melts at about 117 °C.

Solubility: Trientine Hydrochloride USP—Insoluble in chloroform and in ether; slightly soluble in alcohol; soluble in methanol; freely soluble in water.

USP requirements: Trientine Hydrochloride Capsules USP—Preserve in tight containers, and store in a refrigerator. Contain the labeled amount, within ± 10%. Meet the requirements for Identification, Dissolution (80% in 30 minutes in water in Apparatus 2 at 50 rpm), and Uniformity of dosage units.

TRIETHYL CITRATE

Molecular formula: $C_{12}H_{20}O_7$.

Molecular weight: 276.29.

Description: Triethyl Citrate NF—Odorless, practically colorless, oily liquid.

NF category: Plasticizer.

Solubility: Triethyl Citrate NF—Slightly soluble in water; miscible with alcohol and with ether.

NF requirements: Triethyl Citrate NF—Preserve in tight containers. Contains not less than 99.0% and not more than 100.5% of triethyl citrate, calculated on the anhydrous basis. Meets the requirements for Specific gravity (1.135–1.139), Refractive index (1.439–1.441), Acidity, and Water (not more than 0.25%).

TRIFLUOPERAZINE

Chemical group: Phenothiazine derivative of piperazine group.

Chemical name: Trifluoperazine hydrochloride—10*H*-Phenothiazine, 10-[3-(4-methyl-1-piperazinyl)propyl]-2-(trifluoromethyl)-, dihydrochloride.

Molecular formula: Trifluoperazine hydrochloride—$C_{21}H_{24}F_3N_3S \cdot 2HCl$.

Molecular weight: Trifluoperazine hydrochloride—480.42.

Description: Trifluoperazine Hydrochloride USP—White to pale yellow, crystalline powder. Is practically odorless. Melts at about 242 °C, with decomposition.

Solubility: Trifluoperazine Hydrochloride USP—Freely soluble in water; soluble in alcohol; sparingly soluble in chloroform; insoluble in ether.

USP requirements:
Trifluoperazine Hydrochloride Injection USP—Preserve in multiple-dose containers, preferably of Type I glass, protected from light. A sterile solution of Trifluoperazine Hydrochloride in Water for Injection. Contains an amount of trifluoperazine hydrochloride equivalent to the labeled amount of trifluoperazine, within ± 10%. Meets the requirements for Identification, Bacterial endotoxins, pH (4.0–5.0), and Injections.
Trifluoperazine Hydrochloride Oral Solution—Not in USP.
Trifluoperazine Hydrochloride Syrup USP—Preserve in tight, light-resistant containers. Contains an amount of trifluoperazine hydrochloride equivalent to the labeled amount of trifluoperazine, within ± 7%. Meets the requirements for Identification and pH (2.0–3.2).
Trifluoperazine Hydrochloride Tablets USP—Preserve in well-closed, light-resistant containers. Contain an amount of trifluoperazine hydrochloride equivalent to the labeled amount of trifluoperazine, within ± 7%. Meet the requirements for Identification, Dissolution (75% in 30 minutes in 0.1 *N* hydrochloric acid in Apparatus 1 at 50 rpm), and Uniformity of dosage units.

TRIFLUPROMAZINE

Chemical group: Aliphatic.

Chemical name:
Triflupromazine—10*H*-Phenothiazine-10-propanamine, *N,N*-dimethyl-2-(trifluoromethyl)-.
Triflupromazine hydrochloride—10*H*-Phenothiazine-10-propanamine, *N,N*-dimethyl-2-(trifluoromethyl)-, monohydrochloride.

Molecular formula:
Triflupromazine—$C_{18}H_{19}F_3N_2S$.
Triflupromazine hydrochloride—$C_{18}H_{19}F_3N_2S \cdot HCl$.

Molecular weight:
Triflupromazine—352.42.
Triflupromazine hydrochloride—388.88.

Description:
Triflupromazine USP—Viscous, light amber-colored, oily liquid, which crystallizes on prolonged standing into large, irregular crystals.
Triflupromazine Hydrochloride USP—White to pale tan, crystalline powder, having a slight characteristic odor. Melts between 170 and 178 °C.

Solubility:
Triflupromazine USP—Practically insoluble in water.
Triflupromazine Hydrochloride USP—Soluble in water, in alcohol, and in acetone; insoluble in ether.

USP requirements:
Triflupromazine Oral Suspension USP—Preserve in tight, light-resistant, glass containers. Contains an amount of triflupromazine equivalent to the labeled amount of triflupromazine hydrochloride, within ± 10%. Meets the requirement for Identification.
Triflupromazine Hydrochloride Injection USP—Preserve in single-dose or in multiple-dose containers, preferably of Type I glass, protected from light. A sterile solution of Triflupromazine Hydrochloride in Water for Injection. Contains the labeled amount, within −10% to +12%. Meets the requirements for Identification, Bacterial endotoxins, pH (3.5–5.2), and Injections.
Triflupromazine Hydrochloride Tablets USP—Preserve in well-closed, light-resistant containers. Contain the labeled amount, within ± 10%. Meet the requirements for Identification, Dissolution (75% in 45 minutes in 0.1 *N* hydrochloric acid in Apparatus 1 at 100 rpm), and Uniformity of dosage units.

TRIFLURIDINE

Chemical group: Fluorinated pyrimidine nucleoside.

Chemical name: Thymidine, alpha,alpha,alpha-trifluoro-.

Molecular formula: $C_{10}H_{11}F_3N_2O_5$.

Molecular weight: 296.20.

Description: White crystals melting at about 188 °C.

Solubility: Soluble in water and in alcohol.

USP requirements: Trifluridine Ophthalmic Solution—Not in USP.

TRIHEXYPHENIDYL

Chemical group: Synthetic tertiary amine.

Chemical name: Trihexyphenidyl hydrochloride—1-Piperidinepropanol, alpha-cyclohexyl-alpha-phenyl-, hydrochloride.

Molecular formula: Trihexyphenidyl hydrochloride—$C_{20}H_{31}NO \cdot HCl$.

Molecular weight: Trihexyphenidyl hydrochloride—337.93.

Description: Trihexyphenidyl Hydrochloride USP—White or slightly off-white, crystalline powder, having not more than a very faint odor. Melts at about 250 °C.

Solubility: Trihexyphenidyl Hydrochloride USP—Slightly soluble in water; soluble in alcohol and in chloroform.

USP requirements:
Trihexyphenidyl Hydrochloride Extended-release Capsules USP—Preserve in tight containers. Contain the labeled amount, within ± 10%. Meet the requirements for Identification, Drug release (20–50% at 0.25*D* hours, 40–70% at 0.50*D* hours, and not less than 70% at 1.00*D* hours in

water in Apparatus 1 at 100 rpm), and Uniformity of dosage units.

Trihexyphenidyl Hydrochloride Elixir USP—Preserve in tight containers. Contains the labeled amount, within ±10%. Meets the requirements for Identification, pH (2.0–3.0), and Alcohol content (4.5–5.5%).

Trihexyphenidyl Hydrochloride Tablets USP—Preserve in tight containers. Contain the labeled amount, within ±10%. Meet the requirements for Identification, Dissolution (75% in 45 minutes in acetate buffer [pH 4.5] in Apparatus 1 at 100 rpm), and Uniformity of dosage units.

TRIKATES

For *Potassium Acetate, Potassium Bicarbonate,* and *Potassium Citrate*—See individual listings for chemistry information.

USP requirements: Trikates Oral Solution USP—Preserve in tight, light-resistant containers. A solution of Potassium Acetate, Potassium Bicarbonate, and Potassium Citrate in Purified Water. Contains the labeled amount of potassium, within ±10%. Meets the requirement for Identification.

TRILOSTANE

Chemical name: Androst-2-ene-2-carbonitrile, 4,5-epoxy-3,17-dihydroxy-, (4 alpha,5 alpha,17 beta)-.

Molecular formula: $C_{20}H_{27}NO_3$.

Molecular weight: 329.44.

Description: White to nearly white crystalline powder.

Solubility: Practically insoluble in water.

USP requirements: Trilostane Capsules—Not in USP.

TRIMEPRAZINE

Chemical group: Phenothiazine derivative.

Chemical name: Trimeprazine tartrate—10H-Phenothiazine-10-propanamine *N,N*,beta-trimethyl-, [R-(R*,R*)]-2,3-dihydroxybutanedioate (2:1).

Molecular formula: Trimeprazine tartrate—$(C_{18}H_{22}N_2S)_2 \cdot C_4H_6O_6$.

Molecular weight: Trimeprazine tartrate—746.98.

Description: Trimeprazine Tartrate USP—White to off-white, odorless, crystalline powder.

Solubility: Trimeprazine Tartrate USP—Freely soluble in water and in chloroform; soluble in alcohol; very slightly soluble in ether.

USP requirements:

Trimeprazine Tartrate Extended-release Capsules—Not in USP.

Trimeprazine Tartrate Syrup USP—Preserve in tight, light-resistant containers. Contains an amount of trimeprazine tartrate equivalent to the labeled amount of trimeprazine, within ±10%. Meets the requirements for Identification and Alcohol content (4.5–6.5%).

Trimeprazine Tartrate Tablets USP—Preserve in well-closed, light-resistant containers. Contain an amount of trimeprazine tartrate equivalent to the labeled amount of trimeprazine, within ±7%. Meet the requirements for Identification, Dissolution (75% in 45 minutes in 0.1 *N* hydrochloric acid in Apparatus 1 at 100 rpm), and Uniformity of dosage units.

TRIMETHADIONE

Chemical group: Oxazolidinedione.

Chemical name: 2,4-Oxazolidinedione, 3,5,5-trimethyl-.

Molecular formula: $C_6H_9NO_3$.

Molecular weight: 143.14.

Description: Trimethadione USP—White, crystalline granules. Has a slight camphor-like odor.

Solubility: Trimethadione USP—Soluble in water; freely soluble in alcohol, in ether, and in chloroform.

USP requirements:

Trimethadione Capsules USP—Preserve in tight containers, preferably at controlled room temperature. Contain the labeled amount, within ±6%. Meet the requirements for Identification, Dissolution (80% in 30 minutes in water in Apparatus 1 at 100 rpm), and Uniformity of dosage units.

Trimethadione Oral Solution USP—Preserve in tight containers, preferably at controlled room temperature. An aqueous solution of trimethadione. Contains the labeled amount, within ±6%. Meets the requirements for Identification and pH (3.0–5.0).

Trimethadione Tablets USP—Preserve in tight containers, preferably at a temperature not exceeding 25 °C. Contain the labeled amount, within ±6%. Meet the requirements for Identification, Disintegration (30 minutes), and Uniformity of dosage units.

TRIMETHAPHAN

Chemical name: Trimethaphan camsylate—Thieno[1',-2':1,2]thieno[3,4-d]imidazol-5-ium, decahydro-2-oxo-1,3-bis(phenylmethyl)-, salt with (+)-7,7-dimethyl-2-oxobicyclo[2.2.1]heptane-1-methanesulfonic acid (1:1).

Molecular formula: Trimethaphan camsylate—$C_{32}H_{40}N_2O_5S_2$.

Molecular weight: Trimethaphan camsylate—596.80.

Description: Trimethaphan Camsylate USP—White crystals or white, crystalline powder. Is odorless or has a slight odor. Its solution (1 in 10) is clear and practically colorless. Melts at about 232 °C, with decomposition.

Solubility: Trimethaphan Camsylate USP—Freely soluble in water, in alcohol, and in chloroform; insoluble in ether.

USP requirements: Trimethaphan Camsylate Injection USP—Preserve in single-dose or in multiple-dose containers, preferably of Type I glass. Store in a refrigerator, but avoid freezing. A sterile solution of Trimethaphan Camsylate in Water for Injection. Label it to indicate that it is to be appropriately diluted prior to administration. Contains the labeled amount, within ±7%. Meets the requirements for Identification, Bacterial endotoxins, pH (4.9–5.6), Particulate matter, and Injections.

TRIMETHOBENZAMIDE

Chemical group: Structurally related to the substituted ethanolamine antihistamines.

Chemical name: Trimethobenzamide hydrochloride—Benzamide, N-[[4-[2-(dimethylamino)ethoxy]phenyl]methyl]-3,4,5-trimethoxy-, monohydrochloride.

Molecular formula: Trimethobenzamide hydrochloride—$C_{21}H_{28}N_2O_5 \cdot HCl$.

Molecular weight: Trimethobenzamide hydrochloride—424.92.

Description: Trimethobenzamide Hydrochloride USP—White, crystalline powder having a slight phenolic odor.

Solubility: Trimethobenzamide Hydrochloride USP—Soluble in water and in warm alcohol; insoluble in ether.

USP requirements:
Trimethobenzamide Hydrochloride Capsules USP—Preserve in well-closed containers. Contain the labeled amount, within ±10%. Meet the requirements for Identification, Dissolution (75% in 45 minutes in water in Apparatus 1 at 100 rpm), and Uniformity of dosage units.
Trimethobenzamide Hydrochloride Injection USP—Preserve in single-dose or in multiple-dose containers, preferably of Type I glass. A sterile solution of Trimethobenzamide Hydrochloride in Water for Injection. Contains the labeled amount, within ±5%. Meets the requirements for Identification, Bacterial endotoxins, pH (4.5–5.5), and Injections.
Trimethobenzamide Hydrochloride Suppositories—Not in USP.

TRIMETHOPRIM

Chemical name: 2,4-Pyrimidinediamine, 5-[(3,4,5-trimethoxyphenyl)methyl]-.

Molecular formula: $C_{14}H_{18}N_4O_3$.

Molecular weight: 290.32.

Description: Trimethoprim USP—White to cream-colored, odorless crystals, or crystalline powder.

Solubility: Trimethoprim USP—Very slightly soluble in water; soluble in benzyl alcohol; sparingly soluble in chloroform and in methanol; slightly soluble in alcohol and in acetone; practically insoluble in ether and in carbon tetrachloride.

USP requirements: Trimethoprim Tablets USP—Preserve in tight, light-resistant containers. Contain the labeled amount, within ±10%. Meet the requirements for Identification, Dissolution (75% in 45 minutes in 0.01 N hydrochloric acid in Apparatus 2 at 50 rpm), and Uniformity of dosage units.

TRIMIPRAMINE

Chemical group: Dibenzazepine.

Chemical name: Trimipramine maleate—5H-Dibenz[b,f]-azepine-5-propanamine, 10,11-dihydro-N,N,beta-trimethyl-, (Z)-2-butenedioate (1:1).

Molecular formula: Trimipramine maleate—$C_{20}H_{26}N_2 \cdot C_4H_4O_4$.

Molecular weight: Trimipramine maleate—410.51.

Description: Trimipramine maleate—Almost odorless, white or slightly cream-colored, crystalline substance, melting at 140–144 °C.

pka: 8.0.

Solubility: Trimipramine maleate—Very slightly soluble in ether and in water; slightly soluble in ethyl alcohol and in acetone; freely soluble in chloroform and in methanol at 20 °C.

Other characteristics: Tertiary amine.

USP requirements:
Trimipramine Maleate Capsules—Not in USP.
Trimipramine Maleate Tablets—Not in USP.

TRIOXSALEN

Chemical name: 7H-Furo[3,2-g][1]benzopyran-7-one, 2,5,9-trimethyl-.

Molecular formula: $C_{14}H_{12}O_3$.

Molecular weight: 228.25.

Description: Trioxsalen USP—White to off-white or grayish, odorless, crystalline solid. Melts at about 230 °C.

Solubility: Trioxsalen USP—Practically insoluble in water; sparingly soluble in chloroform; slightly soluble in alcohol.

USP requirements: Trioxsalen Tablets USP—Preserve in well-closed, light-resistant containers. Contain the labeled amount, within ±7%. Meet the requirements for Identification, Dissolution (75% in 60 minutes in dilute simulated intestinal fluid [1 in 100 solution] in Apparatus 2 at 100 rpm), and Uniformity of dosage units.

TRIPELENNAMINE

Chemical group: Ethylenediamine derivative.

Chemical name:
Tripelennamine citrate—1,2-Ethanediamine, N,N-dimethyl-N'-(phenylmethyl)-N'-2-pyridinyl-, 2-hydroxy-1,2,3-propanetricarboxylate (1:1).
Tripelennamine hydrochloride—1,2-Ethanediamine, N,N-dimethyl-N'-(phenylmethyl)-N'-2-pyridinyl-, monohydrochloride.

Molecular formula:
Tripelennamine citrate—$C_{16}H_{21}N_3 \cdot C_6H_8O_7$.
Tripelennamine hydrochloride—$C_{16}H_{21}N_3 \cdot HCl$.

Molecular weight:
Tripelennamine citrate—447.49.
Tripelennamine hydrochloride—291.82.

Description:
Tripelennamine Citrate USP—White, crystalline powder. Its solutions are acid to litmus. Melts at about 107 °C.
Tripelennamine Hydrochloride USP—White, crystalline powder. Slowly darkens on exposure to light. Its solutions are practically neutral to litmus.

pKa: 3.9 and 9.0.

Solubility:
Tripelennamine Citrate USP—Freely soluble in water and in alcohol; very slightly soluble in ether; practically insoluble in chloroform.
Tripelennamine Hydrochloride USP—Freely soluble in water, in alcohol, and in chloroform; slightly soluble in acetone; insoluble in ether and in ethyl acetate.

USP requirements:
Tripelennamine Citrate Elixir USP—Preserve in tight, light-resistant containers. Contains, in each 100 mL, not less than 705 mg and not more than 795 mg of tripelennamine citrate. Meets the requirements for Identification and Alcohol content (11.0–13.0%).
Tripelennamine Hydrochloride Tablets USP—Preserve in well-closed containers. Contain the labeled amount, within ±5%. Meet the requirements for Identification, Dissolution (75% in 45 minutes in water in Apparatus 1 at 100 rpm), and Uniformity of dosage units.
Tripelennamine Hydrochloride Extended-release Tablets—Not in USP.

TRIPROLIDINE

Chemical group: Propylamine derivative (alkylamine).

Chemical name: Triprolidine hydrochloride—Pyridine, 2-[1-(4-methylphenyl)-3-(1-pyrrolidinyl)-1-propenyl]-, monohydrochloride, monohydrate, (E)-.

Molecular formula: Triprolidine hydrochloride—$C_{19}H_{22}N_2 \cdot HCl \cdot H_2O$.

Molecular weight: Triprolidine hydrochloride—332.87.

Description: Triprolidine Hydrochloride USP—White, crystalline powder, having no more than a slight, unpleasant odor. Its solutions are alkaline to litmus, and it melts at about 115 °C.

pKa: Triprolidine hydrochloride—3.6 and 9.3.

Solubility: Triprolidine Hydrochloride USP—Soluble in water, in alcohol, and in chloroform; insoluble in ether.

USP requirements:
Triprolidine Hydrochloride Syrup USP—Preserve in tight, light-resistant containers. Contain the labeled amount, within ± 10%. Meets the requirements for Identification, pH (5.6–6.6), and Alcohol content (3.0–5.0%).
Triprolidine Hydrochloride Tablets USP—Preserve in tight, light-resistant containers. Contain the labeled amount, within ± 10%. Meet the requirements for Identification, Dissolution (80% in 30 minutes in acetate buffer [pH 4.0 ± 0.05] in Apparatus 1 at 50 rpm), and Uniformity of dosage units.

TRIPROLIDINE AND PSEUDOEPHEDRINE

For *Triprolidine* and *Pseudoephedrine*—See individual listings for chemistry information.

USP requirements:
Triprolidine Hydrochloride and Pseudoephedrine Hydrochloride Capsules—Not in USP.
Triprolidine Hydrochloride and Pseudoephedrine Hydrochloride Extended-release Capsules—Not in USP.
Triprolidine and Pseudoephedrine Hydrochlorides Syrup USP—Preserve in tight, light-resistant containers. Contains the labeled amounts of triprolidine hydrochloride and pseudoephedrine hydrochloride, within ± 10%. Meets the requirement for Identification.
Triprolidine and Pseudoephedrine Hydrochlorides Tablets USP—Preserve in tight, light-resistant containers. Contain the labeled amounts of triprolidine hydrochloride and pseudoephedrine hydrochloride, within ± 10%. Meet the requirements for Identification, Dissolution (75% of each active ingredient in 45 minutes in water in Apparatus 2 at 50 rpm), and Uniformity of dosage units.

TRIPROLIDINE, PSEUDOEPHEDRINE, AND ACETAMINOPHEN

For *Triprolidine, Pseudoephedrine,* and *Acetaminophen*—See individual listings for chemistry information.

USP requirements: Triprolidine Hydrochloride, Pseudoephedrine Hydrochloride, and Acetaminophen Tablets—Not in USP.

TRIPROLIDINE, PSEUDOEPHEDRINE, AND CODEINE

For *Triprolidine, Pseudoephedrine,* and *Codeine*—See individual listings for chemistry information.

USP requirements:
Triprolidine Hydrochloride, Pseudoephedrine Hydrochloride, and Codeine Phosphate Syrup—Not in USP.
Triprolidine Hydrochloride, Pseudoephedrine Hydrochloride, and Codeine Phosphate Tablets—Not in USP.

TRIPROLIDINE, PSEUDOEPHEDRINE, CODEINE, AND GUAIFENESIN

For *Triprolidine, Pseudoephedrine, Codeine,* and *Guaifenesin*—See individual listings for chemistry information.

USP requirements: Triprolidine Hydrochloride, Pseudoephedrine Hydrochloride, Codeine Phosphate, and Guaifenesin Oral Solution—Not in USP.

TRIPROLIDINE, PSEUDOEPHEDRINE, AND DEXTROMETHORPHAN

For *Triprolidine, Pseudoephedrine,* and *Dextromethorphan*—See individual listings for chemistry information.

USP requirements: Triprolidine Hydrochloride, Pseudoephedrine Hydrochloride, and Dextromethorphan Oral Solution—Not in USP.

TRISULFAPYRIMIDINES

Chemical name:
Sulfadiazine—Benzenesulfonamide, 4-amino-*N*-2-pyrimidinyl-.
Sulfamerazine—Benzenesulfonamide, 4-amino-*N*-(4-methyl-2-pyrimidinyl)-.
Sulfamethazine—Benzenesulfonamide, 4-amino-*N*-(4,6-dimethyl-2-pyrimidinyl)-.

Molecular formula:
Sulfadiazine—$C_{10}H_{10}N_4O_2S$.
Sulfamerazine—$C_{11}H_{12}N_4O_2S$.
Sulfamethazine—$C_{12}H_{14}N_4O_2S$.

Molecular weight:
Sulfadiazine—250.27.
Sulfamerazine—264.30.
Sulfamethazine—278.33.

Description:
Sulfadiazine USP—White or slightly yellow powder. Odorless or nearly odorless. Stable in air, but slowly darkens on exposure to light.
Sulfamerazine USP—White or faintly yellowish white crystals or powder. Odorless or practically odorless. Stable in air, but slowly darkens on exposure to light.
Sulfamethazine USP—White to yellowish white powder, which may darken on exposure to light. Practically odorless.

Solubility:
Sulfadiazine USP—Practically insoluble in water; freely soluble in dilute mineral acids, in solutions of potassium and sodium hydroxides, and in ammonia TS; sparingly soluble in alcohol and in acetone; slightly soluble in human serum at 37 °C.
Sulfamerazine USP—Very slightly soluble in water; sparingly soluble in acetone; slightly soluble in alcohol; very slightly soluble in ether and in chloroform.
Sulfamethazine USP—Very slightly soluble in water and in ether; soluble in acetone; slightly soluble in alcohol.

USP requirements:
Trisulfapyrimidines Oral Suspension USP—Preserve in tight containers, at a temperature above freezing. Its label indicates the presence and proportion of any sodium citrate or sodium lactate and any antimicrobial agent. Contains, in each 100 mL, not less than 3.0 grams and not more than 3.7 grams of sulfadiazine, of sulfamerazine, and of sulfamethazine. May contain either Sodium Citrate or Sodium Lactate, and may contain a suitable antimicrobial agent. Meets the requirement for Identification.

Trisulfapyrimidines Tablets USP—Preserve in well-closed containers. Contain the labeled amount of each of the sulfapyrimidines, consisting of equal amounts of sulfadiazine, sulfamerazine, and sulfamethazine, within ±5%. Meet the requirements for Identification, Dissolution (70% of labeled amount of total sulfapyrimidines in 60 minutes in 0.1 *N* hydrochloric acid in Apparatus 2 at 50 rpm), and Uniformity of dosage units.

TROLAMINE

Chemical name: Ethanol, 2,2',2''-nitrilotris-.

Molecular formula: $C_6H_{15}NO_3$.

Molecular weight: 149.19.

Description: Trolamine NF—Colorless to pale yellow, viscous, hygroscopic liquid, having a slight ammoniacal odor.
NF category: Alkalizing agent; emulsifying and/or solubilizing agent.

Solubility: Trolamine NF—Miscible with water and with alcohol. Soluble in chloroform.

NF requirements: Trolamine NF—Preserve in tight, light-resistant containers. A mixture of alkanolamines consisting largely of triethanolamine containing some diethanolamine and monoethanolamine. Contains not less than 99.0% and not more than 107.4% of alkanolamines, calculated on the anhydrous basis as triethanolamine. Meets the requirements for Identification, Specific gravity (1.120–1.128), Refractive index (1.481–1.486 at 20 °C), Water (not more than 0.5%), Residue on ignition (not more than 0.05%), and Organic volatile impurities.

TROLEANDOMYCIN

Chemical name: Oleandomycin, triacetate (ester).

Molecular formula: $C_{41}H_{67}NO_{15}$.

Molecular weight: 813.98.

Description: White crystalline compound.

Solubility: Insoluble in water; readily soluble and stable in the presence of gastric juice.

USP requirements:
Troleandomycin Capsules USP—Preserve in tight containers. Contain an amount of troleandomycin equivalent to the labeled amount of oleandomycin, within −10% to +20%. Meet the requirements for Identification and Loss on drying (not more than 5.0%).
Troleandomycin Oral Suspension USP—Preserve in tight containers, in a cool place. Contains an amount of troleandomycin equivalent to the labeled amount of oleandomycin, within −10% to +25%. Contains one or more suitable buffers, colors, dispersants, and preservatives. Meets the requirements for Identification, Uniformity of dosage units (single-unit containers), Deliverable volume (multiple-unit containers), and pH (5.0–8.0).

TROMETHAMINE

Chemical name: 1,3-Propanediol, 2-amino-2-(hydroxymethyl)-.

Molecular formula: $C_4H_{11}NO_3$.

Molecular weight: 121.14.

Description: Tromethamine USP—White, crystalline powder, having a slight characteristic odor.

Solubility: Tromethamine USP—Freely soluble in water and in low molecular weight aliphatic alcohols; practically insoluble in chloroform and in carbon tetrachloride.

USP requirements: Tromethamine for Injection USP—Preserve in Containers for Sterile Solids. A sterile, lyophilized mixture of tromethamine with Potassium Chloride and Sodium Chloride. Contains the labeled amount of tromethamine, within ±7%, and the labeled amounts of potassium chloride and sodium chloride, within ±10%. Meets the requirements for Constituted solution, Identification, Bacterial endotoxins, pH (10.0–11.5, in a solution constituted as directed in the labeling), Water (not more than 1.0%), Particulate matter, Potassium chloride content, and Sodium chloride content, and for Sterility tests, Uniformity of dosage units, and Labeling under Injections.

TROPICAMIDE

Chemical name: Benzeneacetamide, *N*-ethyl-alpha-(hydroxymethyl)-*N*-(4-pyridinylmethyl)-.

Molecular formula: $C_{17}H_{20}N_2O_2$.

Molecular weight: 284.36.

Description: Tropicamide USP—White or practically white, crystalline powder, odorless or having not more than a slight odor.

Solubility: Tropicamide USP—Slightly soluble in water; freely soluble in chloroform and in solutions of strong acids.

USP requirements: Tropicamide Ophthalmic Solution USP—Preserve in tight containers, and avoid freezing. A sterile aqueous solution of Tropicamide. Contains the labeled amount, within ±5%. Contains a suitable antimicrobial agent, and may contain suitable substances to increase its viscosity. Meets the requirements for Identification, Sterility, and pH (4.0–5.8).

TRYPSIN

Source: Crystallized trypsin—Proteolytic enzyme crystallized from an extract of the pancreas gland of the ox, *Bos taurus* Linné (Fam. Bovidae).

Description:
Crystallized Trypsin USP—White to yellowish white, odorless, crystalline or amorphous powder.
Crystallized Trypsin for Inhalation Aerosol—White to yellowish white, crystalline or amorphous powder.

USP requirements: Crystallized Trypsin for Inhalation Aerosol USP—Preserve in single-dose containers, preferably of Type I glass, and avoid exposure to excessive heat. It is prepared by cryodesiccation. Contains the labeled potency, within ±10%. Meets the requirements for Identification and Solubility test.

TUAMINOHEPTANE

Chemical name: 2-Heptanamine.

Molecular formula: $C_7H_{17}N$.

Molecular weight: 115.22.

Description: Tuaminoheptane USP—Volatile, colorless to pale yellow liquid, having an amine-like odor. On exposure to air it may absorb carbon dioxide with the formation of a white precipitate of tuaminoheptane carbonate.

Solubility: Tuaminoheptane USP—Sparingly soluble in water; freely soluble in alcohol, in chloroform, and in ether.

USP requirements: Tuaminoheptane Inhalant USP—Preserve in tight containers (inhalers), and avoid exposure to excessive heat. Consists of cylindrical rolls of suitable fibrous material impregnated with Tuaminoheptane (as the carbonate), usually aromatized, and contained in a suitable inhaler. The inhaler contains the labeled amount of tuaminoheptane, within −10% to +25%. Meets the requirement for Identification.

TUBERCULIN

Description: Tuberculin USP—Old Tuberculin is a clear, brownish liquid and has a characteristic odor. Purified Protein Derivative (PPD) of Tuberculin is a very slightly opalescent, colorless solution. Old Tuberculin and PPD concentrates contain 50% of glycerin for use with various application devices. Old Tuberculin and PPD are also dried on the tines of multiple-puncture devices.

Solubility: Tuberculin USP—Old Tuberculin is readily miscible with water.

USP requirements: Tuberculin USP—Preserve at a temperature between 2 and 8 °C. Multiple-puncture devices may be stored at a temperature not exceeding 30 °C. A sterile solution derived from the concentrated, soluble products of growth of the tubercle bacillus (*Mycobacterium tuberculosis* or *Mycobacterium bovis*) prepared in a special medium. It is provided either as Old Tuberculin, a culture filtrate adjusted to the standard potency based on the U.S. Standard Tuberculin, Old, by addition of glycerin and isotonic sodium chloride solution, or as Purified Protein Derivative (PPD), a further purified protein fraction standardized with the U.S. Standard Tuberculin, Purified Protein Derivative. Has a potency, tested by comparison with the corresponding U.S. Standard Tuberculin, on intradermal injection of sensitized guinea pigs, of between 80–120% of that stated on the label. It is free from viable *Mycobacteria* as shown by injection into guinea pigs. Meets the requirement for Expiration date (for concentrated Old Tuberculin containing 50% of glycerin, not later than 5 years after date of issue from manufacturer's cold storage [5 °C, 1 year; or 0 °C, 2 years]; for diluted Old Tuberculin, not later than 1 year after date of issue from manufacturer's cold storage [5 °C, 1 year; or 0 °C, 2 years]; for concentrated PPD containing 50% of glycerin, not later than 2 years after date of issue from manufacturer's cold storage [5 °C, 1 year]; for diluted PPD, not later than 1 year after date of issue by the manufacturer; for Old Tuberculin and PPD dried on multiple-puncture devices, not later than 2 years after date of issue from manufacturer's cold storage [30 °C, 1 year], provided the recommended storage is at a temperature not exceeding 30 °C). Conforms to the regulations of the U.S. Food and Drug Administration concerning biologics.

TUBOCURARINE

Chemical name: Tubocurarine chloride—Tubocuraranium, 7′,12′-dihydroxy-6,6′-dimethoxy-2,2′,2′-trimethyl-, chloride, hydrochloride, pentahydrate.

Molecular formula: Tubocurarine chloride—$C_{37}H_{41}ClN_2O_6 \cdot HCl \cdot 5H_2O$ (pentahydrate); $C_{37}H_{41}ClN_2O_6 \cdot HCl$ (anhydrous).

Molecular weight: Tubocurarine chloride—771.73 (pentahydrate); 681.65 (anhydrous).

Description: Tubocurarine Chloride USP—White or yellowish white to grayish white, crystalline powder. Melts at about 270 °C, with decomposition.

Solubility: Tubocurarine Chloride USP—Soluble in water; sparingly soluble in alcohol.

USP requirements: Tubocurarine Chloride Injection USP—Preserve in single-dose or in multiple-dose containers. A sterile solution of Tubocurarine Chloride in Water for Injection. Contains the labeled amount, within ±7%. Meets the requirements for Identification, Angular rotation (+0.32° to +0.48° for each mg of tubocurarine chloride per mL claimed on the label), Bacterial endotoxins, pH (2.5–5.0), and Injections.

TYLOXAPOL

Chemical name: Phenol, 4-(1,1,3,3-tetramethylbutyl)-, polymer with formaldehyde and oxirane.

Description: Tyloxapol USP—Viscous, amber liquid, having a slight, aromatic odor. May exhibit a slight turbidity.

NF category: Wetting and/or solubilizing agent.

Solubility: Tyloxapol USP—Slowly but freely miscible with water. Soluble in glacial acetic acid, in toluene, in carbon tetrachloride, in chloroform, and in carbon disulfide.

USP requirements: Tyloxapol USP—Preserve in tight containers. A nonionic liquid polymer of the alkyl aryl polyether alcohol type. Meets the requirements for Identification, Cloud point (92–97 °C), pH (4.0–7.0, in a solution [1 in 20]), Residue on ignition (not more than 1.0%), Free phenol, Limit of anionic detergents (not more than 0.075%), Absence of cationic detergents, Limit of formaldehyde (not more than 0.0075%), and Limit of ethylene oxide (not more than 10 ppm).

Note: Precautions should be exercised to prevent contact of Tyloxapol with metals.

TYPHOID VACCINE

Description: Typhoid Vaccine USP—More or less turbid, milky fluid, practically odorless or having a faint odor due to the antimicrobial agent, or white solid having the characteristic appearance of freeze-dried products.

USP requirements: Typhoid Vaccine USP—Preserve at a temperature between 2 and 8 °C. A sterile suspension or solid containing killed typhoid bacilli (*Salmonella typhosa*) of the Ty 2 strain. Label it to state that it is to be well shaken before use and that it is not to be frozen. Has a labeled potency of 8 units per mL. Geometric mean potency, determined by the specific mouse potency test based on the U.S. Standard Typhoid Vaccine using the Ty 2 strain for challenge, from at least 2 assays is not less than 3.9 units per mL. Aqueous vaccine and any constituting fluid supplied with dried vaccine contains a preservative. Dried vaccine contains no preservative. Meets the requirements for Expiration date (not later than 18 months after date of issue from manufacturer's cold storage [5 °C, 1 year]) and Nitrogen content (total not more than 35.0 mcg per mL for non-extracted bacteria preparations and not more than 23.0 mcg per mL for acetone-extracted bacteria preparations). Conforms to the regulations of the U.S. Food and Drug Administration concerning biologics.

TYROPANOATE

Chemical group: Triiodinated benzoic acid derivative.

Chemical name: Tyropanoate sodium—Benzenepropanoic acid, alpha-ethyl-2,4,6-triiodo-3-[(1-oxobutyl)amino]-, monosodium salt.

Molecular formula: Tyropanoate sodium—$C_{15}H_{17}I_3NNaO_3$.

Molecular weight: Tyropanoate sodium—663.01.

Description: Tyropanoate Sodium USP—White, hygroscopic, odorless powder.

Solubility: Tyropanoate Sodium USP—Soluble in water, in alcohol, and in dimethylformamide; very slightly soluble in acetone and in ether.

USP requirements: Tyropanoate Sodium Capsules USP—Preserve in tight, light-resistant containers. Contain the labeled amount, within ±6%. Meet the requirements for Identification, Iodine and iodide, and Uniformity of dosage units.

UNDECYLENIC ACID AND ZINC UNDECYLENATE

Chemical name:
Undecylenic acid—10-Undecenoic acid.
Zinc undecylenate—10-Undecenoic acid, zinc (2+) salt.

Molecular formula:
Undecylenic acid—$C_{11}H_{20}O_2$.
Zinc undecylenate—$C_{22}H_{38}O_4Zn$.

Molecular weight:
Undecylenic acid—184.28.
Zinc undecylenate—431.92.

Description:
Undecylenic Acid USP—Clear, colorless to pale yellow liquid having a characteristic odor.
Zinc Undecylenate USP—Fine, white powder.

Solubility:
Undecylenic Acid USP—Practically insoluble in water; miscible with alcohol, with chloroform, with ether, and with fixed and volatile oils.
Zinc Undecylenate USP—Practically insoluble in water and in alcohol.

USP requirements:
Compound Undecylenic Acid Topical Aerosol Foam—Not in USP.
Compound Undecylenic Acid Topical Aerosol Powder—Not in USP.
Compound Undecylenic Acid Cream—Not in USP.
Compound Undecylenic Acid Ointment USP—Preserve in tight containers, and avoid prolonged exposure to temperatures exceeding 30 °C. Contains not less than 18.0% and not more than 22.0% of zinc undecylenate and not less than 4.5% and not more than 5.5% of free undecylenic acid, in a suitable ointment base.
Compound Undecylenic Acid Topical Powder—Not in USP.
Compound Undecylenic Acid Topical Solution—Not in USP.

URACIL MUSTARD

Chemical name: 2,4(1*H*,3*H*)-Pyrimidinedione, 5-[bis(2-chloroethyl)amino]-.

Molecular formula: $C_8H_{11}Cl_2N_3O_2$.

Molecular weight: 252.10.

Description: Uracil Mustard USP—Off-white, odorless, crystalline powder. Melts at about 200 °C, with decomposition.

Solubility: Uracil Mustard USP—Very slightly soluble in water; slightly soluble in acetone and in alcohol; practically insoluble in chloroform.

USP requirements: Uracil Mustard Capsules USP—Preserve in tight containers. Contain the labeled amount, within ±10% Meet the requirements for Identification, Disintegration (15 minutes, the use of disks being omitted), and Uniformity of dosage units.

UREA

Chemical name: Urea.

Molecular formula: CH_4N_2O.

Molecular weight: 60.06.

Description:
Urea USP—Colorless to white, prismatic crystals, or white, crystalline powder, or small white pellets. Is practically odorless, but may gradually develop a slight odor of ammonia upon long standing. Its solutions are neutral to litmus.
Sterile Urea USP—Colorless to white, prismatic crystals, or white, crystalline powder, or small white pellets. Is practically odorless, but may gradually develop a slight odor of ammonia upon long standing. Its solutions are neutral to litmus.

Solubility:
Urea USP—Freely soluble in water and in boiling alcohol; practically insoluble in chloroform and in ether.
Sterile Urea USP—Freely soluble in water and in boiling alcohol; practically insoluble in chloroform and in ether.

USP requirements: Sterile Urea USP—Preserve in Containers for Sterile Solids. It is Urea suitable for parenteral use. Meets the requirements for Completeness of solution, Constituted solution, and Bacterial endotoxins, for Identification tests, Melting range, Residue on ignition, Alcohol-insoluble matter, Chloride, Sulfate, and Heavy metals under Urea, and for Sterility tests, Uniformity of dosage units, and Labeling under Injections.

UROFOLLITROPIN

Source: A preparation of purified extract of human postmenopausal urine containing follicle-stimulating hormone (FSH).

Chemical name: Urofollitropin.

Description: Urofollitropin for injection—White to off-white powder or pellets.

USP requirements: Urofollitropin for Injection—Not in USP.

UROKINASE

Source: An enzyme obtained from human kidney cells by tissue culture techniques.

Chemical name: Kinase (enzyme-activating), uro-.

Molecular weight: 34,000 and 50,000 daltons.

Description: White powder.

Solubility: Soluble in water.

USP requirements: Urokinase for Injection—Not in USP.

URSODIOL

Source: Ursodeoxycholic acid, a naturally occurring human bile acid found in small quantities in normal human bile and in larger quantities in the biles of certain species of bears.

Chemical name: Cholan-24-oic acid, 3,7-dihydroxy-, (3 alpha,5 beta,7 beta)-.

Molecular formula: $C_{24}H_{40}O_4$.

Molecular weight: 392.58.

Description: White powder.

Solubility: Practically insoluble in water; freely soluble in ethanol, in methanol, and in glacial acetic acid; slightly soluble in ether and in chloroform.

USP requirements: Ursodiol Capsules—Not in USP.

VACCINIA IMMUNE GLOBULIN

Description: Vaccinia Immune Globulin USP—Transparent or slightly opalescent liquid. Practically colorless and practically odorless. May develop a slight granular deposit during storage.

USP requirements: Vaccinia Immune Globulin USP—Preserve at a temperature between 2 and 8 °C. A sterile, non-pyrogenic solution of globulins derived from the blood plasma of adult human donors who have been immunized with vaccinia virus (Smallpox Vaccine). It is standardized for viral neutralizing activity in eggs or tissue culture with the U.S. Reference Vaccinia Immune Globulin and a specified vaccinia virus. Label it to state that it is not intended for intravenous injection. Contains not less than 15 grams and not more than 18 grams of protein per 100 mL, not less than 90.0% of which is gamma globulin. Contains 0.3 *M* glycine as a stabilizing agent, and contains a suitable antimicrobial agent. Meets the requirement for Expiration date (not later than 3 years after date of issue). Conforms to the regulations of the U.S. Food and Drug Administration concerning biologics.

VALPROIC ACID

Chemical name: Pentanoic acid, 2-propyl-.

Molecular formula: $C_8H_{16}O_2$.

Molecular weight: 144.21.

Description: Valproic Acid USP—Colorless to pale yellow, slightly viscous, clear liquid, having a characteristic odor. Refractive index: about 1.423 at 20 °C.

pKa: 4.8.

Solubility: Valproic Acid USP—Slightly soluble in water; freely soluble in 1 *N* sodium hydroxide, in methanol, in alcohol, in acetone, in chloroform, in ether, and in *n*-heptane; slightly soluble in 0.1 *N* hydrochloric acid.

USP requirements:
Valproic Acid Capsules USP—Preserve in tight containers, at controlled room temperature. Contain the labeled amount, within ±10%. Meet the requirements for Identification, Disintegration (15 minutes, determined as directed for Soft Gelatin Capsules), and Uniformity of dosage units.
Valproic Acid Syrup USP—Preserve in tight containers. Contains the labeled amount, within ±10%. It is prepared with the aid of Sodium Hydroxide. Meets the requirements for Identification and pH (7.0–8.0).

VANCOMYCIN

Source: Derived from *Amycolatopsis orientalis* (formerly *Nocardia orientalis*).

Chemical group: High-molecular-weight tricyclic amphoteric glycopolypeptide; not chemically related to currently available antibacterials.

Chemical name: Vancomycin hydrochoride—Vancomycin, monohydrochloride.

Molecular formula: Vancomycin hydrochloride—$C_{66}H_{75}Cl_2$-$N_9O_{24} \cdot HCl$.

Molecular weight: Vancomycin hydrochloride—1485.73.

Description:
Vancomycin Hydrochloride USP—Tan to brown, free-flowing powder, odorless.
Sterile Vancomycin Hydrochloride USP—Tan to brown, free-flowing powder, odorless.

Solubility:
Vancomycin Hydrochloride USP—Freely soluble in water; insoluble in ether and in chloroform.
Sterile Vancomycin Hydrochloride USP—Freely soluble in water; insoluble in ether and in chloroform.

USP requirements:
Vancomycin Hydrochloride Capsules USP—Preserve in tight containers. Contain a dispersion of Vancomycin Hydrochloride in Polyethylene Glycol. Contain an amount of vancomycin hydrochloride equivalent to the labeled amount of vancomycin, within −10% to +15%. Meet the requirements for Identification, Dissolution (85% in 45 minutes in water in Apparatus 1 at 100 rpm), Water (not more than 8.0%), and Uniformity of dosage units.
Vancomycin Hydrochloride for Injection USP—Preserve in Containers for Sterile Solids. A sterile dry mixture of Vancomycin Hydrochloride and a suitable stabilizing agent. It has a potency equivalent to not less than 925 mcg of vancomycin per mg, calculated on the anhydrous basis. In addition, contains an amount of vancomycin hydrochloride equivalent to the labeled amount of vancomycin, within −10% to +15%. Meets the requirements for Constituted solution, Pyrogen, Sterility, Particulate matter, Heavy metals (not more than 0.003%), and Chromatographic purity, for Identification test, pH (2.5–4.5, in a solution containing 50 mg per mL), and Water (not more than 5.0%) under Vancomycin Hydrochloride, and for Uniformity of dosage units and Labeling under Injections.
Vancomycin Hydrochloride for Oral Solution USP—Preserve in tight containers. Contains an amount of vancomycin hydrochloride equivalent to the labeled amount of vancomycin, within −10% to +15%. Meets the requirements for pH (2.5–4.5, for the solution constituted as directed in the labeling) and Water (not more than 5.0%).
Sterile Vancomycin Hydrochloride USP—Preserve in Containers for Sterile Solids. Has a potency equivalent to not less than 900 mcg per mg, calculated on the anhydrous basis and, where packaged for dispensing, contains an amount of vancomycin hydrochloride equivalent to the labeled amount of vancomycin, within −10% to +15%. Meets the requirements for Constituted solution, Bacterial endotoxins, Sterility, Particulate matter, and Heavy metals (not more than 0.003%), for Identification test, pH (2.5–4.5, in a solution containing 50 mg per mL), Water (not more than 5.0%), and Chromatographic purity under Vancomycin Hydrochloride, for Uniformity of dosage units, and for Labeling under Injections.

VANILLA

Description:
Vanilla NF—It has a characteristic, agreeably fragrant odor. NF category: Flavors and perfumes.
Vanilla Tincture NF—NF category: Flavors and perfumes.

NF requirements:
Vanilla NF—Preserve in tight containers, and store in a cold place. The cured, full-grown, unripe fruit of *Vanilla planifolia* Andrews, often known in commerce as Mexican or Bourbon Vanilla, or of *Vanilla tahitensis* J.W. Moore, known in commerce as Tahiti Vanilla (Fam. Orchidaceae). Yields not less than 12.0% of anhydrous diluted

alcohol-soluble extractive. The commercial variety of Vanilla, whether Mexican, Bourbon, or Tahiti, is stated on the label. Note: Do not use Vanilla that has become brittle. Meets the requirements for Botanic characteristics and Test for vanillin.

Vanilla Tincture NF—Preserve in tight, light-resistant containers, and avoid exposure to direct sunlight and to excessive heat.

Prepare Vanilla Tincture as follows: 100 grams of Vanilla cut into small pieces, 200 grams of Sucrose in coarse granules, Alcohol, Diluted Alcohol, and a sufficient quantity of Purified Water to make 1000 mL. Add 200 mL of water to the comminuted Vanilla in a suitable covered container, and macerate for 12 hours, preferably in a warm place. Add 207 mL of Alcohol to the mixture, mix, and macerate for about 3 days. Transfer the mixture to a percolator containing the Sucrose, and drain. Then pack the drug firmly, and percolate slowly, using Diluted Alcohol as the menstruum.

Meets the requirements for Alcohol content (38.0–42.0%) and Organic volatile impurities.

VANILLIN

Chemical name: Benzaldehyde, 4-hydroxy-3-methoxy-.

Molecular formula: $C_8H_8O_3$.

Molecular weight: 152.15.

Description: Vanillin NF—Fine, white to slighty yellow crystals, usually needle-like, having an odor suggestive of vanilla. It is affected by light. Its solutions are acid to litmus.

NF category: Flavors and perfumes.

Solubility: Vanillin NF—Slightly soluble in water; freely soluble in alcohol, in chloroform, in ether, and in solutions of the fixed alkali hydroxides; soluble in glycerin and in hot water.

NF requirements: Vanillin NF—Preserve in tight, light-resistant containers. Contains not less than 97.0% and not more than 103.0% of vanillin, calculated on the dried basis. Meets the requirements for Identification, Melting range (81–83 °C), Loss on drying (not more than 1.0%), and Residue on ignition (not more than 0.05%).

VARICELLA-ZOSTER IMMUNE GLOBULIN

USP requirements: Varicella-Zoster Immune Globulin USP—Preserve at a temperature between 2 and 8 °C. A sterile 15 to 18% solution of pH 7.0 containing the globulin fraction of human plasma consisting of not less than 99% of immunoglobulin G with traces of immunoglobulin A and immunoglobulin M, in 0.3 M glycine as a stabilizer and 1:10,000 thimerosal as a preservative. Derived from adult human plasma selected for high titers of varicella-zoster antibodies. Each unit of blood or plasma has been found non-reactive for hepatitis B surface antigen by a suitable method. The proteins of the plasma pools are fractionated by the cold ethanol precipitation method. The content of specific antibody is not less than 125 units, deliverable from a vial containing not more than 2.5 mL solution. The unit is defined as equivalent to 0.01 mL of a Varicella-Zoster Immune Globulin lot found effective in clinical trials and used as a reference for potency determinations, based on a fluorescent-antibody membrane antigen (FAMA) method for antibody titration. Label it to state that it is to be administered by intramuscular injection, in the recommended dose based on body weight. Meets the requirement for Expiration date (not later than 2 years after date of issue from manufacturer's

cold storage). Conforms to the regulations of the U.S. Food and Drug Administration concerning biologics.

VASOPRESSIN

Chemical name: Vasopressin, 8-L-arginine- (arginine form); Vasopressin, 8-L-lysine- (lysine form).

Molecular formula: $C_{46}H_{65}N_{15}O_{12}S_2$ (arginine form); $C_{46}H_{65}N_{13}O_{12}S_2$ (lysine form).

Molecular weight: 1084.23 (arginine form); 1056.22 (lysine form).

Description: Vasopressin Injection USP—Clear, colorless or practically colorless liquid, having a faint, characteristic odor.

USP requirements:

Vasopressin Injection USP—Preserve in single-dose or in multiple-dose containers, preferably of Type I glass. Do not freeze. A sterile solution, in a suitable diluent, of material containing the polypeptide hormone having the properties of causing the contraction of vascular and other smooth muscle, and of antidiuresis, which is prepared by synthesis or obtained from the posterior lobe of the pituitary of healthy, domestic animals used for food by man. Each mL of Vasopressin Injection possesses a pressor activity stated in the label in USP Posterior Pituitary Units, within −15% to +20%. Meets the requirements for Oxytocic activity, pH (2.5–4.5), and Injections.

Sterile Vasopressin Tannate Oil Suspension—Not in USP.

VECURONIUM

Chemical name: Vecuronium bromide—Piperidinium, 1-[(2 beta,3 alpha,5 alpha,16 beta,17 beta)-3,17-bis(acetyloxy)-2-(1-piperidinyl)androstan-16-yl]-1-methyl-, bromide.

Molecular formula: Vecuronium bromide—$C_{34}H_{57}BrN_2O_4$.

Molecular weight: Vecuronium bromide—637.74.

Description: Vecuronium bromide—White to off-white or slightly pink crystals or crystalline powder.

Solubility: Vecuronium bromide—Solubilities of 9 and 23 mg/mL in water and in alcohol, respectively.

USP requirements: Vecuronium Bromide for Injection—Not in USP.

HYDROGENATED VEGETABLE OIL

Description: Hydrogenated Vegetable Oil NF—Fine, white powder at room temperature, and a pale yellow, oily liquid above its melting temperature.

NF category:
Type I—Tablet and/or capsule lubricant.
Type II—Ointment base.

Solubility: Hydrogenated Vegetable Oil NF—Insoluble in water; soluble in hot isopropyl alcohol, in hexane, and in chloroform.

NF requirements: Hydrogenated Vegetable Oil NF—Preserve in tight containers, in a cool place. A mixture of triglycerides of fatty acids. The melting range, heavy metals limit, iodine value, and saponification value differ, depending on Type, as set forth in the accompanying table.

	Type I	Type II
Melting range	57–70 °C	20–50 °C
Heavy metals	10 ppm	0.001%
Iodine value	0–5	55–80
Saponification value	175–205	185–200

Label it to state whether it is Type I or Type II. Meets the requirements for Loss on drying (not more than 0.1%), Acid value (not more than 4), and Unsaponifiable matter (not more than 0.8%).

VERAPAMIL

Chemical name: Verapamil hydrochloride—Benzeneacetonitrile, alpha-[3-[[2-(3,4-dimethoxyphenyl)ethyl]methylamino]-propyl]-3,4-dimethoxy-alpha-(1-methylethyl)-, monohydrochloride.

Molecular formula: Verapamil hydrochloride—$C_{27}H_{38}N_2O_4 \cdot$ HCl.

Molecular weight: Verapamil hydrochloride—491.07.

Description: Verapamil Hydrochloride USP—White or practically white, crystalline powder. It is practically odorless.

Solubility: Verapamil Hydrochloride USP—Soluble in water; freely soluble in chloroform; sparingly soluble in alcohol; practically insoluble in ether.

USP requirements:
Verapamil Injection USP—Preserve in single-dose containers, preferably of Type I glass, protected from light. A sterile solution of Verapamil Hydrochloride in Water for Injection. Label Injection to state both the content of the active moiety and the content of the salt used in formulating the article. Contains the labeled amount of verapamil hydrochloride, within ±10%. Meets the requirements for Identification, Bacterial endotoxins, pH (4.0–6.5), Particulate matter, Limit for related compounds, and Injections.
Verapamil Tablets USP—Preserve in tight, light-resistant containers. Label Tablets to state both the content of the active moiety and the content of the salt used in formulating the article. Contain the labeled amount of verapamil hydrochloride, within ±10%. Meet the requirements for Identification, Dissolution (75% in 30 minutes in 0.1 N hydrochloric acid in Apparatus 2 at 50 rpm), Limit for related compounds, and Uniformity of dosage units.
Verapamil Hydrochloride Extended-release Capsules—Not in USP.
Verapamil Hydrochloride Extended-release Tablets—Not in USP.

VIDARABINE

Source: Fermentation cultures of *Streptomyces antibioticus*.

Chemical group: Purine nucleoside.

Chemical name: 9*H*-Purin-6-amine, 9-beta-D-arabinofuranosyl-, monohydrate.

Molecular formula: $C_{10}H_{13}N_5O_4 \cdot H_2O$.

Molecular weight: 285.26.

Description: Sterile Vidarabine USP—White to off-white powder.

Solubility: Sterile Vidarabine USP—Very slightly soluble in water; slightly soluble in dimethylformamide.

USP requirements:
Vidarabine Concentrate for Injection USP—Preserve in single-dose or in multiple-dose containers, preferably of Type I glass. Label it to indicate that it is to be solubilized in a suitable parenteral vehicle prior to intravenous infusion. Contains an amount of vidarabine equivalent to the labeled amount of anhydrous vidarabine, within −10% to

+20%, in a sterile, aqueous suspension intended for solubilization with a suitable parenteral vehicle prior to intravenous infusion. Contains suitable buffers and preservatives. Meets the requirements for Depressor substances, Bacterial endotoxins, Sterility, and pH (5.0–6.2, in the undiluted suspension).
Sterile Vidarabine USP—Preserve in tight containers. It has a potency equivalent to not less than 845 mcg and not more than 985 mcg of vidarabine per mg. Meets the requirements for Identification, Specific rotation, Bacterial endotoxins, Sterility, and Loss on drying (5.0–7.0%).
Vidarabine Ophthalmic Ointment USP—Preserve in collapsible ophthalmic ointment tubes. Contains an amount of vidarabine equivalent to the labeled amount of anhydrous vidarabine, within −10% to +20%. Meets the requirements for Sterility, Minimum fill, and Metal particles.

VINBLASTINE

Source: Salt of an alkaloid extracted from *Vinca rosea* Linn, a common flowering herb known as the periwinkle.

Chemical name: Vinblastine sulfate—Vincaleukoblastine, sulfate (1:1) (salt).

Molecular formula: Vinblastine sulfate—$C_{46}H_{58}N_4O_9 \cdot H_2SO_4$.

Molecular weight: Vinblastine sulfate—909.06.

Description:
Vinblastine Sulfate USP—White or slightly yellow, odorless, amorphous or crystalline powder. Is hygroscopic.
Sterile Vinblastine Sulfate USP—Yellowish white solid, having the characteristic appearance of products prepared by freeze-drying.

pKa: 5.4 and 7.4 in water.

Solubility: Vinblastine Sulfate USP—Freely soluble in water.

USP requirements:
Vinblastine Sulfate Injection—Not in USP.
Sterile Vinblastine Sulfate USP—Preserve in Containers for Sterile Solids, in a refrigerator. It is Vinblastine Sulfate suitable for parenteral use. Contains the labeled amount, within ±10%. Meets the requirements for Completeness of solution, Constituted solution, Bacterial endotoxins, Uniformity of dosage units, and Related substances, for Identification test under Vinblastine Sulfate, and for Sterility tests and Labeling under Injections.
Caution: Handle Sterile Vinblastine Sulfate with great care, since it is a potent cytotoxic agent.

VINCRISTINE

Source: Salt of an alkaloid extracted from *Vinca rosea* Linn, a common flowering herb known as the periwinkle.

Chemical name: Vincristine sulfate—Vincaleukoblastine, 22-oxo-, sulfate (1:1) (salt).

Molecular formula: Vincristine sulfate—$C_{46}H_{56}N_4O_{10} \cdot H_2SO_4$.

Molecular weight: Vincristine sulfate—923.04.

Description:
Vincristine Sulfate USP—White to slightly yellow, odorless, amorphous or crystalline powder. Is hygroscopic.
Vincristine Sulfate for Injection USP—Yellowish white solid, having the characteristic appearance of products prepared by freeze-drying.

pKa: 5.1 and 7.5 in water.

Solubility: Vincristine Sulfate USP—Freely soluble in water; soluble in methanol; slightly soluble in alcohol.

USP requirements:

Vincristine Sulfate Injection USP—Preserve in light-resistant, glass containers, in a refrigerator. A sterile solution of Vincristine Sulfate in Water for Injection. The label states: "FATAL IF GIVEN INTRATHECALLY. FOR INTRAVENOUS USE ONLY." Where labeled as containing more than 2 mg, it must also be labeled as a Pharmacy bulk package. The labeling directs that the drug be dispensed only in containers enclosed in an overwrap labeled as directed below. When packaged in a Pharmacy bulk package, it is exempt from the requirement under Injections, that the closure be penetrated only one time after constitution with a suitable sterile transfer device or dispensing set, when it contains a suitable substance or mixture of substances to prevent the growth of microorganisms. When dispensed, the container or syringe (holding the individual dose prepared for administration to the patient) must be enclosed in an overwrap bearing the statement "DO NOT REMOVE COVERING UNTIL MOMENT OF INJECTION. FATAL IF GIVEN INTRATHECALLY. FOR INTRAVENOUS USE ONLY." Contains the labeled amount, within ±10%. Meets the requirements for Identification, pH (3.5–5.5), and Related substances, for Sterility Tests, and for Labeling under Injections.

Caution: Handle Vincristine Sulfate Injection with great care, since it is a potent cytotoxic agent.

Vincristine Sulfate for Injection USP—Preserve in Containers for Sterile Solids, in a refrigerator. A sterile mixture of Vincristine Sulfate with suitable diluents. The label states: "FATAL IF GIVEN INTRATHECALLY. FOR INTRAVENOUS USE ONLY." Where labeled as containing more than 2 mg, it must also be labeled as a Pharmacy bulk package. The labeling directs that the drug be dispensed only in containers enclosed in an overwrap labeled as directed below. When packaged in a Pharmacy bulk package, it is exempt from the requirement under Injections, that the closure be penetrated only one time after constitution with a suitable sterile transfer device or dispensing set, when it contains a suitable substance or mixture of substances to prevent the growth of microorganisms. When dispensed, the container or syringe (holding the individual dose prepared for administration to the patient) must be enclosed in an overwrap bearing the statement "DO NOT REMOVE COVERING UNTIL MOMENT OF INJECTION. FATAL IF GIVEN INTRATHECALLY. FOR INTRAVENOUS USE ONLY." Contains the labeled amount, within ±10%. Meets the requirements for Constituted solution, Identification, Bacterial endotoxins, Related substances, and Uniformity of dosage units, for Sterility tests, and for Labeling under Injections.

Caution: Handle Vincristine Sulfate for Injection with great care since it is a potent cytotoxic agent.

VITAMIN A

Chemical name: Retinol—3,7-Dimethyl-9-(2,6,6-trimethyl-1-cyclohexen-1-yl)-2,4,6,8-nonate-traen-1-ol.

Molecular formula: Retinol—$C_{20}H_{30}O$.

Molecular weight: Retinol—286.46.

Description: Vitamin A USP—In liquid form, a light-yellow to red oil that may solidify upon refrigeration. In solid form, has the appearance of any diluent that has been added. May be practically odorless or may have a mild fishy odor, but has no rancid odor. Is unstable to air and light.

Solubility: Vitamin A USP—In liquid form, insoluble in water and in glycerin; very soluble in chloroform and in ether; soluble in absolute alcohol and in vegetable oils. In solid form, may be dispersible in water.

USP requirements:

Vitamin A Capsules USP—Preserve in tight, light-resistant containers. Label Capsules to indicate the form in which the vitamin is present, and to indicate the vitamin A activity in terms of the equivalent amount of retinol in mg. The vitamin A activity may be stated also in USP Units per Capsule, on the basis that 1 USP Vitamin A Unit equals the biological activity of 0.3 mcg of the all-*trans* isomer of retinol. Contain the labeled amount, within −5% to +20%. Meet the requirements for Uniformity of dosage units, for Identification tests for vitamin A, and for the Absorbance ratio test under Vitamin A.

Vitamin A Injection—Not in USP.

Vitamin A Oral Solution—Not in USP.

Vitamin A Tablets—Not in USP.

VITAMIN E

Molecular formula:

d or *dl*-Alpha tocopherol—$C_{29}H_{50}O_2$.

d or *dl*-Alpha tocopheryl acetate—$C_{31}H_{52}O_3$.

d or *dl*-Alpha tocopheryl acid succinate—$C_{33}H_{54}O_5$.

Description:

Vitamin E USP—Practically odorless. The alpha tocopherols and alpha tocopheryl acetates occur as clear, yellow, or greenish-yellow, viscous oils. *d*-Alpha tocopheryl acetate may solidify in the cold. Alpha tocopheryl acid succinate occurs as a white powder; the *d*-isomer melts at about 75 °C, and the *dl*-form melts at about 70 °C. The alpha tocopherols are unstable to air and to light, particularly when in alkaline media. The esters are stable to air and to light, but are unstable to alkali; the acid succinate is also unstable when held molten.

Vitamin E Preparation USP—The liquid forms are clear, yellow to brownish-red, viscous oils. The solid forms are white to tan-white granular powders.

Solubility:

Vitamin E USP—Alpha tocopheryl acid succinate is insoluble in water; slightly soluble in alkaline solutions; soluble in alcohol, in ether, in acetone, and in vegetable oils; very soluble in chloroform. The other forms of Vitamin E are insoluble in water; soluble in alcohol; miscible with ether, with acetone, with vegetable oils, and with chloroform.

Vitamin E Preparation USP—The liquid forms are insoluble in water; soluble in alcohol; and miscible with ether, with acetone, with vegetable oils, and with chloroform. The solid forms disperse in water to give cloudy suspensions.

USP requirements:

Vitamin E Capsules USP—Preserve in tight containers, protected from light. Contain Vitamin E or Vitamin E Preparation. Vitamin E Capsules meet the requirements for Labeling under Vitamin E Preparation. Contain the labeled amount, within −5% to +20%. Meet the requirements for Identification and Uniformity of dosage units.

Vitamin E Preparation USP—Preserve in tight containers, protected from light. Protect Preparation containing *d*- or *dl*-alpha tocopherol with a blanket of an inert gas. A combination of a single form of Vitamin E with one or more inert substances. May be in a liquid or solid form. Label it to indicate the chemical form of Vitamin E present, and to indicate whether the *d*- or the *dl*-form is present, excluding any different forms that may be introduced as a minor constituent of the vehicle. Designate the quantity of Vitamin E present. Contains the labeled amount of Vitamin E, within −5% to +20%. Vitamin E Preparation labeled to contain a *dl*-form of Vitamin E may contain also a small amount of a *d*-form occurring as a minor constituent of an added substance. Meets the requirements for Identification and Acidity.

Vitamin E Oral Solution—Not in USP.

Vitamin E Tablets—Not in USP.

Vitamin E Chewable Tablets—Not in USP.

VITAMINS A, D, AND C AND FLUORIDE

For *Vitamins A, D* (Calcifediol, Calcitriol, Ergocalciferol), and *C* (Ascorbic Acid) and *Sodium Fluoride*—See individual listings for chemistry information.

USP requirements:

Vitamins A, D, and C and Sodium or Potassium Fluoride Oral Solution—Not in USP.

Vitamins A, D, and C and Sodium or Potassium Fluoride Chewable Tablets—Not in USP.

MULTIPLE VITAMINS AND FLUORIDE

For *Multiple Vitamins* (Ascorbic Acid, Cyanocobalamin, Folic Acid, Niacin, Pyridoxine, Riboflavin, Thiamine, Vitamin A, Vitamin D [Calcifediol, Calcitriol, and Ergocalciferol], and Vitamin E) and *Sodium Fluoride*—See individual listings for chemistry information.

USP requirements:

Multiple Vitamins and Sodium or Potassium Fluoride Oral Solution—Not in USP.

Multiple Vitamins and Sodium or Potassium Fluoride Chewable Tablets—Not in USP.

WARFARIN

Chemical group: Coumarin derivative.

Chemical name: Warfarin sodium—2*H*-1-Benzopyran-2-one, 4-hydroxy-3-(3-oxo-1-phenylbutyl)-, sodium salt.

Molecular formula: Warfarin sodium—$C_{19}H_{15}NaO_4$.

Molecular weight: Warfarin sodium—330.31.

Description: Warfarin Sodium USP—White, odorless, amorphous or crystalline powder. Is discolored by light.

Solubility: Warfarin Sodium USP—Very soluble in water; freely soluble in alcohol; very slightly soluble in chloroform and in ether.

USP requirements:

Warfarin Sodium for Injection USP—Preserve in light-resistant Containers for Sterile Solids. A sterile, freeze-dried mixture of Warfarin Sodium and Sodium Chloride. Contains the labeled amount, within ±5%. Meets the requirements for Completeness of solution, Constituted solution, Bacterial endotoxins, and Water (not more than 4.5%), for Identification tests A and B, pH (7.2–8.3, in a solution [1 in 100]), and Heavy metals (not more than 0.001%) under Warfarin Sodium, and for Sterility tests, Uniformity of dosage units, and Labeling under Injections.

Warfarin Sodium Tablets USP—Preserve in tight, light-resistant containers. Contain the labeled amount, within ±5%. Meet the requirements for Identification, Dissolution (80% in 30 minutes in water in Apparatus 2 at 50 rpm), and Uniformity of dosage units.

WATER

Chemical name: Purified water—Water.

Molecular formula: Purified water—H_2O.

Molecular weight: Purified water—18.02.

Description:

Sterile Water for Inhalation USP—Clear, colorless solution.

Water for Injection USP—Clear, colorless, odorless liquid.

NF category: Solvent.

Bacteriostatic Water for Injection USP—Clear, colorless liquid, odorless, or having the odor of the antimicrobial substance.

NF category: Vehicle (sterile).

Sterile Water for Injection USP—Clear, colorless, odorless liquid.

NF category: Solvent.

Sterile Water for Irrigation USP—Clear, colorless, odorless liquid.

NF category: Solvent.

Purified Water USP—Clear, colorless, odorless liquid.

NF category: Solvent.

USP requirements:

Sterile Water for Inhalation USP—Preserve in single-dose containers. It is water purified by distillation or by reverse osmosis and rendered sterile. Label it to indicate that it is for inhalation therapy only and that it is not for parenteral administration. Contains no antimicrobial agents, except where used in humidifiers or other similar devices and where liable to contamination over a period of time, or other added substances. Meets the requirements for Bacterial endotoxins, Sterility, pH (4.5–7.5), and Chloride (not more than 0.5 ppm), for Sulfate, Calcium, Carbon dioxide, and Heavy metals under Purified Water, and for Ammonia, Oxidizable substances, and Total solids under Sterile Water for Injection.

Note: Do not use Sterile Water for Inhalation for parenteral administration or for other sterile compendial dosage forms.

Water for Injection USP—Where packaged, preserve in tight containers. Where packaged, it may be stored at a temperature below or above the range in which microbial growth occurs. It is water purified by distillation or by reverse osmosis. Contains no added substance. Meets the requirements for Bacterial endotoxins, and of tests under Purified Water, with the exception of the test for Bacteriological purity.

Note: Water for Injection is intended for use as a solvent for the preparation of parenteral solutions. Where used for the preparation of parenteral solutions subject to final sterilization, use suitable means to minimize microbial growth, or first render the Water for Injection sterile and thereafter protect it from microbial contamination. For parenteral solutions that are prepared under aseptic conditions and are not sterilized by appropriate filtration or in the final container, first render the Water for Injection sterile and, thereafter, protect it from microbial contamination.

Bacteriostatic Water for Injection USP—Preserve in single-dose or in multiple-dose containers, preferably of Type I or Type II glass, of not larger than 30-mL size. It is Sterile Water for Injection containing one or more suitable antimicrobial agents. Label it to indicate the name(s) and proportion(s) of the added antimicrobial agent(s). Label it also to include the statement, "NOT FOR USE IN NEWBORNS," in boldface capital letters, on the label immediately under the official name, printed in a contrasting color, preferably red. Alternatively, the statement may be placed prominently elsewhere on the label if the statement is enclosed within a box. Meets the requirements for Antimicrobial agent(s), Bacterial endotoxins, Sterility, pH (4.5–7.0), and Particulate matter, and for Sulfate, Calcium, Carbon dioxide, and Heavy metals under Sterile Water for Injection.

Note: Use Bacteriostatic Water for Injection with due regard for the compatibility of the antimicrobial agent or agents it contains with the particular medicinal substance that is to be dissolved or diluted.

Sterile Water for Injection USP—Preserve in single-dose glass or plastic containers, of not larger than 1-liter size. Glass containers are preferably of Type I or Type II glass, of not larger than 1-liter size. It is Water for Injection sterilized and suitably packaged. Contains no antimicrobial agent or other added substance. Label it to indicate that no antimicrobial or other substance has been added, and that it is not suitable for intravascular injection without its first having been made approximately isotonic by the addition of a suitable solute. Meets the requirements for Bacterial endotoxins, Sterility, Particulate matter, Ammonia, Chloride, Oxidizable substances, and Total solids, and for pH, Sulfate, Calcium, Carbon dioxide, and Heavy metals under Purified water.

Sterile Water for Irrigation USP—Preserve in single-dose glass or plastic containers. Glass containers are preferably of Type I or Type II glass. The container may contain a volume of more than 1 liter, and may be designed to empty rapidly. It is Water for Injection sterilized and suitably packaged. Contains no antimicrobial agent or other added substance. Label it to indicate that no antimicrobial or other substance has been added. The designations "For irrigation only" and "Not for injection" appear prominently on the label. Meets the requirements of all of the tests under Sterile Water for Injection except the test for Particulate matter.

Purified Water USP—Where packaged, preserve in tight containers. It is water obtained by distillation, ion-exchange treatment, reverse osmosis, or other suitable process. It is prepared from water complying with the regulations of the U.S. Environmental Protection Agency with respect to drinking water. Contains no added substance. Where packaged, label it to indicate the method of preparation. Meets the requirements for pH (5.0–7.0), Chloride, Sulfate, Ammonia (not more than 0.3 ppm), Calcium, Carbon dioxide, Heavy metals, Oxidizable substances, Total solids (not more than 0.001%), and Bacteriological purity.

Note: Purified Water is intended for use as an ingredient in the preparation of compendial dosage forms. Where used for sterile dosage forms, other than for parenteral administration, process the article to meet the requirements under Sterility tests, or first render the Purified Water sterile and thereafter protect it from microbial contamination. Do not use Purified Water in preparations intended for parenteral administration. For such purposes use Water for Injection, Bacteriostatic Water for Injection, or Sterile Water for Injection.

CARNAUBA WAX

Description: Carnauba Wax NF—Light brown to pale yellow, moderately coarse powder or flakes, possessing a characteristic bland odor, and free from rancidity. Specific gravity is about 0.99.

NF category: Coating agent.

Solubility: Carnauba Wax NF—Insoluble in water; soluble in warm chloroform and in toluene; slightly soluble in boiling alcohol.

NF requirements: Carnauba Wax NF—Preserve in well-closed containers. It is obtained from the leaves of *Copernicia cerifera* Mart. (Fam. Palmae). Meets the requirements for Melting range (81–86 °C), Residue on ignition (not more than 0.25%), Heavy metals (not more than 0.004%), Acid value (2–7), and Saponification value (78–95).

EMULSIFYING WAX

Description: Emulsifying Wax NF—Creamy white, wax-like solid, having a mild characteristic odor.

NF category: Emulsifying and/or solubilizing agent; stiffening agent.

Solubility: Emulsifying Wax NF—Insoluble in water; freely soluble in ether, in chloroform, in most hydrocarbon solvents, and in aerosol propellants, soluble in alcohol.

NF requirements: Emulsifying Wax NF—Preserve in well-closed containers. A waxy solid prepared from Cetostearyl Alcohol containing a polyoxyethylene derivative of a fatty acid ester of sorbitan. Meets the requirements for Melting range (50–54 °C), pH (5.5–7.0, in a dispersion [3 in 100]), Hydroxyl value (178–192), Iodine value (not more than 3.5), and Saponification value (not more than 14).

MICROCRYSTALLINE WAX

Description: Microcrystalline Wax NF—White or cream-colored, odorless, waxy solid.

NF category: Coating agent.

Solubility: Microcrystalline Wax NF—Insoluble in water; sparingly soluble in dehydrated alcohol; soluble in chloroform, in ether, in volatile oils, and in most warm fixed oils.

NF requirements: Microcrystalline Wax NF—Preserve in tight containers. A mixture of straight-chain, branched-chain, and cyclic hydrocarbons, obtained by solvent fractionation of the still bottom fraction of petroleum by suitable dewaxing or deoiling means. Label it to indicate the name and proportion of any added stabilizer. Meets the requirements for Color, Melting range (54–102 °C), Consistency (0.3–10.0 mm), Acidity, Alkalinity, Residue on ignition (not more than 0.1%), Organic acids, and Fixed oils, fats, and rosin.

WHITE WAX

Description: White Wax NF—Yellowish-white solid, somewhat translucent in thin layers. It has a faint, characteristic odor, and is free from rancidity. Specific gravity is about 0.95.

NF category: Stiffening agent.

Solubility: White Wax NF—Insoluble in water; sparingly soluble in cold alcohol. Boiling alcohol dissolves the cerotic acid and a portion of the myricin, which are constituents of White Wax. Completely soluble in chloroform, in ether, and in fixed and volatile oils. Partly soluble in cold carbon disulfide, and completely soluble at about 30 °C.

NF requirements: White Wax NF—Preserve in well-closed containers. The product of bleaching and purifying Yellow Wax that is obtained from the honeycomb of the bee (*Apis mellifera* Linné [Fam. Apidae]) and that meets the requirements for the Saponification cloud test. Meets the requirements for Melting range (62–65 °C), Saponification cloud test, Fats or fatty acids, Japan wax, rosin, and soap, Acid value (17–24), and Ester value (72–79).

YELLOW WAX

Description: Yellow Wax NF—Solid varying in color from yellow to grayish-brown. It has an agreeable honey-like odor. Somewhat brittle when cold, and presents a dull, granular, noncrystalline fracture when broken. It becomes pliable from the heat of the hand. Specific gravity is about 0.95.

NF category: Stiffening agent.

Solubility: Yellow Wax NF—Insoluble in water; sparingly soluble in cold alcohol. Boiling alcohol dissolves the cerotic acid and a portion of the myricin, which are constituents of Yellow Wax. Completely soluble in chloroform, in ether, in fixed oils, and in volatile oils. Partly soluble in cold carbon disulfide, and completely soluble at about 30 °C.

NF requirements: Yellow Wax NF—Preserve in well-closed containers. The purified wax from the honeycomb of the bee (*Apis mellifera* Linné [Fam. Apidae]). Meets the requirements for Melting range, Saponification cloud test, Fats or fatty acids, Japan wax, rosin, and soap, Acid value, and Ester value under White Wax.

Note: To meet specifications of this monograph, the crude beeswax used to prepare Yellow Wax conforms to the Saponification cloud test.

WHITE LOTION

USP requirements: White Lotion USP—Dispense in tight containers.

Prepare White Lotion as follows: 40 grams of Zinc Sulfate, 40 grams of Sulfurated Potash, and a sufficient quantity of Purified Water to make 1000 mL. Dissolve the Zinc Sulfate and the Sulfurated Potash separately, each in 450 mL of Purified Water, and filter each solution. Add the sulfurated potash solution slowly to the zinc sulfate solution with constant stirring. Then add the required amount of purified water, and mix.

Note: Prepare the Lotion fresh, and shake it thoroughly before dispensing.

XANTHAN GUM

Description: Xanthan Gum NF—Cream-colored powder. Its solutions in water are neutral to litmus.

NF category: Suspending and/or viscosity-increasing agent.

Solubility: Xanthan Gum NF—Soluble in hot or cold water.

NF requirements: Xanthan Gum NF—Preserve in well-closed containers. A high molecular weight polysaccharide gum produced by a pure-culture fermentation of a carbohydrate with *Xanthomonas campestris*, then purified by recovery with Isopropyl Alcohol, dried, and milled. Contains D-glucose and D-mannose as the dominant hexose units, along with D-glucuronic acid, and is prepared as the sodium, potassium, or calcium salt. Yields not less than 4.2% and not more than 5.0% of carbon dioxide, calculated on the dried basis, corresponding to not less than 91.0% and not more than 108.0% of Xanthan Gum. Meets the requirements for Identification, Viscosity (not less than 600 centipoises at 24 °C), Microbial limits, Loss on drying (not more than 15.0%), Ash (6.5–16.0%, calculated on the dried basis), Arsenic (not more than 3 ppm), Heavy metals (not more than 0.003%), Lead (not more than 5 ppm), Isopropyl alcohol (not more than 0.075%), and Pyruvic acid (not less than 1.5%).

XENON Xe 127

Description: Clear, colorless gas.

USP requirements: Xenon Xe 127 USP—Preserve in single-dose vials having leak-proof stoppers, at room temperature. The vials are enclosed in appropriate lead radiation shields. The vial content may be diluted with air and is packaged at atmospheric pressure. A gas suitable for inhalation in diagnostic studies. Xenon 127 is a radioactive nuclide that may be prepared from the bombardment of a cesium 133 target with high-energy protons. Label it to include the following: the name of the preparation; the container volume, MBq (or mCi) of ^{127}Xe per container; the amount of ^{127}Xe expressed as megabecquerels (or millicuries) per mL; the intended route of administration; recommended storage conditions; the date of calibration; the expiration date; the name, address, and batch number of the manufacturer; and the statement "Caution—Radioactive Material"; and a radioactive symbol. The labeling contains a statement of radionuclide purity, identifies probable radionuclidic impurities, and indicates permissible quantities of each impurity. The labeling indicates that in making dosage calculations, correction is to be made for radioactive decay, and also indicates that the radioactive half-life of ^{127}Xe is 36.41 days. Contains the labeled amount of ^{127}Xe, within ±15%, at the calibration date indicated in the labeling. Meets the requirements for Radionuclide identification and Radionuclidic purity.

XENON Xe 133

Chemical name: Xenon, isotope of mass 133.

Description: Xenon Xe 133 Injection USP—Clear, colorless solution.

USP requirements:

Xenon Xe 133 USP—Preserve in single-dose or in multiple-dose vials having leak-proof stoppers, at room temperature. A gas suitable for inhalation in diagnostic studies. Xenon 133 is a radioactive nuclide that may be prepared from the fission of uranium 235. Contains the labeled amount of ^{133}Xe, within ±15%, at the date and time indicated in the labeling. Meets the requirements for Labeling (except for the information specified for Labeling under Injections), for Radionuclide identification, and for Radionuclidic purity under Xenon 133 Injection (except to determine the radioactivity in MBq [or mCi] per container).

Xenon Xe 133 Injection USP—Preserve in single-dose containers that are totally filled, so that any air present occupies not more than 0.5% of the total volume of the container. Store at a temperature between 2 and 8 °C. If there is free space above the solution, a significant amount of the xenon 133 is present in the gaseous phase. Glass containers may darken under the effects of radiation. A sterile, isotonic solution of Xenon 133 in Sodium Chloride Injection suitable for intravenous administration. Xenon 133 is a radioactive nuclide prepared from the fission of uranium 235. Label it to include the following, in addition to the information specified for Labeling under Injections: the time and date of calibration; the amount of xenon 133 expressed as total megabecquerels (or microcuries or millicuries), and concentration as megabecquerels (or microcuries or millicuries) per mL at the time of calibration; the expiration date; the name and amount of any added bacteriostatic agent; and the statement, "Caution—Radioactive Material." The labeling indicates that in making dosage calculations, correction is to be made for radioactive decay, and also indicates that the radioactive half-life of ^{133}Xe is 5.24 days. Contains the labeled amount of Xenon 133, within ±10%, at the date and time stated on the label. Meets the requirements for Radionuclide identification, Bacterial endotoxins, pH (4.5–8.0), Radionuclidic purity, and Injections (except that the Injection may be distributed or dispensed prior to the completion of the test for Sterility, the latter test being started on the day of manufacture, and except that it is not subject to the recommendation on Volume in Container).

XYLITOL

Chemical name: Xylitol.

Molecular formula: $C_5H_{12}O_5$.

Molecular weight: 152.15.

Description: Xylitol NF—White crystals or crystalline powder. Crystalline xylitol has a melting range between 92 and 96 °C.

Solubility: Xylitol NF—One gram dissolves in about 0.65 mL of water. Sparingly soluble in alcohol.

NF requirements: Xylitol NF—Preserve in well-closed containers. Contains not less than 98.5% and not more than 101.0% of xylitol, calculated on the anhydrous basis. Meets the requirements for Identification, Water (not more than 0.5%), Residue on ignition (not more than 0.5%), Arsenic (not more than 3 ppm), Heavy metals (not more than 0.001%), Reducing sugars, Organic volatile impurities, and Limit of other polyols (not more than 2.0%).

XYLOMETAZOLINE

Chemical name: Xylometazoline hydrochloride—1H-Imidazole, 2-[[4-(1,1-dimethylethyl)-2,6-dimethylphenyl]methyl]-4,5-dihydro-, monohydrochloride.

Molecular formula: Xylometazoline hydrochloride—$C_{16}H_{24}N_2 \cdot$ HCl.

Molecular weight: Xylometazoline hydrochloride—280.84.

Description: Xylometazoline Hydrochloride USP—White to off-white, odorless, crystalline powder. Melts above 300 °C, with decomposition.

Solubility: Xylometazoline Hydrochloride USP—Soluble in water; freely soluble in alcohol; sparingly soluble in chloroform; practically insoluble in ether.

USP requirements: Xylometazoline Hydrochloride Nasal Solution USP—Preserve in tight, light-resistant containers. An isotonic solution of Xylometazoline Hydrochloride in Water. Contains the labeled amount, within ±10%. Meets the requirements for Identification and pH (5.0–7.5).

XYLOSE

Chemical name: D-Xylose.

Molecular formula: $C_5H_{10}O_5$.

Molecular weight: 150.13.

Description: Xylose USP—Colorless needles or white crystalline powder. Is odorless.

Solubility: Xylose USP—Very soluble in water; slightly soluble in alcohol.

USP requirements: Xylose USP—Preserve in tight containers at controlled room temperature. Contains not less than 98.0% and not more than 102.0% of xylose, calculated on the dried basis. Meets the requirements for Identification, Specific rotation (+18.2° to +19.4°, calculated on the dried basis), Loss on drying (not more than 0.1%), Residue on ignition (not more than 0.05%), Arsenic (not more than 1 ppm), Iron (not more than 5 ppm), Heavy metals (not more than 0.001%),

Chromatographic impurities, and Organic volatile impurities.

YELLOW FEVER VACCINE

Description: Yellow Fever Vaccine USP—Slightly dull, light-orange colored, flaky or crustlike, desiccated mass.

USP requirements: Yellow Fever Vaccine USP—Preserve in nitrogen-filled, flame-sealed ampuls or suitable stoppered vials at a temperature preferably below 0 °C but never above 5 °C, throughout the dating period. Preserve it during shipment in a suitable container adequately packed in solid carbon dioxide, or provided with other means of refrigeration, so as to insure a temperature constantly below 0 °C. It is the attenuated strain that has been tested in monkeys for viscerotropism, immunogenicity, and neurotropism, of living yellow fever virus selected for high antigenic activity and safety. It is prepared by the culturing of the virus in the living embryos of chicken eggs, from which a suspension is prepared, processed with aseptic precautions, and finally dried from the frozen state. Meets the requirements of the specific mouse potency test in titer of mouse LD_{50} (quantity of virus estimated to produce fatal specific encephalitis in 50% of the mice) or the requirements for plaque-forming units in a suitable cell-culture system, such as a Vero cell system for which the relationship between mouse LD_{50} and plaque-forming units has been established, in which cell monolayers in 35 mm petri dishes are inoculated for a specified time with dilutions of Vaccine, after which the dilutions are replaced with 0.5% agarose-containing medium. Following adsorption and incubation for 5 days an overlay is added of the 0.5% agarose medium containing 1:50,000 neutral red and the plaques are counted on the sixth day following inoculation. Label it to state that it is to be well shaken before use and that the constituted vaccine is to be used entirely or discarded within 1 hour of opening the container. Label it also to state that it is the living yellow fever vaccine virus prepared from chicken embryos and that the dose is the same for persons of all ages, but that it is not recommended for infants under six months of age. It is sterile and contains no human serum and no antimicrobial agent. Yellow Fever Vaccine is constituted, with Sodium Chloride Injection containing no antimicrobial agent, just prior to use. Meets the requirement for Expiration date (not later than 1 year after the date of issue from manufacturer's cold storage [−20 °C, 1 year]). Conforms to the regulations of the U.S. Food and Drug Administration concerning biologics.

YTTERBIUM Yb 169 PENTETATE

Chemical name: Ytterbate (2—)-169Yb, [N,N-bis[2-[bis(carboxymethyl)amino]ethyl]glycinato(5—)]-, disodium.

Molecular formula: $C_{14}H_{18}N_3Na_2O_{10}{}^{169}Yb$.

Description: Ytterbium Yb 169 Pentetate Injection USP—Clear, colorless to light tan, solution.

USP requirements: Ytterbium Yb 169 Pentetate Injection USP—Store in single-dose containers at room temperature. A sterile, isotonic solution of pentetic acid labeled with radioactive 169Yb, suitable for intrathecal injection. Label it to include the following, in addition to the information specified for Labeling under Injections: the date of calibration; the amount of 169Yb as pentetic acid expressed in megabecquerels (or millicuries) and concentration as megabecquerels (or millicuries) per mL at time of calibration; and the statement, "Caution—Radioactive Material." The labeling indicates that in making dosage calculations, correction is to be made for radioactive decay. The radioactive half-life of 169Yb is 32.0

days. Contains the labeled amount of ^{169}Yb, within ±10%, as pentetic acid expressed in megabecquerels (or millicuries) per mL at the time indicated in the labeling. Contains a stabilizing agent and trace quantities of calcium, sodium, and chloride ions as products of the chelating reaction. Other chemical forms of radioactivity do not exceed 2.0% of the total radioactivity. Meets the requirements for Radionuclide identification, Bacterial endotoxins, pH (5.0–7.0), Radiochemical purity, and Injections (except that it is not subject to the recommendation on Volume in Container).

ZEIN

Description: Zein NF—White to yellow powder.
  NF category: Coating agent.

Solubility: Zein NF—Soluble in aqueous alcohols, in glycols, in ethylene glycol ethyl ether, in furfuryl alcohol, in tetrahydrofurfuryl alcohol, and in aqueous alkaline solutions of pH 11.5 or greater. Insoluble in water and in acetone, readily soluble in acetone-water mixtures between the limits of 60% and 80% of acetone by volume; insoluble in all anhydrous alcohols except methanol.

NF requirements: Zein NF—Preserve in tight containers. A prolamine derived from corn (*Zea mays* Linné [Fam. Gramineae]). Meets the requirements for Identification, Microbial limits, Loss on drying (not more than 8.0%), Residue on ignition (not more than 2.0%), Arsenic (not more than 3 ppm), Heavy metals (not more than 0.002%), and Nitrogen content (13.1–17.0%, on the dried basis).

ZIDOVUDINE

Chemical group: Dideoxynucleoside analog; also a thymidine analog.

Chemical name: Thymidine, 3′-azido-3′-deoxy-.

Molecular formula: $C_{10}H_{13}N_5O_4$.

Molecular weight: 267.24.

Description: White to beige, odorless, crystalline solid.

USP requirements:
  Zidovudine Capsules—Not in USP.
  Zidovudine Injection—Not in USP.
  Zidovudine Syrup—Not in USP.

ZINC CHLORIDE

Chemical name: Zinc chloride.

Molecular fomula: $ZnCl_2$.

Molecular weight: 136.29.

Description: Zinc Chloride USP—White or practically white, odorless, crystalline powder, or white or practically white crystalline granules. May also be in porcelain-like masses or molded into cylinders. Very deliquescent. A solution (1 in 10) is acid to litmus.

Solubility: Zinc Chloride USP—Very soluble in water; freely soluble in alcohol and in glycerin. Its solution in water or in alcohol is usually slightly turbid, but the turbidity disappears when a small quantity of hydrochloric acid is added.

USP requirements: Zinc Chloride Injection USP—Preserve in single-dose or in multiple-dose containers, preferably of Type I or Type II glass. A sterile solution of Zinc Chloride in Water for Injection. Label the Injection to indicate that it is to be diluted with Water for Injection or other suitable fluid to appropriate strength prior to administration. Contains an amount of zinc chloride equivalent to the labeled amount of zinc, within ±5%. Meets the requirements for Identification, Bacterial endotoxins, pH (1.5–2.5), Particulate matter, and Injections.

ZINC OXIDE

Chemical name: Zinc oxide.

Molecular formula: ZnO.

Molecular weight: 81.38.

Description: Zinc Oxide USP—Very fine, odorless, amorphous, white or yellowish white powder, free from gritty particles. Gradually absorbs carbon dioxide from air.

Solubility: Zinc Oxide USP—Insoluble in water and in alcohol; soluble in dilute acids.

USP requirements:
  Zinc Oxide Ointment USP—Preserve in well-closed containers, and avoid prolonged exposure to temperatures exceeding 30 °C. Contains not less than 18.5% and not more than 21.5% of zinc oxide.

  Zinc Oxide Ointment may be prepared as follows: 200 grams of Zinc Oxide, 150 grams of Mineral Oil, and 650 grams of White Ointment, to make 1000 grams. Levigate the Zinc Oxide with the Mineral Oil to a smooth paste, and then incorporate the White Ointment.

  Meets the requirements for Identification, Minimum fill, and Calcium, magnesium, and other foreign substances.

  Zinc Oxide Paste USP—Preserve in well-closed containers, and avoid prolonged exposure to temperatures exceeding 30 °C. Contains not less than 24.0% and not more than 26.0% of zinc oxide.

  Zinc Oxide Paste may be prepared as follows: 250 grams of Zinc Oxide, 250 grams of Starch, and 500 grams of White Petrolatum, to make 1000 grams. Mix the ingredients.

  Meets the requirements for Identification and Minimum fill.

ZINC OXIDE AND SALICYLIC ACID

For *Zinc Oxide* and *Salicylic Acid*—See individual listings for chemistry information.

USP requirements: Zinc Oxide and Salicylic Acid Paste USP—Preserve in well-closed containers. Contains not less than 23.5% and not more than 25.5% of zinc oxide, and not less than 1.9% and not more than 2.1% of salicylic acid.

Zinc Oxide and Salicylic Acid Paste may be prepared as follows: 20 grams of Salicylic Acid, in fine powder, and a sufficient quantity of Zinc Oxide Paste to make 1000 grams. Thoroughly triturate the Salicylic Acid with a portion of the paste, then add the remaining paste, and triturate until a smooth mixture is obtained.

Meets the requirements for Identification and Minimum fill.

ZINC SULFATE

Chemical name: Sulfuric acid, zinc salt (1:1), hydrate.

Molecular formula: $ZnSO_4 \cdot xH_2O$.

Molecular weight: 179.46 (monohydrate); 287.54 (heptahydrate); 161.44 (anhydrous).

Description: Zinc Sulfate USP—Colorless, transparent prisms, or small needles. May occur as a granular, crystalline powder. Odorless; efflorescent in dry air. Its solutions are acid to litmus.

Solubility: Zinc Sulfate USP—Very soluble in water; freely soluble in glycerin; insoluble in alcohol.

USP requirements:

Zinc Sulfate Injection USP—Preserve in single-dose or in multiple-dose containers. A sterile solution of Zinc Sulfate in Water for Injection. Label the Injection in terms of its content of anhydrous zinc sulfate and in terms of its content of elemental zinc. Label it to state that it is not intended for direct injection but is to be added to other intravenous solutions. Contains an amount of zinc sulfate equivalent to the labeled amount of zinc, within ±5%. Meets the requirements for Identification, Bacterial endotoxins, pH (2.0–4.0), Particulate matter, and Injections.

Zinc Sulfate Ophthalmic Solution USP—Preserve in tight containers. A sterile solution of Zinc Sulfate in Water rendered isotonic by the addition of suitable salts. Contains the labeled amount, within ±5%. Meets the requirements for Identification, Sterility, and pH (5.8–6.2; or, if it contains sodium citrate, 7.2–7.8).

Section IV

THE MEDICINE CHART

The Medicine Chart presents photographs of the most frequently prescribed medicines in the United States. In general, commonly used brand name products and a representative sampling of generic products have been included. The pictorial listing is not intended to be inclusive and does not represent all products on the market. Only selected solid oral dosage forms (capsules and tablets) have been included. The inclusion of a product does not mean the USPC has any particular knowledge that the product included has properties different from other products, nor should it be interpreted as an endorsement by USPC. Similarly, the fact that a particular product has not been included does not indicate that the product has been judged by the USPC to be unsatisfactory or unacceptable.

The drug products in *The Medicine Chart* are listed alphabetically by generic name of active ingredient(s). To quickly locate a particular medicine, check the product listing index that follows. This listing provides brand and generic names and directs the user to the appropriate page and chart location. In addition, any identifying code found on the surface of a capsule or tablet that might be useful in making a correct identification is included in the parentheses that follow the product's index entry. Please note that these codes may change as manufacturers reformulate or redesign their products. In addition, some companies may not manufacture all of their own products. In some of these cases, the imprinting on the tablet or capsule may be that of the actual manufacturer and not of the company marketing the product.

An inverted cross-index has also been included to help identify products by their identifying codes. These codes may not be unique to a given product; they are intended for use in initial identification only. In this cross-index, the codes are listed first in alpha-numeric order, accompanied by their generic or brand names and page and chart location.

Brand names are in *italics*. An asterisk next to the generic name of the active ingredient(s) indicates that the solid oral dosage forms containing the ingredient(s) are available only from a single source with no generic equivalents currently available in the U.S. Where multiple source products are shown, it must be kept in mind that other products may also be available.

The size and color of the products shown are intended to match the actual product as closely as possible; however, there may be some differences due to variations caused by the photographic process. Also, manufacturers may occasionally change the color, imprinting, or shape of their products, and for a period of time both the "old" and the newly changed dosage form may be on the market. Such changes may not occur uniformly thoughout the different dosages of the product. These types of changes will be incorporated in subsequent versions of the chart as they are brought to our attention.

> Use of this chart is limited to serving as an initial guide in identifying drug products. The identity of a product should be verified further before any action is taken.

Accupril Tablets—
  5 mg (5) MC-20, D6
  10 mg (10) MC-20, D6
  20 mg (20) MC-20, D6
  40 mg (40) MC-20, D6
Accutane Capsules—
  10 mg (10) MC-12, C7
  20 mg (20) MC-12, C7
  40 mg (40) MC-12, C7
Acetaminophen and Codeine .. MC-1, A1–6
  Purepac Tablets—
    300/30 mg (001) MC-1, A3
    300/60 mg (003) MC-1, A3
Achromycin V Capsules—
  250 mg (A3 250) MC-22, B6
  500 mg (A5 500) MC-22, B6
Actigall Capsules—
  300 mg (300 MG) MC-24, B5
Acyclovir.................. MC-1, A7–B1
Adalat Capsules—
  10 mg (811) MC-16, B6
  20 mg (821) MC-16, B6
Albuterol.............. MC-1, B2–6
  Mutual Tablets—
    2 mg (MP 47)............ MC-1, B3
    4 mg (MP 88)............. MC-1, B3
  Schein/Danbury Tablets—
    2 mg (5710) MC-1, B4
    4 mg (5711) MC-1, B4
Aldactazide Tablets—
  25/25 mg (1011) MC-21, C5
  50/50 mg (1021) MC-21, C5

Aldactone Tablets—
  25 mg (1001) MC-21, C1
  50 mg (1041) MC-21, C1
  100 mg (1031) MC-21, C1
Aldomet Tablets—
  125 mg (MSD 135)........ MC-14, C7
  250 mg (MSD 401)........ MC-14, C7
  500 mg (MSD 516)........ MC-14, C7
Aldoril Tablets—
  250/15 mg (MSD 423)...... MC-14, D6
  250/25 mg (MSD 456)...... MC-14, D6
  500/30 mg (MSD 694)...... MC-14, D7
  500/50 mg (MSD 935)...... MC-14, D7
Allopurinol MC-1, B7–C4
  Mutual Tablets—
    100 mg (MP 71) MC-1, C2
    300 mg (MP 80) MC-1, C2
  Mylan Tablets—
    100 mg (M 31)........... MC-1, C3
    300 mg (M 71)........... MC-1, C3
  Schein/Danbury Tablets—
    100 mg (5543) MC-1, C4
    300 mg (5544) MC-1, C4
Alprazolam MC-1, C5
Altace Capsules—
  1.25 mg (1.25 mg)......... MC-21, A4
  2.5 mg (2.5 mg)........... MC-21, A4
  5 mg (5 mg) MC-21, A4
  10 mg (10 mg) MC-21, A4
Alupent Tablets—
  10 mg (BI 74)............. MC-14, B7
  20 mg (BI 72)............. MC-14, B7

Amantadine................. MC-1, C6
Amiloride and
  Hydrochlorothiazide........ MC-1, C7
Amitriptyline MC-1, D1–MC-2, A3
  Geneva Tablets—
    10 mg (GG 40) MC-1, D1
    25 mg (GG 44) MC-1, D1
    50 mg (GG 431) MC-1, D1
    75 mg (GG 451) MC-1, D1
    100 mg (GG 461) MC-1, D1
    150 mg (GG 450) MC-1, D2
  Purepac Tablets—
    10 mg (31) MC-1, D3
    25 mg (32) MC-1, D3
    50 mg (133) MC-1, D3
    75 mg (134) MC-1, D4
    100 mg (135) MC-1, D4
  Rugby Tablets—
    10 mg (3071) MC-1, D5
    25 mg (3072) MC-1, D5
    50 mg (3073) MC-1, D5
    75 mg (3074) MC-1, D5
    100 mg (3075) MC-1, D5
    150 mg (3076) MC-1, D6
  Schein Tablets—
    10 mg (22) MC-1, D7
    25 mg (23) MC-1, D7
    50 mg (24) MC-1, D7
    75 mg (25) MC-1, D7
    100 mg (26) MC-1, D7
    150 mg (M 39)........... MC-2, A1

IV

Amoxicillin MC-2, A4–B1
Amoxicillin and
  Clavulanate MC-2, B2–3
Amoxil
  Capsules—
    250 mg (250) MC-2, A6
    500 mg (500) MC-2, A6
  Chewable Tablets—
    125 mg (125) MC-2, A7
    250 mg (250) MC-2, A7
Ampicillin MC-2, B4–6
Anafranil Capsules—
  25 mg (25 mg) MC-5, D5
  50 mg (50 mg) MC-5, D5
  75 mg (75 mg) MC-5, D5
Anaprox Tablets—
  275 mg (274) MC-16, A6
  500 mg (DS) MC-16, A6
Ansaid Tablets—
  50 mg (50 mg) MC-10, B7
  100 mg (100 mg) MC-10, B7
Antivert
  Tablets—
    12.5 mg (210) MC-14, A4
    25 mg (211) MC-14, A4
    50 mg (214) MC-14, A4
  Chewable Tablets—
    25 mg (212) MC-14, A5
Apresazide Capsules—
  25/25 mg (139) MC-11, A6
  50/50 mg (149) MC-11, A6
  100/50 mg (159) MC-11, A6
Apresoline Tablets—
  10 mg (37) MC-11, A4
  25 mg (39) MC-11, A4
  50 mg (73) MC-11, A4
  100 mg (101) MC-11, A4
Aralen Tablets—
  500 mg (A77) MC-4, D5
Aspirin, Caffeine, and
  Dihydrocodeine MC-2, B7
Aspirin and Codeine MC-2, C1
Astemizole MC-2, C2
Atarax Tablets—
  10 mg (10) MC-11, C5
  25 mg (25) MC-11, C5
  50 mg (50) MC-11, C5
  100 mg (100) MC-11, C5
Atenolol MC-2, C3–6
  Geneva Tablets—
    50 mg (GG 263) MC-2, C3
    100 mg (GG 264) MC-2, C3
  IPR Pharma Tablets—
    50 mg (45) MC-2, C5
    100 mg (90) MC-2, C5
  Lederle Tablets—
    50 mg (A 49) MC-2, C6
    100 mg (A 71) MC-2, C6
Atenolol and Chlorthalidone MC-2, C7
Ativan Tablets—
  0.5 mg (81) MC-13, D7
  1 mg (64) MC-13, D7
  2 mg (65) MC-13, D7
Atropine, Hyoscyamine, Scopolamine, and
  Phenobarbital MC-2, D1–3
Augmentin
  Tablets—
    250/125 mg (250/125) MC-2, B2
    500/125 mg (500/125) MC-2, B2
  Chewable Tablets—
    125/31.25 mg (BMP 189) . . MC-2, B3
    250/62.5 mg (BMP 190) . . . MC-2, B3
Auranofin MC-2, D4
Axid Capsules—
  150 mg (3144) MC-16, D2
  300 mg (3145) MC-16, D2

Azatadine and
  Pseudoephedrine MC-2, D5
Azathioprine MC-2, D6
Azithromycin MC-2, D7
Azulfidine Tablets—
  500 mg (101) MC-21, D3
Azulfidine EN-Tabs Enteric-coated
  Tablets—
    500 mg (102) MC-21, D4
Baclofen MC-3, A1
Bactrim Tablets—
  400/80 mg MC-21, D1
  800/160 mg MC-21, D1
Benadryl Capsules—
  25 mg (P-D 471) MC-7, C7
  50 mg (P-D 473) MC-7, C7
Benazepril MC-3, A2
Bendroflumethiazide MC-3, A3
Bentyl
  Capsules—
    10 mg (10) MC-7, A7
  Tablets—
    20 mg (20) MC-7, B1
Benzphetamine MC-3, A4
Benztropine MC-3, A5–6
  Mutual Tablets—
    1 mg (MP 44) MC-3, A6
    2 mg (MP 142) MC-3, A6
Bepridil MC-3, A7
Betapen VK Tablets—
  250 mg (BL V1) MC-18, B6
  500 mg (BL V2) MC-18, B6
Betaxolol MC-3, B1
Biaxin Tablets—
  250 mg (KT) MC-5, C7
  500 mg (KL) MC-5, C7
Blocadren Tablets—
  5 mg (MSD 59) MC-23, B7
  10 mg (MSD 136) MC-23, B7
  20 mg (MSD 437) MC-23, B7
Brethine Tablets—
  2.5 mg (72) MC-22, B1
  5 mg (105) MC-22, B1
Bromocriptine MC-3, B2–3
Bumetanide MC-3, B4
Bumex Tablets—
  0.5 mg (0.5) MC-3, B4
  1 mg (1) MC-3, B4
  2 mg (2) MC-3, B4
Bupropion MC-3, B5
BuSpar Tablets—
  5 mg (MJ 5) MC-3, B6
  10 mg (MJ 10) MC-3, B6
Buspirone MC-3, B6
Butalbital, Acetaminophen, and
  Caffeine MC-3, B7
Butalbital, Aspirin, and
  Caffeine MC-3, C1–3
  Geneva Tablets—
    50/325/40 mg (GG 119) . . . MC-3, C1
Butalbital, Aspirin, Codeine, and
  Caffeine MC-3, C4
Cafergot Tablets—
  1/100 mg (78-34) MC-8, D7
Calan Tablets—
  40 mg (40) MC-24, D3
  80 mg (80) MC-24, D3
  120 mg (120) MC-24, D3
Calan SR Extended-release Tablets—
  120 mg (SR 120) MC-24, D4
  180 mg (SR 80) MC-24, D5
  240 mg (SR 240) MC-24, D5
Calcitriol MC-3, C5
Capoten Tablets—
  12.5 mg (450) MC-3, C6
  25 mg (452) MC-3, C6
  50 mg (482) MC-3, C7
  100 mg (485) MC-3, C7

Capozide Tablets—
  25/15 mg (338) MC-3, D1
  25/25 mg (349) MC-3, D1
  50/15 mg (384) MC-3, D2
  50/25 mg (390) MC-3, D2
Captopril MC-3, C6–7
Captopril and
  Hydrochlorothiazide MC-3, D1–2
Carafate Tablets—
  1 gram (17 12) MC-21, C6
Carbacephem MC-3, D3
Carbamazepine MC-3, D4–7
  Purepac Tablets—
    200 mg (143) MC-3, D6
  Warner Chilcott Chewable Tablets—
    100 mg (WC 242) MC-3, D7
Carbenicillin MC-4, A1
Carbidopa and Levodopa MC-4, A2
Cardene Capsules—
  20 mg (2437) MC-16, B4
  30 mg (2438) MC-16, B4
Cardizem Tablets—
  30 mg (1771) MC-7, C3
  60 mg (1772) MC-7, C3
  90 mg (90 mg) MC-7, C4
  120 mg (120 mg) MC-7, C4
Cardizem CD Capsules—
  180 mg (180 mg) MC-7, B7
  240 mg (240 mg) MC-7, B7
  300 mg (300 mg) MC-7, C1
Cardizem SR Capsules—
  60 mg (60 mg) MC-7, C2
  90 mg (90 mg) MC-7, C2
  120 mg (120 mg) MC-7, C2
Cardura Tablets—
  1 mg (1 mg) MC-8, A5
  2 mg (2 mg) MC-8, A5
  4 mg (4 mg) MC-8, A5
  8 mg (8 mg) MC-8, A5
Carisoprodol MC-4, A3
Carisoprodol and Aspirin MC-4, A4
Carisoprodol, Aspirin, and
  Codeine MC-4, A5
Carteolol MC-4, A6
Cartrol Tablets—
  2.5 mg (1A) MC-4, A6
  5 mg (1C) MC-4, A6
Catapres Tablets—
  0.1 mg (BI 6) MC-5, D6
  0.2 mg (BI 7) MC-5, D6
  0.3 mg (BI 11) MC-5, D6
Ceclor Capsules—
  250 mg (3061) MC-4, A7
  500 mg (3062) MC-4, A7
Cefaclor MC-4, A7
Cefadroxil MC-4, B1–2
Cefanex Capsules—
  250 mg (7375) MC-4, B7
  500 mg (7376) MC-4, B7
Cefixime MC-4, B3
Ceftin Tablets—
  125 mg (395) MC-4, B4
  250 mg (387) MC-4, B4
  500 mg (394) MC-4, B5
Cefuroxime Axetil MC-4, B4–5
Centrax
  Capsules—
    5 mg (P-D 552) MC-19, B7
    10 mg (P-D 553) MC-19, B7
    20 mg (PD 554) MC-19, B7
Cephalexin MC-4, B6–C3
  Apothecon Capsules—
    250 mg (181) MC-4, B6
    500 mg (239) MC-4, B6
  Biocraft Capsules—
    500 mg (117) MC-4, C1
Cephradine MC-4, C4–6
  Barr Capsules—
    250 mg (550) MC-4, C5
    500 mg (551) MC-4, C5

Cephradine *(continued)*
  Biocraft Capsules—
    250 mg (112) MC-4, C6
    500 mg (113) MC-4, C6
Chlordiazepoxide MC-4, C7–D1
Chlordiazepoxide and
  Amitriptyline MC-4, D2–3
  Mylan Tablets—
    5/12.5 mg (211) MC-4, D2
    10/25 mg (277) MC-4, D2
Chlordiazepoxide and
  Clidinium MC-4, D4
Chloroquine MC-4, D5
Chlorpheniramine and
  Phenylpropanolamine MC-4, D6
Chlorpheniramine, Phenyltoloxamine,
  Phenylephrine, and Phenyl-
  propanolamine..... MC-4, D7–MC-5, A1
  Geneva Extended-release Tablets—
    40/10/15/5 mg (GG
      118) MC-5, A1
Chlorpheniramine and
  Pseudoephedrine MC-5, A2–3
Chlorpheniramine, Pyrilamine, and
  Phenylephrine MC-5, A4
Chlorpromazine......... MC-5, A5–7
  Geneva Tablets—
    100 mg (GG 437)....... MC-5, A5
    200 mg (GG 457)....... MC-5, A5
Chlorpropamide............ MC-5, B1–3
  Geneva Tablets—
    100 mg (GG 61)......... MC-5, B1
    250 mg (GG 144)........ MC-5, B1
  Schein/Danbury Tablets—
    100 mg (5579).......... MC-5, B3
    250 mg (5455).......... MC-5, B3
Chlorthalidone.............. MC-5, B4–6
  Barr Tablets—
    25 mg (267)............ MC-5, B4
    50 mg (268)............ MC-5, B4
Chlorzoxazone............ MC-5, B7–C2
  Barr Tablets—
    500 mg (555 585) MC-5, B7
  Mutual Tablets—
    500 mg (MP 74)........ MC-5, C2
Cimetidine................. MC-5, C3–4
Ciprofloxacin............. MC-5, C5–6
Cipro Tablets—
  250 mg (512)............ MC-5, C5
  500 mg (513)............ MC-5, C6
  750 mg (514)............ MC-5, C6
Clarithromycin............ MC-5, C7
Clemastine................ MC-5, D1
Clemastine and
  Phenylpropanolamine MC-5, D2
Cleocin Capsules—
  75 mg (75 mg) MC-5, D4
  150 mg (150 mg) MC-5, D4
  300 mg (300 mg) MC-5, D4
Clindamycin MC-5, D3–4
  Biocraft Capsules—
    150 mg (149)........... MC-5, D3
Clinoril Tablets—
  150 mg (MSD 941) MC-21, D5
  200 mg (MSD 942) MC-21, D5
Clomipramine MC-5, D5
Clonidine MC-5, D6–MC-6, A5
  Geneva Tablets—
    0.1 mg (GG 81) MC-5, D7
    0.2 mg (GG 82) MC-5, D7
    0.3 mg (GG 83) MC-5, D7
  Lederle Tablets—
    0.1 mg (C 42)........... MC-6, A1
    0.2 mg (C 43).......... MC-6, A1
    0.3 mg (C 44)........... MC-6, A1
  Mylan Tablets—
    0.1 mg (152)........... MC-6, A2
    0.2 mg (186)........... MC-6, A2
    0.3 mg (199)........... MC-6, A2

Clonidine *(continued)*
  Purepac Tablets—
    0.1 mg (127) MC-6, A3
    0.2 mg (128) MC-6, A3
    0.3 mg (129) MC-6, A3
  Schein/Danbury Tablets—
    0.1 mg (DAN 5609)........ MC-6, A4
    0.2 mg (DAN 5612)........ MC-6, A4
    0.3 mg (DAN 5613)........ MC-6, A4
  Warner Chilcott Tablets—
    0.1 mg (443) MC-6, A5
    0.2 mg (444) MC-6, A5
    0.3 mg (WC 445) MC-6, A5
Clonidine and Chlorthalidone .. MC-6, A6–7
  Mylan Tablets—
    0.1/15 mg (M 1) MC-6, A7
    0.2/15 mg (M 27) MC-6, A7
    0.3/15 mg (M 72) MC-6, A7
Clorazepate MC-6, B1–4
  Mylan Tablets—
    3.75 mg (M 30) MC-6, B3
    7.5 mg (M 40) MC-6, B3
    15 mg (M 70) MC-6, B3
  Purepac Tablets—
    3.75 mg (078) MC-6, B4
    7.5 mg (081) MC-6, B4
    15 mg (083)............ MC-6, B4
Clotrimazole MC-6, B5
Cloxacillin MC-6, B6
Clozapine MC-6, B7
Clozaril Tablets—
  25 mg (25).............. MC-6, B7
  100 mg (100)............ MC-6, B7
Cogentin Tablets—
  0.5 mg (MSD 21)......... MC-3, A5
  1 mg (MSD 635)......... MC-3, A5
  2 mg (MSD 60).......... MC-3, A5
Combipres Tablets—
  0.1/15 mg (BI 8) MC-6, A6
  0.2/15 mg (BI 9) MC-6, A6
  0.3/15 mg (BI 10) MC-6, A6
Compazine
  Extended-release Capsules—
    10 mg (SKF C44)....... MC-20, A3
    15 mg (SKF C46)....... MC-20, A3
    30 mg (SKF C47)....... MC-20, A3
  Tablets—
    5 mg (SKF C66)........ MC-20, A4
    10 mg (SKF C67)....... MC-20, A4
    25 mg (SKF C69)........ MC-20, A4
Corgard Tablets—
  20 mg (PPP 232) MC-15, D7
  40 mg (PPP 207) MC-15, D7
  80 mg (PPP 241) MC-15, D7
  120 mg (PPP 208) MC-16, A1
  160 mg (PPP 246) MC-16, A1
Cortef Tablets—
  5 mg (5)............... MC-11, C1
  10 mg (10)............. MC-11, C1
  20 mg (20)............. MC-11, C1
Corzide Tablets—
  40/5 mg (283).......... MC-16, A2
  80/5 mg (284).......... MC-16, A2
Coumadin Tablets—
  2 mg (2)............... MC-24, D6
  2.5 mg (2½)............ MC-24, D6
  5 mg (5)............... MC-24, D6
  7.5 mg (7½)............ MC-24, D6
  10 mg (10)............. MC-24, D6
Cromolyn MC-6, C1
Cyclobenzaprine MC-6, C2–4
  Mylan Tablets—
    10 mg (710)............ MC-6, C3
  Schein/Danbury Tablets—
    10 mg (5658)........... MC-6, C4
Cytotec Tablets—
  0.1 mg (1451) MC-15, D4
  0.2 mg (1461) MC-15, D4

Dalmane Capsules—
  15 mg (15)............. MC-10, B5
  30 mg (30)............. MC-10, B5
Danazol MC-6, C5
Danocrine Capsules—
  50 mg (D 03) MC-6, C5
  100 mg (D 04) MC-6, C5
  200 mg (D 05) MC-6, C5
Dantrium Capsules—
  25 mg (0149 0030)...... MC-6, C6
  50 mg (0149 0031)...... MC-6, C6
  100 mg (0149 0033)..... MC-6, C6
Dantrolene MC-6, C6
Darvocet-N Tablets—
  50/325 mg (50)......... MC-20, B2
  100/650 mg (100) MC-20, B2
Decadron Tablets—
  0.25 mg (MSD 20)....... MC-6, D3
  0.5 mg (MSD 41) MC-6, D3
  0.75 mg (MSD 63) MC-6, D3
  1.5 mg (MSD 95) MC-6, D4
  4 mg (MSD 97) MC-6, D4
  6 mg (MSD 147) MC-6, D4
Deconamine Tablets—
  4/60 mg (184)........... MC-5, A3
Deconamine SR Extended-release Capsules—
  8/120 mg (181)......... MC-5, A2
Deltasone Tablets—
  2.5 mg (2.5)........... MC-19, C6
  5 mg (5).............. MC-19, C6
  10 mg (10)............ MC-19, C6
  20 mg (20)............ MC-19, C6
  50 mg (50)............ MC-19, C6
Demerol Tablets—
  50 mg (D 35) MC-14, B6
  100 mg (D 37) MC-14, B6
Demi-Regroton Tablets—
  0.125/25 mg (32) MC-21, A6
Demulen 1/35-21 Tablets—
  1/0.035 mg (151) MC-9, C5
Demulen 1/35-28 Tablets—
  1/0.035 mg (151) MC-9, C6
  Inert (P)............. MC-9, C6
Demulen 1/50-21 Tablets—
  1/0.05 mg (71) MC-9, C7
Demulen 1/50-28 Tablets—
  1/0.05 mg (71) MC-9, D1
  Inert (P)............. MC-9, D1
Desipramine................ MC-6, C7–D2
  Geneva Tablets—
    100 mg (GG 167)........ MC-6, C7
    150 mg (GG 168)........ MC-6, C7
Desyrel Tablets—
  50 mg (MJ 775) MC-23, D5
  100 mg (MJ 776) MC-23, D5
  150 mg (MJ 778) MC-23, D5
Dexamethasone.............. MC-6, D3–4
DiaBeta Tablets—
  1.25 mg MC-10, C7
  2.5 mg MC-10, C7
  5 mg.................. MC-10, C7
Diabinese Tablets—
  100 mg (393)........... MC-5, B2
  250 mg (394)........... MC-5, B2
Diazepam.......... MC-6, D5–MC-7, A1
  Purepac Tablets—
    2 mg (051)............ MC-6, D5
    5 mg (052)............ MC-6, D5
    10 mg (053)........... MC-6, D5
  Schein/Danbury Tablets—
    2 mg (DAN 5621) MC-7, A1
    5 mg (DAN 5619) MC-7, A1
    10 mg (DAN 5620) MC-7, A1
Diclofenac MC-7, A2
Dicloxacillin................ MC-7, A3–4
Dicyclomine............ MC-7, A5–B1
  Barr
    Capsules—
      10 mg (128)............ MC-7, A5

Dicyclomine *(continued)*
  Barr
    Tablets—
      20 mg (55 126) MC-7, A6
Didrex Tablets—
  25 mg (18) MC-3, A4
  50 mg (50) MC-3, A4
Diethylpropion MC-7, B2–3
Diflucan Tablets—
  50 mg (50) MC-10, A5
  100 mg (100) MC-10, A5
  200 mg (200) MC-10, A5
Diflunisal MC-7, B4
Digoxin MC-7, B5–6
Dilantin
  Capsules—
    30 mg (P-D 365) MC-19, A4
    100 mg (P-D 362) MC-19, A4
  Chewable Tablets—
    50 mg (P-D 007) MC-19, A3
Dilatrate-SR Extended-release Capsules—
  40 mg (0920) MC-12, C3
Diltiazem MC-7, B7–C4
Diphenhist Tablets—
  25 mg (3597) MC-7, D2
Diphenhydramine MC-7, C5–D2
  Barr Capsules—
    25 mg (058) MC-7, C5
    50 mg (059) MC-7, C5
  Geneva Capsules—
    25 mg (GG 533) MC-7, C6
    50 mg (GG 541) MC-7, C6
  Purepac Capsules—
    25 mg (191) MC-7, D1
    50 mg (192) MC-7, D1
Diphenoxylate and Atropine . . . MC-7, D3
Dipyridamole MC-7, D4–7
  Barr Tablets—
    25 mg (252) MC-7, D4
    50 mg (285) MC-7, D4
    75 mg (286) MC-7, D4
  Geneva Tablets—
    25 mg (GG 49) MC-7, D6
    50 mg (GG 45) MC-7, D6
    75 mg (GG 464) MC-7, D6
  Purepac Tablets—
    25 mg (193) MC-7, D7
    50 mg (183) MC-7, D7
    75 mg (185) MC-7, D7
Disopyramide MC-8, A1–4
  Barr Capsules—
    100 mg (331) MC-8, A1
    150 mg (332) MC-8, A1
  Geneva Capsules—
    100 mg (GG 56) MC-8, A2
    150 mg (GG 57) MC-8, A2
Ditropan Tablets—
  5 mg (1375) MC-18, A2
Diulo Tablets—
  2.5 mg (SCS 501) MC-15, B5
  5 mg (SCS 511) MC-15, B5
  10 mg (SCS 521) MC-15, B5
Dolobid Tablets—
  250 mg (MSD 675) MC-7, B4
  500 mg (MSD 697) MC-7, B4
Donnatal
  Capsules—
    0.0194/0.1037/0.0065/16.2 mg
    (AHR 4207) . . . MC-2, D1
  Tablets—
    0.0194/0.1037/0.0065/16.2 mg
    (4250) MC-2, D2
  Extended-release Tablets—
    0.0582/0.3111/0.0195/48.6 mg
    (AHR) MC-2, D3
Doral Tablets—
  7.5 mg (7.5) MC-20, D5
  15 mg (15) MC-20, D5

Doxazosin Mesylate MC-8, A5
Doxepin MC-8, A6–B6
  Geneva Capsules—
    10 mg (GG 576) MC-8, A6
    25 mg (GG 572) MC-8, A6
    50 mg (GG 573) MC-8, A7
    75 mg (GG 574) MC-8, A7
    100 mg (GG 577) MC-8, A7
  Rugby Capsules—
    10 mg (3736) MC-8, B3
    25 mg (3728) MC-8, B3
    50 mg (3729) MC-8, B3
    75 mg (3737) MC-8, B4
    100 mg (3730) MC-8, B4
    150 mg (3738) MC-8, B4
  Schein/Danbury Capsules—
    10 mg (DAN 5629) MC-8, B5
    25 mg (DAN 5630) MC-8, B5
    50 mg (DAN 5631) MC-8, B6
    75 mg (DAN 5632) MC-8, B6
    100 mg (DAN 5633) MC-8, B6
Doxycycline MC-8, B7–C7
  Barr
    Capsules—
      50 mg (296) MC-8, B7
      100 mg (297) MC-8, B7
    Tablets—
      100 mg (295) MC-8, C1
  Purepac Capsules—
    50 mg (194) MC-8, C4
    100 mg (195) MC-8, C4
  Rugby Capsules—
    50 mg (0280) MC-8, C5
    100 mg (0230) MC-8, C5
  Schein/Danbury
    Capsules—
      50 mg (DAN 5535) MC-8, C6
      100 mg (DAN 5440) MC-8, C6
    Tablets—
      100 mg (5553) MC-8, C7
Duricef
  Capsules—
    500 mg (MJ 784) MC-4, B1
  Tablets—
    1 gram (MJ 785) MC-4, B2
Dyazide Capsules—
  50/25 mg (SKF) MC-24, A5
Dyna Circ Capsules—
  2.5 mg (2.5) MC-12, D1
  5 mg (5) MC-12, D1
Dynapen Capsules—
  125 mg (7892) MC-7, A3
  250 mg (7893) MC-7, A3
  500 mg (7658) MC-7, A4
Dyphylline MC-8, D1
E.E.S. Tablets—
  400 mg (EE) MC-9, B3
Elavil Tablets—
  10 mg (MSD 23) MC-2, A2
  25 mg (MSD 45) MC-2, A2
  50 mg (MSD 102) MC-2, A2
  75 mg (MSD 430) MC-2, A2
  100 mg (MSD 435) MC-2, A2
  150 mg (MSD 673) MC-2, A3
Eldepryl Tablets—
  5 mg (JU) MC-21, B2
Empirin with Codeine Tablets—
  325/30 mg (3) MC-2, C1
  325/60 mg (4) MC-2, C1
E-Mycin Delayed-release Tablets—
  250 mg (250mg) MC-9, A6
  333 mg (333mg) MC-9, A6
Enalapril MC-8, D2
Enalapril and
  Hydrochlorothiazide MC-8, D3
Enduron Tablets—
  2.5 mg MC-14, C4
  5 mg MC-14, C4
Entex Capsules—
  5/45/200 mg (0149 0412) MC-18, D7

Entex LA Extended-release Tablets—
  75/400 mg (0149 0436) MC-19, A2
Ergoloid Mesylates MC-8, D4–6
Ergotamine and Caffeine MC-8, D7
Eryc Delayed-release Capsules—
  250 mg (P-D 696) MC-9, A7
EryPed Chewable Tablets—
  200 mg (CHEW EZ) MC-9, B4
Ery-Tab Delayed-release Tablets—
  250 mg (EC) MC-9, A3
  333 mg (EH) MC-9, A3
  500 mg (ED) MC-9, A3
Erythrocin Tablets—
  250 mg (ES) MC-9, B6
  500 mg (ET) MC-9, B6
Erythromycin MC-9, A1–7
  Abbott
    Delayed-release Capsules—
      250 mg (ER) MC-9, A1
    Tablets—
      250 mg (EB) MC-9, A2
      500 mg (EA) MC-9, A2
  Barr Delayed-release Capsules—
    250 mg (584) MC-9, A5
Erythromycin Estolate MC-9, B1–2
Erythromycin Ethylsuccinate . . . MC-9, B3–5
  Barr Tablets—
    400 mg (259) MC-9, B5
Erythromycin Stearate MC-9, B6
Esidrix Tablets—
  25 mg (22) MC-11, B3
  50 mg (46) MC-11, B3
  100 mg (192) MC-11, B3
Eskalith
  Capsules—
    300 mg MC-13, C7
  Tablets—
    300 mg (J09) MC-13, D1
Eskalith CR Extended-release Tablets—
  450 mg (J10) MC-13, D2
Estazolam MC-9, B7
Estrace Tablets—
  1 mg (MJ 755) MC-9, C1
  2 mg (MJ 756) MC-9, C1
Estradiol MC-9, C1
Estrogens, Conjugated MC-9, C2–3
Estropipate MC-9, C4
Ethmozine Tablets—
  200 mg (200) MC-15, D5
  250 mg (250) MC-15, D5
  300 mg (300) MC-15, D6
Ethynodiol Diacetate and Ethinyl
  Estradiol MC-9, C5–D1
Etodolac MC-9, D2
Famotidine MC-9, D3
Feldene Capsules—
  10 mg (322) MC-19, A6
  20 mg (323) MC-19, A6
Felodipine MC-9, D4
Fenoprofen MC-9, D5–MC-10, A3
  Geneva
    Capsules—
      200 mg (GG 558) MC-9, D7
      300 mg (GG 559) MC-9, D7
    Tablets—
      600 mg (GG 254) MC-10, A1
  Purepac Tablets—
    600 mg (317) MC-10, A2
  Schein/Danbury Tablets—
    600 mg (5704) MC-10, A3
Ferrous Sulfate MC-10, A4
  Upsher-Smith Tablets—
    300 mg MC-10, A4
Fioricet Tablets—
  50/325/40 mg (78-84) MC-3, A7
Fiorinal
  Capsules—
    50/325/40 mg (78-103) MC-3, C2
  Tablets—
    50/325/40 mg (78-104) MC-3, C3

Fiorinal with Codeine Capsules—
  50/325/30/40 mg (78-107) ... MC-3, C4
Flagyl Tablets—
  250 mg (1831) MC-15, C5
  500 mg (500) MC-15, C5
Flexeril Tablets—
  10 mg (MSD 931) MC-6, C2
Floxin Tablets—
  200 mg (200 mg) MC-17, C6
  300 mg (300 mg) MC-17, C6
  400 mg (400 mg) MC-17, C7
Fluconazole MC-10, A5
Fluoxetine MC-10, A6
Fluoxymesterone. MC-10, A7
Fluphenazine. MC-10, B1–2
  Mylan Tablets—
    1 mg (4) MC-10, B1
    2.5 mg (4) MC-10, B1
    5 mg (9) MC-10, B1
    10 mg (97) MC-10, B1
Flurazepam MC-10, B3–6
  Barr Capsules—
    15 mg (377) MC-10, B3
    30 mg (378) MC-10, B3
  Purepac Capsules—
    15 mg (R021) MC-10, B4
    30 mg (R022) MC-10, B4
  Schein/Danbury Capsules—
    15 mg (DAN 5614) MC-10, B6
    30 mg (DAN 5615) MC-10, B6
Flurbiprofen. MC-10, B7
Fosinopril. MC-10, C1
Furadantin Tablets—
  50 mg (036) MC-16, C5
  100 mg (037) MC-16, C5
Furosemide MC-10, C2–4
  Barr Tablets—
    20 mg (170) MC-10, C2
    40 mg (555 169) MC-10, C2
    80 mg (555 196) MC-10, C2
  Schein/Danbury Tablets—
    20 mg (M2) MC-10, C4
    40 mg (5575) MC-10, C4
    80 mg (302) MC-10, C4
Gastrocrom Capsules—
  100 mg (101) MC-6, C1
Gemfibrozil. MC-10, C5
Genora 0.5/35-21 Tablets—
  0.5/0.035 mg (0.5/35) ... MC-17, A4
Genora 1/35-28 Tablets—
  1/0.035 mg (1/35). MC-17, A5
  Inert MC-17, A5
Genora 1/50-28 Tablets—
  1/0.05 mg (1/50). MC-17, B5
  Inert MC-17, B5
Geocillin Tablets—
  382 mg (143) MC-4, A1
Glipizide MC-10, C6
Glucotrol Tablets—
  5 mg (411) MC-10, C6
  10 mg (412) MC-10, C6
Glyburide MC-10, C7–D1
Grifulvin V Tablets—
  250 mg (211) MC-10, D2
  500 mg (214) MC-10, D2
Griseofulvin. MC-10, D2
Guanabenz MC-10, D3
Guanfacine MC-10, D4
Halcion Tablets—
  0.125 mg (0.125) MC-24, A6
  0.25 mg (0.25) MC-24, A6
Haldol Tablets—
  0.5 mg (½) MC-11, A1
  1 mg (1) MC-11, A1
  2 mg (2) MC-11, A1
  5 mg (5) MC-11, A1
  10 mg (10) MC-11, A1
  20 mg (20) MC-11, A1

Haloperidol MC-10, D5–MC-11, A3
  Barr Tablets—
    0.5 mg (477) MC-10, D5
    1 mg (478) MC-10, D5
    2 mg (479) MC-10, D5
    5 mg (480) MC-10, D5
    10 mg (481) MC-10, D6
    20 mg (482) MC-10, D6
  Geneva Tablets—
    0.5 mg (105) MC-10, D7
    1 mg (123) MC-10, D7
    2 mg (GG 124) MC-10, D7
    5 mg (GG 125) MC-10, D7
    10 mg (GG 126) MC-10, D7
    20 mg (GG 134) MC-10, D7
  Mylan Tablets—
    0.5 mg (351) MC-11, A2
    1 mg (257) MC-11, A2
    2 mg (214) MC-11, A2
    5 mg (327) MC-11, A2
  Purepac Tablets—
    0.5 mg (289) MC-11, A3
    1 mg (280) MC-11, A3
    2 mg (281) MC-11, A3
    5 mg (282) MC-11, A3
    10 mg (286) MC-11, A3
    20 mg (287) MC-11, A3
Halotestin Tablets—
  2 mg (2) MC-10, A7
  5 mg (5) MC-10, A7
  10 mg (10) MC-10, A7
Hismanal Tablets—
  10 mg (Ast 10) MC-2, C2
Hydergine
  Tablets—
    1 mg. MC-8, D5
  Sublingual Tablets—
    0.5 mg MC-8, D6
    1 mg MC-8, D6
Hydergine LC Capsules—
  1 mg (78-101) MC-8, D4
Hydralazine. MC-11, A4–5
  Lederle Tablets—
    25 mg (H11) MC-11, A5
    50 mg (H12) MC-11, A5
Hydralazine and
  Hydrochlorothiazide. MC-11, A6–7
  Reid Rowell Capsules—
    25/25 mg (0665 4410) MC-11, A7
    50/50 mg (0665 4420) ... MC-11, A7
Hydrochlorothiazide. MC-11, B1–5
  Barr Tablets—
    25 mg (555 19). MC-11, B2
    50 mg (555 20). MC-11, B2
    100 mg (555 192) MC-11, B2
  Geneva Tablets—
    25 mg (GG 28) MC-11, B4
    50 mg (GG 27) MC-11, B4
Hydrocodone and
  Acetaminophen. MC-11, B6–7
Hydrocortisone MC-11, C1
HydroDIURIL Tablets—
  25 mg (MSD 42) MC-11, B5
  50 mg (MSD 105) MC-11, B5
  100 mg (MSD 410) MC-11, B5
Hydroxychloroquine. MC-11, C2
Hydroxyzine MC-11, C3–D1
  Geneva Tablets—
    10 mg (37) MC-11, C3
    25 mg (38) MC-11, C3
    50 mg (39) MC-11, C3
  Rugby Tablets—
    10 mg (3874) MC-11, C6
    25 mg (3875) MC-11, C6
    50 mg (3876) MC-11, C6
  Schein Capsules—
    25 mg (069) MC-11, C7
    50 mg (302) MC-11, C7
    100 mg (324) MC-11, C7

Hydroxyzine *(continued)*
  Schein/Danbury Tablets—
    10 mg (5522) MC-11, D1
    25 mg (5523) MC-11, D1
    50 mg (5565) MC-11, D1
Hygroton Tablets—
  25 mg (22) MC-5, B6
  50 mg (20) MC-5, B6
  100 mg (21) MC-5, B6
Hytrin Tablets—
  1 mg (DF) MC-22, A7
  2 mg (DH) MC-22, A7
  5 mg (DJ) MC-22, A7
  10 mg (DI) MC-22, A7
Ibuprofen. MC-11, D2–MC-12, A3
  Barr Tablets—
    400 mg (419) MC-11, D2
    600 mg (420) MC-11, D2
    800 mg (499) MC-11, D2
  Boots Laboratories Tablets—
    400 mg (IBU 400) MC-11, D3
    600 mg (IBU 600) MC-11, D3
    800 mg (IBU 800) MC-11, D3
  Rugby Tablets—
    300 mg (3976) MC-11, D5
    400 mg (3977) MC-11, D5
    600 mg (3978) MC-11, D5
    800 mg (3979) MC-11, D6
  Schein/Danbury Tablets—
    200 mg (5585) MC-11, D7
    400 mg (5584) MC-11, D7
    600 mg (5586) MC-12, A1
    800 mg (5644) MC-12, A1
Ilosone
  Capsules—
    250 mg (H09) MC-9, B1
  Chewable Tablets—
    125 mg (U05) MC-9, B2
    250 mg (U25) MC-9, B2
Imipramine MC-12, A4–6
Imodium Capsules—
  2 mg. MC-13, D3
Imuran Tablets—
  50 mg (50) MC-2, D6
Indapamide. MC-12, A7
Inderal Tablets—
  10 mg (10) MC-20, C5
  20 mg (20) MC-20, C5
  40 mg (40) MC-20, C5
  60 mg (60) MC-20, C6
  80 mg (80) MC-20, C6
Inderal LA Extended-release Capsules—
  60 mg (60) MC-20, C3
  80 mg (80) MC-20, C3
  120 mg (120) MC-20, C4
  160 mg (160) MC-20, C4
Inderide Tablets—
  40/25 mg (40/25) MC-20, D4
  80/25 mg (80/25) MC-20, D4
Inderide LA Extended-release Capsules—
  80/50 mg (80/50) MC-20, D2
  120/50 mg (120/50) MC-20, D2
  160/50 mg (160/50) MC-20, D3
Indocin Capsules—
  25 mg (MSD 25) MC-12, B2
  50 mg (MSD 50) MC-12, B2
Indocin SR Extended-release Capsules—
  75 mg (MSD 693) MC-12, B3
Indomethacin MC-12, B1–3
  Geneva Capsules—
    25 mg (GG 517) MC-12, B1
    50 mg (GG 518) MC-12, B1
Iodinated Glycerol MC-12, B4
Ionamin Capsules—
  15 mg (15) MC-18, D6
  30 mg (30) MC-18, D6
Isoptin Tablets—
  40 mg (40) MC-24, B7
  80 mg (80) MC-24, B7
  120 mg (120) MC-24, B7

Isoptin SR
Extended-release Tablets—
120 mg (120 SR) MC-24, C1
180 mg (180 MG) MC-24, C2
240 mg MC-24, C2
Isordil
Tablets—
5 mg (4152) MC-12, C4
10 mg (4153) MC-12, C4
20 mg (4154) MC-12, C4
30 mg (4159) MC-12, C4
40 mg (4192) MC-12, C4
Extended-release Tablets—
40 mg (4125) MC-12, C5
Sublingual Tablets—
2.5 mg (25) MC-12, C6
5 mg (5) MC-12, C6
10 mg (10) MC-12, C6
Isosorbide Dinitrate MC-12, B5–C6
Isotretinoin MC-12, C7
Isradipine MC-12, D1
Keflex Capsules—
250 mg (H69) MC-4, C2
500 mg (H71) MC-4, C2
Keftab Tablets—
250 mg (250) MC-4, C3
500 mg (500) MC-4, C3
Kerlone Tablets—
10 mg (10) MC-3, B1
20 mg (20) MC-3, B1
Ketoconazole MC-12, D2
Klor-Con Extended-release Tablets—
600 mg (8) MC-19, B5
750 mg (10) MC-19, B5
Klotrix Extended-release Tablets—
750 mg (MJ 10 mEq 770) ... MC-19, B1
K-Tab Extended-release Tablets—
750 mg. MC-19, A7
Labetalol MC-12, D3–4
Labetalol and
Hydrochlorothiazide....... MC-12, D5–6
Lanoxicaps Capsules—
0.05 mg (A2C) MC-7, B5
0.1 mg (B2C) MC-7, B5
0.2 mg (C2C) MC-7, B5
Lanoxin Tablets—
0.125 mg (Y3B) MC-7, B6
0.25 mg (X3A) MC-7, B6
0.5 mg (T9A) MC-7, B6
Lasix Tablets—
20 mg. MC-10, C3
40 mg (40) MC-10, C3
80 mg (80) MC-10, C3
Ledercillin VK Tablets—
250 mg (L 10) MC-18, C3
500 mg (L 9) MC-18, C3
Levatol Tablets—
20 mg (22) MC-18, B5
Levlen 21 Tablets—
0.15/0.03 mg (21) MC-12, D7
Levlen 28 Tablets—
0.15/0.03 mg (21) MC-13, A1
Inert (28). MC-13, A1
Levonorgestrel and Ethinyl
Estradiol   MC-12, D7–MC-13, A7
Levothyroxine MC-13, B1–6
Rugby Tablets—
0.1 mg (3952) MC-13, B5
0.15 mg (3953) MC-13, B5
0.2 mg (3954) MC-13, B5
0.3 mg (3958) MC-13, B5
Schein/Danbury Tablets—
0.1 mg (832 L01) MC-13, B6
0.15 mg (832 L15) MC-13, B6
0.2 mg (832 L02) MC-13, B6
0.3 mg (832 L03) MC-13, B6
Levoxine Tablets—
0.025 mg (dp 25) MC-13, B3
0.05 mg (dp 50) MC-13, B3
0.075 mg (dp 75) MC-13, B3

Levoxine Tablets (continued)
0.088 mg (dp 88) MC-13, B3
0.1 mg (dp 100) MC-13, B3
0.112 mg (dp 112) MC-13, B4
0.125 mg (dp 125) MC-13, B4
0.15 mg (dp 150) MC-13, B4
0.175 mg (dp 175) MC-13, B4
0.2 mg (dp 200) MC-13, B4
0.3 mg (dp 300) MC-13, B4
Librax Capsules—
5/2.5 mg MC-4, D4
Libritabs Tablets—
5 mg (5) MC-4, D1
10 mg (10) MC-4, D1
25 mg (25) MC-4, D1
Librium Capsules—
5 mg (5) MC-4, C7
10 mg (10) MC-4, C7
25 mg (25) MC-4, C7
Limbitrol Tablets—
5/12.5 mg MC-4, D3
10/25 mg MC-4, D3
Lioresal Tablets—
10 mg (23) MC-3, A1
20 mg (33) MC-3, A1
Lisinopril MC-13, B7–C1
Lisinopril and
Hydrochlorothiazide....... MC-13, C2–3
Lithium MC-13, C4–D2
Roxane
Capsules—
150 mg (54 213) MC-13, C5
300 mg (54 463) MC-13, C5
600 mg (54 702) MC-13, C5
Tablets—
300 mg (54 452) MC-13, C6
Lithobid Extended-release Tablets—
300 mg (65) MC-13, C4
Lodine Capsules—
200 mg (200 mg) MC-9, D2
300 mg (300 mg) MC-9, D2
Loestrin 21 1/20 Tablets—
1/0.02 mg (P-D 915) MC-17, A6
Loestrin 21 1.5/30 Tablets—
1.5/0.03 mg (P-D 916) MC-17, A7
Loestrin Fe 1/20 Tablets—
1/0.02 mg (P-D 915) MC-17, B1
75 mg (P-D 622) MC-17, B1
Loestrin Fe 1.5/30 Tablets—
1.5/0.03 mg (P-D 916) MC-17, B2
75 mg (P-D 622) MC-17, B2
Lomotil Tablets—
2.5/0.025 mg (61) MC-7, D3
Loniten Tablets—
2.5 mg (U 121) MC-15, D3
10 mg (10) MC-15, D3
Lo-Ovral-21 Tablets—
0.3/0.03 mg (78) MC-17, B7
Lo-Ovral-28 Tablets—
0.3/0.03 mg (78) MC-17, C1
Inert (486). MC-17, C1
Loperamide................. MC-13, D3
Lopid Tablets—
600 mg MC-10, C5
Lopressor Tablets—
50 mg (51 51) MC-15, B7
100 mg (71 71) MC-15, B7
Lopressor HCT Tablets—
50/25 mg (35 35) MC-15, C1
100/25 mg (53 53) MC-15, C1
100/50 mg (73 73) MC-15, C1
Lopurin Tablets—
100 mg (0051) MC-1, B7
300 mg (0052) MC-1, B7
Lorabid Capsules—
200 mg (3170) MC-3, D3

Lorazepam MC-13, D4–7
Barr Tablets—
0.5 mg (370)............. MC-13, D4
1 mg (371) MC-13, D4
2 mg (372) MC-13, D4
Purepac Tablets—
0.5 mg (57) MC-13, D5
1 mg (59) MC-13, D5
2 mg (063) MC-13, D5
Schein/Danbury Tablets—
0.5 mg (DAN 5625) MC-13, D6
1 mg (DAN 5624) MC-13, D6
2 mg (DAN 5622) MC-13, D6
Lorelco Tablets—
250 mg (250) MC-19, C7
500 mg (500) MC-19, C7
Lotensin Tablets—
5 mg (5) MC-3, A2
10 mg (10) MC-3, A2
20 mg (20) MC-3, A2
40 mg (40) MC-3, A2
Lovastatin MC-14, A1
Lozol Tablets—
2.5 mg (8) MC-12, A7
Ludiomil Tablets—
25 mg (110) MC-14, A2
50 mg (26) MC-14, A2
75 mg (135) MC-14, A2
Lufyllin Tablets—
200 mg (521) MC-8, D1
400 mg (731) MC-8, D1
Macrodantin Capsules—
25 mg (0149 0007) MC-16, C4
50 mg (0149 0008) MC-16, C4
100 mg (0149 0009) MC-16, C4
Maprotiline MC-14, A2
Maxzide Tablets—
37.5/25 mg (M9).......... MC-24, A3
75/50 mg (M8) MC-24, A3
Meclizine................. MC-14, A3–7
Geneva Tablets—
12.5 mg (GG 141)........ MC-14, A3
25 mg (GG 261) MC-14, A3
Rugby Chewable Tablets—
25 mg (0822 0576) MC-14, A6
Schein Tablets—
12.5 mg (034) MC-14, A7
25 mg (035) MC-14, A7
Meclofenamate.............. MC-14, B1–3
Mylan Capsules—
50 mg (2150) MC-14, B1
100 mg (3000) MC-14, B1
Rugby Capsules—
50 mg (4002) MC-14, B3
100 mg (4003) MC-14, B3
Meclomen Capsules—
50 mg (50 PD) MC-4, B2
100 mg (100 PD) MC-4, B2
Medrol Tablets—
2 mg (2) MC-15, A4
4 mg (4) MC-15, A4
8 mg (8) MC-15, A4
16 mg (16) MC-15, A4
24 mg (155) MC-15, A4
32 mg (32) MC-15, A5
Medroxyprogesterone........ MC-14, B4
Mellaril Tablets—
10 mg (78-2)............. MC-23, A6
15 mg (78-8)............. MC-23, A6
25 mg (78-3)............. MC-23, A6
50 mg (78-4)............. MC-23, A6
100 mg (78-5)............ MC-23, A7
150 mg (78-6)............ MC-23, A7
200 mg (78-7)............ MC-23, A7
Meperidine MC-14, B5–6
Barr Tablets—
50 mg (381) MC-14, B5
100 mg (382) MC-14, B5

Metaprotenerol............... MC-14, B7
Methocarbamol.............. MC-14, C1–2
  Geneva Tablets—
    500 mg (GG 190) MC-14, C1
    750 mg (GG 101) MC-14, C1
Methocarbamol and Aspirin.... MC-14, C3
Methyclothiazide MC-14, C4–5
  Geneva Tablets—
    2.5 mg (GG 244)......... MC-14, C5
    5 mg (GG 242) MC-14, C5
Methyldopa.............. MC-14, C6–D3
  Geneva Tablets—
    125 mg (GG 104) MC-14, C6
    250 mg (GG 111) MC-14, C6
    500 mg (GG 471) MC-14, C6
  Purepac Tablets—
    250 mg (253) MC-14, D1
    500 mg (255) MC-14, D1
  Rugby Tablets—
    250 mg (4021) MC-14, D2
    500 mg (4023) MC-14, D2
  Schein/Danbury Tablets—
    250 mg (5588) MC-14, D3
    500 mg (5587) MC-14, D3
Methyldopa and Hydrochloro-
  thiazide MC-14, D4–MC-15, A1
  Geneva Tablets—
    250/15 mg (GG 219) ... MC-14, D4
    250/25 mg (GG 265) ... MC-14, D4
    500/30 mg (GG 243) ... MC-14, D5
    500/50 mg (GG 289) ... MC-14, D5
  Purepac Tablets—
    250/15 mg (261) MC-15, A1
    250/25 mg (263) MC-15, A1
Methylphenidate.......... MC-15, A2–3
Methylprednisolone MC-15, A4–5
Metoclopramide MC-15, A6–B2
  Purepac Tablets—
    10 mg (269) MC-15, A6
  Rugby Tablets—
    10 mg (4042) MC-15, B1
  Schein/Danbury Tablets—
    10 mg (5589) MC-15, B2
Metolazone MC-15, B3–5
Metoprolol............... MC-15, B6–7
Metoprolol and
  Hydrochlorothiazide..... MC-15, C1
Metronidazole............. MC-15, C2–5
  Geneva Tablets—
    250 mg (GG 103) MC-15, C2
    500 mg (GG 195) MC-15, C2
  Rugby Tablets—
    250 mg (4018) MC-15, C3
    500 mg (4019) MC-15, C3
  Schein/Danbury Tablets—
    250 mg (5540) MC-15, C4
    500 mg (5552) MC-15, C4
Mevacor Tablets—
  20 mg (MSD 731) MC-14, A1
  40 mg (MSD 732)........ MC-14, A1
Micro-K Extended-release Capsules—
  600 mg (AHR 5720)....... MC-19, B2
  750 mg (AHR 5730)....... MC-19, B2
Micronase Tablets—
  1.25 mg (1.25) MC-10, D1
  2.5 mg (2.5) MC-10, D1
  5 mg (5) MC-10, D1
Minipress Capsules—
  1 mg (431) MC-19, C1
  2 mg (437) MC-19, C1
  5 mg (438) MC-19, C1
Minizide Capsules—
  1/0.5 mg (430) MC-19, C4
  2/0.5 mg (432)......... MC-19, C4
  5/0.5 mg (436)......... MC-19, C4
Minocin
  Capsules—
    50 mg (M 45)........ MC-15, C6
    100 mg (M 46).......... MC-15, C6

Minocin (continued)
  Tablets—
    50 mg (M 3)............. MC-15, C7
    100 mg (M 5)............ MC-15, C7
Minocycline............ MC-15, C6–D1
  Warner Chilcott Capsules—
    50 mg (WC 615) MC-15, D1
    100 mg (WC 616) MC-15, D1
Minoxidil.............. MC-15, D2–3
  Schein/Danbury Tablets—
    2.5 mg (DAN 5642) MC-15, D2
    10 mg (DAN 5643)....... MC-15, D2
Misoprostol............... MC-15, D4
Moduretic Tablets—
  5/50 mg (MSD 917)........ MC-1, C7
Monopril Tablets—
  10 mg (158) MC-10, C1
  20 mg (609) MC-10, C1
Moricizine................. MC-15, D5–6
Motrin Tablets—
  300 mg (300mg)......... MC-12, A2
  400 mg (400mg)......... MC-12, A2
  600 mg (600mg)......... MC-12, A3
  800 mg (800mg)......... MC-12, A3
Mycelex Troche Lozenges—
  10 mg (095) MC-6, B5
Mykrox Tablets—
  0.5 mg (½) MC-15, B3
Nadolol MC-15, D7–MC-16, A1
Nadolol and
  Bendroflumethiazide MC-16, A2
Naldecon Extended-release Tablets—
  40/10/15/5 mg (BL N1) MC-4, D7
Nalfon
  Capsules—
    200 mg (H76)....... MC-9, D5
    300 mg (H77)............ MC-9, D5
  Tablets—
    600 mg. MC-9, D6
Nalidixic Acid MC-16, A3–4
Naprosyn Tablets—
  250 mg (250) MC-16, A5
  375 mg (375) MC-16, A5
  500 mg (500) MC-16, A5
Naproxen MC-16, A5
Naproxen Sodium MC-16, A6
Naturetin Tablets—
  5 mg (PPP 606) MC-3, A3
  10 mg (PPP 618) MC-3, A3
Navane Capsules—
  1 mg (571) MC-23, B4
  2 mg (572) MC-23, B4
  5 mg (573) MC-23, B4
  10 mg (574) MC-23, B5
  20 mg (577) MC-23, B5
NegGram Tablets—
  250 mg (N 21) MC-16, A3
  500 mg (N 22) MC-16, A3
  1 gram (N 23) MC-16, A4
Niacin MC-16, A7–B3
Nicardipine MC-16, B4
Nicobid Extended-release Capsules—
  125 mg (125) MC-16, A7
  250 mg (250) MC-16, A7
  500 mg (500) MC-16, B1
Nicolar Tablets—
  500 mg (NE) MC-16, B2
Nicorette Chewing Gum Tablets—
  2 mg. MC-16, B5
Nicotine................. MC-16, B5
Nifedipine MC-16, B6–C2
  Purepac Capsules—
    10 mg (R 497) MC-16, C2
    20 mg (R 530) MC-16, C2
Nimodipine MC-16, C3
Nimotop Capsules—
  30 mg (855) MC-16, C3

Nitrofurantoin.............. MC-16, C4–5
Nitroglycerin............ MC-16, C6–D1
  Geneva Extended-release Capsules—
    2.5 mg (GG 511) MC-16, C6
    6.5 mg (GG 501) MC-16, C6
    9 mg (GG 512) MC-16, C7
Nitrostat Sublingual Tablets—
  0.15 mg................. MC-16, D1
  0.3 mg.................. MC-16, D1
  0.4 mg.................. MC-16, D1
  0.6 mg.................. MC-16, D1
Nizatidine MC-16, D2
Nizoral Tablets—
  200 mg. MC-12, D2
Nolvadex Tablets—
  10 mg (600) MC-22, A2
Nordette-21 Tablets—
  0.15/0.03 mg (75) MC-13, A4
Nordette-28 Tablets—
  0.15/0.03 mg (75) MC-13, A5
  Inert (486). MC-13, A5
Norethindrone and Ethinyl
  Estradiol MC-16, D3–MC-17, A5
Norethindrone Acetate and Ethinyl
  Estradiol MC-17, A6–7
Norethindrone Acetate/Ethinyl Estradiol
  and Ferrous Fumarate..... MC-17, B1–2
Norethindrone and
  Mestranol MC-17, B3–5
Norfloxacin.............. MC-17, B6
Norgestrel and Ethinyl
  Estradiol MC-17, B7–C3
Normodyne Tablets—
  100 mg (244) MC-12, D4
  200 mg (752) MC-12, D4
  300 mg (438) MC-12, D4
Normozide Tablets—
  100/25 mg (235 235) MC-12, D6
  200/25 mg (227 227) MC-12, D6
  300/25 mg (391 391) MC-12, D6
Noroxin Tablets—
  400 mg (MSD 705)........ MC-17, B6
Norpace Capsules—
  100 mg (2752) MC-8, A3
  150 mg (2762) MC-8, A3
Norpace CR Extended-release Capsules—
  100 mg (2732) MC-8, A4
  150 mg (2742) MC-8, A4
Norpramin Tablets—
  10 mg (68-7) MC-6, D1
  25 mg (25) MC-6, D1
  50 mg (50) MC-6, D1
  75 mg (75) MC-6, D2
  100 mg (100) MC-6, D2
  150 mg (150) MC-6, D2
Nortriptyline............. MC-17, C4–5
Ofloxacin................. MC-17, C6–7
Ogen Tablets—
  0.75 mg (LU) MC-9, C4
  1.5 mg (LV) MC-9, C4
  3 mg (LX). MC-9, C4
  6 mg (LY). MC-9, C4
Omeprazole MC-17, D1
Omnipen Capsules—
  250 mg (53) MC-2, B6
  500 mg (309) MC-2, B6
Oretic Tablets—
  25 mg. MC-11, B1
  50 mg. MC-11, B1
Organidin Tablets—
  30 mg (37-4224)............ MC-12, B4
Orinase Tablets—
  250 mg (250) MC-23, C5
  500 mg (500) MC-23, C5
Ornade Extended-release Capsules—
  75/12 mg (SKF) MC-4, D6
Ortho-Novum 1/35-21 Tablets—
  1/0.035 mg (135)........... MC-16, D7

Ortho-Novum 1/35-28 Tablets—
  1/0.035 mg (135)............ MC-17, A1
  Inert....................... MC-17, A1
Ortho-Novum 1/50-21 Tablets—
  1/0.05 mg (150)............. MC-17, B3
Ortho-Novum 1/50-28 Tablets—
  1/0.05 mg (150)............. MC-17, B4
  Inert....................... MC-17, B4
Ortho-Novum 7/7/7-21 Tablets—
  0.5/0.035 mg (535)......... MC-17, A2
  0.75/0.035 mg (75)......... MC-17, A2
  1/0.035 mg (135)........... MC-17, A2
Ortho-Novum 7/7/7-28 Tablets—
  0.5/0.035 mg (535)......... MC-17, A3
  0.75/0.035 mg (75)......... MC-17, A3
  1/0.035 mg (135)........... MC-17, A3
  Inert....................... MC-17, A3
Ovcon 35-21 Tablets—
  0.4/0.035 mg (583)......... MC-16, D3
Ovcon 35-28 Tablets—
  0.4/0.035 mg (583)......... MC-16, D4
  Inert (850)................. MC-16, D4
Ovcon 50-21 Tablets—
  1/0.05 mg (584)............ MC-16, D5
Ovcon 50-28 Tablets—
  1/0.05 mg (584)............ MC-16, D6
  Inert (850)................. MC-16, D6
Ovral-21 Tablets—
  0.5/0.05 mg (56)........... MC-17, C2
Ovral-28 Tablets—
  0.5/0.05 mg (56)........... MC-17, C3
  Inert (445)................. MC-17, C3
Oxacillin....................... MC-17, D2
Oxazepam........ MC-17, D3–MC-18, A1
  Barr
   Capsules—
    10 mg (374)............ MC-17, D3
    15 mg (375)............ MC-17, D3
    30 mg (376)............ MC-17, D3
   Tablets—
    15 mg (373)............ MC-17, D4
  Purepac Capsules—
   10 mg (067)............. MC-17, D5
   15 mg (069)............. MC-17, D5
   30 mg (073)............. MC-17, D5
  Schein/Danbury Capsules—
   10 mg (DAN 5617)....... MC-17, D6
   15 mg (DAN 5616)....... MC-17, D6
   30 mg (DAN 5618)....... MC-17, D6
Oxybutynin...................... MC-18, A2
Oxycodone...................... MC-18, A3
Oxycodone and
  Acetaminophen........... MC-18, A4–6
Oxycodone and Aspirin.... MC-18, A7–B2
Pamelor Capsules—
  10 mg (78-86)............. MC-17, C4
  25 mg (78-87)............. MC-17, C4
  50 mg (78-78)............. MC-17, C5
  75 mg (78-79)............. MC-17, C5
Pancrease Delayed-release Capsules—
  4/12/12*.................. MC-18, B3
  4/20/25* (MT 4)........... MC-18, B3
  10/30/30* (MT 10)......... MC-18, B3
  16/48/48* (MT 16)......... MC-18, B4
  25/75/75* (MT 25)......... MC-18, B4
Pancrelipase............... MC-18, B3–4
Panmycin Capsules—
  250 mg (250 mg).......... MC-22, C2
Parafon Forte DSC Tablets—
  500 mg....................... MC-5, C1
Parlodel
  Capsules—
   5 mg (78-102)............. MC-3, B2
  Tablets—
   2.5 mg (78-17)............ MC-3, B3
Parnate Tablets—
  10 mg...................... MC-23, D4
PCE Delayed-release Tablets—
  333 mg...................... MC-9, A4

Penbutolol................... MC-18, B5
Penicillin V............ MC-18, B6–C5
  Biocraft Tablets—
   250 mg Round (15)....... MC-18, C1
   250 mg Oval (16)........ MC-18, C1
   500 mg Round (17)....... MC-18, C2
   500 mg Oval (49)........ MC-18, C2
Pentazocine and
  Acetaminophen........... MC-18, C6
Pentazocine and Naloxone..... MC-18, C7
Pentoxifylline.............. MC-18, D1
Pen-Vee K Tablets—
  250 mg (59)............... MC-18, C5
  500 mg (390).............. MC-18, C5
Pepcid Tablets—
  20 mg (MSD 963).......... MC-9, D3
  40 mg (MSD 964).......... MC-9, D3
Percocet Tablets—
  5/325 mg.................. MC-18, A4
Percodan Tablets—
  4.88/325 mg............... MC-18, A7
Percodan-Demi Tablets—
  2.44/325 mg............... MC-18, B1
Perphenazine and
  Amitriptyline........... MC-18, D2–3
Persantine Tablets—
  25 mg (BI 17)............. MC-7, D5
  50 mg (BI 18)............. MC-7, D5
  75 mg (BI 19)............. MC-7, D5
Phenaphen with Codeine
  Capsules—
   325/15 mg (AHR 6242).... MC-1, A4
   325/30 mg (AHR 6257).... MC-1, A4
   325/60 mg (AHR 6274).... MC-1, A5
  Tablets—
   650/30 mg (6251)......... MC-1, A6
Phenazopyridine.............. MC-18, D4
Phenergan Tablets—
  12.5 mg (19).............. MC-20, A5
  25 mg (27)................ MC-20, A5
  50 mg (227)............... MC-20, A5
Phenobarbital............... MC-18, D5
  Warner Chilcott Tablets—
   15 mg (WC 699).......... MC-18, D5
   30 mg (WC 700).......... MC-18, D5
   60 mg (WC 607).......... MC-18, D5
   100 mg (WC 698)......... MC-18, D5
Phentermine................. MC-18, D6
Phenylephrine, Phenylpropanolamine, and
  Guaifenesin............. MC-18, D7
Phenylpropanolamine and
  Caramiphen.............. MC-19, A1
Phenylpropanolamine and
  Guaifenesin............. MC-19, A2
Phenytoin................... MC-19, A3
Phenytoin Sodium............ MC-19, A4
Pindolol.................... MC-19, A5
Piroxicam................... MC-19, A6
Plaquenil Tablets—
  200 mg..................... MC-11, C2
Plendil Tablets—
  5 mg (MSD 451)............ MC-9, D4
  10 mg (MSD 452)........... MC-9, D4
Polycillin Capsules—
  250 mg (7992)............. MC-2, B5
  500 mg (7993)............. MC-2, B5
Polymox Capsules—
  250 mg (7278)............. MC-2, A4
  500 mg (7279)............. MC-2, A4
Potassium Chloride..... MC-19, A7–B5
Pravachol Tablets—
  10 mg (10)................ MC-19, B6
  20 mg (20)................ MC-19, B6
Pravastatin................. MC-19, B6
Prazepam.................... MC-19, B7
Prazosin................. MC-19, C1–3
  Purepac Capsules—
   1 mg (500)............... MC-19, C2
   2 mg (501)............... MC-19, C2
   5 mg (502)............... MC-19, C2

Prazosin *(continued)*
  Schein/Danbury Capsules—
   1 mg (DAN 5697)........ MC-19, C3
   2 mg (DAN 5696)........ MC-19, C3
   5 mg (DAN 5693)........ MC-19, C3
Prazosin and Polythiazide.... MC-19, C4
Prednisone.............. MC-19, C5–6
  Rugby Tablets—
   5 mg.................... MC-19, C5
   10 mg (4325)............ MC-19, C5
   20 mg (4326)............ MC-19, C5
   50 mg................... MC-19, C5
Premarin Tablets—
  0.3 mg (0.3).............. MC-9, C2
  0.625 mg (0.625).......... MC-9, C2
  0.9 mg (0.9).............. MC-9, C2
  1.25 mg (1.25)............ MC-9, C3
  2.5 mg (2.5).............. MC-9, C3
Prilosec Delayed-release Capsules—
  20 mg (MSD 742).......... MC-17, D1
Prinivil Tablets—
  5 mg (MSD 19)............ MC-13, B7
  10 mg (MSD 106).......... MC-13, B7
  20 mg (MSD 207).......... MC-13, B7
  40 mg (MSD 237).......... MC-13, B7
Prinzide Tablets—
  20/12.5 mg (MSD 140)..... MC-13, C2
  20/25 mg (MSD 142)....... MC-13, C2
Pro-Banthine Tablets—
  7.5 mg (611).............. MC-20, A7
  15 mg (601)............... MC-20, A7
Probucol.................... MC-19, C7
Procainamide..... MC-19, D1–MC-20, A2
  Geneva
   Capsules—
    250 mg (GG 551)....... MC-19, D1
    375 mg (GG 552)....... MC-19, D1
    500 mg (GG 553)....... MC-19, D1
   Extended-release Tablets—
    250 mg (GG 472)....... MC-19, D2
    500 mg (GG 473)....... MC-19, D2
    750 mg (GG 474)....... MC-19, D2
  Schein/Danbury
   Capsules—
    250 mg (DAN 5026).... MC-20, A1
    375 mg (DAN 5350).... MC-20, A1
    500 mg (DAN 5333).... MC-20, A1
   Extended-release Tablets—
    250 mg (5562)......... MC-20, A2
    500 mg (55 63)........ MC-20, A2
    750 mg (55 64)........ MC-20, A2
Procan SR Extended-release Tablets—
  250 mg (P-D 202)......... MC-19, D3
  500 mg (P-D 204)......... MC-19, D3
  750 mg (P-D 205)......... MC-19, D4
  1 gram (P-D 207).......... MC-19, D4
Procardia Capsules—
  10 mg (260)............... MC-16, B7
  20 mg (261)............... MC-16, B7
Procardia XL Extended-release Tablets—
  30 mg (30)................ MC-16, C1
  60 mg (60)................ MC-16, C1
  90 mg (90)................ MC-16, C1
Prochlorperazine......... MC-20, A3–4
Prolixin Tablets—
  1 mg (PPP 863)............ MC-10, B2
  2.5 mg (PPP 864).......... MC-10, B2
  5 mg (PPP 877)............ MC-10, B2
  10 mg (PPP 956)........... MC-10, B2
Proloprim Tablets—
  100 mg (09A).............. MC-24, B3
  200 mg (200).............. MC-24, B3
Promethazine................ MC-20, A5
Pronestyl
  Capsules—
   250 mg (758)............. MC-19, D5
   375 mg (756)............. MC-19, D5
   500 mg (757)............. MC-19, D5

Pronestyl (continued)
Tablets—
  250 mg (431) MC-19, D6
  375 mg (434) MC-19, D6
  500 mg (438) MC-19, D6
Pronestyl-SR Extended-release Tablets—
  500 mg (PPP 775) MC-19, D7
Propafenone MC-20, A6
Propantheline MC-20, A7
Propoxyphene Napsylate and
  Acetaminophen.......... MC-20, B1–4
  Barr Tablets—
    50/325 mg (317) MC-20, B1
    100/650 mg Pink
      (470) MC-20, B1
    100/650 mg White
      (318) MC-20, B1
  Mylan Tablets—
    100/650 mg Pink
      (155) MC-20, B3
    100/650 mg White
      (521) MC-20, B3
  Purepac Tablets—
    100/650 mg (085) MC-20, B4
Propranolol MC-20, B5–C6
  Geneva Tablets—
    10 mg (GG 71) MC-20, B5
    20 mg (GG 72) MC-20, B5
    40 mg (GG 73) MC-20, B5
    60 mg (GG 74) MC-20, B5
    80 mg (GG 75) MC-20, B5
  Lederle Tablets—
    10 mg (P 44) MC-20, B6
    20 mg (P 45) MC-20, B6
    40 mg (P 46) MC-20, B6
    60 mg (P 65) MC-20, B6
    80 mg (P 47) MC-20, B6
  Purepac Tablets—
    10 mg (27) MC-20, B7
    20 mg (29) MC-20, B7
    40 mg (331) MC-20, B7
    60 mg (321) MC-20, B7
    80 mg (333) MC-20, B7
  Rugby Tablets—
    10 mg (4309) MC-20, C1
    20 mg (4313) MC-20, C1
    40 mg (4314) MC-20, C1
    60 mg (4315) MC-20, C1
    80 mg (4316) MC-20, C1
  Schein/Danbury Tablets—
    10 mg (DAN 5554) MC-20, C2
    20 mg (DAN 5555) MC-20, C2
    40 mg (DAN 5556) MC-20, C2
    60 mg (127) MC-20, C2
    80 mg (DAN 5557) MC-20, C2
Propranolol and
  Hydrochlorothiazide..... MC-20, C7–D4
  Purepac Tablets—
    40/25 mg (358) MC-20, C7
    80/25 mg (360) MC-20, C7
  Rugby Tablets—
    40/25 mg (4402) MC-20, D1
    80/25 mg (4403) MC-20, D1
ProSom Tablets—
  1 mg (UC) MC-9, B7
  2 mg (UD) MC-9, B7
Prostaphlin Capsules—
  250 mg (7977) MC-17, D2
  500 mg (7982) MC-17, D2
Proventil
  Tablets—
    2 mg (252 252)......... MC-1, B5
    4 mg (573 573)......... MC-1, B5
  Extended-release Tablets—
    4 mg (431) MC-1, B6
Provera Tablets—
  2.5 mg (2.5) MC-14, B4
  5 mg (5) MC-14, B4
  10 mg (10) MC-14, B4

Prozac Capsules—
  20 mg (3105) MC-10, A6
Pyridium Tablets—
  100 mg (P-D 180) MC-18, D4
  200 mg (P-D 181) MC-18, D4
Quazepam................. MC-20, D5
Quibron Capsules—
  150/90 mg (516) MC-23, A1
  300/180 mg (515) MC-23, A1
Quibron-T Dividose Tablets—
  300 mg (BL 512) MC-22, C4
Quibron-T/SR Dividose Extended-release
  Tablets—
    300 mg (BL 519) MC-22, C5
Quinaglute Extended-release Tablets—
  324 mg.................. MC-20, D7
Quinapril MC-20, D6
Quinidex Extended-release Tablets—
  300 mg (AHR).......... MC-21, A3
Quinidine
  Gluconate MC-20, D7–MC-21, A1
  Schein/Danbury Extended-release Tab-
    lets—
      324 mg (5538) MC-21, A1
  Quinidine Sulfate MC-21, A2–3
  Mutual Tablets—
    200 mg (MP 108) MC-21, A2
    300 mg (MP 124) MC-21, A2
Ramipril MC-21, A4
Ranitidine MC-21, A5
Reglan Tablets—
  5 mg (5) MC-15, A7
  10 mg (AHR 10) MC-15, A7
Regroton Tablets—
  0.25/50 mg (31).......... MC-21, A7
Reserpine and
  Chlorthalidone MC-21, A6–7
Reserpine, Hydralazine, and
  Hydrochlorothiazide........ MC-21, B1
Restoril Capsules—
  15 mg (78-98) MC-22, A6
  30 mg (78-99) MC-22, A6
Retrovir Capsules—
  100 mg (Y9C 100)......... MC-24, D7
Ridaura Capsules—
  3 mg.................... MC-2, D4
Ritalin Tablets—
  5 mg (7) MC-15, A2
  10 mg (3) MC-15, A2
  20 mg (34) MC-15, A2
Ritalin-SR Extended-release Tablets—
  20 mg (16) MC-15, A3
Robaxin Tablets—
  500 mg (AHR)........... MC-14, C2
  750 mg (750) MC-14, C2
Robaxisal Tablets—
  400/325 mg (AHR)......... MC-14, C3
Rocaltrol Capsules—
  0.25 mcg (.25) MC-3, C5
  0.5 mcg (.5) MC-3, C5
Roxicet Tablets—
  5/325 mg (543) MC-18, A6
  5/500 mg (54 730) MC-18, A6
Roxicodone Tablets—
  5 mg (54 582) MC-18, A3
Roxiprin Tablets—
  4.88/325 mg (54 902) MC-18, B2
Rufen Tablets—
  400 mg (400) MC-11, D4
  600 mg (6) MC-11, D4
  800 mg (8) MC-11, D4
Rynatan Tablets—
  25/8/25 mg (37-0713) MC-5, A4
Rythmol Tablets—
  150 mg (150) MC-20, A6
  300 mg (300) MC-20, A6
Seldane Tablets—
  60 mg MC-22, B2
Seldane-D Tablets—
  60/120 mg MC-22, B3

Selegiline.............. MC-21, B2
Septra Tablets—
  400/80 mg (Y2B) MC-21, C7
  800/160 mg (DS 02C) ... MC-21, C7
Ser-Ap-Es Tablets—
  0.1/25/15 mg (71)......... MC-21, B1
Serax
  Capsules—
    10 mg (51) MC-17, D7
    15 mg (6) MC-17, D7
    30 mg (52) MC-17, D7
  Tablets—
    15 mg (317) MC-18, A1
Sertraline................. MC-21, B3
Simvastatin............... MC-21, B4
Sinemet Tablets—
  10/100 mg (647) MC-4, A2
  25/100 mg (650) MC-4, A2
  25/250 mg (654) MC-4, A2
Sinequan Capsules—
  10 mg (534) MC-8, B1
  25 mg (535) MC-8, B1
  50 mg (536) MC-8, B1
  75 mg (539) MC-8, B2
  100 mg (538) MC-8, B2
  150 mg (537) MC-8, B2
Slo-bid Extended-release Capsules—
  50 mg (WHR 50 mg) MC-22, D2
  75 mg (75) MC-22, D2
  100 mg (WHR 100) MC-22, D2
  125 mg (125) MC-22, D2
  200 mg (WHR 200) MC-22, D3
  300 mg (WHR 300) MC-22, D3
Slo-Niacin Extended-release Tablets—
  250 mg (250) MC-16, B3
  500 mg (500) MC-16, B3
  750 mg (750) MC-16, B3
Slo-Phyllin
  Extended-release Capsules—
    60 mg (WHR 1354) MC-22, D4
    125 mg (WHR 1355) MC-22, D4
    250 mg (WHR 1356) MC-22, D4
  Tablets—
    100 mg (WHR 351) MC-22, D5
    200 mg (WHR 352) MC-22, D5
Slow-K Extended-release Tablets—
  600 mg................. MC-19, B3
Soma Tablets—
  350 mg (37-2001)......... MC-4, A3
Soma Compound Tablets—
  200/325 mg (2103) MC-4, A4
Soma Compound with Codeine Tablets—
  200/325/16 mg (2403) MC-4, A5
Sorbitrate
  Tablets—
    5 mg (770) MC-12, B5
    10 mg (780) MC-12, B5
    20 mg (820) MC-12, B5
    30 mg (773) MC-12, B6
    40 mg (774) MC-12, B6
  Chewable Tablets—
    5 mg (810) MC-12, B7
    10 mg (815) MC-12, B7
  Sublingual Tablets—
    2.5 mg (853) MC-12, C2
    5 mg (760) MC-12, C2
    10 mg (761) MC-12, C2
Sorbitrate SA Extended-release Tablets—
  40 mg (880) MC-12, C1
Spironolactone MC-21, B5–C1
  Geneva Tablets—
    25 mg (GG 85) MC-21, B5
  Mutual Tablets—
    25 mg (MP 35) MC-21, B6
  Purepac Tablets—
    25 mg (388) MC-21, B7
Spironolactone and
  Hydrochlorothiazide....... MC-21, C2–5
  Geneva Tablets—
    25/25 mg (GG 95) MC-21, C2

Spironolactone and Hydrochlorothiazide
  (continued)
    Mutual Tablets—
      25/25 mg (MP 40) MC-21, C3
    Schein/Danbury Tablets—
      25/25 mg (5496) MC-21, C4
Stelazine Tablets—
    2 mg (S04) MC-24, B1
Sucralfate MC-21, C6
Sulfamethoxazole and
  Trimethoprim MC-21, C7–D2
    Schein/Danbury Tablets—
      400/80 mg (5546) MC-21, D2
      800/160 mg (5547) MC-21, D2
Sulfasalazine MC-21, D3–4
Sulindac MC-21, D5–MC-22, A1
    Mutual Tablets—
      150 mg (MP 112) MC-21, D6
      200 mg (MP 116) MC-21, D6
    Schein/Danbury Tablets—
      150 mg (5661) MC-21, D7
      200 mg (5660) MC-21, D7
    Warner Chilcott Tablets—
      150 mg (WC 773) MC-22, A1
      200 mg (WC 774) MC-22, A1
Sumycin
    Capsules—
      250 mg (655) MC-22, B4
      500 mg (763) MC-22, B4
    Tablets—
      250 mg (663) MC-22, B5
      500 mg (603) MC-22, B5
Suprax Tablets—
    200 mg (LL 200) MC-4, B3
    400 mg (400) MC-4, B3
Surmontil Capsules—
    25 mg (4132) MC-24, B4
    50 mg (4133) MC-24, B4
    100 mg (4158) MC-24, B4
Symmetrel Capsules—
    100 mg. MC-1, C6
Synalgos-DC Capsules—
    16/356.4/30 mg (4191) MC-2, B7
Synthroid Tablets—
    0.025 mg (25) MC-13, B1
    0.05 mg (50) MC-13, B1
    0.075 mg (75) MC-13, B1
    0.1 mg (100) MC-13, B1
    0.112 mg (112) MC-13, B1
    0.125 mg (125) MC-13, B2
    0.15 mg (150) MC-13, B2
    0.175 mg (175) MC-13, B2
    0.2 mg (200) MC-13, B2
    0.3 mg (300) MC-13, B2
Tagamet Tablets—
    200 mg (200 SKF) MC-5, C3
    300 mg (300 SKF) MC-5, C3
    400 mg (400 SKF) MC-5, C4
    800 mg (800 SKF) MC-5, C4
Talacen Tablets—
    25/650 mg (T37) MC-18, C6
Talwin Nx Tablets—
    50/0.5 mg (T 51) MC-18, C7
Tamoxifen MC-22, A2
Tavist Tablets—
    1.34 mg (78-75) MC-5, D1
    2.68 mg (78-72) MC-5, D1
Tavist-D Tablets—
    1.34/75 mg (78-221) MC-5, D2
Tegopen Capsules—
    250 mg (7935) MC-6, B6
    500 mg (7496) MC-6, B6
Tegretol
    Tablets—
      200 mg (27 27) MC-3, D4
    Chewable Tablets—
      100 mg (52) MC-3, D5

Temazepam MC-22, A3–6
    Barr Capsules—
      15 mg (487) MC-22, A3
      30 mg (488) MC-22, A3
    Mylan Capsules—
      15 mg (4010) MC-22, A4
      30 mg (5050) MC-22, A4
    Purepac Capsules—
      15 mg (076) MC-22, A5
      30 mg (077) MC-22, A5
Tenex Tablets—
    1 mg (1) MC-10, D4
    2 mg (2) MC-10, D4
Ten-K Extended-release Tablets—
    750 mg. MC-19, B4
Tenoretic Tablets—
    50/25 mg (115) MC-2, C7
    100/25 mg (117) MC-2, C7
Tenormin Tablets—
    25 mg (107) MC-2, C4
    50 mg (105) MC-2, C4
    100 mg (101) MC-2, C4
Tenuate
    Tablets—
      25 mg (25) MC-7, B2
    Extended-release Tablets—
      75 mg (75) MC-7, B3
Terazosin MC-22, A7
Terbutaline MC-22, B1
Terfenadine MC-22, B2
Terfenadine and
  Pseodoephedrine MC-22, B3
Tetracycline MC-22, B4–C3
    Purepac Capsules—
      250 mg (404) MC-22, B7
      500 mg (406) MC-22, B7
    Schein Capsules—
      250 mg Blue/Yellow
        (H 214) MC-22, C1
      250 mg Orange/Yellow
        (DAN 5162) MC-22, C1
      500 mg (H 203) MC-22, C1
    Warner Chilcott Capsules—
      250 mg (WC 407) MC-22, C3
      500 mg (WC 697) MC-22, C3
Thalitone Tablets—
    25 mg (76) MC-5, B5
Theo-24 Extended-release Capsules—
    100 mg (2832) MC-22, D6
    200 mg (2842) MC-22, D6
    300 mg (2852) MC-22, D6
Theobid Extended-release Capsules—
    130 mg. MC-22, D7
    260 mg (260) MC-22, D7
Theo-Dur Extended-release Tablets—
    100 mg (100) MC-22, D1
    200 mg (200) MC-22, D1
    300 mg (300) MC-22, D1
Theo-Dur Sprinkle Extended-release
    Capsules—
      50 mg (50) MC-22, C6
      75 mg (75) MC-22, C6
      125 mg (125) MC-22, C7
      200 mg (200) MC-22, C7
Theophylline MC-22, C4–D7
Theophylline and Guaifenesin .. MC-23, A1
Thioridazine MC-23, A2–B2
    Barr Tablets—
      10 mg (260) MC-23, A2
      25 mg (261) MC-23, A2
      50 mg (262) MC-23, A2
      100 mg (263) MC-23, A2
      150 mg (327) MC-23, A3
      200 mg (328) MC-23, A3
    Geneva Tablets—
      150 mg (GG 35) MC-23, A4
      200 mg (GG 36) MC-23, A4

Thioridazine *(continued)*
    Mylan Tablets—
      10 mg (M 54) MC-23, A5
      25 mg (M 58) MC-23, A5
      50 mg (M 59) MC-23, A5
      100 mg (M 61) MC-23, A5
    Schein/Danbury Tablets—
      10 mg (5566) MC-23, B1
      25 mg (5542) MC-23, B1
      50 mg (5568) MC-23, B1
      100 mg (5569) MC-23, B2
      150 mg (5580) MC-23, B2
      200 mg (5581) MC-23, B2
Thiothixene MC-23, B3–6
    Geneva Capsules—
      1 mg (GG 589) MC-23, B3
      2 mg (GG 596) MC-23, B3
      5 mg (GG 597) MC-23, B3
      10 mg (GG 598) MC-23, B3
    Schein/Danbury Capsules—
      1 mg (5593) MC-23, B6
      2 mg (5592) MC-23, B6
      5 mg (5595) MC-23, B6
      10 mg (5594) MC-23, B6
Thorazine
    Extended-release Capsules—
      75 mg (T64) MC-5, A6
    Tablets—
      25 mg (T74) MC-5, A7
Tigan Capsules—
    100 mg (100) MC-24, B2
    250 mg (250) MC-24, B2
Timolol MC-23, B7–C1
    Mylan Tablets—
      5 mg (M 55) MC-23, C1
      10 mg (M 221) MC-23, C1
      20 mg (715) MC-23, C1
Tocainide MC-23, C2
Tofranil Tablets—
    10 mg (32) MC-12, A6
    25 mg (140) MC-12, A6
    50 mg (136) MC-12, A6
Tofranil-PM Capsules—
    75 mg (20) MC-12, A4
    100 mg (40) MC-12, A4
    125 mg (45) MC-12, A5
    150 mg (22) MC-12, A5
Tolazamide MC-23, C3–4
    Geneva Tablets—
      100 mg (GG 270) MC-23, C3
      250 mg (GG 271) MC-23, C3
      500 mg (GG 272) MC-23, C3
Tolbutamide MC-23, C5
Tolectin Tablets—
    200 mg (200) MC-23, C7
    600 mg (600) MC-23, C7
Tolectin DS Capsules—
    400 mg. MC-23, C6
Tolinase Tablets—
    100 mg (100) MC-23, C4
    250 mg (250) MC-23, C4
    500 mg (500) MC-23, C4
Tolmetin MC-23, C6–D3
    Mutual
    Capsules—
      400 mg (179) MC-23, D1
    Tablets—
      200 mg (MP 50) ... MC-23, D2
    Purepac Capsules—
      400 mg (R 520) MC-23, D3
Tonocard Tablets—
    400 mg (MSD 707) MC-23, C2
    600 mg (MSD 709) MC-23, C2
Toprol XL Extended-release Tablets—
    50 mg (MO) MC-15, B6
    100 mg (MS) MC-15, B6
    200 mg (MY) MC-15, B6
Totacillin Capsules—
    250 mg (BMP 140) MC-2, B4
    500 mg (BMP 141) MC-2, B4

Trandate Tablets—
  100 mg (100) MC-12, D3
  200 mg (200) MC-12, D3
  300 mg (300) MC-12, D3
Trandate HCT Tablets—
  100/25 mg (371) MC-12, D5
  200/25 mg (372) MC-12, D5
  300/25 mg (373) MC-12, D5
Tranxene SD Tablets—
  11.25 mg (TX) MC-6, B1
  22.5 mg (TY) MC-6, B1
Tranxene T-Tab Tablets—
  3.75 mg (TL) MC-6, B2
  7.5 mg (TM) MC-6, B2
  15 mg (TN) MC-6, B2
Tranylcypromine............ MC-23, D4
Trazodone MC-23, D5–7
  Purepac Tablets—
    50 mg (439) MC-23, D6
    100 mg (441) MC-23, D6
  Schein/Danbury Tablets—
    50 mg (5600) MC-23, D7
    100 mg (5599) MC-23, D7
Trental Extended-release Tablets—
  400 mg.................. MC-18, D1
Triamterene and
  Hydrochlorothiazide....... MC-24, A1–5
  Barr Tablets—
    75/50 mg (555 444) MC-24, A1
  Geneva Tablets—
    75/50 mg (GG 172) MC-24, A2
  Schein/Danbury Tablets—
    75/50 mg (DAN
      5682) MC-24, A4
Triavil Tablets—
  2/10 mg (MSD 914)....... MC-18, D2
  2/25 mg (MSD 921)....... MC-18, D2
  4/10 mg (MSD 934)....... MC-18, D2
  4/25 mg (MSD 946)....... MC-18, D3
  4/50 mg (MSD 517)....... MC-18, D3
Triazolam MC-24, A6
Trifluoperazine............ MC-24, A7–B1
  1 mg (GG 51)........... MC-24, A7
  2 mg (GG 53).......... MC-24, A7
  5 mg (GG 55).......... MC-24, A7
  10 mg (GG 58)......... MC-24, A7
Tri-Levlen 21 Tablets—
  0.05/0.03 mg (95) MC-13, A2
  0.075/0.04 mg (96) MC-13, A2
  0.125/0.03 mg (97) MC-13, A2
Tri-Levlen 28 Tablets—
  0.05/0.03 mg (95) MC-13, A3
  0.075/0.04 mg (96) MC-13, A3
  0.125/0.03 mg (97) MC-13, A3
  Inert (11)............. MC-13, A3
Trimethobenzamide.......... MC-24, B2
Trimethoprim MC-24, B3
Trimipramine MC-24, B4
Trimox Capsules—
  250 mg (230) MC-2, A5
  500 mg (231) MC-2, A5
Trinalin Extended-release Tablets—
  1/120 mg (PAA or 703)...... MC-2, D5
Triphasil-21 Tablets—
  0.05/0.03 mg (641) MC-13, A6
  0.075/0.04 mg (642) MC-13, A6
  0.125/0.03 mg (643) MC-13, A6

Triphasil-28 Tablets—
  0.05/0.03 mg (641) MC-13, A7
  0.075/0.04 mg (642) MC-13, A7
  0.125/0.03 mg (643) MC-13, A7
  Inert (650)............. MC-13, A7
Tuss-Ornade Extended-release Capsules—
  75/40 mg MC-19, A1
Tylenol with Codeine Tablets—
  300/7.5 mg (1)............. MC-1, A1
  300/15 mg (2) MC-1, A1
  300/30 mg (3) MC-1, A2
  300/60 mg (4) MC-1, A2
Tylox Capsules—
  5/500 mg MC-18, A5
Ursodiol MC-24, B5
Valium Tablets—
  2 mg (2) MC-6, D7
  5 mg (5) MC-6, D7
  10 mg (10) MC-6, D7
Valrelease Extended-release Capsules—
  15 mg (15) MC-6, D6
Vascor Tablets—
  200 mg (200) MC-3, A7
  300 mg (300) MC-3, A7
  400 mg (400) MC-3, A7
Vaseretic Tablets—
  10/25 mg (MSD 720) MC-8, D3
Vasotec Tablets—
  2.5 mg (MSD 14) MC-8, D2
  5 mg (MSD 712) MC-8, D2
  10 mg (MSD 713) MC-8, D2
  20 mg (MSD 714) MC-8, D2
V-Cillin K Tablets—
  125 mg (125) MC-18, C4
  250 mg (250) MC-18, C4
  500 mg (500) MC-18, C4
Veetids Tablets—
  250 mg (684) MC-18, B7
  500 mg (648) MC-18, B7
Velosef Capsules—
  250 mg (113) MC-4, C4
  500 mg (114) MC-4, C4
Ventolin Tablets—
  2 mg (2) MC-1, B2
  4 mg (4) MC-1, B2
Verapamil MC-24, B6–D5
  Barr Tablets—
    80 mg (425) MC-24, B6
    120 mg (455) MC-24, B6
  Geneva Tablets—
    80 mg (GG 132) MC-24, C3
    120 mg (GG 133) MC-24, C3
  Mutual Tablets—
    80 mg (MP 69) MC-24, C6
    120 mg (MP 76) MC-24, C6
  Purepac Tablets—
    80 mg (473) MC-24, C7
    120 mg (475) MC-24, C7
  Rugby Tablets—
    80 mg (4812) MC-24, D1
    120 mg (4813) MC-24, D1
  Schein/Danbury Tablets—
    80 mg (5601) MC-24, D2
    120 mg (5602) MC-24, D2
Verelan Extended-release Capsules—
  120 mg (V8) MC-24, C4
  180 mg (V7) MC-24, C4
  240 mg (V9) MC-24, C5

Vibramycin Capsules—
  50 mg (094) MC-8, C2
  100 mg (095) MC-8, C2
Vibra-tabs Tablets—
  100 mg (099) MC-8, C3
Vicodin Tablets—
  5/500 mg MC-11, B6
Vicodin ES Tablets—
  7.5/750 mg.............. MC-11, B7
Visken Tablets—
  5 mg (78-111)............. MC-19, A5
  10 mg (78-73).......... MC-19, A5
Vistaril Tablets—
  25 mg (541) MC-11, C4
  50 mg (542) MC-11, C4
  100 mg (543) MC-11, C4
Voltaren Tablets—
  25 mg (25) MC-7, A2
  50 mg (50) MC-7, A2
  75 mg (75) MC-7, A2
Warfarin Sodium............. MC-24, D6
Wellbutrin Tablets—
  75 mg (75) MC-3, B5
  100 mg (100) MC-3, B5
Wymox Capsules—
  250 mg (559) MC-2, B1
  500 mg (560) MC-2, B1
Wytensin Tablets—
  4 mg (73) MC-10, D3
  8 mg (74) MC-10, D3
Xanax Tablets—
  0.25 mg (0.25) MC-1, C5
  0.5 mg (0.5) MC-1, C5
  1 mg (1.0) MC-1, C5
  2 mg (2) MC-1, C5
Zantac Tablets—
  150 mg (150) MC-21, A5
  300 mg (300) MC-21, A5
Zaroxolyn Tablets—
  2.5 mg (2½) MC-15, B4
  5 mg (5) MC-15, B4
  10 mg (10) MC-15, B4
Zestoretic Tablets—
  20/12.5 mg (142)......... MC-13, C3
  20/25 mg (145) MC-13, C3
Zestril Tablets—
  5 mg (130) MC-13, C1
  10 mg (131) MC-13, C1
  20 mg (132) MC-13, C1
  40 mg (134) MC-13, C1
Zidovudine MC-24, D7
Zithromax Capsules—
  250 mg (305) MC-2, D7
Zocor Tablets—
  5 mg (MSD 726) MC-21, B4
  10 mg (MSD 735).......... MC-21, B4
Zoloft Tablets—
  50 mg (50 MG) MC-21, B3
  100 mg (100 MG) MC-21, B3
Zovirax
  Capsules—
    200 mg (200) MC-1, A7
  Tablets—
    800 mg (800) MC-1, B1
Zyloprim Tablets—
  100 mg (100) MC-1, C1
  300 mg (300) MC-1, C1

*In thousands of units of lipase/amylase/protease, respectively.

INVERTED CROSS-INDEX

AHR—*Donnatal* Extended-release Tablets
0.0582/0.3111/0.0195/48.6 mg MC-2, D3
AHR—*Quinidex* Extended-release Tablets 300 mg MC-21, A3
AHR—*Robaxin* Tablets 500 mg MC-14, C2
AHR—*Robaxisal* Tablets 400/325 mg MC-14, C3
AHR 10—*Reglan* Tablets 10 mg MC-15, A7
AHR 4207—*Donnatal* Capsules
0.0194/0.1037/0.0065/16.2 mg MC-2, D1
AHR 5720—*Micro-K* Extended-release Capsules
600 mg MC-19, B2
AHR 5730—*Micro-K* Extended-release Capsules
750 mg MC-19, B2
AHR 6242—*Phenaphen with Codeine* Capsules
325/15 mg MC-1, A4
AHR 6257—*Phenaphen with Codeine* Capsules
325/30 mg MC-1, A4
AHR 6274—*Phenaphen with Codeine* Capsules
325/60 mg MC-1, A5
Ast 10—*Hismanal* Tablets 10 mg MC-2, C2
A2C—*Lanoxicaps* Capsules 0.05 mg MC-7, B2
A3 250—*Achromycin V* Capsules 250 mg MC-22, B6
A5 500—*Achromycin V* Capsules 500 mg MC-22, B6
A 49—Lederle Atenolol Tablets 50 mg MC-2, C6
A 71—Lederle Atenolol Tablets 100 mg MC-2, C6
A77—*Aralen* Tablets 500 mg MC-4, D5
BI 6—*Catapres* Tablets 0.1 mg MC-5, D6
BI 7—*Catapres* Tablets 0.2 mg MC-5, D6
BI 8—*Combipres* Tablets 0.1/15 mg MC-6, A6
BI 9—*Combipres* Tablets 0.2/15 mg MC-6, A6
BI 10—*Combipres* Tablets 0.3/15 mg MC-6, A6
BI 11—*Catapres* Tablets 0.3 mg MC-5, D6
BI 17—*Persantine* Tablets 25 mg MC-7, D5
BI 18—*Persantine* Tablets 50 mg MC-7, D5
BI 19—*Persantine* Tablets 75 mg MC-7, D5
BI 72—*Alupent* Tablets 20 mg MC-14, B7
BI 74—*Alupent* Tablets 10 mg MC-14, B7
BL N1—*Naldecon* Extended-release Tablets
40/10/15/5 mg MC-4, D7
BL V1—*Betapen VK* Tablets 250 mg MC-18, B6
BL V2—*Betapen VK* Tablets 500 mg MC-18, B6
BL 512—*Quibron-T Dividose* Tablets 300 mg MC-22, C4
BL 519—*Quibron-T/SR Dividose* Extended-release
Tablets 300 mg MC-22, C5
BMP 140—*Totacillin* Capsules 250 mg MC-2, B4
BMP 141—*Totacillin* Capsules 500 mg MC-2, B4
BMP 189—*Augmentin* Chewable Tablets
125/31.25 mg MC-2, B3
BMP 190—*Augmentin* Chewable Tablets 250/62.5 mg ... MC-2, B3
B2C—*Lanoxicaps* Capsules 0.1 mg MC-7, B5
CHEW EZ—*EryPed* Chewable Tablets 200 mg MC-9, B4
C2C—*Lanoxicaps* Capsules 0.2 mg MC-7, B5
C 42—Lederle Clonidine Tablets 0.1 mg MC-6, A1
C 43—Lederle Clonidine Tablets 0.2 mg MC-6, A1
C 44—Lederle Clonidine Tablets 0.3 mg MC-6, A1
DAN 5026—Schein/Danbury Procainamide Capsules
250 mg MC-20, A1
DAN 5162—Schein Tetracycline Capsules 250 mg
Orange/Yellow MC-22, C1
DAN 5333—Schein/Danbury Procainamide Capsules
500 mg MC-20, A1
DAN 5350—Schein/Danbury Procainamide Capsules
375 mg MC-20, A1
DAN 5440—Schein/Danbury Doxycycline Capsules
100 mg MC-8, C6
DAN 5535—Schein/Danbury Doxycycline Capsules
50 mg MC-8, C6
DAN 5554—Schein/Danbury Propranolol Tablets
10 mg MC-20, C2
DAN 5555—Schein/Danbury Propranolol Tablets
20 mg MC-20, C2
DAN 5556—Schein/Danbury Propranolol Tablets
40 mg MC-20, C2

DAN 5557—Schein/Danbury Propranolol Tablets
80 mg MC-20, C2
DAN 5609—Schein/Danbury Clonidine Tablets
0.1 mg MC-6, A4
DAN 5612—Schein/Danbury Clonidine Tablets
0.2 mg MC-6, A4
DAN 5613—Schein/Danbury Clonidine Tablets
0.3 mg MC-6, A4
DAN 5614—Schein/Danbury Flurazepam Capsules
15 mg MC-10, B6
DAN 5615—Schein/Danbury Flurazepam Capsules
30 mg MC-10, B6
DAN 5616—Schein/Danbury Oxazepam Capsules
10 mg MC-17, D6
DAN 5617—Schein/Danbury Oxazepam Capsules
15 mg MC-17, D6
DAN 5618—Schein/Danbury Oxazepam Capsules
30 mg MC-17, D6
DAN 5619—Schein/Danbury Diazepam Tablets 5 mg... MC-7, A1
DAN 5620—Schein/Danbury Diazepam Tablets
10 mg MC-7, A1
DAN 5621—Schein/Danbury Diazepam Tablets 2 mg... MC-7, A1
DAN 5622—Schein/Danbury Lorazepam Tablets
2 mg MC-13, D6
DAN 5624—Schein/Danbury Lorazepam Tablets
1 mg MC-13, D6
DAN 5625—Schein/Danbury Lorazepam Tablets
0.5 mg MC-13, D6
DAN 5629—Schein/Danbury Doxepin Capsules
10 mg MC-8, B5
DAN 5630—Schein/Danbury Doxepin Capsules
25 mg MC-8, B5
DAN 5631—Schein/Danbury Doxepin Capsules
50 mg MC-8, B6
DAN 5632—Schein/Danbury Doxepin Capsules
75 mg MC-8, B6
DAN 5633—Schein/Danbury Doxepin Capsules
100 mg MC-8, B6
DAN 5642—Schein/Danbury Minoxidil Tablets
2.5 mg MC-15, D2
DAN 5643—Schein/Danbury Minoxidil Tablets
10 mg MC-15, D2
DAN 5682—Schein/Danbury Triamterene and
Hydrochlorothiazide Tablets 75/50 mg MC-24, A4
DAN 5693—Schein/Danbury Prazosin Capsules
5 mg MC-19, C3
DAN 5696—Schein/Danbury Prazosin Capsules
2 mg MC-19, C3
DAN 5697—Schein/Danbury Prazosin Capsules
1 mg MC-19, C3
DF—*Hytrin* Tablets 1 mg MC-22, A7
DH—*Hytrin* Tablets 2 mg MC-22, A7
DI—*Hytrin* Tablets 10 mg MC-22, A7
DJ—*Hytrin* Tablets 5 mg MC-22, A7
dp 25—*Levoxine* Tablets 0.025 mg MC-13, B3
dp 50—*Levoxine* Tablets 0.05 mg MC-13, B3
dp 75—*Levoxine* Tablets 0.075 mg MC-13, B3
dp 88—*Levoxine* Tablets 0.088 mg MC-13, B3
dp 100—*Levoxine* Tablets 0.1 mg MC-13, B3
dp 112—*Levoxine* Tablets 0.112 mg MC-13, B4
dp 125—*Levoxine* Tablets 0.125 mg MC-13, B4
dp 150—*Levoxine* Tablets 0.15 mg MC-13, B4
dp 175—*Levoxine* Tablets 0.175 mg MC-13, B4
dp 200—*Levoxine* Tablets 0.2 mg MC-13, B4
dp 300—*Levoxine* Tablets 0.3 mg MC-13, B4
DS—*Anaprox* Tablets 500 mg MC-16, A6
DS 02C—*Septra* Tablets 800/160 mg MC-21, C7
D 03—*Danocrine* Capsules 50 mg MC-6, C5
D 04—*Danocrine* Capsules 100 mg MC-6, C5
D 05—*Danocrine* Capsules 200 mg MC-6, C5
D 35—*Demerol* Tablets 50 mg MC-14, B6
D 37—*Demerol* Tablets 100 mg MC-14, B6
EA—Abbott Erythromycin Tablets 500 mg MC-9, A2

EB—Abbott Erythromycin Tablets 250 mg................ MC-9, A2
EC—*Ery-Tab* Delayed-release Tablets 250 mg......... MC-9, A3
ED—*Ery-Tab* Delayed-release Tablets 500 mg......... MC-9, A3
EE—*E.E.S.* Tablets 400 mg.............................. MC-9, B3
EH—*Ery-Tab* Delayed-release Tablets 333 mg......... MC-9, A3
ER—Abbott Erythromycin Delayed-release Capsules
    250 mg.. MC-9, A1
ES—*Erythrocin* Tablets 250 mg MC-9, B6
ET—*Erythrocin* Tablets 500 mg MC-9, B6
GG 27—Geneva Hydrochlorothiazide Tablets 50 mg.... MC-11, B4
GG 28—Geneva Hydrochlorothiazide Tablets 25 mg.... MC-11, B4
GG 35—Geneva Thioridazine Tablets 150 mg MC-23, A4
GG 36—Geneva Thioridazine Tablets 200 mg MC-23, A4
GG 40—Geneva Amitriptyline Tablets 10 mg MC-1, D1
GG 44—Geneva Amitriptyline Tablets 25 mg MC-1, D1
GG 45—Geneva Dipyridamole Tablets 50 mg MC-7, D6
GG 49—Geneva Dipyridamole Tablets 25 mg MC-7, D6
GG 51—Geneva Trifluoperazine Tablets 1 mg MC-24, A7
GG 53—Geneva Trifluoperazine Tablets 2 mg MC-24, A7
GG 55—Geneva Trifluoperazine Tablets 5 mg MC-24, A7
GG 56—Geneva Disopyramide Capsules 100 mg MC-8, A2
GG 57—Geneva Disopyramide Capsules 150 mg MC-8, A2
GG 58—Geneva Trifluoperazine Tablets 10 mg MC-24, A7
GG 61—Geneva Chlorpropamide Tablets 100 mg MC-5, B1
GG 71—Geneva Propranolol Tablets 10 mg MC-20, B5
GG 72—Geneva Propranolol Tablets 20 mg MC-20, B5
GG 73—Geneva Propranolol Tablets 40 mg MC-20, B5
GG 74—Geneva Propranolol Tablets 60 mg MC-20, B5
GG 75—Geneva Propranolol Tablets 80 mg MC-20, B5
GG 81—Geneva Clonidine Tablets 0.1 mg MC-5, D7
GG 82—Geneva Clonidine Tablets 0.2 mg MC-5, D7
GG 83—Geneva Clonidine Tablets 0.3 mg MC-5, D7
GG 85—Geneva Spironolactone Tablets 25 mg MC-21, B5
GG 95—Geneva Spironolactone and
    Hydrochlorothiazide Tablets 25/25 mg............. MC-21, C2
GG 101—Geneva Methocarbamol Tablets 750 mg MC-14, C1
GG 103—Geneva Metronidazole Tablets 250 mg MC-15, C2
GG 104—Geneva Methyldopa Tablets 125 mg......... MC-14, C6
GG 111—Geneva Methyldopa Tablets 250 mg......... MC-14, C6
GG 118—Geneva Phenylpropanolamine, Phenylephrine,
    Phenyltoloxamine, and Chlorpheniramine
    Extended-release Tablets 40/10/15/5 mg MC-5, A1
GG 119—Geneva Butalbital, Aspirin, and Caffeine
    Tablets 50/325/40 mg............................... MC-3, C1
GG 124—Geneva Haloperidol Tablets 2 mg........... MC-10, D7
GG 125—Geneva Haloperidol Tablets 5 mg........... MC-10, D7
GG 126—Geneva Haloperidol Tablets 10 mg........... MC-10, D7
GG 132—Geneva Verapamil Tablets 80 mg............ MC-24, C3
GG 133—Geneva Verapamil Tablets 120 mg........... MC-24, C3
GG 134—Geneva Haloperidol Tablets 20 mg.......... MC-10, D7
GG 141—Geneva Meclizine Tablets 12.5 mg.......... MC-14, A3
GG 144—Geneva Chlorpropamide Tablets 250 mg ... MC-5, B1
GG 167—Geneva Desipramine Tablets 100 mg MC-6, C7
GG 168—Geneva Desipramine Tablets 150 mg MC-6, C7
GG 172—Geneva Triamterene and
    Hydrochlorothiazide Tablets 75/50 mg............. MC-24, A2
GG 190—Geneva Methocarbamol Tablets 500 mg MC-14, C1
GG 195—Geneva Metronidazole Tablets 500 mg MC-15, C2
GG 219—Geneva Methyldopa and
    Hydrochlorothiazide Tablets 250/15 mg............ MC-14, D4
GG 242—Geneva Methyclothiazide Tablets 5 mg MC-14, C5
GG 243—Geneva Methyldopa and
    Hydrochlorothiazide Tablets 500/30 mg............ MC-14, D5
GG 244—Geneva Methyclothiazide Tablets 2.5 mg.... MC-14, C5
GG 254—Geneva Fenoprofen Tablets 600 mg MC-10, A1
GG 261—Geneva Meclizine Tablets 25 mg............ MC-14, A3
GG 263—Geneva Atenolol Tablets 50 mg............. MC-2, C3
GG 264—Geneva Atenolol Tablets 100 mg............ MC-2, C3
GG 265—Geneva Methyldopa and
    Hydrochlorothiazide Tablets 250/25 mg............ MC-14, D4
GG 270—Geneva Tolazamide Tablets 100 mg......... MC-23, C3
GG 271—Geneva Tolazamide Tablets 250 mg......... MC-23, C3
GG 272—Geneva Tolazamide Tablets 500 mg......... MC-23, C3
GG 289—Geneva Methyldopa and
    Hydrochlorothiazide Tablets 500/50 mg............ MC-14, D5

GG 431—Geneva Amitriptyline Tablets 50 mg MC-1, D1
GG 437—Geneva Chlorpromazine Tablets 100 mg MC-5, A5
GG 450—Geneva Amitriptyline Tablets 150 mg MC-1, D2
GG 451—Geneva Amitriptyline Tablets 75 mg MC-1, D1
GG 457—Geneva Chlorpromazine Tablets 200 mg MC-5, A5
GG 461—Geneva Amitriptyline Tablets 100 mg MC-1, D2
GG 464—Geneva Dipyridamole Tablets 75 mg MC-7, D6
GG 471—Geneva Methyldopa Tablets 500 mg MC-14, C6
GG 472—Geneva Procainamide Extended-release
    Tablets 250 mg..................................... MC-19, D2
GG 473—Geneva Procainamide Extended-release
    Tablets 500 mg..................................... MC-19, D2
GG 474—Geneva Procainamide Extended-release
    Tablets 750 mg..................................... MC-19, D2
GG 501—Geneva Nitroglycerin Extended-release
    Capsules 6.5 mg.................................... MC-16, C6
GG 511—Geneva Nitroglycerin Extended-release
    Capsules 2.5 mg.................................... MC-16, C6
GG 512—Geneva Nitroglycerin Extended-release
    Capsules 9 mg...................................... MC-16, C7
GG 517—Geneva Indomethacin Capsules 25 mg MC-12, B1
GG 518—Geneva Indomethacin Capsules 50 mg MC-12, B1
GG 533—Geneva Diphenhydramine Capsules 25 mg ... MC-7, C6
GG 541—Geneva Diphenhydramine Capsules 50 mg ... MC-7, C6
GG 551—Geneva Procainamide Capsules 250 mg MC-19, D1
GG 552—Geneva Procainamide Capsules 375 mg MC-19, D1
GG 553—Geneva Procainamide Capsules 500 mg MC-19, D1
GG 558—Geneva Fenoprofen Capsules 200 mg MC-9, D7
GG 559—Geneva Fenoprofen Capsules 300 mg MC-9, D7
GG 572—Geneva Doxepin Capsules 25 mg............ MC-8, A6
GG 573—Geneva Doxepin Capsules 50 mg............ MC-8, A7
GG 574—Geneva Doxepin Capsules 75 mg............ MC-8, A7
GG 576—Geneva Doxepin Capsules 10 mg............ MC-8, A6
GG 577—Geneva Doxepin Capsules 100 mg........... MC-8, A7
GG 589—Geneva Thiothixene Capsules 1 mg MC-23, B3
GG 596—Geneva Thiothixene Capsules 2 mg MC-23, B3
GG 597—Geneva Thiothixene Capsules 5 mg MC-23, B3
GG 598—Geneva Thiothixene Capsules 10 mg MC-23, B3
H09—*Ilosone* Capsules 250 mg MC-9, B1
H11—Lederle Hydralazine Tablets 25 mg............. MC-11, A5
H12—Lederle Hydralazine Tablets 50 mg............. MC-11, A5
H69—*Keflex* Capsules 250 mg MC-4, C2
H71—*Keflex* Capsules 500 mg MC-4, C2
H76—*Nalfon* Capsules 200 mg MC-9, D5
H77—*Nalfon* Capsules 300 mg MC-9, D5
H 203—Schein Tetracycline Capsules 500 mg MC-22, C1
H 214—Schein Tetracycline Capsules 250 mg
    Blue/Yellow MC-22, C1
IBU 400—Boots Laboratories Ibuprofen Tablets
    400 mg.. MC-11, D3
IBU 600—Boots Laboratories Ibuprofen Tablets
    600 mg.. MC-11, D3
IBU 800—Boots Laboratories Ibuprofen Tablets
    800 mg.. MC-11, D3
JU—*Eldepryl* Tablets 5 mg MC-21, B2
J09—*Eskalith* Tablets 300 mg......................... MC-13, D1
J10—*Eskalith CR* Extended-release Tablets 450 mg ... MC-13, D2
KL—*Biaxin* Tablets 500 mg........................... MC-5, C7
KT—*Biaxin* Tablets 250 mg........................... MC-5, C7
LL 200—*Suprax* Tablets 200 mg....................... MC-4, B3
LU—*Ogen* Tablets 0.75 mg............................ MC-9, C4
LV—*Ogen* Tablets 1.5 mg............................. MC-9, C4
LX—*Ogen* Tablets 3 mg............................... MC-9, C4
LY—*Ogen* Tablets 6 mg............................... MC-9, C4
L 9—*Ledercillin VK* Tablets 500 mg................. MC-18, C3
L 10—*Ledercillin VK* Tablets 250 mg................ MC-18, C3
MJ 5—*BuSpar* Tablets 5 mg MC-3, B6
MJ 10—*BuSpar* Tablets 10 mg MC-3, B6
MJ 10 mEq 770—*Klotrix* Extended-release Tablets
    750 mg.. MC-19, B1
MJ 755—*Estrace* Tablets 1 mg MC-9, C1
MJ 756—*Estrace* Tablets 2 mg MC-9, C1
MJ775—*Desyrel* Tablets 50 mg........................ MC-23, D5
MJ776—*Desyrel* Tablets 100 mg....................... MC-23, D5
MJ778—*Desyrel* Tablets 150 mg....................... MC-23, D5

MJ 784—*Duricef* Capsules 500 mg...................... MC-4, B1
MJ 785—*Duricef* Tablets 1 gram....................... MC-4, B1
MO—*Toprol XL* Extended-release Tablets 50 mg MC-15, B6
MP 35—Mutual Spironolactone Tablets 25 mg MC-21, B6
MP 40—Mutual Spironolactone and
    Hydrochlorothiazide Tablets 25/25 mg............ MC-21, C3
MP 44—Mutual Benztropine Tablets 1 mg MC-3, A6
MP 47—Mutual Albuterol Tablets 2 mg MC-1, B3
MP 50—Mutual Tolmetin Tablets 200 mg MC-23, D2
MP 69—Mutual Verapamil Tablets 80 mg MC-24, C6
MP 71—Purepac Allopurinol Tablets 100 mg MC-1, C2
MP 74—Mutual Chlorzoxazone Tablets 500 mg......... MC-5, C2
MP 76—Mutual Verapamil Tablets 120 mg MC-24, C6
MP 80—Mutual Allopurinol Tablets 300 mg MC-1, C2
MP 88—Mutual Albuterol Tablets 4 mg MC-1, B3
MP 108—Mutual Quinidine Sulfate Tablets 200 mg MC-21, A2
MP 112—Mutual Sulindac Tablets 150 mg MC-21, D6
MP 116—Mutual Sulindac Tablets 200 mg MC-21, D6
MP 124—Mutual Quinidine Sulfate Tablets 300 mg.... MC-21, A2
MP 142—Mutual Benztropine Tablets 2 mg MC-3, A6
MS—*Toprol XL* Extended-release Tablets 100 mg MC-15, B6
MSD 14—*Vasotec* Tablets 2.5 mg MC-8, D2
MSD 19—*Prinivil* Tablets 5 mg MC-13, D7
MSD 20—*Decadron* Tablets 0.25 mg MC-6, D3
MSD 21—*Cogentin* Tablets 0.5 mg MC-3, A5
MSD 23—*Elavil* Tablets 10 mg MC-2, A2
MSD 25—*Indocin* Capsules 25 mg MC-12, B2
MSD 41—*Decadron* Tablets 0.5 mg MC-6, D3
MSD 42—*HydroDIURIL* Tablets 25 mg MC-11, B5
MSD 45—*Elavil* Tablets 25 mg MC-2, A2
MSD 50—*Indocin* Capsules 50 mg MC-12, B2
MSD 59—*Blocadren* Tablets 5 mg MC-23, B7
MSD 60—*Cogentin* Tablets 2 mg MC-3, A5
MSD 63—*Decadron* Tablets 0.75 mg MC-6, D3
MSD 95—*Decadron* Tablets 1.5 mg MC-6, D4
MSD 97—*Decadron* Tablets 4 mg MC-6, D4
MSD 102—*Elavil* Tablets 50 mg MC-2, A2
MSD 105—*HydroDIURIL* Tablets 50 mg MC-11, B5
MSD 106—*Prinivil* Tablets 10 mg MC-13, B7
MSD 135—*Aldomet* Tablets 125 mg MC-14, C7
MSD 136—*Blocadren* Tablets 10 mg MC-23, B7
MSD 140—*Prinzide* Tablets 20/12.5 mg.............. MC-13, C2
MSD 142—*Prinzide* Tablets 20/25 mg MC-13, C2
MSD 147—*Decadron* Tablets 6 mg MC-6, D4
MSD 207—*Prinivil* Tablets 20 mg MC-13, B7
MSD 237—*Prinivil* Tablets 40 mg MC-13, B7
MSD 401—*Aldomet* Tablets 250 mg MC-14, C7
MSD 410—*HydroDIURIL* Tablets 100 mg MC-11, B5
MSD 423—*Aldoril* Tablets 250/15 mg MC-14, D6
MSD 430—*Elavil* Tablets 75 mg MC-2, A2
MSD 435—*Elavil* Tablets 100 mg MC-2, A2
MSD 437—*Blocadren* Tablets 20 mg MC-23, B7
MSD 451—*Plendil* Tablets 5 mg MC-9, D4
MSD 452—*Plendil* Tablets 10 mg MC-9, D4
MSD 456—*Aldoril* Tablets 250/25 mg MC-14, D6
MSD 516—*Aldomet* Tablets 500 mg MC-14, C7
MSD 517—*Triavil* Tablets 4/50 mg MC-18, D3
MSD 635—*Cogentin* Tablets 1 mg MC-3, A5
MSD 673—*Elavil* Tablets 150 mg MC-2, A3
MSD 675—*Dolobid* Tablets 250 mg................... MC-7, B4
MSD 693—*Indocin SR* Extended-release Capsules
    75 mg MC-12, B3
MSD 694—*Aldoril* Tablets 500/30 mg MC-14, D7
MSD 697—*Dolobid* Tablets 500 mg.................. MC-7, B4
MSD 705—*Noroxin* Tablets 400 mg.................. MC-17, B6
MSD 707—*Tonocard* Tablets 400 mg................. MC-23, C2
MSD 709—*Tonocard* Tablets 600 mg................. MC-23, C2
MSD 712—*Vasotec* Tablets 5 mg MC-8, D2
MSD 713—*Vasotec* Tablets 10 mg.................. MC-8, D2
MSD 714—*Vasotec* Tablets 20 mg.................. MC-8, D2
MSD 720—*Vaseretic* Tablets 10/25 mg MC-8, D3
MSD 726—*Zocor* Tablets 5 mg MC-21, B4
MSD 731—*Mevacor* Tablets 20 mg MC-14, A1
MSD 732—*Mevacor* Tablets 40 mg MC-14, A1
MSD 735—*Zocor* Tablets 10 mg MC-21, B4

MSD 742—*Prilosec* Delayed-release Capsules 20 mg ... MC-17, D1
MSD 914—*Triavil* Tablets 2/10 mg MC-18, D2
MSD 917—*Moduretic* Tablets 5/50 mg MC-1, C7
MSD 921—*Triavil* Tablets 2/25 mg MC-18, D2
MSD 931—*Flexeril* Tablets 10 mg.................. MC-6, C2
MSD 934—*Triavil* Tablets 4/10 mg MC-18, D2
MSD 935—*Aldoril* Tablets 500/50 mg MC-14, D7
MSD 941—*Clinoril* Tablets 150 mg MC-21, D5
MSD 942—*Clinoril* Tablets 200 mg MC-21, D5
MSD 946—*Triavil* Tablets 4/25 mg MC-18, D3
MSD 963—*Pepcid* Tablets 20 mg MC-9, D3
MSD 964—*Pepcid* Tablets 40 mg MC-9, D3
MT 4—*Pancrease* Delayed-release Capsules 4/20/25 .. MC-18, B3
MT 10—*Pancrease* Delayed-release Capsules
    10/30/30... MC-18, B3
MT 16—*Pancrease* Delayed-release Capsules
    16/48/48 .... MC-18, B4
MT 25—*Pancrease* Delayed-release Capsules
    25/75/75... MC-18, B4
MY—*Toprol XL* Extended-release Capsules 200 mg ... MC-15, B6
M 1—Mylan Clonidine and Chlorthalidone Tablets
    0.1/15 mg MC-6, A7
M2—Schein/Danbury Furosemide Tablets 20 mg MC-10, C4
M 3—*Minocin* Tablets 50 mg MC-15, C7
M 5—*Minocin* Tablets 100 mg MC-15, C7
M8—*Maxzide* Tablets 75/50 mg MC-24, A3
M9—*Maxzide* Tablets 37.5/25 mg MC-24, A3
M 27—Mylan Clonidine and Chlorthalidone Tablets
    0.2/15 mg MC-6, A7
M 30—Mylan Clorazepate Tablets 3.75 mg MC-6, B3
M 31—Mylan Allopurinol Tablets 100 mg MC-1, C3
M 39—Schein Amitriptyline Tablets 150 mg MC-2, A1
M 40—Mylan Clorazepate Tablets 7.5 mg MC-6, B3
M 45—*Minocin* Capsules 50 mg MC-15, C6
M 46—*Minocin* Capsules 100 mg.................... MC-15, C6
M 54—Mylan Thioridazine Tablets 10 mg MC-23, A5
M 55—Mylan Timolol Tablets 5 mg MC-23, C1
M 58—Mylan Thioridazine Tablets 25 mg MC-23, A5
M 59—Mylan Thioridazine Tablets 50 mg MC-23, A5
M 61—Mylan Thioridazine Tablets 100 mg MC-23, A5
M 70—Mylan Clorazepate Tablets 15 mg MC-6, B3
M 71—Mylan Allopurinol Tablets 300 mg MC-1, C3
M 72—Mylan Clonidine and Chlorthalidone Tablets
    0.3/15 mg MC-6, A7
M 221—Mylan Timolol Tablets 10 mg................ MC-23, C1
NE—*Nicolar* Tablets 500 mg MC-16, B2
N 21—*NegGram* Tablets 250 mg MC-16, A3
N 22—*NegGram* Tablets 500 mg MC-16, A3
N 23—*NegGram* Tablets 1 gram MC-16, A4
P—*Demulen 1/35-28* Tablets Inert MC-9, C6
P—*Demulen 1/50-28* Tablets Inert MC-9, D1
PAA—*Trinalin* Extended-release Tablets 1/120 mg MC-2, D5
PD 554—*Centrax* Capsules 20 mg MC-19, B7
P-D 007—*Dilantin* Chewable Tablets 50 mg MC-19, A3
P-D 180—*Pyridium* Tablets 100 mg MC-18, D4
P-D 181—*Pyridium* Tablets 200 mg................. MC-18, D4
P-D 202—*Procan SR* Extended-release Tablets
    250 mg MC-19, D3
P-D 204—*Procan SR* Extended-release Tablets
    500 mg MC-19, D3
P-D 205—*Procan SR* Extended-release Tablets
    750 mg.. MC-19, D4
P-D 207—*Procan SR* Extended-release Tablets
    1 gram MC-19, D4
P-D 362—*Dilantin* Capsules 100 mg............... MC-19, A4
P-D 365—*Dilantin* Capsules 30 mg................ MC-19, A4
P-D 471—*Benadryl* Capsules 25 mg................ MC-7, C7
P-D 473—*Benadryl* Capsules 50 mg................. MC-7, C7
P-D 552—*Centrax* Capsules 5 mg................... MC-19, B7
P-D 553—*Centrax* Capsules 10 mg................. MC-19, B7
P-D 622—*Loestrin Fe 1/20* Tablets 75 mg.......... MC-17, B1
P-D 622—*Loestrin Fe 1.5/30* Tablets 75 mg......... MC-17, B2
P-D 696—*Eryc* Delayed-release Capsules 250 mg MC-9, A7
P-D 915—*Loestrin Fe 1/20* Tablets 1/0.02 mg........ MC-17, B1
P-D 915—*Loestrin 21 1/20* Tablets 1/0.02 mg MC-17, A6

P-D 916—*Loestrin Fe 1.5/30* Tablets 1.5/0.03 mg MC-17, B2
P-D 916—*Loestrin 21 1.5/30* Tablets 1.5/0.03 mg MC-17, A7
PPP 207—*Corgard* Tablets 40 mg MC-15, D7
PPP 208—*Corgard* Tablets 120 mg MC-16, A1
PPP 232—*Corgard* Tablets 20 mg MC-15, D7
PPP 241—*Corgard* Tablets 80 mg MC-15, D7
PPP 246—*Corgard* Tablets 160 mg MC-16, A1
PPP 606—*Naturetin* Tablets 5 mg MC-3, A3
PPP 618—*Naturetin* Tablets 10 mg MC-3, A3
PPP 775—*Pronestyl-SR* Extended-release Tablets
    500 mg MC-19, D7
PPP 863—*Prolixin* Tablets 1 mg MC-10, B2
PPP 864—*Prolixin* Tablets 2.5 mg MC-10, B2
PPP 877—*Prolixin* Tablets 5 mg MC-10, B2
PPP 956—*Prolixin* Tablets 10 mg MC-10, B2
P 44—Lederle Propranolol Tablets 10 mg MC-20, B6
P 45—Lederle Propranolol Tablets 20 mg MC-20, B6
P 46—Lederle Propranolol Tablets 40 mg MC-20, B6
P 47—Lederle Propranolol Tablets 80 mg MC-20, B6
P 65—Lederle Propranolol Tablets 60 mg MC-20, B6
R021—Purepac Flurazepam Capsules 15 mg MC-10, B4
R022—Purepac Flurazepam Capsules 30 mg MC-10, B4
R 497—Purepac Nifedipine Capsules 10 mg MC-16, C2
R 520—Purepac Tolmetin Capsules 400 mg MC-23, D3
R 530—Purepac Nifedipine Capsules 20 mg MC-16, C2
SCS 501—*Diulo* Tablets 2.5 mg MC-15, B5
SCS 511—*Diulo* Tablets 5 mg MC-15, B5
SCS 521—*Diulo* Tablets 10 mg MC-15, B5
SKF—*Dyazide* Capsules 50/25 mg MC-24, A5
SKF—*Ornade* Extended-release Capsules 75/12 mg . . MC-4, D6
SKF C44—*Compazine* Extended-release Capsules
    10 mg MC-20, A3
SKF C46—*Compazine* Extended-release Capsules
    15 mg MC-20, A3
SKF C47—*Compazine* Extended-release Capsules
    30 mg MC-20, A3
SKF C66—*Compazine* Tablets 5 mg MC-20, A4
SKF C67—*Compazine* Tablets 10 mg MC-20, A4
SKF C69—*Compazine* Tablets 25 mg MC-20, A4
SR 80—*Calan SR* Extended-release Tablets 180 mg . . MC-24, D5
SR 120—*Calan SR* Extended-release Tablets 120 mg . . MC-24, D4
SR 240—*Calan SR* Extended-release Tablets 240 mg . . MC-24, D5
S04—*Stelazine* Tablets 2 mg MC-24, B1
TL—*Tranxene T-Tab* Tablets 3.75 mg MC-6, B2
TM—*Tranxene T-Tab* Tablets 7.5 mg MC-6, B2
TN—*Tranxene T-Tab* Tablets 15 mg MC-6, B2
TX—*Tranxene SD* Tablets 11.25 mg MC-6, B1
TY—*Tranxene SD* Tablets 22.5 mg MC-6, B1
T9A—*Lanoxin* Tablets 0.5 mg MC-7, B6
T37—*Talacen* Tablets 25/650 mg MC-18, C6
T 51—*Talwin Nx* Tablets 50/0.5 mg MC-18, C7
T64—*Thorazine* Extended-release Capsules 75 mg . . . MC-5, A6
T74—*Thorazine* Tablets 25 mg MC-5, A7
UC—ProSom Tablets 1 mg MC-9, B7
UD—ProSom Tablets 2 mg MC-9, B7
U05—*Ilosone* Chewable Tablets 125 mg MC-9, B2
U25—*Ilosone* Chewable Tablets 250 mg MC-9, B2
U 121—*Loniten* Tablets 2.5 mg MC-15, D3
V7—*Verelan* Extended-release Capsules 180 mg MC-24, C4
V8—*Verelan* Extended-release Capsules 120 mg MC-24, C4
V9—*Verelan* Extended-resease Capsules 240 mg MC-24, C5
WC 242—Warner Chilcott Carbamazepine Chewable
    Tablets 100 mg MC-3, D7
WC 407—Warner Chilcott Tetracycline Capsules
    250 mg MC-22, C3
WC 445—Warner Chilcott Clonidine Tablets 0.3 mg . . MC-6, A5
WC 607—Warner Chilcott Phenobarbital Tablets
    60 mg MC-18, D5
WC 615—Warner Chilcott Minocycline Capsules
    50 mg MC-15, D1
WC 616—Warner Chilcott Minocycline Capsules
    100 mg MC-15, D1
WC 697—Warner Chilcott Tetracycline Capsules
    500 mg MC-22, C3

WC 698—Warner Chilcott Phenobarbital Tablets
    100 mg MC-18, D5
WC 699—Warner Chilcott Phenobarbital Tablets
    15 mg MC-18, D5
WC 700—Warner Chilcott Phenobarbital Tablets
    30 mg MC-18, D5
WC 773—Warner Chilcott Sulindac Tablets 150 mg . . . MC-21, A1
WC 774—Warner Chilcott Sulindac Tablets 200 mg . . . MC-21, A1
WHR 50 mg—*Slo-bid* Extended-release Capsules
    50 mg MC-22, D2
WHR 100—*Slo-bid* Extended-release Capsules
    100 mg MC-22, D2
WHR 200—*Slo-bid* Extended-release Capsules
    200 mg MC-22, D3
WHR 300—*Slo-bid* Extended-release Capsules
    300 mg MC-22, D3
WHR 351—*Slo-Phyllin* Tablets 100 mg MC-22, D5
WHR 352—*Slo-Phyllin* Tablets 200 mg MC-22, D5
WHR 1354—*Slo-Phyllin* Extended-release Capsules
    60 mg MC-22, D4
WHR 1355—*Slo-Phyllin* Extended-release Capsules
    125 mg MC-22, D4
WHR 1356—*Slo-Phyllin* Extended-release Capsules
    250 mg MC-22, D4
X3A—*Lanoxin* Tablets 0.25 mg MC-7, B6
Y2B—*Septra* Tablets 400/80 mg MC-21, C7
Y3B—*Lanoxin* Tablets 0.125 mg MC-7, B6
Y9C 100—*Retrovir* Capsules 100 mg MC-24, D7
001—Purepac Acetaminophen and Codeine Tablets
    300/30 mg MC-1, A3
003—Purepac Acetaminophen and Codeine Tablets
    300/60 mg MC-1, A3
0051—*Lopurin* Tablets 100 mg MC-1, B7
0052—*Lopurin* Tablets 300 mg MC-1, B7
0.125—*Halcion* Tablets 0.125 mg MC-24, A6
0.25—*Halcion* Tablets 0.25 mg MC-24, A6
0.25—*Xanax* Tablets 0.25 mg MC-1, C5
0.3—*Premarin* Tablets 0.3 mg MC-9, C2
0.5—*Bumex* Tablets 0.5 mg MC-3, B4
0.5—*Xanax* Tablets 0.5 mg MC-1, C5
0.5/35—*Genora 0.5/35-21* Tablets 0.5/0.035 mg MC-17, A4
0.625—*Premarin* Tablets 0.625 mg MC-9, C2
0.9—*Premarin* Tablets 0.9 mg MC-9, C2
034—Schein Meclizine Tablets 12.5 mg MC-14, A7
035—Schein Meclizine Tablets 25 mg MC-14, A7
036—*Furadantin* Tablets 50 mg MC-16, C5
037—*Furadantin* Tablets 100 mg MC-16, C5
051—Purepac Diazepam Tablets 2 mg MC-6, D5
052—Purepac Diazepam Tablets 5 mg MC-6, D5
053—Purepac Diazepam Tablets 10 mg MC-6, D5
058—Barr Diphenhydramine Capsules 25 mg MC-7, C5
059—Barr Diphenhydramine Capsules 50 mg MC-7, C5
063—Purepac Lorazepam Tablets 2 mg MC-13, D5
067—Purepac Oxazepam Capsules 10 mg MC-17, D5
069—Purepac Oxazepam Capsules 15 mg MC-17, D5
069—Schein Hydroxyzine Capsules 25 mg MC-11, C7
073—Purepac Oxazepam Capsules 30 mg MC-17, D5
076—Purepac Temazepam Capsules 15 mg MC-22, A5
077—Purepac Temazepam Capsules 30 mg MC-22, A5
078—Purepac Clorazepate Tablets 3.75 mg MC-6, B4
081—Purepac Clorazepate Tablets 7.5 mg MC-6, B4
083—Purepac Clorazepate Tablets 15 mg MC-6, B4
085—Purepac Propoxyphene Napsylate and
    Acetaminophen Tablets 100/650 mg MC-20, B4
094—*Vibramycin* Capsules 50 mg MC-8, C2
095—*Mycelex* Troche Lozenges 10 mg MC-6, B5
095—*Vibramycin* Capsules 100 mg MC-8, C2
099—*Vibra-tabs* Tablets 100 mg MC-8, C3
09A—*Proloprim* Tablets 100 mg MC-24, B3
0149 0007—*Macrodantin* Capsules 25 mg MC-16, C4
0149 0008—*Macrodantin* Capsules 50 mg MC-16, C4
0149 0009—*Macrodantin* Capsules 100 mg MC-16, C4
0149 0030—*Dantrium* Capsules 25 mg MC-6, C6
0149 0031—*Dantrium* Capsules 50 mg MC-6, C6
0149 0033—*Dantrium* Capsules 100 mg MC-6, C6

0149 0412—*Entex* Capsules 5/45/200 mg MC-18, D7
0149 0436—*Entex LA* Extended-release Tablets
    75/400 mg MC-19, A2
0230—Rugby Doxycycline Capsules 100 mg MC-8, C5
0280—Rugby Doxycycline Capsules 50 mg MC-8, C5
0665 4410—Reid Rowell Hydralazine and
    Hydrochlorothiazide Capsules 25/25 mg MC-11, A7
0665 4420—Reid Rowell Hydralazine and
    Hydrochlorothiazide Capsules 50/50 mg MC-11, A7
0822 0576—Rugby Meclizine Chewable Tablets
    25 mg MC-14, A6
0920—*Dilatrate-SR* Extended-release Capsules
    40 mg MC-12, C3
½—*Haldol* Tablets 0.5 mg MC-11, A1
½—*Mykrox* Tablets 0.5 mg MC-15, B3
1—*Bumex* Tablets 1 mg MC-3, B4
1—*Haldol* Tablets 1 mg MC-11, A1
1—*Tenex* Tablets 1 mg MC-10, D4
1—*Tylenol with Codeine* Tablets 300/7.5 mg MC-1, A1
1.0—*Xanax* Tablets 1 mg MC-1, C5
1.25—*Micronase* Tablets 1.25 mg MC-10, D1
1.25—*Premarin* Tablets 1.25 mg MC-9, C3
1.25 mg—*Altace* Capsules 1.25 mg MC-21, A4
1/35—*Genora 1/35-28* Tablets 1/0.035 mg MC-17, A5
1/50—*Genora 1/50-28* Tablets 1/0.05 mg MC-17, B5
1A—*Cartrol* Tablets 2.5 mg MC-4, A6
1C—*Cartrol* Tablets 5 mg MC-4, A6
1 mg—*Cardura* Tablets 1 mg MC-8, A5
2—*Bumex* Tablets 2 mg MC-3, B4
2—*Coumadin* Tablets 2 mg MC-24, D6
2—*Haldol* Tablets 2 mg MC-11, A1
2—*Halotestin* Tablets 2 mg MC-10, A7
2—*Medrol* Tablets 2 mg MC-10, D4
2—*Tenex* Tablets 2 mg MC-10, D4
2—*Tylenol with Codeine* Tablets 300/15 mg MC-1, A1
2—*Valium* Tablets 2 mg MC-6, D7
2—*Ventolin* Tablets 2 mg MC-1, B2
2—*Xanax* Tablets 2 mg MC-1, C5
2 mg—*Cardura* Tablets 2 mg MC-8, A5
.25—*Rocaltrol* Capsules 0.25 mcg MC-3, C5
2½—*Coumadin* Tablets 2.5 mg MC-24, D6
2½—*Zaroxolyn* Tablets 2.5 mg MC-15, B4
2.5—*Deltasone* Tablets 2.5 mg MC-19, D6
2.5—*Dyna Circ* Capsules 2.5 mg MC-12, D1
2.5—*Micronase* Tablets 2.5 mg MC-10, D1
2.5—*Premarin* Tablets 2.5 mg MC-9, C3
2.5—*Provera* Tablets 2.5 mg MC-14, B4
2.5 mg—*Altace* Capsules 2.5 mg MC-21, A4
3—*Empirin with Codeine* Tablets 325/30 mg MC-2, C1
3—*Ritalin* Tablets 10 mg MC-15, A2
3—*Tylenol with Codeine* Tablets 300/30 mg MC-1, A1
4—*Empirin with Codeine* Tablets 325/60 mg MC-2, C1
4—*Medrol* Tablets 4 mg MC-15, A4
4—Mylan Fluphenazine Tablets 1 mg MC-10, B1
4—Mylan Fluphenazine Tablets 2.5 mg MC-10, B1
4—*Tylenol with Codeine* Tablets 300/60 mg MC-1, A2
4—*Ventolin* Tablets 4 mg MC-1, B2
4 mg—*Cardura* Tablets 4 mg MC-8, A5
.5—*Rocaltrol* Capsules 0.5 mcg MC-3, C5
5—*Accupril* Tablets 5 mg MC-20, D6
5—*Cortef* Tablets 5 mg MC-11, C1
5—*Coumadin* Tablets 5 mg MC-24, D6
5—*Deltasone* Tablets 5 mg MC-19, C6
5—*Dyna Circ* Capsules 5 mg MC-12, D1
5—*Haldol* Tablets 5 mg MC-11, A1
5—*Halotestin* Tablets 5 mg MC-10, A7
5—*Isordil* Sublingual Tablets 5 mg MC-12, C6
5—*Libritabs* Tablets 5 mg MC-4, D1
5—*Librium* Capsules 5 mg MC-4, C7
5—*Lotensin* Tablets 5 mg MC-3, A2
5—*Micronase* Tablets 5 mg MC-10, D1
5—*Provera* Tablets 5 mg MC-14, B4
5—*Reglan* Tablets 5 mg MC-15, A7
5—*Valium* Tablets 5 mg MC-6, D7
5—*Zaroxolyn* Tablets 5 mg MC-15, B4
5 mg—*Altace* Capsules 5 mg MC-21, A4
6—*Rufen* Tablets 600 mg MC-11, D4
6—*Serax* Capsules 15 mg MC-17, D7
7—*Ritalin* Tablets 5 mg MC-20, D5
7.5—*Doral* Tablets 7.5 mg MC-24, D6
7½—*Coumadin* Tablets 7.5 mg MC-19, B5
8—*Klor-Con* Extended-release Tablets 600 mg MC-19, B5
8—*Lozol* Tablets 2.5 mg MC-12, A7
8—*Medrol* Tablets 8 mg MC-15, A4
8—*Rufen* Tablets 800 mg MC-11, D4
8 mg—*Cardura* Tablets 8 mg MC-8, A5
9—Mylan Fluphenazine Tablets 5 mg MC-10, B1
10—*Accupril* Tablets 10 mg MC-20, D6
10—*Accutane* Capsules 10 mg MC-12, C7
10—*Atarax* Tablets 10 mg MC-11, C5
10—*Bentyl* Capsules 10 mg MC-7, A7
10—*Cortef* Tablets 10 mg MC-11, C1
10—*Coumadin* Tablets 10 mg MC-24, D6
10—*Deltasone* Tablets 10 mg MC-19, C6
10—*Haldol* Tablets 10 mg MC-11, A1
10—*Halotestin* Tablets 10 mg MC-10, A7
10—*Inderal* Tablets 10 mg MC-20, C5
10—*Isordil* Sublingual Tablets 10 mg MC-12, C6
10—*Kerlone* Tablets 10 mg MC-3, B1
10—*Klor-Con* Extended-release Tablets 750 mg MC-19, B5
10—*Libritabs* Tablets 10 mg MC-4, D1
10—*Librium* Capsules 10 mg MC-4, C7
10—*Loniten* Tablets 10 mg MC-15, D3
10—*Lotensin* Tablets 10 mg MC-3, A2
10—*Pravachol* Tablets 10 mg MC-19, B6
10—*Provera* Tablets 10 mg MC-14, B4
10—*Valium* Tablets 10 mg MC-6, D7
10—*Zaroxolyn* Tablets 10 mg MC-15, B4
10 mg—*Altace* Capsules 10 mg MC-21, A4
11—*Tri-Levlen 28* Tablets Inert MC-13, A3
15—Biocraft Penicillin V Tablets 250 mg Round MC-18, C1
15—*Dalmane* Capsules 15 mg MC-10, B5
15—*Doral* Tablets 15 mg MC-20, D5
15—*Ionamin* Capsules 15 mg MC-18, D6
15—*Valrelease* Extended-release Capsules 15 mg ... MC-6, D6
16—Biocraft Penicillin V Tablets 250 mg Oval MC-18, C1
16—*Medrol* Tablets 16 mg MC-15, A4
16—*Ritalin-SR* Extended-release Tablets 20 mg MC-15, A3
17—Biocraft Penicillin V Tablets 500 mg Round MC-18, C2
17 12—*Carafate* Tablets 1 gram MC-21, C6
18—*Didrex* Tablets 25 mg MC-3, A4
19—*Phenergan* Tablets 12.5 mg MC-20, A5
20—*Accupril* Tablets 20 mg MC-20, D6
20—*Accutane* Capsules 20 mg MC-12, C7
20—*Bentyl* Tablets 20 mg MC-7, B1
20—*Cortef* Tablets 20 mg MC-11, C1
20—*Deltasone* Tablets 20 mg MC-19, C6
20—*Haldol* Tablets 20 mg MC-11, A1
20—*Hygroton* Tablets 50 mg MC-5, B6
20—*Inderal* Tablets 20 mg MC-20, C5
20—*Kerlone* Tablets 20 mg MC-3, B1
20—*Lotensin* Tablets 20 mg MC-3, A2
20—*Pravachol* Tablets 20 mg MC-19, B6
20—*Tofranil-PM* Capsules 75 mg MC-12, A4
21—*Hygroton* Tablets 100 mg MC-5, B6
21—*Levlen 21* Tablets 0.15/0.03 mg MC-12, D7
21—*Levlen 28* Tablets 0.15/0.03 mg MC-13, A1
22—*Esidrix* Tablets 25 mg MC-11, B3
22—*Hygroton* Tablets 25 mg MC-5, B6
22—*Levatol* Tablets 20 mg MC-18, B5
22—Schein Amitriptyline Tablets 10 mg MC-1, D7
22—*Tofranil-PM* Capsules 150 mg MC-12, A5
23—*Lioresal* Tablets 10 mg MC-3, A1
23—Schein Amitriptyline Tablets 25 mg MC-1, D7
24—Schein Amitriptyline Tablets 50 mg MC-1, D7
25—*Atarax* Tablets 25 mg MC-11, C5
25—*Clozaril* Tablets 25 mg MC-6, B7
25—*Isordil* Sublingual Tablets 2.5 mg MC-12, C6
25—*Libritabs* Tablets 25 mg MC-4, D1
25—*Librium* Capsules 25 mg MC-4, C7

25—*Norpramin* Tablets 25 mg MC-6, D1
25—Schein Amitriptyline Tablets 75 mg MC-1, D7
25—*Synthroid* Tablets 0.025 mg MC-13, B1
25—*Tenuate* Tablets 25 mg MC-7, B2
25—*Voltaren* Tablets 25 mg MC-7, A2
25 mg—*Anafranil* Capsules 25 mg MC-5, D5
26—*Ludiomil* Tablets 50 mg MC-14, A2
26—Schein Amitriptyline Tablets 100 mg MC-1, D7
27—*Phenergan* Tablets 25 mg MC-20, A5
27—Purepac Propranolol Tablets 10 mg MC-20, B7
27 27—*Tegretol* Tablets 200 mg MC-3, D4
28—*Levlen 28* Tablets Inert MC-13, A1
29—Purepac Propranolol Tablets 20 mg MC-20, B7
30—*Dalmane* Capsules 30 mg MC-10, B5
30—*Ionamin* Capsules 30 mg MC-18, D6
30—*Procardia XL* Extended-release Tablets 30 mg . . MC-16, C1
31—Purepac Amitriptyline Tablets 10 mg MC-1, D3
31—*Regroton* Tablets 0.25/50 mg MC-21, A7
32—*Demi-Regroton* Tablets 0.125/25 mg MC-21, A6
32—*Medrol* Tablets 32 mg MC-15, A5
32—Purepac Amitriptyline Tablets 25 mg MC-1, D3
32—*Tofranil* Tablets 10 mg MC-12, A6
33—*Lioresal* Tablets 20 mg MC-3, A1
34—*Ritalin* Tablets 20 mg MC-15, A2
35 35—*Lopressor HCT* Tablets 50/25 mg MC-15, C1
37—*Apresoline* Tablets 10 mg MC-11, A4
37—Geneva Hydroxyzine Tablets 10 mg MC-11, C3
37-0713—*Rynatan* Tablets 25/8/25 mg MC-5, A4
37-2001—*Soma* Tablets 350 mg MC-4, A3
37-4224—*Organidin* Tablets 30 mg MC-12, B4
38—Geneva Hydroxyzine Tablets 25 mg MC-11, C3
39—*Apresoline* Tablets 25 mg MC-11, A4
39—Geneva Hydroxyzine Tablets 50 mg MC-11, C3
40—*Accupril* Tablets 40 mg MC-20, D6
40—*Accutane* Capsules 40 mg MC-12, C7
40—*Calan* Tablets 40 mg MC-24, D3
40—*Inderal* Tablets 40 mg MC-20, C5
40—*Isoptin* Tablets 40 mg MC-24, B7
40—*Lasix* Tablets 40 mg MC-10, C3
40—*Lotensin* Tablets 40 mg MC-3, A2
40—*Tofranil-PM* Capsules 100 mg MC-12, A4
40/25—*Inderide* Tablets 40/25 mg MC-20, D4
45—IPR Pharma Atenolol Tablets 50 mg MC-2, C5
45—*Tofranil-PM* Capsules 125 mg MC-12, A5
46—*Esidrix* Tablets 50 mg MC-11, B3
49—Biocraft Penicillin V Tablets 500 mg Oval MC-18, C2
50—*Atarax* Tablets 50 mg MC-11, C5
50—*Darvocet-N* Tablets 50/325 mg MC-20, B2
50—*Deltasone* Tablets 50 mg MC-19, C6
50—*Didrex* Tablets 50 mg MC-3, A4
50—*Diflucan* Tablets 50 mg MC-10, A5
50—*Imuran* Tablets 50 mg MC-2, D6
50—*Norpramin* Tablets 50 mg MC-6, D1
50—*Synthroid* Tablets 0.05 mg MC-13, B1
50—*Theo-Dur Sprinkle* Extended-release Capsules
    50 mg MC-22, C6
50—*Voltaren* Tablets 50 mg MC-7, A2
50 mg—*Anafranil* Capsules 50 mg MC-5, D5
50 mg—*Ansaid* Tablets 50 mg MC-10, B7
50 MG—*Zoloft* Tablets 50 mg MC-21, B3
50 PD—*Meclomen* Capsules 50 mg MC-14, B2
51—*Serax* Capsules 10 mg MC-17, D7
51 51—*Lopressor* Tablets 50 mg MC-15, B7
52—*Serax* Capsules 30 mg MC-17, D7
52—*Tegretol* Chewable Tablets 100 mg MC-3, D5
53—*Omnipen* Capsules 250 mg MC-2, B6
53 53—*Lopressor HCT* Tablets 100/25 mg MC-15, C1
54 213—Roxane Lithium Capsules 150 mg MC-13, C5
54 452—Roxane Lithium Tablets 300 mg MC-13, C6
54 463—Roxane Lithium Capsules 300 mg MC-13, C5
54 582—*Roxicodone* Tablets 5 mg MC-18, A3
54 702—Roxane Lithium Capsules 600 mg MC-13, C5
54 730—*Roxicet* Tablets 5/500 mg MC-18, A6
54 902—*Roxiprin* Tablets 4.88/325 mg MC-18, B2

55 63—Schein/Danbury Procainamide
    Extended-release Tablets 500 mg MC-20, A2
55 64—Schein/Danbury Procainamide
    Extended-release Tablets 750 mg MC-20, A2
55 126—Barr Dicyclomine Tablets 20 mg MC-7, A6
56—*Ovral-21* Tablets 0.5/0.05 mg MC-17, C2
56—*Ovral-28* Tablets 0.5/0.05 mg MC-17, C3
57—Purepac Lorazepam Tablets 0.5 mg MC-13, D5
59—*Pen-Vee K* Tablets 250 mg MC-18, C1
59—Purepac Lorazepam Tablets 1 mg MC-13, D5
60—*Inderal LA* Extended-release Capsules 60 mg . . MC-20, C3
60—*Inderal* Tablets 60 mg MC-20, C6
60—*Procardia XL* Extended-release Tablets 60 mg . . MC-16, C1
60 mg—*Cardizem SR* Capsules 60 mg MC-7, C2
61—*Lomotil* Tablets 2.5/0.025 mg MC-7, D3
64—*Ativan* Tablets 1 mg MC-13, D7
65—*Ativan* Tablets 2 mg MC-13, D7
65—*Lithobid* Extended-release Tablets 300 mg MC-13, C4
68-7—*Norpramin* Tablets 10 mg MC-6, D1
71—*Demulen 1/50-21* Tablets 1/0.05 mg MC-9, C7
71—*Demulen 1/50-28* Tablets 1/0.05 mg MC-9, D1
71—*Ser-Ap-Es* Tablets 0.1/25/15 mg MC-21, B1
71 71—*Lopressor* Tablets 100 mg MC-15, B7
72—*Brethine* Tablets 2.5 mg MC-22, B1
73—*Apresoline* Tablets 50 mg MC-11, A4
73—*Wytensin* Tablets 4 mg MC-10, D3
73 73—*Lopressor HCT* Tablets 100/50 mg MC-15, C1
74—*Wytensin* Tablets 8 mg MC-10, D3
75—*Nordette-21* Tablets 0.15/0.03 mg MC-13, A4
75—*Nordette-28* Tablets 0.15/0.03 mg MC-13, A5
75—*Norpramin* Tablets 75 mg MC-6, D2
75—*Ortho-Novum 7/7/7-21* Tablets 0.75/0.035 mg . . MC-17, A2
75—*Ortho-Novum 7/7/7-28* Tablets 0.75/0.035 mg . . MC-17, A3
75—*Slo-bid* Extended-release Capsules 75 mg MC-22, D2
75—*Synthroid* Tablets 0.075 mg MC-13, B1
75—*Tenuate* Extended-release Tablets 75 mg MC-7, B3
75—*Theo-Dur Sprinkle* Extended-release Capsules
    75 mg MC-22, C6
75—*Voltaren* Tablets 75 mg MC-7, A2
75—*Wellbutrin* Tablets 75 mg MC-3, B5
75 mg—*Anafranil* Capsules 75 mg MC-5, D5
75 mg—*Cleocin* Capsules 75 mg MC-5, D4
76—*Thalitone* Tablets 25 mg MC-5, B5
78—*Lo-Ovral-21* Tablets 0.3/0.03 mg MC-17, B7
78—*Lo-Ovral-28* Tablets 0.3/0.03 mg MC-17, C1
78-2—*Mellaril* Tablets 10 mg MC-23, A6
78-3—*Mellaril* Tablets 25 mg MC-23, A6
78-4—*Mellaril* Tablets 50 mg MC-23, A6
78-5—*Mellaril* Tablets 100 mg MC-23, A7
78-6—*Mellaril* Tablets 150 mg MC-23, A7
78-7—*Mellaril* Tablets 200 mg MC-23, A7
78-8—*Mellaril* Tablets 15 mg MC-23, A6
78-17—*Parlodel* Tablets 2.5 mg MC-3, B3
78-34—*Cafergot* Tablets 1/100 mg MC-8, D7
78-72—*Tavist* Tablets 2.68 mg MC-5, D1
78-73—*Visken* Tablets 10 mg MC-19, A5
78-75—*Tavist* Tablets 1.34 mg MC-5, D1
78-78—*Pamelor* Capsules 50 mg MC-17, C5
78-79—*Pamelor* Capsules 75 mg MC-17, C5
78-84—*Fioricet* Tablets 50/325/40 mg MC-3, A7
78-86—*Pamelor* Capsules 10 mg MC-17, C4
78-87—*Pamelor* Capsules 25 mg MC-17, C4
78-98—*Restoril* Capsules 15 mg MC-22, A6
78-99—*Restoril* Capsules 30 mg MC-22, A6
78-101—*Hydergine LC* Capsules 1 mg MC-8, D4
78-102—*Parlodel* Capsules 5 mg MC-3, B2
78-103—*Fiorinal* Capsules 50/325/40 mg MC-3, C2
78-104—*Fiorinal* Tablets 50/325/40 mg MC-3, C3
78-107—*Fiorinal with Codeine* Capsules
    50/325/30/40 mg MC-3, C4
78-111—*Visken* Tablets 5 mg MC-19, A5
78-221—*Tavist-D* Tablets 1.34/75 mg MC-5, D2
80—*Calan* Tablets 80 mg MC-24, D3
80—*Inderal LA* Extended-release Capsules 80 mg . . MC-20, C3
80—*Inderal* Tablets 80 mg MC-20, C6

80—*Isoptin* Tablets 80 mg MC-24, B7
80—*Lasix* Tablets 80 mg MC-10, C3
80/25—*Inderide* Tablets 80/25 mg MC-20, D4
80/50—*Inderide LA* Extended-release Capsules
 80/50 mg MC-20, D2
81—*Ativan* Tablets 0.5 mg MC-13, D7
90—IPR Pharma Atenolol Tablets 100 mg MC-2, C5
90—*Procardia XL* Extended-release Tablets 90 mg MC-16, C1
90 mg—*Cardizem SR* Capsules 90 mg MC-7, C2
90—*Cardizem* Tablets 90 mg MC-7, C4
95—*Tri-Levlen 21* Tablets 0.05/0.03 mg MC-13, A2
95—*Tri-Levlen 28* Tablets 0.05/0.03 mg MC-13, A3
96—*Tri-Levlen 21* Tablets 0.075/0.04 mg MC-13, A2
96—*Tri-Levlen 28* Tablets 0.075/0.04 mg MC-13, A3
97—Mylan Fluphenazine Tablets 10 mg MC-10, B1
97—*Tri-Levlen 21* Tablets 0.125/0.03 mg MC-13, A2
97—*Tri-Levlen 28* Tablets 0.125/0.03 mg MC-13, A3
100—*Atarax* Tablets 100 mg MC-11, C5
100—*Clozaril* Tablets 100 mg MC-6, B7
100—*Darvocet-N* Tablets 100/650 mg MC-20, B2
100—*Diflucan* Tablets 100 mg MC-10, A5
100—*Norpramin* Tablets 100 mg MC-6, D2
100—*Synthroid* Tablets 0.1 mg MC-13, B1
100—*Theo-Dur* Extended-release Tablets 100 mg MC-22, D1
100—*Tigan* Capsules 100 mg MC-24, B2
100—*Tolinase* Tablets 100 mg MC-23, C4
100—*Trandate* Tablets 100 mg MC-12, D3
100—*Wellbutrin* Tablets 100 mg MC-3, B5
100—*Zyloprim* Tablets 100 mg MC-1, C1
100 mg—*Ansaid* Tablets 100 mg MC-10, B7
100 MG—*Zoloft* Tablets 100 mg MC-21, B3
100 PD—*Meclomen* Capsules 100 mg MC-14, B2
101—*Apresoline* Tablets 100 mg MC-11, A4
101—*Azulfidine* Tablets 500 mg MC-21, D3
101—*Gastrocrom* Capsules 100 mg MC-6, C1
101—*Tenormin* Tablets 100 mg MC-2, C4
102—*Azulfidine EN-Tabs* Enteric-coated Tablets
 500 mg MC-21, D4
105—*Brethine* Tablets 5 mg MC-22, B1
105—Geneva Haloperidol Tablets 0.5 mg MC-10, D7
105—*Tenormin* Tablets 50 mg MC-2, C4
107—*Tenormin* Tablets 25 mg MC-2, C4
110—*Ludiomil* Tablets 25 mg MC-14, A2
112—Biocraft Cephradine Capsules 250 mg MC-4, C6
112—*Synthroid* Tablets 0.112 mg MC-13, B1
113—Biocraft Cephradine Capsules 500 mg MC-4, C6
113—*Velosef* Capsules 250 mg MC-4, C4
114—*Velosef* Capsules 500 mg MC-4, C4
115—*Tenoretic* Tablets 50/25 mg MC-2, C7
117—Biocraft Cephalexin Capsules 500 mg MC-4, C1
117—*Tenoretic* Tablets 100/25 mg MC-2, C7
120—*Calan* Tablets 120 mg MC-24, D3
120—*Inderal LA* Extended-release Capsules 120 mg MC-20, C4
120—*Isoptin* Tablets 120 mg MC-24, B7
120 mg—*Cardizem SR* Capsules 120 mg MC-7, C2
120 mg—*Cardizem* Tablets 120 mg MC-7, C4
120 SR—*Isoptin SR* Extended-release Tablets
 120 mg MC-24, C1
120/50—*Inderide LA* Extended-release Capsules
 120/50 mg MC-20, D2
123—Geneva Haloperidol Tablets 1 mg MC-10, D7
125—*Amoxil* Chewable Tablets 125 mg MC-2, A7
125—*Nicobid* Extended-release Capsules 125 mg MC-16, A5
125—*Slo-bid* Extended-release Capsules 125 mg MC-22, D2
125—*Synthroid* Tablets 0.125 mg MC-13, B2
125—*Theo-Dur Sprinkle* Extended-release Capsules
 125 mg MC-22, C7
125—*V-Cillin K* Tablets 125 mg MC-18, C4
127—Purepac Clonidine Tablets 0.1 mg MC-6, A3
127—Schein/Danbury Propranolol Tablets 60 mg MC-20, C2
128—Barr Dicyclomine Capsules 10 mg MC-7, A5
128—Purepac Clonidine Tablets 0.2 mg MC-6, A3
129—Purepac Clonidine Tablets 0.3 mg MC-6, A3
130—*Zestril* Tablets 5 mg MC-13, C1
131—*Zestril* Tablets 10 mg MC-13, C1

132—*Zestril* Tablets 20 mg MC-13, C1
133—Purepac Amitriptyline Tablets 50 mg MC-1, D3
134—Purepac Amitriptyline Tablets 75 mg MC-1, D4
134—*Zestril* Tablets 40 mg MC-13, C1
135—*Ludiomil* Tablets 75 mg MC-14, A2
135—*Ortho-Novum 1/35-21* Tablets 1/0.035 mg MC-16, D7
135—*Ortho-Novum 1/35-28* Tablets 1/0.035 mg MC-17, A1
135—*Ortho-Novum 7/7/7-21* Tablets 1/0.035 mg . . . MC-17, A2
135—*Ortho-Novum 7/7/7-28* Tablets 1/0.035 mg . . . MC-17, A3
135—Purepac Amitriptyline Tablets 100 mg MC-1, D4
136—*Tofranil* Tablets 50 mg MC-12, A6
139—*Apresazide* Capsules 25/25 mg MC-11, A6
140—*Tofranil* Tablets 25 mg MC-12, A6
142—*Zestoretic* Tablets 20/12.5 mg MC-13, C3
143—*Geocillin* Tablets 382 mg MC-4, A1
143—Purepac Carbamazepine Tablets 200 mg MC-3, D6
145—*Zestoretic* Tablets 20/25 mg MC-13, C3
149—*Apresazide* Capsules 50/50 mg MC-11, A6
149—Biocraft Clindamycin Capsules 150 mg MC-5, D3
150—*Norpramin* Tablets 150 mg MC-6, D2
150—*Ortho-Novum 1/50-21* Tablets 1/0.05 mg MC-17, B3
150—*Ortho-Novum 1/50-28* Tablets 1/0.05 mg MC-17, B4
150—*Rythmol* Tablets 150 mg MC-20, A4
150—*Synthroid* Tablets 0.15 mg MC-13, B2
150—*Zantac* Tablets 150 mg MC-21, A5
150 mg—*Cleocin* Capsules 150 mg MC-5, D4
151—*Demulen 1/35-21* Tablets 1/0.035 mg MC-9, C5
151—*Demulen 1/35-28* Tablets 1/0.035 mg MC-9, C6
152—Mylan Clonidine Tablets 0.1 mg MC-6, A2
155—*Medrol* Tablets 24 mg MC-15, A4
155—Mylan Propoxyphene Napsylate and Acetaminophen
 Tablets 100/65 mg Pink MC-20, B3
158—*Monopril* Tablets 10 mg MC-10, C1
159—*Apresazide* Capsules 100/50 mg MC-11, A6
160—*Inderal LA* Extended-release Capsules 160 mg MC-20, C4
160/50—*Inderide LA* Extended-release Capsules
 160/50 mg MC-20, D3
170—Barr Furosemide Tablets 20 mg MC-10, C2
175—*Synthroid* Tablets 0.175 mg MC-13, B2
179—Mutual Tolmetin Capsules 400 mg MC-23, D1
180 mg—*Cardizem CD* Capsules 180 mg MC-7, B7
180 MG—*Isoptin SR* Extended-release Tablets
 180 mg MC-24, C2
181—Apothecon Cephalexin Capsules 250 mg MC-4, B6
181—*Deconamine SR* Extended-release Capsules
 8/120 mg MC-5, A2
183—Purepac Dipyridamole Tablets 50 mg MC-7, D7
184—*Deconamine* Tablets 4/60 mg MC-5, A3
185—Purepac Dipyridamole Tablets 75 mg MC-7, D7
186—Mylan Clonidine Tablets 0.2 mg MC-6, A2
191—*Esidrix* Tablets 100 mg MC-11, B3
192—Purepac Diphenhydramine Capsules 50 mg MC-7, D1
193—Purepac Dipyridamole Tablets 25 mg MC-7, D7
194—Purepac Doxycycline Capsules 50 mg MC-8, C4
195—Purepac Doxycycline Capsules 100 mg MC-8, C4
199—Mylan Clonidine Tablets 0.3 mg MC-6, A2
200—*Diflucan* Tablets 200 mg MC-10, A5
200—*Ethmozine* Tablets 200 mg MC-15, D5
200—*Proloprim* Tablets 200 mg MC-24, B3
200—*Synthroid* Tablets 0.2 mg MC-13, B2
200—*Theo-Dur* Extended-release Tablets 200 mg MC-22, D1
200—*Theo-Dur Sprinkle* Extended-release Capsules
 200 mg MC-22, C7
200—*Tolectin* Tablets 200 mg MC-23, C7
200—*Trandate* Tablets 200 mg MC-12, D3
200—*Vascor* Tablets 200 mg MC-3, A7
200—*Zovirax* Capsules 200 mg MC-1, A7
200 mg—*Floxin* Tablets 200 mg MC-17, C6
200 mg—*Lodine* Capsules 200 mg MC-9, D2
200 SKF—*Tagamet* Tablets 200 mg MC-5, C3
210—*Antivert* Tablets 12.5 mg MC-14, A4
211—*Antivert* Tablets 25 mg MC-14, A4
211—*Grifulvin V* Tablets 250 mg MC-10, D2

211—Mylan Chlordiazepoxide and Amitriptyline
  Tablets 5/12.5 mg MC-4, D2
212—*Antivert* Chewable Tablets 25 mg MC-14, A5
214—*Antivert* Tablets 50 mg MC-14, A4
214—*Grifulvin V* Tablets 500 mg MC-10, D2
214—Mylan Haloperidol Tablets 2 mg MC-11, A2
227—*Phenergan* Tablets 50 mg MC-20, A5
227 227—*Normozide* Tablets 200/25 mg MC-12, D6
230—*Trimox* Capsules 250 mg MC-2, A5
231—*Trimox* Capsules 500 mg MC-2, A5
235 235—*Normozide* Tablets 100/25 mg MC-12, D6
239—Apothecon Cephalexin Capsules 500 mg . . MC-4, B6
240 mg—*Cardizem CD* Capsules 240 mg MC-7, B7
244—*Normodyne* Tablets 100 mg MC-12, D4
250—*Amoxil* Capsules 250 mg MC-2, A6
250—*Amoxil* Chewable Tablets 250 mg MC-2, A7
250—*Ethmozine* Tablets 250 mg MC-15, D5
250—*Keftab* Tablets 250 mg MC-4, C3
250—*Lorelco* Tablets 250 mg MC-19, C7
250—*Naprosyn* Tablets 250 mg MC-16, A5
250—*Nicobid* Extended-release Capsules 250 mg . . MC-16, A7
250—*Orinase* Tablets 250 mg MC-23, C5
250—*Slo-Niacin* Extended-release Tablets 250 mg . . MC-16, B3
250—*Tigan* Capsules 250 mg MC-24, B2
250—*Tolinase* Tablets 250 mg MC-23, C4
250—*V-Cillin K* Tablets 250 mg MC-18, C4
250mg—*E-Mycin* Delayed-release Tablets 250 mg . . MC-9, A6
250 mg—*Panmycin* Capsules 250 mg MC-22, C2
250/125—*Augmentin* Tablets 250/125 mg . . . MC-2, B2
252—Barr Dipyridamole Tablets 25 mg MC-7, D4
252 252—*Proventil* Tablets 2 mg MC-1, B5
253—Purepac Methyldopa Tablets 250 mg . . . MC-14, D1
255—Purepac Methyldopa Tablets 500 mg . . . MC-14, D1
257—Mylan Haloperidol Tablets 1 mg MC-11, A2
259—Barr Erythromycin Ethylsuccinate Tablets
  400 mg MC-9, B5
260—Barr Thioridazine Tablets 10 mg MC-23, A2
260—*Procardia* Capsules 10 mg MC-16, B7
260—*Theobid* Extended-release Capsules 260 mg . . MC-22, D7
261—Barr Thioridazine Tablets 25 mg MC-23, A2
261—*Procardia* Capsules 20 mg MC-16, B7
261—Purepac Methyldopa and Hydrochlorothiazide
  Tablets 250/15 mg MC-15, A1
262—Barr Thioridazine Tablets 50 mg MC-23, A2
263—Barr Thioridazine Tablets 100 mg MC-23, A2
263—Purepac Methyldopa and Hydrochlorothiazide
  Tablets 250/25 mg MC-15, A1
267—Barr Chlorthalidone Tablets 25 mg MC-5, B4
268—Barr Chlorthalidone Tablets 50 mg MC-5, B4
269—Purepac Metoclopramide Tablets 10 mg . . MC-15, A6
274—*Anaprox* Tablets 275 mg MC-16, A6
277—Mylan Chlordiazepoxide and Amitriptyline
  Tablets 10/25 mg MC-4, D2
280—Purepac Haloperidol Tablets 1 mg MC-11, A3
281—Purepac Haloperidol Tablets 2 mg MC-11, A3
282—Purepac Haloperidol Tablets 5 mg MC-11, A3
283—*Corzide* Tablets 40/5 mg MC-16, A2
284—*Corzide* Tablets 80/5 mg MC-16, A2
285—Barr Dipyridamole Tablets 50 mg MC-7, D4
286—Barr Dipyridamole Tablets 75 mg MC-7, D4
286—Purepac Haloperidol Tablets 10 mg MC-11, A3
287—Purepac Haloperidol Tablets 20 mg MC-11, A3
289—Purepac Haloperidol Tablets 0.5 mg . . . MC-11, A3
295—Barr Doxycycline Tablets 100 mg MC-8, C1
296—Barr Doxycycline Capsules 50 mg MC-8, B7
297—Barr Doxycycline Capsules 100 mg MC-8, B7
300—*Ethmozine* Tablets 300 mg MC-15, D6
300—*Rythmol* Tablets 300 mg MC-20, A6
300—*Synthroid* Tablets 0.3 mg MC-13, B2
300—*Theo-Dur* Extended-release Tablets 300 mg . . MC-22, D1
300—*Trandate* Tablets 300 mg MC-12, D3
300—*Vascor* Tablets 300 mg MC-3, A7
300—*Zantac* Tablets 300 mg MC-21, A5
300—*Zyloprim* Tablets 300 mg MC-1, C1
300mg—*Motrin* Tablets 300 mg MC-12, A2

300 MG—*Actigall* Capsules 300 mg MC-24, B5
300 mg—*Cardizem CD* Capsules 300 mg . . . MC-7, C1
300 mg—*Cleocin* Capsules 300 mg MC-5, D4
300 mg—*Floxin* Tablets 300 mg MC-17, C6
300 mg—*Lodine* Tablets 300 mg MC-9, D2
300 SKF—*Tagamet* Tablets 300 mg MC-5, C3
302—Schein/Danbury Furosemide Tablets 80 mg . . MC-10, C4
302—Schein/Danbury Hydroxyzine Capsules 25 mg . . MC-11, C7
305—*Zithromax* Capsules 250 mg MC-2, D7
309—*Omnipen* Capsules 500 mg MC-2, B6
317—Barr Propoxyphene Napsylate and
  Acetaminophen Tablets 50/325 mg MC-20, B1
317—Purepac Fenoprofen Tablets 600 mg . . . MC-10, A2
317—*Serax* Tablets 15 mg MC-18, A1
318—Barr Propoxyphene Napsylate and Acetaminophen
  Tablets 100/650 mg White MC-20, B1
321—Purepac Propranolol Tablets 60 mg MC-20, B7
322—*Feldene* Capsules 10 mg MC-19, A6
323—*Feldene* Capsules 20 mg MC-19, A6
324—Schein/Danbury Hydroxyzine Capsules 50 mg . . MC-11, C7
327—Barr Thioridazine Tablets 150 mg MC-23, A3
327—Mylan Haloperidol Tablets 5 mg MC-11, A2
328—Barr Thioridazine Tablets 200 mg MC-23, A3
331—Barr Disopyramide Capsules 100 mg . . . MC-8, A1
331—Purepac Propranolol Tablets 40 mg MC-20, B7
332—Barr Disopyramide Capsules 150 mg . . . MC-8, A1
333—Purepac Propranolol Tablets 80 mg MC-20, B7
333mg—*E-Mycin* Delayed-release Tablets 333 mg . . MC-9, A6
338—*Capozide* Tablets 25/15 mg MC-3, D1
349—*Capozide* Tablets 25/25 mg MC-3, D1
351—Mylan Haloperidol Tablets 0.5 mg MC-11, A2
358—Purepac Propranolol and Hydrochlorothiazide
  Tablets 40/25 mg MC-20, C7
360—Purepac Propranolol and Hydrochlorothiazide
  Tablets 80/25 mg MC-20, C7
370—Barr Lorazepam Tablets 0.5 mg MC-13, D4
371—Barr Lorazepam Tablets 1 mg MC-13, D4
371—*Trandate HCT* Tablets 100/25 mg MC-12, D5
372—Barr Lorazepam Tablets 2 mg MC-13, D4
372—*Trandate HCT* Tablets 200/25 mg MC-12, D5
373—Barr Oxazepam Tablets 15 mg MC-17, D4
373—*Trandate HCT* Tablets 300/25 mg MC-12, D5
374—Barr Oxazepam Capsules 10 mg MC-17, D3
375—Barr Oxazepam Capsules 15 mg MC-17, D3
375—*Naprosyn* Tablets 375 mg MC-16, A5
376—Barr Oxazepam Capsules 30 mg MC-17, D3
377—Barr Flurazepam Capsules 15 mg MC-10, B3
378—Barr Flurazepam Capsules 30 mg MC-10, B3
381—Barr Meperidine Tablets 50 mg MC-14, B5
382—Barr Meperidine Tablets 100 mg MC-14, B5
384—*Capozide* Tablets 50/15 mg MC-3, D2
387—*Ceftin* Tablets 250 mg MC-4, B4
388—Purepac Spironolactone Tablets 25 mg . . MC-21, B7
390—*Capozide* Tablets 50/25 mg MC-3, D2
390—*Pen-Vee K* Tablets 500 mg MC-18, C5
391 391—*Normozide* Tablets 300/25 mg . . . MC-12, D6
393—*Diabinese* Tablets 100 mg MC-5, B2
394—*Ceftin* Tablets 500 mg MC-4, B5
394—*Diabinese* Tablets 250 mg MC-5, B2
395—*Ceftin* Tablets 125 mg MC-4, B4
400—*Rufen* Tablets 400 mg MC-11, D4
400—*Suprax* Tablets 400 mg MC-4, B3
400—*Vascor* Tablets 400 mg MC-3, A7
400 mg—*Floxin* Tablets 400 mg MC-17, C7
400mg—*Motrin* Tablets 400 mg MC-12, A2
400 SKF—*Tagamet* Tablets 400 mg MC-5, C5
404—Purepac Tetracycline Capsules 250 mg . . MC-22, B7
406—Purepac Tetracycline Capsules 500 mg . . MC-22, B7
411—*Glucotrol* Tablets 5 mg MC-10, C6
412—*Glucotrol* Tablets 10 mg MC-10, C6
419—Barr Ibuprofen Tablets 400 mg MC-11, D2
420—Barr Ibuprofen Tablets 600 mg MC-11, D2
425—Barr Verapamil Tablets 80 mg MC-24, B6
430—*Minizide* Capsules 1/0.5 mg MC-19, C4
431—*Minipress* Capsules 1 mg MC-19, C1

431—*Pronestyl* Tablets 250 mg. MC-19, D6
431—*Proventil* Extended-release Tablets 4 mg MC-19, C4
432—*Minizide* Capsules 2/0.5 mg MC-19, C4
434—*Pronestyl* Tablets 375 mg MC-19, D6
436—*Minizide* Capsules 5/0.5 mg MC-19, C4
437—*Minipress* Capsules 2 mg MC-19, C1
438—*Minipress* Capsules 5 mg MC-19, C1
438—*Normodyne* Tablets 300 mg MC-12, D4
438—*Pronestyl* Tablets 500 mg MC-19, D6
439—Purepac Trazodone Tablets 50 mg MC-23, D6
441—Purepac Trazodone Tablets 100 mg MC-23, D6
443—Warner Chilcott Clonidine Tablets 0.1 mg MC-6, A5
444—Warner Chilcott Clonidine Tablets 0.2 mg MC-6, A5
445—*Ovral-28* Tablets Inert MC-17, C3
450—*Capoten* Tablets 12.5 mg MC-3, C6
452—*Capoten* Tablets 25 mg MC-3, C6
455—Barr Verapamil Tablets 120 mg MC-24, B6
470—Barr Propoxyphene Napsylate and Acetaminophen
    Tablets 100/650 mg Pink MC-20, B1
473—Purepac Verapamil Tablets 80 mg MC-24, C7
475—Purepac Verapamil Tablets 120 mg MC-24, C7
477—Barr Haloperidol Tablets 0.5 mg MC-10, D5
478—Barr Haloperidol Tablets 1 mg MC-10, D5
479—Barr Haloperidol Tablets 2 mg MC-10, D5
480—Barr Haloperidol Tablets 5 mg MC-10, D5
481—Barr Haloperidol Tablets 10 mg MC-10, D6
482—Barr Haloperidol Tablets 20 mg MC-10, D6
482—*Capoten* Tablets 50 mg MC-3, C7
485—*Capoten* Tablets 100 mg MC-3, C7
486—*Lo-Ovral-28* Tablets Inert MC-17, C1
486—*Nordette-28* Tablets Inert MC-13, A5
487—Barr Temazepam Capsules 15 mg MC-22, A3
488—Barr Temazepam Capsules 30 mg MC-22, A3
499—Barr Ibuprofen Tablets 800 mg MC-11, D2
500—*Amoxil* Capsules 500 mg MC-2, A6
500—*Flagyl* Tablets 500 mg MC-15, C5
500—*Keftab* Tablets 500 mg MC-4, C3
500—*Lorelco* Tablets 500 mg MC-19, C7
500—*Naprosyn* Tablets 500 mg MC-16, A5
500—*Nicobid* Extended-release Capsules 500 mg . . . MC-16, B1
500—*Orinase* Tablets 500 mg MC-23, C5
500—Purepac Prazosin Capsules 1 mg MC-19, C2
500—*Slo-Niacin* Extended-release Tablets 500 mg . . . MC-16, B3
500—*Tolinase* Tablets 500 mg MC-23, C4
500—*V-Cillin K* Tablets 500 mg MC-18, C4
500/125—*Augmentin* Tablets 500/125 mg MC-2, B2
501—Purepac Prazosin Capsules 2 mg MC-19, C2
502—Purepac Prazosin Capsules 5 mg MC-19, C2
512—*Cipro* Tablets 250 mg MC-5, C5
513—*Cipro* Tablets 500 mg MC-5, C6
514—*Cipro* Tablets 750 mg MC-5, C6
515—*Quibron* Capsules 300/180 mg MC-23, A1
516—*Quibron* Capsules 150/90 mg MC-23, A1
521—*Lufyllin* Tablets 200 mg MC-8, D1
521—Mylan Propoxyphene Napsylate and
    Acetaminophen Tablets 100/65 mg White MC-8, B1
534—*Sinequan* Capsules 10 mg MC-8, B1
535—*Ortho-Novum 7/7/7-21* Tablets 0.5/0.035 mg . . MC-17, A2
535—*Ortho-Novum 7/7/7-28* Tablets 0.5/0.035 mg . . MC-17, A3
535—*Sinequan* Capsules 25 mg MC-8, B1
536—*Sinequan* Capsules 50 mg MC-8, B1
537—*Sinequan* Capsules 150 mg MC-8, B2
538—*Sinequan* Capsules 100 mg MC-8, B2
539—*Sinequan* Capsules 75 mg MC-8, B2
541—*Vistaril* Capsules 25 mg MC-11, C4
542—*Vistaril* Capsules 50 mg MC-11, C4
543—*Roxicet* Tablets 5/325 mg MC-18, A6
543—*Vistaril* Capsules 100 mg MC-11, C4
550—Barr Cephradine Capsules 250 mg MC-4, C5
551—Barr Cephradine Capsules 500 mg MC-4, C5
555 19—Barr Hydrochlorothiazide Tablets 25 mg . . . MC-11, B2
555 20—Barr Hydrochlorothiazide Tablets 50 mg . . . MC-11, B2
555 169—Barr Furosemide Tablets 40 mg MC-10, C2
555 192—Barr Hydrochlorothiazide Tablets 100 mg . . MC-11, B2
555 196—Barr Furosemide Tablets 80 mg MC-10, C2

555 444—Barr Triamterene and Hydrochlorothiazide
    Tablets 75/50 mg MC-24, A1
555 585—Barr Chlorzoxazone Tablets 500 mg MC-5, B7
559—*Wymox* Capsules 250 mg MC-2, B1
560—*Wymox* Capsules 500 mg MC-2, B1
571—*Navane* Capsules 1 mg MC-23, B4
572—*Navane* Capsules 2 mg MC-23, B4
573—*Navane* Capsules 5 mg MC-23, B4
573 573—*Proventil* Tablets 4 mg MC-1, B5
574—*Navane* Capsules 10 mg MC-23, B5
577—*Navane* Capsules 20 mg MC-23, B5
583—*Ovcon 35-21* Tablets 0.4/0.035 mg MC-16, D3
583—*Ovcon 35-28* Tablets 0.4/0.035 mg MC-16, D4
584—Barr Erythromycin Delayed-release Capsules
    250 mg MC-9, A5
584—*Ovcon 50-21* Tablets 1/0.05 mg MC-16, D5
584—*Ovcon 50-28* Tablets 1/0.05 mg MC-16, D6
600—*Nolvadex* Tablets 10 mg MC-22, A2
600—*Tolectin* Tablets 600 mg MC-23, C7
600mg—*Motrin* Tablets 600 mg MC-12, A3
601—*Pro-Banthine* Tablets 15 mg MC-20, A7
603—*Sumycin* Tablets 500 mg MC-22, B5
609—*Monopril* Tablets 20 mg MC-10, C1
611—*Pro-Banthine* Tablets 7.5 mg MC-20, A7
641—*Triphasil-21* Tablets 0.05/0.03 mg MC-13, A6
641—*Triphasil-28* Tablets 0.05/0.03 mg MC-13, A7
642—*Triphasil-21* Tablets 0.075/0.04 mg MC-13, A6
642—*Triphasil-28* Tablets 0.075/0.04 mg MC-13, A7
643—*Triphasil-21* Tablets 0.125/0.03 mg MC-13, A6
643—*Triphasil-28* Tablets 0.125/0.03 mg MC-13, A7
647—*Sinemet* Tablets 10/100 mg MC-4, A2
648—*Veetids* Tablets 500 mg MC-18, B7
650—*Sinemet* Tablets 25/100 mg MC-4, A2
650—*Triphasil-28* Tablets Inert MC-13, A7
654—*Sinemet* Tablets 25/250 mg MC-4, A2
655—*Sumycin* Capsules 250 mg MC-22, B4
663—*Sumycin* Tablets 250 mg MC-22, B5
684—*Veetids* Tablets 250 mg MC-18, B7
703—*Trinalin* Extended-release Tablets 1/120 mg . . . MC-2, D5
710—Mylan Cyclobenzaprine Tablets 10 mg MC-6, C3
715—Mylan Timolol Tablets 20 mg MC-23, C1
731—*Lufyllin* Tablets 400 mg MC-8, D1
750—*Robaxin* Tablets 750 mg MC-14, C2
750—*Slo-Niacin* Extended-release Tablets 750 mg . . . MC-16, B3
752—*Normodyne* Tablets 200 mg MC-12, D4
756—*Pronestyl* Capsules 375 mg MC-19, D5
757—*Pronestyl* Capsules 500 mg MC-19, D5
758—*Pronestyl* Capsules 250 mg MC-19, D5
760—*Sorbitrate* Sublingual Tablets 5 mg MC-12, C2
761—*Sorbitrate* Sublingual Tablets 10 mg MC-12, C2
763—*Sumycin* Capsules 500 mg MC-22, B4
770—*Sorbitrate* Tablets 5 mg MC-12, B5
773—*Sorbitrate* Tablets 30 mg MC-12, B6
774—*Sorbitrate* Tablets 40 mg MC-12, B6
780—*Sorbitrate* Tablets 10 mg MC-12, B5
800—*Zovirax* Tablets 800 mg MC-1, B1
800mg—*Motrin* Tablets 800 mg MC-12, A3
800 SKF—*Tagamet* Tablets 800 mg MC-5, C4
810—*Sorbitrate* Chewable Tablets 5 mg MC-12, B7
811—*Adalat* Capsules 10 mg MC-16, B6
815—*Sorbitrate* Chewable Tablets 10 mg MC-12, B7
820—*Sorbitrate* Tablets 20 mg MC-12, B5
821—*Adalat* Capsules 20 mg MC-16, B6
832 L01—Schein/Danbury Levothyroxine Tablets
    0.1 mg MC-13, B6
832 L02—Schein/Danbury Levothyroxine Tablets
    0.2 mg MC-13, B6
832 L03—Schein/Danbury Levothyroxine Tablets
    0.3 mg MC-13, B6
832 L15—Schein/Danbury Levothyroxine Tablets
    0.15 mg MC-13, B6
850—*Ovcon 35-28* Tablets Inert MC-16, D4
850—*Ovcon 50-28* Tablets Inert MC-16, D6
853—*Sorbitrate* Sublingual Tablets 2.5 mg MC-12, C2
855—*Nimotop* Capsules 30 mg MC-16, C3

880—*Sorbitrate SA* Extended-release Tablets 40 mg.... MC-12, C1
1001—*Aldactone* Tablets 25 mg MC-21, C1
1011—*Aldactazide* Tablets 25/25 mg MC-21, C5
1021—*Aldactazide* Tablets 50/50 mg MC-21, C5
1031—*Aldactone* Tablets 100 mg MC-21, C1
1041—*Aldactone* Tablets 50 mg MC-21, C1
1375—*Ditropan* Tablets 5 mg MC-18, A2
1451—*Cytotec* Tablets 0.1 mg MC-15, D4
1461—*Cytotec* Tablets 0.2 mg MC-15, D4
1771—*Cardizem* Tablets 30 mg MC-7, C3
1772—*Cardizem* Tablets 60 mg MC-7, C3
1831—*Flagyl* Tablets 250 mg MC-15, C5
2103—*Soma Compound* Tablets 200/325 mg MC-4, A4
2150—Mylan Meclofenamate Capsules 50 mg MC-14, B1
2403—*Soma Compound with Codeine* Tablets 200/325/16 mg MC-4, A5
2437—*Cardene* Capsules 20 mg MC-16, B4
2438—*Cardene* Capsules 30 mg MC-16, B4
2732—*Norpace CR* Extended-release Capsules 100 mg... MC-8, A4
2742—*Norpace CR* Extended-release Capsules 150 mg... MC-8, A4
2752—*Norpace* Capsules 100 mg MC-8, A3
2762—*Norpace* Capsules 150 mg MC-8, A3
2832—*Theo-24* Extended-release Capsules 100 mg MC-22, D6
2842—*Theo-24* Extended-release Capsules 200 mg MC-22, D6
2852—*Theo-24* Extended-release Capsules 300 mg MC-22, D6
3000—Mylan Meclofenamate Capsules 100 mg MC-14, B1
3061—*Ceclor* Capsules 250 mg MC-4, A7
3062—*Ceclor* Capsules 500 mg MC-4, A7
3071—Rugby Amitriptyline Tablets 10 mg MC-1, D5
3072—Rugby Amitriptyline Tablets 25 mg MC-1, D5
3073—Rugby Amitriptyline Tablets 50 mg MC-1, D5
3074—Rugby Amitriptyline Tablets 75 mg MC-1, D5
3075—Rugby Amitriptyline Tablets 100 mg MC-1, D5
3076—Rugby Amitriptyline Tablets 150 mg MC-1, D6
3105—*Prozac* Capsules 20 mg.... MC-10, A6
3144—*Axid* Capsules 150 mg MC-16, D2
3145—*Axid* Capsules 300 mg MC-16, D2
3170—*Lorabid* Capsules 200 mg.... MC-3, D3
3597—*Diphenhist* Tablets 25 mg.... MC-7, D2
3728—Rugby Doxepin Capsules 25 mg MC-8, B3
3729—Rugby Doxepin Capsules 50 mg MC-8, B3
3730—Rugby Doxepin Capsules 100 mg MC-8, B4
3736—Rugby Doxepin Capsules 10 mg MC-8, B3
3737—Rugby Doxepin Capsules 75 mg MC-8, B4
3738—Rugby Doxepin Capsules 150 mg MC-8, B4
3874—Rugby Hydroxyzine Tablets 10 mg MC-11, C6
3875—Rugby Hydroxyzine Tablets 25 mg MC-11, C6
3876—Rugby Hydroxyzine Tablets 50 mg MC-11, C6
3952—Rugby Levothyroxine Tablets 0.1 mg MC-13, B5
3953—Rugby Levothyroxine Tablets 0.15 mg MC-13, B5
3954—Rugby Levothyroxine Tablets 0.2 mg MC-13, B5
3958—Rugby Levothyroxine Tablets 0.3 mg MC-13, B5
3976—Rugby Ibuprofen Tablets 300 mg MC-11, D5
3977—Rugby Ibuprofen Tablets 400 mg MC-11, D5
3978—Rugby Ibuprofen Tablets 600 mg MC-11, D5
3979—Rugby Ibuprofen Tablets 800 mg MC-11, D6
4002—Rugby Meclofenamate Capsules 50 mg MC-14, B3
4003—Rugby Meclofenamate Capsules 100 mg MC-14, B3
4010—Mylan Temazepam Capsules 15 mg MC-22, A4
4018—Rugby Metronidazole Tablets 250 mg MC-15, C3
4019—Rugby Metronidazole Tablets 500 mg MC-15, C3
4021—Rugby Methyldopa Tablets 250 mg MC-14, D2
4023—Rugby Methyldopa Tablets 500 mg MC-14, D2
4042—Rugby Metoclopramide Tablets 10 mg MC-15, B1
4125—*Isordil* Extended-release Tablets 40 mg MC-12, C5
4132—*Surmontil* Capsules 25 mg.... MC-24, B4
4133—*Surmontil* Capsules 50 mg.... MC-24, B4
4152—*Isordil* Tablets 5 mg MC-12, C4
4153—*Isordil* Tablets 10 mg MC-12, C4
4154—*Isordil* Tablets 20 mg MC-12, C4
4158—*Surmontil* Capsules 100 mg.... MC-24, B4
4159—*Isordil* Tablets 30 mg MC-12, C4
4191—*Synalgos-DC* Capsules 16/356.4/30 mg MC-2, B7

4192—*Isordil* Tablets 40 mg MC-12, C4
4250—*Donnatal* Tablets 0.0194/0.1037/0.0065/16.2 mg.... MC-2, D2
4309—Rugby Propranolol Tablets 10 mg.... MC-20, C1
4313—Rugby Propranolol Tablets 20 mg.... MC-20, C1
4314—Rugby Propranolol Tablets 40 mg.... MC-20, C1
4315—Rugby Propranolol Tablets 60 mg.... MC-20, C1
4316—Rugby Propranolol Tablets 80 mg.... MC-20, C1
4325—Rugby Prednisone Tablets 10 mg MC-19, C5
4326—Rugby Prednisone Tablets 20 mg MC-19, C5
4402—Rugby Propranolol and Hydrochlorothiazide Tablets 40/25 mg.... MC-20, D1
4403—Rugby Propranolol and Hydrochlorothiazide Tablets 80/25 mg.... MC-20, D1
4812—Rugby Verapamil Tablets 80 mg.... MC-24, D1
4813—Rugby Verapamil Tablets 120 mg.... MC-24, D1
5050—Mylan Temazepam Capsules 30 mg MC-22, A4
5455—Schein/Danbury Chlorpropamide Tablets 250 mg.... MC-5, B3
5496—Schein/Danbury Spironolactone and Hydrochlorothiazide Tablets 25/25 mg.... MC-21, C4
5522—Schein/Danbury Hydroxyzine Tablets 10 mg MC-11, D1
5523—Schein/Danbury Hydroxyzine Tablets 25 mg MC-11, D1
5538—Schein/Danbury Quinidine Gluconate Extended-release Tablets 324 mg.... MC-21, A1
5540—Schein/Danbury Metronidazole Tablets 250 mg.... MC-15, C4
5542—Schein/Danbury Thioridazine Tablets 25 mg MC-23, B1
5543—Schein/Danbury Allopurinol Tablets 100 mg MC-1, C4
5544—Schein/Danbury Allopurinol Tablets 300 mg MC-1, C4
5546—Schein/Danbury Sulfamethoxazole and Trimethoprim Tablets 400/80 mg.... MC-21, D2
5547—Schein/Danbury Sulfamethoxazole and Trimethoprim Tablets 800/160 mg.... MC-21, D2
5552—Schein/Danbury Metronidazole Tablets 500 mg.... MC-15, C4
5553—Schein/Danbury Doxycycline Tablets 100 mg MC-8, C7
5562—Schein/Danbury Procainamide Extended-release Tablets 250 mg.... MC-20, A2
5565—Schein/Danbury Hydroxyzine Tablets 50 mg MC-11, D1
5566—Schein/Danbury Thioridazine Tablets 10 mg MC-23, B1
5568—Schein/Danbury Thioridazine Tablets 50 mg MC-23, B1
5569—Schein/Danbury Thioridazine Tablets 100 mg MC-23, B2
5575—Schein/Danbury Furosemide Tablets 40 mg MC-10, C4
5579—Schein/Danbury Chlorpropamide Tablets 100 mg.... MC-5, B3
5580—Schein/Danbury Thioridazine Tablets 150 mg ... MC-23, B2
5581—Schein/Danbury Thioridazine Tablets 200 mg ... MC-23, B2
5584—Schein/Danbury Ibuprofen Tablets 400 mg MC-11, D7
5585—Schein/Danbury Ibuprofen Tablets 200 mg MC-11, D7
5586—Schein/Danbury Ibuprofen Tablets 600 mg MC-12, A1
5587—Schein/Danbury Methyldopa Tablets 500 mg.... MC-14, D3
5588—Schein/Danbury Methyldopa Tablets 250 mg.... MC-14, D3
5589—Schein/Danbury Metoclopramide Tablets 10 mg.... MC-15, B2
5592—Schein/Danbury Thiothixene Capsules 2 mg..... MC-23, B6
5593—Schein/Danbury Thiothixene Capsules 1 mg..... MC-23, B6
5594—Schein/Danbury Thiothixene Capsules 10 mg.... MC-23, B6
5595—Schein/Danbury Thiothixene Capsules 5 mg..... MC-23, B6
5599—Schein/Danbury Trazodone Tablets 100 mg MC-23, D7
5600—Schein/Danbury Trazodone Tablets 50 mg MC-23, D7
5601—Schein/Danbury Verapamil Tablets 80 mg MC-24, D2
5602—Schein/Danbury Verapamil Tablets 120 mg MC-24, D2
5644—Schein/Danbury Ibuprofen Tablets 800 mg MC-12, A1
5658—Schein/Danbury Cyclobenzaprine Tablets 10 mg.... MC-6, C4
5660—Schein/Danbury Sulindac Tablets 200 mg MC-21, D7
5661—Schein/Danbury Sulindac Tablets 150 mg MC-21, D7
5704—Schein/Danbury Fenoprofen Tablets 600 mg MC-10, A3
5710—Schein/Danbury Albuterol Tablets 2 mg........ MC-1, B4
5711—Schein/Danbury Albuterol Tablets 4 mg.... MC-1, B4
6251—*Phenaphen with Codeine* Tablets 650/30 mg MC-1, A6
7278—*Polymox* Capsules 250 mg.... MC-2, A4

7279—*Polymox* Capsules 500 mg MC-2, A4
7375—*Cefanex* Capsules 250 mg. MC-4, B7
7376—*Cefanex* Capsules 500 mg. MC-4, B7
7496—*Tegopen* Capsules 500 mg MC-6, B6
7658—*Dynapen* Capsules 500 mg MC-7, A4
7892—*Dynapen* Capsules 125 mg MC-7, A3

7893—*Dynapen* Capsules 250 mg MC-7, A3
7935—*Tegopen* Capsules 250 mg MC-6, B6
7977—*Prostaphlin* Capsules 250 mg MC-17, D2
7982—*Prostaphlin* Capsules 500 mg MC-17, D2
7992—*Polycillin* Capsules 250 mg MC-2, B5
7993—*Polycillin* Capsules 500 mg MC-2, B5

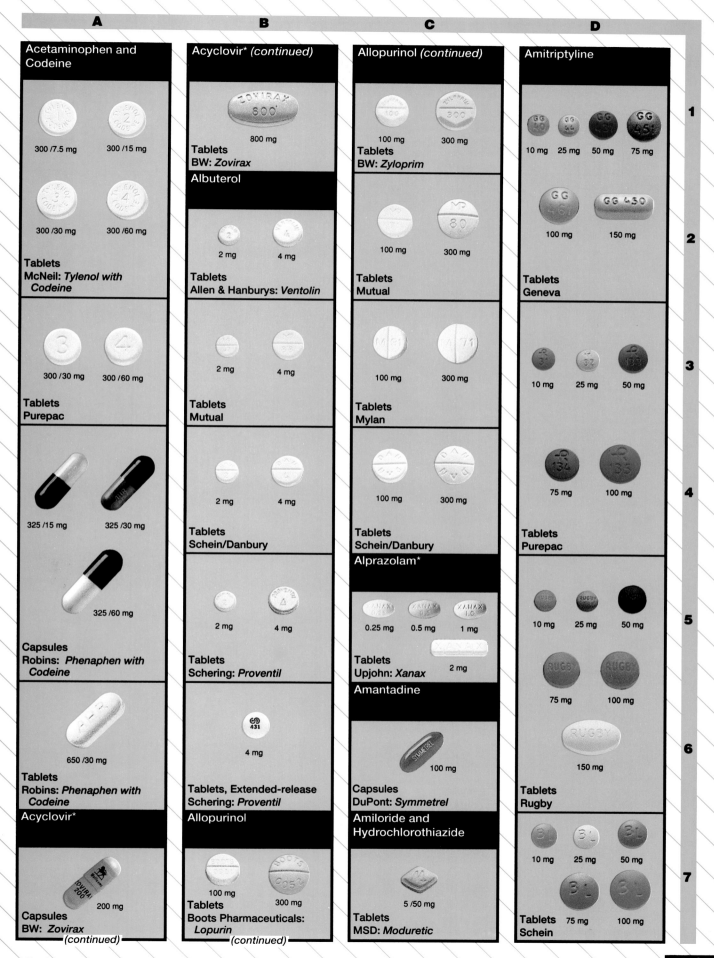

A

Acetaminophen and Codeine

300 /7.5 mg   300 /15 mg

300 /30 mg   300 /60 mg

Tablets
McNeil: *Tylenol with Codeine*

300 /30 mg   300 /60 mg

Tablets
Purepac

325 /15 mg   325 /30 mg

325 /60 mg

Capsules
Robins: *Phenaphen with Codeine*

650 /30 mg

Tablets
Robins: *Phenaphen with Codeine*

Acyclovir*

200 mg

Capsules
BW: *Zovirax*
— *(continued)* —

B

Acyclovir* *(continued)*

800 mg

Tablets
BW: *Zovirax*

Albuterol

2 mg   4 mg

Tablets
Allen & Hanburys: *Ventolin*

2 mg   4 mg

Tablets
Mutual

2 mg   4 mg

Tablets
Schein/Danbury

2 mg   4 mg

Tablets
Schering: *Proventil*

4 mg

Tablets, Extended-release
Schering: *Proventil*

Allopurinol

100 mg   300 mg

Tablets
Boots Pharmaceuticals: *Lopurin*
— *(continued)* —

C

Allopurinol *(continued)*

100 mg   300 mg

Tablets
BW: *Zyloprim*

100 mg   300 mg

Tablets
Mutual

100 mg   300 mg

Tablets
Mylan

100 mg   300 mg

Tablets
Schein/Danbury

Alprazolam*

0.25 mg   0.5 mg   1 mg

2 mg

Tablets
Upjohn: *Xanax*

Amantadine

100 mg

Capsules
DuPont: *Symmetrel*

Amiloride and Hydrochlorothiazide

5 /50 mg

Tablets
MSD: *Moduretic*

D

Amitriptyline

10 mg 25 mg 50 mg 75 mg

100 mg   150 mg

Tablets
Geneva

10 mg 25 mg 50 mg

75 mg   100 mg

Tablets
Purepac

10 mg 25 mg 50 mg

75 mg   100 mg

150 mg

Tablets
Rugby

10 mg 25 mg 50 mg

Tablets 75 mg 100 mg
Schein

1
2
3
4
5
6
7

* Single source product for solid oral dosage forms in the U.S.

© 1993 USPC

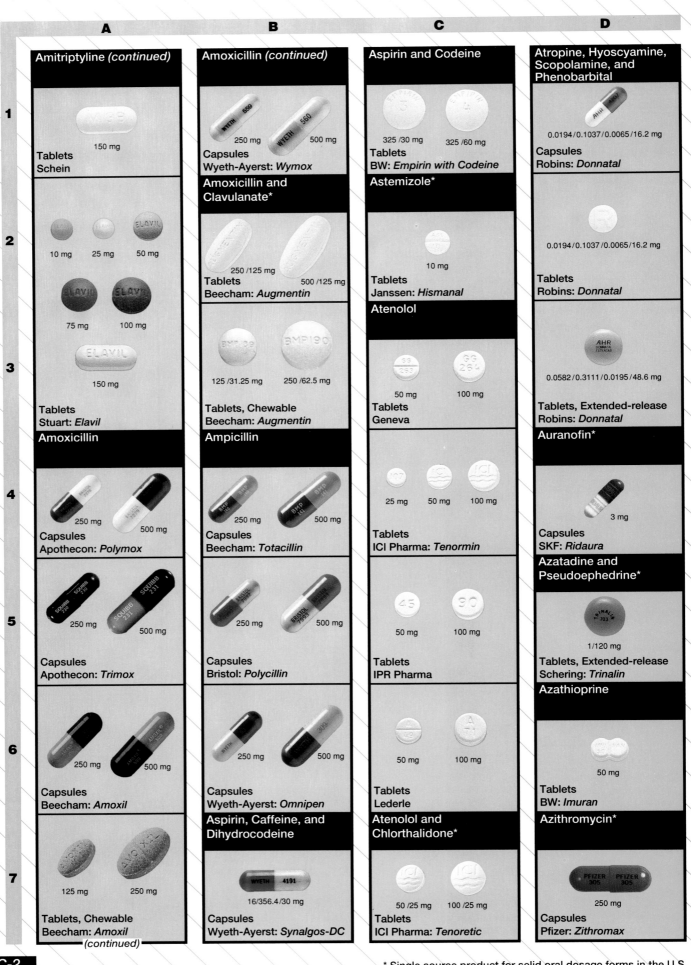

A

Amitriptyline *(continued)*

Tablets
Schein
150 mg

10 mg   25 mg   50 mg

75 mg   100 mg

ELAVIL
150 mg

Tablets
Stuart: *Elavil*

Amoxicillin

Capsules
Apothecon: *Polymox*
250 mg   500 mg

Capsules
Apothecon: *Trimox*
250 mg   500 mg

Capsules
Beecham: *Amoxil*
250 mg   500 mg

125 mg   250 mg

Tablets, Chewable
Beecham: *Amoxil*
—(continued)—

B

Amoxicillin *(continued)*

Capsules
Wyeth-Ayerst: *Wymox*
WYETH 659   250 mg   WYETH 560   500 mg

Amoxicillin and Clavulanate*

Tablets
Beecham: *Augmentin*
250/125 mg   500/125 mg

Tablets, Chewable
Beecham: *Augmentin*
BMP 109   125/31.25 mg   BMP 190   250/62.5 mg

Ampicillin

Capsules
Beecham: *Totacillin*
250 mg   500 mg

Capsules
Bristol: *Polycillin*
250 mg   500 mg

Capsules
Wyeth-Ayerst: *Omnipen*
250 mg   500 mg

Aspirin, Caffeine, and Dihydrocodeine

Capsules
Wyeth-Ayerst: *Synalgos-DC*
WYETH 4191   16/356.4/30 mg

C

Aspirin and Codeine

Tablets
BW: *Empirin with Codeine*
325/30 mg   325/60 mg

Astemizole*

Tablets
Janssen: *Hismanal*
10 mg

Atenolol

Tablets
Geneva
GG 263   50 mg   GG 264   100 mg

Tablets
ICI Pharma: *Tenormin*
25 mg   50 mg   100 mg

Tablets
IPR Pharma
45   50 mg   90   100 mg

Tablets
Lederle
50 mg   100 mg

Atenolol and Chlorthalidone*

Tablets
ICI Pharma: *Tenoretic*
50/25 mg   100/25 mg

D

Atropine, Hyoscyamine, Scopolamine, and Phenobarbital

Capsules
Robins: *Donnatal*
AHR 4207   0.0194/0.1037/0.0065/16.2 mg

Tablets
Robins: *Donnatal*
0.0194/0.1037/0.0065/16.2 mg

Tablets, Extended-release
Robins: *Donnatal*
AHR DONNATAL EXTENTAB   0.0582/0.3111/0.0195/48.6 mg

Auranofin*

Capsules
SKF: *Ridaura*
3 mg

Azatadine and Pseudoephedrine*

Tablets, Extended-release
Schering: *Trinalin*
TRINALIN 703   1/120 mg

Azathioprine

Tablets
BW: *Imuran*
50 mg

Azithromycin*

Capsules
Pfizer: *Zithromax*
PFIZER 305   PFIZER 305   250 mg

© 1993 USPC

* Single source product for solid oral dosage forms in the U.S.

A   **B**   **C**   **D**

1   **2**   **3**   **4**   **5**   **6**   **7**

Column A

Baclofen

10 mg   20 mg

Tablets
Geigy: *Lioresal*

Benazepril

5 mg   10 mg   20 mg

5   10   20

40   40 mg

Tablets
CIBA-GEIGY: *Lotensin*

Bendroflumethiazide

5 mg   10 mg

Tablets
Princeton Pharmaceutical
Products: *Naturetin*

Benzphetamine*

25 mg   50 mg

Tablets
Upjohn: *Didrex*

Benztropine

0.5 mg   1 mg

2 mg

Tablets
MSD: *Cogentin*

1 mg   2 mg

Tablets
Mutual

Bepridil*

200 mg   300 mg

400 mg

Tablets
McNeil: *Vascor*

Column B

Betaxolol*

10 mg   20 mg

Tablets
Searle: *Kerlone*

Bromocriptine*

5 mg

Capsules
Sandoz: *Parlodel*

2.5 mg

Tablets
Sandoz: *Parlodel*

Bumetanide*

0.5 mg   1 mg   2 mg

Tablets
Roche: *Bumex*

Bupropion*

75 mg   100 mg

Tablets
BW: *Wellbutrin*

Buspirone*

5 mg   10 mg

Tablets
Mead Johnson: *BuSpar*

Butalbital, Acetaminophen, and Caffeine

50/325/40 mg

Tablets
Sandoz: *Fioricet*

Column C

Butalbital, Aspirin, and Caffeine

50/325/40 mg

Tablets
Geneva

50/325/40 mg

Capsules
Sandoz: *Fiorinal*

50/325/40 mg

Tablets
Sandoz: *Fiorinal*

Butalbital, Aspirin, Codeine, and Caffeine

50/325/30/40 mg

Capsules
Sandoz: *Fiorinal with Codeine*

Calcitriol*

0.25 mcg   0.5 mcg

Capsules
Roche: *Rocaltrol*

Captopril*

12.5 mg   25 mg

50 mg   100 mg

Tablets
Squibb: *Capoten*

Column D

Captopril and Hydrochlorothiazide*

25/15 mg   25/25 mg

50/15 mg   50/25 mg

Tablets
Squibb: *Capozide*

Carbacephem*

200 mg

Capsules
Lilly: *Lorabid*

Carbamazepine

200 mg

Tablets
Basel: *Tegretol*

100 mg

Tablets, Chewable
Basel: *Tegretol*

200 mg

Tablets
Purepac

100 mg

Tablets, Chewable
Warner Chilcott

---

* Single source product for solid oral dosage forms in the U.S.

© 1993 USPC

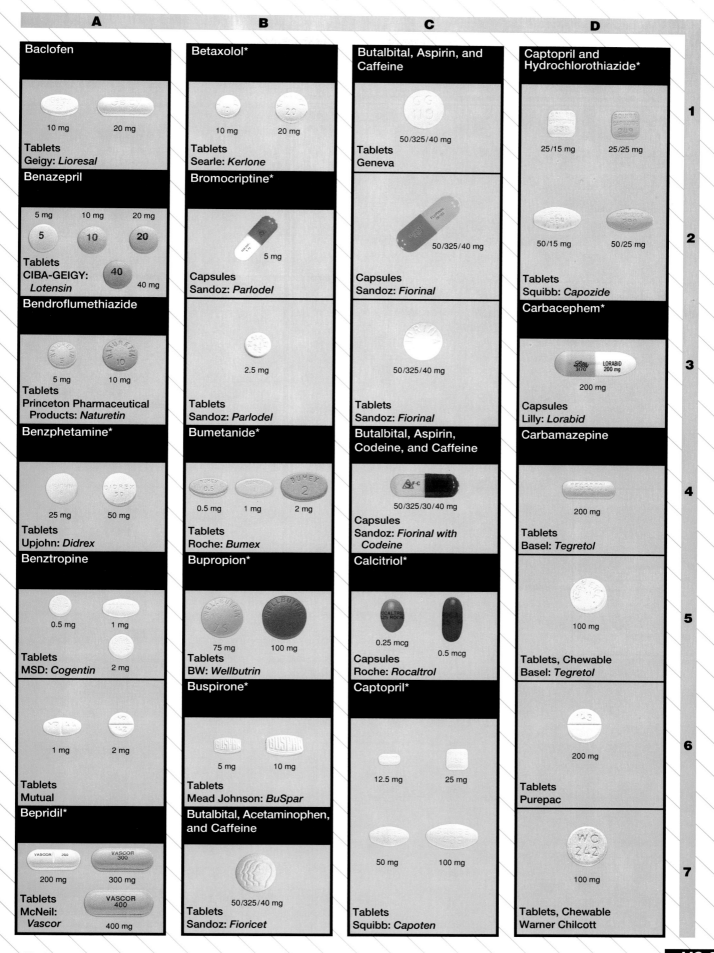

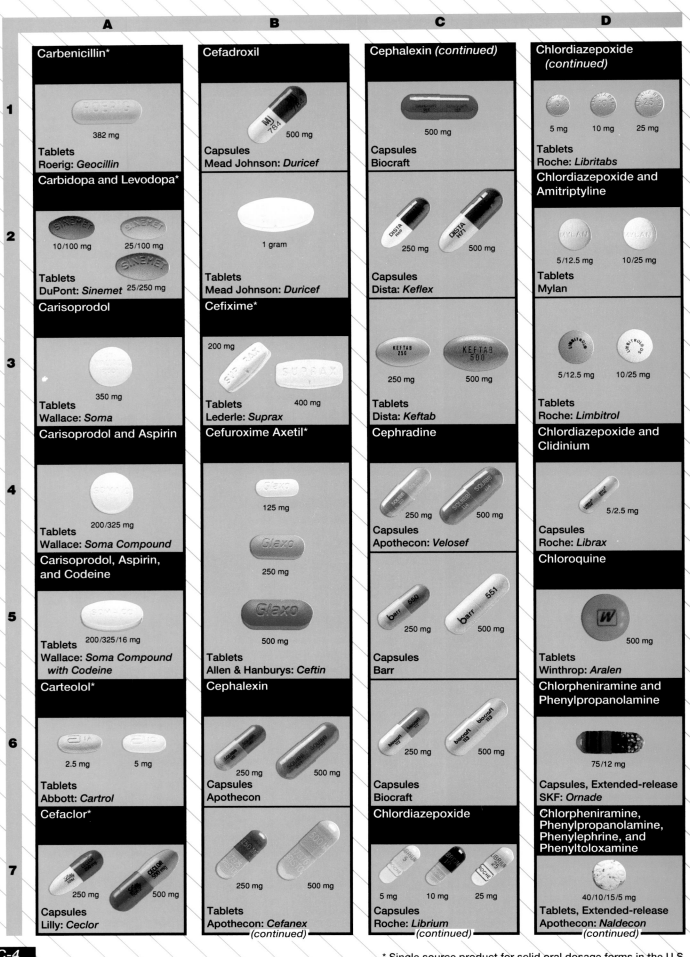

	A	B	C	D
	Carbenicillin*	**Cefadroxil**	**Cephalexin** *(continued)*	**Chlordiazepoxide** *(continued)*
1	382 mg Tablets Roerig: *Geocillin*	500 mg Capsules Mead Johnson: *Duricef*	500 mg Capsules Biocraft	5 mg · 10 mg · 25 mg Tablets Roche: *Libritabs*
	Carbidopa and Levodopa*			**Chlordiazepoxide and Amitriptyline**
2	10/100 mg · 25/100 mg 25/250 mg Tablets DuPont: *Sinemet*	1 gram Tablets Mead Johnson: *Duricef*	250 mg · 500 mg Capsules Dista: *Keflex*	5/12.5 mg · 10/25 mg Tablets Mylan
	Carisoprodol	**Cefixime***		
3	350 mg Tablets Wallace: *Soma*	200 mg · 400 mg Tablets Lederle: *Suprax*	KEFTAB 250 · KEFTAB 500 250 mg · 500 mg Tablets Dista: *Keftab*	5/12.5 mg · 10/25 mg Tablets Roche: *Limbitrol*
	Carisoprodol and Aspirin	**Cefuroxime Axetil***	**Cephradine**	**Chlordiazepoxide and Clidinium**
4	200/325 mg Tablets Wallace: *Soma Compound*	Glaxo 125 mg Glaxo 250 mg Glaxo 500 mg	250 mg · 500 mg Capsules Apothecon: *Velosef*	5/2.5 mg Capsules Roche: *Librax*
	Carisoprodol, Aspirin, and Codeine			**Chloroquine**
5	200/325/16 mg Tablets Wallace: *Soma Compound with Codeine*	Tablets Allen & Hanburys: *Ceftin*	barr 550 · barr 551 250 mg · 500 mg Capsules Barr	500 mg Tablets Winthrop: *Aralen*
	Carteolol*	**Cephalexin**		**Chlorpheniramine and Phenylpropanolamine**
6	2.5 mg · 5 mg Tablets Abbott: *Cartrol*	250 mg · 500 mg Capsules Apothecon	250 mg · 500 mg Capsules Biocraft	75/12 mg Capsules, Extended-release SKF: *Ornade*
	Cefaclor*		**Chlordiazepoxide**	**Chlorpheniramine, Phenylpropanolamine, Phenylephrine, and Phenyltoloxamine**
7	250 mg · 500 mg Capsules Lilly: *Ceclor*	250 mg · 500 mg Tablets Apothecon: *Cefanex* *(continued)*	5 mg · 10 mg · 25 mg Capsules Roche: *Librium* *(continued)*	40/10/15/5 mg Tablets, Extended-release Apothecon: *Naldecon* *(continued)*

© 1993 USPC

* Single source product for solid oral dosage forms in the U.S.

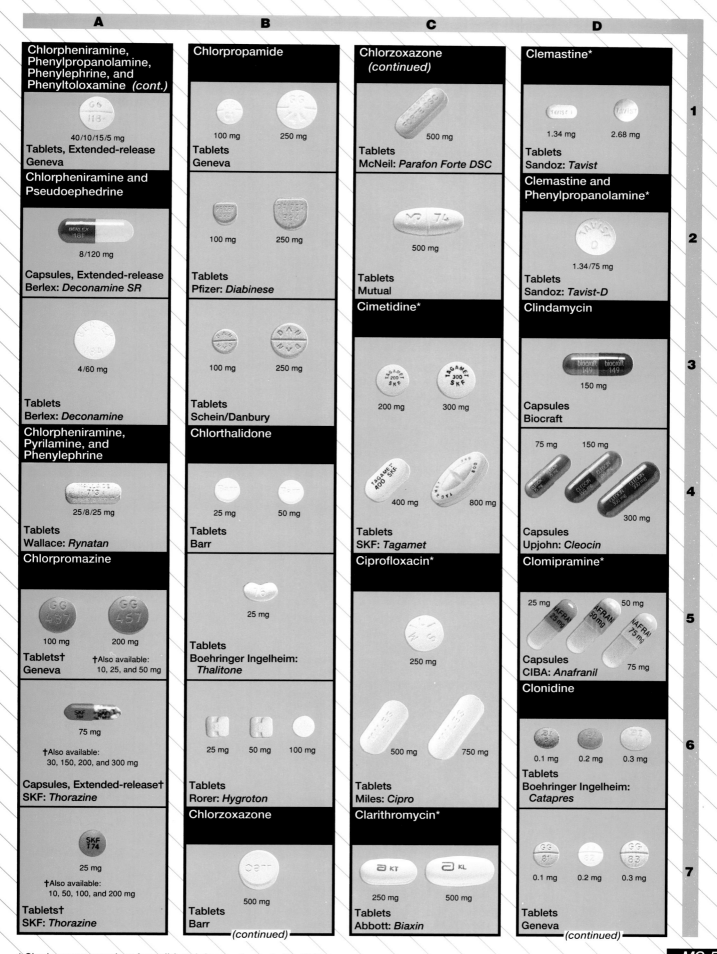

A	**B**	**C**	**D**

A

Chlorpheniramine, Phenylpropanolamine, Phenylephrine, and Phenyltoloxamine *(cont.)*

40/10/15/5 mg
Tablets, Extended-release
Geneva

Chlorpheniramine and Pseudoephedrine

8/120 mg
Capsules, Extended-release
Berlex: *Deconamine SR*

4/60 mg
Tablets
Berlex: *Deconamine*

Chlorpheniramine, Pyrilamine, and Phenylephrine

25/8/25 mg
Tablets
Wallace: *Rynatan*

Chlorpromazine

100 mg   200 mg
Tablets†   †Also available:
Geneva   10, 25, and 50 mg

75 mg
†Also available:
30, 150, 200, and 300 mg

Capsules, Extended-release†
SKF: *Thorazine*

25 mg
†Also available:
10, 50, 100, and 200 mg

Tablets†
SKF: *Thorazine*

B

Chlorpropamide

100 mg   250 mg
Tablets
Geneva

100 mg   250 mg
Tablets
Pfizer: *Diabinese*

100 mg   250 mg
Tablets
Schein/Danbury

Chlorthalidone

25 mg   50 mg
Tablets
Barr

25 mg
Tablets
Boehringer Ingelheim:
Thalitone

25 mg   50 mg   100 mg
Tablets
Rorer: *Hygroton*

Chlorzoxazone

500 mg
Tablets
Barr

(continued)

C

Chlorzoxazone *(continued)*

500 mg
Tablets
McNeil: *Parafon Forte DSC*

500 mg
Tablets
Mutual

Cimetidine*

200 mg   300 mg

400 mg   800 mg
Tablets
SKF: *Tagamet*

Ciprofloxacin*

250 mg

500 mg   750 mg
Tablets
Miles: *Cipro*

Clarithromycin*

250 mg   500 mg
Tablets
Abbott: *Biaxin*

D

Clemastine*

1.34 mg   2.68 mg
Tablets
Sandoz: *Tavist*

Clemastine and Phenylpropanolamine*

1.34/75 mg
Tablets
Sandoz: *Tavist-D*

Clindamycin

150 mg
Capsules
Biocraft

75 mg   150 mg

300 mg
Capsules
Upjohn: *Cleocin*

Clomipramine*

25 mg   50 mg

75 mg
Capsules
CIBA: *Anafranil*

Clonidine

0.1 mg   0.2 mg   0.3 mg
Tablets
Boehringer Ingelheim:
Catapres

0.1 mg   0.2 mg   0.3 mg
Tablets
Geneva

(continued)

* Single source product for solid oral dosage forms in the U.S.

© 1993 USPC

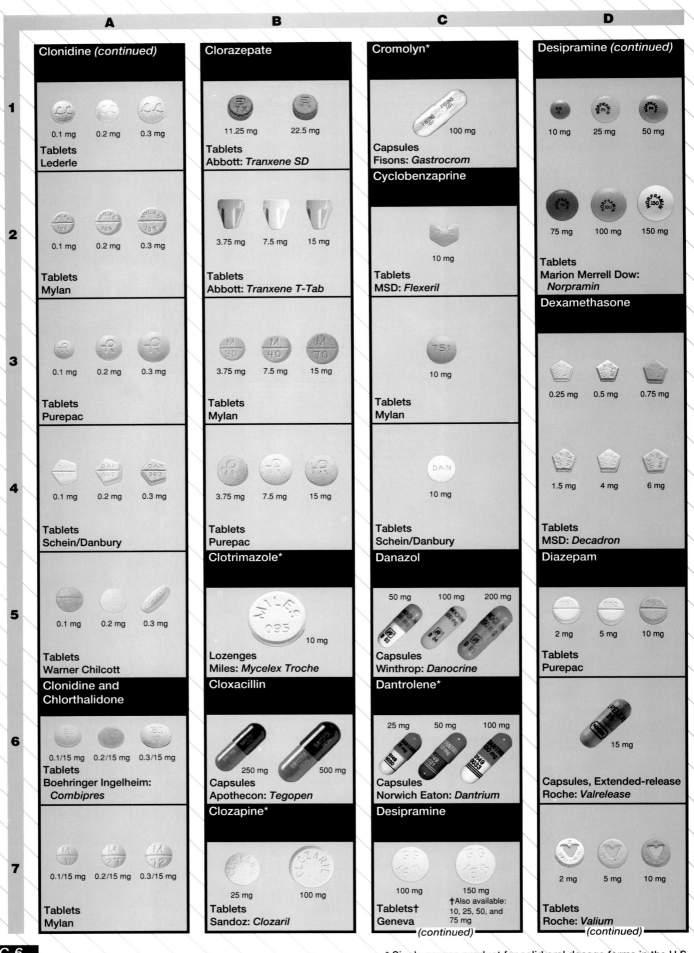

A

Clonidine (continued)

1
0.1 mg   0.2 mg   0.3 mg
Tablets
Lederle

2
0.1 mg   0.2 mg   0.3 mg
Tablets
Mylan

3
0.1 mg   0.2 mg   0.3 mg
Tablets
Purepac

4
0.1 mg   0.2 mg   0.3 mg
Tablets
Schein/Danbury

5
0.1 mg   0.2 mg   0.3 mg
Tablets
Warner Chilcott

Clonidine and Chlorthalidone

6
0.1/15 mg   0.2/15 mg   0.3/15 mg
Tablets
Boehringer Ingelheim:
Combipres

7
0.1/15 mg   0.2/15 mg   0.3/15 mg
Tablets
Mylan

B

Clorazepate

1
11.25 mg   22.5 mg
Tablets
Abbott: *Tranxene SD*

2
3.75 mg   7.5 mg   15 mg
Tablets
Abbott: *Tranxene T-Tab*

3
3.75 mg   7.5 mg   15 mg
Tablets
Mylan

4
3.75 mg   7.5 mg   15 mg
Tablets
Purepac

Clotrimazole*

5
10 mg
Lozenges
Miles: *Mycelex Troche*

Cloxacillin

6
250 mg   500 mg
Capsules
Apothecon: *Tegopen*

Clozapine*

7
25 mg   100 mg
Tablets
Sandoz: *Clozaril*

C

Cromolyn*

1
100 mg
Capsules
Fisons: *Gastrocrom*

Cyclobenzaprine

2
10 mg
Tablets
MSD: *Flexeril*

3
10 mg
Tablets
Mylan

4
10 mg
Tablets
Schein/Danbury

Danazol

5
50 mg   100 mg   200 mg
Capsules
Winthrop: *Danocrine*

Dantrolene*

6
25 mg   50 mg   100 mg
Capsules
Norwich Eaton: *Dantrium*

Desipramine

7
100 mg   150 mg
Tablets†
Geneva
†Also available:
10, 25, 50, and
75 mg
(continued)

D

Desipramine (continued)

1
10 mg   25 mg   50 mg

2
75 mg   100 mg   150 mg
Tablets
Marion Merrell Dow:
Norpramin

Dexamethasone

3
0.25 mg   0.5 mg   0.75 mg

4
1.5 mg   4 mg   6 mg
Tablets
MSD: *Decadron*

Diazepam

5
2 mg   5 mg   10 mg
Tablets
Purepac

6
15 mg
Capsules, Extended-release
Roche: *Valrelease*

7
2 mg   5 mg   10 mg
Tablets
Roche: *Valium*
(continued)

© 1993 USPC

* Single source product for solid oral dosage forms in the U.S.

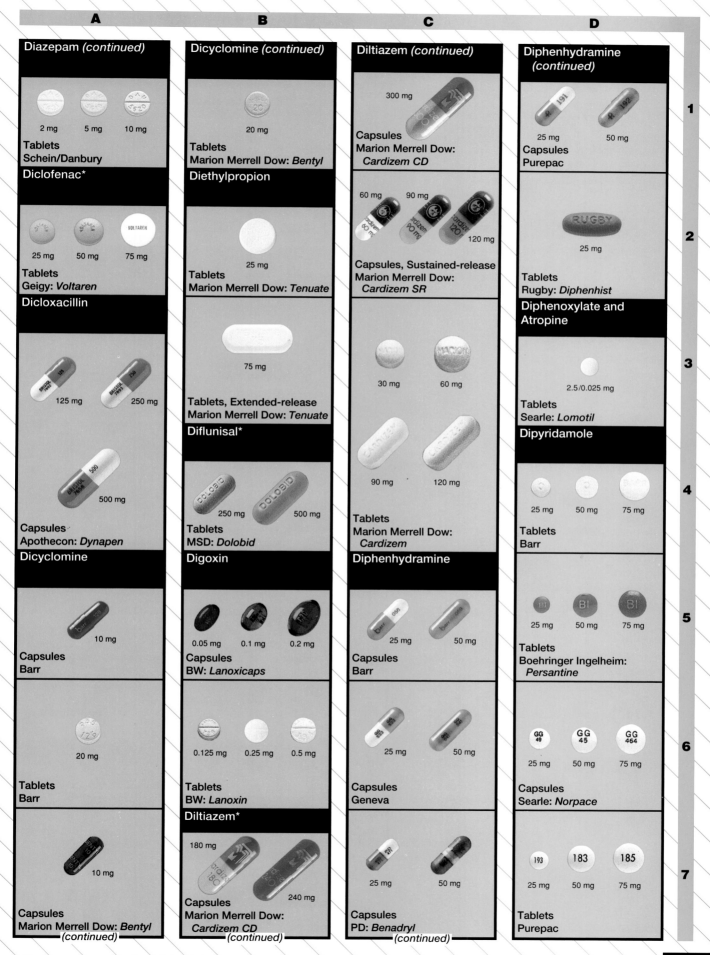

Column A

Diazepam (continued)

2 mg   5 mg   10 mg

Tablets
Schein/Danbury

Diclofenac*

25 mg   50 mg   75 mg

Tablets
Geigy: *Voltaren*

Dicloxacillin

125 mg   250 mg

500 mg

Capsules
Apothecon: *Dynapen*

Dicyclomine

10 mg

Capsules
Barr

20 mg

Tablets
Barr

10 mg

Capsules
Marion Merrell Dow: *Bentyl*
(continued)

Column B

Dicyclomine (continued)

20 mg

Tablets
Marion Merrell Dow: *Bentyl*

Diethylpropion

25 mg

Tablets
Marion Merrell Dow: *Tenuate*

75 mg

Tablets, Extended-release
Marion Merrell Dow: *Tenuate*

Diflunisal*

250 mg   500 mg

Tablets
MSD: *Dolobid*

Digoxin

0.05 mg   0.1 mg   0.2 mg

Capsules
BW: *Lanoxicaps*

0.125 mg   0.25 mg   0.5 mg

Tablets
BW: *Lanoxin*

Diltiazem*

180 mg

240 mg

Capsules
Marion Merrell Dow: *Cardizem CD*
(continued)

Column C

Diltiazem (continued)

300 mg

Capsules
Marion Merrell Dow:
Cardizem CD

60 mg   90 mg

120 mg

Capsules, Sustained-release
Marion Merrell Dow:
Cardizem SR

30 mg   60 mg

90 mg   120 mg

Tablets
Marion Merrell Dow:
Cardizem

Diphenhydramine

25 mg   50 mg

Capsules
Barr

25 mg   50 mg

Capsules
Geneva

25 mg   50 mg

Capsules
PD: *Benadryl*
(continued)

Column D

Diphenhydramine (continued)

25 mg   50 mg

Capsules
Purepac

25 mg

Tablets
Rugby: *Diphenhist*

Diphenoxylate and Atropine

2.5/0.025 mg

Tablets
Searle: *Lomotil*

Dipyridamole

25 mg   50 mg   75 mg

Tablets
Barr

25 mg   50 mg   75 mg

Tablets
Boehringer Ingelheim:
Persantine

25 mg   50 mg   75 mg

Capsules
Searle: *Norpace*

25 mg   50 mg   75 mg

Tablets
Purepac

---

* Single source product for solid oral dosage forms in the U.S.

© 1993 USPC

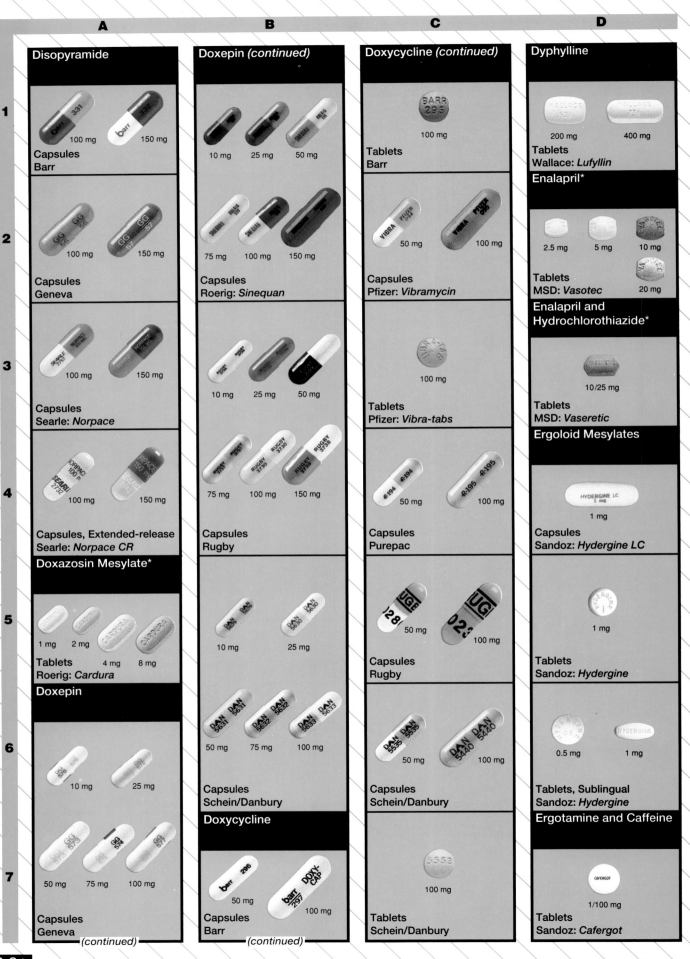

A

Disopyramide

100 mg | 150 mg
Capsules
Barr

100 mg | 150 mg
Capsules
Geneva

100 mg | 150 mg
Capsules
Searle: *Norpace*

100 mg | 150 mg
Capsules, Extended-release
Searle: *Norpace CR*

Doxazosin Mesylate*

1 mg | 2 mg | 4 mg | 8 mg
Tablets
Roerig: *Cardura*

Doxepin

10 mg | 25 mg

50 mg | 75 mg | 100 mg
Capsules
Geneva

(continued)

B

Doxepin *(continued)*

10 mg | 25 mg | 50 mg

75 mg | 100 mg | 150 mg
Capsules
Roerig: *Sinequan*

10 mg | 25 mg | 50 mg

75 mg | 100 mg | 150 mg
Capsules
Rugby

10 mg | 25 mg

50 mg | 75 mg | 100 mg
Capsules
Schein/Danbury

Doxycycline

50 mg | 100 mg
Capsules
Barr

(continued)

C

Doxycycline *(continued)*

100 mg
Tablets
Barr

50 mg | 100 mg
Capsules
Pfizer: *Vibramycin*

100 mg
Tablets
Pfizer: *Vibra-tabs*

50 mg | 100 mg
Capsules
Purepac

50 mg | 100 mg
Capsules
Rugby

50 mg | 100 mg
Capsules
Schein/Danbury

100 mg
Tablets
Schein/Danbury

D

Dyphylline

200 mg | 400 mg
Tablets
Wallace: *Lufyllin*

Enalapril*

2.5 mg | 5 mg | 10 mg

20 mg
Tablets
MSD: *Vasotec*

Enalapril and Hydrochlorothiazide*

10 /25 mg
Tablets
MSD: *Vaseretic*

Ergoloid Mesylates

1 mg
Capsules
Sandoz: *Hydergine LC*

1 mg
Tablets
Sandoz: *Hydergine*

0.5 mg | 1 mg
Tablets, Sublingual
Sandoz: *Hydergine*

Ergotamine and Caffeine

1/100 mg
Tablets
Sandoz: *Cafergot*

© 1993 USPC

* Single source product for solid oral dosage forms in the U.S.

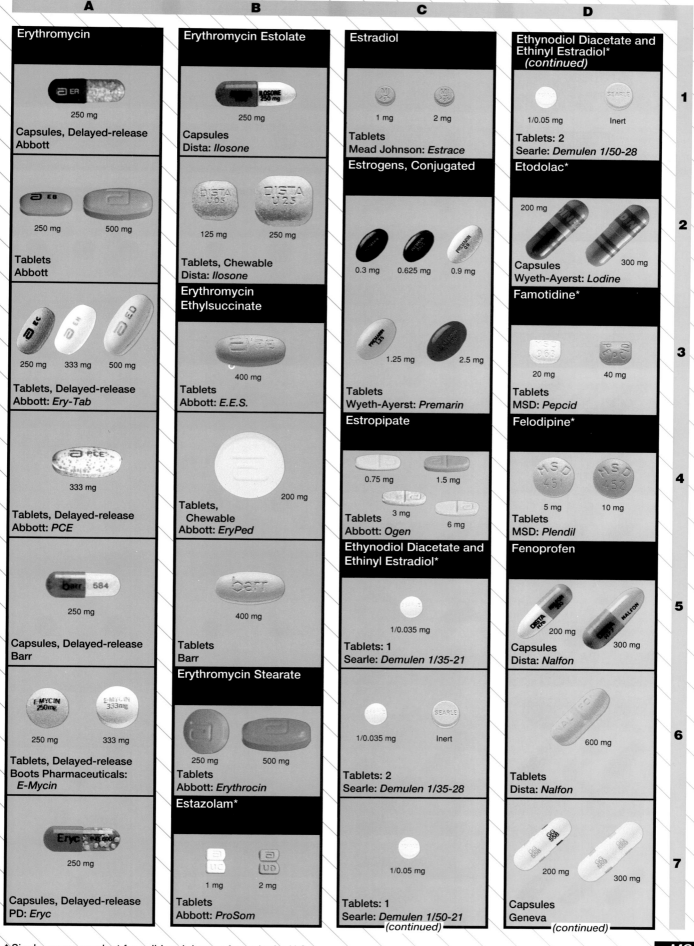

A	B	C	D

A

Erythromycin

250 mg

Capsules, Delayed-release
Abbott

250 mg   500 mg

Tablets
Abbott

250 mg   333 mg   500 mg

Tablets, Delayed-release
Abbott: *Ery-Tab*

333 mg

Tablets, Delayed-release
Abbott: *PCE*

250 mg

Capsules, Delayed-release
Barr

250 mg   333 mg

Tablets, Delayed-release
Boots Pharmaceuticals:
E-Mycin

250 mg

Capsules, Delayed-release
PD: *Eryc*

B

Erythromycin Estolate

250 mg

Capsules
Dista: *Ilosone*

125 mg   250 mg

Tablets, Chewable
Dista: *Ilosone*

**Erythromycin
Ethylsuccinate**

400 mg

Tablets
Abbott: *E.E.S.*

200 mg

Tablets,
Chewable
Abbott: *EryPed*

400 mg

Tablets
Barr

Erythromycin Stearate

250 mg   500 mg

Tablets
Abbott: *Erythrocin*

Estazolam*

1 mg   2 mg

Tablets
Abbott: *ProSom*

C

Estradiol

1 mg   2 mg

Tablets
Mead Johnson: *Estrace*

Estrogens, Conjugated

0.3 mg   0.625 mg   0.9 mg

1.25 mg   2.5 mg

Tablets
Wyeth-Ayerst: *Premarin*

Estropipate

0.75 mg   1.5 mg

3 mg   6 mg

Tablets
Abbott: *Ogen*

**Ethynodiol Diacetate and
Ethinyl Estradiol***

1/0.035 mg

Tablets: 1
Searle: *Demulen 1/35-21*

1/0.035 mg   Inert

Tablets: 2
Searle: *Demulen 1/35-28*

1/0.05 mg

Tablets: 1
Searle: *Demulen 1/50-21*
(continued)

D

**Ethynodiol Diacetate and
Ethinyl Estradiol***
(continued)

1/0.05 mg   Inert

Tablets: 2
Searle: *Demulen 1/50-28*

Etodolac*

200 mg

300 mg

Capsules
Wyeth-Ayerst: *Lodine*

Famotidine*

20 mg   40 mg

Tablets
MSD: *Pepcid*

Felodipine*

5 mg   10 mg

Tablets
MSD: *Plendil*

Fenoprofen

200 mg

300 mg

Capsules
Dista: *Nalfon*

600 mg

Tablets
Dista: *Nalfon*

200 mg   300 mg

Capsules
Geneva   *(continued)*

1
2
3
4
5
6
7

* Single source product for solid oral dosage forms in the U.S.

© 1993 USPC

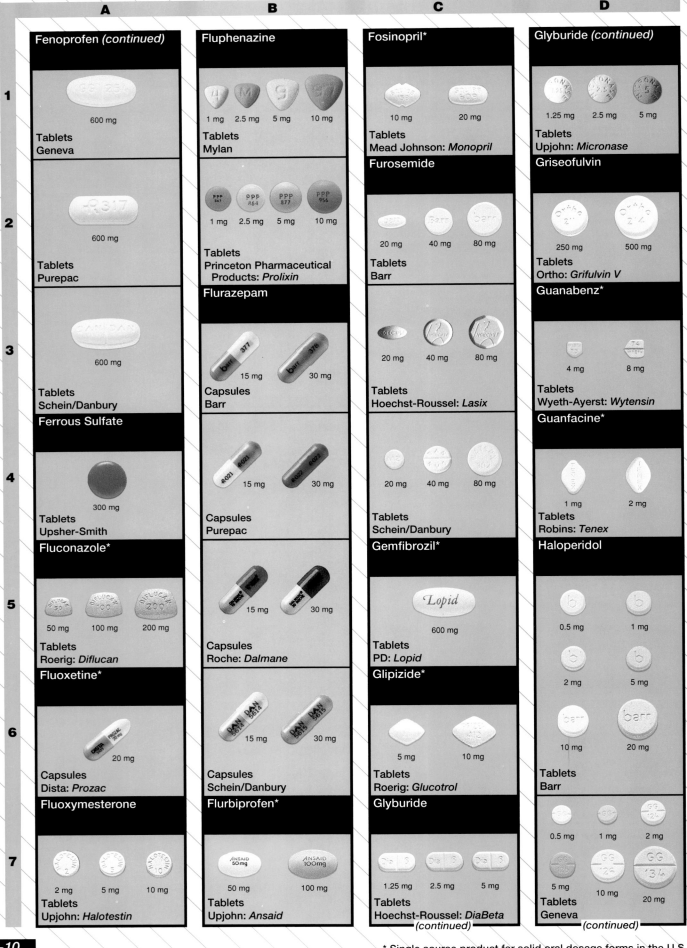

A

Fenoprofen (continued)

600 mg
Tablets
Geneva

600 mg
Tablets
Purepac

600 mg
Tablets
Schein/Danbury

Ferrous Sulfate

300 mg
Tablets
Upsher-Smith

Fluconazole*

50 mg   100 mg   200 mg
Tablets
Roerig: *Diflucan*

Fluoxetine*

20 mg
Capsules
Dista: *Prozac*

Fluoxymesterone

2 mg   5 mg   10 mg
Tablets
Upjohn: *Halotestin*

B

Fluphenazine

1 mg   2.5 mg   5 mg   10 mg
Tablets
Mylan

1 mg   2.5 mg   5 mg   10 mg
Tablets
Princeton Pharmaceutical
  Products: *Prolixin*

Flurazepam

15 mg   30 mg
Capsules
Barr

15 mg   30 mg
Capsules
Purepac

15 mg   30 mg
Capsules
Roche: *Dalmane*

15 mg   30 mg
Capsules
Schein/Danbury

Flurbiprofen*

50 mg   100 mg
Tablets
Upjohn: *Ansaid*

C

Fosinopril*

10 mg   20 mg
Tablets
Mead Johnson: *Monopril*

Furosemide

20 mg   40 mg   80 mg
Tablets
Barr

20 mg   40 mg   80 mg
Tablets
Hoechst-Roussel: *Lasix*

20 mg   40 mg   80 mg
Tablets
Schein/Danbury

Gemfibrozil*

Lopid
600 mg
Tablets
PD: *Lopid*

Glipizide*

5 mg   10 mg
Tablets
Roerig: *Glucotrol*

Glyburide

1.25 mg   2.5 mg   5 mg
Tablets
Hoechst-Roussel: *DiaBeta*
(continued)

D

Glyburide (continued)

1.25 mg   2.5 mg   5 mg
Tablets
Upjohn: *Micronase*

Griseofulvin

250 mg   500 mg
Tablets
Ortho: *Grifulvin V*

Guanabenz*

4 mg   8 mg
Tablets
Wyeth-Ayerst: *Wytensin*

Guanfacine*

1 mg   2 mg
Tablets
Robins: *Tenex*

Haloperidol

0.5 mg   1 mg

2 mg   5 mg

10 mg   20 mg
Tablets
Barr

0.5 mg   1 mg   2 mg

5 mg   10 mg   20 mg
Tablets
Geneva
(continued)

© 1993 USPC

* Single source product for solid oral dosage forms in the U.S.

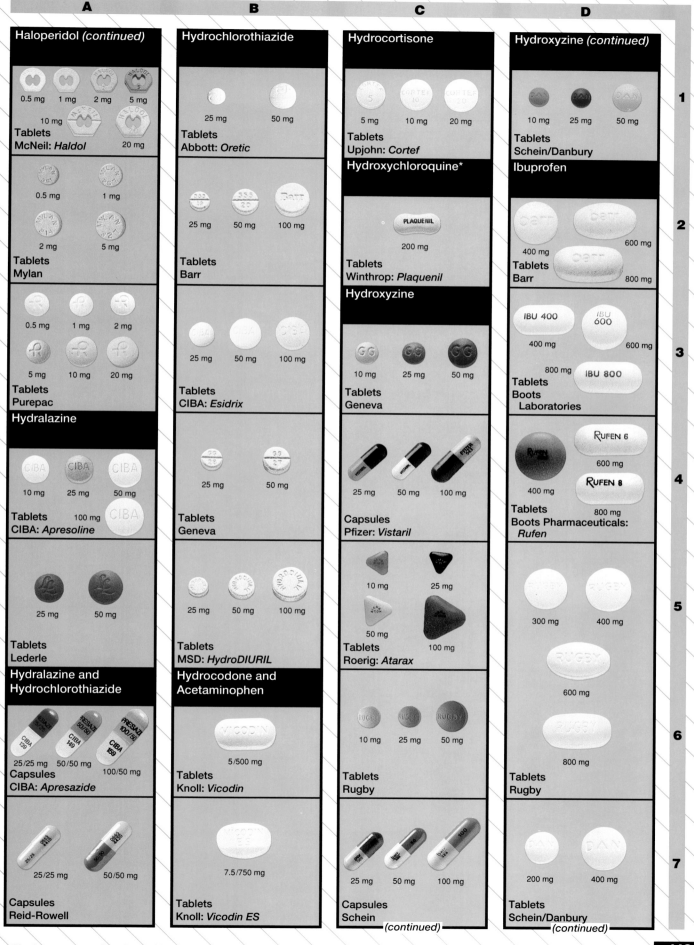

A

Haloperidol (continued)

0.5 mg 1 mg 2 mg 5 mg
10 mg 20 mg
Tablets
McNeil: *Haldol*

0.5 mg 1 mg
2 mg 5 mg
Tablets
Mylan

0.5 mg 1 mg 2 mg
5 mg 10 mg 20 mg
Tablets
Purepac

Hydralazine

10 mg 25 mg 50 mg
100 mg
Tablets
CIBA: *Apresoline*

25 mg 50 mg
Tablets
Lederle

Hydralazine and Hydrochlorothiazide

25/25 mg 50/50 mg 100/50 mg
Capsules
CIBA: *Apresazide*

25/25 mg 50/50 mg
Capsules
Reid-Rowell

B

Hydrochlorothiazide

25 mg 50 mg
Tablets
Abbott: *Oretic*

25 mg 50 mg 100 mg
Tablets
Barr

25 mg 50 mg 100 mg
Tablets
CIBA: *Esidrix*

25 mg 50 mg
Tablets
Geneva

25 mg 50 mg 100 mg
Tablets
MSD: *HydroDIURIL*

Hydrocodone and Acetaminophen

5/500 mg
Tablets
Knoll: *Vicodin*

7.5/750 mg
Tablets
Knoll: *Vicodin ES*

C

Hydrocortisone

5 mg 10 mg 20 mg
Tablets
Upjohn: *Cortef*

Hydroxychloroquine*

200 mg
Tablets
Winthrop: *Plaquenil*

Hydroxyzine

10 mg 25 mg 50 mg
Tablets
Geneva

25 mg 50 mg 100 mg
Capsules
Pfizer: *Vistaril*

10 mg 25 mg
50 mg 100 mg
Tablets
Roerig: *Atarax*

10 mg 25 mg 50 mg
Tablets
Rugby

25 mg 50 mg 100 mg
Capsules
Schein

(continued)

D

Hydroxyzine (continued)

10 mg 25 mg 50 mg
Tablets
Schein/Danbury

Ibuprofen

400 mg 600 mg
800 mg
Tablets
Barr

IBU 400 IBU 600
400 mg 600 mg
IBU 800
800 mg
Tablets
Boots Laboratories

RUFEN 6
400 mg 600 mg
RUFEN 8
800 mg
Tablets
Boots Pharmaceuticals: *Rufen*

300 mg 400 mg
600 mg
800 mg
Tablets
Rugby

200 mg 400 mg
Tablets
Schein/Danbury

(continued)

1

2

3

4

5

6

7

* Single source product for solid oral dosage forms in the U.S.

© 1993 USPC

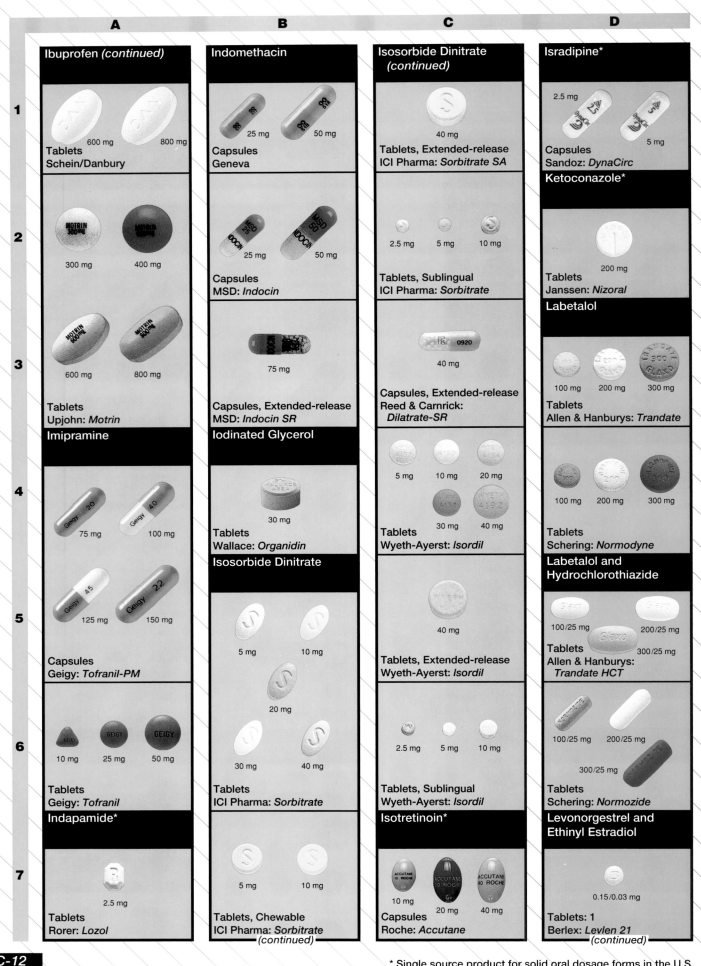

A

Ibuprofen *(continued)*

600 mg   800 mg
Tablets
Schein/Danbury

300 mg   400 mg

600 mg   800 mg
Tablets
Upjohn: *Motrin*

Imipramine

75 mg   100 mg

125 mg   150 mg
Capsules
Geigy: *Tofranil-PM*

10 mg   25 mg   50 mg
Tablets
Geigy: *Tofranil*

Indapamide*

2.5 mg
Tablets
Rorer: *Lozol*

B

Indomethacin

25 mg   50 mg
Capsules
Geneva

25 mg   50 mg
Capsules
MSD: *Indocin*

75 mg
Capsules, Extended-release
MSD: *Indocin SR*

Iodinated Glycerol

30 mg
Tablets
Wallace: *Organidin*

Isosorbide Dinitrate

5 mg   10 mg

20 mg

30 mg   40 mg
Tablets
ICI Pharma: *Sorbitrate*

5 mg   10 mg
Tablets, Chewable
ICI Pharma: *Sorbitrate*
(continued)

C

Isosorbide Dinitrate *(continued)*

40 mg
Tablets, Extended-release
ICI Pharma: *Sorbitrate SA*

2.5 mg   5 mg   10 mg
Tablets, Sublingual
ICI Pharma: *Sorbitrate*

40 mg
Capsules, Extended-release
Reed & Carnrick:
Dilatrate-SR

5 mg   10 mg   20 mg

30 mg   40 mg
Tablets
Wyeth-Ayerst: *Isordil*

40 mg
Tablets, Extended-release
Wyeth-Ayerst: *Isordil*

2.5 mg   5 mg   10 mg
Tablets, Sublingual
Wyeth-Ayerst: *Isordil*

Isotretinoin*

10 mg   20 mg   40 mg
Capsules
Roche: *Accutane*

D

Isradipine*

2.5 mg   5 mg
Capsules
Sandoz: *DynaCirc*

Ketoconazole*

200 mg
Tablets
Janssen: *Nizoral*

Labetalol

100 mg   200 mg   300 mg
Tablets
Allen & Hanburys: *Trandate*

100 mg   200 mg   300 mg
Tablets
Schering: *Normodyne*

Labetalol and Hydrochlorothiazide

100/25 mg   200/25 mg

300/25 mg
Tablets
Allen & Hanburys:
Trandate HCT

100/25 mg   200/25 mg

300/25 mg
Tablets
Schering: *Normozide*

Levonorgestrel and Ethinyl Estradiol

0.15/0.03 mg
Tablets: 1
Berlex: *Levlen 21*
(continued)

© 1993 USPC

* Single source product for solid oral dosage forms in the U.S.

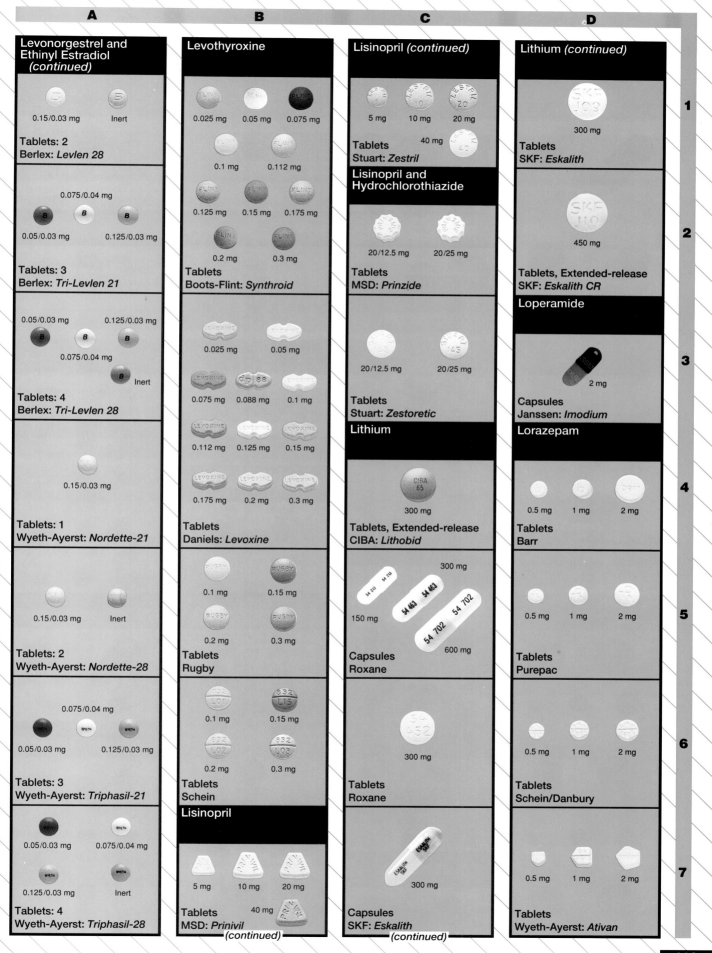

Column A

Levonorgestrel and Ethinyl Estradiol *(continued)*

0.15/0.03 mg   Inert

Tablets: 2
Berlex: *Levlen 28*

0.075/0.04 mg

0.05/0.03 mg   0.125/0.03 mg

Tablets: 3
Berlex: *Tri-Levlen 21*

0.05/0.03 mg   0.125/0.03 mg

0.075/0.04 mg

Inert

Tablets: 4
Berlex: *Tri-Levlen 28*

0.15/0.03 mg

Tablets: 1
Wyeth-Ayerst: *Nordette-21*

0.15/0.03 mg   Inert

Tablets: 2
Wyeth-Ayerst: *Nordette-28*

0.075/0.04 mg

0.05/0.03 mg   0.125/0.03 mg

Tablets: 3
Wyeth-Ayerst: *Triphasil-21*

0.05/0.03 mg   0.075/0.04 mg

0.125/0.03 mg   Inert

Tablets: 4
Wyeth-Ayerst: *Triphasil-28*

Column B

Levothyroxine

0.025 mg   0.05 mg   0.075 mg

0.1 mg   0.112 mg

0.125 mg   0.15 mg   0.175 mg

0.2 mg   0.3 mg

Tablets
Boots-Flint: *Synthroid*

0.025 mg   0.05 mg

0.075 mg   0.088 mg   0.1 mg

0.112 mg   0.125 mg   0.15 mg

0.175 mg   0.2 mg   0.3 mg

Tablets
Daniels: *Levoxine*

0.1 mg   0.15 mg

0.2 mg   0.3 mg

Tablets
Rugby

0.1 mg   0.15 mg

0.2 mg   0.3 mg

Tablets
Schein

Lisinopril

5 mg   10 mg   20 mg

40 mg

Tablets
MSD: *Prinivil*
(continued)

Column C

Lisinopril *(continued)*

5 mg   10 mg   20 mg

40 mg

Tablets
Stuart: *Zestril*

Lisinopril and Hydrochlorothiazide

20/12.5 mg   20/25 mg

Tablets
MSD: *Prinzide*

20/12.5 mg   20/25 mg

Tablets
Stuart: *Zestoretic*

Lithium

300 mg

Tablets, Extended-release
CIBA: *Lithobid*

150 mg   300 mg   600 mg

Capsules
Roxane

300 mg

Tablets
Roxane

300 mg

Capsules
SKF: *Eskalith*
(continued)

Column D

Lithium *(continued)*

300 mg

Tablets
SKF: *Eskalith*

450 mg

Tablets, Extended-release
SKF: *Eskalith CR*

Loperamide

2 mg

Capsules
Janssen: *Imodium*

Lorazepam

0.5 mg   1 mg   2 mg

Tablets
Barr

0.5 mg   1 mg   2 mg

Tablets
Purepac

0.5 mg   1 mg   2 mg

Tablets
Schein/Danbury

0.5 mg   1 mg   2 mg

Tablets
Wyeth-Ayerst: *Ativan*

A   B   C   D

1 2 3 4 5 6 7

* Single source product for solid oral dosage forms in the U.S.

© 1993 USPC

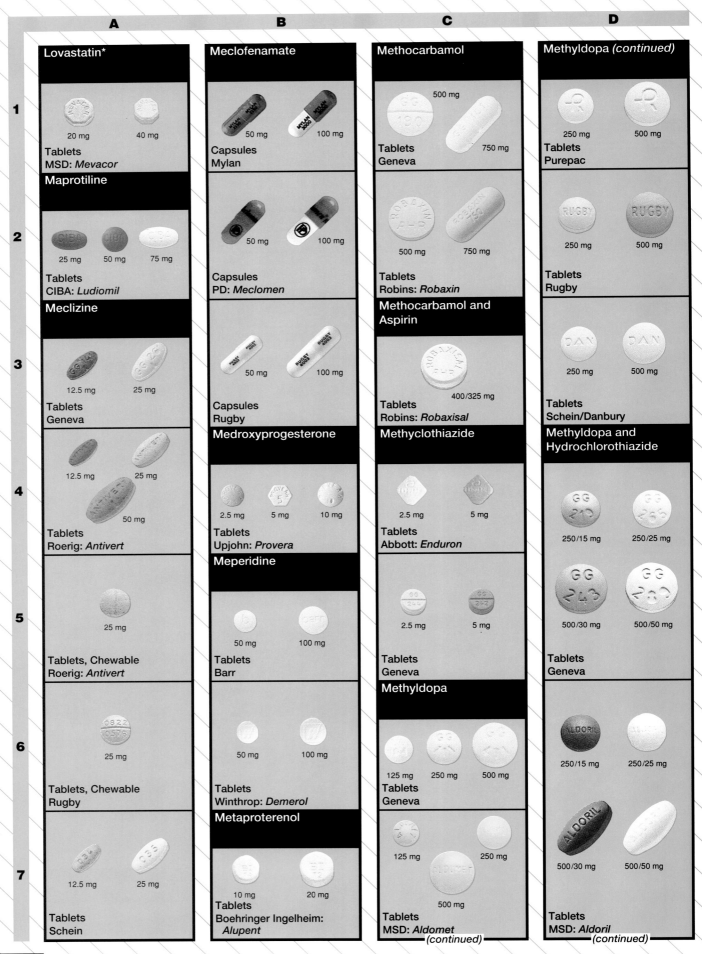

A

Lovastatin*

20 mg | 40 mg
Tablets
MSD: *Mevacor*

Maprotiline

25 mg | 50 mg | 75 mg
Tablets
CIBA: *Ludiomil*

Meclizine

12.5 mg | 25 mg
Tablets
Geneva

12.5 mg | 25 mg | 50 mg
Tablets
Roerig: *Antivert*

25 mg
Tablets, Chewable
Roerig: *Antivert*

25 mg
Tablets, Chewable
Rugby

12.5 mg | 25 mg
Tablets
Schein

B

Meclofenamate

50 mg | 100 mg
Capsules
Mylan

50 mg | 100 mg
Capsules
PD: *Meclomen*

50 mg | 100 mg
Capsules
Rugby

Medroxyprogesterone

2.5 mg | 5 mg | 10 mg
Tablets
Upjohn: *Provera*

Meperidine

50 mg | 100 mg
Tablets
Barr

50 mg | 100 mg
Tablets
Winthrop: *Demerol*

Metaproterenol

10 mg | 20 mg
Tablets
Boehringer Ingelheim:
Alupent

C

Methocarbamol

500 mg | 750 mg
Tablets
Geneva

500 mg | 750 mg
Tablets
Robins: *Robaxin*

Methocarbamol and Aspirin

400/325 mg
Tablets
Robins: *Robaxisal*

Methyclothiazide

2.5 mg | 5 mg
Tablets
Abbott: *Enduron*

2.5 mg | 5 mg
Tablets
Geneva

Methyldopa

125 mg | 250 mg | 500 mg
Tablets
Geneva

125 mg | 250 mg
500 mg
Tablets
MSD: *Aldomet*
(continued)

D

Methyldopa *(continued)*

250 mg | 500 mg
Tablets
Purepac

250 mg | 500 mg
Tablets
Rugby

250 mg | 500 mg
Tablets
Schein/Danbury

Methyldopa and Hydrochlorothiazide

250/15 mg | 250/25 mg
500/30 mg | 500/50 mg
Tablets
Geneva

250/15 mg | 250/25 mg
500/30 mg | 500/50 mg
Tablets
MSD: *Aldoril*
(continued)

© 1993 USPC

* Single source product for solid oral dosage forms in the U.S.

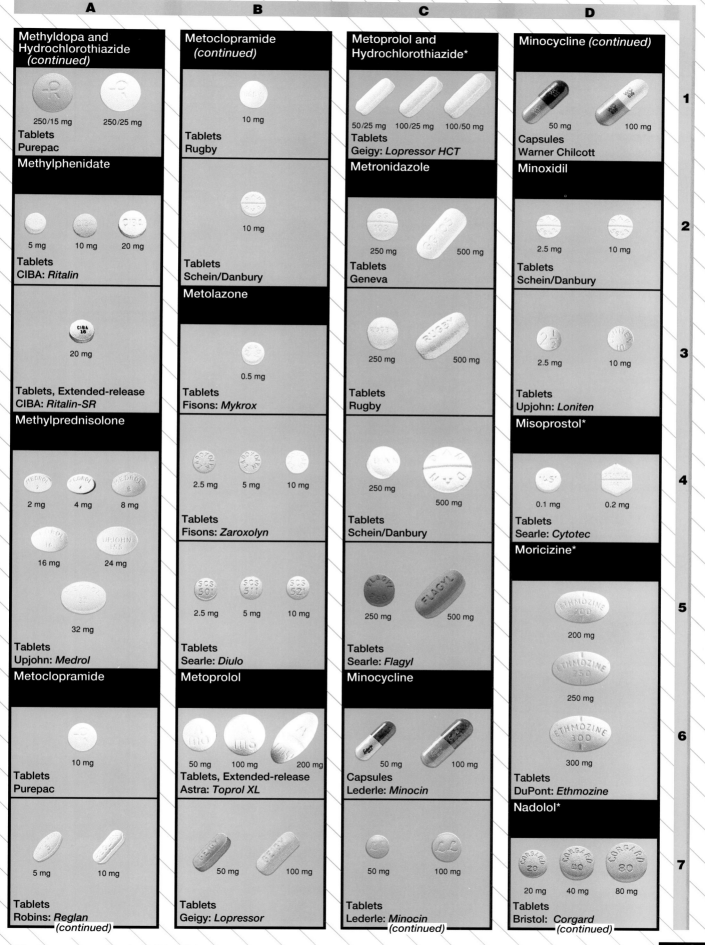

A	**B**	**C**	**D**

A

Methyldopa and Hydrochlorothiazide *(continued)*

250/15 mg 250/25 mg
Tablets
Purepac

Methylphenidate

5 mg 10 mg 20 mg
Tablets
CIBA: *Ritalin*

CIBA 10
20 mg
Tablets, Extended-release
CIBA: *Ritalin-SR*

Methylprednisolone

2 mg 4 mg 8 mg
16 mg 24 mg
32 mg
Tablets
Upjohn: *Medrol*

Metoclopramide

10 mg
Tablets
Purepac

5 mg 10 mg
Tablets
Robins: *Reglan*
(continued)

B

Metoclopramide *(continued)*

10 mg
Tablets
Rugby

10 mg
Tablets
Schein/Danbury

Metolazone

0.5 mg
Tablets
Fisons: *Mykrox*

2.5 mg 5 mg 10 mg
Tablets
Fisons: *Zaroxolyn*

2.5 mg 5 mg 10 mg
Tablets
Searle: *Diulo*

Metoprolol

50 mg 100 mg 200 mg
Tablets, Extended-release
Astra: *Toprol XL*

50 mg 100 mg
Tablets
Geigy: *Lopressor*

C

Metoprolol and Hydrochlorothiazide*

50/25 mg 100/25 mg 100/50 mg
Tablets
Geigy: *Lopressor HCT*

Metronidazole

250 mg 500 mg
Tablets
Geneva

250 mg 500 mg
Tablets
Rugby

250 mg 500 mg
Tablets
Schein/Danbury

250 mg 500 mg
Tablets
Searle: *Flagyl*

Minocycline

50 mg 100 mg
Capsules
Lederle: *Minocin*

50 mg 100 mg
Tablets
Lederle: *Minocin*
(continued)

D

Minocycline *(continued)*

50 mg 100 mg
Capsules
Warner Chilcott

Minoxidil

2.5 mg 10 mg
Tablets
Schein/Danbury

2½ mg 10 mg
Tablets
Upjohn: *Loniten*

Misoprostol*

0.1 mg 0.2 mg
Tablets
Searle: *Cytotec*

Moricizine*

200 mg
250 mg
300 mg
Tablets
DuPont: *Ethmozine*

Nadolol*

20 mg 40 mg 80 mg
Tablets
Bristol: *Corgard*
(continued)

* Single source product for solid oral dosage forms in the U.S.

MC-15

© 1993 USPC

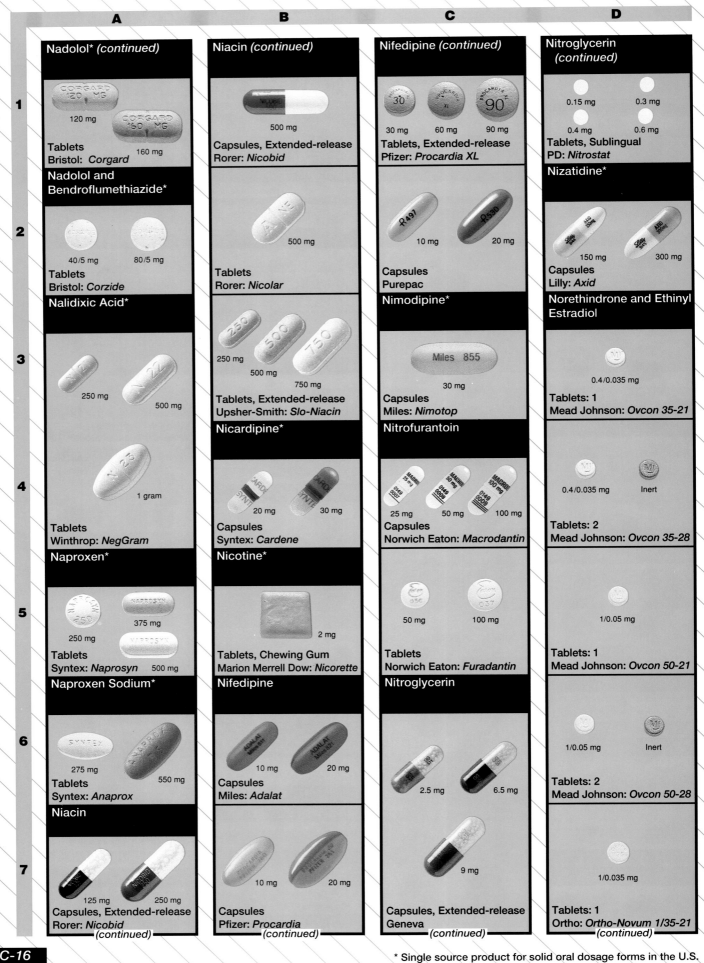

A

Nadolol* *(continued)*

120 mg
160 mg

Tablets
Bristol: *Corgard*

Nadolol and Bendroflumethiazide*

40/5 mg
80/5 mg

Tablets
Bristol: *Corzide*

Nalidixic Acid*

250 mg
500 mg
1 gram

Tablets
Winthrop: *NegGram*

Naproxen*

250 mg
375 mg
500 mg

Tablets
Syntex: *Naprosyn*

Naproxen Sodium*

275 mg
550 mg

Tablets
Syntex: *Anaprox*

Niacin

125 mg
250 mg

Capsules, Extended-release
Rorer: *Nicobid*
(continued)

B

Niacin *(continued)*

500 mg

Capsules, Extended-release
Rorer: *Nicobid*

500 mg

Tablets
Rorer: *Nicolar*

250 mg
500 mg
750 mg

Tablets, Extended-release
Upsher-Smith: *Slo-Niacin*

Nicardipine*

20 mg
30 mg

Capsules
Syntex: *Cardene*

Nicotine*

2 mg

Tablets, Chewing Gum
Marion Merrell Dow: *Nicorette*

Nifedipine

10 mg
20 mg

Capsules
Miles: *Adalat*

10 mg
20 mg

Capsules
Pfizer: *Procardia*
(continued)

C

Nifedipine *(continued)*

30 mg
60 mg
90 mg

Tablets, Extended-release
Pfizer: *Procardia XL*

10 mg
20 mg

Capsules
Purepac

Nimodipine*

Miles 855
30 mg

Capsules
Miles: *Nimotop*

Nitrofurantoin

25 mg
50 mg
100 mg

Capsules
Norwich Eaton: *Macrodantin*

50 mg
100 mg

Tablets
Norwich Eaton: *Furadantin*

Nitroglycerin

2.5 mg
6.5 mg
9 mg

Capsules, Extended-release
Geneva
(continued)

D

Nitroglycerin *(continued)*

0.15 mg
0.3 mg
0.4 mg
0.6 mg

Tablets, Sublingual
PD: *Nitrostat*

Nizatidine*

150 mg
300 mg

Capsules
Lilly: *Axid*

Norethindrone and Ethinyl Estradiol

0.4/0.035 mg

Tablets: 1
Mead Johnson: *Ovcon 35-21*

0.4/0.035 mg
Inert

Tablets: 2
Mead Johnson: *Ovcon 35-28*

1/0.05 mg

Tablets: 1
Mead Johnson: *Ovcon 50-21*

1/0.05 mg
Inert

Tablets: 2
Mead Johnson: *Ovcon 50-28*

1/0.035 mg

Tablets: 1
Ortho: *Ortho-Novum 1/35-21*
(continued)

© 1993 USPC

* Single source product for solid oral dosage forms in the U.S.

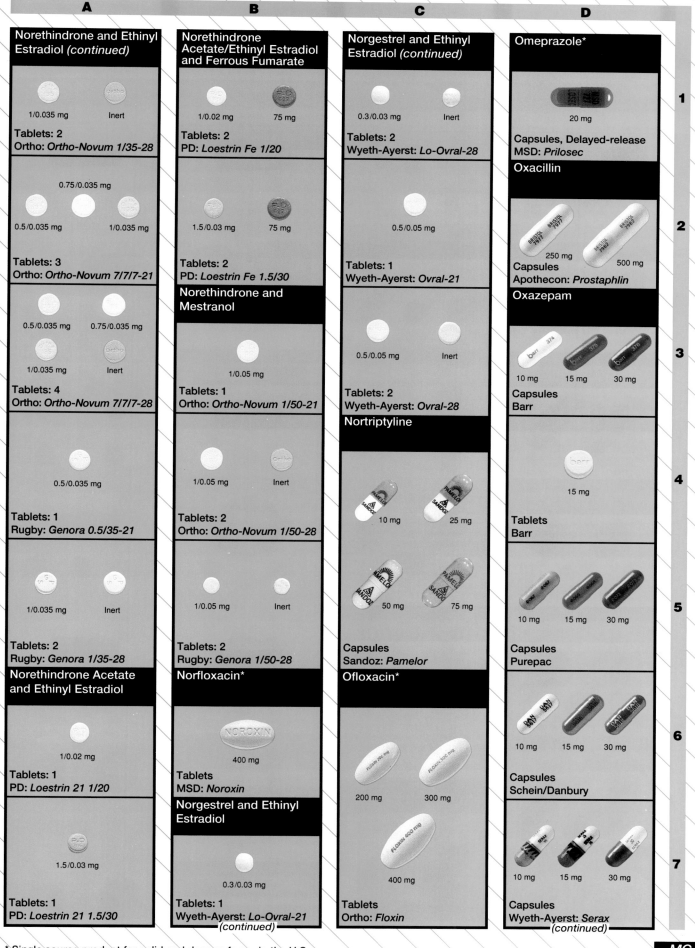

A   **B**   **C**   **D**

Column A

Norethindrone and Ethinyl Estradiol *(continued)*

1/0.035 mg   Inert

Tablets: 2
Ortho: *Ortho-Novum 1/35-28*

0.75/0.035 mg
0.5/0.035 mg   1/0.035 mg

Tablets: 3
Ortho: *Ortho-Novum 7/7/7-21*

0.5/0.035 mg   0.75/0.035 mg
1/0.035 mg   Inert

Tablets: 4
Ortho: *Ortho-Novum 7/7/7-28*

0.5/0.035 mg

Tablets: 1
Rugby: *Genora 0.5/35-21*

1/0.035 mg   Inert

Tablets: 2
Rugby: *Genora 1/35-28*

Norethindrone Acetate and Ethinyl Estradiol

1/0.02 mg

Tablets: 1
PD: *Loestrin 21 1/20*

1.5/0.03 mg

Tablets: 1
PD: *Loestrin 21 1.5/30*

Column B

Norethindrone Acetate/Ethinyl Estradiol and Ferrous Fumarate

1/0.02 mg   75 mg

Tablets: 2
PD: *Loestrin Fe 1/20*

1.5/0.03 mg   75 mg

Tablets: 2
PD: *Loestrin Fe 1.5/30*

Norethindrone and Mestranol

1/0.05 mg

Tablets: 1
Ortho: *Ortho-Novum 1/50-21*

1/0.05 mg   Inert

Tablets: 2
Ortho: *Ortho-Novum 1/50-28*

1/0.05 mg   Inert

Tablets: 2
Rugby: *Genora 1/50-28*

Norfloxacin*

NOROXIN

400 mg

Tablets
MSD: *Noroxin*

Norgestrel and Ethinyl Estradiol

0.3/0.03 mg

Tablets: 1
Wyeth-Ayerst: *Lo-Ovral-21*
(continued)

Column C

Norgestrel and Ethinyl Estradiol *(continued)*

0.3/0.03 mg   Inert

Tablets: 2
Wyeth-Ayerst: *Lo-Ovral-28*

0.5/0.05 mg

Tablets: 1
Wyeth-Ayerst: *Ovral-21*

0.5/0.05 mg   Inert

Tablets: 2
Wyeth-Ayerst: *Ovral-28*

Nortriptyline

10 mg   25 mg

50 mg   75 mg

Capsules
Sandoz: *Pamelor*

Ofloxacin*

200 mg   300 mg

400 mg

Tablets
Ortho: *Floxin*

Column D

Omeprazole*

20 mg

Capsules, Delayed-release
MSD: *Prilosec*

Oxacillin

250 mg   500 mg

Capsules
Apothecon: *Prostaphlin*

Oxazepam

10 mg   15 mg   30 mg

Capsules
Barr

15 mg

Tablets
Barr

10 mg   15 mg   30 mg

Capsules
Purepac

10 mg   15 mg   30 mg

Capsules
Schein/Danbury

10 mg   15 mg   30 mg

Capsules
Wyeth-Ayerst: *Serax*
(continued)

1   2   3   4   5   6   7

* Single source product for solid oral dosage forms in the U.S.

MC-17

© 1993 USPC

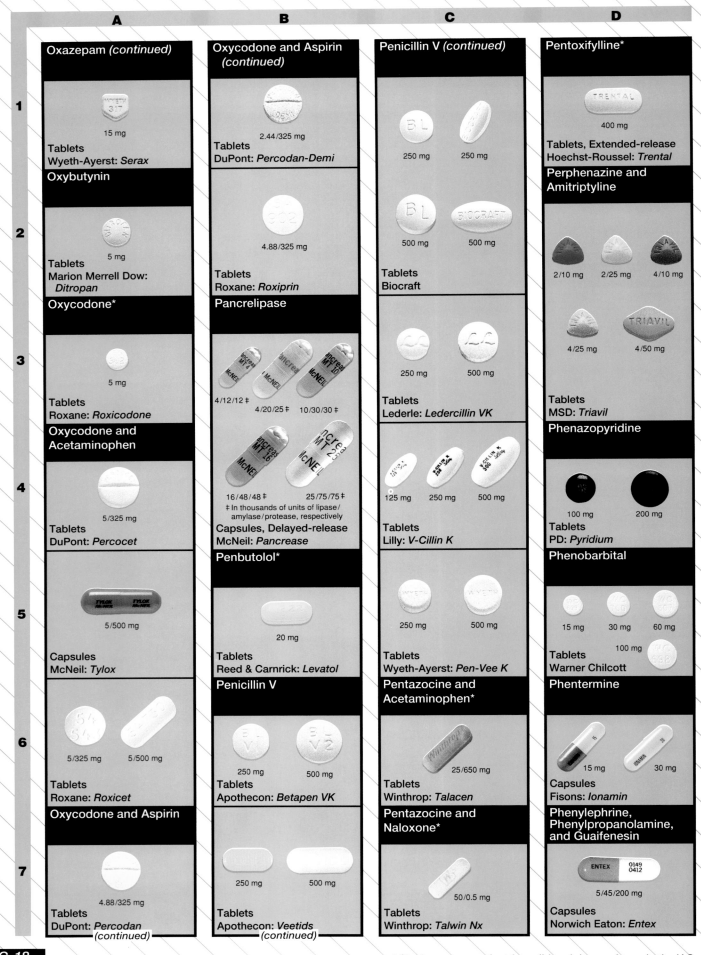

Column A

Oxazepam *(continued)*

15 mg
Tablets
Wyeth-Ayerst: *Serax*

Oxybutynin

5 mg
Tablets
Marion Merrell Dow:
Ditropan

Oxycodone*

5 mg
Tablets
Roxane: *Roxicodone*

Oxycodone and Acetaminophen

5/325 mg
Tablets
DuPont: *Percocet*

5/500 mg
Capsules
McNeil: *Tylox*

5/325 mg   5/500 mg
Tablets
Roxane: *Roxicet*

Oxycodone and Aspirin

4.88/325 mg
Tablets
DuPont: *Percodan*
(continued)

Column B

Oxycodone and Aspirin *(continued)*

2.44/325 mg
Tablets
DuPont: *Percodan-Demi*

4.88/325 mg
Tablets
Roxane: *Roxiprin*

Pancrelipase

4/12/12 ‡   4/20/25 ‡   10/30/30 ‡

16/48/48 ‡   25/75/75 ‡
‡ In thousands of units of lipase/
amylase/protease, respectively
Capsules, Delayed-release
McNeil: *Pancrease*

Penbutolol*

20 mg
Tablets
Reed & Carnrick: *Levatol*

Penicillin V

250 mg   500 mg
Tablets
Apothecon: *Betapen VK*

250 mg   500 mg
Tablets
Apothecon: *Veetids*
(continued)

Column C

Penicillin V *(continued)*

250 mg   250 mg

500 mg   500 mg
Tablets
Biocraft

250 mg   500 mg
Tablets
Lederle: *Ledercillin VK*

125 mg   250 mg   500 mg
Tablets
Lilly: *V-Cillin K*

250 mg   500 mg
Tablets
Wyeth-Ayerst: *Pen-Vee K*

Pentazocine and Acetaminophen*

25/650 mg
Tablets
Winthrop: *Talacen*

Pentazocine and Naloxone*

50/0.5 mg
Tablets
Winthrop: *Talwin Nx*

Column D

Pentoxifylline*

400 mg
Tablets, Extended-release
Hoechst-Roussel: *Trental*

Perphenazine and Amitriptyline

2/10 mg   2/25 mg   4/10 mg

4/25 mg   4/50 mg
Tablets
MSD: *Triavil*

Phenazopyridine

100 mg   200 mg
Tablets
PD: *Pyridium*

Phenobarbital

15 mg   30 mg   60 mg

100 mg
Tablets
Warner Chilcott

Phentermine

15 mg   30 mg
Capsules
Fisons: *Ionamin*

Phenylephrine, Phenylpropanolamine, and Guaifenesin

ENTEX   0149 0412

5/45/200 mg
Capsules
Norwich Eaton: *Entex*

© 1993 USPC

* Single source product for solid oral dosage forms in the U.S.

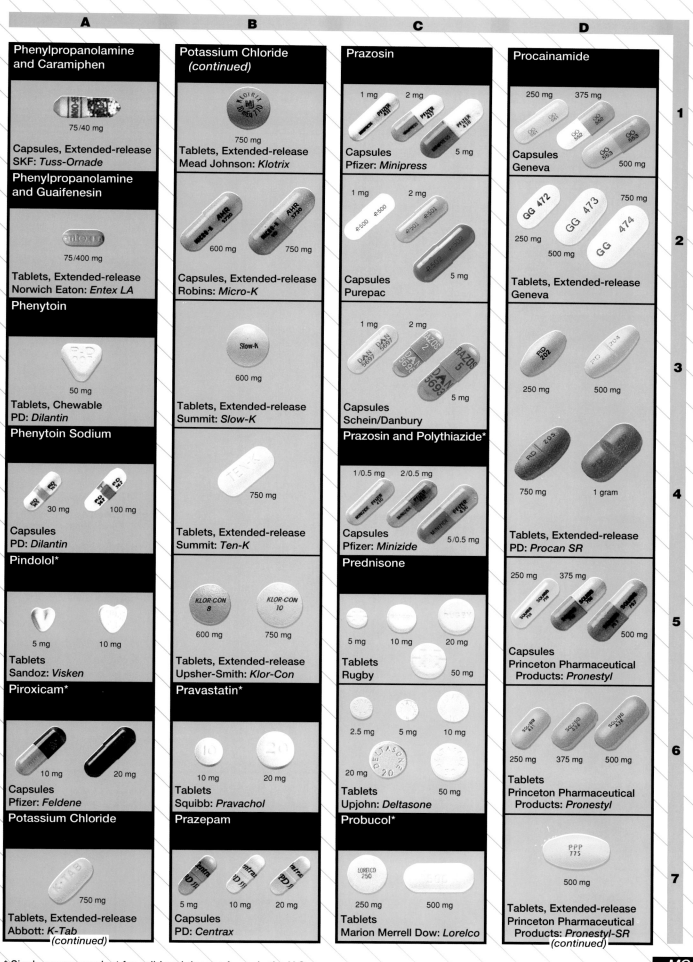

A

Phenylpropanolamine and Caramiphen

75/40 mg
Capsules, Extended-release
SKF: *Tuss-Ornade*

Phenylpropanolamine and Guaifenesin

75/400 mg
Tablets, Extended-release
Norwich Eaton: *Entex LA*

Phenytoin

50 mg
Tablets, Chewable
PD: *Dilantin*

Phenytoin Sodium

30 mg   100 mg
Capsules
PD: *Dilantin*

Pindolol*

5 mg   10 mg
Tablets
Sandoz: *Visken*

Piroxicam*

10 mg   20 mg
Capsules
Pfizer: *Feldene*

Potassium Chloride

750 mg
Tablets, Extended-release
Abbott: *K-Tab*
(continued)

B

Potassium Chloride *(continued)*

750 mg
Tablets, Extended-release
Mead Johnson: *Klotrix*

600 mg   750 mg
Capsules, Extended-release
Robins: *Micro-K*

Slow-K
600 mg
Tablets, Extended-release
Summit: *Slow-K*

750 mg
Tablets, Extended-release
Summit: *Ten-K*

KLOR-CON 8   KLOR-CON 10
600 mg   750 mg
Tablets, Extended-release
Upsher-Smith: *Klor-Con*

Pravastatin*

10 mg   20 mg
Tablets
Squibb: *Pravachol*

Prazepam

5 mg   10 mg   20 mg
Capsules
PD: *Centrax*

C

Prazosin

1 mg   2 mg
5 mg
Capsules
Pfizer: *Minipress*

1 mg   2 mg
5 mg
Capsules
Purepac

1 mg   2 mg
5 mg
Capsules
Schein/Danbury

Prazosin and Polythiazide*

1/0.5 mg   2/0.5 mg
Capsules
Pfizer: *Minizide*
5/0.5 mg

Prednisone

5 mg   10 mg   20 mg
Tablets
Rugby   50 mg

2.5 mg   5 mg   10 mg
20 mg
Tablets
Upjohn: *Deltasone*   50 mg

Probucol*

LORELCO 250
250 mg   500 mg
Tablets
Marion Merrell Dow: *Lorelco*

D

Procainamide

250 mg   375 mg
500 mg
Capsules
Geneva

GG 472   GG 473   750 mg
250 mg   GG 474
500 mg
Tablets, Extended-release
Geneva

250 mg   500 mg

750 mg   1 gram
Tablets, Extended-release
PD: *Procan SR*

250 mg   375 mg
500 mg
Capsules
Princeton Pharmaceutical
Products: *Pronestyl*

250 mg   375 mg   500 mg
Tablets
Princeton Pharmaceutical
Products: *Pronestyl*

PPP 775
500 mg
Tablets, Extended-release
Princeton Pharmaceutical
Products: *Pronestyl-SR*
(continued)

1   2   3   4   5   6   7

* Single source product for solid oral dosage forms in the U.S.

© 1993 USPC

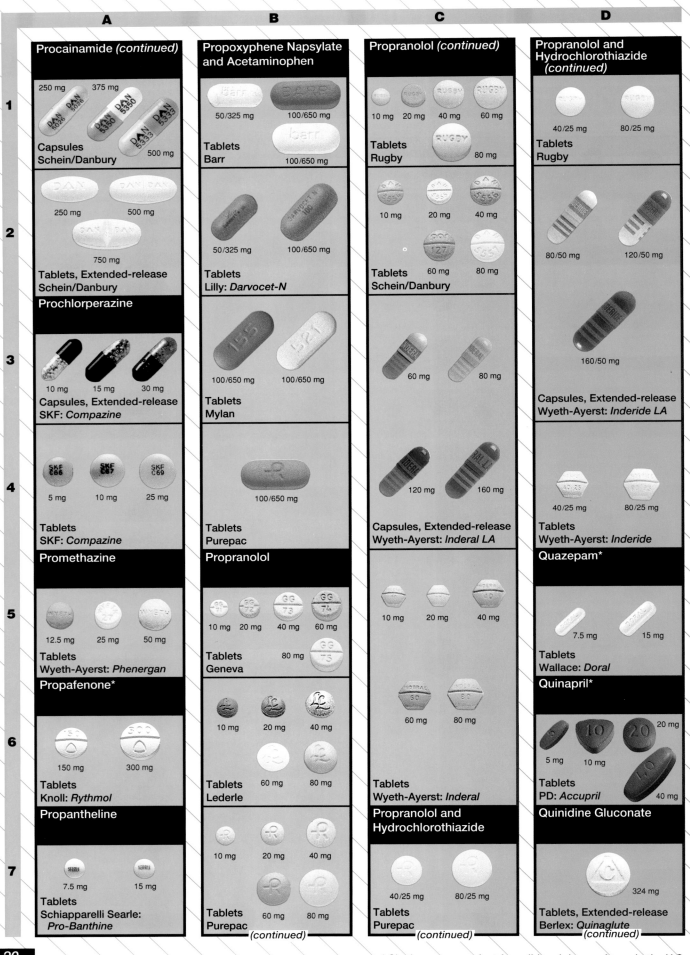

A

Procainamide *(continued)*

250 mg 375 mg
500 mg

Capsules
Schein/Danbury

250 mg 500 mg
750 mg

Tablets, Extended-release
Schein/Danbury

Prochlorperazine

10 mg 15 mg 30 mg

Capsules, Extended-release
SKF: *Compazine*

5 mg 10 mg 25 mg

Tablets
SKF: *Compazine*

Promethazine

12.5 mg 25 mg 50 mg

Tablets
Wyeth-Ayerst: *Phenergan*

Propafenone*

150 mg 300 mg

Tablets
Knoll: *Rythmol*

Propantheline

7.5 mg 15 mg

Tablets
Schiapparelli Searle:
Pro-Banthine

B

Propoxyphene Napsylate and Acetaminophen

50/325 mg 100/650 mg
100/650 mg

Tablets
Barr

50/325 mg 100/650 mg

Tablets
Lilly: *Darvocet-N*

100/650 mg 100/650 mg

Tablets
Mylan

100/650 mg

Tablets
Purepac

Propranolol

10 mg 20 mg 40 mg 60 mg
80 mg

Tablets
Geneva

10 mg 20 mg 40 mg
60 mg 80 mg

Tablets
Lederle

10 mg 20 mg 40 mg
60 mg 80 mg

Tablets
Purepac

(continued)

C

Propranolol *(continued)*

10 mg 20 mg 40 mg 60 mg
80 mg

Tablets
Rugby

10 mg 20 mg 40 mg
60 mg 80 mg

Tablets
Schein/Danbury

60 mg 80 mg

120 mg 160 mg

Capsules, Extended-release
Wyeth-Ayerst: *Inderal LA*

10 mg 20 mg 40 mg

60 mg 80 mg

Tablets
Wyeth-Ayerst: *Inderal*

Propranolol and Hydrochlorothiazide

40/25 mg 80/25 mg

Tablets
Purepac

(continued)

D

Propranolol and Hydrochlorothiazide *(continued)*

40/25 mg 80/25 mg

Tablets
Rugby

80/50 mg 120/50 mg

160/50 mg

Capsules, Extended-release
Wyeth-Ayerst: *Inderide LA*

40/25 mg 80/25 mg

Tablets
Wyeth-Ayerst: *Inderide*

Quazepam*

7.5 mg 15 mg

Tablets
Wallace: *Doral*

Quinapril*

20 mg
5 mg 10 mg
40 mg

Tablets
PD: *Accupril*

Quinidine Gluconate

324 mg

Tablets, Extended-release
Berlex: *Quinaglute*

(continued)

© 1993 USPC

* Single source product for solid oral dosage forms in the U.S.

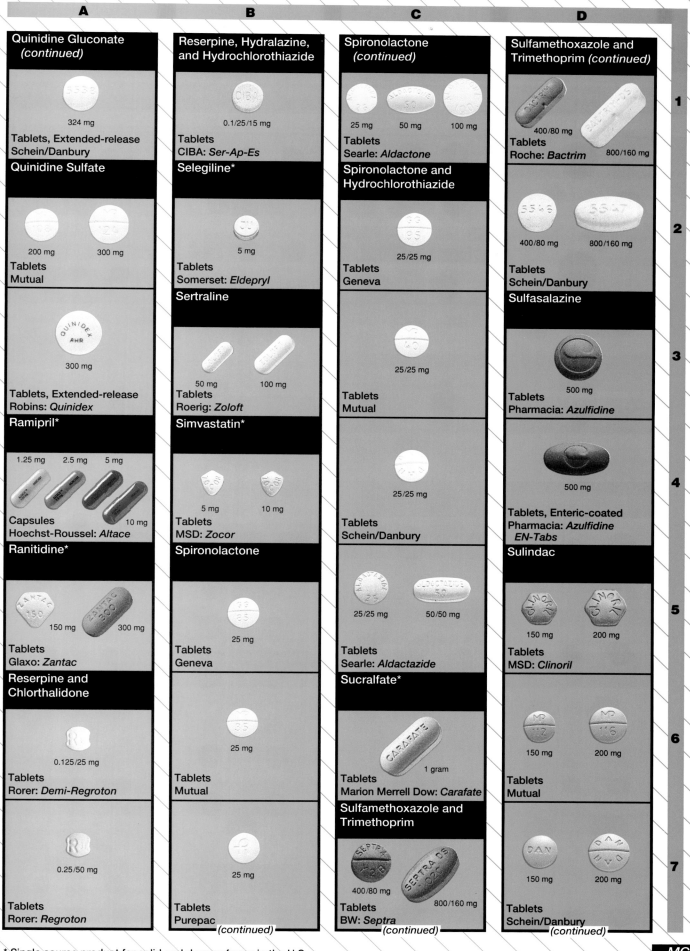

A	B	C	D

A

Quinidine Gluconate (continued)

324 mg
Tablets, Extended-release
Schein/Danbury

Quinidine Sulfate

200 mg   300 mg
Tablets
Mutual

300 mg
Tablets, Extended-release
Robins: *Quinidex*

Ramipril*

1.25 mg   2.5 mg   5 mg   10 mg
Capsules
Hoechst-Roussel: *Altace*

Ranitidine*

150 mg   300 mg
Tablets
Glaxo: *Zantac*

Reserpine and Chlorthalidone

0.125/25 mg
Tablets
Rorer: *Demi-Regroton*

0.25/50 mg
Tablets
Rorer: *Regroton*

B

Reserpine, Hydralazine, and Hydrochlorothiazide

0.1/25/15 mg
Tablets
CIBA: *Ser-Ap-Es*

Selegiline*

5 mg
Tablets
Somerset: *Eldepryl*

Sertraline

50 mg   100 mg
Tablets
Roerig: *Zoloft*

Simvastatin*

5 mg   10 mg
Tablets
MSD: *Zocor*

Spironolactone

25 mg
Tablets
Geneva

25 mg
Tablets
Mutual

25 mg
Tablets
Purepac

(continued)

C

Spironolactone (continued)

25 mg   50 mg   100 mg
Tablets
Searle: *Aldactone*

Spironolactone and Hydrochlorothiazide

25/25 mg
Tablets
Geneva

25/25 mg
Tablets
Mutual

25/25 mg
Tablets
Schein/Danbury

25/25 mg   50/50 mg
Tablets
Searle: *Aldactazide*

Sucralfate*

1 gram
Tablets
Marion Merrell Dow: *Carafate*

Sulfamethoxazole and Trimethoprim

400/80 mg   800/160 mg
Tablets
BW: *Septra*

(continued)

D

Sulfamethoxazole and Trimethoprim (continued)

400/80 mg   800/160 mg
Tablets
Roche: *Bactrim*

400/80 mg   800/160 mg
Tablets
Schein/Danbury

Sulfasalazine

500 mg
Tablets
Pharmacia: *Azulfidine*

500 mg
Tablets, Enteric-coated
Pharmacia: *Azulfidine EN-Tabs*

Sulindac

150 mg   200 mg
Tablets
MSD: *Clinoril*

150 mg   200 mg
Tablets
Mutual

150 mg   200 mg
Tablets
Schein/Danbury

(continued)

1   2   3   4   5   6   7

* Single source product for solid oral dosage forms in the U.S.

MC-21

© 1993 USPC

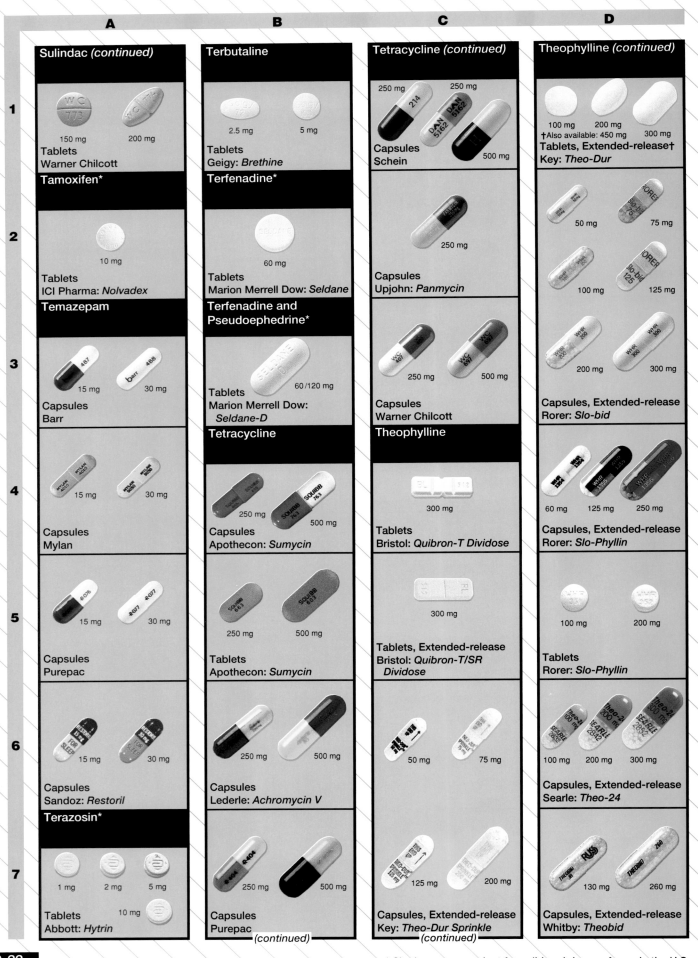

A

Sulindac *(continued)*

150 mg   200 mg
Tablets
Warner Chilcott

Tamoxifen*

10 mg
Tablets
ICI Pharma: *Nolvadex*

Temazepam

15 mg   30 mg
Capsules
Barr

15 mg   30 mg
Capsules
Mylan

15 mg   30 mg
Capsules
Purepac

15 mg   30 mg
Capsules
Sandoz: *Restoril*

Terazosin*

1 mg   2 mg   5 mg
10 mg
Tablets
Abbott: *Hytrin*

B

Terbutaline

2.5 mg   5 mg
Tablets
Geigy: *Brethine*

Terfenadine*

60 mg
Tablets
Marion Merrell Dow: *Seldane*

Terfenadine and Pseudoephedrine*

60/120 mg
Tablets
Marion Merrell Dow:
Seldane-D

Tetracycline

250 mg   500 mg
Capsules
Apothecon: *Sumycin*

250 mg   500 mg
Tablets
Apothecon: *Sumycin*

250 mg   500 mg
Capsules
Lederle: *Achromycin V*

250 mg   500 mg
Capsules
Purepac
(continued)

C

Tetracycline *(continued)*

250 mg   250 mg
500 mg
Capsules
Schein

250 mg
Capsules
Upjohn: *Panmycin*

250 mg   500 mg
Capsules
Warner Chilcott

Theophylline

300 mg
Tablets
Bristol: *Quibron-T Dividose*

300 mg
Tablets, Extended-release
Bristol: *Quibron-T/SR
Dividose*

50 mg   75 mg

125 mg   200 mg
Capsules, Extended-release
Key: *Theo-Dur Sprinkle*
(continued)

D

Theophylline *(continued)*

100 mg   200 mg   300 mg
†Also available: 450 mg
Tablets, Extended-release†
Key: *Theo-Dur*

50 mg   75 mg
100 mg   125 mg
200 mg   300 mg
Capsules, Extended-release
Rorer: *Slo-bid*

60 mg   125 mg   250 mg
Capsules, Extended-release
Rorer: *Slo-Phyllin*

100 mg   200 mg
Tablets
Rorer: *Slo-Phyllin*

100 mg   200 mg   300 mg
Capsules, Extended-release
Searle: *Theo-24*

130 mg   260 mg
Capsules, Extended-release
Whitby: *Theobid*

© 1993 USPC

* Single source product for solid oral dosage forms in the U.S.

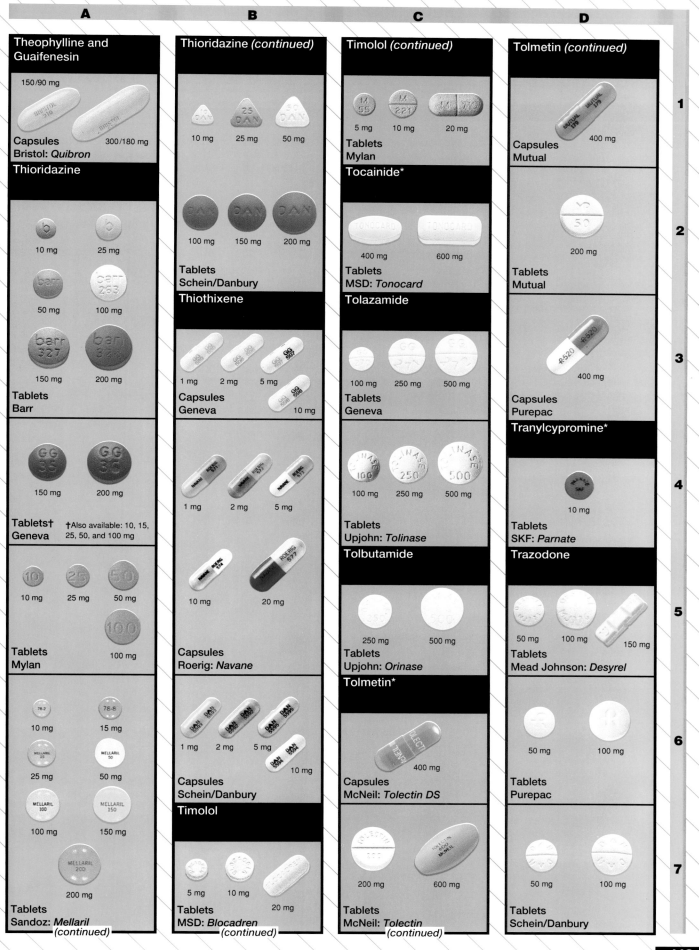

A | B | C | D

Column A

Theophylline and Guaifenesin

150/90 mg

300/180 mg

Capsules
Bristol: *Quibron*

Thioridazine

10 mg 25 mg
50 mg 100 mg
150 mg 200 mg

Tablets
Barr

150 mg 200 mg

Tablets†
Geneva †Also available: 10, 15, 25, 50, and 100 mg

10 mg 25 mg 50 mg
100 mg

Tablets
Mylan

10 mg 15 mg
25 mg 50 mg
100 mg 150 mg
200 mg

Tablets
Sandoz: *Mellaril*
(continued)

Column B

Thioridazine *(continued)*

10 mg 25 mg 50 mg
100 mg 150 mg 200 mg

Tablets
Schein/Danbury

Thiothixene

1 mg 2 mg 5 mg
10 mg

Capsules
Geneva

1 mg 2 mg 5 mg
10 mg 20 mg

Capsules
Roerig: *Navane*

1 mg 2 mg 5 mg
10 mg

Capsules
Schein/Danbury

Timolol

5 mg 10 mg 20 mg

Tablets
MSD: *Blocadren*
(continued)

Column C

Timolol *(continued)*

5 mg 10 mg 20 mg

Tablets
Mylan

Tocainide*

400 mg 600 mg

Tablets
MSD: *Tonocard*

Tolazamide

100 mg 250 mg 500 mg

Tablets
Geneva

100 mg 250 mg 500 mg

Tablets
Upjohn: *Tolinase*

Tolbutamide

250 mg 500 mg

Tablets
Upjohn: *Orinase*

Tolmetin*

400 mg

Capsules
McNeil: *Tolectin DS*

200 mg 600 mg

Tablets
McNeil: *Tolectin*
(continued)

Column D

Tolmetin *(continued)*

400 mg

Capsules
Mutual

200 mg

Tablets
Mutual

400 mg

Capsules
Purepac

Tranylcypromine*

10 mg

Tablets
SKF: *Parnate*

Trazodone

50 mg 100 mg 150 mg

Tablets
Mead Johnson: *Desyrel*

50 mg 100 mg

Tablets
Purepac

50 mg 100 mg

Tablets
Schein/Danbury

---

* Single source product for solid oral dosage forms in the U.S.

MC-23

© 1993 USPC

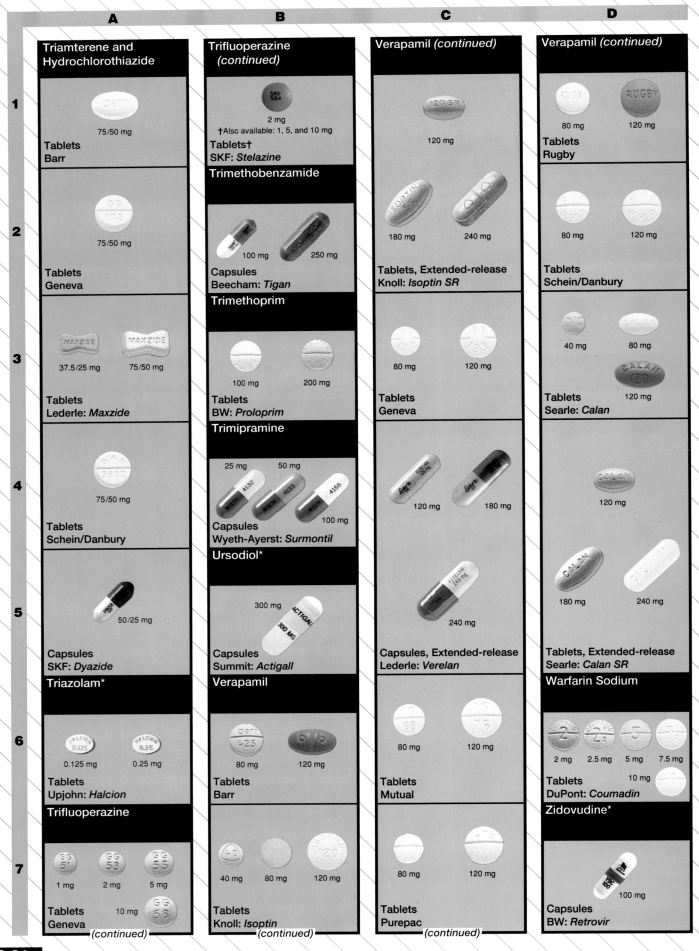

A

Triamterene and Hydrochlorothiazide

75/50 mg
Tablets
Barr

75/50 mg
Tablets
Geneva

37.5/25 mg   75/50 mg
Tablets
Lederle: *Maxzide*

75/50 mg
Tablets
Schein/Danbury

50/25 mg
Capsules
SKF: *Dyazide*

Triazolam*

0.125 mg   0.25 mg
Tablets
Upjohn: *Halcion*

Trifluoperazine

1 mg   2 mg   5 mg
10 mg
Tablets
Geneva

(continued)

B

Trifluoperazine *(continued)*

2 mg
†Also available: 1, 5, and 10 mg
Tablets†
SKF: *Stelazine*

Trimethobenzamide

100 mg   250 mg
Capsules
Beecham: *Tigan*

Trimethoprim

100 mg   200 mg
Tablets
BW: *Proloprim*

Trimipramine

25 mg   50 mg
100 mg
Capsules
Wyeth-Ayerst: *Surmontil*

Ursodiol*

300 mg
Capsules
Summit: *Actigall*

Verapamil

80 mg   120 mg
Tablets
Barr

40 mg   80 mg   120 mg
Tablets
Knoll: *Isoptin*

(continued)

C

Verapamil *(continued)*

120 mg

180 mg   240 mg
Tablets, Extended-release
Knoll: *Isoptin SR*

80 mg   120 mg
Tablets
Geneva

120 mg   180 mg

240 mg
Capsules, Extended-release
Lederle: *Verelan*

80 mg   120 mg
Tablets
Mutual

80 mg   120 mg
Tablets
Purepac

(continued)

D

Verapamil *(continued)*

80 mg   120 mg
Tablets
Rugby

80 mg   120 mg
Tablets
Schein/Danbury

40 mg   80 mg
120 mg
Tablets
Searle: *Calan*

120 mg

180 mg   240 mg
Tablets, Extended-release
Searle: *Calan SR*

Warfarin Sodium

2 mg   2.5 mg   5 mg   7.5 mg
10 mg
Tablets
DuPont: *Coumadin*

Zidovudine*

100 mg
Capsules
BW: *Retrovir*

© 1993 USPC

* Single source product for solid oral dosage forms in the U.S.

Section V

THE USP-PRACTITIONERS' REPORTING NETWORK
(USP-PRN)

USP offers three separate programs under The Practitioners' Reporting Network, designed to collect practitioners' experiences and observations. By participating in these programs you can play an active part in helping to protect your patients from unreliable drug products, defective medical devices, and possible future medication errors.

(1) *The Drug Product Problem Reporting Program*: The USP Drug Product Problem Reporting (DPPR) Program alerts manufacturers, labelers, the FDA, and the USP Committee of Revision to your observations of poor product quality, unclear labeling, defective packaging, therapeutic ineffectiveness, suspected counterfeiting, and possible product tampering.

When you detect a drug product problem, simply submit your report using the convenient USP report form, or call toll free **1-800-638-6725**. There is no charge for using the USP DPPR service.

(2) *The Medication Errors Reporting Program*: Pharmacists who encounter medication errors can greatly improve patient safety and perform a valuable educational service for colleagues by sharing medication error information.

The USP, under a new agreement with the Institute for Safe Medication Practices (ISMP), is now coordinating the Medication Errors Reporting (MER) Program for the Institute.

Contact the Medication Errors Reporting Program whenever you encounter problems with labeling, packaging, actual or potential misadministrations, miscalculations, misinterpretations, drug nomenclature, drug marketing and advertising, medical abbreviations, etc.

The MER Program has already published more than 400 medication error reports received from health professionals nationwide. The MER Program has issued warnings about design flaws as well as potentially dangerous labeling and packaging that could lead to safety hazards.

To report a medication error call **1-800-23ERROR** or submit your report on the form for the Medication Errors Reporting Program.

(3) *The Medical Device and Laboratory Product Problem Reporting Program (PRP)*: The PRP program, funded by the FDA under contract No. 223-91-6001, communicates your medical device problems directly to decision-makers in industry and the government. Use the PRP to express your concerns about malfunctioning medical devices and laboratory equipment.

Collapsing catheters, malfunctioning x-ray equipment, occluded nasal cannulas, plugged needles, defective ventilator valves, and inadequate packaging are examples of the types of reports PRP receives from concerned health care professionals.

When you encounter a medical device problem, call PRP toll free at **1-800-638-6725**. The PRP will forward reported information directly to the FDA as well as to the manufacturer of the product.

Your input can make all the difference. Contact USP-PRN to report a problem or to obtain additional information:

The Practitioners' Reporting Network
United States Pharmacopeia
12601 Twinbrook Parkway
Rockville, Maryland 20852

USP-PRN
CALL US WHEN YOU NEED US.

USP DRUG PRODUCT PROBLEM REPORTING PROGRAM

PRODUCT NAME (brand name and generic name)

DOSAGE FORM (tablet, capsule, injectable, etc.)	SIZE/TYPE OF CONTAINER	STRENGTH	NDC NUMBER

LOT NUMBER(S)	EXPIRATION DATE(S)

NAME AND ADDRESS OF THE MANUFACTURER	NAME AND ADDRESS OF LABELER (if different from manufacturer)

YOUR NAME & TITLE (please type or print)

YOUR PRACTICE LOCATION (include establishment name, address and zip code)

Days and times available_____

PHONE NUMBER AT PRACTICE LOCATION (include area code)	If requested, will the actual product involved be available for examination by the manufacturer or FDA? *(Do not send samples to USP.)* ☐ Yes ☐ No

PLEASE INDICATE TO WHOM USP MAY VOLUNTARILY DISCLOSE YOUR IDENTITY (check box(es) that apply)

You may release my identity to:

☐ The manufacturer and/or labeler as listed above   ☐ The Food and Drug Administration   ☐ Other persons requesting a copy of this report

SIGNATURE OF REPORTER	DATE

PROBLEMS NOTED OR SUSPECTED (If more space is needed, please attach separate page)

Date problem occurred or observed: _____

RETURN TO: **United States Pharmacopeia**
12601 Twinbrook Parkway
Rockville, Maryland 20852
Attention: Joseph G. Valentino

OR

Call Toll Free Anytime

1-800-638-6725

In Maryland, call collect
1-301-881-0256 between 9:00 AM
and 4:30 PM Eastern Time
FAX 1-301-816-8247

File Access Number
Date Received by USP

USPDI

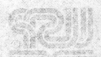

MEDI-CATION ERRORS

REPORTING PROGRAM

MEDICATION ERRORS REPORTING PROGRAM
Coordinated by the United States Pharmacopeial Convention, Inc. for
the Institute for Safe Medication Practices, Inc.
Huntingdon Valley, PA

1. For errors relating to drug labeling, packaging or the naming of drug products, please complete the following:

DRUG #1

Brand Name _____

Generic Name _____

Manufacturer _____

Labeler *(if different from mfr.)* _____

Dosage Form _____

Strength/Concentration _____

Type and Size of Container _____

DRUG #2

Brand Name _____

Generic Name _____

Manufacturer _____

Labeler *(if different from mfr.)* _____

Dosage Form _____

Strength/Concentration _____

Type and Size of Container _____

2. Please describe the medication error or potential error *(if more space is needed, please attach separate page)*
Please note the type of personnel involved *(R.Ph., R.N., M.D., student, etc.)*

3. Please include any pertinent patient information that may be relevant including patient age, sex, diagnosis, etc. *(patient identification not necessary)*

4. Did injury or mortality occur? *(if injury, please be specific)*

5. Date and time incident occurred.

6. When and how was the error discovered?

7. Reports are most useful when materials such as product label, physician's order copy, graphics, etc., can be reviewed by the Institute. Do you have such materials available? ☐ Yes ☐ No
If yes, please specify _____
Please retain these materials/samples if possible for 60 days.

8. This incident has been reported to:
(check all boxes that apply)

☐ Institution *(via incident report)*
☐ Peers
☐ Supervisor
☐ Manufacturer
☐ State regulatory board/department of health
☐ Coroner
☐ Not reported to anyone else
☐ Other _____

This Section Is Optional
The Institute on occasion needs to conduct follow-up analysis on reports. Kindly provide the contact information below. You may use your home address and telephone number should you prefer. The USP and the Institute will not voluntarily disclose your identity in processing this report without your permission.

Name _____
Title _____
May we contact you by mail? ☐ Yes ☐ No
Address to be used: _____
_____

May we contact you by telephone? ☐ Yes ☐ No
Phone number: (_____)_____

9. Do you have any recommendations to prevent recurrence of this error?

RETURN TO:
The Medication Errors Reporting Program
c/o The United States Pharmacopeial
   Convention, Inc.
   12601 Twinbrook Parkway
   Rockville, MD 20852

or call toll free anytime
1-800-23-ERROR
FAX 1-301-816-8247

File Access Number

Date Received by USP

USP DI

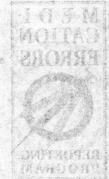

MEDI
CATION
ERRORS
REPORTING
PROGRAM

Reference Number _____
Date Received by USP? _____

USP 01

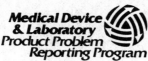

**Medical Device
& Laboratory
Product Problem
Reporting Program**

Form Approved; OMB No. 0910-0143
DATE RECEIVED
ACCESS NO

---

1. PRODUCT IDENTIFICATION:

Name of Product and Type of Device
(Include sizes or other identifying characteristics and attach labeling, if available)

_____

_____

Manufacturer's Name _____

Manufacturer's City, State, Zip Code _____

_____

Is this a disposable item?   YES ☐   NO ☐

Lot Number(s) and Expiration Date(s) (if applicable)

Serial Number(s)

Manufacturer's Product Number and/or Model Number

---

2. REPORTER INFORMATION:

Your Name _____ Today's Date _____

Title and Department _____

Facility's Name _____

Street Address _____

City _____ State _____ Zip _____ Phone ( ) _____ Ext: _____

---

3. PROBLEM INFORMATION:

Date event occurred _____

This event has been reported to: Manufacturer ☐ FDA ☐

Please indicate how you want your identity publicly disclosed:

Other _____

No public disclosure ☐

To the manufacturer/distributor ☐

To the manufacturer/distributor and to anyone who requests a copy of the report from the FDA ☐

If requested, will the actual product involved in the event be available for evaluation by the manufacturer or FDA?   YES ☐   NO ☐

Problem noted or suspected (Describe the event in as much detail as necessary. Attach additional pages if required. Include how and where the product was used. Include other equipment or products that were involved. Sketches may be helpful in describing problem areas.)

RETURN TO

United States Pharmacopeia
12601 Twinbrook Parkway
Rockville, Maryland   20852
Attention: Dr. Joseph G. Valentino

OR

CALL TOLL FREE ANYTIME
800-638-6725*
IN THE CONTINENTAL UNITED STATES
*In Maryland, call collect (301) 881-0256
between 9:00 AM and 4:30 PM

FORM FDA 2519f (3/85)

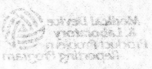

ACCESS NO.	DATE RECEIVED

Your Name

Today's Date

☐ No public disclosure

between 9 AM and 4:30 PM

FORM FDA 2519 (USP)

Section VI: Index

A selected number of brand names *(italicized)* have been included. The inclusion of a brand name does not mean the USPC has any particular knowledge that the brand listed has properties different from other brands of the same drug, nor should it be interpreted as an endorsement by the USPC. Similarly, the fact that a particular brand has not been included does not indicate that the product has been judged to be unsatisfactory or unacceptable. Page numbers for MC-1 through MC-24 refer to the product identification photographs in *The Medicine Chart* (Section IV).

See Appendix A (p. I/405) and Appendix B (p. I/438) of the "Approved Drug Products with Therapeutic Equivalence Evaluations" section of this volume for listings of the products included in the Orange Book.

A

Absorbable Gelatin—See Gelatin, Absorbable
Absorbent Gauze—See Gauze, Absorbent
Acacia
  Acacia NF, III/1
Accupril, IV/MC-20
Accutane, IV/MC-12
Acebutolol Hydrochloride
  Capsules, III/1
  Tablets, III/1
Acetaminophen
  Acetaminophen USP, III/1
  Capsules USP, III/1
  Solution, Oral, USP, III/1
  Suppositories USP, III/1
  Suspension, Oral, USP, III/1
  Tablets USP, III/1
  Wafers, III/1
Acetaminophen and Aspirin
  Tablets USP, III/1
Acetaminophen, Aspirin, and Caffeine
  Capsules USP, III/1
  Powders, Oral, III/1
  Tablets USP, III/1
Acetaminophen, Aspirin, and Caffeine, Buffered
  Tablets, III/1
Acetaminophen, Aspirin, Codeine Phosphate, Magnesium Hydroxide, and Aluminum Hydroxide, Buffered
  Tablets, III/2
Acetaminophen, Aspirin, and Salicylamide, Buffered
  Tablets, III/2
Acetaminophen, Aspirin, Salicylamide, and Caffeine
  Tablets, III/2
Acetaminophen, Aspirin, Salicylamide, Codeine, and Caffeine
  Tablets, III/2
Acetaminophen and Caffeine
  Capsules USP, III/2
  Tablets USP, III/2
Acetaminophen, Calcium Carbonate, Potassium and Sodium Bicarbonates, and Citric Acid
  Tablets for Oral Solution, Effervescent, III/2
Acetaminophen and Codeine Phosphate
  Capsules USP, III/2, IV/MC-1
  Elixir USP, III/2
  Suspension, Oral, III/2
  Tablets USP, III/2, IV/MC-1
Acetaminophen, Codeine Phosphate, and Caffeine
  Capsules, III/2
  Tablets, III/2

Acetaminophen and Diphenhydramine Citrate
  Tablets USP, III/2
Acetaminophen and Salicylamide
  Capsules, III/2
  Tablets, III/2
Acetaminophen, Salicylamide, and Caffeine
  Capsules, III/3
  Tablets, III/3
Acetaminophen, Sodium Bicarbonate, and Citric Acid
  for Solution, Oral, Effervescent, USP, III/3
Acetazolamide
  Acetazolamide USP, III/3
  Capsules, Extended-release, III/3
  Tablets USP, III/3
Acetazolamide Sodium
  Sterile USP, III/3
Acetic Acid
  Acetic Acid NF, III/3
  Glacial USP, III/3
  Irrigation USP, III/3
  Solution, Otic, USP, III/3
Acetohexamide
  Acetohexamide USP, III/3
  Tablets USP, III/3
Acetohydroxamic Acid
  Acetohydroxamic Acid USP, III/4
  Tablets USP, III/4
Acetone
  Acetone NF, III/4
Acetophenazine Maleate
  Acetophenazine Maleate USP, III/4
  Tablets USP, III/4
Acetylcholine Chloride
  Acetylcholine Chloride USP, III/4
  for Solution, Ophthalmic, USP, III/4
Acetylcysteine
  Acetylcysteine USP, III/5
  Injection, III/5
  Solution USP, III/5
Acetylcysteine and Isoproterenol Hydrochloride
  Solution, Inhalation, USP, III/5
Achromycin V, IV/MC-22
Acrisorcin
  Acrisorcin USP, III/5
  Acrisorcin Cream USP, III/5
Actigall, IV/MC-24
Activated Charcoal—See Charcoal, Activated
Actuators, II/10
Acyclovir
  Acyclovir USP, III/5
  Capsules, III/5, IV/MC-1
  Ointment, III/5
  Suspension, Oral, III/5
  Tablets, III/5, IV/MC-1

Acyclovir Sodium
  Sterile, III/5
Adalat, IV/MC-16
Adenine
  Adenine USP, III/5
Adenosine
  Injection, III/6
Adhesive Tape—See Tape, Adhesive
Agar
  Agar NF, III/6
Air, Medical
  Medical Air USP, III/6
Alanine
  Alanine USP, III/6
Albendazole
  Albendazole USP, III/6
Albumin Humin
  Albumin Humin USP, III/6
Albuterol
  Aerosol, Inhalation, III/6
  Albuterol USP, III/6
  Tablets USP, III/6
Albuterol Sulfate
  Albuterol Sulfate USP, III/7
  for Inhalation, III/7
  Injection, III/7
  Solution, Inhalation, III/7
  Solution, Oral, III/7
  Syrup, III/7
  Tablets, Extended-release, III/7, IV/MC-
Alclometasone Dipropionate
  Alclometasone Dipropionate USP, III/7
  Cream USP, III/7
  Ointment USP, III/7
Alcohol
  Alcohol USP, III/7
Alcohol and Acetone
  Lotion, Detergent, III/8
  Pledgets, III/8
Alcohol, Benzyl—See Benzyl Alcohol
Alcohol, Butyl—See Butyl Alcohol
Alcohol, Cetostearyl—See Cetostearyl Alcohol
Alcohol, Cetyl—See Cetyl Alcohol
Alcohol, Dehydrated
  Dehydrated Alcohol USP, III/8
  Injection USP, III/8
Alcohol and Dextrose
  Alcohol in Dextrose Injection USP, III/8
Alcohol, Diluted
  Diluted Alcohol NF, III/8
Alcohol, Isopropyl—See Isopropyl Alcohol
Alcohol, Isopropyl, Azeotropic—See Isopropyl Alcohol, Azeotropic
Alcohol, Isopropyl, Rubbing—See Isopropyl Rubbing Alcohol
Alcohol, Methyl—See Methyl Alcohol
Alcohol, Oleyl—See Oleyl Alcohol

Alcohol, Phenylethyl—See Phenylethyl Alcohol

Alcohol, Polyvinyl—See Polyvinyl Alcohol

Alcohol, Rubbing
Rubbing Alcohol USP, III/8

Alcohols, Lanolin—See Lanolin Alcohols

Alcohol and Sulfur
Gel, III/8
Lotion, III/8

Aldactazide, IV/MC-21

Aldactone, IV/MC-21

Aldomet, IV/MC-14

Aldoril, IV/MC-14

Alfentanil Hydrochloride
Injection, III/9

Alginic Acid
Alginic Acid NF, III/9

Allopurinol
Allopurinol USP, III/9
Tablets USP, III/9, IV/MC-1

Almond Oil
Almond Oil NF, III/9

Aloe
Aloe USP, III/9

Alpha₁-proteinase Inhibitor, Human
for Injection, III/9

Alprazolam
Alprazolam USP, III/9
Tablets USP, III/9, IV/MC-1

Alprostadil
Alprostadil USP, III/10
Injection USP, III/10

Alseroxylon
Tablets, III/10

Altace, IV/MC-21

Alteplase, Recombinant
for Injection, III/10

Altretamine
Capsules, III/10

Alum
Ammonium Alum USP, III/10
Potassium Alum USP, III/10

Alumina and Magnesia
Suspension, Oral, USP, III/11
Tablets USP, III/11

Alumina, Magnesia, and Calcium Carbonate
Suspension, Oral, USP, III/11
Tablets USP, III/11

Alumina, Magnesia, Calcium Carbonate, and
Simethicone
Tablets USP, III/11

Alumina, Magnesia, and Simethicone
Suspension, Oral, USP, III/11
Tablets USP, III/11

Alumina and Magnesium Carbonate
Suspension, Oral, USP, III/11
Tablets USP, III/11

Alumina, Magnesium Carbonate, and Magnesium Oxide
Tablets USP, III/12

Alumina and Magnesium Trisilicate
Suspension, Oral, USP, III/12
Tablets USP, III/12

Alumina, Magnesium Trisilicate, and Sodium Bicarbonate
Tablets, Chewable, III/12

Aluminum Acetate
Solution, Topical, USP, III/12

Aluminum Carbonate, Basic
Capsules, Dried, Gel, USP, III/12
Gel USP, III/12
Tablets, Dried, Gel, USP, III/12

Aluminum Chloride
Aluminum Chloride USP, III/13

Aluminum Hydroxide
Gel USP, III/13

Aluminum Hydroxide, Dried
Capsules, Gel, USP, III/13
Gel USP, III/13
Tablets, Gel, USP, III/13

Aluminum Monostearate
Aluminum Monostearate NF, III/13

Aluminum Phosphate
Gel USP, III/13

Aluminum Subacetate
Solution, Topical, USP, III/14

Aluminum Sulfate
Aluminum Sulfate USP, III/14

Alupent, IV/MC-14

Amantadine Hydrochloride
Amantadine Hydrochloride USP, III/14
Capsules USP, III/14, IV/MC-1
Syrup USP, III/14

Ambenonium Chloride
Tablets, III/14

Amcinonide
Amcinonide USP, III/14
Cream USP, III/14
Lotion, III/14
Ointment USP, III/14

Amdinocillin
Sterile USP, III/15

Amikacin
Amikacin USP, III/15

Amikacin Sulfate
Amikacin Sulfate USP, III/15
Injection USP, III/15

Amiloride Hydrochloride
Amiloride Hydrochloride USP, III/15
Tablets USP, III/15

Amiloride Hydrochloride and Hydrochlorothiazide
Tablets USP, III/15, IV/MC-1

Aminobenzoate Potassium
Aminobenzoate Potassium USP, III/16
Capsules USP, III/16
for Solution, Oral, USP, III/16
Tablets USP, III/16

Aminobenzoate Sodium
Aminobenzoate Sodium USP, III/16

Aminobenzoic Acid
Aminobenzoic Acid USP, III/16
Gel USP, III/16
Solution, Topical, USP, III/16

Aminocaproic Acid
Aminocaproic Acid USP, III/16
Injection USP, III/16
Syrup USP, III/16
Tablets USP, III/16

Aminoglutethimide
Aminoglutethimide USP, III/16
Tablets USP, III/16

Aminohippurate Sodium
Injection USP, III/17

Aminohippuric Acid
Aminohippuric Acid USP, III/17

Aminophylline
Aminophylline USP, III/17
Enema USP, III/17
Injection USP, III/17
Solution, Oral, USP, III/17
Suppositories USP, III/17
Tablets USP, III/17
Tablets, Extended-release, III/17

Aminophylline and Sodium Chloride
Injection, III/18

Aminosalicylate Sodium
Aminosalicylate Sodium USP, III/18
Tablets USP, III/18

Aminosalicylic Acid
Aminosalicylic Acid USP, III/18
Tablets USP, III/18

Amiodarone Hydrochloride
Tablets, III/18

Amitriptyline Hydrochloride
Amitriptyline Hydrochloride USP, III/18
Injection USP, III/18
Tablets USP, III/18, IV/MC-1, MC-2

Amitriptyline Pamoate
Syrup, III/18

Ammonia N 13
Injection USP, III/19

Ammonia Solution, Strong
Strong Ammonia Solution NF, III/19

Ammonia Spirit, Aromatic
Aromatic Ammonia Spirit USP, III/19

Ammoniated Mercury—See Mercury, Ammoniated

Ammonio Methacrylate Copolymer
Ammonio Methacrylate Copolymer NF, III/19

Ammonium Carbonate
Ammonium Carbonate NF, III/20

Ammonium Chloride
Ammonium Chloride USP, III/20
Injection USP, III/20
Tablets, Delayed-release, USP, III/20

Ammonium Molybdate
Ammonium Molybdate USP, III/20
Injection USP, III/20

Ammonium Phosphate
Ammonium Phosphate NF, III/20

Amobarbital
Amobarbital USP, III/20
Tablets USP, III/20

Amobarbital Sodium
Capsules USP, III/20
Sterile USP, III/20

Amodiaquine
Amodiaquine USP, III/21

Amodiaquine Hydrochloride
Amodiaquine Hydrochloride USP, III/21
Tablets USP, III/21

Amoxapine
Amoxapine USP, III/21
Tablets USP, III/21

Amoxicillin
Amoxicillin USP, III/21
Capsules USP, III/21, IV/MC-2
Infusion, Intramammary, USP, III/21
Sterile USP, III/21
Suspension, Oral, USP, III/21
for Suspension, Oral, USP, III/21
for Suspension, Sterile, USP, III/21
Tablets USP, III/21, IV/MC-2

Amoxicillin and Clavulanate Potassium
for Suspension, Oral, USP, III/22
Tablets USP, III/22, IV/MC-2

Amoxil, IV/MC-2

Amphetamine Sulfate
Amphetamine Sulfate USP, III/23
Tablets USP, III/23

Amphotericin B
Amphotericin B USP, III/23
Cream USP, III/23
for Injection USP, III/23
Lotion USP, III/23
Ointment USP, III/23

Ampicillin
Ampicillin USP, III/23
Boluses USP, III/23
Capsules USP, III/23, IV/MC-2
Powder, Soluble, USP, III/23
Sterile USP, III/23
Suspension, Sterile, USP, III/23
for Suspension, Oral, USP, III/23
for Suspension, Sterile, USP, III/23
Tablets USP, III/23

Ampicillin and Probenecid
  Capsules USP, III/24
  for Suspension, Oral, USP, III/24
Ampicillin Sodium
  Sterile USP, III/23
Ampicillin Sodium and Sulbactam Sodium
  Sterile USP, III/25
Amprolium
  Amprolium USP, III/25
  Powder, Soluble, USP, III/25
  Solution, Oral, USP, III/25
Amrinone Lactate
  Injection, III/25
Amylene Hydrate
  Amylene Hydrate NF, III/25
Amyl Nitrite
  Amyl Nitrite USP, III/25
  Inhalant USP, III/25
Anafranil, IV/MC-5
Anaprox, IV/MC-16
ANDA Suitability Petitions, I/388
Anethole
  Anethole NF, III/26
Anileridine
  Anileridine USP, III/26
  Injection USP, III/26
Anileridine Hydrochloride
  Anileridine Hydrochloride USP, III/26
  Tablets USP, III/26
Anisindione
  Tablets, III/26
Anisotropine Methylbromide
  Tablets, III/26
Anistreplase
  for Injection, III/26
Ansaid, IV/MC-10
Antazoline Phosphate
  Antazoline Phosphate USP III/26
Anthralin
  Anthralin USP, III/27
  Cream USP, III/27
  Ointment USP, III/27
Anticoagulant Citrate Dextrose
  Solution USP, III/27
Anticoagulant Citrate Phosphate Dextrose
  Solution USP, III/27
Anticoagulant Citrate Phosphate Dextrose
  Adenine
  Solution USP, III/28
Anticoagulant Heparin
  Solution USP, III/28
Anticoagulant Sodium Citrate
  Solution USP, III/28
Antihemophilic Factor
  Antihemophilic Factor USP, III/28
Antihemophilic Factor, Cryoprecipitated
  Cryoprecipitated Antihemophilic Factor
  USP, III/28
Anti-human Globulin Serum—See Globulin
  Serum, Anti-human
Antimony Potassium Tartrate
  Antimony Potassium Tartrate USP, III/29
Antimony Sodium Tartrate
  Antimony Sodium Tartrate USP, III/29
Antipyrine
  Antipyrine USP, III/29
Antipyrine and Benzocaine
  Solution, Otic, USP, III/29
Antipyrine, Benzocaine, and Phenylephrine
  Hydrochloride
  Solution, Otic, USP, III/29
Antirabies Serum
  Antirabies Serum USP, III/29
Antithrombin III (Human)
  Antithrombin III (Human) for Injection,
  III/29

Antivenin (Crotalidae) Polyvalent
  Antivenin (Crotalidae) Polyvalent USP,
  III/30
Antivenin (Latrodectus Mactans)
  Antivenin (Latrodectus Mactans) USP,
  III/30
Antivenin (Micrurus Fulvius)
  Antivenin (Micrurus Fulvius) USP, III/
  30
Antivert, IV/MC-14
Apomorphine Hydrochloride
  Apomorphine Hydrochloride USP, III/30
  Tablets USP, III/30
Applications for Registration, II/35
Approved Drug Products with Therapeutic
  Equivalence Evaluations, I/1
  ANDA Suitability Petitions, I/388
  Appendix A—Product Name Index, I/
  405
  Appendix B—Product Name Index
  Listed by Applicant, I/438
  Appendix C—Uniform Terms, I/505
  Availability of Internal Policy and Proce-
  dure, I/15
  Availability of the Publication and Up-
  dating Procedures, I/15
  Biopharmaceutic Guidance Availability,
  I/386
  Content and Exclusion, I/6
  Contents of, I/3
  Description of Special Situations, I/14
  Discontinued Drug Product List, I/287
  Drug Product Illustration, I/18
  Drug Products in the Division of Blood
  and Blood Products Approved Under
  Section 505 of the Act, I/283
  Drug Products Lists, I/20
  Drug Products Lists, How to Use the, I/
  17
  Drug Products Which Must Demonstrate
  in vivo Bioavailability Only if Product
  Fails to Achieve Adequate Dissolution,
  I/385
  Exclusivity Terms, I/506
  General Policies and Legal Status, I/8
  Introduction, I/6
  Key Sections for Using the Drug Product
  Lists, I/17
  Orphan Drug and Biological Designations,
  I/364
  OTC Drug Product List, I/273
  Patent and Exclusivity Information Ad-
  dendum, I/506
  Patent and Exclusivity Lists, I/510
  Practitioner's Responsibilities, I/8
  Preface, I/5
  Prescription Drug Product List, I/20
  Product Name Index, I/405
  Product Name Index Listed by Applicant,
  I/438
  Therapeutic Equivalence Code Change for
  a Drug Entity, I/14
  Therapeutic Equivalence Evaluations
  Codes, I/9
  Therapeutic Equivalence Evaluations Illus-
  tration, I/19
  Therapeutic Equivalence-Related Terms,
  I/6
  Uniform Terms, I/505
Apraclonidine
  Solution, Ophthalmic, USP, III/30
Apraclonidine Hydrochloride
  Apraclonidine Hydrochloride USP, III/30
Apresazide, IV/MC-11
Apresoline, IV/MC-11
Aprobarbital
  Elixir, III/31

Aralen, IV/MC-4
Arginine
  Arginine USP, III/31
Arginine Hydrochloride
  Arginine Hydrochloride USP, III/31
  Injection USP, III/31
Aromatic Elixir
  Aromatic Elixir NF, III/31
Ascorbic Acid
  Ascorbic Acid USP, III/31
  Capsules, Extended-release, III/31
  Injection USP, III/31
  Solution, Oral, USP, III/31
  Syrup, III/31
  Tablets USP, III/31
  Tablets, Extended-release, III/31
Ascorbyl Palmitate
  Ascorbyl Palmitate NF, III/32
Asparaginase
  for Injection, III/32
Aspartame
  Aspartame NF, III/32
Aspirin
  Aspirin USP, III/32
  Capsules USP, III/32
  Capsules, Delayed-release, USP, III/32
  Suppositories USP, III/32
  Tablets USP, III/32
  Tablets, Chewing Gum, III/32
  Tablets, Delayed-release, USP, III/32
  Tablets, Extended-release, USP, III/32
Aspirin, Alumina, and Magnesia
  Tablets USP, III/33
Aspirin, Alumina, and Magnesium Oxide
  Tablets USP, III/33
Aspirin, Buffered
  Tablets USP, III/33
Aspirin, Buffered, and Caffeine
  Tablets, III/33
Aspirin and Caffeine
  Capsules, III/33
  Tablets, III/33
Aspirin, Caffeine, and Dihydrocodeine
  Capsules USP, III/33, IV/MC-2
Aspirin and Codeine Phosphate
  Tablets USP, III/34, IV/MC-2
Aspirin, Codeine Phosphate, and Caffeine
  Capsules USP, III/34
  Tablets USP, III/34
Aspirin, Codeine Phosphate, Caffeine, Alu-
  mina, and Magnesia
  Tablets, III/34
Aspirin, Sodium Bicarbonate, and Citric Acid
  Tablets for Solution, Oral, Effervescent,
  USP, III/34
Astemizole
  Suspension, Oral, III/34
  Tablets, III/34, IV/MC-2
Atarax, IV/MC-11
Atenolol
  Injection, III/34
  Tablets, III/34, IV/MC-2
Atenolol and Chlorthalidone
  Tablets, III/34, IV/MC-2
Ativan, IV/MC-13
Atracurium Besylate
  Injection, III/34
Atropine
  Atropine USP, III/34
Atropine Sulfate
  Atropine Sulfate USP, III/34
  Injection USP, III/34
  Ointment, Ophthalmic, USP, III/34
  Solution, Ophthalmic, USP, III/34
  Tablets USP, III/34
  Tablets, Soluble, III/34

Atropine Sulfate, Hyoscyamine, Methena-
    mine, Methylene Blue, Phenyl Salicy-
    late, and Benzoic Acid
    Tablets, III/35
Atropine Sulfate, Hyoscyamine Sulfate (or
    Hyoscyamine Hydrobromide), Scopola-
    mine Hydrobromide, and Phenobarbi-
    tal
    Capsules, III/36, IV/MC-2
    Elixir, III/36
    Tablets, III/36, IV/MC-2
Atropine Sulfate, Hyoscyamine Sulfate, Sco-
    polamine Hydrobromide, and Pheno-
    barbital
    Tablets, Extended-release, III/36, IV/MC-
    2
Atropine Sulfate and Phenobarbital
    Capsules, III/36
    Elixir, III/36
    Tablets, III/36
Attapulgite
    Activated USP, III/36
    Colloidal Activated USP, III/36
    Suspension, Oral, III/36
    Tablets, III/36
Augmentin, IV/MC-2
Auranofin
    Capsules, III/36, IV/MC-2
Aurothioglucose
    Aurothioglucose USP, III/36
    Suspension, Sterile, USP, III/36
Authority to Designate Official Names, II/75
Axid, IV/MC-16
Azaperone
    Azaperone USP, III/36
    Injection USP, III/36
Azatadine
    Azatadine USP, III/36
Azatadine Maleate
    Tablets USP, III/36
Azatadine Maleate and Pseudoephedrine Sul-
    fate
    Tablets, Extended-release, III/37, IV/MC-
    2
Azathioprine
    Azathioprine USP, III/37
    Tablets USP, III/37, IV/MC-2
Azathioprine Sodium
    for Injection USP, III/37
Azithromycin
    Capsules, IV/MC-2
Azlocillin Sodium
    Sterile USP, III/37
Aztreonam
    Aztreonam USP, III/37
    Injection USP, III/37
    for Injection USP, III/37
    Sterile USP, III/37
Azulfidine, IV/MC-21
Azulfidine EN-Tabs, IV/MC-21

B

Bacampicillin Hydrochloride
    Bacampicillin Hydrochloride USP, III/38
    for Suspension, Oral, USP, III/38
    Tablets USP, III/38
Bacillus Calmette-Guérin (BCG) Vaccine
    BCG Live (Connaught Strain), III/38
    BCG Vaccine USP (Tice Strain), III/38
Bacitracin
    Bacitracin USP, III/38
    Ointment USP, III/38
    Ointment, Ophthalmic, USP, III/38
    Sterile USP, III/38

Bacitracin Methylene Disalicylate
    Powder, Soluble, USP, III/38
    Soluble USP, III/38
Bacitracin and Polymyxin B Sulfate
    Aerosol, Topical, USP, III/39
Bacitracin Zinc
    Bacitracin Zinc USP, III/38
    Ointment USP, III/38
    Powder, Soluble, USP, III/38
    Sterile USP, III/38
Bacitracin Zinc and Polymyxin B Sulfate
    Ointment USP, III/39
    Ointment, Ophthalmic, USP, III/39
Baclofen
    Baclofen USP, III/39
    Tablets USP, III/39, IV/MC-3
Bactrim, IV/MC-21
Bandage, Adhesive
    Adhesive Bandage USP, III/40
Bandage, Gauze
    Gauze Bandage USP, III/40
Barium Hydroxide Lime
    Barium Hydroxide Lime USP, III/40
Barium Sulfate
    Barium Sulfate USP, III/40
    for Suspension USP, III/40
Beclomethasone Dipropionate
    Aerosol, Inhalation, III/40
    Aerosol, Nasal, III/40
    Beclomethasone Dipropionate USP, III/
    40
    Cream, III/40
    for Inhalation, III/40
    Lotion, III/40
    Ointment, III/40
Beclomethasone Dipropionate Monohydrate
    Spray, Nasal, III/40
Belladonna
    Leaf USP, III/41
    Tincture USP, III/41
Belladonna Extract
    Belladonna Extract USP, III/41
    Tablets USP, III/41
Belladonna Extract and Butabarbital Sodium
    Elixir, III/41
    Tablets, III/41
Belladonna Extract and Phenobarbital
    Tablets, III/41
Benadryl, IV/MC-7
Benazepril Hydrochloride
    Tablets, IV/MC-3
Bendroflumethiazide
    Bendroflumethiazide USP, III/41
    Tablets USP, III/41, IV/MC-3
Benoxinate Hydrochloride
    Benoxinate Hydrochloride USP, III/41
    Solution, Ophthalmic, USP, III/41
Bentiromide
    Solution, Oral, III/42
Bentonite
    Bentonite NF, III/42
Bentonite Magma
    Bentonite Magma NF, III/42
Bentonite, Purified
    Purified Bentonite NF, III/42
Bentyl, IV/MC-7
Benzaldehyde
    Benzaldehyde NF, III/42
Benzaldehyde, Compound
    Elixir NF, III/42
Benzalkonium Chloride
    Benzalkonium Chloride NF, III/42
    Benzalkonium Chloride Solution NF, III/
    42

Benzethonium Chloride
    Benzethonium Chloride USP, III/43
    Solution, Topical, USP, III/43
    Tincture USP, III/43
Benzocaine
    Aerosol, Topical, (Solution), USP, III/43
    Benzocaine USP, III/43
    Cream USP, III/43
    Gel, III/43
    Jelly, III/43
    Lozenges, III/43
    Ointment USP, III/43
    Paste, Dental, III/43
    Solution, Otic, USP, III/43
    Solution, Topical, USP, III/43
Benzocaine, Butamben, and Tetracaine Hy-
    drochloride
    Aerosol, Topical, Solution, III/44
    Gel, III/44
    Ointment, III/44
    Solution, Topical, III/44
Benzocaine and Menthol
    Aerosol, Topical, Solution, III/44
    Lotion, III/44
Benzoic Acid
    Benzoic Acid USP, III/44
Benzoic and Salicylic Acids
    Ointment USP, III/44
Benzoin
    Benzoin USP, III/44
    Tincture, Compound, USP, III/44
Benzonatate
    Benzonatate USP, III/44
    Capsules USP, III/44
Benzoyl Peroxide
    Bar, Cleansing, III/44
    Benzoyl Peroxide, Hydrous, USP, III/44
    Cream, III/44
    Gel USP, III/44
    Lotion USP, III/44
    Lotion, Cleansing, III/44
    Mask, Facial, III/44
    Stick, III/44
Benzphetamine Hydrochloride
    Tablets, III/45, IV/MC-3
Benzthiazide
    Benzthiazide USP, III/45
    Tablets USP, III/45
Benztropine Mesylate
    Benztropine Mesylate USP, III/45
    Injection USP, III/45
    Tablets USP, III/45, IV/MC-3
Benzyl Alcohol
    Benzyl Alcohol NF, III/45
Benzyl Benzoate
    Benzyl Benzoate USP, III/46
    Lotion USP, III/46
Benzylpenicilloyl Polylysine
    Concentrate USP, III/46
    Injection USP, III/46
Bepridil Hydrochloride
    Tablets, III/46, IV/MC-3
Beta Carotene
    Beta Carotene USP, III/46
    Capsules USP, III/46
    Tablets, III/46
Betaine Hydrochloride
    Betaine Hydrochloride USP, III/46
Betamethasone
    Betamethasone USP, III/46
    Cream USP, III/46
    Syrup USP, III/46
    Tablets USP, III/46
    Tablets, Effervescent, III/46
Betamethasone Acetate
    Betamethasone Acetate USP, III/46

Betamethasone Benzoate
  Betamethasone Benzoate USP, III/46
  Cream, III/46
  Gel USP, III/46
  Lotion, III/46
Betamethasone Dipropionate
  Aerosol, Topical, III/46
  Betamethasone Dipropionate USP, III/46
  Cream USP, III/46
  Gel, III/46
  Lotion USP, III/46
  Ointment USP, III/46
Betamethasone Disodium Phosphate
  Enema, III/46
  Pellets, Dental, III/46
Betamethasone Sodium Phosphate
  Betamethasone Sodium Phosphate USP,
    III/46
  Injection USP, III/46
  Solution, Opthalmic/Otic, III/46
  Tablets, Extended-release, III/46
Betamethasone Sodium Phosphate and Beta-
    methasone Acetate
  Suspension, Sterile, USP, III/46
Betamethasone Valerate
  Betamethasone Valerate USP, III/46
  Cream USP, III/46
  Lotion USP, III/46
  Ointment USP, III/46
Betapen VK, IV/MC-18
Betaxolol
  Solution, Ophthalmic, USP, III/48
Betaxolol Hydrochloride
  Betaxolol Hydrochloride USP, III/48
  Suspension, Ophthalmic, III/48
  Tablets, III/48, IV/MC-3
Bethanechol Chloride
  Bethanechol Chloride USP, III/48
  Injection USP, III/48
  Tablets USP, III/48
Biaxin, IV/MC-5
Bioavailability, II/9
Biological Indicator for Dry-heat Steriliza-
    tion, Paper Strip
  Biological Indicator for Dry-heat Steril-
    ization, Paper Strip USP, III/49
Biological Indicator for Ethylene Oxide Ster-
    ilization, Paper Strip
  Biological Indicator for Ethylene Oxide
    Sterilization, Paper Strip USP, III/49
Biological Indicator for Steam Sterilization,
    Paper Strip
  Biological Indicator for Steam Steriliza-
    tion, Paper Strip USP, III/49
Biotin
  Biotin USP, III/50
  Capsules, III/50
  Tablets, III/50
Biperiden
  Biperiden USP, III/50
Biperiden Hydrochloride
  Biperiden Hydrochloride USP, III/50
  Tablets USP, III/50
Biperiden Lactate
  Injection USP, III/50
Bisacodyl
  Bisacodyl USP, III/50
  Solution, Rectal, III/50
  Suppositories USP, III/50
  Tablets USP, III/50
Bisacodyl and Docusate Sodium
  Tablets, III/50
Bisacodyl Tannex
  Powder for Solution, Rectal, III/50
Bismuth, Milk of
  Bismuth, Milk of, USP, III/51

Bismuth Subgallate
  Bismuth Subgallate USP, III/51
Bismuth Subnitrate
  Bismuth Subnitrate USP, III/51
Bismuth Subsalicylate
  Suspension, Oral, III/51
  Tablets, Chewable, III/51
Bitolterol Mesylate
  Aerosol, Inhalation, III/51
Bleomycin Sulfate
  Sterile USP, III/51
Blocadren, IV/MC-23
Blood Cells, Red
  Red Blood Cells USP, III/53
Blood Grouping Serum, Anti-A
  Serum, Blood Grouping, Anti-A, USP,
    III/52
Blood Grouping Serum, Anti-B
  Serum, Blood Grouping, Anti-B, USP,
    III/52
Blood Grouping Serums
  Serums, Blood Grouping, USP, III/52
Blood Grouping Serums Anti-D, Anti-C,
    Anti-E, Anti-c, Anti-e
  Serums, Blood Grouping, Anti-D, Anti-C,
    Anti-E, Anti-c, Anti-e USP, III/52
Blood Group Specific Substances A, B, and
    AB
  Blood Group Specific Substances A, B,
    and AB USP, III/53
Blood, Whole
  Whole Blood USP, III/53
Boric Acid
  Boric Acid NF, III/54
Botulism Antitoxin
  Botulism Antitoxin USP, III/54
Brethine, IV/MC-22
Bretylium Tosylate
  Injection, III/54
Bretylium Tosylate in 5% Dextrose
  Injection, III/54
Bromazepam
  Tablets, III/54
Bromocriptine Mesylate
  Bromocriptine Mesylate USP, III/54
  Capsules, III/54, IV/MC-3
  Tablets USP, III/54, IV/MC-3
Bromodiphenhydramine Hydrochloride
  Bromodiphenhydramine Hydrochloride
    USP, III/55
  Capsules USP, III/55
  Elixir USP, III/55
Bromodiphenhydramine Hydrochloride and
    Codeine Phosphate
  Syrup, III/55
Bromodiphenhydramine Hydrochloride, Di-
    phenhydramine Hydrochloride, Co-
    deine Phosphate, Ammonium Chlo-
    ride, and Potassium Guaiacolsulfonate
  Solution, Oral, III/55
Brompheniramine Maleate
  Brompheniramine Maleate USP, III/55
  Elixir USP, III/55
  Injection USP, III/55
  Tablets USP, III/55
  Tablets, Extended-release, III/55
Brompheniramine Maleate and Phenyleph-
    rine Hydrochloride
  Elixir, III/56
  Tablets, III/56
Brompheniramine Maleate, Phenylephrine
    Hydrochloride, and Phenylpropanol-
    amine Hydrochloride
  Elixir, III/56
  Solution, Oral, III/56
  Tablets, III/56
  Tablets, Extended-release, III/56

Brompheniramine Maleate, Phenylephrine
    Hydrochloride, Phenylpropanolamine
    Hydrochloride, and Acetaminophen
  Solution, Oral, III/56
  Tablets, III/56
Brompheniramine Maleate, Phenylephrine
    Hydrochloride, Phenylpropanolamine
    Hydrochloride, and Codeine Phos-
    phate
  Tablets, III/56
Brompheniramine Maleate, Phenylephrine
    Hydrochloride, Phenylpropanolamine
    Hydrochloride, Codeine Phosphate,
    and Guaifenesin
  Syrup, III/56
Brompheniramine Maleate, Phenylephrine
    Hydrochloride, Phenylpropanolamine
    Hydrochloride, and Dextromethor-
    phan Hydrobromide
  Elixir, III/56
  Tablets, III/56
Brompheniramine Maleate, Phenylephrine
    Hydrochloride, Phenylpropanolamine
    Hydrochloride, and Guaifenesin
  Syrup, III/56
Brompheniramine Maleate, Phenylephrine
    Hydrochloride, Phenylpropanolamine
    Hydrochloride, Hydrocodone Bitar-
    trate, and Guaifenesin
  Solution, Oral, III/56
Brompheniramine Maleate, Phenylpropanol-
    amine Bitartrate, and Aspirin
  Tablets for Oral Solution, III/57
Brompheniramine Maleate and Phenylpropa-
    nolamine Hydrochloride
  Elixir, III/56
  Tablets, III/56
  Tablets, Extended-release, III/56
Brompheniramine Maleate, Phenylpropanol-
    amine Hydrochloride, and Codeine
    Phosphate
  Syrup, III/57
Brompheniramine Maleate, Phenylpropanol-
    amine Hydrochloride, and Dextro-
    methorphan Hydrobromide
  Syrup, III/57
Brompheniramine Maleate, Phenyltolox-
    amine Citrate, and Phenylephrine Hy-
    drochloride
  Capsules, Extended-release, III/57
Brompheniramine Maleate and Pseudoephed-
    rine Hydrochloride
  Capsules, Extended-release, III/57
  Syrup, III/57
  Tablets, III/57
Brompheniramine Maleate, Pseudoephedrine
    Hydrochloride, and Dextromethor-
    phan Hydrobromide
  Syrup, III/57
Brompheniramine Maleate and Pseudoephed-
    rine Sulfate
  Syrup USP, III/57
Buclizine Hydrochloride
  Tablets, Chewable, III/57
Bumetanide
  Bumetanide USP, III/57
  Injection USP, III/57
  Tablets USP, III/57, IV/MC-3
Bumex, IV/MC-3
Bupivacaine and Dextrose
  Bupivacaine in Dextrose Injection USP,
    III/58
Bupivacaine and Epinephrine
  Injection USP, III/58
Bupivacaine Hydrochloride
  Bupivacaine Hydrochloride USP, III/58
  Injection USP, III/58

Buprenorphine Hydrochloride
  Injection, III/58
Bupropion Hydrochloride
  Tablets, III/58, IV/MC-3
Buserelin Acetate,
  Injection, III/58
  Solution, Nasal, III/58
BuSpar, IV/MC-3
Buspirone Hydrochloride
  Tablets, III/58, IV/MC-3
Busulfan
  Busulfan USP, III/59
  Tablets USP, III/59
Butabarbital
  Butabarbital USP, III/59
Butabarbital Sodium
  Butabarbital Sodium USP, III/59
  Capsules USP, III/59
  Elixir USP, III/59
  Tablets USP, III/59
Butacaine
  Ointment, Dental, III/59
Butalbital
  Butalbital USP, III/59
Butalbital and Acetaminophen
  Capsules, III/60
  Tablets, III/60
Butalbital, Acetaminophen, and Caffeine
  Capsules, III/60
  Tablets USP, III/60, IV/MC-3
Butalbital and Aspirin
  Tablets USP, III/60
Butalbital, Aspirin, and Caffeine
  Capsules, III/60, IV/MC-3
  Tablets, III/60, IV/MC-3
Butalbital, Aspirin, Codeine Phosphate, and
    Caffeine
  Capsules, III/60, IV/MC-3
  Tablets, III/60
Butamben
  Butamben USP, III/60
Butamben Picrate
  Ointment, III/60
Butane
  Butane NF, III/60
Butoconazole Nitrate
  Butoconazole Nitrate USP, III/60
  Cream USP, III/60
Butorphanol Tartrate
  Butorphanol Tartrate USP, III/61
  Injection USP, III/61
Butyl Alcohol
  Butyl Alcohol NF, III/61
Butylated Hydroxyanisole
  Butylated Hydroxyanisole NF, III/61
Butylated Hydroxytoluene
  Butylated Hydroxytoluene NF, III/61
Butylparaben
  Butylparaben NF, III/61

C

Cafergot, IV/MC-8
Caffeine
  Caffeine USP, III/62
  Capsules, Extended-release, III/62
  Tablets, III/62
Caffeine, Citrated
  Injection, III/62
  Solution, III/62
  Tablets, III/62
Caffeine and Sodium Benzoate
  Injection USP, III/62
Calamine
  Calamine USP, III/62
  Lotion USP, III/62

Calamine, Phenolated
  Lotion USP, III/62
Calan
  Tablets, IV/MC-24
Calan SR
  Extended-release Tablets, IV/MC-24
Calcifediol
  Calcifediol USP, III/63
  Capsules USP, III/63
Calcitonin-Human
  for Injection, III/63
Calcitonin-Salmon
  Injection, III/63
Calcitriol
  Capsules, III/63, IV/MC-3
  Injection, III/63
Calcium Acetate
  Calcium Acetate USP, III/63
  Tablets, III/63
Calcium Carbonate
  Calcium Carbonate USP, III/63
  Capsules, III/63
  Chewing Gum, III/63
  Suspension, Oral, USP, III/63
  Tablets USP, III/63
  Tablets (Oyster-shell derived), III/63
  Tablets, Chewable (Oyster-shell derived),
    III/63
Calcium Carbonate and Magnesia
  Tablets USP , III/64
Calcium Carbonate, Magnesia, and Simethi-
    cone
  Tablets USP, III/64
Calcium and Magnesium Carbonates
  Suspension, Oral, III/64
  Tablets USP, III/64
Calcium and Magnesium Carbonates and
    Magnesium Oxide
  Tablets, III/64
Calcium Carbonate and Simethicone
  Suspension, Oral, III/64
  Tablets, Chewable, III/64
Calcium Chloride
  Calcium Chloride USP, III/64
  Injection USP, III/64
Calcium Citrate
  Calcium Citrate USP, III/65
  Tablets, III/65
  Tablets, Effervescent, III/65
Calcium Glubionate
  Syrup USP, III/65
Calcium Gluceptate
  Calcium Gluceptate USP, III/65
  Injection USP, III/65
Calcium Gluconate
  Calcium Gluconate USP, III/65
  Injection USP, III/65
  Tablets USP, III/65
Calcium Glycerophosphate and Calcium
    Lactate
  Injection, III/66
Calcium Hydroxide
  Calcium Hydroxide USP, III/66
  Solution, Topical, USP, III/66
Calcium Lactate
  Calcium Lactate USP, III/66
  Tablets USP, III/66
Calcium Lactobionate
  Calcium Lactobionate USP, III/67
Calcium Levulinate
  Calcium Levulinate USP, III/67
  Injection USP, III/67
Calcium Pantothenate
  Calcium Pantothenate USP, III/67
  Tablets USP, III/67

Calcium Pantothenate, Racemic
  Racemic Calcium Pantothenate USP,
    III/67
Calcium Phosphate, Dibasic
  Dibasic Calcium Phosphate USP, III/68
  Tablets USP, III/68
Calcium Phosphate, Tribasic
  Tribasic Calcium Phosphate NF, III/68
Calcium Polycarbophil
  Calcium Polycarbophil USP, III/68
  Tablets, III/68
  Tablets, Chewable, III/68
Calcium Saccharate
  Calcium Saccharate USP, III/68
Calcium Silicate
  Calcium Silicate NF, III/68
Calcium Stearate
  Calcium Stearate NF, III/69
Calcium Sulfate
  Calcium Sulfate NF, III/69
Camphor
  Camphor USP, III/69
  Spirit USP, III/69
Candicidin
  Candicidin USP, III/69
  Ointment USP, III/69
  Tablets, Vaginal, USP, III/69
Capoten, IV/MC-3
Capozide, IV/MC-3
Capreomycin Sulfate
  Sterile USP, III/69
Capsaicin
  Cream, III/69
Captopril
  Captopril USP, III/69
  Tablets USP, III/69, IV/MC-3
Captopril and Hydrochlorothiazide
  Tablets, III/70, IV/MC-3
Carafate, IV/MC-21
Caramel
  Caramel NF, III/70
Carbacephem
  Capsules, IV/MC-3
Carbachol
  Carbachol USP, III/70
  Solution, Intraocular, USP, III/70
  Solution, Ophthalmic, USP, III/70
Carbamazepine
  Carbamazepine USP, III/71
  Suspension, Oral, III/71
  Tablets USP, III/71, IV/MC-3
  Tablets, Extended-release, III/71
Carbamide Peroxide
  Carbamide Peroxide USP, III/71
  Solution, Topical, USP, III/71
Carbenicillin Disodium
  Sterile USP, III/71
Carbenicillin Indanyl Sodium
  Carbenicillin Indanyl Sodium USP, III/
    71
  Tablets USP, III/71, IV/MC-4
Carbidopa
  Carbidopa USP, III/72
Carbidopa and Levodopa
  Tablets USP, III/72, IV/MC-4
  Tablets, Extended-release, III/72
Carbinoxamine Maleate
  Carbinoxamine Maleate USP, III/72
  Tablets USP, III/72
Carbinoxamine Maleate and Pseudoephed-
    rine Hydrochloride
  Solution, Oral, III/72
  Syrup, III/72
  Tablets, III/72
  Tablets, Extended-release, III/72

Carbinoxamine Maleate, Pseudoephedrine
  Hydrochloride, and Dextromethor-
  phan Hydrobromide
    Solution, Oral, III/72
    Syrup, III/72
Carbinoxamine Maleate, Pseudoephedrine
  Hydrochloride, and Guaifenesin
    Capsules, III/72
    Solution, Oral, III/72
Carbol-Fuchsin
    Solution, Topical, USP, III/72
Carbomer
    Carbomer 910 NF, III/73
    Carbomer 934 NF, III/73
    Carbomer 934P NF, III/73
    Carbomer 940 NF, III/73
    Carbomer 941 NF, III/73
    Carbomer 1342 NF, III/73
Carbon Dioxide
    Carbon Dioxide USP, III/74
Carbon Tetrachloride
    Carbon Tetrachloride NF, III/74
Carboplatin
    Injection, III/74
    for Injection, III/74
Carboprost Tromethamine
    Carboprost Tromethamine USP, III/74
    Injection USP, III/74
Carboxymethylcellulose Calcium
    Carboxymethylcellulose Calcium NF,
      III/74
Carboxymethylcellulose Sodium
    Carboxymethylcellulose Sodium USP,
      III/74
    Paste USP, III/74
    Tablets USP, III/74
Carboxymethylcellulose Sodium 12
    Carboxymethylcellulose Sodium 12 NF,
      III/74
Carboxymethylcellulose Sodium, Casan-
  thranol, and Docusate Sodium
    Capsules, III/75
Carboxymethylcellulose Sodium and Docu-
  sate Sodium
    Capsules, III/75
Cardene, IV/MC-16
Cardizem, IV/MC-7
Cardizem SR, IV/MC-7
Cardura, IV/MC-8
Carisoprodol
    Carisoprodol USP, III/75
    Tablets USP, III/75, IV/MC-4
Carisoprodol and Aspirin
    Tablets USP, III/75, IV/MC-4
Carisoprodol, Aspirin, and Codeine Phos-
  phate
    Tablets USP, III/75, IV/MC-4
Carmustine
    for Injection, III/76
Carnauba Wax—See Wax, Carnauba, NF
Carphenazine Maleate
    Carphenazine Maleate USP, III/76
    Solution, Oral, USP, III/76
Carrageenan
    Carrageenan NF, III/76
Carteolol Hydrochloride
    Tablets, III/76, IV/MC-4
Cartrol, IV/MC-4
Casanthranol
    Casanthranol USP, III/76
    Syrup, III/76
Casanthranol and Docusate Potassium
    Capsules, III/76
Casanthranol and Docusate Sodium
    Capsules, III/76
    Syrup, III/76
    Tablets, III/76

Cascara Sagrada
    Cascara Sagrada USP, III/77
    Extract USP, III/77
    Fluidextract USP, III/77
    Fluidextract, Aromatic, USP, III/77
    Tablets USP, III/77
Cascara Sagrada and Aloe
    Tablets, III/77
Cascara Sagrada Extract and Phenolphtha-
  lein
    Tablets, III/77
Castor Oil
    Capsules USP, III/77
    Castor Oil USP, III/77
    Castor Oil, Aromatic, USP, III/77
    Castor Oil, Hydrogenated, NF, III/77
    Emulsion USP, III/77
Castor Oil, Polyoxyl 35—See Polyoxyl 35
    Castor Oil
Castor Oil, Polyoxyl 40, Hydrogenated—See
    Polyoxyl 40 Hydrogenated Castor Oil
Catapres, IV/MC-5
Ceclor, IV/MC-4
Cefaclor
    Capsules USP, III/78, IV/MC-4
    Cefaclor USP, III/78
    for Suspension, Oral, USP, III/78
Cefadroxil
    Capsules USP, III/78, IV/MC-4
    Cefadroxil USP, III/78
    for Suspension, Oral, USP, III/78
    Tablets USP, III/78, IV/MC-4
Cefamandole Nafate
    for Injection USP, III/78
    Sterile USP, III/78
Cefamandole Sodium
    for Injection, III/78
    Sterile USP, III/78
Cefanex, IV/MC-4
Cefazolin
    Cefazolin USP, III/79
Cefazolin Sodium
    Injection USP, III/79
    Sterile USP, III/79
Cefixime
    Cefixime USP, III/79
    for Suspension, Oral, USP, III/79
    Tablets USP, III/79, IV/MC-4
Cefmenoxime
    for Injection USP, III/80
Cefmenoxime Hydrochloride
    Sterile USP, III/80
Cefmetazole Sodium
    for Injection, III/80
    Sterile USP, III/80
Cefonicid Sodium
    Sterile USP, III/80
Cefoperazone Sodium
    Cefoperazone Sodium USP, III/80
    Injection USP, III/80
    Sterile USP, III/80
Cefocanide
    for Injection USP, III/81
    Sterile, III/81
Cefotaxime Sodium
    Cefotaxime Sodium USP, III/81
    Injection USP, III/81
    Sterile USP, III/81
Cefotetan Disodium
    Sterile USP, III/82
Cefotiam
    for Injection USP, III/82
Cefotiam Hydrochloride
    Sterile USP, III/82

Cefoxitin Sodium
    Cefoxitin Sodium USP, III/82
    Injection USP, III/82
    Sterile USP, III/82
Cefpiramide
    Cefpiramide USP, III/83
    for Injection USP, III/83
Cefprozil
    Suspension, Oral, III/83
    Tablets, III/83
Ceftazidime
    Ceftazidime USP, III/83
    Injection USP, III/83
    for Injection USP, III/83
    Sterile USP, III/83
Ceftin, IV/MC-4
Ceftizoxime Sodium
    Ceftizoxime Sodium USP, III/83
    Injection USP, III/83
    Sterile USP, III/83
Ceftriaxone Sodium
    Ceftriaxone Sodium USP, III/84
    Injection USP, III/84
    Sterile USP, III/84
Cefuroxime Axetil
    Cefuroxime Axetil USP, III/84
    Tablets USP, III/84, IV/MC-4
Cefuroxime Sodium
    Cefuroxime Sodium USP, III/84
    Injection USP III/84
    Sterile USP, III/84
Cellulose Acetate
    Cellulose Acetate NF, III/85
Cellulose Acetate Phthalate
    Cellulose Acetate Phthalate NF, III/85
Cellulose, Hydroxyethyl—See Hydroxyethyl
    Cellulose NF
Cellulose, Hydroxypropyl—See Hydroxypro-
    pyl Cellulose NF
Cellulose, Hydroxypropyl, Low-substituted—
    See Hydroxypropyl Cellulose, Low-
    substituted, NF
Cellulose, Microcrystalline
    Microcrystalline Cellulose NF, III/85
Cellulose, Microcrystalline, and Carboxy-
  methylcellulose Sodium
    Microcrystalline Cellulose and Carboxy-
      methylcellulose Sodium NF, III/86
Cellulose, Oxidized
    Oxidized Cellulose USP, III/86
Cellulose, Powdered
    Powdered Cellulose NF, III/86
Cellulose, Regenerated, Oxidized
    Oxidized Regenerated Cellulose USP,
      III/86
Cellulose Sodium Phosphate
    Cellulose Sodium Phosphate USP (for
      Suspension, Oral), III/86
Centrax, IV/MC-19
Cephalexin
    Capsules USP, III/86, IV/MC-4
    for Suspension, Oral, USP, III/86
    Tablets USP, III/86, IV/MC-4
Cephalexin Hydrochloride
    Cephalexin Hydrochloride USP, III/86
    Tablets, IV/MC-4
Cephalothin Sodium
    Cephalothin Sodium USP, III/87
    Injection USP, III/87
    for Injection USP, III/87
    Sterile USP, III/87
Cephapirin Sodium
    Sterile USP, III/88

Cephradine
  Capsules USP, III/88, IV/MC-4
  Cephradine USP, III/88
  for Injection USP, III/88
  for Suspension, Oral, USP, III/88
  Sterile USP, III/88
  Tablets USP, III/88
Certification
  of Antibiotics, II/74
  of Drugs Containing Insulin, II/73
Cetostearyl Alcohol
  Cetostearyl Alcohol NF, III/88
Cetyl Alcohol
  Cetyl Alcohol NF, III/88
Cetyl Esters Wax
  Cetyl Esters Wax NF, III/89
Cetylpyridinium Chloride,
  Cetylpyridinium Chloride USP, III/89
  Lozenges USP, III/89
  Solution, Topical, USP, III/89
Charcoal, Activated
  Activated Charcoal USP, III/89
  Capsules, III/89
  Suspension, Oral, III/89
  Tablets, III/89
Charcoal, Activated, and Sorbitol
  Suspension, Oral, III/89
Chenodiol
  Tablets, III/89
Child-safety Packaging, II/
Chlophedianol Hydrochloride
  Syrup, III/89
Chloral Hydrate
  Capsules USP, III/90
  Chloral Hydrate USP, III/90
  Suppositories, III/90
  Syrup USP, III/90
Chlorambucil
  Chlorambucil USP, III/90
  Tablets USP, III/90
Chloramphenicol
  Capsules USP, III/90
  Chloramphenicol USP, III/90
  Cream USP, III/90
  Injection USP, III/90
  Ointment, Ophthalmic, USP, III/90
  Solution, Ophthalmic, USP, III/90
  for Solution, Ophthalmic, USP, III/90
  Solution, Oral, USP, III/90
  Solution, Otic, USP, III/90
  Sterile USP, III/90
  Tablets USP, III/90
Chloramphenicol and Hydrocortisone Acetate
  for Suspension, Ophthalmic, USP, III/91
Chloramphenicol Palmitate
  Chloramphenicol Palmitate USP, III/90
  Suspension, Oral, USP, III/90
Chloramphenicol and Polymyxin B Sulfate
  Ointment, Ophthalmic, USP, III/91
Chloramphenicol and Polymyxin B Sulfate,
    and Hydrocortisone Acetate
  Ointment, Ophthalmic, USP, III/91
Chloramphenicol and Prednisolone
  Ointment, Ophthalmic, USP, III/91
Chloramphenicol Sodium Succinate
  Sterile USP, III/90
Chlordiazepoxide
  Chlordiazepoxide USP, III/92
  Tablets USP, III/92, IV/MC-4
Chlordiazepoxide and Amitriptyline Hydrochloride
  Tablets USP, III/92, IV/MC-4

Chlordiazepoxide Hydrochloride
  Capsules USP, III/92, IV/MC-4
  Chlordiazepoxide Hydrochloride USP, III/92
  Sterile USP, III/92
Chlordiazepoxide Hydrochloride and Clidinium Bromide
  Capsules USP, III/92, IV/MC-4
Chlorhexidine Gluconate
  Rinse, Oral, III/92
Chlormezanone
  Tablets, III/92
Chlorobutanol
  Chlorobutanol NF, III/93
Chlorocresol
  Chlorocresol NF, III/93
Chloroform
  Chloroform NF, III/93
Chloroprocaine Hydrochloride
  Chloroprocaine Hydrochloride USP, III/93
  Injection USP, III/93
Chloroquine
  Chloroquine USP, III/93
Chloroquine Hydrochloride
  Injection USP, III/93
Chloroquine Phosphate
  Chloroquine Phosphate USP, III/93
  Tablets USP, III/93, IV/MC-4
Chlorothiazide
  Chlorothiazide USP, III/94
  Suspension, Oral, USP, III/94
  Tablets USP, III/94
Chlorothiazide Sodium
  for Injection USP, III/94
  Sterile USP, III/94
Chlorotrianisene
  Capsules USP, III/94
  Chlorotrianisene USP, III/94
Chloroxine
  Shampoo, Lotion, III/94
Chloroxylenol
  Chloroxylenol USP, III/95
Chlorphenesin Carbamate
  Tablets, III/95
Chlorpheniramine Maleate
  Capsules, Extended-release, USP, III/95
  Chlorpheniramine Maleate USP, III/95
  Injection USP, III/95
  Solution, Oral, III/95
  Syrup USP, III/95
  Tablets USP, III/95
  Tablets, Extended-release, III/95
Chlorpheniramine Maleate, Codeine Phosphate, Aspirin, and Caffeine
  Tablets, III/95
Chlorpheniramine Maleate, Codeine Phosphate, and Guaifenesin
  Syrup, III/95
Chlorpheniramine Maleate and Dextromethorphan Hydrobromide
  Solution, Oral, III/95
Chlorpheniramine Maleate, Dextromethorphan Hydrobromide, and Acetaminophen
  Capsules, III/95
Chlorpheniramine Maleate, Ephedrine Hydrochloride, Phenylephrine Hydrochloride, Dextromethorphan Hydrobromide, Ammonium Chloride, and Ipecac Fluidextract
  Syrup, III/96
Chlorpheniramine Maleate, Ephedrine Sulfate, and Guaifenesin
  Solution, Oral, III/95

Chlorpheniramine Maleate, Phenindamine Tartrate, Phenylephrine Hydrochloride, Dextromethorphan Hydrobromide, Acetaminophen, Salicylamide, Caffeine, and Ascorbic Acid
  Tablets, III/96
Chlorpheniramine Maleate, Phenindamine Tartrate, and Phenylpropanolamine Hydrochloride
  Tablets, Extended-release, III/96
Chlorpheniramine Maleate, Phenindamine Tartrate, Pyrilamine Maleate, Phenylephrine Hydrochloride, Hydrocodone Bitartrate, and Ammonium Chloride
  Syrup, III/96
Chlorpheniramine Maleate, Pheniramine Maleate, Pyrilamine Maleate, Phenylephrine Hydrochloride, Hydrocodone Bitartrate, Salicylamide, Caffeine, and Ascorbic Acid
  Capsules, III/96
Chlorpheniramine Maleate and Phenylephrine Hydrochloride
  Capsules, Extended-release, III/97
  Elixir, III/97
  Syrup, III/97
  Tablets, III/97
  Tablets, Chewable, III/97
Chlorpheniramine Maleate, Phenylephrine Hydrochloride, and Acetaminophen
  Tablets, III/97
Chlorpheniramine Maleate, Phenylephrine Hydrochloride, Acetaminophen, and Caffeine
  Tablets, III/97
Chlorpheniramine Maleate, Phenylephrine Hydrochloride, Acetaminophen, and Salicylamide
  Capsules, III/97
  Tablets, III/97
Chlorpheniramine Maleate, Phenylephrine Hydrochloride, Acetaminophen, Salicylamide, and Caffeine
  Capsules, III/97
Chlorpheniramine Maleate, Phenylephrine Hydrochloride, Codeine Phosphate, Ammonium Chloride, Potassium Guaiacolsulfonate, and Sodium Citrate
  Solution, Oral, III/97
Chlorpheniramine Maleate, Phenylephrine Hydrochloride, Codeine Phosphate, and Potassium Iodide
  Syrup, III/98
Chlorpheniramine Maleate, Phenylephrine Hydrochloride, and Dextromethorphan Hydrobromide
  Solution, Oral, III/98
  Tablets, III/98
Chlorpheniramine Maleate, Phenylephrine Hydrochloride, Dextromethorphan Hydrobromide, Acetaminophen, and Salicylamide
  Tablets, III/98
Chlorpheniramine Maleate, Phenylephrine Hydrochloride, Dextromethorphan Hydrobromide, and Guaifenesin
  Syrup, III/98
Chlorpheniramine Maleate, Phenylephrine Hydrochloride, Dextromethorphan Hydrobromide, Guaifenesin, and Ammonium Chloride
  Solution, Oral, III/98
Chlorpheniramine Maleate, Phenylephrine Hydrochloride, and Guaifenesin
  Solution, Oral, III/98

Chlorpheniramine Maleate, Phenylephrine
Hydrochloride, and Hydrocodone Bi-
tartrate
Solution, Oral, III/98
Syrup, III/98
Chlorpheniramine Maleate, Phenylephrine
Hydrochloride, Hydrocodone Bitar-
trate, Acetaminophen, and Caffeine
Tablets, III/98
Chlorpheniramine Maleate, Phenylephrine
Hydrochloride, and Phenylpropanol-
amine Hydrochloride
Capsules, Extended-release, III/98
Tablets, III/98
Chlorpheniramine Maleate, Phenylephrine
Hydrochloride, Phenylpropanolamine
Hydrochloride, Carbetapentane Ci-
trate, and Potassium Guaiacolsulfon-
ate
Capsules, III/98
Syrup, III/98
Chlorpheniramine Maleate, Phenylephrine
Hydrochloride, Phenylpropanolamine
Hydrochloride, and Codeine Phos-
phate
Syrup, III/99
Chlorpheniramine Maleate, Phenylephrine
Hydrochloride, Phenylpropanolamine
Hydrochloride, and Dextromethor-
phan Hydrobromide
Syrup, III/99
Chlorpheniramine Maleate, Phenylephrine
Hydrochloride, Phenylpropanolamine
Hydrochloride, Dextromethorphan
Hydrobromide, Guaifenesin, and
Acetaminophen
Syrup, III/99
Tablets, III/99
Chlorpheniramine Maleate, Phenylephrine
Hydrochloride, Phenylpropanolamine
Hydrochloride, and Dihydrocodeine
Bitartrate
Syrup, III/99
Chlorpheniramine Maleate, Phenylpropanol-
amine Bitartrate, and Aspirin
for Solution, Oral, III/99
Chlorpheniramine Maleate and Phenylpropa-
nolamine Hydrochloride
Capsules, Extended-release, III/99, IV/
MC-4
Granules, III/99
Solution, Oral, III/99
Syrup, III/99
Tablets, III/99
Tablets, Chewable, III/99
Tablets, Extended-release, III/99
Chlorpheniramine Maleate, Phenylpropanol-
amine Hydrochloride, and Acetamino-
phen
Capsules, III/99
Tablets, III/99
Tablets, Chewable, III/99
Tablets, Effervescent, III/99
Tablets, Extended-release, III/99
Chlorpheniramine Maleate, Phenylpropanol-
amine Hydrochloride, Acetamino-
phen, and Caffeine
Tablets, III/99
Chlorpheniramine Maleate, Phenylpropanol-
amine Hydrochloride, Acetamino-
phen, and Salicylamide
Tablets, Extended-release, III/100
Chlorpheniramine Maleate, Phenylpropanol-
amine Hydrochloride, and Aspirin
for Solution, Oral, III/100
Tablets, III/100

Chlorpheniramine Maleate, Phenylpropanol-
amine Hydrochloride, Aspirin, and
Caffeine
Capsules, III/100
Tablets, III/100
Chlorpheniramine Maleate, Phenylpropanol-
amine Hydrochloride, and Carami-
phen Edisylate
Capsules, Extended-release, III/100
Chlorpheniramine Maleate, Phenylpropanol-
amine Hydochloride, Codeine Phos-
phate, Guaifenesin, and Acetamino-
phen
Syrup, III/100
Tablets, III/100
Chlorpheniramine Maleate, Phenylpropanol-
amine Hydrochloride, and Dextro-
methorphan Hydrobromide
Gel, Oral, III/100
Granules, III/100
Solution, Oral, III/100
Syrup, III/100
Tablets, III/100
Chlorpheniramine Maleate, Phenylpropanol-
amine Hydrochloride, Dextromethor-
phan Hydrobromide, and Acetamino-
phen
Capsules, III/100
Solution, Oral, III/100
Tablets, III/100
Chlorpheniramine Maleate, Phenylpropanol-
amine Hydrochloride, Dextromethor-
phan Hydrobromide, Acetaminophen,
and Caffeine
Capsules, III/101
Chlorpheniramine Maleate, Phenylpropanol-
amine Hydrochloride, Dextromethor-
phan Hydrobromide, and Ammonium
Chloride
Syrup, III/101
Chlorpheniramine Maleate, Phenylpropanol-
amine Hydrochloride, and Guaifene-
sin
Solution, Oral, III/101
Chlorpheniramine Maleate, Phenylpropanol-
amine Hydrochloride, Guaifenesin,
Sodium Citrate, and Citric Acid
Solution, Oral, III/101
Chlorpheniramine Maleate, Phenylpropanol-
amine Hydrochloride, Hydrocodone
Bitartrate, Guaifenesin, and Salicyla-
mide
Tablets, III/101
Chlorpheniramine Maleate, Phenyltolox-
amine Citrate, and Phenylephrine Hy-
drochloride
Capsules, Extended-release, III/101
Tablets, III/101
Chlorpheniramine Maleate, Phenyltolox-
amine Citrate, Phenylephrine Hydro-
chloride, and Phenylpropanolamine
Hydrochloride
Capsules, Extended-release, III/101
Solution, Oral, III/101
Syrup, III/101
Tablets, Extended-release, III/101, IV/
MC-4, MC-5
Chlorpheniramine Maleate, Phenyltolox-
amine Citrate, Phenylpropanolamine
Hydrochloride, Dextromethorphan
Hydrobromide, and Guaifenesin
Syrup, III/102
Chlorpheniramine Maleate, Phenyltolox-
amine Dihydrogen Citrate, Phenylpro-
panolamine Hydrochloride, and
Acetaminophen
Capsules, III/102

Chlorpheniramine Maleate and Pseudo-
ephedrine Hydrochloride
Capsules, III/103
Capsules, Extended-release, III/103, IV/
MC-5
Solution, Oral, III/103
Syrup, III/103
Tablets, III/103, IV/MC-5
Chlorpheniramine Maleate, Pseudoephedrine
Hydrochloride, and Acetaminophen
Capsules, III/103
Solution, Oral, III/103
for Solution, Oral, III/103
Tablets, III/103
Chlorpheniramine Maleate, Pseudoephedrine
Hydrochloride, and Codeine Phos-
phate
Elixir, III/103
Solution, Oral, III/103
Chlorpheniramine Maleate, Pseudoephedrine
Hydrochloride, and Dextromethor-
phan Hydrobromide
Solution, Oral, III/103
Syrup, III/103
Tablets, III/103
Chlorpheniramine Maleate, Pseudoephedrine
Hydrochloride, Dextromethorphan
Hydrobromide, and Acetaminophen
Capsules, III/103
Solution, Oral, III/103
for Solution, Oral, III/103
Tablets, III/103
Chlorpheniramine Maleate, Pseudoephedrine
Hydrochloride, Dextromethorphan
Hydrobromide, Guaifenesin, and As-
pirin
Tablets, III/103
Chlorpheniramine Maleate, Pseudoephedrine
Hydrochloride, and Guaifenesin
Tablets, Extended-release, III/103
Chlorpheniramine Maleate, Pseudoephedrine
Hydrochloride, and Hydrocodone Bi-
tartrate
Solution, Oral, III/104
Chlorpheniramine Maleate and Pseudo-
ephedrine Sulfate
Tablets, III/104
Tablets, Extended-release, III/104
Chlorpheniramine Maleate, Pyrilamine Ma-
leate, Phenylephrine Hydrochloride,
and Acetaminophen
Tablets, III/104
Chlorpheniramine Maleate, Pyrilamine Ma-
leate, Phenylephrine Hydrochloride,
and Phenylpropanolamine Hydrochlo-
ride
Tablets, III/104
Chlorpheniramine Maleate, Pyrilamine Ma-
leate, Phenylephrine Hydrochloride,
Phenylpropanolamine Hydrochloride,
and Acetaminophen
Tablets, III/104
Chlorpheniramine and Phenylpropanolamine
Polistirexes
Suspension, Oral, Extended-release, III/
104
Chlorpheniramine Resin Complex, Phenyltol-
oxamine Resin Complex, Ephedrine
Resin Complex, Codeine Resin Com-
plex, and Guaiacol Carbonate
Suspension, Oral, III/104
Chlorpheniramine Tannate, Ephedrine Tan-
nate, Phenylephrine Tannate, and
Carbetapentane Tannate
Suspension, Oral, III/104
Tablets, III/104

Chlorpheniramine Tannate, Pyrilamine Tannate, and Phenylephrine Tannate
  Suspension, Oral, III/104
  Tablets, III/104, IV/MC-5
  Tablets, Extended-release, III/104
Chlorpromazine
  Chlorpromazine USP, III/104
  Suppositories USP, III/104
Chlorpromazine Hydrochloride
  Capsules, Extended-release, III/104, IV/MC-5
  Chlorpromazine Hydrochloride USP, III/104
  Concentrate, Oral, USP, III/104
  Injection USP, III/104
  Syrup USP, III/104
  Tablets USP, III/104, IV/MC-5
Chlorpropamide
  Chlorpropamide USP, III/104
  Tablets USP, III/104, IV/MC-5
Chlorprothixene
  Chlorprothixene USP, III/105
  Injection USP, III/105
  Suspension, Oral, USP, III/105
  Tablets USP, III/105
Chlortetracyline Bisulfate
  Chlortetracyline Bisulfate USP, III/105
Chlortetracyline Hydrochloride
  Capsules USP, III/105
  Chlortetracyline Hydrochloride USP, III/105
  Ointment USP, III/105
  Ointment, Ophthalmic, USP, III/105
  Powder, Soluble, USP, III/105
  Sterile USP, III/105
  Tablets USP, III/105
Chlortetracyline and Sulfamethazine Bisulfates
  Powder, Soluble, USP, III/106
Chlorthalidone
  Chlorthalidone USP, III/106
  Tablets USP, III/106, IV/MC-5
Chlorzoxazone
  Chlorzoxazone USP, III/106
  Tablets USP, III/106, IV/MC-5
Chlorzoxazone and Acetaminophen
  Capsules, III/106
  Tablets, III/106
Cholecalciferol
  Cholecalciferol USP, III/106
Cholera Vaccine
  Cholera Vaccine USP, III/106
Cholesterol
  Cholesterol NF, III/107
Cholestyramine
  Bar, Chewable, III/107
  Resin USP, III/107
  for Suspension, Oral, USP, III/107
Choline Salicylate
  Solution, Oral, III/107
Choline and Magnesium Salicylates
  Solution, Oral, III/107
  Tablets, III/107
Chorionic Gonadotropin—See Gonadotropin, Chorionic
Chromic Chloride
  Chromic Chloride USP, III/107
  Injection USP, III/107
Chromic Phosphate P 32—See Phosphate P 32, Chromic
Chymopapain
  for Injection, III/108
Chymotrypsin
  Chymotrypsin USP, III/108
  for Solution, Ophthalmic, USP, III/108

Ciclopirox Olamine
  Ciclopirox Olamine USP, III/108
  Cream USP, III/108
  Lotion, III/108
Cilastatin Sodium
  Sterile USP, III/108
Cimetidine
  Cimetidine USP, III/108
  Tablets USP, III/108, IV/MC-5
Cimetidine Hydrochloride
  Injection, III/108
  Solution, Oral, III/108
Cinoxacin
  Capsules USP, III/109
  Cinoxacin USP, III/109
Cinoxate
  Lotion USP, III/109
Cipro, IV/MC-5
Ciprofloxacin
  Injection, III/109
  for Injection, III/109
  Tablets USP, III/109
Ciprofloxacin Hydrochloride
  Ciprofloxacin Hydrochloride USP, III/109
  Tablets USP, IV/MC-5
Cisplatin
  Cisplatin USP, III/109
  Injection, III/109
  for Injection USP, III/109
Citrated Caffeine—See Caffeine, Citrated
Citrate Dextrose, Anticoagulant—See Anticoagulant Citrate Dextrose
Citrate Phosphate Dextrose Adenine, Anticoagulant—See Anticoagulant Citrate Phosphate Dextrose Adenine
Citrate Phosphate Dextrose, Anticoagulant—See Anticoagulant Citrate Phosphate Dextrose
Citric Acid
  Citric Acid USP, III/110
Citric Acid and D-Gluconic Acid
  for Solution, Topical, III/110
Citric Acid, Magnesium Oxide, and Sodium Carbonate
  Irrigation USP, III/110
Clarithromycin
  Tablets, III/110, IV/MC-5
Clavulanate Potassium
  Clavulanate Potassium USP, III/110
Clemastine Fumarate
  Clemastine Fumarate USP, III/111
  Syrup, III/111
  Tablets USP, III/111, IV/MC-5
Clemastine Fumarate and Phenylpropanolamine Hydrochloride
  Tablets, Extended-release, III/111, IV/MC-5
Cleocin, IV/MC-5
Clidinium Bromide
  Capsules USP, III/111
  Clidinium Bromide USP, III/111
Clindamycin Hydrochloride
  Capsules USP, III/111, IV/MC-5
  Clindamycin Hydrochloride USP, III/111
Clindamycin Palmitate Hydrochloride
  Clindamycin Palmitate Hydrochloride USP, III/111
  for Solution, Oral, USP, III/111
Clindamycin Phosphate
  Clindamycin Phosphate USP, III/111
  Gel USP, III/111
  Injection USP, III/111
  Solution, Topical, USP, III/111
  Sterile USP, III/111
  Suspension, Topical, USP, III/111

Clinoril, IV/MC-21
Clioquinol
  Clioquinol USP, III/112
  Cream USP, III/112
  Ointment USP, III/112
  Powder, Compound, III/112
Clioquinol and Flumethasone Pivalate
  Cream, III/112
  Ointment, III/112
  Solution, Otic, III/112
Clioquinol and Hydrocortisone
  Cream USP, III/113
  Lotion, III/113
  Ointment USP, III/113
Clobetasol Propionate
  Cream, III/113
  Ointment, III/113
  Solution, III/113
Clobetasone Butyrate
  Cream, III/113
  Ointment, III/113
Clocortolone
  Clocortolone USP, III/113
Clocortolone Pivalate
  Cream USP, III/113
Clofazimine
  Capsules USP, III/113
  Clofazimine USP, III/113
Clofibrate
  Capsules USP, III/113
  Clofibrate USP, III/113
Clomiphene Citrate
  Clomiphene Citrate USP, III/114
  Tablets USP, III/114
Clomipramine Hydrochloride
  Capsules, III/114, IV/MC-5
  Tablets, III/114
Clonazepam
  Clonazepam USP, III/114
  Tablets USP, III/114
Clonidine Hydrochloride
  Clonidine Hydrochloride USP, III/114
  System, Transdermal, III/114
  Tablets USP, III/114, IV/MC-5, MC-6
Clonidine Hydrochloride and Chlorthalidone
  Tablets USP, III/114, IV/MC-6
Clorazepate Dipotassium
  Capsules, III/115
  Clorazepate Dipotassium USP, III/115
  Tablets, III/115, IV/MC-6
Clotrimazole
  Clotrimazole USP, III/115
  Cream USP, III/115
  Lotion USP, III/115
  Lozenges, III/115, IV/MC-6
  Solution, Topical, USP, III/115
  Tablets, Vaginal, USP, III/115
Clotrimazole and Betamethasone Dipropionate
  Cream USP, III/115
Cloxacillin Benzathine
  Cloxacillin Benzathine USP, III/115
  Infusion, Intramammary, USP, III/115
  Sterile USP, III/115
Cloxacillin Sodium
  Capsules USP, III/115, IV/MC-6
  Cloxacillin Sodium USP, III/115
  Infusion, Intramammary, USP, III/115
  Injection, III/115
  for Solution, Oral, USP, III/115
  Sterile USP, III/115
Clozapine, IV/MC-6
Clozaril, IV/MC-6

Coal Tar
  Bar, Cleansing, III/116
  Coal Tar USP, III/116
  Cream, III/116
  Gel, III/116
  Lotion, III/116
  Ointment USP, III/116
  Shampoo, III/116
  Solution, Topical, USP, III/116
  Suspension, Topical, III/116
Coatings for Tablets, II/19
Cocaine
  Cocaine USP, III/116
Cocaine Hydrochloride
  Cocaine Hydrochloride USP, III/116
  Solution, Topical, III/116
  Solution, Topical, Viscous, III/116
  Tablets for Solution, Topical, USP, III/116
Coccidioidin
  Coccidioidin USP, III/117
Cocoa Butter
  Cocoa Butter NF, III/117
Codeine
  Codeine USP, III/117
Codeine and Calcium Iodide
  Syrup, III/118
Codeine Phosphate
  Codeine Phosphate USP, III/117
  Injection USP, III/117
  Solution, Oral, III/117
  Tablets USP, III/117
  Tablets, Soluble, III/117
Codeine Phosphate and Guaifenesin—See
  Guaifenesin and Codeine Phosphate
Codeine Phosphate and Iodinated Glycerol
  Solution, Oral, III/118
Codeine Sulfate
  Codeine Sulfate USP, III/117
  Tablets USP, III/117
  Tablets, Soluble, III/117
Cod Liver Oil
  Cod Liver Oil USP, III/118
Cogentin, IV/MC-3
Colchicine
  Colchicine USP, III/118
  Injection USP, III/118
  Tablets USP, III/118
Colestipol Hydrochloride
  Colestipol Hydrochloride USP, III/118
  for Suspension, Oral, USP, III/118
Colistimethate Sodium
  Sterile USP, III/119
Colistin Sulfate
  Colistin Sulfate USP, III/119
  for Suspension, Oral, USP, III/119
Colistin and Neomycin Sulfates and Hydro-
    cortisone Acetate
  Suspension, Otic, USP, III/119
Collodion
  Collodion USP, III/119
  Flexible USP, III/119
Colloidal Silicon Dioxide—See Silicon Diox-
    ide, Colloidal
Combipres, IV/MC-6
Compazine, IV/MC-20
Compazine Spansules, IV/MC-20
Compound Benzaldehyde—See Benzalde-
    hyde Compound
Concentrations, II/5
Conjugated Estrogens—See Estrogens, Con-
    jugated
Conjugated Estrogens and Methyltestoster-
    one—See Estrogens, Conjugated, and
    Methyltestosterone
Containers, II/10, 22
Containers—Permeation, II/24

Continuing Records, II/43
Controlled Substances
  Act Regulations, II/30
  Listed in Schedule II, II/48
  Listed in Schedule III and IV, II/49
  Listed in Schedule V, II/51
Copper Gluconate
  Copper Gluconate USP, III/120
  Tablets, III/120
Corgard, IV/MC-15
Corn Oil
  Corn Oil NF, III/120
Cortef, IV/MC-11
Corticotropin
  Injection USP, III/120
  for Injection USP, III/120
  Injection, Repository, USP, III/120
Corticotropin Zinc Hydroxide
  Suspension, Sterile, USP, III/120
Cortisone Acetate
  Suspension, Sterile, USP, III/120
  Tablets USP, III/120
Corzide, IV/MC-16
Cosyntropin
  for Injection, III/121
Cotton
  Purified USP, III/121
Cottonseed Oil
  Cottonseed Oil NF, III/121
Coumadin, IV/MC-24
Creatinine
  Creatinine NF, III/121
Cresol
  Cresol NF, III/121
Cromolyn Sodium
  Aerosol, Inhalation, III/121
  Capsules, III/121, IV/MC-6
  Cromolyn Sodium USP, III/121
  Inhalation USP (Solution), III/121
  for Inhalation USP (Capsules), III/121
  for Insufflation, Nasal, III/121
  Solution, Nasal, USP, III/121
  Solution, Ophthalmic, USP, III/121
Croscarmellose Sodium
  Croscarmellose Sodium NF, III/122
Crospovidone
  Crospovidone NF, III/122
Crotamiton
  Cream USP, III/122
  Crotamiton USP, III/122
  Lotion, III/122
Cupric Chloride
  Cupric Chloride USP, III/122
  Injection USP, III/122
Cupric Sulfate
  Cupric Sulfate USP, III/123
  Injection USP, III/123
Cyanocobalamin
  Cyanocobalamin USP, III/123
  Injection USP, III/123
  Tablets, III/123
Cyanocobalamin Co 57
  Capsules USP, III/123
  Solution, Oral, USP, III/123
Cyanocobalamin Co 60
  Capsules USP, III/124
  Solution, Oral, USP, III/124
Cyclacillin
  Cyclacillin USP, III/124
  for Suspension, Oral, USP, III/124
  Tablets USP, III/124
Cyclandelate
  Capsules, III/124
  Tablets, III/124
Cyclizine
  Cyclizine USP, III/124

Cyclizine Hydrochloride
  Cyclizine Hydrochloride USP, III/124
  Tablets USP, III/124
Cyclizine Lactate
  Injection USP, III/124
Cyclobenzaprine Hydrochloride
  Cyclobenzaprine Hydrochloride USP, III/125
  Tablets USP, III/125, IV/MC-6
Cyclomethicone
  Cyclomethicone NF, III/125
Cyclopentolate Hydrochloride
  Cyclopentolate Hydrochloride USP, III/125
  Solution, Ophthalmic, USP, III/125
Cyclophosphamide
  Cyclophosphamide USP, III/125
  for Injection USP, III/125
  Solution, Oral, III/125
  Tablets USP, III/125
Cyclopropane
  Cyclopropane USP, III/126
Cycloserine
  Capsules USP, III/126
  Cycloserine USP, III/126
Cyclosporine
  Capsules, III/126
  Concentrate for Injection USP, III/126
  Cyclosporine USP, III/126
  Solution, Oral, USP, III/126
Cyclothiazide
  Cyclothiazide USP, III/126
  Tablets USP, III/126
Cyproheptadine Hydrochloride
  Cyproheptadine Hydrochloride USP, III/127
  Syrup USP, III/127
  Tablets USP, III/127
Cysteine Hydrochloride
  Cysteine Hydrochloride USP, III/127
  Injection USP, III/127
Cytarabine
  Cytarabine USP, III/127
  Sterile USP, III/127
Cytotec, IV/MC-15

D

Dacarbazine
  Dacarbazine UPS, III/127
  for Injection USP, III/127
Dactinomycin
  Dactinomycin USP, III/128
  for Injection USP, III/128
Dalmane, IV/MC-10
Danazol
  Capsules USP, III/128, IV/MC-6
  Danazol USP, III/128
Danocrine, IV/MC-6
Danthron and Docusate Sodium
  Capsules, III/128
  Tablets, III/128
Dantrium, IV/MC-6
Dantrolene Sodium
  Capsules, III/129, IV/MC-6
  for Injection, III/129
Dapiprazole
  Powder for Topical Solution, III/129
Dapsone
  Dapsone USP, III/129
  Tablets USP, III/129
Darvocet-N 50, IV/MC-20
Darvocet-N 100, IV/MC-20

Daunorubicin Hydrochloride
    Daunorubicin Hydrochloride USP, III/129
    for Injection USP, III/129
Decadron, IV/MC-6
Deconamine, IV/MC-5
Deconamine SR, IV/MC-5
Deferoxamine Mesylate
    Deferoxamine Mesylate USP, III/129
    Sterile USP, III/129
Definitions, II/61
Dehydrated Alcohol—See Alcohol, Dehydrated
Dehydroacetic Acid
    Dehydroacetic Acid NF, III/130
Dehydrocholic Acid
    Dehydrocholic Acid USP, III/130
    Tablets USP, III/130
Dehydrocholic Acid and Docusate Sodium
    Capsules, III/130
    Tablets, III/130
Dehydrocholic Acid, Docusate Sodium, and Phenolphthalein
    Capsules, III/130
Deltasone, IV/MC-19
Demecarium Bromide
    Demecarium Bromide USP, III/130
    Solution, Ophthalmic, USP, III/130
Demeclocycline
    Demeclocycline USP, III/130
    Suspension, Oral, USP, III/130
Demeclocycline Hydrochloride
    Capsules USP, III/130
    Demeclocycline Hydrochloride USP, III/130
    Tablets USP, III/130
Demeclocycline Hydrochloride and Nystatin
    Capsules USP, III/131
    Tablets USP, III/131
Demerol, IV/MC-14
Demi-Regroton, IV/MC-21
Demulen, IV/MC-9
Denatonium Benzoate
    Denatonium Benzoate NF, III/131
Dental-Type Silica
    Dental-Type Silica NF, III/131
Deserpidine
    Tablets, III/131
Deserpidine and Hydrochlorothiazide
    Tablets, III/131
Deserpidine and Methyclothiazide
    Tablets, III/131
Desipramine Hydrochloride
    Capsules USP, III/132
    Desipramine Hydrochloride USP, III/132
    Tablets USP, III/132, IV/MC-6
Deslanoside
    Deslanoside USP, III/132
    Injection USP, III/132
Desmopressin Acetate
    Injection, III/132
    Solution, Nasal, III/132
Desonide
    Cream, III/132
    Ointment, III/132
Desonide and Acetic Acid
    Solution, Otic, III/132
Desoximetasone
    Cream USP, III/132
    Desoximetasone USP, III/132
    Gel USP, III/132
    Ointment USP, III/132

Desoxycorticosterone Acetate
    Desoxycorticosterone Acetate USP, III/133
    Injection USP, III/133
    Pellets USP, III/133
Desoxycorticosterone Pivalate
    Desoxycorticosterone Pivalate USP, III/133
    Suspension, Sterile, USP, III/133
Desyrel, IV/MC-23
Dexamethasone
    Aerosol, Topical, USP, III/133
    Dexamethasone USP, III/133
    Elixir USP, III/133
    Gel USP, III/133
    Ointment, Ophthalmic, III/133
    Solution, Oral, III/133
    Suspension, Ophthalmic, USP, III/133
    Tablets USP, III/133, IV/MC-6
Dexamethasone Acetate
    Dexamethasone Acetate USP, III/133
    Suspension, Sterile, USP, III/133
Dexamethasone Sodium Phosphate
    Aerosol, Inhalation, USP, III/133
    Aerosol, Nasal, III/133
    Cream USP, III/133
    Dexamethasone Sodium Phosphate USP, III/133
    Injection USP, III/133
    Ointment, Ophthalmic, III/133
    Solution, Ophthalmic, III/133
Dexbrompheniramine Maleate
    Dexbrompheniramine Maleate USP, III/134
Dexbrompheniramine Maleate, Pseudoephedrine Hydrochloride, and Acetaminophen
    Tablets, Extended-release, III/135
Dexbrompheniramine Maleate and Pseudoephedrine Sulfate
    Capsules, Extended-release, III/134
    Syrup, III/134
    Tablets, III/134
    Tablets, Extended-release, III/134
Dexchlorpheniramine Maleate
    Dexchlorpheniramine Maleate USP, III/135
    Syrup USP, III/135
    Tablets USP, III/135
    Tablets, Extended-release, III/135
Dexchlorpheniramine Maleate, Pseudoephedrine Sulfate, and Guaifenesin
    Solution, Oral, III/135
Dexpanthenol
    Dexpanthenol USP, III/135
    Preparation USP, III/135
Dextrates
    Dextrates NF, III/135
Dextrin
    Dextrin NF, III/135
Dextroamphetamine Sulfate
    Capsules USP, III/136
    Capsules, Extended-release, III/136
    Dextroamphetamine Sulfate USP, III/136
    Elixir USP, III/136
    Tablets USP, III/136
Dextromethorphan
    Dextromethorphan USP, III/136
Dextromethorphan Hydrobromide
    Capsules, III/136
    Dextromethorphan Hydrobromide USP, III/136
    Lozenges, III/136
    Syrup USP, III/136
    Tablets, Chewable, III/136

Dextromethorphan Hydrobromide and Guaifenesin
    Capsules, III/136
    Gel, Oral, III/136
    Solution, Oral, III/136
    Syrup, III/136
    Tablets, III/136
Dextromethorphan Hydrobromide, Guaifenesin, Potassium Citrate, and Citric Acid
    Syrup, III/136
Dextromethorphan Hydrobromide and Iodinated Glycerol
    Solution, Oral, III/137
Dextromethorphan Polistirex
    Suspension, Oral, Extended-release, III/136
Dextrose
    Dextrose USP, III/137
    Injection USP, III/137
Dextrose and Electrolytes
    Solution, III/137
    Rehydration Salts, Oral, USP (for Oral Solution), III/137
Dextrose Excipient
    Dextrose Excipient NF, III/137
Dextrose and Sodium Chloride
    Injection USP, III/137
Dextrothyroxine Sodium
    Tablets, III/137
Dezocine
    Injection, III/138
DiaBeta, IV/MC-10
Diabinese, IV/MC-5
Diacetylated Monoglycerides
    Diacetylated Monoglycerides NF, III/138
Diatrizoate Meglumine
    Diatrizoate Meglumine USP, III/138
    Injection USP, III/138
Diatrizoate Meglumine and Diatrizoate Sodium
    Injection USP, III/138
    Solution USP, III/138
Diatrizoate Meglumine and Iodipamide Meglumine
    Injection, III/138
Diatrizoate Sodium
    Diatrizoate Sodium USP, III/138
    Injection USP, III/138
    Solution USP, III/138
    for Solution, III/138
Diatrizoic Acid
    Diatrizoic Acid USP, III/139
Diazepam
    Capsules USP, III/139
    Capsules, Extended-release, USP, III/139, IV/MC-6
    Diazepam USP, III/139
    Emulsion, Sterile, III/139
    Injection USP, III/139
    Solution, Oral, III/139
    Tablets USP, III/139, IV/MC-6, MC-7
Diazoxide
    Capsules USP, III/140
    Diazoxide USP, III/140
    Injection USP, III/140
    Suspension, Oral, USP, III/140
Dibucaine
    Cream USP, III/140
    Dibucaine USP, III/140
    Ointment USP, III/140
Dibucaine Hydrochloride
    Dibucaine Hydrochloride USP, III/140
    Injection, III/140
Dibutyl Sebacate
    Dibutyl Sebacate NF, III/140

Dichlorodifluoromethane
    Dichlorodifluoromethane NF, III/140
Dichlorotetrafluoroethane
    Dichlorotetrafluoroethane NF, III/141
Dichlorphenamide
    Dichlorphenamide USP, III/141
    Tablets USP, III/141
Diclofenac
    Tablets, Delayed-release, III/141
Diclofenac Sodium
    Solution, Ophthalmic, III/141
    Suppositories, III/141
    Tablets, Delayed-release, III/141, IV/
      MC-7
    Tablets, Extended-release, III/141
Dicloxacillin Sodium
    Capsules USP, III/141, IV/MC-7
    Dicloxacillin Sodium USP, III/141
    Sterile USP, III/141
    for Suspension, Oral, USP, III/141
Dicumarol
    Dicumarol USP, III/142
    Tablets USP, III/142
Dicyclomine Hydrochloride
    Capsules USP, III/142, IV/MC-7
    Dicyclomine Hydrochloride USP, III/142
    Injection USP, III/142
    Syrup USP, III/142
    Tablets USP, III/142, IV/MC-7
Didanosine
    for Solution, Oral, III/142
    for Solution, Oral, Buffered, III/142
    Tablets, Chewable/Dispersible, III/142
Didrex, IV/MC-3
Dienestrol
    Cream USP, III/142
    Dienestrol USP, III/142
Diethanolamine
    Diethanolamine NF, III/142
Diethylcarbamazine Citrate
    Diethylcarbamazine Citrate USP, III/
      143
    Tablets USP, III/143
Diethyl Phthalate
    Diethyl Phthalate NF, III/143
Diethylpropion Hydrochloride
    Capsules, Extended-release, III/143
    Diethylpropion Hydrochloride USP, III/
      143
    Tablets USP, III/143, IV/MC-7
    Tablets, Extended-release, III/143, IV/
      MC-7
Diethylstilbestrol
    Diethylstilbestrol USP, III/143
    Injection USP, III/143
    Tablets USP, III/143
Diethylstilbestrol Diphosphate
    Diethylstilbestrol Diphosphate USP, III/
      143
    Injection USP, III/143
    Tablets, III/143
Diethylstilbestrol and Methyltestosterone
    Tablets, III/144
Diethyltoluamide
    Diethyltoluamide USP, III/144
    Solution, Topical, USP, III/144
Difenoxin Hydrochloride and Atropine Sul-
    fate
    Tablets, III/144
Diflorasome Diacetate
    Cream USP, III/144
    Diflorasome Diacetate USP, III/144
    Ointment USP, III/144
Diflucan, IV/MC-10
Diflucortolone Valerate
    Cream, III/145
    Ointment, III/145

Diflunisal
    Diflunisal USP, III/145
    Tablets USP, III/145, IV/MC-7
Digitalis
    Capsules USP, III/145
    Digitalis USP, III/145
    Powdered USP, III/145
    Tablets USP, III/145
Digitoxin
    Capsules, III/145
    Digitoxin USP, III/145
    Injection USP, III/145
    Tablets USP, III/145
Digoxin
    Capsules, III/146, IV/MC-7
    Digoxin USP, III/146
    Elixir USP, III/146
    Injection USP, III/146
    Tablets USP, III/146, IV/MC-7
Digoxin Immune Fab (Ovine)
    for Injection, III/146
Dihydrocodeine Bitartrate
    Dihydrocodeine Bitartrate USP, III/146
Dihydrocodeine Bitartrate, Acetaminophen,
    and Caffeine
    Capsules, III/146
Dihydroergotamine Mesylate
    Injection USP, III/146
Dihydroergotamine Mesylate, Heparin So-
    dium, and Lidocaine Hydrochloride
    Injection USP, III/147
Dihydrostreptomycin Sulfate
    Boluses USP, III/147
    Injection USP, III/147
    Sterile USP, III/147
Dihydrotachysterol
    Capsules USP, III/147
    Solution, Oral, USP, III/147
    Tablets USP, III/147
Dihydroxyaluminum Aminoacetate
    Capsules USP, III/147
    Magma USP, III/147
    Tablets USP, III/147
Dihydroxyaluminum Sodium Carbonate
    Tablets USP, III/148
Diisopropanolamine
    Diisopropanolamine NF, III/148
Dilantin, IV/MC-19
Dilantin Infatabs, IV/MC-19
Dilantin Kapseals, IV/MC-19
Dilatrate-SR
    Extended-release Capsules, IV/MC-12
Diltiazem
    Capsules, Extended-release, III/148, IV/
      MC-7
    Injection, III/148
    Tablets USP, III/148, IV/MC-7
Diluted Alcohol—See Alcohol, Diluted
Dimenhydrinate
    Capsules, III/148
    Capsules, Extended-release, III/148
    Elixir, III/148
    Injection USP, III/148
    Suppositories, III/148
    Syrup USP, III/148
    Tablets USP, III/148
Dimercaprol
    Injection USP, III/148
Dimethicone
    Dimethicone NF, III/149
Dimethyl Sulfoxide
    Irrigation USP, III/149
    Gel, III/149
    Solution, III/149
Dinoprost Tromethamine
    Injection USP, III/149

Dinoprostone
    Gel, Cervical, III/149
    Suppositories, Vaginal, III/149
Dioxybenzone and Oxybenzone
    Cream USP, III/149
Diperodon
    Ointment USP, III/150
Diphemanil Methylsulfate
    Tablets USP, III/150
Diphenhist
    Tablets, IV/MC-7
Diphenhydramine Citrate, Phenylpropanol-
    amine Bitartrate, and Aspirin
    for Solution, Oral, III/150
Diphenhydramine Hydrochloride
    Capsules USP, III/150, IV/MC-7
    Elixir USP, III/150
    Injection USP, III/150
    Syrup, III/150
    Tablets, III/150, IV/MC-7
Diphenhydramine Hydrochloride, Codeine
    Phosphate, and Ammonium Chloride
    Syrup, III/150
Diphenhydramine Hydrochloride, Dextro-
    methorphan Hydrobromide, and Am-
    monium Chloride
    Syrup, III/150
Diphenhydramine Hydrochloride and Pseu-
    doephedrine Hydrochloride
    Solution, Oral, III/150
    Tablets, III/150
Diphenhydramine Hydrochloride, Pseudo-
    ephedrine Hydrochloride, and Aceta-
    minophen
    Solution, Oral, III/151
    Tablets, III/151
Diphenhydramine Hydrochloride, Pseudo-
    ephedrine Hydrochloride, Dextro-
    methorphan Hydrobromide, and
    Acetaminophen
    Solution, Oral, III/151
Diphenhydramine and Pseudoephedrine
    Capsules USP, III/150
Diphenidol Hydrochloride
    Tablets, III/151
Diphenoxylate Hydrochloride and Atropine
    Sulfate
    Solution, Oral, USP, III/151
    Tablets, III/151, IV/MC-7
Diphenylpyraline Hydrochloride
    Capsules, Extended-release, III/151
Diphenylpyraline Hydrochloride, Phenyleph-
    rine Hydrochloride, and Codeine
    Phosphate
    Solution, Oral, III/151
Diphenylpyraline Hydrochloride, Phenyleph-
    rine Hydrochloride, and Dextrometh-
    orphan Hydrobromide
    Syrup, III/152
Diphenylpyraline Hydrochloride, Phenyleph-
    rine Hydrochloride, and Hydrocodone
    Bitartrate
    Solution, Oral, III/152
    Syrup, III/152
Diphenylpyraline Hydrochloride, Phenyleph-
    rine Hydrochloride, Hydrocodone Bi-
    tartrate, and Guaifenesin
    Solution, Oral, III/152
Diphtheria Antitoxin
    Diphtheria Antitoxin USP, III/152
Diphtheria Toxin for Schick Test
    Diphtheria Toxin for Schick Test USP,
      III/152
Diphtheria Toxoid
    Diphtheria Toxoid USP, III/152

Diphtheria Toxoid Adsorbed
    Diphtheria Toxoid Adsorbed USP, III/
    152
Diphtheria and Tetanus Toxoids
    Diphtheria and Tetanus Toxoids USP,
    III/152
Diphtheria and Tetanus Toxoids Adsorbed
    Diphtheria and Tetanus Toxoids Adsorbed USP, III/152
Diphtheria and Tetanus Toxoids and Pertussis Vaccine
    Diphtheria and Tetanus Toxoids and Pertussis Vaccine USP, III/153
Diphtheria and Tetanus Toxoids and Pertussis Vaccine Adsorbed
    Diphtheria and Tetanus Toxoids and Pertussis Vaccine Adsorbed USP, III/
    153
Dipivefrin Hydrochloride
    Solution, Ophthalmic, USP, III/153
Dipyridamole
    Injection, III/153
    Tablets USP, III/153, IV/MC-7
Discontinued Drug Product List, I/287
Disopyramide
    Capsules, III/153
Disopyramide Phosphate
    Capsules USP, III/153, IV/MC-8
    Capsules, Extended-release, USP, III/
    153, IV/MC-8
    Tablets, Extended-release, III/153
Disposal of Controlled Substances, II/53
Disulfiram
    Tablets USP, III/154
Ditropan, IV/MC-18
Diulo, IV/MC-15
Divalproex Sodium
    Capsules, Delayed-release, III/154
    Tablets, Delayed-release, III/154
Dobutamine Hydrochloride
    Injection, III/154
    for Injection USP, III/154
Docusate Calcium
    Capsules USP, III/154
Docusate Calcium and Phenolphthalein
    Capsules, III/155
Docusate Potassium
    Capsules USP, III/154
Docusate Sodium
    Capsules USP, III/154
    Docusate Sodium USP, III/154
    Solution USP (Oral), III/154
    Solution, Rectal, III/154
    Syrup USP, III/154
    Tablets USP, III/154
Docusate Sodium and Phenolphthalein
    Capsules, III/155
    Tablets, III/155
    Tablets, Chewable, III/155
Dolobid, IV/MC-7
Donnatal, IV/MC-2
Donnatal Extentabs, IV/MC-2
Dopamine Hydrochloride
    Injection USP, III/155
Dopamine Hydrochloride and Dextrose
    Injection USP, III/155
Doral, IV/MC-20
Doxacurium
    Injection, III/155
Doxapram Hydrochloride
    Injection, III/155
Doxazosin Mesylate
    Tablets, IV/MC-8
Doxepin Hydrochloride
    Capsules USP, III/156, IV/MC-8
    Solution, Oral, USP, III/156

Doxorubicin Hydrochloride
    Injection USP, III/156
    for Injection USP, III/156
Doxycycline
    for Suspension, Oral, USP, III/156
Doxycycline Calcium
    Suspension, Oral, USP, III/156
Doxycycline Hyclate
    Capsules USP, III/156, IV/MC-8
    Capsules, Delayed-release, USP, III/156
    for Injection USP, III/156
    Sterile USP, III/156
    Tablets USP, III/156, IV/MC-8
Doxylamine Succinate
    Syrup USP, III/157
    Tablets USP, III/157
Doxylamine Succinate, Pseudoephedrine Hydrochloride, Dextromethorphan Hydrobromide, and Acetaminophen
    Solution, Oral, III/157
Dronabinol
    Capsules USP, III/157
Droperidol
    Injection USP, III/157
Dropper, Medicine, II/27
Drug and Dosage Form Information, II/9
Drug and Dosage Form Requirements, II/5
Drugs, Adulterated, II/63
Drugs, Misbranded, II/64
Drugs, New, II/67
Drugs for Rare Diseases or Conditions, II/
    77
Duricef, IV/MC-4
Dusting Powder, Absorbable
    Absorbable Dusting Powder USP, III/
    158
Dyazide, IV/MC-24
Dyclonine Hydrochloride
    Gel USP, III/158
    Lozenges, III/158
    Solution, Topical, Oral, III/158
    Solution, Topical, USP, III/158
Dydrogesterone
    Tablets USP, III/158
DynaCirc, IV/MC-12
Dynapen, IV/MC-7
Dyphylline
    Elixir USP, III/158
    Injection, III/158
    Solution, Oral, III/158
    Tablets USP, III/158, IV/MC-8
Dyphylline and Guaifenesin
    Elixir USP, III/158
    Tablets USP, III/158

E

Echothiophate Iodide
    for Solution, Ophthalmic, USP, III/158
Econazole Nitrate
    Cream, III/159
    Suppositories, Vaginal, III/159
Edetate Calcium Disodium
    Injection USP, III/159
Edetate Disodium
    Edetate Disodium USP, III/159
    Injection USP, III/159
    Solution, Ophthalmic, III/159
Edetic Acid
    Edetic Acid NF, III/159
Edrophonium Chloride
    Injection USP, III/159
Edrophonium Chloride and Atropine Sulfate
    Injection, III/159
E.E.S., IV/MC-9

Eflornithine Hydrochloride
    Concentrate, for Injection, III/160
Elavil, IV/MC-2
Eldepryl, IV/MC-21
Elements, Trace
    Injection USP, III/160
Emetine Hydrochloride
    Injection USP, III/160
Empirin with Codeine No.2, IV/MC-2
Empirin with Codeine No.3, IV/MC-2
Empirin with Codeine No.4, IV/MC-2
E-Mycin, IV/MC-9
Enalaprilat
    Injection, III/160
Enalapril Maleate
    Tablets USP, III/160, IV/MC-8
Enalapril Maleate and Hydrochlorothiazide
    Tablets, III/160, IV/MC-8
Encainide Hydrochloride
    Capsules, III/160
Enduron, IV/MC-14
Enflurane
    Enflurane USP, III/161
Entex, IV/MC-18
Entex LA, IV/MC-19
Ephedrine Hydrochloride and Guaifenesin
    Capsules, III/161
    Syrup, III/161
Ephedrine Hydrochloride and Potassium Iodide
    Syrup, III/161
Ephedrine Sulfate
    Capsules USP, III/161
    Injection USP, III/161
    Solution, Nasal, USP, III/161
    Syrup USP, III/161
    Tablets USP, III/161
Ephedrine Sulfate and Phenobarbital
    Capsules USP, III/161
Epinephrine
    Aerosol, Inhalation, USP, III/161
    Injection USP, III/161
    Solution, Inhalation, USP, III/161
    Solution, Nasal, USP, III/161
    Solution, Ophthalmic, USP, III/161
    Suspension, Sterile, III/161
    Suspension, Sterile, Oil, USP, III/161
Epinephrine Bitartrate
    Aerosol, Inhalation, USP, III/161
    Solution, Ophthalmic, USP, III/161
    for Solution, Ophthalmic, USP, III/161
Epinephryl Borate
    Solution, Ophthalmic, USP, III/162
Epoetin Alfa, Recombinant
    Injection, III/162
Ergocalciferol
    Capsules USP, III/163
    Injection, III/163
    Solution, Oral, USP, III/163
    Tablets USP, III/163
Ergoloid Mesylates
    Capsules, III/163, IV/MC-8
    Solution, Oral, III/163
    Tablets USP, III/163, IV/MC-8
    Tablets, Sublingual, IV/MC-8
Ergonovine Maleate
    Injection USP, III/163
    Tablets USP, III/163
Ergotamine Tartrate
    Aerosol, Inhalation, USP, III/164
    Injection USP, III/164
    Tablets USP, III/164
Ergotamine Tartrate, Belladonna Alkaloids, and Phenobarbital Sodium
    Tablets, III/164
    Tablets, Extended-release, III/164

Ergotamine Tartrate and Caffeine
  Suppositories USP, III/164
  Tablets USP, III/164, IV/MC-8
Ergotamine Tartrate, Caffeine, Belladonna
  Alkaloids, and Pentobarbital
  Suppositories, III/164
Ergotamine Tartrate, Caffeine, Belladonna
  Alkaloids, and Pentobarbital Sodium
  Tablets, III/164
Ergotamine Tartrate, Caffeine Citrate, and
  Diphenhydramine Hydrochloride
  Capsules, III/164
Ergotamine Tartrate, Caffeine, and Dimen-
  hydrinate
  Capsules, III/164
Ergotamine Tartrate, Caffeine Hydrate, and
  Cyclizine Hydrochloride
  Tablets, III/164
Erythrityl Tetranitrate
  Tablets USP, III/164
Eryc, IV/MC-9
EryPed, IV/MC-9
Ery-Tab, IV/MC-9
Erythrocin, IV/MC-9
Erythromycin
  Capsules, Delayed-release USP, III/165,
    IV/MC-9
  Gel, Topical USP, III/165
  Ointment USP, III/165
  Ointment, Ophthalmic, USP, III/165
  Pledgets USP, III/165
  Solution, Topical, USP, III/165
  Tablets USP, III/165, IV/MC-9
  Tablets, Delayed-release, USP, III/165,
    IV/MC-9
Erythromycin and Benzoyl Peroxide
  Gel, Topical, USP, III/166
Erthromycin Estolate
  Capsules USP, III/165, IV/MC-9
  Suspension, Oral, USP, III/165
  for Suspension, Oral, USP, III/165
  Tablets USP, III/165, IV/MC-9
Erythromycin Ethylsuccinate
  Injection USP, III/165
  Suspension, Oral, USP, III/165
  for Suspension, Oral, USP, III/165
  Tablets USP, III/165, IV/MC-9
  Tablets, Chewable, IV/MC-9
Erythromycin Estolate and Sulfisoxazole
  Acetyl
  Suspension, Oral, USP, III/166
Erythromycin Ethylsuccinate and Sulfisoxa-
  zole Acetyl
  for Suspension, Oral, USP, III/166
Erythromycin Gluceptate
  Sterile USP, III/165
Erythromycin Lactobionate
  for Injection USP, III/165
Erythromycin Stearate
  Suspension, Oral, III/165
  for Suspension, Oral, USP, III/165
  Tablets USP, III/165, IV/MC-9
Erythrosine Sodium
  Solution, Topical, USP, III/167
  Tablets, Soluble, USP, III/167
Esidrix, IV/MC-11
Eskalith, IV/MC-13
Eskalith CR, IV/MC-13
Esmolol Hydrochloride
  Injection, III/167
Estazolam
  Tablets, III/167, IV/MC-9
Estrace, IV/MC-9

Estradiol
  Cream, Vaginal, USP, III/167
  Pellets USP, III/167
  Suspension, Sterile, USP, III/167
  System, Transdermal, III/167
  Tablets USP, III/167, IV/MC-9
Estradiol Cypionate
  Injection USP, III/167
Estradiol Valerate
  Injection USP, III/167
Estramustine Phosphate Sodium
  Capsules, III/168
Estrogens, Conjugated
  Cream, Vaginal, III/168
  for Injection, III/168
  Tablets USP, III/168, IV/MC-9
Estrogens, Conjugated, and Methyltestoster-
  one
  Tablets, III/168
Estrogens, Esterified
  Tablets USP, III/168
Estrogens, Esterified, and Methyltestosterone
  Tablets, III/168
Estrone
  Cream, Vaginal, III/168
  Injection USP, III/168
  Suppositories, Vaginal, III/168
  Suspension, Sterile, USP, III/168
Estropipate
  Cream, Vaginal, III/169
  Tablets USP, III/169, IV/MC-9
Ethacrynate Sodium
  for Injection USP, III/169
Ethacrynic Acid
  Solution, Oral, III/169
  Tablets USP, III/169
Ethambutol Hydrochloride
  Tablets USP, III/169
Ethchlorvynol
  Capsules USP, III/169
Ether
  Ether USP, III/169
Ether, Polyoxyl 10 Oleyl—See Polyoxyl 10
  Oleyl Ether
Ether, Polyoxyl 20 Cetostearyl—See Poly-
  oxyl 20 Cetostearyl Ether
Ethinamate
  Capsules USP, III/170
Ethinyl Estradiol
  Tablets USP, III/170
Ethiodized Oil
  Injection USP, III/170
Ethionamide
  Tablets USP, III/170
Ethmozine, IV/MC-15
Ethopropazine Hydrochloride
  Tablets USP, III/170
Ethosuximide
  Capsules USP, III/170
  Syrup, III/170
Ethotoin
  Tablets USP, III/170
Ethyl Acetate
  Ethyl Acetate NF, III/171
Ethylcellulose
  Ethylcellulose NF, III/171
Ethylcellulose Aqueous Dispersion
  Ethylcellulose Aqueous Dispersion NF,
    III/171
Ethylnorepinephrine Hydrochloride
  Injection USP, III/171
Ethyl Oleate
  Ethyl Oleate NF, III/171
Ethylparaben
  Ethylparaben NF, III/171
Ethyl Vanillin
  Ethyl Vanillin NF, III/172

Ethynodiol Diacetate and Ethinyl Estradiol
  Tablets USP, III/172, IV/MC-9
Ethynodiol Diacetate and Mestranol
  Tablets USP, III/172
Etidocaine Hydrochloride
  Injection, III/172
Etidocaine Hydrochloride and Epinephrine
  Injection, III/172
Etidronate Disodium
  Injection, III/172
  Tablets USP, III/172
Etodolac
  Capsules, III/173, IV/MC-9
Etomidate
  Injection, III/173
Etoposide
  Capsules, III/173
  Injection, III/173
Etretinate
  Capsules, III/173
Eucatropine Hydrochloride
  Solution, Ophthalmic, USP, III/173
Eugenol
  Eugenol USP, III/173
Evans Blue
  Injection USP, III/173
Exemptions in Case of Drugs, II/65

F

Factor IX Complex
  Factor IX Complex USP, III/174
Famotidine
  Injection, III/174
  for Suspension, Oral, III/174
  Tablets USP, III/174, IV/MC-9
Fat, Hard
  Hard Fat NF, III/174
Fat Emulsions
  Injection, III/174
Federal Food, Drug and Cosmetic Act Re-
  quirements Relating to Drugs for Hu-
  man Use, II/60
Fees for Registration and Reregistration, II/
  32
Feldene, IV/MC-19
Felodipine
  Tablets, Extended-release, III/175, IV/
    MC-9
Fenfluramine Hydrochloride
  Capsules, Extended-release, III/175
  Tablets, III/175
  Tablets, Extended-release, III/175
Fenoprofen Calcium
  Capsules USP, III/175, IV/MC-9
  Tablets USP, III/175, IV/MC-9, MC-10
Fenoterol Hydrobromide
  Aerosol, Inhalation, III/175
  Solution, Inhalation, III/175
  Tablets, III/175
Fentanyl
  Systems, Transdermal, III/175
Fentanyl Citrate
  Injection USP, III/175
Ferric Oxide
  Ferric Oxide NF, III/176
Ferrous Citrate Fe 59
  Injection USP, III/176
Ferrous Fumarate
  Capsules, III/176
  Capsules, Extended-release, III/176
  Solution, Oral, III/176
  Suspension, Oral, III/176
  Tablets USP, III/176
Ferrous Fumarate and Docusate Sodium
  Tablets, Extended-release, USP, III/176

Ferrous Gluconate
    Capsules USP, III/176
    Elixir USP, III/176
    Syrup, III/176
    Tablets USP, III/176
Ferrous Sulfate
    Capsules (Dried), III/177
    Capsules, Extended-release, III/177
    Elixir, III/177
    Solution, Oral, USP, III/177
    Syrup USP, III/177
    Tablets USP, III/177, IV/MC-10
    Tablets, Enteric-coated, III/177
    Tablets, Extended-release, III/177
    Tablets, Extended-release (Dried), III/
        177
Filgrastim
    Injection, III/177
Fioricet, IV/MC-3
Fiorinal, IV/MC-3
Fiorinal with Codeine No.3, IV/MC-3
Flagyl, IV/MC-15
Flavoxate Hydrochloride
    Tablets, III/177
Flecainide Acetate
    Tablets, III/
Flexeril, IV/MC-6
Floctafenine
    Tablets, III/177
Floxin, IV/MC-17
Floxuridine
    Sterile USP, III/178
Fluconazole
    Injection, III/178
    Tablets, III/178, IV/MC-10
Flucytosine
    Capsules USP, III/178
Fludeoxyglucose F 18
    Injection USP, III/178
Fludrocortisone Acetate
    Tablets USP, III/178
Flumazenil
    Injection, III/178
Flumethasone Pivalate
    Cream USP, III/179
    Ointment, III/179
Flunarizine Hydrochloride
    Capsules, III/179
Flunisolide
    Aerosol, Inhalation, III/179
    Solution, Nasal, USP, III/179
Fluocinolone Acetonide
    Cream USP, III/179
    Ointment USP, III/179
    Solution, Topical, USP, III/179
Fluocinonide
    Cream USP, III/179
    Gel USP, III/179
    Ointment USP, III/179
    Solution, Topical, USP, III/179
Fluorescein
    Injection USP, III/180
Fluorescein Sodium
    Strips, Ophthalmic, USP, III/180
Fluorescein Sodium and Benoxinate Hydro-
        chloride
    Solution, Ophthalmic, USP, III/180
Fluorescein Sodium and Proparacaine Hy-
        drochloride
    Solution, Ophthalmic, USP, III/180
Fluorodopa F 18
    Injection USP, III/180
Fluorometholone
    Cream USP, III/180
    Ointment, Ophthalmic, III/180
    Suspension, Ophthalmic, USP, III/180

Fluorometholone Acetate
    Suspension, Ophthalmic, III/180
Fluorouracil
    Cream USP, III/181
    Injection USP, III/181
    Solution, Topical, USP, III/181
Fluoxetine
    Solution, Oral, III/181
Fluoxetine Hydrochloride
    Capsules, III/181, IV/MC-10
Fluoxymesterone
    Tablets USP, III/181, IV/MC-10
Fluoxymesterone and Ethinyl Estradiol
    Tablets, III/181
Flupenthixol Decanoate
    Injection, III/181
Flupenthixol Dihydrochloride
    Tablets, III/181
Fluphenazine Decanoate
    Injection, III/182
Fluphenazine Enanthate
    Injection USP, III/182
Fluphenazine Hydrochloride
    Elixir USP, III/182
    Injection USP, III/182
    Solution, Oral, USP, III/182
    Tablets USP, III/182, IV/MC-10
Flurandrenolide
    Cream USP, III/182
    Lotion USP, III/182
    Ointment USP, III/182
    Tape USP, III/182
Flurazepam Hydrochloride
    Capsules USP, III/182, IV/MC-10
Flurazepam Monohydrochloride
    Tablets, III/182
Flurbiprofen
    Capsules, Extended-release, III/183
    Tablets, III/183, IV/MC-10
Flurbiprofen Sodium
    Solution, Ophthalmic, III/183
Flutamide
    Capsules, III/183
    Tablets, III/183
Folic Acid
    Injection USP, III/183
    Tablets USP, III/183
Formaldehyde
    Solution USP, III/183
Formulation of Compressed Tablets, II/18
Foscarnet Sodium
    Injection, III/183
Fosinopril
    Tablets, IV/MC-10
Fructose
    Fructose USP, III/184
    Injection USP, III/184
Fructose, Dextrose, and Phosphoric Acid
    Solution, Oral, III/184
Fructose and Sodium Chloride
    Injection USP, III/184
Fumaric Acid
    Fumaric Acid NF, III/184
Furadantin, IV/MC-16
Furazolidone
    Suspension, Oral, USP, III/184
    Tablets USP, III/184
Furosemide
    Bolus, III/184
    Injection USP, III/184
    Solution, Oral, III/184
    Syrup, III/184
    Tablets USP, III/184, IV/MC-10

G

Gadopentetate Dimeglumine
    Injection, III/185
Gallamine Triethiodide
    Injection USP, III/185
Gallium Citrate Ga 67
    Injection USP, III/185
Gallium Nitrate
    Injection, III/185
Ganciclovir Sodium
    Sterile, III/185
Gastrocrom, IV/MC-6
Gauze, Absorbent
    Absorbent Gauze USP, III/185
Gauze, Petrolatum
    Petrolatum Gauze USP, III/186
Gelatin
    Gelatin NF, III/186
Gelatin, Absorbable
    Film USP, III/186
    Sponge USP, III/186
Gemfibrozil
    Capsules USP, III/186
    Tablets, III/186, IV/MC-10
Genora 0.5/35-21, IV/MC-17
Genora 1/35-28, IV/MC-17
Genora 1/50-28, IV/MC-17
Gentamicin and Prednisolone Acetate
    Ointment, Ophthalmic, USP, III/187
    Suspension, Ophthalmic, USP, III/187
Gentamicin Sulfate
    Cream USP, III/187
    Infusion, Uterine, III/187
    Injection USP, III/187
    Ointment USP, III/187
    Ointment, Ophthalmic, USP, III/187
    Powder, Soluble, III/187
    Solution, Ophthalmic, USP, III/187
    Solution, Oral, III/187
    Solution, Otic, III/187
    Sterile USP, III/187
Gentamicin Sulfate in Sodium Chloride
    Injection, III/187
Gentian Violet
    Cream USP, III/187
    Solution, Topical, USP, III/187
    Tampons, Vaginal, III/187
Gentisic Acid Ethanolamide
    Gentisic Acid Ethanolamide NF, III/188
Geocillin, IV/MC-4
Glaze, Pharmaceutical
    Pharmaceutical Glaze NF, III/188
Glipizide
    Tablets, III/188, IV/MC-10
Globulin Serum, Anti-human
    Anti-human Globulin Serum USP, III/
        188
Globulin, Immune
    Immune Globulin USP, III/188
Globulin, Immune, RH₀ (D)
    RH₀ (D) Immune Globulin USP, III/189
Glucagon
    for Injection USP, III/189
Glucose Enzymatic Test Strip
    Glucose Enzymatic Test Strip USP, III/
        189
Glucose, Liquid
    Liquid Glucose NF, III/189
Glucotrol, IV/MC-10
Glutaral
    Concentrate USP, III/189
Glutaral Disinfectant Solution
    Glutaral Disinfectant Solution NF, III/
        189

Glutethimide
  Capsules USP, III/189
  Tablets USP, III/189
Glyburide
  Tablets, III/190, IV/MC-10
Glycerin
  Glycerin USP, III/190
  Solution, Ophthalmic, USP, III/190
  Solution, Oral, USP, III/190
  Solution, Rectal, III/190
  Suppositories USP, III/190
Glyceryl Behenate
  Glyceryl Behenate NF, III/190
Glyceryl Monostearate
  Glyceryl Monostearate NF, III/190
Glycine
  Irrigation USP, III/190
Glycopyrrolate
  Injection USP, III/191
  Tablets USP, III/191
Gold Sodium Thiomalate
  Injection USP, III/191
Gonadorelin Acetate
  for Injection, III/191
Gonadorelin Hydrochloride
  for Injection, III/191
Gonadotropin, Chorionic
  for Injection USP, III/191
Good Manufacturing Practice for Finished
  Pharmaceuticals, II/79
Good Manufacturing Practice for Finished
  Pharmaceuticals, Current, II/80
Good Manufacturing Practices in Manufac-
  turing, Processing, Packing, or Hold-
  ing of Drugs: General, Current, II/79
Goserelin Acetate
  Implants, III/191
  Injection, III/191
Gramicidin
  Gramicidin USP, III/192
Green Soap
  Green Soap USP, III/192
  Tincture USP, III/192
Grifulvin V, IV/MC-10
Griseofulvin
  Capsules USP (Microsize), III/192
  Suspension, Oral, USP (Microsize), III/
  192
  Tablets USP (Microsize), III/192, IV/
  MC-10
  Tablets, Ultramicrosize, USP, III/192
Guaifenesin
  Capsules USP, III/192
  Capsules, Extended-release, III/192
  Solution, Oral, III/192
  Syrup USP, III/192
  Tablets USP, III/192
  Tablets, Extended-release, III/192
Guaifenesin and Codeine Phosphate
  Solution, Oral, III/193
  Syrup USP, III/193
Guanabenz Acetate
  Tablets USP, III/193, IV/MC-10
Guanadrel Sulfate
  Tablets USP, III/193
Guanethidine Monosulfate
  Tablets USP, III/193
Guanethidine Monosulfate and Hydrochloro-
  thiazide
  Tablets, III/193
Guanfacine Hydrochloride
  Tablets, III/193, IV/MC-10
Guide to General Chapters, II/94
Guar Gum
  Guar Gum NF, III/193
Gum, Xanthan—See Xanthan Gum

Gutta Percha
  Gutta Percha USP, III/194

H

Haemophilus b Conjugate Vaccine
  Injection, III/194
Haemophilus b Polysaccharide Vaccine
  for Injection, III/194
Halazepam
  Tablets USP, III/194
Halazone
  Tablets for Solution USP, III/194
Halcinonide
  Cream USP, III/194
  Ointment USP, III/194
  Solution, Topical, USP, III/194
Halcion, IV/MC-24
Haldol, IV/MC-11
Haloperidol
  Injection USP, III/195
  Solution, Oral, USP, III/195
  Tablets USP, III/195, IV/MC-10, MC-
  11
Haloperidol Decanoate
  Injection, III/195
Haloprogin
  Cream USP, III/195
  Solution, Topical, USP, III/195
Halotestin, IV/MC-10
Halothane
  Halothane USP, III/195
Hard Fat—See Fat, Hard
Helium
  Helium USP, III/195
Heparin
  Solution, Lock Flush, USP, III/195
Heparin Calcium
  Injection USP, III/195
Heparin Sodium
  Injection USP, III/195
Heparin Sodium and Dextrose
  Heparin Sodium in Dextrose Injection,
  III/195
Heparin Sodium and Sodium Chloride
  Heparin Sodium in Sodium Chloride In-
  jection, III/195
Hepatitis B Immune Globulin
  Hepatitis B Immune Globulin USP, III/
  196
Hepatitis B Vaccine Recombinant
  Suspension, Sterile, III/196
Hepatitis B Virus Vaccine Inactivated
  Hepatitis B Virus Vaccine Inactivated
  USP, III/196
Hetacillin
  for Suspension, Oral, USP, III/197
  Tablets USP, III/197
Hetacillin Potassium
  Capsules USP, III/197
  Infusion, Intramammary USP, III/197
  Sterile USP, III/197
  Suspension, Oral, USP, III/197
  Tablets USP, III/197
Hexachlorophene
  Emulsion, Cleansing, USP, III/197
  Soap, Liquid, USP, III/197
Hexylcaine Hydrochloride
  Solution, Topical, USP, III/198
Hexylene Glycol
  Hexylene Glycol NF, III/198
Hexylresorcinol
  Lozenges USP, III/198
Hismanal, IV/MC-2
Histamine Phosphate
  Injection USP, III/198

Histoplasmin
  Histoplasmin USP, III/198
Homatropine Hydrobromide
  Solution, Ophthalmic, USP, III/198
Homatropine Methylbromide
  Tablets USP, III/198
Hyaluronidase
  Injection USP, III/199
  for Injection USP, III/199
Hydergine, IV/MC-8
Hydergine LC, IV/MC-8
Hydralazine Hydrochloride
  Injection USP, III/199
  Tablets USP, III/199, IV/MC-11
Hydralazine Hydrochloride and Hydrochlo-
  rothiazide
  Capsules, III/199, IV/MC-11
  Tablets, III/199
Hydrochloric Acid
  Hydrochloric Acid NF, III/199
Hydrochloric Acid, Diluted
  Diluted Hydrochloric Acid NF, III/199
Hydrochlorothiazide
  Solution, Oral, III/200
  Tablets USP, III/200, IV/MC-11
Hydrocodone Bitartrate
  Syrup, III/200
  Tablets USP, III/200
Hydrocodone Bitartrate and Acetaminophen
  Capsules, III/200
  Solution, Oral, III/200
  Tablets, III/200, IV/MC-11
Hydrocodone Bitartrate and Aspirin
  Tablets, III/200
Hydrocodone Bitartrate, Aspirin, and Caf-
  feine
  Tablets, III/200
Hydrocodone Bitartrate and Guaifenesin
  Solution, Oral, III/200
  Syrup, III/200
  Tablets, III/200
Hydrocodone Bitartrate and Homatropine
  Methylbromide
  Syrup, III/200
  Tablets, III/200
Hydrocodone Bitartrate and Potassium
  Guaiacolsulfonate
  Syrup, III/200
Hydrocortisone
  Cream USP, III/201
  Enema USP, III/201
  Gel USP, III/201
  Lotion USP, III/201
  Ointment USP, III/201
  Ointment, Rectal, III/201
  Solution, Topical, III/201
  Solution, Topical Aerosol, III/201
  Solution, Topical Spray, III/201
  Suppositories, III/201
  Suspension, Sterile, USP, III/201
  Tablets USP, III/201, IV/MC-11
Hydrocortisone Acetate
  Aerosol (Foam), Rectal, III/201
  Aerosol (Foam), Topical, III/201
  Cream USP, III/201
  Lotion USP, III/201
  Ointment USP, III/201
  Ointment, Ophthalmic, USP, III/201
  Paste, Dental, III/201
  Suppositories, III/201
  Suspension, Ophthalmic, USP, III/201
  Suspension, Sterile, USP, III/201
Hydrocortisone and Acetic Acid
  Solution, Otic, USP, III/202
Hydrocortisone Butyrate
  Cream USP, III/201
  Ointment, III/201

Hydrocortisone Cypionate
    Suspension, Oral, III/201
Hydrocortisone Sodium Phosphate
    Injection USP, III/201
Hydrocortisone Sodium Succinate
    for Injection USP, III/201
Hydrocortisone and Urea
    Cream, III/201
Hydrocortisone Valerate
    Cream USP, III/201
    Ointment, III/201
HydroDIURIL, IV/MC-11
Hydroflumethiazide
    Tablets USP, III/202
Hydrogen Peroxide
    Concentrate USP, III/202
    Solution, Topical, USP, III/202
Hydromorphone Hydrochloride
    Injection USP, III/203
    Suppositories, III/203
    Tablets USP, III/203
Hydromorphone Hydrochloride and Guai-
    fenesin
    Syrup, III/203
Hydroquinone
    Cream USP, III/203
    Solution, Topical, USP, III/203
Hydroxocobalamin
    Injection USP, III/203
Hydroxyamphetamine Hydrobromide
    Solution, Ophthalmic, USP, III/203
Hydroxyanisole, Butylated—See Butylated
    Hydroxyanisole
Hydroxychloroquine Sulfate
    Tablets USP, III/203, IV/MC-11
Hydroxyethyl Cellulose
    Hydroxyethyl Cellulose NF, III/204
Hydroxyprogesterone Caproate
    Injection USP, III/204
Hydroxypropyl Cellulose
    Hydroxypropyl Cellulose NF, III/204
Hydroxypropyl Cellulose, Low-substituted
    Low-substituted Hydroxypropyl Cellulose
    NF, III/204
Hydroxypropyl Methylcellulose
    Hydroxypropyl Methylcellulose USP,
    III/204
    Solution, Ophthalmic, USP, III/204
Hydroxypropyl Methylcellulose Phthalate
    Hydroxypropyl Methylcellulose Phthalate
    NF, III/205
Hydroxystilbamidine Isethionate
    Hydroxystilbamidine Isethionate NF, III/
    205
    Sterile USP, III/205
Hydroxytoluene, Butylated—See Butylated
    Hydroxytoluene
Hydroxyurea
    Capsules USP, III/205
Hydroxyzine Hydrochloride
    Capsules, III/205
    Injection USP, III/205
    Syrup USP, III/205
    Tablets USP, III/205, IV/MC-11
Hydroxyzine Pamoate
    Capsules USP, III/205, IV/MC-11
    Suspension, Oral, USP, III/205
Hygroton, IV/MC-5
Hyoscyamine
    Tablets USP, III/206
Hyoscyamine Sulfate
    Capsules, Extended-release, III/206
    Elixir USP, III/206
    Injection USP, III/206
    Solution, Oral, USP, III/206
    Tablets USP, III/206

Hyoscyamine Sulfate and Phenobarbital
    Elixir, III/206
    Solution, Oral, III/206
    Tablets, III/206
Hypophosphorous Acid
    Hypophosphorous Acid NF, III/206
Hytrin, IV/MC-22

I

Ibuprofen
    Capsules, III/206
    Ibuprofen USP, III/206
    Suspension, Oral, III/206
    Tablets USP, III/206, IV/MC-11, MC12
Ichthammol
    Ichthammol USP, III/207
    Ointment USP, III/207
Idarubicin
    for Injection, III/207
Idoxuridine
    Idoxuridine USP, III/207
    Ointment, Ophthalmic, USP, III/207
    Solution, Ophthalmic, USP, III/207
Ifosfamide
    Ifosfamide USP, III/207
    for Injection, III/207
    Sterile USP, III/207
Ilosone, IV/MC-9
Imidurea
    Imidurea NF, III/207
Imipenem
    Sterile USP, III/208
Imipenem and Cilastatin Sodium
    for Injection, III/208
    for Suspension, III/208
Imipramine Hydrochloride
    Imipramine Hydrochloride USP, III/208
    Injection USP, III/208
    Tablets USP, III/208, IV/MC-12
Imipramine Pamoate
    Capsules, III/208, IV/MC-12
Imodium, IV/MC-13
Imuran, IV/MC-2
Indapamide
    Indapamide USP, III/208
    Tablets USP, III/208, IV/MC-12
Indecainide
    Tablets, Extended-release, III/208
Inderal, IV/MC-20
Inderal LA, IV/MC-20
Inderide, IV/MC-20
Inderide LA, IV/MC-20
Index to the Portions of Controlled Sub-
    stances Act Presented, II/30
Indigotindisulfonate Sodium
    Indigotindisulfonate Sodium USP, III/
    209
    Injection USP, III/209
Indium In 111 Oxyquinoline
    Solution USP, III/209
Indium In 111 Pentetate
    Injection USP, III/209
Indocin, IV/MC-12
Indocin SR, IV/MC-12
Indocyanine Green
    Sterile USP, III/209
Indomethacin
    Capsules USP, III/210, IV/MC-12
    Capsules, Extended-release, USP, III/
    210, IV/MC-12
    Suppositories USP, III/210
    Suspension, Ophthalmic, III/210
    Suspension, Oral, USP, III/210
Indomethacin Sodium
    Sterile USP, III/210

Influenza Virus Vaccine
    Influenza Virus Vaccine USP, III/210
Information, General, II/31
Ingredients and Processes, II/2
Injections, II/5
Inspections, II/59, 78
Insulin
    Injection USP, III/210
Insulin Human
    Injection USP, III/210
    Injection, Buffered, III/210
Insulin Injection and Isophane Insulin, Hu-
    man Semisynthetic
    Injection, III/210
Insulin, Isophane
    Suspension USP, III/210
    Suspension, Human, III/210
    Suspension, Human, and Insulin Human
    Injection, III/210
    Suspension and Insulin Injection, III/210
Insulin, Protamine Zinc
    Suspension USP, III/210
Insulin Zinc
    Suspension USP, III/210
    Suspension, Human, III/210
Insulin Zinc, Extended
    Suspension USP, III/210
    Suspension, Human, III/210
Insulin Zinc, Prompt
    Suspension USP, III/210
Interferon Alfa-2a, Recombinant
    Injection, III/212
    for Injection, III/212
Interferon Alfa-2b, Recombinant
    for Injection, III/212
Interferon Alfa-n1 (lns)
    Injection, III/212
Interferon Alfa-n3
    Injection, III/212
Interferon Gamma-1b
    Injection, III/213
Inulin
    Injection, III/213
Inulin in Sodium Chloride
    Injection USP, III/213
Inventory Requirements, II/42
Iocetamic Acid
    Tablets USP, III/213
Iodinated Glycerol
    Elixir, III/213
    Solution, Oral, III/213
    Tablets, III/213, IV/MC-12
Iodinated I 125 Albumin
    Injection USP, III/213
Iodinated I 131 Albumin
    Injection USP, III/214
Iodinated I 131 Albumin Aggregated
    Injection USP, III/214
Iodine
    Solution, Topical, USP, III/214
    Tincture USP, III/214
Iodine, Strong
    Solution USP, III/215
    Tincture USP, III/215
Iodipamide Meglumine
    Injection USP, III/215
Iodohippurate Sodium I 123
    Injection USP, III/215
Iodohippurate Sodium I 131
    Injection USP, III/216
Iodoquinol
    Tablets USP, III/216
Iofetamine Hydrochloride I 123
    Injection, III/216
Iohexol
    Injection, III/216
Ionamin, IV/MC-18

Iopamidol
  Injection USP, III/216
Iopanoic Acid
  Tablets USP, III/217
Iophendylate
  Injection USP, III/217
Iothalamate Meglumine
  Injection USP, III/217
Iothalamate Meglumine and Iothalamate Sodium
  Injection USP, III/217
Iothalamate Sodium
  Injection USP, III/217
Ioversol
  Injection, III/218
Ioxaglate Meglumine and Ioxaglate Sodium
  Injection, III/218
Ipecac
  Syrup USP, III/218
Ipodate Calcium
  for Suspension, Oral, USP, III/218
Ipodate Sodium
  Capsules USP, III/218
Ipratropium Bromide
  Aerosol, Inhalation, III/218
  Nasal, Inhalation, III/218
  Solution, Inhalation, III/218
Iron Dextran
  Injection USP, III/219
Iron-Polysaccharide
  Capsules, III/219
  Elixir, III/219
  Tablets, III/219
Iron Sorbitex
  Injection USP, III/219
Isobutane
  Isobutane NF, III/219
Isocarboxazid
  Tablets USP, III/219
Isoetharine
  Solution, Inhalation, USP, III/219
Isoetharine Mesylate
  Aerosol, Inhalation, USP, III/219
Isoflurane
  Isoflurane USP, III/220
Isoflurophate
  Ointment, Ophthalmic, USP, III/220
Isometheptene Mucate, Dichloralphenazone, and Acetaminophen
  Capsules, III/220
Isoniazid
  Injection USP, III/220
  Syrup USP, III/220
  Tablets USP, III/220
Isopropamide Iodide
  Tablets USP, III/220
Isopropyl Alcohol
  Isopropyl Alcohol USP, III/221
Isopropyl Alcohol, Azeotropic
  Azeotropic Isopropyl Alcohol USP, III/221
Isopropyl Alcohol, Rubbing
  Isopropyl Rubbing Alcohol USP, III/221
Isopropyl Myristate
  Isopropyl Myristate NF, III/221
Isopropyl Palmitate
  Isopropyl Palmitate NF, III/221
Isoproterenol
  Solution, Inhalation, USP, III/221
Isoproterenol Hydrochloride
  Aerosol, Inhalation, USP, III/221
  Injection, USP, III/221
  Tablets USP, III/221
Isoproterenol Hydrochloride and Phenylephrine Bitartrate
  Aerosol, Inhalation, USP, III/222

Isoproterenol Hydrochloride and Phenylephrine Hydrochloride
  Aerosol, Inhalation, III/222
Isoproterenol Sulfate
  Aerosol, Inhalation, USP, III/221
  Solution, Inhalation, USP, III/221
Isoptin, IV/MC-24
Isoptin SR, IV/MC-24
Isordil, IV/MC-12
Isosorbide
  Solution, Oral, USP, III/222
Isosorbide Dinitrate
  Capsules, III/222
  Capsules, Extended-release, USP, III/220, IV/MC-12
  Tablets USP, III/222, IV/MC-12
  Tablets, Chewable, USP, III/222, IV/MC-12
  Tablets, Extended-release, USP, III/222, IV/MC-12
  Tablets, Sublingual, USP, III/222, IV/MC-12
Isosorbide Mononitrate
  Tablets, III/222
Isotretinoin
  Capsules, III/223, IV/MC-12
Isoxsuprine Hydrochloride
  Injection USP, III/223
  Tablets USP, III/223
Isradipine
  Capsules, III/223, IV/MC-12
Ivermectin
  for Injection, III/223
  Paste, III/223
  Solution, Oral, III/223
  Tablets, III/223
  Tablets, Chewable, III/223

J

Juniper Tar
  Juniper Tar USP, III/223

K

Kanamycin Sulfate
  Capsules USP, III/224
  Injection USP, III/224
  Sterile USP, III/224
Kaolin
  Kaolin USP, III/224
Kaolin and Pectin
  Suspension, Oral, III/224
Kaolin, Pectin, Hyoscyamine Sulfate, Atropine Sulfate, Scopolamine Hydrobromide, and Opium
  Suspension, Oral, III/224
Kaolin, Pectin, and Paregoric
  Suspension, Oral, III/224
Keflex, IV/MC-4
Keftab, IV/MC-4
Kerlone, IV/MC-3
Ketamine Hydrochloride
  Injection USP, III/224
Ketazolam
  Capsules, III/224
Ketoconazole
  Cream, III/224
  Shampoo, III/224
  Suspension, Oral, III/224
  Tablets USP, III/224, IV/MC-12

Ketoprofen
  Capsules, III/225
  Capsules, Delayed-release, III/225
  Suppositories, III/225
  Tablets, Delayed-release, III/225
  Tablets, Extended-release, III/225
Ketorolac Tromethamine
  Injection, III/225
  Tablets, III/225
Klor-Con 8, IV/MC-19
Klor-Con 10, IV/MC-19
Klotrix, IV/MC-19
Krypton Kr 81m
  Krypton Kr 81m USP, III/225
K-Tab, IV/MC-19

L

Labeling, II/10
Labeling and Packaging Requirements for Controlled Substances, II/40
Labetalol Hydrochloride
  Injection USP, III/225
  Tablets USP, III/225, IV/MC-12
Labetalol Hydrochloride and Hydrochlorothiazide
  Tablets, III/225, IV/MC-12
Lactic Acid
  Lactic Acid USP, III/225
Lactose
  Lactose NF, III/226
Lactulose
  Concentrate USP, III/226
  Solution USP, III/226
Lanolin
  Lanolin USP, III/226
Lanolin Alcohols
  Lanolin Alcohols NF, III/226
Lanolin, Modified
  Modified Lanolin USP, III/226
Lanoxicaps, IV/MC-7
Lanoxin, IV/MC-7
Lasix, IV/MC-10
Laws and Regulations, II/30
Lecithin
  Lecithin NF, III/226
Ledercillin VK, IV/MC-18
Leucovorin Calcium
  Injection USP, III/227
  for Injection, III/227
  for Solution, Oral, III/227
  Tablets, III/227
Leukocyte Typing Serum
  Leukocyte Typing Serum USP, III/227
Leuprolide Acetate
  Injection, III/227
  for Injection, III/227
Levamisole Hydrochloride
  Bolus, III/227
  Paste, III/227
  Powder, Soluble, III/227
  Powder for Drench, Soluble, III/227
  Tablets, III/227
Levatol, IV/MC-18
Levlen 21, IV/MC-12
Levlen 28, IV/MC-13
Levobunolol Hydrochloride
  Solution, Ophthalmic, USP, III/228
Levocarnitine
  Capsules, III/228
  Solution, Oral, USP, III/228
  Tablets, III/228
Levodopa
  Capsules USP, III/228
  Tablets USP, III/228

Levonorgestrel
   Implants, III/228
Levonorgestrel and Ethinyl Estradiol
   Tablets USP, III/228, IV/MC-12, MC-13
Levopropoxyphene Napsylate
   Capsules USP, III/228
   Suspension, Oral, USP, III/228
Levorphanol Tartrate
   Injection, III/229
   Tablets USP, III/229
Levothyroxine Sodium
   Injection, III/229
   for Injection, III/229
   Powder, III/229
   Tablets USP, III/229, IV/MC-13
Levoxine, IV/MC-13
Librax, IV/MC-4
Libritabs, IV/MC-4
Librium, IV/MC-4
Lidocaine
   Aerosol, Topical, USP (Solution), III/229
   Ointment USP, III/229
   Solution, Topical, Oral, USP, III/229
Lidocaine and Epinephrine
   Injection USP, III/230
Lidocaine Hydrochloride
   Injection USP, III/229
   Jelly USP, III/229
   Ointment, III/229
   Solution, Topical, USP, III/229
   Solution, Topical, Oral, USP, III/229
   Sterile USP, III/229
Lidocaine Hydrochloride and Dextrose
   Injection USP, III/230
Lidocaine and Prilocaine
   Cream, III/230
Light Mineral Oil—See Mineral Oil, Light
Limbitrol, IV/MC-4
Limbitrol DS, IV/MC-4
Lime
   Lime USP, III/230
Lime, Sulfurated—See Sulfurated Lime
Lincomycin Hydrochloride
   Capsules USP, III/230
   Injection USP, III/230
   Sterile USP, III/230
   Syrup USP, III/230
Lindane
   Cream USP, III/231
   Lotion USP, III/231
   Shampoo USP, III/231
Lioresal, IV/MC-3
Liothyronine Sodium
   Injection, III/231
   Tablets USP, III/231
Liotrix
   Tablets USP, III/231
Liquid Glucose—See Glucose, Liquid
Lisinopril
   Tablets USP, III/231, IV/MC-13
Lisinopril and Hydrochlorothiazide
   Tablets, III/231, IV/MC-13
Lithium Carbonate
   Capsules USP, III/231, IV/MC-13
   Capsules, Slow-release, III/231
   Tablets USP, III/231, IV/MC-13
   Tablets, Extended-release, USP, III/231, IV/MC-13
Lithium Citrate
   Syrup USP, III/231
Lithobid, IV/MC-13
Lodine, IV/MC-9
Loestrin, IV/MC-17
Loestrin Fe 1/20, IV/MC-17
Loestrin Fe 1.5/30, IV/MC-17

Lomotil, IV/MC-7
Lomustine
   Capsules, III/232
Loniten, IV/MC-15
Lo-Ovral, IV/MC-17
Loperamide Hydrochloride
   Capsules USP, III/232, IV/MC-13
   Solution, Oral, III/232
   Tablets, III/232
Lopid, IV/MC-10
Lopressor, IV/MC-15
Lopressor HCT, IV/MC-15
Lopurin, IV/MC-1
Lorabid, IV/MC-3
Loratadine
   Tablets, III/232
Lorazepam
   Injection USP, III/232
   Solution, Concentrated Oral, USP, III/232
   Tablets USP, III/232, IV/MC-13
   Tablets, Sublingual, III/232
Lorelco, IV/MC-19
Lotensin, IV/MC-3
Lovastatin
   Tablets, III/232, IV/MC-14
Loxapine
   Capsules USP, III/232
Loxapine Hydrochloride
   Injection, III/232
   Solution, Oral, III/232
Loxapine Succinate
   Capsules, III/232
   Tablets, III/232
Lozol, IV/MC-12
Ludiomil, IV/MC-14
Lufyllin, IV/MC-8
Lufyllin-400, IV/MC-8
Lypressin
   Solution, Nasal, USP, III/233

M

Macrodantin, IV/MC-16
Mafenide Acetate
   Cream USP, III/233
   Solution, III/233
Magaldrate
   Suspension, Oral, USP, III/233
   Tablets USP, III/233
Magaldrate and Simethicone
   Suspension, Oral, USP, III/233
   Tablets USP (Chewable), III/233
Magnesium Aluminum Silicate
   Magnesium Aluminum Silicate NF, III/233
Magnesium Carbonate
   Magnesium Carbonate USP, III/234
Magnesium Carbonate and Sodium Bicarbonate
   for Suspension, Oral, USP, III/234
Magnesium Chloride
   Magnesium Chloride USP, III/234
Magnesium Citrate
   Solution, Oral, USP, III/234
Magnesium Gluconate
   Tablets USP, III/234
Magnesium Hydroxide
   Magnesia Tablets USP, III/235
   Milk of Magnesia USP, III/235
   Paste USP, III/235
Magnesium Hydroxide and Mineral Oil
   Milk of Magnesia and Mineral Oil Emulsion, III/235

Magnesium Hydroxide, Mineral Oil, and Glycerin
   Milk of Magnesia, Mineral Oil, and Glycerin Emulsion, III/235
Magnesium Oxide
   Capsules USP, III/235
   Tablets USP, III/235
Magnesium Phosphate
   Magnesium Phosphate USP, III/235
Magnesium Salicylate
   Tablets USP, III/235
Magnesium Silicate
   Magnesium Silicate NF, III/236
Magnesium Stearate
   Magnesium Stearate NF, III/236
Magnesium Sulfate
   (Crystals) USP, III/236
   Injection USP, III/236
   Tablets, III/236
Magnesium Trisilicate
   Tablets USP, III/236
Magnesium Trisilicate, Alumina, and Magnesia
   Suspension, Oral, III/236
   Tablets, Chewable, III/236
Malathion
   Lotion USP, III/237
Malic Acid
   Malic Acid NF, III/237
Maltodextrin
   Maltodextrin NF, III/237
Malt Soup Extract
   Powder, III/237
   Solution, Oral, III/237
   Tablets, III/237
Malt Soup Extract and Psyllium
   Powder, III/237
Manganese Chloride
   Injection USP, III/237
Manganese Sulfate
   Injection USP, III/237
Mannitol
   Injection USP, III/238
   Mannitol USP, III/238
Mannitol and Sodium Chloride
   Mannitol in Sodium Chloride Injection USP, III/238
Manufacture of tablets, II/18
Maprotiline Hydrochloride
   Tablets USP, III/238, IV/MC-14
Maxzide, IV/MC-24
Mazindol
   Tablets USP, III/238
Measles, Mumps, and Rubella Virus Vaccine Live
   Measles, Mumps, and Rubella Virus Vaccine Live USP, III/239
Measles and Mumps Virus Vaccine Live
   Measles and Mumps Virus Vaccine Live USP, III/238
Measles and Rubella Virus Vaccine Live
   Measles and Rubella Virus Vaccine Live USP, III/239
Measles Virus Vaccine Live
   Measles Virus Vaccine Live USP, III/239
Mebendazole
   Tablets USP, III/239
Mecamylamine Hydrochloride
   Tablets USP, III/240
Mechlorethamine Hydrochloride
   for Injection USP, III/240
   Ointment, III/240
   Solution, Topical, III/240

Meclizine Hydrochloride
Capsules, III/240
Tablets USP, III/240, IV/MC-14
Tablets, Chewable, IV/MC-14
Meclocycline Sulfosalicylate
Cream USP, III/240
Meclofenamate Sodium
Capsules USP, III/240, IV/MC-14
Meclomen, IV/MC-14
Medical Air—See Air, Medical
Medicine Chart, IV/1
Medrol, IV/MC-15
Medroxyprogesterone Acetate
Suspension, Sterile, USP, III/241
Tablets USP, III/241, IV/MC-14
Medrysone
Suspension, Ophthalmic, USP, III/241
Mefenamic Acid
Capsules USP, III/241
Mefloquine Hydrochloride
Tablets, III/241
Megestrol Acetate
Tablets USP, III/241
Mellaril, IV/MC-23
Melphalan
Tablets USP, III/241
Menadiol Sodium Diphosphate
Injection USP, III/241
Tablets USP, III/241
Menadione
Injection USP, III/242
Meningococcal Polysaccharide Vaccine
for Injection, III/242
Group A USP, III/242
Groups A and C Combined USP, III/242
Group C USP, III/242
Menotropins
for Injection USP, III/242
Menthol
Menthol USP, III/242
Mepenzolate Bromide
Syrup USP, III/243
Tablets USP, III/243
Meperidine Hydrochloride
Injection USP, III/243
Syrup USP, III/243
Tablets USP, III/243, IV/MC-14
Meperidine Hydrochloride and Acetamino-
phen
Tablets, III/243
Mephentermine Sulfate
Injection USP, III/243
Mephenytoin
Tablets USP, III/243
Mephobarbital
Tablets USP, III/243
Mepivacaine Hydrochloride
Injection USP, III/244
Mepivacaine Hydrochloride and Levonorde-
frin
Injection USP, III/244
Meprobamate
Capsules, Extended-release, III/244
Suspension, Oral, USP, III/244
Tablets USP, III/244
Meprobamate and Aspirin
Tablets, III/244
Meprylcaine Hydrochloride and Epinephrine
Injection USP, III/244
Mercaptopurine
Tablets USP, III/245
Mercury, Ammoniated
Ointment USP, III/245
Ointment, Ophthalmic, USP, III/245

Mesalamine
Suppositories, III/245
Suspension, Rectal, III/245
Tablets, Delayed-release, III/245
Mesna
Injection, III/245
Mesoridazine Besylate
Injection USP, III/245
Solution, Oral, USP, III/245
Tablets USP, III/245
Metaproterenol Sulfate
Aerosol, Inhalation, USP, III/246
Solution, Inhalation, USP, III/246
Syrup USP, III/246
Tablets USP, III/246, IV/MC-14
Metaraminol Bitartrate
Injection USP, III/246
Metaxalone
Tablets, III/246
Methacholine Chloride
for Inhalation, III/246
Methacrylic Acid Copolymer
Methacrylic Acid Copolymer NF, III/246
Methacycline Hydrochloride
Capsules USP, III/247
Suspension, Oral, USP, III/247
Methadone Hydrochloride
Concentrate, Oral, USP, III/247
Injection USP, III/247
Solution, Oral, USP, III/247
Tablets USP, III/247
Methamphetamine
Tablets USP, III/247
Methamphetamine Hydrochloride
Tablets, Extended-release, III/247
Methantheline Bromide
Sterile USP, III/247
Tablets USP, III/247
Metharbital
Tablets USP, III/248
Methazolamide
Tablets USP, III/248
Methdilazine
Tablets USP, III/248
Methdilazine Hydrochloride
Syrup USP, III/248
Tablets USP, III/248
Methenamine
Elixir USP, III/248
Tablets USP, III/248
Methenamine Hippurate
Tablets USP, III/248
Methenamine Mandelate
for Solution, Oral, USP, III/248
Suspension, Oral, USP, III/248
Tablets USP, III/248
Methenamine and Monobasic Sodium Phos-
phate
Tablets USP, III/249
Methicillin Sodium
for Injection USP, III/249
Sterile USP, III/249
Methimazole
Tablets USP, III/249
Methocarbamol
Injection USP, III/249
Tablets USP, III/249, IV/MC-14
Methocarbamol and Aspirin
Tablets, IV/MC-14
Methohexital Sodium
for Injection USP, III/250
for Solution, Rectal, III/250
Methotrexate
Tablets USP, III/250

Methotrexate Sodium
Injection USP, III/250
for Injection USP, III/250
Methotrimeprazine
Injection USP, III/250
Methotrimeprazine Hydrochloride
Solution, Oral, III/250
Syrup, III/250
Methotrimeprazine Maleate
Tablets, III/250
Methoxamine Hydrochloride
Injection USP, III/251
Methoxsalen
Capsules USP, III/251
Solution, Topical, USP, III/251
Methoxyflurane
Methoxyflurane USP, III/251
Methscopolamine Bromide
Tablets USP, III/251
Methsuximide
Capsules USP, III/251
Methychlothiazide
Tablets USP, III/251, IV/MC-14
Methyl Alcohol
Methyl Alcohol NF, III/252
Methylbenzethonium Chloride
Lotion USP, III/252
Ointment USP, III/252
Powder USP, III/252
Methylcellulose
Capsules, III/252
(Granules or Powder) USP, III/252
Solution, Ophthalmic, USP, III/252
Solution, Oral, USP, III/252
Tablets USP, III/252
Methyldopa
Suspension, Oral, USP, III/252
Tablets USP, III/252, IV/MC-14
Methyldopa and Chlorothiazide
Tablets USP, III/253
Methyldopa and Hydrochlorothiazide
Tablets USP, III/253, IV/MC-14, MC-15
Methyldopate Hydrochloride
Injection USP, III/252
Methylene Blue
Injection USP, III/253
Methylene Chloride
Methylene Chloride NF, III/253
Methylergonovine Maleate
Injection USP, III/253
Tablets USP, III/253
Methyl Isobutyl Ketone
Methyl Isobutyl Ketone NF, III/253
Methylparaben
Methylparaben NF, III/254
Methylparaben Sodium
Methylparaben Sodium NF, III/254
Methylphenidate Hydrochloride
Tablets USP, III/254, IV/MC-15
Tablets, Extended-release, USP, III/254, IV/MC-15
Methylprednisolone
Tablets USP, III/254, IV/MC-15
Methylprednisolone Acetate
Cream, III/254
for Enema USP, III/254
Ointment, III/254
Suspension, Sterile, USP, III/254
Methylprednisolone Sodium Succinate
for Injection, III/254
Methyl Salicylate
Methyl Salicylate NF, III/255
Methyltestosterone
Capsules USP, III/255
Tablets USP, III/255

Methyprylon
    Capsules USP, III/255
    Tablets USP, III/255
Methysergide Maleate
    Tablets USP, III/255
Metipranolol Hydrochloride
    Solution, Ophthalmic, III/256
Metoclopramide
    Injection USP, III/256
    Solution, Oral, USP, III/256
    Tablets USP, III/256, IV/MC-15
Metoclopramide Hydrochloride
    Syrup, III/256
Metocurine Iodide
    Injection USP, III/256
Metolazone
    Tablets USP, III/256, IV/MC-15
    Tablets, Prompt, IV/MC-15
Metoprolol Succinate
    Tablets, Extended-release, III/256
Metoprolol Tartrate
    Injection USP, III/256
    Tablets USP, III/256, IV/MC-15
    Tablets, Extended-release, III/256, IV/
       MC-15
Metoprolol Tartrate and Hydrochlorothiazide
    Tablets USP, III/257, IV/MC-15
Metric and Apothecary Dose Equivalents,
    II/29
Metrizamide
    for Injection, III/257
Metronidazole
    Capsules, III/257
    Cream, Vaginal, III/257
    Gel USP, III/257
    Injection USP, III/257
    Suppositories, Vaginal, III/257
    Tablets USP, III/257, IV/MC-15
Metronidazole Hydrochloride
    for Injection, III/257
Metronidazole and Nystatin
    Cream, Vaginal, III/257
    Suppositories, Vaginal, III/257
    Tablets, Vaginal, III/257
Metyrapone
    Tablets USP, III/257
Metyrosine
    Capsules USP, III/258
Mevacor, IV/MC-14
Mexiletine Hydrochloride
    Capsules USP, III/258
Mezlocillin Sodium
    Sterile USP, III/258
Miconazole
    Injection USP, III/258
Miconazole Nitrate
    Cream USP, III/258
    Cream, Vaginal, III/258
    Lotion, III/258
    Powder, Topical, USP, III/258
    Powder, Topical, Aerosol, III/258
    Solution, Topical, Aerosol, III/258
    Suppositories, Vaginal, USP, III/258
    Tampons, Vaginal, III/258
Microcrystalline Wax—See Wax, Microcrys-
    talline
Micro-K, IV/MC-19
Micro-K 10, IV/MC-19
Micronase, IV/MC-10
Midazolam Hydrochloride
    Injection, III/258
Milk of Magnesia—See Magnesium Hydrox-
    ide

Mineral Oil
    Emulsion USP, III/259
    Enema USP, III/259
    Gel, III/259
    Mineral Oil USP, III/259
    Suspension, Oral, III/259
Mineral Oil, Light
    Light Mineral Oil NF, III/259
    Mineral Oil, Topical, Light, USP, III/
       259
Mineral Oil and Cascara Sagrada Extract
    Emulsion, III/259
Mineral Oil, Glycerin, and Phenolphthalein
    Emulsion, III/259
Mineral Oil and Phenolphthalein
    Emulsion, III/259
    Suspension, Oral, III/259
Minipress, IV/MC-19
Minizide, IV/MC-19
Minocin, IV/MC-15
Minocyline Hydrochloride
    Capsules USP, III/259, IV/MC-15
    Sterile USP, III/259
    Suspension, Oral, USP, III/259
    Tablets USP, III/259, IV/MC-15
Minoxidil
    Solution, Topical, III/260
    Tablets USP, III/260, IV/MC-15
Misoprostol
    Tablets, III/260, IV/MC-15
Mitomycin
    for Injection USP, III/260
Mitotane
    Tablets USP, III/260
Mitoxantrone Hydrochloride
    Concentrate, for Injection, USP, III/260
Modification, Transfer, and Termination of
    Registration, II/37
Moduretic, IV/MC-1
Molindone Hydrochloride
    Solution, Oral, III/261
    Tablets, III/261
Mometasone Furoate
    Cream, III/261
    Lotion, III/261
    Ointment, III/261
Monobenzone
    Cream USP, III/261
Mono- and Di-acetylated Monoglycerides
    Mono- and Di-acetylated Monoglycerides
       NF, III/261
Mono- and Di-glycerides
    Mono- and Di-glycerides NF, III/261
Monoethanolamine
    Monoethanolamine NF, III/261
Monooctanoin
    Irrigation, III/262
Monopril, IV/MC-10
Monosodium Glutamate
    Monosodium Glutamate NF, III/262
Monostearate, Glyceryl—See Glyceryl
    Monostearate
Monothioglycerol
    Monothioglycerol NF, III/262
Moricizine Hydrochloride
    Tablets, III/262, IV/MC-15
Morphine Hydrochloride
    Suppositories, III/262
    Syrup, III/262
    Tablets, III/262
    Tablets, Extended-release, III/262

Morphine Sulfate
    Injection USP, III/262
    Solution, Oral, III/262
    Solution (Preservative-free), Sterile, III/
       262
    Suppositories, III/262
    Syrup, III/262
    Tablets, III/262
    Tablets, Extended-release, III/262
    Tablets, Soluble, III/262
Morrhuate Sodium
    Injection USP, III/263
Motrin, IV/MC-12
Moxalactam Disodium
    for Injection USP, III/263
Mumps Skin Test Antigen
    Mumps Skin Test Antigen USP, III/263
Mumps Virus Vaccine Live
    Mumps Virus Vaccine Live USP, III/
       263
Mupirocin
    Ointment, III/264
Muromonab-CD3
    Injection, III/264
Mycelex Troches, IV/MC-6
Mykrox, IV/MC-15
Myristyl Alcohol
    Myristyl Alcohol NF, III/264

N

Nabilone
    Capsules, III/264
Nabumetone
    Tablets, III/264
Nadolol
    Tablets USP, III/264, IV/MC-15, MC-
       16
Nadolol and Bendroflumethiazide
    Tablets USP, III/264, IV/MC-16
Nafcillin Sodium
    Capsules USP, III/264
    Injection USP, III/264
    for Injection USP, III/264
    for Solution, Oral, USP, III/264
    Sterile USP, III/264
    Tablets USP, III/264
Naftifine Hydrochloride
    Cream, III/265
    Gel, III/265
Nalbuphine Hydrochloride
    Injection, III/265
Naldecon, IV/MC-4
Nalfon, IV/MC-9
Nalfon 200, IV/MC-9
Nalidixic Acid
    Suspension, Oral, USP, III/265
    Tablets USP, III/265, IV/MC-16
Nalorphine Hydrochloride
    Injection USP, III/265
Naloxone Hydrochloride
    Injection USP, III/266
Naltrexone Hydrochloride
    Tablets, III/266
Nandrolone Decanoate
    Injection USP, III/266
Nandrolone Phenpropionate
    Injection, III/266
Naphazoline Hydrochloride
    Solution, Nasal, USP, III/266
    Solution, Ophthalmic, USP, III/266
Naprosyn, IV/MC-16

Naproxen
  Suppositories, III/266
  Suspension, Oral, III/266
  Tablets USP, III/266, IV/MC-16
  Tablets, Extended-release, III/266
Naproxen Sodium
  Tablets USP, III/266, IV/MC-16
Natamycin
  Suspension, Ophthalmic, USP, III/267
Naturetin, IV/MC-3
Navane, IV/MC-23
NegGram, IV/MC-16
Neomycin Sulfate
  Cream USP, III/267
  Ointment USP, III/267
  Ointment, Ophthalmic USP, III/267
  Solution, Oral, USP, III/267
  Sterile USP, III/267
  Tablets USP, III/267
Neomycin Sulfate and Bacitracin
  Ointment USP, III/267
Neomycin Sulfate and Bacitracin Zinc
  Ointment USP, III/267
Neomycin Sulfate and Dexamethasone So-
    dium Phosphate
  Cream USP, III/268
  Ointment, Ophthalmic, USP, III/268
  Solution, Ophthalmic, USP, III/268
Neomycin Sulfate and Fluocinolone Aceto-
    nide
  Cream USP, III/268
Neomycin Sulfate and Fluorometholone
  Ointment USP, III/268
Neomycin Sulfate and Flurandrenolide
  Cream USP, III/268
  Lotion USP, III/268
  Ointment USP, III/268
Neomycin Sulfate and Gramicidin
  Ointment USP, III/268
Neomycin Sulfate and Hydrocortisone
  Cream USP, III/268
  Ointment USP, III/268
  Suspension, Otic, USP, III/268
Neomycin Sulfate and Hydrocortisone Ace-
    tate
  Cream USP, III/268
  Lotion USP, III/268
  Ointment USP, III/268
  Ointment, Ophthalmic, USP, III/268
  Suspension, Ophthalmic, USP, III/268
Neomycin Sulfate and Methylprednisolone
    Acetate
  Cream USP, III/269
Neomycin and Polymyxin B Sulfates
  Cream USP, III/269
  Ointment, Ophthalmic, USP, III/269
  Solution, for Irrigation, USP, III/269
  Solution, Ophthalmic, USP, III/269
Neomycin and Polymyxin B Sulfates and
    Bacitracin
  Ointment USP, III/269
  Ointment, Ophthalmic, USP, III/269
Neomycin and Polymyxin B Sulfates, Baci-
    tracin, and Lidocaine
  Ointment USP, III/270
Neomycin and Polymyxin B Sulfates and
    Bacitracin Zinc
  Ointment USP, III/269
  Ointment, Ophthalmic, USP, III/269
Neomycin and Polymyxin B Sulfates, Baci-
    tracin, and Hydrocortisone Acetate
  Ointment USP, III/270
  Ointment, Ophthalmic, USP, III/270
Neomycin and Polymyxin B Sulfates, Baci-
    tracin Zinc, and Hydrocortisone
  Ointment USP, III/270
  Ointment, Ophthalmic, USP, III/270

Neomycin and Polymyxin B Sulfates, Baci-
    tracin Zinc, and Hydrocortisone Ace-
    tate
  Ointment, Ophthalmic, USP, III/270
Neomycin and Polymyxin B Sulfates and
    Dexamethasone
  Ointment, Ophthalmic, USP, III/270
  Suspension, Ophthalmic, USP, III/270
Neomycin and Polymyxin B Sulfates and
    Gramicidin
  Cream USP, III/270
  Solution, Ophthalmic, USP, III/270
Neomycin and Polymyxin B Sulfates, Gram-
    icidin, and Hydrocortisone Acetate
  Cream USP, III/270
Neomycin and Polymyxin B Sulfates and
    Hydrocortisone
  Solution, Otic, USP, III/271
  Suspension, Ophthalmic, USP, III/271
  Suspension, Otic, USP, III/271
Neomycin and Polymyxin B Sulfates and
    Hydrocortisone Acetate
  Cream USP, III/271
  Suspension, Ophthalmic, USP, III/271
Neomycin and Polymyxin B Sulfates and
    Prednisolone Acetate
  Suspension, Ophthalmic, USP, III/271
Neomycin Sulfate and Prednisolone Acetate
  Ointment USP, III/271
  Ointment, Ophthalmic, USP, III/271
  Suspension, Ophthalmic, USP, III/271
Neomycin Sulfate and Prednisolone Sodium
    Phosphate
  Ointment, Ophthalmic, USP, III/271
Neomycin Sulfate, Sulfacetamide Sodium,
    and Prednisolone Acetate
  Ointment, Ophthalmic, USP, III/271
Neomycin Sulfate and Triamcinolone Aceto-
    nide
  Cream USP, III/272
  Ointment, Ophthalmic, USP, III/272
Neostigmine Bromide
  Tablets USP, III/272
Neostigmine Methylsulfate
  Injection USP, III/272
Netilmicin Sulfate
  Injection USP, III/272
Niacin
  Capsules, Extended-release, III/272, IV/
    MC-16
  Injection USP, III/272
  Solution, Oral, III/272
  Tablets USP, III/272, IV/MC-16
  Tablets, Extended-release, III/272, IV/
    MC-16
Niacinamide
  Capsules, III/272
  Gel, III/272
  Injection USP, III/272
  Tablets USP, III/272
Nicardipine Hydrochloride
  Capsules, III/273, IV/MC-16
Niclosamide
  Tablets, Chewable, III/273
Nicobid, IV/MC-16
Nicolar, IV/MC-16
Nicorette, IV/MC-16
Nicotine
  Systems, Transdermal, III/273
Nicotine Polacrilex
  Tablets, Chewing Gum, III/273, IV/MC-
    16
Nicotinyl Alcohol Tartrate
  Tablets, Extended-release, III/273

Nifedipine
  Capsules USP, III/273, IV/MC-16
  Tablets, III/273
  Tablets, Extended-release, III/273, IV/
    MC-16
Nimodipine
  Capsules, III/273, IV/MC-16
Nimotop, IV/MC-16
Nitrazepam
  Tablets, III/273
Nitric Acid
  Nitric Acid NF, III/274
Nitrofurantoin
  Capsules USP, III/274, IV/MC-16
  Suspension, Oral, USP, III/274
  Tablets USP, III/274, IV/MC-16
Nitrofurazone
  Cream USP, III/274
  Ointment USP, III/274
  Solution, Topical, USP, III/274
Nitrogen
  Nitrogen NF, III/274
Nitrogen 13 Ammonia—See Ammonia N 13
Nitrogen 97 Percent
  Nitrogen 97 Percent NF, III/275
Nitroglycerin
  Aerosol, Lingual, III/275
  Capsules, Extended-release, III/275, IV/
    MC-16
  Injection USP, III/275
  Ointment USP, III/275
  Systems, Transdermal, III/275
  Tablets USP (Sublingual), III/275, IV/
    MC-16
  Tablets, Buccal, Extended-release, III/
    275
  Tablets, Extended-release, III/275
Nitromersol
  Solution, Topical, USP, III/275
Nitrostat, IV/MC-16
Nitrous Oxide
  Nitrous Oxide USP, III/275
Nizatidine
  Capsules USP, III/275, IV/MC-16
Nizoral, IV/MC-12
Nolvadex, IV/MC-22
Nonoxynol 9
  Cream, Vaginal, III/276
  Film, Vaginal, III/276
  Foam, Vaginal, III/276
  Gel, Vaginal, III/276
  Jelly, Vaginal, III/276
  Nonoxynol 9 USP, III/276
  Sponge, Vaginal, III/276
  Suppositories, Vaginal, III/276
Nonoxynol 10
  Nonoxynol 10 NF, III/276
Nordette, IV/MC-13
Norepinephrine Bitartrate
  Injection USP, III/276
Norethindrone
  Tablets USP, III/276
Norethindrone Acetate
  Tablets USP, III/276
Norethindrone Acetate and Ethinyl Estradiol
  Tablets USP, III/277, IV/MC-17
Norethindrone Acetate/Ethinyl Estradiol
    and Ferrous Fumarate
  Tablets, IV/MC-17
Norethindrone and Ethinyl Estradiol
  Tablets USP, III/277, IV/MC-16, MC-
    17
Norethindrone and Mestranol
  Tablets USP, III/277, IV/MC-17
Norethynodrel and Mestranol
  Tablets, III/277

Norfloxacin
    Solution, Ophthalmic, III/277
    Tablets USP, III/277, IV/MC-17
Norgestrel
    Tablets USP, III/277
Norgestrel and Ethinyl Estradiol
    Tablets USP, III/278, IV/MC-17
Normodyne, IV/MC-12
Normozide, IV/MC-12
Noroxin, IV/MC-17
Norpace, IV/MC-8
Norpace CR, IV/MC-8
Norpramin, IV/MC-6
Nortriptyline Hydrochloride
    Capsules USP, III/278, IV/MC-17
    Solution, Oral, USP, III/278
Novobiocin Calcium
    Suspension, Oral, USP, III/278
Novobiocin Sodium
    Capsules USP, III/278
Nylidrin Hydrochloride
    Injection USP, III/278
    Tablets USP, III/278
Nystatin
    Cream USP, III/278
    Cream, Vaginal, III/278
    Lotion USP, III/278
    Lozenges USP, III/278
    Ointment USP, III/278
    Powder, Topical, USP, III/278
    Suppositories, Vaginal, USP, III/278
    Suspension, Oral, USP, III/278
    for Suspension, Oral, USP, III/278
    Tablets USP, III/278
    Tablets, Vaginal, USP, III/278
Nystatin and Clioquinol
    Ointment USP, III/279
Nystatin, Neomycin Sulfate, Gramicidin,
        and Triamcinolone Acetonide
    Cream USP, III/279
    Ointment USP, III/279
Nystatin and Triamcinolone Acetate
    Cream USP, III/279
    Ointment USP, III/279

O

Octoxynol 9
    Octoxynol 9 NF, III/279
Octreotide Acetate
    Injection, III/280
Octyldodecanol
    Octyldodecanol NF, III/280
Ofloxacin
    Tablets, III/280, IV/MC-17
Ogen .625, IV/MC-9
Ogen 1.25, IV/MC-9
Ogen 2.5, IV/MC-9
Ogen 5, IV/MC-9
Ointment, Hydrophilic
    Hydrophilic Ointment USP, III/280
Ointments, Ophthalmic, II/8
Ointment, White
    White Ointment USP, III/280
Ointment, Yellow
    Yellow Ointment USP, III/280
Oleic Acid
    Oleic Acid NF, III/280
Oleovitamin A and D
    Capsules USP, III/281
Oleyl Alcohol
    Oleyl Alcohol NF, III/281
Olive Oil
    Olive Oil NF, III/281
Olsalazine Sodium
    Capsules, III/281

Omeprazole
    Capsules, Delayed-release, III/281, IV/
        MC-17
Omnipen, IV/MC-2
Ondansetron Hydrochloride
    Injection, III/281
Ondansetron Hydrochloride Dihydrate
    Injection, III/281
    Tablets, III/281
Opium
    Powdered USP, III/281
    Tincture USP (Laudanum), III/281
Opium Alkaloids Hydrochlorides
    Injection, III/281
Orange Book—See Approved Drug Products
        with Therapeutic Equivalence Evalua-
        tions, I/1
Orange Flower Oil
    Orange Flower Oil NF, III/282
Order Forms, II/44
Oretic, IV/MC-11
Organidin, IV/MC-12
Orinase, IV/MC-23
Ornade Spansules, IV/MC-4
Orphan Drug and Biological Designations, I/
        364
Orphenadrine Citrate
    Injection USP, III/282
    Tablets, Extended-release, III/282
Orphenadrine Citrate, Aspirin, and Caffeine
    Tablets, III/282
Orphenadrine Hydrochloride
    Tablets, III/282
Ortho-Novum 1/35, IV/MC-16, MC-17
Ortho-Novum 1/50, IV/MC-17
Ortho-Novum 7/7/7, IV/MC-17
Osmolarity, II/8
OTC Drug Product List, I/273
Ovcon, IV/MC-16
Ovral, IV/MC-17
Oxacillin Sodium
    Capsules USP, III/282, IV/MC-17
    Injection USP, III/282
    for Injection USP, III/282
    for Solution, Oral, USP, III/282
    Sterile USP, III/282
Oxamniquine
    Capsules USP, III/283
Oxandrolone
    Tablets USP, III/283
Oxazepam
    Capsules USP, III/283, IV/MC-17
    Tablets USP, III/283, IV/MC-17, MC-
        18
Oxidized Cellulose—See Cellulose, Oxidized
Oxprenolol
    Tablets USP, III/283
    Tablets, Extended-release, USP, III/283
Oxtriphylline
    Solution, Oral, USP, III/284
    Syrup, III/284
    Tablets, III/284
    Tablets, Delayed-release, USP, III/284
    Tablets, Extended-release, USP, III/284
Oxtriphylline and Guaifenesin
    Elixir, III/284
    Tablets, III/284
Oxybutynin Chloride
    Syrup USP, III/284
    Tablets USP, III/284, IV/MC-18
Oxycodone
    Tablets USP, III/284, IV/MC-18
Oxycodone and Acetaminophen
    Capsules USP, III/284
    Solution, Oral, III/284
    Tablets USP, III/284

Oxycodone and Aspirin
    Tablets USP, III/285, IV/MC-18
Oxycodone Hydrochloride
    Solution, Oral, USP, III/284
    Suppositories, III/284
Oxycodone Hydrochloride and Acetamino-
        phen
    Capsules USP, IV/MC-18
    Tablets USP, IV/MC-18
Oxygen
    Oxygen USP, III/285
Oxygen 93 Percent
    Oxygen 93 Percent USP, III/285
Oxymetazoline Hydrochloride
    Solution, Nasal, USP, III/285
    Solution, Ophthalmic, USP, III/285
Oxymetholone
    Tablets USP, III/285
Oxymorphone Hydrochloride
    Injection USP, III/286
    Suppositories USP, III/286
Oxyphenbutazone
    Tablets USP, III/286
Oxyphencyclimine Hydrochloride
    Tablets USP, III/286
Oxyquinoline Sulfate
    Oxyquinoline Sulfate NF, III/286
Oxytetracycline
    Injection USP, III/286
    Sterile USP, III/286
    Tablets USP, III/286
Oxytetracycline Calcium
    Suspension, Oral, USP, III/286
Oxytetracycline Hydrochloride
    Capsules USP, III/286
    for Injection USP, III/286
    Sterile USP, III/286
Oxytetracycline Hydrochloride and Hydro-
        cortisone
    Ointment USP, III/287
Oxytetracycline Hydrochloride and Hydro-
        cortisone Acetate
    Suspension, Ophthalmic, USP, III/287
Oxytetracycline Hydrochloride, Phenazopyr-
        idine Hydrochloride, and Sulfamethi-
        zole
    Capsules USP, III/288
Oxytetracycline Hydrochloride and Poly-
        myxin B Sulfate
    Ointment USP, III/288
    Ointment, Ophthalmic, USP, III/288
    Powder, Topical, USP, III/288
    Tablets, Vaginal, USP, III/288
Oxytetracycline and Nystatin
    Capsules USP, III/287
    for Suspension, Oral, USP, III/287
Oxytocin
    Injection USP, III/288
    Solution, Nasal, USP, III/288

P

Packaging—Child-Safety, II/91
Packaging Requirements, II/22
Padimate O
    Lotion USP, III/288
Pamelor, IV/MC-17
Pancrease, IV/MC-18
Pancreatin
    Capsules USP, III/288
    Tablets USP, III/288
Pancreatin, Pepsin, Bile Salts, Hyoscyamine
        Sulfate, Atropine Sulfate, Scopola-
        mine Hydrobromide, and Phenobarbi-
        tal
    Tablets, III/288

Pancrelipase
    Capsules USP, III/289
    Capsules, Delayed-release, III/289, IV/
        MC-18
    Powder, III/289
    Tablets USP, III/289
    Tablets, Delayed-release, USP, III/289
Pancuronium Bromide
    Injection, III/289
Panmycin, IV/MC-22
Pantothenic Acid
    Tablets, III/290
Papain
    Tablets for Solution, Topical, USP, III/
        290
Papaverine Hydrochloride
    Capsules, Extended-release, III/290
    Injection USP, III/290
    Tablets USP, III/290
Parachlorophenol, Camphorated
    Camphorated Parachlorophenol USP,
        III/290
Paraffin
    Paraffin NF, III/290
Paraffin, Synthetic
    Synthetic Paraffin NF, III/290
Parafon Forte DSC, IV/MC-5
Paraldehyde
    Paraldehyde USP, III/291
    Sterile, III/291
Paramethadione
    Capsules USP, III/291
    Solution, Oral, USP, III/291
Paramethasone Acetate
    Tablets USP, III/291
Paregoric
    Paregoric USP, III/291
Pargyline Hydrochloride
    Tablets USP, III/291
Pargyline Hydrochloride and Methylclothia-
        zide
    Tablets, III/292
Parlodel, IV/MC-3
Parnate, IV/MC-23
Paromomycin Sulfate
    Capsules USP, III/292
    Syrup USP, III/292
Patent and Exclusivity Lists, I/510
Peanut Oil
    Peanut Oil NF, III/292
Pectin
    Pectin USP, III/292
PCE Dispertab, IV/MC-9
PEG 3350 and Electrolytes
    for Solution, Oral, USP, III/292
Pegademase Bovine
    Injection, III/292
Pemoline
    Tablets, III/293, 294, 295
    Tablets, Chewable, III/293, 294, 295
Penalties, II/62
Penbutolol Sulfate
    Tablets, III/293, 294, 295, IV/MC-18
Penicillamine
    Capsules USP, III/293, 294, 295
    Tablets USP, III/293, 294, 295
Penicillin G Benzathine
    Sterile USP, III/293, 294, 295
    Suspension, Oral, USP, III/293, 294, 295
    Suspension, Sterile, USP, III/293, 294,
        295
    Tablets USP, III/293, 294, 295
Penicillin G Benzathine and Penicillin G
        Procaine
    Suspension, Sterile, USP, III/293, 294,
        295

Penicillin G Potassium
    Capsules USP, III/293, 294, 295
    Injection USP, III/293, 294, 295
    for Injection USP, III/293, 294, 295
    for Solution, Oral, USP, III/293, 294,
        295
    Sterile USP, III/293, 294, 295
    Tablets USP, III/293, 294, 295
    Tablets for Solution, Oral, USP, III/293,
        294, 295
Penicillin G Procaine
    Infusion, Intramammary, USP, III/293,
        294, 295
    Sterile USP, III/293, 294, 295
    Suspension, Sterile, USP, III/293, 294,
        295
    for Suspension, Sterile, USP, III/293,
        294, 295
Penicillin G Procaine with Aluminum Stea-
        rate
    Suspension, Sterile, USP, III/295
Penicillin G Procaine and Dihydrostreptomy-
        cin Sulfate
    Infusion, Intramammary, USP, III/295
    Suspension, Sterile, USP, III/295
Penicillin G Procaine, Dihydrostreptomycin
        Sulfate, Chlorpheniramine Maleate,
        and Dexamethasone
    Suspension, Sterile, USP, III/295
Penicillin G Procaine, Dihydrostreptomycin
        Sulfate, and Prednisolone
    Suspension, Sterile, USP, III/295
Penicillin G Procaine, Neomycin and Poly-
        myxin B Sulfates, and Hydrocortisone
        Acetate
    Suspension, Topical, USP, III/296
Penicillin G Procaine and Novobiocin So-
        dium
    Infusion, Intramammary, USP, III/296
Penicillin G Sodium
    for Injection USP, III/296
    Sterile USP, III/296
Penicillin V
    for Suspension, Oral, USP, III/296
    Tablets USP, III/296
Penicillin V Benzathine
    Suspension, Oral III/296
Penicillin V Potassium
    for Solution, Oral, USP, III/296
    Tablets USP, III/296, IV/MC-18
Pentaerythritol Tetranitrate
    Capsules, Extended-release, III/297
    Tablets USP, III/297
    Tablets, Extended-release, III/297
Pentagastrin
    Injection, III/297
Pentamidine Isethionate
    for Solution, Inhalation, III/297
    Sterile, III/297
Pentazocine Hydrochloride
    Tablets USP, III/297
Pentazocine Hydrochloride and Acetamino-
        phen
    Tablets, III/297, IV/MC-18
Pentazocine Hydrochloride and Aspirin
    Tablets USP, III/297
Pentazocine Lactate
    Injection USP, III/297
Pentazocine and Naloxone Hydrochlorides
    Tablets USP, III/298, IV/MC-18
Pentetic Acid
Pentetic Acid USP, III/298
Pentobarbital
    Elixir USP, III/298

Pentobarbital Sodium
    Capsules USP, III/298
    Injection USP, III/298
    Suppositories, III/298
Pentostatin
    for Injection, III/298
Pentoxifylline
    Tablets, Extended-release, III/298, IV/
        MC-18
Pen-Vee K, IV/MC-18
Pepcid, IV/MC-9
Peppermint
    Peppermint NF, III/298
Peppermint Oil
    Peppermint Oil NF, III/298
Peppermint Spirit
    Peppermint Spirit USP, III/299
Peppermint Water
    Peppermint Water NF, III/299
Percocet, IV/MC-18
Percodan, IV/MC-18
Percodan-Demi, IV/MC-18
Perfluorochemical Emulsion
    for Injection, III/299
Pergolide Mesylate
    Tablets, III/299
Pericyazine
    Capsules, III/299
    Solution, Oral, III/299
Permethrin
    Lotion, III/299
Perphenazine
    Injection USP, III/299
    Solution, Oral, USP, III/299
    Syrup USP, III/299
    Tablets USP, III/299
Perphenazine and Amitriptyline Hydrochlo-
        ride
    Tablets USP, III/300, IV/MC-18
Persantine, IV/MC-7
Persic Oil
    Persic Oil NF, III/300
Pertussis Immune Globulin
    Pertussis Immune Globulin USP, III/300
Pertussis Vaccine
    Pertussis Vaccine USP, III/300
Pertussis Vaccine Adsorbed
    Pertussis Vaccine Adsorbed USP, III/
        300
Petrolatum
    Petrolatum USP, III/300
Petrolatum Gauze—See Gauze, Petrolatum
Petrolatum, Hydrophilic
    Hydrophilic Petrolatum USP, III/301
Petrolatum, White
    White Petrolatum USP, III/301
Pharmaceutical Dosage Forms, II/9
Pharmaceutical Glaze—See Glaze, Pharma-
        ceutical
Phenacemide
    Tablets USP, III/301
Phenaphen-650 with Codeine, IV/MC-1
Phenaphen with Codeine No.2, IV/MC-1
Phenaphen with Codeine No.3, IV/MC-1
Phenaphen with Codeine No.4, IV/MC-1
Phenazopyridine Hydrochloride
    Tablets USP, III/301, IV/MC-18
Phendimetrazine Tartrate
    Capsules USP, III/301
    Capsules, Extended-release, III/301
    Tablets USP, III/301
    Tablets, Extended-release, III/301
Phenelzine Sulfate
    Tablets USP, III/301
Phenergan, IV/MC-20
Phenindamine Tartrate
    Tablets, III/301

Phenindamine Tartrate, Hydrocodone Bitartrate, and Guaifenesin
Tablets, III/302
Phenindione
Tablets USP, III/302
Pheniramine Maleate, Codeine Phosphate, and Guaifenesin
Syrup, III/302
Pheniramine Maleate, Phenylephrine Hydrochloride, Codeine Phosphate, Sodium Citrate, Sodium Salicylate, and Caffeine Citrate
Syrup, III/302
Pheniramine Maleate, Phenylephrine Hydrochloride, Sodium Salicylate, and Caffeine
Solution, Oral, III/303
Pheniramine Maleate, Phenyltoloxamine Citrate, Pyrilamine Maleate, and Phenylpropanolamine Hydrochloride
Capsules, Extended-release, III/303
Elixir, III/303
Pheniramine Maleate, Pyrilamine Maleate, Hydrocodone Bitartrate, Potassium Citrate, and Ascorbic Acid
Syrup, III/303
Pheniramine Maleate, Pyrilamine Maleate, Phenylephrine Hydrochloride, Phenylpropanolamine Hydrochloride, and Hydrocodone Bitartrate
Solution, Oral, III/304
Pheniramine Maleate, Pyrilamine Maleate, and Phenylpropanolamine Hydrochloride
Solution, Oral, III/305
Tablets, Extended-release, III/305
Pheniramine Maleate, Pyrilamine Maleate, Phenylpropanolamine Hydrochloride, and Aspirin
Tablets, III/305
Pheniramine Maleate, Pyrilamine Maleate, Phenylpropanolamine Hydrochloride, and Codeine Phosphate
Syrup, III/305
Pheniramine Maleate, Pyrilamine Maleate, Phenylpropanolamine Hydrochloride, Codeine Phosphate, Acetaminophen, and Caffeine
Tablets, III/306
Pheniramine Maleate, Pyrilamine Maleate, Phenylpropanolamine Hydrochloride, and Dextromethorphan Hydrobromide
Syrup, III/307
Pheniramine Maleate, Pyrilamine Maleate, Phenylpropanolamine Hydrochloride, Dextromethorphan Hydrobromide, and Ammonium Chloride
Syrup, III/307
Pheniramine Maleate, Pyrilamine Maleate, Phenylpropanolamine Hydrochloride, Dextromethorphan Hydrobromide, and Guaifenesin
Solution, Oral, III/307
Pheniramine Maleate, Pyrilamine Maleate, Phenylpropanolamine Hydrochloride, and Guaifenesin
Solution, Oral, III/308
Pheniramine Maleate, Pyrilamine Maleate, Phenylpropanolamine Hydrochloride, and Hydrocodone Bitartrate
Solution, Oral, III/308
Pheniramine Maleate, Pyrilamine Maleate, Phenylpropanolamine Hydrochloride, Hydrocodone Bitartrate, and Guaifenesin
Solution, Oral, III/309

Phenmetrazine Hydrochloride
Tablets USP, III/309
Phenobarbital
Capsules, III/309
Elixir USP, III/309
Tablets USP, III/309, IV/MC-18
Phenobarbital Sodium
Injection USP, III/309
Sterile USP, III/309
Phenol
Phenol USP, III/310
Phenol, Liquefied
Liquefied Phenol USP, III/310
Phenolphthalein
Gum, Chewing, III/310
Tablets USP, III/310
Wafers, III/310
Phenolsulfonphthalein
Injection, III/310
Phenoxybenzamine Hydrochloride
Capsules USP, III/311
Phenprocoumon
Tablets USP, III/311
Phensuximide
Capsules USP, III/311
Phentermine Hydrochloride
Capsules USP, III/311
Tablets USP, III/311
Phentermine Resin
Capsules, III/311, IV/MC-18
Phentolamine Mesylate
for Injection USP, III/311
Phenylbutazone
Bolus, III/311
Capsules USP, III/311
Granules, III/311
Injection, III/311
Paste, III/311
Tablets USP, III/311
Tablets, Buffered, III/311
Tablets, Delayed-release, III/311
Phenylephrine Hydrochloride
Injection USP, III/312
Jelly, Nasal, USP, III/312
Solution, Nasal, USP, III/312
Solution, Ophthalmic, USP, III/312
Phenylephrine Hydrochloride and Acetaminophen
for Solution, Oral, III/312
Tablets, Chewable, III/312
Phenylephrine Hydrochloride and Dextromethorphan Hydrobromide
Suspension, Oral, III/312
Phenylephrine Hydrochloride, Dextromethorphan Hydrobromide, and Guaifenesin
Syrup, III/312
Phenylephrine Hydrochloride, Dextromethorphan Hydrobromide, Guaifenesin, and Acetaminophen
Tablets, III/312
Phenylephrine Hydrochloride, Guaifenesin, Acetaminophen, Salicylamide, and Caffeine
Tablets, III/312
Phenylephrine Hydrochloride, Hydrocodone Bitartrate, and Guaifenesin
Syrup, III/312
Phenylephrine Hydrochloride, Phenylpropanolamine Hydrochloride, and Guaifenesin
Capsules, III/312, IV/MC-18
Solution, Oral, III/312
Tablets, III/312
Phenylethyl Alcohol
Phenylethyl Alcohol USP, III/312
Phenylmercuric Acetate
Phenylmercuric Acetate NF, III/313

Phenylmercuric Nitrate
Phenylmercuric Nitrate NF, III/313
Phenylpropanolamine Hydrochloride
Capsules, III/313
Capsules, Extended-release, USP, III/313
Tablets, III/313
Tablets, Extended-release, USP, III/313
Phenylpropanolamine Hydrochloride and Acetaminophen
Capsules, III/313
Solution, Oral, III/313
Tablets, III/313
Tablets, Chewable, III/313
Phenylpropanolamine Hydrochloride, Acetaminophen, and Aspirin
Capsules, III/313
Phenylpropanolamine Hydrochloride, Acetaminophen, Aspirin, and Caffeine
Capsules, III/313
Phenylpropanolamine Hydrochloride, Acetaminophen, and Caffeine
Tablets, III/314
Phenylpropanolamine Hydrochloride, Acetaminophen, Salicylamide, and Caffeine
Capsules, III/314
Phenylpropanolamine Hydrochloride and Caramiphen Edisylate
Capsules, Extended-release, III/314, IV/MC-19
Solution, Oral, III/314
Phenylpropanolamine Hydrochloride, Codeine Phosphate, and Guaifenesin
Solution, Oral, III/314
Suspension, Oral, III/314
Syrup, III/314
Phenylpropanolamine Hydrochloride and Dextromethorphan Hydrobromide
Gel, Oral, III/314
Granules, III/314
Lozenges, III/314
Solution, Oral, III/314
Syrup, III/314
Phenylpropanolamine Hydrochloride, Dextromethorphan Hydrobromide, and Acetaminophen
Solution, Oral, III/314
Tablets, III/314
Phenylpropanolamine Hydrochloride, Dextromethorphan Hydrobromide, and Guaifenesin
Solution, Oral, III/314
Syrup, III/314
Phenylpropanolamine Hydrochloride and Guaifenesin
Capsules, Extended-release, III/314
Granules, III/314
Solution, Oral, III/314
Syrup, III/314
Tablets, Extended-release, III/314, IV/MC-19
Phenylpropanolamine Hydrochloride and Hydrocodone Bitartrate
Solution, Oral, III/314
Syrup, III/314
Phenyltoloxamine Citrate, Phenylpropanolamine Hydrochloride, and Acetaminophen
Tablets, Extended-release, III/315
Phenyltoloxamine Polistirex and Hydrocodone Polistirex
Capsules, III/314
Suspension, Oral, III/314
Phenytoin
Suspension, Oral, USP, III/315
Tablets USP, III/315, IV/MC-19

Phenytoin Sodium
  Capsules, Extended, USP, III/315, IV/MC-19
  Capsules, Prompt, USP, III/315
  Injection USP, III/315
Phosphate P 32, Chromic
  Suspension USP, III/315
Phosphate P 32, Sodium
  Solution USP, III/315
Phosphoric Acid
  Phosphoric Acid NF, III/316
Phosphoric Acid, Diluted
  Diluted Phosphoric Acid NF, III/316
Physostigmine Salicylate
  Injection USP, III/316
  Solution, Ophthalmic, USP, III/316
Physostigmine Sulfate
  Ointment, Ophthalmic, USP, III/316
Phytonadione
  Injection USP, III/316
  Tablets USP, III/316
Pilocarpine
  System, Ocular, USP, III/317
Pilocarpine Hydrochloride
  Gel, Ophthalmic, III/317
  Solution, Ophthalmic, USP, III/317
Pilocarpine Nitrate
  Solution, Ophthalmic, USP, III/317
Pimozide
  Tablets USP, III/317
Pindolol
  Tablets USP, III/317, IV/MC-19
Pindolol and Hydrochlorothiazide
  Tablets, III/317
Pipecuronium Bromide
  for Injection, III/317
Piperacetazine
  Tablets USP, III/318
Piperacillin Sodium
  Sterile USP, III/318
Piperazine Adipate
  Capsules, III/318
  Suspension, Oral, III/318
  for Suspension, Oral, III/318
Piperazine Citrate
  Syrup USP, III/318
  Tablets USP, III/318
Piperazine Dihydrochloride
  Powder for Solution, Soluble, III/318
Piperazine Phosphate Monohydrate
  Solution, Oral, III/318
Pipobroman
  Tablets USP, III/318
Pipotiazine Palmitate
  Injection, III/319
Pirbuterol Acetate
  Aerosol, Inhalation, III/319
Pirenzepine Hydrochloride
  Tablets, III/319
Piroxicam
  Capsules USP, III/319, IV/MC-19
  Suppositories, III/319
Pituitary, Posterior
  Injection USP, III/319
Plague Vaccine
  Plague Vaccine USP, III/319
Plantago Seed
  Plantago Seed USP, III/319
Plaquenil, IV/MC-11
Plasma Protein Fraction
  Plasma Protein Fraction USP, III/319
Platelet Concentrate
  Platelet Concentrate USP, III/320
Plendil, IV/MC-9
Plicamycin
  for Injection USP, III/320

Pneumococcal Vaccine Polyvalent
  Injection, III/320
Podophyllum Resin
  Solution, Topical, USP, III/320
Poison Prevention Packaging Act and Regulations, II/92
Poison Prevention Packaging Act of 1970 Regulations, II/93
Polacrilin Potassium
  Polacrilin Potassium NF, III/321
Poliovirus Vaccine
  Poliovirus Vaccine Inactivated USP (Injection), III/321
  Poliovirus Vaccine Inactivated Enhanced Potency (Injection), III/321
Poliovirus Vaccine Live
  Poliovirus Vaccine Live Oral USP (Oral Solution), III/321
Poloxamer
  Poloxamer NF, III/321
Poloxamer 188
  Capsules, III/321
Polycillin, IV/MC-2
Polyethylene Excipient
  Polyethylene Excipient NF, III/322
Polyethylene Glycol
  Polyethylene Glycol NF, III/322
Polyethylene Glycol Monomethyl Ether
  Polyethylene Glycol Monomethyl Ether NF, III/322
Polyethylene Glycol Ointment
  Polyethylene Glycol Ointment NF, III/323
Polyethylene Oxide
  Polyethylene Oxide NF, III/323
Polymox, IV/MC-2
Polymyxin B Sulfate
  Sterile USP, III/323
Polymyxin B Sulfate and Bacitracin Zinc
  Aerosol, Topical, USP, III/324
  Powder, Topical, USP, III/324
Polymyxin B Sulfate and Hydrocortisone
  Solution, Otic, USP, III/324
Polyoxyl 35 Castor Oil
  Polyoxyl 35 Castor Oil NF, III/324
Polyoxyl 20 Cetostearyl Ether
  Polyoxyl 20 Cetostearyl Ether NF, III/324
Polyoxyl 40 Hydrogenated Castor Oil
  Polyoxyl 40 Hydrogenated Castor Oil NF, III/324
Polyoxyl 10 Oleyl Ether
  Polyoxyl 10 Oleyl Ether NF, III/324
Polyoxyl 40 Stearate
  Polyoxyl 40 Stearate NF, III/325
Polyoxyl 50 Stearate
  Polyoxyl 50 Stearate NF, III/325
Polysorbate 20
  Polysorbate 20 NF, III/325
Polysorbate 40
  Polysorbate 40 NF, III/325
Polysorbate 60
  Polysorbate 60 NF, III/325
Polysorbate 80
  Polysorbate 80 NF, III/325
Polythiazide
  Tablets USP, III/326
Polyvinyl Acetate Phthalate
  Polyvinyl Acetate Phthalate NF, III/326
Polyvinyl Alcohol
  Polyvinyl Alcohol USP, III/326
Posterior Pituitary—See Pituitary, Posterior
Potash, Sulfurated
  Sulfurated Potash USP, III/326
Potassium Acetate
  Injection USP, III/326

Potassium Acetate, Potassium Bicarbonate, and Potassium Citrate—See Trikates
Potassium Benzoate
  Potassium Benzoate NF, III/326
Potassium Bicarbonate
  Tablets for Solution, Oral, Effervescent, USP, III/327
Potassium Bicarbonate and Potassium Chloride
  for Solution, Oral, Effervescent, USP, III/327
  Tablets for Solution, Oral, Effervescent, USP, III/327
Potassium Bicarbonate and Potassium Citrate
  Tablets for Solution, Oral, Effervescent, III/327
Potassium Bitartrate and Sodium Bicarbonate
  Suppositories, III/327
Potassium Carbonate
  Potassium Carbonate USP, III/327
Potassium Chloride
  Capsules, Extended-release, USP, III/328, IV/MC-19
  Concentrate, for Injection, USP, III/328
  Potassium Chloride USP, III/328
  Solution, Oral, USP, III/328
  for Solution, Oral, USP, III/328
  for Suspension, Oral, III/328
  Tablets, Extended-release, USP, III/328, IV/MC-19
Potassium Chloride and Dextrose
  Potassium Chloride in Dextrose Injection USP, III/328
Potassium Chloride, Dextrose, and Sodium Chloride
  Potassium Chloride in Dextrose and Sodium Chloride Injection USP, III/328
Potassium Chloride, Lactated Ringer's, and Dextrose
  Potassium Chloride in Lactated Ringer's and Dextrose Injection USP, III/328
Potassium Chloride, Potassium Bicarbonate, and Potassium Citrate
  Tablets for Solution, Oral, Effervescent, USP, III/329
Potassium Chloride and Sodium Chloride
  Potassium Chloride in Sodium Chloride Injection USP, III/329
Potassium Citrate
  Potassium Citrate USP, III/329
  Tablets, III/329
  Tablets, Extended-release, USP, III/329
Potassium Citrate and Citric Acid
  Solution, Oral, USP, III/329
  for Solution, Oral, III/329
Potassium Citrate and Sodium Citrate
  Tablets, III/329
Potassium Citrate, Sodium Citrate, and Citric Acid—See Tricitrates
Potassium Gluconate
  Elixir USP, III/329
  Tablets USP, III/329
Potassium Gluconate and Potassium Chloride
  Solution, Oral, USP, III/330
  for Solution, Oral, III/330
Potassium Gluconate and Potassium Citrate
  Solution, Oral, USP, III/330
Potassium Gluconate, Potassium Citrate, and Ammonium Chloride
  Solution, Oral, USP, III/330
Potassium Guaiacolsulfonate
  Potassium Guaiacolsulfonate USP, III/330

Potassium Hydroxide
  Potassium Hydroxide NF, III/330
Potassium Iodide
  Solution, Oral, USP, III/330
  Syrup, III/330
  Tablets USP, III/330
Potassium Metabisulfite
  Potassium Metabisulfite NF, III/331
Potassium Metaphosphate
  Potassium Metaphosphate NF, III/331
Potassium Permanganate
  Potassium Permanganate USP, III/331
Potassium Phosphate, Dibasic
  Dibasic Potassium Phosphate USP, III/
    331
Potassium Phosphate, Monobasic
  Monobasic Potassium Phosphate NF,
    III/331
Potassium Phosphates
  Capsules for Solution, Oral, III/331
  Injection USP, III/331
  for Solution, Oral, III/331
Potassium and Sodium Bicarbonates and Cit-
  ric Acid
  Tablets for Solution, Oral, Effervescent,
    USP, III/327
Potassium and Sodium Phosphates
  Capsules for Solution, Oral, III/332
  for Solution, Oral, III/332
  Tablets for Solution, Oral, III/332
Potassium and Sodium Phosphates, Monoba-
  sic
  Tablets for Solution, Oral, III/332
Potassium Sodium Tartrate
  Potassium Sodium Tartrate USP, III/332
Potassium Sorbate
  Potassium Sorbate NF, III/332
Povidone
  Povidone USP, III/332
Povidone-Iodine
  Ointment USP, III/332
  Solution, Cleansing, USP, III/332
  Solution, Topical, Aerosol, USP, III/332
Powder, Absorbable Dusting—See Dusting
  Powder, Absorbable
Pralidoxime Chloride
  Sterile USP, III/333
  Tablets USP, III/333
Pramoxine Hydrochloride
  Cream USP, III/333
  Foam, Aerosol, III/333
  Jelly USP, III/333
  Lotion, III/333
  Ointment, III/333
Pramoxine and Pramoxine Hydrochloride
  Suppositories, III/333
Pravachol, IV/MC-19
Pravastatin
  Tablets, IV/MC-19
Pravastatin Sodium
  Tablets, III/333
Prazepam
  Capsules USP, III/333, IV/MC-19
  Tablets USP, III/333
Praziquantel
  Injection, III/334
  Tablets USP, III/334
Prazosin Hydrochloride
  Capsules USP, III/334, IV/MC-19
  Tablets, III/335
Prazosin Hydrochloride and Polythiazide
  Capsules, III/335, IV/MC-19
Prednisolone
  Cream USP, III/335
  Syrup USP, III/335
  Tablets USP, III/335

Prednisolone Acetate
  Suspension, Ophthalmic, USP, III/335
  Suspension, Sterile, USP, III/335
Prednisolone Acetate and Prednisolone So-
  dium Phosphate
  Suspension, Sterile, III/335
Prednisolone Sodium Phosphate
  Injection USP, III/335
  Solution, Ophthalmic, USP, III/335
  Solution, Oral, III/335
Prednisolone Sodium Succinate
  for Injection USP, III/335
Prednisolone Tebutate
  Suspension, Sterile, USP, III/335
Prednisone
  Solution, Oral, USP, III/335
  Syrup USP, III/335
  Tablets USP, III/335, IV/MC-19
Premarin, IV/MC-9
Prescription Balances and Volumetric Appa-
  ratus, II/25
Prescription Drug Product List, I/20
Prescriptions, II/47
Preservation, Packaging, Storage, and Label-
  ing, II/3
Prilocaine and Epinephrine
  Injection USP, III/335
Prilocaine Hydrochloride
  Injection USP, III/335
Prilosec, IV/MC-17
Primaquine Phosphate
  Tablets USP, III/335
Primidone
  Suspension, Oral, USP, III/336
  Tablets USP, III/336
Prinivil, IV/MC-13
Prinzide, IV/MC-13
Pro-Banthine, IV/MC-20
Probenecid
  Tablets USP, III/336
Probenecid and Colchicine
  Tablets USP, III/336
Probucol
  Tablets, III/336, IV/MC-19
Procainamide Hydrochloride
  Capsules USP, III/336, IV/MC-19, MC-
    20
  Injection USP, III/336
  Tablets USP, III/336, IV/MC-19
  Tablets, Extended-release, USP, III/336,
    IV/MC-19, MC-20
Procaine Hydrochloride
  Injection USP, III/337
  Sterile USP, III/337
Procaine Hydrochloride and Epinephrine
  Injection USP, III/337
Procaine and Phenylephrine Hydrochlorides
  Injection USP, III/337
Procaine and Tetracaine Hydrochlorides and
  Levonordefrin
  Injection USP, III/337
Procan SR, IV/MC-19
Procarbazine Hydrochloride
  Capsules USP, III/337
Procardia, IV/MC-16
Procardia XL, IV/MC-16
Procaterol Hydrochloride Hemihydrate
  Aerosol, Inhalation, III/338
Prochlorperazine
  Suppositories USP, III/338
Prochlorperazine Edisylate
  Injection USP, III/338
  Solution, Oral, USP, III/338
  Syrup USP, III/338

Prochlorperazine Maleate
  Capsules, Extended-release, III/338, IV/
    MC-20
  Tablets USP, III/338, IV/MC-20
Prochlorperazine Mesylate
  Injection, III/338
  Syrup, III/338
Procyclidine Hydrochloride
  Elixir, III/338
  Tablets USP, III/338
Progesterone
  Contraceptive, Intrauterine, System, USP,
    III/339
  Injection USP, III/339
  Suppositories, Rectal, III/339
  Suppositories, Vaginal, III/339
  Suspension, Sterile, USP, III/339
Prolixin, IV/MC-10
Proloprim, IV/MC-24
Promazine Hydrochloride
  Injection USP, III/339
  Solution, Oral, USP, III/339
  Syrup USP, III/339
  Tablets USP, III/339
Promethazine Hydrochloride
  Injection USP, III/339
  Suppositories USP, III/339
  Syrup USP, III/339
  Tablets USP, III/339, IV/MC-20
Promethazine Hydrochloride and Codeine
  Phosphate
  Syrup, III/340
Promethazine Hydrochloride and Dextrometh-
  orphan Hydrobromide
  Syrup, III/340
Promethazine Hydrochloride and Phenyleph-
  rine Hydrochloride
  Syrup, III/340
Promethazine Hydrochloride, Phenylephrine
  Hydrochloride, and Codeine Phosphate
  Syrup, III/340
Promethazine Hydrochloride and Pseudo-
  ephedrine Hydrochloride
  Tablets, III/340
Pronestyl, IV/MC-19
Pronestyl-SR, IV/MC-19
Propafenone Hydrochloride
  Tablets, III/340, IV/MC-20
Propane
  Propane NF, III/340
Propantheline Bromide
  Sterile USP, III/340
  Tablets USP, III/340, IV/MC-20
Proparacaine Hydrochloride
  Solution, Ophthalmic, USP, III/340
Propellants, II/10
Propiomazine Hydrochloride
  Injection USP, III/341
Propionic Acid
  Propionic Acid NF, III/341
Propofol
  Injection, III/341
Propoxycaine and Procaine Hydrochlorides
  and Levonordefrin
  Injection USP, III/341
Propoxycaine and Procaine Hydrochlorides
  and Norepinephrine Bitartrate
  Injection USP, III/341
Propoxyphene Hydrochloride
  Capsules USP, III/342
  Tablets, III/342
Propoxyphene Hydrochloride and Acetamino-
  phen
  Capsules, III/342
  Tablets USP, III/342
Propoxyphene Hydrochloride and Aspirin
  Capsules, III/342

Propoxyphene Hydrochloride, Aspirin, and Caffeine
Capsules USP, III/342
Tablets, III/342
Propoxyphene Napsylate
Capsules, III/342
Suspension, Oral, USP, III/342
Tablets USP, III/342
Propoxyphene Napsylate and Acetaminophen
Tablets USP, III/342, IV/MC-20
Propoxyphene Napsylate and Aspirin
Capsules, III/342
Tablets USP, III/342
Propoxyphene Napsylate, Aspirin, and Caffeine
Capsules, III/342
Propranolol Hydrochloride
Capsules, Extended-release USP, III/343, IV/MC-20
Injection USP, III/343
Solution, Oral, III/343
Tablets USP, III/343, IV/MC-20
Propranolol Hydrochloride and Hydrochlorothiazide
Capsules, Extended-release, USP, III/343, IV/MC-20
Tablets USP, III/343, IV/MC-20
Propylene Carbonate
Propylene Carbonate NF, III/343
Propylene Glycol
Propylene Glycol USP, III/343
Propylene Glycol Alginate
Propylene Glycol Alginate NF, III/344
Propylene Glycol Diacetate
Propylene Glycol Diacetate NF, III/344
Propylene Glycol Monostearate
Propylene Glycol Monostearate NF, III/344
Propyl Gallate
Propyl Gallate NF, III/344
Propylhexedrine
Inhalant USP, III/344
Propyliodone
Suspension, Oil, Sterile, USP, III/344
Propylparaben
Propylparaben NF, III/345
Propylparaben Sodium
Propylparaben Sodium NF, III/345
Propylthiouracil
Tablets USP, III/345
ProSom, IV/MC-9
Prostaphlin, IV/MC-17
Protamine Sulfate
Injection USP, III/345
for Injection USP, III/345
Protein Hydrolysate
Injection USP, III/345
Protirelin
Injection, III/346
Protriptyline Hydrochloride
Tablets USP, III/346
Proventil, IV/MC-1
Proventil Repetabs, IV/MC-1
Provera, IV/MC-14
Prozac, IV/MC-10
Pseudoephedrine Hydrochloride
Capsules, III/346
Capsules, Extended-release, III/346
Solution, Oral, III/346
Syrup USP, III/346
Tablets USP, III/346
Pseudoephedrine Hydrochloride and Acetaminophen
Capsules, III/346
Tablets, III/346

Pseudoephedrine Hydrochloride, Acetaminophen, and Caffeine
Capsules, III/346
Pseudoephedrine Hydrochloride and Aspirin
Tablets, III/346
Pseudoephedrine Hydrochloride, Aspirin, and Caffeine
Capsules, III/346
Pseudoephedrine Hydrochloride and Codeine Phosphate
Capsules, III/346
Syrup, III/346
Pseudoephedrine Hydrochloride, Codeine Phosphate, and Guaifenesin
Solution, Oral, III/347
Syrup, III/347
Pseudoephedrine Hydrochloride and Dextromethorphan Hydrobromide
Solution, Oral, III/347
Tablets, Chewable, III/347
Pseudoephedrine Hydrochloride, Dextromethorphan Hydrobromide, and Acetaminophen
Solution, Oral, III/347
Tablets, III/347
Pseudoephedrine Hydrochloride, Dextromethorphan Hydrobromide, and Guaifenesin
Capsules, III/347
Solution, Oral, III/347
Syrup, III/347
Pseudoephedrine Hydrochloride, Dextromethorphan Hydrobromide, Guaifenesin, and Acetaminophen
Solution, Oral, III/347
Tablets, III/347
Pseudoephedrine Hydrochloride and Guaifenesin
Capsules, Extended-release, III/347
Solution, Oral, III/347
Syrup, III/347
Tablets, III/347
Tablets, Extended-release, III/347
Pseudoephedrine Hydrochloride and Hydrocodone Bitartrate
Solution, Oral, III/347
Syrup, III/347
Pseudoephedrine Hydrochloride, Hydrocodone Bitartrate, and Guaifenesin
Solution, Oral, III/347
Syrup, III/347
Tablets, III/347
Pseudoephedrine Hydrochloride and Ibuprofen
Tablets, III/347
Pseudoephedrine Sulfate
Tablets, 346
Tablets, Extended-release, III/346
Psyllium
Caramels, III/347
Granules, III/347
Powder, III/347
Psyllium Husk
Psyllium Husk USP, III/347
Psyllium Hydrophilic Mucilloid
Granules, III/348
Powder, III/348
Powder, Effervescent, III/348
for Suspension, Oral, USP, III/348
Wafers, III/348
Psyllium Hydrophilic Mucilloid and Carboxymethylcellulose Sodium
Granules, III/348
Psyllium Hydrophilic Mucilloid and Senna
Granules, III/348

Psyllium Hydrophilic Mucilloid and Sennosides
Powder, III/348
Psyllium and Senna
Granules, III/348
Pumice
Pumice USP, III/348
Pyrantel Pamoate
Suspension, Oral, USP, III/348
Tablets, III/348
Pyrazinamide
Tablets USP, III/348
Pyrethrins and Piperonyl Butoxide
Gel, III/348
Shampoo, Solution, III/348
Solution, Topical, III/348
Pyridium, IV/MC-18
Pyridostigmine Bromide
Injection USP, III/349
Syrup USP, III/349
Tablets USP, III/349
Tablets, Extended-release, III/349
Pyridoxine Hydrochloride
Capsules, Extended-release, III/349
Injection USP, III/349
Tablets USP, III/349
Pyrilamine Maleate
Tablets USP, III/349
Pyrilamine Maleate, Codeine Phosphate, and Terpin Hydrate
Syrup, III/349
Pyrilamine Maleate, Phenylephrine Hydrochloride, Aspirin, and Caffeine
Tablets, III/349
Pyrilamine Maleate, Phenylephrine Hydrochloride, and Codeine Phosphate
Syrup, III/349
Pyrilamine Maleate, Phenylephrine Hydrochloride, and Dextromethorphan Hydrobromide
Solution, Oral, III/349
Pyrilamine Maleate, Phenylephrine Hydrochloride, Dextromethorphan Hydrobromide, and Acetaminophen
Solution, Oral, III/349
Pyrilamine Maleate, Phenylephrine Hydrochloride, and Hydrocodone Bitartrate
Syrup, III/350
Pyrilamine Maleate, Phenylephrine Hydrochloride, Hydrocodone Bitartrate, and Ammonium Chloride
Syrup, III/350
Pyrilamine Maleate, Phenylpropanolamine Hydrochloride, Acetaminophen, and Caffeine
Tablets, III/350
Pyrilamine Maleate, Phenylpropanolamine Hydrochloride, Dextromethorphan Hydrobromide, Guaifenesin, Potassium Citrate, and Citric Acid
Syrup, III/350
Pyrilamine Maleate, Phenylpropanolamine Hydrochloride, Dextromethorphan Hydrobromide, and Sodium Salicylate
Solution, Oral, III/350
Pyrimethamine
Tablets USP, III/350
Pyrithione Zinc
Shampoo, Bar, III/350
Shampoo, Cream, III/350
Shampoo, Lotion, III/350
Pyrvinium Pamoate
Suspension, Oral, USP, III/350
Tablets USP, III/350

Q

Quazepam
  Tablets, III/351, IV/MC-20
Quibron, IV/MC-23
Quibron-300, IV/MC-23
Quibron-T Dividose, IV/MC-22
Quibron-T/SR Dividose, IV/MC-22
Quinacrine Hydrochloride
  Tablets USP, III/351
Quinaglute Dura-tabs, IV/MC-20
Quinapril Hydrochloride
  Tablets, III/351, IV/MC-20
Quinestrol
  Tablets USP, III/351
Quinethazone
  Tablets USP, III/351
Quinidex Extentabs, IV/MC-21
Quinidine Gluconate
  Injection USP, III/351
  Tablets, III/351
  Tablets, Extended-release, USP, III/351,
    IV/MC-20, MC-21
Quinidine Polygalacturonate
  Tablets, III/351
Quinidine Sulfate
  Capsules USP, III/351
  Injection, III/351
  Tablets USP, III/351, IV/MC-21
  Tablets, Extended-release, USP, III/351,
    IV/MC-21
Quinine Sulfate
  Capsules USP, III/352
  Tablets USP, III/352

R

Rabies Immune Globulin
  Rabies Immune Globulin USP, III/352
Rabies Vaccine
  Rabies Vaccine USP, III/352
Racepinephrine
  Solution, Inhalation, USP, III/352
Ramipril, IV/MC-21
Ranitidine
  Capsules, III/353
  Injection USP, III/353
  Solution, Oral, USP, III/353
  Tablets USP, III/353, IV/MC-21
Ranitidine Hydrochloride
  Syrup, III/353
Ranitidine and Sodium Chloride
  Ranitidine in Sodium Chloride Injection
    USP, III/353
Rauwolfia Serpentina
  Tablets USP, III/353
Rauwolfia Serpentina and Bendroflumethia-
    zide
  Tablets, III/353
Rayon, Purified
  Purified Rayon USP, III/354
Records and Reports of Registrants, II/40
Records of Interstate Shipment, II/78
Registration Requirements, II/76
Reglan, IV/MC-15
Regroton, IV/MC-21
Requirements for Packaging, II/22
Requirements for Registration, II/32
Reserpine
  Elixir USP, III/354
  Injection USP, III/354
  Tablets USP, III/354
Reserpine and Chlorothiazide
  Tablets USP, III/354
Reserpine and Chlorthalidone
  Tablets, III/354, IV/MC-21

Reserpine and Hydralazine Hydrochloride
  Tablets, III/354
Reserpine, Hydralazine Hydrochloride, and
    Hydrochlorothiazide
  Tablets USP, III/354, IV/MC-21
Reserpine and Hydrochlorothiazide
  Tablets USP, III/354
Reserpine and Hydroflumethiazide
  Tablets, III/354
Reserpine and Methyclothiazide
  Tablets, III/354
Reserpine and Polythiazide
  Tablets, III/355
Reserpine and Quinethazone
  Tablets, III/355
Reserpine and Trichlormethiazide
  Tablets, III/355
Resorcinol
  Lotion, III/355
  Ointment, III/355
Resorcinol, Compound
  Ointment, III/355
Resorcinol and Sulfur
  Cake, III/355
  Cream, III/355
  Gel, III/355
  Lotion USP, III/355
  Stick, III/355
Restoril, IV/MC-22
Retrovir, IV/MC-24
Revision of United States Pharmacopeia;
    Development of Analysis and Me-
    chanical and Physical Tests, II/79
Ribavirin
  Solution, for Inhalation, USP, III/355
Riboflavin
  Injection USP, III/355
  Tablets USP, III/355
Rice Syrup Solids and Electrolytes
  Solution, III/355
Ridaura, IV/MC-2
Rifampin
  Capsules USP, III/356
  for Injection USP, III/356
Rifampin and Isoniazid
  Capsules USP, III/356
Ringer's
  Injection USP, III/356
  Irrigation USP, III/356
Ringer's, Lactated
  Injection USP, III/357
Ritalin, IV/MC-15
Ritalin-SR, IV/MC-15
Ritodrine Hydrochloride
  Injection USP, III/357
  Tablets USP, III/357
Robaxin, IV/MC-14
Robaxisal, IV/MC-14
Rocaltrol, IV/MC-3
Rolitetracycline
  for Injection USP, III/357
  Sterile USP, III/357
Rose Bengal Sodium I 131
  Injection USP, III/357
Rose Oil
  Rose Oil NF, III/358
Rose Water
  Ointment USP, III/358
Rose Water, Stronger
  Stronger Rose Water NF, III/358
Roxicet, IV/MC-18
Roxicodone, IV/MC-18
Rubbing Alcohol—See Alcohol, Rubbing
Rubella and Mumps Virus Vaccine Live
  Rubella and Mumps Virus Vaccine Live
    USP, III/358

Rubella Virus Vaccine Live
  Rubella Virus Vaccine Live USP, III/
    358
Rubidium Rb 82
  Injection, III/359
Rufen, IV/MC-11
Rynatan, IV/MC-5
Rythmol, IV/MC-20

S

Saccharin
  Saccharin NF, III/359
Saccharin Calcium
  Saccharin Calcium USP, III/359
Saccharin Sodium
  Saccharin Sodium USP, III/359
  Solution, Oral, USP, III/359
  Tablets USP, III/359
Safflower Oil
  Safflower Oil USP, III/359
Salicylamide
  Salicylamide USP, III/360
Salicylic Acid
  Collodion USP, III/360
  Cream, III/360
  Foam, Topical, USP, III/360
  Gel USP, III/360
  Lotion, III/360
  Ointment, III/360
  Pads, III/360
  Plaster USP, III/360
  Shampoo, III/360
  Soap, III/360
  Solution, Topical, III/360
Salicylic Acid and Sulfur
  Cream, III/360
  Cream, Cleansing, III/360
  Lotion, III/360
  Lotion, Cleansing, III/360
  Shampoo, Cream, III/360
  Shampoo, Lotion, III/360
  Shampoo, Suspension, III/360
  Soap, Bar, III/360
  Suspension, Cleansing, III/360
  Suspension, Topical, III/360
Salicylic Acid, Sulfur, and Coal Tar
  Shampoo, Cream, III/360
  Shampoo, Lotion, III/360
Salsalate
  Capsules USP, III/360
  Tablets, III/360
Sargramostim
  for Injection, III/360
Schedules of Controlled Substances, II/53
Schick Test Control
  Schick Test Control USP, III/361
Scopolamine
  System, Transdermal, III/361
Scopolamine Butylbromide
  Injection, III/361
  Suppositories, III/361
  Tablets, III/361
Scopolamine Hydrobromide
  Injection USP, III/361
  Ointment, Ophthalmic, USP, III/361
  Solution, Ophthalmic, USP, III/361
  Tablets USP, III/361
Secobarbital
  Elixir USP, III/361
Secobarbital Sodium
  Capsules USP, III/361
  Injection USP, III/361
  Sterile USP, III/361

Secobarbital Sodium and Amobarbital So-
    dium
    Capsules USP, III/362
Security Requirements, II/37
Seldane, IV/MC-22
Seldane-D, IV/MC-22
Selected General Notices and Requirements,
    II/1
Selegiline Hydrochloride
    Tablets, III/362, IV/MC-21
Selenious Acid
    Injection USP, III/362
Selenium Sulfide
    Lotion USP, III/362
Selenomethionine Se 75
    Injection USP, III/362
Senna
    Fluidextract USP, III/362
    Granules, III/362
    Solution, Oral, III/362
    Suppositories, III/362
    Syrup USP, III/362
    Tablets, III/362
Senna and Docusate Sodium
    Tablets, III/363
Sennosides
    Tablets USP, III/363
Septra, IV/MC-21
Ser-Ap-Es, IV/MC-21
Serax, IV/MC-17, MC-18
Sertraline Hydrochloride
    Tablets, , IV/MC-21
Sesame Oil
    Sesame Oil NF, III/363
Shellac
    Shellac NF, III/363
Short Title, II/61
Silica, Dental-type—See Dental-type Silica
Siliceous Earth, Purified
    Purified Siliceous Earth NF, III/363
Silicon Dioxide
    Silicon Dioxide NF, III/363
Silicon Dioxide, Colloidal
    Colloidal Silicon Dioxide NF, III/364
Silver Nitrate
    Solution, Ophthalmic, USP, III/364
Silver Sulfadiazine
    Cream USP, III/364
Simethicone
    Capsules USP, III/364
    Emulsion USP, III/364
    Simethicone USP, III/364
    Suspension, Oral, USP, III/364
    Tablets USP, III/364
Simethicone, Alumina, Calcium Carbonate,
    and Magnesia
    Tablets, Chewable, III/365
Simethicone, Alumina, Magnesium Carbon-
    ate, and Magnesia
    Tablets, Chewable, III/365
Simvastatin
    Tablets, III/365, IV/MC-21
Sinemet, IV/MC-4
Sinequan, IV/MC-8
Sisomicin Sulfate
    Injection USP, III/365
Slo-bid Gyrocaps, IV/MC-22
Slo-Niacin, IV/MC-16
Slo-Phyllin, IV/MC-22
Slo-Phyllin Gyrocaps, IV/MC-22
Slow-K, IV/MC-19
Smallpox Vaccine
    Smallpox Vaccine USP, III/365
Soda Lime
    Soda Lime NF, III/365

Sodium Acetate
    Injection USP, III/365
    Sodium Acetate USP, III/365
    Solution USP, III/365
Sodium Alginate
    Sodium Alginate NF, III/366
Sodium Ascorbate
    Injection, III/366
Sodium Benzoate
    Sodium Benzoate NF, III/366
Sodium Benzoate and Sodium Phenylacetate
    Solution, Oral, III/366
Sodium Bicarbonate
    Effervescent, III/366
    Injection USP, III/366
    Powder, Oral, USP, III/366
    Sodium Bicarbonate USP, III/366
    Tablets USP, III/366
Sodium Borate
    Sodium Borate NF, III/367
Sodium Carbonate
    Sodium Carbonate NF, III/367
Sodium Chloride
    Injection USP, III/367
    Injection, Bacteriostatic, USP, III/367
    Irrigation USP, III/367
    Ointment, Ophthalmic, USP, III/367
    Sodium Chloride USP, III/367
    Solution, Inhalation, USP, III/367
    Solution, Ophthalmic, USP, III/367
    Tablets USP, III/367
    Tablets for Solution USP, III/367
Sodium Chloride and Dextrose
    Tablets USP, III/368
Sodium Chromate Cr 51
    Injection USP, III/368
Sodium Citrate
    Sodium Citrate USP, III/368
Sodium Citrate and Citric Acid
    Solution, Oral, USP, III/369
Sodium Dehydroacetate
    Sodium Dehydroacetate NF, III/369
Sodium Fluoride
    Solution, Oral, USP, III/369
    Tablets USP, III/369
Sodium Fluoride and Phosphoric Acid
    Gel USP, III/369
    Solution, Topical, USP, III/369
Sodium Formaldehyde Sulfoxylate
    Sodium Formaldehyde Sulfoxylate NF,
    III/369
Sodium Hydroxide
    Sodium Hydroxide NF, III/369
Sodium Hypochlorite
    Solution USP, III/370
Sodium Iodide
    Sodium Iodide USP, III/370
Sodium Iodide I 123
    Capsules USP, III/370
    Solution USP, III/370
Sodium Iodide I 125
    Capsules USP, III/370
    Solution USP, III/370
Sodium Iodide I 131
    Capsules USP, III/371
    Solution USP, III/371
Sodium Lactate
    Injection USP, III/371
    Solution USP, III/371
Sodium Lauryl Sulfate
    Sodium Lauryl Sulfate NF, III/372
Sodium Metabisulfite
    Sodium Metabisulfite NF, III/372
Sodium Monofluorophosphate
    Sodium Monofluorophosphate USP, III/
    372

Sodium Nitrite
    Injection USP, III/372
Sodium Nitroprusside
    Sterile USP, III/372
Sodium Pertechnetate Tc 99m
    Injection USP, III/372
Sodium Phosphate, Dibasic
    Dibasic Sodium Phosphate USP, III/373
    Effervescent, III/373
Sodium Phosphate, Monobasic
    Monobasic Sodium Phosphate USP, III/
    373
Sodium Phosphate P 32—See Phosphate P
    32, Sodium
Sodium Phosphates
    Enema USP, III/373
    Injection USP, III/373
    Solution, Oral, USP, III/373
Sodium Polystyrene Sulfonate
    Suspension USP, III/374
    (for Suspension) USP, III/374
Sodium Propionate
    Sodium Propionate NF, III/374
Sodium Salicylate
    Tablets USP, III/374
    Tablets, Delayed-release, III/374
Sodium Starch Glycolate
    Sodium Starch Glycolate NF, III/374
Sodium Stearate
    Sodium Stearate NF, III/374
Sodium Stearyl Fumarate
    Sodium Stearyl Fumarate NF, III/375
Sodium Sulfate
    Injection USP, III/375
Sodium Thiosulfate
    Injection USP, III/375
    Sodium Thiosulfate USP, III/375
Solutions, Constituted, II/7
Soma, IV/MC-4
Soma Compound, IV/MC-4
Soma Compound with Codeine, IV/MC-4
Somatrem
    for Injection, III/375
Somatropin, Pituitary-derived
    for Injection, III/375
Somatropin, Recombinant
    for Injection, III/375
Sorbic Acid
    Sorbic Acid NF, III/375
Sorbitan Monolaurate
    Sorbitan Monolaurate NF, III/375
Sorbitan Monooleate
    Sorbitan Monooleate NF, III/376
Sorbitan Monopalmitate
    Sorbitan Monopalmitate NF, III/376
Sorbitan Monostearate
    Sorbitan Monostearate NF, III/376
Sorbitol
    Solution USP, III/376
    Sorbitol NF, III/376
Sorbitrate, IV/MC-12
Sorbitrate SA, IV/MC-12
Sotalol Hydrochloride
    Tablets, III/376
Soybean Oil
    Soybean Oil USP, III/377
Special Exceptions for Manufacture and Dis-
    tribution of Controlled Substances,
    II/52
Spectinomycin Hydrochloride
    Sterile USP, III/377
    for Suspension, Sterile, USP, III/377
Spironolactone
    Tablets USP, III/377, IV/MC-21
Spironolactone and Hydrochlorothiazide
    Tablets USP, III/377, IV/MC-21

Squalane
   Squalane NF, III/377
Stability Considerations in Dispensing Practice, II/19
Stability in Pharmaceutical Dosage Forms, II/9
Stannous Fluoride
   Gel USP, III/377
Stanozolol
   Tablets USP, III/378
Starch
   Starch NF, III/378
Starch, Pregelatinized
   Pregelatinized Starch NF, III/378
Starch, Topical
   Topical Starch, USP, III/378
Stearic Acid
   Stearic Acid NF, III/378
Stearic Acid, Purified
   Purified Stearic Acid NF, III/378
Stearyl Alcohol
   Stearyl Alcohol NF, III/379
Stelazine, IV/MC-24
Streptokinase
   for Injection, III/379
Streptomycin Sulfate
   Injection USP, III/379
   Sterile USP, III/379
Streptozocin
   for Injection, III/379
Strong Iodine—See Iodine, Strong
Succinylcholine Chloride
   Injection USP, III/379
   Sterile USP, III/379
Sucralfate
   Suspension, Oral, III/380
   Tablets, III/380, IV/MC-21
Sucrose
   Sucrose NF, III/380
Sucrose Octaacetate
   Sucrose Octaacetate NF, III/380
Sufentanil Citrate
   Injection, III/380
Sugar, Compressible
   Compressible Sugar NF, III/380
Sugar, Confectioner's
   Confectioner's Sugar NF, III/380
Sugar, Invert
   Injection USP, III/381
Sugar Spheres
   Sugar Spheres NF, III/381
Sulbactam Sodium
   Sterile USP, III/381
Sulfabenzamide
   Sulfabenzamide USP, III/381
Sulfacetamide Sodium
   Ointment, Ophthalmic, USP, III/381
   Solution, Ophthalmic, USP, III/381
Sulfacetamide Sodium and Prednisolone
     Acetate
   Ointment, Ophthalmic, USP, III/382
   Suspension, Ophthalmic, USP, III/382
Sulfacytine
   Tablets, III/382
Sulfadiazine
   Tablets USP, III/382
Sulfadiazine Sodium
   Injection USP, III/382
Sulfadiazine and Trimethoprim
   Suspension, Oral, III/382
   Tablets, III/382
Sulfadoxine and Pyrimethamine
   Tablets USP, III/382
Sulfamerazine
   Tablets USP, III/383

Sulfamethizole
   Suspension, Oral, USP, III/383
   Tablets USP, III/383
Sulfamethoxazole
   Suspension, Oral, USP, III/383
   Tablets USP, III/383
Sulfamethoxazole and Phenazopyridine Hydrochloride
   Tablets, III/383
Sulfamethoxazole and Trimethoprim
   for Injection Concentrate USP, III/383
   Suspension, Oral, USP, III/383
   Tablets USP, III/383, IV/MC-21
Sulfanilamide
   Cream, Vaginal, III/383
   Suppositories, Vaginal, III/383
Sulfanilamide, Aminacrine Hydrochloride,
     and Allantoin
   Cream, Vaginal, III/384
   Suppositories, Vaginal, III/384
Sulfapyridine
   Tablets USP, III/384
Sulfasalazine
   Suspension, Oral, III/384
   Tablets USP, III/384, IV/MC-21
   Tablets, Enteric-coated, IV/MC-21
Sulfathiazole
   Sulfathiazole USP, III/384
Sulfathiazole, Sulfacetamide, and Sulfabenzamide—See Sulfa, Triple
Sulfa, Triple
   Cream, Vaginal, USP, III/381
   Tablets, Vaginal, USP, III/381
Sulfinpyrazone
   Capsules USP, III/384
   Tablets USP, III/384
Sulfisoxazole
   Tablets USP, III/385
Sulfisoxazole Acetyl
   Suspension, Oral, USP, III/385
   Syrup, Oral, III/385
Sulfisoxazole, Aminacrine Hydrochloride,
     and Allantoin
   Cream, Vaginal, III/385
Sulfisoxazole Diolamine
   Injection USP, III/385
   Ointment, Ophthalmic, USP, III/385
   Solution, Ophthalmic, USP, III/385
Sulfisoxazole and Phenazopyridine Hydrochloride
   Tablets, III/385
Sulfobromophthalein Sodium
   Injection USP, III/385
Sulfoxone Sodium
   Tablets USP, III/386
Sulfur
   Cream, III/386
   Lotion, III/386
   Ointment USP, III/386
   Precipitated USP, III/386
   Soap, Bar, III/386
Sulfurated Lime
   Mask, III/386
   Solution, Topical, III/386
Sulfur Dioxide
   Sulfur Dioxide NF, III/386
Sulfuric Acid
   Sulfuric Acid NF, III/386
Sulfur, Sublimed
   Sublimed Sulfur USP, III/386
Sulindac
   Tablets USP, III/387, IV/MC-21, MC-22
Sumycin, IV/MC-22
Suprax, IV/MC-4
Suprofen
   Solution, Ophthalmic, USP, III/387

Surgical Suture, Absorbable
   Absorbable Surgical Suture USP, III/387
Surgical Suture, Nonabsorbable
   Nonabsorbable Surgical Suture USP, III/387
Surmontil, IV/MC-24
Sutilains
   Ointment USP, III/387
Symmetrel, IV/MC-1
Synalgos-DC, IV/MC-2
Synthroid, IV/MC-13
Syrup
   Syrup NF, III/388

T

Tablets
   Chewable, II/18
   Molded, Preparation of, II/18
Tagamet, IV/MC-5
Talacen, IV/MC-18
Talbutal
   Tablets USP, III/388
Talc
   Talc USP, III/388
Talwin-Nx, IV/MC-18
Tamoxifen Citrate
   Tablets USP, III/388, IV/MC-22
   Tablets, Enteric-coated, III/388
Tannic Acid
   Tannic Acid USP, III/388
Tape, Adhesive
   Adhesive Tape USP, III/388
Tartaric Acid
   Tartaric Acid NF, III/389
Tavist, IV/MC-5
Tavist-D, IV/MC-5
Teaspoon, II/27
Technetium Tc 99m Albumin
   Injection USP, III/389
Technetium Tc 99m Albumin Aggregated
   Injection USP, III/389
Technetium Tc 99m Albumin Colloid
   Injection USP, III/389
Technetium Tc 99m Antimony Trisulfide
     Colloid
   Injection, III/390
Technetium Tc 99m Disofenin
   Injection USP, III/390
Technetium Tc 99m Etidronate
   Injection USP, III/390
Technetium Tc 99m Exametazime
   Injection, III/390
Technetium Tc 99m Ferpentetate
   Injection USP, III/390
Technetium Tc 99m Gluceptate
   Injection USP, III/390
Technetium Tc 99m Lidofenin
   Injection USP, III/391
Technetium Tc 99m Mebrofenin
   Injection, III/391
Technetium Tc 99m Medronate
   Injection USP, III/391
Technetium Tc 99m Mertiatide
   Injection, III/391
Technetium Tc 99m Oxidronate
   Injection USP, III/391
Technetium Tc 99m Pentetate
   Injection USP, III/392
Technetium Tc 99m Pyrophosphate
   Injection USP, III/392
Technetium Tc 99m (Pyro- and Trimeta-)
     Phosphates
   Injection USP, III/392

Technetium Tc 99m Sestamibi
  Injection, III/392
Technetium Tc 99m Succimer
  Injection USP, III/392
Technetium Tc 99m Sulfur Colloid
  Injection USP, III/393
Technetium Tc 99m Teboroxime
  Injection, III/393
Tegopen, IV/MC-6
Tegretol, IV/MC-3
Temazepam
  Capsules, III/393, IV/MC-22
  Tablets, III/393
Tenex, IV/MC-10
Ten-K, IV/MC-19
Tenoretic, IV/MC-2
Tenormin, IV/MC-2
Tenuate, IV/MC-7
Tenuate Dospan, IV/MC-7
Terazosin Hydrochloride
  Tablets, III/393, IV/MC-22
Terbutaline Sulfate
  Aerosol, Inhalation, III/393
  Injection USP, III/393
  Tablets USP, III/393, IV/MC-22
Terconazole
  Cream, Vaginal, III/394
  Suppositories, Vaginal, III/394
Terfenadine
  Tablets USP, III/394, IV/MC-22
Terfenadine and Pseudoephedrine Hydro-
    chloride
  Tablets, Extended-release, III/394, IV/
    MC-22
Teriparatide Acetate
  for Injection, III/394
Terpin Hydrate
  Elixir USP, III/394
Terpin Hydrate and Codeine
  Elixir USP, III/394
  Solution, Oral, III/394
Terpin Hydrate and Dextromethorphan Hy-
    drobromide
  Elixir USP, III/394
Testolactone
  Suspension, Sterile, USP, III/394
  Tablets USP, III/394
Testosterone
  Pellets USP, III/395
  Suspension, Sterile, USP, III/395
Testosterone Cypionate
  Injection USP, III/395
Testosterone Cypionate and Estradiol Cypio-
    nate
  Injection, III/395
Testosterone Enanthate
  Injection USP, III/395
Testosterone Enanthate, Benzilic Acid Hy-
    drazone, Estradiol Dienanthate, and
    Estradiol Benzoate
  Injection USP, III/395
Testosterone Enanthate and Estradiol Valer-
    ate
  Injection, III/395
Testosterone Propionate
  Injection USP, III/395
Tests and Assays, II/2
Tetanus Antitoxin
  Tetanus Antitoxin USP, III/396
Tetanus and Diphtheria Toxoids Adsorbed
    for Adult Use
  Tetanus and Diphtheria Toxoids Ad-
    sorbed for Adult Use USP, III/397
Tetanus Immune Globulin
  Tetanus Immune Globulin USP, III/396
Tetanus Toxoid
  Tetanus Toxoid USP, III/396

Tetanus Toxoid Adsorbed
  Tetanus Toxoid Adsorbed USP, III/396
Tetracaine
  Ointment USP, III/397
  Ointment, Ophthalmic, USP, III/397
  Solution, Aerosol, Topical, III/397
Tetracaine Hydrochloride
  Cream USP, III/397
  Injection USP, III/397
  Solution, Ophthalmic, USP, III/397
  Solution, Topical, USP, III/397
  Sterile USP, III/397
Tetracaine Hydrochloride and Dextrose
  Tetracaine Hydrochloride in Dextrose In-
    jection USP, III/397
Tetracaine and Menthol
  Ointment USP, III/398
Tetracycline
  Boluses USP, III/398
  Suspension, Oral, USP, III/398
Tetracycline Hydrochloride
  Capsules USP, III/398, IV/MC-22
  for Injection USP, III/398
  Ointment USP, III/398
  Ointment, Ophthalmic, USP, III/398
  Powder, Soluble, USP, III/398
  for Solution, Topical, USP, III/398
  Sterile USP, III/398
  Suspension, Ophthalmic, USP, III/398
  Tablets USP, III/398, IV/MC-22
Tetracycline Hydrochloride and Novobiocin
    Sodium
  Tablets USP, III/399
Tetracycline Hydrochloride, Novobiocin So-
    dium, and Prednisolone
  Tablets USP, III/399
Tetracycline Hydrochloride and Nystatin
  Capsules USP, III/399
Tetracycline Phosphate Complex
  Capsules USP, III/398
  for Injection USP, III/398
  Sterile USP, III/398
Tetracycline Phosphate Complex and Novo-
    biocin Sodium
  Capsules USP, III/398
Tetrahydrozoline Hydrochloride
  Solution, Nasal, USP, III/399
  Solution, Ophthalmic, USP, III/399
Thalitone, IV/MC-5
Thallous Chloride Tl 201
  Injection USP, III/400
Theo-24, IV/MC-22
Theobid Duracaps, IV/MC-22
Theobid Jr. Duracaps, IV/MC-23
Theo-Dur, IV/MC-22
Theo-Dur Sprinkle, IV/MC-22
Theophylline
  Capsules USP, III/400
  Capsules, Extended-release, USP, III/
    400, IV/MC-22, MC-23
  Elixir, III/400
  Solution, Oral, III/400
  Suspension, Oral, III/400
  Syrup, III/400
  Tablets USP, III/400, IV/MC-22
  Tablets, Extended-release, III/400, IV/
    MC-22
Theophylline in Dextrose
  Injection USP, III/400
Theophylline, Ephedrine, Guaifenesin, and
    Butabarbital
  Capsules, III/400
  Elixir, III/400
Theophylline, Ephedrine Hydrochloride,
    Guaifenesin, and Phenobarbital
  Elixir, III/401
  Tablets, III/401

Theophylline, Ephedrine Hydrochloride, and
    Phenobarbital
  Elixir, III/401
  Suspension, III/401
  Tablets USP, III/401
  Tablets, Extended-release, III/401
Theophylline, Ephedrine Sulfate, Guaifene-
    sin, and Phenobarbital
  Elixir, III/401
  Tablets, III/401
Theophylline, Ephedrine Sulfate, and Hy-
    droxyzine Hydrochloride
  Syrup, III/401
  Tablets, III/401
Theophylline and Guaifenesin
  Capsules USP, III/401, IV/MC-23
  Elixir, III/401
  Solution, Oral, USP, III/401
  Syrup, III/401
  Tablets, III/401
Theophylline Sodium Glycinate
  Elixir USP, III/400
  Tablets USP, III/400
Theophylline Sodium Glycinate and Guai-
    fenesin
  Elixir, III/401
  Syrup, III/401
  Tablets, III/401
Thiabendazole
  Suspension, Oral, USP, III/401
  Suspension, Topical, III/401
  Tablets USP, III/401
Thiamine Hydrochloride
  Elixir USP, III/401
  Injection USP, III/401
  Tablets USP, III/401
Thiamine Mononitrate
  Elixir USP, III/401
Thiamylal Sodium
  for Injection USP, III/402
  for Solution, Rectal, III/402
Thiethylperazine Maleate
  Injection USP, III/402
  Suppositories USP, III/402
  Tablets USP, III/402
Thimerosal
  Aerosol, Topical, USP, III/402
  Solution, Topical, USP, III/402
  Thimerosal USP, III/402
  Tincture USP, III/402
Thioguanine
  Tablets USP, III/403
Thiopental Sodium
  for Injection USP, III/403
  for Solution, Rectal, III/403
  Suspension, Rectal, III/403
Thiopropazate Hydrochloride
  Tablets, III/403
Thioproperazine Mesylate
  Tablets, III/403
Thioridazine
  Suspension, Oral, USP, III/403
Thioridazine Hydrochloride
  Solution, Oral, USP, III/403
  Tablets USP, III/403, IV/MC-23
Thiotepa
  for Injection USP, III/404
Thiothixene
  Capsules USP, III/404, IV/MC-23
Thiothixene Hydrochloride
  Injection USP, III/404
  for Injection USP, III/404
  Solution, Oral, USP, III/404
Thonzonium Bromide
  Thonzonium Bromide USP, III/404
Thorazine, IV/MC-5
Thorazine Spansule, IV/MC-5

Thrombin
　　Thrombin USP, III/404
Thymol
　　Thymol NF, III/405
Thyroglobulin
　　Tablets USP, III/405
Thyroid
　　Tablets USP, III/405
　　Tablets, Enteric-coated, III/405
Thyrotropin
　　for Injection, III/405
Tiaprofenic Acid
　　Tablets, III/405
Ticarcillin Disodium
　　Sterile USP, III/405
Ticarcillin Disodium and Clavulanate Potassium
　　Injection USP, III/406
　　Sterile USP, III/406
Ticarcillin Monosodium
　　Ticarcillin Monosodium USP, III/405
Ticlopidine Hydrochloride
　　Tablets, III/406
Tigan, IV/MC-24
Timolol Maleate
　　Solution, Ophthalmic, USP, III/406
　　Tablets USP, III/406, IV/MC-23
Timolol Maleate and Hydrochlorothiazide
　　Tablets USP, III/406
Tioconazole
　　Cream USP, III/406
　　Ointment, Vaginal, III/406
　　Suppositories, Vaginal, III/406
Tiopronin
　　Tablets, III/406
Titanium Dioxide
　　Titanium Dioxide USP, III/407
Tobramycin
　　Ointment, Ophthalmic, USP, III/407
　　Solution, Ophthalmic, USP, III/407
Tobramycin and Dexamethasone
　　Ointment, Ophthalmic, USP, III/407
　　Suspension, Ophthalmic, USP, III/407
Tobramycin and Fluorometholone Acetate
　　Suspension, Ophthalmic, USP, III/407
Tobramycin Sulfate
　　Injection USP, III/407
　　Sterile USP, III/407
Tocainide Hydrochloride
　　Tablets USP, III/407, IV/MC-23
Tocopherols Excipient
　　Tocopherols Excipient NF, III/408
Tofranil, IV/MC-12
Tofranil-PM, IV/MC-12
Tolazamide
　　Tablets USP, III/408, IV/MC-23
Tolazoline Hydrochloride
　　Injection USP, III/408
　　Tablets USP, III/408
Tolbutamide
　　Tablets USP, III/408, IV/MC-23
Tolbutamide Sodium
　　Sterile USP, III/408
Tolectin, IV/MC-23
Tolectin 600, IV/MC-23
Tolectin DS, IV/MC-23
Tolerances, II/1
Tolinase, IV/MC-23
Tolmetin Sodium
　　Capsules USP, III/409, IV/MC-23
　　Tablets USP, III/409, IV/MC-23

Tolnaftate
　　Cream USP, III/409
　　Gel USP, III/409
　　Powder USP, III/409
　　Powder, Aerosol, Topical, USP, III/409
　　Solution, Topical, III/409
　　Solution, Aerosol, Topical, III/409
Tolu Balsam Syrup
　　Tolu Balsam Syrup NF, III/409
Tolu Balsam Tincture
　　Tolu Balsam Tincture NF, III/409
Tonocard, IV/MC-23
Toprol XL, IV/MC-15
Totacillin, IV/MC-2
Tragacanth
　　Tragacanth NF, III/409
Trandate, IV/MC-12
Trandate HCT, IV/MC-12
Tranexamic Acid
　　Injection, III/410
　　Tablets, III/410
Tranxene-SD, IV/MC-6
Tranxene T-Tab, IV/MC-6
Tranylcypromine Sulfate
　　Tablets, III/410, IV/MC-23
Trazodone
　　Tablets USP, III/410, IV/MC-23, MC-24
Trental, IV/MC-18
Tretinoin
　　Cream USP, III/410
　　Gel USP, III/410
　　Solution, Topical, USP, III/410
Triacetin
　　Triacetin USP, III/410
Triamcinolone
　　Tablets USP, III/410
Triamcinolone Acetonide
　　Aerosol, Inhalation, III/410
　　Aerosol, Nasal, III/410
　　Aerosol, Topical, USP, III/410
　　Cream USP, III/410
　　Lotion USP, III/410
　　Ointment USP, III/410
　　Paste, Dental, USP, III/410
　　Suspension, Sterile, USP, III/410
Triamcinolone Diacetate
　　Suspension, Sterile, USP, III/410
　　Syrup USP, III/410
Triamcinolone Hexacetonide
　　Suspension, Sterile, USP, III/410
Triamterene
　　Capsules USP, III/411
　　Tablets, III/411
Triamterene and Hydrochlorothiazide
　　Capsules USP, III/411, IV/MC-24
　　Tablets USP, III/411, IV/MC-24
Triavil, IV/MC-18
Triazolam
　　Tablets USP, III/412, IV/MC-24
Trichlormethiazide
　　Tablets USP, III/412
Trichloromonofluoromethane
　　Trichloromonofluoromethane NF, III/412
Tricitrates
　　Solution, Oral, USP, III/412
Tridihexethyl Chloride
　　Injection USP, III/412
　　Tablets USP, III/412
Trientine Hydrochloride
　　Capsules USP, III/412
Triethyl Citrate
　　Triethyl Citrate NF, III/412

Trifluoperazine Hydrochloride
　　Injection USP, III/413
　　Solution, Oral, III/413
　　Syrup USP, III/413
　　Tablets USP, III/413, IV/MC-24
Triflupromazine
　　Suspension, Oral, USP, III/413
Triflupromazine Hydrochloride
　　Injection USP, III/413
　　Tablets USP, III/413
Trifluridine
　　Solution, Ophthalmic, III/413
Trihexyphenidyl Hydrochloride
　　Capsules, Extended-release, USP, III/413
　　Elixir USP, III/413
　　Tablets USP, III/413
Trikates
　　Solution, Oral, USP, III/414
Tri-Levlin, IV/MC-13
Trilostane
　　Capsules, III/414
Trimeprazine Tartrate
　　Capsules, Extended-release, III/414
　　Syrup USP, III/414
　　Tablets USP, III/414
Trimethadione
　　Capsules USP, III/414
　　Solution, Oral, USP, III/414
　　Tablets USP, III/414
Trimethaphan Camsylate
　　Injection USP, III/414
Trimethobenzamide Hydrochloride
　　Capsules USP, III/414, IV/MC-24
　　Injection USP, III/414
　　Suppositories, III/414
Trimethoprim
　　Tablets USP, III/415, IV/MC-24
Trimipramine Maleate
　　Capsules, III/415, IV/MC-24
　　Tablets, III/415
Trimox, IV/MC-2
Trinalin Repetabs, IV/MC-2
Trioxsalen
　　Tablets USP, III/415
Tripelennamine Citrate
　　Elixir USP, III/415
Tripelennamine Hydrochloride
　　Tablets USP, III/415
　　Tablets, Extended-release, III/415
Triphasil, IV/MC-13
Triple Sulfa—See Sulfa, Triple
Triprolidine Hydrochloride
　　Syrup USP, III/415
　　Tablets USP, III/415
Triprolidine Hydrochloride and Pseudoephedrine Hydrochloride
　　Capsules, III/416
　　Capsules, Extended-release, III/416
Triprolidine and Pseudoephedrine Hydrochlorides
　　Syrup USP, III/416
　　Tablets USP, III/416
Triprolidine Hydrochloride, Pseudoephedrine Hydrochloride, and Acetaminophen
　　Tablets, III/416
Triprolidine Hydrochloride, Pseudoephedrine Hydrochloride, and Codeine Phosphate
　　Syrup, III/416
　　Tablets, III/416
Triprolidine Hydrochloride, Pseudoephedrine Hydrochloride, Codeine Phosphate, and Guaifenesin
　　Solution, Oral, III/416

Triprolidine Hydrochloride, Pseudoephedrine Hydrochloride, and Dextromethorphan
  Solution, Oral, III/416
Trisulfapyrimidines
  Suspension, Oral, USP, III/416
  Tablets USP, III/416
Trolamine
  Trolamine NF, III/417
Troleandomycin
  Capsules USP, III/417
  Suspension, Oral, USP, III/417
Tromethamine
  for Injection USP, III/417
Tropicamide
  Solution, Ophthalmic, USP, III/417
Trypsin
  Aerosol, for Inhalation, Crystallized, USP, III/417
Tuaminoheptane
  Inhalant USP, III/417
Tuberculin
  Tuberculin USP, III/418
Turbocurarine Chloride
  Injection USP, III/418
Tuss-Ornade Spansules, IV/MC-19
Tylenol with Codeine No.1, IV/MC-1
Tylenol with Codeine No.2, IV/MC-1
Tylenol with Codeine No.3, IV/MC-1
Tylenol with Codeine No.4, IV/MC-1
Tylox, IV/MC-18
Tyloxapol
  Tyloxapol USP, III/418
Typhoid Vaccine
  Typhoid Vaccine USP, III/418
Tyropanoate Sodium
  Capsules USP, III/418

U

Undecylenic Acid and Zinc Undecylenate
  Cream, Compound, III/419
  Foam, Topical, Aerosol, Compound, III/419
  Ointment, Compound, USP, III/419
  Powder, Topical, Aerosol, Compound, III/419
  Powder, Topical, Compound, III/419
  Solution, Topical, Compound, III/419
Units of Potency, II/2
Uracil Mustard
  Capsules USP, III/419
Urea
  Sterile USP, III/419
Urofollitropin
  for Injection, III/419
Urokinase
  for Injection, III/419
Ursodiol
  Capsules, III/419, IV/MC-24
USP General Notices and Requirements, Selected, II/1

V

Vaccinia Immune Globulin
  Vaccinia Immune Globulin USP, III/420
Valium, IV/MC-6
Valproic Acid
  Capsules USP, III/420
  Syrup USP, III/420
Valrelease, IV/MC-6
Valves, II/10

Vancomycin Hydrochloride
  Capsules USP, III/420
  for Injection USP, III/420
  for Solution, Oral, USP, III/420
  Sterile USP, III/420
Vanilla
  Vanilla NF, III/420
Vanilla Tincture
  Vanilla Tincture NF, III/420
Vanillin
  Vanillin NF, III/421
Varicella-Zoster Immune Globulin
  Varicella-Zoster Immune Globulin USP, III/421
Vascor, IV/MC-3
Vaseretic, IV/MC-8
Vasopressin
  Injection USP, III/421
Vasopressin Tannate
  Suspension, Oil, Sterile, III/421
Vasotec, IV/MC-8
V-Cillin K, IV/MC-18
Vecuronium Bromide
  for Injection, III/421
Veetids, IV/MC-18
Vegetable Oil, Hydrogenated
  Hydrogenated Vegetable Oil NF, III/421
Velosef, IV/MC-4
Ventolin, IV/MC-1
Verapamil
  Injection USP, III/422
  Tablets USP, III/422, IV/MC-24
Verapamil Hydrochloride
  Capsules, Extended-release, III/422, IV/MC-24
  Tablets, Extended-release, III/422, IV/MC-24
Verelan, IV/MC-24
Vibramycin, IV/MC-8
Vibra-Tabs, IV/MC-8
Vicodin, IV/MC-11
Vicodin ES, IV/MC-11
Vidarabine
  Concentrate for Injection USP, III/422
  Ointment, Ophthalmic, USP, III/422
  Sterile USP, III/422
Vinblastine Sulfate
  Injection, III/422
  Sterile USP, III/422
Vincristine Sulfate
  Injection USP, III/422
  for Injection USP, III/422
Visken, IV/MC-19
Vistaril, IV/MC-11
Vitamin A
  Capsules USP, III/423
  Injection, III/423
  Solution, Oral, III/423
  Tablets, III/423
Vitamin E
  Capsules USP, III/423
  Preparation USP, III/423
  Solution, Oral, III/423
  Tablets, III/423
  Tablets, Chewable, III/423
Vitamins A, D, and C and Sodium or Potassium Fluoride
  Solution, Oral, III/
  Tablets, III/424
  Tablets, Chewable, III/424
Vitamins, Multiple, and Sodium or Potassium Fluoride
  Solution, Oral, III/424
  Tablets, Chewable, III/424
Voltaren, IV/MC-7

W

Warfarin Sodium
  for Injection USP, III/424
  Tablets USP, III/424, IV/MC-24
Water
  for Inhalation, Sterile, USP, III/424
  for Injection USP, III/424
  for Injection, Bacteriostatic, USP, III/424
  for Injection, Sterile, USP, III/424
  for Irrigation, Sterile, USP, III/424
  for Pharmaceutical Purposes, II/21
  Purified USP, III/424
Wax, Carnauba
  Carnauba Wax NF, III/425
Wax, Emulsifying
  Emulsifying Wax NF, III/425
Wax, Microcrystalline
  Microcrystalline Wax NF, III/425
Wax, White
  White Wax NF, III/425
Wax, Yellow
  Yellow Wax NF, III/426
Weights and Measures, II/5, 25
Weights and Measures, Equivalents of, II/28
Welbutrin, IV/MC-3
White Lotion
  White Lotion USP, III/426
White Ointment—See Ointment, White
White Wax—See Wax, White
Wymox, IV/MC-2
Wytensin, IV/MC-10

X

Xanax, IV/MC-1
Xanthan Gum
  Xanthan Gum NF, III/426
Xenon Xe 127
  Xenon Xe 127 USP, III/426
Xenon Xe 133
  Xenon Xe 133 USP, III/426
  Injection USP, III/426
Xylitol
  Xylitol NF, III/427
Xylometazoline Hydrochloride
  Solution, Nasal, USP, III/427
Xylose
  Xylose USP, III/427

Y

Yellow Fever Vaccine
  Yellow Fever Vaccine USP, III/427
Yellow Ointment—See Ointment, Yellow
Yellow Wax—See Wax, Yellow
Ytterbium Yb 169 Pentetate
  Injection USP, III/427

Z

Zantac, IV/MC-21
Zaroxolyn, IV/MC-15
Zein
  Zein NF, III/428
Zestoretic, IV/MC-13
Zestril, IV/MC-13
Zidovudine
  Capsules, III/428, IV/MC-24
  Injection, III/428
  Syrup, III/428
Zinc Chloride
  Injection USP, III/428

Zinc Oxide
    Ointment USP, III/428
    Paste USP, III/428
Zinc Oxide and Salicylic Acid
    Paste USP, III/428

Zinc Sulfate
    Injection USP, III/428
    Solution, Ophthalmic, USP, III/428
Zithromax, IV/MC-2
Zocor, IV/MC-21

Zoloft, IV/MC-21
Zovirax, IV/MC-1
Zyloprim, IV/MC-1

"Fast-finder" Subject Guide

Approved Drug Products with Therapeutic Equivalence Evaluations

Introduction

How to Use the Drug Product Lists

Prescription Drug Products

OTC Drug Products

Drug Products with Approved Under Section 505 of the Act Administered by the Division of Blood and Blood Products

Discontinued Drug Products

Orphan Drug Product Designations

Drug Products Which Must Demonstrate In vivo Bioavailability Only If Product Fails to Achieve Adequate Dissolution

Biopharmaceutic Guidance Availability

ANDA Suitability Petitions

Product Name Index

Product Name Index Listed by Applicant

Uniform Terms

Patent and Exclusivity Information Addendum

Selected USP General Notices and Chapters

Laws and Regulations

Chemistry and Compendial Requirements

The Medicine Chart

USP Practitioners' Reporting Network

"Fast-finder" Subject Guide

I — Approved Drug Products with Therapeutic Equivalence Evaluations

Introduction

How to Use the Drug Product Lists

Prescription Drug Products

OTC Drug Products

Drug Products with Approved Under Section 505 of the Act Administered by the Division of Blood and Blood Products

Discontinued Drug Products

Orphan Drug Product Designations

Drug Products Which Must Demonstrate *in vivo* Bioavailability Only If Product Fails to Achieve Adequate Dissolution

Biopharmaceutic Guidance Availability

ANDA Suitability Petitions

Product Name Index

Product Name Index Listed by Applicant

Uniform Terms

Patent and Exclusivity Information Addendum

II — Selected USP General Notices and Chapters

Laws and Regulations

III — Chemistry and Compendial Requirements

IV — The Medicine Chart

V — USP-Practitioners' Reporting Network

TO ORDER OTHER USP PUBLICATIONS, USE THIS FORM
See inside of back cover for full listing.

Send orders to:
United States Pharmacopeial Convention, Inc.
Order Processing Department 1141
12601 Twinbrook Parkway, Rockville, MD   20852
Tel. (301) 881-0666   1-800-227-8772 (Toll-free ordering)   FAX: 1-301-816-8148

NO RISK: Full Money Back Guarantee! If for any reason you are not satisfied after receipt of your order, you may return your purchase within 30 days for full refund.

TITLE	CODE #	QTY	PRICE	TOTAL
_____	_____	_____	_____	_____
_____	_____	_____	_____	_____
_____	_____	_____	_____	_____

Add $7 per ship-to address for shipping and handling _____

Order total _____

Maryland residents add 5% sales tax on all items except *About Your Medicines* and *About Your High Blood Pressure Medicines* display cases.

Please allow 2–4 weeks for delivery. Prices subject to change without notice.

Please fill out the reverse side of this form.

Moving?

OUR SUBSCRIBERS' RECORDS and publication labels are computer-generated for efficient service. When you change your address and give us **30 days' notice** together with a recent address label, you assure our mailing to the proper address.

PLEASE SEND your **new** address, and your **latest label**, or an exact copy of it, to: USPC, Inc., Order Processing Dept., 12601 Twinbrook Parkway, Rockville, MD   20852.

THE POSTCARD BELOW is for your convenience if you wish to clip it along the dotted lines, affix postage, and mail it. Or, if you prefer not to clip, please send your **new** address and your **latest label**, or an exact copy of it, in a stamped envelope to the above address.

CHANGE OF ADDRESS

New Address

NAME _____

ADDRESS _____

STATE _____   ZIP CODE _____

COUNTRY _____

Former Address

(attach latest label here)

ALL ORDERS MUST BE PAID IN ADVANCE IN U.S. DOLLARS DRAWN ON A U.S. BANK. Inquire for foreign order shipping charges.

To expedite orders charged to your MasterCard or VISA call Toll-free 1-800-227-8772.

Enclosed is my check or money order made payable to USPC for $_____

Charge my order to: ☐ MasterCard   ☐ VISA   ($20 minimum)

Account Number _____ Expiration Date _____

Signature _____

Name _____

Firm _____

Street Address _____

City _____

State _____ ZIP _____ Phone Number ( ) _____

ATTACH
STAMP
HERE

U. S. Pharmacopeial Convention, Inc.
Order Processing Dept.
12601 Twinbrook Parkway
Rockville, MD   20852